Blaustein's Pathology of the Female Genital Tract

Fifth Edition

Springer
New York
Berlin
Heidelberg
Barcelona
Hong Kong
London
Milan
Paris
Singapore
Tokyo

We shall not cease from exploration
And the end of all our exploring
Will be to arrive where we started
And know the place for the first time

T.S. Eliot

Robert J. Kurman, MD
Richard W. TeLinde Distinguished Professor, Departments of Gynecology, Obstetrics, and Pathology, The Johns Hopkins University School of Medicine, Director of Gynecologic Pathology, The Johns Hopkins Hospital, Baltimore, Maryland

Editor

Blaustein's Pathology of the Female Genital Tract

Fifth Edition

With 1410 Illustrations

Springer

Robert J. Kurman, MD
Richard W. TeLinde Distinguished Professor
Departments of Gynecology, Obstetrics,
and Pathology
The Johns Hopkins University School of Medicine
Director, Gynecologic Pathology
The Johns Hopkins Hospital
Baltimore, MD 21231-2410, USA

Library of Congress Cataloging-in-Publication Data
Blaustein's pathology of the female genital tract.–5th ed./editor, Robert J. Kurman.
p.; cm.
Includes bibliographical references and index.
ISBN 0-387-95203-9 (h/c : alk. paper)
1. Gynecologic pathology. 2. Generative organs, Female–Diseases. I. Title: Pathology of the female genital tract. II. Blaustein, Ancel, 1919-III. Kurman, Robert J.
[DNLM: 1. Genitalia, Female–pathology. WP 100 B645 2001]
RG77.P37 2001
618.1′07–dc21
2001032002

Printed on acid-free paper.

Production coordinated by Chernow Editorial Services, Inc., and managed by Terry Kornak; manufacturing supervised by Jacqui Ashri.
Typeset by Matrix Publishing Services, Inc., York, PA.
Printed and bound by R. R. Donnelley and Sons, Willard OH.
Printed in the United States of America.

9 8 7 6 5 4 3 2 1

ISBN 0-387-95203-9 SPIN 10790770

Springer-Verlag New York Berlin Heidelberg
A member of BertelsmannSpringer Science+Business Media GmbH

To Carole

Preface to the Fifth Edition

With the completion of the fifth edition of *Blaustein's Pathology of the Female Genital Tract*, I am reminded of a statement made by Ibsen after he finished writing one of his plays. "My new play is finished . . . it gives me a curious feeling of emptiness to find myself suddenly separated from a work that has occupied my time and thoughts for several months to the exclusion of everything else. But on the other hand it is good to be done with it. Living every moment of my life with these fictitious characters was beginning to make me a little nervous. . . ."[1] In the case of this text, there were no fictitious characters, as best I could tell, but there were new concepts, ideas, and views with which I and the contributors had to grapple. Work on this book was therefore difficult, but also exhilarating. So, at the completion of this long process, I too feel a certain emptiness but am glad to be done.

Eight years have passed since the last edition of the text was published, and significant progress has occurred in the field of gynecologic pathology. These advances are reflected in this new edition. Since the last edition, the WHO Classification of Tumors of the Ovary has been revised, and these changes have been incorporated into the five chapters on tumors of the ovary. In 2001, The Bethesda System (TBS) for Reporting Cervical/Vaginal Cytology was revised and guidelines for the management of women with cervical abnormalities developed at a subsequently convened consensus meeting. These revisions to TBS and the consensus meeting recommendations have been included in the chapter titled "Precancerous Lesions of the Cervix." The following chapters have been extensively revised as well: "Benign Diseases of the Vulva," "Precursor Lesions of Endometrial Carcinoma," "Endometrial Carcinoma," "Mesenchymal Tumors of the Uterus," "Surface Epithelial Tumors of the Ovary," "Gestational Trophoblastic Disease and Related Lesions," "Immunohistochemistry," and "Molecular Biology." As a result, approximately one third of the book has undergone major revisions. With the widespread availability of computerized searches, it was felt that exhaustive referencing was no longer necessary. Therefore in this edition comprehensive references have been limited to those published in the last decade with the exception of large series that remain clinically relevant and older classic references. The photomicrographs in the fourth edition were carefully reviewed, and those that were not satisfactory were replaced. New photographs were added as necessary to illustrate recently described entities or to provide a more comprehensive description of lesions that had not been adequately illustrated. As a result, there are approximately 375 new photographs in the fifth edition. Very few electron photomicrographs are included in this edition, as it was felt that electron microscopy no longer substantially contributes to our understanding of pathogenesis and is rarely used in diagnosis. Color photomicrographs have not been included because I am not convinced that they are superior to high-quality black-and-white photomicrographs. At first glance they are appealing because they correspond more closely to the H & E stained slide, but on closer inspection, more often than not, they lack the clarity and crispness of good

[1]Letter to translator Mortiz Prozor, Munich, November 20, 1890.

black-and-white photomicrographs. Accordingly, every effort has been made to ensure that the photomicrographs in this edition, which are one of the mainstays of any pathology textbook, are of the highest quality.

Molecular biology is changing the face of pathology, indeed of medicine, but it should be emphasized that advances in our understanding of pathogenesis, which underlie the development of new approaches to diagnosis and treatment, depend on molecular biologic analysis that is guided by morphology. Although much that is new in this edition is based on the contributions of molecular biology, the reader should appreciate that these advances would not have been clinically meaningful had they not been made in conjunction with careful morphologic analysis. New molecular techniques, such as cDNA and oligonucleotide microarrays together with tissue microarrays, are producing prodigious amounts of data, but making sense of these data requires thoughtful analysis by surgical pathologists who are well acquainted with the morphologic and clinical aspects of the disease process. As we begin the twenty-first century, it can be said that in studies aimed at elucidating pathogenesis, morphology without molecular biology is barren but molecular biology without morphology is blind.

As in previous editions, the opportunity to collaborate with an outstanding group of contributors was one of the most gratifying aspects of the entire project. The assistance of the staff at Springer-Verlag, as in the past, has been greatly appreciated. I have been fortunate to work with an outstanding staff in the Division of Gynecologic Pathology at The Johns Hopkins Hospital, notably Drs. Brigitte Ronnett, T-C Wu, Ie-Ming Shih, Richard Roden, and Mark Sherman. My association with these individuals and the fellows and residents who rotate on the Gynecologic Pathology Service has provided continuing intellectual stimulation and an ongoing educational experience for me. Their efforts, directly and indirectly, have contributed to my ability to undertake and execute this project. Finally, I am grateful to my wife Carole, without whose support, patience, and encouragement this endeavor would not have been possible.

Robert J. Kurman, MD
Baltimore, Maryland
2002

Reference

1. Letter to translator Mortiz Prozor, Munich, November 20, 1890

Preface to the First Edition

This text is written for the obstetrician, gynecologist, pathologist, and for residents training in these disciplines. It is a multiauthored book and the editor is aware of the problems this can create, but the expansion of information in the field of gynecologic pathology renders single authorship obsolete.

The format is largely traditional but the contents include topics that have not appeared in past texts. Clear cell adenocarcinoma of the vagina and vaginal and cervical adenoses are discussed in detail in a separate chapter. A chapter on embryology and congenital anomalies is written by an embryologist and the advantage of its inclusion is self evident. Ovarian neoplasms in childhood and adolescence are fortunately rare occurrences, but information concerning them is generally not readily available in existing texts. It is of sufficient importance to deserve a separate chapter. Amniotic fluid analysis for fetal viability is now commonly used and for this reason a detailed discussion of this subject is presented.

A chapter is included on gross description and preparation of gynecologic specimens. It contains the input and review of several directors of gynecologic-pathology laboratories.

The text contains many electron micrographs taken by transmission and scanning electron microscopy. Their inclusion is not an absolute necessity in gynecologic pathology, but is informative because they offer another perspective and are now a commonly used modality for studying tissue. The present day literature is replete with descriptions of specimens by electron microscopy, and it is hoped that the text will enable the readers to familiarize themselves with electron microscopy as used in this specialty.

Experimentation in the field of obstetrics and gynecology has become more sophisticated over the years and for this reason the chapter on animal models of tumors of the ovaries and uterus is included. The contributions that comparative pathology can make to understanding disease mechanisms justify the addition of the chapter on comparative uterine and ovarian tumors in the animal kingdom.

The authors include a mixture of clinicians, pathologists, and basic scientists, and it is hoped that this gives the book the balance between the experience of the clinician and the pathologist.

Ancel Blaustein, MD

Contents

Contributors

NORIO AZUMI, MD, PHD
Associate Professor of Pathology, Medical Director, Molecular Diagnostic Laboratory, Georgetown University School of Medicine, Washington, DC 20007, USA

REX C. BENTLEY, MD
Assistant Professor of Pathology, Duke University Medical Center, Durham, NC 27710, USA

KATHLEEN R. CHO, MD
Associate Professor of Pathology, University of Michigan Medical School, Ann Arbor, MI 48109-0638, USA

PHILIP B. CLEMENT, MD
Clinical Professor of Pathology, University of British Columbia, Vancouver Hospital and Health Sciences Center, Vancouver, BC V5Z 1M9, Canada

BERNARD CZERNOBILSKY, MD
Professor of Pathology, Medical School of Hebrew University and Hadassah, Jerusalem, and Chief, Department of Pathology, Kaplan Hospital, Rehovot 76115, Israel

ALEX FERENCZY, MD
Professor of Pathology and Obstetrics and Gynecology, Department of Pathology, Jewish General Hospital, Montreal, Quebec H3T 1E2, Canada

DEBORAH J. GERSELL, MD
Pathologist, Department of Pathology, St. John's Mercy Medical Center, St. Louis, MO 63141, USA

LORA HEDRICK ELLENSON, MD
Associate Professor of Pathology, Weill Medical College of Cornell University, and Pathologist, New York Hospital, New York, NY 10021, USA

MICHAEL R. HENDRICKSON, MD
Professor of Pathology, Stanford University Medical Center, Stanford University School of Medicine, Stanford, CA 94305, USA

FREDERICK T. KRAUS, MD
Professor (Visiting Staff) of Pathology, Washington University School of Medicine and Director of Placental and Perinatal Pathology, St. John's Mercy Medical Center, St. Louis, MO 63110, USA

ROBERT J. KURMAN, MD
Richard W. TeLinde Distinguished Professor of Gynecologic Pathology, Departments of Gynecology, Obstetrics, and Pathology, The Johns Hopkins University School of Medicine, and Director of Gynecologic Pathology, The Johns Hopkins Hospital, Baltimore, MD 21231-2410, USA

Michael T. Mazur, MD
Clinical Professor of Pathology, SUNY Health Science Center at Syracuse, and Pathologist, Crouse Irving Memorial Hospital, Syracuse, NY 13210, USA

George L. Mutter, MD
Associate Professor, Department of Pathology, Brigham and Women's Hospital, Boston, MA 02115, USA

Stanley J. Robboy, MD
Professor of Pathology, Obstetrics, and Gynecology, and Director, Gynecologic Pathology, Duke University Medical Center, Durham, NC 27710, USA

Brigitte M. Ronnett, MD
Associate Professor of Pathology, The Johns Hopkins University School of Medicine, and Pathologist, The Johns Hopkins Hospital, Baltimore, MD 21231-2410, USA

Peter Russell, MD
Clinical Professor of Pathology, University of Sydney and Royal Prince Alfred Hospital, Sydney, Australia 2050

Mark Schiffman, MD
Clinical Investigator, Environmental Studies Section, Environmental Epidemiology and Biostatistics Program, National Cancer Institute, Rockville, MD 20852, USA

Robert E. Scully, MD
Emeritus Professor of Pathology, Harvard Medical School, and Pathologist, Massachusetts General Hospital, Boston, MA 02114, USA

Jeffrey D. Seidman, MD
Director of Gynecologic Pathology, Washington Hospital Center, Washington, DC 20010, USA

Mark E. Sherman, MD
Environmental Epidemiology Branch, Division of Epidemiology and Genetics, National Cancer Institute, Rockville, MD 20852, USA

Ie-Ming Shih, MD, PhD
Assistant Professor of Pathology, The Johns Hopkins Hospital, Baltimore, MD 21231-2410, USA

Aleksander Talerman, MD, PhD, FRC Path
Peter A. Herbut Professor of Pathology and Cell Biology, Thomas Jefferson University School of Medicine, Philadelphia, PA 19107, USA

James E. Wheeler, MD
Professor of Pathology and Laboratory Medicine, Hospital of the University of Pennsylvania, Philadelphia, PA 19104-4283, USA

Edward J. Wilkinson, MD
Professor and Vice Chairman, Director, Division of Anatomic Pathology, Department of Pathology and Laboratory Medicine, and Adjunct Professor, Department of Obstetrics and Gynecology, University of Florida College of Medicine, Gainesville, FL 32610, USA

Thomas C. Wright, MD
Associate Professor of Pathology, Director, Division of Ob/Gyn Pathology, College of Physicians and Surgeons, Columbia University Presbyterian Medical Center, New York, NY 10032, USA

Dong-lin Xie, MD, PhD
Pathologist, Department of Pathology, DIANON Systems, Tampa, FL 33606, USA

Robert H. Young, MD, FRC Path
Professor of Pathology, Harvard Medical School, and Director of Surgical Pathology, Massachusetts General Hospital, Boston, MA 02114, USA

Richard J. Zaino, MD
Professor of Pathology, M.S. Hershey Medical Center, Pennsylvania State University, Hershey, PA 17033, USA

Charles Zaloudek, MD
Professor of Clinical Pathology, University of California, San Francisco, School of Medicine, San Francisco, CA 94143, USA

PART ONE

Pathology of the Female Genital Tract

1

Embryology of the Female Genital Tract and Disorders of Abnormal Sexual Development

Stanley J. Robboy, M.D., Rex C. Bentley, M.D., and Peter Russell, M.D.

An understanding of the embryologic development of the genital tract provides the background for understanding many pathologic conditions encountered in the female. Among these are disorders of abnormal sexual development, which are closely linked with abnormalities occurring in early embryologic development.

Embryology

Most of the female genital tract is of mesodermal origin. The germ cells are of endodermal origin, and the vulva and the epithelial lining of the vagina are of ectodermal origin. The chronology and sequence of events that underlie the development of the female genital tract are summarized in Table 1.1.

Gonadal Development

In humans and other mammals, the karyotype "XY" genetically defines the sex as male, whereas "XX" defines the female sex. Sex is determined by the presence or absence of a signal from a substance called the *testis determining factor* (TDF), which is found on the Y chromosome. Testes are formed if this gene is expressed by the embryo before the urogenital ridge differentiates. Further male development occurs under the influence of hormones the testes later secrete (Fig. 1.1). Without TDF, the gonads differentiate as ovaries and the embryo develops as a female. The timely expression of TDF is critical to the development of male sex; in its absence, the embryo develops a female phenotype by "default," regardless of genetic sex.

Extensive efforts have been expended during the past two decades to identify TDF and its products.

Table 1.1. Synopsis of stages of normal embryologic development

Crown-rump length (mm)	*Week after ovulation*	*CR length/day*	*Description of event*
3	3.3	2.5/24	Pronephric tubules form; pronephric (mesonephric) duct arises and grows caudad as solid cord
7	4	3–5/27	Pronephros degenerated, but mesonephric duct reaches cloaca
12	5	7–9/33	Cloaca divides into rectum and UGS
18	6	8–11/37	Müllerian ducts appear as funnel-shaped opening of coelomic epithelium; indifferent gonad bulges into coelom
23	7	17/48	Müllerian ducts about 1/2 distance to UGS
		20–30 mm	Testis anatomically distinct with seminiferous tubules
29	8	51 d+	Müllerian ducts elongate and near UGS
		51 d	Ducts approach each other
		23–28 mm/54 d	Ducts in apposition; sinusal tubercle appears
		27–31 mm/56+ d	Ducts fuse and in contact with UGS
43	9	30? mm 56? d	So-called ambisexual stage ends; experimental data for dating müllerian duct regression unclear experimentally, müllerian duct is sensitive to MIS through 25+ mm CR size; ducts in older embryos not sensitive. Clinically, embryos 31–35 mm before effect observed; regression completed by 43–55 mm
			Leydig cells appear
		50? mm	Testes and ovaries acquire capacity to secrete characteristic hormones at same stage of development; testosterone coincides with histologic development of Leydig cells and immediately precedes virilization of genital tract; ovary not yet differentiated; rate-limiting step is appearance of 3-beta-OH-steroid-dehydrogenase, which is 50-fold more abundant in testis than ovary; ovary converts T to estradiol, which testis cannot do; later regulation shifted to pituitary placenta gonadotropins where T → estradiol controlled by conversion of cholesterol to pregnenolone
60	10	56 mm	Müllerian ducts completely fused (entire septum gone); caudal aspect proliferates; epithelium lining canal stratifies (2–3 cells layers thick)
		70 d	Anogenital distance lengthens
71	11	71 d	T synthesis sufficient to induce development of mesonephric duct into definitive structures (epididymis, vas deferens, and seminal vesicle); subsequently, T converted peripherally into 5-DHT, which causes: UGS → prostate Genital tubercle → glans penis Genital folds → penis (only 3.5 mm long) Genital swelling → scrotum
		72–4 d	Fusion of labioscrotal folds
			Closure of median raphe
			Closure of urethral groove
			Phallus in both sexes 3 mm long; thereafter grows in males 0.72 mm/wk and females 0.20 mm/wk
		75 d	Mesonephric ducts regress if not stimulated by T
		60+ mm	Vaginal plate first seen distinctly (complete at 140 mm; wk 17); initially, upper uterovaginal canal is large and oval in cross section, mostly lined by pseudostratified columnar epithelium; extensive growth begins caudally; cells stratify
		68 mm	Uterovaginal canal occluded caudally, progresses cranially
93	12	77 mm	Extensive uterovaginal growth continues caudally
105	13	100–120 mm	Cervical glands appear; wavy, but undifferentiated
		105 mm	Vaginal rudiment approaches vestibule
			True ovarian organogenesis begins with onset of meiotic prophase
116	14		

Table 1.1. Synopsis of stages of normal embryologic development (*Continued*)

Crown-rump length (mm)	*Week after ovulation*	*CR length/day*	*Description of event*
130	15	126 mm	Primary folds of mucosa give uterine lumen "W"-shaped appearance on cross section
		130 mm	Vaginal rudiment reaches level of vestibular glands; uterovaginal canal (15 mm total length) divisible into vagina (3/6ths), cervix (2/6ths), and corpus (1/6th); boundaries ill-defined
			Isthmus readily distinguishable
			Stromal layers of uterus begin definition
			Solid epithelial anlage of anterior and posterior fornices appear
			Vagina begins to show slight estrogen effect
142	16	139 mm	Fallopian tube begins active growth phase, begin to coil
		140 mm	Vaginal plate completed; lower end reaches vestibule; upper end extends into endocervical canal
			Female urogenital sinus becomes shallow vestibule
153	17	151 mm	Vaginal plate longest and begins to canalize; corpus glands appear as slight outpouchings
164	18	160 mm	Palmate folds of cervix appear (forerunner adult cervix)
		162 mm	Mucoid development of cervix begins
			Smooth muscle of uterus appears
			Estrogen effect apparent throughout vagina
		162 mm	Cavitation of vaginal canal completed
177	19	170 mm	Fornices hollow
186	20	185 mm	Dramatic increase in growth and coiling of fallopian tube (about 3 mm/wk to week 34)
197	21		
208	22		
230	24	210 mm	Differentiation of muscular layer of uterus complete
		227 mm	Fundus well marked; uterus assumes adult form
250	26		
270	28		
290	30		
328	34		
362	38	266 d	Birth

UGS, urogenital sinus; MIS, müllerian-inhibiting substance; T, testosterone; d, day; 5-DHT, 5-alpha-dihydrotestosterone; wk, week; CR, crown-rump.

Several candidates have been proposed and later discarded. The candidate now accepted is a gene called SRY (*sex-determining region Y*), located in region 1A1 adjacent to the pseudoautosomal pairing region at the distal end of the short arm of the Y chromosome.[12] The gene, which has a strongly conserved motif,[35] encodes for a DNA-binding protein, the binding activity product (transcriptional switch) that orchestrates the action of other genes. It does so by initiating a cascade of gene expressions that regulate the development of the testis.[12,50] It has been proposed that SRY acts to repress other inhibitory regulators of male development.[110] Some of the target genes also may have been identified.[110] Evidence supporting this thesis includes that the SRY gene is absent from the normal X chromosome, the SRY gene is present on the X chromosome of "sex-reversed" XX human males,[35,56] the homologous gene in the mouse is initially expressed just before sexual differentiation normally occurs,[8] and genetic splicing of the SRY gene into the chromosomally female embryo causes it to develop as a male. Possibly the most important role of SRY is to initiate the indifferent cells in the genital ridge to differentiate into Sertoli cells, which are the first type of cell required to form in the embryonic testis.[97] With monoclonal antibodies, a SRY-specific epitope (protein) has been found in the nuclei of Sertoli cells and

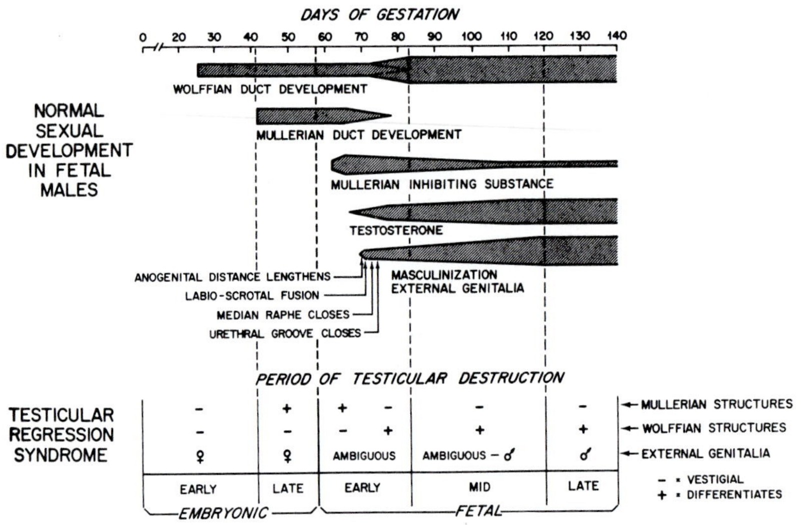

Fig. 1.1. Normal sexual development. Embryologic development is determined by several factors, all of which are time specific during embryogenesis. The abnormalities that accompany the testicular regression syndrome are related to the normal sequence of events. (From Welch and Robboy, ref. 113, with permission of Pediatric Andrology.)

germ cells.[88] Two other genes are thought to be important in Sertoli cell differentiation and function; these include Sox9, an SRY-related gene, and SF-1, a nuclear hormone receptor. Sox9, which the Sertoli cells express, results in XY females when mutations inactivate the gene. SF-1 is also expressed in Sertoli cells and is believed to activate the müllerian inhibiting substance (MIS) gene. (See ref. 110 for an in-depth review of the genes involved in male sex determination.)

During the development of both male and female human embryos, the primordial germ cells, characterized by large clear cells with vesicular nuclei, migrate from the yolk sac to the urogenital ridges via the hindgut approximately 3 weeks after fertilization (Figs. 1.2 and 1.3). The mesodermal epithelium on the medial surface of the urogenital ridge begins to proliferate, resulting in the epithelium of the eventual gonad, while the gonads themselves begin to differentiate. In males, the testis is anatomically distinct with early tubular formation and immature Sertoli cells by day 44. (In this chapter, all dates given are postovulation.) In females, ovarian differentiation, characterized by the development of primordial follicles, begins some 5 weeks later. The initial stages of both testicular and ovarian development appear independent of whether the primordial germ cells are present or absent in the gonad or have proliferated normally.

In the presence of SRY the proliferating surface cells differentiate into so-called sex cords, which are cords of epithelial cells that extend from the surface

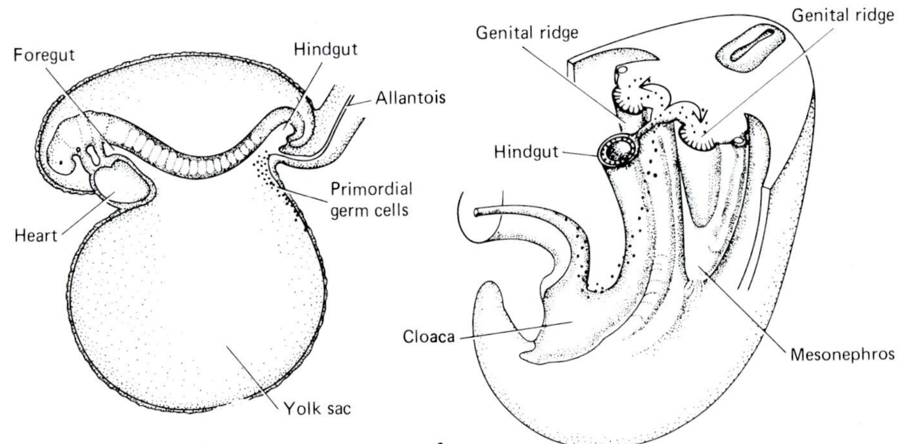

a b

Fig. 1.2. Three-week embryo. a: Curved embryo with primordial germ cells in the wall of the yolk sac, close to the allantoic attachment. **b**: Migration path of primordial germ cells along the wall of the hindgut and dorsal mesentery into the genital ridge. (From Sadler, ref. 88a, with permission of Williams & Wilkins Co.)

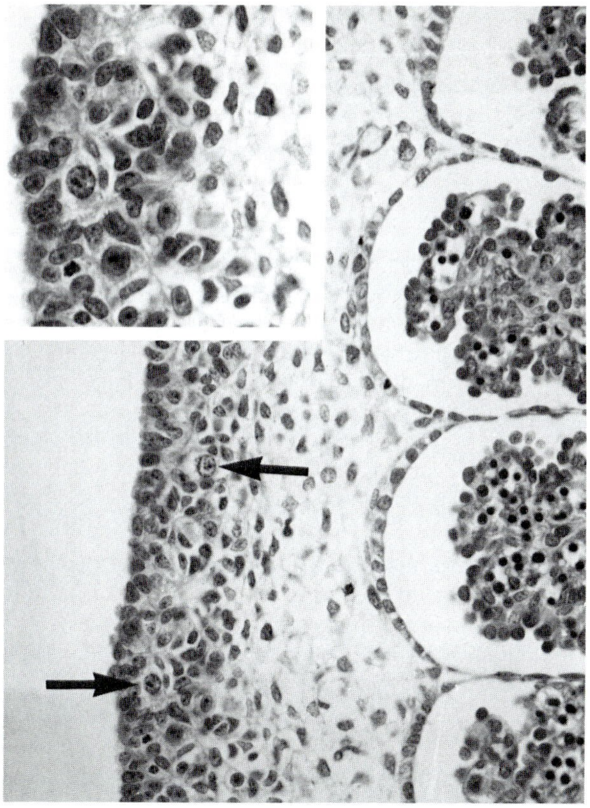

Fig. 1.3. **Urogenital ridge.** A thickened layer of cells that invests two germ cells (*arrows*) lies beneath the surface epithelium. The mesonephric glomeruli are below. *Inset*: A compact layer of cells closely resembling the surface layer surrounds the germ cells.

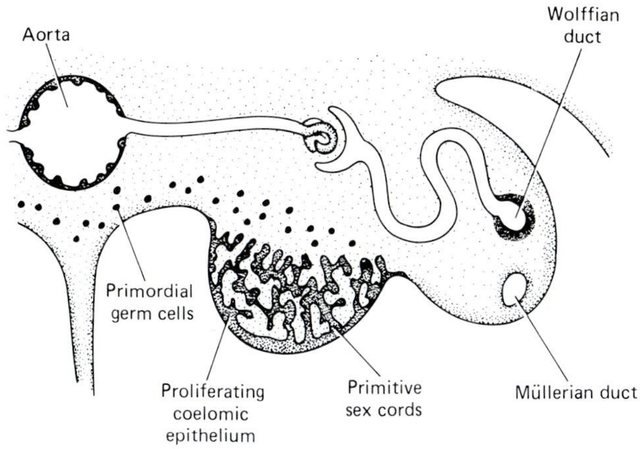

Fig. 1.4. Transverse section through the lumbar region of a 6-week embryo. The indifferent gonad in which the primitive sex cords appear derives from the proliferating coelomic epithelium. Cells of the primitive sex cords surround some of the primordial germ cells. (From Sadler, ref. 88a, with permission of Williams & Wilkins Co.)

of the gonad into the medulla (Fig. 1.4). Subsequently, a capsule (tunica albuginea) develops and separates these epithelial cords from the surface. The cords become the testicular tubules as the epithelial cells differentiate into the tall, clear Sertoli cells of the testis and the gonadal stromal cells become the interstitial or Leydig cells (Fig. 1.5). In normal development, the germ cells are incorporated completely within the tubules. Even in the absence of germ cells, the somatic tissues of the undifferentiated embryonic gonad are capable of developing into a testis, albeit lacking spermatogonia and spermatogenesis.[91]

If SRY is absent (i.e., normal 46 XX females), the dividing germ cells are incorporated into a proliferating mass of surface epithelial cells, which results in a thickened cortex that presages the organization of the adult ovary (Fig. 1.6). From the second to the early third trimester, this thickened cortical mass of

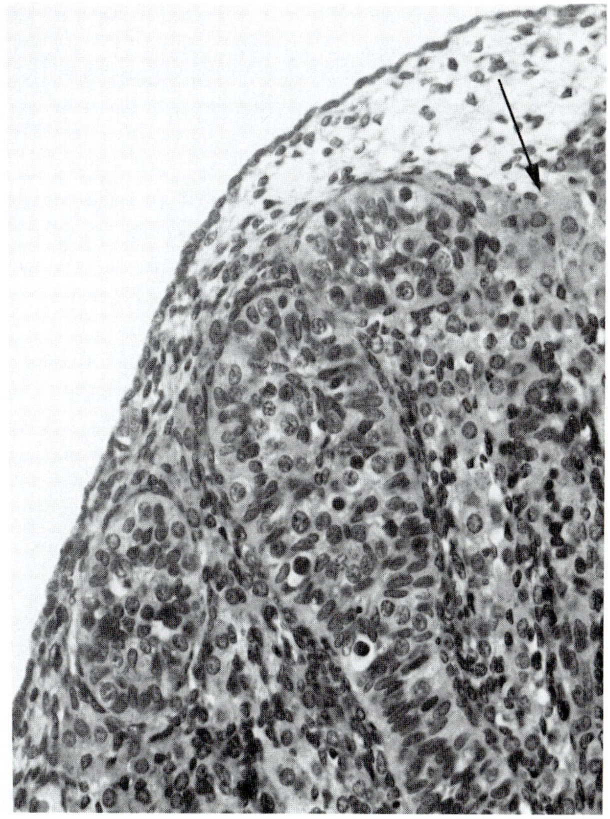

Fig. 1.5. Fetal testis. Epithelial cords are destined to become the testicular tubules and contain Sertoli cells. Interstitial cells, some of which contain abundant eosinophilic cytoplasm characteristic of Leydig cells (*arrow*), lie between the cords. The surface is differentiating into a capsule.

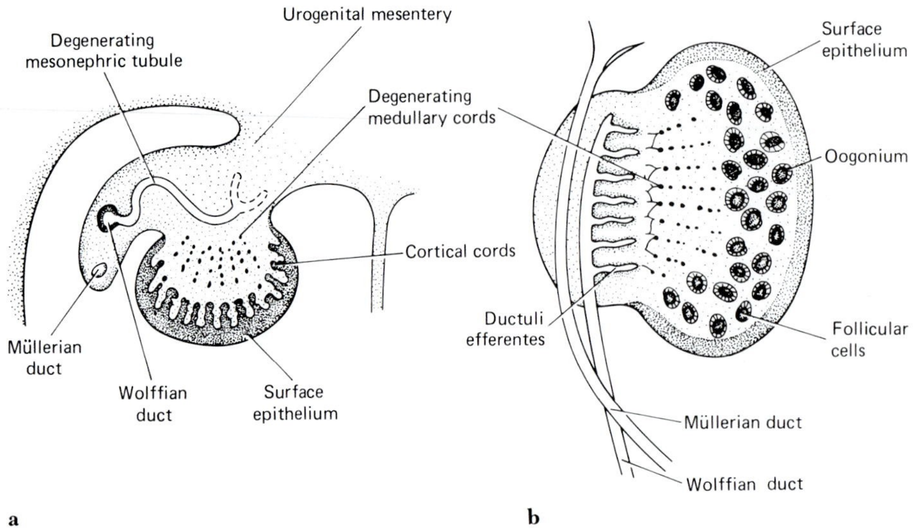

Fig. 1.6. a: Transverse section through the ovary at 7 weeks gestation. The primitive (medullary) sex cords are undergoing degeneration and cortical cords are forming. **b: Five-month fetus.** The ovary and genital ducts have degenerative medullary cords. The excretory mesonephric tubules (ductuli efferentes) lack communication with the rete. Groups of oogonia surrounded by follicular cells lie in the cortical zone of the ovary. (From Sadler, ref. 88a, with permission of Williams & Wilkins Co.)

proliferating epithelial and germ cells divides into small groups demarcated by strands of stromal tissue extending from the medulla to the cortex. The small groups of germ cells and epithelial cells are further subdivided into primordial follicles composed of single germ cells surrounded by a layer of epithelial cells, the primitive granulosa cells. In normal development, each germ cell is characteristically encapsulated in its own (primordial) follicle. Oogonia not so enveloped undergo spontaneous apoptosis, but occasional primordial follicles can contain two, or rarely three, oocytes; this is associated with entry into meiosis and cessation of further proliferation.

If the normal male genetic constitution (46 XY) is present, some of the early epithelial proliferation contributes to the connection between the sex cord and the mesonephric tubules. Where gonads are destined to become ovary, early proliferation degenerates in the ovarian hilum, leaving a few tubules, the rete ovarii. It is these primordial mesonephric cells that are believed to develop and envelop the primordial germ cells and eventually become the follicular granulosa cells. Interstitial (Leydig) cells develop extensively in the stromal tissue of the second-trimester female gonad, but degenerate in most cases by term. The few found in the hilum of the adult ovary are called hilus cells. Thus, the gonad develops primarily from mesodermal tissues, with the exception of the germ cells, which are endodermal in origin.

Müllerian and Wolffian Duct Development

Regardless of genetic sex, the celomic epithelium in both females and males invaginates at several points on the lateral surface of the paired urogenital ridges at the beginning of the fifth week of embryonic life. It coalesces to form the paired tubes termed the müllerian (paramesonephric) ducts (Fig. 1.7). Each of the paired ducts extends caudally in the urogenital ridge immediately lateral to and using the wolffian (mesonephric) duct as a guidewire. For proper müllerian duct migration to occur, it is essential that the wolffian duct be present. Spatially lateral to the cephalad aspect of the wolffian ducts, the müllerian ducts then cross over caudally to lie medial to them as they enter the pelvis (Figs. 1.8 and 1.9). By about the end of the eighth week of embryonic life, the müllerian ducts between the two wolffian ducts fuse to form a single structure, which is the anlage of the common uterovaginal canal (Figs. 1.10 and 1.11). The tip of the müllerian duct abuts on the posterior wall of the urogenital sinus immediately between the two orifices of the wolffian ducts (Fig. 1.12). The point where the tip of the now-fused müllerian duct abuts on the posterior wall of the urogenital sinus defines the site of the

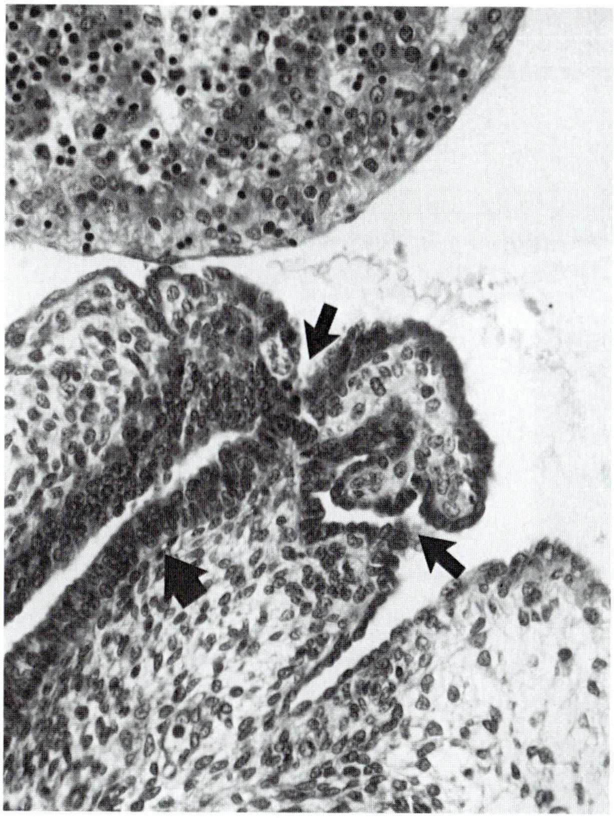

Fig. 1.7. **Lateral surface of the urogenital ridge.** The coelomic epithelium on the surface is proliferating and forming several invaginations (*narrow arrows*), that coalesce to form the müllerian duct (*wide arrow*).

future vaginal introitus, the hymenal membrane (Fig. 1.13). All these developments occur in both female and male fetuses and are completed before the testis, if the embryo is male, begins to secrete MIS. In the presence of MIS, the müllerian tissues regress, remaining only as rudimentary structures in the maturing male urogenital system.

Once the male pathway of development has begun, two hormones produced by the fetal testis then control the differentiation of the male phenotype. The first is MIS, a large glycoprotein that the Sertoli cells produce early during fetal life.[41,83] The gene responsible for this substance is on chromosome 19.[46] The primary function of MIS is to cause regression of the müllerian (paramesonephric) ducts in the male fetus. In the female, MIS is produced in insignificant amounts during fetal life (as there are no testes); in the absence of this substance, the müllerian ducts develop passively to form the fallopian tubes, uterus, and vaginal wall. MIS is first secreted in effective amounts 56 to 62 days after fertilization, and the process of müllerian regression is normally completed by about day 77, after which the müllerian tissue is no longer sensitive to MIS. The MIS receptor in müllerian tissue appears to reside in stromal cells; the mechanism by which müllerian tissue loses its sensitivity to MIS is not understood. MIS has a local action and inhibits development of the ipsilateral fallopian tube. To prevent development of both the uterus and vagina, both testes must se-

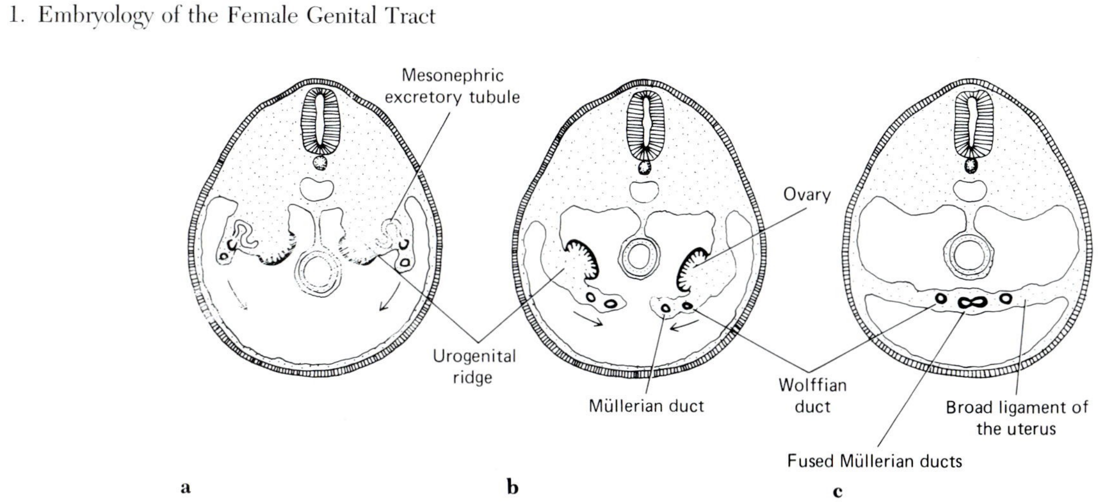

Fig. 1.8. Transverse section through urogenital ridge at progressively lower levels (a,b,c). The müllerian ducts approach each other in the midline and fuse. As a result, a transverse fold, the broad ligament of the uterus, forms in the pelvis. The gonads come to lie at the posterior aspect of the transverse fold. (From Sadler, ref. 88a, with permission of Williams & Wilkins Co.)

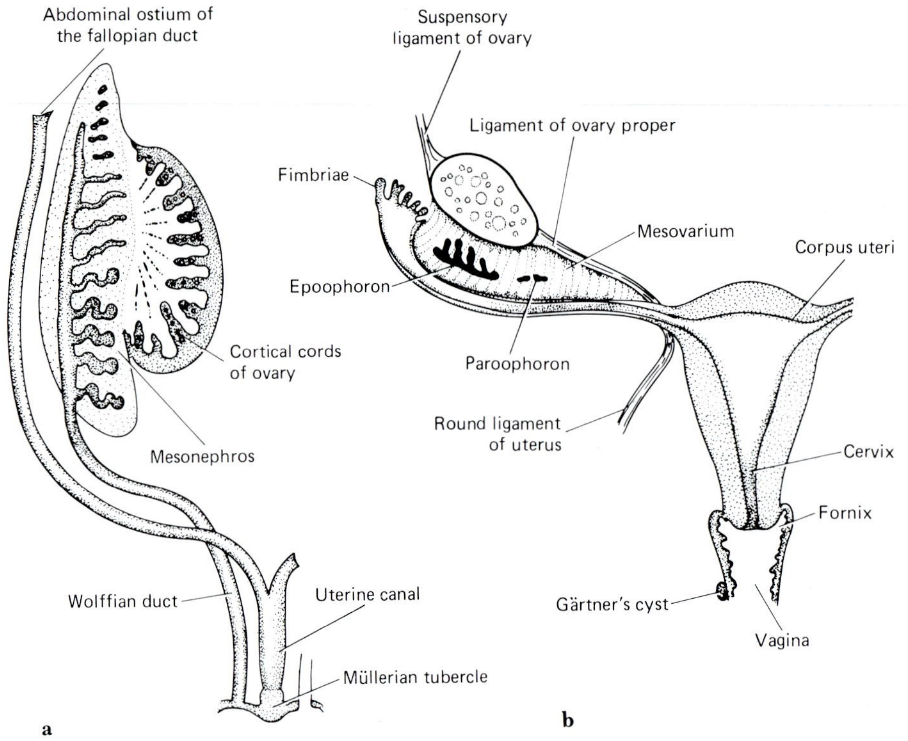

Fig. 1.9. Eight-week female fetus. a: Genital ducts showing the müllerian tubercle and formation of the uterine canal. **b**: Genital ducts after descent of ovary. The only parts of the mesonephric system remaining are the epoophoron, the paroophoron, and Garner cyst. Also present are the suspensory ligament, the ligament of the ovary proper, and the round ligament of the uterus. (From Sadler, ref. 88a, with permission of Williams & Wilkins Co.)

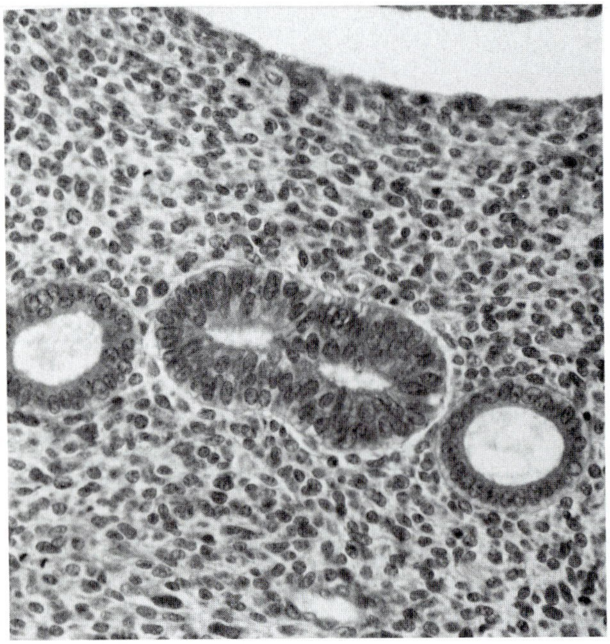

Fig. 1.10. Müllerian and wolffian ducts in a 6-week fetus. Two müllerian ducts lie between the two wolffian ducts and are fusing.

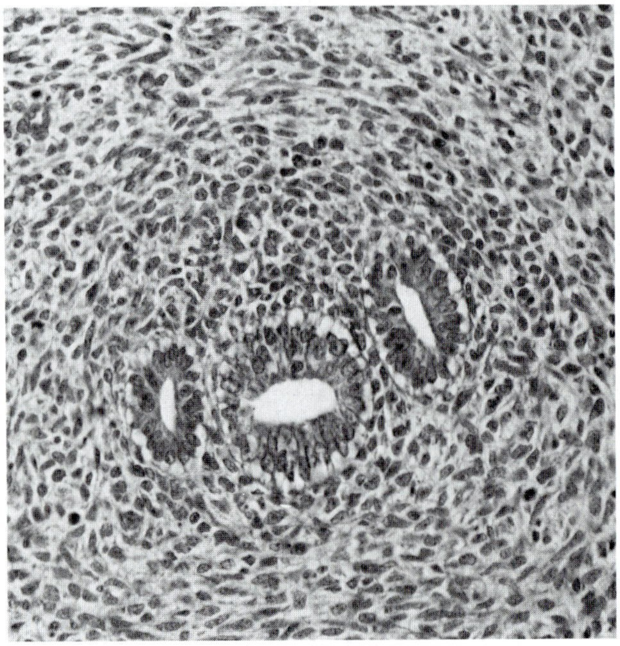

Fig. 1.11. The müllerian and wolffian ducts in a 7-week fetus. The müllerian ducts have fused into a single structure, which lies between the two wolffian ducts.

crete adequate amounts of MIS. Thus, a patient with a testis and a contralateral streak, ovary, or ovotestis generally has a uterus and vagina and a single fallopian tube on the side with the streak or ovary.

Additional functions of MIS have recently been discovered. In the female, ovarian granulosa cells begin producing MIS only after the müllerian-derived tissues (fallopian tubes, uterus, and vagina) are well developed and no longer susceptible to the regressive effects of MIS. Serum MIS levels in girls rise slowly after birth from nearly undetectable levels until they reach a plateau, after 10 years of life, equivalent to the adult male serum MIS concentration. In contrast, the male serum MIS concentration is relatively high at birth, peaks at 4–12 months of age, and then falls progressively to a baseline low adult level by about 10 years of age. A major action of MIS in the young female may be to inhibit oocyte meiosis in the developing follicle. Dramatically high levels of MIS have been found in women with ovarian sex cord tumors, thus serving potentially as a diagnostic marker or method to evaluate the effectiveness of therapy.[47] Secondary actions of MIS in males may be to initiate testicular descent and regulate germ cell maturation.[17]

The second hormone that the fetal testis secretes is testosterone. This androgenic steroid, which is critical for male development, is required for the wolffian (mesonephric) duct to differentiate into the epididymis, vas deferens, and seminal vesicle. Leydig cells appear in the testis around day 54 to 64 and shortly thereafter begin to produce testosterone. Leydig cell activity is probably stimulated by increased production of chorionic gonadotropin by the placenta at that time. Testosterone acts locally on the ipsilateral wolffian duct by binding to a specific high-affinity intracellular receptor protein. This receptor hormone complex binds DNA to regulate transcription of specific genes that govern further development. In the absence of a testis or inability of a testis to produce testosterone in adequate amounts by 10–12 weeks, or with insensitivity of the wolffian duct anlage to testosterone, the epididymis, vas deferens, and seminal vesicle do not differentiate. Only rarely are abnormally elevated testosterone levels reached sufficiently early during embryogenesis in a female fetus to cause the wolffian duct to differentiate into definitive male organs (androgen administration to the mother during pregnancy, or congenital adrenogenital syndrome).

Sometime around the tenth week, the patch of mesodermal urogenital sinus epithelium lying between the orifices of the two wolffian ducts, in response to the apposition of the müllerian duct tip, begins to proliferate. A column of squamous epithelial cells is formed, termed the *vaginal plate*, which displaces the tip of the müllerian duct from the wall of the urogenital sinus. Recent studies suggest that the vaginal plate and müllerian duct are patent early in the second trimester. The vaginal plate gives rise to the epithelium that ultimately lines the vagina.

The development of the stromal component of the genital canal is little studied but is clearly of major importance.[18] In addition to its role in the development of the walls of the tubular muscular organs, there is extensive experimental evidence to indicate that the stroma directs epithelial development as well. Thus, the entire structure of the vagina, cervix, uterus, and tubes is determined by stromal–epithelial interaction.

Smooth muscle appears in the walls of the genital canal between 18 and 20 weeks, and by approximately 24 weeks, the muscular position of the uterine wall is well developed. Vaginal, uterine, and tubal muscular walls develop around the müllerian duct alone, so that the wolffian duct remnants are external to the true wall of the canal. Cervical glands appear at about 15 weeks and rudimentary endometrial glands by 19 weeks, but the endometrium is not well developed even at term in most infants.

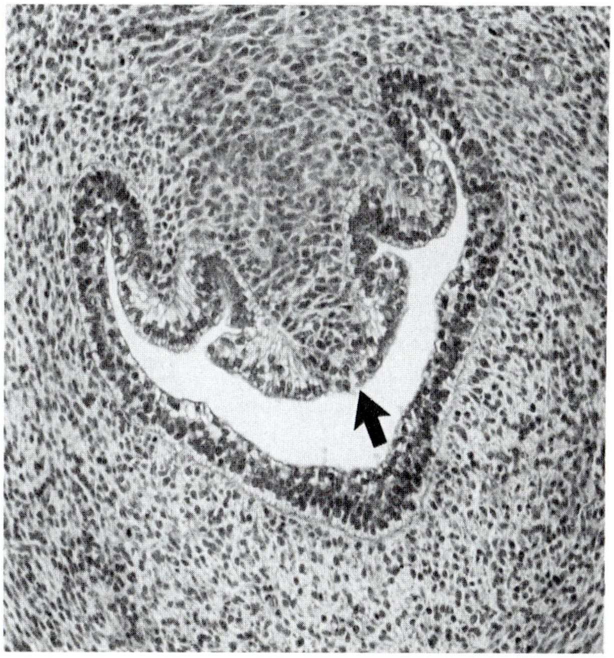

Fig. 1.12. Urogenital sinus at level of the müllerian tubercle. The müllerian ducts contact the urogenital sinus at this site (*arrow*). The epithelium of the anterior and posterior walls of the sinuses is dissimilar.

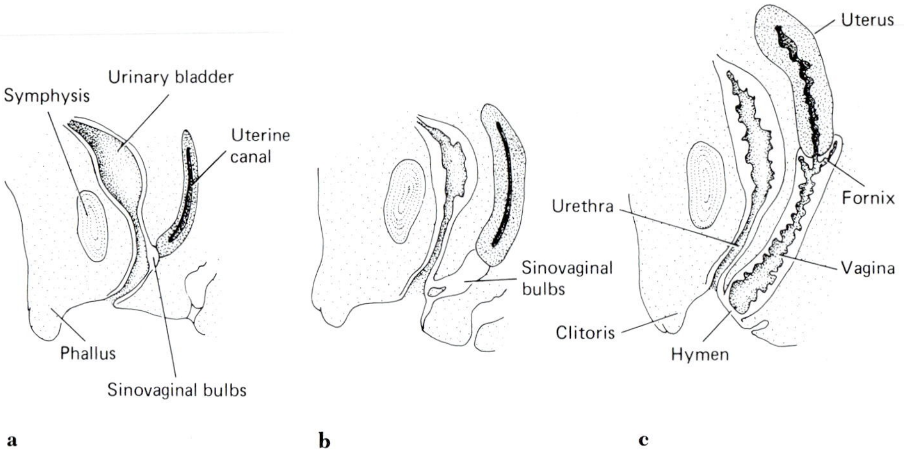

Fig. 1.13. Sagittal sections during different times in the formation of the uterus and vagina. The fused müllerian duct gives rise to the upper third of the vagina, the cervix, and the fundus of the uterus. (From Sadler, ref. 88a, with permission of Williams & Wilkins Co.)

External Genitalia Development

The appearance of the external genitalia is influenced by the systemic hormonal milieu found in the developing fetus beginning about week 15. The genitalia become masculine when exposed to an excess of androgens and female if there is a deficiency of androgens, that is, a relative excess of estrogens. Androgens have a positive influence on the appearance of the external genitalia. Maternal or inappropriate fetal androgens will virilize a female fetus, whereas high levels of circulating estrogens in pregnancy have no effect on the male fetus.

Dihydrotestosterone (DHT), the active androgen that derives from testosterone, is ultimately responsible for initiating masculinization of the external genitalia and differentiation of the prostate. 5-Alpha-reductase, found in the tissues of the external genitalia and urogenital sinus, converts testosterone to DHT. DHT causes (1) the genital tubercle to enlarge and form the glans penis, (2) the genital folds to enlarge and fuse to form the penile shaft with migration of the urethral orifice along the lower border of the shaft to the tip of the glans, (3) the genital swellings to fuse and form a scrotum, and (4) the urogenital sinus tissues to differentiate into prostate. Failure of the external genitalia to develop in males in the presence of testes may be due to a lack of adequate testosterone secretion into the systemic circulation, deficient enzyme (5-alpha-reductase) at the end-organ level to convert testosterone to DHT, or complete end-organ insensitivity (testicular feminization). Lesser degrees of deficiency or end-organ insensitivity may result in partial male development characterized by a small penis, hypospadias, deficient formation of the scrotum, or a persistent urogenital sinus (vaginal opening into urethra). The effects of DHT begin about day 70, with fusion of the labioscrotal folds and closure of the median raphe, and continue at day 74 with closure of the urethral groove. External genital development is complete by day 120–140 (18th–20th week).

The urogenital sinus into which the vagina opens enlarges as the embryo grows, so that it becomes the vestibule of the adult external genitalia. Consequently, the vestibule is lined, except for a variable portion anterior to the urethral orifice, by the endodermal epithelium of the urogenital sinus. This point is clinically important as the endodermal-derived epithelium not only differs morphologically from the mesodermal and ectodermal-derived epithelium but responds differently to a variety of stimuli, notably sex steroids.

The form of the external genitalia results from events that begin during the fourth embryonic week in the mesodermal stroma immediately lateral and ventral to the cloacal plate. Just ventral to the plate, the stroma produces paired elevations of the ectoderm, which fuse to form the genital tubercle (Fig. 1.14). Immediately lateral to the cloacal plate on each side, two parallel folds develop by the same mechanism. The more medial, the urogenital fold, is destined to become the labium minus. The more lateral is the labioscrotal fold, which becomes the labium majus.

The labioscrotal fold extends cranially around

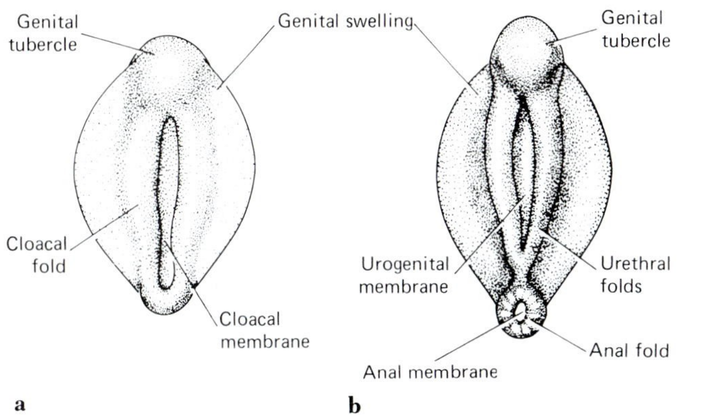

Fig. 1.14. Development of the external genitalis. **a**: The indifferent stage of the external genitalia at approximately 4 weeks. **b**: At approximately 6 weeks. (From Salder, ref. 88a, with permission of Williams & Wilkins Co.)

the genital tubercle and fuses with its partner on the other side, becoming the mons pubis. At the end of the sixth week, the urorectal septum fuses with the cloacal plate, thus dividing this structure into the anal membrane posteriorly and the urogenital membrane ventrally. The lateral folds are distributed primarily in relation to the urogenital membrane. In both the male and female, the lateral folds fuse across the midline in front of the anus. In the male, the fusion moves ventrally in zipper-like fashion.

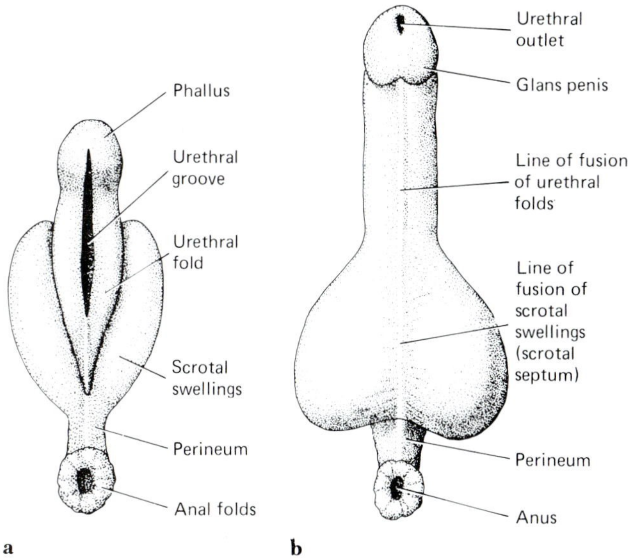

Fig. 1.15. Male external genitalia. **a**: At 10 weeks gestation a deep urethral groove is present that is flanked by urethral folds. **b**: In the newborn. (From Sadler, ref. 88a, with permission of Williams & Wilkins Co.)

The urogenital folds fuse to form a portion of the wall of the penile urethra, and the labioscrotal folds fuse to form the scrotum (Fig. 1.15). As female differentiation reflects the absence of this fusion, it may be difficult to detect, although by the end of the first trimester significant fusion should have occurred in a male fetus.

Summary of Genital Development

In summary, female internal organs and external genitalia develop in the absence of hormones secreted by the fetal ovary, and differentiate even when gonads are absent. Unless interrupted by the regressive influence of MIS, differentiation of the müllerian ducts proceeds cephalocaudally to form fallopian tubes, a uterus, and a vagina. In the absence of the masculinizing effect of DHT, the undifferentiated external genital anlage develops into the vulva. The genital tubercle develops into the clitoris, the genital folds into the labia minora, and the genital swellings into the labia majora. Thus, the infant with ovaries or streak gonads has female internal and external genitalia at birth. Only if the female fetus has systemically elevated levels of androgens before the 10th–12th week of gestation does any degree of internal male development occur. In such cases the external genitalia may appear ambiguous or may resemble that of a normal phenotypic male; the vagina in these instances opens into the membranous portion of the urethra. If the androgens are not elevated until after the 20th week, by which time the external genitalia have fully formed, the only virilizing effect is an enlarged clitoris.

Intersexual Disorders

New insights into the biology of sexual development and advances in chromosome analysis have led to early identification and prompt treatment of the intersexual patient, which facilitates a more normal life for affected individuals. Based on these advances, a classification of abnormal sexual development has been developed that correlates the gonadal and genital anatomy with the chromosomal findings and specific genetic or metabolic defects (Table 1.2). This permits an integrated approach to this complex group of disorders according to the manner by which patients present as well as on the pathophysiologic basis of the defect. The classification also groups patients who are at high risk for development of gonadal neoplasia.

Table 1.2. Classification of intersexual disorders

- Disorders associated with a normal chromosome constitution
  - Female pseudohermaphroditism (Female intersex)
    - Fetal defect
      - Adrenogenital syndrome (testosterone overproduction due to adrenocorticoid insufficiency)
        - 21 Alpha-hydroxylase deficiency
        - 11 Beta-hydroxylase deficiency
      - Placental aromatase defect
    - Maternal influence
      - Maternal ingestion of progestins or androgens
      - Maternal virilizing tumor
  - Male pseudohermaphroditism (male intersex)
    - Gonadal defects
      - Testicular regression syndrome (gonadal destruction)
      - Leydig cell agenesis
        - Defective hCG-LH receptor
      - Defects in testosterone synthesis
        - Testosterone and adrenocorticoid insufficiency
          - 20,22-Demolase deficiency
          - 3-Beta-hydroxylase dehydrogenase deficiency
          - 17-Alpha-hydroxylase deficiency
        - Testosterone insufficiency only
          - 17-20-Desmolase deficiency
          - 17-Beta-hydroxysteroid (17-ketosteroid reductase) dehydrogenase deficiency
    - Persistent müllerian duct syndrome (defect in müllerian inhibiting substance system)
    - End-organ defects
      - Disordered androgen receptor binding
        - Androgen insensitivity syndrome (testicular feminization)
        - Incomplete androgen insensitivity syndrome (Reifenstein syndrome)
      - Disordered testosterone metabolism
        - 5-Alpha-reductase deficiency
    - Defect uncertain
      - Smith–Lemli–Opitz syndrome
- Disorders associated with an abnormal sex chromosome constitution
  - Sexual ambiguity infrequent
    - Klinefelter syndrome
    - Turner syndrome
    - XX male & XY female syndrome (sex reversal)
    - Pure gonadal dysgenesis (some forms)
  - Sexual ambiguity frequent
    - Mixed gonadal dysgenesis (MGD), including
      - Pure gonadal dysgenesis (some forms)
      - Dysgenetic male pseudohermaphroditism
    - True hermaphroditism

hCG, human chorionic gonadotropin; LH, luteinizing hormone.

"Idiopathic" or "unclassified" conditions exist within each major category. We assume that each category of male pseudohermaphroditism with defects in specific protein products or receptors has forms in which the abnormality is total or partial or the defect results from a qualitatively abnormal structure.

Gender Identification Disorders with a Normal Chromosome Constitution

Female Pseudohermaphroditism (Female Intersex)

Female pseudohermaphroditism occurs as a result of relative androgen excess in utero in an individual with two ovaries and two X chromosomes (46 XX). The elevated level of androgen present during embryogenesis usually results in genital ambiguity and may result in the appearance of a phenotypic male. Tumors, if they appear, are virtually always benign.

Adrenogenital Syndrome

Congenital adrenal hyperplasia, unlike all other conditions responsible for the appearance of ambiguous genitalia in the newborn, may be life threatening because of a lack of synthesis of specific adrenal steroids. Prompt diagnosis and institution of appropriate therapy are therefore essential. With early treatment, normal external genitalia and fertility can be achieved. The manifestations of the adrenogenital syndrome in the XX individual are summarized most easily through an understanding of the biosynthetic pathways of mineralocorticoid, glucocorticoid, and sex steroids (Fig. 1.16).[13,66–68] Two enzymes, 21-hydroxylase and 11-beta-hydroxylase, participate in the formation of the glucocorticoids, desoxycorticosterone and cortisol, and the mineralocorticoid, aldosterone, but not of testosterone or the estrogens estrone or estradiol. Deficiency of either enzyme in the 46 XX female leads to elevated adrenocorticotropic hormone (ACTH) products and hence elevated levels of testosterone and other strongly androgenic intermediates, which may result in sexual ambiguity or marked virilization of the newborn's external genitalia.[15,24] 3-Beta-hydroxy-steroid dehydrogenase is required for testosterone formation. In its absence, the principal androgen to form is the weak androgen, dehydroepiandrosterone (DHEA), which has 1/20th the potency of testosterone. Patients with deficiency of this enzyme, therefore, show signs of only mild virilization, usually on clitoral hypertrophy but not with labial fusion or anterior displacement of the urethral orifice.

21-Hydroxylase deficiency is inherited as an autosomal recessive trait caused by an abnormal gene on chromosome 6 that encodes for cytochrome $P_{450}c21$ (i.e., CYP21). It accounts for more than 95% of cases of congenital adrenal hyperplasia, occurring once in 15,000 births. It is high especially in Ashkenazi Jews (1:27 live births). The genetic aberrations responsible for expression of the disease are complicated. This gene exists in tandem with a pseudo-

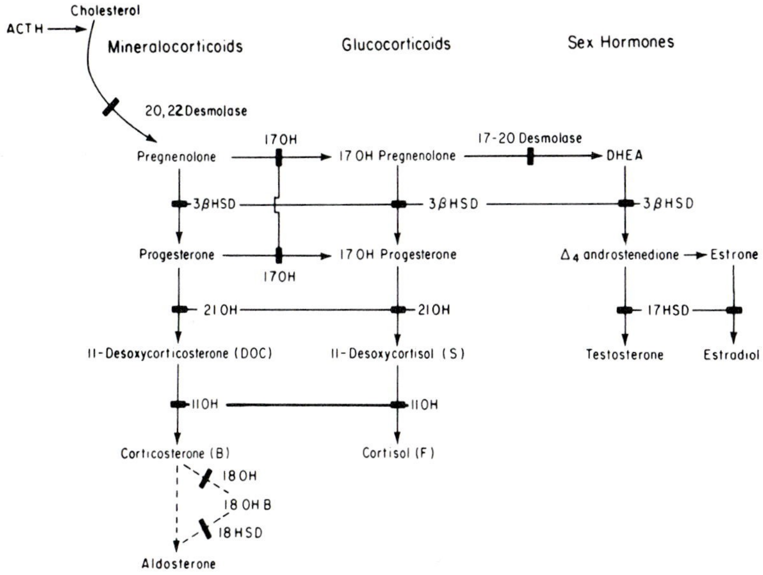

Fig. 1.16. Biosynthesis of mineralocorticoids, glucocorticoids, and sex steroids. (From Saenger et al., ref. 90a, with permission of Pediatric Andrology.)

gene, CYP21P, which is believed to be nontranscribable as it contains a high number of documented mutations.[62] The clinical manifestation depends upon the absence of the single active gene (CYP21, formerly called CYP21B) that actively expresses the 21-hydroxylase enzyme, or of the rearrangements, deletions, or point mutations transferred from the pseudogene present.[13,48,62] Approximately a fourth of cases of classical congenital adrenogenital syndrome are caused by deletion of the CYP21 gene. The remainder are due to nondeleted mutant gene sequences that have been transferred from the pseudogene, rendering the active gene nonfunctional.[13] If the allele carries a defect encoding for a mild defect, then the child will develop a nonclassical form of adrenal hyperplasia, which by definition occurs after birth and is never associated with genital ambiguity.[62] This latter syndrome is common, occurring in 1% of all women, and is thought to be a major cause of adult-onset virilism.

In the congenital form of the adrenogenital syndrome, the extent of virilization depends upon which time during fetal life the disease begins. If the onset follows the 16th week of gestation, the clitoris may be enlarged; if androgen excess occurs earlier, the vagina and urethra may open into a common urogenital sinus. More marked clitoral enlargement and an opening of the urogenital sinus at the clitoral base may mimic penile hypospadias and suggest an even earlier temporal effect. On occasion, the changes have been of such severity that the female infants have been misdiagnosed as cryptorchid males with or without hypospadias.

Males have no evidence of genital ambiguity but may have an enlarged phallus and a hyperpigmented rugated scrotum. Bilateral testicular nodules, composed of interstitial cells resembling Leydig cells or cells of adrenal rest origin, occasionally develop (Fig. 1.17).

Placental Aromatase Defect

Placental aromatase deficiency is a rare cause of maternal virilization during pregnancy and pseudohermaphroditism of the female fetus.[49,92] Mutations in the aromatase gene, CYP19, which cause abnormally low conversion of androstenedione to 17-beta-estradiol and estrone, result in virilization of the mother and her female fetus because of the accumulation of potent androgens. The mothers usually show the onset of progressive virilization during the third trimester. The male fetus has normal genitalia.

Maternal Ingestion of Progestins or Androgens

Maternal ingestion of synthetic progestins was implicated as a cause of female pseudohermaphroditism in the late 1950s when such treatment was employed for threatened or habitual abortion; subsequently, progestins have also been implicated in the development of hypospadias in male offspring. Most cases of female pseudohermaphroditism in this category developed after maternal ingestion of Ethisterone (17-alpha-ethinyl-testosterone) or Norlutin (17-alpha-ethinyl-19-nortestosterone), but occasionally after the ingestion of Enovid, diethylstilbestrol, androgens, or the intramuscular administration of progesterone. Masculinization usually consists of phallic enlargement and variable degrees of labio-

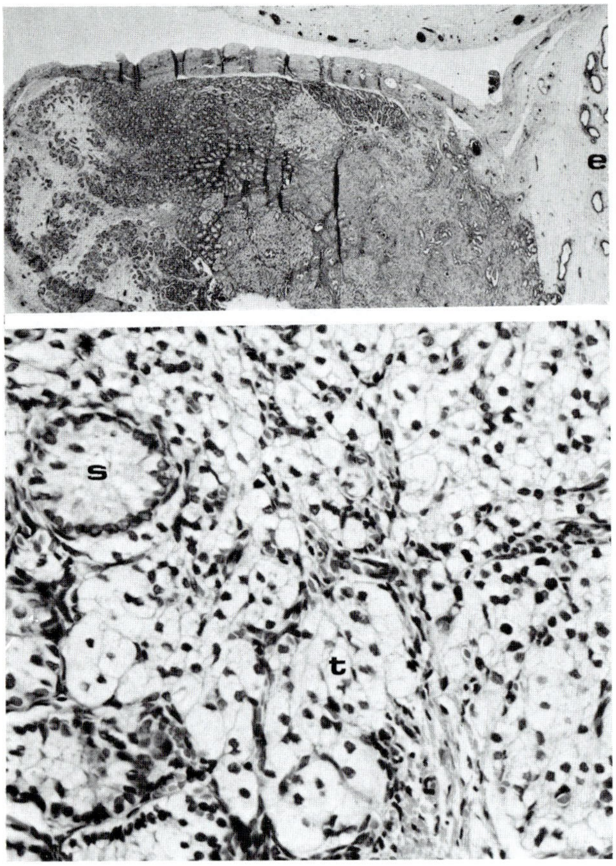

Fig. 1.17. Interstitial cell tumor of the testis in a 4-year-old child with adrenogenital syndrome. The tumor cells (*t*), which are illustrated at high magnification adjacent to immature seminiferous tubules (*s*) in the inset, resemble adrenocortical cells more closely than Leydig cells. The epididymis (*e*) is adjacent to the testis. (From Welch and Robboy, ref. 113, with permission of Pediatric Andrology.)

scrotal fusion, depending on the time during gestation when the therapy was administered. Although the degree of masculinization usually is less than that associated with the adrenogenital syndrome, the sexual ambiguity in female infants has been of such severity in some instances as to result in male sex assignment. The degree of virilization does not progress with age. The gonads and internal genital organs are unaffected, and ovulation, menstruation, and normal secondary female characteristics appear at puberty.

Maternal Virilizing Tumors

A variety of benign and malignant tumors, primary as well as metastatic to the ovary, have been associated on rare occasions with virilization of the mother and her female offspring[27,85,108] (see Chapters 16, 19, 22). The luteoma of pregnancy, by far the most common lesion that causes maternal virilization during pregnancy, is discussed as the prototype of this category. Rarer conditions include Krukenberg tumors arising from primary adenocarcinomas of the stomach and mucinous tumors primary in the ovary. The common thread among all such lesions is the development of hormonally active cells, usually as theca cells, which secrete androgenic hormones.

The *pregnancy luteoma* is a benign hyperplastic lesion of the ovary that is encountered most often as an incidental finding at the time of cesarean section or postpartum sterilization, usually in women who are multiparous. Elevated levels of human chorionic gonadotropin (hCG) are thought to induce hyperplasia of theca-lutein or stroma-lutein cells. A small percentage of the female infants have become masculinized, with mild enlargement of the clitoris and occasionally minimal degrees of labioscrotal fusion or rugate, hyperpigmented ("scrotal") labia. The nature of these changes indicates that the ovarian nodules do not function until the second half of gestation, which is in accord with the occasional onset of masculinization in the mother during the third trimester.

At operation, one and often both maternal ovaries are enlarged by one or more soft, yellow-brown nodules that are well circumscribed but not encapsulated. Although most are less than 2 cm in diameter, they may be as large as 20 cm in greatest dimension. On microscopic examination the nodules consist of large, polygonal cells with granular eosinophilic cytoplasm, which are smaller and more eosinophilic than the luteinized granulosa cells of the corpus luteum but larger than the theca-lutein cells. Intracellular lipid is sparse, if at all present. Mitoses may be observed, but only rarely are they numerous.

Elevated plasma and tissue levels of testosterone, DHT, androstenedione, and DHEA have been detected in virilized patients; the plasma levels return to normal once the tumor is extirpated. Even without treatment, the nodules regress and disappear soon after delivery. Rarely, a functional luteoma may reoccur during a subsequent pregnancy. Other primary functioning tumors of the ovary that may lead to virilization of the female offspring as well as metastatic tumors to the ovary that induce the stroma function during pregnancy are discussed elsewhere in this book.

Male Pseudohermaphroditism

The term *male pseudohermaphroditism* is applied to a heterogeneous group of intersex conditions that are characterized by an intrauterine state of relative functional androgen deficiency, an apparently normal 46 XY karyotype, and either identifiable testes or evidence that testes were present during fetal development. The external genitalia are usually female or ambiguous, although in certain categories (e.g., testicular regression syndrome) they may appear as phenotypically male. The defect may be in the gonad, leading to deficiency in androgens, MIS, or both. Alternatively, end-organ defects in which developing tissues are unresponsive to androgens or MIS may lead to the abnormal phenotype.

Primary Gonadal Defects

A *primary defect of the gonad* in an XY karyotype individual may lead to male pseudohermaphroditism by any one of the following mechanisms: regression (destruction) of the gonads or their anlage during intrauterine life, agenesis of the Leydig cells, a specific enzymatic defect in testosterone to DHT synthesis or receptors to these hormones, or a defect in elaboration or action of MIS.

Testicular Regression Syndrome

Testicular regression follows the irreparable destruction of the testes at a critical stage of fetal development in an XY individual. The phenotype of the affected individual reflects the specific stage of fetal development during which the testes were damaged. In general, gonadal regression that occurs during embryonic life, before the elaboration of MIS and/or androgenic steroids by the testes, leads to a female phenotype. Regression of the testes during late embryonic through mid-fetal life permits a masculine phenotype to develop (see Fig. 1.1). The testicular regression syndrome has a variety of etiologies, some possibly as diverse as inherited genetic defect, intrauterine infection, or infarction. The heterogeneity of presentation of this syndrome and its relative rarity have led to numerous and sometimes confusing terms for this disorder, including *true agonadism*, *testicular dysgenesis*, *rudimentary testis*, *vanishing testis*, and *complete bilateral anorchia*. The terms *pure gonadal dysgenesis* and *Swyer syndrome* have been used for the testicular regression syndrome by some authors. We avoid these latter terms so as not to confuse them with other conditions similarly named and discussed below.

At one end of the spectrum of the testicular regression syndrome, the internal genitalia and gonads are absent and the external genitalia are female.[81] Presumably, the urogenital ridge was destroyed in its entirety during early embryonic life, even before the müllerian ducts began to differentiate (before day 42).

At the other end of the spectrum, which approximates the end point of normal genital development, the patients are phenotypic males with infantile to nearly normal male external genitalia, normally differentiated wolffian duct structures, and completely inhibited müllerian duct development. Often in these cases no genital tissue is identified, but an area of fibrosis, hemorrhage, or hemosiderin deposition is found at the expected site of the gonad near residual vas deferens or epididymis.[14,60,96] Occasionally, atrophic seminiferous tubules may be found amid a fibrous stroma. Testicular regression presumably occurred during the late fetal period (after 120 days), when müllerian structures had already atrophied under the influences of MIS and testosterone and DHT had exerted a major influence on the normal development of internal and external genitalia. Torsion and infarction of improperly descended testes have been suggested.[95]

Intermediate in the spectrum of the testicular regression syndrome are patients with ambiguous genitalia and various combinations of wolffian and/or müllerian duct development. Testes that regressed during the late embryonic period (day 43–59) will have secreted insufficient testosterone to affect the wolffian duct. The production of MIS will have been variable, resulting in poorly differentiated or rudimentary müllerian structures (incomplete inhibition). In the absence of systemic androgens, the external genitalia appear female.

Regression of the testes during the early fetal period (day 59–84) after Sertoli cell (MIS) and Leydig cell (testosterone) function have begun or are about to begin results in an individual with ambiguous external genitalia and various combinations of wolffian and müllerian development, depending on the duration of androgen secretion and müllerian inhibition.

Regression of the testes during the mid-fetal period (day 84–120) results in more advanced masculinization of the external genitalia, although degrees of ambiguity are usually present. Because müllerian duct inhibition is normally completed by day 80, the müllerian structures will have been suppressed and wolffian structures develop.

Leydig Cell Agenesis

Leydig cell agenesis is a very rare cause of male pseudohermaphroditism.[7] Affected individuals have a 46 XY karyotype and testes with interstitial fibrosis, but no mature Leydig cells. Tubules with Sertoli cells and, sometimes, immature spermatogonia are found. The müllerian structures are absent, indicating appropriate testicular production of MIS during fetal life. The wolffian duct system is developed either partially or fully such that identifiable vasa deferentia and epididymides are present. The phenotype varies and is usually female with unremarkable or ambiguous external genitalia, although unambiguous males with evidence of primary hypogonadism have been reported. The presence of wolffian duct development and the variable degrees of masculinization of the external genitalia indicate that some Leydig cells must have differentiated and functioned during early fetal life. Luteinizing hormone levels are elevated in affected individuals. The underlying defect in this disorder is believed to be an absence or defect of the luteinizing hormone (LH)-hCG receptor on the Leydig cell or with some other, unknown, factor arresting Leydig cell development.

Defects in Testosterone Synthesis

Congenital deficiency of any enzyme involved in the production of testosterone in the testis or adrenal gland results in a state of androgen deficiency (relative estrogen excess) (Fig. 1.16). The histologic appearance of the testicular tissue is variable. It has been described occasionally to be "normal," but the photomicrographs in some reports have disclosed large clusters of Leydig cells surrounding tubules lined only by Sertoli cells. In general, the number of gonads studied for any of the conditions and the range of ages studied (infancy, childhood, adulthood) have been limited. Müllerian structures are absent, but wolffian duct structures may be present. The degree to which the external genitalia develop depends on the type and severity of the defect.

Congenital Adrenal Hyperplasia

Several inherited enzymatic defects that cause the syndrome of *congenital adrenal hyperplasia* involve both the synthesis of adrenal mineralocorticoid and glucocorticoid hormones and the adrenal and testicular sex hormones. Because of these genetic defects, one or more adrenal cortical enzymes fail to be synthesized or are defective.[66] The most severe defect, which involves the conversion of cholesterol intermediates to pregnenolone (20,22-desmolase), almost always ends lethally from a salt-wasting crisis if untreated during infancy. Although the external genitalia in the male are ambiguous or female, sufficient testosterone must be secreted during embryogenesis since the internal genitalia are male. The testes in the infant disclose immature seminiferous tubules with spermatogonia. The germ cells disappear by several years of age.

The deficiency of 3-beta-hydroxylase dehydrogenase, like the 20,22-desmolase deficiency, results in decreased synthesis of mineralocorticoid and glucocorticoid hormones as well as adrenal and testicular sex hormones, and may lead to life-threatening salt wasting in infancy. DHEA, which is a weak androgen secreted in high amounts, results in slight clitoral enlargement in the female, but rarely completely masculinizes the external genitalia in males. Hence, the male may be born with ambiguous genitalia and may resemble a virilized female. Males in whom the defect is partial may be born with hypospadias but at puberty develop gynecomastia. The testes in older boys generally are immature, exhibiting seminiferous tubules with spermatogenic arrest and diminished numbers of Leydig cells.

In contrast to the early age of diagnosis in the foregoing two syndromes, the diagnosis in most patients with 17-alpha-hydroxylase deficiency is not suspected until the anticipated time of puberty or later. Recently, however, the detailed steroid analysis of the urine of a newborn male presenting with ambiguous genitalia has shown that the correct diagnosis can be made in the young.

Deficiencies of two enzymes, 17,20-desmolase and 17-hydroxysteroid dehydrogenase (17-ketosteroid reductase), result in deficient testosterone synthesis but do not affect the production of either mineralocorticoids or glucocorticoids. The former defect (conversion of 17-hydroxypregnenolone to DHEA) is extremely rare. The patients reported presented with ambiguous external genitalia and inguinal or intraabdominal testes. Spermatogonia were present in the testis of infants but were absent in the biopsies of their older teenage relatives. All had third-degree hypospadias but normal male internal ductal differentiation.

Genetic males with 17-hydroxysteroid dehydrogenase deficiency have almost all been raised as females because of incomplete masculinization. Most are diagnosed at or after puberty when they fail to menstruate and instead show signs of virilization such as clitoromegaly (enlarged phallus) and hirsutism.[113] Breast development may or may not take place. At surgery, müllerian duct derivatives are absent, consistent with normal anti-müllerian hormone action. Wolffian duct differentiation, indicative of testosterone secretion during embryogenesis, is normal.[5] The testes present in the inguinal canal or labia majora contain rare to no spermatogonia, and may exhibit numerous Leydig cells. 17β-Hydroxysteroid dehydrogenase is under different genetic control from that in extragonadal tissues, and affected males lack testicular 17β-HSD, the extragonadal activity is normal or enhanced. More than

15 mutations have been identified in the responsible gene.[5,10,58]

Defect in Müllerian-Inhibiting Substance (Persistent Müllerian Duct Syndrome)

The persistent *müllerian duct syndrome,* also known as *hernia uteri inguinalis,* is a rare form of male pseudohermaphroditism characterized by the presence of müllerian duct structures in 46 XY phenotypic males. These patients usually present when young with unilateral or bilateral cryptorchid testes, normal or almost normal male external genitalia, and an inguinal hernia into which prolapses an infantile uterus and fallopian tubes. Some patients may be older.[22] The testes are histologically normal, wolffian duct structures are developed, the pubertal development is normal and a rare patient has been fertile. Treatment is surgical consisting of orchiopexy and herniorrhaphy with hysterectomy and bilateral salpingectomy. If at operation any patient has a streak gonad or a tumor rather than bilateral testes, the diagnosis of mixed gonadal dysgenesis should be considered. In most cases of persistent müllerian duct syndrome, the vas deferens is tightly adherent to the residual uterus or upper vagina, and in some cases the müllerian structures must be left intact to preserve the vas deferens. Malignant testicular tumors have been reported in the very rare cases of adult patients with persistent müllerian duct syndrome and uncorrected cryptorchid testes.

The persistent müllerian duct syndrome seems to be a heterogeneous group of disorders, caused by different defects in the müllerian-inhibiting system. Familial cases have been reported. Mutations in the MIS gene are responsible for at least half the cases with persistent müllerian ducts. The remainder appear to be caused by mutations in the receptor for the gene products.[36] Several rare types of receptor alterations have been described.[23] The effect of these abnormalities is that some patients produce no biologically functional MIS, whereas others, who produce normal amounts of biologically active MIS, have end-organ insensitivity to MIS or an abnormality of the timing of MIS secretion. A model for MIS receptor signaling has been proposed and illustrated elsewhere.[46]

End-Organ Defects

The normal development of the wolffian duct derivatives and the external genitalia requires that these structures be responsive to androgen and that the enzyme, 5-alpha-reductase, be present in the anlage of the prostate and external genitalia to convert testosterone to DHT. A molecular defect of the androgen receptor system (e.g., unstable androgen receptor or lack of androgen receptor) leads to impaired development of both wolffian duct structures and external genitalia in 46 XY individuals. If only 5-alpha reductase is absent or defective, the abnormalities in the reproductive tract are confined to the external genitalia and prostate.

Androgen Receptor Disorders (Androgen Insensitivity Syndromes). Disorders of androgen receptor function result in a variety of phenotypes ranging from phenotypic women with intraabdominal testes to individuals with ambiguous genitalia to phenotypic men with minimal clinical abnormalities. Because androgen receptor defects lead to such a variety of different clinical disorders, much nosologic confusion exists in the literature regarding subclassification of the androgen resistance syndromes. In one classification scheme,[54] four categories exist and are, in order of increasing virilization (decreasing feminization), complete and incomplete testicular feminization, Reifenstein syndrome, infertile male syndrome, and undervirilized male syndrome. All share an X-linked recessive inheritance, the result of a defect in the androgen receptor gene, which has been localized to the long arm of the X chromosome, position Xq11.2-q12. A variety of different mutations of this gene have been characterized,[21,32,76,79] many of which are limited to individual families.[42] These mutations may lead to functional absence of the androgen receptor because the primary sequences of the gene are affected. These patients generally present as complete testicular feminization. The more common defect is caused by single amino acid substitutions and is associated with the various other forms of the disease as described next. Rare patients have also been described in whom the androgen receptor disorder has occurred in combination with other unusual karyotypes, e.g., 47,XXY[105] and 47,XYY.[64]

Complete Testicular Feminization

Complete testicular feminization is the most common form of male pseudohermaphroditism. The external genitalia are phenotypically female and, for this reason, the condition is rarely diagnosed before puberty unless an inguinal hernia or labial mass is encountered or unless the disease is known to be familial.[2,111] Primary amenorrhea is the most common complaint leading to evaluation and subsequent diagnosis. The medical history usually reveals that breast development occurred as expected at puberty. Pubic and axillary hair are scant, the vagina is shortened, and the epididymides, vasa differentia, seminal vesicles, and prostate are absent. As a rule, both the cervix and the body of the uterine corpus are absent. A fragment of fallopian tube may be found in up to one-third of cases.[87] The testes are cryptorchid and may be located in the inguinal canal, the pelvis, or rarely the labia. In the complete or almost complete form of the syndrome, the individual exhibits a truly female consciousness gender identity, with normal extragenital erotogenic sensitivity and normal maternal attitude, emphasizing the need to support the patient as a woman, even with reconstructive surgery.[109]

The gonads in infants and young children are relatively normal, but by age 5 years they show abnormalities. By young adulthood, the gonad often is involved with benign or malignant tumors, as described next. If tumors are not present by this age, the gonad is usually small and on section is tan to brown and traversed by thin white bands. A 1- to 2-cm firm, white nodule of hyalinized smooth muscle is usually present at one pole of the testes. Theories regarding what this nodule might represent include an abnormally hypertrophied gubernaculum or rudimentary uterine structure. Microscopic examination of the testicular parenchyma discloses immature seminiferous tubules usually sparsely distributed or clustered in small aggregates. Spermatogonia may be present, but spermatogenesis is absent. The number of spermatogonia that are found is age dependent, diminishing as the patient ages. The interstitium is usually abundant and often resembles ovarian stroma (Fig 1.18). Fetal-type Leydig cells may be abundant. The findings indicate that Leydig cells are active hormone producers. The Leydig cells in individuals with testicular feminization have an ultrastructure typical of cells involved in active hormone synthesis; the systemic androgen levels in these individuals are characteristically elevated. These findings indicate that the pathologic defect in the testicular feminization syndrome is an end-organ defect and not a lack of hormone production by the testes.

Most testes of affected individuals contain multiple benign nodules that are discrete, firm, yellow to brown, and bulge above the sectioned surface (Fig. 1.18). Hamartomatous nodules may be present, usually bilaterally, in virtually every case the authors have examined. The typical size varies from 1 mm to 1 cm, and to 4 cm.[87] The bulk of the nodule usually comprises seminiferous tubules lacking lumina; spermatogonia may be present. Sertoli cell adenomas are hamartomas composed predominantly or exclusively

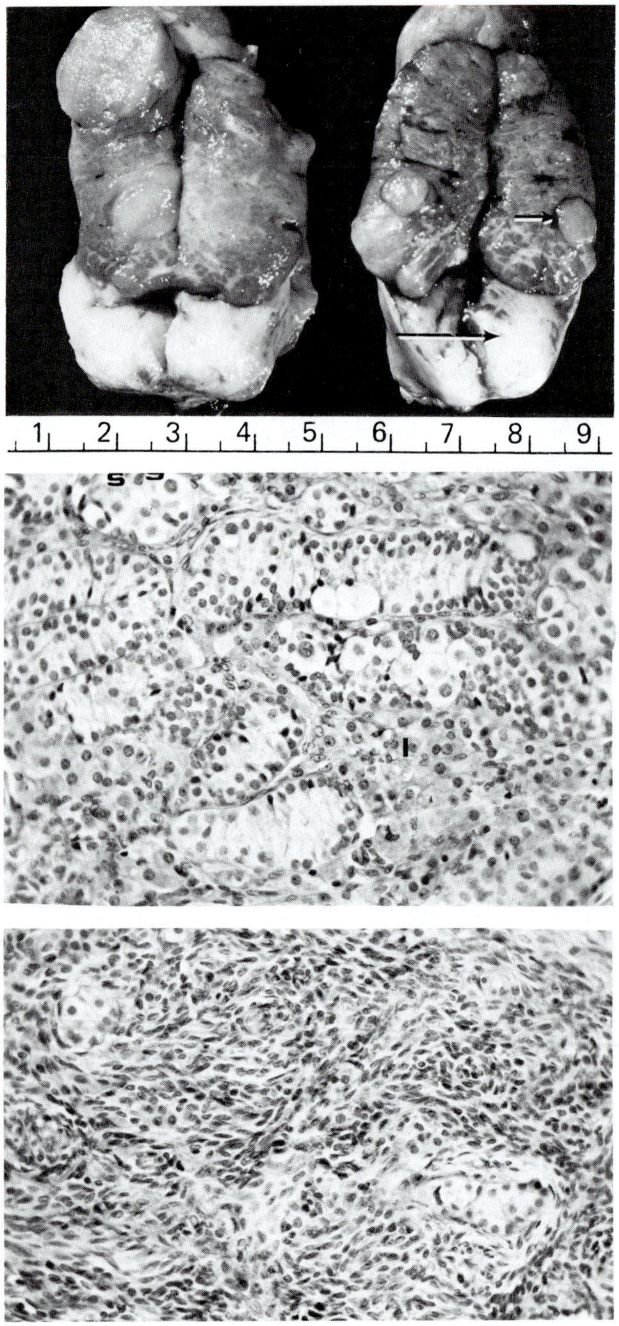

Fig. 1.18. Testis in the complete form of androgen insensitivity (testicular feminization) syndrome. *Top*: Testis in a 17-year-old patient with the complete form of androgen insensitivity (testicular feminization) syndrome. Numerous Sertoli cell adenomas (*short arrows*) are present in the parenchyma. The mass near one pole (*long arrow*) may represent an abnormally hypertrophied gubernaculum. *Middle*: Hamartoma with immature seminiferous tubules (*s*), numerous germ cells (*g*), and numerous Leydig cells (*l*) in the interstitium. *Bottom*: Contralateral testis with scattered immature seminiferous tubules embedded in a dense ovarian-type cortical stroma. Occasional interstitial cells (*arrows*) are present. (From Welch and Robboy, ref. 113, with permission of Pediatric Andrology.)

of closely packed immature seminiferous tubules lacking lumina and lined by immature, uniform Sertoli cells. The adenomas average 3 cm in diameter, ranging up to 25 cm.[31,87] The interstitium in the testes of affected patients often resembles ovarian stroma and frequently contains Leydig cells. On rare occasions, Leydig cell nodules form, and have been considered benign tumors. In summary, the name applied to each type of nodule is somewhat arbitrary and depends largely on the types of components present as well as their number and size. Most nodules are classified as hamartomas, Sertoli cell adenomas, or rarely as Leydig cell tumors.

Malignant gonadal tumors develop with increasing frequency with age in patients with testicular feminization. Seminoma is the most commonly encountered gonadal malignancy in this syndrome. Intratubular germ cell neoplasia is sometimes seen, either independently or in association with seminoma. Other malignant germ cell tumors and malignant sex cord tumors are also rarely encountered. Unlike mixed gonadal dysgenesis, in which tumors develop in young individuals, the risk of malignancy in patients with testicular feminization is only 4% by the age of 25 years, but reaches 33% by 50 years. Because malignant tumors rarely develop before completion of puberty, castration can usually be delayed until after adolescence, thus permitting the patient to undergo a normal pubertal spurt and develop female secondary sex characteristics.

Incomplete Testicular Feminization

About 10% of patients with androgen insensitivity syndrome have *incomplete testicular feminization*.[33,111] It resembles complete testicular feminization except that there is partial fusion of the labioscrotal folds and usually some clitoromegaly at birth. Also, underdeveloped wolffian duct derivatives are often present. If the diagnosis is established during childhood, gonadectomy should be performed before puberty, since virilization may accompany breast development at puberty. Estrogen therapy should be given at the appropriate time to initiate feminization. The pathologic findings are similar to those described for the complete form of testicular feminization.[82]

Other Forms

Reifenstein syndrome, *infertile male syndrome*, and *undervirilized male syndrome* are other forms of incomplete androgen insensitivity in which the phenotype is male. There are few reports describing the microscopic findings of the gonads.

Men with Reifenstein syndrome usually present with gynecomastia and severe hypospadias, and children or teenagers with perineoscrotal hypospadias. However, the phenotypic spectrum is wide, even within the same affected family with a single androgen receptor abnormality in all affected family members. The usual abnormalities include hypospadias, breast development at puberty, female habitus, azoospermia, cryptorchidism, and hypo-plasia or absence of wolffian duct structures. The "infertile male syndrome" is a rare androgen receptor defect characterized by a phenotypically normal man with infertility caused by azoospermia. Finally, in the "undervirilized male syndrome" the individual is a male with gynecomastia, a small penis, decreased beard and body hair, a normal male urethra, a normal sperm density, and an identifiable androgen receptor defect. Most affected individuals are infertile.

Disordered Testosterone Metabolism

5-Alpha-Reductase 2 Deficiency

Deficiency of the enzyme 5-α-reductase 2 impairs the conversion of testosterone to DHT, the hormone that masculinizes the indifferent urogenital sinus and induces development of the prostate.[37,59] The disorder, formerly known as "pseudovaginal perineoscrotal hypospadias," has an autosomal recessive inheritance and is rare. As in other forms of pseudohermaphroditism, some of the abnormality relates to mutations identified in the gene structure.[6,25] The majority of reported cases have come from family clusters found in a number of relatively isolated geographic locations.[1]

Affected males typically are phenotypically female with female to ambiguous external genitalia at birth.[93] The small clitoris-like phallus lacks a urethral orifice. In most affected individuals, the urogenital sinus opens on the perineum, and within the sinus an anterior orifice leads to the urethra and a posterior orifice to a blind vaginal pouch. The testes are in the inguinal canals or labia. The müllerian-derived structures are absent whereas wolffian-derived structures (vas deferens, epididymis, and seminal vesicle), the anlage of which respond to testosterone, are normal.

At puberty, virilization occurs and the breasts fail to develop. The penis lengthens, the bifid scrotum grows and becomes rugated and hyperpigmented, and the testes enlarge and descend. Testicular biopsy specimens reveal spermatogenesis and tubular atrophy in some individuals, complete spermatogenic arrest and Leydig cell hyperplasia in others. The prostate fails to develop and remains impalpable. Erection, ejaculation, and orgasm are possible in some affected individuals; these individuals are not fertile, however.

Neonates with this disorder frequently go unrecognized and are raised as females. After the virilization that accompanies puberty, individuals raised as girls sometimes reverse their sex roles and function as men, often with a stormy period of adjustment. Individuals with a male gender identity benefit from surgical correction of hypospadias and cryptorchidism. High doses of testosterone enhance virilization. Persons raised as females who elect to continue to function as females into adulthood benefit from orchiectomy before the onset of puberty to avoid the accompanying virilization. Estrogen therapy is useful to promote feminization.

Smith–Lemli–Opitz Syndrome

The *Smith–Lemli–Opitz syndrome*, inherited as an autosomal recessive trait, shows ambiguous genitalia, mental retardation, small stature, anteverted nostrils, ptosis, holoprosencephaly, and syndactyly of the second and third toes. The pathogenesis of the ambiguous genitalia reported in some 46 XY patients as well as the morphogenic abnormalities described in general is uncertain, although the syndrome results from an enzymatic defect in the last step of cholesterol metabolism (reduction of 7-dehydrocholesterol due to mutations in the 7-dehydrocholesterol reductase gene).[26,70,72] Studies of testicular function both in vivo and in vitro in a 46 XY patient with ambiguous genitalia and raised as a girl suggested that the fetal testes might have failed to respond to placental hCG at the time of male external genital differentiation.[8] The findings suggest an abnormality in the function of the LH receptor or in the postreceptor message. Testicular histology in this patient was normal for age.

Gender Identification Disorders with an Abnormal Sex Chromosome Constitution

Additions, deletions, or mosaicism of the sex chromosomes characterize individuals in this category. The appearance of the gonads is variable and ranges from the presence of a streak gonad to a nearly normal female or male gonad on both gross and microscopic examination. These disorders are subdivided into two broad categories depending on the frequency with which sexual ambiguity occurs.

Sexual Ambiguity Infrequent Klinefelter Syndrome

Klinefelter syndrome occurs in about 1 of every 1000 live newborn males. The karyotype is usually 47 XXY which, in most cases, results from nondysjunction occurring during meiosis of either paternal or maternal gametes. Less frequently, a 47 XXY/46 XY mosaic karyotype is found, caused by nondysjunction during mitosis of the developing zygote.

Other chromosomal anomalies have also been described.[9] Molecular probe studies have shown that both parents contribute the extra chromosome in about half the incidences. The result is an error in the first paternal meiotic division, but in the mother more than one-fourth occur at the second maternal meiotic division.[34] Unlike trisomy 21, which occurs as a failure of the first maternal meiotic division, the likelihood of Klinefelter's is not increased with advancing maternal age.

The diagnosis is usually first suspected at adolescence when the patient presents with gynecomastia, obesity, or signs of eunuchism. The testes are small. The beard and body hair frequently are sparse. Most patients are tall with long legs, resulting in a diminished upper to lower body segment ratio. Laboratory tests reveal low testosterone levels, elevated gonadotropic levels (postpuberty), and azoospermia. Frequently associated clinical findings include learning disabilities, behavioral disorders, reduced economic striving, and limited sexual drive. The diagnosis also may be established at other stages of life because of evaluation of age-related clinical concerns. Genetic screening programs identify the fetus with Klinefelter syndrome. Although infants with Klinefelter syndrome usually have normal external male genitalia at birth, the syndrome is sometimes discovered during evaluations of newborns with hypospadias, micropenis, and small soft testes or cryptorchidism. In adults, Klinefelter syndrome may be discovered during an evaluation for infertility or malignancy.

The Klinefelter testis is morphologically normal at birth in most cases. Primary spermatogonia are already greatly reduced in number by late childhood. Shortly before the expected time of puberty, the seminiferous tubules begin to degenerate. The absence of elastic fibers in the tubular wall indicates that the process of atrophy began prepubertally. The testes in adult 47 XXY individuals are small and rarely exceed 2 cm in maximal dimension (Fig. 1.19). On microscopic examination, they are largely atrophic, have hyalinized seminiferous tubules, and a relative increase in the number of Leydig cells. Some tubules may be preserved, but lined only by Sertoli cells. Rarely, an occasional seminiferous tubule of the adult

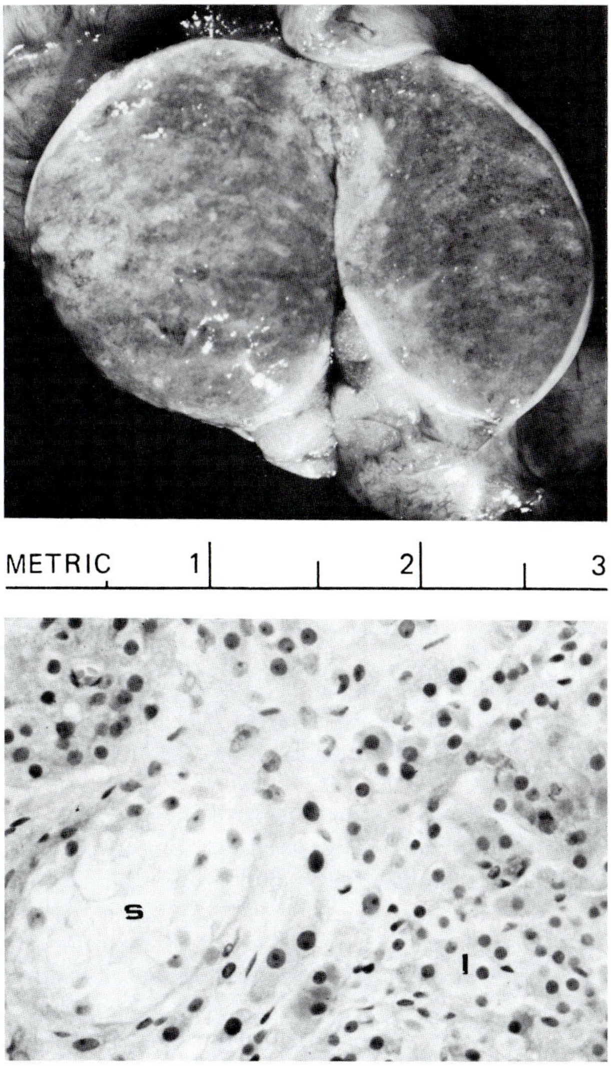

Fig. 1.19. The testis in Klinefelter syndrome. *Top*: The parenchyma of the 2-cm testis is golden yellow to slightly brown. *Bottom*: Clusters of Leydig cells (*l*) surround a seminiferous tubule (*s*). (From Welch and Robboy, ref. 113, with permission of Pediatric Andrology.)

testis contains germ cells in varying stages of maturation. If sperm are detected, mosaicism, most likely of the 46 XY/47 XXY pattern, should be suspected. Patients with this mosaic karyotype are sometimes fertile.

The Leydig cells become pronounced in number sometime after puberty. Although they appear hyperplastic relative to the atrophic appearance of the other elements, it is uncertain whether the absolute volume is greater than in normal testes. Functionally, the Leydig cells are abnormal as evidenced by low levels of serum testosterone in the setting of elevated levels of serum LH and follicle-stimulating hormone (FSH) and subnormal increase in response to administration of hCG.

A variety of neoplasms have been associated with Klinefelter syndrome. Both gonadal and extragonadal germ cell tumors develop with increased frequency. Most extragonadal tumors occur in the mediastinum as teratoma and embryonal cell carcinoma (teratocarcinoma) or choriocarcinoma. In the testis, seminoma, teratoma, and embryonal cell carcinomas have been encountered.[53] Leydig tumors are rare.[71] The risk of breast carcinoma in men with Klinefelter syndrome may be 20% higher than in normal men. Hematologic malignancies have also been reported, including acute leukemia, Hodgkin's disease, malignant lymphoma, and chronic myelogenous leukemia.

Turner Syndrome

In the classic form, *Turner syndrome* is a disorder in which sexually immature phenotypic females of short stature have various congenital anomalies and streak gonads. The cytogenetic hallmark is the 45 X karyotype with a sporadic, nonfamilial pattern of inheritance. Other karyotypes identified less frequently in this syndrome include mosaic 45 X/46 XX and 46 XX with isochrome X (duplication of one arm of the X chromosomes with the loss of the other arm).[39] The X chromosome in 75% of cases is maternal in origin.[39,52] Patients with a 45 X/46 XY mosaic karyotype (considered in mixed gonadal dysgenesis) usually present with obvious sexual ambiguity, but sometimes present as phenotypic females with the clinical stigmata of Turner syndrome. Several recent studies in which conventional cytogenetic analysis disclosed pure X monosomy found hidden "Y" mosaicism or cryptic Y chromosomal material present in 3%[77,112] to about 30%[55,65,74] of the patients after the additional testing was performed. The complex nature of karyotyping is expressed in a recent study in which the blood from a single adult with Turner syndrome was examined in 287 cytogenetic laboratories with many differing results.[73]

A significant difference between patients with 45X/46 XY mosaic karyotype and those with classic 45 X Turner syndrome is that gonadoblastoma and malignant germ cell tumors are common in patients with the former and rare in the latter.[99] Currently, it is common practice to actively exclude Y mosaicism in individuals with Turner syndrome if virilization or a small marker chromosome is seen.[16] In an occasional instance, microscopic gonadoblastoma or other germ cell tumor has been found in some of these Turner-like patients with a cryptic Y chromosome.[38,55]

About 98% of fetuses with a 45 X karyotype abort; the frequency of Turner syndrome is about

1:3000 liveborn females. In the newborn, the overt findings are related to lymph stasis, which manifests itself as edema of the dorsum of the hands or feet or, less frequently, as swellings of the nape of the neck (cystic hygroma). Later in childhood and in adult life, webbing of the neck or elevation of the distal portion of the nails are residua of more marked swellings present during fetal life and may still provide a clue to the correct diagnosis. A rare, but important, major presentation is hydronephrosis due to ureteropelvic stenosis; all female neonates with a ureteropelvic obstruction should have a buccal smear. Congenital anomalies of other organ systems are associated with Turner syndrome and include a short fourth metacarpal, hypoplastic nails, multiple pigmented nevi, and coarctation of the aorta. Growth retardation (short stature) is common.[29] More than 40 somatic anomalies are associated with this condition.

Patients who reach adolescence undiagnosed often present with primary amenorrhea. Examination reveals underdeveloped secondary sex characteristics and a small uterus. Urinary gonadotropins are always elevated and the vaginal smear lacks cornified cells. The buccal smear in a 45 X individual reveals few if any Barr bodies; in those 20% of patients with mosaic karyotype (usually 45 X/46 XX or 45 X/47 XXX, the smear discloses a subnormal number of chromatin positive cells (about 5–15% for a female). Only rare patients with Turner syndrome have become pregnant, and most of these have a 46 XX cell line. Some of these women have mosaic patterns that are found only after extensive search.[51]

At laparotomy, the internal genitalia are female and, although small, are in normal relation to one another. The adult gonads appear as white fibrous streaks, 2–3 cm long and 0.5 cm in diameter, and are located in the position normally occupied by the ovary (Fig. 1.20). On microscopic examination a streak consists of an attenuated cortex, a medulla, and a hilus. The cortex is composed of characteristic ovarian stroma in which the cells are elongated, wavy, and comprise conspicuous nuclei and scant cytoplasm. Rete tubules (rete ovarii) and hilar cells are typically present in the hilus region. Oocytes are almost always absent in adult with Turner syndrome. Oocytes are present in normal numbers in 45 X embryos before the 12th week of gestation. In older fetuses and young children, the number of oocytes falls progressively relative to the normal number for the age until the number reaches zero, usually before the time of normal menarche, thus leading to primary amenorrhea. These findings suggest that the second X chromosome is necessary for

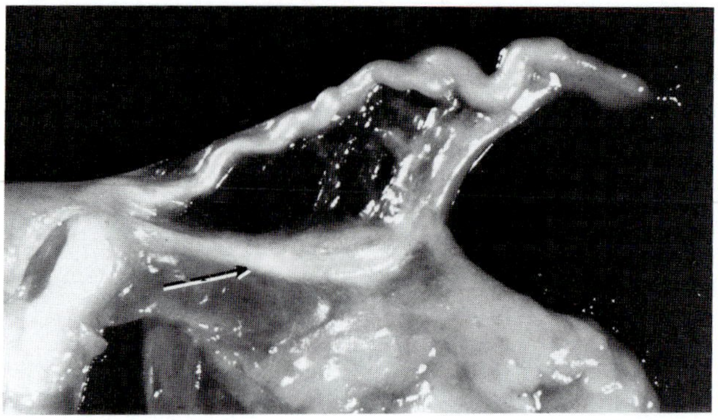

Fig. 1.20. Streak ovary (*arrow*) in Turner syndrome. The streak gonad is thin, fibrous, and lacks germ cells. (From Welch and Robboy, ref. 113, with permission of Pediatric Andrology.)

granulosa cell development and primary follicular formation; in the absence of this X chromosome, granulosa cells fail to differentiate and, as a result, the oocytes degenerate.

Gonadal tumors are exceedingly rare. Tumors of germ cell origin are undoubtedly rare because of the paucity of germ cells. Although occasional germ cell tumors have been reported,[75] care must be exercised because with more sophisticated tools for chromosome analysis, especially newer molecular biologic techniques, cryptic Y-chromosomal fragments have been discovered associated with the tumor tissue.[38,55] Most reported cases with a gonadoblastoma component have had a mosaic pattern with a Y chromosome[55,107] and more appropriately should be considered under the category of mixed gonadal dysgenesis.

Development of neoplasms of the so-called common epithelial type suggest that the coelomic epithelium encapsulating the gonad can undergo malignant change even if the gonad is a streak. Endometrial carcinoma occurred occasionally in those patients who had received long-term, high-dose exogenous unopposed estrogen therapy to foster the appearance of the female secondary sex characteristics. Both natural estrogens and synthetic nonsteroidal estrogens have been implicated, and the duration of usage usually exceeded 3 years. Today, this is exceedingly rare. Extragonadal tumors, most often of neurogenic origin, have been reported in children and young adults.

XX Male Syndrome

The *XX male syndrome* is a disorder characterized by a nearly normal but infertile phenotypic male with a 46 XX karyotype. This syndrome, one of the rarest of all sex chromosome anomalies, occurs in about 1 of 24,000 newborn males.[70] XX males share many characteristics of men with Klinefelter syndrome. Both have a generally masculine appearance, normal or near normal external genitalia, male psychosexual orientation, normal to weak secondary sexual characteristics, normal to low androgen levels, and azoospermia. The testes are small, with prominent Leydig cells and tubules lined only by Sertoli cells. The most common reasons for referral are similar to those with Klinefelter syndrome, namely infertility or abnormal secondary sexual characteristics. XX males also tend to differ clinically from men with Klinefelter syndrome: the former are generally shorter in height, and the frequency of hypospadias and gynecomastia is higher. The frequency of impaired intelligence is not increased in XX males relative to the general population.

The XX male syndrome potentially results from at least three distinctly different mechanisms.[101] About 70% of these patients have a small portion of paternally derived Y chromosome, which contains the SRY gene. The SRY gene normally is found on the short arm of the Y chromosome adjacent to the pseudoautosomal pairing region. During meiosis in the father, an abnormal exchange sometimes leads to the transfer onto the X chromosome of the entire pseudoautosomal region plus the adjacent portion of the Y chromosome with the SRY gene. Inheritance of such an X chromosome from the father leads to the Y(+) XX male syndrome. The inheritance pattern of this form of the syndrome is sporadic. These patients have normal male external genitalia. Hypospadias and ambiguous genitalia are virtually never found. Apparently, the presence of the SRY gene is adequate to lead to normal male phenotype. Azoospermia in these patients results from the lack of other genes normally found on the Y chromosome necessary for sperm development.

Some patients with the XX male syndrome lack Y-derived DNA. Such Y(−) XX males might result by two different mechanisms. The first accounts for the familial transmission of an autosomal dominant or X-linked inheritance of XX maleness. These patients usually have ambiguous genitalia. This indicates that genes exist, probably downstream from TDF, which can trigger testis determination when mutated.[43] A second potential mechanism that might lead to the Y(−) condition is chromosomal mosaicism with a prevalent XX lineage. In such patients, the Y-containing cell line might simply be technically too difficult to identify because of the small number of such cells. Alternatively, a 47 XXY zygote might lose its Y chromosome by nondysjunction early in ontogeny, thus allowing a 46 XX cell line to persist; the 47 XXY cell line may have persisted long enough to induce male gonadal development. Such patients, just as patients with familial Y(−) XX maleness, often present with sexual ambiguity suggesting that patients with Y(−) XX male syndrome are closely related both phenotypically and etiologically to XX true hermaphrodites, who present with both testicular and ovarian tissue.

Pure Gonadal Dysgenesis

Pure gonadal dysgenesis, and its eponym, *Swyer syndrome*, are terms that historically have encompassed a number of diverse conditions, including testicular regression syndrome at one end of the spectrum and mixed gonadal dysgenesis at the other. As used in this chapter, pure gonadal dysgenesis refers to a phenotypic female in whom the internal genitalia include müllerian structures (uterus and fallopian tubes) and generally streak gonads, the constellation of which probably still encompasses a multitude of diverse conditions. The patients may appear phenotypically normal or have hypoplastic external genitalia. The pure gonadal dysgenesis syndrome occurs with both 46 XX and 46 XY karyotypes and has both familial and sporadic patterns of inheritance.

The 46 XX type pure gonadal dysgenesis is usually an autosomal recessive disorder but, less frequently, may be caused by an abnormality of the X chromosome, possibly as a mosaic 45 X cell line confined to the gonad.[61] Deletions of the short or long arm of an X chromosome have been identified in some cases. Such patients have greater ovarian development than those with 46 XY type pure gonadal dysgenesis or Turner syndrome and present more often with signs of ovarian dysfunction (secondary amenorrhea or infertility) rather than primary gonadal failure (primary amenorrhea). Some patients may also have mosaic cell lines with the SRY gene absent in some tissues (peripheral leukocytes), but present in others (testicular tissue).[20]

The 46 XY type pure gonadal dysgenesis is more common than the 46 XX form of the disorder. The syndrome of pure gonadal dysgenesis may be sporadic or familial with either X-linked recessive or autosomal recessive patterns of inheritance.[11,86] Some patients have a mosaic 45 X/46 XY karyotype. The 46 XY type may also involve deletion of the SRY gene, a mutated inactive SRY gene, or a defective cofactor.[89,103,104]

Patients with 46 XX type pure gonadal dysgenesis, as those with Turner syndrome, only rarely develop gonadal tumors. Some have had hilus cell hyperplasia and hilus cell tumors with the usual associated virilizing effects. Epithelial tumors are extremely rare, but of these mucinous tumors occur more frequently than serous.[45] Rare examples of germ cell tumors have been reported,[63] and even though no identifiable Y-chromosome component could be detected in some, the possibility of a cryptic Y fragment cannot be excluded. Patients with 46 XY pure gonadal dysgenesis are at high risk for gonadoblastoma and other germ cell tumors as is true of all patients with streak gonads and a Y chromosome.[104] In one series, 11 of 20 patients had neoplasms in the gonads; 8 patients had gonadoblastomas, half of which were bilateral, and 8 patients had dysgerminoma, all unilateral.[78] On this basis, patients with 46 XY pure gonadal dysgenesis might be considered a subset of the broader condition of mixed gonadal dysgenesis.

Sexual Ambiguity Frequent

Patients in this category exhibit a wide range of phenotypic appearances and internal genitalia. A Y chromosome is often present, usually as part of a mosaic complement. Sexual ambiguity is a common finding.

Mixed Gonadal Dysgenesis

Mixed gonadal dysgenesis (MGD) is a heterogeneous syndrome characterized usually by a 45 X/46 XY or 46 XY karyotype, persistent müllerian duct structures, an abnormal testis, and a contralateral streak gonad.[3] The functional deficit imposed by the abnormal testis is expressed as incomplete inhibition of müllerian development, incomplete differentiation of wolffian duct structures, and incomplete male development of the external genitalia. Often, incomplete mediation of the testicular descent occurs, resulting in both internal and external asymmetry of the genitalia and a mixture of male and female features in an individual in whom neither gonad is normal. About two-thirds of the affected individuals are raised as females and the remainder as males. Some patients with MGD exhibit phenotypic features of Turner syndrome.[4,102] Elsewhere, we have suggested that the syndrome of MGD should be enlarged to incorporate some patients with bilateral streak gonads (described here as 46 XY type pure gonadal dysgenesis) or bilateral abnormal testes with mosaic 45 X/46 XY karyotype (dysgenetic male pseudohermaphroditism), because the clinical, pathological, and chromosomal features of these syndromes closely resemble each other.

The underlying genetic and karyotype abnormalities leading to the syndrome of mixed gonadal dysgenesis are currently under investigation. A variety of different genetic abnormalities appear to result in MGD, thus leading to the phenotypic heterogeneity of MGD. Partial deletions of both the short and long arms of chromosome Y have been detected in these individuals. In most cases in which no detectable Y chromosomal anomaly is observed by conventional chromosome analysis, a Y fragment is found when additional testing is performed.[28]

Clinically, MGD is usually detected in the neonate because of ambiguity of the external genitalia. Frequently, a palpable testis bulges through an indirect inguinal hernia or descends completely into the labioscrotal fold, resulting in asymmetry of the genital swellings. This clinical appearance has prompted some investigators to name the syndrome *asymmetric gonadal dysgenesis*. If the gonads are intraabdominal, the labioscrotal folds may appear as normal labia or as empty scrotal sacs. The condition is likely to go unrecognized unless the clitoris is sufficiently enlarged to mandate investigation, which is common. The gonad that descends is almost always a testis, and the streak gonads are always intraabdominal unless dragged into a "hernia uteri inguinale."

Organs derived from the müllerian duct persist in 95% of cases (Fig. 1.21).[57,84] The uterus is usually infantile or rudimentary. The fallopian tubes are frequently bilateral. If a testis is grossly near normal size and well differentiated, the fimbriated end of the ipsilateral tube may be absent, but in only one-third of cases is the ipsilateral tube entirely absent. Organs of wolffian duct derivation also may be present, but the frequency is variable. The epididymis is identified in two-thirds of cases and is usually present on the side where there is a testis. The vas deferens is encountered less frequently. The seminal vesicle is identified only rarely probably because tissue near the bladder/prostate region is not usually removed.

The gonad may be a testis or a streak. Streak gonads may be partially differentiated toward ovary or testis. Bilateral gross testes, frequently of an asynchronous degree of maturity, are found in about 15% of cases whereas a unilateral gross testis is found in 60%. The testis is consistently abnormal architecturally, its organization being divided into three zones, each of which reflects the quantity and type of cellular components present. The three zones, which are described below in detail, include (1) the region of the tunica albuginea or cortex, which exhibits widely spaced seminiferous tubules or differentiation toward ovary, (2) the medulla, which is composed of normal or near-normal seminiferous tubules and interstitium, and (3) a hilar region with poorly differentiated seminiferous tu-

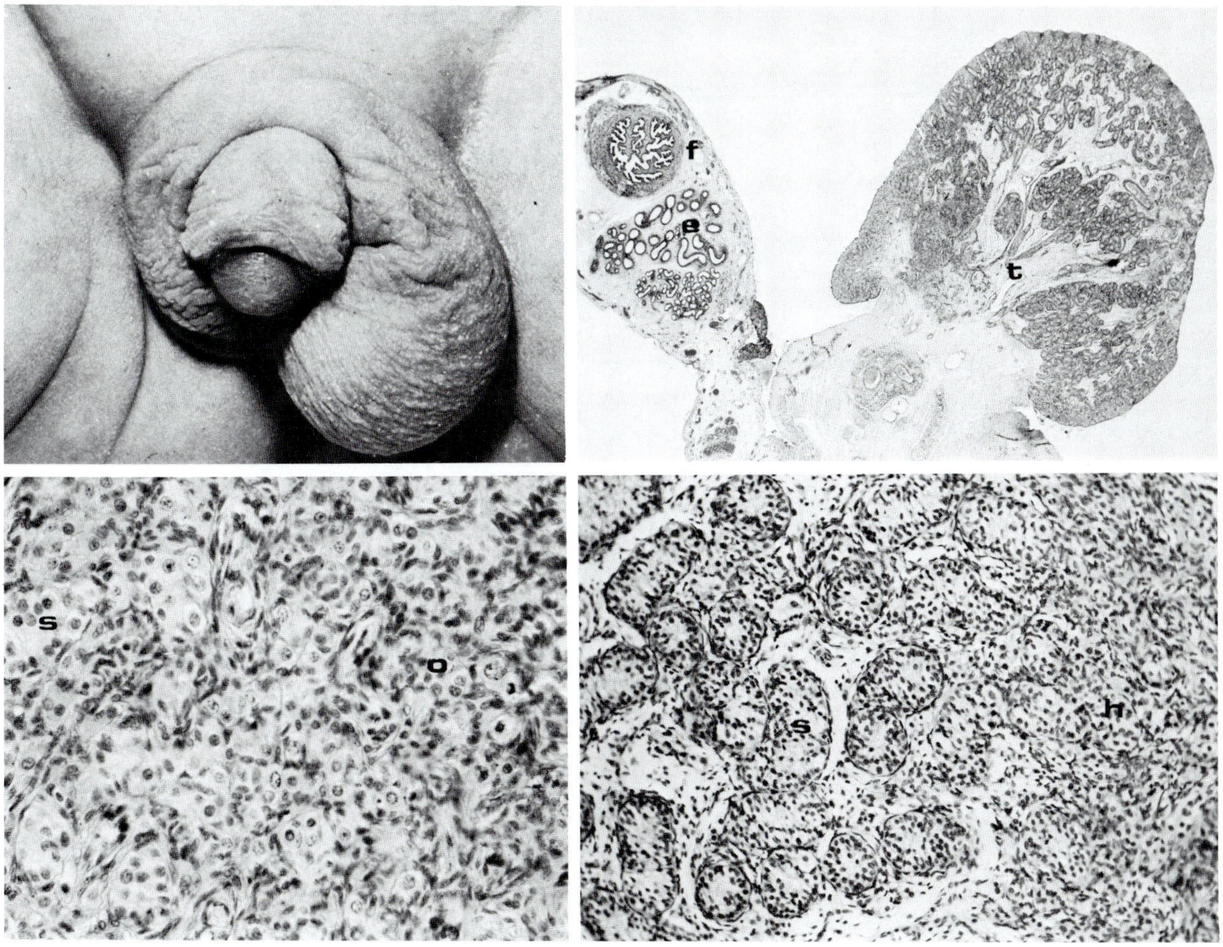

Fig. 1.21. Mixed gonadal dysgenesis. *Top left*: External genitalia in MGD. The left testis had descended into the scrotum; the right streak was in the abdominal cavity. Because of this characteristic appearance, some investigators prefer the name "asymmetric gonadal dysgenesis" rather than mixed gonadal dysgenesis. *Top right*: Testis (*t*) and adjacent fallopian tube (*f*) and epididymis (*e*). The medulla contains immature seminiferous tubules with germ cells and interstitial cells whereas the region nearer the cortex resembles fetal ovary with immature sex cords and rare primordial follicles. *Bottom left*: Cortex of gonad in which testicular seminiferous tubules (*s*) merge into fetal type ovary (*q*). *Bottom right*: The medullary parenchyma of the testis is composed of normal immature seminiferous tubules (*s*) with germ cells and occasional interstitial cells, whereas the parenchyma in the region of the hilus (*h*) near the rete testis appears less committed as testis and is characterized by abnormal, pleomorphic, seminiferous tubules. The photograph is taken at the junction of the two zones. (From Robboy et al., ref. 84, with permission of Human Pathology.)

bules that are only partly differentiated toward testis.

The superficial cortex may contain seminiferous tubules that are often widely separated by edematous, undifferentiated stroma. Sometimes the tubules penetrate the incompletely formed tunica albuginea and open onto the serosa. Occasionally, broad zones of cortex differentiate slightly toward the ovary, even displaying rare primordial follicles. Mice that spontaneously develop chromosomal mosaicism as a result of nondysjunction often show gonads with ovarian tissue at the periphery and seminiferous cords centrally.

The central zone (medulla) of the macroscopic infant testis is architecturally and cytologically normal. Narrow closed seminiferous tubules are lined by Sertoli cells with abundant cytoplasm. The number of spermatogonia vary; advanced forms of spermatogenic maturation are not observed. Leydig cells are present in small clusters of varying size. The nuclei of the Leydig cells contain finely dispersed chromatin, and the cytoplasm varies from minimal and amphophilic or slightly basophilic to abundant and eosinophilic. In older patients, the medulla is atrophic and the tubules are lined only by Sertoli cells (Fig. 1.22). The basement membranes are of-

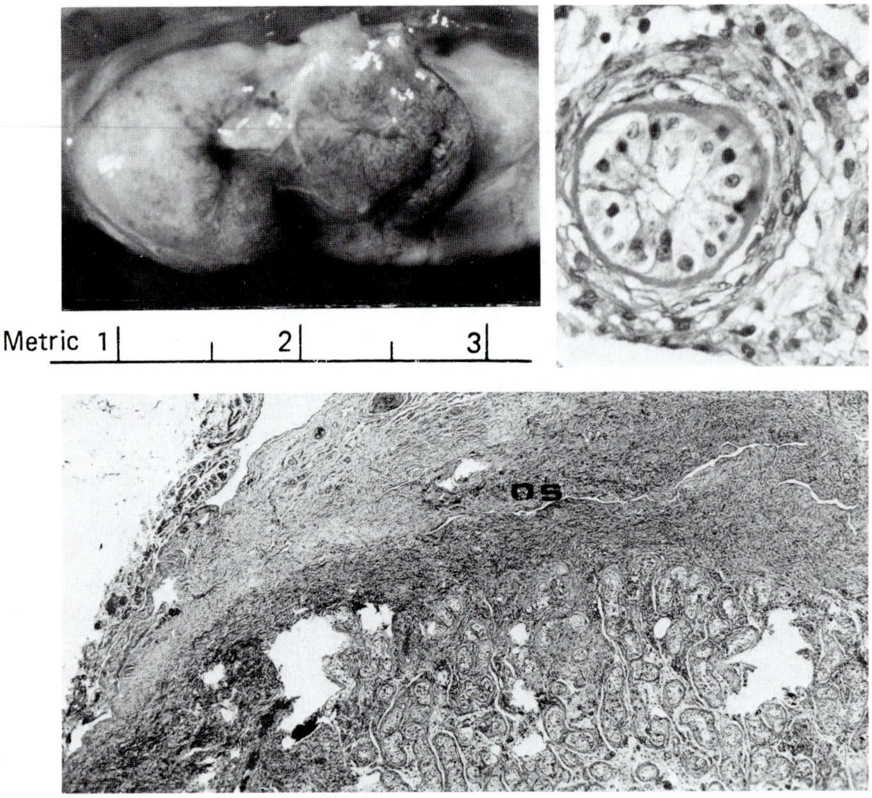

Fig. 1.22. Testis in mixed gonadal dysgenesis. *Upper left*: The tunica albuginea from the testis of a 35-year-old phenotypic man is tan and maximally 1 mm thick; the parenchyma is golden yellow. *Lower*: Cross section of tunica albuginea, which is composed of stroma resembling the stroma of ovarian cortex (*os*) and medulla with seminiferous tubules. *Upper right*: Detail of seminiferous tubules lined only by Sertoli cells. The interstitium is filled with Leydig cells. (From Robboy et al., ref. 84, with permission of Human Pathology.)

ten thickened. Prominent clusters of Leydig cells fill the interstitium.

The architecturally disorganized hilar region discloses seminiferous tubules that are swollen by increased numbers of Sertoli cells and are lined by indistinct basement membranes. These tubules also merge with the surrounding stroma, imparting the appearance of a homogeneous blend of Leydig cells, germ cells, Sertoli cells, and an indeterminate type of interstitial stroma. The region resembles neither fetal ovary nor testis.

The streak gonads appear similar to those found in Turner syndrome. We have not observed a gonad that has been identifiable grossly as an ovary or has been shown microscopically to contain graafian follicles, corpora lutea, or corpora albicantia. The presence of rare primordial follicles or, as in the fetal ovary, aggregates of germ cells partially surrounded by immature granulosa cells are evidence that a streak gonad can differentiate toward the ovary. Morphologic changes may occur over time in the streak gonads. Myriads of germ cells present in a streak of an infant may degenerate and disappear by puberty, resulting in a gonad composed exclusively of fibrous tissue and a few rete tubules (Fig 1.23); similar changes occur in the streak gonads of Turner syndrome (45 X karyotype).

Approximately one-third of patients with MGD develop gonadoblastoma, a tumor found almost exclusively in patients with an intersex syndrome. The tumor virtually always occurs in association with a whole or component of a "Y" chromosome[90] and most likely has its beginnings during prenatal life.[40] Gonadoblastoma accounts for three-fourths of the gonadal tumors arising in dysgenetic gonads and is usually discovered during the first to fourth decades of life. Many of the isolated reports of gonadoblastoma associated with other forms of hermaphroditism described clinically and pathologically actually may be examples of MGD.

About 20% of gonadoblastomas arise in a streak gonad and another 20% arise in a dysgenetic testis; in the remaining cases, the nature of the underlying gonad cannot be determined with certainty because it is replaced by tumor. The gross appearance of the gonad with gonadoblastoma varies according to the

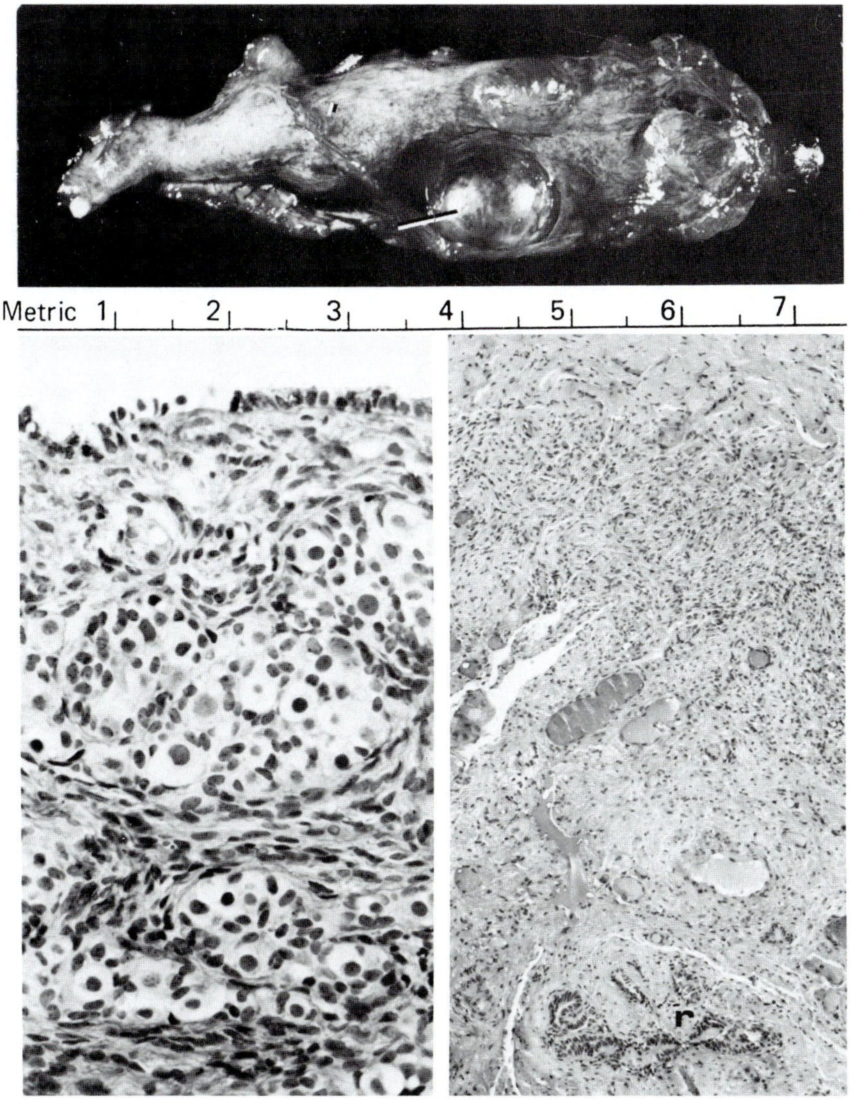

Fig. 1.23. Mixed gonadal dysgenesis. When the patient was an infant, the streak gonad resembled a fetal ovary with germ cells and immature sex cords (*lower left*). When the streak gonad was removed in its entirety 13 years later (*top*; *arrows*), it existed only as several microscopic areas of wispy ovarian-type cortical stroma and rete ovarii (r) (*lower right*). (From Robboy et al., ref. 84, with permission of Human Pathology.)

size of the neoplasm, the presence of calcification, and whether the gonadoblastoma has been overgrown by a malignant form of germ cell tumor (usually germinoma) (Fig. 1.24). Approximately one-fifth of gonadoblastomas are discovered solely because a streak gonad was examined microscopically (Fig. 1.25). The contralateral gonad also contains a gonadoblastoma in more than one-third of patients.

On microscopic examination, the gonadoblastoma appears as circumscribed nests of neoplastic germ cells having the cytologic properties of germinoma (dysgerminoma and seminoma) and that are encompassed individually or in groups by sex cord derivatives with inconspicuous cytoplasm and small round to oval nuclei resembling immature Sertoli cells. The malignant germ cells have large, generally centrally placed nuclei in the cell, obvious macronucleoli that are one to several in number, and copious pale cytoplasm with usually a distinct cytoplasmic membrane. Carcinoma in situ cells express placental-like alkaline phosphatase and the protooncogene, *c-kit*.[40,80] They also react immunocytochemically with several monoclonal antibodies.[40] Inhibin reactivity is also commonly demonstrable, which is in keeping with the sex cord cells (immature Sertoli/granulosa cells) being an integral part of the tumor.[44] Hyaline, composed of basement membrane material, is found along the margin or as nodules within the nests of tumors. In four-fifths of cases the hyaline material is calcified, initially appearing as small, laminated spheres, which eventually fuse and coalesce into large mulberry-like masses. Not infrequently, the only evidence that a dysgerminoma originated in a gonadoblastoma is the presence focally of mulberry-like calcifications. Hormonally active cells that resemble lutein and Leydig cells are found interspersed among the nests of tumor in about two-thirds of cases. These hormonally active cells are found least frequently in nonvirilized phenotypic females, more often in virilized females, and most frequently in phenotypic males. To some degree, their appearance may be related to the postpubertal age of the patient when the gonad is examined.

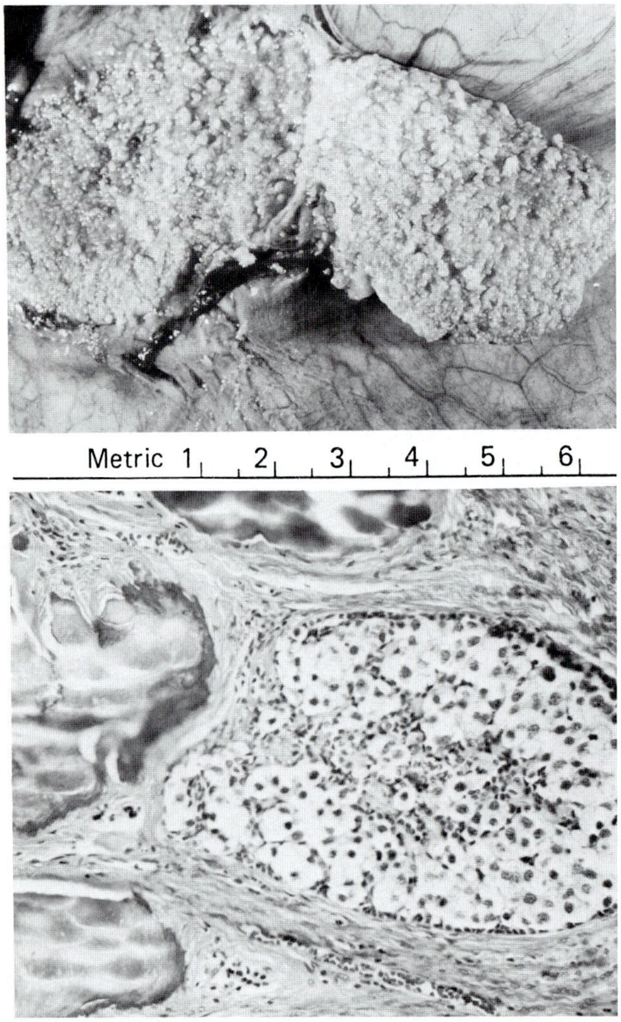

Fig 1.24. Gonadoblastoma in mixed gonadal dysgenesis. *Top*: 15-cm gonadal tumor composed largely of dysgerminoma. At one pole is a 5 × 2 × 0.5 cm calcified gonadoblastoma. *Bottom*: Gonadoblastoma. Multiple mulberry-like calcific masses partially replace the tumor nests composed of germ cells surrounded by sex cord derivatives. (From Welch and Robboy, ref. 113, with permission of Pediatric Andrology.)

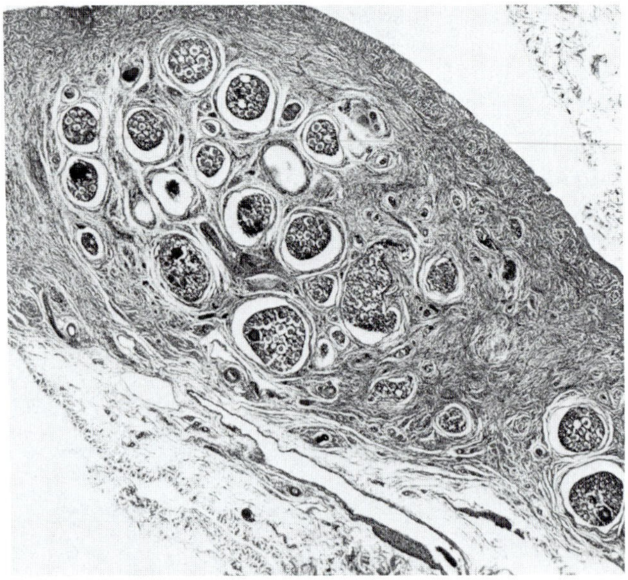

Fig. 1.25. Gonadoblastoma occupying a gonadal streak. (From Scully, ref. 89a, with permission of Cancer.)

Approximately 30% of gonadoblastomas are overgrown by a malignant germ cell tumor, usually the germinoma; 8% are overgrown by endodermal sinus tumor, immature teratoma, embryonal carcinoma, or choriocarcinoma. An occasional gonad may also show proliferative sex cord elements and resemble a Sertoli cell tumor.[69] Although the gonadoblastoma itself does not metastasize and therefore can be considered as an in situ malignancy, the typically malignant behavior of the other tumors makes early prophylactic removal of the gonads in all patients advisable. Also, to avoid the consequences of onset of virilization if the patient is to be raised as a female, it is important that gonadectomy be performed before the patient reaches puberty. Patients who have been treated with long-term administration of estrogen may on occasion develop endometrial carcinoma. Congenital cardiovascular anomalies have also been reported in patients with MGD.

True Hermaphroditism

True hermaphroditism is defined as the presence of both testicular and ovarian tissue in a patient. Affected individuals may have either a female or male phenotype with a variable degree of sexual ambiguity. Because the wavy, cortical-type stroma typically seen in the female gonad can be found in both female and male gonads and therefore is nonspecific, follicular structures must be identified to classify gonadal tissue as ovarian and seminiferous tubules to classify the tissue as testicular. In true hermaphrodites, the gonads may be ovary and testis separately or combined in an ovotestis.

The ovotestis is the most frequently encountered gonad in true hermaphroditism. In four-fifths of cases the ovarian and testicular tissues are arranged in an end-to-end fashion. The ovarian portion of an ovotestis has a convoluted surface whereas the testicular portion is smooth and glistening. Frequently, a distinct line demarcates the two tissues. The firm nature of the palpable ovarian tissue and the soft texture of the testis are valuable clinical signs when evaluating the nature of a gonad in an infant with ambisexual external genitalia.

An ovary, which preferentially develops on the left side, is the second most common gonad in true hermaphrodites. Every patient over 15 years of age in the series of van Niekerk[106] had either a corpus luteum or a corpus albicans. The testis, which is the gonad least often encountered, develops preferentially on the right.

The location of the gonad is influenced by the type and quantity of gonadal tissue present. Increasing amounts of ovarian tissue increase the probability that the gonad will be in an ovarian position. When a gonad with the macroscopic features of an ovary is situated in the inguinal canal or in the labioscrotal fold, the possibility of it being an ovotestis should be seriously considered. The position of the testis is less constant. Most (63%) reside in the scrotum, 14% in the inguinal region, 1% in the internal inguinal ring, and 22% in a normal ovarian position.

The nature of the genital organ adjacent to a gonad in true hermaphroditism depends on the nature of the gonad, which is in contrast to MGD, in which a fallopian tube is often adjacent to the gonad, regardless of whether it is a testis or streak. In true hermaphroditism, a fallopian tube is adjacent to an ovary and an epididymis or vas deferens is adjacent to a testis. Either a müllerian or wolffian structure, but not both, is adjacent to an ovotestis. MIS appears to be functional. Ninety-five percent of fallopian tubes adjacent to ovotestes have closed ostia. Only 10% of uteri are normal; the other patients have absent uteri (13%), unicornuate uteri (10%), absent cervix (14%), or uterine hypoplasia (46%).

The most common karyotypes in true hermaphroditism are 46 XX (60%), 46 XY (12%), and mosaic (28%), usually 46 XX/46 XY, 46 XY/47 XXY, or least frequently 45 X/46 XY. Patients with a "Y" chromosome have a two- to threefold increased frequency of having a testis as opposed to an ovotestis. Nearly 75% of true hermaphrodites with an ovary and ovotestis have a 46 XX karyotype.

As in other disorders of intersex, genetic aberrations appear to play a key role in the development of true hermaphroditism. For example, chromosome Y-specific genes (e.g., SRY) have been detected in some 46 XX true hermaphrodites, suggesting one potential mechanism for the development of XX true hermaphroditism, similar to individuals with XX male syndrome. In some series, however, SRY was undetected in the 46 XX patients,[30] indicating that other mechanisms may also be important. Mutations that mimic the SRY gene have been suggested as one possibility where the SRY gene was absent.[94] One explanation proposed for patients with an XY chromosome is the possibility that the SRY gene, if present, may act at a time too late to stimulate the development of a testis, hence permitting ovarian tissue to develop.

The clinical presentations of true hermaphrodites vary to some extent depending on the patient's age at the time of diagnosis. Until recently, the condition often went undetected until adolescence, when phenotypic male patients were evaluated for gynecomastia and phenotypic female patients were evaluated for amenorrhea or failure to develop secondary sex changes. Thus, in one series,[106] three-fourths of patients were raised as males and one-fourth as females. Many patients, however, menstruated and a few became pregnant. Phenotypic males may experience monthly hematuria because of menstruation into a persistent urogenital sinus. With an increased awareness of intersex states, the condition is recognized more often in infants because of ambiguous genitalia, usually in the form of a small phallus (enlarged clitoris).[19] Like MGD, the scrotum may be asymmetric, with the larger, more normal-appearing hemiscrotum containing a testis. Among 160 patients the external genitalia were asymmetric in three-fourths (labioscrotal folds in 63% and hemiscrotums in 13%).

On microscopic examination, the gonadal tissue often appears normal if the patient is young. In infants the ovarian tissue contains numerous follicles, whereas the testicular parenchyma discloses normal-appearing seminiferous tubules with spermatogonia. Patients in the reproductive years may have ovarian tissue with structures indicative of ovulation, for example, follicles, corpora lutea, and corpora albicantia, but spermatogenesis is rare in the testicular portion. The testicular portion of an ovotestis is usually abnormal with incomplete development, loss of germ cells, and tubular sclerosis. Scrotal testes in these patients show less severe changes, sometimes showing faulty spermatogenesis.

At times, distinction between true hermaphroditism and MGD can be difficult. In the newborn, asymmetric ambiguous genitalia may be observed in both conditions. If a streak gonad from a patient with MGD is serially sectioned, a rare primordial follicle may be encountered in what otherwise appears to be a fetal-type ovary admixed with testis with well developed seminiferous tubules. If the term *true hermaphroditism* is restricted to those patients in whom the ovarian and testicular tissue are both apparent grossly, it should be possible to segregate more clearly those individuals in whom the ovarian tissue may be functional.

Gonadal tumors occur in less than 3% of affected individuals. Germinoma is the most common type of tumor, but gonadoblastomas and a variety of other tumors have been reported.[98] One case has been reported in which the primitive sex-cord cellular elements adjacent to seminiferous tubules in a testis gave rise to cancer in the form of a juvenile granulosa cell tumor.[100]

References

1. Al-Attia HM (1997) Male pseudohermaphroditism due to 5-alpha-reductase-2 deficiency in an Arab kindred. Postgrad Med J 73:802–807
2. Alvarez-Nava F, Gonzalez S, Soto M, Martinez C, Prieto M (1997) Complete androgen insensitivity syndrome: clinical and anatomopathological findings in 23 patients. Genet Couns 8:7–12
3. Alvarez-Nava F, Gonzalez S, Soto M, Pineda L, Morales-Machin A (1999) Mixed gonadal dysgenesis: a syndrome of broad clinical cytogenetic and histopathologic spectrum. Genet Counsel 10:233–243
4. Alvarez-Nava F, Martinez MC, Gonzalez S, Soto M, Borjas L, Rojas A (1999) FISH and PCR analysis of the presence of Y-chromosome sequences in a patient with Xq-isochromosome and testicular tissue. Clin Genet 55:356–361
5. Andersson S, Moghrabi N (1997) Physiology and molecular genetics in 17 beta-hydroxysteroid dehydrogenases. Steroids 62:143–147
6. Anwar R, Gilbey SG, New JP, Markham AF (1997) Male pseudohermaphroditism resulting from a novel mutation in the human steroid 5 alpha-reductase type 2 gene (SRD5A2). J Clin Pathol Mol Pathol 50:51–52
7. Arnhold IJ, Latronico AC, Batista MC, Mendonca BB (1999) Menstrual disorders and infertility caused by inactivating mutations of the luteinizing hormone receptor gene. Fertil Steril 71:597–601
8. Berensztein E, Torrado M, Belgorosky A, Rivarola M (1999) Smith-Lemli-Opitz syndrome: in vivo and in vitro study of testicular function in a prepubertal patient with ambiguous genitalia. Acta Paediatr 88:1229–1232
9. Bertelloni S, Battini R, Baroncelli GI, et al (1999) Central precocious puberty in 48,XXYY Klinefelter syndrome variant. J Pediatr Endocrinol Metab 12: 459–465
10. Bilbao JR, Loridan L, Audi L, Gonzalo E, Castano L (1998) A novel missense (R80W) mutation in 17-beta-hydroxysteroid dehydrogenase type 3 gene associated with male pseudohermaphroditism. Eur J Endocrinol 139:330–333
11. Bilbao JR, Loridan L, Castano L (1996) A novel postzygotic nonsense mutation in SRY in familial XY gonadal dysgenesis. Hum Genet 97:537–539
12. Brennan J, Karl J, Martineau J, et al (1998) Sry and the testis: molecular pathways of organogenesis. J Exp Zool 281:494–500
13. Carlson AD, Obeid JS, Kanellopoulou N, Wilson RC, New MI (1999) Congenital adrenal hyperplasia: update on prenatal diagnosis and treatment. J Steroid Biochem Mol Biol 69:19–29
14. Cendron M, Schned AR, Ellsworth PI (1998) Histological evaluation of the testicular nubbin in the vanishing testis syndrome. J Urol 160:1161–1163
15. Cerame BI, Newfield RS, Pascoe L, et al (1999) Prenatal diagnosis and treatment of 11-beta-hydroxylase deficiency congenital adrenal hyperplasia resulting in normal female genitalia. J Clin Endocrinol Metabol 84:3129–3134
16. Chu C (1999) Y-chromosome mosaicism in girls with Turner's syndrome. Clin Endocrinol 50:17–18
17. Clarnette TD, Sugita Y, Hutson JM (1997) Genital anomalies in human and animal models reveal the mechanisms and hormones governing testicular descent. Br J Urol 79:99–112
18. Cunha GR, Boutin EL, Turner T, Donjacour AA (1998) Role of mesenchyme in the development of the urogenital tract. J Clean Technol Environ Toxicol Occup Med 7:179–194
19. Damiani D, Fellous M, McElreavey K, et al (1997) True hermaphroditism: clinical aspects and molecular studies in 16 cases. Eur J Endocrinol 136: 201–204
20. Dardis A, Saraco N, Mendilaharzu H, Rivarola M, Belgorosky A (1997) Report of an XX male with hypospadias and pubertal gynecomastia, SRY gene negative in blood leukocytes but SRY gene positive in testicular cells. Horm Res (Basel) 47:85–88
21. Dork T, Schnieders F, Jakubiczka S, Wieacker P, Schroeder-Kurth T, Schmidtke J (1998) A new missense substitution at a mutational hot spot of the androgen receptor in siblings with complete androgen insensitivity syndrome. Hum Mutat 11:337–339

22. Erk A, Ozeren S, Ozbay O, Vural B, Elcioglu N (1999) Persistent müllerian duct syndrome: a case report. J Reprod Med 44:135–138
23. Faure E, Gouedard L, Imbeaud S, et al (1996) Mutant isoforms of the anti-müllerian hormone type II receptor are not expressed at the cell membrane. J Biol Chem 271:30571–30575
24. Ferrari P, Obeyesekere VR, Li K, et al (1996) Point mutations abolish 11 beta-hydroxysteroid dehydrogenase type II activity in three families with the congenital syndrome of apparent mineralocorticoid excess. Mol Cell Endocrinol 119:21–24
25. Ferraz LFC, Baptista MTM, Maciel-Guerra AT, Junior GG, Hackel C (1999) New frameshift mutation in the 5 alpha-reductase type 2 gene in a Brazilian patient with 5 alpha-reductase deficiency. Am J Med Genet 87:221–225
26. Fitzky BU, Glossmann H, Utermann G, Moebius FF (1999) Molecular genetics of the Smith-Lemli-Opitz syndrome and postsqualene sterol metabolism. Curr Opin Lipidol 10:123–131
27. Fung MF, Vadas G, Lotocki R, Heywood M, Krepart G (1999) Tubular Krukenberg tumor in pregnancy with virilization. Gynecol Oncol 41:81–84
28. Gibbons B, Tan SY, Yu CC, Cheah E, Tan HL (1999) Risk of gonadoblastoma in female patients with Y chromosome abnormalities and dysgenetic gonads. J Paediatr Child Health 35:210–213
29. Gicquel C, Gaston V, Cabrol S, Le Bouc Y (1998) Assessment of Turner's syndrome by molecular analysis of the X chromosome in growth-retarded girls. J Clin Endocrinol Metab 83:1472–1476
30. Guerra Junior G, de Mello MP, Assumpcao JG, et al (1998) True hermaphrodites in the southeastern region of Brazil: a different cytogenetic and gonadal profile. J Pediatr Endocrinol Metab 11:519–524
31. Hawkyard S, Poon P, Morgan DR (1999) Sertoli tumour presenting with stress incontinence in a patient with testicular feminization. Br J Urol Int 84:382–383
32. Hiort O, Holterhus PM, Nitsche EM (1998) Physiology and pathophysiology of androgen action. Baillieres Clin Endocrinol Metab 12:115–132
33. Hiort O, Sinnecker GH, Holterhus PM, Nitsche EM, Kruse K (1996) The clinical and molecular spectrum of androgen insensitivity syndromes. Am J Med Genet 63:218–222
34. Hunter RHF (1995) Abnormal sexual development in man. In: Hunter RHF (ed) Sex determination, differentiation and intersexuality in placental mammals. Cambridge University Press, Cambridge, pp 204–238
35. Hunter RHF (1995) Mechanisms of sex determination. In: Hunter RHF (ed) Sex determination, differentiation and intersexuality in placental mammals. Cambridge University Press, Cambridge, pp 22–68
36. Imbeaud S, Belville C, Messika-Zeitoun L, et al (1996) A 27 base-pair deletion of the anti-müllerian type II receptor gene is the most common cause of the persistent mullerian duct syndrome. Hum Mol Genet 5:1269–1277
37. Imperato-McGinley J (1997) 5-Alpha-reductase-2 deficiency. Curr Ther Endocrinol Metab 6:384–387
38. Ito K, Kawamata Y, Osada H, Ijichi M, Takano E, Sekiya S (1998) Pure yolk sac tumor of the ovary with mosaic 45X/46X+mar Turner's syndrome with a Y-chromosomal fragment. Arch Gynecol Obstet 262:87–90
39. Jacobs P, Dalton P, James R, et al (1997) Turner syndrome: a cytogenetic and molecular study. Ann Hum Genet 61:471–483
40. Jorgensen N, Muller J, Jaubert F, Clausen OP, Skakkebaek NE (1997) Heterogeneity of gonadoblastoma germ cells: similarities with immature germ cells, spermatogonia and testicular carcinoma in situ cells. Histopathology (Oxf) 30:177–186
41. Josso N, Racine C, di Clemente N, Rey R, Xavier F (1998) The role of anti-müllerian hormone in gonadal development. Mol Cell Endocrinol 145:3–7
42. Kanayama H, Naroda T, Inoue Y, Kurokawa Y, Kagawa S (1996) A case of complete testicular feminization: laparoscopic orchiectomy and analysis of androgen receptor gene mutation. Int J Urol 6:327–330
43. Kolon TF, Ferrer FA, McKenna PH. (1998) Clinical and molecular analysis of XX sex reversed patients. J Urol 160:1169–1172
44. Kommoss F, Oliva E, Bhan AK, Young RH, Scully RE (1998) Inhibin expression in ovarian tumors and tumor-like lesions: an immunohistochemical study. Mod Pathol 11:656–664
45. Lam SK, Yu MY, To KF, Chan MKM, Chun TKH (1996) Ovarian epithelial tumour in gonadal dysgenesis: a case report and literature review. Aust N Z J Obstet Gynaecol 36:106–109
46. Lane AH, Donahoe PK (1998) New insights into müllerian inhibiting substance and its mechanism of action. J Endocrinol 158:1–6
47. Lane AH, Lee MM (1999) Clinical applications of müllerian inhibiting substance in patients with gonadal disorders. Endocrinologist 9:208–215
48. Ludwig M, Beck A, Wickert L, et al (1998) Female pseudohermaphroditism associated with a novel homozygous G-to-A (V370-to-M) substitution in the P-450 aromatase gene. J Pediatr Endocrinol Metab 11:657–664
49. MacGillivray MH, Morishima A, Conte F, Grumbach M, Smith EP (1998) Pediatric endocrinology update: an overview. The essential roles of estrogens in pubertal growth, epiphyseal fusion and bone turnover: lessons from mutations in the genes for aromatase and the estrogen receptor. Horm Res (Basil) 49:2–8
50. MacLean HE, Warne GL, Zajac JD (1997) Intersex disorders: shedding light on male sexual differentiation beyond SRY. Clin Endocrinol 46:101–108

51. Magee AC, Nevin NC, Armstrong MJ, McGibbon D, Nevin J (1998) Ullrich-Turner syndrome: seven pregnancies in an apparent 45,X woman. Am J Med Genet 75:1–3
52. Martinez-Pasarell O, Nogues C, Bosch M, Egozcue J, Templado C (1999) Analysis of sex chromosome aneuploidy in sperm from fathers of Turner synrome patients. Hum Genet 104:345–349
53. Matsuki S, Sasagawa I, Kakizaki H, Suzuki Y, Nakada T (1999) Testicular teratoma in a man with XX/XXY mosaic Klinefelter's syndrome. J Urol 161: 1573–1574
54. McPhaul MJ, Griffin JE (1999) Male pseudohermaphroditism caused by mutations of the human androgen receptor. J Clin Endocrinol Metab 84: 3435–3441
55. Mendes JRT, Strufaldi MWL, Delcelo R, et al (1999) Y-chromosome identification by PCR and gonadal histopathology in Turner's syndrome without overt Y-mosaicism. Clin Endocrinol 50:19–26
56. Mendez JP, Canto P, Lopez M, et al (1999) Scant XYqh- testicular cells with normal SRY was enough to differentiate bilateral testes in a 45,X/46,XYqh- patient. Eur J Obstet Gynecol Reprod Biol 87:159–162
57. Mendez JP, Ulloa-Aguirre A, Kofman-Alfaro S, et al (1993) Mixed gonadal dysgenesis: clinical, cytogenetic, endocrinological, and histopathological findings in 16 patients. Am J Med Genet 46:263–267
58. Mendonca BB, Arnhold IJ, Bloise W, Andersson S, Russell DW, Wilson JD (1999) 17-Beta-hydroxysteroid dehydrogenase 3 deficiency in women. J Clin Endocrinol Metab 84:802–804
59. Mendonca BB, Inacio M, Costa EM, et al (1999) Male pseudohermaphroditism due to steroid 5-alpha-reductase 2 deficiency. Diagnosis, psychological evaluation, and management. Medicine (Baltim) 75:64–76
60. Merry C, Sweeney B, Puri P (1997) The vanishing testis: anatomical and histological findings. Eur Urol 31:65–66
61. Meyers CM, Boughman JA, Rivas M, Wilroy RS, Simpson JL (1996) Gonadal (ovarian) dysgenesis in 46,XX individuals: frequency of the autosomal recessive form. Am J Med Genet 63:518–524
62. Moran C, Knochenhauer ES, Azziz R (1998) Nonclassic adrenal hyperplasia in hyperandrogenism: a reappraisal. J Endocrinol Invest 21:707–720
63. Morimura Y, Nishiyama H, Yanagida K, Sato A (1998) Dysgerminoma with syncytiotrophoblastic giant cells arising from 46,XX pure gonadal dysgenesis. Obstet Gynecol 92:654–656
64. Naguib KK, Al-Etreibi NN, Al-Awadi SA, El-Harbi MK, Kamal AS (1997) Complete testicular feminization syndrome with 47,XYY karyotype: a double hit phenomenon. Med Princ Pract 6:216–221
65. Nazarenko SA, Timoshevsky VA, Sukhanova NN (1999) High frequency of tissue-specific mosaicism in Turner syndrome patients. Clin Genet 56:59–65
66. New MI (1998) Diagnosis and management of congenital adrenal hyperplasia. Ann Rev Med 49:311–328
67. New MI, Newfield RS (1997) Congenital adrenal hyperplasia. Curr Ther Endocrinol Metab 6:179–187
68. Newfield RS, New MI (1997) 21-hydroxylase deficiency. Ann N Y Acad Sci 816:219–229
69. Nomura K, Matsui T, Aizawa S (1999) Gonadoblastoma with proliferation resembling Sertoli cell tumor. Int J Gynecol Pathol 18:91–93
70. Nowaczyk MJ, Whelan DT, Heshka TW, Hill RE (1999) Smith-Lemli-Opitz syndrome: a treatable inherited error of metabolism causing mental retardation. Can Med Assoc J 161:165–170
71. Okada H, Gotoh A, Takechi Y, Kamidono S (1994) Leydig cell tumour of the testis associated with Klinefelter's syndrome and Osgood-Schlatter disease. Br J Urol 73:457
72. Opitz JM (1999) RSH (so-called Smith-Lemli-Opitz) syndrome. Curr Opin Pediatr 11:353–362
73. Park JP, Brothman AR, Butler MG, et al (1999) Extensive analysis of mosaicism in a case of Turner syndrome: the experience of 287 cytogenetic laboratories. College of American Pathologists/American College of Medical Genetics Cytogenetics Resource Committee. Arch Pathol Lab Med 123:381–385
74. Patsalis PC, Sismani C, Hadjimarcou MI, et al (1998) Detection and incidence of cryptic Y chromosome sequences in Turner syndrome patients. Clin Genet 53:249–257
75. Pierga JY, Giacchetti S, Vilain E, et al (1994) Dysgerminoma in a pure 45,X Turner syndrome: report of a case and review of the literature. Gynecol Oncol 55:459–464
76. Quigley CA, DeBellis A, Marschke KB, El-Awady MF, Wilson EM, French FS (1995) Androgen receptor defects: historical, clinical, and molecular perspectives. Endocr Rev 16:271–321
77. Quilter CR, Taylor K, Conway GS, Nathwani N, Delhanty JD (1998) Cytogenetic and molecular investigations of Y chromosome sequences and their role in Turner syndrome. Ann Hum Genet 62:99–106
78. Radakovic B, Jukic S, Bukovic D, Ljubojevic N, Cima I (1999) Morphology of gonads in pure XY gonadal dysgenesis. Coll Antropol 23:203–211
79. Radmayr C, Culig Z, Hobisch A, Corvin S, Bartsch G, Klocker H (1998) Analysis of a mutant androgen receptor offers a treatment modality in a patient with partial androgen insensitivity syndrome. Eur Urol 33:222–226
80. Rajpert-De Meyts E, Jorgensen N, Brondum-Nielsen K, Muller J, Skakkebaek NE (1998) Developmental arrest of germ cells in the pathogenesis of germ cell neoplasia. APMIS 106:198–204
81. Rattanachaiyanont M, Phophong P, Techatraisak K, Charoenpanich P, Jitpraphai P (1999) Embry-

onic testicular regression syndrome: a case report. J Med Assoc Thailand 82:506–510
82. Regadera J, Martinez Garcia F, Paniagua R, Nistal M (1999) Androgen insensitivity syndrome: an immunohistochemical, ultrastructural, and morphometric study. Arch Pathol Lab Med 123:225–234
83. Rey R, Josso N (1996) Regulation of testicular anti-Müllerian hormone secretion. Eur J Endocrinol 135:144–152
84. Robboy SJ, Miller T, Donahoe PK, et al (1982) Dysgenesis of testicular and streak gonads in the syndrome of mixed gonadal dysgenesis: perspective derived from a clinicopathologic analysis of twenty-one cases. Hum Pathol 13:700–716
85. Russell P, Farnsworth A (1997) Surgical pathology of the ovaries, 2nd Ed. Churchill Livingstone, New York
86. Rutgers JL (1991) Advances in the pathology of intersex conditions. Hum Pathol 22:884–891
87. Rutgers JL, Scully RE (1991) The androgen insensitivity syndrome (testicular feminization): a clinicopathologic study of 43 cases. Int J Gynecol Pathol 10:126–144
88. Salas-Cortes L, Jaubert F, Barbaux S, et al (1999) The human SRY protein is present in fetal and adult Sertoli cells and germ cells. Int J Dev Biol 43:135–140
88a. Sadler TW (1985) Langman's medical embryology, 5th Ed. Williams & Wilkins, Baltimore
89. Scherer G, Held M, Erdel M, et al (1998) Three novel SRY mutations in XY gonadal dysgenesis and the enigma of XY gonadal dysgenesis cases without SRY mutations. Cytogenet Cell Genet 80:188–192
89a. Scully RE (1970) Gondoblastoma. A review of 74 cases. Cancer 25:1340–1356
90. Scully RE, Young RH, Clement RB (1998) Tumors of the ovary, maldeveloped gonads, fallopian tube, and broad ligament, 3rd Ed. Atlas of tumor pathology, vol 23. Armed Forces Institute of Pathology, Washington, DC
90a. Saenger P, Levine LS, New MI (1981) Male pseudohermaphroditism due to abnormal testosterone biosynthesis and metabolism. Clon Androl 7:87–97
91. Short RV (1998) Difference between a testis and an ovary. J Exp Zool 281:359–361
92. Shozu M, Akasofu K, Harada T, Kubota Y (1991) A new cause of female pseudohermaphroditism: placental aromatase deficiency. J Clin Endocrinol Metab 72:560–566
93. Sinnecker GH, Hiort O, Dibbelt L, et al (1996) Phenotypic classification of male pseudohermaphroditism due to steroid 5 alpha-reductase 2 deficiency. Am J Med Genet 63:223–230
94. Slaney SF, Chalmers IJ, Affara NA, Chitty LS (1998) An autosomal or X linked mutation results in true hermaphrodites and 46,XX males in the same family. J Med Genet 35:17–22
95. Smith NM, Byard RW, Bourne AJ (1991) Testicular regression syndrome: a pathological study of 77 cases. Histopathology (Oxf) 19:269–272
96. Spires SE (1999) Testicular regression syndrome: histologic recognition among pathologists. Am J Clin Pathol 112:547
97. Swain A, Lovell-Badge R (1997) A molecular approach to sex determination in mammals. Acta Paediatr 86:46–49
98. Talerman A, Verp MS, Senekjian E, Gilewski T, Vogelzang N (1990) True hermaphrodite with bilateral ovotestes, bilateral gonadoblastomas and dysgerminomas, 46,XX/46,XY karyotype, and a successful pregnancy. Cancer (Phila) 66:2668–2672
99. Tanaka Y, Sasaki Y, Tachibana K, et al (1994) Gonadal mixed germ cell tumor combined with a large hemangiomatous lesion in a patient with Turner's syndrome and 45,X/46,X, +mar karyotype. Arch Pathol Lab Med 118:1135–1138
100. Tanaka Y, Sasaki Y, Tachibana K, Suwa S, Terashima K, Nakatani Y (1994) Testicular juvenile granulosa cell tumor in an infant with X/XY mosaicism clinically diagnosed as true hermaphroditism. Am J Surg Pathol 18:316–322
101. Tateno T, Sasagawa I, Ashida J, Nakada T (1999) Deletion of Y chromosome involving the DAZ (deleted in azoospermia) gene in XX males. Arch Androl 42:179–183
102. Telvi L, Lebbar A, Del Pino O, Barbet JP, Chaussain JL (1999) 45,X/46,XY mosaicism: report of 27 cases. Pediatrics 104:304–308
103. Tsutsumi O, Iida T, Nakahori Y, Taketani Y (1996) Analysis of the testis-determining gene SRY in patients with XY gonadal dysgenesis. Horm Res (Basil) 46:6–10
104. Uehara S, Funato T, Yaegashi N, et al (1999) SRY mutation and tumor formation on the gonads of XY pure gonadal dysgenesis patients. Cancer Genet Cytogenet 113:78–84
105. Uehara S, Tamura M, Nata M, et al (1999) Complete androgen insensitivity in a 47,XXY patient with uniparental disomy for the X chromosome. Am J Med Genet 86:107–111
106. van Niekerk WA, Retief AE (1981) The gonads of human true hermaphrodites. Hum Genet 58:117–122
107. Vanderbijl AE, Fleuren GJ, Kenter GG, Dejong D (1994) Unique combination of an ovarian gonadoblastoma, dysgerminoma, and mucinous cystadenoma in a patient with Turners syndrome: a cytogenetic and molecular analysis. Int J Gynecol Pathol 13:267–272
108. Vauthier-Brouzes D, Vanna Lim-You K, Sebagh E, Lefebvre G, Darbois Y (1997) Krukenberg tumor during pregnancy with maternal and fetal virilization: a difficult diagnosis. A case report. J Gynecol Obstet Biol Reprod (Paris) 26:831–833
109. Velidedeoglu HV, Coskunfirat OK, Bozdogan MN, Sahin U, Turkguven Y (1997) The surgical man-

agement of incomplete testicular feminization syndrome in three sisters. Br J Plastic Surg 50:212–216

110. Vilain E, McCabe ERB (1998) Mammalian sex determination: from gonads to brain. Mol Genet Metab 65:74–84

111. Viner RM, Teoh Y, Williams DM, Patterson MN, Hughes IA (1997) Androgen insensitivity syndrome: a survey of diagnostic procedures and management in the UK. Arch Dis Child 77:305–309

112. Vlasak I, Plochl E, Kronberger G, et al (1999) Screening of patients with Turner syndrome for "hidden" Y-mosaicism. Klin Padiatr 211:30–34

113. Welch WR, Robboy SJ (1981) Abnormal sexual development: a classification with emphasis on pathology and neoplastic conditions. Pediatr Androl 7: 71–85

114. Zhu YS, Katz MD, Imperato-McGinley J (1998) Natural potent androgens: lessons from human genetic models. Baillieres Clin Endocrinol Metab 12:83–113

2

Benign Diseases of the Vulva

Edward J. Wilkinson, M.D., and Dong-lin Xie, M.D., Ph.D.

Anatomy

The external female genitalia include the mons pubis, labia majora and minora, prepuce, frenulum, clitoris, and vestibule. The orifices of the paraurethral (Skene) and Bartholin glands, as well as those of the minor vestibular glands and the urethral meatus, open into the vestibule (Fig. 2.1). After menarche, the mons pubis and lateral aspects of the labia majora acquire increased amounts of subcutaneous fat and develop the coarse, curly pubic hair. During adolescence, the labia develop pigmentation and the clitoris undergoes some enlargement. Histologically, the entire vulva, with the exception of the vulvar vestibule, is covered by keratinized, stratified squamous epithelium.[267] The labia majora contain both smooth muscle and fat, whereas the labia minora are devoid of adipose tissue but are rich in elastic fibers and blood vessels.[183] Within the lateral aspects of the labia majora, sebaceous glands are associated with hair follicles but open directly to the surface epithelium toward the medial aspect. Similar sebaceous glands are seen on the perineum posterior to the vestibule. The labia minora typically do not contain glandular elements, except sebaceous glands near the junction with the interlabial sulcus and near the inferior and lateral aspects. The apocrine glands of the labia majora, prepuce, posterior vestibule, and perineal body, like the apocrine glands of the axilla, are activated at menarche, whereas the eccrine sweat glands, primarily involved in heat regulation, function before puberty.[206] The vestibule is bounded medially by the external portion of the hymen ring, posteriorly and laterally by the line of Hart, and anteriorly by the frenulum of the clitoris. The mucosa of the vestibule is glycogenated in women of reproductive age, or under estrogen influence, and resembles vaginal mucosa. The linea vestibularis, seen in approximately one-quarter of newborn female infants, is located in the posterior portion of the vestibule, and is a white streak or spot in the midline of the pos-

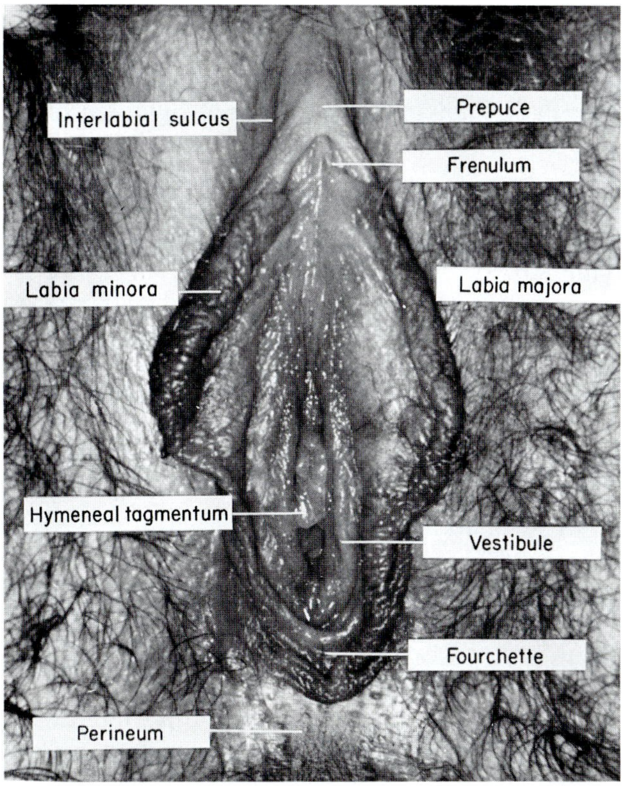

Fig. 2.1. External anatomy of vulva and the Hart's line. The line of Hart is the junction between the nonkeratinized mucous membrane epithelium of the vestibule, the thinly keratinized epithelium of the medial aspects of the labia minora, the posterior aspects of the labia majora, and the perineal body.

terior vestibule extending nearly to the posterior commissure.[115,116] The squamous epithelium of the vestibule merges with the transitional epithelium at the urethral meatus, and with the duct openings of the paraurethral glands (Skene), the major vestibular (Bartholin) glands, and the minor vestibular glands.

The paired Skene's glands, homologues of the prostate in females,[88] are composed of pseudostratified mucus-secreting columnar epithelium, open to the external surface on both sides of the urethral meatus and along the posterior and lateral aspects of the urethra itself. The ducts are lined by transitional epithelium. The major vestibular glands of Bartholin are bilateral racemose, tubuloalveolar glands, with acini composed of simple, columnar, mucus-secreting epithelium (Fig. 2.2). Each gland is drained just external to the hymen ring of the vestibule posterolaterally. The Bartholin duct, approximately 2.5 cm in length, has three types of epithelial linings depending on the location within the duct. It is lined proximally by mucus-secreting epithelium, distally by transitional epithelium, and, at its exit, by squamous epithelium. The minor vestibular glands are composed of acini lined by simple columnar mucus-secreting epithelium. They lie within 1–2.5 mm of the superficial epithelium and communicate with the vestibular surface. Squamous metaplasia often occurs within these glands and may obliterate them completely, resulting in the formation of a vestibular cleft (Fig. 2.3). These minor glands ring the vestibule and extend from the frenulum on both sides of the meatus, around the external base of the hymenal ring, to the fourchette.[40] Specialized anogenital sweat glands (mammary-like) have been found within the vulvar interlabial sulcus, in the medial aspects of the labia majora, and in lesser numbers within the perineum and about the anus. These glands, with long and wide coiled ducts that open to the surface, have a simple columnar epithe-

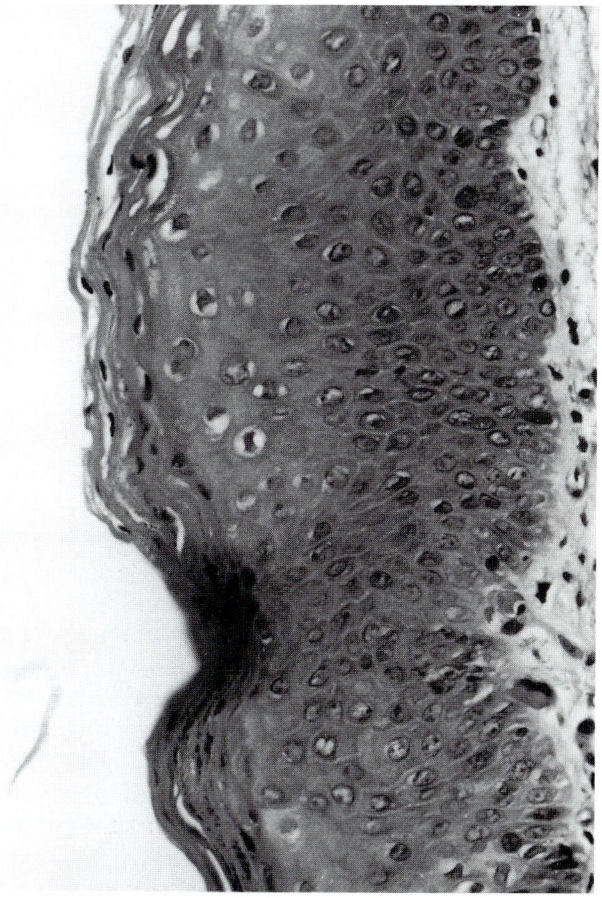

Fig. 2.2. Bartholin duct and gland. The terminal bartholin duct has a transitional epithelial-type lining that merges with the simple columnar mucus-secreting epithelium of the Bartholin's gland acini. The glands are tubuloalveolar and racemose. The surrounding fibrous stroma is somewhat more cellular than the peripheral stroma.

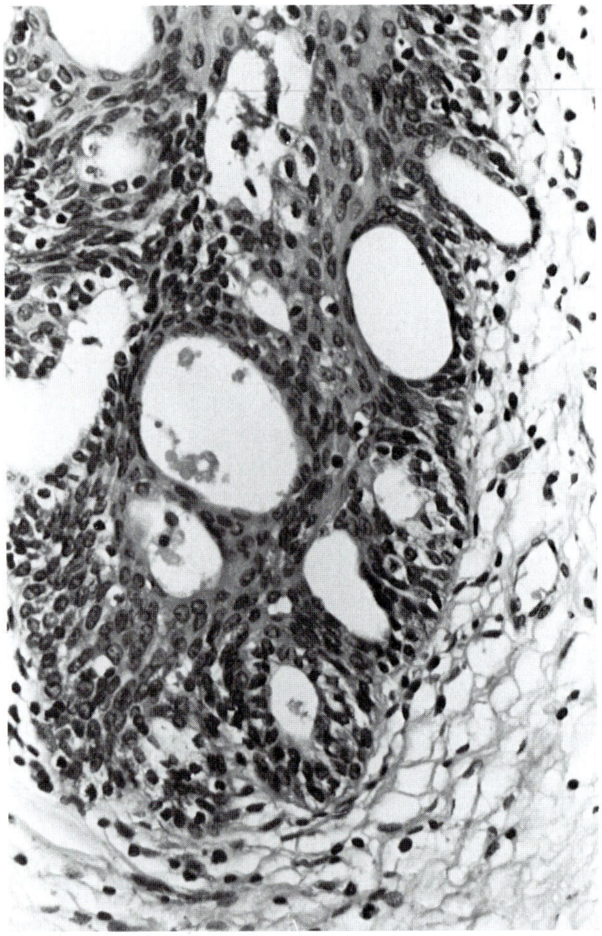

Fig. 2.3. Minor vestibular gland with squamous metaplasia. Some low columnar, mucus-secreting cells line gland lumens and are associated with metaplastic squamous epithelium.

lium with apical snouts and myoepithelium beneath the glandular epithelium.[252–254]

The clitoris, which has no glands, is covered by thinly keratinized stratified squamous epithelium. Within the stroma of the clitoris are two conjoined corpora cavernosa, which branch near the base of the clitoris and lie along the pubic rami as divided crura. They are invested in a loose fibrous sheath containing abundant nerves and with an incomplete center septum. The dermis, subepithelium, and stroma of the vulva are rich in collagen, blood vessels, and myofibroblastic-type cells that are frequently immunoreactive for desmin.[264] Myxoid-like changes are present within the subepithelial stroma and have been reported extending from the ectocervix to the vulva. Atypical-appearing multinucleated cells may be observed in this subepithelial myxoid area.[1] Sparse numbers of inflammatory cells including lymphocytes, a few plasma cells, and mast cells are normally present in the perivascular spaces and interstitium.

The femoral and inguinal lymph nodes receive lymphatic drainage from the entire vulva except the clitoris, which has a minor secondary lymphatic pathway.[104,144] Delicate intercommunicating lymphatic vessels extend to the labia minora, clitoral prepuce, and vestibule, bypassing the clitoris. The lymphatic bed of the labia majora drains in an anterosuperior direction toward the mons, joining the lymphatic vessels from the labia minora and prepuce, and then into the ipsilateral inguinal and femoral nodes. Some contralateral flow also may occur into the superior medial nodes of the femoral group. The superficial inguinal lymph nodes, consisting of 8–10 nodes on each side, divided into a superior oblique and an inferior ventral group, are the major nodes that drain the vulva and therefore are included in a radical vulvectomy.[163] The superior oblique group is found about the Poupart ligament, and the inferior ventral group lies above the junction of the saphenous vein and fascia lata. Lymphatic drainage from the clitoris and midline perineum proceeds bilaterally in more than 67% of cases and may bypass the superficial nodes.[101] A second minor lymphatic pathway from the glans clitoris joins the lymphatics of the urethra, traverses the urogenital diaphragm, and merges with the lymphatic plexus on the anterior surface of the bladder. From there, drainage is into the interiliac, obturator, and external iliac nodes. No direct pathway of lymphatic flow from the clitoris to the pelvic nodes could be demonstrated by in vivo colloid injection.[101] Lymphatic flow from other sites on the vulva usually proceeds to the ipsilateral groin and pelvic lymph nodes. This finding correlates with the observation that in cases of clitoral carcinoma, in which the inguinofemoral lymph nodes are free of tumor, it is highly unlikely that the pelvic nodes are involved.

The superficial and deep external pudendal arteries branch from the femoral artery. The internal pudendal arteries branch from the internal iliac arteries. These branches from the femoral and internal iliac arteries provide the major blood supply to the vulva via the anterior and posterior labial branches. The clitoris, including the crura and corpora cavernosa, is supplied separately by the deep arteries of the clitoris, whereas the anterior vaginal artery supplies blood flow to the vestibule and the Bartholin glands. The venous return parallels the arterial supply. The nerve supply to the vulva includes sensory nerves, special receptors, and autonomic nerves to the vessels and various glands. The major nerves of the vulva derive from the anterior (ilioinguinal) and posterior (pudendal) labial nerves.[131] The clitoris is innervated by the dorsal nerve of the clitoris and the cavernous nerves of the clitoris, which also supply the vestibule.[229]

Developmental Abnormalities

The clitoris in an adult women measures 16.0 ± 4.3 mm in length, with a transverse diameter of 3.4 ± .0 mm and longitudinal diameter of 5.1 ± 1.4 mm. It is slightly larger in parous women. Height and weight do not influence clitoral size.[259] Clitoral hypertrophy may occur as an isolated finding or in association with generalized vulvar enlargement. Clitoral enlargement in a newborn suggests adrenogenital syndrome, exogenous maternal androgen therapy, or some form of hermaphroditism. A clitoral mass from an infant has been identified with chromosomal mosaicism in which the clitoral skin had a hyperdiploid chromosomal abnormality with normal chromosomes being found in the ovary; this is an example of ambiguous genitalia resulting from a somatic cell mutation with maldevelopment of the clitoris.[228] Clitoral enlargement also has been reported associated with lipodystrophy (Lawrence–Seip syndrome).[210] In addition to developmental abnormalities, a variety of tumors including granular cell tumors, hemangiomas, and vascular, neural, and smooth muscle tumors may cause clitoral enlargement.[114,187,237,239]

Hypertrophy and asymmetry of the labia minora may occur without demonstrable etiology and, in some cases, may be associated with chronic irritation, as may be seen in women wearing indwelling urethral catheters. True hypoplasia occurs infrequently and may be a sign of defective steroidogenesis. Slight fusion of the labia minora may be seen in infants without apparent cause and typically responds to topical estrogen cream. Labial fusion, like clitoral hypertrophy, also may be present with intersex disorders. In these situations, the defect is developmental, but such fusion also may be acquired secondary to lichen sclerosus, lichen planus, or inflammatory conditions, with subsequent adhesion formation.[113] A low transverse vaginal septum may occlude the vaginal lumen and result in hematocolpos with the onset of menstruation. Excision of the septum is the usual therapy of choice. Imperforate hymen is remarkably rare, with a reported frequency of 0.014%, and usually is discovered at the onset of menarche between 10 and 18 years of age. Limited surgical excision of the hymen is the usual treatment. Duplication of the vulva is extremely rare and usually is associated with duplication of the internal müllerian system and rectum as well. In müllerian agenesis, the hymen and vagina usually are represented by only a depression in the vestibular area. Congenital absence of the clitoris and external genitalia also have been described. The urethra may open into the vagina rather than into the vestibule. Ectopic urethral orifices are seen occasionally adjacent to the hymen.[113]

Inflammatory Diseases of Vulvar Skin

Inflammatory diseases of vulvar skin can be generally divided into infectious and noninfectious groups (Table 2.1). Further classification of infectious diseases according to etiologic agents is summarized in Table 2.2. The most prevalent infectious diseases of the vulva in North America include human papillomavirus (HPV), typically manifested as condyloma acuminata, herpes genitalis, syphilis, and molluscum contagiosum (Table 2.3). Clinical diagnosis does not necessarily require specific organism characterization in all these conditions.

Human Papillomavirus Infection

General Features

Human papillomvavirus infection (HPV) is responsible for benign tumors, that is, *condylomata acuminata* and precursor lesions of certain types of vulvar carcinoma (i.e., *vulvar intraepithelial neoplasia*, VIN).[58,126,202] (The latter are described in Chapter 3, Premalignant and Malignant Tumors of the Vulva.) Condyloma acuminata (genital warts) are sexually transmitted benign neoplasms that may involve the vulva, vagina, cervix, urethra, anal canal, and perianal skin.[180] The prevalence of HPV infection varies greatly, depending on the population studied. In most studies, clinically evident vulvar involvement is less common than cervical HPV infection.[74,132] Molecular biologic methods have identified HPV-6 as the most common HPV type in typical genital condyloma acuminata. HPV-11 has been found in approximately one-fourth of genital warts.[26,86,87,280]

Table 2.1. Inflammatory disorders of the vulva

Infectious diseases	*Noninfectious dermatoses*
Viral	Papulosquamous disorders
Fungal	Noninfectious bullous dermatoses
Bacterial	Miscellaneous
Parasitic	

Table 2.2. Infectious diseases of vulva skin

Viral infection		
	Human papillomavirus (genital subtype)	
	Herpes virus (simplex and zoster)	
	Molluscum contagiosum	
	Others (rare):	
		Human papillomavirus (nongenital subtype)
		HIV-associated plaques and ulcers
		Cytomegalovirus (CMV)
		Epstein–Barr virus (EBV)-associated ulcer
		Coxsackie virus (hand-foot-mouth disease)
Bacterial infection		
	Syphilis	
	Granuloma inguinale	
	Lymphogranuloma venereum	
	Chancroid	
	Malakoplakia	
	Others	
		Tuberculosis
		Erythrasma
Fungal organisms		
	Dermatophytosis	
	Candidiasis	
Parasitic infestation		
	Scabies	
	Pubic lice	
	Others	
		Enterobius vermicularis
		Schistosomiasis
		Demodex

HIV, human immunodeficiency virus.

Clinical Features

Condylomas present as papillary, verrucous, or papular lesions of the skin and mucous membrane that are nearly always multiple and frequently confluent (Fig. 2.4). Most lesions are asymptomatic unless secondarily infected. Condylomata acuminata are commonly associated with vaginitis, pregnancy, diabetes mellitus, oral contraceptive use, poor perineal hygiene, immunosuppression, and sexual activity with multiple partners or a partner exposed to other partners.[9,42,164,185] Approximately 30–50% of women with vulvar condyloma acuminatum have associated cervical HPV infection.[262] The presence of vulvar condyloma acuminatum in children may be related to sexual abuse.[59,178,279]

Approximately 40%–60% of children with laryngeal papillomatosis are born from mothers with a history of genital HPV infection.[75] However, the true incidence of infection of the larynx of the newborn infant, from a mother with genital papillomavirus infection is unknown but is probably low. No correlation has been shown between the volume of maternal wart tissue and occurrence of infantile laryngeal papillomatosis. Employing DNA hybridization techniques, it has been observed that approximately one-half of laryngeal papillomas contain HPV-11.[60,233] This finding supports the view that laryngeal papillomas of infancy and childhood are acquired at the time of vaginal delivery.

Table 2.3. Infectious diseases of the vulva

Disease	*Causative microorganism*	*Salient histopathological features*	*Diagnostic methods*
Condyloma acuminatum	Papillomavirus	Acanthosis, hyperkeratosis, parakeratosis, papillomatosis, perinuclear halo (koilocyte)	Histopathology Immunohistochemistry Molecular hybridization
Herpes genitalis	Herpes simplex hominis type II	Intranuclear inclusions	Cytopathology, culture, serology
Syphilitic chancre	*Treponema pallidum*	Ulceration, chronic inflammation, vasculitis	Dark-field, fluorescence, silver stain, serology
Condyloma lata	*Treponema pallidum*	Like chancre, with epithelial hyperplasia	Same as syphilitic chancre
Molluscum contagiosum	DNA poxvirus group	Intracytoplasmic inclusions	Cytopathology, histopathology
Granuloma inguinale	*Calymmatobacterium granulomatis*	Donovan bodies, granulomatous reaction without caseation, pseudoepitheliomatous hyperplasia	Giemsa stain, silver stain
Lymphogranuloma venereum	*Chlamydia* (TRIC agent)	Granulomatous reaction without caseation	Serology
Tuberculosis	*Mycobacterium tuberculosis*	Acid-fast bacilli (AFB), granulomatous reaction with caseation	AFB stain, AFB culture
Chancroid	*Hemophilus ducreyi*	Granulomatous reaction without caseation	Culture, Gram stain

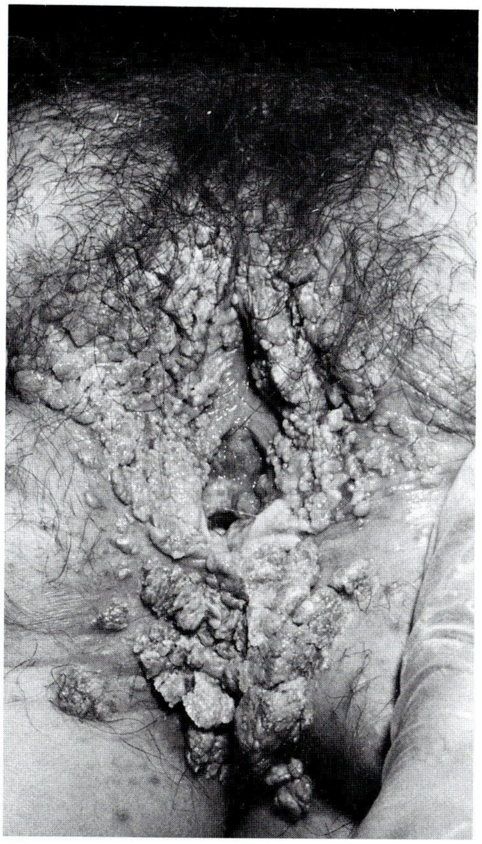

Fig. 2.4. Condylomata acuminata. Widespread involvement of vulva and perianal region.

Gross Findings

Condyloma acuminata usually present as discrete papillary growths, with a central stalk or as large sessile lesions. On the cervix, vagina, or vulva, condyloma acuminata may present as slightly raised rough areas with irregular borders. Small lesions are best appreciated with application of 3%–5% acetic acid for 3–5 minutes on colposcopic examination. Lesions that are detectable by colposcopic magnification only, or by performing HPV testing on the tissue in question, are considered subclinical.[52,97]

Microscopic Findings

Acanthosis, dyskeratosis, parakeratosis, hyperkeratosis, and a prominent granular layer are seen. A superficial chronic inflammatory infiltrate often is present in the dermis. Typical perinuclear cytoplasmic "halos," with "raisinoid" pyknotic nuclei or slightly enlarged nuclei (koilocytosis), are commonly present in the superficial epithelial cells, and binucleated and multinucleated squamous cells often are found (Figs. 2.5 and Fig. 2.6). Parabasalar hyperplasia with accentuated intracellular bridges may be seen. Enlarged parabasal cells with "foamy" or "ground glass"-appearing nuclear chromatin may be present. In situ hybridization studies on cervical tissue have demonstrated the presence of HPV DNA in condylomata.[173]

Differential Diagnosis

Condylomata acuminata at times may be difficult to distinguish from VIN. Condylomata typically are verrucous or papillary and display koilocytosis, parabasal hyperplasia, accentuated intracellular bridges, dyskeratosis, accentuation of the granular layer, and hyperkeratosis. Mitotic figures are infrequently found. In contrast, the presence of flat macular growth, abnormal mitoses, cytologically atypical nuclei, marked variation in nuclear size and shape, and hyperchromasia are characteristics of VIN lesions. Unlike VIN, condylomas usually are diploid; however, atypia may be seen related to tetraploidy or octoploidy. Unlike VIN, this atypia is characterized by large nuclei, with moderate nuclear pleomorphism and some degree of hyperchromasia, but without abnormal mitosis. A high-grade VIN lesion induced by oncogenic HPV often

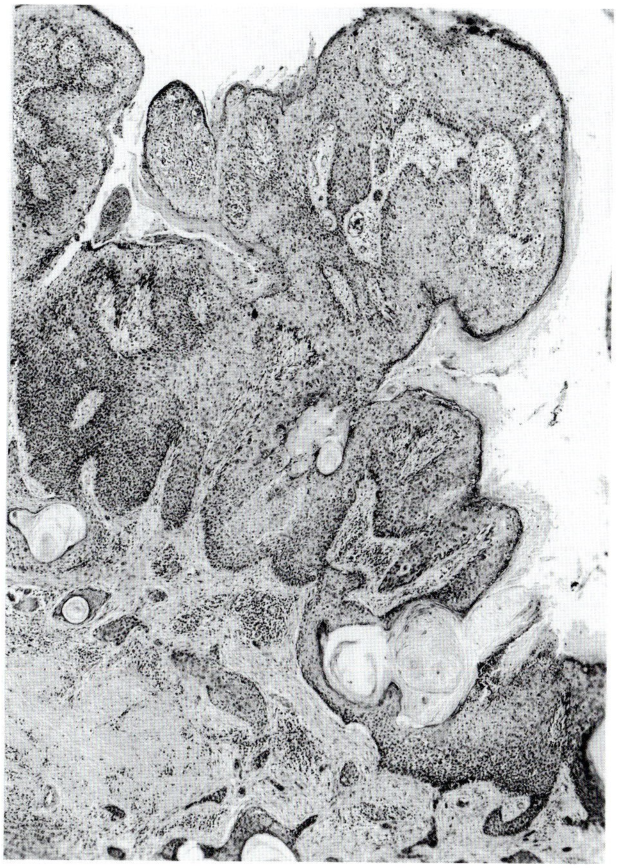

Fig. 2.5. Condyloma acuminatum. Verrucous epidermal hyperplasia with broad rounded papillation. (Courtesy of R.J. Kurman, M.D., Baltimore, MD.)

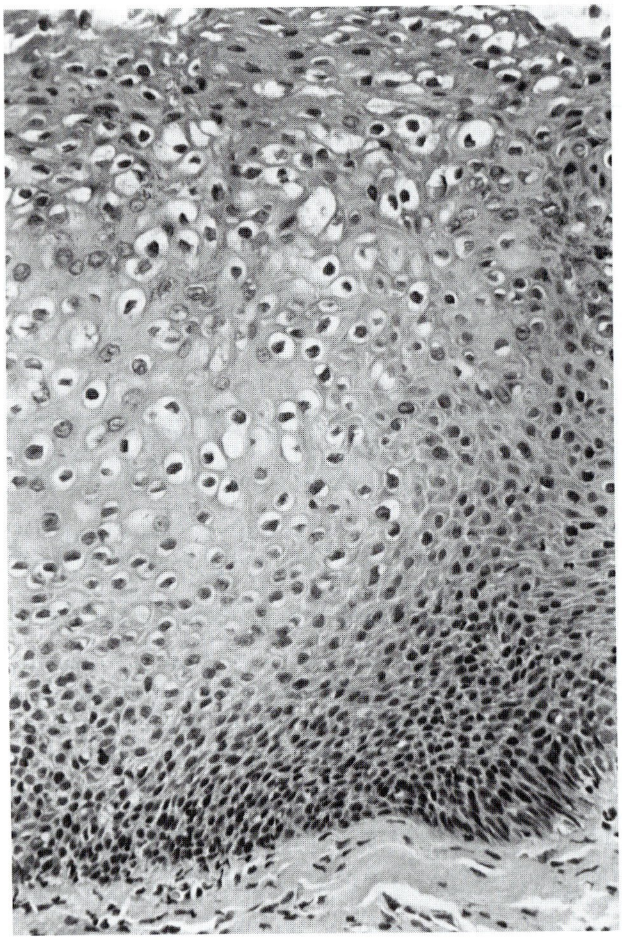

Fig. 2.6. Condyloma acuminatum. Parabasalar hyperplasia is seen with prominent intracellular bridges between some cells. Above the basilar layer, koilocytotic cells with prominent perinuclear halos are found in the more superficial epithelium.

correlates with aneuploidy,[166,211] which is rare in common condyloma.

Typical condylomas will be HPV antigen positive by immunoperoxidase techniques in approximately 50% of cases, whereas VIN will be immunoreactive in less than 10% of cases; however, such testing is not of value in distinguishing these two entities.[105] In a given case of VIN, a spectrum may be found from typical VIN 3 to adjacent changes that may have the morphologic changes of condyloma acuminatum. As a matter of practice, the first diagnosis given on the pathology report is that of the most serious lesion identified, with subsequent diagnosis following. In our present state of understanding, it is acceptable to classify flat condylomata acuminata (condyloma plana) of the vulva as VIN 1 (see Vulvar Intraepithelial Neoplasia in Chapter 3). Regressing or early flat condylomata acuminata also may resemble lichen simplex chronicus or squamous cell hyperplasia; however, the prominent granular layer, accentuated intracellular bridges, parabasalar hyperplasia, and koilocytosis are typically lacking. If this cannot be resolved by histopathologic examination, molecular biologic methods such as polymerase chain reaction (PCR) or in situ hybridization, to detect HPV, may be applicable and are of value in establishing the diagnosis of HPV-associated changes when virus is identified.

Vulvar vestibular papilloma is differentiated from condylomata in that the epithelium lacks hyperkeratosis and other typical microscopic features of condyloma. Moreover, vestibular papilloma are confined to the vulva vestibule.[18,83] Fibroepithelial polyps may have the shape of large condylomas; however, the epithelium also lacks the microscopic features of condyloma. Condylomata lata may resemble condylomata acuminata clinically; however, on biopsy, the deep inflammatory infiltrates with plasma cells and the presence of spirochetes on a Warthin–Starry silver stain distinguishes these lesions.

Clinical Behavior and Treatment

The natural history of HPV infection of the vulva usually is one of a long protracted course and may be influenced by immunologic factors.[7] Regression has been noted after pregnancy. Presentation following radiation therapy has been observed.[185] Progression of condyloma acuminatum of the vulva to VIN and malignant transformation to squamous cell carcinoma have been observed.[247] Oncogenesis secondary to papillomavirus is well recognized in experimental animals. The association of vulvar and vaginal condyloma acuminata with invasive squamous cell carcinoma has been documented in women with immunosuppressive conditions such as Fanconi anemia and Hodgkin disease[264] (see Chapter 3, Premalignant and Malignant Tumors of the Vulva).

The topical application of dilute podophyllin[21] or the judicious application of concentrated halogenated acetic acid (trichloroacetic acid) is the common approach to the treatment of small vulvar condylomata. Electrodesiccation, surgical excision, cryosurgery, hot wire electroloop excision, laser ablation, and interferon have been used for large lesions.[7,24,53,123,223,261]

Herpesvirus Infection

General Features

The causative agent is the herpes simplex virus (HSV) (var. hominis type 2), although in some in-

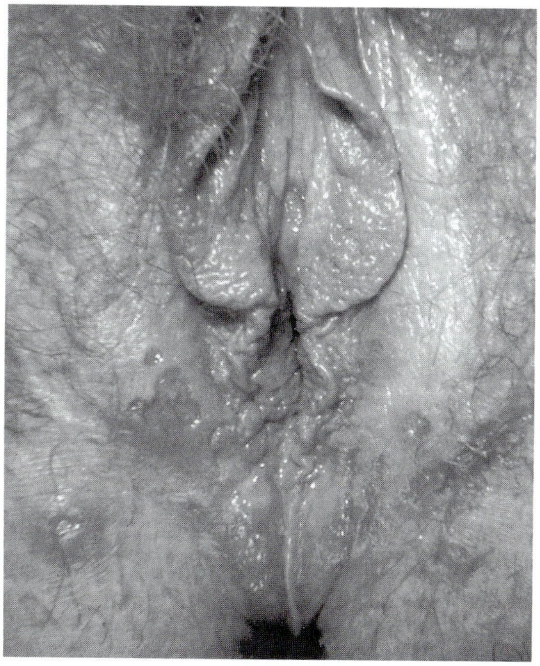

Fig. 2.7. Herpes simplex ulcer. HSV infection, untreated, 7 days after the onset of symptoms. Multifocal ulceration is present.

stances the type I virus may be involved. The incidence of *herpesvirus infection* in the United States has been reported as 126 per 100,000; approximately 600,000 new cases of genital herpes occur each year in the United States. Although approximately 20% of the U.S. population has been infected by HSV 2, the frequency of vulvar involvement is unknown.[135,145,174]

Clinical Features

The initial clinical presentation frequently includes dysuria or urinary retention with vulvar pain that may be incapacitating. Systemic symptoms, including generalized malaise and fever, are frequently seen along with a mild inguinal lymphadenopathy. The sequential appearance of vesicles, pustules, and painful shallow ulcers that often are infected secondarily with bacteria characterize the clinical findings. The vesicles usually are asymptomatic, whereas the ulcers are extremely painful (Fig. 2.7). The lesions can involve the anus, urethra, bladder, cervix, and vagina, as well as the vulva. The acute ulcers heal in approximately 16 days.[145,255] Of the women who are culture positive for HSV, diagnostic genital vesicles and ulcers are present in approximately two-thirds; the remainder of the women have nondetectable or atypical lesions or are asymptomatic.[130,255]

Microscopic Findings

An early intact herpes simplex vesicle extends deeply into the epidermis. The histologic transformation of the HSV-infected epithelial cell begins with a homogenization of the nuclear chromatin resulting in a "ground glass" appearance, which then progresses to the more typical eosinophilic intranuclear inclusion body.[81] The characteristic intranuclear inclusions are seen at the periphery of the lesion (Figs. 2.8 and 2.9). Subsequently, the cells undergo karyorrhexis and lysis. A biopsy taken in the late ulcerative phase, therefore, does not always show the intranuclear inclusions. Cytologic evaluation of the scraping of the base and edges (Tzank preparation) of a fresh ulcer, or freshly opened vesicle, usually will show the multinucleated cells with viral cytopathic effects characteristic of HSV infection. Cytologic examination of vesicular aspirate is an effective method of identifying the cytopathic changes of HSV and is almost as sensitive as virus isolation. Moistening the ulcer with a saline-soaked sponge

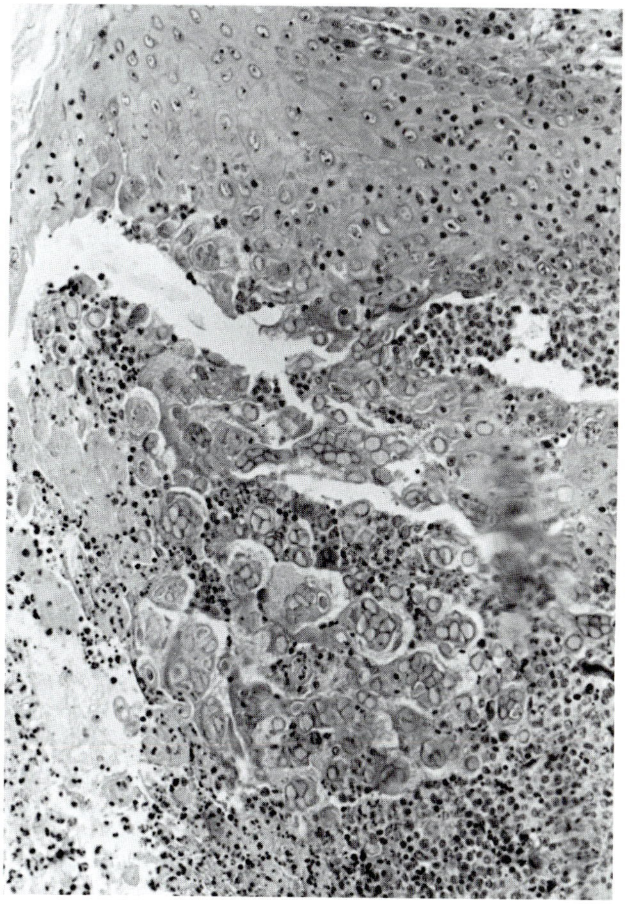

Fig. 2.8. Herpes simplex ulcer. Crater margin shows multinucleated clusters with distinctive intranuclear homogenization and inclusion bodies.

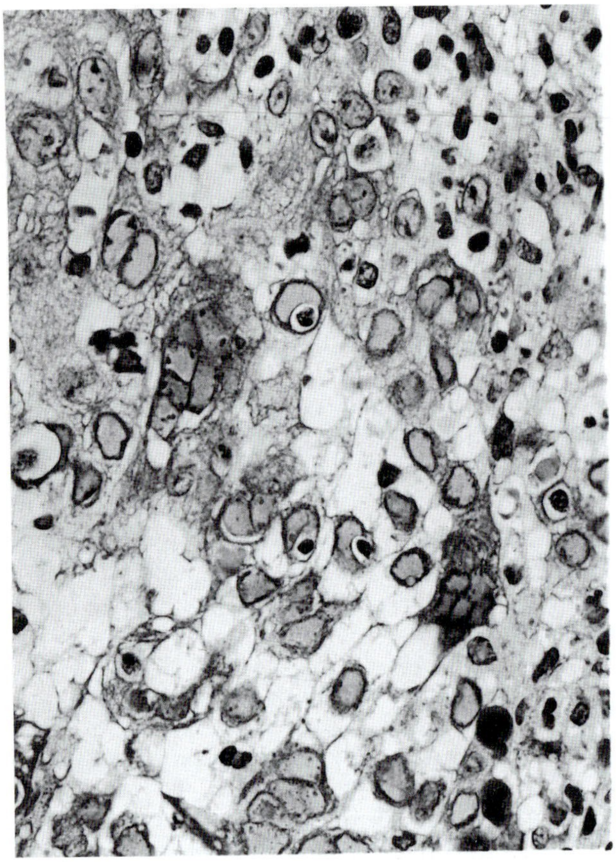

Fig. 2.9. Herpes simplex. High-power view of viral-infected cells with multinucleation and homogenized "ground glass" intranuclear viral inclusions. (Courtesy of R.J. Kurman, M.D., Baltimore, MD.)

and then scraping the ulcer with a wooden spatula may improve the diagnostic yield from ulcerative lesions. Whether the sample is from an ulcer or a freshly opened vesicle, the specimen should be smeared on a clean slide, rapidly fixed in 95% ethanol, or with spray fixative, and stained with Papanicolaou stain. Morphologic changes seen with HSV infection are not reliable in separating primary from secondary infection or in distinguishing HSV type I from type II infection. Furthermore, herpes zoster can involve the vulva and may have similar cytologic findings.

Adjunctive Methods

HSV-specific fluorescein conjugated antiserum may be placed on smears of ulcers or vesicles to identify HSV antigens. Immunoperoxidase techniques, employing HSV-specific antibodies, may be of value if the histopathologic findings are nonspecific and can be employed on paraffin-embedded tissue. Isolation of HSV, whether type I or type II, can be achieved by the inoculation of tissue culture monolayers, such as WI-38 human embryonic lung fibroblasts or monkey kidney cells. Both types of HSV produce characteristic cytopathic changes on these cell lines, which are confirmed by direct immunofluorescence employing monoclonal antibodies to HSV.[130] Virus isolation can be achieved within 4 days.[274] Rapid viral culture over 24 hours, followed by a search for HSV antigen using an immunoperoxidase technique, can give results in less than 2 days.

Polymerase chain reaction (PCR) technique, employing HSV-specific primers, is another approach to the positive identification of HSV infections.[55,216,245] Serologic studies on acute and convalescent serum samples are of value in distinguishing primary from recurrent infection. In primary infection, significant rises (more than fourfold dilution) are found. In recurrent infection the patient is seropositive at presentation and antibody titers will not rise consistently. Serologic methods are not reliable in separating HSV type I from type II.[274] Asymptomatic viral shedding of HSV has been documented in 1.5%–3% of women who are seropositive for HSV type II.[130] HSV infection may have some oncogenic potential; however, this relationship remains to be defined.[107,125]

Clinical Behavior and Treatment

Recurrent episodes of herpatic vulvitis are common after primary infection; recurrences decrease in frequency over time, whether or not acyclovir is given prophylactically. Acyclovir may reduce the severity of infection if given early in the course of illness.[113,145]

Varicella (Herpes Zoster) (Vulvar Shingles)

Varicella infection of the vulva is rare. The prodromal pain within the vulva, without apparent physical findings, may simulate vestibulitis. The subsequent development of vesicles and ulcers assists in making the distinction because vestibulitis is not associated with vesicles and ulcers. The patients usually are postmenopausal or immunosuppressed, and the vesicles are characteristically unilateral.[11,118] The cytologic findings from scrapings of opened vesicles, as well as the histologic findings, are those of a herpesvirus infection. Therapy with famciclovir is reported to reduce pain significantly if begun within 48 hours of the presentation of the rash.[191,250] The protracted neuralgia and recurrent bouts of vesicles are as described for shingles.

Cytomegalovirus Infection

Cytomegalovirus (CMV) vulvitis, like herpes type II vulvitis, presents with an ulcerated vulvovaginitis. The histopathologic findings are similar, although the viral inclusions are both intranuclear and intra-

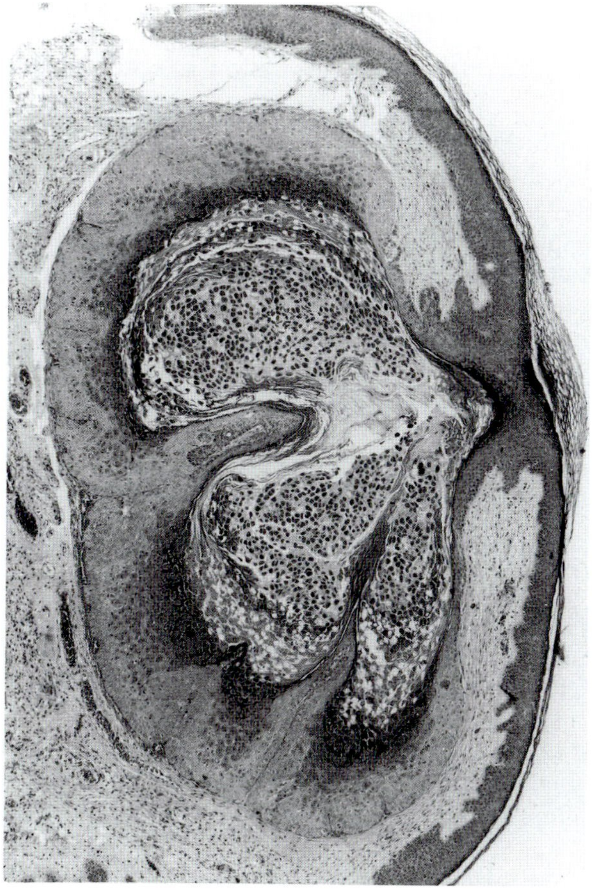

Fig. 2.10. Molluscum contagiosum. Cup-shaped papule under low power shows exo- and endophytic epidermal acanthotic hyperplasia with increasing density of intracytoplasmic inclusions as the surface umbilication is approached.

cytoplasmic. Viral inclusions also may be seen involving vascular endothelial cells, as well as the epithelial cells. CMV infection has been associated with vulvar ulcers in a woman with acquired immunodeficiency syndrome (AIDS). Culture or immunoperoxidase studies using specific antibodies to CMV, or PCR employing CMV-specific primers, are necessary to establish the diagnosis.[77]

Epstein–Barr Virus Infection

Epstein–Barr virus (EBV) has been cultured from painful ulcers on the labia minora during primary infection of infectious mononucleosis. The ulcers slowly healed over a few weeks.[243] EBV infection may be a sexually transmitted disease.[243]

Molluscum Contagiosum

Molluscum contagiosum is a moderately contagious viral disease that, in adults, is often related to intimate or sexual contact.[70] Molluscum contagiosum usually is asymptomatic; however, perianal lesions frequently become pruritic or secondarily infected. The lesions are small, smooth papules (3–6 mm in diameter) with a central punctum or umbilication. They generally are multiple and separate, although they may be single. Rare plaque formations, made up of 50–100 individual clustered lesions, also have been described. The incubation period varies between 14 and 50 days. Clinical diagnosis usually does not require biopsy.

Cytologic identification of the typical eosinophilic intracytoplasmic inclusion bodies (Henderson–Paterson bodies) within scrapings from the interior of the molluscum papule is adequate to confirm the diagnosis. Histologic examination demonstrates marked acanthosis and the characteristic intracytoplasmic viral inclusions in recent infections (Figs. 2.10 and 2.11). With aging, the cytoplasmic bodies take on a more basophilic appearance preceding lysis of the cell.[70] The central dimple of the lesion is seen histologically if the lesion is carefully bisected. Within the dermis there often is a marked vascular response with endothelial proliferation and perivascular inflammation. Electron microscopy has demonstrated that the virus is spherical, ellipsoidal, or brick shaped and contains a DNA core with a two-layered protein coat measuring 210–300 nm.[161] Most lesions regress spontaneously; untreated le-

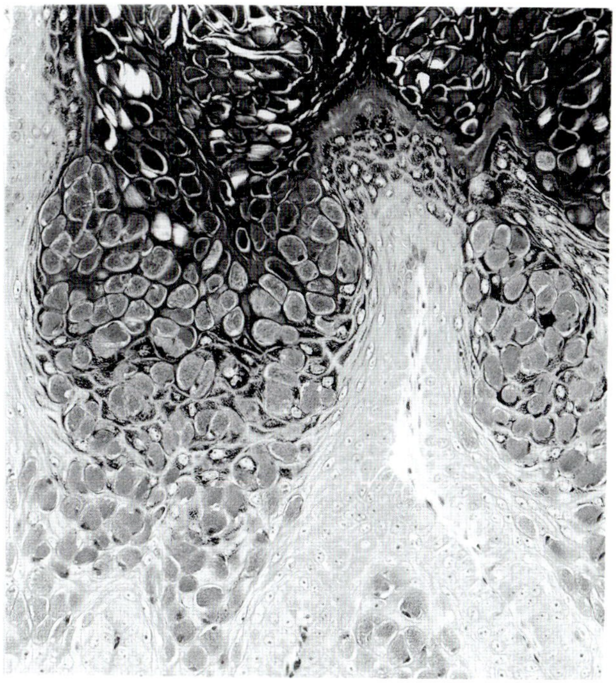

Fig. 2.11. Molluscum contagiosum. High-power view of intracytoplasmic inclusions (molluscum bodies). (Courtesy of R.J. Kurman, M.D., Baltimore, MD.)

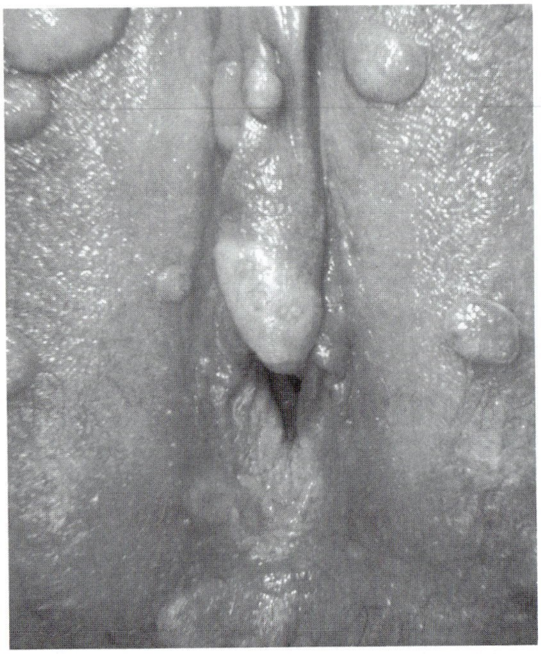

Fig. 2.12. Condyloma lata. Multiple papules are present.

sions may persist for years, during which time they may be spread by close contact or autoinoculation.

Syphilis

Clinical Features

Syphilis is a venereal disease caused by the spirochete *Treponema pallidum*. The primary lesion is the chancre, a painless, indurated, shallow, clean-based ulcer with raised edges. The chancre usually presents within 3 weeks after initial contact; the range, however, is 7–90 days. If secondarily infected, the chancre may become soft and painful and show an ulcerated surface. Although chancres are generally single, they may be multiple. Chancres may occur on inconspicuous surfaces, such as the cervix, anal mucosa, or oral pharynx. In approximately 50% of women and 30% of men the primary lesion is never seen. Lymphadenopathy presents 3–4 days after the chancre. The nodes are nontender, freely movable, and rubbery.[28] Left untreated in the primary phase, the chancre will heal within 2–6 weeks and typically does not leave a scar.[169,266] The secondary stage of the disease will become evident within 6 weeks to 6 months. At this point, the patient may present with a skin rash that often involves mucous membranes as well as the palms of the hands and soles of the feet.[28] On occasion, the secondary lesions are papular, especially about the vulva, presenting as elevated plaques up to 3 cm in diameter. These are known as condylomata lata, which clinically may mimic condylomata acuminata (Fig. 2.12). Such lesions also may occur on other mucocutaneous borders. The tertiary gumma of syphilis is rarely seen on the vulva.

Microscopic Findings

If syphilis were not considered in the clinical differential, the diagnosis may be quite difficult from histologic material alone. The primary chancre is characterized by ulceration of the epidermis with acute and chronic inflammation within the dermis. There is a marked perivascular inflammatory response, characterized by the presence of large numbers of plasma cells. Histologic examination of condylomata lata reveals marked acanthosis and hyperkeratosis (Figs. 2.13 and 2.14). The inflammatory response within the dermis is similar to that in the primary chancre with a marked, predominantly plasma cell inflammatory infiltrate. The arteritis in both lesions may be sufficiently severe to result in obliteration of the smaller vessels. Dieterle, Warthin–Starry, or Steiner stains for spirochetes are always of value if there is any suspicion of syphilis (Fig. 2.15), but may be negative with active infection. Serologic studies for syphilis should be performed if syphilis is considered clinically or from the pathologic findings.[181]

Adjunctive Methods

The primary chancre, as well as the condyloma latum and other secondary lesions, are rich in spirochetes. Therefore, when a chancre or secondary lesion of syphilis is suspected, an attempt to identify

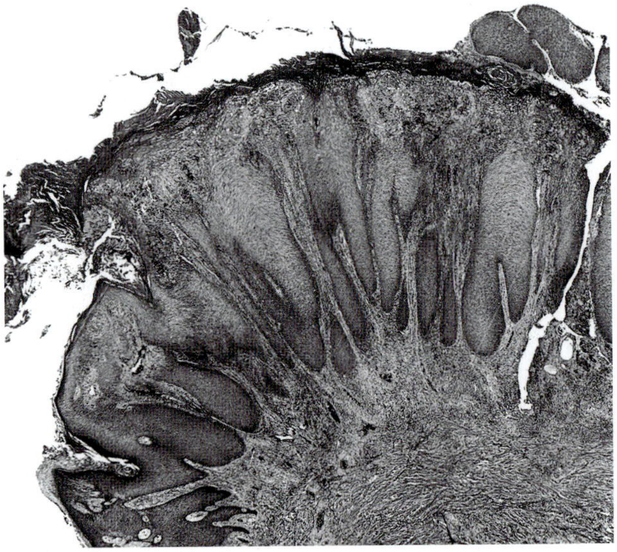

Fig. 2.13. Condyloma latum. Marked psoriasiform epidermal hyperplasia with scales in the cornified layer. (Courtesy of R.J. Kurman, M.D., Baltimore, MD.)

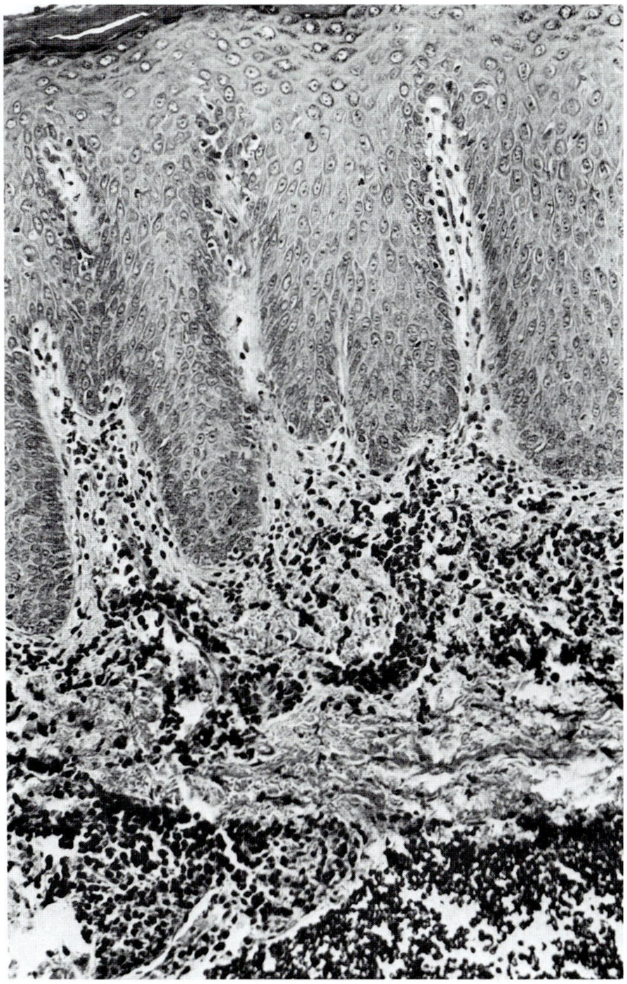

Fig. 2.14. Condyloma latum. Prominent acanthosis is present with a marked dermal perivascular inflammatory cell infiltrate that consists primarily of plasma cells and lymphocytes, with some neutrophils. Vascular endothelial proliferation is present with associated arteritis.

spirochetes within the lesion should be made. This examination is accomplished either through dark-field examination of serum expressed from the base of the ulcer or by the fluorescent conjugated antibody technique, which employs a dried smear preparation. The organism measures up to 15 μm in length and 0.20 μm in thickness; it is spiral in shape, with 6–14 coils. Motility, characterized by flexion, rotation about the long axis, and random movement are noted on dark-field examination of fresh sera from an active lesion. These methods for identification of spirochetes are far more sensitive and specific than is silver stain on paraffin-embedded tissue. The chancre may be present for weeks before serologic tests become reactive. More than 70% of patients with dark-field-positive lesions have a reactive serology at the time of initial diagnosis.

The most common serologic testing methods are based on the identification of reagin. These tests become positive approximately 1 month after the disease is contracted. Common reagin testing methods employ microflocculation testing and include the Venereal Disease Research Laboratory (VDRL) and Rapid Plasma Reagin (RPR).[277] These two tests have similar specificity and can be quantitated to evaluate the course of the disease and response to therapy. The fluorescent *Treponema* antibody, absorbed (FTA-ABS) test, still the "gold standard," is highly sensitive and is ordered if the reagin tests are nonreactive, weakly reactive, or if there is a possibility of a false-positive result. Biologic false positives can occur in lupus erythematosus, virus infection, cirrhosis of the liver, pregnancy, malaria, and other inflammatory or autoimmune diseases. Once the FTA-ABS becomes positive, it can remain so for the life of the patient. Although newer technologies, such as PCR and immunoblotting, have been used in detection of syphilis, serologic tests with RPR/VDRL and FTA-ABS are still the current tests of choice.[277] If the FTA-ABS is positive, spinal fluid serologic evaluation will be necessary to rule out neurosyphilis. A false-positive FTA-ABS is rare and, if detected, requires *T. pallidum* mobilization testing and careful follow-up.[169]

Clinical Behavior and Treatment

Approximately 30% of patients with primary syphilis will undergo spontaneous remission of the

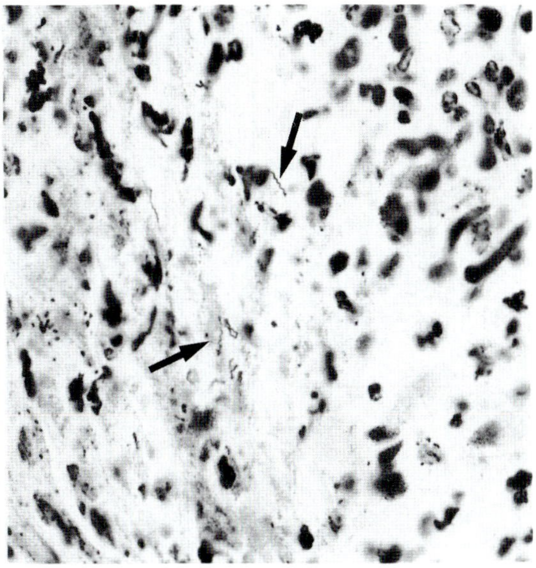

Fig. 2.15. Secondary syphilis. Warthin–Starry stain shows spirochetes in the dermis. (Courtesy of R.J. Kurman, M.D., Baltimore, MD.)

disease. Those who are not treated or who do not achieve spontaneous remission may progress to tertiary syphilis with its well-recognized cardiovascular and central nervous system effects. Untreated syphilis may prove fatal in 10% of those afflicted. Penicillin or another appropriate systemic antibiotic is the treatment of choice.

Granuloma Inguinale

Granuloma inguinale (donovanosis; granuloma venereum) is caused by *Calymmatobacterium granulomatous*, a gram-negative, heavily encapsulated rod considered to be in the bacterial family *Enterobacteriaceae*. Granuloma inguinale occurs with approximately equal frequency in men and women. Primary lesions may occur on the vulva, vagina, or cervix and may present as painless papules or necrotizing ulcers with rolled borders and a friable base. Inguinal adenopathy usually is absent.[27] The lesions usually appear within 1 week to 1 month of exposure; anal coitus or fecal contamination of the vulva or vagina has been incriminated as the mode of transmission.[169,266] Granuloma inguinale extends primarily by local infiltration, although lymphatic permeation may occur during later stages of the disease. Chronic lymphatic infiltration and fibrosis frequently result in a massive brawny edema of the external genitalia. There is controversy as to the true origin of the edema, because dye injection studies suggest that the lymphatic drainage is intact. With involvement of the cervix, the disease may advance via the cervical lymphatics to involve parametrial tissue.[208]

The clinical diagnosis of granuloma inguinale depends on the identification of the Donovan bodies within the tissue; this is best accomplished by preparing smears or a biopsy from the edge of the ulcer and pressing this biopsy tissue between two slides. The tissue imprints are air dried, fixed in methanol, and stained with Giemsa stain. Any antibiotic treatment may obscure the diagnosis, necessitating biopsy at a later date to identify organisms. Histologically, the main portion of the lesion consists of granulation tissue associated with an extensive chronic inflammatory cell infiltrate and endarteritis. An ulcer usually is covered with a fibrinous exudate, and necrosis may be present. The surface epithelium, adjacent to the ulcer, may show prominent pseudoepitheliomatous hyperplasia. Necrosis and microabscesses may be seen within the epidermis.[208] Within the granulation tissue there is a dense mixed inflammatory cell infiltrate, consisting predominantly of plasma cells and mononuclear cells with few lymphocytes, which extends into the dermis. Large vacuolated histiocytes that contain the characteristic encapsulated bacilli, Donovan bodies, within their cytoplasm frequently are present (Fig. 2.16); they can be demonstrated with a Warthin–Starry stain or Giemsa stain. The Donovan bodies may be found extracellularly, as well as intracellularly, and may appear coccoid, coccobacillary, or bacillary.[27,208] Ultrathin plastic-embedded sections, as well as electron microscopy, may be of value in diagnosis.[27,208]

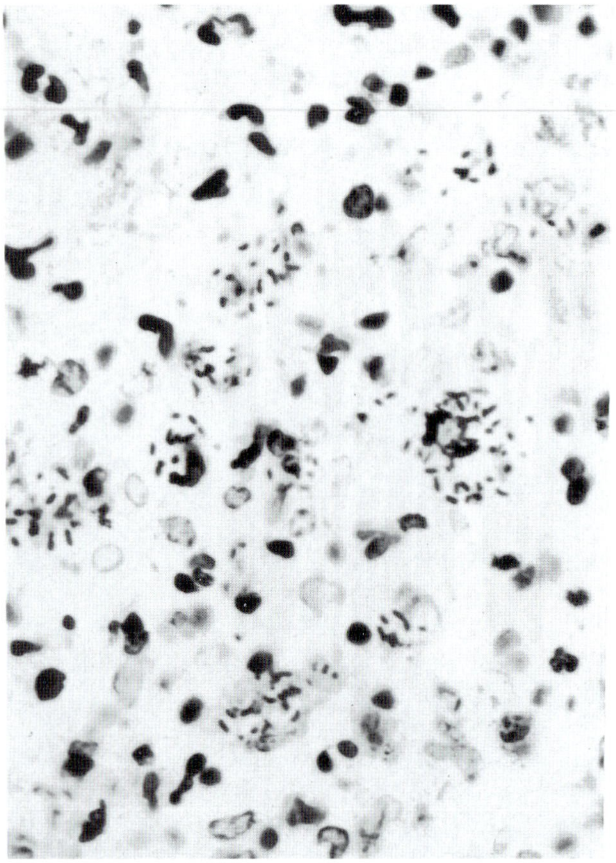

Fig. 2.16. Granuloma inguinale. Giemsa stain shows intracytoplasmic Donovan bodies with characteristic halo around the organisms. (Courtesy of R.J. Kurman, M.D., Baltimore, MD.)

Calymmatobacterium granulomatous may be cultured by special techniques. The diagnosis depends on the clinical findings and documenting the organism within a tissue specimen or by culture. Syphilis, chancroid, and herpesvirus infection usually are included in the differential diagnosis.[69]

Lymphogranuloma Venereum

Lymphogranuloma venereum (LGV) is caused by Chlamydia, and occurs approximately three times more frequently in men than in women. The disease has three phases: (1) erosion of the skin, (2) adenitis, and (3) fibrosis and destruction.[27] Lymphogranuloma venereum is spread primarily via the lymphatics. The initial ulcers, which generally are not tender or painful, often are ignored. Adenitis may evolve into painful superficial groin nodes, or buboes, that frequently rupture through the skin with exudation of a purulent discharge. The third phase of the disease often results in stricture and fibrosis of the vagina and rectum.[269] During this phase, chronic lymphatic obstruction is responsible for the characteristic nonpitting edema of the external genitalia. The histology of LGV is not diagnostic and reveals no characteristic identifiable organisms by the usual modes of investigation. Smears and biopsy specimens should be evaluated for organisms (spirochetes, Donovan bodies, etc.) to rule out other diseases with a similar presentation. Histologically, giant cells may be seen along with lymphocytes and plasma cells (Fig. 2.17). Older lesions may exhibit extensive fibrosis of the dermis and sinus tracts. The diagnosis is based on the typical clinical presentation, along with positive complement fixation tests. Culture, as well as other specific immunohistochemical tests, can assist in the diagnosis of LGV. Treatment is systemic tetracycline or doxycycline.[169,266]

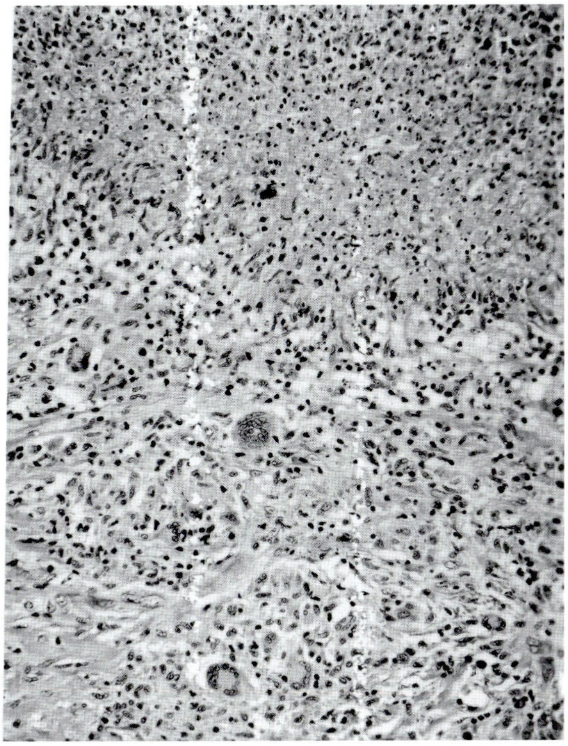

Fig. 2.17. Lymphogranuloma venereum. An intense superficial and deep chronic inflammatory infiltrate is present, composed predominantly of lymphocytes and plasma cells. The lesion has trizonal inflammatory reaction from the surface to deep levels: ulceration and debris, granulation tissue, and intense chronic inflammation. (Courtesy R.J. Kurman, M.D., Baltimore, MD.)

Chancroid

Chancroid is relatively rare and presents with a genital ulcer that usually is tender, nonindurated, and has a friable purulent erythematous base. Primary lesions may be single or multiple and tend to be small, measuring approximately 1–2 mm in diameter. Coalescence of the lesions leads to ulcers approaching 3 cm in diameter. Tender inguinal adenopathy with flocculent nodes may be present. The incubation period may be as short as 10 days.[248] The clinical differential diagnosis includes herpesvirus infection and primary syphilis.[69,248] Chancroid is caused by the organism *Haemophilus ducreyi*, a gram-negative, nonmotile bacillus, which in culture grows in pairs and parallel chains. Skin tests and biopsies may not be diagnostic. Identification of the organism by culture is necessary for accurate diagnosis.[248] Selective agar medium has been developed for the organism, which has improved culture isolation. Recent advances in nonculture diagnostic tests using PCR have enhanced our ability to diagnose chancroid.[186,248] Histologic examination of the tissue demonstrated a granulomatous-type reaction with chronic inflammatory cells consisting primarily of lymphocytes and plasma cells, and the presence of the gram-negative organisms, which may be present in large numbers and in parallel chains.[68]

HIV-Associated Vulva Ulcers

Human immunodeficiency virus (HIV) infection-associated vulva ulcers are usually painful and multiple. A recent study revealed that about 60% of vulva ulcerations have no proven etiologic agent. The rest of the patients are positive for HSV II, unusual or mixed bacteria, and rarely cytomegalovirus, *Chlamydia trachomatis*, and *Gardnerella vaginalis*. Human immunodeficiency virus may play a local role in causation or exacerbation.[134]

Tuberculosis

Tuberculosis of the vulva is rare. It usually is associated with tuberculosis of other genital sites, primarily the fallopian tube, and endometrium. Genital involvement usually is associated with pulmonary

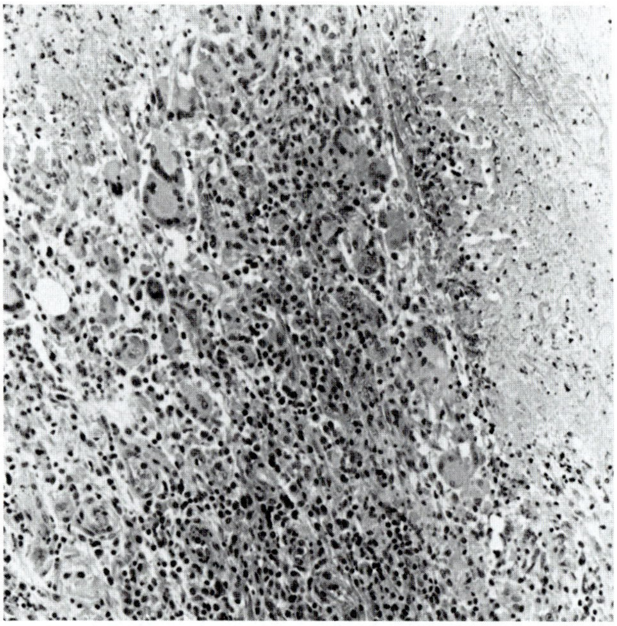

Fig. 2.18. Vulvar tuberculosis. Caseating granulomas with Langhans giant cells.

tuberculosis. Autoinoculation by hematogenous or direct spread therefore is the most common method of transmission to the vulva. Primary inoculation or sexual transmission of tuberculosis is very uncommon. Immunosuppression may play a role in susceptibility, as a case of vulvar tuberculosis has been described in a renal transplant patient.[244] The usual organism is *Mycobacterium tuberculosis*; however, atypical mycobacteria also have been incriminated. Diagnosis usually can be made by biopsy of the involved tissues. Caseating granulomas with Langhans giant cells are found, and acid-fast stains usually reveal the mycobacterium (Fig. 2.18). Confirmation of the diagnosis can be made by culture techniques. Appropriate long-term systemic antibiotics are the recommended therapy. Giant cells of the foreign body type are encountered frequently in vulvar tissues in which a previous biopsy has been performed. These giant cells, associated with noncaseating granulomas, often result from embedded suture occasionally seen in prior biopsied areas, and should not be confused with tuberculosis. Vulvar ulceration, secondary to sarcoidosis, has been reported and should be included in the differential diagnosis of granulomatous ulcerations of the vulva.[121]

Fungal Infection and Miscellaneous Infectious Diseases

Chronic inflammatory conditions of the vulvar and perianal skin without concomitant ulceration often are caused by fungal infections, although a variety of irritants, unrelated to infection, may be responsible.[156] *Candida* and dermatophytes are frequent pathogens. Such conditions rarely require biopsy, and accurate diagnosis generally can be accomplished by microscopic examination of skin scrapings placed in 10% potassium hydroxide, or by appropriate culture methods. Topical antifungal creams are the usual therapy. Chronic and acute vaginitis related to trichomonas, *Chlamydia*, *Candida* species, or other infectious agents may be associated with inflammation of the vulva, especially the vulvar vestibule. The histologic findings usually are not diagnostic. Vulvar candidiasis usually can be diagnosed by employing silver stains for fungus, with recognition of the fungal organisms within the keratin, or superficial epithelium. Bacterial infections may produce clinical findings similar to those seen with fungus infections.

Erythrasma is a chronic bacterial infection of the genitocrural area that shows a coral-red fluorescence under Wood's light. The disease is most common in obese diabetes. Scrapings of these lesions, when stained with Gram stain, demonstrate the causative gram-positive bacteria, *Corynebacterium minutissimum*, in rods, filaments, and coccoid forms.[68]

Parasitic Infections

Enterobius vermicularis (pinworm, seatworm) is a relatively common intestinal parasite. The female worm measures 8–13 mm in length and 0.5 mm in diameter. The male is approximately one-fourth as long as the female, with the same diameter. Infected children frequently present with complaints of severe vulvovaginal pruritus, which may awaken them at night. Other complaints include lower abdominal pain, diarrhea, restlessness, and nocturia. Studies for fungus and bacteria are not diagnostic, and examination of the vulvar vestibule and vagina reveals marked inflammation. Occasionally, an adult female helminth found on the vestibule or perineal areas is brought to the laboratory. More commonly, the pathologist is presented with a cellulose-tape-slide preparation for identification of the typical embryonated eggs of *E. vermicularis*. A granuloma secondary to *Enterobius* eggs has been reported involving the vulva.[241] Vulvar schistosomiasis, usually *Schistosoma mansoni*, is well documented, and primary skin lesions on the vulva from penetration of the infective cercariae may be seen. When biopsied, the parasite may be found within the epidermis.[159] Cutaneous myiasis of the vulva, secondary to infestation of the larval form of the muscoid fly and sarcophaga, has been reported. Recognition of the larva extracted from the vulvar tissues is diagnostic.[46,127]

Noninfectious Papulosquamous Dermatoses

Papulosquamous dermatoses often have a common component of epidermal hyperplasia in which the hyperplasia is somewhat psoriasiform. Table 2.4 summarizes most of the entities in this group.

To establish a standardized system of nomenclature based on histopathological findings, the International Society for the Study of Vulvovaginal Disease (ISSVD) and International Society of Gynecological Pathologists (ISGP) recommended in 1986 that all such lesions be classified as nonneoplastic epithelial disorders and classified as lichen sclerosus, squamous cell hyperplasia, and other dermatoses. Diagnoses as kraurosis vulvae, leukoplakia, and atrophic vulvitis have generally been abandoned. Historically, the term dystrophy was proposed to describe a clinically related group of disorders of vulvar epithelium, which presented as white lesions, and that microscopically were characterized by benign alterations of the epithelial and dermal architecture. Two basic clinical varieties of dystrophy were recognized by the ISSVD in 1976: lichen sclerosus and hyperplastic dystrophy. When both coexisted on different areas of the same vulva, it was recommended that the lesion be classified as a mixed dystrophy. The term mixed dystrophy is now recognized to refer to lichen sclerosus associated with variable degrees of squamous cell hyperplasia (formerly called hyperplastic dystrophy), and this reflects the spectrum of changes seen in lichen sclerosus, rather than the presentation of two distinctive epithelial disorders. The various forms of nonneoplastic epithelial disorders of the vulva cannot be reliably distinguished on the basis of their clinical appearance alone; all may be white, scaly, and fissured (Fig. 2.19). Although biopsy may not be necessary in all cases, especially in children with typical findings of lichen sclerosus, one or more biopsies to sample the entire lesion usually are very informative. On the basis of the histologic findings, the pathologist can separate white lesions of a neoplastic type from nonneoplastic epithelial disorders.

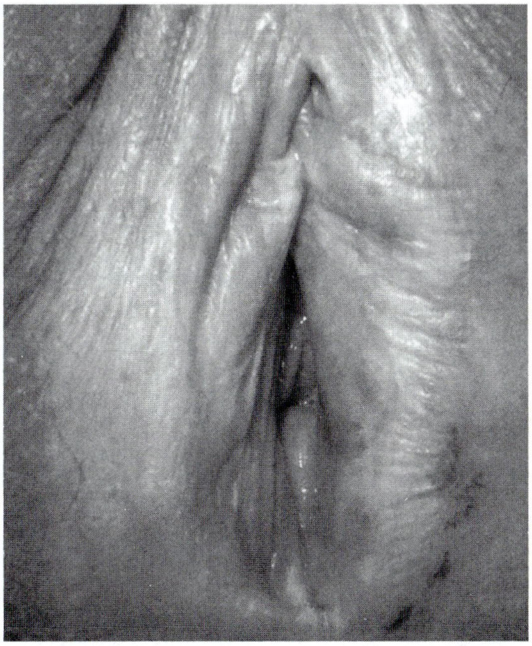

Fig. 2.19. Lichen sclerosus. White epithelium with focal subcutaneous ecchymosis is seen. The labia minora are somewhat atrophic.

Table 2.4. Noninfectious papulosquamous disorder

Psoriasis
Seborrheic dermatitis
Spongiotic dermatitis
Acute, subacute, and chronic atopic/contact dermatitis
Irritant contact dermatitis
Eczema
Nutritional deficiency
Vitamin deficiency-associated dermatitis
Glucoganoma (necrolytic migratory erythema)
Nonneoplastic epithelial disorders
Squamous cell hyperplasia
Lichen simplex chronicus (LSC)
Lichen planus (hypertrophic form)
Lichen sclerosis (hypertrophic form)
Acanthosis nigricans

Lichen Sclerosus (Lichen Sclerosus et Atrophicus)

Clinical Features

In children, symptoms include dysuria, painful defecation, and rectal bleeding.[20,198] *Lichen sclerosus* can lead to anal fissures and strictures and to genital and perianal ulcers, which may resemble evidence of child sexual abuse. In adult women, the clinical findings typically include thinned and whitened epithelium, which usually is symmetric and involves the labia minora, clitoris, prepuce, frenulum, perineal body, and vulvar vestibule. Perirectal involvement is common. In advanced cases, loss and agglutination of the labia minora, frenulum, prepuce, and adhesions of the clitoris are found.[198] Stenosis of the introitus is common. In men, the glands of the penis and prepuce frequently are involved, and distal urethral stricture and phimosis may occur. Under these circumstances, the condition is clinically known as *balanitis xerotica obliterans*.

Gross Findings

The vulvar lesions of lichen sclerosus typically are pale white, flat, plaque-like areas that in advanced cases may be associated with thinned parchment-like epithelium and focal areas of ecchymosis and superficial ulceration (see Fig. 2.19). The vaginal mucosa is not involved.

Microscopic Findings

The microscopic findings of lichen sclerosus can vary considerably, related to age of the lesion, excoriation, and treatment.[34,172] The principal histologic changes show a sandwich appearance, including epidermis with blunting or loss of the rete ridges, a zone of homogeneous collagenized subepithelial edema of variable thickness, and a band of lymphocytic infiltration beneath this zone (Fig. 2.20). The homogeneous zone usually shows a reduction or absence of elastic fibers. The epithelium is thinned, but hyperkeratosis may be present in some cases. The basal cell layer often is disorganized, and spongiosis may be evident. There is both an absence of melanosomes in the keratinocytes and a disappearance of the melanocytes. The lack of pigment, as well as edema, contribute to the white clinical appearance. Mitotic figures are rare or absent. In some cases, the mechanical trauma of rubbing and scratching will have produced bullous areas of lymph edema and subepithelial lacunae filled with erythrocytes. Areas of ulceration and acute inflammation also may be seen.

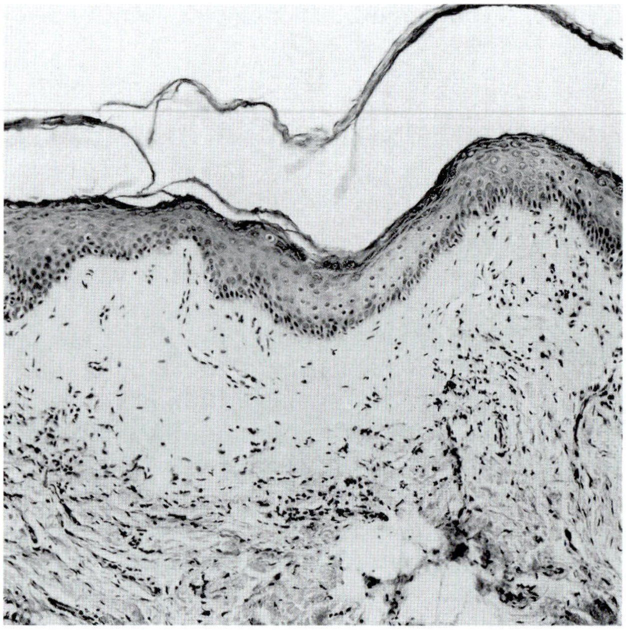

Fig. 2.20. Lichen sclerosus. Hyperkeratosis is present along with loss of rete pegs and homogenization of the dermis. (Courtesy R.J. Kurman, M.D., Baltimore, MD.)

Differential Diagnosis

See Differential under lichen planus.

Ultrastructural Findings

Ultrastructural studies have shown that collagen metabolism is abnormally active and the number of capillaries is reduced. The basal lamina is thickened and discontinuous. Degenerate dermal and collagenous material and formation of a hybrid of elastocollagenous bundles can be found between the cells of the epidermis, and melanocytes are rare.[162]

Immunohistochemical and Related Studies

The presence of an elastase-type protease in vulvar fibroblasts from lichen sclerotic tissue has been reported that may be responsible for the loss of elastic tissue.[91] An increased concentration of collagenase inhibitor also has been reported. Tissue studies of glucose metabolism as well as alkaline phosphatase and adenosine triphosphatase have shown a surprisingly high rate of activity, equal to that seen in hyperplastic specimens and greater than that found in normal menopausal skin. The cell cycle protein Ki-67 is present in the basal and many parabasal epithelial cells involved by lichen sclerosus.[226] An apparent premature maturation of all cells above the basal layer has been reported, based on their high concentration of involucrin.[34] There is a growing body of evidence that an autoimmune mechanism may be involved. Patients with lichen sclerosus have been noted to have an increased number of organ-specific antibodies and more autoimmune disease than the normal population.[31,32] However, the correlation is inconclusive.[225] On a histologic level, direct immunofluorescence studies have shown a deposit of fibrin along the dermoepidermal junction in 75% of the specimens studied.[91,225] With an indirect fluorescent technique, IgM and C3 were concentrated along the basal lamina of the epithelium.[91,225] Studies on activated T cells within lichen sclerosus have identified activated (HLA-DR+) T cells and increased epidermal CD1a+ Langerhans cells, CD57+1μm phocytes, activated lymphoid cells and epidermal antigen-presenting cells, respectively.[32,225]

Clinical Behavior and Treatment

Lichen sclerosus sometimes is associated with vulvar squamous carcinoma; however, it is not considered to be a premalignant intraepithelial neoplasm (see Chapter 3, Premalignant and Malignant Tumors of the Vulva). In a report of vulvar squamous cell carcinoma, 61% had lichen sclerosus. Forty-three of the 47 cases with lichen sclerosus were not recognized to have vulvar lichen sclerosus until the time of the tumor diagnosis.[136] Among patients with symptomatic vulvar lichen sclerosus, 9% developed VIN lesions and 21% invasive squamous cell carcinoma. Symptomatic lichen sclerosus preceded the carcinoma by a mean of 4 years. Squamous cell carcinoma associated with lichen sclerosus occurred in an older age group, were located more commonly on the clitoris, and were of the conventional squamous cell carcinoma type.[34,35] Aneuploidy has been reported, which correlates with elevated p53 expression.[33,34] In cases in which lichen sclerosus is associated with vulvar squamous cell carcinoma, squamous cell hyperplasia usually is observed adjacent to the carcinoma.[215] Differentiated (simplex) type VIN and non-HPV-related squamous cell carcinoma have been associated with vulvar lichen sclerosus.[275]

Traditional management has relied on the long-term topical application of testosterone or progesterone. Recent studies have reported good results with topical, superpotent corticosteroids for a short period.[32,56,67,143] In children, clearing or improvement of the anogenital lesions has been reported at puberty. However, this improvement has not been associated with menarche or pregnancy.[99,142] Topical testosterone has been reported to arrest the symptoms and progress of the disease; however, it cannot be used in children because it is systemically absorbed. It is rarely used today. Current therapy using high-potency topical corticosteroids produces symptomatic relief and, in some cases, resolution of lichen sclerosus.[38] Opinion varies as to the ideal long-term therapy; most advocate high-potency topical corticosteroids, but with reduced frequency. Lichen sclerosus is not a disease that requires vulvectomy or is cured by local excision or ablative treatment, such as laser therapy or cryotherapy. However, women with lichen sclerosus require continued therapy and follow-up because, over time, it is associated with a small but significant risk of vulvar differentiated (simplex) type VIN and squamous cell carcinoma in postmenopausal women. In these cases, tumor development occurs in the field of lichen sclerosus, and typically is associated with visible tumor or hyperplastic changes that indicate biopsy to establish the diagnosis of tumor. With improved therapy, it is expected that the frequency of tumor may be decreased.

Squamous Cell Hyperplasia (Formerly Hyperplastic Dystrophy)

General Features

Squamous cell hyperplasia is an epithelial disorder characterized by acanthosis and variable hyperkeratosis without atypia, significant associated inflammation, or evidence of a specific dermatosis. If significant inflammation is present, a diagnosis of lichen simplex chronicus should be considered. Squamous cell hyperplasia is a descriptive term applicable both clinically and histologically to an epithelial thickening of the vulva that cannot be otherwise specifically classified. It is considered to be a nonspecific response of the genital skin to a wide variety of irritants. A recent study revealed that the expression of retinoid acid receptor-alpha, a modulator of epithelial cell proliferation and differentiation, is decreased and the distribution of the receptor is changed in lichen sclerosus and squamous cell hyperplasia.[17] Squamous cell hyperplasia is typically found in adult women, most commonly occurring in women between 30 and 60 years of age. There is no racial predilection. Clinically, the most common presenting complaint is pruritus confined to a focal area on the vulva that usually can be pointed to by the patient.

Gross Findings

The involved vulvar area usually is not symmetric, as is often seen with lichen sclerosus, and may be confined to a focal area, usually involving the labia majora. The involved area appears gray white or reddened. The skin markings often are accentuated, a sign of intradermal edema and chronic rubbing; excoriation and fissures frequently bear witness to the intensity of the itching. There is no shrinkage, stenosis, or agglutination of the labia, as occurs in lichen sclerosus. The condition is clinically indistinguishable from what has previously been called neurodermatitis or eczema.

Microscopic Findings

The histopathologic features of squamous cell hyperplasia are epidermal acanthosis. Hyperkeratosis and parakeratosis may be present. There typically is no significant inflammatory infiltrate, although some lymphocytes may be seen in the superficial dermis. There is no significant dermal fibrosis or thickening. The changes are otherwise nonspecific, and the diagnosis is arrived at by exclusion of other

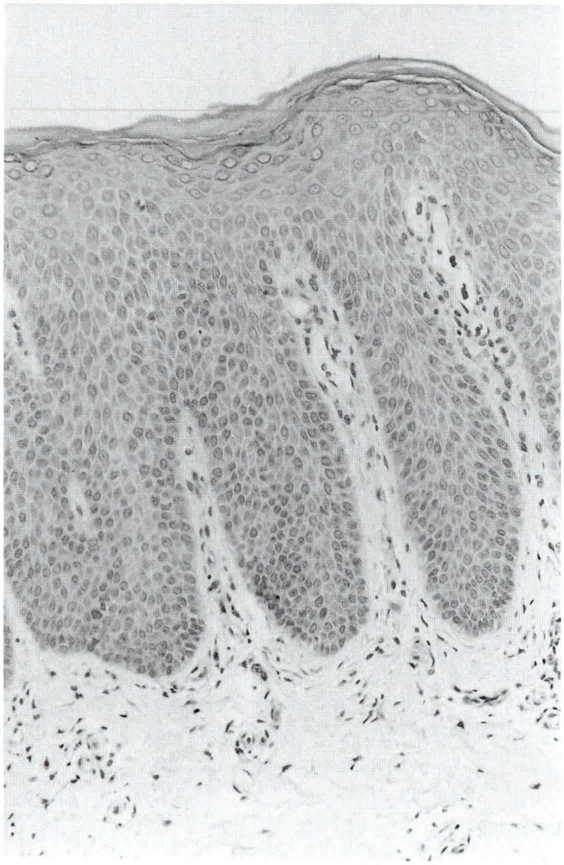

Fig. 2.21. Squamous cell hyperplasia. Epithelial thickening with acanthosis and mild hyperkeratosis is evident. No nuclear atypia is present, and no dermal fibrosis or thickening is identified within the superficial dermis. There is no significant inflammation.

dermatoses (Fig. 2.21). The individual squamous cells are regular with distinct intercellular bridges. The nuclei are round to oval and contain finely distributed chromatin. Nucleoli may be prominent; however, there is progressive maturation of the cells as they approach the superficial layers. Mitotic figures, if present, are normal and confined to the basal layer. Hyperkeratosis may be seen associated with accentuation of the granular layer. Although parakeratosis may be present in otherwise typical areas of hyperplasia, its presence should prompt a careful search for cellular atypia and VIN of the differentiated type (see Vulvar Intraepithelial Neoplasia in Chapter 3). In the absence of atypia or lichen sclerosus, there is no evidence of risk of carcinoma from this process. The diagnosis of squamous hyperplasia is one of exclusion. The differential diagnosis includes lichen simplex chronicus, fungal infection, human papillomavirus infection, and VIN (see differential under Lichen Simplex Chronicus, following).

Clinical Behavior and Treatment

Treatment is based on limiting or preventing exposure of the vulva to potential irritants in conjunction with the use of topical corticosteroids and antipruritics. Symptoms usually abate within 2–3 weeks.[38] Occasionally, local excision or laser ablation of the hyperplastic area may be effective in unresponsive cases. The significance of squamous cell hyperplasia found adjacent to squamous cell carcinoma, as seen in approximately 50% of women with vulvar carcinoma, is not well understood. In some cases, there is associated lichen sclerosus or VIN.[226]

Lichen Simplex Chronicus

Lichen simplex chronicus (LSC) has been considered to be equivalent to squamous cell hyperplasia by some dermatopathologists.[194] The microscopic diagnosis of lichen simplex chronicus, however, includes the finding of a superficial dermal chronic inflammatory infiltrate with vertical collagen streaks in the

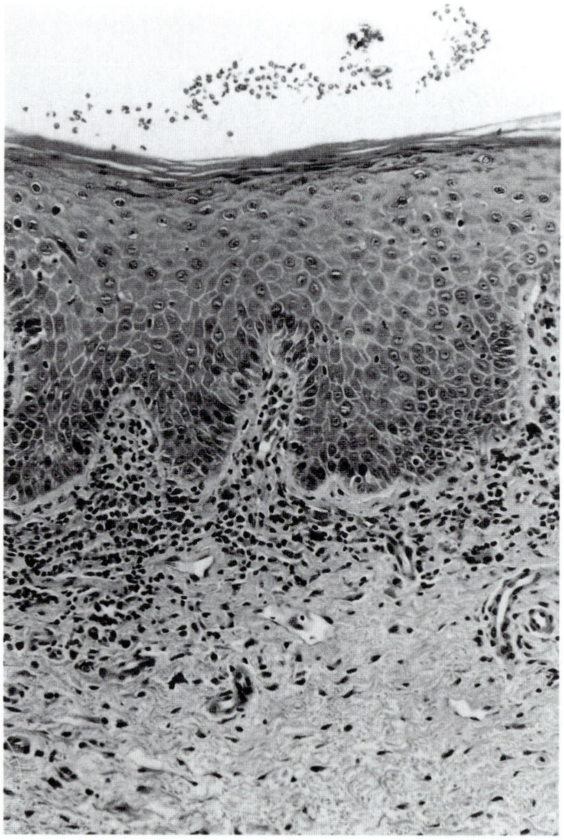

Fig. 2.22. Lichen simplex chronicus. The epithelium is slightly thickened; however, no hyperkeratosis is present. Within the superficial dermis there is a prominent chronic inflammatory cell infiltrate. In this example, there is minimal fibrosis within the superficial dermis.

papillary dermis (Fig. 2.22). The treatment is essentially the same as for squamous cell hyperplasia.

Differential Diagnosis

The differential diagnosis of squamous cell hyperplasia and LSC includes chronic candidiasis or dermatophyte infection of the vulva that usually can be differentiated by a silver stain for fungus or periodic acid–Schiff (PAS) stain for the organisms. The fungal organisms usually are present in the keratin layer. The finding of inflammatory exocytosis, with neutrophils within the epithelium, is a clue for fungal infection. Regressing or early flat condyloma acuminata also may resemble LSC or squamous cell hyperplasia. However, the prominent granular layer, accentuated intracellular bridges, parabasalar hyperplasia, and koilocytosis typically are lacking. If this cannot be resolved by histopathologic examination, molecular biologic methods, such as PCR or in situ hybridization, may be helpful in establishing the diagnosis of HPV-associated changes when virus is identified. Psoriasis or lichen planus may be included in the differential diagnosis; however, they represent distinct entities that are clinically and histologically identifiable.

Lichen Planus

General Features

Lichen planus (LP) has a wide age distribution; however, it presents most commonly in women more than 40 years of age.[139,150] Vulvar pruritis and burning are common symptoms; however, the patient may be asymptomatic. White, lacelike plaques (Wickham's striae) involving the oral and vaginal mucosa also may be present. Involvement of all three sites is referred to as the vulvo-vaginal-gingival syndrome reported by Pelisse. The syndrome is recognized as an erosive form of LP.[189] Patients with this condition experience vulvar pain, dyspareunia, and burning. Postcoital bleeding also has been reported.[146,189] LP can result in severe introital and vaginal adhesions, scarring, and stenosis.

Gross Findings

The clinical appearance may be highly variable on the vulva, ranging from delicate reticulated papules to an erosive desquamative process involving the vagina and vulva. Within the vulva, the erosive process is typically confined to the vulvar vestibule and commonly involves the vagina. With advancing disease, there is loss and agglutination of the labia minora and prepuce, associated with thinned epithelium, postinflammatory hypopigmentation, and shrinkage with stenosis of the vaginal introitus. In advanced stages, it may be difficult to distinguish LP from advanced *lichen sclerosus* (LS). Vaginal involvement with adhesions and synechiae clinically characterizes LP, as does the finding of mucous membrane lesions outside the vulva.

Microscopic Findings

The histopathologic features may be highly variable depending on the age of the lesion as well as its location. Mucous membrane lesions may differ considerably from those occurring on vulvar skin.[68] In the skin, there are two important microscopic features: a bandlike chronic inflammatory infiltrate that is predominantly lymphocytic, with no or rare plasma cells. The inflammation is lichenoid, involving the upper dermis and immediate overlying epidermis (Fig. 2.23). Liquefaction necrosis of the basal

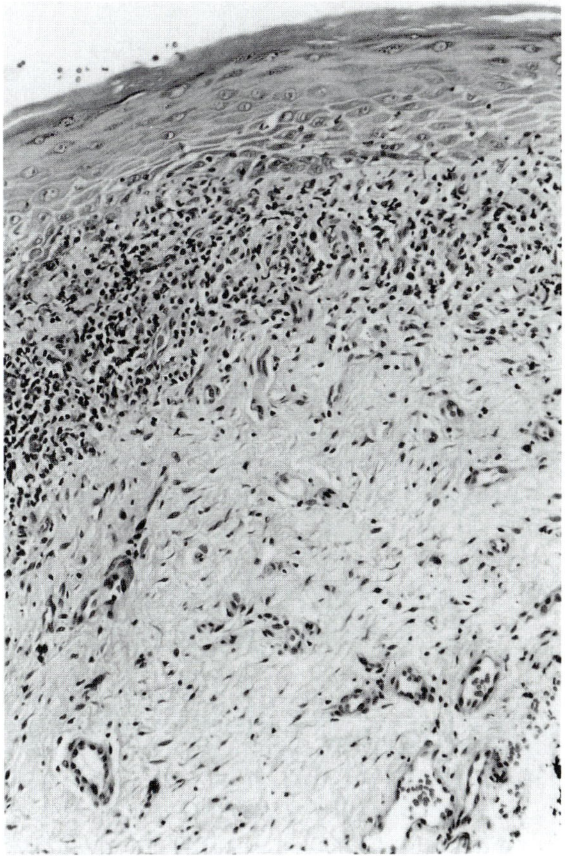

Fig. 2.23. Lichen planus. The epithelium is somewhat thinned with loss of rete ridges. A prominent granular layer is evident without significant hyperkeratosis in this example. There is a prominent bandlike chronic inflammatory infiltrate consisting almost entirely of lymphocytes, which is lichenoid and involves the basal layer. Liquefaction necrosis of the basal cells with colloid body formation is evident. (Courtesy J. L. Thomasen, M.D., Milwaukee, WI.)

epithelial cells is seen, and these cells typically are admixed with chronic inflammatory cells. Degenerated keratinocytes result in the formation of colloid bodies (civatte bodies). Within the vulvar skin, the involved epithelium may show acanthosis, wedge-shaped hypergranulosis, and hyperkeratosis. Usually, parakeratosis is not present. Immunofluorescent studies often reveal fibrin deposition at the dermal–epidermal junction and, occasionally, granular IgM; rarely C3 and IgG deposits are also present. The cluster of necrotic keratinocytes (colloid bodies) positive for IgM in up to 87% of cases and, sometimes, C3 and IgG deposits may be helpful for the diagnosis.[246] The epithelial changes are variable within mucous membranes and include thinning of the epithelium, with ulceration and bullous formation. In contrast to the findings within the skin, plasma cells may be evident with mucosal involvement.

Differential Diagnosis

Well-developed lichen sclerosis (LS) can be distinguished from LP by the absence of the lichenoid inflammatory infiltrate at the dermal–epidermal junction in LS. Colloid bodies also are common in LP. LP typically involves mucosal as well as nonmucosal sites, whereas LS does not involve the vagina or oral mucosa. In advanced cases, mucosal involvement may be the most important distinguishing feature. Cicatricial pemphigoid and LP may both cause scarring and stenosis of the vulvar vestibule and vagina. Lichen planus has the characteristic lichenoid inflammatory pattern with colloid bodies within the epithelium. Cicatricial pemphigoid forms subepithelial blisters and has abundant eosinophils in the vesicles and in the dermis. Immunofluorescence demonstrates linear IgG and C3 deposits, which are usually absent in LP. *Morphea (scleroderma)* may be included in the differential diagnosis in that a band-like chronic inflammatory infiltrate may be seen with epithelial thinning; however, the inflammation is typically perivascular and around skin adnexa in the deep dermis, frequently with plasma cells. The interface liquefaction changes seen in LP typically are not seen in morphea. Morphea usually involves other sites, especially the trunk. Sclerosus of the dermis in morphea results in dermal thickening and loss of fat about skin appendages, as well as loss of skin appendages.

Clinical Behavior and Treatment

Adhesion formation can lead to scarring and agglutination of the labia minora.[139] Topical cortical steroids are the usual form of treatment; fluorinated corticosteroids may be needed initially to provide relief. Additional therapy may include topical or oral cyclosporine, oral dapsone, and oral griseofulvin.[62,139]

Psoriasis

Psoriasis is inherited as an autosomal dominant trait (diathesis) with incomplete penetrance. Psoriasis affects approximately 2% of the population of the United States. On the vulva, the disease typically involves the lateral aspects of the labia majora and genitocrural areas.[209] The lesions present as sharply demarcated, silvery-topped erythematous papules and plaques on skin. When this loose silvery scale is removed, several punctuate bleeding points can be seen (Auspitz sign). In the vulva and other intertrigenous areas, the silvery scales are lost. The sharply demarcated, bright red erythematous plaques are the main clinical finding. The lesions frequently are symmetric and may persist for years. At times, new psoriatic lesions develop at sites of trauma within 7–30 days after the trauma. This is referred to as Koebner phenomenon. Reiter's syndrome of the vulva, which is in the spectrum of psoriasis, rarely affects women.[63]

Microscopic Findings

Hyperkeratosis, parakeratosis, uniform psoriasiform hyperplasia (elongation of the rete ridges to an even length) with club-shaped tips of rete ridges, diminution of the granular layer, and collections of polymorphonuclear leukocytes within the epidermis (Munro abscesses) are the epidermal changes (Fig. 2.24). Mitotic activity increases within the epidermis above the basal layer, reflecting the significantly increased rate of epithelial turnover. The dermal papillae are clubbed and edematous. Prominent tortuous vessels are seen within the papillae, and there is a minimal chronic inflammatory cell infiltrate with the dermis.[68]

Differential Diagnosis

The major differential diagnosis includes seborrheic dermatitis and chronic eczema. The latter two conditions also show psoriasiform hyperplasia; however, the rete ridges typically are not elongated to an even length as in the psoriasis. In seborrheic dermatitis, the subcorneal neutrophils are typically distributed around follicular ostia. Because psoriasis and seborrheic dermatitis have a similar clinical presentation, the differential diagnosis between these two can be very difficult.[209]

Contact Dermatitis

Vulvar *contact dermatitis* may be of an allergic type, which is a cell-mediated response to sensitizing agents such as nickel or rubber, or an irritant related to exposure to chemical or physical agents that damage the skin. Urinary incontinence is a common cause of irritation. Irritant dermatitis is the more

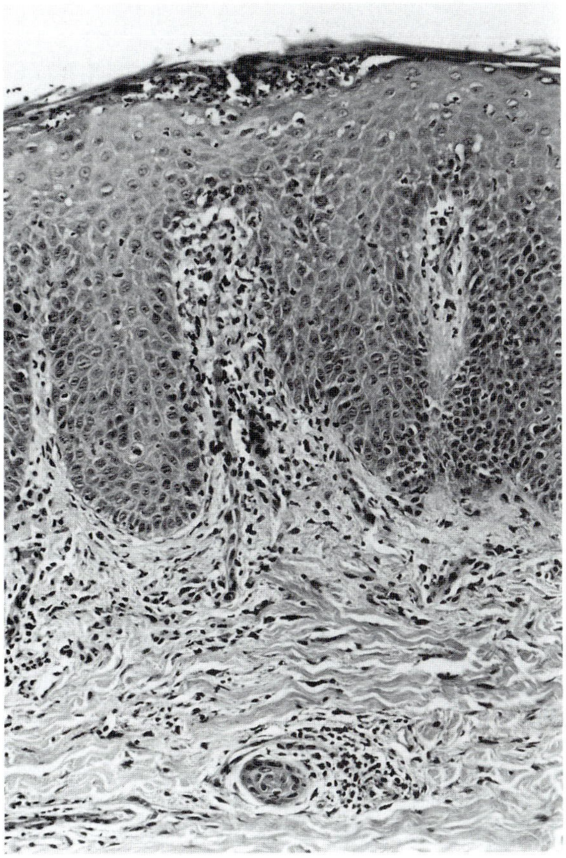

Fig. 2.24. Psoriasis. Prominent uniform acanthosis is present. An intracorneal neutrophil collection (Munro abscess) is evident. The dermal papillae are clubbed and infiltrated by chronic inflammatory cells.

common of the two. The lesions typically are confined to the area of exposure and usually persist for some time after the exposure.[195] The pathologic findings may be quite variable, depending on the severity and duration of the process and whether there is an associated allergic response. The most constant histopathologic findings are spongiosis with microvesiculation. The superficial perivascular inflammatory response consists predominantly of lymphocytes and histiocytes; eosinophils may be present. Superficial erosion or ulceration may be present and, in long-standing contact dermatitis, epithelial thickening with parakeratosis and hyperkeratosis simulating lichen simplex chronicus also occurs.

Atopic Dermatitis

Women with *atopic dermatitis* may have involvement of the vulva, with associated pruritis and burning.[195] The physical findings may be limited to dryness and scaling, but thickening of the skin with localized excoriation may be evident if the vulva has been irritated by scratching. Vulvar biopsies are rarely performed on these patients. The pathologic findings often are typically squamous cell hyperplasia or are nonspecific. Spongiosis can at times be present. Within the dermis, lymphocytes and macrophages are present and the density of the infiltrate tends to correlate with the severity and chronicity of the process. Eosinophils and mast cells also may be identified. Immunofluorescent studies have demonstrated IgE on epidermal Langerhans cells.[182,240]

Fixed Drug Eruption (Dermatitis Medicamentosa)

Fixed drug eruptions constitute a complex group of cutaneous manifestations of drug-hypersensitive reactions that are subclassified as types I through IV. Type I is mediated through IgE antibodies and usually presents as urticaria. Type II is mediated through IgG and IgM antibodies and may be manifested as drug purpura or a bullous drug eruption. Type III is related to immune complexes and may be expressed as a maculopapular eruption, exanthem, urticaria, or vasculitis. Type IV is cell mediated and may be manifested as contact dermatitis, an exanthem, or a maculopapular eruption.

Fixed drug eruptions usually appear at the same place on reexposure to the same drug. Multiple reexposure may elicit lesions at new places in addition to the original locations. After discontinuation of the drug, the lesion may heal with prominent postinflammatory hyperpigmentation on the skin; however, this does not appear on the mucosa. The most common histopathologic findings of a fixed drug reaction are similar to erythema multiforme, that is, interface vacuolar changes with necrotic keratinocytes and scattered eosinophils in the dermis. Histologic findings in drug eruption are usually nonspecific and are only suggestive or supportive of a drug eruption. Patch testing, indirect and direct Coombs tests, and other specific laboratory testing, as well as a detailed clinical history, are necessary to precisely diagnose such cases.[170]

Miscellaneous Inflammatory Dermatoses

A few special *dermatoses*, which are not classified into other categories in this chapter, are summarized in Table 2.5.

Plasma Cell Vulvitis (Vulvitis of Zoon)

Plasma cell vulvitis usually presents with symptoms of pruritus and burning. It is characterized by erythematous macules that usually have focal hemorrhagic areas and may appear orange in color. The

Table 2.5. Miscellaneous inflammatory dermatoses (noninfectious)

Plasma cell vulvitis
Granulomatous diseases
Sarcoidosis
Vulvitis (chelitis) granulomatosa
Crohn disease
Behçet syndrome
Pyoderma gangrenosum
Vulvar vestibulitis (Vulvar vestibular syndrome)
Fox–Fordyce disease
Fixed drug eruption (drug-induced erythema multiforme)

lesions may be multiple.[110,276] On microscopic examination the epithelium is thinned, with flattening of rete ridges and lack of a granular layer or keratinized surface. Parabasal keratinocytes have a horizontal orientation with marked spongiosis. The inflammatory infiltrate is lichenoid in type, consisting predominantly of plasma cells. Prominent dermal blood vessels are evident with associated intradermal hemorrhage and hemosiderin.[68,159] The differential diagnosis includes syphilis, because of the perivascular plasma cell infiltrate, as well as lichen planus and other chronic dermatoses. The etiology is unknown; however, local irritation and poor hygiene may be contributing factors. Perineal hygiene, supportive care, and topical and intralesional corticosteroids are the usual treatment.[276] Use of etretinate has been reported in plasma cell vulvitis.[213]

Fox–Fordyce Disease

Fox–Fordyce disease is a disorder of the apocrine glands; 90% of cases occur in women. The disease generally begins at puberty and presents as a pruritic papular eruption usually involving the axilla, vulva, and perianal regions. On microscopic examination, the center of the papule often contains a hair follicle and apocrine sweat gland duct plugged by keratin. There may be an associated rupture of the intraepithelial portion of the duct with subsequent vesicle formation within the epidermis caused by spongiosis. These vesicles can be seen when serial sections are performed.[204] Transverse histologic sections to make the diagnosis have also been reported.[236] Chronic inflammatory changes are present in the dermis, and there is dilatation of the apocrine gland acini (Fig. 2.25). In addition, there is epidermal acanthosis and spongiosis. Deposition of mucin may be found in the ducts, glands, and tissues surrounding the skin appendages. Fox–Fordyce disease is a chronic condition that may progress somewhat during pregnancy or after menopause; however, no definite therapy is known. In women of reproductive age, oral contraceptives may relieve symptoms and reduce somewhat the severity of the process. Systemic antibiotics and topical, as well as locally injected, corticosteroids and antipruritics relieve symptoms. Isotretinoin has been used in treating this condition.[165] Hidradenitis suppurativa as well as folliculitis may complicate the clinical course.

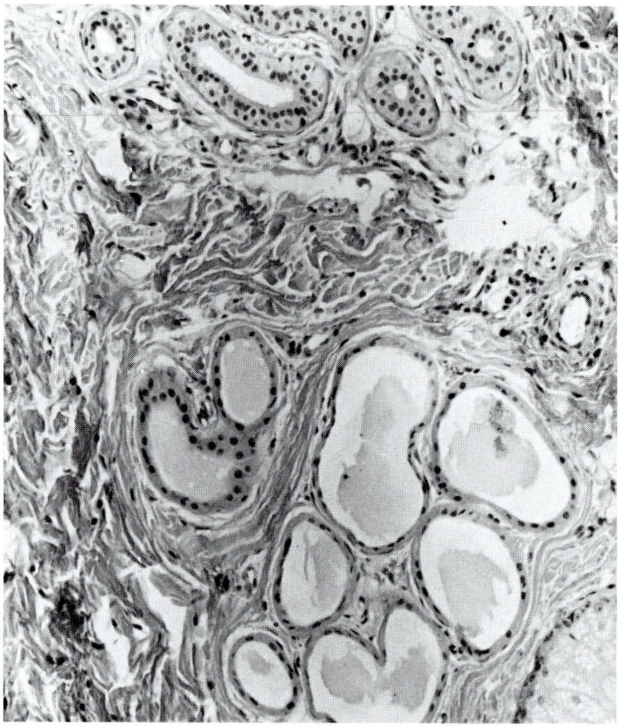

Fig. 2.25. Fox–Fordyce disease. Dilated apocrine glands show inspissated secretion.

Vulvar Vestibulitis (Vulvar Vestibular Syndrome)

General Features

Vulvar vestibulitis, which is a clinical disorder of unknown etiology, has been a subject of significant clinical controversy. As originally described, vulvar vestibulitis is associated with inflammation of the vulvar vestibule, severe vestibular tenderness to pressure, and entry dyspareunia. This condition is characterized clinically by slight edema of the hymen and redness around the gland openings in the vestibule, with marked "pinpoint" tenderness to pressure.[152,153] Bacterial, chlamydial, and viral studies from affected areas have not supported an infectious etiology.[152,158] Vulvar vestibulitis is a clinical complex that represents part of a spectrum of vulvar pain-related disorders. *Chronic candidiasis*, as well as *vulvar papillomatosis*, may be associated with dyspareunia and vulvar pain. A number of vulvar dermatoses may cause vulvar pain. In addition, there is a condition described as *essential vulvodynia* that is of unknown etiology and is a diagnosis of exclusion.[158]

Microscopic Findings

Histopathologic features include areas of mild to moderate inflammatory response, characterized by a superficial chronic inflammatory infiltrate that is composed predominantly of lymphocytes resembling female urethral syndrome.[88] Many cases also have plasma cells within the infiltrate, but leukocytes and eosinophils are rare. The stromal tissue beneath the vestibular epithelium is involved most prominently, and the inflammatory process may surround the minor vestibular glands. Inflammatory cells occasionally are found within the glandular epithelium or within the acini or ductal lumina.[201] These patients rarely have clinically or morphologically evident condyloma acuminatum or VIN.[265]

Adjunctive Methods

Studies for HPV employing PCR have not demonstrated an association with HPV.[154,265] Although there have been studies suggesting some association with normal flora or background contamination, the lack of control groups limits interpretation.[151,251]

Clinical Behavior and Therapy

The natural history of vulvar vestibulitis is poorly understood, and no long-term controlled prospective studies have been reported to date. Local excision of the vestibule has been advocated; however, the recurrence rate, with follow-up for as long as 5 years, reveals that recurrent symptoms after surgery are relatively common, occurring in more than one-half the cases in some series. Biofeedback therapy appears effective in many patients.[89] Antibiotics produce no response, nor can the symptoms be reliably alleviated by corticosteroids. Nonvaporization laser ablation of the superficial submucosal ectatic blood vessels has been proposed, especially in cases having recurrent symptoms after surgery.[152] Interferon has been advocated, with some response.[25] The administration of interferon and biofeedback training of the lower pelvic muscles are treatments used as a first choice before more aggressive treatment.[25] A low-oxalate diet has been proposed but has not been proven to be of value. More than one-half of these patients initially obtain some relief from topical therapy. Management is long term and supportive.

Vulvitis Granulomatosa (Chelitis Granulomatosa)

Vulvitis granulomatosa is of unknown etiology, related to *cheilitis granulomatosa* (Miescher–Melkersson–Rosenthal syndrome) and *Crohn's disease*.[94,95] Clinically, the labia majora are indurated, swollen, and erythematous without tenderness. The labia minora, as well as the perineum and perianal areas, also may be involved. Mild regional lymphadenopathy typically is present. The process remains localized but is slowly progressive. Histopathologic findings include dermal edema and a chronic granulomatous inflammatory infiltrate composed of histiocytes and giant cells, as well as lymphocytes and plasma cells. The infiltrate involves the dermis and extends to the epithelium. The differential diagnosis includes other granulomatous inflammatory processes.[95] Treatment of this condition is with intralesional steroids.

Factitial Vulvitis

Factitial vulvitis is an uncommon disorder that may present as a mild chronic inflammatory process, often with associated superficial ulceration.[195] The pathologic findings often are nonspecific.

Behçet Syndrome

Behçet syndrome refers to the triad of oral aphthous ulcers, genital ulcers, and ophthalmologic inflammation.[220] Ocular changes may be absent in mild cases. Other findings include acne, cutaneous nodules, thrombophlebitis, encephalopathy, and colitis.[220] Behçet syndrome causes deep ulcerations on the vulva that may result in fenestration of the labia and lead to gangrene of the labia. The ulcerations characteristically heal and relapse, and are associated with simultaneous oral ulcers. Histologically, necrotizing arteritis frequently is seen and can be considered a cardinal pathologic finding. A chronic inflammatory infiltrate may be perivascular or involve the vessel wall with homogenization of the arterial media.[68] Endothelial cell swelling also occurs and may result in arteriolar occlusion as well as venous thrombosis.

Crohn's Disease

Crohn's disease is a chronic noncaseating granulomatous disease of unknown etiology that can involve, besides the gastrointestinal tract, the vulva and perineum in adults and children.[249,260] Cutaneous ulcerations occur in areas where there is close apposition of skin, such as the vulva and inframammary areas. When Crohn's disease involves the vulva, the resulting ulcers often are slit shaped, multiple, deep, and secondarily infected. Vulvar and perianal erythema, induration, or ulceration may be the presenting signs.[188,260] Involvement of the colon, rectum, or small bowel is not always present when the vulva is involved. Perianal fistulas, as well as fistulas to other sites in the female genital tract, are complications. When perianal draining sinuses and abscesses occur, they often drain fluid resembling small bowel contents.

Microscopically, the disease is characterized by a noncaseating granulomatous inflammation within the dermis, which usually is deep and associated with fissures and sinus tracts. Studies for acid-fast bacteria and fungi are negative. A marked granulation tissue response frequently is seen surrounding the ulcers, but significant lymphadenitis is rare.[68]

Pyoderma Gangrenosum

Pyoderma gangrenosum is a progressive necrotic and ulcerative condition of the skin, of uncertain etiology. Most case reports of pyoderma gangrenosum occur on the legs and are associated with idiopathic bowel disease such as chronic ulcerative colitis. Other associations include hematologic malignancy, connective tissue disease, and liver disease. Pyoderma gangrenosum of the vulva may present some time after treatment for colitis, ileostomy, or abdominal perineal resection of the colon and rectum.

The microscopic findings reveal epithelial ulceration with severe acute and chronic inflammation. If the biopsy is from the ulcer edge, the sharply demarcated ulcer is adjacent to hyperplastic squamous epithelium. Organisms are not identified within the inflammatory process. Systemic corticosteroid therapy with aggressive local excision, followed by skin grafting, may be necessary in addition to the treatment of the underlying disease.[197]

Necrotizing Fasciitis (Includes Synergistic Bacterial Infection)

Postoperative, posttraumatic, or *necrotizing fasciitis* is a life-threatening condition that usually is secondary to a polymicrobial infection after episiotomy or other types of vaginal, vulvar, or abdominal surgery.[14,238] Diabetes mellitus, arteriosclerosis, obesity, hypertension, and prior irradiation predispose to necrotizing fasciitis.[3] The clinical presentation is that of a rapidly progressing inflammatory process that may initially appear as mild cellulitis or edema with inflammation. Delay in diagnosis without therapy carries a nearly 50% mortality. Prompt radical excision of the infected tissue and broad-spectrum systemic antibiotic therapy offers the only chance of cure.[238]

Hidradenitis Suppurativa

Hidradenitis suppurativa is a chronic inflammatory disorder of the apocrine glands.[92] Deep-seated, painful, subcutaneous nodules are found in areas containing apocrine glands, especially the axilla and vulva. The lesions commonly progress subcutaneously, producing confluent masses that subsequently ulcerate the epidermis and result in draining sinuses and extensive scarring. The condition may coexist with Fox–Fordyce disease. Total excision of involved areas may be necessary in advanced cases, although laser ablation and unroofing the sinuses has been reported to be as effective.[230] Long-term isotretinoin therapy also has been reported to be effective in some cases.[106] Histologically, in the early stage hidradenitis suppurativa demonstrates a perifolliculitis with an acute and chronic inflammatory infiltrate within the dermis. The later stages of the disease result in destruction of the epithelial appendages with sinus tract formation[68] (Fig. 2.26).

Mites and Lice

A variety of mites are capable of producing local and limited chronic skin infections of the perineal area, including scabies.[44,168] Mites must be specifically considered, because definitive diagnosis sometimes is difficult.[44] Mites are small arachnids and belong to the order Acarina; they differ from lice, which are insects. Mites have a fused head and thorax, devoid of primary segmentation, and four pairs of legs. Mites burrow within the subcorneal area of the epidermis, inducing severe pruritus. The overt skin lesions are papular and, when examined under a magnifying lens, reveal an adjacent burrow. Scrapings from the burrow or specimens obtained from the patient's clothing can be fixed in an alcohol-ether-acetic acid-formalin mixture and analyzed microscopically for mites, eggs, and fecal material. Lice are associated with irritation of the skin from secondary infection of feeding sites. The pubic louse, *Phthirius pubis*, class Insecta, is the usual offender and can be diagnosed by identifying the louse and nits on the hair shaft.

Spider Bite

A brown recluse (*Loxosceles reclusa*) spider bite on the vulva has been reported, associated with ulceration and infection of the vulva. Although secondary protracted infection may occur with such ulcers,

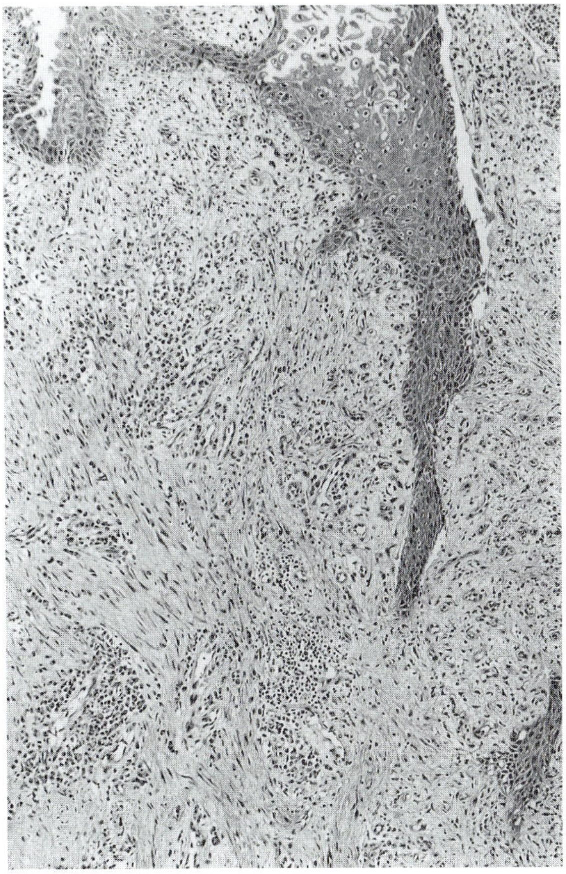

Fig. 2.26. Hidradenitis suppurativa. There is a severe acute and chronic inflammatory cell infiltrate within the dermis with involvement and destruction of the skin appendages. (Courtesy of N. Sisson Hardt, M.D., Gainesville, FL.)

slow and progressive healing over several months is the usual clinical course.[147]

Bullous Diseases

Although virtually any dermatologic disease can involve the vulva, the following *bullous diseases* bear discussion, as they may first be observed and biopsied by the gynecologist. Definitive diagnosis of most bullous diseases requires clinical and pathologic correlation, and in some cases the clinical findings are essential in distinguishing these cutaneous diseases that otherwise have very similar or identical histopathologic findings. Some of the bullous diseases have immunologic components, and others are nonspecific (Table 2.6). The key histopathologic features and differential diagnosis of bullous and bullous-like diseases are summarized in Table 2.7.

Pemphigus (Pemphigus Vulgaris)

Pemphigus vulgaris initially may present on the vulva as recurrent superficial ulcers and erosions. Associated oral lesions usually are present in these patients, and rectal and vaginal lesions may occur.[16,195] The disease was life threatening before the era of steroid treatment. Biopsy of a fresh vulvar vesicle usually is diagnostic. Microscopic findings include acantholysis with suprabasal vesicle formation and eosinophils in the vesicular fluid and superficial dermis (Fig. 2.27). Direct immunofluorescent studies of perilesional skin demonstrate IgG deposited at the epidermal intercellular junctions. Circulating antibodies to epidermal intercellular spaces can be detected with indirect immunofluorescent method against monkey esophageal epithelium; the titer correlates with the clinical activity of the disease. Therapy includes high systemic doses of corticosteroids and cytotoxic agents, plasma pheresis, and supportive measures.[29,93,234]

Pemphigus Vegitans

This rare variant of pemphigus may present as a localized, indurated, inflamed area with vesicles. The pathologic as well as immunofluorescent and immunologic findings are similar to pemphigus vulgaris, although intraepidermal eosinophilic abscesses and verrucous epidermal hyperplasia are prominent.[195,272] The presence of eosinophils, as well as the localized and self-limited character of the disease, distinguish it from pemphigus vulgaris.

Table 2.6. Noninfectious bullous dermatoses

Immunobullous dermatoses	*Nonimmunobullous dermatoses*
Bullous pemphigoid	Benign familial pemphigus (Hailey–Hailey)
Cicatricial pemphigoid	Darier disease (keratosis follicularis)
Pemphigus	Erythema multiforme
Dermatitis herpetiformes	Lichen planus and lichenoid vaginitis
Linear IgA dermatosis	Lichen sclerosus
Herpes gestationis	Pruritus, urticaria, papules and plaques of pregnancy (PUPPP)
Bullous lupus erythematosus	

Table 2.7. Differential diagnosis of vesticular bullous and bullous-like diseases of the vulva

	Location of vesicle				
Disease	*Subepidermal*	*Intraepidermal suprabasal*	*Acantholysis of suprabasal cells*	*Significant systemic manifestations*	*Immunofluorescent localization*
Pemphigus vulgaris	No	Yes	Yes	Yes	IgG Intercellular
Pemphigus vegitans	No	Yes	Yes	No	IgG Intercellular
Pemphigoid (bullous) (cicatricial pemphigoid)	Yes	No	No	Yes, localized scarring (sometimes debilitating)	IgG linear along basement membrane IgA, IgM, C_3, C_5 may be in basement membrane
Herpes gestationis	Yes	No	No	Yes	C_3 Linear along basement membrane. IgG may also be present. IgM, IgA is rare
Polymorphic eruption of pregnancy, pruritic urticarial plaques and papules in pregnancy (PUPPP)	Yes	No	No	Yes	Negative
Darier disease	No	Yes	Yes, 3+ dyskeratosis	Yes	Negative
Warty dyskeratoma	No	Yes	Yes	No	Negative
Erythema multiforme (Stevens–Johnson syndrome)	No	Yes, necrotic keratinocytes, Hydropic degeneration of basal keratinocytes	No	Yes	IgM Complement in and about superficial dermal vessels in some cases
Hailey–Hailey	No	Yes	Yes, 4+ No dyskeratosis	No	Negative
Localized acantholytic disease of the vulva	No	Yes	Yes	No	Negative
Benign chronic bullous disease of childhood (linear IgA disease)	Yes	No	Microabscesses in dermal papillae	No, flu-like symptoms may precede presentation	IgA linear along basement membrane (C_3, IgA, IgG, IgM also may be present)
Dermatitis herpetiformis	Yes	No	No	No, severe pruritus in some cases	IgA deposits in the tips of dermal papillae and/or along the basement membrane

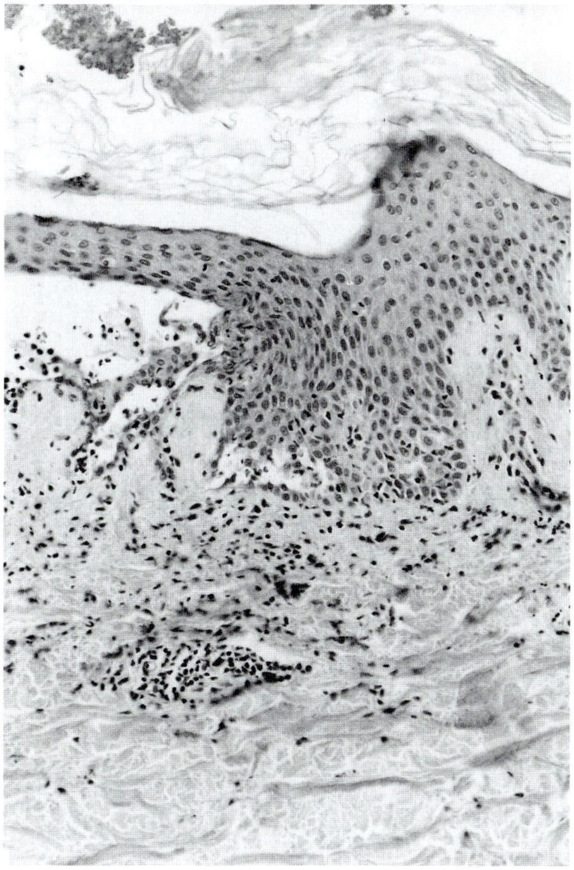

Fig. 2.27. Pemphigus (pemphigus vulgaris). Suprabasal vesicle formation is evident with prominent acantholysis. A small suprabasal acantholytic area is present in the rete, adjacent to the larger vesicle.

Pemphigoid (Bullous Pemphigoid)

Pemphigoid can involve the vulva and is characterized by moist, tender ulcers that involve the labia minora, majora, and perianal areas. At times, fluid-filled tense bullae also are present. Biopsies of fresh ulcers, including normal adjacent skin, typically show the characteristic subepidermal bullae (see Table 2.7). In advanced stages, biopsy of ulcerated areas may show only granulation tissue.[128]

Cicatricial pemphigoid, unlike *bullous pemphigoid*, results in scarring and stenosis. Both bullous pemphigoid and cicatricial pemphigoid can be the result of a drug hypersensitivity reaction.[257] The disease presents as erosions, erythema, and small blisters of the vulva, perianal, and anal mucosa associated with chronic burning pain and painful ulcers. The origin of the recurrent scarring of the vulva may not be apparent until the presentation of ocular involvement secondary to cicatricial pemphigoid.[80] Severe cicatrization with shrinkage, suggesting advanced vulvar lichen sclerosus or lichen planus, characterizes the process. In contrast to lichen sclerosus or lichen planus, cicatricial pemphigoid is associated with small blisters and a positive Nikolsky phenomenon (slippage and detachment of the superficial epidermis from the underlying dermis when the examining finger is slid over the skin surface).

Microscopically, there is subepidermal blister formation with a mixed inflammatory cell infiltrate within the dermis (Fig. 2.28). Eosinophils are prominent. Direct immunofluorescence demonstrates linear IgG, and complement C3, along the basement membrane. Immunoglobulins IgA and IgM may or may not be present.[82,128] Systemic corticosteroids and immunosuppressive drugs may be of value.[93,129] If the condition is drug related, the offending medication should be discontinued.

Herpes Gestationis

This vesiculobullous disease is unique to pregnant women, with an estimated incidence of approximately 0.6 per 100,000 pregnancies. Patients have a strong association with HLA-DR3 and -DR4. Presenting signs and symptoms often are severe pruritus and a macular erythematous rash that leads to blistering and superficial ulcerations. The lesions may involve the vulva and pubic area in addition to the trunk and upper thigh. The process usually presents in the second trimester, and spontaneous regression follows soon after delivery, although regression may occur in the late third trimester.

Histopathologic findings include a subepidermal blister that may contain eosinophils, neutrophils, lymphocytes, and histiocytes. There is a perivascular superficial dermal inflammatory infiltrate that also is rich in lymphocytes and eosinophils. Immunofluorescent studies demonstrate C3 as a linear basement membrane deposit. Serologic studies demonstrate circulating complement-fixing IgG antibodies in 25% of the cases. The antibodies bind to 180-kDa hemidesmosome antigen (BPAg2).[231] The main differential diagnosis is bullous pemphigoid, which is usually not associated with pregnancy. Prurigo of pregnancy, pruritic folliculitis of pregnancy, and polymorphic eruption of pregnancy may be included in the differential of dermatosis associated with pregnancy, but these are not bullous diseases, and the immunofluorescent studies are negative.[159]

Darier Disease (Keratosis Follicularis)

Darier disease is inherited as an autosomal dominant trait with the gene locus mapped to chromosome 12q, although spontaneous cases also may oc-

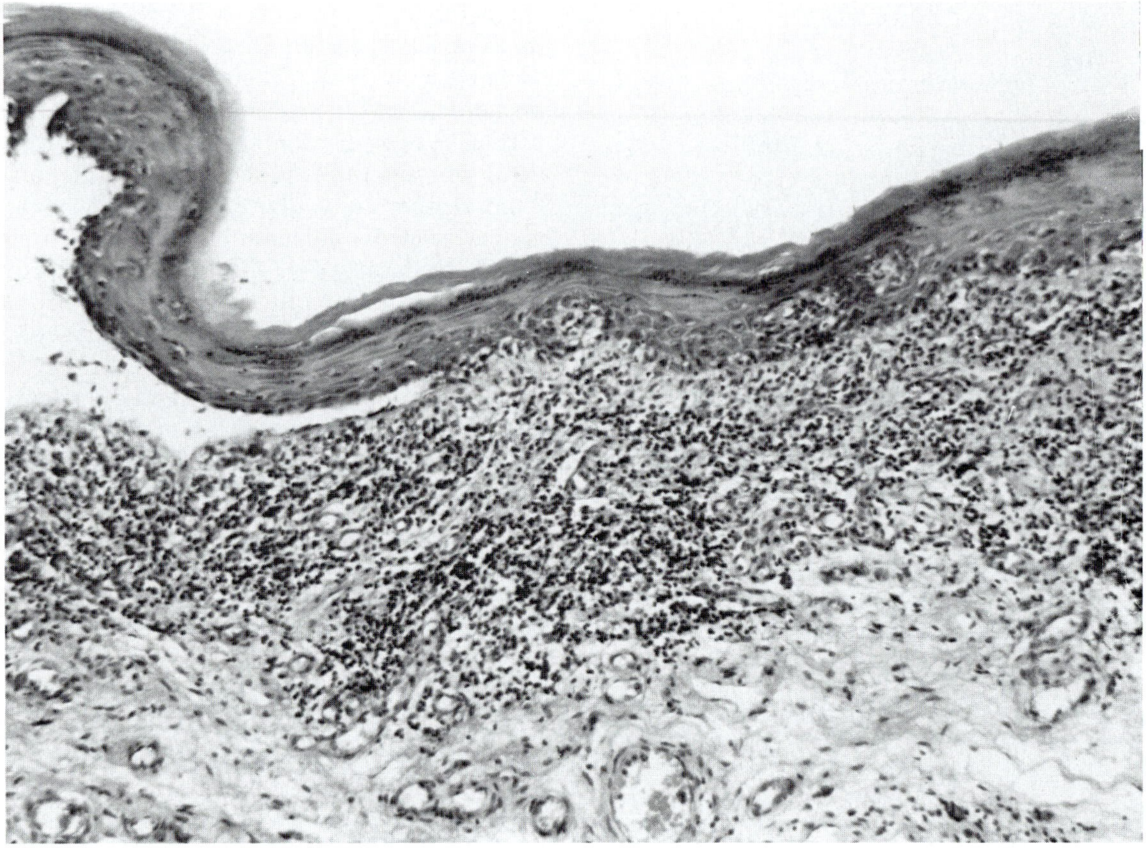

Fig. 2.28. Bullous pemphigoid. A subepidermal bulla is evident, with intact epithelium separated from the underlying dermis. An intense inflammatory infiltrate of lymphocytes, neutrophils, and -eosinophils is seen within the dermis with some inflammatory cells within the bulla.

cur. Patients present anytime after late childhood. The disease has a seborrheic distribution and frequently involves the vulva. Although it usually is not considered a bullous disease, it is listed herein because microscopic intraepidermal acantholysis is a common observation. On clinical examination, the lesions are crusted, hyperkeratotic papules that often appear darker than the surrounding skin. The papules may be secondarily infected.[68,209]

Histologically, acantholysis of the suprabasal epithelial cells results in clefts that extend from the basal layer through the granular layer. Acantholytic cells are seen within the clefts. Corps ronds and nuclear grains can be found in the granular layer along microscopic findings with individual dyskeratotic cells. Hyperkeratosis, acanthosis, and papillomatosis are seen along with keratotic plugs. Rarely, epithelial basal cell budding into the adjacent dermis may be seen. The inflammatory cell infiltration within the dermis usually is minimal, unless the lesions are secondarily infected.[68] The main differential diagnosis is warty dyskeratoma, Hailey–Hailey disease, and localized acantholytic disease of the vulva (see Table 2.7).

Warty Dyskeratoma

Warty dyskeratoma of the vulva typically presents with a histologic picture essentially identical to that of Darier disease. Unlike Darier disease, which is multifocal and may involve the trunk and extremities as well as the face, warty dyskeratoma typically involves the head, neck, or vulva as a solitary lesion. Histologically, warty dyskeratoma has more prominent villous-like projections into the acantholytic space (Fig. 2.29). Other distinguishing clinical features are that Darier disease usually is congenital, and is carried as an autosomal dominant, whereas warty dyskeratoma is not (see Table 2.7).[54]

Erythema Multiforme (Stevens–Johnson Syndrome)

Vulvar involvement has been reported in association with *Stevens–Johnson syndrome*, which is the severe form of *erythema multiforme*. Involvement of the mouth, eyes, and skin, with associated high fever and other systemic symptoms, characterizes the syndrome. The most common cause of the Stevens–

Johnson syndrome is drug therapy. Herpesvirus infection is typically associated with a recurrent minor form of erythema multiforme in which the recurrence may be prevented by prophylactic use of systemic antiviral therapy (e.g., Veltrax). Other causes include mycoplasma infection, malignancy, or radiotherapy.[219]

The histopathologic features are complex, depending on the age of the lesion. Major features include interface vacuolar dermatitis with necrotic keratinocytes and intraepithelial vesicle formation. Separation of the epithelium from the dermis is associated with hydropic degeneration of the basal keratinocytes (see Table 2.7). Within the dermis, there is a prominent chronic inflammatory infiltrate consisting of lymphocytes and histiocytes. Extravasated red blood cells may be present within the dermal inflammatory process, as well as within the epidermis. Nonspecific intravascular complement C3 and IgM deposits may be seen within the superficial dermal vessels by immunofluorescent staining.[159] There are case reports of "introital adenosis" occurring 1–3 years after the diagnosis of Stevens–Johnson syndrome, characterized clinically by erosions within the vulvar vestibule and medial aspects of the labia minora. On histopathologic examination, glandular epithelium has been identified within these areas, associated with submucosal inflammation.[23,155] The epithelium was described in one case as columnar epithelium of tuboendometrial type, having secretory and ciliated-type cells.[155] The term mucinous metaplasia of the vulva has been used to describe these changes, which is consistent with columnar cell metaplasia.[50,61]

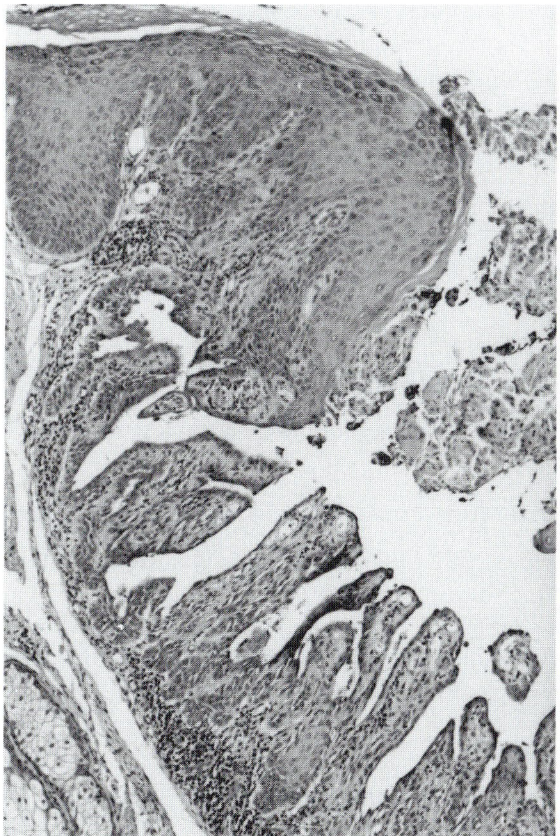

Fig. 2.29. Warty dyskeratoma. Acantholysis of the suprabasal epithelial cells, with intraepithelial clefts extending from the basal layer through the granular layer. Acantholytic dyskeratotic cells are within the clefts and at the surface. A single basal layer is attached to the villous projection of the elongated papillary dermis. (Courtesy of David Dolson, M.D., Tallahassee, FL)

Hailey–Hailey Disease (Familial Benign Pemphigus)

Hailey–Hailey disease is inherited as an autosomal dominant trait with the gene locus mapped to chromosome 3q; approximately one-third of patients, however, have no family history of the disease. Onset of the disease often occurs during adolescence. Intertriginous areas usually are involved, but several cases in which the lesions are confined exclusively to the vulva have been reported.[263] The usual clinical presentation is recurrent clusters of vesicles that develop, rupture, and result in crusted, moist papules that later coalesce to form plaques.

Histologically, there is acantholysis with resultant suprabasalar lacunae. Acantholytic cells that maintain their nuclear details remain attached to each other in the acantholytic space, giving a dilapidated brick-wall appearance. The acantholysis is more marked than in Darier disease (Fig 2.30).[68] Basal cells maintain their orientation to the basement membrane. Rarely, corps ronds are seen in the granular layer. In contrast to Darier disease there is minimal, if any, dyskeratosis in Hailey–Hailey disease. Strands of epidermal cells may proliferate into the dermis, but little dermal inflammatory infiltrate exists unless secondary infection is present. Table 2.7 summarizes the major distinguishing features of Darier disease, Hailey–Hailey disease (familial benign pemphigus), pemphigus vulgaris, pemphigus vegetans, and warty dyskeratoma. Recently, squamous cell carcinoma arising in Hailey–Hailey disease of the vulva has been reported.[48]

Benign Chronic Bullous Disease of Childhood (Linear IgA Disease)

This disease commonly involves the lower abdominal, pelvic, inguinal, and genital areas, presenting as clusters of annular lesions or "clusters of jewels"

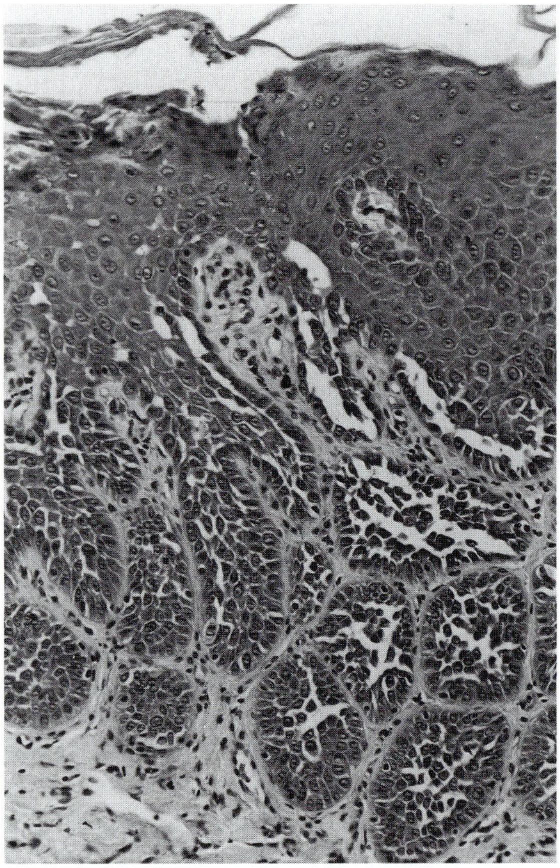

Fig. 2.30. Hailey–Hailey disease (benign familial pemphigus). Acantholysis is present in the suprabasal area and lower dermis. The mid- and upper epidermis remains intact, although some acantholysis is present.

that usually are pruritic and typically evolve over the course of 24 hours. The annular lesions evolve to tense bullae that, if ruptured, ulcerate and become crusted. Patients may have fever and anorexia. In some cases the eruption is proceeded by a bacterial or viral infection,[64,270] and other cases are drug induced, vancomycin being one of the more common offenders.[122] Because of the location and abrupt appearance of the lesions, they may be mistaken for evidence of child abuse. Biopsy of an early bullous lesion reveals subepithelial vesicles that contain predominantly neutrophils within the vesicular fluid. Microabscesses may occur within the epidermis. The diagnostic finding is the identification of a linear deposition of IgA in the basement membrane (see Table 2.7). Other immunoglobulins and complement C3 also may be found.[68] The antigen of the linear IgA disease is a 97-kDa molecule, which is identical to the carboxyl terminal of 180-kDa (BPAg2), located at the basement membrane.[103] The differential diagnosis includes dermatitis herpetiformis and bullous pemphigoid. Dermatitis herpetiformis is distinguished by having granular IgA at the dermal papillae, whereas bullous pemphigoid has linear IgG basement membrane deposits.[68] Therapy includes systemic antiinflammatory drugs including dapsone, colchicine, and intravenous immunoglobulin therapy.[5,120,200]

Depigmentation and Hypopigmented Disorders

In adult women, the vulvar skin, especially that of the perineal body and lateral labia majora, usually is more pigmented than is the general body surface. Biopsies of the normal vulva show dendritic melanocytes scattered along the basal layer of the epithelium as well as squamous keratinocytes containing variable concentrations of melanin granules. Areas of the vulvar skin that appear hypopigmented therefore are clinically remarkable. Three basic conditions result in vulvar hypopigmentation: vitiligo, albinism, and postinflammatory depigmentation (leukoderma).

Vitiligo

Vitiligo is an inherited disorder in which the melanocytes are lost from areas of skin that were previously normally pigmented. This condition frequently affects the vulva, and biopsies from vitiliginous areas show a remarkable absence of both basilar melanocytes and melanin granules. A Fontana stain for melanin pigment in the basal keratinocytes can be used to support the diagnosis.[68]

Albinism

Albinism, an inherited genetic disorder, is characterized by an inability of the melanocytes to produce pigment. There is an absence of melanin granules in the keratinocytes. Large pale cells may be present within the basal layer, representing incompetent melanocytes.

Postinflammatory Depigmentation (Leukoderma)

In areas of previous ulceration, recently healed skin will temporarily lack a normal population of melanocytes, a condition referred to as *postinflammatory depigmentation*, or *leukoderma*. This disorder is common after herpes infection, syphilitic ulceration, burns, and deep laser or cryotherapy. Histologically, the skin appears thinned, metabolically active, and lacks the usual amount of pigment. On careful microscopic inspection, some melanin usually is evident.

Pigment Disorders of Melanocytic Origin and Nevi

In a prospective study of 301 women, 37 (12%) were found to have a pigmented lesion of the vulva. All these women were white, and only 26% of the patients were aware that they had a pigmented lesion. More than 50% of the pigmented lesions were lengito simplex (lengitines); 7 patients had nevi, of which 1 had the histologic features of a dysplastic nevus, 5 patients had postinflammatory hyperpigmentation, 2 cases represented hemangiomas, and 1 patient had a pigmented lesion that proved to be VIN with ulceration.[214]

Lentigo Simplex

The most common hyperpigmented lesion occurring on the vulva is *lentigo simplex* (*lentigines*), which may occur on the mucous membranes as well as the skin. The lesion is typically small, 4 mm or less in diameter, flat, and uniformly pigmented. Clinically, lentigines closely resemble junctional nevi and, therefore, are frequently biopsied. Except for the rare leopard syndrome, in which thousands of lentigines are present all over the body, lentigo simplex is essentially devoid of clinical significance. In contrast to lentigo simplex, solar lentigines usually are seen on sun-exposed areas only.[12]

Histologically, lentigo simplex is a localized circumscribed area of slightly hyperplastic epidermis that contains an increased number of normal-appearing melanocytes along the side and tips of the elongated rete ridges associated with basilar hyperpigmentation. Extreme degrees of epidermal pigmentation may be present, with numerous squamous cells exhibiting cytoplasmic melanin granules, usually in highest concentration near the epithelial–stromal junction (Fig. 2.31). There may be mild acanthosis and slight clubbing of the rete ridges, and heavily pigmented melanophages may be present in the upper dermis. At times, a minimal superficial dermal inflammatory cell infiltrate is noted, but this is by no means constant.

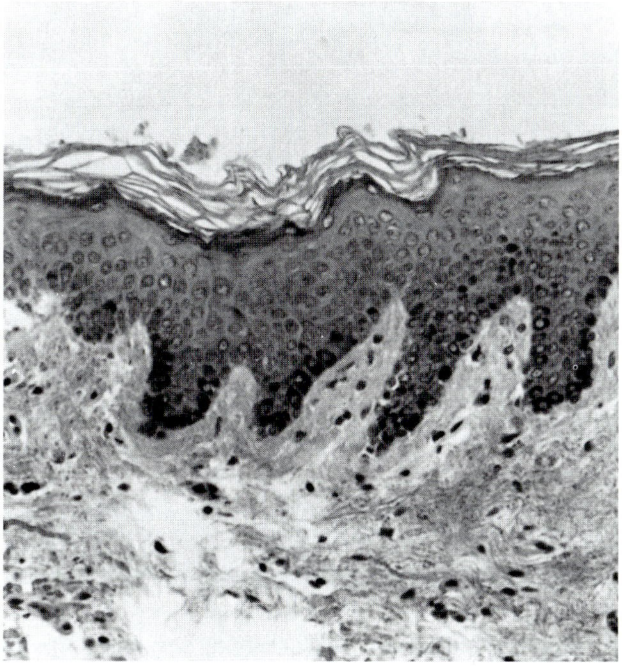

Fig. 2.31. Lentigo simplex. Note the heavy concentration of deeply pigmented basalar keratinocytes at the tips of the accentuated rete ridges. Increased solitary melanocytes along the site of the retes are present.

Vulvar Melanosis

Vulvar melanosis is characterized by prominent brown to black pigmented macular areas with irregular borders that may be solitary or multiple, located on the labia minora or labia majora as well as on the vaginal introitus and perineum. The pigmented areas vary in size and may cover much of the vulva skin. Vulvar melanosis typically occurs in women of reproductive age and is more common on the squamous mucosa portion of the vulva.[72,218]

The microscopic findings are essentially similar to lentigo simplex, with intense basilar keratinocytic hyperpigmentation, although epithelial hyperplasia usually is not seen. The lesions typically are larger than those of lentigo, which characteristically are not more than 4 mm in diameter. The pigmentation may be intense within the basal layer with slight or no increase in the number of melanocytes. The melanocytes are typically arranged in single solitary units within the dermal–epidermal junction.[72,218]

Congenital and Giant Nevomelanocytic Nevi

Congenital nevi are found in approximately 10% of newborns and usually are less than 4 mm in diameter. *Giant nevomelanocytic nevi* (20 cm or more in diameter) (garment type), although rare, carry an increased risk of developing malignant melanoma in prepubertal individuals.

Junctional, Compound, and Intradermal Nevi

Vulvar melanocytic nevi may be junctional, compound, or intradermal. These nevomelanocytic types occur on the vulva with nearly equal distribution.[45] Clinically they usually are well defined, papular, uniformly pigmented, and typically less than 10 mm in diameter.[214] Nevus cells are somewhat larger than melanocytes and have round or ovoid nuclei. Dendrites are not present, and intercellular connections are not visible. The cells may lie singly within the dermis, but more commonly they tend to form nests. Unless they contain melanin, their cytoplasm is clear without granules or fibrils.

In pure junctional nevi, which are identified relatively infrequently on the vulva, the nevus cells are located within the epidermis and at the dermal–epidermal junction. Individual cells, or cell nests, bulge downward from the tips of the rete ridges. There is no connective tissue noted between the nevus cells and the adjacent squamous keratinocytes. Such nevi are young and somewhat undifferentiated.

With age, the nevus becomes a compound nevus with melanocytes located in the epidermis and the dermis (Fig. 2.32). The basement membrane of the epidermis surrounding the nests disappears, and collagen and elastic fibers envelop the nests, pushing the epidermis upward. During this process, the lesion is clinically elevated above the level of the surrounding skin. Further differentiation results in complete enclosure of the nevus cells and nests by connective tissue elements such that they are entirely intradermal; no activity is seen at the dermoepidermal junction. These nevi are referred to as intradermal. Most nevi biopsied on the vulva are either compound or intradermal in type. With time, nevi may regress completely or may result in a fibrous papule or acrochordon.[193]

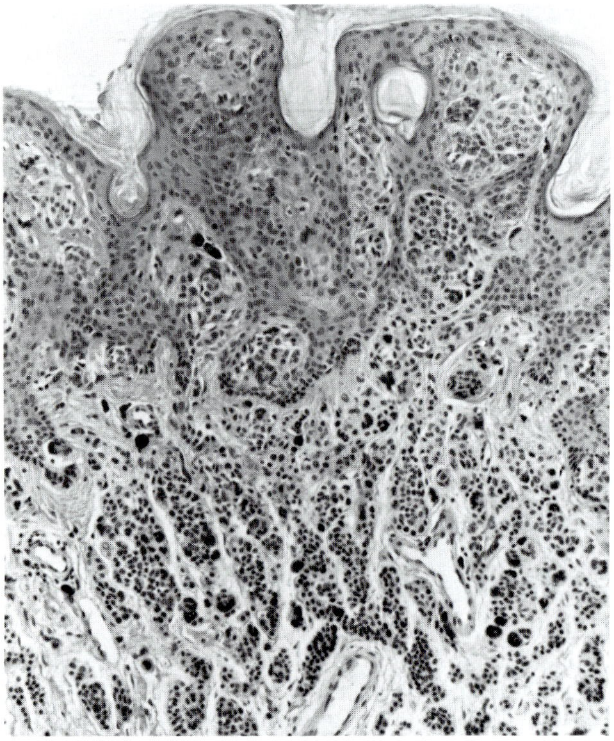

Fig. 2.32. Compound nevus. Nests of nevus cells are evident within the epithelium as well as within the dermis.

Atypical Vulvar Nevi

The so-called *atypical vulvar nevus* has many clinical and histopathologic features in common with acquired dysplastic nevi. The atypical vulvar nevus occurs in young women ranging from 20 to 30 years of age. Although not considered specifically as dysplastic by some authors, or associated with dysplastic nevi in other sites, the atypical vulvar nevus demonstrates prominent variable-sized junctional melanocytic nests. Because of their intertrigenous location, vulvar nevi are subjected to chronic irritation and rubbing, and therefore some of the atypicality is probably reactive. Although some features may suggest a diagnosis of melanoma, the lesion is small, well circumscribed, and lacks pagetoid spread, necrosis, or mitotic activity in the dermis[2,47] (Fig. 2.33).

Dysplastic Nevi

Dysplastic melanocytic nevi are seen most often in young women of reproductive age. Rare on the vulva, they present as pigmented, elevated lesions greater than 0.5 cm in diameter with irregular borders. Microscopic examination reveals large epithelioid or spindle-shaped nevus cells with nuclear pleomorphism and prominent nucleoli. The nevus cells are clustered in intraepithelial nests and are present in skin appendages, including hair shafts and the ducts of sweat glands.[2,47,193] They often have a low-power microscopic appearance of a large junctional nevus, with a dermal component that has spindle- or epithelioid-type nevus cells in nests or isolated within the papillary and reticular dermis. Three features distinguish a dysplastic nevus from melanoma. (1) Symmetric growth, which is evident on microscopic examination of a full cross section of the nevus, can be determined by visualizing a line drawn perpendicular to the surface of the center of the nevus. The halves should be mirror images of each other. (2) The most atypical cells are present in the superficial levels of the nevus, with smaller and more uniform cells in the deeper areas. (3) Rare pagetoid spread of single melanocytes with little or no involvement of the upper one-third of the epithelium is seen and is usually present at the center of the lesion.[2,47,193,207] In addition to malignant melanoma, a lesion of the dysplastic nevus syndrome should be included in the differential diagnosis. Individuals with dysplastic nevus syndrome have multiple large nevi, usually more than 0.5 cm in diameter, which may be found on the vulva and on the trunk and extremities. Individuals with dysplastic nevus syndrome have a high risk of subsequent malignant melanoma, whereas women with isolated atypical nevi of the vulva do not. Vulvar nevi are influenced by hormonal changes. They appear more active or atypical during pregnancy. Quite a few nevi are removed during pregnancy or at the time of the delivery because of the changes in color or size induced by pregnancy.

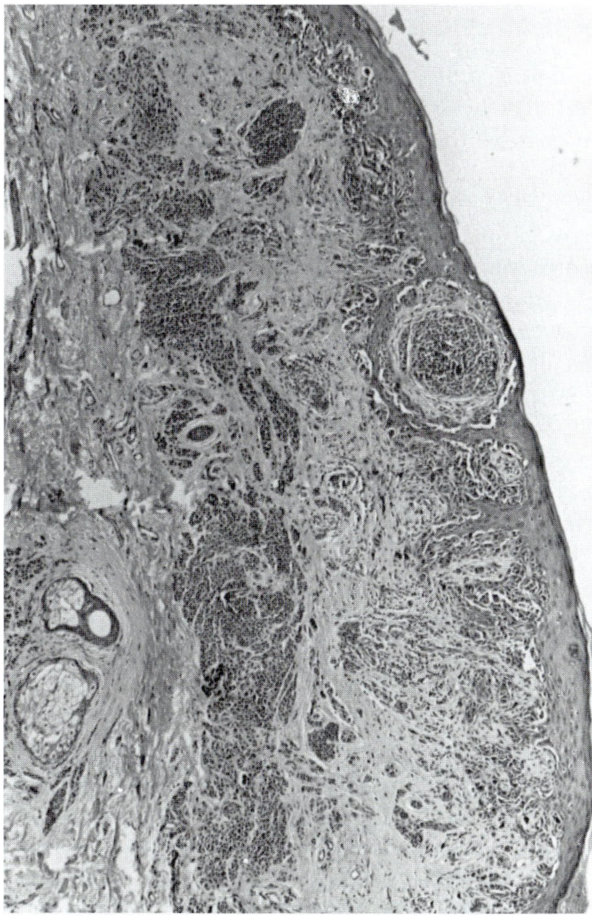

Fig. 2.33. Atypical vulvar nevus. This acquired atypical nevus has marked variation in size and shape of the nests at the dermal epidermal junction with cytologic atypia characterized by scattered hyperchromasia at this power. In the superficial and junctional areas with small, benign-appearing nevus cells within the dermis. (Courtesy of K.K. Pierson, M.D., Gainesville, FL.)

Acanthosis Nigricans and Pseudoacanthosis Nigricans

Acanthosis nigricans has been reported involving the vulva, although other sites where skin folds are found, including the axilla and submammary area, are more commonly involved. The clinical presentation is a diffuse, velvet-like, brown to gray-black skin change that is characteristically symmetric and may involve all the keratinized epithelium of the vulva, including the inguinal gluteal folds as well as the medial aspects of the upper thighs. Within the vulva, the pigmentation usually involves the labia majora and lateral labia minora as well as the pubis.[159] In adults, acanthosis nigricans may be associated with adenocarcinoma of the stomach or other visceral malignancies. Its presentation should prompt the search for gastric and other tumors, especially if it occurs with sudden onset and is associated with pruritis and the appearance of multiple seborrheic keratosis (Leser–Trelet syndrome).[133]

A second variant of this type of skin change recognized in adults is *pseudoacanthosis nigricans*. This lesion has been reported in obese individuals as well as those with autoimmune or endocrine disorders or lipodystrophy.

A third variant of acanthosis nigricans occurs in children. It is not associated with any of the disorders described in adult variants.[224] The microscopic features are characterized by prominent papillomatosis with acanthosis and hyperkeratosis. Keratinous horn cysts may be seen within the epidermis. Increased melanin typically is seen within the basal layer. No significant inflammation or distinctive dermal changes are found.

Cysts

Bartholin Cyst and Abscess

The Bartholin ducts are prone to obstruction at their vestibular orifice. Such obstruction results in subsequent accumulation of secretion with associated cystic dilatation of the duct.[192,221] The content of an uninfected *Bartholin cyst* is a mucoid, clear, translucent

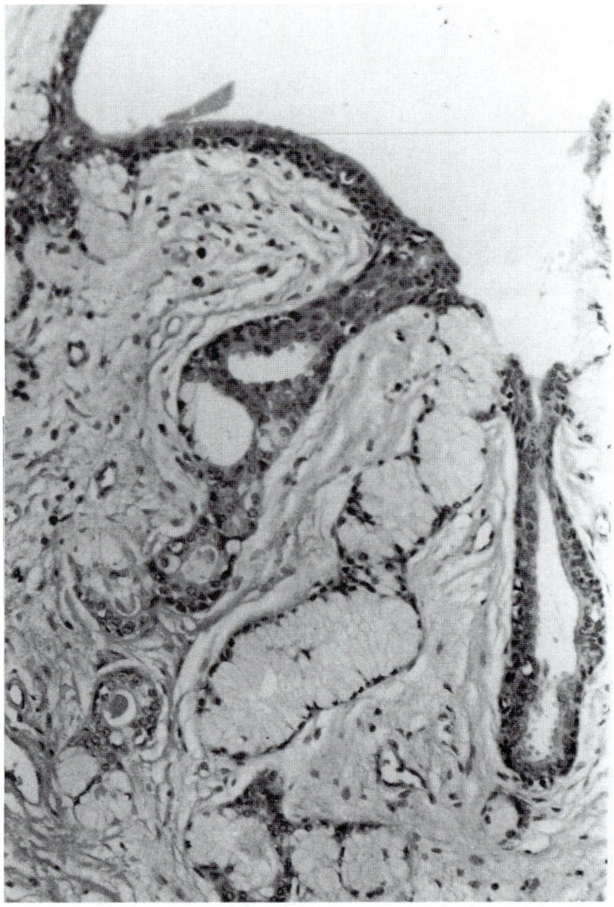

Fig. 2.34. Bartholin cyst. The dilated duct has a flattened transitional epithelial lining. The adjacent tissue has a few scattered inflammatory cells. Bartholin glandular elements are adjacent to the cyst.

liquid that, when cultured, fails to grow bacteria. The secretion stains with mucicarmine, PAS before and after diastase digestion, and Alcian blue at pH 2.5, consistent with sialomucin. The epithelium lining the cyst may be squamous, transitional, or low cuboidal mucinous epithelium. In some cases it is flattened and otherwise not classifiable (Fig. 2.34). Generally, there is minimal, if any, inflammatory response within the adjacent tissue. The epithelium of the cyst is immunoreactive for carcinoembryonic antigen (CEA). Bartholin cysts may be recurrent, and occasionally are associated with primary infection of the Bartholin gland, in which case they require marsupialization. In postmenopausal women, recurrent cysts or a palpable mass after cyst drainage may require excision of the gland because of the possibility of associated carcinoma of the Bartholin gland (see Chapter 3, Premalignant and Malignant Tumors of the Vulva). Bartholin adenocarcinomas, when present, tend to be in the tissues adjacent to the cyst wall.

Bartholin abscess is an acute process often associated with *Neisseria* gonorrheal infection, although it may be related to *Staphylococcus* or to other anaerobic organisms. The patient presents with tenderness and swelling in the Bartholin gland area. Microscopically, the Bartholin duct abscess demonstrates a striking acute inflammatory reaction within the stroma surrounding the duct. A purulent exudate is present within the lumen of the abscess wall. Excision, drainage, and antibiotics are the treatments of choice. Occasionally, the infection subsides without abscess formation or becomes chronic. Bartholin duct cysts, resulting from distal obstruction of the duct secondary to chronic inflammation and scarring, may be a late sequela of chronic infection. Mucocele-like changes have been reported in the Bartholin glands.

Keratinous Cyst (Epithelial Inclusion Cyst)

Keratinous cysts frequently are seen on the vulva; generally, these are located on the labia majora and may involve the clitoris. Typically, they are superficial and range in size from 2 to 5 mm, but may be larger. They may occur at any age, including in newborns. Milium, a type of small keratinous cyst, has been reported in the vulva.[111] Keratinous cysts usually contain a white to pale yellow, grumous or cheesy material without hair. Foreign body-type giant cells may be seen in the tissue adjacent to the cyst wall, secondary to keratinous material leaking into the adjacent dermis. The lining of the cyst is characterized by a relatively flattened, stratified squamous epithelium that is immunoreactive for high molecular weight keratin (Fig. 2.35). Whether these cysts represent primary keratinous cysts, unrelated to sebaceous glands, or are actually occluded sebaceous glands that have undergone squamous metaplasia is debatable. Step sections through the cysts may show communication with the surface epithelium or underlying or adjacent sebaceous glands in some cases. An unusually high frequency of vulvar keratinous cyst has been reported in Nigerian children, related to female circumcision.[98] Such cysts are not considered premalignant, although carcinoma may arise in keratinous cysts. Treatment of asymptomatic small cysts usually is not necessary; however, surgical excision may be necessary for diagnosis or if the cyst is enlarging, symptomatic, or secondarily infected.

Mucous Cyst

Mucous cysts usually are seen within the vestibule and are lined by mucus-secreting, cuboidal to

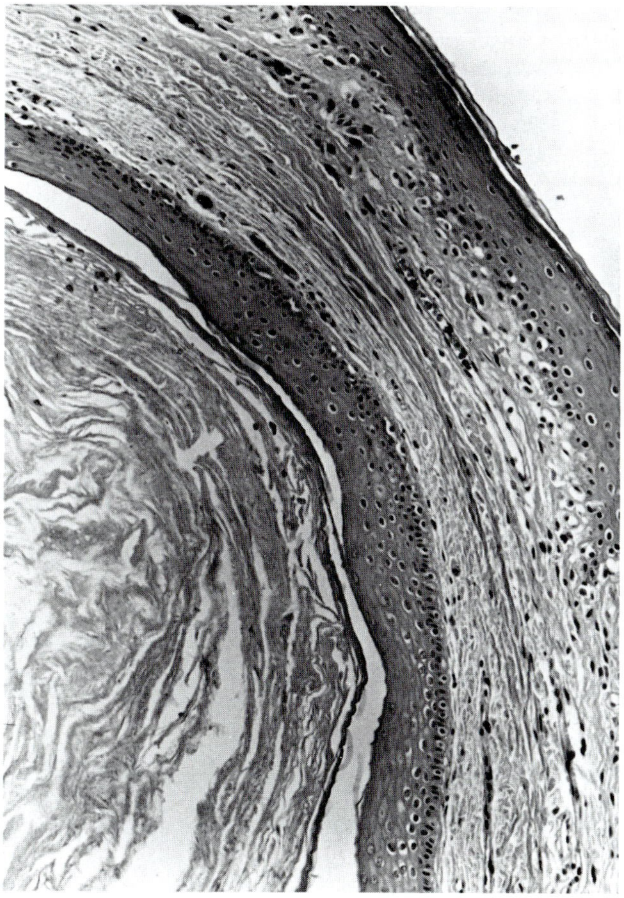

Fig. 2.35. Keratinous cyst. Stratified squamous epithelial lining is evident.

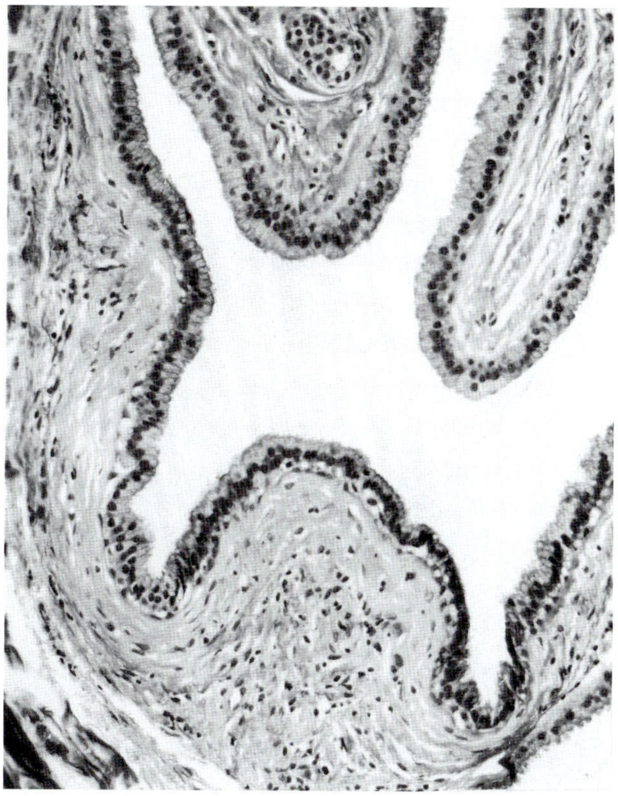

Fig. 2.36. Mucous cyst of the vestibule. Simple columnar mucus-secreting cells rest on the basement membrane. Note absence of underlying smooth muscle layer. (Courtesy of R.J. Kurman, M.D., Baltimore, MD.)

columnar epithelium without peripheral muscle fibers or evidence of myoepithelial cells (Fig. 2.36). Squamous metaplasia may be present. Histochemical studies demonstrate that the epithelial cells lining the cyst stain with both Alcian blue and Mayer mucicarmine, whereas the epithelial lining of cysts of mesonephric origin does not exhibit these reactions.[78,176] The cysts probably develop from occlusion of minor vestibular glands.[78] Electron microscopic studies of mucinous cysts of the vestibule have demonstrated that these cysts have an epithelium consistent with an origin from urogenital sinus endoderm.[212] Because the vulvar vestibule arises embryologically primarily from the urogenital sinus, the origin of these cysts from minor vestibular glands is not inconsistent with a urogenital sinus origin.

Mucinous metaplasia of the vulva has been described, presenting as a solitary depressed red area of the labium minus.[50] In one reported case, this responded to topical estrogen cream. The finding of columnar cell metaplasia of the nonkeratinized squamous epithelium of the vulva vestibule or vagina, to columnar epithelium of mucinous or tuboepithelial type, also has been described after Stevens–Johnson syndrome as well as after laser and 5-fluorouracil (5-FU) therapy.[155]

Apocrine Hidrocystoma/Cystadenoma of the Vulva

Apocrine hidrocystoma is a well-circumscribed cyst, lined by epithelium with apocrine differentiation. The lining cells have abundant pink cytoplasm with apical snoutlike secretion. When the lining cells form micropapillary projections into the cystic space, the lesion is termed *apocrine cystadenoma* (Fig 2.37). The lesion typically arises in the apocrine gland-rich region, which includes the vulva.[90]

Ciliated Cysts of the Vulvar Vestibule: Vestibular Adenosis

Cysts lined with tuboendometrial epithelium resembling mullerian-type epithelium have been reported in the vulvar vestibule in women with

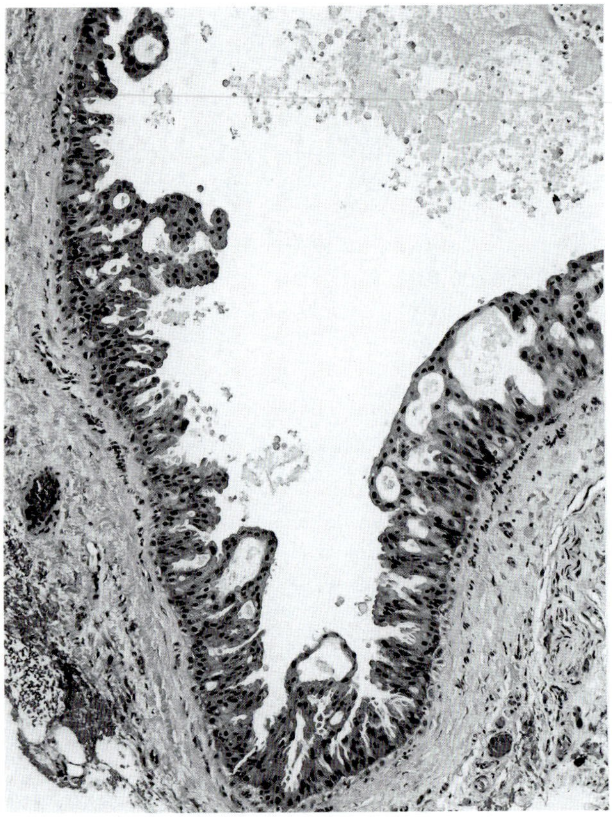

Fig. 2.37. Apocrine cystadenoma. A well-circumscribed cystic space lined by epithelium with apocrine differentiation. The epithelial cells form micropapillary projections into the cystic lumen. (Courtesy of R.J. Kurman, M.D., Baltimore, MD.)

chronic inflammation associated with Stevens–Johnson syndrome or with extensive laser or 5-FU therapy.[112,155,227] The cysts are believed to be acquired as the müllerian system does not contribute to the development of the vestibule. They are distinguished from endometriosis by the absence of associated endometrial stroma or hemosiderin-laden macrophages. In the vagina, such changes, when associated with 5-FU, slowly regress over time by a process of squamous metaplasia. In the vestibule, such cysts may be followed; if persistent or symptomatic, they can be excised.

Mesonephric-Like Cyst (Wolffian-Like Duct Cyst)

Mesonephric-like cysts are encountered occasionally on the lateral aspects of the vulva and vagina. They are thin walled, translucent, and contain clear fluid. The lining epithelium is cuboidal to columnar and is not ciliated. Immunohistochemical techniques show smooth muscle in the submucosal area.[109]

Mammary-Like Cysts (Hidrocystoma)

Hidrocystoma originates in mammary-like glands involving the main collecting duct of anogenital mammary-like sweat glands. It is characterized by a peripheral basal layer of myoepithelial cells and a luminal layer of cuboidal to columnar cells. The luminal layer has discrete apical decapitation secretion. Cutaneous glands, including mammary-like glands, and dartos muscles surround the cysts. The *mammary-like cysts* may have similar alterations resembling eccrine, apocrine, and mammary glands, and most likely represent involution cysts of mammary-like glands.[254]

Cyst of the Canal of Nuck (Mesothelial Cyst)

Cysts of the canal of Nuck are generally found in the superior aspect of the labia majora or inguinal canal and are believed to arise from inclusions of the peritoneum at the inferior insertion of the round ligament into the labia majora. As such, they are analogous to the hydrocele of the spermatic cord. These cysts can achieve substantial size and must be distinguished from an inguinal hernia, with which they are associated in approximately one-third of cases.[222]

Benign Solid Tumors and Tumor-Like Lesions

Benign solid tumors of the vulva are rare. They may be divided into those that are of epithelial origin (squamous and glandular) and those which originate from vulvar soft tissue (mesenchymal origin).

Benign Squamous Epithelial Tumors

Fibroepithelial Polyp (Acrochordon)

A *fibroepithelial polyp*, or "skin tag," is a relatively uncommon benign polypoid tumor of the vulva. In contrast to the vestibular papilloma, the fibroepithelial polyp occurs on the hair-bearing skin of the vulva. These tumors vary in their clinical appearance from small, flesh-colored or hyperpigmented, papillomatous growths resembling condylomata to large pedunculated tumors that often are hypopigmented. On cut section, fibroepithelial polyps are soft and fleshy. Small tumors may resemble intradermal nevi; large lesions may present cosmetic problems but generally are clinically insignificant.

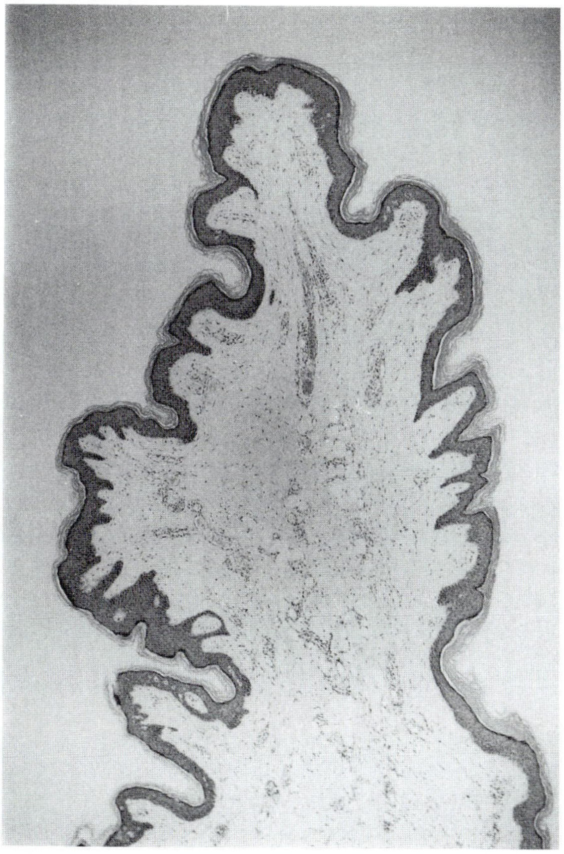

Fig. 2.38. Fibroepithelial polyp. This polyp is primarily stromal, with prominent vessels within the central stalk. The epithelial surface is keratinized, stratified squamous epithelium. No inflammation or glandular elements are evident.

They usually arise in hair-bearing skin but may be found on the labia minora.[37] The origin is most probably from a regressing nevus.

Histologically, fibroepithelial polyps may be of two types, one that is predominantly epithelial and another that is primarily stromal. The epithelial surface varies from a thickened layer with papillomatosis, hyperkeratosis, to an attenuated flattened layer exhibiting multiple primary folds (Fig. 2.38). The connective tissue stalk is composed of loose bundles of collagen with a moderate number of blood vessels. The stroma may be edematous and hypocellular. The stromal cells usually have relatively uniform nuclei; however, marked atypia may be seen in some cases.[37]

Vulvar Vestibular Papilloma (Micropapilloma Labialis)

The *vestibular papilloma* is a benign papillary lesion that is composed of a delicate fibrovascular connective tissue core covered by squamous epithelium (Fig. 2.39), histologically similar to a fibroepithelial polyp. In contrast to a fibroepithelial polyp, vestibular papilloma typically occurs on the vestibule and may be single or multiple. They are relatively common lesions. When multiple, they also may involve the medial aspects of the labia minora and posterior medial labia majora, forming clusters of papules. They occur almost exclusively in women of reproductive age. Vestibular papillae are small, usually less than 5 mm in length, with a diameter of 1–2 mm. Solitary lesions usually are seen adjacent to the hymen, whereas multiple papillomas typically occur in clusters, usually on the lateroposterior aspects of the vestibule. They may be asymptomatic and associated with pruritis. In some cases, they may be seen in women with vulvar vestibulitis. *Vulvar vestibular papilloma*, associated with vestibular pruritus, burning, or dyspareunia, has been identified as a clinical complex. The etiology of

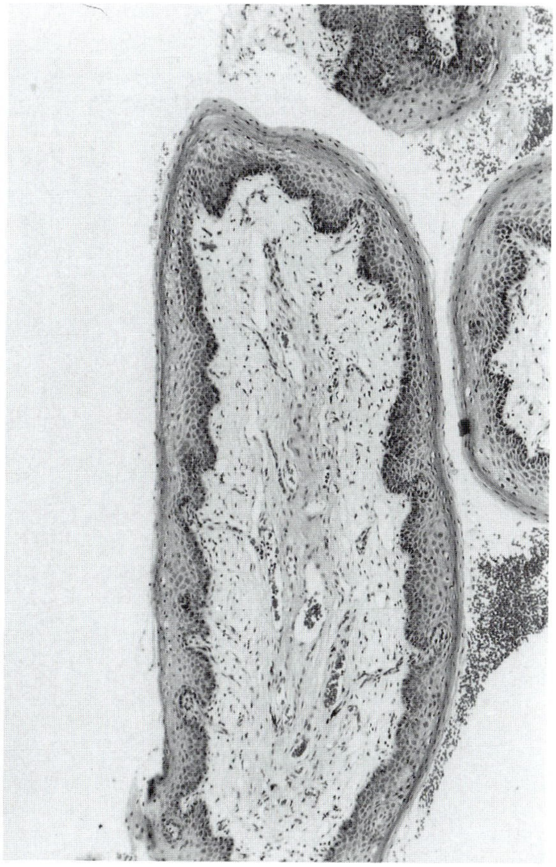

Fig. 2.39. Vestibular papilloma. This papilloma is small and has prominent central nonmuscular vessels oriented to the long axis of the papilloma. The epithelium is nonkeratinized, stratified squamous epithelium. A few lymphocytes are present immediately beneath the epithelium.

vestibular papillomatosis is unknown in most cases. No significant association with HPV has been demonstrated.[18,57,171] These papillae may be an anatomic variant, the female homologue of pearly penile papules.

On microscopic examination, vestibular papillae typically have features of an angiofibroma with stratified nonkeratinized squamous epithelium, which is glycogen-rich in women of reproductive age. They may have a thin keratin layer. The papillae have a fibrovascular core, often with a prominent central vessel (see Fig. 2.39). Usually inflammation is not present. The glycogen-rich squamous epithelium should be distinguished from HPV changes by having normal-sized nuclei whereas the koilocytes have enlarged atypical nuclei. Other features of HPV infection, including dyskeratosis, parabasalar hyperplasia, accentuation of intracellular bridges, and multinucleation, are not identified in glycogen-rich epithelium. In situ hybridization and PCR for HPV may be performed if the findings are equivocal.

Seborrheic Keratosis

Seborrheic keratosis is a benign epithelial growth characterized by acanthosis, papillomatosis, hyperkeratosis, and epithelial invaginations forming horn cysts. The lesions are raised with irregular borders occurring on hair-bearing skin of the vulva. They vary from pale brown to brownish black and appear to be stuck onto the skin surface. Although clinically insignificant, their gross appearance often mimics that of a nevus or melanoma. Seborrheic keratosis of genital skin has been associated in a few studies with human papillomavirus (HPV) infection but is not generally considered a lesion caused by HPV.[140] Multiple seborrheic keratosis presenting over a short period of time may be associated with internal malignancy (Leser–Trelat syndrome).[133] This association is especially strong when associated with acanthosis nigricans.

On low-power examination, the entire lesion appears to be above a straight line drawn from the normal epidermis at one side of the lesion to the

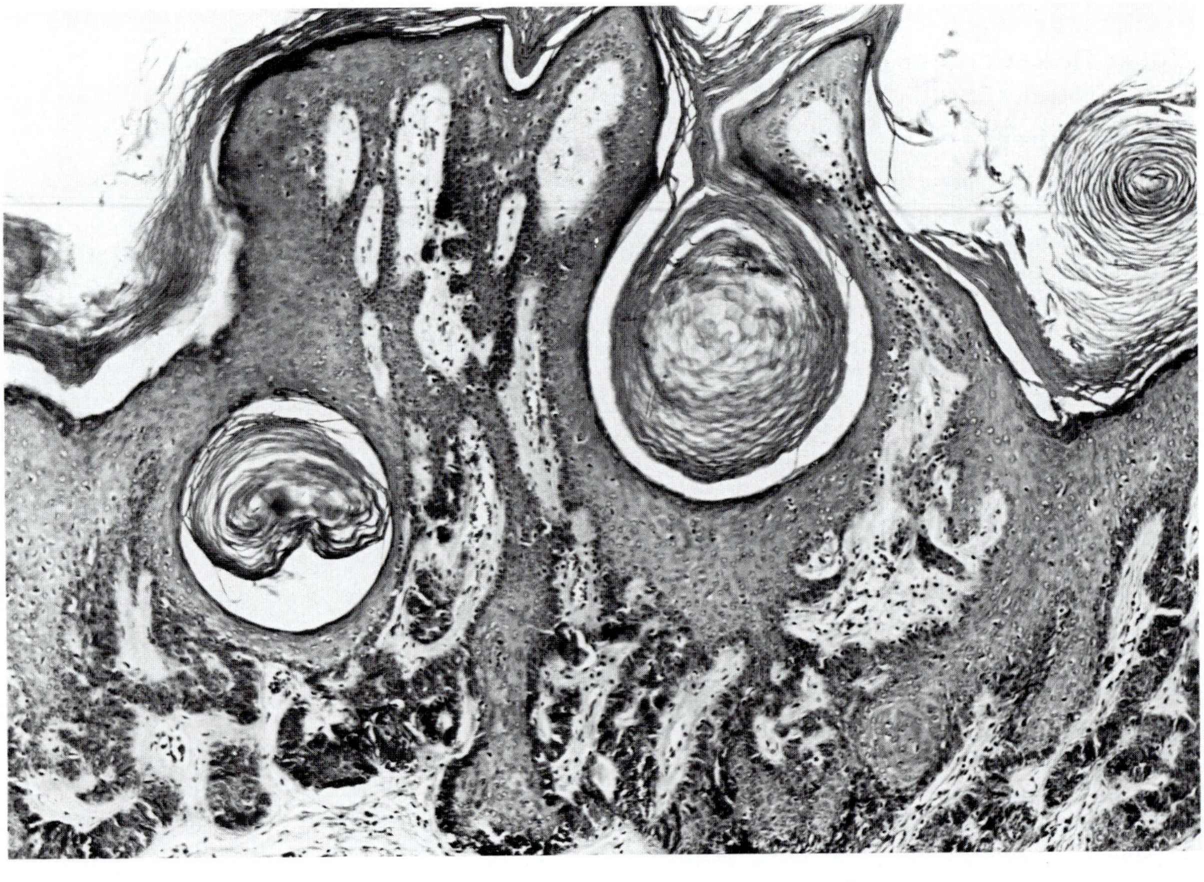

Fig. 2.40. Seborrheic keratosis, pigmented. When pigmented, these lesions may mimic vulvar intraepithelial neoplasia (VIN) or melanoma on the vulva. Note that the diameter of the lesion is substantially greater than its thickness. The melanocytic hyperplasia and hyperpigmentation are present primarily in the basal layers. Keratin pearls are present.

normal epidermis at the other side. Both mature squamous cells and basal type cells are noted in strands and cords surrounding numerous horny keratin cysts (Fig. 2.40). Varying degrees of hyperpigmentation may be present.

Keratoacanthoma

Keratoacanthoma is composed of glassy squamous epithelial proliferation in which horny masses of keratin are pushed upward while tongues of squamous epithelium invade the dermis, resembling squamous cell carcinoma. These tumors commonly occur on sun-exposed skin and may arise on hair-bearing skin of the vulva. They are rapidly growing but are usually self-limited. Keratoacanthoma is generally accepted as a well-differentiated squamous cell carcinoma, keratoacanthoma type. Metastasis of keratoacanthoma has been reported.[68,84] Complete excision with a clear histologic margin is the treatment of choice.

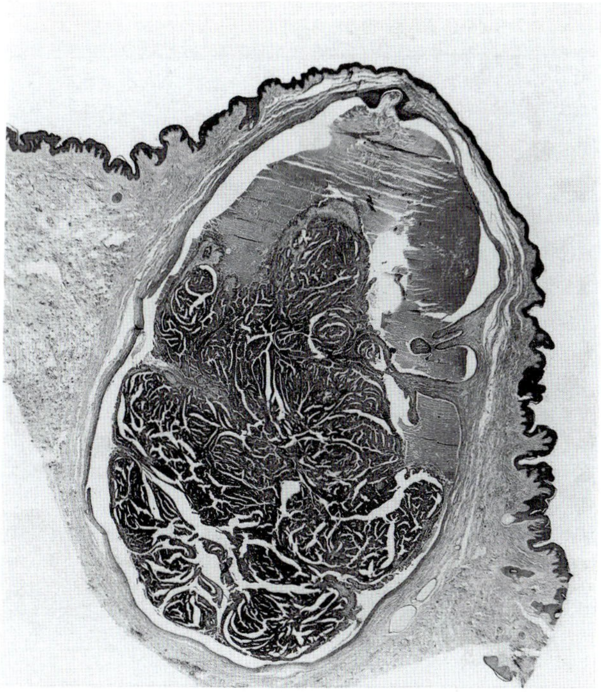

Fig. 2.41. Papillary hidradenoma. This well-circumscribed adenomatous dermal tumor has no connection to skin surface. At low magnification, this benign tumor can be misinterpreted as adenocarcinoma. (Courtesy of R.J. Kurman, M.D., Baltimore, MD.)

Glandular Tumors

Papillary Hidradenoma (Hidradenoma Papilliferum)

Clinical Features

Papillary hidradenoma is a benign tumor of apocrine sweat gland origin, composed of epithelial and myoepithelial cells lining complex delicate fibrovascular branching stalks. Papillary hidradenoma usually presents as a small, dome-shaped tumor less than 2 cm in size. The lesion generally arises from the interlabial sulci, or from the lateral surface of the labia minora. The tumors usually are asymptomatic; however, ulceration of the overlying surface may produce bleeding. Papillary hidradenomas have not been described before puberty, and almost all cases have occurred in Caucasian women.[15] There is evidence that they arise from specialized anogenital mammary-like "sweat" glands.[252,253]

Microscopic Findings

Histologically, under low-power examination, the tumor simulates a well-differentiated adenocarcinoma (Fig. 2.41). Stromal compression often results in the formation of a well-circumscribed pseudocapsule. At times, epithelial cells become entrapped within the compressed connective tissue, creating a pseudoinfiltrative appearance. The tumor is composed of numerous tubules and acini lined by a single or double layer of cuboidal cells, the outer layer representing myoepithelial cells (Fig. 2.42). At times, the cells lining the lumen of the adenomatous structures are large and pale. An inflammatory reaction is unusual unless secondary infection is present. Mitotic figures are rare, and only mild degrees of cellular and nuclear pleomorphism are present.

Clinical Behavior and Treatment

Clinically, the hidradenoma is benign; however, an intraductal carcinoma resembling mammary-type apocrine epithelium has been described arising in a hidradenoma.[190] Local excision, including the base of the mass, is sufficient therapy.

Nodular Hidradenoma

Many names, including *clear cell hidradenoma*, *clear cell myoblastoma*, *solid cystic hidradenoma*, *eccrine acrospiroma*, *eccrine sweat gland adenoma of clear cell type*, and *apocrine hidradenoma*, have all been used for this entity.[68] *Nodular hidradenoma* is generally considered a tumor of eccrine sweat gland origin because it contains eccrine enzymes. Isolated examples of this tumor have been reported on the vulva.

Histologically, nodular hidradenoma is composed of a well-circumscribed lobulated mass with

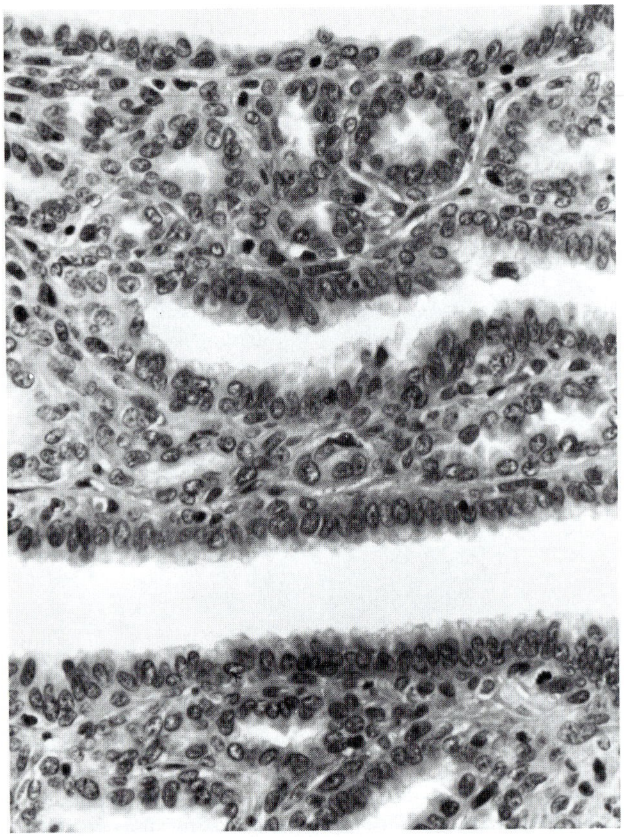

Fig. 2.42. Papillary hidradenoma. High-power examination shows tubules and acini lined with a single or double layer of bland cuboidal to columnar cells.

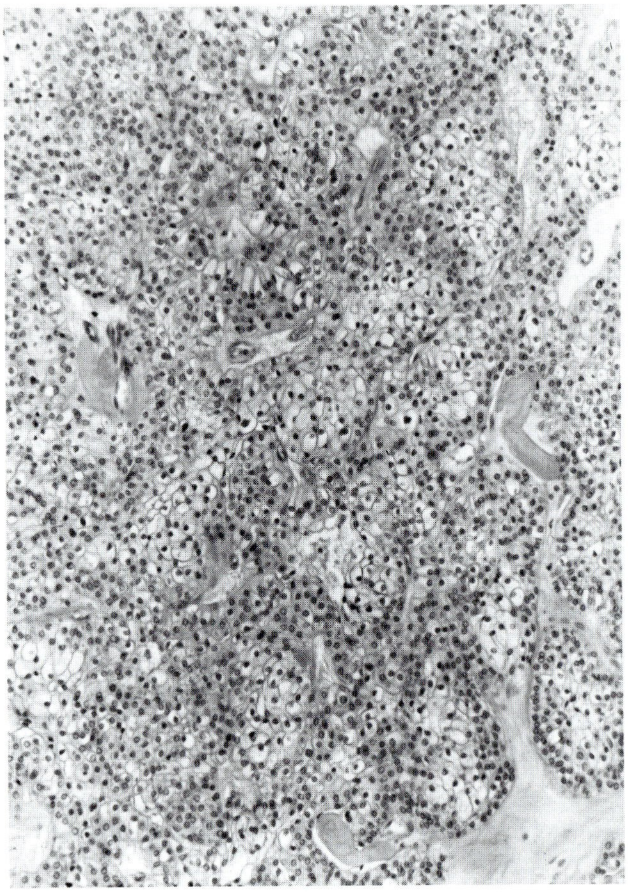

Fig. 2.43. Nodular hidradenoma (clear cell hidradenoma). The sheets of large clear cells are separated by occasional collagen bands and blood vessels.

occasional cystic spaces. Tubular structures, sometimes branching, are often found in the solid areas. The cells are usually the mixtures of pink polyhedral cells and clear cells. The proportion of these two types of cells varies. In addition, secretory cells, dermal and epidermal ductal cells, and immature basaloid cells can be found in this tumor. The relatively small nucleus is round to oval and may exhibit an irregular outline. The chromatin frequently is clumped, and a single small nucleolus often is seen. Mitotic figures are not uncommon (Fig. 2.43).[68] Wide local excision is considered adequate therapy.

Syringoma

The *syringoma* is a benign tumor of eccrine duct origin characterized by multiple, small, relatively uniform epithelial-lined tubules and cysts within a fibrous stroma. It is assumed to be an adenoma of the eccrine ducts. These lesions occur on the vulva as well as the eyelids, cheeks, axillae, and abdomen. Clinically, multiple clustered flesh-colored papules are noted within the deeper skin layers of the labia majora bilaterally. They often are asymptomatic, although pruritis may occur.[36]

Histologically, the tumor lacks a clearly defined border. Within the dermis, numerous small, dilated duct spaces are seen. These spaces usually are lined by two rows of epithelial cells that appear flat, secondary to pressure atrophy. The comma-like formation of these glandular spaces is characteristic (Fig. 2.44). The stroma has a desmoplastic appearance.

Mixed Tumor of the Vulva (Pleomorphic Adenoma, Chondroid Syringoma)

Mixed tumor of the vulva is a rare neoplasm that usually presents as a solid, subcutaneous tumor involving the labia majora or the Bartholin gland area or both. The histopathologic findings are similar to those of mixed tumors of the parotid and other salivary glands. The tumor consists of epithelial cells arranged in tubules or nests, mixed with a fibrous

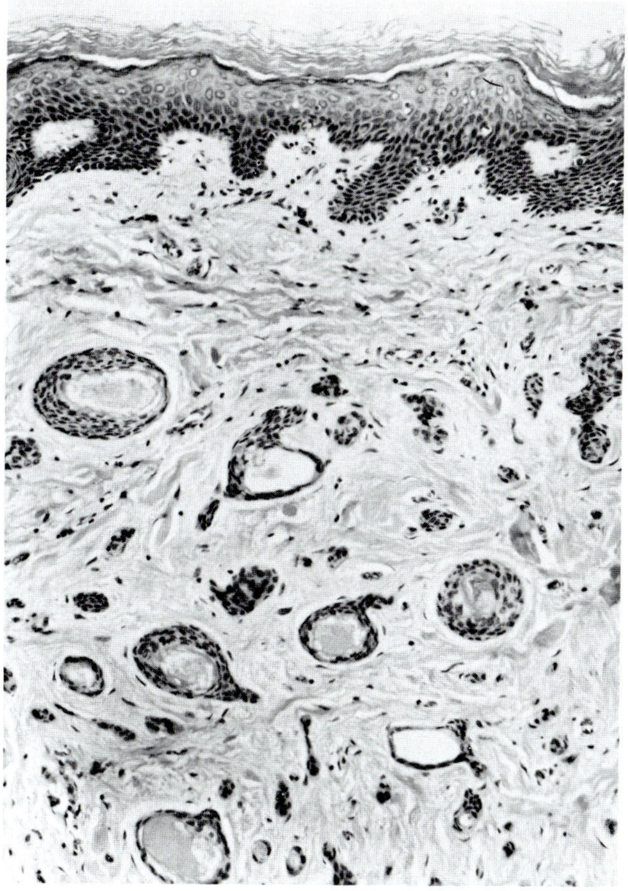

Fig. 2.44. Syringoma. The comma pattern of the eccrine structures is easily appreciated.

stroma containing chondromatous, osseous, and myxoid elements. These stromal-like elements are believed to arise from pluripotential myoepithelial cells that, in the vulva, are found in the Bartholin glands, sweat glands, and accessory breast tissue.[217] These tumors are benign, but local recurrence may occur. Malignant mixed tumors have been reported.[184] When metastasis occurs from a malignant mixed tumor, it is usually composed of only epithelial elements. There are insufficient cases of vulvar mixed tumors to determine its natural history in this site. Wide local excision, with free margins, is the recommended therapy of choice for both the primary tumor and local recurrences.

Trichoepithelioma

Trichoepithelioma is a benign tumor of follicular origin that is rare in the vulva.[43] The tumor presents as single or multiple cutaneous nodules with normal-appearing overlying epithelium. On microscopic examination, the tumor is composed of complex interconnected nests of basaloid cells, which form small cysts containing keratin "horn cysts." The cells in trichoepithelioma are monomorphic without hyperchromasia or nuclear atypia. Occasionally, a granulomatous reaction with giant cells is present next to ruptured horn cysts. Hair or hair-forming elements are rare. Trichoepithelioma is distinguished from basaloid carcinoma or basal cell carcinoma in that it is not infiltrative, contains "horn cysts" and granulomas, may exhibit hair-forming elements, and is not associated with an intraepithelial neoplastic component. Local excision is therapeutic.

Proliferating Trichilemmal Tumor/Cyst (Pilar Tumors)

Proliferating trichilemmal tumor/cyst is rare on the vulva, occurring in the dermis of the labium majus, where it presents as a slowly growing solid mass that may have a cystic cavity in the center of the tumor.[8,203] It is thought to arise from the cells of the outer root sheath of a hair follicle. Microscopic examination reveals a lobulated proliferation of squamous epithelium with a pushing border. The tumor may show no connection with the overlying epithelium. An eosinophilic glassy layer of collagen (vitreous layer) may surround some of the lobules. The tumor cells are palisaded peripherally and have increased cytoplasm in the cells toward the center of the lobules with abrupt changes into eosinophilic amorphous keratin, resembling keratinization of the follicular infundibulum (trichilemmal keratinization). Some degree of nuclear pleomorphism and cytologic atypia, as well as individual cell keratinization, forming squamous "eddies" may be present. Focal calcification within the amorphous keratin may occur.

Trichoblastic fibroma also has been described on the vulva.[85] Local excision is therapeutic.

Adenoma of Minor Vestibular Glands

Adenoma of minor vestibular glands is a rare benign tumor. These lesions are small, ranging from 1–2 mm to 1 cm. The tumor is composed of multiple lobular clusters of small glands lined by mucin-secreting columnar epithelium. Some may represent a nodular hyperplasia. Most cases have been found incidentally in vestibulectomy specimens excised for vulvar vestibulitis.[79,199]

Endometriosis

Vulvar endometriomas develop from ectopic endometrial epithelium. Endometrium implanted in an episiotomy incision at the time of delivery, as well as menstrual endometrium implanting in a small area of trauma, have been implicated in the etiology of this condition (see Chapter 17, Diseases of the Peritoneum). The clinical appearance is variable, ranging from bluish-red cystic masses to amorphous deep-seated nodules. Endometriomas of the vulva usually are located near the posterior fourchette. Cyclic enlargement and regression often are noted. Fine-needle aspiration may be of value in the diagnosis, demonstrating benign glandular and stromal cellular elements.[148]

Histologically, both endometrial glands and stroma are present with a fibrotic response. A foreign body–giant cell reaction and hemosiderin-laden macrophages may be noted, especially in cases in which the onset was preceded by recent surgery.

Mesenchymal Tumors: Vascular Tumors

Capillary Hemangioma (Strawberry Hemangioma, Juvenile Hemangioma, Nevus Vasculosis)

Capillary hemangioma is typically encountered in infants or young children. It is a red to violet, well-demarcated, superficial, slightly elevated lesion that usually has an irregular surface. At times it is ulcerated or is associated with bleeding. The microscopic findings consist of numerous clustered endothelial-lined small capillaries within a fibrous tissue matrix. Biopsy is not indicated because the typical appearance is diagnostic. Because these lesions spontaneously regress, therapy generally is unnecessary.

Cavernous Hemangioma

Cavernous hemangioma is rare on the vulva, although its occurrence in young children has been documented.[175] This benign vascular lesion may be relatively large, complex, and deep in comparison to the capillary hemangiomas. It also may be associated with deep pelvic hemangioma. Distortion of the vulva may occur, and clitoral involvement may resemble clitoral hypertrophy.[175] Association with limb hypertrophy (Klippel–Trenauny syndrome) may be seen in some children. Cavernous hemangioma of the vulva in children, as a rule, does not require therapy because it regresses over time. Like capillary hemangioma, cavernous hemangiomas may ulcerate and bleed, and on rare occasion may require therapy.

Acquired Hemangioma of Adults (Senile Hemangioma)

Acquired hemangioma is far more common than other hemangiomas on the vulva. These are typically multiple, small (1–3 mm), red to purple papules with no known clinical significance. Histologically, acquired hemangiomas have numerous dilated capillaries in the intradermal tissue. The vascular spaces are lined by a single layer of endothelial cells and are separated by connective tissue that may show collagenization.[141] Hemangiomatous-like changes may be found on the vulva after radiotherapy.

The differential diagnosis of hemangiomas includes angiokeratoma, pyogenic granuloma, bacterial angiomatosis, hemangiopericytoma, angiosarcoma, and Kaposi sarcoma. All these lesions are highly vascular and must be differentiated from hemangioma.[49,141] Angiokeratomas typically are dark red to black, raised, warty-appearing lesions that have an acanthotic overlying epithelium which is immediately adjacent to the prominent vascular channels of the angiokeratoma. Pyogenic granuloma usually is an elevated red lesion that histologically resembles granulation tissue and may have a collarette of elevated epithelium surrounding it. Hemangiopericytoma is a solid vascular neoplasm that is composed of staghorn-shaped vessels. In addition, there is a distinctive perivascular pericyte proliferation that can be identified with a reticulin stain. Bacillary angiomatosis resembles Kaposi sarcoma but contains the bacteria *Bartonella* Henselae and Quintana (formerly *Rochalimaea* Henselae and Quintana), which can be identified using a Warthin–Starry stain.[49,205,273] Kaposi sarcoma is a malignant vascular tumor composed of spindle cells, some of which form distinct slitlike vascular spaces containing red blood cells.

Angiokeratoma

The *angiokeratoma* is a variant of hemangioma and occurs almost exclusively on the scrotum and vulva; however, it has been described presenting as an ulcerated tumor of the clitoris.[160] Somewhat larger than senile hemangioma, these lesions often are purple to brown-black in color and occur primarily in women of childbearing age. Their peculiar appearance often prompts excisional diagnostic biopsy, although they have no clinical significance.[51]

Histologically, the dilated endothelial-lined channels are separated by strands and cords of squamous epithelial cells representing downgrowth from the overlying epithelium, which is often hyperkeratotic (Fig. 2.45). Varying degrees of acanthosis and papil-

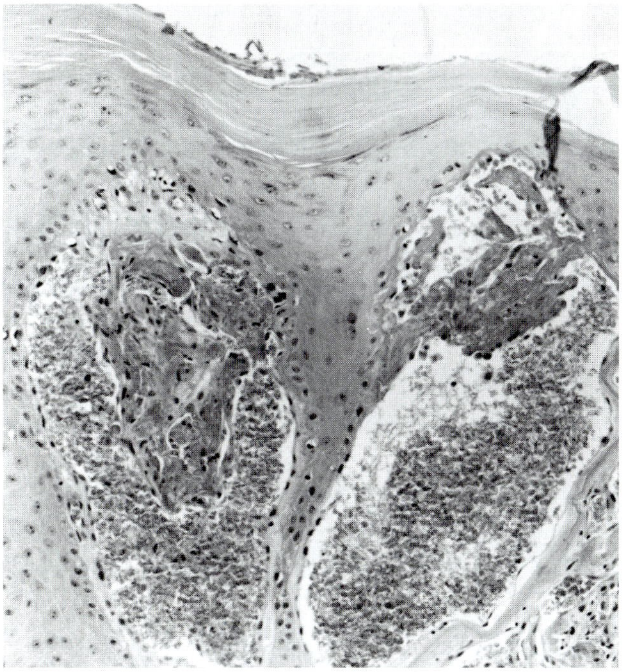

Fig. 2.45. Angiokeratoma. Strands of squamous epithelium surround endothelial-lined vascular spaces.

lomatosis are present, along with a mild inflammatory reaction in the deep dermis. Angiosarcomas and Kaposi sarcoma are included in the differential diagnosis of vascular tumors.[141] These malignant tumors typically are more cellular and have greater cellular atypia. In addition, they have less well formed vascular spaces that are usually slitlike and which are infiltrative with poorly defined margins.

Pyogenic Granuloma (Granuloma Pyogenicum)

The *pyogenic granuloma* is a variant of hemangioma that may occur anywhere on the skin. It is analogous to the epulis tumor of pregnancy. Most of the pyogenic granulomas that occur on the vulva do so during gestation. Although previously thought to be secondary to a superficial wound infection, this tumor is recognized as a form of hemangioma characterized by rapid growth. Because the surface is easily traumatized, the lesion often is secondarily infected. Histologically, a thin ulcerated epidermis is noted covering a mass of granulation tissue. Capillaries are numerous, and secondary inflammatory changes frequently are found within the stroma (Fig. 2.46). Around the periphery of the lesion, there may be a downward growth of the epidermis producing a "collarette." The overall architecture appears lobulated (lobular capillary hemangioma) with a few thickened fibrous septae seperating the vascular proliferation.

Lymphangioma

Vulvar lymphangiomas may be congenital or acquired. Congenital lymphangiomas have been reported associated with lower-extremity lymphangiomas and may be large, cavernous in type, and associated with deep lymphatics.[177] Vulvar lymphangiomas may occur after radiation therapy to the pelvis.

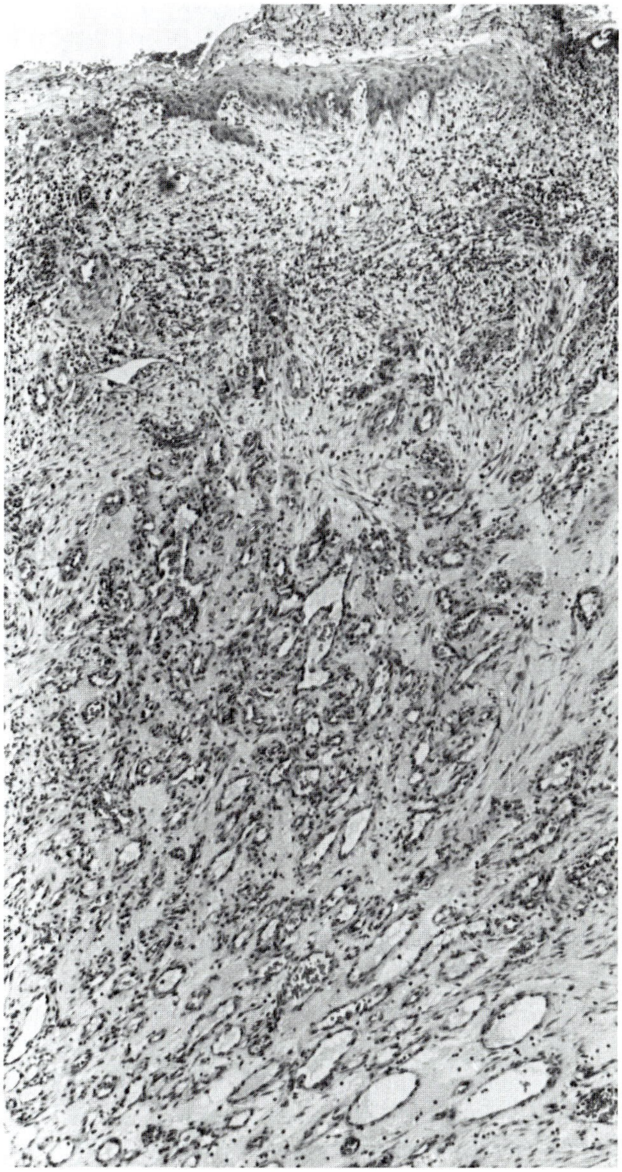

Fig. 2.46. Pyogenic granuloma. Superficial ulceration of the mucosa is present, with a chronic inflammatory infiltrate. Within the submucosa, multiple endothelial-lined vascular spaces are seen surrounded by a delicate fibrous stroma, resembling granulation tissue.

Histologically, lymphangiomas consists of variable-sized lymphatics, lined with endothelial cells within a fibrous connective tissue without associated smooth muscle. Unlike hemangiomas, lymphangiomas characteristically do not contain red blood cells. No therapy is usually necessary; however, surgical excision is applicable in some cases. Secondary infection is a potentially severe complication. Recurrence after therapy does not imply malignant transformation.

Lymphangioma Circumscriptum

Lymphangioma circumscriptum is a relatively rare condition that is benign and thought to be secondary to a localized developmental defect of the dermal lymphatics or a malformation. Initial presentation may be in childhood; however, vulvar cases have been described initially presenting in women in their thirties. The lesion is characterized by multiple clustered blebs and vesicles that are white to purple. The lesions may be small, but may exceed 2 cm in diameter.[39,108] The blebs of lymphangioma circumscriptum may become secondarily infected, ulcerated, and macerated, resulting in pain and cellulitis. The diagnosis usually is made by the clinical appearance and by biopsy.

The microscopic findings reveal distinctive subepidermal cystic spaces containing lymph that is eosinophilic and acellular. These endothelial-lined cysts, which may be multiloculated, are located immediately beneath the basal epithelial layer in the papillary dermis (Fig. 2.47). Dilated lymphatic spaces can be found in the reticular dermis. Some of these deeper lymphatics may be surrounded by a prominent peripheral smooth muscle layer. The overlying epithelium usually is unremarkable but may be eroded or hyperkeratotic. Treatment includes surgical excision or laser therapy.[108]

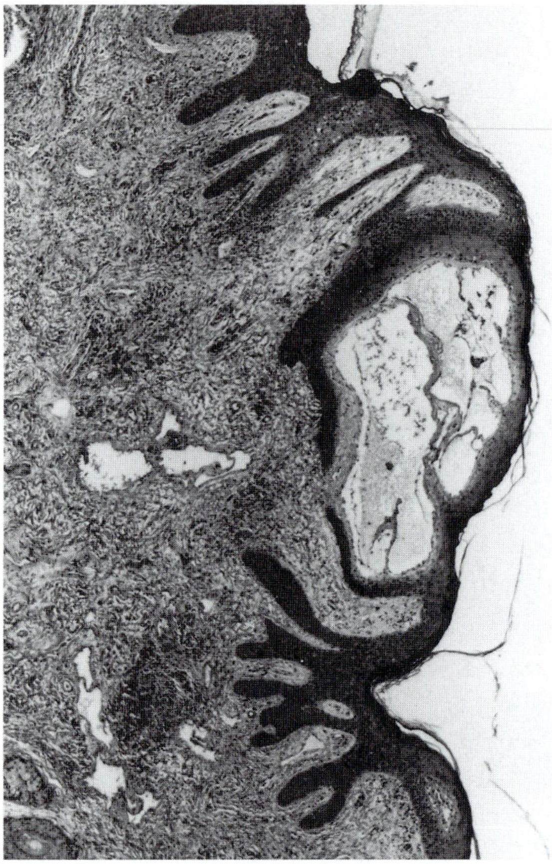

Fig. 2.47. Lymphangioma circumscriptum. Subepidermal multiloculated cystic spaces are seen that are filled with acellular eosinophilic lymph. Some slightly dilated deeper lymphatic channels are evident in the deeper dermis. (Courtesy of G. Segal, M.D., Gainesville, FL.)

Angiomyofibroblastoma

Angiomyofibroblastoma is a benign tumor that may present as a Bartholin cyst or mass measuring from 0.5 to 12 cm in diameter.[76,242] The tumor is well circumscribed and contains numerous capillary-like vessels. It is composed of spindled to oval stromal cells with bland nuclei and eosinophilic cytoplasm. Mitotic figures are absent or rare. Some areas, predominantly around vessels, may be cellular, with adjacent hypocellular areas. Plump stromal cells, especially about vessels, are seen with little stromal mucin (Fig. 2.48). Collagen may be prominent, and mast cells are present in most cases. The stromal cells may be reactive for vimentin and desmin, but lack actin, S-100 protein, and cytokeratin. In contrast to aggressive angiomyxoma, angiomyofibroblastoma is more cellular, has more numerous vessels, and the vessels lack vascular wall thickening and hyalinization. Local excision is the treatment of choice.[66,76]

Mesenchymal Tumors: Muscle Tumors

Leiomyoma

Benign *leiomyomas* are the most common soft tissue tumors of the vulva. They may arise from the smooth muscle elements surrounding the crura of the clitoris. Vulvar leiomyomatosis associated with esophagogastric leiomyomatosis has been reported in children.[73] The tumor is composed of smooth muscle cells having round to oval nuclei with eosinophilic cytoplasm with poorly defined cell borders. Myxoid change may occur, and has been re-

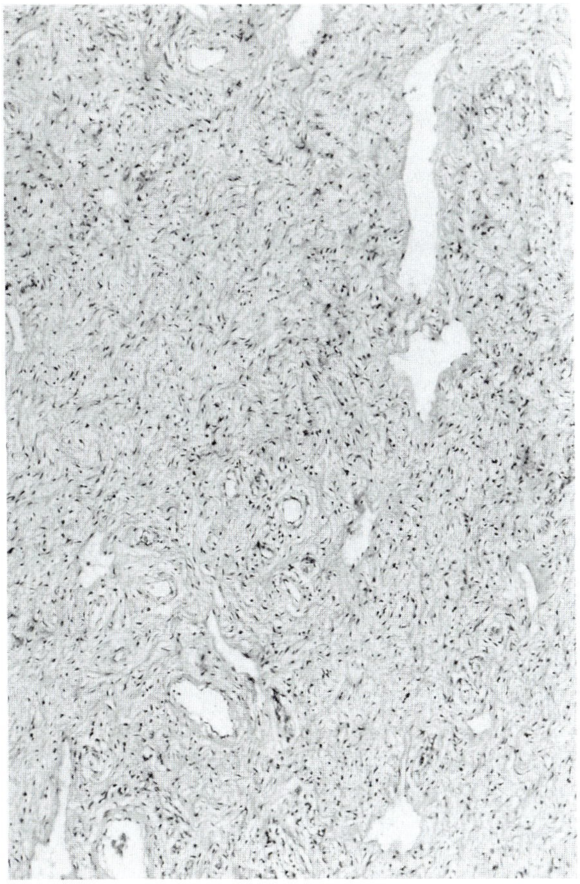

Fig. 2.48. Angiomyofibroblastoma. This benign tumor is composed of spindled and oval stroma cells with relatively uniform, bland-appearing nuclei with eosinophilic cytoplasm and infrequent or no mitosis. Numerous capillary-like vessels are present, with variable shapes. (Courtesy of R.J. Kurman, M.D., Baltimore, MD.)

ported associated with pregnancy. *Epithelioid leiomyoma* also has been reported in pregnancy.[100] Leiomyoma is distinguished from *leiomyosarcoma* by the absent or rare mitotic activity, lack of nuclear hyperchromasia, and pleomorphism (see leiomyosarcoma in Chapter 3). Both are immunoreactive for desmin, myosin, and actin and do not contain myoglobin as do rhabdomyosarcomas and rhabdomyomas.[141] Therapy is local excision. Gonadotropin suppression may be useful in rare cases.[73]

Rhabdomyoma

Rhabdomyoma is a benign tumor of striated muscle origin that, although rare in the vulva, has been reported in women of reproductive age.[268] Rhabdomyoma presents as a polypoid mass. On microscopic examination, the tumor contains mature striated muscle cells intermixed with fibrovascular stroma. Rhabdomyomas of the fetal myxoid type must be differentiated from embryonal rhabdomyosarcomas, which have nuclear pleomorphism, mitotic activity, and are infiltrative.

Mesenchymal Tumors: Neural Tumors

Granular Cell Tumor

The *granular cell tumor* is of peripheral nerve sheath origin and may occur in the vulva in children or adults. Approximately 7% of granular cell tumors in women occur on the vulva.[149] They are multiple in approximately 10%–15% of the cases.[141] The tumor typically presents as a painless, slow-growing, subcutaneous mass, usually involving the labia majora, clitoris, or mons pubis.[149] The tumor may present as a solitary enlargement of the clitoris, mimicking clitoral hypertrophy.[101,271] Priapism of the crus of the clitoris has been reported related to a locally aggressive granular cell tumor.[232]

Histologically, granular cell tumors are not encapsulated and are composed of irregular groups of large polyhedral cells with indistinct cell borders and nuclei that are relatively small and uniform with hyperchromatic chromatin. The cell groups usually are separated by strands of hyalinized stroma. The cytoplasm of these cells is packed with numerous eosinophilic granules (Figs. 2.49 and 2.50). Granular cell tumor contains S-100 protein and myelin basic protein, which can be demonstrated by immunoperoxidase stains.[101] The granules consist of lysozyme and are PAS positive and diastase resistant. Carcinoembryonic antigen and myelin basic protein P0 and P2 also have been identified.[141] In approximately 50% of granular cell tumors, the overlying squamous epithelium exhibits remarkable pseudoepitheliomatous hyperplasia.[271] Extreme degrees of acanthosis are noted, and the nests and cords of hyperplastic squamous cells may mimic an invasive squamous carcinoma.[271] Rapid enlargement of benign granular cell tumors may occur in pregnancy. Malignant vulvar granular cell tumors are rare and usually are not recognized as malignant unless regional aggressive behavior or metastasis is identified.[149] Careful microscopic examination of the margins of the surgical specimen, therefore, is important. Local recurrences are common. Recurrent granular cell tumor shows multilobulation. Malignant granular cell tumor with pulmonary and regional metastasis and with a subsequent fatal outcome has been reported.[149] Wide local excision is the usual treatment for both primary and locally recurrent granular cell tumors.[271]

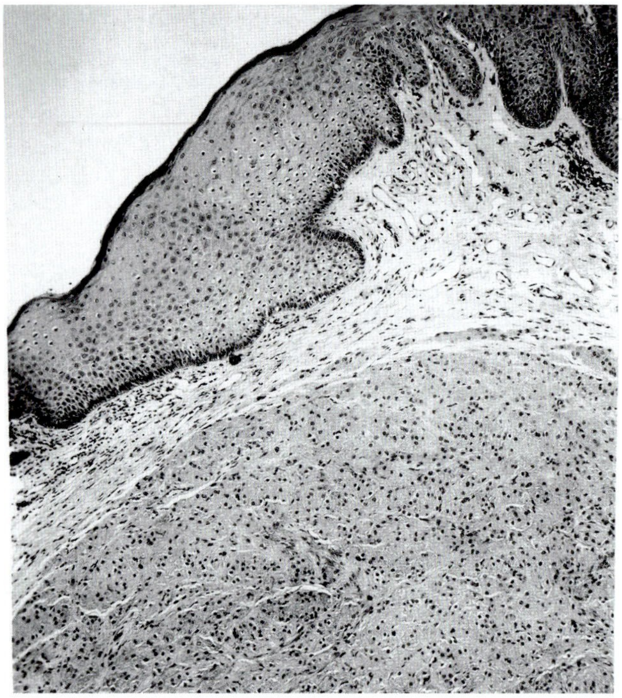

Fig. 2.49. Granular cell tumor. A pseudoepitheliomatous epidermal hyperplasia is overlying the dermal granular cell proliferation. (Courtesy of R.J. Kurman, M.D., Baltimore, MD.)

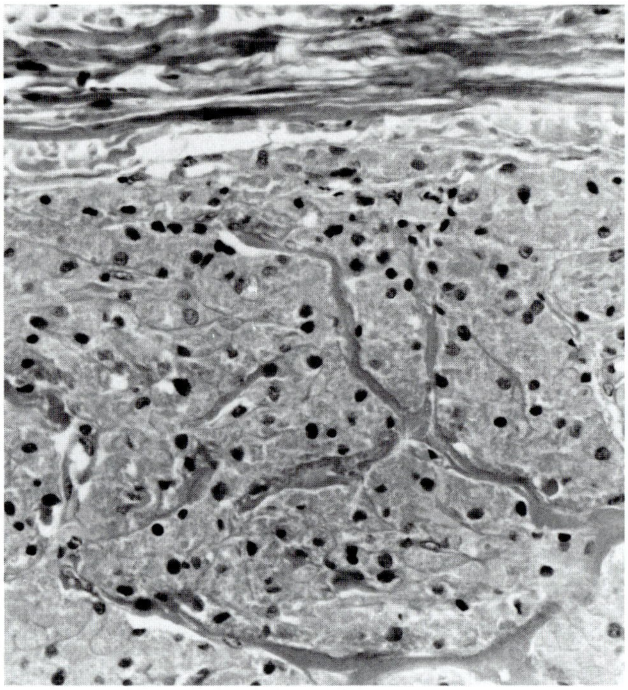

Fig. 2.50. Granular cell tumor. Note nests of polyhedral cells with granular cytoplasm separated by collagenous cords.

Neurofibroma

Neurofibroma is a benign tumor of nerve sheath origin that involves the vulva in approximately 18% of women with von Recklinghausen's disease. Approximately one-half of vulvar neurofibromas are found in women with neurofibromatosis.[96,138] Neurofibromas are generally less than 3 cm in diameter; however, a giant solitary variant of neurofibroma of the labia has been reported.[258] Neurofibromas are rare before puberty. They may grow rapidly, and malignant degeneration to neurofibrosarcoma or malignant schwannoma may occur.

Microscopically, the tumor is composed of whorls and wavy bundles of slender spindle cells that often exhibit a palisaded arrangement of the nuclei. The tumor is not encapsulated and may involve the dermis as well as the underlying fat. The cell borders are indistinct, and strands of collagen-rich stroma, with mast cells, are commonly seen. The nuclei typically are small and have pointed poles; some may have a wavy appearance (Fig. 2.51). Bizarre nuclei with hyperchromatic nuclear chromatin may be seen; this is a benign finding and is referred to as ancient change.[141] Mitosis should not be present in benign neurofibromas, and the presence of only 1 mitotic figure per 10 high-power fields is sufficient evidence for a diagnosis of neurofibrosarcoma.[141] Nerve stains show long, thin nerve fibers scattered throughout the tumor, and occasionally the intervening collagen may undergo a peculiar mucoid degeneration. Neurofibromas contain S-100 antigen.[96] Steroid receptors have been reported in some neural tumors in the pelvis and the vulva.[41] Myxoid neurofibroma is a variant with abundant stromal mucin deposition. In patients with neurofibromatosis, the tumors are multicellular (polyclonal) in origin, unlike neurofibromas in normal individuals, where they are monoclonal in origin.[124] When associated with neurofibromatosis, there generally is no reason to excise vulvar neurofibromas unless they are rapidly enlarging, ulcerated, or symptomatic. In individuals without neurofibromatosis, these tumors present as a subcutaneous mass and excision is both diagnostic and therapeutic. Individuals with hereditary neurofibromatosis also have an increased risk for other tumors, including glioma, ganglioneuroma, pheochromocytoma, meningioma, leukemia, Wilm tumor, and rhabdomyosarcoma.[196]

Schwannoma (Neurilemmoma)

Schwannomas rarely involve the vulva; however, the few cases reported have involved the clitoris and

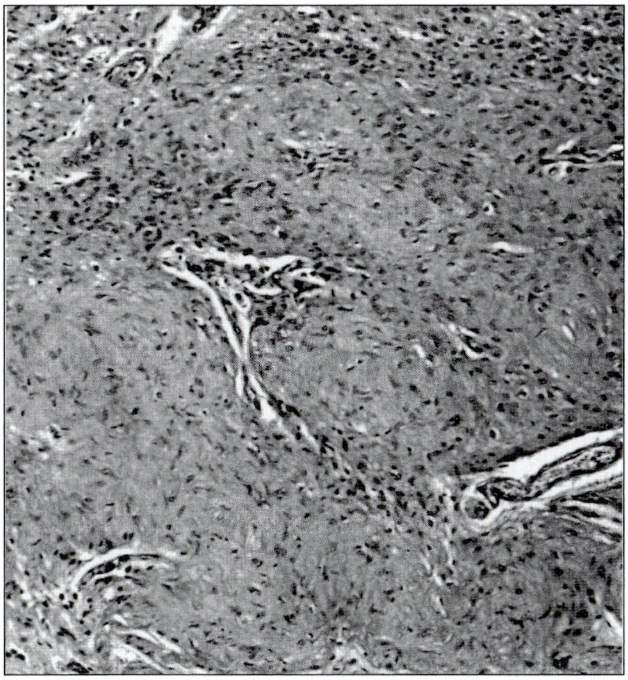

Fig. 2.51. Neurofibroma. Neurofibroma wavy bundles of slender spindle cells with small nuclei and strands of collagen. Some mast cells are present.

may mimic clitoral hypertrophy.[102] These benign tumors arise from the neuroectodermal nerve sheath and usually are solitary. Histologically, they contain both Antoni type A and type B tissue patterns (Fig. 2.52). The cellular (Antoni type A) areas consist of spindle cells with oval or elongated nuclei that have a palisaded and wavy appearance. Verocay bodies, which often are seen in these areas, are formed by alignment of the nuclei in regular rows that are separated by intervening acellular areas. Hypocellular (Antoni type B) areas contain small spindled cells with hyperchromatic nuclear chromatin. Collagen fibers, mast cells, and lipid-laden histiocytes usually are present. A myxomatous matrix is typically present within which small vessels with prominent thickening of the vessel wall are seen. These tumors are immunoreactive for S-100 protein and are distinguished from leiomyomas in that they lack desmin (see Mesenchymal Tumors, Malignant Schwannoma in Chapter 3). Local excision is the treatment of choice.[102]

Glomus Tumor

Glomus tumor of the vulva is rare. However, it has been reported associated with severe introital dyspareunia. The tumor is typically less than 4 cm in diameter and solitary, and the pain is localized to the tumor mass.[235]

Microscopically, the tumor is composed of epithelioid-like cells forming lobules with surrounding vessels. The cells are positive for smooth muscle actin. The stroma about the tumor typically is hyalinized and usually contains identifiable nerves and mast.

Mesenchymal Tumors: Tumors of Fibroblastic or Fibrohistiocytic Origin

Fibroma

Benign *fibromas* may appear as vulvar masses arising from the deeper connective tissues surrounding the vaginal introitus or adjacent to the perineal

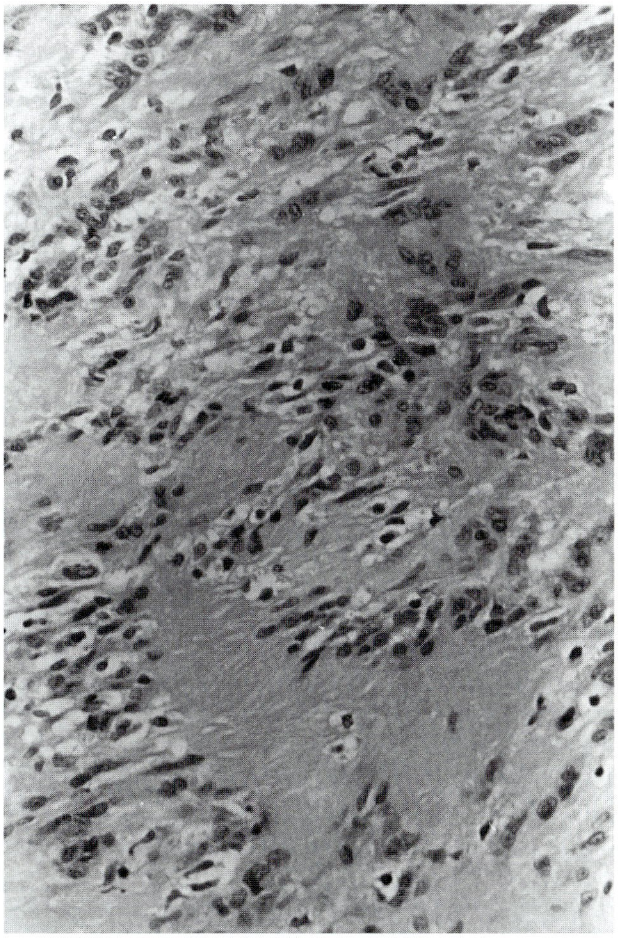

Fig. 2.52. Schwannoma. Densely packed spindle cells from Antoni type A areas are admixed with hypocellular Antoni type B areas.

body. Rarely do such tumors undergo malignant degeneration; left untreated, however, they can grow to substantial size. On cut section, fibromas are firm, smooth, and white or grayish. Yellow striae and a somewhat softer consistency signify the admixture of a lipomatous element, which is not uncommon. They do not involve the overlying epidermis. Histologically, parallel bundles of fibrocytes are seen. With large tumors, hyaline, cystic and hemorrhagic degenerations have been described.[13]

Desmoid Tumor

Desmoid tumors (aggressive fibromatosus) are characterized by increased fibroblasts with thickening and fibrosis of the involved tissue. There is typically no associated inflammatory response. Desmoid tumor of the vulva has been associated with pregnancy.[4,71] Wide local excision is the treatment of choice.

Benign Fibrous Histiocytoma (Dermatofibroma)

Fibrous histiocytomas also have been referred to as *subepidermal nodular fibrosis*, *histiocytoma*, and *sclerosing hemangioma*. The term *dermatofibroma* is reserved for those tumors 1.5 cm or less in diameter. Masses larger than this, or those polypoid in appearance, are referred to as *benign fibrous histiocytoma*.[96] *Cellular dermatofibroma* has been used for cellular lesions, usually polypoid with typical mitoses. This benign tumor rarely occurs on the vulva. The clinical presentation may be a slightly raised, pale brown to red solitary subcutaneous mass.

On microscopic examination, the tumor is composed of fibroblastic-type cells with a fascicular growth pattern that focally may have a storiform appearance. Typically, collagen is evident and may be prominent in some areas, especially at the periphery of the lesion. Lymphocytes, foamy histiocytes, and multinucleated histiocytes may be found. Typically, few if any mitotic figures are present (Fig. 2.53). This benign histiocytic tumor may have associated epithelial hyperplasia; however, it lacks stromal infiltration. In contrast, dermatofibrosarcoma protuberans (DFSP) is characterized by infiltrative growth of spindle cells into the subcutaneous fat. The overlying epithelium is usually attenuated (see Mesenchymal Tumors, Dermatofibrosarcoma Protuberans in Chapter 3). Immunoperoxidase for factor XIIIa is positive in benign fibrohistiocytoma and negative in DFSP. CD34, on the other hand, is positive in DFSP and negative in benign fibrohistiocytoma. The tumor cells are immunoreactive for alpha-1-antichymotrypsin, alpha-1-antitrypsin, and vimentin. Complete local excision is the treatment of choice.

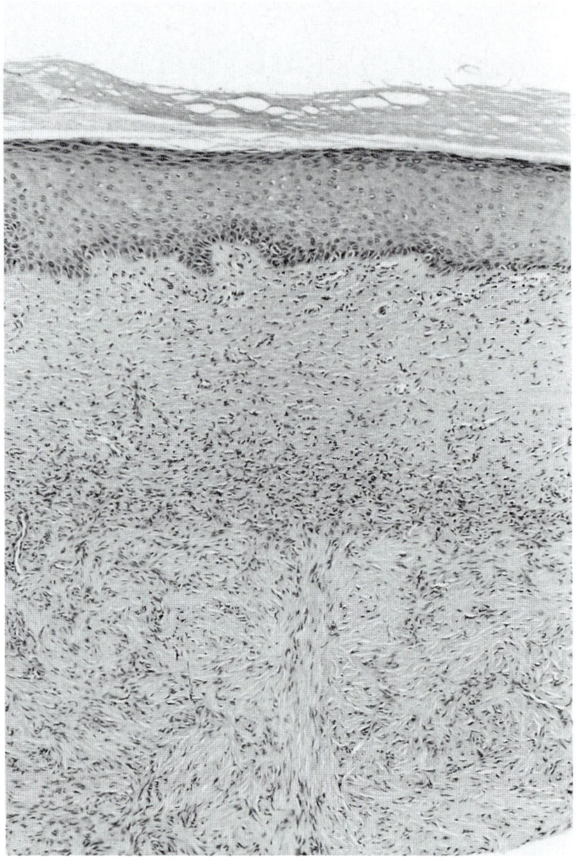

Fig. 2.53. Dermatofibroma. The tumor is beneath the most superficial dermis and is composed of spindled fibroblast-type cells with a fascicular storiform pattern. The cell groups are separated in some areas by collagen.

Miscellaneous Tumors and Tumor-Like Lesions

Lipoma

Lipomas arise from the vulvar fat pads and present as soft, lobulated growths generally attached to the labia majora by a broad-based pedicle. Lipomas of the vulva presenting at birth have been reported.[256] Histologically, mature fat cells are seen, often interspersed with strands of fibrous connective tissue. When the fibrotic element is prominent, the tumor should be called a *fibrolipoma*. When there is a prominent background vasculature with thrombi in some vessels, the tumor is termed *angiolipoma* (Fig. 2.54). Lipocytes are immunoreactive for S-100 antigen.

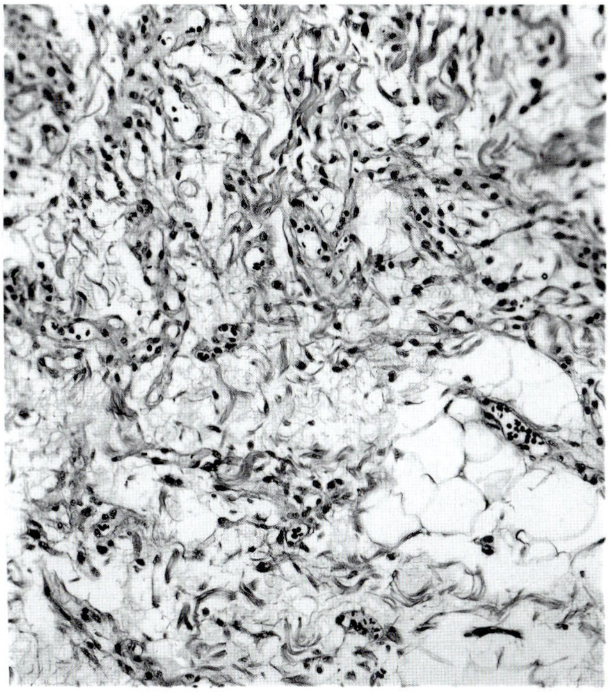

Fig. 2.54. Angiolipoma. Mature adipocytes and an increased capillary background. Thrombosed capillaries are common. (Courtesy of R.J. Kurman, M.D., Baltimore, MD.)

Verruciform Xanthoma

Verruciform xanthoma is a benign lesion that clinically mimics a malignant tumor. It is a tumor of mucosal origin and is most commonly seen in oral cavity and, rarely, in anogenital mucosa as well as in the vulvar mucosa. Histologically, the lesion has verruciform hyperplasia with the expended dermal papillae/submucosa, which is filled with foamy histiocytes.[137] Patients with verruciform xanthoma may have autoimmune diseases.

Nevis Lipomatous Superficialis

This distinctive benign tumor of adipose tissue presents as a nodule within the dermis with normal overlying epithelium. This tumor has been considered a hamartoma of fat. Microscopic examination reveals adipose tissue within the superficial dermis, distinct from the underlying adipose tissue.

Superficial Angiomyxoma

Superficial angiomyxoma is not a well-recognized or widely accepted cutaneous tumor. Clinically, most cases present as papules, nodules, and polypoid lesions arising on the trunk, neck, and lower limbs. In a recent study of 39 patients, 2 patients had lesions located on the vulva. Histologically, this tumor is poorly circumscribed with focal lobular outline. Extensive myxoid stroma, numerous small blood vessels, varying cellularity, acellular mucin pools, stellate or bipolar fibroblasts, muciphages, and a sparse mixed inflammatory cell infiltrate are features of this tumor. Superficial angiomyxoma has a tendency for local recurrence.[30]

Lymphoid Hamartoma

A benign *lymphoid hamartoma* has been described, occurring in the subcutaneous tissue of the labia majora and presenting as a symptomatic subcutaneous cystic mass.[119] The histologic features include lymphoid tissue within an apparent fibrous capsule in the subcutaneous tissue. Unlike a lymph node, no adjacent lymphoid sinusoids are seen. A "whorled" appearance of the epithelioid-like lymphoid element within the mass resembles Hassle capuscles. Chronic anemia with associated hypergammaglobulinemia has been reported with benign lymphoid hamartoma occurring in other sites, but not within the female genital tract. Removal of the mass results in resolution of the laboratory findings. The lesion has a benign clinical course.

Nodular Fasciitis (Pseudosarcomatous Fasciitis, Proliferative Fasciitis)

Nodular fasciitis is not a neoplasm in the strict sense, but it may present as a mass that clinically, as well as pathologically, mimics a sarcoma. Nodular fasciitis may grow locally as a solid subcutaneous mass that may be attached to underlying tissues. The mass usually is solitary, sometimes tender, and may have been present for several years before medical assistance is sought. The histopathologic features of nodular fasciitis show spindle cell-like growth without encapsulation (Fig. 2.55). The mass may have a collagenous or myxoid matrix. Prominent capillaries and chronic inflammatory cells usually are present. Although mitotic figures may be common in the fibroblasts, abnormal mitoses are not seen. Some cytolysis usually is present. Heterologous elements, as well as giant cells, have been reported.[6,179] The mass may be infiltrative and involve muscle. In contrast to smooth muscle tumors, nodular fasciitis is negative for desmin and myoglobin[167] but may show a diffuse weak positivity for HHF-35.

Folliculosebaceous Cystic Hamartoma

Folliculosebaceous cystic hamartoma is a disorganized proliferation of pilosebaceous units that typi-

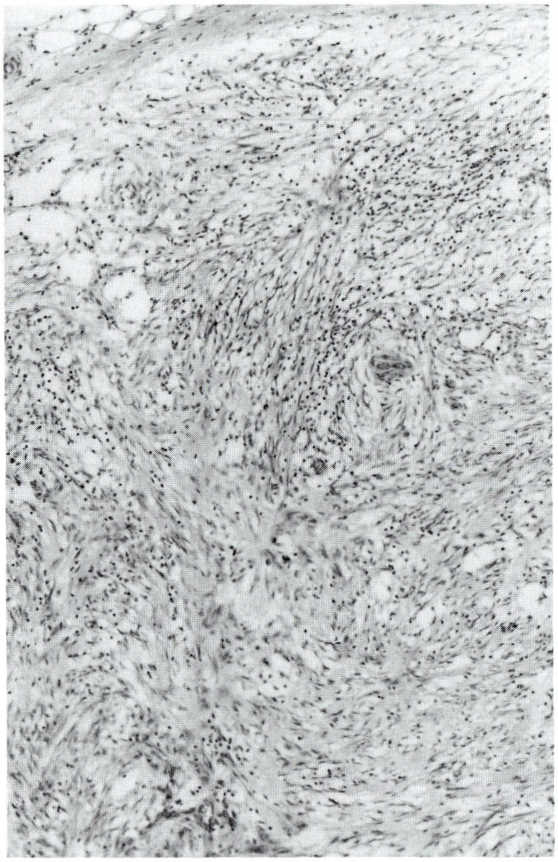

Fig. 2.55. Nodular fasciitis. This nonencapsulated mass is composed of spindle-shaped cells within a somewhat myxoid stroma. Prominent capillaries are within the mass and some lymphocytes are present. (Courtesy of David Dolson, M.D., Philadelphia, PA.)

cally affects the head, neck, and axilla and has been reported in the vulva. Clinically, the lesion presents as asymptomatic papules or nodules. Histologically, it has a central cystic space, lined by squamous epithelium. The cyst is surrounded by abnormally arranged hyperplastic sebaceous glands and fibrous stroma.[22]

Mammary-Like Tissue Within the Vulva

The findings of *mammary-like tissue* in the vulva is not well understood, but it is currently considered to be ectopic in nature.[252,253] Clinically, mammary-like tissue in the vulva may present as an amorphous enlargement of the labia, usually first noted in association with pregnancy.[253] Benign cystic disease (fibrocystic disease), as well as fibroadenomas, lactating adenomas, and intraductal papillomas, have been described.[253] Cystosarcoma phyloides arising in these mammary-like tissues of the vulva is rare (Figs. 2.56 and 2.57). Adenocarcinoma of the mammary-like tissue of the vulva has been reported.[117,253] Surgical removal of symptomatic mammary-like tissue is advocated except when such tissue is discovered during pregnancy, in which case therapy should be deferred until after puerperal regression is complete.

Salivary Glandlike Tissue

Salivary glandlike tissue has been observed in the vulva.[157]

Idiopathic Vulvar Calcinosis

Although not a cystic condition, *vulvar calcinosis* may resemble keratinous cysts on clinical presentation, presenting as small (usually 2 mm or less), firm, subcutaneous nodules involving the majora and fourchette. The vulvar cases reported have occurred predominantly in adolescent women. Histologic examination demonstrates normal-appearing overlying epithelium with basophilic acellular su-

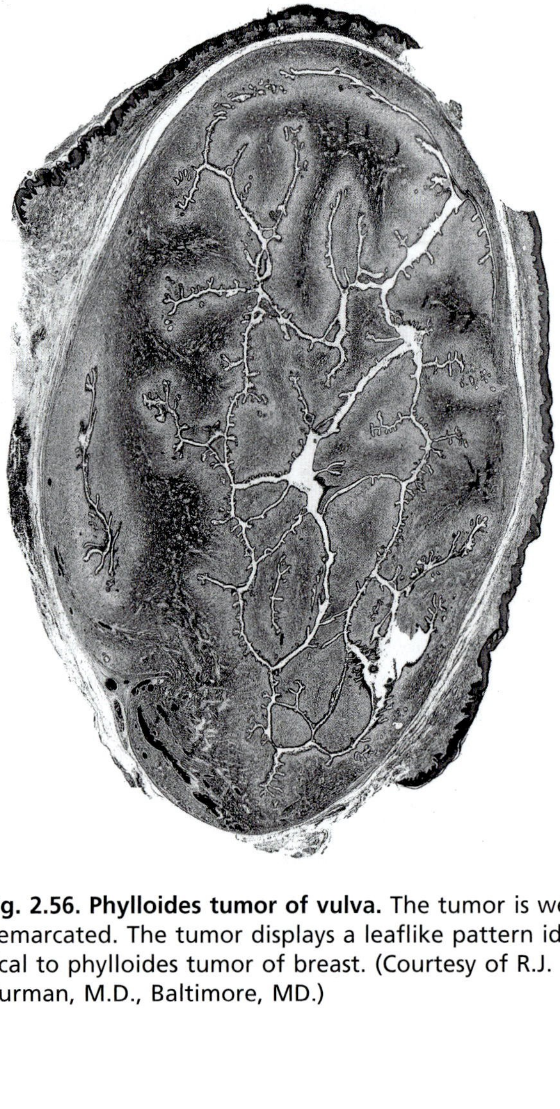

Fig. 2.56. Phylloides tumor of vulva. The tumor is well demarcated. The tumor displays a leaflike pattern identical to phylloides tumor of breast. (Courtesy of R.J. Kurman, M.D., Baltimore, MD.)

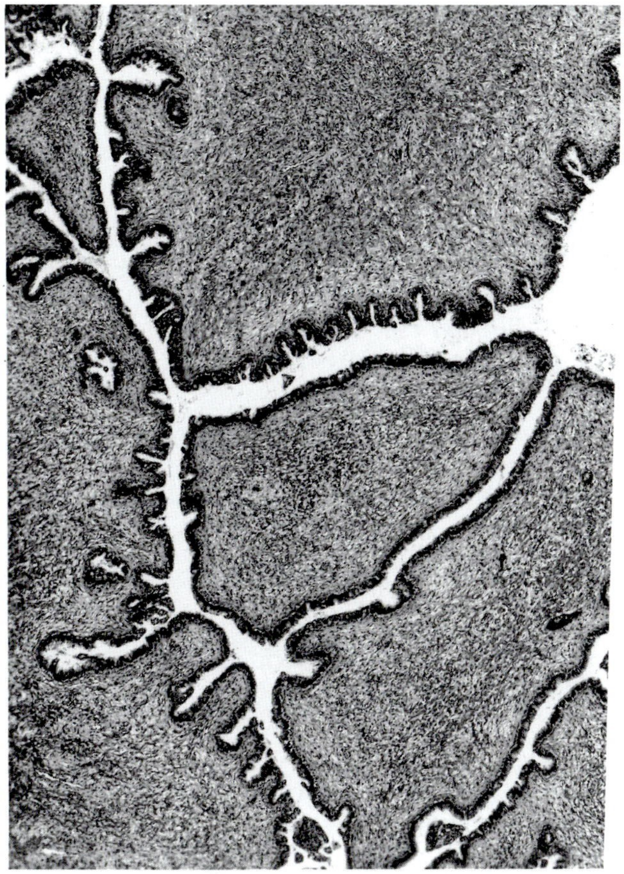

Fig. 2.57. Phylloides tumor of vulva. Marked stromal expansion with spindle cells and proliferation of epithelial cells forming papillary structures. (Courtesy of R.J. Kurman, M.D., Baltimore, MD.)

perficial subcutaneous nodules measuring from less than 0.1 mm to approximately 2 mm, associated with a chronic inflammatory infiltrate, mast cells, and foreign body giant cells. The acellular material stains with Von Kossa stain and contains acid mucopolysaccharides.[10] The process is rare, benign, and of uncertain etiology but appears similar to idiopathic scrotal calcinosis.[19]

Vulvar Amyloidosis

Nodules within the vulva have been described related to involvement of the vulva in a woman with systemic *amyloidosis*, which may mimic giant condyloma.

Benign Lesions of the Urethra

Urethra Prolapse

Prolapse of the urethral mucosa may occur at any age, but it is most common in premenarchal children and in postmenopausal women. Redundancy of the mucosa and laxity of the supporting periurethral fascia contribute to the formation of prolapse, which is aggravated by increased abdominal pressure; it may be related to relative lack of estrogen. The prolapsed urethra may present as a large red polypoid mass covered with urethral mucosa with edematous vascular submucosa, protruding from the urethra and mimicking a urethral neoplasm. Histologically, the urethral mucosa may exhibit ulceration, and the underlying connective tissue is generally filled with an inflammatory infiltrate. Vascular engorgement usually is present. Cryosurgery is an effective method of treatment.[113]

Urethral Caruncles

Caruncles are sessile or polypoid masses that arise at the urethral meatus in postmenopausal women. They may represent localized areas of prolapse, and are by far the most common lesions of the urethra. Caruncles often are asymptomatic but may cause bleeding or dysuria. Clinical differentiation from urethral carcinoma may be impossible; therefore, excision is indicated for diagnosis. Recurrences may be observed.[278] Histologically, the submucosa of the urethral caruncle may contain large venous channels that often are dilated and engorged. A myxomatous or granulomatous pattern may be present in the supporting tissue, which often is densely infiltrated with chronic inflammatory cells. Excision, with hemostatic control of the base of the lesion, is the treatment of choice.

Malacoplakia of the Urethra

Malacoplakia is a chronic granulomatous inflammatory process that usually involves the bladder if the urethra is involved. The lesion presents as a polypoid mass at the urethral meatus.

On microscopic examination the lesion contains foamy histiocytes, lymphocytes, granulocytes, and plasma cells. The diagnostic Michaelis–Gutmann bodies are seen within the cytoplasm of the histiocytes as inclusions having a blue-gray color (Fig. 2.58). The inclusions may appear laminated or targetoid. With PAS stains, the Michaelis–Gutmann bodies usually stain pink to red (see Chapter 4, Diseases of the Vagina). Many of the adjacent histiocytes also contain PAS-positive cytoplasmic material. Excision may be diagnostic and curative for small lesions within the urethra, although recurrences are not uncommon. Antibiotics also may be of value.

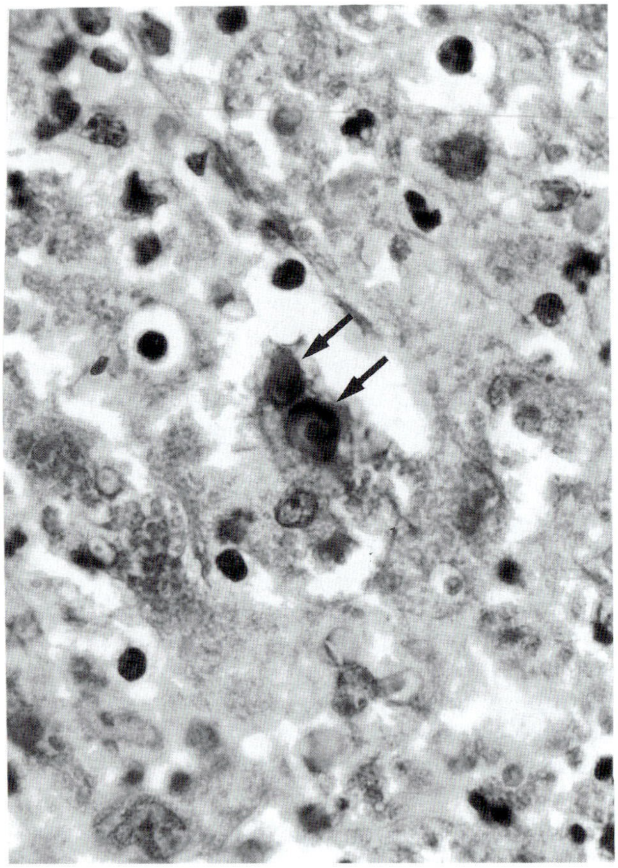

Fig. 2.58. Malacoplakia of the urethra. Round inclusions are present in some of the histiocytes (Michaelis–Gutmann bodies), which are approximately the size of the nuclei of the histiocytes and have a dark periphery and pale center. (Courtesy of R.J. Kurman, M.D., Baltimore, MD.)

Periurethral Cysts

Periurethral cysts can be subclassified according to their epithelial lining, and are similar to cysts of the vulvar vestibule. The cysts can be classified into four types: epithelial inclusion, mucous, mesonephric-like, and urothelial.

Epithelial Inclusion (Keratinous) Cysts

Epithelial inclusion cysts have a squamous epithelial lining, and may arise secondary to trauma or surgical procedures that entrap epithelium.

Mucous Cysts

Mucous cysts have a columnar, endocervical-type epithelial lining and may have associated squamous epithelium, secondary to squamous metaplasia. The cytoplasm of the columnar epithelium contains mucin. These cysts appear essentially identical to the mucous cysts of the vulvar vestibule, although they have been referred to as müllerian cysts.

Mesonephric-Like Cysts

Mesonephric-like cysts have a low cuboidal epithelium that does not stain with mucin.

Urothelial Cysts

Urothelial cysts usually are seen in infants and are rare in adults. They are believed to arise from the Skene ducts or from proximal urothelial ducts. These cysts have a urothelial epithelial lining, although those near the urethra meatus may have a squamous epithelial lining.

Suburethral Diverticulum

Suburethral diverticula originate from the upper two-thirds of the posterior urethral wall and may extend cephalic to involve the region beneath the vesicle neck. Although a congenital etiology has been proposed for some cases, most are thought to begin as an infection in one of the tubular periurethral glands, followed by abscess formation with eventual breakthrough into the urethral lumen.

Urethral Condyloma Acuminatum

Urethral condyloma acuminatum may present like a caruncle or urethral carcinoma, and usually is seen in women of reproductive age and not in older individuals. In children urethral and periurethral condylomata may be polypoid and clinically may suggest sarcoma botryoides. In adult women, they usually are associated with other lower genital infections, especially vulvar vestibular condyloma acuminatum. Some patients may have symptoms of urethritis associated with urethral condyloma acuminatum. In these patients, the condylomas may be in the mid- or upper urethra. On biopsy they have a stratified squamous epithelium within which typical features of mucosal HPV infection are seen, including koilocytosis, multinucleation, and parabasalar hyperplasia. HPV types 6 and 16 have been observed in urethral condylomas.

Leiomyoma of the Urethra

Urethral leiomyoma is a relatively rare, benign, smooth muscle tumor that may be associated with dysuria, hematuria, or infection; approximately one-half of the reported cases present as an external urethral mass. These tumors may enlarge in pregnancy, suggesting that they contain hormonal receptors. Microscopically, the tumor is composed of smooth muscle cells arranged in a whorled pattern. Malignant change has not been reported. Local excision is the treatment of choice and usually is curative.

References

1. Abdul-Karim FW, Cohen RE (1990) Atypical stromal cells of lower female genital tract. Histopathology 17:249–253
2. Ackerman AB, Mihara I (1985) Dysplasia, dysplastic melanocytes, dysplastic nevi, the dysplastic nevus syndrome, and the relation between dysplastic nevi and malignant melanomas. Hum Pathol 16:87–91
3. Adelson MD, Joret DM, Gordon LP, Osborne NG (1991) Recurrent necrotizing fasciitis of the vulva. A case report. J Reprod Med 36:818–822
4. Allen MV, Novotny DB (1997) Desmoid tumor of the vulva associated with pregnancy. Arch Pathol Lab Med 121:512–514
5. Ang P, Tay YK (1999) Treatment of linear IgA bullous dermatosis of childhood with colchicine. Pediatr Dermatol 16:50–52
6. Aranda FI, Laforga JB (1998) Nodular fasciitis of the vulva. Report of a case with immunohistochemical study. Pathol Res Pract 194:805–807
7. Arany I, Tyring SK (1996) Status of local cellular immunity in interferon-responsive and -nonresponsive human papillomavirus-associated lesions. Sex Transm Dis 23:475–480
8. Avinoach I, Zirfkin HJ, Glezerman M (1989) Proliferating trichilemmal tumor of the vulva. Case report and review of the literature. Int J Gynecol Pathol 8:163–168
9. Aziz DC, Ferre F, Robitaille J, Ferenczy A (1993) Human papillomavirus testing in the clinical laboratory. Part II: Vaginal, vulvar, perineal, and penile squamous lesions. J Gynecol Surg 9:9–15
10. Balfour FJT, Vincenti AC (1991) Idiopathic vulvar calcinosis. Histopathology (Oxf) 18:183–184
11. Balfour HH Jr (1991) Varicella-zoster virus infections in the immunocompromised host. Natural history and treatment. Scand J Infect Dis Suppl 80:69–74
12. Barnhill RL, Albert LS, Shama SK, Goldenhersh MA, Rhodes AR, Sober AJ (1990) Genital lentiginosis: a clinical and histopathologic study. J Am Acad Dermatol 22:453–460
13. Basbug M, Tayyar M, Erdogan N (1997) Fibroma of the vulva and uterine leiomyoma. Int J Gynaecol Obstet 59:55–56
14. Basoglu M, Gul O, Yildirgan I, Balik AA, Ozbey I, Oren D (1997) Fournier's gangrene: review of fifteen cases. Am Surg 63:1019–1021
15. Basta A, Madej JG Jr (1990) Hydradenoma of the vulva. Incidence and clinical observations. Eur J Gynecol Oncol 11:185–189
16. Batta K, Munday PE, Tatnall FM (1999) Pemphigus vulgaris localized to the vagina presenting as chronic vaginal discharge. Br J Dermatol 140: 945–947
17. Berger J, Telser A, Widschwendter M, Muller-Holzner E, Daxenbichler G, Marth C, Zeimet AG (2000) Expression of retinoic acid receptors in non-neoplastic epithelial disorders of the vulva and normal vulvar skin. Int J Gynecol Pathol 19:95–102
18. Bergeron C, Ferenczy A, Richart RM, Guralnick M (1990) Micropapillomatosis labialis appears unrelated to human papillomavirus. Obstet Gynecol 76:281–286
19. Bernardo BD, Huettner PC, Merritt DF, Ratts VS (1999) Idiopathic calcinosis cutis presenting as labial lesions in children: report of two cases with literature review. J Pediatr Adolesc Gynecol 12: 157–160
20. Berth-Jones J, Graham-Brown RA, Burns DA (1991) Lichen sclerosus et atrophicus: a review of 15 cases in young girls. Clin Exp Dermatol 16:14–17
21. Beutner KR, von Krogh G (1990) Current status of podophyllotoxin for the treatment of genital warts. Semin Dermatol 9:148–151
22. Bolognia JL, Longley BJ (1998) Genital variant of folliculosebaceous cystic hamartoma. Dermatology (Basel) 197:258–260
23. Bonafe JL, Thibaut I, Hoff J (1990) Introital adenosis associated with the Stevens-Johnson syndrome. Clin Exp Dermatol 15:356–357
24. Bonnez W, Oakes D, Bailey-Farchione A, Choi A, Hallahan D, Pappas P, Holloway M, Corey L, Barnum G, Dunne A, Stoler MH, Demeter LM, Reichman RC (1995) A randomized, double-blind, placebo-controlled trial of systemically administered interferon-alpha, -beta, or -gamma in combination with cryotherapy for the treatment of condyloma acuminatum. J Infect Dis 171:1081–1089
25. Bornstein J, Goldik Z, Alter Z, Zarfati D, Abra-movici H (1998) Persistent vulvar vestibulitis: the continuing challenge. Obstet Gynecol Surv 53:39–44
26. Brown DR, Bryan JT, Cramer H, Fife KH (1993) Analysis of human papillomavirus types in exophytic condylomata acuminata by hybrid capture and Southern blot techniques. J Clin Microbiol 31:2667–2673
27. Brown TJ, Yen-Moore A, Tyring SK (1999) An overview of sexually transmitted diseases. Part I. J Am Acad Dermatol 41:511–532
28. Buntin DM, Rosen T, Lesher JL Jr, Plotnick H, Brademas ME, Berger TG (1991) Sexually transmitted diseases: bacterial infections. Committee on Sexually Transmitted Diseases of the American Academy of Dermatology. J Am Acad Dermatol 25 (pt 1):287–299
29. Bystryn JC, Steinman NM (1996) The adjuvant therapy of pemphigus. An update. Arch Dermatol 132:203–212

30. Calonje E, Guerin D, McCormick D, Fletcher CD (1999) Superficial angiomyxoma: clinicopathologic analysis of a series of distinctive but poorly recognized cutaneous tumors with tendency for recurrence. Am J Surg Pathol 23:910–917
31. Carli P, Bracco G, Taddei G, Sonni L, De Marco A, Maestrini G, Cattaneo A (1994) Vulvar lichen sclerosus. Immunohistologic evaluation before and after therapy. J Reprod Med 39:110–114
32. Carli P, Cattaneo A, Pimpinelli N, Cozza A, Bracco G, Giannotti B (1991) Immunohistochemical evidence of skin immune system involvement in vulvar lichen sclerosus et atrophicus.Dermatologica (Basel) 182:18–22
33. Carlson JA, Grabowski R, Chichester P, Paunovich E, Malfetano J. (2000) Comparative immunophenotypic study of lichen sclerosus epidermotrophic $CD57^+$ lymphocytes are numerous–implications for pathogenesis. Am J Dermatopathol. 22(1):7–16.
34. Carlson JA, Ambros R, Malfetano J, Ross J, Grabowski R, Lamb P, Figge H, Mihm MC Jr (1998) Vulvar lichen sclerosus and squamous cell carcinoma: a cohort, case control, and investigational study with historical perspective; implications for chronic inflammation and sclerosis in the development of neoplasia. Hum Pathol 29:932–948
35. Carlson JA, Lamb P, Malfetano J, Ambros RA, Mihm MC Jr (1998) Clinicopathologic comparison of vulvar and extragenital lichen sclerosus: histologic variants, evolving lesions, and etiology of 141 cases. Mod Pathol 11:844–854
36. Carter J, Elliott P (1990) Syringoma—an unusual cause of pruritus vulvae. Aust N Z J Obstet Gynaecol 30:382–383
37. Carter J, Elliott P, Russell P (1992) Bilateral fibroepithelial polypi of labium minus with atypical stromal cells. Pathology 24:37–39
38. Cattaneo A, Bracco GL, Maestrini G, Carli P, Taddei GH, Colafranceschi M, Marchionni M. (1991) Lichen sclerosus and squamous hyperplasia of the vulva. A clinical study of medical treatment. J Reprod Med 36:301–305
39. Cecchi R, Bartoli L, Brunetti L, Pavesi M, Giomi A (1995) Lymphangioma circumscriptum of the vulva of late onset. Acta Dermato-Venereol 75:79–80
40. Chadha S, Gianotten WL, Drogendijk AC, Weijmar Schultz WC, Blindeman LA, van der Meijden WI (1998) Histopathologic features of vulvar vestibulitis. Int J Gynecol Pathol 17:7–11
41. Chetkowski R, Sakamoto H, MacLusky N, Merino M, Schwartz PE (1985) Solitary pelvic neural tumors with high steroid receptor content. Gynecol Oncol 20:43–52
42. Chiasson MA, Ellerbrock TV, Bush TJ, Sun XW, Wright TC Jr (1997) Increased prevalence of vulvovaginal condyloma and vulvar intraepithelial neoplasia in women infected with the human immunodeficiency virus. Obstet Gynecol 89(pt 1): 690–694
43. Cho D, Woodruff JD (1988) Trichoepithelioma of the vulva. A report of two cases. J Reprod Med 33: 317–319
44. Chosidow O (2000) Scabies and pediculosis. Lancet 355:819–826
45. Christensen WN, Friedman KJ, Woodruff JD, Hood AF (1987) Histologic characteristics of vulvar nevocellular nevi. J Cutan Pathol 14:87–91
46. Cilla G, Pico F, Peris A, Idigoras P, Urbieta M, Perez-Trallero E (1992) Human genital myiasis due to *Sarcophaga*. Rev Clin Esp 190:189–190
47. Clark WH Jr, Hood AF, Tucker MA, Jampel RM (1998) Atypical melanocytic nevi of the genital type with a discussion of reciprocalparenchymal-stromal interactions in the biology of neoplasia. Hum Pathol 29(suppl 1):S1–S24
48. Cockayne SE, Rassl DM, Thomas SE (2000) Squamous cell carcinoma arising in Hailey-Hailey disease of the vulva. Br J Dermatol 142:540–542
49. Cockerell CJ, LeBoit EP (1990) Bacillary angiomatosis: a newly characterized, pseudoneoplastic, infectious, cutaneous vascular disorder. J Am Acad Dermatol 22:501–512
50. Coghill SB, Tyler X, Shaxted EJ (1990) Benign mucinous metaplasia of the vulva. Histopathology (Oxf) 17:373–375
51. Cohen PR, Young AW Jr, Tovell HM (1989) Angiokeratoma of the vulva: diagnosis and review of the literature. Obstet Gynecol Surv 44:339–346
52. Cone R, Beckmann A, Aho M, Wahlstrom T, Ek M, Corey L, Paavonen J (1991) Subclinical manifestations of vulvar human papillomavirus infection. Int J Gynecol Pathol 10:26–35
53. Congilosi SM, Madoff RD (1995) Current therapy for recurrent and extensive anal warts. Dis Colon Rectum 38:1101–1107
54. Cooper PH (1989) Acantholytic dermatosis localized to the vulvocrural area. J Cutan Pathol 16:81–84
55. Coyle PV, Desai A, Wyatt D, McCaughey C, O'Neill HJ (1999) A comparison of virus isolation, indirect immunofluorescence and nested multiplex polymerase chain reaction for the diagnosis of primary and recurrent herpes simplex type 1 and type 2 infections. J Virol Methods 83:75–82
56. Dalziel KL, Mallard R, Wojnarowska F (1991) The treatment of vulvar lichen sclerosus with very potent topical steroid (clobetasol propionate 0.05% cream). Br J Dermatol 124:461–464
57. de Deus JM, Focchi J, Stavale JN, de Lima GR (1995) Histologic and biomolecular aspects of papillomatosis of the vulvar vestibule in relation to human papillomavirus. Obstet Gynecol 86:758–763
58. Della Torre G, Donghi R, Longoni A, Pilotti S, Pasquini G, De Palo G, Pierotti MA, Rilke F, Della Porta G (1992) HPV DNA in intraepithelial neoplasia and carcinoma of the vulva and penis. Diagn Mol Pathol 1:25–30
59. Derksen DJ (1992) Children with condylomata acuminata. J Fam Pract 34:419–423

60. Dickens P, Srivastava G, Loke SL, Larkin S (1991) Human papillomavirus 6, 11, and 16 in laryngeal papillomas. J Pathol 165(3):243–246
61. Dungar CF, Wilkinson EJ (1995) Vaginal columnar cell metaplasia. An acquired adenosis associated with topical 5-fluorouracil therapy. J Reprod Med 40:361–366
62. Edwards L (1992) Desquamative vulvitis. Dermatol Clin 10:325–337
63. Edwards L, Hansen RC (1992) Reiter's syndrome of the vulva. The psoriasis spectrum. Arch Dermatol 128:811–814
64. Egan CA, Zone JJ (1999) Linear IgA bullous dermatosis. Int J Dermatol 38:818–827
65. Egawa K, Honda Y, Ono T (1995) Multiple giant molluscum contagiosa with cyst formation. Am J Dermatopathol 17(4):414–416
66. Elchalal U, Lifschitz-Mercer B, Dgani R, Zalel Y (1992) Aggressive angiomyxoma of the vulva. Gynecol Oncol 47:260–262
67. Elchalal U, Gilead L, Vardy DA, Ben-shachar I, Anteby SO, Schenker JG (1995) Treatment of vulvar lichen sclerosus in the elderly: an update. Obstet Gynecol Surv 50:155–162
68. Kirkham N (1997) Tumors and cysts of the epidermis. In: Elder D, Elenitsas R, Jaworsky C, B Johnson Jr (eds) Lever's histopathology of the skin, 8th Ed. Lippincott-Raven, Philadelphia, pp 685–746
69. Elgart ML (1992) Sexually transmitted diseases of the vulva. Dermatol Clin 10:387–403
70. Epstein WL (1992) Molluscum contagiosum. Semin Dermatol 11:184–189
71. Ergeneli MH, Demirhan B, Duran EH (1999) Desmoid tumor of the vulva. A case report. J Reprod Med 44:748–750
72. Estrada R, Kaufman R (1993) Benign vulvar melanosis. J Reprod Med 38:5–8
73. Faber K, Jones MA, Spratt D, Tarraza HM Jr (1991) Vulvar leiomyomatosis in a patient with esophagogastric leiomyomatosis: review of the syndrome. Gynecol Oncol 41:92–94
74. Ferenczy A, Mitao M, Nagai N, Silverstein SJ, Crum CP (1985) Latent papillomavirus and recurring genital warts. N Engl J Med 313:784–788
75. Fletcher JL Jr (1991) Perinatal transmission of human papillomavirus. Am Fam Physician 43:143–148
76. Fletcher CD, Tsang WY, Fisher C, Lee KC, Chan JK (1992) Angiomyofibroblastoma of the vulva: a benign neoplasm distinct from aggressive angiomyxoma. Am J Surg Pathol 16:373–382
77. Friedmann W, Schafer A, Kretschmer R, Lobeck H (1991) Disseminated cytomegalovirus infection of the female genital tract. Gynecol Obstet Invest 31:56–77
78. Friedrich EG Jr, Wilkinson EJ (1973) Mucous cysts of the vulvar vestibule. Obstet Gynecol 42:407–414
79. Friedrich EG Jr (1987) Vulvar vestibulitis syndrome. J Reprod Med 32:110–114
80. Frith P, Charnock M, Wojnarowska F (1991) Cicatricial pemphigoid diagnosed from ocular features in recurrent severe vulvae scarring. Two case reports. Br J Obstet Gynecol 98:482–484
81. Galloway DA, McDougall JK (1990) Alterations in the cellular phenotype induced by herpes simplex viruses. J Med Virol 31:36–42.
82. Gately LE III, Nesbitt LT Jr (1994) Update on immunofluorescent testing in bullous diseases and lupus erythematosus. Review. Dermatol Clin 12: 133–142
83. Gentile G, Formelli G, Pelusi G, Flamigni C (1997) Is vestibular micropapillomatosis associated with human papillomavirus infection? Eur J Gynaecol Oncol 18:523–525
84. Gilbey S, Moore DH, Look KY, Sutton GP (1997) Vulvar keratoacanthoma. Obstet Gynecol 89(pt 2):848–850.
85. Gilks CB, Clement PB, Wood WS (1989) Trichoblastic fibroma. A clinicopathologic study of three cases. Am J Dermatopathol 11:397–402
86. Gissmann L, deVillers EM, Zur Hausen H (1982) Analysis of human warts (condylomata acuminata) and other genital tumors for human papilloma virus type 6 DNA. Int J Cancer 29:143–146
87. Gissmann L, Wolnik L, Ikenberg H, Koldovsky V, Schnurch HG, Zur Hausen H (1983) Human papillomavirus types 6 and 11 DNA sequences in genital and laryngeal papillomas and in some cervical cancers. Proc Natl Acad Sci USA 80:560–563
88. Gittes RF, Nakamura RM (1996) Female urethral syndrome. A female prostatitis? West J Med 164:435–438
89. Glazer HI, Rodke G, Swencionis C, Hertz R, Young AW (1995) Treatment of vulvar vestibulitis syndrome with electromyographic biofeedback of pelvic floor musculature. J Reprod Med 40:283–290
90. Glusac EJ, Hendrickson MS, Smoller BR (1994) Apocrine cystadenoma of the vulva. J Am Acad Dermatol 31(pt 1):498–499
91. Godeau G, Frances C, Hornebeck W, Brechemier D, Robert L (1982) Isolation and partial characterization of an elastase-type protease in human vulva fibroblasts: its possible involvement in vulvar elastic tissue destruction of patients with lichen sclerosus et atrophicus. J Invest Dermatol 78:270–275
92. Goldberg JM, Buchler DA, Dibbell DG (1996) Advanced hidradenitis suppurativa presenting with bilateral vulvar masses. Gynecol Oncol 60:494–497
93. Groisser DS, Griffiths CE, Ellis CN, Voorhees JJ (1991) A review and update of the clinical uses of cyclosporine in dermatology. Dermatol Clin 9:805 –817
94. Guerrieri C, Ohlsson E, Ryden G, Westermark P (1995) Vulvitis granulomatosa: a cryptogenic chronic inflammatory hypertrophy of vulvar labia related to cheilitis granulomatosa and Crohn's disease. Int J Gynecol Pathol 14:352–359
95. Hackel H, Hartmann AA, Burg G (1991) Vulvitis granulomatosa and anoperineitis granulomatosa. Dermatologica (Basel) 182:128—131

96. Haley JC, Mirowski GW, Hood AF (1998) Benign vulvar tumors. Semin Cutan Med Surg 17:196–204
97. Handsfield HH (1997) Clinical presentation and natural course of anogenital warts. Am J Med 102(5A):16–20
98. Hanly MG, Ojeda VJ (1995) Epidermal inclusion cysts of the clitoris as a complication of female circumcision and pharaonic infibulation. Cent Afr J Med 41:22–24
99. Helm KF, Gibson LE, Muller SA (1991) Lichen sclerosus et atrophicus in children and young adults. Pediatr Dermatol 8:97–101.
100. Hopkins-Luna AM, Chambers DC, Goodman MD (1999) Epithelioid leiomyoma of the vulva. J Natl Med Assoc 91:171–173
101. Horowitz IR, Copas P, Majmudar B (1995) Granular cell tumors of the vulva. Am J Obstet Gynecol 173:1710–1713
102. Huang HJ, Yamabe T, Tagawa H (1983) A solitary neurilemmoma of the clitoris. Gynecol Oncol 15:103–110
103. Ishiko A, Shimizu H, Masunaga T, Yancey KB, Giudice GJ, Zone JJ, Nishikawa T (1998) 97-kDa linear IgA bullous dermatosis antigen localizes in the lamina lucida between the NC16A and carboxyl terminal domains of the 180 kDa bullous pemphigoid antigen. J Invest Dermatol 111:93–96
104. Iversen T, Aas M (1983) Lymph drainage from the vulva. Gynecol Oncol 16:179–189
105. Iwasaki T, Sata T, Sugase M, Sato Y, Kurata T, Suzuki K, Ohmoto H, Iwamoto S (1992) Detection of capsid antigen of human papillomavirus (HPV) in benign lesions of female genital tract using anti-HPV monoclonal antibody. J Pathol 168:293–300
106. Jemec GB (1999) Long-term results of isotretinoin in the treatment of 68 patients with hidradenitis suppurativa. J Am Acad Dermatol 41:658
107. Jha PK, Beral V, Peto J, Hack S, Hermon C, Deacon J, Mant D, Chilvers C, Vessey MP, Pike MC (1993) Antibodies to human papillomavirus and to other genital infectious agents and invasive cervical cancer risk. Lancet 341:1116–1118
108. Johnson TL, Kennedy AW, Segal GH (1991) Lymphangioma circumscriptum of the vulva. A report of two cases. J Reprod Med 36:808–812
109. Junaid TA, Thomas SM (1981) Cysts of the vulva and vagina: a comparative study. Int J Gynecol Obstet 19:239–243
110. Kamarashev JA, Vassileva SG (1997) Dermatologic diseases of the vulva. Clin Dermatol 15:53–65
111. Kanekura T, Kanda A, Higo A, Kanzaki T (1996) Multiple milia localized to the vulva. J Dermatol 23:427–428
112. Kang IK, Kim YJ, Choi KC (1995) Ciliated cyst of the vulva. J Am Acad Dermatol 32:514–515
113. Kaufman RH (1994) Benign diseases of the vulva and vagina, 4th Ed. Mosby-Year Book, St. Louis
114. Kearse WS Jr, Ritchey ML (1993) Clitoral enlargement secondary to neurofibromatosis. Clin Pediatr (Phila) 32:303–304
115. Kellogg ND, Parra JM (1991) Linea vestibularis: a previously undescribed normal genital structure in female neonates. Pediatrics 87:926–929
116. Kellogg ND, Parra JM (1993) Linea vestibularis: follow-up of a normal genital structure. Pediatrics 92: 453–456
117. Kennedy DA, Hermina MS, Xanos ET, Schink JC, Hafez GR (1997) Infiltrating ductal carcinoma of the vulva. Pathol Res Pract 193:723–726
118. Kent HL, Wisniewski PM (1990) Interferon for vulvar vestibulitis. J Reprod Med 35:1138–1140
119. Kernen JA, Morgan ML (1970) Benign lymphoid hamartoma of the vulva. Obstet Gynecol 35:290–292
120. Khan IU, Bhol KC, Ahmed AR (1999) Linear IgA bullous dermatosis in a patient with chronic renal failure: response to intravenous immunoglobulin therapy. J Am Acad Dermatol 40:485–848
121. Klein PA, Appel J, Callen JP (1998) Sarcoidosis of the vulva: a rare cutaneous manifestation. J Am Acad Dermatol 39(pt 1):281–283
122. Klein PA, Callen JP (2000) Drug-induced linear IgA bullous dermatosis after vancomycin discontinuance in a patient with renal insufficiency. J Am Acad Dermatol 42(pt 2):316–323
123. Klutke JJ, Bergman A (1995) Interferon as an adjuvant treatment for genital condyloma acuminatum. Int J Gynaecol Obstet 49:171–174
124. Knudson AG (1985) Hereditary cancer oncogenes, and antioncogenes. Cancer Res 45:1437–1443
125. Koffa M, Koumantakis E, Ergazaki M, Tsatsanis C, Spandidos DA (1995) Association of herpesvirus infection with the development of genital cancer. Int J Cancer 63:58–62
126. Kondi-Paphitis A, Deligeorgi-Politi H, Liapis A, Plemenou-Frangou M (1998) Human papilloma virus in verrucus carcinoma of the vulva: an immunopathological study of the cases. Eur J Gynaecol Oncol 19:319–320
127. Koranantakul O, Lekhakula A, Wansit R, Koranantakul Y (1991) Cutaneous myiasis of vulva caused by the muscoid fly (*Chrysomyia* genus). Southeast Asian J Trop Med Public Health 22:458–460
128. Korman NJ (1998) Bullous pemphigoid. The latest in diagnosis, prognosis, and therapy. Arch Dermatol 134(9):1137–1141
129. Korman NJ (2000) New and emerging therapies in the treatment of blistering diseases. Dermatol Clin 18:127–137, ix–x
130. Koutsky LA, Stevens CE, Holmes KK, Ashley RL, Kiviat NB, Critchlow CW, Corey L (1992) Underdiagnosis of genital herpes by current clinical and viral isolation procedures. N Engl J Med 326:1533–1539
131. Krantz KE (1958) Innervation of the human vulva and vagina. Obstet Gynecol 12:382
132. Kulski JK, Demeter T, Rakoczy P, Sterrett GF, Pixley EC (1989) Human papillomavirus coinfections of the vulva and uterine cervix. J Med Virol 27:244–251

133. Kurzrock R, Cohen PR (1995) Cutaneous paraneoplastic syndromes in solid tumors. Am J Med 99: 662–671
134. LaGuardia KD, White MH, Saigo PE, Hoda S, McGuinness K, Ledger WJ (1995) Genital ulcer disease in women infected with human immunodeficiency virus. Am J Obstet Gynecol 172(pt 1):553–562
135. Lehtinen M, Hakama M, Aaran RK, Aromaa A, Knekt P, Leinikki P, Maatela J, Peto R, Teppo L (1992) Herpes simplex virus type 2 infection and cervical cancer: a prospective study of 12 years of follow-up in Finland. Cancer Causes Control 3:333–338
136. Leibowitch M, Neill S, Pelisse M, Moyal-Baracco M (1990) The epithelial changes associated with squamous cell carcinoma of the vulva: a review of the clinical, histological and viral findings of 78 women. Br J Obstet Gynaecol 97:1135–1139
137. Leong FJ, Meredith DJ (1998) Verruciform xanthoma of the vulva. A case report. Pathol Res Pract 194:661–665; 666–667
138. Lewis FM, Lewis-Jones MS, Toon PG, Rollason TP (1992) Neurofibromatosis of the vulva. Br J Dermatol 127:540–541
139. Lewis FM (1998) Vulval lichen planus. Br J Dermatol 138:569–575
140. Li J, Ackerman AB (1994) "Seborrheic keratoses" that contain human papillomavirus are condylomata acuminata. Am J Dermatopathol 16:398–405
141. LiVolsi VA, Brooks JJ (1987) Soft tissue tumors of the vulva. In: Wilkinson EJ (ed) Contemporary issues in surgical pathology. Pathology of the vulva and vagina, vol 9. Churchill Livingstone, New York, pp 209–238
142. Loening-Baucke V (1991) Lichen sclerosus et atrophicus in children. Am J Dis Child 145:1058–1061
143. Lorenz B, Kaufman RH, Kutzner SK (1998) Lichen sclerosus. Therapy with clobetasol propionate. J Reprod Med 43:790–794
144. Luesley DM (ed) (1999) Cancer and pre-cancer of the vulva. Oxford University Press, New York
145. Maccato ML, Kaufman RH (1992) Herpes genitalis. Dermatol Clin 10:415–422
146. Mann MS, Kaufman RH (1991) Erosive lichen planus of the vulva. Clin Obstet Gynecol 34:605–613
147. Magrina JR, Masterson BJ (1981) Loxosceles reclusa spider bite: a consideration in the differential diagnosis of chronic, nonmalignant ulcers of the vulva. Am J Obstet Gynecol 140:341–343
148. Mahmud N, Kusuda N, Ichinose S, Gyotoku Y, Nakajima H, Ishimaru T, Yamabe J (1992) Needle aspiration biopsy of vulvar endometriois. A case report. Acta Cytol 36:514–516
149. Majmudar B, Castellano PZ, Wilson RW, Siegel RJ (1990) Granular cell tumors of the vulva. J Reprod Med 35:1008–1014
150. Mann MS, Kaufman RH (1991) Erosive lichen planus of the vulva. Clin Obstet Gynecol 34:605–613
151. Mann MS, Kaufman RH, Brown D, Adam E (1992) Vulvar vestibulitis: significant clinical variables and treatment outcome. Obstet Gynecol 79:122–125
152. Marinoff SC, Turner MLC (1991) Vulvar vestibulitis syndrome: an overview. Am J Obstet Gynecol 165:1228–1233
153. Marinoff SC, Turner ML (1992) Vulvar vestibulitis syndrome. Dermatol Clin 10:435–444
154. Marks TA, Shroyer KR, Markham NE, Slocumb JC, Gibbs RS (1995) A clinical, histologic, and DNA study of vulvodynia and its association with humanpapillomavirus. J Soc Gynecol Invest 2:57–63
155. Marquette GP, Su B, Woodruff JD (1985) Introital adenosis associated with Stevens-Johnson syndrome. Obstet Gynecol 66:143–145
156. Marren P, Wojnarowska F (1996) Dermatitis of the vulva. Semin Dermatol 15:6–41
157. Marwah S, Bergman ML (1980) Ectopic salivary gland in the vulva (choristoma): report of a case and review of the literature. Obstet Gynecol 56:389–391
158. McKay M, Frankman O, Horowitz B, Lecart C, Micheletti L, Ridley CM, Turner ML, Woodruff JD (1991) Vulvar vestibulitis and vestibular papillomatosis. Report of the ISSVD Committee on vulvodynia. J Reprod Med 36:413–415
159. McKee PH, Marsden RA, Santa Cruz DJ (1996) Pathology of the skin: with clinical correlations, 2nd Ed. Mosby-Wolfe, London, pp 4.1–4.80
160. McNeely TB (1992) Angiokeratoma of the clitoris. Arch Pathol Lab Med 116:880–881
161. Mihara M (1991) Three-dimensional ultrastructural study of molluscum contagiosum in the skin using scanning-electron microscopy. Br J Dermatol 125:557–560
162. Mihara Y, Mihara M, Hagari Y, Shimao S (1994) Lichen sclerosus et atrophicus. A histological, immunohistochemical and electron microscopic study. Arch Dermatol Res 286:434–442
163. Milbrath JR, Wilkinson EJ, Friedrich EG Jr (1975) Xerographic evaluation of radical vulvectomy specimens. Am J Roentgenol Radiat Ther Nucl Med (AJR) 125:486–488
164. Mindel A (ed) (1995) Genital warts: human papillomavirus infection. Arnold, London.
165. Monk BE (1993). Fordyce spots responding to isotretinoin therapy. Br J Dermatol 129:355
166. Monsonego J, Valensi P, Zerat L, Clavel C, Birembaut P (1997) Simultaneous effects of aneuploidy and oncogenic human papillomavirus on histological grade of cervical intraepithelial neoplasia. Br J Obstet Gynaecol 104:723–727
167. Montgomery EA, Meis JM (1991) Nodular fasciitis. Its morphologic spectrum and immunohistochemical profile. Am J Surg Pathol 15:942–948
168. Moreland AA (1994) Vulvar manifestations of sexually transmitted diseases. Semin Dermatol 13:262–268
169. Morse SA, Moreland AA, Holmes KK (1996) Atlas of sexually transmitted diseases and AIDS, 2nd Ed. Mosby-Wolfe, London
170. Moschella SL, Hurley HJ (1992) Dermatology, 3rd Ed. Saunders, Philadelphia
171. Moyal-Barracco M, Leibowitch M, Orth G (1990) Vestibular papillae of the vulva. Lack of evidence

for human papillomavirus etiology. Arch Dermatol 126:1594–1598
172. Mullins DL, Wilkinson EJ (1994) Pathology of the vulva and vagina. Curr Opin Obstet Gynecol 6: 351–358
173. Multhaupt HA, Rafferty PA, Warhol MJ (1992) Ultrastructural localization of human papilloma virus by nonradioactive in situ hybridization on tissue of human cervical intraepithelial neoplasia. Lab Invest 67:512–518
174. Nettina SM (1998) Herpes genitalis. Lippincotts Prim Care Pract 2:303–306
175. Neubert AG, Golden MA, Rose NC (1995) Kasabach-Merritt coagulopathy complicating Klippel-Trenaunay-Weber syndrome in pregnancy. Obstet Gynecol 85(pt 2):831–833
1776. Newland JR, Fusaro RM (1991) Mucinous cysts of the vulva. Nebr Med J 76:307–310
177. Nishi T (1998) Lymphangioma of the labia minora with deep lymphatic involvement. Br J Obstet Gynaecol 105:926–927
178. Obalek S, Misiewicz J, Jablonska S, Favre M, Orth G (1993) Childhood condyloma acuminatum: association with genital and cutaneous human papillomaviruses. Pediatr Dermatol 10:101–106
179. O'Connell JX, Young RH, Nielsen GP, Rosenberg AE, Bainbridge TC, Clement PB (1997) Nodular fasciitis of the vulva: a study of six cases and literature review. Int J Gynecol Pathol 16:117–123
180. Ogunbiyi OA, Scholefield JH, Robertson G, Smith JH, Sharp F, Rogers K (1994) Anal human papillomavirus infection and squamous neoplasia in patients with invasive vulvar cancer. Obstet Gynecol 83:212–216
181. Olansky S (1972) Serodiagnosis of syphilis. Med Clin North Am 56:1145–1150
182. Olivry T, Moore PF, Affolter VK, Naydan DK (1996) Langerhans cell hyperplasia and IgE expression in canine atopic dermatitis. Arch Dermatol Res 288:579–585
183. O'Rahilly R, Müller F (1996) Human embryology & teratology, 2nd Ed. Wiley-Liss, New York
184. Ordonez NG, Manning JT, Luna MA (1981) Mixed tumor of the vulva: a report of two cases probably arising in Bartholin's gland. Cancer (Phila) 48:181–186
185. Oriel JD (1990) Identification of people at high risk of genital HPV infections. Scand J Infect Dis Suppl 69:169–172
186. Orle KA, Gates CA, Martin DH, Body BA, Weiss JB (1996) Simultaneous PCR detection of *Haemophilus ducreyi*, *Treponema pallidum*, and herpes simplex virus types 1 and 2 from genital ulcers. J Clin Microbiol 34:49–54
187. Ortiz-Hidalgo C, de la Vega G, Moreno-Collado C (1997) Granular cell tumor (Abrikossoff tumor) of the clitoris. Int J Dermatol 36:935–937
188. Patton LW, Elgart ML, Williams CM (1990) Vulvar erythema and induration. Extraintestinal Crohn's disease of the vulva. Arch Dermatol 126:1351–1354
189. Pelisse M (1996) Erosive vulvar lichen planus and desquamative vaginitis. Semin Dermatol 15:47–50
190. Pelosi G, Martignoni G, Bonetti F (1991) Intraductal carcinoma of mammary-type apocrine epithelium arising within a papillary hidradenoma of the vulva. Report of a case and review of the literature. Arch Pathol Lab Med 115:1249–1254
191. Perry CM, Faulds D (1996) Valaciclovir. A review of its antiviral activity, pharmacokinetic properties and therapeutic efficacy in herpesvirus infections. Drugs 52:754–772
192. Peters WA III (1998) Bartholinitis after vulvovaginal surgery. Am J Obstet Gynecol 178:1143–1144
193. Pierson KK (1987) Malignant melanomas and pigmented lesions of the vulva. In: Wilkinson EJ (ed) Contemporary issues in surgical pathology. Pathology of the vulva and vagina, vol 9. Churchill Livingstone, New York, pp 155–179
194. Pincus SH, Stadecker MJ (1987) Vulvar dystrophies and noninfectious inflammatory conditions. In: Wilkinson EJ (ed) Contemporary issues in surgical pathology. Pathology of the vulva and vagina, vol 9. Churchill Livingstone, New York, pp 11–24
195. Pincus SH (1992) Vulvar dermatoses and pruritus vulva. Dermatol Clin 10:297–308
196. Pollack IF, Mulvihill JJ (1997) Neurofibromatosis 1 and 2. Brain Pathol 7:823–836
197. Powell FC, Su WP, Perry HO (1996) Pyoderma gangrenosum: classification and management. J Am Acad Dermatol 34:395–409; 410–412
198. Powell JJ, Wojnarowska F (1999) Lichen sclerosus. Lancet 353:1777–1183
199. Prayson RA, Stoler MH, Hart WR (1995) Vulvar vestibulitis. A histopathologic study of 36 cases, including human papillomavirus in situ hybridization analysis. Am J Surg Pathol 19:154–160
200. Pulimood S, Ajithkumar K, Jacob M, George S, Chandi SM (1997) Linear IgA bullous dermatosis of childhood: treatment with dapsone and co-trimoxazole. Clin Exp Dermatol 22:90–91
201. Pyka RE, Wilkinson EJ, Friedrich EG Jr, Croker BP (1988) The histopathology of vulvar vestibulitis syndrome. Int J Gynecol Pathol 7:249–257
202. Quan MB, Moy RL (1991) The role of human papillomavirus in carcinoma. J Am Acad Dermatol 25: 698–705
203. Ramesh V, Iyengar B (1990) Proliferating trichilemmal cysts over the vulva. Cutis 45:87–189
204. Ranalletta M, Rositto A, Drut R (1996) Fox-Fordyce disease in two prepubertal girls: histopathologic demonstration of eccrine sweat gland involvement. Pediatr Dermatol 13:294–297
205. Reed JA, Brigati DJ, Flynn SD, McNutt NS, Min K, Welch DF, Slater LN (1992) Immunocytochemical identification of *Rochalimaea henselae* in bacillary (epithelioid) angiomatosis, parenchymal bacillary peliosis, and persistent fever with bacteremia. Am J Surg Pathol 16:650–657
206. Requena L, Kiryu H, Ackerman AB (1998) Series: Ackerman's histologic diagnosis of neoplastic skin diseases: neoplasms with apocrine differentiation, with analogues in the breast by Darryl Carter. Lippincott-Raven, Philadelphia, pp 9–28

207. Rhodes AR, Mihm MC Jr, Weinstock MA (1989) Dysplastic melanocytic nevi. A reproducible histologic definition emphasizing cellular morphology. Mod Pathol 2:306–319
208. Richens J (1991) The diagnosis and treatment of donovanosis (granuloma inguinale). Genitourin Med 67:441–452
209. Ridley CM, Neill SM (1999) Non-infective cutaneous conditions of vulva. In: Ridley CM, Neill SM (eds) The vulva, 2nd Ed. Blackwell, Oxford, pp 121–186
210. Ridley CM, Neill SM (1999) The vulva, 2nd Ed. Blackwell, Oxford, pp 1–36
211. Rihet S, Lorenzato M, Clavel C (1996) Oncogenic human papillomaviruses and ploidy in cervical lesions. J Clin Pathol 49:892–896
212. Robboy SJ, Ross JS, Prat J, Keh PC, Welch WR (1978) Urogenital sinus origin of mucinous and ciliated cysts of the vulva. Obstet Gynecol 51:347–351
213. Robinson JB, Im DD, Simmons-O'Brien E, Rosenshein NB (1998) Etretinate: therapy for plasma cell vulvitis. Obstet Gynecol 92(pt 2):706
214. Rock B, Hood AF, Rock JA (1990) Prospective study of vulvar nevi. J Am Acad Dermatol 22:104–106
215. Rodke G, Friedrich EG Jr, Wilkinson EJ (1988) Malignant potential of mixed vulvar dystrophy (lichen sclerosis associated with squamous cell hyperplasia). J Reprod Med 33:545–550
216. Rogers BB, Josephson SL, Mak SK, Sweeney PJ (1992) Polymeras chain reaction amplification of herpes simplex virus DNA from clinical samples. Obstet Gynecol 79:464–469
217. Rorat E, Wallach RC (1984) Mixed tumors of the vulva: clinical outcome and pathology. Int J Gynecol Pathol 3:323–328
218. Rudolph RE (1990) Vulvar melanosis. J Am Acad Dermatol 23:982–984
219. Saitoh A, Ohya T, Yoshida S, Hosoya R, Nishimura K (1995) A case report of Stevens-Johnson syndrome with *Mycoplasma* infection. Acta Paediatr Jpn 37:113–115
220. Sakane T, Takeno M, Suzuki N, Inaba G (1999) Behçet's disease. N Engl J Med 341:1284–1291
221. Sarrel PM, Steege JF, Maltzer M, Bolinsky D (1983) Pain during sex response due to occlusion of the Bartholin gland duct. Obstet Gynecol 62:261–264
222. Schneider CA, Festa S, Spillert CR, Bruce CJ, Lazaro EJ (1994) Hydrocele of the canal of Nuck. N J Med 91:37–38
223. Schoenfeld A, Ziv E, Levavi H, Samra Z, Ovadia J (1995) Laser versus loop electrosurgical excision in vulvar condyloma for eradication of subclinical reservoir demonstrated by assay for 2′5′-oligosynthetase human papillomavirus. Gynecol Obstet Invest 40:46–51
224. Schwartz RA, Janniger CK (1995) Childhood acanthosis nigricans. Cutis 55:337–341
225. Scrimin F, Rustja S, Radillo O, Volpe C, Abrami R, Guaschino S (2000) Vulvar lichen sclerosus: an immunologic study. Obstet Gynecol 95:147–150
226. Scurry J, Beshay V, Cohen C, Allen D (1998) Ki67 expression in lichen sclerosus of vulva in patients with and without associated squamous cell carcinoma. Histopathology 32:399–404
227. Sedlacek TV, Riva JM, Magen AB, Mangan CE, Cunnane MF (1990) Vaginal and vulvar adenosis. An unsuspected side effect of CO_2 laser vaporization. J Reprod Med 35:995–1001
228. Seely JR, Bley R Jr, Altmiller CJ (1984) Localized chromosomal mosaicism as a cause of dysmorphic development. Am J Hum Genet 36:899–903
229. Shafik A, Doss S (1999) Surgical anatomy of the somatic terminal innervation to the anal and urethral sphincters: role in anal and urethral surgery. J Urol 161:85–89
230. Sherman AL, Reid R (1991) CO_2 laser for suppurative hidradenitis of the vulva. J Reprod Med 36:113–117
231. Shornick JK (1993) Herpes gestationis. Dermatol Clin 11:527–533
232. Slavin RE, Christie JD, Swedo J, Powell LC Jr (1986) Locally aggressive granular cell tumor causing priapism of the crus of the clitoris. A light and ultrastructural study, with observations concerning the pathogenesis of fibrosis of the corpus cavernosum in priapism. Am J Surg Pathol 10:497–507
233. Soler C, Allibert P, Chardonnet Y, Cros P, Mandrand B, Thivolet J (1991) Detection of human papillomavirus types 6, 11, 16 and 18 in mucosal and cutaneous lesions by the multiplex polymerase chain reaction. J Virol Methods 35:143–157
234. Sondergaard K, Carstens J, Zachariae H (1997) The steroid-sparing effect of long-term plasmapheresis in pemphigus: an update. Ther Apher 1:155–158
235. Sonobe H, Ro JY, Ramos M, Diaz I, Mackay B, Ordonez NG, Ayala AG (1994) Glomus tumor of the female external genitalia: a report of two cases. Int J Gynecol Pathol 13:359–364
236. Stashower LM, Krivda MS, Turiansky LG (2000) Fox-Fordyce disease: diagnosis with transverse histologic sections. J Am Acad Dermatol 42(pt 1):89–91
237. Stenchever MA, McDivitt RW, Fisher JA (1973) Leiomyoma of the clitoris. J Reprod Med 10:75–76
238. Stephenson H, Dotters DJ, Katz V, Droegemueller W (1992) Necrotizing fasciitis of the vulva. Am J Obstet Gynecol 166:1324–1327
239. Strayer SA, Yum MN, Sutton GP (1992) Epithelioid hemangioendothelioma of the clitoris: a case report with immunohistochemical and ultrastructural findings. Int J Gynecol Pathol 11:234–239
240. Sugiura H, Uehara M, Maeda T (1990) IgE-positive epidermal Langerhans cells in allergic contact dermatitis lesions provoked in patients with atopic dermatitis. Arch Dermatol Res 282:295–299
241. Sun T, Schwartz NS, Sewell C, Lieberman P, Gross S (1991) *Enterobius* egg granuloma of the vulva and peritoneum: review of the literature. Am J Trop Med Hyg 45:249–253
242. Takeshima Y, Shinkoh Y, Inai K (1998) Angiomyofibroblastoma of the vulva: a mitotically active variant? Pathol Int 48:292–296

243. Taylor S, Drake SM, Dedicoat M, Wood MJ (1998) Genital ulcers associated with acute Epstein-Barr virus infection. Sex Transm Infect 74:296–297
244. Tham SN, Choong HL (1992) Primary tuberculous chancre in a renal transplant patient. J Am Acad Dermatol 26:342–344
245. Thomas CA, Smith SE, Morgan TM, White WL, Feldman SR (1994) Clinical application of polymerase chain reaction amplification to diagnosis of herpes virus infection. Am J Dermatopathol 16: 268–274
246. Toussaint S, Kamino H (1997) Noninfectious erythemotous, papular and squamous diseases. In: Elder D (ed) Lever's histopathology of the skin, 8th Ed. Lippincott-Raven, Philadelphia, pp 151–184
247. Traiman P, Bacchi CE, De Luca LA, Uemura G, Nahas Neto J, Nahas EA, Pontes A (1999) Vulvar carcinoma in young patients and its relationship with genital warts. Eur J Gynaecol Oncol 20:191–194
248. Trees DL, Morse SA (1995) Chancroid and *Haemophilus ducreyi*: an update. Clin Microbiol Rev 8: 357–375
249. Tuffnell D, Buchan PD (1991) Crohn's disease of the vulva in childhood. Br J Clin Pract 45:159–160
250. Tyring SK (1998) Advances in the treatment of herpesvirus infection: the role of famciclovir. Clin Ther 20:661–670
251. Umpierre SA, Kaufman RH, Adam E, Wood KV, Adler-Storth ZK (1992) Human papillomavirus DNA in tissue biopsy specimens of vulvar vestibulitis patients treated with interferon. Obstet Gynecol 78:693–695
252. van der Putte SCJ (1991) Anogenital "sweat" glands. Histology and pathology of a gland that may mimic mammary glands. Am J Dermatopathol 13:557–567
253. van der Putte SCJ (1994) Mammary-like glands of the vulva and their disorders. Int J Gynecol 13: 150–160
254. van der Putte SC, van Gorp LH (1995) Cysts of mammarylike glands in the vulva. Int J Gynecol Pathol 14:184–188.
255. Vanderhooft S, Kirby P (1992) Genital herpes simplex virus infection: natural history. Semin Dermatol 11:190–199
256. Van Glabeke E, Audry G, Hervet F, Josset P, Gruner M (1999) Lipoma of the preputium clitoridis in neonate: an exceptional abnormality different from ambiguous genitalia. Pediatr Surg Int 15:147–148
257. Vassileva S (1998) Drug-induced pemphigoid: bullous and cicatricial. Clin Dermatol 16:379–387
258. Venter PF, Rohm GF, Slabber CF (1981) Giant neurofibromas of the labia. Obstet Gynecol 57:128–130
259. Verkauf BS, Von Thron J, O'Brien WF (1992) Clitoral size in normal women. Obstet Gynecol 80:41–44
260. Vettraino IM, Merritt DF (1995) Crohn's disease of the vulva. Am J Dermatopathol 17:410–413
261. Volz LR, Carpiniello VL, Malloy TR (1994) Laser treatment of urethral condyloma: a five-year experience. Urology 43:81–83
262. Walker PG, Colley NV, Grubb C, Tejerina A, Oriel JD (1983) Abnormalities of the uterine cervix in women with vulvar warts. A preliminary communication. Br J Vener Dis 59:120–123
263. Wieselthier JS, Pincus SH (1993) Hailey-Hailey disease of the vulva. Arch Dermatol 129:1344–1345
264. Wilkinson EJ (1992) Normal histology and nomenclature of the vulva, and malignant neoplasms, including VIN. Dermatol Clin 10:283–296
265. Wilkinson EJ, Guerrero E, Daniel R, Shah K, Stone IK, Hardt NS, Friedrich EG, Jr (1993) Vulvar vestibulitis is rarely associated with human papillomavirus infection types 6, 11, 16 or 18. Int J Gynecol Pathol 12:344–349
266. Wilkinson EJ, Stone IK (1995) Atlas of vulvar disease. Williams & Wilkins, Baltimore, pp 129–182
267. Williams PL (ed) (1995) Gray's anatomy: the anatomical basis of medicine and surgery, 38th Ed. Churchill Livingstone, New York.
268. Willis J, Abdul-Karim FW, di Sant'Agnese PA (1994) Extracardiac rhabdomyomas. Semin Diagn Pathol 11(1):15–25
269. Wisdom A (1989) A colour atlas of sexually transmitted diseases, 2nd Ed. Wolfe, London
270. Wojnarowska F, Frith P (1997) Linear IgA disease. Dev Ophthalmol 28:64–72
271. Wolber RA, Talerman A, Wilkinson EJ, Clement PB (1991) Vulvar granular cell tumors with pseudocartinomatous hyperplasia: a comparative analysis with well-differentiated squamous carcinoma. Int J Gynecol Pathol 10:59–66
272. Wong KT, Wong KK (1994) A case of acantholytic dermatosis of the vulva with features of pemphigus vegetans. J Cutan Pathol 21:453–456
273. Wong R, Tappero J, Cockerell CJ (1997) Bacillary angiomatosis and other *Bartonella* species infections. Semin Cutan Med Surg 16:188–199
274. Woods GL (1995) Update on laboratory diagnosis of sexually transmitted diseases. Clin Lab Med 15:665–684
275. Yang B, Hart WR (2000) Vulvar intraepithelial neoplasia of the simplex (differentiated) type: a clinicopathologic study including analysis of HPV and p53 expression. Am J Surg Pathol. 24:429–441
276. Yoganathan S, Bohl TG, Mason G (1994) Plasma cell balanitis and vulvitis (of Zoon). A study of 10 cases. J Reprod Med 39:939–944
277. Young H (1998) Syphilis. Serology. Dermatol Clin 16:691–698
278. Young RH, Oliva E, Garcia JA, Bhan AK, Clement PB (1996) Urethral caruncle with atypical stromal cells simulating lymphoma or sarcoma—a distinctive pseudoneoplastic lesion of females. A report of six cases. Am J Surg Pathol 20:1190–1195
279. Yun K, Joblin L (1993) Presence of human papillomavirus DNA in condylomata acuminata in children and adolescents. Pathology 25:1–3
280. Zhu WY, Leonardi C, Penneys NS (1992) Detection of human papillomavirus DNA in seborrheic keratosis by polymerase chain reaction. J Dermatol Sci 4:166–171

3

Premalignant and Malignant Tumors of the Vulva

Edward J. Wilkinson, M.D.

Squamous Tumors

Vulvar Intraepithelial Neoplasia (Dysplasia, Carcinoma In Situ)

General Features

The incidence of *vulvar intraepithelial neoplasia* (*VIN*) (*dysplasia, carcinoma in situ*) has nearly doubled when comparing recorded cases between 1973–1976 and 1985–1986 and is becoming more frequent in young women 20–35 years of age.[173] The true incidence of VIN probably is higher, because generally only a subset, carcinoma in situ (VIN 3) cases, is reported. Approximately 50% of these women have other neoplasia involving the genital tract, most often *cervical intraepithelial neoplasia* (CIN).[208] Approximately one-half have a history of a preexisting or concomitant sexually transmitted disease, of which *condylomata acuminata* is the most frequent. There is an association between VIN and cigarette smoking. Most patients are symptomatic, often with pruritus. Current terminology

Table 3.1. Classification of squamous intraepithelial lesions of the vulva [vulvar intraepithelial neoplasia (VIN)/dysplasia, carcinoma in situ]

Mild dysplasia (VIN 1): dysplasia confined to the lowest third of the epithelium
Moderate dysplasia (VIN 2): dysplasia involving the lower two-thirds of the epithelium
Severe dysplasia (VIN 3): dysplasia extending into the upper third of the epithelium, but not involving the full thickness
Carcinoma in situ [VIN 3; includes differentiated (simplex) type VIN]: a squamous intraepithelial lesion in which nuclear abnormalities involve the full thickness of the epithelium or in which the lower portion of the epithelium is replaced by a lesion resembling grade 1 squamous cell carcinoma

From ref. 156.

for squamous intraepithelial lesions [dysplasia-carcinoma in situ, vulvar intraepithelial neoplasia (VIN), as proposed by the World Health Organization (WHO)], is summarized in Table 3.1. Lesions of the vulva that are pigmented and papular or verrucoid have been clinically termed *bowenoid papulosis* by some authors, but they are histologically indistinguishable from other forms of intraepithelial neoplasia and behave in a similar fashion. The separate term bowenoid papulosis therefore is not included in the WHO classification.

Clinical Features

The lesions of VIN typically have a raised surface (Figs. 3.1–3.4). Approximately one-quarter are pigmented (Figs. 3.2–3.4). VIN 3 is, in fact, the second most common pigmented vulvar lesion. Pigmented VIN usually occurs in keratinized vulvar skin. Approximately one-half of patients with VIN have white lesions, or lesions that are distinctly acetowhite, after the application of topical 3%–5% acetic acid. The remainder of VIN lesions may be pink, gray, or red. Lesions involving the nonkeratinized mucous membrane of the vestibule appear red. Such red lesions have been called *erythroplasia of Queyrat*, but like bowenoid papulosis are not designated separately and are included within the VIN category. The lesions may be macular (Fig. 3.1) or papular (Fig. 3.2). In approximately three-quarters of cases they are multiple, and in the majority of the remainder of cases VIN is a solitary lesion. This presentation appears to be more common in older women and is more commonly associated with invasive squamous carcinoma.[29] Confluent growth of VIN is relatively uncommon[64,199] (see Figs. 3.1 and 3.4). The anal skin and squamous mucosa of the anal canal are the most frequently involved secondary sites.

Microscopic Findings

The epithelial cells of VIN have a high nuclear:cytoplasmic ratio and lack cytoplasmic maturation

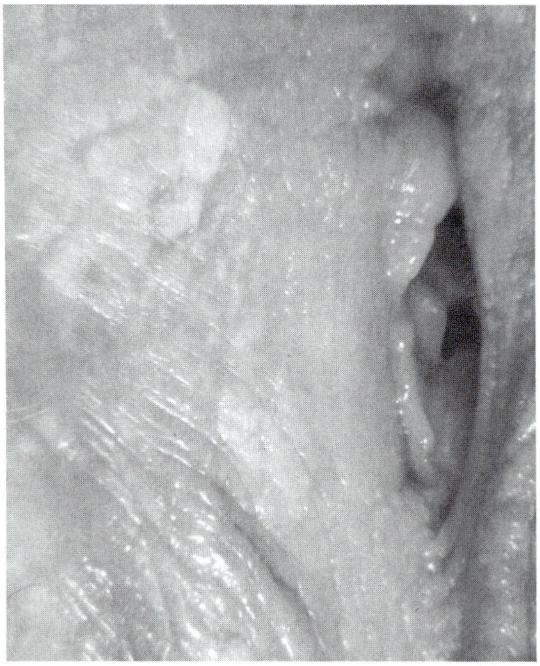

Fig. 3.1. Vulvar intraepithelial neoplasia (VIN). Multiple macular and plaquelike white areas are present on the labia majora.

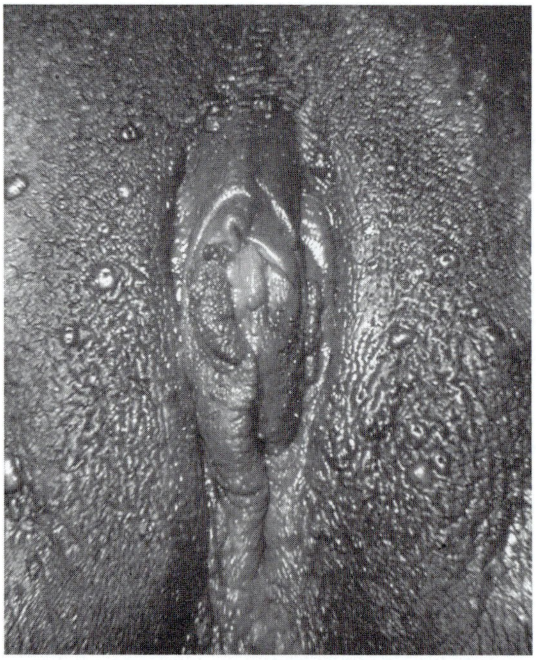

Fig. 3.2. VIN. Multiple pigmented papules are present on the labia majora in this young pregnant woman. Clinically, this lesion has been termed *bowenoid papulosis*.

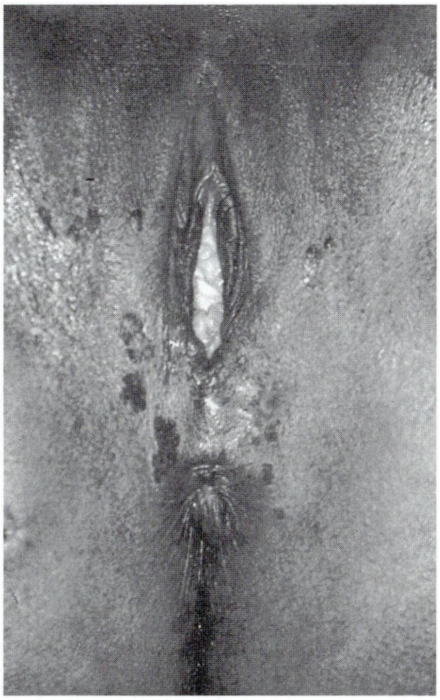

Fig. 3.3. VIN. Multiple pigmented macular areas are present on the vulva and perianal area.

above the basal and parabasal layers. Mitotic activity is present above the basal layer, and the mitotic figures are often abnormal in appearance. Multinucleation and dyskeratosis, including formation of intraepithelial squamous pearls, may be seen (Figs. 3.5 and 3.6a,b). Nuclear pleomorphism and hyperchromasia are present; however, nucleoli are uncommon. Radial dispersion of nuclear chromatin and coarse nuclear chromatin are seen in the epithelial cells of VIN, corresponding to an increased number of interchromatinic and perichromatinic granules. The so-called individual cell keratinization seen within the epithelium is attributed to the presence of aggregated intracytoplasmic tonofilaments that may be produced in the process of abnormal cell division.

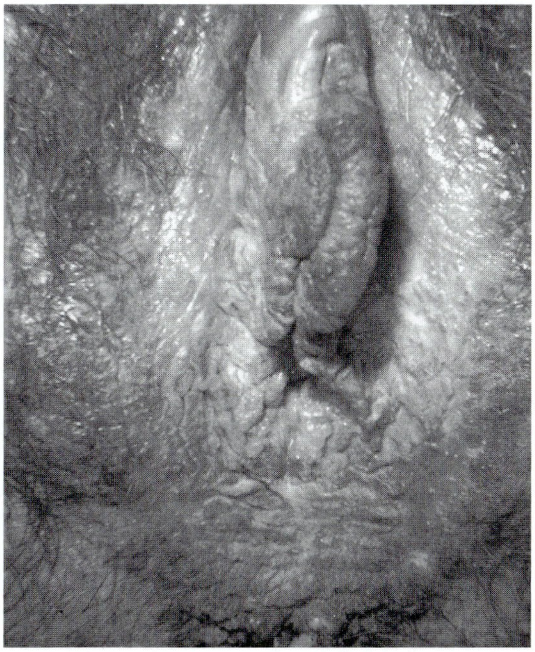

Fig. 3.4. VIN. Confluent distribution of pigmented, slightly raised, rough-surfaced areas involving the labia majora and minora.

Parakeratosis is seen when keratinocytes fail to form granules of prekeratin and retain nuclear material at the epithelial surface. Both intracellular and extracellular pigment granules may be distributed throughout the epidermis. In pigmented VIN lesions, dermal melanophages often are prominent beneath the basal layer and within the dermal papillae. VIN involves the skin appendages in more than 50% of the cases studied. Skin ap-

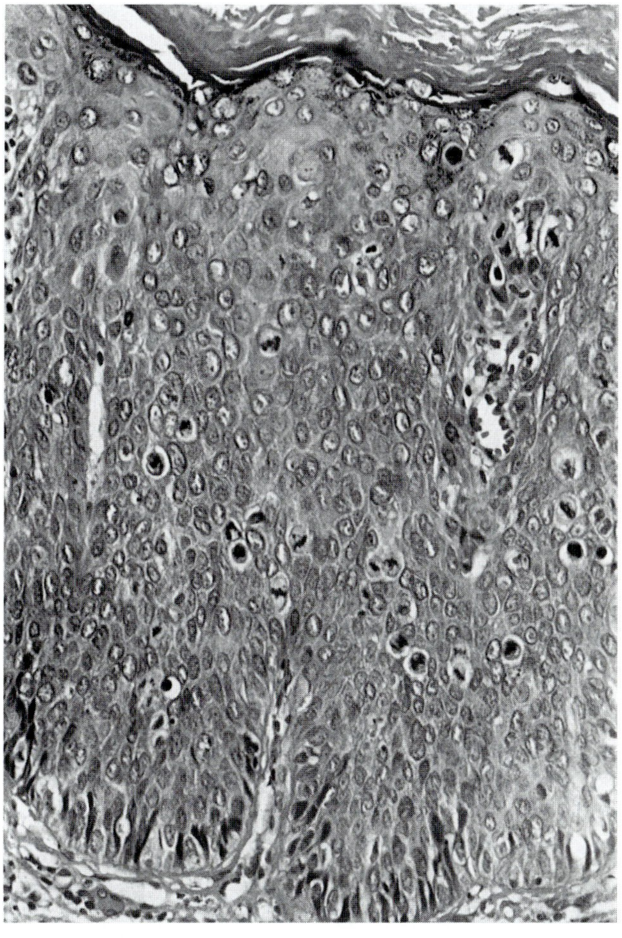

Fig. 3.5. VIN 2. In the lower two-thirds of the epithelium, cells are crowded, vertically oriented, and lack maturation. Nuclei are hyperchromatic and pleomorphic. Many mitotic figures are present, some of which are abnormal.

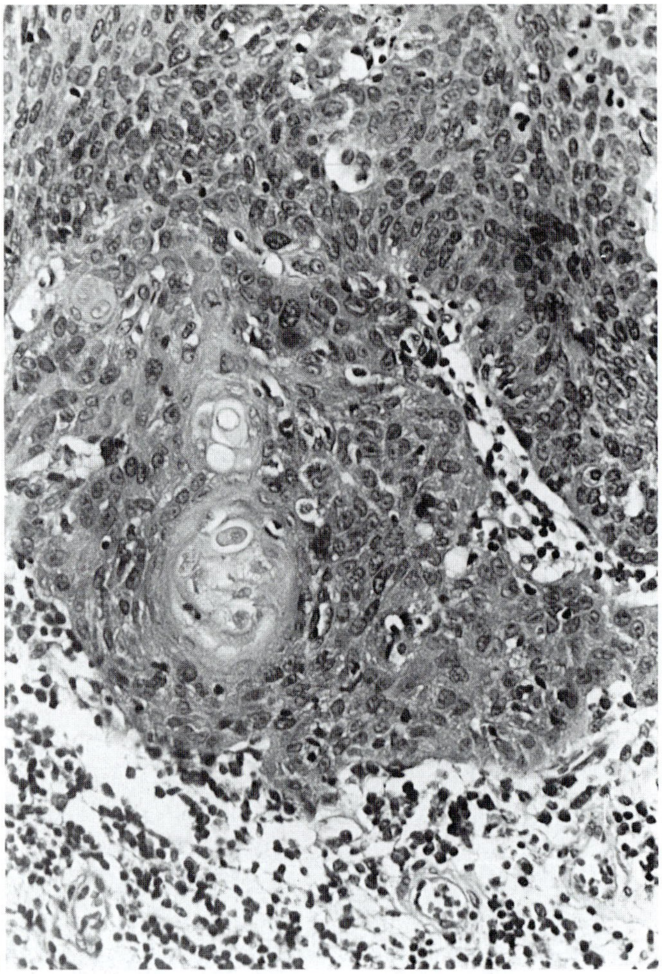

a

Fig. 3.6. a: VIN 3 with superficial invasion. Squamous differentiation within the VIN is manifested by rounded foci of cells with eosinophilic cytoplasm near the basal layer. This is a useful feature in identifying early invasion. **b: VIN 3 with superficial invasion.** Keratinization is present within the VIN. Small clusters of invasive squamous cell carcinoma are present in the superficial dermis. (Courtesy of R.J. Kurman, M.D., Baltimore, MD.) **c: VIN 3 with superficial invasion.** A small focus of invasive squamous carcinoma is noted at the base of the dermal papillae. Note the loss of palisading of the basal cells, as compared to those in the adjacent dermal papillae. (Courtesy of R.J. Kurman, M.D., Baltimore, MD.)

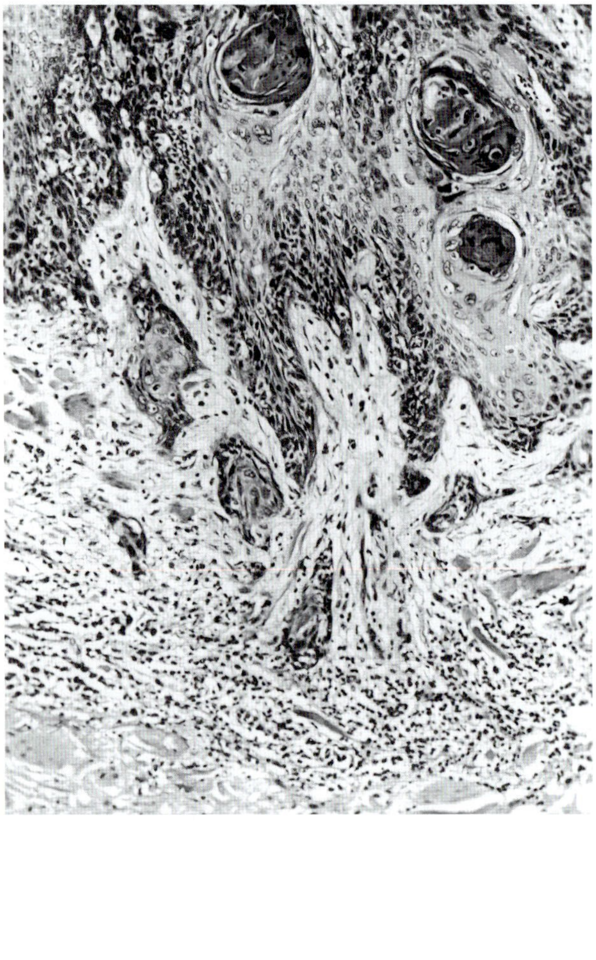

b

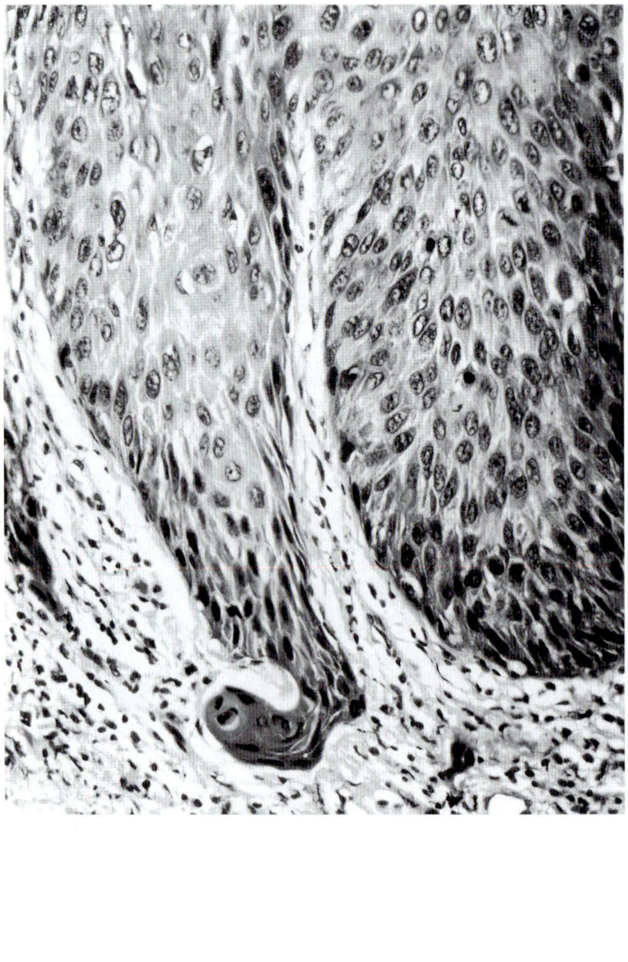

c

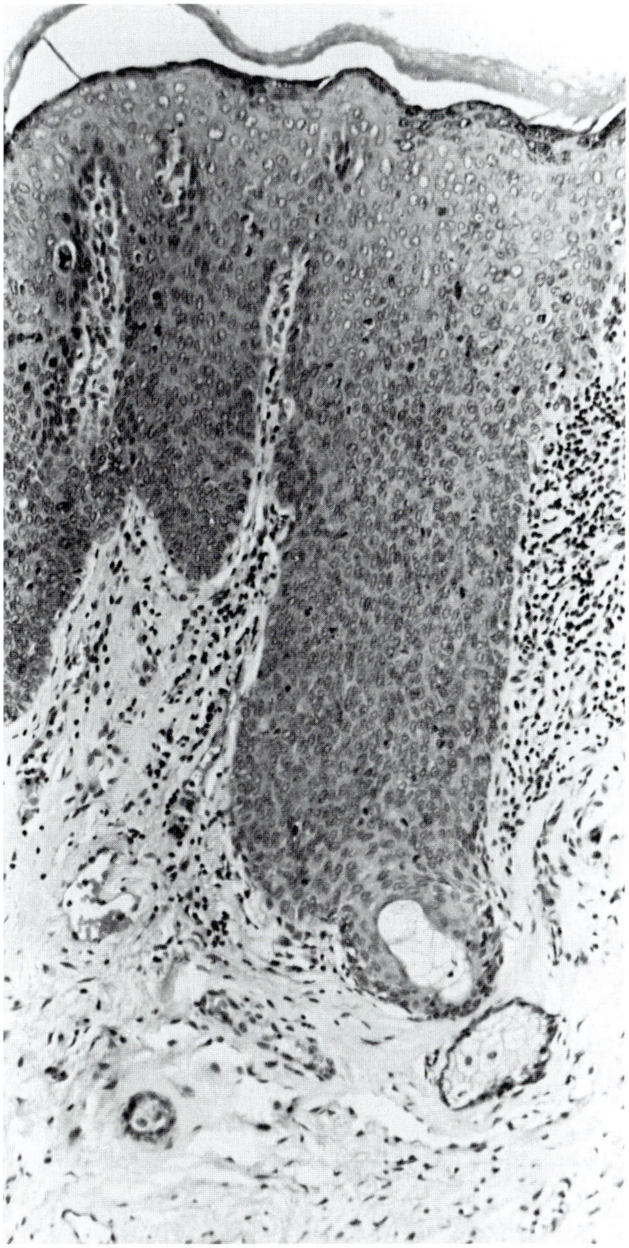

Fig. 3.7. **VIN 3, involving a skin appendage.** Cellular disarray with lack of maturation is seen within the epithelium. Part of a sebaceous gland is present at the base of the lesion.

pendage involvement by VIN should be differentiated from early invasion (compare Figs. 3.6b and 3.6c to Fig. 3.7). Skin appendages as deep as 2.7 mm in hair-bearing areas may be involved with VIN.[160] In non-hair-bearing areas the skin appendages and minor vestibular glands are more superficial. The thickness of the epithelium involved by VIN may range from 0.10 to 1.90 mm, with a mean of 0.52 mm.[14]

Microscopic Grading

As recommended by the World Health Organization on classification, vulva intraepithelial neoplasia is subdivided into three grades: *mild dysplasia/VIN 1*, *moderate dysplasia/VIN 2*, *severe dysplasia/VIN 3*, and *carcinoma in situ/VIN 3*. Differentiated (simplex) VIN is included in the VIN 3 category.[156] When the cellular epithelial abnormalities of VIN are confined to the lower third of the epithelium, VIN 1 (mild dysplasia) is reported (Fig. 3.8). Flat condyloma acuminatum of the vulva may be included in the VIN 1 category because the biologic difference between VIN 1 and flat condyloma is unknown and the morphologic distinction is unreliable. A lesion is classified as VIN 2 if the cellular abnormalities extend through approximately one-half to two-thirds of the epithelium, not including the keratin layer (see Fig. 3.5). If the cellular abnormalities involve more than two-thirds of the epithelial thickness, or are nearly full thickness, not including the surface layers above the granular zone, the diagnosis is VIN 3 (severe dysplasia) or VIN 3 (carcinoma

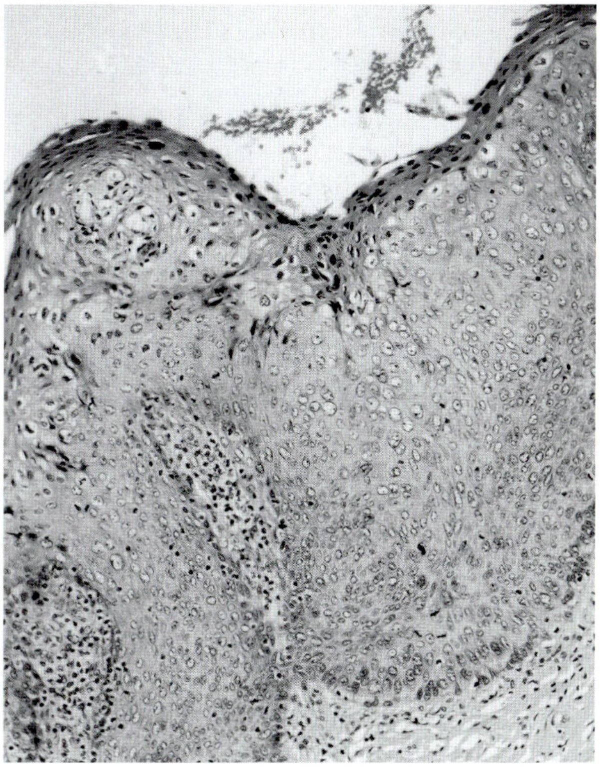

Fig. 3.8. **VIN 1, mild dysplasia.** Crowding of the basal and parabasal cells with some cellular disarray and loss of maturation within the lower one-third of the epithelium. Koilocytotic cells are present on the surface. (Courtesy of R.J. Kurman, M.D., Baltimore, MD.)

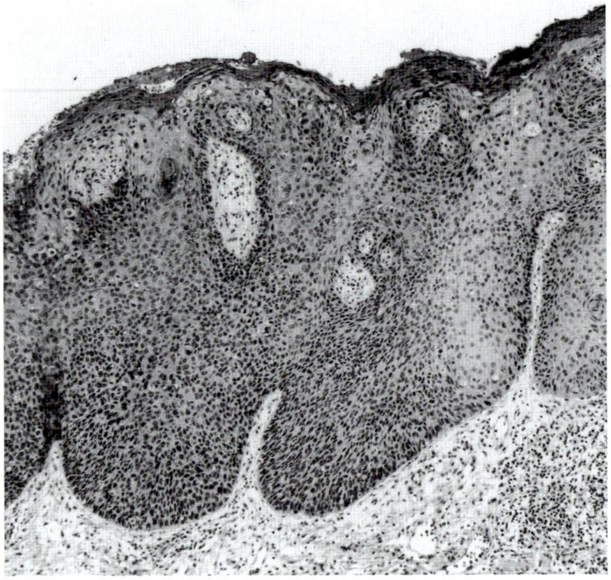

a

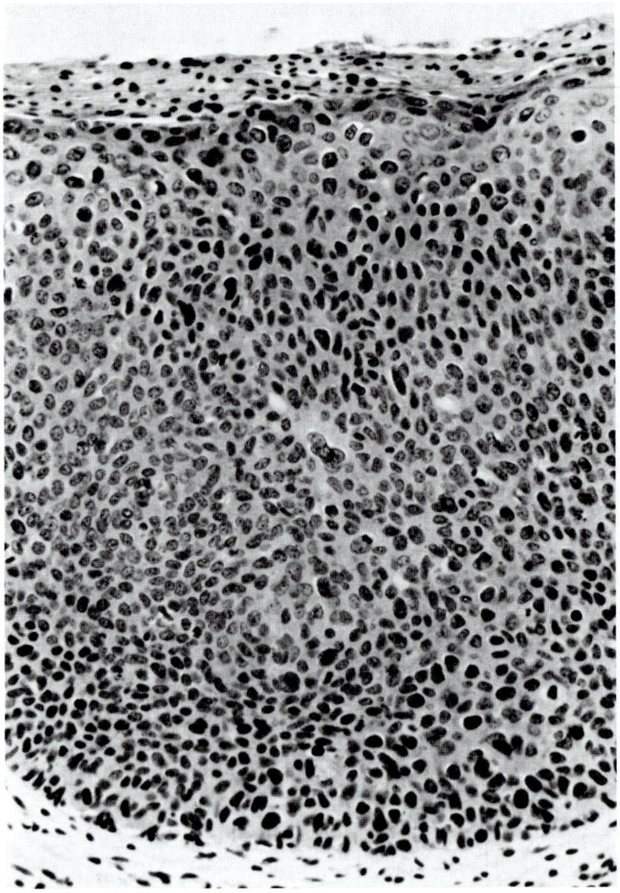

b

Fig. 3.9. a: VIN 3, basaloid type. Prominent acanthosis and basaloid type neoplastic keratinocytes involve nearly the full thickness of the epithelium. (Courtesy of R.J. Kurman, M.D., Baltimore, MD.) **b: VIN 3 (carcinoma in situ), basaloid type.** Complete replacement of the epithelium with overlying parakeratosis resembles carcinoma in situ of the cervix.

in situ) (Figs. 3.9 and 3.10). On rare occasion, cells show prominent eosinophilic cytoplasm with nuclear chromatin changes including chromatin clearing and prominent nucleoli. This lesion is classified as the differentiated VIN and should be classified as a VIN 3 lesion (Fig. 3.11). This cellular change also is commonly seen adjacent to invasive vulvar carcinoma (see Fig. 3.6) (see following, Histologic Subtypes of VIN). Abnormal mitoses are nearly always present in VIN 2 and VIN 3 lesions and may be seen in all but the most superficial layers of the epithelium. Lack of abnormal mitoses, or of mitosis above the basal layer, should raise the question as to whether a lesion belongs in the VIN 2 or 3 category. VIN lesions are predominately VIN 2 or 3; VIN 1 lesions are relatively rare.

There is a trend to employ cytologic "Bethesda terminology" in VIN lesions, wherein the term "high-grade VIN" encompasses VIN 2 and VIN 3, and "low-grade VIN" encompasses VIN 1 and flat condylomas. This terminology is relatively commonly used and is applicable provided one's clinicians understand its use and appropriate ICD9 and other coding are adjusted.

Histologic Subtypes of VIN

VIN has been subclassified into three types—*warty (condylomatous)*, *basaloid*, and *differentiated (simplex)*—on the basis of cellular features. Interobserver reproducibility for subtyping VIN lesions is fair (kappa, 0.31–0.42).[182] Nuclei in VIN may be large and pleomorphic and associated with koilocytes, dyskeratosis, and hyperkeratosis. This lesion is referred to as warty or condylomatous VIN (see Figs. 3.5 and 3.10) The warty type of VIN has larger cells with greater nuclear pleomorphism. The nuclear chromatin is coarse and clumped and nucleoli are not prevalent, although abnormal mitosis usually can be identified. Toward the surface the keratinocytes have features of condyloma acuminatum with koilocytosis and multinucleation. A prominent granular layer, with associated dyskeratosis, parakeratosis, or hyperkeratosis, usually is present[134] (see Fig. 3.10b).

The basaloid type of VIN has relatively small, uniform cells with hyperchromatic and coarse nuclear chromatin. Nucleoli are rare, and abnormal mitoses usually are found. There is little or no mat-

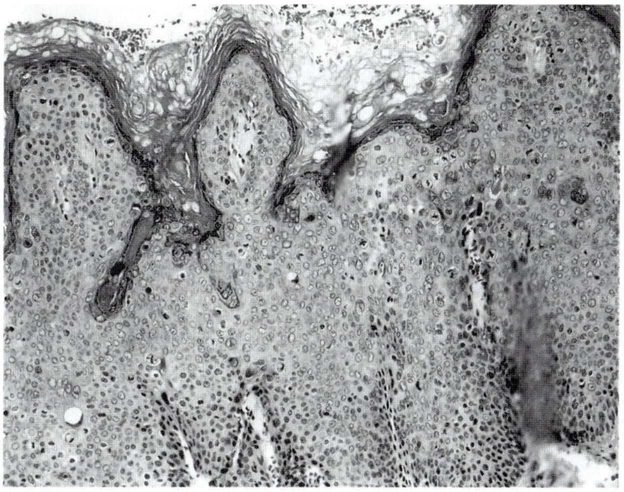

a

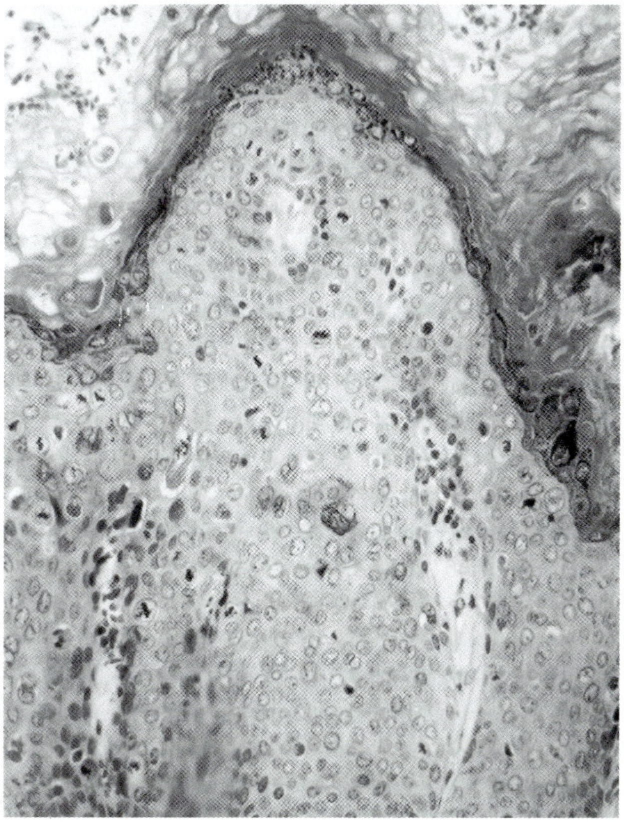

b

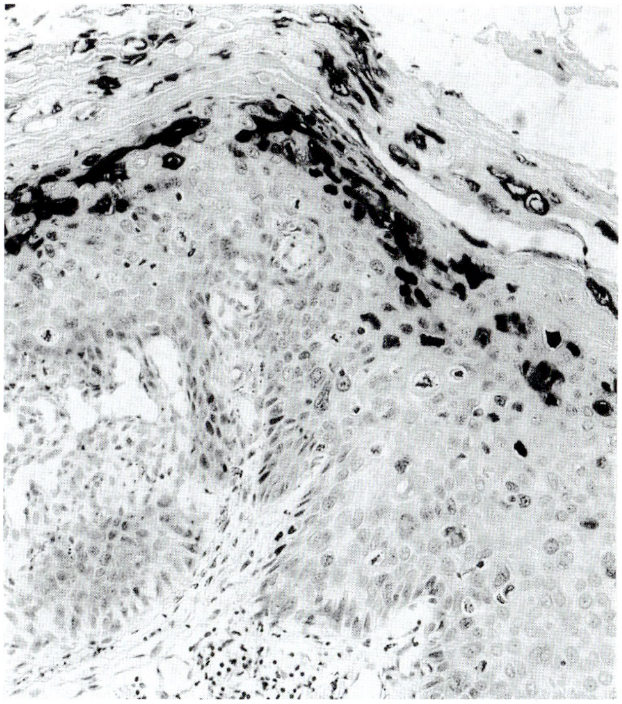

c

Fig. 3.10. a: VIN 3, warty (condylomatous) type. The surface of the lesion is spiked with marked hyperkeratosis. A prominent granular layer is evident. (Courtesy of R.J. Kurman, M.D., Baltimore, MD.) **b: VIN 3, warty (condylomatous) type.** Marked cellular disarray with prominent nuclear pleomorphism. Several multinucleated keratinocytes are present. **c: VIN 3, warty type.** In situ hybridization for HPV 16 demonstrates labeling (*black nuclei*) in the superficial epithelium. (Courtesy of R.J. Kurman, M.D., Baltimore, MD.)

uration of the keratinocytes, similar to carcinoma in situ of the cervix; however, some keratinization or parakeratosis may be seen at the surface (see Fig. 3.9).

The differentiated (simplex) type of VIN has a thickened epithelium that is typically associated with elongation and anastomosis of rete redges. Parakeratosis is usually present, associated with prominent intracellular bridges. The keratinocytes of differentiated VIN are large and pleomorphic with a relatively large amount of eosinophilic cytoplasm, as compared to the other two types of VIN (Fig. 3.11). Keratin pearl formation within the rete may be seen. The nuclear chromatin is vesicular rather than coarse, and the nuclei have prominent nucleoli, usually most prominently in the basal and parabasal keratinocytes. A distinctive feature is the prominent increased eosinophilic cytoplasm within the keratinocytes in the basal and parabasal layer in the base of rete ridges.[109,194,204] In a study of 12 patients with differ-

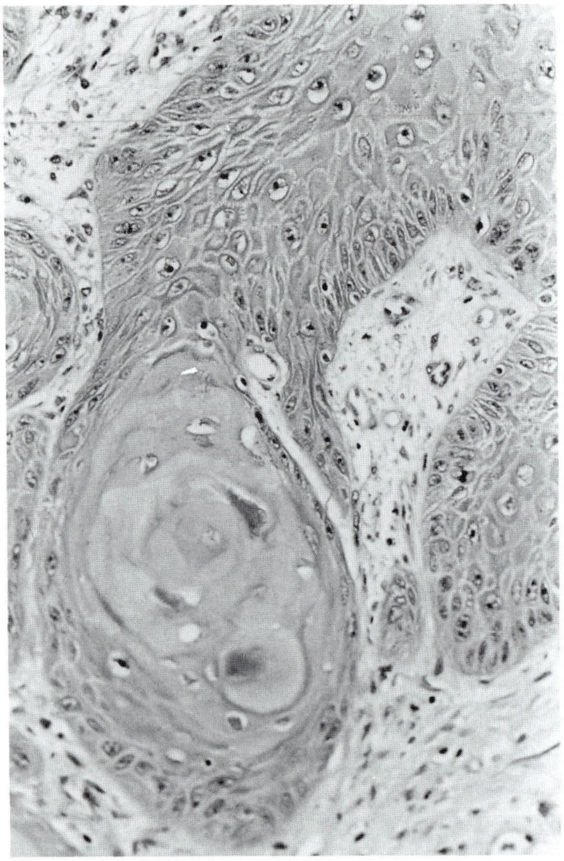

Fig. 3.11. VIN 3, differentiated type. The epithelium has slight cellular disarray and the keratinocytes contain abundant cytoplasm. The nuclei are enlarged and contain prominent nucleoli. Within the parabasal area of the rete ridge, the cells have increased eosinophilic cytoplasm and are dyskeratotic.

entiated VIN, 10 had squamous cell hyperplasia in the epithelium adjacent to the tumor, and 4 patients had associated lichen sclerosus. In this study, only 1 of the 12 patients had evidence of human papillomavirus (HPV); however, p53 was expressed in the suprabasal cells in 10 of the 12 patients.[204] All the patients in this study were postmenopausal; 3 had a prior history of vulvar squamous cell carcinoma, and 1 patient had concurrent superficially invasive vulvar squamous cell carcinoma.

An individual patient may have more than one histologic type in different VIN lesions, and occasionally both basaloid and warty types may be seen in a single lesion. Mixtures of basaloid and warty patterns are particularly frequent, and in some cases both patterns may be seen in a single excised lesion. These "mixed" cases can be classified according to the predominant component or simply as VIN, basaloid/warty type.

Differential Diagnosis

A similar lesion to differentiated VIN, but lacking the distinctive increased eosinophilic cytoplasm of the base of the rete ridges, has been designated by some as *atypical squamous cell hyperplasia* because this lesion has similar nuclear atypia but histologically resembles squamous cell hyperplasia more closely than it does VIN.[108] (See Chapter 2, Benign Diseases of the Vulva.) Despite the association with *keratinizing squamous cell carcinoma*, there are no longitudinal studies demonstrating that squamous cell hyperplasia alone, as already defined here, is a precursor of squamous cell carcinoma. When associated with lichen sclerosus, follow-up studies suggest that associated squamous cell hyperplasia is probably a precursor to squamous cell carcinoma in some cases; however, the association between differentiated VIN, squamous cell hyperplasia, and squamous cell carcinoma requires further study.[151,204] Squamous cell hyperplastic-type lesions do not express p53, and this in part distinguishes these otherwise benign lesions from differentiated VIN.[104]

The differential diagnosis of VIN includes *basal cell carcinoma*, *superficial spreading malignant melanoma*, *Paget disease*, *pagetoid urothelial intraepithelial neoplasia*, and *multinucleated atypia of the vulva*.[34,121,196] Differentiated VIN should also be differentiated from repair or reaction related to erosion or superficial ulceration including pseudoepitheliomatous (pseudocarcinomatous) hyperplasia, trapped epithelium at a prior biopsy site, or granulomatous or decidual change in the immediately adjacent underlying epithelium.

Immunoperoxidase methods to assist in distinguishing melanoma and Paget disease are summarized in Table 3.2. Multinucleated atypia of the vulva is characterized by multinucleated keratinocytes, without significant nuclear atypia, within the lower to middle epithelial layers. The possibility that a podophyllin effect on condylomata acuminata of the vulva could result in these lesions being misinterpreted as VIN is highly improbable because the changes from a single application of podophyllin regress within 1–2 weeks. Mitotic arrest with cells in metaphase seen after podophyllin contrasts with the abnormal mitotic figures seen in VIN. Nuclear karyorrhexis is rarely present in VIN, whereas it is found in at least 90% of condyloma cases.[189] In VIN, in contrast to the podophyllin effect, nuclear size tends to be variable and the nuclear chromatin usually is coarse with little cellular swelling. (See Chapter 2, Benign Diseases of the Vulva.)

Table 3.2. Immunohistochemical studies to differentiate vulvar Paget disease of skin or rectal origin, pagetoid urothelial intraepithelial neoplasia (PUIN), and melanoma

	CK7	*CK20*	*GCDFP-15*	*CEA*	*S-100, HMB-45, and Melan-A*
As a primary skin neoplasm	+	−	+	+	−
Related to rectal carcinoma[a]	+	+	−	+	−
PUIN (pseudopaget's) related to urothelial carcinoma[b]	+	−(+)	−	−	−
Melanoma	0	0	0	0	+

CK 7, cytokeratin 7; CK 20, cytokeratin 20; GCDFP-15, gross cystic disease fluid protein-15; CEA, carcinoembryonic antigen.
[a]From ref. 130.
[b]From ref. 115.

Adjunctive Studies

Most VIN 2 and VIN 3 lesions contain DNA aneuploid populations of cells.[65,199] DNA analysis by microspectrophotometry of multifocal lesions suggests that separate lesions arise from separate stem cells, forming distinguishable clones. Large confluent lesions may result from centrifugal growth from a single cell line or by confluence of separate and distinct clones.[199] In single VIN lesions, approximately half have different stem cells by DNA microspectrophotometry, suggesting that such lesions may undergo clonal evolution.[199]

Evidence for HPV, nearly always type 16, in VIN is predominately found in the warty and basaloid types, based on molecular biologic studies, and has been demonstrated in most cases (see Fig. 3.10c).[21] In differentiated VIN, HPV is infrequent.[44,109,134,152]

Keratin expression provides evidence for the lack of cellular maturation.[59] Immunohistochemical studies for cellular proliferation employing BCL 2 and Ki-67 (MIB-1) have not been demonstrated to be of significant value in the diagnosis of VIN lesions.[188]

Clinical Behavior and Treatment

The clinical course of VIN following treatment has been well studied; however, there are relatively few long-term studies of untreated VIN.[84,102] There is evidence that untreated VIN 3 will progress to invasive squamous cell carcinoma, and this has been reported with invasion being observed within 8 years of the diagnosis of VIN.[102] VIN associated with vulvar invasive squamous cell carcinoma diagnosed within excised VIN lesions is reported in 2%–20% of larger series that have specifically looked for this association.[29,87a,101] In evaluation of epithelial changes adjacent to vulvar squamous cell carcinoma, 60%–80% of superficially invasive carcinomas and 25% of deeply invasive carcinomas have adjacent VIN.[109,209] Differentiated (simplex) VIN was reported associated with vulvar squamous cell carcinoma in 7 of 12 (58%) patients in one study.[204] This study suggests that there is a stronger association between differentiated VIN and squamous cell carcinoma than there is between the other recognized VIN types and invasion. There are no known differences in clinical behavior between warty and basaloid VIN. Squamous cell carcinoma, in the other VIN types, also occurs most commonly in postmenopausal women, although it may occur in women of reproductive age.[77] Spontaneous regression of VIN has been observed in young women; however, no long-term controlled prospective studies have evaluated this event specifically.[35,64] Regression appears to be most common in young women and those who are pregnant, whereas women of advanced age, those who are severely immunosuppressed, and women with Fanconi anemia are at a greater risk for invasion.[27,201]

Conservative therapy is now recommended for VIN, and most cases are managed with local excision; laser ablation also may be appropriate for selected patients, especially when the VIN lesion involves the nonhairy skin or mucous membrane areas (e.g., the vulvar vestibule and perianal areas).[86,194] Recently, topical imiquimod is being used in clinical studies on women with vulvar condyloma acuminatum or VIN 1 lesions. Women who are cigarette smokers appear to have a higher frequency of recurrence of VIN lesions, and cessation of smoking is recommended.[46,197]

Squamous Cell Carcinoma

Vulvar squamous cell carcinoma has an overall incidence of approximately 1.5 per 100,000 women in the United States; this rate increases with advancing age to as high as 20 per 100,000 women.[173,207] Unlike VIN, the incidence of vulvar squamous cell carcinoma in the United States has not increased significantly since 1973.[173] However, in northeastern Scotland there is evidence that the incidence of vulvar carcinoma is increasing.[120]

Current evidence supports the view that women at risk for vulvar carcinoma can be separated into three broad groups: those with VIN, those with known vulvar dermatoses (especially lichen sclerosus), and those related to other conditions, such as chronic granulomatous disease. The first group consists of younger women (mean age, 55 years) who have VIN associated with squamous cell carcinoma. A 12-year-old girl with VIN and superficially invasive vulvar carcinoma has been reported.[146] These women also have a high rate of cervical and vaginal neoplasia, and HPV is detected in approximately 75% of their vulvar squamous carcinomas. These women also tend to be heavy cigarette smokers, and their vulvar squamous cell tumors are predominantly of the warty or basaloid types. Overall, it has been estimated that approximately 30% of all vulvar squamous cell carcinomas are associated with HPV, usually HPV type 16.[134,137,181]

The second population of women with vulvar carcinoma are older (mean age, 77 years) and do not have associated VIN or a history of heavy cigarette smoking. Their tumors rarely contain HPV, and typically they are well-differentiated keratinizing squamous cell carcinomas.[108,181] Suppressed immunocompetence is recognized as a risk factor in these women.[27,201] Women with HPV-related cervical neoplasia with low CD 4 counts who are treated with triple combination antiretroviral therapy can have decreased plasma human immunodeficiency virus-1 (HIV-1) levels, increased CD 4 cell counts, and partially restored immune function. This restored immune function is associated with regression of cervical lesions in these women.[81]

Women with well-differentiated, non-HPV-related vulvar squamous cell carcinoma often have associated vulvar dermatoses, especially lichen sclerosus.[24,44,108] Women with vulvar lichen sclerosus who develop squamous cell carcinoma tend to be older; their primary tumors are more commonly involve the clitoris and typically are not associated with VIN of the warty or basaloid types. VIN was identified in 5% of the cases in one series.[24] Squamous carcinomas associated with lichen sclerosus express tumor suppressor gene product p53 in nearly one-half the cases and cytokine transforming growth factor-beta (TGF-β) in one-third of the cases as compared to 19% and 9%, respectively, for nonlichen sclerosus-related tumors. Approximately one-half of these lichen sclerosus-associated tumors are associated with a prominent fibromyxoid stromal response, as compared to nonlichen sclerosus-related tumors.[24] From a literature review of a cohort of symptomatic women with vulvar lichen sclerosus, it was reported that 9% subsequently presented with VIN and 21% with vulvar squamous cell carcinoma. The carcinoma presented 1–23 years (mean, 4 years) after the onset of symptoms.[24] Primary evidence based on p53 mutation analysis and clonal studies suggests that squamous cell hyperplasia of the vulva is probably not a precursor of non-HPV-related vulvar squamous cell carcinomas.[104]

The third group of women at risk of developing vulvar squamous cell carcinoma includes women with chronic granulomatous disease, most notably granuloma inguinale. In addition to cigarette smoking, other carcinogen exposure, such as topical exposure to arsenicals, also increases risk.[46] Diabetes mellitus, achlorhydria, and poor perineal hygiene have also been associated with a slightly increased risk of vulvar carcinoma. Vulvar carcinoma may occur during pregnancy, although parity does not appear to be a significant risk factor.[162]

Superficially Invasive Squamous Cell Carcinoma (A.J.C.C. and F.I.G.O. Stage IA)

General Features

The majority of vulvar squamous cell carcinomas in the United States are stage 1, being 2 cm or less in diameter and clinically confined to the vulva without evidence of extension to other sites or lymph node metastasis. Stage 1 vulvar carcinomas are divided into two subgroups based on depth of invasion. A stage 1A vulvar carcinoma is a superficially invasive squamous cell carcinoma with a depth of invasion of 1 mm or less and a diameter of 2 cm or less.[4] Stage 1A carcinomas accounted for 16.8% of 238 women with vulvar carcinoma in one study.[117a] The staging of vulvar carcinoma as recommended by the American Joint Commission on Cancer (AJCC) is as summarized in Table 3.3.[4]

A stage 1A (F.I.G.O. Stage 1A; A.J.C.C. T1a) car-

Table 3.3. American Joint Commission on Cancer (AJCC) staging of vulvar carcinoma (FIGO stage)

TX: Primary tumor cannot be assessed
T0: No evidence of primary tumor
Tis: Carcinoma in situ (preinvasive carcinoma, VIN 3)
T1: Tumor confined to the vulva or vulva and perineum, 2 cm or less in greatest dimension. (Stage I, T1 N0 M0)
  T1a: Tumor confined to the vulva or vulva and perineum, 2 cm or less in greatest dimension, and with stromal invasion no greater than 1 mm.*
    (Stage IA, T1 $\leq$ 1 mm)
  T1b: Tumor confined to the vulva or vulva and perineum, 2 cm or less in greatest dimension, and with stromal invasion greater than 1 mm.*
    (Stage IB, T1 > 1 mm)
T2: Tumor confined to the vulva or vulva and perineum, more than 2 cm in greatest dimension (Stage II, T2 N0 M0)
T3: Tumor of any size with adjacent spread to the lower urethra and / or vagina or anus
    (Stage III
    Stage IIIA T3 N0 M0
    IIIB T3 N1 M0
    T2 N1 M0
    T1 N1 M0)
T4: Tumor invades any of the following: upper urethral mucosa, bladder mucosa, rectal mucosa, or is fixed to the pubic bone.
  (Stage IV
  Stage IVA T4 N0 M0
  IVB TX N1 M0
  TX NX M1)
*(The depth of invasion is defined as the measurement of the tumor from the epithelial-stromal junction of the adjacent most superficial dermal papilla to the deepest point of invasion.)

From ref. 4, with permission.

cinoma of the vulva is defined as a single lesion measuring 2 cm or less in diameter with a depth of invasion of 1 mm or less regardless of the presence of vascular invasion. Tumors with more than one site of invasion are not included in this stage.[106,192] It has been suggested that the term *microinvasive carcinoma* not be used in reporting vulvar carcinoma, but rather that the diameter of the tumor, the depth of invasion, the thickness of the tumor, the presence or absence of vascular space involvement, and the status of surgical margins be reported. These findings will influence treatment options.[195]

Gross Findings

Superficially invasive vulvar squamous cell carcinoma may present as an ulcer, a red, brown, or black macule or papule, or a white hyperkeratotic plaque. The invasive carcinoma may be associated with VIN and clinically present as a VIN lesion. Although the presence of invasion associated with VIN may be heralded by the finding of an associated ulcer, irregularly contoured elevated mass, abnormal vascularity, or marked hyperkeratosis, no specific clinical findings definitively separate VIN from VIN with superficial invasion.[29]

Tumor diameter alone in stage 1 vulvar carcinoma is not a reliable predictor of lymph node status. In a study of 190 patients with vulvar carcinomas 2 cm in diameter or smaller, 36 (19%) had lymph node metastasis. Of those with node metastasis, the relative 5-year survival was 78.6%, compared with 97.9% survival at 5 years for those with negative nodes.[87]

Microscopic Findings

In that the staging of a superficially invasive vulvar carcinoma is based upon the depth of invasion of the tumor, measurement of superficially invasive vulvar squamous cell carcinomas should be made to determine both the thickness and the depth of invasion of the tumor (Fig. 3.12). These measurements require a calibrated ocular or comparable measuring device. The measurement from the surface of the tumor, or from the base of the granular layer if a keratin layer is present, to the deepest point of invasion is defined as the "thickness of the tumor." The measurement from the epithelial stromal junction of the adjacent dermal papillae to the deepest point of invasion is defined as the "depth of invasion" (Fig. 3.12). Both measurements are valuable, because in cases in which the tumor is ulcerated the thickness may be 1 mm or less and the depth of in-

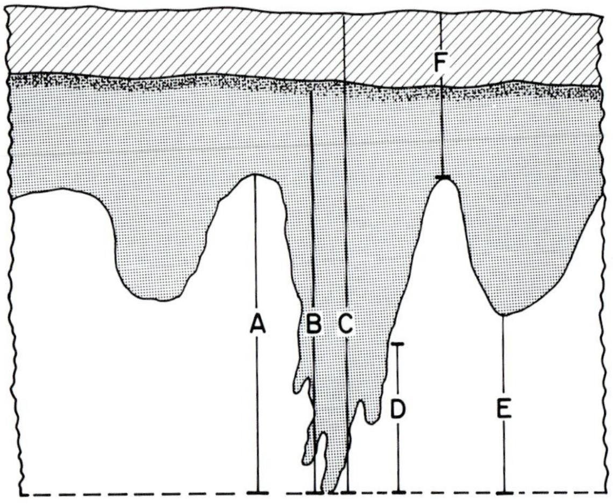

Fig. 3.12. Methods of measuring depth of invasion of squamous cell carcinoma of the vulva. The tumor thickness is defined as the measurement from the granular layer (*B*) or surface if nonkeratinized (*C*) to the deepest point of invasion. The depth of invasion is defined as the measurement from the epithelial stromal junction of the adjacent most superficial dermal papillae to the deepest point of invasion (*A*). Measurement of the depth of invasion also can be accomplished by measuring from the surface to the deepest point of invasion and subtracting the measurement from the surface to the epithelial stromal junction of the most superficial dermal papillae (*F*) ($A = C - F$). Other measurements are from the rete ridge (*D*) and from the deepest tip of the adjacent rete ridge (*E*). (Reprinted by permission of E.J. Wilkinson.)

vasion may be well beyond 1 mm, and a thickness measurement alone would underestimate the depth of invasion. Methods of measurement require a description along with the measurement within the pathology report.[193,195]

The depth of invasion also can be calculated by measuring the thickness of the tumor and subtracting the epithelial measurement from the surface to the epithelial stromal junction of the immediately adjacent dermal papillae.[75,76] In general, both measurements can be made when the tumor is superficial (less than 3 mm in depth), and when the tumor is totally excised and there is intact noninvolved epithelium adjacent to the tumor (Figs. 3.6 and 3.13). In larger tumors, the diameter and dimensions of the tumor may be too great to include an adjacent dermal papillae; however, this often can be overcome by appropriate sectioning. With a partially excised tumor, or when the tumor is superficially biopsied, these tumor measurements cannot be made reliably. When marked acanthosis is present, the thickness of the epithelium may give an overestimate of the depth of invasion. If the tumor is ulcerated, the thickness measurement may underestimate the true tumor size. The College of American Pathologists has recommended that the following information be included in the surgical pathology report.[195]

1. Depth of invasion of the tumor in millimeters and thickness of the tumor in millimeters
2. Method of measurement of the depth of invasion and thickness
3. Presence or absence of vascular space involvement by tumor
4. Diameter of the tumor (as measured from the gross surgical specimen)
5. Clinical measurement of the tumor diameter, when available.[195]

When there is a question as to whether invasion is present and additional sectioning does not resolve the question, it is recommended that invasion not be diagnosed.

Clinical Behavior and Treatment

For patients with stage 1A carcinoma of the vulva (see Table 3.3), the recommended therapy is wide local excision without vulvectomy. Total excision of a lesion suspected of being a superficially invasive carcinoma is necessary to assure that an associated deeper squamous carcinoma is not immediately adjacent to the apparently superficially invasive focus. The surgical specimen typically encompasses the apparent VIN lesion and any associated hyperkeratotic or ulcerative lesions. The specimens are usually not more than 2–3 cm in greatest dimension, usually with 1-cm or less clinically negative margins. Sampling of the ipsilateral groin nodes, or bilateral groin nodes if the tumor is midline, has been suggested. For stage 1A (T1a) vulvar carcinomas, the probability of node metastasis is extremely small, and node sampling or resection is not contributory in most cases[6a,14a,86a,117a,193,200] (Table 3.3). Based on analysis of published series, the current treatment of these patients is local excision without lymphadenectomy.[22,72,117a]

Patients who have had superficially invasive vulvar squamous cell carcinoma that was treated and have recurrence, or have a second primary squamous cell carcinoma of the vulva, risk regional lymph node metastasis and death from recurrence. In a series of 26 women with VIN and associated superficially invasive squamous cell carcinoma, 10 (38%) of these patients experienced recurrence of VIN or superficially invasive squamous cell carcinoma, all within 36 months of treatment.[84] Three of these 10 women subsequently presented with frankly invasive vulvar squamous cell carcinoma. Of

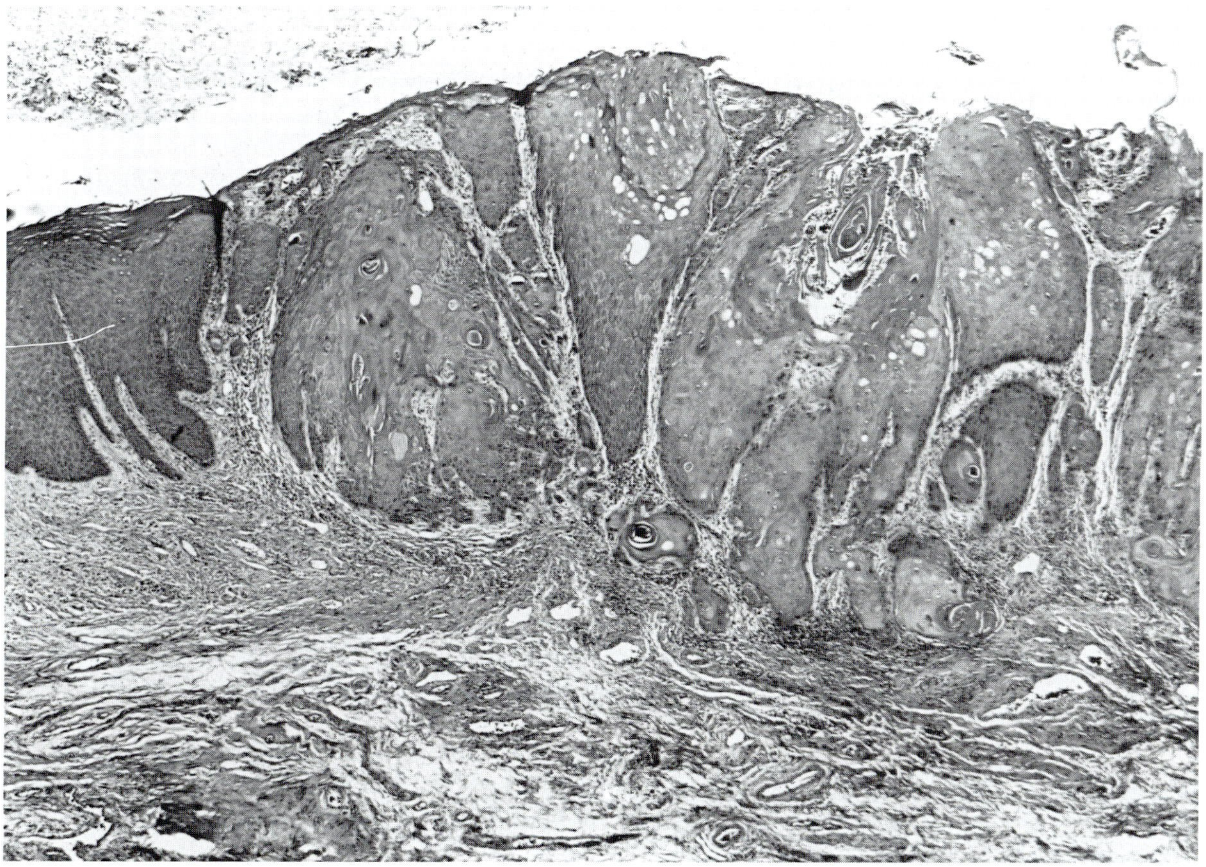

Fig. 3.13. Squamous cell carcinoma. The depth of invasion is 2.7 mm from the most superficial adjacent dermal papillae to the deepest point of invasion.

the patients without recurrence of VIN or superficially invasive carcinoma, none had regional lymph node or distant metastases and none died of tumor.[84] In another study of 40 patients with T1a (stage 1A) vulvar carcinomas, none had regional lymph node metastasis; however, 2 patients had vulvar recurrence, and 1 of them had a groin node metastasis associated with the recurrence.[114]

There are insufficient data specifically evaluating tumors with a depth of invasion of 2 mm or less; however, the risk of lymph node metastasis in these cases appears to be very low. In two small studies specifically examining tumors with invasion of 1–2 mm, without vascular space involvement, none had node metastasis.[15,144] Until more data are available on tumors that invade between 1 and 2 mm, definitive therapeutic recommendations cannot be made.

A 3-mm depth of invasion has been found to be associated with inguinal lymph node metastasis in approximately 10% of cases. Selected patients with tumors of this depth may be treated by wide local excision with ipsilateral regional node dissection.[71] In a study evaluating both depth of invasion and tumor thickness, more than 40% of the cases had groin metastasis when the thickness of the tumor exceeded 4 mm.[15] In a study of patients with vulvar squamous carcinomas with a 5-mm depth of invasion, it was found that approximately 15% of these women had inguinal lymph node metastasis (Fig. 3.14).

For now, it is safe to say there is little risk, if any, of inguinal lymph node metastasis with tumors that are stage 1a (T1a1) with a depth of invasion of 1 mm or less.

Invasive Squamous Cell Carcinoma

Clinical Features

Women presenting with *vulvar carcinoma* may have a wide variety of presenting complaints relevant to the vulvar tumor, especially if the tumor is more advanced. Pruritus, burning, pain, bleeding, discharge, dyspareunia, dysuria, unpleasant odor, or palpation or observation of a mass have all been reported. Mental confusion and disorientation related to hypercalcemia have been reported associated with vulvar squamous cell carcinoma. After the ovary, the

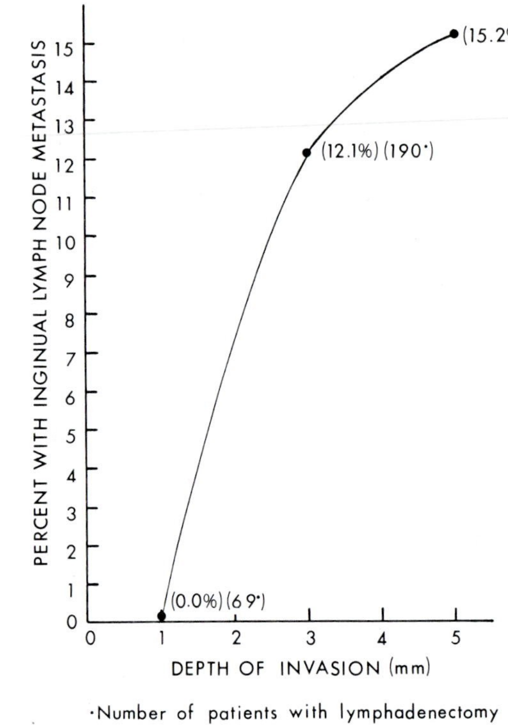

Fig. 3.14. Percent of women who underwent lymphadenectomy with inguinal lymph node metastasis plotted against the depth of invasion of their tumor. The frequency of lymph node metastasis rises rapidly with depth of invasion beyond 1 mm. (Reprinted by permission of E.J. Wilkinson, ref. 200.)

vulva is the second most common gynecologic tumor site associated with hypercalcemia. Vulvar squamous carcinomas with associated hypercalcemia usually are large, well differentiated, and without bony metastasis.[126] Surgical excision of the tumor results in the serum calcium levels returning to normal, and if mental symptoms related to the hypercalcemia were present, these also regress. The hypercalcemia results from secretion by the tumor of parathyroid hormone (PTH) or PTH-like substance.

Invasive squamous carcinoma may present as an exophytic papillomatous mass or as an endophytic ulcer. The tumor usually is located on the labia minora or majora; however, the clitoris is primarily involved in approximately 5%–15% of cases.[75] Typically the tumor is solitary (Fig. 3.15); less than 10% are multifocal.[207]

Microscopic Findings

A number of grading systems for vulvar squamous cell carcinomas have been proposed. However, to date no uniform grading system has been unanimously accepted. An effective grading system must reflect clinical behavior, preferably include three grades only as applied in most other grading systems in gynecologic pathology, and be applicable to the various subtypes of vulvar squamous carcinoma including warty, basaloid, and keratinizing types. To date, none of the grading systems in use achieves these objectives.

The American Joint Committee on Cancer (AJCC) recommends that histopathologic grading of vulvar carcinoma be recorded as follows: GX, grade cannot be assessed; G1, well differentiated; G2, moderately differentiated; G3, poorly differentiated; and G4, undifferentiated.[4] The Gynecologic Oncology Group (GOG) advocates a system according to the percentage of undifferentiated cells. The latter are small cells with scant cytoplasm showing little or no differentiation and infiltrating the stroma in either elongated cords or small clusters.[159] Grade 1 tumors have no undifferentiated cells (Figs. 3.16–3.18), grade 2 tumors contain less than 50% undifferentiated cells, grade 3 tumors (Fig. 3.19) have greater than 50% but less than 100%, and grade 4 is essentially entirely composed of undifferentiated cells. The risk of recurrence is reportedly higher with increasing grade.[89,159]

In addition to tumor staging (as summarized in Table 3.3), the AJCC staging system reports regional lymph node status (as N) and the presence or ab-

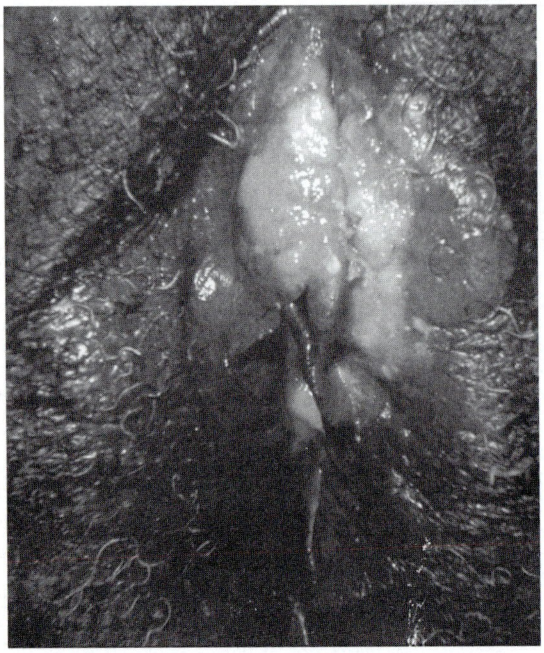

Fig. 3.15. Squamous cell carcinoma. The tumor involves the medial aspect of the left anterior labium majus and clitoris.

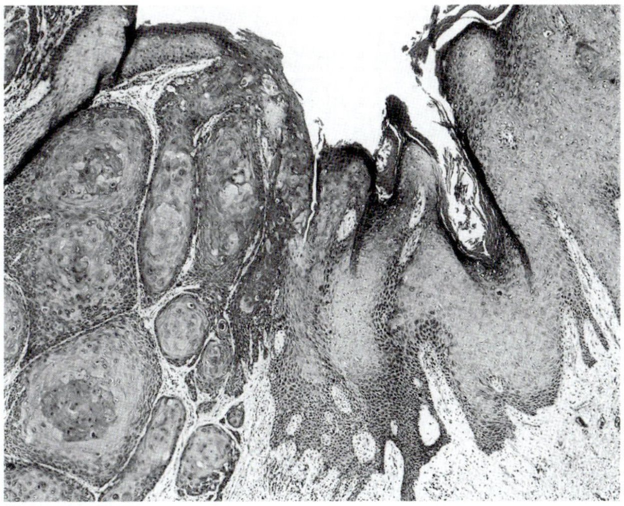

Fig. 3.16. Invasive squamous carcinoma, well differentiated. The tumor is keratinized and has a pushing growth pattern with small nests of tumor in the superficial dermis. Hyperplastic squamous epithelium is adjacent to the tumor. (Courtesy of R.J. Kurman, M.D., Baltimore, MD.)

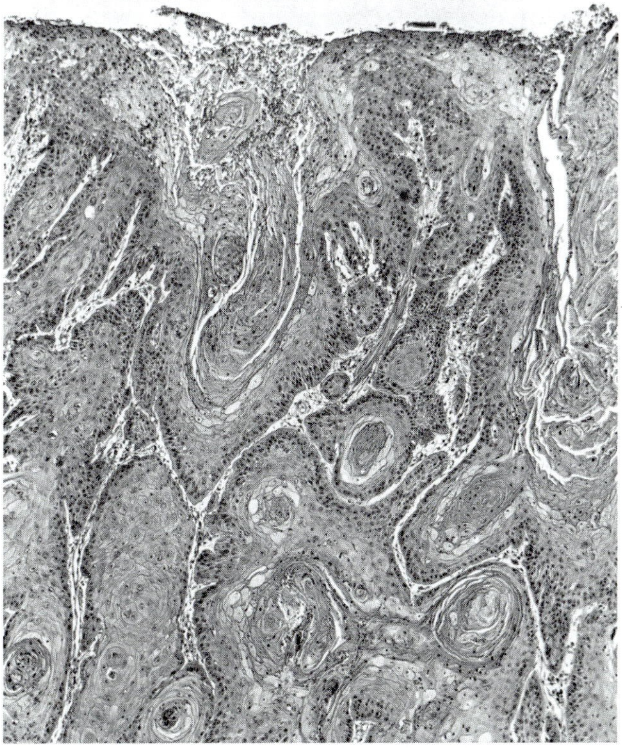

Fig. 3.17 Invasive squamous cell carcinoma, well differentiated. Tongues of well-differentiated squamous epithelium with keratinization are evident.

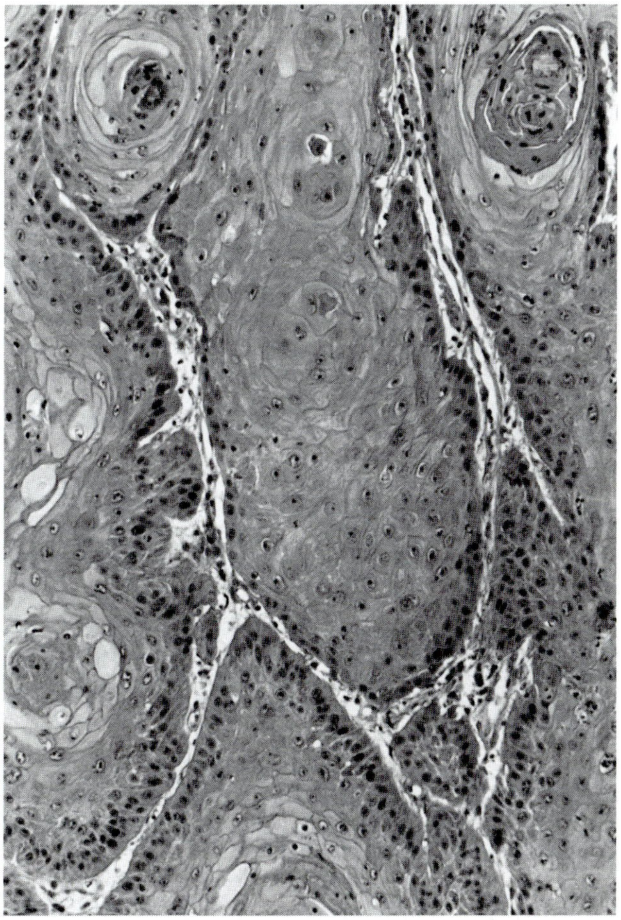

Fig. 3.18. Invasive keratinizing squamous cell carcinoma, well differentiated. The cells have abundant cytoplasm and large, round nuclei with prominent nucleoli.

sence of metastases (as M) (Table 3.4). All lymph node tissue should be submitted for microscopic analysis. The microscopic evaluation of lymph nodes for detection of metastatic cell squamous carcinoma may be augmented by immunohistochemistry using a polyclonal keratin antibody.[9] Pathologic findings included in the College of American Pathologists (CAP) guidelines for evaluation of vulvar squamous cell carcinoma are the same for deep and superficial invasive squamous cell carcinomas (see Superficially Invasive Squamous Cell Carcinoma, Microscopic Findings).[195]

Chromosomal and Immunohistochemical Studies

Cytogenetic studies on vulvar carcinomas have demonstrated that they are genetically complex with multiple chromosomal rearrangements. Nonetheless, they remain karyotypically stable in culture.

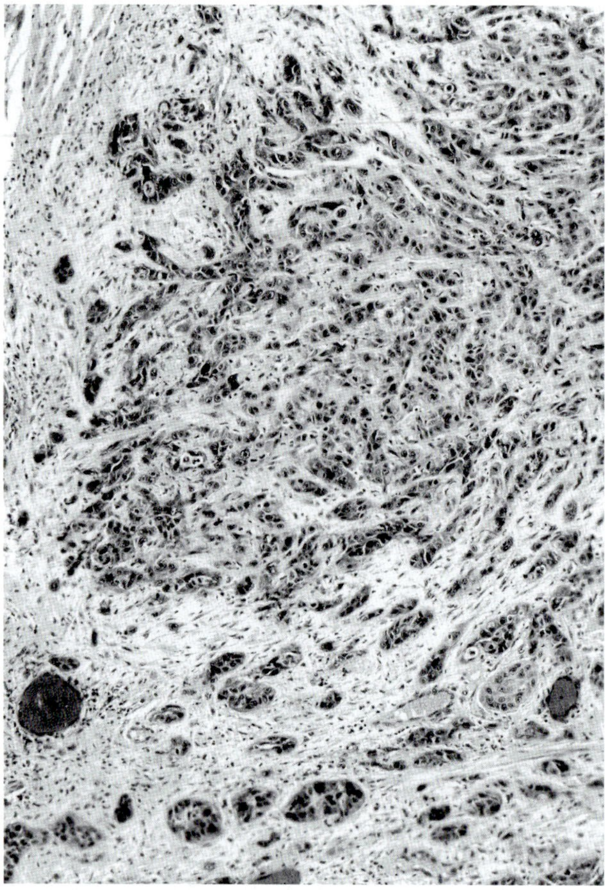

Fig. 3.19. Invasive squamous cell carcinoma, moderately to poorly differentiated. Small nests and cords of invasive squamous cell carcinoma are present without keratinization. (From ref. 108, with permission.)

The tumors typically are heterogeneous with multiple, but closely related, clonal populations. Both development and progression are apparent sequelae of altered gene expression. A study of vulvar carcinomas employing flow cytometry and image analysis demonstrated a high frequency of aneuploidy with a predominance of tumors within the hypotetraploid range.[53]

Table 3.4. Lymph node status and metastasis staging using the American Joint Commission on Cancer (AJCC) staging system

NX: Regional lymph nodes cannot be assessed
(N): no regional lymph node metastasis
N1: unilateral regional lymph node metastasis
N2: bilateral regional lymph node metastasis
With the AJCC system, the presence or absence of metastasis are recorded as (M):
MX: distant metastasis cannot be assessed
M0: no distant metastasis
M1: distant metastasis (includes pelvic node metastasis)

From ref. 4.

Immunohistochemical studies employing monoclonal antibodies to MIB-1 (Ki-67), a proliferation-associated marker, have demonstrated two distinct tumor labeling patterns, diffuse and localized, that appear to be associated with prognosis; the diffuse pattern is associated with poor prognosis.[82] Quantitation of Ki-67 (MIB-1) and Ag-NOR do not appear to predict the presence or absence of inguinofemoral lymph node metastasis, although a correlation was found between the mitotic index and Ki-67 expression.[56] In vulvar squamous cell carcinoma associated with lichen sclerosus, it has been observed that Ki-67 expression is increased in squamous hyperplasia adjacent to the squamous cell carcinoma. These findings may imply premalignancy or a reactive process related to the carcinoma.[157]

Clinical Behavior and Treatment

Factors that may be of significance in prognosis and in the probability of lymph node metastasis include the diameter of the tumor, the presence of vascular space invasion, and tumor ulceration. Confluent growth, defined as anastomosing cords or tumor, or tumor in the dermis exceeding 1 mm^3, does not correlate with the occurrence of node metastasis but is not found in tumors having 1 mm or less of invasion.[193] When controlled for age, survival with vulvar carcinoma decreased with advancing age, higher stage and grade, increasing tumor thickness, prominent fibromyxoid dermal response, inflitrative pattern of growth, and basaloid tumor type.[138]

Inguinofemoral lymph node status[159] and the diameter of the tumor are independent prognostic factors. The overall 5-year relative survival, related to stage, as reported in a series of 588 patients with vulvar carcinoma is as follows: stage I, 98%; stage II, 87%; stage III, 75%; stage IV, 29%.[87] The distance between the tumor and the surgical margin is a significant predictor of local recurrence. A surgical margin of 8 mm or less from the invasive carcinoma is associated with a 50% risk of local recurrence.[80] In a GOG study of 121 patients with stage I vulvar carcinoma with a tumor thickness of 5 mm or less, without vascular space invasion, and with negative lymph nodes, 19 patients (15.7%) experienced recurrence and there were 7 deaths (5.8%) from tumor. Of the 7 deaths, 5 were related to recurrence in the groin nodes.[171] Tumors with a depth of invasion greater than 1 mm require more extensive surgery, including groin node dissection.[23,71,75,103,192] Terminology for surgical proce-

Table 3.5. Surgical procedures and characterization of depth of invasion of vulvar tumors[a]

Vulvectomy
- Partial vulvectomy: removal of a part of the vulvar/perineal integument independent of depth
- Total vulvectomy: removal of the whole vulva and appropriate integument of the perineum independent of depth

Depth of excision
- Superficial: removal of the most superficial layer with a variable amount of dermis and subcutaneous tissue
- Deep: removal of the vulva to the superficial aponeurosis of the urogenital diaphragm and/or pubic periosteum

[a]Developed by the International Society for the Study of Vulvar Disease (ISSVD).

dures and characterization of depth of invasion of vulvar tumors has been developed by the International Society for the Study of Vulvar Disease (ISSVD) and is shown in Table 3.5.[95]

Vulvar carcinoma typically spreads by direct extension and lymphatic metastasis and tends to recur locally. Although distant metastasis is less common, bone metastasis has been reported.[1] The reliability of clinical evaluation in the determination of whether tumor is present in inguinal nodes has a false-positive rate less than 10% but a false-negative rate of approximately 20%.[18] It is recognized that pathologic evaluation of lymph nodes for metastasis also may be falsely negative.

In assessing groin nodes, fine-needle aspiration may be the first step if clinically suspicious nodes are present because the technique is rapid, safe, cost-effective, and will detect gross metastasis.[1] Current therapy attempts to define high- and low-risk groups and requires individualization of therapy.[23,76] Sentinel lymph node identification methods employing technetium-99m-labeled noncolloid have been employed to attempt to select and sample sentinel lymph nodes and possibly avoid inguinfemoral lymph node resection if the sentinel lymph node, or nodes, are free of metastatic tumor[47] (Table 3.6). Many patients are now offered immediate reconstructive surgery as part of the initial procedure.[71] Radiation techniques are now available that allow skin-sparing treatment of the groin nodes and have been used successfully in both primary and adjunctive treatment.[21,116]

Table 3.6. Nodal metastasis in women with stage I vulvar carcinoma with invasion of 1 mm or less

Author and reference number	*Total patients*	*Node metastasis*
Kabulski and Frankman 1978[194]	6	0
Margina et al. 1979[113a]	9	0
Iversen et al. 1981[94a]	23	0
Buscema et al. 1981[23a]	4	0
Wilkinson et al. 1982[200]	5	0
Hacker et al. 1984[75]	24	0
Andreasson and Nyboe 1985[6a]	8	0
Berman et al. 1989[14a]	19	0
Homesley et al. 1993[86a]	38	1 (2.6%)
Magrina et al. 2000[114a]	10	0
Total	146	1 (0.7%)

All patients underwent inguinofemoral lymphadenectomy.

Histologic Subtypes of Vulvar Squamous Cell Carcinoma

Squamous cell carcinoma of the vulva can be subdivided into several morphologically distinct subtypes (Table 3.7). Histologically, invasive squamous cell carcinomas that are not otherwise specified (NOS) usually are well-differentiated tumors, but moderately and poorly differentiated varieties are found in 5%–10% of the cases (see Figs. 3.13 and 3.16–3.19).

Basaloid Carcinoma

An increased prevalence of *human papillomavirus (HPV)*, mainly type 16, has been observed with certain types of invasive squamous carcinomas of the

Table 3.7. Histologic subtypes of squamous vulvar carcinoma

- Squamous cell carcinoma (NOS)
- Basaloid carcinoma
- Warty (condylomatous) carcinoma
- Verrucous carcinoma
- Giant cell carcinoma
- Spindle cell carcinoma
- Acantholytic squamous cell carcinoma (adenoid squamous carcinoma)
- Lymphoepithelioma-like carcinoma
- Basal cell carcinoma
  - Metatypical basal cell carcinoma (basosquamous carcinoma)
  - Adenoid basal cell carcinoma
  - Sebaceous cell carcinoma

NOS, not otherwise specified.

vulva. Among these are *basaloid carcinomas*, which occur in younger women (mean age, 54 years), compared with typical *keratinizing squamous cell carcinomas* (mean age, 77 years). HPV-associated vulvar squamous cell carcinomas can be distinguished histopathologically from non-HPV-related tumors, with agreement between observers noted in 67% of cases.[182] Basaloid carcinomas frequently are associated with adjacent VIN, usually of the basaloid type. In contrast to typical keratinizing squamous cell carcinomas, basaloid carcinomas are associated with synchronous or metachronous squamous neoplasms of the cervix and vagina.[108] On gross examination, basaloid carcinomas are similar to typical keratinizing squamous cell carcinomas. Microscopically, they are characterized by variable-sized nests of immature squamous cells with little, if any, squamous maturation. Some tumors are composed of small, irregularly shaped nests and cords of cells surrounded by a densely hyalinized stroma. The basal-type cells within the nests and cords resemble those in the classic type of *carcinoma in situ of the cervix* (Figs. 3.20–3.22) Characteristically, the cells are ovoid and relatively uniform in size, with scant cytoplasm and a high nuclear cytoplasmic ratio, and therefore they appear undifferentiated. Nuclei contain evenly distributed coarsely granular chromatin, creating a stippled appearance. A moderate degree of mitotic activity usually is evident. Occasionally, the cells in the center of a nest show evidence of maturation and contain more abundant cytoplasm. Small foci of keratinization may be evident in the center of the nests, and keratin pearls occasionally are present. Desmosomes usually are not evident. HPV-16 can be detected in approximately 70% of basaloid squamous carcinomas (Fig. 3.22b).[108] Basaloid carcinoma is reported to be associated with decreased survival in an age-controlled study.[138]

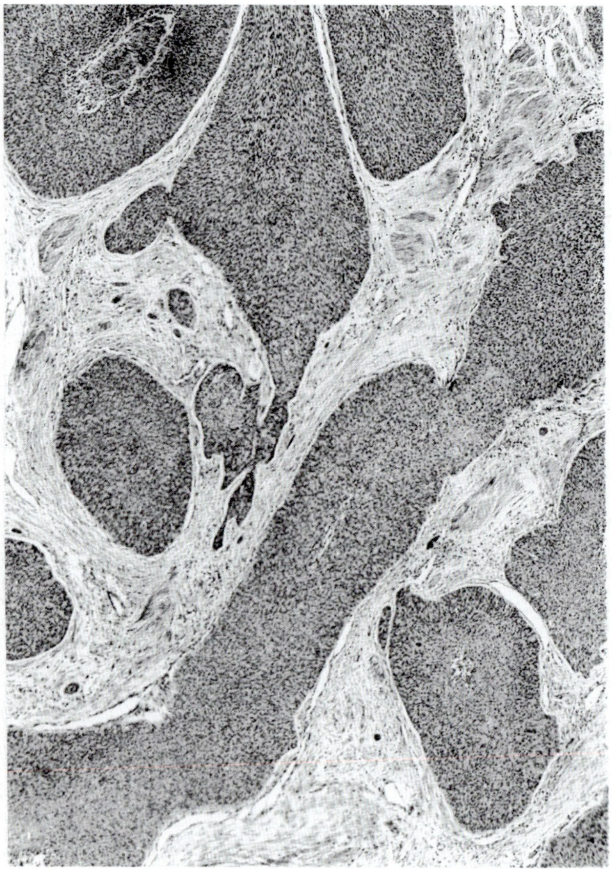

Fig. 3.20. Basaloid carcinoma with a prominent desmoplastic stroma. (From ref. 108, with permission.)

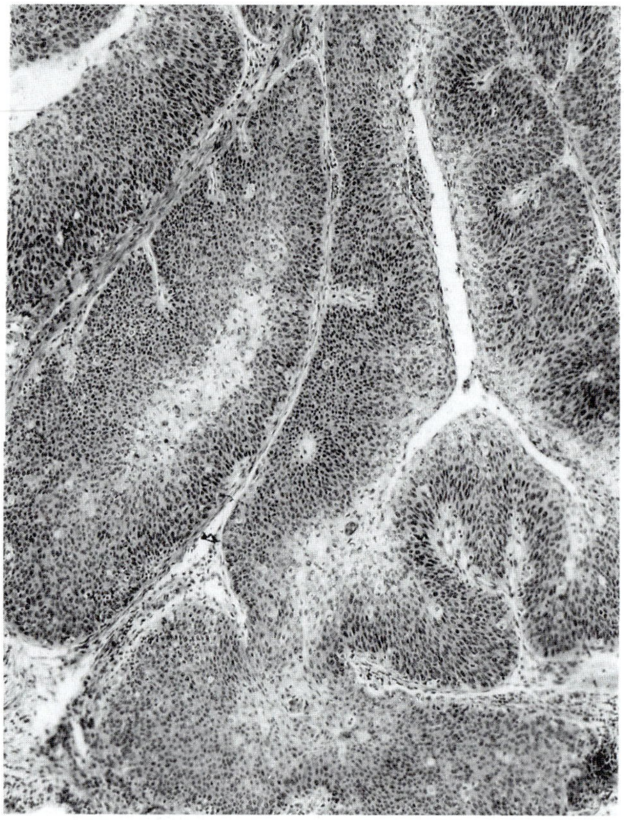

Fig. 3.21. Basaloid carcinoma. The tumor is composed of immature-appearing keratinocytes without significant maturation or keratinization. The surrounding stroma is fibrous. (Courtesy of R.J. Kurman, M.D., Baltimore, MD.)

Basaloid squamous carcinoma must be distinguished from *basal cell carcinoma*, but at times this may be difficult. In contrast to basaloid carcinoma, basal cell carcinomas tend to be more circumscribed and have a lobular appearance. The characteristic palisading of the outermost layer of cells in the nests

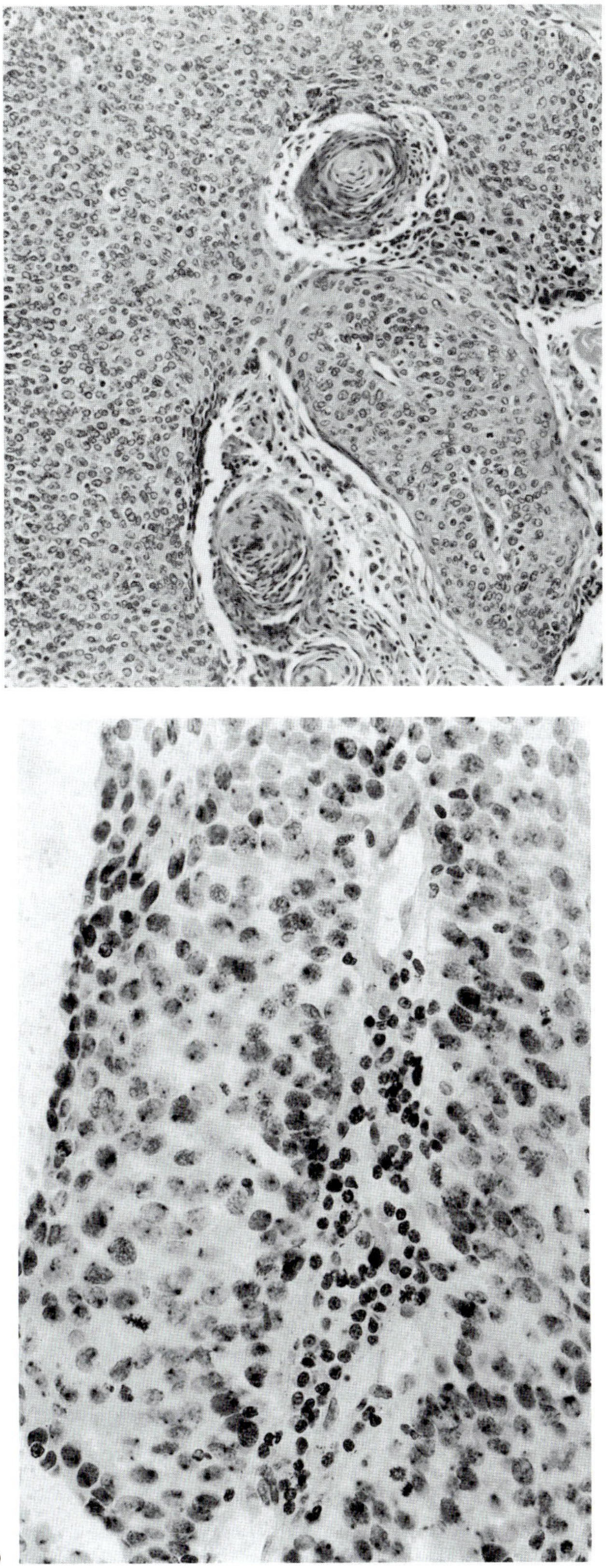

a

b

Fig. 3.22. a: Basaloid carcinoma. The tumor is composed of relatively small cells with hyperchromatic, slightly pleomorphic nuclei. There is cellular disarray throughout the neoplasm; however, some keratinization is evident. (Courtesy of R.J. Kurman, M.D., Baltimore, MD.) **b: Basaloid carcinoma with HPV.** In situ hybridization for HPV 16 demonstrates the dotlike nuclear hybridization pattern, thought to indicate integration of the virus into the host genome. (Courtesy of R.J. Kurman, M.D., Baltimore, MD.)

of basal cell carcinoma is lacking in basaloid carcinoma. The differential diagnosis of basaloid carcinoma also includes *metastatic small cell carcinoma* and *Merkel cell tumor*. These tumors have a more diffusely infiltrative pattern characterized by poorly defined nests, trabeculae, and individual cells invading the stroma rather than the broad anastomosing bands and well-defined nests typical of basaloid carcinoma. Small cell tumors usually are immunoreactive for neuroendocrine markers; Merkel cell tumors have a characteristic perinuclear cytoplasmic "dot" demonstrated by immunohistochemical study with cytokeratins.

Warty Carcinoma (Condylomatous Carcinoma)

Warty carcinoma is found predominantly in younger women (mean age, 55 years) and presents clinically as a verrucoid or papillary tumor that may resemble condyloma acuminatum. Occasionally warty carcinoma or *verrucous carcinoma* may arise in association with condyloma acuminatum.[50,52] On microscopic examination, warty carcinoma has multiple papillary projections with a keratinized epithelial surface and fibrovascular cores (Figs. 3.23 and 3.24). Cytologic atypia is seen, especially within the basal and parabasal cells, where there is nuclear pleomorphism and nuclear hyperchromasia. Multinucleation may be present. Mitotic figures usually can be found and sometimes may be atypical. Cytoplasmic perinuclear clearing similar to koilocytosis in VIN is present in a substantial number of cells; it is the most characteristic feature. At the junction between the exophytic portion of the tumor and the underlying stoma, irregularly shaped nests of epithelium are present that may be associated with keratin pearls and dyskeratotic cells. In this area the tumor resembles a keratinized squamous cell carcinoma. In some cases these areas are small and focal. Warty carcinoma is frequently associated with HPV type 16.[52,108,181]

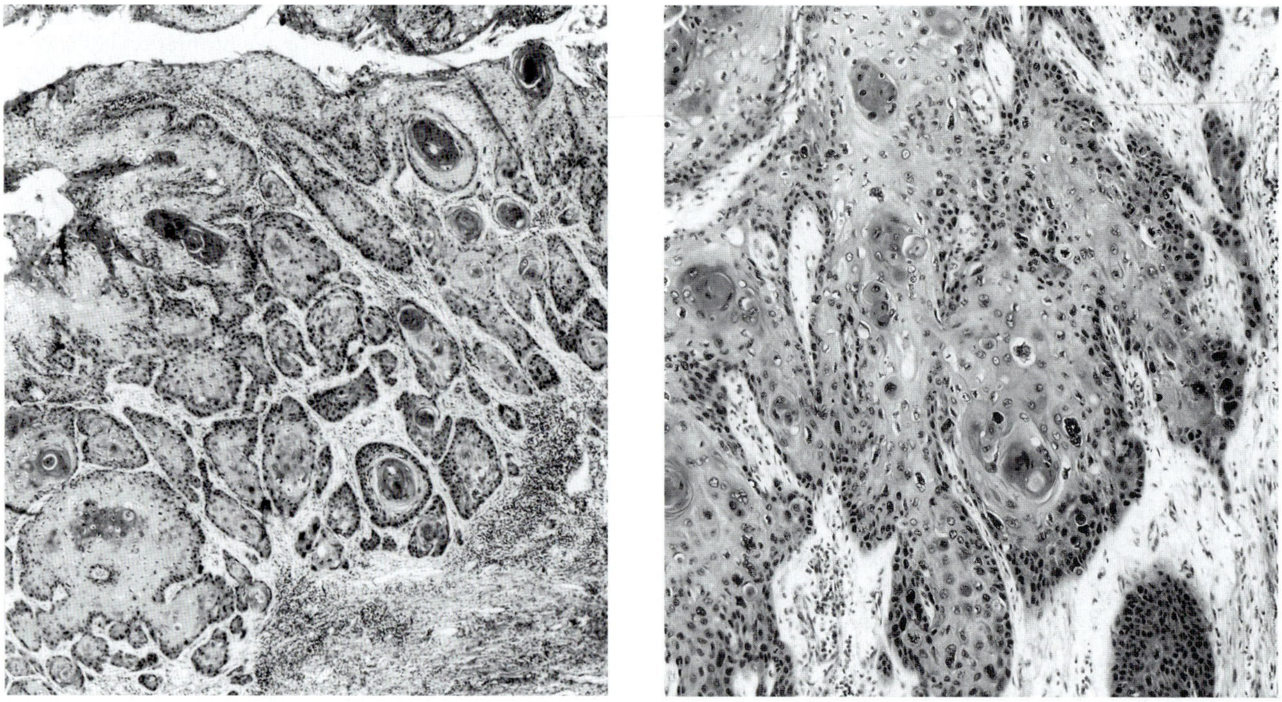

a b

Fig. 3.23. a: Warty (condylomatous) carcinoma. The tumor has well-differentiated neoplastic keratinocytes with keratinization. At the deep margin, the tumor is composed of irregularly shaped, varying sized nests that infiltrate the stroma in a haphazard fashion. (Courtesy of R.J. Kurman, M.D., Baltimore, MD.) **b: Warty (condylomatous) carcinoma.** The cords of neoplastic cells are separated by a fibrovascular stroma. Keratinization is present. (Courtesy of R.J. Kurman, M.D., Baltimore, MD.)

The clinical course of warty carcinoma appears generally good; however, lymph node metastasis may occur. The prognosis appears intermediate between that of verrucous carcinoma and squamous cell carcinoma of the usual type.[181] Approximately 80% of warty and basaloid carcinomas have adjacent warty or basaloid VIN. About one-quarter of the warty and basaloid carcinomas are associated with other genital tract squamous neoplasias.[108]

Verrucous Carcinoma

Verrucous carcinoma is a highly differentiated squamous carcinoma that has a verrucous pattern and invades with a pushing border in the form of bulbous pegs of neoplastic cells.[19,97] The term *giant condyloma of Buschke–Lowenstein* is considered to be a synonym for verrucous carcinoma, but it is confusing and therefore is not recommended. Squamous cell carcinomas at times may have some of the architectural features of verrucous carcinoma, but if they lack a high degree of differentiation, or have a nonpushing pattern of invasion, they should not be designated verrucous carcinoma.[105] Verrucous carcinoma is a papillary exophytic growth that may have the appearance of an exophytic, broad-based condyloma acuminatum and distort or completely obscure the vulva[6] (Fig. 3.25). Condyloma acuminatum may be adjacent to verrucous carcinoma, and rarely the tumor may merge into a typical squamous cell carcinoma.[50,52] Secondary infection may be associated with a malodorous discharge. Regional lymph nodes usually are not enlarged. Verrucous carcinoma has been reported to be associated with HPV, typically type 6 or variants of type 6.

The microscopic features of verrucous carcinoma include prominent acanthosis with a pushing tumor–dermal interface and bland cytologic features (Fig. 3.26) (see Chapter 4, Diseases of the Vagina). Large bulbous nests of squamous epithelium characterize the deep margin. There is minimal nuclear pleomorphism, with the greatest degree of nuclear atypia nearest the dermal interface. The nuclei may have coarse chromatin and variable-sized nucleoli, distinguishing them from normal adjacent keratinocytes. Mitotic figures are rare and when present are normal. The abundant cytoplasm of the tumor cells is eosinophilic, without dyskeratosis. Koilocytosis is not a feature of this tumor.

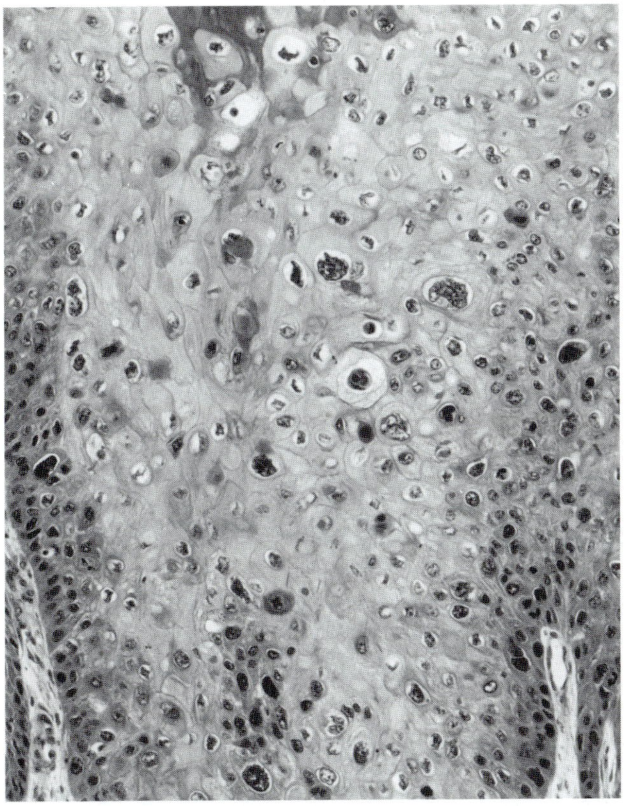

Fig. 3.24. Warty (condylomatous) carcinoma. Cells with pleomorphic nuclei and vacuolated cytoplasm resembling koilocytes are present within the neoplastic epithelium. (Courtesy of R.J. Kurman, M.D., Baltimore, MD.)

Parakeratosis or hyperkeratosis usually is present and may be prominent. There is an absence of fibrovascular cores separating the bulbous epithelial downgrowths. An inflammatory infiltrate within the dermis usually is present. These tumors typically are diploid.

The differential diagnosis includes the typical variety of squamous cell carcinoma, warty carcinoma, and condyloma acuminatum. Squamous cell carcinoma of the usual type (keratinizing squamous carcinoma) has greater nuclear pleomorphism and a more irregular pattern of infiltration of the stroma compared with the bulbous nests of verrucous carcinoma. Warty carcinoma, despite its verruciform appearance, has fibrovascular cores within the papillary fronds, unlike verrucous carcinoma. In addition, these tumors display greater nuclear atypia, "koilocytosis," and, at their deep margin, invade like typical squamous cell carcinomas. Condyloma acuminatum is characterized by a complex branching papillary architecture with vascular papillae,

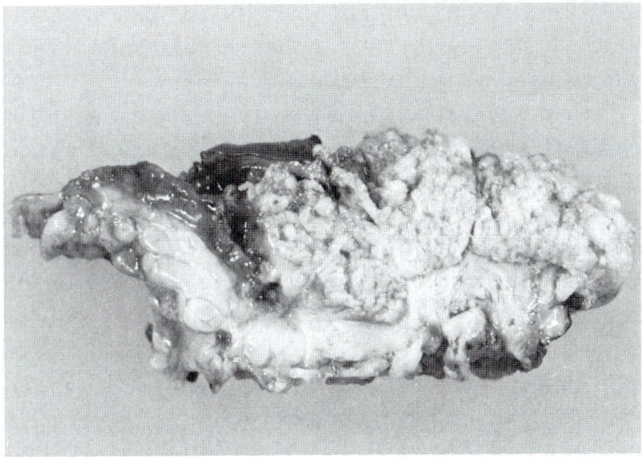

Fig. 3.25. Verrucous carcinoma in cross section. This tumor is 5 cm in diameter and has a broad, well-defined margin of infiltration involving the underlying fibrofatty tissue.

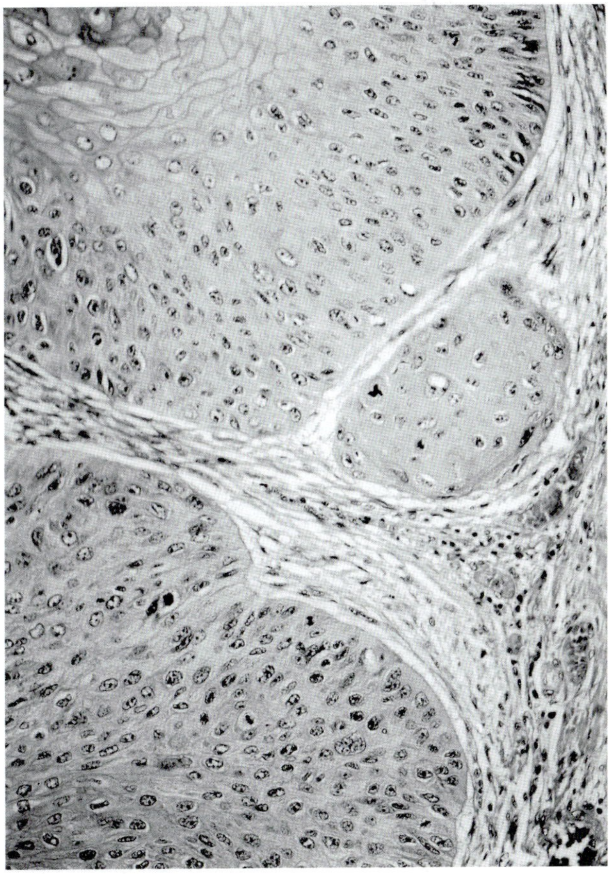

Fig. 3.26. Verrucous carcinoma. There is a well-defined tumor–stromal interface with a pushing, growth pattern. The keratinocytes are very well differentiated, and occasional mitotic figures are present. (Courtesy of R.J. Kurman, M.D., Baltimore, MD.)

lacks bulbous downgrowths, and typically shows koilocytosis, although in vulvar condylomas koilocytosis may be quite subtle.

Verrucous carcinomas may recur locally after excision. Lymph node metastasis is extremely rare, and its presence should prompt reevaluation of the lesion for areas of the usual type of squamous cell carcinoma. Wide local excision and total vulvectomy without lymph node dissection are the most common methods of therapy. If the tumor is excised completely, the prognosis is excellent. The role of radiotherapy in vulvar verrucous carcinomas is not well studied, but it may be applicable in very advanced cases.

Giant Cell Squamous Carcinoma

Squamous cell carcinoma with tumor giant cells is a variant of squamous cell carcinoma characterized by multinucleated tumor giant cells, large nuclei with prominent nucleoli, and prominent eosinophilic cytoplasm (Fig. 3.27). This tumor variant is relatively rare and is associated with a poor prognosis. The most important differential diagnosis is *malignant amelanotic melanoma*, which commonly forms multinucleated tumor giant cells.[198] Melanomas typically have intranuclear inclusions and prominent nucleoli. Unlike giant cell carcinoma, melanomas are typically immunoreactive for S-100, melanoma antigen (HMB 45), and Melan-A and negative for cytokeratin.[198]

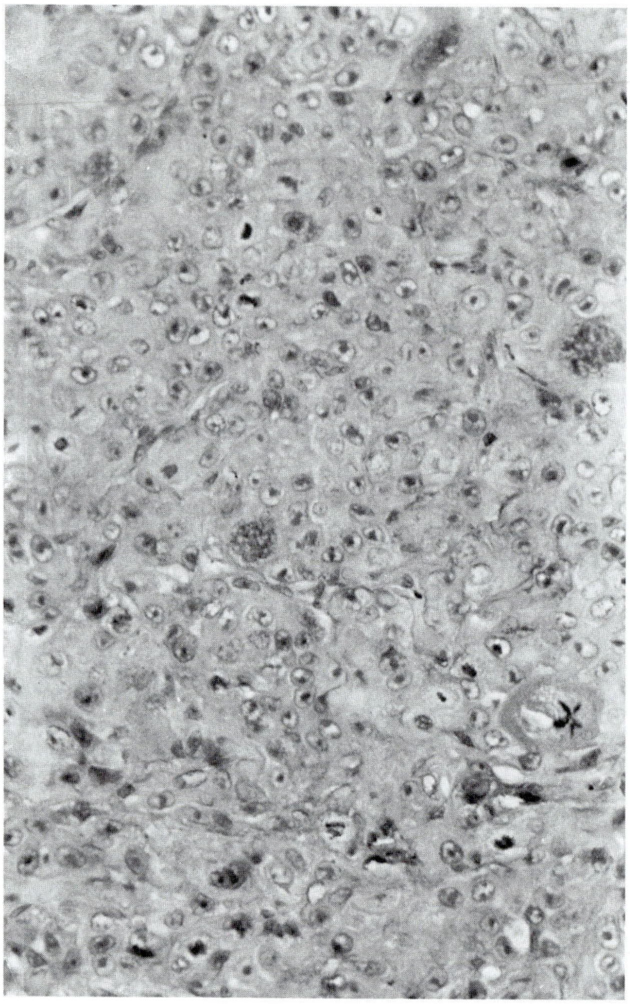

Fig. 3.27. Giant cell carcinoma of the vulva. Multinucleated tumor giant cells are evident. The cells contain nuclei with prominent nucleoli and abundant eosinophilic cytoplasm.

Spindle Cell Squamous Cell Carcinoma

Spindle cell carcinoma of the vulva may mimic a sarcoma or be associated with sarcoma-like stroma.[36,168,169] These tumors must be distinguished from *mesenchymal spindle cell tumors*, including leiomyosarcoma, malignant fibrous histiocytoma, and fibrosarcoma, as well as *spindle cell malignant melanoma* and *transitional cell carcinoma* with spindle cell features. The neoplastic cells of spindle cell carcinoma, unlike all the mesenchymal tumors and melanoma, are immunoreactive for keratin.[153] Spindle cell carcinoma may be associated with tumor giant cells, which are also immunoreactive for keratin.[153]

Acantholytic Squamous Cell Carcinoma (Adenoid Squamous Carcinoma)

The acantholytic squamous tumor forms rounded spaces, or pseudoacini, lined with a single layer of squamous cells. Dyskeratotic and acantholytic cells are sometimes present in the central lumen (Fig. 3.28). These changes are focal in most cases and may occur within otherwise well-differentiated squamous tumors.[100] Acantholytic squamous cell carcinoma appears to have a prognosis similar to squamous carcinoma of the usual type, and the adenoid architecture does not correlate with an increased risk of lymph node involvement or a more adverse clinical outcome.

Lymphoepithelioma-Like Carcinoma

These tumors may occur rarely on the vulva in older individuals.[26] They are composed of nests or syncytial groups of epithelioid-appearing cells mixed with, and surrounded by, a dense lymphocytic infiltrate (see Chapter 8, Carcinoma and Other Tumors of the Cervix). The epithelial cells are im-

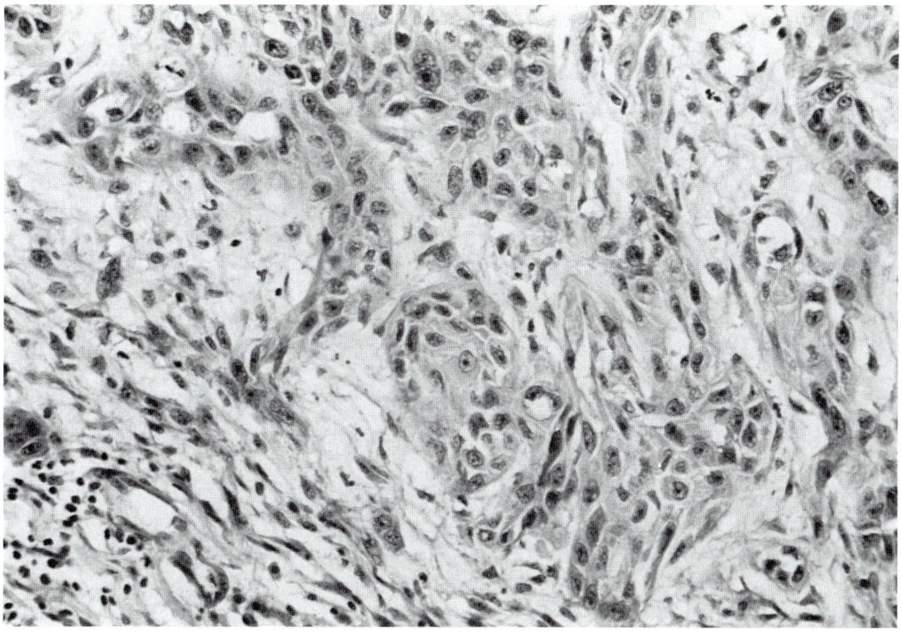

Fig. 3.28. Acantholytic squamous carcinoma. Nests of poorly differentiated squamous cell carcinoma are arranged in a crude acinar manner. Some of the central acini are vacuolated.

munoreactive for high molecular weight cytokeratins, which distinguishes them from inflammatory processes and malignant large cell lymphomas. Lymphomas, including Ki-1 lymphomas, which are immunoreactive for lymphocytic markers, contain an immunophenotypic monoclonal population of neoplastic lymphocytic cells. The therapy is wide local excision with or without local radiation therapy.[26]

Basal Cell Carcinoma

Although *basal cell carcinomas* of the skin are extremely common, they account for only 5%–7% of vulvar carcinomas.[62,140] They are found primarily in elderly white women (mean age, 70–76 years), whose symptomatology consists of pruritus, irritation, soreness, or bleeding. The tumors present as an ulcer, an area of pigmentation or depigmentation, or as a mass.[62,140] Most of these tumors are confined to the labia majora, and approximately one-half are of infiltrative type. Basal cell carcinoma has been reported arising in vulvar Paget disease.[93] Basal cell carcinomas are not associated with human papillomavirus.

The histologic pattern resembles that of basal cell carcinomas occurring elsewhere on the skin (Fig. 3.29). The tumor is composed of small elongated cells with deeply basophilic nuclei and may have a large variety of architectural patterns, ranging from slight palisading of the basal layer of the epidermis to the formation of large club-shaped masses of pleomorphic basal cells. The connective tissue adjacent to the tumor frequently contains a

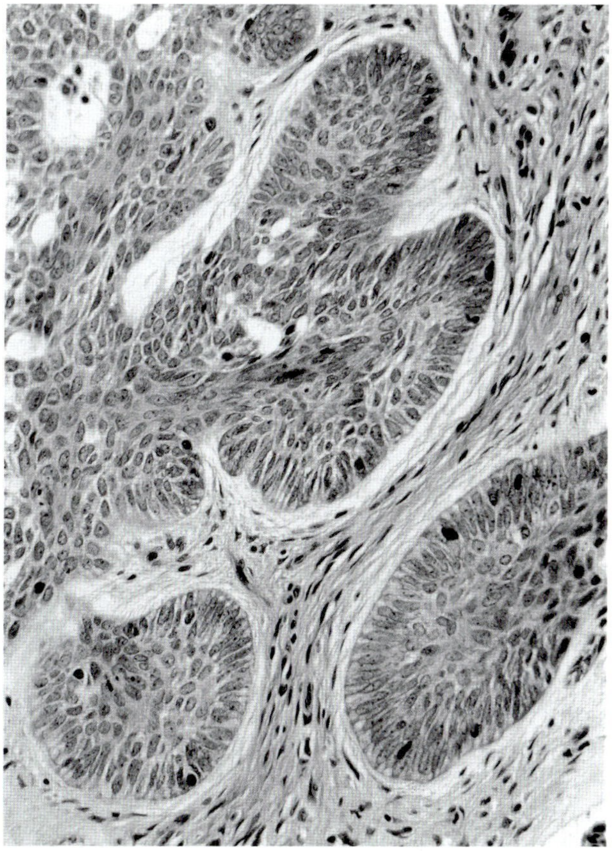

Fig. 3.29. Basal cell carcinoma. The tumor cells are small, uniform, lack maturation, and show characteristic palisading at the periphery of the involved rete ridges. The rete ridges are branched and extend in a pushing manner into the adjacent dermis. (Courtesy of R.J. Kurman, M.D., Baltimore, MD.)

chronic inflammatory cell infiltrate and occasionally shows a mucoid or myxomatous change.

Primary treatment is wide local excision.[139] Local recurrence occurs in approximately 9%–20% of cases.[62,139] Metastasis to regional lymph nodes occurs but is rare.[13,62] The overall prognosis of patients with these tumors is excellent, with only a rare death reported.[13]

Metatypical Basal Cell Carcinoma (Basosquamous Carcinoma)

Metatypical basal cell carcinoma, or *basosquamous carcinoma*, represents a mixture of both squamous and basal cell neoplastic elements (Fig. 3.30). Like basal cell carcinomas, basosquamous carcinomas are locally aggressive and metastasize rarely.

Adenoid Basal Cell Carcinoma

Adenoid basal cell carcinoma is a variant of basal cell carcinoma in which tubular and glandlike differentiation is seen within a tumor that otherwise is a characteristic basal cell carcinoma.

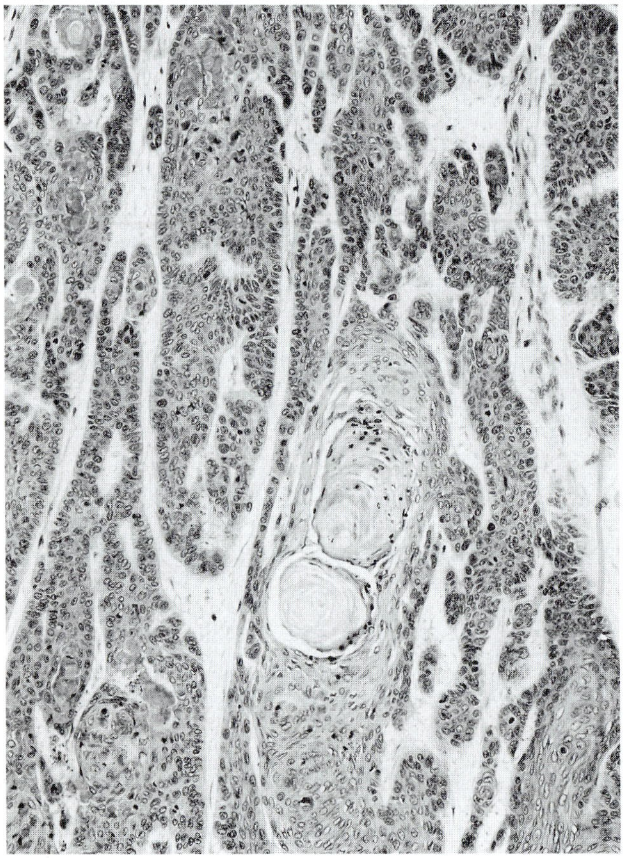

Fig. 3.30. Basosquamous carcinoma (metatypical basal cell carcinoma). The cells show increased cytoplasm in the areas of squamous differentiation. (Courtesy of R.J. Kurman, M.D., Baltimore, MD.)

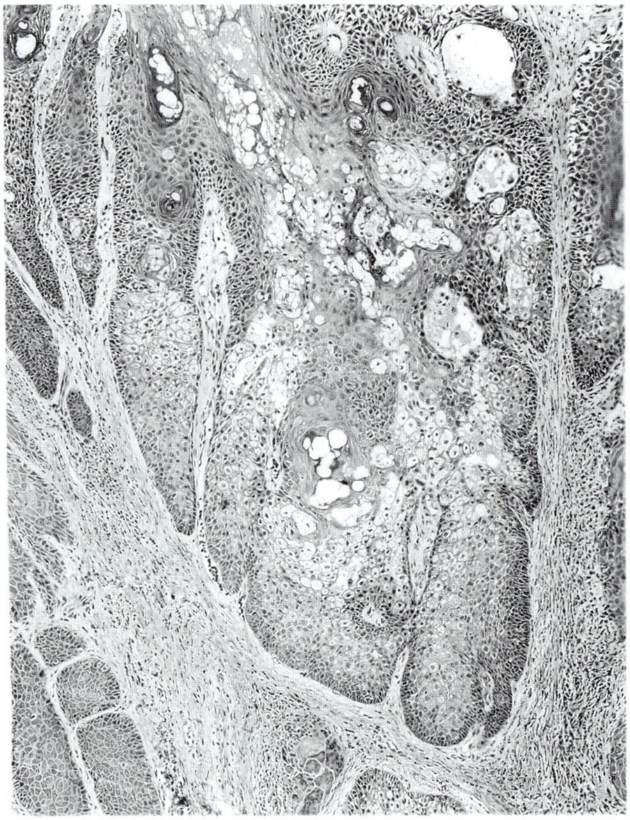

Fig. 3.31. Sebaceous carcinoma. The tumor is composed of cords and nests of basaloid-appearing cells. These cells are associated with sebaceous cells in pagetoid nests in the parabasal areas and in larger clusters near the epithelial surface. (Courtesy of R.J. Kurman, M.D., Baltimore, MD.)

Sebaceous Cell Carcinoma

Sebaceous cell carcinoma is a rare tumor of the vulva.[25] The tumor has features of basosquamous cell carcinoma with sebaceous differentiation (Fig. 3.31). This tumor type has been associated with vulvar intraepithelial neoplasia.[96]

Glandular Tumors

Adenocarcinomas of the vulva are relatively rare. Many previous reports have been shown retrospectively to represent benign hidradenomas or foci of adnexal Paget disease. Most adenocarcinomas of the vulva arise as primary malignant tumors of the Bartholin gland; however, they also may arise from sweat glands or from other skin appendages, the urethra, the Skene gland, and from Paget disease.[178,191] Paget disease and Paget-like neoplastic lesions, including pagetoid urothelial intraepithelial neoplasia (PUIN), are described here.

Paget Disease

Clinical Features

Clinically, *vulvar Paget disease* can present as either an erythematous lesion, often involving the vestibule and adjacent areas, or an eczematous lesion that appears as a red to pink area with white islands of hyperkeratosis and usually involving hair-bearing skin (Fig. 3.32). The extent of involvement can be very focal, or extensive, extending about the anus, medial aspects of the upper thigh, or other contiguous sites. Pruritus is present in more than half the patients, and was present for a median duration of 2 years before the diagnosis in a study of 100 patients.[61] Almost all patients are postmenopausal Caucasian women, with a median age of 70 years,[61] although a case of vulvar Paget disease has been reported in a 24-year-old black woman.[167] The vulvar pruritus or pain may bring the patient to the attention of the physician. Because of its clinical resemblance to a dermatosis, these patients may be treated with various topical medications for some time before the diagnosis is made by biopsy.

Vulvar Paget disease and *pagetoid urothelial intraepithelial neoplasia* (*PUIN*) have recently been subclassified by the author into three distinct types based upon the origin of the neoplastic cells[196] summarized as follows:

Type 1: primary vulvar cutaneous Paget disease
Type 2: Paget disease as a manifestation of an associated adjacent primary anal, rectal, or othernoncutaneous adenocarcinoma
Type 3: pagetoid urothelial intraepithelial neoplasia (PUIN); pseudopaget disease; Paget disease as a manifestation of bladder (urothelial) neoplasia

Type 1, *primary vulvar cutaneous Paget disease*, can be further subclassified as follows. Type 1a Paget disease, *primary vulvar intraepithelial Paget disease*, is characterized by an intraepithelial proliferation of atypical glandular-type cells and may be considered as an adenocarcinoma in situ. Histopathologic features are characterized by relatively large cells, with prominent cytoplasm, which are within the squamous epithelium. These cells are generally larger than the adjacent keratinocytes and have large nuclei with prominent nucleoli. Their cytoplasm is finely granular and amphophilic to basophilic, and may be vacuolated, in contrast to the eosinophilic more homogeneous cytoplasm of keratinocytes. The neoplastic cells are typically clustered in groups or dispersed as single cells within the basal and parabasal areas, and also in various layers within the epithelium, so-called pagetoid spread. They may form small acinar groupings within the surface squamous epithelium and involve the epithelium surrounding hair shafts and skin appendages. Mitotic figures may be present but are not frequent (Figs. 3.33 and 3.34). Paget cells can be identified on cytologic examination of scrapings from saline-moistened areas

In type 1b Paget disease, *primary vulvar intraepithelial Paget disease with invasion* (type 1b), dermal invasion by intraepithelial Paget cells has been well documented and has been reported in 12% in a series of 100 cases.[61] Vulvar Paget disease is therefore properly classified as a form of intraepithelial neoplasia that may become invasive.

In type 1c Paget disease, *vulvar Paget disease presenting as a manifestation of a primary underlying adenocarcinoma of the vulva*, vulvar Paget disease may be associated with underlying invasive adenocarcinoma of the vulva, as has been reported in 4% of vulvar Paget disease cases in one series.[61] Cases with associated adenocarcinoma of the Bartholin gland and squamous cell carcinoma of the vulva have been reported. Primary vulvar adenocarcinoma is identified beneath Paget disease in approximately 10%–20% of the cases reported (see Fig.

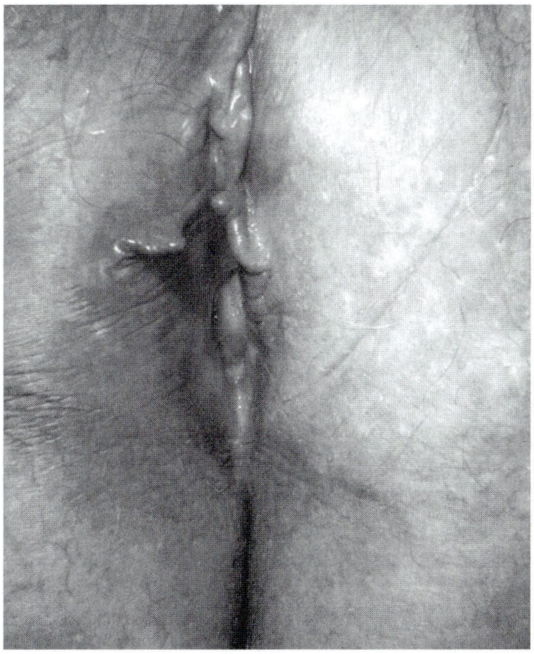

Fig. 3.32. Paget disease. An eczematoid, slightly raised, white area is present on the medial anterior surface of the left labium majus.

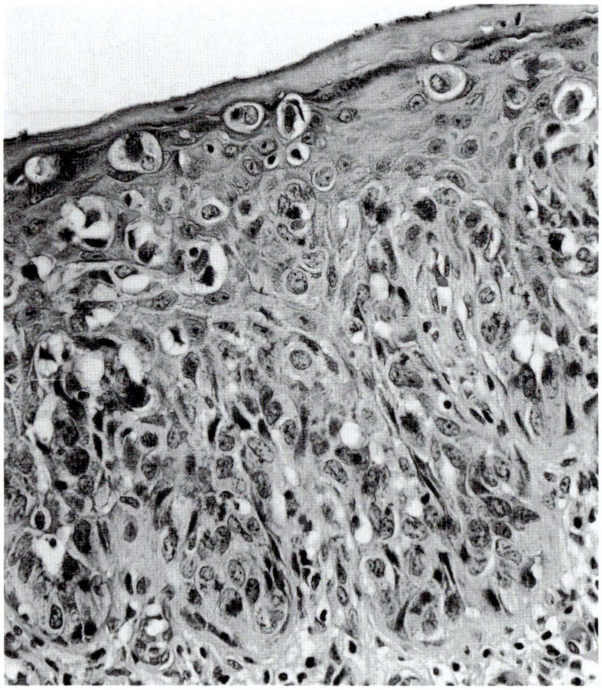

Fig. 3.33. Paget disease. Large numbers of Paget cells within the basal and parabasal areas with isolated Paget cells extending into the upper epithelium. (Courtesy of R.J. Kurman, M.D., Baltimore, MD.)

3.33). Its origin may be from primary invasive Paget disease or adenocarcinoma of the Bartholin gland, specialized anogenital glands, or other vulvar glandular structures. Early investigators noted underlying adnexal adenocarcinoma beneath the skin in the vicinity of Paget disease in many extramammary cases. This finding led some to conclude that Paget cells in the epidermis represented an intradermal migration of neoplastic cells from an underlying cutaneous tumor, as occurs in the breast. The origin of such underlying adenocarcinomas associated with Paget disease does not appear to be sweat gland tumors in that epidermal growth factor (EGF), which is typically present in approximately three-fourths of eccrine or apocrine sweat gland tumors, was absent in vulvar Paget disease in a study of 17 cases.[3]

Cases of type 2 Paget disease, *Paget disease as a manifestation of an associated adjacent primary noncutaneous adenocarcinoma*, include Paget disease associated with in situ or invasive rectal adenocarcinoma or colonic adenocarcinoma, or intraepithelial extension from an adjacent cervical adenocarcinoma. Perianal involvement by Paget disease is associated with a high frequency of adenocarcinoma or squamous carcinoma of the rectum and may present with perianal pruritus, pain and burning, or bleeding after defecation.[130] Primary perianal Paget disease may involve the vulva (Paget type 2) and should be distinguished from primary vulvar Paget disease (types 1a, 1b, or 1c). Although primary vulvar Paget disease (types 1a, 1b, or 1c) involving the perianal area cannot be distinguished by routine histologic examination from primary anal Paget disease involving the vulva (type 2), the distinction can be made employing immunohistochemistry. Primary perianal Paget disease is immunoreactive for cytokeratin 20 and negative for gross cystic disease fluid protein-15 (GCDFP-15). It is also associated with rectal Paget disease and, in most reported cases, with rectal adenocarcinoma (Table 3.7).[130]

Adenocarcinoma of the cervix manifesting as vulvar Paget disease has been reported.[43] In such cases the immunohistochemistry would reflect a cervical adenocarcinoma, depending on cellular type, and

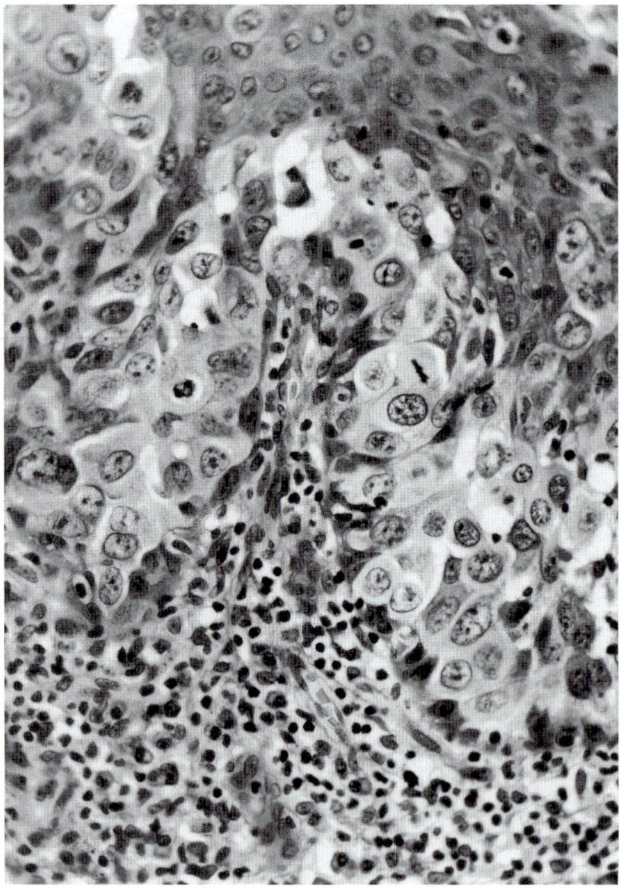

Fig. 3.34. Paget disease. Paget cells are present singly and in nests. Their pale cytoplasm differentiates them from surrounding keratinocytes. The nuclei of the Paget cells are larger, and their nuclear chromatin coarser, than in the adjacent keratinocytes. A mitotic figure is present. (Courtesy of R.J. Kurman, M.D., Baltimore, MD.)

would have a high probability of containing human papillomavirus, especially types 16 or 18. Paget cells typically are HPV negative.

Type 3 Paget disease, pagetoid urothelial intraepithelial neoplasia (PUIN), or pseudopaget disease or Paget disease as a manifestation of bladder (urothelial) neoplasia: urinary tract malignancy has been reported with genital Paget disease, and the original report of extramammary Paget disease by Crocker in 1889 was of a man with penile and scrotal Paget disease associated with bladder carcinoma.[130,143] It has recently been recognized, however, that Paget-like vulvar mucosal and dermal changes associated with urothelial neoplasia can be recognized as a distinct entity. In these cases, there is involvement of the vulvar vestibule, including the periurethral area, which is manifested as an erythematous lesion.

The cells of PUIN have the cytologic features of urothelial carcinoma in situ, with which PUIN is most commonly associated.[115,196] Of key importance regarding the recognition of PUIN (type 3 Paget disease) is that this vulvar neoplasm is a manifestation of bladder urothelial neoplasia and is not associated with underlying adenocarcinoma.

Differential Diagnosis and Adjunctive Studies

The PUIN (Paget type 3) cells do not contain mucin, PAS-positive material, CEA, or GCDFP-15 as do the Paget cells of Paget disease types 1 or 2.[115,196] The cells of PUIN are immunoreactive for cytokeratin 7 and may be cytokeratin 20 positive and uroplakin III positive, as are one-half of the primary urothelial carcinomas (Table 3.2).[124]

Paget cells (types 1 and 2) are positive for PAS (diastase resistant), mucicarmine, aldehydefuchsin, and Alcian blue. The cells stain pink against a background of greenish-blue with Movat stain. In addition, Paget cells of type 1 Paget disease, as well as the cells and secretions of normal eccrine and apocrine glands, are rich in carcinoembryonic antigen (CEA) and gross cystic disease fluid protein-15 (GCDFP-15), and typically are negative for S-100 protein, HMB-45, and Melan-A.[115] Paget cells of type 1 Paget disease are immunoreactive for cytokeratin 7.[43,195] These reactions distinguish typical Paget cells from PUIN, VIN, superficial spreading malignant melanoma, and pagetoid reticulosis. They may also be useful in evaluation of margins in permanent sections.[10,66,115] Melanoma is distinguished by being immunoreactive for S-100, HMB-45, and Melan-A, which are typically not identified in Paget cells.[10] Paget cells, however, may contain granules of melanin, demonstrable with Fontana–Mason stain, probably produced by neighboring melanocytes and engulfed secondarily by the Paget cell. Paget cells have not been demonstrated to be associated with common genital human papillomaviruses.[165] Estrogen receptor expression, p53 immunoreactivity, and DNA ploidy do not appear predictive of clinical behavior or recurrence.[43] However, DNA nondiploid Paget disease has been associated with an increased risk of recurrence, as compared to diploid Paget disease, in one study.[154]

Clinical Behavior and Treatment

The treatment and prognosis of Paget disease of the vulva depends on the type as described herein. For type 1 Paget disease, prognosis depends on whether the lesion is intraepithelial only, or if there is an associated invasive Paget disease. For primary intraepithelial Paget disease (type 1a Paget disease), the lesion is usually a slowly progressive, indolent, superficial process. Accordingly, local excision of the visible lesion to the fascia, with 2-cm clinically visibly clear margins of excision, is sufficient. In cases associated with invasive Paget disease, or with underlying skin appendage or vulvar glandular adenocarcinoma, as determined by histopathologic evaluation, treatment includes ipsilateral inguinofemoral lymphadenectomy. If the tumor extends to the margins of excision, or the excision is deemed inadequate in the face of invasive disease, more extended partial or total vulvectomy may be needed.[43,61,115] Recurrent vulvar Paget disease, occurring peripheral to an excised intraepithelial Paget lesion, does not appear to be associated with any significant risk of underlying adenocarcinoma and can be treated by a more conservative approach, such as superficial excision.[60]

In the patient with vulvar Paget disease (type 1), clinically normal appearing skin may contain Paget cells. A careful topographic study[74] demonstrated that the outline of the histologically involved area was highly irregular and of much greater extent than the visible lesion. In addition, multicentric foci, some occurring in grossly normal-appearing skin, were noted; this accounts for the frequent "recurrences" of disease despite seemingly adequate excision. These clinically normal-appearing areas of skin, however, are not associated with underlying skin appendage adenocarcinoma or invasive Paget disease (type 1). In the author's experience, when invasive Paget disease (type 1b) or underlying skin appendage carcinoma (type 1c) is present, the adenocarcinoma is within the dermis of the skin or mucosa clinically involved with the Paget disease. In such cases, excision to the fascia of these clinically involved areas, to excise the Paget disease and the potential underlying adenocarcinoma, is necessary.

The depth of invasion influences prognosis in such cases. When the depth of dermal invasion was 1 mm or less, no nodal metastasis or death from tumor was observed in 7 such patients, whereas all 3 patients with tumor invasion beyond 1 mm had inguinofemoral node metastasis.[43] Frozen section evaluation of clinically normal-appearing skin margins adjacent to Paget disease (type 1) has not been demonstrated either to improve survival or to reduce recurrence. In a study of 12 patients with involved margins following surgery, 7 (58%) had recurrence, whereas recurrence was seen in 1 of 4 patients (25%) with negative margins.[43] Recurrences of primary intraepithelial Paget disease (type 1a) after excision of the primary lesion have not demonstrated a significant risk of associated underlying adenocarcinoma. Recurrences at the site of the original tumor or remote from it can be treated by local superficial excision. Intraepithelial Paget disease has no significant risk of lymph node metastasis or death.[43,61] The issues regarding margin assessment specifically relate to Paget disease types 1a, 1b, and 1c. Margin assessment for Paget type 2, or PUIN (Paget type 3) needs to be addressed.

In cases of perianal Paget disease, it is necessary to evaluate the rectum and anus to determine if the lesion is a manifestation of underlying rectal Paget disease or rectal or anal adenocarcinoma. In such cases, therapy is directed toward treatment of the rectal or anal carcinoma, and the vulvar Paget disease can be treated as an intraepithelial neoplasm, with local superficial excision, or more conservatively.

In vulvar Paget disease associated with other adjacent adenocarcinomas, such as cervical adenocarcinoma, the treatment is focused on the primary adenocarcinoma and the associated Paget disease is treated as an intraepithelial neoplastic process, with superficial excision. The prognosis in such cases is dependent on the stage and behavior of the associated adenocarcinoma.

Therapy for vulvar PUIN is directed toward the bladder urothelial neoplasm, and the vulvar pagetoid intraepithelial urothelial neoplastic process is treated conservatively, as an intraepithelial neoplasm. Total vulvectomy and excision to the deep fascia is not indicated in this circumstance.[115,196]

Bartholin Gland Tumors

General Features

A wide variety of tumors may arise from the Bartholin gland. The criteria for the diagnosis of a *tumor of Bartholin gland origin* are that the neoplasm must (1) arise at the site of Bartholin gland, (2) be consistent histologically with a primary neoplasm of Bartholin gland, and (3) not be metastatic.[207] Adenocarcinomas account for approximately 40% of Bartholin gland carcinomas, but others include squamous cell carcinoma (40%), adenoid cystic carcinoma (15%), transitional cell carcinoma (less than 5%), adenosquamous carcinoma (less than 5%), and poorly differentiated adenocarcinomas.[48,207]

Clinical Features

Carcinoma of the Bartholin gland usually presents as an enlargement in the gland area and may present as an apparent Bartholin cyst. The average age of women with this tumor is 50 years, with most between 40 and 70 years.

Gross Findings

Bartholin gland tumors are typically solid, deeply infiltrative, and occupy the site of the gland, occasionally obscuring its presence. They range from 1 to 7 cm in diameter.

Microscopic Findings

Adenocarcinomas of the Bartholin gland usually are nonspecific in type, but mucinous and papillary types have been described. The tumors usually contain intracytoplasmic mucin and are immunoreactive for CEA. Fine-needle aspiration cytology may be of value in diagnosis.[91]

Differential Diagnosis

The differential diagnosis of Bartholin gland adenocarcinoma includes adenocarcinoma of skin appendage origin and metastatic adenocarcinoma. These tumors typically do not involve the Bartholin gland, and the tumor type may not be consistent with a primary tumor of the Bartholin gland.

Other Primary Bartholin Gland Carcinomas

Squamous cell carcinomas arising in the Bartholin gland have the same microscopic appearance as those arising elsewhere in the vulva. These tumors are typically immunoreactive for CEA.

Adenoid cystic carcinomas arising in the Bartholin gland are similar to those occurring in salivary glands, the upper respiratory tract, and skin. They are composed of uniform, small cells arranged in cords and nests with a cribriform pattern. Variable-sized cysts filled with an amphophilic or eosinophilic acellular basement membrane-like material also may be encountered (Figs. 3.35 and 3.36). Keratin and S-100 antigen are detectable by im-

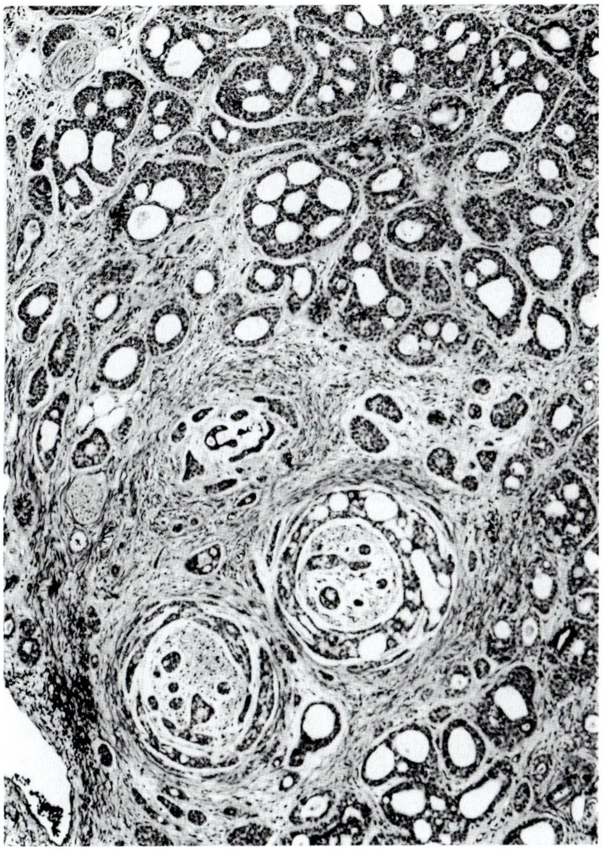

Fig. 3.35. Adenoid cystic carcinoma. The tumor is composed of relatively small hyperchromatic cells arranged in well-circumscribed nests within the stroma. Well-defined cystic spaces are evident in this tumor. The surrounding stroma is desmoplastic. (Courtesy of R.J. Kurman, M.D., Baltimore, MD.)

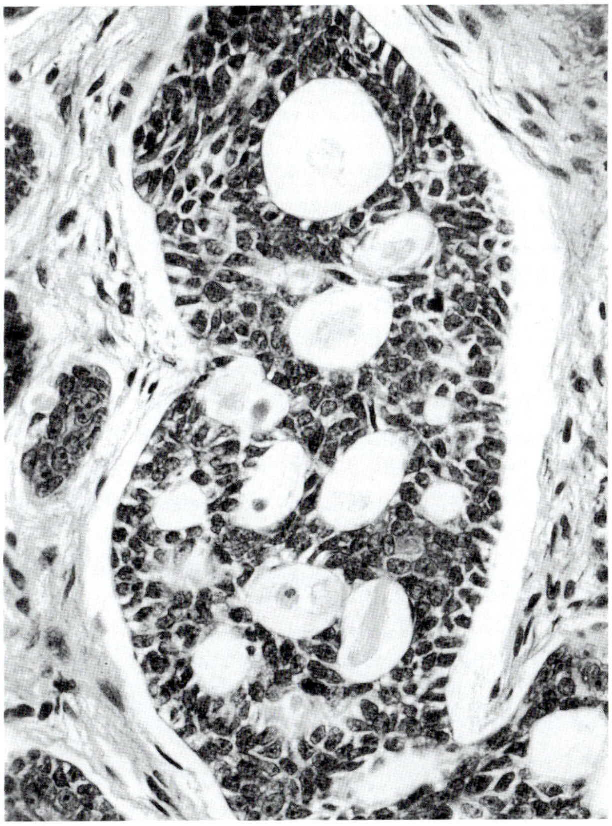

Fig. 3.36. Adenoid cystic carcinoma. Relatively small but somewhat pleomorphic cells surrounding sharply punched-out cystic spaces.

munohistochemical techniques. The S-100 reactivity may demonstrate a myoepithelial cell element.

The differential diagnosis of adenoid cystic carcinoma includes adenocarcinoma, basal cell carcinoma, metastatic atypical carcinoid, and small cell carcinoma. *Metastatic small cell carcinoma* arising in the vagina has been reported as presenting as a Bartholin mass.[123] Adenocarcinomas lack the uniform acinar arrangement and intraluminal basement membrane material of adenoid cystic carcinoma. Basal cell carcinomas are more solid and lack the cystic spaces and the intracystic basement membrane-like material. Metastatic carcinoids and small cell carcinomas are more solid, have fewer lumens, contain argyrophil cells, and stain for neuron-specific enolase in most cases. Carcinoid tumors almost always react with antibodies against chromogranin and other neuroendocrine markers.

Adenosquamous carcinoma of the Bartholin gland contains a mixture of squamous cells with intracellular bridges and glandular cells that typically contain mucin.[100]

Transitional cell carcinoma arising in the Bartholin gland is composed of uniform polyhedral or rounded epithelial cells often lining broad papillary fronds. Rare areas of glandular or squamous differentiation may be found. The differential diagnosis of primary transitional cell carcinoma of the Bartholin gland includes poorly differentiated squamous cell carcinoma and adenocarcinoma. If more than rare foci contain glands or show keratinization, the tumor is of mixed cell type and should be so designated, listing the different tumor types.

Clinical Behavior and Treatment

The primary treatment for a Bartholin gland carcinoma is wide local excision to the fascia, hemivulvectomy, or total vulvectomy. Ipsilateral or bilateral inguinofemoral lymph node dissection is necessary, regardless of the type of primary excision.[40,110,190] Adjunctive radiation therapy to the vulva and regional lymph nodes also has been advocated.[40]

Approximately 20% of carcinomas of the Bartholin gland are associated with metastases to the inguinofemoral lymph nodes. The overall 5-year survival of patients with Bartholin gland carcinomas is approximately 50% when the groin nodes are free of tumor, but decreases to 18% when two or more nodes are involved.[44,190] If the groin nodes are involved there is a 20% probability that pelvic lymph node metastasis also will be present, but if the groin nodes are free of metastasis, there is essentially no risk of pelvic node metastasis.

Therapy for adenoid cystic carcinoma of the Bartholin gland is wide local excision with ipsilateral inguinofemoral lymphadenectomy.[41] Local recurrence is well documented and, when the tumor involves the margin, adjuvant radiotherapy may be beneficial. Survival is better with adenoid carcinoma than with other forms of carcinoma of the Bartholin gland.

The treatment of vulvar adenosquamous carcinoma is similar to that of squamous cell carcinoma. Adenosquamous carcinomas have a poorer prognosis than squamous cell carcinomas, partly because of the higher frequency of lymph node metastasis.

Mammary Glandlike Adenocarcinoma Arising in the Vulva

Specialized anogential mammary-like glands, found typically in the interlabial sulcus, are thought to be the origin of *vulvar mammary-like (breastlike) adenocarcinomas*.[186,187] Other benign and malignant tumors, including *papillary hidradenomas* as well as *fibrocystic-like disease*, have been described within these specialized glands. The origin of these tumors had been previously thought to be ectopic breast tissue; however, current opinion is that these glands are not ectopic tissue, but rather normal anatomic elements composed of specialized anogenital mammary-like glands. The adenocarcinomas arising from these glands have histopathologic features very similar to those of primary mammary adenocarcinomas, and a few have been associated with breast adenocarcinoma. Most have a pattern of growth of infiltrating, well-differentiated adenocarcinoma. In some cases an intraductal carcinoma component has been identified. In one case, an intraductal carcinoma of mammary type was found arising in a papillary hidradenoma of the vulva.[135]

Metastases to inguinal lymph nodes from adenocarcinomas of vulvar mammary-like tumors have been observed. These adenocarcinomas contain secretory material similar to that of breast adenocarcinomas, including alpha-lactalbumin and milk fat globulin protein, and also may contain estrogen and progesterone receptors. *Cystosarcoma phyllodes* arising in the vulva has also been described.[122]

Metastatic adenocarcinoma to the vulva can be distinguished from primary adenocarcinomas if mammary-like glands or in situ adenocarcinoma is present. In the absence of mammary-like tissue, the distinction may not be possible. Treatment of primary adenocarcinoma arising within vulvar specialized anogenital glands is extended wide local excision and ipsilateral inguinofemoral lymphadenectomy.

Carcinomas of Sweat Gland Origin

Carcinomas of vulvar sweat gland origin, including Skene glands, are rare, comprising less than 1% of all vulvar carcinomas.[191] Patients typically present with a painless vulvar mass.[122] In addition to undifferentiated sweat gland adenocarcinomas, *ductal eccrine carcinoma, eccrine porocarcinoma, eccrine hidradenocarcinoma, clear cell hidradenocarcinoma*, and *apocrine carcinomas* have been reported.[37,48,49,191]

Sebaceous carcinoma of the vulva has also been reported, which may be associated with VIN.[58,191] Adenocarcinomas of the vulva may arise from the Skene glands.[178]

Other unusual adenocarcinomas of the vulva include an adenocarcinoma with a tubulovillous pattern resembling colonic adenocarcinoma.[202] A mucinous adenocarcinoma with focal squamous and neuroendocrine differentiation has been reported arising in the labium majus. This tumor expressed chromogranin A, protein gene product 9.5, serotonin, and vasoactive intestinal polypeptide.[73]

Mesenchymal Tumors

Malignant mesenchymal tumors are relatively rare in the vulva; most sarcomas arise from the labia majora.[112] The clinical course is unpredictable and is only somewhat dependent on the histologic type. Patients range in age from 6 to 64 years. The following discussion of these tumors is applicable to the vulva; the reader is referred to the referenced articles or comprehensive texts on soft tissue tumors for a more detailed discussion of these neoplasms. Table 3.8 summarizes some of the differential diagnostic features of myxoid soft tissue tumors that may occur in the vulva. Within the differential diagnosis, some benign tumors should be considered. (See Chapter 2, Benign Diseases of the Vulva.)

Leiomyosarcoma

Leiomyosarcoma is the most common sarcoma involving the vulva.[45] The mean age at presentation is 35 years, with a range from 18 to 66 years. Patients

Table 3.8. Differential histopathologic features of tumors with myxoid change in the vulva

	In children	*Cambium layer*	*Sheets of immature cells*	*Gland elements*	*Prominent vascularity*	*Atypical fibroblasts*	*Nuclear pleomorphism*	*Mitotic figures*	*Cross-striations, straplike muscle cells*
Fetal myxoid rhabdomyoma	−	−	−	−	−	−	−	−	+
Aggressive angiomyxoma	−	−	−	+	+	−	−	±	−
Embryonal rhabdomyosarcoma (sarcoma botyroides)	+	+	+	−	+	−	+	+	+
Benign pseudosarcomatous polyps	−	−	−	−	+	+	±	−	−
Vulvar polyps with myxoid stroma	−	−	−	−	−	+	±	−	−
Leiomyoma with myxoid change (in pregnancy)	−	−	−	−	−	−	±	±	−
Nodular (pseudosarcomatous) fasciitis	±	−	−	−	−	±	−	+	−

+, present; −, absent; ±, occasionally seen.

typically present with a mass.[176] Leiomyosarcoma may arise in the labium majus, Bartholin gland area, the clitoris, or the labium minus, in decreasing order of frequency. The tumors often are 5 cm in diameter or larger at diagnosis. Local pain and an enlarging mass are the most common presenting symptoms.[129,176]

Microscopic Features

Microscopically, leiomyosarcoma is composed of interlacing smooth muscle cells that, when sectioned on the long axis, have a perinuclear clear area, or halo. *Epithelioid leiomyosarcomas* also have been described in this site.[176] Leiomyosarcomas generally are larger, have infiltrative margins, more cellular atypia, and higher mitotic activity than leiomyomas. Generally, leiomyosarcomas will have a mitotic count exceeding 10 mitoses per 10 high-power fields.

Smooth muscle tumors with three or more of the following criteria are considered leiomyosarcomas: a greatest diameter of 5 cm or more, 5 or more mitoses per 10 high power fields, infiltrative margins, and moderate to severe cytologic atypia.[127] Tumors with only one of these features are considered leiomyomas, whereas tumors with only two of these features may be classified as *atypical leiomyomas* but are considered benign.[127,176]

Leiomyosarcoma may recur locally, or metastasize, with pulmonary and hepatic metastasis being the more common sites of distant metastasis.[8] Wide extended local excision is the usual initial clinical approach, and localized radiotherapy may be included.

Embryonal Rhabdomyosarcoma (Sarcoma Botyroides)

Embryonal rhabdomyosarcoma is a malignant tumor of striated muscle that grows in a distinctive polypoid manner. Within the vulva the tumor typically occurs in infants and is rare beyond 10 years of age, although it has been reported in young women.[42] Embryonal rhabdomyosarcoma has been described arising from the labia majora and hymeneal area in infants and usually presents with bleeding, secondary to ulceration.[39,174] In cases in which the tumor involves the vagina as well as the labia minora, the tumor should be considered of vaginal origin. These tumors usually present as a fleshy, violet to skin-colored, grapelike or solid mass.

On microscopic examination, the tumor has an edematous or myxomatous appearance and is covered by thin squamous epithelium (see Chapter 4, Diseases of the Vagina). Within the subepithelial area there is a dense cellular area composed of spindle or round cells that form the "cambium zone." The tumor cells may infiltrate the overlying epithelium. Embryonal rhabdomyoblasts, which are round to spindle shaped with prominent eosinophilic cytoplasm, and hyperchromatic, pleomorphic nuclei are frequently observed. Rhabdomyoblasts with cellular cross-striation are found in approximately 15% of the cases. The cytoplasm of the tumor cells usually is immunoreactive for myoglobin, desmin, actin, and vimentin. Although myoglobin is skeletal muscle specific, it is not always immunoreactive in this tumor.

Local growth with late metastasis to regional nodes and distant sites is the usual pattern of spread. The tumor typically grows rapidly and metastasizes early. Combination systemic chemotherapy, including ifosfamide, actinomycin D, and vincristine, followed by local excision, is highly effective. Brachytherapy has been used as an alternative to radical surgery in patients who do not respond and has provided a high cure rate with preservation of fertility.[85,118] Overall 5-year survival is reported as 85%–97% at 5 years, with disease-free survival reported as 71%–79% at 5 years. Survival is even better with small tumors that are diagnosed early.[39,42,85,118]

Dermatofibrosarcoma Protuberans

Dermatofibrosarcoma protuberans is an aggressive tumor of fibrohistiocytic origin that usually presents as a solitary, firm, brownish, subcutaneous nodular or multinodular mass. It is a relatively uncommon tumor of the vulva but occurs most often in postmenopausal women, with a median age of 54 years.[16,68,155] Clinically, this tumor may resemble a large nevus. Histologically, the tumor is characterized by intradermal growth, with a broad junction between the tumor and the adjacent epithelium, resulting in an elevated surface. The tumor is densely cellular, with the cells arranged in a characteristic storiform pattern. The cells, unlike malignant fibrous histiocytoma, show little cytologic atypia, rare mitosis, and no tumor giant cells.[112] At the base of the tumor an infiltrative growth pattern is seen that may involve the superficial subcutaneous tissue in a "honeycomb" pattern. On immunohistochemical study, the tumor cells are strongly and diffusely reactive for CD 34.[68] Wide local extended excision is the treatment of choice. Local recurrence is not unusual, but distant metastasis is rare.[166] Transformation to fibrosarcoma has been reported, which is also CD 34 immunoreactive.[68,112]

Malignant Fibrous Histiocytoma

Malignant fibrous histiocytoma (*MFH*) arises from histiocytes that have undergone fibroblastic differentiation. It is rare on the vulva, but nonetheless is the second most common sarcoma in this site. It usually presents as a large solitary mass in middle-aged women.[83,177]

Malignant fibrous histiocytoma is typically a solid tumor that is white to yellow on section. Areas of necrosis and focal hemorrhage may be seen. The tumor is typically deep, not immediately beneath the skin, as occurs with dermatofibrosarcoma protuberans. Malignant fibrous histiocytoma is characterized by infiltrative growth and marked nuclear pleomorphism with giant cells and multinucleated cells. Cells with large nuclei containing multiple prominent nucleoli and abundant eosinophilic cytoplasm are admixed with smaller round to spindle-shaped cells with moderate nuclear pleomorphism. Mitotic figures usually are present and commonly atypical. The spindle cells may be arranged in a storiform pattern or in interlacing bundles (Fig. 3.37).

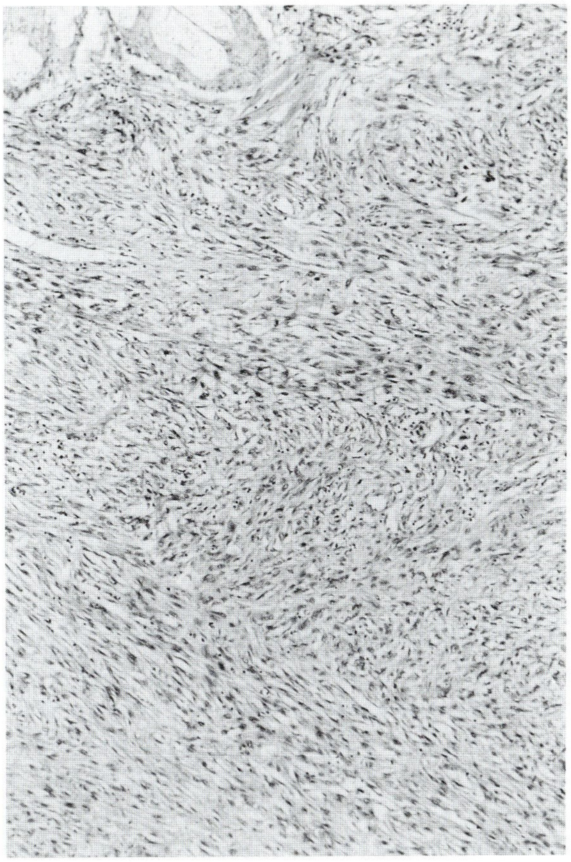

Fig. 3.37. Malignant fibrous histiocytoma. The tumor is deep to the sebaceous glands and is composed of markedly pleomorphic, spindle-shaped cells arranged in an interdigitated "storiform" pattern.

The cells of MFH usually contain alpha-1-antichymotrypsin or alpha-1-antitrypsin, one or both of which can be identified in approximately 80% of cases. A number of subtypes of MFH have been described: these include an inflammatory type, which has many acute inflammatory cells; the giant cell variant (giant cell tumor of soft parts), which contains giant cells with osteoclast-like features but no osteoid or bone; and a myxoid variant, which has a prominent hypocellular myxoid component. *Angiomatoid fibrous histiocytoma* is no longer considered a variant of MFH by the WHO and is classified as a distinct entity. These tumors contain prominent blood vessels and blood-filled spaces.

Characteristically, MFH is locally invasive. Involvement of the underlying fascia increases the risk of local or distant metastasis. The treatment is wide local excision or radical vulvectomy. Lymphadenectomy is reserved for those cases with clinical evidence of regional node involvement. Postoperative radiotherapy is believed of value in reducing local recurrence. An insufficient number of cases have been described in the vulva to permit a definitive statement about the prognosis, but approximately half the patients reported have had recurrences or died of metastatic disease. These tumors should be distinguished from *extraabdominal desmoid of the vulva*, which is rare but has been described involving the labium majus extending into the vaginal wall. These tumors may enlarge with pregnancy and are usually diagnosed following surgical excision for the subcutaneous mass.[57]

Epithelioid Sarcoma

The histogenesis of *epithelioid sarcomas* is obscure. The tumor is believed to arise primarily from the reticular dermis, although it may occur in deeper soft tissue.[78] These tumors typically occur in young individuals and have been observed presenting in the labia majora and in the subclitoral area.

Microscopically, epithelioid sarcoma has a granuloma-like appearance with areas of necrosis. The tumor is composed of polygonal cells arranged in sheets and nests. The cells have abundant eosinophilic cytoplasm, giving some cells an epithelial appearance. Cartilage and bone also may be found, which is thought to reflect metaplasia. There is moderate nuclear pleomorphism, and frequent mitotic figures are generally noted. Epithelioid sarcomas contain keratin by immunoperoxidase study and have immunohistochemical findings essentially the same as those for malignant rhabdoid tumors.[137]

Epithelioid sarcomas usually are indolent, although local recurrence with associated distant metastasis has been seen with unusual frequency compared with other sites, suggesting that vulvar epithelioid sarcoma acts more aggressively. Vascular space invasion is associated with recurrence. Therapy is wide local extended excision with inguinofemoral lymphadenectomy and local radiation therapy.[78]

Malignant Rhabdoid Tumor

Malignant rhabdoid tumor is of uncertain origin and is rare in the vulva. It has been reported as a subcutaneous nodule beneath the labium majus as well as presenting as a Bartholin mass in a young woman.[90,136] The tumor presents as a deep subcutaneous mass that may involve the deep dermis.

On microscopic examination, the tumor has a multinodular, lobulated appearance with poorly defined margins. Areas of hemorrhage and vascularity may be present. The tumor cells are large with pleomorphic nuclei that have vesicular chromatin and prominent nucleoli; mitoses are common. The cytoplasm is eosinophilic, and because of their polygonal shape the cells may resemble squamous cells or rhabdomyoblasts. The cells have a distinctive eosinophilic cytoplasmic inclusion composed of intermediate filaments.[90] Because the inclusion may indent the nucleus, the cells may have a signet-ring appearance. The tumor cells may be immunoreactive to cytokeratins, epithelial membrane antigen, actin, CEA, and human milk fat globulin-2 and typically are not immunoreactive to desmin or S-100 antigen.

The primary differential diagnosis is epithelioid sarcoma, which has the same immunoreactivity but lacks the lobulated growth pattern and the large cells with nuclear pleomorphism and distinctive cytoplasmic inclusions. In addition, a malignant rhabdoid tumor lacks necrosis or the granulomatous appearance of epithelioid sarcoma. The malignant rhabdoid tumor is locally aggressive and may metastasize. Total vulvectomy, or wide local excision, with bilateral inguinofemoral lymphadenectomy has been recommended, although only a few cases have been reported.[136]

Aggressive Angiomyxoma

Although *aggressive angiomyxoma* is included in the category of malignant mesenchymal tumors, it is locally aggressive only and therefore is not a sarcoma. Aggressive angiomyxoma presents as a subcutaneous mass, and may present in the Bartholin gland area. The tumor usually occurs in adult women less than 40 years of age. It may involve contiguous sites including the vagina and buttocks. Aggressive angiomyxoma may arise in the pelvis and present as a vulvar mass as it grows out.[32]

On gross examination, the aggressive angiomyxoma has a soft myxoid appearance, and on cut section, small vessels may be visible (Fig. 3.38). The tumor may appear to have well-defined margins that may prove to be involved on microscopic examination.

On microscopic examination, aggressive angiomyxoma has a distinctive myxoid appearance with numerous muscular medium-sized vessels that are typically clustered. The tumor cells are spindle-shaped fibroblasts and myofibroblasts that lack significant nuclear pleomorphism or mitotic figures (Figs. 3.39 and 3.40). The tumor may contain epithelial elements that form glands and contain mucin. The neoplasm may invade fat and entrap neural elements. The spindle cells are immunore-

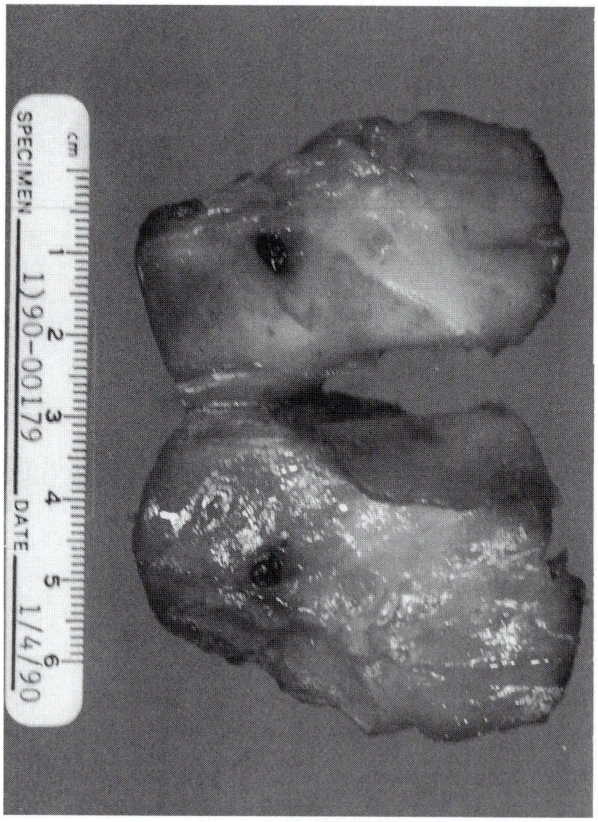

Fig. 3.38. Aggressive angiomyxoma. The tumor has a uniform gelatinous appearance with poorly defined margins. (Courtesy of R.J. Kurman, M.D., Baltimore, MD.)

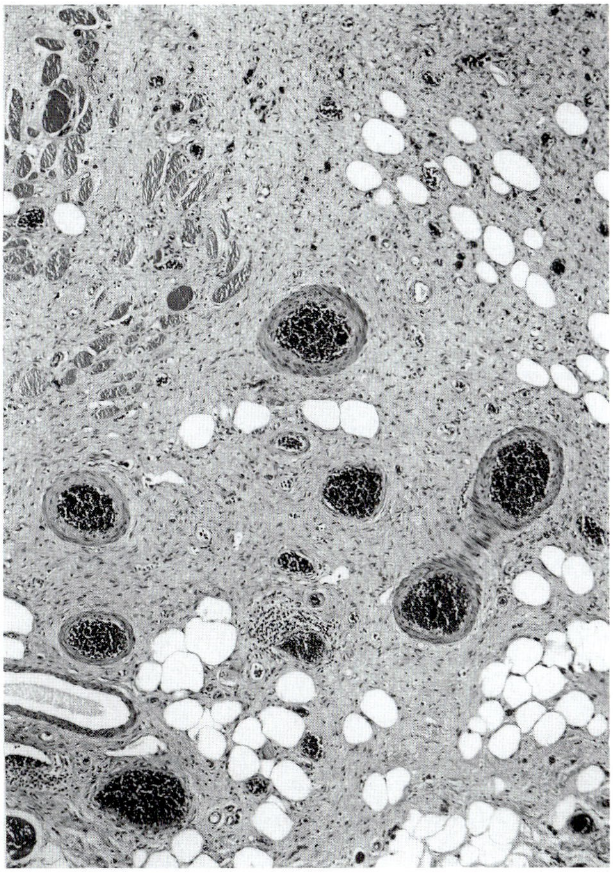

Fig. 3.39. Aggressive angiomyxoma. The tumor has invaded adjacent fat and muscle tissue (*upper left*). Within the tumor, prominent muscular arterioles are present. (Courtesy of R.J. Kurman, M.D., Baltimore, MD.)

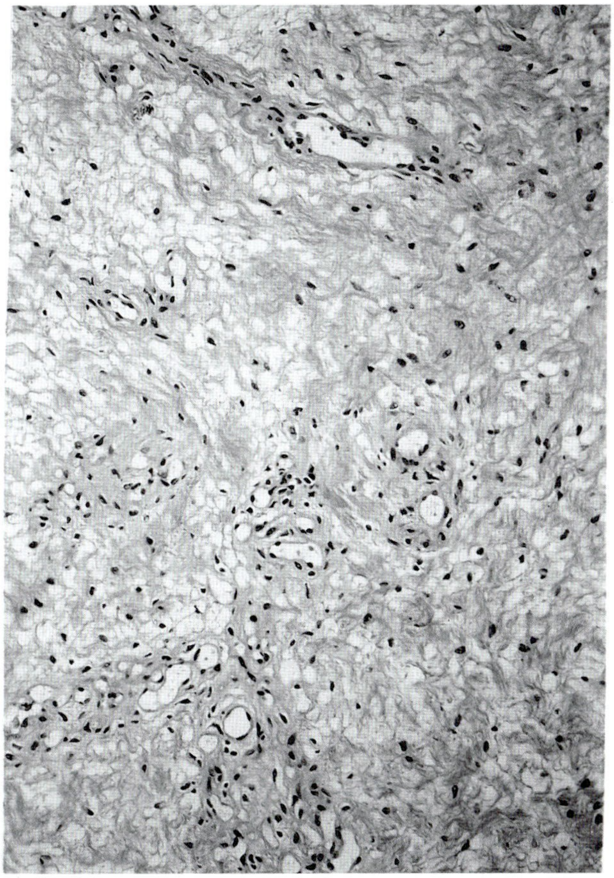

Fig. 3.40. Aggressive angiomyxoma. The tumor is paucicellular and myxoid and contains vessels of varying size. The cells tumor have indistinct cell borders and small spindle-shaped nuclei, with loose, vacuolated appearing cytoplasm. (Courtesy of R.J. Kurman, M.D., Baltimore, MD.)

active to muscle specific actin but are negative for S-100 antigen. Vessels within the tumor are immunoreactive for factor VIII; however, the spindle cell elements do not express this antigen.

The primary differential diagnosis is myxoid MFH and angiomyofibroblastoma. In addition, aggressive angiomyxoma should be distinguished from benign swelling or chronic fibrosis and edema of the labia. Malignant fibrous histiocytoma has a storiform pattern and is immunoreactive for alpha-1-antitrypsin and alpha-1-antichymotrypsin. Angiomyofibroblastoma is more cellular and composed of large epithelioid cells, with well-defined tumor margins without prominent clustered muscular arterioles.

Aggressive angiomyxoma usually has a benign course; however, locally aggressive infiltrative growth and local recurrence are not uncommon. Metastasis has not been reported. Recurrences as early as 1 year and as late as 14 years after surgery have been reported. Wide local excision without lymphadenectomy is the therapy of choice.[11,112,170]

Angiosarcoma and Lymphangiosarcoma

Primary angiosarcoma involving the vulva has been reported as a primary perianal tumor after radiation therapy to the pelvis. *Lymphangiosarcoma* has also been reported in the pubic region related to congenital nonhereditary lymphedema that involved the external genital region and adjacent lower limb.[28] On gross examination these tumors typically are solid, have poorly defined margins, and are usually deep red in color.

On microscopic examination, angiosarcoma is composed of complex slitlike vessels of irregular size lined by cells with large pleomorphic nuclei; mitotic activity usually is evident. In poorly differentiated areas, the tumor may be relatively solid. The tumor cells are typically immunoreactive for factor VIII, CD 31, and usually CD 34. Treatment is extended local excision with radiation therapy to the tumor site following excision.[28]

Angiomyofibroblastoma with Sarcomatous Transformation (Angiomyofibrosarcoma)

Angiomyofibroblastoma has been reported in the vulva associated with a high-grade sarcoma resembling myxoid MFH in an 80-year-old woman. The tumor cells were immunoreactive for vimentin but did not express smooth muscle actin, muscle actin, desmin, keratin, S-100 protein, or CD 34.[128] The tumor should be distinguished from angiomyofibroblastoma, which usually express desmin and lack significant atypia or mitotic activity.[128a]

Hemangiopericytoma

Hemangiopericytoma has been reported as a primary tumor of the vulva. The tumor presents as a subcutaneous, partially cystic mass within the labia majus and fourchette.

Microscopically, the tumor is composed of small spindle-shaped pericytes with slightly eosinophilic cytoplasm and relatively large nuclei with minimal pleomorphism. Nucleoli may be evident. The mitotic count usually is low, with fewer than 4 mitotic figures per 10 high-power fields. There is an associated complex capillary component, with the tumor cells each surrounded by a reticulin network peripheral to the vascular spaces. Necrosis or hemorrhage generally is not present.[112] Currently these tumors are considered malignant and are classified as low grade or high grade on the basis of cellular features. Large size, nuclear pleomorphism, numerous mitoses, high cellularity, and necrosis characterize high-grade tumors whereas low-grade hemangiopericytomas tend to be small, have a mitotic count of fewer than 4 per 10 high-power fields, and lack areas of necrosis or hemorrhage.[112]

The primary differential diagnosis includes *monophasic synovial sarcoma*, *angiosarcoma*, and *metastatic endometrial stromal sarcoma*. The pericytes of hemangiopericytoma are not immunoreactive for cytokeratins or S-100, as seen in synovial sarcoma, or factor VIII, as seen in angiosarcoma.[112] Differentiation from other malignant angiomatous tumors can be facilitated by the use of reticulum stains, which show the pericytes to be external to the reticulin network surrounding the individual blood vessels.[111,112]

Treatment usually is wide local excision.[209] Metastasis to bone 14 years after therapy for vulvar hemangiopericytoma has been observed.[209]

Kaposi Sarcoma

Among the tumors of endothelial origin that may involve the vulva, *Kaposi sarcoma* is important because of its association with acquired immunodeficiency syndrome (AIDS). The tumor is rare in the vulva.[2,112] Over time, the clinical presentation of the tumor evolves from a macule to a plaque to a nodular lesion. Usually more than one skin lesion is present. There remains some debate as to whether this is a primary malignant neoplastic or a reactive process. Herpesvirus type 8 has been described associated with Kaposi sarcoma.

When presenting as a macule, microscopic examination reveals the tumor within the dermis to have increased vascularity with irregularly shaped vascular spaces. Mononuclear cells are seen about the vascular spaces. In later-stage lesions, more numerous vessels are associated with atypical spindle cells within the dermis (Fig. 3.41). In the advanced or nodular stage, the tumor is a highly vascular spindle cell neoplasm.

The differential diagnosis includes *bacillary (epithelioid) angiomatosis*, *tumors of fibrohistiocytic origin*, *benign vascular tumors*, scar, and a variety of other skin changes. Bacillary angiomatosis contains the bacteria *Rochalimaea henselae*. The organism can be identified as bacterial rods using the Warthin-Starry stain or other immunohistochemical techniques on fresh or formalin-fixed tissue, employing bacteria-specific antibodies. The organism also may be cultured.[148]

Tumors of fibrohistiocytic origin typically are immunoreactive for alpha-1-antitrypsin, alpha-1-antichymotrypsin, and antihuman mesothelial cell (HBME-1). Fibrohistiocytic tumors have a storiform appearance, and lack irregular vascular spaces. Benign vascular tumors are well circumscribed and have well-defined vascular spaces. Scars are characterized by lack of skin appendages and a more fibrous and less vascular dermis. The gross appearance is also usually distinctive as compared with Kaposi sarcoma.

Alveolar Soft Part Sarcoma

Alveolar soft part sarcoma has been reported in the labium minus.[161] A metastasis may be the initial presentation. The tumor is characterized by loosely arrayed polygonal cells with granular cytoplasm on delicate to thick fibrovascular and fibrocollagenous stalks. In some areas the tumor cells form alveolar-

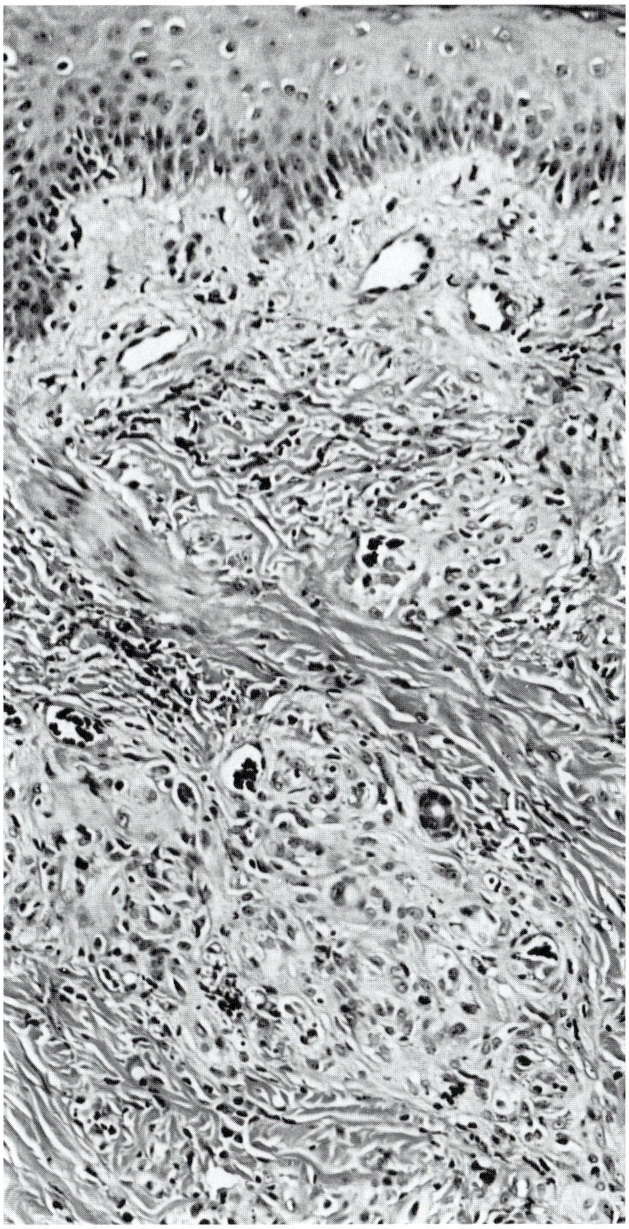

Fig. 3.41. Kaposi sarcoma. Many vessels, some of which are irregularly shaped, are within the dermis. Atypical spindle cells surround the vessels.

like structures. No true glands or secretory products are seen, although the tumor cells do protrude into the tumor luminal spaces. Mitoses are rare and the tumor tends to have a pushing border. Metastatic renal cell or clear cell tumors may mimic this tumor.[112] Metastasis to lymph nodes and distant sites may occur. Local recurrence is reported in approximately one-third of cases, and reported survival ranges from 30% to 50% in nonvulvar sites.[161] Recommended therapy is local extended excision with ipsilateral inguinofemoral lymphadenectomy. Radical surgery does not appear to improve survival, but chemotherapy or immunotherapy may be of value.[161]

Malignant Schwannoma

Malignant schwannoma may arise within the labia minora or labia majora, as well as other sites within the vulva. The tumor characteristically occurs in women of reproductive age. Although this tumor occurs with higher frequency in individuals with von Recklinghausen neurofibromatosis, approximately half the reported cases within the vulva are unrelated to neurofibromatosis.[179] The tumor presents as a subcutaneous, relatively solid, fibrous mass. A nerve trunk typically is associated with the tumor.

On microscopic examination, the tumor is generally cellular with nuclear palisading. Mitotic figures are easily identified. Heterologous elements may be present including cartilage, striated muscle, and epithelial glandular elements. Approximately one-half of the tumors are immunoreactive for S-100 antigen, and those that are reactive are often only weakly reactive. There are insufficient cases reported to determine the prognosis of this tumor in the vulva; however, local recurrence as well as pulmonary metastasis have been reported. Wide local excision of the primary tumor without regional lymphadenectomy or radiation therapy has been advocated for tumors confined to the vulva.[179]

Granular Cell Tumor, Malignant

Malignant granular cell tumor of the vulva has been described. The malignant features are recognized primarily by significant local recurrence and infiltrative growth (see Chapter 2, Benign Diseases of the Vulva).[150]

Liposarcoma

Liposarcoma is a rare tumor within the vulva; it has been observed predominately in middle-aged women.[67,131] Liposarcoma typically presents as a subcutaneous soft tissue tumor, without involvement of the overlying epithelium, and may appear clinically to be lipoma.[20]

On gross examination, well-differentiated liposarcoma may resemble lipoma and be well demarcated on cut section. In contrast, *myxoid liposarcoma* has a gelatinous appearance on cut section.

On microscopic examination, vulvar liposarcoma is usually well differentiated (lipoma-like/sclerosing) and has a lobular growth pattern. The tumor is composed of neoplastic adipocytes with pleomorphic and atypical nuclei. The vessels within liposarcoma are arranged in a "chicken-wire" pattern.[20] In contrast to lipoma, liposarcoma is more cellular and composed of relatively uniform neoplastic adipocytes with prominent eosinophilic cytoplasm.

Liposarcomas classified as myxoid (round cell), pleomorphic, and dedifferentiated are very rare in the vulva. The distribution of these subtypes in the vulva is not well studied, however. Myxoid liposarcoma, on microscopic examination, is composed of small stellate cells with relatively uniform nuclei and occasionally "signet-ring" lipoblasts within an extensively myxoid stroma. A distinct type of liposarcoma described in the vulva is composed of an admixture of bland-appearing neoplastic spindle and round cells with neoplastic adiopcytes of variable size with prominent bivacuolated lipoblasts.[131]

Liposarcoma is often immunoreactive for S-100 antigen, but this is not a uniform finding. Treatment is extended local excision. Local recurrences have been treated successfully with wide local reexcision.[131]

Langerhans Granulomatosis (Histiocytosis X), Including Eosinophilic Granuloma

Langerhans granulomatosis (*histiocytosis X*) is subdivided into three clinical types: Letterer–Siwe disease, Hand–Schuller–Christian disease (a chronic progressive form), and eosinophilic granuloma (a benign localized form).[69] Of these, eosinophilic granuloma has been well documented to involve the vulva.[94,112,145,172,180]

Eosinophilic Granuloma

Eosinophilic granuloma may be localized entirely to the vulva, although most cases reported have involved other sites as well, including the pituitary gland, resulting in diabetes insipidis.[94] The clinical presentation typically is a cutaneous pigmented papule or subcutaneous nodule. The surface of the mass may be ulcerated. The skin lesions typically present between 5 and 13 years of age, although the initial presentation may be in early adulthood.[69] Regional lymphadenopathy, secondary to nodal involvement, may occur; however, systemic symptoms are uncommon.

Microscopic examination reveals a cell population consisting predominantly of Langerhans-type cells intermixed with inflammatory cells. Eosinophils, granulocytes, lymphocytes, and plasma cells may all be present, and an acute inflammatory cell infiltrate may be seen surrounding the mass. Necrosis may be present within the tumor but usually is localized. The Langerhans-type cells within the mass are immunoreactive for S-100 antigen and CD1a. Localized Langerhans cell histiocytosis usually can be treated by radiation therapy. More advanced disease may require chemotherapy.

Malignant Melanoma

General Features

Melanomas account for approximately 9% of all malignant tumors of the vulva, occurring predominantly in white women. The age-specific incidence in a comprehensive Swedish study is 75 years of age or older, occurring in 1.28 per 100,000. In women 60–74 years old, the vulvar melanoma incidence was 0.56; in those 45–59, the incidence was 0.19, in those 30–44 it was 0.08, and in women under 29 years of age, 0.02 or less.[147] Vulvar bleeding was the most common symptom of 198 patients studied, being recorded in 35% of the patients. A vulvar mass was observed in 28%, an ulcer in 5%, and a mole in 5%.[147] Pruritus occurred in 15%, irritation and or burning in 14%, and discomfort with urination in 12%.

Vulvar melanomas may arise from a preexisting benign or atypical pigmented lesion.[125,203] Melanomas occur on the clitoris, labia minora, and labia majora with approximately equal frequency. Of the 182 cases available with data on site within the vulva, 90 melanomas occurred on glabrous skin, 69 on hairy-glabrous skin, and 23 on hairy skin. The mass usually is polypoid or nodular (40%) and, although usually pigmented, was nonpigmented in 27% in one series.[147] Satellite nodules may be present, and were observed in 20% of 198 cases[147] (Fig. 3.42).

Vulvar melanomas are of three distinct histopathologic types: *superficial spreading melanoma* (Fig. 3.43), *nodular melanoma* (Fig. 3.44), and *mucosal/acral lentiginous melanoma* (Fig. 3.45).[12,175] Some vulvar melanomas are mixed or otherwise unclassifiable. This group comprised approximately one-quarter of the cases in one study.[147] The relative frequency of these types differs in various reports. Mucosal/acral lentiginous melanoma was the most common type identified in the Karolinska series, observed in 52% of the cases, where nodular melanoma accounted for 20% and superficial spreading melanoma 4% of the 198 cases reported.

Some of the variation in the type of vulvar melanoma reported may relate to differences in the criteria used to distinguish superficial spreading melanoma from nodular melanoma.[99] Superficial spreading melanoma usually can be differentiated

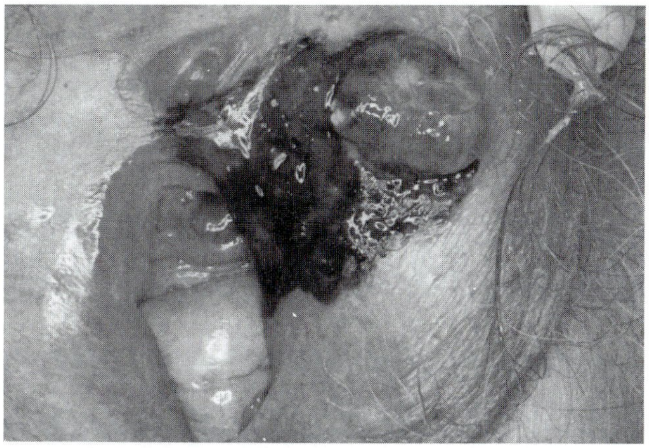

Fig. 3.42. Malignant melanoma. A superficial spreading malignant melanoma with vertical growth within the field of a superficially spreading malignant melanoma. (Courtesy of Linda S. Morgan, M.D., Gainesville, FL.)

from nodular melanoma by evaluating the adjacent epithelium. If the radial growth of a melanoma or atypical melanocytes involves four or more adjacent rete ridges, the tumor should be classified as superficial spreading melanoma (see Fig. 3.43).

There is some variation in the frequency of melanoma type related to the vulvar anatomic site of the tumor. In one large series, mucosal/acral lentiginous melanomas were seen with similar frequency in glabrous, hairy-glabrous, and hairy skin, whereas nodular melanomas were seen primarily in glabrous and hairy-glabrous skin and less frequently in hairy skin. In contrast, superficial spreading melanomas were seen predominately in hairy skin.[147]

Microscopic Findings

Mucosal/acral lentiginous melanomas have both vertical growth, as is seen in nodular melanoma, and radial growth, as is seen in superficial spreading melanoma. Atypical melanocytes usually can be identified within the epithelium adjacent to acral lentiginous and superficial spreading melanomas. Malignant melanomas may consist predominantly of epithelioid, dendritic (nevoid), or spindle cell types, either pure or mixed, within a given tumor. The cells may contain no melanin, or variable amounts, ranging from minimal to very large quantities. The histopathologic features vary considerably, and certain features can be correlated with the subtype of the melanoma. Within the invasive area of a superficial spreading melanoma, the malignant melanocytic cells usually are large and have relatively uniform nuclei with prominent nucleoli. Similar melanocytic cells can be found within the adjacent epithelium, representing the radial growth phase of the tumor. Junctional melanocytes are numerous and distributed within the epithelium in a pagetoid distribution.

In nodular melanomas, an intraepithelial component may be present in addition to an invasive component, but without an adjacent radial growth phase. The cells of nodular melanomas may be polygonal (epithelioid) or spindle shaped. The polygonal cells contain abundant eosinophilic cytoplasm, large nuclei, and prominent nucleoli. The

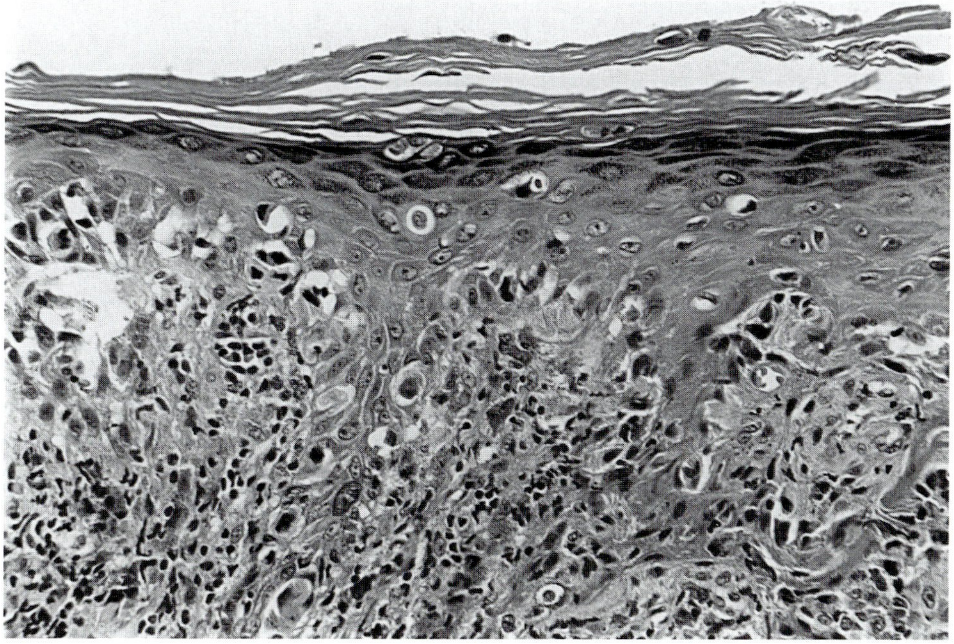

Fig. 3.43. Superficial spreading malignant melanoma. Pagetoid spread of the melanoma cells into the upper third of the epidermis. Markedly atypical melanocytic cells are at the epithelial–stromal junction. No invasion is present. (Courtesy of K.K. Pierson, M.D., Gainesville, FL.)

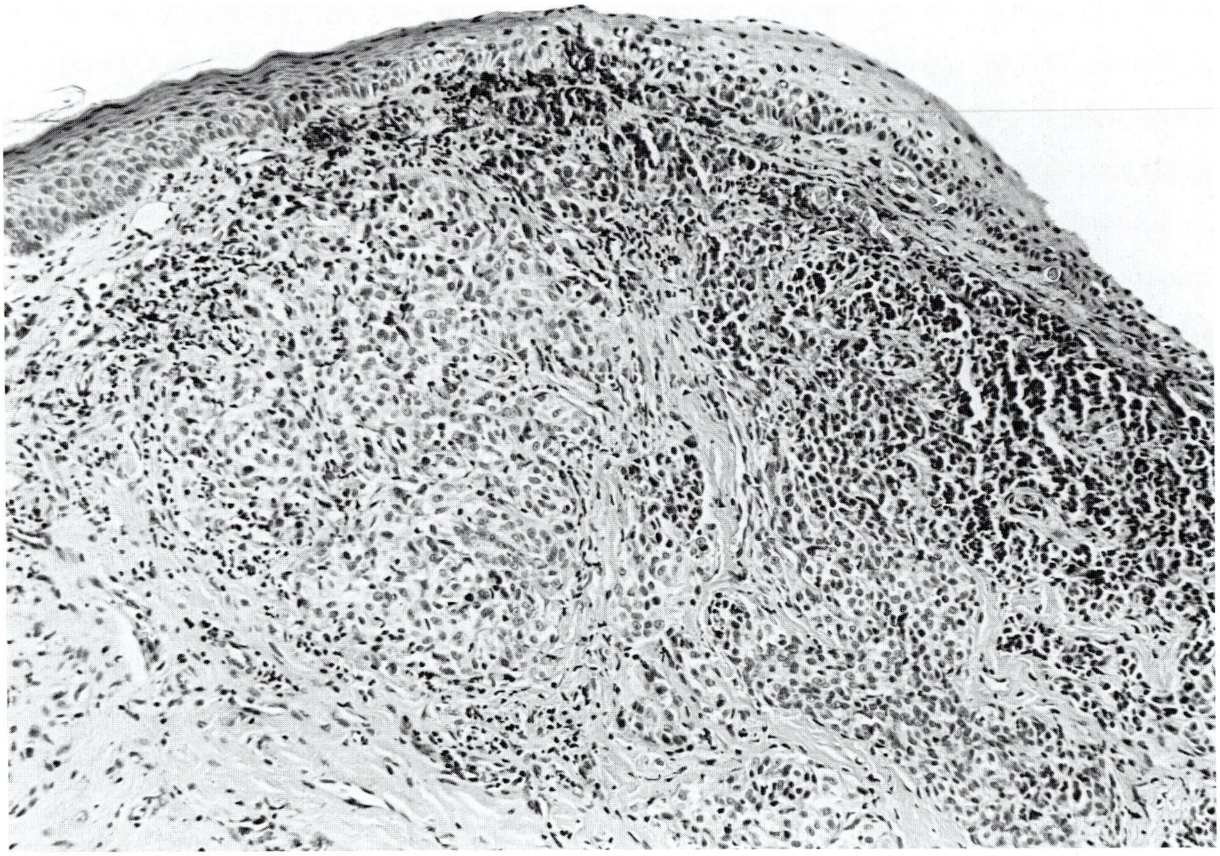

Fig. 3.44. Nodular melanoma. The tumor is entirely within the dermis, with an elevated, intact epithelium above it. The melanoma cells are large, polygonal, and arranged in nests, sheets, and cords within the dermis. (Courtesy of K.K. Pierson, M.D., Gainesville, FL.)

dendritic cells have tapering cytoplasmic extensions resembling nerve cells and show moderate nuclear pleomorphism. Spindle cells have smaller, oval nuclei and may be arranged in sheets or bundles. Mucosal/acral lentiginous melanomas of the vulva arise most commonly within the vestibule. They may show little or no pagetoid spread and are characterized by spindle cells within the junctional zone with extension into the adjacent dermis in a diffuse pattern (see Fig. 3.45). The spindle cells are uniform with little nuclear pleomorphism. Within the subepithelial tissue, the tumor cells usually evoke a desmoplastic response.

Differential Diagnosis

Superficial spreading malignant melanoma must be distinguished from Paget disease, VIN, and dysplastic nevi. The cells of Paget disease usually are larger than superficial spreading melanoma, have more cytoplasm, and are clustered with occasional gland formation. Squamous cell carcinomas with tumor giant cells, or those predominantly composed of spindle cells, may resemble malignant melanoma. Typical squamous cell carcinoma may be identifiable adjacent to the giant cell or spindle cell component, which may establish the diagnosis.[200] Spindle cell tumors of soft tissue origin, large cell lymphomas, and metastatic tumors, including choriocarcinoma, may be included in the differential diagnosis. In these cases, review of the clinical history and physical and radiologic findings, as well as thorough sectioning of the submitted tissue and appropriate immunohistochemical studies, as discussed next, usually will contribute evidence to establish the diagnosis. It should be emphasized that when faced with a poorly differentiated vulvar tumor that defies classification on initial microscopic examination, melanoma should be placed first on the list of the differential diagnosis.

Paget disease can be distinguished from melanoma with histochemical and immunohistochemical studies for mucin, CEA, S-100 protein, HMB-45 (or Melan-A), and cytokeratins. Paget cells [primary cutaneous (type 1) and perianal (type 2)] typically contain cytoplasmic mucin, with mucicarmine stain, and are immunoreactive for CEA and

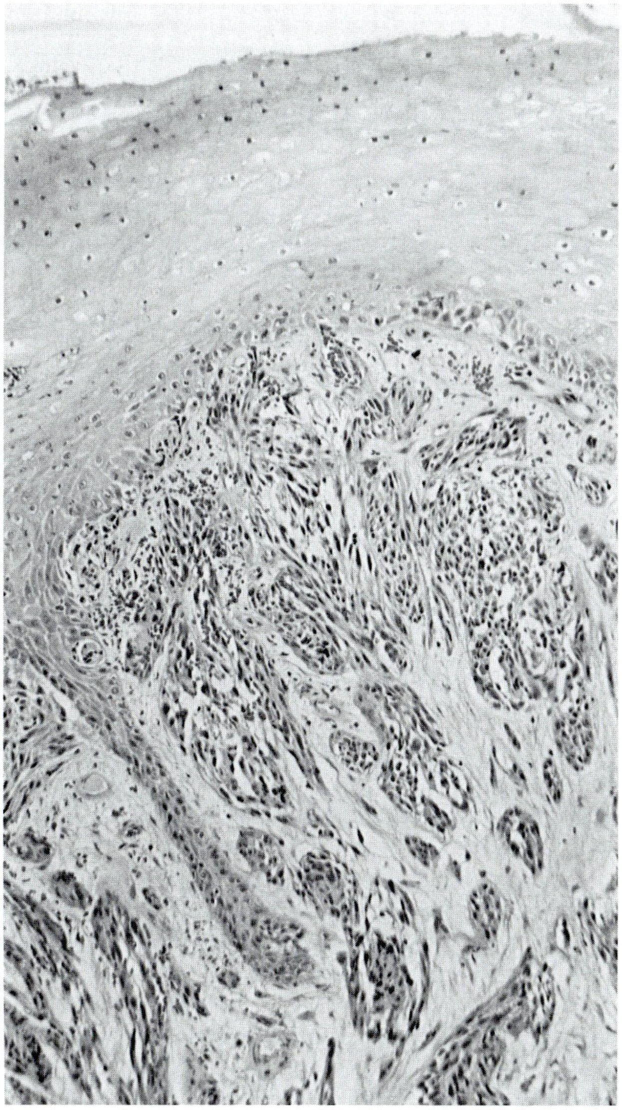

Fig. 3.45. Mucosal/acral lentiginous melanoma. This variant of malignant melanoma is characterized by a radial component with a lentiginous pattern at the mucosal–stromal interface. In this case, spindle cells are present within the submucosa near the junctional zone and within the deeper dermis with an associated desmoplastic response. The cytologic uniformity is characteristic. No pagetoid spread is evident. This type of malignant melanoma usually is found within the vulvar vestibule. (Courtesy of K.K. Pierson, M.D., Gainesville, FL.)

cytokeratin whereas melanomas are not (see Table 3.2). Melanomas usually are immunoreactive for S-100 protein, HMB-45, and Melan-A, whereas the nonmelanocytic tumors, including Paget, PUIN, VIN, squamous cell carcinoma, and bowenoid reticulosis, are negative.[196] When the diagnosis of vulvar melanoma is difficult to resolve, the immunohistochemical studies should include epithelial markers, to identify squamous, glandular, and transitional cell neoplasms (e.g., AE1/3, cytokeratins 7 and 20, EMA, CEA, GCDFP-15); hematopoietic markers, to identify lymphomas including Ki-1 lymphomas, bowenoid reticulosis, etc. (e.g., leukocyte common antigen, LCA); muscle markers for leiomyosarcoma or rhabdomyosarcoma (e.g., desmin, smooth muscle actin); fibrohistiocytic markers (e.g., alpha-1-antitrypsin, alpha-1-antichymotrypsin); neural and neuroendocrine tumor markers (e.g., S-100, chromogranin, synaptophysin); and melanoma markers (e.g., HMB-45, Melan-A, S-100).

Clinical Behavior and Treatment

Both the level of invasion of a malignant melanoma and its thickness have prognostic significance. The Clark classification of cutaneous melanomas into five levels of invasion is well accepted and can be applied to most melanomas of the vulva, with the exception of those arising within mucocutaneous areas. This system has been modified somewhat to accommodate vulvar melanomas (Fig. 3.46). A level I melanoma is a melanoma in situ; level II melanoma extends into the superficial papillary dermis; and level III melanoma fills and expands the papillary dermis; level IV melanoma invades the reticular dermis; and level V melanoma invades beyond the reticular dermis into fat or other deeper tissues.

Thickness measurements for cutaneous malignant melanomas as proposed by Breslow require measurement from the deep border of the granular layer of the overlying epithelium to the deepest point of tumor invasion. If a lesion is less than 0.76 mm

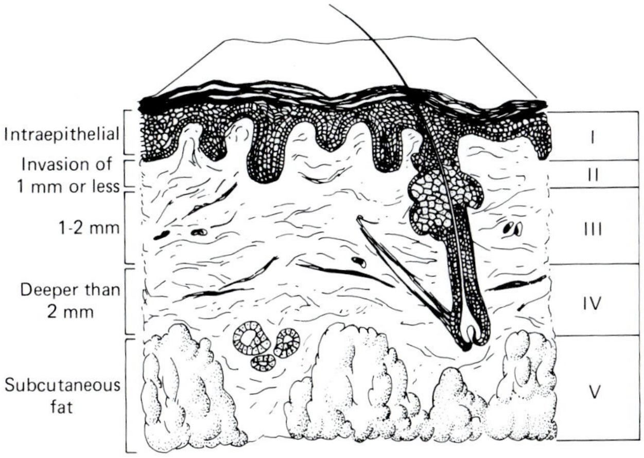

Fig. 3.46. Levels of vulvar melanoma invasion. (Reprinted by permission of The American College of Obstetricians and Gynecologists. Obstetrics and Gynecology 45:638, 1975.)

in thickness, it has little or no metastatic potential. Correlations between the thickness and the level of a vulvar melanoma can be made. Level I melanomas have no measurable thickness. In one study, level II melanomas had a thickness of 1 mm or less, level III melanomas had a thickness from 1 to 2 mm, and level IV melanomas had a thickness exceeding 2 mm, but did not involve subcutaneous fat or adjacent deeper structures.

Factors that adversely influence survival include a tumor thickness exceeding 2 mm, Clark level lV, a mitotic count exceeding $10/mm^2$, surface ulceration, and a minimal or absent inflammatory reaction.[99,185,203] Vascular space invasion and tumor necrosis also are associated with a poorer prognosis and are seen more commonly with large melanomas. No recurrences of vulvar melanoma have been observed when the thickness was 0.75 mm or less.[203] An excellent prognosis has been associated with melanomas at Clark level II or less and those with a thickness of 1.49 mm or less. A tumor volume of less than 100 mm^3 also correlates with an excellent prognosis. Other adverse prognostic factors reported include older age, centrally located tumors, tumor ulceration, vascular space involvement, and a high mitotic rate.[183]

Vulvar melanomas may recur locally, or in the cervix, urethra, vagina, or rectum. Distant metastasis may be the first sign of recurrence. Metastases to the lungs, brain, urinary bladder, bone marrow, and abdominal wall have all been observed.[99] The prognosis after recurrence is guarded, with a 5-year survival of only 5%. The usual treatment for vulvar melanomas with a thickness of 0.75 mm or less is wide local excision with a 1-cm circumferential and 1- to 2-cm-deep margins. Melanomas 1–4 mm thick require 2-cm surgical margins with deep margins of at least 1–2 cm.[183] Melanomas with a thickness greater than 4 mm are usually treated by wide excision to the fascia or partial or total vulvectomy.[184] Depending on the size of the tumor, the surgical procedure may include bilateral inguinal lymphadenectomy.[203] Radical vulvectomy does not appear to improve survival when compared to radical local excision with bilateral groin lymphadenectomy.

Other Malignant Tumors of the Vulva

Yolk Sac Tumor (Endodermal Sinus Tumor)

Endodermal sinus tumor (*EST*) is primarily a germ cell tumor occurring in ovary and testis (see Chapter 20, Germ Cell Tumors of the Ovary). Its occurrence in extragonadal sites is rare. In the vulva, vagina, and pelvis, the tumor is reported primarily in children and young women.[63] The characteristic histopathological features are Schiller–Duval bodies and eosinophilic hyaline droplets. Confusion with adenocarcinoma may occur if these features are not present. Immunoperoxidase studies to demonstrate the presence of alpha-fetoprotein (AFP) and an elevated serum level of AFP confirm the diagnosis. Recommended therapy for vulvar EST is wide local excision and chemotherapy.[63] Platinum-based chemotherapy has markedly improved survival in patients with this tumor.[63]

Primary Malignant Lymphoma

Malignant lymphoma may present as a destructive neoplasm, as clitoral enlargement, or as a mass that can mimic a Bartholin gland neoplasm or other tumor types.[141,185] Kappa-positive *lymphoplasmacytic lymphoma* and *angiocentric small* and *large mixed cell lymphoma*, as well as *plasmocytoma*, have been reported in the vulva.[51,185] The diagnosis of lymphoma is confirmed by immunoperoxidase studies for specific lymphocyte markers to identify the neoplastic cell population. The differential diagnosis includes inflammatory conditions and dermatoses as well as lymphoepithelioma-like carcinoma. Dermatoses and benign inflammatory processes, unlike lymphomas, contain mixed populations of lymphocytes and other inflammatory cells. *Lymphoepithelioma-like carcinomas* contain epithelial cells that express high molecular weight cytokeratins and lack evidence of a monoclonal lymphocytic population.[26] Large cell lymphomas, including Ki-1 lymphomas, may mimic poorly differentiated carcinoma and immunoperoxidase studies, including LCA; and specific lymphocyte markers as well as epithelial markers are of value to distinguish these types. Appropriate aggressive chemotherapy is the treatment of choice for most lymphomas.[185]

Merkel Cell Tumor

Merkel cell tumor of the vulva is rare, and few cases have been reported.[17,30,38,70,88] These tumors typically present as an intradermal nodule or nodules with erythema of the overlying skin.[17,38,88] These tumors may be associated with VIN or squamous cell carcinoma.[17] Both squamous and glandular differentiation has been reported in one case.[158] Three distinctive histopathologic types of Merkel cell tumor are recognized, namely the trabecular or carcinoid-like type, the intermediate cell type, and the small cell or oat cell-like type. The distribution of these types among vulvar tumors has not been determined. The histopathologic features are that of a poorly differentiated neoplasm composed of a diffuse population of relatively small, uniform, hyperchromatic cells usually without prominent nucleoli. Immunocytochemistry demonstrates a distinctive perinuclear cytoplasmic dot with low molecular weight cytokeratin-specific antibodies. The tumors are usually immunoreactive for neuronspecific enolase (NSE).[30,70] Chromogranin may be negative, although these tumors usually contain neurosecretory granules.

Merkel cell tumors are clinically very aggressive, with regional node metastasis and subsequent widespread metastasis often occurring within a year of diagnosis.[30,70] For local disease, therapy includes wide local excision with a 2-cm margin of excision with sentinel lymph node biopsy. If the sentinel node demonstrates metastatic tumor, regional lymphadenectomy and postoperative local radiation therapy to the primary and regional sites is recommended. If there is systemic disease, chemotherapy is recommended.[30,70,164]

Metastatic Tumors

Metastatic tumors comprise approximately 8% of all tumors of the vulva. Tumors from other sites of the genital tract are the most common tumors that metastasize to the vulva, with *squamous carcinoma of the cervix* being the most frequent, followed by *carcinomas of the endometrium and ovary*. Other common primary tumor sites include the bladder and urethra.[119,142] Other primary tumors that have metastasized to the vulva include malignancies of breast, kidney, lung, stomach and gestational choriocarcinoma, melanoma, and neuroblastoma.[119,142]

Metastatic endometrial stromal sarcoma arising in extraovarian endometriosis involving the vulva has been reported; the sarcoma arose in endometriosis involving the round ligament in the canal of Nuck.[92] Malignant lymphomas also may metastasize to the vulva and Bartholin gland.[55,141,209] The vulva may be involved by direct extension of tumors arising in the vagina, urethra, bladder, or rectum. Metastatic tumors typically involve the dermis and overlying epithelium and consequently are often associated with ulceration. Patients with metastatic carcinoma to the vulva have a poor prognosis. Treatment is primarily palliative; radical surgical approaches are not indicated.

Tumors of the Urethra

Urethral Carcinoma

Urethral carcinoma constitutes less than 1% of malignancies affecting the female genitalia and occurs almost exclusively in elderly women.[98] Urethral bleeding, frequency, and dysuria are the most frequent presenting complaints. Tumors in the distal urethra usually give rise to symptoms early in their course. Most of these tumors arise in the distal urethra and are squamous cell carcinomas. Squamous cell carcinomas and transitional cell carcinomas may be papillary, forming papillomas or papillary carcinomas, or nonpapillary, presenting as carcinoma in situ of urothelial or squamous type or as solid high-grade urothelial carcinomas or squamous cell carcinomas. *Urothelial (transitional cell) carcinomas* may be seen in the distal as well as proximal urethra and have been described arising within a urethral diverticulum.

A pagetoid variant of urothelial carcinoma in situ has been described that primarily involves the bladder but is also described in the urethra.[133] Pagetoid urothelial intraepithelial neoplasia (PUIN) involving the urethral meatus and the vulvar vestibule, and clinically resembling vulvar Paget disease, has recently been described (see earlier vulvar Paget section).[196] Primary urothelial carcinomas express cytokeratin 7 and usually cytokeratin 20. In addition, uroplakin III is reported to be expressed in more than one-half of primary urinary tract urothelial carcinoma cases studied and in approximately two-thirds of the metastasis from urinary tract urothelial carcinomas.[124]

Adenocarcinomas of the urethra are relatively rare, accounting for approximately 10% of all primary urethral carcinomas. They occur in the proximal urethra as well as within urethral diverticuli.[5] Histopathologic types of adenocarcinoma include columnar/mucinous, clear cell, and colloid types.[113,206] Of these, clear cell adenocarcinoma of the urethra is of special interest in that this tumor occurs in adults with a wide age range, has distinct immunohistochemical and morphologic features suggesting müllerian differentiation, and appears to have a generally better prognosis, even with more advanced stages.[54] These tumors do not express prostate-specific antigen (PSA) or prostate acid phosphatase, and have tublocystic, papillary, and diffuse patterns of growth similar to clear cell carcinomas of the female genital tract. In one series, two-thirds of the cases arose in a urethral diverticulum.[132]

Primary adenocarcinomas arising in Skene glands have also been reported.[178] These tumors are thought to arise from the luminal secretory cells of these glands and have been demonstrated to express PSA and prostate acid phosphatase, reflecting the homology between Skene periurethral glands and the prostate.[163] Both urethral squamous carcinomas and adenocarcinomas are usually immunoreactive for CEA. The staging system for tumors of the urethra proposed by the AJCC is summarized in Table 3.9.

Table 3.9. American Joint Commission on clinical staging of urethral carcinoma primary tumor (T), urethra

TX: primary tumor cannot be assessed
T0: no evidence of primary tumor
Ta: noninvasive papillary, polypoid, or verrucous carcinoma
Tis: carcinoma in situ
T1: tumor invades subepithelial connective tissue
T2: tumor invades any of the following: corpus spongiosum, prostate periurethral muscle
T3: tumor invades any of the following: anterior vagina, bladder neck
T4: tumor invades other adjacent organs

Regional lymph nodes (N) related to urethral carcinoma are staged as follows:
NX: regional lymph nodes cannot be assessed
NO: no regional lymph node metastasis
N1: metastasis in a single lymph node, 2 cm or less in greatest dimension
N2: metastasis in a single node more than 2 cm in greatest dimension, or in multiple nodes

From ref. 4, with permission.

The prognosis related to urethral carcinoma is relatively poor. The 5-year overall survival for patients with anterior urethral tumors is 51% and for posterior tumors or entire urethral involvement only 6%. The overall survival has been reported to range from 22% to 27%, with a 5-year disease-free survival of only 27%.[207] Survival in urethral carcinoma is influenced by the fact that 20%–50% of women with urethral carcinoma have metastasis to superficial or deep pelvic nodes when first seen. Improved and individualized surgical and radiotherapy techniques may substantially increase survival.

Other Malignant Tumors of the Urethra

Non-Hodgkin's lymphoma,[7] melanoma,[149] carcinosarcoma,[107] and sarcoma have all been reported arising within the urethra.[207] Urethral caruncles with atypical stromal cells, and a florid proliferation of reactive lymphoid cells, are the primary differential diagnosis in regard to lymphomas and sarcomas in this location. Immunohistochemical studies to distinguish lymphocytic populations distinguish these benign processes from lymphoma. The atypical stromal cells in the urethral caruncles are immunoreactive for vimentin in approximately two-thirds of the cases, and express alpha-smooth muscle actin in one-half of cases.[205]

A number of metastatic tumors may involve the urethra, either by direct mucosal growth or by lymphatic or vascular metastasis. Metastatic involvement of the urethra from bladder carcinoma is observed in 8%–16% of cases.[31,117] In one study, direct mucosal-related metastasis was seen in two of 7 patients, and lymphatic metastasis was noted in five of these patients.[117] Bladder neck involvement by the primary bladder carcinoma is the most significant risk factor for urethral involvement.[31] Metastatic tumors from vulvar, vaginal, cervical, or anal carcinomas, as well as endometrial and, rarely, ovarian carcinomas, may occur.[79]

References

1. Abdul-Karim FW, Kida M, Wentz WB, et al (1990) Bone metastasis from gynecologic carcinomas: a clinicopathologic study. Gynecol Oncol 39:108–114
2. Agarossi A, Vago L, Lazzarin A, et al (1991) Vulvar Kaposi's sarcoma: a case report (letter). Ann Oncol 2:609–610
3. Al-Salameh A, Atawil A, Spiegal GW (2000) Absence of epithelial growth factor in anogenital Paget's disease argues against an origin from sweat glands. Mod Pathol 13:120A
4. American Joint Committee on Cancer ACSACoS (1998) AJCC cancer staging handbook. In: AJCC cancer staging manual, 5th Ed. Lippincott-Raven, Philadelphia, pp 171–175
5. Amin MB, Young RH (1997) Primary carcinomas of the urethra. Semin Diagn Pathol 14:147–160
6. Andreasson B, Bock JE, Strom KV, et al (1983) Verrucous carcinoma of the vulvar region. Acta Obstet Gynecol 62:183

6a. Andreasson B, Nyboe J (1985) Predictive factors with reference to low risk of metastases in squamous cell carcinoma of the vulvar region. Gynecol Oncol 21:196–206

7. Atalay AC, Karaman MI, Basak T, et al (1998) Non-Hodgkin's lymphoma of the female urethra presenting as a caruncle. Int Urol Nephrol 30:609–610
8. Audet-Lapointe P, Paquin F, Guerard MJ, et al (1980) Leiomyosarcoma of the vulva. Gynecol Oncol 10:350–355
9. Auger M, Colgan TJ (1990) Detection of metastatic vulvar and cervical squamous carcinoma in regional lymph nodes by use of a polyclonal keratin antibody. Int J Gynecol Pathol 9:337–342
10. Bacchi CE, Goldfogel GA, Greer BE, et al (1992) Paget's disease and melanoma of the vulva: use of a panel of monoclonal antibodies to identify cell type and to microscopically define adequacy of surgical margins. Gynecol Oncol 46:216–221
11. Begin LR, Clement PB, Kirk ME (1985) Aggressive angiomyxoma of pelvic soft parts: a clinico-

pathologic study of nine cases. Hum Pathol 16:621–628
12. Benda JA, Platz CE, Anderson B (1986) Malignant melanoma of the vulva: a clinical pathologic review of 16 cases. Int J Gynecol Pathol 5:202–216
13. Benedet JL, Miller DM, Ehlen TG, et al (1997) Basal cell carcinoma of the vulva: clinical features and treatment results in 28 patients. Obstet Gynecol 90:765–768
14. Benedet JL, Wilson PS, Matisic J (1991) Epidermal thickness and skin appendage involvement in vulvar intraepithelial neoplasia. J Reprod Med 36: 608–612
14a. Berman ML, Soper JT, Creasman WT, et al (1989) Conservative surgical management of superficially invasive stage I vulvar carcioma. Gynecol Oncol 35:352–356
15. Binder SW, Huang I, Fu YS, et al (1990) Risk factors for the development of lymph node metastasis in vulvar squamous cell carcinoma. Gynecol Oncol 37:9–16
16. Bock JE, Andreasson B, Thorn A, et al (1985) Dermatofibrosarcoma protuberans of the vulva. Gynecol Oncol 20:129–135
17. Bottles K, Lacey CG, Goldberg J, et al (1984) Merkle cell carcinoma of the vulva. Obstet Gynecol 63(suppl 3):61S–65S
18. Boyce J, Fruchter RG, Kasambilides E, et al (1985) Prognostic factors in carcinoma of the vulva. Gynecol Oncol 20:364–377
19. Brisigotti M, Moreno A, Murcia C, et al (1989) Verrucous carcinoma of the vulva: a clinicopathologic and immunohistochemical study of five cases. Int J Gynecol Pathol 8:1–7
20. Brooks JJ, LiVolsi VA (1987) Liposarcoma presenting on the vulva. Am J Obstet Gynecol 156: 73–75
21. Bryson SCP, Colgan TJ, Vernon CP (1986) Invasive squamous cell carcinoma of the vulva: delineation of high-risk group requiring adjuvant radiotherapy. J Reprod Med 31:976–976
22. Burke TA, Eifel PJ, McGuire P, et al (2000) The vulva. In: Hoskins WJ, Perez CA, Young RC (eds) Principles and practice of gynecologic oncology, 3rd Ed. Lippincott-Raven, Philadelphia, pp 717–753
23. Burke TW, Stringer CA, Gershenson DM, et al (1990) Radical wide excision and selective inguinal node disection for squamous cell carcinoma of the vulva. Gynecol Oncol 38:328–332
23a. Buscema J, Woodruff JD, Parmley TH, Genadry R (1980) Carcinoma in situ of the vulva. Obstet Gynecol 55:225
24. Carlson JA, Ambros R, Malfetano J, et al (1998) Vulvar lichen sclerosus and squamous cell carcinoma: a cohort, case control, and investigational study with historical perspective; implications for chronic inflammation and sclerosis in the development of neoplasia. Hum Pathol 29:932–948
25. Carlson JW, McGlennen RC, Gomez R, et al (1996) Sebaceous carcinoma of the vulva: a case report and review of the literature. Gynecol Oncol 60: 489–491
26. Carr KA, Bulengo S, Weiss LM, et al (1992) Lymphoepithelioma-like carcinoma of the skin. Am J Surg Pathol 16:909–913
27. Caterson RJ, Furber J, Murray J, et al (1984) Carcinoma of the vulva in two young renal allograft recipients. Transplant Proc 16:559
28. Cerri A, Gianni C, Corbellino M, et al (1998) Lymphangiosarcoma of the pubic region: a rare complication arising in congenital non-hereditary lymphedema. Eur J Dermatol 8:511–514
29. Chafe W, Richards A, Morgan L, et al (1988) Unrecognized invasive carcinoma in vulvar intraepithelial neoplasia (VIN). Gynecol Oncol 31:154–162
30. Chen KT (1994) Merkel's cell (neuroendocrine) carcinoma of the vulva. Cancer (Phila) 73:2186–2191
31. Chen ME, Pisters LL, Malpica A, et al (1997) Risk of urethral, vaginal and cervical involvement in patients undergoing radical cystectomy for bladder cancer: results of a contemporary cystectomy series from M.D. Anderson Cancer Center. J Urol 157:2120–2123
32. Cheung TH, Chan MK, Chang A (1991) Aggressive angiomyxoma of the female perineum: case reports. Aust N Z J Obstet Gynecol 31:285–287
33. Cliby W, Soisson AP, Berchuck A, et al (1991) Stage I small cell carcinoma of the vulva treated with vulvectomy, lymphadenectomy, and adjuvant chemo-therapy. Cancer (Phila) 67:2415–2417
34. Colgan TJ (1998) Vulvar intraepithelial neoplasia: a synopsis of recent developments. J Lower Genital Tract Dis 2:31–36
35. Colgan T (1998) Vulvar intraepithelial neoplasia: a synopsis of recent developments. J Lower Genital Tract Dis 2:31–36
36. Copas P, Dyer M, Comas FV, et al (1982) Spindle cell carcinoma of the vulva. Diagn Gynecol Obstet 4:235–235
37. Copeland LJ, Sneige N, Gershenson DM, et al (1986) Adenoid cystic carcinoma of Bartholin's gland. Obstet Gynecol 67:115
38. Copeland LJ, Cleary K, Sneige N, et al (1985) Neuroendocrine (Merkle cell) carcinoma of the vulva: a case report and review of the literature. Gynecol Oncol 22:367–378
39. Copeland LJ, Gershenson DM, Saul PB, et al (1985) Sarcoma botryoids of the female genital tract. Obstet Gynecol 66:262–266
40. Copeland LJ, Sneige N, Gershenson DM, et al (1986) Bartholin gland carcinoma. Obstet Gynecol 67:794–801
41. Copeland LJ, Sneige N, Gershenson DM, et al (1986) Adenoid cystic carcinoma of Bartholin's gland. Obstet Gynecol 67:115–120
42. Copeland LJ, Sneige N, Stringer CA, et al (1985) Alveolar rhabdomyosarcoma of the female genitalia. Cancer (Phila) 56:849–855

43. Crawford D, Nimmo M, Clement PB, et al (1999) Prognostic factors in Paget's disease of the vulva: a study of 21 cases. Int J Gynecol Pathol 18:351–359
44. Crum CP (1992). Carcinoma of the vulva: epidemiology and pathogenesis. Obstet Gynecol 79: 448–454
45. Curtin JP, Saigo P, Slucher B, et al (1995) Soft-tissue sarcoma of the vagina and vulva: a clinicopathologic study. Obstet Gynecol 86:269–272
46. Daling JR, Sherman KJ, Hislop TG, et al (1992) Cigarette smoking and the risk of anogenital cancer. Am J Epidemiol 135:180–189
47. DeHulla JA, Doting E, Piers DA, et al (1998) Sentinel lymph node identification with technetium-99m-labeled noncolloid in squamous cell cancer of the vulva. J Nuclear Med 39:1381–1385
48. DePasquale SE, McGuinness TB, Mangan CE, et al (1996) Adenoid cystic carcinoma of Bartholin's gland: a review of the literature and report of a patient. Gynecol Oncol 61:122–125
49. Di Bonito L, Patriarca S, Falconieri G (1992) Aggressive "breast-like" adenocarcinoma of vulva. Pathol Res Pract 188:211–214
50. Dinh TV, Powell LC, Hanninan EV, et al (1988) Simultaneously occurring condylomata acuminata, carcinoma in situ and verrucous carcinoma of the vulva and carcinoma in situ of the cervix in a young woman. J Reprod Med 33:510–513
51. Doss LL (1978) Simultaneous extramedullary plasmacytomas of the vagina and vulva. Cancer (Phila) 41:2468–2474
52. Downey GO, Okagaki T, Ostrow RS, et al (1988) Condylomatous carcinoma of the vulva with special reference to human papillomavirus DNA. Obstet Gynecol 72:68–72
53. Drew PA, Al-Abbadi MA, Orlando C, et al (1996) Prognostic factors in carcinoma of the vulva: a clinicopathologic and DNA flow cytometric study. Int J Gynecol Pathol 15:235–241
54. Drew PA, Murphy WM, Civantos F, et al (1996) The histogenesis of clear cell adenocarcinoma of the lower urinary tract. Case series and review of the literature. Hum Pathol 27:248–252
55. Egwuatu VE, Ejeckam GC, Okaro JM (1980) Burkitt's lymphoma of the vulva. Case report. Br J Obstet Gynecol 87:827–830
56. Emanuels AG, Burger MP, Hollema H, et al (1996) Quantitation of proliferation-associated markers Ag-NOR and Ki-67 does not contribute to the prediction of lymph node metastases in squamous cell carcinoma of the vulva. Hum Pathol 27:807–811
57. Ergeneli MH, Demirhan B, Duran EH (1999) Desmoid tumor of the vulva. A case report. J Reprod Med 44:748–750
58. Escalonilla P, Grilli R, Canamero M, et al (1999) Sebaceous carcinoma of the vulva. Am J Dermatopathol 21:468–472
59. Esquius J, Brisigotti M, Matias-Guiu X, et al (1991) Keratin expression in normal vulva, non-neoplastic epithelial disorders, vulvar intraepithelial neoplasia, and invasive squamous cell. Int J Gynecol Pathol 10:341–355
60. Ewing TL (1991) Paget's disease of the vulva treated by combined surgery and laser. Gynecol Oncol 43:137–140
61. Fanning J, Lambert HC, Hale TM, et al (1999) Paget's disease of the vulva: prevalence of associated vulvar adenocarcinoma, invasive Paget's disease, and recurrence after surgical excision. Am J Obstet Gynecol 180:24–27
62. Feakins RM, Lowe DG (1997) Basal cell carcinoma of the vulva: a clinicopathologic study of 45 cases. Int J Gynecol Pathol 16:319–324
63. Flanagan CW, Parker JR, Mannel RS, et al (1997) Primary endodermal sinus tumor of the vulva: a case report and review of the literature. Gynecol Oncol 66:515–518
64. Friedrich EG, Jr, Wilkinson EJ, Fu YS (1980) Carcinoma in situ of the vulva: a continuing challenge. Am J Obstet Gynecol 136:830–843
65. Fu YS, Reagan JW, Townsend DE, et al (1981) Nuclear DNA study of vulvar intraepithelial and invasive squamous neoplasms. Obstet Gynecol 57: 643–652
66. Ganjei P, Giraldo KA, Lampe B, et al (1990) Vulvar Paget's disease. Is immunocytochemistry helpful in assessing the surgical margins? J Reprod Med 35:1002–1004
67. Genton CY, Maroni ES (1987) Vulval liposarcoma. Arch Gynecol 240:63–66
68. Ghorbani RP, Malpica A, Ayala AG (1999) Dermatofibrosarcoma protuberans of the vulva: clinicopathologic and immunohistochemical analysis of four cases, one with fibrosarcomatous change, and review of the literature. Int J Gynecol Pathol 18:366–373
69. Gianotti F, Caputo R (1985) Histiocytic syndromes: a review. J Am Acad Dermatol 13:383–404
70. Gil-Moreno A, Garcia-Jimenez A, Gonzalez-Bosquet J, et al (1997) Merkel cell carcinoma of the vulva. Gynecol Oncol 64:526–532
71. Gordon AN (1991) Current concepts in the treatment of invasive vulvar carcinoma. Clin Obstet Gynecol 34:587–598
72. Gordon AN (2000) Vulvar neoplasms. In: Copeland LJ, Jarrell J (eds) Textbook of gynecology, 2nd Ed. Saunders, Philadelphia, pp 1185–1208
73. Graf AH, Su HC, Tubbs RR, et al (1998) Primary neuroendocrine differentiated mucinous adenocarcinoma of the vulva: case report and review of the literature. Anticancer Res 18:2041–2045
74. Gunn RA, Gallager HS (1980) Vulvar Paget's disease: a topographic study. Cancer (Phila) 46:590–594
75. Hacker NF, Berek JS, Lagasse LD, et al (1984) Individualization of treatment for stage I squamous cell vulvar carcinoma. Obstet Gynecol 63:155–162

76. Hacker NF, Nieberg RK, Berek JS, et al (1983) Superficially invasive vulvar cancer with nodal metastases. Gynecol Oncol 15:65–77
77. Haefner HK, Tate JE, McLachlin CM, et al (1995) Vulvar intraepithelial neoplasia: age, morphological phenotype, papillomavirus DNA, and coexisting invasive carcinoma. Hum Pathol 26:147–154
78. Hall D, Grimes MM, Goplerud DR (1980) Epithelioid sarcoma of the vulva. Gynecol Oncol 9: 237–246
79. Hammadeh MY, Thomas K, Philp T (1996) Urethral caruncle: an unusual presentation of ovarian tumour. Gynecol Obstet Invest 42:279–280
80. Heaps JM, Fu YS, Montz FJ, et al (1990) Surgical-pathologic variables predictive of local recurrence in squamous cell carcinoma of the vulva. Gynecol Oncol 38:309–314
81. Heard I, Kazatchkine MD (1999) Regression of cervical lesions in HIV-infected women receiving HAART. AIDS Reader 9:630–635
82. Hendricks JB, Wilkinson EJ, Kubilis P, et al (1994) Ki-67 expression in vulvar carcinoma. Int J Gynecol Pathol 13;205–210
83. Hensley GT, Friedrich EG (1973) Malignant fibroxanthoma: a sarcoma of the vulva. Am J Obstet Gynecol 116:289–291
84. Herod JJ, Shafi MI, Rollason TP, et al (1996) Vulvar intraepithelial neoplasia with superficially invasive carcinoma of the vulva. Br J Obstet Gynaecol 103:453–456
85. Hicks ML, Piver MS (1992) Conservative surgery plus adjuvant therapy for vulvovaginal rhabdomyosarcoma, diethylstilbestrol clear cell adenocarcinoma of the vagina, and unilateral germ cell tumors of the ovary. Obstet Gynecol Clin North Am 19:219–233
86. Hoffman MS, Pinelli DM, Finan M, et al (1992) Laser vaporization for vulvar intraepithelial neoplasia. III. J Reprod Med 37:135–137
86a. Homesley HD, Bundy BN, Sedlis A, et al (1993) Prognostic factors for groin node metastasis in squamous cell carcinoma of the vulva (a gynecologic onclolgy group study). Gynecol Oncol 49: 279–28
87. Homesley HD, Bundy BN, Sedlis A, et al (1991) Assessment of current international federation of gynecology and obstetrics staging of vulvar carcinoma relative to prognostic factors for survival (a gynecologic oncology group study). Am J Obstet Gynecol 164:997–1004
87a. Husseinzadeh N, Recinto C (1999) Frequency of invasive cancer in surgically excised vulvar lesions with intraepithelial neoplasia (VIN 3). Gyncol Oncol 73:119–120
88. Husseinzadeh N, Wesseler T, Newman N, et al (1988) Neuroendocrine (Merkle cell) carcinoma of the vulva. Gynecol Oncol 29:105–112
89. Husseinzadeh N, Zaino R, Nahhas WA, et al (1983) The significance of histologic findings in predicting nodal metastasis in invasive squamous cell carcinoma of the vulva. Gynecol Oncol 16: 105–111
90. Igarashi T, Sasano H, Konno R, et al (1998) Malignant rhabdoid tumor of the vulva: case report with cytological, immunohistochemical, ultrastructural and DNA ploidy studies and a review of the literature. Pathol Int 48:887–891
91. Imachi M, Tsukamoto N, Shigematsu T, et al (1992) Cytologic diagnosis of primary adenocarcinoma of Bartholin's gland: a case report. Acta Cytol 36:167–170
92. Irvin W, Pelkey T, Rice L, et al (1998) Endometrial stromal sarcoma of the vulva arising in extraovarian endometriosis: a case report and literature review. Gynecol Oncol 71:313–316
93. Ishizawa T, Mitsuhashi Y, Sugiki H, et al (1998) Basal cell carcinoma within vulvar Paget's disease. Dermatology (Basel) 197:388–390
94. Issa PY, Salem PA, Brihi E, et al (1980) Eosinophilic granuloma with involvement of the female genitalia. Am J Obstet Gynecol 137:608–
94a. Iversen T, Abeler V, Aalders J (1981) Individualized treatment of stage I carcinoma of the vulva. Obstet Gynecol 57:85
95. Iversen T, Andreasson B, Bryson SCP, et al (1990) Surgical-procedure terminology for the vulva and vagina: a report of an International Society for the Study of Vulvar Disease Task Force. J Reprod Med 35:1033–1034
96. Jacobs DM, Sandles LG, LeBoit PE (1983) Sebaceous carcinoma arising from bowen's disease of the vulvar. Arch Dermatol 122:1191–1193
97. Japaze H, vanDinh T, Woodruff JD (1982) Verrucous carcinoma of the vulva: study of 24 cases. Obstet Gynecol 60:462–462
98. Johnson DE, O'Connell JR (1983) Primary carcinoma of female urethra. Urology 21:42–45
99. Johnson TL, Kumar NB, White CD, et al (1986) Prognostic features of vulvar melanoma. Int J Gynecol Pathol 5:110–118
100. Johnson WC, Helwig EG (1966) Adenoid squamous cell carcinoma (adenocanthoma). A clinicopathologic study of 155 patients. Cancer (Phila) 19:1639–1660
101. Jones RW, McLean MR (1986) Carcinoma in situ of the vulva: a review of 31 treated and 5 untreated cases. Obstet Gynecol 68:499–503
102. Jones RW, Rowan DM (1994) Vulvar intraepithelial neoplasia. III: A clinical study of the outcome in 113 cases with relation to the later development of invasive vulvar carcinoma [see comments]. Obstet Gynecol 84:741–745
103. Kelley JLI, Burke TW, Tornos C, et al (1992) Minimally invasive vulvar carcinoma: an indication for conservative surgical therapy. Gynecol Oncol 44:240–244
104. Kim YT, Thomas NF, Kessis TD, et al (1996) p53 mutations and clonality in vulvar carcinomas and squamous hyperplasias: evidence suggesting that squamous hyperplasias do not serve as direct pre-

cursors of human papillomavirus-negative vulvar carcinomas. Hum Pathol 27:389–395
105. Kluzak TR, Krause FT (1987) Condylomata, papillomas and verrucous carcinomas of the vulva and vagina. In: Wilkinson EJ (ed) Contemporary issues in surgical pathology. Pathology of the vulva and vagina, vol 9. Churchill Livingstone, New York, pp 49–77
106. Kneale BL (1984) Microinvasive cancer of the vulva: report of the international society for the study of vulvar disease task force, VIIth congress. J Reprod Med 29:454–456
107. Konno N, Mori M, Kurooka Y, et al (1997) Carcinosarcoma in the region of the female urethra. Int J Urol 4:229–231
108. Kurman RJ, Toki T, Schiffman MH (1993) Basaloid and warty carcinomas of the vulva. Distinctive types of squamous cell carcinoma frequently associated with human papillomaviruses. Am J Surg Pathol 17:133–145
109. Leibowitch M, Neill S, Pelisse M, et al (1990) The epithelial changes associated with squamous cell carcinoma of the vulva: a review of the clinical, histological and viral findings in 78 women. Br J Obstet Gynaecol 97:1135–1139
110. Leuchter RS, Hacker NF, Voet RL, et al (1982) Primary carcinoma of the Bartholin gland: a report of 14 cases and review of the literature. Obstet Gynecol 60:361–368
111. Lever WF (1997) Lever's histopathology of the skin, 8th Ed. Lippincott-Raven, Philadelphia
112. LiVolsi VA, Brooks JJ (1987) Soft tissue tumors of the vulva. In: Wilkinson EJ (ed) Contemporary issues in surgical pathology. Pathology of the vulva and vagina, vol 9. Churchill Livingstone, New York, pp 209–238
113. Loo KT, Chan JKC (1992) Colloid adenocarcinoma of the urethra associated with mucosal in situ carcinoma. Arch Pathol Lab Med 116:976–977
113a. Magrina JF, Webb MJ, Gaffey TA, Symmonds RE (1979) Stage I squamous cell cancer of the vulva. Am J Obstet Gynecol 134:453
114. Magrina JF, Gonzalez-Bosquet J, Weaver AL, et al (2000) Squamous cell carcinoma of the vulva stage IA: long-term results. Gynecol Oncol 76:24–27
114a. Magrina JF, Gonzalez-Bosquet J,Weaver AL, et al (2000) Squamous cell carcinoma of the vulva stage 1A: long-term results. Gynecol Oncol 76:24–27
115. Malik SN, Wilkinson EJ (1999) Pseudo-Paget's disease of the vulva: a case report. J Lower Genital Tract Dis 3:201–203
116. Malmstrom H, Janson H, Simonsen E, et al (1990) Prognostic factors in invasive squamous cell carcinoma of the vulva treated with surgery and irradiation. Acta Oncol 29:915–919
117. Maralani S, Wood DP Jr, Grignon D, et al (1997) Incidence of urethral involvement in female bladder cancer: an anatomic pathologic study. Urology 50:537–541
118. Martelli H, Oberlin O, Rey A, et al (1999) Conservative treatment for girls with nonmetastatic rhabdomyosarcoma of the genital tract: a report from the study committee of the International Society of Pediatric Oncology. J Clin Oncol 17:2117–2122
119. Mazur MT, Hsueh S, Gersell DJ (1984) Metastases to the female genital tract: analysis of 325 cases. Cancer (Phila) 53:1978–1984
120. McConnell DT, Miller ID, Parkin DE, et al (1997) p53 protein expression in a population-based series of primary vulval squamous cell carcinoma and immediate adjacent field change. Gynecol Oncol 67:248–254
121. McLachlin CM, Kozakewich H, Craighill M, et al (1994) Histologic correlates of vulvar human papillomavirus infection in children and young adults. Am J Surg Pathol 18:728–735
122. Michael H, Roth L (1987) Congenital and acquired cysts, benign and malignant skin adnexal tumors, and Paget's disease of the vulva. In: Wilkinson EJ (ed) Pathology of the vulva and vagina: contemporary issues in surgical pathology, vol 9. Churchill Livingstone, New York, pp 25–48
123. Mirhashemi R, Kratz A, Weir MM, et al (1998) Vaginal small cell carcinoma mimicking a Bartholin's gland abscess: a case report. Gynecol Oncol 68:297–300
124. Moll R, Wu XR, Lin JH, et al (1995) Uroplakins, specific membrane proteins of urothelial umbrella cells, as histological markers of metastatic transitional cell carcinomas. Am J Pathol 147:1383–1397
125. Morgan LS, Joslyn P, Chafe W, et al (1988) A report on 18 cases of primary malignant melanoma of the vulva. Colpo Laser Surg 4:161–170
126. Niebyl JR, Genadry R, Friedrich EG, et al (1975) Vulvar carcinoma with hypercalcemia. Obstet Gynecol 45:343–348
127. Nielsen GP, Rosenberg AE, Koerner F, et al (1996) Smooth-muscle tumors of the vulva. A clinicopathologic study of 25 cases and review of the literature. Am J Surg Pathol 20:779–793
128. Nielsen GP, Young RH, Dickersin GR, et al (1997) Angiomyofibroblastoma of the vulva with sarcomatous transformation ("angiomyofibrosarcoma"). Am J Surg Pathol 21:1104–1108
128a. Nielsen GP, Rosenberg AE, Young RH, et al (1996) Angiomyofibroblastoma of the vulva and vagina. Mod Pathol 9:284–291
129. Nirenberg A, Slavin J, Ostor AG (1993) Primary vulvar sarcomas. Int J Gynecol Pathol 14(1):55–62
130. Nowak MA, Guerriere-Kovach P, Pathan A, et al (1998) Perianal Paget's disease: distinguishing primary and secondary lesions using immunohistochemical studies including gross cystic disease fluid protein-15 and cytokeratin 20 expression. Arch Pathol Lab Med 122:1077–1081
131. Nucci MR, Fletcher CD (1998) Liposarcoma (atypical lipomatous tumors) of the vulva: a clinicopathologic study of six cases. Int J Gynecol Pathol 17:17–23

132. Oliva E, Young RH (1996) Clear cell adenocarcinoma of the urethra: a clinicopathologic analysis of 19 cases. Mod Pathol 9:513–520
133. Orozco RE, Vander ZR, Murphy WM (1993) The pagetoid variant of urothelial carcinoma in situ. Hum Pathol 24:1199–1202
134. Park JS, Jones RW, McLean MR, et al (1991) Possible etiologic heterogeneity of vulvar intraepithelial neoplasia. A correlation of pathologic characteristics with human papillomavirus detection by in situ hybridization and polymerase chain reaction. Cancer (Phila) 67:1599–1607
135. Pelosi G, Martignoni G, Bonetti F (1991) Intraductal carcinoma of mammary-type apocrine epithelium arising within a papillary hidradenoma of the vulva: report of a case and review of the literature. Arch Pathol Lab Med 115:1249–1254
136. Perrone T, Swanson PE, Twiggs L, et al (1989) Malignant rhabdoid tumor of the vulva: is distinction from epithelioid sarcoma possible? Am J Surg Pathol 13:848–858
137. Pilotti S, Rotola A, D'Amato L, et al (1990) Vulvar carcinomas: search for sequences homologous to human papillomavirus and herpes simplex virus DNA. Mod Pathol 3:442–448
138. Pinto AP, Signorello LB, Crum CP, et al (1999) Squamous cell carcinoma of the vulva in Brazil: prognostic importance of host and viral variables. Gynecol Oncol 74:61–67
139. Piura B, Rabinovich A, Dgani R (1999) Basal cell carcinoma of the vulva. J Surg Oncol 70:172–176
140. Piura B, Rabinovich A, Dgani R (1999) Malignant melanoma of the vulva: report of six cases and review of the literature. Eur J Gynaecol Oncol 20:182–186
141. Plouffe L, Tulandi T, Rosenberg A, et al (1984) Non-Hodgkin's lymphoma in Bartholin's gland: case report and review of literature. Am J Obstet Gynecol 148:608–609
142. Powell CS, Jones PA (1983) Carcinoma of the bladder with a metastasis in the clitoris. Br J Obstet Gynecol 90:380
143. Powell FC, Bjornsson J, Doyle JA, et al (1985) Genital Paget's disease and urinary tract malignancy. J Am Acad Dermatol 13:84–84
144. Preti M, Micheletti L, Barbero M, et al (1993) Histologic parameters of vulvar invasive carcinoma and lymph node metastases. J Reprod Med 38:28–32
145. Prignano F, Domenici L, Carli P, et al (1999) Langerhans cell histiocytosis of the vulva: an ultrastructural study. Ultrastruct Pathol 23:127–132
146. Rabah R, Farmer D (1999) Squamous cell carcinoma of the vulva in a child. J Lower Genital Tract Dis 3:204–206
147. Ragnarsson-Olding BK, Nilsson BR, Kanter-Lewensohn LR, et al (1999) Malignant melanoma of the vulva in a nationwide, 25-year study of 219 Swedish females: predictors of survival. Cancer (Phila) 86:1285–1293
148. Reed JA, Brigati DJ, Flynn SD, et al (1992) Immunocytochemical identification of *Rochalimaea henselae* in bacillary (epithelioid) angiomatosis, parenchymal bacillary peliosis, and persistent fever with bacteremia. Am J Surg Pathol 16: 650–657
149. Rikaniadis N, Konstadoulakis MM, Kymionis GD, et al (1998) Long-term survival of a female patient with primary malignant melanoma of the urethra. Eur J Surg Oncol 24:607–608
150. Robertson AJ, McIntosh W, Lamont P, et al (1981) Malignant granular cell tumor (myoblastoma) of the vulva: report of a case and review of the literature. Histopathology 5:69–79
151. Rodke G, Friedrich EG Jr, Wilkinson EJ (1988) Malignant potential of mixed vulvar dystrophy (lichen sclerosis associated with squamous cell hyperplasia). J Reprod Med 33:545–550
152. Rusk D, Sutton GP, Look KY, et al (1991) Analysis of invasive squamous cell carcinoma of the vulva and vulvar intraepithelial neoplasia for the presence of human papillomavirus DNA. Obstet Gynecol 77:918–922
153. Santeusanio G, Schiaroli S, Anemona L, et al (1991) Carcinoma of the vulva with sarcomatoid features: a case report with immunohistochemical study. Gynecol Oncol 40:160–163
154. Scheistroen M, Trope C, Kaern J, et al (1997) DNA ploidy and expression of p53 and C-erbB-2 in extramammary Paget's disease of the vulva. Gynecol Oncol 64:88–92
155. Schwartz BM, Kuo DYS, Goldberg GL (1999) Dermatofibrosarcoma protuberans of the vulva: a rare tumor presenting during pregnancy in a teenager. J Lower Genital Tract Dis 3:139–142
156. Scully RE, BonfiglioTA, Kurman RJ, Silverberg SG, Wilkenson EJ (1994) Histological typing of female genital tract tumors, World Health Organization international histological classification of tumors, 2 Ed. Springer-Verlag, New York
157. Scurry J, Beshay V, Cohen C, et al (1998) Ki67 expression in lichen sclerosus of vulva in patients with and without associated squamous cell carcinoma. Histopathology (Oxf) 32:399–404
158. Scurry J, Brand A, Planner R, et al (1996) Vulvar Merkel cell tumor with glandular and squamous differentiation. Gynecol Oncol 62:292–297
159. Sedlis A, Homesley H, Bundy BN, et al (1987) Positive groin lymph nodes in superficial squamous cell vulvar cancer: a gynecologic oncology group study. Am J Obstet Gynecol 156:1159–1164
160. Shatz P, Bergeron C, Wilkinson EJ, et al (1989) Vulvar intraepithelial neoplasia and skin appendage involvement. Obstet Gynecol 74:769–774
161. Shen JT, D'ablaing G, Morrow CP (1982) Alveolar soft part sarcoma of the vulva: report of first case and review of literature. Gynecol Oncol 13:120–128
162. Sivanesaratnam V, Pathmanathan R (1990) Carcinoma of the vulva in pregnancy: a rare occurrence. Asia Oceania J Obstet Gynaecol 16:207–210

163. Sloboda J, Zaviacic M, Jakubovsky J, et al (1998) Metastasizing adenocarcinoma of the female prostate (Skene's paraurethral glands). Histological and immunohistochemical prostate markers studies and first ultrastructural observation. Pathol Res Pract 194:129–136
164. Smith DF, Messina JL, Perrott R, et al (2000) Clinical approach to neuroendocrine carcinoma of the skin (Merkel cell carcinoma). Cancer Control 7:72–83
165. Snow SN, DeSouky S, Lo JS, et al (1992) Failure to detect human papillomavirus DNA in extramammary Paget's disease. Cancer (Phila) 69:249–251
166. Soergel TM, Doering DL, O'Connor D (1998) Metastatic dermatofibrosarcoma protuberans of the vulva. Gynecol Oncol 71:320–324
167. Stapleton JJ (1984) Extramammary Paget's disease of the vulva in a young black woman. J Reprod Med 29:444–446
168. Steeper TA, Piscioli F, Rosai J (1983) Squamous cell carcinoma with sarcoma-like stroma of the female genital tract. Cancer (Phila) 52:890–898
169. Steeper TA, Piscioli F, Rosai J (1983) Squamous cell carcinoma with sarcoma-like stroma of the female genital tract. Clinicopathologic study of four cases. Cancer (Phila) 52:890–898
170. Steeper TA, Rosai J (1983) Aggressive angiomyxoma of the female pelvis and perineum. Report of nine cases of a distinctive type of gynecologic soft-tissue neoplasm. Am J Surg Pathol 7:463–475
171. Stehman FB, Bundy BN, Dvoretsky PM, et al (1992) Early stage I carcinoma of the vulva treated with ipsilateral superficial inguinal lymphadenectomy and modified radical hemivulvectomy: a prospective study of the gynecologic oncology group. Obstet Gynecol 79:490–497
172. Stentella P, Cipriano L, Covello R, et al (1997) Langerhans cell histiocytosis of vulva and cervix in a 19-year-old woman. Gynecol Obstet Invest 44:67–69
173. Sturgeon SR, Brinton LA, Devesa SS, et al (1992) In situ and invasive vulvar cancer incidence trends (1973–1987). Am J Obstet Gynecol 166:1482
174. Talerman A (1973) Sarcoma botryoides presenting as a polyp on the labium majorus. Cancer (Phila) 32:994–999
175. Tasseron EW, van der Esch EP, Hart AA, et al (1992) A clinicopathological study of 30 melanomas of the vulva. Gynecol Oncol 46:170–175
176. Tavassoli FA, Norris HJ (1979) Smooth muscle tumors of the vulva. Obstet Gynecol 53:213–217
177. Taylor RN, Bottles K, Miller TR, et al (1985) Malignant fibrous histiocytoma of the vulva. Obstet Gynecol 66:145–148
178. Taylor RN, Lacey CG, Shuman MA (1985) Adenocarcinoma of Skene's duct associated with a systemic coagulopathy. Gynecol Oncol 22:250–256
179. Terada KY, Schmidt RW, Roberts JA (1988) Malignant schwannoma of the vulva. A case report. J Reprod Med 33:969–972
180. Thomas R, Barnhill D, Bibro M, et al (1986) Histiocytosis X in gynecology. A case presentation and review of the literature. Obstet Gynecol 67: 46S-49S
181. Toki T, Kurman RJ, Park JS, et al (1991) Probable nonpapillomavirus etiology of squamous cell carcinoma of the vulva in older women: a clinicopathologic study using in situ. Int J Gynecol Pathol 10:107–125
182. Trimble CL, Diener-West M, Wilkinson EJ, et al (1999) Reproducibility of the histopathological classification of vulvar squamous carcinoma and intraepithelial neoplasia. J Lower Genital Tract Dis 3:98–103
183. Trimble EL (1996) Melanomas of the vulva and vagina. Oncology (Basel) 10:1017–1023
184. Trimble EL, Lewis JL Jr, Williams LL, et al (1992) Management of vulvar melanoma. Gynecol Oncol 45:254–258
185. Tuder RM (1992) Vulvar destruction by malignant lymphoma. Gynecol Oncol 45:52–57
186. Van der Putte SC, van Gorp LH (1994) Adenocarcinoma of the mammary-like glands of the vulva: a concept unifying sweat gland carcinoma of the vulva, carcinoma of supernumerary mammary glands and extramammary Paget's disease. J Cutan Pathol 21:157–163
187. Van der Putte SCJ (1994) Mammary-like glands of the vulva and their disorders. Int J Gynecol Pathol 13:150–160
188. van Hoeven KH, Kovatich AJ (1996) Immunohistochemical staining for proliferating cell nuclear antigen, BCL2, and Ki-67 in vulvar tissues. Int J Gynecol Pathol 15:10–16
189. Wade TR, Kopf AW, Ackerman AB (1979) Bowenoid papulosis of the genitalia. Arch Dermatol 115:306–308
190. Wheelock JB, Goplerud DR, Dunn LJ, et al (1984) Primary carcinoma of the Bartholin gland: a report of ten cases. Obstet Gynecol 63:820–824
191. Wick MR, Goellner JR, Wolfe JT, et al (1985) Vulvar sweat gland carcinoma. Arch Pathol Lab Med 109:43–47
192. Wilkinson EJ, Kneale B, Lynch PJ (1986) Report of the ISSVD Terminology Committee. Proc VIII World Congress, Stockholm, Sweden. J Reprod Med 31:973–974
193. Wilkinson EJ (1991) Superficially invasive carcinoma of the vulva. Clin Obstet Gynecol 34:651–661
194. Wilkinson EJ (1992) Normal histology and nomenclature of the vulva, and malignant neoplasms, including VIN. Dermatol Clin 10:283–296
195. Wilkinson EJ (2000) Protocol for the examination of specimens from patients with carcinomas and malignant melanomas of the vulva: a basis for checklists. Cancer Committee of the American College of Pathologists. Arch Pathol Lab Med 124: 51–56

196. Wilkinson EJ, Brown H (2001) Vulvar pagetoid urothelial intraepithelial neoplasia (PUIN). Mod Pathol 13:134A
197. Wilkinson EJ, Cook JC, Friedrich EG Jr, et al (1988) Vulvar intraepithelial neoplasia: association with cigarette smoking. Colposcopy Gynecol Laser Surg 4:153–159
198. Wilkinson EJ, Croker BP, Friedrich EG Jr, et al (1988) Two distinct pathologic types of giant cell tumor of the vulva: a report of two cases. J Reprod Med 33:519–522
199. Wilkinson EJ, Friedrich EG Jr, Fu YS (1981) Multicentric nature of vulvar carcinoma in situ. Obstet Gynecol 58:69–74
200. Wilkinson EJ, Rico MJ, Pierson KK (1982) Microinvasive carcinoma of the vulva. Int J Gynecol Pathol 1:29–39
201. Wilkinson EJ, Morgan LS, Friedrich EG Jr (1984) Association of Franconi's anemia and squamous-cell carcinoma of the lower female genital tract with condyloma acuminatum. J Reprod Med 29:447–453
202. Willen R, Bekassy, Carlen B, et al (1999) Cloacogenic adenocarcinoma of the vulva. Gynecol Oncol 74:298–301
203. Woolcott RJ, Henry RJ, Houghton CR (1988) Malignant melanoma of the vulva. J Reprod Med 33:699–702
204. Yang B, Hart WR (2000) Vulvar intraepithelial neoplasia of the simplex (differentiated) type: a clinicopathologic study including analysis of HPV and p53 expression. Am J Surg Pathol 24:429–441
205. Young RH, Oliva E, Garcia JA, et al (1996) Urethral caruncle with atypical stromal cells simulating lymphoma or sarcoma—a distinctive pseudoneoplastic lesion of females. A report of six cases. Am J Surg Pathol 20:1190–1195
206. Young RH, Scully RE (1985) Clear cell adenocarcinoma of the bladder and urethra. Am J Surg Pathol 9:816–826
207. Zaino RJ (1987) Carcinoma of the vulva, urethra and Bartholin's gland. In: Wilkinson EJ (ed) Contemporary issues in surgical pathology. Pathology of the vulva and vagina. 1st Ed. Churchill Livingstone, New York, pp 119–154
208. Zaki I, Dalziel K, Solomonsz F, et al (1996) The under-reporting of skin disease in association with squamous cell carcinoma of the vulva. Clin Exp Dermatol 21:334–337
209. ZaKut H, Lotan M, Lipnilsky M (1985) Vulvar hemangiopericytoma: a case report and review of previous cases. Acta Obstet Gynecol Scand 64:619–621

4

Diseases of the Vagina

Richard J. Zaino, M.D., Stanley J. Robboy, M.D., and Robert J. Kurman, M.D.

The vagina, like other orifices that interface between the external environment and the interior milieu, acts as a barrier to many potentially invasive microorganisms. It is thus not surprising that the vagina is the site of a variety of infections, both sexually and nonsexually transmitted, and this, in fact, represents the predominant type of pathology of this organ. In contrast, neoplasms are relatively unusual in this site, which is somewhat unexpected in view of the relationship between infection (e.g., human papilloma virus infection) and the development of carcinoma of the vulva and cervix.

Because of its profound effects on the development of the vagina, the pathology of in utero diethylstilbestrol (DES) exposure has been integrated into the Developmental Disorders and Malignant Neoplasms sections of this chapter. In few other areas of medicine have the interrelationships of embryology, anatomy, physiology, and neoplasia been so well defined. The astute reader will note, however, that the failure to identify many aspects relating to the pathogenesis of many other diseases of the vagina reflects our current state of ignorance.

Development

Debate over the embryologic origins of the vagina has persisted for more than 50 years. These differences reflect the complex and dynamic interrelationship of tissues derived from different germ cell layers and the lack of an animal model that parallels human vaginal development. Nonetheless, the discovery of specific epithelial and stromal abnormalities in the lower genital tract of women exposed to DES in utero emphasizes that pathologic changes in the adult may be a consequence of disordered embryogenesis. A brief review of vaginal development therefore follows (for a more detailed discussion see Chapter 1, Embryology of the Female Genital Tract and Disorders of Abnormal Sexual Development).

It is generally agreed that both the müllerian ducts and the urogenital sinus contribute to the formation of the vagina.[51,271] The müllerian ducts first appear as funnel-shaped openings of the coelomic epithelium in the mesonephric ridge about postconception day 37.[51,76,271] They grow caudally as paired tubes, extending to meet the posterior wall of the urogenital sinus. At about day 54, the caudal portions of the müllerian ducts fuse, forming a straight uterovaginal canal that is lined by simple columnar epithelium. The uterovaginal canal continues to elongate caudally until about day 66. Shortly thereafter, the epithelium from the caudal tip of the canal to the external cervical os changes to a stratified squamous type; this results from a migration of squamous cells from the urogenital sinus, rather than from squamous metaplasia of the native müllerian columnar epithelium.[271] Continued stratification of the squamous epithelial lining progressively occludes the more caudal portion of the canal leading to the development of a solid vaginal plate. In the 16th week, the squamous epithelium of the vagina and ectocervix begins to mature, becoming glycogenated and thickened. Desquamation subsequently results in canalization of the vaginal plate. Vaginal development is essentially complete by the 18th–20th week. A band of subepithelial stroma extending from the endocervix to the vulva has been described, but the role of the vaginal stroma in induction of mucosal changes remains unclear.[51,68,277]

In the past, our knowledge of vaginal embryology was derived from classic dissections of the fetus. Several experiments of nature in humans (in utero exposure to DES, transverse vaginal septation, and partial vaginal agenesis) and in mice (testicular feminization syndrome and agenesis of the lower vagina[51] as well as recent studies using human fetal grafts transplanted into the nude mouse[52,271] have provided the opportunity for elegant studies of altered development. Such studies reaffirm that the vagina is of dual origin, with a native lining of müllerian columnar cells that are retained unless there is a contribution of squamous cells from the urogenital sinus.

Anatomy

The vagina is a partially collapsed, midline, tubular structure that extends from the vestibule of the vulva to the uterine cervix. The vagina is posterior to the urinary bladder and anterior to the rectum, with an angle of more than 90° between the axis of the vagina and that of the uterus (Fig. 4.1). In the adult, the vagina is about 9 cm in length. Its caliber and length are unrelated to sexual activity or symptoms of dyspareunia.[349] The anterior and posterior walls are in contact with each other, with the exception of the cranial (proximal) end where the vagina surrounds the ectocervix. Here, there are vaultlike recesses between the vaginal walls and the cervix termed *fornices*, which are deepest posteriorly. In contrast to the slack anterior and posterior walls, the lateral walls are relatively rigid, resulting in a somewhat compressed lumen with an H shape in transverse sections.[269]

The vagina is in contact anteriorly with the uterine cervix, the base of the bladder, and the urethra. The proximal third of the urethra is separated from the vagina by loose connective tissue; it enters into the vaginal wall distally where their fasciae fuse into a single dense layer. Posteriorly, the upper fourth of the vaginal wall is bounded by peritoneum, and forms the anterior part of the cul-de-sac or pouch of Douglas. The rectovaginal septum connects the adventitia of the middle half of the vagina with the rectum, whereas the perineal body and anal and rectal sphincters separate the remaining more caudal

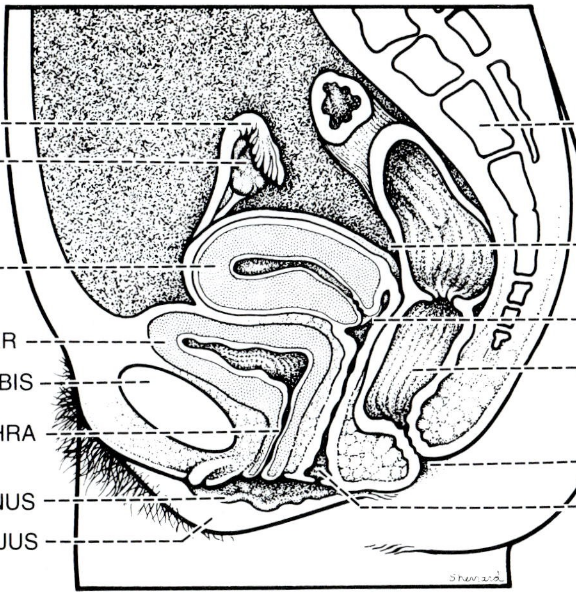

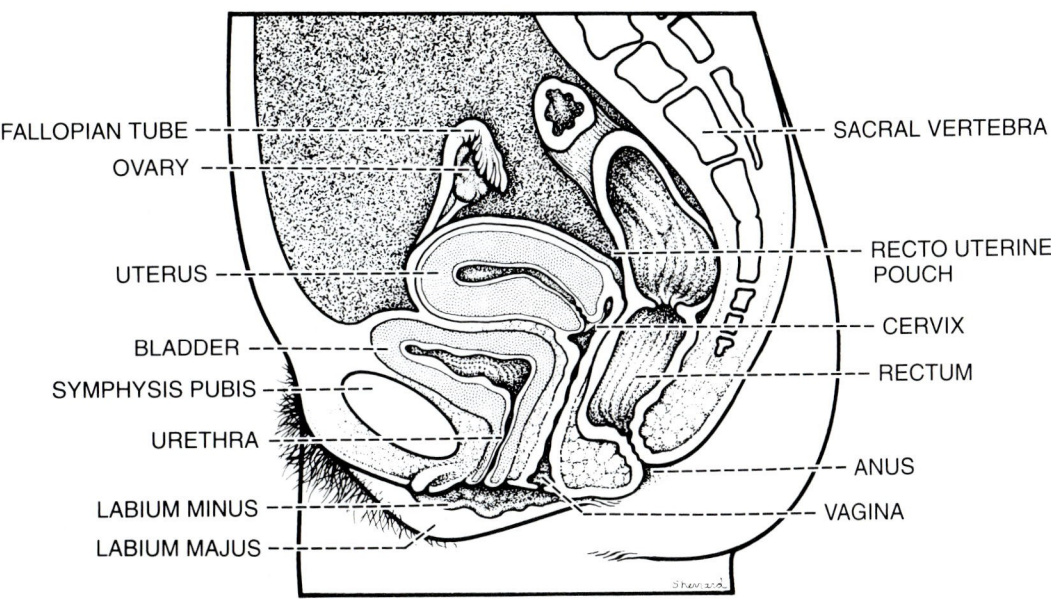

Fig. 4.1. Median sagittal section of the female pelvis.

portion from the anal canal. Laterally, each ureter, crossed by the uterine artery and vein, runs just above the lateral fornix. Caudally (distally), the levator ani and bulbocavernosus muscles partially surround the vagina, which ultimately opens into the vestibule (Fig. 4.2).

Blood is supplied to the vagina primarily by branches of the internal iliac artery, including the uterine, vaginal, middle rectal, and internal pudendal arteries. Extensive anastomoses provide alternate routes of flow, which minimize the possibility of ischemic damage. A complex network of veins

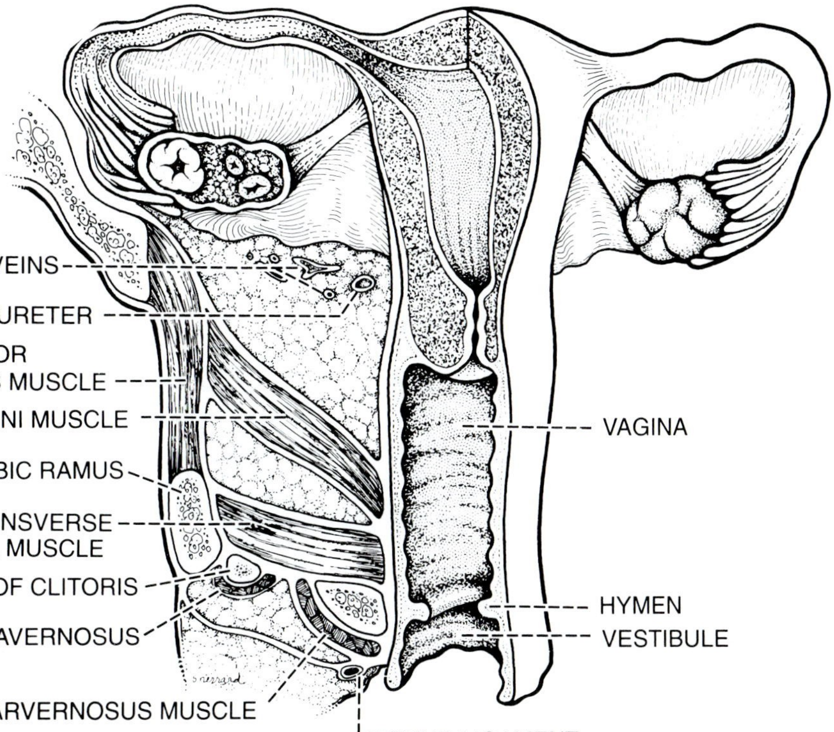

Fig. 4.2. Vagina, uterus, and supporting structures of the pelvis.

surrounds the vagina, forming a plexus with the uterine, pudendal, and rectal veins, which drain into the interior iliac vein.

The lymphatic drainage of the vagina is complex and variable. The lymphatics of the proximal anterior vagina and vaginal vault join those of the cervix and drain primarily into the external iliac lymph nodes. The posterior portion of the vagina drains into the inferior gluteal, sacral, and anorectal lymph nodes, whereas the distal part of the vagina, like the vulva, drains into the femoral lymph nodes. It is important to note that, as a consequence of extensive anastomotic channels, any pelvic, anorectal, or femoral node may be involved in the lymphatic drainage of any part of the vagina.

The innervation of the vagina is principally from the superior hypogastric plexus of the autonomic nervous system. This plexus bifurcates and is joined by branches of the second through fifth sacral nerves, forming the pelvic plexuses.

Histology and Physiology

The vaginal wall consists of three layers: mucosa, muscularis, and adventitia (Fig. 4.3). The vaginal mucosa is thrown into ill-defined laterally oriented folds or rugae of about 2–5 mm in thickness (Fig. 4.4). The thickness of the folds varies according to location and hormonal stimulation. The mucosal lining is a stratified squamous epithelium that is normally glycogenated and nonkeratinizing.[269] Subdivision of the epithelium into layers is somewhat arbitrary but useful as it provides a basis for understanding the variable appearance of squamous cells in vaginal cytologic smears (Fig. 4.5). The basal layer consists of a single layer of columnar cells, with the principal axis of the cells perpendicular to the basement membrane. The nuclei are oval and uniformly hyperchromatic and are surrounded by relatively scant cytoplasm, resulting in a high nuclear/cytoplasmic ratio. The parabasal layer usually consists of two to five layers of cells of cuboidal shape, with a centrally located, round, uniformly hyperchromatic nucleus. Mitoses usually are confined to the basal and parabasal layers. The intermediate layer is of variable thickness. The cells in this layer contain moderate quantities of slightly flattened cytoplasm and oval nuclei with finely dispersed chromatin. The long axis of both nucleus and cytoplasm is parallel to the basement membrane. The superficial layer also varies in thickness. The cells contain pyknotic nuclei, which are small, round, and hyperchromatic. The cytoplasm is abundant, with an orientation similar to intermediate cells. The three-dimensional configuration of these cells is that of a highly attenuated disk, resulting in a flattened appearance when viewed in cross section.

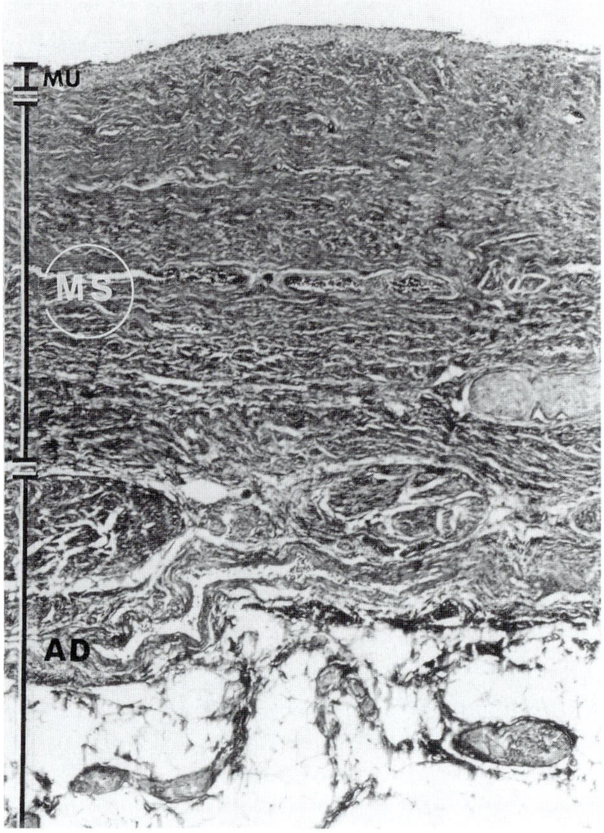

Fig. 4.3. Vaginal wall. Mucosa (*MU*), muscularis (*MS*), and adventitia (*AD*). The smooth muscle bundles are of variable thickness and ill defined. The adventitia contains numerous blood vessels and nerves within adipose tissue.

Variable quantities of glycogen may be present in the intermediate and superficial cell layers. The

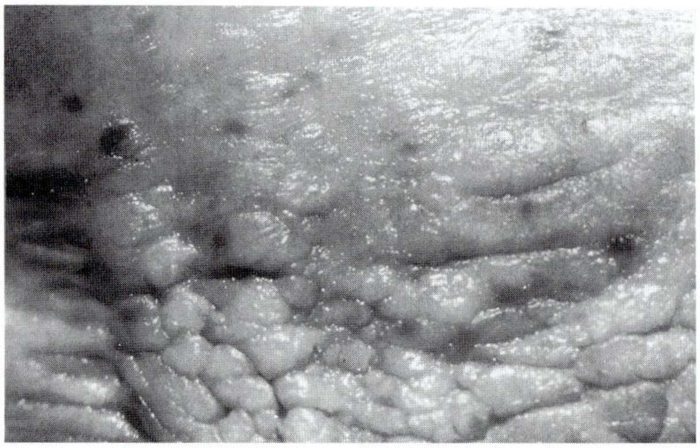

Fig. 4.4. Vaginal mucosa. The mucosa is composed of ill-defined, laterally oriented folds or rugae.

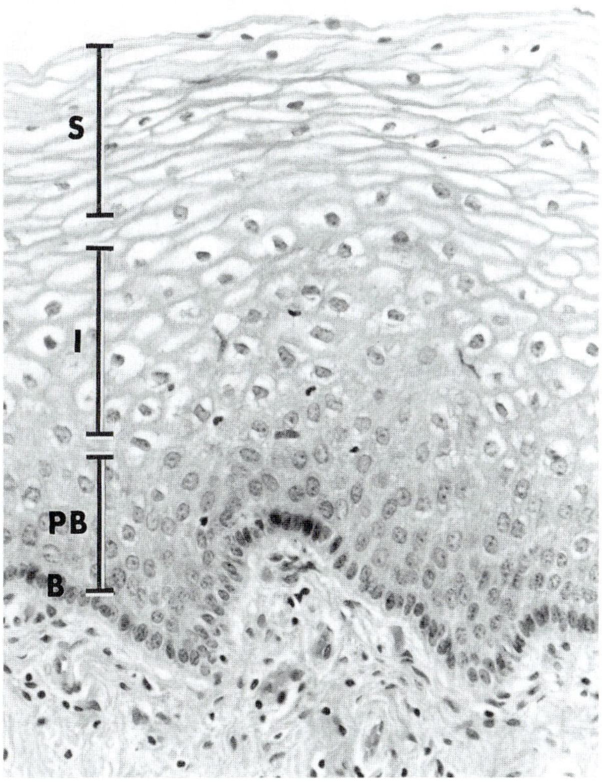

Fig. 4.5. Mature vaginal squamous epithelium. The epithelium is composed of a basal layer (*B*), several layers of parabasal cells (*PB*), and multiple layers of intermediate (*I*) and superficial (*S*) cells that progressively accumulate glycogen.

glycogen accumulates initially in a perinuclear location within intermediate cells, resulting in a clear zone around the nucleus. This appearance may cause confusion with the perinuclear clearing of koilocytes. However, the presence of nuclear membrane irregularity in koilocytes, and the characteristic location of these normal cells in the middle rather than superficial third of the epithelium, are helpful distinguishing features. Melanocytes have been identified as a normal constituent of the basal layer in about 3% of women.[214]

The lamina propria, which lies beneath the squamous epithelium, consists of a loose fibrovascular stroma containing elastic fibers and nerves. A band of stroma extends from the endocervix to the vulva, which contains atypical polygonal to stellate stromal cells with scant cytoplasm. Some of these cells are multinucleated or have multilobulated nuclei (Fig. 4.6 and 4.7).[68] The muscularis consists of poorly delineated, inner circular and outer longitudinal bundles of smooth muscle. Some of the outer longitudinal layers of muscle pass into the lateral pelvic wall to contribute to the inferior portion of the cardinal ligaments,[269] whereas fibers of the bulbocavernosus form a sphincter around the distal vagina. The adventitia is a thin coat of dense connective tissue that merges with the loose connective tissue of the surrounding pelvis, which contains the lymphatic and venous plexuses and nerve bundles.

The squamous cells of the vagina contain intranuclear steroid receptors and represent a target tissue for sex steroids. The thickness and maturation of the epithelium varies throughout the menstrual cycle. Because the vagina is rarely biopsied but frequently sampled cytologically, the latter procedure has contributed greatly to our knowledge of normal and aberrant maturation. During the proliferative phase, the epithelium progressively proliferates and matures fully in response to estrogens. The addition of progesterone during the secretory phase is associated with an arrest of maturation at the intermediate cell level and a decrease in epithelial

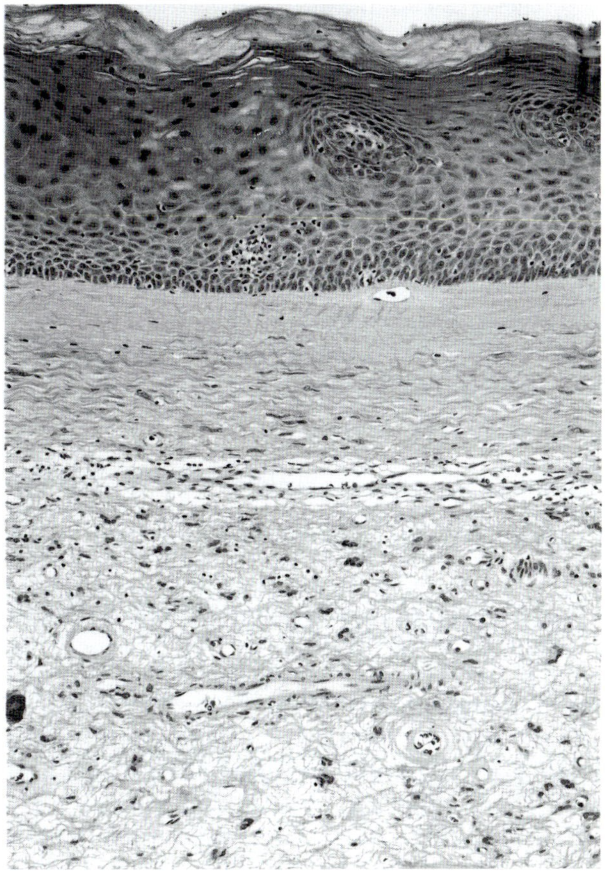

Fig. 4.6. Lamina propria of the vagina. Beneath the squamous epithelium of the vagina is a poorly defined zone containing large, stellate, or spindle stromal cells. This zone extends in irregular fashion from the cervix to the vulva.

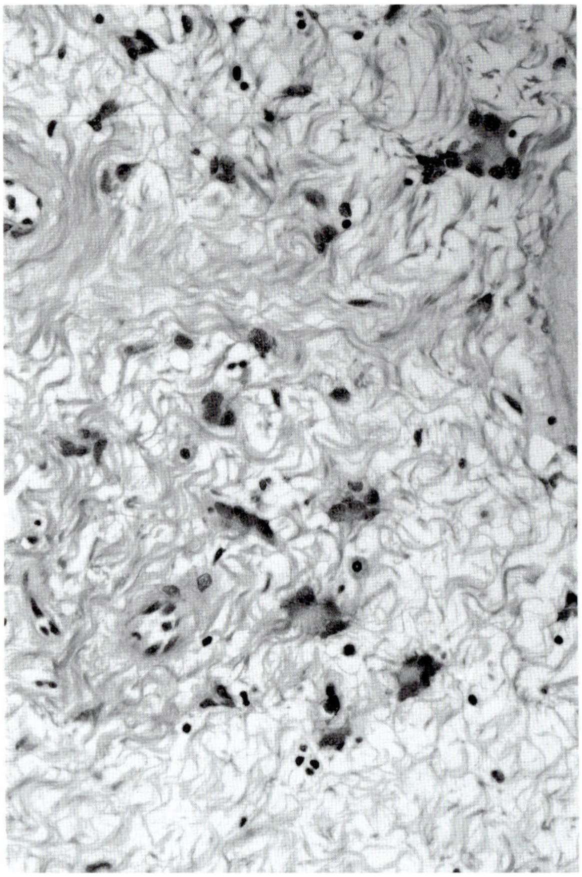

Fig. 4.7. Multinucleate stromal cells of the lamina propria. Scattered bizarre, floret-type multinucleate cells are often admixed with other stellate or spindle cells in the superficial portion of the lamina propria. These may be the source of bizarre cells identified in some vaginal fibroepithelial (mesodermal) stromal polyps.

thickness. Although glycogen is found in the intermediate and superficial cells throughout the menstrual cycle,[106] it is particularly abundant during pregnancy. Transient vaginal atrophy is found in some women postpartum, particularly those who are lactating.[355] After menopause, a gradual reduction in the thickness of the epithelium occurs, first with a loss of superficial cells followed by intermediate cells, such that the mucosa of late menopausal women may be reduced to only six to eight layers of parabasal cells (Fig. 4.8). As a consequence, a normal postmenopausal atrophic pattern may be confused with a high-grade intraepithelial lesion unless care is taken to identify other nuclear abnormalities. Newborn infants, having been exposed to maternal steroids in utero, have a fully mature-appearing epithelium that rapidly regresses to atrophy within about 4 weeks.[226] A gradual maturation of the epithelium follows the onset of menarche.[107] Exposure of the postmenopausal vagina to estrogen leads to squamous maturation comparable to that observed in the proliferative phase of reproductive-age women. It is interesting to note that, in one study, the time required for a vaginal squamous cell to make the transition from progenitor cell through desquamation was about 5 days for both cycling and postmenopausal women.[8]

There are few data concerning vaginal function during coitus or parturition.[195] Distension and lengthening of the proximal two-thirds of the vagina occurs during the early phases of sexual response, followed by constriction of the distal third. The anterior portion of the levator ani, the pubococcygeus muscle, appears to be involved in orgasmic function, but the mechanism is speculative.[102,195] Even the source of vaginal fluids that are present during arousal has been disputed. Glands are not normally present in the vagina, and candidate sources include secretions from sebaceous, sweat, Bartholin and Skene glands, or the endocervix. Fine droplets appear scattered throughout the rugal folds of the vaginal wall during arousal, followed by a rapid coalescence.[195] The fluid is believed to represent a transudate resulting from associated vasoconstriction within the venous plexus.[109,195,269] The fluid usually is acidic, with a pH around 4.6 but the pH rises during the sexual response.[109,143] This fluid contains a variety of enzymes, enzyme inhibitors, and immunoglobulins, which may play a role in liquefaction of coagulated semen and capacitation of spermatocytes or have antimicrobial activity.[109] The

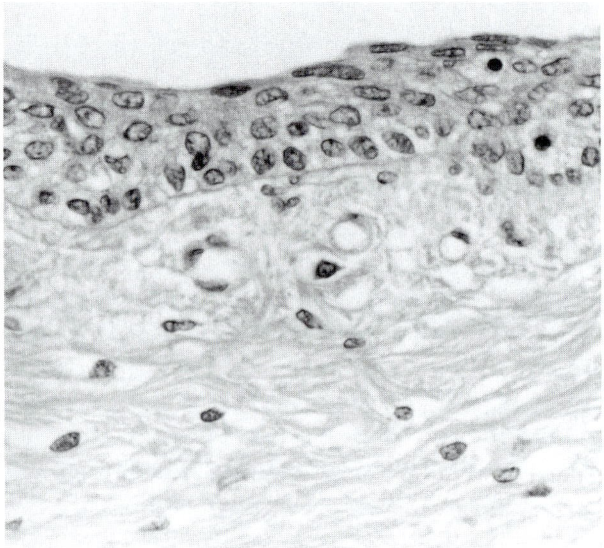

Fig. 4.8. Vaginal atrophy. The epithelium is reduced to only a few layers of parabasal and basal cells.

immunoglobulin A levels are highest during the late proliferative phase,[126] but the significance of this observation is unclear. During pregnancy and immediately postpartum, edema, vascular congestion, and loss of collagen have been noted in the lamina propria, which may serve to increase elasticity of vaginal tissues during delivery.[190]

Developmental Disorders

Lesions Related to In Utero Exposure to DES

Diethylstilbestrol, and the chemically related drugs hexestrol and dienestrol, are synthetic, nonsteroidal estrogens that were administered frequently to gravid women who were thought to be at high risk for early pregnancy loss during the 1940s through the 1960s. An estimated 5 to 10 million Americans received DES during pregnancy or were exposed to the drug in utero.[97] In 1971, the rare development of *clear cell adenocarcinoma of the vagina* in young women was linked to their exposure in utero to these drugs.[122] Subsequently, a number of nonneoplastic changes were identified in the genital tract of DES-exposed daughters, such as *adenosis, cervical ectropion,* various types of *cervicovaginal ridges,* and *structural abnormalities of the uterine corpus and fallopian tube.* DES was soon thereafter withdrawn from the market for use during pregnancy. Consequently, the population exposed in utero now averages about 45 years in age, with the youngest persons about 30 years old.

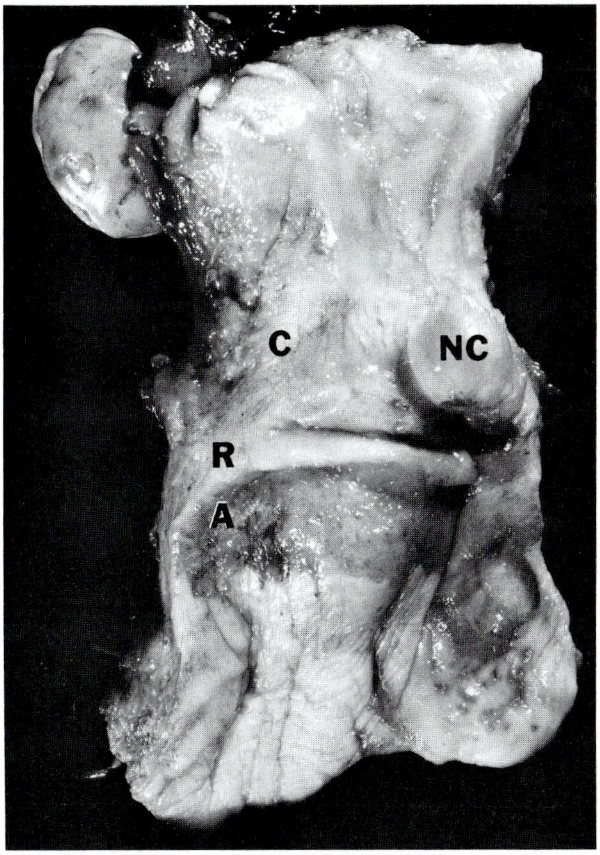

Fig. 4.9. Opened uterus and vagina from a woman exposed to DES in utero. Transverse vaginal ridge (*R*), cervix (*C*), and zone of adenosis (*A*) that macroscopically appears as a red granular patch. Nabothian cyst (*NC*) of cervix is also visible along right margin of specimen. (Reprinted by permission of Herbst et al., N Engl J Med 287:1259–1264, 1972.)

Gross Structural Changes of the Vagina and Cervix

Approximately one-fifth of DES-exposed women demonstrate *gross structural changes* in the cervix or vagina.[121] Descriptive designations have included coxcomb (hood), collar (rim), pseudopolyp, and ridge. The pseudopolyp is caused by a peripheral concentric cervical band that gives the portio vaginalis central to it the appearance of a protruding cervical polyp; however, the presence of the external os at its center differentiates it from a true polyp. The cervix may be hypoplastic, the vaginal fornices may be obliterated, or the vagina may be traversed by a ridge (septum) consisting of fibrous connective tissue covered by squamous epithelium (Fig. 4.9). The natural history of the structural abnormalities is not well understood, although some ridges have been observed to disappear as the cervix and vagina undergo remodeling with age.

Vaginal Epithelial Changes: Adenosis and Squamous Metaplasia

Vaginal adenosis and metaplastic squamous epithelium—vaginal epithelial changes (VECs)—are common in DES-exposed females. During the pre-DES era, vaginal adenosis was a clinical rarity, detected only occasionally in women, usually in their thirties or forties, who often complained of an excessive mucous discharge from the vagina. The demographics are again changing. During the past decade, adenosis caused by DES exposure has become increasingly uncommon. In contrast, multiple occurrences of acquired adenosis in adult women with vaginal dysplasia treated with topical 5-fluorouracil have been reported.[23,66,100] Glandular cells are also more commonly found in vaginal cytology specimens after hysterectomy for malignancy. The adenosis found in non-DES women is identical microscopically to that of young women who were so exposed in utero.[266] Clinically, adenosis should be suspected when the vaginal mucosa contains red granular spots or patches (Fig. 4.9) and does not stain with an iodine solution. On colposcopy, adenosis appears as glandular or metaplastic epithelium replacing the native squamous epithelium of the vaginal mucosa.

Adenosis, with or without squamous metaplasia, involves the upper third of the vagina in 34% of DES-exposed women. The anterior wall is involved most frequently and the posterior wall least frequently. These changes extend into the middle third of the vagina in 9% and the lower third in 2% of exposed women. In unexposed women, adenosis is rare,[341] although during late prenatal life glandular epithelium extends well onto the exocervix in up to a third of females.

Mucinous columnar cells, which by light and electron microscopy resemble those of the normal endocervical mucosa, comprise the glandular epithelium most frequently encountered as adenosis (62% of biopsy specimens with vaginal adenosis).[267] This epithelium, which most frequently lines the surface of the vagina, is the type of glandular epithelium most commonly seen by colposcopy (Fig. 4.10). Commonly, the mucinous columnar cells also line glands in the lamina propria (Fig. 4.11).

Dark cells and light cells, often ciliated and resembling the lining cells of the fallopian tube and endometrium, are found in 21% of specimens with adenosis (Fig. 4.12). These cells usually are found in glands in the lamina propria and not on the surface of the vagina. Although adenosis in the lower vagina is rare, the percentage of biopsy specimens with adenosis that exhibit tuboendometrial cells in comparison with mucinous cells increases markedly in frequency. Mucinous and tuboendometrial cells are found together only occasionally in biopsy material. Intestinal metaplasia has rarely been reported in adenosis.[200]

In most biopsy specimens, metaplastic squamous cells replace adenosis to some degree (Fig. 4.11), indicating the manner by which adenosis regresses. Squamous metaplasia, a reactive and physiologic process, begins as reserve cell proliferation, then progresses through immature and mature stages. The glandular epithelium gradually disappears, and intercellular pools of mucin and droplets remain as the final vestiges of adenosis. When completely replaced by squamous epithelium, obliterated glands appear in the lamina propria as squamous pegs that are continuous with the metaplastic squamous epithelium covering the surface. Eventual maturation of the

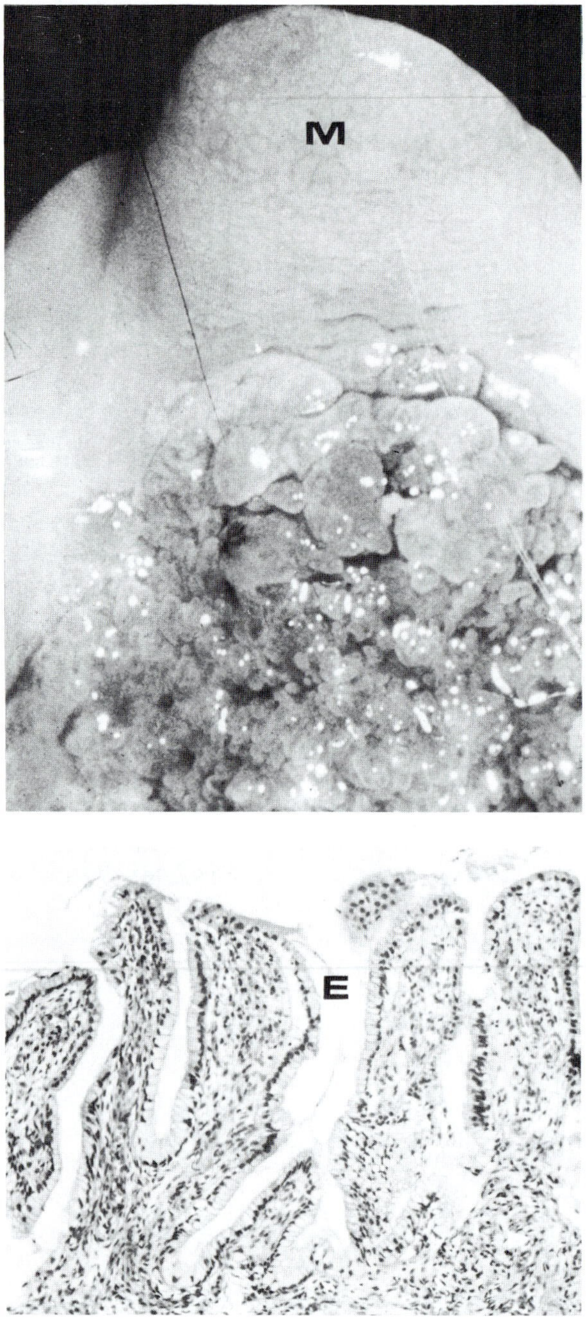

Fig. 4.10. Cervical ectropion. *Top*: Colpophotograph of anterior cervical cockscomb covered with metaplastic squamous epithelium in mosaic pattern (*M*). Grapelike structures along inner half of cervix are composed of fibrovascular cores covered by mucinous columnar epithelium (ectropion). *Bottom*: Photomicrograph of mucinous columnar cells (*E*) lining fibrovascular papillae. Same microscopical pattern in vagina is called *adenosis*.

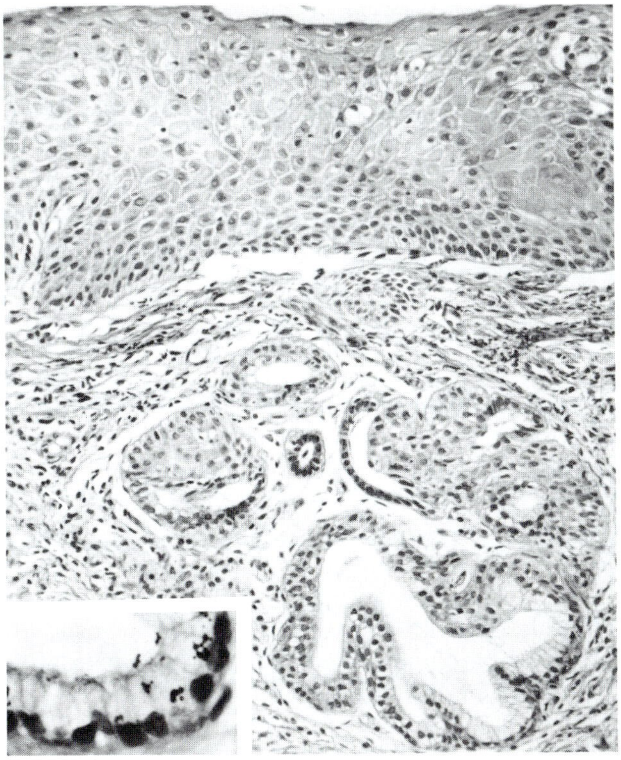

Fig. 4.11. Vaginal adenosis. Mucinous gland with focal squamous metaplasia in lamina propria. *Inset*: Detail of individual mucinous columnar cells.

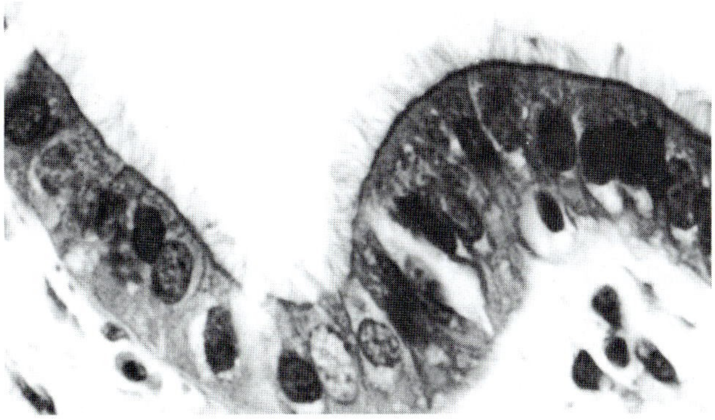

Fig. 4.12. Vaginal adenosis. Detail of ciliated dark (tuboendometrial) cells. Reprinted by permission of Dickersin et al., ref. 63.)

metaplastic squamous epithelium with acquisition of glycogen makes it indistinguishable from the normal (native) squamous epithelium.

Follow-up studies in which the same subjects have been examined repeatedly over a period of several years have indicated that adenosis, structural changes, and VECs may regress spontaneously.[7,219,270] After 3 years of follow-up, the hoods had disappeared in more than half the participants (Fig. 4.13). The extent of VEC did not increase with time. Because VECs disappear spontaneously, they should not be treated.

The Embryologic Basis of Vaginal Adenosis and Cervical Ectropion

The DES experience and the experimental studies it has fostered have provided new insights into the development of the normal lower genital tract and the effects caused by prenatal DES exposure.[264] In brief, the embryonic transitional squamous epithelium of

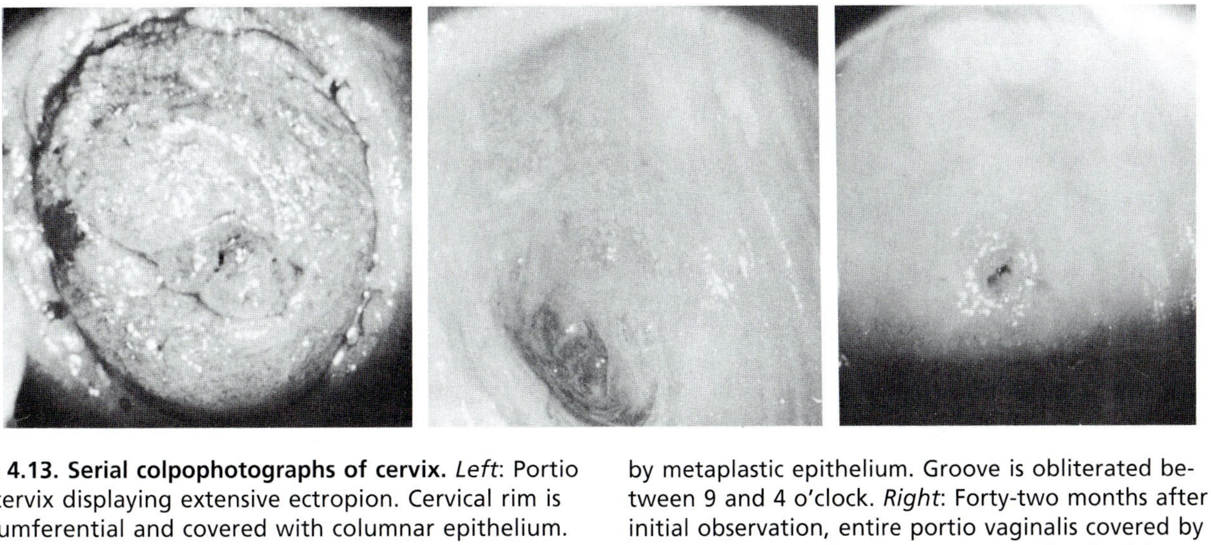

Fig. 4.13. Serial colpophotographs of cervix. *Left*: Portio of cervix displaying extensive ectropion. Cervical rim is circumferential and covered with columnar epithelium. Note prominent groove demarcating it from portio vaginalis. *Middle*: After 24 months, much of rim has disappeared and 70% of the ectropion has been replaced by metaplastic epithelium. Groove is obliterated between 9 and 4 o'clock. *Right*: Forty-two months after initial observation, entire portio vaginalis covered by metaplastic epithelium, with rim completely obliterated. (Reprinted by permission of Antonioli et al., ref. 7.)

the urogenital sinus is now believed to extend up the vagina and exocervix, replacing the original columnar (müllerian) epithelium lining these organs. Estrogen appears to affect the stroma, which then inhibits the upgrowth, and hence leads to the development of adenosis from persistent residual embryonic glandular epithelium. The stroma of the vaginal wall (like the uterine corpus and fallopian tube) induces the growth of a tuboendometrial-type epithelium. The stroma of the superficial endocervix favors mucinous columnar epithelium. In the DES-exposed woman, the embryonic müllerian epithelium that has not been replaced by sinus epithelium differentiates into predominantly mucinous epithelium in the upper vagina and predominantly tuboendometrial epithelium vagina and predominantly tuboendometrial epithelium in the lower vagina. In DES-exposed fetal organs, the stromal components of the uterine wall fail to segregate normally into an outer layer of smooth muscle and an inner layer of endometrial stroma.[271,315] The mechanism by which 5-fluoroucil induces glandular metaplasma in the vagina remains unclear.[23,66,100]

Imperforate Hymen

Imperforate hymen probably represents the most common significant congenital anomaly of the vagina. Its frequency is reported to be about 1 in 2000 female patients. The presence of a thick mucoid secretion that distends the vagina may provide a clue to diagnosis in the neonate, but often an imperforate hymen is not recognized until puberty, when there is retention of menstrual detritus. If it is not corrected promptly, infertility may result from endometriosis and pelvic adhesions associated with retrograde menstruation.[351]

Vaginal Agenesis

Complete vaginal agenesis is relatively rare, occurring in about 1 in 5000 female births.[65,86,334] As an isolated defect it results from incomplete caudal development and fusion of the lower part of the müllerian ducts (müllerian dysgenesis). The external genitalia usually appear normal, except for the introitus, where a short blind pouch may be present.[351] Therapy usually involves construction of an artificial vagina. Although this rarely results in a specimen for pathologic examination, the defect often is associated with the absence of the uterus and fallopian tubes (müllerian agenesis or Mayer–Rokitansky–Kuster–Hauser syndrome)[75] and with anomalies of the urinary tract.[223] The latter syndrome provides insight into embryologic development and demonstrates that an intact mesonephric duct is required for the growth and caudal lengthening of the müllerian duct during fetal life.[185,186] Because the gonads are not of müllerian origin, they usually are normal. About 25% of women with vaginal agenesis have a uterus, and they may have complications from retrograde menstruation.

Transverse Vaginal Septum

A *transverse vaginal septum* is uncommon, with an estimated prevalence of about 1 in 50,000 women,[245] and may occur anywhere within the vagina, but most frequently at the junction of the cranial and middle thirds.[333] It presumably results from incomplete migration or excavation of the vaginal plate. A complete vaginal septum results in obstructive symptoms similar to an imperforate hymen, whereas a partial septum may allow passage of menstrual flow but cause dyspareunia or laceration during childbirth. The microscopic appearance of the septum is typically that of a fibrovascular stroma covered on two surfaces by epithelium. Although the caudal surface is covered by a stratified nonkeratinizing squamous epithelium, the cranial aspect is covered typically by glandular epithelium, as might be predicted from the embryologic development.

Miscellaneous Congenital Disorders

Complete *duplication of the vagina* with a septum including muscularis extending to the introitus is rare, and typically is accompanied by cervical and uterine duplication.[12] Longitudinal septa that lack a muscular layer are more common; they often are clinically asymptomatic. Congenital rectovaginal fistulas often are associated with an imperforate anus. Typically, the anus opens into the posterior caudal portion of the vagina, near the fourchette.[333]

Infectious Inflammatory Disorders

The normal vaginal flora is varied and changes from birth through menarche to menopause. Although it has long been evident that lactobacilli split glycogen to form lactic acid, thus reducing the pH of the vagina, this does not provide a complete explanation for the regulation of the vaginal flora. The ecosystem reflects a delicate balance that includes the interplay of steroid hormones, vascularity, vaginal acidity, and glycogen. It can be upset easily by commonly occurring mechanical, chemical, or hormonal manipulation. Approximately 10^9 obligate anaerobic and 10^8 facultative bacteria are present in a gram of vaginal secretion, of which lactobacilli probably are the most common.[193] Three hundred and forty-five organisms were represented in 52 specimens collected from healthy adults, including the following anaerobes: *Peptococcus, Bacteroides, Peptostreptococcus, Lactobacillus, Eubacterium* spp.; and aerobes: *Stapylococcus epidermidis, Corynebacterium* spp., and *Lactobacillus* sp.[12] The proportion of aerobic organisms decreases about 100 fold during the week before menses. During pregnancy, more lactobacilli and yeast, but fewer anaerobic bacteria, are present.[180] On the third day after parturition, there is a dramatic increase in the number of anaerobic bacteria. Postmenopausal women also have a relatively larger proportion of anaerobes, with more lactobacilli recovered from those treated with estrogen.[172] Organisms that at times are associated with vaginitis may colonize the vagina of healthy, asymptomatic women.

Table 4.1. Sexually transmitted pathogens

Bacterial agents
Neisseria gonorrhoeae
Chlamydia trachomatis
Mycoplasma hominis
Ureaplasma urealyticum
Treponema pallidum
Gardnerella vaginalis
Haemophilus ducreyi
Shigella
Campylobacter
Group B streptococcus
Fungal agents
Candida albicans
Viral agents
Herpes simplex virus
Hepatitis B virus
Cytomegalovirus
Human papilloma virus
Molluscum contagiosum virus
Protozoan agents
Trichomonas vaginalis
Entamoeba histolytica
Ciardia lamblia
Ectoparasites
Pediculus pubis
Sarcoptes scabiei

Vaginitis

Vaginitis is the most common reason for a patient to visit her gynecologist, accounting for more than 10 million office visits each year.[158] Abnormal colonization or invasive infection has been reported for practically all major types of organisms, including viruses, bacteria, fungi, and parasites. It is difficult to determine the most common organism responsible for vaginitis because frequency lists vary according to age, sexual activity, and method of microbial identification.[81,286,299] Currently, more than 20 bacterial, viral, and protozoan agents are considered to be responsible for sexually transmitted diseases (STDs) (Table 4.1). Because notification that one has an STD frequently evokes a strong emotional response, it is important to remember that the distinction between sexually and nonsexually transmitted disease is at times arbitrary. Whereas many infectious agents make use of the opportunity afforded by close apposition of mucous membranes or secretions to spread, there is variability in the stringency of their demands.

The clinical diagnosis of vaginitis frequently is based on the presence of a vaginal discharge. Reliance on this finding alone may lead to overdiagnosis, as the production of vaginal fluid is a physiologic event caused by transudation of fluid through the vaginal wall, with additional contributions by cervical and uterine secretions, exfoliated epithelial cells, bacteria, and bacterial products. This event is particularly noticeable at midcycle when cervical mucus becomes watery and profuse and often is interpreted erroneously as a "discharge." Other relatively nonspecific criteria of vaginitis include subjective assessment of the color, odor, quantity, or quality of the discharge. In contrast to discharge caused by vaginitis, normal vaginal secretions are floccular rather than homogeneous, and neither malodorous nor associated with pruritis. Although accurate diagnosis of vaginitis does not require a biopsy, some infectious agents cause highly specific tissue reactions, with which the pathologist should be familiar.

Candida

Candida albicans probably is the most common potential or active pathogen in the female genital tract.[139] Between 1980 and 1990 the frequency has nearly doubled. *C. albicans* is found frequently in the colon of healthy individuals, and spread from the contaminated perineum probably is the usual method of introduction of the organism into the vagina.[129] Interestingly, fomites from bathtubs or toilet seats do not appear to be a common mechanism for transmission.[6] Sexual transmission plays a role in some patients, resulting from either penile–genital or oral–genital transmission.[31] About 4% of healthy, asymptomatic women harbor *Candida* in the vagina. Factors associated with an increased risk of developing symptomatic infection include pregnancy, oral contraceptive use, antibiotic therapy, diabetes mellitus, and tight-fitting clothes. A deficient cellular immune response has been identified in some women with chronic candidal vaginitis.[314] Changes in the vaginal flora likely play a role in the development of candidiasis.

Vulvar pruritis is the typical presenting symptom, often accompanied by a white, granular, vaginal discharge. The vagina appears reddened, and superficial erosion of the mucosa may be evident after removal of a pseudomembrane of adherent granular debris.

Saline or potassium hydroxide suspensions of a discharge containing blastospores and pseudohyphae permit a presumptive microscopic diagnosis to be made immediately. Unfortunately, the sensitivity of the wet prep exam is only about 65%,[201] and the

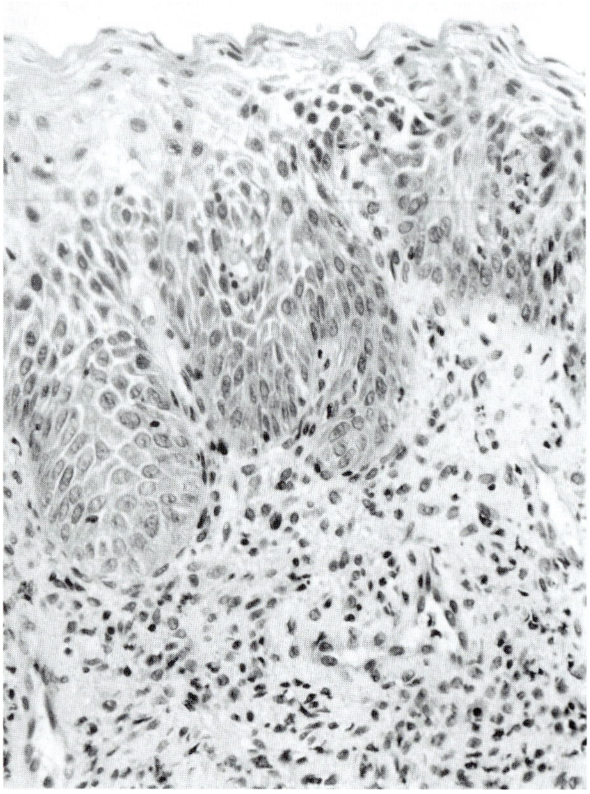

Fig. 4.14. Vaginitis caused by *Candida or Trichomonas*. The histologic changes, including variably dense infiltrates of mononuclear inflammatory cells in the stroma and neutrophils in the epithelium, are similar for both organisms.

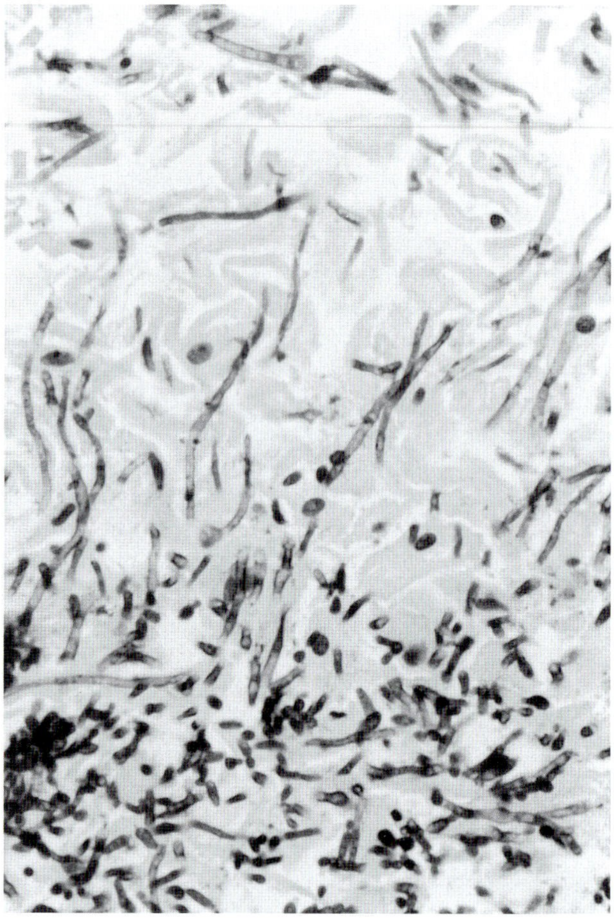

Fig. 4.15. Candidal vaginitis. Yeast and pseudohyphae are present in a mat of exfoliated superficial squamous cells. *Candida* usually are not identified in biopsies of the vagina unless desquamated cells remain aherent to the intact mucosal surface [periodic acid–Schiff (PAS) stain].

morphologic appearance is not entirely specific. In one study, Papanicolaou-stained smears demonstrated the organism in 46% of infected patients, compared with 85% for the wet prep and 94% for culture.[199] In daily practice, it is the experience of the examiner that seems to be the most critical determinant for accurate recognition of the organism. Definitive identification of the fungus is made by culture.

Biopsies, which are rarely obtained, contain relatively dense infiltrates of primarily mononuclear inflammatory cells and congested blood vessels in the stroma, with exocytosis of neutrophils into the overlying epithelium (Fig. 4.14).[152] *Candida* generally are not identifiable unless the discharge remains adherent, where the organisms are visualized as yeast and pseudohyphae intertwined among the desquamated squamous cells (Fig. 4.15).[17] First-line therapy of topical imidazole derivatives, sometimes coupled with initial topical application of gentian violet, has been used for the past 20 years.[81] The recent introduction of triazols permits equally effective therapy of shorter duration.[301] However, recurrence remains common and may result from either failure to respond to medical therapy or endogenous reinfection by the identical strain of organism.[338]

Candidal species other than *C. albicans* are responsible for at least one-third of cases of fungal vaginitis,[137,156] and infection with *C. tropicalis* or *C. glabrata* is associated with a high rate of recurrence.[137] *C. glabrata* typically produces milder symptoms than *C. albicans*,[20] but *C. glabrata* has been reported to cause a severe ulcerative vaginitis simulating malignancy.[39] The microscopic appearances of most *Candida* species are similar, but *C. glabrata* produces only yeasts (blastospores), which are slightly smaller than those of *C. albicans*.[20]

Bacterial Vaginosis

Organisms such as *Trichomonas* and *Candida* have long been known to produce vaginitis; however, until recently there have been a substantial number of women who have a copious vaginal discharge or pruritis in the absence of a readily identifiable pathogen. In the past, this condition was designated nonspecific vaginitis, but the term *bacterial vaginosis* currently is preferred because evidence of inflammation is typically absent.[193] *Gardnerella*, a gram-negative bacillus, has been isolated from women with vaginosis at a higher rate than asymptomatic women and thus was considered to be responsible for nonspecific vaginitis.[91] However, more recent studies cast doubt on this concept, because this organism and "clue" cells have been identified at times with similar frequency in healthy women without vaginal discharge.[304] Currently, it is believed that bacterial vaginosis is not an infection by a single organism, but rather an overgrowth of multiple colonizing bacteria including *Gardnerella* and a variety of anaerobes.[240,324,342] The flora typically found in affected women includes not only disproportionately large numbers of *Gardnerella vaginalis*, but also abundant *Prevotella bivia, Mycoplasma hominis, Mobiluncus mulieris*, and *Mobiluncus curtisii*.[325] In an animal model, the inoculation of *Gardnerella* and *Mobiluncus* together caused the clinical disease, although neither alone was capable of doing so.[194] The diagnosis of bacterial vaginosis is made if three of the following four criteria are present: (1) homogeneous, thin, malodorous discharge, (2) vaginal pH >4.5, (3) vaginal epithelial cells with numerous attached bacteria ("clue" cells), and (4) fishy odor on alkalinization of vaginal secretions.[4,57,287] The diagnosis usually is confirmed by elimination of other pathogens, combined with identification of gram-negative to gram-variable bacilli and "clue" cells on wet mount or smears, or by culture.[322] The identification of squamous cells coated by large numbers of coccobacilli in a cervical vaginal cytology specimen represents a moderately sensitive and highly specific method for screening for bacterial vaginosis.[57,96] No specific histopathologic features have been described.

Efforts to restore the local environment by topical administration of acetic acid, estrogen, or fermented milk products have been ineffective. In contrast, antimicrobial therapy with metronidazole or intravaginal clindamycin produces clinical cure in most women, further supporting the concept that anaerobes acting with *Gardnerella* produce bacterial vaginosis.[304] The initiating cause remains unknown, but sexual transmission occurs in many instances.[173,215] Although bacterial vaginosis was previously thought to carry no appreciable morbidity, it recently has been associated with a 3- to 15-fold increased risk of upper genital tract infection, including salpingitis and endometritis.[128,162,228,311] In addition, the anaerobic bacteria cultured from the endometrium and fallopian tubes of women with asymptomatic endometritis or symptomatic salpingitis were those associated with bacterial vaginosis.[162,302] During pregnancy, bacterial vaginosis significantly increases the likelihood of premature onset of labor and chorioamnionitis.[133,197,212,302]

Trichomonas Vaginalis

Trichomoniasis is responsible for more than 2.5 million infections per year in the United States and about 180 million infections worldwide.[323] It is found in about 10% of asymptomatic women, and almost 50% of those attending STD clinics.[310] The organism is almost always sexually transmitted,[363] although trichomonads reportedly may survive in tap water, soap water, and chlorinated swimming pools.[81] The mechanism by which *Trichomonas* causes disease is unknown, but the organisms are found both in the vaginal lumen and adherent to squamous, but not columnar, epithelial cells.[260] Invasion of the squamous mucosa does not occur. *Trichomonas* is a strict anaerobe and there frequently is an alteration in the associated vaginal flora, with increased anaerobic bacteria.[337] Although the role of sex steroids is unclear, infection is generally lower in women taking oral contraceptives.[25]

Symptoms of infection include vaginal discharge, intense pruritis, and dyspareunia, with exacerbations often temporally related to menses. However, in one study, only 17% of culture-positive women noted pruritis, and more than one-third did not even complain of a vaginal discharge.[198] When present, the vaginal discharge usually is copious, homogeneous, yellow green to gray, and malodorous. Typically, the vaginal mucosa is erythematous and punctate hemorrhages may be present, particularly on the cervical mucosa, leading to what is unfortunately described as a "strawberry cervix."

The diagnosis usually is made by the microscopic identification of motile organisms accompanied by many neutrophils in a saline preparation. The protozoan is ovoid, about 10–20 μm in diameter, with polar flagella. Active motility, in the form of a jerky swaying motion, is provided by the flagella and undulating membrane. If the wet prep diagnosis is based on the presence of motile organisms, the specificity approaches 100%. Trichomonads also may be found in Papanicolaou-stained vaginal smears in about 70% of cases, a sensitivity similar to that of the wet prep.[183] Several recently introduced molecular amplification methods appear to provide both high sensitivity and specificity when applied to distal vaginal secretions.[61,115,189,356] Culture methods are available, expensive, and generally unnecessary. The organism is not detectable in biopsy specimens from culture-positive women, although an inflammatory response of variable intensity may be seen, including dilated vessels in the stroma, accompanied by dense infiltrates of plasma cells and lymphocytes (see Fig. 4.14). The ectocervical as well as vagina mucosa is commonly spongiotic (Fig. 4.15).[160] Neutrophils frequently are present in large numbers among the squamous cells, sometimes forming intraepithelial abscesses. There may be irregular acanthosis of the epithelium, with pseudoepitheliomatous hyperplasia. A fibrinopurulent exudate composed of necrotic debris, neutrophils, and lymphocytes is found in foci of ulceration. Metronidazole provides effective therapy, although recurrence is common if the typically asymptomatic male partner is not also treated. Unfortunately, the frequency of resistance to metronidazole is increasing.[327]

Acquired Immunodeficiency Syndrome

Currently, acquired immunodeficiency virus syndrome (AIDS) is the fourth leading cause of death among American women 25–44 years of age (Fig. 4.16). Between 1981 and 1994, more than 440,000 cases of AIDS were reported in the United States, about 15% of which occurred in females.[36] Although

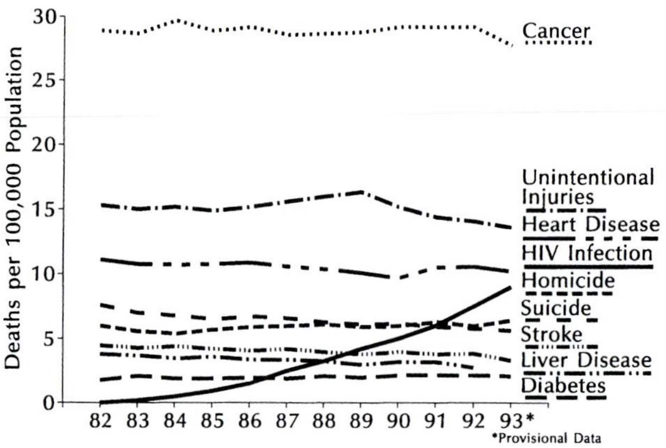

Fig. 4.16. Leading causes of death among women 25–44 years of age in the United States from 1981 through 1992. Data from National Center for Health Statistics. (From Chu SY, Curran J. Epidemiology of HIV in the United States. In DeVita VT Jr, Hellman S, Rosenberg SA (eds) AIDS: Etiology, diagnosis, treatment, and prevention. Lippincott-Raven, Philadelphia, 1997.)

there are no gross or histopathologic changes of AIDS specific to the vagina, the pathologist should be aware that more than one-third of adult women with AIDS have acquired the infection through heterosexual transmission.[37] Worldwide, more than 90% of human immunodeficiency virus (HIV) infection is caused by heterosexual contact, and it is the third most common mode of (HIV) transmission in the United States.[340] In 1994, 62% of the heterosexual AIDS cases in the United States were among women.

Most HIV infections resulting from heterosexual contact have occurred in women who reported only vaginal intercourse.[233] The virus has been identified in both semen and cell-free seminal fluid.[178] Certain sexually transmitted diseases are considered to be risk factors for sexual transmission of HIV, particularly those that cause ulceration of the vaginal mucosa, facilitating HIV exposure to vascular channels, as well as providing a large number of CD4+ lymphocytes and macrophages that contain or could bind HIV at the site of injury.[42] It is estimated that a 5-fold to 10-fold increase in risk of heterosexual transmission of HIV is present in those with genital ulcers.[340] A 2-fold to 5-fold increase in risk is associated with the presence of an inflammatory or exudative STD, presumably reflecting the presence of microscopic ulcerations or increased concentrations of CD4+ lymphocytes in the discharge.[176,340] Recently, localization of simian immunodeficiency virus (SIV) in dendritic cells of the monkey vagina has been demonstrated in an experimental model, suggesting that heterosexual transmission of HIV may occur across an intact mucosa.[203] Nevertheless, the precise mechanism by which heterosexual transmission of HIV occurs remains to be defined.

Group B Streptococcus

Group B streptococci (*Streptococcus agalactiae*) can be found in 5–35% of normal females[135,362] and thus are considered to be part of the normal vaginal flora. These bacteria frequently are sexually transmitted,[126] although they also can ascend from the lower intestinal tract, which may serve as a reservoir.[211] Although group B streptococcal colonization of the vagina or urethra usually causes little morbidity to the adult female, a vaginitis at times may occur.[126] Histopathologic changes resulting from vaginal infection by group B streptococci have not been well described. More significantly, this organism is a frequent cause of abortion, chorioamnionitis, premature rupture of membranes, perinatal death, and intrapartum and postpartum bacteremia.[258,312] For reasons that currently are unknown, only a small proportion of colonized mothers or infants develop symptomatic infection.[312]

Actinomycetes

Actinomycetes have been implicated in upper genital tract infections in women wearing intrauterine contraceptive devices but also are found in the vagina of about one-quarter of women without such devices. These organisms represent part of the normal oral and colonic flora, from which it may be introduced into the vagina. Vaginitis subsequently occurs when overgrowth is favored by the presence of a foreign body.[54] Actinomycetes are recognized in Papanicolaou-stained smears and tissue sections as a dense mass of fine, blue, filamentous bacteria, usually radiating from a central core.

Malacoplakia and Xanthogranulomatous Pseudotumor

Malacoplakia and *xanthogranulomatous pseudotumor* of the vagina are closely related entities resulting from infection by gram-negative bacilli, usually *Escherichia coli*.[179,306] Typically, yellow polypoid nodules arise from the vaginal mucosa, at times accompanied by a discharge. The microscopic findings are identical to those described in other body sites, and include the presence of large collections of histiocytes with abundant granular to pale foamy cytoplasm (von Hansemann cells), with interspersed plasma cells and lymphocytes. Both intracellular and extracellular, concentrically laminated basophilic masses (Michaelis–Gutmann bodies) are present in variable numbers. The clinical suspicion of tumor may lead the pathologist to the misdiagnosis of a rare neoplasm such as a granular cell tumor, unless care is taken to consider this lesion. The correct diagnosis may be confirmed by the finding of numerous gram-negative rodlike bacteria on tissue Gram stain, on silver stain, or by electron microscopy.

Tuberculosis

Genital tract tuberculosis is no longer frequent in the United States but remains a significant problem in Third World nations. The vagina is involved in about only 1% of these women, and patients present with localized ulceration.[216] Characteristic microscopic features include necrotizing granulomata containing Langhans giant cells underlying an ulcerated epithelium.[43]

Emphysematous Vaginitis

Emphysematous vaginitis is a rare entity (about 200 reported cases), characterized by multiple, discrete, gas-filled cystic cavities in the vaginal mucosa. Most patients present with symptoms of vaginal discharge, although some are aware of popping sounds associated with the rupture of the cysts during intercourse. The dramatic presentation and physical findings have prompted an interest disproportionate to the frequency or significance of the disease. There is evidence that it is an unusual manifestation or a common infection in an immunocompromised host.[148,326] No single organism has been identified as the causative agent, although both *Trichomonas vaginalis* and *Gardnerella vaginalis* have been implicated.[92] Chemical analyses of the lesions have disclosed a wide variety of gases, including ammonia, hydrogen sulfide, nitrogen, oxygen, carbonic acid, and trimethylamine. The microscopic findings are variable, with cysts in the stroma lined by either multinucleated giant cells, squamous cells, or both (Fig. 4.17). A scattering of chronic inflammatory cells accompanies the cysts.[92,164] Bacterial or protozoan production of gas with transmucosal passage into the stroma has been suggested, but the pathogenesis remains obscure.[92]

Unusual Types of Bacterial Vaginitis

Occasionally, vaginitis may be caused by bacteria that are commonly pathogenic in other sites. *Shigella vulvogaginitis* has been identified primarily as a cause of a chronic, sanguinous, purulent vagi-

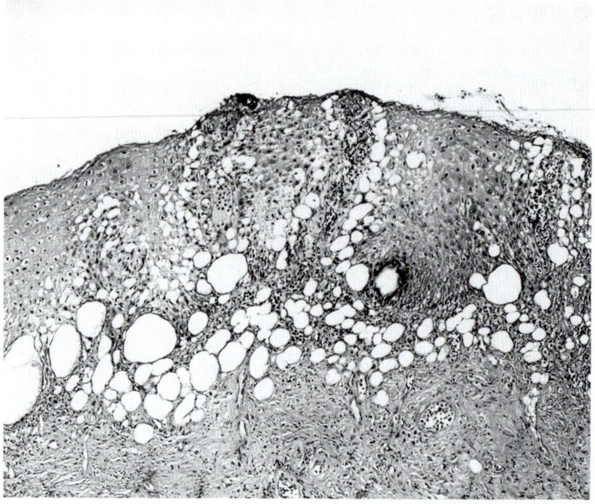

Fig. 4.17. Emphysematous vaginitis. Multiple small cysts without evident lining cells are present in both the superficial stroma and squamous epithelium; these are accompanied by a moderately dense infiltrate of chronic inflammatory cells.

nal discharge in children, unassociated with intestinal infection.[55,256] *Haemophilus influenzae, Corynebacterium diphtheria*, and *Neisseria meningitidis* also rarely cause vaginitis in children,[32,70,71,309] but the histologic changes have not been documented. Staphylococcal infection of the vagina after systemic antibiotic therapy was reported more than 30 years ago and thought to result from a disturbed indigenous flora[171] (see the section on Toxic Shock Syndrome).

Parasitic Vaginitis

Parasitic infection of the vagina, although currently rare in the United States, almost certainly will be encountered more frequently because of more frequent global travel.

Vaginal amebiasis caused by *Entamoeba histolytica* has been reported in Mexico, South Africa, and India, where the infection is endemic.[116,131,207,335] Most patients present with a bloody vaginal discharge. The gross appearance mimics carcinoma, with one or more ulcerated, necrotic growths typically involving the vagina and cervix. Microscopically, the lesions are characterized by ulceration of the epithelium with replacement by a fibrinopurulent exudate containing trophozoites 15–60 μm in diameter. In cytologic preparations they appear somewhat larger than histiocytes, and approximate the size of parabasal cells. Positive staining with periodic acid–Schiff (PAS) stain or acid phosphatase provides further support for the diagnosis.

Eggs of *Enterobius vermicularis* or *Trichuris trichiura* usually are found after incidental contamination of the vagina associated with intestinal infestation by these worms.[206] Eggs and worms of *Schistosoma mansoni* and hematobium have been identified in pelvic tissues including the vagina, presumably reflecting anastomoses between hemorrhoidal and hypogastric veins.[95] They elicit a striking host inflammatory response, ultimately resulting in dense fibrosis.

Toxic Shock Syndrome

General Features

In 1978, Todd et al. described an acute, potentially life-threatening disease characterized by fever, hypotension, headache, confusion, rash, vomiting, diarrhea, and oliguria. The disease was termed *toxic shock syndrome* (TSS) because it was associated with infection with strains of *Staphylococcus* that produced a unique epidermal toxin.[328] By 1980, more than 98% of cases had been related to the use of tampons during menses.[78] The incidence is about 6 cases per 100,000 menstruating women per year. Although *S. aureus* rarely inhabits the vagina normally, it has been isolated from about 75% of women with TSS.[56,197a] More recently it has become evident that children or adults with any focal staphylococcal infection are also at risk for TSS, and about 11% of all reported cases are nonmenstrual.[261]

Pathogenesis

There is a strong relationship between localized infection with *S. aureus* and the development of TSS. Studies of patients with TSS as well as experimental systems have revealed that some staphylococci elaborate a protein of about 22 kDa termed *toxic shock syndrome toxin 1* (or staphylococcal enterotoxin F), which produces essentially all the systemic biologic effects.[18] However, TSS can occur in the absence of this toxin, and other staphylococcal entertotoxins, streptococcal exotoxins, and endotoxins from gram-negative bacteria have been implicated in some cases of TSS.[114,147,261,336] The mechanism by which tampon use during menses predisposes to TSS remains somewhat unclear, but it is believed that microulcerations of the vaginal mucosa caused by tampons (see below, Tampon Ulcer) permit the growth of toxin-producing staphylococci. A diminished host immune response to the toxin, access of toxin through a denuded endometrial mucosa, and the normal menstrual phase decrease in lactobacilli that are inhibitory to the growth of staphylococci may factilitate the process.[78,282] A multifactorial sequence is supported by the observation that some women harbor toxin-producing strains in the vagina without symptoms, whereas other women have recurrent episodes of the illness. A dramatic reduction in the incidence of TTS occurred when Rely superabsorbent tampons were withdrawn from the market in 1980.[166]

Clinical Features

The diagnosis of TSS is based on a constellation of clinical features, as follows: fever, hypotension, palmar or diffuse erythroderma followed by desquamation, hyperemia of conjunctivae or mucous membranes of vagina or pharynx, and multisystem dysfunction: vomiting, diarrhea, impaired renal, cerebral, or hepatic function, cardiopulmonary dysfunction, thrombocytopenia, elevated creatine phosphokinase, and decreased serum calcium and phosphate.[56] Vaginal erythema, erosions, or vaginitis, sometimes accompanied by a purulent exudate, typically are present.[343] Abdominal or bilateral adnexal tenderness is present in about half of cases.[117]

Gross and Microscopic Findings

The disease is systemic, with pathologic abnormalities described in lung, liver, and kidney, as well as genital tract.[1,227] Ulceration and discoloration of the vaginal and cervical mucosa are present focally. Microscopically, there is extensive desquamation of the epithelium, with underlying subacute vasculitis, perivascular inflammatory cell infiltrates, and platelet thrombi.[1,227] Rare gram-positive cocci have been found in the fibrinopurulent exudate associated with ulcers. Deep tissue invasion by the organisms has not been described.[227]

Clinical Behavior and Treatment

The spectrum of severity of TSS varies from a relatively mild to a rapidly fatal illness, with a mortality rate of about 4%.[313] The treatment includes beta-lactamase-resistant antistaphylococcal antibiotics, and aggressive, supportive measures for systemic manifestations related to shock.[261] Intravenous immunoglobulin therapy also has been effective, supporting the concept that the symptoms of TSS result from a toxin that may be neutralized by infused antibodies.[11]

Noninfectious Inflammatory Diseases

The vagina occasionally is the site of involvement by a systemic disease, a generalized disease of squamous mucosa, or by extension from a disease elsewhere in the pelvis.

Desquamative Inflammatory Vaginitis

Desquamative inflammatory vaginitis is the term that has been applied to an unusual process in which bright red, well-delineated areas replace portions of the normal mucosa of the cranial half of the vagina. A pseudomembrane at times replaces the ulcerated mucosa.[153,196] A copious, purulent to hemorrhagic vaginal discharge is present, smears of which display numerous neutrophils and a high proportion of parabasal cells. The women usually are premenopausal and have normal serum estrogen levels. The etiology is unknown, and no single bacterial or viral agent has been identified. Nevertheless, the replacement of long gram-positive bacilli by gram-positive cocci in the vaginal discharge of most affected women suggests an infectious etiology. This hypothesis is reinforced by the observation that intravaginal treatment with clindamycin has resulted in clinical improvement in more than 95% of patients.[300]

Ligneous Vaginitis

Ligneous conjunctivitis is a rare, chronic inflammatory condition of unknown pathogenesis that usually involves the conjunctivae beginning in childhood. In the acute phase there frequently is an associated nasopharyngitis or vulvovaginitis. The chronic phase is characterized by asymptomatic sessile or pedunculated yellow-white to red firm masses on the conjunctiva. Histologically, these represent subepithelial accumulations of eosinophilic material, which may be accompanied by granulation tissue or chronic inflammatory cell infiltrates. Electron microscopic examination reveals electron-dense homogeneous and fibrillary material. Histologically identical lesions have been reported to coexist in the vagina and cervix.[124]

Allergic Reactions to Seminal Fluid

A few women display *allergic reactions* after exposure to seminal fluid.[175] The severity of the response varies from localized vulvovaginal urticarial reactions to generalized urticaria and bronchospasm. The onset of symptoms immediately follows contact with seminal fluid, and the duration of the reaction is between 2 and 72 hours.

Crohn Disease

Rectovaginal fistulas occur in some patients with *Crohn disease*,[72] and in situ squamous carcinoma has been reported in the vaginal and perineal mucosa of a 36-year-old woman with Crohn disease involving the vagina.[250] Vaginal fistulae with the sigmoid colon or cecum after perforation of a diverticulum have been identified in about 1% of women with diverticulosis.[9]

Bullous Dermatoses

Vaginal stenosis may develop as a sequela of severe *bullous erythema multiforme* (Stevens–Johnson syndrome) in which extensive vulvar and vaginal ulceration occurred.[103] Acantholytic intraepithelial bullae may be found when there is vaginal involvement by familial benign chronic pemphigus (Hailey–Hailey disease).[332]

Giant Cell Arteritis

Giant cell arteritis is not always limited to the temporal arteries, and may be associated with either generalized or limited visceral involvement. A panarteritis, with fragmentation and destruction of the internal elastic lamella, and phagocytosis of elastic material by multinucleated giant cells may be seen in the vagina as part of limited female genital tract involvement.[15,285]

Thrombotic Thrombocytopenic Purpura

Massive, acute hemorrhagic necrosis of the vagina has been reported as one of the initial manifestations of *thrombotic thrombocytopenic purpura*.[89] The disease usually is characterized by the pentad of fever, microangiopathic hemolytic anemia, thrombocytopenia, neurologic symptoms, and renal dysfunction. Numerous thrombi are found microscopically in the vaginal stroma, accompanied by superficial hemorrhage and necrosis and sloughing of the epithelium.

Lesions That Follow Trauma, Surgery, and Radiation

Atrophic Vaginitis

Atrophy of the squamous epithelium of the vagina, accompanied by loss of glycogen and an increase in the pH, are physiologic events in postmenopausal women that reflect estrogen deprivation. The response also includes a change in the vaginal flora, with a reduction in the lactobacilli that ordinarily inhibit other potential pathogens. The thin epithelium seems to offer little resistance to an altered flora, which may include streptococci, staphylococci, *E. coli*, and diphtheroids.[14] As a result, minor trauma may facilitate a transition from simple atrophy to atrophic vaginitis. Many patients are asymptomatic, but there may be minor vaginal bleeding, pruritis, dysuria, or dyspareunia, accompanied at times by a watery discharge. Atrophy of the vagina produces a pale-appearing mucosa, with petechiae and loss of rugal folds. Microscopically, there is a variable reduction or loss of the superficial and intermediate cell layers. Small ulcers with acute inflammation and granulation tissue may be interspersed among regions of intact epithelium. Elsewhere, the submucosa is infiltrated by lymphocytes and plasma cells (Fig. 4.18).[153] Although the histologic changes are relatively straightforward, occasionally there is confusion of atrophy with a high-grade squamous intraepithelial lesion (see below, Vaginal Intraepithelial Neoplasia). There usually is a good response to estrogen replacement, with epithelial cell maturation and a return to premenopausal flora and pH. Antibiotic therapy rarely is necessary.

Tampon Ulcer

Although tampons have been in use for 60 years, there had been little interest in their effects on the vagina until about 1980, when *mucosal ulceration* and TSS were related to their use. In several series of cases, the women presented with abnormal vagi-

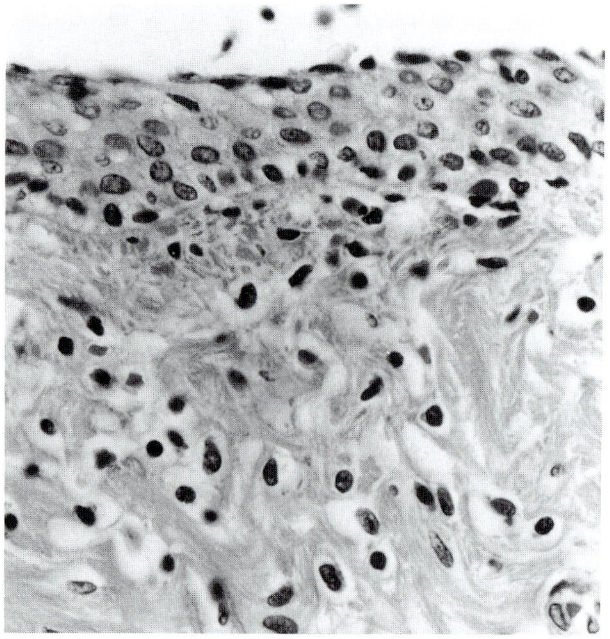

Fig. 4.18. Atrophic vaginitis. In addition to profound atrophy of the epithelium, there is dense infiltration of the stroma by chronic inflammatory cells.

nal discharge or intermenstrual bleeding. Typically, a single ulcer with an irregular border of granulation tissue was identified in one of the vaginal fornices. After neoplasms and infectious etiologies were excluded, a more detailed history revealed the frequent use of tampons. Microscopically, some of the ulcers contained fibrillar foreign bodies within the exudate.[144] The lesions healed spontaneously within 2–3 months after discontinuation of tampon usage.[144] Subsequently, Friedrich studied the vagina during tampon use, and characterized a sequence of clinically asymptomatic, colposcopic, and microscopic changes as follows: (1) mucosal dehydration, (2) layering or intraepithelial cleavage, and (3) microulceration.[80,82] Ultrastructural findings include a widening of the intercellular spaces separating squamous cells and a marked reduction in the number of desmosomes. He suggested that these changes resulted from a fluid shift across the vaginal epithelium due to the absorbent qualities of the tampon. This hypothesis explains the higher frequency of mucosal alteration with the use of superabsorbent tampons. However, this explanation may be incomplete because a recent colposcopic study demonstrated an inverse relationship between vaginal drying and the quantity of blood absorbed by different tampon types.[287] The great frequency with which tampons induce clinically inapparent vaginal microulcerations helps to explain their relationship to superficial staphylococcal infections and the development of TSS.

Postoperative Spindle Cell Nodule

In 1984, Proppe et al. described a lesion of the lower genitourinary tract that closely simulated a sarcoma histologically but was benign.[251] The term *postoperative spindle cell nodule* was applied to the lesion because typically it arose within 1–3 months of surgery in the region, and usually presented as polypoid, poorly defined nodules. The microscopic appearance is characterized by intersecting fascicles of plump spindle cells with a delicate network of small blood vessels, sometimes accompanied by extravasated blood or hemosiderin (Fig. 4.19). Superficial ulceration may be present, and chronic inflammatory cells are scattered in the deeper portions of the lesions. The spindle cells have oval, elongated nuclei with evenly dispersed chromatin and abundant eosinophilic cytoplasm. Because mitotic figures are numerous and the lesions are poorly circumscribed, they may easily be confused with sarcoma (Fig. 4.20). Helpful distinguishing features include the lack of nuclear pleomorphism or nuclear hyperchromasia, absence of abnormal mitotic figures, and the clinical history of a recent surgical procedure in the region of the lesion.[251] Local recurrence has not been reported, even after incomplete resection.[108,251] Lesions of similar histologic appearance have been reported in the urinary tract in the absence of a clinical history of surgery or instrumentation.[360]

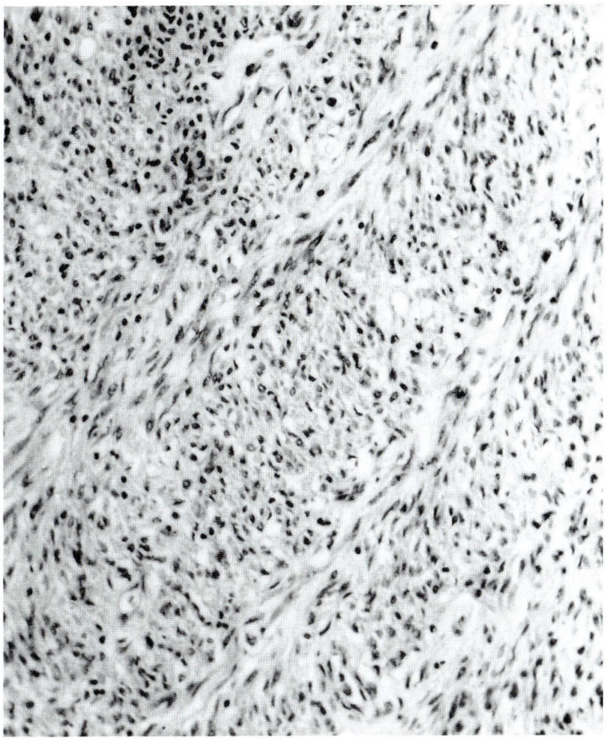

Fig. 4.19. Postoperative spindle cell nodule. The lesion is characterized by intersecting fascicles of plump spindle cells. (Courtesy of Robert E. Scully, M.D., Boston, MA.)

Vaginal Vault Granulation Tissue

Vaginal vault granulation tissue is a common finding after hysterectomy.[105] One or more small, red, granular to polypoid lesions may be seen grossly, which microscopically are composed of ulcerated, edematous, granulation tissue containing numerous neutrophils superficially and lymphocytes and plasma cells in the deeper stroma. Occasionally, scattered bizarre stromal cells may cause confusion with a malignant neoplasm (Fig. 4.21), particularly if the hysterectomy has been performed for a cervical or corpus tumor.

Fistula

Vesicovaginal and *ureterovaginal fistulas* may occur as a complication of hysterectomy, resulting from

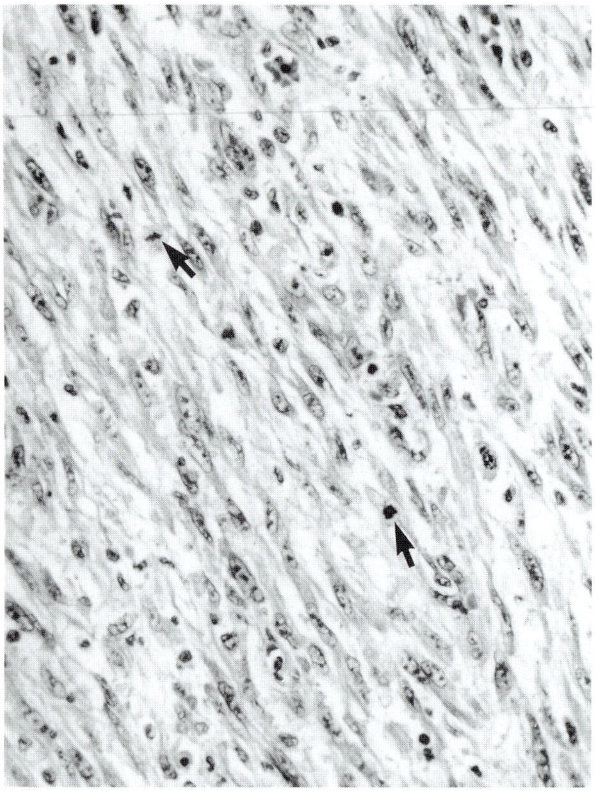

Fig. 4.20. Postoperative spindle cell nodule. The cells contain oval nuclei with delicate chromatin and distinct nucleoli. There are numerous mitotic figures (*arrows*). (Courtesy of Robert E. Scully, M.D., Boston, MA.)

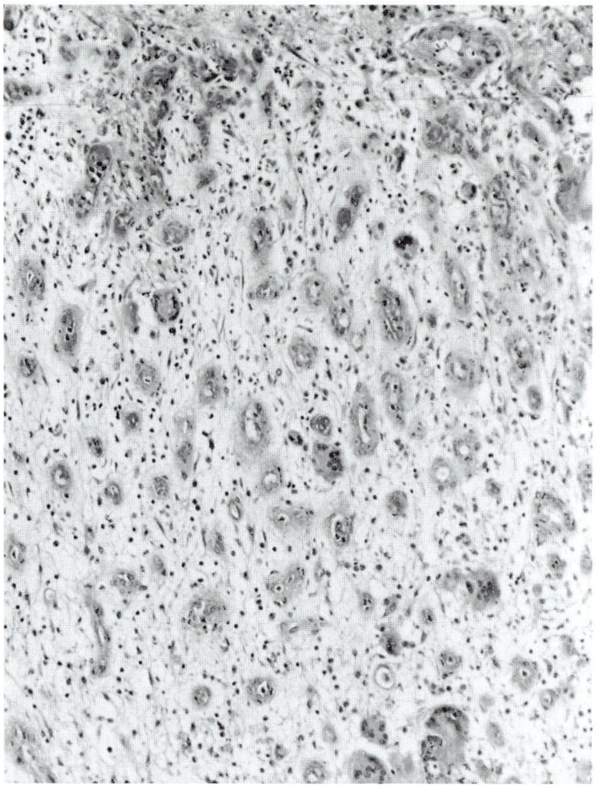

Fig. 4.21. Granulation tissue. Scattered bizarre stromal cells and prominent endothelial cells may simulate adenocarcinoma.

ischemic necrosis secondary to interruption of the vascular supply.[317] The surgical correction usually yields small fragments of tissue with variable amounts of granulation tissue, fibrosis, chronic inflammation, and little or no epithelium. Rarely, calculi are present. These are composed of urinary salts that develop in the vagina because of continuous leakage of urine from a vesicovaginal fistula.[254] Vesicovaginal fistula and vaginal laceration also may be a consequence of coitus.[74,221]

Radionecrosis

Radiation therapy to the vulva, vagina, or uterine cervix may cause *necrosis, ulceration*, or *stenosis* of the vagina.[276] The mechanism by which this injury develops reflects the sensitivity of endothelial cells to radiation, with thrombosis, and subsequent stenosis or obliteration of small blood vessels, stromal fibrosis, and epithelial ulceration. The formation of granular to polypoid masses, particularly in the vaginal vault, may clinically simulate recurrent cervical carcinoma. In addition to the vascular changes, dense infiltrates of plasma cells, granulation tissue, and bizarre stromal cells with pleomorphic, hyperchromatic nuclei may be sprinkled through the stroma. Even in the absence of a gross lesion, one may anticipate extreme atrophy of the vaginal squamous mucosa as a consequence of radiation therapy combined with cessation of ovarian function (Fig. 4.22).[153] Careful examination of nuclear detail helps to distinguish radiation atrophy from intraepithelial carcinoma. Atrophic cells have high nuclear/cytoplasmic ratios such as those of intraepithelial carcinoma, but have a regular, round to oval nuclear shape with a uniform distribution of chromatin that may appear smudged, in contrast to the irregular nuclear contours and clumped chromatin of vaginal intraepithelial neoplasia. Occasionally, radiation may result in partially obliterated vascular channels lined by plump endothelial cells containing large nuclei with vesicular chromatin, which simulate cords of invasive carcinoma. The distinction may be assisted by immunohistochemistry. Although a positive immunostaining reaction is not always present, the localization of factor VIII antigen in the atypical cells coupled with the absence of staining for keratins provides evidence for reactive endothelial rather than epithelial cells.

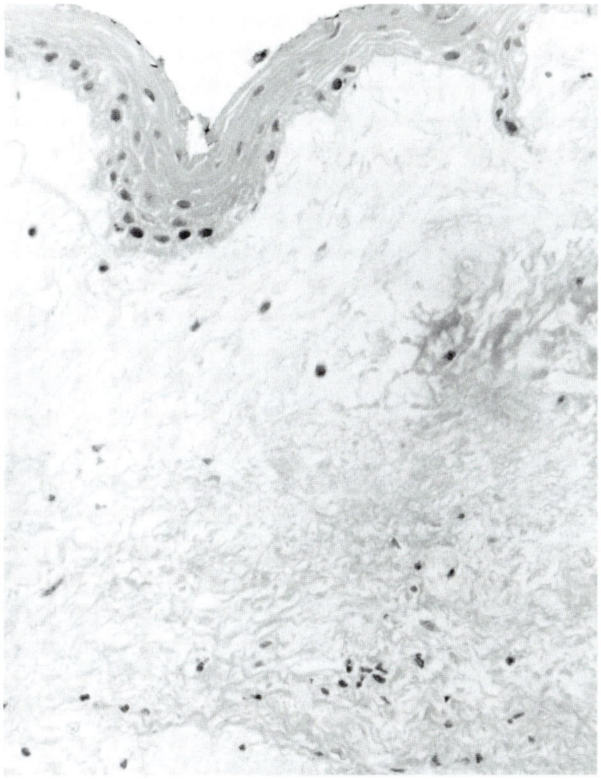

Fig. 4.22. **Radiation change.** Long-term consequences of irradiation to the vagina include atrophy of the squamous epithelium, edema, fibrosis within the stroma, and obliteration of vascular channels.

Vaginal Prolapse

Cystocele, rectocele, and *vaginal prolapse* may occur after multiple vaginal deliveries.[14] The surgical correction may include removal of elliptical fragments of vaginal mucosa in which variable degrees of acanthosis, hyperkeratosis, or parakeratosis are present (Fig. 4.23).

Fallopian Tube Prolapse

Prolapse of the fallopian tube into the vagina is a relatively uncommon complication of either vaginal or abdominal hysterectomy.[296,353] Patients often present with abdominal pain, vaginal discharge, or vaginal bleeding. A red, granular mass usually is present at the vaginal apex, which grossly may be confused with granulation tissue or carcinoma. Manipulation of the prolapsed tube typically causes extreme pain. Microscopically, a complex pattern of tubular, glandular, and papillary structures may be present (Fig. 4.24). Nuclear crowding and stratification are common, and ciliated or secretory columnar cells of typical tubal type may be difficult to locate (Fig. 4.25).[296] There often is associated inflammation and granulation tissue. Fimbriae rarely are identifiable, and both diligence and an awareness of the condition are required to avoid the misdiagnosis of adenocarcinoma.

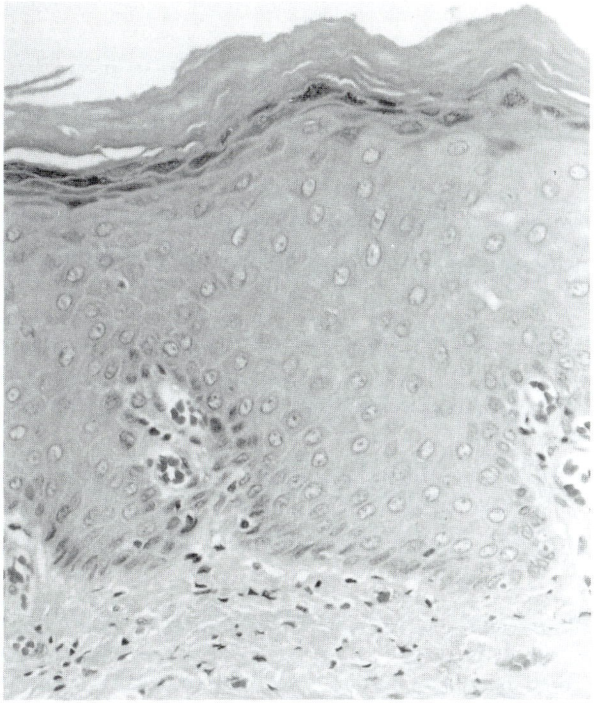

Fig. 4.23. **Vaginal prolapse.** Acanthosis and hyperkeratosis of the squamous epithelium are present.

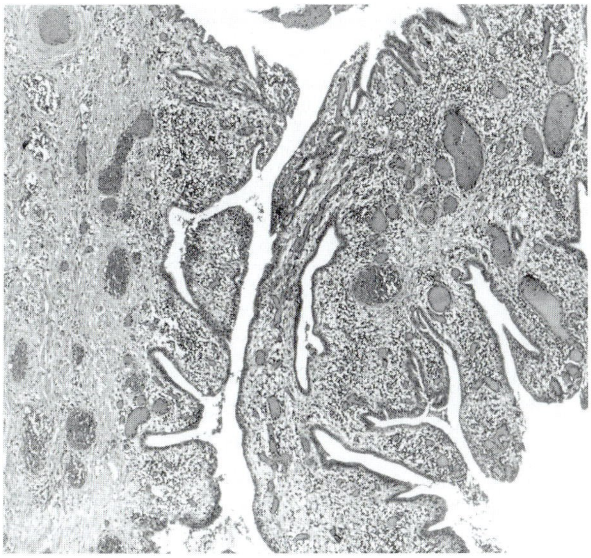

Fig. 4.24. **Fallopian tube prolapse.** When the plicae are blunt, there may be confuson with adenocarcinoma. Note the preserved muscularis visible on the *left*.

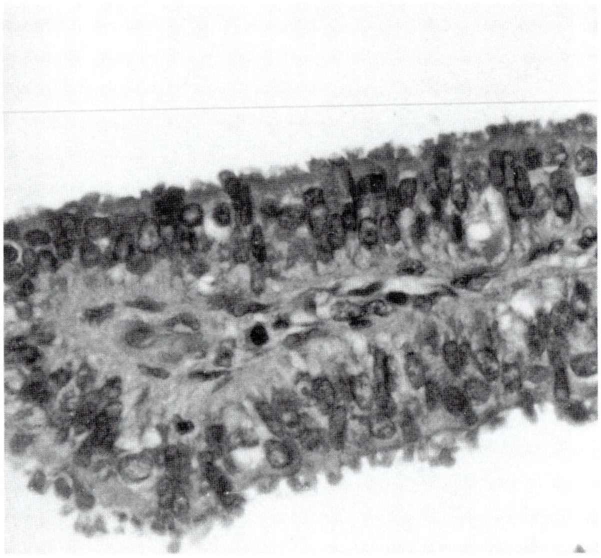

Fig. 4.25. Fallopian tube prolapse. At high magnification, nuclear enlargement and stratification may suggest the possibility of adenocarcinoma. However, many of the cells are ciliated, confirming that the structure is fallopian tube.

Cysts

Cysts of the vagina are relatively uncommon. Several classifications for cystic lesions have been proposed, reflecting a combination of good microscopic descriptions, an incomplete knowledge of embryology, and an assumption that histologic differentiation mirrors histogenesis.[62,154,246] A functional classification scheme follows: squamous inclusion cysts, mesonephric cysts, müllerian cysts, and Bartholin gland cysts.

Squamous Inclusion Cyst

Squamous inclusion cysts probably are the most common of the vaginal cysts, resulting from entrapment of fragments of mucosa during repair of a vaginal laceration or episiotomy.[62,154] These cysts often are asymptomatic and vary from a few millimeters to several centimeters in diameter. The microscopic appearance is that of a cyst wall formed by a stratified squamous epithelium, lacking rete ridges, with a central mass of keratin from desquamated cells.

Mesonephric Cyst

Mesonephric cysts, also termed Gartner's duct cysts, most often are located along the anterolateral wall of the vagina, following the route of the mesonephric duct. It is assumed that mesonephric cysts result from secretion by small isolated epithelial remnants after incomplete regression of the mesonephric duct. Mesonephric cysts are lined by low cuboidal, non-mucin-secreting cells, which are devoid of cytoplasmic mucicarmine or PAS-positive material (Fig. 4.26).

Müllerian Cyst

The genesis of the *müllerian cysts* is poorly understood; perhaps some are derived from islands of adenosis.[154] They are located anywhere within the vagina. Grossly, they are indistinguishable from mesonephric duct cysts, usually less than 2 cm in diameter. The distinction is made on microscopic examination. Müllerian cysts may be lined by any of the epithelia of the müllerian duct, including mucinous endocervical, endometrial, and ciliated tubal types (Fig. 4.27). Tall columnar mucin-secreting cells of endocervical type are most common, and squamous metaplasia may be observed.

Bartholin Gland Cyst

Bartholin gland cysts occur in the region of the ducts of Bartholin glands, near the opening of the primary duct into the vestibule. The pathogenesis is incompletely understood, but usually involves occlusion of the duct, associated with either a highly viscous thick mucoid secretion or infection of the gland.[154] The

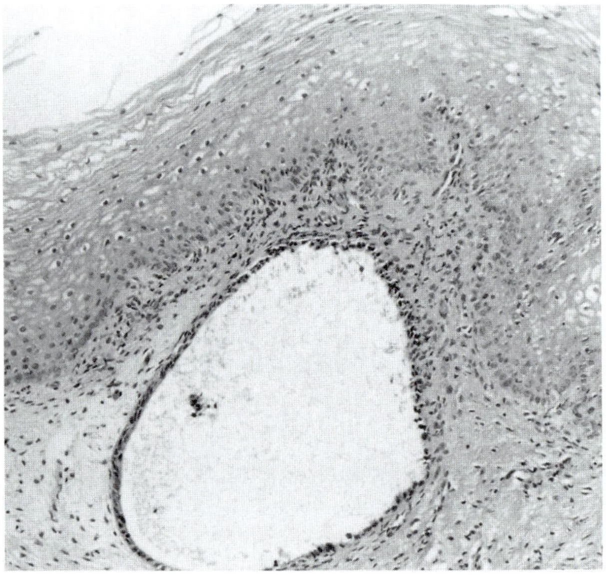

Fig. 4.26. Mesonephric cyst. The cyst is typically small and lined by a simple cuboidal epithelium, lacking cilia or intracellular mucin.

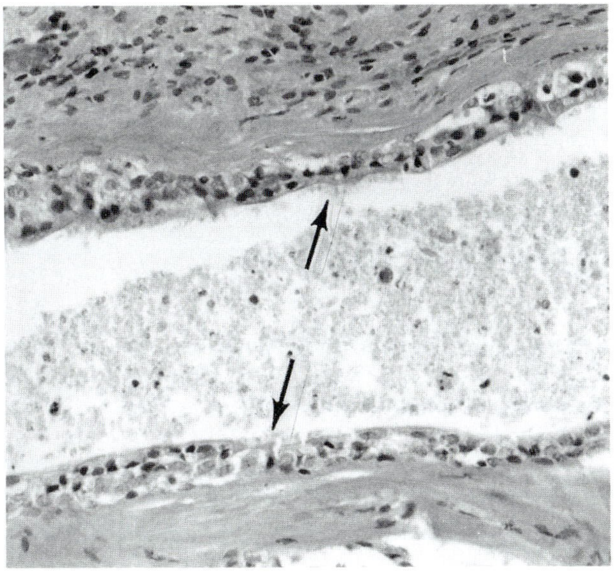

Fig. 4.27. Müllerian cyst. The cyst is lined by cuboidal or columnar cells, which may be endocervical, tubal, or endometrial type. Note the cilia (*arrows*) along the apical border of scattered cells.

cyst may enlarge rapidly and cause dyspareunia. The cyst lining varies from mucin secreting to squamous or "transitional," reflecting the different types of epithelium lining the duct and gland. Histochemical and ultrastructural studies of the mucinous cells of normal Bartholin glands, as well as these cysts, reveal no differences from the cells of the endocervix.[278] The Bartholin gland is of urogenital sinus origin whereas the cervix is of müllerian derivation; therefore, the weakness of a histogenetic classification of vaginal cysts based on histologic features is reinforced further by this observation. Cysts of identical histologic appearance may occur elsewhere in the vestibule, reflecting the presence of numerous minor vestibular glands of urogenital sinus origin.[30,275] The treatment of vaginal cysts usually is excision, although marsupialization may be indicated for some Bartholin gland cysts.[154]

Benign Neoplasms

Squamous Papilloma

Squamous papillomas may be single but frequently are multiple. These lesions usually are only a few millimeters in diameter, and most commonly occur in clusters near the hymenal ring, resulting in a condition referred to as *squamous papillomatosis*.[167] The lesions usually are asymptomatic, but may be associated with vulvar burning or dyspareunia.

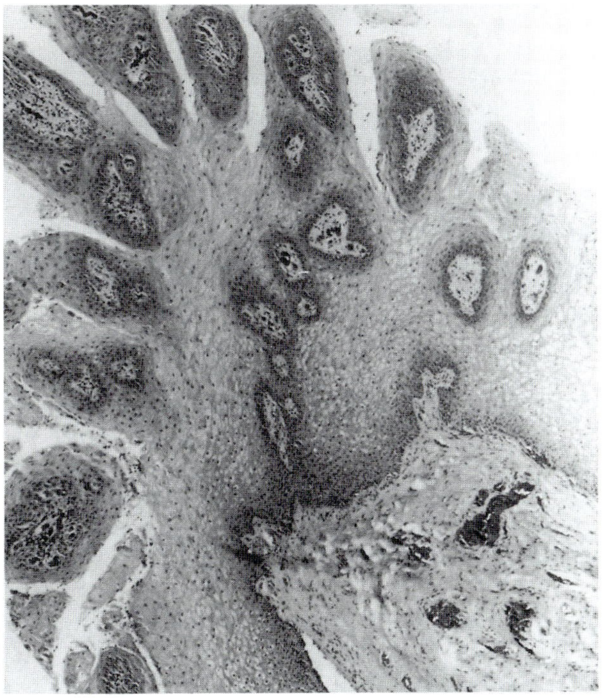

Fig. 4.28. Squamous papilloma. In contrast to a condyloma, this lesion lacks koilocytes and complex branching papillae.

Squamous papillomas may be difficult to distinguish from condylomas by gross inspection. Colposcopic and microscopic examination reveal the squamous papilloma to be composed of a single papillary frond with a central fibrovascular core (Fig. 4.28). It lacks the complex arborizing architecture and koilocytes of the condyloma. In contrast to the condyloma, the squamous papilloma probably is not sexually transmitted or related to infection by human papilloma virus (HPV). However, it is important to note that there may be a time during the evolution of condylomas when koilocytes are not easily identifiable.

Condyloma Acuminatum

An extensive discussion of the features of *condylomas* is provided in Chapter 2, Benign Diseases of the Vulva, and Chapter 6, Benign Diseases of the Cervix. As the biologic and pathologic characteristics of vaginal condylomas are similar to those in the cervix and vulva, they are not described here.

Müllerian Papilloma

Ulbright et al. have described a *papillary tumor* arising in the wall of the upper vagina in a 5-year-old

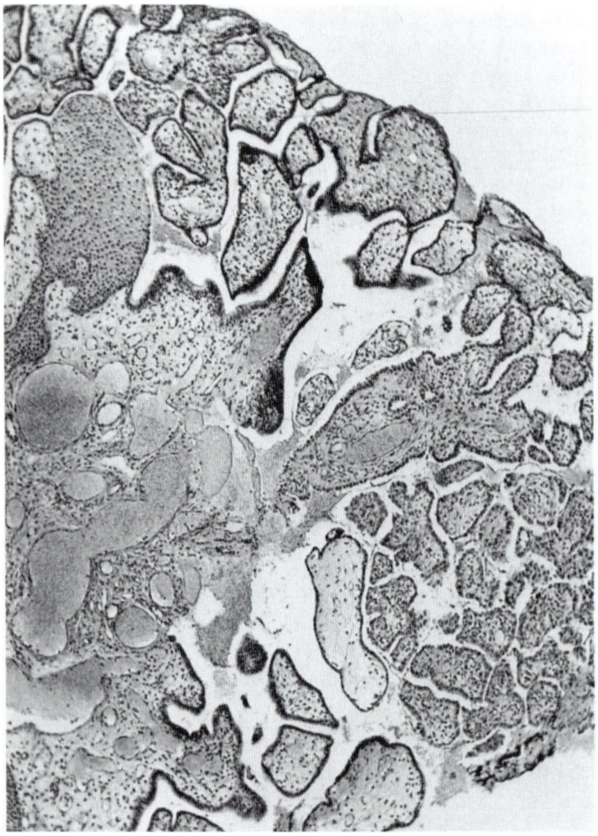

Fig. 4.29. Müllerian papilloma. Complex, branching, thick fibrovascular cores are covered by a bland low columnar epithelium.

girl. Microscopically, it was composed of a complex arborizing fibrovascular core that supported bland-appearing epithelial cells which in some areas formed both solid masses and glandular lumina (Fig. 4.29).[331a] The ultrastructural features, including microvilli, perinuclear arrays of microfilaments, tonofilaments, and complex cytoplasmic interdigitations, were interpreted as evidence of *müllerian origin*. Similar tumors, displaying an exophytic growth pattern and covered by mucin-secreting, hobnail, or eosinophilic cells have been described in both the vagina and cervix of young girls and have been classified as mesonephric müllerian papillomas.[187,284,298] Although their behavior clearly is benign, their embryologic origin remains uncertain.

Fibroepithelial Polyp (Mesodermal Stromal Polyp)

The *fibroepithelial polyp* or *mesodermal stromal polyp* is an uncommon hamartomatous or benign neoplastic polypoid mass of the vagina that evokes a level of interest in pathologists disproportionate to its frequency or significance. Because of the presence of bizarre stromal cells, the lesion also has been referred to as *pseudosarcoma botryoides*, reflecting the potential for confusion with sarcoma botryoides. The mean age at diagnosis is about 40 years, with an age range extending from the newborn to 77 years.[34,202,205,224,252] About 25% of the patients are pregnant at the time of diagnosis. The lesions usually are asymptomatic and are discovered incidentally, during pelvic examination, on the lateral wall of the lower third of the vagina. The size varies from 0.5 to 4 cm, and the gross configuration may be that of a single edematous soft polyp resembling an acrochordon, a papillary lesion with fingerlike projections, or a cerebriform mass (Fig. 4.30). Microscopically, an edematous fibrovascular stroma is covered by stratified squamous epithelium. Within the stroma are variable numbers of fibroblasts. About half the polyps contain large cytologically atypical stromal cells with hyperchromatic, pleomorphic nuclei, and abundant cytoplasm with

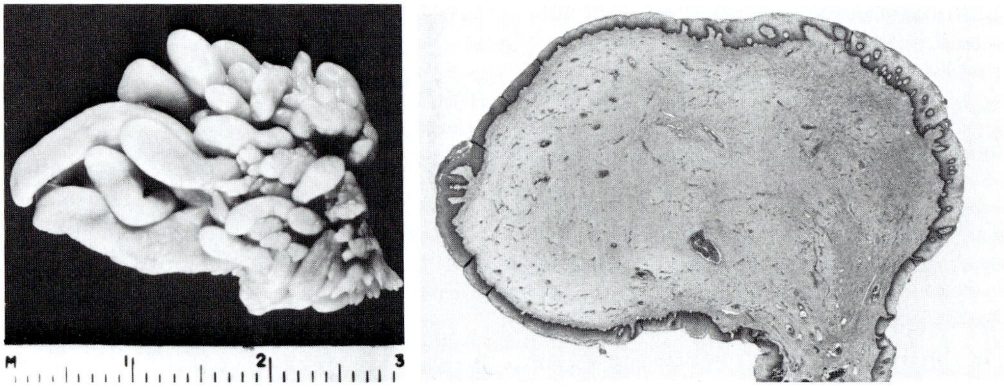

Fig. 4.30. Fibroepithelial polyp. *Left*: Gross; note finger-like projections. *Right*: Microscopic view; note squamous epithelial lining. (Courtesy of Henry J. Norris, M.D., Washington, DC.)

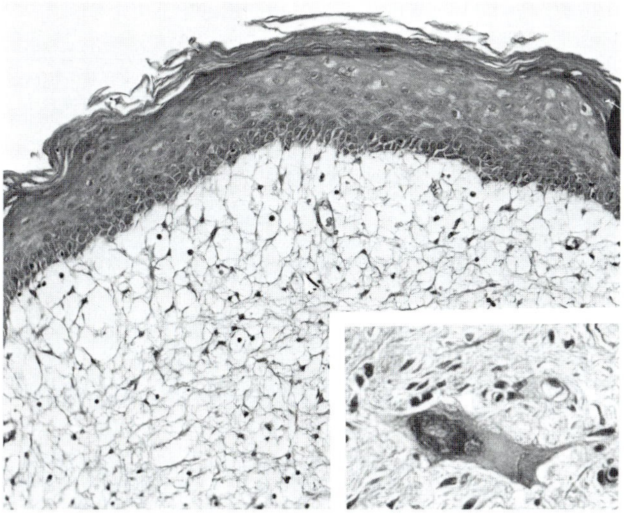

Fig. 4.31. Fibroepithelial polyp. High-power view of an atypical stromal cell. (Courtesy of Henry J. Norris, M.D., Washington, DC.)

sharply tapered cytoplasmic processes (Fig. 4.31). Multinucleated bizarre cells are not uncommon, and mitotic activity is variable, but generally low. Ultrastructural and immunohistochemical studies have shown evidence of fibroblastic or smooth muscle differentiation and localization of desmin but not smooth muscle actin.[112,202,205] Cells with a similar histologic appearance have been described in a bandlike subepithelial stromal zone extending from the endocervix to the vulva of normal females and may represent the origin of these atypical cells.[68] The immunolocalization of steroid receptors in these bizarre cells and frequent relationship to pregnancy raises the possibility that fibroepithelial polyps are hormonally induced.

The bizarre cells may create concern about a malignant mesenchymal neoplasm, particularly sarcoma botryoides; however, the fibroepithelial polyp lacks a "cambium layer," small undifferentiated stromal cells, rhabdomyoblasts, or invasion of the overlying squamous epithelium, which are typical features of sarcoma botryoides. Most fibroepithelial polyps occur in women over the age of 20, whereas sarcoma botryoides is confined almost always to children less than 5 years of age.

A subset of fibroepithelial polyps recently have been designated *cellular pseudosarcomatous fibroepithelial stromal polyps* on the basis of histologic characteristics that raised particular concern about malignancy.[220] These lesions displayed varying combinations of the following features: marked hypercellularity; marked cytologic pleomorphism, more than 10 mitoses per 10 high-power fields, or the

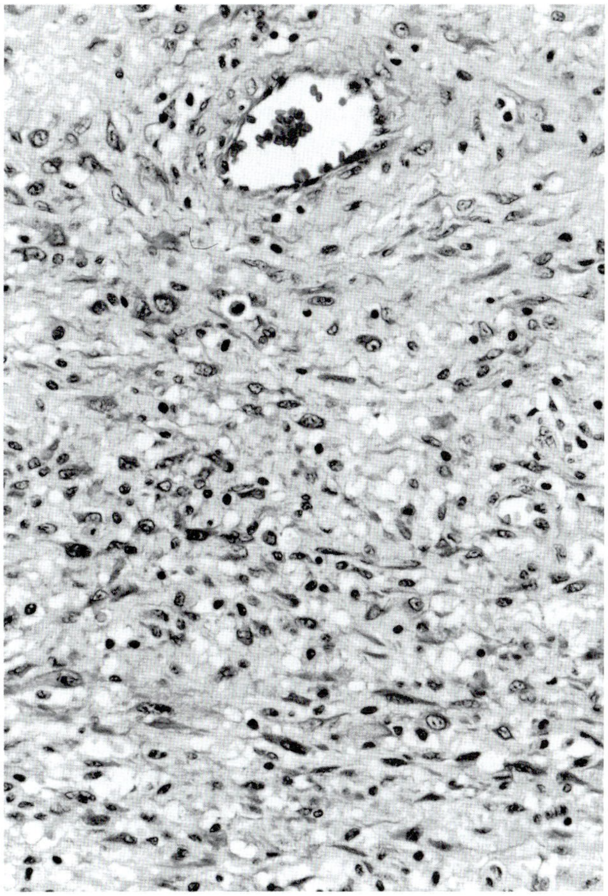

Fig. 4.32. Cellular pseudosarcomatous fibroepithelial stroma polyp. This variant of fibroepithelial polyp is characterized by the presence of marked hypercellularity, marked cytologic pleomorphism, more than 10 mitoses per 10 high-power fields, or the presence of atypical mitoses. Marked cellularity is evident in this example.

presence of atypical mitoses (Fig. 4.32). The median diameter of the polyps was only about 2 cm, and they occurred in the vagina, cervix, or vulva. About half the women were pregnant, and one-quarter had multiple lesions. Fifteen percent developed local, noninvasive recurrences, but none had metastases. The distinction from sarcoma is made primarily on the basis of superficial location, small size, lack of an identifiable lesional margin, extension of abnormal stromal tissue to the mucosal–stromal interface, and the presence of scattered multinucleate stromal cells.[220]

Leiomyoma

The most common mesenchymal neoplasm in the vagina of adult women is the *leiomyoma*.[17,85] The mean age at detection is about 40 years, with a reported range of 19–72 years.[283] The tumor may occur anywhere within the vagina, usually in a submucosal location. Vaginal leiomyomas vary from 0.5 to 15 cm in diameter, averaging about 3 cm.[319] Because most are relatively small, they often are asymptomatic. Larger tumors may produce pain, hemorrhage, dystocia, or dyspareunia.

The gross and microscopic appearances of vaginal leiomyomas resemble those of their uterine counterparts. They are well-circumscribed, firm masses that occasionally may contain foci of necrosis, edema, or hyalinization. Microscopically, they are composed of interlacing fascicles of spindle-shaped cells, with elongated, oval nuclei and little or no mitotic activity or nuclear pleomorphism. Of 60 cases of smooth muscle tumors of the vagina reviewed by Tavassoli and Norris, only 7 contained more than 5 mitoses per 10 high-power fields (HPF). Five patients developed recurrence after local excision. All the recurrent tumors were in the subset with high mitotic activity and generally moderate to marked nuclear atypia.[319] Accordingly, it is recommended that the diagnosis of vaginal leiomyoma be reserved for those tumors with fewer than 5 mitoses per 10 HPF. However, it also should be noted that increased mitotic activity in the absence of aggressive behavior may be present in vaginal leiomyomas during pregnancy.

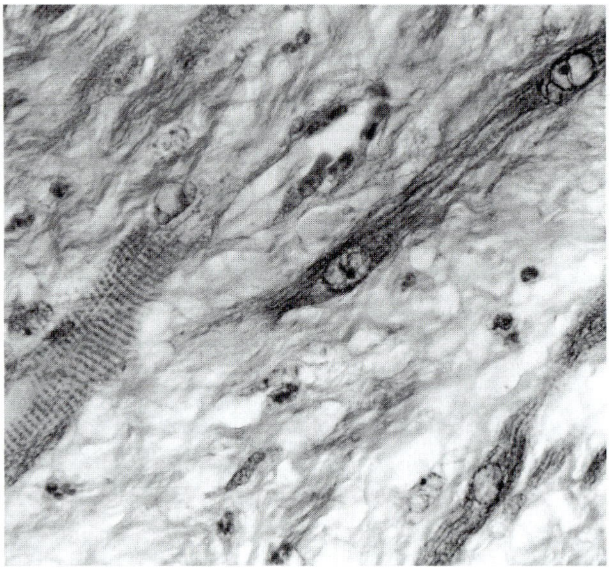

Fig. 4.34. Vaginal rhabdomyoma. At higher magnification, cross-striations are enhanced by staining with PTAH.

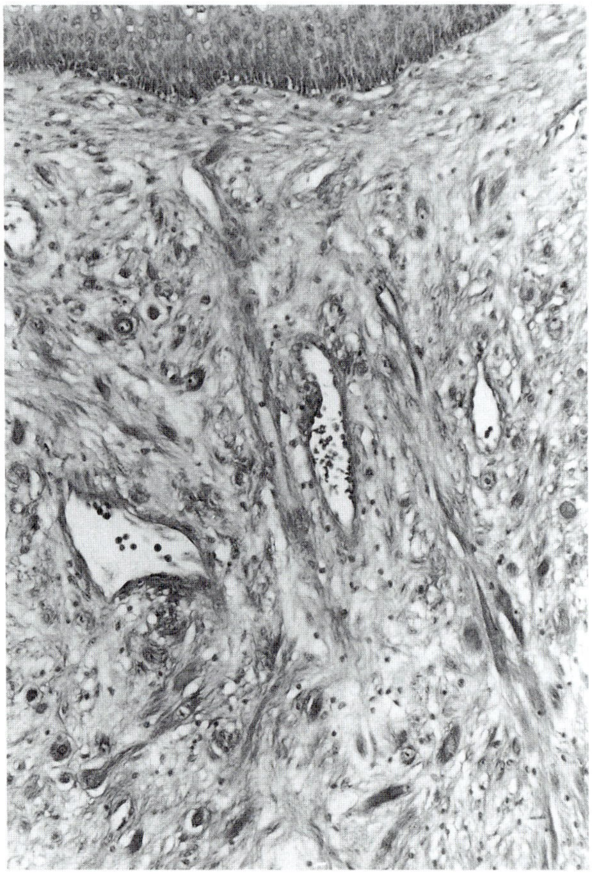

Fig. 4.33. Vaginal rhabdomyoma. At low magnification, a nonencapsulated mass of plump, elongated cells is visible.

Rhabdomyoma

Rhabdomyoma is a rare benign tumor displaying skeletal muscle differentiation, about 20 cases of which have been reported arising within the vagina.[98,141] The average age at diagnosis is about 45 years, with a range extending from 34 to 57 years. Patients typically present with a solitary, polypoid to nodular mass that varies from 1 to 11 cm in diameter. The overlying mucosa usually is intact.

Microscopically, rhabdomyomas are composed of benign-appearing fetal- or adult-type skeletal muscle cells surrounded by variable quantities of fibrous stroma (Fig. 4.33). The cells are of spindle to oval shape, with plump oval nuclei and abundant granular, eosinophilic cytoplasm. Mitotic activity and nuclear pleomorphism are absent. The diagnosis is confirmed by identification of intracytoplasmic fibers with cross-striations (Fig. 4.34), staining for which may be enhanced by phosphotungstic acid hematoxlin (PTAH) or trichrome preparations. Immunohistochemistry and electron microscopy usually are not needed to confirm the presence of skeletal muscle differentiation.[98] It is important not to confuse vaginal rhabdomyoma with embryonal rhabdomyosarcoma, but this is generally

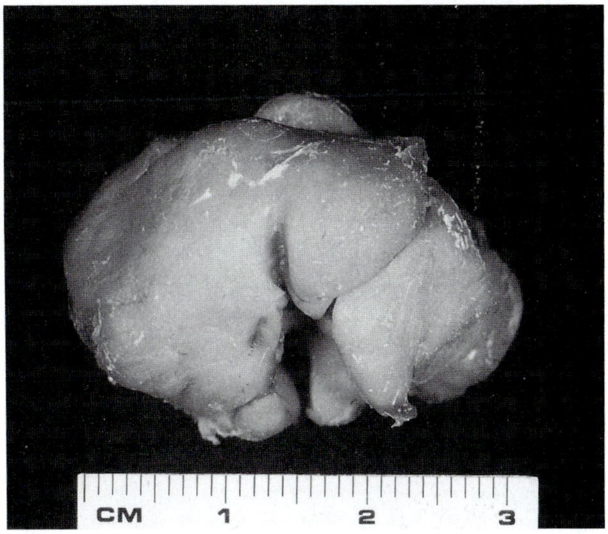

Fig. 4.35. Benign mixed tumor of the vagina. The tumor typically is well circumscribed, but nonencapsulated. (Courtesy of Henry J. Norris, M.D., Washington, DC.)

not difficult because there are differences in the age at presentation and at gross and microscopic appearances (see below, Embryonal Rhabdomyo-sarcoma). The behavior of rhabdomyoma is benign, and local excision provides adequate therapy.

Benign Mixed Tumor

Tumors that histologically bear some resemblance to salivary gland neoplasms are classified as *benign mixed tumors*. These neoplasms are rare, and usually present as a slowly growing painless mass that may occur anywhere in the vagina, but most frequently near the hymenal ring.[26,297] The mean age at diagnosis is 30 years. Because the tumors are well circumscribed but nonencapsulated within the submucosa, they often are diagnosed preoperatively as a polyp or cyst (Fig. 4.35). They range in size from 1.5 to 5 cm.

Microscopically, the neoplasm is characterized by a biphasic proliferation of stromal and epithelial cells (Figs. 4.36 and 4.37). The spindle cells are

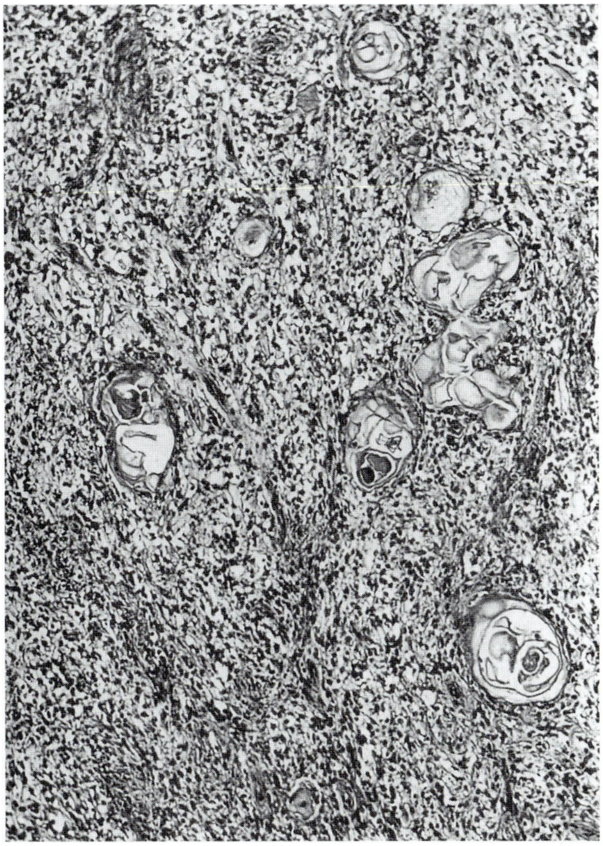

Fig. 4.36. Benign mixed tumor of the vagina. Nests of stratified squamous cells are surrounded by irregular fascicles of spindle stromal cells.

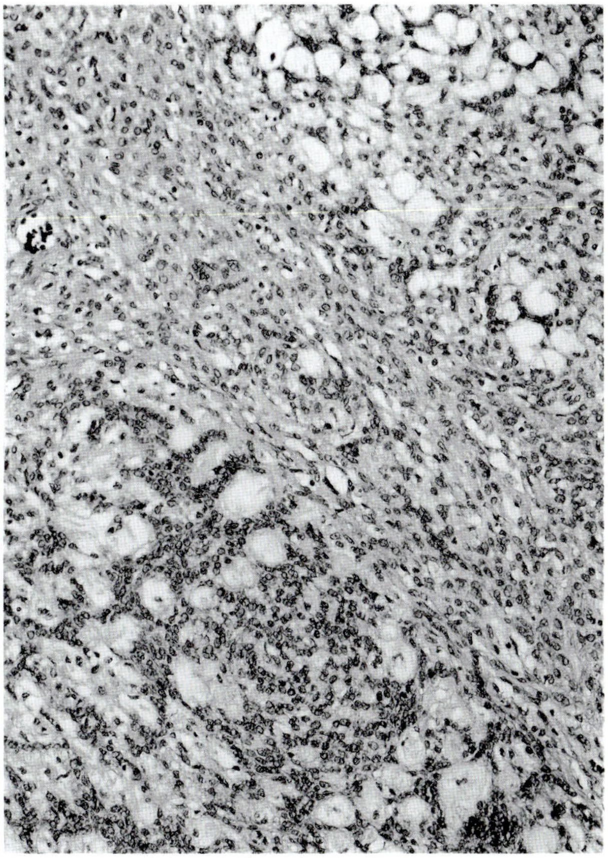

Fig. 4.37. Benign mixed tumor of the vagina. Although a mixture of spindle cells and squamous cell nests predominate in most benign mixed tumors, some contain mucin-secreting glands or glandlike structures.

arranged in intersecting fascicles and contain small, oval nuclei with finely granular chromatin and usually only rare mitotic figures. The epithelial component includes nests of bland-appearing glycogenated, stratified squamous cells and occasional glands lined by a mucin-secreting epithelium.[87] The behavior is benign, and recurrences have not been reported after local excision.

Endometriosis

It is not uncommon for *endometriosis* to involve the vagina, either superficially implanted in the squamous mucosa or involving the deep stroma, particularly of the rectovaginal septum.[90,159,191,339,354] A complete discussion of endometriosis is provided in Chapter 17, Diseases of the Peritoneum.

Miscellaneous Benign Tumors and Tumor-Like Lesions

In addition to those tumors that are highly characteristic for the vagina, sporadic cases of benign neoplasms and tumor-like processes have been reported, including adenomatoid tumor,[182] villous adenoma (Fig. 4.38),[77] mature cystic teratoma,[168] Brenner tumor,[33] hemangioma,[99] granular cell tumor,[163] neurofibroma,[59] paraganglioma,[239] glomus tumor,[305] blue nevus,[327] and eosinophilic granuloma.[364] Thyroid and parathyroid glands have been described in the vaginal wall of a 3-year-old girl, but probably these represented monodermal differentiation within a benign vaginal teratoma.[168]

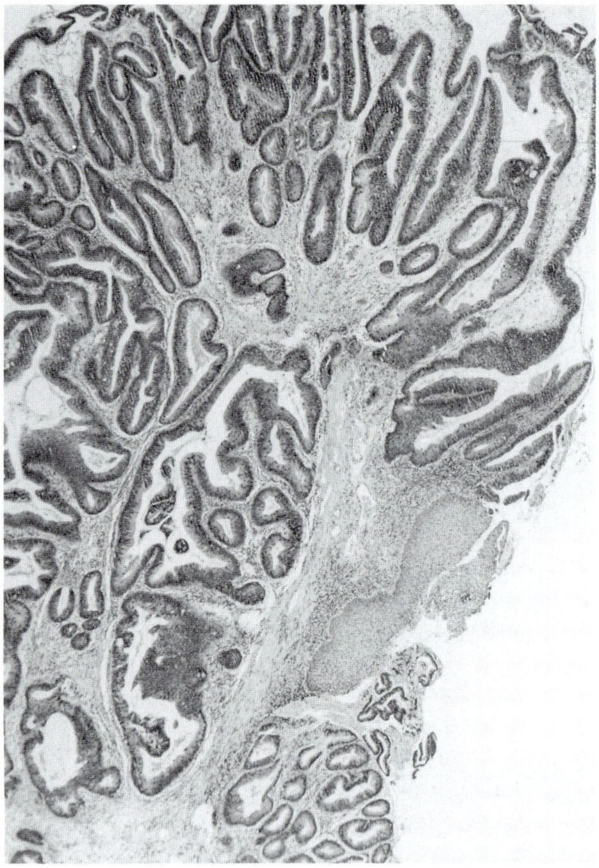

Fig. 4.38. Villous adenoma of the vagina. The lesion presented as a polypoid mass. It is histologically identical to villous adenoma in the colon.

Malignant Neoplasms

Vaginal Intraepithelial Neoplasia

In contrast to the high prevalence of intraepithelial lesions of the cervix and vulva, *vaginal intraepithelial neoplasia* (*VAIN*) is relatively rare. The reason for this discrepancy is unknown, but may prove pivotal to understanding carcinogenesis involving the squamous epithelium of the lower female genital tract. The terminology for intraepithelial neoplasia of the vagina continues to evolve, reflecting conceptual refinements, and parallels that for the cervix and vulva.

General Features

The incidence of in situ carcinoma of the vagina is reported to be about 0.20 cases per 100,000 in Caucasian females and 0.31 cases per 100,000 in black females; this is less than 1% of the incidence for the same disease in the cervix.[48,118] The highest incidence rates are observed in women over the age of 60, with the mean age at diagnosis of VAIN 3 about 53 years. These figures are 10 or more years greater than the age of detection of cervical intraepithelial neoplasia (CIN) 3.[138] Risk factors for the development of VAIN include immunosuppression, HPV infection or squamous neoplasia elsewhere in the lower genital tract, irradiation, and in utero exposure to DES.[27] Almost 75% of women with VAIN have preceding or coexisting squamous carcinomas of the cervix or vulva.[16,150,151,174,294] These observations have generated the concept of a field effect, in which the squamous epithelium of the entire lower female genital tract is at risk for neoplastic transformation. This hypothesis is appealing, because the squamous epithelia of these sites do share a common embryonic derivation from the urogenital sinus, and all are susceptible to infection by various HPVs.

Radiation therapy for cervical carcinoma results in exposure of the vagina to ionizing radiation, and women who have had pelvic radiation for benign as well as malignant diseases are at increased risk for development of VAIN.[16,93,174]

During the mid-1970s, it was first suggested that DES-exposed offspring might be at risk for increased rates of dysplasia because of the extent of metaplastic tissue present in both the cervix and vagina. Multiple studies of prevalence rates subsequently conducted indicated that the frequency of dysplasia in both the exposed and unexposed populations was approximately the same. In 1984, the DESAD Project amplified its findings on the frequency of dysplasia. The incidence rates were slightly higher in exposed women. The new occurrence of squamous cell dysplasia in women under observation developed twice as frequently in DES-exposed women in contrast to those that were never exposed in utero.[22,268] Some believe that the DESAD findings may not be valid and that the increased rates of dysplasia, especially of mild form, may be caused by over- or misinterpretation of the HPV-infected tissue for dysplasia,[263] especially as the DESAD study was conducted before many of the histologic intricacies of HPV infection were fully appreciated. Regardless of interpretation, DES itself is not believed to be the etiologic cause of dysplasia. Possibly, the metaplastic squamous epithelium, which is more extensive in the vagina in DES-exposed women, may be more susceptible to agents that give rise to dysplasia, but even this is speculative.

Recent reports have suggested that in utero exposure to DES may impair the immune system and that this may influence development of squamous cell lesions.[22] Treatment of mice with DES introduces a significant long-term inhibitory effect of all components of the immune system, especially on the natural killer (NK) cell system. Clinical studies have reported that exposed women also have biochemical alterations.[217,347] It has been suggested that a selective suppression of the immune system might allow for the development of squamous cell neoplasia in the cervix and vagina by permitting higher susceptibility to infection with HPV and herpes simplex virus. Without further evidence, such consideration must be viewed as speculative.

Gross Findings

Women with VAIN usually are asymptomatic, and in most instances there is no grossly identifiable lesion in the vagina. Occasionally, the epithelium appears raised, roughened, and white or pink. More often, the diagnosis is made by a colposcopically directed biopsy (Fig. 4.39) subsequent to an abnormal cytologic diagnosis in which sampling of the vagina as well as the cervix has been performed, or in vaginal samples after hysterectomy. The process is multifocal or diffuse in almost half of the cases, and usually is located in the upper third of the vagina.[16,174,204,281]

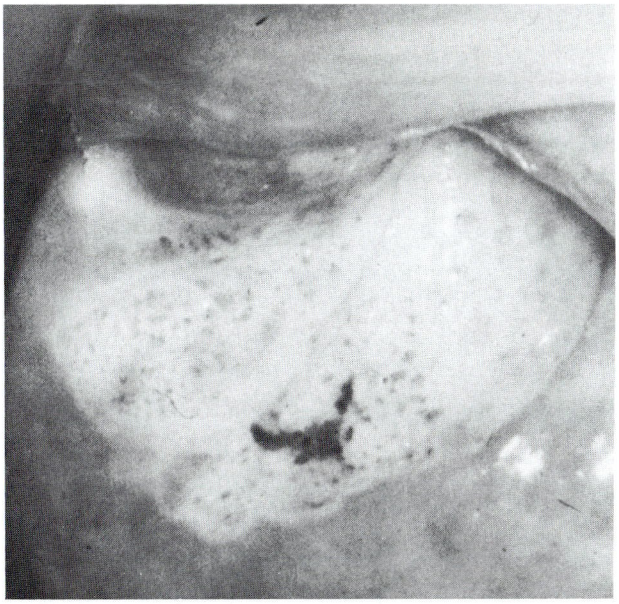

Fig 4.39. VAIN 3 of the vaginal vault, colposcopic appearance. The lesion was detected after a hysterectomy for cervical intraepithelial neuroplasia. It appears as a raised white plaque with a punctate pattern resulting from engorged subepithelial capillaries. (Reprinted by permission of Frederick Sillman, M.D., New York, NY.)

Microscopic Findings

The microscopic features of VAIN are analogous to those of CIN (see Chapter 7, Precancerous Lesions of the Cervix). VAIN is characterized histologically by the presence of nuclear abnormalities including enlargement with irregular shape, hyperchromasia, and irregular condensation of chromatin. Lesions are graded from VAIN 1 to 3 (corresponding to mild, moderate, and severe dysplasia, carcinoma in situ) or as LSIL and HSIL. The grade is inversely related to the retention of the ability of the cells to differentiate as they progress through the epithelium, as manifested by acquisition of cytoplasmic organelles, appropriate cell polarity, and loss of mitotic activity (Figs. 4.40–4.43). SIL (VAIN) lesions nearly always display some loss of squamous maturation as well as disordered maturation, frequently including increased mitotic activity, abnormal mitotic figures, acanthosis, and dyskeratosis.

The differential diagnosis of SIL (VAIN) includes atrophy, radiation change, and immature squamous metaplasia in women with adenosis, all of which may display loss of glycogen and a relative increase in cellularity. The distinction rests primarily on the characteristic nuclear features of SIL (VAIN), which are absent in the other conditions. Radiation changes include nuclear enlargement, smudged chromatin, multinucleation, and vacuolization of cytoplasm, with lack of mitotic activity.[84] Occasionally, there may be significant nuclear atypia associated with inflammatory and reactive processes, but usually this is expressed as regular nuclear enlargement with vesicular chromatin and moderate-sized nucleoli. Such changes are referred to as *reactive squamous atypia* (Fig. 4.44).

Clinical Behavior and Treatment

The natural history of SIL (VAIN) is uncertain. In one study, about 5% of SIL (VAIN) progressed to invasive carcinoma, with sequential changes documented by serial biopsies,[281] but this figure probably significantly underestimates the biologic potential of VAIN because many lesions were treated.[295] Therapy generally is local excision, although topical 5-fluorouracil, laser vaporization, vaginectomy, and irradiation also have been successfully used.[188,307,357] In a study of 94 women with VAIN, 70% achieved remission after a single treatment of any type, but 24% required additional therapy with chemosurgery or upper vaginectomy; 5% progressed to invasive squamous carcinoma in spite of therapy and close follow-up.[295]

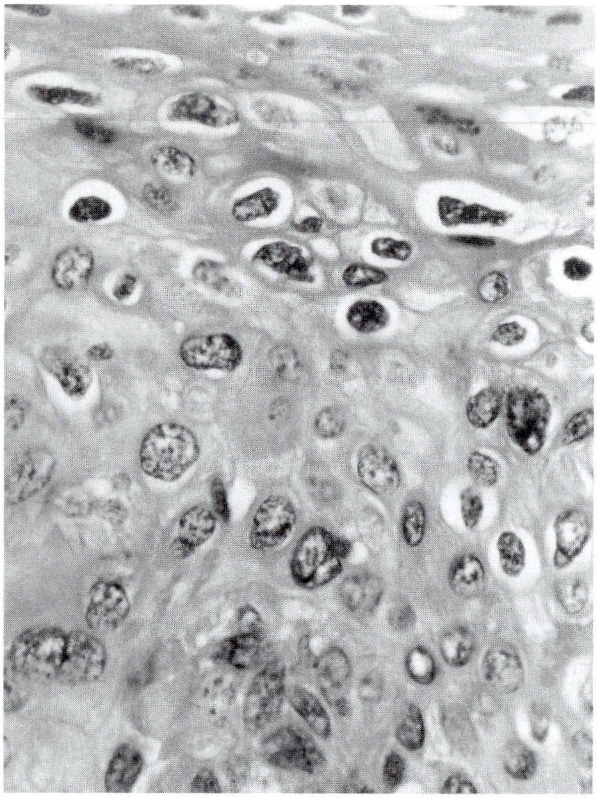

Fig. 4.41. Low-grade SIL (VAIN I). At high magnification, the nuclear features of intraepithelial neoplasia are evident. This includes nuclear enlargement, pleomorphism, coarse chromatin, and irregular nuclear contours. Koilocytosis is also evident.

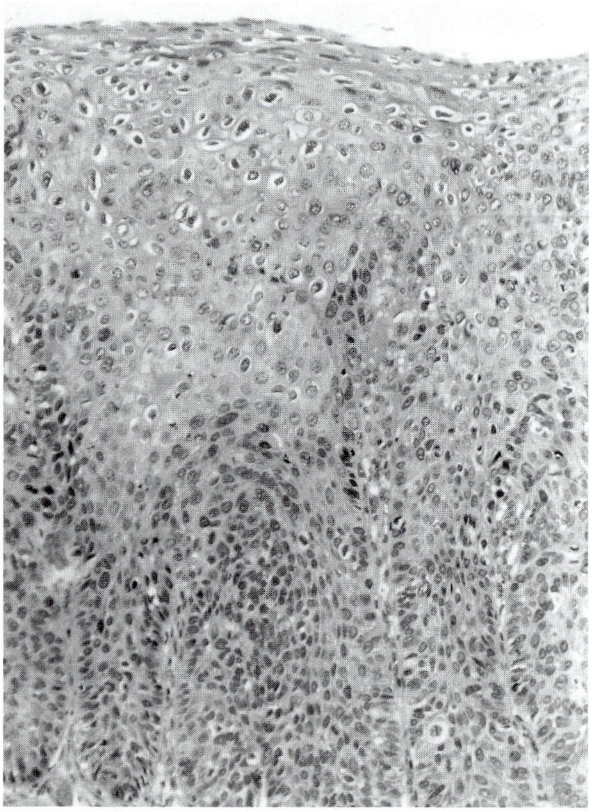

Fig. 4.40. Low-grade SIL (VAIN I). There is irregular acanthosis of this epithelium in addition to koilocytosis and nuclear features of intraepithelial neoplasia. The extensive cytoplasmic differentiation is diagnostic of VAIN I (low-grade SIL).

Squamous Cell Carcinoma

General Features

Squamous cell carcinoma represents about 80% of malignant neoplasms primary to the vagina.[49,242] The incidence in the United States is about 1000 cases each year. The incidence is 0.42 cases per 100,000 in Caucasian women and 0.93 per 100,000 in black women,[48,242] which is about one-fiftieth the incidence of cervical squamous cell carcinoma.[208] Only 1% of malignant neoplasms of the female genital tract are classified as squamous cell carcinoma originating in the vagina.[242] The incidence reflects both the relative rarity of squamous cell carcinoma

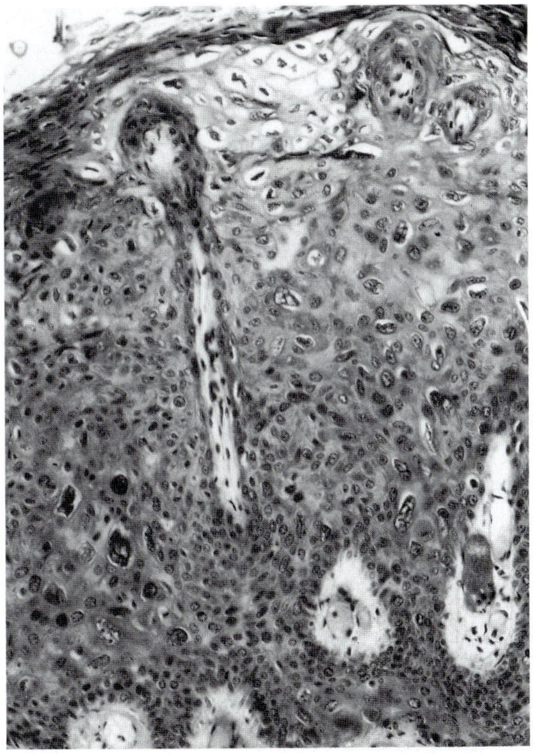

Fig. 4.42. High-grade SIL (VAIN 2). This intraepithelial process is characterized by enlargement and pleomorphism of nuclei, but preservation of some features of cytoplasmic differentiation is noted in cells of the intermediate and superficial layers. (Reprinted by permission of Kurman et al., ref. 167.)

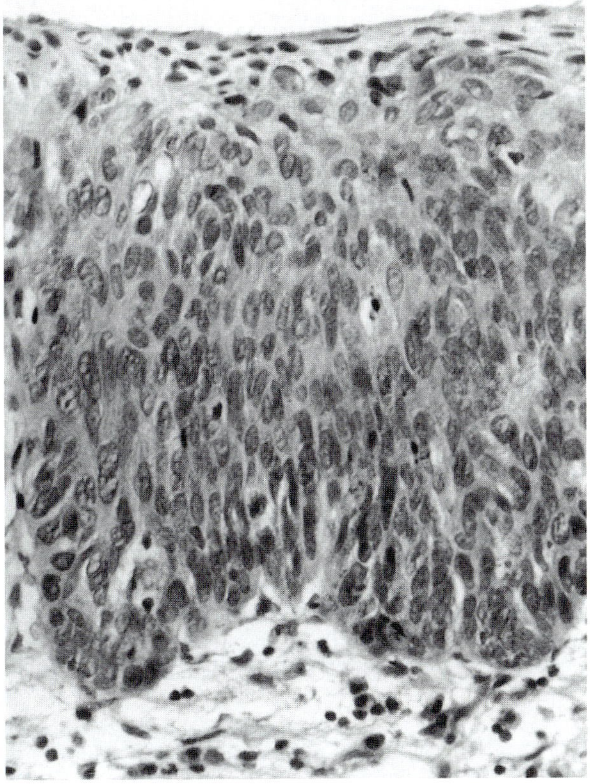

Fig. 4.43. High-grade SIL (VAIN 3). Cytoplasmic differentiation is limited to the uppermost layers of the squamous epithelium. The remaining cells have a high nuclear/cytoplasmic ratio, with a longitudinal nuclear axis perpendicular to the basement membrane.

at this site and the extremely rigid criteria for diagnosis of vaginal as compared with cervical carcinoma, which results in underestimation of its true frequency. The International Federation of Gynecology and Obstetrics (FIGO) staging of vaginal cancer is analogous to that of cervical cancer and is based on clinical rather than pathologic examination (Table 4.2). To be considered a primary tumor of the vagina the neoplasm must be located in the vagina, without clinical or histologic evidence of involvement of the cervix or vulva. Thus, bulky tumors located in the upper vagina that have extended onto the portio vaginalis of the cervix are classified as primary cervical carcinoma. Similarly, squamous cell carcinoma occurring in the vagina within 5 years of therapy for cervical carcinoma is considered to be recurrent cervical carcinoma rather than a new primary carcinoma of the vagina.[235] It is thus not surprising that only 10–20% of vaginal malignancies are classified as primary neoplasms of the vagina.[84] The risk factors for invasive squamous carcinoma of the vagina are the same as those for SIL (VAIN).[27,281] In a case control study of VAIN and in-

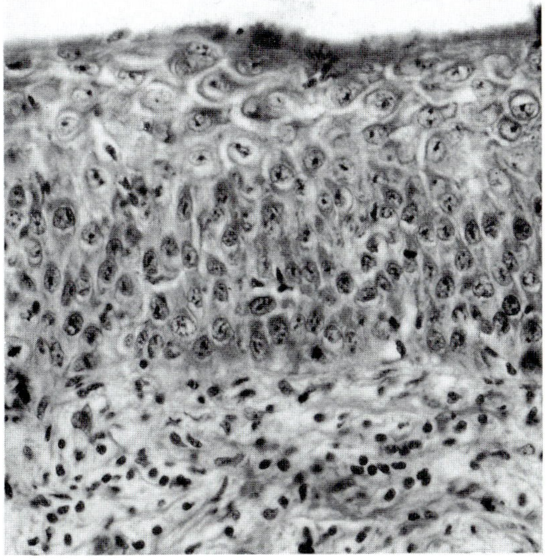

Fig. 4.44. Reactive squamous atypia. The cells have enlarged, oval nuclei with vesicular chromatin, and prominent nucleoli. (Reprinted by permission of Kurman et al., ref. 167.)

Table 4.2. FIGO staging of vaginal carcinoma (1978)

Stage	*Clinical status*
0	Intraepithelial
I	Limited to vaginal wall
II	Extends to subvaginal tissue but not to pelvic side wall
III	Extends to pelvic side wall
IV	Extends beyond the true pelvis or involves mucosa of the bladder or rectum (bullous edema does not consign the patient to stage IV)
IVa	Adjacent organs involved
IVb	Distant organs involved

vasive squamous carcinoma of the vagina, significant risk factors also included prior vaginal discharge, condyloma acuminata, or irritation, prior abnormal cervical vaginal cytology, and prior hysterectomy. Surprisingly, early age at first intercourse, multiple sexual partners, and a history of smoking were not associated with an elevated risk of neoplasia.[27] Occasionally, squamous cell carcinomas also have been reported in young women with congenital absence of the vagina 8 to 25 years after the creation of a neovagina.[136,280]

Clinical Features

The mean age at diagnosis of invasive vaginal squamous carcinoma is 64 years.[167] The presenting symptoms usually are painless vaginal bleeding or discharge, dysuria, or frequency.[3] There is a relationship between duration of symptoms and the size and spread of tumor. Unfortunately, about 20% of patients with vaginal cancer delay more than 7 months from onset of symptoms to initiation of therapy.[244]

Most of the tumors arise in the upper third of the vagina,[244] with 57% involving the posterior wall and 27% located on the anterior wall.[243]

Gross Findings

Vaginal squamous carcinomas vary in size from clinically occult to larger than 10 cm. The gross configuration is similarly variable and includes polypoid, fungating, indurated, and ulcerated lesions.

Microscopic Findings

Squamous cell carcinomas of the vagina resemble those arising in the cervix (Fig. 4.45). Histologic grade using either the method of Broders or Reagen and Wentz has not been related to prognosis.[64,229] Microinvasive carcinoma is not currently a defined entity in the vagina; however, superficially invasive tumors, with less than 3 mm of stromal invasion and no vascular space invasion, appear to have a low likelihood of nodal metastasis.[236] The distinction of early invasive carcinoma from intraepithelial carcinoma is based on a constellation of findings, including the presence of angulated narrow cords of squamous cells at the stromal interface, frequently with acquisition of more abundant eosinophilic cytoplasm, and a desmosplastic or inflammatory host response. Unfortunately, these features are not present in every case of early invasive squamous carcinoma.

Clinical Behavior and Treatment

Historically, the survival rates for women with squamous cell carcinoma of the vagina were low. However, recent studies indicate a considerably better prognosis, with rates comparable to those of cervical carcinoma when corrected for stage of disease.[64,230,248] In a review of 300 women with vaginal carcinoma treated over a 40-year interval at one institution, the overall 5- and 10-year survival rates were 60% and 49%, respectively.[38] The most important prognostic indicators included FIGO stage, tumor size, and location in the vagina (with better outcomes for those with lesions in the upper

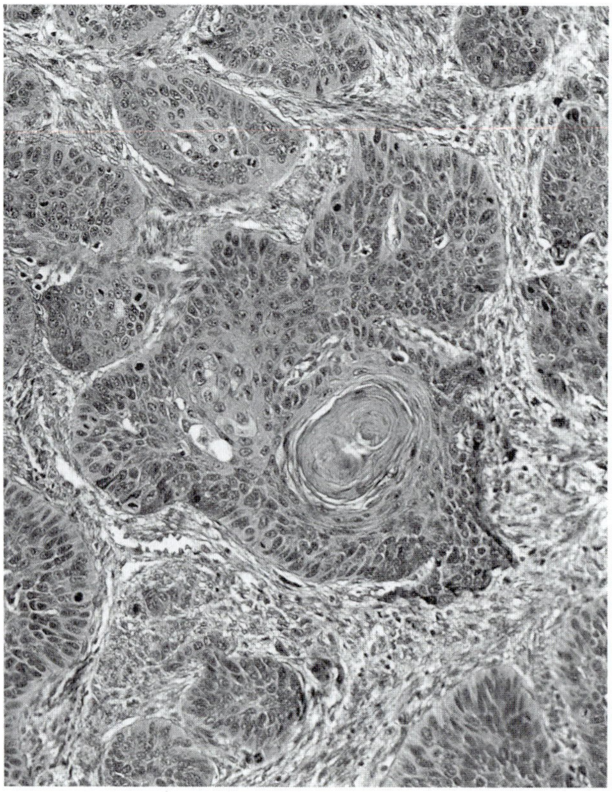

Fig. 4.45. Squamous cell carcinoma of the vagina. Keratin pearl formation is evident.

vagina). Results from the National Cancer Data Base between 1985 and 1994 support the prognostic importance of stage. The relative 5-year survival rate for stage I disease was 73%, 53% for stage II tumors, and only 36% for stages III and IV.[49] Unfortunately, relatively few women are diagnosed with tumors confined to the vagina. Direct spread into the soft tissues of the pelvis or to the mucosa of the bladder or rectum occurs early because the wall of the vagina is thin and is separated from these organs by only a few millimeters of connective tissue. Consequently, at initial diagnosis, most tumors have invaded the soft tissues surrounding the vaginal wall and about 20% extend to the pelvic sidewall.[38]

As discussed in the section on anatomy, the lymphatic drainage of the vagina is complex and variable, and any of the inguinal or pelvic lymph nodes may be the site of metastasis, although there is some relationship to the location of the tumor within the vagina.[192]

Radiation therapy, including brachytherapy and external beam radiation, is the modality used primarily to treat vaginal squamous carcinoma, although radical vaginectomy may be indicated in selected instances. Although metastases may be discovered ultimately in the lungs or supraclavicular lymph nodes, recurrent disease typically is local and occurs within 2 years of diagnosis.[167] In one large study, local recurrences were identified at 5 years in 23% and distant metastases in 15% of patients.[38] Only 12% of the women who suffered a recurrence survived for 5 years.

Verrucous Carcinoma

The use of the term *verrucous carcinoma* should be reserved for those rare vaginal tumors that display the characteristic features described by Ackerman.[2,50] Grossly, they are exophytic, fungating masses with a coarsely granular or undulating surface. Microscopically, the characteristic feature of verrucous carcinoma is the presence of squamous cells with bland cytologic features. At the deep margin of the tumor, the squamous cells invade in a pushing fashion as broad bulbous masses, creating a so-called baggy pants appearance (Fig. 4.46) (See also Fig. 3.26). On the surface of the tumor, hyperkeratosis and acanthosis are common. The distinction of verrucous carcinoma from condyloma or pseudoepitheliomatous hyperplasia may be difficult and may not be possible in a superficial biopsy specimen. Some authors have indicated that verrucous carcinoma does not display the koilocytosis or surface papillae formed of fibrovascular cores covered by squamous cells, which are typical of condylomata or warty carcinomas,[142,167] but other investigators disagree.[67,184] This issue, however, is not of primary importance because the diagnosis rests on the presence of bland cytologic features in the broad bulbous masses of squamous cells at the stromal interface. Verrucous carcinomas display a relatively indolent growth potential, with frequent local recurrence after incomplete excision. Lymph node metastasis occurs rarely, if ever. Because verrucous carcinomas not only are resistant to therapeutic irradiation but actually may transform to conventional squamous carcinoma after radiation therapy, the treatment usually is wide local or radical surgery.[2,165] Tumors with a mixed pattern of both verrucous and conventional squamous carcinomas behave with the aggressiveness of typical squamous cancer and should be classified as such.

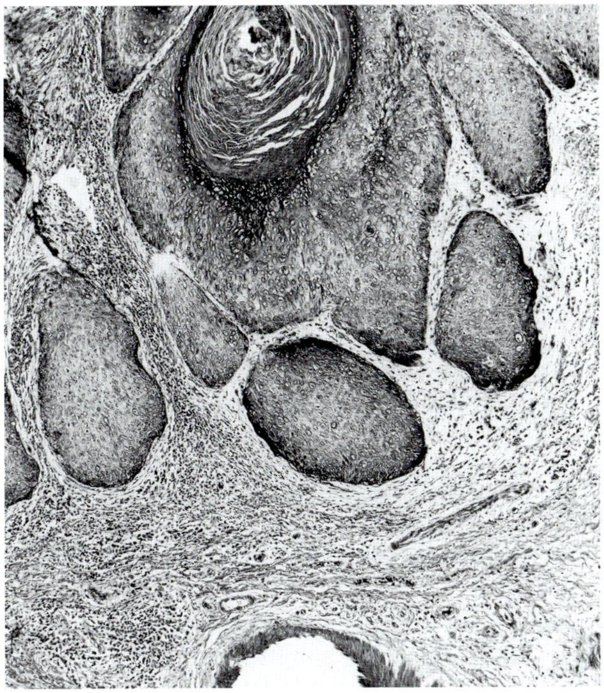

Fig. 4.46. Verrucous carcinoma. The tumor is characterized by a proliferation of cytologically bland squamous cells arranged in broad bulbous masses, which have a smooth interface with the stoma.

Warty Carcinoma

Squamous cell carcinomas in which many of the cells contain nuclear abnormalities and perinuclear cytoplasmic cavitation similar to the koilocytes in intraepithelial neoplasms have been designated *warty carcinoma*. These changes are not typically present in verrucous carcinoma. In addition, warty carcinomas have greater nuclear pleomorphism than verrucous carcinomas, as well as multinucleation, and an infiltrative pattern at the stromal interface. A detailed clinicopathologic analysis of warty carcinomas in the vagina has not been reported. Preliminary data from similar tumors in the vulva indicate that they behave in a low-grade malignant fashion, although metastases to regional lymph nodes occur occasionally (see Chapter 3, Premalignant and Malignant Tumors of the Vulva).[169]

Papillary Squamotransitional Cell Carcinoma

During the past decade, there has been increased recognition that lesions involving the lower genital tract may bear a close resemblance to those arising from urothelium. In addition to transitional cell metaplasia,[351] malignant neoplasms have been reported, primarily in the cervix,[161,255] but with occasional cases originating in the vagina.[13,73,279] The diagnostic terminology has been varied, including *papillary squamous carcinoma, transitional cell carcinoma*, and *mixed squamous* and *transitional* (*squamotransitional*) *cell carcinoma*, reflecting the less than unambiguous histologic features that discriminate such epithelia.[161] Immunohistochemical studies have usually demonstrated the presence of cytokeratin CK-7 and the frequent absence of CK-20 in the papillary genital tract tumors, unlike the profile of transitional cell carcinomas of the urinary bladder, which typically react with both CK-7 and CK-20.[161]

The presenting symptom of papillary squamotransitional cell carcinoma is usually either abnormal bleeding or abnormal cervical–vaginal cytology. The gross tumor configuration is described as papillary, polypoid, or exophytic. The neoplasm is characterized microscopically by the presence of predominantly narrow fibrovascular cores covered by a multilayered epithelium that may resemble either transitional cells, squamous cells, or both. Cytologic atypia is usually present in cells having oval nuclei, with frequent hyperchromasia and the occasional presence of longitudinal intranuclear grooves. Koilocytosis is rare, but mitoses are distributed throughout the epithelium. Often, stromal invasion is not identifiable within the papillae of a superficial biopsy and must be sought at the deeper stromal interface. The invasive component may be identical to either conventional squamous or transitional cell carcinoma and usually elicits a desmoplastic host response.

The biologic behavior remains incompletely defined and has been described as either indolent or similar to that of conventional squamous carcinoma.[161,255] Some of the cases have followed treatment of primary papillary transitional cell carcinomas of the urinary tract or have been associated with transitional cell metaplasia, suggesting the possibility of an extended urogenital field at risk for transitional cell neoplasia.[73]

Clear Cell Adenocarcinoma

General Features

During the 1970s through the 1990s, most cases of vaginal clear cell adenocarcinoma occurred in young women with a documented history of DES exposure in utero. Consequent to the removal of DES from the market for the treatment of high-risk pregnancy in 1971, the exposed population has aged, and fewer DES-associated cases are currently identified in the United States. Data from a national registry in the Netherlands, as well as those from the United States, indicate a bimodal age distribution for clear cell adenocarcinoma.[111,242] The first peak occurred at a mean age of 26 years and the second peak occurred at a mean age of 71 years.[111] None in the older peak had been born during the era of DES use in the Netherlands, whereas about two-thirds of the younger women had a history of DES exposure in utero. Two-thirds of the younger women had clear cell carcinoma of the vagina; two-thirds of the older women had tumors arising in the cervix. Consequently, pathologists should be aware that many of the current cases of clear cell adenocarcinoma of the vagina are diagnosed in older, non-DES-exposed women. Nevertheless, there is concern that, as the DES-exposed cohort ages further, the frequency of clear cell carcinoma may again rise. Because the most exhaustive studies of vaginal clear cell adenocarcinoma have focused on the DES-exposed population, these data are emphasized in the following section.

Slightly more than 700 cases of clear cell adenocarcinoma of the cervix or vagina had been accessioned worldwide by 1999 to the Registry for Research on Hormonal Transplacental Carcinogenesis, with an estimate that about 25–50 new cases develop each year.[123] Approximately 60% of the patients have had documented exposure in utero to DES, hexestrol, or dienestrol; another 12% were exposed to an unknown form of medication, usually for a high-risk pregnancy.

The median age at the time of diagnosis in the DES-exposed U.S. population is 19 years. Although a rare patient has been as young as 7 years of age, only after the age of 14 years does the age–incidence curve rise sharply. It plateaus between ages 17 and 21 years and then declines rapidly. Clear cell adenocarcinoma develops in about 0.014–0.14% of exposed girls and women up to the age of 24 years. The rarity of the neoplasm has been confirmed in multiple studies in which no tumors were encountered among large groups of women specifically examined because of their history of prenatal DES ex-

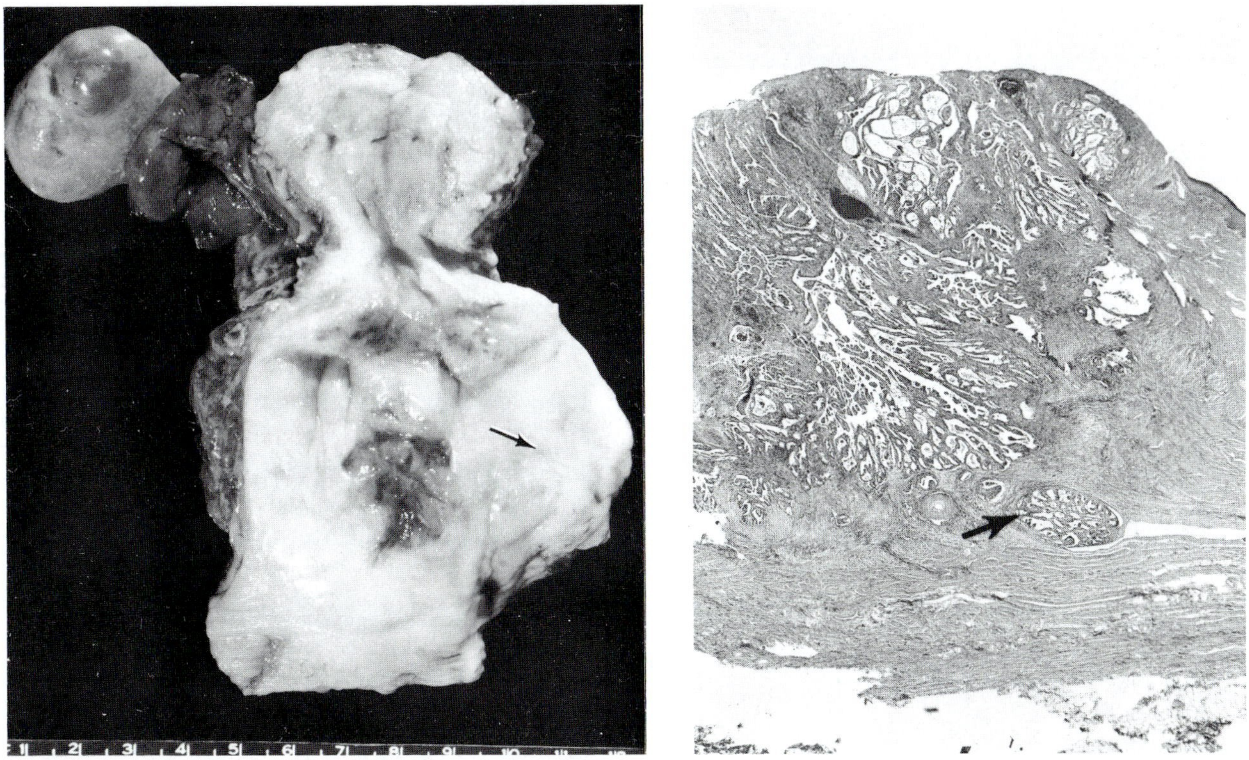

Fig. 4.47. Flat clear cell carcinoma of vagina. *Left*: In addition to tumor, several patches of adenosis (*arrow*) are present in the vagina. Vaginal adenosis and extensive ectropion of the cervix appear red in the fresh state. *Right*: Cross section of the vagina with deeply invasive tumor and vascular invasion (*arrow*).

posure.[218,241] The greatest number of DES-exposed patients with these tumors were born in 1951–1953, the years when the drug was prescribed most frequently for pregnancy support. The risk of tumor development is higher when the drug was started early in pregnancy.

Recent molecular studies have demonstrated a high frequency of microsatellite instability in vaginal clear cell adenocarcinoma.[24] Overexpression of wild-type p53 is also very common, frequently accompanied by a strong expression of BCL-2 and little evidence of apoptosis. These observations suggest that overexpression of BCL-2 can inhibit p53-induced apoptosis.[345,346] Nevertheless, our understanding of DES-mediated carcinogenesis remains incomplete.

Clinical Features

The tumor may involve any portion of the vagina and/or cervix. Approximately 60% of lesions have been confined to the vagina (Fig. 4.47). The remainder have been limited to the cervix or involved both the cervix and vagina. Most vaginal tumors arise on the anterior wall, usually in the upper third, corresponding to the most frequent site of adenosis.

Tumors also have been found on the wall opposite the main tumor, presumably a result of implantation ("kissing lesions"). Unlike the larger tumors, which almost always cause symptoms such as vaginal bleeding or discharge, many small tumors are asymptomatic and have been detected only as more young women have sought examination because of their known exposure to DES.

Gross Findings

Tumors have varied in size from microscopic to large. Most of the larger cancers are polypoid and nodular, but some are flat or ulcerated, having a granular or indurated surface. Small tumors, currently being seen more frequently, usually are palpable. They may be invisible on colposcopic examination if confined to the lamina propria and if covered by intact, normal, or metaplastic squamous epithelium. Although most cancers are superficial and invade only a few millimeters into the vaginal or cervical wall (Fig. 4.48), some penetrate far more deeply or extend more centrifugally than might be anticipated on gross examination.

Microscopic Findings

By light and electron microscopy, the DES-associated clear cell adenocarcinoma is identical to the clear cell adenocarcinoma of the ovary and endometrium, which occur sporadically in older women. Several histologic patterns may be observed, either alone or

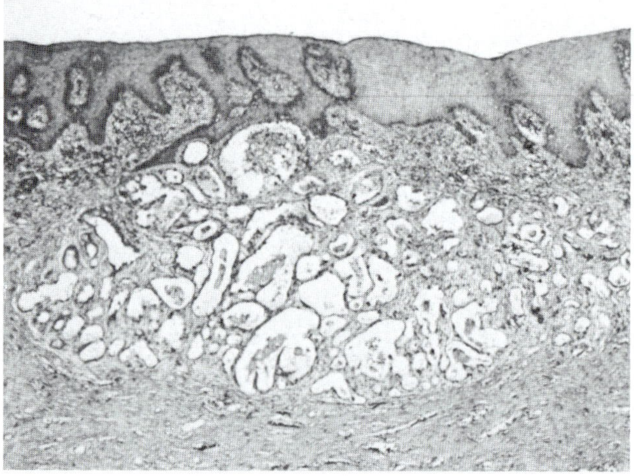

Fig. 4.48. Clear cell carcinoma confined to lamina propria. The tumor is palpable, but cannot be seen with the colposcope.

in combination. A characteristic pattern, for which the tumor is named, consists of solid sheets of clear cells (Fig. 4.49), the clear appearance of the cytoplasm being caused by the dissolution of glycogen when the specimen is processed for microscopic examination. A second (and the most frequent) pattern, the tubulocystic pattern (see Fig. 4.47), is characterized by tubules and cysts lined by hobnail cells, by flat cells, or by cells that resemble müllerian type epithelium to varying degrees. The hobnail cell is characterized by a bulbous nucleus that protrudes into the lumen beyond the apparent cytoplasmic limits of the cell. Flat cells often appear innocuous. When only this type of epithelium is present in a small biopsy it may be difficult to differentiate tumor from adenosis.[288] Less common patterns include a papillary pattern (Fig. 4.50), a tubular pattern resembling endometrial carcinoma (Fig. 4.51) and a pattern composed of cords of cells with eosinophilic cytoplasm (Fig. 4.52). Mitoses usually are rare. In any of these patterns, the lumen may contain mucin. The cytoplasm, however, is mucin free.

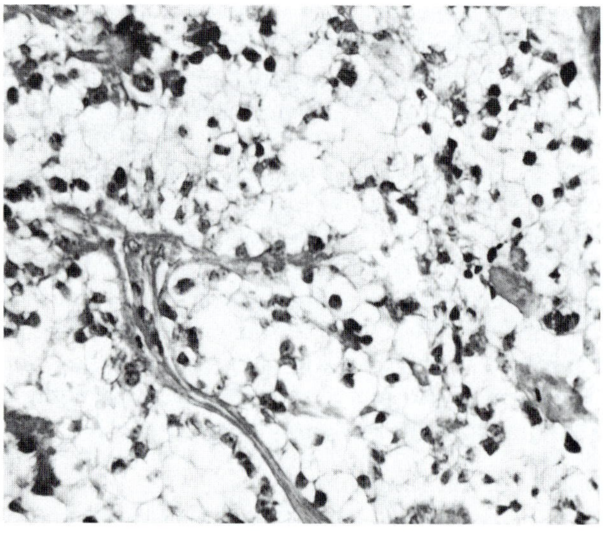

Fig. 4.49. Clear cell carcinoma. Solid pattern of tumor, resembling clear cell carcinoma of ovary and endometrium. (Reprinted by permission of Scully et al. Ann Clin Lab Sci 4:222–233, 1974.)

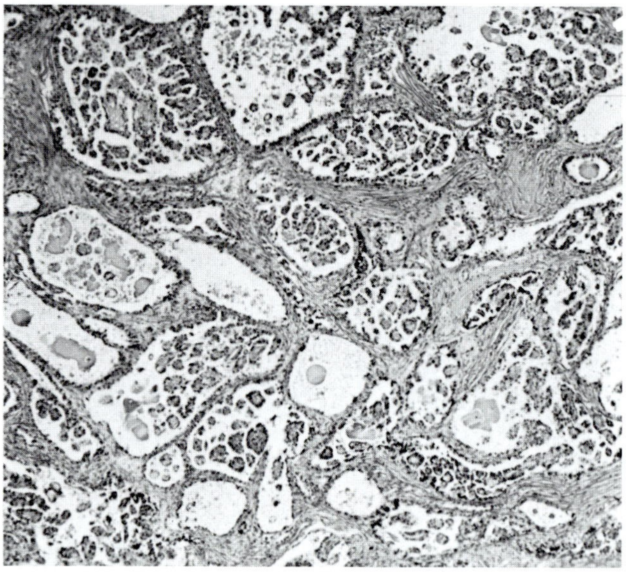

Fig. 4.50. Clear cell carcinoma. Papillary pattern of tumor.

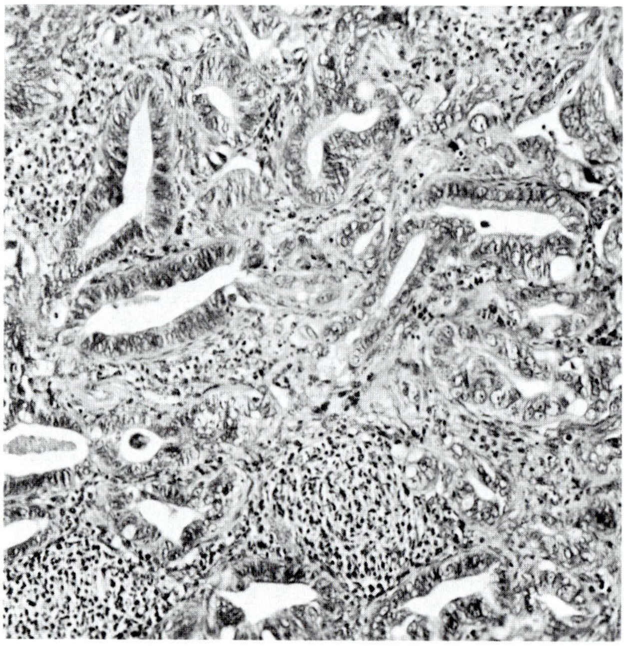

Fig. 4.51. Clear cell carcinoma. The tumor is composed of tubules lined by stratified columnar cells resembling endometrial carcinoma. This is a very rare pattern.

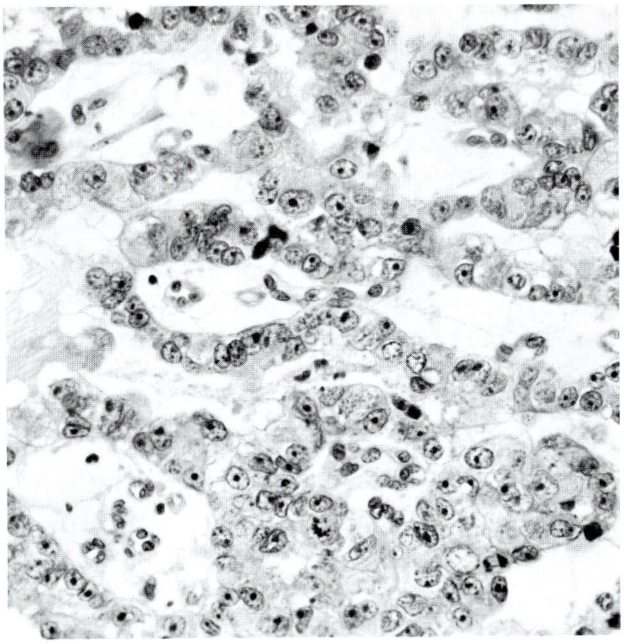

Fig. 4.52. Clear cell carcinoma. Cords and solid masses of cell with deeply eosinophilic cytoplasm and nuclei with prominent nucleoli. This is a rare pattern.

Atypical adenosis, characterized by glands with cellular stratification, nuclear pleomorphism, hyperchromasia, and prominent nucleoli (Fig. 4.53), has been identified near the periphery of most clear cell carcinomas in which the excised vagina has been serially blocked for microscopic examination.

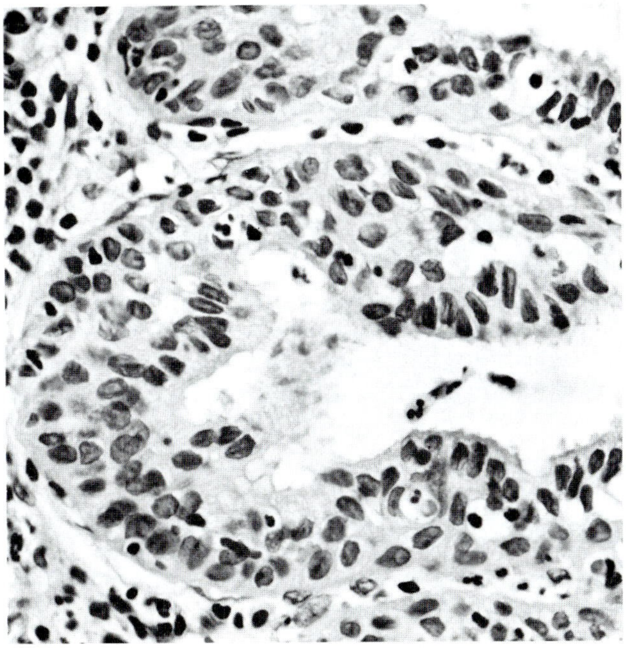

Fig. 4.53. Atypical adenosis. Nuclei vary both in size and shape; cells are stratified.

Atypical cells with nuclei that are larger and more irregular in outline than those seen in normal endocervical cells or the cells lining the glands of the adenosis have been identified in approximately 0.5% of cervical and vaginal smears from DES-exposed women.[265,270] The frequent finding of the tuboendomentrial type of glandular cell and the rarity of the mucinous type of cell adjacent to the tumors suggest that the clear cell adenocarcinoma arises from the tuboendometrial cells.[273,274] The studies of nuclear DNA content show that (1) atypical forms of tuboendometrial-type cells may have an aneuploid pattern, (2) tuboendometrial cells demonstrate greater proliferative activity (more often in a tetraploid state) than do endocervical-type cells, and (3) polyploid patterns are associated with active-appearing vaginal adenosis. However, there has been no case yet in which, over time, microscopically proven atypical adenosis has progressed to carcinoma and, consequently, proof that atypical adenosis is a precursor of clear cell carcinoma is lacking.

Differential Diagnosis

Microglandular hyperplasia is a benign condition that can resemble adenocarcinoma on gross and microscopic examination. Usually associated with the use of oral contraceptives or occasionally with pregnancy, it is rarely observed in their absence. Although microglandular hyperplasia almost always develops in the cervix, cases also have been described arising in foci of vaginal adenosis. Most of the young women had histories of exposure prenatally to DES.[272] Initially, the lesions were misinterpreted as a clear cell adenocarcinoma. Grossly, the lesion is soft, granular, tan yellow, and usually flat (Fig. 4.54). Microscopic examination demonstrates many small, closely packed glands devoid of intervening stroma (see Chapter 6, Benign Diseases of the Cervix). The presence of extensive nests of metaplastic squamous cells with pale eosinophilic cytoplasm may make the lesion difficult to distinguish from the solid pattern of clear cell carcinoma. A clue to the diagnosis is the presence of clefts lined by mucinous epithelium that course through the metaplastic squamous epithelium. The lesion generally is reversed when oral contraceptives are discontinued.

The Arias–Stella reaction (see Chapter 9, Anatomy and Histology of the Uterine Corpus) usually occurs in pregnant women and must be distinguished from clear cell adenocarcinoma. Although usually seen in the endometrium, the Arias–Stella reaction has been observed occasionally in vaginal adenosis of the tuboendometrial type. Characteristically, hypersecretory glands are lined by cells with markedly enlarged nuclei resembling hobnail cells. However, in clear cell adenocarcinoma, the presence of sheets

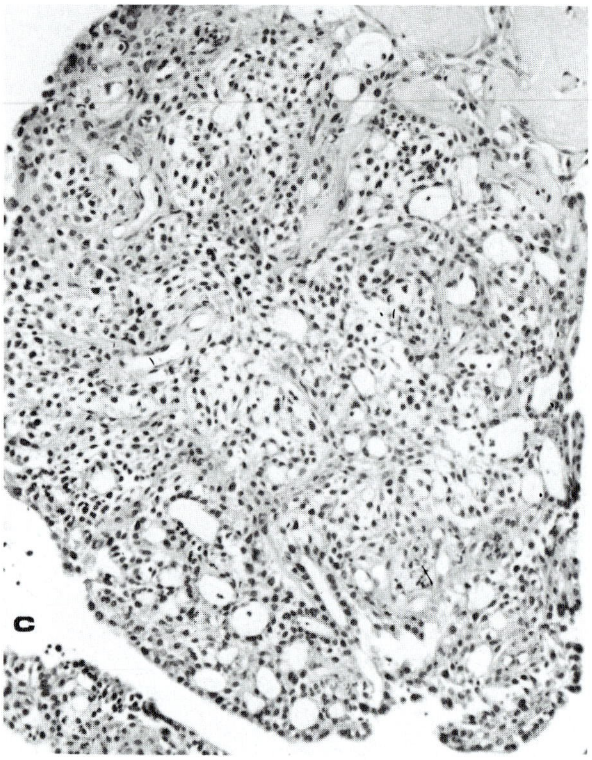

Fig. 4.54. Microglandular hyperplasia. Nests composed largely of metaplastic squamous cells. (Reprinted by permission of Robboy et al., ref. 272.)

of clear cells or prominent papillae should enable the two lesions to be distinguished. In addition, the hobnail-like nuclei in the Arias–Stella reaction commonly are smudged, lack mitotic activity, and appear to be degenerative.

Clinical Behavior and Treatment

The tumor spreads locally and also metastasizes via lymphatics and blood vessels. Approximately one-sixth of tumors confined clinically to the vagina or cervix (stage I) are discovered on exploration to have metastasized to the pelvic lymph nodes. The frequency of nodal involvement reaches approximately 50% when stage II tumors are considered. Clear cell carcinoma extends outside the abdominal cavity more frequently than does squamous cell carcinoma of the vagina or cervix. Thirty-six percent of the initial recurrences of clear cell carcinomas are in the lung or a supraclavicular lymph node, in contrast to less than 10% for squamous cell carcinomas.

The 5-year actuarial survival rates for all patients with clear cell adenocarcinoma is high. It is about 93% at 5 years and 87% at 10 years when the tumor is stage I.[119] When tumors cause no symptoms or are discovered during the course of an examination because of a history of DES exposure, survival with appropriate therapy approaches 100%. Other factors associated with a better prognosis are an older age (19 years or older) at the time of diagnosis and a tubulocystic microscopic pattern. Large size and/or deep invasion into the wall are associated with a poorer prognosis, but small or superficial tumors also may recur or metastasize. The presence of aneuploidy appears to have no effect on prognosis,[352] but nuclear atypia may be associated with a worse prognosis.[110] Pregnancy at the time of diagnosis does not appear to affect outcome adversely.[289] Recurrences develop most often within 3 years after primary therapy; however, recurrences as late as 19 years after treatment have been observed.[29] After treatment of the recurrence, approximately one-fifth of the patients survive an additional 3 years or more.

The prognosis for women with clear cell adenocarcinoma who have known exposure to DES in utero is significantly better than for those who have no history of DES exposure (5-year survival rates of 84% and 69%, respectively).[344] Although some of this difference could reflect earlier detection in the intensively screened exposed population, the survival advantage persists even when the comparison is adjusted for stage of disease. Metastases to the lungs or supraclavicular lymph nodes are more frequent in the non-DES-exposed group.

Embryonal Rhabdomyosarcoma (Sarcoma Botryoides)

General Features

The most common malignant neoplasm of the vagina in infants and children is *embryonal rhabdomyosarcoma*, most of which are of the subtype designated *sarcoma botyroides*.[47,49,213] Nearly 90% of cases are diagnosed before 5 years of age.[49,79] This is a rare tumor of unknown etiology and pathogenesis. Certainly the distribution of embryonal rhabdomyosarcomas does not correlate with the mass of skeletal muscle, as most of these neoplasms arise in or near the mucosa of either the head and orbit or the lower urogenital system.

Clinical Features

The mean age at diagnosis is 2 years, with a range extending from birth to 41 years.[79] Most children present with symptoms of a vaginal mass or bleeding. The tumors usually are located along the anterior wall of the vagina, and appear as papillae, small nodules, or pedunculated or sessile soft, polypoid masses with an intact overlying mucosa. Larger tumors may protrude through the introitus (Fig. 4.55). The tumors usually are staged according to a modification of the Intergroup Rhabdomyosarcoma Study (IRS) classification, which is based on combined features of extent of disease, resectibility, and

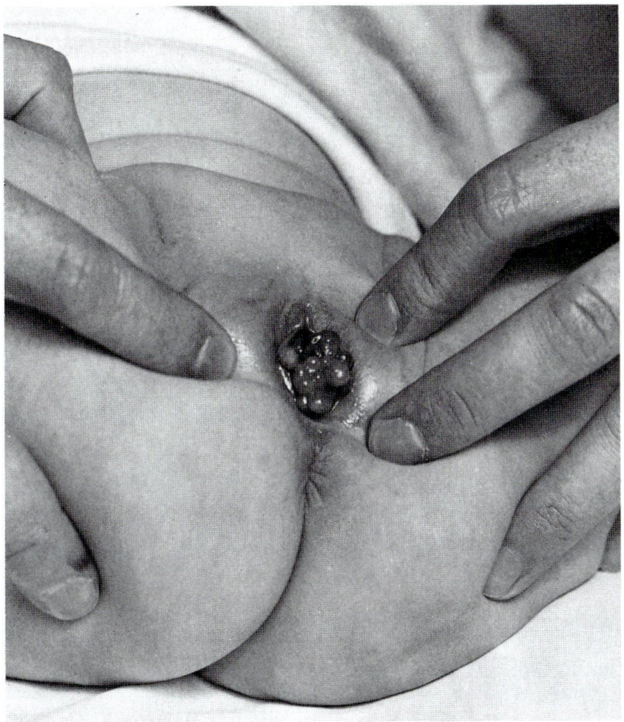

Fig. 4.55. Sarcoma botryoides of the vagina. The gross appearance is that of a polypoid mass protruding through the vaginal introitus and resembling a bunch of grapes. (Reprinted by permission of Hilgers R. Malkasian GD Jr, Soule EH (1970) Embryonal rhabdomyosarcoma (botyroid type) of the vagina: A clinicopathologic review. Am J Obstet Gynecol 107:484.)

microscopic evaluation of margins of excision (Table 4.3).

Gross Findings

Soft gray or tan, edematous, and nodular tumors are typical. The polypoid gross configuration is thought to result from relatively unrestricted growth into the lumen of a hollow organ (Fig. 4.56).

Microscopic Findings

The distinction of sarcoma botryoides from the spindle or nonspecialized variants of embryonal rhabdomyosarcoma is based on the presence of a cambium tumor cell layer underlying an intact epithelium in at least one microscopic field.[253] The cambium layer is defined as the condensed subepithelial layer of rhabdomyoblasts that are scattered in a loose myxoid or dense collagenous stroma (Fig. 4.57). The term *cambium* was chosen as an analogy to the peripheral, actively growing layer in tree trunks and branches, which it mimics at a microscopic level. The histologic criteria are more important in establishing the diagnosis than the gross demonstration of a polypoid or "grapelike" pattern of tumor growth. The cells in the cambium layer often are polyhedral, with little discernible cytoplasm, but extensive rhabdomyoblastic differentiation, with a spindled configuration of tumor cells, may predominate in this or other portions of the tumor. The tumor cells are of round to spindle shape, with oval nuclei, an open chromatin pattern, and inconspicuous nucleoli.[331]

Focal evidence of rhabdomyogenesis may be evident in any of the patterns, with eosinophilic cytoplasm containing fibers in which cross-striations are present (Fig. 4.58). However, in cases that lack such features, ultrastructural examination is useful for identification of both thick and thin fibrils, and occasionally Z bands.[85] Immunohistochemical staining with antibodies directed against muscle-specific actin, desmin, or myoglobin also may be helpful in establishing the diagnosis.[10,28,69,167,253] Although the first two antibodies are more sensitive than myoglobin, they are not specific for skeletal muscle differentiation. It is important not to be misled to the erroneous diagnosis of melanoma by the presence of immunoreactivity for S-100 protein, which has been reported in about 20% of cases of rhabdomyosarcoma.[253]

Table 4.3. International classification of rhabdomyosarcoma[a]

Diagnosis	*Histology*	*Incidence (all sites) (%)*[b]	*Five-year survival (%)*	*Prognosis*
Embryonal, botryoid	Favorable	6	95	Superior
Embryonal, spindle cell	Favorable	3	88	Superior
Embryonal, not otherwise specified (NOS)	Favorable	49	66	Intermediate
Alveolar, NOS or solid variant	Unfavorable	31	53	Poor
Anaplasia, diffuse	Unfavorable	2	45	Poor
Undifferentiated sarcoma	Unfavorable	3	44	Poor

[a]With the addition of IRSG-defined anaplastic variant.
[b]Total incidence is only 94%; some 6% of accepted cases fall into the sarcoma NOS category because of insufficient or inadequate tissue to make a more specific diagnosis.

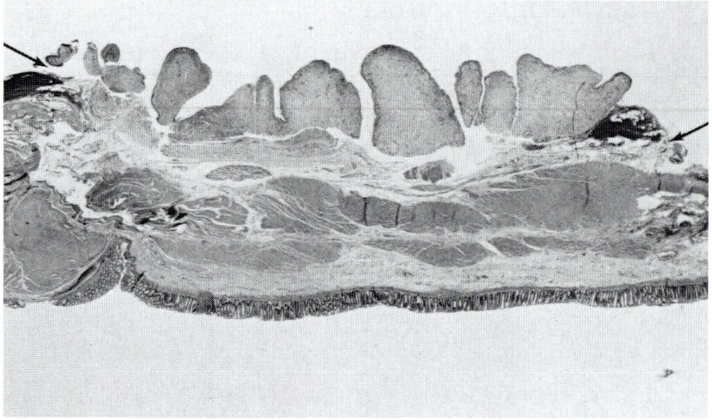

Fig. 4.56. Sarcoma botryoides of the rectovaginal septum. Note the polypoid appearance of the tumor outlined by *arrows*.

The differential diagnosis includes fibroepithelial polyps, müllerian papillomas, and rhabdomyomas. The correct diagnosis can be made by considering the age at presentation and the microscopic features as described above. After radiation or chemotherapy, occasionally there is difficulty in determining whether scattered mature-appearing skeletal muscle fibers represent residual tumor cells that are refractory to therapy, or radiated benign muscle fibers of the pelvis. A recent study suggests that differentiation occurs more frequently with the botryoid variant of rhabdomyosarcoma following therapy and that it is associated with a favorable outcome.[45]

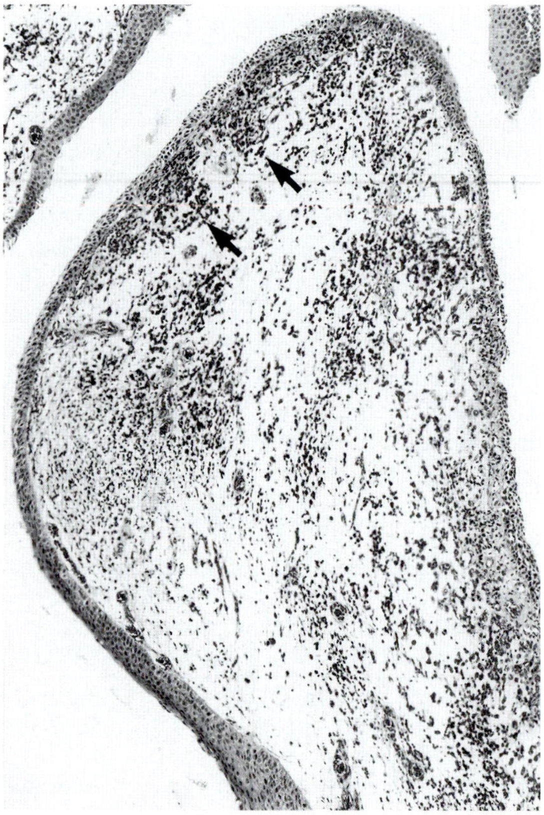

Fig. 4.57. Embryonal rhabdomyosarcoma, botryoid type. The cambium layer is recognized as a condensed subepithelial layer of rhabdomyoblasts that are scattered in a loose myxoid or dense collagenous stroma.

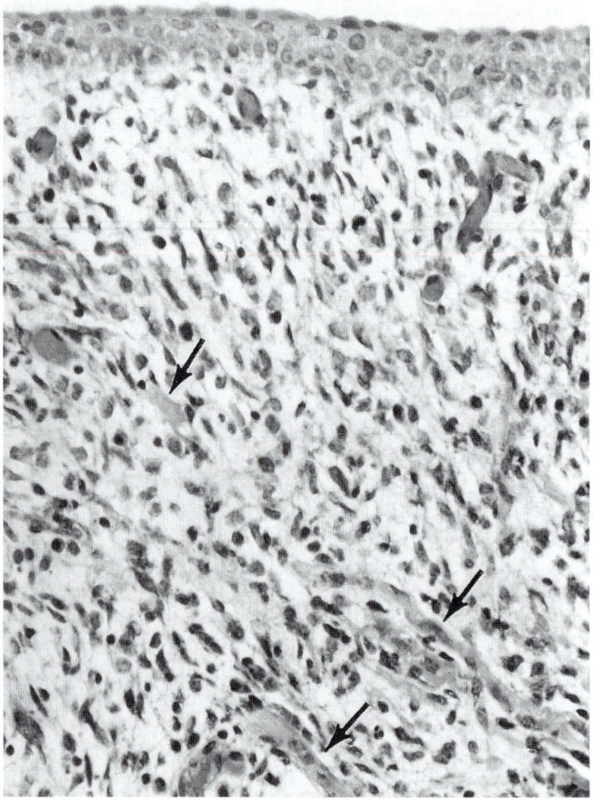

Fig 4.58. Embryonal rhabdomyosarcoma, botryoid type. In contrast to the vaginal rhabdomyoma, the embryonal rhabdomyosarcoma contains densely cellular regions composed of small primitive cells. Interspersed strap cells (*arrows*) confirm the skeletal muscle differentiation.

Clinical Behavior and Treatment

The tumor initially grows into the vaginal wall and soft tissue of the pelvis, bladder, or rectum and subsequently metastasizes to lymph nodes, lungs, liver, and bone. Historically, the prognosis after radical surgery was poor, with survival rates of less than 20%.[44] The introduction of combined multiagent chemotherapy with vincristine and actinomycin, in addition to surgery, has dramatically improved the probability of survival.[44,213]

A consensus classification of rhabdomyosarcoma, based upon a review of 800 cases from all anatomic sites from the Intergroup Rhabdo-myosarcoma Study, was published in 1995 (see Table 4.3).[253] This classification, coupled with other prognostic factors including primary site, clinical group (Table 4.4), and tumor size, represents an advance in the prediction of survival. Fortunately, the botryoid type, the variant of embryonal rhabdomyosarcoma found most frequently in the vagina, has a superior prognosis, with a survival rate of 95%. The spindle cell variant, which is more common in the paratesticular region, shares a favorable prognosis although survival drops to 66% for the nonspecialized embryonal rhabdomyosarcoma.[253] Other recent studies confirm the relatively favorable outcome for vaginal rhadomyosarcoma, with a 90% or greater survival rate.[116a,204]

Table 4.4. Intergroup Rhabdomyosarcoma Clinical Group stage system for rhabdomyosarcoma

Clinical group		*Extent of disease/surgical result*
I	A	Localized tumor, confined to site of origin, completely resected
	B	Localized tumor, infiltrating beyond site of origin, completely resected
II	A	Localized tumor, gross total resection, but with microscopic residual disease
	B	Locally extensive tumor (spread to regional lymph nodes), completely resected
	C	Locally extensive tumor (spread to regional lymph nodes), gross total resection, but microscopic residual disease
III	A	Localized or locally extensive tumor, gross residual disease after biopsy only
	B	Localized or locally extensive tumor, gross residual disease after major resection (>50% debulking)
IV		Any size primary tumor, with or without regional lymph node involvement, with distant metastases, without respect to surgical approach to primary tumor

Melanoma

General Features

More than 155 cases of vaginal melanoma have been reported, representing less than 5% of the malignant neoplasms of the vagina and less than 1% of all melanomas.[49,60,94,140,238] The mean age at diagnosis is 57 years, with a range from 22 to 83 years.[177,238] Presenting symptoms include vaginal bleeding, discharge, and a mass. Although the tumors may arise anywhere within the vagina, there is a predilection for the distal third.[37] The etiology and pathogenesis are unknown, but a disproportionately large number of vaginal melanomas have occurred in Japanese women, followed in frequency by Caucasian and then black women.[37,49,177] In one autopsy study, melanocytes were identified in the basal layer of the vagina of 3 of 100 women.[214] It has been suggested that such a condition, referred to as *benign melanosis*, is the setting from which melanoma occasionally may arise,[113] and we have seen localized regions of melanosis in the vagina remote from melanomas. Unfortunately, the term *melanosis* also has been used to designated melanophages in the stroma and lentigo malignum-like lesions in mucosal tissues, further obscuring interpretation of the scant available literature.

Gross Findings

Melanomas may appear as nodular, polypoid, or fungating gray or black soft masses that vary from 0.5 to 8 cm in diameter.[37,181] Frequently, there is ulceration of the overlying epithelium.

Microscopic Findings

Vaginal melanomas have no microscopic characteristics that are distinctive for this site. The diagnosis usually rests on a constellation of features. In addition to junctional activity, the presence of highly atypical melanocytes, either singly or in clusters, extending through the squamous epithelium is common (Fig. 4.59). The infiltrating neoplastic cells may be epithelioid, spindled, or mixed (Fig. 4.59 and 4.60). Melanin is common within both neoplastic melanocytes and benign melanophages. The lateral spread is typically of the lentiginous type, with single, spindled cells containing pleomorphic nuclei at the epithelial-stromal interface.[37] Rarely, a pagetoid junctional component consisting of epithelioid melanocytes in nests is present.[37]

Because Clark's levels are not appropriate for mucosal sites of melanoma, a system based entirely on tumor thickness has been proposed by Chung et al., as follows: level I, tumor confined to the surface epithelium; level II, invasion of 1 mm or less; level III, invasion of 1–2 mm; and level IV, invasion greater

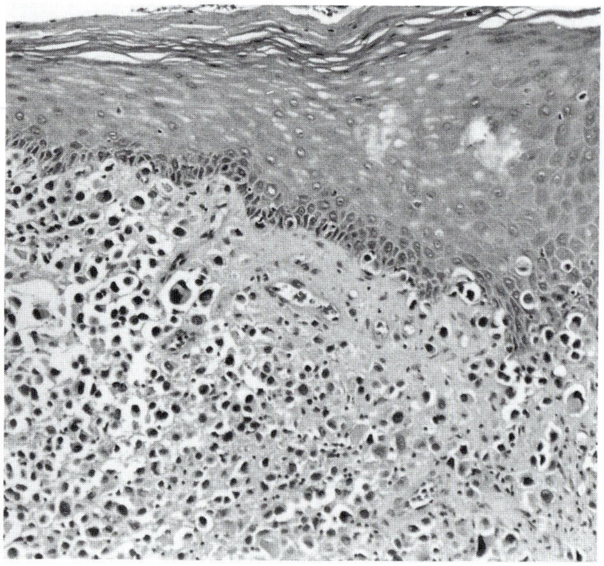

Fig. 4.59. Melanoma. Junctional involement (right side of field) is frequently identified peripheral to ulcerated or intact central region of deep stromal invasion in primary vaginal melanomas.

than 2 mm.[37] Unfortunately, most of the tumors are deeply invasive. In a group of 19 patients, only 1 was at level III; the remainder were at level IV.[37]

Differential Diagnosis

The diagnosis usually is straightforward as most vaginal melanomas are large, with gross and microscopic pigmentation. The differential diagnosis may include melanoma metastatic from other sites, poorly differentiated squamous carcinoma, sarcoma, and blue nevus. Because primary vaginal melanoma is rare, it is important to rule out metastasis from other sites. The presence of an extensive lateral junctional component is typical in melanomas arising in the vagina but relatively uncommon in metastases. A complete history is essential, and some cases can be confirmed only by postmortem examination. When large ulcerated lesions are devoid of pigment, immunohistochemistry and ultrastructural examination may permit discrimination of melanoma from other poorly differentiated neoplasms. Positive staining of malignant cells with antibodies directed against S-100 protein is a sensitive, but not specific, marker of melanocytic or neural differentiation. HMB-45 is a less-sensitive but more-specific indicator of melanoma, and staining for keratin or desmin should be absent. Ultrastructural findings include premelanosomes and melanosomes, as well as abundant rough and smooth endoplasmic reticulum.[113] A high degree of nuclear atypia and numerous mitotic figures usually permit discrimination of melanoma from the rare benign vaginal nevus.

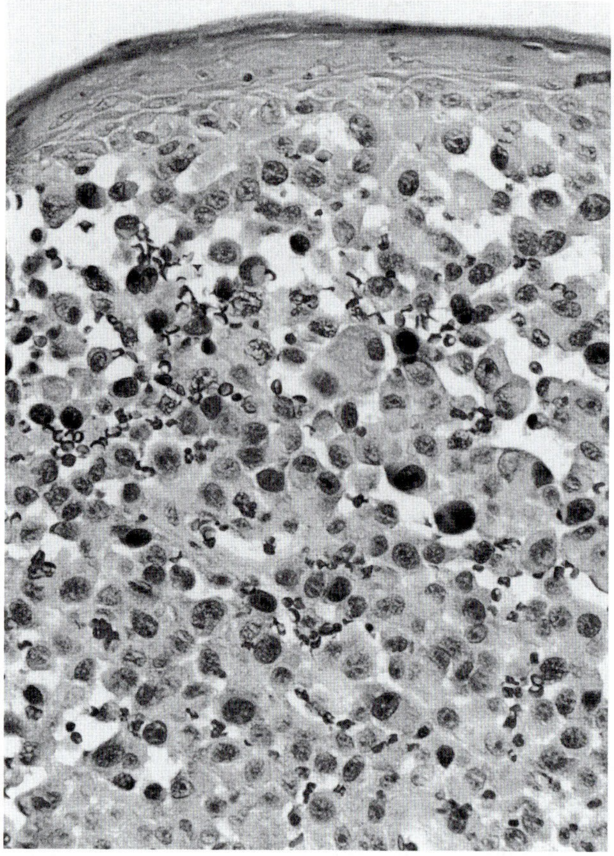

Fig. 4.60. Melanoma. The neoplastic cells may be of polyhedral or spindle configuration and may be confused in routinely stained sections with either squamous carcinoma or sarcoma, particularly if the overlying epithelium is ulcerated. Immunohistochemistry can help to resolve the diagnosis.

Clinical Behavior and Treatment

The prognosis for vaginal melanoma is poor, with 5-year survival rates of less than 10–20%.[37,49,177,350] Undoubtedly, this reflects the inherent aggressiveness of melanoma coupled with the typically deep invasion found at the time of diagnosis.[37,49,60,259] In one study, survival was inversely related to the mitotic activity.[21] Both lymphatic and hematogenous metastases are common, with the vagina and groin being the most common initial sites of spread. Primary therapy usually includes radical local excision, although pelvic exenteration has been suggested as treatment for tumors greater than 3 mm in thickness. The value of groin node dissection, radiation, and chemotherapy remains unknown.[177,231]

Yolk Sac Tumor

Although the *yolk sac tumor* (*endodermal sinus tumor* [*EST*]) usually arises in the gonads, about 57 cases have been reported in the vagina.[41] It is appealing to

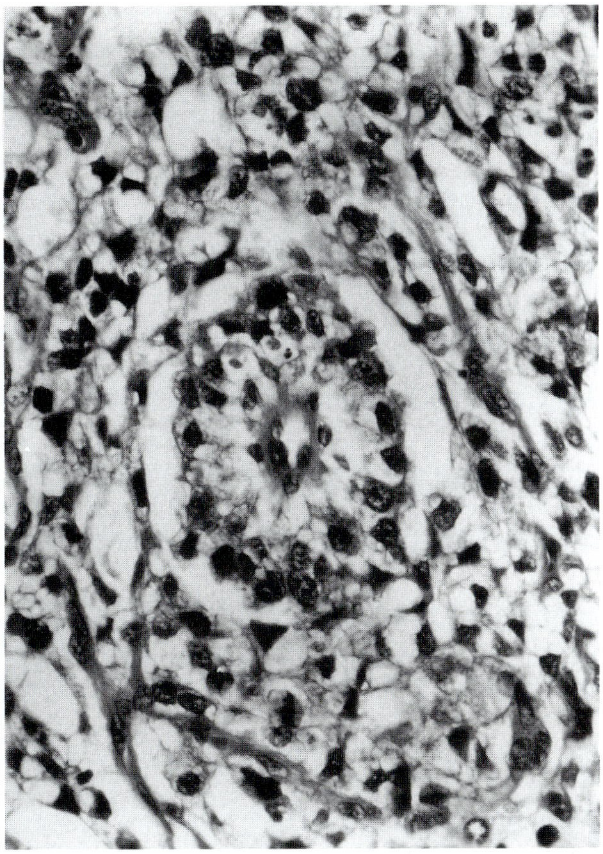

Fig. 4.61. Yolk sac tumor. The centrally located Schiller-Duval body is charactreized by a papillary arrangement of columnar cells separated from a central vascular core by a zone of acellular connective tissue. (Courtesy of Henry J. Norris, M.D., Washington, DC.)

consider that these tumors originate from germ cells that have failed to complete migration normally in the embryo from the hindgut to the gonad. However, this hypothesis does not provide an obvious explanation for the absence of other malignant germ cell tumors in the vagina, or the predilection of EST for the vagina.

Most vaginal ESTs have been diagnosed in children less than 4 years of age. The presenting symptom usually is a bloody vaginal discharge. The gross and microscopic features of vaginal EST closely resemble those of ovarian origin. Polypoid or sessile, soft, tan or white vaginal masses 1–5 cm in diameter are typical.[167] A variety of histologic patterns may be present including the microcystic, reticular, papillary, and solid types of EST. Schiller–Duval bodies, composed of papillary arrangements of columnar cells separated from central vascular channels by an acellular zone of connective tissue, are characteristic findings (Fig. 4.61). Extracellular hyaline droplets also are common. Although the histologic findings usually are typical, the diagnosis may not be considered initially because of the rarity of EST in the vagina. The differential diagnosis includes clear cell adenocarcinoma, from which EST may be distinguished by the younger age and positive immunohistochemical reactions for alpha-fetoprotein and alpha-1-antitrypsin.[359]

EST is an extremely aggressive tumor. In the past, the median survival was 11 months, and the survival rate at 5 years was less than 25%.[46,231] Most patients developed recurrence and died within 2 years, even after radical surgery.[46,167] The addition of multiagent chemotherapy, usually consisting of vincristine, actinomycin, and cyclophosphamide, since 1970 has resulted in a 95% disease-free survival at 2 years.[5,46,359] Preliminary data suggest that combination chemotherapy and conservative surgery may permit preservation of future sexual function and fertility as well as an excellent cure rate.[231]

Leiomyosarcoma

About 65 *leiomyosarcomas* of the vagina have been reported.[49,53,234] The frequency and behavior have been difficult to establish because the pathologic criteria separating benign from malignant smooth muscle tumors have varied. Currently, it is recommended that smooth muscle tumors of greater than 3 cm diameter, with five or more mitotic figures per 10 HPFs, moderate or marked cytologic atypia, and infiltrating margins be classified as leiomyosarcoma (Fig. 4.62).[319] The age range extends from 25 to 86 years. Vaginal bleeding is the most common presenting symptom. The gross and microscopic features resemble those of uterine leiomyosarcoma, but the spread of tumor is by local invasion and hematogenous metastasis. The 5-year survival rate is about

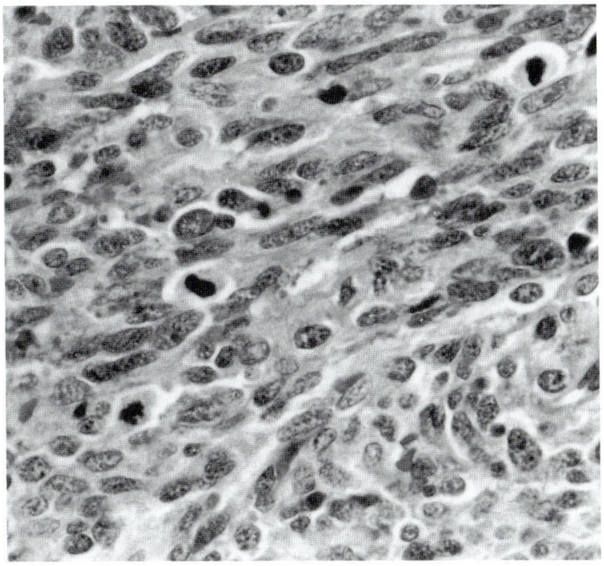

Fig. 4.62. Vaginal leiomyosarcoma. The tumor resembles that of uterine origin, with fascicles of spindle cells having moderate or marked nuclear pleomorphism with increased mitotic activity.

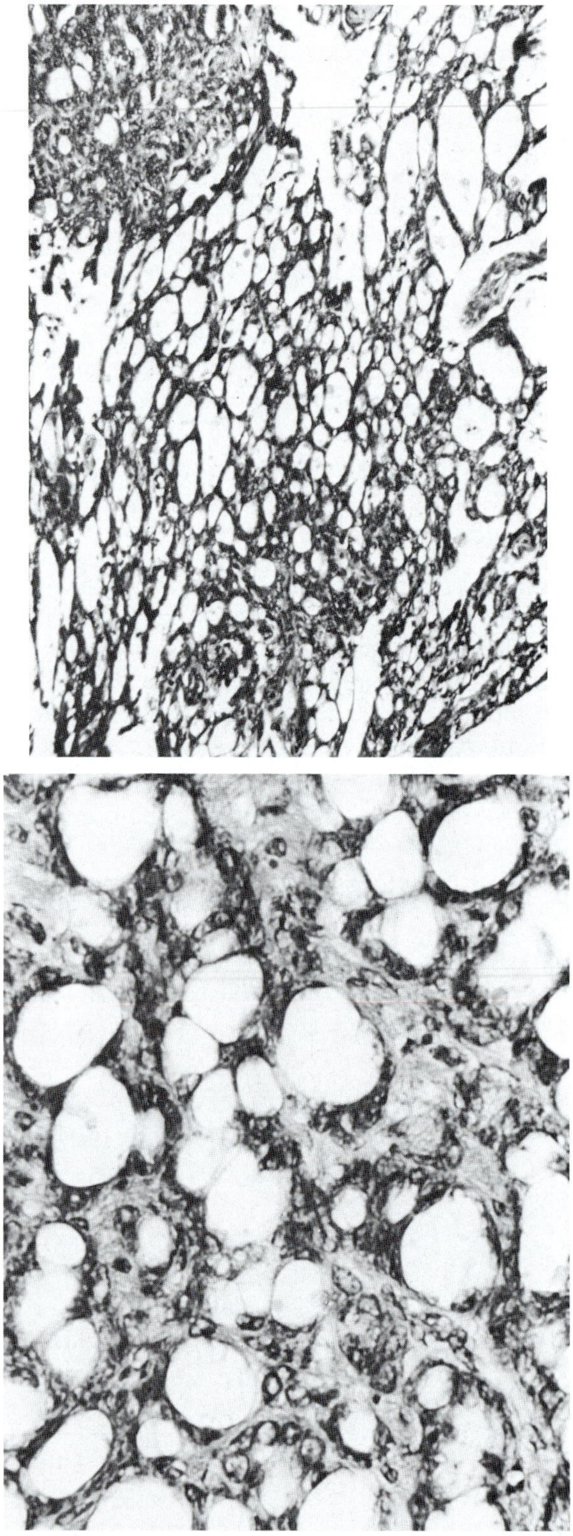

Fig. 4.63. **Malignant tumor of the vagina resembling synovial sarcoma.** *Top*: In this area, the tumor is predominantly acinar. Mucin stains showed positive reactions in inspissated material in lumina and in some of the cells. *Bottom*: High-power view of the acini. The nuclei of cells are prominent, whereas cytoplasmic borders are indistinct. (Reprinted by permission of Okagaki et al., ref. 222.)

35%, and the stage of the disease is the most important prognostic indicator.[234] The primary therapy is surgical, and exenteration may be required to provide an adequate margin around larger tumors.

Malignant Mixed Tumor

Probably unrelated to the benign vaginal mixed tumor is the reportedly *malignant mixed tumor*, which resembles either synovial sarcoma or a malignant tumor arising from mesonephric rests.[222,292,316] Two of these rare tumors occurred in women 24 and 33 years old, who presented with a polypoid nodule in the lateral vaginal fornix. The microscopic appearance is of an intact vaginal squamous mucosa with a subjacent mixture of solid nests of polyhedral-shaped cells and flattened epithelial cells in acinar or tubular arrays, bordered peripherally by smaller bundles of spindle cells resembling fibro-blasts (Fig. 4.63). Ultrastructural features resembling synovial sarcoma were noted in one case.[222,292] The presence of mitotic activity as great as eight mitoses per 10 HPFs coupled with nuclear pleomorphism and moderate-sized nucleoli suggested that the process was malignant. How-

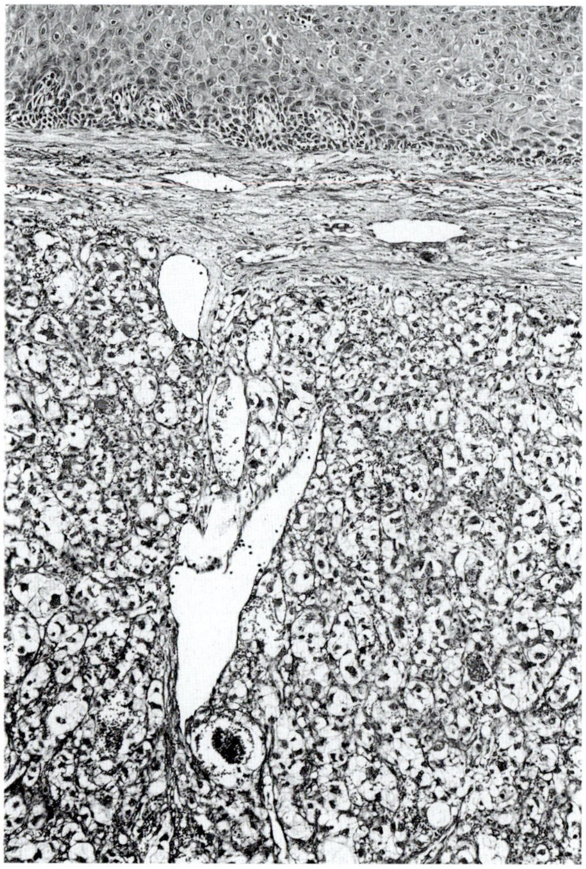

Fig. 4.64. Metastatic renal cell carcinoma. Solid masses of polygonal cells with clear cytoplasm are separated from each other by delicate fibrovascular septa.

ever, the biologic potential remains uncertain in the absence of long-term follow-up.

Secondary Neoplasms

Although primary neoplasms of the vagina are quite rare, *secondary spread of malignant neoplasms* to the vagina by direct extension or lymphatic or hematogenous metastasis is quite common. Fu and Reagan found that only 58 (16%) of 355 invasive carcinomas involving the vagina represented primary neoplasms.[85] Spread from primary carcinoma of the cervix was most common (32%), followed by endometrium (18%), colon and rectum (9%), ovary (6%), vulva (6%), and urinary tract (4%). Even among the squamous carcinomas found in the vagina, only a minority prove to be primary to this site. About 75% are secondary, arising in either the cervix (79%) or vulva (14%).[85]

About 70 cases of vaginal metastases from renal cell carcinoma have been reported (Fig. 4.64).[318,330,357] Metastases from clear cell carcinoma of the kidney may be very difficult to distinguish histologically from primary clear cell carcinoma of the vagina. This difficulty is complicated by the observation that in some instances the identification of the metastatic lesion has preceded the diagnosis of the renal tumor.[330] A young age, history of DES exposure in utero, prior or concurrent vaginal adenosis, and foci of neoplastic clear cells with a tubulocystic or papillary architecture are features that favor a vaginal primary, whereas older age and regions of granular, cytoplasm or sarcomatoid differentiation are more common in tumors which originate in the kidney. In rare cases, the histologic distinction of clear cell carcinoma of the vagina from a renal metastasis may be impossible.

Miscellaneous Malignant Neoplasms

Endometrioid adenocarcinomas, stromal sarcomas, and *malignant mixed müllerian tumors* occasionally originate in the vagina, at times arising from a background of endometriosis (Fig. 4.65).[101,210,234] In addition, there are occasional reported cases of primary vaginal adenocarcinoma in situ,[40] intestinal-type adenocarcinoma,[83] adenosquamous carcinoma,[262,290,308] adenocarcinoma arising in mesonephric duct remnants,[130,361] adenoid basal cell carcinoma,[209] adenoid cystic carcinoma (Fig. 4.66),[167]

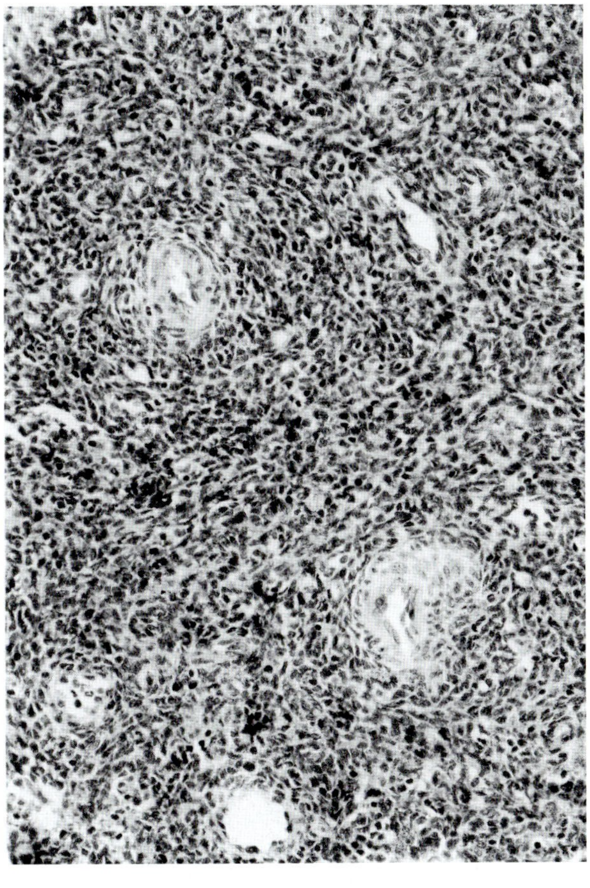

Fig 4.65. Low-grade endometrial stromal sarcoma. This tumor is characterized by a dense mass of compact cells with oval nuclei, coarse chromatin, inconspicuous nucleoli, and scant cytoplasm. A stromal matrix is not apparent, but small-caliber arteries and arterioles are often abundant.

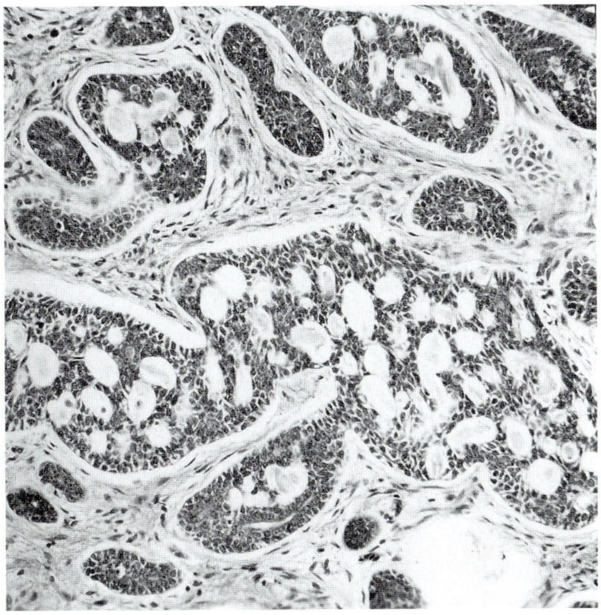

Fig. 4.66. Adenoid cystic carcinoma of the vagina. The tumor resembles that found in the uterine cervix, with solid and cribriform arrangements of well-delineated cell masses. (Courtesy of Henry J. Norris, M.D., Washington, DC.)

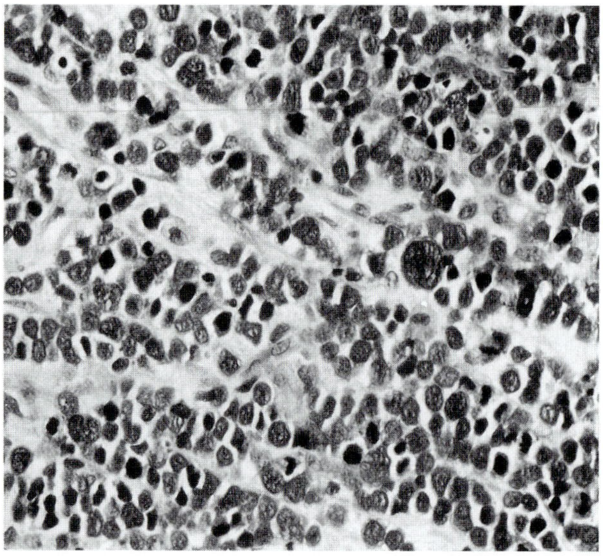

Fig. 4.67. Small cell carcinoma of the vagina. The tumor shares histologic features with small cell carcinomas arising elsewhere. The cell of origin remains unknown. (Reprinted by permission of Kurman et al., ref. 167.)

carcinoid tumor,[88] small cell carcinoma (Fig. 4.67),[145,247] malignant schwannoma,[58] fibrosarcoma,[225] malignant fibrous histiocytoma,[348] angiosarcoma,[249,329] alveolar soft part sarcoma.[31,170]

References

1. Abdul-Karim FW, Lederman MM, Carter JR, et al (1981) Toxic shock syndrome: clinicopathologic findings in a fatal case. Hum Pathol 12:16–22
2. Ackerman LV (1948) Verrucous carcinoma of the oral cavity. Surgery (St. Louis) 23:670–678
3. Al-Durdi M, Monaghan JM (1977) Thirty-two years experience in management of primary tumors of the vagina. Br J Obstet Gynecol 127:513
4. Amsel R, Totten PA, Spiegel CA, et al (1983) Nonspecific vaginitis: diagnostic criteria and microbial and epidemiologic associations. Am J Med 74:14–22
5. Anderson WA, Sabio H, Durso N, et al (1985) Endodermal sinus tumor of the vagina. The role of primary chemotherapy. Cancer (Phila) 56:1025–1027
6. Andrew DE, Bumstead K, Kempton AG (1975) The role of fomites in the transmission of vaginitis. Can Med Assoc J 112:1181–1183
7. Antonioli DA, Burke L, Friedman EA (1980) Natural history of diethylstilbestrol-associated genital lesions: cervical ectopy and cervicovaginal hood. Am J Obstet Gynecol 137:847
8. Averette HE, Weinstein GD, Frost P (1970) Autoradiographic analysis of cell proliferation kinetics in human genital tissues. I. Normal cervix and vagina. Am J Obstet Gynecol 108:8–17
9. Bacon HE, Ross ST, Malvar P (1972) Sigmoidovaginal and cecovaginal fistula as a complication of peridiverticulitis: Report of eight cases. Dis Colon Rectum 15:41–48
10. Bale PM, Parsons RE, Stevens MM (1983) Diagnosis and behavior of juvenile rhabdomyosarcoma. Hum Pathol 14:596–611
11. Barry W, Hudgins L, Donta ST, Pesanti EL (1992) Intravenous immunoglobulin therapy for toxic shock syndrome. JAMA 267:3315–3316
12. Bartlett JG, Onderdonk AB, Drude E, et al (1977) Quantitative bacteriology of the vaginal flora. J Infect Dis 136:271–277
13. Bass P, Birch B, Smart C, Theaker J, Wells M (1994) Low grade transitional cell carcinoma of the vagina—an unusual cause of vaginal bleeding. Histopathology (Oxf) 24:581–583
14. Beecham CT (1980) Classification of vaginal relaxation. Am J Obstet Gynecol 136:957–958
15. Bell DA, Mondschein M, Scully RE (1986) Giant cell arteritis of the female genital tract. A report of three cases. Am J Surg Pathol 10:696–701
16. Benedet JL, Sanders BH (1984) Carcinoma in situ of the vagina. Am Obstet Gynecol 148:695–700
17. Bennett HG, Ehrlich HM (1941) Myoma of the vagina. Am J Obstet Gynecol 42:314
18. Bergdoll MS, Reiser RF, Crass BA, et al (1981) A new staphylococcal enterotoxin, enterotoxin F, associated with toxic-shock-syndrome staphylococcus aureus isolates. Lancet 1:1017–1021
19. Berger BJ, Kolton S, Zenilman JM, Cummings MC, Feldman J, McCormack WM (1995) Bacterial vaginosis in lesbians: a sexually transmitted disease. Clin Infect Dis 21(6):1402–1405
20. Boquet-Jiménez E, Alvarez San Cristóbal A (1978) Cytologic and microbiologic aspects of vaginal torulopsis. Acta Cytol 22:331–334
21. Borazjani G, Prem KA, Okagaki T, et al (1990) Primary malignant melanoma of the vagina: a clinicopathological analysis of 10 cases. Gynecol Oncol 37:264–267
22. Bornstein J, Adam E, Adler-Storthz K, Kaufman RH (1988) Development of cervical and vaginal squamous cell neoplasia as a late consequence of in utero exposure to diethylstilbestrol. Obstet Gynecol Surv 43:15–21
23. Bornstein J, Sova Y, Atad J, Lurie M, Abramovici H (1993) Development of vaginal adenosis following combined 5-fluorouracil and carbon dioxide laser treatments for diffuse vaginal condylomatosis. Obstet Gynecol 81(5 pt 2):896–898
24. Boyd J, Takahashi H, Waggoner SE, et al (1996) Molecular genetic analysis of clear cell adenocarcinomas of the vagina and cervix associated and unassociated with diethylstilbestrol exposure in utero. Cancer (Phila) 77(3):507–513
25. Bramley M, Kinghorn G (1979) Do oral contraceptives inhibit *Trichomonoas vaginalis*? Sex Transm Dis 6:261–263
26. Branton PA, Tavassoli FA (1993) Spindle cell ep-

ithelioma, the so-called mixed tumor of the vagina. Am J Surg Path 17:509–515
27. Brinton LA, Nasca PC, Mallin K, et al (1990) Case-control study of in situ and invasive carcinoma of the vagina. Gynecol Oncol 38:49
28. Brooks JJ (1982) Immunohistochemistry of soft tissue tumors. Myoglobin as a tumor marker for rhabdomyosarcoma. Cancer 50:1757
29. Burks RT, Schwarz AM, Wheeler JE, Antoniolli D (1990) Late recurrence of clear cell adenocarcinoma of the cervix: Case report. Obstet Gynecol 76:525–527
30. Carinelli SG, Carinelli I, Merlo D-N (1984) Mucinous cysts of the vulva. Cervix 2:143–148
31. Chapman GW, Benda JO, Williams T (1984) Alveolar soft part sarcoma of the vagina. Gynecol Oncol 18:125–129
32. Charles V, Charles SX (1978) A case of vulvo-vaginal diphtheria in a girl of seven years. Indian J Pediatr 15:257–258
33. Chen KTK (1981) Brenner tumor of the vagina. Diagn Gynecol Obstet 3:255
34. Chirayil SJ, Tobon H (1981) Polyps of the vagina: a clinicopathologic study of 18 cases. Cancer (Phila) 47:2904–2907
35. Chu SY, Berkelman RL, Curran JW (1992) Epidemiology of HIV in the United States. In: DeVita VT, Hellman S, Rosenberg SA (eds) AIDS: Etiology, diagnosis, treatment, and prevention. Lippincott, Philadelphia, pp 99–109
36. Chu Y, Curran J (1997) Epidemiology of human immunodeficiency virus infection in the United States. In: DeVita V Jr, Hellman S, Rosenberg S (eds) AIDS: biology, diagnosis, treatment and prevention, 4th Ed. Lippincott-Raven, Philadelphia, pp 137–145
37. Chung AF, Casey MJ, Flannery JT, et al (1980) Malignant melanoma of the vagina: report of 19 cases. Obstet Gynecol 55:720–727
38. Chyle V, Zagars GK, Wheeler JA, Wharton JT, Delclos L (1996) Definitive radiotherapy for carcinoma of the vagina: outcome and prognostic factors. Int J Radiat Oncol Biol Phys 35(5):891–905
39. Clark JFJ, Faggett T, Peters B, Sampson CC (1978) Ulcerative vaginitis due to torulopsis glabrata: a case report. J Natl Med Assoc 70:913–914
40. Clement PB, Benedet JL (1979) Adenocarcinoma in situ of the vagina. A case report. Cancer (Phila) 43:2479–2485
41. Clement PB, Young RH, Scully RE (1988) Extraovarian pelvic yolk sac tumors. Cancer (Phila) 62:620–626
42. Clemetson D, Moss G, Willerford D (1993) Detection of HIV DNA in cervical and vaginal secretions. JAMA 269:2860–2863
43. Coetzee LF (1972) Tuberculous vaginitis. South Afr Med J 46:1225–1226
44. Coffin CM, Dehner LP (1992) The soft tissue. In: Stocker JT, Dehner LP (eds) Pediatric pathology, vol 2. Lippincott, Philadelphia, pp 1091–1132
45. Coffin C, Rulon J, Smith L, Bruggers C, White F (1997) Pathologic features of rhabdomyosarcoma before and after treatment: a clinicopathologic and immunohistochemical analysis. Mod Pathol 10:1175–1187
46. Copeland LJ, Sneige N, Ordonez NG (1985) Endodermal sinus tumor of the vagina and cervix. Cancer (Phila) 55:2558–2565
47. Copeland LJ, Sneige N, Stringer CA, et al (1985) Alveolar rhabdomyosarcoma of the female genitalia. Cancer (Phila) 56:849–855
48. Cramer DW, Cutler SJ (1974) Incidence and histopathology of malignancies of the female genital organs in the United States. Am J Obstet Gynecol 118:443–460
49. Creasman WT, Phillips JL, Menck HR (1998) The National Cancer Data Base report on cancer of the vagina. Cancer (Phila) 83(5):1033–1040
50. Crowther ME, Lowe DG, Shepherd JH (1988) Verrucous carcinoma of the female genital tract: a review. Obstet Gynecol Surv 43:263–280
51. Cunha GR (1975) The dual origin of vaginal epithelium. Am J Anat 143:387–392
52. Cunha GR, Taguchi O, Namikawa R, et al (1987) Teratogenic effects of clomiphene, tamoxifen, and diethylstilbestrol on the developing human female and genital tract. Hum Pathol 18:1132–1143
53. Curtin JP, Saigo P, Slucher B, Venkatraman ES, Mychalczak B, Hoskins WJ (1995) Soft-tissue sarcoma of the vagina and vulva: a clinicopathologic study. Obstet Gynecol 86(2):269–272
54. Curtis EM, Pine L (1981) Actinomyces in the vaginas of women with and without intrauterine contraceptive devices. Am J Obstet Gynecol 140:880–884
55. Davis TC (1975) Chronic vulvovaginitis in children due to *Shigella flexneri*. Pediatrics 56:41–44
56. Davis JP, Chesney PJ, Wand PJ, LaVenture M (1980) Toxic-shock syndrome. Epidemiologic features, recurrence, risk factors, and prevention. N Engl J Med 303:1429–1435
57. Davis JD, Connor EE, Clark P, Wilkinson EJ, Duff P (1997) Correlation between cervical cytologic results and Gram stain as diagnostic tests for bacterial vaginosis. Am J Obstet Gynecol 177(3):532–535
58. Davos I, Abell MR (1976) Sarcomas of the vagina. Obstet Gynecol 47(3):342–350
59. Dekel A, Avidan D, Bar-ziv J, et al (1988) Neurofibroma of the vagina presenting with urinary retention. Review of the literature and report of a case. Obstet Gynecol Surv 43:325–327
60. De Matos P, Tyler D, Seigler HF (1998) Mucosal melanoma of the female genitalia: a clinicopathologic study of forty-three cases at Duke University Medical Center. Surgery (St. Louis) 124(1): 38–48
61. De Meo LR, Draper DL, McGregor JA, et al (1996) Evaluation of a deoxyribonucleic acid probe for the detection of *Trichomonas vaginalis* in vaginal secretions. Am J Obstet Gynecol 174(4):1339–1342

62. Deppisch LM (1975) Cysts of the vagina: classification and clinical correlations. Obstet Gynecol 45:632–637
63. Dickersin GR, Welch WR, Erlandson R, Robboy SJ (1980) Ultrastructure of 16 cases of clear cell adenocarcinoma of the vagina and cervix in DES-exposed young women. Cancer (Phila) 45:1615.
64. Dixit S, Singhal S, Baboo HA (1993) Squamous cell carcinoma of the vagina: A review of 70 cases. Gynecol Oncol 48:80–87
65. Droegemueller W, Herbst AL, Mishell DR Jr, Stenchever MA (1987) Comprehensive gynecology. Mosby, St. Louis, p 974
66. Dungar C, Wilkinson E (1995) Vaginal columnar cell metaplasia. An acquired adenosis associated with topical 5-fluorouracil therapy. J Reprod Med 40(5):361–366
67. Dvoretsky PM, Bonfiglio TA (1986) The pathology of vulvar squamous cell carcinoma and verrucous carcinoma. In: Sommers SC, Rosen PP, Fechner RE (eds) Pathology annual, part 2, vol 21. Appleton-Century-Crofts, Norwalk, pp 23–45
68. Elliott GB, Elliott JDA (1973) Superficial stromal reactions of lower genital tract. Arch Pathol 95: 100–101
69. Eusebi V, Ceccarelli C, Gorza L, et al (1986) Immunocytochemistry of rhabdomyosarcoma. The use of four different markers. Am J Surg Pathol 10:293
70. Fallon RJ, Robinson ET (1974) Meningococcal vulvovaginitis. Scand J Infect Dis 6:295–296
71. Farrand RJ (1971) *Haemophilus influenzae* infections of the genital tract. J Med Microbiol 4:357–358
72. Faulconer HT, Muldoon JP (1975) Rectovaginal fistula in patients with colitis: review and report of a case. Dis Colon Rectum 18:413–415
73. Fetissof F, Haillot O, Lanson Y, Arbeille B, Lansac J (1990) Papillary tumor of the vagina resembling transitional cell carcinoma. Pathol Res Pract 186: 358–364
74. Fish SA (1956) Vaginal injury due to coitus. Am J Obstet Gynecol 72:544–548
75. Fliegner JR (1987) Congenital atresia of the vagina. Surg Gynecol Obstet 165:387–391
76. Forsberg J-G (1973) Cervicovaginal epithelium: Its origin and development. Am J Obstet Gynecol 7:1025–1043
77. Fox H, Wells M, Harris M, et al (1988) Enteric tumors of the lower female genital tract: a report of three cases. Histopathology (Oxf) 12:167–176
78. Friedell S, Mercer LJ (1986) Nonmenstrual toxic shock syndrome. Obstet Gynecol Surv 41:336–341
79. Friedman M, Peretz BA, Nissenbaum M, Paldi E (1986) Modern treatment of vaginal embryonal rhabdomyosarcoma. Obstet Gynecol Surv 41:614–618
80. Friedrich EG (1981) Tampon effects on vaginal health. Clin Obstet Gynecol 24:395–406
81. Friedrich EG (1985) Vaginitis. Am J Obstet Gynecol 152:247–251
82. Friedrich EG, Siegesmund KA (1980) Tampon-associated vaginal ulcerations. Obstet Gynecol 55: 149–156
83. Frick HC, Jacox HW, Taylor HC (1968) Primary carcinoma of the vagina. Am J Obstet Gynecol 101:695–703
84. Fu YS, Reagan JW (1989) Pathology of the uterine cervix, vagina, and vulva. Saunders, Philadelphia, pp 193–224
85. Fu YS, Reagan JW (1989) Pathology of the uterine cervix, vagina, and vulva. Saunders, Philadelphia, pp 336–379
86. Fujimoto V, Miller J, Klein N, Soules M (1997) Congenital cervical atresia: report of seven cases and review of the literature. Am J Obstet Gynecol 177(6):1419–1425
87. Fukunaga M, Endo Y, Ishikawa E, Ushigome S (1996) Mixed tumour of the vagina. Histopathology (Oxf) 28(5):457–461
88. Fukushima M, Twiggs LB, Okagaki T (1986) Mixed intestinal adenocarcinoma-argentaffin carcinoma of the vagina. Gynecol Oncol 23:387–394
89. Gallup DC, Nolan TE, Martin D, et al (1991) Thrombotic thrombocytopenic purpura first seen as massive vaginal necrosis. Am J Obstet Gynecol 165:413–415
90. Gardner HL (1966) Cervical and vaginal endometriosis. Clin Obstet Gynecol 9:358–372
91. Gardner HL (1980) *Haemophilus vaginalis* vaginitis after twenty-five years. Am J Obstet Gynecol 137:385–391
92. Gardner HL, Fernet P (1964) Etiology of vaginitis emphysematosa. Report of ten cases and review of literature. Am J Obstet Gynecol 88:680–694
93. Geelhoed GW, Henson DE, Taylor PT, et al (1976) Carcinoma in situ of the vagina following treatment for carcinoma of the cervix. A distinctive clinical entity. Am J Obstet Gynecol 124:510
94. Geisler JP, Look KY, Moore DA, Sutton GP (1995) Pelvic exenteration for malignant melanomas of the vagina or urethra with over 3 mm of invasion. Gynecol Oncol 59(3):338–341
95. Gelfand M, Ross MD, Blair DM, Weber MC (1972) Distribution and extent of schistosomiasis in female pelvic organs, with special reference to the genital tract, as determined at autopsy. Am J Trop Med Hyg 20:846–849
96. Giacomini G, Calcinai A, Moretti D, Cristofani R (1998) Accuracy of cervical/vaginal cytology in the diagnosis of bacterial vaginosis. Sex Transm Dis 25(1):24–27
97. Giusti RM, Iwamoto K, Hatch EE (1995) Diethylstilbestrol revisited: a review of the long-term health effects. Ann Intern Med 122(10):778–788
98. Gold JH, Bossen EH (1976) Benign vaginal rhabdomyoma. A light and electron microscopic study. Cancer (Phila) 37:2283–2294

99. Gompel C, Silverberg SG (1977) Pathology in gynecology and obstetrics. Lippincott, Philadelphia.
100. Goodman A, Zukerberg LR, Nikrui N, Scully RE (1991) Vaginal adenosis and clear cell carcinoma after 5-fluorouracil treatment for condylomas. Cancer (Phila) 68(7):1628–1632.
101. Goyert G, Budev H, Wright C, et al (1987) Vaginal müllerian stromal sarcoma. A case report. J Reprod Med 32:129–130
102. Graber B, Kline-Graber G (1979) Female orgasm: role of pubococcygeus muscle. J Clin Psychiatry 40:348–351
103. Graham-Brown RAC, Cochrane GW, Swinhoe JR, et al (1981) Vaginal stenosis due to bullous erythema multiforme (Stevens-Johnson syndrome). Br J Obstet Gynaecol 88:1156–1157
104. Grant TD, Mace KD (1977) Quantitation of secretory immunoglogulin A in vaginal secretions. J Am Coll Health 26:81–84
105. Greenhalf JO (1972) Vaginal vault granulation tissue following total abdominal hysterectomy. Br J Clin Pract 26:247–249
106. Gregoire AT, Kandil O, Ledger WJ (1971) The glycogen content of human vaginal epithelial tissue. Fertil Steril 22:64–68
107. Gompel C, Silverberg SG (1985) Pathology in gynecology and obstetrics, 3rd Ed. Lippincott, Philadelphia.
108. Guillou L, Gloor E, De Grandi P, Costa J (1989) Postoperative pseudosarcoma of the vagina. A case report. Pathol Res Pract 185:245–248
109. Hafez ESE (1977) The vagina and human reproduction. Am J Obstet Gynecol 129:573–584
110. Hanselaar AG, Van Leusen ND, De Wilde PCM, Vooijs GP (1991) Clear cell adenocarcinoma of the vagina and cervix. A report of the Central Netherlands Registry with emphasis on early detection and prognosis. Cancer (Phila) 67(7):1971–1978
111. Hanselaar A, van Loosbroek M, Schuurbiers O, Helmerhorst T, Bulten J, Bernhelm J (1997) Clear cell adenocarcinoma of the vagina and cervix. An update of the Central Netherlands registry showing twin age incidence peaks. Cancer (Phila) 79(11):2229–2236
112. Hartmann C-A, Sperling M, Stein H (1990) So-called fibroepithelial polyps of the vagina exhibiting an unusual but uniform antigen profile characterized by expression of desmin and steroid hormone receptors but no muscle-specific actin or macrophage markers. Am J Clin Pathol 93:604–608
113. Hasumi K, Sakamoto G, Sugano H, et al (1978) Primary malignant melanoma of the vagina. Study of four autopsy cases with ultrastructural findings. Cancer (Phila) 42:2675–2686
114. Hauser AR (1998) Another toxic shock syndrome. Streptococcal infection is even more dangerous than the staphylococcal form. Postgrad Med 104(6):31–34, 39, 43–44
115. Heine RP, Wiesenfeld HC, Sweet RL, Witkin SS (1997) Polymerase chain reaction analysis of distal vaginal specimens: a less invasive strategy for detection of *Trichomonas vaginalis*. Clin Infect Dis 24(5):985–987
116. Heinz KPW (1973) Amoebic infection of the female genital tract. A report of three cases. South Afr Med J 47:1795–1798
116a. Hays DM, Shimada H, et al (1985) Sarcomas of the vagina and the uterus: The Intergroup Rhabdomyosarcoma Study. J Pediatr Surg 20:718
117. Helms CM, Lengeling RW, Pinsky RL, et al (1981) Toxic shock syndrome: a retrospective study of 25 cases from Iowa. Am J Med Sci 282:50–60
118. Henson D, Tarone R (1977) An epidemiologic study of cancer of the cervix, vagina, and vulva based on the Third National Cancer Survey in the United States. Am J Obstet Gynecol 129:525–532
119. Herbst AL (1992) Vaginal clear cell cancer: incidence, survival and screening. In: Long-term effects of exposure to diethylstilbestrol (DES) (NIH Workshop), April 23–24. Falls Church, VA, pp 19–20
120. Herbst AL, Anderson S, Hubby MM, et al (1986) Risk factors for the development of diethylstilbestrol-associated clear cell adenocarcinoma: a case-control study. Am J Obstet Gynecol 154:814–822
121. Herbst AL, Poskanzer DC, Robboy SJ, et al (1975) Prenatal exposure to stilbestrol: a prospective comparison of exposed female offspring with unexposed control. N Engl J Med 292:334
122. Herbst AL, Ulfelder H, Poskanzer DC (1971) Adenocarcinoma of the vagina: association of maternal stilbestrol therapy with tumor appearance in young women. N Engl J Med 284:878
123. Herbst AL (2000) Behavior of estrogen-associated female genital tract cancer and its relation to neoplasia following intrauterine exposure to diethylstilbestrol (DES). Gynecol Oncol 76:147–156
124. Hidayat AA, Riddle PJ (1987) Ligneous conjunctivitis: a clinicopathologic study of 17 cases. Ophthalmology 94:949–959
125. Hilgers RD, Malkasian GD Jr, Soule EH (1970) Embryonal rhabdomyosarcoma (botryoid type) of the vagina: a clinicopathologic review. Am J Obstet Gynecol 107:484
126. Hill HR (1984) Group B streptococal infections. In: Holmes KK, Mårdh P-A, Sparling PF, Wiesner PJ (eds) Sexually transmitted diseases. McGraw-Hill, New York, pp 397–407
127. Hillier SL, Critchlow CW, Stevens CE, et al (1991) Microbiological, epidemiological and clinical correlates of vaginal colonisation by *Mobiluncus* species. Genitourin Med 67:26–31.
128. Hillier SL, Kiviat NB, Hawes SE, et al (1996) Role of bacterial vaginosis-associated microorganisms in endometritis. Am J Obstet Gynecol 175(2):435–441
129. Hilton AL, Warnock DW (1975) Vaginal candidiasis and the role of the digestive tract as a source of infection. Br J Obstet Gynaecol 82:922–926

130. Hinchey WM, Silva EG, Guarda LA, et al (1983) Paravaginal wolffian duct (mesonephros) adenocarcinoma: a light and electron microscopic study. Am J Clin Pathol 80:539–544
131. Hingorani V, Mahapatra LN (1964) Amebiasis of vagina and cervix. J Int Coll Surg 42:662–667
132. Hoffkes HG, Schumann A, Uppenkamp M, et al (1995) Primary non-Hodgkin's lymphoma of the vagina. Case report and review of the literature. Ann Hematol 70(5):273–276
133. Holst E, Goffeng AR, Andersch B (1994) Bacterial vaginosis and vaginal microorganisms in idiopathic premature labor and association with pregnancy outcome. J Clin Microbiol 32(1):176–186
134. Hood M. Janney A, Dameron G (1961) Beta hemolytic streptococcus group B associated with problems of the perinatal period. Am J Obstet Gynecol 82:809
135. Hoogkamp-Korstanje JAA, Gerrards LJ, Cats BP (1982) Maternal carriage and neonatal acquisition of group B streptococci. J Infect Dis 145:800–803
136. Hopkins MP, Morley GW (1987) Squamous cell carcinoma of the neovagina. Obstet Gynecol 69: 525–527
137. Horowitz BJ, Edelstein SW, Lippman L (1985) *Candida tropicalis* vulvovaginitis. Obstet Gynecol 66:229–232
138. Hummer WK, Mussey E, Decker DG, Dockerty MB (1970) Carcinoma in situ of the vagina. Am J Obstet Gynecol 108:1109–1116
139. Hurley R, Leask B, Faktor JA, de Fonseka CJ (1973) Incidence and distribution of yeast species and of trichomonas vaginalis in the vagina of pregnant women. J Obstet Gynaecol Br Commonw 80:252
140. Irvin WP Jr, Bliss SA, Rice LW, Taylor PT Jr, Andersen WA (1998) Malignant melanoma of the vagina and locoregional control: radical surgery revisited. Gynecol Oncol 71(3):476–480
141. Iversen UM (1996) Two cases of benign vaginal rhabdomyoma. Case reports. APMIS 104(7-8): 575–578
142. Japaze H, Dinh TV, Woodruff JD (1982) Verrucous carcinoma of the vulva: study of 24 cases. Obstet Gynecol 60:462–466
143. Jaszczak S, Hafez ESE (1978) The vagina and infertility. In: Hafez ESE, Evans TN (eds) The human vagina. Elsevier/North-Holland, Amsterdam, p 223
144. Jimerson SD, Becker JD (1980) Vaginal ulcers associated with tampon usage. Obstet Gynecol 56: 97–99
145. Joseph RE, Enghardt MH, Doering DL, et al (1992) Small cell neuroendocrine carcinoma of the vagina. Cancer (Phila) 70:784–789
146. Joesoef MR, Schmid GP (1995) Bacterial vaginosis: review of treatment options and potential clinical indications for therapy. Clin Infect Dis 20(1):S72–S79
147. Jorup-Ronstrom C, Hofling M, Lundberg C, Holm S (1996) Streptococcal toxic shock syndrome in a postpartum woman. Case report and review of the literature. Infection 24(2):164–167
148. Josey WE. Campbell WG (1990) Vaginitis emphysematosa. J Reprod Med 35:974–977
149. Kahn HJ, Yeger H, et al (1983) Immunohistochemical and electron microscopic assessment of childhood rhabdomyosarcoma: increased frequency of diagnosis over routine laboratory methods. Cancer (Phila) 51:1897
150. Kalogirou D, Antoniou G, Karakitsos P, Botsis D, Papadimitriou A, Giannikos L (1997) Vaginal intraepithelial neoplasia (VAIN) following hysterectomy in patients treated for carcinoma in situ of the cervix. Eur J Gynaecol Oncol 18(3):188–191
151. Kanbour AI, Klionski B, Murphy AI (1974) Carcinoma of the vagina following cervical cancer. Cancer (Phila) 34:1838–1841
152. Kaufman RH (1980) The origin and diagnosis of "nonspecific vaginitis." N Engl J Med 303:637–638
153. Kaufman RH, Friedrich EG, Gardner HL (1989) Atrophic, desquamative, and postradiation vulvovagnitis. In: Benign diseases of the vulva and vagina, 3rd Ed. Year Book, Chicago, pp 419–434
154. Kaufman RH, Friedrich EG, Gardner HL (1989) Cystic tumors. In: Benign diseases of the vulva and vagina, 3rd Ed. Year Book, Chicago, pp 237–285
155. Kawauchi S, Fukuda T, Tsuneyoshi M (1998) Case report: a mixed tumor of the vagina. J Obstet Gynaecol Res 24(3):223–229
156. Kearns PR, Gray JE (1963) Mycotic vulvovaginitis. Incidence and persistence of specific yeast species during infection. Obstet Gynecol 22:621–625
157. Keltz M, Berger S, Comite F, Olive D (1994) Duplicate cervix and vagina associated with infertility, endometriosis, and chronic pelvic pain. Obstet Gynecol 84(4 pt 2):701–703
158. Kent HL (1991) Epidemiology of vaginitis. Am J Obstet Gynecol 165:1168
159. Keyzer C, Lilford R, Gordon W, Bloch B (1982) Pyoderma gangrenosum, vesicovaginal fistula and endometriosis. A case report. South Afr Med J 61: 843–845
160. Kiviat NB, Paavonen JA, Wølner-Hanssen P, et al (1990) Histopathology of endocervical infection caused by *Chlamydia trachomatis*, *herpes simplex* virus, *Trichomonas vaginalis*, and *Neisseria gonorrhoeae*. Hum Pathol 21:831–837
161. Koenig C, Turnicky R, Kankam C, Tavassoli F (1997) Papillary squamotransitional cell carcinoma of the cervix: a report of 32 cases. Am J Surg Pathol 21:915–921
162. Korn AP, Bolan G, Padian N, Ohm-Smith M, Schachter J, Landers DV (1995) Plasma cell endometritis in women with symptomatic bacterial vaginosis. Obstet Gynecol 85(3):387–390
163. Koskela O (1964) Granular cell myoblastoma of the vagina. Ann Chir Gynaecol Fenn 53:270–273
164. Kramer K, Tobin H (1987) Vaginitis emphysematosa. Arch Pathol Lab Med 111:746–749

165. Kraus FT, Perez-Mesa C (1966) Verrucous carcinoma. Clinical and pathologic study of 105 cases involving oral cavity, larynx and genitalia. Cancer (Phila) 19:26–38
166. Krause RM (1992) The origin of plagues: old and new. Science 257:1073–1078
167. Kurman RJ, Norris HJ, Wilkinson E (1992) Tumors of the vagina. In: Atlas of tumor pathology, 3rd series, fasc 4. Tumors of the cervix, vagina, and vulva. Armed Forces Institute of Pathology, Washington DC, pp 141–178
168. Kurman RJ, Prabha AC (1973) Thyroid and parathyroid glands in the vaginal wall: Report of a case. Am J Clin Pathol 59:503–507
169. Kurman RJ, Toki T, Schiffman MH (1993) Basaloid and warty carcinomas of the vulva. Distinctive types of squamous cell carcinoma frequently associated with human papillomaviruses. Am J Surg Pathol 17(2):133–145
170. Lakshminarasimhan S, Doval DC, Rajashekhar U, et al (1996) Preleukemic granulocytic sarcoma of vagina. A case report with review of literature. Indian J Cancer 33(3):145–148
171. Lang WR, Israel SL, Fritz MA (1958) Staphylococcal vulvovaginitis. A report of two cases following antibiotic therapy. Obstet Gynecol 11:352–354
172. Larsen B, Galask RP (1980) Vaginal microbial flora: practical and theoretic relevance. Obstet Gynecol 55:100S–113S
173. Larsson P-G, Platz-Christensen J-J, Sundström E (1991) Is bacterial vaginosis a sexually transmitted disease? Int J STD AIDS 2:362–364
174. Lenehan PM, Meffe F, Lickrish GM (1986) Vaginal intraepithelial neoplasia: biologic aspects and management. Obstet Gynecol 68:333–337
175. Levine BB, Sriaganian RP, Schenkein I (1973) Allergy to human seminal plasma. N Engl J Med 288:894
176. Levine WC, Pope V, Bhoomkar A, et al (1998) Increase in endocervical CD4 lymphocytes among women with nonulcerative sexually transmitted diseases. J Infect Dis 177(1):167–174
177. Levitan Z, Gordon AN, Kaplan AL, Kaufman RH (1989) Primary malignant melanoma of the vagina: report of four cases and review of the literature. Gynecol Oncol 33:85–90
178. Lifson AR (1992) Transmission of the human immunodeficiency virus. In: DeVita VT, Hellman S, Rosenberg SA (eds) AIDS: Etiology, diagnosis, treatment, and prevention. Lippincott, Philadelphia, pp 111–117
179. Lin JI, Caracta PF, Chang CH, et al (1979) Malacoplakia of the vagina. South Med J 72:326–328
180. Lindner JGEM, Plantema FHF, Hoogkamp-Korstanje JAA (1978) Quantitative studies of the vaginal flora of healthy women and of obstetric and gynaecologic patients. J Med Microbiol 11: 233
181. Liu L-Y, Hou Y-J, Li J-Z (1987) Primary malignant melanoma of the vagina: A report of seven cases. Obstet Gynecol 70:569–572
182. Lorenz G (1978) Adenomatoid tumor of the ovary and vagina. Zentbl Gynakkol 100:1412–1416
183. Lossick JG, Kent HL (1991) Trichomoniasis: trends in diagnosis and management. Am J Obstet Gynecol 165:1217–1222
184. Lucas WE, Benirschke K, Lebherz TB (1974) Verrucous carcinoma of the female genital tract. Am J Obstet Gynecol 119:435–440
185. Ludwig K (1998) The Mayer-Rokitansky-Kuster syndrome. An analysis of its morphology and embryology. Part I: Morphology. Arch Gynecol Obstet 262(1-2):1–26
186. Ludwig K (1998) The Mayer-Rokitansky-Kuster syndrome. An analysis of its morphology and embryology. Part II: Embryology. Arch Gynecol Obstet 262(1-2):27–42
187. Luttges JE, Lubke M (1994) Recurrent benign müllerian papilloma of the vagina. Immunohistological findings and histogenesis. Arch Gynecol Obstet 255(3):157–160
188. MacLeod C, Fowler A, Dalrymple C, Atkinson K, Elliott P, Carter J (1997) High-dose-rate brachytherapy in the management of high-grade intraepithelial neoplasia of the vagina. Gynecol Oncol 65(1):74–77
189. Madico G, Quinn TC, Rompalo A, McKee KT Jr, Gaydos CA (1998) Diagnosis of *Trichomonas vaginalis* infection by PCR using vaginal swab samples. J Clin Microbiol 36(11):3205–3210
190. Manabe Y, Yoshida Y (1986) Collagenolysis in human vaginal tissue during pregnancy and delivery: a light and electron microscopic study. Am J Obstet Gynecol 155:1060–1066
191. March CM, Israel R (1976) Rectovaginal endometriosis: an isolated engima. Am J Obstet Gynecol 125:274–275
192. Marcus SL (1960) Primary carcinoma of the vagina. Obstet Gynecol 15:673
193. Mårdh P-A (1991) The vaginal ecosystem. Am J Obstet Gynecol 165:1163–1168
194. Mårdh P-A, Holst E, Moller BR (1984) The Grivet monkey as a model for study of vaginitis. In: Mårdh P-A, Taylor-Robinson D (eds) Bacterial vaginosis. Almquist and Wiksell International, Stockholm, p 201
195. Masters WH (1960) The sexual response cycle of the human female. I. Gross anatomic considerations. West J Surg, Obstet Gynecol (Jan-Feb), pp 57–72
196. McCormack WM (1990) Unusual vulvovaginal conditions: Interstitial cystitis, focal vulvitis and desquamative inflammatory vaginitis. In: Sobel JD (ed) Vulvovaginal infections: current concepts in diagnosis and therapy. Academy Professional Information Services. New York, pp 149–160
197. McGregor JA, French JI, Jones W, et al. (1994) Bacterial vaginosis is associated with prematurity and vaginal fluid mucinase and sialidase: results of a controlled trial of topical clindamycin cream.

Am J Obstet Gynecol 170(4):1048–1059; discussion 1059–1060.

197a. McKenna UG, Meadows JA, Brewer NS, et al (1980) Toxic shock syndrome, a newly recognized disease entity. Report of 11 cases, Mayo Clin Proc 55:663–672

198. McLellan R, Spence MR, Brockman M, et al (1982) The clinical diagnosis of trichomoniasis. Obstet Gynecol 60:30

199. McLennan MT, Smith JM, McLennan CE (1972) Diagnosis of vaginal mycosis and trichomoniasis: reliability of cytologic smear, wet smear and culture. Obstet Gynecol 40:231–234

200. Merchant WJ, Gale J (1993) Intestinal metaplasia in stilboestrol-induced vaginal adenosis. Histopathology (Oxf) 23(4):373–376

201. Merkus JMWM, Bisschop MPJM, Stolte LAM (1985) The proper nature of vaginal candidosis and the problem of recurrence. Obstet Gynecol Surv 40:493–504

202. Miettinen M, Wahlström T, Vesterinen E, Saksela E (1983) Vaginal polyps with pseudosarcomatous features. A clinicopathologic study of seven cases. Cancer (Phila) 51:1148–1151

203. Miller CJ, Vogel P, Alexander NJ (1992) Localization of SIV in the genital tract of chronically infected female rhesus macaques. Am J Pathol 141: 655–660

204. Minucci D, Cinel A, Insacco E, Oselladore M (1995) Epidemiological aspects of vaginal intraepithelial neoplasia (VAIN). Clin Exp Obstet Gynecol 22(1):36–42

205. Mucitelli DR, Charles EZ, Kraus FT (1990) Vulvovaginal polyps. Histologic appearance, ultrastructure, immunocytochemical characteristics and clinicopathologic correlations. Int J Gynecol Pathol 9:20–40

206. de Mundi Zamorano A, del Alamo CM, de Blas LL, San Cristobal AA (1978) Egg of *Trichuris trichiura* in a vaginal smear. Acta Cytol 22:119–120

207. Munguia H, Franco E, Valenzuela P (1966) Diagnosis of genital amebiasis in women by the standard Papanicolaou technique. Am J Obstet Gynecol 94:181–188

208. Murad TM, Durant JR, Maddox WA, Dowling EA (1975) The pathologic behavior of primary vaginal carcinoma and its relationship to cervical cancer. Cancer (Phila) 35:787–794

209. Naves AE, Monti JA, Chichoni E (1980) Basal cell-like carcinoma of the upper third of the vagina. Am J Obstet Gynecol 137:136–137

210. Neesham D, Kerdemelidis P, Scurry J (1998) Primary malignant mixed müllerian tumor of the vagina. Gynecol Oncol 70(2):303–307

211. Newton ER, Butler MC, Shain RN (1996) Sexual behavior and vaginal colonization by group B streptococcus among minority women. Obstet Gynecol 88(4 pt 1):577–582

212. Newton ER, Piper J, Peairs W (1997) Bacterial vaginosis and intraamniotic infection. Am J Obstet Gynecol 176(3):672–677

213. Newton WA, Soule EH, Hamoudi AB, et al (1988) Histopathology of childhood sarcomas, intergroup rhabdomyosarcoma studies I and II: clinicopathologic correlation. J Clin Oncol 6:67–75

214. Nigogosyan G, de la Pava S, Pickren JW (1964) Melanoblasts in vaginal mucosa: origin for primary malignant melanoma. Cancer (Phila) 17:912–913

215. Nilsson U, Hellberg D, Shoubnikova M, Nilsson S, Mardh PA (1997) Sexual behavior risk factors associated with bacterial vaginosis and *Chlamydia trachomatis* infection. Sex Transm Dis 24(5):241–246

216. Nogales-Ortiz F, Tarancón I, Nogales F (1979) The pathology of female genital tuberculosis. Obstet Gynecol 53:422–428

217. Noller KL, Blair PB, O'Brien PC, et al (1988) Increased occurrence of autoimmune disease among women exposed in utero to DES. Fertil Steril 49:1080–1082

218. Noller KL (1990) DES update. Clin Pract Gynecol 2:149

219. Noller KL, Townsend DE, Kaufman RH, et al (1983) Maturation of vaginal and cervical epithelium in women exposed in utero to diethylstilbestrol (DESAD) Project). Am J Obstet Gynecol 146: 279

220. Nucci M, Young R, Fletcher C (2000) Cellular pseudosarcomatous fibroepithelial stromal polyps of the lower female genital tract: an underrecognized lesion often misdiagnosed as sarcoma. Am J Surg Pathol 24:231–240

221. O'Collins JP, Butler B (1973) Vesico-vaginal fistula after sexual intercourse. Med J Aust 1:299

222. Okagaki T, Ishida T, Hilgers RD (1976) A malignant tumor of the vagina resembling synovial sarcoma. A light and electron microscopic study. Cancer (Phila) 37:2306–2320

223. Opitz JM (1987) Editorial comment: Vaginal atresia (von Mayer-Rokitansky-Küster or MRK anomaly) in hereditary renal adysplasia (HRA). Am J Med Genet 26:873–876

224. Östör AG, Fortune DW, Riley CB (1988) Fibroepithelial polyps with atypical stromal cells (pseudosarcoma botryoides) of vulva and vagina. A report of 13 cases. Int J Gynecol Pathol 7:351–360

225. Palmer JP, Biback SM (1954) Primary cancer of the vagina. Am J Obstet Gynecol 67:377–397

226. Parker CE, Johnson FC (1963) The effect of maternal estrogens on the vaginal epithelium of the newborn. Clin Pediatr 2:374–377

227. Paris AL, Herwaldt LA, Blum D, et al (1982) Pathologic findings in twelve fatal cases of toxic shock syndrome. Ann Intern Med 96:852–857

228. Peipert JF, Montagno AB, Cooper AS, Sung CJ (1997) Bacterial vaginosis as a risk factor for upper genital tract infection. Am J Obstet Gynecol 177(5):1184–1187

229. Perez CA, Arneson AN, Dehner LP, et al (1974) Radiation therapy in carcinoma of vagina. Obstet Gynecol 44:862

230. Perez CA, Camel HM, Galakatos AE, et al (1988) Definitive irradiation in carcinoma of the vagina: Long-term evaluation of results. Int J Radiat Oncol Biol Phys 15:1283
231. Perez CA, Gersell DJ, Hoskins WJ, McGuire WP III (1992) Vagina. In: Hoskins WJ, Perez CA, Young RC (eds) Principles and practice of gynecologic oncology. Lippincott, Philadelphia, pp 567–590
232. Perez C, Gersell D, McGuire W, Morris M (1997) Vagina. In: Hoskins W, Perez C, Young R (eds) Principles and practice of gynecologic oncology, 2nd Ed. Lippincott-Raven, Philadelphia, pp 753–783
233. Peterman TA, Stoneburner RL, Allen JR, et al (1988) Risk of human immunodeficiency virus transmission from heterosexual adults with transfusion-associated infections. JAMA 259:55
234. Peters WA, Kumar NB, Anderson WA, Morley GW (1985) Primary sarcoma of the adult vagina: a clinicopathologic study. Obstet Gynecol 65:699–704
235. Peters WA, Kumar NB, Morley GW (1985) Carcinoma of the vagina: factors influencing treatment outcome. Cancer (Phila) 55:892
236. Peters WA, Kumar NB, Morley GW (1985) Microinvasive carcinoma of the vagina: a distinct clinical entity? Am J Obstet Gynecol 153:505–507
237. Petrin D, Delgaty K, Bhatt R, Garber G (1998) Clinical and microbiological aspects of *Trichomonas vaginalis*. Clin Microbiol Rev 11(2): 300–317
238. Petru E, Nagele F, Czerwenka K, et al (1998) Primary malignant melanoma of the vagina: long-term remission following radiation therapy. Gynecol Oncol 70(1):23–26
239. Pezeshkpour G (1981) Solitary paraganglioma of the vagina. Report of a case. Am J Obstet Gynecol 139:219–221
240. Pheifer TA, Forsyth PS, Durfee MA, et al (1978) Nonspecific vaginitis. Role of *Haemophilus vaginalis* and treatment with metronidazole. N Engl J Med 298:1429–1434
241. Piver MS, Lele SB, Baker TR, Sandecki A (1988) Cervical and vaginal cancer detection at a regional diethylstilbestrol (DES) screening clinic. Cancer Detect Prevent 11:197–202
242. Platz C, Benda J (1995) Female genital tract cancer. Cancer (Phila) 75:270–294
243. Plentl AA, Friedman EA (1971) Lymphatic system of the female genitalia. The morphologic basis of oncologic diagnosis and therapy. Saunders, Philadelphia pp 51–74
244. Podczaski E, Herbst AL (1986) Cancer of the vagina and fallopian tube. In: Knapp RC, Berkowitz RS (eds) Gynecologic oncology, Macmillan, New York, pp 399–424
245. Polasek P, Erickson L, Stanhope C (1995) Transverse vaginal septum associated with tubal atresia. Mayo Clin Proc 70(10):965–968
246. Pradhan S, Tobon H (1986) Vaginal cysts: a clinicopathological study of 41 cases. Int J Gynecol Pathol 5:35–46
247. Prasad CJ, Ray JA, Kessler S (1992) Primary small cell carcinoma of the vagina arising in a background of atypical adenosis. Cancer (Phila) 70: 2484–2487
248. Premptee T, Amornmarn R (1985) Radiation treatment of primary carcinoma of the vagina: Patterns of failure after definitive therapy. Acta Radiol Oncol 24:51
249. Premptee T, Tang C-K, Hatef A, et al (1983) Angiosarcoma of the vagina: A clinicopathologic report. Cancer (Phila) 51:618–622
250. Prezyna AP, Kalyanaraman U (1977) Bowen's carcinoma in vulvovaginal Crohn's disease (regional enterocolitis). Report of first case. Am J Obstet Gynecol 128:914–916
251. Proppe KH, Scully RE, Rosai J (1984) Postoperative spindle cell nodules of genitourinary tract resembling sarcomas. A report of eight cases. Am J Surg Pathol 8:101–108
252. Pul M, Yilmaz N, Gürses N, Ozoran Y (1990) Vaginal polyp in a newborn—a case report and review of the literature. Clin Pediatr 29:346
253. Qualman S, Coffin C, Newton W, et al (1998) Intergroup rhabdomyosarcoma study: update for pathologists. Pediatr Dev Pathol 1:550–561
254. Raghavaiah NV, Devi AI (1980) Primary vaginal stones. J Urol 123:771–772
255. Randall M, Andersen W, Mills S, Kim J-A (1986) Papillary squamous cell carcinoma of the uterine cervix. Int J Gynecol Pathol 5:1–10
256. Rajkumar S, Narayanaswamy G, Laude TA (1979) Shigella vulvovaginitis in childhood: a case report. J Natl Med Assoc 71:1005–1006
257. Raudrant D, Landrivon G, Frappart L, De Haas P, Champion F, Ecochard R (1995) Comparison of the effects of different menstrual tampons on the vaginal epithelium: a randomised clinical trial. Eur J Obstet Gynecol Reprod Biol 58(1):41–46
258. Regan JA, Klebanoff MA, Nugent RP, et al (1996) Colonization with group B streptococci in pregnancy and adverse outcome. VIP Study Group. Am J Obstet Gynecol 174(4):1354–1360
259. Reid GC, Schmidt RW, Roberts JA, et al (1989) Primary melanoma of the vagina: a clinicopathologic analysis. Obstet Gynecol 74:190–199
260. Rein MF, Müller M (1990) *Trichomonas vaginalis*. In: Holmes KK, Mårdh P-A, Sparling PF, Wiesner PJ (eds) Sexually transmitted diseases, 2nd Ed. McGraw-Hill, New York
261. Resnick SD (1990) Toxic shock syndrome: recent developments in pathogenesis. J Pediatr 116:321–328
262. Rhatigan RM, Mojadidi Q (1973) Adenosquamous carcinomas of the vulva and vagina. Am J Clin Pathol 59:208–217
263. Richart RM (1986) The incidence of cervical and vaginal dysplasia after exposure to DES. JAMA 255:36–37
264. Robboy SJ (1983) A hypothetic mechanism of diethylstilbestrol (DES)-induced anomalies in prenatally exposed women. Hum Pathol 14:831

265. Robboy SJ, Friedlander LM, Welch WR, et al (1976) Cytology of 575 young females exposed prenatally to diethylstilbestrol (DES). Obstet Gynecol 48:511
266. Robboy SJ, Hill EC, Sandberg EC, Czernobilsky B (1986) Vaginal adenosis in women born prior to the diethylstilbestrol (DES) era. Hum Pathol 17:488
267. Robboy SJ, Kaufman RH, Prat J, et al (1979) Pathologic findings in young women enrolled in national cooperative diethylstilbestrol adenosis (DESAD) project. Obstet Gynecol 53:309
268. Robboy SJ, Noller KL, O'Brien P, et al (1984) Increased incidence of cervical and vaginal dysplasia in 3,980 diethylstilbestrol (DES)-exposed young women: Experience of the National Collaborative DES-Adenosis (DESAD) Project. JAMA 252:2979
269. Robboy SJ, Prade M, Cunha G (1992) Vagina. In: Sternberg SS (ed) Histology for pathologists. Raven Press, New York, pp 881–892
270. Robboy SJ, Szyfelbein WM, Goellner JR, et al. (1981) Dysplasia and cytologic findings in 4,589 young women enrolled in diethylstilbestrol-adenosis (DESAD) project. Am J Obstet Gynecol 140:579
271. Robboy SJ, Taguchi O, Cunha GR (1982) Normal development of the human female reproductive tract and alterations resulting from experimental exposure to diethylstilbestrol. Hum Pathol 13:190–198
272. Robboy SJ, Welch WR (1977) Microglandular hyperplasia in vaginal adenosis associated with oral contraceptives and prenatal diethylstilbestrol (DES) exposure. Obstet Gynecol 49:430
273. Robboy SJ, Welch WR, Young RH, et al (1982) Topographic relation of adenosis, clear cell adenocarcinoma and other related lesions of the vagina and cervix in DES-exposed progeny. Obstet Gynecol 60:546
274. Robboy SJ, Young RH, Welch WR, et al (1984) Atypical (dysplastic) adenosis: forerunner and transitional state to clear cell adenocarcinoma in young women exposed in utero to diethylstilbestrol. Cancer (Phila) 54:869
275. Robboy SJ, Ross JS, Prat J, et al (1978) Urogenital sinus origin of mucinous and ciliated cysts of the vulva. Obstet Gynecol 51:347–351
276. Roberts WS, Hoffman MS, LaPolla JP, et al (1991) Management of radionecrosis of the vulva and distal vagina. Am J Obstet Gynecol 164:1235–1238
277. Roberts DK, Walker NJ, Parmley TH, Horbelt DV (1988) Interaction of epithelial and stromal cells in vaginal adenosis. Hum Pathol 19:855–861
278. Rorat E, Ferenczy A, Richart RM (1975) Human Bartholin gland, duct, and duct cyst. Histochemical and ultrastructural study. Arch Pathol 99:367–374.
279. Rose P, Stoler M, Abdul-Karim F (1998) Papillary squamotransitional cell carcinoma of the vagina. Int J Gynecol Pathol 17:372–375
280. Rotmensch J, Rosenshein N, Dillon M, et al (1983) Carcinoma arising in the neovagina: case report and review of the literature. Obstet Gynecol 61:534
281. Rutledge F (1967) Cancer of the vagina. Am J Obstet Gynecol 97:635–655
282. Sanders CC, Sanders WE, Fagnant JE (1982) Toxic shock syndrome: an ecologic imbalance within the genital microflora of women? Am J Obstet Gynecol 142:977–982
283. Sangwan K, Khosla AH, Hazra PC (1996) Leiomyoma of the vagina. Aust N Z J Obstet Gynaecol 36(4):494–495
284. Schmedding A, Zense M, Fuchs J, Gluer S (1997) Benign papilloma of the cervix in childhood: immunohistochemical findings and review of the literature. Eur J Pediatr 156(4):320–322
285. Schneider V (1981) Visceral giant cell arteritis limited to the female genital tract. A case report. J Reprod Med 26:328–331
286. Schneider GT, Geary WL (1971) Vaginitis in adolescent girls. Clin Obstet Gynecol 14:1057–1076
287. Schwebke JR, Hillier SL, Sobel JD, McGregor JA, Sweet RL (1996) Validity of the vaginal Gram stain for the diagnosis of bacterial vaginosis. Obstet Gynecol 88(4 pt 1):573–576
288. Scurry J, Planner R, Grant P (1991) Unusual variants of vaginal adenosis: a challenge for diagnosis and treatment. Gynecol Oncol 41(2):172–177
289. Senekjian EK, Hubby M, Bell DA, et al (1986) Clear cell adenocarcinoma (CCA) of the vagina and cervix in association with pregnancy. Gynecol Oncol 24:207–219
290. Sheets JL, Dockerty MD, Decker DG, Welch JS (1964) Primary epithelial malignancy in the vagina. Am J Obstet Gynecol 89:121–128
291. Shenker L, Blaustein A (1963) Emphysematous vaginitis. A theory of its pathogenesis and report of a case. Obstet Gynecol 22:295–300
292. Shevchuk MM, Fenoglio CM, Lattes R (1978) Malignant mixed tumor of the vagina probably arising in mesonephric rests. Cancer (Phila) 42:214–223
293. Shy SW, Lee WH, Chen D, Ho SY (1995) Rhabdomyosarcoma of the vagina in a postmenopausal woman: report of a case and review of the literature. Gynecol Oncol 58(3):395–399
294. Sillman FH, Sedlis A, Boyce JG (1985) A review of lower genital intraepithelial neoplasia and the use of topical 5-fluorouracil. Obstet Gynecol Surv 40:190–220
295. Sillman FH, Fruchter RG, Chen YS, Camilien L, Sedlis A, McTigue E (1997) Vaginal intraepithelial neoplasia: risk factors for persistence, recurrence, and invasion and its management. Am J Obstet Gynecol 176(1 pt 1):93–99
296. Silverberg SG, Frabler WJ (1974) Prolapse of fallopian tube into vaginal vault after hysterectomy. Histopathology, cytopathology, and differential diagnosis. Arch Pathol 97:100–103
297. Sirota RL, Dickerson GR, Scully RE (1981) Mixed tumors of the vagina: A clinicopathologic analysis of eight cases. Am J Surg Pathol 5:413–422
298. Smith YR, Quint EH, Hinton EL (1998) Recurrent

benign mullerian papilloma of the cervix. J Pediatr Adolesc Gynecol 11(1):29–31

299. Sobel JD (1990) Vaginal infections in adult women. Med Clin North Am 74:1573–1602
300. Sobel JD (1994) Desquamative inflammatory vaginitis: a new subgroup of purulent vaginitis responsive to topical 2% clindamycin therapy. Am J Obstet Gynecol 171(5):1215–1220
301. Sobel JD, Brooker D, Stein GE, et al (1995) Single oral dose fluconazole compared with conventional clotrimazole topical therapy of *Candida* vaginitis. Fluconazole Vaginitis Study Group. Am J Obstet Gynecol 172(4 pt 1):1263–1268
302. Soper DE, Brockwell NJ, Dalton HP, Johnson D (1994) Observations concerning the microbial etiology of acute salpingitis. Am J Obstet Gynecol 170(4):1008–1014; discussion 1014–1017
303. Spencer LM, Straatsma BR, Foos RY (1968) Ligneous conjunctivitis. Arch Ophthal 80:365–367
304. Spiegel CA, Amsel R, Eschenbach D, et al (1980) Anaerobic bacteria in nonspecific vaginitis. N Engl J Med 303:601–607
305. Spitzer M, Molho L, Seltzer VL, et al (1985) Vaginal glomus tumor: Case presentation and ultrastructural findings. Obstet Gynecol 66:86S–88S
306. Strate SM, Taylor WE, Forney JP, Silva FG (1983) Xanthogranulomatous pseudotumor of the vagina: evidence of a local response to an unusual bacterium (mucoid *Escherichia coli*). Am J Clin Pathol 79:637–643
307. Stuart GCE, Flagler EA, Nation JG, et al (1988) Laser vaporization of vaginal intraepithelial neoplasia. Am J Obstet Gynecol 158:240–243
308. Sulak P, Barnhill D, Heller P, et al (1988) Nonsquamous cancer of the vagina. Gynecol Oncol 29: 309–320
309. Sunderland WA, Harris HH, Spence DA, Lawson HW (1972) Meningococcemia in a newborn infant whose mother had meningococcal vaginitis (Letter to the Editor). J Pediatr 81:856
310. Sweet RL, Gibbs RS (1985) Infectious vulvovaginitis. In: Infectious diseases of the female genital tract. Williams & Wilkins, Baltimore, pp 89–96
311. Sweet RL (1995) Role of bacterial vaginosis in pelvic inflammatory disease. Clin Infect Dis 20(2): S271–S275
312. Sweet RL, Gibbs RS (1985) Perinatal infections. In: Infectious diseases of the female genital tract. Williams & Wilkins, Baltimore, pp 206–214
313. Sweet RL, Gibbs RS (1985) Toxic shock syndrome. In: Infectious diseases of the female genital tract. Williams & Wilkins, Baltimore, pp 78–88
314. Syverson RE, Buckley H, Gibian J, Ryan GM (1979) Cellular and humoral immune status in women with chronic *Candida vaginitis*. Am J Obstet Gynecol 134:624–627
315. Taguchi O, Cunha GR, Robboy SJ (1983) Experimental study of the effect of diethylstilbestrol (DES) on the development of the human female reproductive tract. Biol Res Prac 4:56
316. Takehara M, Hayakawa O, Itoh E, Sagae S, Suzuki T, Kudo R (1998) A case of a malignant mixed tumor in the vagina. J Obstet Gynaecol Res 24(1):7–11
317. Tancer ML (1980) The post-total hysterectomy (vault) vesicovaginal fistula. J Urol 123:839–840
318. Tarraza HM Jr, Meltzer SE, De Cain M, Jones MA (1998) Vaginal metastases from renal cell carcinoma: report of four cases and review of the literature. Eur J Gynaecol Oncol 19(1):14–18
319. Tazvassoli FA, Norris HJ (1979) Smooth muscle tumors of the vagina. Obstet Gynecol 53:689–693
320. Teo C, Kwong L, Benn R (1987) Incidence of motile, curved anaerobic rods (Mobiluncus species) in vaginal secretions. Pathology 19:193–196
321. The Working Group on Severe Streptococcal Infections (1993) Defining the Group A streptococcal toxic shock syndrome. Rationale and consensus definition. JAMA 269:390–391
322. Thomason JL, Anderson RJ, Gelbart SM, et al (1992) Simplified Gram stain interpretive method for diagnosis of bacterial vaginosis. Am J Obstet Gynecol 167:16–19
323. Thomason JL, Gelbart SM (1989) *Trichomonas vaginalis*. Obstet Gynecol 74:536–541
324. Thomason JL, Gelbart SM, Anderson RJ, et al (1990) Statistical evaluation of diagnostic criteria for bacterial vaginosis. Am J Obstet Gynecol 162:155–160
325. Thorsen P, Jensen IP, Jeune B, et al (1998) Few microorganisms associated with bacterial vaginosis may constitute the pathologic core: a population-based microbiologic study among 3596 pregnant women. Am J Obstet Gynecol 178(3):580–587
326. Tjugum J, Jonassen F, Olsson JH (1986) Vaginitis emphysematosa in a renal transplant patient. Acta Obstet Gynecol Scand 65:377, 378
327. Tobon H, Murphy AI (1977) Benign blue nevus of the vagina. Cancer (Phila) 40:3174
328. Todd J, Fishaut M, Kapral F, Welch T (1978) Toxic-shock syndrome associated with phage-group-I staphylococci. Lancet 2:1116–1118
329. Tohya T, Katabuchi H, Fukuma K, et al (1991) Angiosarcoma of the vagina. A light and electronmicroscopy study. Acta Obstet Gynecol Scand 70: 169–172
330. Torne A, Pahisa J, Castelo-Branco C, Fabregues F, Mallofre C, Iglesias X (1994) Solitary vaginal metastasis as a presenting form of unsuspected renal adenocarcinoma. Gynecol Oncol 52(2):260–263
331. Tsokos M, Webber BL, Parham DM, et al (1992) Rhabdomyosarcoma. A new classification scheme related to prognosis. Arch Pathol Lab Med 116:847–855

331a. Ulbright TM, Alexander RW, Kraus FT (1981) Intramural papilloma of the vagina: evidence of müllerian histogenesis. Cancer 48:2260–2266

332. Václavínková V, Neumann E (1981) Vaginal involvement in familial benign chronic pemphigus (morbus Hailey-Hailey). Acta Dermatovenereal (Stockh) 62:80–81
333. Valdes CT, Malinak LR, Franklin RR (1989) Developmental anomalies of the vulva and vagina. In: Kaufman RH, Friedrich EG, Gardner HL (eds)

Benign diseases of the vulva and vagina, 3rd Ed. Year Book, Chicago, pp 26–54
334. Van Lingen B, Reindollar R, Davis A, Gray M (1998) Further evidence that the WT1 gene does not have a role in the development of the derivatives of the mullerian duct. Am J Obstet Gynecol 179(3 pt 1):597–603
335. van Coeverden de Groot HA (1963) Amoebic vaginitis. South Afr Med J 37:246–247
336. van den Broek N, Emmerson C, Dunlop W (1996) Benign mixed tumour of the vagina: an unusual cause for postmenopausal bleeding. Eur J Obstet Gynecol Reprod Biol 69(2):143–144
337. van der Meijden WI, Duivenvoorden HJ, Both-Patoir HC, et al (1988) Clinical and laboratory findings in women with bacterial vaginosis and trichomoniasis versus controls. Eur J Obstet Gynecol Reprod Biol 28:39–52
338. Vazquez JA, Sobel JD, Demitriou R, Vaishampayan J, Lynch M, Zervos MJ (1994) Karyotyping of *Candida albicans* isolates obtained longitudinally in women with recurrent vulvovaginal candidiasis. J Infect Dis 170(6):1566–1569
339. Venter PF, Anderson JD, Van Velden DJJ (1979) Postmenopausal endometriosis. A case report. South Afr Med J 56:1136–1138
340. Vermund S (1997) Transmission of HIV-1 among adolescents and adults. In: DeVita V Jr, Hellman S, Rosenberg S (eds) AIDS: biology, diagnosis, treatment and prevention. Lippincott-Raven, Philadelphia, pp 147–165
341. de Virgiliis G, Sideri M, Rossi A, et al (1985) "DES-Like" anomalies. I. Biological and clinical problems. A study on 12,285 cases. Cervix Low Female Genital Tract 3:297–312
342. Vontver LA, Eschenbach DA (1981) The role of gardnerella vaginalis in nonspecific vaginitis. Clin Obstet Gynecol 24:439–460
343. Wager GP (1983) Toxic shock syndrome: a review. Am J Obstet Gynecol 146:93–102
344. Waggoner SE, Mittendorf R, Biney N, Anderson D, Herbst AL (1994) Influence of in utero diethylstilbestrol exposure on the prognosis and biologic behavior of vaginal clear-cell adenocarcinoma. Gynecol Oncol 55(2):238–244
345. Waggoner SE, Anderson SM, Luce MC, Takahashi H, Boyd J (1996) p53 protein expression and gene analysis in clear cell adenocarcinoma of the vagina and cervix. Gynecol Oncol 60(3):339–344
346. Waggoner SE, Baunoch DA, Anderson SA, Leigh F, Zagaja VG (1998) Bcl-2 protein expression associated with resistance to apoptosis in clear cell adenocarcinomas of the vagina and cervix expressing wild-type p53. Ann Surg Oncol 5(6): 544–547
347. Ways SC, Mortola JF, Zvaifler NJ, et al (1987) Alterations in immune responsiveness in women exposed to diethylstilbestrol in utero. Fertil Steril 48:193–197
348. Webb MJ, Symmonds RE, Weiland LH (1974) Malignant fibrous histiocytoma of vagina. Am J Obstet Gynecol 119:190–192
349. Weber A, Walters M, Schover L, Mitchinson A (1995) Vaginal anatomy and sexual function. Obstet Gynecol 86(6):946–949
350. Weinstock MA (1994) Malignant melanoma of the vulva and vagina in the United States: patterns of incidence and population-based estimates of survival. Am J Obstet Gynecol 171(5):1225–1230
351. Weir M, Bell D, Young R (1997) Transitional cell metaplasia of the uterine cervix and vagina: an underrecognized lesion that may be confused with high-grade dysplasia. Am J Surg Pathol 21:510–517
352. Welch WR, Fu YS, Robboy SJ, Herbst AL (1983) Nuclear DNA content of clear cell adenocarcinoma of the vagina and cervix and its relations to prognosis. Gynecol Oncol 15:230
353. Wheelock JB, Schneider V, Goplerud DR (1985) Prolapsed fallopian tube masquerading as adenocarcinoma of the vagina in a postmenopausal woman. Gynecol Oncol 21:369–375
354. Williams GA (1965) Postsurgical and post-traumatic tumors. Clin Obstet Gynecol 8:1020–1034
355. Wisniewski PM, Wilkinson EJ (1991) Postpartum vaginal atrophy. Am J Obstet Gynecol 165:1249–1254
356. Witkin SS, Inglis SR, Polaneczky M (1996) Detection of *Chlamydia trachomatis* and *Trichomonas vaginalis* by polymerase chain reaction in introital specimens from pregnant women. Am J Obstet Gynecol 175(1):165–167
357. Wooduff JD, Parmley TH, Julian CG (1975) Topical 5-fluorouracil in the treatment of vaginal carcinoma in situ. Gynecol Oncol 3:124–125
358. Yokoyama Y, Sato S, Kawaguchi T, Saito Y (1998) A case of concurrent uterine cervical adenocarcinoma and renal-cell carcinoma, and subsequent vaginal metastasis from the renal-cell carcinoma. J Obstet Gynaecol Res 24(1):37–43
359. Young RH, Scully RE (1984) Endodermal sinus tumor of the vagina: a report of nine cases and review of the literature. Gynecol Oncol 18:380–392
360. Young RH, Scully RE (1987) Pseudosarcomatous lesions of the urinary bladder, prostate gland, and urethra. A report of three cases and review of the literature. Arch Pathol Lab Med 111:354–358
361. Yousem HL (1961) Adenocarcinoma of Gartner's duct cyst presenting as a vaginal lesion. A case report. Sinai Hosp J. pp 112–114
362. Yow MD, Leeds LJ, Thompson PK, et al (1980) The natural history of group B streptococcal colonization in the pregnant woman and her offspring. I. Colonization studies. Am J Obstet Gynecol 137:34–38
363. Zhang ZF (1996) Epidemiology of trichomonas vaginalis. A prospective study in China. Sex Transm Dis 23(5):415–424
364. Zinkham WH (1976) Multifocal eosinophilic granuloma. Natural history, etiology and management. Am J Med 60:457

5

Anatomy and Histology of the Cervix

Thomas C. Wright, M.D., and
Alex Ferenczy, M.D.

Gross Anatomy

The uterus is divided into the corpus, isthmus, and cervix. The cervix (term taken from the Latin, meaning *neck*) is the most inferior portion of the uterus, protruding into the upper vagina. The transition between the endocervix and the lower portion of the uterine corpus is termed the *isthmus* or *lower uterine segment*. The latter is used for descriptive purposes during gestation and labor and is an important landmark for the pathologist when describing cancers of the uterine corpus. The muscular layer in the region of the isthmus is less well developed than in the corpus, a feature that facilitates effacement and dilation during labor. The vagina is fused circumferentially and obliquely to the distal part of the cervix and is divided into an upper, supervaginal, and lower vaginal portion. The cervix measures 2.5–3.0 cm in length in the adult nulligravida, and when normally positioned is angled slightly downward and backward. The vaginal portion (portio vaginalis) of the cervix, also referred to as the *exocervix*, is delimited by the anterior and posterior vaginal fornices; it has a convex elliptical surface. The portio may be divided into anterior and posterior lips, of which the anterior is shorter and projects lower than the posterior lip. In the center of the exocervix is the external os. The external os is circular in the nulligravida and slitlike in the parous woman (Fig. 5.1). The external os is connected to the isthmus uterine by the cervical canal (endocervix). The canal is an elliptical cavity, measuring 8 mm in greatest diameter, and contains longitudinal mucosal ridges, the plicae palmatae (Fig. 5.2).

The blood supply of the cervix is provided by the descending branches of the uterine arteries, reaching the lateral walls along the upper margin of the paracervical ligaments (cardinal ligaments of Mackenrodt) (Fig. 5.3). These ligaments and the uterosacral ligaments, which attach the supervaginal portion of the cervix to the second through fourth sacral vertebrae, are the main sources of fixation, support, and suspension of the organ.

The venous drainage parallels the arterial system, with communication between the cervical plexus and neck of the urinary bladder. The lymphatics of the cervix have a dual origin: coursing beneath the mucosa and deep in the fibrous stroma. Both systems collect into two lateral plexuses in the region of the isthmus and give origin to four efferent channels running toward the external iliac and obturator nodes, the hypogastric and common iliac nodes, the sacral nodes, and the nodes of the posterior wall of the urinary bladder (Fig. 5.3). The innervation of the cervix is chiefly limited to the endocervix and peripheral deep portion of the exocervix. This distribution is responsible for the relative insensitivity to pain of the inner two-thirds of the portio vaginalis. The cervical nerves are derived from the pelvic autonomic system, the superior, middle, and inferior hypogastric plexuses.

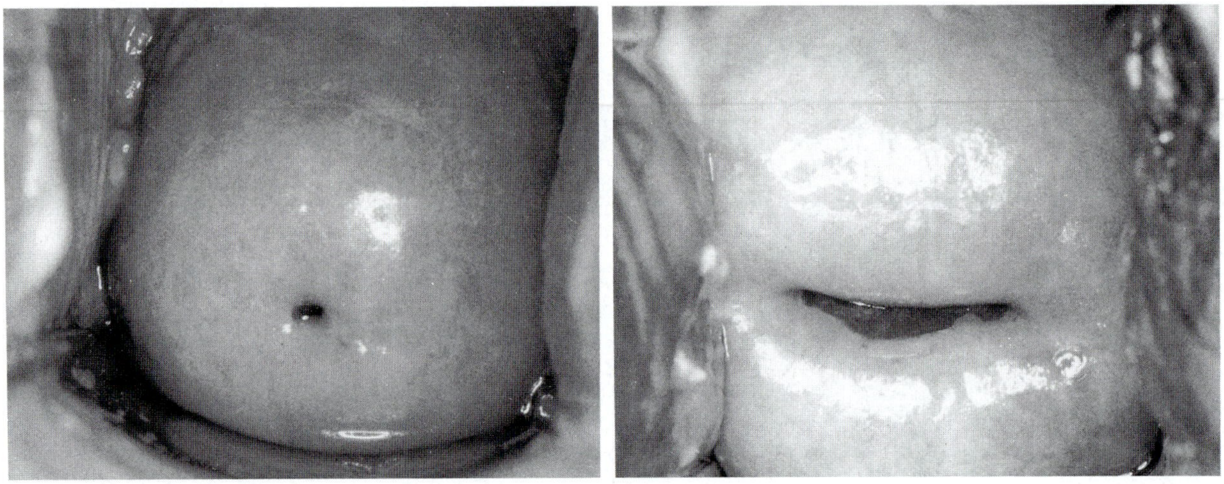

Fig. 5.1. Normal cervix uteri. *Left*: Nulliparous cervix with a circular external os. *Right*: Parous cervix with a slitlike external os.

Histology and Physiology

The cervix is composed of an admixture of fibrous, muscular, and elastic tissue and is lined by columnar and squamous epithelium. Fibrous connective tissue is the predominant component. Smooth muscle comprises 15% of the substance and is located mainly in the endocervix, the portio vaginalis being nearly devoid of smooth muscle fibers. In contrast, at the isthmus, 50%–60% of the supportive tissue consists of concentrically arranged smooth muscle that acts as a sphincter.

Squamous Epithelium

Histology

The mature nonkeratinized *squamous epithelium* of the exocervix is similar to the vaginal epithelium but under normal circumstances lacks the rete pegs seen in the vagina. It is divided into three zones: the basal/parabasal or germinal cell layer, which is responsible for continuous epithelial renewal; the midzone or stratum spinosum, the dominant portion of the epithelium; and the superficial zone, containing the most mature cell population (Fig. 5.4).

The basal/parabasal or germinal layer contains

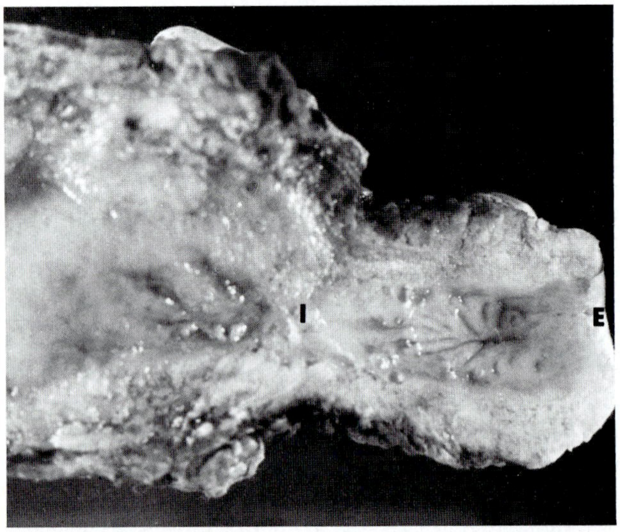

Fig. 5.2. Normal cervix uteri. Transected multiparous uterus. The endocervical canal is delimited by the isthmus (*I*) and external os (*E*). Note prominent mucosal folds of endocervical canal.

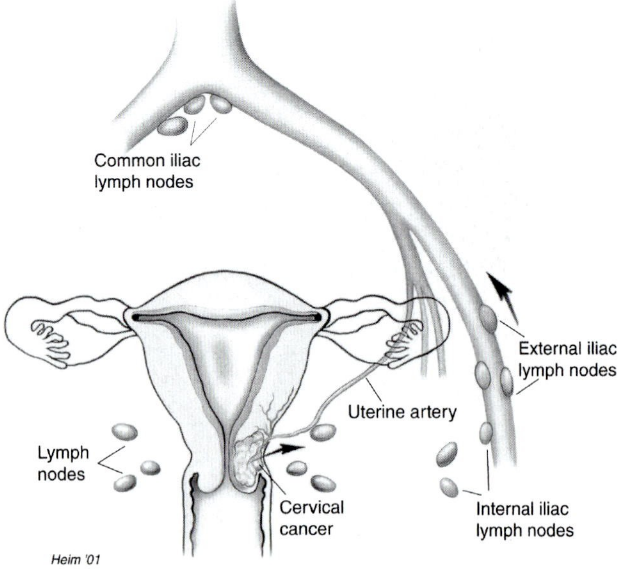

Fig. 5.3. Anatomy of the cervix. The blood supply and lymphatic drainage of the cervix are demonstrated.

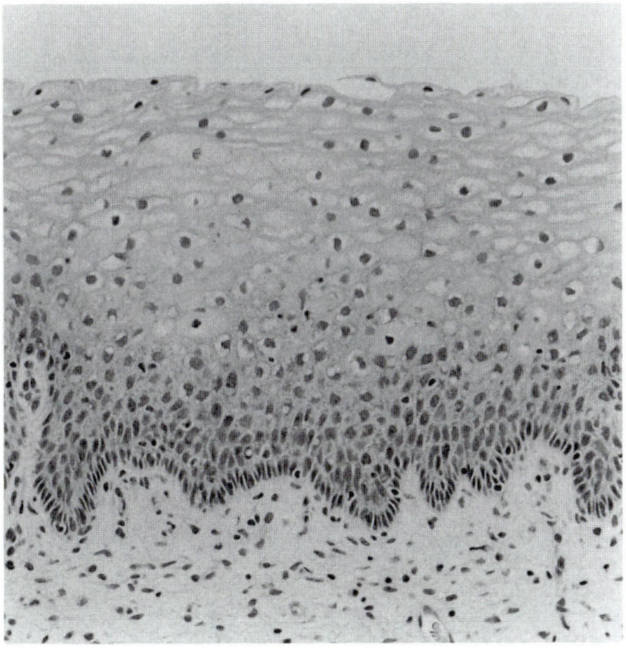

Fig. 5.4. Normal squamous epithelium. The mature squamous epithelium of the portio of the cervix shows a gradual ascending maturation, vacuolization of midzone cells, and a single layer of basal cells in which the nuclei are perpendicularly oriented to the basal lamina. The stromal–epithelial junction contains a finger-like, fibrovascular stromal papilla penetrating the lower portion of the epithelium.

two types of cells. One type is the true *basal cell,* which is about 10 μm in diameter, with scant cytoplasm and oval nuclei oriented perpendicularly to the underlying basal lamina (Fig. 5.4). The other type of cell is termed the *parabasal cell* because of its geographic placement. Parabasal cells are larger than basal cells and have more cytoplasm. Parabasal cells typically form a layer that is one to two cells thick.

Epithelial regeneration appears to be the major function of the basal/parabasal layer. Accordingly, epidermal growth factor receptors and HER-2/neu, which is a growth factor receptor structurally related to the epidermal growth factor receptor, and receptors for estrogen and progesterone are found predominantly in the basal and parabasal cells (Table 5.1).[4,26] The number of growth factor receptors becomes reduced as the squamous epithelial cells differentiate and move into the intermediate cell layer. Basal cells appear to act as stem or reserve cells whereas parabasal cells comprise the actively replicating compartment. This view is supported by the following: (1) mitotic figures are usually found in parabasal but not basal cells; (2) radioautography studies demonstrate a high uptake of tritiated thymidine, one of the best markers for DNA proliferation, in the parabasal but not in the basal cell layer[3]; and (3) other markers for actively proliferating cells such as Ki-67 antigen, proliferating cell nuclear antigen (PCN), and other cyclins are

Table 5.1. Immunohistochemical staining patterns of normal cervical tissues

	Cells of stratified squamous epithelium				*Reserve cells/ squamous metaplasia*	*Endocervical columnar cells*
Antibody	*Basal*	*Parabasal*	*Intermediate*	*Superficial*		
Growth factors/ receptors						
Her 2/ neu[4]	+	+	−	−	+	+
EGF receptor[4]	+	+	−	−	+	−
Estrogen receptor[18,26,47]	+/−	+	+	−	+	+
Progesterone receptor[18,26,47]	−	+[a]	−	−	+	+
Cell cycle proteins						
PCN[1,27,44,48]	−	+	−	−	NA	+
MIB-1 (Ki-67)[35,51]	−	+/−	−	−	−	−
bcl-2[47,51]	+		−	−	+	+/−
Cyclin B1[26]	−	+	−	−	?	?
Cyclin D1[5]	+	+	−	−	+	+
Other proteins						
CD44[22]	+	+	−	−	+	−
CEA	−	−	−	−	−	+

[a]Expressed during luteal phase of menstrual cycle and during pregnancy.

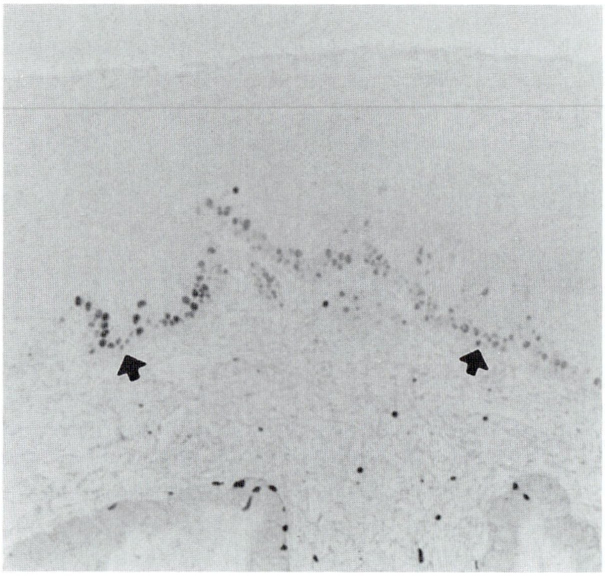

Fig. 5.5. Normal squamous epithelium. Markers for proliferating cells are restricted to the parabasal cell layer (*arrows*) of the exocervical stratified squamous epithelium. Immunohistochemical staining using antibodies against proliferating cell nuclear antigen (PCN).

localized to parabasal cells (Fig. 5.5 and Table 5.1).[5,28,44] Ki-67 antigen is a nuclear antigen expressed in all phases of the cycle except G_0, and PCN is a cellular protein that is present only in the nucleus of cycling cells, not in resting cells. These antigens are excellent markers for cells that are actively replicating. In contrast, bcl-2, which is a cellular protein that protects against apoptosis and which is identified in stem cells and cells of the proliferating compartment in self-renewing epithelium, is found only in the basal cell layer.[47]

The midzone is occupied by cells that are undergoing maturation, characterized by a gradual increase in the volume of the cytoplasm. Nuclear size, however, remains stable up to the most superficial cell level. These cells are referred to as *intermediate cells* when they exfoliate. They do not divide. Intermediate cells have abundant periodic acid–Schiff reagent (PAS)-positive, diatase-labile intracellular glycogen, which is responsible for the clear, vacuolated appearance of their cytoplasm.

The superficial zone forms the most differentiated compartment of the squamous epithelium. These cells are flattened and have a larger area of cytoplasm (50 μm in diameter) and smaller pyknotic nuclei than the underlying intermediate cells (Fig. 5.6). The pink, eosinophilic cytoplasm has abundant intermediate filaments, which provide rigidity (Fig. 5.6, inset). Superficial cells also contain occasional membrane-bound keratinosomes. The abundant intermediate filaments form a complex network of microridges seen on the surface of the most superficial and mature cells. The function of the cornified surface is to protect the underlying epithelial cells and subepithelial vasculature from trauma and infection. The microridges are believed to enhance surface adhesion (Fig. 5.7). The paucity of desmosomes between the upper superficial cells explains their loose attachment and easy desquamation.

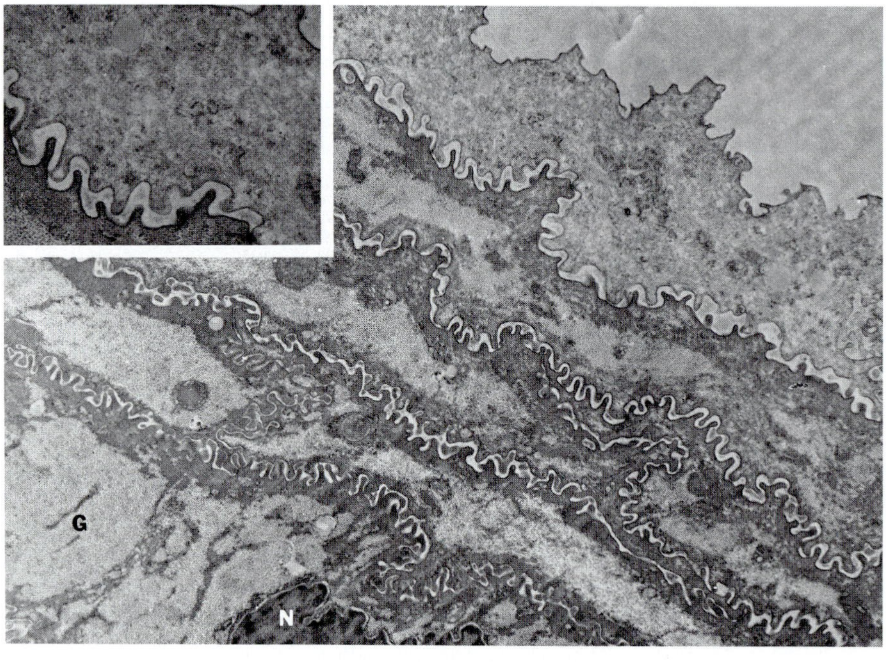

Fig. 5.6. Normal squamous epithelium. Electron microscopy of the superficial cells, which have pyknotic nuclei (*N*) and flattened cytoplasm packed with glycogen (*G*). The most superficial cells are rich in microfilaments and contain irregular surface membrane projections. Note the lack of desmosomal attachments between the most superficial cells, a feature facilitating desquamation. ×4,795. *Inset*: Higher magnification of intracytoplasmic microfilaments in the most superficial cells. ×11,370.

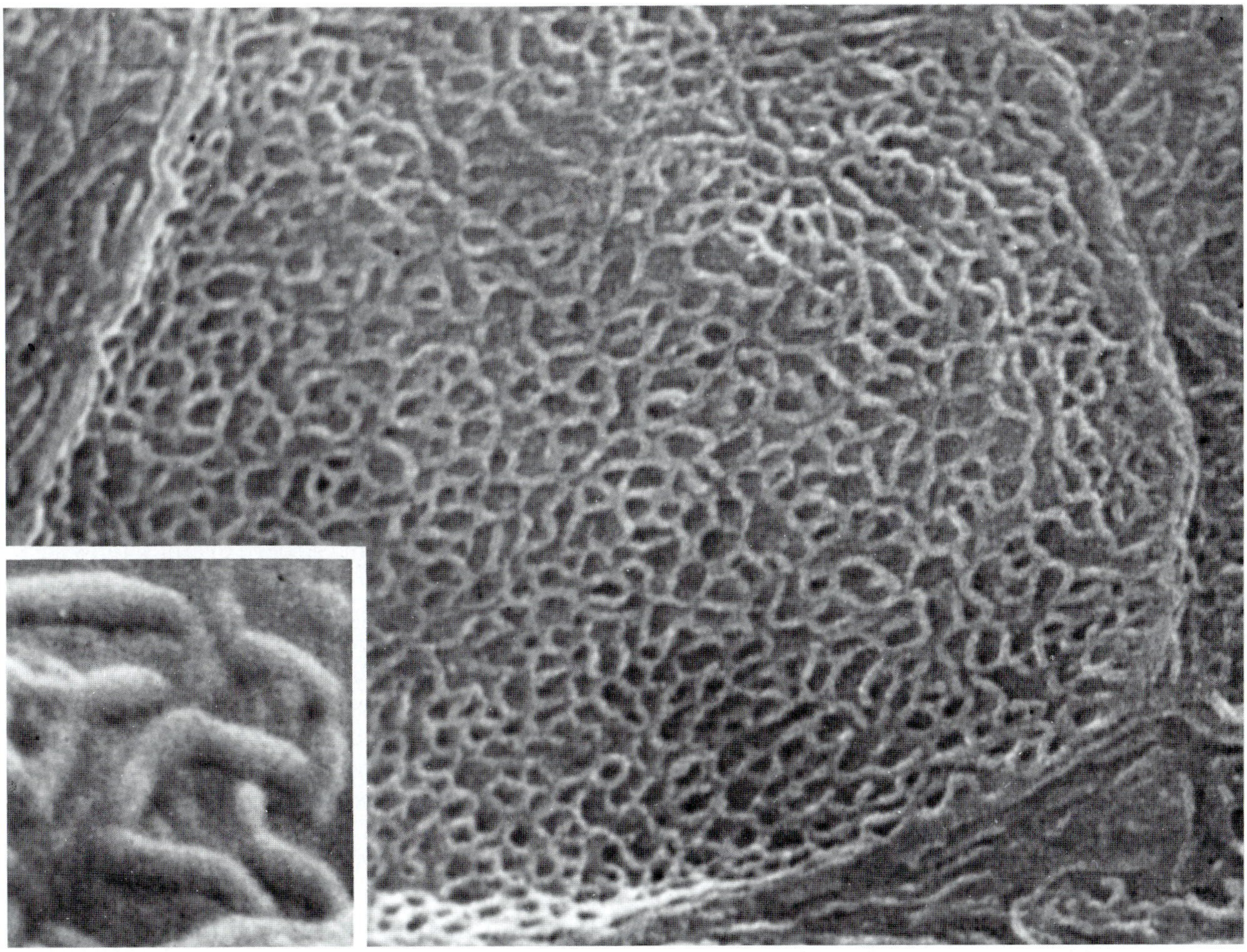

Fig. 5.7. Normal squamous epithelium. Scanning electron photomicrograph of the most superficial cells of the native squamous portio epithelium. The surface contains an intricate system of microridges. ×8,240. *Inset*: Higher magnification of microridges representing nodular evaginations of the surface plasma membrane. ×22,660.

The squamous epithelium of the portio is supported by fibrous connective tissue, devoid of endocervical glands. There is a well-developed capillary network at the stromal–epithelial junction, with occasional finger-like extensions into the epithelium, the stromal papillae (see Fig. 5.4). The penetrating vessels within the papillae supply the epithelial cells with nutrients and oxygen. In addition to connective tissue fibers and capillaries, occasional free nerve endings are seen entering the stromal papilla.

In postmenopausal women, who no longer produce ovarian hormones, the squamous epithelium is atrophic with little or no intracytoplasmic glycogen (Fig. 5.8). Surface epithelial maturation and stromal papillae are absent. These cellular alterations should not be confused with cervical intraepithelial neoplasia (see Chapter 7, Precancerous Lesions of the Cervix). The atrophic epithelial covering does not adequately protect the subepithelial vasculature against trauma, a situation that frequently leads to bleeding and inflammation.

Biochemical and immunohistochemical analysis of the squamous epithelium of the cervical portio has demonstrated the presence of cytoplasmic proteins specific for terminally differentiated squamous cells corresponding to the orderly vertical maturation process seen histologically and ultrastructurally. Although large bundles of intermediate filaments are identified ultrastructurally in only superficial cells, all cell layers of the stratified squamous epithelium of the cervix express intermediate-sized filaments of the cytokeratin type.[9,17,39] The cytokeratin family of intermediate filaments consists of at least 20 cytokeratin polypeptides with molecular weights between 40 and 70 kDa and isoelectric

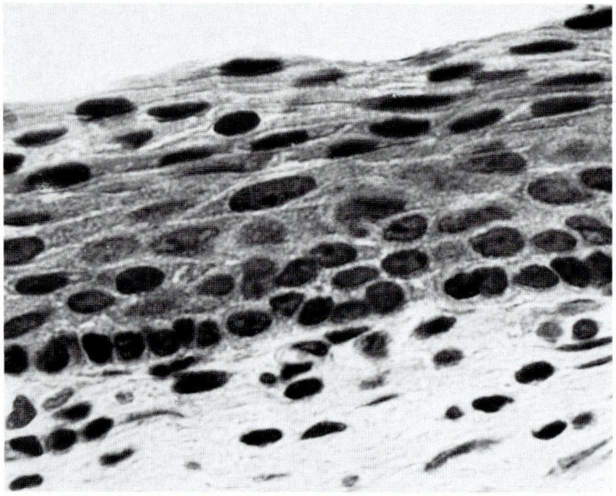

Fig. 5.8. Atrophic squamous epithelium. The epithelium is thin and devoid of glycogen-rich vacuolated cells. The cells in the lower half of the epithelium have prominent nuclei and nucleoi, but cellular cohesion is normal and cytologic atypia is absent.

points between pH 7.8 and 4.9. The expression of different cytokeratin polypeptides can serve as a marker for the state of epithelial differentiation. In the exocervix, the expression of cytokeratin polypeptides is positionally regulated. Immunohistochemical studies using monoclonal antibodies directed against specific cytokeratin polypeptides have shown that basal cells express cytokeratins characteristic of simple (nonstratified) types of epithelium.[9,17,50] These are specifically cytokeratins 18 and 19. Cells in the parabasal, intermediate, and superficial cell layers do not stain with monoclonal antibodies directed against cytokeratins 18 and 19, but do react with monoclonal antibodies directed against cytokeratins 4 and 13, which are characteristic of certain types of stratified epithelium.[9,17,50] A number of other cytokeratin polypeptides are also expressed in the stratified epithelium of the cervix, but in varying amounts depending on the location. Thus, near the squamocolumnar junction, large amounts of cytokeratins 4, 5, 6, 13, 14, and 15 are expressed together with minor amounts of cytokeratins 16, 17, and 19. In contrast, closer to the vagina additional cytokeratins, including 1, 2, 10, and 11, are also expressed.[17]

Effect of Estrogen and Progesterone

The epithelium of the exocervix is remodeled by proliferation, maturation, and desquamation during the reproductive period. The epithelium is completely replaced by a new population of cells every 4–5 days; the process of squamous epithelial maturation can be accelerated to 3 days by the administration of estrogenic compounds.[29,30] Estrogen receptors have been localized to nuclei in the basal, parabasal, and intermediate cell layers.[26,28,32] Compared to the endometrium where marked variations in estrogen receptor content occur during the menstrual cycle, much less cyclic variation of estrogen receptor expression occurs in the cervix. Only a small increase in levels of estrogen receptor occurs during the follicular as compared to the luteal phase. In atrophic and highly inflamed exocervical epithelium, the amount of estrogen receptor is reduced. No, or only low levels of, progesterone receptors are detected immunohistochemically in the exocervical epithelium during the follicular phase of the menstrual cycle, whereas during the luteal phase and during pregnancy, progesterone receptors appear in the parabasal cell layer.[28] Both estrogen and progesterone receptors can be detected in stromal fibroblast-like cells of the exocervix throughout the menstrual cycle.

In general, estradiol-17β stimulates epithelial proliferation, maturation, and desquamation, whereas progesterone inhibits maturation at the upper midzone level of the epithelium. Accordingly, the portio epithelium during the postnatal period is fully mature and contains large amounts of glycogen as a result of maternal estrogen stimulation. Maturation ceases and glycogen rapidly disappears as the serum hormone levels fall. The epithelium remains atrophic during childhood until menarche when, under the stimulatory effect of ovarian hormones, maturation occurs again and glycogen reappears. During pregnancy, when progesterone levels are elevated, superficial cell maturation is absent.

Effect of Retinoids

In addition to estrogen and progesterone, the human cervical epithelium also responds to retinoids. Retinoids are a class of steroid molecules that includes naturally occurring compounds with vitamin A activity, as well as synthetic analogues of retinol that may or may not have biologic activity. Retinoids play important roles in regulating the growth and differentiation of a variety of epithelia. Their role in regulating cellular differentiation may be especially important in the cervix because retinoids modulate squamous and mucinous differentiation. In some target epithelia, vitamin A deficiency results in squamous metaplasia and excessive keratinization, whereas vitamin A excess promotes the formation of mucinous epithelium.[53] Epidemiologic studies have found that women with high dietary intakes of vitamin A and closely related compounds have a reduced risk of developing cervical cancer.[8] Other studies have demonstrated that the topical administration of certain forms of retinoic acid or retinyl acetate can cause regression of squamous intraepithelial lesions (SIL), cervical intraepithelial neoplasia (CIN), and affect cervical cancers.[34,37] Retinoid action in target epithelium is mediated by both cellular binding proteins and nuclear receptors.[42] Immunohistochemical studies have localized a binding protein for retinoic acid called *cellular retinoic acid-binding protein* (CRABP) and a binding protein for retinol called *cellular retinol-binding protein* (CRBP) in the stratified squamous epithelium of the cervix.[20] CRABP is localized predominantly to the basal layer of the epithelium, whereas CRBP is present throughout all layers of the cervical epithelium (Fig. 5.9).

Columnar Epithelium

Histology

The mucosa of the cervical canal (endocervix) is composed of a single layer of mucin-secreting, columnar epithelium that lines both the surface and the underlying glandular structures. The latter are traditionally called *compound, tubular racemose, endocervical glands*. Fluhmann, however, using three-dimensional plastic reconstructions from serial histologic sections, demonstrated that the endocervical glands actually represent deep, cleftlike infoldings of the surface epithelium with numerous blind, tunnel-like collaterals (Fig. 5.10).[16] Because of the complex architecture of these clefts, or grooves, including oblique, transverse, and longitudinal arrangements, they appear as isolated glands in histologic sections. The epithelium lining the clefts is identical with that lining the surface, and consequently the endocervical mucin-producing apparatus is not considered glandular but a complex infolding mucinous membrane. True glands, in contrast, have different epithelial lining in their secretory apparatus compared to their ductal and surface epithelial portions.

Especially in multiparous and older women, endocervical glands can appear in histologic sections

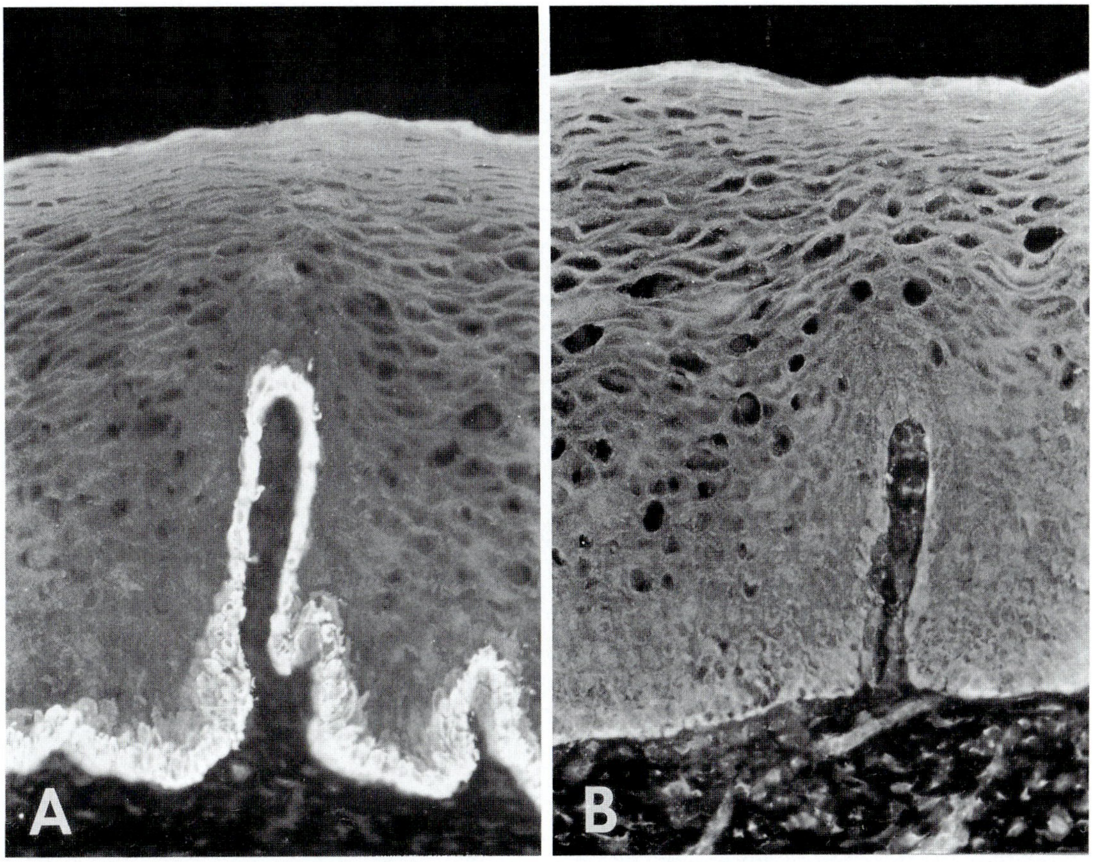

Fig. 5.9. Normal squamous epithelium. Cellular retinoic acid-binding protein and cellular retinol-binding protein can be identified in exocervical stratified squamous epithelium using indirect immunofluorescence. **A**: Cellular retinoic acid-binding protein (CRABP) is present in the basal cells. **B**: Cellular retinol-binding protein (CRBP) is present throughout the entire epithelial thickness. (Reproduced with permission by Hillemanns et al., ref. 20.)

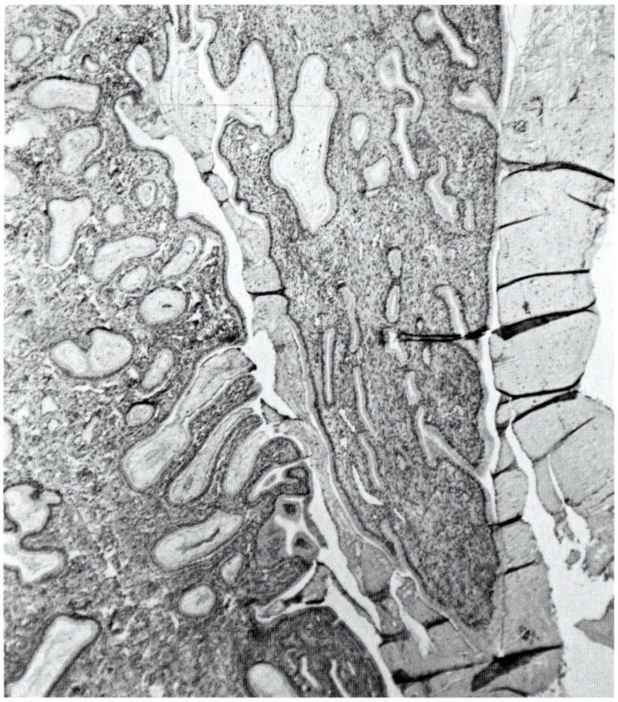

Fig. 5.10. Endocervical mucosa. There are cleftlike infoldings and tunnel-like collaterals. The neighboring glandlike structures represent tangentially sectioned cleft–tunnel complexes.

as distinct clusters of as many as 50 small glands (Fig. 5.11). Connections between these glands and the endocervical surface may not be apparent. The glands in these clusters are frequently distended by inssipated mucus. Because of distention of the glands by mucus, the lining columnar epithelium is frequently quite flattened. Fluhmann used the term *tunnel clusters* to refer to these benign clusters of endocervical glands.[16] It is important not to confuse these structures with well-differentiated, invasive endocervical adenocarcinoma (see Chapter 8, Carcinoma and Other Tumors of the Cervix).

The columnar epithelial cells characteristically have basally placed nuclei and tall, uniform, finely granular cytoplasm filled with mucinous droplets (Fig. 5.12). The droplets have great affinity for Alcian blue stains, reflecting their sulfated, sialic acid, mucopolysaccharide content.[11] Cells lining the luminal surface have been termed *picket cells* because of their resemblance to a picket fence (Fig. 5.12). Occasionally, nonsecretory cells with cilia are observed (Fig. 5.12, inset), the main function of which appears to relate to the distribution and mobilization of endocervical mucus.[19] Isolated neuroendocrine epithelial cells of argyrophil and argentaffin type may also be identified within the endocervical epithelium by histochemical stains.[14,15] The argentaffin-positive

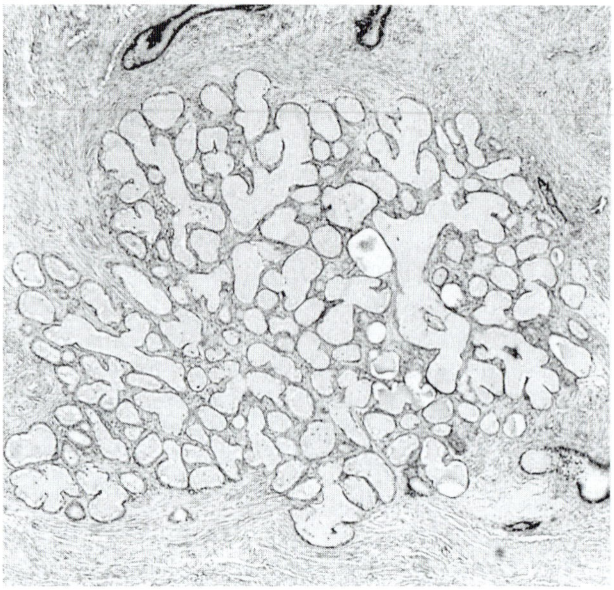

Fig. 5.11. Endocervical tunnel clusters. Small clusters of endocervical glands can develop in the stroma of the older patient and are called *endocervical tunnel clusters*.

cells often contain serotonin, as demonstrated by immunoperoxidase techniques. The physiologic purpose of these rare endocrine endocervical cells is obscure. Biochemically and immunohistochemically, the columnar cells of the endocervix have fea-

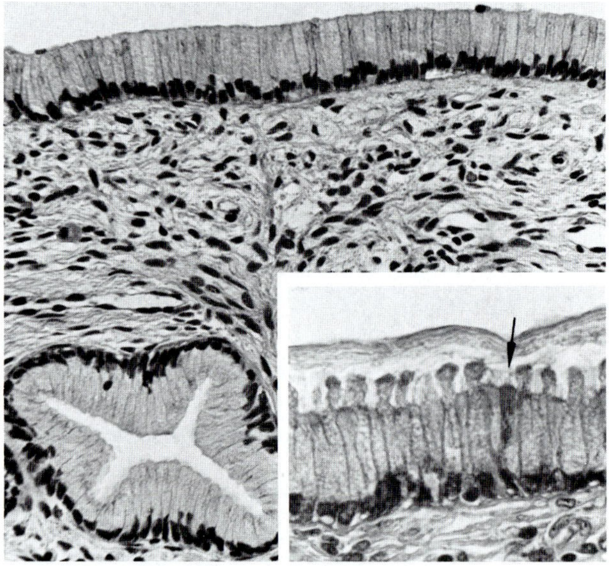

Fig. 5.12. Endocervical mucosa. Tall columnar mucin-filled endocervical cells with basal nuclei. *Inset*: Endocervical cells engaged in apocrine secretion whereby portions of apical cytoplasm are expelled. Ciliated cells are present (*arrow*).

tures of simple epithelia characterized by the presence of only low molecular weight cytokeratins, including cytokeratins 7, 8, 18, and 19.[17] However, endocervical cells are not completely homogeneous with regards to cytokeratin expression, and occasional endocervical cells express cytokeratin 4, which is usually associated with stratified epithelium.

Mitoses in the columnar epithelium are rarely observed. It is not known whether regeneration occurs from the underlying subcolumnar reserve cells, which under normal circumstances are seldom seen even at the ultrastructural level, or from the persisting mature endocervical cells.[19] Unlike the attenuated vascular stromal papillae of the original squamous portio epithelium, the subepithelial capillary network in the endocervical mucosa is well developed.

The stroma of the endocervix is comparatively better innervated than that of the exocervix. Fibers run parallel to muscle bundles, but sensory free endings have not been clearly demonstrated. True lymphoid follicles, with or without germinal centers, are encountered in the subepithelial stroma of both the exocervix and the endocervix.

Effects of Estrogen and Progesterone

The cervical mucus is subject to profound cyclic changes. Under estrogenic stimulation, the endocervical secretions are profuse, watery, and alkaline, facilitating sperm penetration. During the postovulatory phase, secretions are scant, thick, and acid, containing numerous leukocytes, and act as a barrier to sperm penetration. Biochemical and ultrastructural analyses have shown that cervical mucus is composed of a heterogeneous micellar network of glycoproteins.[6,43] The intermicellar space occupied by cervical plasma is rich in sodium chloride and potassium, the ions of which are responsible for the crystallization of mucus or ferning (arborization) reaction. Under estrogenic influence, the glycoprotein micelles are arranged parallel to each other at a distance of 5–15 μm, creating a channel system that is favorable to sperm penetration. During progesterone stimulation, the micellar channel system is replaced by a dense network composed of interlacing micellar fiber bridges that preclude sperm penetration. Ultrastructurally, endocervical secretory activity operates by both the apocrine and the merocrine type of expulsion of secretory products.[13] In the former, a portion of apical cytoplasm packed with secretory granules is detached (Fig. 5.13), whereas in the latter secretory products are released from apical granules through porelike openings of the surface cytoplasmic membrane.

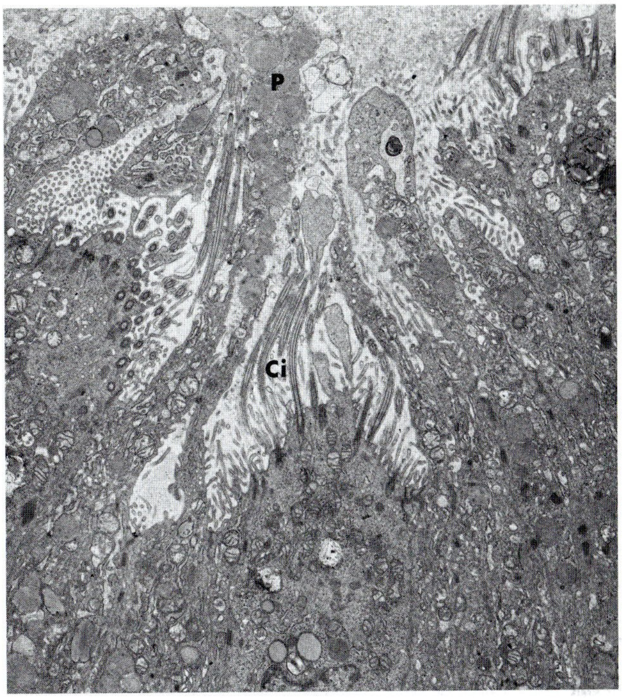

Fig. 5.13. Endocervical mucosa. Electron photomicrograph of mucin-containing endocervical cells alternating with ciliated cells (*Ci*). Secretion is of the apocrine type, as indicated by intraluminal protrusions (*P*) of apical cytoplasmic substance packed with mucinous droplets and various organelles. ×4030.

Lymphoid-Derived Cells

Mucosal immunity is an important component of the host's defense mechanism against viral and bacterial pathogens. Components of the secretory (IgA antibody-mediated) and humoral (IgG antibody-mediated) systems, as well as the cellular immune systems, are present in the cervix. Cellular local immune responses may be particularly important in determining the outcome of human papillomavirus (HPV) infections in the cervix and in modulating the shedding of human immunodeficiency virus (HIV) into genital tract secretions and the susceptibility of women to infection by HIV. A variety of lymphocyte and dendritic macrophage subsets are present in the epithelium of both the exo- and endocervix as well as the subepithelial stroma. *Dendritic cells* are antigen-presenting cells that are found in all tissues and are characterized by long cytoplasmic processes (Fig. 5.14). They are critical for maintaining cellular immunity at mucosal surfaces because they have a high antigen capture and processing potential and the capacity to present antigen peptides in conjunction with major histocompatibility complex (MHC) class II antigens to T lymphocytes after migration to the re-

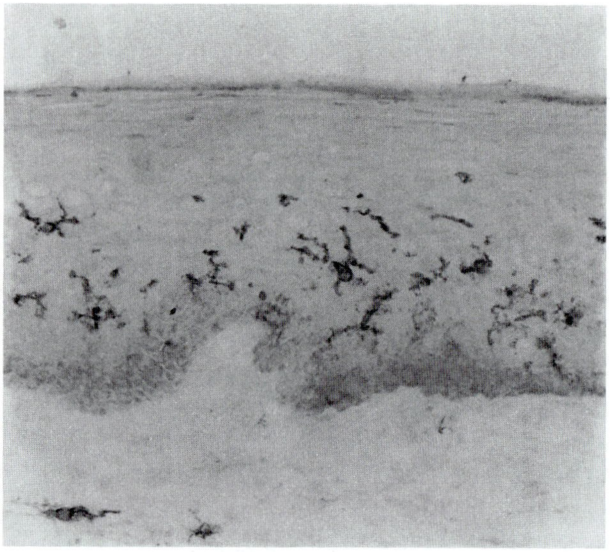

Fig. 5.14. Normal squamous epithelium. Leu 6-positive dendritic macrophages (Langerhans cells) can be localized used immunohistochemistry and are present predominantly in the intermediate cell layers of the epithelium.

gional lymph nodes. In the cervix, these cells display both topographic and phenotypic heterogeneity.[10,46] Dendritic cells include both mature and immature forms. *Langerhans cells* are a type of immature dendritic cell that express MHC class II antigens and the CD4 receptor on their surface. They also express surface CD1a and coexpress P55, a 55-kDa, intracytoplasmic actin-binding protein termed fascin. Only a small subset of all cervical dendritic macrophages are Langerhans cells, and the Langerhans cells are primarily located in the stratified squamous epithelium in the suprabasal cell layers.[10,46] Under normal conditions, basal cells express tumor necrosis factor-alpha (TNF-α), which is a potent activator of Langerhans cells.[40] In the rhesus macaque, Langerhans cells extend cell processes to the mucosal surface and, together with other types of dendritic cells, appear to be the initial site of infection with simian immunodeficiency virus (SIV).[21]

Large numbers of T lymphocytes are also present in the cervix under normal conditions.[24] CD3+ T lymphocytes are concentrated in a band directly beneath both the squamous epithelium of the exocervix and the columnar epithelium of the endocervix.[24,38] These cells are predominately cytotoxic T lymphocytes (e.g., CD8+), although helper T lymphocytes (e.g., CD4+) are also present. Variable numbers of B lymphocytes and plasma cells are also found in the lamina propria of the cervix.[24] Because the presence of lymphocytes in the cervix is a normal finding, the diagnosis of chronic cervicitis should be reserved for specimens showing a marked infiltration of lymphocytes. It should also be pointed out that cervical epithelial cells may play an as yet undefined role in mucosal immunity. Although MHC class II antigens are not expressed by ectocervical keratinocytes under baseline conditions, keratinocytes in squamous intraepithelial lesions (SIL) can express HLA-DR on their surfaces.[2,41]

The Transformation Zone

The squamocolumnar junction of the cervix is defined as the border between the stratified squamous epithelium and the mucin-secreting columnar epithelium of the endocervix. Morphogenetically, there are two different squamocolumnar junctions (Fig. 5.15). One is termed the *original* squamocolumnar junction and is the site at which the native squamous covering of the exocervix abuts the endocervical columnar epithelium at the time of birth. At birth, most females have some mucin-secreting columnar endocervical epithelium present on the portio surface of the cervix, which forms an *ectropion* or cervical *ectopy*. The exact location of the original squamocolumnar junction and, therefore, the amount of endocervical ectopy present at birth depends on the extent of inward migration of squamous epithelium from the lower third of the vagina. In women exposed to diethylstilbestrol (DES) in utero, the normal migration of the squamous epithelium is prematurely halted and the original squamocolumnar junction is often located in the vagina rather than on the exocervix.[45] In these DES-exposed women, the entire cervical portio can be covered with endocervical columnar epithelium.

At about the age of 1 year, the cervix begins to elongate, which results in migration of the squamocolumnar junction toward the external os. This migration is frequently incomplete, and one colposcopic study of prepubertal girls between the ages of 1 and 13 years found endocervical ectopy in 43% of these girls.[33] Hormonal and other physical factors influence the size and distribution of the cervical ectopy by altering the shape and volume of the cervical lips. At the time of menarche or during pregnancy, both the uterus and the cervix enlarge. Enlargement of the cervix is accompanied by alterations in its shape, which result in more of an "eversion" or rolling outward of endocervical columnar epithelium onto the portio (see Fig. 5.15). As a result, in most women during the reproductive period, cervical ectopy is present and the size of the ectopy is most extensive in younger women (under 20 years of age), following the first pregnancy. Cer-

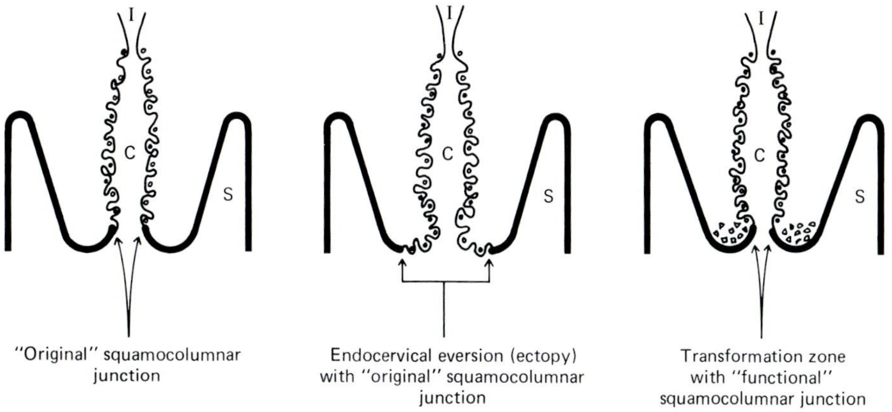

Fig. 5.15. The transformation zone. Schematic representation of original and functional squamocolumnar junctions and three basic types of portios. *Left*: Diagram of a portio completely covered with native squamous epithelium. The squamocolumnar junction is at the external os. *Middle*: Denotes cervical ectopy, with the squamocolumnar junction being located on the exocervix below the external os. *Right*: Indicates areas of cervical ectopy that have become covered with squamous epithelium. This area is the cervical transformation zone. The new, or functional, squamocolumnar junction of the transformation zone is at the external os. *S*, squamous epithelium: *C*, endocervical columnar epithelium; *I*, uterine isthmus.

vical ectopy occurs twice as commonly on the anterior as on the posterior lip, but both lips maybe involved simultaneously. Factors that influence the amount of cervical ectopy include age, which is associated with decreased ectopy, parity, which is associated with increased ectopy, and the length of time a woman has been sexually active, which is associated with reduced ectopy.[23,31] Recent studies have shown that neither oral contraceptives nor injectible progestational agents are associated with a reduction in ectopy.[23,31]

When viewed with the naked eye, the endocervical mucosa appears as a red, velvety zone, sharply contrasting with the neighboring pink, translucent squamous portio epithelium (Fig. 5.16A). Because of its gross appearance, the term *cervical erosion* is often used by clinicians to refer to this columnar epithelium. This term is incorrect, however, because there is no epithelial denudation (true erosion). Instead, the red appearance is caused by papillary excrescences of varying size, resembling a bunch of grapes when viewed with the colposcope. Histologically, these are blunt-ended papillae, lined by endocervical columnar epithelium and supported by a fibrovascular stroma containing numerous chronic inflammatory cells. The cervical ectopy is a normal physiologic finding and should not be construed as a pathologic abnormality.

Over time, the columnar epithelium that composes the cervical ectopy is remodeled and replaced by metaplastic squamous epithelium. As this occurs, the histologic squamocolumnar junction moves toward the exocervical os. This newly formed squamocolumnar junction is called the *physiologic, functional,* or *new* squamocolumnar junction. The original squamocolumnar junction is usually quite abrupt (Fig. 5.17), whereas the junction between the columnar and squamous epithelium at the physiologic or functional squamocolumnar junction can be either abrupt or gradual. The region between the original squamocolumnar junction and the postpubertal functional squamocolumnar junction is termed the *transformation zone*. The transformation zone is histologically characterized by the presence of metaplastic epithelium. The concept of the transformation zone is extremely important for understanding the pathogenesis of squamous cell carcinomas of the cervix and its precursors, because virtually all cervical squamous neoplasia begins at the new squamocolumnar junction and because the extension and limits of cervical cancer precursors coincide with the distribution of the transformation zone. It is also important to remember that during the childbearing years and during pregnancy the transformation zone is located, in almost all instances, on the exposed portion of the cervix. Consequently, most cervical neoplasias can be sampled for histologic diagnosis by punch biopsy.

The transformation zone may be difficult to visualize with the naked eye. Its localization, however, is greatly enhanced with the application of a 5% solution of acetic acid and the use of the colposcope (see Chapter 7, Precancerous Lesions of the Cervix). Colposcopically the T-zone is characterized by smooth, translucent, slightly white tissue that corresponds to metaplastic squamous epithelium with circular open-

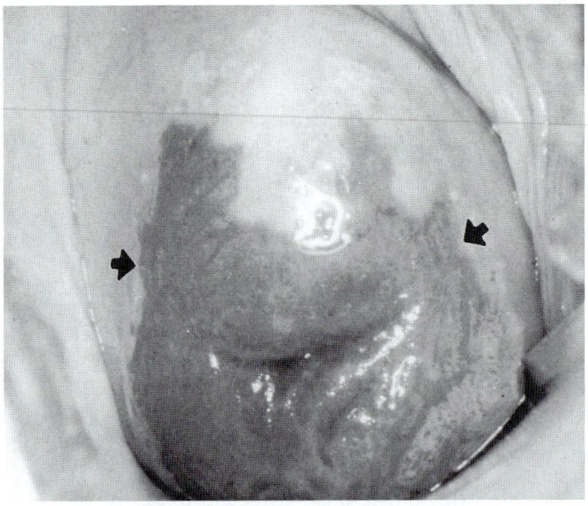

a

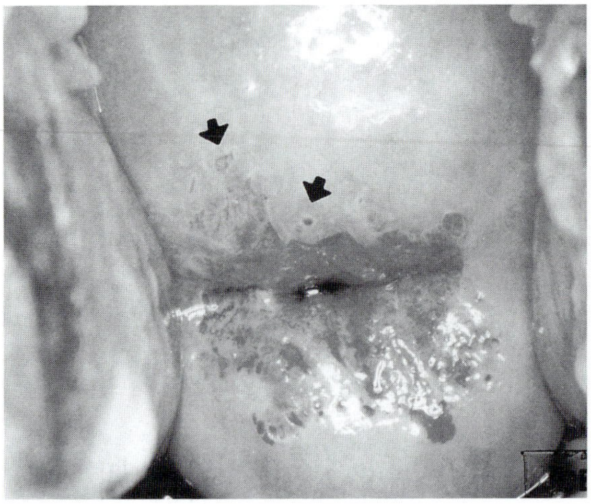

b

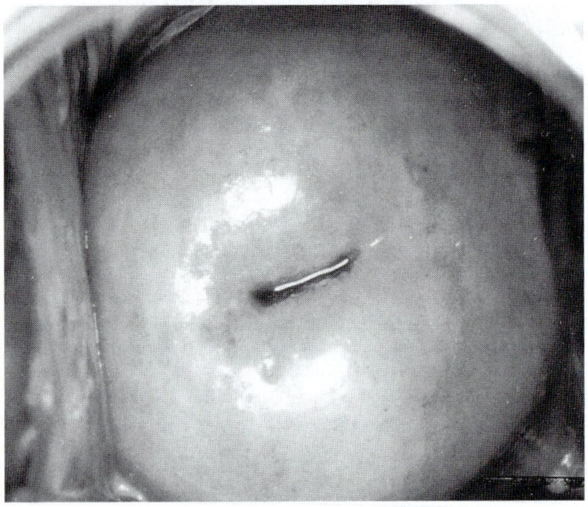

b

Fig. 5.16. The transformation zone. Colpophotographs of endocervical eversion of the transformation zone. **A:** Endocervical mucosa is everted on both the anterior and the posterior lip and surrounds the anatomic external os. The original squamocolumnar junction (*SCJ*) is on the portio of the cervix (*arrows*). **B:** Squamous metaplasia is occurring, and the new SCJ is now internal to the original SCJ. The area between the original and new SCJ is the transformation zone. Residual endocervical gland mouths are represented by the circular openings (*arrows*). **C:** The transformation zone is completely mature and the SCJ is inside the endocervical canal. No endocervical gland mouths are present.

ings and spherical bumps of 2–4 mm, which correspond to the underlying endocervical glands and nabothian cysts, respectively (see Fig. 5.16B). Nabothian cysts are formed when the mouths of endocervical clefts become obliterated by the proliferating surface metaplastic squamous epithelium. As the flow of mucus is blocked, the secretory products accumulate, leading to cystic glandular dilations, or nabothian cysts. Microscopically, the cystic spaces are lined by low columnar endocervical cells, supported by a distended basal lamina (Fig. 5.18).

Movement of the functional squamocolumnar junction continues throughout the reproductive years. Therefore, in older and postmenopausal women, the functional squamocolumnar junction is nearly always located above the external os (see Fig. 5.16C).

Squamous Metaplasia

Metaplasia is defined as the replacement of one type of mature tissue by another equally mature type of tissue. In the cervix, *squamous metaplasia* is the replacement of the mucin-producing columnar epithelium by stratified squamous epithelium and appears to occur by two different mechanisms (Fig. 5.19). One mechanism consists of direct ingrowth from the native portio epithelium bordering the columnar epithelium, a process frequently referred to as "squamous epithelialization." The second mechanism involves a proliferation of undifferentiated subcolumnar reserve cells of the endocervical epithelium, which differentiate into squamous epithelium. This process has been termed *squamous metaplasia*, but such names as *epidermidization* and *squamous prosoplasia* are also used.[16] The latter term, derived from the Greek meaning *forward* and *to form*, was proposed by Fluhmann and is probably the most accurate one, although rarely used today.

The process of squamous epithelialization has been documented by histologic, colposcopic, colpomicroscopic, and electron microscopic observations, which have shown that tongues of native squamous epithelium of the portio grow beneath the adjacent columnar epithelium and expand between the mucinous epithelium and its basement mem-

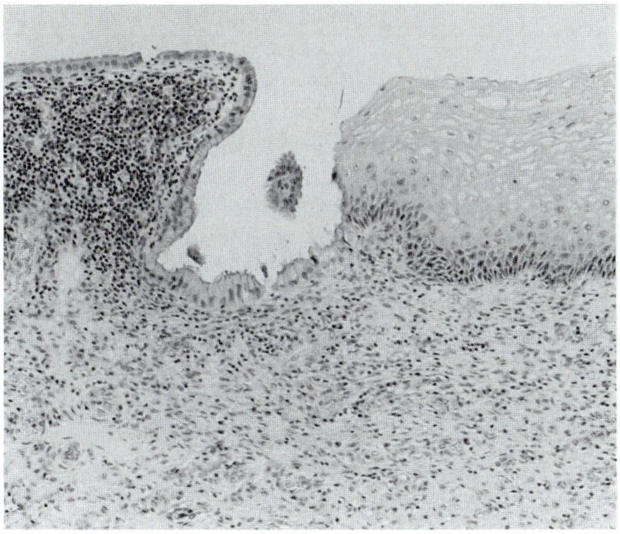

Fig. 5.17. Squamocolumnar junction. Endocervical columnar epithelium meets the native squamous portio epithelium. Note the abrupt transition between the mature squamous epithelium of the portio and the endocervical mucosa. A similar sharp demarcation may be seen at the squamocolumnar junction of the mature transformation zone. The lamina propria of the columnar epithelium is frequently obscured by a chronic inflammatory exudate.

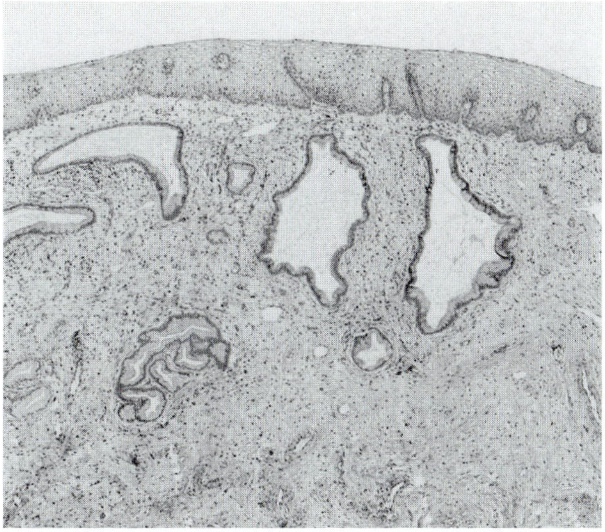

Fig. 5.18. Transformation zone. Microscopic appearance of the outer portio limit of the transformation zone. Mature squamous epithelium covers underlying endocervical glands that are distended with mucin.

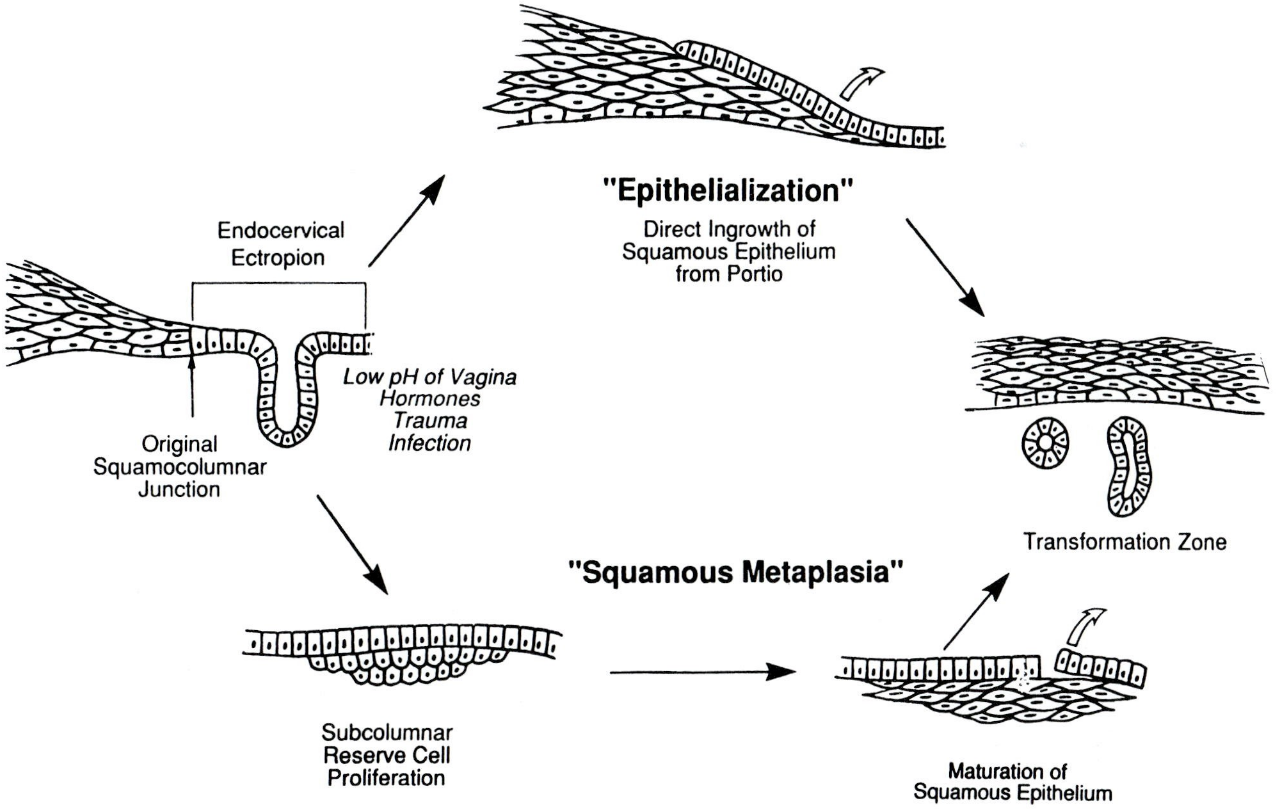

Fig. 5.19. Squamous metaplasia. There are two histogenic mechanisms by which the endocervical mucosa is replaced by squamous epithelium. The first is the direct ingrowth of squamous epithelium from the portio, which is referred to as squamous epithelialization (*top*). The other is through proliferation of subcolumnar reserve cells and their subsequent maturation into a squamous epithelium, which is called squamous metaplasia (bottom). Both result in a mature squamous epithelium overlying endocervical mucus-producing glands (*right*).

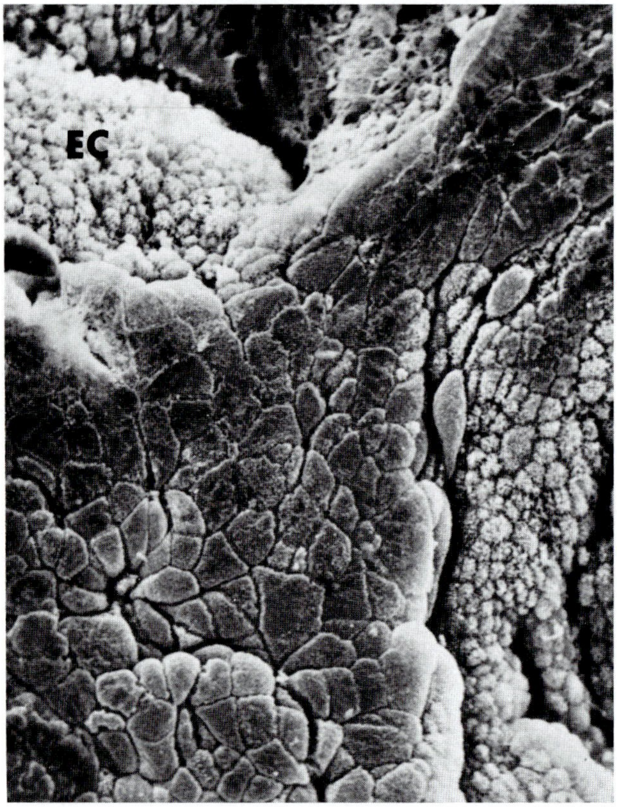

Fig. 5.20. Squamous metaplasia. Scanning electron microscopic appearance of the outer edge of the early transformation zone. Narrow tongues of squamous epithelium with a pavement-like surface pattern extend onto the everted endocervical mucosa (*EC*). ×4280.

brane (Fig. 5.20).[7,12] As the squamous cells expand and mature, the endocervical cells are gradually displaced upward, degenerate, and eventually are sloughed (Fig. 5.21, top). A similar process is observed in the reepithelialization of true pathologic erosion of the endocervix, the so-called ascending healing of Meyer.[36] The progression of squamous transformation of the endocervical ectropion has been hypothesized to be primarily dependent on local (vaginal) environmental factors, with the initial stimulus being the low (acid) pH of the vagina after puberty.[7] Trauma, chronic irritation, or cervical infection also play a role in development and maturation of the transformation zone by stimulating repair and remodeling; eventually, the ectocervix is covered by a protective surface of mature squamous epithelium (see Fig. 5.18). The process of squamous epithelialization is thought to be responsible for the obliteration of the outer two-thirds of endocervical ectopy. Rapid squamous reepithelialization of the columnar epithelium of the transformation zone may also be produced iatrogenically by electrocautery, cryosurgery, or laser surgery.

The second mechanism involved in replacement of columnar epithelium by a squamous epithelium and the function of the transformation zone is squamous metaplasia (i.e., squamous prosoplasia). This process has been thoroughly documented by Fluhmann and others.[7,16] The first stage of squamous metaplasia is the appearance of small cuboidal cells beneath the columnar mucinous epithelium, the so-called subcolumnar reserve cells (Fig. 5.21, bottom). *Reserve cells* have large, uniformly shaped, round nuclei with faintly granular chromatin and occasional aggregates of chromatin (i.e., chromocenters

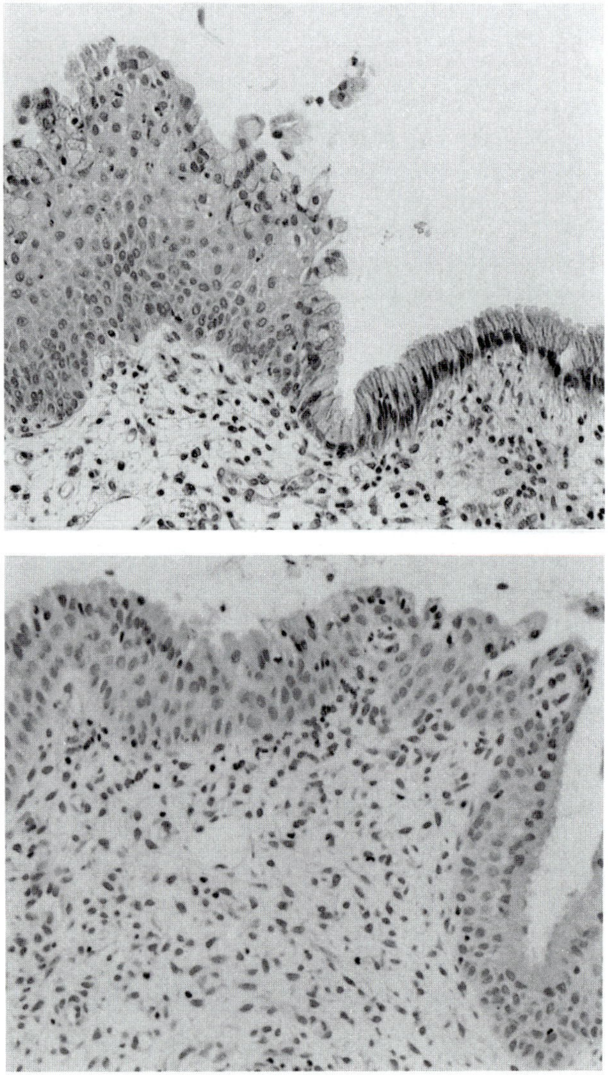

Fig. 5.21. Squamous metaplasia. *Top*: During squamous epithelialization, a narrow tongue of squamous epithelium from the portio grows under the everted endocervical mucosa and lifts it off the basement membrane. The endocervical cells then degenerate and are sloughed. *Bottom*: During squamous metaplasia, a layer of cuboidal reserve cells develops between the columnar endocervical cells and the basal lamina.

of reserve cells). The cell borders are poorly defined and the cells have only scant amounts of cytoplasm. There is an increased rate of nucleic acid synthesis in reserve cells when examined by autoradiography, and their fine ultrastructural characteristics are similar to those of the basal cells of the mature squamous portio epithelium.[19] The origin of subcolumnar reserve cells is controversial. Some investigators suggest a direct derivation from columnar mucinous secretory cells, whereas others favor an origin from the basal cells of the squamous portioepithelium, embryonal rests of urogenital origin, or stromal cells as possible sources. Cell culture and implantation experiments in vitro and in vivo combined with immunohistochemical studies show that human endocervical cells can differentiate reversibly and give rise to both CK7- and CK18-positive endocervical mucin-secreting cells and CK13-positive reserve cells. In these experiments, reserve cells were identified to be the origin of squamous metaplastic cells.[52] Progressive growth and stratification of reserve cells (subcolumnar reserve cell hyperplasia), followed by differentiation into immature squamous metaplasia, result in the formation of a fully mature squamous epithelium indistinguishable from the native portio epithelium (see Fig. 5.18).

Immature squamous metaplastic epithelium is distinguished from its mature counterpart by a lack of surface maturation and inconspicuous intracytoplasmic glycogen. It is, characteristically, sharply demarcated from the native portion epithelium by a perpendicular or oblique line to the surface (Fig. 5.22). As a result, the uninitiated observer may mistake immature squamous metaplasia for a squamous intraepithelial lesion (SIL), particularly when the process also involves the underlying glands (Fig. 5.23). In contrast to neoplastic epithelium, the immature squamous metaplastic epithelium maintains cell organization and cohesion, nuclear atypia is absent, and, frequently, a single row of endocervical cells overlies the squamous cells. Ultrastructurally, the immature, squamous metaplastic cells resemble the parabasal cells of the portio epithelium. The superficial cells of the immature transformation zone

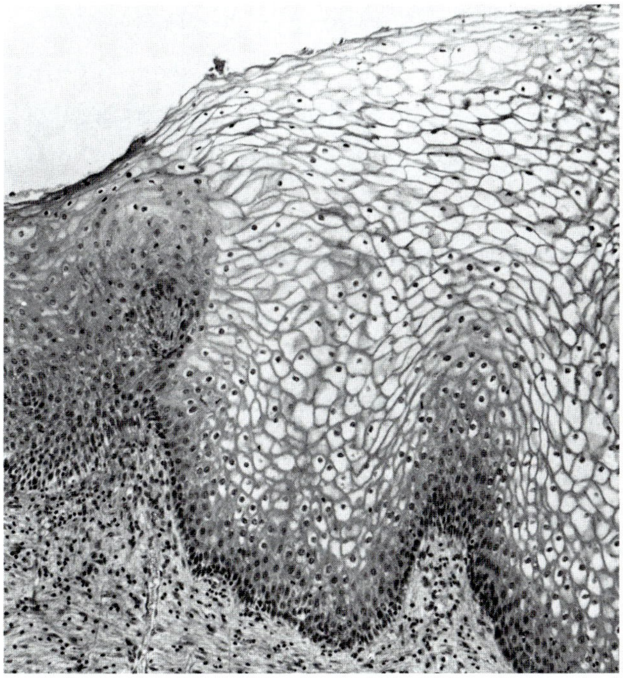

Fig. 5.22. Transformation zone epithelium. On the *right*, the epithelium has achieved full maturation and is identical with normal native portio epithelium, whereas on the *left*, squamous differentiation, including glycogenation, is incomplete.

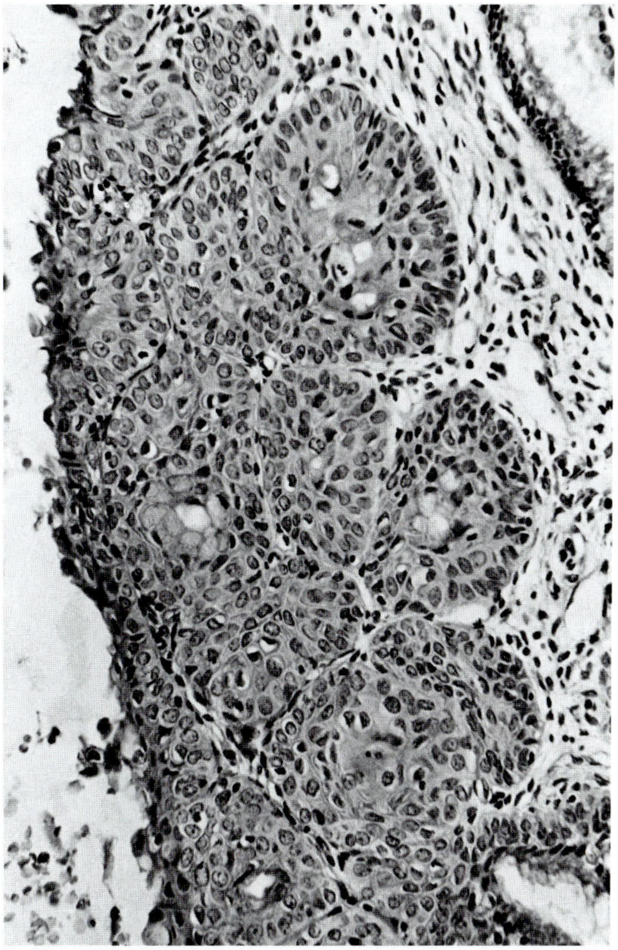

Fig. 5.23. Immature squamous metaplasia. Immature squamous metaplasia can involve both the surface and the deeper endocervical glands. Note trapped mucinous endocervical cells in the center of the metaplastic foci. Unlike squamous intraepithelial lesions (SIL) with gland involvement, in squamous metaplasia nuclear atypia is minimal and there is normal cellular cohesion.

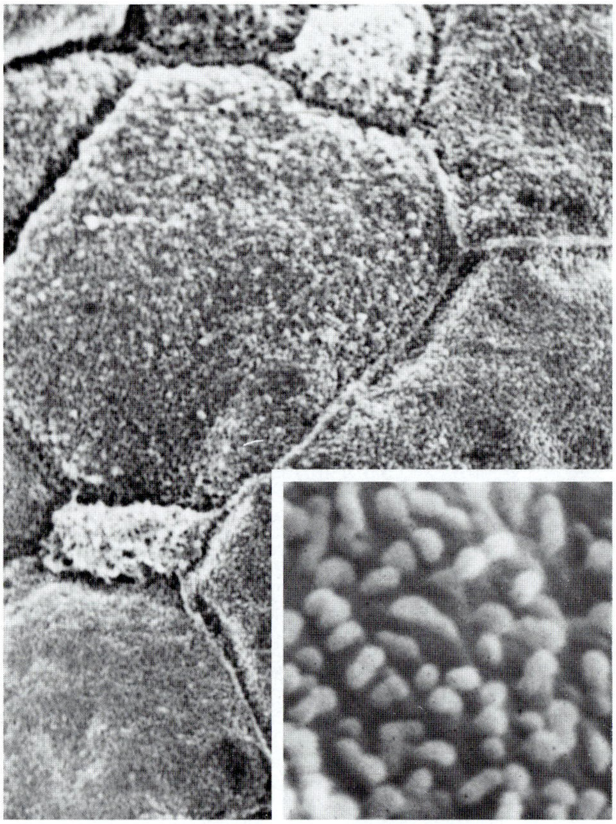

Fig. 5.24. Immature squamous metaplasia. Scanning electron microscopy of immature squamous metaplastic cells with well-developed terminal bars. In contrast to the superficial cells of the mature squamous epithelium, which are covered by microridges, the superficial cells of the immature transformation zone are covered by microvilli. Among the squamous cells is an entrapped endocervical cell (*lower left*). ×2,400. *Inset*: Higher magnification of surface microvilli. ×15,000.

epithelium are covered by numerous microvillous projections rather than surface microridges (Fig. 5.24).[13] Unlike squamous epithelialization, which involves the peripheral regions of the endocervical tissue, squamous metaplasia has a random distribution within the ectropion, reflecting its asynchronous development. The patchy, uneven distribution of squamous metaplasia within the ectropion may be caused by the presence of circumscribed, focal stimuli or differing rates of cell transition and maturation.[12]

Biochemically and immunohistochemically, immature squamous metaplasia shares features of both the mature squamous epithelium and the columnar mucinous epithelium. The keratin intermediate filaments of metaplastic squamous cells are similar to those of terminally differentiated squamous cells but are less complex and fewer in number.[9,39] Focal mucin production may be demonstrated by cytoplasmic mucicarmine positivity. The bipotential nature of immature metaplasia is further corroborated ultrastructurally by the finding of individual cells, within islands of metaplasia, that demonstrate both squamous and columnar mucinous features. Cilia may occasionally persist in otherwise mature squamous cells.

With the aid of the colposcope, islands of squamous metaplastic epithelium are seen on the tips of endocervical papillae, expanding centripetally and developing delicate epithelial bridges that fuse with neighboring epithelial proliferations (Fig. 5.16, middle). Further growth, expansion, and interanastomosis between squamous epithelial islands eventually lead to complete obliteration of the underlying columnar epithelium (Fig. 5.16, bottom).

Pregnancy and Puerperium

The morphologic alterations that occur in the antepartum or postpartum cervix are not pathognomonic of pregnancy or parturition but are seen more commonly at these times than in the nonpregnant postpartum state. They are related to the stimulatory effects of elevated steroid hormones. The spongy enlargement of the pregnant cervix is caused by increased vascularity and edema of the stroma, accompanied by acute inflammation. The massive destruction of collagen fibers and accumulation of ex-

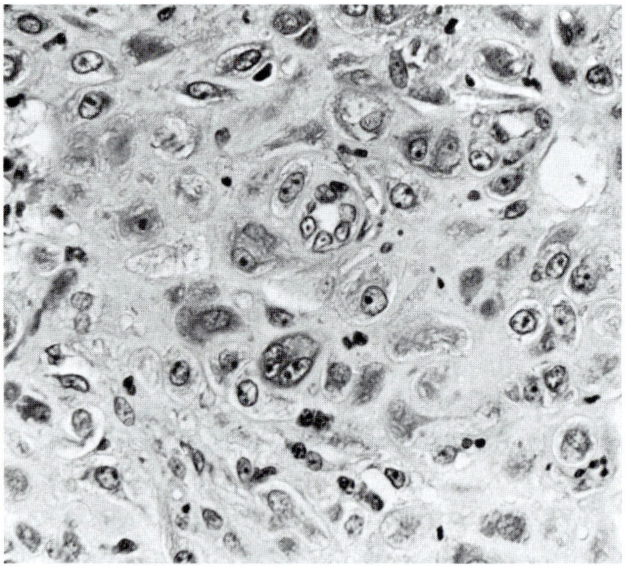

Fig. 5.25. Decidual reaction. A decidual reaction of cervical stromal cells can occur during pregnancy. The cells are identical with gestational decidual cells of the endometrium. Decidual change in the cervix should be distinguished from poorly differentiated invasive squamous cell carcinoma or undifferentiated carcinoma.

tracellular glycoprotein ground substance before labor result in cervical softening and effacement, facilitating dilation of the cervix to about 10 cm during labor. Decidualization of the stroma, either patchy or diffuse, occurs in about one-third of the cervices examined histologically (Fig. 5.25) and disappears by 2 months postpartum.[25] It is presumably mediated by the high levels of progesterone during pregnancy.

Gestational cervical mucus is thick, tenacious, rich in leukocytes, and forms a mucous plug that obliterates the cervical canal, sealing the endometrial cavity from the vagina and thus preventing bacterial invasion. Squamous metaplasia and lobules of tightly packed, small endocervical glandular units forming polypoid protrusions into the canal are often seen. The term *microglandular endocervical hyperplasia* is used for the latter type of lesion (see *Chapter 6, Benign Diseases of the Cervix*). The marked proliferation of endocervical mucinous cells is associated with enlargement and softening of the portio during the course of gestation and leads to a more exaggerated protrusion of the endocervical ectropion onto exocervix. It is rapidly replaced by immature squamous epithelium of both native portio and subcolumnar reserve cell origin postpartum. As a result, in most primigravidas an immature cervical transformation zone is seen that often persists for long periods of time. The squamocolumnar junction of the transformation zone is nearly always located distal to the external os. Subsequent active remodeling of the transformation zone occurs to a comparatively lesser extent in subsequent pregnancies. Postpartum injuries, such as lacerations produced during labor, are frequently seen in primiparous and half of multiparous patients, with a distribution of 2:1 in favor of the anterior lip.[49] The denuded areas are subsequently reepithelialized by ingrowing native squamous epithelium on the exocervix.

References

1. Al-Nafussi AI, Klys HS, Rebello G, et al (1993) The assessment of proliferating cell nuclear antigen (PCNA) immunostaining in the uterine cervix and cervical squamous neoplasia. Int J Gynecol Cancer 3:154–158
2. al-Saleh W, Giannini SL, Jacobs N, et al (1998) Correlation of T-helper secretory differentiation and types of antigen-presenting cells in squamous intraepithelial lesions of the uterine cervix. J Pathol 184:283–290
3. Averette HE, Weinstein GD, Frost P (1970) Autoradiographic analysis of cell proliferation kinetics in human genital tissues. I. Normal cervix and vagina. Am J Obstet Gynecol 108:8–17
4. Berchuck A, Rodriguez G, Kamel A, et al (1990) Expression of epidermal growth factor receptor and HER-2/Neu in normal and neoplastic cervix, vulva and vagina. Obstet Gynecol 76:381–387
5. Cho NH, Kim YT, Kim JW (1997) Correlation between G1 cyclins and HPV in the uterine cervix. Int J Gynecol Pathol 16:339–347
6. Chretien FC, Gernigon C, David G, et al (1973) The ultrastructure of human cervical mucus under scanning electron microscopy. Fertil Steril 24:746–757
7. Coppleson M, Pixley E, Reid B (1971) Colposcopy. A scientific and practical approach to the cervix in health and disease. Thomas, Springfield
8. Cuzick J, De Stavola BL, Russell MJ, et al (1990) Vitamin A, vitamin E and the risk of cervical intraepithelial neoplasia. Br J Cancer 62:651–652
9. Czernobilsky B, Moll R, Franke WW, et al (1984) Intermediate filaments of normal and neoplastic tissues of the female genital tract with emphasis on problems of differential diagnosis. Pathol Res Pract 179:31–37
10. Edwards JN, Morris HB (1985) Langerhans' cells and lymphocyte subsets in the female genital tract. Br J Obstet Gynecol 92:974–982
11. Fand SB (1973) The histochemistry of human cervical epithelium. In: Blandau RJ, Moghissi K (eds) The biology of the cervix. University of Chicago Press, Chicago pp 103–124
12. Feldman D, Romney SL, Edgecomb J, et al (1984) Ultrastructure of normal, metaplastic and abnormal human uterine cervix: use of montages to study the topographical relationship of epithelial cells. Am J Obstet Gynecol 150:573–688
13. Ferenczy A, Richard RM (1974) Female reproductive system. Dynamics of scan and transmission electron microscopy. Wiley, New York
14. Fetissof F, Berger G, Dubois MP, et al (1985) Endocrine cells in the female genital tract. Histopathology (Oxf) 9:133–145
15. Fetissof F, Serres G, Arbeille B, et al (1991) Argyrophilic cells and ectocervical epithelium. Int J Gynecol Pathol 10:177–190
16. Fluhmann FC (1961) The cervix uteri and its diseases. Saunders, Philadelphia
17. Franke WW, Moll R, Achstaetter T, et al (1986) Cell typing of epithelial and carcinomas of the female genital tract using cytoskeletal proteins as markers. In: Peto R, zur Hausen H (eds) Viral etiology of cervical cancer. Banbury Report, vol. 21, Cold Spring Harbor Laboratory, pp. 121–148
18. Fujiwara H, Tortolero-Luna G, Mitchell MF, et al (1997) Adenocarcinoma of the cervix. Expression and clinical significance of estrogen and progesterone receptors. Cancer (Phila) 79:505–512
19. Gould PR, Barter RA, Papadimitriou JM (1979) An ultrastructural, cytochemical and autoradiographic study of the mucous membrane of the human cervical canal with reference to subcolumnar cells. Am J Pathol 95:1–16
20. Hillemanns P, Tannous-Khouri L, Koulos JP, et al (1992) Localization of cellular retinoid-binding proteins in human cervical intraepithelial neoplasia and invasive carcinoma. Am J Pathol 141:973–979
21. Hu J, Gardner MB, Miller CJ (2000) Simian immunodeficiency virus rapidly penetrates the cer-

vicovaginal mucosa after intravaginal inoculation and infects intraepithelial dendritic cells. J Virol 74: 6087–6095
22. Ibrahim EM, Blackett AD, Tidy JA, et al (1999) CD44 is a marker of endocervical neoplasia. Int J Gynecol Pathol 18:101–108
23. Jacobson DL, Peralta L, Farmer M, et al (1999) Cervical ectopy and the transformation zone measured by computerized planimetry in adolescents. Int J Gynaecol Obstet 66:7–17
24. Johansson EL, Rudin A, Wassen L, et al (1999) Distribution of lymphocytes and adhesion molecules in human cervix and vagina. Immunology 96:272–277
25. Johnson LD (1973) Dysplasia and carcinoma in situ in pregnancy. In: Norris HJ, Hertig AT, Abell MR (eds) The uterus. International Academy of Pathology Monographs. Williams & Wilkins, Baltimore, pp 382–412
26. Kanai M, Shiozawa T, Xin L, et al (1998) Immunohistochemical detection of sex steroid receptors, cyclins, and cyclin-dependent kinases in the normal and neoplastic squamous epithelia of the uterine cervix. Cancer (Phila) 82:1709–1719
27. Karakitsos P, Kyroudes A, Apostolaki C, et al (1994) The evaluation of PCNA/cyclin expression in cervical intraepithelial lesions. Gynecol Oncol 55:101–107
28. Konishi I, Fujii S, Nonogaki H, et al (1991) Immunohistochemical analysis of estrogen receptors, Ki-67 antigen, and human papillomavirus DNA in normal and neoplastic epithelium of the uterine cervix. Cancer (Phila) 68:1340–1350
29. Koss LG (1992) Diagnostic cytology and its histopathologic basis. Lippincott, New York
30. Krantz KE (1973) The anatomy of the human cervix, gross and microscopic. In: Blandau RJ, Moghissi K (eds) The biology of the cervix. University of Chicago Press, Chicago
31. Kuhn L, Denny L, Pollack AE, et al (1999) Prevalence of visible disruption of cervical epithelium and cervical ectopy in African women using Depo-Provera. Contraception 59:363–367
32. Kupryjanczyk J, Moller P (1988) Estrogen receptor distribution in the normal and pathologically changed human cervix uteri: an immunohistochemical study with use of monoclonal anti-ER antibody. Int J Gynecol Pathol 7:75–85
33. Linhartova A (1978) Extent of columnar epithelium on the ectocervix between the ages of 1 and 13 years. Obstet Gynecol 52:451–455
34. Lippman SM, Lotan R (2000) Advances in the development of retinoids as chemopreventive agents. J Nutr 130:479S–482S
35. McCluggage WG, Buhidma M, Tang L, et al (1996) Monoclonal antibody MIB1 in the assessment of cervical squamous intraepithelial lesions. Int J Gynecol Pathol 15:131–136
36. Meyer R (1941) The basis of the histological diagnosis of carcinoma with special reference to carcinoma of the cervix and similar lesions. Surg Gynecol Obstet 73:14
37. Meyskens FL, Surwit E, Moon TE, et al (1994) Enhancement of regression of cervical intraepithelial neoplasia II (moderate dysplasia) with topically applied all-*trans*-retinoic acid: a randomized trial. J Natl Cancer Inst 86:539–543
38. Miller CJ, McChesney M, Moore PF (1992) Langerhans cells, macrophages and lymphocyte subsets in the cervix and vagina of rhesus macaques. Lab Invest 67:628–634
39. Moll R, Levy R, Czernobilsky B, et al (1983) Cytokeratins of normal epithelial and some neoplasms of the female genital tract. Lab Invest 49:599–610
40. Mota F, Rayment N, Chong S, et al (1999) The antigen-presenting environment in normal and human papillomavirus (HPV)-related premalignant cervical epithelium. Clin Exp Immunol 116:33–40
41. Mota FF, Rayment NB, Kanan JH, et al (1998) Differential regulation of HLA-DQ expression by keratinocytes and Langerhans cells in normal and premalignant cervical epithelium. Tissue Antigens 52: 286–293
42. Noy N (2000) Retinoid-binding proteins: mediators of retinoid action. Biochem J 348:481–495
43. Odeblad E (1968) The functional structure of human cervical mucus. Acta Obstet Gynecol Scand 47:57–79
44. Raju GC (1994) Expression of the proliferating cell nuclear antigen in cervical neoplasia. Int J Gynecol Pathol 13:337–341
45. Robboy SJ, Taguchi O, Cunha GR (1982) Normal development of the human female reproductive tract and alterations resulting from experimental exposure to diethylstilbestrol. Hum Pathol 13:190–198
46. Roncalli M, Sideri M, Gie P, et al (1988) Immunophenotypic analysis of the transformation zone of human cervix. Lab Invest 58:141–149
47. Saegusa M, Takano Y, Hashimura M, et al (1995) The possible role of bcl-2 expression in the progression of tumors of the uterine cervix. Cancer (Phila) 76:2297–2303
48. Shurbaji MS, Brooks SK, Thurmond TS (1993) Proliferating cell nuclear antigen immunoreactivity in cervical intraepithelial neoplasia and benign cervical epithelium. Am J Clin Pathol 100:22–26
49. Singer A (1976) The cervical epithelium during pregnancy and the puerperium. In: Jordan JA, Singer A (eds) The cervix. Saunders, London, pp 105–127
50. Smedts F, Ramekers F, Troyanovsky S, et al (1992) Basal-cell keratins in cervical reserve cells and a comparison to their expression in cervical intraepithelial neoplasia. Am J Pathol 140:601–612
51. ter Harmsel B, Kuijpers J, Smedts F, et al (1997) Progressing imbalance between proliferation and apoptosis with increasing severity of cervical intraepithelial neoplasia. Int J Gynecol Pathol 16:205–211
52. Tsutsumi K, Sun Q, Yasumoto S, et al (1993) In vitro and in vivo analysis of cellular origin of cervical squamous metaplasia. Am J Pathol 143:1150–1158
53. Wolbach SB, Howe PR (1925) Tissue changes following deprivation of fat-soluble A vitamin. J Exp Med 42:753–757

6

Benign Diseases of the Cervix

Thomas C. Wright, M.D., and Alex Ferenczy, M.D.

Inflammatory Diseases

Cervicitis can be divided into two categories, based on whether the etiology of the disorder is noninfectious or infectious. Whatever the etiology, the tissue response of the cervix to injury is limited and reflects the basic mechanisms of inflammation and repair. Two types of morphologic changes, however, that are often encountered in association with a variety of inflammatory diseases deserve specific attention: these are atypia of repair and hyperkeratosis and parakeratosis.

Atypia of Repair

In cases of severe, acute long-standing chronic inflammation or infection with epithelial injury of any kind—true erosion, biopsy, or conization—the squamous and endocervical epithelia undergo reactive changes characterized by epithelial disorganization and nuclear atypia (Fig. 6.1). These changes are often confused, histologically and cytologically, with intraepithelial neoplasia. In *reactive atypia*, the cytoplasmic membrane is well defined, the nuclei are uniform in shape and size, and the chromatin is aggregated in prominent aggregates or clumps. The epithelium is often infiltrated with migrating inflammatory cells. Mitotic figures are normal and are confined to the proliferative basal and parabasal cell populations. Characteristically, the cells in the upper half of the epithelium are normal, and maturation occurs in an orderly fashion. In the endocervical columnar cells, the reparative morphologic alterations include nuclear enlargement and hyperchromasia with irregularity of nuclear size and shape and smudgy chromatin. There can also be cytoplasmic eosinophilia and loss of mucinous droplets (Fig. 6.1).

The combination of endocervical cell enlargement with dense, eosinophilic, focally vacuolated cytoplasm and varying degrees of nuclear atypia has been referred to as "atypical oxyphilic (eosinophilic) metaplasia".[58] Although this type of glandular epithelium appears highly atypical, the changes are focal, alternating with normal mucinous columnar cells, and are confined to areas with inflammation or mucosal injury. In addition, the deep cytoplasmic eosinophilia, when it is present, and the absence

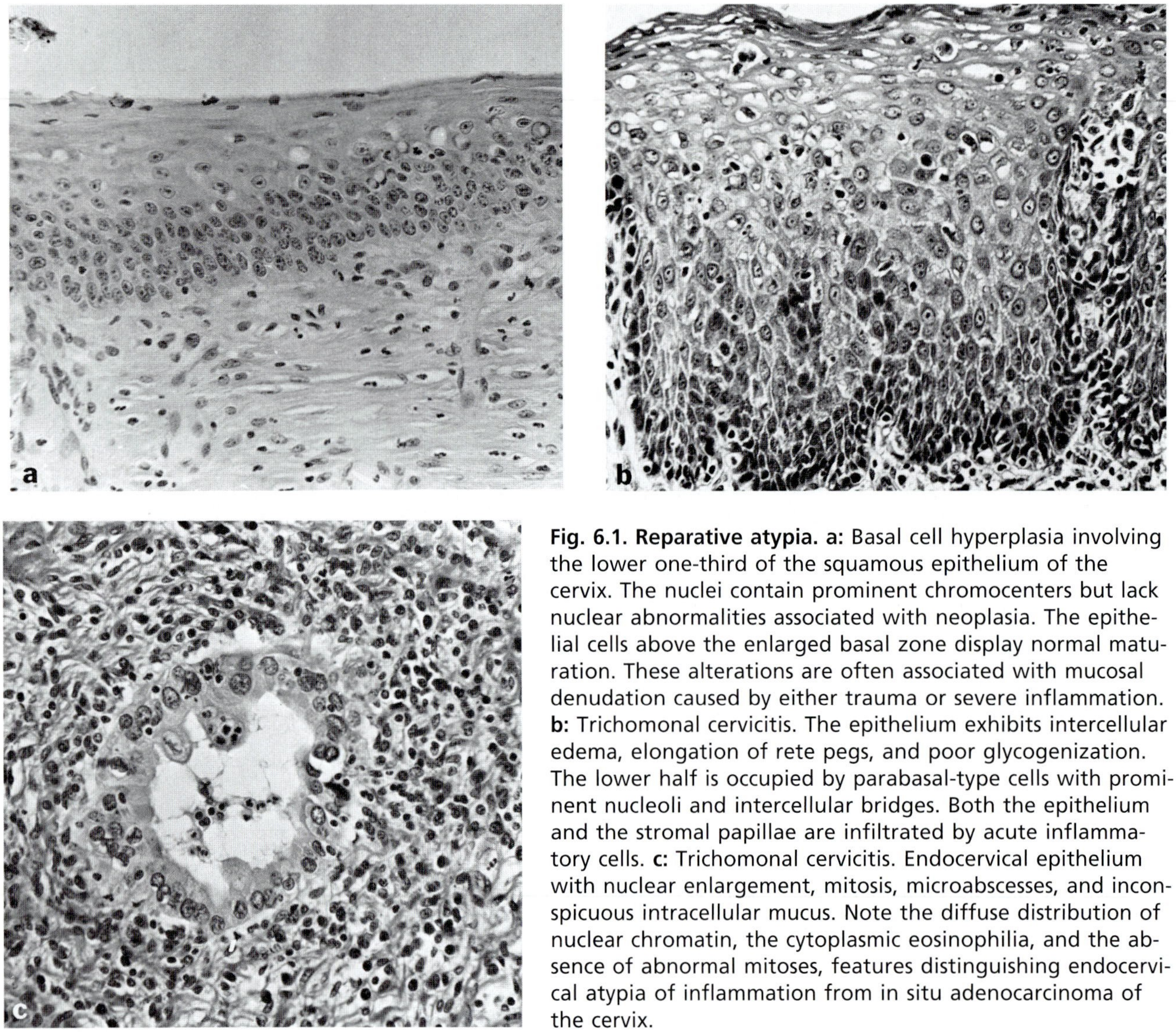

Fig. 6.1. Reparative atypia. a: Basal cell hyperplasia involving the lower one-third of the squamous epithelium of the cervix. The nuclei contain prominent chromocenters but lack nuclear abnormalities associated with neoplasia. The epithelial cells above the enlarged basal zone display normal maturation. These alterations are often associated with mucosal denudation caused by either trauma or severe inflammation. **b:** Trichomonal cervicitis. The epithelium exhibits intercellular edema, elongation of rete pegs, and poor glycogenization. The lower half is occupied by parabasal-type cells with prominent nucleoli and intercellular bridges. Both the epithelium and the stromal papillae are infiltrated by acute inflammatory cells. **c:** Trichomonal cervicitis. Endocervical epithelium with nuclear enlargement, mitosis, microabscesses, and inconspicuous intracellular mucus. Note the diffuse distribution of nuclear chromatin, the cytoplasmic eosinophilia, and the absence of abnormal mitoses, features distinguishing endocervical atypia of inflammation from in situ adenocarcinoma of the cervix.

of abnormal mitoses are features that distinguish the inflammatory lesions from an in situ adenocarcinoma of the endocervix.

Radiation-Induced Atypia

Treatment of the cervix with therapeutic levels of radiation can cause morphologic changes in both the squamous and glandular epithelium. The *atypical squamous cells* that develop post radiation have nuclear enlargement and can be multinucleated. The cells can have abundant amounts of vacuolated cytoplasm and are usually detected in cervical cytologic preparations. Radiation-induced changes in the endocervical glandular epithelium include cellular enlargement, a loss of polarity of nuclei, and dense eosinophilic, enlarged nucleoli that can be multiple.[71] The stroma in women who have received therapeutic radiation is frequently fibrotic, often with hyalinization. Blood vessels often have intimal hyaline thickening and can be totally occluded. "Radiation fibroblasts" are usually not present.[71] These morphologic changes can exist up to 17 years after radiation therapy.

Hyperkeratosis and Parakeratosis

Hyperkeratosis and *parakeratosis* can be detected cytologically in up to 8% of all women undergoing routine Pap smear screening.[55] Both hyperkeratosis and parakeratosis have the gross appearance of a thickened, white epithelium and can be either focal or diffuse. When diffuse, the entire portio is covered by a thickened, white, and wrinkled epithelial membrane. When focal, a slightly raised white plaque is present. The etiology of cervical hyperkeratosis is

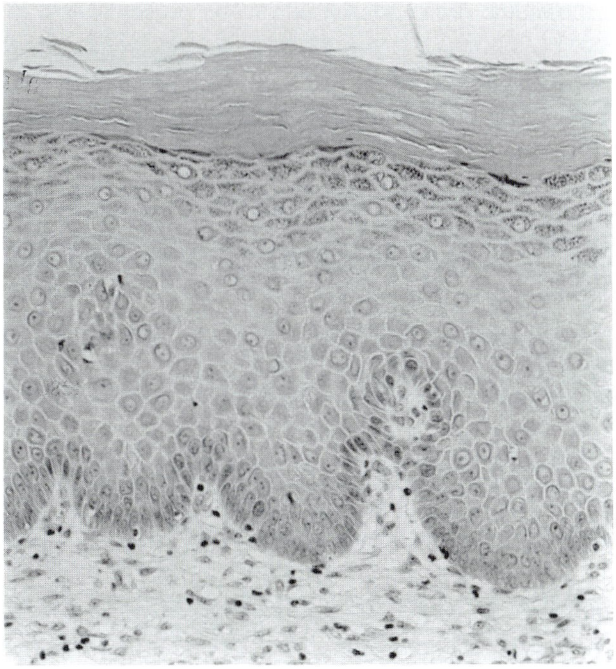

Fig. 6.2. Hyperkeratosis of the cervix. A superficial layer of anucleated, keratinized squamous cells, which frequently is accompanied by a thickened granular layer.

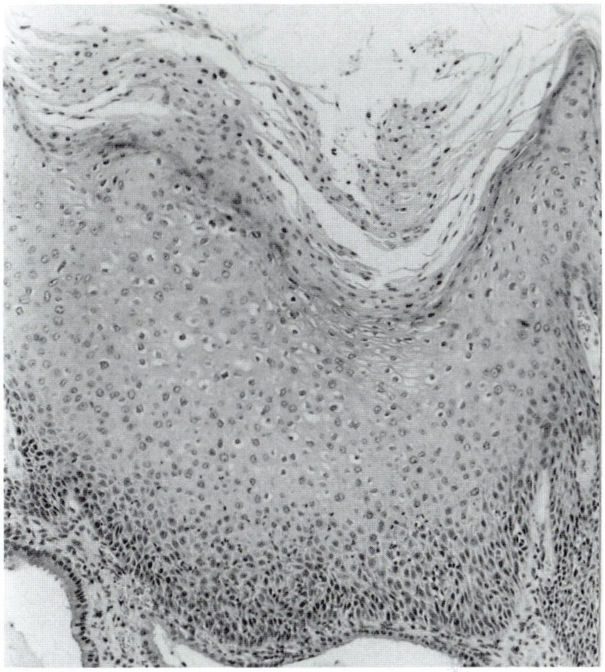

Fig. 6.3. Parakeratosis of the cervix. Pyknotic nuclei are retained in the superficial cell layer. Parakeratosis is frequently accompanied by hyperkeratosis, and both are present in this patient with a low-grade squamous intraepithelial lesion (SIL) (cervical intraepithelial neoplasm, CIN 1).

poorly understood, but in some cases it appears to be related to chronic irritation. For example, most patients with diffuse hyperkeratosis have prolapsed uteri. Focal areas of hyperkeratosis can be associated with a local chronic irritation, such as seen in women who wear a diaphragm or pessary, and in women with cervical neoplasia. However, in most cases there is no known cause.

Microscopically, the whitish plaque corresponds to the presence of a thick keratin layer (hyperkeratosis) that may or may not contain pyknotic nuclei (parakeratosis) (Figs. 6.2 and 6.3). The epithelium is often acanthotic and has a well-developed granular layer, prominent intercellular bridges, and elongated rete pegs. Characteristically, the epithelial cells contain sparse glycogen, but cytologic atypia is absent. Epithelial hyperplasia and chronic inflammation are frequent.

Although there is neither morphologic nor clinical evidence that hyperkeratosis or parakeratosis represent precursor lesions to cervical neoplasia, both hyperkeratosis and parakeratosis can occur in association with a squamous intraepithelial lesion (SIL) (also referred to as cervical intraepithelial neoplasia, or CIN) and invasive cervical cancer. Therefore, there is controversy surrounding the need for further evaluation of women in whom hyperkeratosis or parakeratosis is detected on an otherwise negative Pap smear. Because of the association of hyperkeratosis and parakeratosis with SIL (CIN) and cervical cancer, some experts have suggested that all women with Pap smears demonstrating these findings need colposcopy. However, several studies have reported that less than 4% of women with hyperkeratosis or parakeratosis without nuclear atypia on an otherwise negative Pap smear had SIL (CIN) and that in all instances the SIL was low grade, suggesting that routine colposcopic evaluation is unnecessary in such women.[8,18,55] It should be emphasized, however, that because hyperkeratosis may occasionally overlie invasive carcinomas, all grossly visible white plaques on the portio vaginalis or vaginal epithelium should be biopsied.

Noninfectious Cervicitis

Noninfectious cervicitis is, for the most part, chemical or mechanical in nature, and the inflammatory response is nonspecific. Common causes include chemical irritation secondary to douching or local trauma produced by foreign bodies, including tampons, diaphragms, pessaries, and intrauterine contraceptive devices. Surgical instrumentation and therapeutic intervention are common iatrogenic

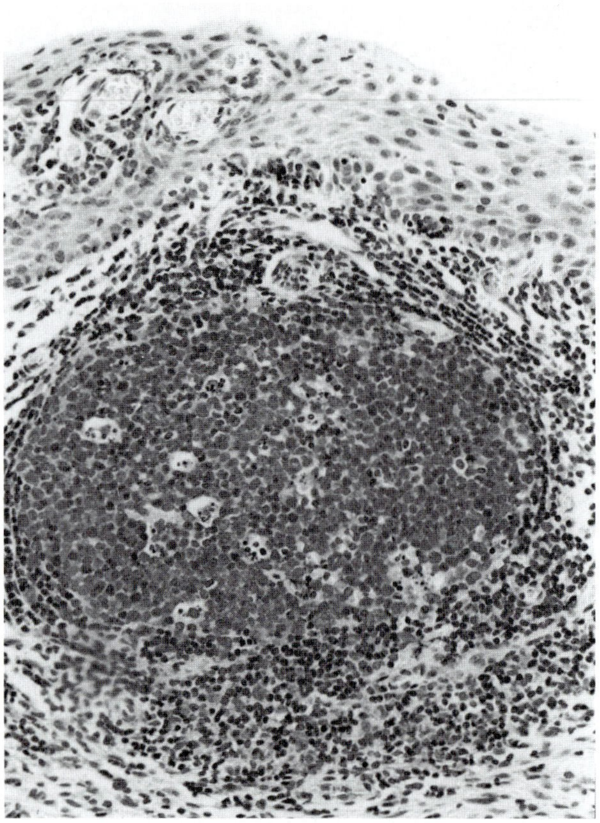

Fig. 6.4. Chronic cervicitis. A subepithelial lymphoid follicle with a prominent germinal center is present. When lymphoid follicles are numerous, the condition is referred to as *follicular cervicitis.*

causes of cervical tissue injury and inflammation. Stromal edema, vascular congestion, and neutrophilic infiltration of the stroma and epithelium characterize acute cervicitis. Clinically, the cervix appears swollen, erythematous, and friable, and there may be an associated purulent endocervical discharge. Prolonged or severe acute inflammation eventually leads to degenerative changes in the epithelial surface, loss of endocervical secretory activity, and ulceration.

In chronic cervicitis, round cells, including lymphocytes, plasma cells, and histiocytes, predominate in the inflammatory infiltrate and are associated with varying amounts of granulation tissue and stromal fibrosis. On gross and colposcopic examination, the cervical mucosa is hyperemic because of an increased number of terminal vessels and may contain true epithelial erosions (ulceration) or lacerations. The cervical stroma contains a normal, physiologic population of inflammatory cells, and the diagnosis of chronic cervicitis should be reserved for cases where there is definite clinical and histologic evidence of a significant chronic inflammatory process. Otherwise, a histologic diagnosis based on the presence of scattered lymphocytes has no clinical significance and is meaningless. Occasionally, lymphoid follicles with germinal centers are found beneath the epithelium in noninfectious cervicitis (Fig. 6.4). The presence of lymphoid follicles beneath the cervical epithelium is frequently referred to as *follicular cervicitis*. In some instances, the lymphoid inflammatory reactions may produce lymphoma-like lesions, raising the question of lymphoma (see following).[108]

Infectious Cervicitis

Table 6.1 summarizes some of the important or pathologically significant etiologic organisms of *infectious cervicitis*. It is apparent from this listing that infectious cervicitis is important because of its epidemic proportions and because of its central role in the pathogenesis of pelvic inflammatory disease and endometrial infections. In our current understanding of the pathogenesis of pelvic inflammatory disease, infectious cervicitis is the initial event; it is also the primary infectious focus in related syndromes, such as postpartum and postabortal endometritis. Spontaneous abortion, premature delivery, chorioamnionitis, stillbirth, and neonatal pneumonia and septicemia have been directly related to concurrent bacterial infection of the cervix. Even when asymptomatic, infectious cervicitis can be clinically important because it can act as a source for sexual transmission to male partners, as well as ascending

Table 6.1. Microorganisms causing infectious cervicitis

Bacteria, *Chlamydia*, Mycobacteria, polymicrobial, endogenous vaginal aerobes and anaerobes
Chlamydia trachomatis
Neisseria gonorrhoeae
Mycoplasma hominis
Group B *Streptococcus*
Ureaplasma ureolyticum
Gardnerella vaginalis
Actinomyces israelii
Mycobacterium tuberculosis
Treponema pallidum
Viruses
Herpes simplex virus
Human papillomavirus
Fungi
Candida
Aspergillus
Protozoa and parasites
Trichomonas vaginalis
Ameba
Schistosomes

infection in the female, and vertical transmission during pregnancy.

Infectious cervicitis can affect either the endocervical-type columnar epithelium, producing *endocervicitis* (mucopurulent cervicitis), or the stratified squamous epithelium of the exocervix, producing *exocervicitis*.[51] The infectious agents that cause endo- and exocervicitis tend to differ, although some agents can cause both. When discussing infectious cervicitis, it is important that clear criteria be used to define the disease and to distinguish clinically apparent disease from asymptomatic disease. Clinically apparent endocervicitis (mucopurulent cervicitis) is defined principally by the presence of a yellow endocervical discharge containing large numbers of polymorpholeukocytes, erythema, and friability of the cervical ectropion.[51] Exocervicitis is manifested by either ulceration and necrosis or the diffuse punctated erythema (colpitis macularis) associated with *Trichomonas vaginalis* infections.

Bacterial and Chlamydial Cervicitis

Bacterial and chlamydial infections of the cervix are the most common cause of infectious cervicitis and are associated with a nonspecific inflammatory response. The columnar epithelium of the endocervix is much more susceptible to bacterial and chlamydial infections than is the surrounding squamous epithelium, and endocervicitis is characteristic. Consequently, patients with a large columnar ectropion, as is seen in young women or during pregnancy, are at higher risk for bacterial and chlamydial infections and for developing acute endocervicitis.[28,50,51] Although some degree of cervical involvement commonly occurs in women with bacterial vaginosis, the cervical involvement is rarely important clinically. The infectious agents that most commonly cause clinically significant mucopurulent cervicitis are *Chlamydia trachomatis* and *Neisseria gonorrhoea*. Infection with either of these two agents requires no predisposing factors and is primarily dependent on exposure and size of the inoculum. Although chlamydial and bacterial infections of the cervix are infrequent in older postmenopausal women and are unusual before menarche, both *N. gonorrhoea* and *C. trachomatis* are occasionally reported in children and may affect the atrophic vaginal epithelium as well as the cervix, producing cervicovaginitis. The prevalence of *C. trachomatis* cervical infection ranges from 3% to 5% of asymptomatic women and as many as 20% of women attending sexually transmitted disease (STD) clinics.[2,51] Infection rates are greatest in women 15–21 years of age.[98] In pregnant women and young women less than 22 years of age, isolation rates for *C. trachomatis* from cervices of asymptomatic patients are as high as 11%.[2] Slightly more than one-third of women with cervical chlamydial infections are symptomatic.[98] Symptomatic women with acute mucopurulent cervicitis, defined by the presence of a visible, yellow-green, endocervical exudate or by the presence of 10 or more neutrophils per (1000×) field in a smear of endocervical mucus have culture-positive *C. trachomatis* infection in 58% of cases. Generalized lower genital tract infection is common, often involving the urethra (so-called urethral syndrome) and the rectum.[14] The high risk of exposure of these patients to multiple sexually transmitted diseases is highlighted by the frequent finding of other concurrent bacterial infections, principally gonorrhea.

Inflammatory and reactive colposcopic patterns in women with *C. trachomatis* cervicitis include hypertrophied cervical ectropion and an atypical transformation zone epithelium that may be confused colposcopically with a low-grade squamous intraepithelial lesion.[28,47] Histologically, follicular cervicitis is frequently found in patients with *C. trachomatis* infection, and *C. trachomatis* is now presumed to be a major cause of this condition in younger women (see Fig. 6.4).[47] *C. trachomatis* cervicitis has also been associated with a dense, diffuse inflammatory exudate as well as reactive squamous and endocervical atypia (Fig. 6.5).[29] Intracytoplasmic inclusions in endocervical columnar or metaplastic cells may be identified in some cases. Immunohistochemical studies have demonstrated that these inclusions are composed of aggregated chlamydial organisms at different stages of development (Fig. 6.5).[29] However, it should be stressed that the identification of these cytoplasmic epithelial inclusions in cervical Papanicolaou smears and biopsies is too insensitive and nonspecific to be of use diagnostically.[41,63]

C. trachomatis cervicitis is most accurately diagnosed by culture or molecular diagnostic methods such as polymerase chain reaction (PCR) or ligase chain reaction (LCR). Other methods, such as direct immunofluorescence staining of smears using monoclonal antibodies or by enzyme-linked immunoabsorbant assay (EIA) on cervical swabs, are less sensitive. Because endometritis and salpingitis (see Chapter 10, Benign Diseases of the Endometrium, and Chapter 14, Diseases of the Fallopian Tube) complicate *C. trachomatis* cervicitis in approximately 40% and 11% of cases, respectively, and are often subclinical, the patient with *C. trachomatis* cervicitis and her sexual partner(s) should be

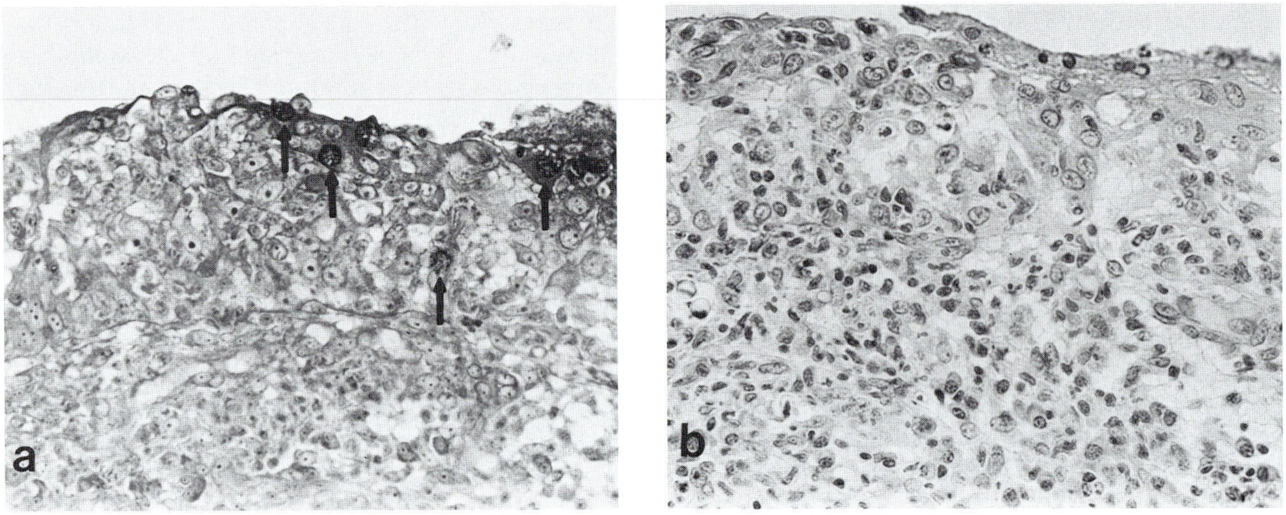

Fig. 6.5. Chlamydial cervicitis. a: Immunoperoxidase staining for chlamydial antigens shows several rounded cytoplasmic inclusions. **b:** The epithelium and stroma are infiltrated by acute and chronic inflammatory cells, partially obscuring the epithelial–stromal junction. The metaplastic epithelium displays reactive atypia. Scattered cytoplasmic vacuoles are present, but the finding is not specific for the definitive diagnosis of chlamydia infection. (Courtesy of C.P. Crum, M.D., Boston, MA.)

treated.[1] Postinfectious sequelae include pelvic inflammatory disease, tubal infertility, and neonatal pneumonia. Symptomatic infection in the male is more commonly manifested as acute urethritis, but the infection may be asymptomatic.

Actinomycosis

Actinomyces israelii is a frequent commensual organism found in the female lower genital tract. Culture and immunofluorescence studies of cervical and vaginal secretions indicate that 3%–27% of asymptomatic women without obvious risk factors are infected with *Actinomyces israelii*.[72] Aggregates of bacteria with the morphologic appearance of actinomyces have been reported to occur in approximately 0.13% of all Papanicolaou smears.[80] The organism is more commonly identified in women wearing intrauterine devices (IUDs) than in women in the general population, and detection is related to the length of time that the IUD has been in place.[30,72,80] Structures resembling the "sulfur granules" observed in *A. israelii* infections are sometimes identified in endocervical curettings of asymptomatic women. In the majority of cases these are "pseudoactinomycotic radiate granules," which are nonspecific collections of bacteria or foreign material, glycoproteins, and lipids rather than actual collections of *A. israelii*.[12]

The identification of *A. israelii* in asymptomatic women has little clinical significance and does not warrant antibiotic therapy.[72] Rarely, *A. israelii* can be associated with pelvic abscesses. A recent review reported a single case of pelvic actinomycosis from among 126,313 women discharged from hospitals in Buffalo, NY, and Seattle, WA, between 1983 and 1997.[72] When abscesses do occur, the diagnosis is made by demonstrating the organism in the center of large abscesses, occasionally with granuloma formation. The lesions appear yellow and granular to the naked eye, hence the term *sulfur granules*. Sulfur granules are composed of branching, gram-positive filaments with peripheral palisading clubs.

Tuberculosis

Tuberculosis of the cervix is almost invariably secondary to tuberculous salpingitis and endometritis and is typically associated with pulmonary tuberculosis (see Chapter 10, Benign Diseases of the Endometrium and Chapter 14, Diseases of the Fallopian Tube).[85] The prevalence of cervical tuberculosis in a population with genital tuberculosis varies between 2% and 82%.[6,19,85] Macroscopically, the cervix may appear normal, inflamed, or simulate invasive carcinoma. Histologically, tuberculous infection of the cervix is recognized by the presence of multiple granulomas or tubercles characterized by central caseous necrosis, epithelioid histiocytes, and multinucleated Langhans giant cells. The periphery of the tubercle contains a heavy lymphoplasmocytic infiltrate (Fig. 6.6). Granulomas typically disappear after successful antitubercular therapy.[6] Tuberculous cervicitis may appear as

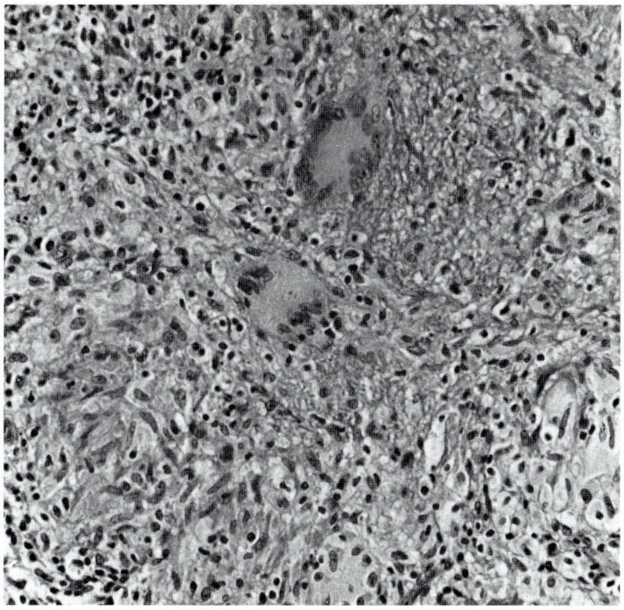

Fig. 6.6. Tuberculous cervicitis. Typical granuloma with palisading epithelial cells, Langerhans giant cells, and central caseous necrosis. Acid-fast stain for *Mycobacterium tuberculosis was positive.*

a noncaseating, granulomatous lesion. Because caseating, nontuberculous granulomas caused by lymphogranuloma venereum or sarcoidosis may be encountered in the cervix, the unequivocal diagnosis of tuberculous cervicitis requires demonstration of acid-fast *Mycobacterium tuberculosis*, a straight, rod-shaped bacillus, by Ziehl–Neelsen-stained sections, or by culture.[34] Because culture yields far better results than staining of tissue sections, unfixed biopsy material should be obtained for microbiologic testing whenever tuberculosis is suspected. The most common granulomatous lesions to be distinguished from tuberculous cervicitis include foreign body giant cell granulomas secondary to sutures, crystals, or cotton, lymphogranuloma venereum, schistosomiasis, and sarcoidosis. Cervical granuloma may occasionally develop after a biopsy or operation as a reaction to local tissue necrosis.[34]

Other Granulomatous Infections

Certain venereally transmitted diseases commonly encountered in the vulva may also involve the cervix (see Chapter 3, Diseases of the Vulva): these include *syphilis*, either as the primary chancre, secondary mucous patches, or tertiary gumma, *lymphogranuloma venereum*, *granuloma inguinale*, and *chancroid*.[64] All these conditions may resemble carcinoma clinically. This resemblance is particularly a problem with granuloma inguinale, which is endemic in areas of Africa that have a high prevalence of invasive cervical cancer. As many as 50% of women with granuloma inguinale may be initially misdiagnosed as having carcinoma of the cervix. Many of these women are thought to have high-stage tumors because of spread of the infection to the parametrial tissue.[52] In addition to characteristic morphologic features, specific bacteriologic and immunologic techniques are available for identifying each of these diseases.

Viral Diseases

In contrast to bacterial infections of the cervix, the most common cervical viral infections—*human papillomavirus* (HPV) and *herpes simplex virus* (HSV)—have a predilection for the squamous epithelium and produce characteristic morphologic changes. *Cytomegalovirus*, although often isolated from cervical secretions, is not typically associated with cervicitis, and its role in cervical infection is poorly understood.

Herpesvirus Infection (HSV)

Although the precise prevalence of cervical HSV infection (*herpes genitalis*) is not known, it is far greater than generally recognized. HSV can be isolated from the genital tract in 1.6%–10% of women attending STD clinics.[27] Up to 70% of HSV-2 infections appear to be asymptomatic; this results in wide discrepancies between the prevalence of serologic evidence of infection and clinically recognized infections. HSV-2 antibodies are detected in approximately 20%–30% of women in the United States.[27] In the United States, serologic evidence of HSV-2 infection is much greater in blacks than in whites, but symptomatic infections are more common in whites. The prevalence of serum antibodies to HSV-2 is strongly associated with socioeconomic status and increases with age. The prevalence of genital HSV infections increased markedly between the 1960s and 1990s in the United States, Europe, Australia, and parts of Africa. Initial visits to physicians in the United States for genital HSV infections increased 10 fold from approximately 20,000 in the 1960s to approximately 200,000 during the mid-1990s.[2] Genital herpesvirus infections are caused chiefly by HSV-2. Between 1% and 30% of primary genital HSV outbreaks are caused by HSV-1.[88]

Herpes simplex viruses types 1 and 2 have several common features, including architecture, size, envelope, mode of multiplication, and double-stranded DNA genetic content that measures 150 nm in diameter. The virions are surrounded by a hexagonal protein capsid and the capsid, in turn, is enveloped by an inner glycoprotein-rich and outer lipid-rich membrane. Viral particles are thought to replicate within the host cell nuclei, where they synthesize viral proteins necessary for replication of viral DNA. HSV-1 is chiefly found in the oropharyngeal region (herpes buccalis) and has different biologic properties and a different distribution than does HSV-2 virus. HSV-2 is acquired through sexual contact. Primary herpetic infections produce symptoms within 3–7 days after exposure. When the vulva is involved, symptoms include severe vulvar pain, tenderness, painful urination, and profuse watery vaginal discharge. The symptoms of recurrent herpes genitalis are comparatively less severe than those experienced during the primary infection.

The disease is characterized by the development of multiple, painful vesicles involving the vulva, perineum, vagina, and cervix that rapidly evolve into shallow, painful ulceration. Cervical involvement can be detected in 70%–90% of women with primary genital HSV-2 infections.[11,26] In contrast, only 15%–20% of women with recurrent genital herpetic lesions involving the external genitalia have cervical involvement.[27] In most women with cervical involvement, the cervical lesions are readily observable on the cervix (Fig. 6.7). Occasionally, the ulceronecrotic process is so extensive that a fungating, necrotic mass appears on the cervical portio that can be mistaken for carcinoma. Shedding of herpesvirus from asymptomatic, clinically unapparent cervical lesions occurs frequently and serves as a hidden reservoir for propagation of infection.[67] One study of women attending a STD clinic in Seattle, WA, found that HSV was isolated from the cervix of 4% of the attendees. Of these, one-half had a first episode of genital lesions. More than one-third of the women from whom HSV was isolated from cervical samples had no colposcopically visible cervical lesions.[68]

Herpesvirus infection may be confirmed by viral cultures, HSV DNA detection by PCR, or HSV antigen detection by either enzyme-linked immunoabsorbant assay (EIA) or fluorescence. In the Papanicolaou smear, large multinucleated cells with the characteristic intranuclear ground glass viral inclusions can be observed. Approximately 60% of the women with visible HSV-associated cervical lesions have cytologic evidence of a HSV infection.[68] Occasionally, during the vesicular phase of a cervical lesion, a biopsy may reveal the presence of suprabasal intraepidermal vesicles filled with serum, degenerated epidermal cells, and multinucleated giant cells, some containing eosinophilic, intranuclear inclusions surrounded by a clear halo (Fig. 6.8). Diagnostic yield by isolation and cytology is most efficient within 2–3 days after the onset of symptoms.

Herpes genitalis has two important clinical implications. First, it may result in spontaneous abortion, fetal morbidity, and fetal mortality. Second, be-

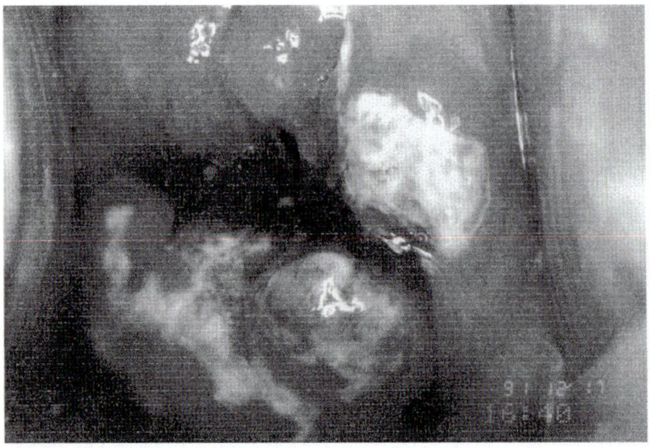

Fig. 6.7. Herpetic cervicitis. A large ulceration is present on the cervix. When extensive, these lesions can sometimes be mistaken for invasive carcinoma.

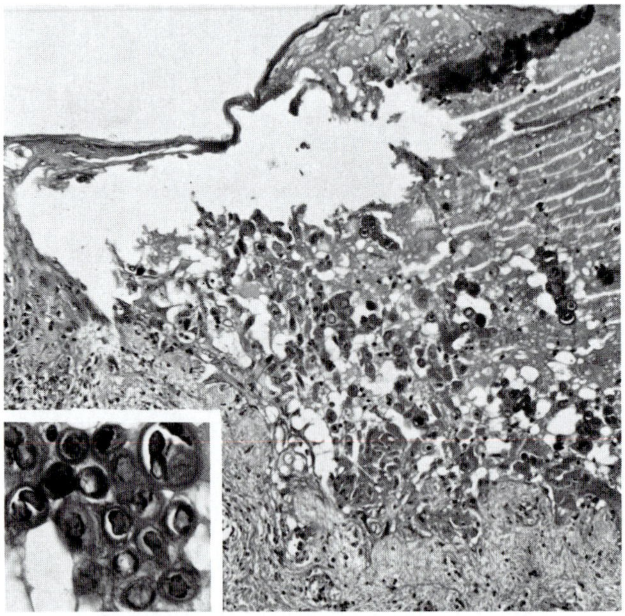

Fig. 6.8. Herpetic cervicitis. Suprabasal vesicle in squamous epithelium of the portio. *Inset*: High-power view of acantholytic intravesicular epithelial cells with ground glass intranuclear viral inclusions.

cause it is a chronic infection, it is associated with significant long-term morbidity and psychological consequences.

Herpes-Like Lesions

Vesicular and bullous lesions of the cervical squamous mucous membrane, other than herpetic cervicitis, have been reported.[15] *Pemphigus vulgaris* of the cervix is a common finding in women with generalized disease.[61] Microscopically, there are multiple intraepithelial bullae in a suprabasal location containing the characteristic acantholytic Tzanck cells.

Isolated arteritis of the cervix, histologically identical but clinically unrelated to polyarteritis nodosa, may rarely be encountered.[70] The etiology of this condition is unknown. It may be asymptomatic or may be associated with bleeding and may clinically resemble cancer.

Human Papillomavirus (HPV)

Human papillomavirus (HPV) is a double-stranded DNA tumor virus that is a member of the family Papovaviridae. More than 35 of the more than 100 different types of HPV can infect the lower anogenital tract, and the resulting infections can produce a variety of gross and histological lesions (see Chapter 7, Precancerous Lesions of the Cervix). Exophytic condyloma acuminata are one of the common manifestations of HPV infection of the lower anogenital tract and are usually caused by HPV types 6 and 11.[101] When florid condylomas of the vulva are identified, multicentric disease can occur, and internal vaginal or cervical exophytic condylomas can be occasionally identified.[16,92] Exophytic condylomas of the cervix are commonly multifocal and may involve the mature squamous epithelium of the native cervical portio as well as the immature squamous epithelium of the transformation zone, including metaplastic squamous epithelium replacing endocervical glands. Extension into the endocervical canal may occur. Grossly and colposcopically, condyloma acuminata appears white, and the degree of whiteness depends largely on the thickness of associated surface hyperkeratosis (Fig. 6.9). Other configurations of cervical exophytic condylomas include a myriad of minute, maculopapular, only slightly raised, condylomas involving the vagina and the cervix.

Microscopically, the histological features of exophytic cervical condyloma acuminata include architectural alterations such as papillomatosis, acanthosis, parakeratosis, and hyperkeratosis as well as cytologic alterations including koilocytosis (manifested by perinuclear cytoplasmic cavitation), nuclear enlargement, and atypia (Fig. 6.10). Multinucleation is also frequently observed (see Chapter 2, Benign Diseases of the Vulva, and Chapter 7, Precancerous Lesions of the Cervix).

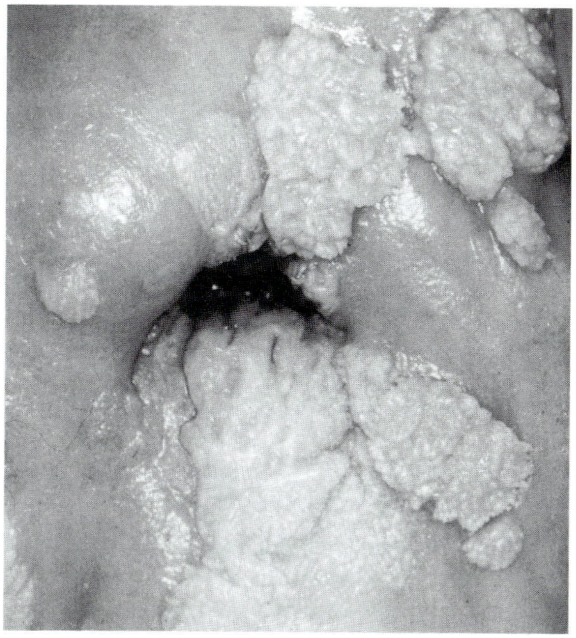

Fig. 6.9. Exophytic condyloma acuminata. The lesions are multifocal and form raised white papillary projections.

The natural history of exophytic cervical condyloma accuminata is one of spontaneous regression, good response to conservative therapy, unpredictable recurrence, and sometimes persistence. Lesion regression or apparent cure following biopsy is fairly common. The natural history of genital condylomas in general may be modified by host factors, notably immunosuppression and steroid hormone levels. For example, women who are infected with HIV-1 have an approximately seven-fold increased risk of having or developing condyloma accuminata of the lower genital tract, including the cervix, compared to women not infected with HIV-1.[20,21] Recurrence of condylomas during early and midtrimester pregnancy is reported commonly, with the lesions increasing in size and multifocality until term.[79] After delivery, spontaneous regression of the condylomas is the rule.[79] There is increasing concern about genital HPV infection during pregnancy because of the possibility of vertical transmission of infection to the fetus and neonate. There are anecdotal reports of infants born with genital condylomas or developing them in the immediate postnatal period. Of even greater concern is the risk of development

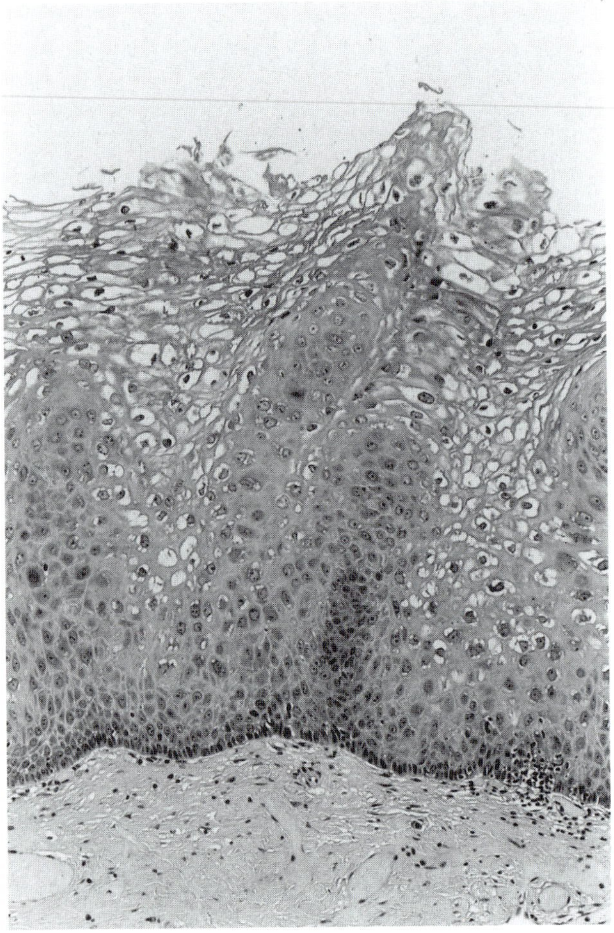

Fig. 6.10. Exophytic condyloma acuminata. The classic histologic features are papillomatosis with acanthosis, parakeratosis, and hyperkeratosis as well as cytologic alterations including multinucleation, koilocytosis, and nuclear atypia.

of juvenile onset of respiratory papillomatosis (JORP) because of the morbidity and mortality associated with this disease.[60] Although correlated with similar genital HPV types and linked causally to infection in the mother, the factors requisite for the development of JORP are not fully understood. The estimated incidence of clinically apparent disease is approximately 0.12–2.3 per 100,000 children less than 18 years of age in the United States.[9]

Fungal Diseases

Cervical fungal infection by *Candida albicans* usually occurs as part of a generalized lower genital tract infection involving the vagina and vulva. Antibiotic therapy, poorly controlled diabetes mellitus, and immunosuppression all favor fungal overgrowth.[96] Typically, a *Candida* infection is associated with a viscous vaginal discharge containing white flakes, often accompanied by vulvar pruritus. Cervical candidal infections can be associated with increased numbers of polymorpholeukocytes present in the upper layers of the epithelium and fungal hyphae that can be identified by periodic acid–Schiff (PAS) stains both at the surface of the epithelium and within the superficial layers of the epithelium.

Protozoal and Parasitic Diseases

Cervical infestation by *Trichomonas vaginalis* is quite frequent and most often associated with concurrent trichomonal vaginitis. A foamy, yellow-green vaginal discharge is typically described. *Acute trichomonal cervicitis* may provoke an intense inflammatory response with prominent reparative atypia in exfoliated squamous and endocervical cells, with corresponding gross and colposcopic abnormalities. Diagnosis is usually made by wet mount, culture using Diamond's medium, or identification of the organism on Papanicolaou smear (see Chapter 4, Diseases of the Vagina, and Chapter 25, Immunohistochemistry).

Rare instances of *parasitic infestations*, such as echinococcosis or hydatid cysts, Chagas' disease, and ulceronecrotic amebiasis, have been encountered in the cervix (Fig. 6.11).[25,64,104] In contrast, schistosomiasis (bilharziasis) of the cervix, generally caused by *Schistosoma mansoni*, is very common in Africa (Egypt), South America, Puerto Rico, and several Asian countries.[82] A large number of cases of cervical schistosomiasis are associated with urinary schistosomiasis and sterility. Microscopically, noncaseating granulomas (pseudotubercles) with ova surrounded by multinucleated giant cells are seen, and the ova are often calcified (Fig. 6.12). *S. mansoni* has a long lateral spine, whereas *Schistosoma haematobium* has a short spine extending from one of its poles. Cervical schistosomiasis may be associated with extensive pseudoepitheliomatous hyperplasia of the cervical squamous epithelium, masquerading both clinically and histologically as carcinoma. Although it was previously thought that chronic, untreated cervical schistosomiasis plays a role in the genesis of cervical carcinoma in populations where schistosomiasis is prevalent, there is now evidence indicating no association between schistosomiasis and cervical cancer.[74,83]

Cervicovaginitis Emphysematosa

Multiple, blue-gray, subepithelial cysts of the portio vaginalis and vagina characterize this unusual disease.[40] In rare cases the cysts have been misdiagnosed as an invasive cervical cancer.[7] The cause of

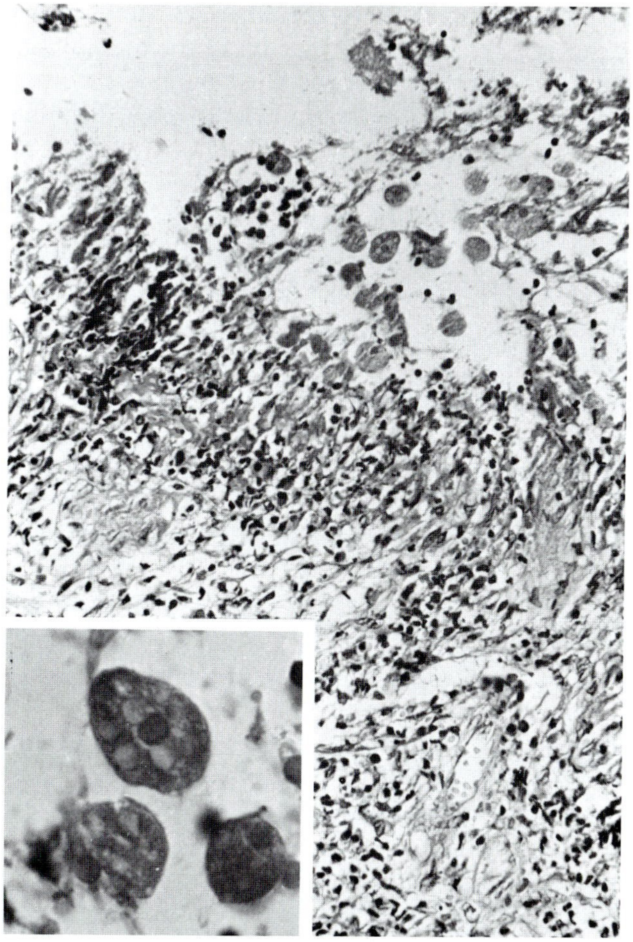

Fig. 6.11. Ulceronecrotic amebiasis of cervix. Numerous amebae are present in the superficial exudate. *Inset*: Detail of *Entamoeba histolytica* with vacuolated cytoplasm.

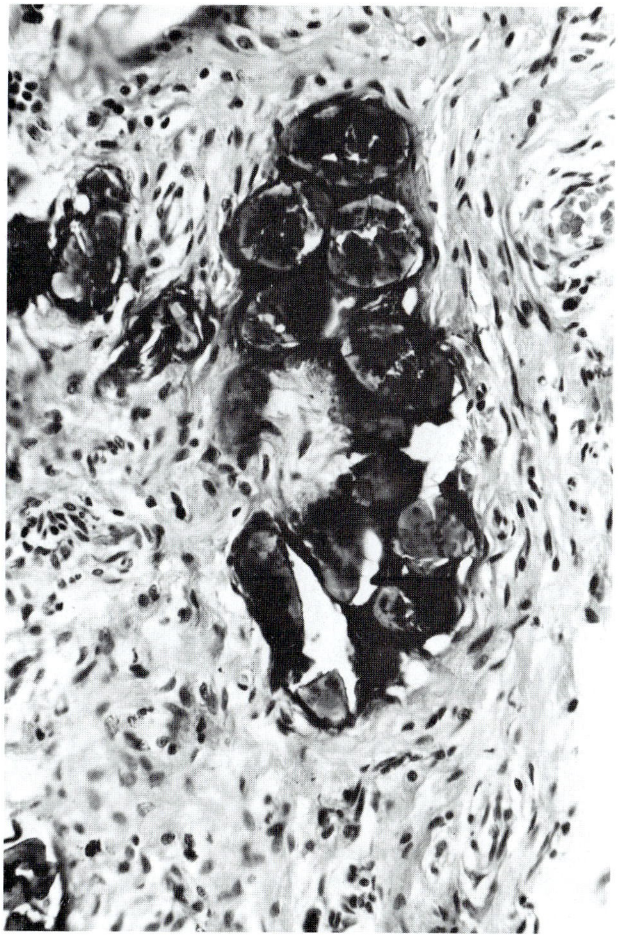

Fig. 6.12. Cervical schistosomiasis. Note calcified *Schistosoma haematobiium* ova.

this condition is unknown, but it is often associated with trichomoniasis.[40] Gas-forming bacteria have never been identified within the cysts. The cysts are dilated connective tissue spaces without lining epithelium that contain air and carbon dioxide. Multinucleated foreign body giant cells surround some of the cysts, and often the subepithelial veins and lymphatics are dilated.

Metaplasias, Hyperplasias, and Endometriosis

Tubal Metaplasia

Tubal metaplasia refers to endocervical glands that are lined by a müllerian-type epithelium that closely resembles that of the fallopian tube. In pure tubal metaplasia, the endocervical glands are lined by an epithelium that more closely resembles that of the fallopian tube and contains many more ciliated cells than are normally present in the endocervical epithelium as well as tubal-type secretory cells and reserve or intercalary cells (Fig. 6.13).[56,76,102] Tubal metaplasia can be found in up to 31% of patients and does not appear to be related to the phase of menstrual cycle, the presence of inflammatory changes, or low-grade SIL.[56]

Tubal metaplasia can be quite extensive and can occasionally be mistaken for endocervical glandular neoplasia. However, the bland cytologic features, lack of mitotic activity, and prominent cilia seen at the apical surfaces of tubal metaplasia usually allow it to be differentiated from a neoplastic lesion. Other features that can aid in distinguishing between tubal metaplasia and glandular neoplasia are the location and shape of the glands and the surrounding stroma. Glands demonstrating tubal metaplasia are typically confined to the superficial third of the cervical wall (i.e., they extend less than 7 mm into the cervical

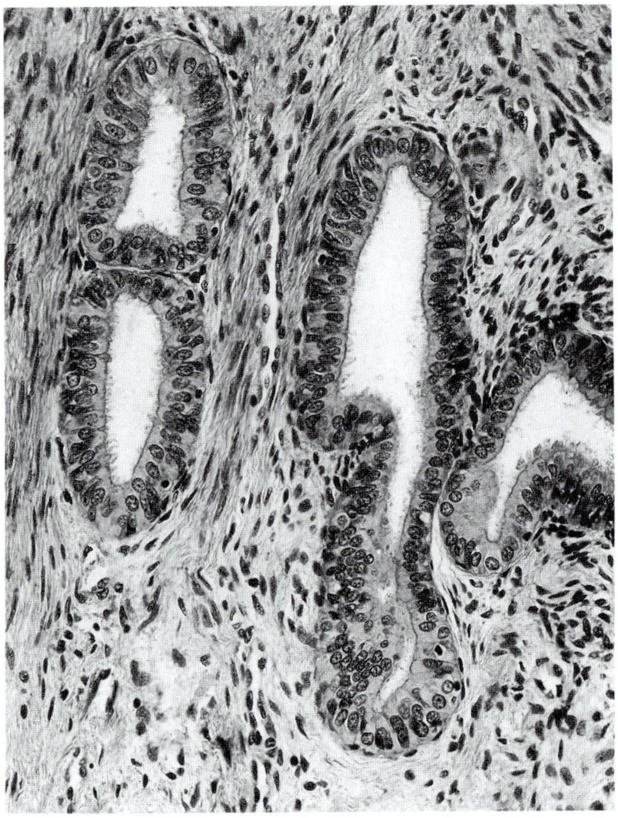

Fig. 6.13. Tubal metaplasia. The columnar, mucus-producing epithelium has been replaced by a tubal-type epithelium with ciliated, secretory, and intercalated cells.

stroma) and typically show only slight variation in size and shape. Moreover, the stroma surrounding glands involved by tubal metaplasia is usually normal appearing and is neither desmoplastic nor edematous appearing. Cases of tubal metaplasia demonstrating glandular architectural abnormalities or hypercellularity of the adjacent stroma can present diagnostic difficulties.[77]

Atypical tubal metaplasia is a form of tubal metaplasia in which the glands are lined by ciliated and nonciliated cells that are crowded and have larger, more hyperchromatic nuclei than observed in typical tubal metaplasia (Fig. 6.14). The cells of atypical tubal metaplasia are frequently pseudostratified. Atypical tubal metaplasia frequently presents a diagnostic problem because histologically it can be confused with adenocarcinoma in situ. Differentiation from adenocarcinoma in situ is based on a lack of significant mitotic activity and the absence of architectural abnormalities such as cribiforming and papillary projections. However, it should be cautioned that atypical tubal metaplasia can occur in association with adenocarcinoma in situ of the cervix, including both tubal and nontubal types (see Chapter 7, Precancerous Lesions of the Cervix). Because of its frequent association with adenocarcinoma in situ, it has been suggested recently that atypical tubal metaplasia represents a transition lesion between benign tubal metaplasia and adenocarcinoma in situ.[86]

Tuboendometrioid Metaplasia

Tuboendometrioid metaplasia of the cervix is a type of metaplasia that is histologically similar to the tubal metaplasia which can develop in the endometrium in patients with unopposed estrogenic stimulation. Endocervical glands demonstrating tuboendometrioid metaplasia are lined by a pseudostratified epithelium composed of columnar cells with a higher nuclear:cytoplasmic ratio (Fig. 6.15). Many of these cells are ciliated or have secretory features with apical snouts, but the glands lack an associated endometrial stroma. Tuboendometrioid metaplasia occurs commonly after cervical conization and has been interpreted as a form of aberrant differentiation following cervical injury.[54] Because of the pseudostratification and high nuclear:cytoplasmic ratio, these glands can be misinterpreted as representing adenocarcinoma in situ. As with tubal metaplasia, the features that indicate a metaplastic, as opposed to a neoplastic, process are the location and shape of the glands and lack of a desmoplastic or edematous stromal response.

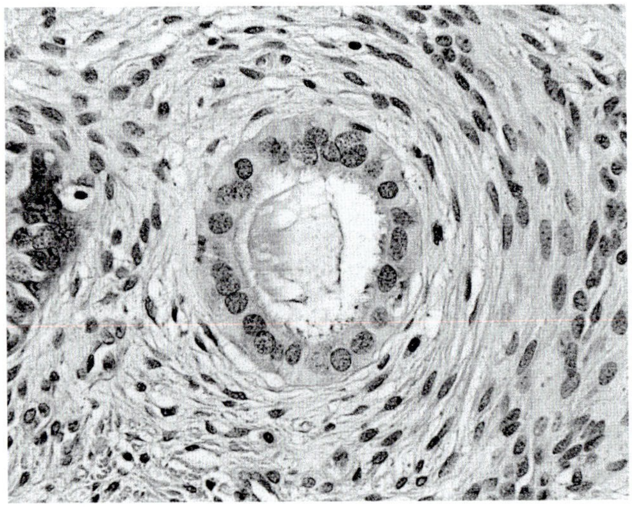

Fig. 6.14. Atypical tubal metaplasia. The epithelium is more crowded than seen in typical tubal metaplasia and has larger, hyperchromatic nuclei. Ciliated cells are present, but mitotic figures are uncommonly seen.

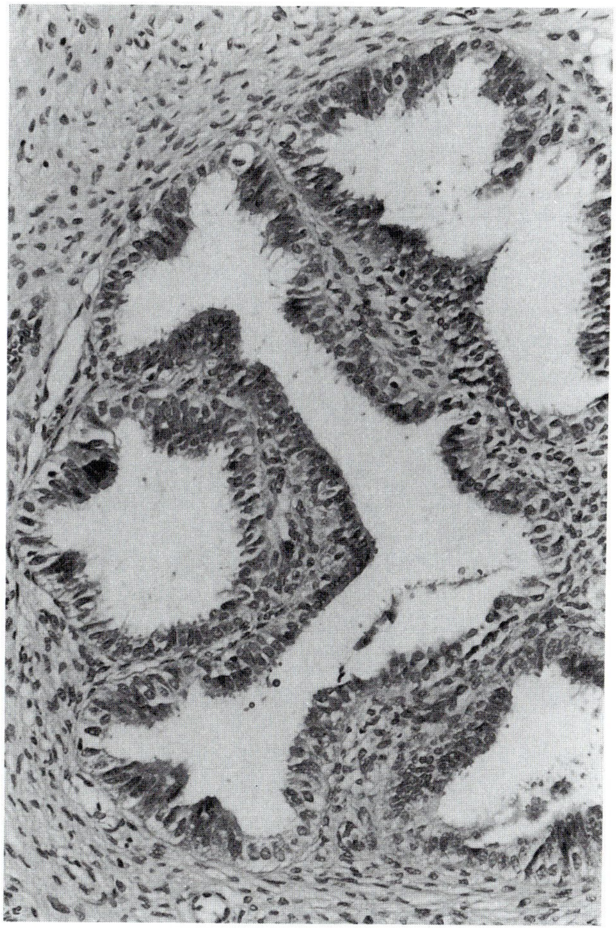

Fig. 6.15. Tuboendometrioid metaplasia. The columnar, mucus-producing epithelium has been replaced by a pseudostratified epithelium with a high nuclear:cytoplasmic ratio and cilia or apical snouting.

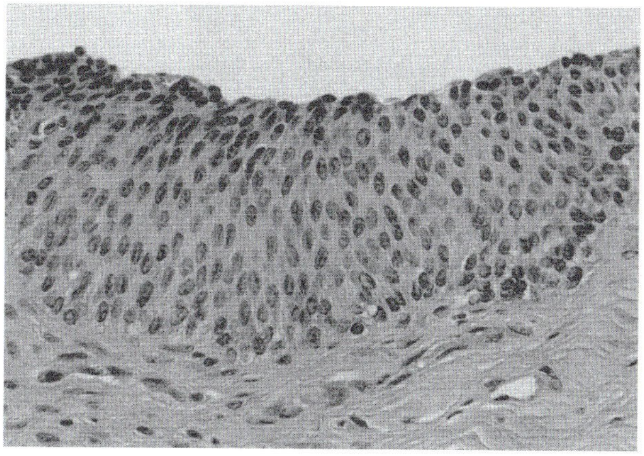

Fig. 6.16. Transitional cell metaplasia. The squamous epithelium in this postmenopausal patient is more than 10 layers thick and is disorganized. This type of change is referred to by some as *transitional cell metaplasia*.

Transitional Cell Metaplasia

Transitional cell metaplasia refers to a controversial type of metaplasia in which the surface of the cervix and endocervical crypts is lined by a epithelium that is interpreted by some to resemble a hyperplastic urothelium.[31,32,57,105] The epithelium in regions interpreted as demonstrating transitional cell metaplasia is composed of more than 10 layers of cells that have oval to spindle-shaped nuclei and are oriented vertically in the deeper layers (Fig. 6.16). The usual "picket fence" orientation of the basal cell layer observed in normal or metaplastic cervical squamous epithelia is missing, and the epithelium has a "disordered" appearance.[32] The cells of the superficial layer often resemble the umbrella cells of the normal urothelium and have horizontally oriented nuclei.

The controversy surrounding transitional cell metaplasia revolves around whether it represents a unique histopathologic entity that has a specific biology or whether it simply represents a biologically insignificant histologic variation of other well-described histologic entities. Almost all the reported examples of transitional cell metaplasia have been identified in postmenopausal women. In the two largest series, the mean ages of women with the lesion were 60 and 67.8 years.[32,105] Some of these women have had previous abnormal Papanicolaou smears, and it has been suggested that some of the cases may represent atrophic high-grade CIN (SIL).[65,66] In addition to arising in the transformation zone, transitional cell metaplasia can also be identified in the exocervix and the vagina.[105] This finding suggests that in some cases transitional cell metaplasia may simply represent a histological variant of atrophy, either of the original squamous epithelium or of a fully mature metaplastic squamous epithelium, in which the number of cell layers is not reduced. Recent immunohistochemical studies using cytokeratin antibodies have shown that foci of transitional cell metaplasia express cytokeratins 13, 17, and 18, which are expressed in normal urothelium, but do not express cytokeratin 20 and the asymmetric unit membrane, which are related to urothelial differentiation.[49]

Arias–Stella Reaction

During pregnancy, the *gestational Arias–Stella reaction* can develop in both endocervical glands and in ectopic endometrial glands within the cervix. In one study of 191 gravid hysterectomy specimens, an Arias–Stella reaction of endocervical glands was seen, at least focally, in 9% of the cases.[87] The Arias–Stella reaction of the endocervix is usually focal and is more commonly present in the proximal portion of the endocervix involving superficial as opposed to deeply situated glands. Microscopically, the Arias–Stella reaction that occurs in the endocervical glands during pregnancy is identical to that which occurs in the endometrium. The cells within the affected glands are markedly enlarged with irregular, frequently hyperchromatic nuclei that can project into the glandular lumen in a hobnail pattern. The cells are pseudostratified and have hypersecretory cytoplasmic features with abundant vacuolated cytoplasm (Fig. 6.17). Papillary processes with fibrovascular cores lined by enlarged epithelial cells can project into the endocervical gland lumen. The Arias–Stella reaction can occasionally be mistaken for clear cell carcinoma or adenocarcinoma in situ of the cervix. Differentiation from clear cell carcinoma is made by the lack of a mass lesion and clear-cut stromal invasion as well as by the absence of the classic tubular and papillary areas typical of clear cell carcinoma. The cells in adenocarcinoma in situ have more uniform nuclei and less cytoplasmic vacuolization. The Arias–Stella reaction lacks mitotic activity whereas both clear cell carcinoma and adenocarcinoma in situ are mitotically active.

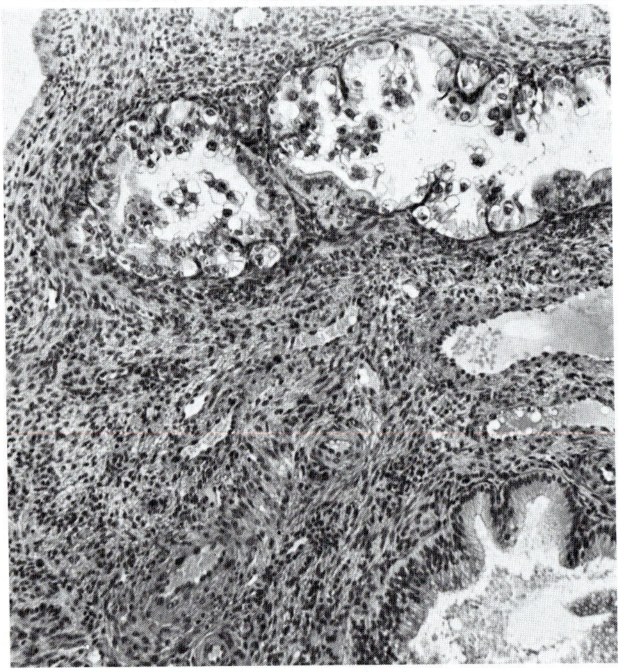

Fig. 6.17. Arias–Stella reaction. The Arias–Stella reaction should not be confused with clear cell adenocarcinoma of the cervix.

Because of the possibility of confusing Arias–Stella reaction with clear cell carcinoma or adenocarcinoma in situ, the diagnosis of the later two entities should be made with caution in the pregnant patient.

Microglandular Endocervical Hyperplasia

Microglandular endocervical hyperplasia is a benign proliferation of endocervical glands. Microglandular hyperplasia is frequently detected as an incidental finding on a cervical biopsy, cone biopsy, or a hysterectomy specimen. If clinically apparent, it most often resembles a cervical polyp measuring 1–2 cm in size. These patients may complain of postcoital bleeding or spotting. Microglandular hyperplasia is most common in women of reproductive ages and has been detected in up to 27% of cone biopsies or hysterectomy specimens.[13] Early studies reported that microglandular hyperplasia typically occurs in patients with a history of recent progesterone exposure, as a result of either oral contraceptive use or pregnancy, and have concluded that it represents a progestin-induced lesion.[17,103,106] However, a number of cases have been reported in which there is no associated hormonal history, and a recent comprehensive study did not find a relationship between microglandular hyperplasia and progestin exposure.[44] Therefore, the role of progestin exposure in the pathogenesis of this lesion is currently unclear.

Histologically, microglandular hyperplasia may present in a single focus or be distributed in multiple foci. It may involve the surface or deeper portions of endocervical clefts. Two histologic types of microglandular hyperplasia were originally recognized. The most common form, initially termed *microglandular hyperplasia*, consists of tightly packed glandular or tubular units of varying size lined by flattened to cuboidal cells with eosinophilic granular cytoplasm containing small quantities of mucin (Fig. 6.18). The glands vary in size and shape from round and small to large, irregularly dilated cystic structures. The stroma separating the glands is usually infiltrated with acute and chronic inflammatory cells. The nuclei of the endocervical cells are uniform, with occasional pleomorphism and hyperchromasia, but mitotic activity is quite low with only 1 mitotic figure per 10 high-power fields.[110] Associated squamous metaplasia and subcolumnar reserve cell hyperplasia are seen in a large number of cases. Foci with a solid proliferation of cells, including signet ring cells, can also be present.

A second form of microglandular hyperplasia was originally described by Taylor et al. and desig-

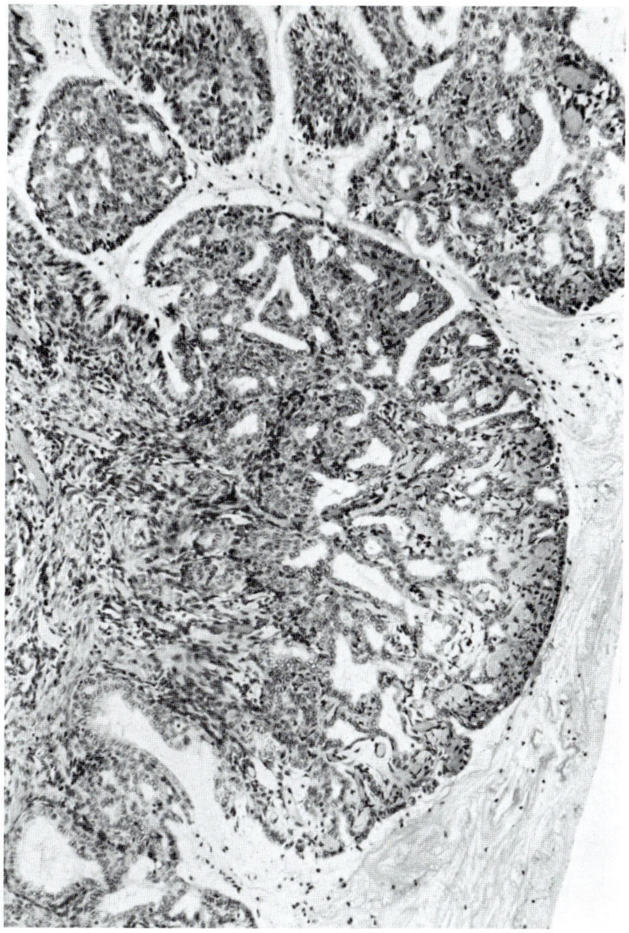

Fig. 6.18. Microglandular hyperplasia. This lesion was associated with oral contraceptive use. There is an adenomatous pattern with cuboidal lining cells and focal squamous metaplasia.

nated *endocervical hyperplasia*.[103] This is a florid form of microglandular proliferation that is simply classified as part of the histologic spectrum of microglandular hyperplasia by most contemporary authors.[110] In florid forms of microglandular hyperplasia, the glandular elements are arranged in a reticulated or solid pattern with areas of nuclear hyperchromasia and pleomorphism (Fig. 6.19). These lesions clearly appear to be benign as no patients have yet been reported to have developed malignant tumors during long-term follow-up. The significance of the florid forms of microglandular hyperplasia is that the irregularly arranged glands can impart an infiltrative appearance and thus they can be mistaken for adenocarcinoma; in particular, clear cell adenocarcinoma. Microglandular hyperplasia with solid areas, especially when the solid component predominates or when signet ring cells are present, can also be difficult to distinguish from adenocarcinomas.[110] The benign nature of these florid lesions is usually demonstrable by a lack of clear-cut stromal invasion and the low mitotic activity of microglandular hyperplasia as compared to endocervical adenocarcinoma. More importantly, unlike clear cell carcinoma, microglandular hyperplasia lacks intracellular glycogen and usually contains intracellular mucin. In addition, florid forms of microglandular hyperplasia almost always contain areas with the more typical histologic features of microglandular hyperplasia. Immunohistochemistry does not appear to be particularly useful for distinguishing microglandular hyperplasia from adenocarcinoma. Although the majority of cases of microglandular hyperplasia do not react with antibodies against carcinoembryonic antigen (CEA), occasional cases of invasive adenocarcinomas of the cervix can also be CEA negative, and in others the

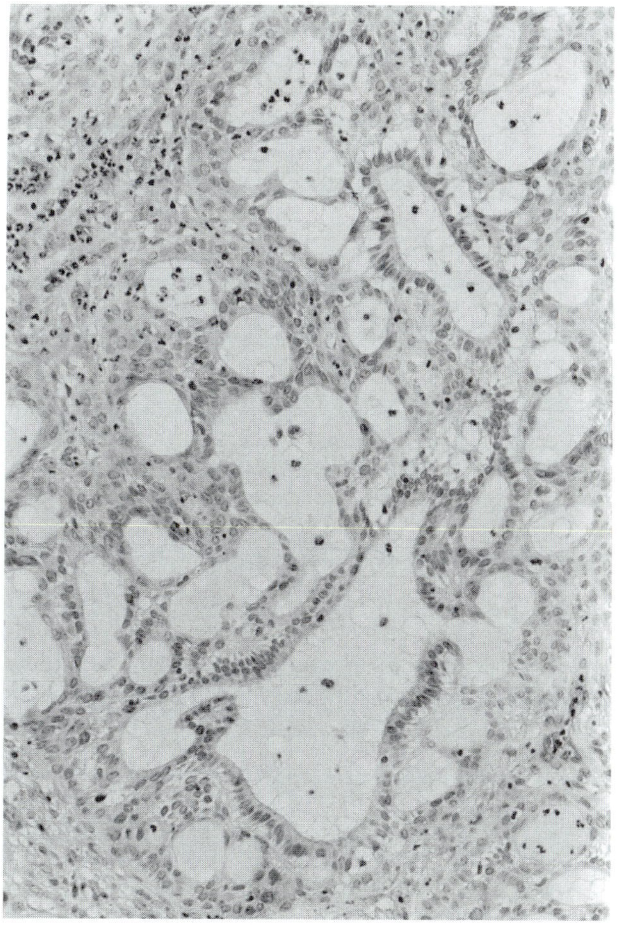

Fig. 6.19. Microglandular hyperplasia. The hyperplastic cells form a reticular pattern of florid microglandular hyperplasia. Note extensive vacuolization, which is caused by cystic dilation of intercellular spaces. There is a paucity of intracellular mucin. Squamous metaplasia surrounds several glands.

positivity may be focal and quite weak (see Chapter 8, Carcinoma and Other Tumors of the Cervix).[42,97,99]

Mesonephric Hyperplasia and Mesonephric Remnants

The vestigial elements of the distal ends of the *mesonephric ducts* are found in 1%–22% of adult cervices and in up to 40% of the cervices of newborns and children.[53,95] The wide variation in the reported prevalence of these remnants appears to be a function of how extensively the cervix is sampled and the site of sampling.[35] *Mesonephric remnants* are most commonly present in the lateral aspects of the cervix, a region that is usually not sampled on routine hysterectomy specimens. They consist of small tubules or cysts that are usually located deep in the lateral cervical wall. Characteristically, the tubules are arranged in small clusters or have an orderly distribution reminiscent of the ampullary portion of the fetal mesonephric duct. The tubules are lined by nonciliated, low columnar or cuboidal epithelium. The lining cells contain no glycogen or mucin, features that distinguish mesonephric from endocervical epithelium (Fig. 6.20). The tubular lumen, however, is often filled with pink, homogeneous, PAS-positive secretions.

Mesonephric remnants may become hyperplastic, resulting in a florid, tubuloglandular proliferation with transmural involvement of the cervix (Fig. 6.21). Based on the architecture of the glandular structures, mesonephric hyperplasia has been classified by some authors into different histologic types.[35,90] The most common type is called the lobular type and is characterized by clustered mesonephric tubules, with or without a centrally placed duct. The lobular form tends to occur at a younger age, is less extensive, and tends to arise deeper in the cervical stroma. The less common type is called the diffuse type and is characterized by a nonclustered diffuse pattern or proliferation of mesonephric tubules. The histologic subdivision of mesonephric hyperplasia into different forms does not have clinical significance.

Mesonephric hyperplasia is almost always asymptomatic and is detected on either cervical biopsy, cone biopsy, or hysterectomy specimens. Histologic differentiation between *mesonephric hyperplasia* and mesonephric remnants is quite arbitrary and of little clinical importance. Mesonephric hyperplasia is a benign condition that is of pathologic significance because it can be misinterpreted as a minimal deviation adenocarcinoma of the endocervix (see Chapter 8, Carcinoma and Other Tumors of the Cervix). Mesonephric hyperplasia is distinguished from carcinoma by lack of a complex glandular pattern, mitosis, intracellular mucin, and periglandular stromal edema. In contrast to most cervical adenocarcinomas, carcinoembryonic antigen (i.e., CEA) is absent in mesonephric hyperplasia, and these lesions have low Ki-67 staining indices.[22,69] In addition, normal mesonephric remnants are usually admixed with the hyperplastic tubules.

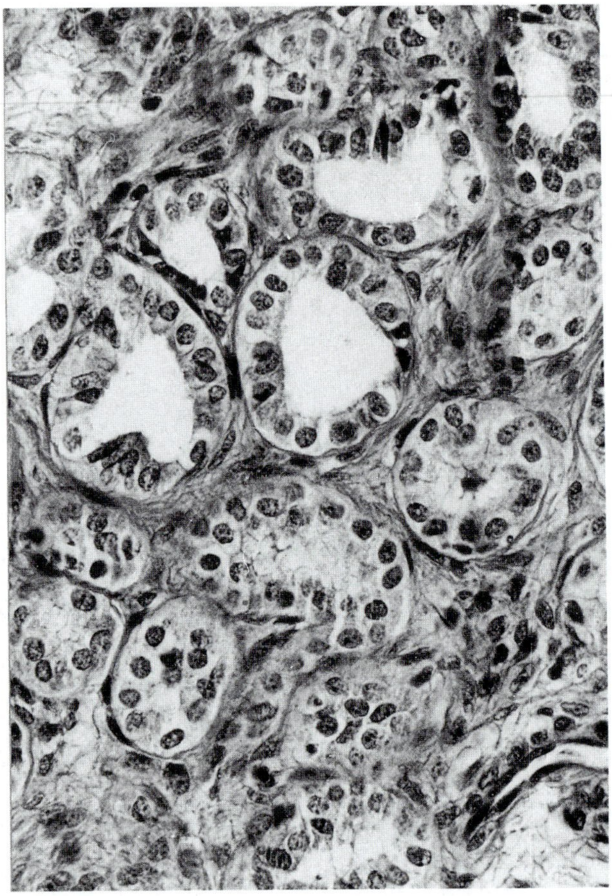

Fig. 6.20. Mesonephric remnants. The mesonephric tubules are lined by cuboidal epithelium with bland nuclei. Occasional tubules contain pink, homogeneous intraluminal secretions. (Courtesy of R.J. Kurman, M.D., Baltimore, MD.)

Endometriosis

Endometriosis refers to lesions that are composed of ectopic endometrial glands and stroma (see Chapter 17, Diseases of the Peritoneum) whereas *tuboendometrioid metaplasia* refers to endocervical glands that are lined by ciliated cells or secretory-type cells with apical snouts that resemble those that can be seen in the endometrium but which lack endome-

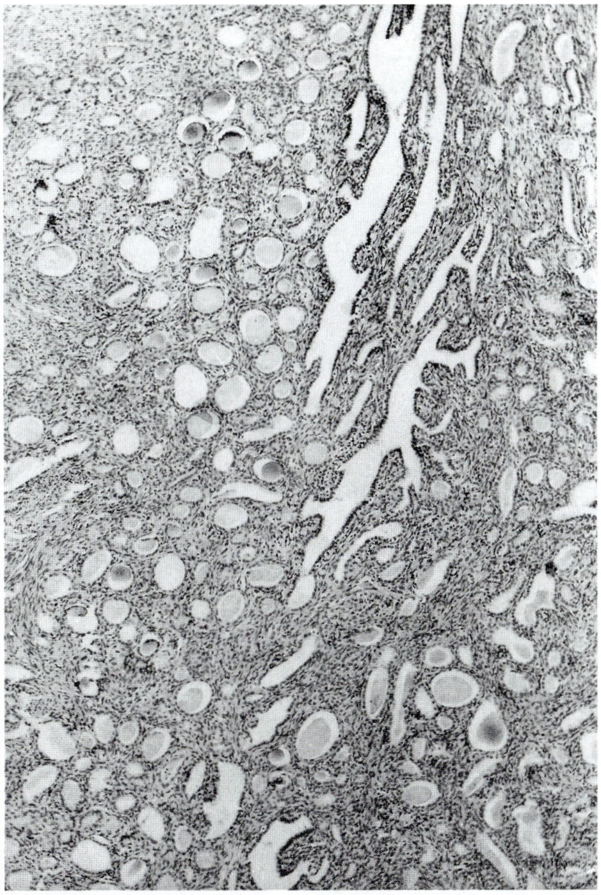

Fig. 6.21. Florid mesonephric hyperplasia. Extensive mesonephric tubular–ductal proliferation in the deeper portion of the cervix, resembling an invasive adenocarcinoma. Unlike the latter, the lobular architecture is maintained in hyperplasia. Note mesonephric duct in center surrounded by a proliferation of small tubules. (Courtesy of R.J. Kurman, M.D., Baltimore, MD.)

trial stroma. Endometriosis of the cervix may occur on the portio or in the endocervical canal. The process is usually confined to the superficial third of the cervical wall.[10] Most areas of endometriosis of the exocervix appear as one or more, small, blue or red nodules measuring a few millimeters in diameter. Occasionally, however, the lesion may be larger or cystic and may produce abnormal vaginal bleeding. Histologically, the glands and stroma resemble proliferative endometrium. Rarely, the glands are secretory. Decidua may be seen in pregnancy or with progestin therapy (Fig. 6.22).

The mechanism responsible for the development of endometriosis is unknown but it is clear that cervical endometriosis frequently develops following cervical trauma. Gardner reported that cervical endometriosis developed in 5%–15% of patients undergoing cervical cautery or cone biopsy, and a more recent analysis of 42 cervices after cone biopsy detected endometriosis in 43%.[39,54] This association has been interpreted by some investigators as evidence supporting the implantation theory of endometriosis. According to this theory, endometrial tissue is implanted into the cervical mucosa or submucosa following postmenstrual cauterization or during delivery. However, the frequent occurrence of posttraumatic endometriosis could also be interpreted as supporting the view that cervical endometriosis represents a reparative/metaplastic process. Support for the concept that cervical endometriosis develops as a metaplastic process, as opposed to direct implantation, also comes from the frequent demonstration of glands with either *tuboendometrioid* or pure *tubal metaplasia* in posttraumatic cervices.

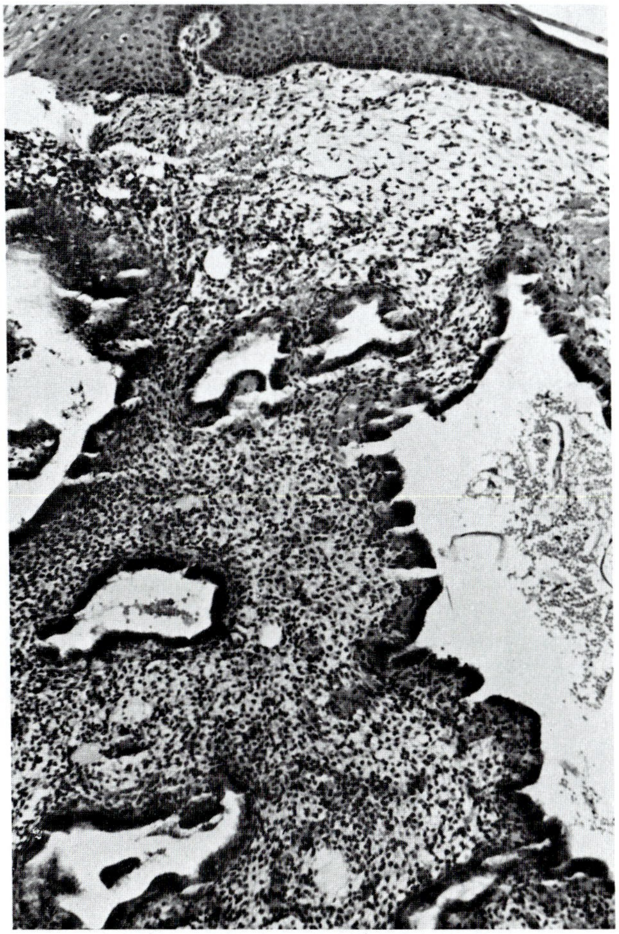

Fig. 6.22. Endometriosis of the cervix. Both typical endometrial glands and stroma are present beneath the squamous portio epithelium.

Benign Tumors

Endocervical Polyps

Endocervical polyps constitute the most common new growths of the uterine cervix. Cervical polyps are focal, hyperplastic protrusions of endocervical folds, including the epithelium and substantia propria. Cervical polyps are most often found during the fourth to sixth decades and in multigravidas. They may present with profuse leukorrhea caused by hypersecretion of mucus from inflamed endocervical epithelium or abnormal bleeding from ulceration of the surface epithelium. Clinically, cervical polyps are rounded or elongated with a smooth or lobulated surface that is often reddened because of increased vascularity. Most polyps are single and measure from a few millimeters to 2–3 cm. In rare instances, they may reach gigantic dimensions, protruding beyond the introitus and resembling carcinoma. Various cervical lesions with a polypoid gross appearance are presented in Table 6.2. Microscopically, cervical polyps display a variety of patterns that vary according to the preponderance of one or another of the tissue components. The most common type is the endocervical mucosal polyp. It is composed of mucinous epithelium that lines crypts, with or without cystic changes (Fig. 6.23). Occasionally, they may be mainly fibrous, representing an overgrowth of the connective tissue stroma of the portio. In other cases, blood vessels predominate and the lesion is called a *vascular polyp*. Squamous metaplasia involving the surface or glandular epithelium of polyps is frequently observed. The supporting connective tissue of polyps is generally loose, with centrally placed feeding vessels, and is almost always infiltrated by a chronic inflammatory infiltrate. Occasionally, such infiltration may be so extensive as to be the principal tissue constituent of the polyp. In these cases, polypoid granulation tissue devoid of surface epithelium is observed (Fig. 6.24). Polyps originating in the isthmus often have an admixture of endocervical- and endometrial-type epithelial components and are referred to as *mixed polyps* (Fig. 6.25).

Table 6.2. Differential clinical diagnosis of polypoid lesions of the cervix

Polyp
Microglandular endocervical hyperplasia
Decidua
Granulation tissue
Leiomyoma
Adenomyoma
Fibroadenoma
Squamous papilloma
Condyloma acuminatum
Papillary adenofibroma
Squamous cell carcinoma
Adenocarcinoma
Sarcoma, primary or secondary

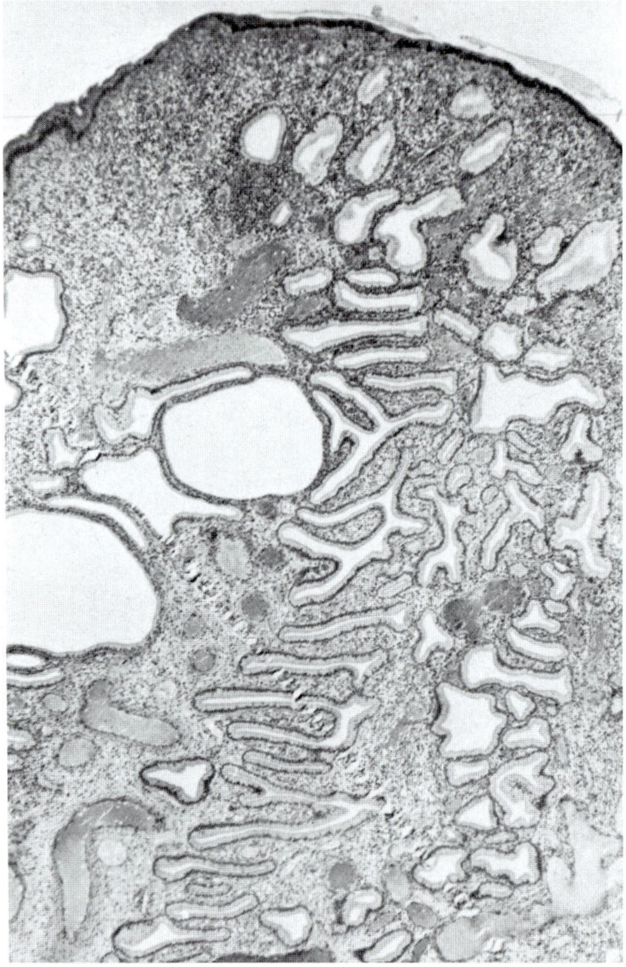

Fig. 6.23. Endocervical polyp. This is the most common histologic type of endocervical polyp. Endocervical-type, tall columnar, mucinous epithelium covers the surface and crypts.

It is extremely uncommon for either in situ or invasive carcinoma (adeno or squamous) to arise in cervical polyps. Endocervical polyps with adenocarcinomatous changes must be differentiated from polypoid adenocarcinoma of the endocervix and from endocervical polyps that are secondarily involved by adjacent adenocarcinoma (Fig. 6.26). The most useful criterion for differentiating between the two is to determine whether the base of the pedicle of the polyp is involved by carcinoma. The base of a polyp that harbors a primary tumor is free of dis-

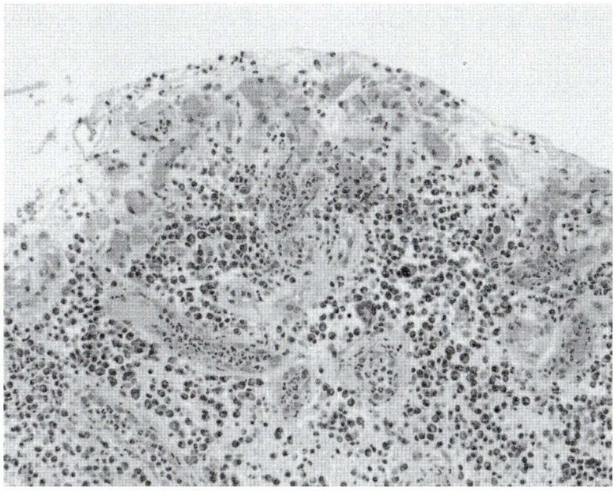

Fig. 6.24. Granulation tissue. Polypoid nodules of granulation tissue can grossly resemble an endocervical polyp. This type of lesion often leads to bleeding.

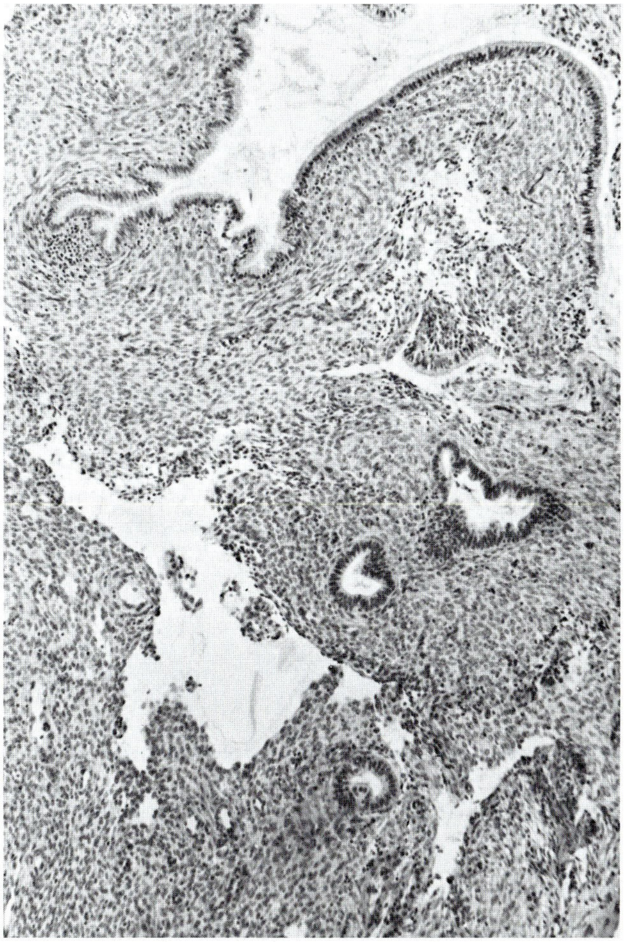

Fig. 6.25. Mixed endocervical–endometrial polyp. This polyp developed from the uterine isthmus. There is endometrial stroma with endometrial glands admixed with mucinous endocervical epithelium (*top*).

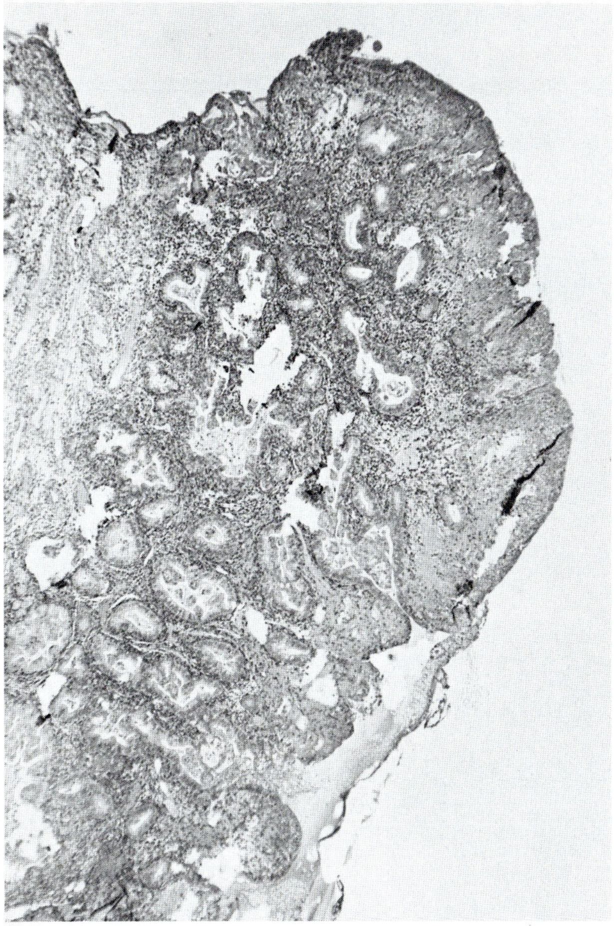

Fig. 6.26. Adenocarcinoma in situ within endocervical polyp. The adenocarcinoma in situ is confined to the superficial area of the polyp.

ease and the carcinoma usually has a focal distribution within an otherwise benign polyp. In a polypoid carcinoma, the entire mass is malignant, including its base and neighboring areas. A focus of carcinoma in a cervical polyp without involvement of its base but associated with similar carcinoma in the adjacent regions should be regarded as a secondary rather than a primary focus. Adenocarcinoma confined to a polyp has an excellent prognosis.[4]

Mesodermal Stromal Polyp (Pseudosarcoma Botryoides)

Mesodermal stromal polyps are benign, exophytic proliferations of stroma and epithelium that can occur in the vagina and cervix of women of reproductive age. These lesions are seen most frequently in pregnant patients and arise more commonly from the vagina than from the cervix.[75] Histologically,

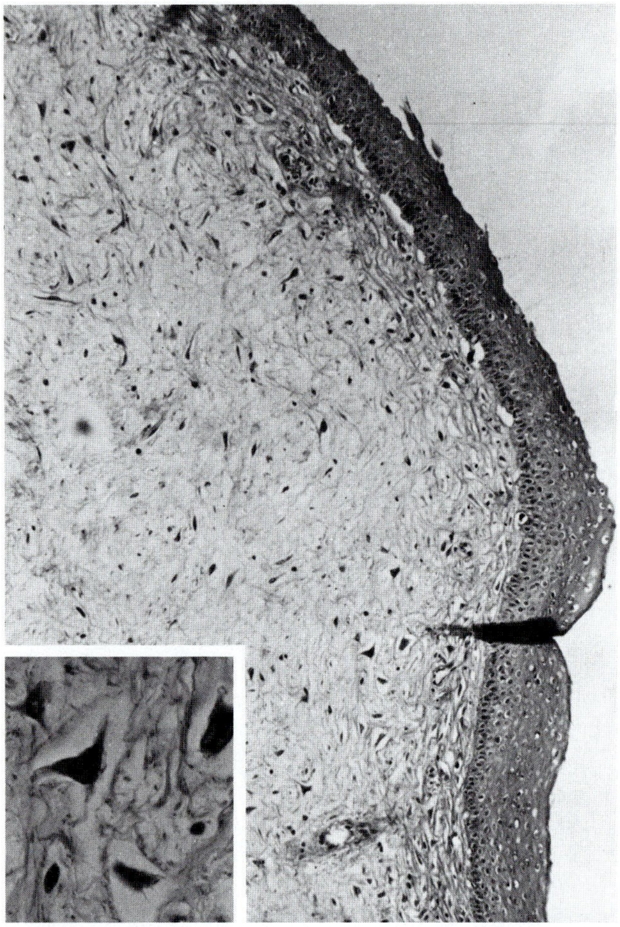

Fig. 6.27. Mesodermal stromal polyp (pseudosarcomatous) of cervix. Spindle-shaped and stellate fibroblasts are embedded in a loose myxoid stroma simulating sarcoma botryoides. Note absence of subepithelial cambium layer. *Inset*: High magnification of stellate atypical fibroblasts.

these polyps are composed of an edematous stroma that is covered by a benign-appearing, stratified squamous epithelium (Fig. 6.27). The stromal component is usually composed of bland-appearing, plump stromal fibroblasts. However, in some cases there can be focal areas of bizarre fibroblasts with irregular, occasionally multinucleated hyperchromatic nuclei that resemble the fibroblasts in radiation reactions.[23] Occasional multinucleated stromal giant cells can be identified in approximately 25% of cone biopsy or hysterectomy specimens when a careful search is made.[48] These cells stain negatively for cytokeratin, desmin, factor VIII, and S-100 protein, but stain positively for vimentin and alpha-1-antichymotrypsin. When stromal polyps contain large numbers of these cells, they can appear quite alarming and simulate the appearance of sarcoma botryoides (Fig. 6.27).[33] However, careful inspection allows these lesions to be differentiated from sarcoma botryoides by the absence of mitotic figures, lack of rhabdomyoblasts, and lack of a cambium layer.

Placental Site Trophoblastic Nodule

Placental site trophoblastic nodules can be found in the endocervix, immediately beneath the epithelium. These lesions are histologically identical to early implantation sites that can be detected in the endometrium of women of reproductive age.[109] Microscopically, placental site trophoblastic nodules are well-defined lesions that have a hyalinized appearance and contain intermediate trophoblasts and inflammatory cells (see Chapter 24, Gestational Trophoblastic Disease and Related Lesions). The intermediate trophoblast cells are frequently degenerated and have extensive cytoplasmic vacuolization but lack significant nuclear atypia, lack mitotic activity, and have very low Ki-67 labeling indices.[93] Intermediate trophoblast stains positively with antibodies against cytokeratins, human placental lactogen, and Mel-CAM, a cell adhesion molecule of the immunoglobulin gene superfamily.[93] The lack of significant nuclear atypia and mitotic activity, as well as staining with antibodies against human placental lactogen, allow these lesions to be microscopically differentiated from invasive nonkeratinizing squamous cell carcinomas.

Leiomyoma

Cervical leiomyomas are much less common than uterine myomas. They usually occur singly and produce unilateral enlargement of the cervical portio. At times the lesion may protrude from the canal, resembling an endocervical polyp, and in pregnancy may produce dystocia. Cervical leiomyomas are similar grossly, microscopically, and ultrastructurally to those observed in the myometrium; a variety of histologic patterns may be encountered, including *atypical leiomyoma*, which contains cells with bizarre nuclei (see Chapter 13, Mesenchymal Tumors of the Uterus).

Adenomyoma and Papillary Adenofibroma

These neoplasms are rare and are composed of an admixture of fibroconnective tissue and smooth muscle elements intermingling with glands lined by a predominately endocervical-type epithelium. The

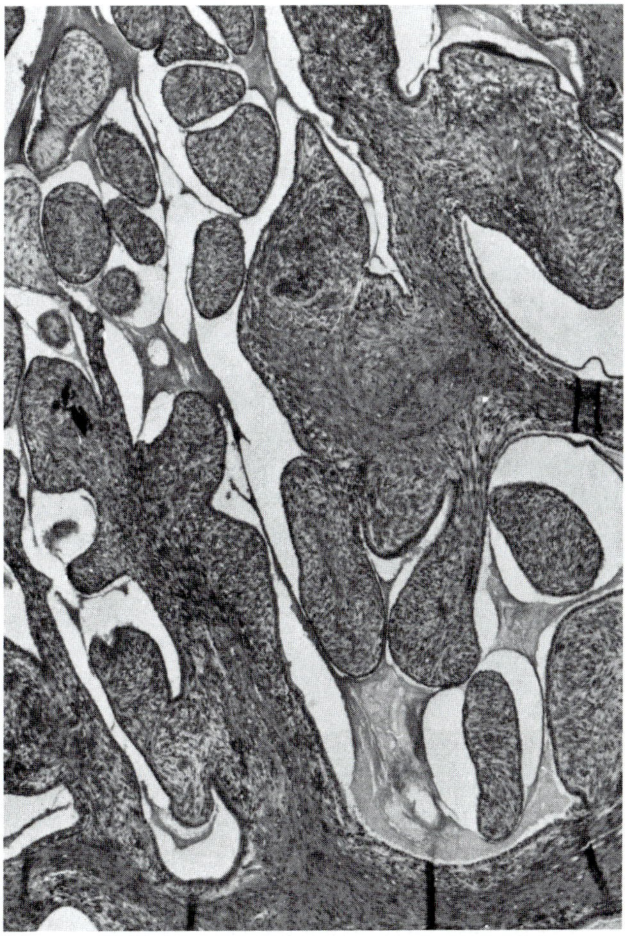

Fig. 6.28. **Papillary adenofibroma of the endocervix.** Fibroepithelial papillae project into cystic spaces. The endocervical lining epithelium produces abundant mucin.

tumors typically measure 1.3–8.0 cm in diameter and usually present as asymptomatic cervical polyps.[43] The epithelial component is typically composed of irregular, large glands that may be accompanied by smaller glands in a lobular arrangement. These tumors can be distinguished from endocervical adenocarcinomas by the lack of invasion of the stromal component by the epithelial component, lack of nuclear atypia, and minimal mitotic activity. Adenomyomas can persist or recur, but there are no reported instances of extracervical spread or metastasis.[43]

Papillary adenofibromas are a rare benign neoplasm with histologic characteristics similar to the *ovarian adenofibroma*. Only several cases have been reported in the literature; these consist of an admixture of fibroconnective tissue and glands lined by either endocervical-type epithelium or a tubal-type epithelium. The fibroconnective tissue usually forms papillary projections (Fig. 6.28).[3,38,73]

Miscellaneous Tumors

Hemangiomas are rarely found in the cervix. They may be of capillary or cavernous type.[45] A single instance of *cervical lymphangioma* was reported by Stout, and several cases of lipoma of the cervix are on record.[100] Neoplasms of neurogenic derivation arising in the cervix are extremely rare and include *neurofibroma* and *ganglioneuroma*. *Benign blue nevi* of the endocervix, indistinguishable from those arising in the dermis, are seen occasionally[78]; these are composed of melanin-containing fusiform cells with dendritic cytoplasmic processes, located in the stroma of the endocervix. *Cervical melanosis* is an uncommon finding characterized by hyperpigmentation of the cervical basal epithelium. It is reported to occur either with or without accompanying basal melanocytes.[107]

Cysts

Nabothian Cyst

Nabothian cysts are the most common type of cyst of the cervix and develop within the transformation zone secondary to squamous metaplasia covering over and obstructing endocervical glands. Grossly, these lesions appear as yellow-white cysts that are frequently multiple and can measure up to 1.5 cm in diameter. Microscopically, they are lined by a somewhat flattened, single layer of mucin-producing endocervical epithelium (Fig. 6.29). In some

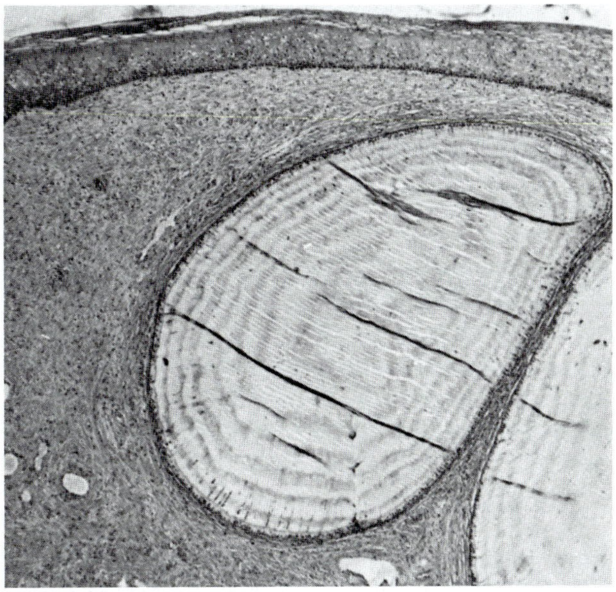

Fig. 6.29. **Nabothian cysts.** Nabothian cysts are lined by a flattened layer of mucin-producing epithelium.

cases squamous metaplasia of the lining epithelium occurs. The lining epithelium is almost always at least focally positive with mucicarimine stains, allowing these lesions to be distinguished from traumatic inclusion cysts and mesonephric duct cysts. Although nabothian cysts are usually confined to the superficial portion of the cervix, they have been reported to extend through the wall of the cervix.[24]

Tunnel Clusters

Endocervical tunnel clusters are benign collections of endocervical glands that are usually located close to the surface epithelium of the cervix. Tunnel clusters are quite common and become more prevalent with increasing age. In Fluhmann's original description, they were detected in 8% of all adult women and 13% of postmenopausal women.[36] They appear to be more common in pregnant women. These lesions are asymptomatic and are detected as incidental findings in either hysterectomy specimens or cone biopsies obtained for unrelated reasons.[89]

Two types of tunnel clusters were originally described. One type represents a cluster of closely packed glands that are noncystic and are lined by tall columnar epithelium; the other type is grossly cystic and lined by a cuboidal or flattened epithelium (Fig. 6.30). These collections of glands have a clustered appearance with a rounded margin and do not invade into the deep cervical stroma. The importance of tunnel clusters is that they are occasionally misinterpreted as minimal deviation adenocarcinomas of the cervix.[59,89] However, tunnel clusters do not have nuclear atypia or mitotic activity and, most importantly, do not invade into the deep cervical stroma.

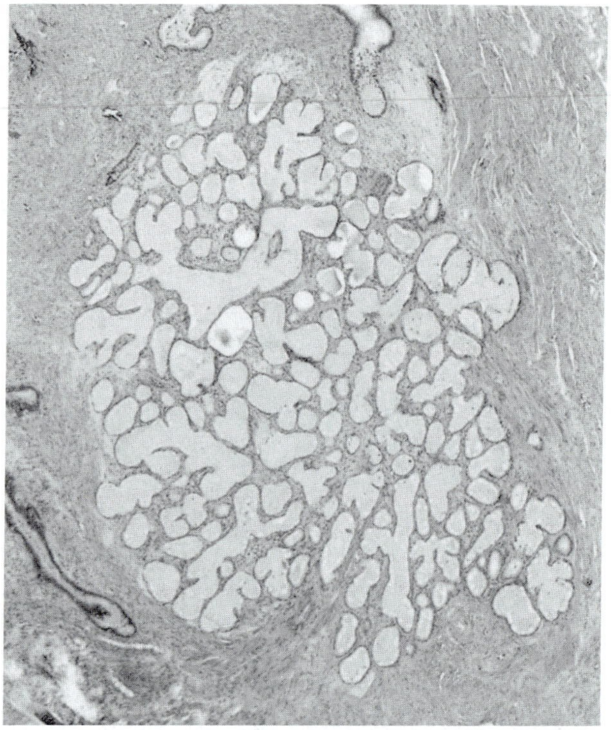

Fig. 6.30. Endocervical tunnel cluster. Closely packed cystically dilated glands lined by a flattened epithelium. The lesion is well demarcated and does not extend beyond the depth of the normal endocervical glands.

Inclusion Cyst

Traumatic inclusion cysts are a form of epidermal inclusion cysts that commonly occur in the vagina at sites of surgical repair of episiotomies or vaginal intrapartum lacerations (see Chapter 4, Diseases of the Vagina). They are thought to develop from viable fragments of epithelium that become entrapped within the stroma at the time of obstetric trauma or subsequent surgical repair. Inclusion cysts are uncommonly found on the cervix. Grossly, they present as unilocular cystic structures measuring 1–2 cm in diameter beneath the native portio epithelium.[37] Microscopically, traumatic inclusion cysts are lined by a stratified squamous epithelium similar to that of the vaginal mucosa but usually somewhat thinner. The epithelium shows normal maturation with the basal cells oriented away from the cyst cavity that is filled with desquamated epithelial cells. The cyst contents are identical to those of epidermal inclusion cysts at other sites and are thick, white, and cheesy.

Tumor-Like Lesions

Decidual Pseudopolyp and Decidualization

During gestation, the stroma of the cervix can undergo *focal decidual changes*. This decidual change is identical to that which occurs in the lamina propria of the fallopian tube or on the serosal surface of the uterus during pregnancy. Histologically, the decidualized cells are present just underneath the surface epithelium and have oval, bland nuclei with large amounts of pale eosinophilic granular cytoplasm and prominent cytoplasmic membranes (Fig. 6.31). The gross appearance of the decidual change depends on the site. If the change occurs on the exocervix, it frequently presents as a raised plaque or pseudopolyp that can be mistaken for invasive carcinoma both colposcopically and microscopically. During gestation, cervical polyps may also contain

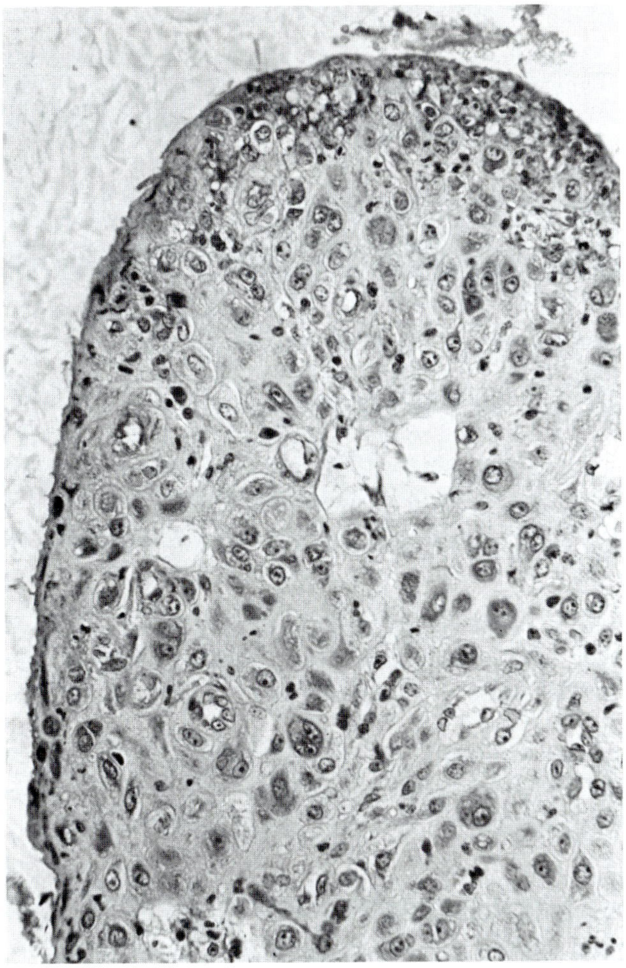

Fig. 6.31. Decidual pseudopolyp. These pseudopolyps develop during pregnancy and are composed of typical decidual cells.

focal stromal decidual changes, and rarely massive decidualization of endocervical stroma occurs producing a polypoid protrusion from the endocervix. Clinically, *decidualized polyps* need to be differentiated from extruded fragments of decidua that may indicate an impending miscarriage. Distinction is made by identifying a stalk for the decidualized polyp, whereas expulsed fragments of decidua lack a stalk. Areas of decidualization are microscopically differentiated from invasive nonkeratinizing squamous cell carcinoma by the lack of significant nuclear atypia, as well as lack of mitotic figures, a coexisting squamous intraepithelial lesion (SIL), and continuity with the surface epithelium. In difficult cases, immunohistochemistry using antibodies against cytokeratin proteins can be used to differentiate cytokeratin-negative decidual reactions from cytokeratin-positive nonkeratinizing squamous cell carcinoma.

Müllerian Papilloma

Rare instances of a benign, papillary growth of the cervix in children have been described[91] that are composed of complex papillary projections lined by flat cuboidal epithelium with cores of loose fibrovascular tissue. Cytologic atypia and mitoses are absent. In the past the lesions were thought to be of mesonephric duct origin, although they have not been encountered in association with mesonephric remnants. Although the histogenesis of these lesions remains uncertain, recent studies favor a müllerian origin.

Postoperative Spindle Cell Nodule and Inflammatory Pseudotumor

Postoperative spindle cell nodules of the cervix are clinically and histologically identical to their more common counterparts of the vulva and vagina.[62,81] These lesions may develop after a cervical biopsy or some other form of trauma. They resemble nodular fasciitis and are composed of actively proliferative spindle cells with oval nuclei arranged in interlacing bundles (see Chapter 4, Diseases of the Vagina). The cells may vary slightly in size, and mitotic figures are often present. A characteristic feature is the presence of neutrophils and erythrocytes in the lesion, giving it the appearance of granulation tissue.

Inflammatory pseudotumor refers to a lesion closely related to postoperative spindle cell nodule that occurs in the absence of a known history of trauma.[5] Inflammatory pseudotumor is a proliferative process of an unknown etiology with a polymorphic morphology. The lesions contain two cellular components: a fibrohistiocytic component consisting of fibroblasts, myofibroblasts, and histiocytes and a polymorphous inflammatory component consisting of lymphocytes and plasma cells. The lesion can be differentiated from other neoplastic processes by the lack of atypia and mitoses and the presence of a polymorphous inflammatory infiltrate.

Lymphoma-Like Lesions

Lymphoma-like lesions (*pseudolymphomas*) are marked inflammatory lesions of the cervix, extensive enough to cause confusion with a lymphoproliferative lesion.[108] Lymphoma-like lesions are composed of a superficial band of large lymphoid cells admixed with mature lymphocytes and plasma cells. The lymphoid infiltrates commonly include macrophages and germinal centers that help to distinguish them from lymphomas (Fig. 6.32). Another feature that helps to distinguish lymphoma-like lesions

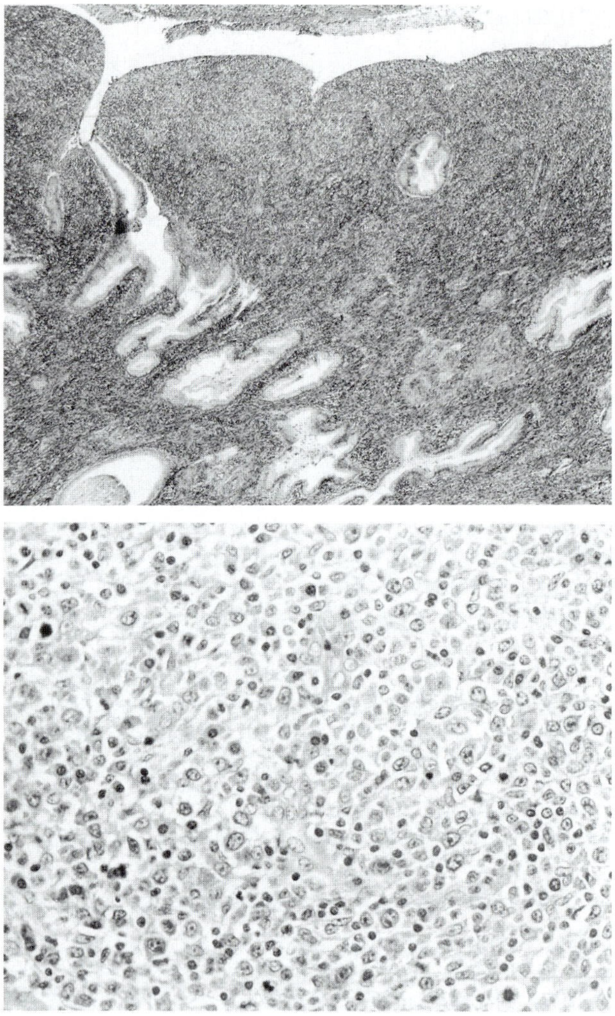

Fig. 6.32. Lymphoma-like lesion. a: This lesion is distinguished from lymphoma by its superficial location and the presence of macrophages and germinal centers. **b:** Higher magnification view of the infiltrate. (Photograph courtesy of Dr. R. Young, Boston, MA.)

from lymphomas is the superficial localization of the infiltrate. Lymphoma-like lesions rarely infiltrate deeper than 3 mm from the surface epithelium whereas lymphomas of the cervix usually extend beyond the depth of the endocervical glands (see Chapter 8, Carcinoma and Other Tumors of the Cervix).

Heterologous Tissue

Glia

There are 15 recorded cases of *neuroglial tissue* in the cervix or the endometrium (see Chapter 10, Benign Disease of the Endometrium).[94] Although the term *glioma* is used for this condition, the high degree of differentiation of the glial tissue, the absence of mitoses, and the absence of recurrence mean it is unlikely that the condition is neoplastic (Fig. 6.33). The lesion should not be confused with a pure heterologous sarcoma or a teratoma. The neural tissue is believed to represent either implantation of fetal cerebral glia at the time of instrumentation of the gravid uterus or heterotopic maldevelopment during embryogenesis. When the cervix is involved, the lesion usually appears as a polyp that bleeds readily.

Skin

Among the pathologic curiosities of the cervix are cases of true epidermidization of the cervical mucosa. In these instances sebaceous glands, hair, and sweat glands are found. The presence of these ectodermal structures, which are normally appendages of the epidermis, on a mucous membrane of mesodermal derivation is difficult to explain. It is conceivable, however, that stratified squamous epithelium under certain circumstances, such as long-standing chronic inflammation, can form the appendages of its epidermal analogue.

Cartilage

Four cases of *heterotopic mature cartilage* in the cervix are on record.[84] The finding of these struc-

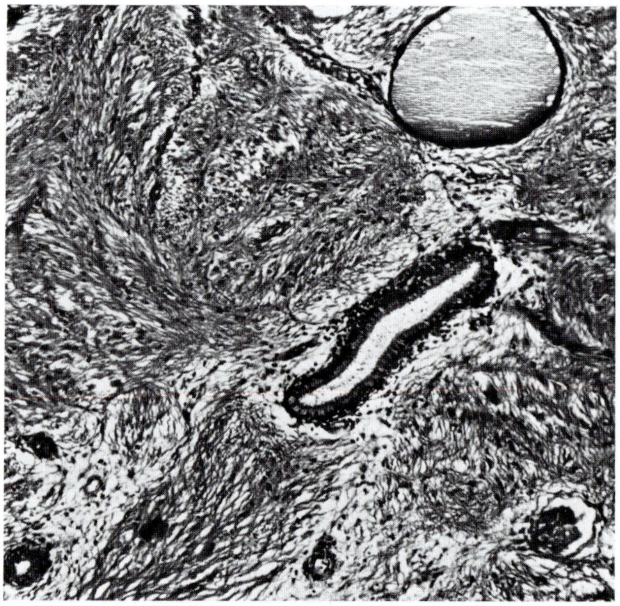

Fig. 6.33. Glioma of the endocervix. Bundles of well-differentiated neuroglial tissue intermingle with normal endocervical epithelium. (Courtesy of Dr. Y. Boivin, Montreal, Quebec.)

tures alone has no clinical significance. They should not be confused with a malignant mixed mesodermal tumor.

References

1. CDC (1998) 1998 Guidelines for treatment of sexually transmitted diseases. Morb Mortal Wkly Rep 47(RR-1):95–98
2. CDC (1999) 1997 Sexually transmitted disease surveillance report. Centers for Disease Control and Prevention, Atlanta, GA. http://www.cdc.gov/nchstp/dstd/Stats_Trends/1997_Surveillance_Report.pdf: Division of Sexually Transmitted Disease Prevention, United States Department of Health and Human Services, Public Health Service, Centers for Disease Control and Prevention, Atlanta GA
3. Abell MR (1971) Papillary adenofibroma of the uterine cervix. Am J Obstet Gynecol 110:990–993
4. Abell MR, Gosling RG (1962) Gland cell carcinoma (adenocarcinoma) of the uterine cervix. Am J Obstet Gynecol 83:729
5. Abenoza P, Shek YH, Perrone T (1994) Inflammatory pseudotumor of the cervix. Int J Gynecol Pathol 13:80–86
6. Agarwal J, Gupta JK (1993) Female genital tuberculosis—a retrospective clinico-pathologic study of 501 cases. Indian J Pathol Microbiol 36:389–397
7. Akang EE, Matiluko AA, Omigbodun AO, et al (1997) Cervicovaginitis emphysematosa mimicking carcinoma of the cervix: a case report. Afr J Med Med Sci 26:99–100
8. Andrews S, Miyazawa K (1989) The significance of a negative Papanicolaou smear with hyperkeratosis or parakeratosis. Obstet Gynecol 73:751–753
9. Armstrong LR, Preston EJ, Reichert M, et al (2000) Incidence and prevalence of recurrent respiratory papillomatosis among children in Atlanta and Seattle. Clin Infect Dis 31:107–109
10. Baker PM, Clement PB, Bell DA, et al (1999) Superficial endometriosis of the uterine cervix: a report of 20 cases of a process that may be confused with endocervical glandular dysplasia or adenocarcinoma in situ. Int J Gynecol Pathol 18:198–205
11. Barton IG, Kinghorn GR, Walker MJ, et al (1981) Association of HSV-1 with cervical infection. Lancet 2:1108
12. Bhagavan BS, Ruffier J, Shinn B (1982) Pseudoactinomycotic radiate granules in the lower female genital tract: relationship to the Splendore-Hoeppli phenomenon. Hum Pathol 13:898–904
13. Brown LJR, Wells M (1986) Cervical glandular atypia associated with squamous intraepithelial neoplasia: a premalignant lesion? J Clin Pathol 39:22–28
14. Brunham RC, Paavonen J, Stevens CE, et al (1984) Mucopurulent cervicitis—the ignored counterpart in women of urethritis in men. N Engl J Med 311:1–6
15. Burd LI, Easterly JR (1971) Vesicular lesions of the uterine cervix. Am J Obstet Gynecol 110:887–888
16. Byrne MA, Walker MM, Leonard J, et al (1989) Recognising covert disease in women with chronic vulval symptoms attending an STD clinic: value of detailed examination including colposcopy. Genitourin Med 65:46–49
17. Candy J, Abell MR (1968) Progestogen-induced adenomatous hyperplasia of the uterine cervix. JAMA 203:323
18. Cecchini S, Iossa A, Ciatto S, et al (1990) Colposcopic survey of Papanicolaou test-negative cases with hyperkeratosis or parakeratosis. Obstet Gynecol 76:857–859
19. Chakraborty P, Roy A, Bhattacharya S, et al (1995) Tuberculous cervicitis: a clinicopathological and bacteriological study. J Indian Med Assoc 93: 167–168
20. Chiasson MA, Wright TC (1997) The gynecologic manifestations of HIV. In: Mandel GL, Mildvan D (eds) Atlas of infectious diseases, vol 1. Churchill Livingstone, Edinburgh, pp 12.1–12.5
21. Chiasson MA, Ellerbrock TV, Bush TJ, et al (1997) Increased prevalence of vulvovaginal condyloma and vulvar intraepithelial neoplasia in women infected with the human immunodeficiency virus. Obstet Gynecol 89:690–694
22. Cina SJ, Richardson MS, Austin RM, et al (1997) Immunohistochemical staining for Ki-67 antigen, carcinoembryonic antigen, and p53 in the differential diagnosis of glandular lesions of the cervix. Mod Pathol 10:176–180
23. Clement PB (1985) Multinucleated stromal giant cells of the uterine cervix. Arch Pathol Lab Med 109:200–202
24. Clement PB, Young RH (1989) Deep nabothian cysts of the uterine cervix. A possible source of confusion with minimal-deviation adenocarcinoma (adenoma malignum). Int J Gynecol Pathol 8:340–348
25. Concetti H, Retegui M, Perez G, et al (2000) Chagas' disease of the cervix uteri in a patient with acquired immunodeficiency syndrome. Hum Pathol 31:120–122
26. Corey L, Holmes KK (1983) Clinical course of genital herpes simplex virus infections in men and women. Ann Intern Med 48:973–983
27. Corey L, Wald A (1999) Genital herpes simplex virus infections. In: Holmes KK, Sparling PF, Mardh P-A, et al (eds) Sexually transmitted diseases. McGraw-Hill, New York, pp 285–312
28. Critchlow CW, Wolner-Hanssen P, Eschenbach DA, et al (1995) Determinants of cervical ectopia and of cervicitis: age, oral contraception, specific cervical infection, smoking, and douching. Am J Obstet Gynecol 173:534–543
29. Crum CP, Mitao M, Winkler B, et al (1984) Localizing chlamydial infection in cervical biopsies with the immunoperoxidase technique. Int J Gynecol Pathol 3:191–197

30. Curtis EM, Pine L (1981) Actinomyces in the vaginas of women with and without intrauterine contraceptive devices. Am J Obstet Gynecol 140:880–884
31. Duggan MA (2000) Cytologic and histologic diagnosis and significance of controversial squamous lesions of the uterine cervix. Mod Pathol 13:252–260
32. Egan AJ, Russel P (1997) Transitional (urothelial) cell metaplasia of the uterine cervix: morphological assessment of 31 cases. Int J Gynecol Pathol 16:89–98
33. Elliott GB, Elliott JDA (1973) Superficial stromal reactions of the lower genital tract. Arch Pathol 95:100–101
34. Evans CS, Goldman RL, Klein HZ, et al (1984) Necrobiotic granulomas of the uterine cervix. A probable postoperative reaction. Am J Surg Pathol 8:841–844
35. Ferry JA, Scully RE (1990) Mesonephric remnants, hyperplasia, and neoplasia in the uterine cervix. A study of 49 cases. Am J Surg Pathol 14:1100–1111
36. Fluhmann CF (1961) Focal hyperplasia (tunnel clusters) of the cervix uteri. Obstet Gynecol 17: 206–214
37. Fluhmann CF (1961) The cervix uteri and its diseases. Saunders, Philadelphia
38. Fratini D, Cavaliere A (1996) Papillary adenofibroma of the uterine cervix. A case report. Pathologica (Genoa) 88:135–136
39. Gardner HL (1966) Cervical and vaginal endometriosis. Clin Obstet Gynecol 9:358
40. Gardner HL, Fernet P (1964) Etiology of vaginitis emphysematosa. Am J Obstet Gynecol 88:680
41. Giampaolo C, Murphy J, Benes S, et al (1983) How sensitive is the Papanicolaou smear in the diagnosis of infections with *Chlamydia trachomatis*? Am J Clin Pathol 80:844–849
42. Gilks CB, Young RH, Aguirre P, et al (1989) Adenoma malignum (minimal deviation adenocarcinoma) of the uterine cervix. A clinicopathological and immunohistochemical analysis of 26 cases. Am J Surg Pathol 13:717–729
43. Gilks CB, Young RH, Clement PB, et al (1996) Adenomyomas of the uterine cervix of endocervical type: a report of ten cases of a benign cervical tumor that may be confused with adenoma malignum. Mod Pathol 9:220–224
44. Greeley C, Schroeder S, Silverberg SG (1995) Microglandular hyperplasia of the cervix: a true "pill" lesion? Int J Gynecol Pathol 14:50–54
45. Gudson JT (1965) Hemangioma of the cervix. Am J Obstet Gynecol 91:204
46. Hacker NF, Berek JS, Lagasse LD, et al (1982) Carcinoma of the cervix associated with pregnancy. Obstet Gynecol 59:735–746
47. Hare MJ, Toone E, Taylor-Robinson D, et al (1981) Follicular cervicitis—colposcopic appearances and association with *Chlamydia trachomatis*. Br J Obstet Gynaecol 88:174–180
48. Hariri J, Ingemanssen JL (1993) Multinucleated stromal giant cells of the uterine cervix. Int J Gynecol Pathol 12:228–234
49. Harnden P, Kennedy W, Andrew AC, et al (1999) Immunophenotype of transitional metaplasia of the uterine cervix. *Int J Gynecol Pathol* 18:125–129
50. Harrison HR, Costin M, Meder JB, et al (1985) Cervical *Chlamydia trachomatis* infection in university women: relationship to history, contraception, ectopy, and cervicitis. Am J Obstet Gynecol 153:244–251
51. Holmes KK, Stamm WE (1999) Lower genital tract infections in women. In: Holmes KK, Sparling PF, Mardh P-A, et al (eds) Sexually transmitted diseases. McGraw-Hill, New York, pp 761–782
52. Hoosen AA, Draper G, Moodley J, et al (1990) Granuloma inguinale of the cervix: a carcinoma lookalike. Genitourin Med 66:380–382
53. Huffman JW (1948) Mesonephric remnants in the cervix. Am J Obstet Gynecol 56:23–40
54. Ismail SM (1991) Cone biopsy causes cervical endometriosis and tubo-endometrioid metaplasia. Histopathology (Oxf) 18:107–114
55. Johnson CA, Lorenzetti LA, Liese BS, et al (1991) Clinical significance of hyperkeratosis on otherwise normal Papanicolaou smears. J Fam Pract 33:354–358
56. Jonasson JG, Wang HH, Antonioli DA, et al (1992) Tubal metaplasia of the uterine cervix: a prevalence study in patients with gynecologic pathologic findings. Int J Gynecol Pathol 11:89–95
57. Jones MA (1998) Transitional cell metaplasia and neoplasia in the female genital tract: an update. Adv Anat Pathol 5:106–113
58. Jones MA, Young RA (1997) Atypical oxyphilic metaplasia of the endocervical epithelium: a report of six cases. Int J Gynecol Pathol 16:99–102
59. Jones MA, Young RH (1996) Endocervical type A (noncystic) tunnel clusters with cytologic atypia. A report of 14 cases. Am J Surg Pathol 20:1312–1318
60. Kashima HK, Mounts P, Shah K (1996) Recurrent respiratory papillomatosis. In: Lorincz A, Reid R (eds) Obstetrics and gynecology clinics of North America, vol 23. Saunders, Philadelphia, pp 699–706
61. Kaufman RH, Watts JM, Gardner HL (1969) Pemphigus vulgaris genital involvement. Obstet Gynecol 33:264
62. Kay S, Schneider V (1985) Reactive spindle cell nodule of the endocervix simulating uterine sarcoma. Int J Gynecol Pathol 4:255–257
63. Kiviat NB, Paavonen JA, Brockway J, et al (1985) Cytologic manifestations of cervical and vaginal infections. I. Epithelial and inflammatory cellular changes. JAMA 253:989–996
64. Koller AB (1975) Granulomatous lesions of the cervix uteri in black patients. S Afr Med J 49:1228–1232
65. Koss LG (1998) Traditional cell metaplasia of cervix: a misnomer. Am J Surg Pathol 22:774–776

66. Koss LG (1998) Transitional cell metaplasia. Adv Anat Pathol 5:202–203
67. Koutsky LA, Ashley RL, Holmes KK, et al (1990) The frequency of unrecognized type 2 herpes simplex virus infection among women. Implications for the control of genital herpes. Sex Transm Dis 17:90–94
68. Koutsky LA, Stevens CE, Holmes KK, et al (1992) Underdiagnosis of genital herpes by current clinical and viral-isolation procedures. N Engl J Med 326:1533–1539
69. Lang G, Dallenbach-Hellweg G (1990) The histogenetic origin of cervical mesonephric hyperplasia and mesonephric adenocarcinoma of the uterine cervix studied with immunohistochemical methods. In J Gynecol Pathol 9:145–157
70. Laurtizen AF, Meinecke G (1987) Isolated arteritis of the uterine cervix. Acta Obstet Gynecol Scand 66:659–660
71. Lesack D, Wahab I, Bilks CB (1996) Radiation-induced atypia of endocervical epithelium: a histological, immunohistochemical and cytometric study. Int J Gynecol Pathol 15:242–247
72. Lippes J (1999) Pelvic actinomycosis: a review and preliminary look at prevalence. Am J Obstet Gynecol 180:265–269
73. Mohan H, Punia RS, Mohan P (1999) Papillary adenofibroma of cervix. J Indian Med Assoc 97:524
74. Moubayed P, Lepere JF, Mwakyoma H, et al (1994) Carcinoma of the uterine cervix and schistosomiasis. Int J Gynaecol Obstet 45:133–139
75. Norris HJ, Taylor HB (1966) Polyps of the vagina: a benign lesion resembling sarcoma botryoides. Cancer (Phila) 19:226
76. Novotny DB, Maygarden SJ, Johnson DE, et al (1992) Tubal metaplasia. A frequent potential pitfall in the cytologic diagnosis of endocervical glandular dysplasia on cervical smears. Acta Cytol 36:1–10
77. Oliva E, Clement PB, Young RH (1995) Tubal and tubo-endometrioid metaplasia of the uterine cervix. Unemphasized features that may cause problems in differential diagnosis: a report of 25 cases. Am J Clin Pathol 103:618–623
78. Patel DS, Bhagavan BS (1985) Blue nevus of the uterine cervix. Hum Pathol 16:79–86
79. Patsner B, Baker DA, Orr JW Jr (1990) Human papillomavirus genital tract infections during pregnancy. Clin Obstet Gynecol 33:258–267
80. Petitti DB, Yamamoto D, Morgenstern N (1983) Factors associated with actinomyces-like organisms on Papanicolaou smear in users of intrauterine contraceptive devices. Am J Obstet Gynecol 145:338–341
81. Proppe KH, Scully RE, Rosai J (1984) Postoperative spindle cell nodules of geniturinary tract resembling sarcomas. A report of eight cases. Am J Surg Pathol 8:101–108
82. Rand RJ, Lowe JW (1998) Schistosomiasis of the uterine cervix. Br J Obstet Gynaecol 105:1329–1331
83. Riffenburgh RH, Olson PE, Johnstone PA (1997) Association of schistosomiasis with cervical cancer: detecting bias in clinical studies. East Afr Med J 74:14–16
84. Roth E, Taylor HB (1966) Heterotopic cartilage in the uterus. Obstet Gynecol 27:838
85. Schaefer G (1970) Tuberculosis of female genital tract. Clin Obstet Gynecol 13:965–998
86. Schlesinger C, Silverberg SG (1999) Endocervical adenocarcinoma in situ of tubal type and its relation to atypical tubal metaplasia. Int J Gynecol Pathol 18:1–4
87. Schneider V (1981) Arias-Stella reaction of the endocervix: frequency and location. Acta Cytol 25:224–228
88. Schomogyi M, Wald A, Corey L (1998) Herpes simplex virus-2 infection. An emerging disease? Infect Dis Clin North Am 12:47–61
89. Segal GH, Hart WR (1990) Cystic endocervical tunnel clusters: a clinicopathologic study of 29 cases of so-called adenomatous hyperplasia. Am J Surg Pathol 14:895–903
90. Seidman JD, Tavassoli FA (1995) Mesonephric hyperplasia of the uterine cervix: a clinicopathologic study of 51 cases. Int J Gynecol Pathol 14:293–299
91. Selzer F, Nelson HM (1982) Benign papilloma (polypoid tumor) of the cervix uteri in children: report of two cases. Am J Obstet Gynecol 84:165
92. Sfameni SF, Ostor AG, Chanen W, et al (1986) The association between vulvar condylomata acuminata, cervical wart virus infection and cervical intraepithelial neoplasia. Aust N Z J Obstet Gynaecol 26:149–151
93. Shih IM, Kurman RJ (1998) Ki-67 labeling index in the differential diagnosis of exaggerated placental site, placental site trophoblastic tumor, and choriocarcinoma: a double immunohistochemical staining technique using Ki-67 and Mel-CAM antibodies. Hum Pathol 29:27–33
94. Slavutin L (1979) Uterine gliosis and ossification. Am J Diagn Gynecol Obstet 1:351
95. Sneeden VD (1958) Mesonephric lesions of the cervix. A practical means of demonstration and a suggestion of incidence. Cancer (Phila) 11:334–336
96. Sobel JD (1997) Vaginitis. N Engl J Med 337:1896–1903
97. Speers WC, Picaso LG, Silverberg SG (1983) Immunohistochemical localization of carcinoembryonic antigen in microglandular hyperplasia and adenocarcinoma of the endocervix. Am J Clin Pathol 79:105–107
98. Stamm WE (1999) *Chlamydia trachomatis* infections of the adult. In: Holmes KK, Sparling PF, Mardh P-A, et al (eds) Sexually transmitted diseases. McGraw-Hill, New York, pp 407–422
99. Steeper TA, Wick MR (1986) Minimal deviation adenocarcinoma of the uterine cervix. An immunohistochemical comparison with microglandular endocervical hyperplasia and conventional adenocarcinoma. Cancer (Phila) 58:1131–1138
100. Stout AP (1943) Hemangioendothelioma: a tumor of blood vessels featuring vascular endothelial cells. Ann Surg 118:445

101. Sugase M, Moriyama S, Matsukura T (1991) Human papillomavirus in exophytic condylomatous lesions on different female genital regions. J Med Virol 34:1–6
102. Suh KS, Silverberg SG (1990) Tubal metaplasia of the uterine cervix. Int J Gynecol Pathol 9:122–128
103. Taylor HB, Irey NS, Norris HJ (1967) Atypical endocervical hyperplasia in women taking oral contraceptives. JAMA 202:637–639
104. Veliath AJ, Bansal R, Sankaran V, et al (1987) Genital amebiasis. Int J Gynaecol Obstet 25:249–256
105. Weir MM, Bell DA, Young RH (1997) Transitional cell metaplasia of the uterine cervix and vagina: an underrecognized lesion that may be confused with high-grade dysplasia. A report of 59 cases. Am J Surg Pathol 21:510–517
106. Wilkinson E, Dufour DR (1976) Pathogenesis of microglandular hyperplasia of the cervix uteri. Obstet Gynecol 47:189–195
107. Yilmaz AG, Chandler P, Hahm GK, et al (1999) Melanosis of the uterine cervix: a report of two cases and discussion of pigmented cervical lesions. Int J Gynecol Pathol 18:73–76
108. Young RH, Harris NL, Scully RE (1985) Lymphoma-like lesions of the lower female genital tract: a report of 16 cases. Int J Gynecol Pathol 4:289–299
109. Young RH, Kurman RJ, Scully RE (1988) Proliferations and tumors of intermediate trophoblast of the placental site. Semin Diagn Pathol 5:223–237
110. Young RH, Scully RE (1989) Atypical forms of microglandular hyperplasia of the cervix simulating carcinoma. Am J Surg Pathol 13:50–56

7

Precancerous Lesions of the Cervix

Thomas C. Wright, M.D., Robert J. Kurman, M.D., and Alex Ferenczy, M.D.

Precursors of Squamous Cell Carcinoma

Terminology and Historical Perspective

The histopathologic classification of a disease should reflect current concepts of its pathogenesis as well as its clinical behavior. During the past 50 years, our understanding of the pathobiology and behavior of cervical cancer precursors has evolved considerably. As a result, the terminology used to classify preinvasive lesions of the cervix has frequently changed. Although these changes in nomenclature and the resulting lack of a uniform terminology have been an ongoing source of confusion to both gynecologists and pathologists, each change has actually reduced the number of specific pathologic categories and has made clinical decision making more straightforward.

The existence of precursor lesions for invasive cervical cancer has been recognized for more than half a century. As early as 1886, Sir John Williams commented on the presence of noninvasive epithelial abnormalities adjacent to invasive squamous cell carcinomas of the cervix.[302] The spatial relationships and histologic appearance of these noninvasive epithelial lesions were better described by Cullen in 1900, who recognized that these intraepithelial lesions histologically resembled the adjacent invasive cancers.[64] In the 1930s, Broders reintroduced the term *carcinoma in situ* that was first used by Schottlander and Kermauner to refer to these intraepithelial cervical lesions.[34] A temporal relationship between carcinoma in situ and invasive cancer was subsequently reported by Smith and Pemberton, as well as by Galvin, Jones, and Telinde, who diagnosed carcinoma in situ in several patients months to years before the development of invasive cervical cancer.[218] The recognition that there was both a spatial and temporal relationship between carcinoma in situ and invasive squamous cell carcinoma led to the hypothesis that invasive squamous cell carcinoma develops from a histologically well-defined precursor lesion.[34] This hypothesis was subsequently substantiated by long-term follow-up studies, which clearly demonstrated that a significant proportion of untreated patients with carcinoma in situ subsequently develop invasive squamous cell carcinoma.[150,154]

Once it was accepted that carcinoma in situ was a precursor to invasive squamous cell carcinoma, population-based cytologic screening programs were begun to detect and treat precursor lesions before the actual development of cancer. As large numbers of women were screened for cervical disease, it became apparent that many women had cervical epithelial abnormalities that were cytologically/histologically less severe than carcinoma in situ. These lesions formed a histologic spectrum that ranged from lesions in which the majority of the cells had the cytologic features of carcinoma in situ to those in which the degree of atypicality was much less. In 1956, Reagan and coworkers introduced the term *dysplasia* to refer to this spectrum of cervical abnormalities with features intermediate between those of carcinoma in situ and normal cervical epithelium.[227] Dysplasia actually means "abnormality of development." Reagan used the term to describe a proliferation of abnormal squamous cells that superficially resemble those of the basal layer but which have nuclear atypia and there is enlargement resulting in an altered nuclear:cytoplasmic ratio; in addition, a disorganized arrangement and loss of normal cellular polarity occur. Depending on the extent to which the thickness of the epithelium displayed these changes, dysplasia was subclassified as mild, moderate, or severe. This classification was thought to reflect the biologic potential of the lesions for progressing to carcinoma in situ and, eventually, invasive squamous cell carcinoma.

In 1961, at the First International Congress on Exfoliative Cytology, the Committee on Histological Terminology for Lesions of the Uterus Cervix defined carcinoma in situ as follows: "Only those cases should be classified as carcinoma in situ which, in the absence of invasion, show a surface lining epithelium in which, throughout its whole thickness, no differentiation takes place. The process may involve the lining of the cervical glands. It is recognized that the cells of uppermost layers may show some slight flattening. The very rare case of an otherwise characteristic carcinoma in situ that shows a greater degree of differentiation belongs to the exceptions for which no classification can provide." Dysplasia of the cervix was defined as ". . . all other (than carcinoma in situ) disturbances of differentiation of the squamous epithelial lining of surface and glands. . . . They may be characterized as of high or low degree, terms which are preferable to suspicious and non-suspicious, as the proposed terms describe the histological appearance and do not express an opinion."[297] Therefore, the key distinguishing feature of dysplasia was that the atypical cells did not extend through the full thickness of the epithelium or invade the basement membrane. Although most pathologists used the term dysplasia, occasionally, lesions with this histology were termed *basal cell hyperplasia* or *atypical hyperplasia*. In the cytologic nomenclature, dysplasia was considered to be a benign to possibly malignant squamous epithelial atypia, whereas carcinoma in situ was designated as positive for malignant cells.

The separation of noninvasive cervical lesions into two groups, dysplasia and carcinoma in situ, implied that there was a biologic distinction between these two entities and that the two could be reproducibly distinguished from each other. In most centers dysplasia was considered to be a potentially reversible process and therefore was either ignored, followed, or treated depending on a variety of clinical factors whereas carcinoma in situ was considered to be a highly significant lesion such that patients with this diagnosis were usually treated with hysterectomy. This classification of noninvasive precursor lesions into dysplastic and carcinoma in situ lesions was based solely on arbitrary histologic differences that were often quite subtle.[38,152] For example, the diagnosis of severe dysplasia as opposed to carcinoma in situ was based on the presence of a single layer of flattened epithelial cells on the surface of the lesion and, on the basis of the appearance of this single layer of cells, a patient might either be treated conservatively or by hysterectomy. In the 1960s, several studies of inter- and intraobserver variability of histologic diagnosis demonstrated that pathologists could not reproducibly distinguish between severe dysplasia and carcinoma in situ.[58,144] This realization called into question the justification of such marked differences in clinical management based solely on subjective histologic criteria.

Subsequently, a number of studies in the late 1960s suggested that the cellular changes of dysplasia and carcinoma in situ were qualitatively similar and remained constant throughout the histologic spectrum. Both dysplasia and carcinoma in situ were found to be monoclonal proliferations of abnormal squamous epithelial cells with an aneuploid nuclear DNA content.[93] On the basis of these descriptive biologic studies, Richart introduced the concept that all types of precursor lesions to squamous cell carcinoma of cervix represented a single disease process, which he termed cervical intraepithelial neoplasia (CIN).[232]

The CIN terminology divided cervical cancer precursors into three groups. CIN 1 corresponded to lesions previously diagnosed as mild dysplasia, CIN 2 corresponded to moderate dysplasia, and CIN 3 to both severe dysplasia and carcinoma in situ, because pathologists could not reproducibly distinguish between the two. At the time of its introduction, CIN was thought to define a spectrum of histologic changes that shared a common etiology, biology, and natural history. Furthermore, the diagnostic term CIN implied that such lesions, if untreated, had a significant, albeit individually unknown risk of developing into invasive carcinoma in the future. As a corollary, it was presumed that when the histologic changes of CIN were diagnosed and the lesion adequately treated, the development of invasive cancer could be prevented. Although the CIN terminology allowed lesions to be subdivided into three separate categories, it was anticipated that the use of a unified concept of a single disease process would deemphasize lesion grade as a determinate of clinical management.[232,235]

The CIN terminology became the most widely used histologic terminology for cervical cancer precursors in the 1970s and the 1980s. However, during the past two decades there has been an explosion of information about the etiology of cervical cancer and its precursor lesions. It is now widely accepted that both invasive squamous cell carcinomas and adenocarcinomas of the cervix, as well as their respective precursor lesions, are caused by specific types of human papillomavirus (HPV) that infect the anogenital tract. More importantly, as our understanding of the pathogenesis of cervical cancer precursors has grown, it has become clear that the basic premise underlying the CIN terminology is incorrect; the spectrum of histologic changes that are referred to as CIN do not represent a single disease process at different stages in its development but instead two distinct biologic entities, one a productive viral infection and the other a true neoplastic process confined to the epithelium.

Productive HPV infections of the cervical squamous epithelium are self-limited in the majority of patients and commonly result in flat lesions and less frequently in exophytic ones (condylomata acuminata). The flat lesion can be caused by any of the more than 40 different types of HPV that infect the human anogenital tract.[17,137,169,174] Flat lesions in which there is productive viral infection display cytoplasmic cavitation and nuclear abnormalities. These lesions have been designated in the past *koilocytotic atypia, koilocytosis, flat condyloma, mild dysplasia*, or *CIN 1*.[83]

The other entity subsumed within the morphologic CIN spectrum is histologically "high grade." High-grade lesions are frequently aneuploid and represent true intraepithelial neoplasia with a potential to progress to invasive squamous cell carcinoma if left untreated. High-grade lesions are composed of proliferating basal-type atypical cells with a high nuclear:cytoplasmic ratio and have been designated *moderate dysplasia, severe dysplasia, carcinoma in situ*, or *CIN 2 or 3*. In contrast to low-grade intraepithelial lesions, which are very heterogeneous with regard to associated HPV types, high-grade intraepithelial lesions are usually associated with a limited number of high oncogenic risk HPV types including HPV 16, 18, 31, 45, and 56.[17,86,137,169,174] There is a common misconception that low-grade lesions are "viral" whereas high-grade lesions are not. The prevalence of HPV in both low- and high-grade lesions is similar, approximately 90%. In low-grade lesions large numbers of viral particles are produced, whereas in high-grade lesions viral DNA is present but infectious viral particles are produced in comparatively lower amounts.

Because of our increased understanding of the pathogenesis of cervical cancer precursors, it has been suggested that the terminology used to refer to these lesions be changed to better reflect the biologic processes that underlie the histologic patterns. The most widely accepted modification is the terminology that has been incorporated into the Bethesda System of cytologic diagnosis. This terminology uses the term *"low-grade squamous intraepithelial lesion"* (LSIL) for lesions previously classified as koilocytotic atypia and CIN 1 and *"high-grade squamous intraepithelial lesion"* (HSIL) for lesions previously called CIN 2 and CIN 3.[172,202] For histopathologic reporting, it has been suggested that the terms low-grade squamous intraepithelial lesion (LSIL) and high-grade squamous intraepithelial lesion (HSIL) also be used.[308] In this chapter, we have adopted the use of the Bethesda Terminology for reporting histopathology, as well as cytopathology. The rationale for adapting the two-tiered terminology for histopathology is the same as for using a two-tiered terminology for cytology. First, low-grade SIL (previously referred to as CIN 1) represent a biologically distinct group compared to high-grade SIL (previously referred to as CIN 2 and CIN 3). Low-grade SIL are heterogeneous with respect to associated HPV types, clonality, ploidy, and loss of heterozygosity at specific chromosomal loci, whereas high-grade SIL are heterogeneous with respect to these parameters. Moreover, the natural history of low-grade SIL is characterized by higher rates of spontaneous regression and lower rates of progression than compared to high-grade SIL.

In our opinion, using the term lesion rather than neoplasia better reflects the natural history of these histopathologic entities, because the majority of what were previously considered to be cervical cancer precursors are histologically low grade and represent

Table 7.1. Terminologies for cervical cancer precursor lesions

WHO/ISGYP classification*	*Bethesda System terminology*
Mild dysplasia (CIN 1)	Low-grade squamous intraepithelial lesion (Low-grade SIL)
Moderate dysplasia (CIN 2)	High-grade squamous intraepithelial lesion (High-grade SIL)
Severe dysplasia/Carcinoma in situ (CIN 3)	

*World Health Organization and International Society of Gynecological Pathologists.

self-limited HPV infections that spontaneously resolve in the absence of therapy. "Intraepithelial lesion" better describes these low-grade viral infections than does the term "intraepithelial neoplasia." Proponents of the CIN terminology contend that the use of the term lesion is imprecise when referring to what they consider to be high-grade neoplasia, which is frequently aneuploid and has the potential for progressing to invasive cancer.[233] Use of the term intraepithelial lesions to describe the low-grade abnormalities and intraepithelial neoplasia when referring to the high-grade precursors would be more precise, but would lead to confusion among clinicians accustomed to considering cervical cancer precursors as a histologic and cytologic continuum. The advantages of the two-tiered SIL terminology are that it reflects the biology of the lesions as we currently understand it, it can be used for both cytologic and histologic diagnosis, and it reflects current clinical management, because many clinicians now follow selected patients with low-grade SIL but treat patients with high-grade SIL. The use of a uniform terminology for both cytologic and histologic diagnoses should minimize the misunderstanding that inevitably occurs when different terminologies are used for cytologic and histologic diagnosis. Correlations between this system and the previous terminologies are shown in Table 7.1. It should be noted that because older studies utilized either the dysplasia/carcinoma in situ or the CIN terminology, in many places in this chapter we have used the older terminology.

General Features

Prevalence

SIL is predominantly a disease of women in their reproductive years, with a large population impact and risk factors characteristic of a sexually transmitted disease (STD). The prevalence of SIL in different countries and populations within a country varies widely depending on the underlying risk factors in the population and the extent of cytologic screening. Although SIL is not a reportable disease, good estimates of the prevalence of SIL in women undergoing screening in the United States are available from a number of sources. One of the most comprehensive surveys is the College of American Pathologists "Q-Probes" study, which compiles rates of cytologic abnormalities diagnosis from more than 300 U.S. cytology laboratories.[133] According to this survey, in 1997, 1.97% of all Papanicolaou tests were reported as LSIL and 0.5% as HSIL. In 1993, a similar survey reported rates of 1.83% and 0.45% for a cytologic diagnosis of LSIL and HSIL, respectively.[132]

Another large national program that compiles statistics of cytologic abnormalities among women in the United States is the National Breast and Cervical Cancer Early Detection Program (NBCCEDP). This program is designed to increase access to cancer screening for low-income and uninsured women. The overall rates of cytologic abnormalities in this program is 2.9% for LSIL and 0.8% for HSIL, reflecting the high-risk nature of the women being screened.[167] The prevalence of cytologically detected SIL among women enrolled in the NBCCEDP decreases with increasing age (Fig. 7.1), as do the rates of biopsy-confirmed low-grade SIL and high-grade SIL (Fig. 7.2). In contrast, the rate of biopsy-confirmed invasive cervical cancer increases until 64 years of age. Similar age-related decreases in the prevalence of cytologic abnormalities have been reported among attendees of Planned Parenthood clinics in the United States.[245] Among women attending Planned Parenthood clinics, the prevalence of cytologically diagnosed CIN 1 and 2 peaked at 2.6% in women 25–29% years of age and decreased to 0.9% in women over the age of 50 years. The peak prevalence of CIN 3 was 0.5%, which occurred in Papanicolaou tests from women 35–39 years old. Among women undergoing screening at Kaiser Permanente in Northern California, the rate of biopsy high-grade SIL has been reported to be 0.92% in women under the age of 40 years and 0.21% in women over the age of 40 years.[143] Only 5% of all cases of high-grade SIL were found in women under the age of 20 years. Approximately 40% of all cases were detected among women 20–29 years of age and 40% in women 30–39 years of age.

Estimates of the prevalence of CIN 3 in the

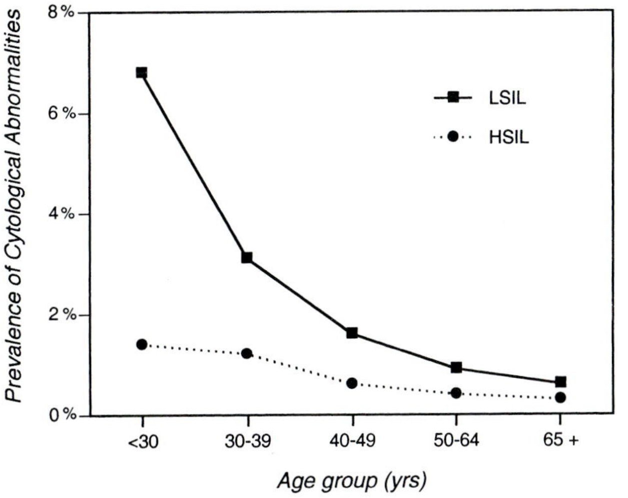

Fig. 7.1. Impact of age on rates of cytological abnormalities. Data from the National Breast and Cervical Cancer Early Detection Program demonstrates a reduction in the prevalence of cytological abnormalities with increasing age. Data from ref. 167.

United States as a whole can be obtained from the Surveillance, Epidemiology, and End Results (SEER) Program, which is a population-based tumor registry that accrues data from several locations in the United States. Although the SEER data set probably underestimates the true prevalence of CIN 3 because not all centers report both severe "dysplasia" and carcinoma in situ, these are the best data available at the national level. According to the

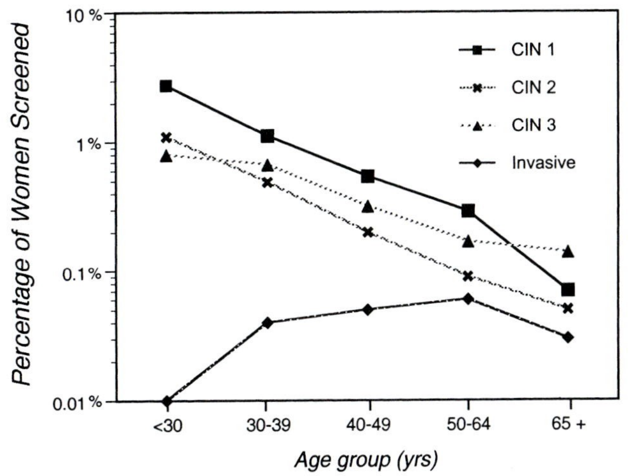

Fig. 7.2. Impact of age on the prevalence of biopsy-confirmed cervical lesions. Data from the National Breast and Cervical Cancer Early Detection Program demonstrates a reduction in the prevalence of both low-grade SIL and high-grade SIL with increasing age. The prevalence of invasive cervical cancer increases until age 64 years. Data from ref. 167.

SEER data set, the average annual age-adjusted incidence rate per 100,000 females for CIN 3 in 1986–1987 was 31.5 for white females and 31.2 for black females.[89]

The clinical scope and epidemiology of SIL has undergone dramatic changes over the past few decades. SIL appears to be becoming increasingly common. A review of Papanicolaou tests over a 10-year period at one medical center from southern Australia found that the prevalence of cytologic evidence of low-grade SIL increased from 0.6% in 1978 to 5.6% in 1988.[77] The mean age at diagnosis of high-grade SIL has decreased, and both the incidence and prevalence of high-grade SIL have increased in teenagers and women under 30.[10,244] In studies from the 1950s, dysplasia was rarely documented in women younger than 25 years of age and the mean age of patients with CIN 3 ranged between 35 and 40.[57,217] Cytologic evidence of high-grade SIL can now be found in women under the age of 15 years, and the age-specific incidence for CIN 3 currently peaks in the 25- to 29-year-old group and decreases with advancing age thereafter.[248] The prevalence of SIL of all grades in teenagers and young adults of age 15–19 years has been reported to be as high as is 18.8 per 1000.[244] Similarly, studies of Jewish Israeli women have indicated a substantial increase in the incidence of SIL and invasive cervical cancer in that population, historically at low risk for the development of cervical malignancy. The incidence of cervical cancer in all ages of Israeli-born Jewish women rose from 2.7/100,000 in 1960–1966 to 4.6/100,000 in 1972–1976.[275] These epidemiologic changes have been attributed to changes in sexual behavior patterns and corroborate previous epidemiologic data suggesting a direct causal relationship between sexual activity and the pathogenesis of cervical neoplasia.

Etiology

Epidemiologic studies have identified a number of possible risk factors for the development of both cervical cancer and its precursor lesions that include early age at first intercourse, age at first pregnancy, number of sexual partners, a history of cigarette smoking, oral contraceptive use, socioeconomic class, interval since the last Pap test, a history of abnormal Pap tests, parity, nutritional variables, immunosuppression, and infection with a variety of sexually transmitted infections including *Chlamydia trachomatis*, herpes simplex virus type 2, or specific types of human papillomavirus (i.e., types 16 and 18) (Table 7.2).[250,314] Although the risk factors for cervical cancer and its precursors are similar, the strength of association between these risk factors and cervical

Table 7.2. Risk factors associated with SIL in various epidemiological studies

Sexual activity
number of sexual partners
early sexual activity (especially less than 16 years of age)
Sexually transmitted diseases
human papillomavirus
herpes simplex virus
Chlamydia trachomatis
Early age of first pregnancy
Parity
Low socioeconomic class
Cigarette smoking
Human immunodeficiency virus
Immunosuppression from any cause
Vitamin deficiencies
Interval since last Pap smear
Oral contraceptive use

SIL: squamous intraepithelial lesion.

cancer is generally stronger than the strength of association between the risk factors and SIL. The major independent risk factors in recent case-control studies of cervical cancer precursors have been HPV infection, lifetime number of sexual partners, and a history of cigarette smoking.[214,247] Some studies, but not others, have identified early sexual activity during the period of active development of the cervical transformation zone to be an important risk factor.[214] There are also a large number of covariables that are believed to be secondarily related to the incidence of cervical carcinoma because they are a common feature of the population that has early, multiple sexual contacts.

The concept that cervical cancer (and presumably its precursors) is a sexually transmitted disease is further substantiated by the epidemiologic characterization of the high-risk male. These studies document the relevance of the male partner's sexual history in determining a woman's risk for the development of cervical carcinoma and support the concept that a transmissible agent is responsible, in part, for the pathogenesis of cervical cancer.[27] A comparison of the ratio of sexual partners of males with the incidence of invasive cervical cancer in different countries indicates a statistically significant association (Fig. 7.3). A variety of sexually transmitted pathogens including *Chlamydia trachomatis, Neisseria gonorrhoeae, Gardnerella vaginalis, Mycoplasma hominis, Trichomonas vaginalis*, and cytomegalovirus have been proposed over the years as being the etiologic agent for cervical cancer. Recently, a case-control study from Finland tested banked serum from women who subsequently developed cervical cancer and found a strong association between antibodies for *Chlamydia* and cervical cancer.[8] However, other studies, including a number of case-control studies, of the prevalence of these pathogens in women with cervical cancer precursors have not found a relationship between other sexually transmitted pathogens and cervical cancer when controlled for sexual activity. Therefore, it is generally thought that the association between sexually transmitted pathogens other than that of HPV and cervical cancer and its precursors reflects the sexual history of the population at risk rather than an etiologic role of the agents themselves.[156,314]

Human Papillomaviruses

In the late 1970s, based on theoretical considerations, zur Hausen suggested that there might be an

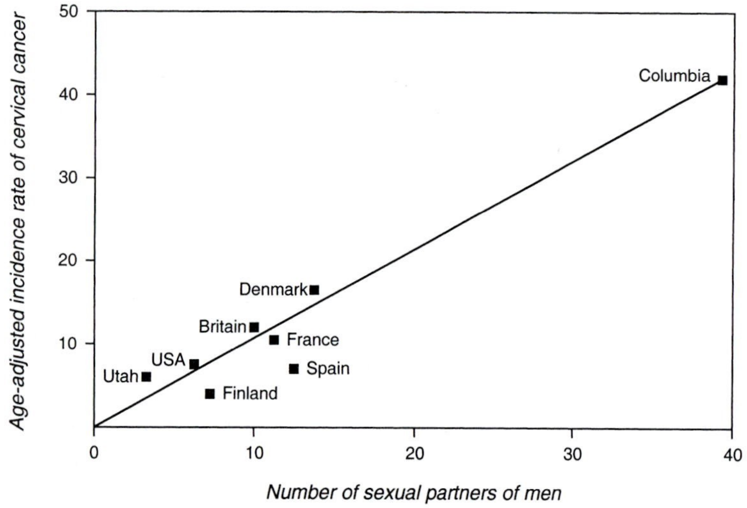

Fig. 7.3. Relationship between number of sexual partners of men and cervical cancer incidence. There is a strong correlation between the average number of sexual partners that men living in a country have and the incidence of invasive cervical cancer in that country. (Modified from ref. 27, with permission.)

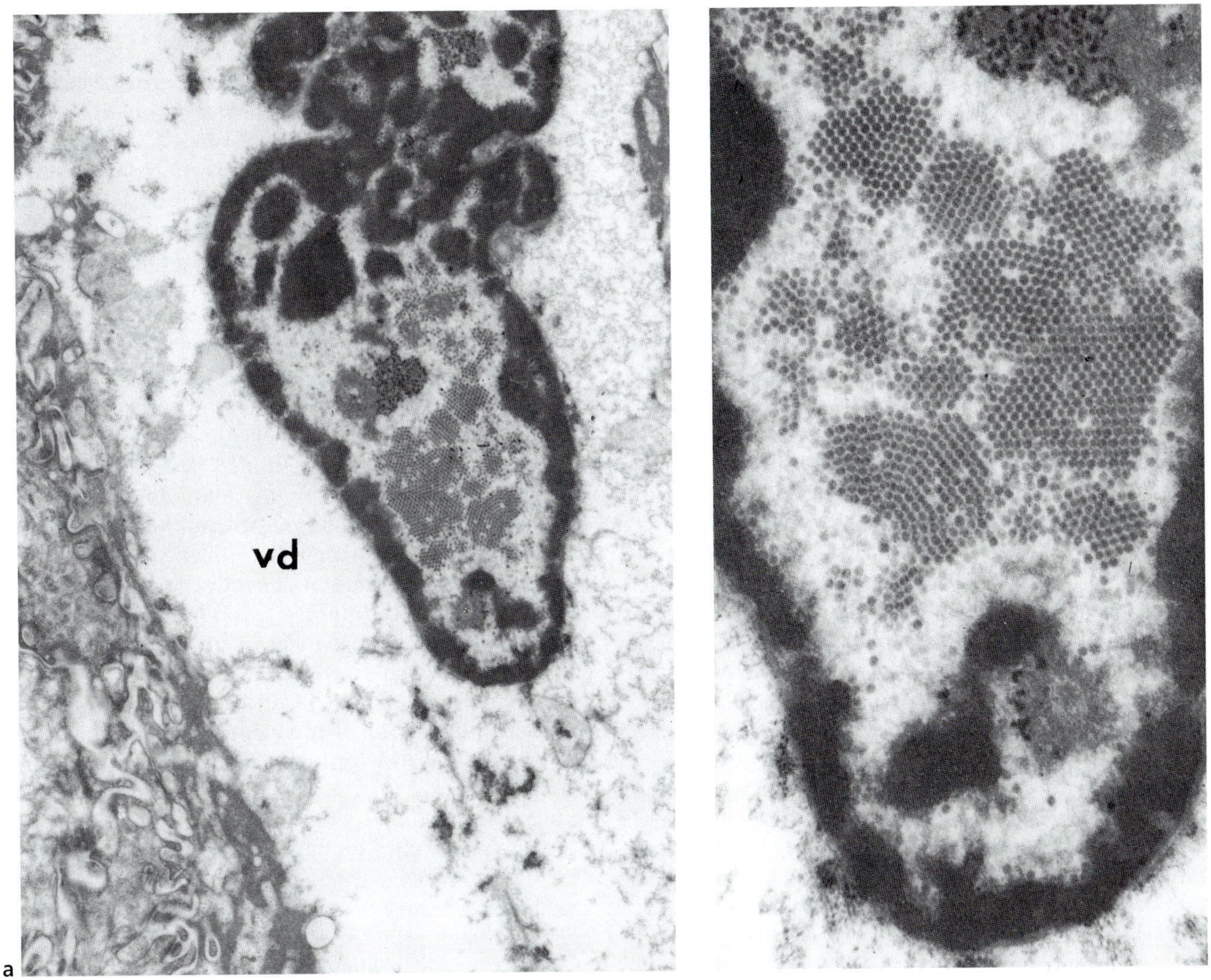

Fig. 7.4. HPV-infected cells. Electron microscopy of cells productively infected with HPV. **a**: There are intranuclear aggregates of HPV in a koilocytotic, superficial cell of a low-grade SIL. The marginated nuclear chromatin is agglutinated, and the cytoplasmic substance displays vacuolar degeneration (vd). The latter corresponds to koilocytotic ballooning on light microscopy. **b**: Higher magnification of HPV particles in the nucleus.

association between HPV and cervical cancer.[317] A large number of epidemiologic, clinicopathologic, and molecular studies have subsequently linked the presence of specific types of HPV to the development of anogenital cancers and their precursors, and it is now accepted that HPVs play a critical role in the pathogenesis of most cervical cancers and their precursor lesions.[123,197]

Koss and Durfee coined the term *koilocytotic atypia* in 1956 to describe abnormal squamous epithelial cells that were characterized by prominent perinuclear vacuolization (*koilocytes*) and were detected in Pap tests of patients with dysplasia and invasive carcinoma.[151] In 1976 both Meisels and coworkers, as well as Purola and Savia, published papers suggesting that the cells in condyloma acuminata that contained viral particles compatible with HPV by electron microscopy were cytologically identical to the "koilocytes" that had been described by Koss and Durfee.[183,225] Soon after this, several groups detected viral particles using electron microscopy or HPV capsid proteins using immunohistochemistry in low-grade SIL (Fig. 7.4).[166] With the application of molecular techniques to the study of cervical disease, rapid progress was made in understanding the relationships between HPV and cervical cancer. zur Hausen and coworkers were the first to isolate new types of HPV from anogenital lesions and to demonstrate that specific types of HPV DNA could be identified by Southern blot hybridization in the majority of invasive squamous cell carcinomas of the cervix and a substantial number of cervical cancer precursors.[73] Shortly thereafter, HPV DNA was isolated in tissues from metastatic cervical carcinoma[164] and in tumor cell lines established from cervical carcinoma, indicating that the HPV was an integral component of the tumors.[30] Since these initial studies, similar findings have been reported from numerous laboratories throughout the world.

Classification of HPV and Association with Specific Types of Anogenital Lesions

Papillomaviruses are classified as members of the A genus of the family Papovaviridae, which includes simian virus 40 (SV 40) and polyoma virus as well as the papillomaviruses. All members of Papovaviridae are double-standard DNA tumor viruses that are dissimilar in size, lack shared antigens, and have only limited DNA sequence homologies. However, as more is learned about their biologic properties, it is becoming apparent that the actions of the different members of Papovaviridae on their target cells are similar. The characteristic features of human papillomaviruses that set them apart from other members of Papovaviridae are a double-stranded DNA genome of approximately 8000 base pairs in length, a nonenveloped virion that measures 45–55 nm in diameter, and an icosahedral capsid composed of 72 capsomers. Papillomaviruses are widely distributed throughout nature. There are bovine, canine, avian, rabbit, deer, and human papillomaviruses. They are all highly species-specific viruses that infect only one species. Within a given species, many types and subtypes of papillomaviruses may exist. Unlike many other viruses in which specific viral isolates have capsid proteins with different antigenic structures, the capsid proteins of papillomavirus are highly conserved, and antibodies directed against BPV capsid proteins cross-react with human papillomaviruses.[129] Therefore, specific types of HPV cannot be identified serologically (serotypes), and DNA sequence is used to classify different viral types (genotypes).

Originally, DNA hybridization under stringent conditions was used to define new HPV types.[52] More recently, DNA sequence analysis has been used to classify the papillomaviruses. To be considered a distinct type, the L1, E6, and E7 gene sequences (approximately one-third of the genome) must differ by more than 10% from those of other, known HPV types.[288] In humans, 85 types of papillomaviruses have been characterized and fully sequenced and more than 120 putative novel types have been partially characterized.[318] Approximately 40 types of HPV can infect the epithelium of the anogenital tract. Although the different types of HPV are quite similar structurally, they have significant specificity with regard to the anatomic location of the epithelia that they infect and the type of lesions that they produce at the site of infection.[69] In addition to types, there also are subtypes or variants of specific types, such as HPV-16. To be considered a subtype or variant, a virus must differ by 2–5% from the original isolate. Different subtypes of HPV-16 have been shown to have different biologic potential, and in some, but not other, studies specific variants appear to more likely to be associated with invasive cervical cancers than others.[23,206]

Papillomaviruses are epitheliotrophic viruses that predominantly infect skin and mucous membranes and produce characteristic epithelial proliferations at the sites of infection.[121] These benign epithelial proliferations or papillomas have the capacity to undergo malignant transformation under certain circumstances. Examples of this in animals include the papillomas induced in domestic rabbits by the cottontailed rabbit papillomavirus (CRPV), which can progress to invasive squamous cell carcinomas when treated with topical applications of methylcholantrene, and alimentary tract papillomas induced in cattle by bovine papillomavirus (BPV), which undergo malignant transformation when the animals eat radiomimetic bracken ferns.[121] In humans, HPV infections occur on the skin and mucous membranes, on the conjunctiva, oral cavity, larynx, tracheobronchial tree, esophagus, bladder, anus, and genital tract of both sexes. HPVs appear to be fastidious in their growth requirements and replicate only in the nucleus of infected cells. Therefore, only limited success has been achieved in obtaining viral replication in model systems.

In addition to being species specific, papillomaviruses are also relatively tissue- and site specific. For example, HPV-1 preferentially infects the stratified squamous epithelium of the sole of the foot and produces plantar warts (verruca plantaris), whereas HPV-2 and HPV-4 preferentially infect the stratified epithelium of the fingers to produce common warts termed verruca vulgaris. Other types, such as 6 and 11, almost exclusively infect the stratified epithelium of mucosal surfaces of the oral and anogenital tract, producing laryngeal papillomatosis and condyloma acuminata, respectively.

The more than 100 types of HPV that have been isolated can be divided into three general groups (Table 7.3). A mucocutaneous group contains types that infect the skin and the oral epithelium. Another group includes viruses isolated from patients with epidermodysplasia verruciformis, a rare genetic disorder of cellular immunity in which patients fre-

Table 7.3. Classification of human papillomaviruses

HPV type	*Lesion*
Mucocutaneous Group	
1	Verruca plantaris
2	Verruca vulgaris verruca plantaris
3	Verruca plana
4	Verruca vulgaris verruca plantaris
7	Butcher's warts
13	Focal epithelial hyperplasia (oral)
26, 27	Verruca vulgaris immunosuppressed
28	Verruca plana
29	Verruca vulgaris
32	Focal epithelial hyperplasia (oral)
36	Actinic keratosis
37	Keratoacanthoma
38	Verruca vulgaris
41	Squamous carcinoma
Epidermodysplasia Verruciformis	
5, 15, 47; 8, 17; 9, 19; 12, 36; 14, 36	Macular warts
Genital Lesions	
6, 11	Condyloma acuminatum low-grade SIL
16	All grades of SIL squamous cell carcinoma
18	All grades of SIL adeno- and squamous carcinoma
31, 33, 34, 35	All grades of SIL squamous cell carcinoma
39	All grades of SIL rarely in squamous cell carcinoma
40	All grades of SIL
42	Flat penile lesions low-grade SIL
43, 44	Low-grade SIL occasionally high-grade SIL
45	All grades of SIL squamous cell carcinoma
51, 52	All grades of SIL
53, 54	All grades of SIL
56, 58, 59, 61, 66, 68	All grades of SIL squamous cell carcinoma
70	All grades of SIL
72	All grades of SIL squamous cell carcinoma

Modified from refs. 47, 69, 121, 169, 239.

quently develop HPV-associated skin lesions that can progress to invasive squamous cell carcinomas when exposed to the sun. The third group of more than 40 types of HPV infects the anogenital tract. These target cell associations are not absolute, however, and some cutaneous HPVs such as type 2 can also infect mucosal epithelium, and HPV-16, which is considered to be a genital-type HPV, has been found in association with squamous cell carcinomas of the conjunctiva and subungual region.[181,196] The specific associations of 23 of the most commonly encountered anogenital HPV types are shown in Table 7.3.

Based on their associations with specific types of lesions, the most prevalent anogenital HPVs have been divided into three "oncogenic risk" groups (Table 7.4). The low oncogenic risk group includes HPVs 6 and 11. These viruses are considered to be of low oncogenic risk because they are usually associated with condyloma acuminata of the anogenital tract and occasionally associated with low-grade SIL, but only rarely associated with high-grade SIL and almost never associated with invasive squamous cell carcinomas of the cervix. HPV types 42, 43, and 44 are included in the low oncogenic risk viruses because they have the same distribution as HPVs 6 and 11. The high oncogenic risk HPVs are types 16, 18, 45, 56, and 58; these are considered high oncogenic risk viruses because they are the type most frequently associated with invasive squamous cell carcinomas of the anogenital tract.[47,112,204] In addition, there are a number of other HPV types that also have many features of high oncogenic risk viruses because they can be found in association with invasive cervical cancers, although less frequently than the typical high oncogenic risk viruses. These viruses include types 31, 33, 35, 39, 51, 52, 59, and 68 and have been sometimes referred to as "intermediate" oncogenic risk viruses. However, recent studies indicate that anogenital infection with these viruses confer similar relative risks for high-grade SIL or cancer as does infection with the prototypical high oncogenic risk viruses, so we consider types 31, 33, 35, 39, 51, 52, 59, and 68 to also be high oncogenic risk viruses.

When this grouping was originally proposed, it was anticipated that histology would predict HPV type

Table 7.4. Oncogenic-risk grouping of anogenital human papillomavirus

Low oncogenic risk:	6, 11, 42, 43, 44, 53
High oncogenic risk:	16, 18, 45, 56, 58
Other high risk types:	31, 33, 35, 39, 51, 52, 59, 68

Table 7.5. HPV associated with low-grade SIL

	No. (%) HPV-DNA + lesions associated with specific HPV types					
Reference	*6/11*	*16*	*18*	*30s*	*Other*[a]	*Multiple*[b]
Bergeron et al.	0	11 (21)	2 (4)	10 (19)	28 (53)	5 (9)
Genest et al.	6 (17)	2 (3)	3 (9)	3 (9)	19 (54)	2 (5)
Kadish et al.	5 (11)	3 (6)	5 (11)	5 (11)	32 (68)	ND
Kalantari et al.	20 (20)	25 (25)	17 (17)	17 (17)	22 (22)	19 (19)
Lungu et al.	15 (15)	16 (16)	3 (3)	18 (18)	26 (26)	22 (22)
Willett et al.	7 (27)	8 (31)	1 (4)	3 (12)	7 (25)	ND
Mean percentage	(21)	(14)	(5)	(13)	(40)	(14)

ND, not determined
[a]Includes both other known HPV types and "novel" or unknown HPV types.
[b]Multiple HPV types represent lesions containing more than a single type of HPV.
Modified from refs. 17, 95, 136, 137, 174, 301.

and that low-grade SIL lesions of the cervix would usually be associated with low oncogenic risk HPVs.[61,170] However, it is now known that low-grade SIL lesions are extremely heterogeneous with regard to their associated HPV types. A study of Lungu et al. that used PCR to detect and type HPV DNA in 278 cervical biopsies from SIL lesions of all grades found that 22% of low-grade SIL were associated with multiple HPV types (Table 7.5).[174] Only 15% of low-grade SIL were associated with low oncogenic risk HPVs (6, 11, 42, 43, and 44), 19% were associated with unknown or "novel" HPV types, and 29% with HPV 16, 18, and 33. Very similar results have been reported by others. For example, Bergeron et al. used high-stringency Southern blots with a large number of type-specific probes to type 188 cervical biopsies (Table 7.5); low oncogenic risk HPV types were very infrequently associated with low-grade SIL. HPV 16 and 18 were detected in 25% of the low-grade SIL, novel HPV types in 25%, and multiple types in 9%. In the recent National Cancer Institute ASCUS LSIL Triage Study (ALTS) clinical trial, it was found that 83% of women presenting with a LSIL Pap test had a high oncogenic risk HPV type detected using the Hybrid "capture" II HPV DNA assay, which detects HPV types 16, 18, 31, 33, 35, 39, 45, 51, 52, 56, 58, 59, and 66. These studies clearly indicate that low-grade SIL can be associated with either low-risk or high-risk types of HPV.

In contrast, there is a much closer correlation between histology and associated HPV type in high-grade SIL (Table 7.6). In the polymerase chain reaction (PCR) study of Lungu et al., only 7% of high-grade SIL contained more than one HPV type and 88% were associated with HPV types 16, 18, or 33.[174] Similar results were reported by Willet et al. and by Franquemont et al., who used in situ hybridization to type HPV and detected HPV-16 in more than 70% of high-grade SIL.[86,301] Bergeron et al. detected HPV 16 and 18 in 61% of high-grade SIL using high-stringency Southern blot hybridization.[17]

Table 7.6. HPV types associated with high-grade SIL

	No. (%) HPV-DNA + lesions associated with specific HPV types					
Reference	*6/11*	*16*	*18*	*30s*	*Others*[a]	*Multiple*[b]
Bergeron et al.	0	30 (57)	2 (4)	4 (8)	15 (29)	2 (4)
Franquemont et al.	0	20 (77)	0	0	0	0
Genest et al.	2 (5)	15 (38)	1 (3)	10 (25)	10 (25)	2 (5)
Kadish et al.	3 (2)	38 (30)	8 (6)	19 (15)	53 (42)	ND
Kalantari et al.	7 (5)	58 (43)	12 (9)	30 (22)	21 (21)	28 (21)
Lungu et al.	1 (1)	127 (72)	6 (3)	19 (11)	9 (5)	13 (7)
Willett et al.	3 (27)	20 (71)	0	0	1 (4)	ND
Mean percentage	(2)	(58)	(4)	(12)	(2)	(4)

ND, not determined.
[a]Includes both other known HPV types and "novel" or unknown HPV types.
[b]Multiple HPV types represent lesions containing more than a single type of HPV.
Modified from refs. 17, 86, 95, 136, 137, 174, 301.

The only HPV assay that is commercially available in the United States (Hybrid Capture II) combines the 13 most common intermediate and high-risk viruses together into a single "high risk" probe mixture; these are HPV types 16, 18, 31, 33, 35, 39, 45, 51, 52, 56, 58, 59, and 68. Therefore the commercially available assay cannot distinguish lesions associated with the prototypical high-risk types of HPV (e.g., 16, 18, 45, 56, and 58) from these associated with other high-risk viruses.

Genomic Organization of HPV

The genomic organization of the different types of HPV appears to be similar (Fig. 7.5). The viral genome can be divided into three regions: the upstream regulatory region (also referred to as the long central region or LCR), the early region, and the late region. The upstream regulatory region (URR) is a noncoding region of the viral genome that is important in regulating viral replication and transcription of downstream sequences in the early region. Both the early region and the late region contain a series of open reading frames (ORFs), which are regions of the genome lacking stop codons and, therefore, are potentially translated into proteins. The early region is transcribed early in the viral life cycle (hence its name) and encodes predominately for proteins that are important in viral replication, whereas the late region encodes for viral structural proteins that are produced late in the viral life cycle.

The URR is a highly complex regulatory region of approximately 400 base pairs that contains a complex array of overlapping binding sites for a number of different transcriptional activators and repressors[285]; these include activator protein 1 (AP-1), a nuclear factor (NF-I/CTF), Oct 1, Sp1, and YY1, as well as virally derived transcriptional factors and keratinocyte-specific factors such KRF-1.[14,285,315,316] Binding of these and other transcriptional factors regulates transcription of the early region open reading frames (ORFs) and maintains differentiation-dependent transcription programs. This region may also play a central role in determining the host range of specific types of HPV.

The early-region ORFs encode for proteins required for viral replication and maintenance of a high viral copy number in infected cells.[121] The early region also includes the transforming regions of the HPV genome. Six different ORFs, which are designated E1, E2, E4, E5, E6, and E7, have been identified in the early region of HPV. The E1 ORF encodes for two distinct proteins that play a role in the extrachromosomal replication of the virus. The E1 protein of HPV has been shown to have ATPase

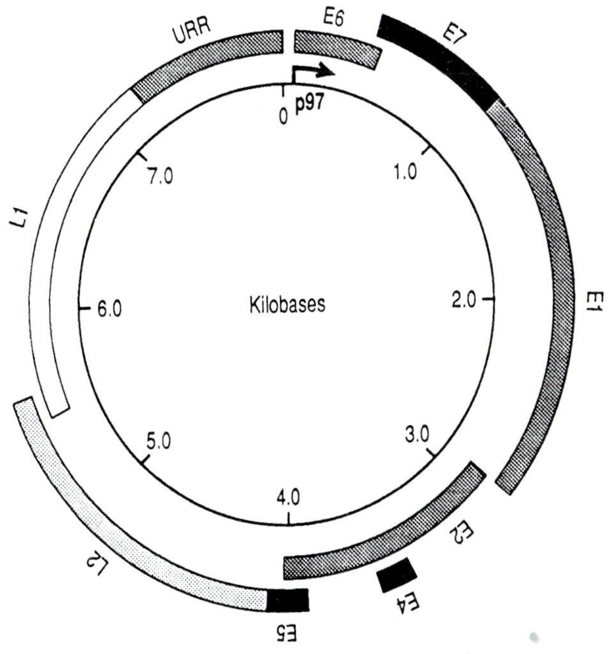

Fig. 7.5. HPV genome. HPV is a double-stranded, circular, DNA tumor virus whose genome can be divided into three regions; the upstream regulatory region (URR), the early region, and the late region.

activity.[175] The E2 ORF encodes for two proteins that are DNA-binding proteins that regulate transcription.[296] One of the E2 proteins has important transcriptional regulatory activities. This E2 protein promotes the assembly of enzymatically active E1 complexes at the HPV origin or origin of replication (ori). The complexes between E1, E2, and ori are required for initiation of viral DNA replication.[179] The E2 proteins are also important for regulating the expression of the early-region ORFs.[19] Two of the key proteins that are regulated by E2 are E6 and E7; the E6 and E7 ORFs encode for the major transforming genes of HPV (see following). Expression of E2 represses the E6/E7 promotor, resulting in reduction of E6 and E7 within the cells. Overexpression of E2 in cells also results in apoptosis.[85,298]

The E5 ORF of HPV encodes a protein with weak transforming activity. The E4 ORF encodes for a series of proteins that appear to be important for maturation of the virus and viral replication. The function of the E4 protein is not fully understood. E4 has many characteristics of a structural protein, and E4 is similar to the protein products of the late region. Like the L1 and L2 late-region capsid proteins, E4 is expressed late during the viral life cycle, at a time when viral production is occurring. The function of E4 may be to disrupt the cornified cell envelope, allowing viral particles to be released from the cells.[37] HPV E4 can also associate with the keratinocyte intermediate filament network and can cause disruption of the network in some cases.[237]

The late region of HPV is downstream of the early region and contains two ORFs, termed L1 and L2, which encode capsid proteins. The L1-encoded protein is the major capsid protein and is highly conserved among papillomaviruses from all species. The L2-encoded protein is a minor capsid protein that is much more variable among viral types. Transcription from the L1 and L2 ORFs occurs as a late event in the viral life cycle at a time when infectious virus is being produced.[82] Transcription from the late region appears to be regulated by cell-derived, transcriptional regulators that are produced only by the differentiated cells of the intermediate and superficial layers of the squamous epithelium. Therefore, large amounts of L1- and L2-encoded capsid proteins can be detected in condyloma acuminata and in low-grade SIL, but these proteins are present in only small amounts in high-grade SIL or cervical cancers. L1 and L2 capsid proteins produced in in vitro culture systems are capable of associating and forming viral-like particles (VLPs) that are similar to native virions but lack the viral genome. VLPs are currently being tested as prophylactic HPV vaccines.[251]

Life Cycle of HPV

Although the HPV life cycle is not completely characterized, the rough outlines of the process are known (Fig. 7.6).[121] The initial site of infection is thought to be either basal cells or primitive "basal-like" cells of the immature squamous epithelium, which may result from the presence of specific receptors for HPV on the basal cells. One potential receptor that has been localized to the basal cells of stratified squamous epithelium are integrin complexes containing $alpha_6$ integrin complexed with either beta 1 or beta 2 integrins.[76] Once HPV enters into the basal cells, it can exist within the cells in two distinct biologic states. One is as a nonproductive infection in which HPV DNA continues to reside in the basal cells but infectious virions are not produced. In the literature, nonproductive HPV infections have frequently been referred to as *latent infections*. In nonproductive latent infections, a small number of copies of the HPV genome usually remain in the nucleus in a free circular form called an *episome*. Replication of the episomal DNA in latent infections is tightly coupled to

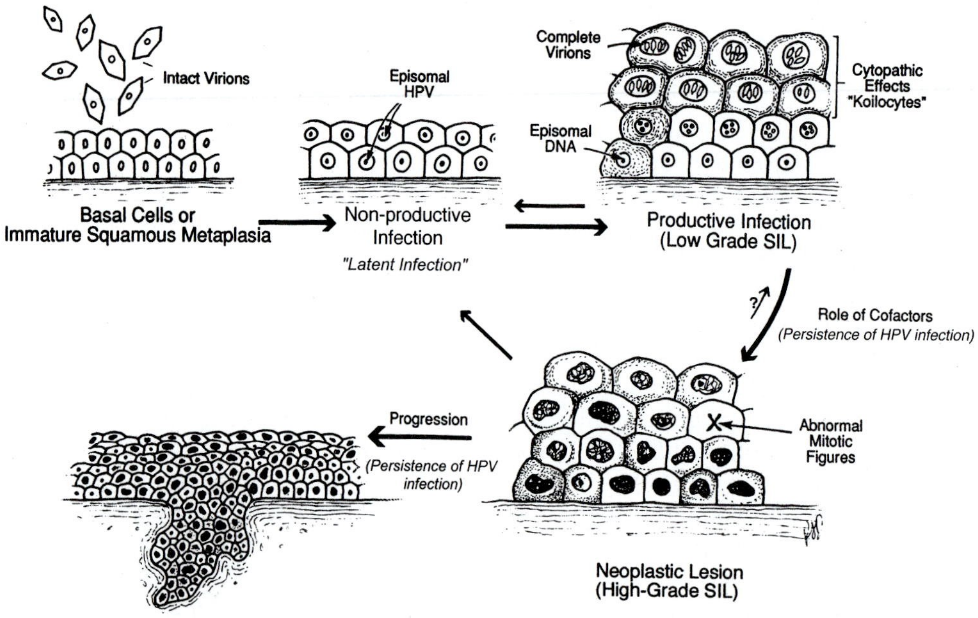

Fig. 7.6. Lifecycle of HPV. The first step in an HPV infection is contact of intact virions with basal cells or immature squamous metaplastic cells. This can produce either a nonproductive infection or a productive infection. In a nonproductive infection HPV DNA remains as an episomal form in the nucleus of the infected basal cell. In productive infections, viral replication becomes uncoupled from cellular DNA synthesis and large amounts of viral DNA and proteins are made in the intermediate and superficial cell layers of the epithelium, producing the characteristic cytopathic effects of HPV. During the development of high-grade SIL and invasive squamous cancers, additional cellular and viral events take place resulting in the formation of a "true" cancer precursor. These can include the generation of aneuploid stemlines and integration of HPV DNA into the chromosomal DNA.

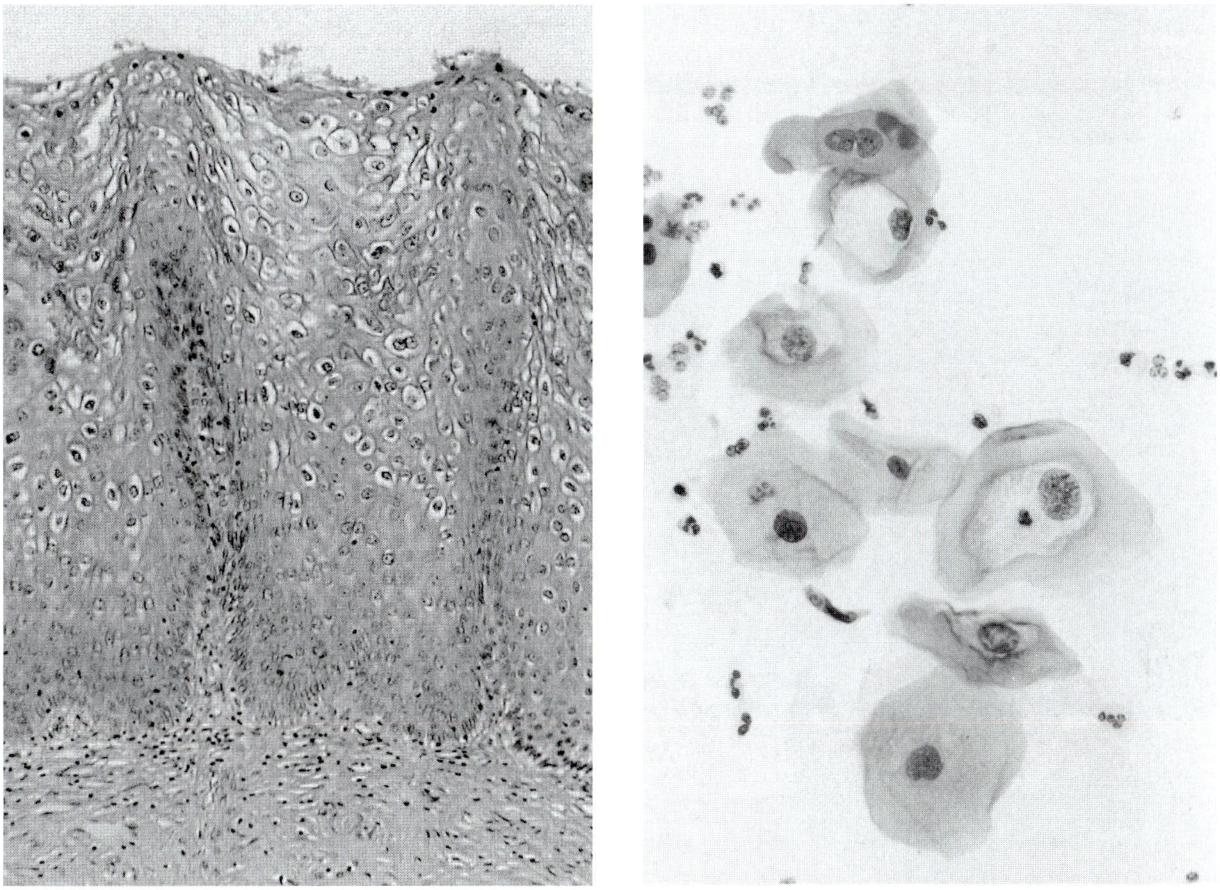

a b

Fig. 7.7. Cytopathic effects of HPV. The cytopathic effects of HPV include nuclear enlargement, nuclear pyknosis or hyperchromaticity, anisocytosis, multinucleation, and perinuclear cytoplasmic vacuolization. **a**: Histological features on cervical biopsy. This lesion is classified as a low-grade SIL. **b**: Cytological features on Papanicolaou smear.

the replication of the epithelial cells and only occurs in concert with replication of the host cell chromosomal DNA. Because complete viral particles are presumably not produced in latent infections, the characteristic cytopathic effects of a HPV infection are not present and HPV can only be identified using molecular methods. Latently infected epithelium displays no morphologic abnormality. The use of the term latent to characterize HPV infections in which there is no gross or microscopic evidence of a HPV-induced epithelial lesion, but in which HPV DNA is detected utilizing molecular tests, is often confusing to clinicians accustomed to using the term latent for viral infections in which virus cannot be detected with routine detection methods.

The other form of HPV infection is a *productive viral infection*. In productive viral infections, viral DNA replication occurs independently of host chromosomal DNA synthesis. This independent viral DNA replication produces large amounts of viral DNA and results in infectious virions. Viral DNA replication takes place predominantly in the intermediate and superficial cell layers of the stratified squamous epithelium. As the virally infected epithelial cells mature and move toward the epithelial surface, cell-derived, differentiation-specific transcriptional factors produced by the epithelium stimulate the production of viral capsid proteins. This process allows large amounts of intact virions to be formed (see Fig. 7.4) and produces the characteristic cytopathic effects of HPV that can be detected cytologically and histologically (Figs. 7.7 and 7.8). These cytopathic effects include acanthosis, cytoplasmic vacuolization, koilocytosis, multinucleation, and nuclear atypia.

Epidemiology of HPV Infections

Epidemiologic studies show that the prevalence of anogenital HPV infections in virgins is extremely low but that large numbers of young women come in contact with anogenital HPVs once they initiate sexual intercourse. In a prospective study of 100 virgins from Denmark, all were found at enrollment to

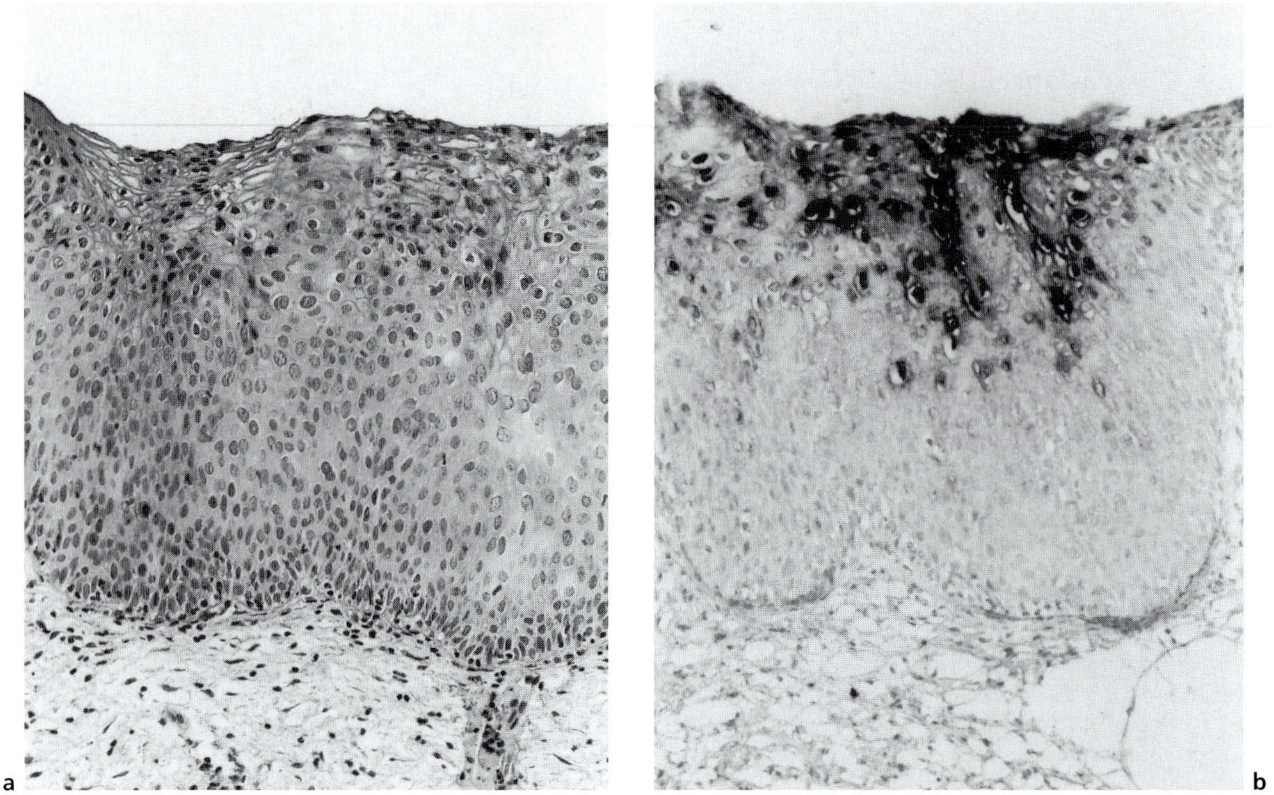

Fig. 7.8. Productive HPV infection. In productive HPV infections large amounts of viral DNA and capsid proteins are produced in the intermediate and superficial cell layers resulting in the characteristic cytopathic effects. **a**: Histological and cytological features of productive HPV infections include acanthosis, cytoplasmic vacuolization, nuclear atypia (koilocytosis), and multinucleation. **b**: In situ hybridization using a probe directed against HPV DNA detects large amounts of viral DNA in the superficial epithelial cells that demonstrate cytopathic effects.

be HPV DNA negative and seronegative for antibodies against HPV 16.[146] In another recent study of college-age women who were followed at regular intervals during a 3-year period using HPV DNA testing and cytology, it was found that 26% of the women were HPV DNA positive at entry into the study.[115] After 3 years of follow-up, HPV DNA was detected in cervicovaginal samples of an additional 43% of the women. Therefore, the cumulative rate of detection of HPV DNA in these young, sexually active college women was 69%. The risk of acquiring an anogenital HPV infection increased with number of lifetime sexual partners and with having a large number of sex partners over a short interval. Other studies have confirmed high rates of anogenital infections in sexually active young women. In a study of college women from the University of California, Bauer et al. reported that 46% of the women had anogenital HPV infections detected using PCR.[13] These prevalence figures may underestimate the number of infected women because shedding of sufficient quantities of HPV DNA to be detected with the currently available molecular methods occurs only transiently in many young women. For example, using PCR Wheeler et al. examined a group of college students from the University of New Mexico weekly over a 10-week period. Only 26% of the women were HPV DNA positive at the first examination, but the cumulative prevalence of HPV DNA positivity was 44% after 10 weeks.[299]

In general, anogenital HPV infections tend to be transient and of relatively short duration in both young and older women. In the study by Ho et al. of college women, the median duration of HPV infections was only 8 months, and by 24 months of follow-up, 91% of HPV-infected women had become HPV DNA negative.[115] The duration of infection was longer for women infected with high-risk types of HPV than for women infected with low-risk types of HPV. Similarly, in a study of young women from San Francisco, Moscicki et al. reported that approximately 70% of young women positive for HPV experienced regression of their infections by 24 months.[194] Women with low-risk HPV type infections were also more likely to show HPV regression than were women with high-risk HPV type infection in this study. In another study of older women from New York City, it was found that persistent HPV infections (defined as the same type of HPV detected twice over a 12-month period) occurred in only 16% of the women who were HPV DNA positive at enrollment. In the New York City study, persistence was more common among women infected with high-risk HPV types compared to low-risk HPV types.[274] Because most HPV-infected women spontaneously resolve their infections, the prevalence of HPV infections decreases with increasing age (Table 7.7).

Therefore, the natural history of HPV infections is that most sexually active young women are exposed to the virus at some point after initiating sexually activity.[13,115,146,194] Most of these women develop transient HPV infections that are of relatively short duration, and eventually most of these HPV-infected women will become HPV DNA negative. Only a small proportion of women exposed to HPV become persistently infected and continue to have detectable levels of HPV DNA in the genital epithelium. It is these persistently infected women who are at risk for having persistent high-grade SIL and of developing invasive cervical cancer.[75,120,294] Although the exact factors that regulate the clearance of an anogenital HPV infection are unknown, immunologic factors and viral type are important. The role of immunologic factors is demonstrated by the finding that persistence of HPV infections is more common in HIV-infected compared to HIV-uninfected women and that rates of persistence in this population increase with increasing levels of immunosuppression.[274] A possible role for humoral immunity in the loss of infection is suggested by the finding that 67% of women enrolled in a prospective follow-up study who developed an incident HPV 16 infection subsequently developed serum antibodies against HPV 16.[42] The median time to seroconversion was 8.3 months, which is similar to the median duration of incident HPV infections in most studies.[42]

Evidence supporting a central role for persistence of infection with high-risk types of HPV in the pathogenesis of high-grade SIL and invasive cervical cancer comes from two types of studies. One is case-control studies of women developing high-grade SIL or invasive cervical cancer in which archived conventional Papanicolaou tests have been tested for the presence of HPV using sensitive PCR-based methods. These case-control studies have shown that women who are persistently infected with high-risk types of HPV are at least 30 times more likely to develop high-grade SIL than women who are high-risk HPV DNA negative. Also, women who are persistently infected with HPV DNA are up to 213 times more likely to develop invasive cervical cancer than are women who are not infected with HPV.[135,294,311] Long-term prospective follow-up studies have also documented a central role for HPV persistence in the pathogenesis of SIL. Hopman et al. followed 68 women who were cytologically negative, but HPV DNA positive, using cytology, colposcopy, and HPV DNA testing for 34 months. During follow-up, 17 (25%) of these women subsequently developed an abnormal Papanicolaou test and 8 (12%) developed biopsy-confirmed high-grade SIL. Of the women developing a cervical abnormality, 94% had a persistent high-risk HPV DNA infection.[120] Similar findings were reported by Ellerbrock et al., who found that 12% of cytologically and colposcopically normal women who had high-risk HPV infections subsequently developed biopsy-confirmed SIL during 36 months of follow-up.[75] Women who were persistently infected with high-risk types of HPV were significantly more likely to develop incident SIL on follow-up than were women who were transiently infected with high-risk types of HPV.

Table 7.7. Prevalence of high-risk HPV DNA by age

Country	*<25 yrs*	*25–34 yrs*	*35–44 yrs*	*45+ yrs*
Netherlands*^	13%	10%	2%	2%
Costa Rica*^	10%	6%	3%	3%
Newfoundland$^{\Psi\pi}$	17%	12%	5%	4%
United Kingdom$^{\Psi\Lambda}$		3%	3%	5%
France$^{\Psi\pi}$	21%	20%	13%	11%

*Only women with negative Papanicolaou tests.
$^{\Psi}$All women (including those with and without abnormal Papanicolaou tests).
$^{\Lambda}$Detected using PCR.
$^{\pi}$High-risk HPV types detected using Hybrid Capture II.
Modified from refs. 51, 66, 112, 126, 226.

Mechanism of Malignant Transformation

Molecular studies using tissue culture cells have provided insight into the mechanism by which HPV *transforms* (i.e., induces the properties of malignancy in) the cervical epithelium. High-risk types of

HPV such as HPV-16 and -18 produce three proteins with growth-stimulating and transforming proteins, E5, E6, and E7. E5 is not essential for transformation as the E5 region is frequently deleted in cervical carcinoma cells.[253] E5 encodes for a small hydrophobic protein usually found in association with cell membranes. The E5 protein has weak transforming activity in vitro and induces both protein kinase C (PKC) -mediated and PKC-independent activation of membrane kinases.[62] The E6 and E7 ORFs represent the principal transforming genes of HPV.[318] Expression of the E6 and E7 ORFs from high oncogenic risk HPVs such as 16 and 18, but not of low oncogenic risk HPVs such as 6 and 11, in established tissue culture cell lines causes the cells to become completely transformed.[318] A high efficiency of transformation of these already immortalized (i.e., have already have acquired an infinite life span in culture) tissue culture cell lines requires that both E6 and E7 be present. The E6 and E7 genes complement each other and are only weakly active when introduced alone. In addition to having in vitro transforming activity, both E6 and E7 are almost always actively transcribed in cervical cancers, suggesting that the over- or unregulated expression of these genes is required for the maintenance of the transformed malignant phenotype. This finding has been confirmed by studies demonstrating that inhibition of E6 and E7 expression by antisense mRNA leads to reversion to a nontransformed phenotype.[59]

HPV E7 Oncoprotein

The E7 protein accounts for the major transforming and immortalizing activity in high-risk types of HPV.[16,220] E7 is a small zinc-binding protein composed of approximately 100 amino acids that is phosphorylated in the native state and lacks enzymatic activity. The amino acid sequences of HPV 16 E7 protein and that of proteins made by other DNA-transforming viruses of the family Papovaviridae show a high degree of similarity between E7 and the conserved domains 1 and 2 of the adenovirus E1A polypeptides as well as the SV40 and polyoma large T antigens and the *myc* oncogene.[74,220] The conserved domains 1 and 2 of adenovirus E1A* gene are important in inducing host cellular DNA synthesis, in repressing viral transcription, and in cooperating with an activated *ras* oncogene for transforming cells. The HPV 16 E7 protein can also cooperate with activated *ras* oncogenes for transformation and can transactivate the adenovirus E2 promoter.[220] Another common feature between the conserved regions of the adenovirus E1A and E7 is that they both contain a casein kinase II-mediated serine phosphorylation consensus sequence and a binding site for the product of the retinoblastoma (*Rb*) gene, as well as the Rb-related pocket proteins p130 and p107.[11,74] These proteins (Rb, p130, and p170) play critical regulation roles in cell proliferation.[52,90]

Although the exact mechanism of action of Rb and the Rb-related pocket proteins within cells has not been fully established, it is clear that the binding of the HPV E7 protein to this class of proteins blocks the cell proliferation–inhibitory function of these endogenous tumor suppressors. Rb helps to regulate cell proliferation by undergoing various degrees of phosphorylation during the cell cycle (Fig. 7.9). During the G_0 and G_1 phases of the cell cycle, Rb exists in a hypophosphorylated form that binds to a cellular transcription factor called E2F-1 which plays a critical role in regulating the temporal expression of other cell cycle regulatory genes such as *c-myc*. Binding of Rb (and presumably the other Rb-related pocket proteins) to E2F-1 disrupts the E2F-1 function and blocks cells from entering into the S-phase of the cell cycle. Initiation of DNA synthesis and transition of the cell from G_1 into S-phase requires removal of this block, which occurs when Rb becomes hyperphosphorylated. Hyperphosphorylated Rb no longer binds to E2F-1, and the resultant high level of unbound E2F-1 stimulates the expression of other cellular regulatory genes and causes cell proliferation. Binding of HPV E7 to Rb and other Rb-related pocket proteins blocks their ability to interact with E2F-1, and unregulated cell proliferation occurs. pRb also inhibits transcription of a cyclin-dependent kinase inhibitor gene *p16* (*INK 4A*) that plays a role in cell cycle proliferation. Blocking pRb function allows overexpression of *p16* (*INK 4A*) within cells. It has recently been suggested that increased expression of *p16* (*INK 4A*) may be a marker for SIL associated with high-risk types of HPV.[148]

Binding of E7 to Rb and Rb-related pocket proteins may be but one of many ways in which E7 proteins can affect cell proliferation and may not be essential for cell transformation.[130] E7 can interact with a variety of other cellular proteins that play important roles in cellular proliferation (Table 7.8). Binding of E7 to cyclin E and cyclin A complexes has been reported and results in activation of kinase activity. Cyclin E is a G_1-phase cyclin that is synthesized late in G_1-phase and is present until cells enter S-phase. Cyclin E forms complexes with cyclin-dependent kinase 2 (CDK2), which phosphorylates Rb, resulting in release of E2F and the subsequent initiation of cellular DNA synthesis. Cyclin A is a S-phase cyclin that forms associations with

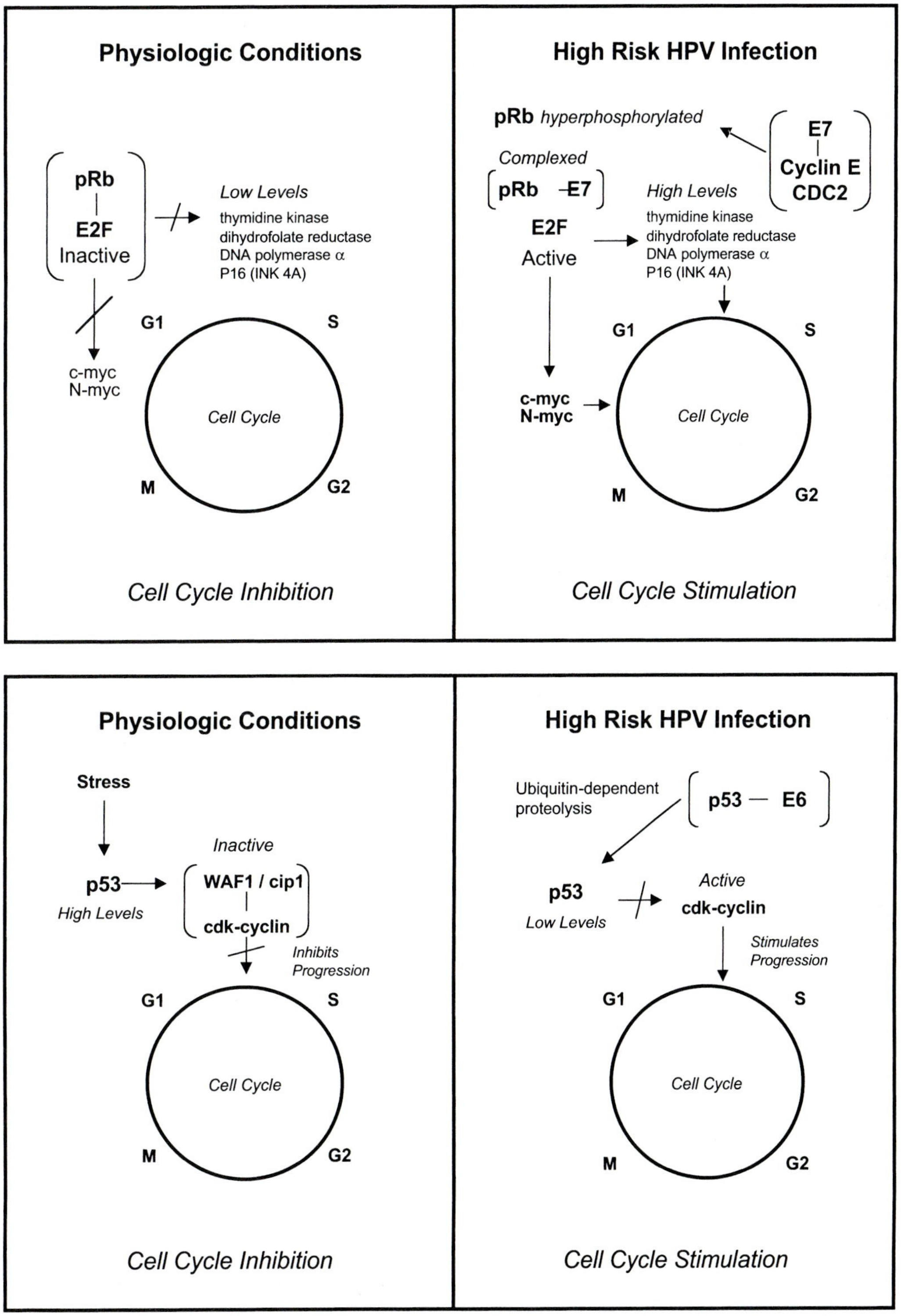

Fig. 7.9. Interactions of HPV E6 and E7 in the cell cycle.

CDK2. Although the mechanism of action of cyclin A during S-phase is unknown, blocking its kinase activity produces a halt in DNA synthesis.[263]

E7 proteins also disrupt the control of cellular proliferation by inactivating the cyclin-dependent kinase inhibitors p21 CIP-1 and p27 KIP-1. Inactivating p21 CIP-1 and p27 KIP-1 uncouples cyclin-dependent kinase activities from their endogenous cell regulators and could lead to unchecked cellular proliferation. E7 also sensitizes p53-reactive cells to

Table 7.8. Host cell cycle proteins that interact with E6 and E7

Interact with E6	*Interact with E7*
p53	Retinoblastoma protein (*Rb*)
E6-associated protein	Retinoblastoma-related pocket proteins
Paxillin	E2F/cyclin A complex
Bak	Cyclin E
ERC55	Histone H1 kinase
c-jun	

Modified from ref. 318.

undergo apoptosis and enhances the mutagenicity of chemical carcinogens.[124,176]

HPV E6 Oncoprotein

HPV E6 has relatively weak independent transforming and immortalizing activity compared to HPV E7. However, the presence of E6 significantly enhances the immortalizing and transforming activities of E7 oncoproteins of high oncogenic risk HPV types. The HPV E6 protein is a small zinc-binding protein (approximately 150 amino acids long) that exerts its effects through interactions with cell cycle regulatory proteins and lacks endogenous enzymatic activity. E6 has sequence homology with both adenovirus E1B protein and SV40 large T antigen. These proteins all have the capacity to bind to a variety of important regulatory proteins such as p53 (see Table 7.8; see Fig. 7.9). Binding of E6 to p53 is mediated by the E6-associated protein (E6-AP) ligase.[246] *p53* is a key cellular regulatory gene that acts as a transcriptional activator and has the characteristics of a tumor suppressor gene. Loss of wild-type *p53* expression is associated with the development of malignancy. In addition, *p53* has characteristics of an oncogene, because mutant forms of this gene can act as a dominant transforming gene. In noninfected cells, *p53* levels increase in response to cellular or DNA damage or aberrant cell proliferation signals. High levels of *p53* induce expression of *p53*-responsive genes such as $p21^{cip\ 1}$ to increase, causing the cells to undergo growth arrest in the G_1 phase of the cell cycle. G_1 growth arrest provides an opportunity for cells to either repair DNA damage caused by the stress before the next round of DNA synthesis or for the cells to be eliminated through programmed cell death (*apoptosis*).

In HPV-infected cells, p53 levels are low because E6-associated protein-mediated binding of *p53* to the E6 proteins of high oncogenic risk HPVs results in the rapid proteolytic degradation of the bound *p53* through an ubiquitin-dependent pathway[246]; this reduces the amount of p53 present within the cell and causes a loss of the p53 repair mechanism. Interactions between E6 and E6-AP also produce other consequences, including blocking of ubiquitination and degradation of the SRC family tyrosine kinase Blk,[208] which could result in the stimulation of cell proliferation. E6 also interacts with a variety of other known proteins including the focal adhesion protein paxillin and the calcium-binding protein ERC 55.[45,282] E6 also has an anti-apoptotic effect that is mediated in part through degradation of *p53* and Bak.[281] Another possible important role of E6 is telomerase activation. Telomerase is a cellular ribonucleoprotein reverse transcriptase whose activation may play a role in the growth of transformed cells.[102] Activation of telomerase by E6 may occur through the activation of the *myc* oncogene.

Role of E2, E6, and E7 in Transformation

Mutational analysis of E6 and E7 indicates that the capacity to bind *Rb* and *p53*, respectively, is important for the transforming and immortalizing function of these oncoproteins.[117] E7 proteins from high oncogenic risk HPV types such as HPV-16 avidly bind to *Rb* whereas the E7 proteins of low oncogenic risk HPV types such as HPV-6 bind *Rb* with much lower affinity. In a manner analogous to that described for E7–Rb interactions, the E6 proteins of high oncogenic risk viruses have much higher *p53*-binding affinities than the E6 of low oncogenic risk viruses.

Both E6 and E7 play important roles in productive viral infection and the life cycle of HPV. Both proteins evolved as a mechanism whereby the virus could stimulate intermediate and superficial squamous epithelial cells to reenter the cell cycle, allowing the virus to co-opt the host DNA replicative pathway. Therefore, malignant transformation should be considered as an aberration of the viral life cycle rather than an inherent characteristic of HPV. During the viral life cycle, E2-derived proteins act as important regulators of the expression of the E6 and E7 ORFs.[287] In most infected epithelia, E2 appears to inhibit transcription from the E6 and E7 ORFs, which helps maintains some regulation of cellular proliferation.[296]

In most low-grade cervical cancer precursor lesions, HPV DNA exists as a closed circular form termed an *episome*. In the episomal form, the E2 ORF is physically intact, and transcription from the E6 and E7 ORFs is presumed to be well regulated. However, in some high-grade precursor lesions, 75% of HPV-16-associated carcinomas, and almost all HPV-18-associated carcinomas, the HPV genome becomes physically integrated into the host chromosomal DNA.[63,67] Integration into the host chromosomal DNA appears to be a random event that does not lead to the consistent activation of specific cellular oncogenes. However, integration requires that the episomal viral genome breaks, and this break frequently leads to disruption of the E2 ORF.[49] Disruption of the E2 ORF with retention of the E6 and E7 ORFs could result in the unregulated expression of the E6 and E7 ORFs and uncontrolled cell proliferation.

This model of cervical cancer pathogenesis based on E2 inactivation secondary to integration with resultant E6 and E7 overexpression does not fully explain the development of cervical cancer. For example, even though in most cervical cancers HPV DNA is integrated into the cellular DNA, in some invasive cancers only episomal HPV DNA is detected.[63] Likewise, fusion of HPV-associated transformed cervical epithelial cells with nontransformed cells results in the formation of nonmalignant hybrids despite the fact that there is continued overexpression of the E6 and E7 ORFs.[268] In vivo, there is, on average, a 10-year delay between an initial HPV infection and the development of cancer. Moreover, only a small fraction of the patients exposed to high oncogenic risk HPVs subsequently develop cancer. In vitro, cultured human epithelial cells expressing the E6 and E7 ORFs are nonmalignant at early passages but become fully malignant at later passages.[107] This finding suggests that additional events or factors, which may include induction of chromosomal instability with the development of aneuploidy, are probably important for the development of cervical cancer. Loss of heterozygosity (LOH) studies of cervical cancers have detected frequent allelic loss of loci on chromosomes 3p, 4p, 4q, and 11q.[191] Cytogenetic, nonrandom deletions in the 3p 14-p21 region appear to be quite frequent, and this location may contain a tumor suppressor gene important for cervical cancer.[165]

Epidemiologic Evidence Linking HPV to the Development of Cervical Cancer and Its Precursors

There is now consistent and compelling epidemiologic evidence that HPV infection plays a central role in the development of cervical cancer precursors and invasive cervical cancers, and it is now accepted that high-risk HPV is the major etiologic agent in the development of cervical cancer. Evidence that supports this idea includes the following: the temporal sequence between infection and the development of cancer is correct, the associations between specific types of HPV and cervical cancer are specific, and the natural history and biologic behavior of HPV infections and cervical cancer are consistent with a causal association. Recent studies that have analyzed tissue from invasive cervical cancers from different countries using sensitive PCR-based methods to detect HPV infections have found that the DNA of high-risk types of HPV can be identified in more than 93% of invasive cervical cancers.[28,47,204] Moreover, these studies have found that the same types of HPV are identified in cervical cancers, irrespective of geographic area (Table 7.9). When HPV DNA-negative samples from these studies were reexamined using more sensitive HPV DNA detection methods, HPV DNA was identified in almost all the HPV DNA-negative samples, and the overall HPV DNA detection rate was more than 99%.[293]

Consistent associations between infection with high-risk types of HPV and either invasive cervical cancer or cervical cancer precursors have been identified in a number of large case-control studies. Case-control studies of HPV and SIL have found that more than 75% of SIL can be attributed to HPV infection. When HPV infection was controlled for in these studies, traditional risk factors such as number of sexual partners and a history of sexually transmitted diseases frequently disappear, suggesting that sexual behavior is a surrogate of HPV infection.[249] For example, a case-control study of women with high-grade SIL enrolled from the southwestern United States reported an odds ratio of 20.8 for HPV DNA positivity.[15] Case-control studies of cervical cancer and HPV have also consistently reported strong associations between the detection of high-risk HPV and invasive cervical cancer with odds ratios greater than 10 in the majority of studies. In a case-control study of 436 women with cervical cancer and 387 control women enrolled in Columbia and Spain, Bosch et al. found that HPV DNA positivity was the single strongest risk factor for the development of cervical cancer (odds ratio, 23.8).[27,29] After controlling for HPV DNA positivity, the number of sexual partners, but not age at first intercourse, disappeared as a risk factor. In another case-control study of women with invasive cervical cancer from the Philippines, the odds ratio observed for the association between HPV DNA positivity and cervical cancer was 151.[204] In a case-control study from Thailand, the fraction of risk attributable to HPV in the population was 95% for invasive squamous cell carcinoma of the cervix.[47]

A number of recent prospective studies of women negative colposcopically and by cytology have demonstrated that HPV infection occurs before the development of the lesions. Thus, the temporal associations between HPV infection and the development of cervical cancer precursors or invasive cer-

Table 7.9. Prevalence of specific types of HPV in invasive cervical cancer by geographic region

	Geographic Region									
	Africa		*Latin America*		*Southeast Asia*		*Europe*		*North America*	
HPV Type	*No.*	*%*	*No.*	*%*	*No.*	*%*	*No.*	*%*	*No.*	*%*
HPV 16 and associated										
HPV 16	79	43%	255	51%	42	43%	56	65%	33	58%
HPV 31	5	3%	35	7%	1	1%	5	6%	3	5%
HPV 33	5	3%	18	4%	2	2%	1	1%	0	
HPV 35	4	2%	10	2%	1	1%	1	1%	0	
HPV 52	4	2%	16	3%	2	2%	3	4%	0	
HPV 58	5	3%	11	2%	2	2%	1	1%	0	
HPV 18 and associated										
HPV 18	33	18%	48	10%	31	32%	7	8%	9	16%
HPV 39	0		13	3%	1	1%	0		0	
HPV 45	23	12%	37	7%	8	8%	2	2%	8	14%
HPV 59	0		14	2.8%	1	1%	0		0	
HPV 68										
Other										
HPV 56	6	3%	3	1%	3	3%	2	2%	2	4%
Miscellaneous	5	3%	16	3%	4	4%	1	1%	0	
Undetermined	2	1%	8	2%	0		1	1%	1	2%
HPV negative	19	10%	36	7%	7	3%	4	5%	4	7%
Total samples	186		505		98		86		57	

Modified from ref. 28.

vical cancer support a role for HPV in the pathogenesis of these lesions. In a study of young women enrolled from a sexually transmitted diseases clinic in Seattle, Koutsky et al. found that 36% of women who were positive for either HPV 16 or 18 at entry into the study subsequently developed biopsy-confirmed high-grade SIL over a 24-month period.[157] In a study of colposcopically negative "high-risk" women enrolled from methadone clinics and sexually transmitted disease clinics in New York City, Ellerbrock et al. reported that 12% of women who were infected with HPV 16 or 18 at entry developed biopsy-confirmed SIL of any grade over a 36 month follow-up period compared to 3% of HPV DNA negative women.[75] Almost identical rates of incident SIL were reported in HPV DNA-positive and -negative women by Rozendaal et al. in the Netherlands.[242]

Taken together, these epidemiologic studies demonstrate that there is a clear and consistent association between infection with specific types of HPV and invasive cervical cancer and its precursor lesions. Moreover, epidemiologic studies have demonstrated that exposure to HPV precedes the development of cervical disease. When combined with the strong molecular evidence identifying the molecular pathways by which HPV could cause cervical cancer, these findings clearly indicate that HPV infection, acquired through sexual contact, is causal in the development of both SIL and invasive cervical cancer. Based on these data, the International Agency for Research on Cancer (IARC) of the World Health Organization have classified HPV 16 and HPV 18 as carcinogens in humans.[123]

However, it should be stressed that although infection with specific high-risk types of HPV is necessary for the development of invasive cervical cancer, it is not sufficient for the development of cervical cancer. The long latency between the initial exposure to HPV and the development of cervical cancer as well as the fact that only a small fraction of women exposed to HPV develop cervical disease suggest that other cofactors are necessary in the pathogenesis of cervical neoplasia. For example, in a recent case-control study of women with cervical cancer in the Philippines, high parity, low socioeconomic status, and smoking continued to be significantly associated with invasive cervical cancer even after controlling for HPV DNA status.[204] Similarly, in a case-control study from Thailand, limited socioeconomic status, increasing number of sexual partners, and a history of sexually transmitted diseases continued to be significant risk factors for invasive cervical cancer, even after controlling for infection with HPV.[47]

Other Infections Agents

Herpes simplex virus type 2 (HSV-2) previously received considerable attention in relation to the etiology of cervical neoplasia, with studies linking HSV-2 to SIL and cervical carcinoma biologically and epidemiologically.[141,198] Herpes virus antigens have been detected by immunofluorescence in exfoliated cervical squamous carcinoma cells,[241] and the virus has been identified sporadically at the ultrastructural level in cervical carcinoma cells grown in tissue culture. However, whole viral particles consistent with HSV-2 virions have not been observed in genital tract carcinoma. A number of studies that have been utilized in situ hybridization have reported occasionally finding portions of the HSV genome in cervical cancer cells.[71] However, HSV is much less commonly detected in cervical cancer than is HPV, and it is now generally accepted that HSV does not play a central role in the development of cervical cancer, although it may be important as a cofactor in certain patients.

Well-controlled, retrospective seroepidemiologic studies have shown that patients with invasive and noninvasive cancers of the cervix have a higher frequency of neutralizing antibodies against HSV-2 than do controls matched for race, age, and socioeconomic status.[114] A case-control study of 766 women with invasive cervical carcinoma and 1532 controls of women from Latin America found a possible interaction between HPV-16/18 and HSV-2 in the development of invasive cervical carcinoma. The presence of HSV-2 antibodies alone was associated with a relative risk of 1.6 for the development of invasive cervical cancer.[114] Although this relative risk was much less than that associated with the presence of HPV-16 or HPV-18 DNA, it persisted independently of other risk factors. Most importantly, patients who had antibodies against HSV-2 and who were also HPV-16/18 DNA positive had a twofold greater risk for developing cervical cancer than patients who were only HPV-16/18 DNA positive, suggesting a possible interaction between the two viruses.

Another herpesvirus that has recently been detected in some invasive cervical cancers and SIL is human herpesvirus 6 (HHV-6).[43] HHV-6 has the capacity to infect human cervical epithelial cells and to enhance the expression of HPV when cells are infected with both viruses. However, because HHV-6 is only occasionally identified in association with cervical neoplasia, it is more likely to act as a cofactor in selected patients than as a causal factor.

Immunosuppression and Human Immunodeficiency Virus

Our understanding of carcinogenesis is now based on the interaction of initiators and promoters, with neoplastic transformation developing as the result of a series of multiple, synergistic events. The host immune system plays an important role in this multifactorial process. Immunosuppression provides a background for the development of neoplasia by predisposing to infection by oncogenic viruses and by allowing neoplastic proliferations to escape immune surveillance and other host regulatory mechanisms. With respect to cervical carcinogenesis, there is clear evidence for an interaction with the immune system. HPV infection occurs more frequently in immunosuppressed individuals, and condylomas in immunosuppressed patients tend to be larger in size, multicentric, and refractory to treatment.[46,258,272] Vulvovaginal neoplasia, SIL, and cervical carcinoma are also more common in patients on immunosuppressive therapy.[104] It has been proposed that the cytostatic and cytotoxic effects of therapeutic agents, such as azathioprine, corticosteroids, and alkylating agents, potentiate the effects of the already compromised immune system.[303] In renal transplant patients, the relative risk (RR) of cervical cancer is increased by 5.4. This increased relative risk for cervical cancer should be compared to a 1.5- to 2.5-fold-increased relative risk for the development of epithelial cancers on other mucosal surfaces that are unassociated with a viral etiology.[219]

A number of studies have clearly documented that there is a high prevalence of cytologic abnormalities in women infected with the human immunodeficiency virus (HIV), and cervical cancer has been classified as an AIDS (acquired immunodeficiency syndrome) case-defining illness by the Centers for Disease Control and Prevention of the United States.[160] Strong and consistent associations between HIV infection and SIL have now been demonstrated. Several large, well-controlled studies have observed substantially increased risks of biopsy-confirmed SIL in HIV-infected women. One of the largest of these studies, from New York City, used both cytology and colposcopy to evaluate a cohort of HIV-infected and uninfected women. Biopsy-confirmed low-grade SIL was identified in 13% of the 398 HIV-infected women and in 4% of the 307 HIV-uninfected women ($p < 0.001$).[306] High-grade SIL was detected in 7% of the HIV-infected group and in 1% of the HIV-uninfected group ($p < 0.001$). Another study from Italy that had a similar study design reported an even higher rate of SIL in HIV-infected women.[54] In the Italian study, 115 (42%) of the 273 HIV-infected women had biopsy-confirmed SIL of any grade, of which 51% was high-grade SIL, compared to 13 (8%) of the 161 HIV-uninfected women.

In the study from New York City, demographic information and SIL risk factor information were analyzed to determine whether other behavioral and biologic factors that occur commonly in HIV-infected women could explain their increased risk of SIL. HIV infection emerged as a strong predictor of biopsy-confirmed SIL in this cohort of women independent of other risk factors for SIL. As expected, HIV-infected women with more profound immunosuppression (CD4+ T-lymphocyte counts, <200 cells/μl) were at greater risk of SIL than HIV-infected women with less profound levels, but even HIV-infected women with relatively intact immune function (defined by CD4+ counts) were at greater risk than uninfected women.[306] Other studies have documented high rates of HPV infection and also of persistence of HPV infections among HIV-infected women, but the types of HPV associated with cervical disease appear to be identical in HIV-infected and uninfected women.[212,274] Prospective follow-up studies of the cohort from New York City have now demonstrated that the incidence of SIL is 4.6 fold greater among HIV-infected compared to HIV-uninfected women.[75]

Although it has been clearly shown that HIV-infected women are at increased risk for developing preinvasive cervical lesions, fewer cases of invasive cervical cancer have occurred in HIV-infected women than was initially expected. Data from the Sentinel Hospital Surveillance System for HIV Infection in the United States observed the prevalence of invasive cervical cancer to be only modestly higher for HIV-infected women (10.4 cases per 1000 women) than for HIV-uninfected women (6.2 cases per 1000 women) [relative risk, 1.7; 95% confidence interval (CI), 1.1–2.5].[48] Data from the National Cancer Institute's AIDS—Cancer Registry Match Study has found a fivefold-elevated risk of invasive cervical cancer during the early pre-AIDS period but weaker (elevated but nonsignificant) risks after AIDS.[97] Aggressive screening for and treatment of precancerous lesions in HIV-infected women under intense medical scrutiny may prevent most cases of invasive cervical cancer from developing.

Smoking, Diet, and Oral Contraceptives

In addition to *sexual behavior* and *parity*, several other *risk factors such as cigarette smoking, low social economic class, diet*, and *contraceptive use* have been associated with the development of cervical cancer.[15,33,100] Szarewski completed a comprehensive review of the literature and concluded that a positive association between cigarette smoking and the development of cervical cancer had been reported by the majority of studies designed to address this question.[277] In a recent large case-control study of women with high-grade SIL from Sweden, the association between smoking and high-grade SIL had an odds ratio of 2.6 (95% CI, 1.7–4.0); the effect was dose dependent and was not affected by adjusting for HPV status.[147] It has been proposed that there are several mechanisms that could account for the association between cervical cancer and cigarette smoking. One is the secretion of cigarette smoke by-products, such as nicotine and cotinine, in the cervical mucous of tobacco users and women passively exposed to cigarette smoke.[180] Structurally altered DNA sequences (e.g., DNA adducts) are identified significantly more frequently in the cervical epithelium of smokers than in nonsmokers, and it has been suggested that the secretion of cigarette smoke by-products might have a direct mutagenic effect on the cervical epithelium.[259] Another possible mechanism that could explain the association between smoking and cervical cancer is the effect of cervical smoke by-products on local immune responses in the cervix. A reduction in the number of Langerhans cells in the cervices of smokers compared to nonsmokers has been described, and this reduction may result in a decreased level of local immunity to HPV.[12]

Only a few studies have focused on relationships between diet and cervical cancer, but several studies have reported data suggesting that a diet low in either vitamin A or C may be associated with an increased risk.[211,290] However, other studies have not detected an association between dietary intake of beta-carotene or retinol and SIL.[68,147] Folate deficiency has also been considered as a potential risk factor. A recent case-control study reported that folate deficiency enhances the effects of other risk factors such as parity, HPV-16 infection, and cigarette smoking on the development of SIL.[40] In general, it appears that the impact of nutritional factors is small compared to the effects of other risk factors such as HPV infection and smoking. A case-control study of women with incident SIL that measured micronutrient levels using both a food frequency questionnaire and blood samples found slight, but nonstatistical, protection from SIL among women in the upper tertile of lycopene and vitamin A intake.[138] Other similar studies have found that mean plasma lycopene and total cryptoxanthin are lower in women with SIL than in controls, also suggesting weak protective effects.[99] However, in another large nested case-control study of women with low-grade SIL and equivocal SIL, no protective role for any micronutrient was observed after controlling for HPV.[300]

The use of combined oral contraceptives has also been found to be a risk factor for the development of cervical cancer and its precursors in some studies. Several comprehensive reviews have concluded that oral contraceptive use of 5 years or more is associated with an approximately twofold residual excess risk, even after controlling for sexual behavior and Papanicolaou test screening history.[100,213] However, it should be cautioned that the apparent association between cervical disease and oral contraceptive use is so weak that it could possibly be explained by either bias or confounding.[32] In a recent case-control study of women with high-grade SIL from Sweden, the association observed between oral contraceptive use and high-grade SIL disappeared after taking HPV status into account.[147] There are also some studies suggesting that oral contraceptive use may accelerate the progression of SIL from low grade to high grade or to invasive cancer.[291] Associations between exogenous hormones and cervical disease could be explained by a number of mechanisms, including the direct promoting effects of estrogens and progestins on the HPV genome, as well as by indirect effects such as a reduction in blood folate levels that is occasionally observed in women on oral contraceptives.[40] Whether there is an association between endogenous hormone levels and invasive cervical cancer is even more controversial.

There is no association between age at menarche or age of menopause and the risk of invasive cervical squamous cell carcinoma. The strong association observed between early age of first parity and risk for cervical cancer in most studies most likely reflects risk of exposure to a sexually transmitted agent at an early age, rather than an influence of endogenous hormones.[26] Other studies have shown no effect of the initiation of hormone replacement therapy in postmenopausal women on the frequency with which HPV DNA is detected in cervical samples.[80] Barrier methods of contraception, particularly condoms and diaphragms, appear to decrease the risk of cervical neoplasia.[229]

Correlations between prenatal diethylstilbestrol (DES) exposure and cervicovaginal intraepithelial neoplasia (CIN) have been similarly conflicting. Despite early observations to the contrary,[236] a study by the Diethylstilbestrol Adenosis (DESAD) Project of 3899 DES-exposed women in the United States described a twofold-increased incidence rate of SIL in DES progeny compared to matched controls (relative risk, 2.12; 95% CI, 1.2–3.8).[106] These studies must be interpreted with caution because immature squamous metaplasia in the DES offspring is often confused with SIL, even by expert pathologists. Such diagnostic pitfalls might have contributed to the relatively high SIL incidence in the DES offspring. However, recent data from the Netherlands DES Information Center have shown that DES-exposed daughters have triple the risk of invasive cervical cancer compared to unexposed women in the general population.[289]

Clinical Features

SIL occurs on the anterior lip of the cervix twice as commonly as on the posterior lip and is rarely seen at the lateral cervical angles. This distribution is similar to the distribution of both the everted endocervical epithelium and the transformation zone during the postpartum period.[230] SIL may expand horizontally and involve the entire transformation zone, but it stops abruptly at the junction with the native portio epithelium. The area of the transformation zone, therefore, predetermines the distribution and extent of SIL on the exposed portion of the cervix. The endocervical extension of SIL is not restricted, and extension along the entire endocervical canal and into the uterus can rarely occur. The size and endocervical distribution of SIL tend to vary directly with increasing severity of lesion grade. High-grade SIL usually has the largest surface area and more frequently involves the endocervical canal.

The mechanism by which SIL grows and extends into normal squamous epithelium and into the columnar epithelium of the endocervix is a matter of contention. In the 1960s and early 1970s, many investigators studied this process, and two separate theories were developed. One view was that SIL is multicellular in origin and spreads by transformation of cells from normal to neoplastic in a vertical direction.[55,228] This multicellular theory predicts that SIL will arise in predetermined areas containing an abnormal cell population. The primary lesion grows and expands by transforming the adjacent normal epithelium into neoplastic epithelium or by the coalescence of multiple predetermined neoplastic fields, producing a larger lesion.[55,228] The contrasting theory was that SIL is unicellular in origin and begins in a single cell or at most in an extremely circumscribed group of cells. According to the unicellular theory, SIL spreads horizontally along the basement membrane by mechanically lifting the adjacent normal squamous and endocervical columnar cells.[230] The concept that SIL has a unicellular origin was supported by studies of the distribution of glucose-6-phosphatase within lesions. Glucose-6-phosphatase is an X-chromosome-linked enzymatic marker. Because of random X-chromosome inactivation, the individual cells of women who are heterozygous for this marker express only a single form of the enzyme. Studies that have analyzed cases of SIL from women who are heterozygous for glucose-6-phosphatase reported that only a single isoenzyme was present within a lesion, supporting a unicellular origin.[260] Other chromosomal studies have also supported a unicellular origin of SIL.[265]

These theories were both developed before the recognition that the biology/virology of low-grade SIL and high-grade SIL are quite different. In light of our current understanding of the pathogenesis of SIL, it would be expected that low-grade SIL would be frequently multicellular in origin, because it develops within a field of latently infected cervical epithelium and frequently is associated with multiple types of HPV. In contrast, high-grade SIL is usually associated with only a single type of HPV, is frequently aneuploid, and may contain integrated HPV DNA. Therefore, high-grade SIL would be expected to be unicellular in origin. More recent studies that have utilized PCR-based detection methods to identify X-chromosome-linked genetic markers have shown that SIL can be either monoclonal or polyclonal. Park et al. analyzed clonality by evaluating inactivation of the human androgen receptor gene that is located in the X-chromosome.[215] They found that low-grade SIL associated with low-risk HPV types are typically polyclonal, whereas low-grade SIL associated with high-risk HPV types are typically monoclonal, as are almost all high-grade SIL lesions. This finding indicates that low-grade SIL associated with low-risk or novel types of HPV are biologically different at their inception from lesions that are histologically low grade, but associated with high-risk HPV types. Similarly, other studies that have looked at loss of heterozygosity (LOH) at specific chromosomal loci have found low rates of LOH in low-grade SIL but frequent LOH in high-grade SIL.[50,165]

There is no unanimous opinion on the cellular origin of SIL. Three cellular sites of origin have been proposed: basal cells of the squamous epithelium of the portio, basal cells of the transformation zone epithelium, and reserve cells of the endocervix.[131] Most SIL begins at the squamocolumnar junction of the transformation zone, with one edge of the lesion bordering the endocervical columnar epithelium. Only about 10% of SIL involves the endocervical canal without involving the squamocolumnar junction.[3,84,224] In general, the portion of SIL on the exocervical portio surface is low grade whereas the portion of SIL that extends into the endocervical canal is high grade (Fig. 7.10). From these observations it is now thought that most SIL arises in the basal cells of the transformation zone epithelium, which is formed by the coalescence of squamous metaplastic epithelium with native squamous epithelium.

Pathologic Findings

Squamous epithelial lesion (SIL) is characterized by *abnormal cellular proliferation, maturation*, and *cytologic atypia*. The cytologic abnormalities include hyperchromatic nuclei, abnormal chromatin distribution, nuclear pleomorphism, and increased nuclear:cytoplasmic ratio. Nuclear atypia is the hallmark of SIL. The nuclear borders are irregular, and the chromatin is coarse, granular (salt and pepper), or filamentous throughout the nuclear mass. The nuclear alterations are found in all levels of the epithelium regardless of the degree of cytoplasmic maturation. Increased mitotic activity at all epithelial levels and the presence of morphologically abnormal mitotic figures are also typical of SIL.[195,221]

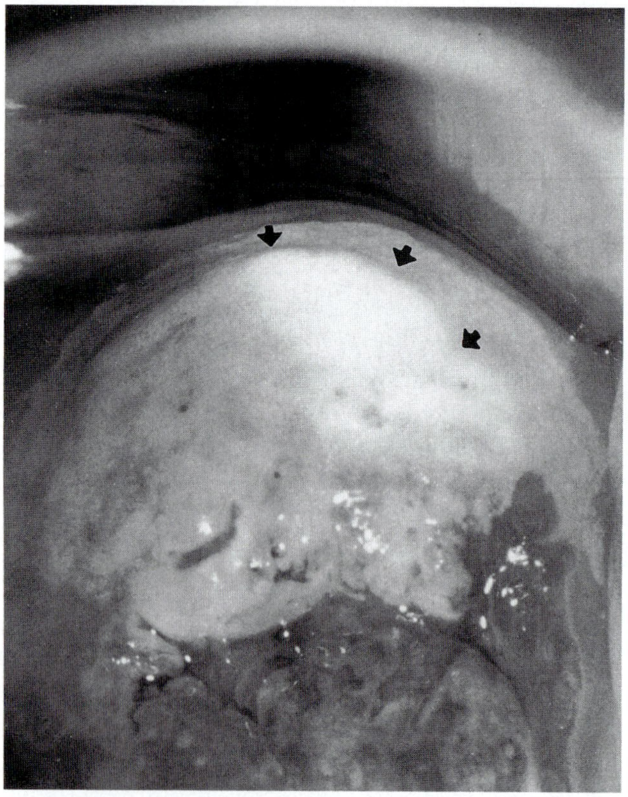

Fig. 7.10. High-grade SIL. Colposcopic appearance of high-grade SIL arising within a low-grade SIL. High-grade SIL usually develops internally to the low-grade SIL, presents with an internal margin, and extends into the endocervical canal.

Ultrastructurally, both the nuclear and cytoplasmic alterations of SIL are consistent with a progressive lack of normal differentiation.[257] There is a decrease in glycogen, tonofilaments, desmosomes, and specialized junctional units with increasing histologic dedifferentiation. These alterations are correlated with a progressive decrease in cellular adhesion, basal pseudopodia, and cell contact inhibition demonstrated by time-lapse cinematography in cells grown in vitro.[234] The surface ultrastructure of cervical cancer precursors also differs from the normal architecture. The most outstanding feature is the absence of surface microridges and the presence of abundant microvilli.

The traditional grading of intraepithelial neoplasia was based on the proportion of the epithelium occupied by basaloid, undifferentiated cells, reflecting a progressive loss of epithelial maturation and decreasing glycogenization with increasing lesion severity. The spectrum of epithelial alterations that constitutes SIL were therefore semiquantitatively classified into three categories: CIN grade 1, neoplastic, basaloid cells occupying the lower third of the epithelium; CIN grade 2, basaloid cells occupying the lower third to two-thirds of the epithelium; and CIN grade 3, basaloid cells occupying two-thirds to full thickness of the epithelium (Fig. 7.11). Adoption of the Bethesda System nomenclature to histologic classification results in a two-tier rather than a three-tier grading system.

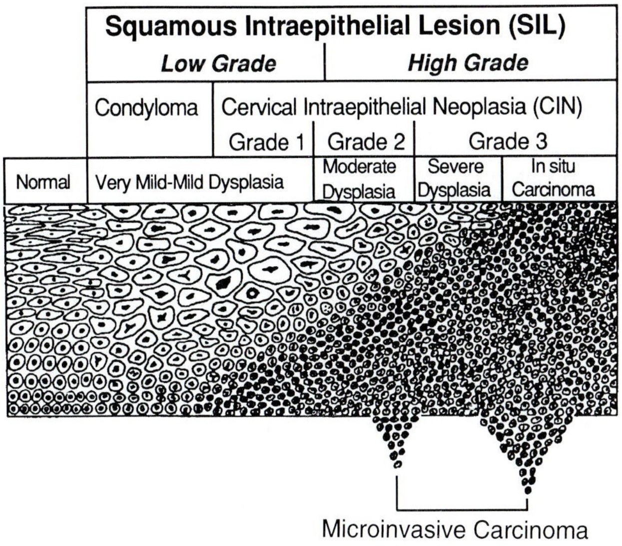

Fig. 7.11. Cervical squamous carcinoma precursors. Schematic representation of cervical cancer precursors and the different terminologies that have been used to refer to them. The risk of developing microinvasion from different states of SIL is arbitrarily represented and is not necessarily proportional to that illustrated in this scheme.

Low-Grade Squamous Intraepithelial Lesion

In 1977, Meisels et al. introduced the term *flat condyloma* to describe a flat HPV-induced cervical lesion that closely resembled the typical exophytic appearance of a cervical condyloma acuminatum.[184] Implicit in the use of this term was the belief that flat cervical condylomata could be distinguished from CIN 1 on a histologic basis and that there was a different distribution of HPV types in the two lesions; flat condylomas, like exophytic condylomas, would contain HPV-6 and -11; and CIN 1 would contain HPV-16, like carcinoma. Flat condylomata were defined as lesions with a marked HPV cytopathic effect and an orderly basal cell layer, whereas CIN 1 lesions had a marked HPV cytopathic effect accompanied by a loss of polarity, crowding, overlapping, and disorganization of the basal cell layer.[185,186]

To clarify possible differences between cervical "flat condyloma" and CIN 1 lesions, several studies analyzed these lesions for nuclear DNA content and associated HPV type. Using computerized imaging cytometry, Fu and coworkers compared ploidy levels in cervical lesions diagnosed as either cervical condyloma or CIN 1 and found similar ploidy levels in both.[91] All lesions histologically classified as flat condyloma and 67% of lesions histologically classified as CIN 1 had diploid, and occasionally polyploid, DNA patterns.[91] Similarly, Jakobsen et al., using flow cytometry, reported diploid DNA patterns in almost all lesions classified as mild and moderate dysplasia.[127] Although early studies suggested differences in HPV distribution in these lesions, several subsequent studies have reported that there were no differences in the HPV types associated with "flat condylomas" and CIN 1 (see "Human Papillomavirus"), indicating that lesions with the histological appearances of "flat condyloma" or CIN 1 should be grouped into a single entity, that is, low-grade SIL.[301]

The associated architectural abnormalities indicating that lesions with the histologic appearances of "flat condyloma" or CIN 1 should be grouped with low-grade SIL are a result of proliferation of basal and parabasal cells in the infected epithelium. The resultant hyperplasia can be highly variable and takes many forms but is most commonly characterized by papillomatosis and acanthosis. One of the more common patterns of the acanthosis is that of moderate epithelial thickening and an undulating, slightly raised surface (Fig. 7.12). In the older literature, cervical lesions with HPV-associated cyto-

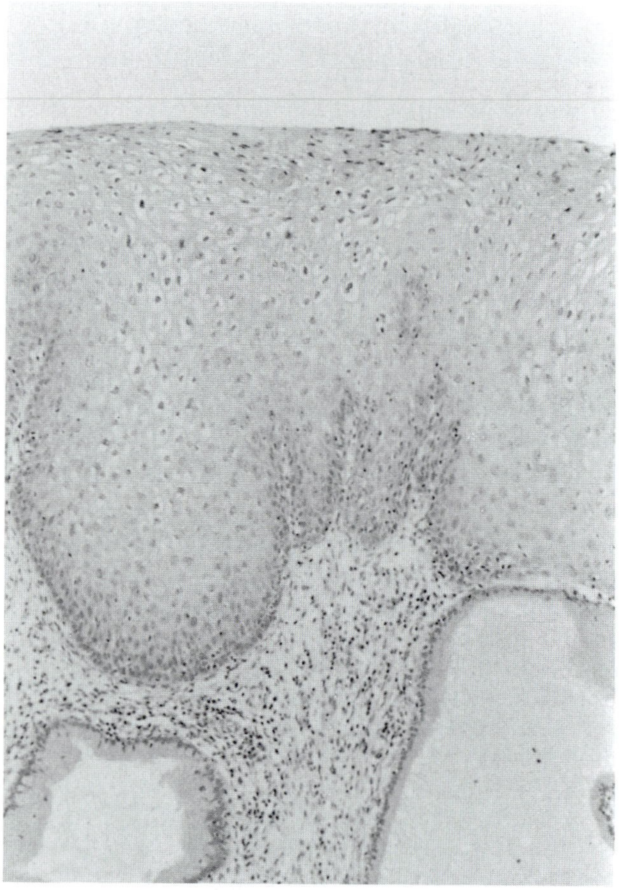

Fig. 7.12. **Low-grade SIL.** Acanthosis is frequently found in low-grade SIL. Most commonly acanthosis is manifested as a slightly thickened epithelium with an undulating surface.

pathic effects and only a moderate degree of epithelial thickening were referred to as *condyloma planum*. Using the Bethesda terminology, such lesions, when they occur on the cervix, are designated low-grade SIL. Other types of epithelial hyperplasia that can occur in productive HPV infection are multiple papillary fronds containing fibrovascular cores and pointed epithelial spikes (Fig. 7.13). Colposcopically, the latter have prominent, fine surface spikes and are frequently referred to in the colposcopic literature as *spiked condyloma*. The surface of low-grade SIL frequently has a layer of parakeratosis and somewhat less commonly hyperkeratosis with an associated granular layer (Fig. 7.13). When gland involvement by the HPV-infected epithelium and acanthosis predominate, the histologic pattern appears endophytic and superficially resembles that of an inverted nasal papilloma (Fig. 7.14).

It is now recognized that low-grade SIL is the morphologic manifestation of productive HPV infections of the cervical squamous epithelium that can be caused by any of the anogenital types of HPV. In productive HPV infection, many viral particles are produced in the superficial epithelium. If in situ hybridization is used to identify HPV DNA within the squamous epithelium, high numbers of HPV DNA copies can be seen in superficial squamous cells (see Fig. 7.8). The infected squamous cells usually demonstrate the *cytopathic effects* of HPV. These cytopathic effects are considered the most characteristic cytologic/histologic features of low-grade SIL and include perinuclear cytoplasmic cavitation with thickening of the cytoplasmic membrane, nuclear atypia, and anisocytosis (see Fig. 7.7). Nuclear atypia is characterized by enlargement, hyperchromasia, and irregularity and wrinkling of the nuclear membrane. Cells near the surface may have nuclei that are somewhat smaller and pyknotic. The combination of nuclear atypia and cytoplasmic cavita-

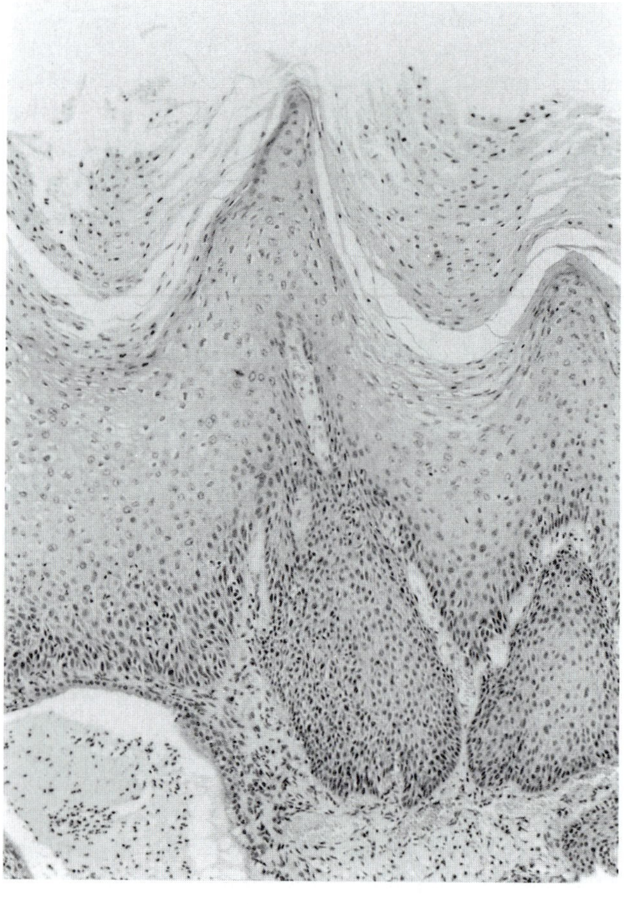

Fig. 7.13. **Low-grade SIL.** Papillomatosis, acanthosis, parakeratosis, and hyperkeratosis are frequently present. Acanthosis and papillomatosis also can produce pointed spikes with fibrovascular cores, the so-called "spiked condyloma."

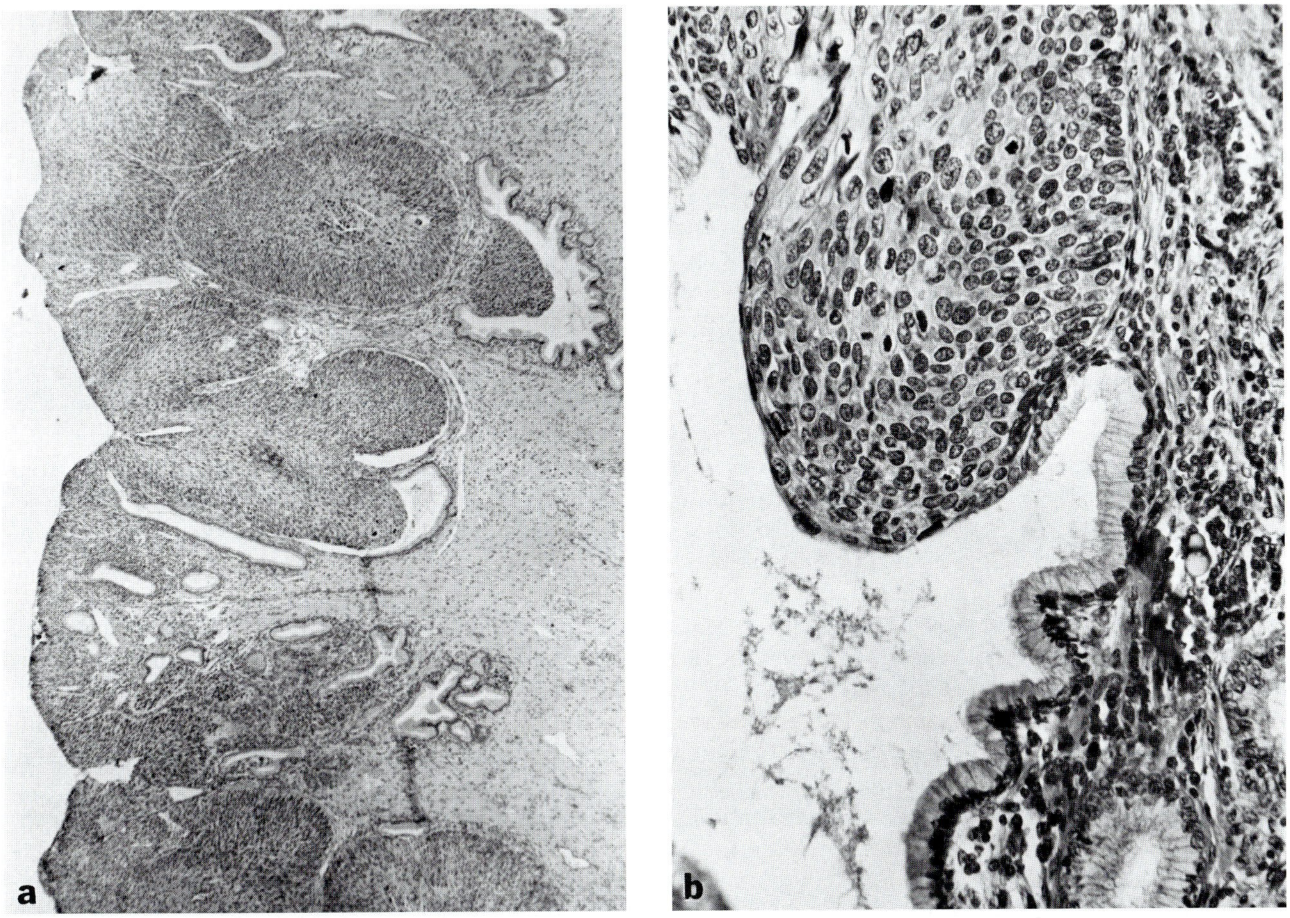

Fig. 7.14. Low-grade SIL. a: SIL can grow into and distend endocervical clefts. Note the smooth margins of ingrowing SIL retaining the normal configuration of endocervical mucosa. **b**: SIL grows between the endocervical epithelium and its basal lamina.

tion has been termed *koilocytosis* or *koilocytotic atypia*. The cells productively infected with HPV typically are polyploid, and many are also binucleated or multinucleated.[91] Polyploid cells are cytologically atypical and are readily recognized as being "abnormal" on either cytology or histology. This atypia is characterized predominantly by anisonucleosis; to a lesser extent, there is nuclear enlargement and an increase in nuclear:cytoplasmic ratio. Taken together, the histologic and cytologic features of koilocytosis, nuclear atypia, architectural abnormalities, and multinucleation are pathognomonic of an HPV-infected epithelium at any site in the lower genital tract and are especially prominent in low-grade SIL lesions. It must be emphasized that nuclear abnormalities need to be present to diagnose low-grade SIL.

The microscopic features of low-grade SIL are a direct result of productive HPV infection, which induces cytoskeletal abnormalities that may lead to the cytoplasmic cavitation that is one of the features of koilocytosis. Mitotic spindle abnormalities that occur in productive HPV infections appear to interfere with mitosis and cytokinesis; this leads to the polyploidy and bi- or multinucleated cells that are usually present in productive HPV infections. Although the mechanism responsible for the interference of mitosis and cytokinesis by HPV is unknown, it has been shown that the capsid proteins of a closely related DNA tumor virus, polyoma, directly bind to the mitotic spindle of infected cells and may interfere with mitosis through this mechanism.[278]

Differential Diagnosis

The most common problem in the differential diagnosis of low-grade SIL is the overinterpretation of koilocytosis and flat condyloma, largely because of the indiscriminant use of this term for squamous epithelium showing the slightest hint of "cytoplasmic vacuolization" in the absence of nuclear atypia.

Table 7.10. Variability in histopathological diagnoses in ALTS

	Quality control panel review diagnosis				
Initial DX	*WNL*	*ASCUS*	*LSIL*	*HSIL*	*Total*
WNL	91%	22%	4%	3%	685
ASCUS	77%	10%	9%	4%	184
LSIL	44%	4%	43%	13%	887
HSIL	7%	2%	14%	77%	481

Modified from ref. 271.

Normal metaplastic squamous epithelium with prominent glycogen vacuolization is often confused with low-grade SIL. In contrast to the focal distribution of koilocytes in low-grade SIL, cells of normal squamous epithelium that have perinuclear clearing are not sharply demarcated, the nuclei are not enlarged or atypical, and multinucleated cells are infrequent. Cytoplasmic vacuolization in the absence of nuclear atypia is a nonspecific change that may occur as a reflection of atrophy-related vacuolar degeneration in non-HPV-related infections such as trichomoniasis, *Gardnerella vaginalis*, and candidiasis. In addition to the absence of nuclear atypia, normal stratification and maturation are maintained in such conditions, whereas in HPV-associated lesions, there is some degree of cellular disorganization, particularly near the surface, and there is disturbance in the normal pattern of maturation.

Studies measuring interobserver variability of histologic diagnosis of cervical lesions demonstrate that although agreement between pathologists is excellent for invasive lesions and moderately good for high-grade SIL, it is poor for low-grade SIL.[125,238,271] In the NCI-sponsored ALTS multicenter study, 2237 colposcopically-directed biopsies that had been initially diagnosed at the clinical performance sites were reviewed by a quality control panel of pathologists. Only 43% of the biopsies initially diagnosed as low-grade SIL were classified as low-grade SIL after review (Table 7.10). The most significant discrepancies are in the ability of the pathologists to distinguish low-grade SIL from reactive squamous proliferations, suggesting that the morphologic criteria routinely used to distinguish these two lesions have serious shortcomings. The importance of nuclear atypia in the distinction of low-grade SIL from reactive lesions is confirmed by a number of studies. Correlation of HPV DNA with specific cytologic/histologic findings have uniformly found that perinuclear halos in the absence of significant nuclear atypia are nonspecific features.[86,192,295] Therefore, the diagnosis of low-grade SIL should be made only when significant nuclear atypia accompanies perinuclear halos.

High-Grade Squamous Intraepithelial Lesion

In high-grade SIL, immature basal-type cells should occupy more than the lower third of the epithelium. In addition there is nuclear crowding, pleomorphism, and loss of the normal cell polarity (Fig. 7.15). The nuclei of the immature basal-type cells are enlarged when compared to the nuclei of cells at comparable levels of the normal epithelium. This nuclear enlargement is frequently most pronounced in the lower half of the epithelium, although in all cases the superficial cells demonstrate some degree of nuclear enlargement. As in low-grade SIL, the nuclei are hyperchromatic and the chromatin is finely to coarsely granular. Prominent nuclei or chromocenters are uncommon. Normal and abnormal mitotic figures are present. Cytoplasm is usually scant, resulting in an increase in the nuclear:cytoplasmic ratio. Cell borders between the primitive cells are usually indistinct. The cells overlying the basal-type cells also have atypical nuclei but have more cytoplasm and therefore lower nuclear:cytoplasmic ratios and more distinct cell boundaries, and also can have prominent HPV cytopathic effects including perinuclear halos and bi- or multinucleation. In the superficial layers of the epithelium, individual

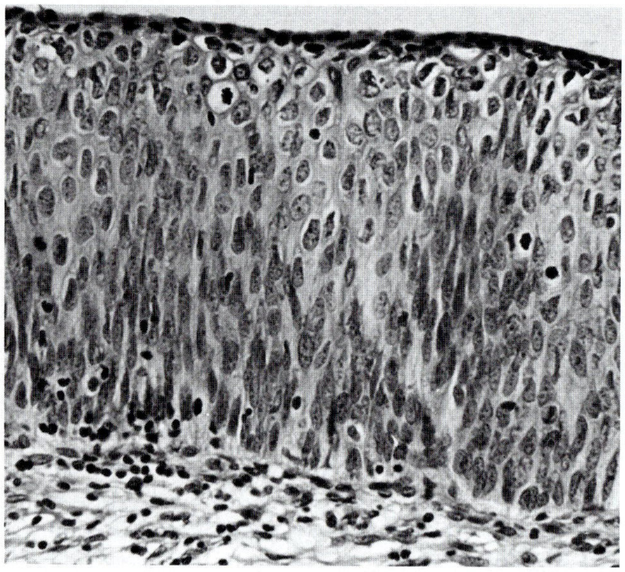

Fig. 7.15. High-grade SIL. Undifferentiated neoplastic cells replace 50–70% of the epithelium. The nuclear:cytoplasmic ratio is high, and the cytoplasmic membranes and the basal layer are indistinct. A few koilocytes are present in the superficial layers.

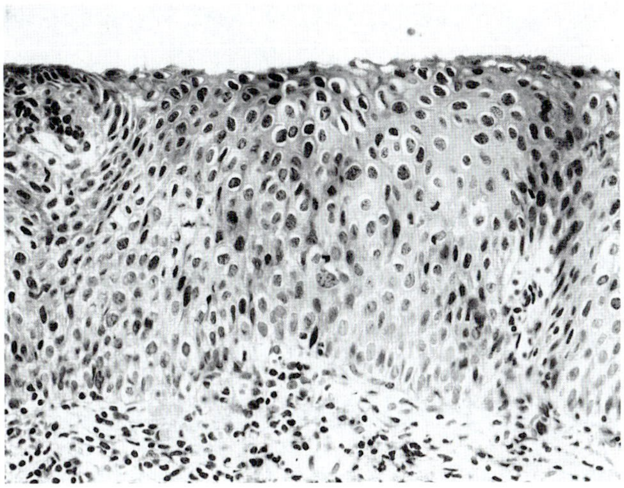

Fig. 7.16. High-grade SIL. This lesion would previously have been referred to as a CIN 2 lesion. Immature basaloid cells occupy the lower half of the epithelium and mitotic figures are present in the middle-third of the epithelium.

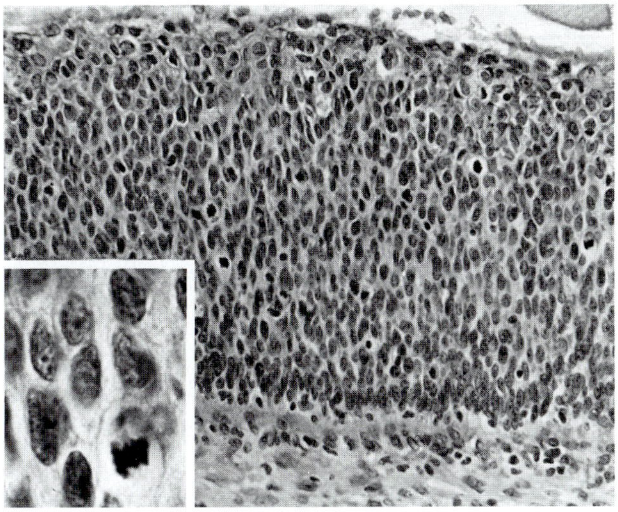

Fig. 7.17. High-grade SIL. The full thickness of the epithelium is composed of small, undifferentiated neoplastic cells. This is the classic *small cell carcinoma in situ*. Note numerous mitotic figures, loss of cellular maturation and organization, and lack of koilocytes. *Inset*: Aggregated nuclear chromatin and mitosis. Characteristically, cell membranes are ill-defined.

dyskeratotic cells may be seen. These cells are small with pyknotic hyperchromatic nuclei and dense acidophilic cytoplasm.

Another characteristic feature of high-grade SIL is the variability in nuclear size (anisonucleolis). It should be stressed, however, that this is a variable histologic feature. In some high-grade SIL lesions, particularly those that were previously termed carcinoma in situ, the nuclei at first glance appear relatively uniform in size, although careful scrutiny will reveal some variation in nuclear size and shape. The CIN terminology subdivides high-grade SIL into two categories, CIN 2 and CIN 3. This distinction is made on the basis of the proportion of the epithelial thickness occupied by undifferentiated neoplastic cells. In CIN 2, the immature basaloid-type cells occupy up to two-thirds of the epithelial thickness but do not extend into the upper third of the epithelium (Fig. 7.16). Similarly, mitoses are found in the lower two-thirds of the epithelium but not in the upper third. In CIN 3 lesions, immature basaloid-type cells occupy the upper third of the epithelium and mitoses can be present at any level. Studies of the reproducibility of the histopathologic diagnosis of different grades of cervical cancer precursors have shown that diagnosis of CIN 2 is not reproducible.[125,238] The lack of reproducibility of the diagnosis of CIN 2 is a result of the subjective criteria used to separate the different grades of CIN and the fact that the thickness of the epithelium occupied by immature basaloid-type cells varies considerably, even in cervical biopsy specimens.

A subset of high-grade SIL has been further subdivided by some investigators into three cytologic subtypes: small cell anaplastic, large cell keratinizing, and large cell nonkeratinizing dysplasia.[217] The small cell variety is usually found within the external os or endocervical canal and is composed of small, undifferentiated, malignant cells of the basal cell type (Fig. 7.17). The large cell keratinizing lesion originates on the exposed portion of the cervix and displays prominent intercellular bridges, macronucleoli, and extensive surface keratinization (Fig. 7.18). Large cell nonkeratinizing lesions are by far the most frequent of all intraepithelial carcinomas of the cervix and are found within the cervical transformation zone. The epithelium is composed of undifferentiated cells the size of normal parabasal cells (Fig. 7.19). Individual cell keratinization may be encountered. Because accurate studies concerning the invasive potential of each of these subtypes are lacking, prediction of the likelihood of progression to invasive carcinoma should not be based on this subclassification.

In most tissues, aneuploidy is a marker of malignant potential. Chromosomal karyotyping studies as well as studies directly measuring the DNA content of lesional tissue support the concept that aneuploid SIL lesions are true cervical cancer precursors. By either Feulgen microspectroscopy or flow cytometry, the majority of low-grade SIL are diploid or polyploid whereas the majority of high-grade SIL

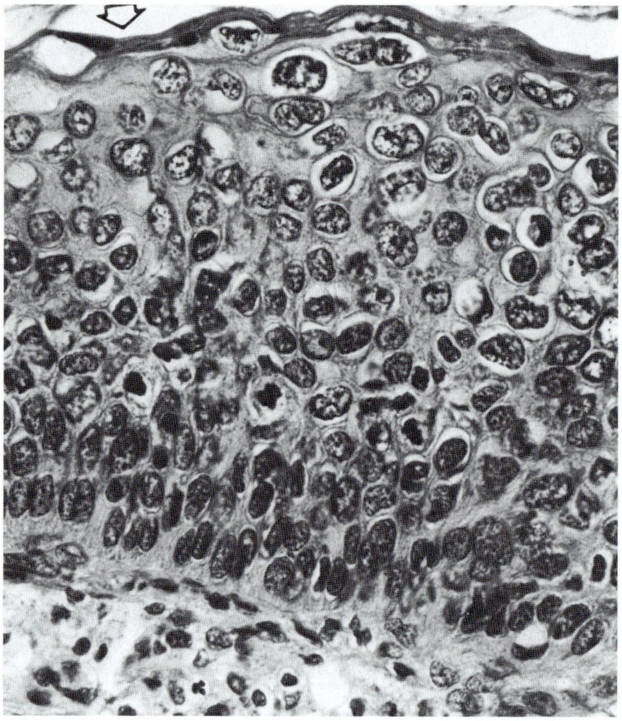

Fig. 7.18. High-grade SIL. This type of high-grade SIL has been referred to as *large cell keratinizing carcinoma in situ*. Note cellular prominence, well-defined cytoplasmic membranes, occasional koilocytes, and fine surface keratinization (*arrow*).

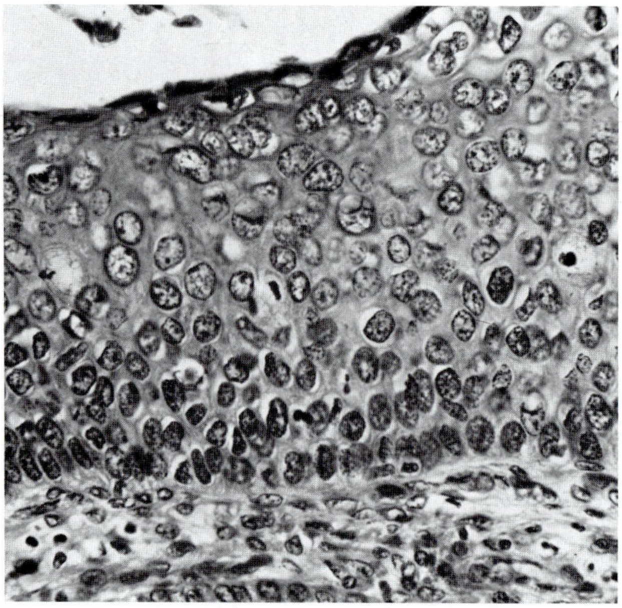

Fig. 7.19. High-grade SIL. This type of high grade SIL has been referred to as *large cell nonkeratinizing carcinoma in situ*. The neoplastic cells have hyperchromatic nuclei with clumping of chromatin. There is a high degree of cellular disorder, and cytoplasmic membranes are indistinct.

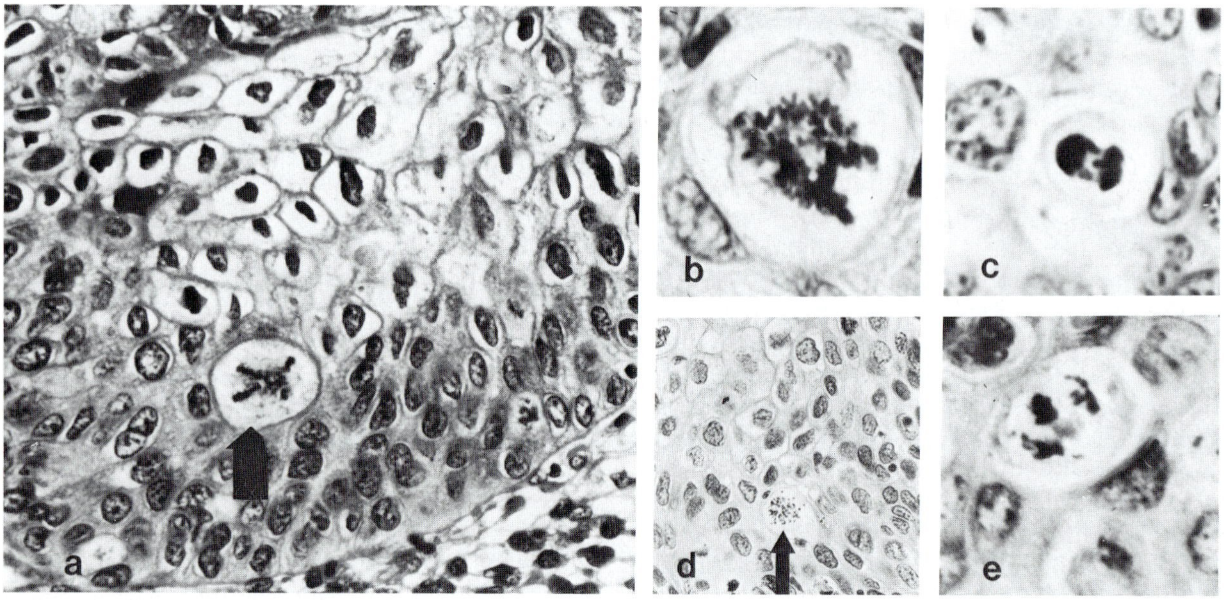

Fig. 7.20. Abnormal mitotic figures. Morphologic variability of abnormal mitotic figures in aneuploid CIN lesions. **a**: Quadripolar mitotic figure (*arrow*) in a lesion with extensive koilocytosis. **b**: Bizarre mitotic figure with Y shape and numerous poorly organized chromosomes. **c**: Two-group metaphase. **d**: Dispersed mitotic figure (arrow) with finely distributed chromosomes. **e**: Three-group metaphase.

are aneuploid.[92,127] In both prospective and retrospective studies, ploidy has been a good predictor of clinical behavior; the majority of SIL that progress or persist have been aneuploid whereas the majority of those that regress are diploid or polyploid.[111] A number of studies have compared histologic features with ploidy levels and found that cervical lesions with diploid or polyploid DNA contents generally retain polarity of the basal cell layer and lack abnormal mitotic figures, whereas aneuploid lesions have more marked nuclear atypia and more cellular disorganization. The best histologic correlate of aneuploid is *abnormal mitotic figures* (AMF) (Fig. 7.20).[18,92]

Some authors, therefore, have suggested that AMFs other than multipolar and dispersed metaphases are an accurate histologic surrogate of aneuploidy and can be used as a histological determinate for discriminating between low-grade SIL and high-grade SIL.[233] However, AMFs should not be used as the sole criterion for discriminating between low-grade SIL and high-grade SIL for several reasons: (1) AMFs can be difficult to distinguish from karyorrhexis; (2) detection of AMFs is influenced by variables that are independent of ploidy level, including size of biopsy, quality of fixation, quality of the microscopic section, and number of levels examined; and (3) some high-grade SIL lesions, and even some invasive cancers, lack AMFs and are not aneuploid.[21,105,195] Therefore, although a lesion showing these features with unequivocal AMFs should be classified as high-grade SIL, the converse is not true. Lesions with the other histologic features of a high-grade SIL should be classified as such even in the absence of AMFs. It is also important to point out that using these criteria some high-grade lesions have cells with prominent HPV cytopathic effects similar to those seen in low-grade SIL (Fig. 7.21). The presence of such cells should not be taken as evidence that the lesion is low grade if other features of a high-grade lesion are present. Therefore, the criteria that are used for distinguishing low-grade SIL from high-grade SIL include other features such as the distribution of immature, basal-type cells, the level at which mitotic figures in the epithelium are identified, the extent of abnormalities of differentiation and polarity, and the degree of nuclear atypia (Table 7.11).

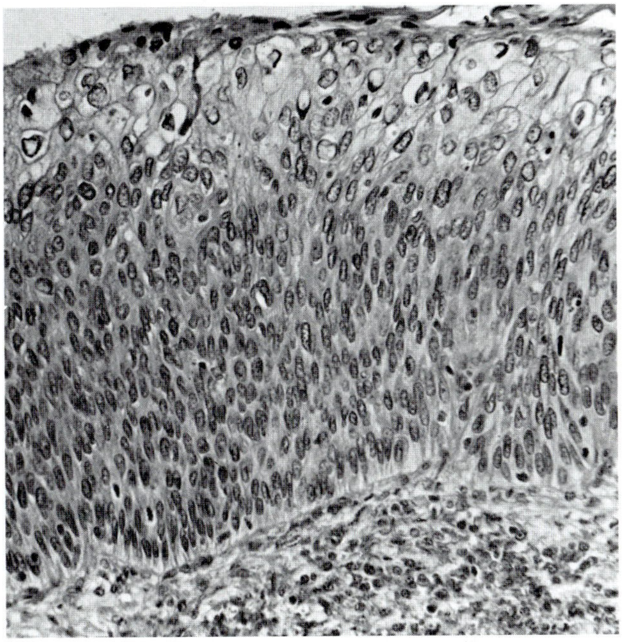

Fig. 7.21. High-grade SIL. Even though the upper third of the epithelium is occupied by single and multinucleated koilocytes, this is a high-grade SIL with undifferentiated basal-type cells replacing approximately two-thirds of the epithelium.

Differential Diagnosis

Immature metaplasia and atrophy are the lesions most commonly mistaken for high-grade SIL. In immature metaplasia, the full thickness of the epithelium is composed of immature parabasal cells with a high nuclear:cytoplasmic ratio (Fig. 7.22). The cells usually are vertical, and the nuclei are only slightly hyperchromatic. The most helpful feature in distinguishing high-grade SIL from immature metaplasia is the absence of nuclear pleomorphism in

Table 7.11. Distinguishing features of low-grade SIL and high-grade SIL

Feature	*Low-grade SIL*	*High-grade SIL*
HPV types	Any anogenital HPV	High-risk types*
Koilocytosis	Frequently present	Occasionally present
Ploidy	Mostly diploid or polyploid	Usually aneuploid
Abnormal Mitotic Figures	Absent	Frequent
Location of undifferentiated cells and mitotic figures	Lower third	Upper two-thirds

*High risk types of HPV include 16, 18, 45, 56, 58.

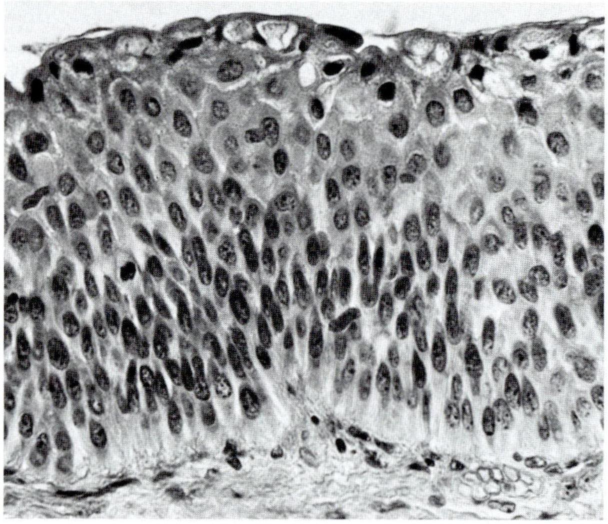

Fig. 7.22. Immature squamous metaplastic epithelium. Metaplastic squamous cells proliferate beneath the mucinous endocervical cells. These may be confused with koilocytes; however, their vacuolar features are due to mucinous-vacuolar degeneration secondary to their separation from the basal lamina rather than papillomavirus infection. Note the hyperplasia of the basal cells with occasional mitotic divisions and attempt at cytoplasmic maturation in the upper half of the epithelium. The cells in the upper strata of the epithelium are regularly orientated, with uniformly disposed nuclear chromatin and cellular borders. Intercellular bridges are well defined.

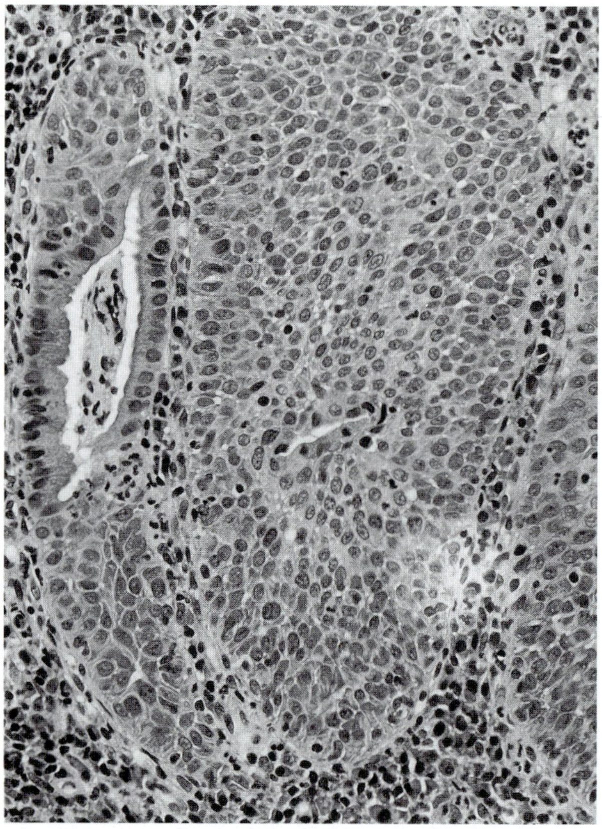

Fig. 7.24. Atypical immature metaplasia. This lesion is composed of proliferating metaplastic squamous cells that have nuclear atypia, but to a lesser degree than usually associated with SIL.

the latter. Immature metaplasia may have mitotic activity, but abnormal mitotic figures are not present. The chromatin in metaplastic squamous epithelium is finer and more evenly distributed than in high-grade SIL. In addition, cellular polarity is

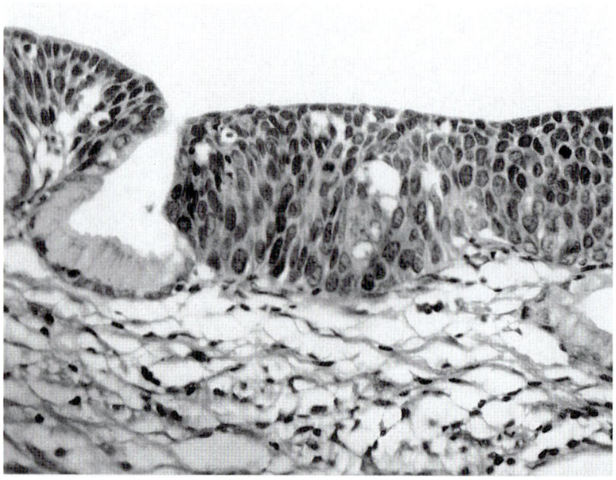

Fig. 7.23. Immature squamous metaplastic epithelium. The nuclei of the metaplastic squamous cells vary somewhat in size and shape, but lack coarse clumped chromatin and abnormal mitotic figures.

retained, cell membranes are clearly defined, and cellular crowding is not marked. Finally, mucinous epithelium is often present on the surface of immature metaplastic squamous epithelium but rarely overlies SIL (Fig. 7.23). Sometimes there may be nuclear atypia within immature metaplasia (Fig. 7.24); such lesions are designated by some as *atypical immature metaplasia*.[60] The use of this term is not generally recommended unless clarified with a note because it is not widely accepted and may be confusing to clinicians.

Reparative processes may also be misinterpreted as high-grade SIL (Fig. 7.25). In reparative processes atypical basal cells occupy the lower half of the epithelium but the cells have a regular nuclear outline, prominent nucleoli, and usually have distinct cell membranes. In addition, dense acute and chronic inflammatory infiltrates are usually present. Atrophic epithelium is occasionally difficult to distinguish from high-grade SIL because it is composed of basal and parabasal cells showing no differentiation. Although there is a high nuclear:cytoplasmic ratio, atrophic epithelium is thin and shows no nuclear pleomorphism, mitotic ac-

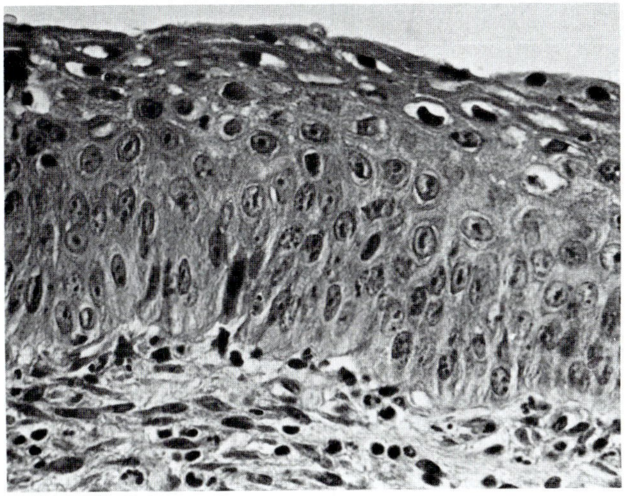

Fig. 7.25. Atypia of repair. Note abnormal maturation. Atypical basal cells occupy the lower half of the epithelium, simulating a high-grade SIL lesion with koilocytosis. Unlike SIL however, the basal cells in atypia of repair have a regular nuclear outline, prominent nucleoli, and distinct cell membranes. Additionally, cells in the upper half of the epithelium are not koilocytotic but contain degenerative perinuclear elliptoid-shaped halos.

tivity, atypia, or lack of polarity. In older women, in whom it is difficult to distinguish atrophy from a high-grade SIL, immunohistochemical staining using Ki-67 is frequently quite helpful. Atrophic epithelium shows either absent or minimal staining with Ki-67 whereas SIL stains strongly. Another approach that can be taken in difficult cases is to obtain a repeat biopsy after a course of topical, daily estrogen that includes maturation in the atrophic epithelium. In contrast, estrogen administration does not alter the appearance of SIL. Finally, high-grade SIL, particularly with extensive gland involvement, may be confused with microinvasive carcinoma (see Chapter 8, Carcinoma and Other Tumors of the Cervix).

Clinical Behavior

The behavior of SIL has been studied extensively using two types of studies, prospective, clinical follow-up studies of individual women with cervical lesions and epidemiologic studies linking cytology records with cancer registries. Large-scale prospective clinical studies with follow-up using cytology with colposcopy, without biopsy, are particularly useful.

Studies of the "natural history" or behavior of different grades of dysplasia have provided widely varying estimates of the rate of progression and regression the different lesions (Table 7.12). This result is not surprising because various studies have used different entry criteria, different diagnostic criteria for categorizing lesions as SIL, and different study designs. For example, some studies have used punch biopsy and endocervical curettage to establish the diagnosis. These diagnostic methods may remove (treat) lesions and therefore may interfere with long-term analysis by increasing the frequency of spontaneous regression and decreasing the frequency of progression.[200]

One of the largest long-term clinical follow studies of women with SIL was carried out in Sweden by Nasiell and coworkers. In this study, 555 women with mild dysplasia and 894 women with moderate dysplasia were followed on average for 39 and 78 months, respectively.[200,201] In 62% of the women with mild dysplasia, regression to normal occurred; in 22%, there was persistence of mild or moderate dysplasia; and in 16% there was progression of mild dysplasia to severe dysplasia or "carcinoma in situ." In women with moderate dysplasia followed without biopsy for an average of 51 months, spontaneous regression occurred in 28% and progression to severe dysplasia or carcinoma in situ occurred in 50%. Many other prospective follow-up studies of low-grade SIL have found rates of regression, progression, and persistence similar to those reported by Nasiell et al. (see Table 7.12). Taken together, these

Table 7.12. Natural history of low-grade SIL

Study	*No. of pts.*	*Regressed*	*Persisted*	*Progressed*
Campion et al.	100	7%	67%	26%
Greenberg et al.	176	46%	46%	9%
Heinzl et al.	2417	46%	44%	10%
Kataja et al.	532	43%	39%	16%
Nasiell et al.	555	62%	22%	16%
Robertson et al.	1347	57%	27%	15%
Total	5337	51%	36%	13%

*Includes both CIN 1 and CIN 2.
Modified from refs. 41, 102, 110, 140, 201, 239.

Table 7.13. Toronto long-term follow-up of abnormal cervical cytology

Grade of lesion	*2 years*	*10 years*
Regression rates[A]		
mild dysplasia	44%	88%
moderate dysplasia	33%	83%
Progression rates		
mild dysplasia	0.6%	12%
moderate dysplasia	1.5%	17%
severe dysplasia	2.8%	21%

[A]Regression to within normal limits.
*Progression to carcinoma in situ or worse.
Modified from ref. 118.

studies clearly demonstrate that although approximately 15% of low-grade SIL lesions have the potential for progressing to high-grade SIL and about 46% persist, many of these lesions (approximately 44%) regress spontaneously if left untreated.

Another informative study recently evaluated the records of the largest cytology laboratory serving the Toronto (Canada) region and linked these records with the Ontario Tumor Registry for the years 1962–1980.[118] During this time, most women with dysplasia who were evaluated by this laboratory were managed conservatively and did not undergo treatment. This study provides an unique insight into the long-term natural history of untreated SIL (Table 7.13). The key findings of this study were that after 10 years of follow-up only 12% of untreated mild dysplasia and 17% of untreated moderate dysplasia progressed to carcinoma in situ. At 10 years, 88% of the mild dysplasia and 83% of cases of moderate dysplasia had regressed.[118]

High-grade SIL has a much greater potential for progressing than does low-grade SIL (Table 7.14). In a prospective analysis reported by McIndoe et al., carcinoma in situ progressed to invasive carcinoma in 29% of patients followed from 1 to 20 years, and the rate of progression increased directly with the length of follow-up, peaking at 34.6% in patients followed for 14 years.[182] In another study, Kottmeier reported that 71% of women with carcinoma in situ developed invasive carcinoma during a minimum follow-up period of 12 years.[155] Other long-term retrospective studies have demonstrated progression of carcinoma in situ to invasive cancer in 22–72% of cases.

The prevalence of low-grade SIL proportionally decreases with age.[38,269] Mathematical calculations derived from incidence rates suggest that new lesions arise in the form of low-grade instead of high-grade SIL. There is a 1000 to 2000 fold higher annual incidence of high-grade SIL in women with previously documented low-grade SIL than in those with normal cytologic findings.[38,269] In animals, cervical lesions also develop through progressive stages of SIL to frankly invasive carcinoma.[243] Therefore, it has been believed that high-grade SIL always develops from low-grade SIL. Richart and coworkers contend that high-grade SIL usually begins as a small focus within a low-grade SIL.[231] This small focus then gradually expands and replaces the low-grade SIL. According to this theory, the transition from a low-grade SIL to a high-grade SIL represents a monoclonal event within an HPV-infected epithelium. That such transitions can occur has been shown by a chromosomal study of SIL and microinvasive carcinoma in a single patient that demonstrated that both lesions had a similar abnormal modal number and marker chromosomes.[265]

It should be pointed out, however, that several lines of evidence suggest that high-grade SIL may develop as an independent event without progressing from low-grade SIL. Based primarily on mapping studies, Burghart and coworkers, as well as Koss, have argued that high-grade SIL does not develop by a direct transformation from low-grade SIL.[38,153] Instead, they have suggested that high-grade SIL develops de novo from the epithelium adjacent to low-grade SIL. Prospective follow-up studies also suggest that at least some high-grade SIL lesions can develop independently from low-grade SIL. In a study of women visiting an STD clinic, Koutsky et al. found that most cases of high-grade

Table 7.14. Natural history of carcinoma in situ (CIS)

Study	*No. of pts.*	*Follow-up*	*Regressed*	*Persisted*	*Progressed*
Gad	16	0.5–17 yrs	31%	41%	
Kottmeier	30	>12 yrs			72%
Koss et al.	67	6 yrs	25%	61%	6%
McIndoe et al.	131	1–28 yrs	8%	69%	22%
Sorensen et al.	127	>5 yrs		35%	
Spriggs et al.	37	>2 yrs	41%	60%	

Modified from refs. 94, 154, 155, 182, 262, 265A.

SIL arose de novo in this population in the absence of a cytologically detectable, low-grade SIL.[157] In another study of women infected with high-risk and HPV types, Nobbenhuis et al. found that 88% of the incident cases of SIL were first identified as high-grade SIL.[207] On the basis of these and other data, some authors have challenged the entire concept that low-grade SIL is a precursor to high-grade SIL.[145]

Management

Current management of SIL depends on a combination of cytology, colposcopy, and directed biopsy, as outlined in Fig. 7.26.[4,162,235] This management protocol provides a logical approach to therapy based on lesion size, distribution, and grade. The primary objectives both for the clinician treating the patient and the pathologist examining the specimens are (1) to rule out invasive cancer and (2) to determine the extent and distribution of noninvasive lesions. Once these objectives have been met, the clinician treating the patient may select from a variety of options for managing women with SIL. Although an extensive discussion of the workup and management of women with cervical disease is beyond the purview of this chapter, pathologists should have a basic understanding of this workup if they are to provide information that will facilitate patient management.

Colposcopy and Cervical Biopsy

If the clinician believes that a woman with an abnormal Pap test has a significant chance of having a high-grade SIL, a glandular lesion, or cancer, colposcopy is generally performed. The risk of an individual patient having a significant cervical lesion varies proportionally with the degree of cytologic abnormality and is influenced by other factors such as the patient's age, immune status, and previous medical history. In general, women with atypical squamous cells of undetermined significance have only a 5–10% risk of having a high-grade SIL or invasive cancer of the cervix. Therefore, these women can be followed up in a variety of ways, ranging from repeating the Papanicolaou test at intervals of 4–6 months until two consecutive Papanicolaou tests within normal limits are obtained, testing the patient for high-risk HPV types and performing colposcopy if a high-risk HPV type is identified, or performing colposcopy (see Fig. 7.26).

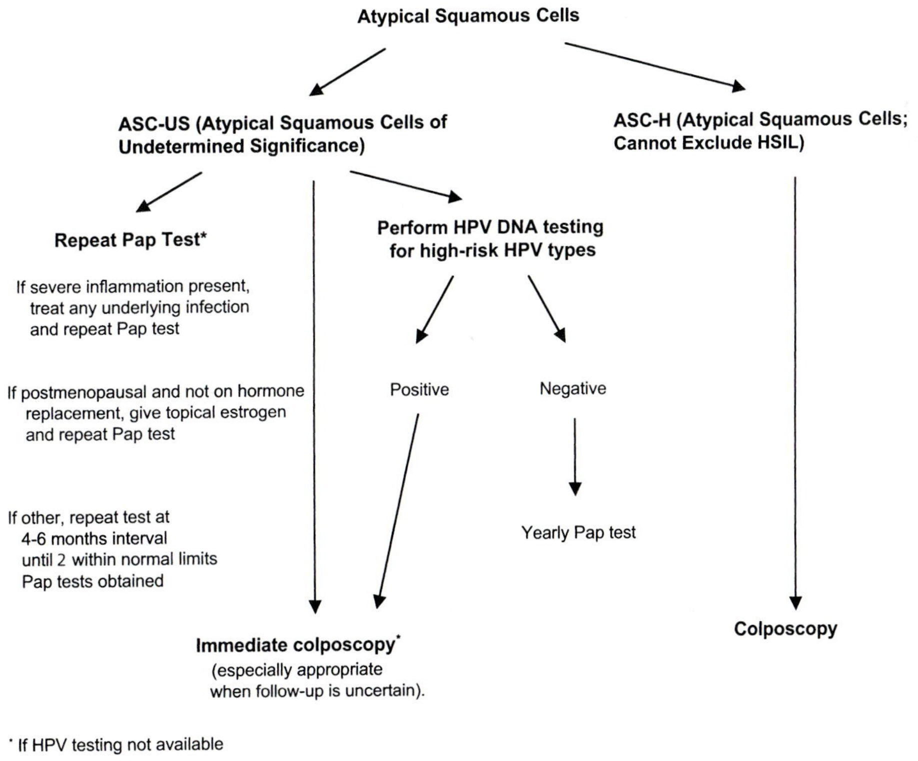

Fig. 7.26. Diagnostic evaluation, treatment, and follow-up of patients with abnormal cytology: Three different options.

(continues on next page)

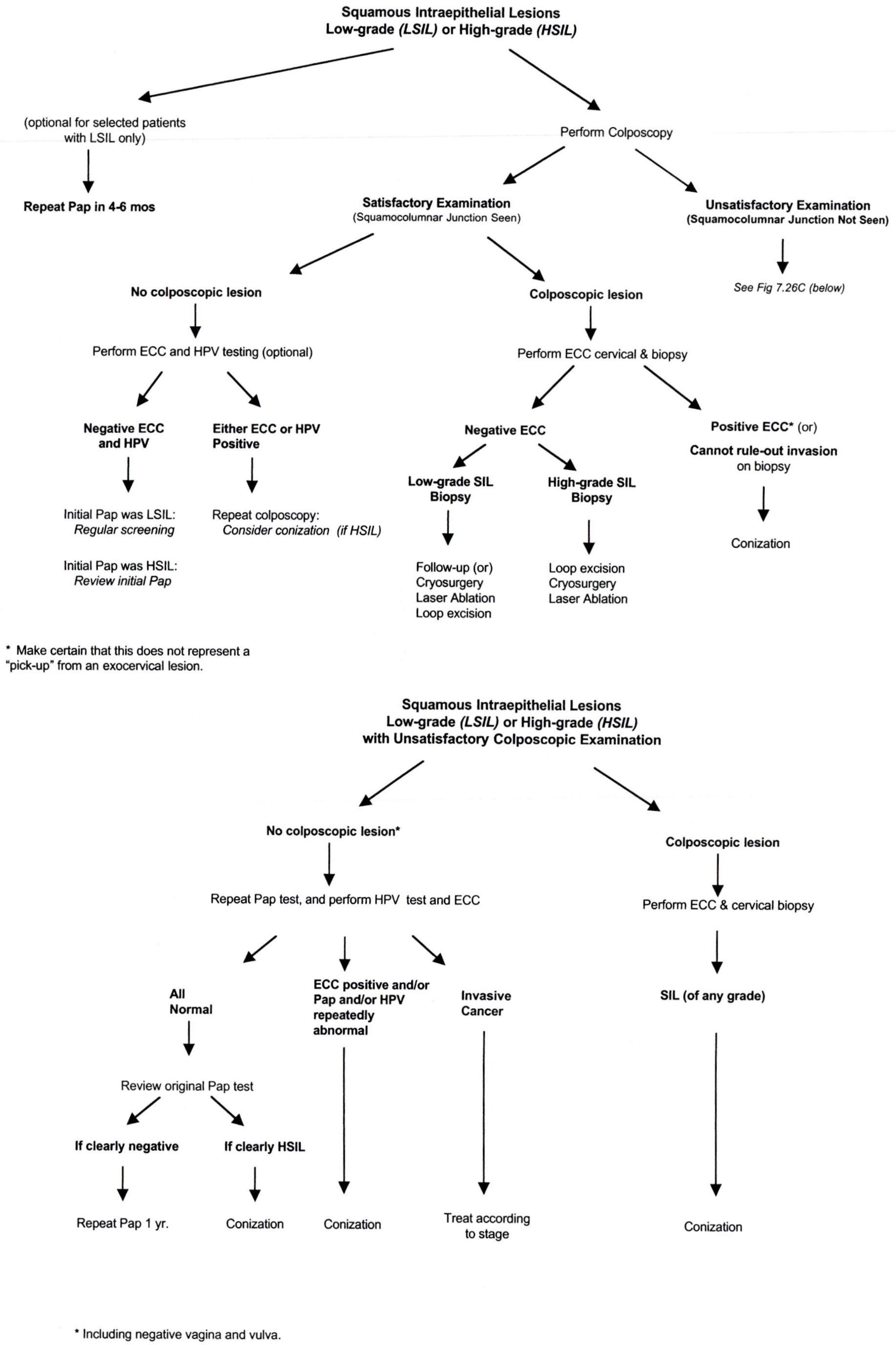

Squamous Intraepithelial Lesions
Low-grade (LSIL) or High-grade (HSIL)
(optional for selected patients with LSIL only)
Repeat Pap in 4-6 mos
Perform Colposcopy
Satisfactory Examination
(Squamocolumnar Junction Seen)
Unsatisfactory Examination
(Squamocolumnar Junction Not Seen)
See Fig 7.26C (below)
No colposcopic lesion
Perform ECC and HPV testing (optional)
Negative ECC and HPV
Initial Pap was LSIL: Regular screening
Initial Pap was HSIL: Review initial Pap
Either ECC or HPV Positive
Repeat colposcopy: Consider conization (if HSIL)
Colposcopic lesion
Perform ECC cervical & biopsy
Negative ECC
Low-grade SIL Biopsy
Follow-up (or)
Cryosurgery
Laser Ablation
Loop excision
High-grade SIL Biopsy
Loop excision
Cryosurgery
Laser Ablation
Positive ECC* (or)
Cannot rule-out invasion on biopsy
Conization
* Make certain that this does not represent a "pick-up" from an exocervical lesion.
Squamous Intraepithelial Lesions
Low-grade (LSIL) or High-grade (HSIL)
with Unsatisfactory Colposcopic Examination
No colposcopic lesion*
Repeat Pap test, and perform HPV test and ECC
All Normal
Review original Pap test
If clearly negative
Repeat Pap 1 yr.
If clearly HSIL
Conization
ECC positive and/or Pap and/or HPV repeatedly abnormal
Conization
Invasive Cancer
Treat according to stage
Colposcopic lesion
Perform ECC & cervical biopsy
SIL (of any grade)
Conization
* Including negative vagina and vulva.

Fig. 7.26. (*Continued*) Diagnostic evaluation, treatment, and follow-up of patients with abnormal cytology: Three different options.

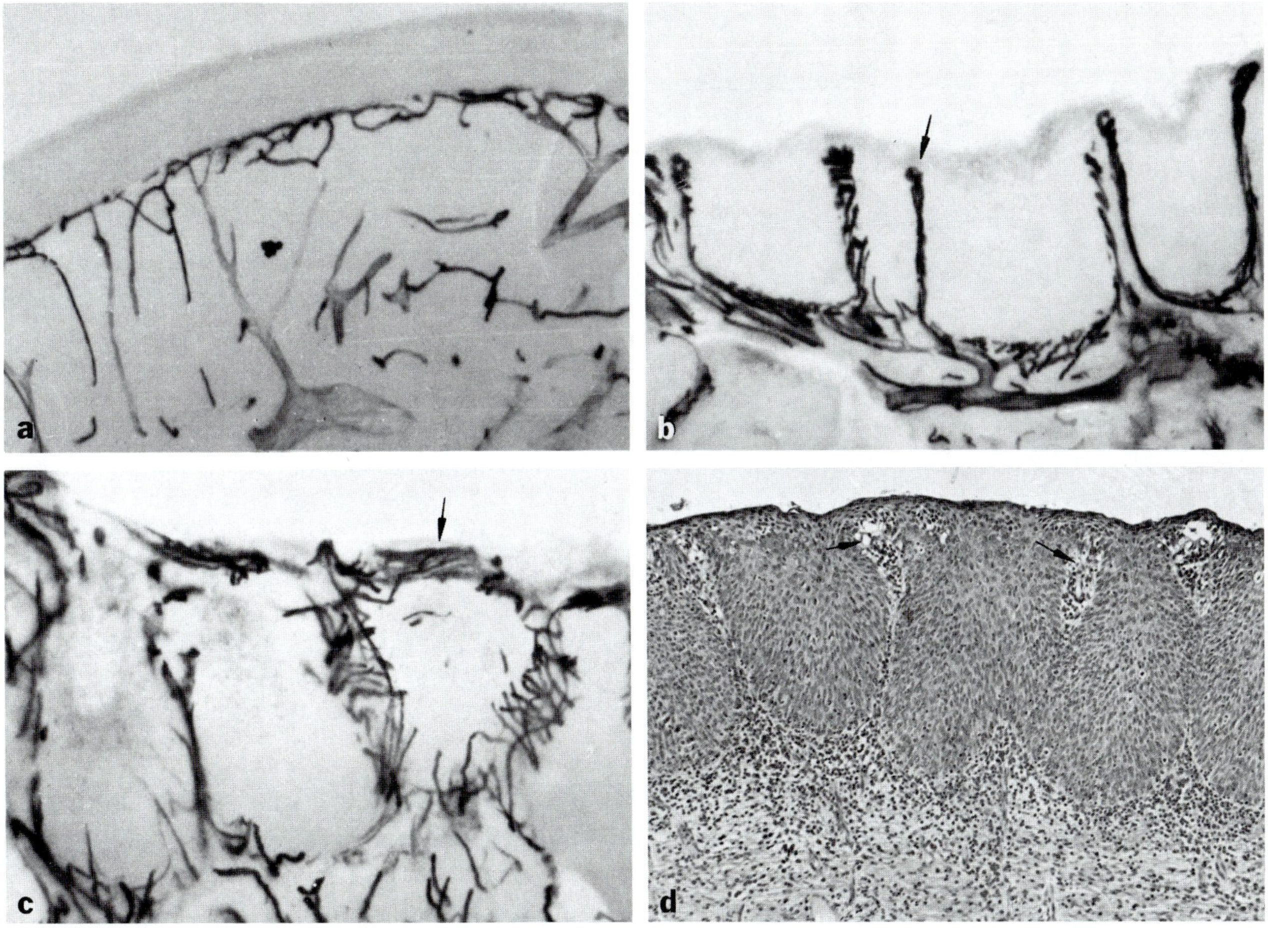

Fig. 7.27. Histochemical preparations of the terminal vascular network of the cervix. a: Flat capillary network beneath normal squamous epithelium. b: Abnormal vascular growth (*arrow*) in advanced SIL, producing colposcopic mosaic pattern. c: Abnormal horizontal vascular pattern (*arrow*) in early invasive carcinoma of cervix. d: Histology of high-grade SIL in which the vascular stroma papillae are compressed vertically by masses of neoplastic cells, with extension near the surface (*arrows*) producing a colposcopic pattern of punctation. (Courtesy of Dr. A. Stafl, Milwaukee.)

The colposcope is a stereoscopic binocular magnifying instrument that provides a three-dimensional image of the tissue surfaces examined. Morphologic changes of the epithelium and the vascular pattern that accompany SIL and invasive cancer can be visualized and magnified from 4 to 40 times. Before colposcopic examination, a 3–5% solution of acetic acid is applied to the cervix to remove mucus and dehydrate cells; in areas that microscopically display abnormal surface keratinization, epithelial hyperplasia, or nuclear crowding, the mucosa appears white.

Colposcopic examination of the cervix is limited to the portio and outer third of the endocervical canal. It is inadequate for the evaluation of endocervical neoplasia. The entire transformation zone and lesion, if present, must be visualized for the colposcopic examination to be considered satisfactory. Colposcopic diagnosis is based on the evaluation of the surface contour, color tone (degree of opacity), and border of the lesions.[7,39] In addition to epithelial abnormalities, the subepithelial vascular network undergoes profound alterations in association with SIL.[266] The flat capillary network, which is found beneath the normal cervical epithelium, becomes tortuous and compressed vertically by the actively growing epithelium, with extension close to the surface (Fig. 7.27) producing a colposcopic pattern of punctation (Fig. 7.28). Further proliferation and interconnection of proliferating masses of epithelium result in compression of the vascular network into basket-like structures around the abnormal epithelium, producing a colposcopic mosaic pattern (see Fig. 7.27). Because of severe compression, some of the capillaries eventually disappear, resulting in an increase in the intercapillary dis-

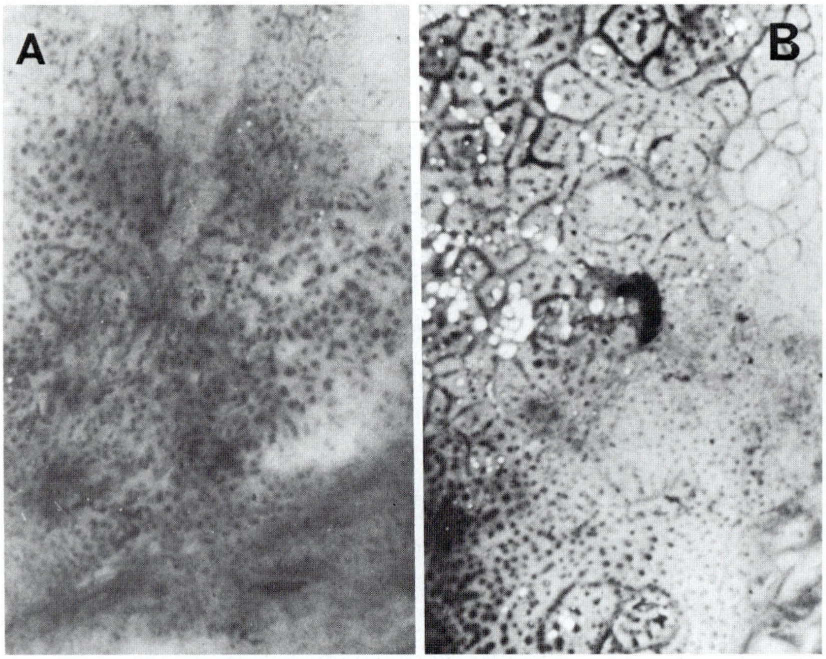

Fig. 7.28. Colposcopic appearances of SIL. a: Colposcopic pattern of punctation. Note variation in size of punctate vessels and intercapillary distance. b: Colposcopic pattern of mosaic. The epithelium is compartmentalized into irregular baskets and is associated with a coarse punctation pattern.

tance. In early invasive carcinoma, a system of new capillaries is generated running parallel to the surface of the abnormal epithelium; this is the so-called horizontal capillary network. These vascular changes and variation in the intercapillary distance are the most important diagnostic colposcopic criteria that serve to distinguish noninvasive from invasive cervical squamous carcinoma.[7,39] Areas with the most pronounced colposcopic abnormality are sampled using a small punch biopsy instrument, such as the square-jawed Kevorkian biopsy punch.

Endocervical Sampling

Many clinicians perform an endocervical sampling during colposcopic evaluation of the cervix. Endocervical sampling is performed to evaluate lesion distribution and morphology within the endocervical canal and to exclude the presence of invasive carcinoma, unsuspected cervical adenocarcinoma in situ, and invasive adenocarcinoma. Endocervical sampling contributes to the diagnostic accuracy of the colposcopic evaluation, particularly in patients in whom no exocervical lesion can be visualized or in whom the squamocolumnar junction is within the endocervical canal.[108,116,149] The endocervical curettage (ECC) specimen consists of endocervical tissue fragments, blood, mucus, and, when positive, strips of atypical epithelium (Fig. 7.29). To avoid the loss of tiny tissue fragments during processing, the clinician should collect and concentrate the sample, including mucus and blood, on a small square of lens paper or using a cytobrush and immediately place it in the fixative. By this method, even the smallest tissue fragments can be recovered easily in the laboratory, embedded, and sectioned in their entirety.

In most instances, when atypical epithelium is detected in the endocervical curettage it lacks underlying stroma and orientation is not possible. As a result, the pathologist can neither rule out underlying invasion nor grade an intraepithelial lesion. In other cases in which the atypical epithelium is well oriented, the pathologist is able to grade the lesion and can, if desired. However, it should be emphasized that a basic principle of colposcopy is that unless a SIL lesion is visualized in its entirety during the examination, cancer has not been ruled out and a cone biopsy is required regardless of the grade of the SIL. It is also helpful if the pathologist conveys an estimate of the amount of atypical epithelium that is present in the endocervical curettage. If only a few small fragments of atypical epithelium are present in the endocervical curettage, these may represent "pick-ups" from a lesion that is actually confined to the portio and does not extend into the endocervical canal. In such cases it is preferable to reexamine the patient with the colposcope rather than proceeding directly with conization. If the lesion is fully visualized, the endocervical curettage should be repeated under colposcopic visualization to avoid lesional tissue on the portio. The second, carefully performed curettage frequently yields no atypical epithelium, and the patient may be managed on a conservative, outpatient basis. Conversely, the pathologist should be careful not to discount or

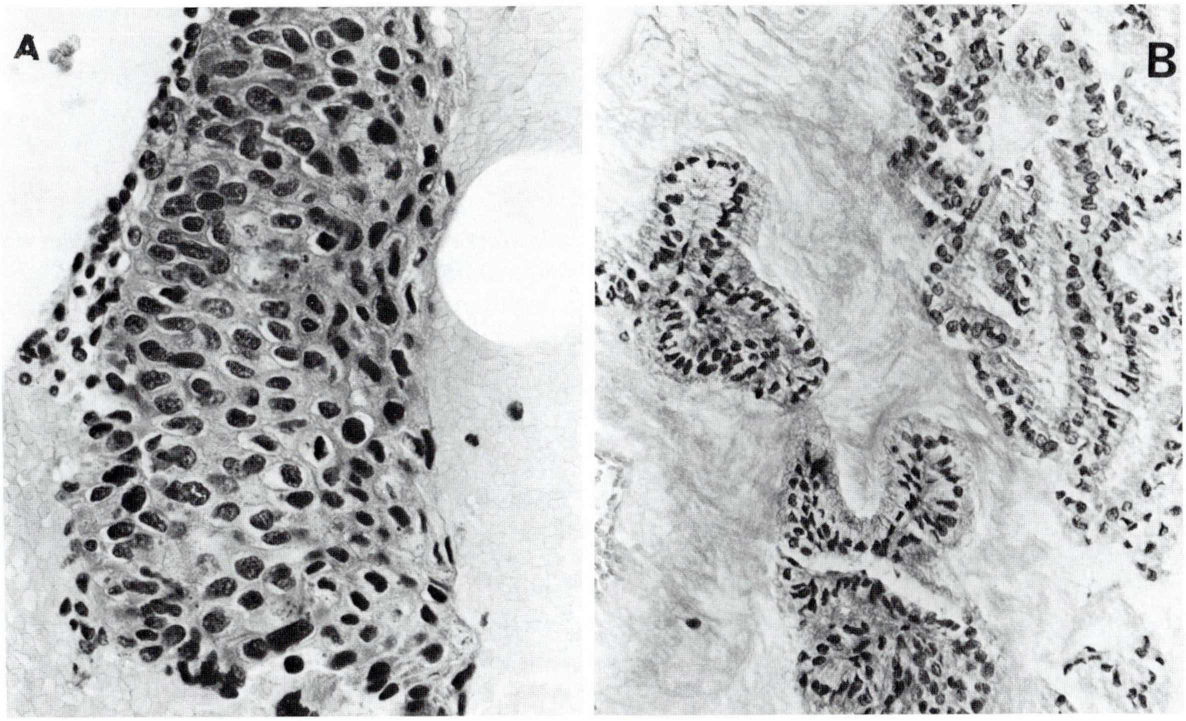

Fig. 7.29. Endocervical curettings. **a**: Positive endocervical curetting with a strip of atypical epithelium. The latter lacks orientation and underlying stroma. As a result, grading cannot be performed, and invasion cannot be ruled out. **b**: Negative endocervical curetting with fragments of endocervical epithelium.

overlook a few fragments or even a single fragment of atypical epithelium in an endocervical curettage. In a review of 21 women who developed invasive cancer after cryotherapy, 7 of 18 endocervical curettages taken before cryotherapy were found on review to contain SIL that had been missed at the time of original diagnosis.[252]

Cervical Conization

Cervical conization is performed as a diagnostic procedure under a number of different circumstances (Table 7.15). A cervical conization specimen represents a conically shaped section of cervix performed for both diagnostic and therapeutic purposes. The cone size varies according to lesion distribution and corresponding operative plan: shallow conization for a predominantly exocervical lesion or a deep cone for a predominantly endocervical lesion. The apex and base of the sample represent the endocervical and exocervical margins, respectively. The technique for processing the specimen is discussed in Chapter 28, Gross Description, Processing, and Reporting of Gynecologic and Obstetric Specimens.

Treatment

It should be stressed that the observations on the behavior of SIL described previously apply only to a population and provide no objective means to predict the potential of regression, persistence, or progression of SIL in the individual patient. Because it is impossible to predict which patients will progress to invasion with a given SIL at a given time, many clinicians think that these lesions, once detected, regardless of degree or morphologic severity, should be treated to prevent the development of invasive carcinoma. However, as increasing numbers of young patients are diagnosed with low-grade SIL, other clinicians are now taking a more conservative approach and are following patients with low-grade

Table 7.15. Indications for cone biopsy

Normal colposcopy,[a] persistent abnormal cytology or positive endocervical curettage
Abnormal cytology, squamocolumnar junction not visualized
Limits of lesion not visualized
Microinvasive carcinoma on biopsy or colposcopy suspicious of invasive carcinoma
Adenocarcinoma in situ on biopsy or endocervical curettage
Lack of significant correlation among cytologic, colposcopic, and histologic findings

[a]Including the vagina, vulva, and urethra.

SIL.[162,235] However, in the United States in most instances a diagnosis of high-grade SIL results in the patient being treated with ablative (cryosurgical or laser surgical) or excisional (electrosurgical loop excision or cone biopsy) therapy.

Cryosurgery as a method for ablating SIL was introduced in the 1970s and is one of the most frequently used techniques for treating lesions limited to the portio. The failure or residual rate (5–15%) and the long-term recurrence rate (1 of 1000 women per year develops a new SIL following successful cryotherapy) in experienced hands do not exceed that of therapeutic conization.[190,283] Cure rates are not affected by the grade of lesion treated, with only lesion size and quality of freeze proving to be prognostic variables of statistical significance.[79,283] Furthermore, the complications and costs of cryosurgery are negligible compared to those of conization. Cryodestruction of cervical tissue is caused by freezing tissue below −22°C with a cryoprobe applied to the cervix. Intracellular and extracellular crystallization leads to dehydration of cells, which results in high electrolyte concentrations that produce biochemical injury associated with lysosomal enzyme release and cell destruction. The only significant endpoint for successful cryosurgical management of SIL is that the margins of the ice ball extend 5 mm and preferably 10 mm beyond the limits of the lesion. Postcryotherapy cervical epithelium quickly sloughs, and healing is generally completed with 4–6 weeks.

The carbon dioxide (CO_2) laser is another treatment modality for noninvasive neoplasia of the cervix, vagina, and vulva. Unlike conventional light, which is emitted in all directions and has low energy, laser light is composed of parallel beams of uniform wave lengths (10.6 μm). The laser beam thus can be directed onto a small spot where it produces a very high energy density. In the CO_2 laser, a mixture of CO_2, nitrogen, and helium is excited by an electrical discharge, and the excited CO_2 molecules give off photons of light energy in the infrared (invisible) part of the spectrum. The light energy is amplified, focused, and directed by a luminous spot of the target beam. Energy output ranges from 1 to 100 W. The laser beam energy is absorbed by the intracellular and extracellular water in tissues, and tissue temperatures rise instantaneously above 100°C. The tissue fluids boil and expand, and the exploded cells are evaporated. As a result, CO_2 laser treatment produces considerably less necrosis than cryosurgery. Evaporation of tissues permits more rapid healing with less vaginal discharge than is associated with cryosurgery.[267] The failure and recurrence rates of laser treatment of cervical lesions are similar to those of cryosurgery.[283] The cost of the equipment is its major disadvantage when compared to cryotherapy. Extensive cervical lesions and associated vaginal or vulvar lesions can be more easily and appropriately treated by laser surgery than by cryotherapy.[79]

The loop electrosurgical excision procedure is a technique that is being increasingly used to treat patients with SIL.[223,307] With this technique, a tissue specimen is obtained using thin wire loop electrodes that simultaneously cut and coagulate the tissue. Because a tissue specimen is obtained each time the procedure is performed, the technique is both diagnostic as well as therapeutic. As with cervical biopsies, the role of pathologic examination of this specimen is to rule out invasive cancer and rule in the presence of SIL. Because this technique is performed under colposcopic guidance, the colposcopist can determine whether the "true" surgical margin of excision is free of disease at the time the procedure is performed, and the pathologist need not report margins.

Clinical Uses of HPV Testing

During the past 5 years, a number of studies have evaluated HPV DNA testing using the Hybrid Capture II assay as a form of intermediate triage to determine which women with ASCUS Pap smears should be referred for colposcopy and which women can be returned to routine cytologic screening. These studies have found that HPV DNA testing identifies more cases of high-grade SIL than does a single repeat Papanicolaou smear but refers approximately equivalent numbers of women for colposcopy.[51,56,178,261,273,309] In a study of women with an ASCUS referred for colposcopy, Wright et al. found that high-risk HPV DNA testing correctly identified 89% of the cases of biopsy-confirmed high-grade SIL and would have referred a total of 62% of women to colposcopy.[309] A repeat Papanicolaou test (liquid-based) correctly identified 70% of the cases of high-grade SIL and would have referred 56% of the women to colposcopy. Using receiver–operator curves (ROC) analysis, HPV DNA testing was found to be less useful in women younger than 30 years of age. It also was much less useful in women referred with a LSIL Papanicolaou test than among women referred with an ASCUS Papanicolaou test because the underlying rate of HPV DNA positivity in the absence of disease was quite high in these two groups of women.

Similar results were reported by Manos et al. in a study of women undergoing routine cytologic screening enrolled from the prepaid Kaiser Permanente Northern California Region health plan.[178] In that study, 46,009 women underwent cytologic screening, and a sample was collected for possible subsequent HPV DNA testing. A total of 995 (3.5%) of the women were diagnosed with ASCUS and were subsequently referred for colposcopy. Testing for high-risk HPV types using Hybrid Capture II identified 89% of the cases of biopsy-confirmed high-grade SIL and would have referred 40% of the women with ASCUS to colposcopy. A repeat conventional Pap smear would have correctly identified 76% of the cases of high-grade SIL and referred 39% of all women to colposcopy.

Recently, the initial results of the large NCI-sponsored ALTS (ACUS/LSIL Triage Study) have become available. These results confirm that HPV DNA testing is not useful for determining which women with LSIL Papanicolaou tests should be referred to colposcopy because 83% of the women diagnosed as having LSIL were also high-risk HPV DNA by Hybrid Capture II.[1] Among women diagnosed with ASCUS, HPV DNA testing identified more women with biopsy-confirmed high-grade SIL than did a repeat liquid-based cytology, but both triage methods would have referred approximately equal numbers of women to colposcopy.[261]

When conventional glass Pap smears are used for cytologic screening, women with a diagnosis of ASCUS must return to the clinic or office for a cervical sample to be collected for HPV DNA testing. However, when liquid-based cervical cytology is used for primary screening, the residual cellular material remaining in the vial after the initial cytology preparation has been made can be utilized for HPV DNA testing. This method is referred to as "reflex HPV DNA testing" and eliminates the need for a separate clinical visit simply to collect a specimen for HPV DNA testing.[309] Thus, the clinician can immediately notify a patient with an ASCUS Papanicolaou test whether colposcopy is warranted.

Precursors of Cervical Adenocarcinoma

During the past three decades, endocervical glandular lesions have received increasing attention for a variety of reasons. One factor is a perception that the prevalence of adenocarcinomas of the cervix and its precursor lesions is increasing. There has been a documented absolute increase in the prevalence of invasive adenocarcinomas in specific groups of women in both the United States and Europe. This increase may result in part from the increased routine use of cytobrushes in screening and the widespread adoption of excisional methods for treating SIL lesions such as the loop electrosurgical excision procedure (LEEP), which permit pathologic examination of the entire transformation zone. In addition, there is an increased recognition of these lesions by pathologists and an awareness by colposcopists that certain types of glandular lesions are difficult to recognize colposcopically.

Terminology and Historical Perspective

In 1957, Stewart stated that "every infiltrative cervical cancer must come from in situ cancer, there being no other thing it could come from."[270] Although this statement is universally accepted, more than four decades after it was made little is known about the natural history of precursors of invasive endocervical adenocarcinoma. The first indication that precursor lesions exist came in 1952 when Helper described highly atypical neoplastic cells lining architecturally normal endocervical glands adjacent to frankly invasive endocervical adenocarcinomas.[109] Shortly thereafter, Friedell and McKay described two patients with atypical glandular lesions of the cervix and designated these lesions *adenocarcinoma in situ (AIS)* because of their histologic resemblance to invasive endocervical adenocarcinoma.[87] One of these patients had a coexistent invasive adenocarcinoma of the cervix and one had squamous "carcinoma in situ." Although endocervical glandular lesions with this morphology had been alluded to by Hauser in 1894 and Meyer in 1930, before the descriptions by Helper and Friedell and McKay, these lesions were not considered to be precursors of endocervical adenocarcinomas.

By analogy to squamous cell cervical cancer precursors that demonstrate a wide spectrum of histologic changes, some authors have proposed parallel classification schemas for endocervical adenocarcinoma precursors that include lesions with a lesser degree of abnormality than AIS.[31,36,96,171] Such low-grade putative glandular precursor lesions were originally termed *endocervical dysplasia* by Bousfield et al.,[31] but other terms such as *atypical hyperplasia* are also used to refer to lesions that resemble AIS but have a somewhat lesser degree of nuclear atypia and mitotic activity. Gloor and associates have suggested that the term *cervical intraepithelial glandular neoplasia (CIGN)* be used to refer to both endocervical glandular dysplasia and AIS and that endocervical glandular dysplasia be classified as either CIGN grade 1 or 2 and AIS be classified as CIGN grade 3.[96] Because of the relative rarity of endocervical glandular dysplasia, the subjective nature of the morphologic criteria used to distinguish it from AIS and the infrequent coexistence of endocervical glandular dysplasia with AIS, the significance of endocervical glandular dysplasia is not known.[98,119] Because glandular dysplasia implies a relationship to AIS and invasive carcinoma that has not been documented, we prefer the more noncommittal term *endocervical glandular atypia* for these atypical proliferations that fall short of AIS.

Epidemiology and Etiology

The prevalence of AIS is not known but it is considerably less common than SIL. In most series, the ratio between AIS and high-grade SIL has ranged from 1:26 to 1:237. One of the best estimates for the prevalence of AIS comes from the Kentucky Cervical Cancer Tumor Registry, a population-based tumor registry encompassing 4,877,301 patient-years at risk that includes 4,350 cervical "cancers" (including 2,391 cases of squamous "carcinoma in situ").[88] In this registry, only 16 cases of AIS are documented; 9 occurred in association with squamous "carcinoma in situ" and 7 occurred as pure AIS. For comparison, there were 121 invasive adenocarcinomas of the cervix. Estimates for the United States as a whole are available in the Surveillance Epidemiology and End Results (SEER) public database, which contains data from patients entered into the database between 1973 and 1995.[2] In the SEER registry, there are a total of 149,178 women with either in situ or invasive cervical cancer. Of these, 96% have squamous lesions and 4% have glandular lesions. Of all cervical lesions, 121,793 (82%) were classified as in situ and of these, 120,317 (99%) were squamous cell carcinoma in situ and only 1,476 (1%) were adenocarcinoma in situ. For comparison, of the 27,385 women with invasive cervical cancer, 4,369 (16%) had invasive adenocarcinoma. The 1995 age-adjusted incidence rate in SEER was 0.61 cases per 100,000 for adenocarcinoma in situ and 27.93 cases per 100,000 for squamous cell carcinoma in situ.[222]

Although no population-based data are available on the prevalence of endocervical glandular atypia, in the first large histologic study of this lesion, it was detected in 15% of 105 cone biopsies or hysterectomies performed for CIN 3 (high-grade SIL).[36] In that study, endocervical glandular atypia was 16 times more common than AIS. This prevalence is considerably higher than that reported in most other series in which the majority of patients with endocervical glandular atypia also have AIS.[96,171]

The mean age at diagnosis for endocervical glandular atypia is 37 years.[36,171] The mean age at diagnosis of women with AIS in the SEER registry is 28.8 years, and it is 51.7 years for invasive adenocarcinoma of the cervix.[222] The age relationship between AIS and invasive adenocarcinoma is similar to that of high-grade SIL (CIN 3) and invasive squamous cell carcinoma, suggesting that AIS is a precursor lesion.[222] However, unlike squamous lesions of the cervix in which high-grade precursors occur more frequently than invasive cancer, exactly the opposite relationship exists for AIS and invasive adenocarcinoma of the cervix. The incidence of invasive glandular lesions is higher than that of noninvasive glandular lesions in all age groups.[222] A number of reasons have been proposed for this apparent discrepancy, including the fact that AIS is more difficult to detect both cytologically and colposcopically than is SIL and, therefore, might not be detected before the development of invasive adenocarcinoma. The experience reported for both Finland and Australia indicates that few women with endocervical adenocarcinoma are identified through screening.[189,205]

Additional support implicating AIS as a precursor of invasive adenocarcinoma comes from several anecdotal case reports and two small series of patients who had cytologic or histologic evidence of AIS several years before the detection of invasive adenocarcinoma.[22,25,139] In a cytologic study, Boddington et al. found that 6 of 13 women with invasive adenocarcinoma had previous Pap tests containing atypical endocervical cells 2–8 years before the diagnosis of cancer.[22] Similarly, Boon et al. found that 5 of 18 women with invasive adenocarcinomas had unrecognized AIS on cervical biopsies 3–7 years before detection of the invasive lesion.[25] Although these studies have been interpreted as indicating that AIS is a precursor lesion, it is conceivable that an unrecognized invasive cancer was present at the time of the original Pap test or cervical biopsy.

The proportion of AIS that occurs in association with SIL ranges from 24% to 75%.[6,53,70] This finding suggests that the two types of lesions may share a common etiology. Moreover, many of the risk factors are similar between glandular and squamous lesions; these include multiple sex partners, use of oral contraceptives, early onset of sexual activity, and low socioeconomic class.[286] Both squamous and glandular lesions also appear to be associated with high-risk types of HPV. Using in situ hybridization, Tase and coworkers examined 8 cases of AIS for the presence of HPV DNA and found that 5 of the cases contained HPV but that, unlike SIL lesions analyzed with the same method, the majority of AIS was associated with HPV-18 as opposed to HPV-16 in SIL.[279] Since this initial report, other groups have analyzed AIS for the presence of HPV DNA and it appears clear that most AIS is associated with HPV DNA. Farnsworth et al. detected HPV DNA in 89% of AIS, and the ratio of HPV-18 to HPV-16 in positive cases was 2:1.[78] In a series of 8 cases Griffin et al., using PCR, detected HPV in 63% of AIS but HPV-18 was not detected.[103] Duggan analyzed a series of 37 cases of AIS using PCR with dot blot enhancement and identified HPV-18 in 43% of cases and HPV-16 in 23%.[72] HPV DNA positivity was not correlated with any clinical variable in that series. Associations between endocervical glandular atypia and HPV are more controversial. In the original study by Tase et al., only 2 of 36 cases of endocervical glandular atypia contained HPV DNA.[280] However, in another study, Higgins et al. reported that 94% of endocervical glandular atypia were associated with HPV DNA and 75% were associated with HPV 18.[113] Recently, Anciaux et al. evaluated a group of endocervical glandular atypia both with and without associated squamous lesions, finding a low prevalence of HPV DNA positivity in the cases of glandular atypia not associated with SIL.[5] Moreover, they used in situ hybridization to identify the cells containing HPV DNA in the cases of HPV DNA-positive endocervical glandular atypia that were associated with SIL and found that, in all cases, HPV DNA was only identified in the squamous component.

Clinical Features

Up to 83% of women with AIS or endocervical glandular atypia are asymptomatic, and the lesions are detected either during cytologic screening or fortuitously on an endocervical curettage, cervical punch biopsy, cone, or loop excisional biopsy performed during the workup for SIL. In women who are symptomatic, the most common complaint is abnormal vaginal bleeding, either postcoital, postmenopausal, or out of phase. Rarely, symptomatic patients present with an abnormal discharge.

AIS and endocervical glandular atypia are difficult to detect both cytologically and colposcopically. In a recent histologic study of 42 women with AIS, only 45% of the women had atypical glandular cells detected cytologically on the prediagnosis Pap tests.[70] The other cases were detected fortuitously on biopsies taken to evaluate SIL. Similarly, in another study of 36 women with AIS, glandular abnormalities were detected on the prediagnosis Pap test in only one-half the women.[6] The detection of AIS on endocervical curettage can also be difficult.[6]

The distribution of AIS in the cervix is important for determining the most appropriate clinical management of these patients. AIS involves both the surface and glands in almost all cases. In 65% of cases, AIS involves the transformation zone[6,20] and in most cases it is unifocal. AIS can extend for a distance as great as 3 cm into the endocervical canal.[20,65]

Pathologic Findings

AIS is characterized by the presence of endocervical glands lined by atypical columnar epithelial cells that cytologically resemble the cells of invasive adenocarcinoma but which occur in the absence of invasion (Fig. 7.30). These cells have elongated, cigar-shaped, hyperchromatic nuclei with coarse granular chromatin (Fig. 7.31). The amount of cytoplasm is greatly reduced and there is only minimal intracellular mucin, which produces an increased nuclear:cytoplasmic ratio. The cells are crowded and

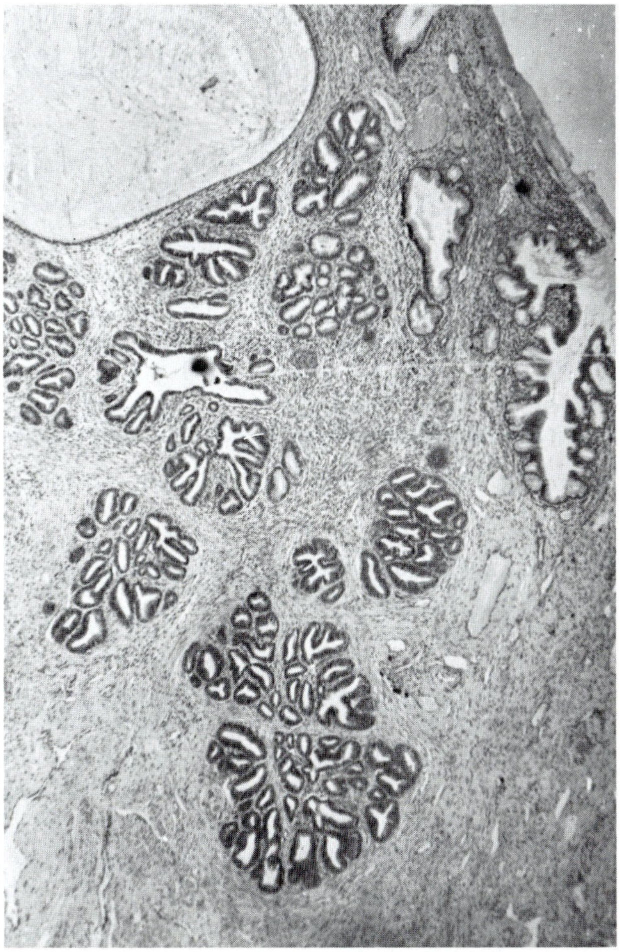

Fig. 7.30. Adenocarcinoma in situ. AIS is characterized at low magnification by the presence of endocervical glands that have numerous outpouchings and some complex papillary infoldings.

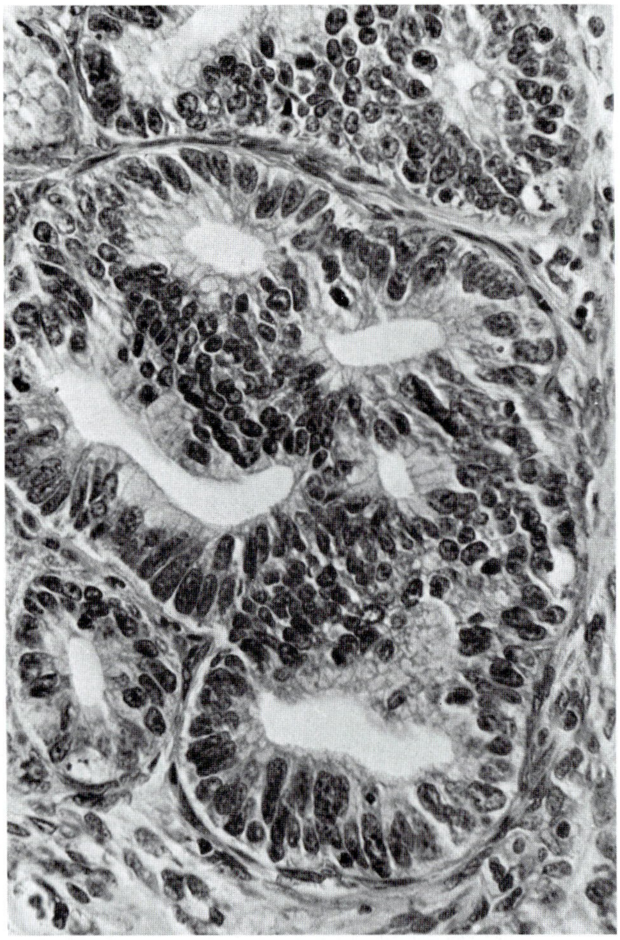

Fig. 7.31. Adenocarcinoma in situ. The endocervical glands are lined by atypical columnar pseudostratified cells with elongated, hyperchromatic nuclei, coarse granular chromatin and frequent mitotic figures. A cribriform appearance can be focally present.

pseudostratified, forming two or more rows. AIS may involve glands either focally, multifocally or diffusely. Typically, some glands show an abrupt transition between normal epithelium and AIS (Fig. 7.32). Mitotic figures including AMFs are common. Apoptotic bodies are commonly seen in the epithelium, usually subadjacent to the nucleus. Architecturally, the glands of AIS can have numerous outpouchings and complex papillary infoldings and may display a cribriform pattern focally (Fig. 7.33).

Ostor et al. have described two histologic types of AIS[210]: one is the typical endocervical-type of AIS already described, and the other has features of a colonic, as opposed to endocervical, mucosa with prominent goblet cells (Fig. 7.34). The colonic type is uncommon and usually occurs in association with typical endocervical AIS. The goblet cells in colonic AIS contain O-acetylated sialomucin, which is a marker of intestinal differentiation. Some intestinal types of AIS also contain argentaffin and Paneth cells.[284] Endometrioid types of AIS and, more rarely, adenosquamous and clear cell AIS also occur.[128]

Carcinoembryonic antigen (CEA) is expressed cytoplasmically in 67% of AIS, whereas the normal columnar epithelium of the endocervix is either negative or demonstrates only luminal as opposed to cytoplasmic staining.[122] A monoclonal antibody referred to as IC5 raised against a cervical adenocarcinoma cell line is reported to react with 75% of AIS but to not react with normal endocervical glands.[159] Most AIS show cytoplasmic reactivity with antibodies against CA-125 and HMFG1, an antibody reactive against a mucin-type glycoprotein, whereas normal endocervical glands show only luminal staining.[35,199]

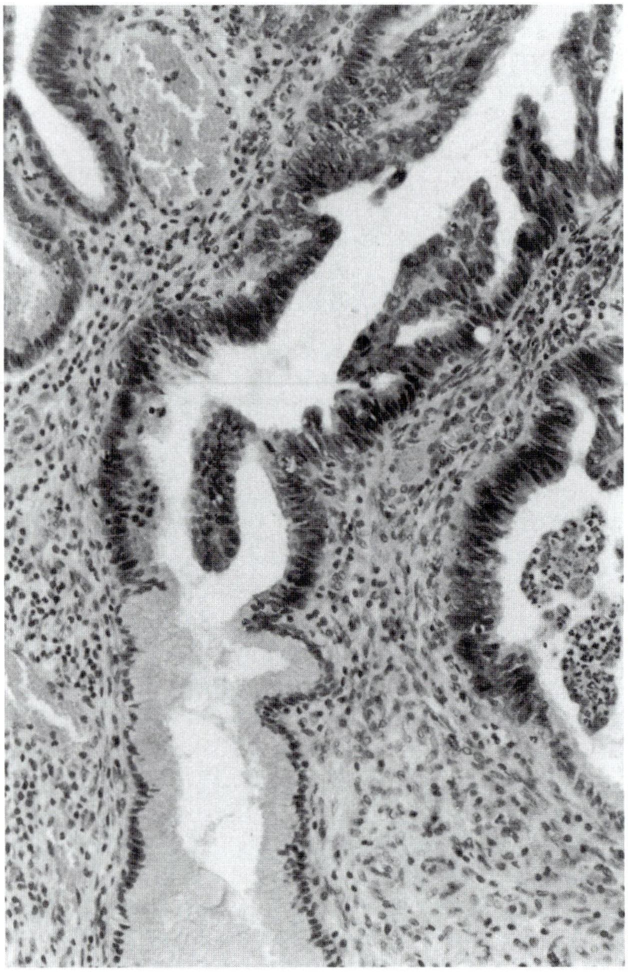

Fig. 7.32. Adenocarcinoma in situ. AIS frequently demonstrates abrupt changes within single glands between neoplastic (*top*) and normal appearing glandular epithelium (*bottom*).

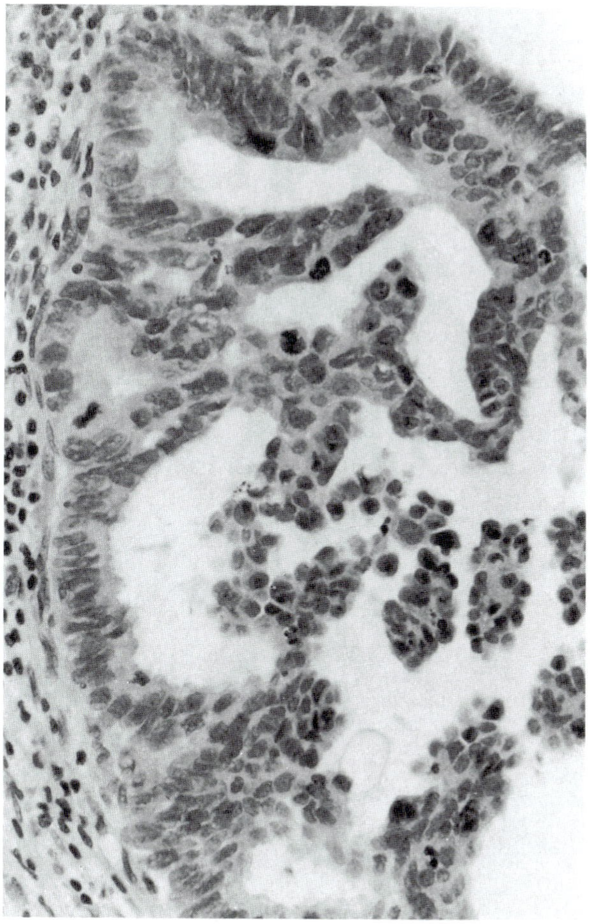

Fig. 7.33. Adenocarcinoma in situ. The glands of AIS may have complex papillary infoldings and a cribriform appearance focally.

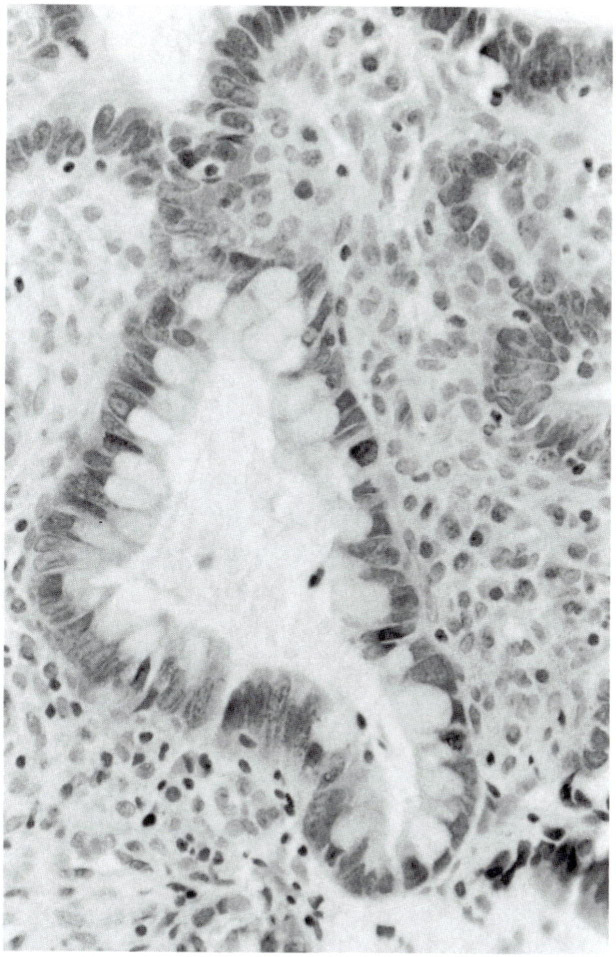

Fig. 7.34. Adenocarcinoma in situ. Colonic-type AIS contains prominent goblet cells and usually occurs in association with typical endocervical adenocarcinoma in situ.

Invasion should be suspected if the involved glands extend beyond the glandular field or beyond the deepest uninvolved endocervical crypt. In addition, in AIS there should be no desmoplasia or stromal reaction around the involved glands. Other worrisome features that can be associated with invasion are exuberant glandular budding, an extensive cribiform pattern, foci in which the glands become confluent or appear back to back, and the formation of papillary projections from the endocervical surface.[158]

The histologic criteria used for diagnosing endocervical glandular atypia include hyperchromatic nuclei with only occasional mitotic figures and minimal pseudostratification (Fig. 7.35). Endocervical glandular atypia usually lacks cribiform areas and papillary projections. Some authors have suggested that the number of glands involved in the process is a distinguishing feature between AIS and endocervical glandular atypia.[163] If only a single gland is involved, even if there is marked nuclear atypia, a diagnosis of endocervical glandular atypia rather than AIS is made. The use of this criterion may decrease the possibility of overdiagnosing reactive, reparative endocervical processes as AIS.

Differential Diagnosis

The differential diagnosis of AIS and endocervical glandular atypia includes reparative/reactive glandular atypias secondary to inflammation, radiation, or viral infections, Arias–Stella reaction, microglandular hyperplasia, endometriosis, tubal metaplasia, mesonephric remnants, and invasive adenocarcinoma. Endocervical glands may display a wide range of cytologic and architectural changes in response to inflammation and radiation. In reactive/reparative atypia, the nuclei become enlarged and have prominent nucleoli but have nuclear clearing and lack hyperchromasia (Fig. 7.36). Nuclei may be

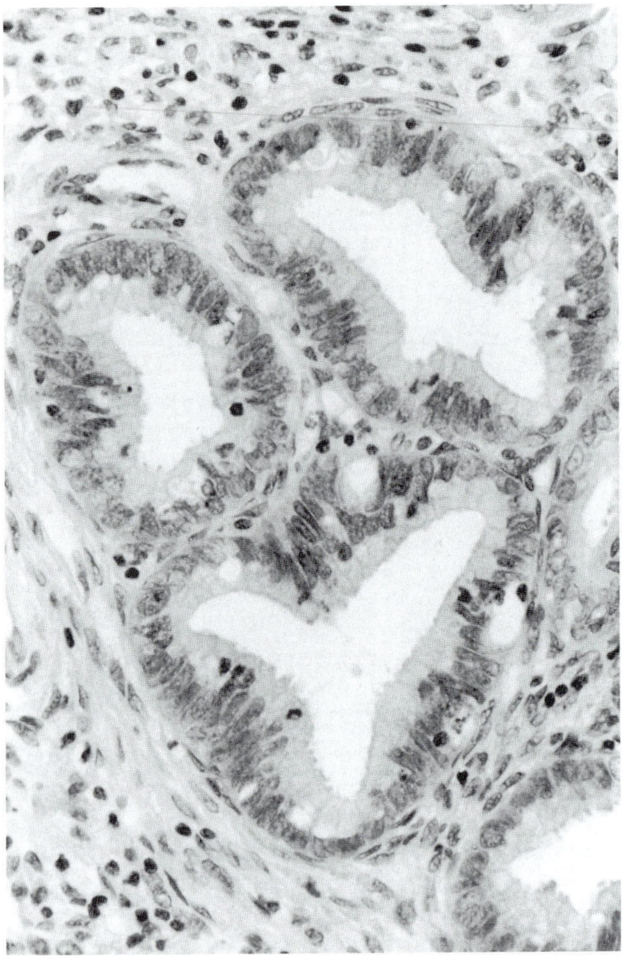

Fig. 7.35. Endocervical glandular atypia. Compared with AIS, endocervical glandular atypia has less pseudostratification (usually only two rows of cells) and fewer mitotic figures. Endocervical glandular atypia also lacks cribriform areas and papillary projections.

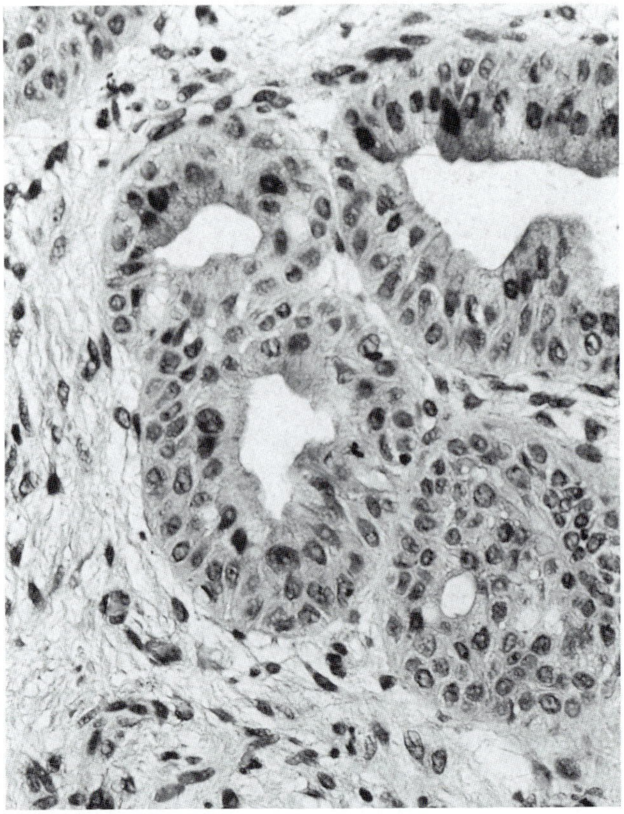

Fig. 7.36. Reactive endocervical atypia. The nuclei are enlarged but the chromatin is smudged. Mitotic activity is either absent or minimal.

pleomorphic but the chromatin is usually smudged and degenerative in appearance. Mitotic activity is usually absent or minimal, as is pseudostratification. Care must be taken to distinguish between true pseudostratification and tangential sectioning through glands that can appear as pseudostratification. Although intraglandular papillary projections should not occur in reactive/reparative processes, exaggerated endocervical papillary projections that project into the endocervical canal can occur. These stromal projections contain infiltrates of chronic inflammatory cells and are lined by a single layer of endocervical cells. This entity has been termed *papillary endocervicitis*.[312] Endocervical atypia secondary to repair characteristically has a dense acute and chronic inflammatory infiltrate surrounding the glands, and polymorphonuclear leukocytes may infiltrate into the epithelium.

Reactive glandular atypia secondary to irradiation is characterized by nuclear enlargement and pleomorphism, but the cytoplasm is frequently vacuolated or granular. Pseudostratification and mitotic figures are absent. Atypia caused by irradiation has greater cell-to-cell variation in size and shape than AIS or endocervical glandular atypia (Fig. 7.37). Glands with the Arias–Stella reaction have a single layer of hyperchromatic, enlarged nuclei that frequently protrude into the gland lumen (i.e., hobnail cells). Typically, the Arias–Stella reaction involves only a portion of a gland and a mitotic activity is absent. Although microglandular hyperplasia can occasionally be confused with AIS, microglandular hyperplasia lacks significant nuclear atypia, lacks pseudostratification, and has few mitotic figures. Moreover, microglandular hyperplasia has a characteristic pattern of closely packed, small, uniform glands. Atypical forms of microglandular hyperplasia have been described that form solid masses of epithelium and have significant degrees of cytologic atypia.[313] These lesions almost always contain areas of typical microglandular hyperplasia that allow them to be identified as atypical forms of micro-

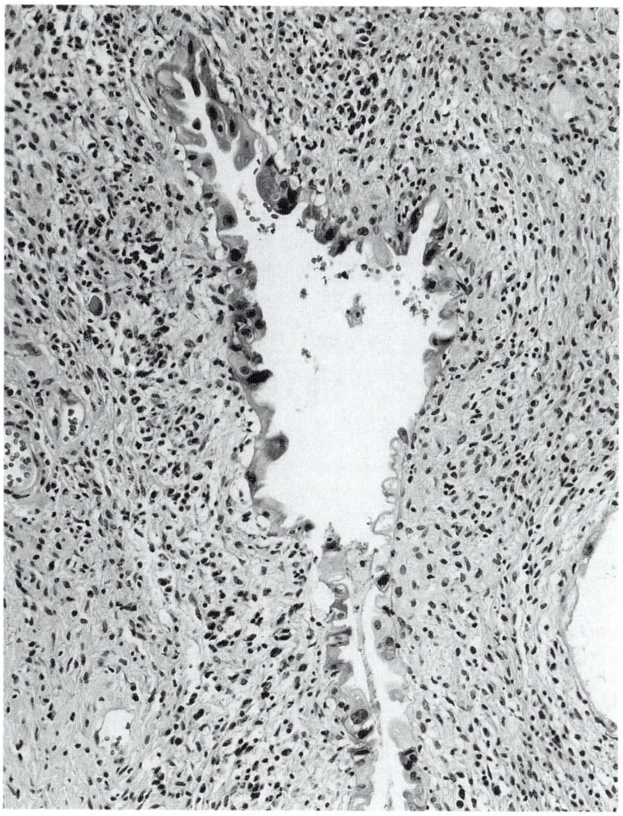

Fig. 7.37. Radiation-induced endocervical atypia. Endocervical atypia induced by irradiation lacks pseudostratification and mitotic figures. In addition it is accompanied by degenerative cytoplasmic changes and more cell to cell variation than AIS.

glandular hyperplasia (see Chapter 6, Benign Diseases of the Cervix). Similarly, endometriosis of the cervix is usually readily recognizable and easily distinguished from AIS. Typical endometriosis consists of glands and endometrial-type stroma. The cells lining the glands are basally located endometrial type cells that can be pseudostratified and mitotically inactive. Both tubal metaplasia and mesonephric remnants should not be mistaken for AIS because they have bland, nonmitotically active nuclei and typical histologic features that allow them to be recognized (see Chapter 6, Benign Diseases of the Cervix).

Clinical Behavior and Treatment

Because of the relatively rarity of AIS, no natural history studies have been published and therefore the evidence that these lesions are precursors for invasive endocervical adenocarcinoma remains circumstantial. Despite this, until recently the treatment of choice was simple hysterectomy. Recently, however, there have been several series of patients with AIS who have been followed after cone biopsy (Table 7.16). These studies have generally shown modest rates of recurrence among women treated by means of a cone biopsy, provided the endocervical margin is negative. Women with positive endocervical margins are at significant risk for having an undiagnosed invasive cervical adenocarcinoma or for developing recurrent AIS. Based on these studies, conservative management by cone biopsy alone is now considered to be an option in women with AIS desirous of maintaining their fertility if the cone biopsy margins are negative.

Cervical Cytology

Strengths and Limitations of the Papanicolaou Test

Although it was introduced more than a half century ago, cervical cytologic screening continues to be the most effective cancer prevention test available. Cytologic screening has never been tested in a prospective double-blind study; however, during the half century since it was introduced, so many epidemiologic and modeling data have accumulated demonstrating the effectiveness of cytology that it has become the index by which all other cancer screening tests are compared. Cytologic screening performed only twice in a woman's lifetime can re-

Table 7.16. Impact of cone biopsy margin status in adenocarcinoma in situ

	Negative margin		*Positive margin*	
Author	*Total*	*No. recurrent (%)*	*Total*	*No. recurrent (%)*
Wolf et al.	21	7 (33%)	19	10 (53%)
Denehy et al.	7	2 (29%)	10	7 (70%)
Azodi et al.	16	1 (6%)	16	6 (38%)
Shin et al.	16	1 (6%)	21	13 (62%)
Ostor et al.	8	2 (20%)	12	19 (75%)

Modified from refs. 9, 70, 209, 256, 304.

duce her risk for invasive cervical cancer by as much as 43%, and yearly screening is estimated to reduce a woman's risk by 93%.[216] However, despite the effectiveness of cytologic screening, it is important to remember that no screening, diagnostic, or therapeutic technique used in medicine is perfect, and the Papanicolaou test is no exception. Some women develop invasive cervical cancer despite annual cytologic screening.

During the past decade, numerous advances have been made in cervical cytology collection techniques, the way cytologic preparations are evaluated, and the classification systems used for reporting cytologic diagnosis. One of the most important advances has been the recent introduction of liquid-based cytology. With liquid-based cytology, the cells collected from the cervix are transferred directly to a liquid fixation solution that is shipped to the cytology laboratory where the slide is prepared. The advantages of liquid-based cytology compared to conventional cytology are its increased sensitivity for detecting both low-grade SIL and high-grade SIL, a reduction in the number of specimens with obscuring blood and inflammation, and, in many series, an increase in the LSIL:ASC ratio. Table 7.17 compares the results obtained with conventional glass Papanicolaou tests and liquid-based cytology in recent studies. Another advantage is that HPV DNA testing can be performed directly from liquid-based specimens when a diagnosis of ASC is made (i.e., "reflex" HPV DNA testing).

Because of the advances just described, routine cervical cytology is more effective today than it has ever been. However, cervical cytology continues to have inherent limitations, which include nonrepresentative sampling of the cervix and transference of cells from the collection device to the glass slide or liquid media; the fact that neoplastic cells can be obscured by blood, inflammatory cells, or mucus, especially when conventional Pap tests are used; and, most importantly, that the cytologic features of neoplasia can be subtle, making it difficult to identify the cells cytologically.

The Bethesda System (TBS) Terminology

In 1988, the Bethesda System (TBS) for reporting cervical/vaginal cytologic diagnoses was developed to provide uniform guidelines for reviewing and reporting gynecologic Papanicolaou tests.[202] The Bethesda System classification, subsequently modified in 1991 and 2001,[305] is now the most widely used classification for cervical cytology in the United States. There are two distinct parts to the report: a statement of specimen adequacy, and a general categorization (Table 7.18). In addition, in many instances a descriptive diagnosis is provided designed to assist clinicians by answering three basic questions: (1) Was the sample adequate? (2) Was the Papanicolaou test normal? (3) If the test was not completely normal, what specifically was wrong?

Specimen Adequacy

The Papanicolaou test is a cancer-screening test. Therefore, a normal Papanicolaou test is generally

Table 7.17. Comparison of liquid-based cytology with conventional Pap smears

			Change in detection: liquid vs conventional			
Author	*Comparison*	*No. cases*	*SBLB*	*ASCUS*	*LSIL*	*HSIL*
ThinPrep Pap Test						
Lee	Split sample*	7,360	−40%	−5%	−28%	−1.8%
Corkill	Split sample	1,583	NA	−37%	134%	54%
Papillo	Historical	16,314	−52%	−27%	88%	55%
Dupree	Historical	19,351	NA	−6%	44%	33%
Bolick	Concurrent	10,694	−35%	NA	181%	171%
Guidos	Concurrent	9,583	−97%	NA	267%	233%
AutoCyte PREP						
Howell	Split sample	852	−11%	−10%	−36%	−21%
Bishop	Split sample	8,983	−78%	−3%	46%	6%
Vassilakos	Concurrent	32,655	−83%	−57%	275%	100%
Saurel	Concurrent	134,870	NA	−41%	28%	66%
Rondez	Concurrent	17,000	NA	−21%	85%	144%

*Conventional specimen prepared first and residual used to make liquid preparation.
Modified from ref. 310.

Table 7.18. The Bethesda System 2001 Classification*

SPECIMEN TYPE: *Conventional of Liquid-based*

SPECIMEN ADEQUACY

- Satisfactory for evaluation (*describe presence or absence of T-zone component or other quality indicators*)
- Unsatisfactory for evaluation . . . (*specify reason*)
  - Specimen rejected/not processed
  - Specimen processed and examined, but unsatisfactory

GENERAL CATEGORIZATION (*optional*)

- Negative for intraepithelial lesion or malignancy
- Epithelial Cell Abnormality: *See Interpretation/Result*
- Other: See Interpretation/Result

Automated Review: (*If done specify*)

Ancillary Testing: (*If done specify*)

INTERPRETATION/RESULT

Negative for Intraepithelial Lesion or Malignancy

- Organisms
  - *Trichomonas vaginalis*
  - Fungal organisms consistent with *Candida* spp
  - Shift in flora suggestive of bacterial vaginosis
  - Bacteria morphologically consistent with Actinomyces
  - Cellular change consistent with Herpes simplex
- Other non-neoplastic findings (*optional, not inclusive*)
  - Reactive cellular changes
  - Glandular cells status post hysterectomy
  - Atrophy

Other

- Endometrial cells in women ≥40 yrs of age

Epithelial Cell Abnormalities

- ***Squamous Cell***
- Atypical squamous cells
  - of undetermined significance (ASC-US)
  - cannot exclude HSIL (ASC-H)
- Low grade squamous intraepithelial lesion (LSIL)
- High grade squamous intraepithelial lesion (HSIL)
  - with features suspicious for invasion (*if suspected*)
- Squamous cell carcinoma
- ***Glandular Cell***
- ***Atypical***
  - endocervical cells (NOS *or specify in comments*)
  - endometrial cells (NOS *or specify in comments*)
  - glandualr cells (NOS *or specify in comments*)
- Atypical
  - endocervical cells, favor neoplastic
  - glandualr cells, favor neoplastic
- Endocervical adenocarcinoma *in situ*
- Adenocarcinoma (*specify type or NOS*)
- **Other Malignant Neoplasms (*specify*)**

EDUCATIONAL NOTES AND SUGGESTIONS (*optional*)

*Modified from http://Bethesda2001.cancer.gov

interpreted as indicating that the patient does not have cervical cancer. However, 20–50% of Papanicolaou tests obtained from women with high-grade disease and invasive cancer are classified as "within normal limits." There are a number of reasons for these false-negative Papanicolaou tests.[24,187,292] A proportion of false-negative Papanicolaou tests is attributable to laboratory error, approximately 30%. In these cases atypical or malignant cells are present on the slide but were overlooked or misinterpreted by the cytologist. A greater proportion, approximately 70%, is a result of sampling error. In these Papanicolaou tests atypical or malignant cells cannot be identified on the slide, which can be caused by the sampling device not contacting the lesion, tumor cells not exfoliating from the lesion, or blood, inflammation, or poor preservation obscuring the atypical cells present on the slide. A specimen that has been obtained poorly or is of low quality because of obscuring blood, inflammation, or poor preservation is more difficult for the cytologist to interpret. Because poor-quality Papanicolaou tests may have a false-negative rate that is higher than usual, it is important that cytologists inform clinicians of the limited quality of these cases so that the Papanicolaou test can be repeated.

The 2001 Bethesda System requires that every Papanicolaou test be assessed with respect to its adequacy. Papanicolaou tests are classified into one of two specimen adequacy categories: "satisfactory for evaluation" or "unsatisfactory for evaluation."

Satisfactory for Evaluation

Conventional glass slide preparations that are "satisfactory for evaluation" are defined as having an estimated minimum of approximately 8,000–12,000 well-preserved and well-visualized squamous cells. For liquid-based cytology preparations it is recommended that there be a minimum of 5,000 well-visualized and well-preserved squamous cells. Although the presence or absence of endocervical cells is a widely used indicator of the quality of a Papanicolaou test, it is controversial among pathologists as to whether the presence or absence of identifiable columnar cells has a major bearing on the adequacy of a cervical sample.[264] Several studies have reported a higher prevalence of cytologically detected SIL among Papanicolaou tests that contain endocervical cells compared with those that do not.

For example, Boon et al. reported that when Papanicolaou tests obtained using a modified Ayre spatula were compared to slides obtained using both a spatula and cytobrush, the rate of detection of either endocervical cells or squamous metaplastic cells increased from 84% to 98% and the detection rate of CIN 3 or greater increased from 0.39% to 0.75%.[24] However, other studies have failed to identify increased rates of cytologic abnormalities among women with prior Papanicolaou tests lacking endocervical cells.

In a study that compared different collection devices in the same population of women contemporaneously, Szarewski et al. found that despite large differences between techniques with regards to the presence or absence of endocervical cells, no differences were found in the detection of SIL.[276] Therefore, there is considerable evidence to support Mitchell an Medley's conclusion that when the detection rate of endocervical cells is relatively high, for example, when cytobrushes are used, the presence of endocervical cells is not an important determinant of whether a slide is adequate.[188]

In the 2001 Bethesda System, a specimen does not have to have a transformation zone component (i.e., squamous metaplastic cells or columnar epithelial cells) to be classified as satisfactory for evaluation. However, it is recommended that the presence or absence of a transformation zone component be clearly stated in the cytology report. The minimum criterion for endocervical cells or squamous metaplastic cells in either conventional or liquid-based cytology is 10 well-preserved cells occurring either individually or in groups (Fig. 7.38). In liquid-based cytology preparations, endocervical cell groups are often more three dimensional and endocervical cell nuclei may appear more "reactive" than in conventional glass slides. Squamous metaplastic cells tend to round up in liquid-based preparations and appear smaller and rounder than in conventional smears. A statement should also be made whenever 50–75% of the cells on the slide are obscured by blood, inflammation, or other factors. In cases with obscuring blood or inflammation, an attempt should be made to quantitate the number of visualized cells. Therefore a typical 2001 Bethesda System report might read as follows: "Satisfactory for evaluation: No transformation zone component identified, approximately 60% of the cells are obscured by inflammation."

Unsatisfactory for Evaluation

When a Papanicolaou test is classified as "unsatisfactory for evaluation," no diagnosis can be rendered. This category is reserved for conventional glass

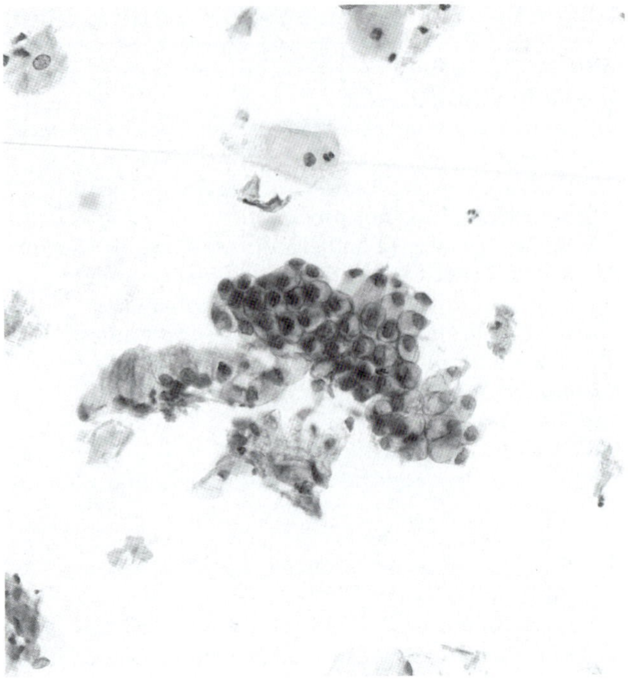

Fig. 7.38. Endocervical cells. The columnar endocervical cells have basally located nuclei and abundant apical cytoplasm. This imparts a "picket-fence" appearance to strips of endocervical cells. When seen *en face*, the cell sheets have a honeycomb appearance.

Papanicolaou tests that have estimated fewer than 8,000–12,000 well-preserved and well-visualized squamous epithelial cells and liquid-based preparations that have fewer than 5,000 well-preserved and well-visualized squamous cells. Moreover, a Papanicolaou test is considered unsatisfactory is more than 75% of the cells are obscured. It is important to note that if atypical cells are identified on a slide, it should not be reported as "unsatisfactory for evaluation."

General Categorization

Papanicolaou tests that are reported using the 2001 Bethesda System are classified into one of three general categorizations: "Negative for Intraepithelial Lesion or Malignancy," "Epithelial Cell Abnormalities," and "Other" (see Table 7.18).

Negative for Intraepithelial Lesion or Malignancy

Papanicolaou tests that are diagnosed as "negative for intraepithelial lesion or malignancy" lack cytologic evidence of SIL or malignancy. In addition to superficial and intermediate squamous cells (Fig. 7.39), immature squamous metaplastic cells are often present. The type and percentage of squamous cells vary with the hormonal status of the patient. Superficial cells

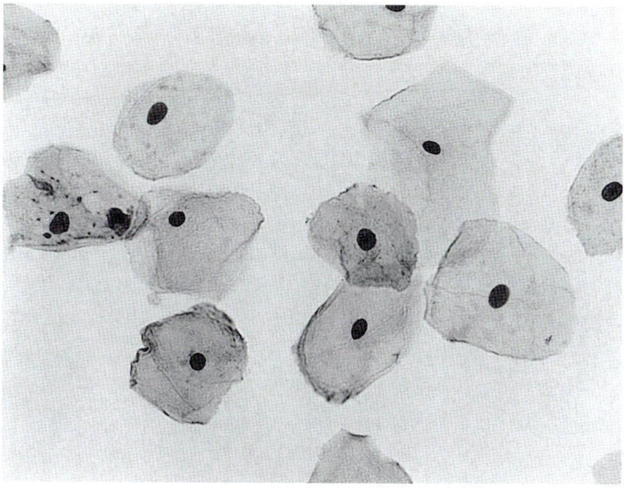

Fig. 7.39. Superficial and intermediate squamous cells. The cells with small pyknotic nuclei are superficial squamous cells. Cells with somewhat larger nuclei and darker cytoplasm on the Papanicolaou stain are intermediate cells.

predominate at the time of ovulation (day 14) when estrogen levels are highest, and intermediate cells predominate in the late luteal phase of the cycle when progestin levels are highest.

A number of common conditions that previously were classified as "benign cellular changes" are now classified as "negative for intraepithelial lesion or malignancy." With the 2001 Bethesda System, these include reactive/reparative cellular changes, responses to radiation, changes secondary to intrauterine devices, and specific organisms. In addition, common conditions such as cytolysis, parakeratosis, hyperkeratosis, and atrophy are retained in the "negative for intraepithelial lesion or malignancy" category. These reactive or other nonneoplastic changes can be mentioned in the report along with the "negative for intraepithelial lesion or malignancy" diagnosis. Specific organisms that are identified can also be included in the report.

Benign-Appearing Endometrial Cells. Benign-appearing endometrial cells are typically observed in Papanicolaou tests obtained during menses. In normally cycling women without endometrial pathology, occasional clusters of benign-appearing endometrial cells can be identified at any point during the first half of the menstrual cycle. These normal endometrial cells can appear in two forms in Papanicolaou tests: one is as a menstrual aggregate (Fig. 7.40), and another is as a sheet or cluster of stromal cells. Benign-appearing endometrial cells occurring in a postmenopausal patient are also placed in this general category. The clinical significance of finding benign-appearing endometrial cells in a postmenopausal patient is debated. Most recent studies have found a relatively low prevalence of significant endometrial lesions in such women. For example, in a recent report of 93 cases occurring in asymptomatic postmenopausal women receiving hormone replacement therapy who underwent subsequent endometrial sampling. Montz found only 1 case of adenocarcinoma and 1 case of atypical hyperplasia.[193] However, a considerable number of women had either endometrial hyperplasia without atypia (8%) or endometrial polyps (8%). In another study of 297 postmenopausal women with benign-appearing endometrial cells, 132 of the women underwent endometrial sampling and only 3 significant lesions were identified (2 typical hyperplasia and 1 adenocarcinoma).[44]

Specific Infections. Specific infectious agents can be identified on Papanicolaou tests including *Trichomonas vaginalis*, fungal organisms, *Actinomyces*, an overabundance of coccobacilli reflecting bacterial vaginosis, herpes simplex virus (HSV), and human papillomavirus (HPV). Because of their close association with squamous intraepithelial lesions (SIL), HPV infections are classified together with mild dysplasia as a low-grade squamous intraepithelial lesion (LSIL) rather than as a benign cellular change.

Trichomonas vaginalis is a common cause of benign cellular changes. *Trichomonas* appears as round

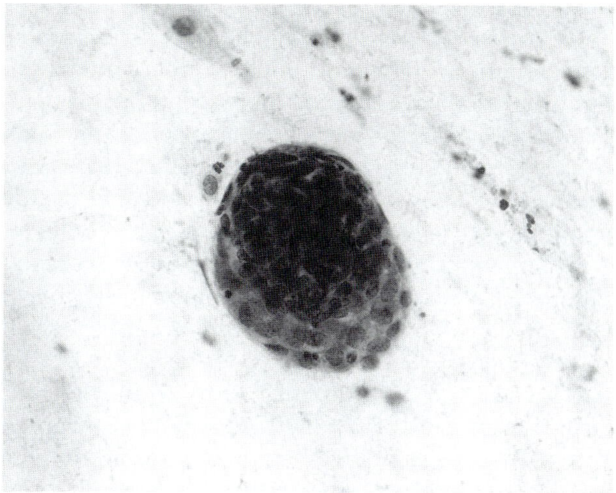

Fig. 7.40. Endometrial cells. Normal endometrial cells forming a menstrual aggregate. Degenerated stromal cells form the center of the aggregate and epithelial cells form the outer layer. Appearance resembles that of endometrial stomal breakdown in curettage specimens.

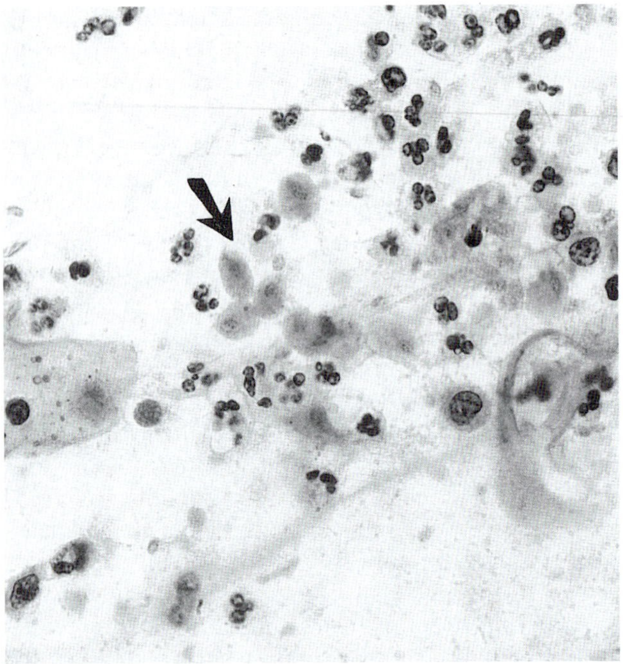

Fig. 7.41. ***Trichomonas vaginalis.*** The organisms are the small gray-blue, pear-shaped structures seen at the arrow. Considerable number of inflammatory cells are present in the background.

to oval, pale gray-blue structures 10–25 μm in diameter (Fig. 7.41). In liquid-based preparations, trichomonads appear smaller than when seen in conventional glass Papanicolaou tests. Leptotrichia, large filamentous bacteria-like organisms that appear as gray hairlike structures, frequently coexist with *T. vaginalis*. Typically in trichomonal infections, the squamous epithelial cells demonstrate reactive changes with mild nuclear enlargement and small perinuclear halos. Proteinaceous debris that imparts a "broken glass" appearance in the background of the slide is frequently seen. There is often a dense neutrophilic infiltrate, and neutrophils frequently form large aggregates sometimes referred to as "cannonballs" or "pus balls"; these represent squamous cells covered by trichomonal organisms that have been phagocytosed by macrophages and neutrophils.

The most common fungal infection of the lower genital tract is *Candida albicans* and closely related organisms. Yeast appears as both pseudohyphae and blastospores (budding yeast forms) in Papanicolaou tests. The pseudohyphae can form arborized branching structures that typically intermingle with exfoliated squamous epithelial cells (Fig. 7.42). The squamous cells frequently demonstrate mild nuclear enlargement and hyperchromasia. A considerable amount of inflammation can accompany a yeast infection. *Candida albicans, Torulopsis glabrata*, and other yeast forms look similar on Papanicolaou tests. Therefore, the 2001 Bethesda System uses the terminology "fungal organisms morphologically consistent with *Candida* species" to describe all yeast infections detected cytologically.

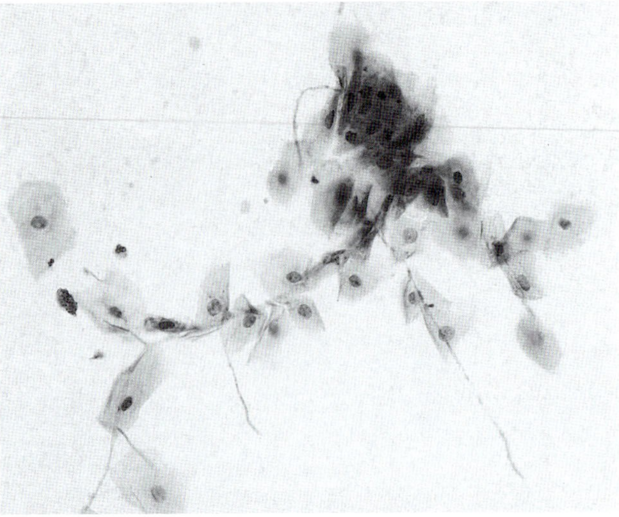

Fig. 7.42. ***Candida albicans.*** The yeast is identified as long branching pseudohypae intermingled with squamous cells. The squamous cells have hyperchromatic, slightly enlarged nuclei.

The terminology "shift in vaginal flora suggestive of bacterial vaginosis" is used in the 2001 Bethesda System to describe the cytologic findings associated with bacteria vaginosis. As on wet mounts, the "clue cell" is the characteristic feature of bacterial vagi-

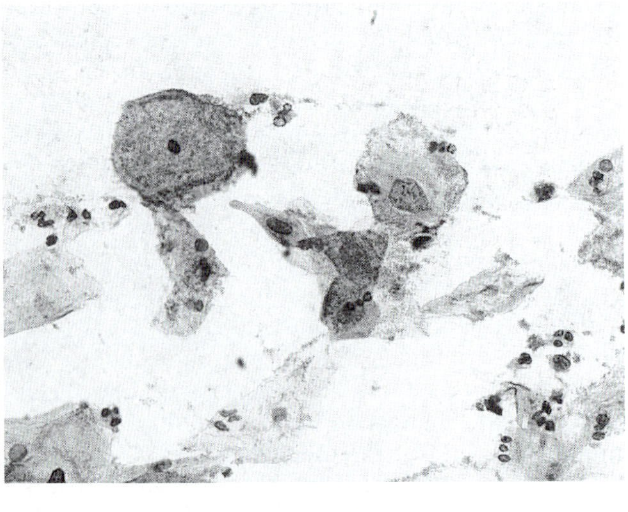

Fig. 7.43. ***Bacterial vaginosis.*** Clue cells are mature squamous epithelial cells that are covered with coccibacilli. This makes the cells appear gray and granular on the Papanicolaou stain.

nosis seen on the Papanicolaou test. Clue cells appear gray-blue and are superficial squamous cells coated with coccobacilli. Typically, bacteria extend beyond the cell margin of clue cells (Fig. 7.43). Additionally, characteristic clumps of small rodlike bacteria are seen in the background of the slide, and lactobacilli are absent or reduced in numbers.

Actinomyces israelii is an organism taxonomically close to hyphae bacteria. It is considered part of the normal vaginal flora, and identification of organisms does not indicate that clinical disease is present.[168] However, actinomyces is typically found in association with foreign bodies such as intrauterine devices (IUDs), pessaries, or retained vaginal tampons. On Papanicolaou tests, actinomyces appear as aggregates of poorly defined blue-gray, thick, filamentous organisms; the aggregates are considerably larger than superficial squamous cells and are more dense at the center than at the periphery (Fig. 7.44).

Herpes simplex virus produces a characteristic cellular change in infected squamous cells. Infected cells are enlarged, multinucleated, have nuclear molding, and develop either a "ground glass" appearance of their nuclear chromatin or large, eosinophilic intranuclear inclusions (Fig. 7.45). The large intranuclear viral inclusions are referred to as Cowdry type A inclusions. Herpetic infections are usually accompanied by marked inflammation and reparative changes of squamous cells.

Reactive Cellular Changes. All benign epithelial changes associated with inflammation, intrauterine devices, radiation therapy, and unknown causes are classified as "negative for intraepithelial lesion or malignancy" in the 2001 Bethesda System. Reactive cellular changes include reparative changes that are by definition "typical" and nonneoplastic. Reactive changes can occur in both squamous and endocervical cells. The characteristic cytologic features of reactive or reparative change include nuclear enlargement and the development of prominent nucleoli. However, the cells have a bland chromatin pattern and abundant cytoplasm and, as a result, the nuclear:cytoplasmic ratio is not increased to levels seen in neoplasia (Fig. 7.46). In addition,

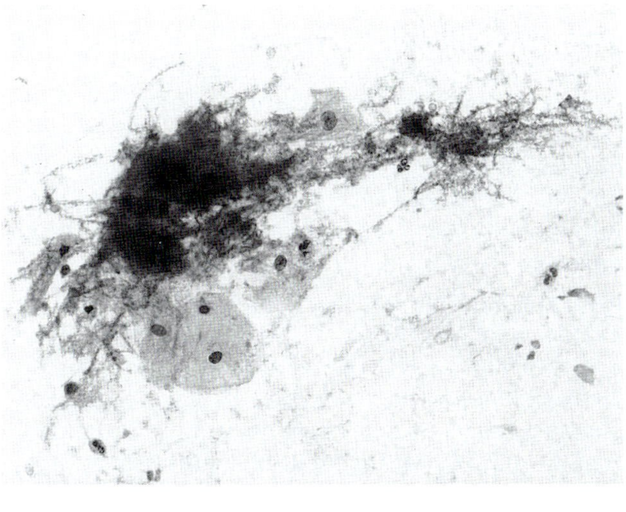

Fig. 7.44. *Actinomyces israelii.* The organisms are identified as aggregates of thick filaments.

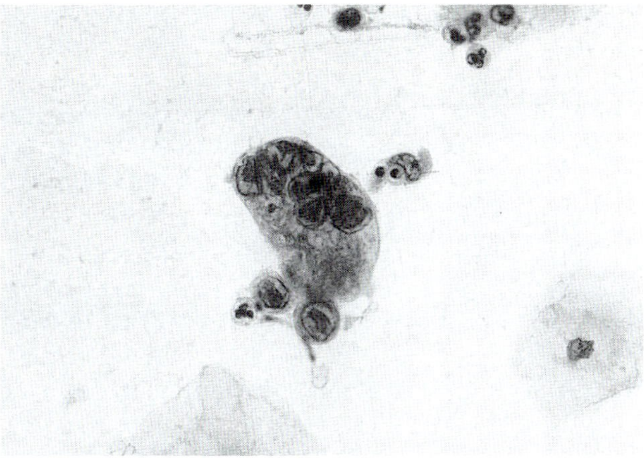

Fig. 7.45. Herpes simplex virus. Infected squamous epithelial cells become multinucleated and demonstrate nuclear molding. In this example of a liquid-based cytology specimen, Cowday type A intranuclear inclusions are present in the infected cells.

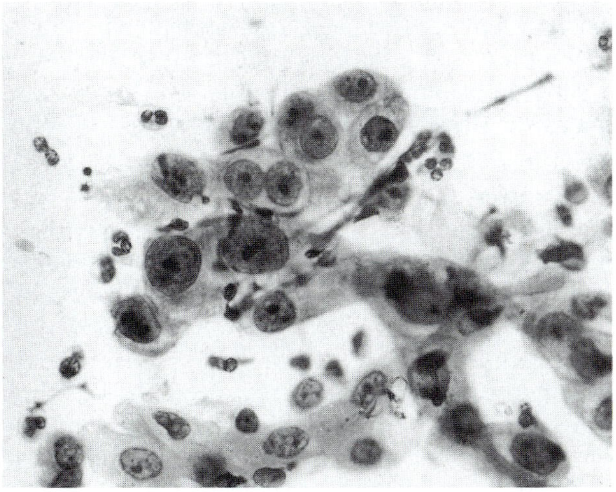

Fig. 7.46. Reactive cellular changes. The reactive cells have enlarged nuclei with prominent nuclei. The cytoplasm is abundant and the cells form a sheet with indistinct cell membranes. An inflammatory background is present.

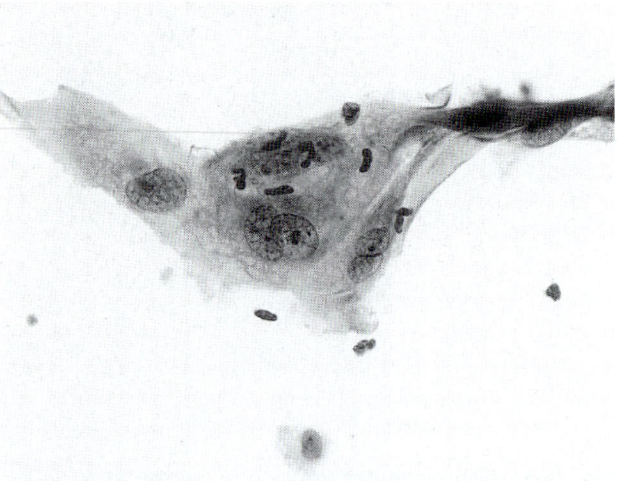

Fig. 7.47. Radiation-induced changes. Several squamous cells are enlarged and quite atypical. The cytoplasm of these cells is vacuolated, indicating the changes are secondary to radiation.

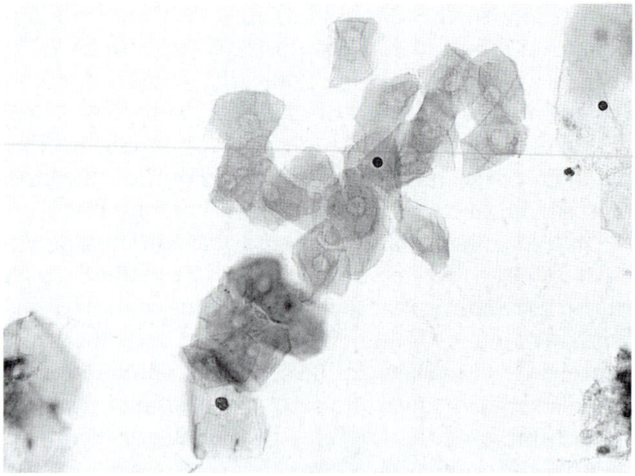

Fig. 7.48. Hyperkeratosis. Enucleated squamous cells that stain deep orange–yellow on the Papanicolaou stain. When hyperkeratosis occurs as an isolated finding, it has little clinical significance.

reactive epithelial cells frequently form loose sheets or syncytium-like arrangements. Mitoses can be observed in the cellular sheets. In most cases, the etiology of reparative/reactive changes is unknown. However, in some cases patients have a history of recent cryosurgery, laser ablation, pregnancy, or a voluntary abortion.

Radiation therapy produces dramatic, but usually transient, cellular changes in most patients. Cells become quite enlarged and frequently multinucleated. Cytoplasmic vacuolization and cellular degeneration often occur (Fig. 7.47). These changes can make it difficult to determine whether malignant cells are still present in a woman undergoing radiation therapy for cervical cancer. IUDs can occasionally produce cytologic changes that are misinterpreted as neoplastic.

Other Cellular Changes. Other cytologic changes that are included in the "negative for intraepithelial lesion and malignancy" category are hyperkeratosis, parakeratosis, cytolysis, and atrophy. Hyperkeratosis presents as anucleated, orange-staining squamous cells (Fig. 7.48). Although SIL or invasive squamous cell cancer can be associated with hyperkeratosis, hyperkeratosis is most commonly an insignificant cytologic finding. Hyperkeratosis and parakeratosis are frequently associated with epithelial damage, such as occurs in women with uterine prolapse. Parakeratosis presents as small keratinized cells with pyknotic nuclei. When parakeratosis lacks nuclear atypia, it is a benign finding.

Cytolysis is a degeneration of the epithelial cells that causes them to appear poorly defined or "fuzzy." Any marked increase in lactobacilli, such as during pregnancy and in some nonpregnant women, often produces extensive cytolysis of the epithelial cells. Because of a deficiency of estrogen, Papanicolaou tests from postpartum or postmeno-pausal women are usually atrophic. Atrophic smears vary widely in their appearance depending the amount of estrogen to which the epithelium is exposed. When low, but measurable, levels of estrogen are present, the slide contains large numbers of intermediate cells. When estrogen levels have been reduced for prolonged periods of time, the Papanicolaou test contains numerous parabasal cells that occur singly and as syncytial-like sheets.

"Epithelial Cell Abnormalities"

All other epithelial cytologic abnormalities are reported as "epithelial cell abnormalities." The category epithelial cell abnormalities is subdivided into abnormalities of squamous cells and abnormalities involving glandular cells, either endocervical or endometrial. Cytologic changes previously classified as mild squamous cytological atypia and atypical endocervical cells are also included in this category.

Squamous Cell Abnormalities

Atypical Squamous Cells (ASC)

The ASC category is used to designate cytologic changes suggestive of a squamous intraepithelial lesion that are quantitatively or qualitatively insufficient for a definitive diagnosis of SIL. Several points need to be made with respect to ASC. First, a diagnosis of ASC is one of exclusion; the cells are abnormal, but they do not warrant a diagnosis of SIL.

Second, a diagnosis of ASC should not be used when the underlying process is inflammatory or reactive; such slides should be classified as "negative for intraepithelial lesion or malignancy" rather than ASC. Third, although the ASC category is sometimes disparagingly referred to as a "cytological wastebasket," there are specific criteria that should be used for making this diagnosis. If these criteria are adhered to, the rate of ASC in a routine cytology laboratory should be no greater than about 5% of all Papanicolaou tests and the ASC rate should be approximately twice the SIL rate.

The 2001 Bethesda System subdivides the ASC category into two subdivisions. Atypical Squamous Cells of Undetermined Significance (ASCUS) refers to samples in which the cytologic changes are suggestive of LSIL but lack sufficient cytologic abnormalities to allow a definitive diagnosis. Atypical Squamous Cells; Cannot Exclude HSIL (ASCH) refers to samples in which the cytologic changes are suggestive of HSIL but the cytologic abnormalities are insufficient to allow a definitive interpretation.[255]

The specific criteria used to diagnose ASC are given in Table 7.19. One of the major criteria used to distinguish ASCUS from benign cellular changes is nuclear size. In ASCUS, the nuclei are typically two or three times the size of a normal intermediate cell. In addition to changes in nuclear size, the nuclei in ASCUS are somewhat irregular and frequently hyperchromatic (Fig. 7.49). However, the degree of nuclear changes considered sufficient to warrant a diagnosis of ASCUS is highly subjective and varies among cytologists; this introduces a degree of uncertainty with respect to a diagnosis of ASCUS, and studies have shown that a diagnosis of ASCUS is nonreproducible among pathologists.[254,261] In the recent NCI-sponsored ALTS trial, only 55% of the referral

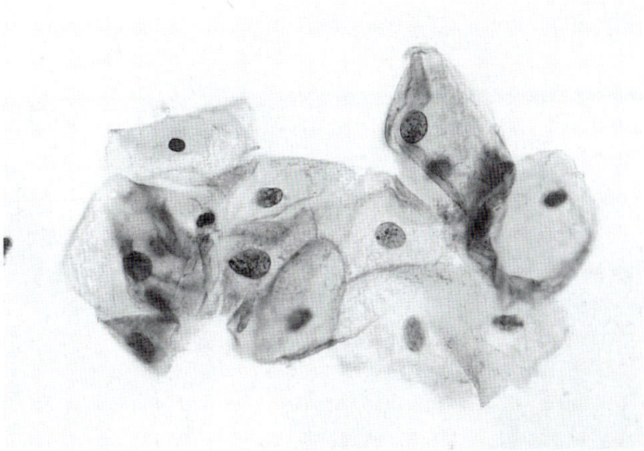

Fig. 7.49. Atypical squamous cells undetermined significance (ASCUS). Superficial squamous epithelial cells demonstrate nuclear enlargement, hyperchromasia, and small perinuclear halos. No organisms or inflammatory changes were identified on the smear. At colposcopy the patient was found to be high risk HPV DNA-positive using Hybrid Capture, but no lesion was identified colposcopically.

Papanicolaou tests originally classified as ASCUS were classified as ASCUS by the pathology quality control panel.[271] Only 5–16% of women with a diagnosis of ASC have a high-grade SIL of the cervix identified when colposcopy is performed.[81,178,261,309] It should also be noted that a diagnosis of ASCUS is also sometimes made when there are cells with some, but not all of the criteria necessary for a diagnosis of LSIL (Fig. 7.50).

In ASCH, the cells resemble parabasal or basal cells in size and configuration; these cells frequently

Table 7.19. Criteria used to diagnosis atypical squamous cells (ASC)

Atypical squamous cells of undetermined significance (ASCUS)
Cells resemble superficial or intermediate squamous cells in size and configuration
Nuclei are 2–3 times the size of a normal intermediate cell
Nuclei are round to oval with minimal irregularities
Nuclei are normochromatic to slightly hyperchromatic
Atypical squamous cells; cannot exclude HSIL (ASCH)
Cells resemble parabasal or basal cells in size and configuration
Nuclei often have uneven chromatin and are hyperchromatic
Nuclear contour is often irregular

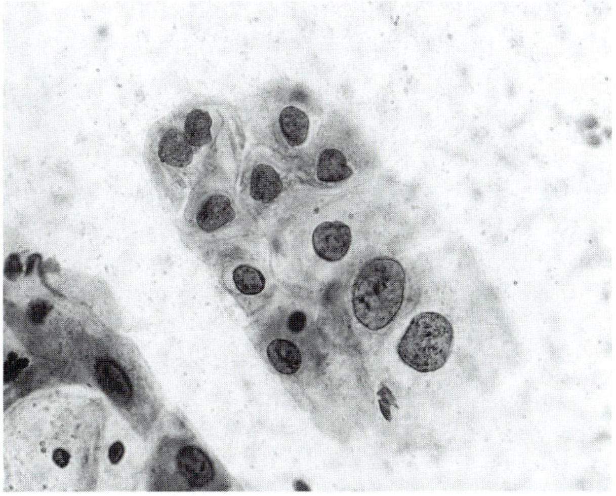

Fig. 7.50. Atypical squamous cells undetermined significance (ASCUS). Nuclei are enlarged with irregular contours and clumped chromatin. Changes closely approach those necessary for a diagnosis of LSIL.

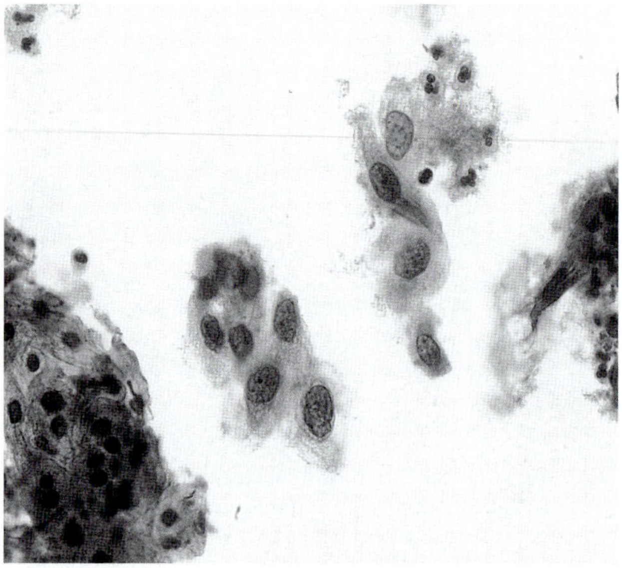

Fig. 7.51. Atypical squamous cells: cannot exclude HSIL (ASC-H). A cluster of atypical metaplastic type cells is present. The cells have enlarged nuclei with an increased N:C ratio, hyperchromasia, and slightly irregular nuclei. At colposcopy a high-grade SIL was diagnosed.

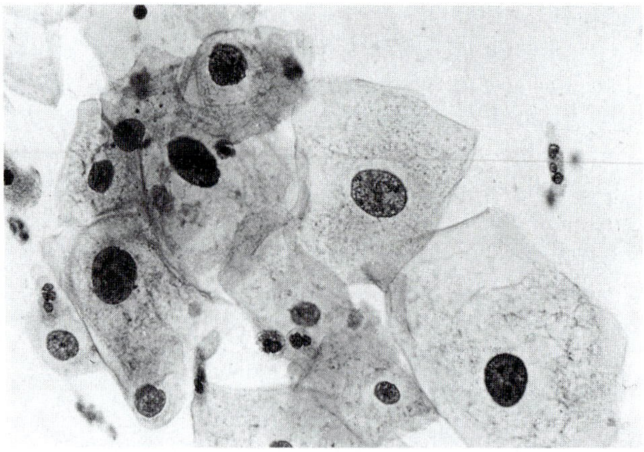

Fig. 7.52. Low-grade SIL. Cells from this lesion demonstrate less koilocytosis than seen in many low-grade SIL. However, the atypical cells are of the intermediate cell type and demonstrate increased nuclear size and increased N:C ratios, nuclear hyperchromasia, and coarse clumped chromatin.

have irregular nuclear contours and uneven chromatin (Fig. 7.51). There are varying degrees of hyperchromasia. The differential diagnosis in such cases is between atypical immature squamous metaplasia and HSIL. Women who have ASCH have been found to be at increased risk for having a high-grade SIL compared to women with ASCUS detected when colposcopy is performed.[177,255]

Low-Grade Squamous Intraepithelial Lesions (LSIL)

The low-grade squamous intraepithelial lesion category in the Bethesda System includes both HPV effects and mild dysplasia (CIN 1). The classic studies of Reagan and others identified the key cytologic features of mild dysplasia (CIN 1) (Table 7.20).[227] The cells of LSIL are of the superficial or intermediate cell type. They have enlarged nuclei that are four to six times the size of a normal intermediate cell nucleus (Fig. 7.52), but many vary in size, and in LSIL with marked HPV cytopathic effects the nuclei are often only two times the size of a normal intermediate cell nucleus (Fig. 7.53). In LSIL, the nuclei are usually hyperchromatic, and multinucleation is common. The chromatin is finely granular and uniformly distributed. The cells typically occur as individual cells or as sheets of cells with well-defined cell borders.

Table 7.20. Criteria used to diagnosed squamous epithelial cell abnormalities

Bethesda system	*LSIL*	*HSIL*		
CIN terminology	*CIN 1*	*CIN 2*	*CIN 3*	
WHO terminology	*Mild dysplasia*	*Moderate dysplasia*	*Severe dysplasia*	*CIS*
Cell type	Superficial or intermediate	Parabasal	Basal	Basal, spindle, pleomorphic
Cell arrangement	Singly or sheets	Singly or sheets	Singly or sheets	Singly or sheets or syncitia
Number abnormal cells	+	++	+++	++++
Koilocytosis	+++	+	+/−	+/−
Nuclear size	+++	++	+	+
Hyperchromasia	+	++	+++	++++
Nuclear:cytoplasmic ratio	+	++	+++	++++

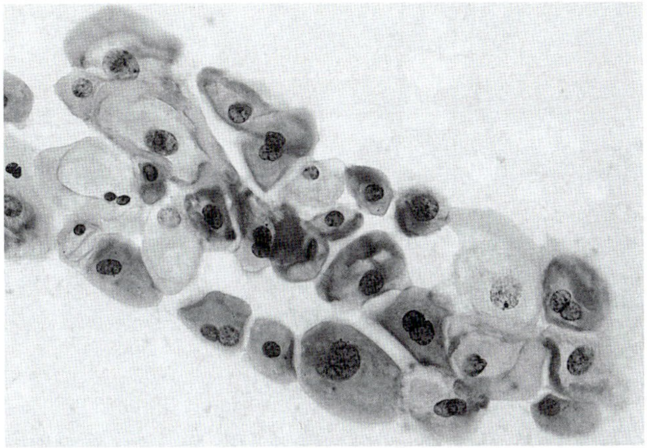

Fig. 7.53. Low-grade SIL. The cells are the superficial type and demonstrate prominent koilocytosis.

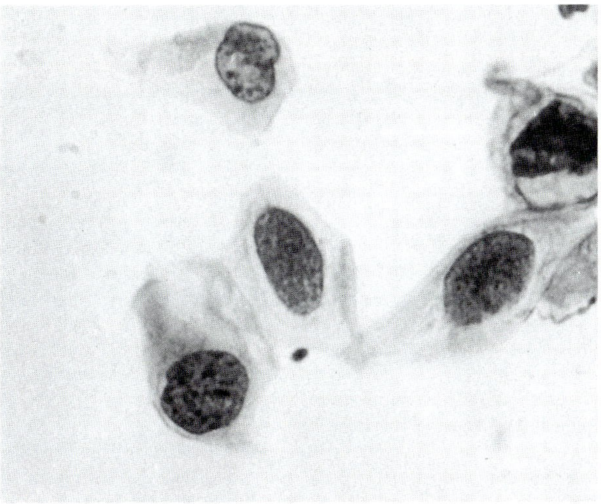

Fig. 7.54. High-grade SIL. High-grade SIL of the type previously referred to as moderate dysplasia. These are enlarged hyperchromatic nuclei with irregular nuclear contour and an increase in the nuclear cytoplasmic ratio.

High-Grade Squamous Intraepithelial Lesions (HSIL)

Because the Bethesda System combines moderate and severe dysplasia together with carcinoma in situ in the high-grade squamous intraepithelial lesion (HSIL) category, there is a wide variation in the cytologic appearance of HSIL. As the severity of the lesion increases, the degree of differentiation and the amount of cytoplasm decreases, the nuclear: cytoplasmic ratio increases, and the degree of nuclear atypia increases (see Table 7.20). HSIL of the moderate dysplasia type typically contains cells similar to those seen in LSIL, as well as atypical immature cells of the parabasal type (Fig. 7.54). The nuclei of these cells are more hyperchromatic and irregular than typically seen in LSIL. In severe dysplasia, the overall size of the cells is reduced compared to mild and moderate dysplasia, but because the cells demonstrate minimal differentiation the nuclear:cytoplasmic ratio is greatly increased (Fig. 7.55). In severe dysplasia, there are usually greater numbers of neoplastic cells compared to mild and moderate dysplasia, and individual dysplastic cells are frequently found. In liquid-based cytology preparations, the cells of HSIL frequently appear smaller than in conventional Papanicolaou preparations (Fig. 7.56).

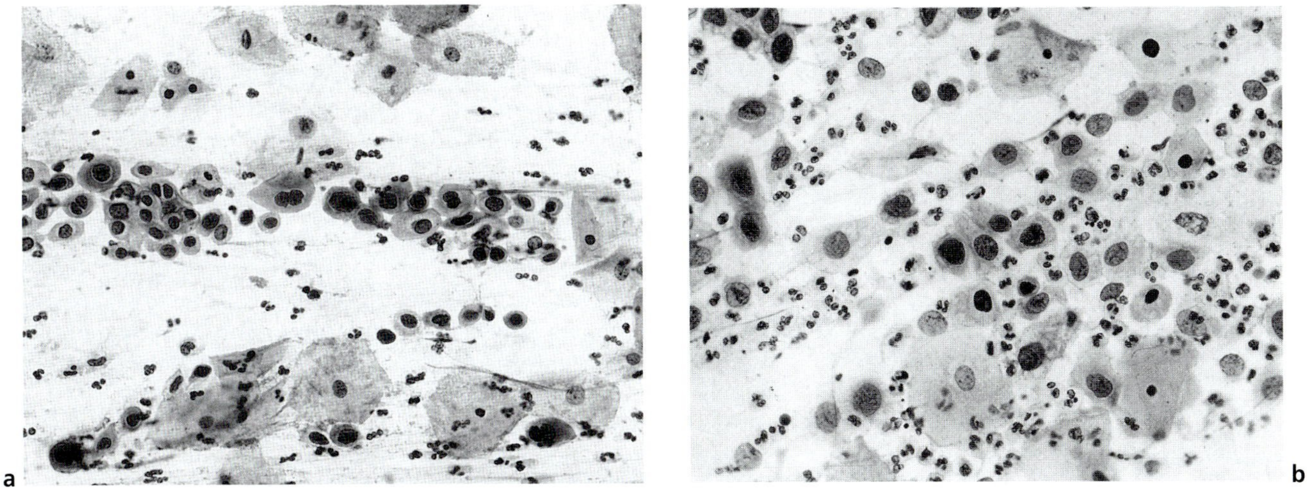

Fig. 7.55. High-grade SIL. High-grade SIL of the type previously referred to as severe dysplasia. **a**: Low magnification showing the typical pattern of high-grade SIL on a conventional Papanicolaou test. **b**: High magnification of a high-grade SIL with many small cells with hyperchromatic nuclei and scant cytoplasm.

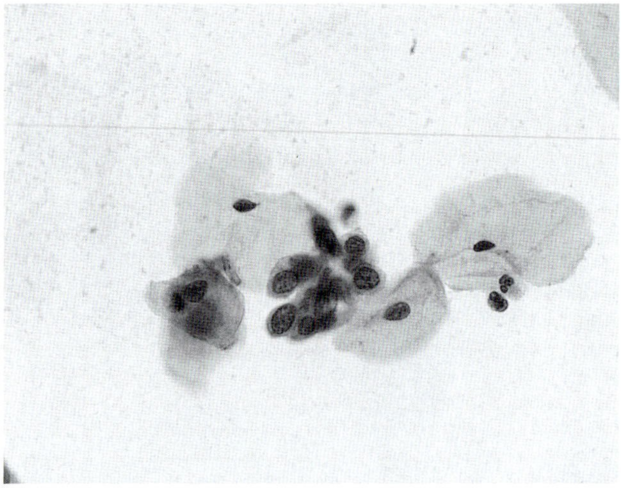

a

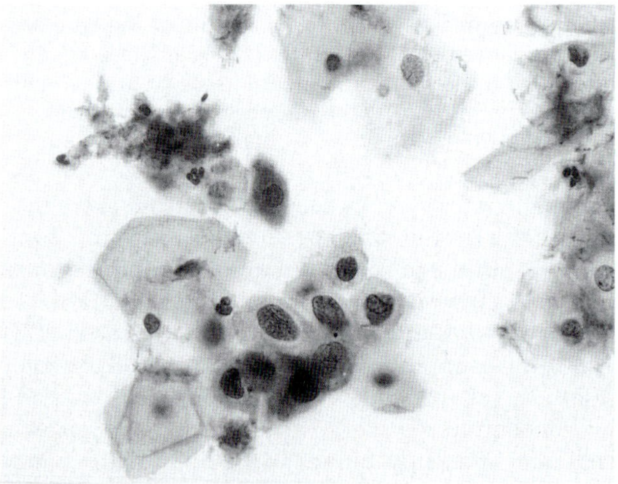

b

Fig. 7.56. High-grade SIL. Liquid-based cytology with high-grade SIL of the type previously referred to as severe dysplasia. **a:** At low magnification the cells appear quite small and sometimes can be overlooked. **b:** At higher magnification the nuclei are seen to be quite enlarged, hyperchromatic, and irregular.

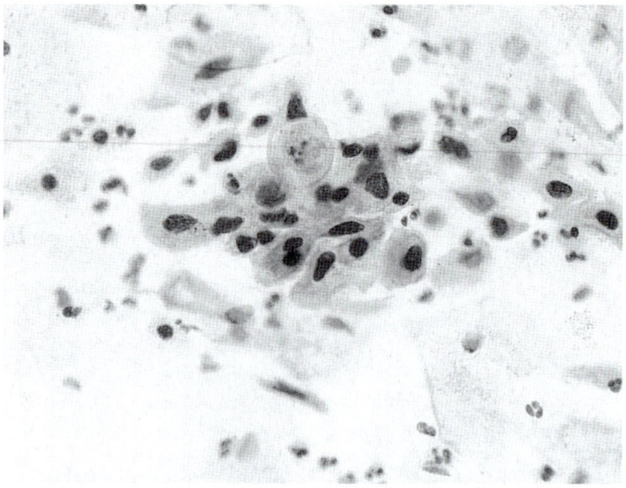

Fig. 7.57. High-grade SIL. High-grade SIL with focal keratinization.

Carcinoma in situ can be of the small cell type, the large cell nonkeratinizing type, or the large cell keratinizing (pleomorphic) type, although separation of carcinoma in situ into these three different cytologic types has no clinical significance. Small cell lesions consist of small basal-type cells similar to those seen in severe dysplasia but which demonstrate even less cytoplasm and higher nuclear: cytoplasmic ratios. Because of their small size, these cells can be easily overlooked during routine screening, and these cases account for a disproportionate percentage of false-negative Papanicolaou tests. The cells of large cell nonkeratinizing lesions typically form syncytial-like cell sheets in which individual cell membranes are difficult to identify. These cells have enlarged, hyperchromatic nuclei and minimal amounts of cytoplasm. The keratinizing large cell type of carcinoma in situ is composed of pleomorphic, highly atypical cells, many of which have thick orangophilic, keratinized cytoplasm (Fig. 7.57). These cells are often spindled or "tadpole" shaped and have extremely dense nuclear chromatin.

Invasive Squamous Cell Carcinoma

Squamous cell carcinomas of the cervix are subdivided into keratinizing and nonkeratinizing types. Nonkeratinizing carcinomas typically have large numbers of malignant cells that form loose cell sheets and syncytial arrangements. The cells have enlarged nuclei that are two to three times the size of a normal intermediate cell nucleus, coarsely clumped chromatin, prominent macronucleoli, and foal chromatin clearing (Fig. 7.58). These cells are often smaller than those of mild or moderate dysplasia. A key cytologic feature is the presence of a "dirty" background on conventional Papanicolaou tests containing blood, cellular debris, fibrin, and necrotic material (Fig. 7.58), often referred to as a tumor diathesis. This characteristic background is usually less prominent in liquid-based cytology specimens. However, in liquid-based cytology there is often a distinctive necrotic background that is easy to recognize because it surrounds the cellular material in a "clumped" appearance and large, necrotic tissue fragments are sometimes present (Fig. 7.59).

Papanicolaou tests from women with keratinizing carcinomas contain malignant cells demonstrating a variety of cell shapes and sizes (Fig. 7.60). Some of the cells are pleomorphic or tadpole shaped. These cells have abundant organophilic cytoplasm, and abundant hyperkeratosis and parakeratosis are frequent. The nuclei are irregular in

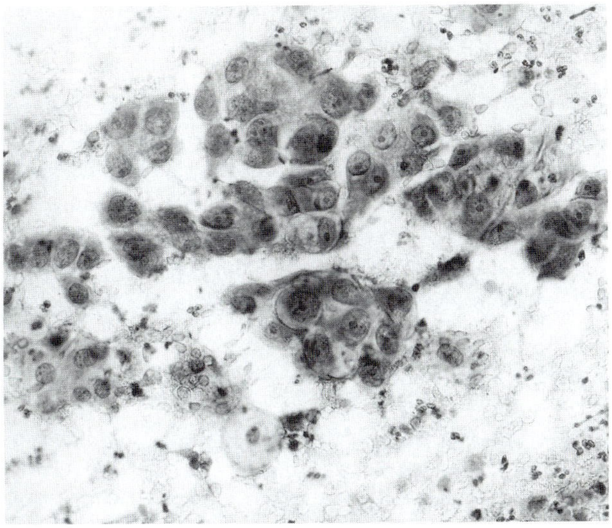

Fig. 7.58. Squamous cell carcinoma. Malignant squamous cells displaying irregularly shaped nuclei with thickened rims and prominent nucleoli. Note tumor diathesis.

shape and quite hyperchromatic; sometimes the nuclei are degenerated, appearing as opaque masses or "ink blots." Unlike nonkeratinizing squamous cell carcinoma, keratinizing squamous cell carcinomas usually do not have a "dirty" background or evidence of tumor diathesis.

Glandular Cell Abnormalities

In the 2001 Bethesda System, all types of glandular cell abnormalities, including both atypical endocervical and endometrial cells, are combined in a single entity referred to as glandular cell abnormalities. Benign-appearing endometrial cells occurring in postmenopausal women are now classified in a separate "other" category. Glandular cell abnormalities are divided into three categories: atypical glandular cells, either unqualified or favor neoplastic; adenocarcinoma in situ; and invasive adenocarcinoma.

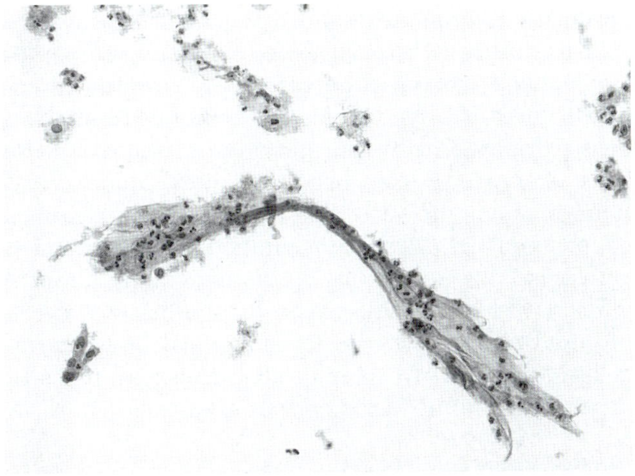

Fig. 7.59. Tumor diathesis. Liquid-based cytology preparation from a woman with squamous cell carcinoma. There is a large fragment of necrotic tissue with a few inflammatory cells. In liquid-based cytology preparations, hemorrhage and inflammation is much less marked than in conventional Papanicolaou tests.

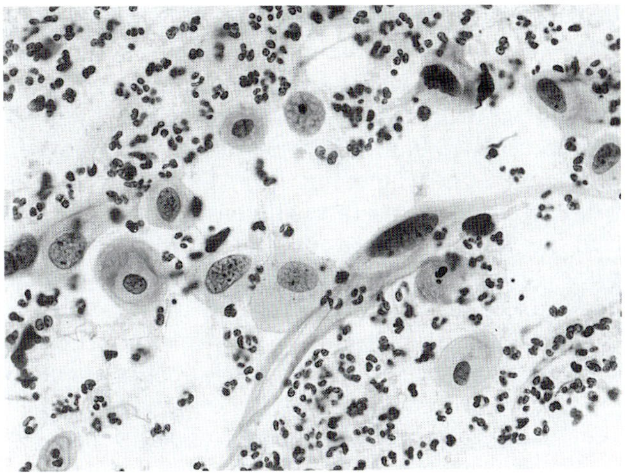

Fig. 7.60. Squamous cell carcinoma. The cells are quite pleomorphic and include bizarre forms. The nuclei of some cells are extremely hyperchromatic.

Atypical Glandular Cells (AGC)

All atypical glandular cells lacking the diagnostic features of adenocarcinoma, irrespective of whether they are of endometrial or endocervical origin, are classified by the 2001 Bethesda System as atypical glandular cells with a specification as to whether they are endocervical, endometrial, or of uncertain origin. There are two categories of AGC: the first is atypical glandular cells (either endocervical, endometrial, or unclassified) that are not qualified, and the second is atypical glandular cells, favor neoplastic.

Glandular cytologic abnormalities are considerably less common than squamous abnormalities, and most cytologists tend to be less comfortable recognizing and diagnosing them. In addition, the criteria used to differentiate reactive endocervical changes, endocervical dysplasia, endocervical adenocarcinoma in situ, and invasive endocervical adenocarcinoma are less well established than those used for squamous lesions. Cytologists even have difficulty in differentiating atypical endocervical cells from cases of high-grade SIL that have extended into endocervical crypts. This difficulty accounts for the high prevalence of squamous abnormalities (approximately 30%) detected in women referred for AGC to colposcopy.[142,240]

The cytologic features of atypical endocervical cells vary depending on the degree of the underlying histopathologic abnormality. Cases of the type designated by cytopathologists as atypical endocervical cells–NOS have minor degrees of variability in nuclear size and shape (Fig. 7.61). Endocervical cells from dense two- or three-dimensional aggregates that have minor degrees of nuclear overlapping. In some cases, the chromatin is somewhat granular and nuclear feathering can be seen at the periphery of the cellular aggregates. "Atypical endocervical cells, favor neoplasia" includes those cases in which

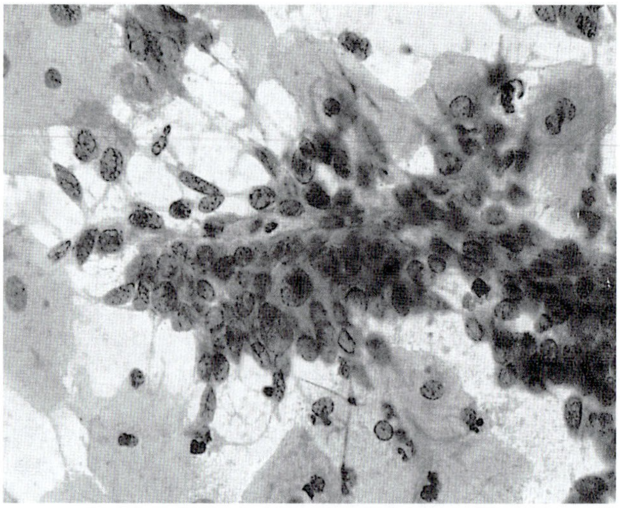

Fig. 7.62. Adenocarcinoma in-situ. These endocervical cells are from a patient with adenocarcinoma in-situ. The nuclei are hyperchromatic and the chromatin is coarsely clumped. Nuclear protrusion (e.g., "feathering") is present at the edge of the group.

the cytologic features suggest adenocarcinoma in situ but are insufficient to allow a definitive diagnosis. These cases typically have more nuclear hyperchromasia, variability in nuclear size, and granularity of the cytoplasm than is observed in cases of atypical endocervical cells, unqualified.

The AGC category also encompasses atypical endometrial cells lacking the cytologic features of adenocarcinoma. Therefore, cells spontaneously exfoliated from both atypical and nonatypical endometrial hyperplasia are classified as atypical endometrial cells. The atypical endometrial cells form a cytologic spectrum ranging from normal to frankly invasive that is similar to that observed with atypical endocervical cells. As one progresses from simple to complex to atypical hyperplasia, the number of atypical cells exfoliated from the uterus increases. Both the cells and the nuclei become larger, micro- and macronucleoli are seen, and the chromatin becomes coarser and less evenly distributed. However, most cytologists have difficulty in distinguishing atypical from nonatypical hyperplasia on the basis of cytology and simply use the term atypical endometrial cells–unqualified to refer to all grades and types of atypical but noninvasive endometrial cells.

a

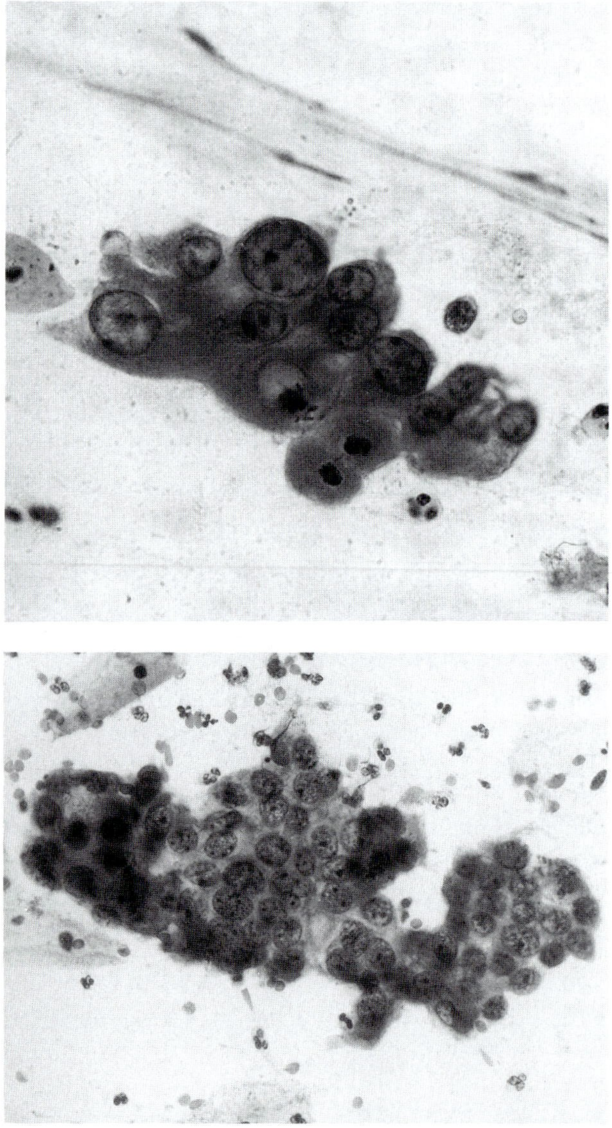

b

Fig. 7.61. Atypical endocervical cells. a: NOS. Granual cells display marked anisokaryosis and mitotic figures. Follow-up studies have been negative. **b:** Favor neoplasin. These endocervical cells are crowded and form a sheet. They have enlarged nuclei, prominent nucleoli, and vary somewhat in size and shape.

Adenocarcinoma In Situ

In cases of adenocarcinoma in situ, there are usually a larger number of atypical glandular cells that form crowded cellular clusters (Fig. 7.62). The sheets are usually three dimensional. The cells within these sheets occasionally form rosettes and have extensive feathering of the cells at the periphery. Individual endocervical cells are highly atypical with enlarged round, oval, or elongated nuclei that vary in size from cell to cell. In most cases, the chromatin is coarsely clumped and multiple mitoses are seen. Sometimes it is difficult for the cytologist to determine whether the atypical cells represent atypical glandular cells or high-grade SIL cells that have extended into an endocervical crypt or "gland." In these cases, highly atypical nuclei are identified in the center of a cell aggregate, and some of the cells at the periphery of the aggregate appear to be endocervical cells.

Adenocarcinoma

The Bethesda System subclassifies invasive adenocarcinomas into "adenocarcinoma-endocervical type," "adenocarcinoma-endometrial type," "adenocarcinoma-extrauterine type," and "adenocarcinoma-not otherwise specified." The cytologic diagnosis of invasive adenocarcinoma is relatively straightforward. Adenocarcinoma cells from either an endocervical or an endometrial primary have enlarged nuclei, high nuclear:cytoplasmic ratios, coarsely clumped chromatin, and prominent nucleoli (Fig. 7.63). They can occur singly or in clusters.

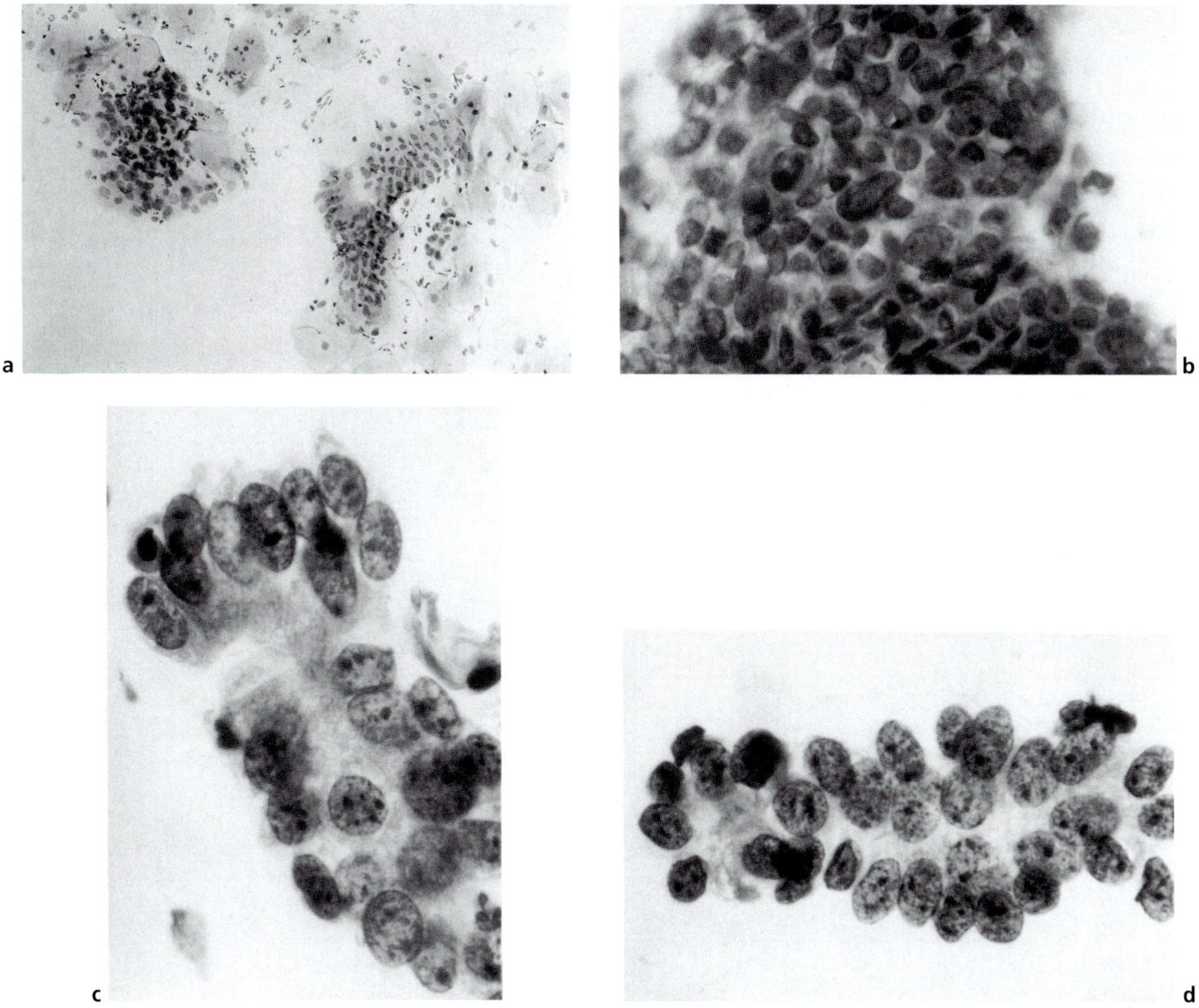

Fig. 7.63. Endocervical adenocarcinoma. a: Sheet of endocervical adenocarcinoma (upper left) displaying cellular overlapping and nuclear hyperchromasia contrasts with benign glandular cells (upper right). **b:** Endocervical adenocarcinoma cells possess pleomorphic nuclei with loss of polarity. **c:** Cellular palisading typical of endocervical adenocarcinoma. Cells have prominent nucleoli which are partially obscured by dense chromatin. **d:** Poorly formed rosette is present. These endocervical cells have the features of frank adenocarcinoma. The nuclei are quite enlarged, the chromatin is coarsely clumped and marginated, and there are prominent nucleoli. (Figs. **a, c,** and **d** courtesy of Bruce Werness, M.D., Washington, DC.)

Cytologists should try to distinguish between endometrial and endocervical primary adenocarcinomas whenever possible. Key features that allow discrimination between endometrial and endocervical origin in cytology include number of abnormal cells, size of the cells, retention of columnar configuration, appearance of cytoplasm, and unclear structure.[203] Typically, adenocarcinoma of the cervix shows considerably larger numbers of cells than does endometrial adenocarcinoma. Cells derived from endocervical adenocarcinoma typically retain a columnar configuration that is lost in most endometrial carcinomas. The cytoplasm of cells exfoliated from endocervical adenocarcinoma are typically eosinophilic and granular, whereas the cytoplasm from cells of endometrial adenocarcinoma is typically finely vacuolated cytoplasm and cyanophilic. The nuclei of cells of endometrial adenocarcinoma have less granular chromatin, are less hyperchromatic, are smaller, and less frequently have multiple nucleoli than do the nuclei of cells of endocervical adenocarcinoma.

References

1. Anonymous (2000) Human papillomavirus testing for triage of women with cytologic evidence of low-grade squamous intraepithelial lesions: baseline data from a randomized trial. The Atypical Squamous Cells of Undetermined Significance/Low-Grade Squamous Intraepithelial Lesions Triage Study (ALTS) Group. J Natl Cancer Inst 92:397–402
2. Anonymous (2001) SEER Program—National Cancer Institute, USA. http://www-seer.ims.nci.nih.gov/ScientificSystems/
3. Abdul-Karim FW, Fu YS, Reagan JW, et al (1982) Morphometric study of intraepithelial neoplasia of the uterine cervix. Obstet Gynecol 60:210–214
4. ACOG (1993) Cervical cytology: evaluation and management of abnormalities. ACOG Technical Bulletin, Washington DC
5. Anciaux D, Lawrence WD, Gregoire L (1997) Glandular lesions of the uterine cervix: prognostic implications of human papillomavirus status. Int J Gynecol Pathol 16:103–110
6. Andersen ES, Arffmann E (1989) Adenocarcinoma in situ of the uterine cervix: a clinico-pathologic study of 36 cases. Gynecol Oncol 35:1–7
7. Anderson M, Jordan J, Morse A, et al (1991) A text and atlas of integrated colposcopy. Mosby Year Book, St Louis
8. Anttila T, Saikku P, Koskela P, et al (2001) Serotypes of *Chlamydia trachomatis* and risk for development of cervical squamous cell carcinoma. JAMA 285:47–51
9. Azodi M, Chambers SK, Rutherford TJ, et al (1999) Adenocarcinoma in situ of the cervix: management and outcome. Gynecol Oncol 73:348–353
10. Bamford PN, Barber M, Beilby JOW (1982) Letter to the editor. Changing patterns of cervical intraepithelial neoplasia seen in a family planning clinic. Lancet i:747–827
11. Barbosa MS, Edwards C, Fisher C, et al (1990) The region of the HPV E7 oncoprotein homologous to adenovirus E1A and SV40 large T antigen contains separate domains for Rb binding and casein kinase II phosphorylation. EMBO J 9:153–160
12. Barton SE, Maddox PH, Jenkins D, et al (1988) Effect of cigarette smoking on cervical epithelial immunity: a mechanism for neoplastic change? Lancet i:652–654
13. Bauer HM, Ting Y, Greer CE, et al (1991) Genital human papillomavirus infection in female university students as determined by a PCR-based method. JAMA 265:472–477
14. Bauknecht T, See RH, Shi Y (1996) A novel C/EBP beta-YY1 complex controls the cell-type-specific activity of the human papillomavirus type 18 upstream regulatory region. J Virol 70:7695–7705
15. Becker TM, Wheeler CM, McGough NS, et al (1994) Sexually transmitted diseases and other risk factors for cervical dysplasia among Southwestern hispanic and non-hispanic white women. JAMA 271:1181–1188
16. Bedell MA, Jones KH, Laimins LA (1987) The E6-E7 region of human papillomavirus type 18 is sufficient for transformation of NIH 3T3 and rat-1 cells. J Virol 61:3635–3640
17. Bergeron C, Barrasso R, Beaudenon S, et al (1992) Human papillomaviruses associated with cervical intraepithelial neoplasia. Great diversity and distinct distribution in low- and high-grade lesions. Am J Surg Pathol 16:641–649
18. Bergeron C, Ferenczy A, Shah K, et al (1987) Multicentric human papillomavirus infections of the female genital tract. Correlation of viral types with abnormal mitotic figures, colposcopic presentation, and location. Obstet Gynecol 69:736–742
19. Bernard BA, Bailly C, Lenoir MC, et al (1989) The human papillomavirus type 18 (HP18) E2 gene product is a repressor of the HPV18 regulatory region in human keratinocytes. J Virol 63:4317–4324
20. Bertrand M, Lickrish GM, Colgan TJ (1987) The anatomic distribution of cervical adenocarcinoma in situ: implications for treatment. Am J Obstet Gynecol 157:21–25
21. Bibbo M, Dytch HE, Alenghat E, et al (1989) DNA ploidy profiles as prognostic indicators in CIN lesions. Am J Clin Pathol 92:261–265
22. Boddington MM, Spriggs AI, Cowdell RH (1976) Adenocarcinoma of the uterine cervix: cytological evidence of a long preclinical evolution. Br J Obstet Gynecol 83:900–903
23. Bontkes HJ, van Duin M, de Gruijl TD, et al (1998) HPV 16 infection and progression of cervical intraepithelial neoplasia: analysis of HLA polymor-

phism and HPV 16 E6 sequence variants. Int J Cancer 78:166–171
24. Boon ME, Alons-van Kordelaar JJM, Rietveld-Scheffers PEM (1986) Consequences of the introduction of combined spatula and Cytobrush sampling for cervical cytology: improvements in smear quality and detection rates. Acta Cytol 30:264–270
25. Boon ME, Baak JPA, Kurver PJH, et al (1981) Adenocarcinoma in situ of the cervix: an underdiagnosed lesion. Cancer (Phila) 48:768–773
26. Bornstein J, Rahat MA, Abramovici H (1995) Etiology of cervical cancer: current concepts. Obstet Gynecol Surv 50:146–154
27. Bosch FX, de Sanjose S, Castellsague X, et al (1997) Geographical and social patterns of cervical cancer incidence. In: Franco E, Monsonego J (eds) New developments in cervical cancer screening and prevention. Blackwell, London, pp 23–33
28. Bosch FX, Manos MM, Munoz N, et al (1995) Prevalence of human papillomavirus in cervical cancer: a worldwide perspective. International Biological Study on Cervical Cancer (IBSCC) Study Group. J Natl Cancer Inst 87:779–780
29. Bosch FX, Munoz N, de Sanjose S, et al (1992) Risk factors for cervical cancer in Colombia and Spain. Int J Cancer 52:750–758
30. Boshart M, Gissman L, Ikenberg H, et al (1984) A new type of papillomavirus DNA, its presence in genital cancer biopsies and in cell lines derived from cervical cancer. EMBO J 3:1151–1157
31. Bousfield L, Pacey F, Young Q, et al (1980) Expanded cytologic criteria for the diagnosis of adenocarcinoma in situ of the cervix and related lesions. Acta Cytol 24:283–296
32. Brinton LA (1991) Oral contraceptives and cervical neoplasia. Contraception 43:581–595
33. Brinton LA (1992) Epidemiology of cervical cancer-an overview. In: Munoz N, et al (eds) The epidemiology of cervical cancer and human papillomavirus. IARC, Lyon, pp 3–23
34. Broders AC (1932) Carcinoma in situ contrasted with benign penetrating epithelium. JAMA 99: 1670–1674
35. Brown LJ, Griffin NR, Wells M (1987) Cytoplasmic reactivity with the monoclonal antibody HMFG-1 as a marker of cervical glandular atypia. J Pathol 151:203–208
36. Brown LJR, Wells M (1986) Cervical glandular atypia associated with squamous intraepithelial neoplasia: a premalignant lesion? J Clin Path 39: 22–28
37. Bryan JT, Brown DR (2000) Association of the human papillomavirus type 11 E1()E4 protein with cornified cell envelopes derived from infected genital epithelium. Virology 277:262–269
38. Burghardt E (1991) Colposcopy-cervical pathology. Thieme Medical Publishers, New York
39. Burke L, Antonioli DA, Ducatman BS (1991) Colposcopy: text and atlas, 1st Ed. Appleton and Lange, Norwalk, CT, p 228
40. Butterworth CEJ, Hatch KD, Macaluso M, et al (1992) Folate deficiency and cervical dysplasia. JAMA 267:528–533
41. Campion MJ, McCance DJ, Cuzick J, et al (1986) Progressive potential of mild cervical atypia: prospective cytological, colposcopic, snd virologic study. Lancet ii:237–240
42. Carter JJ, Koutsky LA, Wipf GC, et al (1996) The natural history of human papillomavirus type 16 capsid antibodies among a cohort of university women. J Infect Dis 174:927–936
43. Chan PK, Chan MY, Li WW, et al (2001) Association of human beta-herpesviruses with the development of cervical cancer: bystanders or cofactors. J Clin Pathol 54:48–53
44. Chang A, Sandweiss L, Bose S (2001) Cytologically benign endometrial cells in the Papanicolaou smears of postmenopausal women. Gynecol Oncol 80:37–43
45. Chen JJ, Reid CE, Band V, et al (1995) Interaction of papillomavirus E6 oncoproteins with a putative calcium-binding protein. Science 269:529–531
46. Chiasson MA, Ellerbrock TV, Bush TJ, et al (1997) Increased prevalence of vulvovaginal condyloma and vulvar intraepithelial neoplasia in women infected with the human immunodeficiency virus. Obstet Gynecol 89:690–694
47. Chichareon S, Herrero R, Munoz N, et al (1998) Risk factors for cervical cancer in Thailand: a case-control study. J Natl Cancer Inst 90:50–57
48. Chin KM, Sidhu JS, Janssen RS, et al (1998) Invasive cervical cancer in human immunodeficiency virus-infected and uninfected hospital patients. Obstet Gynecol 92:83–87
49. Choo K-B, Pan C-C, Han S-H (1987) Integration of human papillomavirus type 16 into cellular DNA of cervical carcinoma: preferential deletion of the E2 gene and invariable retention of the long control region and the E6/E7 open reading frames. Virology 161:259–261
50. Chung TK, Cheung TH, Lo WK, et al (2000) Loss of heterozygosity at the short arm of chromosome 3 in microdissected cervical intraepithelial neoplasia. Cancer Lett 154:189–194
51. Clavel C, Masure M, Bory JP, et al (1999) Hybrid capture ii-based human papillomavirus detection, a sensitive test to detect in routine high-grade cervical lesions: a preliminary study on 1518 women. Br J Cancer 80:1306–1311
52. Cobrinik D, Dowdy SF, Hinds PW (1992) The retinoblastoma protein and the regulation of cell cycling. Trends Biol Sci 17:312
53. Colgan TJ, Lickrish GM (1990) The topography and invasive potential of cervical adenocarcinoma in situ, with and without associated squamous dysplasia. Gynecol Oncol 36:246–249
54. Conti M, Agarossi A, Parazzini F, et al (1993) HPV, HIV infection, and risk of cervical intraepithelial neoplasia in former intravenous drug abusers. Gynecol Oncol 49:344–348

55. Coppleson M (1970) The origin and nature of premalignant lesions of the cervix uteri. Int J Gynecol Obstet 8:539
56. Cox T, Lorincz AT, Schiffman MH, et al (1995) Human papillomavirus testing by hybrid capture appears to be useful in triaging women with a cytologic diagnosis of atypical squamous cells of undetermined significance. Am J Obstet Gynecol 172:946–954
57. Cramer DW, Cutler SJ (1974) Incidence and histopathology of malignancies of the female genital organs in the United States. Am J Obstet Gynecol 118:443
58. Crocker J, Fox H, Langley FA (1968) Consistency in the histological diagnosis of epithelial abnormalities of the cervix uteri. J Clin Pathol 21:67–70
59. Crook T, Morgenstern JP, Crawford L, et al (1989) Continued expression of HPV 16 E7 protein is required for maintenance of the transformed phenotype of cells co-transformed by HPV 16 plus EJ-ras. EMBO J 8:513–519
60. Crum CP, Egawa K, Fu YS, et al (1983) Atypical immature metaplasia (AIM): a subset of human papillomavirus infection of the cervix. Cancer (Phila) 51:2214–2219
61. Crum CP, Nagai N, Mitao M, et al (1985) Histological and molecular analysis of early cervical neoplasia. In: Howley P, Broker T (eds) Papillomaviruses: molecular and clinical aspects. Cold Spring Harbor, New York, pp 19–29
62. Crusius K, Auvinen E, Alonso A (1997) Enhancement of EGF- and PMA-mediated MAP kinase activation in cells expressing the human papillomavirus type 16 E5 protein. Oncogene 15:1437–1444.
63. Cullen AP, Reid R, Campion M, et al (1991) Analysis of the physical state of different human papillomavirus DNAs in intraepithelial and invasive cervical neoplasia. J Virol 65:606–612
64. Cullen TS (1900) Cancer of the uterus. Appleton, New York
65. Cullimore JE, Luesley DM, Rollason TP, et al (1992) A prospective study of conization of the cervix in the management of cervical intraepithelial glandular neoplasia (CIGN)—a preliminary report. Br J Obstet Gynaecol 99:314–318
66. Cuzick J, Beverley E, Ho L, et al (1999) Hpv testing in primary screening of older women. Br J Cancer 81:554–558
67. Das BC, Sharma JK, Gopalakrishna V, et al (1992) Analysis by polymerase chain reaction of the physical state of human papillomavirus type 16 in cervical preneoplastic and neoplastic lesions. J Gen Virol 73:2327–2336
68. de Vet HC, Knipschild PG, Grol ME, et al (1991) The role of beta-carotene and other dietary factors in the aetiology of cervical dysplasia: results of a case control study. Int J Epidemiol 20:603–610
69. de Villiers EM (1992) Hybridization methods other than PCR: an update. In: Munoz N, et al (eds) The epidemiology of human papillomavirus and cervical cancer. IARC, Lyon, pp 111–119
70. Denehy TR, Gregori CA, Breen JL (1997) Endocervical curettage, cone margins, and residual adenocarcinoma in situ of the cervix. Obstet Gynecol 90:1–6
71. DiPaolo JA, Jones C (1999) The role of herpes simplex 2 in the development of HPV-positive cervical carcinoma. Papillomavirus Rep 10:1–8
72. Duggan MA, Benoit JL, McGregor SE, et al (1994) Adenocarcinoma in situ of the endocervix: human papillomavirus determination by dot blot hybridization and polymerase chain reaction amplification. Int J Gynecol Pathol 13:143–149
73. Durst M, Kleinheinz A, Hotz M, et al (1985) The physical state of human papillomavirus type 16 DNA in benign and malignant genital tumors. J Gen Virol 66:1515–1522
74. Dyson N, Howley PM, Munger K, et al (1989) The human papillomavirus 16 E7 oncoprotein is able to bind to the retinoblastoma gene product. Science 243:934–937
75. Ellerbrock TV, Chiasson MA, Bush TJ, et al (2000) Incidence of cervical squamous intraepithelial lesions in HIV-infected women. JAMA 283:1031–1037
76. Evander M, Frazer IH, Payne E, et al (1997) Identification of the alpha6 integrin as a candidate receptor for papillomaviruses. J Virol 71:2449–2456
77. Evans S, Dowling K (1990) The changing prevalence of cervical human papillomavirus infection. Aust N Z J Obstet Gynecol 30:375–377
78. Farnsworth A, Laverty C, Stoler MH (1989) Human papillomavirus messenger RNA expression in adenocarcinoma in situ of the uterine cervix. Int J Gynecol Pathol 8:321–330
79. Ferenczy A (1985) Comparison of cryo- and carbon dioxide laser therapy for cervical intraepithelial neoplasia. Obstet Gynecol 66:793–798
80. Ferenczy A, Gelfand MM, Franco E, et al (1997) Human papillomavirus infection in postmenopausal women with and without hormone therapy. Obstet Gynecol 90:7–11
81. Ferris DG, Wright TC Jr, Litaker MS, et al (1998) Triage of women with ASCUS and LSIL on Pap smear reports: management by repeat Pap smear, HVP DNA testing, or colposcopy? J Fam Pract 46:125–134
82. Firzlaff JM, Kiviat NB, Beckmann AM, et al (1988) Detection of human papillomavirus capsid antigens in various squamous epithelial lesions using antibodies directed against the L1 and L2 open reading frames. Virology 164:467–477
83. Fletcher S (1983) Histopathology of papillomavirus infection of the cervix uteri: the history, taxonomy, nomenclature and reporting of koilocytic dysplasias. J Clin Pathol 36:616–624
84. Foote FW, Stewart FW (1948) The anatomical distribution of intraepithelial epidermoid carcinomas of cervix. Cancer (Phila) 1:431–440

85. Francis DA, Schmid SL, Howley PM (2000) Repression of the integrated papillomavirus E6/E7 promoter is required for growth suppression of cervical cancer cells. J Virol 74:2679–2686
86. Franquemont DW, Ward BE, Anderson WA, et al (1989) Prediction of "high-risk" cervical papillomavirus infection by biopsy morphology. Am J Clin Pathol 92:577–582
87. Friedell GH, McKay DG (1953) Adenocarcinoma in situ of endocervix. Cancer (Phila) 6:887–897
88. Friedell GH, Ross FE, Tucker TC, et al (2000) Cervical cancer in Kentucky. J Ky Med Assoc 98:398–405
89. Friedell GH, Tucker TC, McManmon E, et al (1992) Incidence of dysplasia and carcinoma of the uterine cervix in an Appalachian population. J Natl Cancer Inst 84:1030–1032
90. Friend SH, Dryja T, Weinberg RA (1988) Oncogenes and tumor-suppressing genes. N Engl J Med 318:618–622
91. Fu YS, Braun L, Shah KV, et al (1983) Histologic, nuclear DNA, and human papillomavirus studies of cervical condylomas. Cancer (Phila) 52:1705–1711
92. Fu YS, Huang I, Beaudenon S, et al (1988) Correlative study of human papillomavirus DNA, histopathology and morphometry in cervical condyloma and intraepithelial neoplasia. Int J Gynecol Pathol 7:297–307
93. Fu YS, Reagan JW, Richart RM (1983) Precursors of cervical cancer. Cancer Surv 2:359–382
94. Gad C (1976) The management and natural history of severe dysplasia and carcinoma in situ of the uterine cervix. Br J Obstet Gynecol 83:554–559
95. Genest DR, Stein L, Cibas E, et al (1993) A binary (bethesda) system for classifying cervical cancer precursors: criteria, reproducibility, and viral correlates. Hum Pathol 24:730–736
96. Gloor E, Hurlimann J (1986) Cervical intraepithelial glandular neoplasia (adenocarcinoma in situ and glandular dysplasia). A correlative study of 23 cases with histologic grading, histochemical analysis of mucins and immunohistochemical determination of the affinity for four lectins. Cancer (Phila) 58:1272–1280
97. Goedert JJ, Cote TR, Virgo P, et al (1998) Spectrum of AIDS-associated malignant disorders. Lancet 351:1833–1839
98. Goldstein NS, Ahmad E, Hussain M, et al (1998) Endocervical glandular atypia: does a preneoplastic lesion of adenocarcinoma in situ exist? Am J Clin Pathol 110:200–209
99. Goodman MT, Kiviat N, McDuffie K, et al (1998) The association of plasma micronutrients with the risk of cervical dysplasia in Hawaii. Cancer Epidemiol Biomark Prev 7:537–544
100. Gram IT, Macaluso M, Stalsberg H (1992) Oral contraceptive use and the incidence of cervical intraepithelial neoplasia. Am J Obstet Gynecol 167: 40–44
101. Greenberg MD, Reid R, Schiffman M, et al (1999) A prospective study of biopsy-confirmed cervical intraepithelial neoplasia grade 1: colposcopic, cytological, and virological risk factors for progression. J Lower Gen Tract Dis 3:104–110
102. Grieder CW (1999) Telomerase activation: one step on the road to cancer? Trends Genet 15:109–112
103. Griffin NR, Dockey D, Lewis FA, et al (1991) Demonstration of low frequency of human papillomavirus DNA in cervical adenocarcinoma and adenocarcinoma in situ by the polymerase chain reaction and in situ hybridization. Int J Gynecol Pathol 10:36–43
104. Halpert R, Fruchter RG, Sedlis A, et al (1986) Human papillomavirus and lower genital neoplasia in renal transplant patients. Obstet Gynecol 150:251–258
105. Hanselaar AG, Vooijs GP, Oud PS, et al (1988) DNA ploidy patterns in cervical intraepithelial neoplasia grade III, with and without synchronous invasive squamous cell carcinoma: measurements in nuclei isolated from paraffin-embedded tissue. Cancer (Phila) 62:2537–2545
106. Hatch E, Herbst A, Hoover R, et al (2000) Incidence of squamous neoplasia of the cervix and vagina in DES-exposed daughters. Ann Epidemiol 10:467
107. Hawley-Nelson P, Vousden KH, Hubbert NL, et al (1989) HPV16 E6 and E7 proteins cooperate to immortalize human foreskin keratinocytes. EMBO J 8:3905–3910
108. Helmerhorst TJM (1992) Clinical significance of endocervical curettage as part of colposcopic evaluation. A review. Int J Gynecol Cancer 2:256–262
109. Helper TK, Dockerty MB, Randall LM (1952) Primary adenocarcinoma of the cervix. Am J Obstet Gynecol 63:800–808
110. Heinzl S, Szalmay G, Jochum L, et al (1982) Observations on the development of dysplasia. Acta Cytol 26:453–456
111. Hering B, Horn LC, Nenning H, et al (2000) Predictive value of DNA cytometry in CIN 1 and 2. Image analysis of 193 cases. Anal Quant Cytol Histol 22:333–337
112. Herrero R, Hildesheim A, Bratti C, et al (2000) Population-based study of human papillomavirus infection and cervical neoplasia in rural Costa Rica. J Natl Cancer Inst 92:464–474
113. Higgins GD, Phillips GE, Smith LA, et al (1992) High prevalence of human papillomavirus transcripts in all grades of cervical intraepithelial glandular neoplasia. Cancer (Phila) 70:136–146
114. Hildesheim A, Mann V, Brinton LA, et al (1991) Herpes simplex virus type 2: a possible interaction with human papillomavirus types 16/18 in the development of invasive cervical cancer. Int J Cancer 49:335–340
115. Ho GY, Bierman R, Beardsley L, et al (1998) Natural history of cervicovaginal papillomavirus infection in young women. N Engl J Med 338:423–428
116. Hoffman MS, Sterghos S, Gordy LW, et al (1993) Evaluation of the cervical canal with the endocervical brush. Obstet Gynecol 82:573–577

117. Hollingworth RE, Lee W-H (1991) Tumor suppression genes: new prospects for cancer research. J Natl Cancer Inst 83:91–96
118. Holowaty P, Miller AB, Rohan T, et al (1999) Natural history of dysplasia of the uterine cervix. J Natl Cancer Inst 91:252–258
119. Hopkins MP, Roberts JA, Schmidt RW (1988) Cervical adenocarcinoma in situ. Obstet Gynecol 71:842–844
120. Hopman EH, Rozendaal L, Voorhorst FJ, et al (2000) High risk human papillomavirus in women with normal cervical cytology prior to the development of abnormal cytology and colposcopy. Br J Obstet Gynaecol 107:600–604
121. Howley PM (1991) Papillomavirinae and their replication. In: Fields BN, Knipe DM (eds) Fundamental virology. Raven Press, New York, pp 743–770
122. Hurlimann J, Gloor E (1984) Adenocarcinoma in situ and invasive adenocarcinoma of the uterine cervix. An immunohistologic study with antibodies specific for several epithelial markers. Cancer (Phila) 54:103–109
123. IARC (1995) Human papillomaviruses. 64:407
124. Iglesias M, Yen K, Gaiotti D, et al (1998) Human papillomavirus type 16 E7 protein sensitizes cervical keratinocytes to apoptosis and release of interleukin-1alpha. Oncogene 17:1195–1205
125. Ismail SM, Colelough AB, Dinnen JS, et al (1989) Observer variation in histopathological diagnosis and grading of cervical intraepithelial neoplasia. Br Med J 298:707–710
126. Jacobs MV, Walboomers JM, Snijders PJ, et al (2000) Distribution of 37 mucosotropic hpv types in women with cytologically normal cervical smears: the age-related patterns for high-risk and low-risk types. Int J Cancer 87:221–227
127. Jakobsen A, Kristensen PB, Poulsen HK (1983) Flow cytometric classification of biopsy specimens from cervical intraepithelial neoplasia. Cytometry 4:166–169
128. Jaworski RC, Pacey NR, Greenberg ML, et al (1988) The histologic diagnosis of adenocarcinoma in situ and related lesions of the cervix uteri. Adenocarcinoma in situ. Cancer (Phila) 61:1171–1181
129. Jenson AB, Rosenthal JD, Olson C, et al (1980) Immunologic relatedness of papillomavirus from different species. J Natl Cancer Inst 64:495–500
130. Jewers RJ, Hildebrandt P, Ludlow JW, et al (1992) Regions of human papillomavirus type 16 E7 oncoprotein required for immortalization of human keratinocytes. J Virol 66:1329–1335
131. Johnson LD (1969) The histopathological approach to early cervical neoplasia. Obstet Gynecol Surv 24:735–767
132. Jones BA (1995) Rescreening in gynecologic cytology. Arch Pathol Lab Med 119:1097–1103
133. Jones BA, Novis DA (2000) Follow-up of abnormal gynecologic cytology: a college of American pathologists Q-probes study of 16132 cases from 306 laboratories. Arch Pathol Lab Med 124:665–671
134. Jones CJ, Brinton LA, Hamman RF, et al (1990) Risk factors for in situ cervical cancer: results from a case-control study. Cancer Res 50:3657–3662
135. Josefsson AM, Magnusson PK, Yitalo N, et al (2000) Viral load of human papilloma virus 16 as a determinant for development of cervical carcinoma in situ: a nested case-control study. Lancet 355:2189–2193
136. Kadish AS, Hagan RJ, Ritter DB, et al (1992) Biologic characteristics of specific human papillomavirus types predicted from morphology of cervical lesions. Hum Pathol 23:1262–1269
137. Kalantari M, Karlsen F, Johansson B, et al (1997) Human papillomavirus findings in relation to cervical intraepithelial neoplasia grade: a study on 476 stockholm women, using pcr for detection and typing of hpv. Hum Pathol 28:899–904
138. Kantesky PA, Gammon MD, Mandelblatt J, et al (1998) Dietary intake and blood levels of lycopene: association with cervical dysplasia among non-Hispanic, black women. Nutr Cancer 31:31–40
139. Kashimura M, Shinohara M, Oikawa K, et al (1990) An adenocarcinoma *in situ* of the uterine cervix that developed into invasive adenocarcinoma after 5 years. Gynecol Oncol 36:128–133
140. Kataja V, Syrjanen S, Mantyjarvi R, et al (1992) Prognostic factor in cervical human papillomavirus infections. Sex Transm Dis 19:154–160
141. Kessler II (1974) Perspectives on the epidemiology of cervical cancer with special reference to the herpes virus hypothesis. Cancer (Phila) 34:1091
142. Kim TJ, Kim HS, Park CT, et al (1999) Clinical evaluation of follow-up methods and results of atypical glandular cells of undetermined significance (AGUS) detected on cervicovaginal Pap smears. Gynecol Oncol 73:292–298
143. Kinney WK, Manos MM, Hurley LB, et al (1998) Where's the high-grade cervical neoplasia? The importance of minimally abnormal Papanicolaou diagnoses. Obstet Gynecol 91:973–976
144. Kirkland JA (1963) Atypical epithelial changes in the uterine cervix. J Clin Pathol 16:150–154
145. Kiviat NB, Critchlow CW, Kurman RJ (1992) Reassessment of the morphological continuum of cervical intraepithelial lesions; does it reflect different stages in the progression to cervical carcinoma? In: Munoz N, et al (eds) The epidemiology of cervical cancer and human papillomavirus. I.A.R.C., Lyons, pp 59–66
146. Kjaer SK, Chackerian B, van den Brule AJ, et al (2001) High-risk human papillomavirus is sexually transmitted: evidence from a follow-up study of virgins starting sexual activity (intercourse). Cancer Epidemiol Biomark Prev 10:101–106
147. Kjellberg L, Hallmans G, Ahren AM, et al (2000) Smoking, diet, pregnancy and oral contraceptive use as risk factors for cervical intraepithelial neo-

plasia in relation to human papillomavirus infection. Br J Cancer 82:1332–1338
148. Klaes R, Friedrich T, Spitkovsky D, et al (2001) Overexpression of p16(INK4A) as a specific marker for dysplastic and neoplastic epithelial cells of the cervix uteri. Int J Cancer 92:276–284
149. Klam S, Arseneau J, Mansour N, et al (2000) Comparison of endocervical curettage and endocervical brushing. Obstet Gynecol 96:90–94
150. Kolstad P, Klem V (1979) Long-term follow-up of 1121 cases of carcinoma in situ. Obstet Gynecol 48:125–133
151. Koss L, Durfee GR (1956) Unusual patterns of squamous epithelium of uterine cervix: cytologic and pathologic study of koilocytotic atypia. Ann NY Acad Sci 63:1245–1261
152. Koss LG (1978) Dysplasia. A real concept or a misnomer? Obstet Gynecol 51:374–379
153. Koss LG (1992) Diagnostic cytology and its histopathologic basis. Vol. 1, 4th ed. Lippincott, Philadelphia, pp 383–387
154. Koss LG, Stewart FW, Foote FW, et al (1963) Some histological aspects of behavior of epidermoid carcinoma in situ and related lesions of the uterine cervix. Cancer (Phila) 16:1160–1211
155. Kottmeier HL (1961) Evolution et traitment des epitheliomas. Rev Fr Gynecol Obstet 56:821–826
156. Koutsky LA, Galloway DA, Holmes KK (1988) Epidemiology of genital human papillomavirus infection. Epidemiol Rev 10:122–163
157. Koutsky LA, Holmes KK, Critchlow CW, et al (1992) A cohort study of the risk of cervical intraepithelial neoplasia grade 2 or 3 in relation to papillomavirus infection. N Engl J Med 327:1272–1278
158. Kudo R, Sagai S, Hayakawa O, et al (1991) Morphology of adenocarcinoma in situ and microinvasive adenocarcinoma of the uterine cervix. Acta Cytol 35:109–116
159. Kudo R, Sasano H, Koizumi M, et al (1990) Immunohistochemical comparison of new monoclonal antibody IC5 and carcinoembryonic antigen in the differential diagnosis of adenocarcinoma of the uterine cervix. Int J Gynecol Pathol 9:325–336
160. Kuhn L, Sun X-W, Wright TC (1999) Human immunodeficiency virus infection and female lower genital tract malignancy. Curr Opin Obstet Gynecol 11:35–41
161. Kurman R, Soloman D (1994) The Bethesda system for reporting cervical/vaginal cytologic diagnoses. Springer-Verlag, New York
162. Kurman RJ, Henson DE, Herbst AL, et al (1994) Interim guidelines for management of abnormal cervical cytology. The 1992 National Cancer Institute workshop. JAMA 271:1866–1869
163. Kurman RJ, Norris HJ, Wilkinson E (1992) Tumors of the cervix, vagina and vulva. Armed Forces Institute of Pathology, Washington DC
164. Lancaster WD, Castellano C, Santos C, et al (1986) Human papillomavirus deoxyribonucleic acid in cervical carcinoma from primary and metastic sites. Am J Obstet Gynecol 154:115–119
165. Larson AA, Kern S, Curtiss S, et al (1997) High resolution analysis of chromosome 3p alterations in cervical carcinoma. Cancer Res 57:4082–4090
166. Laverty CR, Russell P, Hills E, et al (1978) The significance of noncondylomatous wart virus infection of the cervical transformation zone: a review with discussion of two illustrative cases. Acta Cytol 22:195–201
167. Lawson HW, Lee NC, Thames SF, et al (1998) Cervical cancer screening among low-income women: results of a national screening program, 1991–1995. Obstet Gynecol 92:745–752
168. Lippes J (1999) Pelvic actinomycosis: a review and preliminary look at prevalence. Am J Obstet Gynecol 180:265–269
169. Lorincz AT, Reid R, Jenson AB, et al (1992) Human papillomavirus infection of the cervix: relative risk associations of 15 common anogenital types. Obstet Gynecol 79:328–337
170. Lorincz AT, Temple GF, Kurman J, et al (1987) Oncogenic association of specific human papillomavirus types with cervical neoplasia. J Natl Cancer Inst 79:671–677
171. Luesley DM, Jordan JA, Woodman CBJ, et al (1987) A retrospective review of adenocarcinoma-in-situ and glandular atypia of the uterine cervix. Br J Obstet Gynaecol 94:699–703
172. Luff RD (1992) The Bethesda System for reporting cervical/vaginal cytologic diagnoses: report of the 1991 Bethesda Workshop. Hum Pathol 23:719–721
173. Lungu O, Crum CP, Silverstein S (1991) Biologic properties and nucleotide sequence analysis of human papillomavirus type-51.
174. Lungu O, Sun XW, Felix J, et al (1992) Relationship of human papillomavirus type to grade of cervical intraepithelial neoplasia. JAMA 267:2493–2496
175. Ma T, Zou N, Lin BY, et al (1999) Interaction between cyclin-dependent kinases and human papillomavirus replication-initiation protein E1 is required for efficient viral replication. Proc Natl Acad Sci USA 96:382–387
176. Magal SS, Jackman A, Pei XF, et al (1998) Induction of apoptosis in human keratinocytes containing mutated p53 alleles and its inhibition by both the E6 and E7 oncoproteins. Int J Cancer 75:96–104
177. Malik SN, Wilkinson EJ, Drew PA, et al (1999) Do qualifiers of ASCUS distinguish between low- and high-risk patients? Acta Cytol 43:376–380
178. Manos MM, Kinney WK, Hurley LB, et al (1999) Identifying women with cervical neoplasia: using human papillomavirus DNA testing for equivocal Papanicolaou results. JAMA 281:1605–1610
179. Masterson PJ, Stanley MA, Lewis AP, et al (1998) A C-terminal helicase domain of the human papillomavirus E1 protein binds E2 and the DNA polymerase alpha-primase p68 subunit. J Virol 72: 7407–7419

180. McCann MF, Irwin DE, Walton LA, et al (1992) Nicotine and cotinine in the cervical mucus of smokers, passive smokers, and nonsmokers. Cancer Epidemiol Biomark Prev 1:125–129
181. McDonnell JM, Mayr AJ, Martin WJ (1989) DNA of human papillomavirus type 16 in dysplastic and malignant lesions of the conjunctiva and cornea. N Engl J Med 320:1442–1446
182. McIndoe WA, McLean MR, Jones RW, et al (1984) The invasive potential of carcinoma in situ of the cervix. Obstet Gynecol 64:451–458
183. Meisels A, Fortin R (1976) Condylomatous lesions of the cervix and vagina. I. Cytologic patterns. Acta Cytol 20:505–509
184. Meisels A, Fortin R, Roy M (1977) Condylomatous lesions of the cervix: II. Cytologic, colposcopic and histopathologic study. Acta Cytol 21:379–390
185. Meisels A, Morin C, Casas-Cordero M (1982) Human papillomavirus infection of the uterine cervix. Int J Gynecol Pathol 1:75–94
186. Meisels A, Roy M, Fortier M, et al (1979) Condylomatous lesions of the cervix: morphologic and colposcopic diagnosis. Am J Diagn Gynecol Obstet 1:109–116
187. Mitchell H, Medley G (1991) Longitudinal study of women with negative cervical smears according to endocervical status. Lancet 337:265–267
188. Mitchell H, Medley G (1992) Influence of endocervical status on the cytologic prediction of cervical intraepithelial neoplasia. Acta Cytol 36:875–880
189. Mitchell H, Medley G, Gordon I, et al (1995) Cervical cytology reported as negative and risk of adenocarcinoma of the cervix: no strong evidence of benefit. Br J Cancer 71:894–897
190. Mitchell MF, Tortolero-Luna G, Cook E, et al (1998) A randomized clinical trial of cryotherapy, laser vaporization, and loop electrosurgical excision for treatment of squamous intraepithelial lesions of the cervix. Obstet Gynecol 92:737–744
191. Mitra AB, Murty VV, Li RG, et al (1994) Allelotype analysis of cervical carcinoma. Cancer Res 54:4481–4487
192. Mittal KR, Chan W, Demopoulos RL (1990) Sensitivity and specificity of various morphological features of cervical condylomas. Arch Pathol Lab Med 114:1038–1041
193. Montz FJ (2001) Significance of "normal" endometrial cells in cervical cytology from asymptomatic postmenopausal women receiving hormone replacement therapy. Gynecol Oncol 81:33–39
194. Moscicki AB, Shiboski S, Broering J, et al (1998) The natural history of human papillomavirus infection as measured by repeated DNA testing in adolescent and young women. J Pediatr 132:277–284
195. Mourits MJE, Pieters WJ, Hollema H, et al (1992) Three-group metaphase as a morphologic criterion of progressive cervical intraepithelial neoplasia. Am J Obstet Gynecol 167:591–595
196. Moy RL, Eliezri YD, Nuovo GJ, et al (1989) Human papillomavirus type 16 DNA in periungual squamous cell carcinomas. JAMA 261:2669–2673
197. Munoz N (2000) Human papillomavirus and cancer: the epidemiological evidence. J Clin Virol 19: 1–5
198. Nahmias AJ, Roizman B (1973) Infection with herpes-simplex viruses 1 and 2. N Engl J Med 289: 667–674, 719–725, 781–789
199. Nanbu Y, Fujii S, Konishi I, et al (1988) Immunohistochemical localizations of CA 125, carcinoembryonic antigen, and CA 19-9 in normal and neoplastic glandular cells of the uterine cervix. Cancer (Phila) 62:2580–2588
200. Nasiell K, Nasiell M, Vaclavinkova V (1983) Behavior of moderate cervical dysplasia during long-term follow-up. Obstet Gynecol 61:609–614
201. Nasiell K, Roger V, Nasiell M (1986) Behavior of mild cervical dysplasia during long-term follow-up. Obstet Gynecol 67:665–669
202. NCI (1989) National Cancer Institute Workshop: the 1988 Bethesda system for reporting cervical/vaginal cytologic diagnoses. JAMA 262:931–934
203. Ng A (1993) Glandular diseases of the uterus. In: Keebler CM, Somrak TM (eds) The manual of cytotechnology. American Society of Clinical Pathologists, Chicago
204. Ngelangel C, Munoz N, Bosch FX, et al (1998) Causes of cervical cancer in the Philippines: a case-control study. J Natl Cancer Inst 90:43–49
205. Nieminen P, Kallio M, Hakama M (1995) The effect of mass screening on incidence and mortality of squamous and adenocarcinoma of cervix uteri. Obstet Gynecol 85:1017–1021
206. Nindl I, Rindfleisch K, Lotz B, et al (1999) Uniform distribution of HPV 16 E6 and E7 variants in patients with normal histology, cervical intra-epithelial neoplasia and cervical cancer. Int J Cancer 82: 203–207
207. Nobbenhuis MA, Walboomers JM, Helmerhorst TJ, et al (1999) Relation of human papillomavirus status to cervical lesions and consequences for cervical-cancer screening: a prospective study. Lancet 354: 20–25
208. Oda H, Kumar S, Howley PM (1999) Regulation of the Src family tyrosine kinase Blk through E6AP-mediated ubiquitination. Proc Natl Acad Sci USA 96:9557–9562
209. Ostor AG, Duncan A, Quinn M, et al (2000) Adenocarcinoma in situ of the uterine cervix: an experience with 100 cases. Gynecol Oncol 79:207–210
210. Ostor AG, Pagano R, Davoren RAM, et al (1984) Adenocarcinoma *in situ* of the cervix. Int J Gynecol Pathol 3:179–190
211. Palan PR, Mikhail M, Basu J, et al (1988) Decreased plasma B-carotene levels in women with uterine cervical dysplasias and cancer. J Natl Cancer Inst 80:454–455
212. Palefsky JM, Minkoff H, Kalish LA, et al (1999) Cervicovaginal human papillomavirus infection in human immunodeficiency virus-1 (HIV)-positive and

high-risk HIV-negative women. J Natl Cancer Inst 91:226–236
213. Parazzini F, La Vecchia C, Negri E, et al (1990) Oral contraceptive use and invasive cervical cancer. Int J Epidemiol 19:259–263
214. Parazzini F, LaVecchia C, Negri E, et al (1992) Risk factors for cervical intraepithelial neoplasia. Cancer (Phila) 69:2276–2282
215. Park TJ, Richart RM, Sun X-W, et al (1996) Association between HPV type and clonal status of cervical squamous intraepithelial lesions (SIL). J Natl Cancer Inst 88:355–358
216. Parkin DM (1991) Screening for cervix cancer in developing countries. In: Miller AB, et al (eds) Cancer screening. Cambridge University Press, Cambridge, pp 184–198
217. Patten SF (1978) Diagnostic cytopathology of the uterine cervix.
218. Pemberton FA, Smith GV (1929) The early diagnosis and prevention of carcinoma of the cervix: a clinical pathologic study of borderline cases treated at the Free Hospital for women. Am J Obstet Gynecol 17:165
219. Penn I (1986) Cancers of the anogenital region in renal transplant recipients. Cancer (Phila) 58:611–616
220. Phelps WC, Yee CL, Munger K, et al (1988) The human papillomavirus type 16 E7 gene encodes transactivation and transforming functions similar to those of adenovirus E1A. Cell 58:539–547
221. Pieters WJ, Koudstaal J, Ploem-Zaajer JJ, et al (1992) The three group metaphase as morphologic indicator of high ploidy cells in cervical intraepithelial neoplasia. Anal Quant Cytol Histol 14: 227–232
222. Plaxe SC, Saltzstein SL (1999) Estimation of the duration of the preclinical phase of cervical adenocarcinoma suggests that there is ample opportunity for screening. Gynecol Oncol 75:55–61
223. Prendiville W, Cullimore J, Norman S (1989) Large loop excision of the transformation zone (LLETZ). A new method of management for women with cervical intraepithelial neoplasia. Br J Obstet Gynecol 96:1054–1060
224. Przybora LA, Plutowa A (1959) Histological topography of carcinoma in situ of cervix uteri. Cancer (Phila) 12:263–277
225. Purola E, Savia E (1977) Cytology of gynecologic condyloma acuminatum. Acta Cytol 21:26–31
226. Ratnam S, Franco EL, Ferenczy A (2000) Human papillomavirus testing for primary screening of cervical cancer precursors. Cancer Epidemiol Biomarkers Prevent 9:945–951
227. Reagan JW, Hamonic MJ (1956) Dysplasia of the uterine cervix. Ann NY Acad Sci 63:662–682
228. Reagan JW, Ng ABP, Wentz WB (1969) Concepts of genesis and development in early cervical neoplasia. Obstet Gynecol Surv 24:860–874
229. Richardson AC, Lyon JB (1981) The effect of condom use on squamous cell cervical intraepithelial neoplasia. 140:909–913
230. Richart M (1965) Colpomicroscopic studies of the distribution of dysplasia and carcinoma in-situ on the exposed portion of the human uterine cervix. Cancer (Phila) 18:950
231. Richart RM (1966) Colpomicroscopic studies of cervical intraepithelial neoplasia. Cancer (Phila) 19:395–405
232. Richart RM (1973) Cervical intraepithelial neoplasia: a review. In: Sommers SC (ed) Pathology annual. Appleton-Century-Crofts, East Norwalk, pp 301–328
233. Richart RM (1990) A modified terminology for cervical intraepithelial neoplasia. Obstet Gynecol 75: 131–133
234. Richart RM, Lerch V, Baron B (1967) A time-lapse cinematographic study in vitro of mitosis in normal human cervical epithelium, dysplasia and carcinoma in situ. J Natl Cancer Inst 39:571
235. Richart RM, Wright TC (1993) Controversies in the management of low grade cervical intraepithelial neoplasia. Cancer (Phila) 71:1413–1421
236. Robboy SJ, Szyfelbein WM, Goellner JR, et al (1981) Dysplasia and cytologic findings in 4,489 young women enrolled in diethylstillbesterol-adenosis (DESAD) project. Am J Obstet Gynecol 140:579
237. Roberts S, Ashmole I, Rookes SM, et al (1997) Mutational analysis of the human papillomavirus type 16 E1–E4 protein shows that the C terminus is dispensable for keratin cytoskeleton association but is involved in inducing disruption of the keratin filaments. J Virol 71:3554–3562
238. Robertson AJ, Anderson JM, Beck JS, et al (1989) Observer variability in histopathological reporting of cervical biopsy specimens. J Clin Pathol 42: 231–238
239. Robertson JH, Woodend BE, Crozier EH, et al (1988) Risk of cervical cancer associated with mild dyskaryosis. Br Med J 297:18–21
240. Ronnett BM, Manos MM, Ransley JE, et al (1999) Atypical glandular cells of undetermined significance (AGUS): cytopathologic features, histopathologic results, and human papillomavirus DNA detection. Hum Pathol 30:816–825
241. Royston I, Aurelian L (1970) Immunofluorescent detection of herpesvirus antigens in exfoliated cells from human cervical carcinoma. Proc Natl Acad Sci USA 67:204
242. Rozendaal L, Walboomers JM, van der Linden JC, et al (1996) PCR-based high-risk HPV test in cervical cancer screening gives objective risk assessment of women with cytomorphologically normal cervical smears. Int J Cancer 68:766–769
243. Rubio CA, Lagerlof B (1974) Studies on the histogenesis of experimentally induced cervical carcinoma. Acta Pathol Microbiol Scand 82:153
244. Sadeghi SB, Hsieh EW, Gunn SW (1984) Prevalence of cervical intraepithelial neoplasia in sexually active teenagers and young adults. Am J Obstet Gynecol 148:726

245. Sadeghi SB, Sadeghi A, Robboy SJ (1988) Prevalence of dysplasia and cancer of the cervix in a nationwide Planned Parenthood population. Cancer (Phila) 61:2359–2361
246. Scheffner M, Huibregtse JM, Vierstra RD, et al (1993) The HPV-16 E6 and E6-AP complex functions as a ubiquitin-protein ligase in the ubiquitination of p53. Cell 75:495–505
247. Schiffman M, Herrero R, Hildeschein A, et al (2000) HPV DNA testing in cervical cancer screening: results from a high-risk provence in Costa Rica. JAMA 283:87–93
248. Schiffman MH (1992) Recent progress in defining the epidemiology of human papillomavirus infection and cervical neoplasia. J Natl Cancer Inst 84:394–398
249. Schiffman MH, Bauer HM, Hoover RN, et al (1993) Epidemiologic evidence that human papillomavirus infection causes most cervical intraepithelial neoplasia. J Natl Cancer Inst 85:958–964
250. Schiffman MH, Brinton LA (1995) The epidemiology of cervical carcinogenesis. Cancer (Phila) 76: 1888–1901
251. Schiller JT, Hidesheim A (2000) Developing HPV virus-like particle vaccines to prevent cervical cancer: a progress report. J Clin Virol 19:67–74
252. Schmidt C, Pretorius RG, Bonin M, et al (1992) Invasive cervical cancer following cryotherapy for cervical intraepithelial neoplasia or human papillomavirus infection. Obstet Gynecol 80:797–800
253. Schwarz E, Freese UK, Gissman L, et al (1985) Structure and transcription of human papillomavirus sequences in cervical carcinoma cells. Nature 314:111–114
254. Sherman ME, Schiffman MH, Erozan YS, et al (1992) The Bethesda System. A proposal for reporting abnormal cervical smears based on the reproducibility of cytopathologic diagnoses. Arch Pathol Lab Med 116:1155–1158
255. Sherman ME, Tabbara SO, Scott DR, et al (1999) "ASCUS, rule out HSIL": cytologic features, histologic correlates, and human papillomavirus detection. Mod Pathol 12:335–342
256. Shin CH, Schorge JO, Lee KR, et al (2000) Conservative management of adenocarcinoma in situ of the cervix. Gynecol Oncol 79:6–10
257. Shingleton HM, Richart RM, Wiener J, et al (1968) Human cervical intraepithelial neoplasia. Fine structure of dysplasia and carcinoma in situ. Cancer Res 28:695–706
258. Sillman F, Stanek A, Sedlis A, et al (1984) The relationship between human papillomavirus and lower genital intraepithelial neoplasia in immuno-suppressed women. Am J Obstet Gynecol 150:300–308
259. Simons AM, Phillips DH, Coleman DV (1993) Damage to DNA in cervical epithelium related to smoking tobacco. Br Med J 306:1444–1448
260. Smith JW, Townsend DE, Spark RS (1971) Genetic variants of glucose-6-phosphate dehydrogenase in the study of carcinoma of the cervix. Cancer (Phila) 28:529–532
261. Solomon D, Schiffman M, Tarrone R (2001) Comparison of three management strategies for patients with atypical squamous cells of undetermined significance: baseline results from a randomized trial. J Natl Cancer Inst 93:293–299
262. Sorensen HM, Petersen O, Nielsen J, et al (1964) The spontaneous course of premalignant lesions of the vaginal portion of the uterus. Acta Obstet Gynecol Scand 43:103–104
263. Southern SA, Herrington CS (2000) Disruption of cell cycle control by human papillomaviruses with special reference to cervical carcinoma. Int J Gynecol Cancer 10:263–274
264. Spires S, Banks E, Weeks J, et al (1993) Specimen adequacy according to the Bethesda system: interobserver and intraobserver reproducibility. Acta Cytol 37:778
265. Spriggs AI, Bowey CE, Cowdell RH (1971) Chromosomes of precancerous lesions of the cervix uteri. Cancer (Phila) 27:1239
265a. Spriggs AI (1971) Follow-up of untreated carcinoma-in-situ of the cervix uteri. Lancet 2:599–600
266. Stafl A, Mattingly RF (1975) Angiogenesis of cervical neoplasia. Am J Obstet Gynecol 121:845–852
267. Stafl A, Wilkinson EJ, Mattingly RF (1977) Laser treatment of cervical and vaginal neoplasia. Am J Obstet Gynecol 128:128–136
268. Stanbridge EJ (1990) Human tumor suppressor genes. Annu Rev Genet 24:615–657
269. Stern E, Neely PM (1963) Carcinoma and dysplasia of the cervix. A comparison of rates for new and returning populations. Acta Cytol 7:357–361
270. Stewart FW (1957) Factors influencing curability of cancer. In: Conference proceedings of the third national cancer conference. Lippincott, Philadelphia, pp 62–73
271. Stoler MH, Schiffman M (2001) Interobserver reproducibility of cervical cytologic and histologic interpretations: realistic estimates from the ASCUS-LSIL Triage Study. JAMA 285:1500–1505
272. Sun X-W, Ellerbrock RV, Lungu O, et al (1995) Human papillomavirus infection in human immunodeficiency virus-seropositive women. Obstet Gynecol 85:680–686
273. Sun X-W, Ferenczy A, Johnson D, et al (1995) Evaluation of the hybrid capture HPV DNA detection test. Am J Obstet Gynecol 173:1432–1437
274. Sun XW, Kuhn L, Ellerbrock TV, et al (1997) Human papillomavirus infection in HIV-seropositive women; natural history and variability of detection. N Engl J Med 337:1343–1349
275. Suprun HZ, Schwartz J, Spira H (1985) CIN and associated condylomatous lesions. A preliminary report on 4,764 women from northern Israel. Acta Cytol 29:334–340
276. Szarewski A, Curran G, Edwards R, et al (1993) Com-

parison of four cytologic sampling techniques in a large family planning center. Acta Cytol 37:457–460
277. Szarewski A, Cuzick J (1998) Smoking and cervical neoplasia: a review of the evidence. J Epidemiol Biostat 3:229–256
278. Talmage DA, Freund R, Dubensky T, et al (1992) Heterogeneity in state and expression of viral DNA in polyoma virus-induced tumors of the mouse. Virology 187:734–747
279. Tase T, Okagaki T, Clark BA, et al (1989) Human papillomavirus DNA in adenocarcinoma in situ, microinvasive adenocarcinoma of the uterine cervix and coexisting cervical squamous intraepithelial neoplasia. Int J Gynecol Pathol 8:8–17
280. Tase T, Okagaki T, Clark BA, et al (1989) Human papillomavirus DNA in glandular dysplasia and microglandular hyperplasia: presumed precursors of adenocarcinoma of the uterine cervix. Obstet Gynecol 73:1005–1008
281. Thomas M, Banks L (1998) Inhibition of Bak-induced apoptosis by HPV-18 E6. Oncogene 17: 2943–2954
282. Tong X, Howley PM (1997) The bovine papillomavirus E6 oncoprotein interacts with paxillin and disrupts the actin cytoskeleton. Proc Natl Acad Sci USA 94:4412–4417
283. Townsend E, Richart RM (1983) Cryotherapy and carbon dioxide laser management of cervical intraepithelial neoplasia: a controlled comparison. Obstet Gynecol 61:75–78
284. Trowell JE (1985) Intestinal metaplasia with argentaffin cells in the uterine cervix. Histopathology (Oxf) 9:561–569
285. Turek LP (1994) The structure function and regulation of papillomaviral genes in infection and cervical cancer. Adv Virol Res 44:305–356
286. Ursin G, Pike MC, Preston-Martin S, et al (1996) Sexual, reproductive, and other risk factors for adenocarcinoma of the cervix: results from a population-based case-control study (California, United States). Cancer Causes Control 7:391–401
287. Ustav E, Ustav M (1998) E2 protein as the master regulator of extrachromosomal replication of the papillomaviruses. Papillomavirus Rep 9:145–150
288. Van Ranst MS, Tachezy R, Delius H, et al (1993) Taxonomy of the human papillomaviruses. Papillomavirus Rep 4
289. Verloop J, Rookus MA, van Leeuwen FE (2000) Prevalence of gynecologic cancer in women exposed to diethylstilbestrol in utero. N Engl J Med 342:1838–1839
290. Verreault R, Chu J, Mandelson M, et al (1989) A case control study of diet and invasive cervical cancer. Int. J Cancer 43:1050–1054
291. Vessey MF (1984) Exogenous hormones in the aetiology of cancer in women. J R Soc Med 77:542
292. Vooijs GP, Elias A, van der Graaf Y, et al (1986) The influence of sample takers on the cellular composition of cervical smears. Acta Cytol 30:251–257
293. Walboomers JM, Jacobs MV, Manos MM, et al (1999) Human papillomavirus is a necessary cause of invasive cervical cancer worldwide. J Pathol 189: 12–19
294. Wallin KL, Wiklund F, Angstrom T, et al (1999) Type-specific persistence of human papillomavirus DNA before the development of invasive cervical cancer. N Engl J Med 341:1633–1638
295. Ward BE, Burkett BA, Peterson C, et al (1990) Cytological correlates of cervical papillomavirus infection. Int J Gynecol Pathol 9:297–305
296. Ward P, Coleman AD, Malcolm DB (1989) Regulatory mechanisms of the papillomaviruses. Trends Genet 5:92–98
297. Weid GL (1961) Proceedings of the First International Congress on Exfoliative Cytology.
298. Wells SI, Francis DA, Karpova AY, et al (2000) Papillomavirus E2 induces senescence in HPV-positive cells via pRB- and p21(CIP)-dependent pathways. EMBO J 19:5762–5771
299. Wheeler CM, Greer CE, Becker TM, et al (1996) Short-term fluctuations in the detection of cervical human papillomavirus DNA. Obstet Gynecol 88: 261–268
300. Wideroff L, Potischman N, Glass AG, et al (1998) A nested case-control study of dietary factors and the risk of incident cytological abnormalities of the cervix. Nutr Cancer 30:130–136
301. Willett GD, Kurman RJ, Reid R, et al (1989) Correlation of the histological appearance of intraepithelial neoplasia of the cervix with human papillomavirus types. Int J Gynecol Pathol 8:18–25
302. Williams J (1888) Cancer of the uterus: Harveian lectures for 1886.
303. Winkler B, Norris HJ, Fenoglio CM (1982) The female genital tract. In: Ridell RH (ed) Pathology of drug-induced and toxic diseases. Churchill Livingstone, New York
304. Wolf JK, Levenback C, Malpica A, et al (1996) Adenocarcinoma in situ of the cervix: significance of cone biopsy margins. Obstet Gynecol 88:82–86
305. Workshop NCI (1991) The revised Bethesda System for reporting cervical/vaginal cytologic diagnoses. Report of the 1991 Bethesda Workshop. JAMA 267:1892
306. Wright TC, Ellerbrock TV, Chiasson MA, et al (1994) Cervical intraepithelial neoplasia in women infected with human immunodeficiency virus: prevalence, risk factors, and validity of Papanicolaou smears. Obstet Gynecol 84:591–597
307. Wright TC, Gagnon MD, Richart RM, et al (1992) Treatment of cervical intraepithelial neoplasia using the loop electrosurgical excision procedure. Obstet Gynecol 79:173–178
308. Wright TC, Kurman RJ (1994) A critical review of the morphologic classification systems of preinvasive lesions of the cervix: the scientific basis of the paradigm. Papillomavirus Rep 5:175–181
309. Wright TC, Lorincz AT, Ferris DG, et al (1998) Re-

flex HPV DNA testing in women with abnormal Papanicolaou smears. Am J Obstet Gynecol 178:962–966
310. Wright TC (2000) Pathogenesis and diagnosis of preinvasive lesions of the lower genital tract. WJ Hoskins, CA Perez, et al (eds) Principles and practice of gynecologic oncology, 3rd ed. Lippincott Williams and Wilkins, Philadelphia, pp 710–775
311. Ylitalo N, Sorensen P, Josefsson AM, et al (2000) Consistent high viral load of human papillomavirus 16 and risk of cervical carcinoma in situ: a nested case-control study. Lancet 355:2194–2198
312. Young RH, Clement PB (1991) Pseudoneoplastic glandular lesions of the uterine cervix. Semin Diagn Pathol 8:234–249
313. Young RH, Scully RE (1989) Atypical forms of microglandular hyperplasia of the cervix simulating carcinoma. Am J Surg Pathol 13:50–56
314. Zenilman JM (2001) *Chlamydia* and cervical cancer: a real association? JAMA 285:81–83
315. Zhao W, Chow LT, Broker TR (1999) A distal element in the HPV-11 upstream regulatory region contributes to promoter repression in basal keratinocytes in squamous epithelium. Virology 253: 219–229
316. Zhao W, Noya F, Chen WY, et al (1999) Trichostatin A up-regulates human papillomavirus type 11 upstream regulatory region-E6 promoter activity in undifferentiated primary human keratinocytes. J Virol 73:5026–5033
317. zur Hausen H (1977) Human papillomaviruses and their possible role in squamous cell carcinomas. Curr Top Microbiol Immunol 78:1–30
318. zur Hausen H (2000) Papillomaviruses causing cancer: evasion from host-cell control in early events in carcinogenesis. J Natl Cancer Inst 92:690–698

8

Carcinoma and Other Tumors of the Cervix

Thomas C. Wright, M.D., Alex Ferenczy, M.D., and Robert J. Kurman, M.D.

Invasive Carcinoma

The World Health Organization (WHO) classification for tumors of the cervix has been revised recently in collaboration with the International Society of Gynecological Pathologists. Three general categories of invasive carcinoma of the cervix are now recognized: squamous cell carcinoma, adenocarcinoma, and "other" epithelial tumors (Table 8.1).[251] The later category encompasses adenosquamous carcinoma and glassy cell carcinoma, tumors that have been grouped in the past with mucoepidermoid carcinoma and classified as "mixed" carcinomas. The "other epithelial tumor" category also includes adenoid basal cell carcinoma and adenoid cystic carcinomas, which previous classifications have classified as adenocarcinomas, as well as typical and atypical carcinoids and small cell carcinoma, which were previously classified as neuroendocrine carcinoma (Table 8.1). The relative proportions of these different types of carcinoma varies from study to study, but in general approximately 60–80% of invasive carcinomas of the cervix are classified as squamous cell carcinomas.[38,41,58,62,263,290]

The most widely accepted staging system for tumors of the cervix is that of the International Federation of Gynecologists and Obstetricians (FIGO) (Table 8.2). This staging system divides invasive tumors into four stages. Stage I includes all tumors confined to the cervix and is divided into two broad categories: those that invade 5 mm or less into the stroma and are macroscopically not visible, and those that either invade more than 5 mm or are macroscopically visible.[223] Stage II tumors extend beyond the cervix, but not to the pelvic sidewall, and do not involve the lower third of the vagina. Stage

Table 8.1. Modified World Health Organization histological classification of invasive carcinomas of the uterine cervix

Squamous cell carcinoma
Microinvasive squamous cell carcinoma
Invasive squamous cell carcinoma
Verrucous carcinoma
Warty (condylomatous) carcinoma
Papillary squamous cell (transitional) carcinoma
Lymphoepithelioma-like carcinoma
Adenocarcinoma
Mucinous adenocarcinoma
Endocervical type
Intestinal type
Signet-ring type
Endometrioid adenocarcinoma
Endometrioid adenocarcinoma with squamous metaplasia
Clear cell adenocarcinoma
Minimal deviation adenocarcinoma
Endocervical type (adenoma malignum)
Endometrioid type
Well-differentiated villoglandular adenocarcinoma
Serous adenocarcinoma
Mesonephric carcinoma
Other epithelial tumors
Adenosquamous carcinoma
Glassy cell carcinoma
Clear cell adenosquamous carcinoma
Mucoepidermoid carcinoma
Adenoid cystic carcinoma
Adenoid basal carcinoma
Typical carcinoid tumor
Atypical carcinoid tumor
Large cell neuroendocrine carcinoma
Small cell carcinoma
Undifferentiated carcinoma

III tumors include those that extend to the pelvic sidewall, cause hydronephrosis or a nonfunctioning kidney, or involve the lower third of the vagina. Stage IV tumors extend beyond the true pelvis or have clinically involved the mucosa of the bladder or rectum.

Squamous Cell Carcinoma

Microinvasive Squamous Cell Carcinoma

The concept of *microinvasive carcinoma* (*MICA*) of the cervix was first introduced in 1847 by Mestwerdt.[198] Microinvasive carcinoma is considered a preclinical stage in the progressive spectrum of *squamous intraepithelial lesions* (*SIL*), previously referred to as cervical intraepithelial neoplasia (CIN) and frank clinical invasive carcinoma of the cervix uteri. The most appropriate definition of MICA remains controversial despite numerous studies. The main subjects of contention are the maximum depth of permissible stromal invasion and the significance of vascular invasion, tumor volume, and confluency of neoplastic epithelium, as related to the frequency of pelvic lymph node metastasis, vaginal recurrence, and survival. Most patients who die of disseminated squamous cell carcinoma have either lymphatic channel involvement, tumors that invade more than 5 mm into the cervical stroma, or tumors more than 2.5 cm^3 in volume. Accordingly, FIGO has defined stage IA tumors as tumors that invade to a depth of *not more than 5 mm taken from the base of the epithelium, either surface or glandular, from which it originates and a second dimension, the horizontal spread, must not exceed 7 mm* (see Table 8.2). Tumors that qualify as stage IA are further subdivided into those that invade no more than 3 mm into the cervical stroma (stage IA1) and those that invade more than 3 mm, but no more than 5 mm, into the stroma (stage IA2). Stage IA1 tumors frequently are referred to as *microinvasive carcinoma (MICA)*.

The Society of Gynecological Oncologists (SGO) in the United States has proposed a more restricted definition of MICA. The definition of MICA proposed in 1974 by the Committee on Nomenclature for the SGO states: *A microinvasive lesion should be defined as one in which neoplastic epithelium invades the stroma in one or more places to a depth of 3 mm or less below the basement membrane of the epithelium and in which lymphatic or blood vascular involvement is not demonstrated.*[68] According to this definition, histologically detected lesions with vascular space invasion, but less than 3.1-mm-deep stromal invasion, are not considered MICA. Lesions that fulfill the SGO definition of MICA have virtually no potential for either metastases or recurrence, and therefore this definition appears to be the most appropriate one for guiding clinical management of patients. It is important to stress that because the lesion cannot be visualized on gross inspection, the diagnosis of MICA is *always* based on histologic examination of a cone biopsy specimen that *includes the entire lesion*.

General Features

The majority of MICA occurs in women 35–46 years of age, between two extremes of age, the early twenties and the seventies. According to various investigators, the frequency of MICA in patients with SIL (CIN) varies from less than 1% to more than 50%. This wide variation in prevalence reflects differences

Table 8.2. 2000 modification of FIGO staging of carcinoma of the cervix uteri

Stage	*Definition*
0	Carcinoma in situ (preinvasive carcinoma)
I	Cervical carcinoma confined to uterus (extension to the corpus should be disregarded)
IA	Invasive carcinoma diagnosed only by microscopy; all macroscopically visible lesions, even with superficial invasion, are stage IB
IA1	Stromal invasion no greater than 3.0 mm in depth and 7.0 mm or less in horizontal spread
IA2	Stromal invasion more than 3.0 mm and not more than 5.0 mm with a horizontal spread of 7.0 mm or less[a]
IB	Clinically visible lesion confined to the cervix or microscopic lesion greater than IA2
IB1	Clinically visible lesion 4.0 cm or less in greatest dimension
IB2	Clinically visible lesion more than 4.0 cm in greatest dimension
II	Tumor invades beyond the uterus but not to pelvic wall or to lower third of the vagina
IIA	Without parametrial invasion
IIB	With parametrial invasion
III	Tumor extends to the pelvic wall and/or involves lower third of vagina and/or causes hydronephrosis or nonfunctioning kidney
IIIA	Tumor involves lower third of vagina with no extension to pelvic wall
IIIB	Tumor extends to pelvic wall and/or causes hydronephrosis or nonfunctioning kidney
IVA	Tumor invades mucosa of bladder or rectum and/or extends beyond true pelvis[b]
IV	Distant metastasis

[a]The depth of invasion should not be more than 5 mm taken from the base of the epithelium, either surface or glandular, from which it originates. The depth of invasion is defined as the measurement of the tumor from the epithelial–stromal junction of the adjacent most superficial epithelial papilla to the deepest point of invasion. Vascular space involvement, venous or lymphatic, does not affect classification.
[b]The presence of bullous edema is not sufficient to classify a tumor as T4.
From: Staging classifications and clinical practice guidelines of gynecologic cancers by FIGO Committee on Gynecologic Oncology, September 2000. In: J Gynecol Obstet (2000) 70:207–312.

in the definition of MICA, methods of sampling of cervical specimens, and the criteria used for diagnosing invasion. A 4% prevalence of MICA has been demonstrated in serial step sections of specimens with SIL.[12,33,162] It is important to note, however, that patients included in these series were treated with traditional cold knife cone biopsy and usually had high-grade SIL (CIN 2,3) that extended into the endocervical canal. For example, in Anderson's series of patients treated with cold knife cone biopsies, 91% of the patients were classified as having CIN 3.[12] Estimates of the prevalence of MICA in the general population can be obtained from population-based cervical cancer registries. A population-based registry from British Columbia, Canada, estimates the prevalence of MICA to be 4.8 per 100,000 women screened. In this same registry, the prevalence of carcinoma in situ was 316 per 100,000 women screened.[24]

With the widespread adoption of shallow laser excisional conization and the loop electrosurgical excision procedure (LEEP) as methods for treating SIL, better estimates of the prevalence of MICA in patients with all grades of SIL have been obtained. In an analysis of shallow laser excisional conization specimens from 196 patients with SIL that did not extend into the endocervical canal, McIndoe et al. detected colposcopically unsuspected MICA in 2 (1%) patients.[196] Larger studies of specimens obtained by loop electrosurgical excision have reported colposcopically undetected MICA in 0.4–3% of all patients with biopsy-confirmed SIL.[127,187,206] In assessing the probability of MICA developing in women with SIL, the size as well as grade of the lesion seems to be important. Microinvasive squamous cell carcinoma appears to be most commonly associated with extensive biopsy-confirmed, high-grade SIL involving the endocervical crypts.[280]

Clinical Features

Most patients with MICA are asymptomatic, and the tumors generally are discovered on a routine cervical smear. The cervix demonstrates a grossly normal appearance or nonspecific findings, such as chronic cervicitis or true erosion. A definitive diagnosis of microinvasion is made on histologic evaluation of cervical tissue removed by conization or at hysterectomy. For many years, it has been taught that cytopathologists and colposcopists are able to predict early stromal invasion with a high degree of accuracy. Ng et al., on the basis of cellular characteristics in Pap smears, correctly predicted 27 of 31 patients with proved MICA, an accuracy of 87%.[209] However, more recent cytologic studies have failed to accurately predict the presence of microinvasion.[169,244] For example, in a study of 536 women undergoing laser conization, cytology predicted the presence of invasion in only 27.3% of women with MICA.[11]

Colposcopically, areas of MICA usually display dense acetowhitening consistent with high-grade SIL and may contain one or more foci of bizarre surface branching vessels (Fig. 8.1). However, microinvasion frequently cannot be accurately detected using colposcopy or cytology. For example, in a study that correlated colposcopic appearances with histologic findings of a large number of loop excision specimens, Murdoch et al. demonstrated that the accurate colposcopic detection of MICA requires invasion of more than 1 mm into the cervical stroma.[206] Because it is difficult to colposcopically identify MICA, many colposcopists routinely treat all large biopsy-confirmed, high-grade SIL using excisional methods such as loop excision. It should be stressed, however, that a diagnosis of MICA should only be made after a conization (either a cold knife, laser, or loop electrosurgical) has been performed to exclude more advanced disease. The cone is completely, and serially, sampled for microscopic examination, and the pathologist evaluates the surgical margins, depth of stromal invasion, greatest lateral extent of the lesion, and whether vascular space invasion is present.

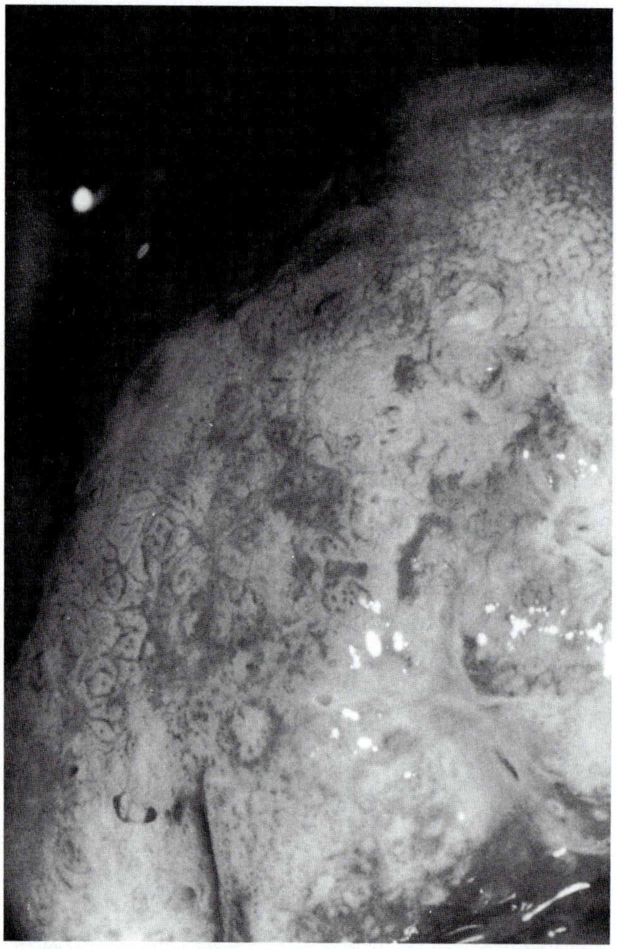

Fig. 8.1. Microinvasive squamous cell carcinoma of the cervix. The colposcopic lesion is densely acetowhite with a prominent mosaic vascular pattern and coarse branching vessels. (Photograph courtesy of Dr. Duane Townsend, Park City, UT.)

Pathologic Features

The diagnosis of MICA is based on the presence of one or more tongues of malignant cells penetrating through the basement membrane of the squamous epithelium (Fig. 8.2a). The latter invariably demonstrates a SIL of varying severity, and in most instances the underlying endocervical glands are extensively replaced by the intraepithelial disease. Typically, in the microinvasion foci, the cells are better differentiated with abundant eosinophilic cytoplasm and prominent nucleoli as compared to the associated SIL. Occasionally, small foci of keratinization are seen within the microinvasive foci. Because of focal disruption of the basement membrane, the margin of the invading nests is ragged, flanked by intact basement membrane on either side (Fig. 8.2b). This irregular contour is probably the most reliable criterion for the diagnosis of MICA. It is easily distinguished from the smooth and regular contour or masses of neoplastic cells that represent endocervical gland involvement by high-grade SIL. There is often a conspicuous lymphoplasmacytic infiltrate surrounding the tips of the invasive epithelial prongs, and frequently there is a desmoplastic response in the adjacent stroma. Two additional histologic features that are reported to be helpful for diagnosing MICA, particularly when there is a marked inflammatory infiltrate, are apparent duplication or folding of the neoplastic epithelium and scalloping of the margins of the epithelium at the dermal–epidermal interface (Fig. 8.3).[70]

Roche and Norris defined lymphatic space invasion as endothelial-lined (capillary-like) spaces containing tumor cells that are contiguous with the stroma (Fig. 8.4).[241] Identification of early lymphatic and vascular space invasion, particularly in the cervical stroma adjacent to the overlying epithelium, may be difficult and is often hampered by technical processing artifacts (Fig. 8.5). Staining endothelial cells either using antibodies against factor VIII or with *Ulex agglutinin* is sometimes helpful for distinguishing between true lymphvascular space involvement and processing artifacts. In view of the diffi-

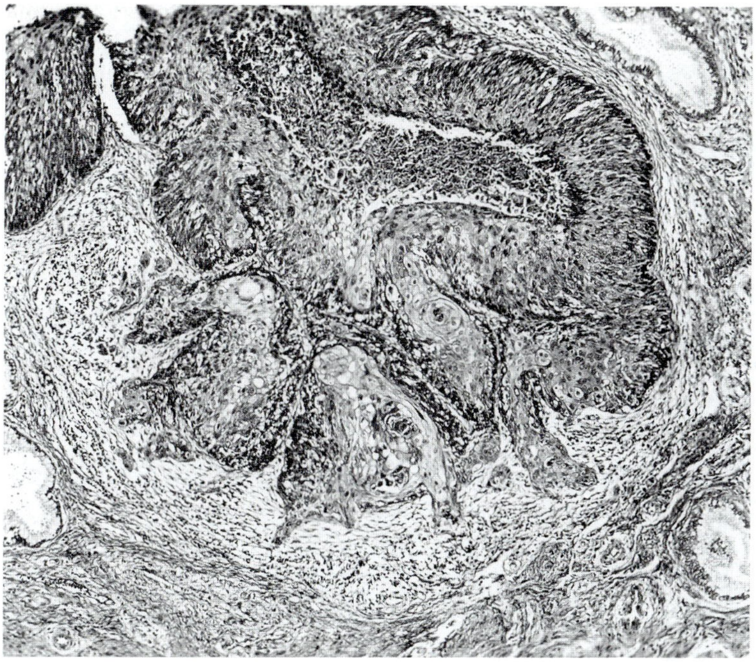

a

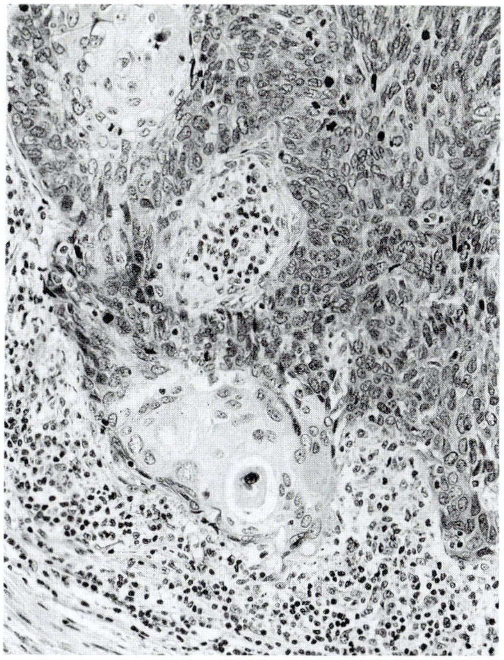

b

Fig. 8.2. Microinvasive squamous carcinoma of the cervix. a: Tongues of neoplastic epithelium project into the stroma from an area of high-grade SIL that has replaced a preexisting endocervical gland. Stromal extension is less than 1 mm in depth. **b**: Higher magnification of the microinvasive focus, which characteristically displays an irregular margin and better-differentiated neoplastic cells than those above the basal lamina. The stromal–epithelial junction of the invasive focus is typically infiltrated by chronic inflammatory cells. (Reprinted with permission from Kurman et al., ref. 174.)

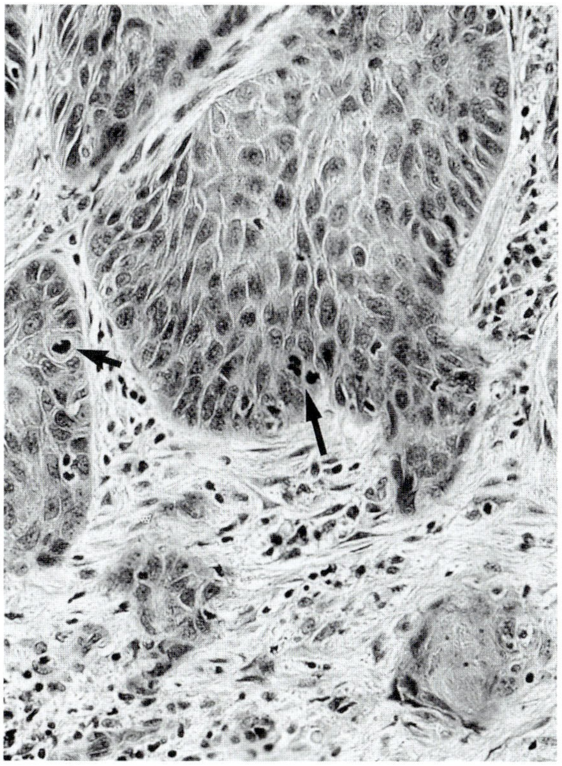

Fig. 8.3. Microinvasive squamous cell carcinoma of the cervix. Scalloping of the junction between the epithelium and the stroma with loss of cellular polarity is a feature of microinvasion. Note abnormal mitotic figures (*arrows*). (Reprinted with permission from ref. 70.)

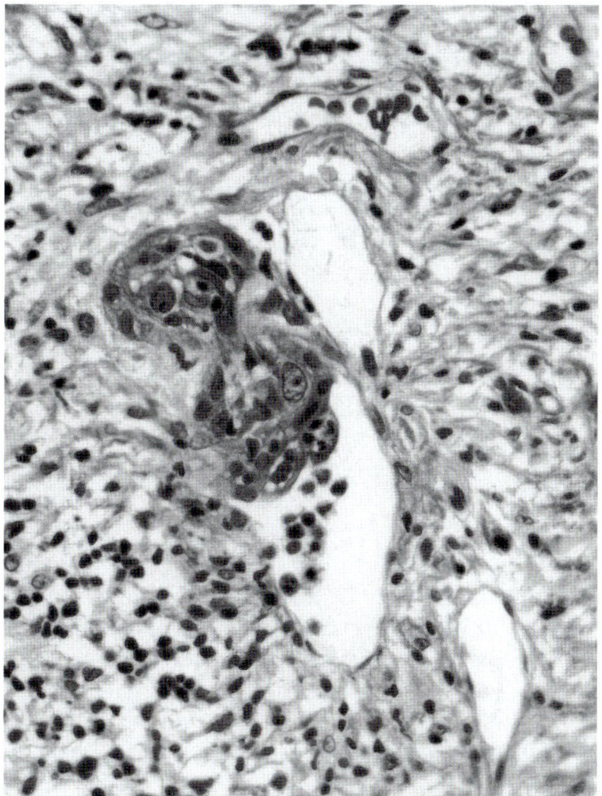

Fig. 8.4. Microinvasive squamous cell carcinoma of the cervix. Neoplastic cells adhere to the endothelial lining of a lymphatic capillary space.

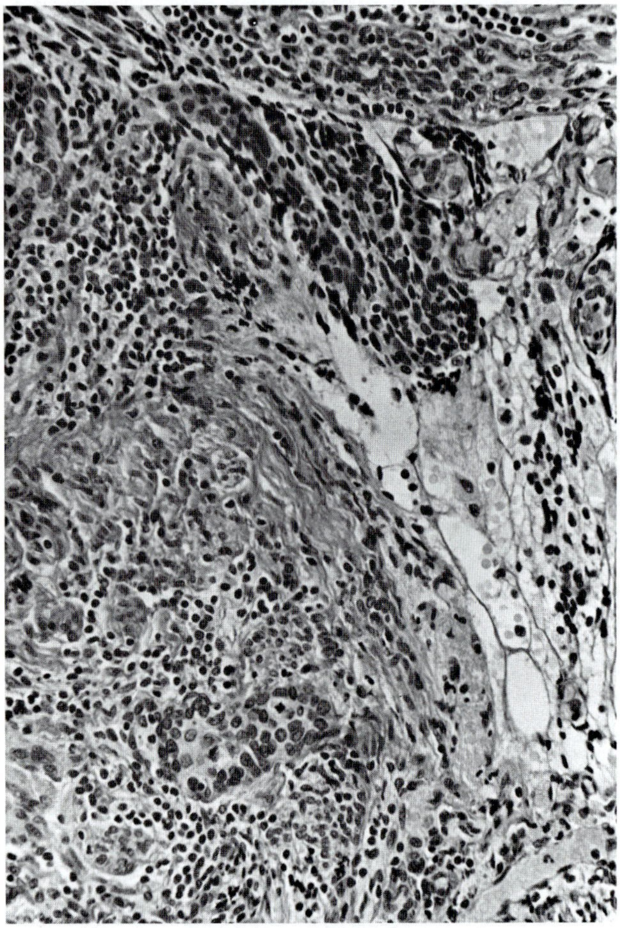

Fig. 8.5. Squamous intraepithelial lesion (SIL). Implanted nests of neoplastic epithelium are present at the site of previous biopsy. Note artifact of shrinkage characterized by irregular outline and absence of endothelial lining of the space surrounding tumor cells. Edema, extravasated red blood cells, and inflammatory exudate indicate response to injury.

culties in distinguishing small blood vessels and capillaries from small lymphatic channels, the term *lymphvascular space(s) (LVSI)* is used in this chapter.

For consistency in the measurement of the depth of stromal invasion, the following guidelines are recommended. The depth of neoplastic projections should be measured from the initial site of invasion, either from the basal lamina of the surface epithelium or from endocervical glands replaced by intraepithelial neoplasia (Figs. 8.6 and 8.7). There are cases, however, in which a direct histologic continuity between invasive foci and SIL cannot be demonstrated, even in deeper cuts of the paraffin block. In such instances, it is assumed that invasion originated from the basal cells of the overlying SIL. Therefore, depth of invasion is arbitrarily measured from the basal lamina of the surface SIL (Fig. 8.6).

The most accurate method to measure the depth of stromal penetration is with a calibrated slide or ocular micrometer. A more convenient, but perhaps less accurate, method of establishing the size and depth of penetrating foci consists of direct microscopic visualization with a transparent metric ruler. The depth of penetration also depends on the angle at which sections are prepared, and efforts should be made to secure vertically sectioned tissue samples. The lateral extent of MICA is measured as described for the depth of stromal penetration. Measurements are made between the two farthest lateral points where invasion is identified.

Immunohistochemistry

At the site of initial stromal invasion, disruption of the basement membrane has been identified using electron microscopy. Therefore, a number of studies have attempted to use immunohistochemistry and antibodies directed against basement membrane constituents such as laminin or type IV collagen as a way of enhancing the recognition of early stromal invasion in cervical lesions.[21] However, small basement membrane disruptions (as defined by laminin and type IV collagen staining) frequently occur both in the normal cervical epithelium and in squamous intraepithelial lesions that lack microinvasion, especially in areas with severe stromal inflammatory infiltrates.[74,291] In addition, foci of basement membrane staining frequently occur in areas of invasion, and the amount of staining tends to increase as the degree of differentiation of the in-

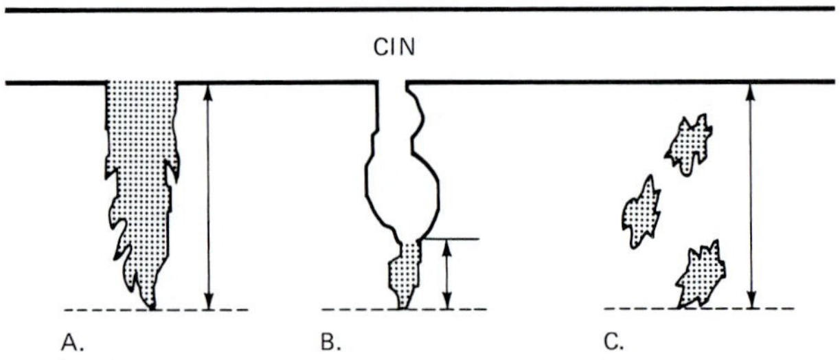

Fig. 8.6. Methods of measuring depth of invasion of microinvasive squamous cell carcinoma of the cervix. The pattern of stromal invasion determines the stromal depth measurement that is most appropriate. **a**: Origin of invasion at surface SIL: depth of stromal invasion is measured from point of origin of invasion downward to the last cell of the invasive focus. **b**: Origin of invasion at SIL with gland involvement: depth of stromal invasion is measured from site of origin downward to the last cell of the invasive focus. **c**: Origin of invasion not seen: depth of stromal invasion is measured from basal lamina of surface SIL downward to the last cell of the invasive focus.

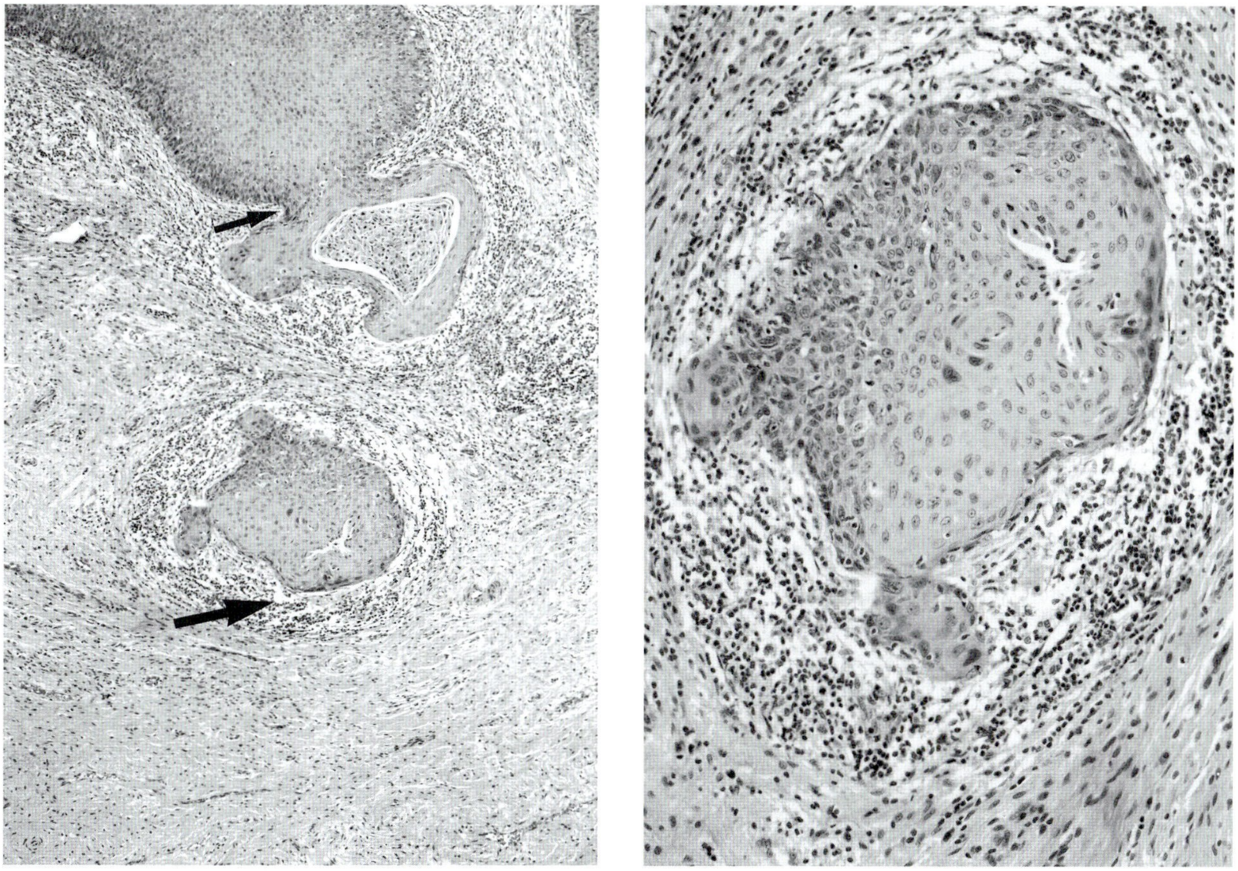

Fig. 8.7. Microinvasive squamous cell carcinoma of the cervix. **a**: A tongue of neoplastic epithelium projects into the stroma from the base of an endocervical gland that has been replaced by high-grade SIL (*small arrow*). The invasive focus contains a central space filled with desquamated keratinized cells. Beneath the upper focus of invasion is another nest of invasive cells. Depth of invasion in this case would be measured from the *upper small arrow* to the *lower large arrow*. **b**: Higher magnification of the lower focus of invasion shows the stromal edema and conspicuous inflammatory infiltrate at the epithelial–stromal junction that is typical of microinvasion.

vading tumor increases. Therefore, immunohistochemistry appears to be of limited value in assessing questionable early stromal invasion.[270]

Differential Diagnosis

MICA is frequently misdiagnosed. Of 265 purported cases of MICA submitted to a group of reference pathologists of the Gynecologic Oncology Group (GOG), 132 cases (approximately 50%) were rejected.[252] Another recent study from the United Kingdom that reviewed 286 cases initially diagnosed as MICA found that 41% were incorrectly diagnosed.[202] Special attention should be paid to the interpretation of recently biopsied conization specimens as these often harbor individual nests of neoplastic epithelium buried within the cervical stroma at the site of a previous punch biopsy (see Fig. 8.5). Such nests represent clusters of intraepithelial disease that may be disrupted and incorporated into the stroma by the punch biopsy and masquerade as MICA. Therefore, a diagnosis of microinvasion should be made with caution when such a phenomenon is seen at or near a recent biopsy site. Both SIL and immature squamous metaplasia with extensive gland involvement should also be distinguished from MICA. A prominent stromal desmoplastic response, abundant eosinophilic cytoplasm, and an irregular margin or scalloping of the epithelial nest are features associated with invasive foci.

Risk Factors

Factors that have been reported to increase an individual's risk for nodal metastases, recurrence, and death are (1) depth of stromal invasion, (2) presence of lymphvascular space involvement, (3) tumor volume, and (4) status of the resection margin. However, the lack of a uniform definition and methodology for measuring the depth of invasion together with different follow-up time and treatment methods make interpretation of the published data difficult. For example, the maximal depth of stromal invasion in studies of MICA varies from 1 to 5 mm. Some studies characterize microinvasion by the absence of confluency of invasive foci or the absence of vascular permeation, whereas in others lymphatic involvement and confluency do not exclude the diagnosis of MICA. It is not surprising, therefore, that the frequency of pelvic node metastasis associated with MICA varies from 0% to 7%.[26,30]

Depth and Pattern of Invasion

Depth of stromal invasion is a major factor in determining the outcome of patients with MICA. Early studies reported that no residual carcinoma was detected in the subsequent hysterectomy specimen when MICA invaded 1 mm or less in the cone biopsy. In contrast, residual carcinoma was detected in a significant proportion of cases when MICA detected in the cone biopsy invaded 3 mm or more into the stroma. Pathologic analysis of lymph nodes removed at the time of radical surgery demonstrates a clear relationship between the depth of stromal invasion and the presence of lymph node metastases (Table 8.3).[43,63,64,68,78,115,132,190,259,274,287] Lymph node metastases are very uncommon in patients with stromal invasion of 3 mm or less. In contrast, the prevalence of lymph node metastases is 5.8% in women with 3.1–5 mm of invasion, 15.8% in women with stage 1B invasive cervical squamous cell carcinoma invading to a depth of 6–10 mm, and 23.5% in women with stage 1B carcinoma invading to a depth of 11–15 mm.

The development of recurrent disease or death from cervical cancer in women with less than 1 mm of stromal invasion who have been managed with either a cone biopsy or a simple hysterectomy is infrequent.[17,63,64,68,167] In three long-term follow-up studies involving 403 women, not a single patient with less than 1 mm of stromal invasion treated with a cone biopsy or simple hysterectomy died of their tumor (Table 8.4).[48,64,167] Similarly, recurrent disease occurs in approximately 1% of patients when tumors invade less than 3 mm (Table 8.5).[63,68,190,252,256,259] Recurrence occurs in approximately 5% of patients when there is 3.1–5 mm of invasion (Table 8.5).

Confluency of neoplastic epithelium in MICA has not been associated with pelvic node metastases, vaginal recurrence, or cancer death in most series.[115,179,241,259] In addition, a reproducible definition of what constitutes a confluent pattern of invasion has been difficult to achieve.[23] Therefore, clinical outcome is strongly influenced by the depth but not the pattern of invasion.

Table 8.3. Pelvic node metastasis with early invasive carcinoma according to depth of stromal penetration

Depth of invasion (mm)[a]	*No. of patients*	*Percent (%) of patients with (+) lymph nodes*
≤3	464	0.6
3.1–5	566	5.8
5.1–10	329	15.8
10.1–15	179	23.5
15.1–20	121	38.0

[a]Depth of stromal invasion regardless of presence or absence of vascular invasion and confluency.
Modified from refs. 40, 63, 68, 78, 115, 123, 179, 190, 256, 259, 274, 287.

Table 8.4. Outcome of women with microinvasive squamous cell carcinoma with 1 mm or less invasion managed by cone biopsy or simple hysterectomy

Author	*No. of patients*	*No. of deaths from tumor*
Burghardt et al.	259	0
Coppleson et al.	54	0
Koldstad	90	0
Total	403	0

Modified from refs. 48, 64, 167.

Table 8.5. Invasive cancer recurrences after any type of therapy for early invasive squamous cell carcinoma of the cervix with differing depths of invasion

Author	*No. of patients with recurrent invasive cancer/total patients (%)*	
	<3.0 mm of invasion[a]	*3.1–5.0 mm of invasion*[a]
Copeland et al.	8/552 (1.4%)	3/121 (2.5%)
Maiman et al.	0/65	0/30
Sedlis et al.	1/111 (0.9%)	1/21 (4.7%)
Sevin et al.	0/7	4/36 (11%)
Simon et al.	0/43	0/26
van Nagell et al.	2/145 (1.4%)	6/32 (19%)
Total	11/923 (1.2%)	14/266 (5.3%)

[a]Irrespective of presence or absence of lymphvascular space involvement or horizontal extent of tumor.
Modified from refs. 63, 190, 252, 256, 259, 287.

Table 8.6. Relationship between depth of invasion and presence of lymphvascular space involvement

Depth of invasion (mm)	*No. of patients*	*Percentage of specimens showing lymphvascular space involvement*	
		Mean	*Range*
<1.0	353	3%	0–8%
1.0–3.0	416	16%	9–29%
3.1–5.0	406	25%	12–43%

Adopted from refs. 43, 63, 68, 167, 179, 190, 252.

Lymphvascular Space Involvement

The relationship between lymphvascular space involvement and clinical outcome in women with early invasive squamous cell carcinoma is less clear cut than the relationship between depth of invasion and lymph node metastases. Lymphvascular space involvement is reported to occur in 0–8% of early squamous cell carcinomas that invade less than 1 mm into the stroma and in 9–29% of tumors invading 1–3 mm into the stroma (Table 8.6).[47,68,167,179,252,256] The large variation between the different reports results from several factors, including the number of pathologic sections evaluated and interobserver variability in determining lymphvascular space involvement. Shrinkage of stroma surrounding invasive nests can result in the formation of artifactual spaces that can be erroneously interpreted as vascular invasion. One study of early invasive squamous cell carcinoma reported that the frequency of detection of lymphvascular space involvement increased from 30% to 57% when step sections were cut through the site of invasion.[241] Despite the problems with recognizing lymphvascular space involvement, most studies have found a relationship between increasing depth of invasion and an increased frequency of lymphvascular space invasion (Table 8.6).

The clinical significance, however, of lymphvascular space involvement in patients with early invasive cervical cancer is controversial. Although several series of patients with 5 mm or less invasion have reported no direct relationship between the presence of lymphvascular space involvement and the presence of lymph node metastases, other studies have found lymphvascular space involvement to be an adverse prognostic indicator.[48,179,290,252,287] For example, in a study by Burghardt et al., 3 of 4 patients with 3 mm or less of invasion who developed recurrent disease after simple hysterectomy or cone biopsy had lymphvascular space involvement.[48] Similarly, in a study by Buckley et al. of 94 patients with stage 1A2 squamous cell carcinoma, 3 of 4 patients who died of recurrent cancer after therapy had lymphvascular space involvement.[43] Vascular invasion also appears to be a predictor of the presence of invasive carcinoma in the subsequent hysterectomy specimen.[78] Invasive carcinoma has been found in 80% of subsequent hysterectomy specimens when vascular invasion was present in the cone biopsy. Therefore, it is the prevailing opinion in the United States that lymphvascular space involvement should be assessed in women with early invasive squamous cell carcinoma and that the presence of lymphvascular space involvement excludes a diagnosis of MICA.

Tumor Volume and Horizontal Extent

In recent years, the morphologic evaluation of the volume of MICA has been emphasized by some authors. Burghardt and Holzer have introduced the concept of tumor as applied to MICA and have reported no pelvic node metastases in patients with 420 mm^3 of cancer or less, with the exception of one case in which vascular invasion was noted.[49] However, their method of measuring volume by serially sectioning cone specimens is both cumbersome and time-consuming and is unlikely to become a routine laboratory method. Other investigators and FIGO have used lateral extent of spread as a surrogate for measuring tumor volume. The lateral extent of spread of early invasive squamous cell carcinoma has been correlated with the frequency of residual neoplasia in the postcone hysterectomy specimens (Table 8.7).[252] In a study of 402 patients with stromal invasion of 5 mm or less, Takeshima et al. found that 18% had greater than 7 mm of horizontal spread.[274] As depth of invasion increased, there was an increase in horizontal spread. Only 6.3% of le-

Table 8.7. Residual invasive tumor in postconization hysterectomy specimens according to lateral extent of carcinoma with as much as 5 mm stromal invasion

Lateral extent of invasion (mm)	*No. of patients*	*Percent (%) with residual disease in postconization hysterectomy specimen*
<4	55	2
4–8	26	27
>8	23	35

Adapted from ref. 252.

Table 8.8. Relationship between status of cone biopsy margin in patients with early invasive squamous cell carcinoma of the cervix and residual disease in the postcone hysterectomy specimen

	Negative margins		*Positive margins*[a]	
Author	*No. patients*	*(% with residual cancer)*	*No. pts.*	*(% with residual cancer)*
Creasman et al.	45	(4.4)	13	(77)
Greer et al.	17	(24)	33	(82)
Jones et al.	25	(4)	46	(35)
Leman et al.	24	(0)	23	(39)
Sedlis et al.	85	(4)	15	(80)
Total	196	(5.1)	130	(57)

[a]Positive margin includes either microinvasive carcinoma or high-grade SIL at the margin.
Adapted from refs. 68, 105, 144, 179, 252.

sions with 3 mm of invasion or less had greater than 7 mm horizontal spread, whereas 61% of those with 3–5 mm of invasion had more than 7 mm lateral spread.[274]

Surgical Margins

Perhaps one of the most important contributions of the pathologist to the appropriate management of early invasive squamous cell carcinoma is evaluating surgical margins of conization specimens.[68,105,179,252,254] In fact, the status of cone margins may well be the most important single parameter in deciding the therapeutic approach to patients with early invasive squamous cell carcinoma. In most studies, women with cone margins positive for either SIL or invasive disease are much more likely to have residual invasive disease in the hysterectomy specimens than are women with a negative margin. Furthermore, the residual invasion may actually be deeper than that found in the cone biopsy specimen (Table 8.8).

Treatment

The therapy for MICA is more conservative than that for stage IA2 and greater cancers, with attempts at individualization of treatment based on (1) the definition of the lesion, (2) lateral extent, and (3) involvement of cone margins. The data on risk factors for nodal metastases, recurrence, and death, although incomplete, suggest that lesions with 3 mm or less stromal penetration, measured from the point of origin in invasion and without lymphvascular space involvement, have virtually no potential for metastasis or recurrences. On the other hand, those invading 3 mm or less but with vascular invasion may potentially metastasize, although the risk is small, about 3.5%. Therefore, most authorities believe that women with less than 3 mm of stromal invasion and lacking lymphvascular space involvement can be managed with procedures less radical than those required for stage IB invasive squamous cell carcinomas.[25] Patients who are to be managed with less radical procedures should not have colposcopically overt carcinoma and should have had a diagnostic conization that removed the entire lesional tissue with negative lines of resection together with a negative endocervical curettage obtained at the time of conization.

At most centers the recommended therapy for MICA that fulfills the SGO definition is a simple hysterectomy. Most authorities now agree that women with MICA who are desirous of maintaining fertility can be safely managed with conization provided they are willing to undergo careful, periodic follow-up and provided they clearly understand that there is a measurable (albeit low) risk of developing pelvic lymph node metastases or recurrent disease.[25]

Invasive Squamous Cell Carcinoma

General Features

Despite advances in its detection and management, cervical cancer continues to be a significant health problem on a worldwide scale. In 1990, cervical cancer was the second most frequent cancer in women throughout the world.[220] It has been estimated that 390,000 cases of invasive cervical cancer occurred throughout the world in 1990.[226] Because of widespread differences in the availability of screening programs and the prevalence of risk factors, there continue to be marked differences in the relative frequency of cervical cancer in developed and undeveloped countries. Cervical cancer is the most frequent type of cancer in women in many developing countries whereas it is the seventh most frequent type in much of the developed world.[220] The regions of the world where the incidence is greatest include sub-Saharan Africa, Central and South America, and Southeast Asia. The highest incidence rate is in Central America, where there is an age-standardized rate of 31.2.[220] The lowest reported incidence rates are from Eastern Asia (China) and Western Asia, with age-standardized incidence rates of 4.4 and 4.1, respectively, and in Northern Africa, 7.3.[220]

The average age of patients with invasive squamous cell carcinoma is 51.4 years, 15–23 years older than patients with high-grade SIL and 8 years older than patients with microinvasive carcinoma.[66] Cervical cancer occurs, however, at almost any age between 17 and 90 years. In recent years there has been increasing recognition that cervical cancer can occur in women under the age of 35 years. Women under the age of 35 years account for 22.1% of all patients with invasive cervical cancer in the United States.[208] In the United Kingdom, an increase in the incidence of, and death from, invasive cervical cancer in women in this age group has been observed over the last several decades.[221,289] The increase observed in the United Kingdom is most likely related to multiple factors including a failure to provide adequate cytologic screening programs for sexually active young women and changes in the demographics of the population being screened.[221,289] However, intensification of cytologic screening efforts in the United Kingdom has recently reversed this trend and produced a fall in mortality for cervical cancer in young women.[221]

There is little doubt that cytologic screening programs play a major role in reducing both the incidence and mortality of invasive cervical cancer, as has been most conclusively demonstrated by data from the Nordic countries, Canada, and parts of Scotland. The incidence of cervical cancer in the Nordic countries between 1945 and 1980 is directly correlated with the extent of cytologic screening.[108] Cytologic screening was introduced into Iceland and Finland in the mid-1960s and was rapidly accepted and widely used. In both these countries, a marked decrease in the incidence of cervical cancer occurred after the introduction of screening programs. In contrast, Denmark and Sweden introduced widespread screening more slowly and less uniformly and experienced less of a decline in the incidence of cervical cancer. In Norway, no cytologic screening program was introduced, and the incidence of invasive cervical cancer actually increased during this time period.

Reductions in the incidence and mortality of invasive cervical cancer have also occurred in the United States and Canada since the widespread introduction of cytologic screening. According to the American Cancer Society, in 1961 only 30% of all U.S. women had ever had a Pap smear, but this number increased to 87% by 1987 (Fig. 8.8).[228] In 1940, the incidence of invasive cervical cancer in the United States was 32.6 per 100,000 women, which is similar to that currently seen in the developing world, whereas by 1984 the incidence was 8.3 per 100,000 women. The reduction in incidence was paralleled by a reduction in mortality.[80] In 2000, there were only 12,800 cases of invasive cervical cancer diagnosed in the United States and 4,600 cervical cancer deaths according to the American Cancer Society.[2] Despite the low incidence of invasive cervical cancer in the United States, cervical cancer continues to be a problem among selected

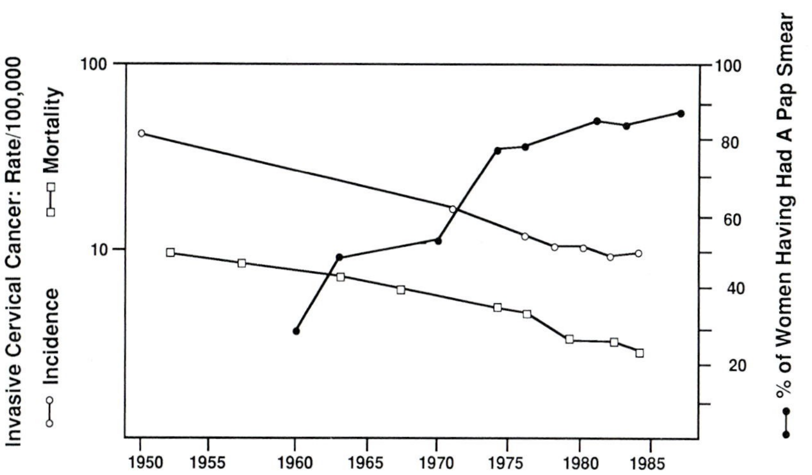

Fig. 8.8. Rate of cytological screening (*curve with black dots*) versus the incidence and mortality of invasive cervical cancer in the United States, 1940–1984. As the rate of screening increased, the incidence and mortality of invasive cancer decreased. (Modified from refs. 80, 228.)

groups of women. The incidence among black women is almost 50% higher than the incidence of white women in the United States, and the incidence among Hispanic women is more than twice that of white women.[3] A significant proportion of the remaining cases of invasive cervical carcinoma in the United States could be prevented if all women at risk underwent routine cytologic screening and colposcopic evaluation of significant cytologic abnormalities. In the United States, approximately half of the women who developed invasive cervical cancer had not had a Pap smear in the preceding 3 years.[135,163]

Histogenesis and Etiology

Because of the integration of information from multiple disciplines during the past 15 years, we now know much about the etiology and histogenesis of cervical cancer. There is a considerable body of evidence indicating that invasive squamous cell carcinoma develops from SIL and, as a result, women with invasive squamous cell carcinoma have similar epidemiologic characteristics to those with preinvasive precursor lesions (see Chapter 7, Precancerous Lesions of the Cervix). Like women with SIL, the majority of women with invasive cancer of the cervix are from lower socioeconomic groups, began heterosexual activity early in life, married early, are multiparous, and have many sexual partners.[217] These associations suggest a role for a sexually transmitted agent(s) in the etiology of cervical cancer and, based on recent molecular and epidemiologic studies, we now recognize that cervical cancer is caused by specific, high-risk types of human papillomavirus (HPV).

Almost all the recent studies from well-established laboratories analyzing tissues for multiple types of HPV have detected HPV DNA in more than 90% of invasive squamous cell carcinomas and have found that, irrespective of geographic location, most invasive cervical cancers are associated with the same high-risk types of HPV, predominantly HPV 16, 18, 45, and 58.[32,54,130,210,293] The failure to detect HPV DNA in a small subset of invasive squamous cell carcinomas appears to be caused by a number of factors including failure to adequately sample the lesion, presence of a HPV type other than those assayed for, and loss of part of the HPV genome from the malignant cells. A recent study that thoroughly investigated, with multiple molecular techniques, a group of supposedly HPV DNA-negative tumors detected HPV DNA in most of the cases and concluded that the worldwide prevalence of HPV in cervical carcinomas is 99.7%.[293] In patients with metastatic cervical carcinoma, HPV DNA can also be identified in lymph node metastases, with viral DNA hybridization patterns frequently, but not always, matching those of the primary cervical tumor.[131] Based on the strength of the molecular and epidemiologic evidence linking HPV to invasive squamous cell carcinoma of the cervix, select types of high-risk HPV have been classified as human carcinogens by the World Health Organization.[130]

There is also considerable epidemiologic evidence indicating that factors other than HPV are important in the development of invasive squamous cell carcinoma of the cervix. Two of the most recent of these studies found that even after controlling for HPV, there continued to be a significant associations between cervical cancer and number of sexual partners, smoking, and histories of venereal disease.[54,210] These studies have been interpreted as suggesting that other sexually associated cofactors, in addition to HPV, play a role in the histogenesis of cervical cancer.

It has been estimated that only approximately 1–5% of untreated low-grade SIL eventually progress to invasive cancer.[201,216] In the Ontario Cancer Registry study of more than 17,000 women with a history of abnormal Pap smears, the actual rate of untreated low-grade SIL progressing to carcinoma in situ or invasive cervical cancer was 2.8% for women followed more than 10 years.[121] The percentage of carcinoma in situ that has progressed to invasive squamous cell carcinoma has been between 6% and 74% in the various follow-up series (see Chapter 7, Precancerous Lesions of the Cervix). The estimated average duration of preclinical microinvasive disease to overt clinical carcinoma is about 10 years.[235]

Clinical Features

The presenting symptoms of patients with invasive carcinoma of the cervix of all histologic types appear to be dependent on the size and stage of the lesion.[228] Early series from the 1950s through the 1970s were composed predominantly of patients with bulky, late-stage disease. Nearly all these patients had clinically visible cancers and nearly all complained of abnormal vaginal bleeding. The most significant and common feature was bleeding following intercourse or douching. Intermittent spotting, serosanguinous discharge, and frank hemorrhage were also frequently encountered; 10–20% of the patients complained of bloody malodorous discharge and pain, often radiating to the sacral region. More recent studies include a much higher percentage of patients with stage I disease. Patients with stage I disease are frequently asymptomatic and detected on the basis of an abnormal Pap smear.[228] Weakness, pallor, weight loss, edema of the lower extremities, rectal pain, and hematuria are symptoms and signs of either locally advanced or metastatic disease.

Means for accurate detection and diagnosis of frank invasive carcinoma include cytology, colposcopy, and colposcopically directed punch biopsy.[268] Rectovaginal examination, intravenous pyelography (IVP), cystoscopy, proctosigmoidoscopy, and skeletal survey are used to assess the clinical stage of the disease. Other investigations including barium enema, lymphangiogram, CT scan, and MRI or sonogram are frequently performed.[25]

Invasive carcinoma of either the squamous or glandular type develops in the cervical stump that remains following subtotal hysterectomy in 0.1–1.9% of patients.[161,299] In a study of 173 women with carcinoma of the cervical stump, Wolff et al. divided their patients into those in whom the neoplasm was found within 2 years of the subtotal hysterectomy and those in whom the lesion appeared more than 2 years after the operation.[299] The 5-year survival of patients of the first group was worse (30%) than either those of the second group (49%) or those with cancer of the cervix in general. Based on these observations, it has been suggested that cervical stump cancers occurring within the first 2 years following surgery represent residual malignancy, whereas those discovered after 2 years are "new" cancers arising de novo from the cervical stump.

Although 3–10% of cervical cancers occur in pregnant women and cervical cancer is the most common gynecologic cancer found during pregnancy, invasive carcinoma of the cervix is relatively uncommon during gestation, occurring approximately once in 2200 pregnancies.[31,111,145] Nevertheless, routine cervical cytology should be part of the initial prenatal examination. The mean age of pregnant women with invasive cervical cancer is 32 years, which is considerably lower than that of women in the general population with invasive cervical cancer, and women who are pregnant usually present with early-stage tumors.[145] In one series of pregnant patients with invasive cervical disease, 83% were stage I.[145] The treatment of pregnant patients with invasive cervical cancer depends on the clinical stage of the disease and gestational age. In general, prognosis is not altered by pregnancy.

Pathologic Findings

Gross Appearances

Invasive squamous cell carcinoma displays a wide range of gross appearances. Early lesions may be fo-

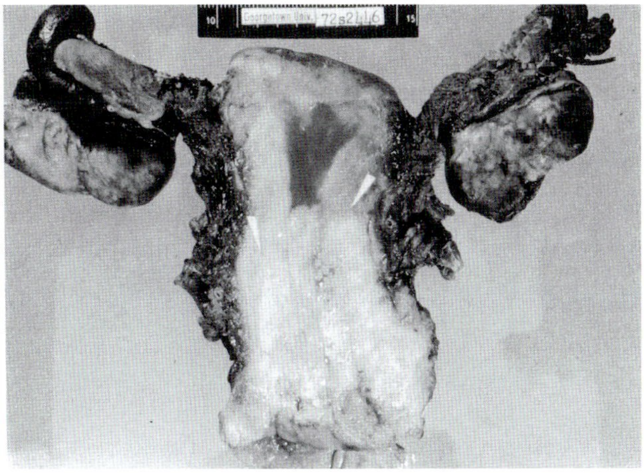

Fig. 8.9. Squamous carcinoma of the cervix. This endophytic tumor has totally replaced the endocervix and extends to the lower uterine segment, producing a "barrel-shaped" cervix. (Reprinted with permission from Kurman et al., ref. 174.)

cally indirated, ulcerated, or present as a slightly elevated and granular area that bleeds readily on touch. Colposcopic examination usually reveals atypical, tortuous vessels varying widely in size and configuration. Approximately 98% of early carcinomas are localized within the transformation zone, with variable degrees of encroachment onto the neighboring native portio. More advanced tumors have two major types of gross appearance: endophytic and exophytic. Endophytic carcinomas are either ulcerated or nodular (Fig. 8.9); they tend to develop within the endocervical canal and frequently invade deeply into the cervical stroma to produce an enlarged, hard, barrel-shaped cervix. In some patients with endophytic carcinomas, the cervix grossly appears normal. The exophytic varieties of cervical carcinomas have a polypoid or papillary appearance (Fig. 8.10).

Microscopic Appearance

Microscopically, invasive squamous cell carcinomas have considerable heterogeneity. Many cases are characterized by anastomosing tongues or cords of neoplastic epithelium infiltrating the fibrous stroma of the cervix (Fig. 8.11). Characteristically, the contour of the infiltrating nests and clusters is irregular and ragged. In other cases, the tumor invades either as individual cells or almost completely replaces the stroma with large masses of neoplastic squamous cells. Cells in the center of the invading nests frequently become necrotic or undergo extensive keratinization (Fig. 8.12). Individual cells are generally polygonal or oval with eosinophilic cyto-

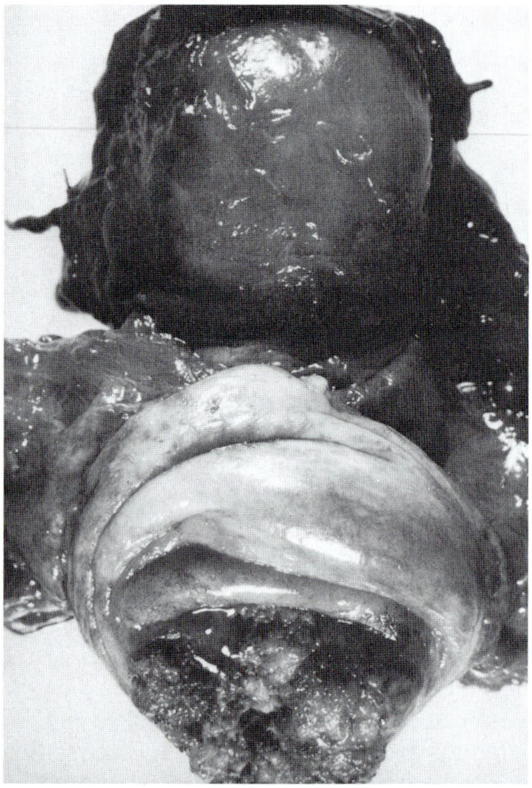

Fig. 8.10. Squamous carcinoma of the cervix. A bulky friable exophytic mass projects from the external os. (Courtesy of Dr. B.K. Chun, Washington, DC.)

plasm and prominent cellular membranes. Intracellular bridges may or may not be visible. In some cases, the nuclei are relatively uniform, whereas in others they are quite pleomorphic. In most cases, the chromatin is coarse and clumped, and mitotic figures, including abnormal forms, commonly are encountered.

Histological Typing

One of the earliest approaches to classifying cervical squamous cell carcinomas was based on the predominant cell type.[234] The classification separated squamous cell carcinomas into large cell keratinizing, large cell nonkeratinizing, and small cell nonkeratinizing. In the experience of Wentz and Reagan, the best 5-year survival rate after radiation therapy was associated with large cell nonkeratinizing carcinomas (68.3%), followed by the large cell keratinizing type (41.7%), whereas small cell carcinomas had a 20% 5-year survival rate.[297] Because there has been frequent confusion between the small cell nonkeratinizing squamous cell carcinomas described by Wentz and Reagan and small cell undifferentiated carcinomas with neuroendocrine features similar to those described in the lung, the current WHO classification of invasive cervical cancers places small cell undifferentiated carcinoma with neuroendocrine features in a separate category and divides invasive squamous cell carcinomas into two groups, keratinizing and nonkeratinizing.[251]

Keratinizing carcinomas are characterized by the presence of well-differentiated squamous cells that are arranged in nests or cords which vary greatly in size and configuration. One of the most characteristic features of keratinizing carcinomas is the presence of keratin "pearls" within the epithelium (see Fig. 8.12). These "pearls" are composed of clusters of squamous cells that have undergone keratinization and are arranged in a concentric nest. The presence of a single keratin "pearl" is sufficient to classify a tumor as a keratinizing carcinoma. The neoplastic squamous cells not forming keratin "pearls" frequently have abundant eosinophilic cytoplasm and prominent intracellular bridges. The nuclei are often enlarged, but mitotic figures are not numerous.

Nonkeratinizing squamous cell carcinomas are characterized by nests of neoplastic squamous cells

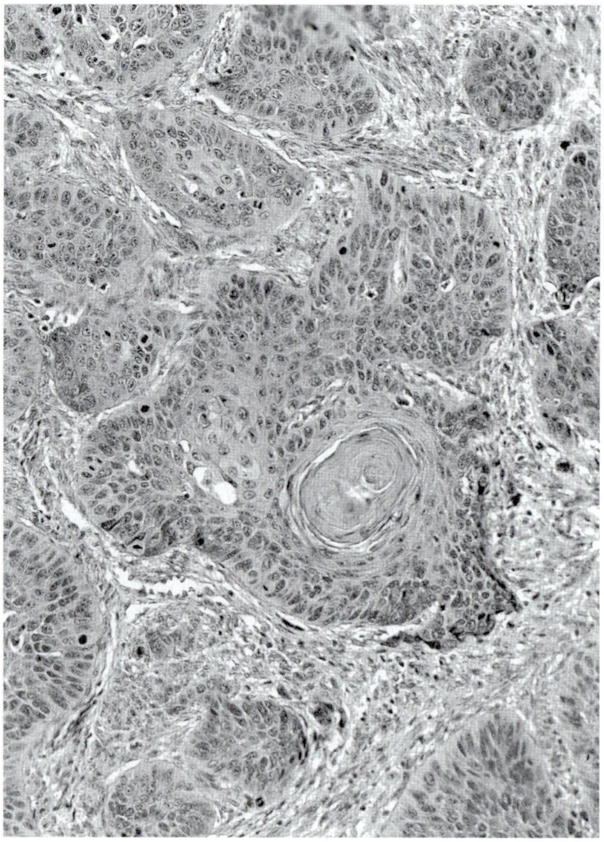

Fig. 8.11. Invasive squamous carcinoma of the cervix. Note the irregular contour of infiltrative nests. A keratin pearl is present in the center of the next.

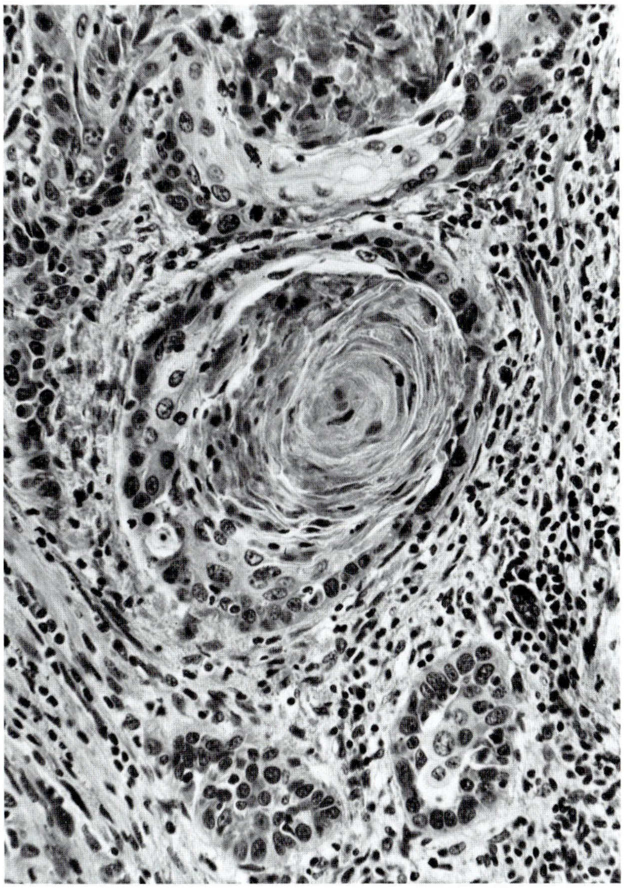

Fig. 8.12. Well-differentiated (grade I) invasive squamous carcinoma of the cervix. Keratin pearl formation is evident.

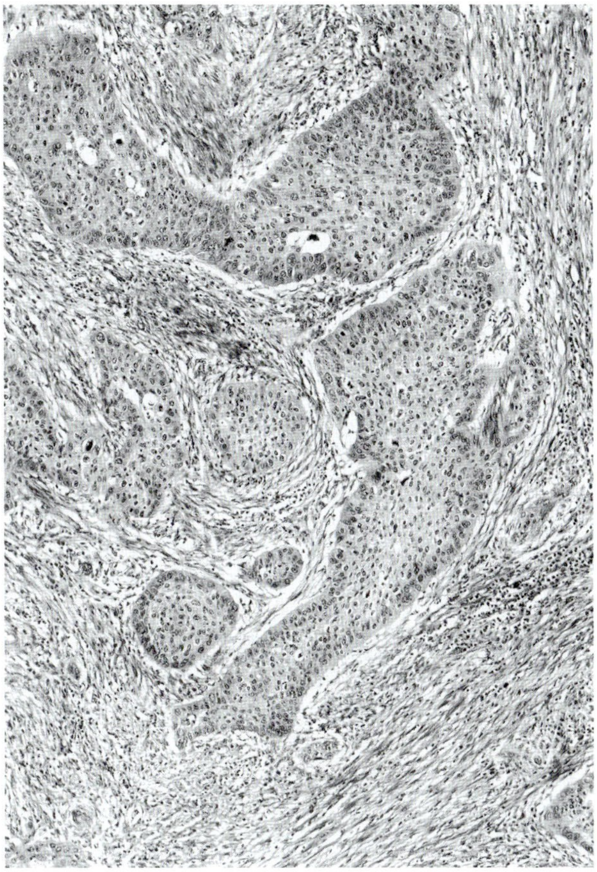

Fig. 8.13. Moderately differentiated (grade 2) squamous carcinoma of the cervix. Irregular nests of squamous neoplasia invade into the stroma. There is a prominent inflammatory infiltrate surrounding the nests.

that frequently undergo individual cell keratinization but, by definition, do not form keratin "pearls" (Fig. 8.13). These cells have relatively indistinct cell borders. The nuclei tend to be round to oval with coarsely clumped chromatin (Fig. 8.14). Mitotic figures are frequent. Other nonkeratinizing squamous cell carcinomas are composed of masses and nests of small basaloid cells with scant cytoplasm and hyperchromatic uniform nuclei with frequent mitotic activity. These tumors are similar to the basaloid carcinomas of the vulva and vagina.

Although some investigators have reported that this classification has prognostic significance in patients being treated with radiotherapy,[92,232,272] others have found no significant difference in prognosis between patients with large cell nonkeratinizing and large cell keratinizing squamous carcinomas when treated with radical surgery.[271,277,307]

Microscopic Grading

Several attempts have been made to classify cervical carcinomas according to the degree of differentiation. The first method used for grading squamous cell carcinomas of the cervix was that originally proposed in the 1920s by Broders for grading squamous cell carcinomas of the lip.[39] This method was based on the proportion of the tumor that was undergoing keratinization with the formation of squamous pearls and the number of mitoses. A modification of the Broders's method that is based on the degree of differentiation is currently the most widely used histologic grading system. Using this method, squamous cell carcinomas are graded as well differentiated (grade 1), moderately differentiated (grade 2), and poorly differentiated (grade 3). Most squamous cell carcinomas are moderately differentiated (grade 2), followed by poorly differentiated (grade 3) and well differentiated (grade 1).

In well-differentiated (grade 1) tumors, the most striking feature is abundant keratin, which is deposited as concentric whorls (keratin pearls) in the centers of neoplastic epithelial nests (see Fig. 8.12).

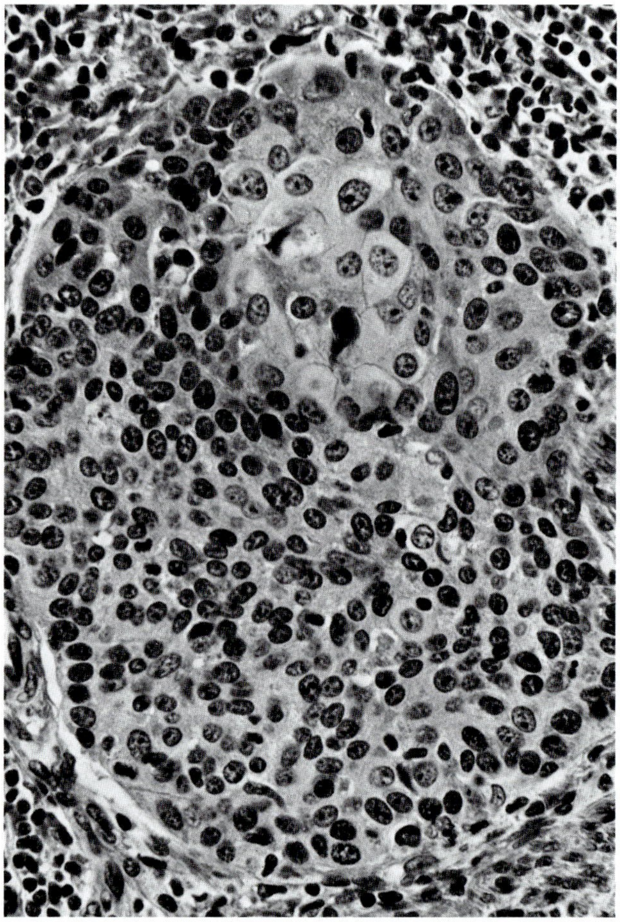

Fig. 8.14. Moderately differentiated (grade 2) squamous carcinoma of the cervix. Abortive keratinization but no pearl formation. Accordingly, this tumor can be classified as a nonkeratinizing squamous carcinoma.

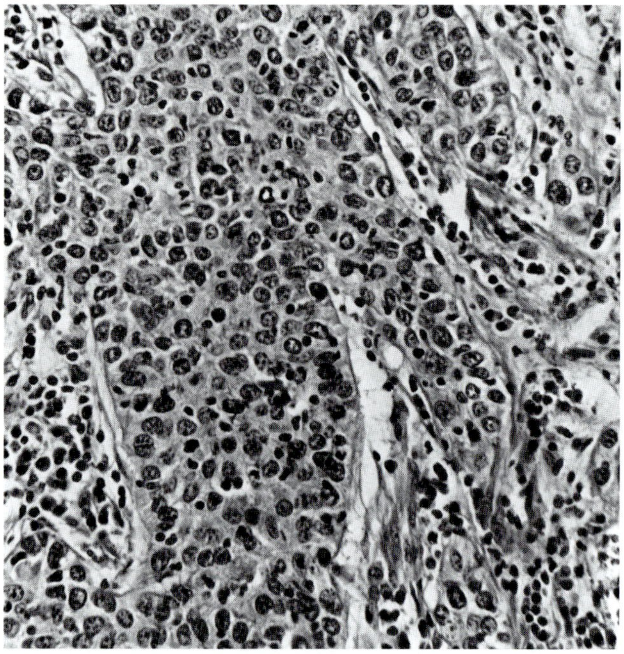

Fig. 8.15. Poorly differentiated (grade 3) squamous carcinoma. There is anisonucleosis, scant cytoplasm, and indistinct cell membranes.

The cells appear mature, with abundant eosinophilic cytoplasm. Individual cell keratinization (dyskeratosis) characterized by intense cytoplasmic eosinophilia may also be present. The cells are tightly packed and have well-developed intercellular bridges. The nuclei are large, irregular, and hyperchromatic, with numerous chromocenters. Mitotic figures are present, with maximum concentration at the periphery of the advancing epithelial nests. The stroma is often infiltrated by chronic inflammatory cells, and occasionally a foreign body giant cell reaction is observed.

In moderately differentiated (grade 2) squamous cell carcinomas, the neoplastic cells are more pleomorphic than in grade 1 tumors, are characterized by large irregular nuclei, and have less abundant cytoplasm. The cellular borders, as well as intercellular bridges, appear indistinct. Keratin pearl formation is virtually nonexistent, but individual cell keratinization is seen in the center of nests of tumor cells. Mitotic figures are more numerous than in grade 1 carcinomas (see Fig. 8.13).

Poorly differentiated (grade 3) squamous cell carcinomas are generally composed of cells with hyperchromatic oval nuclei and scant indistinct cytoplasm, resembling the malignant cells of high-grade SIL (Fig. 8.15). Clear-cut squamous differentiation manifested by keratinization may be difficult to find. Mitoses and areas of necrosis are abundant. Poorly differentiated lesions are occasionally composed of large, pleomorphic cells with giant, bizarre nuclei and abnormal mitotic figures. In rare instances, the neoplastic cells assume a spindle-shaped configuration resembling a sarcoma (Fig. 8.16). Immunohistochemical staining for epithelial membrane antigen (EMA) and cytokeratins demonstrates the epithelial nature of the spindle cell component in these cases.

Studies analyzing the effect of tumor grade on prognosis are difficult to compare because of wide differences in the stage of the patients and the therapies used. A study by Chung et al. of early-stage squamous cell carcinomas found that poorly differentiated tumors were associated with a higher incidence of tumor recurrence and a poorer 2-year survival.[56] Although this finding has been confirmed by some,[262,271] most studies have failed to confirm that histopathologic grade, as determined by the degree of differentiation, influences clinical outcome.[77,277,309]

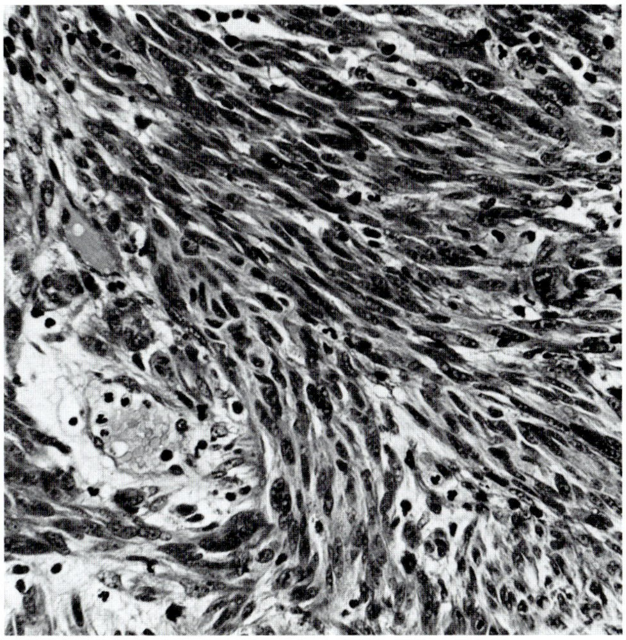

Fig. 8.16. Invasive squamous carcinoma with spindle-shape features. Note fusiform configuration of cells, resembling a sarcoma. This area was merged with moderately differentiated squamous carcinoma.

For example, a study from the Gynecologic Oncology Group (GOG) evaluated a number of different tumor grading systems including those proposed by Warren, Reagan, and Broder in surgically treated stage IB cervical cancers.[307] Although there was good reproducibility between observers (76–92%), none of the grading systems had prognostic significance. In addition, nuclear grade, degree of keratinization, mitotic activity, pattern of infiltration, and degree of lymphoid response all lacked prognostic significance. Because histopathologic grade has failed to predict clinical outcome in many studies, more comprehensive grading systems have been developed that take into account the tumor–host interactions, including the degree of tumor keratinization, nuclear differentiation, number of mitoses, cell size, nuclear: cytoplasmic ratio, inflammatory response to the tumor, stromal response to the tumor, vascular invasion, and the pattern of invasion of the tumor into the underlying stroma. This approach was found to be of highly significant prognostic value in early studies.[268,269] However, even these more comprehensive methods of determining tumor grade have provided none, or only minimal, prognostic information in other large, well-controlled studies.[69,171] In summary, there has been no conclusive demonstration that a histologic grading or histologic typing system (see above) reliably predicts prognosis.

Immunohistochemistry

Squamous cell carcinomas of the cervix express a complex variety of keratins differing in pattern and number depending on the grade of histologic differentiation.[73,261] Differentiated, keratinizing cervical carcinomas have the most complex pattern of keratin intermediate filaments and contain polypeptides characteristic of terminally differentiated cervical keratinocytes, including 4, 5, 6, 8, 13, 14, 16, 17, 18, and 19. Nonkeratinizing cervical squamous cell carcinomas express keratins 6, 14, 17, and 19 in all cases and keratins 4, 5, 7, 8, 10, 13, 16, and 18 occasionally. The heterogeneous intermediate filament patterns expressed in cervical carcinoma indicate that some sets of keratin polypeptides are conserved during malignant transformation whereas the expression of other keratin polypeptides reflects a selection of a minor cell type or clone during carcinogenesis or even de novo expression. The distribution of keratin polypeptides in invasive squamous cell carcinomas of the cervix has not yet been shown to assist in histologic diagnosis.

Monoclonal antibodies derived from cervical carcinomas include a tumor-associated antigen, referred to as squamous cell carcinoma antigen or TA-4, which is a glycoprotein of 48,000 molecular weight. This protein is a member of the high molecular weight serine proteinase inhibitor (e.g., serpin) superfamily. Elevations of serum squamous cell carcinoma antigen have been observed in women with cervical carcinoma and can be used to monitor the effects of therapy, detect tumor recurrence, and identify patients at high risk for having nodal metastases.[18,182] In tissue sections, TA-4 is localized in the cytoplasm of differentiated and keratinized cells in normal cervical squamous epithelium and malignant tumors.[285] Antigen expression in carcinomas is linked to differentiation and cannot be identified in small cell undifferentiated tumor.

Cathepsin D is a lysosomal acid protease whose overexpression is thought to increase the metastatic potential of tumor cells. About half of stage IB squamous cell carcinomas stain positively for cathepsin D, and these tumors demonstrate lower relapse-free survival rates.[172] Studies have also found that tumors that show increased immunostaining for the epidermal growth factor receptor (EGFR) also have lower rates of relapse-free survival.[172] For additional discussion of immunohistochemical findings, see Chapter 25, Immunohistochemistry.

Ultrastructure

The ultrastructural hallmarks of neoplastic cells of squamous origin include intracytoplasmic bundles of tonofilaments, desmosome–tonofilament complexes, and finger-like intercellular microvilli.[87] These alterations are readily identified in well- and moderately differentiated neoplasms.[87] The tonofilaments may be aggregated and form large globular masses. In the lesser-differentiated lesions, tonofilaments and desmosomal plates are reduced and poorly developed. Loss of desmosomal attachments and separation of desmosomal–tonofilament complexes lead to loss of cellular cohesion. Another characteristic feature of squamous carcinoma cells is the profound decrease in gap junction nexuses compared to normal cervical squamous epithelium.

Differential Diagnosis

Histologically, the lesions most commonly confused with invasive squamous cell carcinomas are squamous metaplasia and high-grade SIL with extensive endocervical gland involvement, gestational decidual reaction with degenerative features, condylomata acuminata, and reparative changes associated with chronic granulomatous diseases such as lymphogranuloma venereum and granuloma inguinale. With the exception of high-grade SIL, these lesions can all be differentiated from invasive squamous cell carcinomas by the absence of significant nuclear atypia and their low mitotic activity.

Both squamous metaplasia and high-grade SIL are frequently extensive and extend into endocervical glands. Even though a low level of mitotic activity can be present in squamous metaplasia, careful evaluation of the cytologic appearance of the metaplastic cells reveals their benign nature because the cells are relatively uniform in size and shape and lack significant nuclear atypia. Moreover, the borders of endocervical glands involved with either squamous metaplasia or high-grade SIL are rounded and distinct and lack the irregular margins, scalloping, and the desmoplasia and dense inflammatory infiltrate that occasionally contains foreign body giant cells in the stroma adjacent to the nests (Fig. 8.17). A decidual reaction with degenerative features lacks mitotic activity and in difficult cases can be differentiated from invasive squamous cell carcinomas by the use of immunohistochemical staining because decidual cells do not contain cytokeratin. Placental site nodules or plaques represent incompletely resorbed hyalinized implantation sites and appear as well-circumscribed nodules or plaques containing intermediate trophoblastic cells. These cells lack mitotic activity and are arranged in nests surrounded by hyaline material. Again, in difficult cases immunohistochemistry can be used to determine the true nature of these lesions because the intermediate trophoblasts within these well-circumscribed nodules usually contain placental

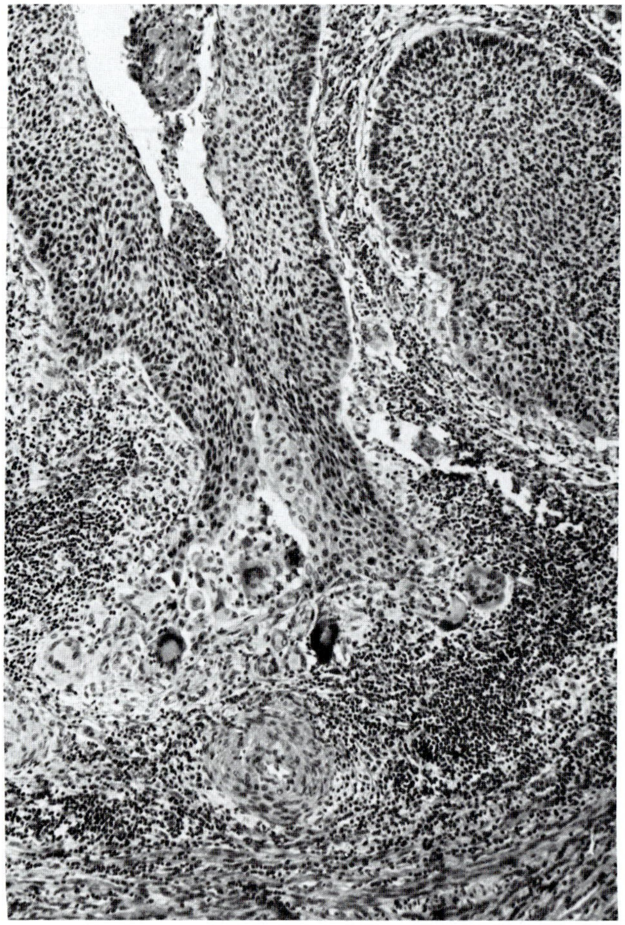

Fig. 8.17. Moderately differentiated (grade 2) squamous carcinoma of the cervix. Note foreign body giant cell reaction to infiltrating tumor cells.

lactogen. (See *Chapter 24*, Gestational Trophoblastic Disease and Related Lesions.)

Squamous cell carcinomas that contain large amounts of cytoplasmic glycogen can sometimes be confused with clear cell carcinomas (Fig. 8.18). Like clear cell carcinomas, cells in these tumors have clear cytoplasm and distinct cell membranes. However, squamous cell carcinoma with clear cytoplasm lacks the characteristic hobnail cells and the papillary or tubulocystic areas that are typical of clear cell carcinomas. In squamous cell carcinoma, a careful search of multiple sections will usually detect areas with unambiguous squamous differentiation.

It can also be difficult to distinguish between poorly differentiated squamous cell carcinomas composed of small, basaloid cells and small (oat) cell carcinomas of the neuroendocrine type. Small cell carcinomas of the neuroendocrine type typically invade the stroma diffusely as individual cells or as small discohesive nests and show extensive crush artifact; they frequently form rosettes or trabeculae and the cells characteristically have smudged in-

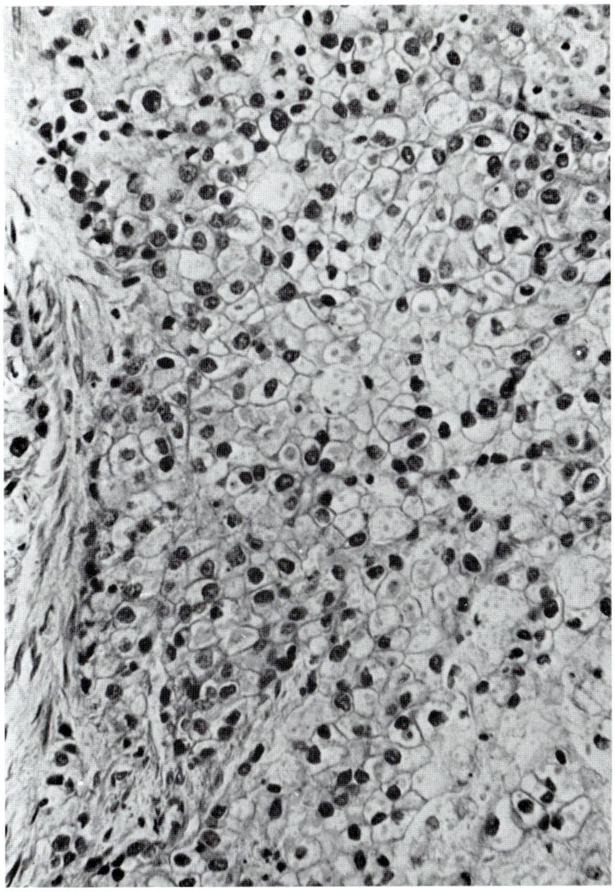

Fig. 8.18. Invasive squamous carcinoma of the cervix with clear cell features. The cells are rich in glycogen, which results in their clear cytoplasmic appearance. The cellular borders are well defined.

tensely hyperchromatic nuclei and lack nucleoli. In contrast, poorly differentiated squamous cell carcinomas invade as cohesive nests, and the cells have oval nuclei with granular chromatin. In difficult cases, electron microscopy or immunohistochemistry can be used to demonstrate neurosecretory granules in small cell carcinomas of the neuroendocrine type. Unfortunately, there is overlap of this feature between the two types of neoplasm. In the final analysis, conventional microscopic features are the most useful in distinguishing these tumors.[10]

Histopathologic Prognostic Features

Stage is the most important prognostic factor in cervical carcinoma. Histologic typing and grading have little direct influence on survival within any stage (see "Microscopic Grading"). Within a particular stage, the most significant pathologic prognostic factors in women with surgically treated stage IB and IIA squamous cell carcinoma are tumor size, depth of invasion, parametrial involvement, and nodal status.[77,171,271,277,307] For example, a study of 188 women undergoing radical hysterectomy with bilateral pelvic lymphadenectomy for stage IB squamous cell carcinoma found that patients with tumors measuring less than 2 cm in diameter and patients with larger tumors that invaded less than 10 mm into the cervical stroma had a 5-year-disease-free survival of 95%. In contrast, all other patients had a 5-year-disease-free survival of 52%.[171] In the Gynecological Oncology Group (GOG) series of stage IB squamous cell carcinomas treated surgically, patients whose tumors invaded the inner third of the cervical stroma had a 98% 5-year progression-free rate, whereas it was 63% for those whose tumors invaded the outer third.[307] In most series of surgically treated stage IB cancers, lymph-vascular space involvement has proven to be somewhat less important than tumor size and depth of invasion. In the Gynecological Oncology Group (GOG) series of stage IB squamous cell carcinomas, the 5-year progression-free interval was 70% in tumors with lymphvascular space involvement compared to 83% in cases without lymphvascular space involvement.[307] Similarly, in the series of Stockler et al. of surgically treated stage IB and IIA cancers that lacked nodal metastases, lymphvascular space involvement was found to be associated with a 2.5-fold increase in the risk of relapse.[271] Accordingly, in reporting squamous cell carcinomas, the depth of invasion (in millimeters or the proportion of the wall invaded), the presence or absence of vascular invasion, and the size of the tumor (greatest tumor dimension) should be reported. In contrast, histologic grading and typing into keratinizing and nonkeratinizing are of lesser clinical value.

Another factor that may influence prognosis is patient age. In 1952, Lindell demonstrated that survival of women with cervical cancer increases with increasing age.[183] This finding was later confirmed by others, who also reported poorer survival rates for young women with cervical cancer. However, there are a number of other large studies, including one of Meanwell et al. from the United Kingdom that analyzed more than 10,000 women with invasive cervical cancer, that have actually reported younger women to have a better prognosis than older women.[147,197] In general, it appears that there is little difference in prognosis between younger and older women with stage I or IIA tumors, but that younger women with higher-stage disease have a poorer survival.[224,245]

HPV DNA Status

Several studies have assessed the role of HPV type on outcome, and there appears to be a significant correlation between specific types of HPV (e.g., HPV 18) and a poor prognosis. In one study of 30 patients, 83% of tumors associated with HPV 18 were poorly differentiated.[19] In that study, weaker associations were noted between the presence of HPV 18 and lymph node involvement and young age. Walker et al. analyzed 100 invasive cervical cancers for HPV DNA using Southern blot and found that 45% of the tumors associated with HPV 18 recurred compared to a 16% recurrence rate in HPV 16-associated tumors.[295] Women with HPV 18-associated tumors were 8 years younger than women whose tumors were associated with HPV 16, but HPV status was not significantly associated with tumor size, presence of parametrial involvement, or lymph node status. An effect of HPV type on outcome has been confirmed in several recent large series. In a study of 148 surgically treated stage IB and IIA cancers, Rose et al. found that HPV 18 DNA positivity was a significant risk factor for tumor recurrence.[242] Similar results were reported by Burger et al., who studied 171 women with all stages of surgically treated cervical cancer, and by Nakagawa et al.[45,46]

DNA Ploidy

The clinical importance of tumor ploidy is currently unclear. Using flow cytometry, 33%–80% of invasive cervical carcinomas have an aneuploid DNA distribution.[83,113,136,156] There is little agreement, however, as to whether DNA ploidy level is an independent prognostic factor. Although several studies have demonstrated associations between aneuploidy and poor prognostic indicators such as lymph node metastases, higher stage, or increased age, other flow cytometry studies have all failed to demonstrate any significant effect (independent of stage) of DNA ploidy status on clinical outcome.[136,137,156] When considering DNA ploidy measurements made by flow cytometry, it must be pointed out that tumors that are "diploid" by flow usually have chromosomal aberrations and are therefore actually aneuploid (but at a level too low to be detected by flow cytometry). Large cytogenetic studies have found that all invasive cervical cancers contain chromosomal aneuploidy when defined as numerical or structural aberrations and that euploid cervical cancers either do not exist or are extremely uncommon.[15,265]

Cellular Oncogenes

Alterations in either the expression or function of cellular genes that control cell growth and differentiation are being actively investigated as prognostic markers in cervical cancer (see Chapter 26, Molecular Biology). Currently, there is little consensus in the literature on the prognostic implications of alterations in the genes in cervical cancer. Both specific point mutations of the first exon of *ras* genes as well as amplifications of *ras* genes occur in invasive carcinomas of the cervix. Using immunohistochemical methods, overexpression of *ras* genes is found in a considerable proportion of squamous cell carcinomas.[260] Overexpression of the *ras* gene product, p21, has been associated with a poor prognosis and an increased frequency of lymph node involvement in some studies.[117,246] Overexpression of p21 appears to be caused by amplification of Ha-*ras* genes, which occurs in 66% of cervical squamous cell carcinomas. Mutations and loss of heterozygosity of Ha-*ras* genes have been reported to occur in invasive cervical carcinomas in some series and to be associated with a poor prognosis.[238] However, other more recent studies have failed to detect mutations of Ha-, Ki-, and N-*ras* genes in squamous cell carcinomas of the cervix.[213] Mutations of the Ki-*ras* gene have been detected in a small percentage of invasive cervical adenocarcinomas, but are not significantly associated with stage, grade, or survival.[170]

Alterations in the c-*myc* oncogene also have been associated with a poor prognosis in some studies. The c-*myc* oncogene is amplified from 3 to 30 times in 21% of cervical squamous cell carcinomas and is more frequent in high-stage (stage III and IV) tumors than in low-stage tumors.[237] Overexpression of c-*myc* has been associated with a worse clinical outcome in some, but not other, studies of early-stage disease.[79,158,239]

Increased cytoplasmic expression of *bcl-2*, a gene involved in the control of apoptosis, has been associated with an increased 5-year survival in women with cervical cancer.[81] Increased expression of the tumor suppressor gene p53 has been associated with decreased survival in some studies but not in others.[67,81] Similarly, there are conflicting reports of differential expression of p53 in squamous cell carcinomas compared to adenocarcinomas. Mutations of p53 have been detected in 13.5% of cervical carcinomas.[276] Increased expression of c-*erbB-2*, a member of the epidermal growth factor receptor family, has been reported to be associated with an increased incidence of lymph node metastases and a poor prognosis in women with adenocarcinoma but not with squamous cell carcinoma.[191]

Spread and Metastases

Squamous cell carcinoma of the cervix spreads principally by direct local invasion of adjacent tissues and lymphatics and less commonly through blood vessels. Initially, the tumor grows by extending along tissue spaces of least resistance, such as the perineural and perivascular tissues, into the paracervical and parametrial areas, and into the cardinal and uterosacral ligaments. Ultimately, lateral spread may reach the bony pelvis, encompassing and obstructing one or both ureters. Direct extension may also involve the uterine cavity and vagina, with extension into the urinary bladder and rectum, resulting in vesicovaginal and rectovaginal fistulas.

The spread of cervical cancer via lymphatics occurs relatively early in the course of the disease, occurring in 25%–50% of patients with stage IB and II carcinomas. The most common sites of lymph node metastases are the internal iliac, obturator, external iliac, and common iliac lymph nodes. Later in the course of the disease, extension to the lateral sacral, paraaortic, and inguinal nodes can occur. Isolated invasion of the sacral, external iliac, and hypogastric nodes is occasionally observed. Distant lymph node metastases above the diaphragm including the supraclavicular lymph nodes are uncommon and are a feature of widespread disease. In these cases, cancer cells are transported from the paraaortic nodes into the mediastinum and then into the thoracic duct. Hematogenous dissemination is the least common metastatic pathway of cervical carcinoma. Blood-borne metastases to the lung, liver, bone, heart, skin, and brain are generally seen in stage IV tumors or when the local growth has previously been irradiated.

Ureteral obstruction caused by tumor invasion of the ureteral wall or by compression due to tumor in periureteral lymphatics leads to hydroureter, hydronephrosis, hydronephrotic renal atrophy, pyelonephritis, and loss of renal function. Obstruction of both ureters results in uremia and is a leading cause of death. Although the frequency of ureteral involvement was unchanged between the 1930s–1960s period and the 1970s, advances in radiation therapy that occurred in the 1970s have reduced the number of patients dying of ureteral obstruction and uremia from 28% to 6.7%.[155] Peritonitis caused by obstruction and perforation of large or small bowel, respiratory failure associated with pulmonary metastasis, or massive edema, hemorrhage, cardiac failure, massive venous thrombosis, pulmonary embolism, and complications of radiation therapy represent the major causes of death.

Treatment

The three basic therapeutic modalities for squamous cell carcinoma are radiation, surgery, and combinations of radiation and surgery or radiation with concurrent chemotherapy. At present, radical hysterectomy with pelvic lymphadenectomy is considered the most appropriate therapeutic approach for most stage IA2 squamous cell carcinomas of the cervix and stage IA1 tumors with lymphvascular space involvement. The operative death rate has declined considerably since the introduction of radical surgery and now approaches zero. In stage IB and early stage II cases, radical hysterectomy with bilateral pelvic lymphadenectomy and radiation therapy produce almost identical results. Recently, a large randomized Gynecological Oncology Group (GOG) trial compared radiation therapy followed by adjunctive extrafascial hysterectomy for bulky stage IB cervical cancers with radiation therapy combined with concurrent cisplatin chemotherapy and adjunctive extrafascial hysterectomy.[160] The concurrent use of cisplatin and radiation significantly improved survival. Other recent trials that have incorporated combinations of combined external and intracavitary radiotherapy with concurrent platinum-based chemotherapy for stage II and stage III cancers have also shown significant improvements in survival with the addition of chemotherapy compared to radiation alone.[204,243]

Radiation of invasive squamous cell carcinoma of the cervix produces a decrease in tumor size and eventual regression. In one study, 90% of 493 patients of all stages had no gross tumor 12 weeks after termination of combined external radiation (^{60}Co, 5000 R) and intracavitary radium (4000 R) therapy.[192] Tumor regression is generally faster in neoplasms of small size and in those confined to the cervix (stage I) than in larger advanced stage lesions. The rapidity of tumor regression is apparently unrelated to histologic patterns and degree of differentiation.

Morphologic changes in cervical squamous carcinoma cells that are considered evidence of response to ionizing radiation are cellular differentiation with keratinization, cell degeneration with cytoplasmic vacuolization, pyknosis, and nucleomegaly. Nuclear polyploidy, i.e., generation of multiple double sets of DNA, is the result of arrest of mitotic activity caused by radiation. Radiation-induced changes in adenocarcinoma of the cervix include nuclear shrinkage and pyknosis, cytoplasmic vacuolization, decrease in mucin synthesis, and a striking abundance of intracytoplasmic cytophagosomes.

Modern techniques of radiotherapy use a variety of intracavitary radium applicators and low-intensity needles combined with external beam irradiation. The most common complications, in decreasing frequency, are proctitis, vault necrosis, hemorrhagic cystitis, peritonitis resulting from obstruction, perforation, necrosis of the bowel, vesicovaginal fistula, and profuse hemorrhage.[267] The frequency of major complications associated with radical surgery is about 3% and includes ureterovaginal and vesicovaginal fistulas, bladder atony and hypotonic bladder dysfunction, ureteral strictures, thrombophlebitis, cuff abscesses, and hematoma.

Chemotherapy using a variety of regimens, most of which use cisplatin either alone or in combination with other drugs, has been recommended by the National Cancer Institute for concurrent therapy in women with cervical cancer undergoing radiation therapy.[1] In addition, chemotherapy is used for patients with metastatic or recurrent cancer previously treated with surgery or radiation therapy. Although 40%–70% of such patients being treated for the first time will respond to cisplatin-containing regimens, the proportion of patients with prolonged responses is considerably less.

Prognosis

The 5-year survival for treated Stage I patients is 90%–95%, 50%–70% for stage II, 30% for stage III, and less than 20% for patients with stage IV disease.[25] The survival rates are reduced even in patients with low-stage disease when metastases to lymph nodes are present, and survival rate appears to correlate with the number of positive nodes.[133] Metastatic node involvement occurs in 8%–25% of stage I, 21%–38% of stage II, and 32%–46% of stage III lesions.[159,211] Typically, the majority of recurrences appear within 2 years after initial therapy.

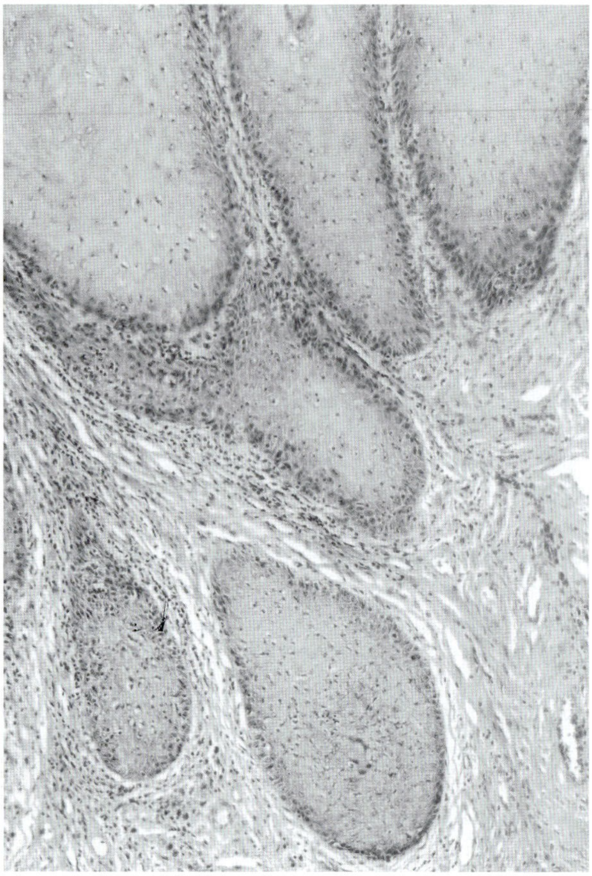

Fig. 8.19. Verrucous carcinoma. Broad tongues of mature-appearing squamous cells with minimal nuclear atypia invade into the stroma.

Verrucous Carcinoma

Verrucous carcinoma is a rare variant of squamous cell carcinoma. In the female genital tract, the region most commonly involved is the vulva, but well-documented cases have been described in the cervix.[86,154,281] In the past, this tumor has been reported as *giant condyloma acuminatum of Buschke and Lowenstein*, but the implication that this tumor is a type of condyloma is erroneous and confusing and therefore the term is no longer used. Clinically, verrucous carcinoma appears as a large, sessile tumor that grossly resembles a condyloma. Verrucous carcinoma is a slow-growing, locally invasive malignant tumor. Because it is frequently diagnosed incorrectly, it may become quite advanced and lead to death. Five of eight patients in one series died of verrucous carcinoma shortly after the diagnosis was made.[185] Histologically, cervical verrucous carcinomas are identical to the more common vulvar tumors and are predominately exophytic and characterized by frondlike papillae with or without surface keratinization (Fig. 8.19) (see Figs. 3.26 and 4.46). The epithelium lacks significant cytologic atypia and mitotic activity, although in some cases mitoses may be found in the deep layers. The base of the tumor is composed of invasive nests of epithelium that are broad and expansile with a well-circumscribed pushing margin. There is a conspicuous inflammatory reaction at the epithelial stromal junction.

Verrucous carcinoma should be distinguished from warty carcinoma (see following) and condyloma acuminata. Unlike condyloma acuminatum, verrucous carcinoma lacks the central fibroconnective tissue cores in the epithelial papillae that are characteristic of condylomata. Typically, these tumors recur locally but do not metastasize unless they are inadequately radiated, in which case accelerated growth and metastasis may occur.[86,154,281] The most appropriate therapy is wide local excision, if possible. However, these lesions can frequently be deeply invasive, even extending into the endometrium or adjacent pelvic tissue.[185,273] Regional lymph nodes are rarely involved, and distant metastases are exceedingly rare.[185]

Warty (Condylomatous) Carcinoma

Warty (condylomatous) carcinoma is a variant of squamous cell carcinoma of the cervix that has

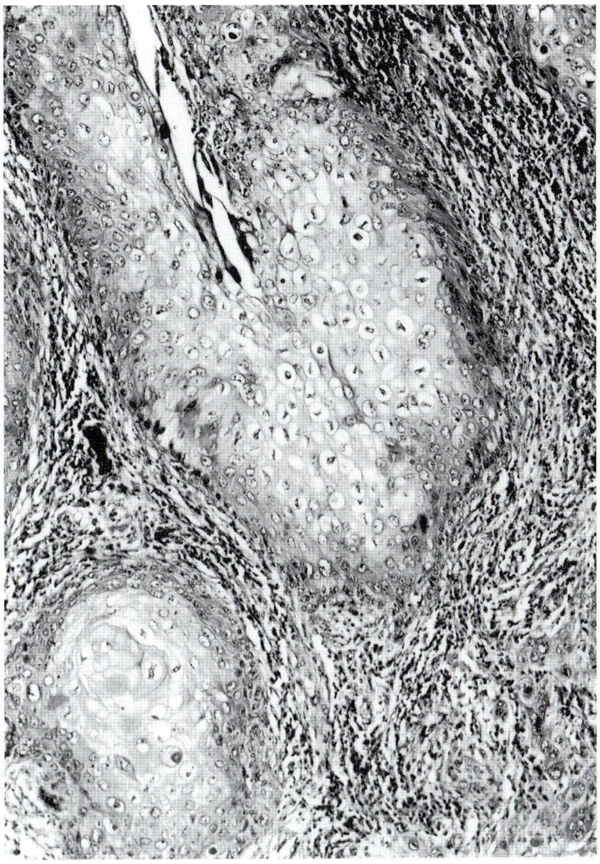

Fig. 8.20. Warty (condylomatous) carcinoma. This variant of squamous cell carcinoma contains squamous cells demonstrating koilocytotic atypia similar to those seen in low-grade SIL.

marked condylomatous changes.[174] These tumors have been recently described and are histologically identical to the warty carcinoma of the vulva.[233] Unlike verrucous carcinoma, warty carcinomas demonstrate features of a typical squamous cell carcinoma at the deep margin. In addition, many of the malignant cells have cytoplasmic vacuolization and nuclear changes closely resembling koilocytotic atypia (Fig. 8.20). Although clinical experience with these tumors is very limited, they appear to behave less aggressively than typical well-differentiated squamous cell carcinomas of the cervix. In one study, multiple types of HPV including low-risk types were identified in two-thirds of these tumors.[55]

Papillary Squamous Cell (Transitional) Carcinoma

Papillary squamous cell carcinoma is a rare variant of squamous cell carcinoma of the cervix. These tumors were initially described by Randall et al., who reported that they had a histologic resemblance to transitional cell carcinoma of the bladder.[231] Albores-Saavedra and Young described three aggressive tumors involving the cervix that histologically resembled high-grade transitional cell carcinomas of the urinary bladder.[8] They referred to these tumors as transitional cell carcinomas and suggested that they be distinguished from papillary squamous cell carcinomas.

A comprehensive study from the Armed Forces Institute of Pathology of 32 cases of papillary cervical carcinomas reported that these papillary tumors of the cervix can be subdivided into three groups based on their histologic appearance: predominately squamous, predominantly transitional, and mixed squamous and transitional.[166] However, all three histologic subdivisions demonstrated similar immunohistochemical staining patterns for cytokeratin 7 and 20. The tumors were typically positive for cytokeratin 7 and negative for cytokeratin 20, which is a pattern more typical of cervical squamous lesions than of transitional cell tumors of the urinary tract. Follow-up was available for 12 patients, and 3 were reported to have died of their disease.[166] However, no apparent differences were observed in the clinical behavior of the three subtypes. Therefore, it appears that papillary squamous cell carcinomas of the cervix present with a spectrum of histologic appearances with some tumors appearing more squamous and others more transitional. Because they demonstrate a spectrum of histologic appearances, these tumors have been referred to as papillary squamotransitional carcinomas.[166] HPV 16 has been identified in three cases of papillary squamous cell carcinoma of the cervix.[36]

Histologically, papillary squamous cell carcinomas are composed of papillary projections that are covered by several layers of atypical epithelial cells. In cases that appear more transitional, the cells are oval with their long axis oriented perpendicular to the surface and there is minimal flattening of the cells as they reach the surface. In cases with more squamous differentiation, the cells are more basaloid and resemble those of a high-grade SIL (Fig. 8.21). The cells have hyperchromatic oval nuclei and minimal amounts of cytoplasm. Mitoses are frequent. Focally, there are usually areas of squamous differentiation. Typical invasive squamous cell carcinoma can often be identified at the base of the tumor, appearing as well-circumscribed nests of epithelium in continuity with papillae that extend deeply into the stroma. Focal invasion of the papillae themselves also sometimes occurs. The behavior of papillary squamous cell carcinoma is similar to that of invasive squamous cell carcinoma with the exception that late recurrences have been reported in the larger series.[231]

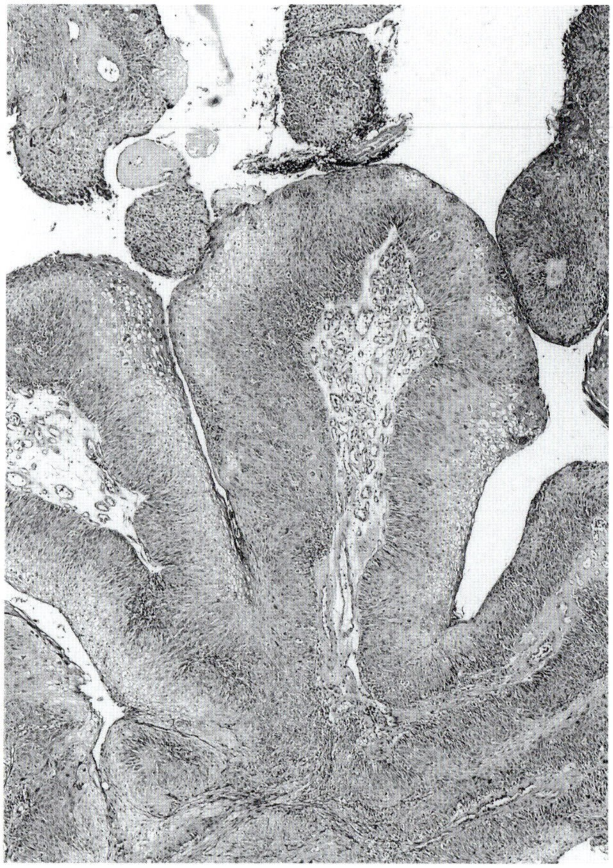

Fig. 8.21. Papillary squamous (transitional) cell carcinoma. The tumor is composed of papillary projections covered by neoplastic cells resembling high-grade SIL. There are koilocytotic changes in the superficial squamous cells lining the projections.

Papillary squamous cell carcinoma can be mistaken for a papillary squamous cell carcinoma in situ on a superficial biopsy. Because papillary squamous cell carcinoma is capable of acting aggressively and metastasizing, it is important that a cone biopsy be performed to rule out invasion whenever a papillary squamous cell carcinoma in situ is diagnosed. These tumors can also be mistakenly diagnosed as verrucous carcinoma or as condyloma accuminatum with atypia. Papillary squamous cell carcinomas lack the condylomatous changes and degree of cytoplasmic differentiation present in the other lesions.

Lymphoepithelioma-Like Carcinoma

Lymphoepithelioma-like carcinomas are a distinctive subset of squamous cell carcinomas of the cervix that are typically well circumscribed and composed of undifferentiated cells surrounded by a marked stromal inflammatory infiltrate.[107,110] These tumors are reported to have a better prognosis than typical squamous cell carcinomas and to have a higher incidence in Asia than in the West.[283] These tumors account for up to 5.5% of cervical cancers in some series from Asia and are histologically similar to lymphoepitheliomas arising in the nasopharynx, salivary glands, breast, and thymus. A recent study of 15 cases of lymphoepithelioma-like carcinoma of the cervix identified Epstein–Barr virus (EBV) genomes in 73% of the cases compared to 27% of typical cervical squamous cell carcinomas.[283] In addition, HPV 16 or HPV 18 DNA was identified in only 20% of the cases of lymphoepithelioma-like carcinomas compared to 80% of typical squamous cell carcinomas.

The cells composing lymphoepithelioma-like carcinomas are relatively undifferentiated but have abundant cytoplasm and uniform vesicular nuclei (Fig. 8.22). The cell borders tend to be indistinct and form what has been described as a syncytium. The

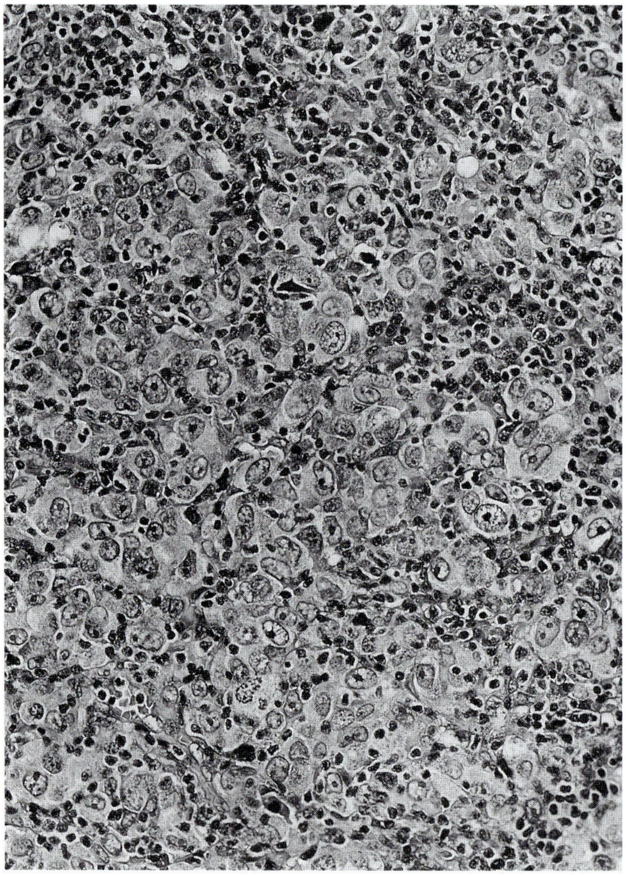

Fig. 8.22. Lymphoepithelioma-like carcinoma. The tumor is composed of sheets of undifferentiated cells surrounded by a stromal inflammatory infiltrate. The individual cells have abundant cytoplasm, indistinct cell borders, and uniform vesicular nuclei.

nests of undifferentiated cells are surrounded by a marked chronic inflammatory infiltrate composed of lymphocytes, plasma cells, and eosinophils.

Lymphoepithelioma-like carcinomas can be mistaken for either glassy cell carcinomas or true lymphoproliferative disorders. Glassy cell carcinomas have a very poor prognosis and are characterized by prominent cell borders, ground glass cytoplasm, and prominent nucleoli. Lymphoproliferative disorders can be easily differentiated from lymphoepithelioma-like carcinoma through the use of immunohistochemical staining with antibodies against leukocyte common antigen, cytokeratin, and epithelial membrane antigen.

Adenocarcinoma

Adenocarcinomas of the cervix comprise a heterogeneous group of neoplasms that display a variety of histologic patterns (see Table 8.1). Because these cell types and patterns are frequently admixed, the histologic classification of these tumors is based on the predominate cell type. If additional histologic components comprise at least 10% of the tumor, some authors recommend classifying the tumor according to the predominant pattern and listing the individual components as part of the diagnosis.

The most commonly encountered type of cervical adenocarcinoma is the mucinous type.[96,129,165,278] In one series of 136 invasive adenocarcinomas, mucinous adenocarcinomas accounted for 57% of the tumors, endometrioid adenocarcinomas for 30%, and clear cell adenocarcinomas for 11%; the other types combined accounted for only 3% of the tumors.[247] Although some studies have found endometrioid adenocarcinomas to be more prevalent than endocervical adenocarcinomas, in almost all series these two histologic types taken together account for between 45% and 90% of all invasive cervical adenocarcinomas.

Prevalence

The relative proportions and absolute incidences of squamous cell carcinomas and adenocarcinomas of the cervix have been changing in the United States and Western Europe during the past 40 years since the introduction of widespread cytologic screening programs. In the 1950s and 1960s, approximately 95% of all invasive cervical carcinomas were classified as squamous cell carcinomas and only 5% as adenocarcinomas.[118,200] However, series of invasive cervical cancers published since the early 1970s have found that squamous cell carcinomas account for only 75%–80% of the cases while the remainder, 20%–25%, include various types of adenocarcinomas, adenosquamous carcinomas, and undifferentiated carcinomas.[76,124] In the clinical series of Shingleton et al., the percentage of adenocarcinomas to total cervical cancers increased from 7% in the period from 1974 to 1978 to 19% in the 1979–1980 period.[257] Similarly, in the clinical series of Hopkins and Morley, the percentage of adenocarcinomas to total cervical cancers increased from 19% in 1970–1973 to 27% in 1982–1985.[122]

Cancer registries from the United States, Finland, and Norway have all reported increases in the ratio of adenocarcinomas to squamous cell carcinomas during the same period.[3,9,180,218,222] In the Finnish Cancer Registry, 88% of all cervical cancers were classified as squamous cell carcinoma and 6% as adenocarcinoma in 1953–1957 whereas 81% were classified as squamous cell carcinoma and 17% as adenocarcinoma in 1978–1982.[180] Between 1973 and 1996 in the United States, the overall age-adjusted incidence of invasive cervical cancer decreased by 36.9%. However, the age-adjusted incidence rates for adenocarcinoma increased by 29.1% and the proportion of adenocarcinoma relative to squamous cell carcinoma increased by 95%.[263] The Norwegian Cancer registry also showed an increase in the incidence of invasive adenocarcinoma of the cervix, and the increase was greatest in women 35 years old and younger.[9] A recent review of time trends in the incidence of cervical adenocarcinomas in 60 cancer registries from 25 countries found wide geographic variations.[290] Cumulative incidence rates were higher for women born after 1935 for whites and Hispanics in the United States and for all women in Australia, New Zealand, England, Scotland, Denmark and Sweden. However, a decrease in incidence was seen in Finland, France, and Italy. Registries from 24 other countries showed no change in the incidence of cervical adenocarcinomas.[290]

Histogenesis and Risk Factors

The cell of origin of invasive cervical adenocarcinoma is thought to be the pluripotential subcolumnar reserve cell of the columnar endocervical epithelium, and adenocarcinoma in situ is regarded as the immediate precursor to invasive endocervical adenocarcinoma (see Chapter 7, Precancerous Lesions of the Cervix). Many of the epidemiologic risk factors for the development of adenocarcinoma of the cervix are similar to those described for invasive squamous cell carcinomas.[38,219] Both are frequently associated with SIL and both are associated with an interval of more than 5 years since the last Pap smear (relative risk of 2.7 and 3.6 for adenocarcinoma and squamous cell carcinomas, respectively), multiple sexual partners (more than 10 partners has a relative risk of 10.9 and 2.9, respectively, for adenocarcinoma and squamous cell carcinoma), and a young age at first intercourse (intercourse before the age of 15 has a relative risk of 2.0 for both adenocarcinoma and squamous cell carcinoma).[164] In addition, HPV, particularly type 18, has been found in association with the majority of invasive adenocarcinomas.[32,71,134,184,286]

Even though the use of oral contraceptives for more than 10 years, particularly those with a large progestational component, has been shown to be a risk factor for invasive cervical adenocarcinoma in some studies, these findings have not been confirmed by others.[72,141,175,225] Most recent studies comparing the risk factors for invasive adenocarcinomas with those of squamous cell carcinomas have revealed no significant differences in oral contraceptive usage between the two groups of women after controlling for HPV and sexual factors.[37,38,122,175] It should also be noted that one recent case-control study has reported a significant association between the use of hormone replacement therapy in older women and invasive adenocarcinomas of the cervix.[176]

A genetic predisposition to invasive cervical adenocarcinoma has been documented in women with Peutz–Jeghers syndrome in whom minimal deviation adenocarcinoma of the cervix occurs more frequently than in the general population.[195,227] It also appears that a generalized predisposition to the development of adenocarcinoma of the ovary and cervix can occur because dual primary cervical and ovarian adenocarcinomas develop in some women.[302] Mucinous tumors of the ovary appear to be particularly prevalent in women with minimal deviation mucinous adenocarcinomas of the cervix.[153]

Clinical Features

The presenting symptoms of invasive cervical adenocarcinoma is abnormal vaginal bleeding in about 75% of patients.[129,180] Occasional women present with vaginal discharge or with pelvic pain. The majority of invasive cervical adenocarcinomas arise in the transformation zone, and on gross examination 50% of patients have a fungating, polypoid, or papillary mass.[278] In approximately 15% of patients, the cervix is either diffusely enlarged or nodular. In another 15%, no gross lesions are visible. Although the majority of patients with grossly inapparant tumors have early-stage adenocarcinomas, some have deep invasion because the carcinoma arose deep within the endocervical canal.[247] Adenocarcinoma of the cervix is confined to the cervix (stage I) or the parametrium/vagina (stage II) in 80% of women at the time of diagnosis.[129] The diagnostic accuracy of cytopathology in the detection of cervical adenocarcinoma varies according to the expertise of the pathologist and the sampling techniques used. Although in some series only a minority of the tumors has been detected through cytologic screening, in most large series the majority of patients with cervical adenocarcinomas have cytologic abnormalities.[13,180,247]

Microinvasive Adenocarcinoma

Definition

Although the FIGO staging system for cervical cancer applies to both squamous cell carcinoma and adenocarcinoma, there is considerable controversy as to whether stage IA adenocarcinomas exist as a histologically recognizable entity. One reason for the controversy is that the irregular distribution and architecture of the normal endocervical crypts in the cervical stroma make it difficult to differentiate between early stromal invasion and adenocarcinoma in situ. Another reason is that such lesions, if they exist, would be relatively uncommon, have been treated surgically with either a simple or radical hysterectomy, and would be expected to behave in a relatively nonaggressive manner, making it difficult to make clinicopathologic correlation.

Pathologic Features

In the largest study of *microinvasive adenocarcinoma*, Ostor et al. analyzed 77 cases.[215] The first histologic sign of invasion was thought to be the presence of a finger-like extension of epithelium with abundant pink cytoplasm into the stroma from a gland demonstrating the histologic features of adenocarcinoma in situ (Fig. 8.23).[215] More advanced areas of invasion showed glands that lack the lobular architecture of crypts involved by adenocarcinoma in situ. These glands are often separated by stroma and may be within the zone of normal endocervical mucosa. There may or may not be a stromal response with edema, inflammation, and desmoplasia. Lee and Flynn recently evaluated 40 cases of what they classified as early invasive adenocarcinoma of the cervix and described five histologic patterns they considered indicative of invasion[178]; these included (1) small detached tumor cell islands adjacent to adenocarcinoma in situ that elicit a stromal response, (2) closely packed collections of glands that have lost their smooth outlines, and (3) smooth-contoured, dilated glands with complex intraglandular cribiform or papillary growth patterns. In both series, most of the patients had a coexisting adenocarcinoma in situ and some also had SIL.

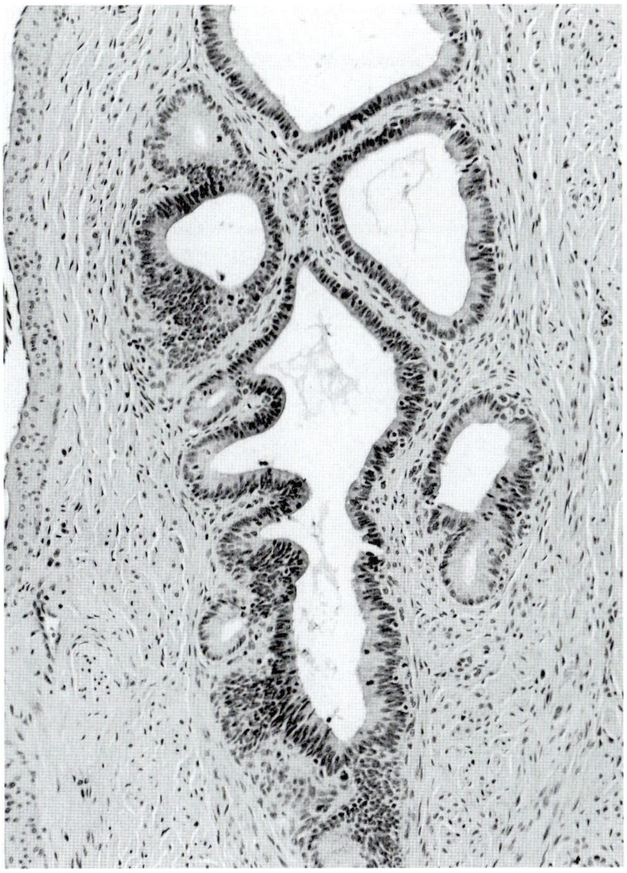

Fig. 8.23. Microinvasive adenocarcinoma of the cervix. Tongues of atypical glandular epithelium extend from a gland into the stroma. The gland is lined by endocervical adenocarcinoma and was located at a depth of less than 2 mm from the surface.

Clinical Outcomes

The average age in the two series just described was 39 and 41 years. Lymphvascular space involvement was observed in 9% of the cases in one series and 5% in the other. Clinical follow-up is available in the series of Ostor et al.[215] At least 5 years of follow-up was available for 29 women who received a variety of treatments ranging from cone biopsy alone to radical hysterectomy. Pelvic node dissections were available for 48 women (many of whom had invasion of 3.1–5 mm), and no nodal metastases were identified. One patient developed a vaginal vault recurrence after a total abdominal hysterectomy and external pelvic radiation. Another series of 30 cases of early adenocarcinoma of the cervix by Kaku et al. correlated depth of invasion with nodal metastases and clinical outcome, with a median follow-up of 79 months.[149] All but one of the women were treated with at least a simple hysterectomy and bilateral salpingo-oophorectomy. Pelvic nodes were evaluated in 25. None of the patients had nodal metastases and none with less than 3 mm of invasion developed recurrent tumor. Two (22%) of 9 patients with tumors invading to a depth of 3.0–4.9 mm. developed vaginal recurrences.

Mucinous Adenocarcinoma

Pathologic Findings

Mucinous adenocarcinoma is the most common type of invasive cervical adenocarcinoma.[9,96,129] There are three histologic variants of mucinous adenocarcinomas that can occur either alone or as an admixture. One type is composed of cells that resemble the columnar cells of the normal endocervical mucosa and is referred to as the *endocervical type*. Endocervical-type adenocarcinomas are composed of cells that have basal nuclei and abundant pale granular cytoplasm which stains positively with mucicarmine stains. The majority of the endocervical-type mucinous adenocarcinomas are well to moderately differentiated, and the glandular elements are arranged in a complex, racemose, glandular pattern simulating the cleft–tunnel configuration of the normal endocervical mucosa (Figs. 8.24 and 8.25). Complex papillary projections may project into the

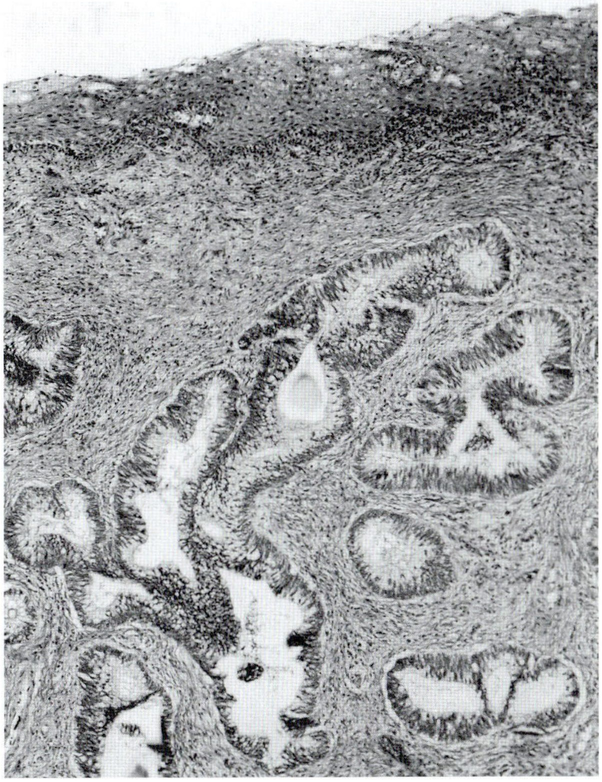

Fig. 8.24. Adenocarcinoma of endocervical type. The tumor invades in the stroma underneath an intact surface epithelium. The tumor is composed of complex glandular structures.

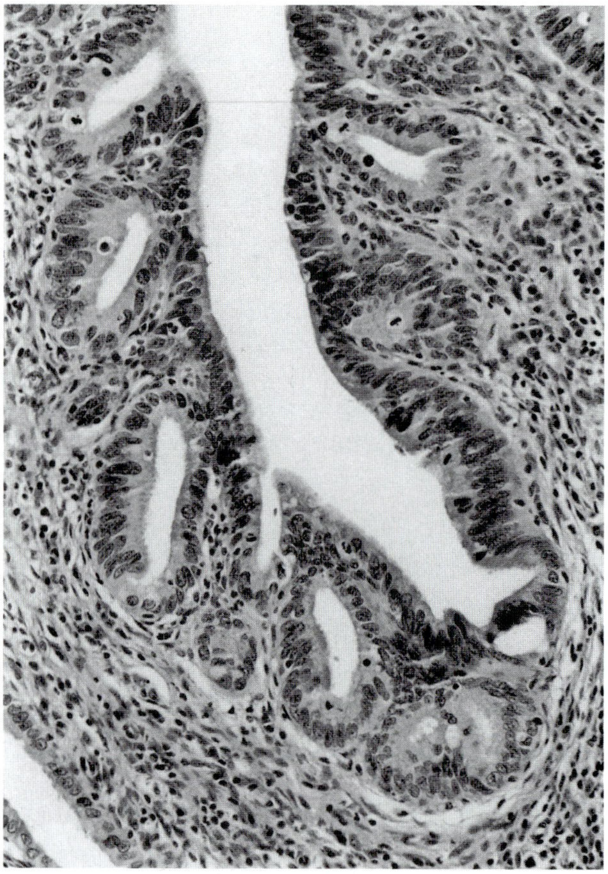

Fig. 8.25. Adenocarcinoma of endocervical type. The cells lining the glands are pseudostratified and have hyperchromatic nuclei with coarse chromatin, mitosis, and reduced intracytoplasmic mucin.

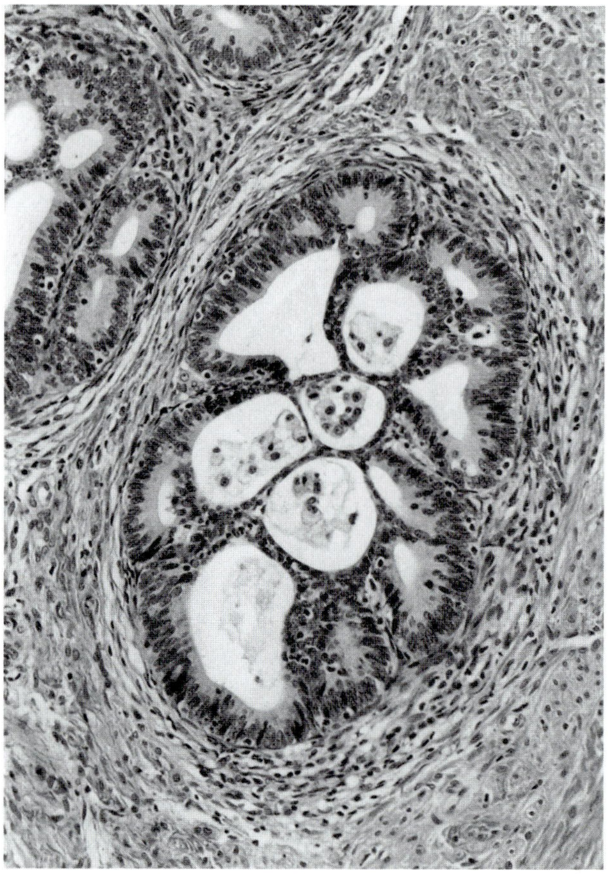

Fig. 8.26. Adenocarcinoma of endocervical type. Invasive glands may have a cribriform arrangement and be surrounded by an altered, desmoplastic stroma.

gland lumens and from the surface of the tumor (Fig. 8.26). In less-differentiated tumors, the cells contain less cytoplasm but usually still form recognizable glandular structures. Cells are typically stratified, and there may be considerable nuclear atypia with variation in nuclear size, coarsely clumped chromatin, and prominent nucleoli (Fig. 8.25). Mitoses are usually numerous. Large amounts of mucin may be found in the stroma, forming mucin lakes or pools.

The second type of mucinous adenocarcinoma of the cervix is termed the *intestinal type* and is composed of cells similar to those present in adenocarcinomas of the large intestine (Fig. 8.27). These tumors frequently contain goblet cells and more rarely argentaffin cells and Paneth cells. In the intestinal type, the tumor cells tend to be pseudostratified and contain only small amounts of intracellular mucin (Fig. 8.28). They can either form glands with papillae or infiltrate throughout the stroma in a pattern similar to that of colonic adenocarcinoma. The third form of mucinous adenocarcinoma is designated the *signet-ring* form (Fig. 8.29). Signet-ring carcinomas rarely occur in a pure form and are usually admixed with intestinal or endocervical adenocarcinomas.

Mucinous adenocarcinomas of the cervix are graded either on the basis of architectural features, in a manner similar to that used for endometrial adenocarcinomas, or on the basis of nuclear grade.[27,129,174] Using an architectural grading system, well-differentiated tumors are defined as those in which less than 10% of the tumor volume is composed of solid sheets of cells, the remainder of the tumor being glandular; in moderately differentiated tumors, 11–50% of the tumor is composed of solid sheets of cells; and in poorly differentiated tumors, more than 50% of the tumor is solid.

Immunohistochemistry

Because it can be difficult to distinguish between primary endometrial and cervical adenocarcinomas on the basis of histologic parameters alone, a num-

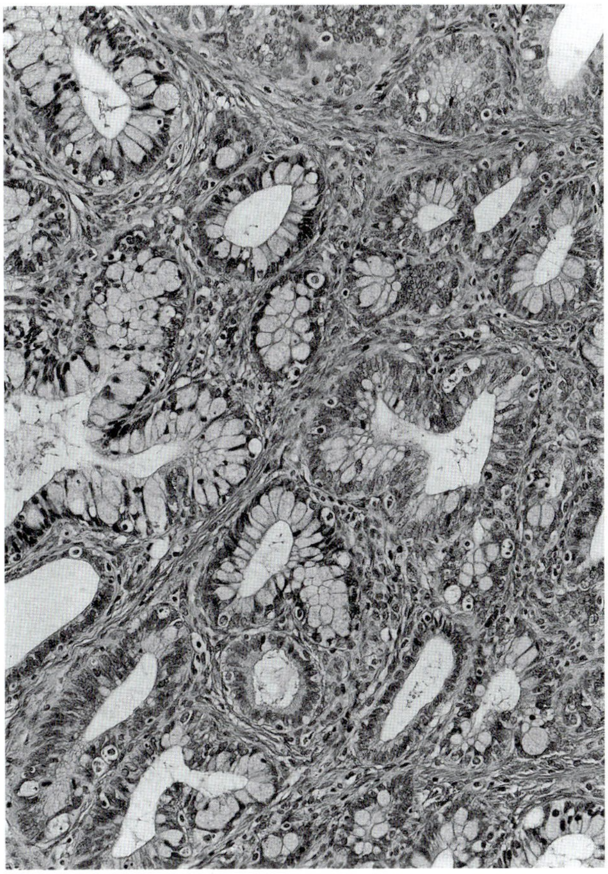

Fig. 8.27. Adenocarcinoma of intestinal type. The invasive glands have goblet cells interspersed throughout the epithelium.

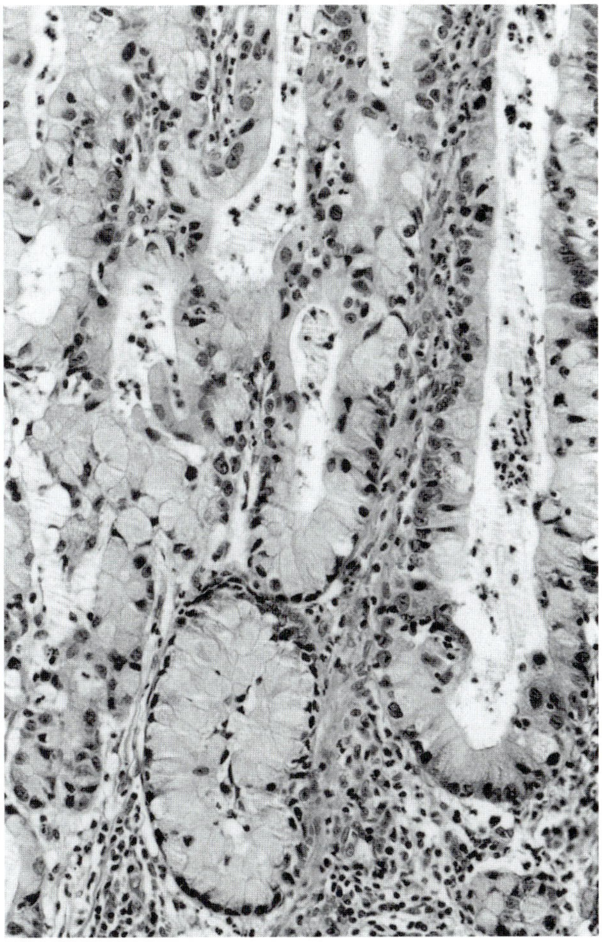

Fig. 8.28. Adenocarcinoma of intestinal type. The neoplastic glands are lined by goblet cells with abundant intracellular mucus.

ber of investigators have studied the utility of special strains for mucin and immunohistochemistry for discriminating between these two types of tumors. It is now clear that even though more cervical adenocarcinomas than endometrial adenocarcinomas stain strongly positive with alcian blue, there is sufficient overlap between the staining patterns of the two tumors to render alcian blue staining of little diagnostic value (Table 8.9).[61] Immunostaining patterns with carcinoembryonic antigen (CEA) have also been suggested as a way of discriminating between endometrial and cervical primaries. In one early study, 80% of endocervical tumors stained positively with CEA composed to 8% of primary endometrial adenocarcinomas.[292] More recent studies, however, have found CEA staining to be of limited value in distinguishing an endocervical from an endometrial primary in the individual case (Table 8.9).[173,188] CEA immunocytochemistry is also of limited value for distinguishing invasive adenocarcinomas from atypical, but benign, glandular lesions of the endocervix, because CEA positivity can be detected in squamous metaplasia and in normal cervical glandular epithelium and some endocervical adenocarcinomas are negative or only weakly positive.[93,199,264] A recent study has found that estrogen receptors (ER) and progesterone receptors (PR) are rarely expressed in cervical as compared to endometrial carcinoma whereas HPV can be detected by in situ hybridization in most cervical adenocarcinomas but not in endometrial carcinoma.[266]

Several other immunohistochemical stains may be of value in distinguishing primary cervical adenocarcinomas from metastatic carcinomas (see Table 8.9). Primary cervical adenocarcinomas stain relatively weakly with antibodies directed against vimentin whereas approximately 60% of primary endometrial adenocarcinomas stain strongly.[75,275] IC5 is a monoclonal antibody developed against a human cervical adenocarcinoma cell line. The IC5 antibody stains 90% of cervical adenocarcinomas cytoplasmically but does not stain the cytoplasm of

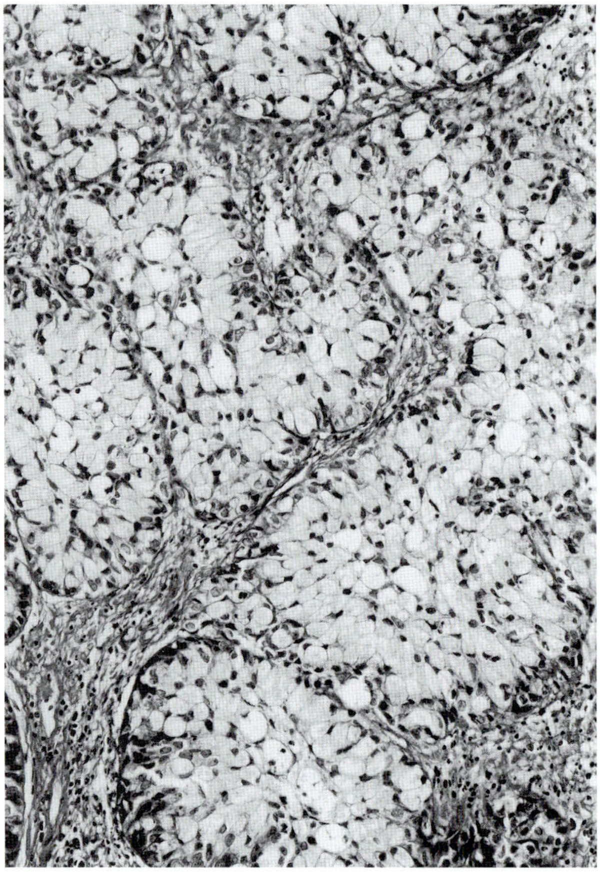

Fig. 8.29. Adenocarcinoma of the signet-ring type. This uncommon type of endocervical adenocarcinoma is composed of nests of signet-ring cells.

endometrial adenocarcinomas.[173] Instead, staining of endometrial adenocarcinomas is restricted to the luminal surface cell membrane and occurs in only 40% of the tumors. Panels of monoclonal antibodies directed against the mucus-specific antigens M1, M2, and M3 may also be helpful in selected cases. One study demonstrated that 56% of cervical adenocarcinomas contain both the M1 and M3 mucus-associated antigens whereas no primary endometrial adenocarcinomas stained for both types of antigen (Table 8.9).[188]

Ultrastructure

Transmission electron microscopy confirms the light microscopic and histochemical observations of a gradual decrease and an eventual loss of mucin production in increasingly dedifferentiated adenocarcinoma of the cervix.[87]

Differential Diagnosis

The major benign lesions that must be distinguished from invasive mucinous adenocarcinoma of the cervix are microglandular hyperplasia, hyperplastic mesonephric remnants, and the Arias–Stella reaction. Microglandular hyperplasia tends to occur in younger women and is frequently polypoid. Unlike invasive adenocarcinomas that extend beyond the depth of normal endocervical glands, microglandular hyperplasia should be confined to the normal endocervical glands.[303] In addition, microglandular hyperplasia is composed of relatively uniform, small glands lined by a simple layer of bland epithelium with few mitoses. Mesonephric remnants are tubular, retain a clustered arrangement associated with a mesonephric duct, and are usually deep in the cervical stroma. The epithelium lining the tubules is usually cuboidal and not stratified. Cytologic atypia is minimal.[90] The Arias–Stella reaction is distinguished from clear cell adenocarcinoma by the distinctive cytonucleomegaly and lack of mitoses. In addition, the clear cytoplasmic appearance of Arias–Stella reaction is not caused by an accumulation of glycogen but by an increased cytoplasmic matrix in which the organelles are dispersed. The presence of other changes of pregnancy, such as decidua, confirms the diagnosis.

The malignant lesions that must be distinguished from invasive adenocarcinoma of the cervix include adenocarcinoma in situ (AIS), primary endometrial adenocarcinoma with extension into the endocervical canal, and metastatic adenocarcinoma. Adenocarcinoma in situ of the cervix is distinguished from invasive cervical adenocarcinoma by the lack of extension beyond the depth to which normal endocervical glands extend, lack of desmoplasia surrounding the glands, and lack of foci of closely packed glands. The normal endocervical glandular architecture is maintained in adenocarcinoma in

Table 8.9. Differentiating primary endometrial from primary cervical adenocarcinomas

	Per cent of primary tumors that stain	
Stain or antigen	*Endocervical*	*Endometrial*
Alcian blue[188]	100	77
CEA[173,188,292]	59–80	8–50
Vimentin[275]	0	66
IC5[173]	90 (cytoplasmic)	40 (luminal)
Mucus antigens M1 and M3[188]	56	0

CEA, carcinoembryonic antigen; M1, M3, and IC5, monoclonal antibodies derived against either endocervical adenocarcinoma cells or mucus-associated proteins.
Adapted from refs. 173, 188, 275, 292.

situ. Metastatic adenocarcinoma of the cervix usually occurs in the setting of a patient with a known, widely metastatic primary lesion and is histologically characterized by a lack of surface involvement and widespread lymphvascular involvement. In assessing whether a carcinoma is of primary endocervical origin or is metastatic in the cervix, the pathologist should evaluate the following morphologic features: (1) neoplastic growth pattern, (2) coexistent in situ changes, (3) cell type, and (4) immunohistochemical characteristics. Transition between in situ and invasive carcinoma provides the strongest evidence for a primary origin and is found in up to 43% of primary cervical adenocarcinomas.[5,229]

Risk Factors

Major prognostic indicators for cervical adenocarcinoma include tumor diameter, depth of invasion, involvement of lymphvascular spaces, stage, age, and presence or absence of lymph node metastases.[13,16,27,84,85,230] Depth of invasion can be expressed either in millimeters of distance from the endocervical lumen or as percentage of the total thickness of the wall that is involved.

Poor prognostic features include tumor size greater than 3 cm, uterine enlargement, and high grade. Ploidy level (nuclear DNA content) has been correlated with histologic grade and may have prognostic significance. Low ploidy level, with stem cell modal values less than triploid, are associated with well-differentiated adenocarcinoma, whereas poorly differentiated adenocarcinomas are associated with high ploidy, greater than triploid stem cell modal values. Moreover, women with hypotriploid tumors have a significantly higher survival rate (45%–55%) than women with hypertriploid tumors (10%–18%).[94] Young age at presentation has been associated with a good prognosis in one series.[16]

Clinical Behavior and Treatment

Adenocarcinoma of the cervix spreads in a fashion similar to squamous cell carcinoma and, in general, both squamous and adenocarcinomas are treated similarly. The most commonly used therapeutic modalities for stage I and II adenocarcinoma are radiation alone, radiation with concurrent chemotherapy, radiation followed by simple hysterectomy, or radical surgery.[267] Only a few studies have directly compared the therapeutic results achieved with invasive squamous cell and adenocarcinomas over the same time period and from the same institution, and these studies have produced conflicting data. In one report, Hopkins and Morley found that local extension as well as lymph node metastases occurred comparatively earlier in adenocarcinomas than in squamous cell carcinoma.[124] Similar results have been reported by others who have found that the overall 5-year survival rates are lower for adenocarcinoma (48%–65%) than for squamous cell carcinoma patients (68%).[27,84,122] In a study of 1538 stage IB squamous cell carcinomas of the cervix and 229 adenocarcinomas initially treated with radiation therapy, Eifel et al. observed a worse outcome in women with adenocarcinoma.[84] A large retrospective analysis of 3678 cases of cervical cancer from Taiwan found that the difference in survival between adenocarcinomas and squamous cell carcinomas appeared to be predominantly the result of a poorer outcome in early-stage lesions.[53] In data from the United States, reported survival is lower for adenocarcinoma versus squamous cell carcinoma for stage II disease but not for stage I or stage III or IV disease.[263] Other comparison studies, as well as several population-based studies, have failed to confirm that prognosis and survival are affected by histologic type.[14,109,180]

Endometrioid Adenocarcinoma

As in endometrial and ovarian neoplasms, *endometrioid adenocarcinomas of the cervix* are defined as tumors composed of cells that resemble those of primary adenocarcinomas of the uterine corpus. Endometrioid carcinomas account for up to 30% of endocervical adenocarcinomas. The cells of endometrioid adenocarcinomas tend to be stratified and have oval nuclei that are arranged with their long axis perpendicular to the basement membrane of the gland (Fig. 8.30). The cells do not contain mucin and have less cytoplasm than do the cells of mucinous adenocarcinomas. Endometrioid adenocarcinomas frequently contain small foci of squamous epithelium. However, at times it can be difficult to differentiate endometrioid adenocarcinoma from less well differentiated mucinous adenocarcinomas of the endocervical type, and many tumors classified as endometrioid adenocarcinomas may actually represent poorly differentiated mucinous tumors that have lost their capacity to produce mucin.

It can also be difficult to differentiate between an endometrioid carcinoma primary in the cervix and a primary endometrial adenocarcinoma. Primary uterine corpus tumors are usually bulky tumors that have invaded the myometrium by the time they extend to the cervix and therefore cause uterine enlargement. In contrast, primary cervical adenocarcinomas often cause cervical enlargement in the absence of uterine enlargement. Even with large, destructive primary cervical adenocarcinomas, dif-

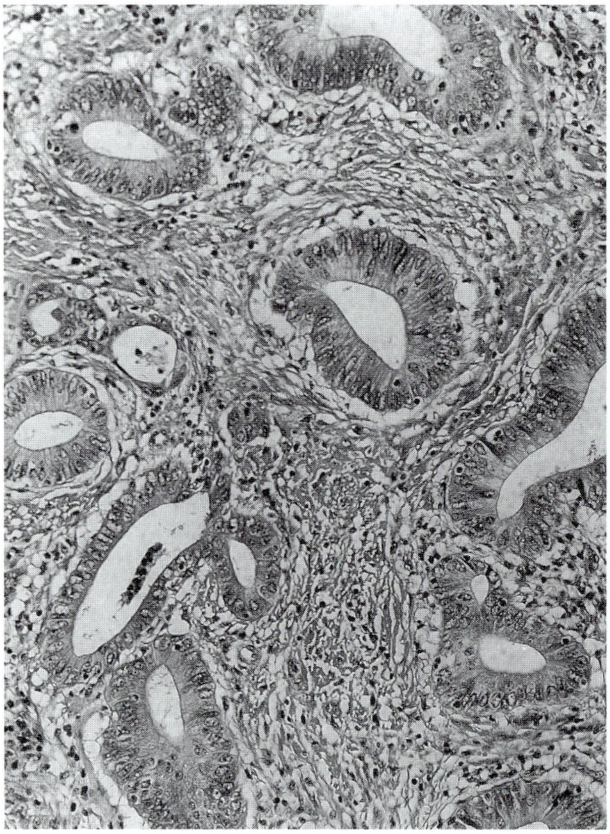

Fig. 8.30. Adenocarcinoma of endometrioid type. These tumors are similar to the typical primary endometrial adenocarcinoma.

ferentiation from primary endometrial adenocarcinomas can be made if normal endometrium is present either on a fractional dilation and curettage or on an endometrial biopsy. Contamination, however, of the endometrial sample can occur while passing the curette or biopsy instrument through the involved endocervical canal. In these cases a careful search through multiple sections may reveal atypical endometrial hyperplasia in primary endometrial tumors and either AIS, SIL, or foci with features of a typical endocervical carcinoma in primary endocervical tumors.

Clear Cell Adenocarcinoma

Clear cell carcinomas account for approximately 4% of adenocarcinomas of the cervix.[212] Although clear cell adenocarcinoma of the cervix has been reported in young women with a history of in utero exposure to diethylstilbestrol (DES), these tumors can also develop in the absence of exposure to DES.[112,114,119,151,240] Tumors that develop in the absence of DES exposure occur most commonly in postmenopausal women whereas those which occur in women exposed to DES tend to occur in young women.[112] The sporadically developing tumors arise in either the exocervix or endocervix, whereas the tumors developing in DES-exposed women develop predominately on the exocervix. The cumulative incidence rate of clear cell carcinoma in DES-exposed women is 1.5 per 1000 exposed women.[116] The microscopic features of clear cell carcinoma, developing in women with or without DES exposure, are the same and are described in detail in Chapter 4, Diseases of the Vagina. There are three basic microscopic patterns; solid, tubulocystic, and papillary. The cells comprising the tumor have abundant clear cytoplasm due to the accumulation of glycogen or granular eosinophilic cytoplasm, with prominent nuclei that can be quite hyperchromatic and pleomorphic and project into the lumen of the cysts and tubules to form "hobnail cells" (Figs. 8.31 and 8.32).

The differential diagnosis of clear cell carcinomas includes other types of cervical adenocarcinomas as well as benign processes such as Arias–Stella

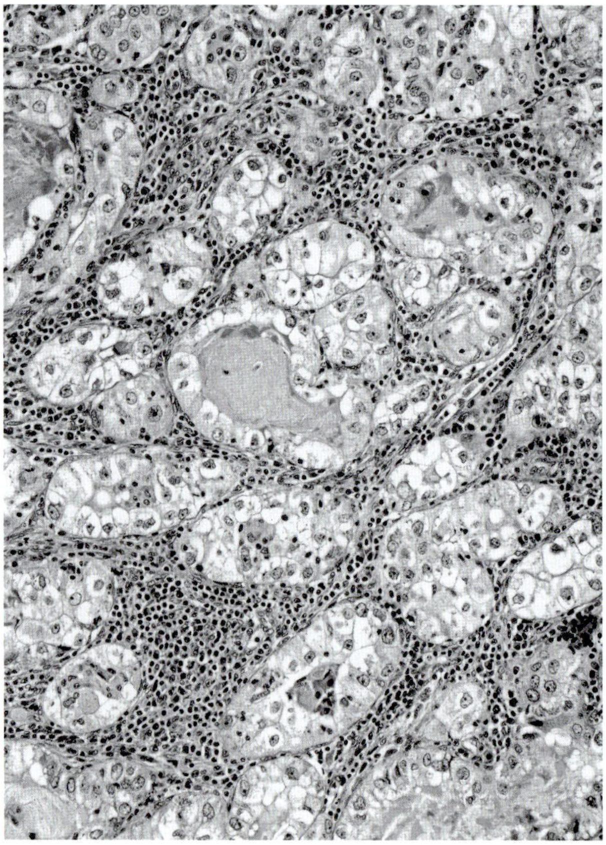

Fig. 8.31. Clear cell carcinoma of the cervix. Infiltrating nests of clear cells with abundant vacuolated cytoplasm and variably sized, highly atypical nuclei are present.

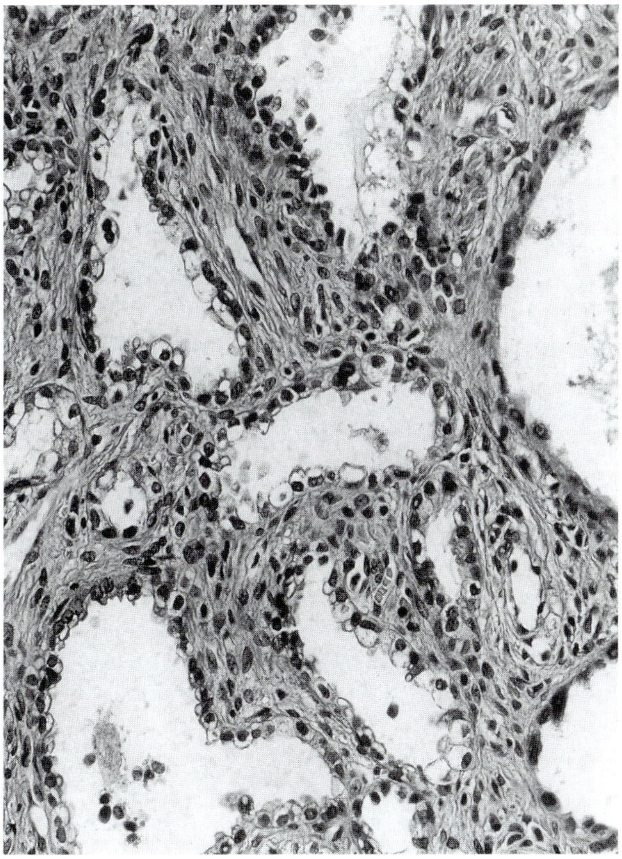

Fig. 8.32. Clear cell carcinoma of the cervix. Clear cells and hobnail cells are seen lining tubules and cysts.

reaction and microglandular hyperplasia. Distinguishing between these entities can be difficult, especially on small biopsy samples. Microglandular hyperplasia usually lacks the degree of nuclear atypica of clear cell carcinoma and it usually contains mucin. Arias–Stella reactions can be differentiated on the basis of lack of mitotic activity, lack of the classic patterns of clear cell carcinoma, and the clinical history of pregnancy.

Minimal Deviation Adenocarcinoma

Minimal deviation adenocarcinoma is an extremely well-differentiated variant of cervical adenocarcinoma in which the cells composing the tumor lack the typical cytologic features of malignancy. These tumors were originally referred to as *adenoma malignum*. Because of their close cytologic resemblance to normal endocervical glands, in 1975 Silverberg and Hurt introduced the term *minimal deviation adenocarcinoma* (*MDA*) for these lesions.[258] Although all the tumors in the original description were extremely well differentiated mucin-producing adenocarcinomas, more recently MDA has been expanded to include endometrioid and clear cell variants.[152,278,305]

Minimal deviation adenocarcinomas are uncommon tumors and account for only 1%–3% of all cervical adenocarcinomas.[152] These tumors are more likely than other types of cervical adenocarcinomas to either precede or develop coincidentally with an ovarian carcinoma. The ovarian neoplasms with which MDA is most likely to be associated include mucinous adenocarcinomas and sex cord tumors with annular tubules. Both MDA of the cervix and ovarian sex cord tumors with annular tubules have been strongly associated with Peutz–Jeghers syndrome.[195,306] In one series, 4 of 27 women with Peutz–Jeghers syndrome developed MDA.[306] Therefore, close clinical surveillance of women with Peutz–Jeghers syndrome is recommended, including careful endocervical cytologic examination and periodic endocervical curettage.

Minimal deviation adenocarcinomas are frequently associated with a profuse watery, mucinous vaginal discharge or abnormal vaginal bleeding and some cases are associated with abnormal endocervical cells on Pap smear.[120] Grossly and colposcopically, cervices with early forms of MDA can appear normal. In more advanced cases, polypoid lesions or irregularities of the cervix can sometimes be noted. In other cases, there is cervical ulceration or only cervical stenosis without any obvious lesion.

The characteristic microscopic features of MDA are the presence of cytologically low-grade but architecturally atypical glands that vary in size, shape, and location (Fig. 8.33). In the mucin-producing forms, the glands are lined by a single layer of tall columnar epithelium that usually has minimal, if any, nuclear atypia (Fig. 8.34). The nuclei are bland, lack prominent nucleoli, and are located at the base of the epithelium. In the endometrioid type, the cells lining the glands resemble either normal proliferative or hyperplastic endometrium. Although the glands may exhibit a branching arrangement similar to that of the normal endocervical glands, characteristically glands with bizarre angular outpouchings, which vary greatly in size, are present.[100,148,199] Desmoplasia is frequently present surrounding the angular outpouchings of MDA. Young and Scully have described five minimal deviation endometrioid adenocarcinomas of the cervix that were characterized by a benign-appearing proliferation of glands and cysts which were for the most part unassociated with a stromal reaction.[305] The cells comprising these tumors were of the type seen in tuboendometrioid metaplasia and were ciliated in four cases, but had moderate cytologic atypicality and occasional mitotic figures.

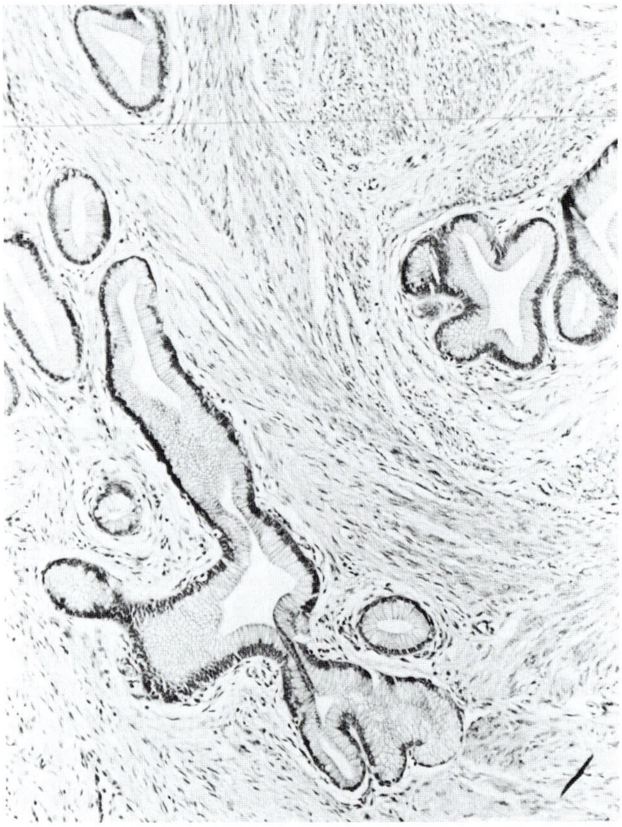

Fig. 8.33. Minimal deviation adenocarcinoma. There is an irregular glandular, branching pattern that differs from normal endocervical glands despite close resemblance of lining cells to normal endocervical epithelium. A discrete rim of periglandular stromal edema is present around the glands.

The most reliable criterion to assess the malignant nature of MDA is the haphazard arrangement of glands that extend beyond the level of normal endocervical glands and the presence of occasional mitoses in glandular cells. Mitoses are quite uncommon in the normal, nonneoplastic, endocervical epithelium, and the presence of mitoses should alert the pathologist to the possible presence of MDA. However, occasional mitotic figures in otherwise normal-appearing glands should not be taken as sufficient for a diagnosis of MDA. Minimal deviation adenocarcinoma often involves more than two-thirds of the thickness of the cervical stroma and should be regarded as invasive because the normal endocervical crypts and tunnels do not extend beyond 5–7 mm.[100,152] Because the depth of penetration of the glands is an essential histologic feature of MDA, in most cases the diagnosis cannot be made on a superficial cervical biopsy, but instead requires either a cone biopsy or hysterectomy specimen. Immunohistochemical studies using CEA have found a highly variable staining of MDA with only focal areas of positivity, and CA 125 staining is significantly reduced compared to normal endocervical glands.[44,100,282] Immunohistochemical staining for estrogen and progesterone receptors is uniformly negative in MDA, and this criterion can be used to help differentiate these tumors from variants of normal endocervical glands.[282]

The differential diagnosis of MDA includes several conditions in which nonneoplastic glands extend beyond 7 mm from the surface. These conditions include endocervical tunnel clusters, deeply situated nabothian cysts, endocervicosis of the cervical wall, and mesonephric hyperplasia.[301] The glands of endocervical tunnel clusters, mesonephric hyperplasia, and deep nabothian cysts are usually much more uniform in size than are the glands of MDA and lack the bizarre branching and irregular outpouchings that are characteristic of the glands of MDA. The benign processes also lack a desmoplastic response.

Although earlier reports, and several of the more recent studies, have suggested an extremely poor prognosis for women with MDA, other series have found

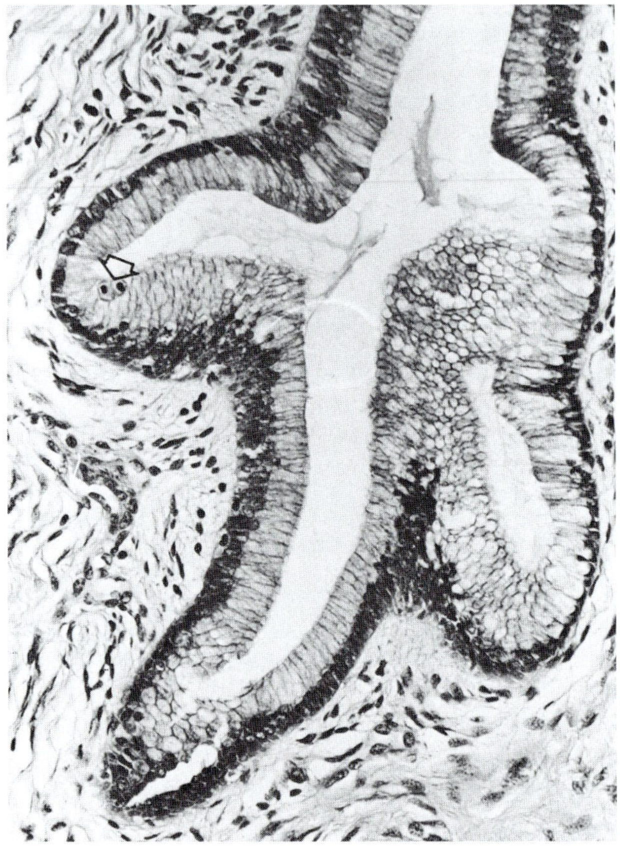

Fig. 8.34. Minimal deviation adenocarcinoma. Slightly enlarged nuclei in a basal position and occasional mitotic figures (*arrow*) are present.

survival rates similar to those of women with well-differentiated ordinary adenocarcinoma.[100,148,258] For example, a recent series of six cases from Japan reported a 5-year disease-free survival of 83% in treated cases.[120] The discrepancy in observations may be caused by a number of factors, including undertreatment of MDA because deep invasion by the tumor was not appreciated. In some cases, minimal deviation adenocarcinomas have not been correctly diagnosed, even in hysterectomy specimens, before the development of recurrent disease.

Serous Adenocarcinoma

Serous adenocarcinoma of the cervix is an uncommon form of cervical adenocarcinoma that histologically is identical to serous adenocarcinomas arising in the ovary or endometrium. In one large series, pure or mixed papillary serous adenocarcinomas accounted for 1% of cervical adenocarcinomas.[96] These tumors are composed of papillary tufts and complex papillae lined by cells with pleomorphic, high-grade nuclei (Figs. 8.35 and 8.36).[99] This histological variant has been associated with a poor prognosis.[65,99]

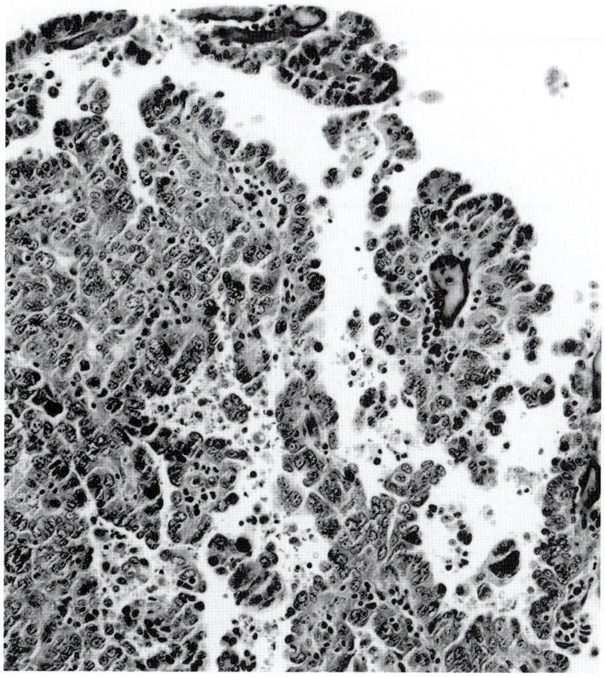

Fig. 8.36. Serous adenocarcinoma of the cervix. At higher magnification, the marked cellular pleomorphism characteristic of serous carcinoma is apparent.

Mesonephric Carcinoma

Mesonephric duct remnants are detected in up to 20% of cervices removed during routine hysterectomy, and adenocarcinomas can rarely develop in these remnants.[128] *Mesonephric carcinomas* are very rare and in the past were confused with clear cell carcinomas of the cervix. Only 14 cases of mesonephric carcinoma are reported in the literature, 10 of which are pure adenocarcinomas; 4 have adenocarcinoma mixed with a malignant spindle cell component. In most cases, gross inspection of the cervix reveals a mass that can be exophytic or endophytic. In contrast to the superficial location of cervical clear cell adenocarcinomas, true mesonephric adenocarcinomas develop deep in the lateral wall of the cervix, in a site corresponding to the location of mesonephric duct remnants. Therefore, they often extend into the outer third of the cervical wall. The tumors can be either pure adenocarcinomas or adenocarcinomas that are mixed with a spindle cell component; they vary in histologic appearance.[57,59] The most common appearance has been termed the ductal pattern and consists of tubular glands that vary in size and are lined by one to several layers of columnar cells (Figs. 8.37 and 8.38). Some of the gland lumens contain PAS-positive, diastase-resistant secretions. Other patterns that have been described include a retiform pattern, a tubular pattern, and a sex cord pattern.[59]

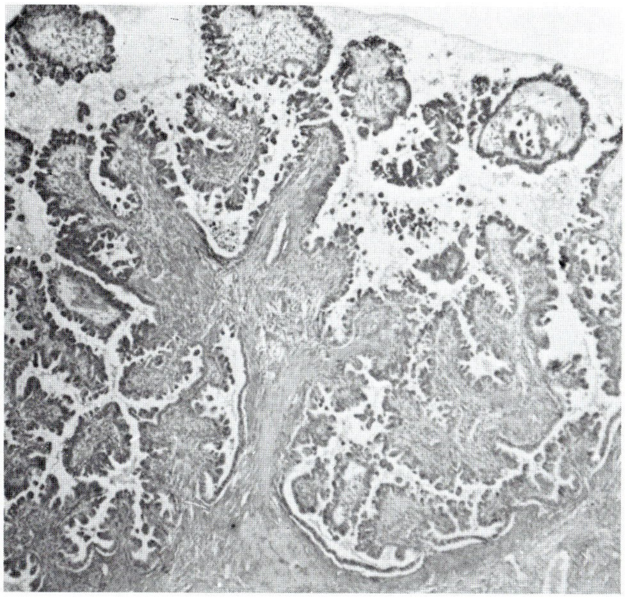

Fig. 8.35. Serous adenocarcinoma of the cervix. There are branching papillae lined by atypical epithelium and supported by connective tissue stroma resembling papillary serous carcinoma of the ovary.

When a spindle cell component occurs, it appears as closely packed oval to spindle cells that can resemble an endometrial stromal sarcoma. A diag-

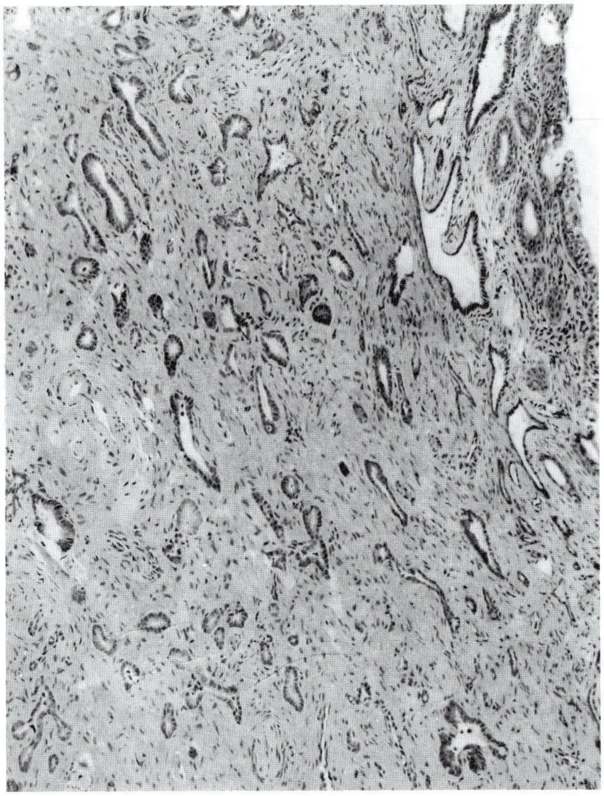

Fig. 8.37. Mesonephric carcinoma of the cervix. The tumor is composed of tubular glands that diffusely infiltrate the stroma.

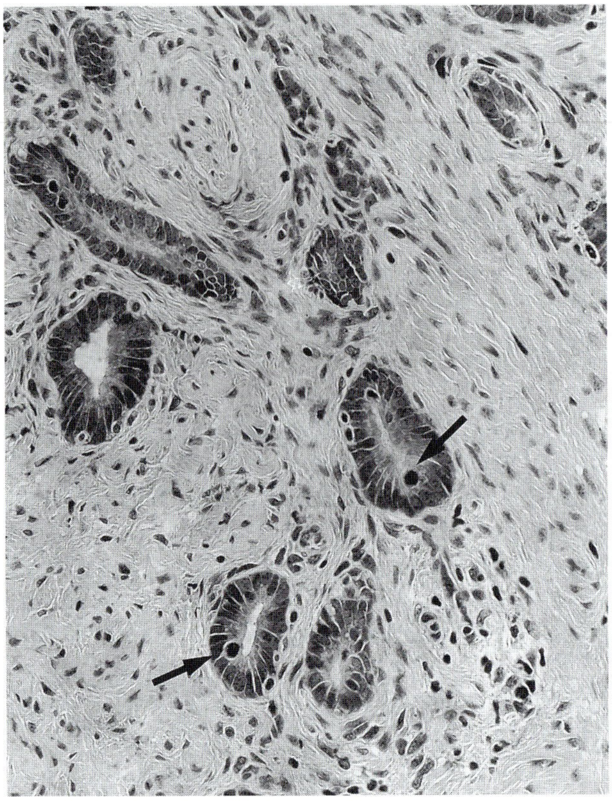

Fig. 8.38. Mesonephric carcinoma of the cervix. Haphazardly arranged tubular glands with minimal nuclear atypia. Note mitotic activity (*arrows*).

nosis of mesonephric carcinoma should only be made if the tumor is located deep in the wall of the cervix, the endocervical mucosa is uninvolved, and there is no evidence that the patient was exposed to DES. Distinguishing mesonephric carcinoma from florid mesonephric hyperplasia can be difficult because the majority of carcinomas develop in the setting of a diffuse form of mesonephric hyperplasia (see Chapter 6, Benign Diseases of the Cervix).[90] In contrast to mesonephric hyperplasia, the carcinoma does not have a lobular architecture and the nuclei appear cytologically malignant. Although there are only limited published data on clinical presentation and outcome, the mean age of patients at presentation is 50 years and most present with abnormal vaginal bleeding. Some mesonephric carcinomas have metastasized.

Well-Differentiated Villoglandular Adenocarcinoma

Villoglandular adenocarcinoma is a well-differentiated form of cervical adenocarcinoma that occurs predominantly in young women and has an excellent prognosis.[125,142,304] The characteristic features of this tumor are a surface component that is composed of papillae lined by epithelium that has only mild cytologic atypia (Figs. 8.39 and 8.40). The epithelial cells lining the papillae can have either endocervical, endometrioid, or intestinal features (including goblet cells). Because of the large number of surface papillae, these tumors frequently form an exophytic, friable tumor mass. Most of the papillae have central cores containing spindle-shaped stromal cells resembling those of the normal cervical stroma and a variable number of inflammatory cells. The papillae can be either long and thin or thick and short. Small papillary tufts composed entirely of epithelial cells of the type characteristic of serous carcinomas of the ovary are absent. Beneath the papillary surface, the infiltrating portion of the tumor is composed of irregular branching glands that are typically surrounded by only a minimal desmoplastic response.

The differential diagnosis of these tumors includes papillary endocervicitis, papillary adenofibromas of the cervix, and müllerian papillomas.[304] All three of these lesions lack the degree of cellular

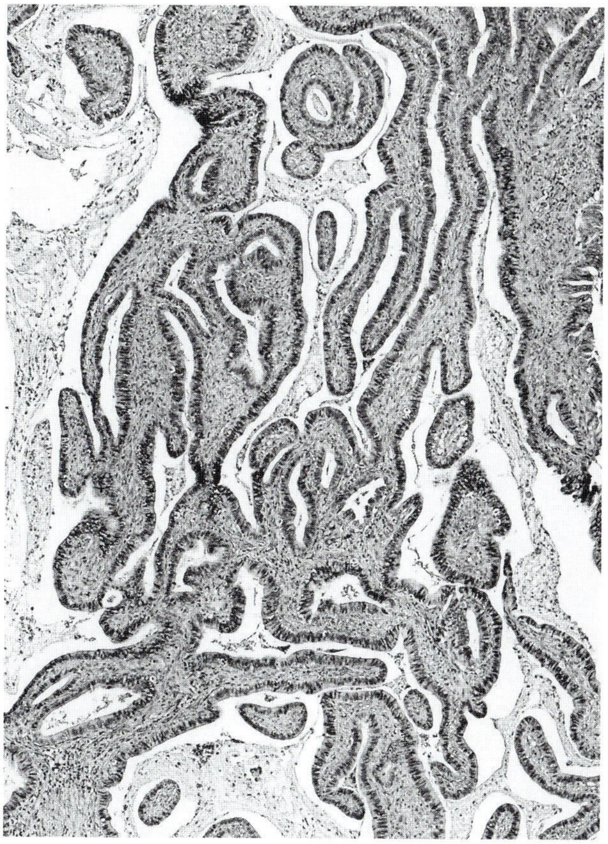

Fig. 8.39. Well-differentiated villoglandular adenocarcinoma. The tumor is composed of long, thin papillae. (Used with permission from ref. 142.)

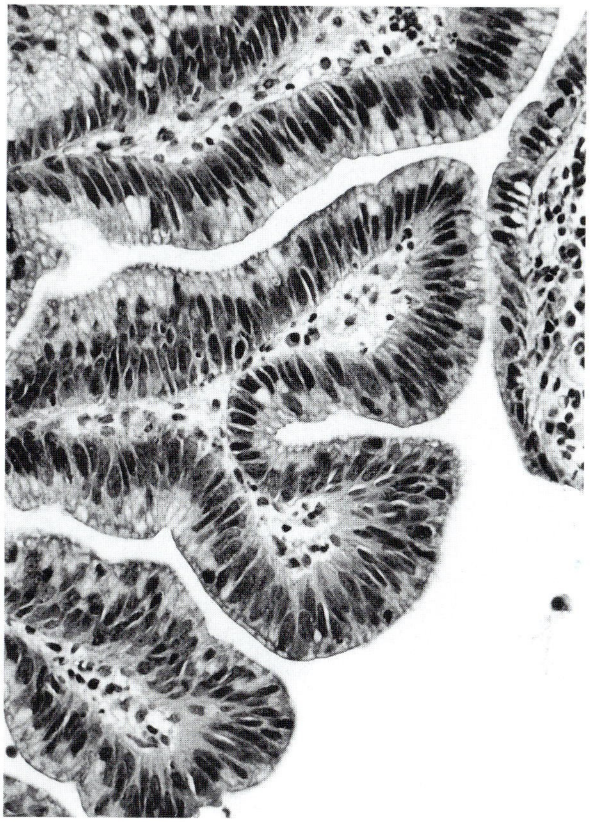

Fig. 8.40. Well-differentiated villoglandular adenocarcinoma. The cells lining the papillae are pseudostratified and have minimal cytological atypia. (Used with permission from ref. 142.)

atypia that is present in villoglandular adenocarcinomas. The müllerian papilloma is a lesion of children, whereas the age of patients with villoglandular adenocarcinomas ranges from 23 to 54 years, with a mean of 37 in one series. These tumors must also be distinguished from serous papillary carcinomas of the cervix. Serous papillary carcinomas have more irregular papillae that are lined by cells with marked nuclear atypia and high mitotic counts which frequently form cellular tufts.

Villoglandular adenocarcinomas have been associated with the use of oral contraceptives before diagnosis and are frequently associated with high-risk types of HPV.[139,142] In the majority of cases, the tumor is superficially invasive, although deep invasion with extension into the uterine corpus may occur. In most of the cases published to date, the clinical outcome of patients with villoglandular adenocarcinomas has been excellent. In the two largest series, all patients, including those who were treated by simple excisional biopsy or cone biopsy, were alive and well with no evidence of recurrent disease after 7–77 months of follow-up.[143,304] However, a recent series of seven cases from Japan reported the presence of lymphvascular space involvement in two villoglandular adenocarcinomas, which was associated with lymph node metastases in both cases and death in one patient.[150] Rarely, villoglandular carcinomas may be mixed with other types of carcinomas. The authors are aware of two such cases in which lymph node metastasis has occurred (unpublished observations).

Other Epithelial Tumors

Adenosquamous Carcinoma

Adenosquamous carcinomas are defined as tumors that contain an admixture of histologically malignant squamous and glandular cells. Glucksmann and Cherry, who originally emphasized the importance of adenosquamous carcinomas, used the term *mixed cervical carcinomas* to refer to adenosquamous carcinomas as well as glassy cell carcinomas and signet-ring carcinomas.[102] In the most recent

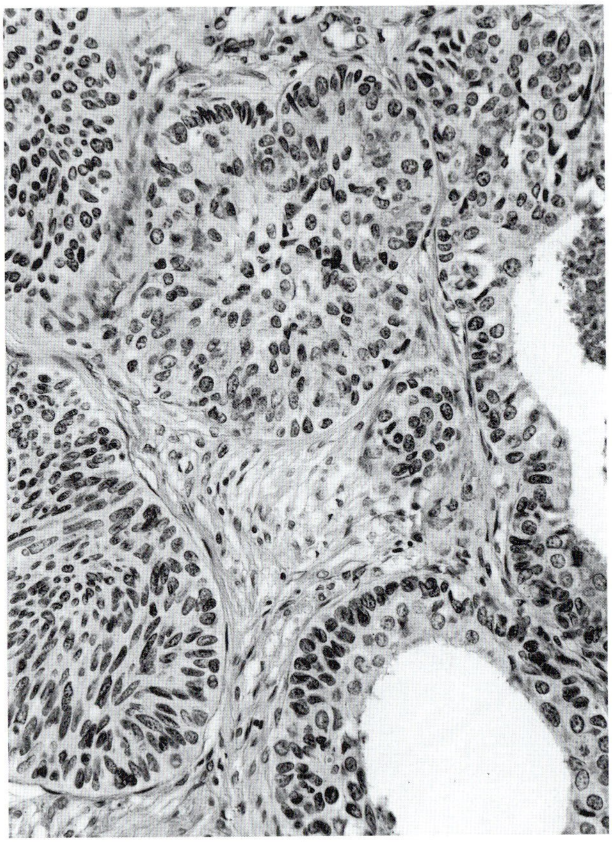

Fig. 8.41. Adenosquamous carcinoma of the cervix. Malignant glandular elements are present on the *right* and malignant squamous elements with spindle cell features are present on the *left*.

WHO classification, the term mixed carcinomas has been deleted and adenosquamous carcinomas are now classified under *other epithelial tumors*.[251]

Adenosquamous carcinomas account for between 5% and 25% of all cervical cancers.[38,109,232,300] They occur in both young and old women and can be associated with pregnancy. The squamous component generally includes areas that are well differentiated and contain either keratin "pearls" or sheets of cells with individual cell keratinization. To make the diagnosis of adenosquamous carcinoma, there must be sufficient differentiation of the adenocarcinomatous component so that glands are histologically recognizable (Fig. 8.41). Although the well-differentiated forms are usually easily recognized, when the adenocarcinomatous component is less well differentiated and is present in relatively small amounts, it can easily be overlooked. The term *adenosquamous carcinoma* is not used for adenocarcinomas that contain bland (nonmalignant)-appearing squamous differentiation. Instead, such tumors are classified as endometrioid adenocarcinomas of the cervix with squamous metaplasia (see "Endometrioid Carcinoma," earlier).

Lesions with mixed patterns of epithelial differentiation are thought to arise from the pluripotential subcolumnar reserve cells of the endocervical mucous membrane and represent biphasic differentiation.[40] The epidemiologic risk factors associated with adenosquamous carcinomas of the cervix are more similar to those of squamous cell carcinomas than of adenocarcinomas.[38] The prevalence of adenosquamous carcinomas may be increased in young women, and these tumors metastasize to pelvic lymph nodes twice as frequently as squamous cell carcinomas or adenocarcinomas.[28,109,288] Despite the increase in pelvic lymph node metastases, the prognosis in patients with adenosquamous carcinomas has not been significantly worse than that of patients with squamous cell carcinomas in some studies, although other series have reported a poorer prognosis associated with these tumors.[28,29,97,109,288,300]

Glassy Cell Carcinoma

A poorly differentiated form of adenosquamous carcinoma has been referred to as *glassy cell carcinoma*. Glassy cell carcinoma comprise less than 1% of cervical cancers and has been reported to have an extremely aggressive clinical course, with a poor response to radiation and surgery.[97,189,253] Although the existence of poorly differentiated adenosquamous carcinomas with this histology is widely ac-

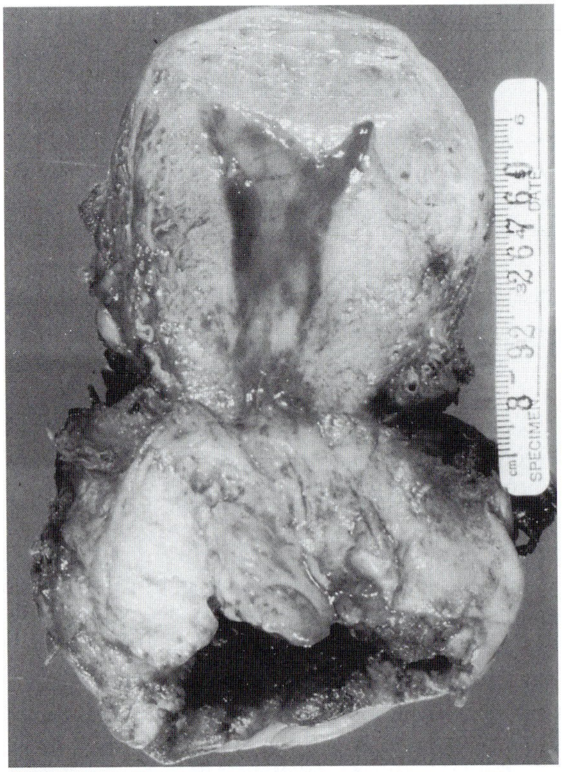

Fig. 8.42. Glassy cell carcinoma. The tumor has diffusely infiltrated the cervix to form a barrel-shaped cervix.

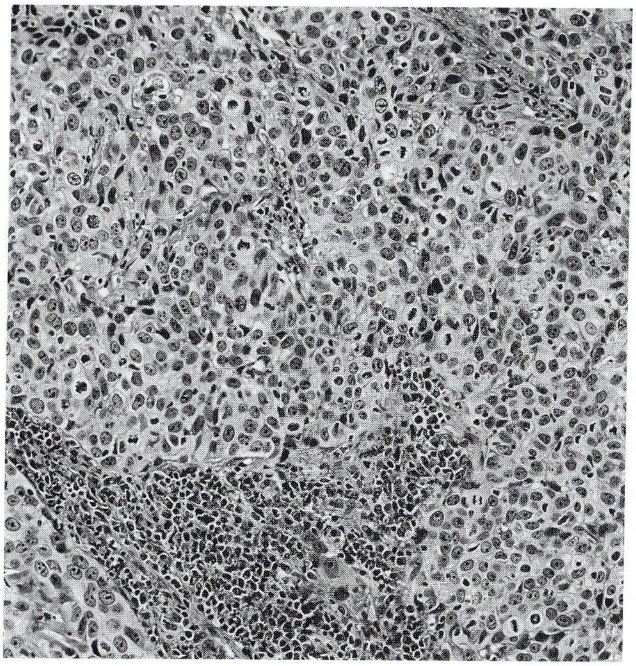

a

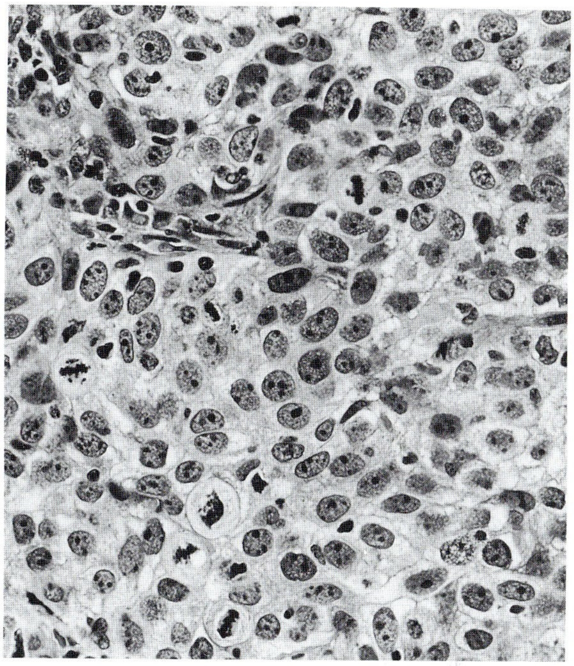

b

Fig. 8.43. Glassy cell carcinoma. **a**: The tumor has neither apparent squamous nor glandular differentiation and is arranged in lobules. The stroma contains an abundant chronic inflammatory exudate. **b**: The neoplastic cells have a granular glassy cytoplasm, well-defined cytoplasmic membranes, and prominent nucleoli.

cepted, it has been argued that classifying these tumors as a separate entity is unwarranted because, compared to other types of poorly differentiated carcinomas, these tumors do not have a significantly different clinical course.[189,296]

On gross examination these tumors are commonly large and produce a barrel-shaped cervix (Fig. 8.42). The major microscopic features of glassy cell carcinomas include (1) uniform large polygonal cells with finely granular ground glass-type cytoplasm (hence the name *glassy cell*), (2) distinct cell membranes, and (3) prominent nucleoli (Fig. 8.43). In addition, the cells lack intercellular bridges, dyskeratosis, and intracellular glycogen. Mitotic figures are abundant. The stroma is characteristically heavily infiltrated by lymphoplasmacytic and eosinophilic inflammatory cells. Occasionally, areas of keratin pearl and abortive lumen formation are seen together with signet-ring cells and intracellular mucin. The overlying surface squamous epithelium may be normal or may contain SIL. Ultrastructurally, the adenosquamous nature of glassy cell carcinoma is evidenced by rare abortive glandular lumen formation together with well-developed tonofilament–desmosomal complexes, interdigitating microvilli, and cytoplasmic microfilaments.[236]

Clear Cell Adenosquamous Carcinoma

Recently a variant of adenosquamous carcinoma has been described that was referred to as *clear cell adenosquamous carcinoma*.[95] It has been suggested that clear cell adenosquamous carcinoma should be distinguished from adenosquamous carcinoma because of their association with HPV 18 and aggressive clinical behavior. The characteristic histologic features of these tumors are sheets of cohesive cells with prominent cell borders and a vacuolated or clear cytoplasm containing large amounts of glycogen (Fig. 8.44). The cohesive sheets are frequently subdivided by connective tissue septa, which can have a prominent lymphocytic infiltrate that produces a lobulated appearance. The tumors demonstrate focal gland formation and stain positively with a mucin stain such as mucicarmine. In some clear cell adenosquamous carcinomas there are spindle-shaped cells suggesting squamous differentiation. Clear cell adenosquamous carcinomas need to be distinguished from clear cell carcinomas and glassy cell carcinoma of the cervix. Unlike clear cell carcinomas, clear cell adenosquamous carcinomas lack papillary or tubulocystic areas and hobnail cells. Moreover, clear cell carcinomas lack focal mucin production and distinct cell borders. Glassy cell carcinomas have an eosinophilic or granular cytoplasm and large oval nuclei with prominent nucleoli, which are not features of clear cell adenosquamous carcinoma.

The mean age of the 11 patients in the literature is 43 years (range, 24–74 years). Of 11 reported patients, all were associated with HPV 18. The re-

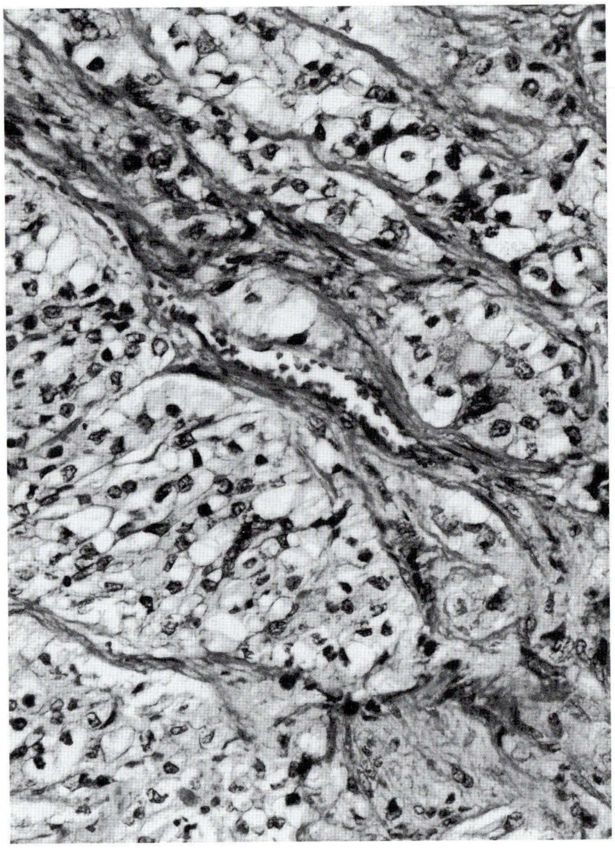

Fig. 8.44. Clear cell adenosquamous carcinoma. The tumor is composed of sheets of vacuolated cells that are subdivided into lobules by connective tissue septa which in some cases contain a prominent inflammatory infiltrate.

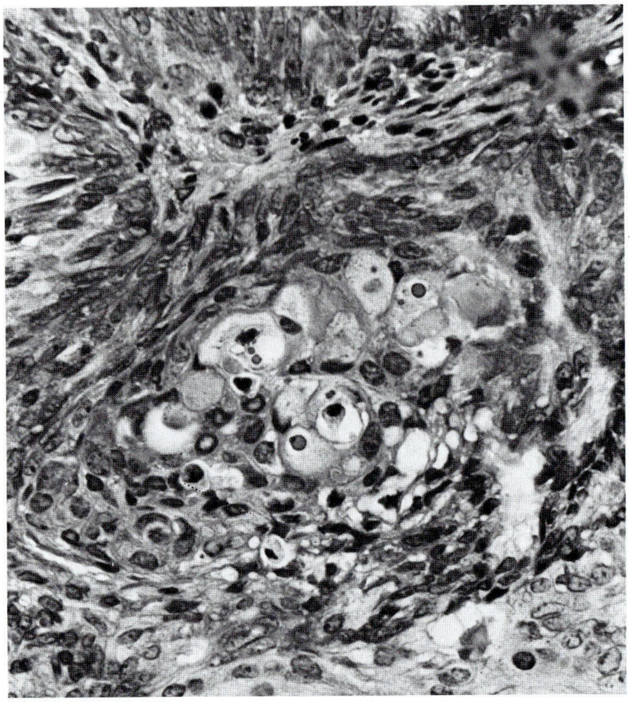

Fig. 8.45. Mucoepidermoid carcinoma of the cervix. There are pale, mucin-containing cells within masses of neoplastic squamous cells.

ported cases of clear cell adenosquamous carcinoma have tended to behave aggressively. Seven (64%) of the 11 patients died of their disease, including 3 (60%) of 5 patients with stage IB disease.[95]

Mucoepidermoid Carcinoma

Buckley and Fox have argued that all cervical carcinomas should be stained with a mucin stain such as mucicarmine before classification because a considerable number of cervical squamous cell carcinomas lacking recognizable glands still produce mucin that can be detected with special stains.[40,41] They and others use the term *mucoepidermoid carcinoma* to refer to these mixed squamous cell carcinomas that produce mucin but lack recognizable glands.[40,41,279] Mucoepidermoid carcinomas are a very common form of cervical carcinoma, accounting for up to 36% of cervical carcinomas in some series.[22,62,248] In mucoepidermoid carcinoma, the squamous component is usually large cell nonkeratinizing or focally keratinizing, and the mucin-producing cells are frequently localized in the center of nests of squamous cell carcinoma (Fig. 8.45). The mucinous component includes goblet or signet-ring type cells that contain mucinocarminophilic, periodic acid–Schiff (PAS)-positive, diastase-resistant mucopolysaccharides. The mucin from these cells is extruded into the intercellular spaces or fibrous stroma, where it may collect in small or large lakes.

In some studies, mucoepidermoid carcinomas have been more common in younger patients and have been associated with an increased risk of lymph node metastases.[22,42,109] This association has led some authors to propose that these tumors have a distinctive clinical presentation and contribute to a subset of young women with highly aggressive cervical cancers. However, most studies have failed to detect a significant clinical difference between patients with mixed carcinomas and those with pure squamous cell carcinomas of the cervix.[22,51,62,248,288] Therefore, these tumors are not incorporated as a separate entity in the most recent WHO classification of cervical tumors but are included within the category of adenosquamous carcinoma.

Adenoid Cystic Carcinoma

Adenoid cystic carcinoma of the cervix is a relatively uncommon tumor accounting for less than 1% of all cervical adenocarcinomas. It is characterized by nests of small basaloid cells of varying size with high

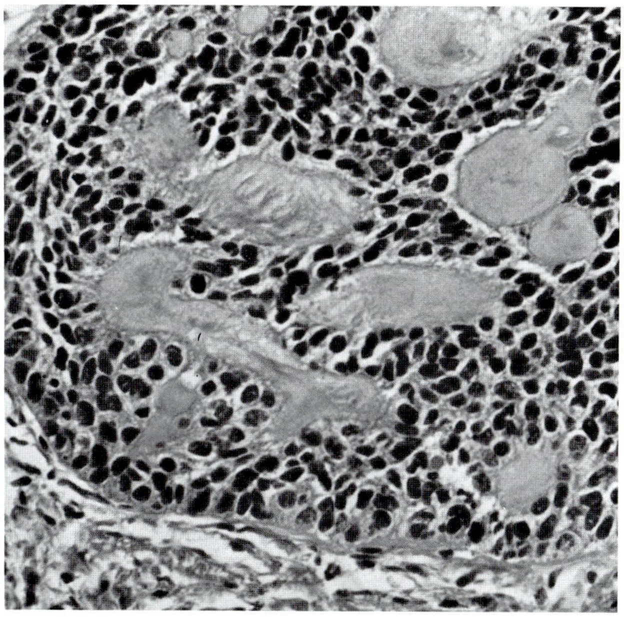

Fig. 8.46. Adenoid cystic carcinoma of the cervix. Cylindrical hyaline bodies are present within solid nests of basaloid tumor cells.

nuclear-to-cytoplasmic ratios that have a cribiform appearance due to cylindrical hyaline bodies or small acini or cysts.[194,207] The nuclei of the cells are small, only mildly pleomorphic, and there are occasional mitotic figures. There is frequently peripheral palisading of the cells. Focal squamous differentiation and necrosis may be present. Most tumors also contain infiltrating anastomosing cords of cells. In cross section, the hyaline cylinders appear round or ovoid, giving the neoplasm a sievelike appearance (Fig. 8.46). At the electron microscopic level, the hyaline material is partly composed of coalesced masses of basal lamina produced by the epithelial tumor cells and partly of fine precollagen and collagen fibers of fibroblastic origin.[194] This material stains positively on immunohistochemistry for laminin and type IV collagen.[104,203] However, unlike adenoid cystic carcinomas of other sites, cervical adenoid cystic carcinomas contain few myoepithelial cells as detected by electron microscopy or S-100 and actin immunohistochemical stains. The basaloid cells stain positively on immunohistochemistry with MNF 116 and CAM 5.2 (low molecular weight cytokeratin).[104]

Adenoid cystic carcinoma may be associated with squamous adenocarcinoma of the cervix.[89] The tumor is most often seen in patients between the sixth and seventh decades (mean age of 71 years in the largest series) and is more common in blacks than whites.[89,104] The tumors are associated with high-risk types of HPV[103]; they are also commonly associated with mucinous ovarian neoplasms. Adenoid cystic carcinoma often forms hard palpable masses in the cervix that can be ulcerated or friable. Lymphatic involvement is common, and the tumor behaves aggressively with frequent local recurrences or metastatic spread. Adenoid cystic carcinoma of the cervix should be differentiated from adenoid basal carcinoma of the cervix (see following).

Adenoid Basal Carcinoma

Adenoid basal carcinoma can be confused with adenoid cystic carcinoma because they have common histologic features. Adenoid basal carcinomas are composed of small uniform cells that resemble basal cell carcinomas of the skin and lack significant nuclear atypia. These cells are arranged in small nests and cords with a rounded or lobulated appearance (Fig. 8.47). At the periphery of the nests palisading of the nuclei is seen, and some of the nests have central cystic spaces that can be filled with necrotic debris. In the center of the nests there also can be either squamous or glandular differentiation (Fig. 8.48). Adenoid cystic carcinomas can usually be distinguished from adenoid cystic carcinomas by the lack of the characteristic intraluminal hyaline ma-

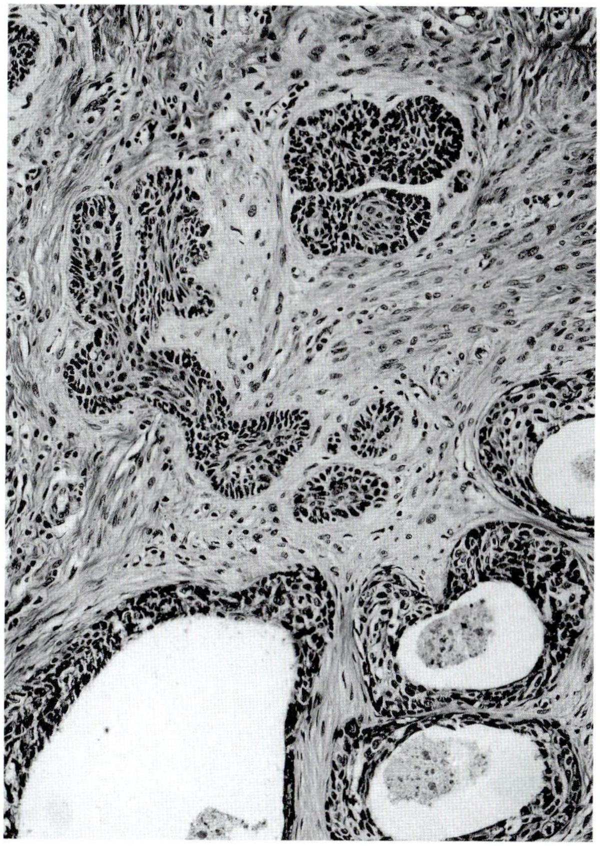

Fig. 8.47. Adenoid basal carcinoma of the cervix. Small uniform cells display palisading of the nuclei at the periphery of the nests. The appearance simulates basal cell carcinoma.

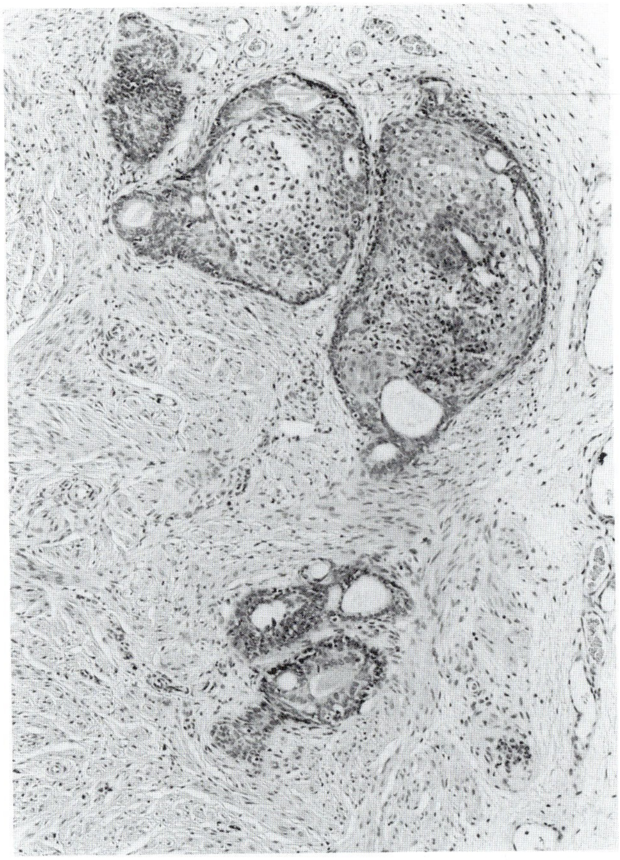

Fig. 8.48. Adenoid basal carcinoma of the cervix. The cells in the center of the nests have abundant cytoplasm and appear squamoid. There are gland lumens within the nests.

terial frequently present in adenoid cystic carcinomas, the presence of smaller, less pleomorphic nuclei, and less mitotic activity than is characteristic of adenoid cystic carcinomas.[82,89] Both adenoid basal and adenoid cystic carcinomas are frequently associated with SIL and can have squamous differentiation in the center of the invading nests of cells. Therefore, these features should not be used to distinguish between the two types of tumors.

Adenoid basal carcinomas are uncommon neoplasms that account for less than 1% of cervical adenocarcinomas and usually are found in postmenopausal, especially black, women.[82,89] The mean age of patients with adenoid basal carcinoma is approximately 64 years. Adenoid basal carcinomas have been shown to be associated with high-risk types of HPV.[138] Adenoid basal carcinoma behaves much less aggressively than adenoid cystic carcinoma. Because of their usual benign behavior, it has recently been suggested that they be referred to as *adenoid basal epitheliomas* of the cervix.[35] However, it should be cautioned that adenoid basal carcinomas can be found in association with adenoid cystic carcinomas, adenosquamous cell carcinomas, and squamous cell carcinomas of the cervix.[88]

Patients with adenoid basal carcinoma are usually asymptomatic without grossly detectable masses. Adenoid basal carcinomas are usually detected as unexpected findings in patients undergoing hysterectomy or cone biopsy for a coexistent SIL or another reason. Although the tumors can penetrate into the wall of the cervix and almost half the reported cases are classified as stage IB, the tumors rarely metastasize. There are several reported cases in the literature that acted aggressively (one was metastatic), but these tumors differ morphologically from the usual adenoid basal carcinoma. Aggressive tumors typically have irregularly shaped nests of basaloid cells that infiltrate into the stroma and elicit a stromal reaction analogous to morphoeic basal cell carcinoma of the skin.[88,104]

Neuroendocrine Tumors

Neuroendocrine tumors of the cervix are relatively rare, and the terminology that has been used to describe endocrine tumors of the cervix is confusing because multiple terms have been used to describe this group of tumors; these include *carcinoid tumor, carcinoid tumor with squamous cell carcinoma or adenocarcinoma, argyrophil cell carcinoma, apudoma, small cell tumor with neuroepithelial features*, and many others. The most recent histologic typing of female genital tract tumors of the World Health Organization recognizes only two types of endocrine tumors, small cell carcinomas and carcinoid tumors.[251]

Recently, the College of American Pathologists and the National Cancer Institute held a workshop to develop a more comprehensive terminology for these tumors. Because the morphologic features of neuroendocrine tumors occurring in the cervix are similar to those of endocrine tumors of the lung, this workshop proposed using the same classification for cervical tumors as used for the lung.[6] This workshop recognized four general categories of endocrine tumors of the cervix: (1) typical (classical) carcinoid tumor, (2) atypical carcinoid tumor, (3) large cell neuroendocrine carcinoma, and (4) small (oat) cell carcinoma.

The exact cellular origin of neuroendocrine tumors of the cervix is unknown. Small numbers of argyrophil cells are present in the exocervical epithelium of approximately 40% of women and in the endocervical epithelium in about 20% of women.[91] Argyrophil cells are also detected in about 60% of minimal deviation adenocarcinomas of the cervix and in 14% of other types of cervical adenocarcinomas or adenosquamous carcinomas.[250]

Typical (Classical) Carcinoid Tumor

Tumors that have been categorized as *well-differentiated carcinoid tumors of the cervix* were originally described by Albores-Saavedra et al. and were classified as carcinoid tumors because they contained neuroendocrine granules and were histologically similar to intestinal carcinoid tumors.[7,20] Microscopically these well-differentiated tumors grow in trabecular, nodular, or cordlike patterns (Figs. 8.49 and 8.50). Rosette-like structures are common, but follicles with eosinophilic material are uncommon. The neoplastic cells have round to oval spindle-shaped nuclei and finely granular cytoplasm. Mitoses are quite rare. More than 70% of these tumors are argyrophilic, and most stain positively using immunohistochemistry for synaptophysin, chromogranin A, and neuron-specific enolase. Neurosecretory granules can be identified in these tumors by electron microscopy.

Typical carcinoid tumors are quite uncommon. In a recent series of 15 neuroendocrine tumors of the cervix, only a single typical carcinoid tumor was encountered.[298] Some of the tumors that have been previously described in the literature as well-differentiated cervical carcinoid tumors actually appear to be adenocarcinomas of the cervix that focally resemble carcinoid tumors of the intestinal tract and have neuroendocrine differentiation. It should be noted that neurosecretory granules can be identified in many carcinomas of the cervix if a diligent search is made. Although early reports suggested that these tumors had a relatively good prognosis, more recent reports clearly demonstrate that these tumors can act in a malignant fashion with local and distant metastasis. To date, none of the published cases has been associated with the carcinoid syndrome.

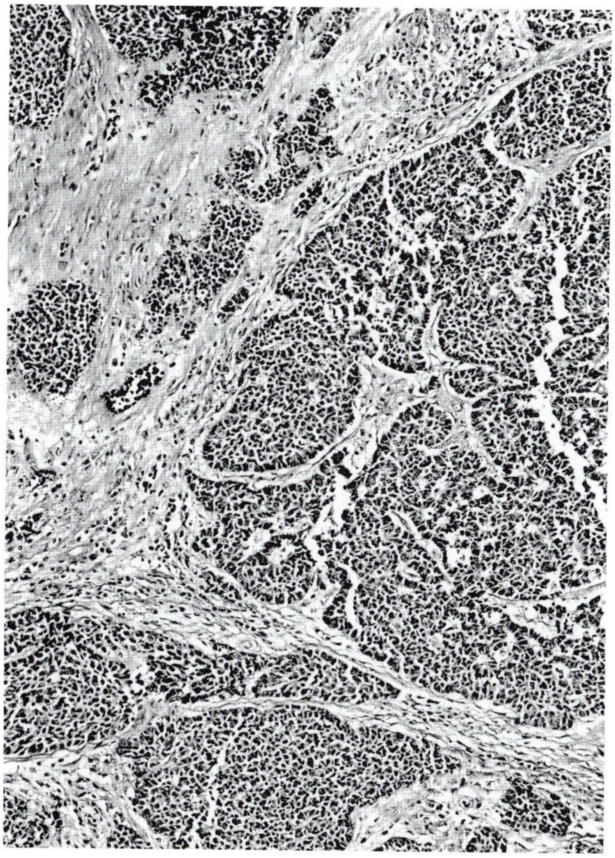

Fig. 8.49. Typical carcinoid tumor of the cervix. Solid masses and acini composed of small uniform cells.

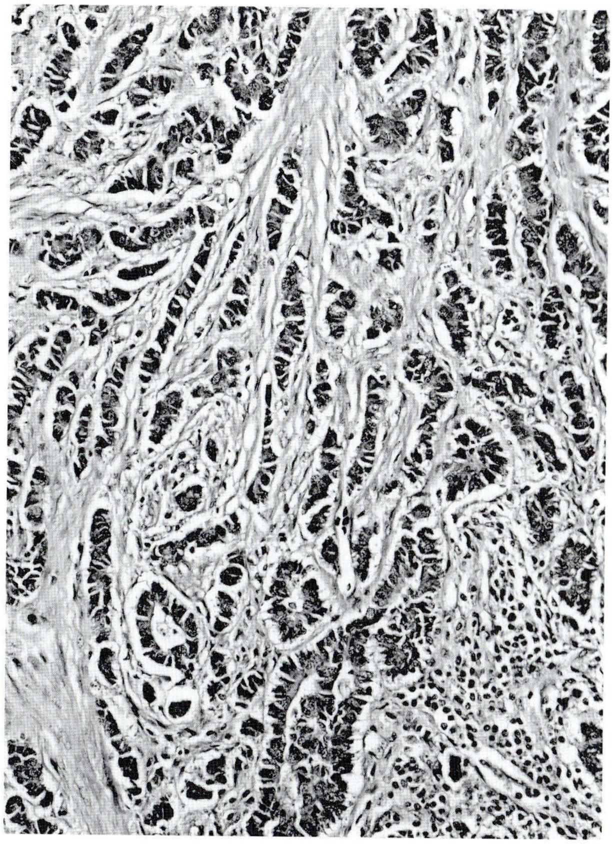

Fig. 8.50. Typical carcinoid tumor of the cervix. Small uniform cells in a trabecular pattern.

Atypical Carcinoid Tumor and Large Cell Neuroendocrine Carcinoma

Atypical carcinoids share the same architectural patterns of growth as typical carcinoids, but are much more cellular than typical carcinoids and have increased mitotic activity (5–10 mitoses/10 high-power fields) and focal areas of necrosis.[6] *Large cell neuroendocrine carcinomas* are poorly differentiated tumors that typically grow in organoid, trabecular, or cordlike patterns, although some cases only grow in sheets (Fig. 8.51). Peripheral palisading of the cells and geographic patterns of necrosis are frequently present. The tumors often have glandular differentiation and form small gland lumens. The

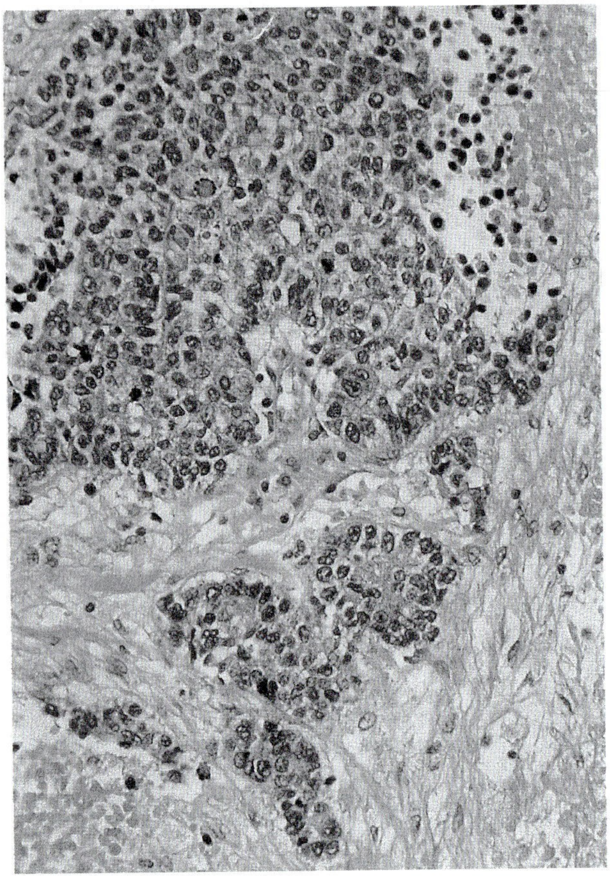

Fig. 8.51. Large cell neuroendocrine carcinoma. The tumor is composed of large cells with marked nuclear atypia and many mitoses that grow in a trabecular arrangement.

cells of large cell neuroendocrine carcinomas are large with abundant eosinophilic cytoplasm, and small eosinophilic cytoplasmic granules can sometimes be identified on hematoxylin and eosin-stained sections. The cells have vesicular high-grade nuclei with prominent nucleoli. Mitotic figures are quite numerous (>10 mitoses/10 high-power fields). Both atypical carcinoid tumors and large cell neuroendocrine carcinomas are argyrophilic and usually stain for neuron-specific enolase, chromogranin A, and synaptophysin. Large cell neuroendocrine carcinomas are often associated with glandular lesions. In the series of Gilks et al., 66% of large cell neuroendocrine carcinomas had a coexisting adenocarcinoma in situ and 25% had a coexisting cervical adenocarcinoma.[101]

Atypical carcinoids and large cell neuroendocrine carcinomas can be distinguished based on mitotic activity, nuclear atypia, and degree of necrosis (Table 8.10).[6] It is more difficult to differentiate between large cell neuroendocrine carcinoma and poorly differentiated cervical adenocarcinomas or squamous cell carcinomas. Large cell neuroendocrine tumors frequently have glandular differentiation and sometimes coexist with components of typical adenocarcinomas. Therefore, it is important that trabecular and insular growth patterns be looked for in poorly differentiated cervical tumors and that stains for neuroendocrine markers be used whenever there is an indication of neuroendocrine differentiation. It should be cautioned, however, that occasional typical cervical adenocarcinomas and adenosquamous carcinomas can stain focally with neuroendocrine markers or contain occasional argyrophilic cells.[20,249]

Large cell neuroendocrine carcinomas are highly aggressive neoplasms.[4] In one recent study, 7 (64%) of 11 cases died with disease within 2 years of diagnosis.[101]

Small (Oat) Cell Carcinoma

Small (oat) cell carcinomas of the cervix are histologically identical to their counterparts at other sites

Table 8.10. Histologic features used for distinguishing neuroendocrine tumors of the cervix

Tumor	*Patterns*	*Mitoses*	*Nuclear atypia*	*Neurosecretory granules*[a]	*Necrosis*
Typical carcinoid tumor	Trabecular, insular, sheetlike	Rare	No	Yes	No
Atypical carcinoid tumor	Trabecular, insular, sheetlike	5–10/10 HPF	Moderate	Yes	Focal
Large cell neuroendocrine carcinoma	Sheets, organoid trabecular, cordlike	>10/10 HPF	Marked	Yes	Moderate
Small cell carcinoma	Sheets, nests, trabecular, cordlike	>10/10 HPF	Moderate	Sometimes	Extensive

HPF, high-power fields.
[a]By electron microscopy or immunohistochemistry.
Adapted from refs. 6, 101.

such as the lung.[106] These tumors are characterized by small anaplastic cells that have scant amounts of cytoplasm, finely stippled chromatin, and inconspicuous nucleoli. They should be distinguished from adenocarcinomas with carcinoid features and poorly differentiated nonkeratinizing squamous cell carcinomas composed of small cells. These tumors account for between 2% and 5% of all cervical tumors. In one of the larger series, patients ranged in age from 25 to 87 years with a median age of 42 years.[98] In another study comparing small cell carcinoma to nonkeratinizing squamous carcinoma composed of small cells, the mean age of women with small cell carcinoma was 36 years compared to 50 years for the squamous carcinomas.[10] Grossly, these lesions range in size from small, clinically inapparent lesions to large ulcerated lesions measuring more than 6 cm in diameter.[98] Small cell carcinomas are more frequently deeply infiltrative than are squamous or adenocarcinomas, and a barrel-shaped cervix is commonly present.[174]

Microscopically, small cell carcinomas are composed of sheets and cords of closely packed, small scant cells with inconspicuous cytoplasm, closely resembling the cells of "oat cell" carcinoma of the lung. The cells have hyperchromatic nuclei, high nuclear:cytoplasmic ratios, and a high mitotic rate with three or more mitoses present in most high-power fields (Fig. 8.52). The nuclear shape varies from round to spindled, and nuclear molding is a characteristic feature. Nuclear detail and nucleoli are frequently obscured by smudging of the nucleus and, as with their pulmonary counterparts, histologic sections frequently demonstrate extensive crush artifact. Small areas of either squamous or glandular differentiation can be present but should account for less than 5% of the total tumor volume.[98]

Neuroendocrine dense-core granules can be detected using Grimelius staining or electron microscopy in most cases. Although these tumors have been associated with ectopic ACTH, insulin, and gastrin production, this appears to be an uncommon event.[98] By immunohistochemistry, neuroendocrine markers such as neuron-specific enolase, chromogranin, or synaptophysin are present in many cases; however, calcitonin, insulin, somatostatin, and serotonin are only uncommonly detected.

Small cell carcinoma of the cervix is a highly aggressive tumor.[4,255] The prognosis for this tumor is comparatively worse than that of its well-differentiated carcinoid counterpart and is worse than that of stage-comparable, poorly differentiated squamous carcinoma.[7,10,106] In the series of Walker et al., 9 of 12 patients died as a direct result of their tumor, and the median duration of survival of those dying of disease was only 12.5 months.[294] Similarly, in the series of Gersell et al., 10 of 15 patients died as a direct result of their tumor.[98] Comparison of the distribution of HPV 16 to that of HPV 18 in small cell carcinoma and nonkeratinizing squamous cell carcinomas composed of small cells revealed that HPV 16 was found more frequently in the squamous carcinomas (56% versus 20%), whereas small cell carcinoma had a higher frequency of HPV 18 (60% versus 36%).[10] Another study that utilized archival material and polymerase chain reaction (PCR) reported that 10 of 24 small cell carcinomas were HPV DNA positive and all 10 contained HPV 18.[184]

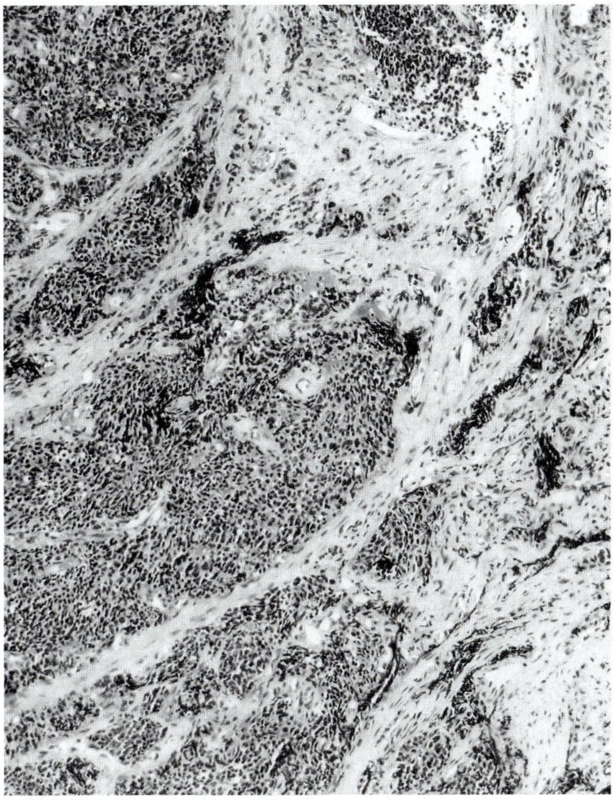

Fig. 8.52. Small cell carcinoma of the cervix. Small cells with hyperchromatic nuclei and scant, indistinct cytoplasm diffusely infiltrate the stroma. A characteristic type of crush artifact is present in the center and right.

Differentiation between small cell carcinoma and nonkeratinizing squamous carcinoma with small cells can be difficult. The diagnosis of small cell carcinoma should be reserved to tumors composed of small cells in which squamous or glandular differentiation is absent or minor. Women with small cell carcinoma tend to be younger than women with nonkeratinizing squamous carcinoma with small cells. Histologically, cells of nonkeratinizing squamous carcinoma with small cells resemble those of high-grade SIL and lack the nuclear molding and extensive crush artifact present in most small cell carcinomas. Small cell carcinomas invade the stroma diffusely in trabeculae and poorly defined nests. In contrast, nonkeratinizing squamous carcinoma with small cells invade the stroma in discrete nests. In an individual case immunocytochemistry for neuroendocrine markers may not be helpful because 40% of nonkeratinizing squamous carcinoma with small cells are positive for neuroendocrine markers and 40% of small cell carcinomas are positive for cytokeratins.[10] Immunohistochemical staining with antibodies against leukocyte common antigen and neuroendocrine markers can be useful for differentiating between small cell carcinoma from lymphoproliferative disorders.

Mixed Epithelial and Mesenchymal Tumors and Mesenchymal Tumors

Malignant mesenchymal tumors that can arise in the cervix include leiomyosarcoma, endocervical stromal sarcoma, embryonal rhabdomyosarcoma (botryoid type), alveolar soft part sarcoma, malignant schwannomas, and osteosarcomas (see Chapter 13, Mesenchymal Tumors of the Uterus). Primary cervical sarcomas are rare, and the most common form is the leiomyosarcoma.

Primary cervical mixed epithelial and mesenchymal tumors include *müllerian adenosarcomas* and *malignant müllerian mixed tumors* (MMMT) of the cervix. Approximately 30 cases of primary cervical MMMT have been reported in the literature. These cervical tumors are similar to their much more common uterine counterparts in some ways but differ in other ways.[60] Both usually occur in postmenopausal women and both typically form polypoid or pedunculated masses. The mean age of cervical tumors was 65 years in the largest published series.[60] However, cervical MMMTs differ in their histologic appearance from MMMTs arising in the uterus. The most common carcinomatous pattern in cervical tumors is a basaloid pattern that consists of anastomosing densely cellular trabeculae composed of small cells with scant cytoplasm and peripheral palisading. Other epithelial patterns include typical squamous cell carcinoma and endometrioid adenocarcinoma. Adenoid basal and adenoid cystic components have also been reported in several cases.[193] The sarcomatous element is typically homologous and frequently has the appearance of a fibrosarcoma or endometrial stromal sarcoma. The sarcomatous element is frequently high grade and may have myxoid change. Although the number of reported cases is small, cervical MMMT cases may have a better prognosis than their uterine counterparts.

Only a relative small number of cases of müllerian adenosarcomas of the cervix have been reported. However, this tumor may occur more frequently than reported in the literature because it is frequently misdiagnosed.[140,157] Müllerian adenosarcomas appear as broad-based polyps arising from the cervix. Microscopically, they usually demonstrate thick papillae covered with a typical endocervical-type endothelium. The appearance of the sarcomatous component can vary considerably between cases. In some, it consists of mitotically active, plump, spindle cells that form periglandular cuffs and a cambrium layer under the surface epithelium (Fig. 8.53). In other cases, the stromal component contains foci that are more embryonic in appear-

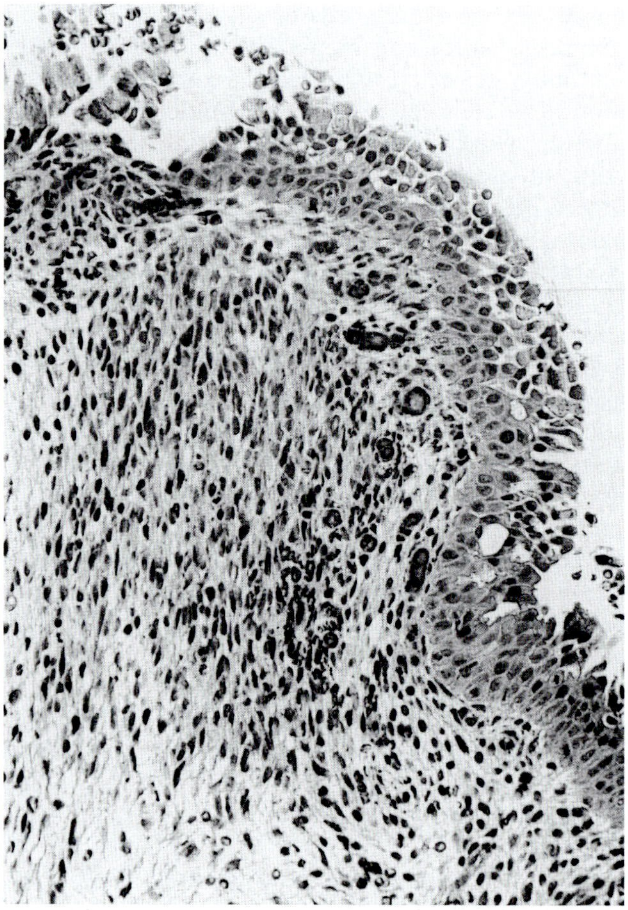

Fig. 8.53. Adenosarcoma of the cervix. The stroma of what initially appeared to be an endocervical polyp contains mitotically active plump spindle cells with hyperchromatic nuclei that coalesce under the epithelium.

ance, with small undifferentiated round cells that are mitotically active. Heterologous sarcomatous elements including strap cells, lipoblasts, cartilage, and osteoid can be present.

Adenosarcomas can occur in women between the ages of 14 and 67 years, and mean age in the two large series has been 37 and 39 years.[140,157] Women typically present with vaginal bleeding or recurrent cervical polyps. Prognosis is typically good after surgical therapy, although several patients have died of disease or developed recurrent tumor.

Miscellaneous Tumors

Examples of *synchronous adenocarcinoma and squamous cell carcinoma* occurring independently in the cervix have been reported.[299] They may be either invasive or in situ. In the invasive form, one carcinoma often invades the other, resulting in a collision tumor. Although such lesions closely resemble adenosquamous carcinomas, the different neoplastic components remain histologically distinct, separated from each other by narrow stroma or their respective basal lamina. Because direct transition from one cell type into another, as occurs in adenosquamous carcinoma, is not seen, these tumors are best considered separate primary carcinomas.

Primary malignant melanoma is among the least common of the malignant tumors that arise in the cervix; 27 patients have been reported.[50] The prognosis of primary malignant melanoma is quite poor, with only a 40% 5-year survival rate for patients with stage I disease and 14% 5-year survival for patients with higher-stage disease.[146] Most cases are stage I or II at diagnosis. Common presenting signs include vaginal bleeding, frequently of short duration. In most instances, the lesion is pigmented and dark brown. The diagnosis of primary melanoma of the cervix is based on the histologic demonstration of junctional changes in the squamous epithelium and the absence of similar lesions elsewhere in the body. Morphologically, it is identical to melanoma arising in the skin and extragenital mucous membranes; it frequently contains intracytoplasmic melanin pigment granules. The pathogenesis of malignant melanoma of the cervix is unclear, although its origin may be ascribed to the melanin-containing cells from the schwannian sheath in the normal cervix.

Primary choriocarcinoma in the cervix is rare and presumably results from a preexisting cervical pregnancy or displaced intrauterine molar tissue.[284] The gross and microscopic appearance, as well as the clinical course, are identical with those found in the uterine corpus.

Lymphomas and *leukemias* both can involve the cervix. More often these disorders are secondary, a manifestation of systemic disease. Leukemic infiltration of the cervix, especially of the granulocytic type, is a rather common occurrence at autopsy in women with leukemia.[186] Granulocytic sarcomas, which are well-demarcated extramedullary tumors composed of malignant granulocytic precursor cells, have also been reported in the cervix.[214] Granulocytic sarcomas should be differentiated from granulocytic leukemic infiltrates and can either accompany or proceed the development of acute myelogenous leukemia. Secondary lymphomatous involvement of the cervix is reported in 6% of women dying with generalized disease.[177] Primary lymphomas can occasionally arise in the cervix and usually present in premenopausal women as abnormal vaginal bleeding; 70% of these tumors are of the diffuse large cell type and 20% are lower-grade follicular lymphomas.[205]

Primary cervical germ cell tumors have been described: these include both the mature teratomas and yolk sac tumors. There are also case reports of primitive neuroectodermal tumors (PNET) of the cervix.[52,126] These tumors appear to be identical to PNETs occurring at other sites, and in some cases have stained positive on immunohistochemistry for the restricted surface antigen MIC-2 and contained the EWS/FLI-1 chimeric mRNA transcript characteristic of PNET/Ewing's sarcoma family.

Secondary Tumors

Direct extension from local pelvic tumor is the most common source of cervical involvement by *secondary carcinoma*, often originating in the endometrium, rectum, or bladder. Intrapelvic and intragenital, lymphatic or vascular metastases to the cervix occur less often but are associated with ovarian carcinoma, endometrial adenocarcinoma, and uncommonly with transitional cell carcinoma of the bladder.[34,168,181,308] Another lesion that has a relatively high rate of cervical metastasis is choriocarcinoma. Sarcomas of the uterine corpus may also involve the cervix. Metastases to the cervix from distant primary foci are rare, the most common sites being the gastrointestinal tract (colon and stomach), the ovary, and the breast. Instances of metastatic carcinoma from the kidney, gall bladder, pancreas, lung, thyroid, and malignant melanoma have also been described. On occasion, metastases may occur primarily as cervical involvement and pose a differential diagnostic problem. Unusual gross appearance or histologic patterns, e.g., signet-ring cell carcinoma or clear cell carcinoma, may provide a clue to the possibility of origin in a distant primary site.

References

1. National Cancer Institute (1999) Concurrent chemoradiation for cervical cancer. Clinical announcement, February 22, 1999. NCI, Washington, DC
2. ACS (2000) American Cancer Society: cervical cancer facts and figures. http://www.cancer.org/cancerinfo
3. NCI (2001) SEER Program: National Cancer Institute, USA. http://www-seer.ims.nci.nih.gov/ScientificSystems/
4. Abeler VM, Holm R, Nesland JM, et al (1994) Small cell carcinoma of the cervix. A clinicopathologic study of 26 patients. Cancer (Phila) 73:672–677
5. Abell MR, Gosling JRG (1962) Gland cell carcinoma (adenocarcinoma) of the uterine cervix. Am J Obstet Gynecol 83:729
6. Albores-Saavedra J, Gersell D, Gilks CB, et al (1997) Terminology of endocrine tumors of the uterine cervix: results of a workshop sponsored by the College of American Pathologists and the National Cancer Institute. Arch Pathol Lab Med 121:34–39
7. Albores-Saavedra J, Larraza O, Poucell S, et al (1976) Carcinoid tumors of the uterine cervix. Cancer (Phila) 38:2328–2342
8. Albores-Saavedra J, Young RH (1995) Transitional cell neoplasms (carcinomas and inverted papillomas) of the uterine cervix. A report of five cases. Am J Surg Pathol 19:1138–1145
9. Alfsen GC, Thoresen SO, Kristensen GB, et al (2000) Histopathologic subtyping of cervical adenocarcinoma reveals increasing incidence rates of endometrioid tumors in all age groups. Cancer (Phila) 89:1291–1299
10. Ambros RA, Park J-S, Shah KV, et al (1991) Evaluation of histologic, morphometric, and immunohistochemical criteria in the differential diagnosis of small cell carcinomas of the cervix with particular reference to human papillomavirus types 16 and 18. Mod Pathol 4:586–593
11. Andersen ES, Nielsen K, Pedersen B (1995) The reliability of preconization diagnostic evaluation in patients with cervical intraepithelial neoplasia and microinvasive carcinoma. Gynecol Oncol 59:143–147
12. Anderson MC (1987) Are we vapourising microinvasive lesions? Colposcopy Gynecol Laser Surg 3: 33–36
13. Angel C, DuBeshter B, Lin JY (1992) Clinical pre sentation and management of stage I cervical adenocarcinoma: a 25 year experience. Gynecol Oncol 44:71–78
14. Anton-Culver H, Bloss JD, Bringman D, et al (1992) Comparison of adenocarcinoma and squamous cell carcinoma of the uterine cervix: a population based epidemiologic study. Am J Obstet Gynecol 166: 1507–1514
15. Atkin NB, Baker MC, Fox MF (1990) Chromosome changes in 43 carcinomas of the cervix uteri. Cancer Genet Cytogenet 44:229–241
16. Attanoos R, Nahar K, Bigrigg A, et al (1995) Primary adenocarcinoma of the cervix. A clinical pathologic study of prognostic variables in 55 cases. Int J Gynecol Cancer 5:179–186
17. Averette HE, Nelson JH, Ng AP, et al (1976) Diagnosis and management of microinvasive (stage IA) carcinoma of the uterine cervix. Cancer (Phila) 38: 414–425
18. Barnes RC, Coulter J, Worrall DM (2000) Immunoreactivity of recombinant squamous cell carcinoma antigen and leupin/SCCA-2: implications for tumor marker detection. Gynecol Oncol 78:62–66
19. Barnes W, Delgado G, Kurman RJ, et al (1988) Possible prognostic significance of human papillomavirus type in cervical cancer. Gynecol Oncol 29: 267–273
20. Barrett RJ, Davos I, Leuchter RS, et al (1987) Neuroendocrine features in poorly differentiated and undifferentiated carcinomas of the cervix. Cancer (Phila) 60:2325–2330
21. Barsky SH, Siegel GP, Jannotta F, et al (1983) Loss of basement membrane components by invasive tumors but not by their benign counterparts. Lab Invest 49:140–147
22. Benda JA, Platz CE, Bushsbaum H, et al (1985) Mucin production in defining mixed carcinoma of the uterine cervix: a clinicopathologic study. Int J Gynecol Pathol 4:314–327
23. Benedet JL, Anderson GH (1996) Stage IA carcinoma of the cervix revisited. Obstet Gynecol 87: 1052–1059
24. Benedet JL, Anderson GH, Boyes DA (1985) Colposcopic accuracy in the diagnosis of microinvasive and occult invasive carcinoma of the cervix. Obstet Gynecol 65:557–562
25. Benedet JL, Bender H, Jones H III, et al (2000) FIGO staging classifications and clinical practice guidelines in the management of gynecologic cancers. FIGO Committee on Gynecologic Oncology. Int J Gynaecol Obstet 70:209–262
26. Benson WL, Norris HJ (1977) A critical review of the frequency of lymph node metastasis and death from microinvasive carcinoma of the cervix. Obstet Gynecol 49:632–638
27. Berek JS, Hacker NF, Fu YS, et al (1985) Adenocarcinoma of the uterine cervix: histologic variables associated with lymph node metastases and survival. Obstet Gynecol 65:46–52
28. Berkowitz RS, Ehrmann RL, Lavizzo-Mourey R, et al (1979) Invasive cervical carcinoma in young women. Gynecol Oncol 8:311–316
29. Bethwaite P, Yeong ML, Holloway L, et al (1992) The prognosis of adenosquamous carcinomas of the uterine cervix. Br J Obstet Gynecol 99:745–750

30. Bohm JW, Krupp PJ, Lee FYL, et al (1976) Lymph node metastasis in microinvasive epidermoid cancer of the cervix. Obstet Gynecol 48:65–67
31. Bokhman JV, Urmancheyeva AF (1989) Cervix uteri cancer and pregnancy. Eur J Gynaecol Oncol 10: 406–411
32. Bosch FX, Manos MM, Munoz N, et al (1995) Prevalence of human papillomavirus in cervical cancer: a worldwide perspective. International biological study on cervical cancer (IBSCC) Study Group. J Natl Cancer Inst 87:779–780
33. Boyes DA, Worth AJ, Fidler HK (1970) The results of treatment of 4389 cases of preclinical squamous carcinoma. J Obstet Gynecol Br Commonw 77:769
34. Brady LW, O'Neill EA, Farber SH (1977) Unusual sites of metastasis. Semin Oncol 4:59–64
35. Brainard JA, Hart WR (1998) Adenoid basal epitheliomas of the uterine cervix: a reevaluation of distinctive cervical basaloid lesions currently classified as adenoid basal carcinoma and adenoid basal hyperplasia. Am J Surg Pathol 22:965–975
36. Brinck U, Jakob C, Bau O, et al (2000) Papillary squamous cell carcinoma of the uterine cervix: report of three cases and a review of its classification. Int J Gynecol Pathol 19:231–235
37. Brinton LA, Huggins GR, Lehman HF, et al (1986) Long-term use of oral contraceptives and risk of invasive cervical cancer. Int J Cancer 38:399–344
38. Brinton LA, Tashima KT, Lehman HF, et al (1987) Epidemiology of cervical cancer by cell type. Cancer Res 47:1706–1711
39. Broders AC (1920) Squamous-cell epithelioma of the lip: a study of five hundred and thirty-seven cases. JAMA 74:656–664
40. Buckley CF, Fox H (1992) Pathology of clinically invasive cervical cancer. In: Coppleson M (ed) Gynecological oncology. Churchill Livingstone, Edinburgh, pp 649–662
41. Buckley CH, Beards CS, Fox H (1988) Pathological prognostic indicators in cervical cancer with particular reference to patients under the age of 40 years. Br J Obstet Gynecol 95:47–56
42. Buckley JD, Harris RW, Doll R, et al (1981) Case-control study of the husbands of women with dysplasia or carcinoma of the cervix uteri. Lancet ii: 1010–1015
43. Buckley SL, Tritz DM, Van Le L, et al (1996) Lymph node metastases and prognosis in patients with stage IA2 cervical cancer. Gynecol Oncol 63:4–9
44. Bulmer JN, Griffin NR, Bates C, et al (1990) Minimal deviation adenocarcinoma (adenoma malignum) of the endocervix: a histochemical and immunohistochemical study of two cases. Gastroenterology 36:139–146
45. Burger JPM, Hollema H, Gouw ASH, et al (1993) Cigarette smoking and human papillomavirus in patients with reported cervical cytological abnormality. Br Med J 306:749
46. Burger RA, Monk BJ, Kurosaki T, et al (1996) Human papillomavirus type 18: association with poor prognosis in early stage cervical cancer. J Natl Cancer Inst 88:1361–1368
47. Burghardt E, Baltzer J, Tulusan H, et al (1992) Results of surgical treatment of 1028 cervical cancers studied with volumetry. Cancer (Phila) 70:648–655
48. Burghardt E, Girardi F, Lahousen M, et al (1991) Microinvasive carcinoma of the uterine cervix (International Federation of Gynecology and Obstetrics stage IA). Cancer (Phila) 67:1037–1045
49. Burghardt E, Holzer E (1977) Diagnosis and treatment of microinvasive carcinoma of the uterine cervix. Obstet Gynecol 49:641–653
50. Cantuaria G, Angioli R, Nahmias J, et al (1999) Primary malignant melanoma of the uterine cervix: case report and review of the literature. Gynecol Oncol 75:170–174
51. Carmichael JA, Clarke DH, Moher D, et al (1986) Cervical carcinoma of women aged 34 and younger. Am J Obstet Gynecol 154:264–269
52. Cenacchi G, Pasquinelli G, Montanaro L, et al (1998) Primary endocervical extraosseous Ewing's sarcoma/PNET. Int J Gynecol Pathol 17:83–88
53. Chen RJ, Lin YH, Chen CA, et al (1999) Influence of histologic type and age on survival rates for invasive cervical carcinoma in Taiwan. Gynecol Oncol 73:184–190
54. Chichareon S, Herrero R, Munoz N, et al (1998) Risk factors for cervical cancer in Thailand: a case-control study. J Natl Cancer Inst 90:50–57
55. Cho NH, Joo HJ, Ahn HJ, et al (1998) Detection of human papillomavirus in warty carcinoma of the uterine cervix: comparison of immunohistochemistry, in situ hybridization and in situ polymerase chain reaction methods. Pathol Res Pract 194:713–720
56. Chung CK, Stryker JA, Ward SP, et al (1981) Histologic grade and prognosis of carcinoma of the cervix. Obstet Gynecol 57:636–642
57. Clement PB, Scully RE (1974) Mullerian adenosarcoma of the uterus. A clinicopathologic analysis of ten cases of a distinctive type of mullerian mixed tumor. Cancer (Phila) 34:1138–1149
58. Clement PB, Scully RE (1982) Carcinoma of the cervix: histologic types. Semin Oncol 9:251–264
59. Clement PB, Young RH, Keh P, et al (1995) Malignant mesonephric neoplasms of the uterine cervix. A report of eight cases, including four with a malignant spindle cell component. Am J Surg Pathol 19:1158–1171
60. Clement PB, Zubovits JT, Young RH, et al (1998) Malignant mullerian mixed tumors of the uterine cervix: a report of nine cases of a neoplasm with morphology often different from its counterpart in the corpus. Int J Gynecol Pathol 17:211–222
61. Cohen C, Shulman G, Budgeon LR (1982) Endocervical and endometrial adenocarcinoma. Am J Surg Pathol 6:151–157
62. Colgan TJ, Auger M, McLaughlin JR (1993) Histopathologic classification of cervical carcinomas and recognition of mucin-secreting squamous carcinoma. Int J Gynecol Pathol 12:64–69

63. Copeland LJ, Silva EG, Gershenson DM, et al (1992) Superficially invasive squamous cell carcinoma of the cervix. Gynecol Oncol 45:307–312
64. Coppleson M (1992) Early invasive squamous and adenocarcinoma of the cervix (FIGO stage Ia): clinical features and management. In: Coppleson M (ed) Gynecological oncology. Churchill Livingstone, Edinburgh, pp 631–648
65. Costa MJ, McIlnay KR, Trelford J (1995) Cervical carcinoma with glandular differentiation: histological evaluation predicts disease recurrence in clinical stage I or II patients. Hum Pathol 26:829–837
66. Cramer DW (1974) The role of cervical cytology in the declining morbidity and mortality of cervical cancer. Cancer (Phila) 34:2018–2027
67. Crawford RA, Caldwell C, Iles RK, et al (1998) Prognostic significance of the bcl-2 apoptotic family of proteins in primary and recurrent cervical cancer. Br J Cancer 78:210–214
68. Creasman WF, Fetter BF, Clarke-Pearson DL, et al (1985) Management of stage IA carcinoma of the cervix. Am J Obstet Gynecol 153:164–172
69. Crissman JD, Budhraja M, Aron BS, et al (1987) Histopathologic prognostic factors in stage II and III squamous cell carcinoma of the uterine cervix: an evaluation of 91 patients treated primarily with radiation therapy. Int J Gynecol Pathol 6:97–103
70. Crum CP (1993) Papillomavirus-related changes and premalignant and malignant squamous lesions of the uterine cervix. In: Clement PB, Young RH (eds) Tumors and tumorlike lesions of the uterine corpus and cervix. Churchill Livingstone, New York, pp 51–83
71. Cuzick J, Terry G, Ho L, et al (2000) Association between high-risk HPV types, HLA DRB1* and DQB1* alleles and cervical cancer in British women. Br J Cancer 82:1348–1352
72. Czernobilsky B, Kessler I, Lancet M (1974) Cervical adenocarcinoma in a woman on long-term contraceptives. Obstet Gynecol 1974:517–521
73. Czernobilsky B, Moll R, Franke WW, et al (1984) Intermediate filaments of normal and neoplastic tissues of the female genital tract with emphasis on problems of differential diagnosis. Pathol Res Pract 179:31–37
74. D'Ardenne AJ (1989) Use of basement membrane markers in tumour diagnosis. J Clin Pathol 42: 449–457
75. Dabbs DJ, Geisinger KR, Norris HT (1986) Intermediate filaments in endometrial and endocervical carcinomas. Am J Surg Pathol 10:568–576
76. Davis JR, Moon LB (1975) Increased incidence of adenocarcinoma of uterine cervix. Obstet Gynecol 45:79–83
77. Delgado G, Bundy B, Zaino R, et al (1990) Prospective surgical-pathological study of disease-free interval in patients with stage IB squamous cell carcinoma of the cervix: a Gynecologic Oncology Group study. Gynecol Oncol 38:352–357
78. Delgado G, Bundy BN, Fowler WCJ, et al (1989) A prospective surgical pathological study of stage I squamous carcinoma of the cervix: a Gynecologic Oncology Group Study. Gynecol Oncol 35:314–320
79. Dellas A, Schultheiss E, Holzgreve W, et al (1997) Investigation of the bcl-2 and c-myc expression in relationship to the ki-67 labelling index in cervical intraepithelial neoplasia. Int J Gynecol Pathol 16: 212–218
80. Devesa SS, Young JL Jr, Brinton LA, et al (1989) Recent trends in cervix uteri cancer. Cancer (Phila) 64:2184–2190
81. Dimitrakakis C, Kymionis G, Diakomanolis E, et al (2000) The possible role of p53 and bcl-2 expression in cervical carcinomas and their premalignant lesions. Gynecol Oncol 77:129–136
82. Dinh TV, Woodruff JD (1985) Adenoid cystic and adenoid basal carcinomas of the cervix. Obstet Gynecol 65:705–709
83. Dyson JED, Joslin CAF, Rothwell RI, et al (1987) Flow cytofluorometric evidence for the differential radioresponsiveness of aneuploid and diploid cervix tumors. Radiother Oncol 8:263–272
84. Eifel PJ, Burke RW, Morris M, et al (1995) Adenocarcinoma as an independent risk factor for disease recurrence in patients with stage 1B cervical carcinoma. Gynecol Oncol 59:38–44
85. Eifel PJ, Morris M, Oswald MJ, et al (1990) Adenocarcinoma of the uterine cervix. Prognosis and patterns of failure in 367 cases. Cancer (Phila) 65: 2507–2514
86. Faaborg LL, Smith ML, Newland JR (1979) Case report: uterine cervical and vaginal verrucous squamous cell carcinoma. Gynecol Oncol 8:104–109
87. Ferenczy A, Richard RM (1974) Female reproductive system. Dynamics of scan and transmission electron microscopy. John Wiley & Sons, New York
88. Ferry JA (1997) Adenoid basal carcinoma of the uterine cervix: evolution of a distinctive clinicopathologic entity. Int J Gynecol Pathol 16:299–300
89. Ferry JA, Scully RE (1988) "Adenoid cystic" carcinoma and adenoid basal carcinoma of the uterine cervix. A study of 28 cases. Am J Surg Pathol 12: 134–144
90. Ferry JA, Scully RE (1990) Mesonephric remnants, hyperplasia, and neoplasia in the uterine cervix. A study of 49 cases. Am J Surg Pathol 14:1100–1111
91. Fetissof F, Berger G, Dubois MP, et al (1985) Endocrine cells in the female genital tract. Histopathology (Oxf) 9:133–145
92. Finck FM, Denk M (1970) Cervical carcinoma: relationship between histology and survival following radiation therapy. Obstet Gynecol 116:339–343
93. Flint A, McCoy JP, Schade W, et al (1988) Cervical carcinoma antigen: distribution in neoplastic lesions of the uterine cervix and comparison to other tumor markers. Gynecol Oncol 30:63–70
94. Fu YS, Regan JW, Fu AS, et al (1982) Adenocarcinoma and mixed carcinoma of the uterine cervix. II. Prognostic value of nuclear DNA analysis. Cancer (Phila) 49:2571–2577

95. Fujiwara H, Mitchell MF, Arseneau J, et al (1995) Clear cell adenosquamous carcinoma of the cervix. An aggressive tumor associated with human papillomavirus 18. Cancer (Phila) 76:1591–1600
96. Fujiwara H, Tortolero-Luna G, Mitchell MF, et al (1997) Adenocarcinoma of the cervix. Expression and clinical significance of estrogen and progesterone receptors. Cancer (Phila) 79:505–512
97. Gallup DG, Harper RH, Stock RJ (1985) Poor prognosis in patients with adenosquamous cell carcinoma of the cervix. Obstet Gynecol 65:416–422
98. Gersell DJ, Mazoujian G, Mutch DG, et al (1988) Small-cell undifferentiated carcinoma of the cervix. A clinico-pathologic, ultrastructural, and immunocytochemical study of 15 cases. Am J Surg Pathol 12:684–698
99. Gilks CB, Clement PB (1992) Papillary serous adenocarcinoma of the uterine cervix: a report of three cases. Mod Pathol 5:426–431
100. Gilks CB, Young RH, Aguirre P, et al (1989) Adenoma malignum (minimal deviation adenocarcinoma) of the uterine cervix. A clinicopathological and immunohistochemical analysis of 26 cases. Am J Surg Pathol 13:717–729
101. Gilks CB, Young RH, Gersell DJ, et al (1997) Large cell neuroendocrine carcinoma of the uterine cervix: a clinicopathologic study of 12 cases. Am J Surg Pathol 21:905–914
102. Glucksmann A, Cherry CP (1956) Incidence, histology and response to radiation of mixed carcinomas (adenocanthomas) of the uterine cervix. Cancer (Phila) 9:971
103. Grayson W, Taylor L, Cooper K (1996) Detection of integrated high risk human papillomavirus in adenoid cystic carcinoma of the uterine cervix. J Clin Pathol 49:805–809
104. Grayson W, Taylor LF, Cooper K (1999) Adenoid cystic and adenoid basal carcinoma of the uterine cervix: comparative morphologic, mucin, and immunohistochemical profile of two rare neoplasms of putative 'reserve cell' origin. Am J Surg Pathol 23:448–458
105. Greer BE, Figge DC, Tamimi HK, et al (1990) Stage IA2 squamous carcinoma of the cervix: a difficult diagnosis and therapeutic dilemma. Am J Obstet Gynecol 162:1406–1411
106. Groben P, Reddick R, Askin F (1985) The pathologic spectrum of small cell carcinoma of the cervix. Int J Gynecol Pathol 4:42–57
107. Hafix MA, Kragel PJ, Toker C (1985) Carcinoma of the uterine cervix resembling lymphoepithelioma. Obstet Gynecol 66:829–831
108. Hakama M (1997) Screening for cervical cancer: experience of the Nordic countries. In: Franco E, Monsonego J (eds) New developments in cervical cancer screening and prevention. Blackwell, London, pp 190–199
109. Hale RJ, Wilcox FL, Buckley CH, et al (1991) Prognostic factors in uterine cervical carcinoma: a clinicopathological analysis. Int J Gynecol Cancer 1: 19–23
110. Halpin TF, Hunter RE, Cohen MB (1989) Lymphoepithelioma of the uterine cervix. Gynecol Oncol 34:101–105
111. Hannigan EV (1990) Cervical cancer in pregnancy. Clin Obst Gynecol 33:837–845
112. Hanselaar A, van Loosbroek M, Schuurbiers O, et al (1997) Clear cell adenocarcinoma of the vagina and cervix. An update of the central Netherlands registry showing twin age incidence peaks. Cancer (Phila) 79:2229–2236
113. Hanselaar AG, Vooijs GP, Oud PS, et al (1988) DNA ploidy patterns in cervical intraepithelial neoplasia grade III, with and without synchronous invasive squamous cell carcinoma: Measurements in nuclei isolated from paraffin-embedded tissue. Cancer (Phila) 62:2537–2545
114. Hart WR, Norris HJ (1972) Mesonephric adenocarcinomas of the cervix. Cancer (Phila) 29:106–113
115. Hasumi K, Sakamoto A, Sugano H (1980) Microinvasive carcinoma of the uterine cervix. Cancer (Phila) 45:928–931
116. Hatch EE, Palmer JR, Titus-Ernstoff L, et al (1998) Cancer risk in women exposed to diethylstilbestrol in utero. JAMA 280:630–634
117. Hayashi Y, Hachisuga T, Iwasaka T, et al (1991) Expression of ras oncogene product and EGF receptor in cervical squamous cell carcinomas and its relationship to lymph node involvement. Gynecol Oncol 40:147–151
118. Helper TK, Dockerty MB, Randall LM (1952) Primary adenocarcinoma of the cervix. Am J Obstet Gynecol 63:800–808
119. Herbst AL, Cole P, Norusis MJ, et al (1979) Epidemiologic aspects and factors related to survival in 384 registry cases of clear cell adenocarcinoma of the vagina and cervix. Am J Obstet Gynecol 135: 876–886
120. Hirai Y, Takeshima N, Haga A, et al (1998) A clinicocytopathologic study of adenoma malignum of the uterine cervix. Gynecol Oncol 70:219–223
121. Holowaty P, Miller AB, Rohan T, et al (1999) Natural history of dysplasia of the uterine cervix. J Natl Cancer Inst 91:252–258
122. Hopkins MP, Morley GW (1991) A comparison of adenocarcinoma and squamous cell carcinoma of the cervix. Obstet Gynecol 77:912–917
123. Hopkins MP, Morley GW (1991) Stage 1B squamous cell cancer of the cervix: clinicopathologic features related to survival. Am J Obstet Gynecol 164:1520–1529
124. Hopkins MP, Schmidt RW, Roberts JA, et al (1988) Gland cell carcinoma (adenocarcinoma) of the cervix. Obstet Gynecol 72:789–795
125. Hopson L, Jones MA, Boyce CR, et al (1990) Papillary villoglandular carcinoma of the cervix. Gynecol Oncol 39:221–224
126. Horn LC, Fishcer U, Bilek K (1997) Primitive neuroectodermal tumor of the cervix uteri. A case report. Gen Diagn Pathol 142:227–230

127. Howe DT, Vincenti AC (1991) Is large loop excision of the transformation zone (LLETZ) more accurate than colposcopically directed punch biopsy in the diagnosis of cervical intraepithelial neoplasia? Br J Obstet Gynecol 98:588–591
128. Huffman JW (1948) Mesonephric remnants in the cervix. Am J Obstet Gynecol 56:23–40
129. Hurt WG, Silverberg SG, Frable WJ, et al (1977) Adenocarcinoma of the cervix: histopathologic and clinical features. Am J Obstet Gynecol 129:304–315
130. IARC (1995) Human papillomaviruses. IARC, Lyons. 64:407
131. Ikenberg H, Teufel G, Schmitt B, et al (1993) Human papillomavirus DNA in distant metastases of carcinoma cancer. Gynecol Oncol 48:56–60
132. Inoue T (1984) Prognostic significance of the depth of invasion relating to nodal metastases, parametrial extension and cell types. A study of 628 cases with stage Ib, IIa, and IIB cervical carcinoma. Cancer (Phila) 54:3035–3042
133. Inoue T, Morita K (1990) The prognostic significance of number of positive nodes in cervical carcinoma stages IB, IIA, and IIB. Cancer (Phila) 65: 1923–1927
134. Iwasawa A, Nieminen P, Lehtinen M, et al (1996) Human papillomavirus DNA in uterine cervix squamous cell carcinoma and adenocarcinoma detected by polymerase chain reaction. Cancer (Phila) 77:2275–2279
135. Janerich DT, Hadjimichael O, Schwarz PE, et al (1995) The screening histories of women with invasive cervical cancer, Connecticut. Am J Public Health 85:791–794
136. Jarrell MA, Heintz N, Howard P, et al (1992) Squamous cell carcinoma of the cervix: HPV 16 and DNA ploidy as predictors of survival. Gynecol Oncol 46:361–366
137. Jelen I, Valente PT, Gautreaux L, et al (1994) Deoxyribonucleic acid ploidy and S-phase fraction are not significant prognostic factors for patients with cervical cancer. Am J Obstet Gynecol 171:1511–1516
138. Jones MW, Kounelis S, Papadaki H, et al (1997) The origin and molecular characterization of adenoid basal carcinoma of the uterine cervix. Int J Gynecol Pathol 16:301–306
139. Jones MW, Kounelis S, Papadaki H, et al (2000) Well-differentiated villoglandular adenocarcinoma of the uterine cervix: oncogene/tumor suppressor gene alterations and human papillomavirus genotyping. Int J Gynecol Pathol 19:110–117
140. Jones MW, Lefkowitz M (1995) Adenosarcoma of the uterine cervix: a clinicopathological study of 12 cases. Int J Gynecol Pathol 14:223–229
141. Jones MW, Silverberg SG (1989) Cervical adenocarcinoma in young women: possible relationship to microglandular hyperplasia and use of oral contraceptives. Obstet Gynecol 73:984–989
142. Jones MW, Silverberg SG, Kurman RJ (1992) Well-differentiated villoglandular adenocarcinoma of the uterine cervix: A clinicopathological study of 24 cases. Int J Gynecol Pathol 12:1–7
143. Jones MW, Silverberg SG, Kurman RJ (1993) Well differentiated villoglandular adenocarcinoma of the uterine cervix: a clinicopathological study of 24 cases. Int J Gynecol Pathol 12:1–7
144. Jones WB, Mercer GO, Lewis JL, et al (1993) Early invasive carcinoma of the cervix. Gynecol Oncol 51: 26–32
145. Jones WB, Shingleton HM, Russell A, et al (1996) Cervical carcinoma and pregnancy. A national patterns of care study of the American College of Surgoens. Cancer (Phila) 77:1479–1488
146. Jones WH, Droegemueller W, Makowski ELA (1971) A primary melanocarcinoma of the cervix. Obstet Gynecol 111:959
147. Junor EJ, Symonds RP, Watson ER, et al (1989) Survival of younger cervical carcinoma patients treated by radical radiotherapy in the West of Scotland 1964–1984. Br J Obstet Gynecol 92:522–528
148. Kaku T, Enjoji M (1983) Extremely well-differentiated adenocarcinoma ("adenoma malignum") of the cervix. Int J Gynecol Pathol 2:28–41
149. Kaku T, Kamura T, Sakai K, et al (1997) Early adenocarcinoma of the uterine cervix. Gynecol Oncol 65:281–285
150. Kaku T, Kamura T, Shigematsu T, et al (1997) Adenocarcinoma of the uterine cervix with predominantly villoglandular papillary growth pattern. Gynecol Oncol 64:147–152
151. Kaminski PF, Maier RC (1983) Clear cell adenocarcinoma of the cervix unrelated to diethylstilbestrol exposure. Obstet Gynecol 62:720–727
152. Kaminski PF, Norris HJ (1983) Minimal deviation carcinoma (adenoma malignum) of the cervix. Int J Gynecol Pathol 2:141–152
153. Kaminski PF, Norris HJ (1984) Coexistence of ovarian neoplasms and endocervical adenocarcinoma. Obstet Gynecol 64:553–556
154. Kashimura M, Tsukamoto N, Matsukuma K, et al (1984) Verrucous carcinoma of the uterine cervix: report of a case with follow-up of $6^1/_2$ years. Gynecol Oncol 19:204–215
155. Katz HJ, Davies JNP (1980) Death from cervix uteri carcinoma: the changing pattern. Gynecol Oncol 9: 86–89
156. Kenter GG, Cornelisse CJ, Aartsen EJ, et al (1990) DNA ploidy levels as prognostic factor in low stage carcinoma of the uterine cervix. Gynecol Oncol 39:181–185
157. Kerner H, Lichtig C (1993) Mullerian adenosarcoma presenting as cervical polyps: a report of seven cases and review in the literature. Obstet Gynecol 81:655–659
158. Kersemaekers AM, Fleuren GJ, Kenter GG, et al (1999) Oncogene alterations in carcinomas of the uterine cervix: overexpression of the epidermal growth factor receptor is associated with poor prognosis. Clin Cancer Res 5:577–586
159. Ketcham AS, Hoye RC, Taylor PT, et al (1971) Radical hysterectomy and pelvic lymphadenectomy for carcinoma of the uterine cervix. Cancer (Phila) 28: 1272–1277

160. Keys HM, Bundy BN, Stehman FB, et al (1999) Cisplatin, radiation, and adjuvant hysterectomy compared with radiation and adjuvant hysterectomy for bulky stage IB cervical carcinoma. N Engl J Med 340:1154–1161
161. Kilkku P, Gronroos M (1982) Perioperative electrocoagulation of endocervical mucosa and later carcinomas of the cervical stump. Acta Obstet Gynecol Scand 61:265–267
162. Killackey MA, Jones WB, Lewis JL (1986) Diagnostic conization of the cervix: review of 460 consecutive cases. Obstet Gynecol 67:766–770
163. Kinney W, Sung HY, Kearney KA, et al (1998) Missed opportunities for cervical cancer screening of HMO members developing invasive cervical cancer (ICC). Gynecol Oncol 71:428–430
164. Kjaer SK, Brinton LA (1993) Adenocarcinomas of the uterine cervix: the epidemiology of an increasing problem. Epidemiol Rev 15:486–498
165. Kleine W, Rau K, Schwoeorer D, et al (1989) Prognosis of the adenocarcinoma of the cervix uteri: a comparative study. Gynecol Oncol 35:145–149
166. Koenig C, Turnicky RP, Kankam CF, et al (1997) Papillary squamotransitional cell carcinoma of the cervix: a report of 32 cases. Am J Surg Pathol 21:915–921
167. Kolstad P (1989) Follow-up study of 232 patients with stage IA1 and 411 patients with stage IA2 squamous cell carcinoma of the cervix (microinvasive carcinoma). Gynecol Oncol 33:265–272
168. Korhonen M and Stenback F (1984) Adenocarcinoma metastatic to the uterine cervix. Gynecol Obstet Invest 17:57–65
169. Koss LG (1992) Diagnostic cytology and its histopathologic basis, vol 1. JB Lippincott, New York
170. Koulos J, Wright TC, Follen MM, et al (1993) Relationships between cKi-ras mutations, HPV types and prognostic indicators in invasive endocervical adenocarcinomas. Gynecol Oncol 48:364–369
171. Kristensen GB, Abeler VM, Risberg B, et al (1999) Tumor size, depth of invasion, and grading of the invasive tumor front are the main prognostic factors in early squamous cell cervical carcinoma. Gynecol Oncol 74:245–251
172. Kristensen GB, Holm R, Abeler VM, et al (1996) Evaluation of the prognostic significance of cathepsin D, epidermal growth factor receptor, and c-erbB-2 in early cervical squamous cell carcinoma. An immunohistochemical study. Cancer (Phila) 78: 433–440
173. Kudo R, Sasano H, Koizumi M, et al (1990) Immunohistochemical comparison of new monoclonal antibody IC5 and carcinoembryonic antigen in the differential diagnosis of adenocarcinoma of the uterine cervix. Int J Gynecol Pathol 9:325–336
174. Kurman RJ, Norris HJ, Wilkinson E (1992) Atlas of tumor pathology, third series, fas 4. Tumors of the cervix, vagina and vulva. Armed Forces Institute of Pathology, Washington, DC
175. Lacey JV Jr, Brinton LA, Abbas FM, et al (1999) Oral contraceptives as risk factors for cervical adenocarcinomas and squamous cell carcinomas. Cancer Epidemiol Biomark Prev 8:1079–1085
176. Lacey JV Jr, Brinton LA, Barnes WA, et al (2000) Use of hormone replacement therapy and adenocarcinomas and squamous cell carcinomas of the uterine cervix. Gynecol Oncol 77:149–154
177. Lathrop JC (1967) Views and reviews: malignant pelvic lymphomas. Obstet Gynecol 30:137
178. Lee KR, Flynn CE (2000) Early invasive adenocarcinoma of the cervix. Cancer (Phila) 89:1048–1055
179. Leman MH, Benson WL, Kurman RJ, et al (1976) Microinvasive carcinoma of the cervix. Obstet Gynecol 48:571
180. Leminen A, Paavonen J, Forss M, et al (1990) Adenocarcinoma of the uterine cervix. Cancer (Phila) 65:53–59
181. Lemoine NR, Hall PA (1986) Epithelial tumors metastatic to the uterine cervix. A study of 33 cases and review of the literature. Cancer (Phila) 57: 2238
182. Lin H, Chang Chien CC, Huang EY, et al (2000) The role of pretreatment squamous cell carcinoma antigen in predicting nodal metastasis in early stage cervical cancer. Acta Obstet Gynecol Scand 79:140–144
183. Lindell A (1952) Carcinoma of the uterine cervix: incidence and influence of age. A statistical study. Acta Radiol Suppl 92:1–102
184. Lizano M, Berumen J, Guido MC, et al (1997) Association between human papillomavirus type 18 variants and histopathology of cervical cancer. J Natl Cancer Inst 89:1227–1231
185. Lucas WE, Benirschke K, Lebherz RB (1974) Verrucous carcinoma of the female genital tract. Am J Obstet Gynecol 119:435–440
186. Lucia SP, Mills H, Lowenhaupt E, et al (1952) Visceral involvement in primary neoplastic diseases of the reticuloendothelial system. Cancer (Phila) 5: 1193
187. Luesley DM, Cullimore J, Redman CWE, et al (1990) Loop diathermy excision of the cervical transformation zone in patients with abnormal cervical smears. Br Med J 300:1690–1693
188. Maes G, Fleuren GJ, Bara J, et al (1988) The distribution of mucins, carcinoembryonic antigen, and mucus-associated antigens in endocervical and endometrial adenocarcinomas. Int J Gynecol Pathol 7:112–122
189. Maier RC, Norris HJ (1982) Glassy cell carcinoma of the cervix. Obstet Gynecol 60:219–224
190. Maiman M, Fruchter RG, DiMaio TM, et al (1988) Superficially invasive squamous cell carcinoma of the cervix. Obstet Gynecol 72:399–403
191. Mandai M, Konishi I, Koshiyama M, et al (1995) Altered expression of nm23-H1 and *c*-erbB-2 proteins have prognostic significance in adenocarcinoma but not in squamous cell carcinoma of the uterine cervix. Cancer (Phila) 75:2523–2529
192. Marcial WA, Bosch A (1970) Radiation-induced tumor regression in carcinoma of the uterine

cervix. Prognostic significance. Am J Roentgenol 108:113–124
193. Mathoulin-Portier MP, Penault-Llorca F, Labit-Bouvier C, et al (1998) Malignant mullerian mixed tumor of the uterine cervix with adenoid cystic component. Int J Gynecol Pathol 17:91–92
194. Mazur MT, Battifora HA (1982) Adenoid cystic carcinoma of the uterine cervix: ultrastructure, immunofluorescence and criteria for diagnosis. Am J Clin Pathol 77:494–500
195. McGowan L, Young RH, Scully RE (1980) Peutz-Jeghers syndrome with "adenoma malignum" of the cervix. A report of two cases. Gynecol Oncol 10: 125–133
196. McIndoe GA, Robson MS, Tidy JA, et al (1989) Laser excision rather than vaporization: the treatment of choice for cervical intraepithelial neoplasia. Obstet Gynecol 74:165–168
197. Meanwell CA, Kelly KA, Wilson S, et al (1988) Young age as a prognostic factor in cervical cancer: analysis of population based data from 10,022 cases. Br Med J 296:386–391
198. Mestwerdt G (1947) Probeexzision und kolpposkopie in des fruhdiagnose des portiokarcinoms. Zentralb Gynaekol 4:326
199. Michael H, Grawe L, Kraus FT (1984) Minimal deviation endocervical adenocarcinoma: clinical and histologic features, immunohistochemical staining for carcinoembryonic antigen, and differentiation from confusing benign lesions. Int J Gynecol Pathol 3:261–276
200. Mikuta JJ, Celebre JA (1969) Adenocarcinoma of the cervix. Obstet Gynecol 33:753–756
201. Mitchell MF, Tortolero-Luna G, Wright T, et al (1996) Cervical human papillomavirus infection and intraepithelial neoplasia: a review. J Natl Cancer Inst Monogr 21:17–25
202. Morgan PR, Anderson MC, Buckley CH, et al (1993) The Royal College of Obstetricians and Gynaecologists micro-invasive carcinoma of the cervix study: preliminary results. Br J Obstet Gynaecol 100: 664–668
203. Morimura Y, Honda T, Hoshi K, et al (1995) A case of uterine cervical adenoid cystic carcinoma: immunohistochemical study for basement membrane material. Obstet Gynecol 85:903–905
204. Morris M, Eifel PJ, Lu J, et al (1999) Pelvic radiation with concurrent chemotherapy compared with pelvic and para-aortic radiation for high-risk cervical cancer. N Engl J Med 340:1137–1143
205. Muntz HG, Ferry JA, Flynn D, et al (1991) Stage IE primary malignant lymphomas of the uterine cervix. Cancer (Phila) 68:2023–2032
206. Murdoch JB, Grimshaw RN, Morgan PR, et al (1992) The impact of loop diathermy on management of early invasive cervical cancer. Int J Gynecol Cancer 2:129–133
207. Musa AG, Hughes RR, Coleman SA (1985) Adenoid cystic carcinoma of the cervix: a report of 17 cases. Gynecol Oncol 22:167–173
208. NCI (2000) SEER Cancer Statistics Review: 1973–1996. 2000
209. Ng ABP, Reagan JW, Lindner EA (1972) The cellular manifestations of microinvasive squamous cell carcinoma of the uterine cervix. Acta Cytol 16:5–13
210. Ngelangel C, Munoz N, Bosch FX, et al (1998) Causes of cervical cancer in the Philippines: a case-control study. J Natl Cancer Inst 90:43–49
211. Nogales F, Bottela-Llusia J (1965) The frequency of invasion of the lymph nodes in cancer of the uteri cervix: a study of the degree of extension in relation to the histological type of tumor. Am J Obstet Gynecol 93:91
212. Noller KL, Decker GG, Dockerty MB, et al (1974) Mesonephric (clear cell) carcinoma of the vagina and cervix. a retrospective analysis. Obstet Gynecol 640–644
213. O'Leary JJ, Landers RJ, Silva I, et al (1998) Molecular analysis of ras oncogenes in CIN III and in stage I and II invasive squamous cell carcinoma of the uterine cervix. J Clin Pathol 51:576–582
214. Oliva E, Ferry JA, Young RH, et al (1997) Granulocytic sarcoma of the female genital tract: a clinicopathologic study of 11 cases. Am J Surg Pathol 21:1156–1165
215. Ostor A, Rome R, Quinn M (1997) Microinvasive adenocarcinoma of the cervix: a clinicopathologic study of 77 women. Obstet Gynecol 89:88–93
216. Ostor AG (1993) Natural history of cervical intraepithelial neoplasia: a critical review. Int J Gynecol Pathol 12:186–192
217. Parazzini F, Franceschi S, La Vecchia C, et al (1997) The epidemiology of female genital tract cancers. Int. J. Gynecol. Cancer (Phila) 7:169–181
218. Parazzini F, La Vecchia C (1990) Epidemiology of adenocarcinoma of the cervix. Gynecol Oncol 39: 40–46
219. Parazzini F, La Vecchia C, Negri E, et al (1988) Risk factors for adenocarcinoma of the cervix: a case-control study. Br J Cancer 57:201–204
220. Parkin DM, Pisani P, Ferlay J (1999) Estimates of the worldwide incidence of 25 major cancers in 1990. Int J Cancer 80:827–841
221. Patnick J (1997) Has screening for cervical cancer been successful? Br J Obstet Gynaecol 104:876–878
222. Patnick J (2000) Cervical cancer screening in England. Eur J Cancer 36:2205–2208
223. Pecorelli S, Benedet JL, Creasman WT, et al (1999) FIGO staging of gynecologic cancer. 1994–1997 FIGO Committee on Gynecologic Oncology. International Federation of Gynecology and Obstetrics. Int J Gynaecol Obstet 64:5–10
224. Peel KR, Khoury GG, Joslin CAF, et al (1991) Cancer of the cervix in women under 40 years of age, a regional survey, 1975–1984. Br J Obstet Gynecol 98:993–1000
225. Peters RK, Chao A, Mack TM, et al (1986) Increased frequency of adenocarcinoma of the uterine cervix in young women in Los Angeles County. J Natl Cancer Inst 76:423–428

226. Pisani P, Parkin DM, Bray F, et al (1999) Estimates of the worldwide mortality from 25 cancers in 1990. Int J Cancer 83:18–29
227. Podczaski E, Kaminski PF, Pees RC, et al (1991) Peutz-Jeghers syndrome with ovarian sex cord tumor with annular tubules and cervical adenoma malignum. Gynecol Oncol 42:74–78
228. Pretorius R, Semrad N, Watring W, et al (1991) Presentation of cervical cancer. Gynecol Oncol 42: 48–53
229. Qizilbash A-H (1975) In situ and microinvasive adenocarcinoma of the uterine cervix. J. Clin. Pathol 64:155–170
230. Raju KS, Kjorstad KE, Abeler V (1991) Prognostic factors in the treatment of stage 1B adenocarcinoma of the cervix. Int J Gynecol Cancer 1:69–74
231. Randall ME, Andersen WA, Mills SE, et al (1986) Papillary squamous cell carcinoma of the uterine cervix: a clinicopathologic study of nine cases. Int J Gynecol Pathol 5:1–10
232. Randall ME, Constable WC, Hahn SS, et al (1988) Results of the radiotherapeutic management of carcinoma of the cervix with emphasis on the influence of histologic classification. Cancer (Phila) 62:48–53
233. Rastkar G, Okagaki T, Twiggs LB, et al (1982) Early invasive and in situ warty carcinoma of the vulva: clinical, histologic, and electron microscopic study with particular reference to viral association. Am J Obstet Gynecol 143:814–820
234. Reagan JW, Ng ABP (1973) The cellular manifestations of uterine carcinogenesis. In: Norris NJ, et al (eds) The uterus. Williams & Wilkins, Baltimore, pp 320–347
235. Report TW (1982) Report of the Task Force of the Department of Health and Welfare of Canada. Cervical Cancer Screening Programs. The Walton Report. Can Med Assoc J 127:581
236. Richard L, Guralnick M, Ferenczy A (1981) Ultrastructure of glassy cell carcinoma of cervix. 3:31–38
237. Riou G, Barrois M, Le MG, et al (1987) c-myc protooncogene expression and prognosis in early carcinoma of the uterine cervix. Lancet i:761–763
238. Riou G, Barrois M, Sheng ZM, et al (1988) Somatic deletions and mutations of c-Ha-*ras* gene in human cervical cancers. Oncogene 3:329–333
239. Riou GF (1988) Protooncogenes and prognosis in early carcinoma of the uterine cervix. Cancer Surv 7:441–456
240. Robboy SJ, Herbst AL, Scully RE (1974) Clear-cell adenocarcinoma of the vagina and carcinoma in young females: analysis of 37 tumors that persisted or recurred after primary therapy. Cancer (Phila) 34:606–614
241. Roche WD, Norris HJ (1975) Microinvasive carcinoma of the cervix. The significance of lymphatic invasion and confluent patterns of stromal growth. Cancer (Phila) 36:180–186
242. Rose BR, Thompson CH, Simpson JM, et al (1995) Human papillomavirus deoxyribonucleic acid as a prognostic indicator in early-stage cervical cancer: a possible role for type 18. Am J Obstet Gynecol 173:1461–1468
243. Rose PG, Bundy BN, Watkins EB, et al (1999) Concurrent cisplatin-based radiotherapy and chemotherapy for locally advanced cervical cancer. N Engl J Med 340:1144–1153
244. Rubio CA (1974) Cytologic studies in cases with carcinoma in situ and microinvasive carcinoma of the uterine cervix. Acta Pathol Microbiol Scand 82: 161–181
245. Rutledge FN, Mitchell MF, Munsell M, et al (1992) Youth as a prognostic factor in carcinoma of the cervix: a matched analysis. Gynecol Oncol 44:123–130
246. Sagae S, Kuzumaki N, Hisada T, et al (1989) ras oncogene expression and prognosis of invasive squamous cell carcinomas of the uterine cervix. Cancer (Phila) 63:1577–1582
247. Saigo PE, Cain JM, Kim WS, et al (1986) Prognostic factors in adenocarcinoma of the uterine cervix. Cancer (Phila) 57:1584–1593
248. Samlal RA, Ten Kate FJ, Hart AA, et al (1998) Do mucin-secreting squamous cell carcinomas of the uterine cervix metastasize more frequently to pelvic lymph nodes? A case-control study? Int J Gynecol Pathol 17:201–204
249. Savargaonkar PR, Hale RJ, Mutton A, et al (1996) Neuroendocrine differentiation in cervical carcinoma. J Clin Pathol 49:139–141
250. Scully RE, Aguirre P, DeLellis RA (1984) Argyrophilia, serotonin, and peptide hormones in the female genital tract and its tumors. Int J Gynecol Pathol 3:51–70
251. Scully RE, Bonfiglio TA, Kurman RJ, et al (1994) Histological typing of female genital tract tumors, 2nd ed. Springer-Verlag, Berlin
252. Sedlis A, Sall S, Tsukada Y, et al (1979) Microinvasive carcinoma of the uterine cervix: a clinical-pathologic study. Am J Obstet Gynecol 133:64–74
253. Seltzer V, Sall S, Castadot MJ, et al (1979) Glassy cell cervical carcinoma. Gynecol Oncol 8:141–151
254. Seski JC, Abell MR, Morley GW (1977) Microinvasive squamous carcinoma of the cervix. Definition, histologic analysis, late results of treatment. Obstet Gynecol 50:410–414
255. Sevin BU, Method MW, Nadji M, et al (1996) Efficacy of radical hysterectomy as treatment for patients with small cell carcinoma of the cervix. Cancer (Phila) 77:1489–1493
256. Sevin BU, Nadji M, Averette HE, et al (1992) Microinvasive carcinoma of the cervix. Cancer (Phila) 70:2121–2128
257. Shingleton HM, Gore H, Bradley DH, et al (1981) Adenocarcinoma of the cervix. I. Clinical evaluation and pathologic features. Am J Obstet Gynecol 139:799–814
258. Silverberg SG, Hurt WG (1975) Minimal deviation adenocarcinoma ("adenoma malignum") of the cervix: a reappraisal. Am J Obstet Gynecol 121: 971–975

259. Simon NL, Gore H, Shingleton HM, et al (1986) Study of superficially invasive carcinoma of the cervix. Obstet Gynecol 68:19–24
260. Skomedal H, Kristensen GB, Lie AK, et al (1999) Aberrant expression of the cell cycle associated proteins TP53, MDM2, p21, p27, cdk4, cyclin D1, RB, and EGFR in cervical carcinomas. Gynecol Oncol 73:223–228
261. Smedts F, Ramaekers F, Troyanovsky S, et al (1992) Keratin expression in cervical cancer. Am J Pathol 141:497–511
262. Smiley LM, Burke TW, Silva EG, et al (1991) Prognostic factors in stage IB squamous cervical cancer patients with low risk for recurrence. Obstet Gynecol 77:271–275
263. Smith HO, Tiffany MF, Qualls CR, et al (2000) The rising incidence of adenocarcinoma relative to squamous cell carcinoma of the uterine cervix in the United States—a 24-year population-based study. Gynecol Oncol 78:97–105
264. Speers WC, Picaso LG, Silverberg SG (1983) Immunohistochemical localization of carcinoembryonic antigen in microglandular hyperplasia and adenocarcinoma of the endocervix. Am J Clin Pathol 79:105–107
265. Sreekantaiah C, De Braekeleer M, Haas O (1991) Cytogenetic findings in cervical carcinoma. A statistical approach. Cancer Genet Cytogenet 53:75–81
266. Staebler , and Ronnett BM (2001) (in press)
267. Stehman FB, Perez CA, Kurman RJ, et al (2000) Uterine cervix In: Hoskins W, et al (eds) Principles and practice of gynecologic oncology. Lippincott, Philadelphia, pp 841–918
268. Stendahl U, Willen H, Willen R (1979) Classification and grading of invasive squamous cell carcinoma of the uterine cervix. Acta Radiol Oncol 18:481–496
269. Stendahl U, Willen H, Willen R (1980) Invasive squamous cell carcinoma of the uterine cervix. I. Definition of parameters in a histopathologic malignancy grading system. Acta Radiol Oncol 19:467–480
270. Stewart CJR, McNicol AM (1992) Distribution of type IV collagen immunoreactivity to assess questionable early stromal invasion. J Clin Pathol 45:9–15
271. Stockler M, Russell P, McGahan S, et al (1996) Prognosis and prognostic factors in node-negative cervix cancer. Int J Gynecol Cancer 6:477–482
272. Swan DS, Roddick JW (1973) A clinical-pathological correlation of cell type classification for cervical cancer. Am J Obstet Gynecol 116:666–670
273. Szczepulska E, Nasierowska-Guttmejer A, Bidzinski M (1999) Cervical verrucous carcinoma involving endometrium. Case report. Eur J Gynaecol Oncol 20:35–37
274. Takeshima N, Yanoh K, Tabata T, et al (1999) Assessment of the revised International Federation of Gynecology and Obstetrics staging for early invasive squamous cervical cancer. Gynecol Oncol 74: 165–169
275. Tamimi HK, Gown AM, Kim-Deobald J, et al (1992) The utility of immunocytochemistry in invasive adenocarcinoma of the cervix. Am J Obstet Gynecol 166:1655–1662
276. Tenti P, Pavanello S, Padovan L, et al (1998) Analysis and clinical implications of p53 gene mutations and human papillomavirus type 16 and 18 infection in primary adenocarcinoma of the uterine cervix. Am J Pathol 152:1057–1063
277. ter Harmsel B, van Muyden R, Smedts F, et al (1998) The significance of cell type and tumor growth markers in the prognosis of unscreened cervical cancer patients. Int J Gynecol Cancer 8:
278. Teshima S, Shimosata Y, Kishi K, et al (1985) Early stage adenocarcinoma of the uterine cervix. Histopathologic analysis with consideration of histogenesis. Cancer (Phila) 56:167–172
279. Thelmo WL, Nicastri AD, Fruchter R, et al (1990) Mucoepidermoid carcinoma of the uterine cervix stage IB. Long-term follow-up, histochemical and immunohistochemical study. Int J Gynecol Pathol 9:316–324
280. Tidbury P, Singer A, Jenkins D (1992) CIN 3: the role of lesion size in invasion. Br J Obstet Gynaecol 99:583–586
281. Tiltman AJ, Atad J (1982) Verrucous carcinoma of the cervix with endometrial involvement. Int J Gynecol Pathol 1:221–226
282. Toki T, Shiozawa T, Hosaka N, et al (1997) Minimal deviation adenocarcinoma of the uterine cervix has abnormal expression of sex steroid receptors, CA125, and gastric mucin. Int J Gynecol Pathol 16:111–116
283. Tseng CJ, Pao CC, Tseng LH, et al (1997) Lymphoepithelioma-like carcinoma of the uterine cervix: association with Epstein-Barr virus and human papillomavirus. Cancer (Phila) 80:91–97
284. Tsukamoto N, Nakamura M, Kashimura M, et al (1980) Primary cervical choriocarcinoma. Gynecol Oncol 9:99–107
285. Uemura Y, Pak SC, Luke C, et al (2000) Circulating serpin tumor markers SCCA1 and SCCA2 are not actively secreted but reside in the cytosol of squamous carcinoma cells. Int J Cancer 89: 368–377
286. van Muyden RC, ter Harmsel BW, Smedts FM, et al (1999) Detection and typing of human papillomavirus in cervical carcinomas in Russian women: a prognostic study. Cancer (Phila) 85:2011–2016
287. van Nagell JR, Greenwell N, Powell DF, et al (1983) Microinvasive carcinoma of the cervix. Am J Obstet Gynecol 145:981–991
288. Vesterinen E, Forss M, Nieminen U (1989) Increase of cervical adenocarcinoma: a report of 520 cases of cervical carcinoma including 112 tumors with glandular elements. Gynecol Oncol 33:49–53
289. Vizcaino AP, Moreno V, Bosch FX, et al (2000) International trends in incidence of cervical cancer: II. Squamous-cell carcinoma. Int J Cancer 86: 429–435
290. Vizcaino AP, Moreno V, Bosch FX, et al (1998) International trends in the incidence of cervical can-

cer: I. Adenocarcinoma and adenosquamous cell carcinomas. Int J Cancer 75:536–545
291. Vogel HP, Mendelsohn G (1987) Laminin immunostaining in hyperplastic, dysplastic, and neoplastic lesions of the endometrium and uterine cervix. Obstet Gynecol 69:794–799
292. Wahlstrom T, Lindgren J, Korhonen M, et al (1979) Distinction between endocervical and endometrial adenocarcinoma with immunoperoxidase staining of carcinoembryonic antigen in routine histological tissue specimens. Lancet 2:1159–1160
293. Walboomers JM, Jacobs MV, Manos MM, et al (1999) Human papillomavirus is a necessary cause of invasive cervical cancer worldwide. J Pathol 189:12–19
294. Walker AN, Mills SE, Taylor PT (1988) Cervical neuroendocrine carcinoma; a clinical and light microscopic study of 14 cases. Int J Gynecol Pathol 7:64–74
295. Walker J, Bloss JD, Liao SY, et al (1989) Human papillomavirus genotype as a prognostic indicator in carcinoma of the uterine cervix. Obstet Gynecol 74:781–785
296. Wells M, Brown LJR (1986) Glandular lesions of the uterine cervix: the present state of our knowledge. Histopathology (Oxf) 10:777–792
297. Wentz WB, Reagan JW (1959) Survival in cervical cancer with respect to cell type. Cancer (Phila) 12: 384–388
298. Wistuba II, Thomas B, Behrens C, et al (1999) Molecular abnormalities associated with endocrine tumors of the uterine cervix. Gynecol Oncol 72:3–9
299. Wolff JP, Lacour J, Chassagne D, et al (1972) Cancer of the cervical stump. A study of 173 patients. Obstet Gynecol 39:10–16
300. Yazigi R, Sandstad J, Munoz AK, et al (1990) Adenosquamous carcinoma of the cervix: prognosis in stage IB. Obstet Gynecol 75:1012–1015
301. Young JJ, Percy C, Asire A (1981) Surveillance, epidemiology, and end results: incidence and mortality data, 1973–1977. NIH publication 81, Washington, DC
302. Young RH, Scully RE (1988) Mucinous ovarian tumors associated with mucinous adenocarcinomas of the cervix. A clinicopathological analysis of 16 cases. Int J Gynecol Pathol 7:99–111
303. Young RH, Scully RE (1989) Atypical forms of microglandular hyperplasia of the cervix simulating carcinoma. Am J Surg Pathol 13:50–56
304. Young RH, Scully RE (1989) Villoglandular papillary adenocarcinoma of the uterine cervix. A clinicopathologic analysis of 13 cases. Cancer (Phila) 63:1773–1779
305. Young RH, Scully RE (1993) Minimal deviation endometrioid adenocarcinoma of the uterine cervix: a report of five cases of a distinctive neoplasm that may be misinterpreted as benign. Am J Surg Path 17:660–665
306. Young RH, William R, Welch WR, et al (1982) Ovarian sex cord tumor with annular tubules. Review of 74 cases including 27 with Peutz-Jeghers syndrome and four with adenoma malignum of the cervix. Cancer (Phila) 50:1384–1402
307. Zaino RJ, Ward S, Delgado G, et al (1992) Histopathologic predictors of the behavior of surgically treated stage IB squamous cell carcinoma of the cervix. Cancer (Phila) 69:1750–1758
308. Zhang YC, Zhang PF, Wei YH (1983) Metastatic carcinoma of the cervix uteri from the gastrointestinal tract. Gynecol Oncol 15:287–290
309. Zreik TG, Chambers JT, Chambers SK (1996) Parametrical involvement, regardless of nodal status: a poor prognostic factor for cervical cancer. Obstet Gynecol 87:741–746

9

Anatomy and Histology of the Uterine Corpus

George L. Mutter, M.D., and Alex Ferenczy, M.D.

Embryology and Anatomy

The *endometrium* and *myometrium* are of mesodermal origin, and both structures are formed secondary to fusion of the müllerian ducts between the 8th and 9th postovulatory weeks.[70] Until the 20th week of gestation, the endometrium is composed of a single layer of columnar epithelium supported by a thick layer of fibroblastic stroma. By the 20th gestational week, the surface epithelium invaginates into the underlying stroma, forming glandular structures that extend toward the underlying myometrium. At birth the uterus measures about 4 cm in length, much of which is made up of the cervix (Fig. 9.1A). The endometrial surface and glands are lined by a low columnar to cuboidal epithelium, which in general is devoid of either proliferative or secretory changes; it resembles the inactive endometrium in menopausal or in castrated premenopausal women (Fig. 9.1B). The endometrial mucosa measures less than 0.5 mm in thickness.

During the prepubertal period, the endometrial mucosa remains inactive, and the cervix comprises the predominant portion of the uterus. In the reproductive years, the size and weight of a normal uterus vary according to parity. In nulliparous women, it measures 8 cm in length, 5 cm in width at the fundus level, and 2.5 cm in thickness, and weighs between 40 and 100 g. Multigravid uteri (four deliveries or more) measure about 10–12 cm × 5–7 cm × 2.5–3.5 cm and weigh up to 250 g.[60] The corpus uterus is divided into fundus, corpus, and isthmus regions. The uterus is located between the rectum (posteriorly) and urinary bladder (anteriorly); it is supported by the round and utero-ovarian ligaments and is covered by the pelvic peritoneum. The endometrium during the reproductive period undergoes cyclic morphologic changes, which are particularly evident in the upper two-thirds of the mucosa, the so-called functionalis layer. Morphologic alterations are minimal in the lower one-third of the basalis layer. In postmenopausal life, the endometrium recapitulates the neonatal–fetal period, being thin with relatively few glands and lined by cuboidal epithelium that is devoid of proliferative or secretory activity (see section on "Inactive and Atrophic Endometrium").

Vascular Anatomy

The endometrial mucosa has an abundant vascular supply originating from the radial arteries of the underlying myometrium (Fig. 9.2). These arteries penetrate the endometrium at regular intervals and give rise to the basal arteries; these in turn divide into

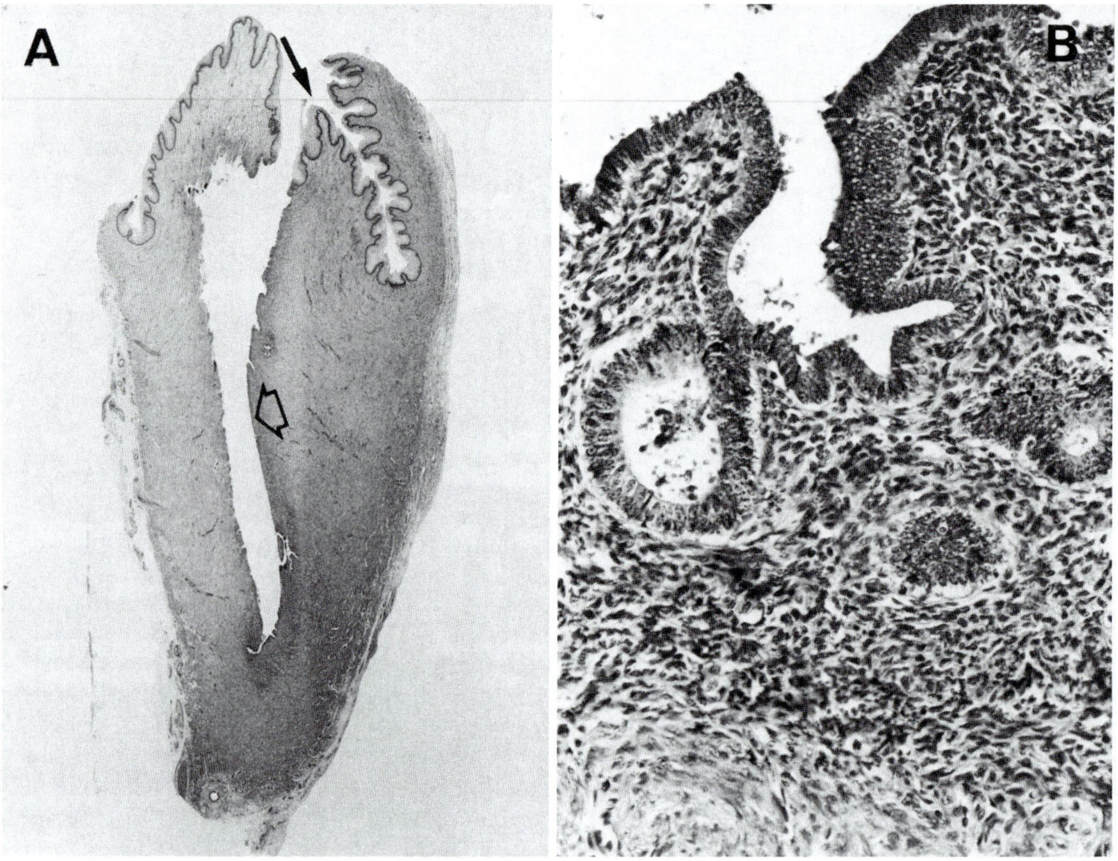

Fig. 9.1. Neonatal uterus. A: Whole mount section of a 4-day-old baby's uterus. The cervix (*narrow and open arrows*) is the dominant part of the uterus. **B**: The endometrium is thin and has few glands. The endometrial lining epithelium is of the inactive type. The stroma is dense and compact, resembling the basalis layer of the endometrium during the postpubertal period.

horizontal and vertical branches, the former providing the blood supply to the basal layer of the endometrium and the latter to the overlying functionalis layer. The endometrial vessels in the functionalis layer are referred to as *spiral arterioles* (Fig. 9.2). Their development and arborization near the surface and their connections with the subsurface epithelial precapillary system, as well as extreme coiling during the menstrual cycle (Figs. 9.2 and 9.3), are influenced by the ovarian steroid hormones and, presumably, prostaglandins.[7]

Histologically, the feature differentiating the endometrial and myometrial arteries is the absence of subendothelial elastica in the endometrial arteries, except for the basal portion, and its presence in the myometrial arteries (Fig. 9.4). Veins and lymphatics are closely associated with the endometrial arteries and glands, respectively. Uterine lymphatics drain from subserosal uterine plexuses to the pelvic and periaortic lymph nodes.

Steroid Hormone, Receptor, and Immunopeptide Interactions in the Endometrial Cycle

The *endometrial cycle* in women follows a series of morphologic and physiologic events characterized by proliferation, secretory differentiation, degeneration, and regeneration of the uterine lining (Fig. 9.5). These alterations are controlled by cyclically released ovarian estradiol (E_2) and progesterone (P). The endometrium thus is a highly sensitive indicator of the hypothalamopituitary—ovarian axis and serves to determine whether the infertile patient has ovulatory cycles.[68] Steroid hormone control of endometrial, epithelial, stromal, and presumably endothelial cells is mediated by estrogen receptors (E_2R) and progesterone receptors (PgR). These steroid receptors are proteins concentrated in the nuclei of endometrial cells that have high affinity to bind E_2 and P, re-

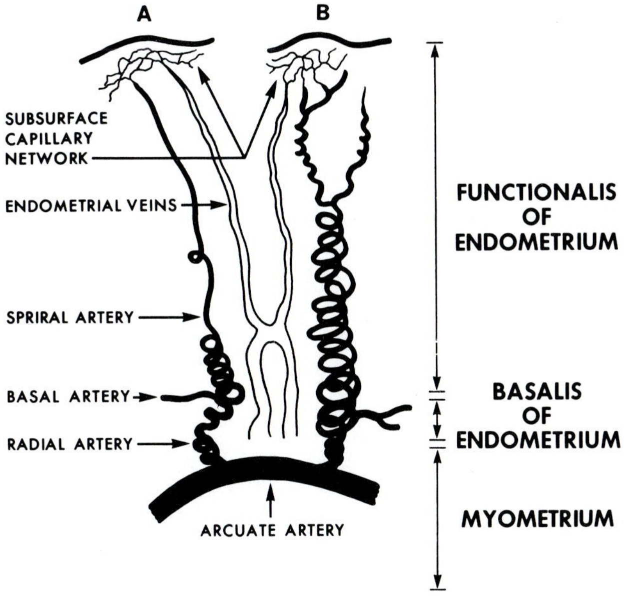

Fig. 9.2. Endometrial vessels. The coiled endometrial spiral arteries originate from the myometrial arcuate arteries and have connections with the subsurface capillary network, which in turn is drained by dilated veins. Arborization and coiling of spiral arteries are amplified in the postovulatory period (**B**) compared with the preovulatory phase (**A**) of the menstrual cycle.

spectively.[54] Because they are sex steroid hormone (ligand) specific, a particular receptor may display high affinity for a closely related class of hormones, and the same class may compete for available binding sites. For example, E_2R effectively binds not only E_2 but also estrone (E_1), as well as synthetic estrogens, such as diethylstilbestrol (DES).

Although E_2 has a crucial role in the proliferation of endometrial cells in vivo, E_2 alone is not able to induce proliferation of endometrial cells in primary culture. Recent studies suggest that the mitogenic action of E_2 is mediated indirectly (paracrine) by a polypeptide growth factor, epidermal growth factor (EGF).[99] EGF promotes the transition of cells from G_0 to G_1 phase of the cell cycle.[37,84] Human endometrial cells have EGF receptors and mRNA for EGF. EGF-like immunoreactivity is seen in both the endometrial glands and stromal cells, with higher concentrations in the glands than stroma, and parallels the fluctuation of cyclic sex steroids during the menstrual cycle. It appears that the regulation of EGF receptor content is regulated by ovarian estradiol and progesterone secretion (autocrine control).[110] Indeed, EGF alone fails to influence cell proliferation, but in combination with E_2 it increases mean gland but not stromal cell counts more than 50% in vitro. The immunolocalization of EGF

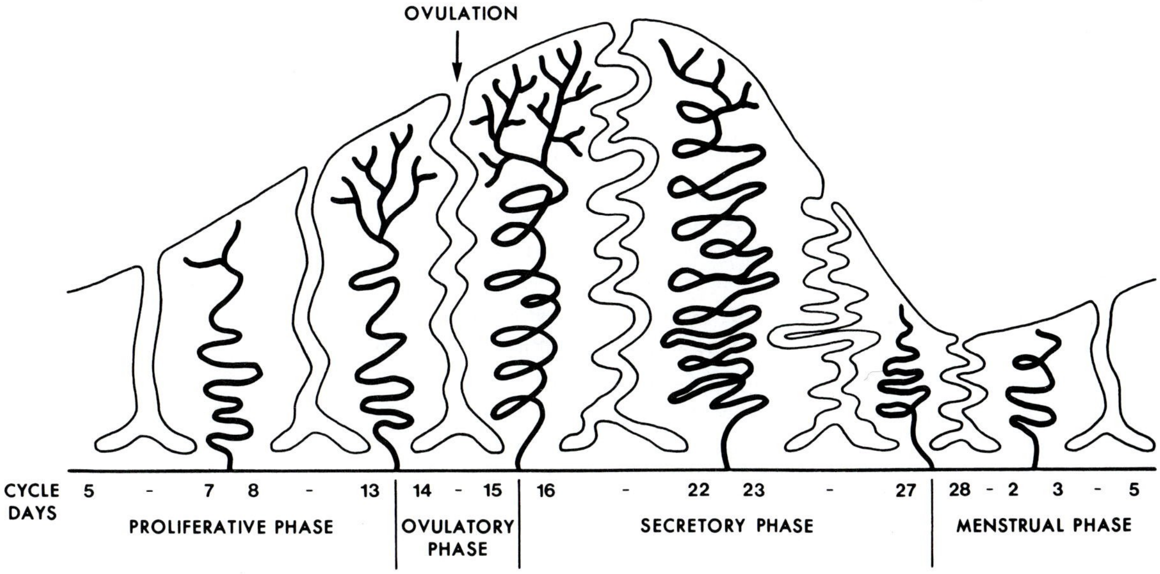

Fig. 9.3. Diagrammatic representation of endometrial vascular alterations during the menstrual cycle. There is a gradual increase in the arborization and coiling of spiral arteries during the preovulatory–ovulatory and postovulatory periods up to cycle days 23–25. The spiral arterial growth parallels the gradual increase in length and coiling of endometrial glands (*hollow tubules*). During the late-secretory phase and menstrual period, collapse of the vascular and glandular systems predominates, whereas both the vessels and glands remain essentially unchanged in the lower one-third of the basal layer throughout the menstrual cycle.

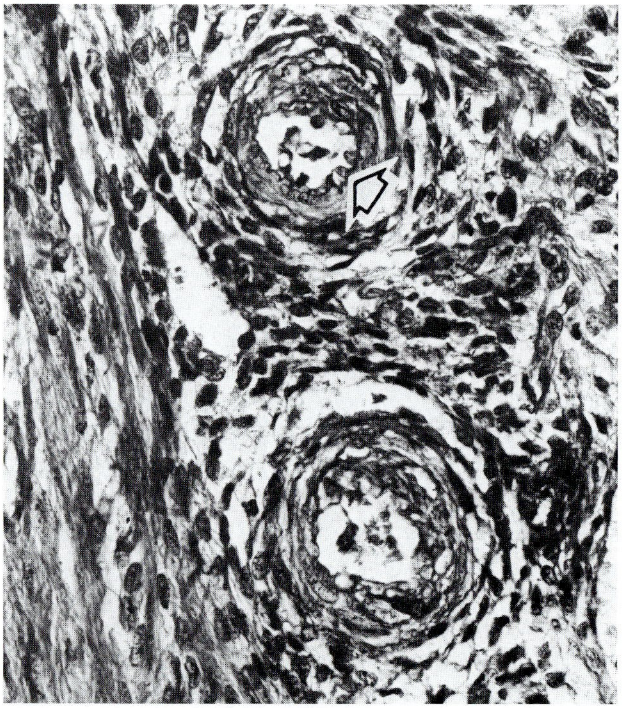

Fig. 9.4. Basal endometrial and myometrial arcuate arteries. Both arterial systems contain fine Weigert stain-positive elastic membranes (*arrow*) that presumably contribute to vascular constriction and ischemic necrosis during periods of menstruation. Elastica is absent in arteries of the endometrial functionalis.

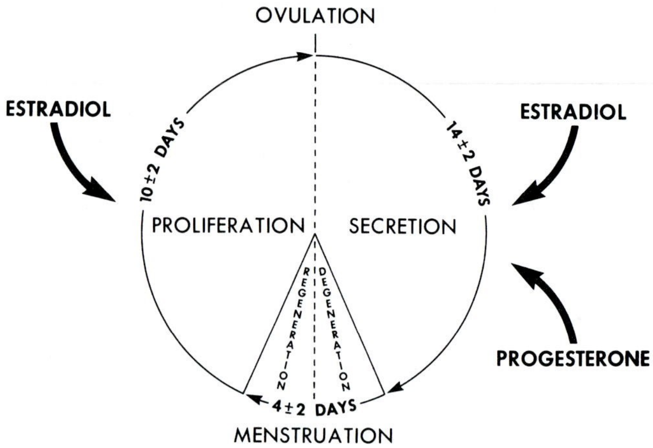

Fig. 9.5. Schematic representation of steroid hormone—morphologic interactions during the endometrial cycle. Estradiol promotes endometrial proliferation, whereas after ovulation progesterone converts estradiol-primed endometrium into secretory tissue. Postovulatory estradiol amplifies the progesterone effect, and after withdrawal of both estradiol and progesterone, the endometrial mucosa degenerates and regenerates within the period of menstruation. [Reprinted by permission of Ferenczy A, Guralnick M (1983) Endometrial microstructure: structure function relationships throughout the menstrual cycle. Semin Reprod Endocrinol 1: 205.]

in normal human endometrium (Table 9.1) and the stimulation of gland cell proliferation in cultures by EGF and E_2 provide support for a role of EGF in uterine growth.[43,99]

Dynamic remodeling of the endometrium results from a delicate balance of proliferation and programmed cell death within specific subpopulations of stromal and glandular cells, a process that likely is modulated by steroid hormones. A ladder pattern of DNA cleavage characteristic of apoptosis is seen in the late-secretory and menstrual to early-proliferative phases.[90] Localization of apoptotic subpopulations using in situ assays for DNA breakage have shown that the majority of apoptotic cells are glandular elements of the basalis, and these become increasingly numerous throughout the secretory phase before peaking during menses.[98] The apoptotic effects of steroid hormones are likely mediated through a complex network of inhibitors and initiators.[97] Progestins have been shown to decrease endometrial secretion of the apoptosis inhibitor bcl-2,[39] a process that is reversed upon administration of antiprogestins.[17] Progestins may also positively promote apoptosis by increasing levels of the apoptosis inducer gene BAK.[100]

The concentrations of E_2R and PgR in the normal endometrium vary during the normal menstrual cycle according to fluctuating plasma levels of E_2 and P. The highest values of E_2R (400 fmol/mg protein) and PgR (1000 fmol/mg protein) concentrations occur during the mid-proliferative phase (8th–10th day of the cycle)[42,105] and correspond to rising plasma levels of E_2 during the preovulatory and early postovulatory secretory phases of the cycle. E_2 promotes the synthesis of both E_2R and PgR,[54] whereas P inhibits the synthesis of E_2R. Mono-clonal antibodies to E_2R (estrophilin) derived from MCF-7 human breast cancer cell lines permit[40] the precise intracellular localization of E_2R by means of immunohistochemistry in frozen tissue sections.[10] Most of E_2R is localized in the nuclei rather than the cytoplasm of endometrial epithelial and stromal cells (Fig. 9.6). Endothelial cells fail to stain with antiestrophilin antibody. The concept of the mechanisms of sex steroid hormone–receptor action in target cells illustrated in Fig. 9.7 includes the following major steps: (1) circulating and unbound (from sex hormone-binding globulin) steroid hormone molecules are taken up from the cytoplasmic membrane, presumably by cytoplasmic receptors; (2) the hormone molecules enter the nucleus, which contains most (90–95%) of the cellular

Table 9.1. Immunoreactivity of human endometrium during the menstrual cycle[a]

	Proliferative phase		*Secretory phase*		
Antigen	*Glands*	*Stroma*	*Glands*	*Stroma*	*Presumed function*
E_2R	+	+	+	+	Proliferation
PgR	+	+	+	+ (decidual +++)	Secretory differentiation
EGF	+	+	±	+	Proliferation
IGF-1	+	+	±	+	Proliferation
Ki-67	+	±	+ (POD 3)	+ (decidua +++)	Proliferation
1BE12	+	−	−	−	Proliferation
pHER-2/neu	+	−	±	−	Proliferation
Cathespin	+	−	±	−	Proliferation
p.myc/RAS	−	−	−	−	
HLA-DR	+	−	−	−	Proliferation
VLA-1	−	−	+	+ (decidua +++)	Proliferation
B72.3 (TAG-72)	−	−	+	−	Secretory differentiation
Placental protein 14	−	−	+	−	
Carbohydrate—type 3 chains (ABO)					Secretory differentiation (glycolysation)
A	+	−	−	−	
H	+	−	+	−	Secretory differentiation (glycolysation)
Sialyl T	+	−	+	−	Secretory differentiation (glycolysation)
Sialyl TN	−	−	+	−	Secretory differentiation (glycolysation)
Relaxin	+	−	+	+ (decidual +++)	Collagenolysis
CD13, CD10	−	+	−	+ (decidual +++)	Immunomodulators
Keratins (AE 1/3, CAM 5.2)	+	−	+	−	Cytoplasmic support
EMA	+	−	+	−	Epithelial differentiation
Vimentin	+	+	+	+	Cytoplasmic support
Desmin	−	+	−	+	
MSA	−	+	−	+	Mesenchymal cell migration and integrity?
α-SMA	−	+	−	+	Mesenchymal cell migration and integrity?
S-100	−	−	−	−	Mesenchymal cell migration and integrity?

[a]Heterogeneous distribution.
MSA, muscle-specific actin; α-SMA, smooth muscle actin; IGF-1, insulin-like growth factor 1 (evaluated in rats).
E_2R, estrogen receptor; PgR, progesterone receptor; EGF, epidermal growth factor; EMA, epithelial membrane antigen.

receptors; (3) the intranuclear hormone molecules induce conversion of the inactive (nonfunctional) 4S form of receptor to active (functional) 5S form of receptor; (4) the hormonally activated 5S receptor binds to acceptor genes in the nucleus and influences gene expression by stimulating RNA polymerase and thus messenger RNA (mRNA) transcription; and (5) the newly formed mRNA is transported to the cytoplasm, where it is translated into proteins, including anabolic and catabolic enzymes as well as new receptors (receptor replenishment). According to this concept, the most significant effect of sex hormones is intranuclear activation of receptors that in turn initiate a sequence of events which lead to alterations in physiologic functions of target cells.

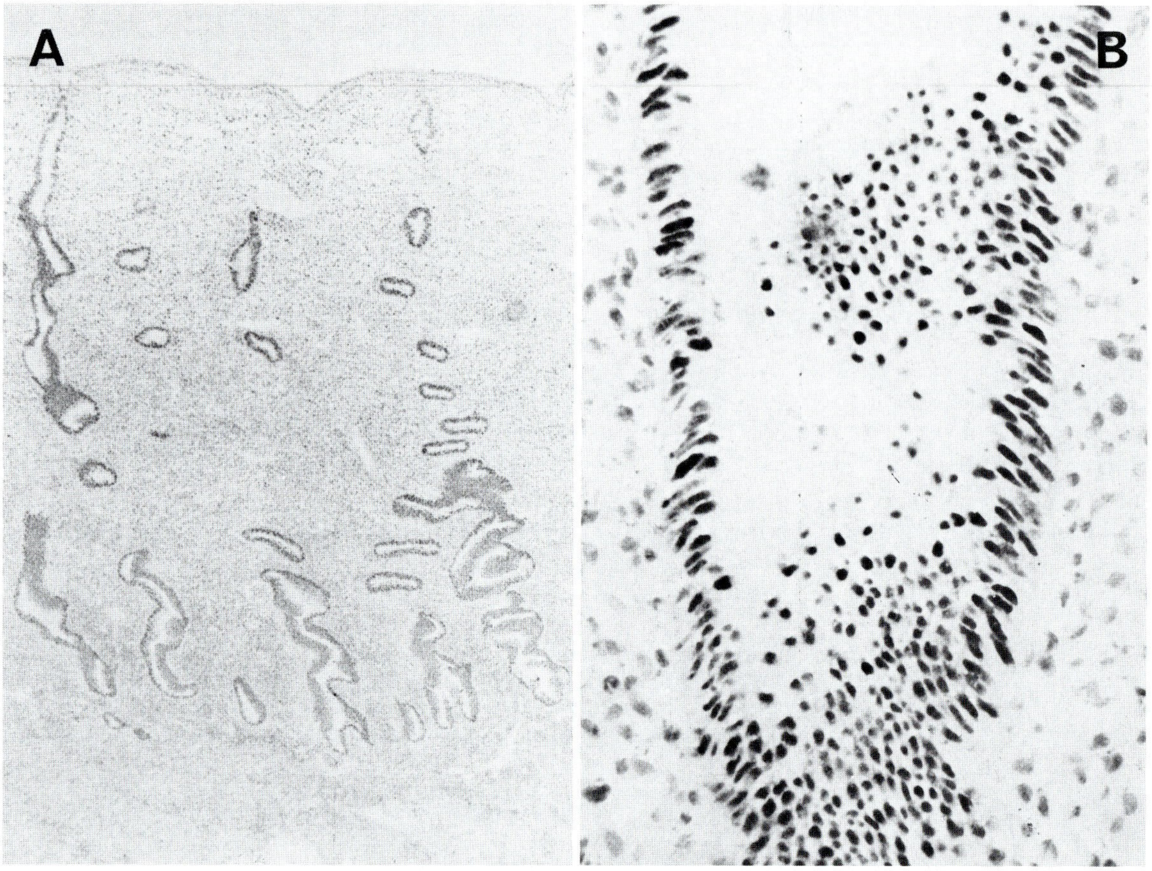

Fig. 9.6. Immunohistochemical localization of estrogen receptor (estrophilin). A: Estrogen receptors are present in midproliferative-phase endometrium, as indicated by the dark (*gray to black*) diaminobenzidine reaction product within cell nuclei. B: Receptors are localized to epithelial and stromal cell nuclei, although the intensity of specific staining is stronger in most epithelial cell nuclei than in most stromal cell nuclei. (Reprinted by permission of Press et al., ref. 77.)

Morphology and Physiology of the Normal Endometrium

An awareness of the morphologic variation of the endometrium throughout the cycle is essential for documenting whether ovulation has occurred and to diagnose specific causes of infertility such as luteal-phase defect. Endometrial dating, even in expert hands, is not highly reproducible. A discrepancy of 1–2 days in endometrial dating in relation to the calendar day on which subsequent menses occurs is generally acceptable. Unfortunately, in less-experienced hands, diagnostic inconsistencies between evaluators of the same biopsies may be as high as 65%; the same pathologist even may be inconsistent in reading the same biopsy at different times as many as in 27% of cases.[38] To avoid bias, the pathologist should read the clinical information, including the date of the last menstrual period, after evaluating the histologic section. The first day of bleeding is considered day 1 of the cycle (Fig. 9.8).[68]

The major morphologic features that occur in the endometrium throughout the cycle are shown in Fig. 9.8 and Table 9.2. During the proliferative phase, daily morphologic alterations are not sufficiently obvious to permit accurate dating. On the other hand, the daily changes in the endometrium during the postovulatory period are sufficiently distinct to permit accurate evaluation of the endometrial cycle.[44,68]

Proliferative Phase

The preovulatory endometrium is characterized by proliferation of gland cells, stromal cells, and vascular endothelial cells, leading to an increase in the volume of the uterine mucosa. Synthesis of nuclear DNA is increased[27] (Fig. 9.9A), and mitoses are numerous (Fig. 9.9B). As a result, the straight glands in the early proliferative phase (Fig. 9.9C)

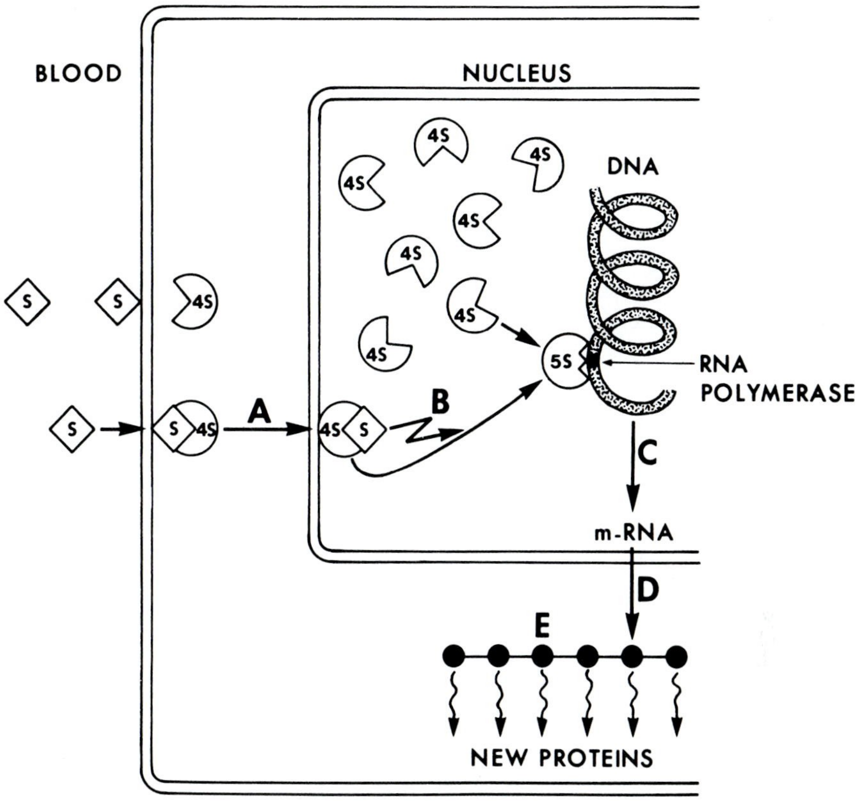

Fig. 9.7. Schematic representation of sex steroid hormone–receptor interaction in target cells. Circulating, free hormone molecule(s) following their passage through cell membranes are bound to cytoplasmic 4S receptors; the hormone–receptor complex is transported (*A*) to and in the nucleus, where the biologically active 5S steroid receptor complex is formed (*B*) from either the inactive 4S cytoplasmic steroid–receptor complex or by interaction of the 4S nuclear receptor with the steroid dissociated from 4S cytoplasmic receptor. The 5S receptor stimulates RNA polymerase and transcription (*C*) of messenger RNA; mRNA is transported (*D*) to cytoplasm, where it is translated (*E*) into new proteins related to physiologic cell functions. Most cellular receptors are intranuclear and are in equilibrium with small amounts of cytoplasmic receptors.

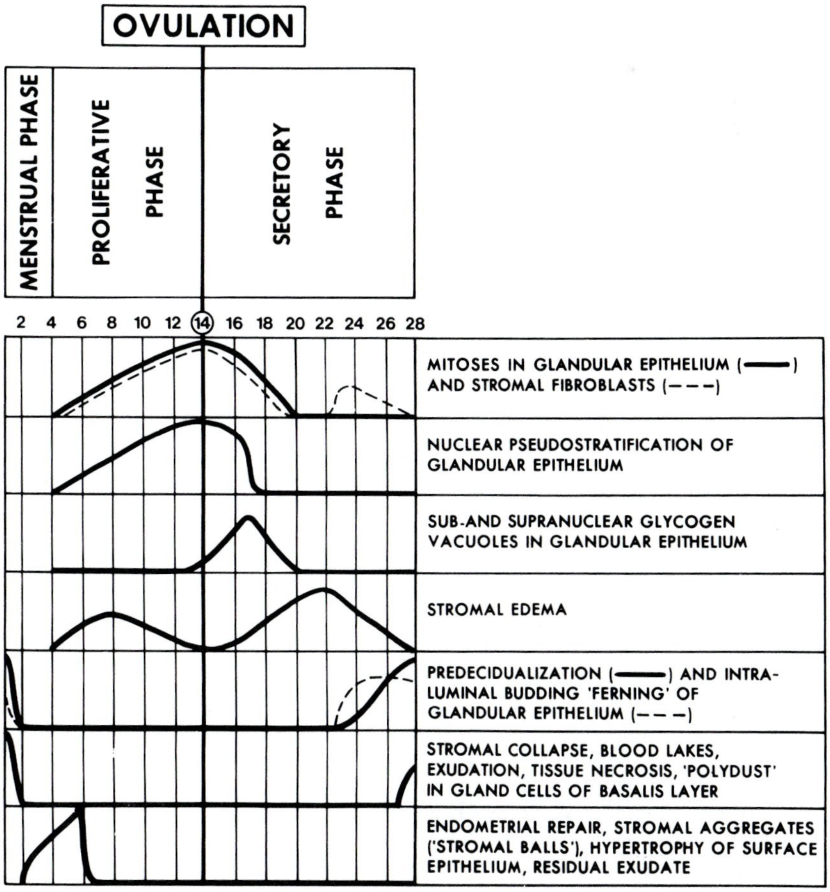

Fig. 9.8. Endometrial morphologic alterations during the menstrual cycle. (Adapted by permission of Noyes et al., ref. 68.)

Table 9.2. Sequential landmarks useful for endometrial dating

Cycle day	*Phase*	*Glands/epithelium*	*Stroma*	*Comments*
1–4	Ovulatory Menstrual	Secretory changes	Breakdown	
4–6	Late menstrual-Early Proliferative	Thin reparative functionalis with occasional mitoses	Scant breakdown	Ovulation in preceding cycle cannot be confirmed
6–15	Proliferative	Mitoses, no vacuoles	No breakdown	
16	Interim	Irregular basal vacuoles and pseudostratified nuclei, many mitoses		
17	Early Secretory	Even basal vacuoles and aligned nuclei, occasional mitoses		First day ovulation confirmed
18	Early Secretory	Basal and luminal vacuoles with pseudostratified nuclei, mitoses rare		
19	Early Secretory	Straight glands with luminal secretions but no vacuoles and no mitoses		
20–21	Early Secretory		Stromal edema increases	Hard to resolve from 19 Days
22	Mid Secretory		Perivascular clustering "naked" stromal of nuclei	
23	Mid Secretory		Individual vessels cuffed by predecidua	
24	Mid Secretory		Vascular groups bridged by predecidua	
25	Late Secretory		Focal predecidua under uterine lining	
26	Late Secretory		Predecidua under most of uterine lining	
27	Late Secretory		Predecidua under uterine lining and extending deep between vessels. Stromal granulocytes	
28	Late Secretory		Predecidua begins condensing into aggregates	

become progressively more voluminous and tortuous (Fig. 9.10) during the mid- and late phases of proliferation. Increased nuclear DNA synthesis and mitotic activity in gland cells correlates with high levels of nucleolar organizer regions (NORs). These NORs can be demonstrated by silver stains and are found on chromosomes 13–15, 21, and 22 as loops of DNA.[112] They are transcribed to ribosomal RNA and serve as an index of gland cell growth. The changes are under the influence of E_2, which stimulates the DNA promoter enzyme thymidylate synthetase.[27]

The endometrium demonstrates zonal variations in its response to hormonal stimuli. For example, DNA synthesis is greater in the upper two-thirds of the functionalis of the fundus and corpus than in the lower third, the isthmic and cornual regions, and the basalis layer.[27] Both Ki-67 and HLA-DR, as detected by immunostaining, parallel the mitotic activity in gland cells during the preovulatory cycle and until the third postovulatory day. Expression of Ki-67 is comparatively greater in the functionalis than the basalis endometrium, whereas HLA-DR, one of the major class II histocompatibility antigens, is more evident in the basalis.[96] The geographic variation in the sensitivity of the endometrium to hor-

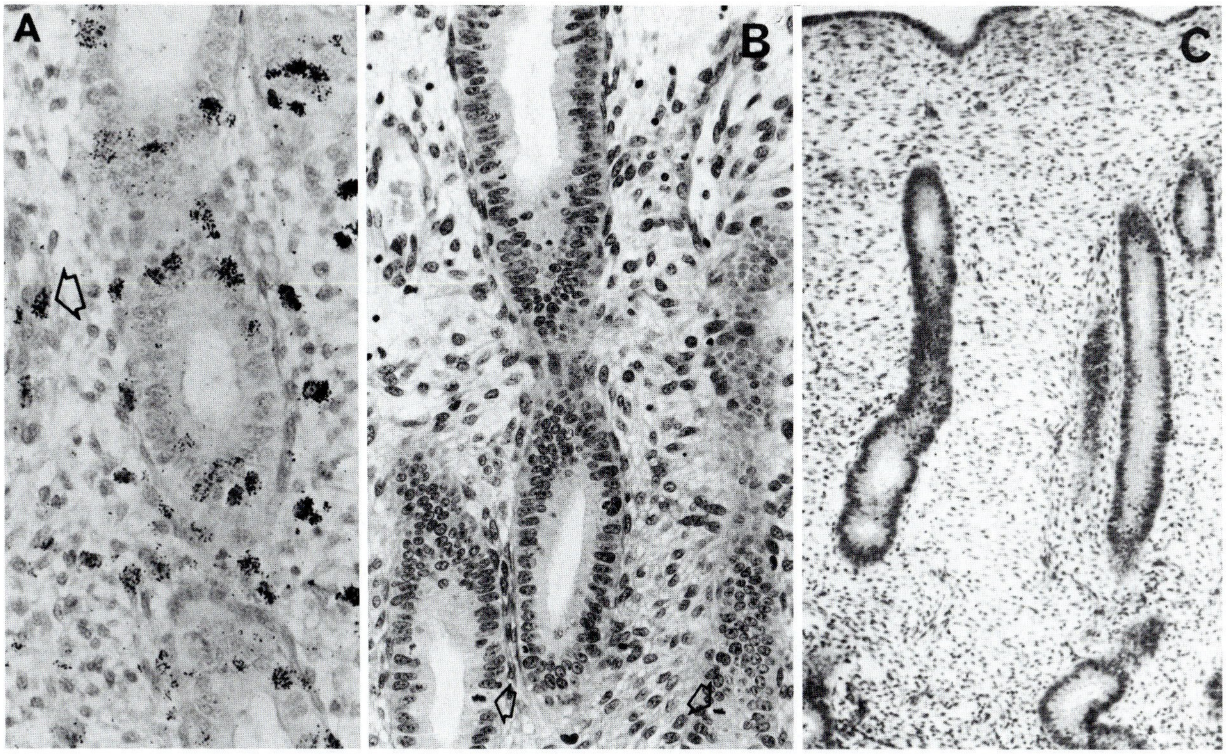

Fig. 9.9. Proliferative endometrium. A: Historadioautography of proliferative endometrium, cycle day 12. Radiothymidine granules are heavily incorporated into the nuclei of endometrial gland cells, stromal fibroblasts, and capillary endothelium (*arrow*). **B**: Routine histologic staining of proliferative glands lined by columnar cells with pseudostratified, pencil-shaped nuclei. Mitoses (arrows) are seen. (Reprinted by permission of Ferenczy and Guralnick (1983) Endometrial microstructure: structure function relationships throughout the menstrual cycle. Semin Reprod Endocrinol 1:205.) **C**: Cycle day 8. Straight glands with narrow lumens oriented perpendicular to the surface. The stroma is edematous and well vascularized.

monal stimulation correlates with different biologic functions. The upper functional layer serves as the implantation site, providing an appropriate metabolic and physical environment for the implanted blastocyst. The lower functionalis provides the integrity of the endometrial mucosa. The maximum number of endometrial cells engaged in DNA synthesis is seen between cycle days 8 and 10 (Fig. 9.11) and corresponds to maximal mitotic activity, peak plasma E_2 levels, and maximum concentration of E_2R. The decline in the E_2-promoted DNA activity by days 11–14 (Fig. 9.11) when P levels are low is possibly related to endometrial refractoriness to relative hyperstimulation of the preovulatory endometrium by E_2. In addition to E_2, insulin-like growth factor (IGF-1), as well as agents that increase intracellular cyclic adenosine monophosphate (cAMP), stimulate PgR synthesis.[4]

Experimental studies[95] in animals reveal that sex steroid molecules may be transported from the cytoplasm into the nucleus by endometrial lysosomes that migrate into the nucleus. Some aspects of the glycosylation pattern in normal cyclic endometrium have been investigated by the use of monoclonal antibodies against mucin type 3 chain ABO-related antigens and their precursors.[81] Expression of these antigens is influenced not only by the erythrocyte ABO blood type but also by the secretory genes (SE, *se*) and, in the endometrium, they may be hormonally regulated. Glands in the functionalis of proliferative endometrium express type 3 chain A, H, and sialated T antigens, whereas sialyl-T and sialyl TN antigens are observed in secretory glands (see Table 9.1). Antigen expression is focal and is consistent with the increased synthesis of galactose, mannose, sialic acid, fucose, etc., and with the apocrine and merocrine secretion of carbohydrates in glands in the secretory phase of the cycle.[81]

Characteristically, both the proliferative- and secretory-type epithelial cells stain positively for cytokeratin and vimentin (AE 1-3 and CAM 5.2),[19] although vimentin is absent in glands of the late secretory-phase endometrium (Table 9.1; Fig. 9.12). Unlike endometrial epithelial cells, stromal cells do not react with cytokeratin but only with vimentin (Fig. 9.12) and smooth muscle-related

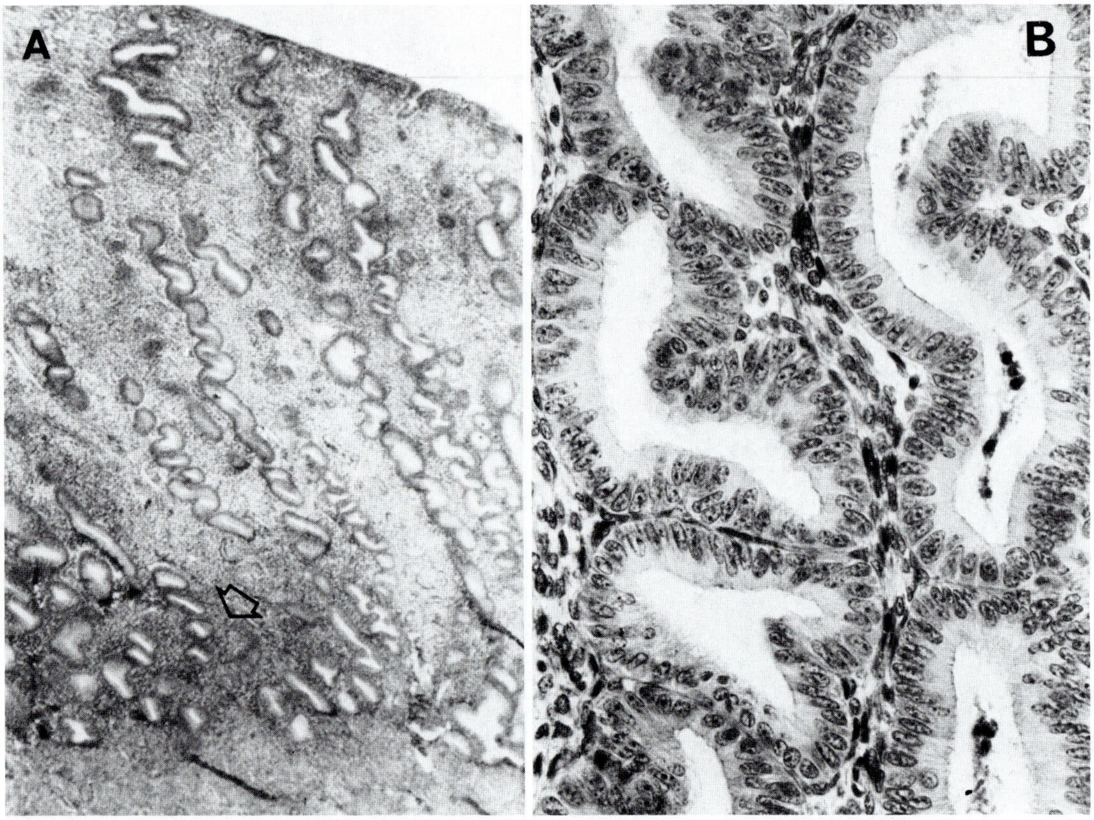

Fig. 9.10. Proliferative endometrium, cycle day 12. A: Rows of voluminous, tortuous glands arranged at regular intervals characterize the preovulatory endometrium. The somewhat edematous stroma of the functionalis layer contrasts with the dense, compact stroma of the lower basalis layer (*arrow*). **B**: The glands have an S-shaped configuration, are closely apposed, and the lining cells have pseudostratified nuclei.

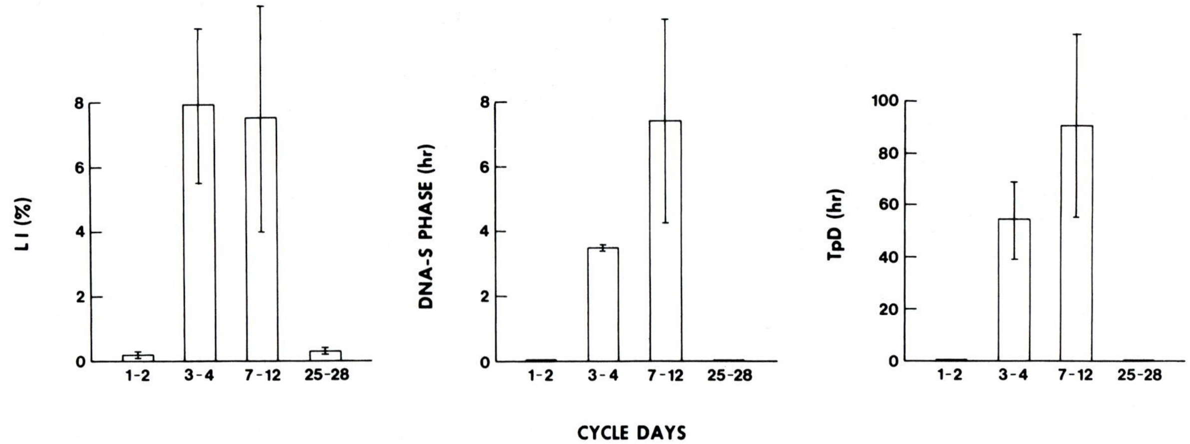

Fig. 9.11. Kinetic characteristics of the endometrium during the menstrual cycle according to in vitro historadioautography using the double-labeling technique with ^{3}H-thymidine. Labeling index (*LI*), DNA synthesis phase (*DNA-S phase*), and potential doubling time (*TpD*) are negligible during the premenstrual and early menstrual periods. Note the sudden increase in LI and shortening of the DNA-S phase and tissue turnover time during the regenerative period on cycle days 3–4. The postregenerative period (cycle day 5 on) is characterized by prolongation of both the DNA-S phase and tissue turnover time. (Reprinted by permission of Ferenczy, ref. 26.)

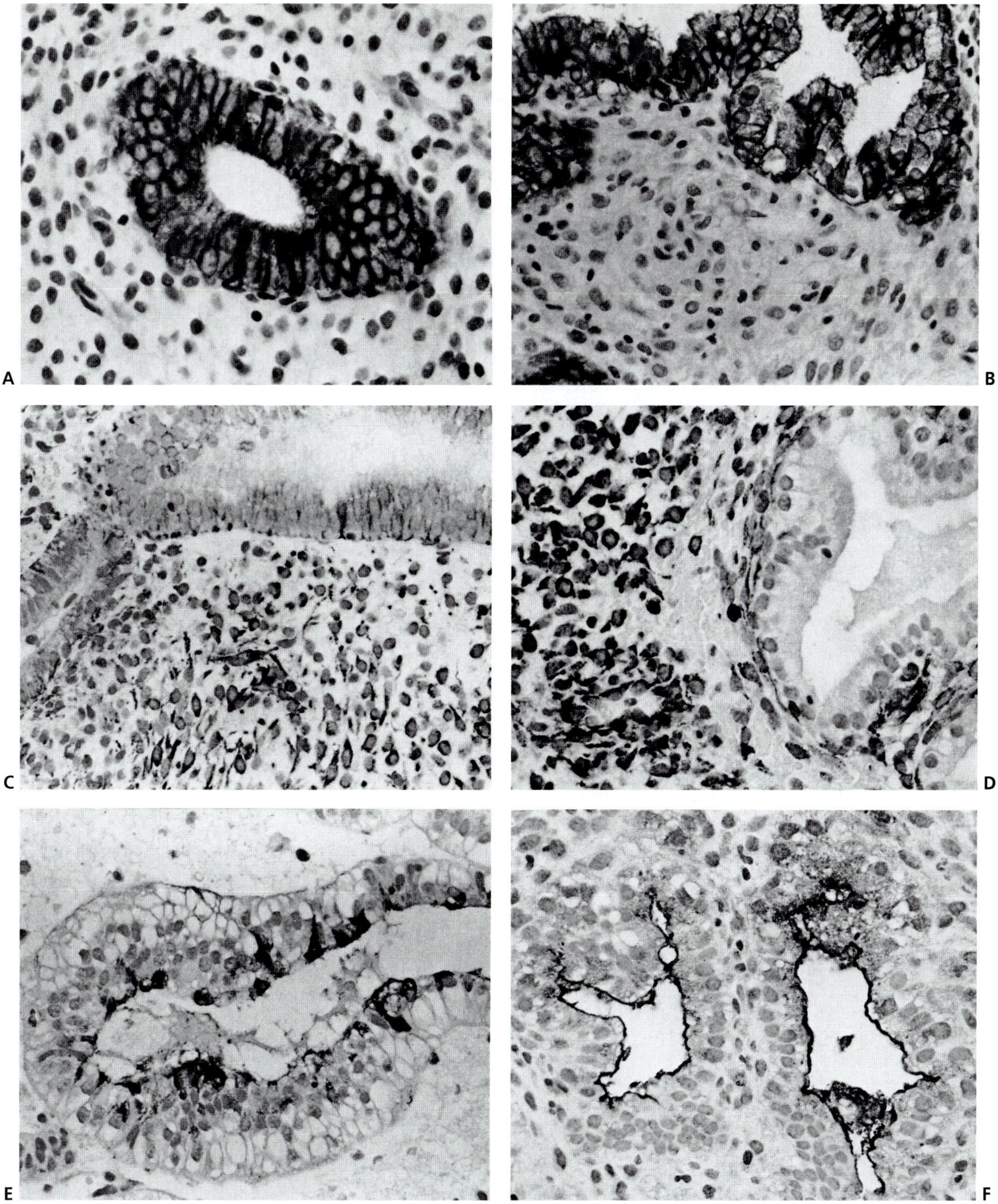

Fig. 9.12. Immunohistochemistry of cyclic endometrium. Cytokeratin AE1/3 (**A**, **B**), vimentin (**C**, **D**), and B72.3 (**E**, **F**) staining in cycling endometrium. **A**: Proliferative endometrium; intense cytokeratin transepithelial staining is observed only in gland cells. **B**: Secretory endometrium, cycle day 25 (POD 11); staining remains intense in the glands, whereas none is found in the adjacent predecidual cells. **C**: In the proliferative endometrium, all elements including stromal fibroblasts, vessels, and, to a lesser extent, the base of gland cells, demonstrate vimentin immunostaining. **D**: Secretory endometrium, cycle day 26 (POD 12). Staining is confined to predecidual and endothelial cells. **E**: Early secretory endometrium, 17th day (POD 3). B72.3 staining is prominent in the apical portion of some gland cells. (×500). **F**: Secretory endometrium, cycle day 26 (POD 12). Immunostaining is confined to the luminal surface membranes of gland cells.

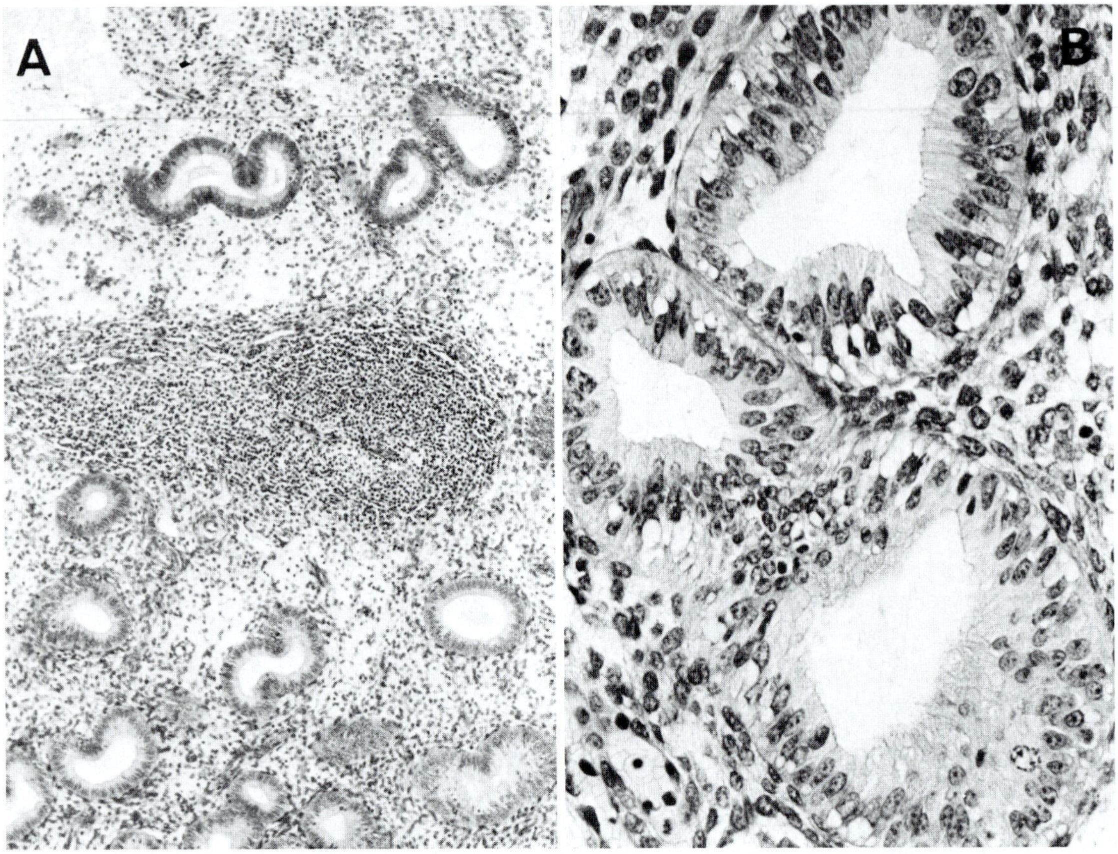

Fig. 9.13. Proliferative endometrium. A: Aggregates of mature lymphocytes forming lymphoid follicle-like structures in the basalis layer of the endometrium. **B**: Day 16 endometrium. Gland cells with small, abortive, subnuclear glycogen vacuoles. Many gland cells are devoid of vacuoles, and nuclear pseudostratification is maintained. The overall histology is that of glands of the late-proliferative rather than the postovulatory phase. Similar changes may be seen in anovulatory endometrium.

antigens (Table 9.1). Also, the surface and gland cells acquire numerous cilia and microvilli. Ciliary shafts have a strong forward and slow recovery ciliary beat pattern, and cilia are particularly numerous around gland openings.[23,24,26] These findings are consistent with their role in facilitating mobilization and distribution of endometrial secretions during the progestational phase of the menstrual cycle.[28]

Lymphoid aggregates resembling follicles (Fig. 9.13A) may be seen in the endometrial stroma, particularly during the proliferative phase of the cycle. Although they stain for IgA, IgM, or IgG, they are unlikely to play a significant role, if any, in the local secretory immune system. Indeed, endometrial epithelial cells synthesize negligible amounts of immunoproteins,[82] have few Langerhans' cells, and IgG-containing plasma cells are absent in normal endometria. The observations are consistent with the sterile nature of normal endometrium.

Secretory Phase

Postovulation Days 1–3

After ovulation, under the influence of P, the E_2-primed endometrium undergoes rapid secretory differentiation.[27,68] The morphologic alterations that are used to date the endometrium are shown in Table 9.3. During cycle days 14 and 15 (postovulation day [POD] 1), the morphology of the endometrium is not significantly different from that seen in the late proliferative phase of the menstrual cycle. On the 16th day (POD 2) of the cycle, small cylindrical vacuoles appear in the base of the gland cells in the functional layer. Otherwise, the epithelium is indistinguishable from that of the late proliferative phase; the gland cells remain tall and the nuclei pseudostratified (Fig. 9.13B). Similar changes may be produced by estrogens alone in the absence of ovulation. As a result, incomplete or abortive subnuclear vacuolization is not considered specific to ovulation. Coinciding with the appearance of sub-

Table 9.3. Morphologic evidence of ovulation

Morphology	*Cycle days*
Nucleolar channel system* in gland cells	15–25
Subnuclear vacuolization with nuclear palisading of gland cells	17–18
Stromal edema with ferning of glandular epithelium	22–23
Perivascular and stroma; predecidualization	23–28
Diffuse predecidual and glandular necrosis, inflammation, and vascular thrombosis	1–2
Inflammatory exudate, aggregates of stromal cells (stromal balls) with or without hypertrophic surface epithelial cells, diffuse	2–4

*At transmission electron microscope level.

nuclear vacuoles, the secretory gland endometrium acquires B72.3 and the very late antigen-1 (see Table 9.1). The latter are heterodimers, belong to the integrin receptor superfamily, and are related to maintaining cell shape, function, and integrity. Very late antigen-1 also is demonstrated in the predecidual cells during the secretory phase of the cell cycle. The first reliable histologic alterations that are considered specific to ovulation are seen on the 17th day (POD 3) of the cycle[68]; these include well-developed subnuclear glycogen vacuoles in gland-lining cells and palisading of gland cell nuclei. Both phenomena involve every cell in a given gland (Fig. 9.14A,B).

Ultrastructurally[27] and histochemically,[81] the vacuoles correspond to pools of glycogen granules. Accumulation of glycogen and its synthesis are unique phenomena of the endometrium in that this occurs in the absence of excessive glycogen intake or exercise. Mitochondrial gigantism, with increased numbers of cristae, occurs in response to the increased demand for energy for glycogen metabolism.[113] The intracellular glycogen is broken down by enzymes of oxidative phosphorylation into glycoproteins and synthesized via the Golgi complex in the supranuclear region.

At the ultrastructural level, ovulation is manifested by the appearance of giant mitochondria and the so-called nucleolar channel system (NCS) formed by the helical infolding of the nuclear mem-

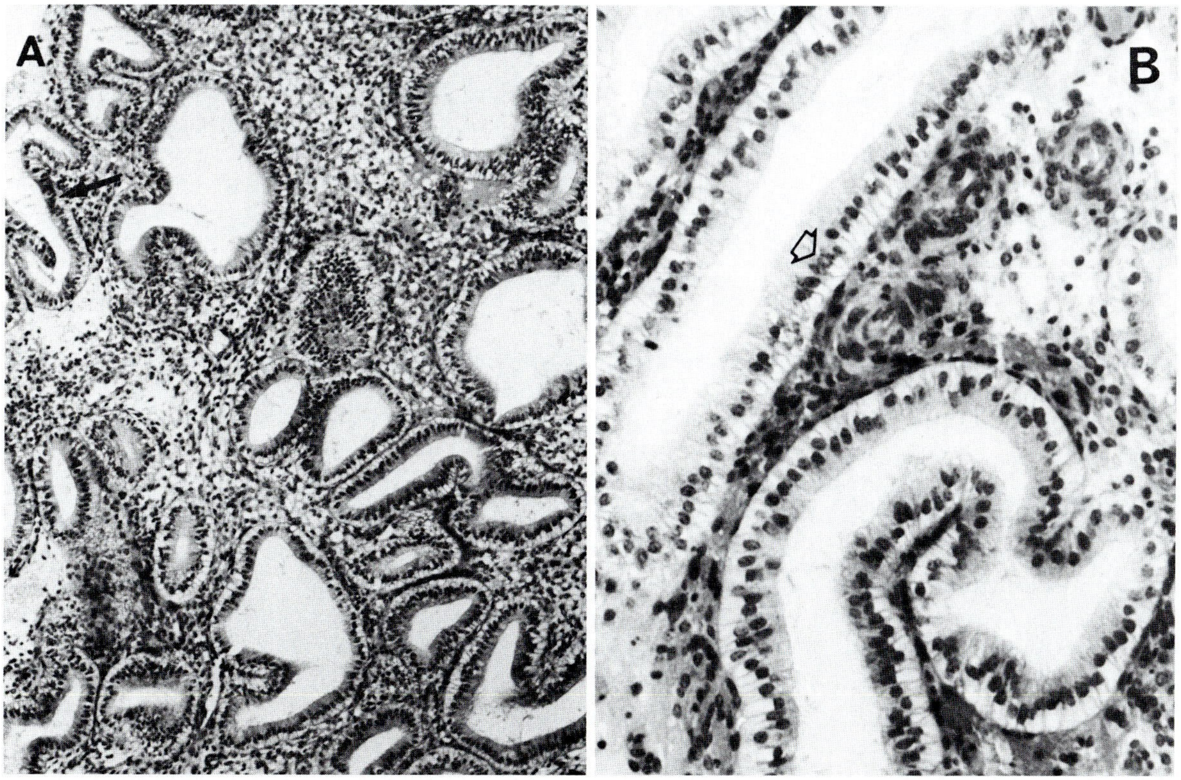

Fig. 9.14. Postovulatory, secretory endometrium. A: Many glands on cycle day 17 (POD 3) have S-shaped configurations, conspicuous subnuclear vacuolization, and nuclear palisading. The stroma is relatively edematous. **B**: Detailed view of the 17th day secretory endometrium. Each gland cell has a well-developed subnuclear vacuole. As a result, the nuclei are pushed up to the center of the cells, producing nuclear palisading (*arrow*). These are the first morphologic features in the menstrual cycle that are indicative of ovulation.

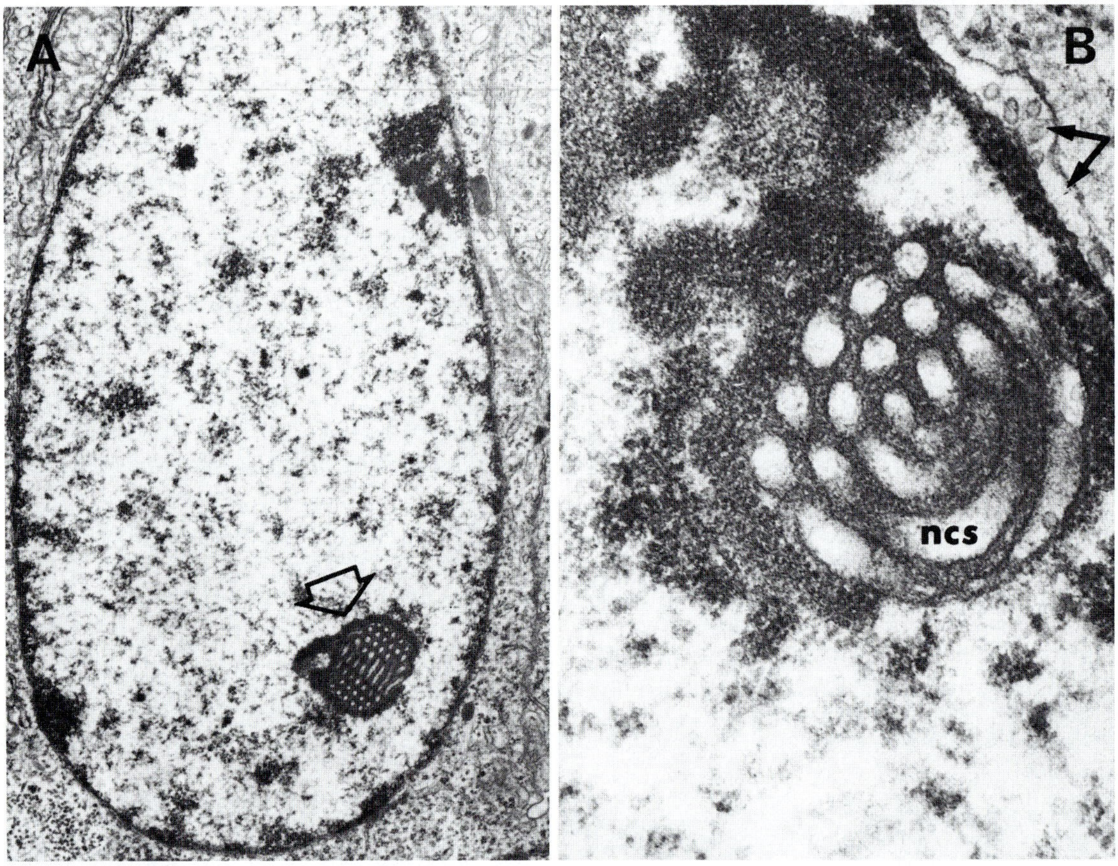

Fig. 9.15. Postovulatory secretory endometrium, cycle day 17 (POD 3). A: Gland cell with a nucleolar channel system (*arrow*), subnuclear glycogen, and giant mitochondria enveloped by parallel membranes of glandular endoplasmic reticulum. These ultrastructural features are typical of postovulatory endometrium. ×8000. **B**: Detailed view of nucleolar channel system (**ncs**) made of hollow, membrane-bound tubules embedded in dark granular nucleolonema. Vesicular structures seen in ncs are also seen between the inner and outer nuclear membrane (*arrows*). ×60,000.

branes into the nuclear or nucleolar substance[67] in gland cells (Table 9.1; Fig. 9.15A,B). NCS is seen as early as the 15th day of the cycle, but its significance is not known. These structures are unique to women and are seen only during the postovulatory phase.[113] However, NCS may be produced both in vivo and in vitro by progesterone or its synthetic variants[78] and has been described in two cases of pelvic endometriosis.[49]

MAb B72.3 recognizes an epitope associated with a high molecular weight, mucin-like glycoprotein TAG-72[104]; intense B72.3 immunoreactivity is observed in the fundal endometrium only during the postovulatory phase of the cycle (Fig. 9.12), whereas staining is sporadic in the lower uterine segment (Table 9.1). In the latter, immunoreactivity is unrelated to cycle days. TAG72/B72.3 is thus a marker of ovulation in cyclic endometrium.[72] Another protein marker of secretory endometrium is placental protein 14 (PP 14), which is synthesized in the endometrial glandular cells.[109]

Postovulation Days 4–6

On cycle day 18 (POD 4), supranuclear vacuolization is established (Fig. 9.16A), and between days 19 and 20 (POD 5 and 6) the glycoprotein-rich and mucopolysaccharide-rich supranuclear cytoplasmic products are expelled into the glandular lumen by apocrine-type secretion.[113] This event is characterized by protrusion and eventual detachment of the apical portion of cells (Fig. 9.16B). Uterine secretory fluids also contain plasma transudates derived from circulating blood in the endometrial mucosa. The peak of intraglandular secretions coincides with the time of implantation of the free blastocyst, on cycle day 21 (POD 7) if fertilization takes place.

DNA synthesis and cell divisions in gland cells cease (Figs. 9.11, 9.16B) concomitantly with the ini-

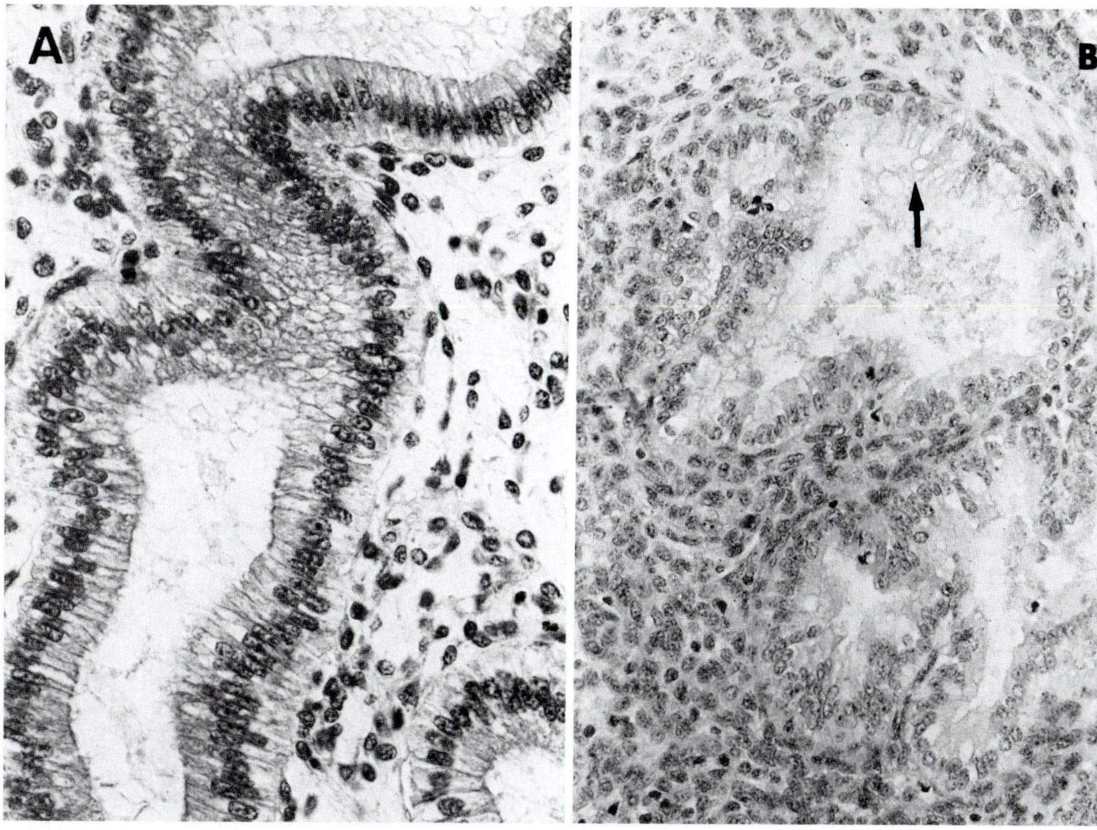

Fig. 9.16. Postovulatory secretory endometrium, cycle day 18 (POD 4). A: Endometrial gland cells have well developed sub- and supranuclear vacuoles, and nuclear palisading is evident. Many cells contain finely granular cytoplasmic substance, and intraluminal vacuolated secretory products are abundant. **B:** Historadioautograph of secretory endometrium. Lack of uptake of radiothymidine by gland cells coincides with conspicuous apocrine secretory activity (*arrow*) and accumulation of intraluminal secretory products.

tiation of apocrine secretory activity by day 19.[27] Mitosis is inhibited further by the rising levels of postovulatory P. Progesterone antagonizes the action of E_2 by interfering with either the recycling or replenishment or both of cytoplasmic E_2R[54] and through the action of the P-specific enzyme 17β-hydroxy dehydrogenase (E_2DH).[42] E_2DH converts the potent uterotropic E_2 into relatively weak E_1, which rapidly leaves the cell without significantly stimulating the nuclei of target cells. As a result, an increase in E_2DH lowers the intracellular concentration of E_2 and its receptors. Progesterone prevents the epithelial cells from entering the premitotic (G_1 and S) phases of the cell cycle.[117]

Postovulation Days 7–10

From cycle day 20 on, the changes in the stroma rather than the glands are evaluated in dating the endometrium (see Table 9.1). The changes are edema (days 20–23), coiling of spiral arterioles (days 22–25), and predecidualization of the stroma (days 23–28). These alterations are mediated by prostaglandin F_2 (PGF_2) and PGE_2.[94] The elevated concentrations of midluteal phase E_2 on cycle day 22 (POD 8) increase the synthesis of the enzyme, cyclooxygenase, responsible for PG production.[1] PGE_2 in turn promotes capillary permeability,[26] leading to maximal stromal edema on day 22 (POD 10) (Fig. 9.17A). Experimental studies have shown that PGE_2 and leukotrienes (LTs) are potent vasoactive agents that promote vascular permeability as well as stromal decidualization in progesterone-primed endometrium. PGE_2, LTC_4, or both elicit a marked decidual/vascular response in hypophysectomized progesterone-primed pseudopregnant rats; conversely, inhibitors of PGs and LTs such as indomethacin and FPL 55712, respectively, reduce decidualization.[101] E_2 triggers production of PGE_2 and leukotrienes.[102] The increasing concentration of E_2 in the early to midpostovulatory period may play a role in preparing the endometrium for implantation of the blastocyst through these arachidonate metabolites.[94] Endometrial vascular arborization is best visualized by factor VIII immunostaining. PGE_2

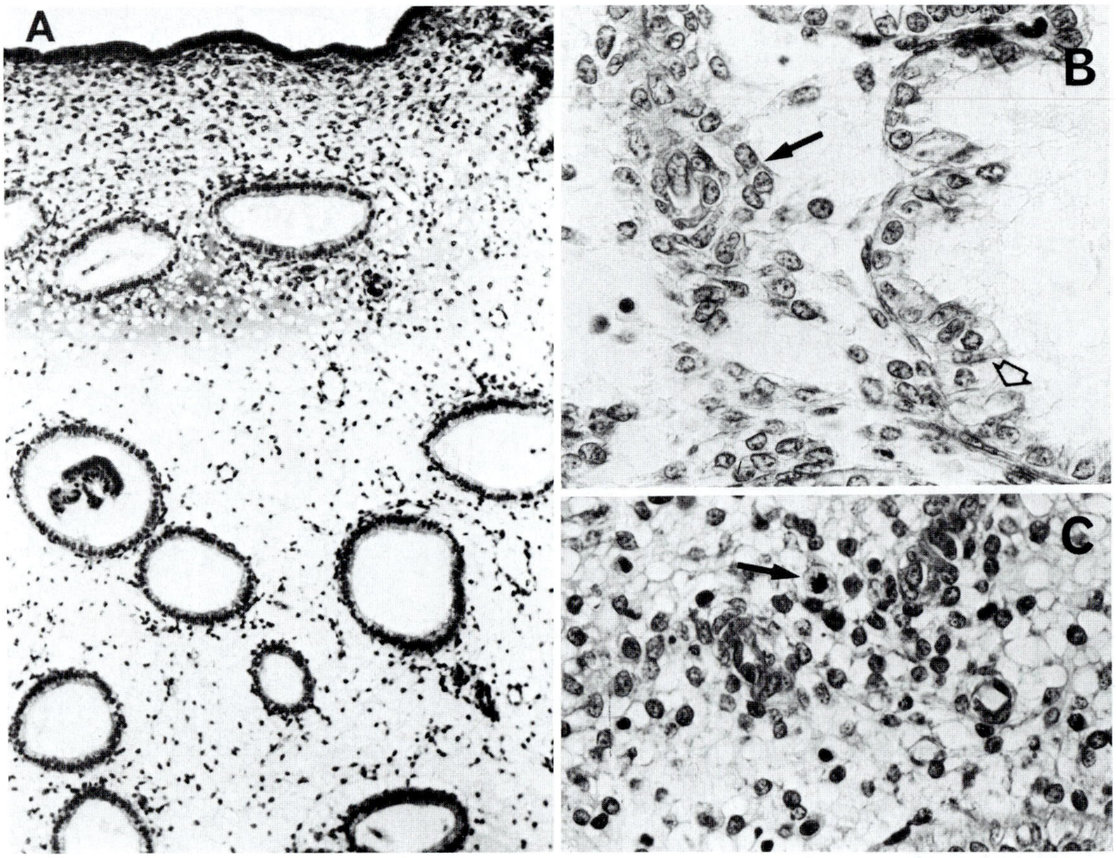

Fig. 9.17. Postovulatory, secretory endometrium, cycle day 22 (POD 8). **A**: There is marked stromal edema producing a naked gland–stromal cell pattern. The glands have somewhat dilated lumens with secretions, and the lining epithelium is low, columnar, and devoid of intraluminal projections. **B**: Detailed view of perivascular thickening caused by hypertrophy of perivascular stromal cells (*arrow*). The gland cells are low columnar to cuboidal and have apical apocrine secretory protuberances (*open arrow*). **C**: Mitoses (*arrow*) in perivascular stromal cells reappear on late 22nd–early 23rd day of the menstrual cycle.

presumably also promotes vascular endothelial mitotic activity, perivascular concentrations of filaments (Fig. 9.17B), and mitoses that are first seen in the postovulatory endometrium on day 22 of the cycle (Fig. 9.17C). Endothelial proliferation leads to coiling of the arterial system of the endometrium, a phenomenon that produces vascular clusters in the upper functionalis layer, seen in histologic sections. The PGE-mediated vascular growth concept is substantiated further by the fact that immunohistochemically the vascular endothelium is devoid of receptors of estradiol and progesterone.[74]

Vascular permeability and edema of the stroma are the essential prerequisites for the predecidual transformation (Fig. 9.18) of uncommitted stromal cells.[87] The role of endometrial histamine,[16] bradykinin, and serotonin[106] in these biologic events is not completely understood.

In rare instances, endocrine-type cells with positive immunostaining for serotonin and somatostatin are encountered in proliferative- and secretory-phase endometrial glands.[88] In experimental animal systems, release of histamine from mast cells and the subsequent edematous response occur within a few hours of E_2 stimulation, and histamine has been implicated as a cofactor in estrogen-primed cell growth and proliferation.[41,52] The human endometrium contains few mast cells even when the endometrium is fixed in basic lead citrate and stained with toluidine blue for 4–5 days.[18] These cells are located chiefly in the basal layer; their number is unchanged through the cycle but drops with age, with a marked decrease in the menopause. Although they contain heparin-rich granules and mast cells are increased in endometria with an intrauterine contraceptive device (IUCD) in place, they have no relationship with abnormal uterine bleeding. In addition, antihistamines do not prevent stromal edema, whereas indomethacin does.[16] These observations, and dose-dependent histamine induction of prostaglandin

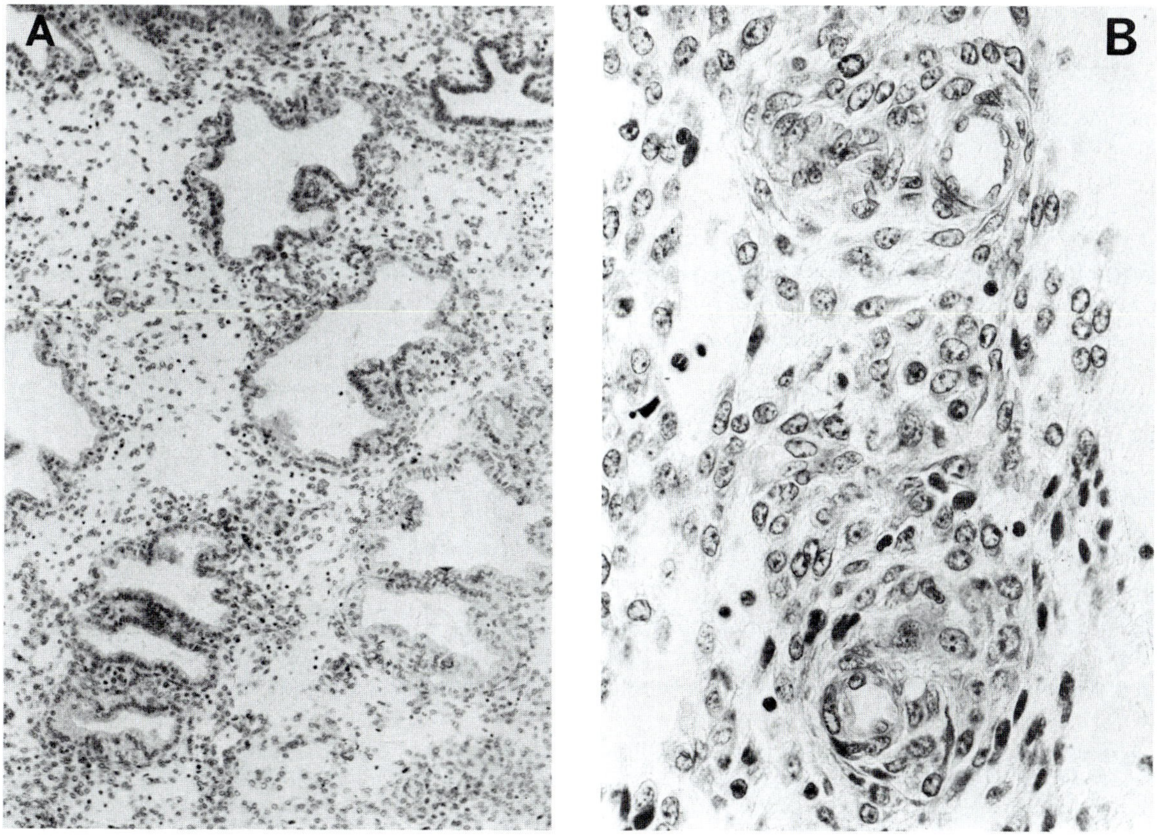

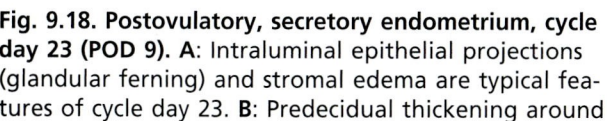

Fig. 9.18. Postovulatory, secretory endometrium, cycle day 23 (POD 9). A: Intraluminal epithelial projections (glandular ferning) and stromal edema are typical features of cycle day 23. **B**: Predecidual thickening around spiral arteries can better be appreciated on cycle day 23; this is caused by enlargement and rounding of the cytoplasm and nuclei of perivascular stromal cells.

release by cultured decidual cells, suggest that histamine may act on the endometrium indirectly by the production of PG.[52,89] Endometrial cell membranes and blastocyst membranes in the rabbit and rat, respectively, have receptors for histamine.[52] Pharmacologic inhibition of histamine release by mast cells has no effect on implantation efficiency in rats.[86] In contrast, an increased number of endometrial mast cells seems to have a negative impact on human gestation, as spontaneous abortions have a dramatically increased density of endometrial mast cells compared to normal pregnancies.[64] Endometrial vascular proliferation at the implantation site is related to the blastocyst rather than to histamine or PGE_2. The blastocyst has a unique biologic property that is shared only with tumor cells producing the so-called angiogenesis factor, a substance capable of inducing growth of new capillaries.[32]

An important immunosuppressive mechanism that operates at the chorio–decidual interface is provided by trophoblast-derived E_2 and P. The concentrations of both sex steroids are increased at this area, and P has been shown to effectively suppress interleukin-2-activated lymphocyte cytotoxicity.[76] This paracrine immunosuppressive effect of P is dose dependent and confers resistance to lysis to trophoblast by cytotoxic mononuclear cells.[22] Because cytotoxic cells are stimulated by IL-1 and because P suppresses in vitro IL-1 production by monocytes, P-related immunosuppression may operate by decreasing macrophage IL-1 production and the subsequent activation of cytotoxic lymphocytes.[22]

EGF (and its receptor, EGFR) are immunolocalized predominantly in the cytoplasm of syncytiotrophoblast but also in intermediate trophoblast during human implantation.[48] EGF has a differentiating effect on trophoblast, stimulating synthesis and secretion of human chorionic gonadotropin (hCG), human placental lactogen (hPL), and P. EGFR is similar to ERB-B oncogene,[83,92,93] and it is possible that it also contributes to the controlled trophoblastic invasion of the decidua.

Stromal predecidualization (not pseudodecidualization; the prefix "pre" refers to decidual transformation of stromal cells before their further decidual development during pregnancy) begins by day 22–23 (POD 8–9) (see Table 9.2) around spiral arterioles and capillaries of the functional layer (Fig. 9.18). Coinciding with the beginning of the predecidual reaction on cycle day 23, the glands form intraluminal epithelial projections, so-called ferning (see Table 9.2; Fig. 9.18). Perivascular predecidualization is more obvious on day 24 (POD 10) and is characterized by the conversion of uncommitted spindle-shaped stromal cells into plump epithelial-like cells with enlarged nuclei and increased cytoplasm.

Predecidual cells increase in size not only by cellular hypertrophy but also by mitosis and endoreduplication. The latter may be recognized by enlarged nuclei or double nucleation (tetraploidy). Proliferation of predecidual cells is mediated by growth-related peptides, as well as prostaglandins[9] and presumably Ki-67. Predecidual cells are devoid of E_2 receptors by immunohistochemistry[10]; their growth thus seems not to be stimulated by circulatory E_2. Progesterone receptors, on the other hand, are present,[10] which together with the high midsecretory-phase serum progesterone levels may play a role in cytoplasmic differentiation of predecidual cells. Ki-67 is expressed only in the nucleus of cycling proliferative but not in resting cells,[36] and its expression is upregulated by progesterone.[96] In endometrial stromal cells, PgR is expressed in both the proliferative and secretory phases of the cycle; however, Ki-67 immunoreactivity in endometrial stromal cells is weak during the proliferative phase but is increased in secretory-phase endometrium (Table 9.1). Decidualized cells show strong reactivity both for PR and often for Ki-67 (Fig. 9.19). Decidual transformation also may occur in extrauterine locations, chiefly during periods of pregnancy, in the subcoelomic mesenchyme of the pelvic peritoneum, ovary, and omentum.[46] Decidualization also can be triggered by electrical, mechanical, or chemical stimulation in progesterone-primed rodent uteri and fallopian tubes.[58,116]

Ultrastructurally, predecidual cells lack the typical features of epithelial cells, such as bundles of intermediate tonofilaments, glandular lumens, or desmosomal connections. On the other hand, they have intercellular gap junction nexuses. The latter are composed of hexagonal microtubules forming an open-channel system between adjacent cells that facilitates passage of electrolytes and molecules and plays a role in cell contact inhibition.[61,112] Histochemically, the predecidual cells contain glycogen and periodic acid–Schiff (PAS)-positive mucosubstances. Despite their epithelial-like appearance, predecidual cells often stain with vimentin (see Fig. 9.12) and desmin but not with cytokeratins or epithelial membrane antigen (see Table 9.1). The immunoreactivity of predecidual cells is consistent with their stromal cell derivation. Predecidual cells represent precursor forms of gestational decidual cells (decidua vera). The cells have several metabolic functions related either to pregnancy or, if conception has not occurred, to menstrual breakdown of the endometrium; for example, the decidual cells have phagocytotic properties and digest extracellular collagen matrix.[61] Decidual phagocytosis may facilitate the development of the decidual reaction by removing collagen from the endometrial stroma. The latter may represent a mechanical obstacle to proliferating and expanding predecidual cells. If conception does not occur, predecidual cells, by removing collagen, may contribute to menstrual breakdown of the endometrial stroma.

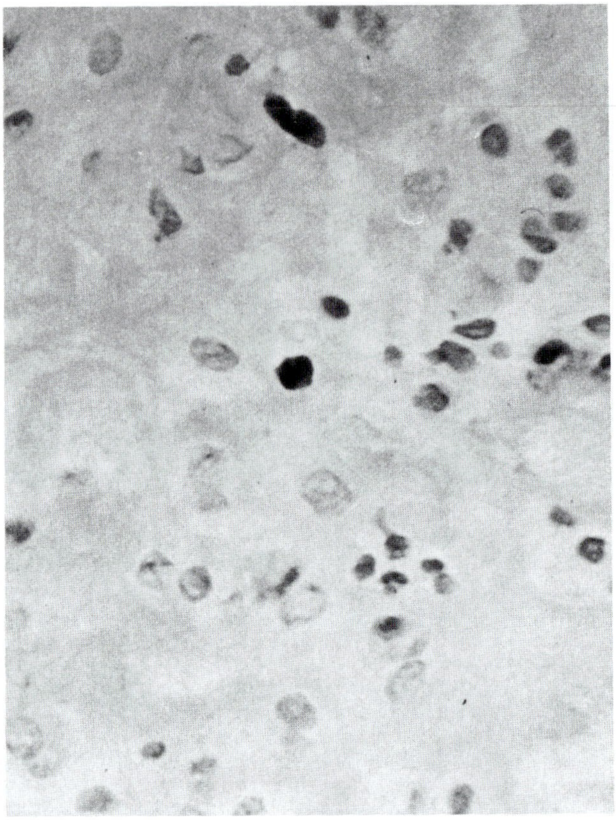

Fig. 9.19. Occasional gestational decidual cells have intense nuclear staining with Ki-67. (Courtesy of Shingo Fujii, M.D., Matsumoto, Japan.)

Postovulation Days 11–13

Predecidual transformation of stromal cells under the surface epithelium is achieved by day 25 (POD 11), producing the compacta layer (Fig. 9.20). On days 26 and 27 (POD 12 and 13), the upper two-thirds of the functionalis becomes predecidualized,

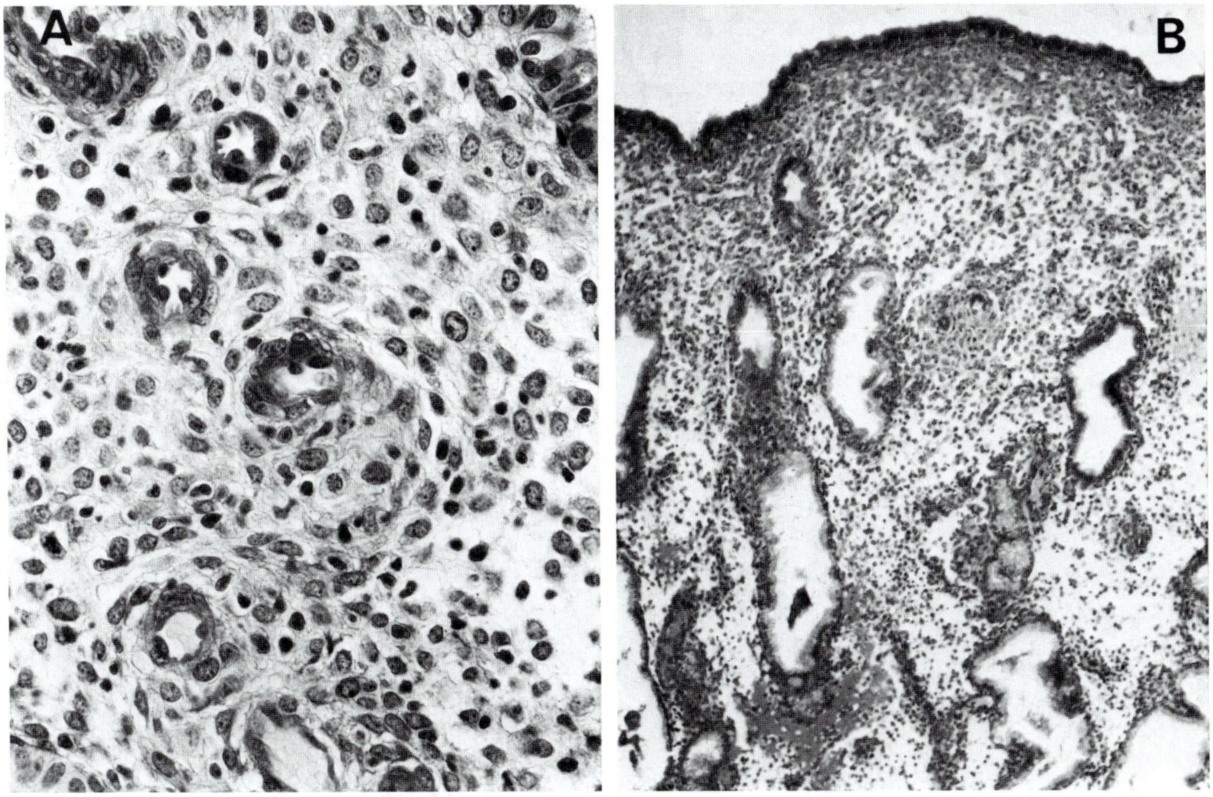

Fig. 9.20. Postovulatory, secretory endometrium, cycle days 24 and 25. A: On cycle day 24 (POD 10), predecidual transformation of perivascular stromal cells is evident. Note the well-defined cytoplasmic membranes and round nuclei of predecidual cells resembling epithelial cells. **B**: On cycle day 25 (POD 11), predecidualization of fibroblasts beneath the surface epithelium produces a bandlike cellular plate, the so-called compacta layer.

and the glands demonstrate coiling and ferning (Fig. 9.21A). The endometrial stroma during days 26 and 27 is infiltrated by extravasated polymorphonuclear leukocytes and the so-called metrial cells or granulocytes (Fig. 9.21B) Metrial granulocytes resemble eosinophils, except that they have a single, kidney-shaped nucleus (Fig. 9.21B). Endometrial stromal granulocytes (EGs), also named Kadornchenzellen or "K" cells, are abundant in the late-secretory phase of the menstrual cycle, more so in early pregnancy, after which they decline in number and are virtually absent at term.[12] Histologically, it was suggested by immunofluorescence technique that EGs derived from undifferentiated endometrial cells and their secretory granules contained relaxin.[20] However, later studies failed to support the view that EGs are a source of relaxin, and more recently immunohistochemical evidence has been presented that EGs are in fact members of the large granular lymphocyte series.[12] In both formalin-fixed and acetone-fixed decidual tissues, EGs stain positive with LCA, CD 2, MT 1, UCHL 1, and Leu-19 but fail to stain with CD

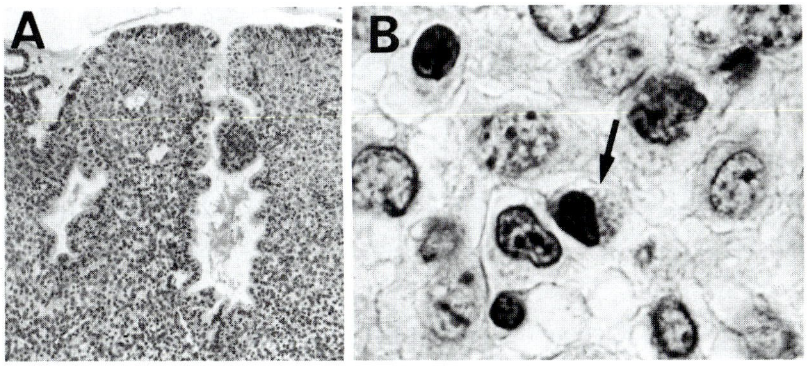

Fig. 9.21. Postovulatory, secretory endometrium, cycle day 26 (POD 12). A: The entire functionalis layer is occupied by predecidual cells secondary to expansion and confluency between the surface epithelial predecidual compacta and perivascular predecidua. The glands demonstrate secretory exhaustion, with inspissated intraglandular secretions. **B**: Granular lymphocyte (*arrow*) with a unilobar nucleus and eosinophilic granular cytoplasm.

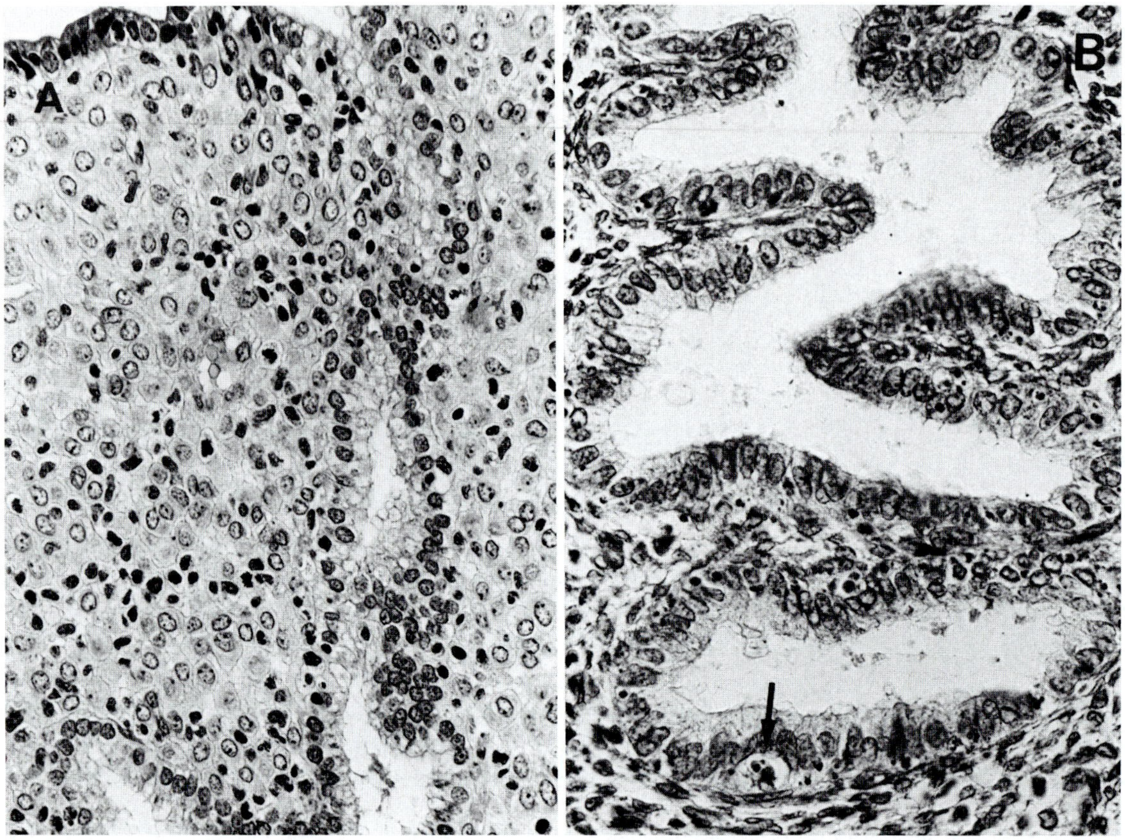

Fig. 9.22. Postovulatory secretory endometrium, cycle day 27 (POD 13). A: The predecidua is scattered with inflammatory cells; they are more conspicuous on cycle day 27 than day 26. **B**: Polydust (*arrow*) in gland cells and the stroma is a typical feature of impending (cycle day 28) or ongoing (cycle days 1 and 2) menstrual degeneration. Polydust has been phagocytosed by gland cells of the lower functionalis and basal layers.

16, Leu-7, CD 3, CD 5, CD 7, and HLA-DR. In view of the gradual increase in the number of EGs during the postovulatory secretory phase of the menstrual cycle and their maximum concentration during the first trimester of pregnancy, they are believed to be under hormonal control, and their immunocompetent phenotypic characteristics suggest that they may play an important role in implantation and placentation.

Relaxin (disulfide homologue of insulin) is considered to be an autocrine/paracrine hormone believed to be involved in collagenolysis. Monoclonal antibodies to human relaxin and polyclonal antiserum to porcine relaxin identified this hormone predominantly in the glands of both proliferative- and secretory-phase endometria. The predecidual cells in the late-secretory phase, and particularly early-gestational decidua parietalis, stain heavily, and relaxin genes appear to be transcribed in both the endometrial glands and stroma.[11,85] Whether they are translated as well has to be determined, but if so, they may be involved in the preparation and maintenance of early pregnancy by increasing collagenase and tissue plasminogen activators to break down collagen. Relaxin also is produced by syncytiotrophoblast, and trophoblast-derived relaxin also may facilitate penetration of decidua; this may cause weakening, rupture, and eventual detachment of fetal membranes, as well as contribute to cervical dilation.[30] If conception does not occur, relaxin may affect the endometrial stroma, facilitating breakdown of menstrual tissue. Degenerated nuclear debris of acute and chronic inflammatory cell origin often is seen to be phagocytosed by intact gland cells of the lower spongiosa and basalis layers on cycle days 28, 1, and 2 (Fig. 9.22B).

Menstrual Phase

A normal menstrual period lasts 4 ± 1 days. During this time, the endometrial mucosa rapidly degenerates, and 50% of the menstrual detritus is expelled in the first 24 hours of menses. Tissue shedding is

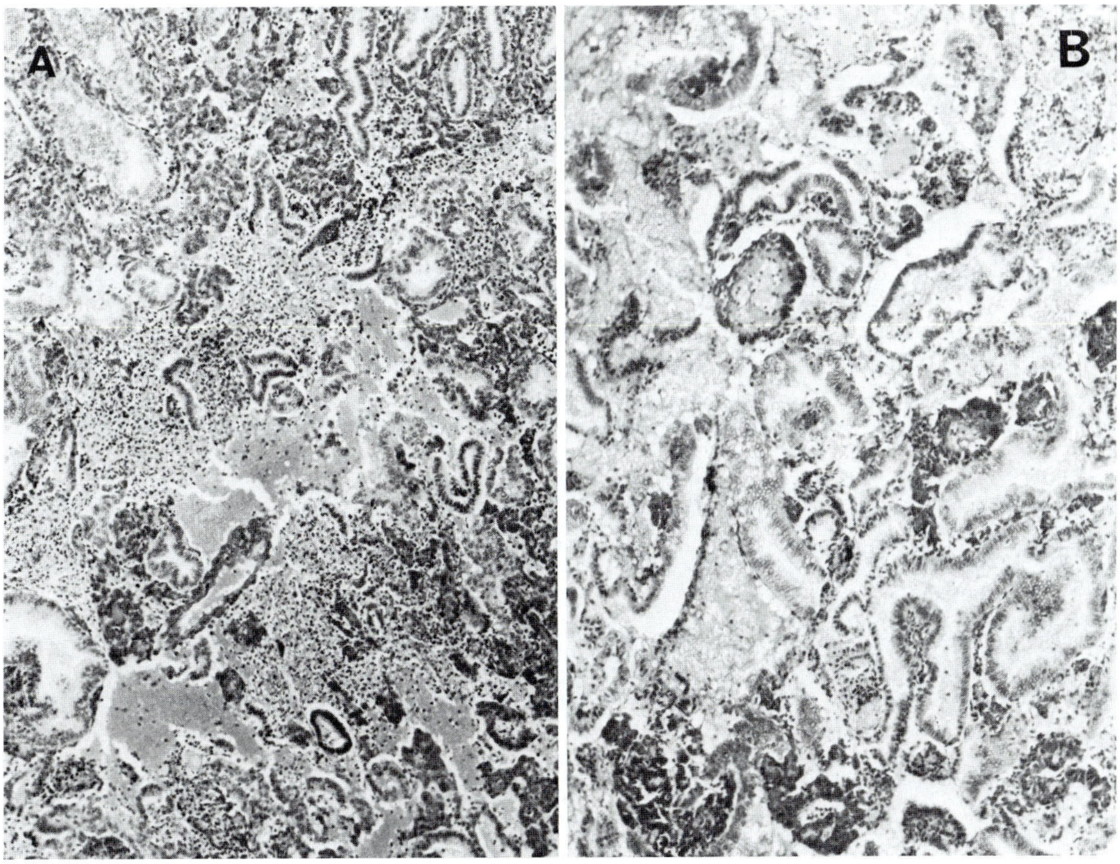

Fig. 9.23. Menstrual endometrium, degenerative phase. **A**: On cycle days 1–2, the endometrium contains collapsed stroma, ruptured glands with secretory exhaustion, degenerated predecidua, and inflammatory cells. **B**: Menstrual endometrium in a 42-year-old woman. The glands are larger and less exhausted than in **A**; however, degeneration is diffuse, a feature typical of estrogen–progestogen withdrawal type of bleeding endometrium.

followed by regeneration. The upper two-thirds of the endometrium on cycle days 28–2 contains fissures and degenerative predecidual cells admixed with epithelial glandular cells as well as acute and chronic (lymphoid) inflammatory cells (Figs. 9.23 and 9.24).

The mechanisms by which degeneration occurs are shown in Fig. 9.25. During endometrial proliferation, E_2 stimulates the development of Golgi-derived, primary lysosomes in the epithelial, stromal, and endothelial cells of the functional layer of the endometrium.[26,45] These lysosomes contain highly potent proteolytic enzymes. During the first half of the postovulatory period, lytic enzymes, including acid phosphatase, are confined to membrane-bound lysosomes by the action of P that stabilizes lysosomal membranes.[111] Coinciding with the fall of E_2 and P by day 25, the integrity of lysosomal membrane is no longer maintained. As a result, lysosomal enzymes are released intracellularly as well as into the intercellular space. Acid hydrolases digest the cytoplasmic elements, intercellular desmosomes, and ultimately the entire cellular system.[45] Lysosomal autodigestion destroys the glandular and stromal cells and also the vascular endothelium. Vascular luminal surface membrane injury promotes platelet deposits.[15] These alterations presumably are mediated by prostaglandin–thromboxane, and the final results are manifest by multiple minute foci of ischemic tissue necrosis.[15,71] In addition, acute swelling of the endothelial cells of endometrial arterioles contributes to obliteration of the vascular lumen.[45]

Paralleling these events, PGE_2 and particularly PGF_2 significantly increase in the late-secretory endometrium and reach maximum concentrations during the menstrual period.[30] It has been speculated that the high levels of PGF_2 also may release acid hydrolases from lysosomes and, during menstruation, stimulate the onset of ischemic necrosis via vasoconstriction of myometrial and basal arteries. Expulsion of degenerated endometrium is en-

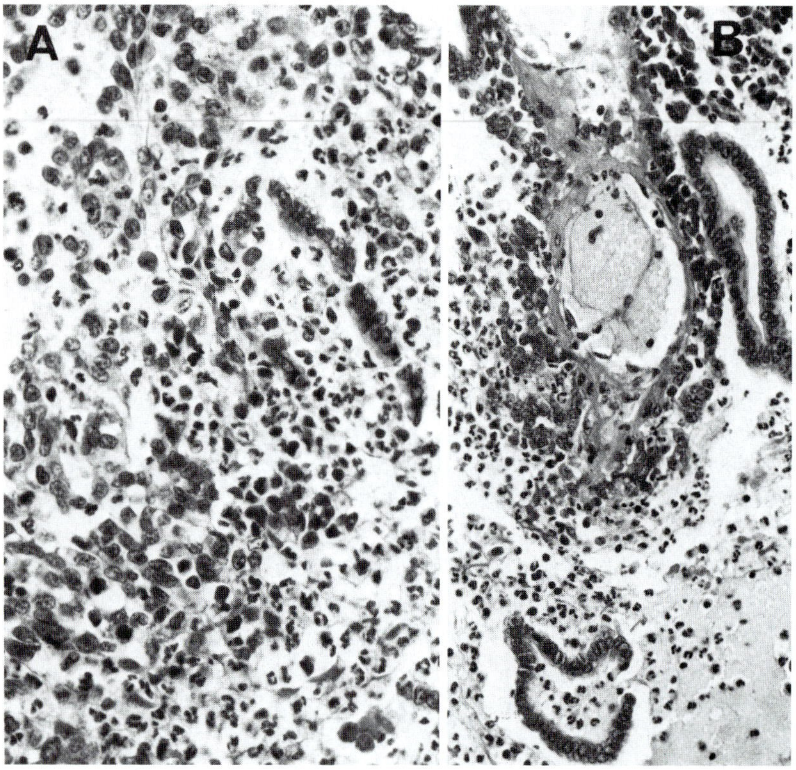

Fig. 9.24. Menstrual endometrium, degenerative phase. A: Ruptured, collapsed, exhausted glands and degenerative stromal cells intermingling with acute inflammatory cells, edema, and red blood cells. **B**: Ruptured endometrial vessel with fibrinoid deposit surrounded by degenerated predecidua and polymorphs.

hanced by PGF2-mediated myometrial contractions.[30] The menstrual fluid is composed of autolyzed tissue admixed with a heavy polymorphonuclear exudate, red blood cells, and proteolytic enzymes.[8] One of the latter is blood protease plasmin, a potent fibrinolytic agent that prevents clotting of menstrual blood and facilitates expulsion of the degenerated functionalis. The fibrinolytic activity of the endometrium, which characteristically disappears during the implantation period (cycle day

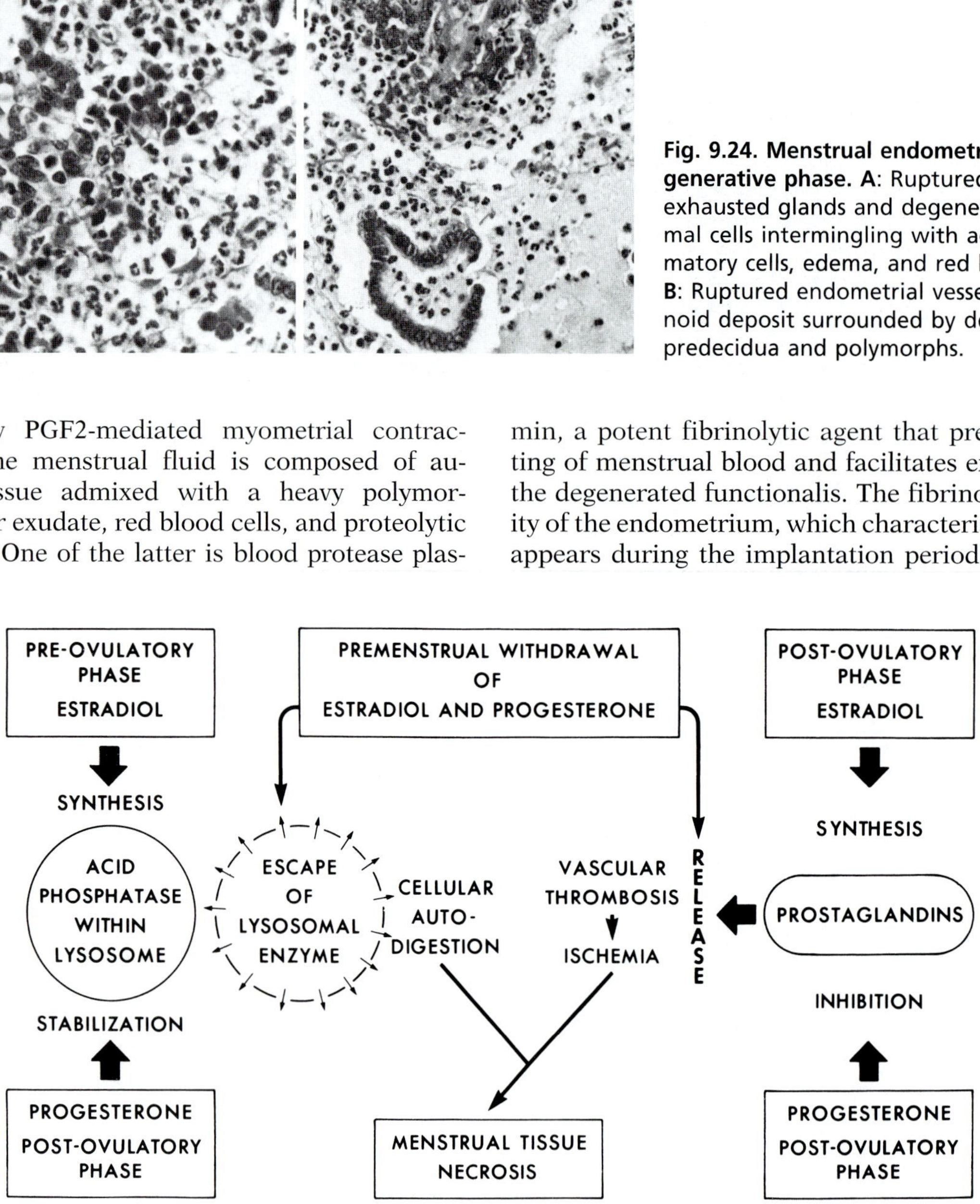

Fig. 9.25. Schematic representation of the morphobiochemical events that lead to the menstrual breakdown of the endometrium. The *large arrows* indicate the stimulatory effects of ovarian hormones. [Reprinted by permission of Ferenczy (1981) Contemp Obstet Gynecol 18:115.]

21), may play a role in preventing this process from occurring during the menstrual period. Plasminogen activators, which convert plasminogen into plasmin, are found in and released from degenerated endometrial vascular endothelium.[57]

Menstrual bleeding is controlled by vasoconstriction of the ruptured basal arteries in the denuded basal layer and radial and arcuate arteries in the myometrium. Rapid denudation of the basal layer reduces menstrual blood loss considerably. The arteries of the functionalis layer lack elastin and consequently cannot contract. In addition, they are shed with the functionalis and fail, therefore, to contribute to uterine hemostasis.[15]

On days 2–4, the functionalis becomes gradually detached from the underlying basalis.[23–26,68] Detachment starts from the fundus and slowly extends toward the isthmus, as observed by hysteroscopy.[63] The cleaved mucosa rolls on itself until it is detached from the basalis and is shed from the endometrial cavity. Shedding is most prominent during the first 2 days of the menstrual period, and endometrial biopsy or curettage yields abundant tissue. On the other hand, the next 2 days are dominated by proliferation of the residual basal gland epithelium in areas of complete denudation,[23–26] and the material obtained for histology during these days is generally scant. Reepithelialization occurs by extension of the residual glandular epithelium over the denuded surface. Essentially similar phenomena are observed in the spontaneously menstruating monkey and in the rabbit[25] in which the endometrium has been artificially denuded. The peripheral regions of the endometrial cavity, such as the isthmus and peritubal ostium, both of which remain intact during the menstrual period,[23,24] also contribute to resurfacing the epithelium. These converging epithelial proliferations interanastomose, leading to a new surface epithelium by cycle day 5. Bleeding ceases when the surface has been completely reepithelialized.

Epithelial cell migration followed by replication characterizes the biodynamics of endometrial surface repair.[26] Normal proliferative- and secretory-phase stromal cells are immunopositive for vimentin, muscle-specific actin (MSA), alpha-smooth muscle actin (α-SMA), and rarely desmin (see Table 9.1). None of the epithelial-type antibodies (i.e., cytokeratin, epithelial membrane antigen) react with stromal cells.[34] The immunohistochemical findings indicate the potential for smooth muscle differentiation of endometrial stromal cells. The light microscopic, immunohistochemical, and ultrastructural features of endometrial stromal cells are consistent with their similarity to myofibroblasts. Both stromal cells and myofibroblasts participate in normal wound healing. Endometrial stromal cells of the basal layer proliferate to replace shed endometrium and later in the cycle play a supportive role in maintaining endometrial integrity. The first-generation, resurfacing epithelial cells are flattened and have abundant surface microvilli, intracellular intermediate filaments, microtubules, and pseudopodial projections. These alterations reflect ameboid motility promoted by cyclic adenosine monophosphate and by the interaction of actin-containing filaments with myosin-containing plasma membranes. Nuclear and nucleolar enlargement (Fig. 9.26C) in regenerative cells also promotes cellular motility by providing increased DNA and RNA, respectively.

After the initial epithelial spread, mitosis and migration operate simultaneously until a confluent surface layer has been regenerated on cycle day 5. The sudden increase in DNA synthesis and the shortened DNA synthesis phase of regenerative cells provide for accelerated tissue turnover (see Fig. 9.11). The cellular migration and the rapid wound healing capability observed in the human endometrium together with the kinetic and ultrastructural data do not support the view that new endometrial surface and glandular epithelium are regenerated directly from persistent, secretory spongiosa[31] or stromal cells.[6] The latter are believed to contribute to endometrial epithelial repair[25] indirectly, presumably by their positive influence on growth factors[99] and by providing cellular support to the newly resurfacing surface epithelial cells. The latter event is recognized by aggregates of stromal cells beneath resurfacing epithelial cells. These so-called stromal "blue" balls (Fig. 9.26B,C) are typical features of endometrial stromal breakdown after uterine bleeding associated with tissue regeneration (see Fig. 9.8). The deep blue staining characteristic of aggregated stromal cells with H&E stain results from their prominent nuclei and scant cytoplasm. Tenascin, an extracellular matrix protein, has been immunolocalized around proliferative gland cells and vessels but not secretory-type glands.[107] Tenascin is thought to enhance epithelial migration and proliferation during periods of postmenstrual repair by inhibiting cell attachment to fibronectin.[13] Experimental studies have demonstrated that epithelial growth is stimulated and maintained by the adjacent or subjacent supportive fibroblasts.[13] The stromal aggregates are not pathognomonic of postovulatory menstrual regeneration, because they are also seen in endometrium after anovulation, estrogen or progestogen breakthrough bleeding, or withdrawal of exogenous estrogen and progestogens.

Postmenstrual endometrium repair is not induced by E_2. During cycle days 3 and 4, despite in-

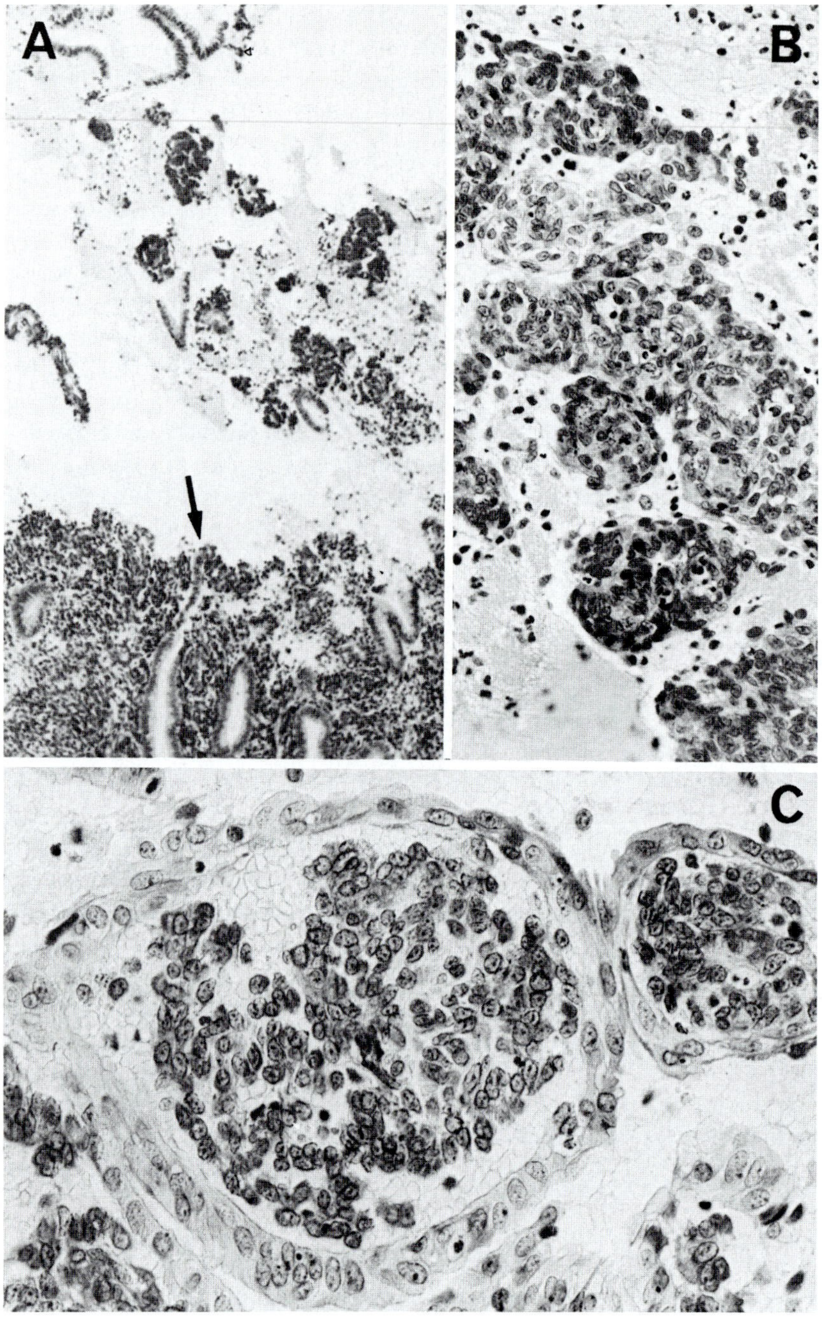

Fig. 9.26. Menstrual endometrium, regenerative phase. A: After expulsion of the functionalis layer, the basalis appears denuded (*arrow*) and is cleaved from the upper residual degenerated endometrial mucosa. The latter is composed of stromal aggregates, ruptured glands, and inflammatory cells. **B**: Aggregates of residual stromal fibroblasts (stromal balls) are typical of late degenerative–early regenerative phase endometrium. **C**: Endometrial stromal fibroblasts forming the stromal balls are surrounded by resurfacing regenerative epithelial cells, which typically have flattened cytoplasm, enlarged nuclei and nucleoli consistent with repair, and nuclear polyploidy.

creased DNA synthesis, circulating estrogens and receptors for E_2 and P are low, unchanged from the premenstrual values.[26] In experimental endometrial regeneration in the rabbit, similar proliferative and morphologic patterns are observed, regardless of whether the animals are ovariectomized or have intact ovaries.[25] On cycle days 7–12, however, there is a marked increase in DNA synthesis (see Fig. 9.11) and mitotic activity in all cell components of the regenerated human endometrium; this coincides with an increase in plasma estrogens and E_2R–PgR concentrations and a slight decrease in serum pituitary hormones. These alterations reflect target cell sensitivity and response to preovulatory E_2.

Morphology of Gestational Endometrium

Glandular Epithelium

If pregnancy occurs, the secretory-phase endometrium undergoes further morphophysiologic development and achieves its raison d'etre, that is,

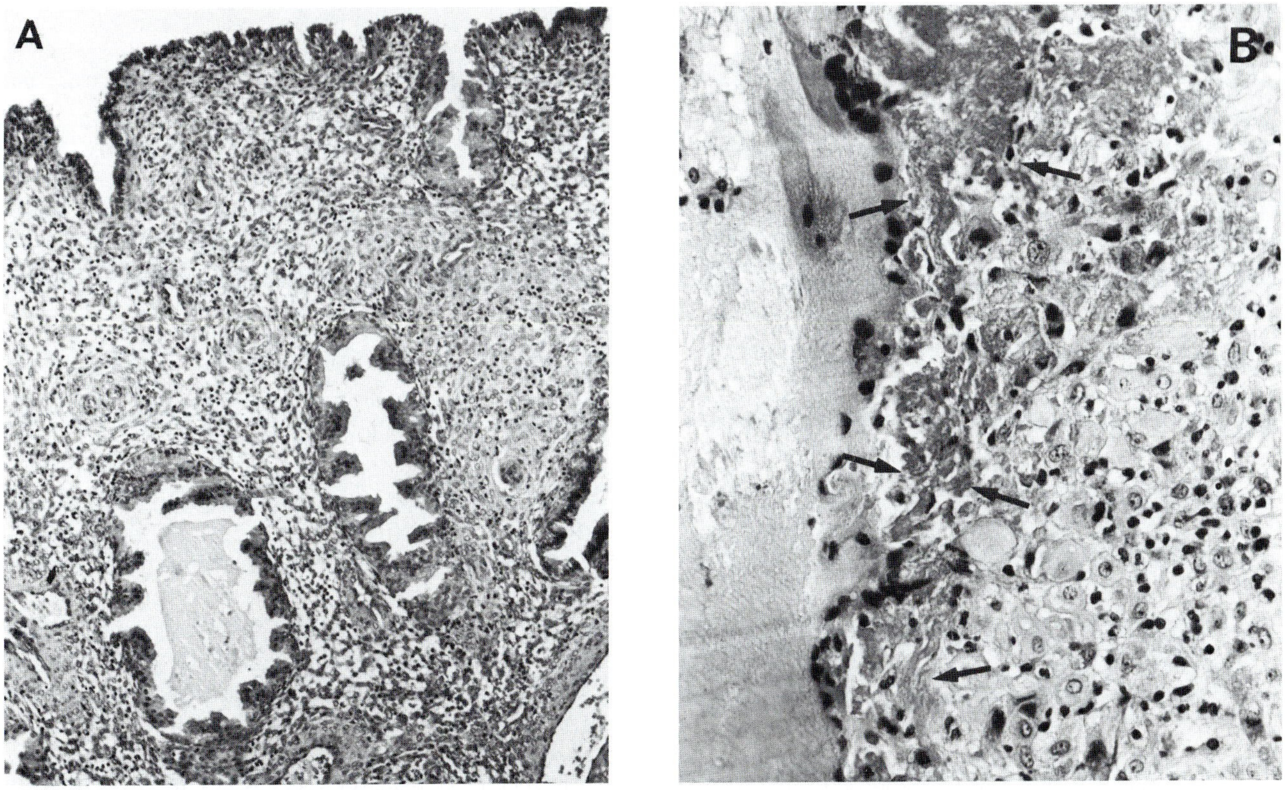

Fig. 9.27. Gestational endometrium. A: Voluminous secretory glands with numerous, prominent intraluminal epithelial projections and secretions are associated with dense predecidua (*right*), stromal edema (*left*), and a well-developed arterial system. When these changes are seen in the upper one-third of the spongiosa layer, they are suggestive but not diagnostic of early gestation. **B**: Fibrinoid (Nitabuch's) layer (*arrows*), with placental site multinucleated syncytial cells on one side (*left*) and gestational decidua vera cells on the other side (*right*), is pathognomonic of intrauterine pregnancy.

to provide an appropriate environment for the conceptus. Between days 22 and 28, the endometrium displays hypertrophic and hypersecretory features that many refer to as "gestational hyperplasia."[47] The endometrium is characterized by (1) glandular ferning with epithelial and intraluminal secretions, (2) stromal edema and vascular congestion, and (3) transmucosal predecidual reaction devoid of inflammatory exudate (Fig. 9.27A). The changes are similar to but quantitatively exaggerated from nongestational 22- to 26-day secretory endometrium. In the latter, each of these alterations is prominent on a given day of the secretory phase, whereas during early pregnancy they occur simultaneously. However, gestational hyperplasia is not diagnostic of early pregnancy unless an ovum of POD 9–13 is seen implanted in the endometrium or elevated serum hCG is detected.[5,44] The presence of fibrinoid with syncytial giant cells representing the placental site is diagnostic. Indeed, morphologic modification similar to gestational hyperplasia also may be found in association with double (twin) corpora lutea[47] and persistent corpus luteum cyst.[44] The only pathognomonic feature of intrauterine pregnancy is chorionic tissue, embryonic tissue, or a fibrinoid layer with trophoblastic cells (Fig. 9.27B).

The gestational endometrium becomes distinctive by the fourth week of gestation. Many gestational glands display intraluminal epithelial projections (ferning), and often they are lined with large cells with clear or eosinophilic cytoplasm and nuclei of varying size (Fig. 9.28). Exaggeration of these cytonuclear alterations produces the so-called Arias—Stella reaction (ASR),[3] characterized by voluminous cells with large hyperchromatic nuclei and irregular nuclear membranes. The cytoplasm often is clear and vacuolated. ASR, when extensive, may be confused with clear cell carcinoma. Unlike clear cell carcinoma, ASR is typically focal, and the adjacent endometrium shows normal gestational changes, that is, a prominent decidual reaction. In addition, in the malignant clear cells, there is a high nucleocytoplasmic (N/C) ratio, whereas ASR cells have normal N/C ratios, both the cytoplasm and nu-

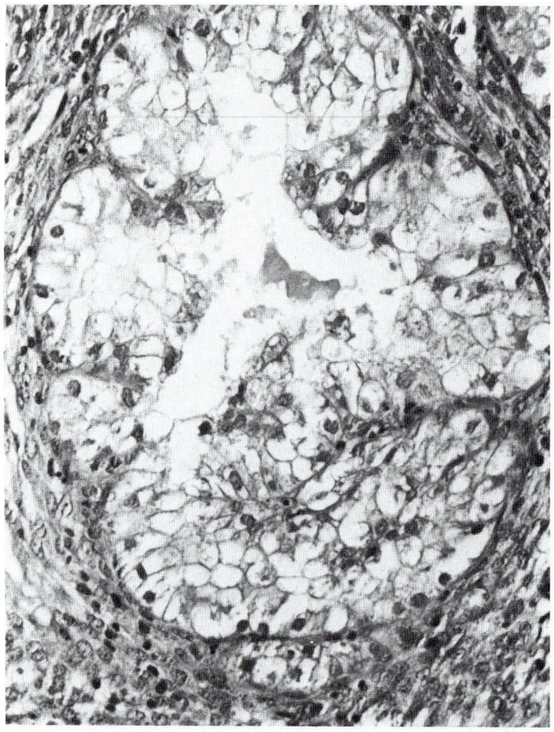

Fig. 9.28. Hypersecretory gland with thickened, hypertrophic, pseudostratified cells with clear cytoplasm and blunt-ended epithelial projections into the lumen. The nuclei are round, and unlike those in the Arias–Stella reaction, are small. Both the glandular and cellular alterations are suggestive but not pathognomonic of early pregnancy.

cleus being enlarged (cytonucleomegaly) (Fig. 9.29). Nuclear enlargement in ASR is a consequence of nuclear polyploidy, which presumably occurs by endomitosis and subsequent fusion of divided nuclei[108]; this is in contrast with the near-diploid or aneuploid nuclear DNA content of endometrial carcinoma. ASR is a hormonally related gland cell hypertrophy associated with intra- or extrauterine pregnancy or trophoblastic disease.[91] The hormones involved are presumably chorionic gonadotropin, estrogen, and progesterone. ASR also may be seen in the glandular epithelium of the cervix, the fallopian tube, endometriosis, or vaginal adenosis.[91] In spontaneous abortion or later gestation, ASR demonstrates nuclear aberrations consistent with degenerative features, including agglutinated nuclear DNA, cytoplasmic vacuolization, and apical nuclear position (hobnail cells) (Fig. 9.29). These observations suggest that ASR in endometrial gland cells results from hyperstimulation induced by high levels of gestational hormones. These changes regress and disappear after withdrawal of hormonal stimulation.

Another distinctive feature in endometrial gland cells associated with intrauterine pregnancy and trophoblastic disease is nuclear vacuolization, so-called optically clear nuclei (Fig. 9.30), resembling the ground glass appearance of herpes virus inclusions.[65] Ultrastructurally, however, nuclear clearing corresponds to strands of filaments 70 to 80 Å thick, which in turn may correspond to a filamentous presentation of nuclear chromatin, secondary to gestational hormonal hyperstimulation.

Stroma

As discussed earlier, the predecidual cells are transformed into larger epithelioid decidual cells termed decidua vera. These cells are particularly prominent in the upper one-third of the endometrium and produce the compacta layer. Ultrastructurally, gestational decidual cells contain comparatively more organelles, including intermediate filaments, cigar-shaped mitochondria, and granular endoplasmic reticulum, than their predecidual nongestational counterparts.[61,113] Although predecidual cells are interconnected by tight junctional nexuses, the gestational variant has nexuses between cytoplasmic filopodial projections. The gestational decidual reaction is not pathognomonic of intrauterine pregnancy in general, because similar changes may be seen in ectopic pregnancy or as a result of exogenous progestational therapy.

Near the implantation site, cells resembling decidual cells often contain significant nuclear atypia. However, immunohistochemistry localizes human placental lactogen in these cells, indicating that they are intermediate-type trophoblast rather than decidual cells (see Chapter 23, Diseases of the Placenta and Chapter 24, Gestational Trophoblastic Disease and Related Lesions)[59]; this is also true for the so-called placental site reaction, which is produced by trophoblastic cells infiltrating the decidua near the implantation site. In both instances, the atypical cytologic features often are those of degeneration with agglutinated nuclear DNA and are focal. The neighboring endometrium contains gestational decidual cells and displays glandular secretory features. Occasionally, however, cytologic atypia seems to be a reflection of active trophoblastic cells that extend into the decidua. The decidual cells have phagocytic properties and digest the extracellular collagen matrix.[61] Decidual phagocytosis may facilitate the development of the decidual reaction by removing collagen from the endometrial stroma, which may represent a mechanical obstacle to proliferating and expanding decidual cells and also infiltrating trophoblastic cells.

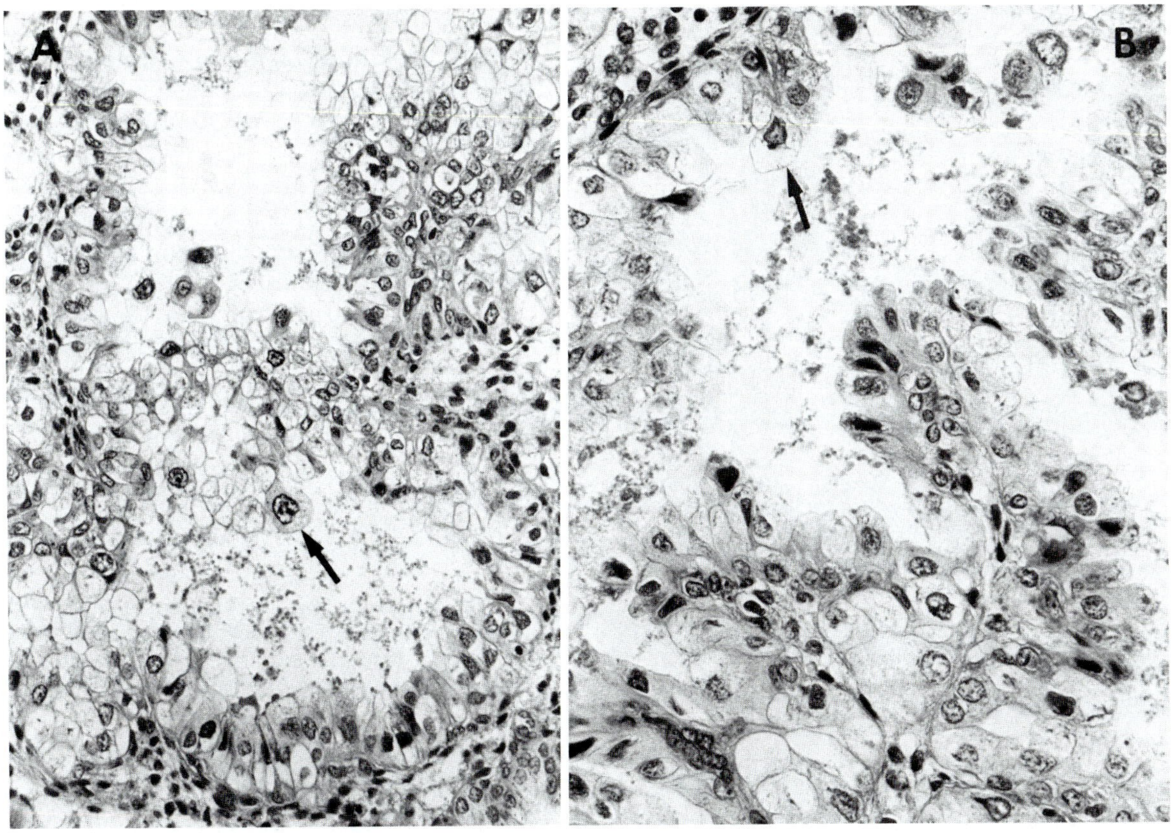

Fig. 9.29. Gestational endometrium with Arias–Stella reaction (ASR). A: Voluminous gland in which some of the lining cells demonstrate ASR (*arrow*), characterized by cytonucleomegaly, hyperchromatic nuclei, and enlarged nucleoli. Note the well-preserved, finely granular cytoplasmic substance and nuclear chromatin of ASR cells, seen in the early developmental phase of ASR. **B**: ASR cells with shrunken, degenerated nuclei and vacuolated cytoplasm (*arrow*); this is the degenerative phase of ASR and is seen in missed abortions.

Another important function of decidual cells is related to the maintenance of the fetal allograft (fetus).[73] Indeed, it is likely that decidual cells control the invasive nature of the normal trophoblast. Lack of a decidual reaction in the endometrium as occurs in the isthmus or in the fallopian tubal mucosa is accompanied by deep myometrial implantation of the placenta (placenta accreta) and invasion of the myosalpinx, respectively. An abdominal pregnancy may be viable because the subcoelomic mesenchymal cells of the pelvic and abdominal peritoneum are capable of decidual transformation.[69] The factors that control decidual transformation in different sites are unknown; however, immunologic mechanisms may be involved.[11] Soon after implantation, decidual cells develop direct contact with semiallogenic fetal antigens and are considered to play an important role(s) in maintaining successful implantation and pregnancy. Both endometrial stromal cells and decidual cells have been shown immunohistochemically to express hemopoietic cell-associated CD 13 and CD 10 antigens in all respects similar to granulocytes, monocytes, and lymphoid cells (see Table 9.1).[51] CD 13 and CD 10 antigens are peptidases; CD 13 is an ectoenzyme identical to aminopeptidase, which also is found in intestinal and kidney brush border membrane. It hydrolyzes peptides such as bradykinin and enkephalin. CD 10 antigen is similar to endopeptidase and is expressed in lymphoid and kidney cells; it also is an ectopeptidase. It has been speculated that endometrial met-enkephalin and interleukin-1 (IL-1),[76] an immunomodulator and an inhibitor of decidualization, respectively,[75] may be degraded by CD 13 or CD 10, thereby contributing to a favorable environment for successful pregnancy.[51] The immunologic role of decidua is suggested by its suppression of the antibody response of spleen cultures to DNP-polylysine, as well as its suppression of the mixed lymphocyte reaction and proliferative response of lymphocytes to allogeneic graft cells and to T-cell mitogens.[55]

Earlier studies using hemopoietic cell-associated antigens suggested the bone marrow derivation of

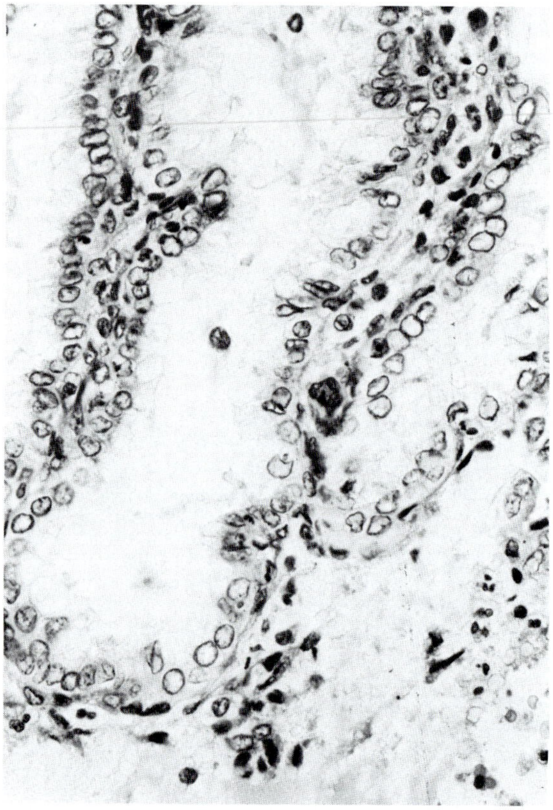

Fig. 9.30. Gestational endometrium. Intranuclear clearing resembling the ground glass appearance of nuclei with herpes simplex virus inclusions. In gestational endometrial gland cells, however, the nuclei contain threadlike filaments rather than viral particles.

decidual cells.[55] However, most recent studies provide evidence that this may not be the case.[33,51] Both endometrial stromal cells and decidual cells express CD 13 and CD 10 surface antigens in all respects similar to granulocytes, monocytes, and lymphoid cells (see Table 9.1); however, they are clearly distinguished from the latter by immunohistochemical tracing studies.[51] Also, decidual cells fail to express specific surface antigens of hematopoietic cells such as CD 2, CD 20, CD 11b, and CD 14.[53] The human nongestational and, particularly, gestational decidua also has been reported to have endocrinologic functions,[11] which apparently synthesize and release prolactin (PRL) that is immunologically identical to pituitary PRL.

Although decidual cells lack ultrastructural similarity to pituitary cells and are devoid of secretory granules, prolactin was localized both in the predecidua and decidua in vitro by immunoblotting, and its production is stimulated by progesterone and relaxin.[50] Furthermore, prolactin production was demonstrated exclusively in nongestational stromal cell cultures, but not in gland cell cultures, and is induced and maintained by P and E_2.[80] Earlier observations identified gestational decidua synthesizing de novo prolactin as the source of amniotic fluid prolactin.[83] The basement membrane of decidual cells resembles other basement membranes in the body and may contribute to the formation of the laminin-rich Nitabuch's layer in the placental implantation site. Both predecidual cells and cytotrophoblast produce laminin-containing basement membrane[55,56] and intermediate intracytoplasmic fibroblasts,[115] providing for their rigidity and supportive role to endometrial glands. Decidual cells also are suspected of synthesizing PGF_2 from arachidonic acid released from intracellular stores of phospholipids.[30] Phospholipase A_2 that releases arachidonic acid is found in intracytoplasmic lysosomes. Release of PGF_2 from gestational decidual cells may play a role in the initiation of labor.

Spiral arteries are larger and their walls are thicker than those found in nongestational secretory endometrium. Some of them display acute atherosis, with concentric intimal proliferation of myofibroblasts and foamy cells (Fig. 9.31). These alterations apparently occur in response to trophoblastic invasion of endometrial vessels; they are focal and are more frequent in primigravidas.[103] Such

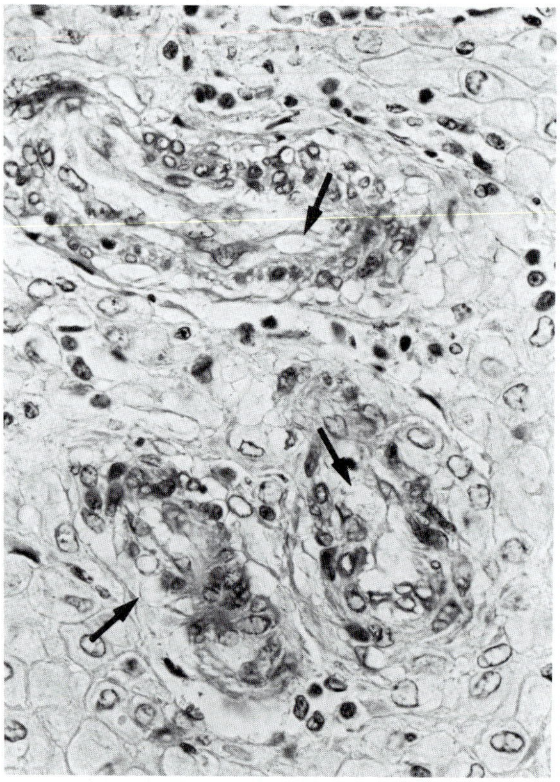

Fig. 9.31. Gestational endometrium. Atherosis of endometrial vessels with foamy vacuolization (*arrows*) of endothelial cells.

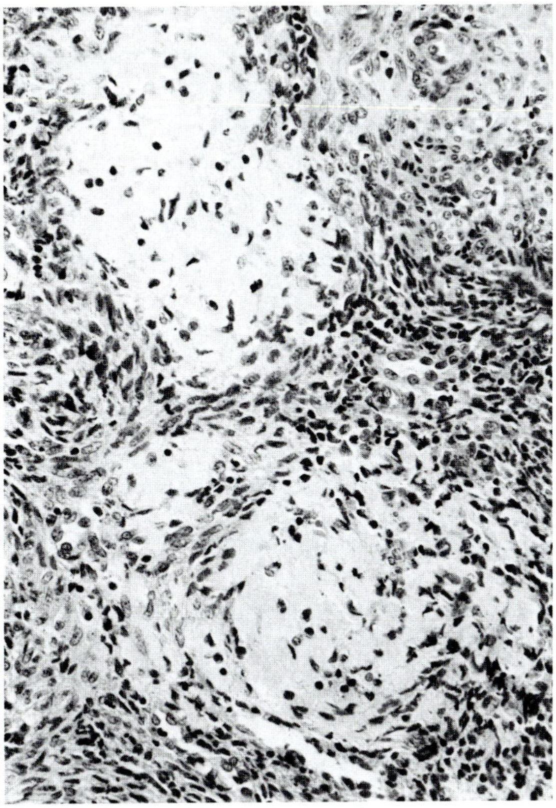

Fig. 9.32. Fibrohyaline nodules scattered with fibroblasts. These structures represent obliterated endometrial arteries at a previous placental site. This patient delivered 8 weeks before a curettage for postpartum bleeding.

changes are not associated with preeclampsia, eclampsia, diabetes, or hypertension.[62] After delivery, the endometrial vessels near the implantation site undergo thrombosis and later hyalinization, as does the surrounding decidua. These alterations produce fibrohyaline nodules, so-called placental site nodules, typical of recent to remote (several years) intrauterine pregnancy (Fig. 9.32). When the placental site becomes acutely or chronically inflamed, the partially hyalinized and thrombosed vessels cannot contract, which leads to postpartum bleeding of the subinvoluting uterus.

Morphology of Inactive and Atrophic Endometrium

An endometrium that is as thick as early- to mid-proliferative-phase endometrium but is devoid of morphologic features of either active proliferation or secretion may be considered inactive as far as its response to hormonal stimuli is concerned. The glands and stroma resemble proliferative endometrium, but the glands usually are oriented parallel rather than perpendicular to the surface epithelium. The surface epithelium as well as that lining the glands is columnar to cuboidal and contains pseudostratified nuclei without mitoses, and occasional ciliated cells are seen. The stroma generally is dense throughout, without a clear-cut separation between the basalis and functionalis layer (Fig. 9.33). Such endometrial changes are found in most menopausal and postmenopausal women,[2] in whom ovarian hormonal stimuli have decreased to levels not sufficient to induce endometrial proliferation. Nuclear DNA synthesis and E_2R are maintained in the senescent or inactive but not in the severely atrophic endometrium.[77] This phenomenon explains why exogenous estrogens can "revitalize" the inactive endometrium and both glandular and stromal cells acquire receptors for P. As a result, unopposed estrogens in the menopause may lead to hyperplasia,[35] whereas P therapy either may convert hyperplasia to secretory endometrium or prevent the development of hyperplasia.[29]

There are several morphologic manifestations of atrophic endometrium, but all have in common a thin mucosa that measures about half or less of the thickness of a basal layer of cyclic endometrium (less than 0.5 mm). Typically, in the curettings, the entire atrophic endometrial mucosa, including its basalis layer, can be seen within a microscopic field of ×250. There is a further decrease in the number and volume, respectively, of glands and stroma, and most commonly the glands are oriented parallel to the surface (Fig. 9.34). The lining epithelium of both the surface and glands is low and cuboidal and devoid of cilia, although cilia may be quite frequent in surface epithelial cells. The stroma often is collagenized and resembles the stroma of the isthmus or lower uterine segment in premenopausal women. Endometrial vascular alterations are seldom seen in women with atrophic endometrium, including those with abnormal uterine bleeding. In fact, in more than 50% of patients, no pathology is found in the uterus.[14,66] The most frequent morphologic changes that can be related to clinical bleeding are (1) arteriosclerosis of the myometrial arteries, including the arcuate and radial arteries, with medial hypertrophy and calcification and narrowing of the lumen, and (2) rupture of dilated and engorged endometrial veins secondary to uterine prolapse or compression by dilated atrophic endometrial cysts.[14,66] The former condition when associated with cardiovascular collapse may lead to hemorrhagic necrosis of the endometrial mucosa, producing apoplexia uteri.[21] At other times, coexistent chronic endometritis, submucous leiomyomata, or endometrial polyps may be the organic causes of uterine bleeding.

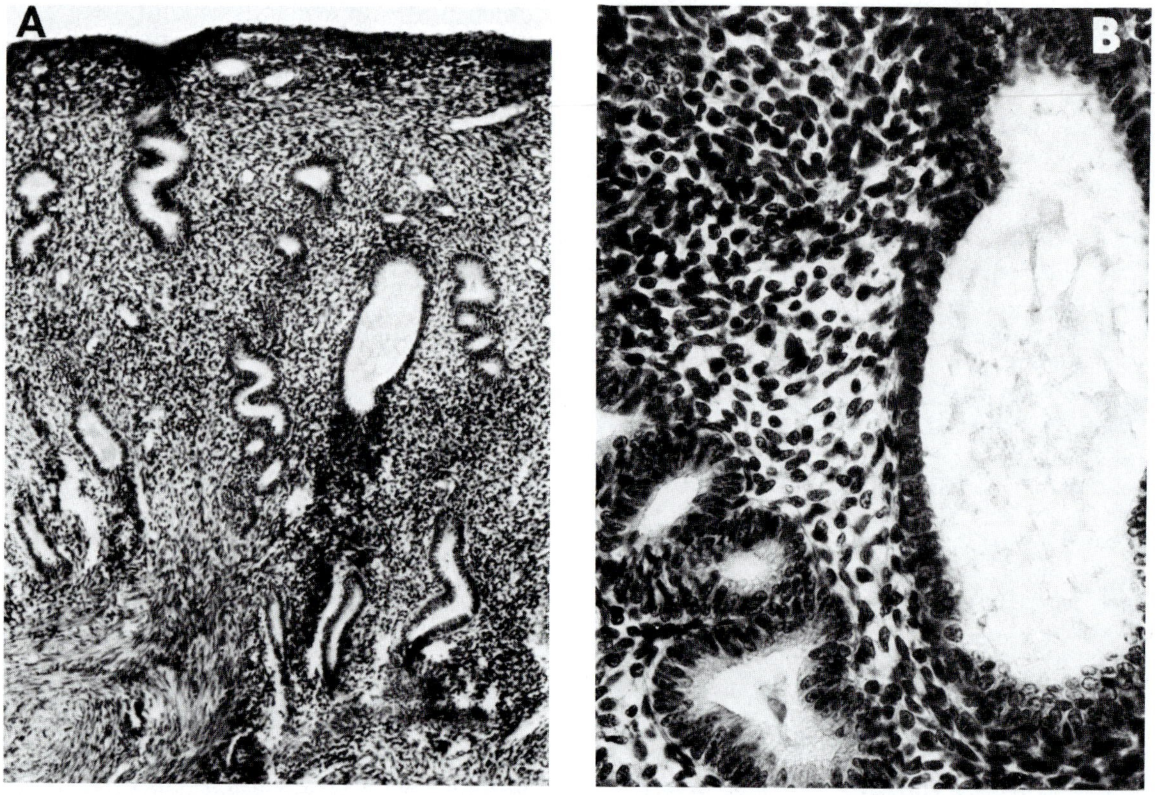

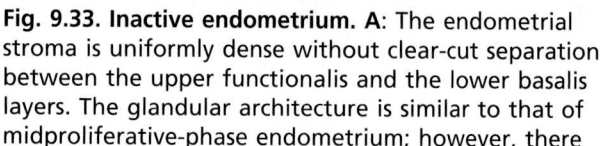

Fig. 9.33. Inactive endometrium. A: The endometrial stroma is uniformly dense without clear-cut separation between the upper functionalis and the lower basalis layers. The glandular architecture is similar to that of midproliferative-phase endometrium; however, there are fewer glands, and some of them are oriented parallel to the surface. **B**: Inactive glandular epithelium has pseudostratified nuclei devoid of mitoses, and the surrounding stroma is dense and cellular, resembling the stroma of the basalis layer of cyclic endometrium.

Atrophic endometrium often has cystically dilated glands. Whether these represent the atrophic variants of cystically dilated glands that are seen in the lower functionalis in virtually all women aged 35 years and over[54] is not clear. However, the condition is often referred to as cystic atrophy (Fig. 9.35A). Cystically dilated glands also are seen in cystic glandular hyperplasia with retrogressive atrophy. In this case, the endometrial mucosa retains the thickness of an otherwise active hyperplasia, but the glandular epithelium is atrophic and the stroma is collagenized (see Fig. 9.33B). On occasion, both the surface and glandular epithelium is composed of tall columnar to cuboidal cells, including ciliated cells resembling those seen in hyperplasia. Unlike true hyperplasia, this form of atrophy lacks mitotic figures, the mucosa is thin, and the stroma is relatively rich in collagen fibers (Fig. 9.36A). It is possible that the changes reflect the estrogenic response of otherwise atrophic endometrial epithelium that has been under either endogenous or exogenous estrogenic stimulation. The morphologic changes, furthermore, appear to be confined to the epithelial cells without stromal cell participation. In extreme atrophy, there is endometrial stromal fibrosis, and only the surface epithelium and rare glands remain lined by low cuboidal cells (Fig. 9.36B). In such cases, the isthmic ostium (internal os), as well as the external cervical os, may be completely stenotic, resulting in pyometra. In response to long-standing irritation by the chronic inflammatory exudate, the surface epithelium may undergo squamous metaplasia, which in extreme cases lines the entire endometrial cavity, resulting in the condition referred to as ichthyosis or psoriasis uteri.

Technical Consideration and Pitfalls in Interpretation of Biopsies

Accurate morphologic interpretation is achieved when either the biopsy sample or the curetting is taken from the body or fundus region and fixed immediately in either 10% buffered formalin or Bouin's solution. Formalin is superior to Bouin's solution if one plans DNA or immunohistochemical studies, whereas the excellent preservation of cyto-

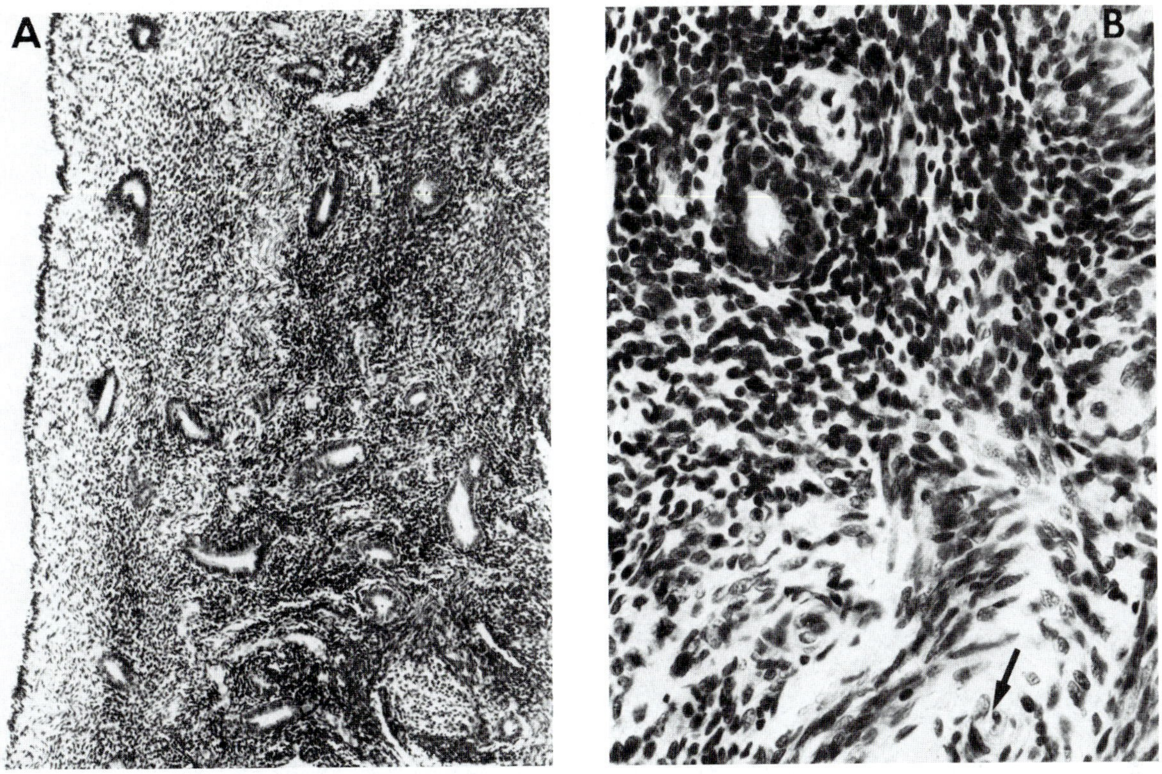

Fig. 9.34. Atrophic endometrium. A: The endometrial mucosa is thin and made of dense fibrocellular stroma and a few small glands with narrow lumens. **B**: Detailed view of endometrial arteries in basalis layer shows severe obliterative endarteritis with minute lumens (*arrow*). The gland in the *upper left* is the size of a capillary, has a narrow lumen, and is lined by low cuboidal cells.

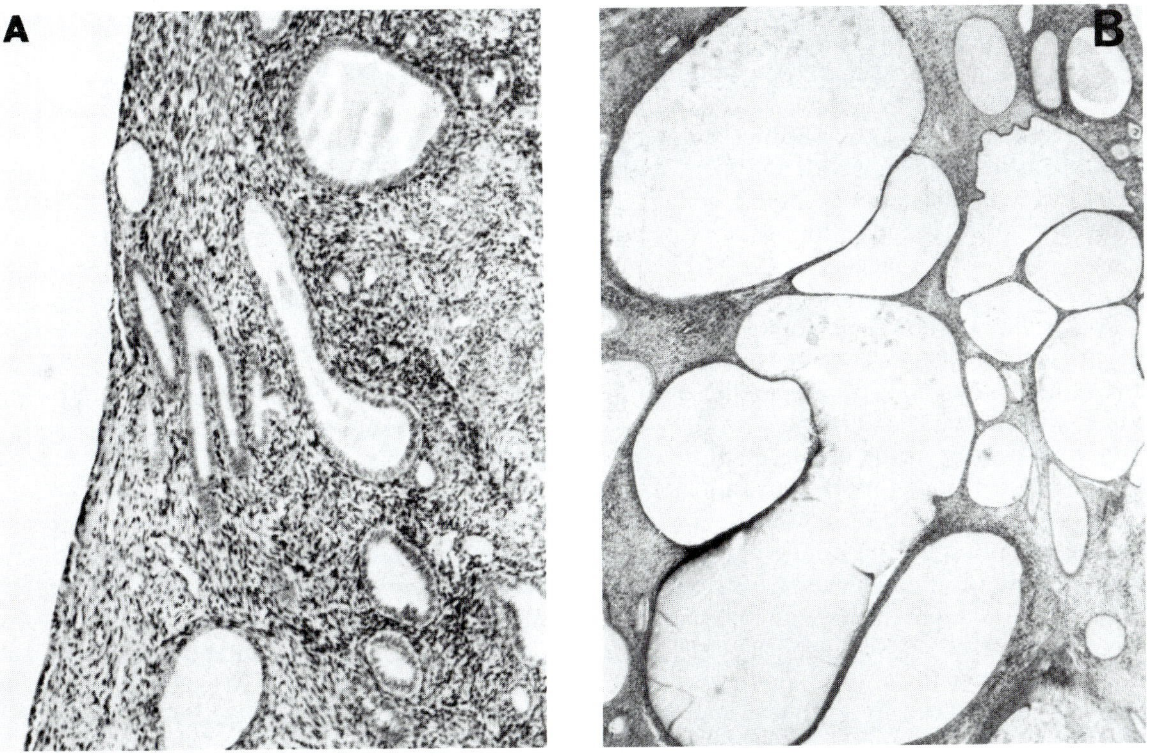

Fig. 9.35. Atrophic endometrium. A: Several cystically dilated glands, particularly at the endomyometrial junction, are often seen in otherwise atrophic endometrium. Their significance, if any, is unknown, but they are not considered to reflect previous hyperplasia. **B**: Cystic glandular dilation characterized by a relatively tall endometrial mucosa in which there are multiple cystic spaces lined by atrophic epithelium and surrounded by dense fibrous stroma.

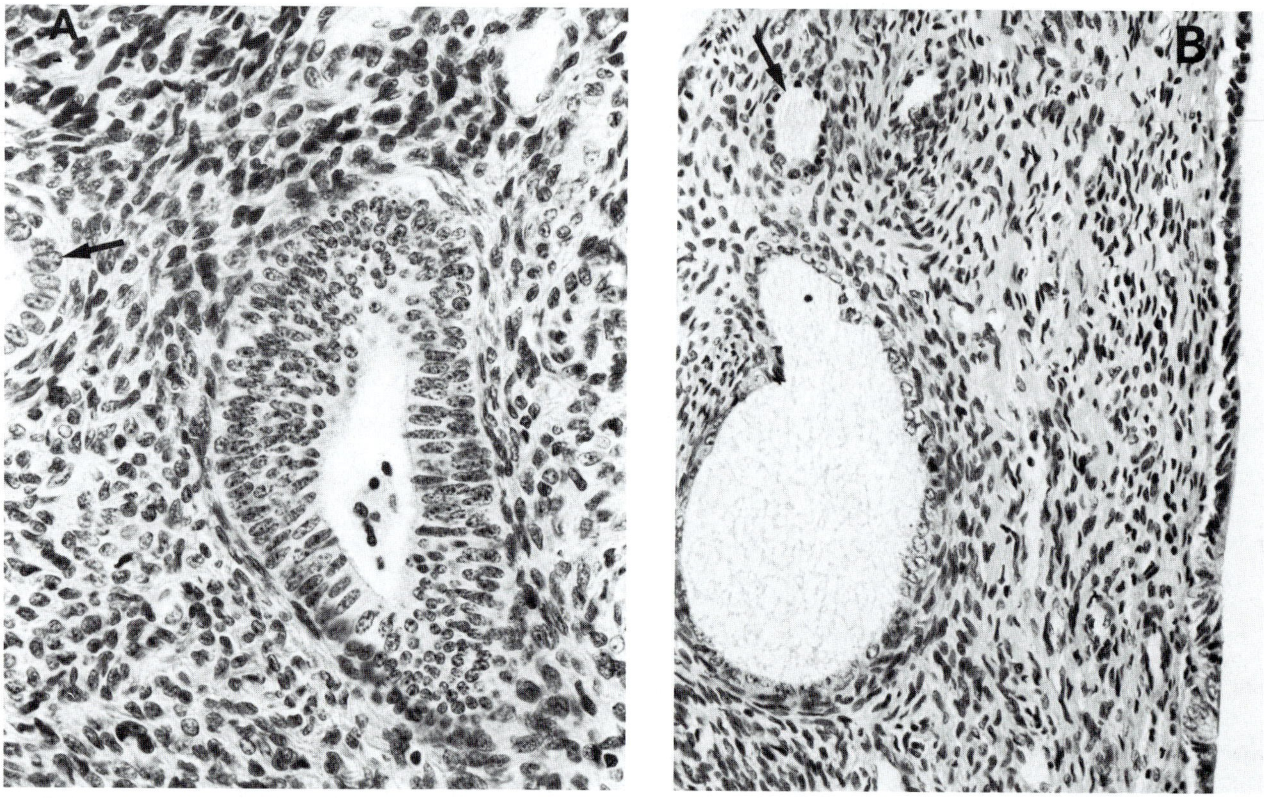

Fig. 9.36. Atrophic endometrium. A: The gland-lining cells are tall, columnar, with pencil-shaped pseudostratified nuclei and cilia resembling those found in endometrial hyperplasia. However, the endometrium is thin, and the stroma is dense, with many glands lined by atrophic epithelium (*arrow*). **B**: On the other end of the spectrum, in severe glandulostromal atrophy, both the surface- and gland-lining epithelium is low, cuboidal, and the stroma is collagenous. Some of the glands resemble capillaries (*arrow*).

logic characteristics afforded by Bouin's solution is preferred by some pathologists. If Bouin's solution is used, the jaw of the curette should not be immersed in the fixative, because Bouin's solution contains highly corrosive glacial acetic acid, which quickly blunts the cutting edge of the curette. Instead, the specimen should be removed from the curette with forceps, placed on a lens paper, and immersed in the fixative. The specimen adheres to the lens paper, thereby minimizing the possibility that the tissue may be lost during processing (see Chapter 27, Gross Description, Processing, and Reporting of Gynecologic and Obstetric Specimens).

Morphologic interpretation, including dating of the endometrium, is based on the assessment of the functionalis of the endometrium, which is identified by its covering surface epithelium (see Figs. 9.20B and 9.21A). An endometrial specimen devoid of surface epithelium may lead to an inaccurate diagnosis because, in many instances, such endometrium represents the basalis layer, which does not respond to cyclic hormonal stimuli, and the specimen cannot be dated. In addition, because it often contains voluminous glands and compact stroma, with clusters of basal arteries (Fig. 9.37A), it may be confused with an endometrial polyp or hyperplasia. The endometrium in hysterectomy specimens often contains autolytic artifacts, which result from the high proteolytic enzyme content of the endometrium.[8,57] This high enzyme content quickly produces autolytic changes if the specimen is not fixed immediately after removal of the uterus. The major morphologic autolytic artifacts include gland and stromal cell retractions (Fig. 9.37B). The best time to confirm ovulation is on cycle day 22 (POD 8) or later.

Some investigators, including the authors, advocate endometrial sampling at the onset of uterine bleeding.[5] By obtaining samples at the time of early uterine bleeding, the pathologist is able to determine whether the bleeding is caused by breakdown of postovulatory, secretory endometrium, focal necrosis of the endometrium associated with anovulation or other pathologic states, or exogenous sex steroid hormone administration. In addition, as with a few exceptions (inadequate luteal phase) the secretory

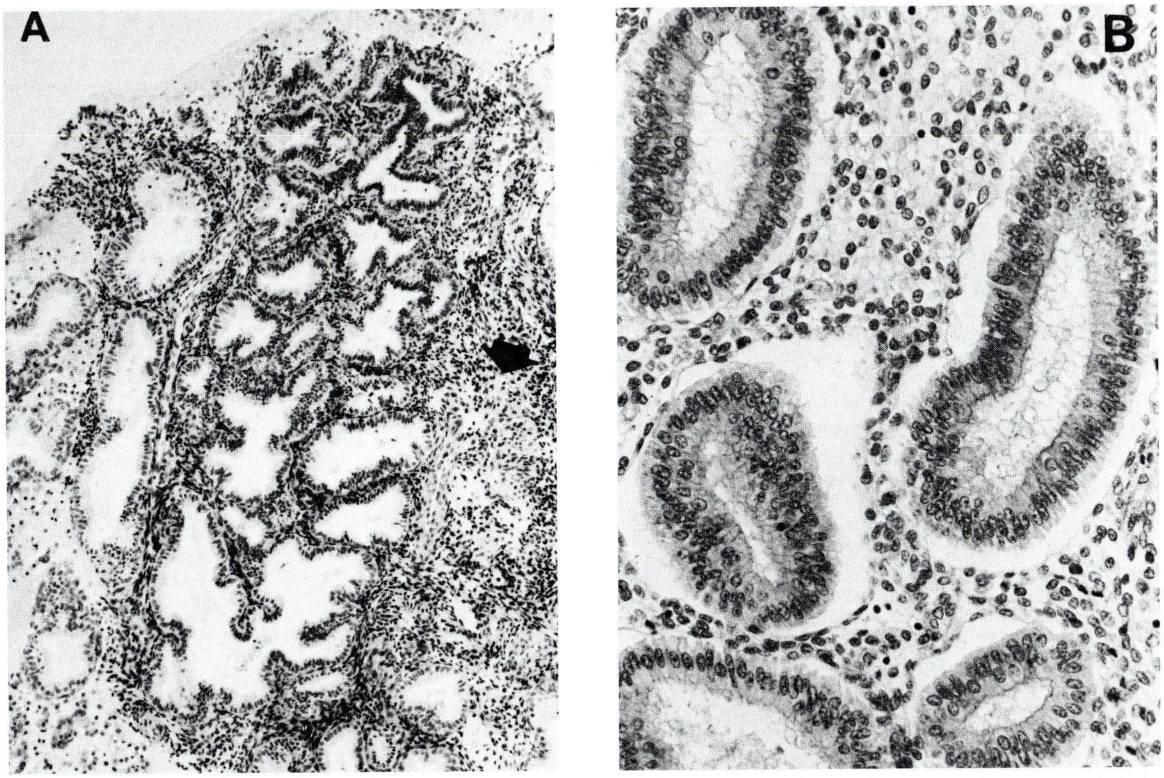

Fig. 9.37. Basalis endometrium. A: Clusters of tortuous glands in a back-to-back position masquerading as hyperplasia. The glandular aggregate is focal and flanked by clusters of basal arteries (*right*) (*arrow*) and degenerative spongiosa (*left*). Note the absence of surface epithelium. **B**: Delayed fixation artifact of endometrial specimens results in separation of glands from the supportive stroma, producing periglandular spaces. Such endometrium is difficult to date accurately.

phase of the cycle is constant in length (14 ± 2 days), the time of ovulation can be estimated if the endometrium is of the normal menstrual type. During the period of bleeding, both the external os and the lower uterine segment are dilated, facilitating introduction of an endometrial aspirator into the endometrial cavity, thereby minimizing the discomfort associated with the endometrial biopsy. When the pathologist is confronted often with the morphology of menstrual endometrium, his diagnostic expertise of this condition is considerably improved, and this in turn prevents the confusion of menstrual endometrium with endometrial carcinoma. Such a mistake is seen somewhat frequently in routine pathology practice.[114] Secretory endometrium may be relatively more difficult to date precisely than menstrual endometrium. Indeed, secretory endometrium often demonstrates subtle changes and combinations of morphologic patterns that may result in errors of ±4–5 days; this can be improved to ±2 days, however, by basing the date on the endometrial alterations that represent the most advanced phase of the menstrual cycle. For example, an endometrial biopsy may show changes consistent with the 16th, 17th, and 18th days of the cycle; the diagnosis should be based on the most advanced date and, therefore, reported as 18th-day secretory endometrium instead of averaging cycle days and reporting 17th-day secretory endometrium.

References

1. Abel MH, Baird DT (1980) The effect of 17β-estradiol and progesterone on prostaglandin production by human endometrium maintained in organ culture. Endocrinology 106:1599
2. Archer DF, McIntyre-Seltman K, Wilborn WW, et al (1991) Endometrial morphology in asymptomatic postmenopausal women. Am J Obstet Gynecol 165:317–322
3. Arias-Stella J (1972) Atypical endometrial changes produced by chorionic tissue. Hum Pathol 3:450
4. Aronica SM, Katzenellenbogen BS (1991) Progesterone receptor regulation in uterine cells: stimulation by estrogen, cyclic adenosine 3″,5″-monophosphate, and insulin-like growth factor I and suppression by antiestrogens and protein kinase. Endocrinology 128:2045–2052
5. Arronet GH, Berquist GA, Parekh MC, et al (1973)

Evaluation of endometrial biopsy in the cycle of conception. Int J Fertil 18:220
6. Baggish MS, Pauerstein CJ, Woodruff JD (1967) Role of stroma in regeneration of endometrial epithelium. Am J Obstet Gynecol 99:453
7. Bartelemez GW (1957) The form and the functions of the uterine blood vessels in the rhesus monkey. Contrib Embryol Carnegie Inst Wash 36:153
8. Beller FK, Schweppe KW (1979) Review on the biology of menstrual blood. In: Beller FK, Schaumacher GFB (eds) The biology of the fluids of the female genital tract. Elsevier-North Holland, Amsterdam, pp 231–245
9. Berchuck A, Soisson AP, Olt GJ, et al (1989) Reactivity of epidermal growth factor receptor monoclonal antibodies with human uterine tissues. Arch Pathol Lab Med 113:1155–1158
10. Bergeron C, Ferenczy A, Toft DO, Schneider W, Shyamala G (1988) Immunocytochemical study of progesterone receptors in the human endometrium during the menstrual cycle. Lab Invest 59:862–869
11. Bryant-Greenwood GD (1991) The human relaxins: consensus and dissent. Mol Cell Endocrinol 79: C125—C132
12. Bulmer JN, Hollings D, Ritson A (1987) Immunocytochemical evidence that endometrial stromal granulocytes are granulated lymphocytes. J Pathol 153:281–288
13. Chiquet-Ehrismann R, Kalla P, Pearson CA (1989) Participation of tenascin and TGF-beta in reciprocal epithelial-mesenchymal interactions of MCF 7 cells and fibroblasts. Cancer Res 49:4322–4325
14. Choo YC, Mak KC, Hsu C, Wong TS, Ma HK (1985) Postmenopausal uterine bleeding of nononcogenic cause. Obstet Gynecol 66:225
15. Christiaens GCML, Sixma JJ, Haspels AA (1980) Morphology of haemostasis in menstrual endometrium. Br J Obstet Gynecol 87:425
16. Clark KE, Farley DB, Van Orden DE, Brody MJ (1977) Estrogen-induced uterine hyperemia and edema persist during histamine receptor blockade. Proc Soc Exp Biol Med 156:411
17. Critchley HO, Tong S, Cameron ST, Drudy TA, Kelly RW, Baird DT (1999) Regulation of bcl-2 gene family members in human endometrium by antiprogestin administration in vivo. J Reprod Fertil 115:389–395
18. Crow J, Wilkins M, Howe S, More L, Helliwell P (1991) Mast cells in the female genital tract. Int J Gynecol Pathol 10:230–237
19. Dabbs DJ, Geisinger KR, Norris HT (1986) Intermediate filaments in endometrial and endocervical carcinomas: the diagnostic utility of vimentin patterns. Am J Surg Pathol 10:568–576
20. Dallenbach FD, Dallenbach G (1964) Immunohistologische untersuchungen zur lokalisation des relaxins in menschlichen placenta und decidua. Virchows Arch [Pathol Anat] 337:301
21. Daly JJ, Balogh K Jr (1968) Hemorrhagic reaction of the senile endometrium ("apoplexia uteri"). Relation to superficial hemorrhagic necrosis of the bowel. N Engl J Med 278:709
22. Feinberg BB, Tan NS, Gonik B, Brath PC, Walsh SW (1991) Increased progesterone concentrations are necessary to suppress interleukin-2-activated human mononuclear cell cytotoxicity. Am J Obstet Gynecol 165:1872–1876
23. Ferenczy A (1976) Studies on the cytodynamics of human endometrial regeneration: I. Scanning electron microscopy. Am J Obstet Gynecol 124:64–74
24. Ferenczy A (1976) Studies on the cytodynamics of human endometrial regeneration: II. Transmission electron microscopy and histochemistry. Am J Obstet Gynecol 124:582–595
25. Ferenczy A (1977) Studies on the cytodynamics of experimental endometrial regeneration in the rabbit. Historadioautography and ultrastructure. Am J Obstet Gynecol 128:536–545
26. Ferenczy A (1980) Regeneration of the human endometrium. In: Fenoglio CM, Wolff M (eds) Progress in surgical pathology, vol 1. Masson, New York, pp 157–173
27. Ferenczy A, Bertrand G, Gelfand MM (1979) Proliferation kinetics of human endometrium during the normal menstrual cycle. Am J Obstet Gynecol 133:859–867
28. Ferenczy A, Richart RM, Agate FJ Jr, Purkerson ML, Dempsey EW (1972) Scanning electron microscopy of the endometrial surface. Fertil Steril 23:515–521
29. Ferenczy A, Gelfand M (1989) The biologic significance of cytologic atypia in progestogentreated endometrial hyperplasia. Am J Obstet Gynecol 160: 126–131
30. Fitzpatrick RL, Liggins GC (1980) Effects of prostaglandins on the cervix of pregnant women and sheep. In: Naftolin F, Stubblefield PF (eds) Dilatation of the uterine cervix. Raven Press, New York, pp 287–300
31. Flowers CE Jr, Wilborn WH (1978) New observations on the physiology of menstruation. Obstet Gynecol 51:14–16
32. Folkman J (1976) The vascularization of tumors. Sci Am 234:58
33. Fowlis DJ, Ansell JD (1985) Evidence that decidual cells are not derived from bone marrow. Transplantation 39:445–446
34. Franquemont DW, Frierson HF, Mills SE (1991) An immunohistochemical study of normal endometrial stroma and endometrial stromal neoplasms. Am J Surg Pathol 15:861–870
35. Gelfand MM, Ferenczy A (1989) A prospective 1-year study of estrogen and progestin in postmenopausal women. Effects on the endometrium. Obstet Gynecol 74:398–401
36. Gerdes GL, Lemke H, Baisch H, et al (1984) Cell cycle analysis of a cell proliferation associated human nuclear antigen defined by the monoclonal antibody Ki67. J Immunol 133:1710–1715
37. Gerdes J, Pickartz H, Brotherton J, et al (1987)

Growth fractions and estrogen receptors in human breast cancers as determined in situ with monoclonal antibodies. Am J Pathol 129:486–492
38. Gibson M, Badger GJ, Byrn F, et al (1991) Error in histologic dating of secretory endometrium: variance component analysis. Fertil Steril 56:242–247
39. Gompel A, Sabourin JC, Martin A, Yaneva H, Audouin J, Decroix Y, Poitout P (1994) Bcl-2 expression in normal endometrium during the menstrual cycle. Am J Pathol 144:1195–1202
40. Greene GL, Nolan C, Engner JP, Jensen EW (1980) Monoclonal antibodies to human estrogen receptors. Proc Natl Acad Sci USA 77:5115
41. Gunin AG, Sharov AA (1998) Role of mast cells in oestradiol effects on the uterus of ovariectomized rats. J Reprod Fertil 113:61–68
42. Gurpide E, Tseng L, Gusberg SB (1977) Estrogen metabolism in normal and neoplastic endometrium. Am J Obstet Gynecol 129:809
43. Haining REB, Cameron IT, van Papendorp C, et al (1991) Epidermal growth factor in human endometrium: proliferative effects in culture and immunocytochemical localization in normal and endometriotic tissues. Human Reprod 6:1200–1205
44. Hendrickson MR, Kempson RL (1980) Surgical pathology of the uterine corpus. In: Bennington JL (ed) Major problems in pathology, vol 12. Saunders, Philadelphia, pp 36–98
45. Henzl MR, Smith RE, Boost G, Tyler ET (1972) Lysosomal concept of menstrual bleeding in humans. J Clin Endocrinol Metab 34:860
46. Herr J (1978) Decidual cells in the human ovary at term. Am J Anat 152:7–28
47. Hertig AT (1964) Gestational hyperplasia of endometrium. A morphologic correlation of ova, endometrium and corpora lutea during pregnancy. Lab Invest 13:1153
48. Hofmann GE, Drews MR, Scott RT (1992) Epidermal growth factor and its receptor in human implantation trophoblast: immunohistochemical evidence for autocrine/paracrine function. J Clin Endocrinol Metab 74:981–988
49. Horbelt DV, Roberts DK, Walker N, Delmore JE (1986) Nucleolar canalicular structure in extrauterine endometriosis. Human Pathol 17:924–925
50. Huang JR, Tseng L, Bischof P, Janne OA (1987) Regulation of prolactin production by progestin, estrogen and relaxin in human endometrial stromal cells. Endocrinology 121:2011–2017
51. Imai K, Maeda M, Fujiwara H, et al (1992) Human endometrial stromal cells and decidual cells express cluster of differentiation (CD) 13 antigen/aminopeptidase N and CD10 antigen/neutral endopeptidase. Biol Reprod 46:328–334
52. Johnson DC, Dey SK (1980) Role of histamine in implantation: dexamethasone inhibits estradiol-induced implantation in the rat. Biol Reprod 22:1136
53. Kamat BR, Isaacson PG (1987) The immunocytochemical distribution of leukocytic subpopulations in human endometrium. Am J Pathol 127:66–73
54. Katzenellenbogen BS (1980) Dynamics of steroid hormone receptor action. Annu Rev Physiol 42:17
55. Kearns M (1983) Life history of decidual cells: a review. Am J Reprod Immunol 3:78–82
56. Kliman HJ, Coutifaris C, Feinberg RF, Strauss JF III, Haimowitz JE (1989) In: Yoshinaga K (ed) Blastocyst implantation. Adams, Boston, pp 19–83
57. Kok P (1979) Separation of plasminogen activators from human plasma and a comparison with activators from human uterine tissue and urine. Thromb Haemost 4:734
58. Krehbiel RH (1937) Cytochemical studies of the decidual reaction in the rat during early pregnancy and in the production of deciduomata. Physiol Zool 10:212–235
59. Kurman RJ, Young RH, Norris HJ, et al (1984) Immunocytochemical localization of placental lactogen and chorionic gonadotropin in the normal placenta and trophoblastic tumors, with emphasis on intermediate trophoblast and the placental site trophoblastic tissue. Int J Gynecol Pathol 3:101
60. Langlois PL (1970) The size of the normal uterus. J Reprod Med 4:220
61. Lawn AM, Wilson EW, Finn CA (1971) The ultrastructure of human decidual and predecidual cells. J Reprod Fertil 26:85
62. Lichtig C, Deutch M, Barnes J (1984) Vascular changes of endometrium in early pregnancy. Am J Clin Pathol 81:702
63. Lindeman HJ (1979) Hysteroscopic data during menstruation. In: Beller FK, Schaumacher GFB (eds) The biology of the fluids of the female genital tract. Elsevier-North Holland, Amsterdam, pp 225–229
64. Marx L, Arck P, Kieslich C, Mitterlechner S, Kapp M, Dietl J (1999) Decidual mast cells might be involved in the onset of human first- trimester abortion. Am J Reprod Immunol 41:34–40
65. Mazur MT, Hendrickson MR, Kempson RL (1983) Optically clear nuclei: an alteration of endometrial epithelium in the presence of trophoblast. Am J Surg Pathol 7:415
66. Meyer WC, Malkasian GD, Dockerty MB, Decker DG (1971) Postmenopausal bleeding from atrophic endometrium. Obstet Gynecol 38:731
67. More IAR, Armstrong EM, McSeveney D, Chatfield WR (1974) The morphogenesis and fate of the nucleolar channel system in the human endometrial glandular cells. J Ultrastruc Res 47:74
68. Noyes RW, Hertig AT, Rock J (1950) Dating the endometrial biopsy. Fertil Steril 1:3
69. Ober WB (1979) Carcinosarcoma of the ovary. Case report, review of literature and comment on the subcoelomic mesenchyme. Am J Diagn Gynecol Obstet 1:73
70. O'Rahilly R (1977) Prenatal human development. In: Wynn RM (ed) Biology of the uterus. Plenum Press, New York, pp 35–57
71. Orcel L, Smadja A, Roland J, Minh HN (1973) Nouvelle hypothagese sur le mechanisme intime de la menstruation. Rev Fr Gynecol 68:477

72. Osteen KG, Anderson TL, Schwartz K, Hargrove JT, Gorstein F (1992) Distribution of tumor-associated glycoprotein-72 (TAG-72) expression throughout the normal female reproductive tract. Int J Gynecol Pathol 11:216–220
73. Parhar RS, Kennedy TG, Lala PK (1988) Suppression of lymphocyte alloreactivity by early gestational human decidua. Cell Immunol 116:392–410
74. Perrot-Applanat M, Groyer-Picard MT, Garcia E, Lorenzo F, Milgrom E (1988) Immunocytochemical demonstration of estrogen and progesterone receptors in muscle cells of uterine arteries in rabbits and humans. Endocrinology 123:1511–1519
75. Pierart ME, Najdovski T, Appelboom TE, Deschodt-Lanckman MM (1988) Effect of human endopeptidase 24.11 ("enkephalinase") on IL-1 induced thymocyte proliferation activity. J Immunol 140:3808–3811
76. Polan ML, Loukides J, Nelson P, et al (1989) Progesterone and estradiol modulate interleukin-1 beta messenger ribonucleic acid levels in cultured human peripheral monocytes. J Clin Endocrinol Metab 69:1200–1206
77. Press MF, Nousek-Goebl N, King WJ, Herbst AL, Greene GL (1984) Immunohistochemical assessment of estrogen receptor distribution in the human endometrium throughout the menstrual cycle. Lab Invest 51:495–503
78. Pryse Davies J, Ryder TA, Mackenzie ML (1979) In vivo production of the nucleolar channel system in postmenopausal endometrium. Cell Tissue Res 203: 493
79. Ramsey EM (1977) History. In: Wynn RM (ed) Biology of the uterus. Plenum Press, New York, pp 1–34
80. Randolph JF Jr, Peegel H, Ansbacher R, Menon KMJ (1990) In vitro induction of prolactin production and aromatase activity by gonadal steroids exclusively in the stroma of separated proliferative human endometrium. Am J Obstet Gynecol 162: 1109–1114
81. Ravn V, Teglbjaerg CS, Visfeldt J (1992) Mucin-type carbohydrates (type 3 chain antigens) in normal cycling human endometrium. Int J Gynecol Pathol 11:38–46
82. Rebello R, Green FHY, Fox H (1975) A study of the secretory immune system of the female genital tract. Br J Obstet Gynaecol 82:812
83. Riddick DH, Kusmik WF (1977) Decidua: a possible source of amniotic fluid prolactin. Am J Obstet Gynecol 127:187–190
84. Sainsbury JRC, Farndon JR, Needham GK, Malcolm AJ, Harris AL (1987) Epidermal growth factor receptor status as predictor of early recurrence of and death from cancer. Lancet i:1398–1402
85. Sakbun V, Ali SM, Greenwood FC, Bryant-Greenwood GD (1990) Human relaxin in the amnion, chorion, decidua parietalis, basal plate and placental trophoblast by immunocytochemistry and northern analysis. J Clin Endocrinol Metab 70: 508–514
86. Salamonsen LA, Jeziorska M, Newlands GF, Dey SK, Woolley DE (1996) Evidence against a significant role for mast cells in blastocyst implantation in the rat and mouse. Reprod Fertil Dev 8:1157–1164
87. Sananes N, Baulieu EE, LeGoascogne C (1976) Prostaglandin(s) as inductive factor of decidualization in the rat uterus. Mol Cell Endocrinol 6:153
88. Satake T, Matsuyama M (1987) Argyrophil cells in normal endometrial glands. Virchows Arch A 410: 449–454
89. Schrey MP, Hare AL, Ilson SL, Walters MP (1995) Decidual histamine release and amplification of prostaglandin F2 alpha production by histamine in interleukin-1 beta-primed decidual cells: potential interactive role for inflammatory mediators in uterine function at term. J Clin Endocrinol Metab 80: 648–653
90. Shikone T, Kokawa K, Yamoto M, Nakano R (1997) Apoptosis of human ovary and uterine endometrium during the menstrual cycle. Horm Res (Basel) 48(suppl 3):27–34
91. Silverberg SG, Arias-Stella J (1972) Phenomenon in spontaneous and therapeutic abortion. Am J Obstet Gynecol 112:777
92. Slamon DJ, Clark GM, Wong SG, et al (1987) Human breast cancer: correlation of relapse and survival with amplification of the HER-2/neu protooncogene. Science 235:177–182
93. Slamon DJ, Goldolphin W, Jones LA, et al (1989) Studies of the HER -/neu protooncogene in human breast and ovarian cancer. Science 244:707–712
94. Smith SK, Abel MH, Baird DT (1984) Effect of 17β-estradiol and progesterone on the levels of prostaglandin $F_{2\alpha}$ and E_2 in human endometrium. Prostaglandins 27:591–597
95. Szego CM (1972) Lysosomal membrane stabilization and antiestrogen action in specific hormonal target cells. Gynecol Invest 3:63
96. Tabibzadeh S (1990) Immunoreactivity of human endometrium: correlation with endometrial dating. Fertil Steril 54:624–631
97. Tabibzadeh S (1995) Signals and molecular pathways involved in apoptosis, with special emphasis on human endometrium. Hum Reprod Update 1: 303–323
98. Tabibzadeh S, Kong Q, Satyaswaroop P, Zupi E, Marconi D, Romanini C, Kapur S (1994) Distinct regional and menstrual cycle dependent distribution of apoptosis in human endometrium. Potential regulatory role of T cells and TNF-alpha. Endocrinol J 2:87–95
99. Taketani Y, Masahiko M (1991) Evidence for direct regulation of epidermal growth factor receptors by steroid hormones in human endometrial cells. Human Reprod 6:1365–1369
100. Tao XJ, Sayegh RA, Tilly JL, Isaacson KB (1998) Elevated expression of the proapoptotic BCL-2 family member, BAK, in the human endometrium

coincident with apoptosis during the secretory phase of the cycle. Fertil Steril 70:338–343
101. Tawfik OW, Huet YM, Malathy PV, Johnson DC, Dey SK (1987) Release of prostaglandins and leukotrienes from the rat uterus is an early estrogenic response. Prostaglandins 34:805–814
102. Tawfik OW, Sagrillo C, Johnson DC, Dey SK (1987) Decidualization in the rat: role of leukotrienes and prostaglandins. Prostagland Leukot Med 29:221–227
103. Taylor PV, Hancock KW (1975) Antigenicity of trophoblast and possible antigen-marking effects during pregnancy. Immunology 28:973
104. Thor A, Viglione MJ, Muraro R, et al (1987) Monoclonal antibody B72.3 reactivity with human endometrium: a study of normal and malignant tissues. Int J Gynecol Pathol 6:235–247
105. Tseng L (1979) Physiologic changes in binding and metabolism of estradiol and progesterone in human endometrium during the menstrual cycle. Obstet Gynecol Annu 8:1
106. Van Orden DE, Clancey CJ, Farley DB (1981) Uterine serotonin and receptor blockage during estrogen-induced uterine hyperemia. Proc Soc Exp Biol Med 167:469
107. Vollmer G, Siegal GP, Chiquet-Ehrismann R, et al (1990) Tenascin expression in the human endometrium and in endometrial adenocarcinomas. Lab Invest 62:725–730
108. Wagner D, Richart RM (1968) Polyploidy in the human endometrium with the Arias–Stella reaction. Arch Pathol 85:475
109. Waites GT, James RFL, Bell SC (1988) Immunohistological localization of the human endometrial secretory protein pregnancy-associated endometrial alpha 1-globulin, an insulin-like growth factor-binding protein during the menstrual cycle. J Clin Endocrinol Metab 67:1100–1104
110. Watson H, Franks S, Bonney RC (1996) Regulation of epidermal growth factor receptor synthesis by ovarian steroids in human endometrial cells in culture. J Reprod Fertil 107:199–205
111. Weissman G (1964) Labilization and stabilization of lysosomes. Fed Proc 23:1038
112. Wilkinson N, Buckley CH, Chawner L, Fox H (1990) Nucleolar organiser regions in normal, hyperplastic and neoplastic endometrium. Int J Gynecol Pathol 9:55–59
113. Wynn RM (1977) Histology and ultrastructure of the human endometrium. In: Wynn RM (ed) Biology of the uterus. Plenum Press, New York, pp 341–376
114. Winkler B, Alvarez S, Richart RM, Crum CP (1984) Pitfalls in the diagnosis of endometrial neoplasia. Obstet Gynecol 64:185
115. Winter S, Yarrasch ED, Schmid E, Franke WW (1980) Differences in polypeptide composition of cytokeratin filaments, including filaments from different epithelial tissues and cells. Eur J Cell Biol 22:371
116. Zaytsev P, Taxy JB (1987) Pregnancy-associated ectopic decidua. Am J Surg Pathol 11:526–530
117. Zhinkin LD, Samoshkina NA (1967) DNA synthesis and cell proliferation during formation of deciduomata in mice. J Embryol Exp Morphol 17:598

10

Benign Diseases of the Endometrium

Mark E. Sherman, M.D., Michael T. Mazur, M.D., and Robert J. Kurman, M.D.

Accurate histopathologic diagnosis is important in the management of benign endometrial conditions and lesions. Although many functional disorders do not produce specific morphologic changes, pathologic examination plays a critical role by excluding entities that do. Because the histopathologic appearance of the endometrium reflects a women's hormonal milieu, endometrial tissue studies may be useful in diagnosing abnormalities of the hypothalamic–pituitary axis or assessing the effects of exogenous hormones. The two main indications for endometrial biopsy or curettage are to elucidate the etiology of abnormal uterine bleeding or infertility. Basic clinical terms used to characterize abnormal uterine bleeding are summarized in Table 10.1. Readers may consult reviews

Table 10.1. Clinical characterization of abnormal bleeding

Oligomenorrhea	Infrequent bleeding (more than every 35 days)
Polymenorrhea	Frequent bleeding (less than every 21 days)
Hypomenorrhea	Decreased flow (regular periodicity)
Menorrhaghia	Excessive bleeding (amount and number of days)
Metrorrhagia	Irregular bleeding (amount may be normal or increased)
Menometrorhagia	Excessive, irregular bleeding (frequent and prolonged)

for an overview of the differential diagnosis.[25] This chapter considers benign, congenital, and acquired conditions involving the uterine corpus. For a more comprehensive discussion of the diagnosis of these diseases in endometrial biopsies and curettings, the reader is directed to texts that specifically address these issues.[166,316]

Congenital Abnormalities

Congenital abnormalities of the uterus are uncommon.[18] Many of these abnormalities are due to the effects of exogenous hormones, such as diethylstilbestrol (DES)[130] in utero or imbalances in endogenous hormones associated with abnormal gonads and chromosomal defects. The latter group of congenital disorders is described in Chapter 1, Embryology of the Female Genital Tract and Disorders of Abnormal Sexual Development, and the upper and lower genital tract structural abnormalities associated with in utero DES exposure are discussed in Chapter 4, Diseases of the Vagina. Genotypically normal females with normal gonads may also have müllerian duct abnormalities. These developmental aberrations, such as defects in the fusion of the müllerian ducts, are caused by errors in embryogenesis. The etiology of these developmental errors is unknown, but hormonal imbalances or genetic abnormalities may be involved. These disorders are frequently associated with malformations in the urinary system and the distal gastrointestinal tract (see Chapter 1). For practical purposes, these müllerian duct abnormalities can be divided into two categories: (1) abnormalities of fusion and (2) abnormalities caused by atresia.

Fusion Defects of the Müllerian Ducts

Normally, the upper one-third of the vagina and the uterus are formed by fusion of the paired müllerian ducts. After fusion, the intervening wall degenerates, forming to endometrial cavity and upper vaginal canal.[233] Nonfusion of the müllerian ducts results in uterus bicornis (Figs. 10.1c and 10.2). If the ducts fuse but the wall between the two lumens persists, an abnormal septate uterus results. If the defect is minor or confined to the fundus, the uterus is referred to as arcuatus (Fig. 10.1b). If the full length of the uterus and upper vagina is divided by a septum, the condition results in uterus didelphys with a partially double vagina (Fig. 10.1a). These congenital anomalies may cause infertility or spontaneous abortion and therefore require surgical correction.[97,290]

Atresia of the Müllerian Ducts and Vagina

Atresia of the müllerian ducts and vagina may be partial or complete. The etiology of these conditions is obscure, although a genetic cause is suggested in families with multiple affected siblings. The pattern of inheritance may be autosomal recessive or dominant.[304,305] If just one of the müllerian ducts is involved, only the fimbriae and a small muscular mass at the pelvic sidewall will form. Occasionally, a rudimentary structure remains as an appendage attached to the unaffected side, giving rise to what is referred to as uterus bicornis unicollis with a rudimentary horn (Fig. 10.1d). With bilateral atresia, the upper genital tract may consist of bilateral noncanalized standards of muscular tissue located on the lateral pelvic walls. In Rokitansky–Kuster–Hauser syndrome, a severe defect characterized by müllerian and vaginal aplasia, patients may have urinary tract anomalies such as a pelvic kidney or anephria. Vertebral and other skeletal abnormalities may also be present, suggesting a more generalized morphogenetic abnormality.

Patients with these conditions are endocrinologically normal and develop normal gonads. Lindenman and colleagues have postulated that activating mutations affecting the gene coding for antimüllerian hormone or its receptor may be related to the development of this syndrome.[154] If the anomaly is associated with obstruction of the vagina and func-

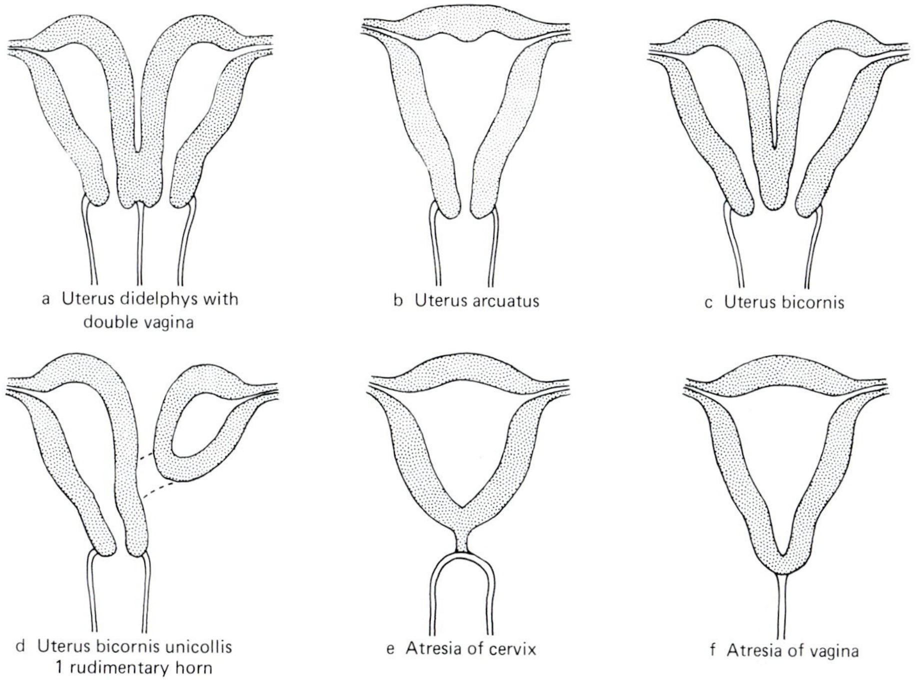

Fig. 10.1. Schematic representation of the main congenital abnormalities of the uterus and vagina. These abnormalities are caused by persistence of the uterine septum or obliteration of the lumen of the uterine canal. (Reprinted by permission of Salder, ref. 233.)

tional endometrial tissue is present, hydrocolpos may be present at birth, or patients may present with primary amenorrhea. A uterus bicornis unicollis may develop in women with one affected müllerian duct, resulting in a pelvic mass and cyclic pelvic pain associated with menses. A number of multiple malformation syndromes have been associated with müllerian or vaginal agenesis. Winter syndrome, a genetically inherited autosomal recessive disorder, is characterized by vaginal agenesis, renal agenesis, and middle ear anomalies.[305] Treatment of patients with complete vaginal atresia requires surgery to create a neovagina. If the anomaly is isolated vaginal atresia (Fig. 10.1f), as most commonly occurs, the patient usually will be fertile if a normal uterus and fallopian tubes are present.

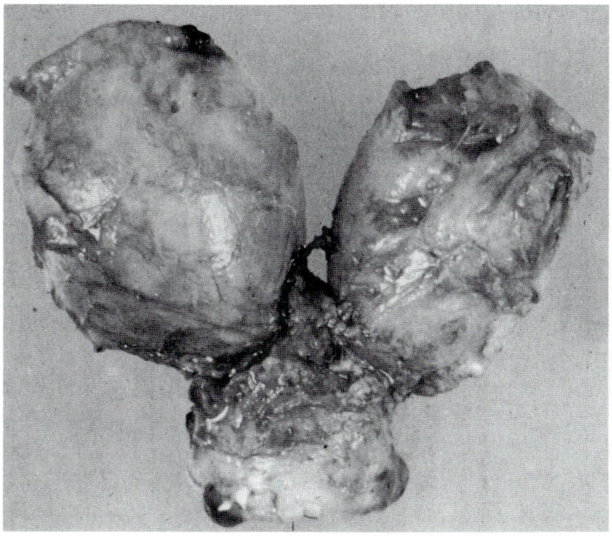

Fig. 10.2. Bicornuate uterus. The specimen is unopened.

Inflammation

Endometritis is histopathologically classified as *acute or chronic* depending on the type of inflammatory cells present; however, these designations do not necessarily reflect the duration of disease. In some cases of endometritis, a specific etiologic agent or a distinctive inflammatory pattern (e.g., granulomatous) can be recognized, whereas in others the findings are nonspecific. The diagnosis of endometritis is sometimes challenging because specific types of leukocytes are present in normal endometrium in defined distributions that vary with menopausal status and the phase of the cycle.

Normal Hematopoietic Cells of the Endometrium

Immunohistochemical studies have demonstrated that B lymphocytes are present mainly in aggregates in the basalis and are rarely found in the functionalis.[32] Occasional lymphoid follicles can be found in otherwise normal endometria.[207] T lymphocytes are relatively uncommon in the proliferative phase but increase during the secretory and menstrual phases.[32] CD 44, an adhesion molecule that may be involved in lymphocyte homing, was detected in all four midsecretory and 9 of 11 late-secretory endometria in one study.[310] Granulated lymphocytes with the phenotype CD 2+, CD 3− may be found in predecidual tissue that is present in mid- and late-secretory endometrium. Formerly, these cells were designated as endometrial stromal granulocytes.[31,135] In addition, polymorphonuclear leukocytes (PMNs) are present in small numbers throughout the cycle but do not become evident in large numbers before the tissue breakdown and necrosis associated with menses occurs.[214] In contrast to lymphocytes and PMNs, plasma cells are not normally present in the endometrium. Rare mast cells demonstrable with toluidine blue staining may be found in the endometrium, primarily within the basalis. Mast cells are also found in the myometrium, endometrial polyps, and leiomyomas.[54] The number of mast cells present in the endometrium and myometrium tends to decrease with advancing age. The significance of mast cells in the development of endometrial pathology has not been established.[54]

Acute and Chronic (Nonspecific) Endometritis

Although the cervix acts as a barrier to the entry of microorganisms into the endometrial cavity, most types of endometritis result from ascending infection. Endometritis related to bacteremia or secondary spread to the uterus from a primary salpingitis (e.g., tuberculosis) is unusual. During menses, abortion, parturition, and instrumentation (curettage, insertion of an intrauterine device, cervical conization), the cervical barrier to infection is breached, allowing normal vagina flora access to the endometrial cavity, but colonization and infection are uncommon. A study analyzing the histologic findings in the endometrium of women with documented upper genital tract infection (UGTI) and laparoscopically confirmed acute salpingitis suggests that classification of endometritis into "acute" and "chronic" forms based on the type of inflammatory infiltrate may not be valid.[137] This study found that the endometria of women with acute salpingitis usually did not contain large numbers of PMNs in the stroma. In fact, PMNs comprising at least 30% of the inflammatory cells occurred in only 27% of the cases. PMNs were found in the superficial endometrium, but numerous lymphocytes and plasma cells were identified in the stroma. Therefore, these women would have been classified histopathologically as having chronic endometritis. Possibly, these patients may have had acute salpingitis superimposed on an occult low-grade, chronic endometritis.

Clinical Features

Clinically significant *acute endometritis* is usually associated with pregnancy or abortion. The complex clinical aspects of postpartum and postabortal endometritis are described elsewhere.[148,177] Most acute endometritis is caused by hemolytic *Streptococcus*, *Staphylococcus*, *Neisseria gonorrhoeae*, and *Clostridium welchii*.

Pathologic Findings

Chronic endometritis has been observed in 3–10% of women undergoing an endometrial biopsy for investigation of irregular bleeding.[98,228] Patients may have menometrorrhagia, mucopurulent cervical discharge, uterine tenderness, or an elevated erythrocyte sedimentation rate and/or leukocytosis, but some women are asymptomatic. Chronic endometritis has been associated with an abortion in 41%, with salpingitis in 25%, with an intrauterine device in 14%, and with a recent pregnancy in 12%.[34] It also is associated with necrotic tissue, such as an infarcted polyp or carcinoma, or cervical stenosis secondary to radiation or cryosurgery. Endometritis associated with pregnancy and abortion is characterized by an acute inflammatory infiltrate. Based on a study of 111 women with cervical in-

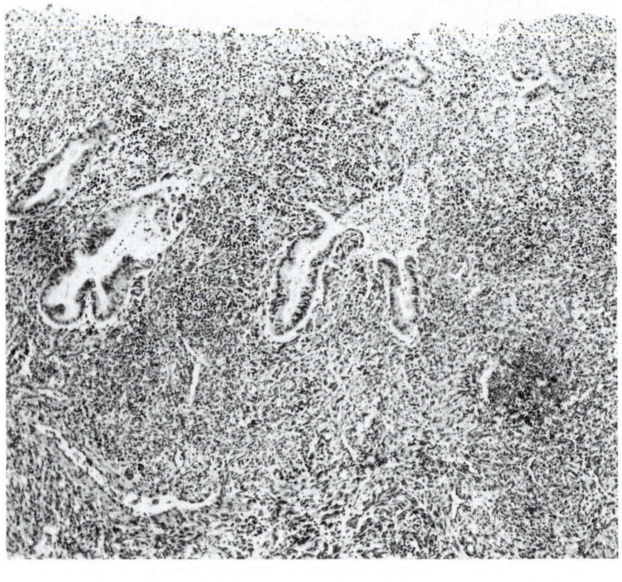

Fig. 10.3. Acute endometritis. A profuse infiltrate of polymorphonuclear leukocytes destroys and fills gland lumens. A microabscess is present on *right*.

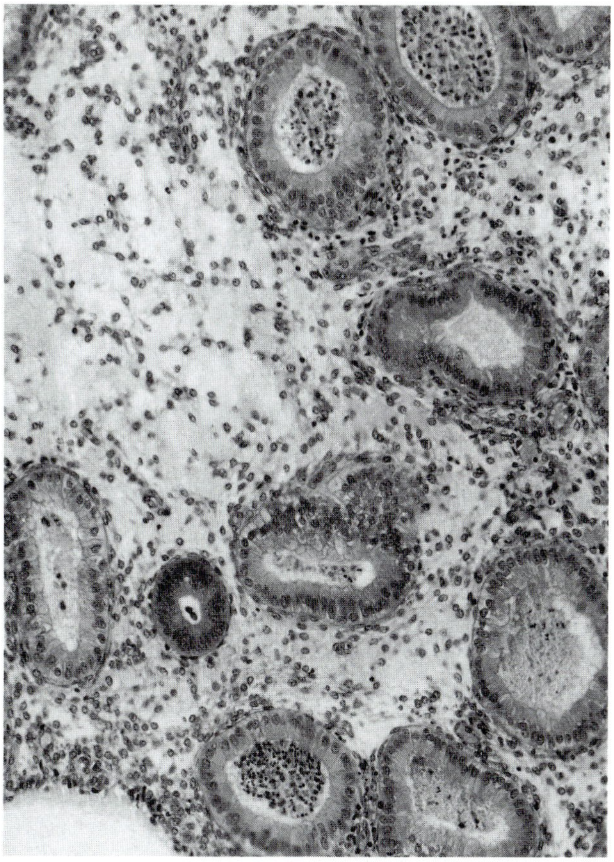

Fig. 10.4. Endometrial glands with luminal debris. Tubular glands near the surface contain neutrophils and debris in the lumens. There was no evidence of endometritis in the specimen. This change should not be misinterpreted as acute endometritis.

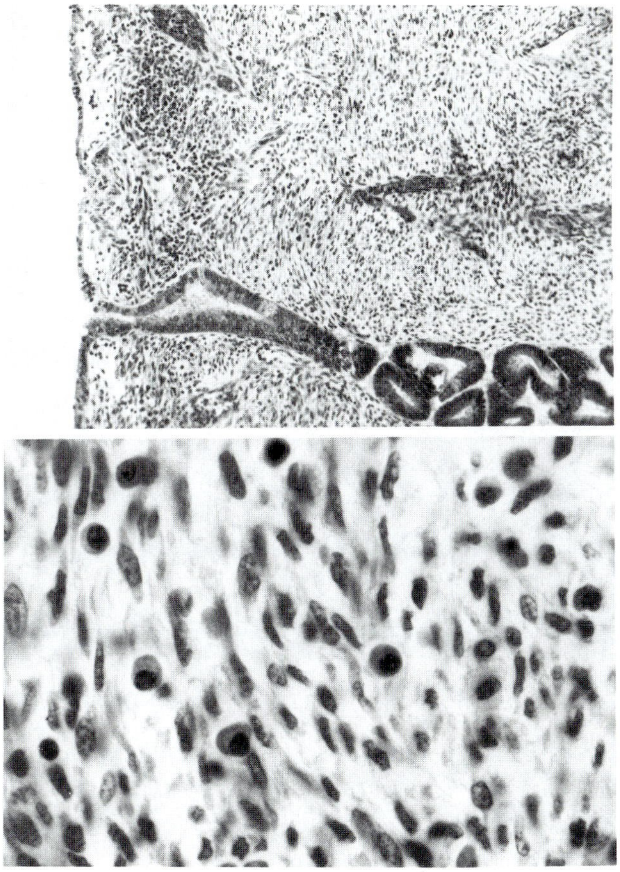

Fig. 10.5. Chronic endometritis. *Top*: Chronic endometritis characterized by aggregates of lymphocytes and plasma cells. *Bottom*: Plasma cells with eccentrically placed nuclei and clockface chromatin pattern.

fections caused by gonorrhea, *Chlamydia*, or bacterial vaginosis and 24 controls, Korn et al. reported that women with proliferative endometrium had a fourfold increased risk for having signs of upper genital tract disease. The authors postulated that hormonal effects or loss of barrier function after menses may render the endometrium susceptible to infection.[140]

Currently, identification of a specific microorganism is based on culture. Criteria for the histologic diagnosis of acute endometritis include identification of moderate to large numbers of PMNs in nonbleeding endometrium, aggregates of PMNs in the stroma, (microabscesses) or filling and disruption of glands by PMNs.[214] These findings must be distinguished from necrosis, hemorrhage, and infiltrates of PMNs occurring as a normal physiologic event in menstrual endometrium (Fig. 10.3). Occasionally, isolated glands in otherwise normal endometrium contain PMNs and debris (Fig. 10.4), reflecting entrapped menstrual detritus. This focal findings is not diagnostic of acute endometritis, which is typically a diffuse process.

The diagnosis of chronic endometritis rests on the identification of plasma cells, but lymphocytes, macrophages, and rare PMNs may be present (Fig. 10.5).[28,34,72,228] Plasma cells may be difficult to distinguish from lymphocytes and endometrial stromal cells possessing an eccentric nucleus. Diagnostic plasma cells contain an eccentric nucleus with a characteristic clumped chromatin pattern and a paranuclear pale-staining area representing the Golgi apparatus. Routine use of special stains to identify rare plasma cells is not recommended, and examination under high magnification should be reserved for biopsies that are suspicious at low power. Specifically, spindle cell alteration of the stroma (Fig. 10.6) or secretory endometrium that is difficult to date should prompt closer study. The spindle cell alteration is characterized by a tendency of the endometrial stromal cells to palisade around glands in a pinwheel arrangement. The nuclei of the stromal

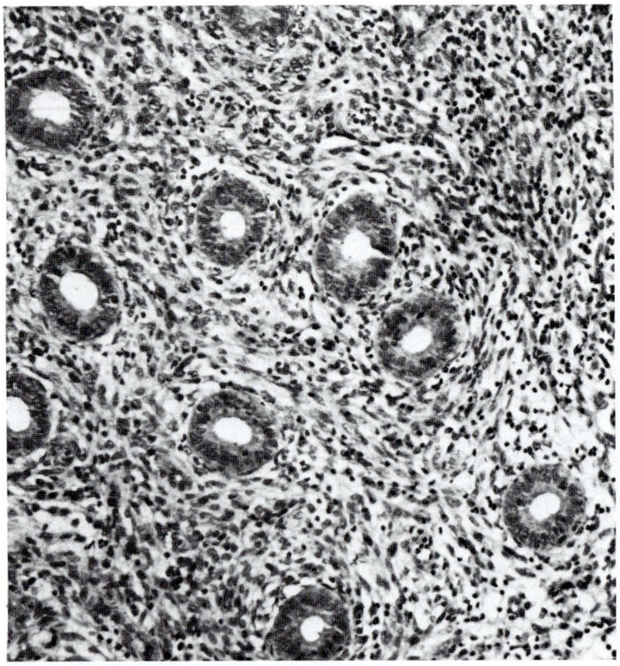

Fig. 10.6. Chronic endometritis. Note the spindle-shaped stromal cells surrounding glands in a pinwheel arrangement.

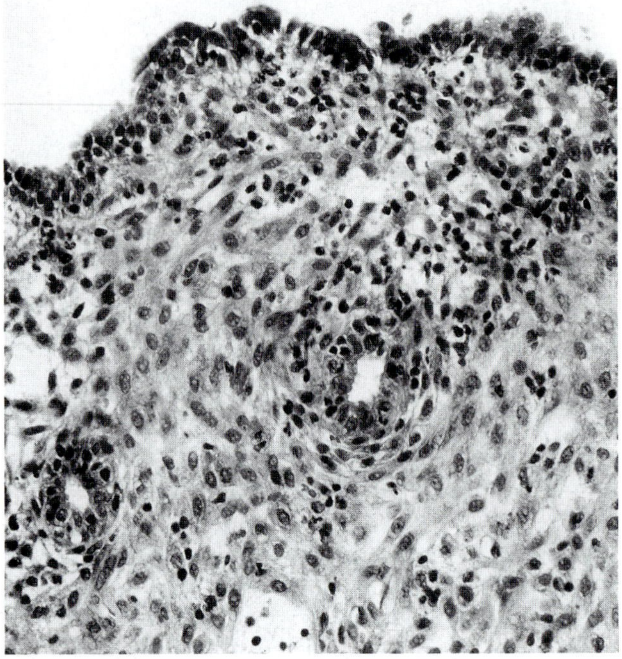

Fig. 10.7. Chronic endometritis. Numerous neutrophils in addition to lymphocytes are present involving the surface of the endometrium, glands, and stroma. Plasma cells were present elsewhere in the specimen.

cells may appear more elongated and slightly enlarged. Frequent problems with dating include glands and stroma that are not consistent with the same menstrual date, inactive glands that are difficult to classify as proliferative or secretory, and extensive fragmentation; the latter finding has been associated with *N. gonorrhoeae*.[137] Glandular cells may be stratified, with karyomegaly and prominent nucleoli, and both glands and stroma may show increased mitotic activity. Occasionally these cells may be identified in cervical cytology specimens, prompting an interpretation of atypical glandular cells of undetermined significance. Rarely, the surface epithelium in chronic endometritis shows squamous metaplasia.

One study of women with acute salpingitis and laparoscopically confirmed upper genital tract infection (UGTI) found that small numbers of plasma cells had low specificity for the diagnosis of endometritis.[137] In this study, identification of one or more plasma cells in the endometrial stroma per 120× field and five or more PMNs per 400× field in the surface epithelium (Fig. 10.7) had a sensitivity of 94% and a specificity of 85%, respectively, for the diagnosis of UGTI. The authors questioned the clinical significant of finding rare plasma cells in endometrial biopsies obtained from asymptomatic women because, in an unpublished series of 29 biopsies performed as part of an infertility workup, they found rare plasma cells in two women who had normal hysterosalpingograms and negative *Chlamydia trachomatis* serology. Korn et al. also demonstrated that the concordance between clinical findings diagnostic of endometritis, histopathologic plasma cell endometritis, and microbiologic detection of *N. gonorrhoeae* and *Chlamydia* was poor.[141] These authors also identified plasma cell endometritis in 2 (9%) of 11 controls, noting that the significance of this finding in women who do not meet standard diagnostic criteria is unclear. Accordingly, if chronic endometritis is diagnosed exclusively on the basis of the detection of extremely rare plasma cells, the cells in question should have typical morphology and the modifier "mild" may be added. Our understanding of the clinical significance of pathologic diagnoses of endometritis has been limited historically by our inability to use pathologic samples to identify and localize pathogens to endometrial tissue. It is hoped that these problems can be overcome with newer techniques.[267]

Clinical Behavior and Treatment

Chlamydia trachomatis and *N. gonorrhoeae* are the most common upper genital tract pathogens cultured from the endometrium, tubes, or cul-de-sac concurrently with the histopathologic diagnosis of chronic endometritis. Other less common isolates include *Escherichia coli*, *Streptococcus agalactiae*, and *Peptostreptococcus magnus*.[137] Accordingly, endocervical cultures for gonococci and *Chlamydia* may be indicated after the histologic diagnosis of chronic endometritis is rendered. The histologic diagnosis of endometritis often is associated with pelvic inflammatory disease. In a study comparing endometrial biopsy, clinical examination, and laparoscopy in the diagnosis of acute pelvic inflammatory disease, Paavonen et al. found that a biopsy diagnosis of chronic endometritis was associated with acute salpingitis at laparoscopy in 89% of patients, whereas endometritis was confirmed in only 67% of women with an abnormal bimanual examination.[206] The association of mucopurulent cervicitis, endometritis, and salpingitis suggests that chronic endometritis may represent an intermediate stage of pelvic inflammatory disease between ascending cervicitis and salpingitis. The importance of the endometrial biopsy as a predictor of pelvic inflammatory disease is underscored by the observation that significant pelvic adhesions can be found at laparoscopy despite normal hysterosalpingography.[159] Because chronic endometritis may be found without salpingitis, it is conceivable that early endometritis can cause infertility.[206] Thus, the endometrial biopsy can serve as a method for directing specific therapy or indicating the need for laparoscopy.

Chronic Endometritis: Specific Types

Chlamydia

Clinical Features

Data from several Western European countries and the United States indicate that *C. trachomatis* infection, defined by culture or a high serologic antibody titer, is associated with 50–60% of cases of salpingitis.[104] The risk of infertility after an episode of salpingitis rises from 11% after one episode to 54% after three or more episodes.[297] Most patients undergoing tuboplasty for tubal stenosis or adhesions that appears to have an infectious etiology have never had pain, bleeding, or any clinical sign that would have suggested the diagnosis.[104] This finding suggests that *C. trachomatis*, possibly in association with other microorganisms, can cause an acute salpingitis or a chronic "silent" salpingitis that is recognized only during the course of an infertility workup.

Pathogenesis

Animal experiments have convincingly demonstrated that *C. trachomatis* by itself can cause salpingitis and tubal obstruction. In one study of 100 guinea pigs, unilateral salpingitis and pyosalpinx developed in all the animals following an inoculation of *C. trachomatis* into the tube.[238]

Pathologic Findings

Findings at surgery in women with culture-proven *C. trachomatis* include adhesions and a viscous effusion in the pouch of Douglas, shiny red peritoneal surfaces suggesting inflammation, and mesothelial cysts ranging from a few millimeters to macroscopic in size (see Chapter 17, Diseases of the Peritoneum). Cytologic examination of the peritoneal fluid reveals numerous lymphocytes and plasma cells and clusters of reactive mesothelial cells. The fallopian tubes can show a wide range of findings from acute to chronic salpingitis (see Chapter 14, Diseases of the Fallopian Tube). Chronic endometritis caused by *C. trachomatis* displays a mixed inflammatory infiltrate composed of plasma cells, lymphocytes, and PMNs (see "Acute and Chronic Endometritis"). One study has suggested that *C. trachomatis*-associated endometritis is associated with a denser plasma cell infiltrate than gonococcal endometritis.[137] In addition, lymphoid follicles containing transformed lymphocytes were found with *Chlamydia* infection but not with gonococcal infection. Similarly, in a study using immunohistochemistry to detect *Chlamydia*, the organism was found in only 4% of 90 endometrial biopsies showing chronic endometritis as compared to 57% in biopsies showing severe chronic endometritis and superimposed acute inflammation.[303] Chlamydial endometritis was associated with stromal necrosis and reparative cytologic atypia in the glandular and surface epithelium. Chlamydial inclusions were difficult to identify because of obscuring inflammation. In another study, *C. trachomatis* elementary bodies were identified by direct immunofluorescence in 75% of cases, and typical intracellular *Chlamydia* inclusions were found in more than 60%.[136] Stern et al. detected chlamydial DNA in only 1 of 43 samples tested using a sensitive technique, which prompted them to concluded that *Chlamydia* plays a limited role, if any, in mild or moderate endometritis.[267] Chlamydia has also been detected in 9 (11.7%) of 77 fallopian tubes showing chronic salpingitis using a polymerase chain reaction-based method in combination with enzyme immunoassay.[107]

Clinical Behavior and Treatment

Chlamydia cultures performed after a histologic diagnosis of chronic endometritis may facilitate early treatment, thereby minimizing the risk of tubal damage and infertility. Patients undergoing tuboplasty should be cultured and treated before microsurgery to improve the chances of successful intrauterine pregnancy.[104] *Chlamydia* infections usually respond to tetracycline therapy.

Mycoplasma

Mycoplasma infection of the endometrium has been associated with infertility and fetal wastage.[28,279,280] Three species, *Mycoplasma hominis*, *Mycoplasma fermentans*, and *Ureaplasma urealyticum*, have been demonstrated in the lower female genital tract.[39,84,85,204,279] Most infections are transmitted by sexual contact, but the organisms have been cultured from prepubertal girls and women who have not reported sexual contact, suggesting that the anal canal or other sites may represent the source of infection in some cases.[72] Although mycoplasma species, especially *U. urealyticum*, may play a role in some cases of unexplained infertility, the relationship of this organism to endometrial infection is controversial.[39,40,99] Data regarding both the culture of the organism from the endometrium and the association of positive cultures with an inflammatory endometrial response have been conflicting.[39,40,99,112] The differences in isolated rates among infertile women may be due to cervical contamination because mycoplasmas frequently colonize the lower genital tract. However, Andrews et al. reported a threefold risk for endometritis in women undergoing cesarean section, which presumably permitted culture of placental tissue without cervical contamination.[7]

Significant endometrial infection with *U. urealyticum* should cause an identifiable inflammatory response. Horne et al. have described a lesion termed subacute focal inflammation (SFI) consisting of focal collections of lymphocytes, plasma cells, and rarely PMNs that they have identified in these patients.[112] The lymphoid aggregates characteristic of SFI are most easily identified in the secretory phase from the 20th to the 23rd days (postovulation day 6–9) of the cycle, when there is maximal stromal edema. The lymphoid aggregates generally lack germinal centers and tend to be localized immediately beneath the surface endometrium, adjacent to glands, or around spiral arterioles. Our experience with SFI is limited. The link between *U. ureaplasma* infection and infertility is not well understood and may be indirect. For example, in a study of 262 patients, 87% of women with SFI reportedly had laparoscopically detected pelvic adhesions compared to only 11% who did not have SFI ($p = 0.0001$).[33] One speculation is that ureaplasmas, if truly pathogenic, may act by producing adhesions or increasing the risk for developing more severe adhesions. Cervicovaginal isolation of *U. urealyticum* was associated with male factor infertility in one study, suggesting that the organism may produce more significant pathology in men, by interfering with spermatogenesis and reducing spermatozoa motility, rather than producing endometritis.[40]

Anaerobic Gram-Negative Rods

Anaerobic gram-negative rods, such as those associated with bacterial vaginosis, may represent endometrial pathogens. Studies evaluating the etiologic role of these organisms in endometritis have been hampered by difficulties related to assessing the frequency of vaginal colonization and bacterial vaginosis. Peipert et al. found that bacterial vaginosis was associated with a threefold risk of having laparoscopic, histologic, or microbiologic evidence of upper genital tract disease.[208] In contrast, Hillier et al. found that only recovery of gram-negative rods from the endometrium was associated with endometritis, whereas clinical bacterial vaginosis was not significantly associated in a multivariate analysis.[106] In addition, this study found agreement between species identified in the endometrium and the fallopian tube. Finally, Korn et al. reported that 10 of 22 patients with bacterial vaginosis had endometritis compared to only 1 of 19 controls.[139] Although further evaluation of the role of these organisms in upper genital tract infection is needed, accumulated data suggest a possible role.

Tuberculosis

Endometritis caused by *Mycobacterium tuberculosis* is a manifestation of a systemic disease; its frequency is proportionate to that of pulmonary tuberculosis in a population, but it is considerably more rare, with very low rates in most developed countries.[24,120,182,194,271] Tuberculous endometritis may be found in women of any age. Clinical presentation includes a pelvic mass, lower abdominal pain, and infertility. The diagnosis may not be made until a hysterectomy is performed and pathologic examination reveals typical caseating granulomas. The endometrium is the second most commonly infected site in the female genital tract after the fallopian tubes, and it is involved in one-half to three-quarters of patients with genital tuberculosis.[194] Endometrial involvement is generally secondary to seeding by organisms draining from an infected fallopian tube. Salpingitis in turn is usually secondary to hematogenous or, rarely, lymphatic spread from a primary infection in the lungs or gastrointestinal tract.[103] The extent of the inflammatory involvement in tuberculous endometritis varies from a focal

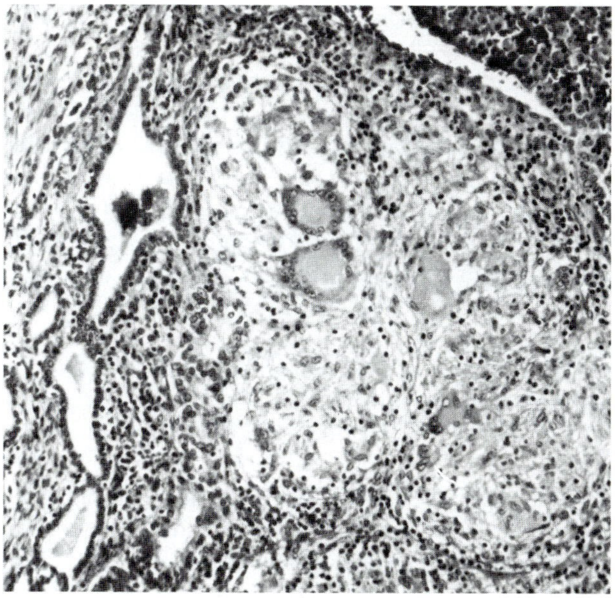

Fig. 10.8. Tuberculous endometritis. Tuberculous endometritis with a nonnecrotizing granuloma containing Langhans' giant cells.

process with very few granulomas to a diffuse process with ulceration of the mucosa and extensive caseous necrosis. Typical granulomatous inflammation with Langhans' giant cells (Fig. 10.8) may be present, but sometimes nonspecific endometritis with focal or diffuse infiltrates of plasma cells and lymphocytes and glandular microabscess is the only pathologic finding.[60]

The inflammation usually is confined to the superficial and intermediate portion of the endometrium, with transmural involvement occurring only in very severe infections.[194] As with any severe inflammatory process, the epithelium may show reactive proliferative changes with cellular stratification, mild nuclear atypia, and squamous metaplasia that mimic a neoplastic process. Histologic diagnosis of tuberculosis is difficult because granulomas are often focal and take up to 2 weeks to develop, and the functionalis, where granulomas usually occur, is shed every 4 weeks.[194] Thus, if tuberculosis is suspected, a curettage, rather than an endometrial biopsy, should be performed during the late-secretory or menstrual phase of the cycle. Specific diagnosis requires culture or identification of acid-fast organisms, because other microorganisms and noninfectious processes may be associated with granulomatous inflammation. Acid-fast bacilli are rarely demonstrated, even when cultures are positive.[194] Patients with tuberculous endometritis are nearly always sterile because they also have severe tubal infections. After appropriate antimicrobial therapy, granulomas become hyalinized, but the inflammatory infiltrate may persist for years. In fertile patients there is a high risk of tubal implantation, and intrauterine pregnancy may terminate in fatal miliary tuberculosis.

Sarcoidosis

Granulomatous endometritis has been reported in patients with *systemic sarcoidosis*.[108,277] In contrast to tuberculosis, granulomas in sarcoidosis are typically noncaseating and acid-fast bacilli are not identified. Because classic caseating granulomas may not be identified in tuberculous endometritis and identification of organisms may be difficult, patients with granulomatous endometritis must be carefully evaluated.

Fungal Infections

Blastomycosis (*Blastomyces dermatitidis*)[75] and coccidioidomycosis (*Coccidioides immitis*)[101,236] may produce granulomatous endometritis as part of a disseminated infection. There have been case reports of mycotic infection consistent with *Candida*[225] and cryptococcosis (*Cryptococcus glabratus*)[212] in the endometrium. The Gomori silver-methenamine and periodic acid–Schiff (PAS) stain are helpful for identifying these organisms.

Viral Infections

Herpes simplex virus (HSV),[2,73,95,222,241] *cytomegalovirus* (CMV),[63,167,293] and *human immunodeficiency virus* (HIV)[211,306] are known to infect the endometrium. Human papillomavirus (HPV) infection of the endometrium is controversial. In a study that used a combination of polymerase chain reaction (PCR) and in situ methods, HPV DNA was not detected in normal endometrium but was identified in endometrial carcinomas, as has been previously reported.[202]

Both acute[2,95,241] and latent[222] HSV infection have been reported. Acute herpes endometritis may result from an ascending infection or a disseminated viremia.[2,73,241] In acute herpes infection, the glandular cell have ground glass nuclei that are enlarged and contain round eosinophilic inclusions surrounded by a halo. There are associated patchy necrosis, acute inflammation, and multinucleated giant cells.[73,241] In latent herpes infection, immunohistochemistry may demonstrate HSV-specific virion and nonvirion antigens.[222] The clinical significance of "latent" infection is unknown. HSV-1 and HSV-2 were also identified in 13 (72%) of 18 cases of endometritis in HIV-infected women as compared to 2 (11%) of 18 HIV-negative controls.[306]

Cervical cultures detect CMV infection in about 14% of women during pregnancy.[179] In contrast, CMV represents an unusual incidental microscopic finding in nonpregnant healthy women.[293] CMV endometritis has been reported in immunocompromised women with systemic CMV infection[26,237] and as a primary infection in nonimmunocompromised patients.[167] CMV may infect the endometrium during pregnancy and may be linked to spontaneous abortion.[73] Because of its occult presentation, the frequency of CMV infection of the endometrium is probably underestimated. CMV infection is characterized by an inflammatory infiltrate composed of lymphocytes and plasma cells. The endometrial epithelial cells are markedly enlarged and contain large, round basophilic nuclear and cytoplasmic inclusions (Fig. 10.9). CMV DNA has also been detected in paraffin blocks using the polymerase chain reaction in a case of chronic endometritis with ill-defined nonnecrotizing granulomas but without any of the other features of CMV infection.[83] The patient had systemic CMV infection and CMV in the endocervix. The Arias–Stella reaction (see Chapter 9, Anatomy and Histology of the Uterine Corpus) may be confused with CMV because both lesions show marked nuclear enlargement. In the Arias–Stella reaction, however, cells typically display a hobnail arrangement and cytoplasmic vacuolization, associated with luminal secretions and changes consistent with gestational endometrium (i.e., decidua). CMV endometritis lacks these features and typically is associated with a plasma cell infiltrate.

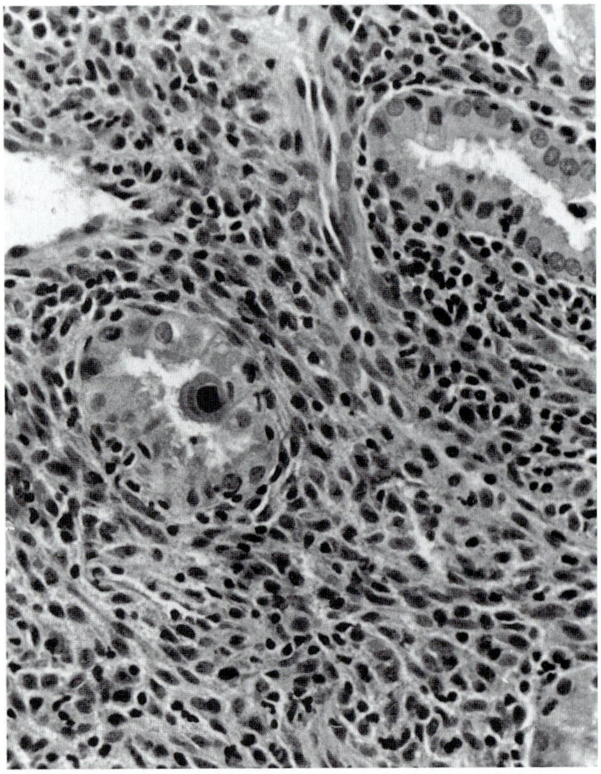

Fig. 10.9. Cytomegalovirus endometritis. An enlarged glandular cell contains a large, round, basophilic inclusion.

HIV has been detected using immunohistochemistry and in situ hybridization within cells demonstrating monocyte/macrophage differentiation located in endometrial stroma.[211] In a study comparing 12 endometrial samples from HIV-infected women to matched controls, HIV-infected patients with menstrual symptoms showed an increase in lymphocytes (CD 45) and T cells (CD 3), prompting the suggestion that nonclassical forms of chronic endometritis may be common in advancing HIV disease.[123]

Parasitic Infections

Schistosoma,[20,181,301] *Enterobius vermicularis*,[239] and *Echinococcus granulosus*[291] are rare causes of endometritis in the United States, but *schistosomiasis* is endemic in Central America, Africa, the Middle East, and the Far East. Patients usually present with amenorrhea and infertility. The infection may be mild or severe and is characterized by granulomatous inflammation with lymphocytes, plasma cells, eosinophils, and histiocytes closely simulating a tubercle. The endometrial surface may ulcerate and be replaced by granulation tissue. Diagnosis is made by identifying the ova in tissue sections or in smears of vaginal secretions. Toxoplasmosis (*Toxoplasma gondii*)[219,268] evokes a nonspecific inflammatory reaction in the endometrium. The microorganism can be identified by immunofluorescence. Fragmentary data implicate this organism in the endometrium as a cause of congenital toxoplasmosis and habitual abortion.

Xanthogranulomatous Inflammation

There have been several reported cases of *xanthogranulomatous or histiocytic endometritis*.[29,30,231,247] The lesion involves the endometrium, but may extend into the myometrium, and is characterized by an extensive accumulation of foamy histiocytes. The condition has been reported in postmenopausal women, some of whom have been radiated previously for endometrial or cervical carcinoma. Presentations include vaginal bleeding, vaginal discharge, cervical stenosis, and pyometria. It has been suggested that the lesion results from obstruction as-

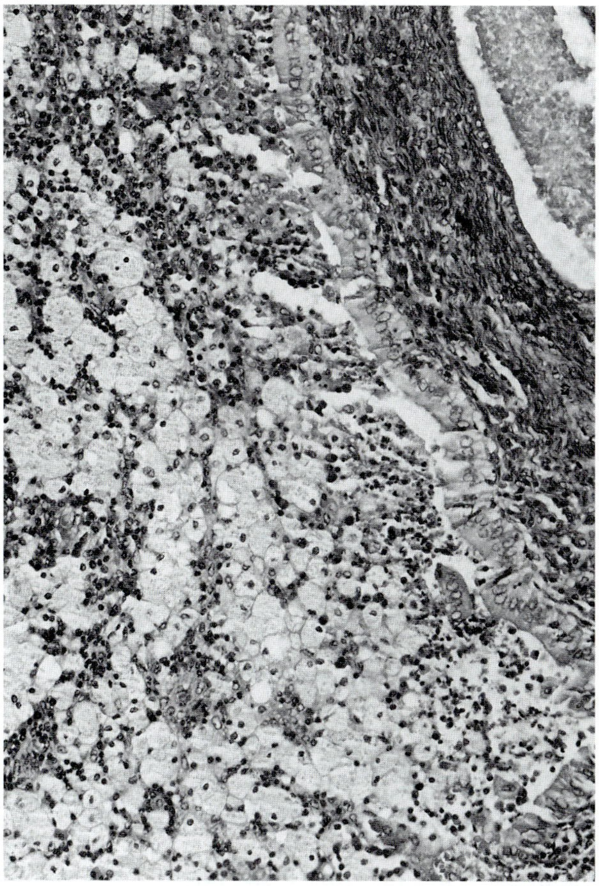

Fig. 10.10. Xanthogranulomatous endometritis. Large numbers of endometrial stromal cells with foamy cytoplasm. Lymphocytes and plasma cells also are present.

sociated with hematometria, inflammation, and perhaps some factors specifically related to radiation-induced tumor necrosis, such as the generation of free radicals and lipid peroxidation.[231] Microscopically, xanthogranulomatous endometritis is characterized by numerous histiocytes with foamy, glandular, or eosinophilic cytoplasm and variable numbers of multinucleated giant cells, lymphocytes, and plasma cells (Fig. 10.10). The foam cells are distended with lipid, hemosiderin, or ceroid resulting from erythrocyte breakdown following nonphysiologic hemorrhage. PAS stains are positive at times. Cholesterol crystals, calcification, and necrotic debris typically are present.

Miscellaneous Infections

Two rare forms of endometritis of probable bacterial origin that produce specific morphologic changes are *pneumopolycystic endometritis*[209] and *malakoplakia*.[216,285] The former is characterized by the presence of multiple thin-walled cysts and vesicles lined by flattened cells. Multinucleated giant cells occasionally are present. A similar condition can be seen in the vagina (see Chapter 4, Diseases of the Vagina). The disease in the vagina is thought to result from infection by *Haemophilus vaginalis* or *Trichomonas*, but the etiologic agent in the endometrium is unknown. Malakoplakia most often involves the urinary bladder; the genital tract is rarely affected.[41,43,131,177,216,281,285,288,300] Patients with malakoplakia involving the genital tract range widely in age and may present with vaginal bleeding. Grossly, the lesions appear as soft, yellow, gray-brown plaques and nodules. Microscopically, the lesions are composed of a monomorphic population of histiocytes containing eosinophilic or clear cytoplasm (Von Hansemann cells), which may mimic xanthogranulomatous endometritis or clear cell carcinoma. The diagnosis of malakoplakia is made by the identification of intracellular and extracellular calcified spherules (Michaelis–Gutman bodies). *Escherichia coli* has been isolated most frequently from these lesions, but *Klebsiella* and *Proteus* spp. have also been identified. Malakoplakia may be related to a defect in the phagocytic function of monocytes–macrophages that leads to persistence of bacteria, which calcify to form Michaelis–Gutman bodies. Management consists of antibiotic treatment and surgical excision, but lesions may recur.

Dysfunctional Uterine Bleeding

During the reproductive years, the endometrium proliferates, differentiates, and sheds in a cyclic, predictable fashion in response to physiologic fluctuations in estrogen and progesterone levels. In ovulatory cycles, the luteal phase is 14 days in length, whereas the follicular phase is variable and may range from 10 to 20 days, yielding a wide range of cycle lengths among normal, ovulating women. Early after menarche, cycles tend to be long and irregular. After 5–7 years, cycles shorten to assume a regular pattern that is maintained until the perimenopause. In the fifth decade, cycles gradually lengthen, ceasing in the perimenopausal years. Data from a twin study suggest that genetics are a major determinant of both age at menarche and age at menopause, although these ages seem unrelated and probably are controlled by different genes.[255] Cycle length is based on the rate of follicular growth and maturation, which in turn is influenced by follicle-stimulating hormone (FSH) and inhibin secretion.[151] Abnormalities along the hypothalamic–pituitary–ovarian axis may result in a derangement of follicular maturation, ovulation, or corpus luteum development, with subsequent abnormal hormone secretion. These alterations in the normal hormonal patterns may cause abnormal uterine bleeding, infertility, or both.

Dysfunctional uterine bleeding (*DUB*) is a clinical term used to describe bleeding not attributable to an underlying organic pathologic condition.[4,5,16,119,128,195,215,242,256] DUB is a diagnosis of exclusion rendered only after known causes of abnormal bleeding such as endometrial polyps, adenomyosis, leiomyomas, endometritis, atrophy, intrauterine devices, oral contraceptive use, abortion, ectopic pregnancy, hyperplasia, malignant tumors, gestational trophoblastic disease, blood dyscrasias, certain drugs (particularly anticoagulants), severe renal or liver disease, and hypothyroidism and hyperthyroidism have been ruled out.[166] Therefore, DUB is generally ascribed to poorly understood derangements in the functional effects of hormones on the endometrium.[262,263] Some, however, have also loosely applied this term to heavy, prolonged bleeding at the time of menses (i.e., menorrhagia). Bleeding resulting from anovulatory cycles is probably the most common cause of DUB in women of reproductive age. Also, either early decline or persistence of the corpus luteum may result in abnormal progesterone stimulation of the endometrium, causing DUB. Bleeding from breakdown of normal-appearing atrophic endometrium is the most common cause of postmenopausal uterine bleeding and is often discussed with DUB, although purists might consider this condition an explained source of bleeding. Finally, menorrhagia (if considered a form of DUB) is generally ascribed to local coagulation abnormalities associated with enhanced fibrinolysis and prostaglandin-mediated inhibition of platelet aggregation rather than the hormonally mediated mechanisms postulated in DUB.

Glandular and Stromal Breakdown Associated with Anovulation

In anovulatory cycles, one or more follicles develop in the ovary without the development of a corpus luteum. In these cycles, estradiol synthesized by follicular granulosa and theca cells stimulates endometrial proliferation, but stromal and glandular differentiation typical of the secretory phase fails to develop because progesterone is lacking. The follicles may persist and continue to produce estradiol, or they may regress, ending estrogen production. When estrogen levels decline, the endometrium can no longer be maintained, and bleeding ensues. The level of estrogenic stimulation is roughly linked to the pattern of bleeding. Relatively minimal estrogenic stimulation results in intermittent spotting that may be prolonged. Sustained endometrial stimulation by high levels of estrogen leads to prolonged amenorrhea followed by precipitous onset of heavy bleeding. Both these patterns have been referred to as estrogen breakthrough bleeding.[262,263]

Clinical Features

DUB related to anovulatory cycles typically occurs at menarche and at menopause but can occur at any time during the reproductive years.[195,284] In the first year after menarche, nearly 60% of cycles are anovulatory. Ovulatory cycles soon develop in most women, but some never establish normal cycles.[260] Women in this latter group may have infrequent, irregular periods or heavy bleeding, re-

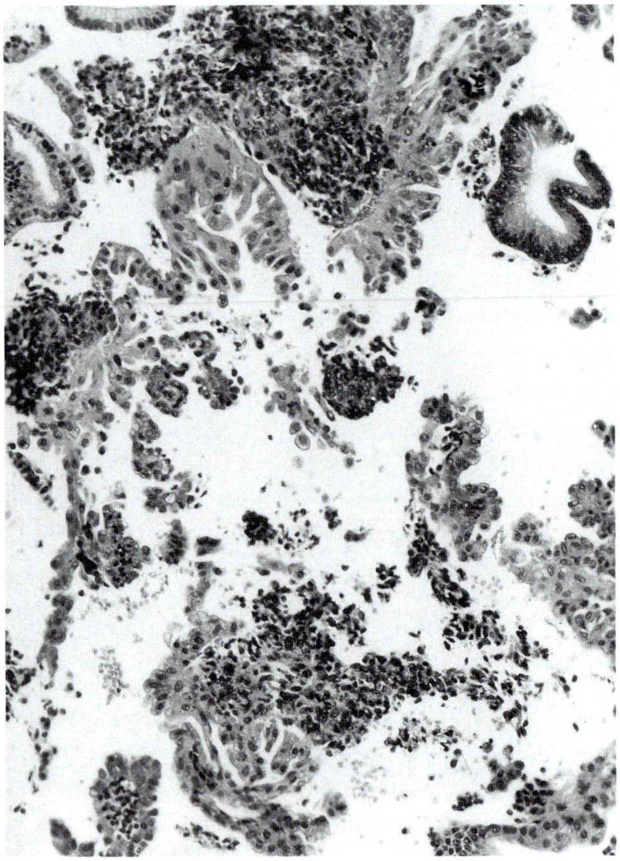

Fig. 10.11. Endometrial glandular and stromal breakdown. There is extensive fragmentation of endometrial glands. Strips of surface epithelium showing eosinophilic syncytial change are present in the *upper part* of the field. The stromal cells are condensed into tight clusters. These findings are typically found in association with anovulatory cycles.

quiring hospitalization. Some of these women display stigmata of polycystic ovarian disease, including obesity, infertility, and hirsutism (Stein–Leventhal syndrome) (see Chapter 16, Nonneoplastic Lesions of the Ovary). Many women in the reproductive age group with anovulatory cycles, however, do not manifest these classic clinical features. Although patients with polycystic ovarian disease are often anovulatory, up to 25% of cycles in these women may result in ovulation and formation of a corpus luteum.

Pathologic Findings

Histologic examination of endometrial tissue removed at the time of bleeding may be scant or abundant, depending on the duration and amount of bleeding that preceded the curettage. The glands are proliferative, but the degree of proliferation depends mainly on the duration of exposure to unopposed estrogen. Metaplasia, hyperplasia, and carcinoma may develop over a period of months or years (see Chapter 11, Precursor Lesions of Endometrial Carcinomas and Chapter 12, Endometrial Carcinoma). If estrogenic stimulation has been limited, the endometrium may appear extensively fragmented (Fig. 10.11), which can compromise the evaluation of glandular architecture, prompting both overdiagnosis and underdiagnosis of hyperplasia. In these cases, the glands should be carefully examined for features such as abnormal shape, cellular stratification, and nuclear atypia that may reflect concurrent breakdown and hyperplasia. Small fragments containing intact glands and stroma resembling typical proliferative endometrium may be seen (Fig. 10.12). As the ground substance undergoes dissolution, stromal cells condense and form compact nests of cells with hyperchromatic nuclei and little or no cytoplasm. The normal architecture collapses, and isolated, fragmented glands lie in haphazard disarray without surrounding stroma. Frequently, dark cytoplasmic granules may be identified in glandular cells, representing nuclear debris from necrotic cells. In combination, these features are referred to as glandular and stromal breakdown, and when present in a background of proliferative endometrium, suggest anovulatory bleeding. In cases with stronger estrogenic effects, the endometrium is less fragmented and more typical of normal proliferative endometrium with only focal areas of glandular and stromal breakdown (Fig. 10.13). If foci of dilated irregularly shaped glands with focal outpouchings and branching are present, the en-

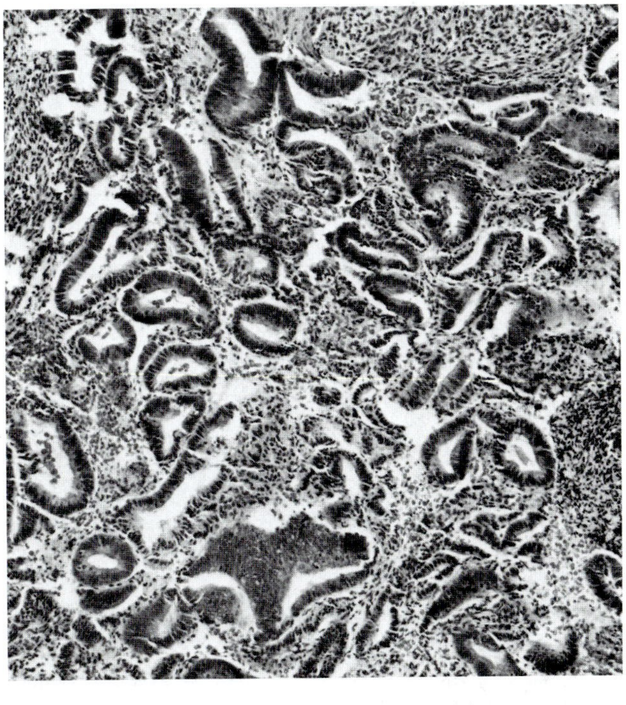

Fig. 10.12. Endometrial glandular and stromal breakdown. There is extensive fragmentation of proliferative glands, stromal necrosis, and hemorrhage.

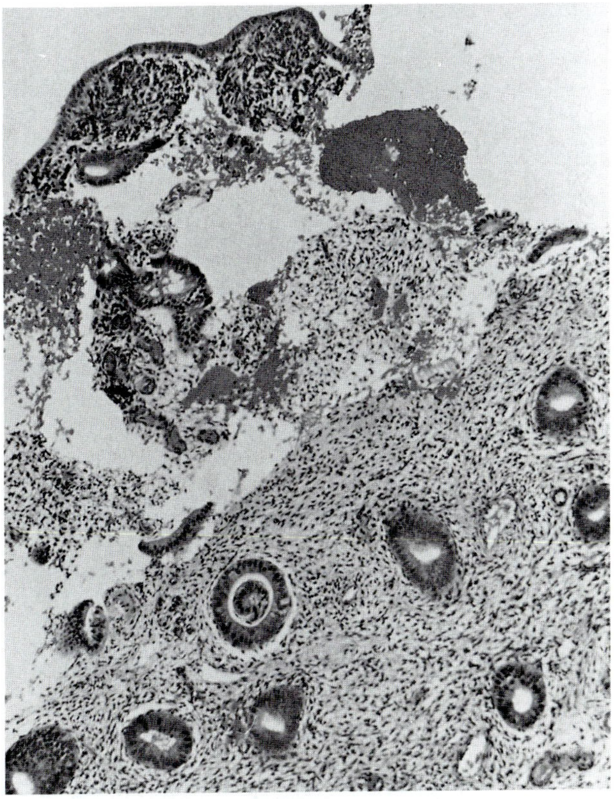

Fig. 10.13. Proliferative endometrium with focal breakdown. Most of the endometrium is in the proliferative phase. A focal area of breakdown is present on the surface in the *upper part* of the field.

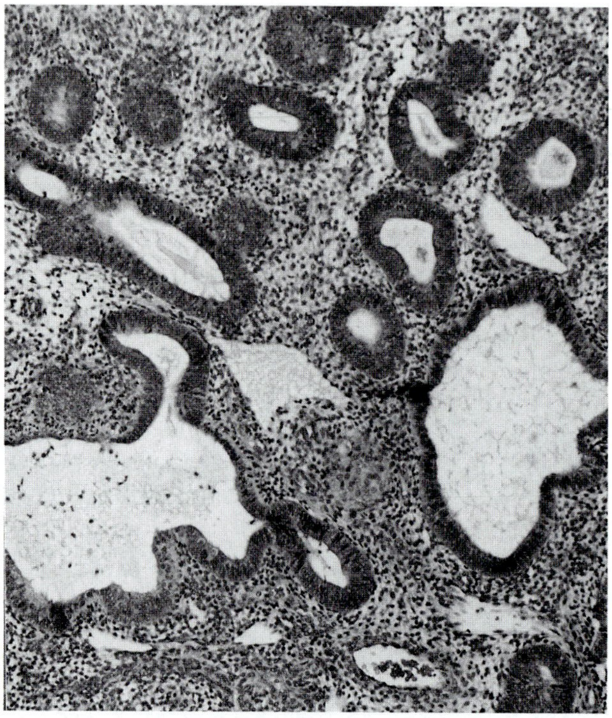

Fig. 10.14. **Disordered proliferative phase.** A few glands are enlarged and irregularly shaped.

dometrium is classified as disordered proliferative phase (Figs. 10.14 and 10.15).[103] Qualitatively, disordered proliferative phase resembles simple hyperplasia but the process is focal rather than diffuse (see Chapter 11, Precursor Lesions of Endometrial Carcinomas). Rare crowded glands with complex invaginations (Fig. 10.16) in an otherwise normal endometrium may represent an artifact that should not be confused with disordered proliferative phase or "focal" hyperplasia.

Papillary syncytial metaplasia is an epithelial alteration that is associated with stromal breakdown and bleeding. Because this lesion probably reflects a degenerative–regenerative process rather than a metaplastic one and formation of true papillae are lacking, alternative terms such as eosinophilic syncytial change, papillary syncytial change, or surface syncytial change have been proposed[317] (see Chapter 11, Precursor Lesions of Endometrial Carcinomas). These lesions typically involve the surface but glands may also be involved. Typically, cells with eosinophilic cytoplasm, indistinct cell membranes, and moderately prominent nucleoli form microscopic mounds on the endometrial surface overlying condensed stromal cells (Figs. 10.11 and 10.17).

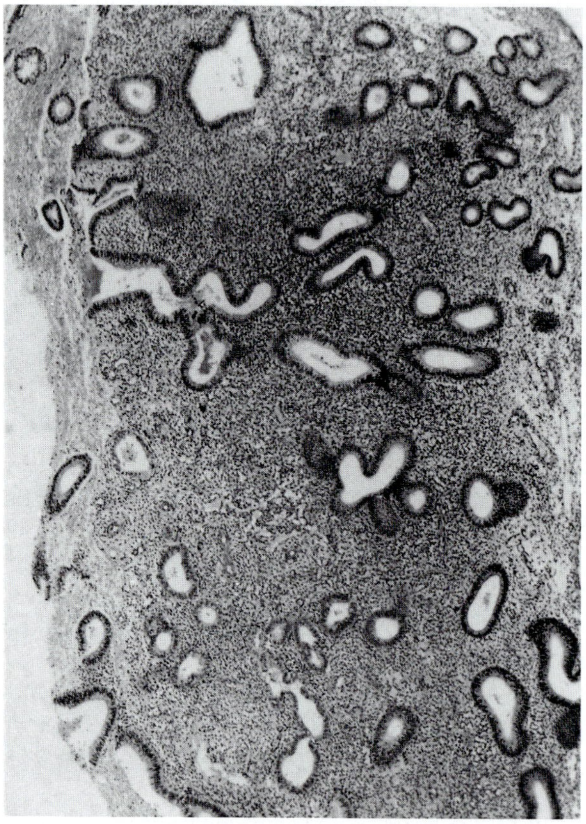

Fig. 10.15. **Disordered proliferative phase.** Most of the endometrium is in the proliferative phase but a few scattered glands that are enlarged and irregularly shaped are present.

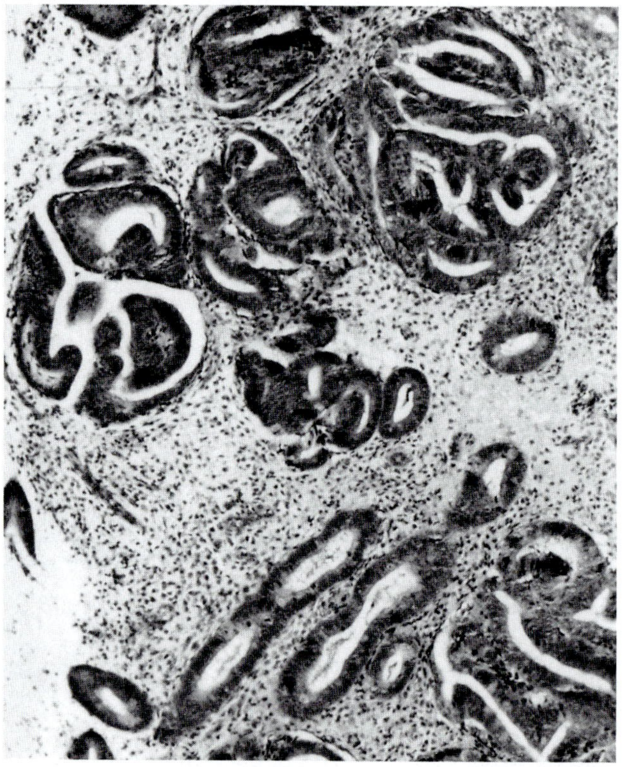

Fig. 10.16. **Focal glandular crowding.** The endometrium is in the proliferative phase. The crowding and the convoluted appearance of the glands are artifactual changes.

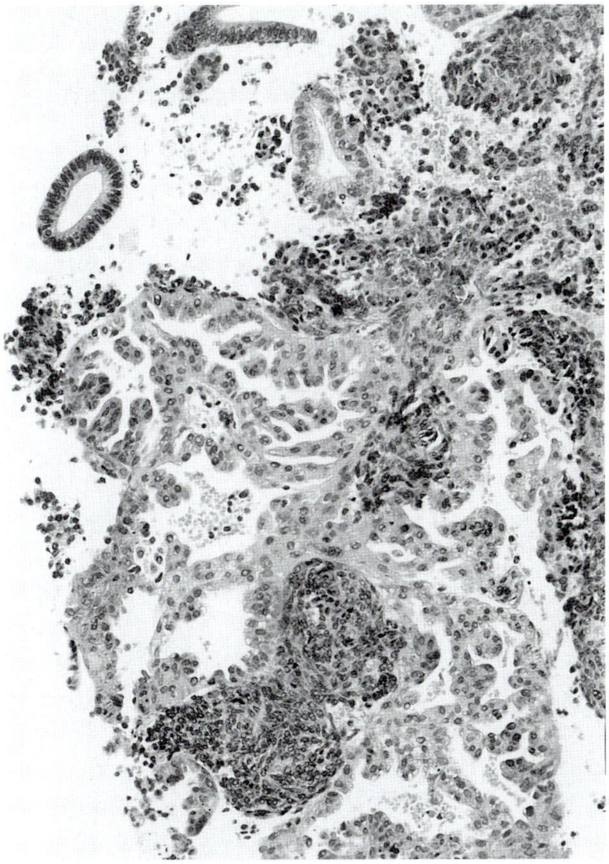

Fig. 10.17. Eosinophilic syncytial change. Cells with eosinophilic cytoplasm form a syncytium that envelops clusters of stromal cells.

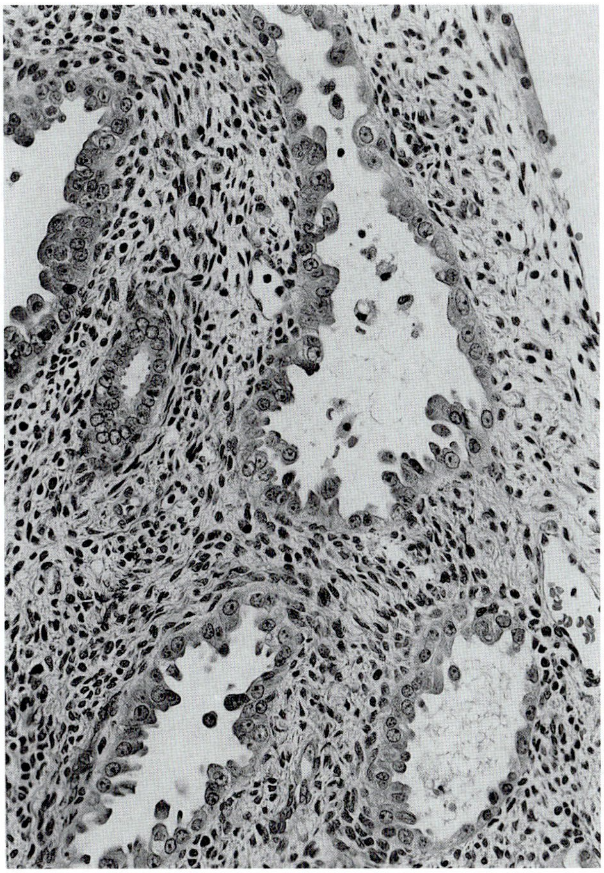

Fig. 10.18. Eosinophilic and hobnail cell change. Cells have enlarged, rounded nuclei, some of which contain small nucleoli. This change should not be interpreted as "atypia." Some cells protrude into the lumen (hobnail change).

Microcysts containing PMNs and nuclear debris may be present within the cell masses.

Another common finding associated with bleeding and breakdown is termed *eosinophilic change* or *eosinophilic metaplasia*. This change is characterized by cells with abundant eosinophilic cytoplasm, nucleolar prominence, or mitoses reflecting epithelial regeneration or smudgy, hyperchromatic chromatin reflecting degeneration (Fig. 10.18). Eosinophilic change, also referred to as eosinophilic syncytial change when the cell borders of the cells are not evident, may mimic the significant atypia found in endometrial intraepithelial carcinoma or atypical endometrial hyperplasia. However, the changes in papillary syncytial metaplasia are usually more delimited than in precursor lesions and the degree of nuclear enlargement, pleomorphism, and irregularity is comparatively modest. Eosinophilic syncytial change may be associated with other cytoplasmic alterations (metaplasias) including squamous, mucinous, and ciliated change (see Chapter 11).

In abnormal shedding, the endometrium often displays thin-walled ectatic venules that may contain prominent fibrin thrombi (Fig. 10.19), a feature seldom encountered in normal menstrual endometrium. Bleeding during a normal menstrual cycle is a consequence of rhythmic vasospasm and relaxation of the spiral arterioles, resulting in a complete, yet self-limited sloughing of the functionalis (see Chapter 9, Anatomy and Histology of the Uterine Corpus).[224] In anovulatory cycles, spiral arterioles fail to develop adequately, and the dilated, thin-walled venules undergo thrombosis. Stromal necrosis involving random portions of the endometrium results in incomplete shedding. Consequently, the bleeding pattern is asynchronous and highly variable in duration.

Differential Diagnosis

Artifactual glandular crowding secondary to stromal collapse may superficially resemble hyperplasia or carcinoma (Fig. 10.20). However, the glands in glandular and stromal breakdown typically have normal shapes and the epithelium lacks stratifica-

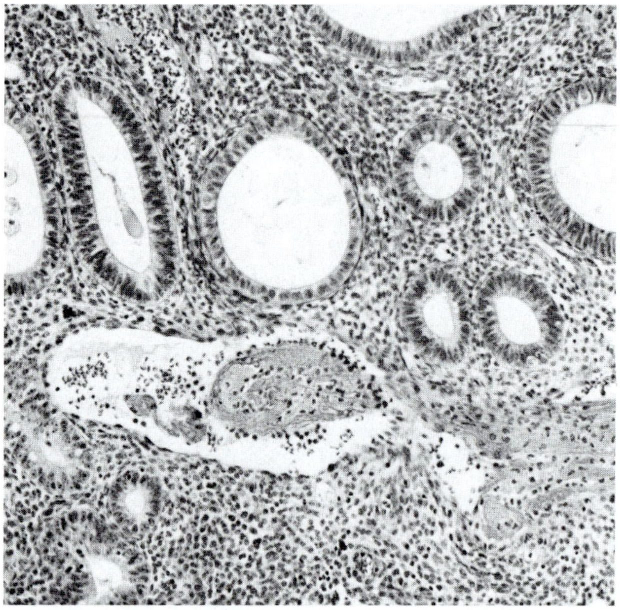

Fig. 10.19. Fibrin thrombi in association with glandular and stromal breakdown. Dysfunctional bleeding associated with anovulatory cycles may result in mild irregularities in proliferative glands and in the development of thin-walled blood vessels. Bleeding is caused, in part, by disruption of the capillaries that contain fibrin thrombi.

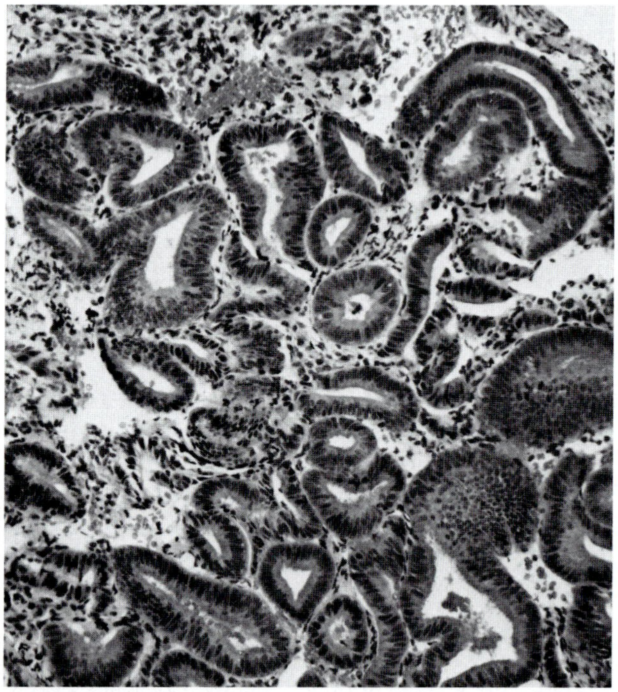

Fig. 10.20. Pseudoglandular crowding in glandular and stromal breakdown. The glandular crowding results from breakdown and dissolution of the intervening stroma; this should not be confused with crowding as a result of hyperplasia.

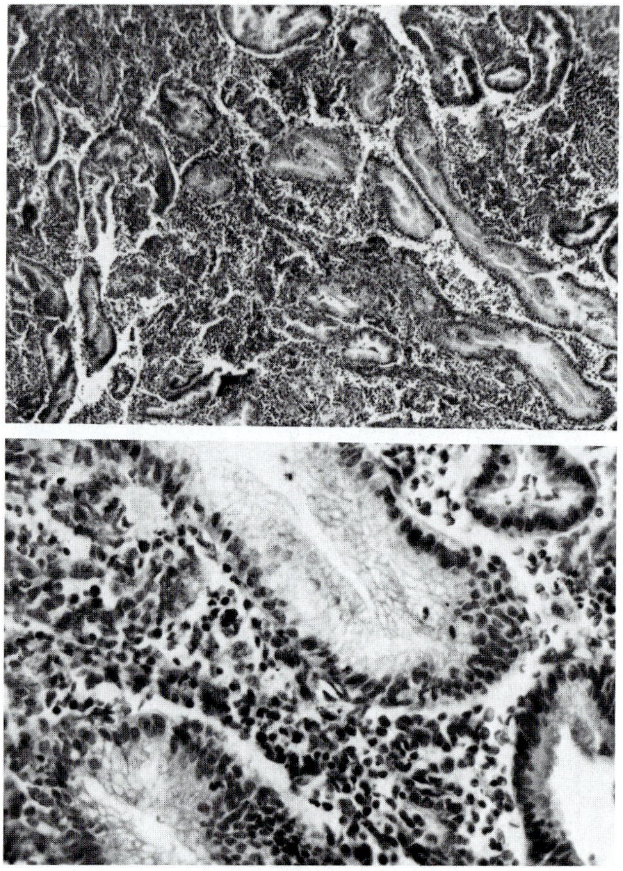

Fig. 10.21. Menstrual endometrium. *Top*: Diffuse hemorrhage, necrosis, and stromal breakdown. *Bottom*: Numerous glands containing vacuolated cytoplasm.

tion, atypia, and significant mitotic activity. In menstrual endometrium, a predecidual reaction is present and the glands are typically dilated and filled with secretions (Fig. 10.21). Degenerative cytoplasmic vacuolization may be seen in either.

Treatment

Treatment depends on the age of the patient. An acute bleeding episode in a woman under 35 years of age may respond to a short course of low-dose combination monophasic birth control pills.[262,263] The progestin stabilizes the uterine vasculature, differentiates the glands and stroma, and results in a complete shedding of the endometrium when therapy is discontinued. Bleeding may be heavy, but it is self-limited. In women over 35 years old and in young women with bleeding not controlled by hormones, an endometrial biopsy to rule out organic pathology should be considered. In young women with recurrent anovulatory cycles who are not immediately desirous of childbearing, a week's course of oral medroxyprogesterone acetate (Provera) every

2 months will prevent excessive endometrial buildup and should give controlled withdrawal bleeding. If bleeding occurs in an anovulatory patient who is infertile, successful induction of ovulation with clomiphene may achieve normal ovulatory cycles and menstrual shedding. Bleeding that cannot be controlled by medical treatment requires surgical intervention. Options include hysterectomy and endometrial ablation using a laser or resectoscope with a loop or rolling ball electrode.[160]

Atrophy

Bleeding associated with *endometrial atrophy* related to insufficient estrogen stimulation may develop in women taking oral contraceptives, in postmenopausal women with naturally occurring atrophy, in young women with premature ovarian failure, or following radiation for cervical cancer. Typically, patients complain of vaginal spotting. Atrophy may account for up to 82% of postmenopausal vaginal spotting or bleeding.[44,87,153,172,229,240] The microscopic appearance of atrophic endometrium is different in hysterectomy and biopsy specimens.[166,316] In hysterectomy specimens, the endometrium is thin and composed of variably sized glands that are often cystic and surrounded by a diminished amount of compact stroma compared with endometria from reproductive age women. The glands are lined by a single layer of flattened or cuboidal cells containing bland nuclei without mitoses. Under low magnification, cystically dilated atrophic glands may mimic simple hyperplasia, but the epithelial cells are not stratified, mitotic figures are absent, and the cells possess little cytoplasm. Biopsy or curettage specimens of atrophic endometrium typically consist of scant mucus with rare fragments and strips of cuboidal or columnar cells. Intact glands may be absent (Fig. 10.22), and only small clusters of stromal cells with dark ovoid nuclei resembling those seen in anovulatory bleeding are observed. Cases containing scant epithelium may be considered adequate provided that the cells can be definitively recognized as atrophic endometrium and not endocervical. These specimens should not be diagnosed as being insufficient for diagnosis because this amount of tissue generally is all that is present, even after a thorough curettage. Such specimens should be given a descriptive diagnosis, for example, "scant fragments of atrophic endometrial tissue."

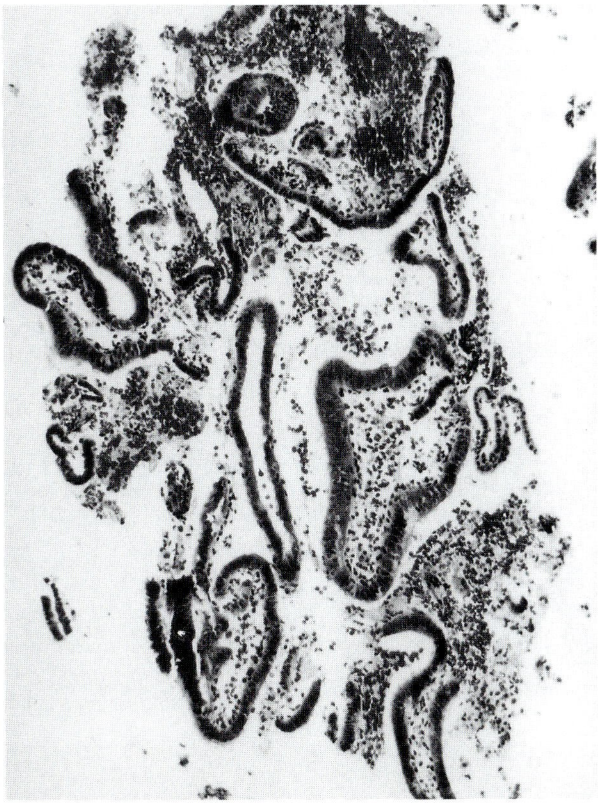

Fig. 10.22. Atrophy. Atrophic endometrium in curettings is characterized by strips of surface endometrium, fragmented glands, and minimal stroma.

Inadequate Luteal Phase

Inadequate luteal phase, or *luteal-phase defect* (*LPD*), is thought to result from inadequate progesterone secretion by the corpus luteum and is usually diagnosed during an evaluation for infertility or abnormal bleeding. The pathogenesis of LPD is complex and poorly understood. In many cases, LPD develops when the corpus luteum either fails to develop adequately or regresses prematurely. It is postulated that a poorly formed corpus luteum may be caused by inappropriately low FSH levels during the follicular phase or low FSH and luteinizing hormone (LH) peaks at midcycle, leading to deficient luteinization of the granulosa cells.[262,263] Elevated prolactin levels may also lead to LPD by suppressing progesterone release by the granulosa cells. Any of these processes could reduce total progesterone secretion by the corpus luteum. Studies suggest that LPD may reflect an end-organ receptor defect, in view of the finding of a reduced number of endometrial progesterone receptor-binding sites in some patients with LPD.[145,264] As a result, menses occurs 6–9 days after the LH surge.[124,125,180]

Clinical Features

In most studies, LPD is found in only 3–5% of infertile women,[295] and its significance remains controversial because controlled studies are lacking. LPD may also contribute to early habitual spontaneous abortions and to abnormal uterine bleeding.[113] The diagnosis of LPD requires the demonstration of the diagnostic findings in at least two consecutive cycles because similar changes occur sporadically in normal women.[126] Endometrial biopsy is considered one of the best methods of establishing the diagnosis,[8,61,294] but basal body temperature graphs showing a temperature rise that is sustained for less than 10 days and low serum progesterone levels are valuable adjuncts.[57,61,226,262]

Pathologic Findings

Exact pathologic criteria for the diagnosis of LPD have not been definitively established. Characteristically, the endometrium resembles normal secretory endometrium but shows an appearance that is consistent with a date that is at least 2 days earlier than expected (in two consecutive cycles), according to the basal body temperature graph and the onset of menses after biopsy (e.g., a day 24 pattern on day 26).[180,259] In normally cycling women, endometrial dating is, at best, an approximation, with variation from one microscopic field to another and between observers. Reproducibility of endometrial dating is within 2 days of the expected date in about 80% of cases.[196] The secretory pattern in LPD varies with the patient's hormone balance, and dating is often impossible due to a discordant appearance of the glands and stroma.[60] For example, glands may show secretory changes but lack the complex tortuosity expected, or the stroma may fail to show edema or predecidual changes in an endometrium that otherwise resembles late-secretory phase. The pathologic changes in benign secretory endometrium attributable to hormonal imbalances have not been well characterized. Consequently, abnormal-appearing secretory-phase endometrium may reflect LPD, but the changes are not diagnostic.

Treatment

Various treatments have been used for LPD. If low FSH and LH levels are implicated, clomiphene citrate or human menopausal gonadotropin is used to cause an elevation of FSH.[71,262] Progesterone vaginal suppositories administered after the midcycle temperature rise have also been tried in an attempt to alleviate a presumptive deficiency of progesterone in LPD.[125,259,296] Alternatively, human chorionic gonadotropin (hCG) may be administered to patients with hyperprolactinemia to stimulate the corpus luteum to produce progesterone,[262] or bromocriptine, to inhibit prolactin secretion.[65]

Irregular Shedding

Irregular shedding is diagnosed when endometrial tissue obtained at least 5 days after the onset of bleeding shows a mixture of secretory and proliferative patterns (Fig. 10.23). It is a rare cause of abnormal bleeding in women between 24 and 50 years of age.[168,284] It is characterized by prolonged, heavy bleeding at the time of menses, sometimes lasting longer than 2 weeks.[169,254] Irregular shedding may occur at every menstrual period or only once, such as with a persistent corpus luteum cyst. The mechanism underlying irregular shedding with a persistent corpus luteum is presumably prolonged exposure to progesterone because injecting small doses

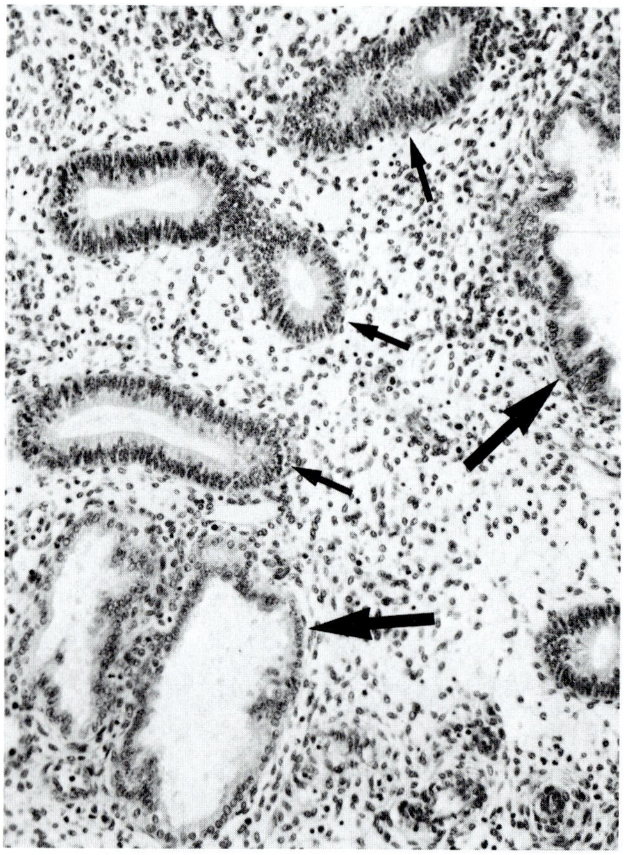

Fig. 10.23. Irregular shedding. Glands showing secretory exhaustion (*large arrows*) are immediately adjacent to proliferative glands (*small arrows*) in an edematous, secretory-type stroma.

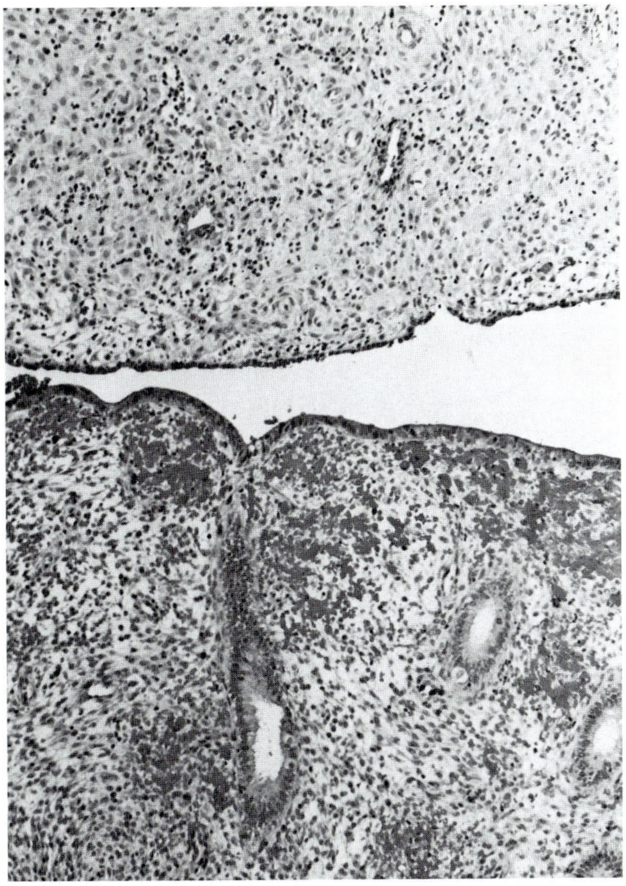

Fig. 10.24. Irregular shedding. *Top*: A secretory pattern with a predecidual reaction. *Bottom*: A proliferative pattern.

of progesterone during the menstrual phase of the cycle produces similar effects.[111] Microscopically, a diverse array of endometrial fragments containing irregular star-shaped secretory glands admixed with early proliferative glands are seen.[60] The stroma around proliferative glands is dense and compact. In areas containing secretory-type glands, the stroma is edematous and the stromal cells may be converted into predecidual cells (Fig. 10.24). Fibrin thrombi may be present. In addition, there is frequent evidence of glandular and stromal breakdown. In contrast to LPD, which shows only secretory changes, irregular shedding demonstrates secretory and proliferative changes. Other endometrial disorders, including abortions, polyps, and chronic endometritis, may produce bleeding patterns that mimic irregular shedding. In addition, there are abnormal secretory patterns with superimposed bleeding for which there are no specific clinical correlations. Accordingly, these abnormal secretory patterns are best given a descriptive diagnosis.

Unexplained Menorrhagia

In contrast to DUB related to hormonal imbalances, some unexplained menorrhagia may be related to abnormal mechanisms of local hemostasis.[114,287] Ultrastructurally, clots in women with menorrhagia appear different than those in normal women, and abnormal platelet aggregation related to alterations in prostaglandin synthesis have been suggested.[3,35] Enhanced fibrinolysis has also been proposed as a mechanism in these women.[93,232] Studies have found that women with essential menorrhagia have higher levels of tissue plasminogen activator activity in the menstrual phase and higher levels of the corresponding antigen in both the late-secretory and menstrual phases than controls. Accordingly, treatment with prostaglandin synthetase inhibitors may be highly effective in reducing bleeding in these women. Use of progesterone-releasing intrauterine devices may also be effective.

Effects of Drugs

Estrogens

The endometrium is sensitive to low concentrations of *estrogen*, with most pathologic effects more strongly related to duration of exposure rather than the dose. In rabbits, prolonged estrogen exposure induces endometrial carcinoma,[171] whereas high doses in monkeys result in atrophy.[102] In humans, prolonged administration of estrogens may produce hyperplasia and endometrioid adenocarcinoma (see Chapter 11, Precursor Lesions of Endometrial Carcinomas, and Chapter 12, Endometrial Carcinoma).[199] Estrogen may also result in proliferative-phase patterns and in glandular and stromal breakdown resembling the findings in DUB caused by anovulatory cycles. In addition to inducing proliferation, estrogens, probably in combination with other hormones, may promote epithelial differentiation, including formation of cilia (tubal metaplasia) and cytoplasmic eosinophilia[103] (see Chapter 11).

Tamoxifen

Tamoxifen acts as a partial estrogen receptor agonist and antagonist. In the endometrium, the former properties dominate, whereas the antiestrogenic properties are responsible for the effectiveness of tamoxifen as a breast cancer treatment and its possible use in chemoprevention. Results from the National Surgical Adjuvant Breast and Bowel Project Breast Cancer Prevention Trial (P-1) demonstrated that 5 years of tamoxifen use at a dose of 20 mg/day reduced breast cancer risk in high-risk women by 49%. It is unclear how much of this benefit reflected true chemoprevention or simply suppression of cancers already present at study enrollment. Tamoxifen recipients had a risk ratio of 2.5 for the development of endometrial carcinoma. All the tumors were stage I, and there were no reported deaths related to these tumors.[77]

In a case-control study of 309 women diagnosed with malignant endometrial tumors after a diagnosis of breast carcinoma and 860 matched breast cancer controls, Bergman et al. found that tamoxifen use was associated with a relative risk of 1.5 for the development of endometrial cancer.[19] Risk was strongly associated with duration of use, with a relative risk of 6.9 for women receiving 5 years or more of treatment. Treatment for 2 years or more was associated with a higher frequency of advanced stage tumors, sarcomas, malignant mixed müllerian tumors, and shortened survival. Cancer risk was associated with cumulative dose but not with daily dose. Kedar et al. reported, in a randomized trial of 111 healthy women with family histories of breast cancer given tamoxifen or placebo, that patients receiving tamoxifen had thicker endometria and significantly more often developed endometrial pathology. Most notably, endometrial hyperplasia was identified in 16% of the treated group compared to none of the controls.[132] Fornander et al. also reported that tamoxifen users have a relative risk of 6.4 at 3–4 years for developing endometrial carcinoma compared to nonusers[80] (see Chapter 12, Endometrial Carcinoma). These results are concordant with the bulk of evidence suggesting that tamoxifen use is causally related to the development of endometrial proliferation, hyperplasia, and carcinoma.[118]

Although some studies suggest that tamoxifen-associated carcinomas tend to be more aggressive and skewed toward high-risk types,[161,250] there is at least equal evidence that these carcinomas are similar in grade, stage, type, and behavior to cancers arising in nonusers.[14,118] However, studies have been small and some may not have accounted fully for all prognostic variables. Some studies suggesting an overrepresentation of aggressive tumor types compared to the general population have included patients receiving 40 mg/day instead of 20 mg/day of famoxifen (usual dose for adjuvant treatment of breast cancer in the United States) or may have reflected a referral bias because the research was conducted at tertiary centers.[161,250]

Other uterine abnormalities that have been associated with tamoxifen use include endometrial polyps, hyperplasia, sarcomas, adenomyosis, endometriosis, and leiomyomas.[66,86,188] The appearance of endometrial polyps in tamoxifen-treated patients is generally similar to those occurring spontaneously.[51] Stromal decidualization may reflect concurrent administration of progesterone. Tamoxifen-associated endometrial polyps tend to be large and multiple. These polyps often have a myxoid or edematous stroma and staghorn gland that may be polarized along the long axis of the polyp. Metaplasias and carcinomas may occur in these polyps.[49a,133a]

Tamoxifen has also consistently been associated with an increased incidence of endometrial polyps,[49,147] but potentially important confounding factors such as baseline endometrial status and body fat distribution were not taken into account.[188] Raloxifen is a benzo-thiophene-selective estrogen-receptor modulator that may also reduce breast cancer risk, but in contrast to tamoxifen, raloxifen does not seem to increase endometrial thickness, produce bleeding, or induce endometrial proliferation or hyperplasia.[48,96] The STAR trial (study of tamoxifen and raloxifen) should shed light on the potential value of these agents in chemoprevention.

Estrogen and Progesterone Therapy in Postmenopausal Women

Hormone replacement therapy has been administered to many postmenopausal women to alleviate menopausal symptoms, including abnormal bleeding, and to reduce the risk of osteoporotic fractures and death from coronary artery disease.[62,74] Use of hormone replacement had increased dramatically in the United States. During the period 1982–1992, progesterone prescriptions increased 2.3 fold and those for progesterone 4.9 fold.[309] Data from the Postmenopausal Estrogen/Progestin Interventions (PEPI) Trial have demonstrated that estrogen or estrogen/progestin combination therapy has salutary effects on lipoprotein levels.[282] However, it is unclear whether improvement in lipid profiles translates into reduced cardiovascular mortality. In the PEPI Trial, estrogen alone demonstrated the highest elevation in the cardioprotective high-density lipoprotein cholesterol, but 34% of recipients developed adenomatous (complex) or atypical hyperplasia, making this regimen suitable only for women without a uterus.[283] Medical intervention was successful in reversing these lesions in all but 2 of 10 women with atypical hyperplasia. The reported occurrence of endometrial hyperplasia in women taking estrogen alone is similar to that reported in other studies.[47] The risk of endometrial carcinoma is also greater in women on unopposed estrogen as compared with untreated women.[289] After 1 year of treatment, risk of endometrial carcinoma may remain increased for more than 10 years after discontinuation of therapy. Accordingly, a progestational agent given either continuously with estrogen or sequentially for 10–14 days in the latter half of the cycle is usually included in hormonal replacement therapies. By adding a synthetic progestational agent or natural progesterone, the rate of hyperplasia is reduced substantially when the dose and duration of treatment are optimized.[47,269,299]

Effects of progesterone depend on type, dose, and duration of use, as reviewed by Song and Fraser.[257] Salient effects include inhibition of glandular proliferation, stromal decidualization, stromal necrosis, and recruitment of leukocytes. Based on screening results of 2964 peri- and postmenopausal candidates for hormone replacement therapy showing only 0.6% with hyperplasia and 0.07% with adenocarcinoma, Korhoneen et al. suggested that biopsy before initiating hormone replacement therapy is not required in asymptomatic women.[138] The average age of women in this study was 52 years, with a last menstrual period 29 months before enrollment. Sequential regimens originally were used in doses that were high enough to induce secretory transformation and result in cyclic withdrawal bleeding. Many postmenopausal women, however, find regular bleeding objectionable and consequently compliance is poor with this regimen. A continuous regimen employing reduced doses of estrogen and progesterone that results in an atrophic endometrium and amenorrhea has also been used. Cases of hyperplasia or carcinomas were not identified in a study of 236 women treated for more than 5 years with this combined therapy, and mitotic activity was low.[185] The amount of tissue obtained via endometrial biopsy in this study was associated with the dose of estrogen and progesterone used and the bleeding pattern. Recovery of endometrial tissue was 100% with high doses but only 18% with low doses. Tissue was not obtained in 83% of amenorrheic patients but was collected in 93% of women with regular withdrawal bleeding. Hysteroscopic examination confirmed the presence of endometrial atrophy in women with scant specimens. This study demonstrated that low doses of progesterone inhibit endometrial proliferation, resulting in endometrial atrophy and amenorrhea without inducing secretory maturation. Protection from hyperplasia equaled the higher-dose regimens, which resulted in regular bleeding (Moyer, personal communication).[185]

Williams et al. investigated the effects of giving 0.625 mg/day estradiol with 10 mg/day medroxyprogesterone acetate in three different regimens: 14 days of progestational treatment every 28 days, 14 days every 84 days, or 28 days every 84 days.[302] Women receiving the least amount of progesterone in the 84-day period had the least bleeding. Simple hyperplasia was recognized in 1% of each group. Nand et al. reported that among 568 postmenopausal women receiving 1.25 mg/day estrone sulfate and either 2.5, 5.0, or 10.0 mg/day medroxyprogesterone acetate, 80% became amenorrheic at 6 months and none developed hyperplasia.[187] Similarly, in a randomized, double-masked multicenter trial of 1176 postmenopausal women, 14.6% of patients receiving 1 mg/day estradiol developed hyperplasia within 1 year compared to less than 1% of those given combination treatment with norethindrone acetate at doses as low as 0.1 mg daily.[143] Although both the sequential and combined hormone replacement regimens and oral contraceptives contain estrogen and progesterone, hormone replacement regimens contain much lower doses and produce different histologic effects.

The histologic appearance of the endometrium in women receiving hormone replacement varies depending on the dosage, duration of use, regimen (combined or sequential), status of the endometrium before therapy, and the time in the cycle when the biopsy is obtained. Possible appearances include normal-appearing proliferative or secretory endometrium, mixed proliferative and secretory endometrium, abnormal secretory patterns, and atrophy. Secretory endometria can show variable secretory activity with or without predecidual change (Figs. 10.25 and 10.26). In addition, disordered proliferative phase, hyperplasia, and various types of cytoplasmic changes (metaplasias) can be observed.[64] Low-dose preparations produce endometrial atrophy or secretory changes that are not as fully developed as those in the normal luteal phase.[166] In postmenopausal women, decidualization usually reflects the use of a relatively high-dose hormone replacement regimen; idiopathic decidual reactions in postmenopausal women have been reported rarely.[45] Arias–Stella reaction has also been reported in nonpregnant patients, especially in the setting of exogenous hormone administration including progestational agents.[116]

Contraceptive Steroids (Progestin-Estrogen Agents)

The chemical composition, metabolism, and effects of *contraceptive steroids* differ from those of naturally occurring hormones. Naturally occurring estrogens are inactivated when administered orally, but oral contraceptives contain an orally active agent, 17-alpha-ethinylestradiol, produced by adding

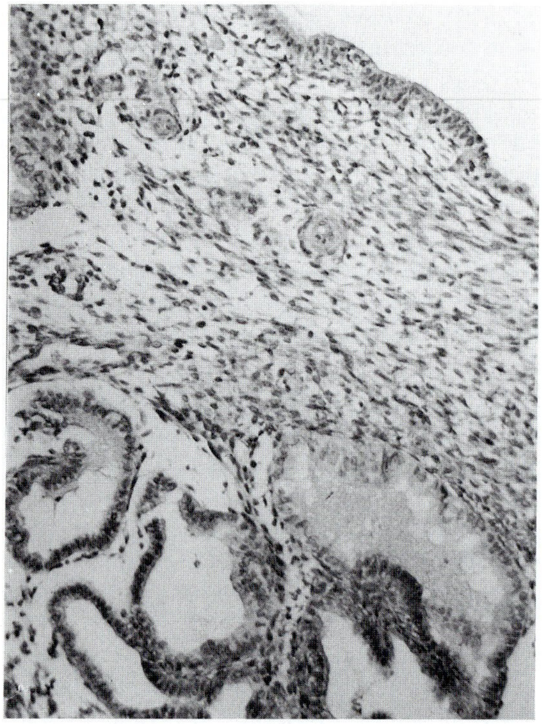

Fig. 10.25. Estrogen and progesterone hormone replacement therapy. The glands are variable in appearance. One gland contains secretory material in the lumen and the others are lined by nondescript epithelium, which represent a weak secretory response. The stroma is composed of spindle-shaped cells. There is no evidence of a predecidual reaction. (Courtesy of Dr. Dean Moyer, Los Angeles, CA.)

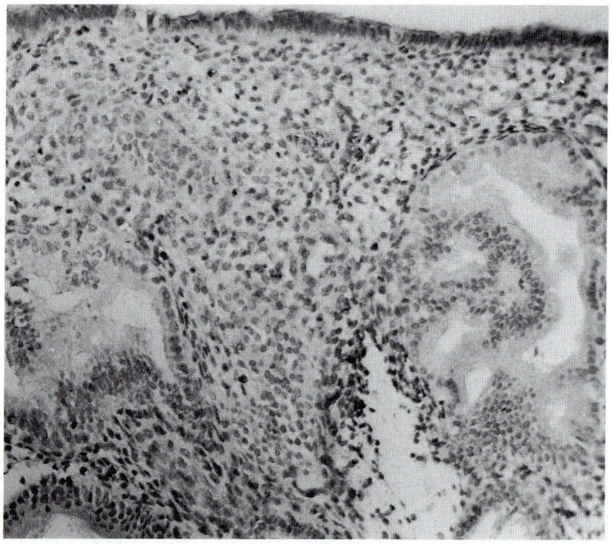

Fig. 10.26. Estrogen and progesterone hormone replacement therapy. The endometrium shows full secretory maturation. Glands show secretory exhaustion, and the stroma has undergone a predecidual change. (Courtesy of Dr. Dean Moyer, Los Angeles, CA.)

an ethinyl group to position 17. The less potent 3-methyl ether derivative of ethinylestradiol, mestranol, is also used as the estrogenic component of oral contraceptives. Some oral contraceptives have profound progestational activity, which may be 50 times more potent that natural progesterone. Also, some progestational agents are metabolized to estrogenic compounds in the body.[262] Potency of different progestins varies considerably, and biologic effects depend mainly on potency rather than on dosage. The progestational agents in the combination pill prevent ovulation by inhibiting LH secretion through a negative feedback effect on the hypothalamus. Although the estrogen component in the pill exerts a similar effect on FSH, its primary function is to stimulate endometrial proliferation, thereby preventing breakthrough bleeding. Estrogen also potentiates the negative feedback action of the progestational agent, permitting the use of a lower dose of the latter. This effect is attributed to estrogen increasing the intracellular concentration of progesterone receptors.[262,263]

Clinical Features

In the past, contraceptive steroids were administered either as a sequential regimen in which estrogen alone was taken for 14–16 days, followed by 5–6 days during which the estrogen and progestin were given in a single tablet, or as a combined regimen in which a synthetic estrogen was combined with a synthetic progestin in a single tablet taken on day 5 of the cycle and continued for 21 days. The sequential regimen was introduced with the expectation that it would be tolerated better because it more closely simulated a woman's natural endocrine milieu. However, sequential pills proved to be less reliable contraceptive agents, with breakthrough ovulations reported in about 8% of women.[170] These agents were withdrawn from the market in the United States and Canada in 1976 after reports linking them to endometrial cancer surfaced.[133,158,251,252] Notably, 83% of sequential pill users who developed endometrial carcinoma used Oracon.[158,251] and the elevation in risk was supported by an epidemiologic study.[292] This study also suggested that endometrial carcinoma risk is reduced in women taking combined oral contraceptives, as would be expected from the suppressive effect of progestin-dominated combined regimens. The carcinogenic effect of Oracon does not seem to have been attributable simply to the effects of unopposed estrogen because other sequential pills were not associated with the development of endometrial carcinoma. Oracon, however, used a high dose (100 μg) of the potent estrogen ethinylestradiol combined with a weak progestin, which insufficiently opposed the estrogenic effect.

Continued use of oral contraceptives, particularly the low-dose preparations (20–35 μg ethinylestradiol), may result in breakthrough bleeding or amenorrhea.[176] Secondary amenorrhea may occur because the low estrogen content of the pill frequently is inadequate to stimulate endometrial growth. Consequently, there is insufficient tissue to produce withdrawal bleeding at the end of a pill cycle. A pill with a slightly higher estrogen content helps in this situation. Prolonged use of oral contraceptives results in the development of thin-walled vascular sinusoids located beneath the endometrial surface, which become ectatic and undergo thrombosis. The endometrial vessels become disrupted and bleed and the surrounding tissue shrinks but is not shed completely, which is manifested clinically as breakthrough bleeding. A 7-day course of conjugated estrogens or ethinylestradiol daily will build up the endometrium and result in uniform withdrawal bleeding.[262,263]

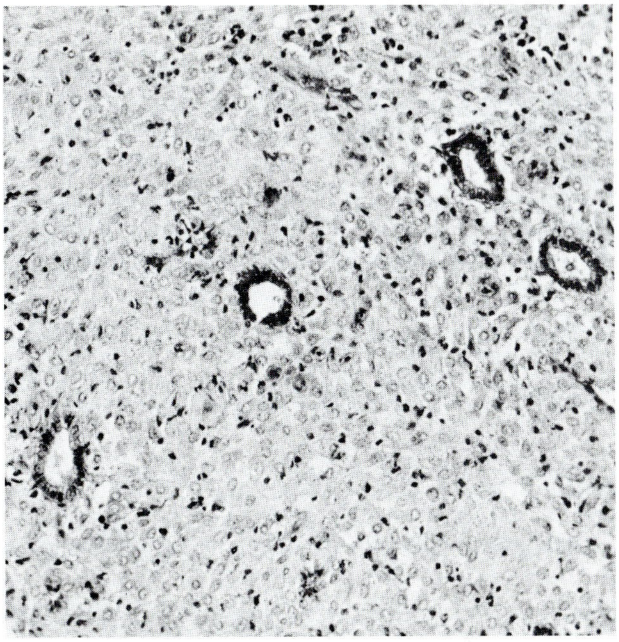

Fig. 10.28. Oral contraceptive therapy. After several cycles of oral contraceptives, the endometrium shows a marked decidual reaction. Glands are small and lined by inactive epithelium.

Pathologic Findings

The histologic alterations produced by oral contraceptives on the endometrium are a function of (1) whether the drugs are administered in the combined or sequential regimen, (2) the dose and duration of drug used, (3) the morphologic appearance of the endometrium before the start of therapy, and (4) the time of the cycle when the tissue is obtained for study.[105,166,197,198] During the first cycle of the combined regimen in women who had previously been ovulating normally, the proliferative phase is markedly shortened, with an arrest in both the growth and differentiation of the glandular epithelium. The glands remain straight and are lined by a single layer of low, inactive columnar epithelium. Glycogen vacuoles appear prematurely and tend to be randomly distributed (Fig. 10.27). Glandular growth is inhibited, and secretory changes develop minimally, if at all. Stromal edema, which can be striking early in therapy, gives way to a distinct decidual change, and numerous granular lymphocytes appear (Fig. 10.28). After long-term contraceptive use, there is no evidence of secretory activity. The endometrium undergoes atrophy and is composed of sparse, narrow glands.[42] The remaining glands are composed of flattened epithelial cells. In addition, thin-walled vascular sinusoids develop and the stroma is decreased. A decidual reaction may not be evident. This is the usual appearance of the endometrium in women using the low-dose formulations.

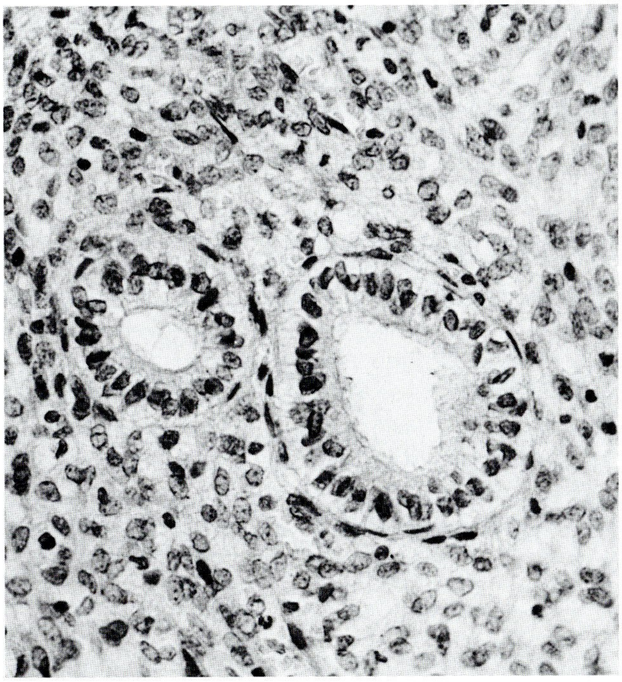

Fig. 10.27. Oral contraceptive therapy. Secretory vacuoles appear prematurely in endometrial glands early during the course of combined oral contraceptive administration.

Progestins, Including Norplant

Progestin-type drugs alone produce effects on the endometrium similar to those described for combined oral contraceptives, but atrophy develops earlier. A marked decidual reaction and glandular suppression of the endometrium may be induced with intramuscular injection of medroxyprogesterone acetate (Depo-Provera). A similar effect is observed with intrauterine devices (IUDs) impregnated with progesterone, but the effect is confined to the superficial endometrium. High-dose progestin therapy has been used in the medical treatment of endometrial hyperplasia in young women who wish to retain their fertility or in older women who are poor surgical candidates. Glands with abnormal shapes and crowding typical of hyperplasia may persist but the glandular cells show secretory changes, including the presence of vacuoles. Mitotic activity is decreased, and the stroma becomes decidualized. Typically, the initial findings are patchy with only some foci showing suppression of the hyperplastic process. Accordingly, patients treated in this manner must undergo repeated curettages, both to remove hyperplastic tissue and to monitor treatment response.

An unusual type of stromal atypia, referred to as pseudomalignant[69] or pseudosarcoma,[56] has been reported in women receiving high-dose progestational oral contraceptives (Fig. 10.29). Although this lesion is rarely seen now because of the use of low-dose oral contraceptives, the change may be seen in women being treated with progestational agents for endometrial hyperplasia because of the high doses that are used. Norplant is a long-acting, reversible contraceptive method that is introduced under the skin and releases small amounts of levonorgesterol at a relatively constant rate for as long as 5 years. The pregnancy rate during the first 3 years of use is comparable to tubal sterilization.[248] As with other progestins, the mechanism of action may be multifactorial: suppression of ovulation, increase in the viscosity of cervical mucus, and suppression of endometrial growth. The main endometrial change is gland atrophy and stromal decidualization.[55] As with other progestin-only contraceptives, pregnancies that do occur are often ectopic (20–30%) because progestins inhibit tubal motility.

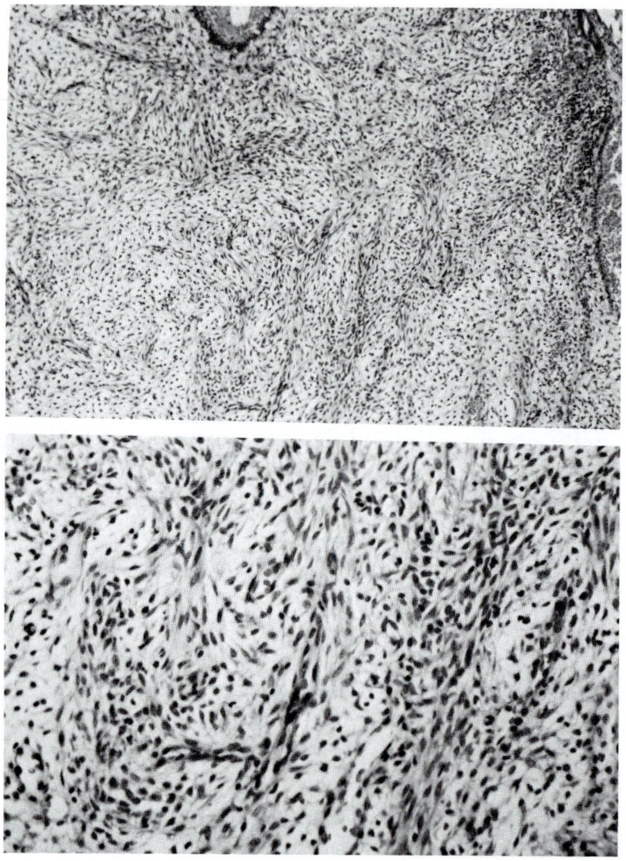

Fig. 10.29. High-dose progesterone effect showing a "pseudosarcomatous" change. *Top*: Low magnification shows a hypercellular spindle cell stroma. *Bottom*: High magnification shows minimal atypia and an absence of mitotic activity. The lesion mimics low-grade endometrial stromal sarcoma, but the stromal cells lack the intimate relationship to small blood vessels characteristic of low-grade stromal sarcoma.

Clomiphene Citrate

Clomiphene citrate is an orally active nonsteroidal compound that is structurally similar to diethylstilbestrol (DES) and binds to estrogen receptors. Clomiphene reduces the number of estrogen receptors in the hypothalamus by inhibiting the process of receptor replacement, thereby stimulating the hypothalamus to respond as if estrogen levels were low by secreting gonadotropin-releasing hormone, which leads to pituitary secretion of FSH and LH. When clomiphene is used to induce ovulation, the endometrium usually displays histologic changes reflecting a hypoestrogenic state, presumably related to competitive binding of clomiphene to estrogen receptors. Based on a review of 710 biopsies, Benda found that clomiphene induced specific alterations in secretory endometrium, including a reduction in the gland/stroma ratio and a decrease in size and tortuosity of the glands.[17] Secretory activity and stromal decidualization were diminished. Sereepapong et al. also reported a similar diminution in gland density and diameter.[243] Deligdisch reported a dyssynchrony in glandular–stromal maturation with the glands appearing consistent with a date about 7 days earlier in the menstrual cycle than the stroma.[64] Not all studies have shown consistent effects on secretory development.

Gonadotropin-Releasing Hormone Agonists

Gonadotropin-releasing hormone agonists (*GnRH*) are used mainly to suppress the endometrium before resectoscopic ablation or to decrease the size of leiomyomas before myomectomy. After GnRH treatment the endometrium becomes markedly atrophic.[27] GnRH is sometimes combined with progestins, which results in secretory changes.[150]

Human Menopausal Gonadotropin/ Human Chorionic Gonadotropin

Human menopausal gonadotropin (*hMG*) (Pergonal) and *chorionic gonadotropin* (*hCG*) have been used to treat infertile, anovulatory women with polycystic ovarian disease. The two hormones used together enhance the LH surge after initial treatment with clomiphene. The histologic effects on the endometrium are unclear. Some studies have reported retarded secretory maturation,[37,220] whereas others have described more highly developed secretory changes than expected for the chronologic date of the cycle.[89,244] There are no specific morphologic changes that can be correlated with the effects of these hormones.

Emergency Contraceptives and Abortifacients

Emergency contraceptives include high-dose estrogens, danazaol, levonorgesterel, IUD insertion, combined estrogen and progesterone (Yuzpe regimen), and mifepristone (RU-486).[109] Assessing the efficacy of emergency contraception is difficult because the percentage of pregnancies prevented by an intervention can only be approximated. Available data on the histopathologic changes induced by emergency contraceptive measures are limited. Although post-treatment endometrial samples are rarely submitted for pathologic diagnosis, it is important for pathologists to distinguish normal gestational changes and organic pathology from treatment effects. Currently, high-dose estrogen therapy and danazol are rarely used because of the unacceptable side effects for the former and contraceptive failures in the latter.

The Yuzpe regimen consists of two doses of combined pills, typically consisting of 100 μg ethinyl estradiol and 1 mg norgestrel, administered within a 12-hour interval.[315] It is estimated that this treatment prevents 74% of pregnancies, effectiveness declining as the postcoital interval lengthens. Nausea and vomiting are frequent compared to treatment with mifepristone, which is now approved for use in the United States. Proposed mechanisms of action for the Yupze regimen include inhibition of ovulation, disruption of endometrial maturation, producing an unfavorable environment for implantation, and alteration in the expression of hormone receptors or other molecules required for implantation. The effect of the Yuzpe regimen on endometrial histopathology has been assessed in several small investigations with slightly different study designs. Some investigators have reported little or no specific histologic change, whereas others have reported dyssynchronous maturation of glands and stroma.[155,217,273] In one study using a masked histopathologic review, glandular–stromal discordance for dates was not identified and the only significant difference between treated women and controls was an increase in supranuclear vacuoles in endometrial glands.[217] Other findings in this study included a reduction in MUC-1 expression (normally present in midsecretory endometrium), an increase in estrogen receptor expression, low luteal-phase serum estrogen, and reduced endometrial thickness.

Mifepristone is a synthetic steroid that produces a high-affinity progesterone receptor blockade. Mifepristone is approved for use as a single-dose *abortifacient*.[189] Mifepristone may also have utility as a contraceptive agent and, possibly, as a treatment for endometrial hyperplasia.[36] The ability of RU-486 to inhibit endometrial glandular proliferation is paradoxical, suggesting a dose-dependent antiestrogenic effect in addition to progesterone inhibition. Histologic alterations ascribed to RU-486 include inhibition of secretory activity, acceleration of degenerative changes in glandular epithelium, alteration of stromal blood vessels, and an increase in stromal mitoses.[36,152,265,272] Ultrastructural studies suggest that RU-486 inhibits the development of the nucleolar channel system and mitochondria, which are typical changes found in postovulatory endometrium.[70]

Prostaglandins

Endometrial production of *prostaglandins* increases through the secretory phase. Primary dysmenorrhea is thought to be caused by myometrial contractions induced by prostaglandins, which may account for the association between dysmenorrhea and ovulatory cycles. This mechanism could explain the beneficial effect of oral contraceptives on primary dysmenorrhea because oral contraceptives produce endometrial atrophy and thereby reduce prostaglandin levels. The morphologic effects of prostaglandins on the human endometrium have not been well described. In rats, prostaglandins appear to induce decidualization.[274–276]

Effects of Intrauterine Devices

The histologic effects of *IUDs* on the endometrium are device specific. Plastic devices induce a focal inflammatory response (Fig. 10.30) composed of polymorphonuclear leukocytes, lymphocytes, plasma cells, macrophages, and, rarely, foreign body giant cells.[183,184,200] A significant degree of chronic inflammation is observed in 25–40% of IUD users and may be related to the duration of use.[200] Other findings include squamous metaplasia and premature predecidualization, which may represent a reaction to injury.[200,307,308] The endometrium immediately beneath the device may show pressure atrophy and focal fibrosis, whereas surrounding regions are unaffected. Inflammatory reactions occur slightly less frequently with copper-containing devices. Leukocytes are commonly confined to the gland lumens, with exudation on the endometrial surface and sparing of the endometrial stroma. Progesterone-impregnated devices release hormones in a slow, continuous fashion, producing a sharply localized area of decidualization immediately adjacent to the device.[164] Copper-containing devices may induce endothelial degeneration, necrosis, and formation of defects between endothelial cells and basement membranes. This effect, together with the increase in vessel density, may account for the increased bleeding associated with IUD use.[110,245]

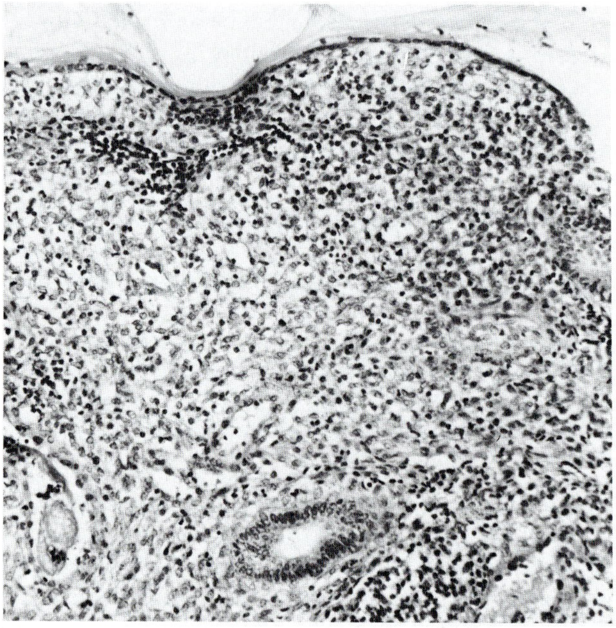

Fig. 10.30. Intrauterine device effect. Endometrium in the vicinity of an intrauterine device shows chronic inflammation.

Mechanism of Action

Three possible mechanisms proposed to explain the contraceptive effects of IUD include (1) inhibition of sperm transport from the cervix to the tube, (2) inhibition of sperm capacitation, and (3) interference with implantation.[6] Only the last hypothesis is plausibly explained by IUD-induced changes in the endometrium. For the plastic devices, the inflammatory reaction, in conjunction with an asynchronous premature decidual reaction, results in an unfavorable local environment for implantation of the blastocyst. Release of copper ions from impregnated devices may inhibit normal metabolism in endometrial cells.[205] Decidualization associated with progesterone-releasing devices may hinder implantation and render cervical mucus impermeable to sperm.

Complications

The IUD, unlike barrier methods, does not protect against sexually transmitted diseases. There is an increased risk of pelvic infection shortly after IUD insertion, probably related to the introduction of bacteria, but these organisms are cleared within 24 hours and endometrial cultures obtained 30 days after insertion are sterile.[174] IUD users may develop upper genital tract infections after this period related to sexually transmitted diseases, but these infections appear unrelated to the IUD per se[134,149] because the risk of infertility among IUD users who are monogamous is not elevated.[53] Pregnancy rates after IUD removal resemble those associated with discontinued use of other contraceptive devices.[221,235]

IUD use of any duration predisposes patients to colonization or infection with *Actinomyces*, a gram-positive anaerobic bacteria.[100] Actinomycotic infections are characterized by typical sulfur granules, composed of a dense central basophilic mass of tangled hyphae surrounded by peripheral radiating filaments (Figs. 10.31 and 10.32). The organism can be demonstrated in Papanicolaou-stained cervical vaginal smears[21] and IUD scrapings obtained after removal of the device. *Actinomyces* must be distinguished from the Splendore–Hoeppli phenomenon, a nonspecific tissue reaction, in which debris, fibrin, immunoglobulin, and complement form eosinophilic masses that may closely resemble the branching structures of *Actinomyces* but lack true filamentous bacilli.[186]

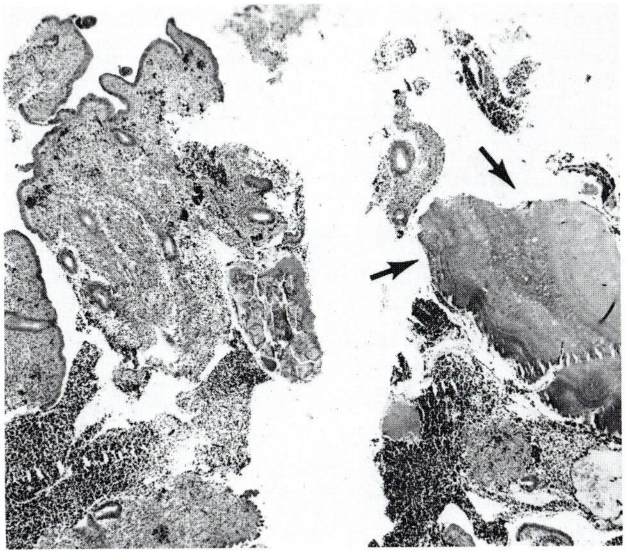

Fig. 10.31. *Actinomyces* in a patient with an intrauterine device. Sulfur granules (*arrows*) can be identified under low magnification in endometrial curettings infected with *Actinomyces.*

Actinomyces is not normally found in the cervix and vagina but is part of the normal flora of the oral cavity and gastrointestinal tract. It is likely that the organism is introduced into the lower genital tract during coitus. *Actinomyces* does not ordinarily invade mucosal surfaces, but the IUD acts as a foreign body and the associated tissue injury associated with its placement may create an anaerobic microenvironment that permits colonization by *Actinomyces* and other anaerobic organisms. Tubo-ovarian abscesses occurring in this setting tend to be unilateral.[191] However, bilateral tubo-ovarian abscesses, especially when associated with bowel or bladder involvement, may mimic ovarian carcinoma. Leukocytosis, long-term IUD use, and normal CA-125 levels provide clues to the diagnosis, and frozen section interpretation at the time of surgery may avert unnecessary procedures.[186] A serious but rare complication of the IUD is uterine perforation, with secondary involvement of the omentum and possible bowel obstruction. Copper devices produce a greater peritoneal reaction than plastic IUDs and are more often implicated in bowel obstruction. In one study, all seven copper devices that perforated into the abdominal cavity required laparotomy for removal, whereas other devices were removed laparoscopically.[203] Finally, there is a 2–3% risk among IUD users that a pregnancy will be ectopic.[274]

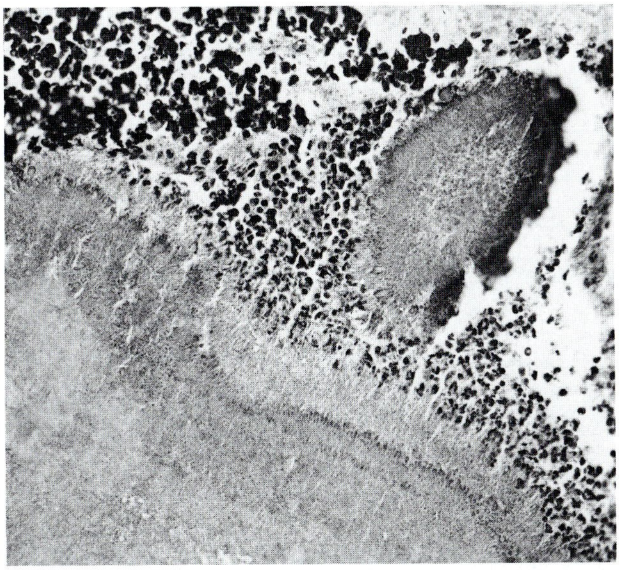

Fig. 10.32. *Actinomyces* in a patient with an intrauterine device. Sulfur granules are composed of a dense central basophilic mass of tangled hyphae surrounded by peripheral radiating filaments.

Effects of Curettage

Curettage evokes transient inflammatory and regenerative changes in the endometrium.[122] Three days after curettage, the endometrial surface consists of flattened attenuated cells. The basalis contains a serosanguinous exudate containing PMNs that clears completely in 7–9 days. In one large study, more than 83% of women had normally timed menses after a curretage, whereas in 10% it was delayed and in 7% it was early.[125,127] Eosinophilic endomyometritis following curettage has also been reported.[23,68,173] In the endometrium, the inflammatory cells form dense aggregates containing a mixed population of inflammatory cells, especially lymphocytes, whereas in the myometrium, the inflammatory infiltrate percolates through the connective tissue between muscle bundles and perivascular tissue.[68] The eosinophilic component of the infiltrate may be recruited by chemotactic factors released from mast cells in the myometrium in response to injury.[173]

Asherman syndrome is a specific posttraumatic condition associated with hypomenorrhea or amenorrhea and infertility following endometrial injury.[11,38,117,121] Inciting events include postpartum or postabortal curettage, particularly if infection is present, and more rarely, tuberculous endometritis or myomectomy. The diagnosis of Asherman syndrome is made by identifying bands of fibrous tissue or smooth muscle traversing or rarely, obliterating the endometrial cavity. Curettings obtained

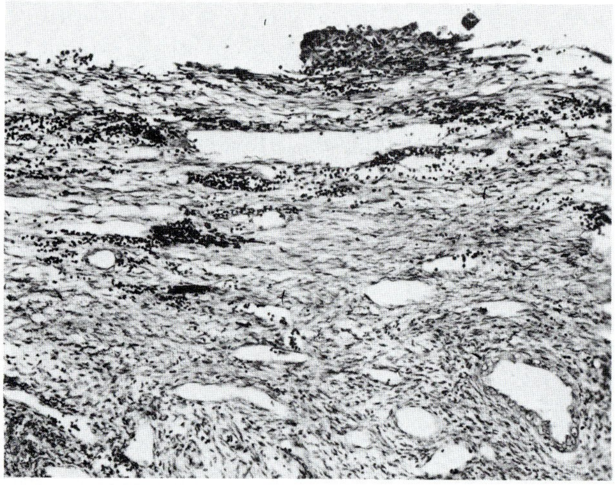

Fig. 10.33. Asherman syndrome. The endometrium is characterized by atrophy and fibrosis.

from women with Asherman syndrome usually are scant (Fig. 10.33).[79] Physiologic alterations may be severe in cases in which mild if any alterations are recognized clinically.[286] It has been postulated that the intrauterine adhesions reflect a more widespread process in which the endomyometrium is replaced by fibrous tissue.[311] Treatment of Asherman syndrome consists of curettage to break the synechiae, placement of an IUD to separate the endometrial surfaces, and cyclic estrogen-medroxyprogesterone treatment to induce endometrial proliferation.[38] This form of treatment is curative in most patients, but occasionally intrauterine adhesions recur.[286]

Effects of Laser Surgery

Endometrial ablation using the Nd:YAG laser and resection using a modified rectoscope have proven effectiveness in treating dysfunctional uterine bleeding uncontrolled by hormonal treatment.[201] Histologic descriptions of laser effects are limited and may reflect a biased subset removed for intractable bleeding.[94,218] Reepithelization of the endometrium seems to require about 3–5 months and is associated with only mild acute or chronic inflammation and foreign body giant cells surrounding carbon particles. Glandular regeneration and replacement of the endometrium by a simple cuboidal epithelium overlying a fibrous stroma or directly applied to the myometrium may be seen in the same uterus. The appearance is similar to that of Asherman's syndrome (see foregoing). Pathologic specimens obtained within 3 months of electrosurgical ablation may show necrotic myometrium, spicules of damaged muscle, florid giant cell reactions, and varying degrees of acute inflammation. After 3 months, specimens show endometrial fibrosis and a persistent giant cell reaction that may be confused with other forms of granulomatous endometritis.[50] Biopsy before treatment may be indicated to exclude the presence of hyperplasia or carcinoma.

Effects of Radiation

The morphologic changes induced by *radiation* are presented in Chapter 12, Endometrial Carcinoma, and elsewhere.[142] Briefly, cells are often enlarged, assume unusual shapes and display vacuolated cytoplasm. Nuclear changes include enlargement, pleomorphism, and hyperchromasia with poorly preserved chromatin (Fig. 10.34).

Benign Tumors

Endometrial Polyps

Endometrial polyps are benign, localized overgrowths of endometrial glands and stroma that are covered by epithelium and project above the adjacent surface epithelium. Polyps may arise from hyperplasia in the basalis because focal glandular proliferations and thick-walled feeder vessels are often identified at the base of these lesions.

Clinical Features

The prevalence of polyps in the general population is about 24%. Polyps are common in women over 40

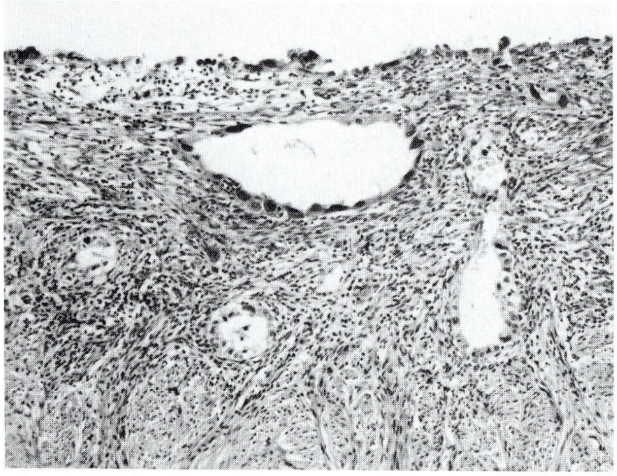

Fig. 10.34. Radiation effect. The glands and the surface endometrium are lined by cells showing nuclear atypia.

years of age and extremely rare before menarche. The most common presentations are intermenstrual bleeding or menometrorrhagia in younger women and postmenopausal bleeding in older patients. Polyps may also present as a cause of infertility.[81,290] A polyp should always be considered if abnormal bleeding persists after curettage because polyps that contain a delicate, pliable stalk may elude the curette.

Pathologic Findings

Polyps may be broad based and sessile, pedunculated, or attached to the endometrium by a slender stalk. Polyps vary in size from 1.0 mm to large masses filling and expanding the endometrial cavity (Fig. 10.35). Large pedunculated polyps may extend into the endocervical canal and project through the cervical os, producing as a visible mass on physical examination. Usually polyps have a tan, glistening surface, but irritated or infarcted polyps may appear hemorrhagic. About 20% of uteri contain multiple polyps. Polyps may originate anywhere in the uterine cavity, including the lower uterine segment, but most occur in the fundus, commonly in the cornal region. Upper endocervical polyps and mixed endometrial–endocervical polyps contain glandular epithelium from both components.

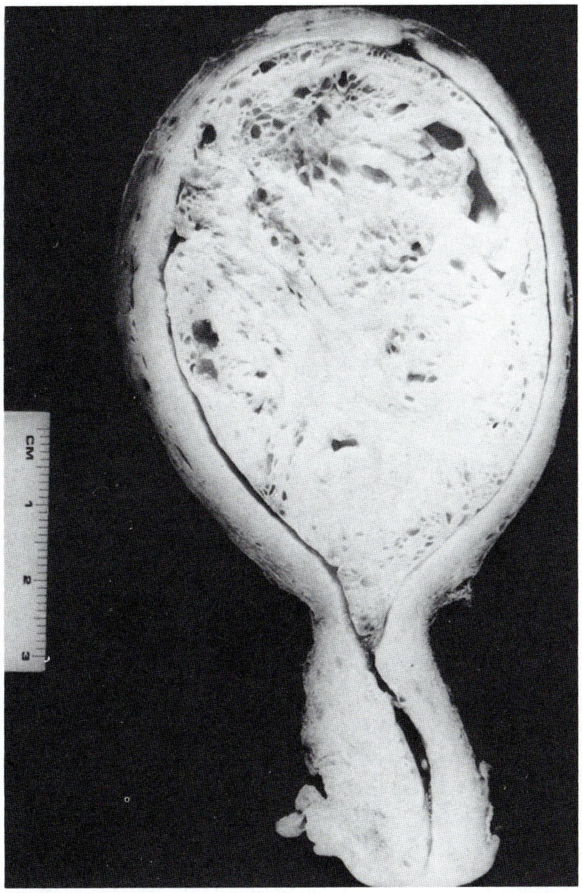

Fig. 10.35. Large endometrial polyp. The polyp entirely fills and distends the endometrial cavity.

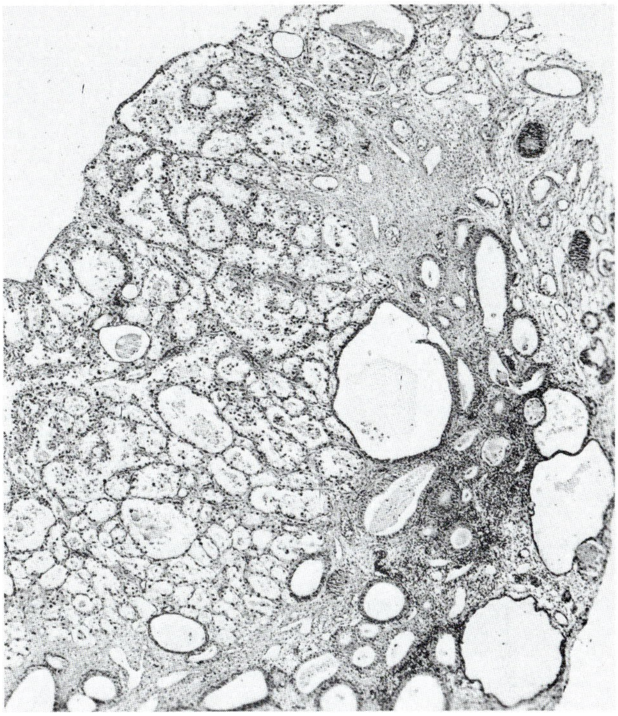

Fig. 10.36. Clear cell carcinoma in the tip of an endometrial polyp. The tumor shows a tubulocystic pattern and is confined to an endometrial polyp. (Reprinted by permission of Kurman and Scully, ref. 144.)

Glands in polyps often fail to cycle normally; secretory changes may be weak or absent in contrast to the surrounding endometrium or the glands may appear dilated and inactive. Squamous metaplasia may be present. The mesenchymal component of polyps may consist of endometrial stroma, fibrous tissue, or smooth muscle, but generally the stroma appears more fibrous than normal fundic endometrium. Decidualization is uncommon in women not receiving exogenous hormones.[103] Polyps containing a significant amount of smooth muscle are referred to as adenomyomatous. Hyperplasia, carcinoma (any type) (Fig. 10.36), and carcinosarcoma may involve or be entirely confined to a polyp.[15,67,129,144,246,249,253,298] Although the base of a polyp usually contains thick-walled vessels, abundant dilated vessels may be present, simulating a hemangioma.

Polyps are morphologically diverse lesions that are difficult to subclassify; however, most can be categorized as hyperplastic, atrophic, or functional.

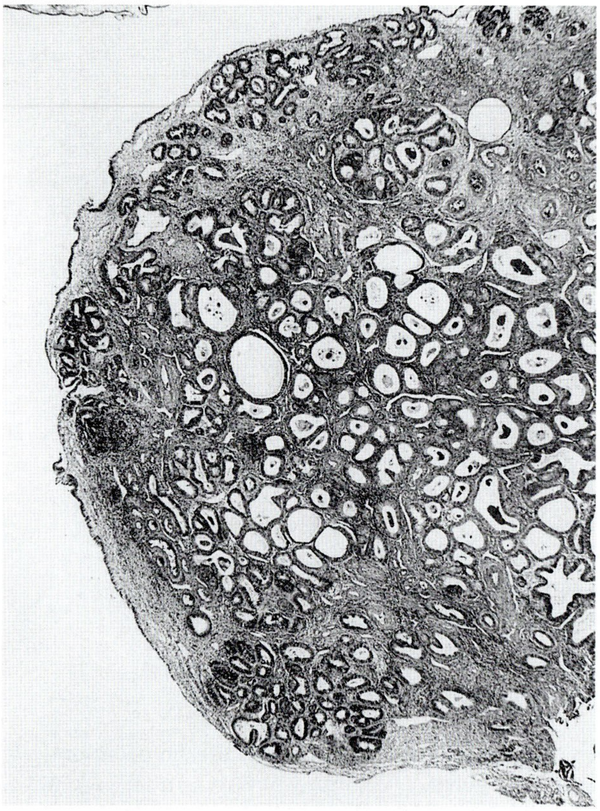

Fig. 10.37. Hyperplastic polyp. The polyp is broad based and composed of irregularly shaped, crowded, hyperplastic glands.

Hyperplastic polyps contain proliferating, irregularly shaped glands resembling diffuse, nonpolypoid endometrial hyperplasia (Figs. 10.37 and 10.38). These polyps, like diffuse endometrial hyperplasia, are probably etiologically related to hormone imbalances. There is no evidence that these have the same significance as diffuse hyperplasia, however, so it is generally best to avoid the subcategorization, i.e., hyperplastic, in the diagnosis. Atrophic polyps consist of low columnar or cuboidal cells lining cystically dilated glands. These polyps are typically found in postmenopausal patients and may represent regression of hyperplastic or functional polyps. Functional polyps containing glands resembling normally cycling endometrium are relatively uncommon (Fig. 10.39).

Polyps may be difficult to recognize in curettage specimens.[166,316] Ideally, they appear as polypoid-shaped fragments of tissue, with epithelium on three sides. However, these criteria may be difficult to appreciate if lesions are fragmented or partially removed. In addition, normal endometrium has an irregular surface that may appear as a polypoid fragment with epithelium on three sides when sectioned tangentially; therefore, identification of fingerlike tissue fragments alone is insufficient for diagnosis. Identification of tissue fragments containing irregular glands, dense or fibrous stroma (Fig. 10.40), or thick-walled vessels that contrast with the appearance of the surrounding endometrium suggest a polyp. However, these criteria should be appreciated in tissue fragments lined with attached surface epithelium because normal basalis can show some of these features. Molecular studies have demonstrated that polyps are clonal and may contain abnormalities on chromosome 6.[58,59,261]

Differential Diagnosis

The differential diagnosis of polyps includes hyperplasias, polypoid adenocarcinomas, adenofibromas, and adenosarcomas. Florid hyperplasias may mimic polyps because they can assume a polypoid configuration; however, these are diffuse abnormalities that should involve most or all fragments in a specimen, whereas true polyp fragments generally com-

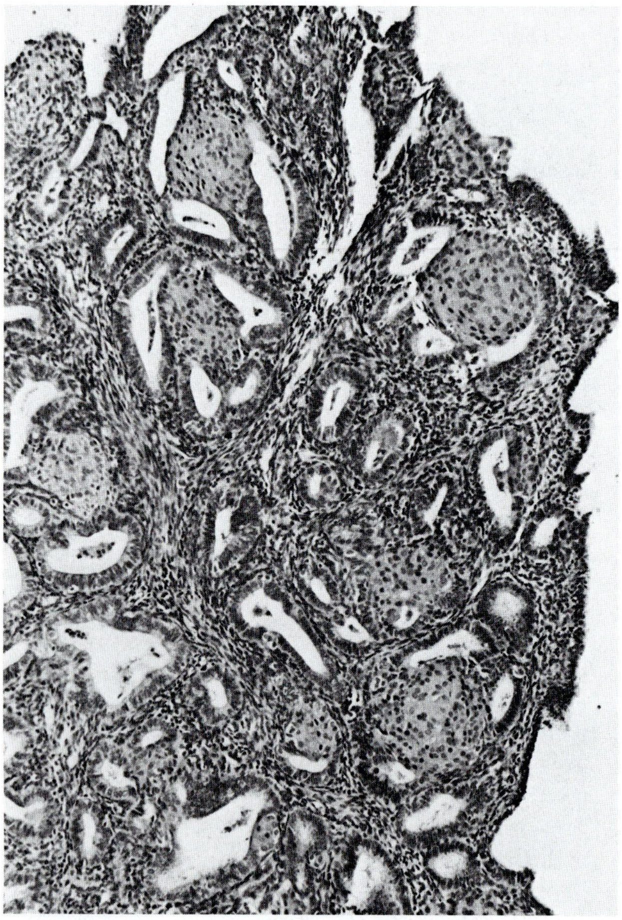

Fig. 10.38. Hyperplastic polyp. This polyp contains crowded irregular glands, some of which show squamous change.

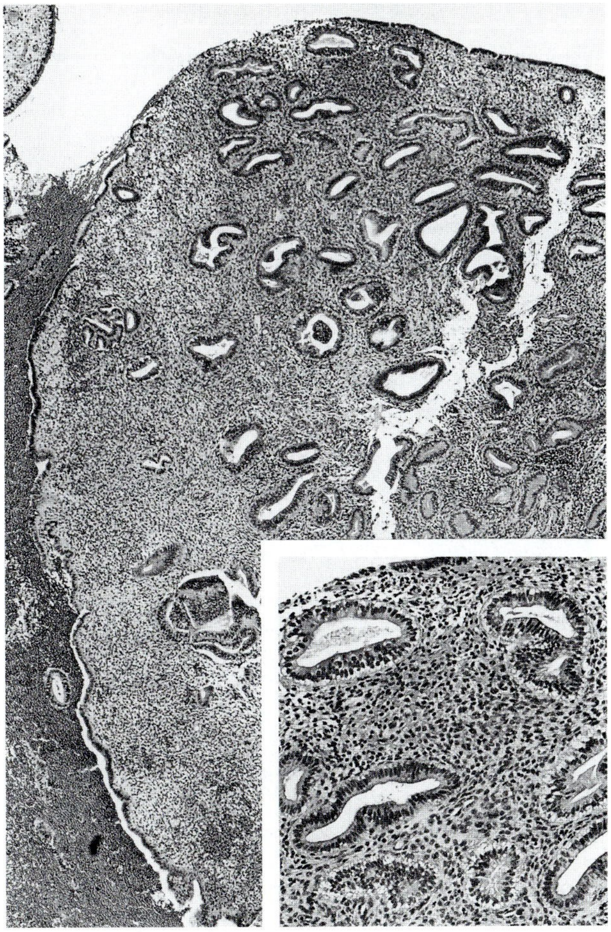

Fig. 10.39. Functional polyp. This polyp contains secretory glands surrounded by dense stroma. *Inset*: Secretory glands with subnuclear vacuoles.

prise only a portion of such tissue. Adenocarcinomas with polypoid growth will retain diagnostic features of malignancy. Adenosarcoma is distinguished from a benign polyp because the stromal cells demonstrate increased mitotic activity, cytologic atypia, and a tendency to encircle glands. Preserved fragments of adenosarcoma may display a characteristic leaflike pattern at low magnification that would not be found in a typical benign polyp (see Chapter 13, Mesenchymal Tumors of the Uterus).

Clinical Behavior and Treatment

At most, 5% of polyps contain carcinoma; however, 12%–34% of uteri containing endometrial carcinoma also contain a polyp.[210,234] A long-term prospective study of patients with endometrial polyps found that endometrial carcinoma ultimately developed in 3.5% of the patients, but nearly one-half the women who developed carcinoma had been treated with intracavitary radium.[10] Polyps may represent a marker of increased cancer risk because they reflect a tendency for the endometrium to develop proliferative lesions. However, there is no evidence to suggest that polyps themselves have a significantly greater propensity for developing carcinoma than adjacent endometrium. In general, polyps containing atypical hyperplasia or carcinoma should be treated similarly to comparable flat lesions. Polyps containing lesser degrees of hyperplasia are often treated by polypectomy and curettage. In young women with atypical hyperplasia or carcinoma confined to a polyp, polypectomy can be considered as a treatment to preserve fertility, provided that the entire endometrial cavity has been vigorously curetted (hysteroscopically confirmed) and the nonpolypoid endometrium appears normal. Endometrial intraepithelial carcinoma (EIC), the presumed precursor of serous carcinoma, may be identified as a malignant surface change in atrophic polyps removed from elderly women.[246,298] Staging should be

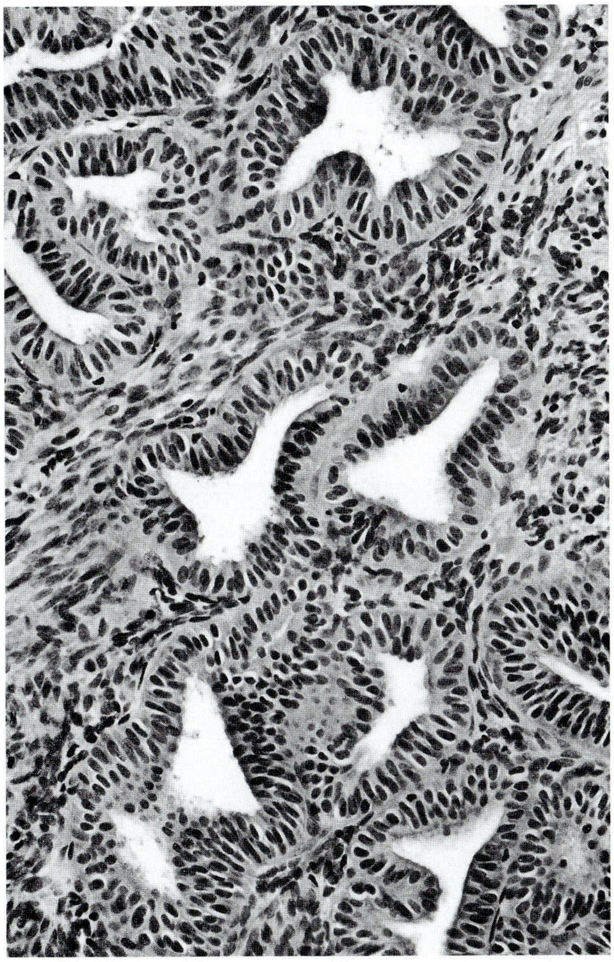

Fig. 10.40. Endometrial polyp. The stroma of a polyp typically is fibrotic.

considered for all women with EIC or small amounts of serous carcinoma in the uterus ("minimal uterine serous carcinoma") because some of these patients have disseminated disease.[298]

Atypical Polypoid Adenomyoma

Atypical polypoid adenomyomas (*APA*) are typically detected during the reproductive and perimenopausal period. In a series of 55 cases, Longacre et al. reported that 96% of patients were premenopausal with a median age of 39 years.[157] Among patients with complete histories, 28 were nulliparous, 15 had a history of infertility, and 13 were obese, suggesting that these lesions may share risk factors with type I endometrial carcinomas. The lesion has also been reported in patients with Turner's syndrome who have been on estrogen replacement therapy.[46] APAs, like other polyps, usually present with abnormal uterine bleeding.

The APA grossly resembles a typical endometrial polyp (Fig. 10.41) and often involves the lower uterine segment. Microscopically, the APA is composed of irregularly shaped hyperplastic glands arranged haphazardly within stroma containing abundant smooth muscle[165] (Fig. 10.42). Extensive morular squamous metaplasia, sometimes showing central necrosis, may exaggerate the appearance of glandular crowding and raise concerns regarding the possibility of carcinoma. The glandular cells display nuclear atypia, loss of polarity, and cytoplasmic eosinophilia (Fig. 10.43). The smooth muscle is arranged in short interlacing fascicles, rather than elongated muscle bundles typical of normal myometrium. The lesion may be difficult to identify in curettings and must be distinguished from hyperplasia, infiltrating carcinoma, or a malignant mixed mesodermal tumor. The focal nature of APA and the intimate admixture of smooth muscle and glands distinguish this lesion from atypical hyperplasia (see Chapter 11). In contrast to adenocarcinoma, desmoplastic reactive stroma resembling chronically inflamed granulation tissue is not found (see Chapter 12).

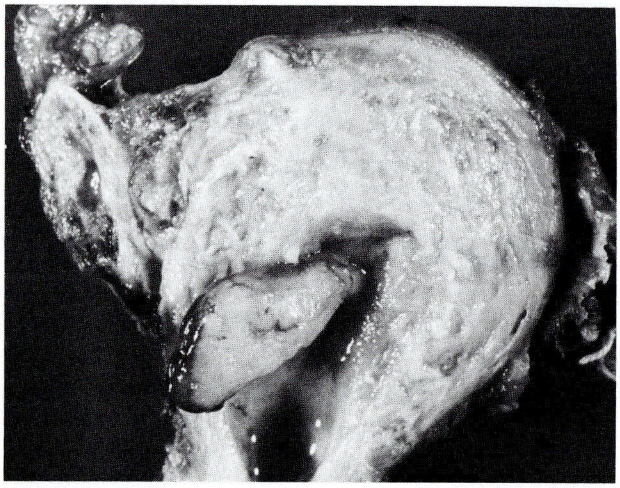

Fig. 10.41. Atypical polypoid adenomyoma. The lesion is a discrete pedunculated polypoid mass within the uterine cavity.

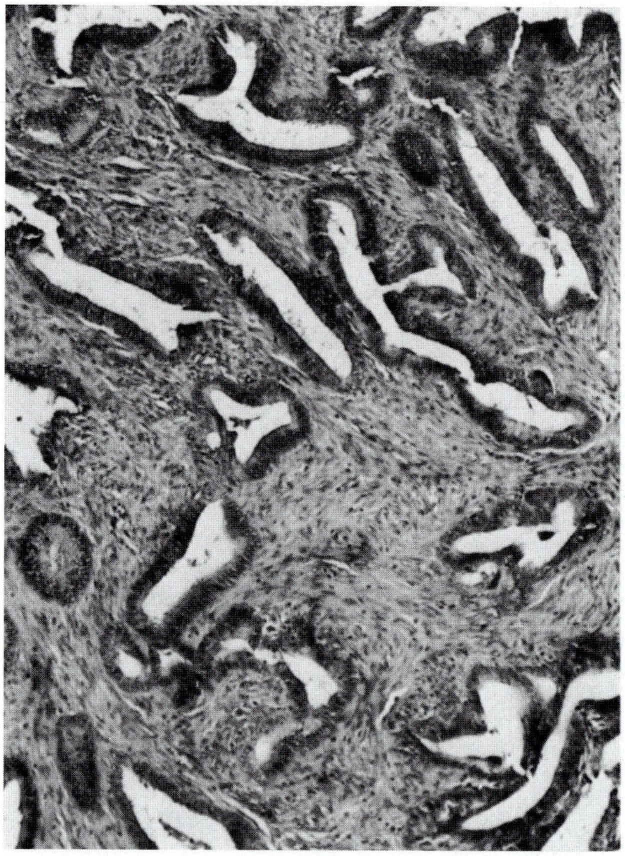

Fig. 10.42. Atypical polypoid adenomyoma. Large and atypical glands are surrounded by smooth muscle. (Reprinted by permission of Mazur, ref. 165.)

Compared to most APAs, carcinomas generally show greater cytologic atypia and more glandular crowding and architectural complexity. Because myometrial invasion is rarely demonstrable in curettings of carcinoma, the diagnosis of APA should be strongly considered whenever atypical glands surrounded by obvious bundles of smooth muscle on routine stains are identified. However, studies demonstrate that the stroma in these lesions contains a mixture of smooth muscle cells, fibrous tissue, and endometrial stroma, which has prompted some authors to propose the alternative term *atypical polypoid adenomyofibroma* to emphasize the stromal heterogeneity.[157,258] Furthermore, immunohistochemical studies have demonstrated that the stroma in APA and adenocarcinoma may show sim-

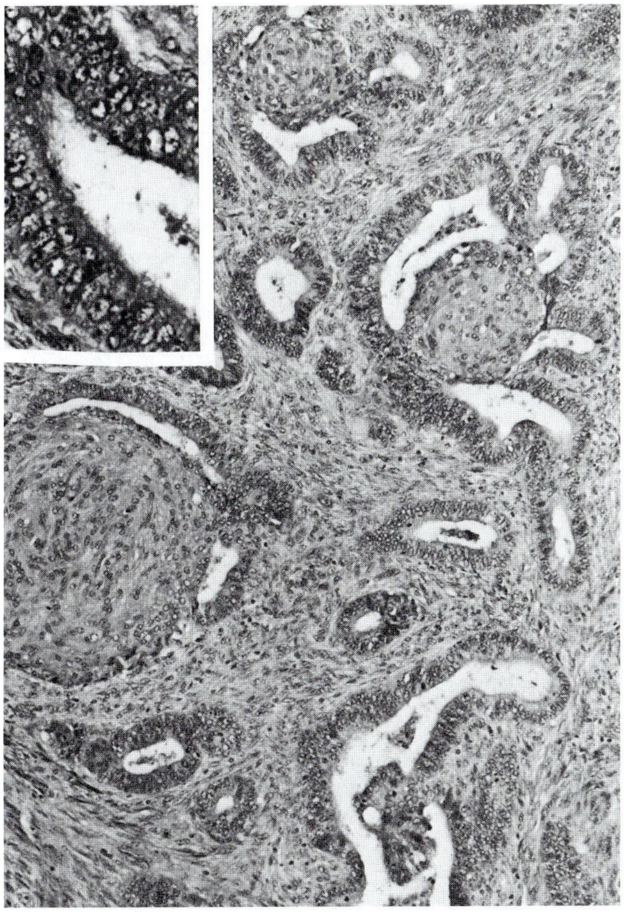

Fig. 10.43. Atypical polypoid adenomyoma. The lesion contains irregular glands with foci of squamous differentiation. Smooth muscle surrounds the glands. *Inset*: Cytologic atypia is characterized by enlarged nuclei with prominent nucleoli.

ilar markers including smooth muscle actin, desmin, and CD 34, underscoring the possible limited utility of these stains in differential diagnosis. Squamous cells with mild atypia can be found in both adenocarcinomas and APA (Fig. 10.43); therefore, this feature is not helpful in separating these entities. Another related differential diagnosis is uterine adenomyoma, a lesion composed of glands and stroma consisting predominantly of smooth muscle with a minor component of endometrial stroma. The glands usually resemble proliferative endometrium but may show focal dilatation, mucinous, tubal or squamous differentiation. Because the endometrial stroma tends to encircle the glands, these lesions may be confused with adenosarcoma. However, atypia and mitoses are generally not identified in these stromal cells. The smooth muscle component may be cellular or demonstrate occasional mitoses.[91]

In rare instances, it may not be possible to distinguish an APA from a well-differentiated carcinoma, and a hysterectomy will be necessary. Based on data suggesting that APAs with marked architectural complexity have an increased tendency to recur following conservative treatment and may be associated with invasive carcinoma, Longacre has proposed designating these lesions as *low malignant potential*. Although the smooth muscle in APA may show some mitotic activity (generally less than two mitoses per 10 high-power fields), the cytologic atypia and more frequent mitoses found in malignant smooth muscle are not seen (Chapter 13, Mesenchymal Tumors of the Uterus).[157] APA is a benign lesion that can be cured by curettage, permitting premenopausal women to preserve their fertility and become pregnant.[165,314] However, Longacre reported that 45% of lesions treated conservatively recurred clinically, although none progressed to a fatal invasive carcinoma. APAs associated with adenocarcinoma have been rarely reported, and criteria used for the diagnosis of carcinoma presented here should be applied, recognizing that the majority of errors in this area result from overdiagnosis.[175,266,270]

Teratoma

Primary benign teratomas of the uterus are extremely rare,[146,163,278] and immature teratomas are even more unusual.[103] Teratomas must be distinguished from more common entities such as metaplasia and implantation of fetal tissues. Therefore, sufficient sampling to exclude the presence of a remnant embryo or placental and decidual tissue is required. Most cases reported in the older literature are of dubious authenticity. Nicholson concluded in 1956 that only four cases were acceptable, and since then rare additional cases have been reported.[192] Microscopically, uterine teratomas resemble those found in the ovary. Typically, these neoplasms contain squamous and respiratory-type epithelium, adipose tissue, and sebaceous glands.[163]

Brenner Tumor

An example of a *Brenner tumor* that appeared to arise from metaplasia of the uterine serosa and involved the subjacent myometrium has been described.[9] Brenner tumors have also been identified in paracervical tissue.

Papillary Serous Tumor

Small *papillary tumors* lined by tubal-type epithelium resembling ovarian serous surface tumors may occur in the endometrium (Fig. 10.44). The rare cases that we have seen behaved in a benign fashion.

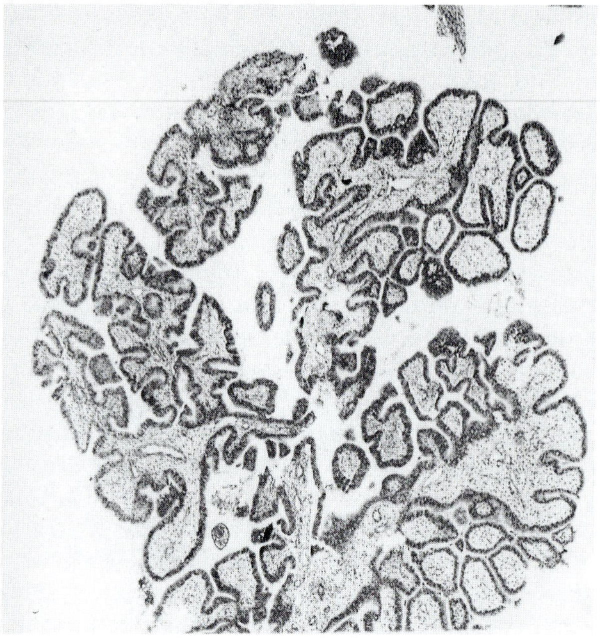

Fig. 10.44. Benign serous tumor. The lesion is composed of papillary fronds lined by bland-appearing tubal-type epithelium. The lesion resembles a serous surface tumor of the ovary.

Miscellaneous Lesions

Inflammatory Pseudotumor

Inflammatory pseudotumor, also referred to as *plasma cell granuloma* or *inflammatory myofibroblastic tumor*, are uncommon lesions that are generally viewed as non-neoplastic proliferations that may simulate neoplasms in many different organs. Uterine lesions are particularly uncommon.[92] These lesions may contain bland spindle cells representing fibroblasts or myofibroblasts, resulting in a leiomyoma-like appearance. Studied examples have demonstrated immunoreactivity for actin and vimentin and ultrastructural features of myofibroblasts. Mitotic figures are rare. A marked inflammatory infiltrate composed mainly of plasma cells with large numbers of PMNs and small and large lymphocytes is usually present. Eosinophils and mast cells may also be present. Two reported patients with uterine lesions were alive and well after 4 years of follow-up.[92]

Postoperative Spindle-Cell Nodule

Postoperative spindle-cell nodules are composed of dense proliferations of spindle cells, small blood vessels, and inflammatory cells, representing an exuberant reparative response at a site of injury. The high level of mitotic activity may raise the differential diagnosis of sarcoma, but cytologic atypia is lacking. This lesion is more common in the vagina (see Chapter 4, Diseases of the Vagina) but has been described in the endometrium[46] (see Chapter 13, Mesenchymal Tumors of the Uterus).

Lymphoma-Like Lesion

A *lymphoma-like lesion* characterized by aggregates of large lymphoid cells with only rare plasma cells and PMNs has been described in the cervix (see Chapter 6, Benign Diseases of the Cervix).[313] The aggregates of lymphoid cells resemble reactive germinal centers but lack a peripheral layer of mature lymphocytes. The large lymphoid cells include cleaved and noncleaved follicular center cells and immunoblasts. A mixed inflammatory infiltrate is present at the periphery of the aggregates. Typically, the lesions arise on a background of chronic endometritis. The polymorphism of the infiltrate with associated germinal centers, the background of chronic endometritis, and the absence of a gross mass assist in the distinction of this lesion from a true malignant lymphoma (see Chapter 13, Mesenchymal Tumors of the Uterus).

Massive Lymphocytic Infiltration in Leiomyomas

Massive lymphocytic infiltration in leiomyomas has been reported.[76] In addition to a moderate to dense infiltration of small lymphocytes, plasma cells, rare eosinophils, and occasional germinal centers are present. The inflammatory process does not involve the endometrium and adjacent myometrium. The underlying cause of this condition is unknown, and the patients reported were apparently disease free after 12 years of follow-up. The gross and microscopic findings of this lesion distinguish it from lymphoma. In contrast to a lymphoma, which is soft, fleshy, and poorly circumscribed, a leiomyoma with a dense lymphocytic infiltrate has the gross appearance of a typical leiomyoma, being firm and well circumscribed. Microscopically, the leiomyoma is associated with an infiltrate containing small lymphocytes, plasma cells, and occasionally eosinophils, whereas uterine lymphomas are typically composed of large monomorphous atypical cells.

Langerhans' Cell Histiocytosis

Langerhans' cell histiocytosis can either involve the female genital tract as part of a systemic disease or be limited to the genital tract. The endometrium is rarely involved; the vulva is the most common site of genital tract involvement.[12] The lesion is characterized by clusters and sheets of Langerhans' cells with grooved and folded vesicular nuclei. There is no correlation between the clinical presentation, extent of involvement, histologic appearance, and outcome of the genital lesions, which may undergo complete regression, persistence, or recurrence.

Intravascular Menstrual Endometrium

Occasionally, menstrual detritus consisting of clusters of epithelial and/or spindle cells can be identified in uterine and parametrial blood vessels. The benign appearance of the cells distinguishes this finding from intravascular tumor.[13]

Giant Cell Arteritis

Giant cell arteritis typically is a localized process with clinical consequences reflecting the site of organ involvement. The uterus was involved in 12 of 17 cases involving the female genital tract in one report.[162] Systemic disease was identified in 11 of these patients, and 6 did not have systemic symptoms. Uterine lesions are most common in postmenopausal women and are asymptomatic. Microscopically, large numbers of vessels show narrowing and complete obliteration of the lumens by a marked inflammatory infiltrate. The inflammatory infiltrate is sharply localized to the blood vessels and consists of epithelioid histiocytes, lymphocytes, eosinophils, occasional neutrophils, and giant cells (Fig. 10.45). Fibrinoid necrosis is not identified. Asymptomatic patients with no laboratory abnormalities may not require treatment, but steroids may help symptomatic patients.[156] In contrast to giant cell arteritis, acute necrotizing arteritis in the female genital tract is characterized by fibrinoid necrosis, a more acute inflammatory infiltrate, and an absence of giant cells. Isolated necrotizing arteritis is usually an incidental finding characterized by small- and medium-sized arteries demonstrating fibrinoid necrosis associated with mononuclear infiltrates and rare PMNs. Immune complexes are demonstrable using immunohistochemistry in many cases. The lesion is most common in the cervix but can occur anywhere in the genital tract. Possible etiologies of the lesion include a drug reaction, a response to a foreign body, and an immune reaction to vessels following injury. Patients may present with menorrhagia or postmenopausal bleeding. A systemic vasculitis should be excluded clinically.[82]

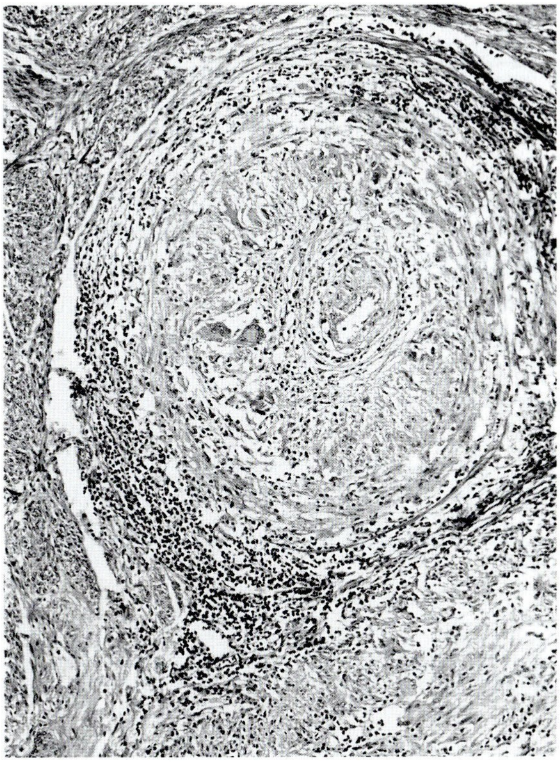

Fig. 10.45. Giant cell arteritis. Marked chronic inflammatory infiltrate consisting mainly of lymphocytes with scattered giant cells involving an artery.

Arteriovenous Malformations

Uterine arteriovenous malformations are vascular fistulas composed of an admixture of arterial, venous, and capillary-like channels involving the myometrium and sometimes the endometrium. These lesions may be either congenital or acquired.[78] Although most are considered to represent hamartomas, many patients have had a prior curettage, suggesting a possible etiologic relationship to this procedure. These lesions usually present in adults with heavy vaginal bleeding. Curettage does not successfully control the hemorrhage and may in fact result in exacerbation of the bleeding. Clinical examination is generally unrevealing, but pelvic angiography or ultrasonography can facilitate the diagnosis. Microscopically, the lesions may be circumscribed or diffuse in the myometrium with or without endometrial involvement. Arteriovenous malformations are composed of a varying proportion of thick- and thin-walled vessels. The thick-walled muscular vessels often show fibrous intimal thickening and represent both arteries and veins. Lesions may erode into the endometrium, producing an obvious source of bleeding, but in some cases with minor bleeding the malformation is entirely intramural. Hysterectomy usually is necessary to control bleeding, although some cases have been managed successfully by intra-arterial embolization.[213]

Heterologous Tissues

Heterologous tissues including bone,[52,88,90,115,190] cartilage,[1,90,190,227] smooth muscle,[22] and glial tissue[190,193,223,318] have been reported in the endometrium. Two theories advanced to account for the presence of these tissues include metaplastic transformation of the endometrial stromal cell and implantation of fetal tissue after abortion and instrumentation, with the fetal tissue persisting and growing as a homograft. Before classifying heterologous tissue as benign, the pathologist should exclude the possibility that the tissue in question is not a deceptively bland-appearing component of a malignant mixed mesodermal tumor or an adenosarcoma. Heterotopic bone in the endometrium is characteristically found in women with a history of repeated abortions and endometritis.[52,88,115,190] In rare instances, the bone may represent metaplasia of the endometrial stroma, triggered by inflammation. In most cases, the association with prior pregnancy, the immaturity of the heterologous element, and the rarity of osseous metaplasia in other types of endometritis indicate that it represents implantation from fetal parts.

Heterotopic cartilage in the endometrium (Fig. 10.46) frequently is associated with a history of prior abortion and is, therefore, caused by implantation of fetal tissue.[190] A few patients have no history of pregnancy and, furthermore, in the series reported by Roth and Taylor[227] one of the patients was 52 years old. Microscopically, the cartilage was mature, and a transition from endometrial stromal cells to chondrocytes was found in some, suggesting a metaplastic process. Smooth muscle is only considered heterologous when it is localized in the endometrium. Benign heterologous smooth muscle may form fascicles or nodules within the endometrium and sometimes appears continuous with the underlying myometrium. This tissue may develop from endometrial stromal cells that have undergone metaplasia, as the two have a common anlage.[22]

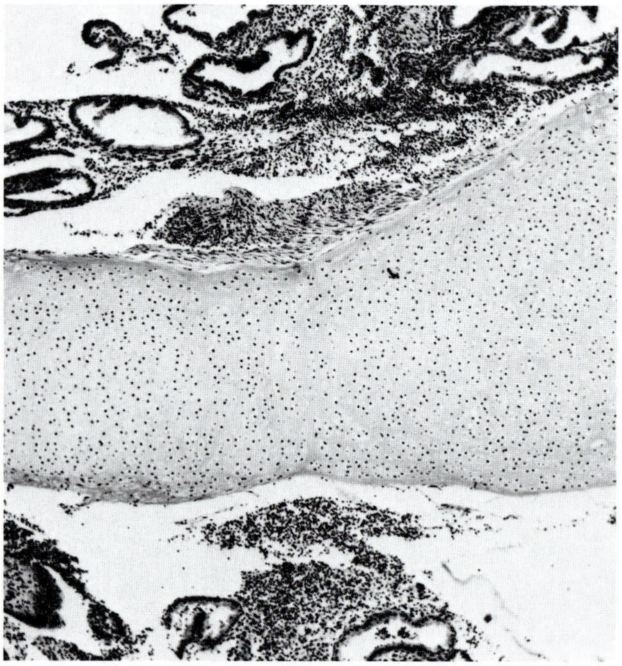

Fig. 10.46. Heterotopic cartilage. A well-circumscribed fragment of cartilage is surrounded by otherwise normal-appearing endometrium.

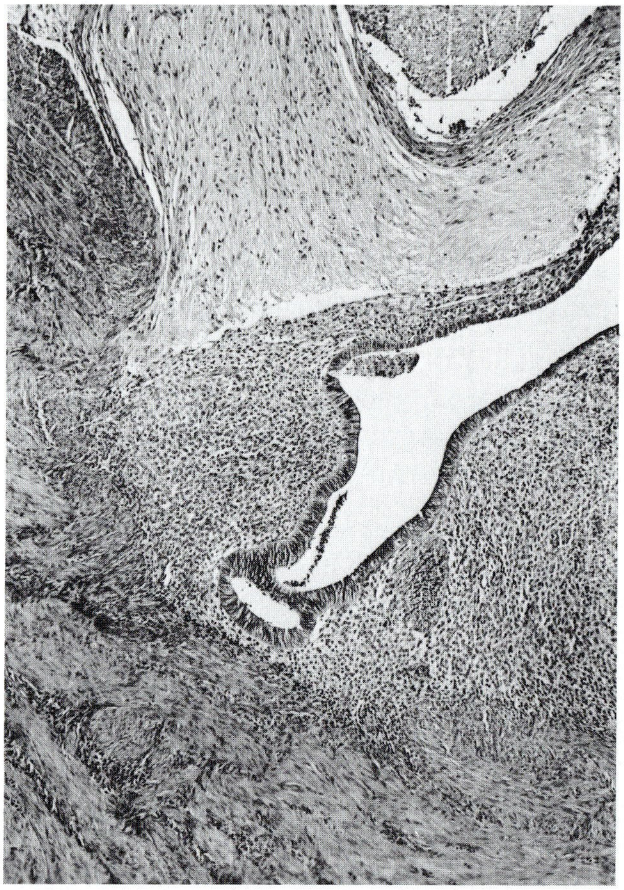

Fig. 10.47. Mature glia. A well-circumscribed glial implant is present in the *top* of the field just above an endometrial gland.

The occurrence of multiple microscopic foci of mature glial tissue in the endometrium is well recognized.[46,193,223,318] These foci are composed of cells lacking mitoses and are often surrounded by a lymphocytic and plasma cell infiltrate, resembling graft rejection (Fig. 10.47). Most cases have a history of instrumented termination of pregnancy. This history, together with the unlikely development of monotypic heterologous glial tissue in the uterus, suggests that these lesions represent remnant fetal tissue. Theoretically, gliomas of the uterus may occur, and in one reported case the follow-up was uneventful.[312] Other rare heterologous tissues that have been found in the endometrium include skin, retina, skeletal muscle, liver, and kidney.[46,278] Like

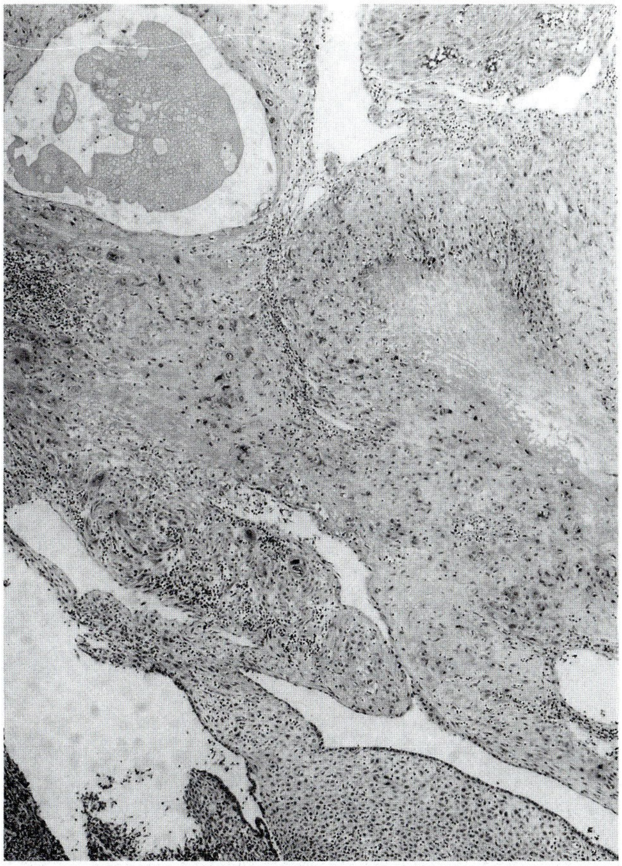

Fig. 10.48. Subinvolution of the uterus. A partially involuted placental site composed of enlarged vessels with intermediate trophoblastic cells and fibrinoid replacing the vascular walls. The underlying endometrium has enlarged, dilated glands and a decidualized stroma.

the previously described heterotopic tissues, these probably represent fetal tissue remaining after an abortion. Bone, squamous cell, and muscular metaplasia may represent underrecognized causes of infertility.[230]

Subinvolution of the Uterus

After delivery of the placenta, the uterus normally decreases dramatically in size over a period of 6–8 weeks. Failure of the uterus to return to its normal size is referred to as subinvolution. On physical examination, the subinvoluted uterus is typically enlarged to 6- to 8-week size, soft, and boggy rather than firm and normal in size. Occasionally the uterus is considerably more enlarged. Grossly, the serosa may have a slightly bluish cast. The cut surface reveals a thickened wall with enlarged blood vessels projecting from the surface. Microscopically, remnants of the placental site, containing intermediate trophoblastic cells and enlarged vessels enmeshed in eosinophilic fibrinoid along with necrotic deciduas and inflammation, are present (Fig. 10.48). A retained placental site may serve as a nidus for infection and the subsequent development of postpartum endometritis.

References

1. Aabye R (1955) Cartilage in the endometrium. Acta Obstet Gynecol Scand 34:105
2. Abraham AA (1978) Herpesvirus hominis endometritis in a young woman wearing an intrauterine contraceptive device. Am J Obstet Gynecol 3:340
3. Adelanto JM, Rees MRP, Lopez Bernal A, et al (1988) Increased uterine prostaglandin E receptors in menorrhagic women. Br J Obstet Gynaecol 99:162
4. Aksel S, Jones GS (1974) Etiology and treatment of dysfunctional uterine bleeding. Obstet Gynecol 44:1
5. Altchek A (1977) Dysfunctional uterine bleeding in adolescence. Clin Obstet Gynecol 20:633
6. Alvarez F, Brache V, Fernandez E, et al (1988) New insights on the mode of action of intrauterine contraceptive devices in women. Fertil Steril 49:768–773
7. Andrews WM, Shah SR, Goldenberg RL, et al (1995) Association of post-cesarean delivery endometritis with colonization of the chorioamnion by *Ureaplasma urealyticum*. Obstet Gynecol 85:509–514
8. Amos T, Thompson IE, Taymor ML (1980) Luteal phase deficiency and infertility: difficulties encountered in diagnosis and treatment. Obstet Gynecol 55:705
9. Arhelger RB, Bocian JJ (1976) Brenner tumor of the uterus. Cancer (Phila) 38:1741
10. Armenia CC (1967) Sequential relationship between endometrial polyps and carcinoma of the endometrium. Obstet Gynecol 30:524
11. Asherman JG (1948) Amenorrhoea traumatica (atretica). J Obstet Gynaecol Br Emp 55:23
12. Axiotis CA, Merino MJ, Duray PH (1991) Langerhans cell histiocytosis of the female genital tract. Cancer (Phila) 67:1650–1660
13. Banks ER, Mills SE, Frierson HF Jr (1991) Uterine intravascular menstrual endometrium simulating malignancy. Am J Surg Pathol 15:407–412
14. Barakat RR, Wong G, Curtin JP, et al (1994) Tamoxifen use in breast cancer patients who subsequently develop corpus cancer is not associated with a higher incidence of adverse histologic features. Gynecol Oncol 55:164–168
15. Barwick KW, LiVolsi VA (1979) Heterologous mixed mullerian tumor confined to an endometrial polyp. Obstet Gynecol 53:512–514
16. Beer AE (1970) Differential diagnosis and clinical analysis of dysfunctional uterine bleeding. Clin Obstet Gynecol 13:434

17. Benda JA (1992) Clomiphene's effect on endometrium in infertility. Int J Gynecol Pathol 11: 273–282
18. Benirschke K (1973) Congenital anomalies of the uterus with emphasis on genetic causes. In: Norris HT, Hertig AT, Abel MR (eds) The uterus. International Academy of Pathology monograph no. 14. Williams and Wilkins, Baltimore, pp 68–79
19. Bergman L, Beelen MLR, Gallee MPW, et al (2000) Risk and prognosis of endometrial cancer after tamoxifen for breast cancer. Lancet 356:881–887
20. Berry A (1966) A cytopathological and histopathological study of biharziasis of the female genital tract. J Pathol Bacteriol 91:325
21. Bhagavan BS, Gupta PK (1978) Genital actinomycosis and intrauterine contraceptive devices. Hum Pathol 9:567
22. Bird CC, Willis RA (1965) The production of smooth muscle by the endometrial stroma of the adult human uterus. J Pathol Bacteriol 90:75
23. Bjersing L, Borglin NE (1962) Eosinophilia in the myometrium of the human uterus. Acta Pathol Microbiol Scand 54:353–364
24. Botella-Llusia J (1967) Tuberculosis of the endometrium. In: Bertelli A, Houck JC (eds) Proceedings of the 5th World Congress on Fertility and Sterility, Stockholm 1966. International Congress Series 188. Excerpta Medica, Amsterdam, p 514
25. Brenner PF (1996) Differential diagnosis of abnormal uterine bleeding. Am J Obstet Gynecol 175:766–769
26. Brodman M, Deligdisch L (1986) Cytomegalovirus endometritis in a patient with AIDS. Mt Sinai J Med (NY) 53:673–675
27. Brooks PG, Serden SP, Davos I (1991) Hormonal inhibition of the endometrium for rectoscopic endometrial ablation. Am J Obstet Gynecol 164: 1601–1608
28. Brudenell JM (1955) Chronic endometritis and plasma cell infiltration of the endometrium. J Obstet Gynaecol Br Emp 62:269
29. Buckley CH, Fox H (1980) Histiocytic endometritis. Histopathology 4:105
30. Budny NN (1972) Pyometra with massive foam cell reaction: a case report. Am J Obstet Gynecol 112:126
31. Bulmer JN, Hollings D, Ritson A (1987) Immunocytochemical evidence that endometrial stromal granulocytes are granulated lymphocytes. J Pathol 153:281–288
32. Bulmer JN, Lunny DP, Hagin SV (1988) Immunohistochemical characterization of stromal leucocytes in nonpregnant human endometrium. Am J Reprod Immunol Microbiol 17:83–90
33. Burke RK, Hertig AT, Miele CA (1985) Prognostic value of subacute focal inflammation of the endometrium, with special reference to pelvic adhesions as observed on laparoscopic examination. An eight-year review. J Reprod Med 30:646
34. Cadena D, Cavanzo FJ, Leone CL, et al (1973) Chronic endometritis. A comparative clinicopathologic study. Obstet Gynecol 41:733
35. Cameron IT, Kelly RW, Baird DT (1985) Prostaglandins in the human uterus: an interaction between endometrium and myometrium. Prostaglandins Leukot Med 17:329
36. Cameron ST, Critchley HOD, Thong KJ, et al (1996) Effects of daily low dose mifepristone on endometrial maturation and proliferation. Hum Reprod 11:2518–2526
37. Campbell BF, Phipps WR, Nagel TC (1988) Endometrial biopsies during treatment with subcutaneous pulsatile gonadotrophin releasing hormone and luteal phase human chorionic gonadotropins. Int J Fertil 33:329
38. Carmichael DE (1970) Asherman's syndrome. Obstet Gynecol 36:922
39. Cassell GH, Cole BC (1981) Mycoplasms as agents of human disease. N Engl J Med 304:80
40. Cassell GH, Younger JB, Brown MB, et al (1983) Microbiologic study of infertile women at the time of diagnostic laparoscopy. N Engl J Med 308:502
41. Chadha S, Vuzevski VD, ten Kate FJW (1985) Malakoplakia of the endometrium: a rare cause of postmenopausal bleeding. Eur J Obstet Gynecol Reprod Biol 20:181
42. Charles D (1964) Iatrogenic endometrial patterns. J Clin Pathol 17:205
43. Chen KTK, Hendricks EJ (1985) Malakoplakia of the female genital tract. Obstet Gynecol 65:84s
44. Choo YC, Mak KC, Hsu C, et al (1985) Postmenopausal uterine bleeding of nonorganic cause. Obstet Gynecol 66:225–228
45. Clement PB, Scully RE (1988) Idiopathic postmenopausal decidual reaction of the endometrium. Int J Gynecol Pathol 7:152–161
46. Clement PB (1993) Tumor-like lesions of the uterine corpus. In: Clement PB, Young RH (eds) Tumors and tumor-like lesions of the uterine corpus and cervix. Churchill Livingstone, New York, pp 139–179
47. Clisham PR, Cedars MI, Greendale G, Fu YS, et al (1992) Long-term transdermal estradiol therapy: effects on endometrial histology and bleeding patterns. Obstet Gynecol 79:196–201
48. Cohen FJ, Watts S, Shah A, et al (2000) Uterine effects of 3-year raloxifene therapy in postmenopausal women younger than age 60. Obstet Gynecol 95:104–110
49. Cohen I, Rosen DJ, Shapria J, et al (1993) Endometrial changes in postmenopausal women treated with tamoxifen for breast cancer. Br J Obstet Gynaecol 106:567–570

49a. Cohen I, Bernheim J, Azaria R, et al (1999) Malignant endometrial polyps in postmenopausal breast cancer tamoxifen-treated patients. Gynecol Oncol 75:136

50. Colgan TJ, Shah R, Leyland N (1999) Post-hys-

teroscopic ablation reaction: a histopathologic study of the effects of electrosurgical ablation. Int J Gynecol Pathol 18:325–331
51. Corley D, Rowe J, Curtis MT, et al (1992) Postmenopausal bleeding from unusual endometrial polyps in women on chronic tamoxifen therapy. Obstet Gynecol 79:111–116
52. Courpas AS, Morris JD, Woodruff JD (1964) Osteoid tissue in utero. Report of 3 cases. Obstet Gynecol 24:636
53. Cramer DW, Schiff I, Schoenbaum SC, et al (1985) Tubal infertility and the intrauterine device. N Engl J Med 312:941–947
54. Crow J, Wilkins M, Howe S, et al (1991) Mast cells in the female genital tract. Int J Gynecol Pathol 10:230–237
55. Croxatto HD, Diaz S, Pavez M, et al (1984) The endometrium during continuous use of levonorgestrel. In: Zatuchni GI, Goldsmith A, Shelton JD, Sciarra JJ (eds) Long-acting contraceptive delivery systems. Harper & Row, Philadelphia, p 290
56. Cruz-Aquino M, Shenker L, Blaustein A (1967) Pseudosarcoma of the endometrium. Obstet Gynecol 29:93
57. Cumming DC, Honore LH, Scott JZ, Williams KP (1985) The late luteal phase in infertile women: Comparison of simultaneous endometrial biopsy and progesterone levels. Fertil Steril 43:715
58. Dal Cin P, Brosens I, Van Den Berghe H (1991) Involvement of 6p in an endometrial polyp. Cancer Genet Cytogenet 51:279–280
59. Dal Cin P, De Wolf F, Klerckx P, van den Berghe H (1992) The 6p21 chromosome region is nonrandomly involved in endometrial polyps. Gynecol Oncol 46:393–396
60. Dallenbach-Hellweg G (1981) Histopathology of the endometrium, 3rd Ed. Springer, New York
61. Daly DC, Walters CA, Soto-Albors CE, et al (1983) Endometrial biopsy during treatment of luteal phase defects is predictive of therapeutic outcome. Fertil Steril 40:305
62. Dawson-Hughes B (1991) Calcium supplementation and bone loss. A review of controlled clinical trials. Am J Clin Nutrition 54(1):274S–280S
63. Dehner LP, Askin FB (1975) Cytomegalovirus endometritis. Report of a case associated with spontaneous abortion. Obstet Gynecol 45:211–214
64. Deligdisch L (1993) Effects of hormone therapy on the endometrium. Mod Pathol 6:94
65. Del Pozo E, Wyss H, Tolis G, et al (1979) Prolactin and deficiency luteal function. Obstet Gynecol 53:282
66. De Muylder X, Neven P, De Somer M, et al (1991) Endometrial lesions in patients undergoing tamoxifen therapy. Int J Gynecol Obstet 36:127–130
67. Dinh TV, Slavin RE, Bhagavan BS, et al (1989) Mixed mullerian tumors of the uterus: a clinicopathologic study. Obstet Gynecol 74:388–392
68. Divack DM, Janovski NA (1962) Eosinophilia encountered in female genital organs. Am J Obstet Gynecol 84:761–763
69. Dockerty MB, Smith RA, Symmonds RE (1950) Pseudomalignant endometrial changes induced by administration of new synthetic progestins. Proc Mayo Clin 34:321
70. Dockery P, Ismail RMJ, Li TC, et al (1997) The effect of a single dose of mifepristone (RU486) on the fine structure of the human endometrium during the early luteal phase. Hum Reprod 12:1778–1784
71. Downs KA, Gibson M (1983) Basal body temperature graph and the luteal phase defect. Fertil Steril 40:466
72. Dumoulin JG, Hughesdon PE (1951) Chronic endometritis. J Obstet Gynaecol Br Emp 58:222
73. Duncan DA, Varner RE, Mazur MT (1989) Uterine herpes virus infection with multifocal necrotizing endometritis. Hum Pathol 20:1021–1024
74. Evans RA, Somers NM, Dunstan CR, Royle H, Kos S (1993) The effect of low-dose cyclical ethidronate and calcium on bone mass in early postmenopausal women. Osteoporosis Int 3:71–75
75. Farber ER, Leahy MS, Meadows TR (1968) Endometrial blastomycosis acquired by sexual contact. Obstet Gynecol 32:195
76. Ferry JA, Harris NL, Scully RE (1989) Uterine leiomyomas with lymphoid infiltration simulating lymphoma. Int J Gynecol Pathol 8:263–270
77. Fisher B, Constantino JP, Wickerham DL, et al (1998) Tamoxifen for prevention of breast cancer: report of the National Surgical Adjuvant Breast and Bowel Project P-1 Study. J Natl Cancer Inst 90:1371–1388
78. Fleming H, Ostor AG, Pickel H, et al (1989) Arterio-venous malformations of the uterus. Obstet Gynecol 73:209
79. Foxi A, Bruno RO, Davison T, et al (1966) The pathology of post-curettage intrauterine adhesions. Am J Obstet Gynecol 96:1027
80. Fornander T, Rutqvist LE, Cedermark B, et al (1989) Adjuvant tamoxifen in early breast cancer. Occurrence of new primary cancers. Lancet i:117–120
81. Foss BA, Home HW, Hertig AT (1958) The endometrium and sterility. Fertil Steril 9:193
82. Francke M-L (1998) Isolated necrotizing arteritis of the female genital tract: a clinicopathologic and immunohistochemical study of 11 cases. Int J Gynecol Pathol 17:193–200
83. Frank TS, Himebaugh KS, Wilson MD (1992) Granulomatous endometritis associated with histologically occult cytomegalovirus in a healthy patient. Am J Surg Pathol 16(7):716–720
84. Friberg J (1978) Genital mycoplasma infections. Am J Obstet Gynecol 132:573
85. Friberg J (1980) Mycoplasmas and ureaplasmas in infertility and abortion. Fertil Steril 33:351
86. Gal D, Kopel S, Bashevkin M, Lebowicz J, et al

(1991) Oncogenic potential of tamoxifen on endometria of postmenopausal women with breast cancer—preliminary report. Gynecol Oncol 42: 120–123
87. Gambrell RD (1974) Postmenopausal bleeding. J Am Geriatr Soc 22:337–343
88. Ganem KJ, Parsons L, Friedell GH (1982) Endometrial ossification. Am J Obstet Gynecol 83: 1592
89. Garcia JE, Acosta AA, Hsiu J-G, Jones HW Jr (1984) Advanced endometrial maturation after ovulation induction with human menopausal gonadotropin/human chorionic gonadotropin for in vitro fertilization. Fertil Steril 41:31–35
90. Gerbie AB, Greene RR, Reis RA (1958) Heteroplastic bone and cartilage in the female genital tract. Obstet Gynecol 11:573
91. Gliks CB, Clement PB, Hart WR, et al (2000) Uterine adenomyomas excluding atypical polypoid adenomyomas and adenomyomas of endocervical type: a clinicopathologic study of 30 cases of an underemphasized lesion that may cause diagnostic problems with brief consideration of adenomyomas of other female genital tract sites. Int Gynecol Pathol 19:195–205
92. Gilks CB, Taylor GP, Clement PB (1987) Inflammatory pseudotumor of the uterus. Int J Gynecol Pathol 6:275–286
93. Gleeson NC (1994) Cyclic changes in endometrial tissue plasminogen activator and plasminogen activator inhibitor type 1 in women with normal menstruation and essential mennorrhagia. Am J Obstet Gynecol 171:178–183
94. Goldfarb HA (1990) A review of 35 endometrial ablations using the Nd:YAG laser for recurrent menometrorrhagia. Obstet Gynecol 76:833–836
95. Goldman RL (1970) Herpetic inclusions in the endometrium. Obstet Gynecol 36:603
96. Goldstein SR, Scheele WH, Rajagopalan SK, et al (2000) A 12-month comparative study of raloxifene, estrogen, and placebo on the postmenopausal endometrium. Obstet Gynecol 95:95–103
97. Gray SW, Skandalakis JE (1972) Embryology for surgeons: The embryological basis for the treatment of congenital defects. Saunders, Philadelphia, pp 633–664
98. Greenwood SM, Moran JJ (1981) Chronic endometritis: Morphologic and clinical observations. Obstet Gynecol 58:176
99. Gump DW, Gibson M, Ashikaga T (1984) Lack of association between genital mycoplasmas and infertility. N Engl J Med 310:927
100. Hager WD, Douglas B, Majmudar B, et al (1979) Pelvic colonization with Actinomyces in women using intrauterine contraceptive devices. Am J Obstet Gynecol 135:680
101. Hart WR, Prins RP, Tsai JC (1976) Isolated coccidioidomycosis of the uterus. Hum Pathol 7:235
102. Hartman CG, Geschikter GF, Speert H (1941) Effects of continuous estrogen administration in very large doses. Anat Rec 79(suppl 2):31
103. Hendrickson MR, Kempson RL (1980) The approach to endometrial diagnosis: a system of nomenclature. In: Bennington JL (ed) Surgical pathology of the uterine corpus. Saunders, Philadelphia, pp 99–157
104. Henry-Suchet J (1988) Chlamydia trachomatis infection and infertility in women. J Reprod Med 33:912
105. Hilliard GD, Norris JH (1979) The pathologic effects of oral contraceptives. In: Lingeman C (ed) Recent results in cancer research. Carcinogenic steroids, vol 66. Springer-Verlag, New York, pp 49–71
106. Hillier SL, Kiviat NB, Hawes SE, et al (1996) Role of bacterial vaginosis-associated microorganisms in endometritis. Am J Obstet Gynecol 175:435–441
107. Hinton EL, Bobo LD, WU T-C, et al (2000) Detection of *Chlamydia trachomatis* deoxyribonucleic acid in archival paraffinized specimens from chronic salpingitis cases using the polymerase chain reaction. Fertil Steril 74:152–157
108. Ho KH (1979) Sarcoidosis of the uterus. Hum Pathol 20:219
109. Ho PC (2000) Emergency contraception: methods and efficacy. Curr Opin Obstet Gynecol 12:175–179
110. Hohnman WR, Shaw ST Jr, Macaulay L, Moyer DL (1977) Vascular defects in human endometrium caused by intrauterine contraceptive devices. Contraception 16:507
111. Holmstrom EG, McLennan CE (1947) Menorrhagia associated with irregular shedding of the endometrium. Am J Obstet Gynecol 53:727
112. Horne HW Jr, Hertig AT, Knudsin RB (1973) Subclinical endometrial inflammation and T-mycoplasma. Int J Fertil 18:226
113. Horta JLH, Fernandez IG, Soto de Leon B, Cortes Gallegos V (1977) Direct evidence of luteal insufficiency in women with habitual abortion. Obstet Gynecol 49:705
114. Hourihan HM, Sheppard BL, Bonnar J (1989) The morphologic characteristics of menstrual hemostasis in patients with unexplained menorrhagia. Int J Gynecol Pathol 8:221–229
115. Hsu C (1975) Endometrial ossification. Br J Obstet Gynaecol 82:836
116. Huettner PC, Gersell DJ (1994) Arias-Stella reaction in nonpregnant women: a clinicopathologic study of nine cases. Int J Gynecol Pathol 13:241–247
117. Hunt JE, Wallach EE (1974) Uterine factors in infertility: an overview. Clin Obstet Gynecol 17:44
118. Ingle JN (1994) Editorial. Tamoxifen and endometrial cancer: new challenges for an "old" drug. Gynecol Oncol 55:161–163
119. Israel R, Mishell DR Jr, Labudovich M (1970) Mechanisms of normal and dysfunctional uterine bleeding. Clin Obstet Gynecol 13:386

120. Israel SL, Roitman HB, Clancy C (1963) Infrequency of unsuspected endometrial tuberculosis. JAMA 183:63
121. Jewelewicz R, Khalaf S, Neuwirth RS, Vande Wiele RL (1976) Obstetric complications after treatment of intrauterine synechiae (Asherman's syndrome). Obstet Gynecol 47:701
122. Johannisson E, Fournier K, Riotton G (1981) Regeneration of the human endometrium and presence of inflammatory cells following diagnostic curettage. Acta Obstet Gynecol Scand 60:451–457
123. Johnstone FD, Williams ARW, Bird GA, et al (1994) Immunohistochemical characterization of endometrial lymphoid cell populations in women infected with human immunodeficiency virus. Obstet Gynecol 83:586–593
124. Jones GS (1972) Luteal phase insufficiency. Clin Obstet Gynecol 16:255
125. Jones GS (1975) Luteal phase defects. In: Behrman SJ, Kistner RW (eds) Progress in infertility, 2nd Ed. Little Brown, Boston, pp 299–324
126. Jones GS, Aksel S, Wentz AC (1974) Serum progesterone values in the luteal phase defects. Effects of chorionic gonadotropin. Obstet Gynecol 44:26
127. Jorgensen V, Enevoldsen B (1964) The occurrence of the first menstruation after curettage. Acta Obstet Gynecol Scand 42(Suppl 6):159
128. Judd HL (1978) Endocrinology of polycystic ovarian disease. Clin Obstet Gynecol 21:99
129. Kahner S, Ferenczy A, Richart RM (1975) Homologous mixed mullerian tumors (carcinosarcoma) confined to endometrial polyps. Am J Obstet Gynecol 121:278
130. Kaufman RH, Binder GL, Gray PN, et al (1977) Upper genital tract changes associated with exposure in utero to diethylstilbestrol. Am J Obstet Gynecol 128:51
131. Kawai K, Fukuda K, Tsuchiyama H (1988) Malacoplakia of the endometrium: an unusual case studied by electron microscopy and a review of the literature. Acta Pathol Jpn 38:531
132. Kedar RP, Bourne TH, Powles TJ, et al (1994) Effects of tamoxifen on uterus and ovaries of postmenopausal women in a randomized breast cancer prevention trial. Lancet 343:1318–1321
133. Kelly HW, Miles PA, Buster JE, Scragg WH (1976) Adenocarcinoma of the endometrium in women taking sequential oral contraceptives. Obstet Gynecol 47:200
133a. Kennedy MM, Baigrie CF, Manek S (1999) Tamoxifen and the endometrium: review of 102 cases and comparison with HRT-related and non-HRT-related endometrial pathology. Int J Gynecol Pathol 18:130
134. Kessel E (1989) Pelvic inflammatory disease with intrauterine device use: a reassessment. Fertil Steril 51:1–11
135. King A, Wellings V, Gardner L, Loke YW (1989) Immunocytochemical characterization of the unusual large granular lymphocytes in human endometrium throughout the menstrual cycle. Hum Immunol 24:195–205
136. Kiviat NB, Wolner-Haussen P, Peterson M, et al (1986) Localization of *Chlamydia trachomatis* infection by direct immunofluorescence and culture in pelvic inflammatory disease. Am J Obstet Gynecol 154:865–873
137. Kiviat NB, Eschenbach DA, Paavonen JA, Critchlow CW, Moore DE (1990) Endometrial histopathology in patients with culture-proved upper genital tract infection and laparoscopically diagnosed acute salpingitis. Am J Surg Pathol 14(2):167–175
138. Korhoneen MO, Symons JP, Hyde BM, et al (1997) Histologic classification and pathologic findings for endometrial biopsy specimens obtained from 2964 perimenopausal and postmenopausal women undergoing screening for continuous hormones as replacement therapy (CHART 2 study). Am J Obstet Gynecol 176:377–380
139. Korn AP, Bolan G, Padian N, et al (1995) Plasma cell endometritis in women with symptomatic bacterial vaginosis. Obstet Gynecol 85:387–390
140. Korn AP, Hessol NA, Padian NS, et al (1998) Risk factors for plasma cell endometritis among women with cervical *Neisseria gonorrhoeae*, cervical *Chlamydia trachomatis*, or bacterial vaginosis. Am J Obstet Gynecol 178:987–990
141. Korn AP, Hessol N, Padian N, et al (1995) Commonly used diagnostic criteria for pelvic inflammatory disease have poor sensitivity for plasma cell endometritis. Sex Transm Dis 22:335–341
142. Kraus FT (1973) Irradiation changes in the uterus. In: Hertig AT, Norris HJ, Abell MR (eds) International Academy of Pathology monograph no. 14. The uterus. Williams & Wilkins, Baltimore, pp 457–488
143. Kurman RJ, Felix JC, Archer DF, et al (2000) Norethindrone acetate and estradiol-induced endometrial hyperplasia. Obstet Gynecol 96:373–379
144. Kurman RJ, Scully RE (1976) Clear cell carcinoma of the endometrium. An analysis of 21 cases. Cancer (Phila) 37:872–882
145. Laatikainen T, Anderson B, Karkkainen I, et al (1983) Progestin receptor levels in endometria with delayed or incomplete secretory changes. Obstet Gynecol 62:592
146. Lackner JE, Krohn L (1932) Report of a case of teratoma of the uterus. Am J Obstet Gynecol 25: 735
147. Lahti E, Blanco G, Kauppila A, Apaja-Sarkkinen M, Taskinen PJ, Laatikainen T (1993) Endometrial changes in postmenopausal breast cancer patients receiving tamoxifen. Obstet Gynecol 81: 660–664
148. Ledger WJ (1977) Infection in the female. Lea & Febiger, Philadelphia
149. Lee NC, Rubin GL, Borucki R (1988) The intrauterine device and pelvic inflammatory disease revisited: new results from the Women's Health Study. Obstet Gynecol 72:1–6

150. Lemay A, Jean C, Faure N (1987) Endometrial histology during intermittent intranasal luteinizing hormone-releasing hormone (LH-RH) agonist sequentially combined with an oral progestogen as an antiovulatory contraceptive approach. Fertil Steril 48(5):775–782
151. Lenton EA, Landgren B, Sexton L, Harper R (1984) Normal variation in the length of the follicular phase of the menstrual cycle. Effect of chronological age. Br J Obstet Gynecol 91:681
152. Li T-C, Dockery P, Thomas P, et al (1988) The effects of progesterone receptor blockade in the luteal phase of normal fertile women. Fertil Steril 50:732–742
153. Lidor A, Ismajovich B, Confino E, David MP (1983) Histopathological findings in 226 women with postmenopausal uterine bleeding. Acta Obstet Gynecol Scand 65:41–43
154. Lindenman E, Shepard MK, Pescovitz OH (1997) Clinical commentary. Müllerian agenesis: an update. Obstet Gynecol 90:307–312
155. Ling WY, Wrixon W, Zayid I, et al (1983) Mode of action of *dl*-norgestrel and ethinylestradiol combination in postcoital contraception. II. Effect of post-ovulatory administration on ovarian function and endometrium. Fertil Steril 39:292
156. Lombard CM, Moore MH, Seifer DB (1986) Diagnosis of systemic polyarteritis nodosa following total abdominal hysterectomy and bilateral salpingo-oophorectomy: a case report. Int J Gynecol Pathol 5:63–68
157. Longacre TA, Chung MH, Rouse RV, et al (1996) Atypical polypoid adenomyofibromas (atypical polypoid adenomyomas) of the uterus. Am J Surg Pathol 20:1–20
158. Lyon FA, Frisch MJ (1976) Endometrial abnormalities occurring in young women on long-term sequential oral contraception. Obstet Gynecol 47: 639
159. Maathius JB, Horbach JGM, Hall EV (1972) A comparison of the result of hysterosalpingography and laparoscopy in the diagnosis of fallopian tube dysfunction. Fertil Steril 23:428
160. Magos AL, Baumann R, Lockwood GM, Turnbull AC (1991) Experience with the first 250 endometrial resections for menorrhagia. Lancet 337: 1074–1078
161. Magriples U, Naftolin F, Schwartz PE, et al (1993) High-grade endometrial carcinoma in tamoxifen-treated breast cancer patients. J Clin Oncol 11:485–490
162. Marrogi AJ, Gersell DJ, Kraus FT (1991) Localized asymptomatic giant cell arteritis of the female genital tract. Int J Gynecol Pathol 10:51–58
163. Martin E, Scholes J, Richart RM, Fenoglio CM (1979) Benign cystic teratoma of the uterus. Am J Obstet Gynecol 135:429
164. Martinex-Manautou J, Maqueo M, Aznar R, Phariss BB, Zaffaroni A (1975) Endometrial morphology in women exposed to intrauterine systems releasing progesterone. Am J Obstet Gynecol 121: 175
165. Mazur MT (1981) Atypical polypoid adenomyoma of the endometrium. Am J Surg Pathol 5:473
166. Mazur MT, Kurman RJ (1994) Diagnosis of endometrial biopsies and curettings: a practical approach. Springer-Verlag, New York
167. McCracken AW, D'Agostino AN, Brucks AB, Kingsly WB (1974) Acquired cytomegalovirus infection presenting as viral endometritis. Am J Clin Pathol 61:556–560
168. McKelvey JL (1942) Irregular shedding of the endometrium. Lancet 2:434
169. McLennan CE (1952) Current concepts of prolonged or irregular endometrial shedding. Am J Obstet Gynecol 64:988
170. Mears E (1965) Handbook on oral contraception. Churchill Livingstone, London
171. Meissner WA, Sommers SC, Sherman G (1957) Endometrial hyperplasia, endometrial carcinoma, and endometriosis produced experimentally by estrogen. Cancer (Phila) 10:500
172. Meyer WC, Malkasian KGD, Dockerty MB, Decker DG (1971) Postmenopausal bleeding from atrophic endometrium. Obstet Gynecol 38:731–738
173. Miko TL, Lampe LG, Thomazy VA, Molnar TP, Endes P (1988) Eosinophilic endomyometritis associated with diagnostic curettage. Int J Gynecol Pathol 7:162–172
174. Mishell DR Jr, Moyer DL (1969) Association of pelvic inflammatory disease with the intrauterine device. Clin Obstet Gynecol 12:179
175. Mittal KR, Peng XC, Wallach RC, et al (1995) Coexistent atypical polypoid adenomyoma and endometrial adenocarcinoma. Hum Pathol 26:584–576
176. Moghissi KS (1975) Endometrium and endosalpinx of women treated with microdose progestogens. J Reprod Med 14:217
177. Molnar JT, Poliak A (1983) Recurrent endometrial malakoplakia. Am J Clin Pathol 80:762
178. Monif GRR (1974) Infectious diseases in obstetrics and gynecology. Harper & Row, New York
179. Mortgomery R, Youngblood L, Medearis DN (1972) Recovery of cytomegalovirus from the cervix in pregnancy. Pediatrics 49:524–531
180. Moszkowski E, Woodruff JD, Jones GS (1962) The inadequate luteal phase. Am J Obstet Gynecol 83: 363
181. Mouktar M (1966) Functional disorders due to bilharzial infection of the female genital tract. J Obstet Gynecol Br Commonw 73:307
182. Moyer DL (1975) Endometrial lesions in infertility. In: Behrman SJ, Kistner RW (eds) Progress in infertility, 2nd Ed. Little, Brown, Boston, pp 91–115
183. Moyer DL, Mishell DR Jr (1971) Reactions of human endometrium to the intrauterine foreign body. II. Long-term effects on the endometrial histology and cytology. Am J Obstet Gynecol 111:66

184. Moyer DL, Mishell DR Jr, Bell J (1970) Reactions of human endometrium to the intrauterine device. I. Correlation of the endometrial histology with the bacterial environment of the uterus following short-term insertion of the IUD. Am J Obstet Gynecol 106:799
185. Moyer DL, de Lignieres B, Driguez P, et al (1993) Prevention of endometrial hyperplasia by progesterone during long-term estradiol replacement: Influence of bleeding pattern and secretory changes. Fertil Steril 59:992–997
186. Muller-Holzner E, Ruth NR, Abfalter E, et al (1995) IUD-associated pelvic actinomycosis: a report of five cases. Int J Gynecol Pathol 14:70–74
187. Nand SL, Webster MA, Baber R, et al (1998) Bleeding pattern and endometrial changes during continuous combined replacement therapy. The Ogen/Provera Study Group. Obstet Gynecol 91: 678–684
188. Neven P (1993) Tamoxifen and endometrial lesions. Lancet 342:452
189. Newhall EP, Winikoff B (2000) Abortion with mifepristone and misoprostol: regimens, efficacy, acceptability and future directions. Am J Obstet Gynecol 183:S44–S53
190. Newton CW III, Abell MR (1973) Iatrogenic fetal implants. Obstet Gynecol 40:686
191. Niebyl JR, Parmley TH, Spence MR, Woodruff JD (1978) Unilateral ovarian abscess associated with the intrauterine device. Obstet Gynecol 52:165
192. Nicholson GW (1956) Studies of tumour formation: polypoid teratoma of the uterus. Guy's Hosp Rep 205:157
193. Niven PAR, Stansfeld AG (1973) "Glioma" of the uterus: a fetal homograft. Am J Obstet Gynecol 115:434
194. Nogales-Ortiz F, Taranco I, Nogales FF Jr (1979) The pathology of female genital tuberculosis. A 31-year study of 1436 cases. Obstet Gynecol 53:422
195. Novak E (1933) Recent advances in the physiology of menstruation. Can menstruation occur without ovulation? JAMA 94:833
196. Noyes RW, Haman JO (1954) Accuracy of endometrial dating. Fertil Steril 4:504
197. Ober WB (1966) Synthetic progesten-oestrogen preparations and endometrial morphology. J Clin Pathol 19:138
198. Ober WB (1977) Effects of oral and intrauterine administration of contraceptives on the uterus. Hum Pathol 8:513
199. Ober WB, Bronstein SB (1967) Endometrial morphology following oral administration of quinestrol. Int J Fertil 23:210
200. Ober WB, Sobrero AJ, Kurman R, Gold S (1968) Endometrial morphology and polyethylene intrauterine devices. A study of 200 endometrial biopsies. Obstet Gynecol 32:782
201. O'Connor H, Magos A (1996) Endometrial resection for the treatment of mennorrhagia. N Engl J Med 335:151–156
202. O'Leary JJ, Landers RJ, Crowley M, et al (1998) Human papillomavirus and mixed epithelial tumors of the endometrium. Hum Pathol 29:383–389
203. Osborne JL, Bennett MJ (1978) Removal of intraabdominal intrauterine contraceptive devices. Br J Obstet Gynecol 85:868
204. Osborne NG (1977) The significance of mycoplasma in pelvic infection. J Reprod Med 19:39
205. Oster G, Salgo MP (1975) The copper intrauterine device and its mode of action. N Engl J Med 293:432
206. Paavonen J, Aine R, Teisala K, et al (1985) Comparison of endometrial biopsy and peritoneal fluid cytologic testing with laparoscopy in the diagnosis of acute pelvic inflammatory disease. Am J Obstet Gynecol 151:645
207. Payan H, Daino J, Kish M (1964) Lymphoid follicles in endometrium. Obstet Gynecol 23:570
208. Peipert JF, Montagno AB, Cooper AS, et al (1997) Bacterial vaginosis as a risk factor for upper genital tract infection. Am J Obstet Gynecol 177:1184–1187
209. Perkins MB (1960) Pneumopolycystic endometritis. Am J Obstet Gynecol 80:332
210. Peterson WF, Novak ER (1956) Endometrial polyps. Obstet Gynecol 8:40
211. Peuchmaur M, Emilie D, Vazeux R, et al (1989) HIV-associated endometritis AIDS 3:239–241
212. Plaut A (1950) Human infection with *Cryptococcus glabratus*. Report of case involving uterus and fallopian tube. Am J Clin Pathol 20:377
213. Poppe W, Van Assche FA, Wilms G, Favril A, Baert A (1987) Pregnancy after transcatheter embolization of a uterine arteriovenous malformation. Am J Obstet Gynecol 156:1179–1180
214. Poropatich C, Rojas M, Silverberg SG (1987) Polymorphonuclear leukocytes in the endometrium during the normal menstrual cycle. Int J Gynecol Pathol 6:230–234
215. Povey WG (1970) Abnormal uterine bleeding at puberty and climacteric. Clin Obstet Gynecol 13: 474
216. Rao NB (1969) Malacoplakia of broad ligament, inguinal region and endometrium. Arch Pathol 88: 85
217. Raymond EG, Lovely LP, Chen-Mok M, et al (2000) Effect of the Yuzpe regimen of emergency contraception on markers of endometrial receptivity. Hum Reprod 15:2351–2355
218. Reid PC, Thurrell W, Smith JHF, et al (1992) Nd:YAG laser endometrial ablation: Histological aspects of uterine healing. Int J Gynecol Pathol 11:174–179
219. Remington JS (1973) Toxoplasmosis. In: Charles D, Finland M (eds) Obstetric and perinatal infections. Lea & Febiger, Philadelphia, pp 27–74
220. Reshef E, Segars JH, Hill GA, et al (1990) Endometrial inadequacy after treatment with human menopausal gonadotropin/human chorionic gonadotropin. Fertil Steril 54:1012–1016

221. Rioux JE, Cloutier D, Dupont P, Lamonde D (1986) Pregnancy after IUD use. Adv Contracept 2:185–192
222. Robb JA, Benirschke K, Barmeyer R (1986) Intrauterine latent herpes simplex virus infection: I. Spontaneous abortion. Hum Pathol 17:1196–1209
223. Roca AN, Guajardo M, Estrada WJ (1980) Glial polyp of the cervix and endometrium. Report of a case and review of the literature. Am J Clin Pathol 73:718
224. Rock J, Garcia CR, Menkin MF (1959) A theory of menstruation. Ann NY Acad Sci 75:831
225. Rodriguez M, Okagaki T, Richart RM (1972) Mycotic endometritis due to *Candida*. A case report. Obstet Gynecol 39:292
226. Rosenfeld DL, Chudow S, Bronson RA (1980) Diagnosis of luteal phase inadequacy. Obstet Gynecol 56:193
227. Roth E, Taylor HB (1966) Heterotopic cartilage in uterus. Obstet Gynecol 27:838
228. Rotterdam H (1978) Chronic endometritis: a clinicopathologic study. Pathol Annu 13:209
229. Rubin SC (1987) Postmenopausal bleeding: etiology, evaluation, and management. Med Clin North Am 71:59–69
230. Ruiz-Velasco V, Gonzalez AG, Pliego SL, et al (1997) Endometrial pathology and infertility. Fertil Steril 67:687–692
231. Russack V, Lammers RJ (1990) Xanthogranulomatous endometritis. Arch Pathol Lab Med 114: 929–932
232. Rybo G (1966) Plasminogen activators in the endometrium. Acta Obstet Gynecol Scand 45:411
233. Sadler TW (1985) Langman's medical embryology, 5th Ed. Williams & Wilkins, Baltimore
234. Salm R (1972) The incidence and significance of early carcinomas in endometrial polyps. J Pathol 108:47
235. Sandmire HF, Cavanaugh RA (1985) Long-term use of intrauterine contraceptive devices in a private practice. Am J Obstet Gynecol 152:169–175
236. Saw EC, Smale LE, Einstein H, Huntington RW (1975) Female genital coccidioidomycosis. Obstet Gynecol 45:199
237. Sayage L, Gunby R, Gonwa T, Husberg B, Goldstein R, Klintmalm G (1990) Cytomegalovirus endometritis after liver transplantation. Transplantation 49:815–817
238. Schachter J, Banks J, Sung M, et al (1982) Hydrosalpinx as a consequence of chlamydial salpingitis in the guinea pig. In: Mardh PA (ed) Chlamydial infections. Elsevier, Amsterdam, pp 371–374
239. Schenken JR, Tamisica J (1956) *Enterobius vermicularis* (pinworm) infection of the endometrium. Am J Obstet Gynecol 72:913
240. Schindler AE, Schmidt G (1980) Postmenopausal bleeding: a study of more than 1000 cases. Maturitas 2:269–274
241. Schneider V, Behm FG, Mumaw VR (1982) Ascending herpetic endometritis. Obstet Gynecol 59: 259
242. Scommegna A, Dmowski WP (1973) Dysfunctional uterine bleeding. Clin Obstet Gynecol 16:221
243. Sereepapong W, Suwajanakom S, Triratanachat S, et al (2000) Effects of clomiphene citrate on the endometrium of regularly cycling women. Fertil Steril 73:287–291
244. Sharma V, Whitehead M, Mason B, et al (1990) Influence of superovulation on endometrial and embryonic development. Fertil Steril 53:822–829
245. Shaw ST, Maucaulay LK, Hohman WR (1979) Vessel density in endometrium of women with and without intrauterine contraceptive devices. A morphometric evaluation. Am J Obstet Gynecol 135:101
246. Sherman ME, Bitterman P, Rosenshein NB, Delgado G, Kurman RJ (1992) Uterine serous carcinoma. A morphologically diverse neoplasm with unifying clinicopathologic features. Am J Surg Pathol 16:600–610
247. Shintaku M, Sasaki M, Baba Y (1991) Ceroid-containing histiocytic granuloma of the endometrium. Histopathology (Oxf). 8:169
248. Shoupe D, Mishell DR Jr, Bopp BL, Fielding M (1991) The significance of bleeding patterns in Norplant implant users. Obstet Gynecol 77:256
249. Silva EG, Jenkins R (1990) Serous carcinoma in endometrial polyps. Mod Pathol 3:120–128
250. Silva EG, Tornos CS, Follen-Mitchell M (1994) Malignant neoplasms of the uterine corpus in patients treated for breast carcinoma: the effects of tamoxifen. Intl J Gynecol Pathol 13:248–258
251. Silverberg SG, Makowski EL (1975) Endometrial carcinoma in young women taking oral contraceptive agents. Obstet Gynecol 46:503
252. Silverberg SG, Makowski EL, Roche WD (1977) Endometrial carcinoma in young women under 40 years of age: comparison of cases in oral contraceptive users and nonusers. Cancer (Phila) 39:592
253. Silverberg SG, Major FJ, Blessing JA, et al (1990) Carcinosarcoma (malignant mixed mesodermal tumor) of the uterus. A gynecologic oncology group pathologic study of 203 cases. Int J Gynecol Pathol 9:1–19
254. Sinykin MB, Goodlin RC, Barr MM (1956) Irregular shedding of the endometrium. Am J Obstet Gynecol 71:990
255. Snieder H, MacGregor AJ, Spector TD (1998) Genes control the cessation of a woman's reproductive life: a twin study of hysterectomy and age at menopause. J Clin Endocrinol Metab 83:1875–1880
256. Sobrino LG, Kase N (1970) Endocrinologic aspects of dysfunctional uterine bleeding. Clin Obstet Gynecol 13:400
257. Song JY, Fraser IS (1995) Effects of progestogens on human endometrium. Obstet Gynecol Surv 50:385–394

258. Soslow RA, Chung MH, Rouse RV, et al (1996) Atypical polypoid adenomyofibroma (APA) versus well-differentiated endometrial carcinoma with prominent stromal matrix: an immunohistochemical study. Int J Gynecol Pathol 15:209–216
259. Soules MR, Wiebe RH, Aksel S, Hammond CB (1977) The diagnosis and therapy of luteal phase deficiency. Fertil Steril 28:1033
260. Southam AL, Richart RM (1966) The prognosis for adolescents with menstrual abnormalities. Am J Obstet Gynecol 94:637
261. Speleman F, Dal Cin P, Van Roy N, et al (1991) Is t(6;20)(p21;q13) a characteristic chromosome change in endometrial polyps? Genes Chromosomes Cancer 3:318–319
262. Speroff L, Glass RH, Kase NG (1983) Clinical gynecological endocrinology and infertility, 3rd Ed. Williams & Wilkins, Baltimore, pp 467–492
263. Speroff L, Glass RH, Kase NG (1989) Clinical gynecologic endocrinology and infertility, 4th Ed. Williams & Wilkins, Baltimore
264. Spirtos NJ, Yurewicz EC, Moghisii KS, et al (1985) Pseudocorpus luteum insufficiency: a study of cytosol progesterone receptors in human endometrium. Obstet Gynecol 65:535
265. Spitz IM, Bardin CW (1993) Mifepristone (RU 486)—a modulator of progestin and glucocorticoid action. N Engl J Med 329:404–412
266. Staros EB, Shilkitus WF (1991) Atypical polypoid adenomyoma with carcinomatous transformation. A case report. Surg Pathol 4:157–166
267. Stern RA, Svoboda-Newman S, Frank TS (1996) Analysis of chronic endometritis for *Chlamydia trachomatis* by polymerase chain reaction. Hum Pathol 27:1085–1088
268. Stray-Pedersen B, Lorentzen-Styr A-M (1977) Uterine toxoplasma infections and repeated abortions. Am J Obstet Gynecol 128:716
269. Sturdee DW, Wade-Evans T, Paterson MEL, Thom M, Studd JW (1978) Relations between bleeding pattern, endometrial histology, and oestrogen treatment in menopausal women. Br Med J 1: 1575–1577
270. Sugiyama T, Ohta S, Nishida T, et al (1998) Two cases of endometrial adenocarcinoma arising from atypical polypoid adenomyoma 71:141–144
271. Sutherland AM (1958) Tuberculosis of endometrium: a report of 250 cases with results of drug treatment. Obstet Gynecol 11:527
272. Swahn ML, Bygdeman M, Cekan S, et al (1990) The effect of RU 486 administered during the early luteal phase on bleeding pattern, hormonal parameters and endometrium. Hum Reprod 5:402–408
273. Swalin M-L, Westlund P, Johannisson E, et al (1996) Effect of post-coital contraceptive methods on the endometrium and the menstrual cycle. Acta Obstet Gynecol 75:738–744
274. Tatum JH, Schmidt FH, Jain AK (1976) Management and outcome of pregnancies associated with the Copper T intrauterine contraceptive device. Am J Obstet Gynecol 126:869–879
275. Tawfik OW, Huet YM, Malathy PV, Johnson DC, Dey SK (1987) Release of prostaglandins and leukotrienes from the rat uterus is an early estrogenic response. Prostaglandins 34:805–814
276. Tawfik OW, Sagrillo C, Johnson DC, Dey SK (1987) Decidualization in the rat: role of leukotrienes and prostaglandins. Prostaglandins Leuko Med 29:221–227
277. Taylor AB (1960) Sarcoidosis of the uterus. J Obstet Gynecol Br Emp 67:32
278. Taylor RN, Welch KL, Sklar DM, et al (1984) Heterotopic skin in the uterus. A report of an unusual case. J Reprod Med 29:837
279. Taylor-Robinson D, McCormack WM (1980) The genital mycoplasmas. Part 1. N Engl J Med 302: 1003
280. Taylor-Robinson D, McCormack WM (1980) The genital mycoplasmas. Part 2. N Engl J Med 302:1063
281. Tesluk H, Munn RJ (1984) Malacoplakia of the uterus (letter). Arch Pathol Lab Med 108:692
282. The Writing Group for the PEPI Trial (1995) Effects of estrogen and estrogen/progestin regimens on heart disease risk factors in postmenopausal women. The postmenopausal estrogen/progestin interventions (PEPI) trial. JAMA 273:199–208
283. The Writing Group for the PEPI Trial (1996) Effects of hormone replacement therapy on endometrial histology in postmenopausal women. JAMA 275:370–375
284. Thiery M (1955) Irregular shedding of the endometrium. Gynaecologia (Basel) 139:1
285. Thomas W Jr, Sadeghieh B, Fresco R, Rubenstone AI, Stepto RC, Carasso B (1978) Malacoplakia of the endometrium, a probable cause of postmenopausal bleeding. Am J Clin Pathol 69:637
286. Toaff R, Ballas S (1978) Traumatic hypomenorrhea-amenorrhea (Asherman's syndrome). Fertil Steril 30:379
287. Van Eijkeren MA, Christiaens GCML, Gueze JJ, Haspels AA, Sixma JJ (1991) Morphology of menstrual hemostasis in essential menorrhagia. Lab Invest 64:284
288. Villaneuva DL (1992) Malakoplakia of the urogenital tract. The Female Patient 17:July:37–38
289. Voigt LF, Weiss NS, Chu J, Daling JR, McKnight B, VanBelle G (1991) Progestogen supplementation of exogenous oestrogens and risk of endometrial cancer. Lancet 338:274–277
290. Wallach EE (1972) The uterine factor in infertility. Fertil Steril 23:138
291. Weicker ML, Kaneb GD, Goodale RH (1940) Primary echinococcal cyst of the uterus. N Engl J Med 223:574
292. Weiss NS, Sayvetz TA (1980) Incidence of endometrial cancer in relation to the use of oral contraceptives. N Engl J Med 302:551
293. Wenckelbach GFC, Curry B (1976) Cytomegalovirus infection of the female genital tract. Histo-

logic findings in three cases and review of the literature. Arch Pathol Lab Med 100:1609–1612
294. Wentz AC (1980) Endometrial biopsy in the evaluation of infertility. Fertil Steril 33:121
295. Wentz AC (1982) Diagnosing luteal phase inadequacy. Fertil Steril 37:334
296. Wentz AC, Herbert CM, Maxson WS, Garner CH (1984) Outcome of progesterone treatment of luteal phase inadequacy. Fertil Steril 41:856
297. Westrom L (1980) Incidence, prevalence and trends of acute pelvic inflammatory disease and its consequences in industrialized countries. Am J Obstet Gynecol 138:880
298. Wheeler DT, Bell KA, Kurman RJ, et al (2000) Minimal uterine serous carcinoma: diagnosis and clinicopathologic correlation. Am J Surg Pathol 24: 797–806.
299. Whitehead MI, King RJB, McQueen J, Campbell S (1979) Endometrial histology and biochemistry in climacteric women during oestrogen and oestrogen/progestogen therapy. J R Soc Med 72:322–327
300. Willen R, Stendahl U, Willen H, Trope C (1983) Malacoplakia of the cervix and corpus uteri: a light microscopic, electron microscopic, and x-ray microprobe analysis of a case. Int J Gynecol Pathol 2:201
301. Williams A (1967) Pathology of schistosomiasis of the uterine cervix due to *S. haematobium*. Am J Obstet Gynecol 98:784
302. Williams DB, Voigt BJ, Fu YS, et al (1994) Assessment of less than monthly progestin therapy in postmenopausal women given estrogen replacement. Obstet Gynecol 84:787–793
303. Winkler B, Reumann W, Mitao M (1984) Chlamydial endometritis. A histological and immunohistochemical analysis. Am J Surg Pathol 8:771
304. Winter JD, Faiman C, Reyes FI (1978) Normal and abnormal pubertal development. Clin Obstet Gynecol 21:67
305. Winter JD, Kohn G, Mellinin WJ, et al (1968) A familial syndrome of renal, genital, and middle ear anomalies. J Pediatr 72:88
306. Wright CA, Haffajee Z, van Iddekinge B, et al (1995) Detection of herpes simplex virus DNA in spontaneous abortions from HIV-positive women using nonisotopic in situ hybridization. J Pathol 176:399–402
307. Wynn RM (1967) Intrauterine devices: effects on ultrastructure of human endometrium. Science 156:1508
308. Wynn RM (1968) Fine structural effects of intrauterine contraceptives on the human endometrium. Fertil Steril 19:867
309. Wysowski DK, Golden L, Burke L (1995) Use of menopausal estrogens and medroxyprogesterone in the United States, 1982–1992. Obstet Gynecol 85:6–10
310. Yaegashi N, Fujita N, Yajima A, et al (1995) Menstrual cycle dependent expression of CD44 in normal human endometrium. Hum Pathol 26:862–865.
311. Yaffe H, Ron M, Polishuk WZ (1978) Amenorrhea, hypomenorrhea, and uterine fibrosis. Am J Obstet Gynecol 130:599
312. Young RH, Kleinman GM, Scully RE (1981) Glioma of the uterus. Am J Surg Pathol 5:695
313. Young RH, Harris NL, Scully RE (1985) Lymphoma-like lesions of the lower female genital tract: a report of 16 cases. Int J Gynecol Pathol 4:289–299
314. Young RH, Treger T, Scully RE (1986) Atypical polypoid adenomyoma of the uterus. A report of 27 cases. Am J Clin Pathol 86:139
315. Yuzpe AA, Thurlow HJ, Ramzy I, et al (1974) Post coital contraception—a pilot study. J Reprod Med 13:53–57
316. Zaino RJ (1996) Interpretation of endometrial biopsies and curettings. Lippincott-Raven, Philadelphia
317. Zaman SS, Mazur MT (1993) Endometrial papillary syncytial change. Am J Clin Pathol 99:741–745
318. Zettergren L (1973) Glial tissue in the uterus. Am J Pathol 171:419

11

Precursor Lesions of Endometrial Carcinoma

Brigitte M. Ronnett, M.D., and
Robert J. Kurman, M.D.

Endometrial carcinoma is the most common malignant neoplasm of the female genital tract. Factors associated with unopposed estrogenic stimulation, such as obesity, exogenous hormone use, and endometrial hyperplasia, are related to the development of the most common form of endometrial carcinoma, that is, the endometrioid subtype.[14] More recent studies have confirmed this association by demonstrating elevated serum estrogen levels in patients with endometrioid carcinoma.[15,69] It also has been recognized that some forms of endometrial carcinoma appear to be unrelated to hormonal factors and hyperplasia.[80] Serous carcinoma is the prototypic endometrial carcinoma that is not related to estrogenic stimulation. In the past two decades, clinicopathologic, immunohistochemical, and molecular genetic studies have provided additional data to allow for the development of a dualistic model of endometrial carcinogenesis. In this model, two types of precursor lesions are proposed for the two pathways of endometrial carcinogenesis. Atypical hyperplasia (AH) is recognized as the precursor for the endometrioid type of endometrial carcinoma and endometrial intraepithelial carcinoma (EIC) as the precursor for serous carcinoma, the most common nonendometrioid subtype of endometrial carcinoma. The following discussion summarizes current knowledge about the relationship of these precursor lesions to the various forms of endometrial carcinoma.

Endometrial Hyperplasia

Definition and Classification

In the past, the terms *adenomatous hyperplasia* and *atypical hyperplasia* were used to denote proliferative lesions of the endometrium with varying degrees of architectural complexity and cytologic atypia.[16,17,31–33,38,39,67,92,94] In addition, the term *carcinoma in situ* was proposed to describe small lesions, with or without glandular crowding, having the cytologic features of carcinoma but lacking invasion.[16,38,39,90,92,94] However, because carcinoma in situ was never clearly defined the term was abandoned and, in retrospect, many of these lesions would be classified today as hyperplasia with eosinophilic change. Recently, the term has been applied to an entirely different set of lesions that are associated with serous carcinoma (see following), adding further ambiguity to the confusion surrounding its clinical and biologic significance. In summary, pathologists have recognized for decades that endometrial cancer precursors are morphologically and biologically heterogeneous. However, early studies designed to clarify the significance of these lesions were limited by the lack of standardized diagnostic criteria, failure to consider cytologic and architectural features separately, and inclusion of irradiated patients, which may have altered the natural history of the lesions studied.[12,19,31,32,38,39,61,92,94] Many of these limitations have been addressed in more recent studies (see "Behavior of Hyperplasia").

Endometrial hyperplasia is defined as a proliferation of glands of irregular size and shape with an increase in the gland/stroma ratio compared with proliferative endometrium. The process is generally diffuse but may also be focal. Endometrial hyperplasia is subdivided into two broad categories, hyperplasia without cytologic atypia and hyperplasia with cytologic atypia (atypical hyperplasia). These proliferative lesions are classified further into simple or complex according to the extent of glandular complexity and crowding. Thus, both types of hyperplasia, nonatypical and atypical, are classified further as either simple or complex based on the degree of glandular crowding. The rationale for this classification is based on the natural history of the disease as shown in long-term follow-up studies.[8,25,52] Fewer than 2% of hyperplasias without cytologic atypia progress to carcinoma, whereas 23% of hyperplasias with cytologic atypia (atypical hyperplasia) progress to carcinoma. Increasing degrees of glandular complexity and crowding (architectural abnormalities) appear to increase the likelihood of progression to carcinoma but not to the extent that cytologic atypia does. The classification proposed by the World Health Organization (WHO) (Table 11.1), therefore, takes into account both cytologic and architectural abnormalities.[76]

For practical purposes, it is reasonable to classify noninvasive proliferative lesions of the endometrium as either hyperplasia without atypia or atypical hyperplasia. This simplified approach is recommended for several reasons. First, simple atypical hyperplasia is relatively rare and thus most atypical hyperplasias are complex. Second, there is some difficulty in reproducibly distinguishing varying degrees of glandular crowding. Finally, there is minimal, if any, clinical relevance in distinguishing simple from complex hyperplasia or simple atypical from complex atypical hyperplasia because it is the presence of cytologic atypia that confers a significantly increased risk of progression to carcinoma.

Table 11.1. Classification of endometrial hyperplasia

Simple hyperplasia
Complex hyperplasia (adenomatous)
Simple atypical hyperplasia
Complex atypical hyperplasia (adenomatous with atypia)

From World Health Organization.

Clinical Features

Patients with endometrial hyperplasia typically have abnormal bleeding. Occasionally, the lesion is detected fortuitously by endometrial biopsy performed during the course of an infertility workup or before the start of hormone replacement therapy in postmenopausal women. Hyperplasia develops as a result of unopposed estrogenic stimulation, and consequently most patients with hyperplasia have a history of either persistent anovulation or exogenous unopposed estrogen usage. Although anovulation occurs at menarche and in perimenopausal women, hyperplasia is not usually encountered in young women, probably because bleeding in menarchial women is seldom evaluated by an endometrial biopsy. The youngest patient reported with hyperplasia was 16 years old.[55] During the reproductive years, hyperplasia is relatively uncommon, typically occurring in women with polycystic ovarian disease (Stein–Leventhal syndrome). In the original description of this syndrome, the women were reported to be anovulatory, obese, infertile, and exhibit hirsutism, but many women with this disorder lack some of these features. Conversely, women who are obese but who do not have polycystic ovarian disease may have hyperplasia, presumably as a result of peripheral conversion of androstenedione to estrogen in adipose tissue.

The findings of diabetes mellitus and hypertension described in association with endometrial carcinoma may occur in women with hyperplasia, but often none of these associated disorders is present. Most hyperplasias that occur in perimenopausal women are associated with anovulation. Postmenopausal women who develop hyperplasia usually are on unopposed estrogen hormone replacement therapy. In these women, the hyperplasia is almost invariably manifested by abnormal bleeding. Although hyperplasia or carcinoma should always be suspected in a postmenopausal woman with bleeding, atrophy is by far the most common cause of abnormal uterine bleeding in this age group. In one study of postmenopausal women with bleeding, 7% had endometrial cancer, 15% had various types of hyperplasia, and 56% had atrophy.[56] Typically, women with hyperplasia or carcinoma have moderate or heavy vaginal bleeding compared with women with atrophic endometria who present with spotting.

Pathologic Findings

Hyperplastic endometrium is not distinctive grossly. In hysterectomy specimens, hyperplasia usually presents a velvety, knobby surface of pale, spongy tissue with vague borders. Diffuse thickening is typical, but focal overgrowth may occur and simulate a polyp. The volume of tissue obtained in curettings is usually increased, but it may be quite variable and less than that obtained during the secretory phase of the normal cycle. A diagnosis of hyperplasia, therefore, depends on the histologic pattern and not on the volume of tissue. A small volume of tissue may reflect inadequate sampling.

Hyperplasia Without Cytologic Atypia

Hyperplasia is characterized by an increased gland/stroma ratio and a variety of abnormal architectural patterns. Glands typically vary in size and shape. Dilatation and outpouching of glandular epithelium into the stroma characterize the lesser degrees of architectural abnormalities. Thus, in *simple hyperplasia* the glands are cystically dilated, with occasional outpouchings surrounded by an abundant cellular stroma. In other instances, the glands are only minimally dilated but focally crowded. Admixtures of the various patterns frequently occur (Figs. 11.1 and 11.2). The cells lining the glands are pseudostratified and columnar with amphophilic cytoplasm. Mitotic activity is variable.

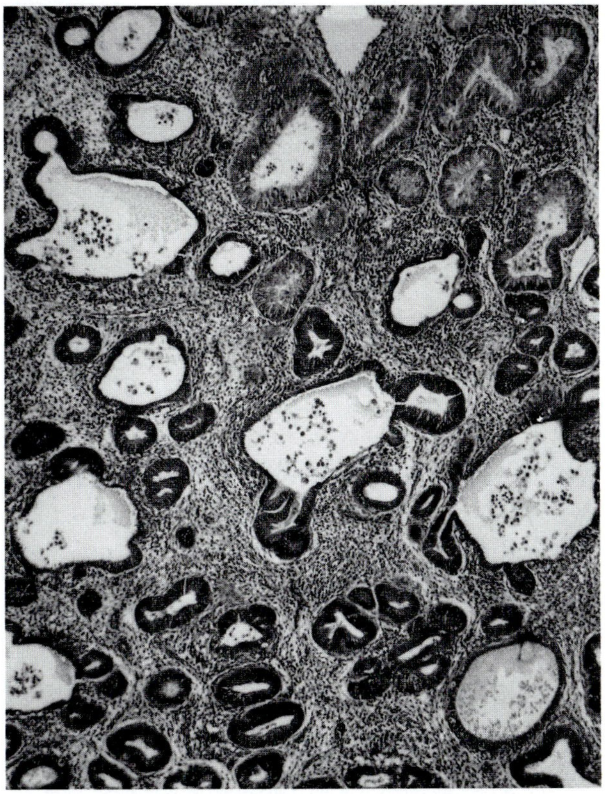

Fig. 11.1. Simple hyperplasia. The lesion is characterized by dilated glands with glandular outpouchings. (Reprinted by permission of Kurman et al., ref. 52.)

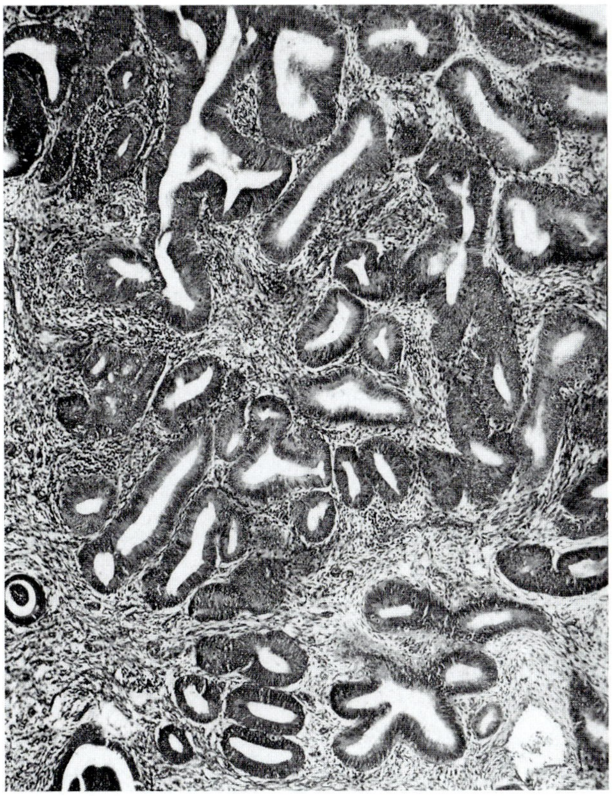

Fig. 11.2. Simple hyperplasia. There is slight crowding of glands that are abnormally branched. (Reprinted by permission of Kurman et al., ref. 52.)

With increasing degrees of architectural abnormality, glands become complex and branched with irregular outlines and papillary infoldings into the lumens. In addition, with increased proliferation glands become crowded, compressing the intervening stroma, resulting in "back-to-back" glandular crowding. Thus, *complex hyperplasia* is composed of crowded glands with little intervening stroma[52] (Figs. 11.3 and 11.4). Usually the glandular outlines are highly complex but at times are tubular. Epithelial stratification and mitotic activity generally parallel the architectural complexity, but sometimes they are discordant. Epithelial stratification can range from two to four layers, but some glands may exhibit little or no stratification. Mitotic activity is variable and is usually less than five mitotic figures

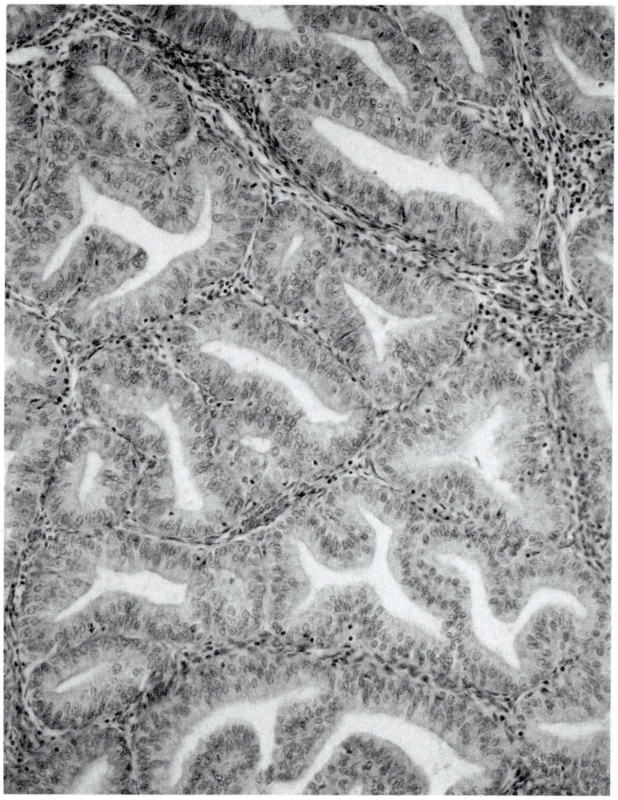

Fig. 11.3. Complex hyperplasia. There is marked glandular crowding resulting in a "back-to-back" appearance.

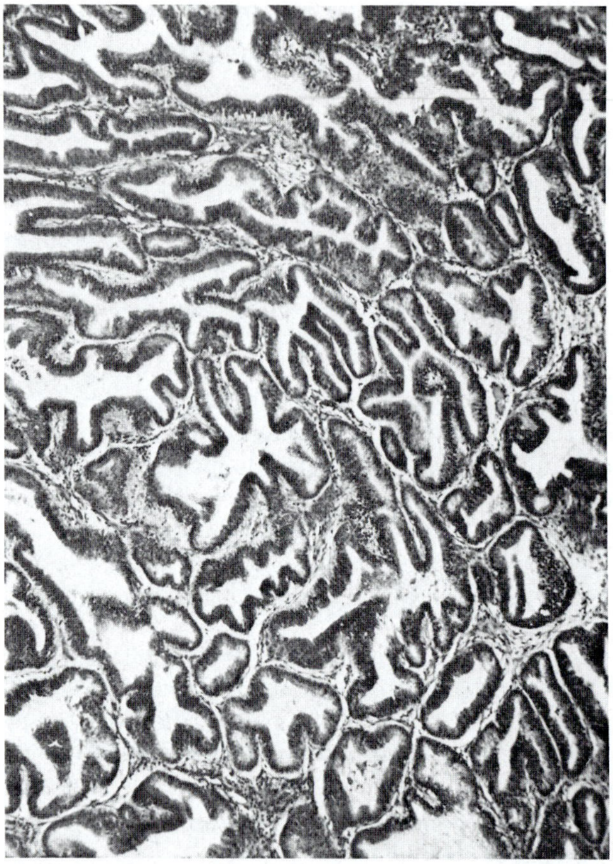

Fig. 11.4. Complex hyperplasia. The lesion is characterized by glands with complex glandular outlines that are markedly crowded. There is no cytologic atypia. (Reprinted by permission of Kurman et al., ref. 52.)

per 10 high power fields. Even in highly complex hyperplasia with marked stratification, mitotic figures may be inconspicuous. Cells of a hyperplasia lacking nuclear atypia contain oval, basally oriented bland nuclei with smooth, uniform contours resembling those in normal proliferative glands (Fig. 11.5).

In simple hyperplasia, the stromal cells are more densely packed than in proliferative endometrium. The cells retain their spindle shape but are plump, with enlarged nuclei and indistinct cytoplasm. Mitotic activity in endometrial stromal cells is variable but may be increased. Cytologic atypia is rarely observed. In the complex forms of hyperplasia, the stromal cells are spindle shaped and become compressed by the glandular proliferation. In addition to densely packed stromal cells, clusters of foamy, lipid-laden cells (Fig. 11.6) can occur in the stroma of simple and complex hyperplasias, atypical hyperplasias, and well-differentiated adenocarcinomas.[21,73,74,82] Foam cells have small pyknotic nuclei and cytoplasm that contain lipid droplets but no mucin. The foam cells have been shown to be histiocytes by immunohistochemistry.[82] These histiocytic cells may also be observed in atrophic and nonneoplastic endometria. The isolated finding of histiocytes in the cervicovaginal smears of asymptomatic postmenopausal women has not been associated with an increased likelihood of detecting endometrial hyperplasia or carcinoma.[34] The presence of histiocytes alone in cervicovaginal smears from postmenopausal women with abnormal uterine bleeding also has not been shown to predict the presence of either endometrial hyperplasia or carcinoma. However, the finding of histiocytes containing phagocytosed acute inflammatory cells or normal endometrial cells in postmenopausal women with abnormal uterine bleeding has been associated with a three- to fourfold greater likelihood of coexistent endometrial carcinoma or hyperplasia.[65]

Atypical Hyperplasia

The most important feature in the evaluation of endometrial hyperplasia is the presence or absence of *nuclear atypia.* Cells with nuclear atypia are stratified and show loss of polarity and an increase in the

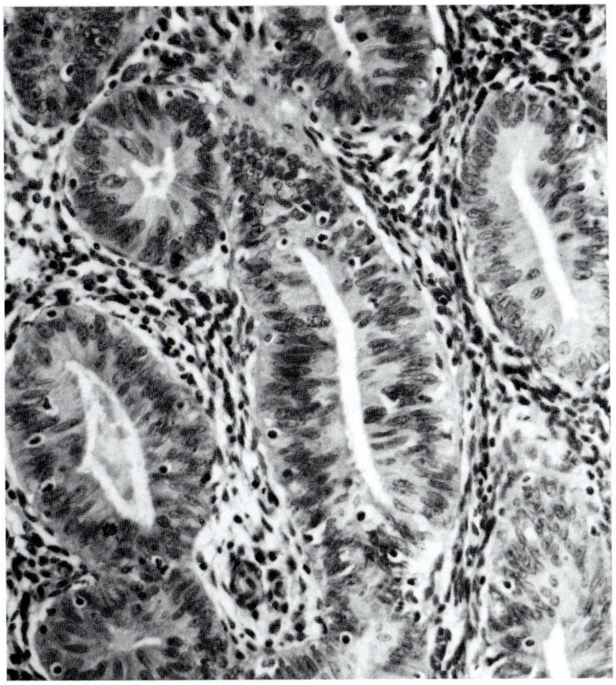

Fig. 11.5. Hyperplasia without atypia. The cells contain nuclei that are cigar shaped and resemble those in proliferative endometrium.

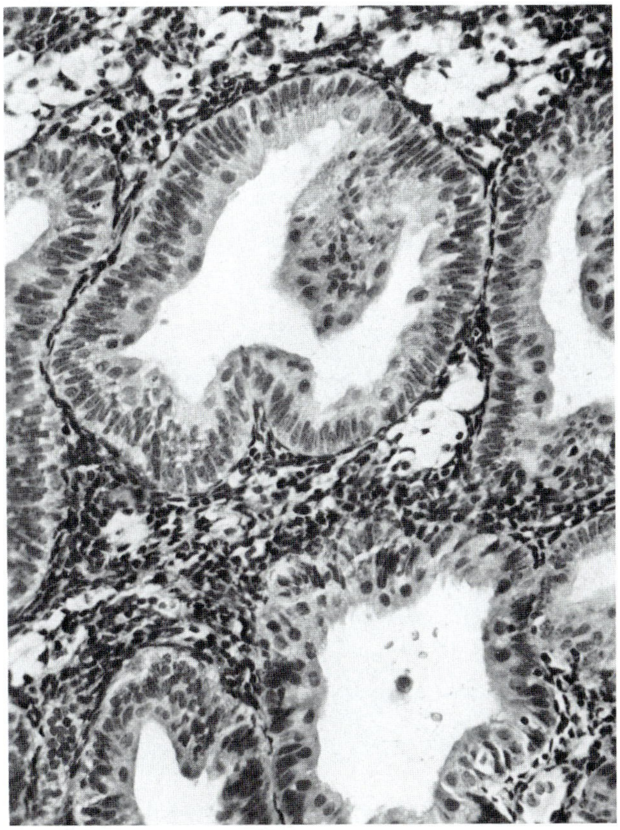

Fig. 11.6. Complex hyperplasia. Clusters of foamy, lipid-laden histiocytes are present in the stroma.

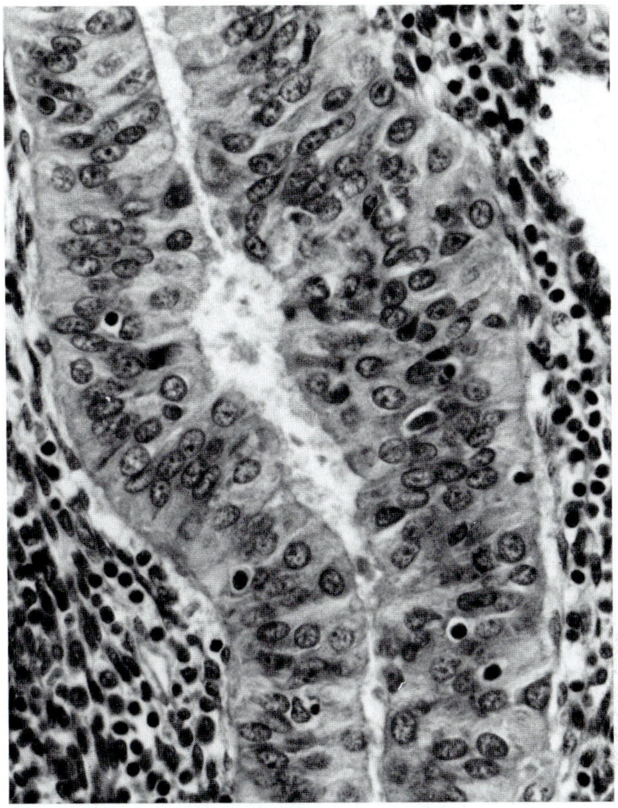

Fig. 11.7. Hyperplasia with atypia. The cells are stratified with loss of polarity. Nuclei are rounded, with granular chromatin, and appear vesicular.

nuclear/cytoplasmic ratio (Fig. 11.7). The nuclei are enlarged, irregular in size and shape, with coarse chromatin clumping, a thickened irregular nuclear membrane, and prominent nucleoli. Nuclei tend to be round as compared with the oval nuclei of proliferative endometrium and hyperplasia without atypia. As a result, the nuclei often have a cleared or vesicular appearance with condensation of the chromatin around the nuclear membrane. Nuclear atypia is variable, both qualitatively and quantitatively. Not all glands contain atypical cells, and in an individual gland some cells are atypical and others are not. Rare atypical cells should be ignored, but if cellular atypia is evident without a diligent search, the diagnosis of atypical hyperplasia should be made. Grading atypia as mild, moderate, or severe is subjective and not reproducible.

The architectural features of atypical simple and complex hyperplasia are similar to their nonatypical counterparts. The glandular outlines in simple atypical hyperplasia may be relatively simple with minimal complexity or they may be more irregular with intraglandular tufting. They are separated by abundant stroma; back-to-back glands are absent

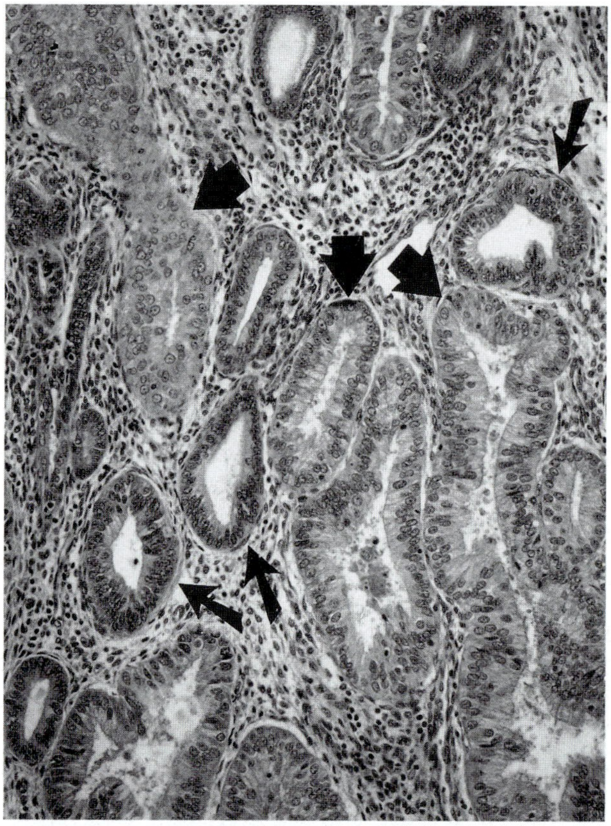

Fig. 11.8. Simple atypical hyperplasia. The glands are lined by atypical cells (*broad arrows*) that are separated by fairly abundant endometrial stroma from glands with no cytologic atypia (*narrow arrows*). (Reprinted by permission of Kurman et al., ref. 52.)

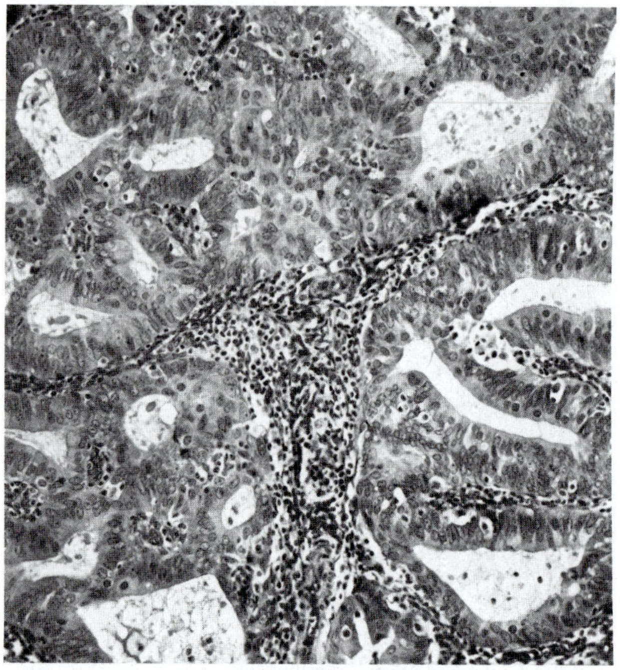

Fig. 11.9. Complex atypical hyperplasia. The lesion is characterized by glands with a complex pattern. The cells lining the glands show cytologic atypia.

(Fig. 11.8). In complex atypical hyperplasia, the glands almost invariably demonstrate marked structural complexity with irregular outlines and back-to-back crowding (Fig. 11.9). Epithelial stratification, and mitotic activity are variable. Papillary infoldings also are seen. Some atypical hyperplasias may have little stratification, and mitotic activity may be inconspicuous.

Differential Diagnosis

Simple and complex hyperplasia must be distinguished from disordered proliferative phase, polyps, ciliated cell change (tubal metaplasia), cystic atrophy, and endometrial glandular and stromal breakdown. *Disordered proliferative phase* is similar qualitatively to simple hyperplasia but is a focal lesion (Fig. 11.10). Disordered proliferative phase is characterized by irregularly shaped and enlarged glands that are focally interspersed among normal proliferative glands. The latter may be focally crowded. The key feature that distinguishes disordered proliferative phase from simple hyperplasia is the focal

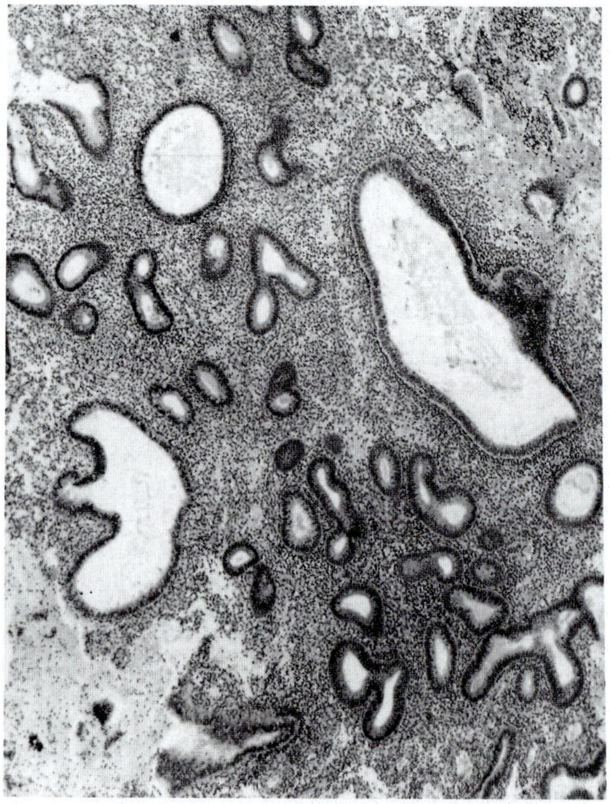

Fig. 11.10. Disordered proliferative phase. The lesion is characterized by occasional cystically dilated glands with outpouchings intermixed with normal proliferative endometrial glands.

nature of the glandular abnormality in disordered proliferative phase. The fragments of endometrium containing the disordered glands should not have the appearance of a polyp. Hyperplastic endometrial polyps often contain areas of simple and complex hyperplasia that are confined to one or just a few fragments of polypoid tissue. The polyp usually stands out as a large rounded tissue fragment in sharp contrast to the remainder of the uninvolved endometrium. Polyps typically have dense fibrous stroma and contain clusters of thick-walled blood vessels near the center of the fragment. The fragments usually are covered on three sides by surface endometrium (see Chapter 10, Benign Diseases of the Endometrium).

Endometrial glands with ciliated cell change are often found in association with simple and complex hyperplasia. When found with hyperplasia, the presence of ciliated cell change does not need to be specified. Ciliated glands are usually slightly dilated. When a few isolated glands show ciliated cell change in the absence of hyperplasia, a diagnosis of ciliated cell change (tubal metaplasia) is justified (see following).

Distinction of cystic atrophy from simple hyperplasia is seldom a problem in curettings because atrophic glands are separated by little intervening stroma and collapse during the procedure. In hysterectomy specimens, glands are not collapsed but are dilated and lined by a single layer of cells that are often flattened. Mitotic activity is not present. In contrast, in simple hyperplasia there is pseudostratification of columnar epithelial cells. Mitotic activity is variable but present in hyperplasia.

In endometrial glandular and stromal breakdown caused by estrogen withdrawal, proliferative-type glands appear back to back because of loss of intervening endometrial stroma. Glands are often fragmented, and nuclear dust typically is present in the cytoplasm. Clusters of stromal cells and fragmented glands surrounded by blood are consistent features (see Chapter 10, Benign Diseases of the Endometrium). In contrast, in complex hyperplasia the glandular outlines are more irregular and complex than the tubular, proliferative-type glands in breakdown. Furthermore, glandular fragmentation, nuclear dust, and clusters of stromal cells are usually absent in hyperplasia.

Atypical hyperplasia must be distinguished from an atypical polypoid adenomyoma and from well-differentiated adenocarcinoma. The *atypical polypoid adenomyoma* is composed of glands that show variable architectural complexity and some cytologic atypia. Squamous differentiation in the form of squamous morules is an almost constant feature of the atypical polypoid adenomyoma. Characteristically, the glands in the atypical polypoid adenomyoma are surrounded by smooth muscle in contrast with the dense proliferative stroma found in hyperplasia and the altered or desmoplastic stroma found in association with well-differentiated carcinoma (Fig. 11.11).

Most endometrial carcinomas are readily identified, but it may be difficult to distinguish some *well-differentiated carcinomas* from atypical hyperplasia. The two conditions can be separated if specific criteria are used to reduce the subjectivity of the appraisal. The stroma interacts with invasive carcinoma,[41,57] and the morphologic changes it undergoes can serve as a means of identifying carcinoma. The stromal and epithelial alterations associated with invasive carcinoma are referred to collectively as endometrial stromal invasion. There are three useful criteria, any of which identifies stromal invasion: (1) an irregular infiltration of glands associated with an altered fibroblastic stroma (desmoplastic response); (2) a confluent glandular

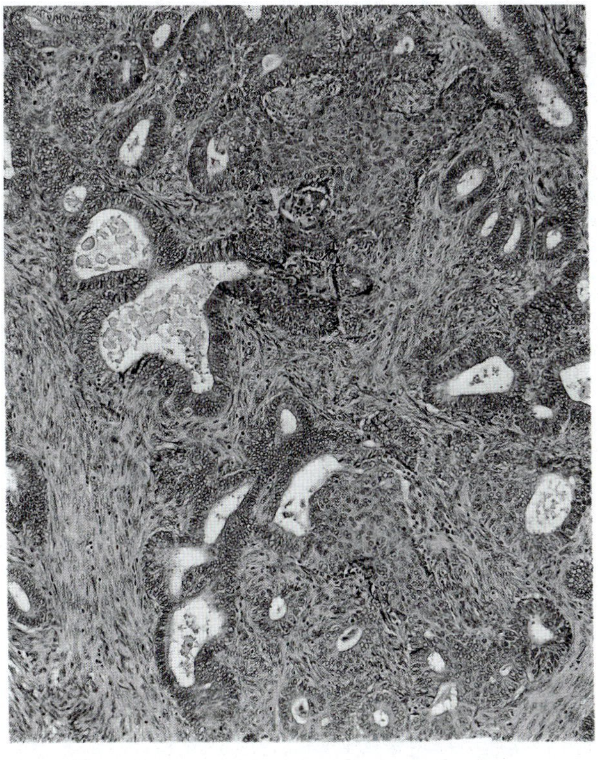

Fig. 11.11. Atypical polypoid adenomyoma. The stroma is composed of smooth muscle and myofibroblasts in bundles and fascicles simulating the desmoplastic response in invasive carcinoma. The glands are crowded and irregular and contain squamous morules.

pattern in which individual glands, uninterrupted by stroma, merge at times creating a cribriform pattern; and (3) an extensive papillary pattern. A process manifesting the features of invasion must be sufficiently extensive to involve half (2.1 mm) of a low-power field 4.2 mm in diameter to have value in predicting the presence of a biologically significant carcinoma in the uterus.[53,66] This criterion, however, should not be applied too rigidly in view of the potential of missing a carcinoma in small samples. If unequivocal evidence of stromal invasion is present in an area measuring less than one-half a low-power field, a diagnosis of well-differentiated carcinoma should be made. The quantification criterion does not apply to moderately or poorly differentiated carcinomas. The three criteria for the identification of stromal invasion are described in greater detail next.

1. The altered stroma that reflects invasion contains parallel, densely arranged fibroblasts with more fibrosis than normal endometrial stroma and disrupts the usual glandular pattern (Fig. 11.12). The stromal cells are more spindle shaped than are the stromal cells of proliferative endometrium, with more elongated nuclei. Collagen compresses the stromal cells so that they have an eosinophilic and wavy appearance (Fig. 11.13), compared with the basophilic naked-nucleus appearance of stromal cells found in proliferative endometrium and hyperplasia (Figs. 11.14 and 11.15). In some curettings, fragments of fibrous, relatively glandular polyps, or stroma from the lower segment of the uterus may have a similar appearance, making distinction of hyperplasia from carcinoma difficult or impossible. Atypical polypoid adenomyomas (see Chapter 10, Benign Diseases of the Endometrium) contain smooth muscle and may simulate myometrial invasion (see Fig. 11.11).[60] In contrast with the atypical polypoid adenomyoma, smooth muscle is rarely identified in curettings of well-differentiated carcinoma even when there is deep myometrial invasion because only the exophytic portion of the tumor is removed in biopsies and curettings.

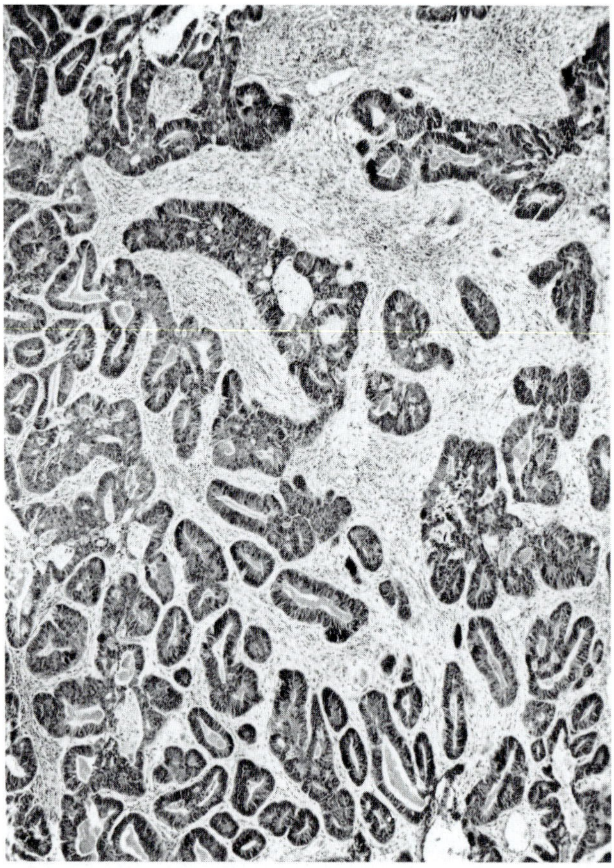

Fig. 11.12. Well-differentiated carcinoma. An altered stroma (desmoplastic stromal response) results in a haphazard glandular pattern.

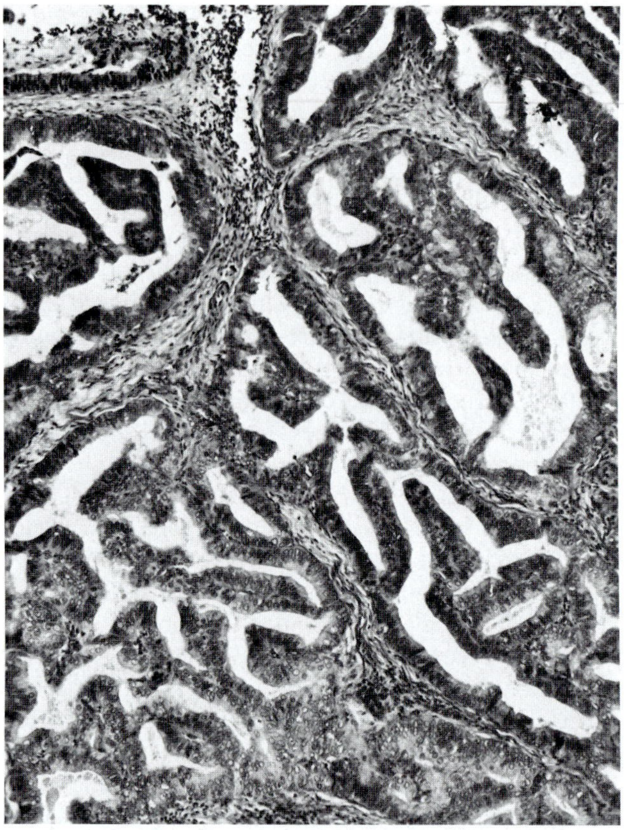

Fig. 11.13. Well-differentiated carcinoma. The altered stroma contains parallel fibroblasts that produce collagen and have an eosinophilic, wavy appearance.

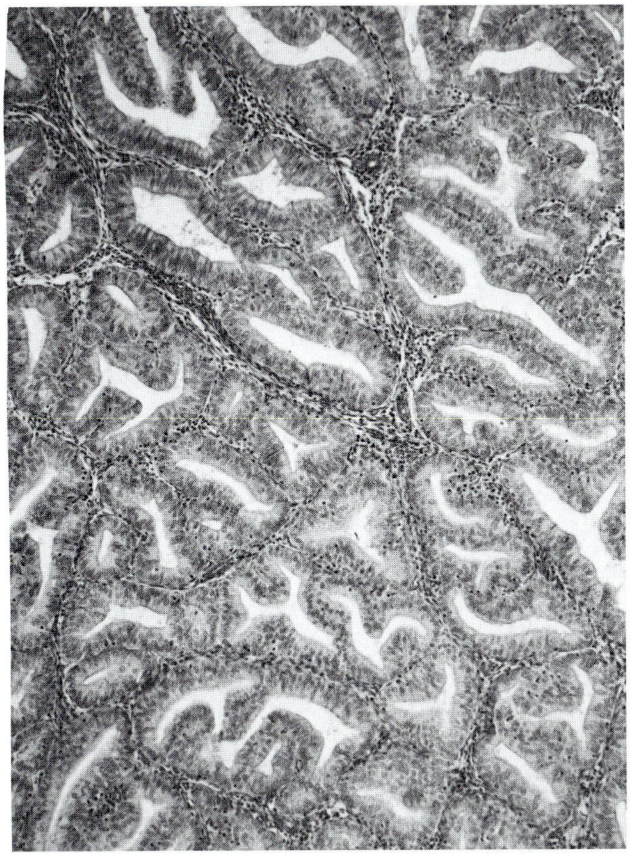

Fig. 11.14. Atypical hyperplasia. There is marked glandular crowding resulting in compression of the endometrial stroma. The stromal cells are spindle shaped.

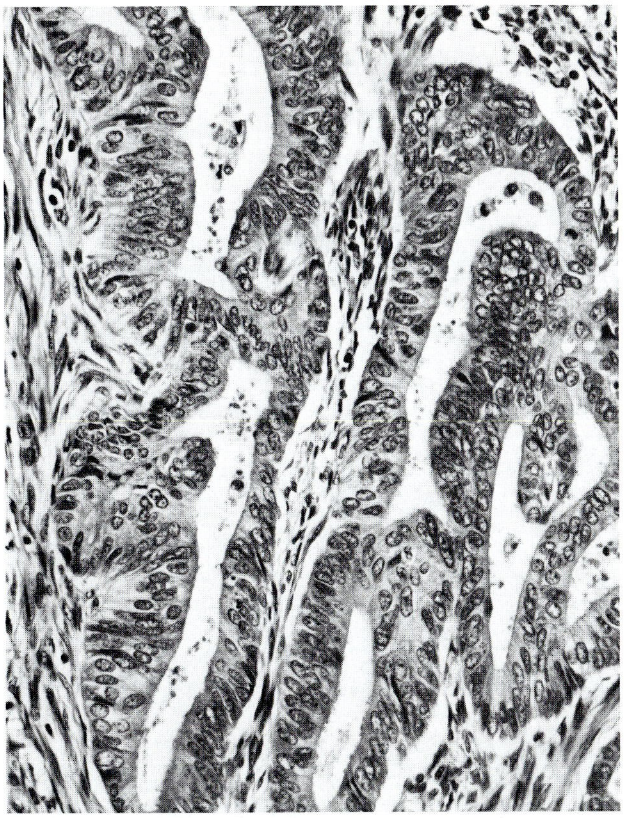

Fig. 11.15. Atypical hyperplasia. The endometrial stromal cells are spindle shaped with scant cytoplasm similar to that found in proliferative endometrium.

2. Confluent glandular aggregates without intervening stroma reflect stromal invasion (Fig. 11.16). Confluent patterns are characterized by glandular configurations in which individual glands are not surrounded by stroma. Instead, glands appear to merge into one another to form a complex labyrinth. Some proliferations are cribriform, resulting from proliferation and bridging of epithelium (Fig. 11.17).
3. Complex papillary patterns represent stromal invasion if multiple, branching, thin fibrous processes lined by epithelium are present (Fig. 11.18). At times, these may create a villoglandular pattern. Epithelial papillations lacking a fibrovascular core do not qualify as a feature of invasion.

In the past, the presence of masses of *squamous epithelium* replacing the endometrial stroma was considered a feature of invasion.[53] Masses of squamous epithelium with minimal nuclear atypia that extensively replace the endometrium (over a 2-mm^2 area) reflect stromal invasion only if they are asso-

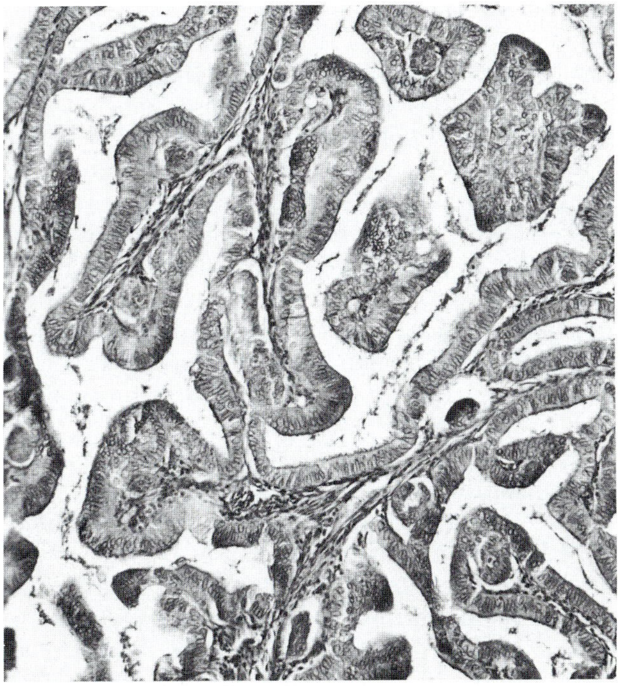

Fig. 11.16. Well-differentiated carcinoma. Stromal invasion is manifested by a confluent glandular pattern in which glandular epithelium interconnects one gland with another.

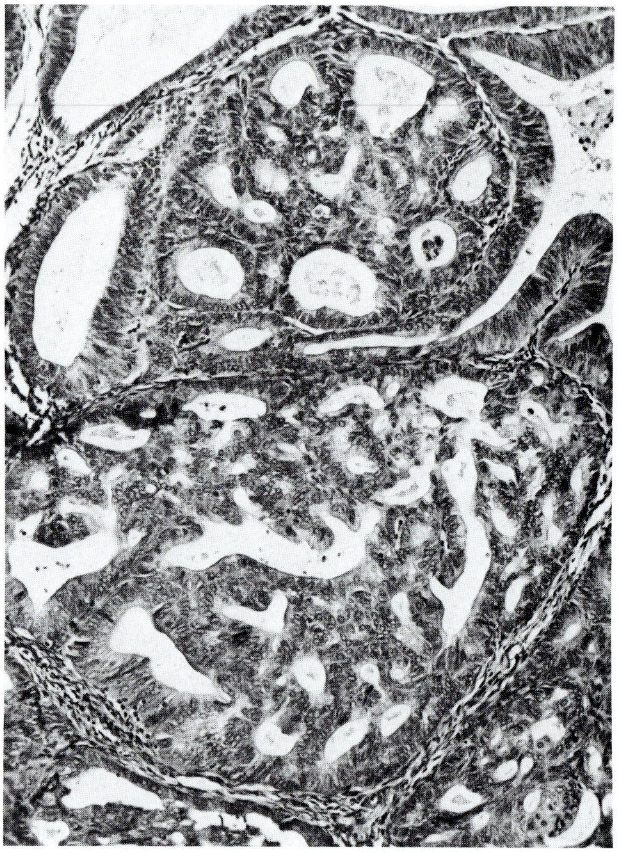

Fig. 11.17. Well-differentiated carcinoma. A confluent glandular pattern of stromal invasion creating a cribriform arrangement. (Reprinted by permission of Kurman and Norris, ref. 53.)

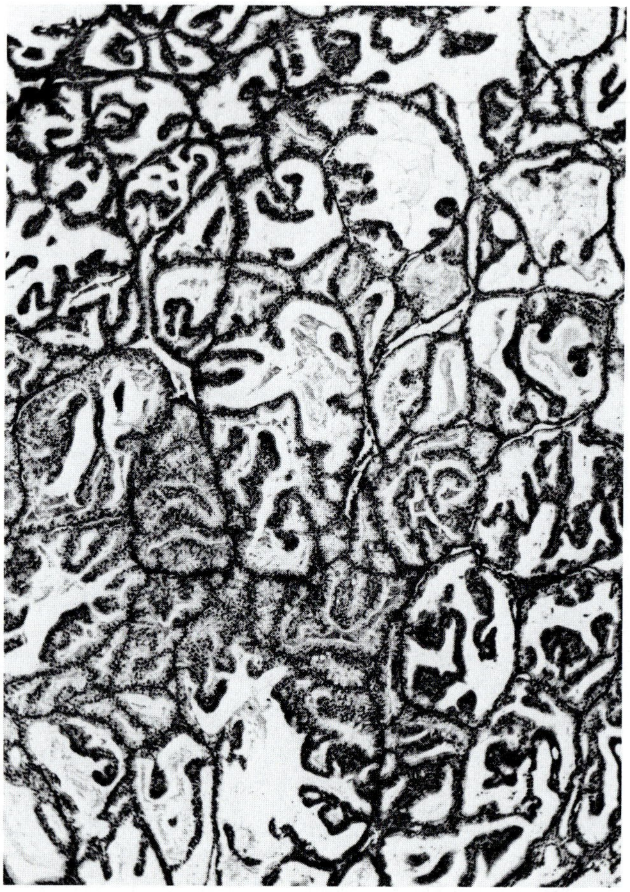

Fig. 11.18. Well-differentiated carcinoma. The complex papillary pattern is extensive enough to indicate stromal invasion.

ciated with a desmoplastic response (Fig. 11.19) or a confluent glandular pattern (Fig. 11.20).

Increasing degrees of nuclear atypia, mitotic activity, and stratification of cells in curettings are associated with a higher frequency of carcinoma in the uterus but are of limited value because even a mild degree of these changes is associated with carcinoma in nearly one-third of cases.[53] Even with mild atypia, low mitotic activity, and lesser degrees of stratification in curettings, 20% of residual carcinomas in the resected uterus are moderately or poorly differentiated, and 10% deeply invade the myometrium. These other features in curettings, although useful, therefore are not sufficiently accurate to predict whether a biologically significant lesion is present in the uterus. Unfortunately, assessing varying degrees of nuclear atypia in this borderline group of lesions is subjective and not easily reproduced. In contrast, when stromal invasion is absent in curettings, carcinoma is found in the uterus in only 17% of cases, and all the carcinomas are well differentiated and either confined to the endometrium or only superficially invasive (Table 11.2).

If stromal invasion is present in curettings, residual carcinoma is found in the uterus in half; more than one-third of the carcinomas are moderately or poorly differentiated, and a fourth of them invade deeply into the myometrium (Table 11.3). A small proportion (7%) of patients with invasion in curettings will have extrauterine metastases at hysterectomy, and half with metastasis will die of tumor.[53] Thus, the absence of stromal invasion provides the basis for distinguishing atypical hyperplasia from a biologically significant, well-differentiated carcinoma.[48,53] Two more recent studies, however, found higher frequencies of endometrial carcinoma (43% and 50%) in hysterectomy specimens following a diagnosis of atypical hyperplasia.[42,96] Of the carcinomas detected in both studies, 43% were stage 1C or greater. These studies included patients who had been diagnosed by either curettage or biopsy, but there were no significant differences in the frequencies with which carcinoma was detected at hysterectomy in those patients who received a curettage compared to those who had been biopsied. However, in one of these studies, the biopsy and

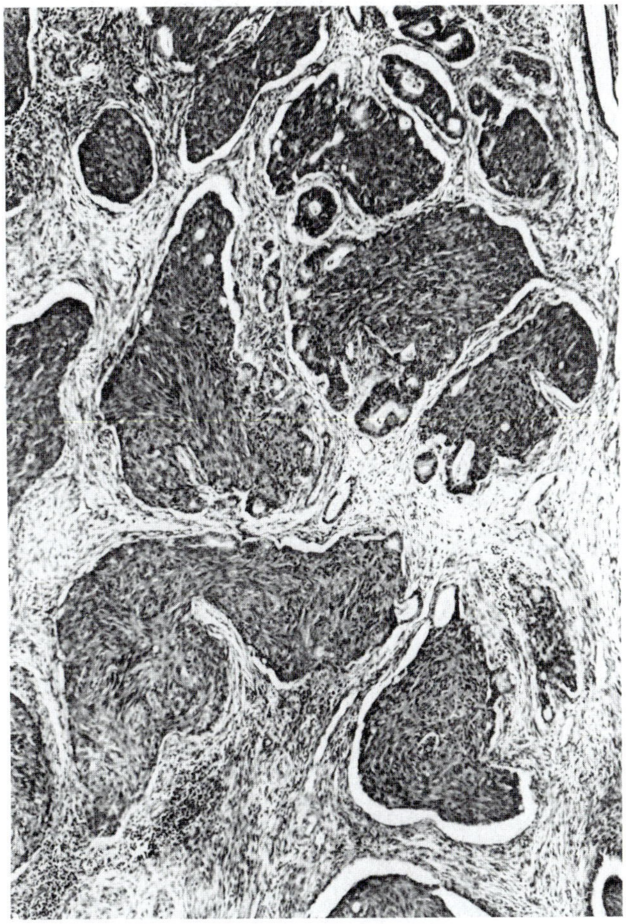

Fig. 11.19. Well-differentiated carcinoma with squamous differentiation (squamous metaplasia). The squamous cells expand out of gland lumens into the surrounding stroma. The diagnosis of stromal invasion is based on the desmoplastic reaction in the stroma.

curettage specimens were not reviewed to confirm that features of stromal invasion were absent in these specimens.[42] More recently, another study has demonstrated that clinically significant endometrial proliferations, that is, those that have a high likelihood of myometrial invasion, can be recognized when either sufficient architectural complexity or nuclear atypia, including prominence of nucleoli, is present.[58] In addition, the strong association of a desmoplastic stromal response with a myoinvasive lesion was confirmed.

The identification of stromal invasion in curettings has two advantages: (1) it is semiquantitative and, therefore, less subjective than other criteria; and (2) it delineates a biologically significant lesion, one having a much greater likelihood of metastasis than one in which invasion is absent. Experimental studies of neoplasms from the breast, colon, pancreas, and lung lend support to the division of endometrial proliferations into noninvasive and invasive forms based on the histologic alterations observed in the endometrial stroma. These studies demonstrate profound molecular and structural alterations in the stroma adjacent to invasive as

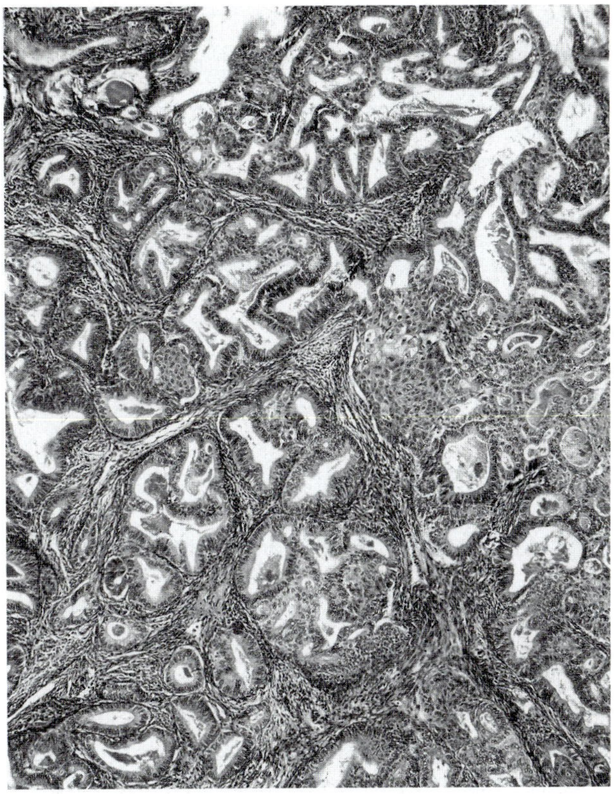

Fig. 11.20. Well-differentiated carcinoma with squamous differentiation. The diagnosis of carcinoma is based on the confluent glandular pattern and altered stroma (desmoplastic response).

Table 11.2. Hysterectomy findings when atypical hyperplasia[a] is present in curettings (89 patients)

Finding	*No. (%)*
Carcinoma	15 (17)
Grade	
Well differentiated	15 (100)
Moderately differentiated	0
Poorly differentiated	0
Myometrial invasion	
None	8 (53)[b]
Inner one-third	7 (47)[b]
1 mm or less	5
2–4 mm	2

[a]A diagnosis of atypical hyperplasia based on cytological atypia in the absence of endometrial stromal invasion.
[b]The percentages refer to the proportion of carcinomas in the hysterectomy specimen.
Adapted with permission from Kurman and Norris, ref. 53.

Table 11.3. Hysterectomy findings when well-differentiated carcinoma[a] is present in curettings (115 patients)

Finding	*No. (%)*
Carcinoma	58 (50)
Grade	
Well differentiated	38 (66)[b]
Moderately differentiated	14 (24)[b]
Poorly differentiated	6 (10)[b]
Myometrial invasion	42 (72)[b]
Inner-one-third	28 (48)[b]
Middle and outer third	14 (24)[b]

[a]A diagnosis of well-differentiated carcinoma based on identification of endometrial stromal invasion.
[b]The percentages refer to the proportion of carcinomas in the hysterectomy specimen.
Adapted with permission from Kurman and Norris, ref. 53.

compared with noninvasive tumors.[41,57,75,77] Invasive tumors can induce a conversion of stromal fibroblasts into myofibroblasts, which elaborate extracellular matrix components, such as type V collagen and proteoglycans, that are increased in desmoplasia and are readily observed by light microscopy using the criteria for stromal invasion as outlined. It has been shown that tumor cells produce growth factors such as platelet-derived growth factor,[72] epidermal-derived growth factor, and insulin-like growth factor,[51] which may play a role in stimulating the growth of stromal cells surrounding tumors.[37]

Adjunctive Techniques in the Classification of Endometrial Hyperplasias and Prediction of Coexistent Carcinoma

Few studies have addressed the reproducibility of the diagnosis of endometrial hyperplasia and its distinction from well-differentiated carcinoma. One study that compared diagnostic reproducibility using the 1975 and 1994 WHO classifications of endometrial hyperplasia and carcinoma found that interobserver agreement was fair to moderate with both systems.[84] A subsequent study of 100 endometrial biopsy and curettage specimens ranging from proliferative endometrium to well-differentiated carcinoma found substantial interobserver agreement for diagnoses of hyperplasia and well-differentiated carcinoma but only moderate agreement for the diagnosis of atypical hyperplasia.[46] Several histologic features, including nuclear enlargement, vesicular change, nuclear pleomorphism, chromatic irregularities, loss of polarity, nuclear rounding, and presence of nucleoli, were associated with a diagnosis of atypical hyperplasia by univariable logistic regression analysis. However, of the histologic features evaluated, the only feature that was associated with the distinction of atypical hyperplasia from hyperplasia without atypia in multivariable logistic regression analysis was the presence of nucleoli.

The features that were associated with the distinction of carcinoma from atypical hyperplasia in both univariable and multivariable analysis included stromal alteration (stromal desmoplasia) and glandular confluence. A more recent study found similar values for intraobserver agreement and slightly lower values for interobserver agreement.[11] In addition, the study confirmed that the category of atypical hyperplasia has the lowest diagnostic reproducibility of the various categories. Similar histologic features were found to be useful for distinguishing the various diagnostic categories, although the utility of the presence of nucleoli for diagnosing atypical hyperplasia and of stromal alteration for diagnosing well-differentiated carcinoma were somewhat less, as evidenced by lower mean interobserver agreement values for these features. Thus, interobserver agreement is lowest for the diagnostic category of atypical hyperplasia, indicating that further refinement of the histologic criteria used to make the diagnosis of atypical hyperplasia is needed.

Some investigators have attempted to use computerized morphometric analyses of endometrial hyperplasias to predict coexistent carcinoma in hysterectomy specimens.[3,5–7,24] Nuclear morphometry alone has been shown to be insufficiently sensitive and specific to properly distinguish hyperplasias that are associated with carcinoma from those that are not.[3,5] In contrast, the combination of architectural and nuclear morphometric features has been shown to be useful for predicting risk of endometrial carcinoma in patients with hyperplasia.[6,7,24] In particular, the morphometric analysis of endometrial lesions involves the calculation of a score (D-score) that predicts the likelihood of finding coexistent carcinoma or future progression to carcinoma. The D-score incorporates volume percentage stroma, standard deviation of the shortest nuclear axis, and gland outer surface density. Studies have demonstrated that the D-score is more sensitive and specific than the WHO classification for predicting risk of progression of endometrial hyperplasia to carcinoma.[8,9,24] Although morphometric analysis has been shown to be reproducible, it is more labor-intensive and costly than is practical for many laboratories.

More recently, investigators have proposed that endometrial proliferations be broadly divided into two categories based on the molecular genetic analysis of clonality.[62–64] Proliferations that are polyclonal are regarded as a response to an abnormal hormonal environment—either unopposed estrogenic stimulation associated with anovulatory cycles or exogenous estrogenic stimulation—and are designated "hyperplasia." Monoclonal lesions, on the other hand, are associated with an increased risk of progression to carcinoma and are designated "endometrial intraepithelial neoplasia" (EIN). The rationale cited for this approach is that therapy for hyperplasia should be aimed at treating the suspected cause and symptoms, whereas EIN should be removed or ablated. However, because clonality cannot routinely be performed on diagnostic specimens in most laboratories, it has been proposed that the diagnosis of EIN be made when glandular crowding results in a volume percentage of stroma less than 55%. Ideally, this parameter would be assessed by morphometric analysis (calculation of D-score), (calculation of D-score), which has been shown to separate hyperplasias, particularly those classified as non-atypical by light microscopic assessment, into monoclonal and polyclonal lesions.[63] For practicality, routine light microscopic assessment aided by an ocular graticule and a web-based tutorial that correlates patterns of endometrial proliferations with clonality data has been proposed as an alternative to morphometry. However, it is not clear how volume percentage stroma as a measure of glandular crowding in the hyperplasia–EIN system differs from the back-to-back glandular crowding that is required for a diagnosis of complex atypical hyperplasia (CAH) in the WHO classification. In addition, the diagnostic reproducibility of the light microscopic assessment of volume percentage stroma has not been determined. Finally, cytologic atypia that allegedly differs from atypia as shown in the WHO classification is required for the diagnosis of EIN but criteria for its diagnosis have not been published. Thus, when compared to a simplified version of the WHO classification system that collapses the four categories into two (hyperplasia and atypical hyperplasia), it is not clear that these new categories of hyperplasia and EIN differ from the WHO categories of hyperplasia and atypical hyperplasia. In the future, molecular genetic data will undoubtedly play a role in the classification of these lesions. At present, however, the proposed hyperplasia–EIN classification system is not recommended for clinical practice.

Behavior of Endometrial Hyperplasia

It has been noted[94] that most older studies[16,17,19,32,33,38,39,61,67] designed to determine the fate of untreated hyperplasia did not consider cytologic and architectural abnormalities separately. This shortcoming was avoided in a retrospective analysis of 170 patients with endometrial hyperplasia in curettings who were followed (mean, 13.4 years) without a hysterectomy being performed for at least 1 year.[52] Various histologic features were evaluated, and cytologic and architectural abnormalities were analyzed independently in an effort to delineate the histologic features associated with an increased risk of progression to carcinoma. A third of the patients with both nonatypical and atypical hyperplasia were asymptomatic after the diagnostic curettage and required no further treatment. Only 2 (2%) of 122 patients with hyperplasia lacking cytologic atypia, one with simple and one with complex hyperplasia (Tables 11.4 and 11.5), progressed to carcinoma. The two cases of hyperplasia that progressed underwent an alteration to atypical hyperplasia before developing into carcinoma. In contrast, 11 (23%) of the 48 women with atypical hyperplasia progressed to carcinoma ($p = 0.001$) (Table 11.6); 8% of patients with simple atypical hyperplasia and 29% of patients with complex atypical hyperplasia

Table 11.4. Chronological sequence of progression of simple hyperplasia to carcinoma over 11 years in one patient

Age (yr) of patient	*Diagnosis, treatment, follow-up*
21	Simple hyperplasia; no treatment
26	Term pregnancy
28	Atypical hyperplasia; no treatment
32	Grade 2 adenocarcinoma; TAH
60	Alive and well

TAH, total abdominal hysterectomy.
Adapted with permission from Kurman et al., ref. 52.

Table 11.5. Chronological sequence of progression of complex hyperplasia to carcinoma over 8 years in one patient

Age (yr) of patient	*Diagnosis, treatment, follow-up*
22	Complex hyperplasia Obese, infertile menometrorrhagia Clomid, Pergonal, bilateral wedge resection of ovaries No pregnancy
26	Atypical hyperplasia; no treatment
30	Grade 1 adenocarcinoma with squamous differentiation; TAH
43	Alive and well

TAH, total abdominal hysterectomy.
Adapted with permission from Kurman et al., ref. 52.

Table 11.6. Follow-up of hyperplasia and atypical hyperplasia in 170 patients

		Regressed		*Persisted*		*Progressed to carcinoma*	
Type of hyperplasia	*No. of patients*	*No.*	*(%)*	*No.*	*(%)*	*No.*	*(%)*
Hyperplasia	122	97	(80)	23	(19)	2	(2)
Atypical hyperplasia	48	29	(60)	8	(17)	11	(23)

Adapted with permission from Kurman et al., ref. 52.

progressed to carcinoma (Table 11.7). The presence of glandular complexity and crowding superimposed on atypia, therefore, appears to place the patient at greater risk than does cytologic atypia alone. The differences in progression to carcinoma among the four subgroups, however, were not statistically significant. Thus, cytologic atypia is the most useful feature in identifying a lesion that might progress to carcinoma. Similar findings have been reported by other investigators.[8,25]

The carcinomas that develop in patients with hyperplasia are relatively innocuous.[32,52] The mean duration of progression of hyperplasia without atypia to carcinoma is nearly 10 years, and it takes a mean of 4 years to progress from atypical hyperplasia to clinically evident carcinoma.[52] A comparison of the clinicopathologic features and behavior of the carcinomas developing after a diagnosis of atypical hyperplasia in women 40 years or younger compared with women over the age of 40 years is shown in Table 11.8. Although all but one of the carcinomas that developed from atypical hyperplasia were well differentiated and minimally invasive, one well-differentiated tumor that extended into the endocervix metastasized to the pelvic peritoneum and a paraaortic lymph node. After abdominal radiation the patient was disease free 19 years later. These findings and others[10] suggest that carcinomas associated with hyperplasia are relatively innocuous compared with carcinomas not associated with it.

It has been shown that 17–25% of women with atypical hyperplasia in curettings will have a well-differentiated carcinoma in the uterus if a hysterectomy is performed within 1 month of the curettage.[48,90] Increasing degrees of nuclear atypia, mitotic activity, and stratification of cells in curettings are associated with a higher frequency of carcinoma in the uterus. With long-term follow-up, however, only 11–23% of women with atypical hyperplasia develop carcinoma if a hysterectomy is not done.[32,52] Thus, the lesion designated as well-differentiated carcinoma usually remains stable for a long period of time. Several reasons may account for the relatively low rate of progression to carcinoma in untreated patients with atypical hyperplasia. First, there is a general tendency for the highest grade of atypical hyperplasia to be selected for hysterectomy, leaving the lesser degree of atypia for conservative management. Second, atypical hyperplasia may not be the precursor of all forms of endometrial cancer, but only of a type that is slowly progressive.

A more recent study of the behavior of endometrial hyperplasia found that most cases of endometrial hyperplasia without atypia regressed spontaneously whereas those with complex atypical hyperplasia were much more likely to persist.[91] Another recent study confirmed the significance of cy-

Table 11.7. Follow-up of simple and complex hyperplasia and atypical hyperplasia in 170 patients

		Regressed		*Persisted*		*Progressed to carcinoma*	
Type of hyperplasia	*No. of patients*	*No.*	*(%)*	*No.*	*(%)*	*No.*	*(%)*
Simple	93	74	(80)	18	(19)	1	(1)
Complex	29	23	(80)	5	(17)	1	(3)
Simple atypical	13	9	(69)	3	(23)	1	(8)
Complex atypical	35	20	(57)	5	(14)	10	(29)

Adapted with permission from Kurman et al., ref. 52.

Table 11.8. Clinical and pathological findings from 11 "untreated" women with progression of atypical hyperplasia to carcinoma

	40 years and younger (8 patients)	*Over 40 years (3 patients)*
Age range	23–40 years	43–50 years
Polycystic ovarian disease	4 (50%)	0
Obese	4 (50%)	1
Mean time of progression	3.3 years	7.8 years
Grade 1 adenocarcinoma	8 (100%)	2 (66%)
Grade 2 adenocarcinoma	0	1 (33%)
Carcinoma confined to endometrium or superficially invasive	8 (100%)	3 (100%)
Metastatic carcinoma	1[a]	0

[a]Grade 1 adenocarcinoma with squamous differentiation that extended to the endocervix subsequently metastasized to pelvic peritoneum and a paraaortic lymph node. Patient was treated with abdominal radiation and is alive and well 19 years later.
Adapted with permission from Kurman et al., ref. 52.

tologic atypia in predicting increased risk of associated endometrial carcinoma in hysterectomy specimens.[40] Because most atypical hyperplasias have complex architecture, it is complex atypical hyperplasia that is associated with a significant risk of persistence and progression to carcinoma. Hence, this lesion is regarded as a direct precursor of well-differentiated endometrioid carcinoma of the endometrium. However, hyperplasia is identified in a prior endometrial specimen or in the hysterectomy specimen in only 35–75% of women with endometrial carcinoma.[4,10,14,22,30,43] In those reports that specified the number of hyperplasias that were classified as atypical, 14–36% of women with endometrial carcinoma had associated atypical hyperplasia.[30,43] It is unclear whether failure to identify an associated atypical hyperplasia in all cases of endometrioid carcinoma reflects overgrowth of a preexisting hyperplasia by carcinoma or the development of carcinoma through a different pathway.

Management of Endometrial Hyperplasia

Management of patients with endometrial hyperplasia is based on a consideration of clinical factors in addition to the microscopic findings,[49] which include the desire to preserve fertility in young women and associated medical conditions that render older women at high risk for a surgical procedure.

Premenopausal Women (Less Than 40 Years of Age)

Most premenopausal women who present with abnormal bleeding have nonspecific hormonal disorders that are self-limited. These women are at low risk of having carcinoma (Table 11.9). In a study of 460 women 40 years of age and younger, 6 (1.3%) had "mild" hyperplasia (simple hyperplasia) but none had atypical hyperplasia or carcinoma.[45] Therefore, most women in this age group with abnormal bleeding do not require an endometrial biopsy. Women with risk factors for endometrial cancer, such as polycystic ovarian disease or obesity, and women with persistent bleeding should have an endometrial biopsy performed. Traditionally, evaluation of such patients has been by curettage in the operating room but it has been shown that office-based endometrial sampling devices such as the Pipelle device are comparable and are substantially less expensive, with 96% agreement between the biopsy and hysterectomy findings.[29,81,88] Even a curettage removes less than half of the endometrium in 60% of cases assessed immediately after the curettage by hysterectomy.[87]

If a diagnosis of simple or complex hyperplasia is made, the patient can be treated conservatively because these lesions have an extremely low risk (1–2%) of progression to carcinoma. Because the transit time to carcinoma is approximately 10 years and hyperplasia without cytologic atypia first progresses through atypical hyperplasia before becoming carcinoma (see Tables 11.4 and 11.5), follow-up and periodic endometrial biopsies suffice.[52] Conservative management of young women with simple hyperplasia and complex hyperplasia resulted in subsequent pregnancies in 29% and 20% of these women, respectively, in one study (Table 11.10).[52]

Table 11.9. Pertinent findings in endometrium in women with abnormal bleeding according to age

	Age					
	Premenopausal[a] *<40 years (n = 460)*		*Perimenopausal*[a] *40–55 years (n = 748)*		*Postmenopausal*[b] *>55 years (n = 226)*	
Finding in endometrial specimen[d]	*No.*	*(%)*	*No.*	*(%)*	*No.*	*(%)*
Carcinoma	0	(—)	3	(0.4)	15	(7)
Atypical hyperplasia	0	(—)	5	(0.7)	NK[c]	
Hyperplasia	6	(1)	41	(6)	34	(15)
Atrophy	7	(2)	51	(7)	127	(56)
Polyp	6	(1)	13	(2)	19	(8)
Proliferative	139	(29)	273	(36)	31	(14)
Secretory	241	(50)	287	(38)	0	(—)

NK, not known.
[a]Kaminski and Stevens, ref. 45.
[b]Lidor et al., ref. 56.
[c]A category of atypical hyperplasia was not specified in this study.
[d]Not all the endometrial findings in the study by Kaminski and Stevens are listed and therefore percentages do not total 100%.

Women with atypical hyperplasia on an endometrial biopsy who wish to preserve their fertility should be treated with progestin suppression. In view of the very similar accuracy of endometrial biopsy and curettage and the low risk of an associated endometrial carcinoma in women younger than 40 years of age, a curettage need not be performed to exclude carcinoma but close follow-up and periodic endometrial biopsies are necessary. A conservative plan of management is justified because the risk of progression to carcinoma in young women is low and the carcinomas that do develop tend to be innocuous (Fig. 11.21; Table 11.11); 20% of those women less than 40 years of age can subsequently become pregnant and have normal deliveries.[70]

Conservative management also can be considered for women diagnosed with well-differentiated carcinoma. A recent study of progestin treatment of atypical hyperplasia and well-differentiated carcinoma in women under age 40 found that 75% of women with carcinoma and 95% with atypical hyperplasia had regression of their lesions.[70] In addition, all patients were alive without evidence of progressive disease during the follow-up period. The median duration of progestin treatment necessary to effect regression was 9 months. In another study, 62% of women under 40 years treated with pro-gestins alone for endometrial carcinoma responded to the hormonal therapy, although 23% of these later developed recurrent disease.[47] Ninety percent of the patients were alive without evidence of disease during the follow-up period. The lower frequency of responders in this study may have been a result of the relatively short duration of the hormonal therapy. Thus, in premenopausal women, atypical hyperplasia and well-differentiated carcinoma can be regarded as a single clinicopathologic entity for management purposes. Histologic distinction of atypical hyperplasia from well-differentiated carcinoma is not critical because both lesions are highly responsive to progestin therapy. If conservative management is elected, magnetic resonance imaging (MRI) must be performed to ex-

Table 11.10. Subsequent pregnancies in "untreated" women with hyperplasia and atypical hyperplasia

Diagnosis	*No. of patients <40*	*No. of patients who became pregnant*	*No. of full-term pregnancies*
Simple hyperplasia	35	10 (29%)	19
Complex hyperplasia	15	3 (20%)	4
Atypical hyperplasia (simple and complex)	24	3 (13%)	4

Adapted from Kurman et al., ref. 52.

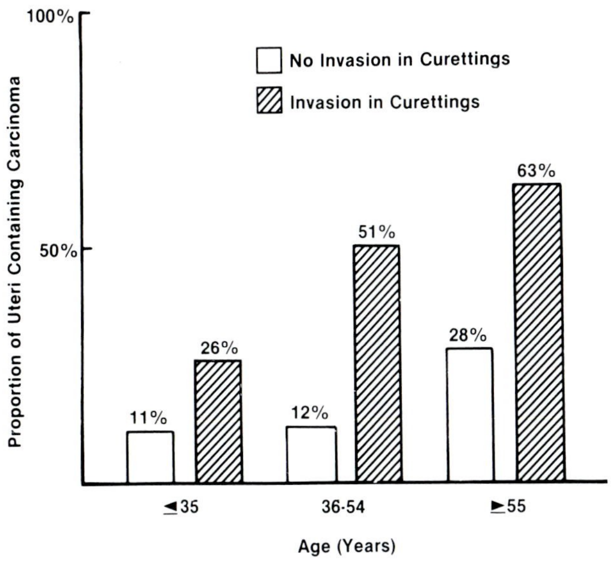

Fig. 11.21. Carcinoma in uterus according to age and presence of stromal invasion in curettings of 204 patients. There is a striking increase in residual carcinoma in the uteri of patients with atypical hyperplasia and well-differentiated adenocarcinoma in curettings with advancing age. (Adapted by permission of Kurman and Norris, ref. 53.)

clude deep myometrial invasion or the presence of a coexisting ovarian neoplasm.

PERIMENOPAUSAL WOMEN (40 TO 55 YEARS OF AGE)

Abnormal bleeding in the perimenopausal age group can be managed in a similar fashion as in younger women because perimenopausal women also are at low risk of having carcinoma (see Table 11.9). Most simple and complex hyperplasias in the 40- to 55-year-old age group are related to anovulation and are self-limited. Nonetheless, a biopsy is usually performed to exclude carcinoma. Patients with a diagnosis of atypical hyperplasia can be treated with progestins or a hysterectomy.

Nearly 60% of atypical hyperplasias regress, but the likelihood of residual carcinoma in the uterus after a curettage increases with age (see Fig. 11.21). For patients in the 40- to 55-year age range, treatment should be individualized. Regression occurs frequently, and the risk of residual carcinoma is lower than in older women. Therefore, observation or suppression with progestins monitored by endometrial biopsies every 3 months suffices. If the lesion persists, a hysterectomy may have to be performed.

Table 11.11. Hysterectomy findings according to the presence of atypical hyperplasia or well-differentiated adenocarcinoma in curettings in women under 40 years of age

	Curettings	
Hysterectomy findings	*Atypical hyperplasia (n = 17) No.*	*Well-differentiated carcinoma (n = 35) No.*
Carcinoma	2 (12%)	13 (37%)
Grade 1	2	10
Grade 2	0	3
Myometrial invasion		
Endometrium only	2	3
Inner one-third	0	9
Middle one-third	0	1

Adapted from Kurman and Norris, ref. 53.

POSTMENOPAUSAL WOMEN (OVER 55 YEARS OF AGE)

Women in the postmenopausal age group who have abnormal bleeding have a significant risk of having either carcinoma or atypical hyperplasia (see Table 11.9). Accordingly, abnormal bleeding requires immediate evaluation with an endometrial biopsy. A diagnosis of hyperplasia or atypical hyperplasia should be evaluated with a fractional curettage. If the curettings demonstrate hyperplasia without atypia, conservative management is an option because these types of hyperplasia are related to unopposed estrogenic stimulation, either from exogenous hormone treatment or because of peripheral conversion of androgens to estrogen in adipose tissue. Most (80%) hyperplasias treated with cyclic medroxyprogesterone acetate at 10 mg/day for 14 days regress; none progressed to carcinoma in a prospective study of 65 postmenopausal women.[25] Conservative management, either observation only or treatment with medroxyprogesterone to produce a medical curettage, therefore, is adequate. Repeated episodes of irregular bleeding that are not responsive to hormone treatment require a hysterectomy. Hysterectomy is the treatment of choice for a diagnosis of atypical hyperplasia based on a curettage. In postmenopausal women with surgical risk factors that preclude a hysterectomy, continuous treatment with 20–40 mg/day megestrol acetate can be used effectively to avoid surgery. In a study of 70 women with complex hyperplasia (38 women) and atypical hyperplasia (32 women), surgery was avoided in 93% of patients. The hyperplasias (atypical and nonatypical) completely regressed in 85% after a mean follow-up of more than 5 years. None of the lesions progressed to carcinoma.[27]

For postmenopausal women with hyperplasia or atypical hyperplasia who are receiving exogenous estrogen, termination of the estrogen usually suffices even for atypical hyperplasia, because these proliferations regress after the stimulus for their growth has been removed. Alternatively, the addition of cyclically or continuous administered medroxyprogesterone in women being treated with estrogen can be considered because the use of even low doses of progestins substantially reduces the risk of development of endometrial hyperplasia and carcinoma.[1] Using a 7- to 14-day regimen of orally administered 10 mg medroxyprogesterone to postmenopausal women receiving estrogen, five endometrial carcinomas were detected in 5402 woman-years of continuous estrogen therapy.[28] This incidence is not greater than that of untreated postmenopausal women, in whom the expected incidence of endometrial cancer is 1 to 2 per 1000 woman-years, that is, 5.4 to 9.8 cases. The addition of continuous low doses norethindrone acetate to estradiol therapy also reduces the incidence of endometrial hyperplasia in postmenopausal women. Hyperplasia developed in 15% of women receiving unopposed estradiol therapy compared to less than 1% of those receiving continuous low doses of norethindrone combined with estradiol.[51]

Endometrial Cellular Changes: Metaplasia, Cellular Differentiation

In contrast to hyperplasia, which is a proliferative response to estrogenic stimulation, metaplasia represents cytoplasmic differentiation. The cytoplasmic alterations (metaplasia) are manifested by eosinophilic, ciliated cell (tubal), squamous, secretory/clear, and mucinous differentiation. Metaplasias develop most commonly in response to estrogenic and progestational stimulation, although these changes may develop in response to various other stimuli as well. Thus, the morphologic response of the endometrium to hormonal stimulation is complex and is reflected by a combination of architectural, nuclear, and cytoplasmic alterations. Although classifications separate hyperplasia and the various metaplasias, both are usually intimately associated and cannot always be separately classified.

Definitions and Classification

Metaplasia is defined as replacement of one type of adult tissue by another type that is not normally found in that location. In the endometrium, most of the changes that are designated as metaplasia represent a variety of cytoplasmic alterations or forms of differentiation that are not encountered in normal proliferative endometrium but do not qualify as true metaplasia. Accordingly, it has been suggested that a more appropriate term is change.[83] Use of the term change also has the advantage of providing a descriptive designation without employing a specific mechanism of development. In this chapter, the terms metaplasia, change, and differentiation are used interchangeably. The various forms of cellular differentiation are typically focal when unaccompanied by hyperplasia but can be diffuse when hyperplasia is present.

The WHO classification subdivides endometrial metaplasia as follows: squamous, mucinous, ciliary, hobnail, clear cell, eosinophilic, surface syncytial,

Table 11.12. Classification of endometrial cellular (cytoplasmic) changes

Eosinophilic (including syncytial change)
Squamous (squamous metaplasia)
Ciliated cell (tubal metaplasia)
Secretory and clear cell
Mucinous

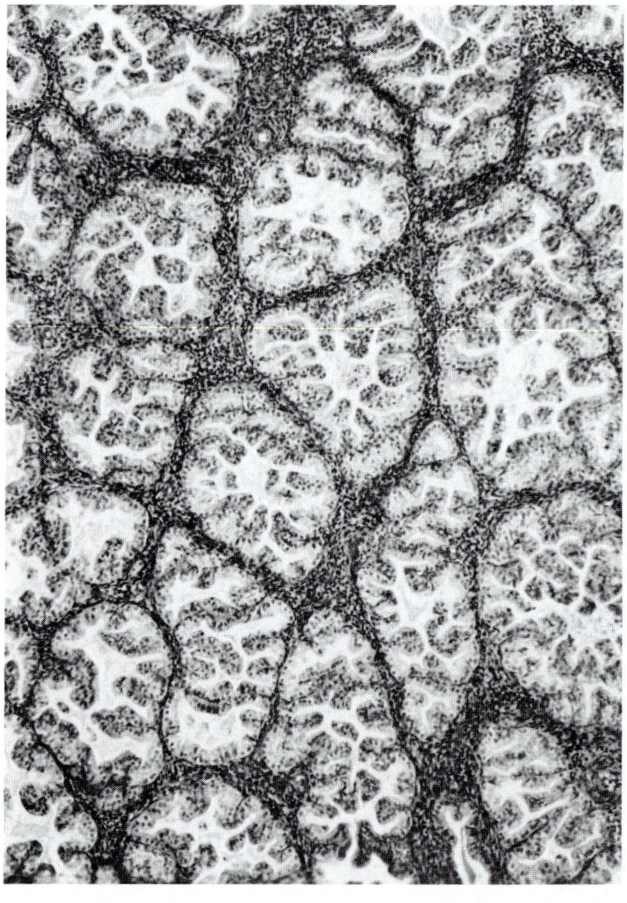

Fig. 11.22. Eosinophilic cell change in an atypical hyperplasia. The cells lining the glands form intraglandular tufts.

papillary proliferation, and Arias–Stella effect.[76] This classification combines both cytologic and architectural alterations, some of which have different etiologies. As previously noted, the endometrial epithelium can undergo a variety of cytoplasmic changes in response to different stimuli that can be observed in both benign and malignant conditions. A simplified classification of these is shown in Table 11.12. It is important to recognize the various cytoplasmic changes because they are benign and can be confused with hyperplasia. When hyperplasia and the cytoplasmic alterations coexist, as they often do, the hyperplasia should be classified, but it is not necessary to describe the cytoplasmic changes because they do not influence prognosis (see "Behavior").

Clinical Features

The frequent association of the various endometrial cytoplasmic changes with hyperplasia is probably because both result from a hyperestrogenic state. More than 70% of perimenopausal and postmenopausal women with metaplasia had received exogenous estrogen in one study.[35] In addition, most young women with metaplasia have clinical manifestations of persistent anovulation and primary infertility, features of polycystic ovarian disease.[13,20,35] Metaplasia also may occur in various benign conditions, including polyps, endometritis, trauma, and vitamin A deficiency.[20,26,35,36]

Pathologic Findings

The various types of endometrial cytoplasmic changes have no distinctive gross features.

Eosinophilic Change

Eosinophilic change is the most common cytoplasmic alteration. Several types of eosinophilic cytoplasmic transformation occur, all of them innocuous. Ciliated cells, squamous cells, oncocytes, and papillary and surface syncytial change all may have eosinophilic cytoplasm. However, eosinophilic cells also occur in association with hyperplasia, particularly atypical hyperplasia (Fig. 11.22).

Glands may be partially or completely lined by eosinophilic cells. Eosinophilic cells that line glands can show considerable variation in shape. They may be columnar when associated with atypical hyperplasia, rounded when associated with ciliated cells, or polygonal, forming pavement-like aggregates, when they merge with cells that show squamous differentiation (Fig. 11.23). In hyperplastic lesions ag-

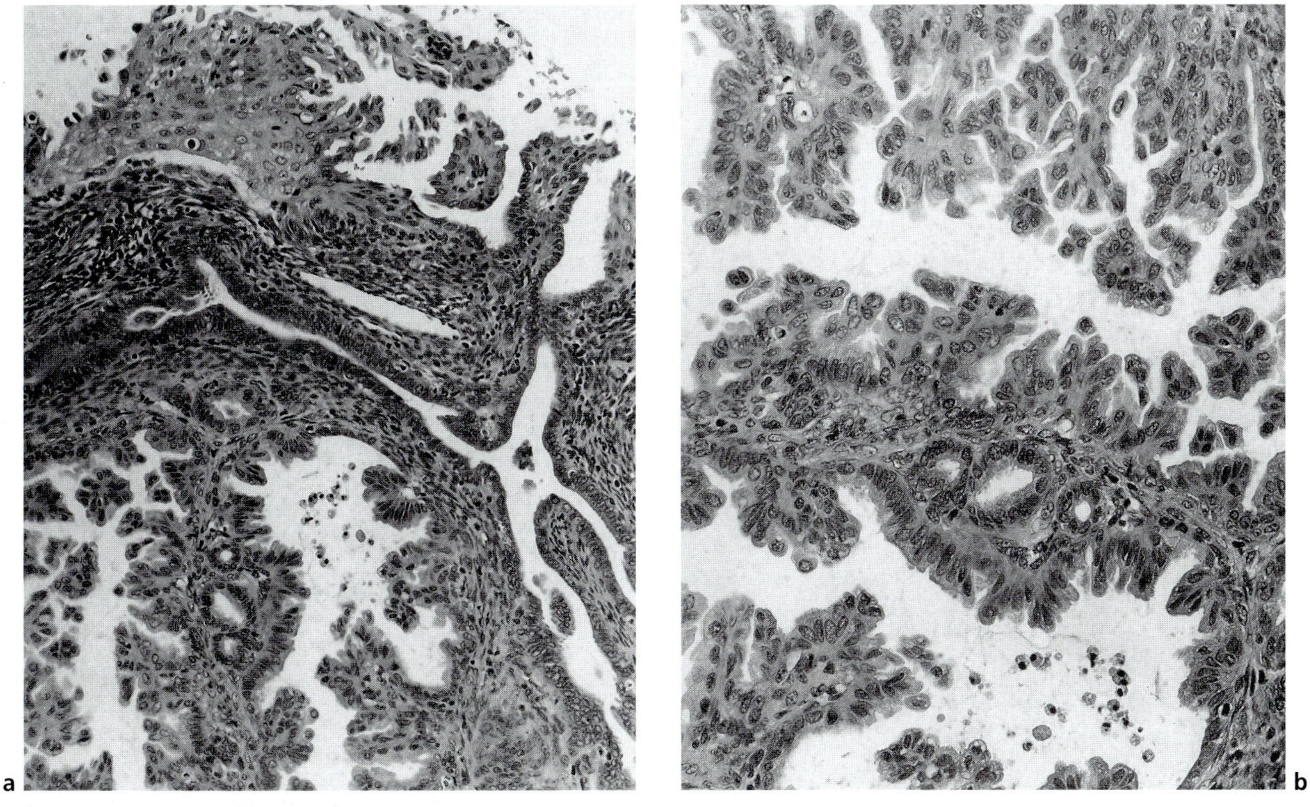

Fig. 11.23. Eosinophilic syncytial change. a: On the surface of the endometrium, the eosinophilic cells have a squamous appearance. Papillary procsses involve the surface and the glands. **b**: The eosinophilic cells form complex intraglandular papillary tufts. There is no cytologic atypia.

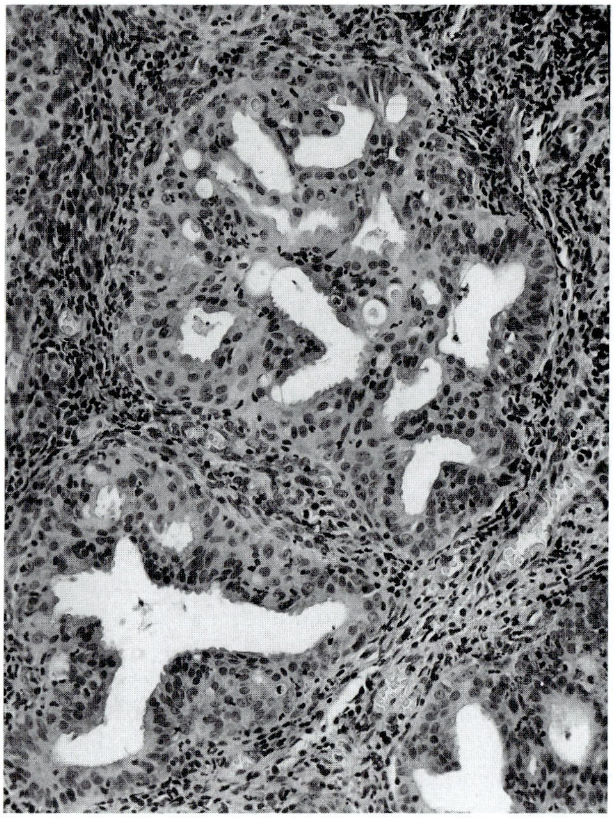

Fig. 11.24. Eosinophilic change in complex hyperplasia. The cells bridge gland lumens simulating a cribriform pattern (compare with Fig. 11.17).

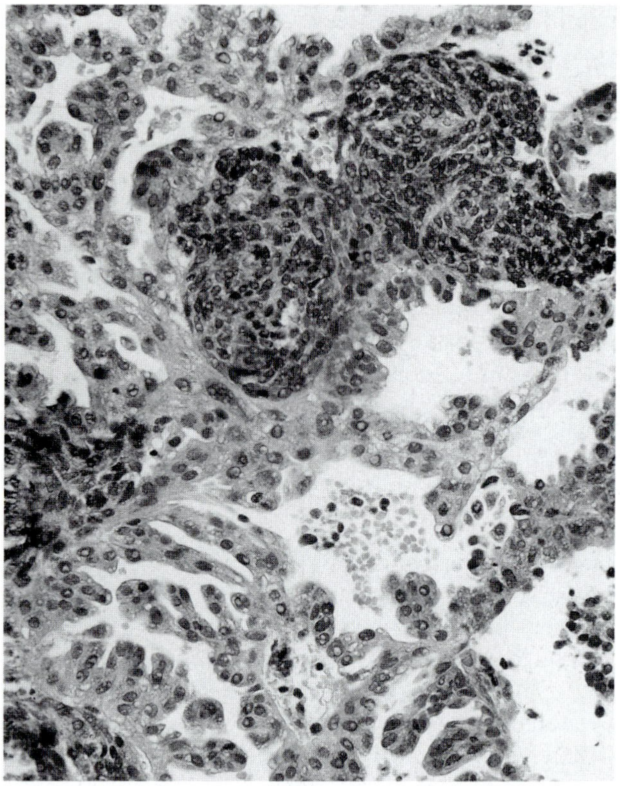

Fig. 11.25. Eosinophilic syncytial change. The cells with eosinophilic cytoplasm display mild vacuolization, merging to form a syncytium within glands and extending onto the surface. The eosinophilic change envelopes condensed stromal cells (*upper, center*). The latter is a common manifestation of endometrial stromal breakdown.

gregates of eosinophilic cells often form intraglandular papillary tufts (Fig. 11.23) and bridges (Fig. 11.24), thus simulating carcinoma. Eosinophilic cells contain variable amounts of cytoplasm that at times can be partially vacuolated (Figs. 11.25 and 11.26). The nuclei tend to be round and somewhat stratified. In most instances, the nuclei are smaller, more uniform, and lack the irregular nuclear membrane, coarse chromatin, and nucleoli that characterize cells with true cytologic atypia. Occasionally, the nuclei can be enlarged and contain a single prominent nucleolus. Mitotic figures are rarely present. On the endometrial surface, cells with eosinophilic cytoplasm typically merge into a syncytium that either can be flat or more commonly form papillary processes (see Fig. 11.23).[71] Typically, the papillary processes lack connective tissue support and contain small cystic spaces filled with polymorphonuclear leukocytes. This lesion has been referred to as surface syncytial change, papillary syncytial change, or papillary metaplasia.[36,83] We prefer the term eosinophilic syncytial change because the lesion is characteristically composed of eosinophilic cells forming a syncytium and can involve glands as well as the surface. Eosinophilic syncytial change is commonly associated with endometrial stromal breakdown (see Fig. 11.25) or inflammation, suggesting that it is a degenerative or a reparative process.[97] The nuclei within the syncytium are arranged haphazardly and piled up; they generally are small and bland but at times may be round and vesicular and display alterations in shape and chromatin texture. Mitotic figures are rare. Hyperchromatic nuclei with smudged chromatin and irregular nuclear membranes appear degenerated whereas enlarged, vesicular nuclei with a prominent nucleolus and smooth nuclear membranes appear reactive (Fig. 11.26). These degenerative and reparative changes should not be interpreted as nuclear atypia. Eosinophilic change can be seen in combination with hobnail secretory change on occasion (Fig. 11.27)

Squamous Differentiation (Squamous Metaplasia)

Squamous differentiation may occur in all forms of

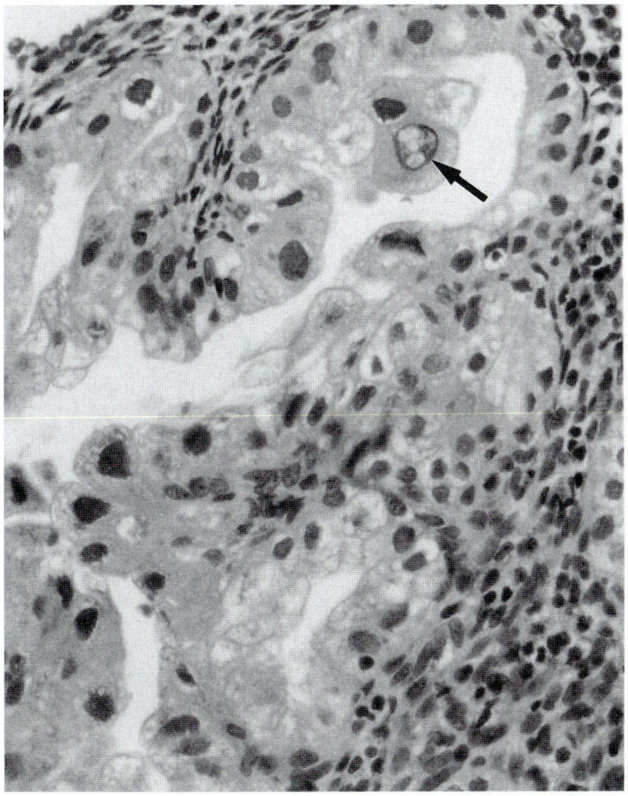

Fig. 11.26. Eosinophilic change. The cells display varying degrees of cytoplasmic vacuolization and nuclear alterations. Some nuclei are enlarged and hyperchromatic with smudged chromatin and irregular borders. One cell in the *upper part* of the field has an enlarged, "moth-eaten" nucleus (*arrow*) with chromatin that is indistinct and partially smudged.

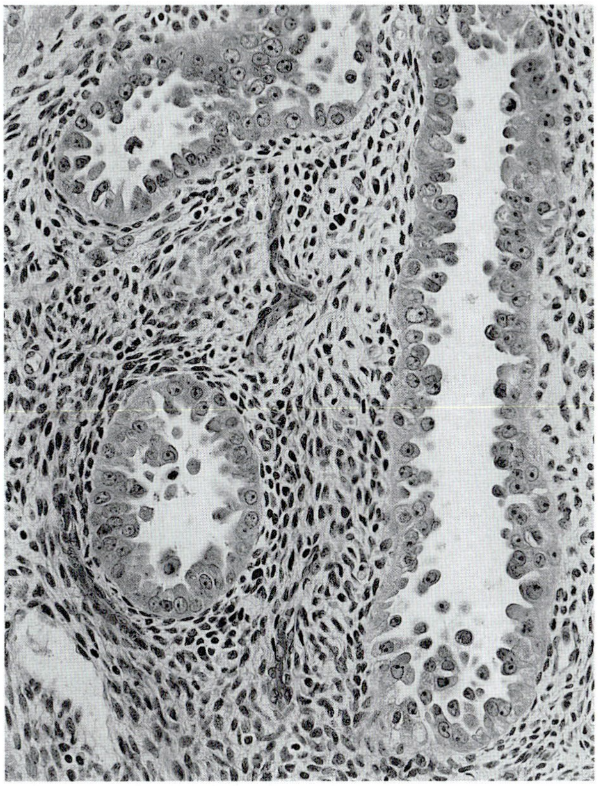

Fig. 11.27. Eosinophilic cell and hobnail change. The glandular cells within an endometrial polyp display abundant eosinophilic cytoplasm. The nuclei are vesicular, have prominent nucleoli, and bulge into the glandular lumen. This change is distinguished from endometrial intraepithelial carcinoma by the smooth nuclear membranes, even chromatin, relatively uniform nuclear size, and absence of mitotic figures. In addition, the nuclei were negative for p53 and the Ki-67 proliferation index was very low.

hyperplasia as well as in carcinoma. It is especially common in the more atypical endometrial proliferations (Fig. 11.28) and is rare in normally cycling endometrium or in simple and complex hyperplasias (Fig. 11.29). The squamous cells are usually cytologically bland. The degree of nuclear atypia, when present, generally parallels that of the glandular cells. Typically, the squamous cells have a moderate amount of eosinophilic cytoplasm and are surrounded by a well-defined cell membrane. Often they merge with eosinophilic cells that qualify as eosinophilic change. The squamous cells tend to be rounded or polygonal but may be spindle shaped, forming a circumscribed nest (squamous morule) within the gland lumen (Fig. 11.28). Morules reflect immature or incomplete squamous differentiation. The cells are smaller and the cytoplasm is less prominent than in more completely differentiated squamous cells. Central keratinization and necrosis rarely occur. Eventually, proliferation results in protrusion of the squamous cells into the lumen, leading to replacement of the lumen by nests of squamous cells and coalescence with neighboring glands undergoing the same process. Mitotic activity is rare.

Ciliated Cell Change (Tubal Metaplasia)

Cilia are not usually evident microscopically in proliferative endometrial glandular cells, although they may be observed on the endometrial surface.[59] Ciliated cells occasionally are observed in isolated glands in atrophic or inactive endometria or in polyps in the absence of hyperplasia. The presence of a significant number of ciliated glandular cells is referred to as *ciliated cell change* or *tubal metaplasia* because of the resemblance to the epithelium of the fallopian tube. The ciliated cells are often round and slightly enlarged, but the nuclear membranes are smooth and uniform and the chromatin is fine and evenly dis-

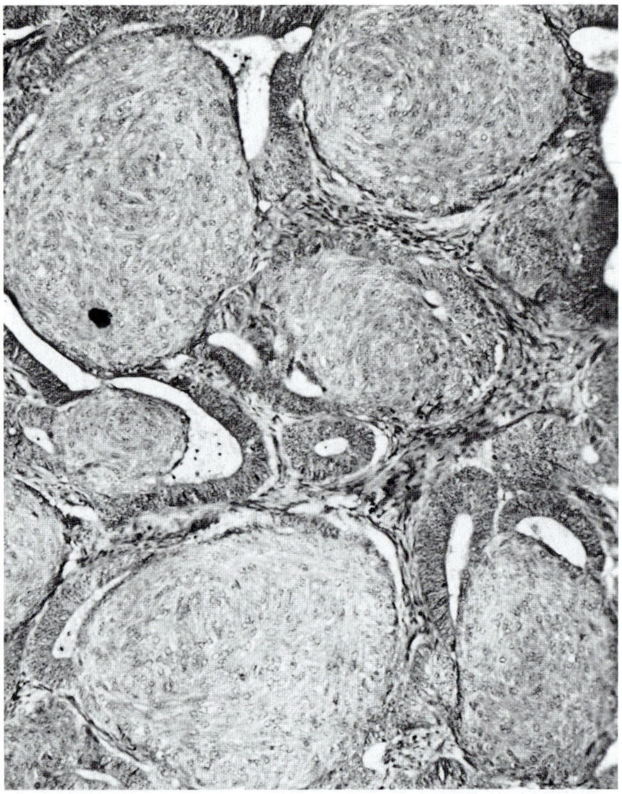

Fig. 11.28. Squamous change (metaplasia) in atypical hyperplasia. The squamous cells have almost entirely obliterated gland lumens.

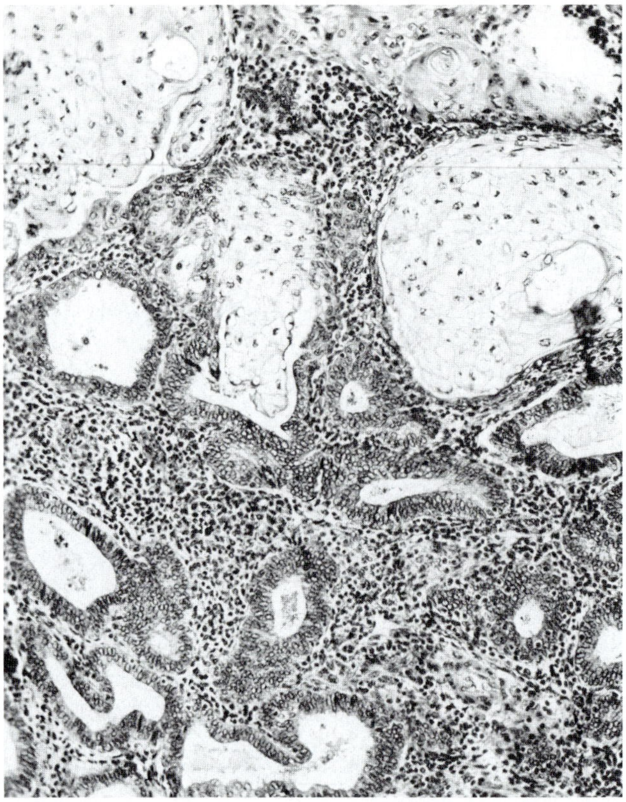

Fig. 11.29. Squamous change (metaplasia) in simple hyperplasia. Both squamous and glandular cells lack cytologic atypia.

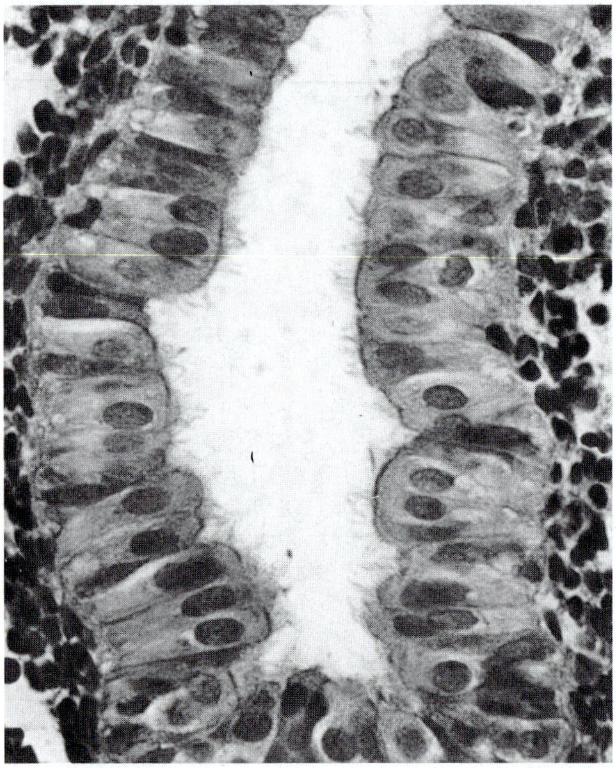

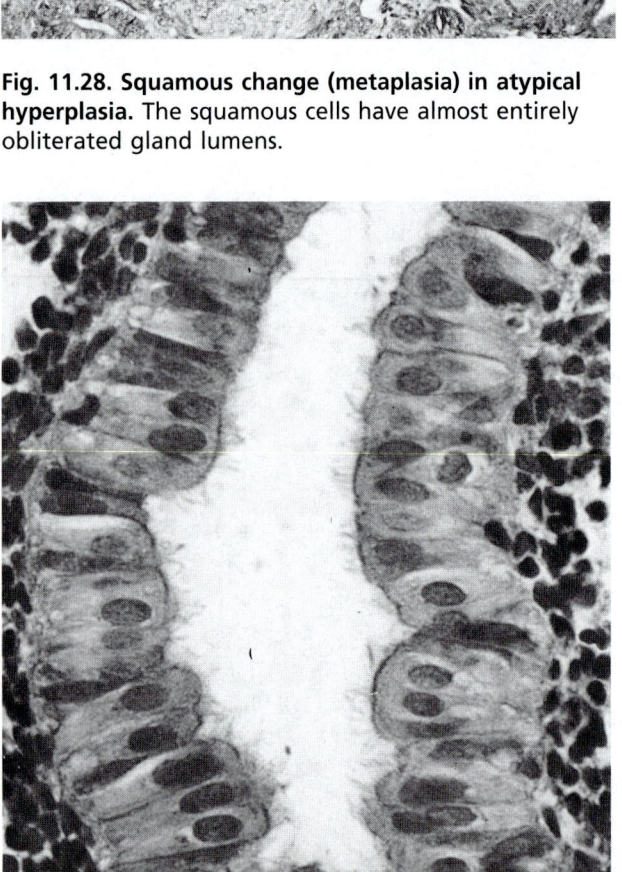

Fig. 11.30. Ciliated cell change. This type of change is characterized by ciliated cells along with intercalated (peg) cells closely resembling the epithelium of the fallopian tube.

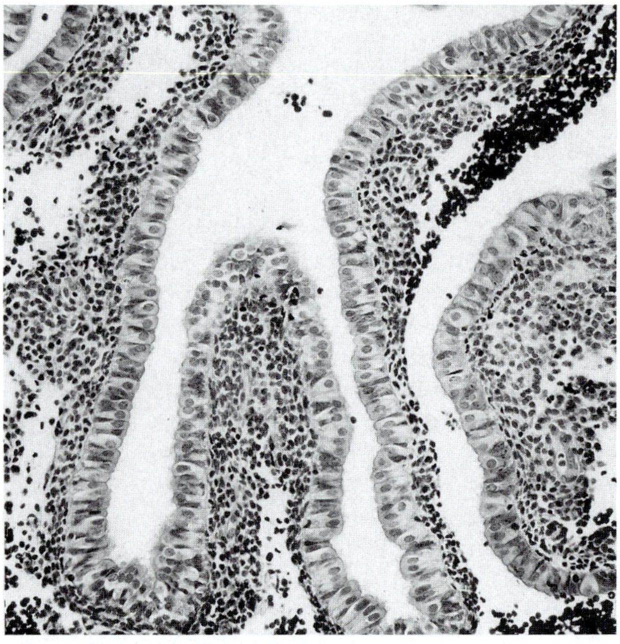

Fig. 11.31. Ciliated cell change. Ciliated cells are present in an enlarged gland with an irregular outline.

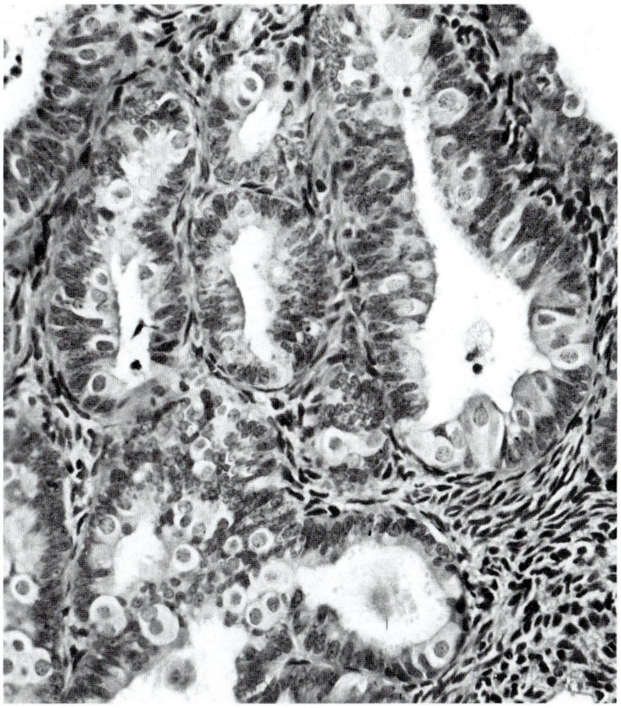

Fig. 11.32. Ciliated change in complex hyperplasia. Numerous ciliated cells with round, bland nuclei and clear cytoplasmic halos are present.

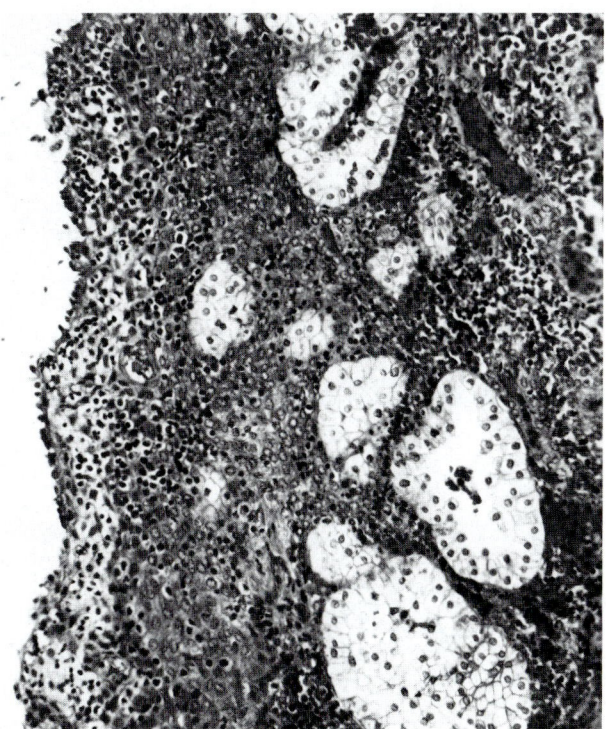

Fig. 11.33. Clear cell change. The clear cells lining endometrial glands contain glycogen.

persed (Fig. 11.30). There is no nuclear atypia. The ciliated cells may be interspersed singly or in small groups among nonciliated cells, or they may line a larger segment of a gland (Fig. 11.31). Mitotic activity is limited to the adjacent nonciliated cells. Ciliated cell change may occur in glands in the absence of hyperplasia. Dilated venous sinusoids are also frequently present. All these changes reflect a mild degree of estrogenic stimulation. Ciliated cell change frequently accompanies simple, complex, or atypical hyperplasia (Fig. 11.32).

Secretory, Clear Cell, and Hobnail Change

On rare occasions, polygonal cells with clear cytoplasm containing glycogen and bland nuclei are found in glands or on the surface of the endometrium and have been referred to as *clear cell metaplasia* (Fig. 11.33).[35] In contrast, *secretory effect* is characterized by columnar cells with sub- or supranuclear vacuoles containing clear glycogenated cytoplasm resembling the glandular cells of early secretory endometrium. These cells also can be observed in nonneoplastic endometria but are seen more often in association with hyperplasia or carcinoma (Fig. 11.34).[50,54] Rarely, the cells in secretory change can display *hobnail morphology* reminiscent of the Arias–Stella reaction (Fig. 11.35). At times secretory change can result from progestational stimulation, but often there is no such

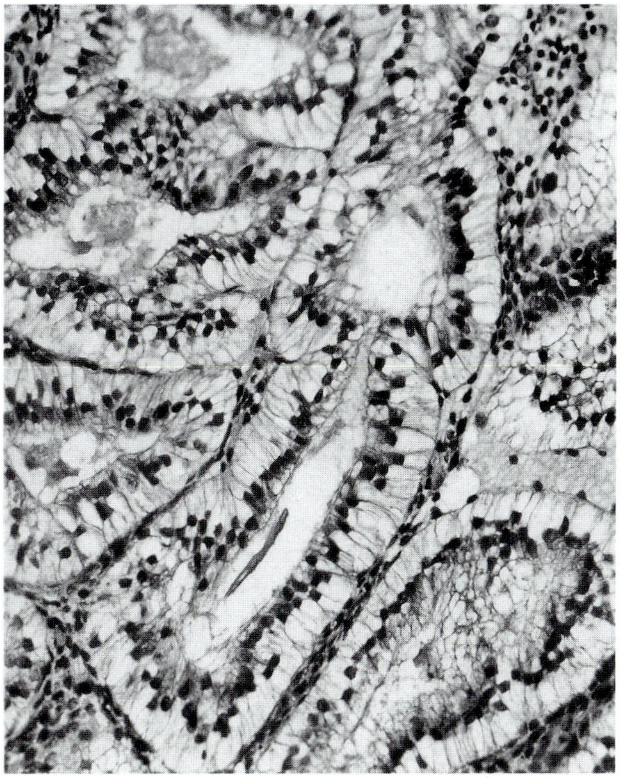

Fig. 11.34. Secretory change in complex hyperplasia. The glands are markedly crowded with little intervening stroma. The cells are columnar with subnuclear vacuoles, and the nuclei show no cytologic atypia.

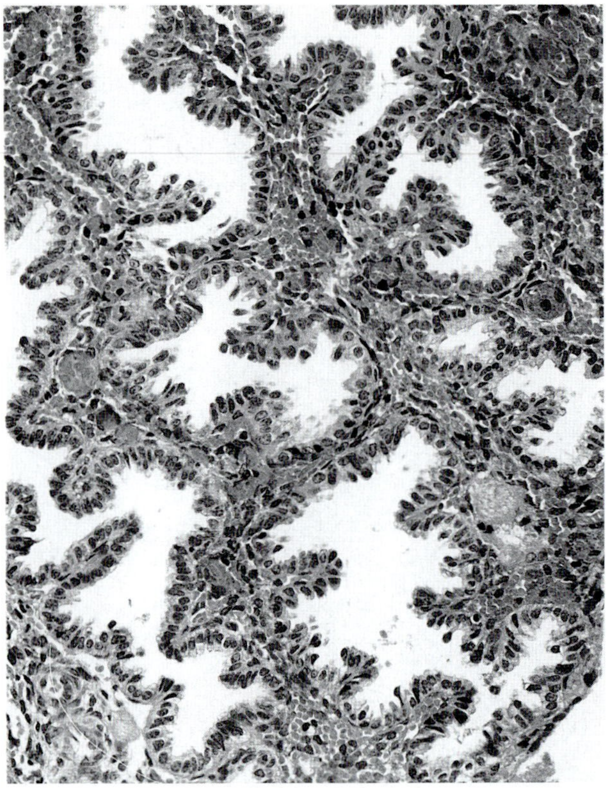

Fig. 11.35. Hobnail change. The glands are lined by cells with inconspicuous cytoplasm and nuclei that bulge into the lumen. This change resembles the Arias–Stella reaction.

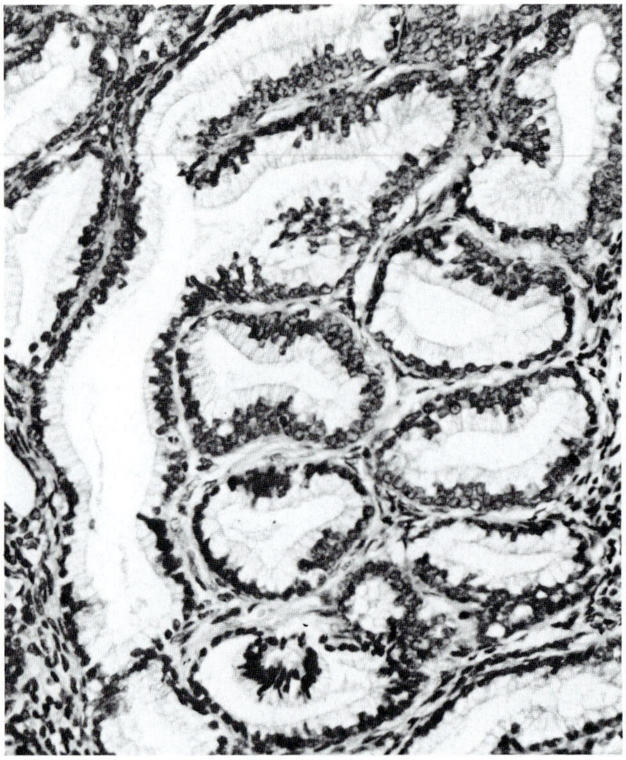

Fig. 11.36. Mucinous changes in complex hyperplasia. The nuclei of the glandular cells are closely applied to the basement membrane. The cytoplasm is clear and intensely positive with mucicarmine stains but contains no stainable glycogen.

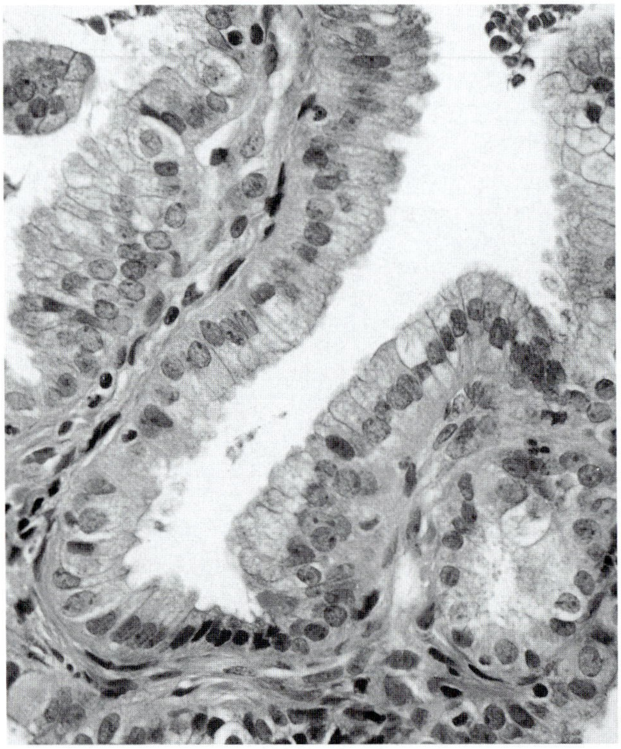

Fig. 11.37. Mucinous change. The mucinous cells form a single layer of columnar epithelium with bland nuclei and granular cytoplasm. The cytoplasm is positive with mucicarmine stains.

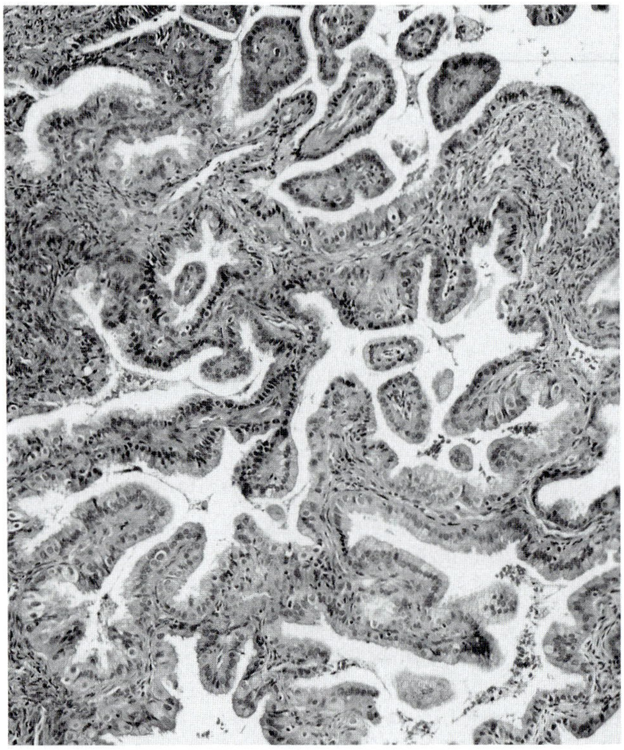

Fig. 11.38. Complex hyperplasia with papillary proliferation. The lesion involves the surface of the endometrium (*top of field*). Most of the glandular epithelium is mucinous.

association. Columnar cells with secretory change may merge with polygonal-shaped clear cells and with squamous cells containing clear glycogenated cytoplasm. As the accumulation of glycogen can occur in the cytoplasm of a variety of cell types, it is thus a cytoplasmic alteration rather than a true metaplasia.

Mucinous Change

Mucinous change is characterized by mucinous epithelium resembling that of the endocervix cytologically, histochemically, and ultrastructurally.[23] It is one of the least commonly encountered cytoplasmic alterations. The mucinous epithelium tends to be distributed focally and is composed of tall columnar cells with bland, basally oriented nuclei and clear, slightly granular cytoplasm (Figs. 11.36 and 11.37). At times mucinous change is accompanied by a papillary proliferation. The papillary processes contain normal but compressed stromal cells and are lined by nonstratified columnar epithelium, which is mucinous in areas (Fig. 11.38). Mitotic figures are rare. The cytoplasm is clear in hematoxylin and eosin (H&E) stains because it contains mucin, which is periodic acid–Schiff (PAS) positive and diastase resistant and stains with mucicarmine, toluidine blue, and alcian blue. In contrast to mucinous epithelium, the vacuolated cytoplasm of secretory endometrium contains glycogen. On rare occasion the mucinous epithelium may contain goblet cells and is referred to as intestinal metaplasia.

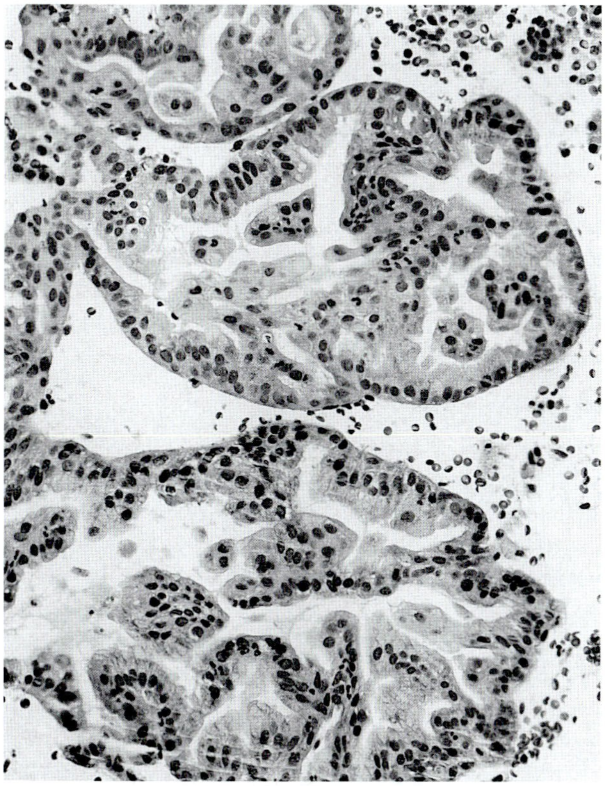

Fig. 11.39. Mucinous change in a complex endometrial proliferation (curettage specimen). Complex glands devoid of surrounding stroma display intraluminal tufts and mucinous differentiation with minimal cytologic atypia. The hysterectomy specimen demonstrated complex atypical hyperplasia.

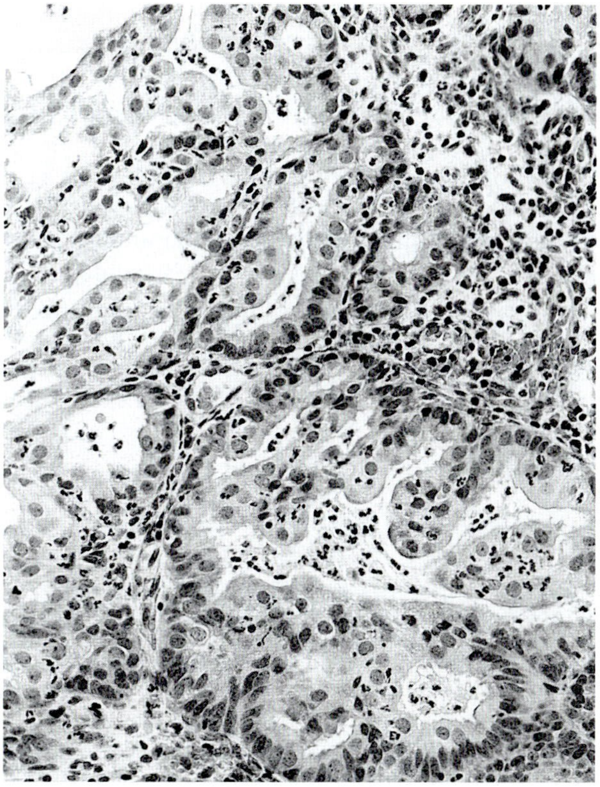

Fig. 11.40. Mucinous change in a complex endometrial proliferation (curettage specimen). Crowded glands with intraluminal tufts display mucinous cytoplasmic differentiation and moderate cytologic atypia. The hysterectomy specimen contained a grade 1, stage 1A endometrioid carcinoma.

Mucinous differentiation can be seen in a spectrum of epithelial proliferations ranging from benign to malignant. A recent study found that the likelihood of finding carcinoma associated with mucinous proliferations of the endometrium varies according to the degrees of architectural complexity and cytologic atypia of the lesions.[68] Architecturally simple lesions with papillary projections into luminal spaces and no cytologic atypia were found to have carcinoma on follow-up only when the initial specimen also contained atypical hyperplasia; otherwise, none of these simple mucinous proliferations was associated with carcinoma on follow-up. More complex proliferations with microglandular or cribriform patterns and minimal cytologic atypia, often presenting as endometrial surface lesions without coexistent atypical hyperplasia, were found to have well-differentiated noninvasive or minimally invasive carcinoma on follow-up in 65% of cases (Figs. 11.39 and 11.40). Highly complex proliferations with glandular budding, cribriform growth, and branching of villous structures that also displayed moderate to severe cytologic atypia were invariably associated with carcinoma on follow-up. Also, 80% of the study patients were over age 50. Thus, in perimenopausal and postmenopausal women with complex mucinous proliferations, including those with and without cytologic atypia, the risk of finding coexistent carcinoma is quite high.

Mixed Cellular Changes

Mixtures of different *types of cellular changes* are common. Most are closely related and represent different morphologic responses to a variety of stimuli, including estrogenic stimulation.[35] For example, eosinophilic change, especially eosinophilic syncytial change, may resemble squamous epithelium and often is associated with squamous metaplasia. Likewise, eosinophilic and ciliated cell change share many morphologic features and commonly occur together.

Differential Diagnosis

The most important aspect of the evaluation of the various metaplasias and cellular changes is not to confuse them with hyperplasia or carcinoma, which is best accomplished by evaluating the glandular architecture and cytological features. In hyperplasia, the glandular outlines are irregular and complex and there is stratification of the epithelium reflecting a proliferative process. In contrast, in the various cytoplasmic changes the glandular outlines are regular and have a tubular configuration, although cystic dilatation and slight glandular irregularity occasionally can occur.

Although the various cellular changes may be accompanied by slight nuclear enlargement, the cells lack the abnormal chromatin patterns that characterize the nuclei in atypical hyperplasia. At times the various cellular changes may look ominous and suggest carcinoma, but evidence of stromal invasion is lacking and therefore a diagnosis of carcinoma is not justified. For example, extensive squamous metaplasia may suggest a diagnosis of carcinoma but without a desmoplastic response or a confluent glandular pattern a diagnosis of carcinoma should not be made (Fig. 11.41). Eosinophilic change associated with hyperplasia can fill and bridge gland lumens but lacks a true confluent or cribriform pattern (Fig. 11.42). Mucinous change at times can form complex papillary processes, but the stroma of the papillae are composed of normal endometrial stroma and the epithelium lacks cytologic atypia (Figs. 11.38 and 11.43).

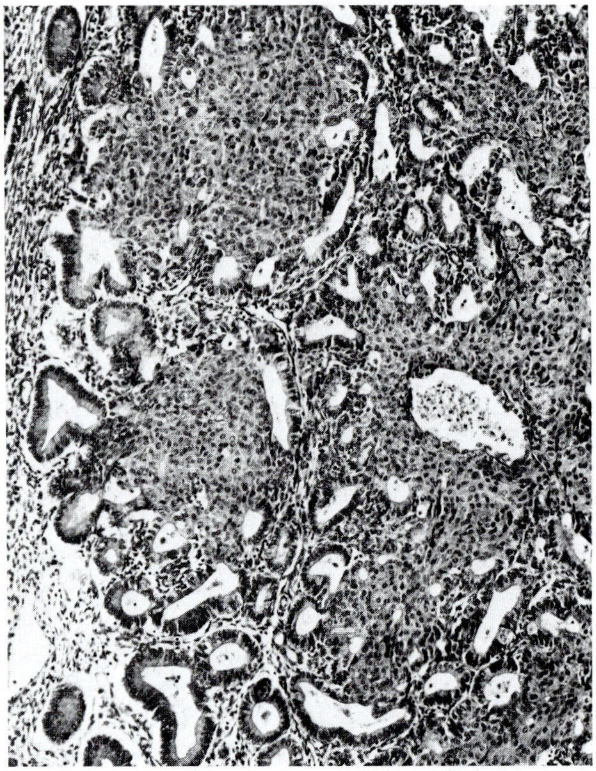

Fig. 11.41. Complex hyperplasia with squamous change. There is extensive replacement of the stroma by squamous epithelium. In the absence of an altered (desmoplastic) stroma or a confluent glandular pattern, a diagnosis of carcinoma should not be made.

Behavior

Cytoplasmic changes, other than eosinophilic syncytial change, rarely occur in the absence of hyperplasia or carcinoma.[44] In the absence of hyperplasia these changes (metaplasia) had no clinical significance in one study of 89 patients.[35] In a long-term follow-up study of endometrial hyperplasia, 5 of 11 patients with atypical hyperplasia and associated squamous metaplasia eventually developed carcinoma, indicating that atypical hyperplasia with squamous metaplasia has malignant potential.[52] Inasmuch as the cytoplasmic changes by themselves have no prognostic significance, the importance of recognizing them lies in not confusing these benign processes with hyperplasia or carcinoma.

Management

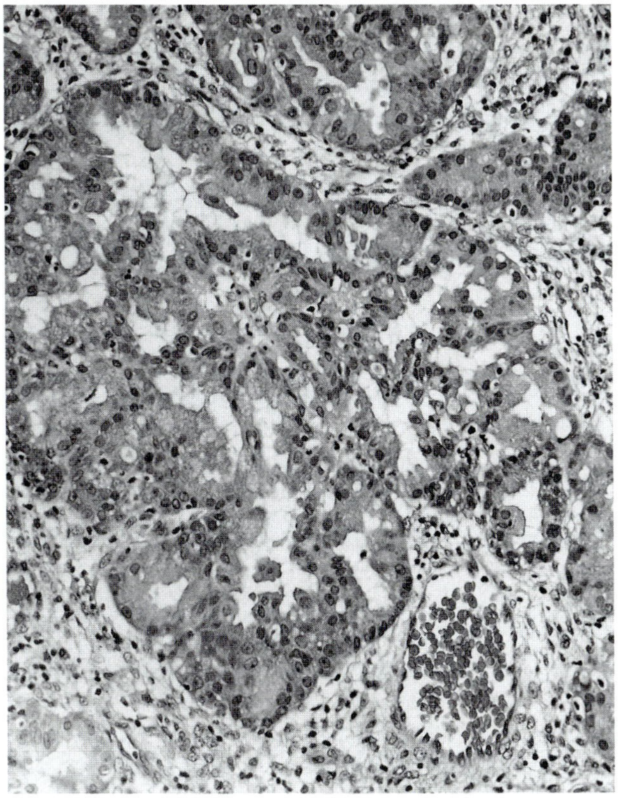

Fig. 11.42. Eosinophilic cell change. Cells with eosinophilic cells fill and bridge the glandular lumen. The microcystic spaces that result lack the punched-out, hard outlines of a cribriform pattern (compare with Fig. 11.17).

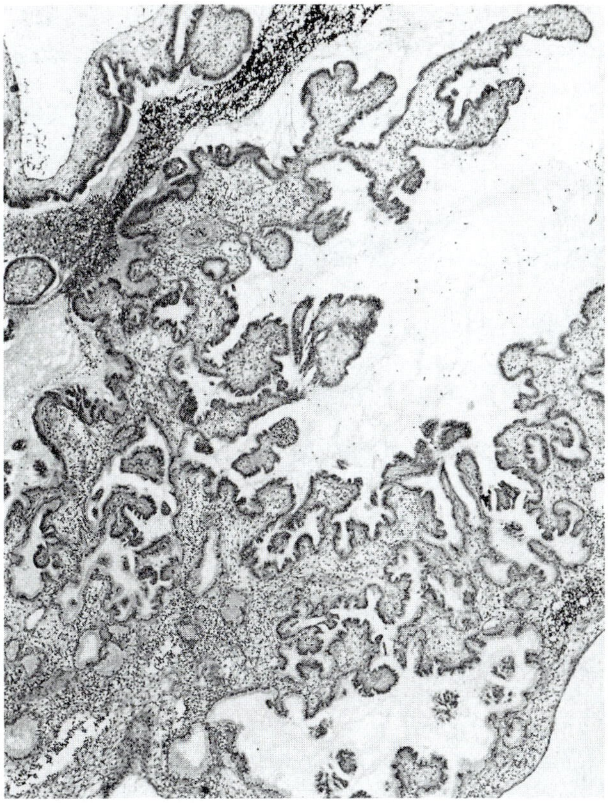

Fig. 11.43. Papillary mucinous change. In contrast to the delicate fibrovascular cores of a well-differentiated (endometrioid) carcinoma, the papillae in the papillary mucinous change contain normal endometrial stroma and the epithelial cells are bland.

The management of endometrial cytoplasmic changes depends entirely on the nature of the associated proliferative process. If hyperplasia is present it should be managed accordingly. Endometrial cytoplasmic changes without hyperplasia do not require treatment.

Endometrial Intraepithelial Carcinoma

Definition and Pathologic Findings

Serous carcinoma is the prototypic endometrial carcinoma that is not related to estrogenic stimulation and typically occurs in the setting of endometrial atrophy. Serous carcinoma is frequently associated with a putative precursor lesion, termed "endometrial intraepithelial carcinoma" (EIC). EIC is characterized by markedly atypical nuclei, identical to those of invasive serous carcinomas, lining the surfaces and glands of the atrophic endometrium (Figs.

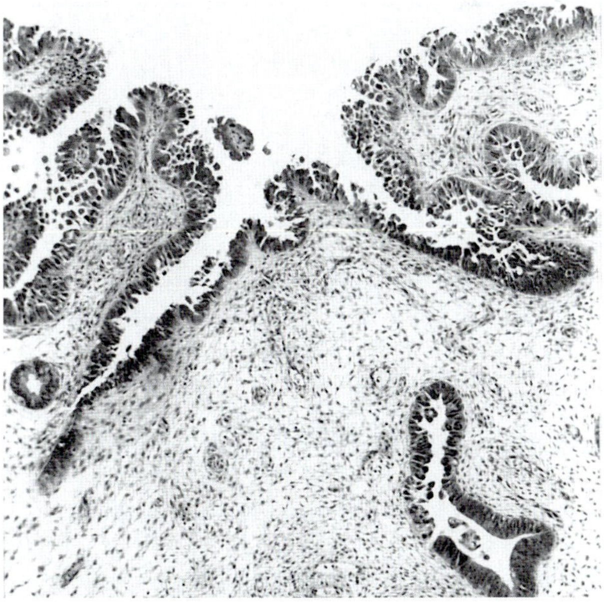

Fig. 11.44. Endometrial intraepithelial carcinoma. An atypical papillary proliferation lines the endometrial surface and a portion of an underlying gland. There is no stromal invasion.

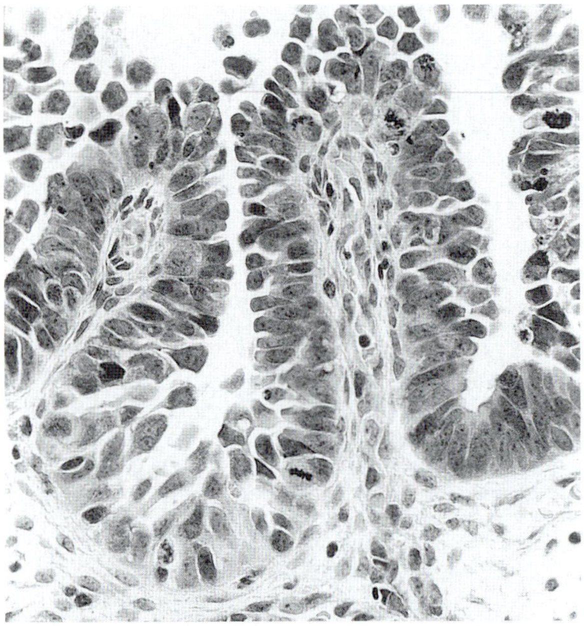

Fig. 11.45. Endometrial intraepithelial carcinoma. Higher magnification of the case illustrated in Fig. 11.44 demonstrates the atypical surface proliferation characterized by cells with enlarged nuclei, some of which have hobnail morphology with smudged, hyperchromatic nuclei. Numerous mitotic figures are seen.

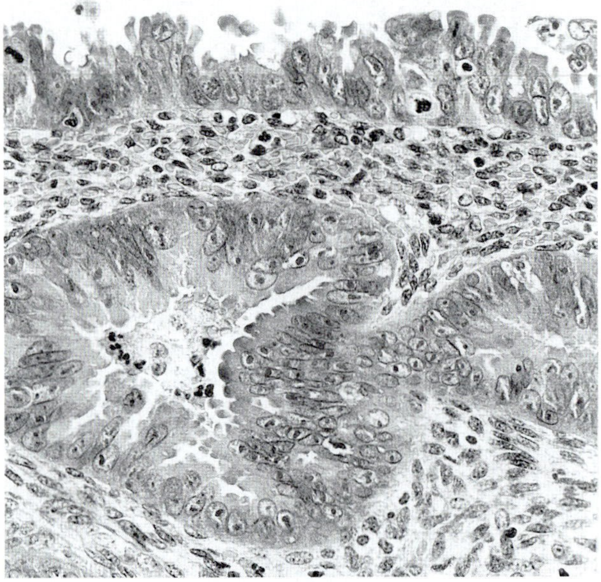

Fig. 11.46. Endometrial intraepithelial carcinoma. Markedly enlarged, atypical nuclei with vesicular chromatin and prominent nucleoli line the endometrial surface and an underlying gland.

11.44–11.47).[2,78] The surface often demonstrates a slightly papillary contour and some cells display hobnail morphology and smudged, hyperchromatic nuclei (Fig. 11.44 and 11.45). The nuclei are enlarged, with granular or vesicular chromatin, and frequently display enlarged eosinophilic nucleoli (Figs. 11.46 and 11.47). Numerous mitotic figures, including atypical ones, are present (Fig. 11.45). On occasion, the abnormal proliferation can be seen involving only a portion of an endometrial gland (Fig. 11.48). This lesion also has been referred to as "carcinoma in situ"[86] and "uterine surface carcinoma."[98] We prefer the term EIC to carcinoma in situ (CIS) because EIC can be associated with metastatic disease (see following), whereas the term CIS implies a lesion that does not have metastatic potential. EIC also can be found in uteri without evidence of an invasive serous carcinoma, frequently on the surface of a polyp in an atrophic endometrium (Figs. 11.49 and 11.50).

Molecular genetic evidence supports the concept that EIC is a precursor lesion of serous carcinoma. Recent studies have demonstrated immunohistochemical overexpression of p53 protein, loss of heterozygosity of chromosome 17p, and corresponding p53 gene mutations in a high proportion of serous carcinomas and EIC (Figs 11.51 and 11.52).[79,89] The finding of diffuse, intense staining for p53 is highly

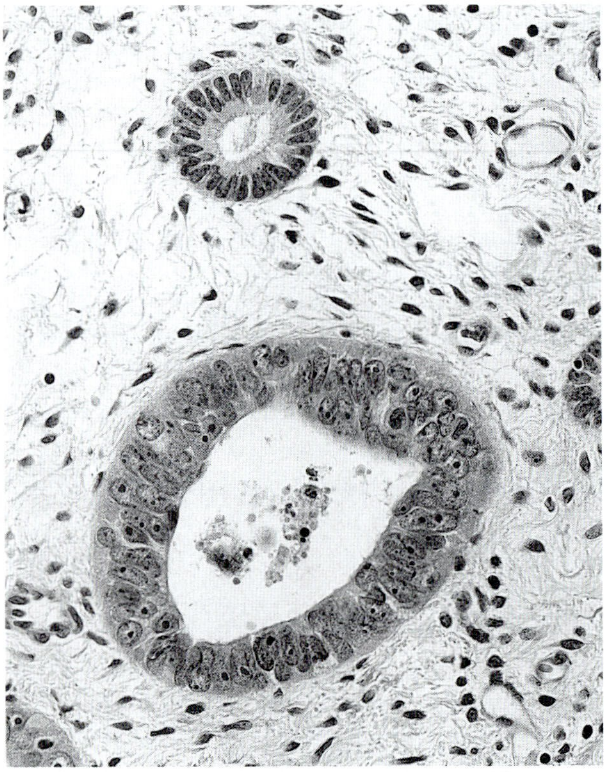

Fig. 11.47. Endometrial intraepithelial carcinoma (EIC). An endometrial gland involved by EIC is seen adjacent to an atrophic gland. The nuclei in EIC are markedly enlarged, with grainy to vesicular chromatin, and display prominent nucleoli.

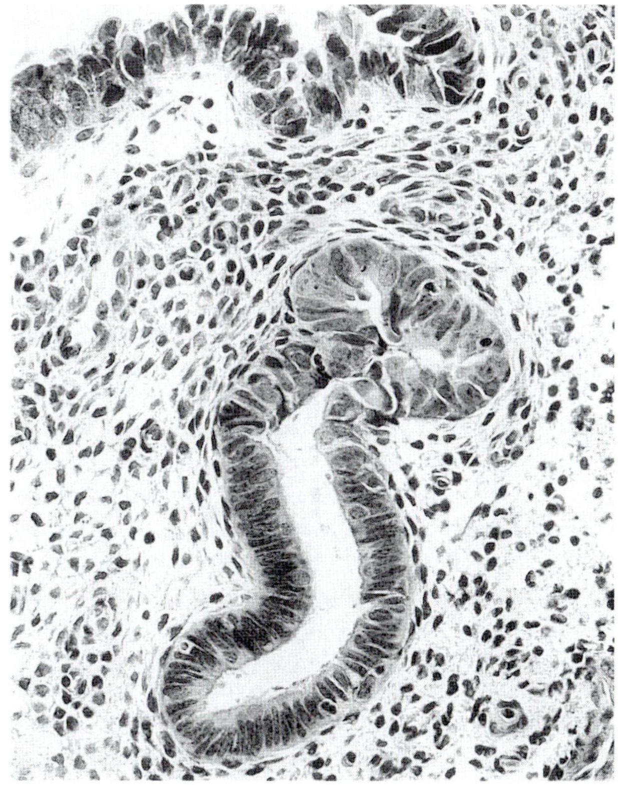

Fig. 11.48. Endometrial intraepithelial carcinoma. Atypical cells line the endometrial surface and a portion of the underlying gland.

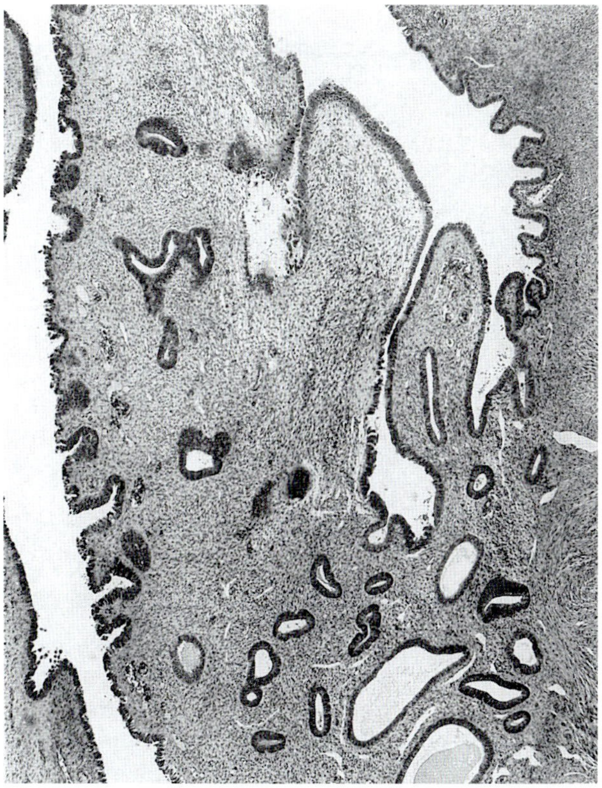

Fig. 11.49. Endometrial polyp with endometrial intraepithelial carcinoma (EIC). The surface epithelium lining the polyp, best seen in the *left portion of the field*, is involved by EIC.

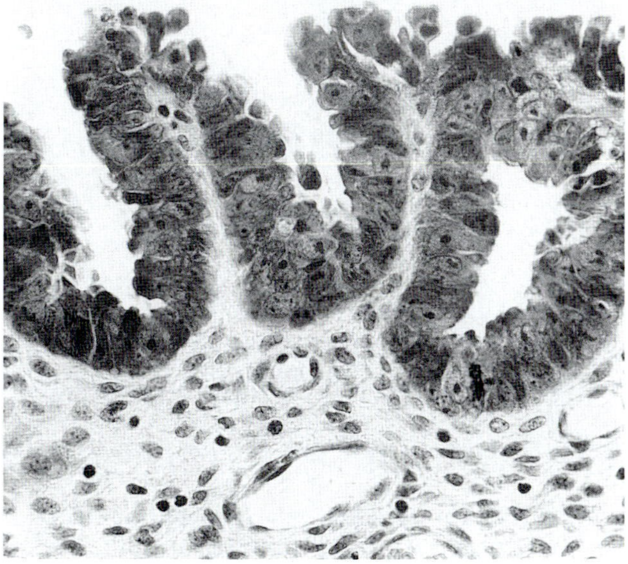

Fig. 11.50. Endometrial polyp with endometrial intraepithelial carcinoma (EIC). Higher magnification of Fig. 11.49 demonstrates the crowded atypical cells of EIC.

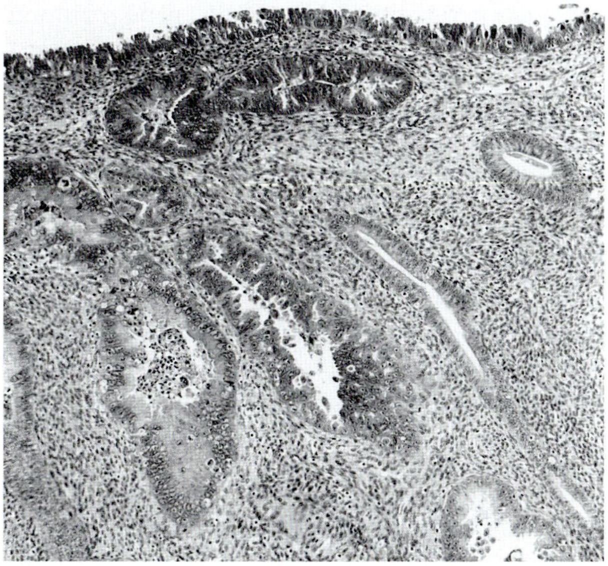

Fig. 11.51. Endometrial intraepithelial carcinoma (EIC). EIC involves the endometrial surface and the underlying glands in the *left portion of the field.* Glands in the *right portion of the field* are not involved.

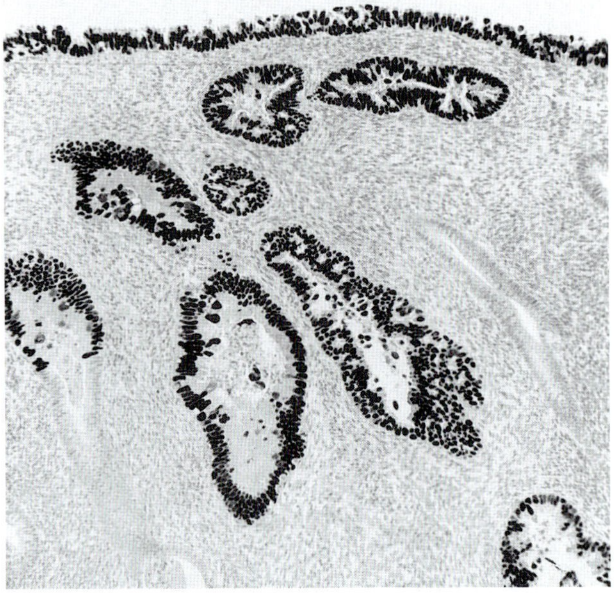

Fig. 11.52. Endometrial intraepithelial carcinoma (EIC). Immunohistochemical stain for p53 performed on the section adjacent to that in Fig. 11.51 demonstrates diffuse, strong nuclear positivity in EIC on surface and in underlying glands, including a partially involved gland at the *left*. Adjacent normal glands are negative.

correlated with identification of p53 mutation in these cases. Lack of immunoreactivity for p53, however, does not exclude the presence of a mutation in p53 because mutations have been detected in a small number of serous carcinomas that were nonreactive for p53 due to the formation of a truncated or unstable protein.[89] Identical p53 gene mutations have been found in the EIC and adjacent serous carcinoma in several cases. Examples of pure EIC unassociated with serous carcinoma also have been shown to contain p53 mutations. In addition, a case of pure EIC has been shown to contain p53 mutation in the absence of loss of heterozygosity of chromosome 17p, suggesting that p53 mutation occurs early in the evolution of serous carcinoma.[89] The finding of EIC unassociated with invasive carcinoma and the presence of identical p53 mutations in both lesions support the view that EIC is the precursor lesion of serous carcinoma.

Differential Diagnosis

The distinction of extensive EIC from early serous carcinoma has not been well defined. Crowded glands involved by EIC within a polyp or within the endometrium should be classified as extensive EIC when the proliferation lacks a confluent glandular pattern, demonstrates no evidence of stromal desmoplasia (stromal invasion), and is less than 1 cm in greatest dimension (Fig. 11.53). When either glandular confluence or stromal invasion is present and the proliferation exceeds 1 cm in greatest dimension, the lesion qualifies as serous carcinoma. Lesions with glandular confluence or stromal invasion but measuring less than 1 cm can be subclassified as minimal uterine serous carcinoma (Fig. 11.53; see following). It is important to note, however, that metastatic serous carcinoma can be found in other sites in the genital tract and in the abdomen in the absence of demonstrable invasion in uteri with EIC, indicating that EIC is capable of metastasizing without first invading the stroma of the endometrium.[85,93]

EIC must be distinguished from benign metaplastic endometrial lesions that can mimic the nuclear changes seen in EIC, which include eosinophilic cell change, hobnail change, and tubal metaplasia. At times eosinophilic cell change and hobnail change can display enlarged, smudged, hyperchromatic nuclei, but these nuclei usually have a degenerative appearance and typically lack the prominent nucleoli seen in EIC. On occasion, however, the nuclei can appear more overtly atypical, with prominent nucleoli, suggesting EIC (see Fig. 11.27).

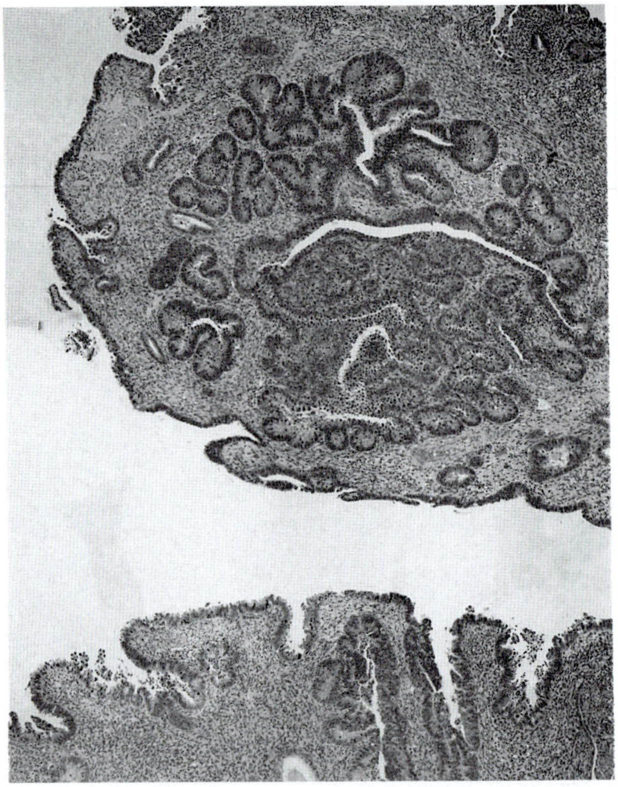

Fig. 11.53. Extensive endometrial intraepithelial carcinoma (EIC)/minimal uterine serous carcinoma. Crowded glands, measuring less than 1 cm in greatest dimension, within an endometrial polyp are involved by EIC. The glandular proliferation is partially confluent, suggesting early stromal invasion. Endometrium in the *lower portion of the field* is also involved by EIC.

Tubal metaplasia typically displays enlarged, hyperchromatic nuclei, but these are admixed with other cell types, including ciliated cells and intercalated cells, and nucleoli are usually not prominent. Immunohistochemistry for Ki-67, a proliferation marker, is very useful for distinguishing EIC from eosinophilic cell change and tubal metaplasia in that EIC typically displays a very high proliferation index (virtually all the nuclei express Ki-67), whereas the metaplasias have very low proliferation indices. In addition, EIC is usually diffusely and strongly positive for p53, whereas eosinophilic metaplasia is typically negative or occasionally displays weak or scattered moderate nuclear staining.

A recent study reported strong expression of p53 in surface endometrial lesions that lacked marked nuclear atypia diagnostic of EIC.[98] The authors suggested that the definition of EIC be expanded to include surface epithelium containing less atypical cells that are strongly positive for p53 by immunohistochemistry. These investigators proposed the term "uterine surface carcinoma" for this lesion. We have made similar observations but are reluctant to render a definitive diagnosis of carcinoma for lesions that lack the morphologic features of carcinoma on routine hematoxylin and eosin stains despite strong immunohistochemical expression of p53. A variety of metaplastic and reactive processes can display substantial cytologic atypia and closely resemble EIC. Preliminary data based on a small number of cases indicate that these lesions do not strongly overexpress p53.[98] However, a larger number of cases needs to be analyzed by immunohistochemical and molecular genetic methods before these minimally atypical, p53-positive lesions are classified as early manifestations of serous carcinoma.

Behavior and Treatment

There are limited data on the behavior of pure EIC. A recent study found that patients with pure EIC, and those with minimal uterine serous carcinoma (less than 1 cm of carcinoma in the endometrium) lacking myometrial or vascular invasion and no evidence of extrauterine disease, had an overall survival of 100% after a mean follow-up of 27 months.[95] The majority of these patients received no treatment after hysterectomy. In addition, the few patients with involvement of endocervical glands by EIC (stage IIA disease) were also alive without evidence of disease at intervals ranging from 12 to 54 months. Similarly, in another study of stage IA serous carcinoma, 11 of 13 patients were alive without evidence of disease after a median follow-up of 38 months.[18] In contrast, patients with either EIC or minimal serous carcinoma and evidence of extrauterine disease (even microscopic disease) all died of disease despite intensive chemotherapy.[95] Accordingly, patients with a diagnosis of EIC in an endometrial biopsy or curettage specimen should undergo careful surgical staging at the time of hysterectomy.

References

1. The Postmenopausal Estrogen/Progestin Interventions (PEPI) Trial. The Writing Group for the PEPI Trial (1996) Effects of hormone replacement therapy on endometrial histology in postmenopausal women. JAMA 275:370–375
2. Ambros RA, Sherman ME, Zahn CM, Bitterman P, Kurman RJ (1995) Endometrial intraepithelial carcinoma: a distinctive lesion specifically associated with tumors displaying serous differentiation. Hum Pathol 26:1260–1267
3. Ausems EW, van der Kamp JK, Baak JP (1985) Nuclear morphometry in the determination of the prognosis of marked atypical endometrial hyperplasia. Int J Gynecol Pathol 4:180–185
4. Ayhan A, Yarali H (1991) Endometrial carcinoma: a pathologic evaluation of 142 cases with and without associated endometrial hyperplasia. J Surg Oncol 46:182–184
5. Baak JPA (1986) Further evaluation of the practical applicability of nuclear morphometry for the prediction of the outcome of atypical endometrial hyperplasia. Anal Quant Cytol Histol 8:46–48
6. Baak JPA, Nauta JJ, Wisse-Brekelmans EC, Bezemer PD (1988) Architectural and nuclear morphometrical features together are more important prognosticators in endometrial hyperplasias than nuclear morphometrical features alone. J Pathol 154:335–341
7. Baak JPA, Wisse-Brekelmans EC, Fleege JC, van der Putten HW, Bezemer PD (1992) Assessment of the risk on endometrial cancer in hyperplasia, by means of morphological and morphometrical features. Pathol Res Pract 188:856–859
8. Baak JPA, Orbo A, van Diest PJ, Jiwa M, deBruin P, Broeckaert M, Snijders W, Boodt PJ, Fons G, Birger C, Verheijen RHM, Houben PWH, The HS, Kenemans P (2001) Prospective multicenter evaluation of the morphometric D-score for prediction of the outcome of endometrial hyperplasias. Am J Surg Pathol 25:930–935
9. Baak JPA, Kuik DJ, Bezemer PD (1994) The additional prognostic value of morphometric nuclear arrangement and DNA-ploidy to other morphometric and stereologic features in endometrial hyperplasias. Int J Gynecol Cancer 4:289–297
10. Beckner ME, Mori T, Silverberg SG (1985) Endometrial carcinoma: nontumor factors in prognosis. Int J Gynecol Pathol 4:131–145
11. Bergeron C, Nogales FF, Masseroli M, Abeler V, Duvillard P, Muller-Holzner E, Pickartz H, Wells M (1999) A multicentric European study testing the reproducibility of the WHO classification of endometrial hyperplasia with a proposal of a simplified

working classification for biopsy and curettage specimens. Am J Surg Pathol 23:1102–1108
12. Beutler HK, Dockerty MB, Randall LM (1963) Precancerous lesions of the endometrium. Am J Obstet Gynecol 86:433–443
13. Blaustein A (1982) Morular metaplasia misdiagnosed as adenoacanthoma in young women with polycystic ovarian disease. Am J Surg Pathol 6:223–228
14. Bokhman JV (1983) Two pathogenetic types of endometrial carcinoma. Gynecol Oncol 15:10–17
15. Brinton LA, Berman ML, Mortel R, Twiggs LB, Barrett RJ, Wilbanks GD, Lannom L, Hoover RN (1992) Reproductive, menstrual, and medical risk factors for endometrial cancer: results from a case-control study. Am J Obstet Gynecol 167:1317–1325
16. Buehl IA, Vellios F, Carter JE, Huber CP (1964) Carcinoma in situ of the endometrium. Am J Clin Pathol 42:594–601
17. Campbell PE, Barter RA (1961) The significance of atypical hyperplasia. J Obstet Gynaecol Br Commonw 68:668–672
18. Carcangiu ML, Tan LK, Chambers JT (1997) Stage IA uterine serous carcinoma. A study of 13 cases. Am J Surg Pathol 21:1507–1514
19. Chamlian DL, Taylor HB (1970) Endometrial hyperplasia in young women. Obstet Gynecol 36:659–666
20. Crum CP, Richart RM, Fenoglio CM (1981) Adenoacanthosis of endometrium: a clinicopathologic study in premenopausal women. Am J Surg Pathol 5:15–20
21. Dawagne MP, Silverberg SG (1982) Foam cells in endometrial carcinoma—a clinicopathologic study. Gynecol Oncol 13:67–75
22. Deligdisch L, Cohen CJ (1985) Histologic correlates and virulence implications of endometrial carcinoma associated with adenomatous hyperplasia. Cancer (Phila) 56:1452–1455
23. Demopoulos RI, Greco MA (1983) Mucinous metaplasia of the endometrium: ultrastructural and histochemical characteristics. Int J Gynecol Pathol 1: 383–390
24. Dunton CJ, Baak JP, Palazzo JP, van Diest PJ, McHugh M, Widra EA (1996) Use of computerized morphometric analyses of endometrial hyperplasias in the prediction of coexistent cancer. Am J Obstet Gynecol 174:1518–1521
25. Ferenczy A, Gelfand M (1989) The biologic significance of cytologic atypia in progestogen-treated endometrial hyperplasia. Am J Obstet Gynecol 160: 126–131
26. Fluhman CF (1954) Comparative studies of squamous metaplasia of the cervix uteri and endometrium. Am J Obstet Gynecol 68:1447–1463
27. Gal D (1986) Hormonal therapy for lesions of the endometrium. Semin Oncol 13:33–36
28. Greenblatt RB, Gambrell RDJ, Stoddard LD (1982) The protective role of progesterone in the prevention of endometrial cancer. Pathol Res Pract 174: 297–318
29. Grimes DA (1982) Diagnostic dilation and curettage: a reappraisal. Am J Obstet Gynecol 142:1–6
30. Gucer F, Reich O, Tamussino K, Bader AA, Pieber D, Scholl W, Haas J, Petru E (1998) Concomitant endometrial hyperplasia in patients with endometrial carcinoma. Gynecol Oncol 69:64–68
31. Gusberg SB (1947) Precursors of corpus carcinoma estrogens and adenomatous hyperplasia. Am J Obstet Gynecol 54:905–927
32. Gusberg SB, Kaplan AL (1963) Precursors of corpus cancer. IV. Adenomatous hyperplasia as Stage 0 carcinoma of the endometrium. Am J Obstet Gynecol 87:662–678
33. Gusberg SB, Moore DB, Martin F (1954) Precursors of corpus cancer II. A clinical and pathological study of adenomatous hyperplasia. Am J Obstet Gynecol 68:1472–1481
34. Hall TE, Stapleton JJ, McCance JM (1982) The isolated finding of histiocytes in Papanicolaou smears from postmenopausal women. J Reprod Med 27: 647–650
35. Hendrickson MR, Kempson RL (1980) Endometrial epithelial metaplasias: proliferations frequently misdiagnosed as adenocarcinoma. Report of 89 cases and proposed classification. Am J Surg Pathol 4:525–542
36. Hendrickson MR, Kempson RL (1980) Surgical pathology of the uterine corpus, vol 12. Saunders, Philadelphia
37. Herlyn M, Malkowicz SB (1991) Regulatory pathways in tumor growth and invasion. Lab Invest 65: 262–271
38. Hertig AT, Sommers SC (1949) Genesis of endometrial carcinoma. I. Study of prior biopsies. Cancer (Phila) 2:946–956
39. Hertig AT, Sommers SC, Bengloff H (1949) Genesis of endometrial carcinoma. III. Carcinoma in situ. Cancer (Phila) 2:964–971
40. Hunter JE, Tritz DE, Howell MG, DePriest PD, Gallion HH, Andrews SJ, Buckley SB, Kryscio RJ, van Nagell JR Jr (1994) The prognostic and therapeutic implications of cytologic atypia in patients with endometrial hyperplasia. Gynecol Oncol 55:66–71
41. Iozzo RV (1984) Proteoglycans and neoplastic–mesenchymal cell interactions. Hum Pathol 15:2–10
42. Janicek MF, Rosenshein NB (1994) Invasive endometrial cancer in uteri resected for atypical endometrial hyperplasia. Gynecol Oncol 52:373–378
43. Kaku T, Tsukamoto N, Hachisuga T, Tsuruchi N, Sakai K, Hirakawa T, Amada S, Saito T, Kamura T, Nakano H (1996) Endometrial carcinoma associated with hyperplasia. Gynecol Oncol 60:22–25
44. Kaku T, Tsukamoto N, Tsuruchi N, Sugihara K, Kamura T, Nakano H (1992) Endometrial metaplasia associated with endometrial carcinoma. Obstet Gynecol 80:812–816
45. Kaminski PF, Stevens CW (1985) The value of endometrial sampling in abnormal uterine bleeding. Am J Gynecol Health II:33–36
46. Kendall BS, Ronnett BM, Isacson C, Cho KR, Hedrick L, Diener-West M, Kurman RJ (1998) Reproducibility of the diagnosis of endometrial hyper-

plasia, atypical hyperplasia, and well-differentiated carcinoma. Am J Surg Pathol 22:1012–1019
47. Kim YB, Holschneider CH, Ghosh K, Nieberg RK, Montz FJ (1997) Progestin alone as primary treatment of endometrial carcinoma in premenopausal women. Report of seven cases and review of the literature. Cancer (Phila) 79:320–327
48. King A, Seraj IM, Wagner RJ (1984) Stromal invasion in endometrial adenocarcinoma. Am J Obstet Gynecol 149:10–14
49. Kraus FT (1985) High-risk and premalignant lesions of the endometrium. Am J Surg Pathol 9:31–40
50. Kumar NB, Hart WR (1982) Metastases to the uterine corpus from extragenital cancers. A clinicopathologic study of 63 cases. Cancer (Phila) 50:2163–2169
51. Kurman RJ, Felix JC, Archer DF, Nanavati N, Arce J, Moyer DL (2000) Norethindrone acetate and estradiol-induced endometrial hyperplasia. Obstet Gynecol 96:373–379
52. Kurman RJ, Kaminski PF, Norris HJ (1985) The behavior of endometrial hyperplasia. A long-term study of "untreated" hyperplasia in 170 patients. Cancer (Phila) 56:403–412
53. Kurman RJ, Norris HJ (1982) Evaluation of criteria for distinguishing atypical endometrial hyperplasia from well-differentiated carcinoma. Cancer (Phila) 49:2547–2559
54. Kurman RJ, Scully RE (1976) Clear cell carcinoma of the endometrium: an analysis of 21 cases. Cancer (Phila) 37:872–882
55. Lee KR, Scully RE (1989) Complex endometrial hyperplasia and carcinoma in adolescents and young women 15 to 20 years of age. A report of 10 cases. Int J Gynecol Pathol 8:201–213
56. Lidor A, Ismajovich B, Confino E, David MP (1986) Histopathological findings in 226 women with postmenopausal uterine bleeding. Acta Obstet Gynecol Scand 65:41–43
57. Liotta LA, Rao CN, Barsky SH (1983) Tumor invasion and the extracellular matrix. Lab Invest 49:636–649
58. Longacre TA, Chung MH, Jensen DN, Hendrickson MR (1995) Proposed criteria for the diagnosis of well-differentiated endometrial carcinoma. Am J Surg Pathol 19:371–406
59. Masterton R, Armstrong EM, More IA (1975) The cyclical variation in the percentage of ciliated cells in the normal human endometrium. J Reprod Fertil 42:537–540
60. Mazur MT (1981) Atypical polypoid adenomyomas of the endometrium. Am J Surg Pathol 5:473–482
61. McBride JM (1959) Pre-menopausal cystic hyperplasia and endometrial carcinoma. J Obstet Gynaecol Br Emp 66:288–296
62. Mutter GL (2000) Endometrial intraepithelial neoplasia (EIN): will it bring order to chaos? The Endometrial Collaborative Group. Gynecol Oncol 76: 287–290
63. Mutter GL, Baak JP, Crum CP, Richart RM, Ferenczy A, Faquin WC (2000) Endometrial precancer diagnosis by histopathology, clonal analysis, and computerized morphometry. J Pathol 190:462–469
64. Mutter GL, Chaponot ML, Fletcher JA (1995) A polymerase chain reaction assay for non-random X chromosome inactivation identifies monoclonal endometrial cancers and precancers. Am J Pathol 146: 501–508
65. Nguyen TN, Bourdeau JL, Ferenczy A, Franco EL (1998) Clinical significance of histiocytes in the detection of endometrial adenocarcinoma and hyperplasia. Diagn Cytopathol 19:89–93
66. Norris HJ, Tavassoli FA, Kurman RJ (1983) Endometrial hyperplasia and carcinoma. Diagnostic considerations. Am J Surg Pathol 7:839–847
67. Novak E, Rutledge F (1948) Atypical endometrial hyperplasia simulating adenocarcinoma. Am J Obstet Gynecol 55:46–63
68. Nucci MR, Prasad CJ, Crum CP, Mutter GL (1999) Mucinous endometrial epithelial proliferations: a morphologic spectrum of changes with diverse clinical significance. Mod Pathol 12:1137–1142
69. Potischman N, Hoover RN, Brinton LA, Siiteri P, Dorgan JF, Swanson CA, Berman ML, Mortel R, Twiggs LB, Barrett RJ, Wilbanks GD, Persky V, Lurain JR (1996) Case-control study of endogenous steroid hormones and endometrial cancer. J Natl Cancer Inst 88:1127–1135
70. Randall TC, Kurman RJ (1997) Progestin treatment of atypical hyperplasia and well-differentiated carcinoma of the endometrium in women under age 40. Obstet Gynecol 90:434–440
71. Rorat E, Wallach RC (1984) Papillary metaplasia of the endometrium: clinical and histopathologic considerations. Obstet Gynecol 64:90S–92S
72. Rozengurt E, Sinnett-Smith J, Taylor-Papadimitriou J (1985) Production of PDGF-like growth factor by breast cancer cell lines. Int J Cancer 36:247–252
73. Salm R (1962) Macrophages in endometrial lesions. J Pathol Bacteriol 83:405–409
74. Salm R (1980) Ultrastructure of endometrial stromal foam cells [letter]. Am J Clin Pathol 73:731–732
75. Sawhney N, Garrahan N, Douglas-Jones AG, Williams ED (1992) Epithelial–stromal interactions in tumors. A morphologic study of fibroepithelial tumors of the breast. Cancer (Phila) 70:2115–2120
76. Scully RE, Bonfiglio TA, Kurman RJ, Silverberg SG, Wilkinson EJ (1994) Histologic typing of female genital tract tumours (international histological classification of tumours), 2nd Ed. Springer-Verlag, New York, pp 1–189
77. Seemayer TA, Lagace R, Schurch W, Tremblay G (1979) Myofibroblasts in the stroma of invasive and metastatic carcinoma: a possible host response to neoplasia. Am J Surg Pathol 3:525–533
78. Sherman ME, Bitterman P, Rosenshein NB, Delgado G, Kurman RJ (1992) Uterine serous carcinoma. A morphologically diverse neoplasm with unifying clinicopathologic features. Am J Surg Pathol 16:600–610
79. Sherman ME, Bur ME, Kurman RJ (1995) p53 in endometrial cancer and its putative precursors: evidence for diverse pathways of tumorigenesis. Hum Pathol 26:1268–1274
80. Sherman ME, Sturgeon S, Brinton LA, Potischman

N, Kurman RJ, Berman ML, Mortel R, Twiggs LB, Barrett RJ, Wilbanks GD (1997) Risk factors and hormone levels in patients with serous and endometrioid uterine carcinomas. Mod Pathol 10:963–968
81. Silver MM, Miles P, Rosa C (1991) Comparison of Novak and Pipelle endometrial biopsy instruments. Obstet Gynecol 78:828–830
82. Silver SA, Sherman ME (1998) Morphologic and immunophenotypic characterization of foam cells in endometrial lesions. Int J Gynecol Pathol 17:140–145
83. Silverberg SG, Kurman RJ (1992) Atlas of tumor pathology. Tumors of the uterine corpus and gestational trophoblastic disease, third series, fascicle 3. Armed Forces Institute of Pathology, Washington, DC
84. Skov BG, Broholm H, Engel U, Franzmann MB, Nielsen AL, Lauritzen AF, Skov T (1997) Comparison of the reproducibility of the WHO classifications of 1975 and 1994 of endometrial hyperplasia. Int J Gynecol Pathol 16:33–37
85. Soslow RA, Pirog E, Isacson C (2000) Endometrial intraepithelial carcinoma with associated peritoneal carcinomatosis. Am J Surg Pathol 24:726–732
86. Spiegel GW (1995) Endometrial carcinoma in situ in postmenopausal women. Am J Surg Pathol 19: 417–432
87. Stock RJ, Kanbour A (1975) Prehysterectomy curettage. Obstet Gynecol 45:537–541
88. Stovall TG, Ling FW, Morgan PL (1991) A prospective, randomized comparison of the Pipelle endometrial sampling device with the Novak curette. Am J Obstet Gynecol 165:1287–1290
89. Tashiro H, Isacson C, Levine R, Kurman RJ, Cho KR, Hedrick L (1997) p53 gene mutations are common in uterine serous carcinoma and occur early in their pathogenesis. Am J Surg Pathol 150:177–185
90. Tavassoli FA, Kraus FT (1978) Endometrial lesions in uteri resected for atypical endometrial hyperplasia. Am J Clin Pathol 70:770–779
91. Terakawa N, Kigawa J, Taketani Y, Yoshikawa H, Yajima A, Noda K, Okada H, Kato J, Yakushiji M, Tanizawa O, Fujimoto S, Nozawa S, Takahashi T, Hasumi K, Furuhashi N, Aono T, Sakamoto A, Furusato M (1997) The behavior of endometrial hyperplasia: a prospective study. Endometrial Hyperplasia Study Group. J Obstet Gynaecol Res 23: 223–230
92. Vellios F (1974) Endometrial hyperplasia and carcinoma in situ. Gynecol Oncol 2:152–161
93. Baergen RN, Warren CD, Isacson C, Ellenson LH (2001) Early uterine serous carcinoma: clonal origin of extrauterine disease. Int J Gynecol Pathol 20: 214–219
94. Welch WR, Scully RE (1977) Precancerous lesions of the endometrium. Hum Pathol 8:503–512
95. Wheeler DT, Bell KA, Kurman RJ, Sherman ME (2000) Minimal uterine serous carcinoma: diagnosis and clicopathologic correlation. Am J Surg Pathol 24:797–806
96. Widra EA, Dunton CJ, McHugh M, Palazzo JP (1995) Endometrial hyperplasia and the risk of carcinoma. Int J Gynecol Cancer 5:233–235
97. Zaman SS, Mazur MT (1993) Endometrial papillary syncytial change. A nonspecific alteration associated with active breakdown [see comments]. Am J Clin Pathol 99:741–745
98. Zheng W, Khurana R, Farahmand S, Wang Y, Zhang ZF, Felix JC (1998) p53 immunostaining as a significant adjunct diagnostic method for uterine surface carcinoma. Am J Surg Pathol 22:1463–1473

12

Endometrial Carcinoma

Brigitte M. Ronnett, M.D., Richard J. Zaino, M.D., Lora Hedrick Ellenson, M.D., and Robert J. Kurman, M.D.

Epidemiology and Etiology

Endometrial carcinoma is the most common invasive neoplasm of the female genital tract and the fourth most frequently diagnosed cancer in women in the United States. In 2000, it is estimated there will have been 36,100 new cases and 6,500 deaths resulting from this neoplasm. These figures represent an estimated 6% of the new cancer cases and 2% of the cancer deaths in women.[13] Worldwide, approximately 150,000 cases are diagnosed each year, making endometrial carcinoma the fifth most common cancer in women.[253,255] The incidence of endometrial cancer varies widely throughout the world. The highest rates occur in North America and Europe, whereas rates in developing countries and Japan are four to five times lower. The incidence is also about twice as high in whites compared to blacks.

Hormonal Stimulation

The strong association between replacement estrogen therapy and the development of endometrial cancer was demonstrated in a number of case-control studies in the late 1970s.[123,125,213,222,296,307,366] Recent reviews summarize the data generated by numerous studies of hormonal therapy and risk of endometrial cancer and confirm the increased risk of unopposed estrogen therapy.[26,265] A recent study of endogenous hormones and endometrial cancer demonstrated that the risk associated with elevated levels of unopposed estrogen varies according to menopausal status.[270] In particular, high estrone and albumin-bound estradiol levels were associated with increased risk in postmenopausal women, but high levels of total, free, and albumin-bound estradiol were unrelated to increased risk in premenopausal women. In addition, high circulating levels of androstenedione were identified as a risk factor in both pre- and postmenopausal women. In both age groups, the risk associated with obesity was not affected by adjustment for hormones. Factors that lower the exposure of the endometrium to unopposed estrogen reduce the risk of endometrial cancer; these include the addition of progestin to hormone replacement regimens, the use of oral contraceptives, and smoking.[15,20,26,97,105,124,174,204,254,265,345] It has been shown that women using unopposed estrogen for more than 2 years have a two- to threefold increase in the risk of endometrial cancer, whereas women receiving progestins in conjunction with estrogen have no increased risk.[258] One large case-control study demonstrated that the use of oral contraceptives for at least 1 year reduces the risk of endometrial carcinoma by 50% and that protection persists at least 15 years after discontinuation.[15]

The data on the risk of endometrial cancer in patients on tamoxifen are conflicting.[294] Tamoxifen is a nonsteroidal compound that acts by competing with estrogen for estrogen receptors. In reproductive age women it therefore has an antiestrogenic effect, but in postmenopausal (hypoestrogenic) women it has weak estrogenic effects. Some large studies have reported that there is a significantly increased risk of endometrial cancer, apparently related to dose and duration of use, whereas others have not shown a significant risk.[14,29,58,93,94,96,173,273,279,280,316,337] In addition, some studies have reported a higher proportion of high-risk types of carcinomas in tamoxifen-treated women whereas others have found predominantly low-grade carcinomas.[23,94,216,303] Thus, some investigators are convinced that tamoxifen confers an increased risk of endometrial cancer while others believe the evidence is inconclusive.[66,149,152,162,185,214]

Constitutional Factors

Obesity, like estrogen replacement therapy, is a well-defined risk factor for endometrial cancer, with reported relative risks ranging from 2 to 10.[253,255] The risk can be explained by the increased availability of peripheral estrogens as a result of aromatization of androgens to estrogens in adipose tissue and lower concentrations of sex hormone-binding globulins in obese women.[86] Diabetes has been repeatedly associated with an increased risk of endometrial cancer, ranging from 1.2 to 2.1, and this risk appears to be independent of other frequently associated variables such as obesity.[35,253,255] Other factors that have been associated with an increased risk of endometrial cancer include early age of menarche, later age of menopause, and nulliparity. The association with nulliparity appears to be primarily on the basis of infertility due to chronic anovulation in which unopposed estrogenic stimulation occurs.[35,253] The protective effect of pregnancy appears to be related and restricted to the first full-term pregnancy because abortions and increasing numbers of births do not influence the risk.

Diet

Endometrial cancer risk is correlated with total caloric intake, total protein intake, and frequency of consumption of meat, eggs, milk, fats, and oils. These dietary factors, as well as decreased energy expenditure and physical exercise associated with a sedentary lifestyle, are major determinants of obesity, which is an established risk factor. The independent contribution of specific dietary factors to endometrial cancer risk has not been clearly established.[206,253]

Classification

In the past two decades, clinicopathologic, immunohistochemical, and molecular genetic studies have provided data to allow for the development of a dualistic model of endometrial carcinogenesis. In this model, there are two types of endometrial carcinoma that have been designated, type I and type II (Table 12.1). As discussed, factors associated with unopposed estrogenic stimulation, such as obesity and exogenous hormone use, as well as the presence of endometrial hyperplasia, are related to the development of the most common form of endometrial carcinoma, that is, the endometrioid subtype that represents the type I carcinomas.[30] More recent studies have confirmed this association by demonstrating elevated serum estrogen levels in patients

Table 12.1. Pathogenetic forms of endometrial carcinoma

Form	*Type I*	*Type II*
Unopposed estrogen	Present	Absent
Menopausal status	Pre- and perimenopausal	Postmenopausal
Precursor lesion	Atypical hyperplasia	Endometrial intraepithelial carcinoma
Tumor grade	Low	High
Myometrial invasion	Variable, often minimal	Variable, often deep
Histologic subtypes	Endometrioid	Serous and clear cell
Behavior	Indolent	Aggressive
Genetic alterations	*PTEN* mutation Microsatellite instability K-*ras* mutation	*P53* mutation

Table 12.2. Classification of endometrial carcinoma[a]

Endometrioid adenocarcinoma
Villoglandular
Secretory
Ciliated cell
Endometrioid adenocarcinoma with squamous differentiation
Serous carcinoma
Clear cell carcinoma
Mucinous carcinoma
Squamous carcinoma
Mixed types of carcinoma
Undifferentiated carcinoma

[a]Modified World Health Organization and International Society of Gynecological Pathologists Histologic Classification of Endometrial Carcinoma.

with endometrioid carcinoma.[35,270] It also has been recognized that some forms of endometrial carcinoma appear to be unrelated to hormonal factors and hyperplasia.[300] Serous carcinoma is the prototypic endometrial carcinoma that is not related to estrogenic stimulation and represents the type II carcinoma. Most of the other subtypes of endometrial carcinoma can be classified as variants of either type I or II on the basis of clinicopathologic and immunohistochemical features. Thus, other low-grade carcinomas, which are associated with endometrial hyperplasia and estrogenic stimulation, such as mucinous, ciliated cell, or low-grade endometrioid with squamous differentiation, are type I carcinomas. In contrast, clear cell carcinoma shares features with serous carcinoma and is considered a type II carcinoma.

A modified version of the recent World Health Organization (WHO) and International Society of Gynecological Pathologists (ISGYP) classification of endometrial carcinoma is shown in Table 12.2.[293] This classification has certain limitations. The WHO classification uses the term papillary in the designation of serous carcinoma. Although uterine serous carcinomas often demonstrate papillary growth, a papillary pattern can be seen in other carcinomas, including villoglandular, mucinous, and clear cell carcinomas. Thus, papillary growth is not specifically associated with serous differentiation. Hence, its use in designating subtypes of endometrial carcinoma should be avoided. Malignant mesodermal mixed tumors (MMMTs, carcinosarcomas) are classified as mixed epithelial and nonepithelial tumors in the WHO classification of uterine tumors but as epithelial tumors in the ovarian tumor classification. This inconsistency reflects the confusion over the histogenesis and classification of carcinosarcomas in different anatomic sites. Recent molecular genetic data support the concept that both components in these biphasic tumors are clonally derived from a transformed epithelial cell. Accordingly, many investigators now consider these neoplasms as poorly differentiated carcinomas that display sarcomatous differentiation (see following).

Clinical and Pathologic Features of Specific Types of Carcinomas

Endometrioid Carcinoma

Endometrioid carcinoma is the most common form of endometrial carcinoma, accounting for more than three-fourths of all cases. These tumors are referred to as endometrioid because they resemble proliferative-phase endometrium and to maintain consistency with the terminology used for describing tumors with the same histologic appearance in the cervix, ovary, or fallopian tube. The tumors in this category, by definition, do not contain areas showing more than 10% of squamous, serous, mucinous, or clear cell differentiation. Such foci are common in endometrioid carcinoma and are designated as mixed (see "Mixed Types of Carcinoma").

Clinical Features

Patients with endometrioid carcinoma range in age from the second to the eighth decade, with a mean age of 59 years. Most women are postmenopausal, as the disease is relatively uncommon in young women. Only 1–8% of endometrial carcinomas occur in women under 40 years.[67,75,118,175,262] A small number of cases have been reported in women under the age of 30 years, the youngest being 15 years.[91,199] In young women, the tumor is generally low grade and minimally invasive. In most series, the majority of patients have had clinical evidence of polycystic ovary disease (irregular menses, infertility, obesity, or hirsuitism) but in some reports the patients lacked these features. Rarely, endometrioid carcinoma occurs during pregnancy.[143] In pregnant women, endometrial carcinomas are nearly always low grade, superficially invasive or noninvasive, and have an excellent prognosis. The tumors generally do not show histologic evidence of progesterone-induced changes.

The initial manifestation of endometrial carcinoma usually is abnormal vaginal bleeding, although rarely the patient is asymptomatic and the diagnosis is made fortuitously. In one study 24 asymptomatic women with unsuspected endometrial carcinoma were detected among 8998 women dying of unrelated causes who were autopsied at the Yale–New Haven and Massachusetts General Hospitals.[146] The estimated rates of undetected endometrial carcinoma were 22 and 31 per 10,000, respectively. These rates were four to five times higher than the diagnosis of endometrial carcinoma recorded by the Connecticut State Tumor Registry, indicating that a number of endometrial carcinomas may be asymptomatic and are undetected during life.

A number of studies have evaluated cytologic screening of endometrial cancer. Both direct endometrial sampling as well as examination of cervical cytologic smears for the presence of endometrial carcinoma have been performed. In a study of 2586 asymptomatic women the prevalence of occult carcinoma using endometrial cytological sampling was 6.96 per 1000; however, 4 cases were missed.[187] In addition, the investigators emphasized that endometrial smears were difficult to interpret and that the detection methods were only moderately reliable. About a third of the cases would have been detected using a vaginal pool specimen. In a population-based study from Australia, it was found that when a cervical smear was reported as showing endometrial carcinoma, the lesion was confirmed histologically in only 64% of cases.[227] Conversely, among women with endometrial carcinoma a cervical smear performed in the 2 years preceding the diagnosis predicted the presence of endometrial carcinoma in only 28% of cases. Because the sensitivity and specificity of cytologic examination for the detection of endometrial carcinoma is low in asymptomatic women, it is not a cost-effective screening tool for endometrial cancer. In an attempt to use cytologic screening in specific high-risk populations, it was reported that among 597 asymptomatic women over the age of 45 with diabetes and/or hypertension the diabetic women had a significantly higher rate of atypical hyperplasia compared with women with hypertension, suggesting that screening might be useful in diabetic patients.[128] In another study of endometrial cytology in 541 women, all 16 carcinomas were detected by cytologic examination; however, because all but 1 patient were symptomatic, the ability to detect cancers in asymptomatic women could not be assessed.[330] Similarly, endometrial brush sampling detected all but 1 of 13 cancers in 1042 symptomatic patients in another study.[181] Cytologic detection methods in symptomatic women are thus of little value as women with abnormal vaginal bleeding are evaluated by either endometrial biopsy or curettage, which yields a more easily interpreted specimen.

Gross Findings

The gross appearance of endometrioid carcinoma is similar to the various other types of endometrial carcinoma with the possible exception of serous carcinoma (see "Serous Carcinoma"). The endometrial surface is shaggy, glistening, and tan and may be focally hemorrhagic. Endometrioid carcinoma is almost uniformly exophytic even when deeply invasive (Fig. 12.1). The neoplasm may be focal or diffuse. At times the tumor may appear to be composed of separate polypoid masses. Necrosis usually is not evident macroscopically in well-differentiated carcinomas but may be seen in poorly differentiated tumors, sometimes in association with ulcerated or firm areas. Myometrial invasion by carcinoma may result in enlargement of the uterus, but a small atrophic uterus may harbor carcinoma diffusely invading the myometrium. Myometrial invasion appears as well-demarcated, firm, gray-white tissue with linear extensions beneath an exophytic mass or as multiple, white nodules with yellow areas of necrosis within the uterine wall. Extension into the lower uterine segment is common, whereas involvement of the cervix occurs in approximately 20% of cases.

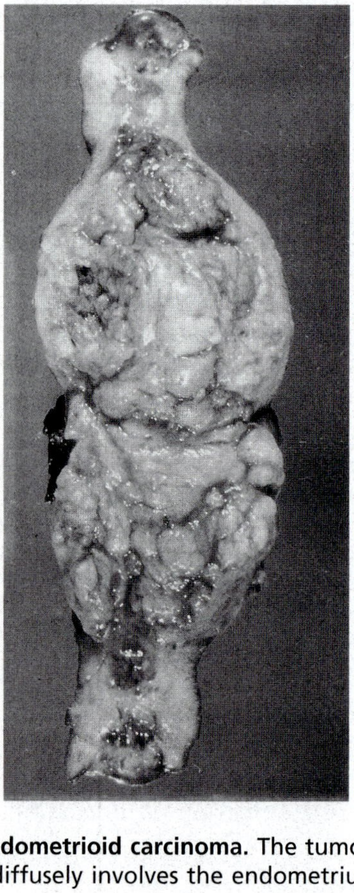

Fig. 12.1. Endometrioid carcinoma. The tumor is exophytic and diffusely involves the endometrium.

Table 12.3. Architectural grading of endometrial carcinoma

Grade 1	No more than 5% of the tumor is composed of solid masses
Grade 2	6–50% of the tumor is composed of solid masses
Grade 3	More than 50% of the tumor is composed of solid masses

Microscopic Findings: Grading

The microscopic appearance of endometrioid carcinoma is determined by the grade of the tumor. Grading is based on the architectural pattern, nuclear features, or both. The architectural grade is determined by the extent to which the tumor is composed of solid masses of cells as compared with well-defined glands (Table 12.3; Figs. 12.2–12.4). In endometrioid carcinomas with squamous differentiation, it is important to exclude masses of squamous epithelium in determining the amount of solid growth (see following). The nuclear grade is determined by the variation in nuclear size and shape, chromatin distribution, and size of the nucleoli (Figs. 12.5–12.7). Grade 1 nuclei are oval, mildly enlarged, and have evenly dispersed chromatin. Grade 3 nuclei are markedly enlarged and pleomorphic, with irregular, coarse chromatin and prominent eosinophilic nucleoli. Grade 2 nuclei have features intermediate to grades 1 and 3. Mitotic activity is an independent histologic variable, but it is generally increased with increasing nuclear grade, as are abnormal mitotic figures.

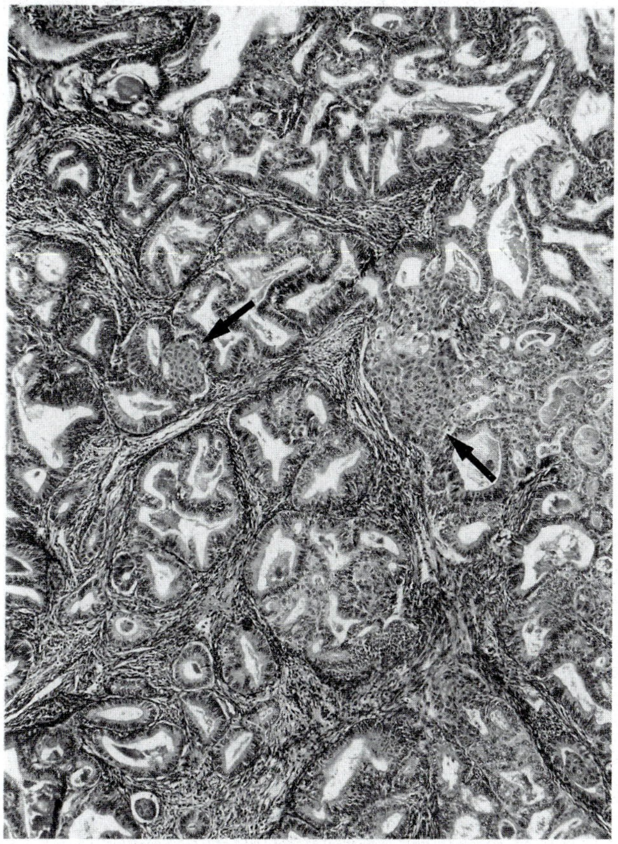

Fig. 12.2. Endometrioid carcinoma, architectural grade 1. The tumor is composed exclusively of well-formed glands. Two small foci of squamous differentiation (*arrows*) are present but because these contribute less than 10% of the tumor, their presence need not be specified.

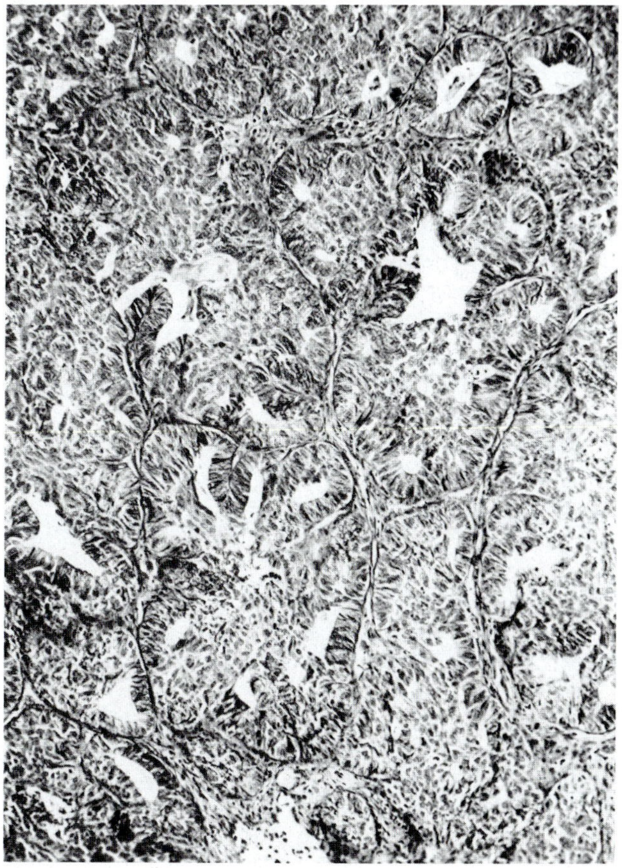

Fig. 12.3. Endometrioid carcinoma, architectural grade 2. A combination of well-formed glands and masses of solid epithelium. The latter comprises 6–50% of the tumor.

The most recent revision of the FIGO (International Federation of Gynecology and Obstetrics) Staging System (Table 12.4) and the WHO Histopathologic Classification of uterine carcinoma recommend that tumors be graded using both architectural and nuclear criteria.[65,293] The grade of tumors that are architecturally grade 1 or 2 should be increased by one

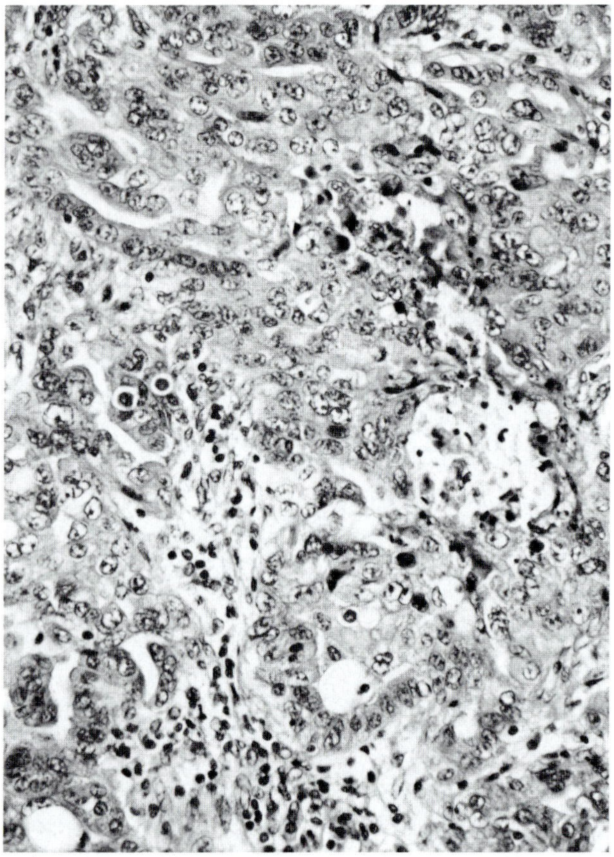

Fig. 12.4. Endometrioid carcinoma, architectural grade 3. Only rare gland lumens are present in an otherwise solid proliferation of epithelium.

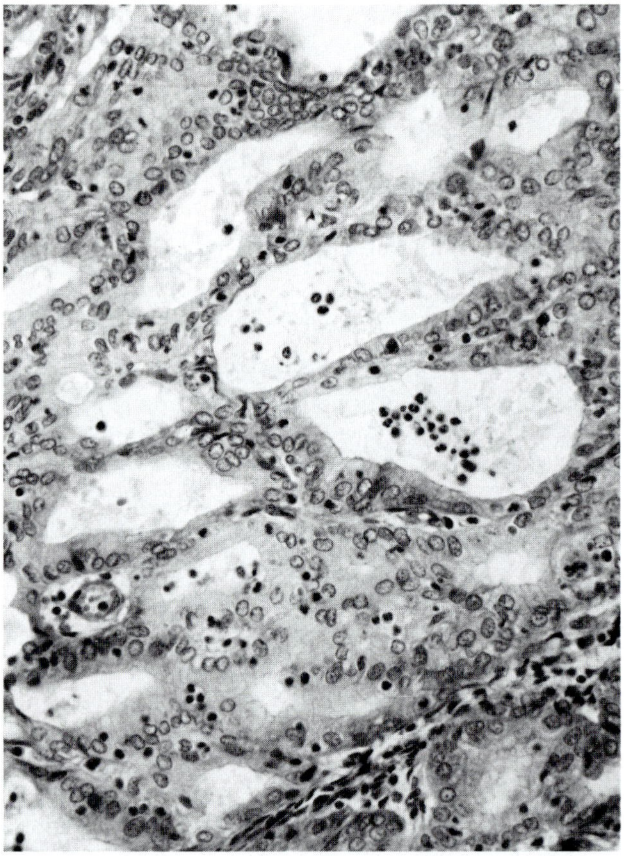

Fig. 12.5. Endometrioid carcinoma, nuclear grade 1. The nuclei are uniform in size, with finely dispersed chromatin.

grade in the presence of "notable" nuclear atypia, defined as grade 3 nuclei.[359] For example, a tumor that is grade 2 by architecture but in which there is marked nuclear atypia (nuclear grade 3) should be upgraded to grade 3. Thus, tumors are graded primarily by their architecture, with the overall grade modified by the nuclear grade when there is discordance. Marked discordance between nuclear and architectural grade is unusual in endometrioid carcinoma and should raise suspicion that the tumor is a serous carcinoma (see "Serous Carcinoma"). For a further discussion of grading, see following ("Histologic Grade").

Marked differences in architectural grade can be seen within a tumor. It is not unusual to see well-formed glandular elements immediately adjacent to solid masses of cells. When a tumor displays this type of heterogeneity, the architectural grade should be based on the overall appearance. The heterogeneity in differentiation accounts for the differences in grade that can be observed between the endometrial curettings and the hysterectomy specimen. Discordance between the curettage and hysterectomy specimens occurs in 15–25% of cases.[70,193,251]

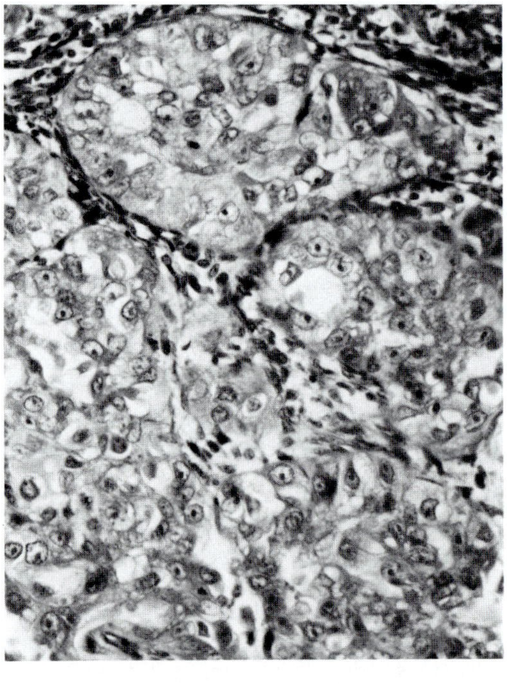

Fig. 12.6. Endometrioid carcinoma, nuclear grade 2. Nuclei are enlarged relative to nuclear grade 1, and prominent nucleoli are present. The degree of pleomorphism and chromatin clumping is less than nuclear grade 3.

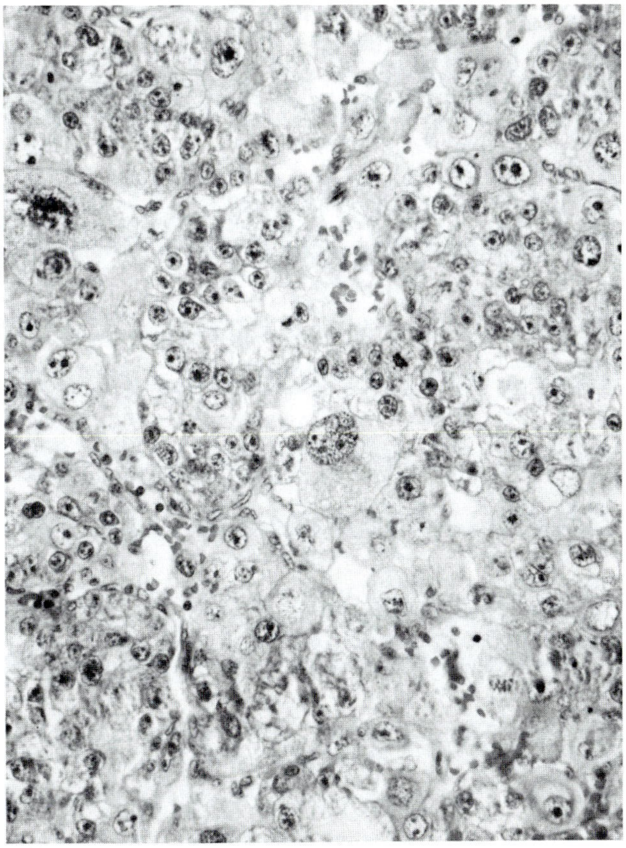

Fig. 12.7. Endometrioid carcinoma, nuclear grade 3. The nuclei are markedly enlarged and pleomorphic with large prominent nucleoli and irregular coarse chromatin.

Differential Diagnosis

The main problem in the differential diagnosis of low-grade endometrioid carcinoma is the distinction from atypical hyperplasia, the atypical polypoid adenomyoma, hyperplasia with various types of cytoplasmic alterations (metaplasias), the Arias-Stella reaction and menstrual endometrium. The distinction from the first three conditions is discussed in Chapter 11. At times an extremely atypical Arias-Stella reaction may simulate adenocarcinoma. In the reproductive age group, Arias–Stella reaction is a much more likely possibility than carcinoma, especially if the clinical history indicates a recent pregnancy. Nonetheless, carcinoma can occur in young women and also in pregnancy. In contrast to a carcinoma, the Arias–Stella reaction tends to be multifocal and is admixed with secretory glands and decidua. The glands in the Arias–Stella reaction may be complex and tortuous but lack confluent or papillary patterns. The stroma does not show a desmoplastic response. The nuclei in the glandular epithelium of the Arias–Stella reaction may be markedly enlarged, but the chromatin appears degenerated and smudged and mitotic figures are very unusual.

Menstrual endometrium can be confused with adenocarcinoma because of the extensive tissue breakdown characterized by tissue fragmentation and hemorrhage. The pattern of stromal breakdown results in fragmented glands of varying size and compact clusters of stromal cells haphazardly mixed with blood,

Table 12.4. International Federation of Gynecology and Obstetrics Staging of Endometrial Cancer, 1988

IA	G123	Tumor limited to the endometrium
IB	G123	Invasion to $\leq 1/2$ myometrium
IC	G123	Invasion to $> 1/2$ myometrium
IIA	G123	Endocervical glandular involvement only
IIB	G123	Cervical stromal invasion
IIIA	G123	Tumor invades serosa and/or adnexae and/or positive peritoneal cytology
IIIB	G123	Vaginal metastases
IIIC	G123	Metastases to pelvic and/or para-aortic lymph nodes
IVA	G123	Tumor invasion of bladder and/or bowel mucosa
IVB	G123	Distant metastases including intraabdominal and/or inguinal lymph nodes

G1, 5% or less of a nonsquamous or nonmorular solid growth pattern; G2, 6–50% of a nonsquamous or nonmorular solid growth pattern; G3, more than 50% of a nonsquamous or nonmorular solid growth pattern.

Rules on staging:

1. Corpus cancer is now surgically staged. Those patients who do not undergo a surgical procedure should be staged according to the 1971 FIGO clinical staging.
2. Ideally, the thickness of the myometrium should be measured along with the depth of tumor invasion.

Notes on grading:

1. Notable nuclear atypia, inappropriate for the architectural grade, raises a grade 1 or grade 2 tumor by one.
2. In serous adenocarcinomas, clear cell adenocarcinomas, and squamous cell carcinomas, nuclear grading takes precedence.
3. Adenocarcinomas with squamous differentiation are graded according to the nuclear grade of the glandular component.

which can appear ominous. The glandular epithelium, however, is bland and shows evidence of secretory activity. Adjacent intact fragments of endometrium with associated predecidual change usually can be identified and assist in the differential diagnosis.

Another problem in differential diagnosis is the distinction of an endometrial from an endocervical primary. Both endometrioid and mucinous carcinomas can arise in either location. The presence of associated endometrial hyperplasia favors a primary site in the endometrium whereas the presence of adenocarcinoma in situ favors endocervical origin. In addition, well to moderately differentiated endometrioid carcinomas usually express estrogen and progesterone receptors whereas endocervical adenocarcinomas are usually negative for hormone receptors by immunohistochemistry.[99,196,219] Carcinoembryonic antigen (CEA) is more commonly expressed in endocervical than in typical endometrioid endometrial adenocarcinomas, whereas vimentin is less commonly expressed in endocervical than endometrial adenocarcinomas.[69] However, immunohistochemistry for CEA is not particularly useful for distinguishing endometrial mucinous carcinomas from endocervical adenocarcinomas because both have a high frequency of positivity. Detection of human papilloma virus (HPV) DNA by either polymerase chain reaction (PCR) or in situ hybridization also can be used to distinguish some endometrial and endocervical carcinomas because endocervical adenocarcinomas usually contain HPV DNA whereas endometrial adenocarcinomas are thought to be etiologically unrelated to HPV infection.[78,145,158,324]

A related problem is the distinction of a primary endometrial carcinoma from a metastasis from an extrauterine site, discussed in "Tumors Metastatic to the Endometrium." A high-grade endometrioid carcinoma at times may be difficult to distinguish from a malignant mesodermal mixed tumor (MMMT). The diagnosis of an MMMT depends on the identification of malignant epithelial and mesenchymal components. The latter is characterized by highly atypical spindle cells with increased cellularity and high mitotic activity. The spindle cells may be intimately associated with the carcinomatous component but should in areas be distinct from it. In these cases, immunostaining for keratin can be helpful. Although occasional spindle cells may be keratin positive in an MMMT, it is unusual for most of the spindle cells to be positive, as they would be in a diffusely infiltrating, poorly differentiated endometrioid adenocarcinoma. The diagnosis of an MMMT usually is not difficult if heterologous elements such as cartilage or rhabdomyoblasts are present. However, rare foci of heterologous tissue, such as cartilage (Fig. 12.8), in

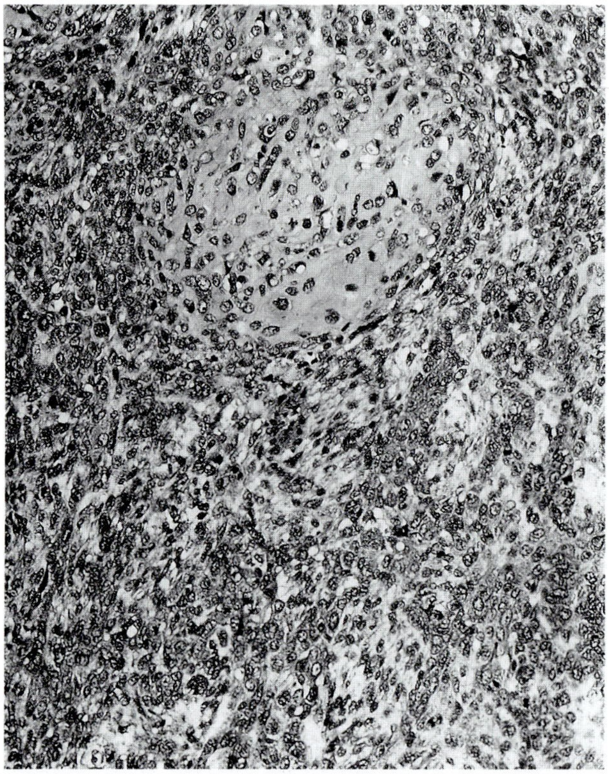

Fig. 12.8. Endometrioid carcinoma, FIGO grade 3. A small focus of cartilage is present in the *upper part of the field.* In view of its small size and the absence of a "sarcomatous"-appearing mesenchymal component, a diagnosis of malignant mixed mesodermal tumor is not justified.

what is otherwise a typical endometrioid carcinoma are insufficient for the diagnosis of an MMMT because the latter has a malignant spindle cell component in addition to the heterologous elements. If heterologous elements are not present, the diagnosis of an MMMT depends on clear-cut demonstration of biphasic epithelial and mesenchymal components.

Prognostic Factors

Based largely on a series of Gynecologic Oncology Group (GOG) studies, it has been shown that the risk factors for endometrial carcinoma can be divided into uterine and extrauterine factors.[32,64,233] Uterine factors include (1) histologic type, (2) grade, (3) depth of myometrial invasion, (4) cervical involvement, (5) vascular invasion, (6) presence of atypical endometrial hyperplasia, (7) hormone receptor status, and (8) DNA ploidy and S-phase fraction. Extrauterine factors include (1) adnexal involvement, (2) intraperitoneal metastasis, (3) positive peritoneal cytology, and (4) pelvic and paraaortic lymph node metastasis. Patients with no evidence of extrauterine disease, no cervical involvement, and no evidence of vascular invasion are at a low overall risk of recurrence. For these patients the grade and depth of invasion are important prognostic factors. In contrast to this low-risk group of patients, women with evidence of extrauterine disease, cervical involvement, or vascular invasion constitute a high-risk group. If one of these three factors is positive, the frequency of recurrence is 20%, increasing to 43% for two positive factors and 63% for three factors.[233]

Clinical Factors

Age, race, and socioeconomic status are prognostic factors in endometrial cancer. Some studies have shown that age is the most important prognostic factor followed by FIGO stage, tumor grade, race, and socioeconomic status.[27,107] Younger women tend to have lower-grade and less invasive tumors, but age remains an important independent risk factor. It has also been demonstrated that women age 45 or less have a better prognosis than women over age 45 because of a significantly higher proportion of early-stage disease and less myometrial invasion.[352] Another recent study also demonstrated that age is a significant prognostic factor, with decreased survival for women over age 50 unrelated to surgical stage or grade of carcinoma.[92] Although there is a lower prevalence of endometrial cancer in African-American woman as compared with white women, white women have a significant survival advantage as compared with African-American women even after controlling for other clinicopathologic and socioeconomic factors.[25,56,142] Some studies have shown that African-American women have a higher proportion of high-grade tumors and less favorable histologic subtypes and tend to present with higher-stage tumors compared to white women.[56,142] In addition, they are treated less often at every stage of disease. Another study showed that the incidence of high-risk tumors is the same in African-American and white women, whereas the incidence of low-risk tumors is significantly lower in African-American women.[268]

Histologic Grade

Grading methods have already been discussed. Numerous studies have confirmed the value of grading.[6,52,83,186,202,357,359] In a study of more than 600 women with clinical stage I or occult stage II endometrioid adenocarcinoma, the 5-year relative survival was as follows: grade 1, 94%; grade 2, 84%; and grade 3, 72%.[357] According to a population-based study from the Norwegian Radium Hospital involving nearly 2000 patients, the 5- and 10-year survival rates for patients with grade 1 tumors were 88% and 80%, respectively; with grade 2 tumors, 77% and 62%; and with grade 3 tumors, 60% and 49%.[6]

A study of the reproducibility of the FIGO grading method found that interobserver reproducibility was acceptable for the architectural grade but unacceptably low for the assessment of notable nuclear atypia.[239] A more recent study comparing FIGO grading to pure nuclear grading of endometrioid carcinoma demonstrated fair interobserver reproducibility for FIGO grading but only poor interobserver reproducibility for nuclear grading.[198] Using a database of 715 patients with low clinical stage endometrial carcinomas (excluding serous and clear cell types), the utility of the FIGO grading system using arbitrary definitions for three nuclear grades was examined.[359] Patients with architectural grade 1 or 2 adenocarcinomas but with predominantly grade 3 nuclei were moved up one grade. This change resulted in upgrading 44 patients for whom the risk of recurrence and death from tumor was similar to that of the other patients in the grade into which they were reassigned. This study provided support for the FIGO modification of architectural grade based on inappropriate nuclear atypia and reinforced the need for a uniform definition of nuclear grade.

Histologic grade is highly correlated with other prognostic factors such as age, stage, and depth of myometrial invasion, so its prognostic utility must also be examined in multivariate analyses. In such studies, the significance of histologic grade in the prediction of survival or recurrence is diminished after adjustment for the other factors, suggesting that grade primarily provides information about the probability of local or disseminated spread of tumor.[6,360] Nevertheless, even for patients with metastatic (stage III) tumor, the histologic grade is significant in predicting outcome after multivariate analysis.[126]

Recently, a two-tiered system for assessing uterine tumor grade was proposed, based on a study of 85 patients with stage I and II endometrial cancer.[323] Separation of tumors into two groups based on the amount of solid growth identified those that recurred as having greater than 20% solid growth. The two-tiered grading system yielded a higher degree of interobserver agreement than the three-tiered FIGO system. Another recent study proposed a binary architectural grading system based on the presence of greater than 50% solid growth, a diffusely infiltrative rather than pushing pattern of invasion, and tumor cell necrosis.[198] High-grade tumors displayed at least two of these three features whereas low-grade tumors had at most one (Figs. 12.9–12.12). The binary system stratified patients into three distinct prognostic groups. Patients with stage I low-grade tumors with invasion confined to the inner half of the myometrium (stages IA and IB)

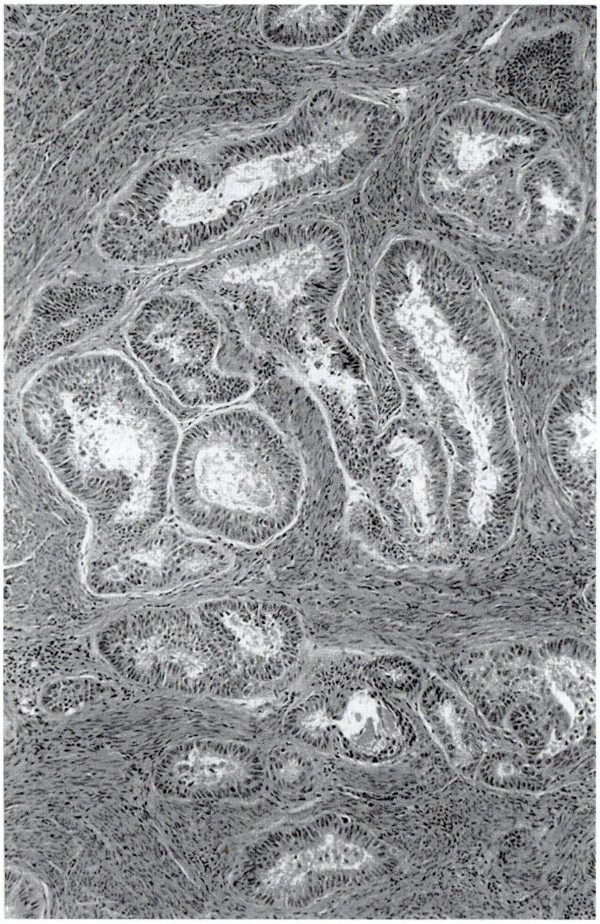

Fig. 12.9. Endometrioid carcinoma, low grade. The carcinoma is entirely glandular and has an expansile rather than infiltrative growth pattern; there is no necrosis.

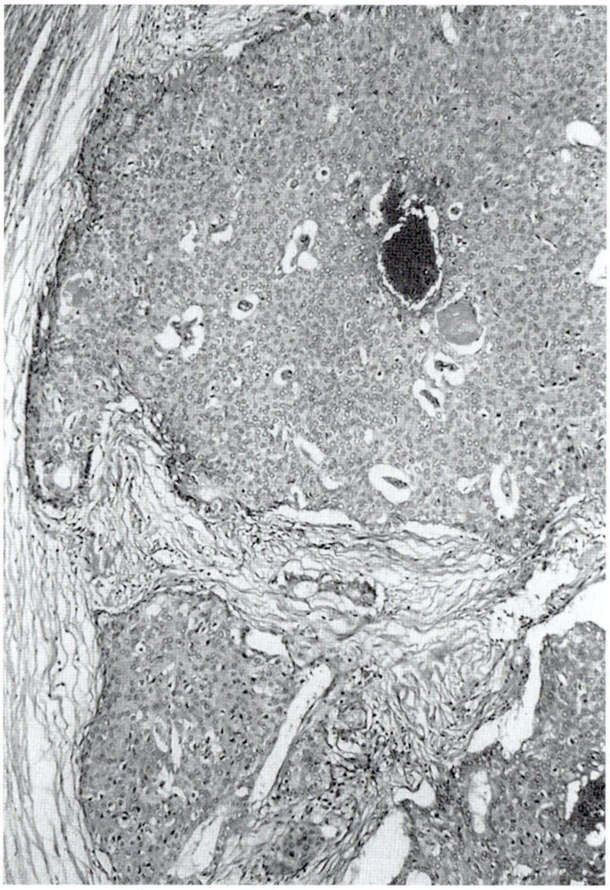

Fig. 12.10. Endometrioid carcinoma, low grade. The carcinoma is virtually entirely solid but the growth pattern is expansile and there is no necrosis.

had a 100% 5-year survival rate. Patients with low-grade tumors that invaded into the outer half of the myometrium or beyond (stages IC-IV) had a 5-year survival rate of 67%. Similarly, those with high-grade tumors with invasion confined to the myometrium (stages IA-IC) had a 5-year survival rate of 76%. Patients with advanced-stage (stages II–IV) high-grade tumors had a 26% 5-year survival rate. In addition, greater intra- and interobserver reproducibility were demonstrated for the binary system in comparison with the FIGO system and pure nuclear grading. There are several advantages of the binary system over the FIGO system. The assessment of solid growth does not require distinction of squamous from nonsquamous growth, small amounts of solid growth (around 5%) need not be recognized, and nuclear grading is not necessary. This system should be tested in other studies to verify its utility.

Surgical–Pathological Staging (FIGO Staging)

The stage reflects the extent of disease at the time of diagnosis. It is useful to determine prognosis and plan treatment as well as to provide a standardized method of reporting data among different investigators. Effective in 1989, FIGO revised the previous clinical staging to a surgical–pathological system (Table 12.5).[65,256] The revision in the staging system was based on studies showing that endometrial carcinoma was frequently under- or overstaged clinically and on data demonstrating the importance of a variety of histopathologic risk factors.[6] The staging system requires hysterectomy as well as assessment of the pelvic and paraaortic lymph nodes, adnexae, and peritoneal fluid cytology. Pathologic analysis includes evaluation of the grade of the tumor, depth of myometrial invasion, and determination of endocervical involvement; therefore, it is essential that all this information be communicated clearly in the surgical pathology report.

The prognostic utility of surgical–pathologic stage has been confirmed in multiple studies of large numbers of patients using both univariate and multivariate analysis.[6,32,64,104,144,186,348,358–360] The prognostic significance of the individual components of FIGO staging is discussed next.

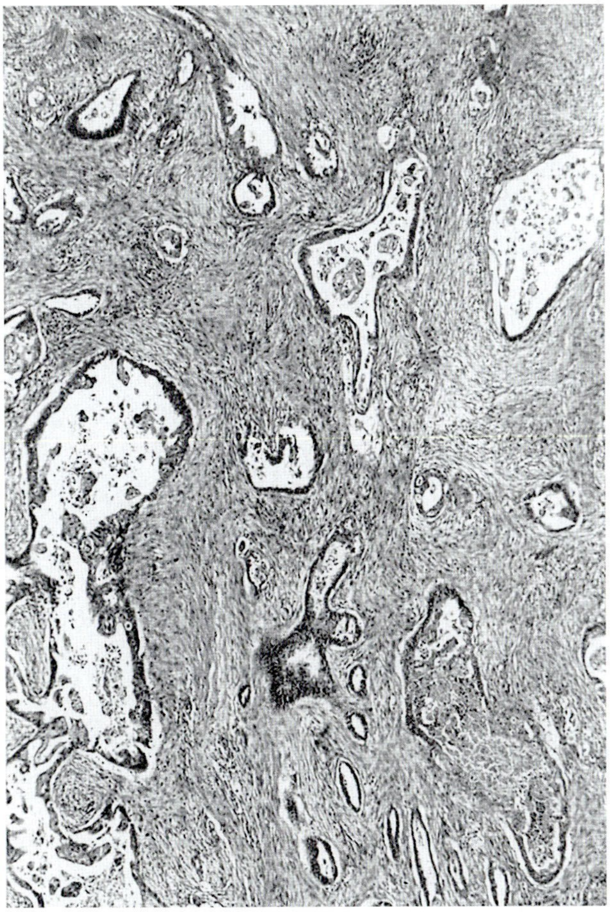

Fig. 12.11. Endometrioid carcinoma, high grade. The carcinoma is entirely glandular but the growth pattern is infiltrative and there is necrosis within the large gland in the *lower right of the field.*

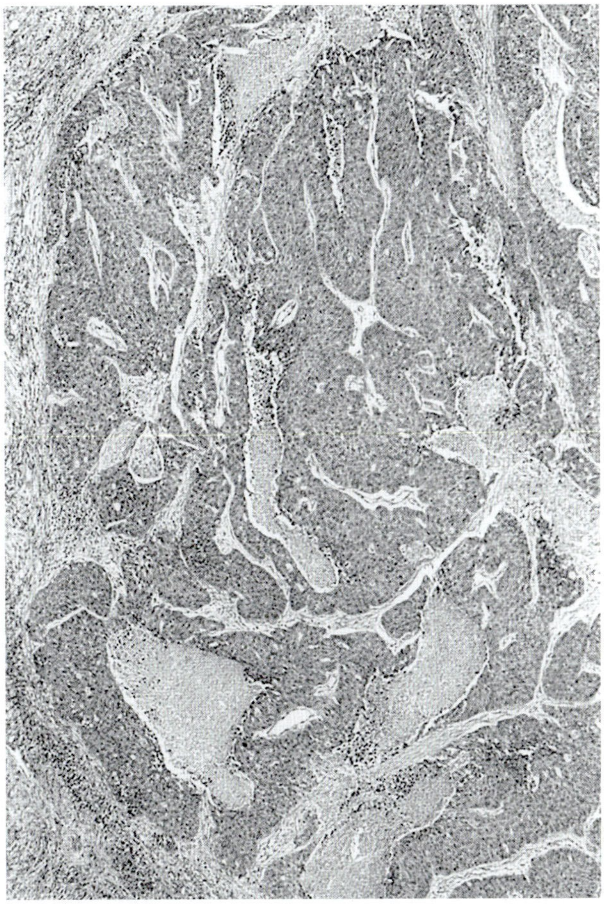

Fig. 12.12. Endometrioid carcinoma, high grade. The carcinoma has an expansile growth pattern but it is entirely solid, and there are areas of central necrosis within some of the solid nests in the *lower half of the field.*

Myometrial Invasion

In the past, depth of myometrial invasion has been reported as the proportion of the uterine wall invaded by tumor and expressed in thirds. More recently, the revised FIGO staging of endometrial carcinoma limited to the uterine corpus (stage I) incorporates depth of myometrial invasion expressed as inner or outer half. Tumors confined to the endometrium are stage IA, those involving the inner half of the myometrium are stage IB, and those involving more than half the uterine wall thickness are stage IC. In addition, we recommend measuring the maximum depth of invasion in millimeters and expressing this as a percentage of the myometrial thickness. For example, 2 mm of myometrial invasion in a uterus measuring 1 cm thick would be 20% invasion. Tumor in vascular spaces beyond the deepest point of invasion should not be used for this measurement.

Endometrial carcinoma may manifest different forms of myometrial invasion. It can invade along a broad pushing front or it can infiltrate the myometrium diffusely as masses, cords, or clusters of cells and individual glands. When it invades along a broad front it may be difficult to determine whether invasion is in fact present unless it can be

Table 12.5. Statistical model of survival predicted by myometrial invasion and vascular invasion-associated changes

		Survival	
Score	*No. of cases*	*No.*	*%*
<1	20	19	95
1–2	45	39	87
2–2.6	17	12	70
>2.6	20	7	35

Score = 0.695 [myometrial invasion (1 if not present, 2 if inner half, 3 if outer half)] + 1.8972 [vascular invasion associated changes (0 if absent, 1 if present)]. Reprinted by permission of Ambros RA and Kurman RJ, ref. 10.

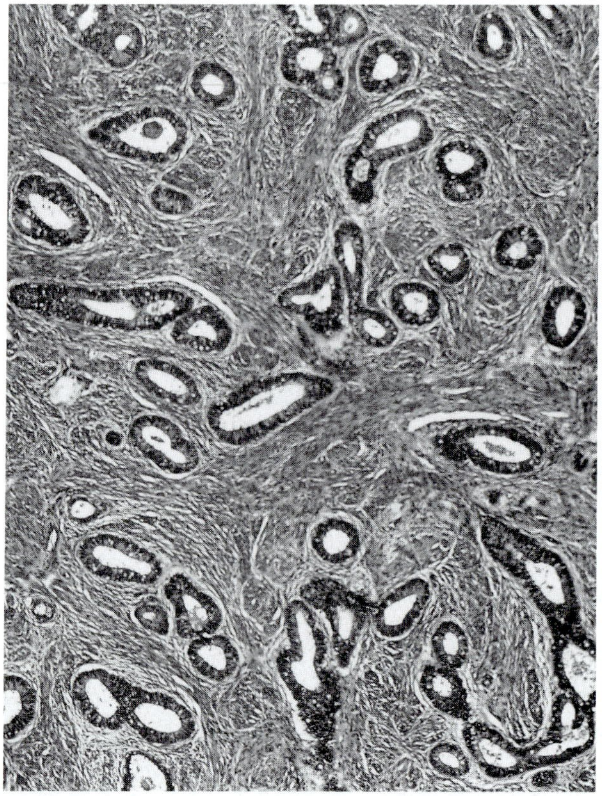

Fig. 12.13. Endometrioid carcinoma, FIGO grade 1. Well-formed glands diffusely invade the myometrium. Surrounding reactive change is minimal.

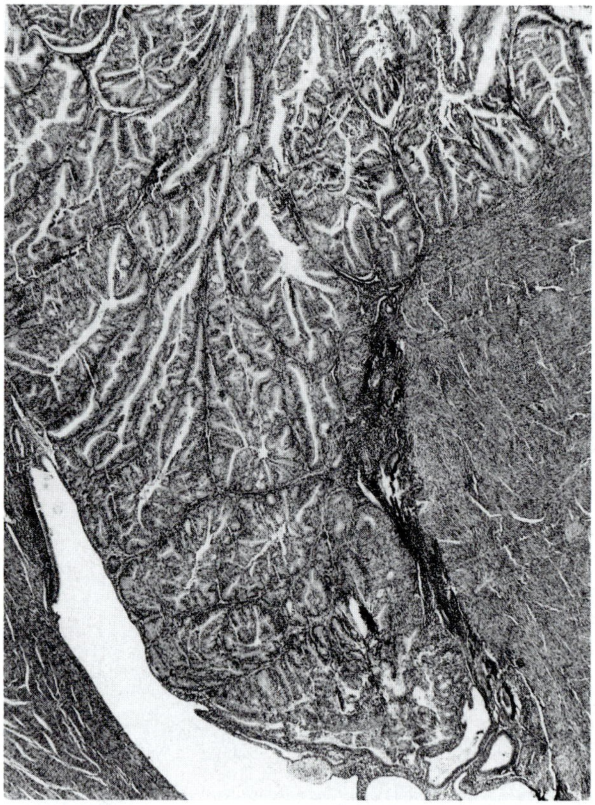

Fig. 12.14. Endometrioid carcinoma, FIGO grade 1. The tumor is involving endometrial glands that appear to be in the myometrium; this is because of the irregular endomyometrial junction. The tumor in this case is in the cornual region, heightening the appearance of myometrial invasion.

compared to the adjacent uninvolved endomyometrium. When the tumor diffusely invades the myometrium the neoplastic glands usually elicit a reactive stromal response characterized by loose fibrous tissue accompanied by a chronic inflammatory infiltrate that surrounds the glands. Occasionally, well-differentiated carcinomas may be deeply invasive with glands directly in contact with surrounding myometrium in the absence of a stromal response (diffusely infiltrative or adenoma malignum pattern of invasion) (Fig. 12.13).[210] In these cases, when myometrial invasion is superficial the presence of invasion can be identified if a haphazard glandular arrangement is present. Usually this pattern of invasion is found in deeply invasive tumors, however, and therefore recognizing myometrial invasion is not a problem. Endometrioid carcinomas with the diffusely infiltrative pattern of invasion share the same prognostic indicators of clinically aggressive disease as those having the more conventional pattern of myometrial invasion.[210] Finally, carcinoma may be confined to the endometrium and invade preexisting endometrial glands that are beyond the basalis and are in the myometrium. It is important to remember that the endomyometrial junction is typically irregular, and it is not unusual for endometrial glands to appear to be in the myometrium (Fig. 12.14); this can be especially confusing in the cornual area, because of tangential sectioning. Tumors that involve these superficial glands should be reported as being confined to the endometrium.

It may be difficult to distinguish myometrial invasion from extension of the carcinoma into adenomyosis. The distinction, however, is important because the presence of carcinoma in adenomyosis deeper than the maximum depth of true tumor invasion does not worsen the prognosis.[131,140,159,228] When the carcinoma is surrounded by endometrial stroma and residual benign glands are present in these foci, the diagnosis of carcinoma extending into adenomyosis is straightforward (Fig. 12.15). At times, however, the distinction from myometrial invasion may be extremely difficult, particularly in older women in whom adenomyosis may have very minimal stroma as a result of fibrosis and atrophy.

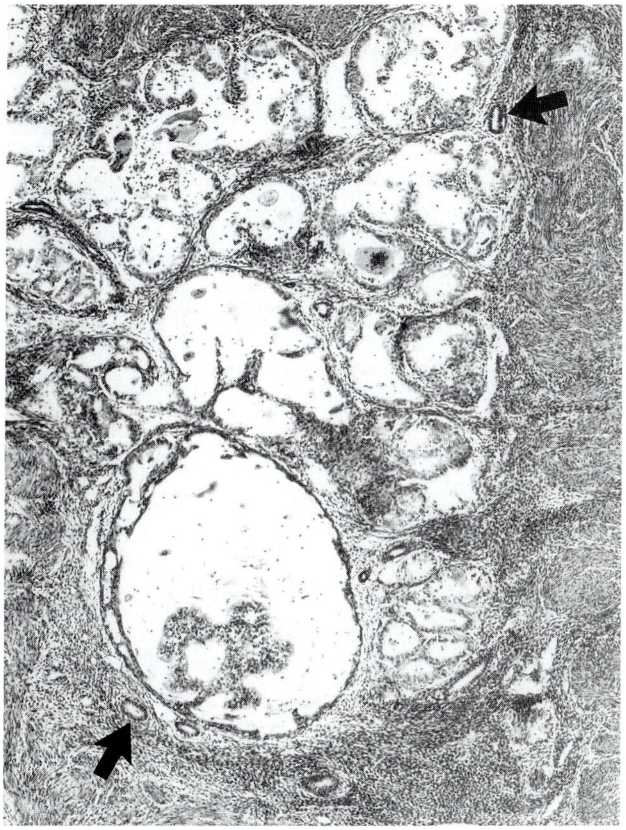

Fig. 12.15. Endometrioid carcinoma, FIGO grade 1, involving adenomyosis. The presence of small uninvolved glands (*arrows*) at the periphery of the carcinoma facilitates recognition of the adenomyosis. (Reprinted by permission of Jacques and Lawrence, ref. 159.)

In these cases it is necessary to evaluate additional features such as the presence of desmoplasia, surrounding edema and inflammation, and the shape of the glands.[159] In contrast to carcinoma involving adenomyosis, true myometrial invasion is characterized by desmoplasia or loosening of the myometrium surrounding the glands. Often there is accompanying chronic inflammation and the glandular outline is jagged and irregular, as compared to carcinoma involving adenomyosis in which the glands have a smooth, rounded outline and desmoplasia and inflammation are lacking (Fig. 12.16). A diagnosis of carcinoma involving adenomyosis should be made only when there is evidence of adenomyosis uninvolved by carcinoma or residual adenomyosis within foci involved by carcinoma in the uterus because some endometrioid carcinomas invade the myometrium without eliciting a stromal response (see foregoing). A recent study noted that adenocarcinoma involving adenomyosis frequently is associated with preceding estrogen use, low tumor grade, and an excellent prognosis.[228]

Myometrial invasion, independent of tumor grade, is an important predictor of prognosis. In fact, it probably is the single most important predictor of behavior in stages I and II disease and has been shown to be an independent predictor of outcome for women with early-stage endometrial carcinoma.[1,9,32,52,83,202,233,360] For example, in the GOG experience, recurrence developed in only 1 of 99 (1%) patients with no myometrial invasion compared with 15 of 196 (7.7%) with inner-third, 8 of 55 (14.5%) with middle-third, and 6 of 40 (15%) with outer-third invasion when grade was not corrected.[233] In another GOG study it was shown that the 5-year relative survival for endometrioid carcinoma confined to the endometrium was 94%; involving the inner third, 91%; involving the middle third, 84%; and involving the outer third, 59%.[357]

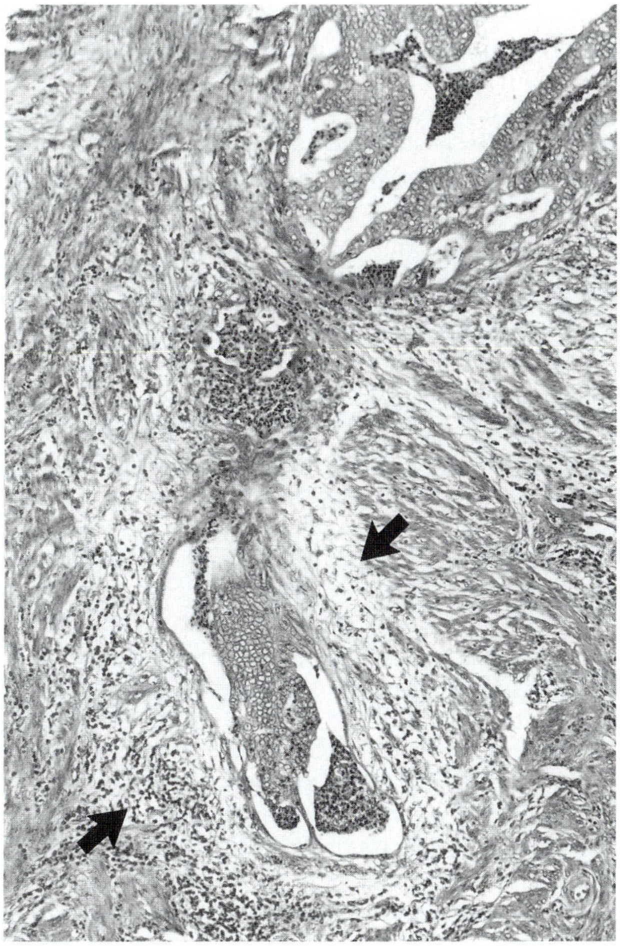

Fig. 12.16. Endometrioid carcinoma invading the myometrium in association with adenomyosis. In contrast to carcinoma involving adenomyosis, glands that invade the myometrium are surrounded by a loose stroma with inflammatory cells (*arrows*). (Reprinted by permission of Jacques and Lawrence, ref. 159.)

The frequency of lymph node metastasis also is related to the depth of myometrial invasion. In clinical stage I endometrial carcinoma, inner-third myometrial invasion is associated with lymph node metastasis in 5% of cases, middle-third invasion with metastasis in 23%, and outer-third invasion with metastasis in 33%. When grade and myometrial invasion are analyzed together, grade 1 tumors invading the inner third of the myometrium do not have pelvic node metastasis, but with outer-third invasion, pelvic node metastasis occurs in 25%. A similar trend occurs with higher-grade tumors.

Cervical Involvement

Cervical involvement also has been incorporated into the new FIGO staging system. Tumors confined to the uterus but involving the cervix are stage II. These neoplasms are then staged as IIA if tumor is confined to the surface epithelium or glands and stage IIB if the tumor invades the adjacent stroma. Cervical stromal involvement is characterized by carcinoma that is not confined to the surface epithelium or preexisting endocervical glands and typically elicits a stromal reaction. Cervical involvement is associated with a somewhat elevated risk of recurrence, with an overall relapse rate of 16% in the absence of extrauterine disease.[233] Generally, cervical involvement is associated with increasing grade, depth of invasion, and tumor volume so the higher recurrence is not surprising.

Peritoneal Cytology

Between 5% and 15% of patients have positive peritoneal cytology as their only manifestation of extrauterine spread of tumor. The presence of malignant cells identified cytologically in a peritoneal fluid sample is the basis for classification of a patient as stage IIIA. The significance of a positive peritoneal cytology has been the subject of several studies.[62,127,134,164,176,319,332,353,360] Some studies have reported the significance of positive peritoneal cytology, including one in which almost 40% of clinical stage I patients with positive peritoneal cytology suffered tumor recurrence compared with 10% of those with negative washings.[62,134,332] Other studies, however, have reported a lack of significance of peritoneal cytology in predicting the probability of recurrence or death from endometrial adenocarcinoma.[127,353] Positive peritoneal cytology has been associated with other risk factors for recurrence, such as high grade, deep myometrial invasion, or extrauterine spread.[127,134,176] One recent study, however, found that positive peritoneal cytology did not correlate with histologic subtype, FIGO grade, depth of myometrial invasion, or vascular invasion and was only significantly associated with stage III and IV disease.[129] Nonetheless, in a study of 567 patients with clinical stage I and II disease, a statistically significant difference in survival between patients with and without positive peritoneal cytology was found that persisted when the data were subjected to multivariate analysis.[332] Only 7% of patients with negative cytology recurred, while 32% of those with positive peritoneal cytology suffered a recurrence. Another study also found a threefold increase in the risk of death from tumor for a similar population using a multivariate analysis that adjusted for other risk factors.[360] Thus the weight of evidence in large studies with multivariate analysis supports the presence of malignant cells in peritoneal washings as a significant indicator of poor prognosis.

Vascular Invasion and Lymph Node Metastases

Venous or lymphatic capillary invasion is defined by the presence of neoplastic cells within endothelial-lined channels. Although artifactual retraction of stroma around aggregates of neoplastic cells may simulate vascular invasion, capillary invasion can usually be reliably assessed in the myometrium peripheral to the bulk of the tumor mass. Also, the presence of perivascular lymphocytic infiltrates in the myometrium (Fig. 12.17), but not lymphocytic infiltrate at the tumor–myometrial junction, is frequently associated with vascular invasion and hence is a useful marker of vascular invasion.[10] Vascular invasion is relatively uncommonly seen in endometrioid adenocarcinoma of the uterus, but the frequency increases with deeper myometrial invasion, aggressive cell types, and decreasing histologic differentiation.[2,133,306] Nonetheless, some studies have revealed a significant correlation between vascular invasion and tumor recurrence independent of differentiation and depth of myometrial invasion. In one investigation of FIGO stage I endometrial adenocarcinomas, 9 of 15 patients with lymphatic invasion died of tumor, while none of the 78 without identified vascular invasion died of cancer.[103] In a similar study of stage I cases, it was found that lymphatic invasion represented a strong predictor of tumor recurrence and extrapelvic metastasis, which was independent of depth of invasion or histologic differentiation.[133]

In an analysis of stage I, grade 1 endometrioid adenocarcinomas with a poor outcome, vascular invasion in addition to myometrial invasion, mitotic index, and absence of progesterone receptor were significant factors that predicted aggressive behavior.[328] In another study aimed at comparing the significance of various pathologic risk factors in stage

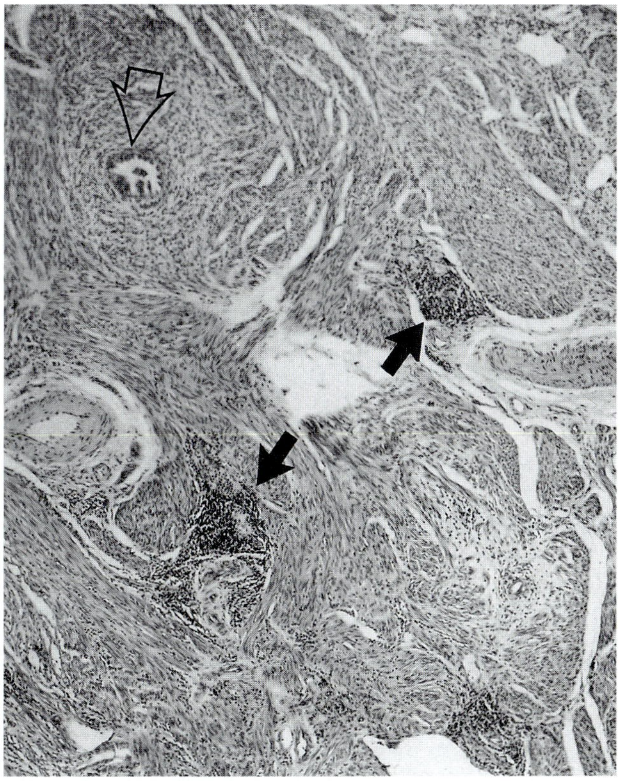

Fig. 12.17. Vascular invasion-associated changes. Perivascular lymphocytic infiltration (*dark arrows*) in the myometrium is a useful marker for vascular invasion. An invasive gland is present in the myometrium (*open arrow*).

I endometrioid carcinoma, univariate analysis showed that vascular invasion was more important than grade and depth of myometrial invasion in predicting prognosis.[10] Another study examined specimens with probable lymphatic invasion using immunoperoxidase with an antibody directed against factor VIII.[202] A greatly increased risk of recurrence was present in those with definite vascular invasion but not in those in whom the lining of the spaces failed to stain. Another study found that vascular invasion was a statistically significant indicator of death from tumor in early clinical stage tumors, but not for surgical stage I and II endometrial adenocarcinoma.[360] This finding suggests that lymphatic invasion may help to identify patients likely to have spread to lymph nodes or distant sites, but that its importance is diminished for those in whom thorough sampling of nodes has failed to identify metastases. Others have also found that vascular invasion was a significant prognosticator by univariate analysis but less important after adjusting for other variables.[2] Nevertheless, one study found that among women with lymph node metastases the presence or absence of vascular invasion in the primary tumor was associated with different survival rates.[150]

Among the extrauterine risk factors, the presence of positive aortic lymph nodes is most important in predicting prognosis.[233] Only 36% of patients with positive aortic nodes were free of tumor at 5 years compared with 85% with negative aortic nodes. The highest correlation of positive paraaortic lymph nodes is with pelvic lymph nodes. Nearly a third of patients with positive pelvic lymph nodes have positive paraaortic lymph nodes. Other features that correlate with positive aortic nodes are vascular invasion (19%), deep myometrial invasion (17%), positive peritoneal cytology (16%), cervical involvement (12%), and grade 3 tumors (8%).

Endometrial Hyperplasia and Metaplasia

Among nontumor risk factors, the presence of atypical endometrial hyperplasia and various metaplasias, especially ciliated cell and eosinophilic change, are important in identifying patients with a favorable prognosis. The presence of atypical hyperplasia and metaplasia correlates with low tumor grade and lack of myometrial invasion.[25,168] In contrast, high-grade tumors are associated more often with an atrophic endometrium.[49]

Ploidy

About two-thirds of endometrial adenocarcinomas are composed of cells that are diploid at the level of flow or static cytometry. This statement is qualified, as the sensitivity of the technique is limited and the addition or deletion of DNA equivalent to one average chromosome would not alter the assessment of a cell as diploid. Similar to many of the other prognostic factors, diploid tumors tend to be more frequently associated with less aggressive cell type, superficial invasion, and better histologic differentiation.[36,109,156,309,315,335] Survival has generally been higher for women with diploid tumors.[36,156,335] One study of stage I patients demonstrated 94% progression-free survival for those with diploid tumors versus 64% for those with aneuploid cancers, but these results have not been universally reproducible.[129–131,133] However, in more recent larger studies employing multivariate analysis, ploidy has almost always remained a strong predictor of outcome.[132,211,245,263,265,317,329,361] Thus, DNA content can be considered a prognostic indicator of demonstrated utility for endometrial adenocarcinoma.

Steroid Receptors

During the past decade, there has been a dramatic shift in the methodology for assessing estrogen (ER) and progesterone receptor (PR) expression in tissues, with immunohistochemistry almost universally supplanting biochemical measurements. Immunohistochemical analysis on formalin-fixed tissues is the preferred method because it allows visualization of the distribution and intensity of staining in both neoplastic and surrounding normal tissues. It has been demonstrated that biochemical assays can yield false-positive results because of contamination of normal tissues.[334] The studies that have employed immunohistochemical methods to assess receptor content in formalin-fixed paraffin-embedded tumor tissues have demonstrated that endometrioid carcinomas frequently express ER and PR whereas serous and clear cell carcinomas are almost always negative.[165,195,196] In most studies, the presence and quantity of steroid receptors have been correlated with histologic differentiation, FIGO stage, and survival.[43,72,109,110,165,221]

Several studies have reported variable results regarding the correlation of hormone receptor expression and prognosis. One study found that the presence of ER, but not PR, was predictive of survival.[259] Another found that the presence of PR was a favorable prognosticator.[328] Yet another found that both ER and PR were predictive of survival, but also strongly related to the clinical stage, histologic grade, and the absence of vascular invasion.[109] In contrast, another study reported that recurrence was related to the absence of ER or PR, and that response to progestin therapy was more common in PR-positive tumors, but noted that survival for patients with surgical stage I or II disease was not related to ER or PR.[81] Others have found that ER and PR were not independently predictive of lymph node metastasis.[232] However, PR persisted as a significant prognosticator of survival in two studies using multivariate analyses.[101,250] Given the disparity in results and the relationship with other strong risk factors, hormone receptor expression is best considered a prognostic indicator of potential utility.

BCL-2 and Markers of Apoptosis

BCL-2 is a proto-oncogene that inhibits programmed cell death, which is manifest morphologically as apoptosis. In the endometrium, BCL-2 expression assessed by immunohistochemistry varies during the menstrual cycle and is highly expressed in the proliferative phase, with downregulation during the secretory phase.[119] Given this cyclic regulation of endometrial growth, differentiation, and shedding, it is not surprising that during the past few years there has been significant interest in apoptosis-related events, with more than a dozen immunohistochemical studies of BCL-2 in abnormal endometrium. In general, the observations support the concept that BCL-2 protein expression persists at high levels in simple hyperplasia but progressively diminishes in atypical hyperplasia and with decreasing differentiation in invasive endometrial adenocarcinoma.[44,48,112,137,151,243,286,322,351] Apoptotic cells and apoptotic bodies are also increased in poorly differentiated endometrioid carcinomas, clear cell carcinomas, and serous carcinomas compared with well-differentiated endometrioid adenocarcinomas.[135,136] Loss of BCL-2 expression has also been associated with other features of poor prognosis including increasing depth of invasion, negative PR status, increasing FIGO stage, and aggressive cell types.[112,232,283,322,365] In two studies that used multivariate analysis to adjust for other prognostic factors, loss of BCL-2 expression was significantly related to the probability of lymph node metastasis or tumor recurrence.[112,286]

Markers of Proliferation

Various aspects of proliferation within tissues can now be assessed directly or indirectly by a multitude of modalities in tissue sections and cell suspensions. These methods include the determination of mitotic indices; AgNOR counting; S-phase fraction; proliferating cell nuclear antigen (PCNA); and Ki-67-, Ki-S5-, or MIB-1-positive cell populations by immunohistochemistry. As is discussed next, each assessment provides slightly different information about the number and type of cells in different parts of the cell cycle. Standardized methods for detection, enumeration, and determination of levels of significance do not exist for most of these parameters, however, and need to be established before the assays can be considered clinically useful.

Antibodies (Ki-67, Ki-S5, and MIB-1) directed against the DNA-binding nuclear protein, Ki-67 antigen, identify cells in most of G_1 and all of S, G_2, and M phases of the cell cycle, but not in the G_0, or quiescent, phase. In one study, MIB-1 staining correlated with grade and mitotic activity but did not predict short-term outcome.[240] Ki-S5 staining has been shown to be a significant predictor of survival by univariate but not multivariate analysis.[31] However, in a prospective study of 115 women with endometrial adenocarcinoma, immunohistochemical staining with Ki-67 was related to FIGO stage, cell type, histologic subtype, and probability of survival by univariate analysis; and, in addition, using multivariate analysis, only Ki-67 expression and stage remained as significant independent prognosticators.[288] Thus, Ki-67 could be considered a prognosticator of potential utility, but further corroboration is needed.

Proliferating cell nuclear antigen (PCNA) is a nuclear protein that is expressed in the late G_1 phase, peaks in the S phase, and persists in the G_2M phases of the cycle. A high PCNA index has failed to discriminate outcome in several studies but has been predictive of decreased survival by univariate analysis in other studies, although not by multivariate analysis.[106,132,171,177]

Flow cytometry can be used to distinguish populations of cells in the S phase or G_2 and M phases of the cycle. The prognostic value of flow cytometry to identify endometrial cancers composed of increased percentages (either 10% or 20%) of cells in the S phase of the cell cycle also has been variable. One study demonstrated a nonsignificant trend toward decreased survival whereas others have shown either significance by univariate analysis alone or significance by multivariate analysis.[169,263,266,288]

Silver-stained proteins of interphase nucleolar organizer regions (AgNORs), which are associated with ribosomal genes, are selectively stained with silver and can be visualized in paraffin embedded sections. The quantity of AgNOR proteins (measured as either area of nucleus or number of discrete dots) is generally related to the rapidity of cell proliferation and has been shown to increase sequentially in specimens from proliferative endometrium through hyperplasia, atypical hyperplasia, and adenocarcinoma.[30] The AgNOR staining was correlated with MIB-1 staining, mitotic index, and histologic grade but not with outcome in one study but has been related to likelihood of recurrence and diminished probability of survival by univariate analyses in two other investigations.[226,240,329] There are insufficient data at present to determine the prognostic utility of AgNOR staining in endometrial adenocarcinoma.

Tumor Suppressor Genes and Oncogenes

The p53 gene is classified as a tumor suppressor gene, the product of which is a protein involved in the regulation of the cell cycle at the G_1 checkpoint. Mutations of the p53 gene often result in a protein with a longer half-life that accumulates in the cell. Upregulation of wild type (i.e., nonmutated) p53 may occur after DNA damage and also result in overexpression detected by immunohistochemistry. Mutations or overexpression of p53 in endometrial carcinoma has been examined in more than two dozen studies. Overexpression of p53 protein has been generally related to higher FIGO stage, aggressive cell types (particularly serous carcinoma), increased histologic grade, and depth of myometrial invasion.[12,59,113,132,161,177,179,184,195,211,242,245,321,322,351] There is a surprisingly high degree of concordance in the observation that p53 overaccumulation is associated with a decreased probability of survival by univariate analysis, and this is true even by multivariate analysis in at least eight studies.[21,113,132,153,155,161,179,183,184,211,241,242,266,351] These results support the classification of p53 expression as a prognostic indicator of proven utility.

HER-2/neu is a proto-oncogene, the product of which is a transmembrane growth factor receptor, p185erb-2, which shares some homology with the epidermal growth factor receptor. It is normally expressed at low levels in the cycling endometrium. Gene amplification or overexpression occurs in about 20–40% of endometrial carcinomas. Overexpression of HER-2/neu protein has been associated with advanced stage, decreased differentiation, aggressive cell types, particularly including clear cell type, and increased depth of myometrial invasion.[27,177,272,277] Reports of its utility as a predictor of survival have been mixed, with no apparent association of overexpression to outcome identified in several studies, but a statistically significant relationship was shown in most others.[22,132,141,211,236,241,242,266,272,277,285] In several investigations, the significance of HER-2/neu amplification or overexpression as a prognosticator has remained after adjusting for other known risk factors.[132,236,277] At present, HER-2/neu overexpression is a prognostic factor of potential utility.

The activation of *ras* proto-oncogenes through either point mutations or gene amplification has been identified in various malignant tumors. Mutations in codon 12 of K-*ras* appear to occur in only 10–15% of endometrial carcinomas, and in most studies they have not been related to stage, grade, depth of invasion, or survival, although one study found mutations predictive of recurrence and death by univariate analysis.[39,88,154,161,295] K-*ras* mutations currently represent a prognostic marker of unlikely utility.

Angiogenesis and Vascular Endothelial Growth Factor

Angiogenesis in the form of proliferation of new capillaries from preexisting vessels is necessary to permit tumor growth. This neovascularization potentially could result from stimulation by a variety of factors released from neoplastic cells, host cells responding to the neoplasm, or supporting matrix. In the endometrium, it appears that stromal vascularity is greater in the secretory phase than proliferative phase, but it is greater in the stroma of carcinoma than in cycling endometrium.[231] This difference may reflect stimulation by vascular endothelial growth factor (VEGF) RNA and its protein product, which have been found in high concentration in neoplastic cells but not in benign atrophic endometrial glandular cells.[130] Although tumor vascularity has been associated with increased stage, decreased differentiation, and lymphatic invasion, high microvessel counts have been a statistically significant predictor of decreased survival independent of other common risk factors in several studies.[167,252,341] Microvessel density thus represents a prognostic marker of potential utility.

Models for Predicting Prognosis

Recent studies reveal that the behavior of a tumor is based on a complex interaction of a number of different factors. Accordingly, models have been developed that assess several factors and permit more accurate prognostication than simply considering one factor alone. For example, by multivariate analysis, the depth of invasion and presence of vascular invasion-associated changes were found to provide a highly reliable model for predicting outcome (see Table 12.5).[10] The model was better able to define patients who were at low and high risk of recurrence as compared with the traditional risk factors using grade and depth of invasion. Inclusion of ploidy in the model permitted even better discrimination of high- and low-risk patients. In a subset of pathologic stage I endometrioid carcinoma in whom ploidy analysis was performed, multivariate analysis showed that only the depth of invasion, DNA ploidy, and vascular invasion-associated changes were significant risk factors.[9] A statistical model based on these features permitted stratification of patients into four risk groups with 93%, 67%, 38%, and 10% survival, respectively (Table 12.6).

In an analysis of 819 women with clinical stage I and occult stage II adenocarcinoma of the endometrium entered on a GOG protocol, multivariate analysis demonstrated that age, cell type, architectural grade, depth of myometrial invasion, vascular space involvement, and peritoneal cytology were independent risk factors for recurrence and death from tumor.[360] From these data it appears possible to create a model for assignment of the relative risk of death from tumor for individual patients based solely on information gathered by pathologic examination of the hysterectomy specimen. For example, a woman with grade 1 endometrioid carcinoma, with tumor confined to the endometrium and no vascular invasion, is arbitrarily assigned a risk of 1. Relative to this baseline risk, a woman with a grade 2 endometrioid carcinoma that invades superficial myometrium and lacks vascular space involvement has a relative risk of 2.6. Similarly, a woman with a grade 3 endometrioid carcinoma, with middle-third myometrial invasion and positive vascular space involvement, has a relative risk of 10. The probability of disease-free survival at 5 years for these three women would be approximately 95%, 90%, and 65%, respectively. Knowledge of the specific risk for each patient would allow better prognostication and, potentially, individually tailored therapy.

Table 12.6. Statistical model of survival predicted by depth of myometrial invasion, vascular invasion-associated changes, and tumor ploidy

		Survival	
Score	*No. of cases*	*No.*	*%*
<2.2	27	25	93
2.2–2.3	12	8	67
2.4–4.0	8	3	38
>4	10	1	10

Score = 1.91 (vascular invasion associated changes [0 if absent, 1 if present]) + 0.982 [DNA ploidy (0 if peridiploid, 1 if aneuploid)] + 1.13 [depth of myometrical involvement (0 if none, 1 if <50%, 2 if >50%)]
Reprinted by permission of Ambros RA and Kurman RJ, ref. 9.

Behavior and Treatment

Endometrioid adenocarcinoma spreads by lymphatic and vascular dissemination, direct extension to contiguous organs, and transperitoneal and transtubal seeding. Lymphatic metastasis is more common than hematogenous spread, but involvement of the lungs without metastasis to mediastinal lymph nodes suggests that hematogenous spread may occur early in the course of disease. Endometrial carcinoma tends to spread to the pelvic lymph nodes before involving paraaortic lymph nodes. The relative frequency of metastasis to lymph node groups and various organs is shown in Tables 12.7 and 12.8, respectively.

The standard treatment for endometrial carcinoma is hysterectomy and bilateral salpingo-oophorectomy. Over the years, preoperative or postoperative radiotherapy and chemotherapy have been used in addition to hysterectomy. The current approach is to treat all patients when feasible by hysterectomy supplemented by surgical staging and to administer postoperative radiation to patients with poor prognostic factors that put them at high risk of recurrence. Postoperative estrogen replacement therapy has been advocated for patients with early stage disease and no significant poor prognostic factors.[63] One study showed that survival is not compromised in patients with low tumor grade (grades 1 and 2), less than 50% myometrial invasion, and no metastases to lymph nodes or other organs.[200] Given the prognostic significance of pelvic

Table 12.7. Sites of lymph node metastasis from endometrial carcinomas at autopsy

Lymph nodes	*Relative frequency (%)*
Para-aortic	64
Hypogastric	61
External iliac	48
Common iliac	40
Obturator	37
Sacral	22
Mediastinal	18
Inguinal	16
Supraclavicular	12

From Hendrickson E (1975) The lymphatic dissemination in endometrial carcinoma. A study of 188 necropsies. Am J Obstet Gynecol 123:570.

and paraaortic lymph node status, these nodes should be sampled in patients when any of the following is present: greater than 50% myometrial invasion, grade 3 tumor, cervical involvement, extrauterine spread, serous, clear cell, or undifferentiated carcinoma, or palpably enlarged lymph nodes. In a GOG study only a quarter of patients had these findings, but they accounted for the majority of patients with positive aortic lymph nodes.[233] Several studies have shown that the depth of myometrial invasion can be assessed by gross inspection and intraoperative frozen section.[76,249,301]

Table 12.8. Sites of metastasis from endometrial carcinoma at autopsy

Organ site	*Relative frequency (%)*
Lung	41
Peritoneum and omentum	39
Ovary	34
Liver	29
Bowel	29
Vagina	25
Bladder	23
Vertebra	20
Spleen	14
Adrenal	14
Ureter	8
Brain or skull	5
Vulva	4
Breast	4
Hand	Rare
Femur	Rare
Tibia	Rare
Pubic bone	Rare
Skin	Rare

From Hendrickson E (1975) The lymphatic dissemination in endometrial carcinoma. A study of 188 necropsies. Am J Obstet Gynecol 123:570.

Postoperatively, patients are classified as low, intermediate, or high risk based on surgical pathologic staging. Patients with grade 1 or 2 tumors that are confined to the endometrium or are minimally invasive are defined as low risk and require no further therapy. Patients with pelvic or paraaortic lymph node metastases or involvement of the adnexa or intraperitoneal sites are high risk and receive postoperative radiation (vaginal cuff, pelvis, paraaortic area, or whole abdominal). Radiation appears to be of benefit because the 5-year survival rate for women with positive aortic lymph nodes who were treated with postoperative radiation is nearly 40%.[233] Despite treatment with surgery and radiotherapy, 50% of stage III tumors recur. Half of these patients die with distant metastasis, although local control also is a major problem. About 4% of patients with endometrial carcinoma have stage IV disease. Spread to the lungs occurs in 36% of patients. Patients who do not qualify as low or high risk are intermediate in risk. A decision as to whether or not these patients should receive postoperative radiation should be individualized because there are no conclusive data demonstrating a survival benefit for these patients treated with postoperative radiotherapy. Studies evaluating the use of adjuvant hormonal or cytotoxic chemotherapy have shown no improvement in survival over surgery and radiation, and consequently these methods currently are not recommended as standard treatment. In contrast, radiation, hormone, and cytotoxic chemotherapy are used for management of patients with recurrent tumor; 50% of patients with isolated vaginal vault recurrence treated by irradiation are alive at 3 years.[269]

Histologic Effects of Treatment

Radiation

The histologic changes in neoplastic tissues after intracavitary radiation are nonspecific and variable, showing minor to major alterations from their preirradiated state. Similarly, nonneoplastic endometrial or endocervical glands may be affected only minimally or show nuclear and cytoplasmic changes that are indistinguishable from those found in neoplastic cells. Because the cytologic changes in both neoplastic and nonneoplastic tissue are similar, identification of carcinoma depends largely on the recognition of histologic patterns and signs of invasion. Irradiated carcinoma generally retains a haphazard glandular pattern, but nonirradiated, nonneoplastic glands tend to maintain their normal

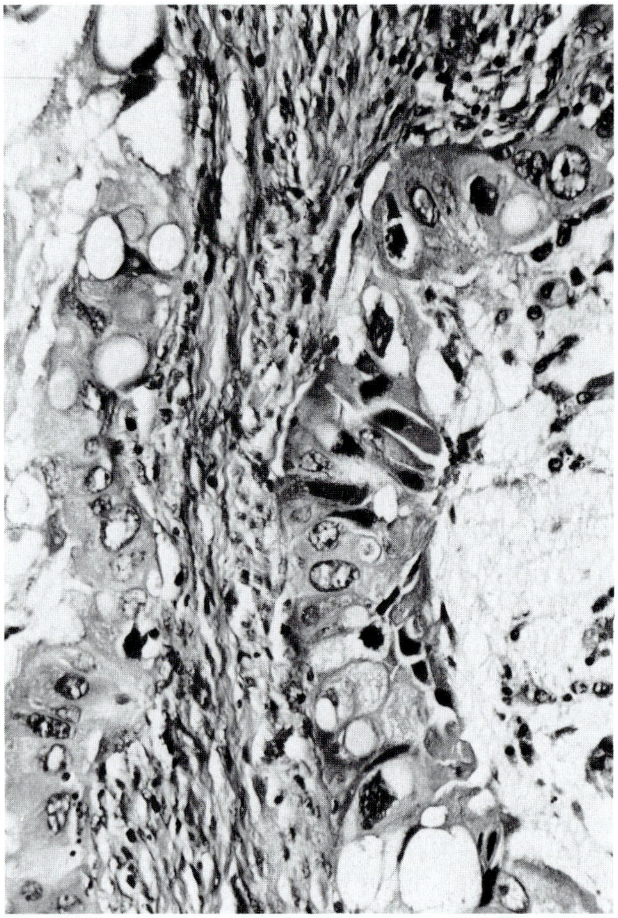

Fig. 12.18. Endometrioid carcinoma with radiation effect. There is marked vacuolation, nuclear hyperchromasia, and pleomorphism within the glandular cells.

architectural arrangement despite radiation effects in the endometrial stroma and myometrium. When radiation effect is evident, nuclei tend to be enlarged, highly pleomorphic, and hyperchromatic, with coarsely clumped chromatin. The cytoplasm often is granular and swollen. Vacuolation can be present in both the nucleus and the cytoplasm (Fig. 12.18). The nuclear changes result from replication of DNA without cell division.

Cytoplasmic vacuolation results from dilatation of various organelles and possible lysis caused by damaged lysosomal membranes. In some instances, radiation may enhance cellular differentiation. Occasionally, poorly differentiated carcinomas without squamous differentiation in the curettings may have nests of squamous epithelium in the resected uterus after radiation. It is in mitosis and the S phase of the cell cycle that a cell is most susceptible to radiation injury. Thus, the difference in radiosensitivity of tumor cells and benign cells is due largely to the increased mitotic activity of the neoplastic cells and the better reparative capacity of nonneoplastic cells. In view of the variable morphologic response to irradiation, it is often difficult to determine whether irradiated tumor cells are viable. On a practical basis, if tumor cells are evident after irradiation, it should be assumed that some retain the capacity to persist however abnormal they appear.

Radiation changes in the endometrial stroma and myometrium are greatest in the vicinity of the radiation source. The stromal cells are first converted to giant fibroblasts. Early vascular effects include damage to endothelial cells, resulting in thrombosis. The stroma undergoes progressive hyalinization, resulting in a collagenous scar. Elastic tissue often is fragmented and frayed, and blood vessels are thickened and sclerotic. Occasionally, changes similar to those found in atherosclerosis may be present in the intima of blood vessels. Foam cells occur in the intima, and myometrial cells may appear granular and swollen, especially in areas close to the radium source. Scarring, atrophy, and

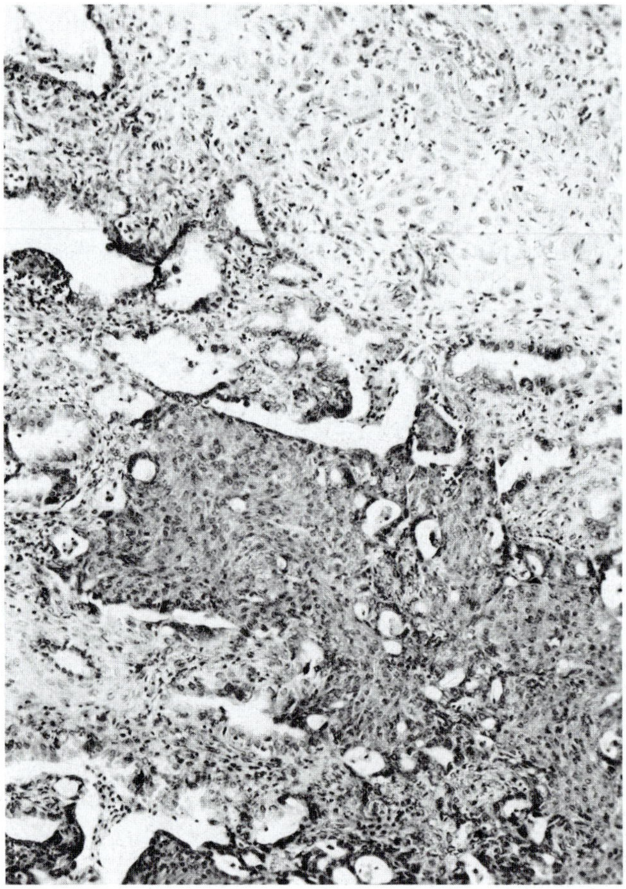

Fig. 12.19. Endometrioid carcinoma with progestin effect. A marked decidual reaction is present in the stroma (*upper portion of field*) after 1 month of high-dose progestin treatment.

sclerosis of vessels characterize long-standing radiation effects. The endometrium is thin and easily traumatized, and small blood vessels in the stroma are thin walled and ectatic. Some blood vessels form plaques of lipid-filled clear cells in the media.

PROGESTINS

Progestin-induced changes include secretory differentiation of glandular cells, mitotic arrest, conversion of spindle-shaped stromal cells to decidual cells, decrease in estrogen-related cellular changes such as ciliogenesis, and development or enlargement of squamous areas (Fig. 12.19).[274,284] The earliest evidence of progestin effect is subnuclear vacuolization, observed within 2–3 days of treatment. The vacuoles are a manifestation of glycoprotein synthesis, which is followed by an apocrine-type secretion in which the apical portion of the cytoplasm of the cell is discharged into the gland lumen, with reduction in the size of the cell.

Villoglandular Carcinoma

Villoglandular carcinoma is a variant of endometrioid carcinoma that displays a papillary architecture in which the papillary fronds are composed of a delicate fibrovascular core covered by columnar cells that generally contain bland nuclei.[46,138] The median age is 61 years, similar to that of women with typical endometrioid carcinoma. In all other respects, women with these tumors are similar to patients with low-grade endometrioid carcinoma.

The microscopic appearance of villoglandular carcinoma is characterized by thin, delicate fronds covered by stratified columnar epithelial cells with oval nuclei that generally display mild to moderate (grade 1 or 2) atypia (Figs. 12.20 and 12.21). Occasionally, more atypical (grade 3) nuclei may be observed. Mitotic activity is variable, and abnormal mitotic figures are rare.[46,138] Myometrial invasion usually is superficial.

The main consideration in the differential diagnosis is serous carcinoma because both villoglandular and serous carcinomas have a prominent papillary pattern. In contrast to serous carcinomas, villoglandular carcinomas have long delicate papillary fronds and are covered by columnar cells with only mild to moderate nuclear atypia. The cells look distinctly endometrioid with a smooth, luminal border. To have significance as a distinctive entity, the

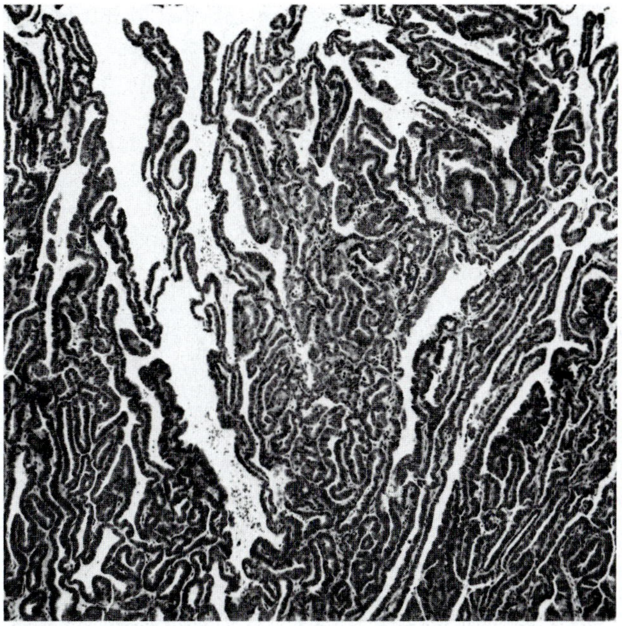

Fig. 12.20. Villoglandular carcinoma, FIGO grade 1. The tumor is composed of delicate papillary fronds covered by columnar epithelium that has an endometrioid appearance.

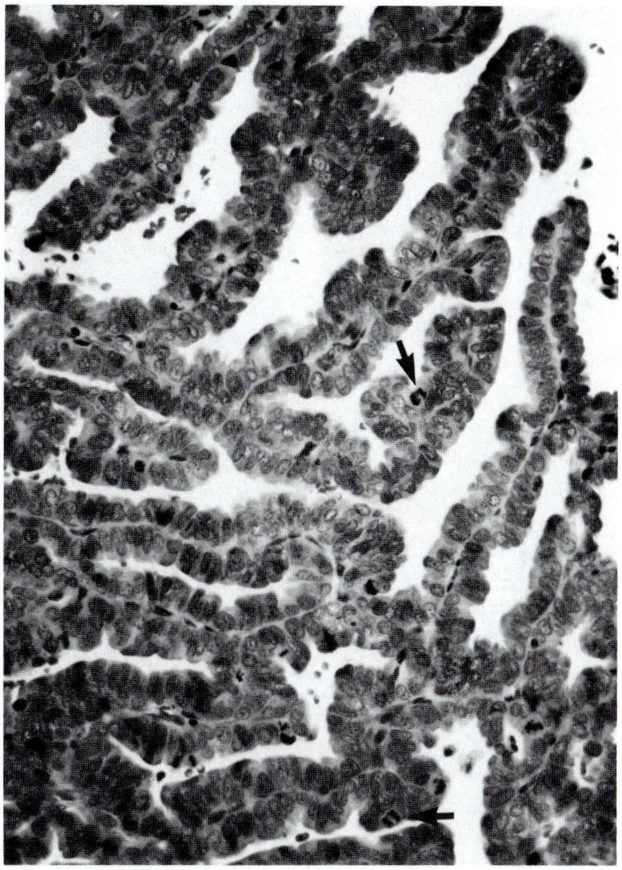

Fig. 12.21. Villoglandular carcinoma, FIGO grade 1. The cells covering the fibrovascular cores resemble those in endometrioid carcinoma. There is minimal nuclear atypia. Mitotic activity is present (*arrows*).

diagnosis is reserved for tumors in which most of the neoplasm has a villoglandular appearance. In contrast to villoglandular carcinomas, serous carcinomas tend to have shorter, thick, densely fibrotic papillary fronds. Probably the most important distinguishing feature is the cytologic appearance. The cells of serous carcinoma tend to be rounder, forming small papillary clusters that are detached from the papillary fronds, a finding that is often referred to as papillary tufts (see Figs. 12.32, 12.33 later in this chapter). As a consequence, the luminal border has a scalloped appearance. The nuclei of serous carcinomas are highly pleomorphic and atypical (grade 3). Macronucleoli typically are present. Many of the cells have a hobnail appearance, often with smudged, hyperchromatic nuclei (see Figs. 12.34 and 12.36, later in this chapter). It should be noted that considerable nuclear heterogeneity can be observed.

Villoglandular carcinomas are generally better differentiated than typical endometrioid carcinomas but are not significantly different with respect to depth of invasion or frequency of nodal metastases.[362] In addition, villoglandular carcinomas are frequently admixed with typical endometrioid carcinoma. In view of the frequent admixture of the two patterns and similar prognosis, villoglandular carcinoma is considered a variant of endometrioid carcinoma. Treatment is the same as for endometrioid carcinoma of comparable stage, grade, and depth of invasion.

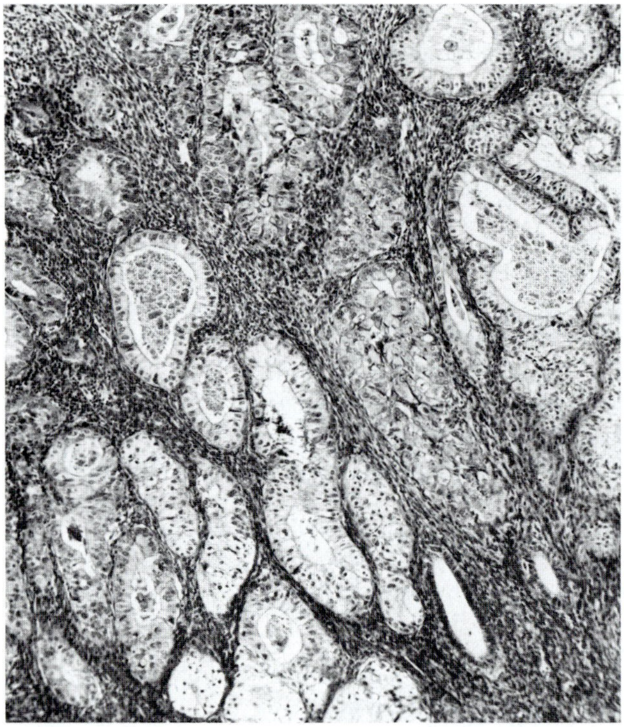

Fig. 12.22. Secretory carcinoma, FIGO grade 1. The tumor is composed of crowded, irregularly shaped glands lined by cells with relatively bland nuclei. The subnuclear and supranuclear vacuolization is similar to that found in secretory endometrium 2–6 days after ovulation.

Secretory Carcinoma

Secretory carcinoma is a variant of typical endometrial carcinoma in which the majority of cells exhibit subnuclear or supranuclear cytoplasmic vacuoles resembling early secretory endometrium. A rare pattern, it represents only 1–2% of endometrial carcinomas.[191,327] The age range is from 35 to 79 years, with a mean age of 55–58.[50,327] Most patients are postmenopausal and experience abnormal bleeding. This histologic subtype also may be seen rarely after progestin treatment of an endometrioid carcinoma. In all other respects, including the association of obesity, hypertension, diabetes mellitus, and exogenous estrogen administration, patients with secretory carcinoma are similar to women with endometrioid carcinoma.

Microscopically, secretory carcinoma displays a well-differentiated glandular pattern and is composed of columnar cells, often unstratified, with subnuclear or supranuclear vacuolization closely resembling day 17–22 secretory endometrium (Fig. 12.22).[191,327] Usually the nuclei are grade 1. The secretory pattern may be focal or diffuse, and it is frequently admixed with endometrioid adenocarcinoma. The endometrium adjacent to secretory carcinoma in young women typically shows a secretory pattern that is more advanced than 17 days, and a corpus luteum is found in most premenopausal patients when a hysterectomy and bilateral salpingo-oophorectomy are performed. Nonetheless, a relationship to progesterone stimulation is not always demonstrable, and most of the women are postmenopausal. The secretory activity in the tumor may be transient because it has been observed in curettings but not in the later hysterectomy specimen.[50] Secretory carcinoma may occur spontaneously in postmenopausal women without exogenous or abnormal levels of progesterone. It is important to distinguish secretory carcinoma from clear cell carcinoma in view of the excellent prognosis of the former and unfavorable prognosis of the latter. Although both tumors are composed of cells with clear, glycogen-rich cytoplasm, the histologic features are distinctive. At times a secretory carcinoma that has a predominantly glandular pattern can become solid and simulate clear cell carcinoma

(Figs. 12.23 and 12.24). The tumors are distinguished by their architectural and cytologic appearance. Secretory carcinoma displays a glandular architecture like endometrioid carcinoma, is rarely papillary or cystic, and usually is not solid.

Clear cell carcinoma, in contrast, frequently has a papillary or solid pattern and typically is associated with serous differentiation. A well-formed glandular pattern is unusual. The cells of secretory carcinoma are columnar with supranuclear or subnuclear vacuoles. The cells are similar to those in endometrioid carcinoma except for the presence of vacuoles (Fig. 12.24). In contrast, the cells in a clear cell carcinoma are more rounded and the nucleus is generally centrally located; hobnail cells are characteristic. Nuclear atypia is more marked (grade 3) in clear cell carcinoma. Cells with clear cytoplasm also may be seen in the squamous component of an endometrioid adenocarcinoma with squamous differentiation. The clear appearance of these cells is also due to the presence of glycogen. Clear squamous cells tend to be polygonal and usually merge with more typical squamous cells with abundant eosinophilic cytoplasm. The distinction of secretory carcinoma from atypical hyperplasia with secretory effect can be difficult and is based on the presence of stromal invasion in the carcinoma (see Chapter 11). Treatment is the same as that for endometrioid carcinoma of the same stage and grade. Secretory carcinoma usually is low grade with a good prognosis.[327] Death from recurrent disease occurs rarely.[50]

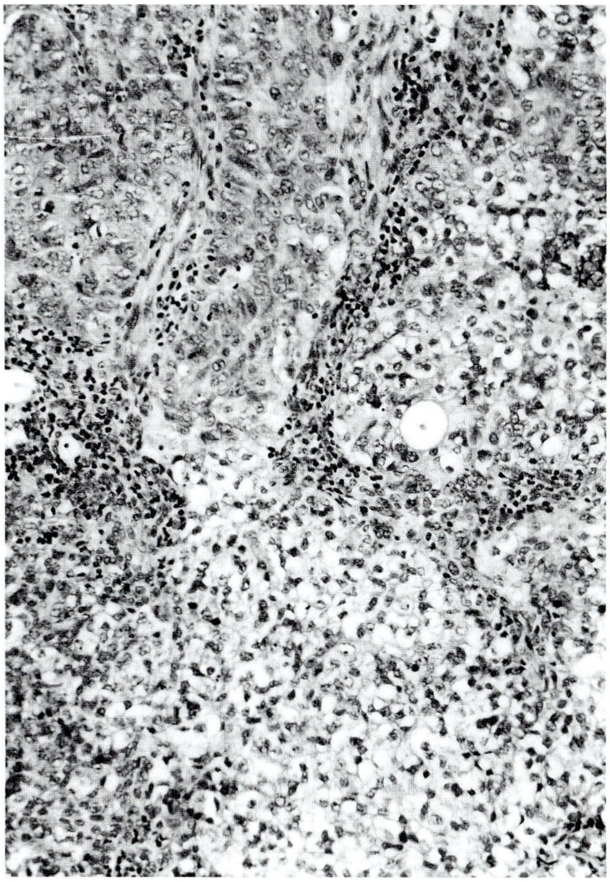

Fig. 12.23. Mixed endometrioid and secretory carcinoma. Secretory carcinoma in the *lower part of the field* is solid and merges with endometrioid carcinoma in the *left upper part of field.*

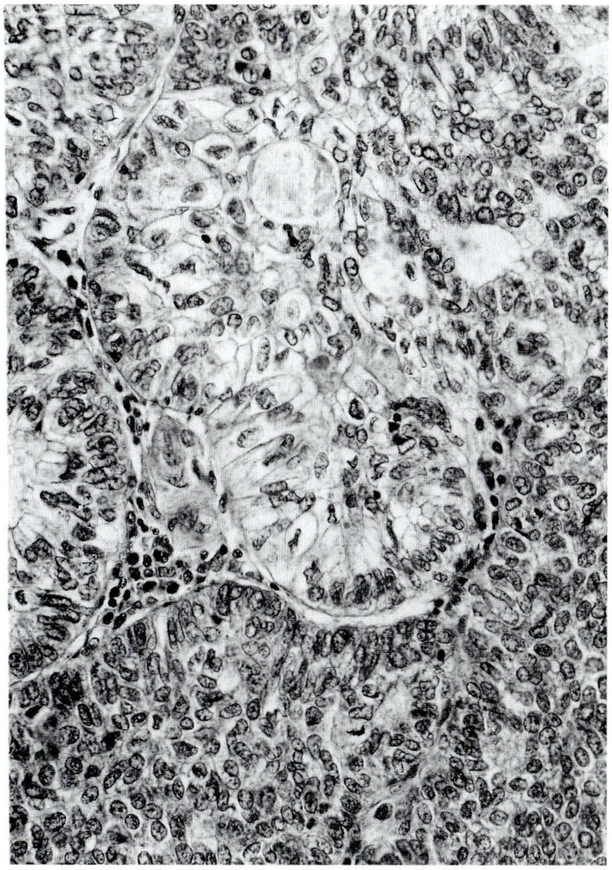

Fig. 12.24. Mixed endometrioid and secretory carcinoma. Higher magnification of another field of the same case illustrated in Fig. 12.23. The cells of the secretory carcinoma are columnar with sub- and supranuclear vacuoles. The secretory cells merge with endometrioid carcinoma in the *lower part of the field.*

Ciliated Carcinoma

Ciliated carcinoma is a rare form of differentiation in low-grade endometrioid carcinoma.[139] It does not need to be classified separately from endometrioid carcinoma; its only importance is to remind the pathologist that endometrial proliferations with cilia may still be carcinomas. Estrogen induces cilia formation in the normal endometrium. Despite the

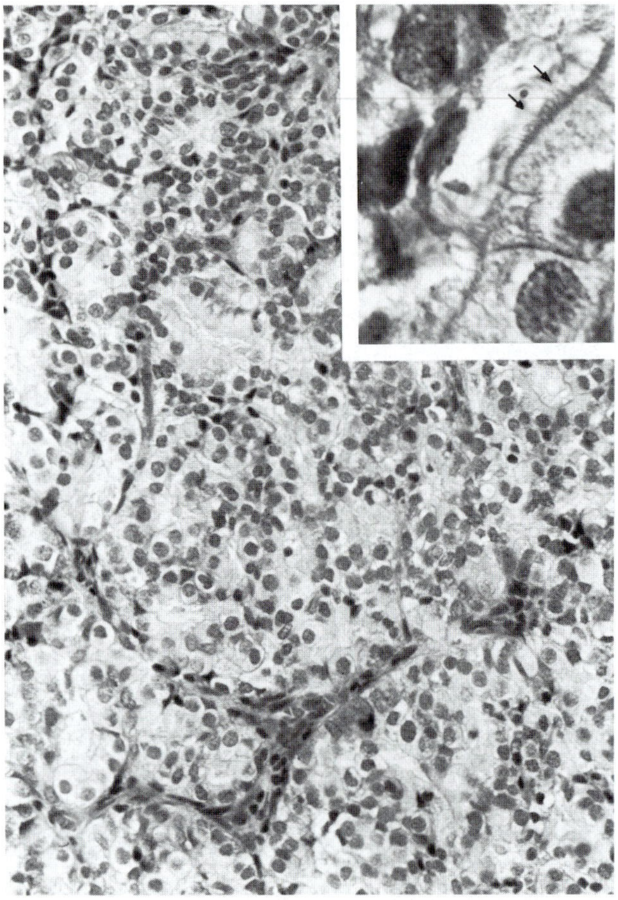

Fig. 12.25. Ciliated carcinoma. The tumor is composed of well-differentiated glands. *Inset*: Cells with minimal nuclear atypia containing cilia (*arrows*) on the luminal surface. The tumor invaded two-thirds into the myometrium. (Courtesy of Michael R. Hendrickson, M.D., Palo Alto, CA.)

prevalence of estrogen use, ciliated carcinoma is an extremely rare carcinoma, and most endometrial proliferations in which cilia are observed represent hyperplasias associated with eosinophilic or ciliated change. Patients range in age from 42 to 79 years, are often postmenopausal, and present with bleeding. Ciliated carcinoma has an association with exogenous estrogen treatment. Microscopically, ciliated carcinoma is almost always well differentiated and often displays a cribriform pattern. The gland lumens in the cribriform areas are lined by cells with prominent eosinophilic cytoplasm and cilia (Fig. 12.25). The nuclei of ciliated cells generally have an irregular nuclear membrane and display coarse nuclear chromatin with prominent nucleoli. In most cases, ciliated carcinoma is admixed with nonciliated endometrioid carcinoma and occasionally areas of mucinous carcinoma. Although some ciliated carcinomas are moderately differentiated and invade to the middle third of the myometrium, none of the patients has developed recurrence or died of disease. Thus, the presence of cilia in a bona fide carcinoma identifies a low-grade neoplasm.

Endometrioid Carcinoma with Squamous Differentiation

Many endometrioid adenocarcinomas contain squamous epithelium, but the amount of squamous epithelium can vary widely. In a well-sampled neoplasm, the squamous element should constitute at least 10% of a tumor to qualify as an *adenocarcinoma with squamous differentiation*. Adenocarcinomas with squamous elements were formerly divided into those with benign-appearing squamous elements and favorable prognosis, designated adenoacanthoma (AA), and those with malignant-appearing squamous epithelium and a worse prognosis, termed adenosquamous carcinoma (AS).[8,237] Recent studies indicate that the difference in behavior be-

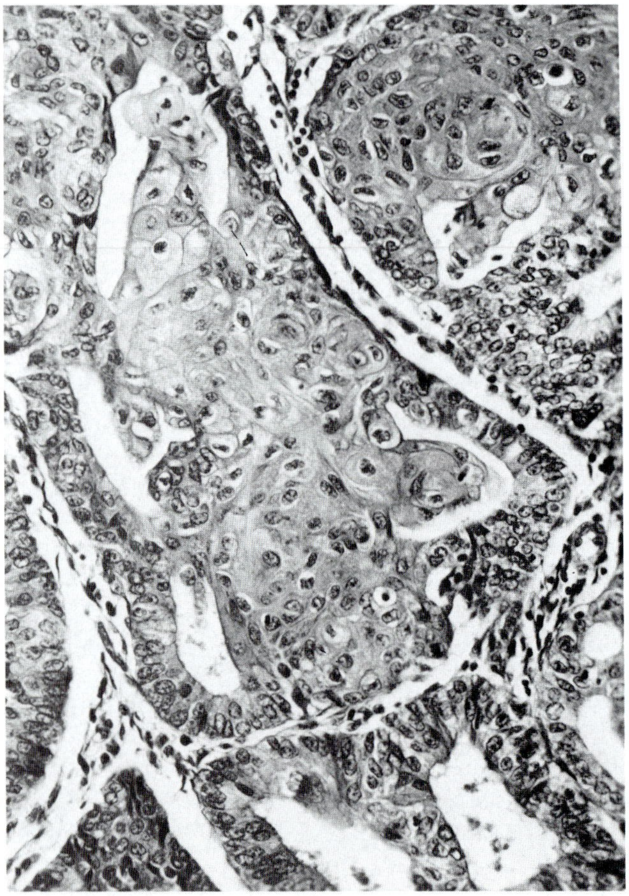

Fig. 12.26. Endometrioid carcinoma with squamous differentiation, FIGO grade 1. Both the glandular and squamous elements are grade 1. The squamous nests are confined to the gland lumens.

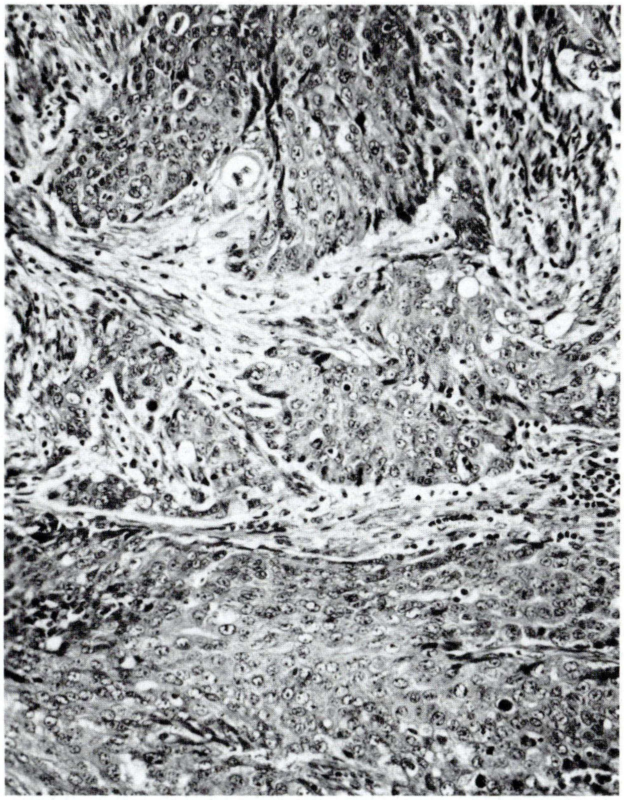

Fig. 12.27. Endometrioid carcinoma with squamous differentiation, FIGO grade 3. Sheets of malignant-appearing squamous epithelium diffusely infiltrate the myometrium.

tween AA and AS mainly reflects the difference in the grade of these respective neoplasms.[5,356,357] Thus, categorization of carcinomas with squamous epithelium according to the depth of myometrial invasion and the grade of the glandular component provides more useful prognostic information than the division into AA or AS because the grade of the glandular component generally parallels that of the squamous element.[357] This understanding had led to the view that AA and AS reflect a continuum in the degree of differentiation of the squamous epithelium that parallels the differentiation of the glandular component. Accordingly, it is recommended that endometrioid carcinomas with squamous epithelium be classified simply as endometrioid carcinoma with squamous differentiation and graded, on the basis of the glandular component, as well, moderately, or poorly differentiated (grade 1, 2, or 3, respectively).

There are no differences in the clinical features of adenocarcinoma containing squamous epithelium and endometrioid adenocarcinoma. Thus, there are no differences in the frequency of obesity, hypertension, diabetes, and nulliparity among the large series in which this has been analyzed.[8,57]

Gross and Microscopic Findings

These tumors have no distinctive gross findings. Low-grade tumors (grade 1) are composed of glandular and squamous elements but generally the glandular component predominates; the nests of squamous epithelium are confined to gland lumens (Fig. 12.26). The squamous epithelium resembles metaplastic squamous cells of the cervical transformation zone. Frequently, nests of cells with a prominent oval to spindle cell appearance, referred to as morules, are observed. Intercellular bridges can be identified within the squamous epithelium, and keratin formation is common. The nuclei of the squamous cells are bland, uniform, and lack prominent nucleoli. Mitotic figures are rare. In higher-grade tumors, the squamous element is cytologically more atypical and is not confined to gland lumens but often extends out from the glands (Fig. 12.27). At times the squamous cells have a spindle appearance simulating a sarcoma (Fig. 12.28). They may not be in

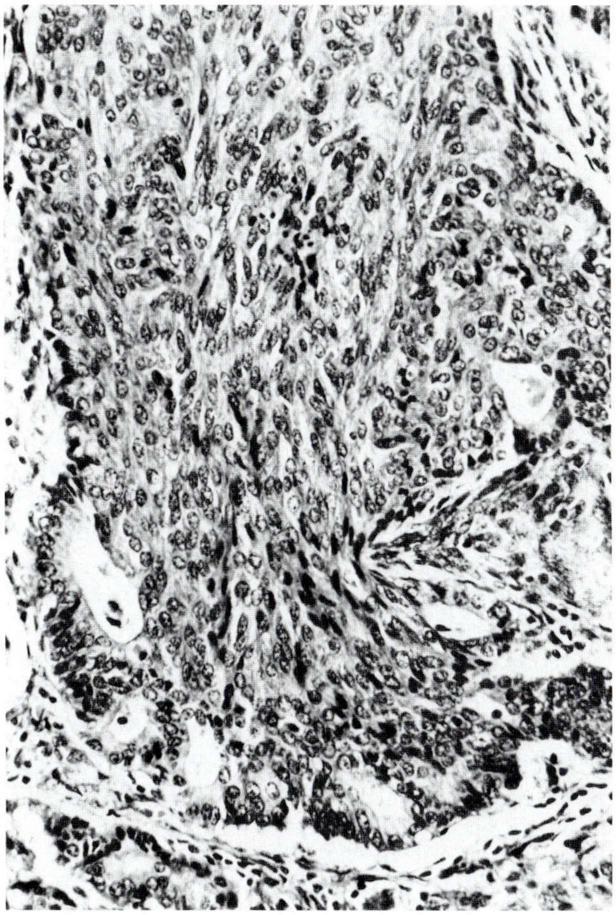

Fig. 12.28. Endometrioid carcinoma with squamous differentiation, FIGO grade 2. The squamous cells have a prominent spindle cell appearance. This spindle cell appearance should not be confused with sarcoma.

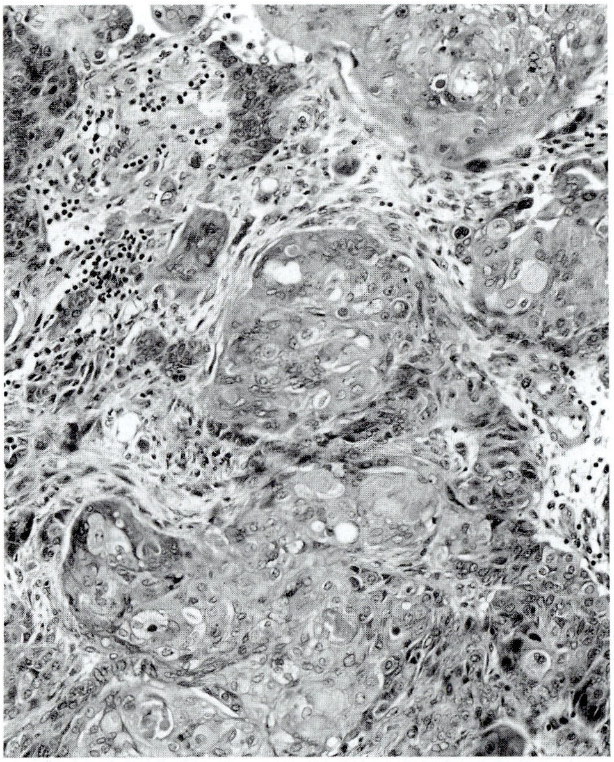

Fig. 12.29. Endometrioid carcinoma with squamous differentiation, FIGO grade 3. Isolated nests of squamous epithelium are diffusely infiltrating the myometrium. (Reprinted by permission of Zaino and Kurman, ref. 356)

direct continuity with the glandular epithelium, appearing in isolated nests within the myometrium (Fig. 12.29) or in vascular spaces. Keratinization and pearl formation occur to varying degrees.

Generally, the glandular component predominates, but masses of undifferentiated cells that may represent poorly differentiated glandular or squamous cells lie between glands. This undifferentiated epithelium should be considered glandular unless intercellular bridges are demonstrated or the cells have prominent eosinophilic cytoplasm, well-defined cytoplasmic borders, and a sheetlike proliferation without evidence of gland formation. Both the glandular and squamous components display grade 2 or 3 nuclear atypia, an increased nuclear cytoplasmic ratio, and increased mitotic activity. The glandular architecture usually is poorly differentiated. Tumors of intermediate differentiation are common. These neoplasms contain glandular and solid areas in which the squamous cells display a moderate degree of nuclear atypia, defying separation into a "benign" and "malignant" category.

A rare finding in patients with adenocarcinoma with squamous differentiation is the presence of keratin granulomas that may involve a wide variety of sites in the peritoneal cavity including the ovaries, tubes, omentum, and serosa of the uterus and bowel.[45,180] Microscopically, these lesions consist of a central mass of keratin and necrotic squamous cells surrounded by a foreign body granulomatous reaction. A proliferation of mesothelial cells also may be present. The granulomas probably result from exfoliation of necrotic cells from the tumor, followed by transtubal spread and implantation on peritoneal surfaces. It is important to distinguish pure keratin granulomas from lesions with both viable-appearing tumor cells and keratin accompanied by a foreign body-type giant cell reaction because the former lesions have not been associated with an unfavorable prognosis.

Differential Diagnosis

The most common problem in the differential diagnosis of the low-grade tumors is with atypical hyperplasia showing squamous metaplasia. To distinguish between the two, the criteria for identifying endometrial stromal invasion should be employed (see Chapter 11). At times, a low-grade tumor may be confused with a high-grade carcinoma because the masses of squamous epithelium are misconstrued as a solid proliferation of neoplastic cells. The nuclear grade is high in poorly differentiated carcinoma, however. Occasionally, squamous morules may be confused with granulomas, but the presence of foreign body giant cells and an inflammatory infiltrate helps identify the latter. For high-grade adenocarcinomas with squamous epithelium, the major problem in differential diagnosis in curettings is distinguishing a primary carcinoma of the endometrium from an adenosquamous carcinoma arising in the endocervix. In the cervix, the squamous component usually predominates, whereas in the endometrium the glandular component predominates. A profusion of cell types, especially mucinous or signet ring cells, is more characteristic of an endocervical neoplasm.

Behavior and Treatment

As already described, when stratified according to stage, grade, and depth of myometrial invasion, there are few differences in the behavior of carcinomas with squamous epithelium compared with endometrioid carcinomas without squamous epithelium.[5,356,357] As occurs with endometrioid carcinomas, the low-grade carcinomas with squamous epithelium tend to be only superficially invasive and seldom invade vascular channels. In contrast, high-grade tumors have a high frequency of deep myometrial invasion, vascular space involvement, and pelvic and paraaortic lymph node metastasis. Metastasis of high-grade tumors occurs widely throughout the pelvis and abdomen, involving bowel, mesentery, liver, kidney, spleen, and lymph nodes. Distant metastasis may involve the lungs, heart, skin, and bones. Nearly two-thirds of metastases contain both glandular and squamous elements, but pure adenocarcinoma or squamous carcinoma is encountered in 20% and 8%, respectively.[237] Often it is the squamous component that is identified in vascular channels. Accordingly, the treatment for carcinomas with squamous epithelium is the same as that for endometrioid carcinomas of comparable stage.

Mucinous Carcinoma

This uncommon type of endometrial carcinoma has an appearance similar to *mucinous carcinoma of the endocervix*.[68,326] *Mucinous carcinoma* represents the dominant cellular population in only 1–9% of endometrial carcinomas.[224,278] To qualify as a mucinous carcinoma, more than one-half the cell population of the tumor must contain periodic acid–Schiff- (PAS-) positive, diastase-resistant intracytoplasmic mucin.

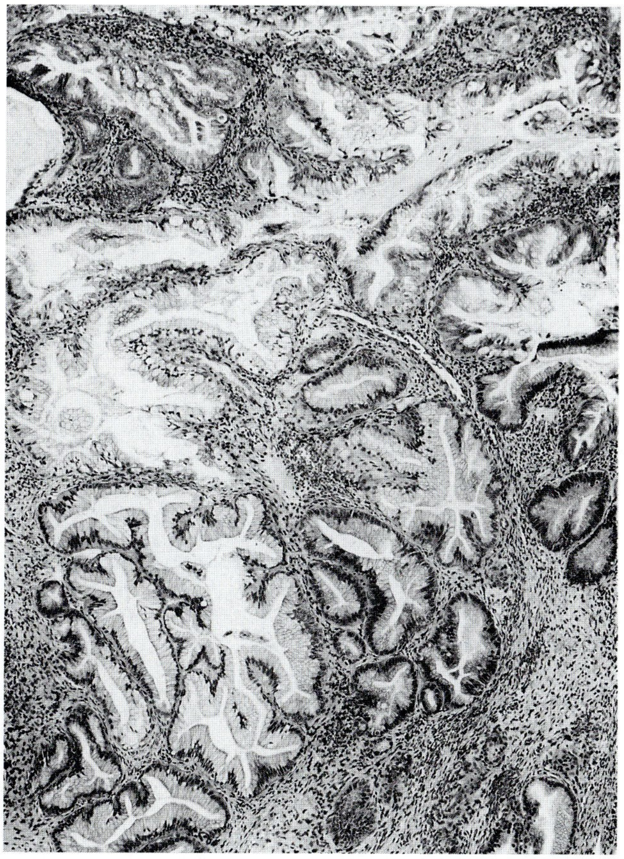

Fig. 12.30. Mucinous carcinoma, FIGO grade 1. The tumor is composed of irregularly shaped glands invading the myometrium. Uniform columnar cells with basally oriented nuclei can be seen even at this magnification.

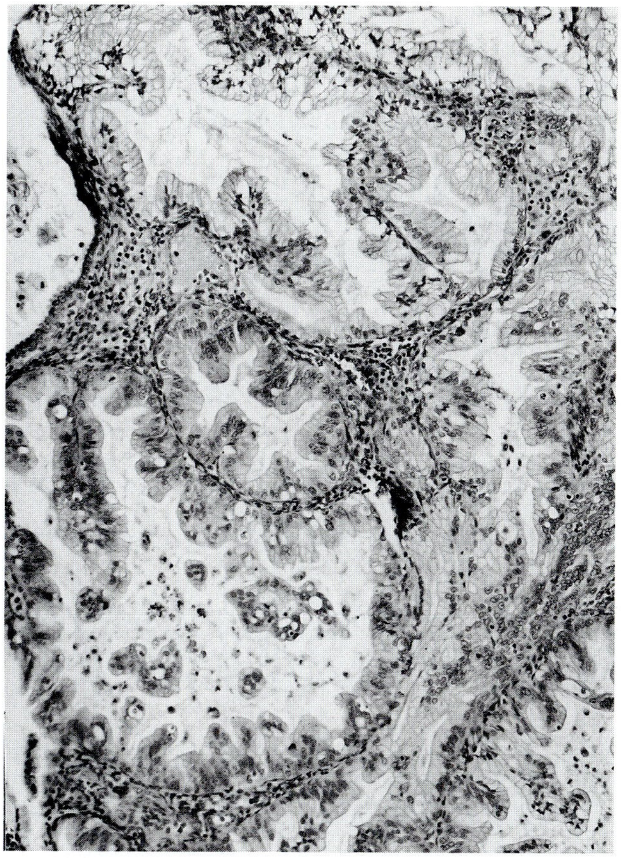

Fig. 12.31. Mucinous carcinoma, FIGO grade 1. Higher magnification of same case shown in Fig. 12.30. Papillary projections extend into gland lumens. The latter contain neutrophils. Nuclear atypia is minimal.

Judging from the few published cases, the clinical features of patients with mucinous carcinoma of the endometrium do not differ from those with endometrioid carcinoma. Patients range in age from 47 to 89 years and typically present with vaginal bleeding. In one study, more than 40% had a history of receiving exogenous estrogens.[224] Most patients present with stage I disease.

These tumors do not have distinctive gross features. The most frequent architectural pattern is glandular, often in a villoglandular configuration. The epithelial cells lining the glands and papillary processes tend to be uniform columnar cells with minimal stratification (Fig. 12.30). Cribriform areas are unusual; cystically dilated glands filled with mucin and papillary fronds surrounded by extracellular lakes of mucin, containing neutrophils, are typical (Fig. 12.31). Curiously, mucinous differentiation sometimes is associated with squamous differentiation. Nuclear atypia is mild to moderate, and mitotic activity is not prominent. Hyperplasia and mucinous metaplasia sometimes are present in the adjacent endometrium. One study reported that the carcinoma was present in a polyp in 27% of the cases.[224] The presence of intracytoplasmic mucin can be identified on hematoxyin and eosin (H&E) stains by its distinctive granular, foamy, or bubbly appearance and can be confirmed by PAS, mucicarmine, or alcian blue stains. The intracytoplasmic mucin is variable in both the distribution of mucinous cells in the tumor and in the location of the mucin within individual cells. Mucin may be diffusely present in the cytoplasm, confined to the apical area, or show a combination of both patterns.

Endocervical epithelium merges with the endometrium in the lower uterine segment, so it is not surprising that the distinction of primary endocervical from endometrial mucinous carcinoma in curettings can be difficult. There is no histochemical difference in the mucin at either site.[278] The distinction of endocervical from endometrial adenocarcinomas has been discussed earlier (see differential diagnosis section for endometrioid carcinoma).

The distinction of mucinous carcinoma of the endometrium from clear cell or secretory carcinoma is made on the basis of morphology and PAS and mucin stains. The cells in secretory carcinoma are clear (not granular or foamy) because of the presence of glycogen, which is PAS positive and is removed by diastase treatment. Mucin in these tumors is focal at most. Clear cell carcinoma is almost always papillary or solid in contrast to the glandular pattern of mucinous carcinoma. The cells in clear cell carcinoma tend to be polygonal rather than columnar and hobnail cells are almost invariably present, a cytologic feature that is absent in mucinous carcinoma.

Rarely, a mucinous carcinoma or a mixed mucinous and endometrioid carcinoma may contain areas that simulate microglandular hyperplasia of the cervix.[355,363] Such foci are characterized by cells showing mucinous and eosinophilic change with microcystic spaces containing acute inflammatory cells. The patients are in their fifties and sixties, in contrast to women with microglandular hyperplasia, who are young. The complexity of the glandular pattern and the degree of cytologic atypia distinguish this type of carcinoma from microglandular hyperplasia.

When stratified by stage, grade, and depth of myometrial invasion, mucinous tumors behave as do endometrioid carcinomas.[278] Mucinous carcinomas, however, tend to be low grade and minimally invasive and therefore as a group have an excellent prognosis. Treatment is the same as for endometrioid carcinoma. Because most of the tumors are stage I, low grade, and minimally invasive, total abdominal hysterectomy and bilateral salpingo-oophorectomy usually suffice.

Serous Carcinoma

The existence of papillary patterns within endometrial carcinoma has been recognized since the turn of the century. In the past two decades, several reports have described the morphologic similarity of *serous carcinomas* of the endometrium, which frequently display papillary architecture, to ovarian serous carcinomas and identified them as a highly aggressive type of endometrial carcinoma.[50,138,194,342] Although papillary architecture is a common finding in serous carcinoma, most other types of endometrial carcinoma can display papillary architecture but are usually not highly aggressive tumors. What distinguishes serous carcinoma from these other types is the uniformly marked cytologic atypia. Thus, the designation "serous carcinoma," rather than "papillary serous carcinoma," is preferred so that cell type rather than architecture is emphasized.

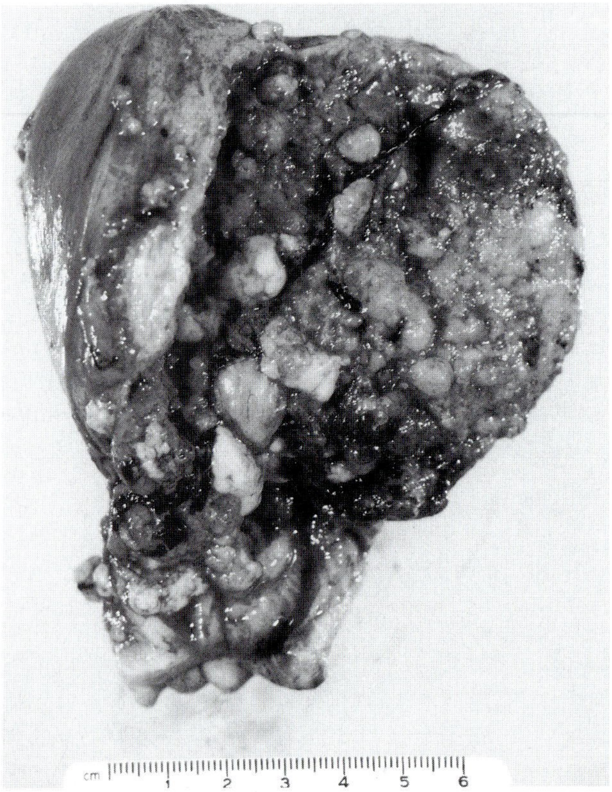

Fig. 12.32. Serous carcinoma. The tumor is exophytic, markedly papillary, and deeply invades the myometrium and cervix.

Clinical Features

The prevalence of serous carcinomas reported from referral centers usually is about 10%; however, in a population-based study from Norway it was only 1%.[1] Patients with serous carcinoma range in age from 39 to 93 years but typically are postmenopausal and, in contrast to women with endometrioid carcinoma, are older (reported median and mean ages are in the late sixties). In addition, they are less likely to have received estrogen replacement therapy and are more likely to have abnormal cervical cytology. There are some data to suggest that women with this neoplasm are less likely to be obese and that a higher proportion of women are black.[79] In other respects, they appear similar.

Gross Findings

On gross examination, uteri containing these tumors often are small and atrophic. Generally the tumor is exophytic (Fig. 12.32) and has a papillary appearance. Depth of invasion is difficult to assess on macroscopic examination. It is not unusual to find a benign-appearing polyp containing the carcinoma in the hysterectomy specimen after a diagnosis of serous carcinoma or endometrial intraepithelial carcinoma has been made on a curetting because these tumors frequently develop within a polyp (see Chapter 11, Precursor Lesions of Endometrial Carcinoma).[40,42,298,302,310,346]

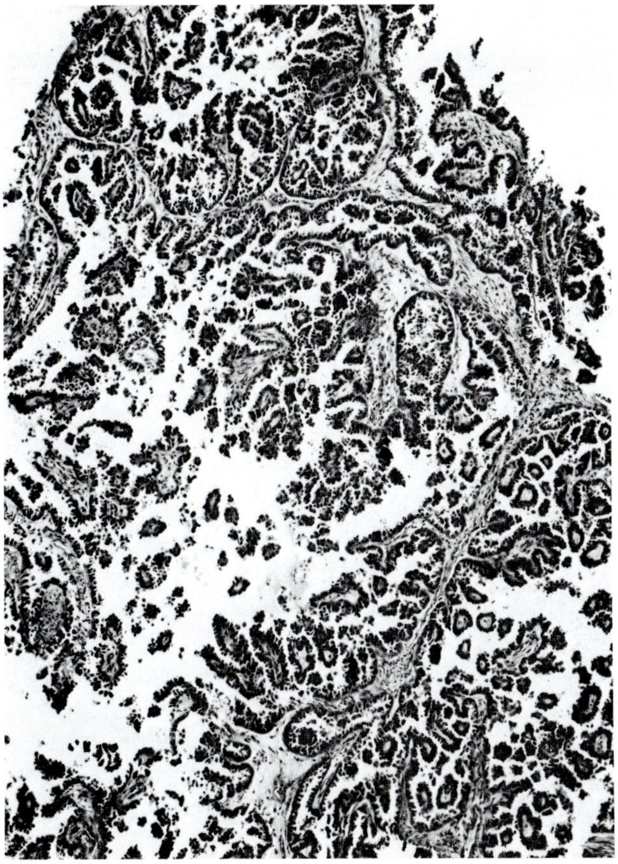

Fig. 12.33. Serous carcinoma. The tumor is characterized by a complex papillary architecture resembling serous carcinoma of the ovary.

Microscopic Findings

As experience with serous carcinoma has increased, it has become apparent that this neoplasm demonstrates considerable diversity in its architectural features. Although a papillary pattern typically predominates, glandular and solid patterns also occur.[138,201,298] Serous carcinoma originally was described as having thick, short papillae, but subsequent studies have shown that thin papillae may be present in more than half of them. The cytologic features of these tumors also are quite varied. Polygonal cells with eosinophilic and clear cytoplasm often are seen, but hobnail cells are among the most frequently observed cells. Marked nuclear atypia is always present and is required for a tumor to qualify as serous carcinoma. Thus, serous carcinoma is defined by the discordance between its architecture, which appears well differentiated (papillary or glandular pattern), and its nuclear morphology, which is high grade (grade 3 nuclei).[73] Areas containing clear cells do not preclude the diagnosis of serous carcinoma.

Microscopically, the exophytic component of a serous carcinoma typically has a complex papillary architecture resembling serous carcinoma of the ovary (Fig. 12.33). The papillary fronds may be either short and densely fibrotic (Fig. 12.34) or thin and delicate (Fig. 12.33). The cells covering the papillae and lining the glands form small papillary tufts, many of which are detached and float freely in spaces between the papillae and in gland lumens (Fig. 12.34). The cells are cuboidal or hobnail shaped (Fig. 12.35) and contain abundant granular eosinophilic or clear cytoplasm. The cells tend to be loosely cohesive. There may be considerable cytologic variability throughout the tumor, as many cells tend to show marked cytologic atypia manifested by nuclear pleomorphism, hyperchromasia, and macronucleoli whereas others are small and not so ominous in appearance. Multinucleated cells, giant nuclei, and bizarre forms occur in half the tumors. Lobulated nuclei with smudged chromatin also are frequently encountered (Fig. 12.35). Mitotic activity usually is high and abnormal mitotic figures are easily identified. Psammoma bodies are encountered in a third of cases. The invasive component of the neoplasm can show contiguous down-

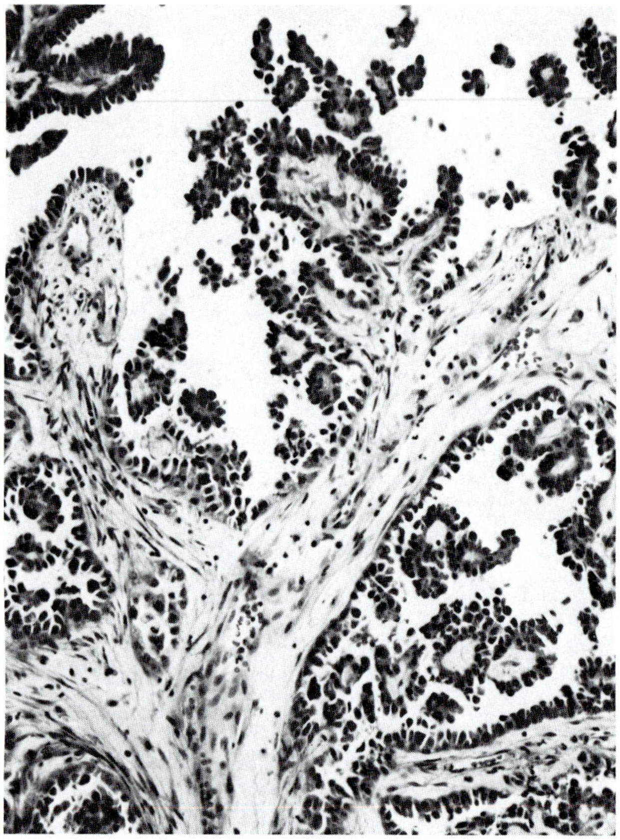

Fig. 12.34. Serous carcinoma. Dense fibrotic fibrovascular cores are covered by papillary tufts with many cells having a hobnail appearance. Most of the nuclei in this field are grade 2.

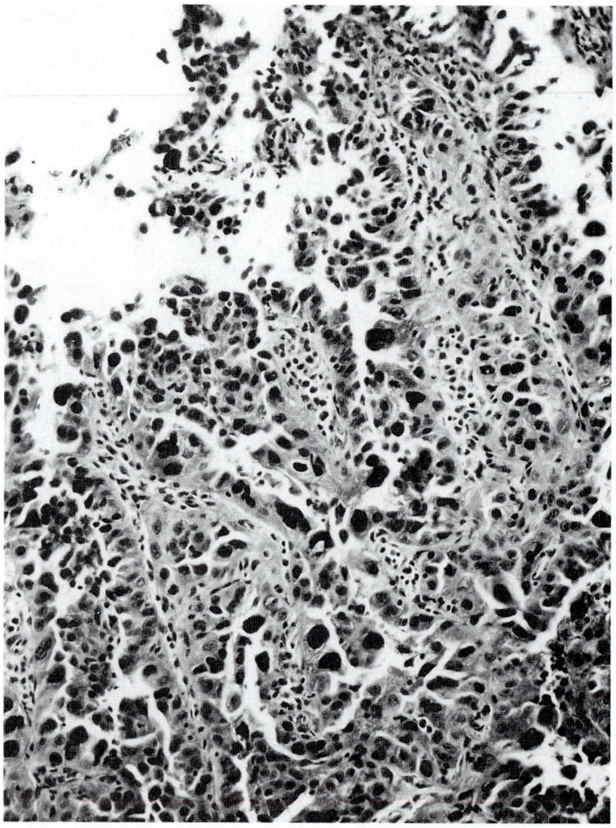

Fig. 12.35. Serous carcinoma. Most of the cells covering the papillae are hobnail cells showing marked nuclear atypia (grade 3). Bizarre-shaped nuclei with marked hyperchromasia and smudged chromatin are evident.

growth; of papillary processes, or solid masses or glands, the latter often have a gaping appearance. Nests of cells within vascular spaces are commonly found (Fig. 12.36).

The adjacent endometrium in hysterectomy specimens with serous carcinoma is atrophic in almost all cases. Hyperplasia, generally without atypia, is present in less than 10% of cases.[40,298,312] In nearly 90% of cases, the surface endometrium adjacent to the carcinoma or at other sites away from the neoplasm is replaced by one or several layers of highly atypical cells that overlie atrophic endometrium and extend into normal glands. These cells are identical to those of the invasive carcinoma and at times form micropapillary processes. This lesion, which has been designated *endometrial intraepithelial carcinoma* (*EIC*) (Figs. 12.37 and 12.38), is discussed in detail in Chapter 11.[11,312] The intraepithelial carcinoma can extensively replace the surface endometrium and underlying glands without stromal invasion (Fig. 12.39). The clinicopathologic features and distinction of extensive EIC from early invasive serous carcinoma has been reported recently.[346] It has been proposed that EIC and serous carcinoma measuring 1 cm or less should be designated minimal uterine serous carcinoma because these lesions are difficult to distinguish and they behave in a similar fashion when confirmed as stage IA by meticulous surgical staging. It is important to recognize that patients whose uteri demonstrate only EIC, without evidence of invasive serous carcinoma in the completely sampled endometrium, can have metastatic serous carcinoma in the ovary, peritoneum, or omentum, presumably as a result of exfoliation and implantation of the loosely cohesive tumor cells.[310,346]

Differential Diagnosis

Serous carcinoma must be distinguished from villoglandular carcinoma, which also has papillary architecture. Unlike serous carcinoma, villoglandular carcinoma is characterized by the predominance of long, delicate papillary fronds that do not display papillary tufting. In addition, the cells are columnar, resembling cells in endometrioid carcinoma and lack high-grade nuclear atypia (see "Villoglandular Car-

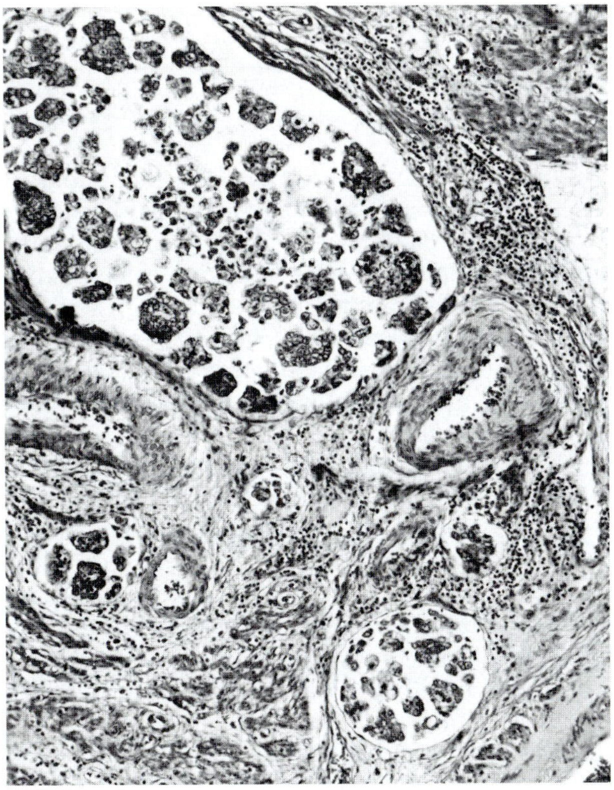

Fig. 12.36. Serous carcinoma. The tumor extensively involves vascular channels within the myometrium far removed from the tumor mass. The papillary architecture is retained in the intravascular component.

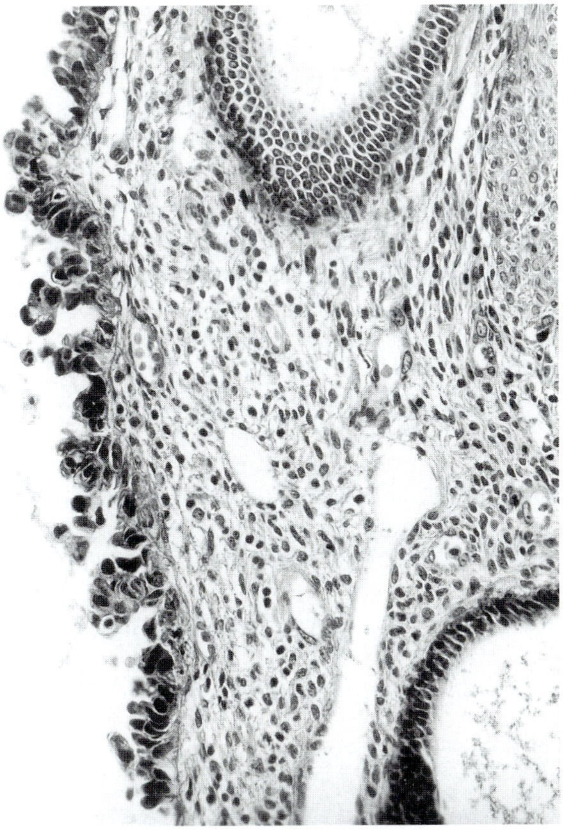

Fig. 12.38. Endometrial intraepithelial carcinoma. Another focus of intraepithelial carcinoma on the endometrial surface (*left side of field*) at a site remote from the invasive carcinoma.

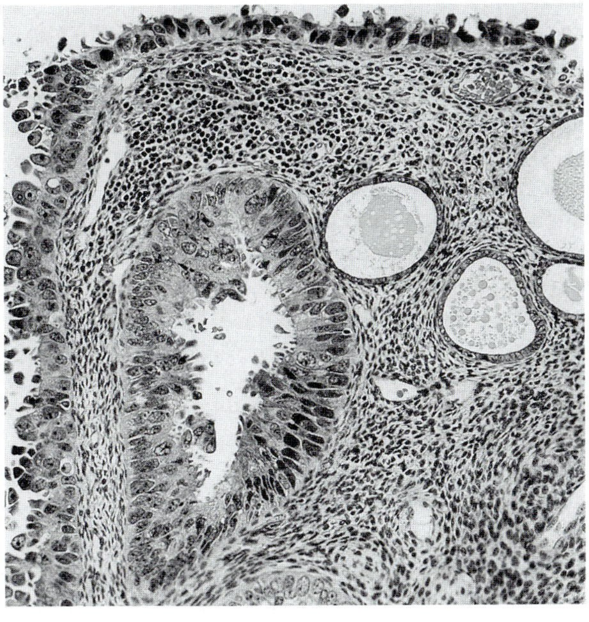

Fig. 12.37. Endometrial intraepithelial carcinoma. Highly atypical cells identical to those in serous carcinoma replace the surface epithelium overlying atrophic glands and extend into normal glands (*left side of field*). This lesion was immediately adjacent to an invasive serous carcinoma. (Reprinted by permission of Sherman et al., ref. 298.)

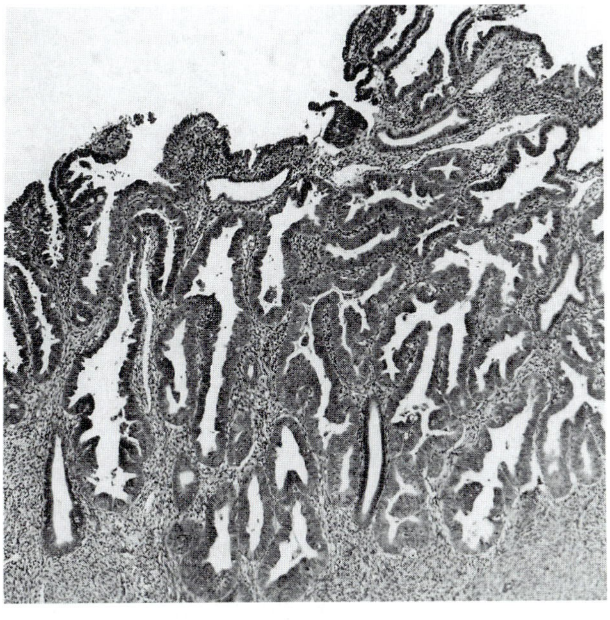

Fig. 12.39. Endometrial intraepithelial carcinoma. The neoplasm extensively replaces glands but does not invade the stroma. Elsewhere, an invasive serous carcinoma was present. This appearance can easily be confused with endometrioid carcinoma.

cinoma"). A serous carcinoma with a prominent glandular pattern that lacks prominent papillary features may be confused with an endometrioid carcinoma. In this case it is predominantly the nuclear morphology that aids in the distinction. The glands in an endometrioid carcinoma have a smooth luminal border and are lined by columnar cells with nuclei that are grade 1 or 2. Endometrioid carcinomas with grade 3 nuclei are almost always solid, not glandular. In contrast, the glands in a serous carcinoma are lined by cells with high-grade nuclei, some of which are hobnail shaped, thus imparting a scalloped luminal border to the glands (Fig. 12.40). In addition, in most cases papillary tufts project or lie detached in the gland lumens. Immunohistochemical analysis can aid in the distinction of glandular serous carcinoma from endometrioid carcinoma. Several studies have demonstrated a very high frequency of strong, diffuse positivity for p53 in serous carcinomas, and this pattern of staining is correlated with the presence of mutations in the p53 gene (see "Molecular Genetics of Endometrial Carcinoma").[189,197,229,299,321] In addition, most serous carcinomas demonstrate a lack of expression of estrogen and progesterone receptors and very high proliferation indices as measured by immunohistochemical expression of Ki-67.[41,195] In contrast, endometrioid carcinomas (particularly grade 1 and 2 tumors) frequently express hormone receptors and have lower proliferation indices.[41,195,196] In addition, strong, diffuse immunohistochemical expression of p53 is confined to a subset of grade 3 endometrioid carcinomas and is not encountered in lower-grade endometrioid carcinomas.[195,196] Hence, glandular carcinomas with high-grade cytology for which the differential diagnosis includes grade 2 endometrioid carcinoma and serous carcinoma can be distinguished by immunohistochemistry for p53, Ki-67, and hormone receptors. The distinction of serous carcinoma from clear cell carcinoma is discussed later (see "Clear Cell Carcinoma").

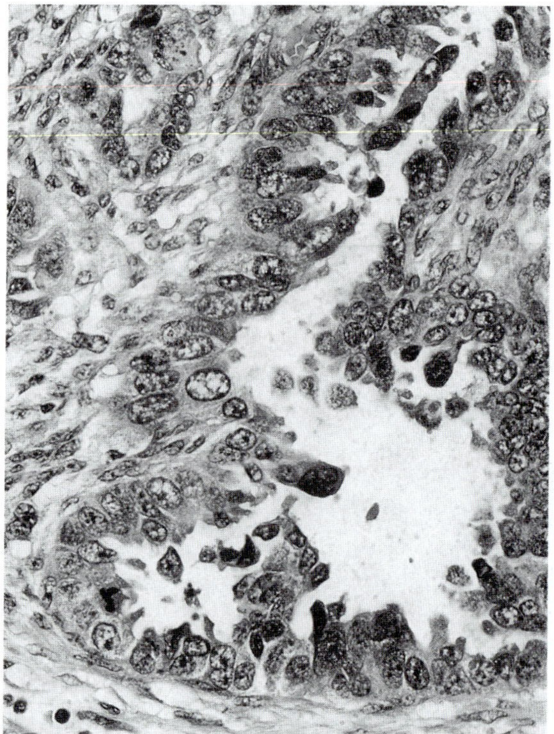

Fig. 12.40. Serous carcinoma. A gaping gland lined by cells with high-grade nuclei. Several of the cells are hobnail cells. The high-grade nuclear morphology distinguishes serous carcinoma with a prominent glandular pattern from an endometrioid carcinoma. Endometrioid carcinoma with grade 3 nuclei nearly always displays a solid rather than a glandular architecture.

At times papillary syncytial eosinophilic change, particularly in a small curettage specimen in an older patient, may be difficult to distinguish from serous carcinoma. The papillary processes in eosinophilic change lack fibrovascular support and the cells that form these processes are small and lack significant nuclear atypia or mitotic activity. Typically, small microcystic spaces containing neutrophils are present in the syncytial masses (see Chapter 11, Precursor Lesions of Endometrial Carcinoma). At times it may not be clear if a serous carcinoma involving the endometrium is primary or metastatic from the ovary. More often than not the uterus is the primary site, even when invasion cannot be demonstrated in the hysterectomy specimen.[343] In these cases the ovarian involvement is typically bilateral and characterized by small foci of tumor on the ovarian surface or nodules of tumor in the parenchyma with clusters of tumor cells in hilar vascular spaces.

Behavior and Treatment

Serous carcinoma has a propensity for myometrial and lymphatic invasion (see Fig. 12.36). The hysterectomy specimen often discloses tumor in lymphatics extensively within the myometrium, cervix, broad ligament, fallopian tube, and ovarian hilus. In addition, intraepithelial carcinoma similar to that involving the endometrium has been reported on the surfaces of the ovaries, peritoneum, and mucosa of the endocervix and fallopian tube in the absence of gross disease in these sites.[298,346] Involvement of peritoneal surfaces in the pelvis and abdomen, as in ovarian serous carcinoma, occurs early in the course of disease. Not surprisingly, most studies report that uterine serous carcinoma is clinically understaged in approximately 40% of cases.[40,79] In addition to intraperitoneal spread, serous carcinoma can metastasize to the liver, brain, and skin.

The 5- and 10-year actuarial survival rates for all stages were 36% and 18%, respectively, in a study from Norway[1]; 5-year survival for pathologic stage I serous carcinoma was 40% in one study.[40] A recent study of stage I and II serous and clear cell carcinomas demonstrated a 5-year survival rate of 57% for patients with stage IA tumors, which was similar to that for patients with stage IB and IC tumors (53%).[55] In addition, prognostic factors for shorter survival included age greater than 60 years, vascular invasion, and greater than 50% myometrial invasion. Nearly half the serous carcinomas and 40% of the clear cell carcinomas in this study population that were thought to be early stage (clinical stage I and II) were upstaged to surgical stage III or IV despite the finding that the majority of these tumors had invaded only the inner third of the myometrium.[54] In addition, 13% of the serous carcinomas that were confined to the endometrium had paraaortic lymph node metastases. Patients with mixed endometrial carcinomas containing a component of serous carcinoma that accounted for as little as 25% of the tumor have the same survival as patients with pure serous carcinoma, underscoring the importance of identifying areas of serous carcinoma in uterine carcinomas.[298]

The current approach to treatment is hysterectomy and bilateral salpingo-oophorectomy along with omentectomy and careful surgical staging, including peritoneal cytology and pelvic and paraaortic lymph node sampling. In view of the highly aggressive behavior, adjuvant therapy should be considered for all tumors except those that qualify as minimal uterine serous carcinoma. In a recent study of 21 cases with pure EIC or minimal uterine serous carcinoma (less than 1 cm of carcinoma in the endometrium), all 14 patients whose tumors lacked myometrial or vascular invasion and who had no evidence of extrauterine disease at staging had an overall survival of 100% after a mean follow-up of 27 months.[346] The majority of these patients received no treatment after hysterectomy. Included among these cases were a few patients with involvement of endocervical glands by EIC (stage IIA disease) who were also alive without evidence of disease at intervals ranging from 12 to 54 months. In contrast, the patients with either EIC or minimal serous carcinoma and evidence of extrauterine disease (even microscopic disease) all died of disease despite intensive chemotherapy. In another study of stage IA serous carcinoma, 11 of 13 patients were alive without evidence of disease after a median follow-up of 38 months.[42] Another recent study of 16 noninvasive serous carcinomas of the endometrium found that 6 tumors were stage IA and the remaining 10 had metastases identified at staging.[168] Two of the 6 patients with stage IA disease experienced a recurrence but none died of disease during the follow-up period, which ranged from 2 to 73 months. Three patients with stage IIA disease also were alive without evidence of disease at intervals ranging from 37 to 61 months.

The finding of advanced-stage disease in the absence of myometrial invasion in 10 patients emphasizes the need for complete staging of all patients with serous carcinoma. Another study of 8 patients with serous or clear cell carcinoma confined to endometrial curettings without evidence of residual high-grade carcinoma (serous, clear cell, or FIGO grade 3 endometrioid) or vascular invasion in the hysterectomy specimen were without evidence of recurrence after a median follow-up of 3 years.[16] Unfortunately, no satisfactory adjuvant therapy is available. In a study evaluating cisplatin, doxorubicin (Adriamycin), and cyclophosphamide (PAC) chemotherapy, which has a 70% response rate in previously untreated ovarian serous carcinoma, the response rate for uterine serous carcinoma was only 20%, suggesting that there are inherent differences in uterine and ovarian serous carcinomas.[205] Another study of platinum-based chemotherapy found that 8 of the 12 treated women were alive without evidence of disease, including 4 patients with advanced-stage disease and mean follow-up of 23 months, suggesting a possible role for chemotherapy.[117] These tumors are unresponsive to hormonal treatment because they almost always lack expression of hormone receptors.

Molecular Genetics of Endometrial Carcinoma

Endometrial carcinoma can be broadly divided into two types (see section on "Classification") based on clinical, epidemiologic, immunohistochemical, and molecular genetic features. In addition to confirming this subdivision, the molecular studies have provided insights into the genetic events involved in the development and progression of endometrial carcinoma. For conceptual and practical reasons, this section does not attempt to provide an exhaustive list of the cancer-causing genes that have been studied but rather is intended to provide the reader with an overview of the current understanding of the molecular genetics of endometrial carcinoma.

Since the initial clinical observation of endometrial carcinoma as two broad disease entities, it has been recognized by pathologists that there is a general correlation of the clinical type with the morphologic features of the endometrial tumor. For the most part, type I tumors are associated with endometrioid features and arise in the setting of hyperplasia, whereas type II tumors are often of serous type and present in a background of endometrial atrophy. Although somewhat oversimplified, this histologic distinction is important to the understanding of endometrial carcinoma at the molecular level. For this reason, the two tumor types are discussed separately, recognizing that many molecular studies have not clearly classified the tumors by morphologic type. For explanation of terms or concepts included in this section that are unfamiliar to the reader, refer to Chapter 26 (Molecular Biology).

Endometrioid Carcinoma

During the past decade, a number of cancer-causing genes have been analyzed in endometrial carcinoma. Recently, several studies have shown that the most frequently altered gene in endometrioid carcinoma is the *PTEN* tumor suppressor gene, which is mutated in 30–50% of cases.[275,320] *PTEN* is located on chromosome 10q23.3 and encodes a phosphatase.[208] The primary target is the lipid molecule phosphatidylinositol 3,4,5-triphosphate (PIP3) that is involved in a signal transduction pathway that regulates cell growth and apoptosis.[215] The frequency of mutation of the gene is similar in all three grades of endometrioid carcinoma, and it is also mutated in approximately 20% of atypical and nonatypical hyperplasias.[207,220] These findings suggest that inactivation of this gene is important early in the pathogenesis of endometrioid carcinoma. In addition, an immunohistochemical study found that the majority of endometrioid carcinomas show loss of PTEN expression, indicating that it may play a central role in the development of this tumor type.[234] Furthermore, this study and a subsequent molecular study found loss of PTEN expression and PTEN genetic alterations (mutations, deletions) in clusters of otherwise benign-appearing endometrial glands, suggesting that *PTEN* inactivation may occur before the development of a recognizable histopathologic lesion.[234a] Clearly, understanding *PTEN* and its role in the development of endometrioid carcinomas may provide novel markers for detecting endometrial glands predisposed to progress to malignancy and provide targets for therapeutic intervention before the development of malignant disease.

The *p53* tumor suppressor gene has been extensively studied in endometrial cancer, as in other tumors. *p53* encodes a DNA-binding phosphoprotein that is involved in cell cycle control and apoptosis. Mutations in *p53* are found in approximately 10% of all endometrioid carcinomas, with most occurring in grade 3, and occasionally in grade 2, tumors. Overall, *p53* mutations occur in approximately 50% of grade 3 tumors, and they have not been identified in grade 1 tumors or endometrial hyperplasia.[254] This finding is consistent with a role for *p53* in the progression, but not the initiation, of endometrioid carcinoma.

Another molecular alteration in endometrioid carcinomas that has received substantial attention is the molecular phenotype called microsatellite instability. Microsatellite instability is defined as alterations in the length of short, repetitive DNA sequences, called microsatellites, in tumors when compared to DNA prepared from the same patient's normal tissue. This molecular phenotype is detected in tumors that lack an intact DNA mismatch repair system, a fundamental cellular mechanism for preventing DNA alterations that are created largely during DNA replication. In tumors that display microsatellite instability, the DNA mismatch repair system has been inactivated either through mutation or "silencing" by promoter hypermethylation of one of the DNA mismatch repair genes.[89] The consequence of inactivating the DNA mismatch repair system is an increase in the rate at which mutations occur, a factor that clearly contributes to tumori-genesis. Microsatellite instability is found in tumors from patients affected by hereditary nonpolyposis colorectal carcinoma (HNPCC), a syndrome in which endometrial carcinoma is the most common noncolorectal malignancy.[87] Microsatellite instability also is present in approximately 20% of sporadic endometrial cancers and can be found in complex atypical hyperplasias that are associated with cancers that demonstrate instability.[77,207,235] It has not, however, been found in lesser degrees of hyperplasia. It remains unclear exactly when in the development of endometrial neoplasia the DNA mismatch repair system becomes inactivated.[90] Further studies of endometrial hyperplasia are warranted to address this important biologic and potentially clinically relevant question.

During the past decade several oncogenes have been studied in endometrial carcinomas, but only a few are altered in a significant number of cases. Mutations in the K-*ras* proto-oncogene have been identified consistently in 10–30% of endometrial cancers in several studies.[34,85,197] The mutations have been found in all grades of endometrioid carcinoma and have been reported in complex atypical hyperplasia, suggesting a relatively early role for K-*ras* mutations in this tumor type. K-*ras* encodes a guanine nucleotide-binding protein of 21 kDa that plays a role in the regulation of cell growth and differentiation by transducing signals from activated transmembrane receptors. In the mutant form, K-*ras* is constitutively "on" even in the absence of an activated receptor. Other oncogenes that have been found to be overexpressed or amplified are c-*myc*, *HER-2/neu*, *bcl-2*, and c-*fms*.[33,141,203,322] Most recently, mutations in the *β-catenin* gene have been found in approximately 15–20% of endometrioid carcinomas.[100,182,291] Additional studies on these genes are needed to more definitively determine their role in endometrial cancer.

Serous Carcinoma

Compared to endometrioid carcinoma, relatively little is known about serous carcinoma at the molecular level, partly because of its relative infrequency and because this tumor type is not analyzed separately in many molecular studies. Although a number of candidate cancer genes have been analyzed in serous carcinoma, only the p53 tumor suppressor gene has been shown to be altered in a significant number, with mutations identified in almost 90% of cases.[229,321] In fact, there are few other tumor types that demonstrate a mutation frequency in a single gene as high as that of p53 in serous endometrial carcinoma. Furthermore, approximately 75% of endometrial intraepithelial carcinomas, the putative precursor of serous carcinoma, have mutations in p53.[321] In this setting, it has been shown that intense, diffuse immunohistochemical staining for p53 correlates well with p53 mutation. These findings suggest that in serous carcinoma p53 mutations occur relatively early and are central to the development of this tumor type; this is in contrast to endometrioid carcinoma, in which p53 mutations are relatively uncommon and, when they do occur, they are largely confined to grade 3 tumors. Thus, it is possible that the mutation of p53 early in the pathogenesis of serous carcinoma is an important factor that accounts for its aggressive behavior. In addition, the fact that p53 mutations occur most commonly in grade 3 endometrioid and serous carcinomas most likely explains the finding that it is an independent indicator of tumors that behave aggressively.[308]

In contrast to endometrioid carcinoma, mutations in K-*ras* and *PTEN* appear to be very uncommon in serous carcinoma, and microsatellite instability has not definitively been described in this tumor type.[197] Studies have suggested that there is amplification and overexpression of c-*myc* and *Her-2/neu*; however, it is not clear from the literature what percentage of serous carcinomas demonstrate these alterations.

As is clear from this discussion, relatively little is known about the molecular pathogenesis of the two major types of endometrial carcinoma and almost nothing is known about the more uncommon histologic types of endometrial carcinoma. However, it is evident from the studies just described that endometrioid and serous carcinoma of the endometrium are distinct biologic entities. As in other tumor systems, the molecular studies of endometrial cancer support the notion that epithelial-derived tumors often develop from preinvasive precursors that accumulate a combination of genetic alterations, thus providing the cell with the attributes necessary for unregulated growth. In endometrioid carcinoma it appears that *PTEN* alterations may be central to the initiation of proliferative lesions that then acquire mutations in other cancer-causing genes (e.g., DNA mismatch repair genes, K-*ras*, *p53*) in the progression to malignancy. On the other hand, p53 mutations appear to be important in the conversion of relatively quiescent, atrophic endometrium to an intraepithelial form of serous carcinoma that then sets the stage for the accumulation of alterations in yet unidentified cancer-causing genes.

The genes that have been described to play a role in endometrial cancer to date have been genes discovered in other tumor systems that have subsequently been found to have alterations in endometrial cancer. Hopefully, with the technologic advances occurring in human genetics and the information being provided by the human genome project, novel genes that are involved in endometrial carcinogenesis will be identified.

Clear Cell Carcinoma

In the past, *clear cell carcinoma* was regarded as mesonephric in origin because of its resemblance to renal carcinoma, but the occurrence of clear cell carcinoma in the endometrium, a müllerian derivative, is evidence of its müllerian origin.[191] The prevalence of clear cell carcinoma ranges from 1% to 6% in most series. Almost all studies report that women with clear cell carcinoma are older than women with endometrioid carcinoma (mean age in late sixties).[4,50,172,264,344] Some studies have reported a higher likelihood of abnormal cytology, a lower frequency of some of the associated constitutional symptoms, such as obesity and diabetes mellitus, and a lack of association of estrogen replacement therapy compared with endometrioid carcinomas, but this has not been confirmed by other studies.

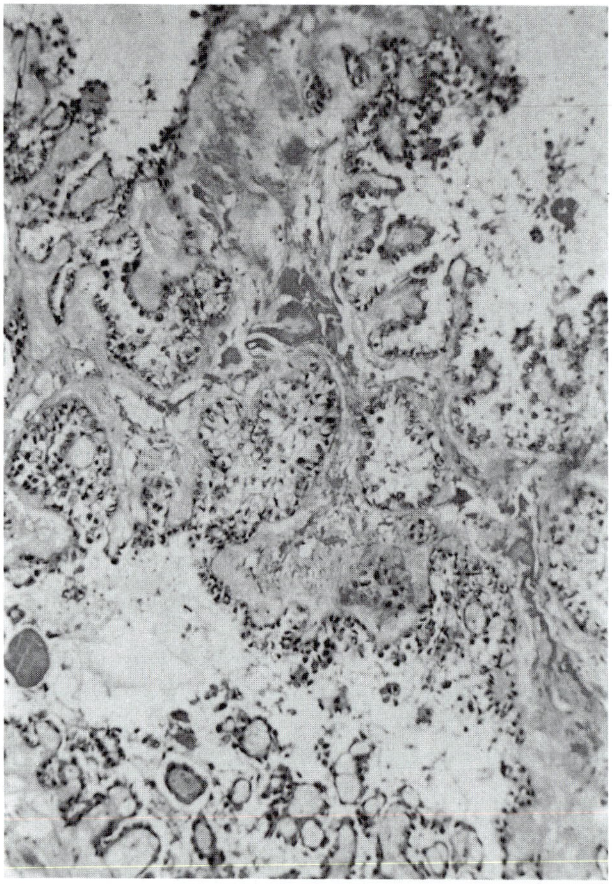

Fig. 12.41. Clear cell carcinoma. The tumor displays a papillary pattern resembling serous carcinoma.

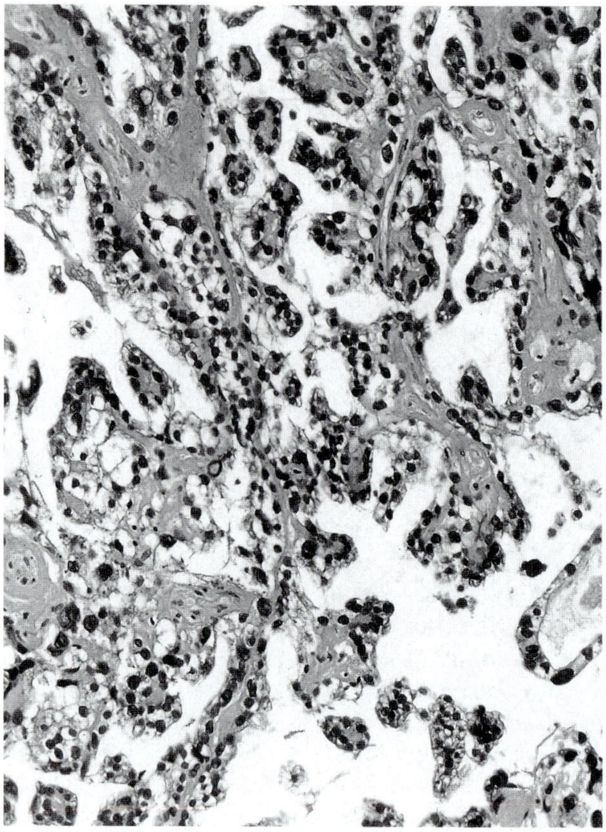

Fig. 12.42. Clear cell carcinoma. The papillae in this neoplasm have hyalinized cores. This feature is seen more frequently in papillary clear cell as compared with serous carcinoma.

These tumors do not have distinctive gross features. Clear cell carcinoma may exhibit solid, papillary, tubular, and cystic patterns (Figs. 12.41–12.45). The solid pattern is composed of masses of clear cells intermixed with eosinophilic cells, whereas papillary, tubular, and cystic patterns are composed predominantly of hobnail-shaped cells with interspersed clear and eosinophilic cells. Cystic spaces frequently are lined by flattened cells. Psammoma bodies can be found in association with papillary areas within the tumor. The cells typically are large, with clear or lightly stained eosinophilic cytoplasm. The clear cytoplasm results from the presence of glycogen, demonstrated with a PAS stain and diastase digestion. Cells that have discharged their glycogen and lost most of their cytoplasm are characterized by a naked nucleus, the hobnail cell. Nuclear atypia generally is marked, manifested by pleomorphic, often large, multiple nuclei with prominent nucleoli (Fig. 12.45). Mitotic activity is high, and abnormal mitoses are readily seen. PAS-positive, diastase-resistant intracellular and extracellular hyaline bodies, similar to those in endodermal sinus tumors, can be found in nearly

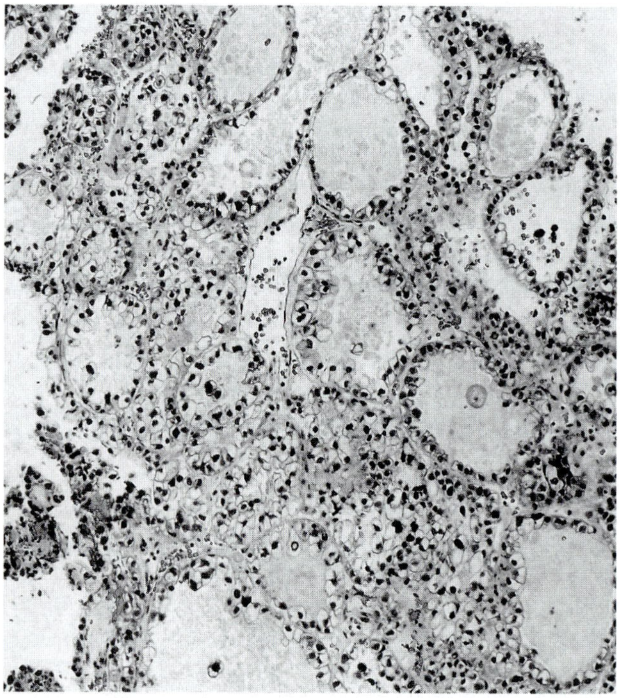

Fig. 12.43. Clear cell carcinoma. The tumor displays a tubulocystic pattern resembling endometrioid carcinoma.

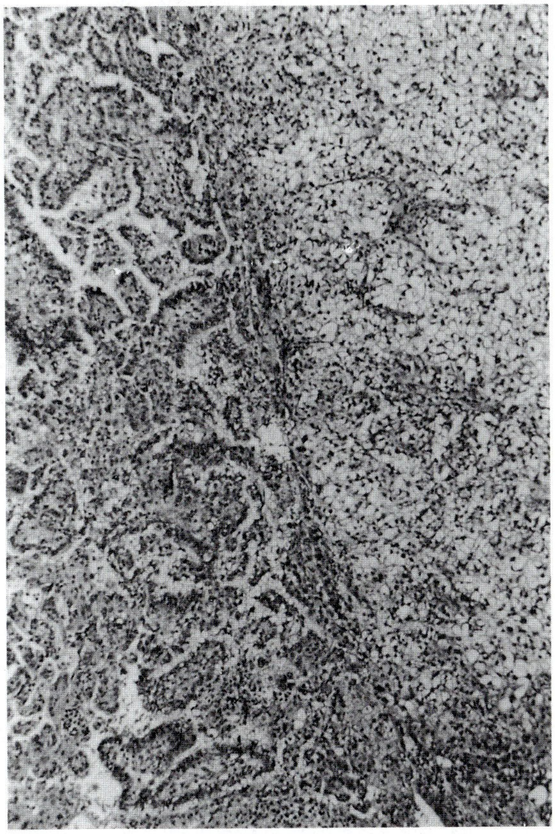

Fig. 12.44. Clear cell carcinoma. The tumor displays a solid and papillary pattern.

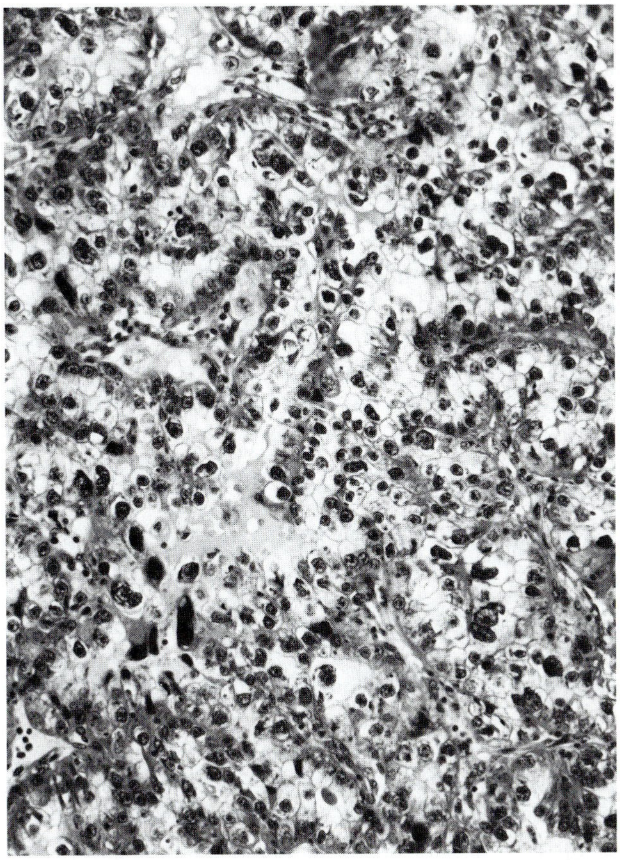

Fig. 12.45. Clear cell carcinoma. The tumor is composed of sheets of large clear cells with enlarged, pleomorphic nuclei.

two-thirds of clear cell carcinomas and serve as a useful identifying feature.

The differential diagnosis of clear cell carcinoma includes secretory carcinoma, serous carcinoma, and yolk sac tumor. The differential diagnosis of the first tumor has been discussed (see "Secretory Carcinoma"). Clear cell carcinoma can be distinguished from serous carcinoma by architectural and cytoplasmic rather than nuclear features because both tumors display similar high-grade nuclear features, including vesicular nuclei with prominent nucleoli, hobnail cells, and cells with hyperchromatic, smudged nuclei. Serous carcinomas do not display the tubulocystic or solid growth patterns, clear cytoplasm, and hyalinized stroma that are characteristic of clear cell carcinomas. The distinction of clear cell carcinoma from serous carcinoma is not clinically relevant because their behavior is similar. In some cases, mixtures of both types are found. Nonetheless, clear cell carcinomas are probably distinct from serous carcinomas based on the significantly less frequent expression of p53 by immunohistochemistry.[195] Yolk sac tumors occur rarely in the endometrium but the patients are young, in contrast to women with clear cell carcinoma, who are almost always postmenopausal. Microscopically, yolk sac tumors often have a microcystic pattern that can resemble the tubulocystic pattern of clear cell carcinoma. Characteristically, the yolk sac tumor contains Schiller–Duval bodies, which are lacking in clear cell carcinoma. Yolk sac tumors are associated with elevated serum alpha-fetoprotein (AFP) levels, and AFP can be identified in the tumor by immunohistochemistry.

Clear cell carcinoma tends to be high grade, deeply invasive, and to present in an advanced stage. Similar to serous carcinoma, clear cell carcinomas are more frequently associated with deep myometrial invasion, high nuclear grade, lymphvascular space invasion, and pelvic lymph node metastasis compared to endometrioid carcinomas.[287] Occasionally they are confined to a polyp.[172] The reported survival of patients with clear cell carcinoma differs considerably as reported in various series, ranging from 21% to 75%.[4,50,191,264,344] In one series, none of the patients with tumor beyond stage I survived for 5 years, and even in stage I the 5-year survival was only 44%.[50] Another report of low-stage tumors demonstrated better survival, with an estimated survival rate of 71%.[217] In a series of nearly

97 patients the 5-year crude survival was 42% and the 10-year survival, 31%.[4] Another study reported 5- and 10-year actuarial disease-free survival rates of 43% and 39%.[7] (See "Serous Carcinoma," "Behavior and Treatment" for additional data.) The wide range in survival reported in these different series suggests that different investigators may be applying different criteria for the diagnosis of clear cell carcinoma, resulting in a heterogeneous group of cases being studied. Treatment is the same as that for endometrioid carcinoma. The role of adjuvant radiation or chemotherapy is not established at present. In view of the poor prognosis and because these tumors often have high nuclear grade and invade the myometrium deeply, adjuvant therapy often is administered.

Mixed Types of Carcinoma

An endometrial carcinoma may show combinations of two or more of the pure types. By convention, a *mixed carcinoma* has at least one other component comprising at least 10% of the tumor. For example, an endometrioid carcinoma containing a clear cell carcinoma that constitutes 10% of the tumor is classified as an endometrioid carcinoma with areas of clear cell carcinoma. Except for a few studies evaluating the significance of foci of serous carcinoma admixed with endometrioid carcinoma, there are no data that can be used as a basis for making valid recommendations concerning what proportion of an additional component justifies being separately classified. Mixed serous and endometrioid carcinomas containing as little as 25% of a serous component behave as pure serous carcinomas.[298] Except for serous and possibly clear cell components, it is likely that the combination of other tumor types has little, if any, clinical significance.

Malignant Mesodermal Mixed Tumor (MMMT)/Carcinosarcoma

These tumors represent less than 5% of malignant neoplasms of the uterine corpus.[304] By definition, they are composed of malignant epithelial and mesenchymal components as recognized by light microscopy. Because of the biphasic appearance of *MMMTs*, there has been considerable controversy about their histopathogenesis. Recent clinicopathologic, immunohistochemical, and molecular genetic studies have provided compelling evidence that MMMTs should be classified as variants of carcinoma. One study demonstrated that both patients with MMMTs and those with endometrial carcinomas have similar risk factor profiles, consistent with the concept that the pathogenesis of the two tumor types is similar.[364] These factors include body weight, exogenous estrogen use, and nulliparity, all of which are associated with increased risk of developing either tumor type, as well as oral contraceptive use and current smoking, which are associated with decreased risk. It has also been observed that MMMTs respond better to cisplatin-based chemotherapy, which is used for the treatment of carcinomas and thus targets the carcinomatous component, than to regimens directed at the sarcomatous component.[338]

These observations support the view that MMMTs are high-grade variants of carcinoma. It has also been shown that the microvessel density in the carcinomatous component of MMMTs is significantly higher than in the sarcomatous component, suggesting that the former is responsible for the aggressive biologic behavior of these neoplasms.[354] Several immunohistochemical studies have demonstrated that the mesenchymal components of MMMTs express cytokeratins and epithelial membrane antigen in the majority of cases, supporting the view that these portions of the tumor arise from the carcinomatous areas via divergent differentiation.[19,28,60,71,111,114,223,271]

There have been a small number of molecular studies suggesting that the majority of MMMTs show common molecular alterations in both components, supporting a monoclonal origin. One study demonstrated identical p53 mutations in the epithelial and mesenchymal components of 9 MMMTs, consistent with the concept that MMMTs are monoclonal neoplasms in which both components arise from a common precursor cell and subsequently manifest different phenotypes.[188] Another study demonstrated monoclonality of the epithelial and mesenchymal components of 3 tumors using three different methods for determining clonality.[325] Yet another study demonstrated identical patterns of chromosome X inactivation in the epithelial and mesenchymal components of 21 of 25 MMMTs, and those cases with K-*ras* or *p53* mutations also shared identical mutations in the two components, consistent with a monoclonal origin.[340] Only 3 tumors were thought to represent "collision" tumors as a result of the finding of discordant patterns of X inactivation in the epithelial and mesenchymal components of these tumors.

A recent study that analyzed allelic status of 17 MMMTs demonstrated shared allelic losses and retentions among multiple individual carcinomatous and sarcomatous foci within each tumor in 16 cases, supporting the concept of a monoclonal origin for these neoplasms.[98] Studies using cell lines also support the theory of a single cell origin of

MMMTs.[84,121,122] In sum, most molecular studies support a monoclonal origin of MMMTs with subsequent divergent differentiation. In conjunction with the observations that the behavior of these tumors is dictated by the carcinomatous component and immunohistochemical stains commonly demonstrate keratin expression in the mesenchymal components, it has been proposed that MMMTs be classified as aggressive variants of carcinoma rather than as sarcomas.

Clinical Features

Most women with MMMTs are postmenopausal and the most common symptom is postmenopausal bleeding.[53,166,212,247,248,261,297,347] An enlarged irregular uterus with tumor protruding through the cervical os is commonly encountered.[248,257] Some tumors are associated with a history of prior pelvic irradiation.[53,102,225,246,257,261,297,339,347] Women with postirradiation MMMTs are younger than those without a history of irradiation and tend to present with advanced-stage disease.

Gross Findings

MMMTs are frequently polypoid and usually fill the entire endometrial cavity (Fig. 12.46).[24,297,292] Many invade the myometrium but some are confined to polyps.[304] Because they are often polypoid, the tumors often protrude through the cervical os, simulating a cervical neoplasm. The protruding tip of the mass is often necrotic, making diagnosis based on biopsy of this portion of the tumor difficult. In approximately a quarter of the cases the uterine tumor extends into the endocervix.[304] The tumors are variably soft to firm and tan with areas of necrosis and hemorrhage.[24,247]

Microscopic Findings

MMMTs are composed of an intimate admixture of histologically malignant epithelial and mesenchymal components.[24,53,248] The most common type of epithelial component is endometrioid carcinoma, which is often accompanied by squamous differentiation. Serous, clear cell, mucinous, squamous, and undifferentiated carcinoma also can be found as the epithelial component.[28,74,192,238,247,248,257,304] Approximately half the cases demonstrate a homologous type of stromal component, which is high-grade endometrial stromal sarcoma or fibrosarcoma in most and only occasionally leiomyosarcoma (Figs. 12.47 and 12.48).[304] When heterologous elements are present, rhabdomyosarcoma and chondrosarcoma are the most common types encountered (Figs. 12.49 and 12.50).[24,74,212,238,304] Rhabdomyosarcoma can be identified by finding round or elongated cells with granular or fibrillar eosinophilic cytoplasm. On occasion, striated rhabdomyoblasts can be found.

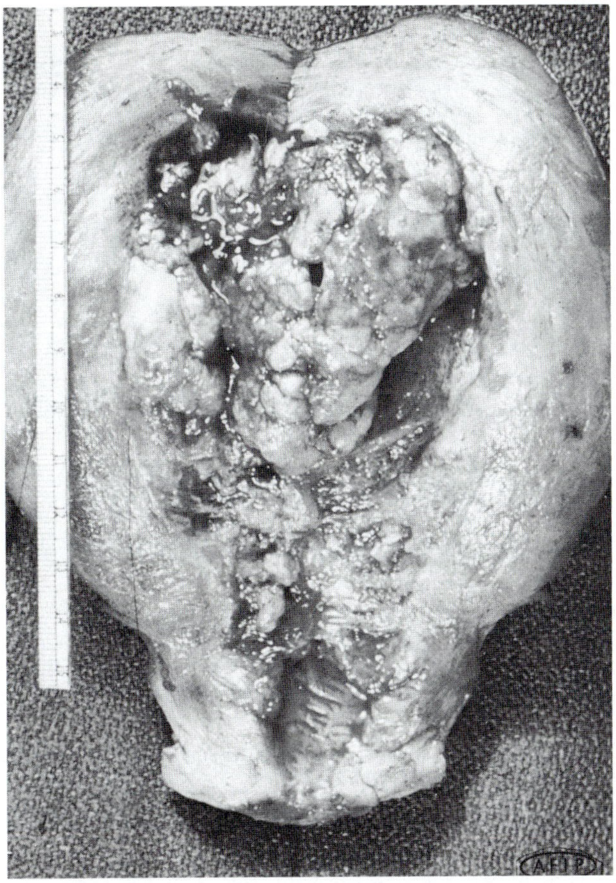

Fig. 12.46. Carcinosarcoma (malignant mixed mesodermal tumor). The tumor fills the endometrial cavity and invades the myometrium and cervix. (Reprinted by permission from The American College of Obstetricians and Gynecologists. Obstet Gynecol 1966;28:57.)

MMMTs metastasize to pelvic and paraaortic lymph nodes, pelvic soft tissues, the vagina, peritoneal surfaces of the upper abdomen, and the lungs.[53,95,247] The histologic appearance of metastases is variable. Three studies on metastases of MMMTs have demonstrated that invasive foci in lymphatic or vascular spaces are always pure carcinoma and metastatic lesions are most commonly purely carcinoma; occasionally, mixtures of carcinoma and sarcoma are found and only rarely is pure sarcoma encountered.[28,304,314] Another study, however, found biphasic metastases to be the most common type.[114]

By immunohistochemistry, the carcinomatous components of MMMTs are always strongly and diffusely positive for cytokeratins and epithelial membrane antigen (EMA) and variably immunoreactive for vimentin in the minority of cases.[19,28,111,114,223,271]

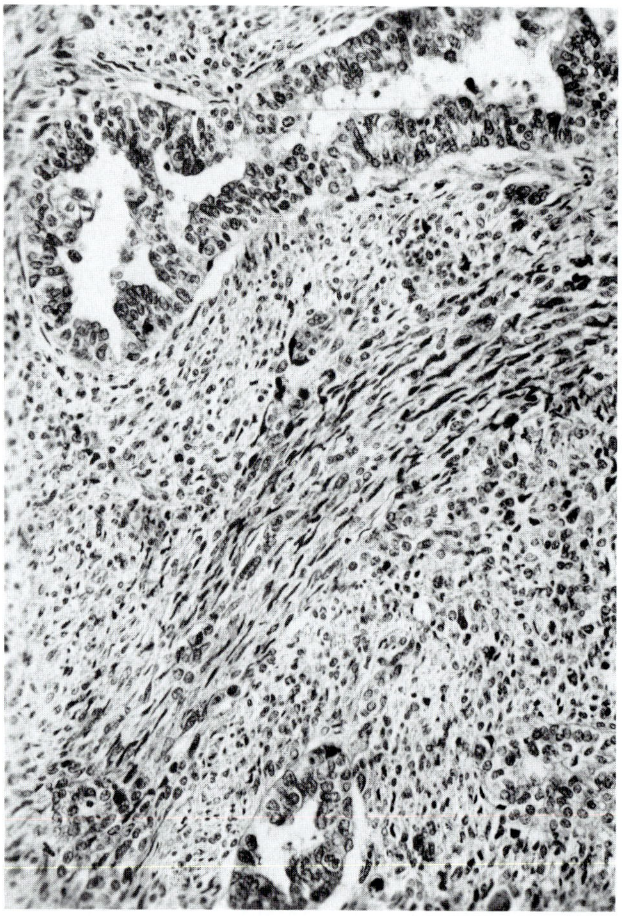

Fig. 12.47. Carcinosarcoma (malignant mixed mesodermal tumor). Carcinomatous glands are admixed with a homologous sarcomatous stroma.

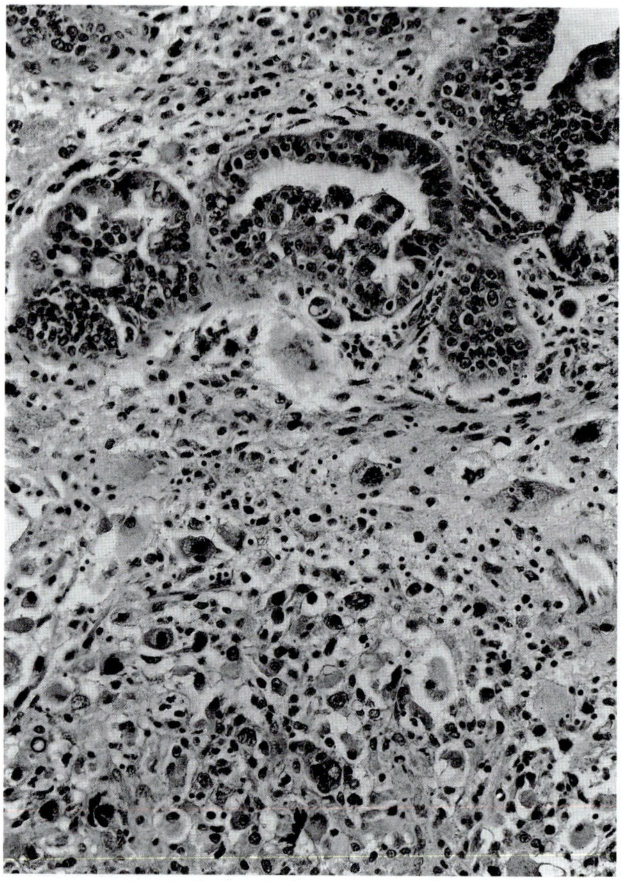

Fig. 12.48. Carcinosarcoma (malignant mixed mesodermal tumor). Tumor is composed of carcinomatous glands (*upper half*) and a poorly differentiated stromal component consistent with sarcomatous differentiation.

The mesenchymal components are diffusely positive for vimentin and occasionally express muscle-specific actin and alpha-smooth muscle actin. In addition, there is often patchy staining for cytokeratins and EMA. When the mesenchymal component displays the histologic features of rhabdomyosarcoma, immunoreactivity of this component for desmin confirms the presence of this heterologous element.[19,114] Usually, areas of rhabdomyosarcoma and chondrosarcoma can be recognized easily by light microscopy.

Behavior and Treatment

When compared to pure endometrial carcinomas, the behavior of MMMTs is significantly worse than FIGO grade 3 endometrial carcinomas, serous carcinomas, and clear cell carcinomas. In addition, the presence of this tumor type is an independent predictor of survival after other factors such as pathologic stage, depth of myometrial invasion, and vascular invasion have been taken into account.[115] Surgical stage is the most important prognostic factor, and extrauterine extension and deep myometrial invasion are independent predictors of survival in multivariate analysis.[18,24,80,102,166,212,218,238,244,289,292,297,349,350] The 5-year survival for patients with early-stage disease (stages I and II) is 40–60%.[61,192,257,292,311] Patients with tumor confined to the uterine corpus have a somewhat better prognosis, with 5-year survival rates of 60–75%.[337] In contrast, the 5-year survival for patients with advanced-stage disease is only 15–30%.[324,327,340]

Even though small MMMTs confined to the tip of a polyp can have a favorable prognosis, such tumors can metastasize and be fatal.[74,304] In one large study of clinical stage I and II tumors, there was a significant difference in extent of myometrial invasion between cases with and without metastatic disease.[304] Nonetheless, some cases without evident myometrial invasion had extrauterine metastases at surgery. In addition, lymphatic or vascular space invasion was a significant predictor of metastatic disease at initial

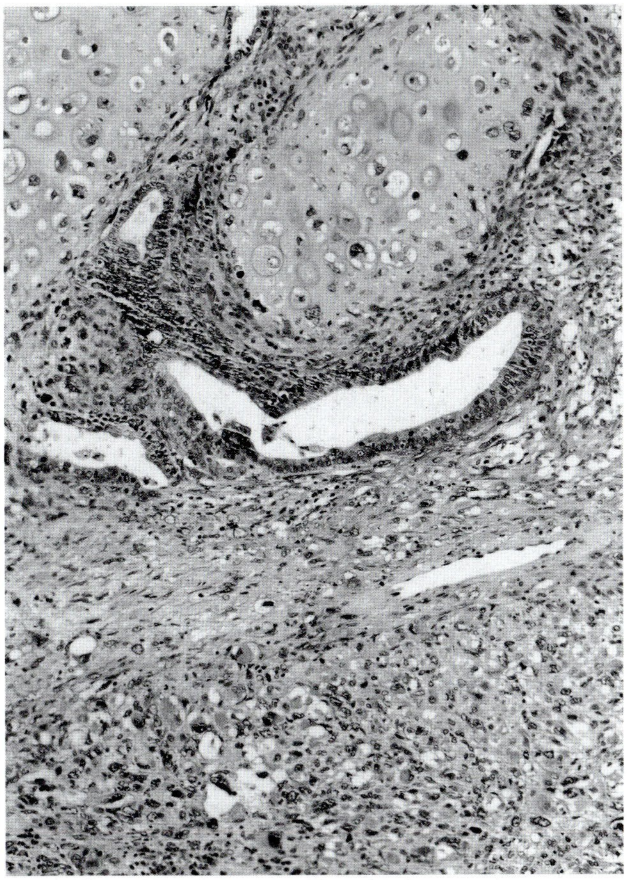

Fig. 12.49. Carcinosarcoma (malignant mixed mesodermal tumor). A few carcinomatous glands are admixed with heterologous sarcomatous elements that include chondrosarcoma (*upper portion of field*) and rhabdomyosarcoma (*lower portion of field*).

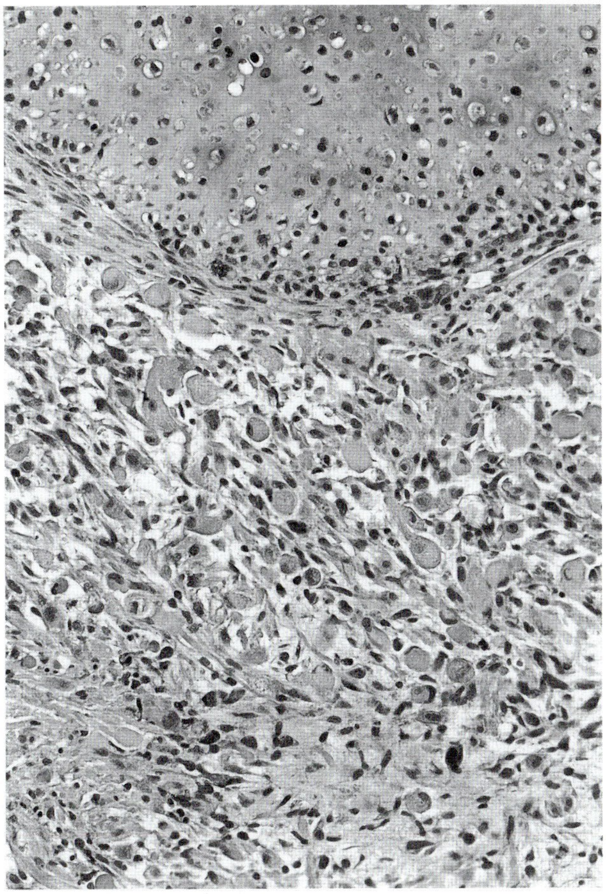

Fig. 12.50. Carcinosarcoma (malignant mixed mesodermal tumor). Higher magnification of Fig. 12.49 illustrates chondrosarcoma (*upper portion of field*) and rhabdomyosarcoma (*lower portion of field*); the latter is characterized by round and elongated cells with abundant granular eosinophilic cytoplasm.

surgery. Cases in which the carcinomatous component was serous or clear cell carcinoma had a significantly greater tendency to be associated with metastatic disease, whereas the presence of heterologous elements was not associated with an increased frequency of metastatic disease. The histologic appearance of the sarcomatous component (homologous versus heterologous, type of heterologous element, grade of sarcoma) of MMMTs does not appear to have any prognostic significance.[102,192,212,304,311,347]

MMMTs are treated by total abdominal hysterectomy and bilateral salpingo-oophorectomy with staging. In one study, adjuvant radiotherapy reduced local recurrence rates but only improved distant failure rates and survival in stage I and II disease.[116] However, another study of whole pelvic irradiation demonstrated only a trend in improved pelvic control without improved distant recurrence or survival rates for patients with stage I and II disease.[47] A Gynecologic Oncology Group study of ifosfamide with or without cisplatin for the treatment of advanced, persistent, or recurrent MMMT demonstrated that the addition of cisplatin provided a small improvement in progression-free survival but no significant survival benefit.[318]

Undifferentiated Carcinoma

Tumors that fail to show evidence of either glandular or squamous differentiation are regarded as *undifferentiated carcinomas*. The prevalence is 1—2%. The mean age of patients with undifferentiated carcinoma is 64 years. The clinical features of women with undifferentiated carcinoma, insofar as age, parity, hypertension, and diabetes are concerned, are similar to those of endometrioid carcinoma.

In a study of 31 undifferentiated carcinomas, these tumors were divided into large cell and small cell/intermediate types (Fig. 12.51).[3] Some small cell

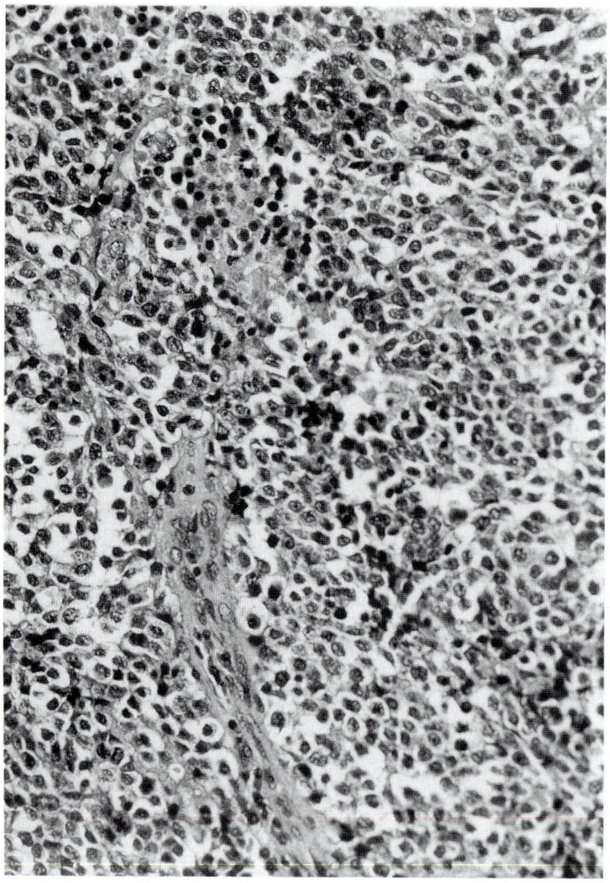

Fig. 12.51. Small cell carcinoma. The tumor is composed of undifferentiated small cells resembling neuroendocrine-type small cell carcinoma in other organs.

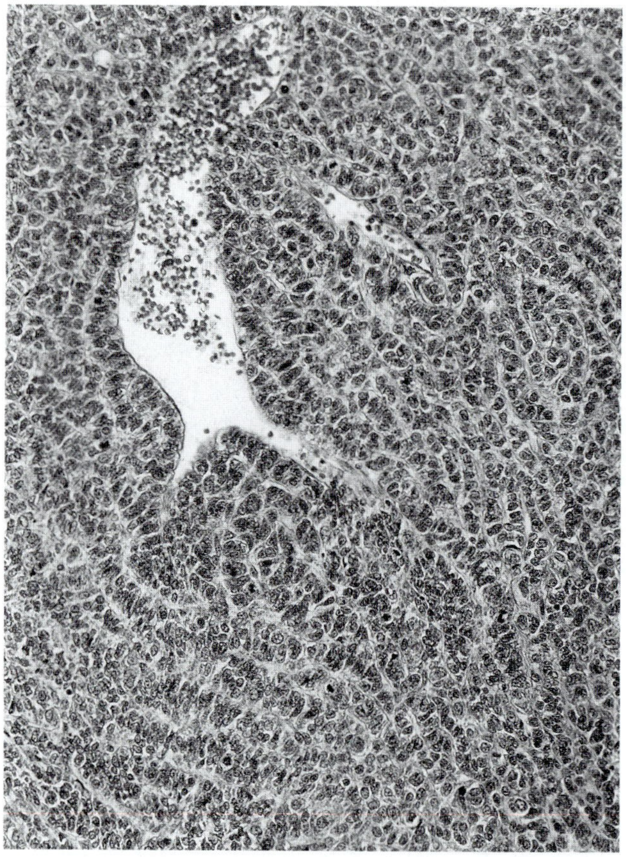

Fig. 12.52. Small cell carcinoma. Same case as illustrated in Fig. 12.51. The tumor has a trabecular pattern simulating carcinoid.

carcinomas display a trabecular pattern simulating a carcinoid tumor (Fig. 12.52). Not infrequently these tumors are found admixed with adenocarcinoma, adenocarcinoma with squamous differentiation, or malignant mesodermal mixed tumor (Fig. 12.53).[148,336] Both large and small cell undifferentiated carcinomas have been reported to be positive for cytokeratin.[344] The small cell carcinomas are positive for neuroendocrine markers such as neuron-specific enolase, synaptophysin, chromogranin, or leu-7.[148,336] In our experience, small cell carcinomas have been cytokeratin negative and neuron-specific enolase positive. The survival difference of the large cell compared with the small or intermediate cell carcinomas was not statistically significant (54% versus 64%, respectively, at 5 years).[3] As a group, the survival rates for patients with undifferentiated carcinoma at 5 and 10 years were 58% and 48%, respectively, which was similar to grade 3 endometrioid carcinoma. Recent studies have confirmed the aggressive behavior of small cell carcinoma of the endometrium.[148,336]

Miscellaneous Epithelial Tumors

A number of rare examples of unusual neoplasms arising in the endometrium have been reported, but the data consist largely of case reports precluding a detailed clinicopathologic analysis. Some of these are discussed next.

Squamous Cell Carcinoma

Squamous carcinoma develops in the endometrium, but it is extremely rare. In a population-based study from Norway the prevalence was 0.1%.[6] To qualify as primary squamous carcinoma of the endometrium, three criteria must be met: (1) adenocarcinoma is not present in the endometrium, (2) the squamous carcinoma in the endometrium does not have any connection with the squamous epithelium of the cervix, and (3) squamous carcinoma is not present in the cervix. By these criteria, only 56 cases of primary squamous carcinoma of the endometrium have been reported.[120] The mean age of patients is 67 years. There is a strong association with cervical

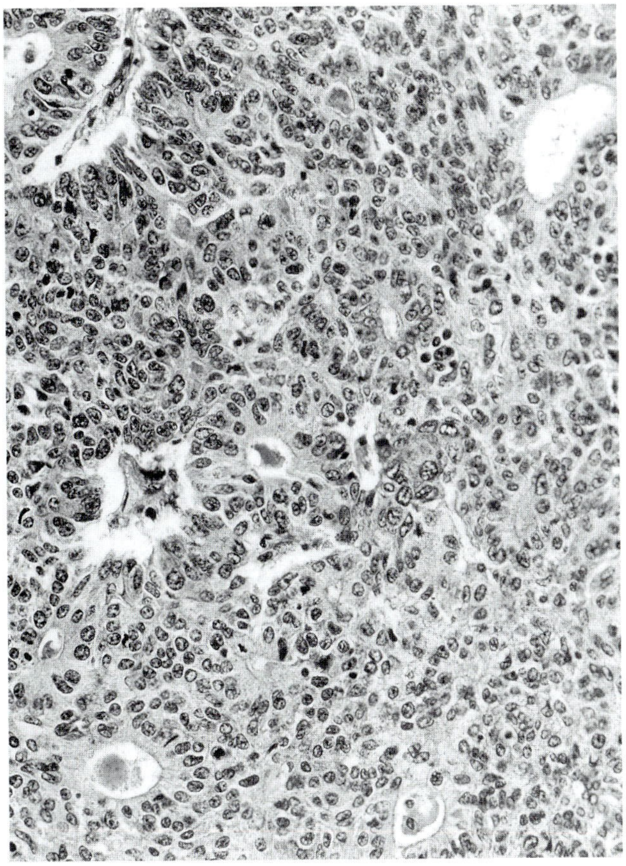

Fig. 12.53. **Small cell carcinoma.** Same case as illustrated in Fig. 12.51. The small cell carcinoma forms glandular structures resembling a poorly differentiated endometrioid carcinoma.

stenosis, pyometra, chronic inflammation, and nulliparity. The tumor may arise from ichthyosis uteri, a condition in which the endometrium is replaced by keratinized squamous epithelium. In the past, this condition was considered a sequela of the use of steam as treatment for endometritis. With the abandonment of this procedure, ichthyosis uteri has become quite rare.

Microscopically, squamous carcinomas of the endometrium resemble those in the cervix; however, at times they can be extremely well differentiated and therefore difficult to diagnose with certainty in curettings. Sometimes the diagnosis is not established until a hysterectomy is performed (Fig. 12.54).

In addition to typical squamous cell carcinoma, verrucous carcinoma may arise as a primary tumor in the endometrium (Fig. 12.55).[281] The prognosis of squamous cell carcinoma is related to stage at diagnosis. In a review of the reported cases, 80% of stage I patients survived whereas survival for patients with stage III disease was only 20%.[120]

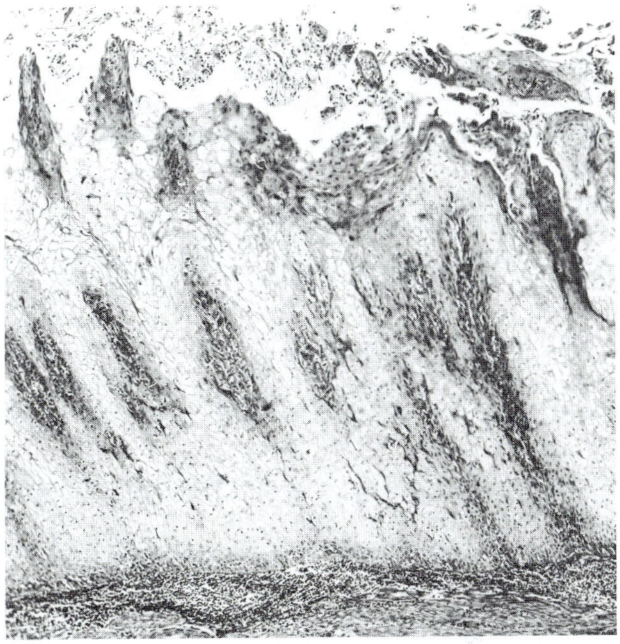

Fig. 12.54. **Squamous cell carcinoma.** There is complete replacement of the surface endometrium. Elsewhere, the tumor deeply invaded the myometrium.

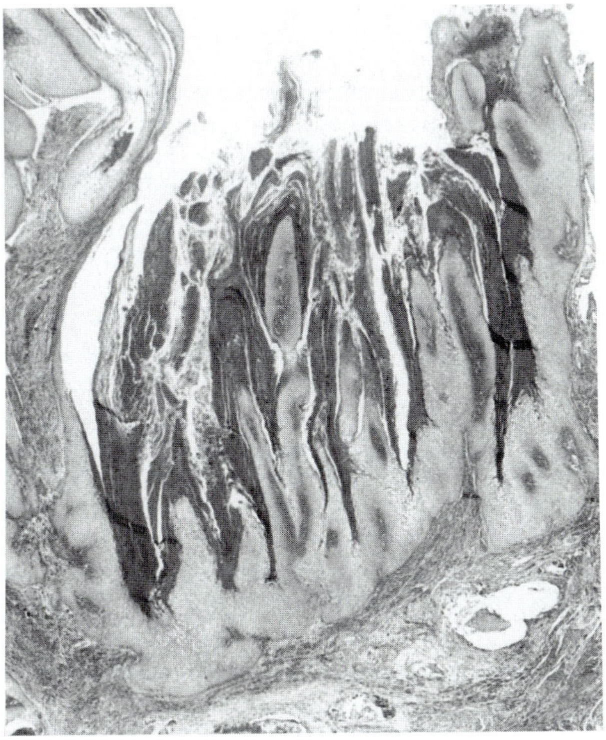

Fig. 12.55. **Verrucous carcinoma.** This tumor arose in endometrial glands and invaded the myometrium superficially. There was no tumor in the cervix, vagina, or vulva.

Glassy Cell Carcinoma

Glassy cell carcinoma is regarded as a variant of a mixed adenosquamous carcinoma and rarely occurs in the endometrium.[17,51] First described in the cervix, glassy cell carcinoma is a poorly differentiated neoplasm with little or no glandular or squamous differentiation and is composed of masses and nests of characteristic polygonal cells separated by a fibrous stroma that often contains an abundance of inflammatory cells. The cells have well-defined borders and granular eosinophilic or amphophilic cytoplasm, giving a ground glass appearance. The nuclei are enlarged and round, with centrally placed, prominent, eosinophilic nucleoli. Mitotic activity, including the presence of abnormal mitotic figures, is high. The behavior, based on a small series of cases, is highly aggressive.

Yolk Sac Tumor

Four cases of primary *yolk sac tumor* of the endometrium have been reported.[163] Three of the patients have been in their twenties, and one was 42 years of age. Light microscopic, immunohistochemical, and ultrastructural studies have shown features similar to yolk sac tumor of the ovary. AFP is elevated in the serum preoperatively and is localized within the cytoplasm of tumor cells. It is thought that these tumors arise in the uterus as a result of aberrant migration of primordial germ cells. All four patients were treated with hysterectomy followed by adjuvant multiagent chemotherapy. Two patients are long-term survivors, and two died of disease.

Giant Cell Carcinoma

Rare primary endometrial carcinomas may contain multinucleated giant cells resembling *giant cell carcinomas* in other sites such as the lung, thyroid, pancreas, and gallbladder. In a report of six cases, the giant cells accounted for a substantial part of the tumor.[160] The remainder of the neoplasm contained undifferentiated carcinoma and areas of more differentiated endometrioid carcinoma. Immunohistochemical studies demonstrated positive immunoreactivity for cytokeratin and epithelial membrane antigen in the giant cell component. Vimentin, desmin, and smooth muscle actin were negative. Four of the six patients in whom the tumor invaded more than superficially developed recurrent tumor, and three patients died of disease within 3 years. Tumors with cells resembling osteoclast-like giant cells also have been observed in the endometrium (Fig. 12.56).

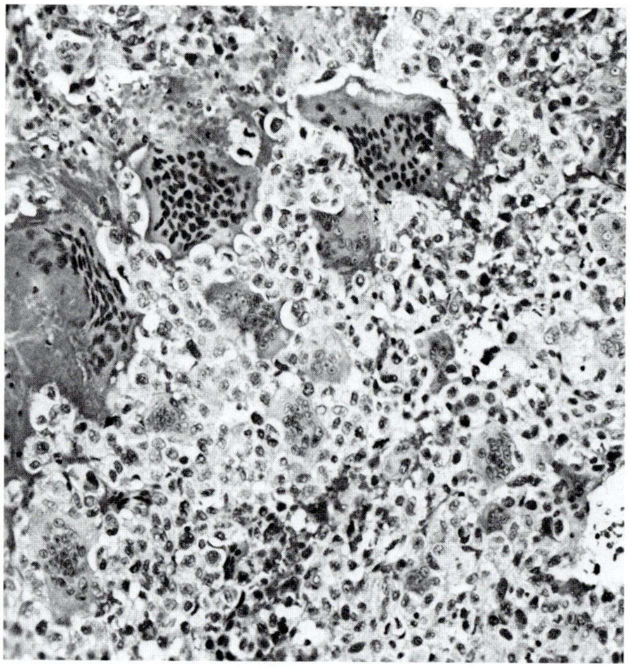

Fig. 12.56. Undifferentiated carcinoma with giant cells. The multinucleated giant cells resemble osteoclastic giant cells.

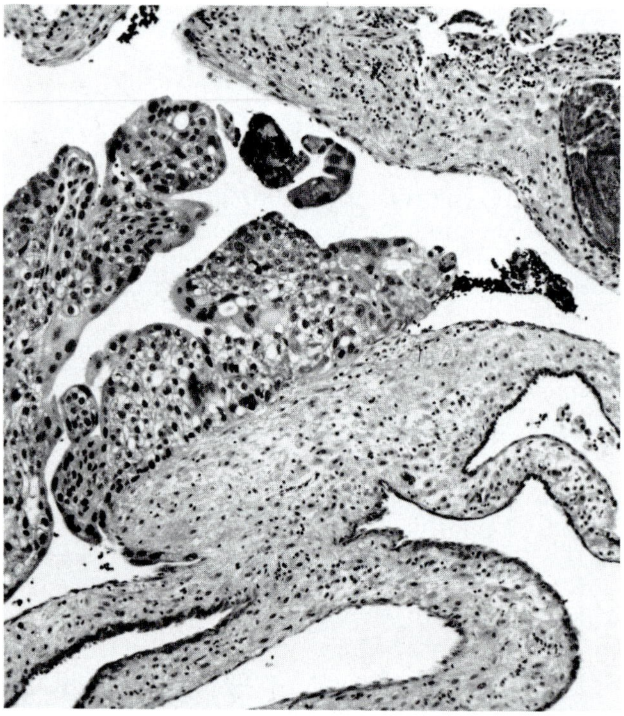

Fig. 12.57. Primary choriocarcinoma. This neoplasm developed in a 64-year-old woman. The tumor appeared to arise from an endometrioid carcinoma with squamous differentiation, FIGO grade 3. The endometrial stroma has undergone a decidual reaction.

Choriocarcinoma

Rarely, primary *choriocarcinoma* of the endometrium may develop in a postmenopausal woman (Figs. 12.57 and 12.58), representing a form of differentiation of a carcinoma derived from somatic cells rather than germ cells or trophoblasts. Six patients ranging in age from 48 to 78 years have been reported.[170,260,290,331] Most patients had elevated serum human chorionic gonadotropin (hCG) levels and/or hCG detected in the syncytiotrophoblastic element in the tumor. A case of choriocarcinoma associated with a carcinosarcoma (malignant mesodermal mixed tumor) has been reported, and we have observed one such case as well.[178] These tumors appear to behave in an aggressive fashion.

Transitional Cell Carcinoma

Ten cases of *transitional cell carcinoma* of the endometrium have been reported.[209,313] Patients have ranged in age from 41 to 83 years, with a mean of 62. The tumors are typically polypoid and present with uterine bleeding. The tumors often are papillary and resemble transitional cell carcinomas of other organs. The tumors are invariably admixed with other patterns of endometrial carcinoma, including endometrioid, squamous, and serous components. The overall prognosis does not appear to be worse than expected for the stage of disease, but the transitional cell component seems to be the more aggressive subtype among the patterns with which it is admixed.[209]

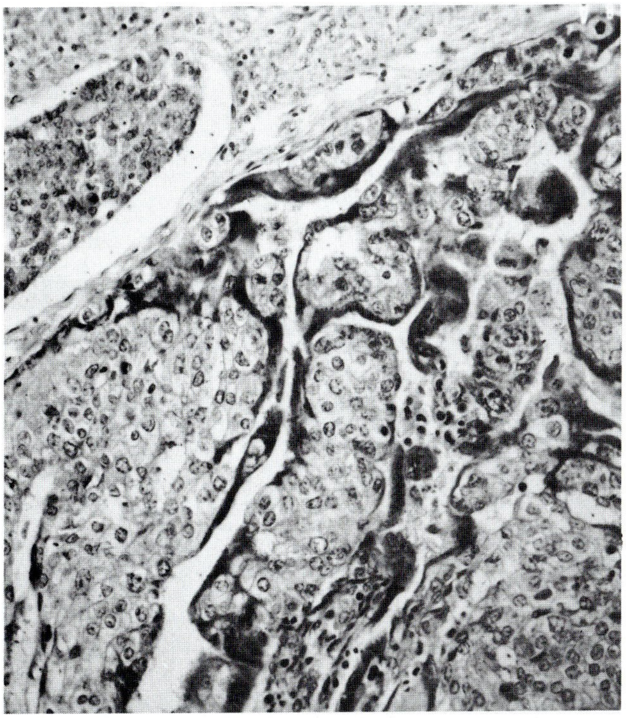

Fig. 12.58. Choriocarcinoma. Same case as illustrated in Fig. 12.57. Localization of human chorionic gonadotropin (hCG) (*dark black reaction product*) is seen in syncytiotrophoblast.

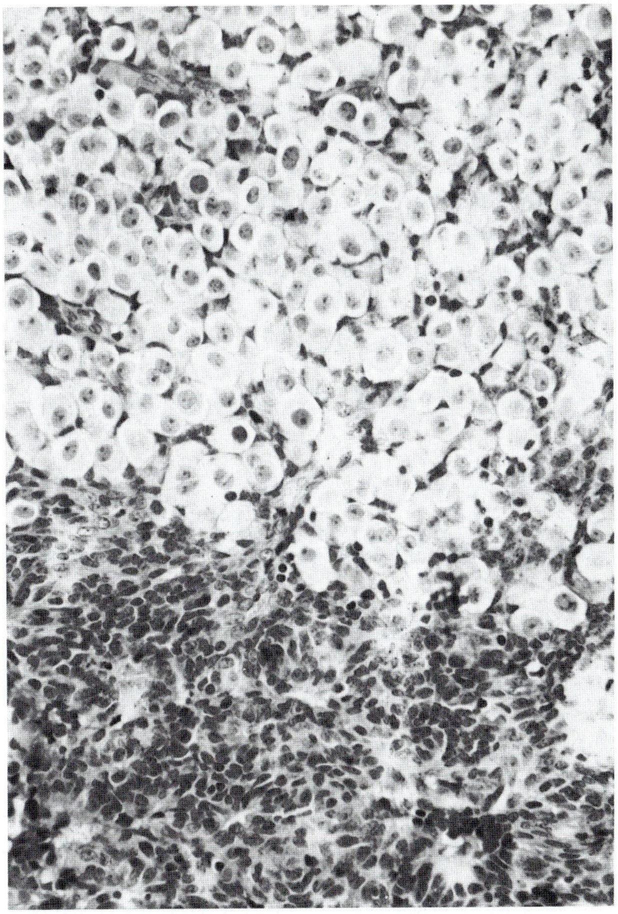

Fig. 12.59. Metastatic breast carcinoma. The tumor cells are uniform in size and diffusely infiltrate the endometrium. Metastatic carcinoma should not be mistaken for primary, undifferentiated carcinoma of the endometrium.

Other Rare Variants

Other rare types of carcinomas of the endometrium that have been reported include an oxyphilic variant of endometrioid carcinoma, a primary signet-ring cell carcinoma, and an alpha-fetoprotein-secreting hepatoid adenocarcinoma associated with endometrioid carcinoma.[147,230,267] In addition, an endometrioid carcinoma associated with Ewing sarcoma/peripheral primitive neuroectodermal tumor has been reported.[305]

Tumors Metastatic to the Endometrium

Ovarian Carcinoma

Simultaneous cancers involving the endometrium and the ovary may represent (1) metastasis from the endometrium to the ovary, (2) metastasis from the ovary to the endometrium, or (3) independent primary tumors (see Chapter 22, Metastatic Tumors of the Ovary). The distinction is important because the prognosis and treatment differ. It has been suggested that when the endometrial carcinoma is small and minimally invasive, the two neoplasms should be considered independent. One study found that if the two carcinomas have an endometrioid pattern, the prognosis is good, and therefore the two neoplasms probably are independent.[82] When serous or clear cell carcinoma is found, the prognosis is poor and a primary tumor with metastasis is likely. The primary neoplasm is identified by its larger size or more advanced stage.

Another study proposed that tumors be classified as primary in the endometrium with metastasis to the ovaries when there is multinodular ovarian involvement or at least two of the following criteria are met: (1) small (<5 cm) ovaries, (2) bilateral ovarian involvement, (3) deep myometrial invasion, (4) vascular invasion, or (5) fallopian tube involvement.[333] When these criteria are used, there is a significant difference in the frequency of distant metastasis in the group classified as metastatic versus the group classified as an independent primary. Metastasis from the endometrium to the ovary occurs more often than the reverse. About a third of the cases are independent tumors involving both sites simultaneously. Independent tumors display either well-differentiated endometrioid or nonendometrioid patterns, whereas grade 3 endometrioid carcinoma and MMMTs generally are primary in one organ and metastatic to the other when detected.

Carcinomas from Extragenital Sites

When an extragenital tumor metastasizes to the uterus, it usually is a manifestation of obvious dissemination. The diagnosis in curettings may, on rare occasion, be the first clue of an occult primary tumor. The mean age of patients is 60 years. Metastatic breast cancer is the most frequent extragenital tumor that metastasizes to the uterus (47%), followed by stomach (29%), cutaneous melanoma (5%), lung (4%), colon (3%), pancreas (3%), and kidney (3%).[190] Metastatic neoplasms to the endometrium frequently infiltrate the endometrium diffusely, sparing the glands (Fig. 12.59). Most neoplasms metastatic to the endometrium are poorly differentiated and lack squamous differentiation, unlike primary endometrial carcinoma. The myometrium can contain metastatic nodules as well.

References

1. Abeler VM, Kjorstad KE (1990) Serous papillary carcinoma of the endometrium: a histopathological study of 22 cases. Gynecol Oncol 39:266–271
2. Abeler VM, Kjorstad KE (1991) Endometrial adenocarcinoma in Norway. A study of a total population. Cancer (Phila) 67:3093–3103
3. Abeler VM, Kjorstad KE, Nesland JM (1991) Undifferentiated carcinoma of the endometrium. A histopathologic and clinical study of 31 cases. Cancer (Phila) 68:98–105
4. Abeler VM, Kjorstad KE (1991) Clear cell carcinoma of the endometrium: a histopathological and clinical study of 97 cases. Gynecol Oncol 40:207–217
5. Abeler VM, Kjorstad KE (1992) Endometrial adenocarcinoma with squamous cell differentiation. Cancer (Phila) 69:488–495
6. Abeler VM, Kjordstad K, Berle E (1992) Carcinoma of the endometrium in Norway: a histopathological and prognostic survey of a total population. Int J Gynecol Cancer 2:9–22
7. Abeler VM, Vergote IB, Kjorstad KE, Trope CG (1996) Clear cell carcinoma of the endometrium. Prognosis and metastatic pattern. Cancer (Phila) 78:1740–1747
8. Alberhasky RC, Connelly PJ, Christopherson WM (1982) Carcinoma of the endometrium. IV. Mixed adenosquamous carcinoma. A clinical-pathological study of 68 cases with long-term follow-up. Am J Clin Pathol 77:655–664
9. Ambros RA, Kurman RJ (1992) Identification of patients with stage I uterine endometrioid adenocarcinoma at high risk of recurrence by DNA ploidy, myometrial invasion, and vascular invasion. Gynecol Oncol 45:235–239
10. Ambros RA, Kurman RJ (1992) Combined assessment of vascular and myometrial invasion as a model to predict prognosis in stage I endometrioid adenocarcinoma of the uterine corpus. Cancer (Phila) 69:1424–1431
11. Ambros RA, Sherman ME, Zahn CM, Bitterman P, Kurman RJ (1995) Endometrial intraepithelial carcinoma: a distinctive lesion specifically associated with tumors displaying serous differentiation. Hum Pathol 26:1260–1267
12. Ambros RA, Sheehan CE, Kallakury BV, Ross JS, Malfetano J, Paunovich E, et al (1996) MDM2 and p53 protein expression in the histologic subtypes of endometrial carcinoma. Mod Pathol 9:1165–1169
13. American Cancer Society (2000) 2000 cancer statistics. CA Cancer J Clin 50:(1)1–64

14. Andersson M, Storm HH, Mouridsen HT (1991) Incidence of new primary cancers after adjuvant tamoxifen therapy and radiotherapy for early breast cancer. J Natl Cancer Inst 83:1013–1017
15. Anonymous (1987) Combination oral contraceptive use and the risk of endometrial cancer. The Cancer and Steroid Hormone Study of the Centers for Disease Control and the National Institute of Child Health and Human Development. JAMA 257:796–800
16. Aquino-Parsons C, Lim P, Wong F, Mildenberger M (1998) Papillary serous and clear cell carcinoma limited to endometrial curettings in FIGO stage 1a and 1b endometrial adenocarcinoma: treatment implications. Gynecol Oncol 71:83–86
17. Arends JW, Willebrand D, DeKoning GH, Swaen GJ, Bosman FT (1984) Adenocarcinoma of the endometrium with glassy-cell features—immunohistochemical observations. Histopathology (Oxf) 8: 873–879
18. Arrastia CD, Fruchter RG, Clark M, Maiman M, Remy JC, Macasaet M, et al (1997) Uterine carcinosarcomas: incidence and trends in management and survival. Gynecol Oncol 65:158–163
19. Auerbach HE, LiVolsi VA, Merino MJ (1988) Malignant mixed Mullerian tumors of the uterus. An immunohistochemical study. Int J Gynecol Pathol 7:123–130
20. Austin H, Drews C, Partridge EE (1993) A case-control study of endometrial cancer in relation to cigarette smoking, serum estrogen levels, and alcohol use. Am J Obstet Gynecol 169:1086–1091
21. Backe J, Gassel AM, Hauber K, Krebs S, Bartek J, Caffier H, et al (1997) p53 protein in endometrial cancer is related to proliferative activity and prognosis but not to expression of p21 protein. Int J Gynecol Pathol 16:361–368
22. Backe J, Gassel AM, Krebs S, Muller T, Caffier H (1997) Immunohistochemically detected HER-2/neu-expression and prognosis in endometrial carcinoma. Arch Gynecol Obstet 259:189–195
23. Barakat RR, Wong G, Curtin JP, Vlamis V, Hoskins WJ (1994) Tamoxifen use in breast cancer patients who subsequently develop corpus cancer is not associated with a higher incidence of adverse histologic features. Gynecol Oncol 55:164–168
24. Barwick KW, LiVolsi VA (1979) Malignant mixed mullerian tumors of the uterus. A clinicopathologic assessment of 34 cases. Am J Surg Pathol 3:125–135
25. Beckner ME, Mori T, Silverberg SG (1985) Endometrial carcinoma: nontumor factors in prognosis. Int J Gynecol Pathol 4:131–145
26. Beral V, Banks E, Reeves G, Appleby P (1999) Use of HRT and the subsequent risk of cancer. J Epidemiol Biostat 4:191–210
27. Berchuck A, Rodriguez G, Kinney RB, Soper JT, Dodge RK, Clarke-Pearson DL, et al (1991) Overexpression of HER-2/neu in endometrial cancer is associated with advanced stage disease. Am J Obstet Gynecol 164:15–21
28. Bitterman P, Chun B, Kurman RJ (1990) The significance of epithelial differentiation in mixed mesodermal tumors of the uterus. A clinicopathologic and immunohistochemical study. Am J Surg Pathol 14:317–328
29. Boccardo F, Rubagotti A, Amoroso D, Sismondi P, Genta F, Nenci I, et al (1992) Chemotherapy versus tamoxifen versus chemotherapy plus tamoxifen in node-positive, oestrogen-receptor positive breast cancer patients. An update at 7 years of the 1st GROCTA (Breast Cancer Adjuvant Chemo-Hormone Therapy Cooperative Group) trial. Eur J Cancer 28:673–680
30. Bokhman JV (1983) Two pathogenetic types of endometrial carcinoma. Gynecol Oncol 15:10–17
31. Bonatz G, Luttges J, Hedderich J, Inform D, Jonat W, Rudolph P, et al (1999) Prognostic significance of a novel proliferation marker, anti-repp 86, for endometrial carcinoma: a multivariate study. Hum Pathol 30:949–956
32. Boronow RC, Morrow CP, Creasman WT, Disaia PJ, Silverberg SG, Miller A, et al (1984) Surgical staging in endometrial cancer: clinical-pathologic findings of a prospective study. Obstet Gynecol 63:825–832
33. Borst MP, Baker VV, Dixon D, Hatch KD, Shingleton HM, Miller DM (1990) Oncogene alterations in endometrial carcinoma. Gynecol Oncol 38:364–366
34. Boyd J, Risinger JI (1991) Analysis of oncogene alterations in human endometrial carcinoma: prevalence of ras mutations. Mol Carcinog 4:189–195
35. Brinton LA, Berman ML, Mortel R, Twiggs LB, Barrett RJ, Wilbanks GD, et al (1992) Reproductive, menstrual, and medical risk factors for endometrial cancer: results from a case-control study. Am J Obstet Gynecol 167:1317–1325
36. Britton LC, Wilson TO, Gaffey TA, Lieber MM, Wieand HS, Podratz KC (1989) Flow cytometric DNA analysis of stage I endometrial carcinoma. Gynecol Oncol 34:317–322
37. Brustmann H, Riss P, Naude S (1995) Nucleolar organizer regions as markers of endometrial proliferation: a study of normal, hyperplastic, and neoplastic tissue. Hum Pathol 26:664–667
38. Burks RT, Kessis TD, Cho KR, Hedrick L (1994) Microsatellite instability in endometrial carcinoma. Oncogene 9:1163–1166
39. Caduff RF, Johnston CM, Frank TS (1995) Mutations of the Ki-ras oncogene in carcinoma of the endometrium. Am J Pathol 146:182–188
40. Carcangiu ML, Chambers JT (1992) Uterine papillary serous carcinoma: a study on 108 cases with emphasis on the prognostic significance of associated endometrioid carcinoma, absence of invasion, and concomitant ovarian carcinoma. Gynecol Oncol 47:298–305
41. Carcangiu ML, Chambers JT, Voynick IM, Pirro M, Schwartz PE (1990) Immunohistochemical evaluation of estrogen and progesterone receptor content in 183 patients with endometrial carcinoma.

Part I: Clinical and histologic correlations. Am J Clin Pathol 94:247–254
42. Carcangiu ML, Tan LK, Chambers JT (1997) Stage IA uterine serous carcinoma. A study of 13 cases. Am J Surg Pathol 21:1507–1514
43. Chambers JT, Carcangiu ML, Voynick IM, Schwartz PE (1990) Immunohistochemical evaluation of estrogen and progesterone receptor content in 183 patients with endometrial carcinoma. Part II: Correlation between biochemical and immunohistochemical methods and survival. Am J Clin Pathol 94:255–260
44. Chan WK, Mole MM, Levison DA, Ball RY, Lu QL, Patel K, et al (1995) Nuclear and cytoplasmic bcl-2 expression in endometrial hyperplasia and adenocarcinoma. J Pathol 177:241–246
45. Chen KT, Kostich ND, Rosai J (1978) Peritoneal foreign body granulomas to keratin in uterine adenocanthoma. Arch Pathol Lab Med 102:174–177
46. Chen JL, Trost DC, Wilkinson EJ (1985) Endometrial papillary adenocarcinomas: two clinicopathological types. Int J Gynecol Pathol 4:279–288
47. Chi DS, Mychalczak B, Saigo PE, Rescigno J, Brown CL (1997) The role of whole-pelvic irradiation in the treatment of early-stage uterine carcinosarcoma. Gynecol Oncol 65:493–498
48. Chieng DC, Ross JS, Ambros RA (1996) bcl-2 expression and the development of endometrial carcinoma. Mod Pathol 9:402–406
49. Christopherson WM, Alberhasky RC, Connelly PJ (1982) Carcinoma of the endometrium. I. A clinicopathologic study of clear-cell carcinoma and secretory carcinoma. Cancer (Phila) 49:1511–1523
50. Christopherson WM, Alberhasky RC, Connelly PJ (1982) Carcinoma of the endometrium. II. Papillary adenocarcinoma: a clinical pathological study of 46 cases. Am J Clin Pathol 77:534–540
51. Christopherson WM, Alberhasky RC, Connelly PJ (1982) Glassy cell carcinoma of the endometrium. Hum Pathol 13:418–421
52. Christopherson WM, Connelly PJ, Alberhasky RC (1983) Carcinoma of the endometrium. V. An analysis of prognosticators in patients with favorable subtypes and stage I disease. Cancer (Phila) 51:1705–1709
53. Chuang JT, Van Velden DJ, Graham JB (1970) Carcinosarcoma and mixed mesodermal tumor of the uterine corpus. Review of 49 cases. Obstet Gynecol 35:769–780
54. Cirisano FDJ, Robboy SJ, Dodge RK, Bentley RC, Krigman HR, Synan IS, et al (1999) Epidemiologic and surgicopathologic findings of papillary serous and clear cell endometrial cancers when compared to endometrioid carcinoma. Gynecol Oncol 74:385–394
55. Cirisano FDJ, Robboy SJ, Dodge RK, Bentley RC, Krigman HR, Synan IS, et al (2000) The outcome of stage i–ii clinically and surgically staged papillary serous and clear cell endometrial cancers when compared with endometrioid carcinoma. Gynecol Oncol 77:55–65
56. Connell PP, Rotmensch J, Waggoner SE, Mundt AJ (1999) Race and clinical outcome in endometrial carcinoma. Obstet Gynecol 94:713–720
57. Connelly PJ, Alberhasky RC, Christopherson WM (1982) Carcinoma of the endometrium. III. Analysis of 865 cases of adenocarcinoma and adenoacanthoma. Obstet Gynecol 59:569–575
58. Cook LS, Weiss NS, Schwartz SM, White E, McKnight B, Moore DE, et al (1995) Population-based study of tamoxifen therapy and subsequent ovarian, endometrial, and breast cancers. J Natl Cancer Inst 87:1359–1364
59. Coppola D, Fu L, Nicosia SV, Kounelis S, Jones M (1998) Prognostic significance of p53, bcl-2, vimentin, and S100 protein-positive Langerhans cells in endometrial carcinoma. Hum Pathol 29:455–462
60. Costa MJ, Khan R, Judd R (1991) Carcinoma (malignant mixed mullerian [mesodermal] tumor) of the uterus and ovary. Correlation of clinical, pathologic, and immunohistochemical features in 29 cases. Arch Pathol Lab Med 115:583–590
61. Covens AL, Nisker JA, Chapman WB, Allen HH (1987) Uterine sarcoma: an analysis of 74 cases. Am J Obstet Gynecol 156:370–374
62. Creasman WT, Disaia PJ, Blessing J, Wilkinson RHJ, Johnston W, Weed JCJ (1981) Prognostic significance of peritoneal cytology in patients with endometrial cancer and preliminary data concerning therapy with intraperitoneal radiopharmaceuticals. Am J Obstet Gynecol 141:921–929
63. Creasman WT, Henderson D, Hinshaw W, Clarke-Pearson DL (1986) Estrogen replacement therapy in the patient treated for endometrial cancer. Obstet Gynecol 67:326–330
64. Creasman WT, Morrow CP, Bundy BN, Homesley HD, Graham JE, Heller PB (1987) Surgical pathologic spread patterns of endometrial cancer. A Gynecologic Oncology Group Study. Cancer (Phila) 60:2035–2041
65. Creasman WT (1989) Announcement. FIGO stages: 1988 revision. Gynecol Oncol 35:125–127
66. Creasman WT (1997) Endometrial cancer: incidence, prognostic factors, diagnosis, and treatment. Semin Oncol 24:S1–S1
67. Crissman JD, Azoury RS, Barnes AE, Schellhas HF (1981) Endometrial carcinoma in women 40 years of age or younger. Obstet Gynecol 57:699–704
68. Czernobilsky B, Katz Z, Lancet M, Gaton E (1980) Endocervical-type epithelium in endometrial carcinoma: a report of 10 cases with emphasis on histochemical methods for differential diagnosis. Am J Surg Pathol 4:481–489
69. Dabbs DJ, Sturtz K, Zaino RJ (1996) The immunohistochemical discrimination of endometrioid adenocarcinomas. Hum Pathol 27:172–177
70. Daniel AG, Peters WA (1988) Accuracy of office and operating room curettage in the grading of endometrial carcinoma. Obstet Gynecol 71:612–614
71. de Brito PA, Silverberg SG, Orenstein JM (1993)

Carcinosarcoma (malignant mixed mullerian (mesodermal) tumor) of the female genital tract: immunohistochemical and ultrastructural analysis of 28 cases. Hum Pathol 24:132–142

72. Deligdisch L, Holinka CF (1986) Progesterone receptors in two groups of endometrial carcinoma. Cancer (Phila) 57:1385–1388
73. Demopoulos RI, Genega E, Vamvakas E, Carlson E, Mittal K (1996) Papillary carcinoma of the endometrium: morphometric predictors of survival. Int J Gynecol Pathol 15:110–118
74. Dinh TV, Slavin RE, Bhagavan BS, Hannigan EV, Tiamson EM, Yandell RB (1989) Mixed mullerian tumors of the uterus: a clinicopathologic study. Obstet Gynecol 74:388–392
75. Dockerty MB, Lovelady SB, Foust GT (1951) Carcinoma of the corpus uteri in young women. Am J Obstet Gynecol 61:966–981
76. Doering DL, Barnhill DR, Weiser EB, Burke TW, Woodward JE, Park RC (1989) Intraoperative evaluation of depth of myometrial invasion in stage I endometrial adenocarcinoma. Obstet Gynecol 74: 930–933
77. Duggan BD, Felix JC, Muderspach LI, Tourgeman D, Zheng J, Shibata D (1984) Microsatellite instability in sporadic endometrial carcinoma. J Natl Cancer Inst 86:1216–1221
78. Duggan MA, Benoit JL, McGregor SE, Nation JG, Inoue M, Stuart GCE (1993) The human papillomavirus status of 114 endocervical adenocarcinoma cases by dot blot hybridization. Hum Pathol 24:121–125
79. Dunton CJ, Balsara G, McFarland M, Hernandez E (1991) Uterine papillary serous carcinoma: a review. Obstet Gynecol Surv 46:97–102
80. Echt G, Jepson J, Steel J, Langholz B, Luxton G, Hernandez W, et al (1990) Treatment of uterine sarcomas. Cancer (Phila) 66:35–39
81. Ehrlich CE, Young PC, Stehman FB, Sutton GP, Alford WM (1988) Steroid receptors and clinical outcome in patients with adenocarcinoma of the endometrium. Am J Obstet Gynecol 158:796–807
82. Eifel P, Hendrickson M, Ross J, Ballon S, Martinez A, Kempson R (1982) Simultaneous presentation of carcinoma involving the ovary and the uterine corpus. Cancer (Phila) 50:163–170
83. Eifel PJ, Ross J, Hendrickson M, Cox RS, Kempson R, Martinez A (1983) Adenocarcinoma of the endometrium. Analysis of 256 cases with disease limited to the uterine corpus: treatment comparisons. Cancer (Phila) 52:1026–1031
84. Emoto M, Iwasaki H, Kikuchi M, Shirakawa K (1993) Characteristics of cloned cells of mixed mullerian tumor of the human uterus. Carcinoma cells showing myogenic differentiation in vitro. Cancer (Phila) 71:3065–3075
85. Enomoto T, Fujita M, Inoue M, Rice JM, Nakajima R, Tanizawa O, et al (1993) Alterations of the p53 tumor suppressor gene and its association with activation of the c-K-*ras*-2 protooncogene in premalignant and malignant lesions of the human uterine endometrium. Cancer Res 53:1883–1888
86. Enriori CL, Reforzo-Membrives J (1984) Peripheral aromatization as a risk factor for breast and endometrial cancer in postmenopausal women: a review. Gynecol Oncol 17:1–21
87. Eshleman JR, Markowitz SD (1995) Microsatellite instability in inherited and sporadic neoplasms. Curr Opin Oncol 7:83–89
88. Esteller M, Garcia A, Martinez-Palones JM, Xercavins J, Reventos J (1997) The clinicopathological significance of K-ras point mutation and gene amplification in endometrial cancer. Eur J Cancer 33:1572–1577
89. Esteller M, Levine R, Baylin SB, Ellenson LH, Herman JG (1998) MLH1 promoter hypermethylation is associated with the microsatellite instability phenotype in sporadic endometrial carcinomas. Oncogene 17:2413–2417
90. Esteller M, Catasus L, Matias-Guiu X, Mutter GL, Prat J, Baylin SB, et al (1999) hMLH1 promoter hypermethylation is an early event in human endometrial tumorigenesis. Am J Pathol 155:1767–1772
91. Farhi DC, Nosanchuk J, Silverberg SG (1986) Endometrial adenocarcinoma in women under 25 years of age. Obstet Gynecol 68:741–745
92. Farley JH, Nycum LR, Birrer MJ, Park RC, Taylor RR (2000) Age-specific survival of women with endometrioid adenocarcinoma of the uterus. Gynecol Oncol 79:86–89
93. Fisher B, Costantino JP, Redmond CK, Fisher ER, Wickerham DL, Cronin WM (1994) Endometrial cancer in tamoxifen-treated breast cancer patients: findings from the National Surgical Adjuvant Breast and Bowel Project (NSABP) B-14. J Natl Cancer Inst 86:527–537
94. Fisher B, Costantino JP, Wickerham DL, Redmond CK, Kavanah M, Cronin WM, et al (1998) Tamoxifen for prevention of breast cancer: report of the National Surgical Adjuvant Breast and Bowel Project P-1 Study. J Natl Cancer Inst 90:1371–1388
95. Fleming WP, Peters WA III, Kumar NB, Morley GW (1984) Autopsy findings in patients with uterine sarcoma. Gynecol Oncol 19:168–172
96. Fornander T, Rutqvist LE, Cedermark B, Glas U, Mattsson A, Silfversward C, et al (1989) Adjuvant tamoxifen in early breast cancer: occurrence of new primary cancers. Lancet 1:117–120
97. Franks AL, Kendrick JS, Tyler CWJ (1987) Postmenopausal smoking, estrogen replacement therapy, and the risk of endometrial cancer. Am J Obstet Gynecol 156:20–23
98. Fujii H, Yoshida M, Gong ZX, Matsumoto T, Hamano Y, Fukunaga M, et al (2000) Frequent genetic heterogeneity in the clonal evolution of gynecological carcinosarcoma and its influence on phenotypic diversity. Cancer Res 60:114–120
99. Fujiwara H, Tortolero-Luna G, Mitchell MF, Koulos JP, Wright TCJ (1997) Adenocarcinoma of the

cervix. Expression and clinical significance of estrogen and progesterone receptors. Cancer (Phila) 79:505–512
100. Fukuchi T, Sakamoto M, Tsuda H, Maruyama K, Nozawa S, Hirohashi S (1998) Beta-catenin mutation in carcinoma of the uterine endometrium. Cancer Res 58:3526–3528
101. Fukuda K, Mori M, Uchiyama M, Iwai K, Iwasaka T, Sugimori H (1998) Prognostic significance of progesterone receptor immunohistochemistry in endometrial carcinoma. Gynecol Oncol 69:220–225
102. Gagne E, Tetu B, Blondeau L, Raymond PE, Blais R (1989) Morphologic prognostic factors of malignant mixed müllerian tumor of the uterus: a clinicopathologic study of 58 cases. Mod Pathol 2:433–438
103. Gal D, Recio FO, Zamurovic D, Tancer ML (1991) Lymphvascular space involvement—a prognostic indicator in endometrial adenocarcinoma. Gynecol Oncol 42:142–145
104. Gal D, Recio FO, Zamurovic D (1992) The new International Federation of Gynecology and Obstetrics surgical staging and survival rates in early endometrial carcinoma. Cancer (Phila) 69:200–202
105. Gambrell RDJ, Bagnell CA, Greenblatt RB (1983) Role of estrogens and progesterone in the etiology and prevention of endometrial cancer: review. Am J Obstet Gynecol 146:696–707
106. Garzetti GG, Ciavattini A, Goteri G, de Nictolis M, Romanini C (1996) Proliferating cell nuclear antigen in endometrial carcinoma: pretreatment identification of high-risk patients. Gynecol Oncol 61:16–21
107. Gasparini GS, Fea RP (1992) Multivariate analysis of prognostic factors in 232 patients with clinical stage I endometrial carcinoma using the new FIGO surgical staging system. Int J Oncol 1:665–672
108. Gehrig PA, Groben PA, Fowler WC, Walton LA, Van Le L (2001) Noninvasive papillary serous carcinoma of the endometrium. Obstet Gynecol 97:153–157
109. Geisinger KR, Homesley HD, Morgan TM, Kute TE, Marshall RB (1986) Endometrial adenocarcinoma. A multiparameter clinicopathologic analysis including the DNA profile and the sex steroid hormone receptors. Cancer (Phila) 58:1518–1525
110. Geisinger KR, Marshall RB, Kute TE, Homesley HD (1986) Correlation of female sex steroid hormone receptors with histologic and ultrastructural differentiation in adenocarcinoma of the endometrium. Cancer (Phila) 58:1506–1517
111. Geisinger KR, Dabbs DJ, Marshall RB (1987) Malignant mixed mullerian tumors. An ultrastructural and immunohistochemical analysis with histogenetic considerations. Cancer (Phila) 59:1781–1790
112. Geisler JP, Geisler HE, Wiemann MC, Zhou Z, Miller GA, Crabtree W (1998) Lack of bcl-2 persistence: an independent prognostic indicator of poor prognosis in endometrial carcinoma. Gynecol Oncol 71:305–307
113. Geisler JP, Wiemann MC, Zhou Z, Miller GA, Geisler HE (1996) p53 as a prognostic indicator in endometrial cancer. Gynecol Oncol 61:245–248
114. George E, Manivel JC, Dehner LP, Wick MR (1991) Malignant mixed mullerian tumors: an immunohistochemical study of 47 cases, with histogenetic considerations and clinical correlation. Hum Pathol 22:215–223
115. George E, Lillemoe TJ, Twiggs LB, Perrone T (1995) Malignant mixed mullerian tumor versus high-grade endometrial carcinoma and aggressive variants of endometrial carcinoma: a comparative analysis of survival. Int J Gynecol Pathol 14:39–44
116. Gerszten K, Faul C, Kounelis S, Huang Q, Kelley J, Jones MW (1998) The impact of adjuvant radiotherapy on carcinosarcoma of the uterus. Gynecol Oncol 68:8–13
117. Gitsch G, Friedlander ML, Wain GV, Hacker NF (1995) Uterine papillary serous carcinoma. A clinical study. Cancer (Phila) 75:2239–2243
118. Gitsch G, Hanzal E, Jensen D, Hacker NF (1995) Endometrial cancer in premenopausal women 45 years and younger. Obstet Gynecol 85:504–508
119. Gompel A, Sabourin JC, Martin A, Yaneva H, Audouin J, Decroix Y, et al (1994) Bcl-2 expression in normal endometrium during the menstrual cycle. Am J Pathol 144:1195–1202
120. Goodman A, Zukerberg LR, Rice LW, Fuller AF, Young RH, Scully RE (1996) Squamous cell carcinoma of the endometrium: a report of eight cases and a review of the literature. Gynecol Oncol 61:54–60
121. Gorai I, Doi C, Minaguchi H (1993) Establishment and characterization of carcinosarcoma cell line of the human uterus. Cancer (Phila) 71:775–786
122. Gorai I, Yanagibashi T, Taki A, Udagawa K, Miyagi E, Nakazawa T, et al (1997) Uterine carcinosarcoma is derived from a single stem cell: an in vitro study. Int J Cancer 72:821–827
123. Gray LAS, Christopherson WM, Hoover RN (1977) Estrogens and endometrial carcinoma. Obstet Gynecol Surv 32:619–621
124. Greenblatt RB, Gambrell RDJ, Stoddard LD (1982) The protective role of progesterone in the prevention of endometrial cancer. Pathol Res Pract 174: 297–318
125. Greenwald P, Caputo TA, Wolfgang PE (1977) Endometrial cancer after menopausal use of estrogens. Obstet Gynecol 50:239–243
126. Greven KM, Lanciano RM, Corn B, Case D, Randall ME (1993) Pathologic stage III endometrial carcinoma. Prognostic factors and patterns of recurrence. Cancer (Phila) 71:3697–3702
127. Grimshaw RN, Tupper WC, Fraser RC, Tompkins MG, Jeffrey JF (1990) Prognostic value of peritoneal cytology in endometrial carcinoma. Gynecol Oncol 36:97–100
128. Gronroos M, Salmi TA, Vuento MH, Jalava EA, Tyrkko JE, Maatela JI, et al (1993) Mass screening for endometrial cancer directed in risk groups of

patients with diabetes and patients with hypertension. Cancer (Phila) 71:1279–1282
129. Gu M, Shi W, Barakat RR, Thaler HT, Saigo PE (2000) Peritoneal washings in endometrial carcinoma. A study of 298 patients with histopathologic correlation. Acta Cytol 44:783–789
130. Guidi AJ, Abu-Jawdeh G, Tognazzi K, Dvorak HF, Brown LF (1996) Expression of vascular permeability factor (vascular endothelial growth factor) and its receptors in endometrial carcinoma. Cancer (Phila) 78:454–460
131. Hall JB, Young RH, Nelson JHJ (1984) The prognostic significance of adenomyosis in endometrial carcinoma. Gynecol Oncol 17:32–40
132. Hamel NW, Sebo TJ, Wilson TO, Keeney GL, Roche PC, Suman VJ, et al (1996) Prognostic value of p53 and proliferating cell nuclear antigen expression in endometrial carcinoma. Gynecol Oncol 62:192–198
133. Hanson MB, van NJJ, Powell DE, Donaldson ES, Gallion H, Merhige M, et al (1985) The prognostic significance of lymph-vascular space invasion in stage I endometrial cancer. Cancer (Phila) 55:1753–1757
134. Harouny VR, Sutton GP, Clark SA, Geisler HE, Stehman FB, Ehrlich CE (1988) The importance of peritoneal cytology in endometrial carcinoma. Obstet Gynecol 72:394–398
135. Heatley MK (1995) Association between the apoptotic index and established prognostic parameters in endometrial adenocarcinoma. Histopathology 27:469–472
136. Heatley MK (1997) A high apoptotic index occurs in subtypes of endometrial adenocarcinoma associated with a poor prognosis. Pathology 29:272–275
137. Henderson GS, Brown KA, Perkins SL, Abbott TM, Clayton F (1996) bcl-2 is down-regulated in atypical endometrial hyperplasia and adenocarcinoma. Mod Pathol 9:430–438
138. Hendrickson MR, Ross J, Eifel P, Martinez A, Kempson R (1982) Uterine papillary serous carcinoma: a highly malignant form of endometrial adenocarcinoma. Am J Surg Pathol 6:93–108
139. Hendrickson MR, Kempson RL (1983) Ciliated carcinoma—a variant of endometrial adenocarcinoma: a report of 10 cases. Int J Gynecol Pathol 2: 1–12
140. Hernandez E, Woodruff JD (1980) Endometrial adenocarcinoma arising in adenomyosis. Am J Obstet Gynecol 138:827–832
141. Hetzel DJ, Wilson TO, Keeney GL, Roche PC, Cha SS, Podratz KC (1992) HER-2/neu expression: a major prognostic factor in endometrial cancer. Gynecol Oncol 47:179–185
142. Hicks ML, Phillips JL, Parham G, Andrews N, Jones WB, Shingleton HM, et al (1998) The National Cancer Data Base report on endometrial carcinoma in African-American women. Cancer (Phila) 83:2629–2637
143. Hoffman MS, Cavanagh D, Walter TS, Ionata F, Ruffolo EH (1989) Adenocarcinoma of the endometrium and endometrioid carcinoma of the ovary associated with pregnancy. Gynecol Oncol 32:82–85
144. Homesley HD, Zaino R (1994) Endometrial cancer: prognostic factors. Semin Oncol 21:71–78
145. Hording U, Daugaard S, Visfeldt J (1997) Adenocarcinoma of the cervix and adenocarcinoma of the endometrium: distinction with PCR-mediated detection of HPV DNA. APMIS 105:313–316
146. Horwitz RI, Feinstein AR, Horwitz SM, Robboy SJ (1981) Necropsy diagnosis of endometrial cancer and detection-bias in case/control studies. Lancet 2:66–68
147. Hoshida Y, Nagakawa T, Mano S, Taguchi K, Aozasa K (1996) Hepatoid adenocarcinoma of the endometrium associated with alpha-fetoprotein production. Int J Gynecol Pathol 15:266–269
148. Huntsman DG, Clement PB, Gilks CB, Scully RE (1994) Small-cell carcinoma of the endometrium. A clinicopathological study of sixteen cases. Am J Surg Pathol 18:364–375
149. Ingle JN (1994) Tamoxifen and endometrial cancer: new challenges for an "old" drug. Gynecol Oncol 55:161–163
150. Inoue Y, Obata K, Abe K, Ohmura G, Doh K, Yoshioka T, et al (1996) The prognostic significance of vascular invasion by endometrial carcinoma. Cancer (Phila) 78:1447–1451
151. Ioffe OB, Papadimitriou JC, Drachenberg CB (1998) Correlation of proliferation indices, apoptosis, and related oncogene expression (bcl-2 and c-erbB-2) and p53 in proliferative, hyperplastic, and malignant endometrium. Hum Pathol 29:1150–1159
152. Ismail SM (1996) The effects of tamoxifen on the uterus. Curr Opin Obstet Gynecol 8:27–31
153. Ito K, Watanabe K, Nasim S, Sasano H, Sato S, Yajima A, et al (1994) Prognostic significance of p53 overexpression in endometrial cancer. Cancer Res 54:4667–4670
154. Ito K, Watanabe K, Nasim S, Sasano H, Sato S, Yajima A, et al (1996) K-ras point mutations in endometrial carcinoma: effect on outcome is dependent on age of patient. Gynecol Oncol 63:238–246
155. Ito K, Sasano H, Matsunaga G, Sato S, Yajima A, Nasim S, et al (1997) Correlations between p21 expression and clinicopathological findings, p53 gene and protein alterations, and survival in patients with endometrial carcinoma. J Pathol 183:318–324
156. Iversen OE (1986) Flow cytometric deoxyribonucleic acid index: a prognostic factor in endometrial carcinoma. Am J Obstet Gynecol 155:770–776
157. Iwasa Y, Haga H, Konishi I, Kobashi Y, Higuchi K, Katsuyama E, et al (1998) Prognostic factors in uterine carcinosarcoma: a clinicopathologic study of 25 patients. Cancer (Phila) 82:512–519
158. Iwasawa A, Nieminen P, Lehtinen M, Paavonen J (1996) Human papillomavirus DNA in uterine cervix squamous cell carcinoma and adenocarci-

noma detected by polymerase chain reaction. Cancer (Phila) 77:2275–2279
159. Jacques SM, Lawrence WD (1990) Endometrial adenocarcinoma with variable-level myometrial involvement limited to adenomyosis: a clinicopathologic study of 23 cases. Gynecol Oncol 37:401–407
160. Jones MA, Young RH, Scully RE (1991) Endometrial adenocarcinoma with a component of giant cell carcinoma. Int J Gynecol Pathol 10:260–270
161. Jones MW, Kounelis S, Hsu C, Papadaki H, Bakker A, Swalsky PA, et al (1997) Prognostic value of p53 and K-*ras*-2 topographic genotyping in endometrial carcinoma: a clinicopathologic and molecular comparison. Int J Gynecol Pathol 16:354–360
162. Jordan VC, Morrow M (1994) Should clinicians be concerned about the carcinogenic potential of tamoxifen? Eur J Cancer 30A:1714–1721
163. Joseph MG, Fellows FG, Hearn SA (1990) Primary endodermal sinus tumor of the endometrium. A clinicopathologic, immunocytochemical, and ultrastructural study. Cancer (Phila) 65:297–302
164. Kadar N, Homesley HD, Malfetano JH (1992) Positive peritoneal cytology is an adverse factor in endometrial carcinoma only if there is other evidence of extrauterine disease. Gynecol Oncol 46:145–149
165. Kadar N, Malfetano JH, Homesley HD (1993) Steroid receptor concentrations in endometrial carcinoma: effect on survival in surgically staged patients. Gynecol Oncol 50:281–286
166. Kahanpaa KV, Wahlstrom T, Grohn P, Heinonen E, Nieminen U, Widholm O (1986) Sarcomas of the uterus: a clinicopathologic study of 119 patients. Obstet Gynecol 67:417–424
167. Kaku T, Kamura T, Kinukawa N, Kobayashi H, Sakai K, Tsuruchi N, et al (1997) Angiogenesis in endometrial carcinoma. Cancer (Phila) 80:741–747
168. Kaku T, Silverberg SG, Tsukamoto N, Tsuruchi N, Kamura T, Saito T, et al (1993) Association of endometrial epithelial metaplasias with endometrial carcinoma and hyperplasia in Japanese and American women. Int J Gynecol Pathol 12:297–300
169. Kaleli S, Kosebay D, Bese T, Demirkiran F, Oz UA, Arvas M, et al (1997) A strong prognostic variable in endometrial carcinoma: flow cytometric S-phase fraction. Cancer (Phila) 79:944–951
170. Kalir T, Seijo L, Deligdisch L, Cohen C (1995) Endometrial adenocarcinoma with choriocarcinomatous differentiation in an elderly virginal woman. Int J Gynecol Pathol 14:266–269
171. Kallakury BV, Ambros RA, Hayner-Buchan AM, Sheehan CE, Malfetano JH, Ross JS (1998) Cell proliferation-associated proteins in endometrial carcinomas, including papillary serous and endometrioid subtypes. Int J Gynecol Pathol 17:320–326
172. Kanbour-Shakir A, Tobon H (1991) Primary clear cell carcinoma of the endometrium: a clinicopathologic study of 20 cases. Int J Gynecol Pathol 10:67–78
173. Katase K, Sugiyama Y, Hasumi K, Yoshimoto M, Kasumi F (1998) The incidence of subsequent endometrial carcinoma with tamoxifen use in patients with primary breast carcinoma. Cancer (Phila) 82:1698–1703
174. Kaufman DW, Shapiro S, Slone D, Rosenberg L, Miettinen OS, Stolley PD, et al (1980) Decreased risk of endometrial cancer among oral-contraceptive users. N Engl J Med 303:1045–1047
175. Kempson RL, Pokorny GE (1968) Adenocarcinoma of the endometrium in women aged forty and younger. Cancer (Phila) 21:650–662
176. Kennedy AW, Peterson GL, Becker SN, Nunez C, Webster KD (1987) Experience with pelvic washings in stage I and II endometrial carcinoma. Gynecol Oncol 28:50–60
177. Khalifa MA, Mannel RS, Haraway SD, Walker J, Min KW (1994) Expression of EGFR, HER-2/neu, P53, and PCNA in endometrioid, serous papillary, and clear cell endometrial adenocarcinomas. Gynecol Oncol 53:84–92
178. Khuu HM, Crisco CP, Kilgore L, Rodgers WH, Conner MG (2000) Carcinosarcoma of the uterus associated with a nongestational choriocarcinoma. South Med J 93:226–228
179. Kihana T, Hamada K, Inoue Y, Yano N, Iketani H, Murao S, et al (1995) Mutation and allelic loss of the p53 gene in endometrial carcinoma. Incidence and outcome in 92 surgical patients. Cancer (Phila) 76:72–78
180. Kim KR, Scully RE (1990) Peritoneal keratin granulomas with carcinomas of endometrium and ovary and atypical polypoid adenomyoma of endometrium. A clinicopathological analysis of 22 cases. Am J Surg Pathol 14:925–932
181. Klemi PJ, Alanen KA, Salmi T (1995) Detection of malignancy in endometrium by brush sampling in 1042 symptomatic patients. Int J Gynecol Cancer 5:222–225
182. Kobayashi K, Sagae S, Nishioka Y, Tokino T, Kudo R (1999) Mutations of the beta-catenin gene in endometrial carcinomas. Jpn J Cancer Res 90:55–59
183. Kohlberger P, Gitsch G, Loesch A, Tempfer C, Kaider A, Reinthaller A, et al (1996) p53 protein overexpression in early stage endometrial cancer. Gynecol Oncol 62:213–217
184. Kohler MF, Carney P, Dodge R, Soper JT, Clarke-Pearson DL, Marks JR, et al (1996) p53 overexpression in advanced-stage endometrial adenocarcinoma. Am J Obstet Gynecol 175:1246–1252
185. Kommoss F, Karck U, Prompeler H, Pfisterer J, Kirkpatrick CJ (1998) Steroid receptor expression in endometria from women treated with tamoxifen. Gynecol Oncol 70:188–191
186. Kosary CL (1994) FIGO stage, histology, histologic grade, age and race as prognostic factors in determining survival for cancers of the female gynecological system: an analysis of 1973–87 SEER cases of cancers of the endometrium, cervix, ovary, vulva, and vagina. Semin Surg Oncol 10:31–46
187. Koss LG, Schreiber K, Oberlander SG, Moussouris HF, Lesser M (1984) Detection of endometrial car-

cinoma and hyperplasia in asymptomatic women. Obstet Gynecol 64:1–11
188. Kounelis S, Jones MW, Papadaki H, Bakker A, Swalsky P, Finkelstein SD (1998) Carcinosarcomas (malignant mixed mullerian tumors) of the female genital tract: comparative molecular analysis of epithelial and mesenchymal components. Hum Pathol 29:82–87
189. Kovalev S, Marchenko ND, Gugliotta BG, Chalas E, Chumas J, Moll UM (1998) Loss of p53 function in uterine papillary serous carcinoma. Hum Pathol 29:613–619
190. Kumar NB, Hart WR (1982) Metastases to the uterine corpus from extragenital cancers. A clinicopathologic study of 63 cases. Cancer (Phila) 50: 2163–2169
191. Kurman RJ, Scully RE (1976) Clear cell carcinoma of the endometrium: an analysis of 21 cases. Cancer (Phila) 37:872–882
192. Larson B, Silfversward C, Nilsson B, Pettersson F (1990) Mixed mullerian tumours of the uterus—prognostic factors: a clinical and histopathologic study of 147 cases. Radiother Oncol 17:123–132
193. Larson DM, Johnson KK, Broste SK, Krawisz BR, Kresl JJ (1995) Comparison of D&C and office endometrial biopsy in predicting final histopathologic grade in endometrial cancer. Obstet Gynecol 86:38–42
194. Lauchlan SC (1981) Tubal (serous) carcinoma of the endometrium. Arch Pathol Lab Med 105:615–618
195. Lax SF, Pizer ES, Ronnett BM, Kurman RJ (1998) Clear cell carcinoma of the endometrium is characterized by a distinctive profile of p53, Ki-67, estrogen, and progesterone receptor expression. Hum Pathol 29:551–558
196. Lax SF, Pizer ES, Ronnett BM, Kurman RJ (1998) Comparison of estrogen and progesterone receptor, Ki-67, and p53 immunoreactivity in uterine endometrioid carcinoma and endometrioid carcinoma with squamous, mucinous, secretory, and ciliated cell differentiation. Hum Pathol 29:924–931
197. Lax SF, Kendall B, Tashiro H, Slebos RJ, Hedrick L (2000) The frequency of p53, K-ras mutations, and microsatellite instability differs in uterine endometrioid and serous carcinoma: evidence of distinct molecular genetic pathways. Cancer (Phila) 88:814–824
198. Lax SF, Kurman RJ, Pizer ES, Wu L, Ronnett BM (2000) A binary architectural grading system for uterine endometrial endometrioid carcinoma has superior reproducibility compared with FIGO grading and identifies subsets of advance-stage tumors with favorable and unfavorable prognosis. Am J Surg Pathol 24:1201–1208
199. Lee KR, Scully RE (1989) Complex endometrial hyperplasia and carcinoma in adolescents and young women 15 to 20 years of age. A report of 10 cases. Int J Gynecol Pathol 8:201–213
200. Lee RB, Burke TW, Park RC (1990) Estrogen replacement therapy following treatment for stage I endometrial carcinoma. Gynecol Oncol 36:189–191
201. Lee KR, Belinson JL (1991) Recurrence in noninvasive endometrial carcinoma. Relationship to uterine papillary serous carcinoma. Am J Surg Pathol 15:965–973
202. Lee KR, Vacek PM, Belinson JL (1994) Traditional and nontraditional histopathologic predictors of recurrence in uterine endometrioid adenocarcinoma. Gynecol Oncol 54:10–18
203. Leiserowitz GS, Harris SA, Subramaniam M, Keeney GL, Podratz KC, Spelsberg TC (1993) The proto-oncogene c-*fms* is overexpressed in endometrial cancer. Gynecol Oncol 49:190–196
204. Lesko SM, Rosenberg L, Kaufman DW, Helmrich SP, Miller DR, Strom B, et al (1985) Cigarette smoking and the risk of endometrial cancer. N Engl J Med 313:593–596
205. Levenback C, Burke TW, Silva E, Morris M, Gershenson DM, Kavanagh JJ, et al (1992) Uterine papillary serous carcinoma (UPSC) treated with cisplatin, doxorubicin, and cyclophosphamide (PAC). Gynecol Oncol 46:317–321
206. Levi F, Franceschi S, Negri E, La Vecchia C (1993) Dietary factors and the risk of endometrial cancer. Cancer (Phila) 71:3575–3581
207. Levine RL, Cargile CB, Blazes MS, van Rees B, Kurman RJ, Ellenson LH (1998) PTEN mutations and microsatellite instability in complex atypical hyperplasia, a precursor lesion to uterine endometrioid carcinoma. Cancer Res 58:3254–3258
208. Li J, Yen C, Liaw D, Podsypanina K, Bose S, Wang SI, et al (1997) PTEN, a putative protein tyrosine phosphatase gene mutated in human brain, breast, and prostate cancer [see comments]. Science 275:1943–1947
209. Lininger RA, Ashfaq R, Albores-Saavedra J, Tavassoli FA (1997) Transitional cell carcinoma of the endometrium and endometrial carcinoma with transitional cell differentiation. Cancer (Phila) 79: 1933–1943
210. Longacre TA (1999) Diffusely infiltrative endometrial adenocarcinoma. An adenoma malignum pattern of myoinvasion. Am J Surg Pathol 23:69–78
211. Lukes AS, Kohler MF, Pieper CF, Kerns BJ, Bentley R, Rodriguez GC, et al (1994) Multivariable analysis of DNA ploidy, p53, and HER-2/neu as prognostic factors in endometrial cancer. Cancer (Phila) 73:2380–2385
212. Macasaet MA, Waxman M, Fruchter RG, Boyce J, Hong P, Nicastri AD, et al (1985) Prognostic factors in malignant mesodermal (mullerian) mixed tumors of the uterus. Gynecol Oncol 20:32–42
213. Mack TM, Pike MC, Henderson BE, Pfeffer RI, Gerkins VR, Arthur M, et al (1976) Estrogens and endometrial cancer in a retirement community. N Engl J Med 294:1262–1267
214. MacMahon B (1997) Overview of studies on endometrial cancer and other types of cancer in hu-

mans: perspectives of an epidemiologist. Semin Oncol 24:S1–S1

215. Maehama T, Dixon JE (1998) The tumor suppressor, PTEN/MMAC1, dephosphorylates the lipid second messenger, phosphatidylinositol 3,4,5–trisphosphate. J Biol Chem 273:13375–13378
216. Magriples U, Naftolin F, Schwartz PE, Carcangiu ML (1993) High-grade endometrial carcinoma in tamoxifen-treated breast cancer patients. J Clin Oncol 11:485–490
217. Malpica A, Tornos C, Burke TW, Silva EG (1995) Low-stage clear-cell carcinoma of the endometrium. Am J Surg Pathol 19:769–774
218. Marchese MJ, Liskow AS, Crum CP, McCaffrey RM, Frick HC (1984) Uterine sarcomas: a clinicopathologic study, 1965–1981. Gynecol Oncol 18:299–312
219. Masood S, Rhatigan RM, Wilkinson EW, Barwick KW, Wilson WJ (1993) Expression and prognostic significance of estrogen and progesterone receptors in adenocarcinoma of the uterine cervix. An immunocytochemical study. Cancer (Phila) 72:511–518
220. Maxwell GL, Risinger JI, Gumbs C, Shaw H, Bentley RC, Barrett JC, et al (1998) Mutation of the PTEN tumor suppressor gene in endometrial hyperplasias. Cancer Res 58:2500–2503
221. McCarty KSJ, Barton TK, Fetter BF, Creasman WT, McCarty KSS (1979) Correlation of estrogen and progesterone receptors with histologic differentiation in endometrial adenocarcinoma. Am J Pathol 96:171–183
222. McDonald TW, Annegers JF, O'Fallon WM, Dockerty MB, Malkasian GDJ, Kurland LT (1977) Exogenous estrogen and endometrial carcinoma: case-control and incidence study. Am J Obstet Gynecol 127:572–580
223. Meis JM, Lawrence WD (1990) The immunohistochemical profile of malignant mixed mullerian tumor. Overlap with endometrial adenocarcinoma. Am J Clin Pathol 94:1–7
224. Melhem MF, Tobon H (1987) Mucinous adenocarcinoma of the endometrium: a clinico-pathological review of 18 cases. Int J Gynecol Pathol 6:347–355
225. Meredith RF, Eisert DR, Kaka Z, Hodgson SE, Johnston GA Jr, Boutselis JG (1986) An excess of uterine sarcomas after pelvic irradiation. Cancer (Phila) 58:2003–2007
226. Miller B, Morris M, Silva E (1994) Nucleolar organizer regions: a potential prognostic factor in adenocarcinoma of the endometrium. Gynecol Oncol 54:137–141
227. Mitchell H, Giles G, Medley G (1993) Accuracy and survival benefit of cytological prediction of endometrial carcinoma on routine cervical smears. Int J Gynecol Pathol 12:34–40
228. Mittal KR, Barwick KW (1993) Endometrial adenocarcinoma involving adenomyosis without true myometrial invasion is characterized by frequent preceding estrogen therapy, low histologic grades, and excellent prognosis. Gynecol Oncol 49:197–201
229. Moll UM, Chalas E, Auguste M, Meaney D, Chumas J (1996) Uterine papillary serous carcinoma evolves via a p53–driven pathway. Hum Pathol 27:1295–1300
230. Mooney EE, Robboy SJ, Hammond CB, Berchuck A, Bentley RC (1997) Signet-ring cell carcinoma of the endometrium: a primary tumor masquerading as a metastasis. Int J Gynecol Pathol 16:169–172
231. Morgan KG, Wilkinson N, Buckley CH (1996) Angiogenesis in normal, hyperplastic, and neoplastic endometrium. J Pathol 179:317–320
232. Morris PC, Anderson JR, Anderson B, Buller RE (1995) Steroid hormone receptor content and lymph node status in endometrial cancer. Gynecol Oncol 56:406–411
233. Morrow CP, Bundy BN, Kurman RJ, Creasman WT, Heller P, Homesley HD, et al (1991) Relationship between surgical-pathological risk factors and outcome in clinical stage I and II carcinoma of the endometrium: a Gynecologic Oncology Group study. Gynecol Oncol 40:55–65
234. Mutter GL, Lin MC, Fitzgerald JT, Kum JB, Baak JP, Lees JA, et al (2000) Altered PTEN expression as a diagnostic marker for the earliest endometrial precancers. J Natl Cancer Inst 92:924–930
234a. Mutter GL, Inca TA, Baak JPA, Kust GA, Zhan XP, Eng C (2001) Molecular Identification of Latent precursors in histologically normal endometrium. Cancer Res 61:4311–4314
235. Mutter GL, Boynton KA, Faquin WC, Ruiz RE, Jovanovic AS (1996) Allelotype mapping of unstable microsatellites establishes direct lineage continuity between endometrial precancers and cancer. Cancer Res 56:4483–4486
236. Nazeer T, Ballouk F, Malfetano JH, Figge H, Ambros RA (1995) Multivariate survival analysis of clinicopathologic features in surgical stage I endometrioid carcinoma including analysis of HER-2/neu expression. Am J Obstet Gynecol 173:1829–1834
237. Ng AB, Reagan JW, Storaasli JP, Wentz WB (1973) Mixed adenosquamous carcinoma of the endometrium. Am J Clin Pathol 59:765–781
238. Nielsen SN, Podratz KC, Scheithauer BW, O'Brien PC (1989) Clinicopathologic analysis of uterine malignant mixed mullerian tumors. Gynecol Oncol 34:372–378
239. Nielsen AL, Thomsen HK, Nyholm HC (1991) Evaluation of the reproducibility of the revised 1988 International Federation of Gynecology and Obstetrics grading system of endometrial cancers with special emphasis on nuclear grading. Cancer (Phila) 68:2303–2309
240. Nielsen AL, Nyholm HC, Engel P (1994) Expression of MIB-1 (paraffin Ki-67) and AgNOR morphology in endometrial adenocarcinomas of endometrioid type. Int J Gynecol Pathol 13:37–44
241. Nielsen AL, Nyholm HC (1994) p53 protein and c-erbB-2 protein (p185) expression in endometrial adenocarcinoma of endometrioid type. An immunohistochemical examination on paraffin sections. Am J Clin Pathol 102:76–79
242. Nielsen AL, Nyholm HC (1996) The combination of

p53 and age predict cancer specific death in advanced stage (FIGO Ic-IV) of endometrial carcinoma of endometrioid type. An immunohistochemical examination of growth fraction: Ki-67, MIB-1 and PC10; suppressor oncogene protein: p53; oncogene protein: p185 and age, hormone treatment, stage, and histologic grade. Eur J Obstet Gynecol Reprod Biol 70:79–85
243. Niemann TH, Trgovac TL, McGaughy VR, Vaccarello L (1996) bcl-2 expression in endometrial hyperplasia and carcinoma. Gynecol Oncol 63:318–322
244. Nordal RR, Kristensen GB, Stenwig AE, Nesland JM, Pettersen EO, Trope CG (1997) An evaluation of prognostic factors in uterine carcinosarcoma. Gynecol Oncol 67:316–321
245. Nordstrom B, Strang P, Lindgren A, Bergstrom R, Tribukait B (1996) Carcinoma of the endometrium: do the nuclear grade and DNA ploidy provide more prognostic information than do the FIGO and WHO classifications? Int J Gynecol Pathol 15:191–201
246. Norris HJ, Taylor HB (1965) Postirradiation sarcomas of the uterus. Obstet Gynecol 26:689–694
247. Norris HJ, Roth E, Taylor HB (1966) Mesenchymal tumors of the uterus. II. A clinical and pathologic study of 31 mixed mesodermal tumors. Obstet Gynecol 28:57–63
248. Norris HJ, Taylor HB (1966) Mesenchymal tumors of the uterus. III. A clinical and pathologic study of 31 carcinosarcomas. Cancer (Phila) 19:1459–1465
249. Noumoff JS, Menzin A, Mikuta J, Lusk EJ, Morgan M, LiVolsi VA (1991) The ability to evaluate prognostic variables on frozen section in hysterectomies performed for endometrial carcinoma. Gynecol Oncol 42:202–208
250. Nyholm HC, Christensen IJ, Nielsen AL (1995) Progesterone receptor levels independently predict survival in endometrial adenocarcinoma. Gynecol Oncol 59:347–351
251. Obermair A, Geramou M, Gücer F, Denison U, Graf AH, Kapshammer E, et al (1999) Endometrial cancer: accuracy of the finding of a well differentiated tumor at dilation and curettage compared to the findings at subsequent hysterectomy. Int J Gynecol Cancer 9:383–386
252. Obermair A, Tempfer C, Wasicky R, Kaider A, Hefler L, Kainz C (1999) Prognostic significance of tumor angiogenesis in endometrial cancer. Obstet Gynecol 93:367–371
253. Parazzini F, La Vecchia C, Bocciolone L, Franceschi S (1991) The epidemiology of endometrial cancer. Gynecol Oncol 41:1–16
254. Parazzini F, La Vecchia C, Negri E, Moroni S, Chatenoud L (1995) Smoking and risk of endometrial cancer: results from an Italian case-control study. Gynecol Oncol 56:195–199
255. Parazzini F, Franceschi S, La Vecchia C, Chatenoud L, Di Cintio E (1997) The epidemiology of female genital tract cancers. Int J Gynecol Cancer 7:169–181
256. Pecorelli S, Benedet JL, Creasman WT, Shepherd JH (1999) FIGO staging of gynecologic cancer. 1994–1997 FIGO Committee on Gynecologic Oncology. International Federation of Gynecology and Obstetrics. Int J Gynaecol Obstet 65:243–249
257. Perez CA, Askin F, Baglan RJ, Kao MS, Kraus FT, Perez BM, et al (1979) Effects of irradiation on mixed mullerian tumors of the uterus. Cancer (Phila) 43:1274–1284
258. Persson I, Adami HO, Bergkvist L, Lindgren A, Pettersson B, Hoover R, et al (1989) Risk of endometrial cancer after treatment with oestrogens alone or in conjunction with progestogens: results of a prospective study. Br Med J 298:147–151
259. Pertschuk LP, Masood S, Simone J, Feldman JG, Fruchter RG, Axiotis CA, et al (1996) Estrogen receptor immunocytochemistry in endometrial carcinoma: a prognostic marker for survival. Gynecol Oncol 63:28–33
260. Pesce C, Merino MJ, Chambers JT, Nogales F (1991) Endometrial carcinoma with trophoblastic differentiation. An aggressive form of uterine cancer. Cancer (Phila) 68:1799–1802
261. Peters WA, III, Kumar NB, Fleming WP, Morley GW (1984) Prognostic features of sarcomas and mixed tumors of the endometrium. Obstet Gynecol 63:550–556
262. Peterson EP (1968) Endometrial carcinoma in young women. A clinical profile. Obstet Gynecol 31: 702–707
263. Pfisterer J, Kommoss F, Sauerbrei W, Rendl I, Kiechle M, Kleine W, et al (1995) Prognostic value of DNA ploidy and S-phase fraction in stage I endometrial carcinoma. Gynecol Oncol 58:149–156
264. Photopulos GJ, Carney CN, Edelman DA, Hughes RR, Fowler WCJ, Walton LA (1979) Clear cell carcinoma of the endometrium. Cancer (Phila) 43: 1448–1456
265. Pickar JH, Thorneycroft I, Whitehead M (1998) Effects of hormone replacement therapy on the endometrium and lipid parameters: a review of randomized clinical trials, 1985 to 1995. Am J Obstet Gynecol 178:1087–1099
266. Pisani AL, Barbuto DA, Chen D, Ramos L, Lagasse LD, Karlan BY (1995) HER-2/neu, p53, and DNA analyses as prognosticators for survival in endometrial carcinoma. Obstet Gynecol 85:729–734
267. Pitman MB, Young RH, Clement PB, Dickersin GR, Scully RE (1994) Endometrioid carcinoma of the ovary and endometrium, oxyphilic cell type: a report of nine cases. Int J Gynecol Pathol 13:290–301
268. Plaxe SC, Saltzstein SL (1997) Impact of ethnicity on the incidence of high-risk endometrial carcinoma. Gynecol Oncol 65:8–12
269. Podczaski E, Kaminski P, Gurski K, MacNeill C, Stryker JA, Singapuri K, et al (1992) Detection and patterns of treatment failure in 300 consecutive cases of "early" endometrial cancer after primary surgery. Gynecol Oncol 47:323–327
270. Potischman N, Hoover RN, Brinton LA, Siiteri P,

Dorgan JF, Swanson CA, et al (1996) Case-control study of endogenous steroid hormones and endometrial cancer. J Natl Cancer Inst 88:1127–1135
271. Ramadan M, Goudie RB (1986) Epithelial antigens in malignant mixed Müllerian tumours of endometrium. J Pathol 148:13–18
272. Reinartz JJ, George E, Lindgren BR, Niehans GA (1994) Expression of p53, transforming growth factor alpha, epidermal growth factor receptor, and c-erbB-2 in endometrial carcinoma and correlation with survival and known predictors of survival. Hum Pathol 25:1075–1083
273. Ribeiro G, Swindell R (1992) The Christie Hospital adjuvant tamoxifen trial. J Natl Cancer Inst Monogr 84:121–125
274. Richart RM, Ferenczy A (1974) Endometrial morphologic response to hormonal environment. Gynecol Oncol 2:180–197
275. Risinger JI, Hayes AK, Berchuck A, Barrett JC (1997) PTEN/MMAC1 mutations in endometrial cancers. Cancer Res 57:4736–4738
276. Risinger JI, Berchuck A, Kohler MF, Watson P, Lynch HT, Boyd J (1993) Genetic instability of microsatellites in endometrial carcinoma. Cancer Res 53:5100–5103
277. Rolitsky CD, Theil KS, McGaughy VR, Copeland LJ, Niemann TH (1999) HER-2/neu amplification and overexpression in endometrial carcinoma. Int J Gynecol Pathol 18:138–143
278. Ross JC, Eifel PJ, Cox RS, Kempson RL, Hendrickson MR (1983) Primary mucinous adenocarcinoma of the endometrium. A clinicopathologic and histochemical study. Am J Surg Pathol 7:715–729
279. Rutqvist LE, Johansson H, Signomklao T, Johansson U, Fornander T, Wilking N (1995) Adjuvant tamoxifen therapy for early stage breast cancer and second primary malignancies. Stockholm Breast Cancer Study Group. J Natl Cancer Inst 87:645–651
280. Ryden S, Ferno M, Moller T, Aspegren K, Bergljung L, Killander D, et al (1992) Long-term effects of adjuvant tamoxifen and/or radiotherapy. The South Sweden Breast Cancer Trial. Acta Oncol 31:271–274
281. Ryder DE (1982) Verrucous carcinoma of the endometrium—a unique neoplasm with long survival. Obstet Gynecol 59:78S-80S
282. Saegusa M, Kamata Y, Isono M, Okayasu I (1996) Bcl-2 expression is correlated with a low apoptotic index and associated with progesterone receptor immunoreactivity in endometrial carcinomas. J Pathol 180:275–282
283. Saegusa M, Okayasu I (1997) Bcl-2 is closely correlated with favorable prognostic factors and inversely associated with p53 protein accumulation in endometrial carcinomas: immunohistochemical and polymerase chain reaction/loss of heterozygosity findings. J Cancer Res Clin Oncol 123:429–434
284. Saegusa M, Okayasu I (1998) Progesterone therapy for endometrial carcinoma reduces cell proliferation but does not alter apoptosis. Cancer (Phila.) 83:111–121
285. Saffari B, Jones LA, el-Naggar A, Felix JC, George J, Press MF (1995) Amplification and overexpression of HER-2/neu (c-erbB2) in endometrial cancers: correlation with overall survival. Cancer Res 55:5693–5698
286. Sakuragi N, Ohkouchi T, Hareyama H, Ikeda K, Watari H, Fujimoto T, et al (1998) Bcl-2 expression and prognosis of patients with endometrial carcinoma. Int J Cancer 79:153–158
287. Sakuragi N, Hareyama H, Todo Y, Yamada H, Yamamoto R, Fujino T, et al (2000) Prognostic significance of serous and clear cell adenocarcinoma in surgically staged endometrial carcinoma. Acta Obstet Gynecol Scand 79:311–316
288. Salvesen HB, Iversen OE, Akslen LA (1998) Identification of high-risk patients by assessment of nuclear Ki-67 expression in a prospective study of endometrial carcinomas. Clin Cancer Res 4:2779–2785
289. Sartori E, Bazzurini L, Gadducci A, Landoni F, Lissoni A, Maggino T, et al (1997) Carcinosarcoma of the uterus: a clinicopathological multicenter CTF study. Gynecol Oncol 67:70–75
290. Savage J, Subby W, Okagaki T (1987) Adenocarcinoma of the endometrium with trophoblastic differentiation and metastases as choriocarcinoma: a case report. Gynecol Oncol 26:257–262
291. Schlosshauer PW, Pirog EC, Levine RL, Ellenson LH (2000) Mutational analysis of the CTNNB1 and APC genes in uterine endometrioid carcinoma. Mod Pathol 13:1066–1071
292. Schweizer W, Demopoulos R, Beller U, Dubin N (1990) Prognostic factors for malignant mixed mullerian tumors of the uterus. Int J Gynecol Pathol 9:129–136
293. Scully RE, Bonfiglio TA, Kurman RJ, Silverberg SG, Wilkinson EJ (1994) Histologic typing of female genital tract tumours: International histological classification of tumours, 2nd Ed. Springer, Berlin
294. Seidman JD, Kurman RJ (1999) Tamoxifen and the endometrium. Int J Gynecol Pathol 18:293–296
295. Semczuk A, Berbec H, Kostuch M, Cybulski M, Wojcierowski J, Baranowski W (1998) K-ras gene point mutations in human endometrial carcinomas: correlation with clinicopathological features and patients' outcome. J Cancer Res Clin Oncol 124:695–700
296. Shapiro S, Kaufman DW, Slone D, Rosenberg L, Miettinen OS, Stolley PD, et al (1980) Recent and past use of conjugated estrogens in relation to adenocarcinoma of the endometrium. N Engl J Med 303:485–489
297. Shaw RW, Lynch PF, Wade-Evans T (1983) Mullerian mixed tumour of the uterine corpus: a clinical histopathological review of 28 patients. Br J Obstet Gynaecol 90:562–569
298. Sherman ME, Bitterman P, Rosenshein NB, Del-

gado G, Kurman RJ (1992) Uterine serous carcinoma. A morphologically diverse neoplasm with unifying clinicopathologic features. Am J Surg Pathol 16:600–610
299. Sherman ME, Bur ME, Kurman RJ (1995) p53 in endometrial cancer and its putative precursors: evidence for diverse pathways of tumorigenesis. Hum Pathol 26:1268–1274
300. Sherman ME, Sturgeon S, Brinton LA, Potischman N, Kurman RJ, Berman ML, et al (1997) Risk factors and hormone levels in patients with serous and endometrioid uterine carcinomas. Mod Pathol 10:963–968
301. Shim JU, Rose PG, Reale FR, Soto H, Tak WK, Hunter RE (1992) Accuracy of frozen-section diagnosis at surgery in clinical stage I and II endometrial carcinoma. Am J Obstet Gynecol 166:1335–1338
302. Silva EG, Jenkins R (1990) Serous carcinoma in endometrial polyps. Mod Pathol 3:120–128
303. Silva EG, Tornos CS, Follen-Mitchell M (1994) Malignant neoplasms of the uterine corpus in patients treated for breast carcinoma: the effects of tamoxifen. Int J Gynecol Pathol 13:248–258
304. Silverberg SG, Major FJ, Blessing JA, Fetter B, Askin FB, Liao SY, et al (1990) Carcinosarcoma (malignant mixed mesodermal tumor) of the uterus. A Gynecologic Oncology Group pathologic study of 203 cases. Int J Gynecol Pathol 9:1–19
305. Sinkre P, Albores-Saavedra J, Miller DS, Copeland LJ, Hameed A (2000) Endometrial endometrioid carcinomas associated with Ewing sarcoma/peripheral primitive neuroectodermal tumor. Int J Gynecol Pathol 19:127–132
306. Sivridis E, Buckley CH, Fox H (1987) The prognostic significance of lymphatic vascular space invasion in endometrial adenocarcinoma. Br J Obstet Gynaecol 94:991–994
307. Smith DC, Prentice R, Thompson DJ, Herrmann WL (1975) Association of exogenous estrogen and endometrial carcinoma. N Engl J Med 293:1164–1167
308. Soong R, Knowles S, Williams KE, Hammond IG, Wysocki SJ, Iacopetta BJ (1996) Overexpression of p53 protein is an independent prognostic indicator in human endometrial carcinoma. Br J Cancer 74:562–567
309. Sorbe B, Risberg B, Frankendal B (1990) DNA ploidy, morphometry, and nuclear grade as prognostic factors in endometrial carcinoma. Gynecol Oncol 38:22–27
310. Soslow RA, Pirog E, Isacson C (2000) Endometrial intraepithelial carcinoma with associated peritoneal carcinomatosis. Am J Surg Pathol 24:726–732
311. Spanos WJ Jr, Wharton JT, Gomez L, Fletcher GH, Oswald MJ (1984) Malignant mixed Mullerian tumors of the uterus. Cancer (Phila) 53:311–316
312. Spiegel GW (1995) Endometrial carcinoma in situ in postmenopausal women. Am J Surg Pathol 19:417–432
313. Spiegel GW, Austin RM, Gelven PL (1996) Transitional cell carcinoma of the endometrium. Gynecol Oncol 60:325–330
314. Sreenan JJ, Hart WR (1995) Carcinosarcomas of the female genital tract. A pathologic study of 29 metastatic tumors: further evidence for the dominant role of the epithelial component and the conversion theory of histogenesis. Am J Surg Pathol 19:666–674
315. Stendahl U, Strang P, Wagenius G, Bergstrom R, Tribukait B (1991) Prognostic significance of proliferation in endometrial adenocarcinomas: a multivariate analysis of clinical and flow cytometric variables. Int J Gynecol Pathol 10:271–284
316. Stewart HJ (1992) The Scottish trial of adjuvant tamoxifen in node-negative breast cancer. Scottish Cancer Trials Breast Group. J Natl Cancer Inst Monogr 117–120
317. Susini T, Rapi S, Savino L, Boddi V, Berti P, Massi G (1994) Prognostic value of flow cytometric deoxyribonucleic acid index in endometrial carcinoma: comparison with other clinical-pathologic parameters. Am J Obstet Gynecol 170:527–534
318. Sutton G, Brunetto VL, Kilgore L, Soper JT, McGehee R, Olt G, et al (2000) A phase III trial of ifosfamide with or without cisplatin in carcinosarcoma of the uterus: a gynecologic oncology group study [In Process Citation]. Gynecol Oncol 79:147–153
319. Szpak CA, Creasman WT, Vollmer RT, Johnston WW (1981) Prognostic value of cytologic examination of peritoneal washings in patients with endometrial carcinoma. Acta Cytol 25:640–646
320. Tashiro H, Blazes MS, Wu R, Cho KR, Bose S, Wang SI, et al (1997) Mutations in PTEN are frequent in endometrial carcinoma but rare in other common gynecological malignancies. Cancer Res 57:3935–3940
321. Tashiro H, Isacson C, Levine R, Kurman RJ, Cho KR, Hedrick L (1997) p53 gene mutations are common in uterine serous carcinoma and occur early in their pathogenesis. Am J Pathol 150:177–185
322. Taskin M, Lallas TA, Barber HR, Shevchuk MM (1997) bcl-2 and p53 in endometrial adenocarcinoma. Mod Pathol 10:728–734
323. Taylor RR, Zeller J, Lieberman RW, O'Connor DM (1999) An analysis of two versus three grades for endometrial carcinoma. Gynecol Oncol 74:3–6
324. Tenti P, Romagnoli S, Silini E, Zappatore R, Spinillo A, Giunta P, et al (1996) Human papillomavirus types 16 and 18 infection in infiltrating adenocarcinoma of the cervix: PCR analysis of 138 cases and correlation with histologic type and grade. Am J Clin Pathol 106:52–56
325. Thompson L, Chang B, Barsky SH (1996) Monoclonal origins of malignant mixed tumors (carcinosarcomas). Evidence for a divergent histogenesis. Am J Surg Pathol 20:277–285
326. Tiltman AJ (1980) Mucinous carcinoma of the endometrium. Obstet Gynecol 55:244–247
327. Tobon H, Watkins GJ (1985) Secretory adenocar-

cinoma of the endometrium. Int J Gynecol Pathol 4:328–335
328. Tornos C, Silva EG, el-Naggar A, Burke TW (1992) Aggressive stage I grade 1 endometrial carcinoma. Cancer (Phila) 70:790–798
329. Trere D, Melchiorri C, Chieco P, Marabini A, Derenzini M (1994) Interphase AgNOR quantity and DNA content in endometrial adenocarcinoma. Gynecol Oncol 53:202–207
330. Tsuda H, Kawabata M, Yamamoto K, Inoue T, Umesaki N (1997) Prospective study to compare endometrial cytology and transvaginal ultrasonography for identification of endometrial malignancies [published erratum appears in Gynecol Oncol 1998;68(3):307]. Gynecol Oncol 65:383–386
331. Tunc M, Simsek T, Trak B, Uner M (1998) Endometrium adenocarcinoma with choriocarcinomatous differentiation: a case report. Eur J Gynaecol Oncol 19:489–491
332. Turner DA, Gershenson DM, Atkinson N, Sneige N, Wharton AT (1989) The prognostic significance of peritoneal cytology for stage I endometrial cancer. Obstet Gynecol 74:775–780
333. Ulbright TM, Roth LM (1985) Metastatic and independent cancers of the endometrium and ovary: a clinicopathologic study of 34 cases. Hum Pathol 16:28–34
334. Umpierre SA, Burke TW, Tornos C, Ordonez N, Levenback C, Morris M (1994) Immunocytochemical analysis of uterine papillary serous carcinomas for estrogen and progesterone receptors. Int J Gynecol Pathol 13:127–130
335. van der Putten HW, Baak JP, Koenders TJ, Kurver PH, Stolk HG, Stolte LA (1989) Prognostic value of quantitative pathologic features and DNA content in individual patients with stage I endometrial adenocarcinoma. Cancer (Phila) 63:1378–1387
336. van Hoeven KH, Hudock JA, Woodruff JM, Suhrland MJ (1995) Small cell neuroendocrine carcinoma of the endometrium. Int J Gynecol Pathol 14:21–29
337. van Leeuwen FE, Benraadt J, Coebergh JW, Kiemeney LA, Gimbrere CH, Otter R, et al (1994) Risk of endometrial cancer after tamoxifen treatment of breast cancer. Lancet 343:448–452
338. Van Rijswijk REN, Tognon G, Burger CW, Baak JP, Kenemans P, Vermorken JB (1994) The effect of chemotherapy on the different components of advanced carcinomas (malignant mixed mesodermal tumors) of the female genital tract. Int J Gynecol Cancer 4:52–60
339. Varela-Duran J, Nochomovitz LE, Prem KA, Dehner LP (1980) Postirradiation mixed mullerian tumors of the uterus: a comparative clinicopathologic study. Cancer (Phila) 45:1625–1631
340. Wada H, Enomoto T, Fujita M, Yoshino K, Nakashima R, Kurachi H, et al (1997) Molecular evidence that most but not all carcinosarcomas of the uterus are combination tumors. Cancer Res 57:5379–5385
341. Wagatsuma S, Konno R, Sato S, Yajima A (1998) Tumor angiogenesis, hepatocyte growth factor, and c-Met expression in endometrial carcinoma. Cancer (Phila) 82:520–530
342. Walker AN, Mills SE (1982) Serous papillary carcinoma of the endometrium. A clinicopathologic study of 11 cases. Diagn Gynecol Obstet 4:261–267
343. Warren CD, Horak C, Isacson C, Hedrick Ellenson L (1998) Extrauterine serous tumors in minimally invasive USC are metastatic. Mod Pathol 11:116A
344. Webb GA, Lagios MD (1987) Clear cell carcinoma of the endometrium. Am J Obstet Gynecol 156: 1486–1491
345. Weir HK, Sloan M, Kreiger N (1994) The relationship between cigarette smoking and the risk of endometrial neoplasms. Int J Epidemiol 23:261–266
346. Wheeler DT, Bell KA, Kurman RJ, Sherman ME (2000) Minimal uterine serous carcinoma: Diagnosis and clicopathologic correlation. Am J Surg Pathol 24:797–806
347. Wheelock JB, Krebs HB, Schneider V, Goplerud DR (1985) Uterine sarcoma: analysis of prognostic variables in 71 cases. Am J Obstet Gynecol 151:1016–1022
348. Wolfson AH, Sightler SE, Markoe AM, Schwade JG, Averette HE, Ganjei P, et al (1992) The prognostic significance of surgical staging for carcinoma of the endometrium. Gynecol Oncol 45:142–146
349. Wolfson AH, Wolfson DJ, Sittler SY, Breton L, Markoe AM, Schwade JG, et al (1994) A multivariate analysis of clinicopathologic factors for predicting outcome in uterine sarcomas. Gynecol Oncol 52:56–62
350. Yamada SD, Burger RA, Brewster WR, Anton D, Kohler MF, Monk BJ (2000) Pathologic variables and adjuvant therapy as predictors of recurrence and survival for patients with surgically evaluated carcinosarcoma of the uterus. Cancer (Phila) 88: 2782–2786
351. Yamauchi N, Sakamoto A, Uozaki H, Iihara K, Machinami R (1996) Immunohistochemical analysis of endometrial adenocarcinoma for bcl-2 and p53 in relation to expression of sex steroid receptor and proliferative activity [published erratum appears in Int J Gynecol Pathol 1996;15(4):369]. Int J Gynecol Pathol 15:202–208
352. Yamazawa K, Seki K, Matsui H, Kihara M, Sekiya S (2000) Prognostic factors in young women with endometrial carcinoma: a report of 20 cases and review of literature. Int J Gynecol Cancer 10:212–222
353. Yazigi R, Piver MS, Blumenson L (1983) Malignant peritoneal cytology as prognostic indicator in stage I endometrial cancer. Obstet Gynecol 62:359–362
354. Yoshida Y, Kurokawa T, Fukuno N, Nishikawa Y, Kamitani N, Kotsuji F (2000) Markers of apoptosis and angiogenesis indicate that carcinomatous components play an important role in the malignant behavior of uterine carcinosarcoma [In Process Citation]. Hum Pathol 31:1448–1454

355. Young RH, Scully RE (1992) Uterine carcinomas simulating microglandular hyperplasia. A report of six cases. Am J Surg Pathol 16:1092–1097
356. Zaino RJ, Kurman RJ (1988) Squamous differentiation in carcinoma of the endometrium: a critical appraisal of adenoacanthoma and adenosquamous carcinoma. Semin Diagn Pathol 5:154–171
357. Zaino RJ, Kurman R, Herbold D, Gliedman J, Bundy BN, Voet R, et al (1991) The significance of squamous differentiation in endometrial carcinoma. Data from a Gynecologic Oncology Group study. Cancer (Phila) 68:2293–2302
358. Zaino RJ (1995) Pathologic indicators of prognosis in endometrial adenocarcinoma. Selected aspects emphasizing the GOG experience. Gynecologic Oncology Group. Pathol Annu 30(pt 1):1–28
359. Zaino RJ, Kurman RJ, Diana KL, Morrow CP (1995) The utility of the revised International Federation of Gynecology and Obstetrics histologic grading of endometrial adenocarcinoma using a defined nuclear grading system. A Gynecologic Oncology Group study. Cancer (Phila) 75:81–86
360. Zaino RJ, Kurman RJ, Diana KL, Morrow CP (1996) Pathologic models to predict outcome for women with endometrial adenocarcinoma: the importance of the distinction between surgical stage and clinical stage—a Gynecologic Oncology Group study [published erratum appears in Cancer 1997;79(2):422]. Cancer (Phila) 77:1115–1121
361. Zaino RJ, Davis AT, Ohlsson-Wilhelm BM, Brunetto VL (1998) DNA content is an independent prognostic indicator in endometrial adenocarcinoma. A Gynecologic Oncology Group study. Int J Gynecol Pathol 17:312–319
362. Zaino RJ, Kurman RJ, Brunetto VL, Morrow CP, Bentley RC, Cappellari JO, et al (1998) Villoglandular adenocarcinoma of the endometrium: a clinicopathologic study of 61 cases. A Gynecologic Oncology Group study. Am J Surg Pathol 22:1379–1385
363. Zaloudek C, Hayashi GM, Ryan IP, Powell CB, Miller TR (1997) Microglandular adenocarcinoma of the endometrium: a form of mucinous adenocarcinoma that may be confused with microglandular hyperplasia of the cervix. Int J Gynecol Pathol 16:52–59
364. Zelmanowicz A, Hildesheim A, Sherman ME, Sturgeon SR, Kurman RJ, Barrett RJ, et al (1998) Evidence for a common etiology for endometrial carcinomas and malignant mixed müllerian tumors. Gynecol Oncol 69:253–257
365. Zheng W, Cao P, Zheng M, Kramer EE, Godwin TA (1996) p53 overexpression and bcl-2 persistence in endometrial carcinoma: comparison of papillary serous and endometrioid subtypes. Gynecol Oncol 61:167–174
366. Ziel HK, Finkle WD (1975) Increased risk of endometrial carcinoma among users of conjugated estrogens. N Engl J Med 293:1167–1170

13

Mesenchymal Tumors of the Uterus

Charles Zaloudek, M.D., and
Michael R. Hendrickson, M.D.

This chapter considers neoplasms of the uterus in which there is mesenchymal differentiation. Purely mesenchymal tumors, such as those derived from smooth muscle and endometrial stroma, are considered, as are some benign and malignant neoplasms in which there are mixtures of epithelium and connective tissue.

The capacity of neoplasms arising in the uterus to form heterologous mesenchymal elements is a reflection of the potentiality of the uterine primordium, which is formed from an anlage of coelomic lining cells and subjacent mesenchymal cells. Within the mesodermal primordium that is to become the uterus, the distinction between duct epithelium and mesenchyme is lost. The müllerian duct epithelial cells seem to form part of the mesenchyme accompanying the duct before the formation of the uterus (see Chapter 1, Embryology of the Female Genital Tract and Disorders of Abnormal Sexual Development). A distinction between the precursors of the endometrium and myometrium is not possible. Neoplasms that subsequently arise in the uterus may express the bipotentiality of their ancestry by forming a mixture of epithelial and mesodermal components as in the biphasic adenofibroma, adenosarcoma, and

Table 13.1. Classification of mesenchymal and mixed tumors of the uterus

Smooth muscle tumors
Leiomyoma
Mitotically active leiomyoma
Cellular leiomyoma
Hemorrhagic cellular leiomyoma
Atypical leiomyoma
Epithelioid leiomyoma
Myxoid leiomyoma
Vascular leiomyoma
Lipoleiomyoma
Smooth muscle tumor of uncertain malignant potential
Leiomyosarcoma
Epithelioid leiomyosarcoma
Myxoid leiomyosarcoma
Other smooth muscle tumors
Metastasizing leiomyoma
Intravenous leiomyomatosis
Disseminated peritoneal leiomyomatosis
Endometrial stromal tumors
Stromal nodule
Low-grade endometrial stromal sarcoma
High-grade endometrial stromal sarcoma
Mixed endometrial stromal–smooth muscle tumors
Adenomatoid tumor
Other mesenchymal tumors (benign and malignant)
Homologous
Heterologous
Mixed epithelial–nonepithelial tumors
Benign
Adenofibroma
Adenomyoma
Atypical polypoid adenomyoma
Malignant
Adenosarcoma (homologous or heterologous)
Mixed müllerian tumor (carcinosarcoma)
Homologous or heterologous
Miscellaneous tumors
Sex cord-like tumors
Neuroectodermal tumors
Lymphoma
Other

mixed müllerian tumor (the latter is discussed in Chapter 12, Endometrial Carcinoma).

Mesenchymal tumors of the uterus, other than leiomyomas, are uncommon. Sarcomas, for example, comprise only 3% of uterine malignancies. A comprehensive classification of nonepithelial neoplasms of the uterus developed by the World Health Organization (WHO) is shown in Table 13.1.[261]

Proper pathologic study of a mesenchymal tumor of the uterus is predicated on careful gross examination and adequate sectioning. The tumor should be examined thoroughly, and one block of tissue should be taken for each centimeter of tumor diameter, except from grossly typical leiomyomas; even the latter may have to be examined extensively if the microscopic appearance is unusual. Three major goals of the pathologic examination of potentially malignant mesenchymal tumors are to determine the type of tumor margin (expansile or infiltrating), to evaluate the depth of myometrial invasion, and to determine whether the tumor involves the serosa or extends beyond the uterus. Tissue samples should be taken with these requirements in mind.

Smooth Muscle Tumors

Smooth muscle neoplasms of the uterus are extremely common, and most are leiomyomas. These tumors may be incidental in uteri removed for other reasons but they are also frequently responsible for a variety of common gynecologic and obstetric difficulties. Histologically, almost all leiomyomas are easily identified as being of smooth muscle origin and benign. A small percentage of uterine smooth muscle neoplasms are leiomyosarcomas, which, by modern diagnostic criteria, are highly malignant neoplasms. Most leiomyosarcomas are easily recognized both as showing smooth muscle differentiation and as malignant. A small number of uterine smooth muscle proliferations pose difficult diagnostic challenges for a variety of reasons.

Our discussion of smooth muscle neoplasms first presents a general approach to the evaluation of uterine smooth muscle neoplasms, detailing the individual features that need to be assessed: the type of differentiation, the degree of cellularity, the mitotic index, the presence and degree of cytologic atypia, and the presence of necrosis and its pattern. Second, we gather the facts of epidemiology, pathology, molecular biology, cytogenetics, natural history and treatment around a discussion of each of the named smooth muscle entities.

Evaluation of Smooth Muscle Neoplasms

The most effective way of distinguishing clinically benign from clinically malignant uterine smooth muscle neoplasms is through the use of multivariate criteria; that is, criteria that involve considering several microscopic features as an ensemble. These features include differentiated cell type, the presence and type of necrosis, the degree of cytologic atypia, the mitotic index, and the relationship of the process to surrounding normal structures, including extrauterine sites.

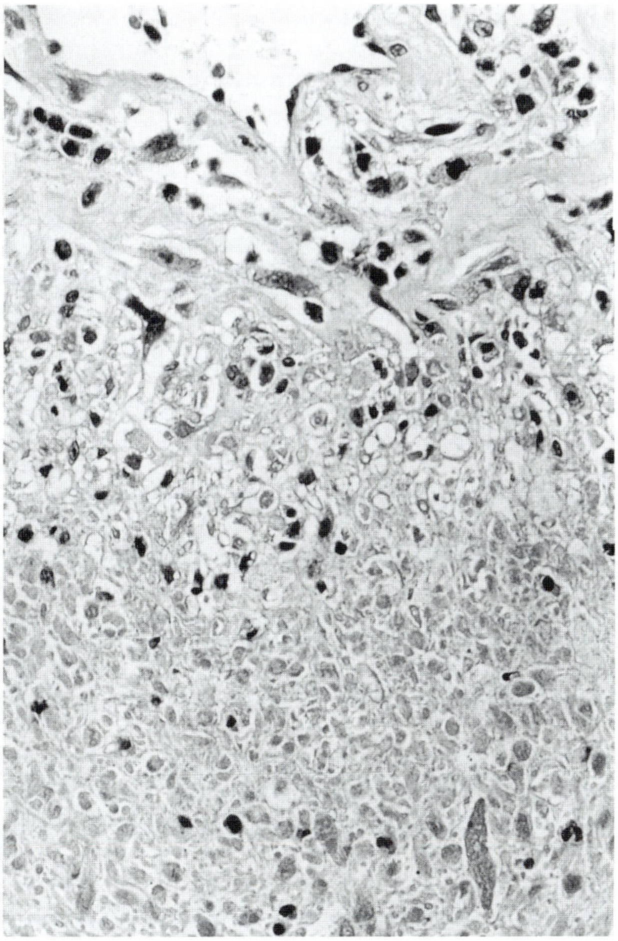

Fig. 13.1. Coagulative tumor cell necrosis. Viable cells are present only around the blood vessel on the top. Ghostlike outlines of necrotic atypical tumor cells can still be discerned.

Differentiated Cell Type

The term *usual smooth muscle differentiation* denotes a pattern of differentiation recapitulating that of the constituent cells of the normal myometrium. Usual smooth muscle cells are elongated, possess distinct cell membranes, and have readily apparent eosinophilic, sometimes fibrillar cytoplasm. These cells grow in a fascicular arrangement.

Epithelioid smooth muscle cells are round or polygonal and have eosinophilic to colorless cytoplasm. They may have perinuclear cytoplasmic vacuoles or there may be a perinuclear rim of eosinophilic cytoplasm although the rest of the cytoplasm is clear. When the cytoplasm is completely clear, the label *clear cell* is used.

Myxoid smooth muscle proliferations feature widely spaced stellate cells with inapparent cytoplasm embedded in a myxoid matrix. Malignant myxoid smooth muscle neoplasms exhibit varying degrees of cytologic atypia and often have an appearance reminiscent of myxoid malignant fibrous histiocytoma of the soft tissues.

Less common types of differentiation, such as fat and skeletal muscle, are discussed later (see "Leiomyomas with Heterologous Elements").

Patterns of Necrosis

The presence or absence and type of necrosis are powerful predictors of clinical behavior.[19] Two patterns of necrosis in uterine smooth muscle tumors are diagnostically important: *coagulative tumor cell necrosis* and *hyalinizing (or "infarction") necrosis*.[124]

In coagulative tumor cell necrosis, there is an abrupt transition between necrotic and preserved cells (Fig. 13.1). The hematoxyphilia of the nuclei is often retained in the necrotic cells, and usually there is no associated inflammation. The characteristic low-power microscopic pattern is one of blood vessels cuffed by viable cells surrounded by a sea of necrotic tumor. Coagulative tumor cell necrosis is commonly present in clinically malignant smooth muscle neoplasms. In contrast, hyalinizing necrosis has a distinctly zonal pattern with central necrosis, a more peripheral zone of granulation tissue, and, at the periphery, a variable amount of hyaline eosinophilic collagen interposed between the central degenerated region and peripheral preserved smooth muscle cells (Fig. 13.2). This pattern is highly reminiscent of an infarction in various stages of evolution. When shadow cells or nuclei are discernible in the necrosis, there is little hyperchromasia or nuclear pleomorphism. Another pattern of necrosis that may be seen in ulcerated submucous leiomyomas features acute inflammatory cells and an associated peripheral reparative process.

Cytologic Atypia

Several studies have demonstrated a relationship between *cytologic atypia* and clinical behavior in uterine smooth muscle neoplasms.[19,32,208,226] The problem, as always, is defining "significant atypia" in a way that is reproducible and can be communicated to others. Bell et al. found that a two-tiered scheme of absent to mild atypia and moderate to severe atypia is reasonably reproducible.[19] They defined moderate to severe atypia as follows: nuclear hyperchromatism and pleomorphism that is obvious at scanning power (Fig. 13.3). Enlarged and sometimes abnormal mitotic figures are a frequent finding. Most commonly, moderate to severe atypia is diffusely present throughout the neoplasm but it can, occasionally, be present only focally. In contrast, absent or mild atypia features uniform cells with no more than mild nuclear pleomorphism (Fig.

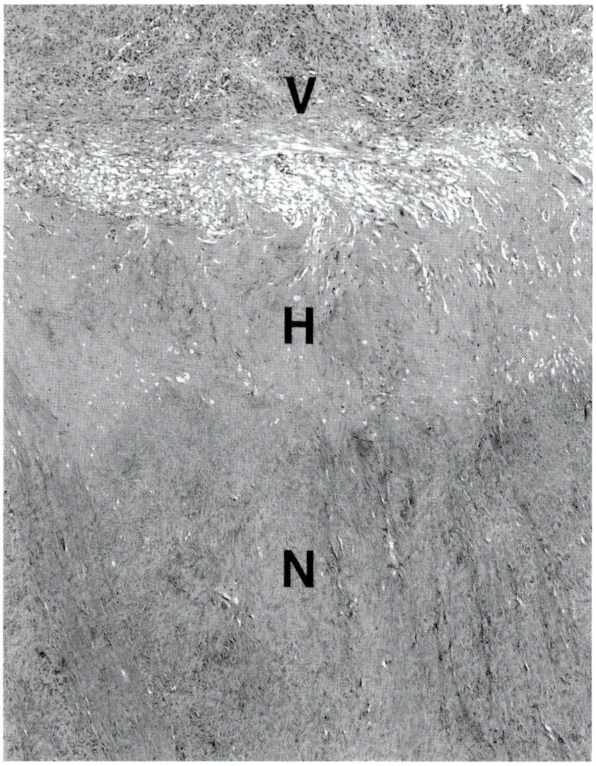

Fig. 13.2. Hyaline necrosis. An area of bland necrosis (*N*) is separated from viable spindle-shaped tumor cells (*V*) by a zone of hyalinized collagen (*H*).

13.3). The chromatin of the constituent cells is typically fine to granular. The nuclei may be enlarged in comparison to those of the cells comprising the surrounding myometrium, but the enlargement is uniform throughout the tumor. More than one or two enlarged abnormal mitotic figures place the tumor in the moderate to severe atypia group.

MITOTIC INDEX

The *mitotic index* is expressed in terms of the number of definite mitotic figures per 10 high-power fields.[131,299] Compulsive mitosis counting, fortunately, is not always necessary; the required level of compulsiveness depends on associated features such as significant atypia or tumor cell necrosis. The mitotic index is determined by first finding the area with the highest density of mitotic figures and then counting them in that area. The slide is searched at low magnification for the most mitotically active area. Then, mitotic counts are performed at high magnification in four sets of 10 randomly chosen contiguous fields. The mitotic index is expressed as the average number of mitotic figures per 10 high-power fields. Care must be taken not to count lymphocytes, karyorrhectic debris, precipitated hematoxylin, or mast cells as mitotic figures. Most reliable are mitotic figures in metaphase, anaphase, or telophase. A critical review of mitotic counting has been recently presented.[209]

RELATIONSHIP TO SURROUNDING NORMAL STRUCTURES AND THE ANATOMIC DISTRIBUTION OF THE PROCESS

It is important to note the relationship of the smooth muscle neoplasm to the surrounding myometrium and uterine vessels and to determine whether there is any extrauterine extension. Infiltrative margins, intravascular growth, and extrauterine spread, although commonly encountered in uterine malignancies are not, when seen as isolated findings, diagnostic of sarcoma. It is important to be aware of some relatively rare smooth muscle proliferations that are either benign or clinically low-grade processes that mimic leiomyosarcoma by virtue of their relationship to normal uterine structures or their extrauterine extension.

Leiomyoma

Leiomyomas are the most common uterine neoplasms.[304] They are noted clinically in 20–30% of women over 30 years of age, and are found in as many as 75% of hysterectomy specimens when a systematic search is conducted.[63] Most leiomyomas are detected in middle-aged women. They are uncommon in women less than 30 years of age; however, the youngest patient on record was 13 years old. Some leiomyomas apparently shrink after the menopause, but their frequency does not decrease.[63] Leiomyomas are more common in black women than in white women.[154]

The growth of leiomyomas is affected by the hormonal milieu.[6] Leiomyomas contain estrogen and progesterone receptors, which can be demonstrated biochemically and immunohistochemically.[303] Leiomyomas may increase in size during estrogen therapy, and most decrease in size when the patient is treated with a gonadotropin-releasing hormone (GnRH) agonist.[4,240,269,279,298] Progestins, progesterone, hormone replacement therapy, clomiphene use, and pregnancy occasionally are associated with a rapid increase in the size of leiomyomas and sometimes produce hemorrhagic degeneration.[268]

Nonrandom inactivation of the X chromosome, demonstrated by glucose-6-phosphate dehydrogenase isoform expression and other techniques, indicates that leiomyomas are a proliferation of a single clone of smooth muscle cells. Each one of the multiple leiomyomas in a particular uterus appears to be a distinct clone.[128,181,236] Cytogenetic studies provide further evidence of the clonal nature of the

a

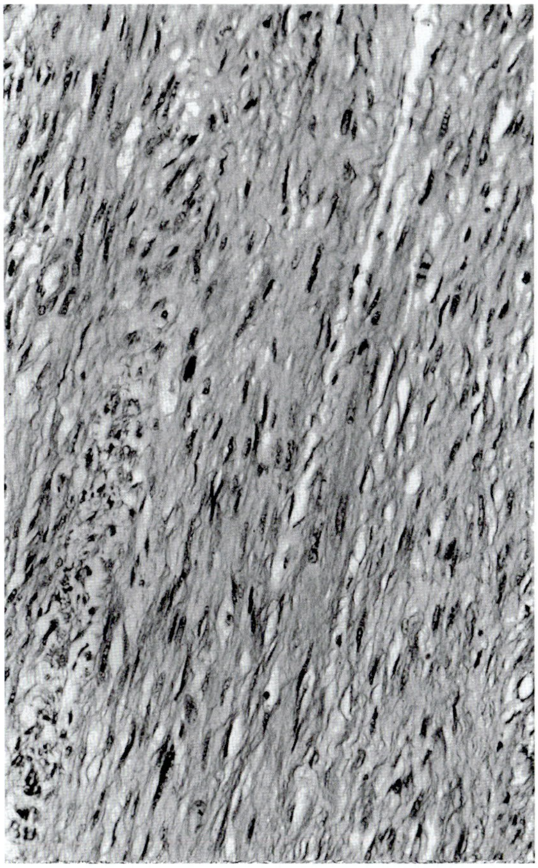

b

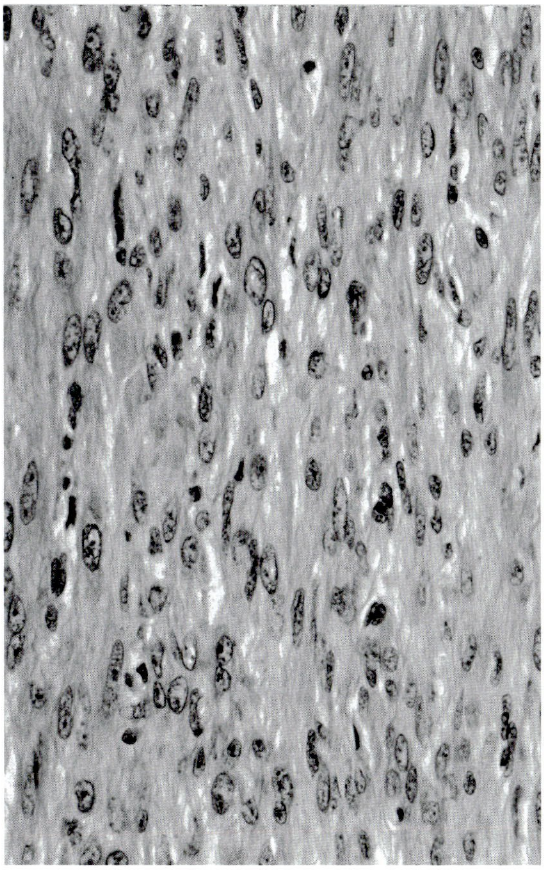

c

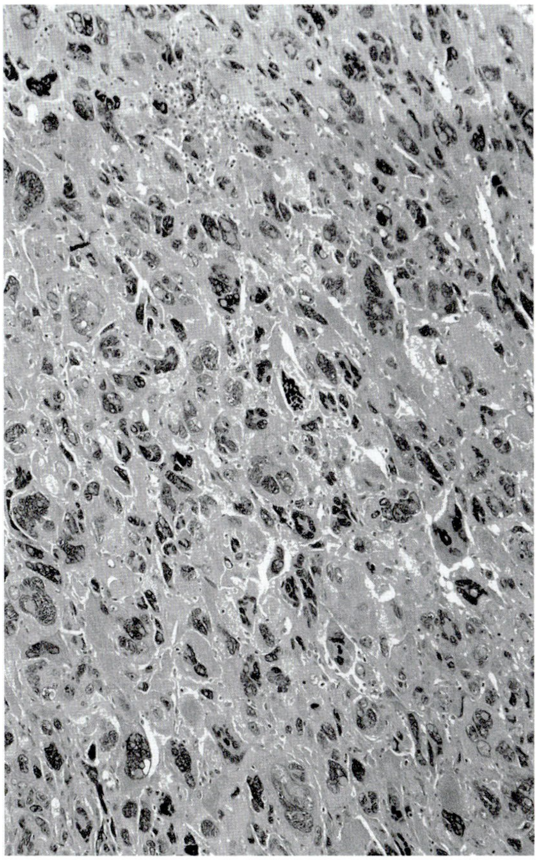

Fig. 13.3. Nuclear atypia in smooth muscle tumors of the uterus. a: Diffuse mild atypia. Uniform mild atypia characterizes this infiltrating smooth muscle neoplasm. **b**: Diffuse mild atypia. This example is at the high end of mild atypia and is associated with a scattering of inflammatory cells. **c**: Severe atypia. Nuclear pleomorphism against a background of diffuse severe atypia of spindled cells.

smooth muscle cell proliferation in many leiomyomas.[236]

Clinical Features

The clinical presentation of leiomyomas depends on their size and location.[172] Leiomyomas cause many signs and symptoms, the most common of which are pain, a sensation of pressure, and abnormal uterine bleeding. Even small leiomyomas, when submucosal, can cause bleeding due to compression of the overlying endometrium and compromise of its vascular supply. In some instances, infertility is attributed to the presence of leiomyomas. Large tumors can be detected during pelvic examination because they produce uterine enlargement or an irregular uterine contour. Some leiomyomas are pedunculated and protrude through the cervical os. On rare occasions, subserosal pedunculated leiomyomas undergo torsion, infarction, and separation from the uterus. Secondary infection of leiomyomas can result in fever, leukocytosis, and an elevated sedimentation rate. Among the complications of pregnancy ascribed to leiomyomas are spontaneous abortion, premature rupture of membranes, dystocia, inversion of the uterus, and postpartum hemorrhage.

Gross Findings

Despite the variety of histologic subtypes of leiomyoma, all are grossly similar. Multiple leiomyomas are present in two-thirds of women with these neoplasms.[63] Leiomyomas are spherical and firm; they bulge above the surrounding myometrium from which they are easily shelled out. The cut surfaces are white to tan, with a whorled trabecular pattern (Fig. 13.4). Leiomyomas can be located anywhere in the myometrium. Submucosal leiomyomas compress the overlying endometrium. As they enlarge, they bulge into the endometrial cavity. Rare examples become pedunculated and prolapse through the cervix. Intramural leiomyomas are the most common. Subserosal leiomyomas can become pedunculated and, if there is torsion and necrosis of the pedicle, the leiomyoma can lose its connection with the uterus. Very rarely, some become attached to another pelvic structure (parasitic leiomyoma). The appearance of a leiomyoma is commonly altered by degenerative changes. Submucosal leiomyomas are frequently ulcerated and hemorrhagic. Hemorrhage and necrosis can be observed in leiomyomas, particularly if they are large or occur in women who are pregnant or undergoing high-dose progestin therapy. Dark red areas represent hemorrhage, and sharply demarcated yellow areas reflect necrosis. The damaged smooth muscle is replaced eventually by firm white or translucent collagenous tissue. Cystic degeneration also occurs, and some leiomyomas become extensively calcified.

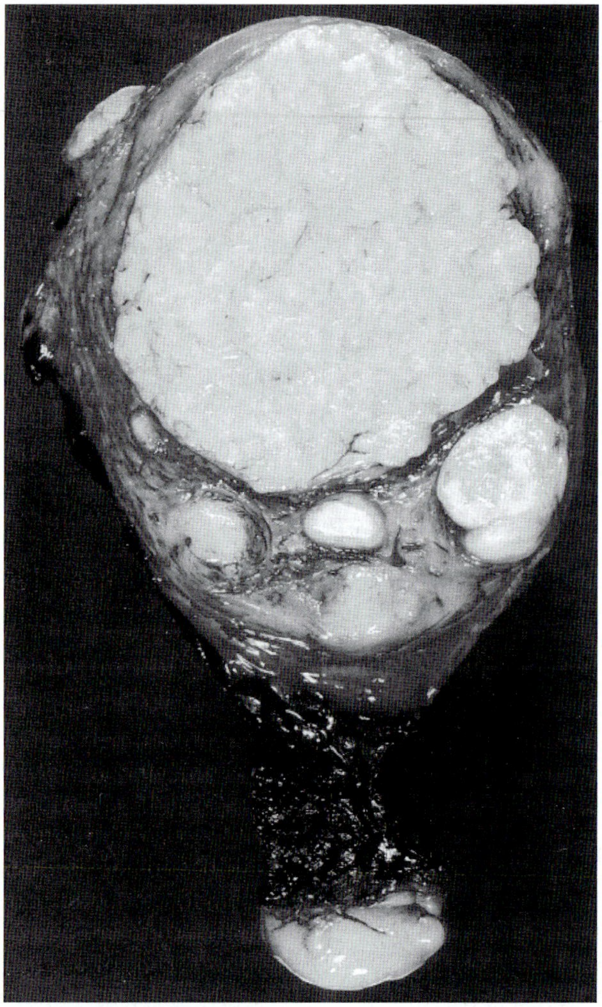

Fig. 13.4. Enlarged uterus containing multiple leiomyomas. The leiomyomas have a whorled white-tan cut surface that bulges above the surrounding myometrium.

Microscopic Findings

Typical leiomyomas are composed of whorled, anastomosing fascicles of uniform fusiform smooth muscle cells. The spindle-shaped cells have indistinct borders and abundant fibrillar eosinophilic cytoplasm (Fig. 13.5). Nuclei are elongated with blunt or tapered ends and have finely dispersed chromatin and small nucleoli. Mitotic figures usually are infrequent. Most leiomyomas are more cellular than the surrounding myometrium; those that are not are identified by their nodular circumscription and by the disorderly arrangement of the smooth muscle fascicles within them, which are out of align-

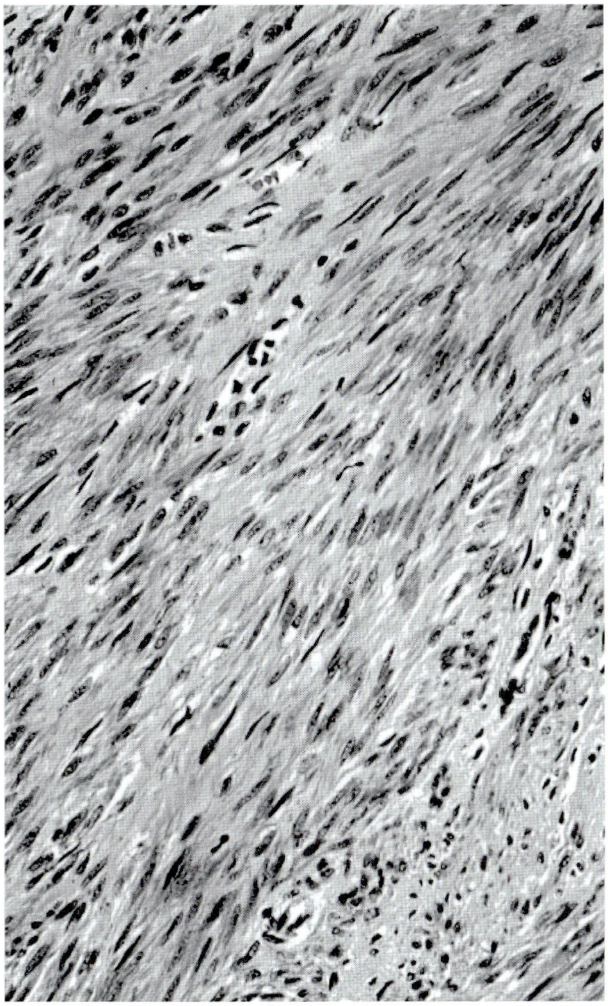

Fig. 13.5. Leiomyoma of the uterus. The spindle-shaped tumor cells have cytologically bland relatively uniform fusiform nuclei with fine chromatin and small nucleoli. The cytoplasm is abundant, eosinophilic, and fibrillar.

ment with the surrounding myometrium. Degenerative changes are common in leiomyomas. Hyaline fibrosis is present in more than 60%, particularly in postmenopausal women.[62] Edema is present in about 50% of leiomyomas and, on occasion, marked hydropic change can mimic the appearance of a myxoid smooth muscle tumor or produce a pattern that can be confused with intravenous leiomyomatosis.[56,57] There are significant areas of hemorrhage, which tend to be zonal and sharply demarcated, in about 10% of leiomyomas, and cystic degeneration and microcalcification each occur in about 4%. Hemorrhage, edema, myxoid change, hypercellular foci, and cellular hypertrophy occur in leiomyomas in women who are pregnant or taking progestins (see following, "Hemorrhagic Cellular Leiomyoma"). Progestational agents are associated with a slight increase in mitotic activity, but not to the level observed in a leiomyosarcoma.

The margins of most leiomyomas are microscopically circumscribed, but some benign tumors interdigitate with the surrounding myometrium, occasionally extensively (see following, "Dissecting Leiomyomas"). Submucous leiomyomas, particularly if they protrude into the endometrial cavity, may display extensive necrosis, often with acute inflammatory cells. Not infrequently, there is increased mitotic activity in the tumor cells near areas of necrosis. On the other hand, the coagulative tumor cell necrosis common in leiomyosarcoma is not often associated with acute inflammation. In addition, the outlines of cells are prominent in the latter whereas they are inconspicuous or absent in submucous necrosis. Also, the mitotic figures seen in conjunction with inflammatory necrosis have normal morphology.

Immunohistochemistry

Smooth muscle cells in the myometrium and within smooth muscle tumors react with antibodies to muscle-specific actin, alpha-smooth muscle actin, desmin, and caldesmon.[87] There is immunoreactivity with vimentin, but the intensity of staining and the proportion of cells that stain are less than with the muscle-specific antibodies.[87] Cytokeratin immunoreactivity is frequently observed in myometrium and in smooth muscle tumors, the extent and intensity of reactivity depending on the antibodies used and the fixation of the specimen.[29,31,87,116] Epithelial membrane antigen is usually negative in smooth muscle tumors (see Chapter 25, Immunohistochemistry).

Cytogenetics

A large literature has appeared in recent years concerning the cytogenetic abnormalities in leiomyomas. Approximately 40% of uterine leiomyomas have chromosomal abnormalities detectable by conventional cytogenetic analysis, including t(12;14)(q15;q23-24), rearrangements involving the short arm of chromosome 6, and interstitial deletions of the long arm of chromosome 7.[236,277] This growing body of literature may in time shed some light on the development of this extremely common neoplasm but, to date, has little diagnostic relevance.

Clinical Behavior and Treatment

Most leiomyomas are asymptomatic, and only a minority require treatment. Therapy is indicated only if leiomyomas are symptomatic, interfere with fertility, enlarge rapidly, or pose diagnostic problems.[172] Sometimes they can be excised (myomectomy) but if they are large or multiple, a hysterectomy may be required.[309,314] Treatment with leuprolide acetate or another gonadotropin-releasing hormone agonist (GnRHa) results in shrinkage of leiomyomas, a decrease in uterine volume, and alleviation of the patient's symptoms.[4,269,279] The maximum effect is noted after 8 to 12 weeks. The leiomyomas increase in size again with cessation of the GnRH agonist therapy. Such therapy can be used before surgery to decrease uterine size (facilitating myomectomy or permitting treatment by vaginal rather than abdominal hysterectomy) and to reduce the risk of hemorrhage during surgery. A discussion of alternative pharmacological strategies, including the antiprogesterone RU-486, has recently been presented.[82]

Specific Subtypes of Leiomyoma

Most subtypes of leiomyoma are chiefly of interest in that they mimic malignancy in one or more respects. These subtypes are *mitotically active leiomyoma, cellular leiomyoma, hemorrhagic cellular leiomyoma, leiomyoma with bizarre nuclei, epithelioid leiomyoma,* and *myxoid leiomyoma.* Other leiomyoma variants—*vascular leiomyoma, leiomyoma with other elements,* and *leiomyomas with hematopoietic elements* are more curiosities than diagnostic problems.

Mitotically Active Leiomyoma

Occasionally, a typical-appearing leiomyoma in a premenopausal woman will have 5 or more mitotic figures (MF) per 10 high-power fields (HPF) (Fig. 13.6); these are designated as *mitotically active leiomyomas.*[19,208,226,234] The number of mitotic figures is usually 5–9 MF/10 HPF, but occasional mitotically active leiomyomas with 10–20 MF/10 HPF have been reported. The clinical evolution is benign, even if the neoplasm is treated by myomectomy.[19,208,226,234] It is imperative that this diagnosis not be used for neoplasms that exhibit moderate to severe nuclear atypia, for those that contain abnormal mitotic figures, or for those that demonstrate zones of tumor cell necrosis.

Leiomyomas removed during the secretory phase of the menstrual cycle have a significantly increased mitotic index compared to those removed during menses or during the proliferative phase.[150] Also, leiomyomas removed from women who are taking progestins have a higher mitotic rate than that observed in women who are taking a combination of estrogen and progestin or who are not taking any exogenous hormones.[293] The patient's hormonal status may play a role in the increased number of mitotic figures seen in mitotically active leiomyomas.[234] No studies of gonadotropin-releasing hormone agonists (GnRHa) have demonstrated a difference in mitotic index between treated and untreated patients, although an increase may be seen several weeks after cessation of treatment.[262] In one study comparing leiomyomas removed from treated patients with tumors from untreated controls, cellular proliferation (Ki-67 and proliferating cell nuclear antigen [PCNA] labeling indices), estrogen receptors, and progesterone receptors were decreased in tumors from treated patients, but a statistically significant decrease in the mitotic index was not observed.[306]

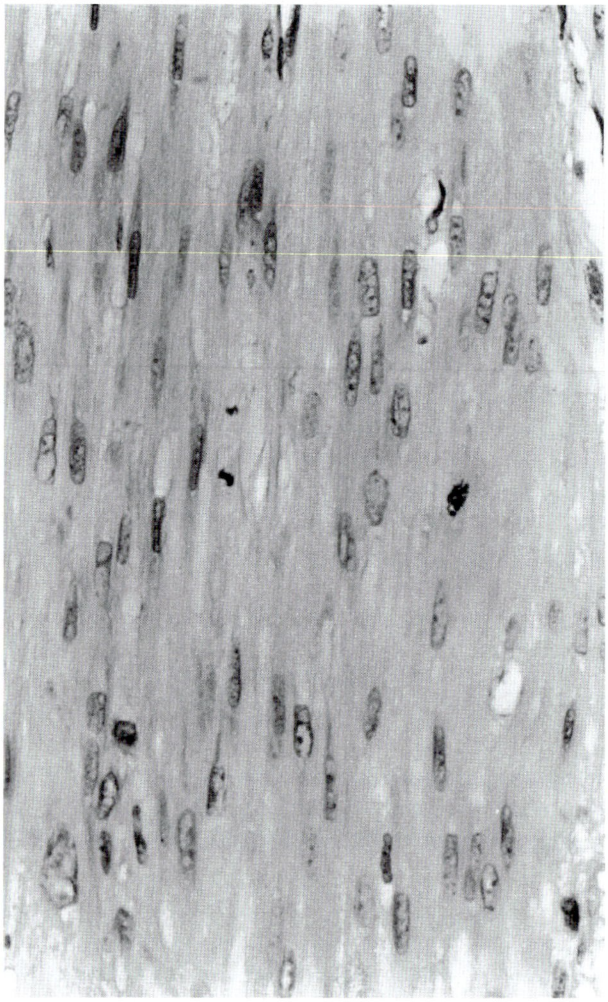

Fig. 13.6. Mitotically active leiomyoma. The tumor is not hypercellular and there is no nuclear atypia, but two mitotic figures (*center*) are present in this high-power field.

Cellular Leiomyoma

According to the WHO definition, a *cellular leiomyoma* is one in which the cellularity is "significantly" greater than the surrounding myometrium; "significantly" translates, operationally, into a use of the modifier "cellular" in less than 5% of leiomyomas.[261] The isolated finding of hypercellularity may suggest a diagnosis of leiomyosarcoma, but cellular leiomyoma lacks tumor cell necrosis, has few mitotic figures, and lacks the moderate to severe cytologic atypia seen in leiomyosarcoma.[19,32,42] Palisading of nuclei, reminiscent of those seen in the Verocay bodies of a neurilemoma, is present in some cellular leiomyomas.[86,110] The ultrastructural appearance of these tumors, however, is that of the ordinary leiomyoma.[86,110,183] Prolapse of submucosal leiomyomas may result in accentuated cellularity.[185] A cellular leiomyoma composed of small cells with scanty cytoplasm can be confused with an endometrial stromal tumor. This problem becomes particularly difficult with what has been termed the highly cellular leiomyoma (Fig. 13.7).[214]

Features that help distinguish a cellular leiomyoma from a stromal tumor are the spindled shape of the cells, the fusiform shape of the nuclei, the reticulin pattern, and the absence of a plexiform vasculature. Reticulin fibers tend to parallel the fascicles of cells in a leiomyoma, but the reticulin network surrounds individual tumor cells in an endometrial stromal tumor. Additionally, Oliva et al. emphasized the presence of large thick-walled muscular vessels (Fig. 13.7) as features that serve to distinguish a highly cellular leiomyoma from a stromal proliferation.[214] Although some authors have reported that smooth muscle cells and stromal cells have immunophenotypic similarities,[89,100] marked diffuse staining with muscle markers, particularly desmin, is more suggestive of a smooth muscle tumor than of a stromal neoplasm.[214] In a hysterectomy specimen, the relationship of the proliferation to the surrounding normal structures can be appreciated. In the absence of myoinvasion or vascular invasion, the differential lies between two benign conditions: highly cellular leiomyoma and stromal nodule. When there is intravascular tumor, the distinction between endometrial stromal and smooth muscle differentiation becomes clinically relevant as the differential diagnosis lies between stromal sarcoma and intravenous leiomyomatosis.

Care must be taken to consider benign alternatives to stromal sarcoma when a cellular mesenchymal proliferation is recovered in an endometrial sampling. Thus, three issues need to be considered in this setting: (1) what differentiation does the proliferation exhibit (smooth muscle or endometrial stromal); (2) are the criteria of malignancy evaluable; and, finally, (3) are the criteria of malignancy met? In a "low penalty" hysterectomy (older women; young women who have no interest in having children) setting, the issue is usually resolved by what amounts to a diagnostic hysterectomy. In the "high penalty" hysterectomy (young women wishing to retain their fertility; older women who are poor surgical candidates) setting, diagnostic modalities should be considered (e.g., hysteroscopy, imaging studies, repeat sampling) that might clarify the situation without the need of hysterectomy. Again, the important point is that not all cellular, spindle cell proliferations recovered in a curettage are stromal sarcoma; the clinically in-

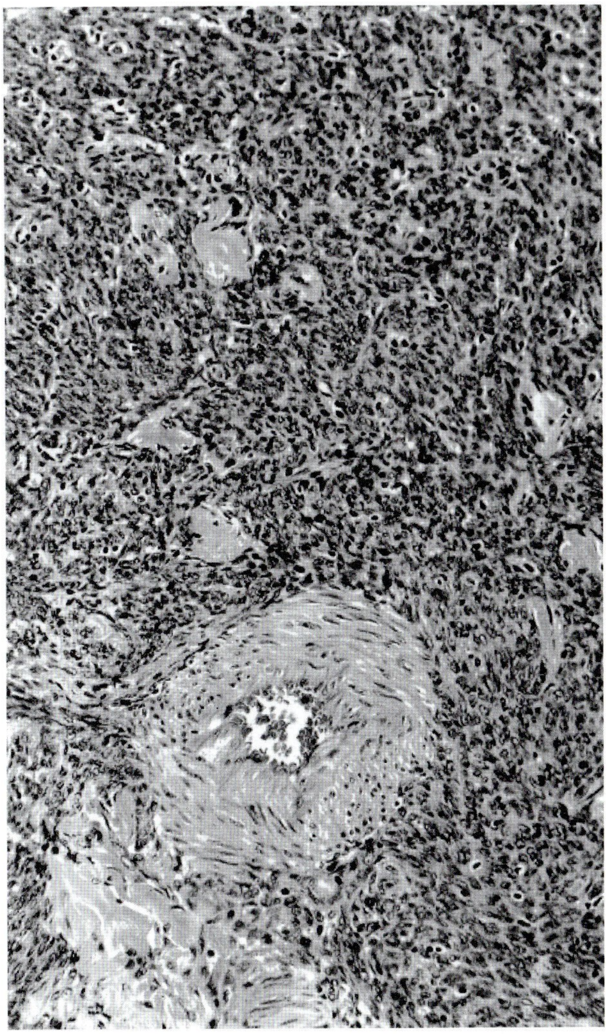

Fig. 13.7. Highly cellular leiomyoma. The tumor is markedly cellular, and the cells are small and rounded. The large blood vessel is a feature that suggests a smooth muscle tumor.

nocuous cellular leiomyoma is a highly probable alternative. Rarely, some uterine neoplasms appear to be composed of a mixture of stromal and smooth muscle cells.[19,212]

Hemorrhagic Cellular Leiomyoma and Hormone-Induced Changes

Hemorrhagic cellular leiomyoma, or "apoplectic" leiomyoma, is a form of cellular leiomyoma that is found in women who are taking oral contraceptives or who are either pregnant or postpartum.[198,204] Multifocal stellate hemorrhages are present grossly (Fig. 13.8). Microscopically, the leiomyoma is cellular and contains patchy areas of hemorrhage and edema. Necrosis generally is not present. Mitotic figures, which may be slightly increased in number, are detected mainly within a narrow zone resembling granulation tissue around areas of hemorrhage. In contrast to leiomyosarcoma, neither atypical mitotic figures nor significant cytologic atypia are present, and the neoplasm has a circumscribed, compressive margin.

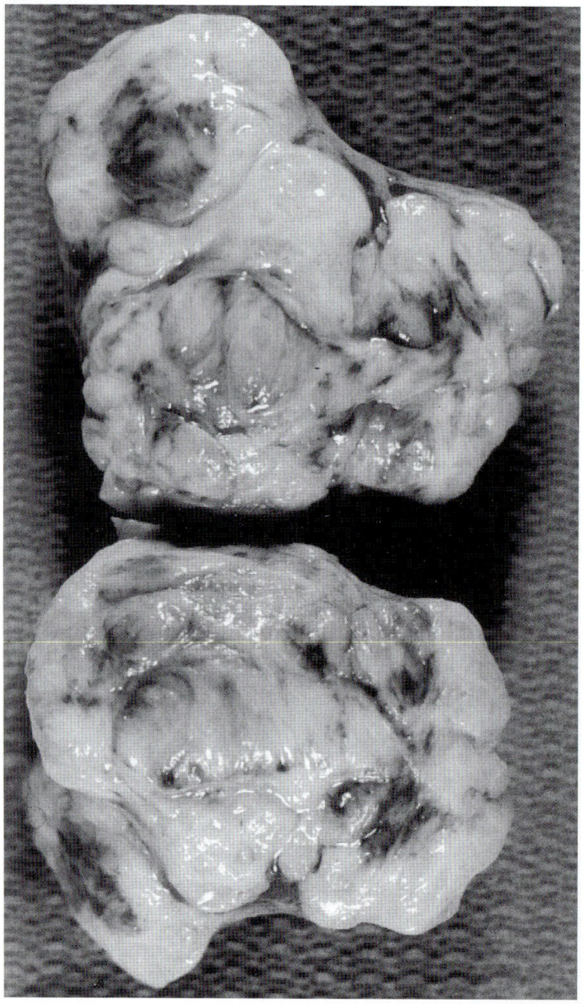

Fig. 13.8. Hemorrhagic cellular leiomyoma. Multiple foci of hemorrhage are visible on the cut surfaces of a myomectomy specimen.

With the advent of gonadotropin-releasing hormone agonist (GnRHa) therapy to shrink leiomyomata, a substantial body of literature has accumulated concerning the mechanism of shrinkage and the histologic correlates of this process. Some workers have found no differences between GnRHa-treated and untreated leiomyomas,[119,278] whereas others have been able to detect changes in tumor vasculature, pattern of necrosis, proliferation index, and cellularity.[58,59,64,72,144,249,306] None of these differences are sufficiently striking to be of practical importance in distinguishing leiomyoma from leiomyosarcoma. On rare occasions, leiomyosarcomas have been discovered in patients undergoing GnRHa therapy.[188,189]

Leiomyomas with Bizarre Nuclei (Atypical Leiomyoma)

As an isolated finding, cytologic atypia, even when severe, is an unreliable criterion for the diagnosis of clinically malignant uterine smooth muscle tumors because it can be seen in clinically benign, otherwise banal smooth muscle neoplasms.[19,76] A leiomyoma that exhibits moderate to severe cytologic atypia is designated an *atypical leiomyoma*. The atypical cells may be distributed throughout the leiomyoma or may be focal; they have enlarged hyperchromatic nuclei with prominent chromatin clumping and, often, smudging (Fig. 13.9). Large cytoplasmic pseudonuclear inclusions are often present. Multinucleated tumor giant cells can be numerous and prompt the name "bizarre" or "symplastic" leiomyoma. These changes have been noted in leiomyomas excised from women taking progestins.[90,232] By definition, mitotic figures cannot be present in numbers in excess of 10 MF/10 HPF in an atypical leiomyoma, and tumor cell necrosis must be absent. A mitotic index higher than 10 MF/10 HPF in such a tumor is diagnostic of malignancy (Table 13.2).[19] A smooth muscle tumor featuring diffuse moderate to severe atypia and coagulative tumor cell necrosis should be considered a leiomyosarcoma regardless of the mitotic index.

It is worth noting that leiomyosarcomas can vary greatly in appearance and may contain areas that lack the typical features of hypercellularity, cytologic atypia, and increased mitotic activity. Thus, extensive sampling is important to rule out leiomyosarcoma; atypical leiomyoma is a diagnosis of exclusion. The age of the patient must also be considered, as atypical leiomyoma is less common in postmenopausal women. A careful search for other features of

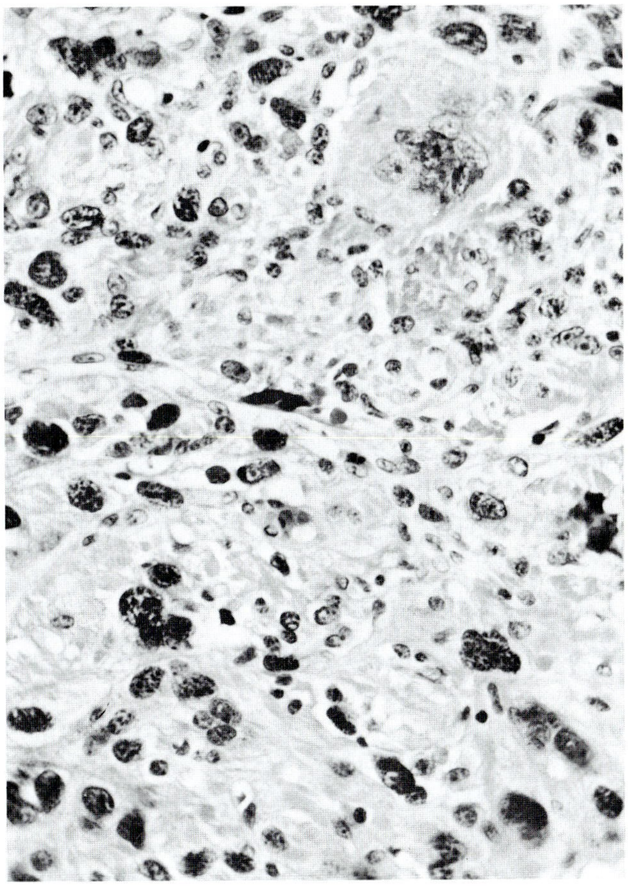

Fig. 13.9. Atypical leiomyoma. Tumor cells have single or multiple pleomorphic hyperchromatic nuclei with coarse, smudged chromatin.

leiomyosarcoma is indicated when a smooth muscle tumor containing atypical cells is detected in an older woman.

The natural history of smooth muscle neoplasms featuring mitotic indices of less than 10 MF/10 HPF, that lack tumor cell necrosis, and that exhibit diffuse moderate to severe atypia remains controversial. Downes and Hart reported a benign clinical course in their series of 24 cases of atypical leiomyoma.[76] On the other hand, Bell et al. found 1 clinically malignant tumor in 43 cases (2%), all of which had at least 2 years follow-up.[19] These workers considered the entire group of neoplasms with moderate to severe atypia, a mitotic index less than 10 MF/10 HPF, and without tumor cell necrosis as "atypical leiomyomas with a low risk of recurrence." The differences in the findings probably are related to differences in sample size in a neoplastic process with a low recurrence rate. Peters et al. reported a series of 15 smooth muscle tumors of uncertain malignant potential (STUMP) and confirmed both the low failure rate in this category and the slow tempo of disease when recurrence did occur.[228] Although necrosis was not recorded, at least some of the tumors in their group would qualify as atypical leiomyomas using the Bell et al. criteria. In a recent study, Downes and Hart found that the combination of aneuploidy and high MIB-1 activity served to distinguish leiomyosarcoma from atypical leiomyoma.[77]

Epithelioid Leiomyoma

This category includes *leiomyoblastoma, clear cell leiomyoma*, and *plexiform leiomyoma*.[158] Epithelioid smooth muscle tumors have the same histologic appearance in the uterus as in other sites in the body. The mean age of women with *epithelioid leiomyoma* is in the fifth decade, with a range of 30–78 years.[10,158,213,233] Epithelioid leiomyomas are yellow or gray and may contain areas of hemorrhage. They tend to be softer than the usual leiomyoma. Most are solitary, and they can occur in any part of the uterus. The median diameter is 6–7 cm.

Table 13.2. Histologic criteria for the diagnosis of uterine smooth muscle tumors with standard smooth muscle differentiation

Tumor cell necrosis	*Atypia*	*Mitotic index, MF/10 HPF*	*Diagnosis*
Present	Diffuse moderate to severe	Any level	Leiomyosarcoma
	None to mild	Greater than 10	Leiomyosarcoma
		Less than 10	Leiomyosarcoma (R/O, recent infarction of leiomyoma, due, for example, to torsion)
Absent	Diffuse moderate to severe	Greater than 10	Leiomyosarcoma
		Less than 10	Atypical leiomyoma with low risk of recurrence
	None to mild	Less than 10	Leiomyoma
		Greater than 10	Mitotically active leiomyoma
	Focal moderate to severe	Less than 15	Leiomyoma with limited experience or if MI>15, "STUMP"

MF, mitotic figure; HPF, high-power field; MI, mitotic index; STUMP, smooth muscle tumor of uncertain potential.

Microscopically, the cells are round or polygonal rather than spindle shaped, and they are arranged in clusters or cords. The nuclei are round, relatively large, and centrally positioned. There are three basic subtypes of epithelioid leiomyoma: leiomyoblastoma,[30,158,164] clear cell leiomyoma,[35,138,158,184,250] and plexiform leiomyoma.[86,158] Mixtures of the various patterns are common, providing the basis for designating all of these as epithelioid leiomyomas. Leiomyoblastoma is composed of round cells with eosinophilic cytoplasm (Fig. 13.10) rather than spindle cells. The cells in clear cell leiomyoma are polygonal and have abundant clear cytoplasm and well-defined cell membranes (Fig. 13.11). The cells may contain glycogen, but there is minimal lipid and mucin is absent. The nucleus sometimes is displaced to the periphery of the cell, resulting in a signet-ring appearance. Plexiform leiomyoma is characterized by cords or nests of round cells with scanty to moderate amounts of cytoplasm. Transition to more typical spindled smooth muscle cells is often identified within an epithelioid leiomyoma. Immunohistochemical study confirms the myogenous phenotype of the tumor cells.[30,73,138,242] Ultrastructural study reveals features of smooth muscle differentiation such as parallel cytoplasmic filaments, dense bodies, and basal lamina production.[35,138,139,184] The cells in some clear cell leiomyomas contain numerous mitochondria or cytoplasmic vacuoles.

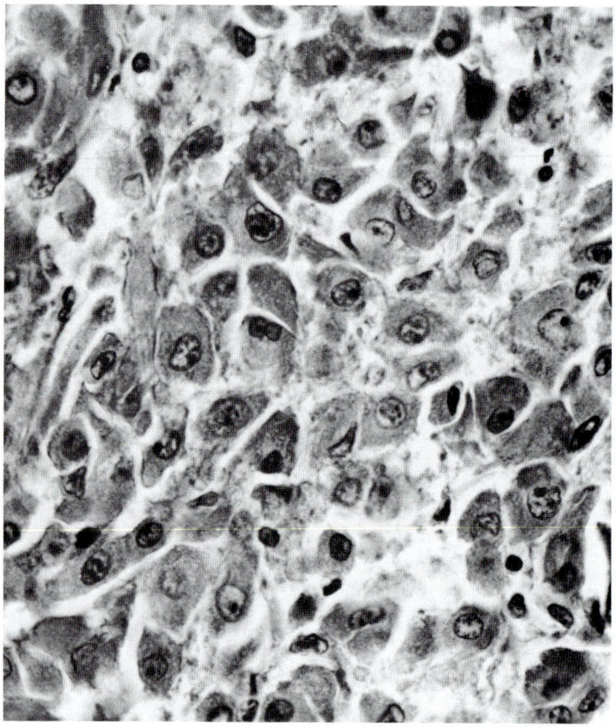

Fig. 13.10. Epithelioid leiomyoma, leiomyoblastoma type. Cellular tumor composed of poorly cohesive polygonal cells with abundant eosinophilic cytoplasm. (Reprinted from Cancer 37; 1976: 1853–1865. Copyright © 1976 American Cancer Society. Reprinted by permission of Wiley-Liss, Inc., a subsidiary of John Wiley & Sons, Inc.)

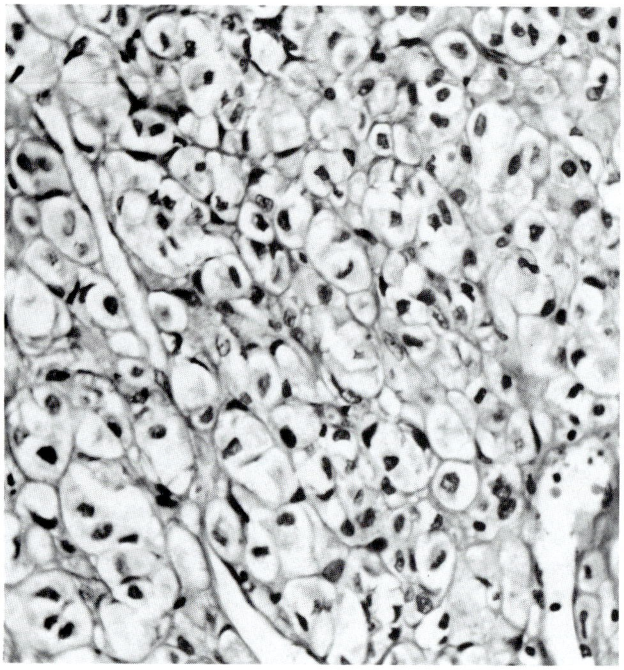

Fig. 13.11. Epithelioid leiomyoma, clear cell type. Nests of cells with abundant clear cytoplasm. (Reprinted from Cancer 37; 1976: 1853–1865. Copyright © 1976 American Cancer Society. Reprinted by permission of Wiley-Liss, Inc., a subsidiary of John Wiley & Sons, Inc.)

Small plexiform leiomyomas that are detected only on microscopic examination are referred to as plexiform tumorlets (Fig. 13.12).[145] These lesions were formerly thought to be angiomas or endometrial stromal tumors, but ultrastructural examination revealed myofilaments and other features of smooth muscle cells,[145,207] and the cells have a myogenous immunophenotype.[73] Plexiform tumorlets usually are solitary and submucosal, but they can occur anywhere in the myometrium and even in the endometrium. Multiple tumorlets are present in some patients.[264]

The behavior of epithelioid smooth muscle neoplasms of the uterus, like that of similar tumors elsewhere in the body, is difficult to predict.[10,47,158,213,233] Small tumors that lack cytologic atypia, tumor cell necrosis, and an elevated mitotic index can be safely regarded as benign.[158,233] Plexiform tumorlets invariably are benign.[145] Epithelioid leiomyomas with circumscribed margins, extensive hyalinization, and predominance of clear

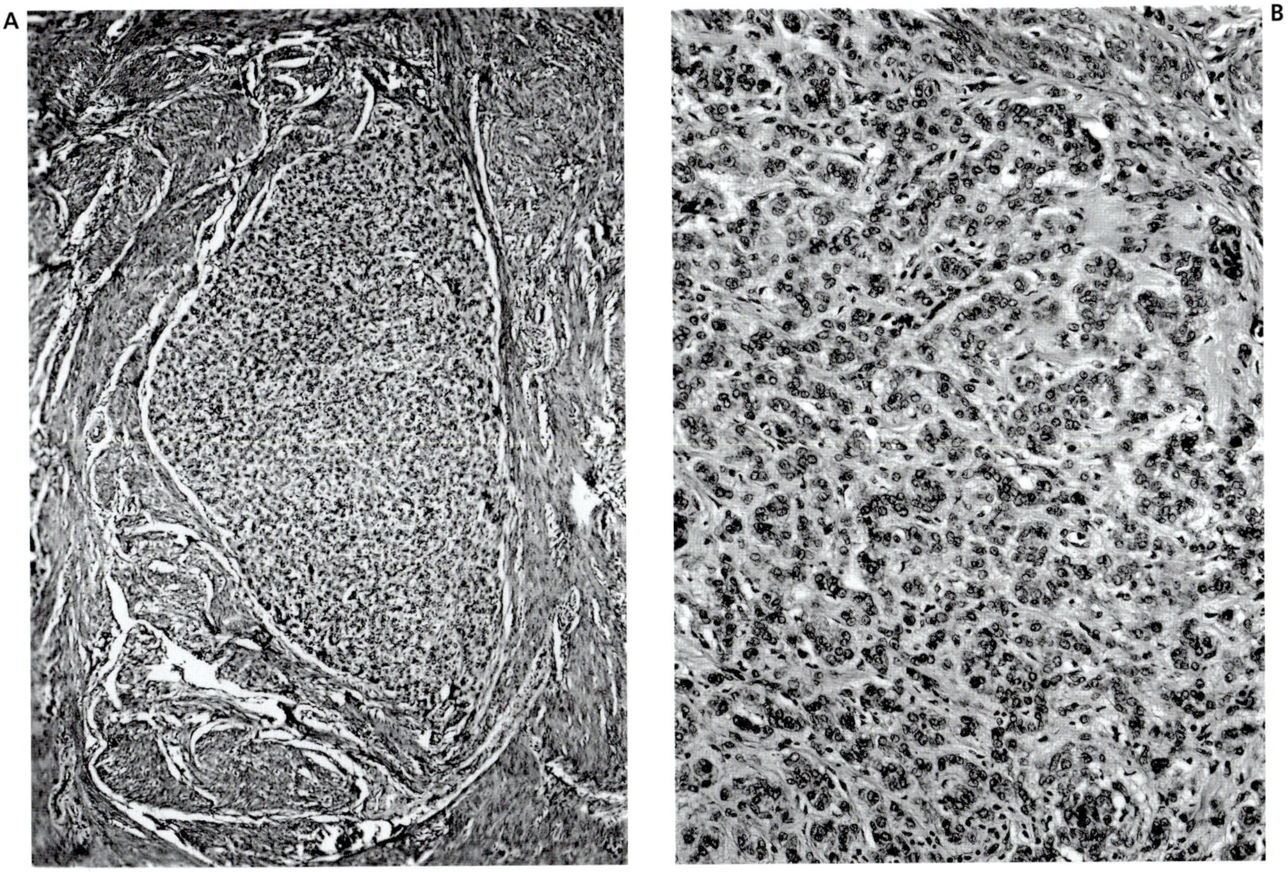

Fig. 13.12. Plexiform tumorlet. This microscopic tumor is completely surrounded by normal myometrium (**A**) and consists of serpiginous cords of epithelioid smooth muscle cells (**B**).

cells generally are benign.[158] The behavior of epithelioid leiomyomas with two or more of the following features is not well established: large size (greater than 6 cm), moderate mitotic activity (2–4 MF/10 HPF), moderate to severe cytologic atypia, and necrosis.

The accumulated experience with epithelioid tumors as a group is limited and discourages dogmatism in predicting clinical course. Those neoplasms with moderate to severe atypia, without necrosis and with MI <5 should be classified as STUMP because experience is too limited to be certain about their aggressive potential. Careful follow-up is warranted. Neoplasms with 5 or more MF/10 HPF metastasize with sufficient frequency that all should be regarded as epithelioid leiomyosarcoma.[35,158] Epithelioid differentiation in more than just a few foci of a uterine smooth muscle tumor is a worrisome finding because the absence of cytologic atypia and tumor cell necrosis is no guarantee of a clinically benign course when the tumor contains more than 5 MF/10 HPF,[141] although the failure rate is probably quite low. All epithelioid tumors with tumor cell necrosis in the Stanford series were clinically malignant.[10] On the other hand, all seven epithelioid tumors in this study with MI < 5, with at most minimal cytologic atypia, and without necrosis behaved in a benign fashion. Most malignant epithelioid smooth muscle tumors are of the leiomyoblastoma type, although clear cell leiomyosarcoma has been reported.[273] The epithelioid appearance of these neoplasms raises a broad differential including carcinoma and epithelioid variants of gestational trophoblastic disease.[215,266,270,319]

Myxoid Leiomyoma

Myxoid leiomyomas are soft and translucent. Microscopically, there is abundant amorphous myxoid material between the smooth muscle cells.[11,183] The margins of a myxoid leiomyoma are circumscribed, and neither cytologic atypia nor mitotic figures are present. We diagnose *leiomyoma with myxoid stroma* when the cells are small and uniform, atypia is absent or at most mild, and the MI < 2 MF/10 HPF. Areas of ordinary leiomyoma should be present focally. Large myxoid smooth muscle tumors and those in which an infiltrating margin, cytologic atypia, or mitotic activity are observed microscopically should be regarded with suspicion. Some myxoid smooth muscle tumors exhibiting these features are clinically malignant even though they do not meet standard criteria for a diagnosis of leiomyosarcoma. Myxoid differentiation coupled with enlarged and atypical cells is an ominous finding. Four of seven such uterine tumors failed in the Stanford series.[11] We diagnose myxoid leiomyosarcoma in the presence of moderate to marked atypia with or without necrosis and with any mitotic index. The tumor margins are usually infiltrating.

Vascular Leiomyoma

Vascular leiomyomas contain numerous large-caliber vessels with muscular walls. It can be difficult to distinguish a vascular leiomyoma from a hemangioma or an arteriovenous malformation if the vascular component predominates. Vascular leiomyomas are well defined, circumscribed neoplasms that contain at least foci of typical spindled smooth muscle cells. Hemangiomas are very rare in the uterus and are usually of the cavernous type. Hemangiomas and arteriovenous malformations tend to be poorly defined grossly and microscopically and lack the sharp circumscription of a leiomyoma.

Leiomyoma with Other Elements

Some benign uterine neoplasms are composed of a mixture of smooth muscle cells and other elements. Endometrial stromal cells are prominent in some *mixed tumors*.[212] The natural history of these rare neoplasms is incompletely documented, although it appears that the rules for assessing malignancy in endometrial stromal tumors applies to mixed tumors as well. Infiltrative margins and/or vascular invasion are associated with a malignant clinical course, and the absence of these features with a benign one.[212,254]

It is not uncommon to find scattered adipocytes in an otherwise typical leiomyoma. A leiomyoma that contains a striking amount of fat is called a *lipoleiomyoma* (Fig. 13.13); if a vascular component is also present, it is designated as an *angiolipoleiomyoma*. Most such tumors occur in middle-aged or elderly women and may arise in any part of the uterus, including the cervix.[73,134,272] They average 6 cm in diameter and have soft yellow areas on the cut surface. Fat cells are generally found in circumscribed areas within the leiomyoma but may be present diffusely. Brown fat, skeletal muscle, and cartilage

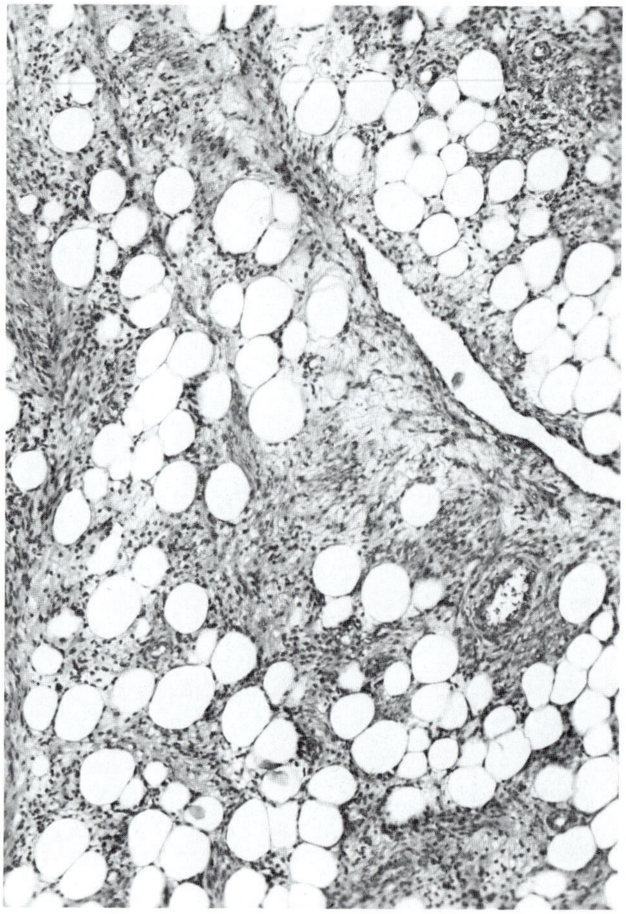

Fig. 13.13. Lipoleiomyoma. The tumor is composed of an intermixture of fat cells, smooth muscle, and collagen.

have been identified in leiomyomas.[38,97,180,305,315] In most instances, the smooth muscle component predominates and is composed of spindled cells. Other types of leiomyoma, such as epithelioid leiomyoma,[30] may also have a lipomatous component and fatty change is common in intravenous leiomyomatosis. The vascular component of an angiolipoleiomyoma may be venous, arterial, or indeterminate. Only a few pure lipomas have been described in the uterus.[75,231] Complex cytogenetic abnormalities have been described in a case of lipoleiomyoma.[225]

Leiomyoma with Hematopoietic Cells

Large numbers of *hematopoietic cells*, which sometimes have no obvious etiology, may infiltrate leiomyomas. Leiomyomas may develop abscesses in the setting of bacterial infection.[235] Peculiar infiltrates include extramedullary hematopoiesis in the absence of systemic disease[257], a prominent histiocytic infiltrate[5], a prominence of mast cells or eosinophils,[65,176,219] and, most importantly, a dense lymphoid infiltrate that can mimic lymphoma.[94]

Smooth Muscle Proliferations with Unusual Growth Patterns

Diffuse Leiomyomatosis and Myometrial Hypertrophy

Diffuse leiomyomatosis is an unusual condition in which innumerable small smooth muscle nodules produce symmetric enlargement of the uterus (Fig. 13.14). The uterus may be greatly enlarged, weighing up to 1000 g. The smooth muscle nodules range from microscopic to 3 cm in size but most are less than 1 cm in diameter. They are composed of uniform, bland, spindled smooth muscle cells and are less circumscribed than typical leiomyomas. The clinical course may be complicated by hemorrhage, but the condition is benign.[47,118,160,196] *Myometrial hypertrophy* is a condition in which the myometrium is thickened and the uterus is symmetrically enlarged. No specific gross or microscopic abnormality is noted; the uterus is abnormal in size only. Uterine weight increases with age and with increasing parity until the menopause. The average uterine weight decreases after the menopause. The weight beyond which the uterus is abnormally large, indicative of myometrial hypertrophy, is 130 g for the nulliparous uterus, 210 g for parity 1–3, and 250 g for parity of 4 and above.[161]

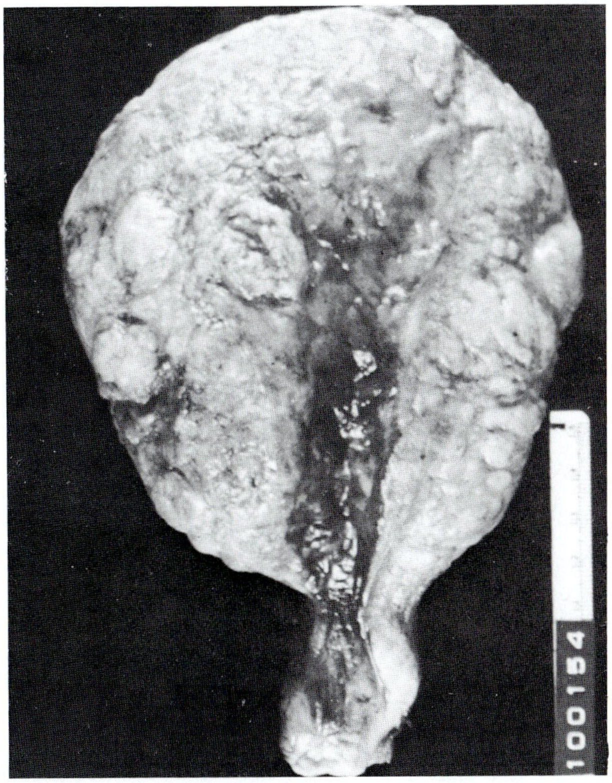

Fig. 13.14. Diffuse leiomyomatosis. The uterus is markedly enlarged, weighing 945 g, and contains innumerable small smooth muscle nodules. (Reprinted from Obstet Gynecol 53; 1979: 82s-84s. Copyright © 1979 American College of Obstetricians and Gynecologists. Reprinted by permission of Elsevier Science, Inc.)

Dissecting Leiomyoma

Dissecting leiomyoma refers to a benign smooth muscle proliferation with a border marked by the dissection of compressive tongues of smooth muscle into the surrounding myometrium and, occasionally, into the broad ligament and pelvis.[245] This pattern of infiltration may also be seen in intravenous leiomyomatosis (see following). When edema and congestion are prominent, a uterine dissecting leiomyoma with extrauterine extension may resemble placental tissue, hence the name *cotyledonoid dissecting leiomyoma*.[103,246,247]

Intravenous Leiomyomatosis and Leiomyoma with Vascular Invasion

Intravenous leiomyomatosis is a very rare smooth muscle tumor characterized by nodular masses of histologically benign smooth muscle cells growing within venous channels.[45,197,200,205] Women with intravenous leiomyomatosis have a median age of 45 years; few are younger than 40 years. There is no racial predisposition, history of infertility, or decreased parity. The main symptoms are abnormal bleeding and pelvic discomfort. Most patients have a pelvic mass. Grossly, intravenous leiomyomatosis is a complex coiled or nodular growth within the myometrium with convoluted, wormlike extensions into the uterine veins in the broad ligament or into other pelvic veins (Fig. 13.15). The growth extends into the vena cava in more than 10% of patients, and in some it reaches as far as the heart.[45,60,248,282,294] The wormlike masses vary from soft and spongy to rubbery and firm, and their color is pink-white or gray.

Microscopically, tumor is found within venous channels lined by endothelium. Arteries are not involved. The histologic appearance is highly variable, even within the same tumor. The cellular composition of some examples of intravenous leiomyomatosis is similar to a leiomyoma, but most contain prominent zones of fibrosis or hyalinization (Fig. 13.16). Smooth muscle cells may be inconspicuous and difficult to identify. The intravenous

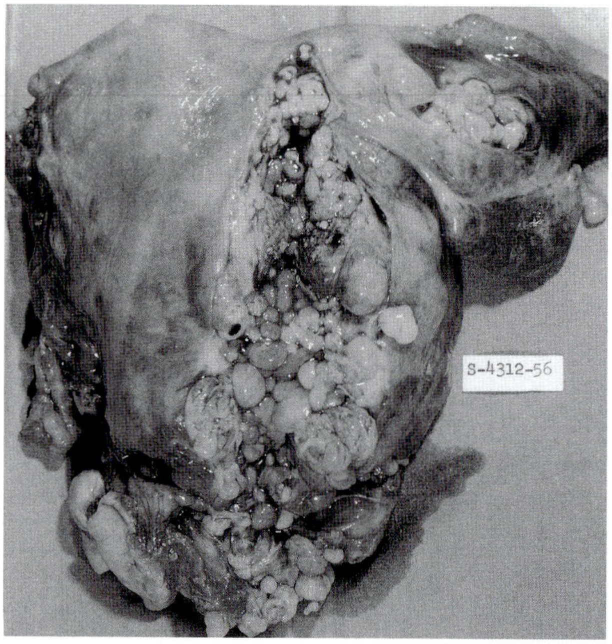

Fig. 13.15. Intravenous leiomyomatosis. Tumor replaces most of the uterus and extends into both broad ligaments and the uterine veins.

growth is itself highly vascular (Fig. 13.17), and in some cases contains so many small and large blood vessels that the process may resemble a vascular tumor. Any type of smooth muscle differentiation that occurs in a leiomyoma can be present in intravenous leiomyomatosis.[55] Cellular, atypical, epithelioid, and lipoleiomyomatous growth patterns have all been described; these have the same behavior and prognosis as ordinary intravenous leiomyomatosis.[28,55,121]

Intravenous leiomyomatosis originates in vascular smooth muscle in some cases.[205] The tumor is predominantly or entirely intravascular in this situation (Figs. 13.16 and 13.17), and there are many sites of attachment to the vein walls. Other examples develop by intravascular extension from a leiomyoma.[200,205] In these cases the bulk of the tumor is extravascular and sites of origin from a vein wall are not found. Treatment is by total abdominal hysterectomy and bilateral salpingo-oophorectomy together with excision of any extrauterine extensions. Intravenous leiomyomatosis

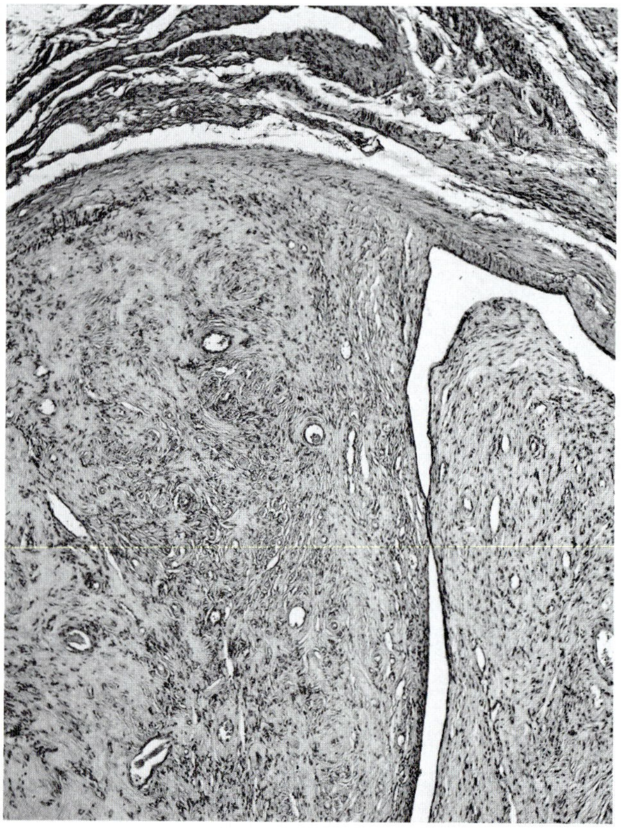

Fig. 13.16. Intravenous leiomyomatosis. Nearly the entire tumor was within the vascular spaces. Note that the intravascular tumor is highly vascular and extensively hyalinized.

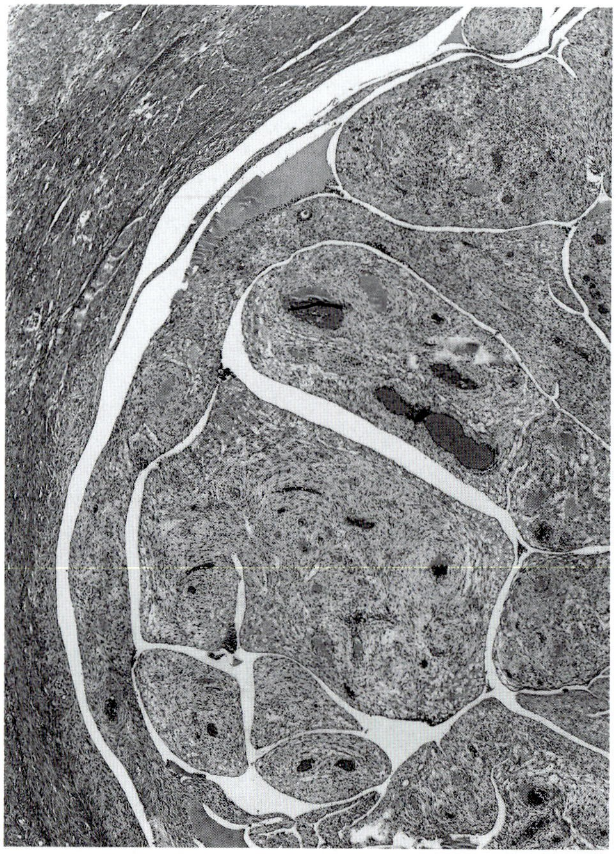

Fig. 13.17. Intravenous leiomyomatosis. This predominantly intravascular tumor contains numerous small and large blood vessels. Normal myometrium is present at the *left.*

has a favorable prognosis even when it is incompletely excised.[197] Pelvic recurrence is infrequent and usually is amenable to surgical excision.[84,205] Residual pelvic tumor may remain stable but progressive growth is possible. Intravenous leiomyomatosis is a hormonally dependent tumor, and progression is more likely in women whose treatment does not include bilateral salpingo-oophorectomy.[45,84,200,205] Long-term survival is possible after removal of plugs of tumor from the vena cava or right atrium or excision of nodules from the lung. In one case, leuprolide acetate induced tumor regression and rendered debulking surgery feasible in a patient with previously unresectable, widespread, retroperitoneal intravascular leiomyomatosis.[296]

Benign Metastasizing Leiomyoma

Benign metastasizing leiomyoma is a nebulous condition in which "metastatic" smooth muscle tumor deposits in the lung, lymph nodes, or abdomen appear to be derived from a benign leiomyoma of the uterus. Reports of this condition are often difficult to assess. Almost all cases of benign metastasizing leiomyoma occur in women, most of whom have a history of pelvic surgery. The primary neoplasm, typically removed years before the metastatic deposits are detected, often has been inadequately studied. In some cases, the primary tumor was not examined histologically by the reporting author and, in others, the cytologic appearance, including mitotic counts, is not recorded for either the primary tumor or the alleged metastasis. A few examples may represent deportation metastases from intravenous leiomyomatosis that reach the lungs, where they become implanted and grow as multiple intrapulmonary nodules of smooth muscle (Fig. 13.18). Others may represent a multifocal smooth muscle proliferation involving the uterus and extrauterine sites.[41] Most examples of "benign metastasizing leiomyoma," however, appear to be either a primary benign smooth muscle lesion of the lung in a woman with a history of uterine leiomyoma or pulmonary metastases from a morphologically noninformative smooth muscle neoplasm of the uterus.[19,106,312] The findings of a recent cytogenetic study were most consistent with a monoclonal origin of both uterine and pulmonary tumors and the interpretation that the pulmonary tumors were metastatic.[292] The hormone dependence of this proliferation is suggested by the finding of estrogen and progesterone receptors in metastatic deposits[140] and the regression of tumor during pregnancy,[137] after the menopause, and after oophorectomy.[3]

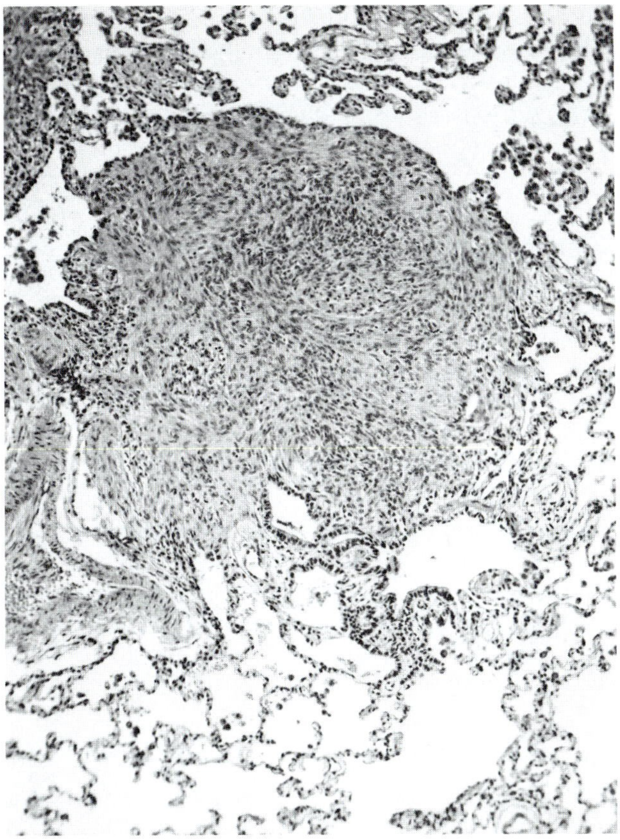

Fig. 13.18. Smooth muscle tumor in lung. The diagnosis was leiomyoma metastatic to lung (benign metastasizing leiomyoma) until the uterus, removed years earlier, was reexamined and found to contain intravenous leiomyomatosis.

Peritoneal Leiomyomas ("Parasitic" Leiomyomas)

On rare occasions, leiomyomas have been reported to "detach" from their initial subserosal location and "attach" to some other pelvic site. This improbable event presumably occurs through the mediation of a combination of infarction and inflammatory adhesions. A diagnosis of *parasitic leiomyoma* should be made with great caution because clinically malignant smooth muscle neoplasms arising in the retroperitoneum or gastrointestinal tract are notorious for being bland and having a low mitotic index.

Disseminated Peritoneal Leiomyomatosis

Disseminated peritoneal leiomyomatosis (*DPL*) is a rare condition characterized by the presence of multiple smooth muscle, myofibroblastic, and fibroblastic nodules on the peritoneal surfaces of the pelvic and abdominal cavities in women of reproductive age.[9,78,113,193,290] This condition is discussed in connection with leiomyoma of the uterus because it must be distinguished from metastatic leiomyosarcoma. Most cases are associated with pregnancy, an estrinizing granulosa tumor, or oral contraceptive use.[78,290] The most common presentation is as an unexpected finding at the time of cesarean section. DPL appears as multiple, small, granular white or tan nodules on the pelvic and abdominal peritoneum, on the surfaces of the uterus, adnexa, intestines, and in the omentum (Fig. 13.19). The nodules are distributed randomly, and most of them are less than 1 cm in diameter; this contrasts with metastatic leiomyosarcoma, in which the nodules tend to be fewer, larger, and invasive into adjacent tissues. Microscopically, the nodules consist of collagen, fibroblasts, myofibroblasts, smooth muscle cells, and, in pregnancy or the postpartum period, decidual cells (Fig. 13.20). Spindled cells usually dominate, raising the possibility that disseminated peritoneal leiomyomatosis may be confused with a metastatic sarcoma.

The clinical setting is quite different, however, as is the morphology of the cells. Mitotic figures are infrequent in DPL, and nuclear atypia and pleomorphism are minimal or absent. Electron microscopic studies have shown that most nodules are composed of smooth muscle and decidual cells, although some are mixtures of decidua and fibroblasts or myofibroblasts.[113,199,229,290] A recent cytogenetic study assessed the clonality of 42 tumorlets and 15 normal tissues from four women with DPL by analyzing X chromosome inactivation as indicated by the methylation status of the androgen receptor gene (HUMARA). In each of the four patients, the same parental X chromosome was nonrandomly inactivated in all tumorlets, consistent with a metastatic unicentric neoplasm or, alternatively, selection for an X-linked allele in clonal multicentric lesions.[237] Disseminated peritoneal leiomyomatosis is initiated or promoted by hormonal factors in most cases. Estrogen and progesterone receptors may be demonstrated within DPL by biochemical or immunohistochemical methods.[79] DPL generally regresses or remains static after removal of the hormonal stimulus (i.e., after delivery), so radical attempts at excision are unnecessary.[9,290] In keeping with a hormonally dependent process, DPL may regress during therapy with a GnRH agonist.[120] The peritoneal smooth muscle nodules may enlarge again when the GnRH agonist is discontinued or if the patient becomes pregnant.[120,290] Five cases of malignant DPL have been reported and recently reviewed.[18] Four of these cases were distinguished from typical cases of DPL by not having an exposure to estrogen or associated uterine leiomyomas and by absence of estrogen and progesterone receptors in their tumors.

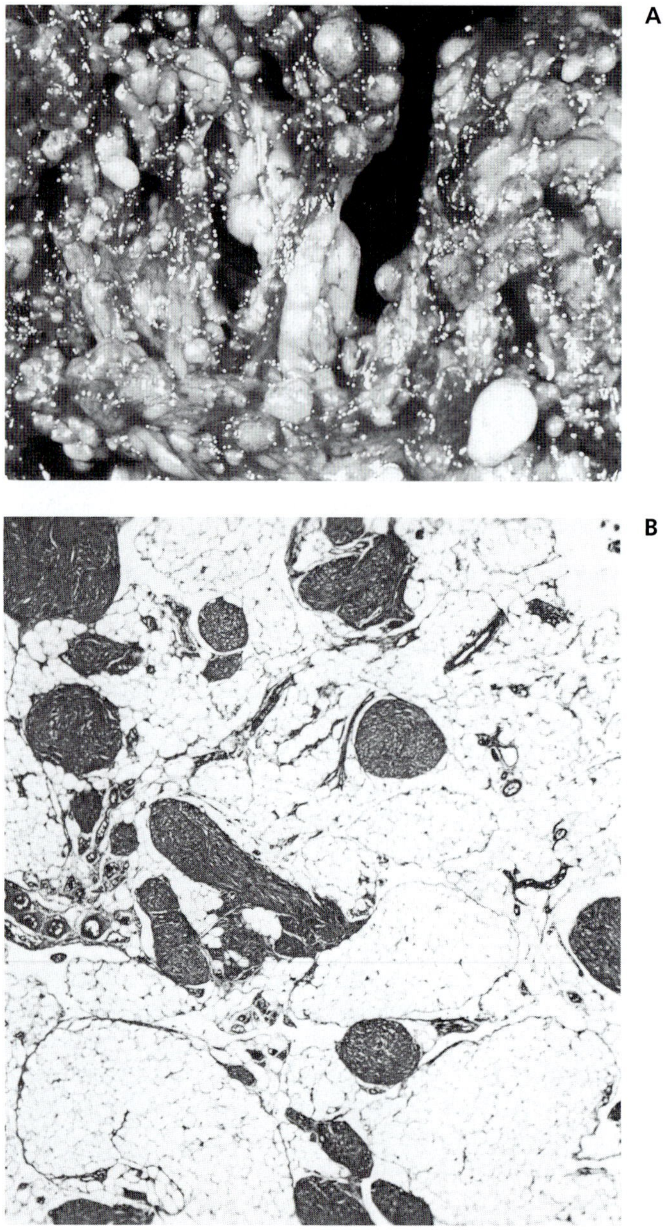

Fig. 13.19. Disseminated peritoneal leiomyomatosis. A: Gross photo showing innumerable small nodules in the omentum. **B:** Low power photomicrograph illustrates multiple small nodules of smooth muscle cells surrounded by omental fat.

Leiomyosarcoma

Leiomyosarcoma represents about 1.3% of uterine malignancies and about one-third of uterine sarcomas. Approximately 1 of every 800 smooth muscle

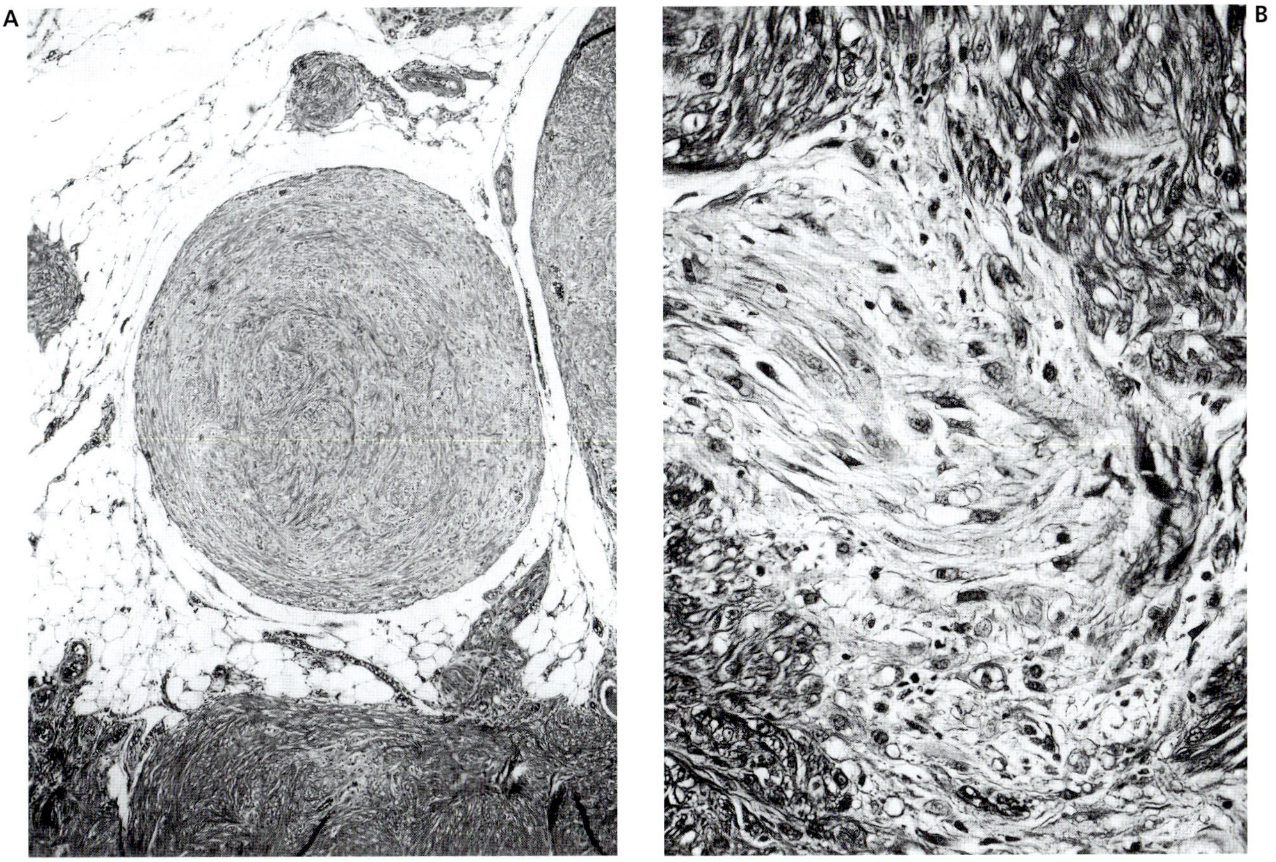

Fig. 13.20. Disseminated peritoneal leiomyomatosis (DPL). A: Nodules of spindle-shaped smooth muscle cells surrounded by fat. **B**. The tumor nodules in DPL contain variable mixtures of decidualized cells (*center*), smooth muscle cells (*top* and *bottom*), and fibroblasts (not shown).

tumors of the uterus is a leiomyosarcoma, but less than 1% of women thought clinically to have leiomyoma prove to have leiomyosarcoma.[166]

Clinical Features

Women with leiomyosarcoma average 52 years of age, nearly a decade older than women with leiomyomas, although the disease is well known to occur in women in the third decade of life.[17,61,125,259,310] There is no consistent racial predisposition nor is there a relationship with gravidity or parity. The clinical presentation is nonspecific. The main symptoms are abnormal vaginal bleeding, lower abdominal pain, or a pelvic or abdominal mass.[61,125,163,253] The average duration of symptoms before diagnosis is 5 months.[163] There appears to be little support for the clinical dictum that a rapidly enlarging uterine smooth muscle neoplasm is indicative of leiomyosarcoma. In a recent study, only 1 of 371 women with this finding proved to have a leiomyosarcoma.[222] Unlike mixed müllerian tumor, leiomyosarcoma is seldom associated with a history of pelvic radiation.[301]

Gross Findings

Most leiomyosarcomas are intramural, and 50–75% are solitary masses.[32,86,259,301] A higher proportion involve the cervix than is the case with leiomyoma. Leiomyosarcoma averages 6–9 cm in diameter and is soft or fleshy with poorly defined margins.[17] The cut surface is gray-yellow or pink with areas of necrosis and hemorrhage. Leiomyosarcoma tends to be larger and softer than leiomyoma; it has a more irregular margin, and it is more likely to be hemorrhagic and necrotic (Table 13.3).

Microscopic Findings

The usual leiomyosarcoma is composed of fascicles of spindle cells with abundant eosinophilic cytoplasm (Fig. 13.21). Longitudinal cytoplasmic fibrils, best appreciated with a trichrome stain, are frequently present. The nuclei are fusiform, usually have rounded ends, and are hyperchromatic with coarse chromatin and prominent nucleoli. Cellular pleomorphism can be marked in poorly differentiated neoplasms (Fig.

Table 13.3. Comparison of the gross pathology of leiomyoma and leiomyosarcoma

Leiomyoma	*Leiomyosarcoma*
Usually multiple	Usually solitary (50–75%)
Variable size, usually 3–5 cm	Large, often >10 cm
Firm, whorled cut surface	Soft, fleshy cut surface
White	Yellow or tan
Hemorrhage and necrosis (infarction type) infrequent	Hemorrhage and necrosis (coagulative type) frequent

13.22). Multinucleated tumor cells are found in 50% of leiomyosarcomas. Giant cells resembling osteoclasts occasionally are present[67,86,179,307] and, rarely, xanthoma cells may be prominent.[117] Many leiomyosarcomas invade the surrounding myometrium, but a leiomyosarcoma with a circumscribed margin can give rise to metastases. Vascular invasion is identified in 10–22% of leiomyosarcomas.[32,174,182,203] Tumor cell necrosis is typically prominent but need not be present. In a recently published series, the mitotic index was in excess of 15 MF/10 HPF in 80% of cases.[174] The main criteria used to diagnose leiomyosarcoma of the uterus are the presence of nuclear atypia, a high mitotic index, and coagulative tumor cell necrosis (see Table 13.2).

Myxoid leiomyosarcoma is a large, gelatinous neoplasm that usually appears circumscribed on

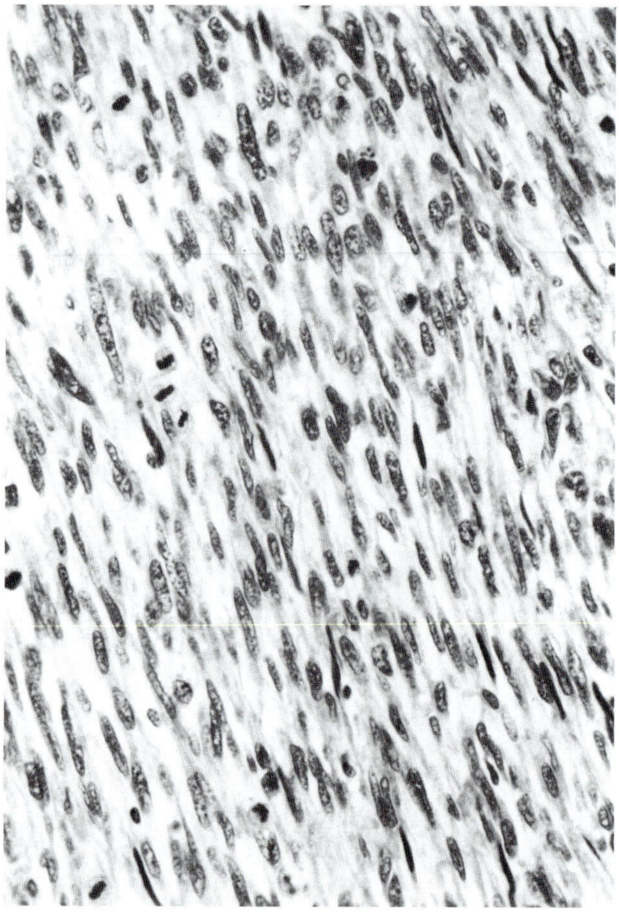

Fig. 13.21. Leiomyosarcoma. The tumor cells are spindle shaped with eosinophilic cytoplasm. The nuclei are fusiform, hyperchromatic, and atypical, and there are many mitotic figures.

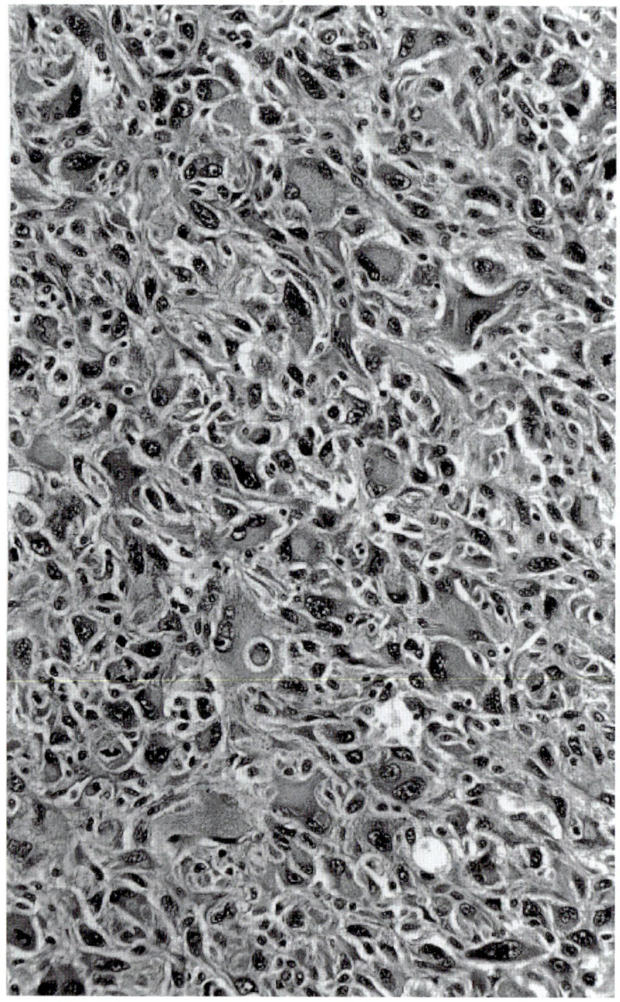

Fig. 13.22. Pleomorphic leiomyosarcoma. The tumor cells vary in size and shape and have markedly atypical pleomorphic nuclei.

A B

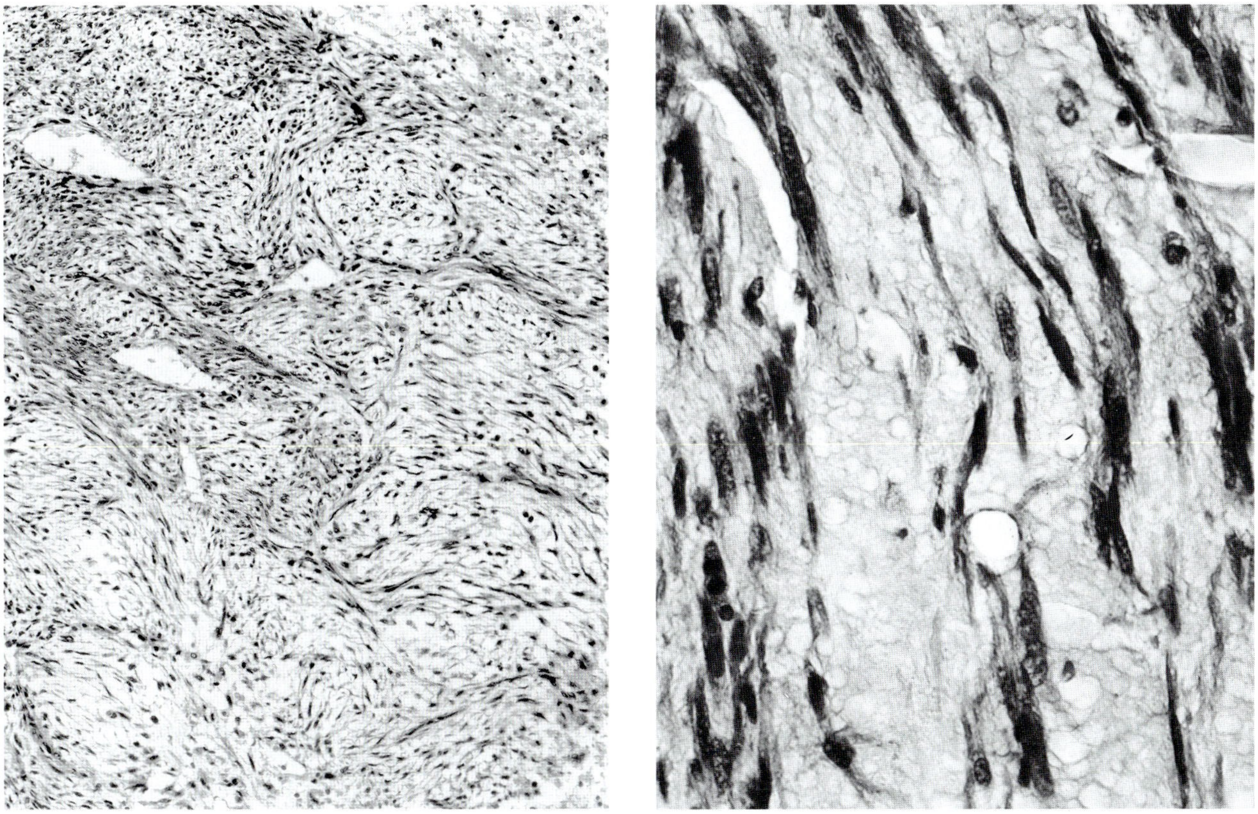

Fig. 13.23. Myxoid leiomyosarcoma. A: The abundant myxoid stroma widely separates the bundles of smooth muscle cells, resulting in a hypocellular appearance. **B**: As shown here, the degree of nuclear atypia can be deceptively bland, and, because the tumor cells are widely separated by myxoid stroma, the number of mitotic figures per 10 HPF is often low.

gross examination.[11,37,153,224] Microscopically, the smooth muscle cells are usually widely separated by myxoid material (Fig. 13.23). The characteristic low cellularity partly accounts for the low mitotic index in most myxoid leiomyosarcomas. Sometimes, however, the mitotic index is high and there is a high degree of atypia.[157,258] In addition to the myxoid appearance, other microscopic features that help identify the tumor as a leiomyosarcoma include myometrial infiltration and vascular invasion. Despite the low mitotic counts, myxoid leiomyosarcoma has the same unfavorable prognosis as typical leiomyosarcoma. Myxoid smooth muscle tumors of the uterus must be regarded with suspicion. It is critical to distinguish the myxoid differentiation found in myxoid leiomyosarcomas from the vastly more prevalent hydropic changes seen in degenerating leiomyomas.[56] In addition, myxoid leiomyosarcoma must be differentiated from an inflammatory myofibroblastic tumor (see "Inflammatory Myofibroblastic Tumor"). In myxoid leiomyosarcoma, not only is the stroma myxoid but the cells are enlarged with hyperchromatic nuclei and pleomorphism is usually obvious. The usual case of myxoid leiomyosarcoma bears a striking resemblance to soft tissue myxoid malignant fibrous histiocytoma.

Epithelioid leiomyosarcomas exhibit one of the patterns of epithelioid differentiation in addition to the usual features of malignancy seen in the more conventional leiomyosarcoma: cytologic atypia, tumor cell necrosis, and a high mitotic index.[10,47,141,148,158,213,233]

Finally, there is the rare, otherwise conventional smooth muscle tumor with a low mitotic count that proves to be clinically malignant. Unless the tumor is invasive or contains abnormal mitotic figures or areas of tumor cell necrosis, there are no good grounds for suspecting that it is a leiomyosarcoma until it announces itself by metastasizing. Doubtless, the pulmonary metastases from some "benign metastasizing leiomyomas" originate from neoplasms in this category.

Flow Cytometry

Reports of flow cytometric analysis of malignant uterine smooth muscle tumors are limited and some are difficult to evaluate. One group observed that women with stage I DNA diploid leiomyosarcoma had a significantly more favorable prognosis than did those whose tumors were DNA nondiploid.[297] Their microscopic diagnostic criteria were unclear, however, and their finding that most leiomyosarcomas were tetraploid or polyploid (versus diploid or aneuploid) suggests a technical problem. Several other reports indicate that most leiomyosarcomas are DNA aneuploid.[175,227] A recent multivariate analysis showed that DNA ploidy did not achieve statistical significance when categorized as diploid/nondiploid. Patients with tumors with multiple aneuploid cell populations had a very poor prognosis. When categorized as multiple aneuploidy versus all other ploidy groups, DNA ploidy was marginally significant in multivariate analysis.[203]

Cytogenetics

The cytogenetics of leiomyosarcoma are even more complicated and varied than those of leiomyoma, but no specific diagnostically useful differences have emerged.[122,236,238]

Clinical Behavior and Treatment

The staging system for uterine corpus carcinoma is used for uterine sarcomas. Most leiomyosarcomas are clinically confined to the uterus on presentation; when extrauterine disease is present it is likely to involve the lung.[112] Leiomyosarcoma spreads intraperitoneally, to regional lymph nodes, and hematogenously, particularly to the lungs, liver, brain, kidney, and bone. Recurrences in a recent large series of stage I and II leiomyosarcomas were hematogenous in 57% and pelvic in 20%. The incidence of lymph node metastasis varies from series to series, but it is substantially lower than that found in clinical stage I and II high risk endometrial carcinomas. In the Gynecologic Oncology Group (GOG) study, 83% of 59 clinical stage I and II leiomyosarcoma patients were surgical stage I; 2 of 59 (3%) had lymph node involvement, 2 had adnexal involvement, and 1 had positive peritoneal cytology.[174] Because patients in this series underwent lymph node sampling rather than lymph node dissection, these figures probably somewhat underestimate the true incidence of lymph node involvement. Lymph node involvement is higher in series reporting advanced-stage leiomyosarcoma, and figures as high as 44% are reported in autopsy series.[96,112,243] Goff et al. found in their series of 15 surgically staged patients that lymph nodes were involved only when there was peritoneal disease. Moreover, a high percentage of lymph node-negative patients failed.[112] In view of this, there would appear to be little role for lymph node sampling in this disease.

Leiomyosarcoma is a highly malignant neoplasm; survival rates are poorer for this disease than for carcinosarcoma.[174,211] For postmenopausal women, primary therapy for early-stage leiomyosarcoma is total abdominal hysterectomy and bilateral salpingo-oophorectomy. Therapy in premenopausal women is more controversial. The ovaries are only rarely the site of metastatic disease in clinically low-stage leiomyosarcoma; in the GOG study, only 2 of 59 patients had this finding. Moreover, there is no evidence that oophorectomy influences the results of therapy.[20,107,163] Accordingly, ovarian conservation is reasonable in premenopausal women. On the other hand, patients with low-grade smooth muscle neoplasms metastatic to the lung have responded to oophorectomy alone.[3]

The literature provides conflicting reports on the efficacy of radiotherapy in the management of leiomyosarcoma. Two series reported no effect,[20,136] whereas the GOG series did show a lower relapse rate in patients with early-stage leiomyosarcoma when they were treated with combined radiation and surgery compared to patients treated with surgery alone (none versus 17%).[174] The role of radiotherapy would appear to be limited given the conflicting reports on the radiosensitivity of leiomyosarcoma and its noncontroversial tendency to spread hematogenously.[194] Advocates of adjuvant radiotherapy have argued that although survival is not changed, pelvic radiation prevents local and regional recurrences and thus is associated with an improvement in the quality of remaining life.[107,136]

Recurrent or metastatic leiomyosarcoma is very difficult to treat. A minority of patients respond to chemotherapy with doxorubicin.[20,283] Localized pelvic or abdominal recurrences and solitary pulmonary metastases occasionally are amenable to surgical resection.[167] Given the poor results obtained by surgery alone in early-stage leiomyosarcoma, there is an urgent need for effective adjuvant chemotherapy; unfortunately, no active regimen has been identified.[17,129,216,217]

The variation in survival rates reported historically for leiomyosarcoma is largely a result of the use of different criteria for its diagnosis. Overall 5-year survival rates in series using modern criteria range from 15% to 25%.[17,20,32,86,163,301,310] When only stage I and II tumors are considered, the 5-year survival rate is 40–70%.[25,104,142,163,178,182,201,203,223,313] The 3-year progression-free interval was 31% in a GOG series of 59 early-stage leiomyosarcomas; the first recurrence was in the pelvis in 14% of cases and in the lung in 41%.[174] Most recurrences are detected within 2 years.[20,32,125,142]

The prognosis of leiomyosarcoma depends chiefly on stage.[25,104,142,178,201,203,313] For stage I tumors, some investigators have found the size of the neoplasm to be an important prognostic factor.[86,203] In Evans' series, all patients with tumors larger than 5 cm died of disease, while only three of eight patients with tumors smaller than 5 cm died of disease.[86] In another series of metastasizing leiomyosarcomas, only 20% were less than 5 cm.[141] Premenopausal women have had a more favorable outcome in some series[104,142,163,182,301,313] but not in others.[17,125] Several recent series, including the large GOG study of early-stage leiomyosarcoma, have found mitotic index to be of prognostic significance[104,163,174,223] whereas others have not.[86] A modification of the classification of Bell et al.[19] was employed as a grading scheme in one study and found to provide independent prognostic information.[25] In another study, a grading scheme designed for soft tissue neoplasms was applied to uterine sarcomas but was not found to be of prognostic significance.[223]

What should be incorporated in the pathology report in the face of these conflicting claims about prognostically relevant features? We do not grade leiomyosarcomas, as no universally agreed-upon grading scheme exists, but do comment on the features listed here: maximum tumor diameter, mitotic index, the presence or absence of necrosis and its extent if present, and the presence or absence of vascular space involvement.

Smooth Muscle Tumor of Uncertain Malignant Potential (STUMP)

This diagnosis is used when there is significant doubt about the failure rate associated with a particular combination of histologic features. With the acquisition of more clinicopathologic information about smooth muscle neoplasms, the size of this category has diminished. Some of the situations for which we currently employ this designation include the following.

1. The available clinicopathologic information about a differentiated type is scant and there is, for whatever reason, some chance that the neoplasm might not be benign; this is true of myxoid and epithelioid neoplasms that lack tumor cell necrosis, have midrange atypia, and have moderately high mitotic indices.
2. There is uncertainty concerning the type of smooth muscle differentiation present, which would make a difference in the prediction of its clinical behavior.
3. There is uncertainty about the mitotic index, which would make a difference in the prediction made about the clinical behavior of the neoplasm. This situation most frequently occurs in smooth muscle neoplasms with standard smooth muscle differentiation that lack tumor cell necrosis, have moderate to severe atypia, have a mitotic index is in the neighborhood of 10 MF/10 HPF, and have structures that could be regarded either as abnormal mitotic figures or smudged karyorrhectic nuclei, because counting them as mitotic figures would result in a leiomyosarcoma diagnosis and as smudged nuclei would result in a diagnosis of atypical leiomyoma.
4. There is uncertainty about the presence of tumor cell necrosis. Sometimes the distinction between hyaline/infarction necrosis and tumor cell necrosis is ambiguous. There may be widespread individual cell necrosis or a pattern that could represent either early infarction or tumor cell necrosis.

Endometrial Stromal Tumors

Endometrial stromal tumors are rare and can be benign or malignant. Benign endometrial stromal tumors are called *stromal nodules*; they are circumscribed, expansile, and do not invade the myometrium. Malignant stromal tumors are called *endometrial stromal sarcomas*.[261] Formerly, some were termed endolymphatic stromal myosis or stromatosis.[206,291] Endometrial stromal sarcomas infiltrate the myometrium, invade vascular spaces, and have the capability to invade adjacent tissues and metastasize. Several variants of endometrial stromal tumors exist, including uterine tumors with histologic features reminiscent of ovarian sex cord–stromal tumors and combined smooth muscle–stromal tumors. Most endometrial stromal tumors originate in the uterus, but rare examples arise outside the uterus, presumably from endometriosis.[13,34,102,155,318]

Endometrial Stromal Nodule

Endometrial stromal nodules are rare. They represent less than a quarter of endometrial stromal tumors.[33,92]

Clinical Features

Endometrial stromal nodules have been reported in women from 23 to 75 years of age.[289] The median age is 47 years, and about 75% of patients are premenopausal. There is no racial predisposition. The main symptoms are abnormal vaginal bleeding and menorrhagia.[289] The bleeding is occasionally severe enough to cause anemia. Pelvic or abdominal discomfort is a frequent complaint. The average duration of symptoms before diagnosis is about 2 months. About 10% of patients are asymptomatic, and their tumors are found incidentally in uteri from hysterectomies performed for other conditions.

Gross Findings

Endometrial stromal nodules have a circumscribed contour (Fig. 13.24) and range from 0.8 to 15 cm in diameter; the average diameter is 4–5 cm.[214,289] Many stromal nodules are polypoid and protrude into the uterine cavity, but nearly half grow entirely within the myometrium with no apparent connection to the endometrium.[92] They have fleshy yellow or tan cut surfaces and tend to bulge above the surrounding myometrium. Occasional tumors are cystic, but foci of necrosis and hemorrhage are rare. About 5% of patients have two or more nodules. The cervix is seldom involved.

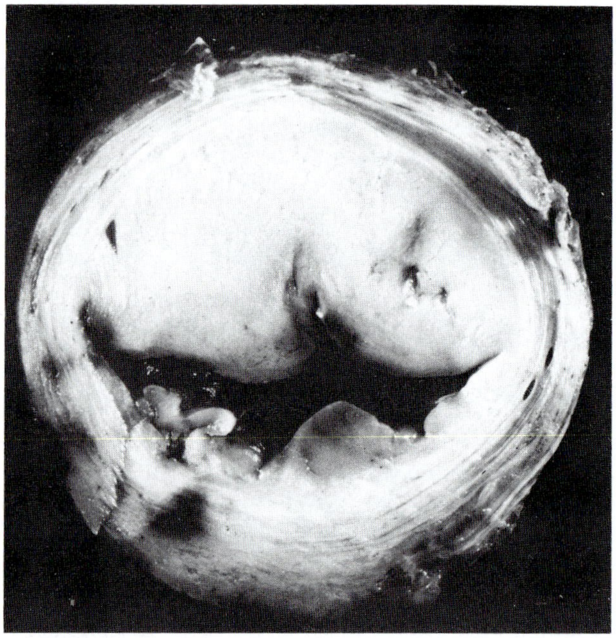

Fig. 13.24. Endometrial stromal nodule. The nodule has a homogenous tan cut surface and there is focal cystic change. (Reprinted with permission from *Progress in Surgical Pathology, Volume III*, edited by C. M. Fenoglio and M. Wolff, New York: Masson Publishing USA, Inc., 1981, pp. 1–35.)

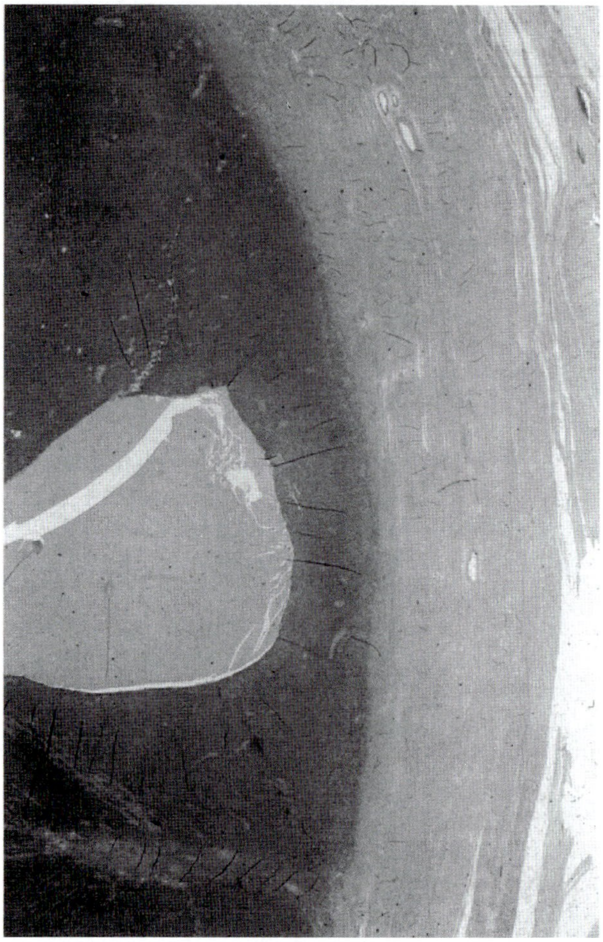

Fig. 13.25. Endometrial stromal nodule. Note the circumscribed, expansile margin. A noninvasive pattern of growth characterizes a stromal nodule.

Microscopic Findings

Stromal nodules have expansile, noninfiltrative margins that compress the surrounding endometrium and myometrium (Fig. 13.25). Minor irregularities of the margin are common, but invasion of the surrounding myometrium indicates that the tumor is a stromal sarcoma, not a stromal nodule. Endometrial stromal nodules consist of cells that closely resemble normal proliferative-phase endometrial stromal cells. The tumor cells have uniform, small, darkly staining round or oval nuclei with finely granular chromatin and inconspicuous nucleoli (Fig. 13.26). The cytoplasm varies from scanty to moderate, and cell borders tend to be poorly defined. A reticulin network encircles individual cells. Mitotic activity ranges from none to 15 MF/10 HPF but it is usually low (<3 MF/10 HPF).[81] Mitotic figures cannot be identified in about 50% of stromal nodules, and more than 5 MF/10 HPF are

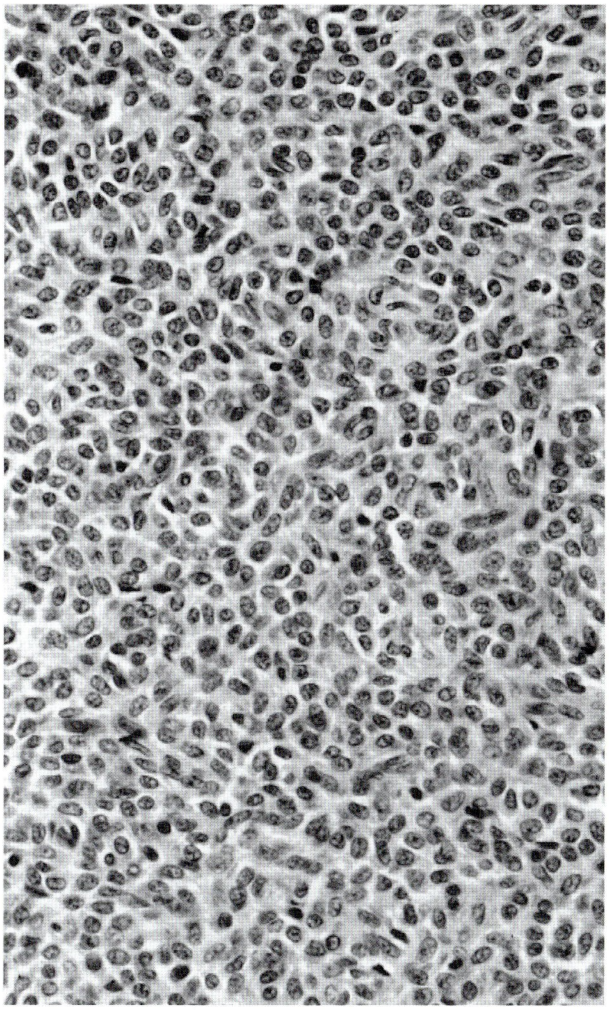

Fig. 13.26. Endometrial stromal nodule. Typical pattern, in which the nodule is composed of sheets of endometrial stromal cells with small, uniform, round to oval nuclei and scanty cytoplasm.

detected in only 5–10% of them.[289] Stromal nodules are highly vascular, with small arterioles distributed throughout. Epithelial or sex cord-like arrangements of cells, such as cords or trabeculae of tumor cells or glandlike structures, are present in some stromal nodules (Fig. 13.27).[92,289,324] Uncommon findings that are occasionally noted in stromal nodules include decidual changes, aggregates of foam cells, cysts, small areas of necrosis, and calcifications. Minor foci of smooth muscle differentiation are found in about 10% of stromal nodules,[289] sometimes associated with starburst-like aggregates of hyalinized collagen. If extensive smooth muscle differentiation is present (>30%), the tumor should be classified as a combined stromal–smooth muscle tumor.[212,289] Immunohistochemistry can help to differentiate a stromal nodule from a highly cellular leiomyoma. The cells in both tumors express vimentin. Stromal nodules exhibit variable, but often weak and patchy, staining for smooth muscle actin and are typically desmin negative.[214] In contrast, there is strong cytoplasmic staining for both actin and desmin in highly cellular leiomyomas.

Clinical Behavior and Treatment

All stromal nodules reported to date have had a benign clinical evolution.[33,81,127,289,291] Nevertheless, hysterectomy is usually the appropriate therapy because the periphery of the tumor must be thoroughly evaluated to be certain that it is completely circumscribed and noninvasive. As already discussed in the section on cellular leiomyomas, endometrial stromal tumors must be differentiated from highly cellular leiomyomas because this distinction may significantly affect the treatment. In occasional cases, usu-

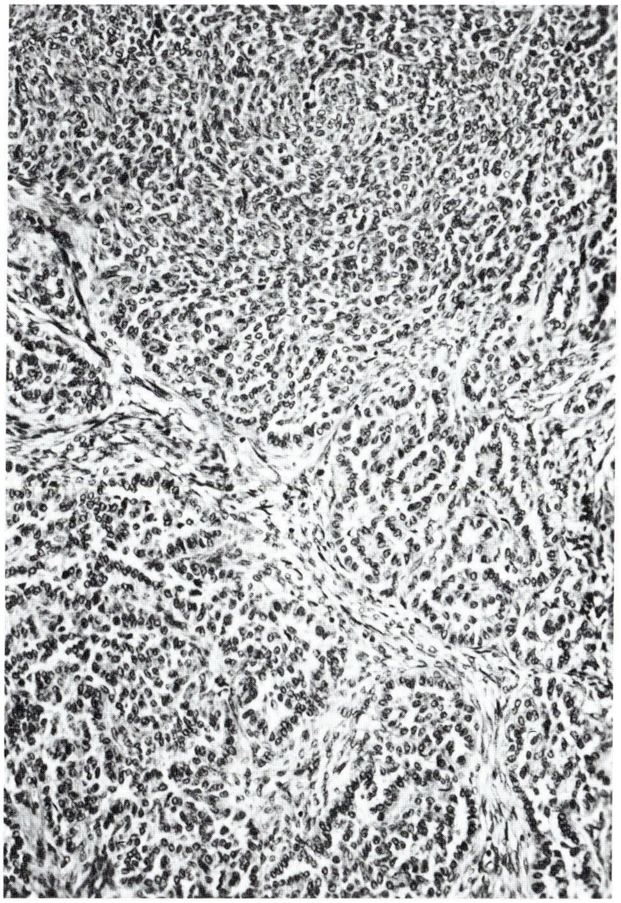

Fig. 13.27. Endometrial stromal nodule. Typical pattern on top, sex cord-like pattern on bottom. (Reprinted from Histopathology 5;1981:1–10. Copyright © 1981 Blackwell Science, Ltd. Reprinted by permission of Blackwell Science, Ltd.)

ally involving tumors occurring in young women, small nodules that can be completely excised by polypectomy or myomectomy may be treated by local excision rather than hysterectomy.[256] Six of the 60 patients reported by Tavassoli and Norris were treated in this fashion and none had a recurrence.[289] Neither minor irregularities of the margin nor the presence of frequent mitotic figures appear to imply an unfavorable prognosis.

Endometrial Stromal Sarcoma

Endometrial stromal sarcoma (*ESS*) is a tumor of endometrial stromal cells that invades the myometrium.[261] ESS has traditionally been divided into two categories, low-grade stromal sarcoma (LGSS) and high-grade stromal sarcoma (HGSS), although the criteria for and validity of this division have recently been questioned. The prevalence of endometrial stromal sarcoma is difficult to estimate. The distinction between low-grade and high-grade stromal sarcomas has been made in some reports but not in others; some reports have included pleomorphic homologous müllerian sarcomas and others benign stromal nodules. Despite these limitations, it is clear that in most large studies endometrial stromal sarcomas comprise less than 20% of uterine sarcomas and that most are LGSS.[36,93,162,174]

Clinical Features

Endometrial stromal sarcoma occurs at an earlier age than most other uterine malignancies. The mean age is between 42 and 53 years, and more than 50% of patients are premenopausal.[21,33,36,81,105,127,177,230] Rare examples occur in young women or girls.[33,190,316] There is no association with any of the endometrial carcinoma risk factors, but a few patients have a history of prior pelvic irradiation. A few cases of LGSS have been reported in women treated for breast cancer with tamoxifen.[80,221] The main symptoms are abnormal vaginal bleeding, cyclic menorrhagia that gradually becomes more severe, and abdominal pain.[149,177] The uterus is typically enlarged and has an irregular contour. A few women have bulky polypoid tumors that protrude from the cervical os. The usual clinical impression is that the patient has a uterine leiomyoma that is causing an exceptional degree of bleeding. Occasional patients present with abdominal or pulmonary metastases; metastatic deposits that are detected before the uterine primary is diagnosed or long afterward often cause diagnostic problems.[2] LGSS usually cannot be detected on Papanicolaou smears because the cells lack sufficient atypia to permit their differentiation from benign endometrial stromal cells.

Stromal tumors that involve the endometrium can be recognized in endometrial biopsies and curettings. A definitive diagnosis of stromal sarcoma can be made if myometrial invasion is identified in the tissue fragments or with imaging studies, but a hysterectomy is usually required to permit the thorough evaluation of the tumor margin necessary to distinguish a stromal sarcoma from a benign stromal nodule. Because stromal sarcomas are considerably more common than stromal nodules, a stromal tumor found in an endometrial biopsy or curettage is likely to be malignant. As discussed earlier in the section on cellular leiomyomas, endometrial stromal tumors must be differentiated from highly cellular leiomyomas because the treatment of these tumors is quite different. At surgery, LGSS may resemble intravenous leiomyomatosis or a leiomyoma that has extended into the parametrium or broad ligament. These entities can usually be distinguished on frozen section examination.

Gross Findings

Endometrial stromal sarcoma usually involves the endometrium, sometimes extensively. It forms soft, tan, smooth-surfaced polyps that are occasionally partly infarcted and hemorrhagic. By definition, ESS invades the myometrium. There are three main patterns of growth within the myometrium. In the first, the myometrium is diffusely thickened, but a clearly defined tumor is not evident. In the second, there is a nodular tumor with soft, tan or yellow-orange cut surfaces, as opposed to the white, whorled, firm surface of a leiomyoma. In the third, and most frequent, pattern of growth, the myometrium is permeated by poorly demarcated pink, tan, or yellow cords and nodules of tumor (Fig. 13.28). High-grade tumors grow as soft, fleshy, polypoid tumors that bulge into, and often fill, the endometrial cavity.[316] Multiple masses of soft, white-to-tan tumor invade the underlying myometrium on a broad front. Hemorrhage and necrosis are frequently present.[162]

ESS grows beyond the uterus as infiltrating masses of tan or white tumor that can be palpated as firm cords in the parauterine tissues. Pink or tan strands of tumor protrude from the cut surface of the infiltrated tissues and sometimes can be pulled from tissue spaces and vessels.

Microscopic Findings

Endometrial stromal sarcoma cells resemble proliferative phase or hyperplastic endometrial stromal cells.[85,127] Most ESS are low-grade tumors with cells of relatively uniform size and shape, imparting a monotonous appearance to the tumor. The tumor cells have round or ovoid nuclei with finely granu-

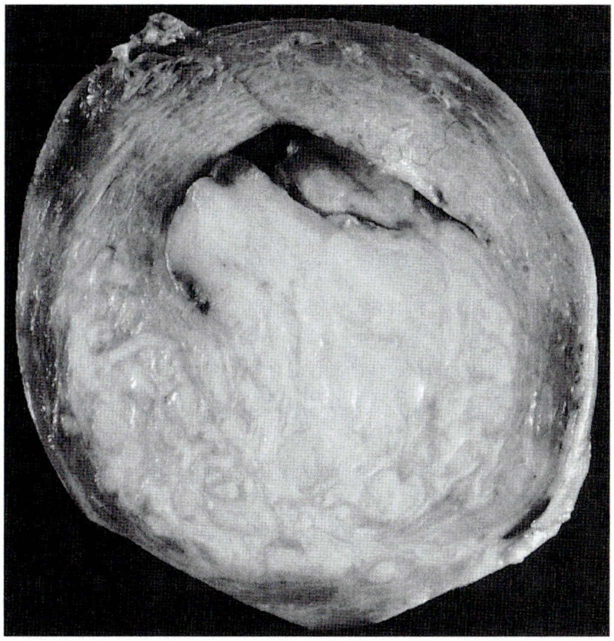

Fig. 13.28. Low-grade endometrial stromal sarcoma. Fleshy tan polypoid tumor projects into the endometrial cavity, and cordlike or trabecular masses of tumor extensively infiltrate the myometrium in the lower half of the uterus.

lar dispersed chromatin and small, inconspicuous nucleoli (Fig. 13.29). The cytoplasm is amphophilic, and the cell borders are poorly defined. Rare LGSS consist predominantly of spindle-shaped cells that are fibroblastic in appearance with fusiform nuclei and elongated cell bodies.[215] Reticulin fibers surround individual cells or small groups of cells in a basket-weave pattern. Mitotic activity is low in most LGSS. There are typically less than 3 MF/10 HPF, but there can be greater mitotic activity in neoplasms that are otherwise typical of LGSS; occasionally there are more than 10 MF/10 HPF. Proliferation of small vessels and arterioles resembling the endometrial spiral arterioles is a characteristic finding (Fig. 13.30). The arterioles tend to be uniformly distributed among the stromal cells, and capillaries and small veins are often conspicuous as well. In the past, the prominent vascularity occasionally led to a mistaken diagnosis of hemangiopericytoma. Plaques and zones of hyaline fibrosis are common in LGSS, and aggregates of foam cells or foci of necrosis are occasionally noted. Rarely, abundant myxoid stroma widely separates the tumor cells.[215] The stromal cells can show focal or diffuse decidual change in patients who are pregnant or taking exogenous progestins. Limited smooth muscle differentiation is occasionally present in LGSS[33,92,127]; only when the proportion of smooth muscle cells exceeds 30% is the tumor classified as a combined stromal–smooth muscle tumor.[212]

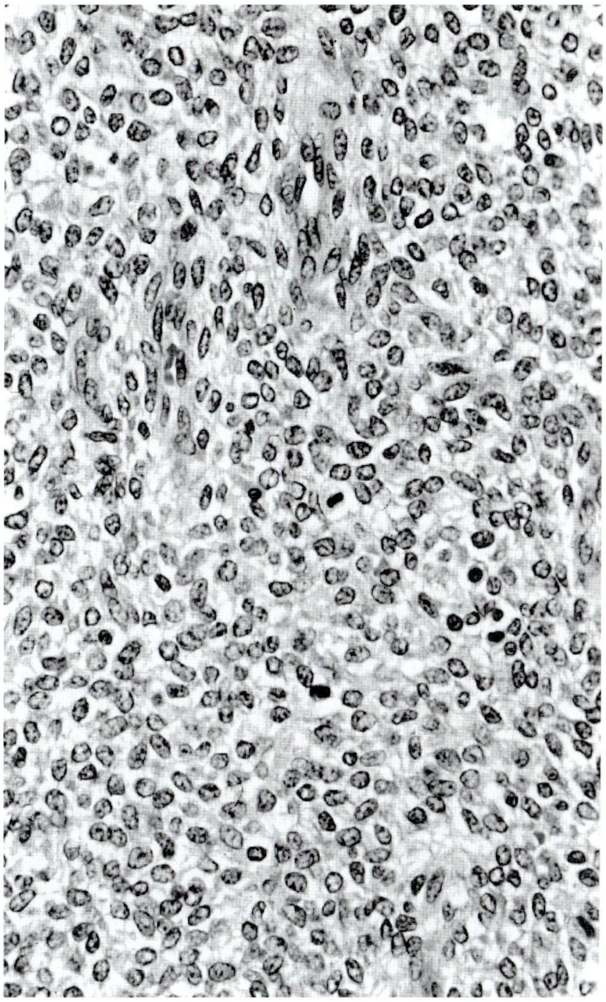

Fig. 13.29. Low grade endometrial stromal sarcoma. The tumor cells have uniform round or oval nuclei and scanty cytoplasm with ill-defined cell borders. Note the absence of mitotic activity.

LGSS invades the myometrium and may extensively permeate it (Fig. 13.31). Invasion of lymphatic and vascular channels is a characteristic finding (Fig. 13.32) that at one time led pathologists to call the tumor endolymphatic stromal myosis.[149] Epithelial-like differentiation occurs in about 25% of LGSS. It is highly variable in its appearance and can take the form of trabecular cords of epithelioid cells, mesothelial-like tubules lined by cuboidal or low columnar cells with eosinophilic cytoplasm, endometrial-type glands, or glands lined by clear or vacuolated cells (Fig. 13.33).[206] The epithelial-like pattern is reminiscent of an ovarian sex cord tumor in some instances,[50] and, in others, there is en-

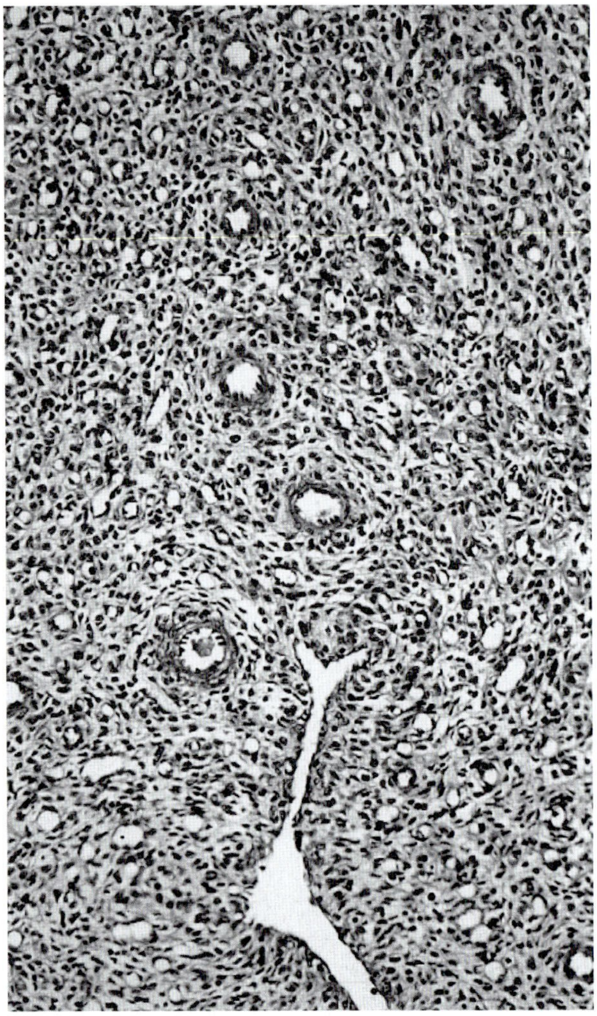

Fig. 13.30. Low-grade endometrial stromal sarcoma. Note the numerous small blood vessels distributed relatively uniformly among the tumor cells.

dometrial glandular differentiation that can make it difficult to recognize that the tumor is a stromal sarcoma.[54]

Most ESS are low-grade tumors, but some appear to be of higher grade, based on the nuclear size, degree of nuclear atypia, or mitotic activity. The former have traditionally been designated as low-grade ESS and the latter as high-grade ESS. The criteria for differentiating between LGSS and HGSS are controversial, and some pathologists think that it would be more appropriate to classify HGSS as pleomorphic or undifferentiated sarcomas rather than as a type of ESS.[33,85,151] Most, however, continue to use the term HGSS, and that is the approach used in this chapter. Norris and Taylor initially proposed using the mitotic count to differentiate LGSS from HGSS.[206] Tumors with less than 10 MF/10 HPF were classified as LGSS and those with 10 or more as HGSS. More recently, several authors have noted that occasional tumors that are otherwise typical of LGSS have more than 10 MF/10 HPF and some HGSS have fewer than 10 MF/10 HPF.[21,26,33,70,85,286,291] Chang et al. have shown that the mitotic count is not a statistically valid method for dividing ESS into low and high-grade types.[33] In the WHO monograph *Histological Typing of Female Genital Tract Tumours*, HGSS is defined as "a sarcoma without specific features or heterologous elements but with an infiltrating pattern that suggests an origin from endometrial stromal cells."[261]

In this chapter, the more restrictive definition adopted by Silverberg and Kurman in the AFIP fascicle *Tumors of the Uterine Corpus and Gestational Trophoblastic Disease* is used. HGSS is defined as "an infiltrative tumor composed of anaplastic and mitotically active cells bearing at least some morphologic resemblance to endometrial stromal cells."[274] Compared to LGSS, the cells in HGSS have larger, more vesicular nuclei (Fig. 13.34) in which chromatin clumps are coarser and more prominent

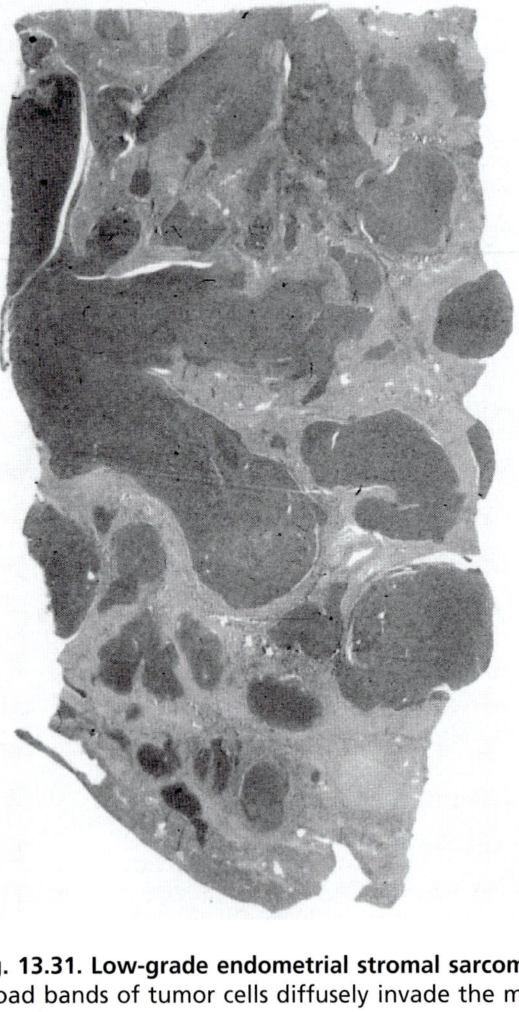

Fig. 13.31. Low-grade endometrial stromal sarcoma. Broad bands of tumor cells diffusely invade the myometrium.

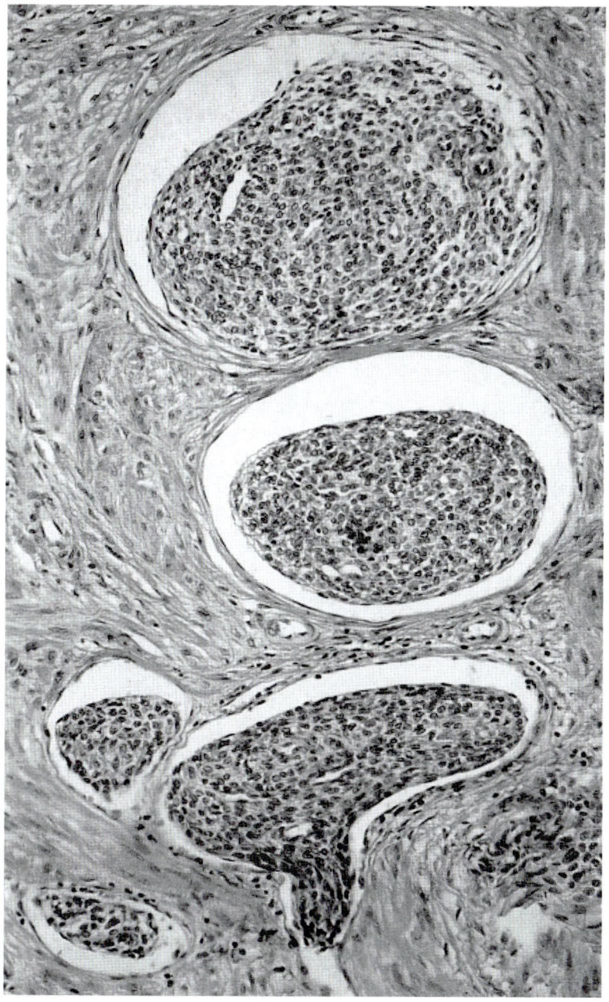

Fig. 13.32. Low grade endometrial stromal sarcoma. Plugs of tumor grow within lymphovascular spaces in the myometrium. (Reprinted with permission from Progress in Surgical Pathology, Volume III, edited by C. M. Fenoglio and M. Wolff, New York: Masson Publishing, Inc., 1981, pp. 1–35.)

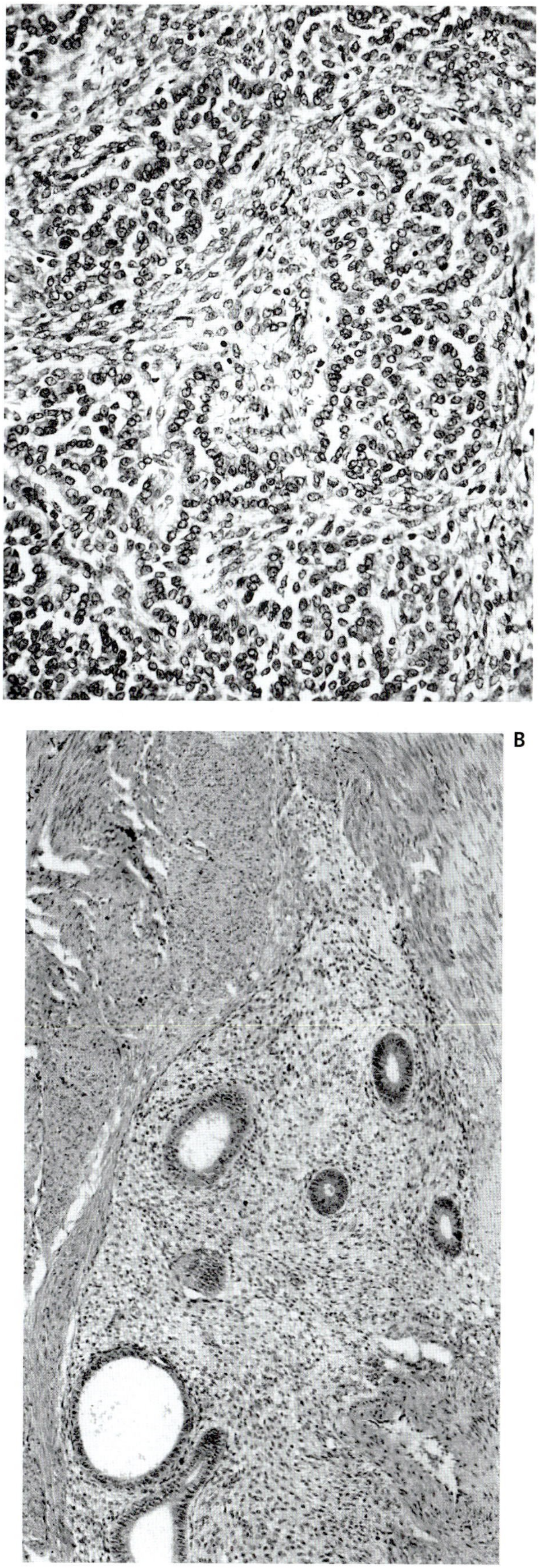

Fig. 13.33. Patterns of epithelial-like differentiation in low-grade endometrial stromal sarcoma. Trabeculae and tubules reminiscent of ovarian sex cords are present in some tumors (**A**). Rare tumors contain endometrial-type glands within myoinvasive nests of endometrial stromal cells (**B**).

and nucleoli are more conspicuous.[149,316] The tumor cells tend to be larger, with eosinophilic or amphophilic cytoplasm and indistinct cell borders (Fig. 13.35). The mitotic count cannot be used as the sole criterion to differentiate HGSS from LGSS, but a high mitotic count is characteristic of HGSS. There are almost always 10 or more MF/10 HPF, and not uncommonly there are 20 or more MF/10 HPF in the most active areas. Flow cytometric studies usually reveal a DNA aneuploid pattern and a high percentage of cells in S phase.[81,260] A destructive pattern of myometrial invasion with areas of hemorrhage and necrosis is indicative of HGSS, as is an irregular and pleomorphic vascular pattern. Various other features have been proposed as adjuncts for grading and can be considered in difficult cases (Table 13.4). It remains a matter of dispute whether LGSS and HGSS should be viewed as low- and high-grade variants of a single type of neoplasia or two essentially unrelated tumor types. The finding of occasional cases in which both low- and high-grade elements are intermixed (see Fig. 13.34) indicates that, at least occasionally, a LGSS can evolve into a higher-grade sarcoma.[39,88,316]

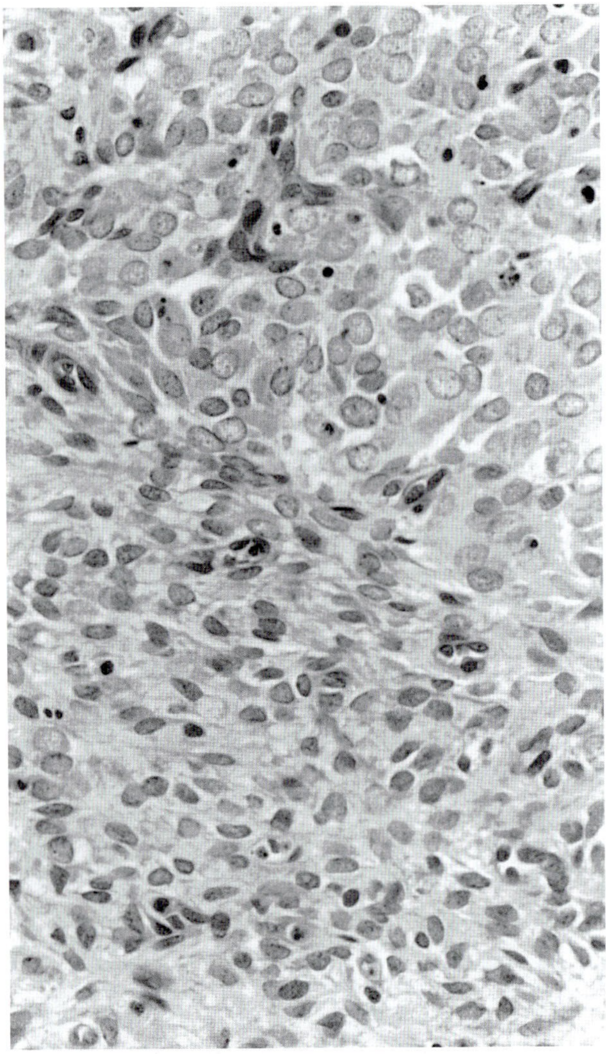

Fig. 13.34. High-grade endometrial stromal sarcoma. This stromal sarcoma has both high-grade (HGSS, *top*) and low-grade (LGSS, *bottom*) areas. The HGSS cells have significantly larger, more vesicular nuclei, and apoptotic bodies and mitotic figures are more numerous.

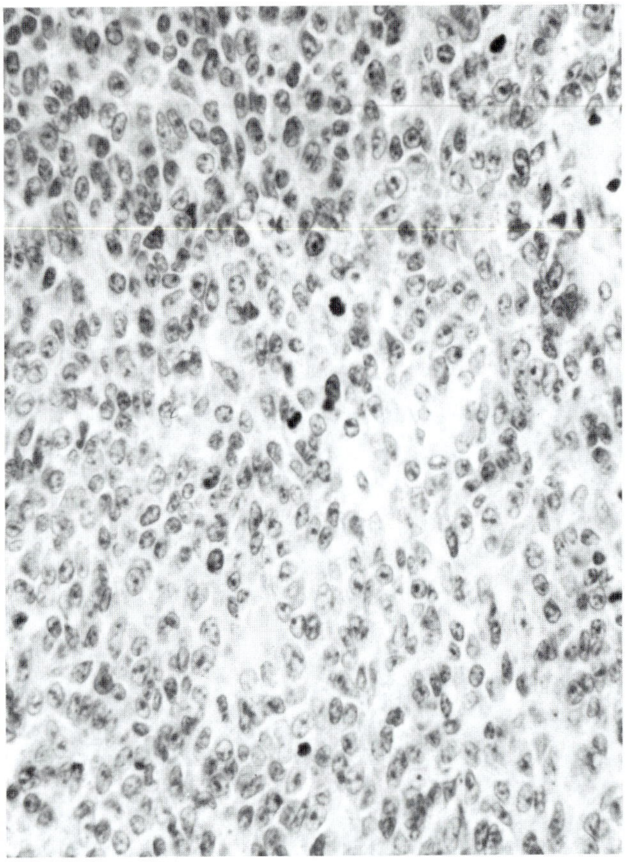

Fig. 13.35. High-grade endometrial stromal sarcoma. The stromal cells are atypical and there are frequent mitotic figures.

There are a limited number of reports describing the cytogenetics of LGSS, but these include some describing a recurrent translocation involving chromosomes 7 and 17 [t(7;17)(p15;q21)]. Koonz et al recently identified two genes, which they called JAZF1 (*J*uxtaposed with *A*nother *Z*inc *F*inger gene, at 7p15) and JJAZ1 (*J*oined to *JAZF1*, at 17q21), which are fused in most endometrial stromal tumors.[155a] The fusion was detected in all stromal nodules and LGSS tested, and in 3/7 HGSS. They commented that 2 of the HGSS would be classified as "undifferentiated endometrial stromal sarcomas" by some, and that of these two, one showed the fusion and the other did not. The function of the genes involved and the significance of the absence of the fusion in some HGSS remain to be determined.

Table 13.4. Typical pathologic findings in endometrial stromal tumors

Diagnosis	*MF/10 HPF*	*Atypia*	*Vascular pattern*	*Ploidy*	*S phase (%)*	*ER/PR*
Stromal nodule	<3[a]	0–1+	Prominent, regular	Diploid	Low	+
LGSS	<3[a]	0–1+	Prominent, regular	Diploid	Low	+
HGSS	>10[b]	2+–3+	Inconspicuous, irregular	Aneuploid	High	–

MF, mitotic figures; HPF, high-power field; ER, estrogen receptor; PR, progesterone receptor; LGSS, low-grade endometrial stromal sarcoma; HGSS, high-grade endometrial stromal sarcoma.
[a]Some have more mitotic figures, including >10 MF/10 HPF in occasional tumors.
[b]Occasional tumors in this category have <10 MF/10 HPF.

Immunohistochemistry

Immunostains for cytoplasmic thin and intermediate filaments can be useful in the diagnosis of ESS. Although stromal sarcoma cells are immunoreactive for vimentin, other tumors in the differential diagnosis, such as smooth muscle tumors, are also vimentin positive.[73] Staining for vimentin is therefore mainly used to verify that a tumor is adequately preserved for immunohistochemical testing. Immunoreactivity for actin and desmin has been reported in ESS,[89,100] but our experience, like that of others,[23,73] is that most ESS either lack these filaments or express them only weakly. Actin, as detected by antibodies to muscle-specific actin or smooth muscle actin, is the more likely of the two to be expressed, and occasional tumors exhibit diffuse strong staining for actin filaments. ESS cells generally either do not stain for desmin or show only focal and weak reactivity. Diffuse strong staining for both actin and desmin suggests that the tumor is a small cell smooth muscle tumor that simulates a stromal neoplasm or, if the staining is focal, a mixed endometrial stromal–smooth muscle tumor. Immunostains for caldesmon, a recently developed marker of smooth muscle differentiation, are reported to be negative in ESS.[206a,248a] Stromal sarcoma cells are typically negative for cytokeratin, but positive staining is occasionally noted, either diffusely or in the epithelial-like structures seen in some LGSS.[23,89] Staining for epithelial membrane antigen is negative. Immunostains for the CD10 antigen appear to be a useful marker for LGSS, as the tumor cell cytoplasm is strongly stained in LGSS but not in smooth muscle tumors.[5a,43,185a] The epithelial-like structures that are present in about a quarter of LGSS have a mixed epithelial–myogenic phenotype.[169] They may stain for cytokeratin but not for epithelial membrane antigen. They also tend to stain strongly for vimentin, muscle-specific actin, and, in some instances, desmin. Occasionally, these epithelial-like structures stain for calretinin, and the ones that resemble sex cord derivatives can be immunoreactive for inhibin (see "Uterine Tumor Resembling an Ovarian Sex Cord Tumor").[14]

Immunostains for proliferation markers such as Ki-67 (MIB-1) stain the nuclei of cycling tumor cells; the percentage of positive nuclei generally correlates with the degree of mitotic activity. Estrogen receptors can be demonstrated in a majority of LGSS, and virtually all express progesterone receptors.[241,251] Positive immunohistochemical staining for hormone receptors can be used to guide therapy in those instances in which the clinician is contemplating treatment with progestins or some other form of hormonal therapy. Immunohistochemistry is most often used as an aid in the differential diagnosis between LGSS and smooth muscle tumors such as highly cellular leiomyoma and intravenous leiomyomatosis. A panel of immunostains that can help with this differential diagnosis is shown in Table 13.5. In general, immunohistochemistry is not as effective in evaluating HGSS, because reactivity for many antigens, especially hormone receptors, is lost in these poorly differentiated tumors. Staining for actin and desmin can help in the differential diagnosis between HGSS and leiomyosarcoma as the latter is often immunoreactive for these filaments whereas the former is typically negative. Strong pos-

Table 13.5. Immunohistochemical findings in endometrial stromal and smooth muscle tumors

Antibody	*Stromal tumor*	*Smooth muscle tumor*
Smooth muscle actin	0–++	++–+++
Desmin	0–+	++–+++
Caldesmon	0	++–+++
CD 10	++–+++	0–+
Vimentin	+++	+++

itive staining for actin and/or desmin therefore favors leiomyosarcoma, but negative staining is uninformative, because a significant proportion of poorly differentiated leiomyosarcomas also fail to stain for these filaments.

Clinical Behavior and Treatment

The extent of tumor, the type of surgical intervention, and, possibly, the tumor grade determine the risk of recurrence. The tumor stage is the most significant prognostic factor.[81,85] Hysterectomy and bilateral salpingo-oophorectomy is the standard treatment for stage I stromal sarcoma, with debulking of extrauterine tumor performed in more advanced cases. Some gynecologic oncologists remove the adnexa, even in young women, because adnexal spread (Fig. 13.36) is not always visible at surgery, LGSS generally contain estrogen receptors and the residual tumor cells might be stimulated by estrogen secreted by the ovaries, and some studies have suggested that recurrence is more frequent when the adnexal structures are conserved.[21,162] Others, however, do not recommend a salpingo-oophorectomy for young women whose adnexa appear normal and have not observed an adverse outcome in women whose ovaries were conserved.[177,206] Conservative approaches to treatment are sometimes considered in young women when preservation of fertility is an important consideration. If the uterus is small, and if the tumor is low grade and circumscribed or delimited on hysteroscopy or MRI, gynecologic oncologists sometimes attempt to treat ESS by local excision. Unfortunately, our experience has been that this is rarely successful and the tumor tends to recur within a year or two.

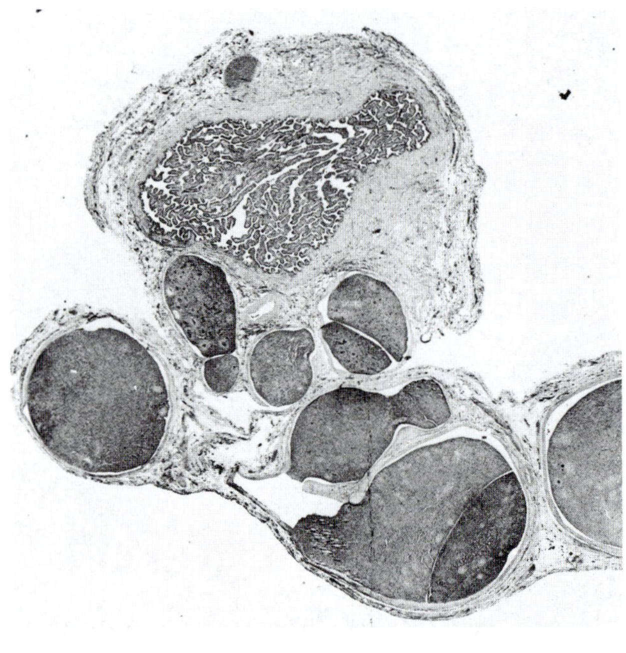

Fig. 13.36. Low-grade endometrial stromal sarcoma. The tumor has spread to the adnexa and grows in the lymphatics of the mesosalpinx and fallopian tube wall.

Even when the tumor appears confined to the uterus (stage I), there is a high risk of pelvic recurrence, ranging from 25% to 50%.[21,105,112,162,230] The risk of recurrence is even greater in patients with advanced-stage tumors. Some oncologists recommend postoperative progestin therapy for LGSS with the hope of reducing the risk of recurrence, but many patients are unable to tolerate long-term treatment. LGSS grows slowly, and recurrences are often not detected until many years after initial treatment. Most recurrences are in the pelvis and involve the pelvic soft tissues, ureters, bladder, vagina, or bowel. Metastases in the abdomen involve the peritoneal surfaces or omentum. A few patients develop pulmonary metastases.[2,21,112,127,177] Recurrent or metastatic LGSS can be stabilized or suppressed with progestational agents in more than 50% of patients.[85,149,230,291] Tumors with a high level of progesterone receptors are most likely to respond to progestin therapy. Treatment with gonadotropin-releasing hormone agonists has been used in a few cases.[187,260] Recurrent or metastatic low-grade ESS that do not respond to treatment with progestins can sometimes be treated surgically or with radiotherapy.[21] Chemotherapy tends to be ineffective.[230] Low-grade ESS is a slowly progressive disease and, in those patients who ultimately die of tumor, the median time from diagnosis to death ranges up to about 11 years. Despite the high frequency of recurrences, women with stage I low grade ESS have a survival rate in excess of 80%.[33,202,230] The outcome is less favorable for women with advanced-stage tumors, for whom 5-year survival rates of 40–50% have been reported.[33,162]

High-grade ESS is relatively uncommon, and its clinical behavior is difficult to evaluate because of differences in diagnostic criteria and because many reported series have included other types of high-grade sarcomas.[70] Reported 5-year survival rates vary.[85,177,202] The best survival rates in stage I HGSS exceed 50% and, as mentioned earlier, some authors have been unable to document a difference in survival between low- and high-grade stage I ESS.[21,33,162] The survival is less favorable when there is advanced disease at presentation (0–50% 5-year survival for HGSS versus 40–50% for low grade ESS).[21,105,186] HGSS can be more rapidly growing than LGSS, with recurrences often presenting within 2 years of initial treatment.[105,177,316] Pelvic recurrences are fewer, and survival is better in patients with low-stage disease who are treated with combined surgery and radiotherapy. Recurrence outside the radiation field is the most common reason for treatment failure in a patient who has had combined therapy. An effective chemotherapy regimen is not available and high grade ESS usually does not express progesterone receptors or respond to progestin therapy.[177,284,316]

Endometrial Stromal Tumor Variants

There are two types of neoplasms containing endometrial stroma that can be viewed as variants of endometrial stromal nodules or sarcomas. One is a tumor that resembles, at least focally, an ovarian sex cord tumor; the other is a combined smooth muscle–stromal tumor.

Uterine Tumor Resembling an Ovarian Sex Cord Tumor

The tumors in this category were initially described by Clement and Scully, who separated them into two types.[50] Type I tumors are endometrial stromal nodules or sarcomas in which there are significant areas of epithelial-like structures that have an appearance reminiscent of an *ovarian sex cord–stromal tumor*. The epithelial-like cells range from small, cuboidal, or polygonal cells with scanty amphophilic or eosinophilic cytoplasm to plump polygonal cells with pale foamy or granular eosinophilic cytoplasm (Fig. 13.37). Their nuclei often resemble those of the surrounding stromal cells. The epithelial-like cells grow in cords, trabeculae, or nests, or form tubules (Fig. 13.37). Immunohistochemical tests to elucidate their nature yield variable results. There is most often a mixed epithelial–myoid phenotype, with immunoreactivity for cytokeratin and actin, and, in some cases, desmin.[14,169] Immuno-stains for EMA are almost always negative. In accord with the resemblance to a sex cord tumor, immunoreactivity for inhibin and CD 99 is detected in the epithelial-like structures in about a third of type I tumors.[14]

Type II tumors tend to be surrounded by myometrium and lack an identifiable site of origin from the endometrium. They have a circumscribed or slightly irregular periphery. The tumor cells form plexiform cords, trabeculae, and nests, and may line

A

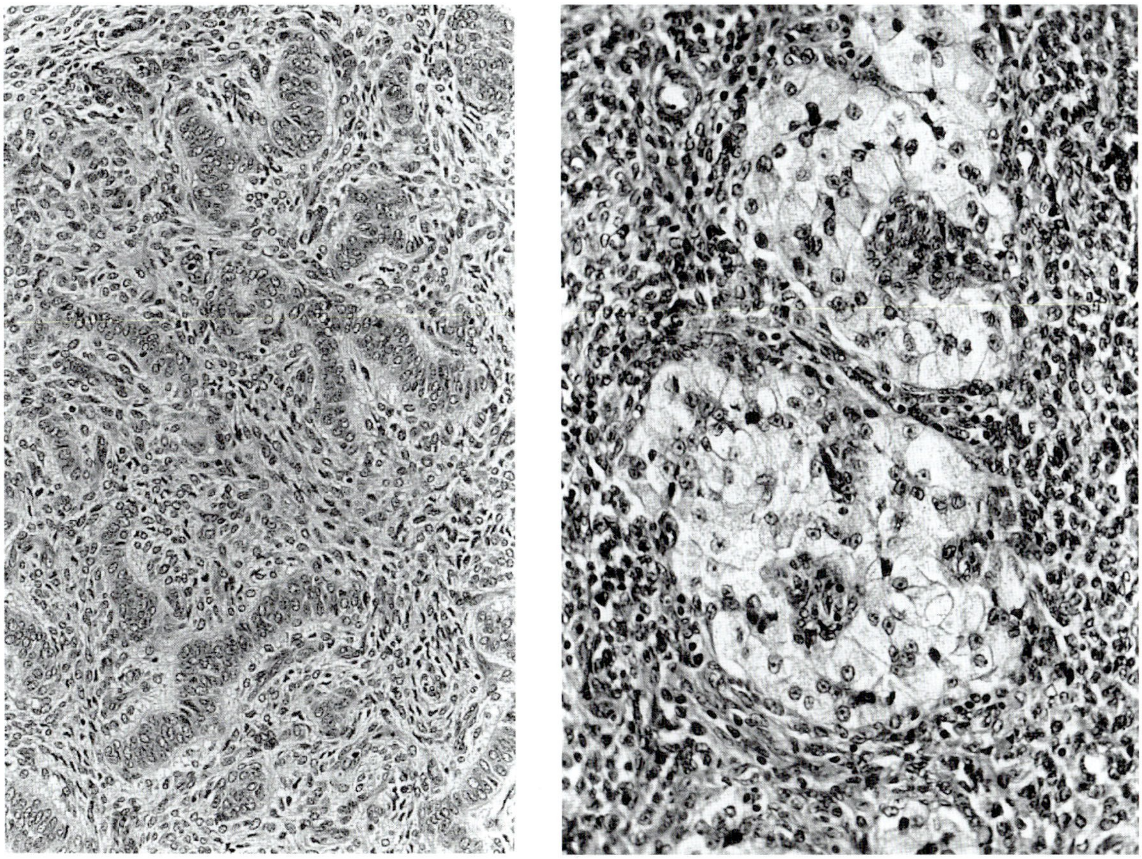

B

Fig. 13.37. Uterine tumor resembling an ovarian sex cord tumor. Type I tumors in which sex cord-like trabeculae composed of small cells (**A**) or polygonal cells with pale, foamy cytoplasm (**B**) are surrounded by neoplastic endometrial stromal cells.

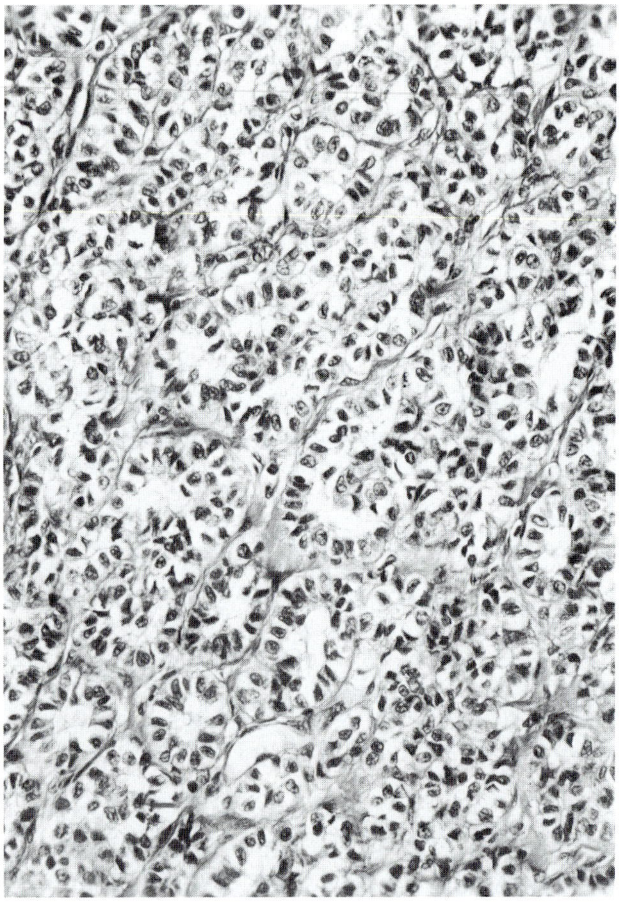

Fig. 13.38. Uterine tumor resembling an ovarian sex cord tumor. Type II tumor, in which the cells grow in a tubular pattern with scanty stroma.

well-formed tubules with lumens (Fig. 13.38).[50,156] The tumor cells have uniform small bland nuclei with inconspicuous nucleoli, and mitotic figures are rare. The cytoplasm varies from scant to moderate and eosinophilic to abundant and foamy, and the cells are cuboidal or columnar in shape. The stroma accounts for less than 50% of the tumor, and ranges from endometrial-like to hyaline or fibrous; stroma is scanty in some type II tumors. The nature of type II tumors is unclear, but since the epithelial-like structures in many of them are similar to those that occur in type I tumors, some or all may be of endometrial stromal cell origin.[50] Diverse immunohistochemical results have been described in case reports of tumors of this type, but recently two small series of type II cases have revealed that the sex cord-like structures are usually immunoreactive for vimentin, cytokeratin, inhibin, CD 99, Melan-A, and, often, smooth muscle actin.[14,156] Immunostains for EMA are negative,[14] but estrogen and progesterone receptors are usually present.[156] An aggregate of filaments resembling Charcot–Böttcher filaments was observed in a sertoliform type II tumor studied with the electron microscope, but the case was unusual in that tumor was also present in the ovary and there were omental metastases.[146] The immunophenotype, together with the absence of heterologous mesenchymal elements and clear-cut carcinoma, helps to differentiate these rare tumors from mixed müllerian tumor.

Clinically, uterine tumors resembling ovarian sex cord tumors occur in middle-aged women; the average age is around 50. The main symptom is abnormal bleeding or pelvic pain. Most patients have an enlarged uterus or a palpable uterine mass. Although type I and II tumors have a similar presentation, the clinical behavior differs. Type I tumors are endometrial stromal tumors with a focal sex cord pattern; those with circumscribed margins are benign, but those with infiltrating margins behave as low-grade endometrial stromal sarcomas. In Clement and Scully's initial report, three of five patients with follow-up had recurrences and two died.[50] In their review of the literature, Baker et al. found that about 15% of reported cases were known to have recurred.[14] Type II tumors, on the other hand, usually have a benign clinical evolution.[50]

Combined Stromal–Smooth Muscle Tumor

Focal areas of smooth muscle differentiation are commonly observed in endometrial stromal tumors, but tumors with extensive areas of both smooth muscle and endometrial stromal differentiation are rare. *Combined smooth muscle–stromal tumors* have been arbitrarily defined as those having at least 30% of each component.[47,212,289] The components tend to be sharply demarcated, although they occasionally merge into each other. Tumors with circumscribed margins are more common than those with infiltrating margins. The stromal elements are typical of endometrial stromal neoplasms and consist of uniform small cells with round nuclei and scanty cytoplasm. Small thin-walled blood vessels are scattered uniformly throughout the stromal component, and epithelial-like structures are present in some tumors.

The immunophenotype of the stromal cells is identical to that observed in other endometrial stromal tumors. In most tumors, the stromal cells do not stain for desmin, or only scattered cells stain. Staining for smooth muscle actin shows a similar pattern, although in some tumors staining is more extensive or more intense. The smooth muscle elements grow in fascicles, irregular circumscribed aggregates of spindle cells surrounded by stromal cells, or nodules within which the tumor cells are embedded in a collagenous stroma, sometimes resulting in a "starburst"-like appearance. The smooth muscle cells vary in appearance from typical spindle-shaped smooth muscle cells with abundant eosinophilic cytoplasm in the fascicles and aggregates to rounded epithelioid cells with clear or amphophilic cytoplasm in the nodules. Despite their variable appearance, the smooth muscle cells have a typical immunophenotype and show uniform strong positive staining for smooth muscle actin and desmin. Large, thick-walled blood vessels are typically present in the smooth muscle areas.

The clinical evolution of combined smooth muscle–stromal tumors is poorly documented, but tumors with an infiltrative margin are endometrial stromal sarcomas capable of recurrence or metastasis whereas those with a circumscribed margin are benign endometrial stromal nodules.[47,212] Tumors in which the smooth muscle elements show features of leiomyosarcoma such as significant nuclear atypia, a high mitotic rate, and necrosis presumably have the potential to metastasize, but no case of this type with documented metastases has been reported to date. Some neoplasms that were reported as "stromomyomas" are endometrial stromal tumors in which there are trabeculae and cords of cells that exhibit ultrastructural features of smooth muscle differentiation.[288] This finding is not surprising because the epithelial-like structures commonly seen in endometrial stromal tumors often have a myogenous immunophenotype, and such tumors are best classified as endometrial stromal tumors, not combined neoplasms.[14,169] It remains unclear whether immunophenotypic evidence of extensive smooth muscle differentiation (i.e., strong positive staining for desmin and smooth muscle actin) in an otherwise typical endometrial stromal tumor should be viewed as indicative of a combined smooth muscle–stromal tumor. At present, the diagnosis of a combined tumor is based solely on the presence of significant amounts of both elements as recognized by routine light microscopy.[47]

Mixed Epithelial–Mesenchymal Tumors

Mixed epithelial–mesenchymal tumors contain both epithelial and mesenchymal elements as active participants in the neoplastic process (Table 13.6). The tumors in this group are morphologically, but perhaps not histogenetically, related. The mixed epithelial–mesenchymal tumor group includes adenofibroma and adenosarcoma. Mixed müllerian tumor (MMT) or carcinosarcoma is included in this group in many classifications of uterine tumors, including the one published by the WHO (see Table 13.1).[261] Recent biologic and clinical studies suggest a close relationship between mixed müllerian tumor and endometrial carcinoma, and MMT is often considered to be a special type of sarcomatoid or metaplastic carcinoma. It is discussed in Chapter 12, Endometrial Carcinoma, in this volume.

Adenofibroma

Adenofibroma is a benign biphasic neoplasm that typically occurs in the endometrium, although occasionally it arises in the cervix or in an extrauterine location.[1,302,323]

Clinical Features

Women with adenofibroma tend to be elderly.[323] The median age is 68 years, and most patients are peri- or postmenopausal. Despite a predilection for the elderly, adenofibroma occurs in women of all ages, from less than 20 years to more than 80 years.[267] There is no known association with race, nor does adenofibroma have the epidemiologic features of endometrial carcinoma. Abnormal vaginal bleeding is the most frequent complaint. Less common findings include abdominal pain, abdominal enlargement, or a polypoid tumor projecting from the cervix. Some patients have a history of prior removal of polyps.

Table 13.6. Classification of mixed epithelial–mesenchymal tumors of the uterus

Tumor	*Malignant potential*	*Epithelium*	*Mesenchymal component*
Adenofibroma	None	Benign	Benign, homologous
Adenosarcoma	Low[a]	Benign	Low-grade sarcoma, homologous or heterologous[b]
Mixed müllerian tumor (carcinosarcoma)[c]	High	Carcinoma	High-grade sarcoma, homologous or heterologous

[a,b]Uncommon tumors with sarcomatous stromal overgrowth are more aggressive and have high-grade sarcomatous elements.
[c]Mixed müllerian tumor is discussed in Chapter 12, Endometrial Carcinoma.

Gross Findings

Adenofibroma is a lobulated polypoid tumor that can arise anywhere in the uterus or in the cervix. It varies from soft to firm and is tan or brown. About 50% of adenofibromas contain small cysts that give the cut surface a spongy or mucoid appearance. The tumor ranges from 2 to 20 cm in maximum diameter, with a median of 7 cm. A large adenofibroma may fill the endometrial cavity and enlarge the uterus.

Microscopic Findings

Adenofibroma contains a mixture of histologically bland epithelium and mesenchyme. It originates in the endometrium or cervix. Broad papillary fronds covered by epithelium project from the surface of the neoplasm and extend into cystic spaces within it (Fig. 13.39). Columnar or cuboidal epithelial cells, most often of endometrioid type, line cysts and cleft-like spaces. A mixture of various types of epithelia, including endocervical, tubal, and squamous, often occurs within the same neoplasm. The epithelium can be hyperplastic and stratified, but when this is the case the possibility that the tumor might be an atypical polypoid adenomyoma should be carefully considered.[170] Malignant epithelium has been reported to occur in adenofibroma, but such tumors are best viewed as variants of endometrial adenocarcinoma and treated accordingly.[191]

The mesenchymal component is usually fibroblastic, but endometrial stromal cells or mixtures of stromal cells and fibroblasts are present in some neoplasms. Rarely, histologically benign heterologous elements such as fat or skeletal muscle are present.[135,275] The fibrotic stroma is more cellular and uniform than it is in polyps. The hypercellular periglandular stroma that characterizes adenosarcoma is not present in adenofibromas. Stromal cell atypia is generally absent or mild, and markedly atypical mesenchymal cells are not present. Mitotic figures are rare. There are invariably fewer than 4 MF/10 HPF,[323] and some regard the presence of virtually any detectable mitotic activity as indicative of adenosarcoma.[53] Adenofibromas are usually confined to the endometrium or cervical mucosa and do not invade the underlying myometrium or cervical stroma (Fig. 13.40). Two unique adenofibromas that invaded the myometrium, and, in one case, myometrial veins, have, however, been reported.[52]

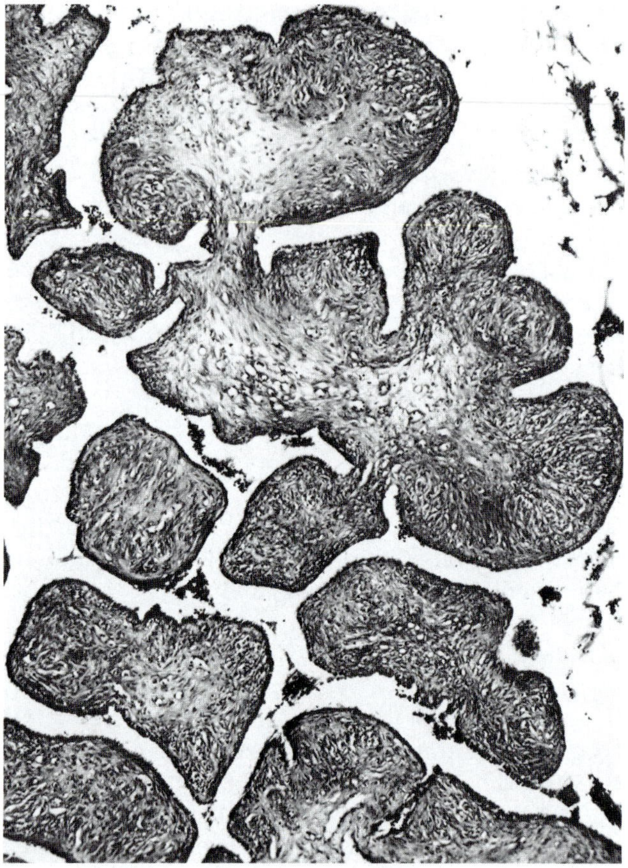

Fig. 13.39. Adenofibroma. The papillary growth projects from the surface and into cystic spaces. It has a hypocellular, collagenous stroma and is lined by cytologically bland cuboidal to low columnar epithelium. (Reprinted from Cancer 48;1981:354–366. Copyright © 1981 American Cancer Society. Reprinted by permission of Wiley-Liss, Inc., a subsidiary of John Wiley & Sons, Inc.)

Clinical Behavior and Treatment

Hysterectomy is the preferred treatment for an adenofibroma because the neoplasm may recur if it is incompletely curetted or excised.[220,267] Hysterectomy ensures complete removal, and also permits the thorough sampling needed to exclude an adenosarcoma. Conservative therapy, such as hysteroscopy with repeat curettage, can be considered in situations in which hysterectomy is not the first choice of treatment, such as in a young woman who wishes to preserve her fertility. Adenofibroma is benign and no tumor-related deaths have been reported. Both the previously mentioned patients with myoinvasive adenofibromas were well after hysterectomy, but the prognosis is less clear cut when an adenofibroma exhibits unusual gross or microscopic features.

Adenosarcoma

Initially reported by Clement and Scully in 1974, *adenosarcoma* is a biphasic tumor composed of benign epithelial elements and a sarcomatous stroma.[49] It most often occurs in the endometrium

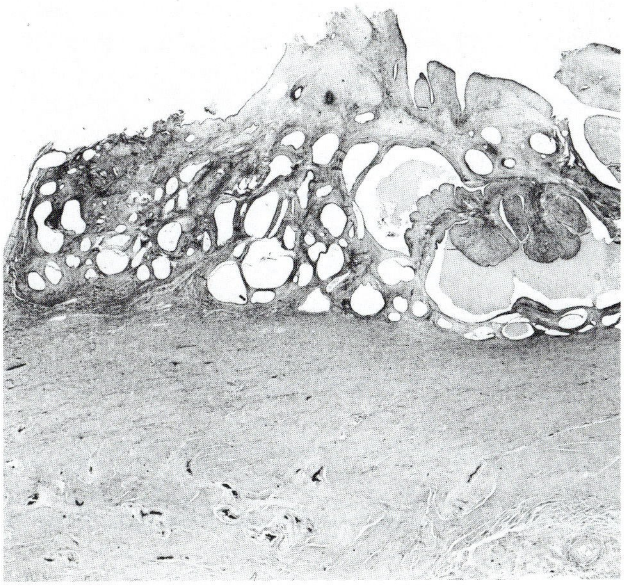

Fig. 13.40. Adenofibroma. A typical superficial tumor that is limited to the endometrium and does not invade the myometrium. (Reprinted from Cancer 48;1981: 354–366. Copyright © 1981 American Cancer Society. Reprinted by permission of Wiley-Liss, Inc., a subsidiary of John Wiley & Sons, Inc.)

but it is also found in the cervix and in extrauterine pelvic locations, such as the fallopian tube, ovary, and paraovarian tissues.

Clinical Features

Adenosarcoma occurs in women of all ages. The median age is 57–59 years, with a range of 15 to 90 years.[7,24,53,143,265,323] Extrauterine adenosarcoma occurs in younger women and is more aggressive than its uterine counterpart.

There is no association of adenosarcoma with obesity or hypertension. A few patients have a history of prior pelvic radiation.[53] Occasional patients are diabetic. Adenosarcoma has been reported in women undergoing tamoxifen therapy for breast cancer.[48,195,265] Some patients have had a history of surgery for removal of cervical or endometrial polyps.

The most common presenting symptom is abnormal vaginal bleeding. Vaginal discharge, pain, nonspecific urinary symptoms, a palpable pelvic mass, and a tumor protruding from the cervix are other common signs and symptoms. Most patients have stage I tumors at the time of diagnosis.[24,53,285]

Gross Findings

Adenosarcoma is a polypoid endometrial neoplasm that grows into the cavity and can enlarge the uterus.[53] Rare tumors arise in the myometrium, presumably from adenomyosis,[53,115,210] and 5–10% of adenosarcomas occur in the cervix.[143,152] Adenosarcoma is usually a polypoid neoplasm averaging about 5 cm in maximum dimension, but it sometimes grows as multiple papillary or polypoid masses.[53,143] It can be either soft or firm. The cut surface is tan, brown, or gray, and zones of hemorrhage and necrosis are observed in about 25% of adenosarcomas. Small cysts are present in most tumors.

Microscopic Findings

Tubular glands and cleftlike spaces are dispersed throughout the stroma, and papillary stromal fronds covered by epithelium project from the surface and into cysts (Fig. 13.41).[53,323] The most common type of epithelium resembles inactive or proliferative endometrial epithelium. Many other types of epithelium also occur in adenosarcoma, including secretory, hyperplastic, atypical hyperplastic endometrioid, mucinous, squamous, and clear cell.[98] The epithelium typically is cytologically bland, but slight atypia

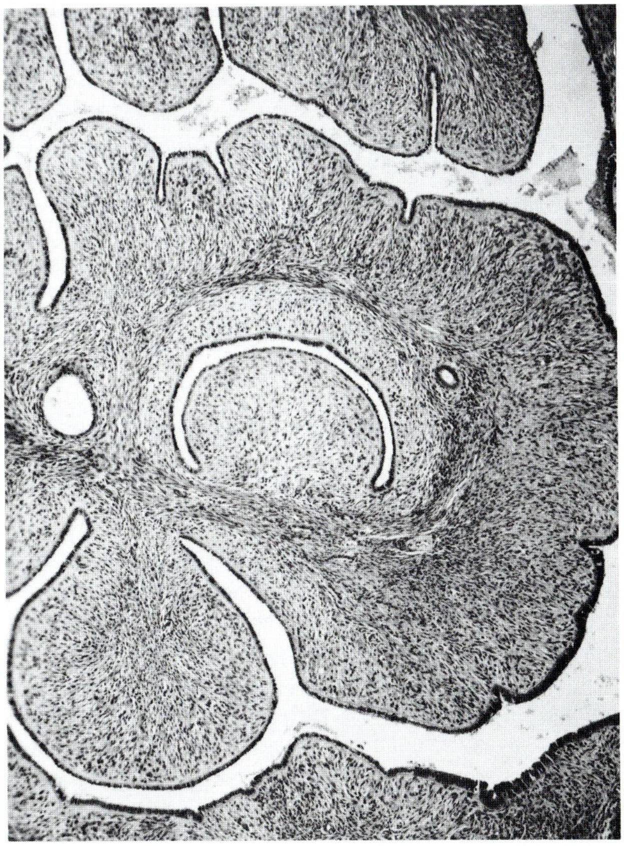

Fig. 13.41. Adenosarcoma. This polypoid tumor is lined by bland epithelium and exhibits dense stromal cellularity. The high cellularity contrasts with the low degree of stromal cellularity seen in adenofibroma (compare with Fig. 13.39).

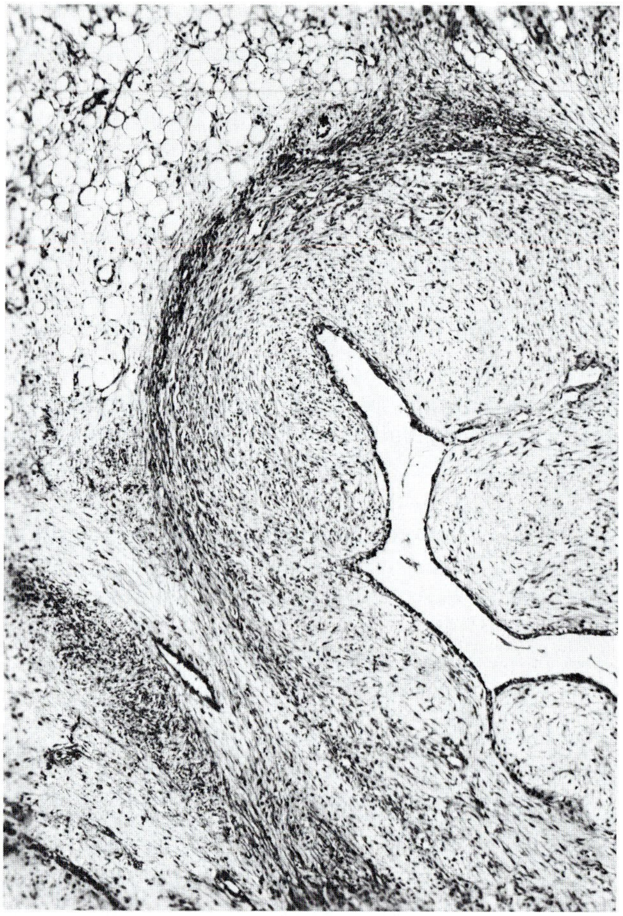

Fig. 13.42. Adenosarcoma. Note the periglandular stromal hypercellularity, a feature that is characteristic of adenosarcoma. Fat is present in the *upper left*. Smooth muscle, cartilage, and striated muscle also occur in adenosarcoma but are not seen here.

is occasionally noted.[53] By definition, carcinoma is not present in adenosarcoma (see Table 13.6), but it is occasionally noted in the adjacent endometrium.[53,265] Glands and stroma can both be present in areas of myometrial invasion, which are observed in 15–52% of adenosarcomas,[143] suggesting that the epithelium is an actively proliferating part of the neoplasm.

The mesenchymal component of an adenosarcoma generally is a homologous sarcoma such as stromal sarcoma or fibrosarcoma[53]; smooth muscle is also present in some tumors.[91] Periglandular stromal hypercellularity is a characteristic feature of adenosarcoma (Figs. 13.41 and 13.42). The mesenchymal cells show a variable degree of nuclear atypia, but only mild to moderate atypia is present in most tumors. Mitotic figures are readily identified in most tumors and generally number 4/10 HPF or more.[143,323] Rare neoplasms with an atypical cellular stroma characteristic of adenosarcoma, but in which mitotic activity is inconspicuous, recur or metastasize.[53] Therefore, a neoplasm with an atypical, hypercellular stroma that is condensed around the epithelial elements should be diagnosed as an adenosarcoma even if there are only 1–3 MF/10 HPF.[53]

Adenosarcomas often contain bland areas indistinguishable from adenofibroma, so extensive microscopic study may be required to identify a sarcomatous component.[98] Trabecular, insular, or tubular arrangements of plump epithelial-like cells, some having abundant foamy cytoplasm, can be found in about 5% of adenosarcomas (Fig. 13.43).[51,132] These structures, which are designated as sex cord-like elements, resemble the epithelial-like structures commonly seen in endometrial stromal tumors. Heterologous mesenchymal elements are present in 20–25%

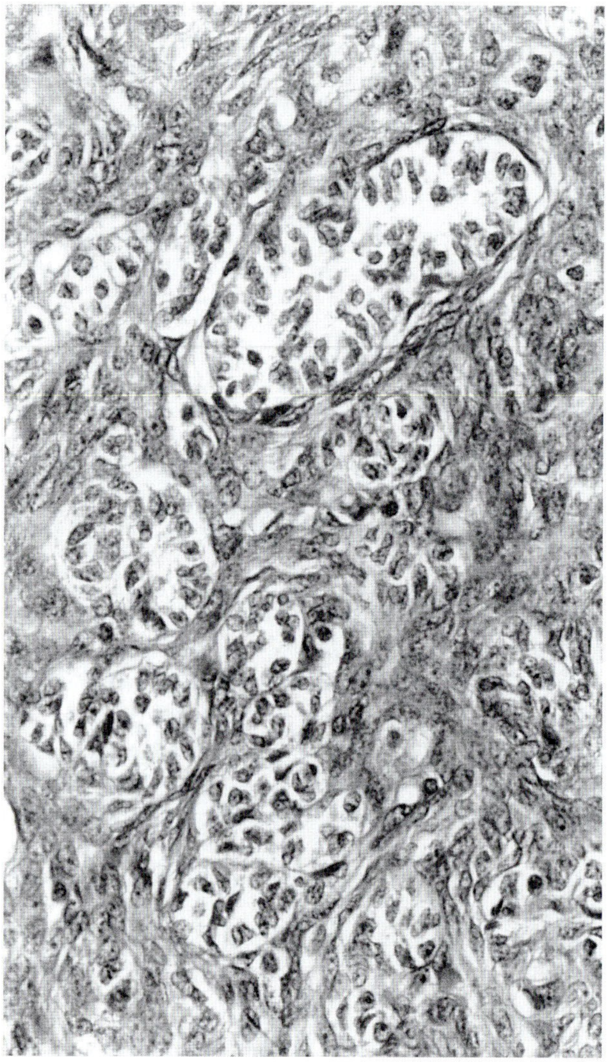

Fig. 13.43. Adenosarcoma. Tubular structures reminiscent of sex cord elements are present in the stroma.

of adenosarcomas. Striated muscle (rhabdomyosarcoma) is the most common heterologous element, but cartilage, fat (Fig. 13.42), and other elements are occasionally observed.[159] The differential diagnosis of adenosarcoma of the cervix with rhabdomyosarcomatous mesenchymal elements includes embryonal rhabdomyosarcoma of the cervix. The latter occurs in teenagers and young adults, and when a botryoid pattern is present, the appearance can mimic adenosarcoma.[69] Rhabdomyosarcoma lacks an epithelial component, and the mesenchymal elements are more monomorphic.

Sarcomatous overgrowth, seen in 10% of adenosarcomas, is said to occur when the sarcomatous component of the tumor occupies 25% or more of the total tumor volume.[24,46,143] Epithelial elements are absent in the region of sarcomatous overgrowth. The mesenchymal component is typically of higher grade in the region of sarcomatous overgrowth, with increased cellularity and mitotic activity and greater nuclear atypia (Fig. 13.44). It can be stromal sarcoma, fibrosarcoma, or leiomyosarcoma, or a mixture of elements.[91,143] Heterologous elements, particularly rhabdomyosarcoma, may occur in and be limited to the zone of sarcomatous overgrowth.[143] Lymphovascular space invasion, when it occurs in adenosarcoma, is most often found in zones of sarcomatous overgrowth.[143]

Clinical Behavior and Treatment

Adenosarcoma is usually treated by hysterectomy and bilateral salpingo-oophorectomy, although a few young patients have been treated by local excision of the tumor.[53,111,323] Occasional patients whose tumors show sarcomatous overgrowth have pelvic lymph node metastases.[143,265] The role of postoperative pelvic radiation and chemotherapy is unclear. Adenosarcoma is not as aggressive as mixed müllerian tumor, but it recurs in 25–40% of patients and occasionally follows an aggressive course.[15,24,143,220,265] Recurrence is generally in the pelvis or vagina, but distant metastases occur in 5% of patients.[24,53,98] Recurrences typically consist exclusively of the sarcomatous component,[15,24,115] but both epithelium and stroma are occasionally present.[53] Pathologic features of the primary tumor that are associated with an increased risk of recurrence or metastasis are extrauterine spread at diagnosis; myometrial invasion, especially into the outer half of the myometrium; and sarcomatous overgrowth of the mesenchymal component.[53,143,323] Invasion of capillary–lymphatic spaces in the myometrium or the presence of rhabdomyosarcoma in zones of sarcomatous overgrowth also portend an unfavorable outcome.[143] There is no clear correlation between the prognosis and the mitotic rate in the mesenchymal component.[53,323] Extended clinical observation is necessary because there is typically a long (3.5–5 years) interval between treatment and recurrence.[53,323] About a quarter of patients with adenosarcoma die of tumor, often more than 5 years after initial diagnosis.

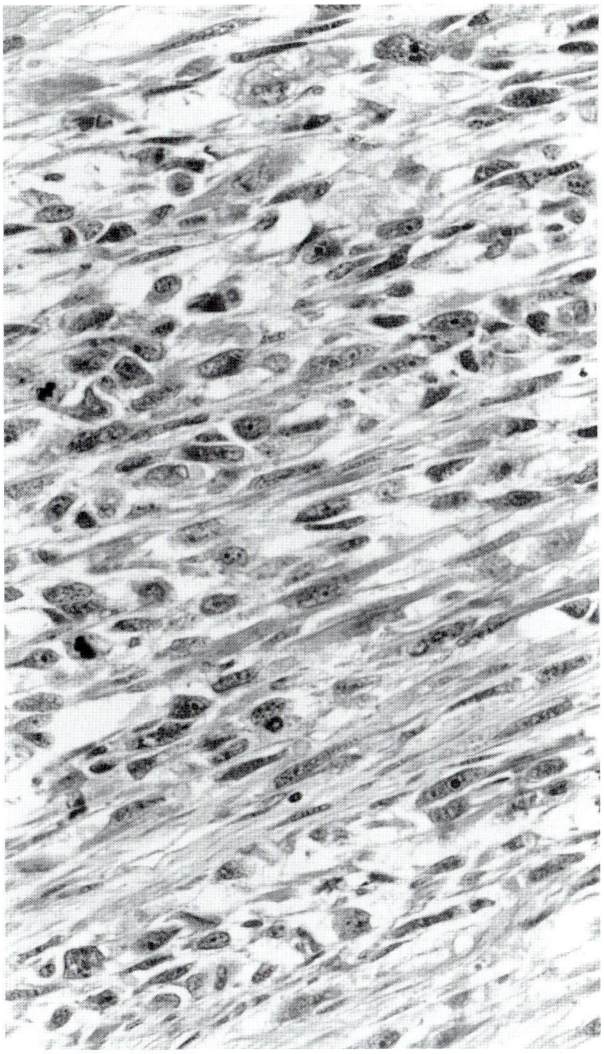

Fig. 13.44. Adenosarcoma with sarcomatous stromal overgrowth. The mesenchymal cells and spindle shaped and have atypical, hyperchromatic nuclei. Several mitotic figures are present.

Miscellaneous Mesenchymal Tumors and Conditions

Adenomyosis and Adenomyoma

Adenomyosis is a common condition, detected in 15–30% of hysterectomy specimens.[263] It is characterized by the presence of endometrial glands and stroma within the myometrium.

Clinical Features

Patients are typically pre- or perimenopausal women who present with abnormal bleeding and dysmenorrhea.[12] Symptoms tend to be more severe in women with deep myometrial involvement.[168] The uterus is enlarged. Adenomyosis is usually most extensive in the posterior wall, which may be thickened. A clinical diagnosis of adenomyosis can often be confirmed by such imaging studies as transvaginal ultrasonography and MRI.[27]

Pathologic Findings

On gross examination, the cut surface of the myometrium is trabeculated and contains hemorrhagic foci, but a distinct tumor nodule is not present. Small blood-filled cysts may be noted. Microscopically, foci of endometrial glands and stroma are present within the myometrium (Fig. 13.45).

The lower border of the endometrium is irregular and dips into the superficial myometrium. To avoid misclassifying a normal histologic finding as adenomyosis, it is advisable to make the diagnosis only when the distance between the lower border of the endometrium and the adenomyosis exceeds one-half of a low-power field (about 2.5 mm). Adenomyosis exhibits a varied functional response to ovarian hormones. Proliferative glands and stroma generally are observed in the first half of the menstrual cycle. Adenomyosis may not respond to physiologic levels of progesterone, and secretory changes frequently are absent or incomplete during the second half of the cycle.

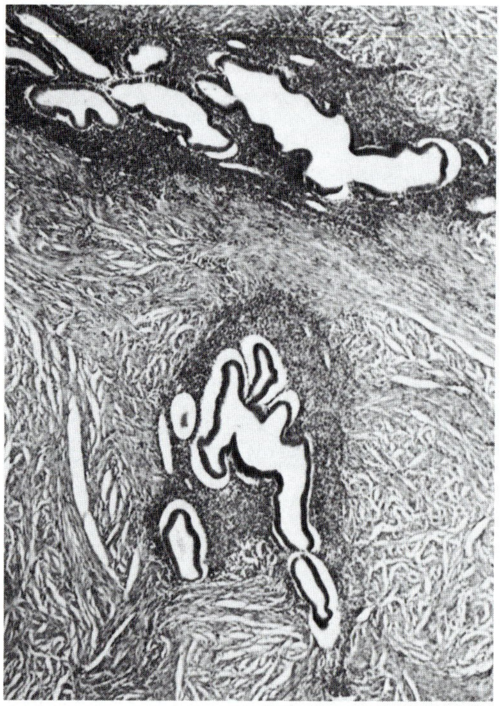

Fig. 13.45. Adenomyosis. Endometrial glands and stroma are present within the myometrium.

There are two variants of adenomyosis that pathologists should be aware of as they can suggest a malignant tumor. In one, endometrial tissue protrudes into myometrial vessels, simulating vascular invasion by a neoplasm. Intravascular endometrial tissue, consisting of endometrial stroma and glands or endometrial stroma alone, can be found in as many as 20% of uteri with adenomyosis.[252] It usually appears to arise in the perivascular region and push into the vessel lumen. In another variant of adenomyosis, which tends to occur in elderly women, glands are sparse and some adenomyotic foci consist mainly or exclusively of endometrial stromal cells.[114] Careful evaluation reveals that these variants of adenomyosis lack features of malignancy. When present, glands are dispersed, uncrowded, and lined by cytologically benign cells. The stromal cells are mitotically inactive and show no evidence of myometrial invasion. These variants are almost always accompanied by foci of typical adenomyosis and are not part of a more widespread malignant process.

An adenomyoma is a circumscribed, nodular aggregate of smooth muscle, endometrial glands, and, usually, endometrial stroma.[108] It may be located within the myometrium or it may involve or originate in the endometrium and grow as a polyp. About 2% of endometrial polyps are adenomyomas. A rare variant of an adenomyomatous polyp, the atypical polypoid adenomyoma, has atypical hyperplastic glands that usually contain foci of squamous metaplasia. Atypical polypoid adenomyoma occurs most often in premenopausal women (see Chapter 10, Benign Diseases of the Endometrium).[101,170,321]

Adenomatoid Tumor

Adenomatoid tumors are distinctive genital tract neoplasms of mesothelial origin that occur in both men and women.[71] In women they occur in the uterus, the fallopian tube, and the ovary.[320,322]

Clinical Features

Adenomatoid tumors typically occur in women of reproductive age; the median age is 42 years. There is no evidence that they impair fertility, and they are usually incidental findings in uteri removed for other causes. Adenomatoid tumors are found in about 1% of hysterectomy specimens, but no specific symptoms have been attributed to them. The tumor is benign. Rarely, an adenomatoid tumor merges with another type of mesothelioma that has the potential for recurrence.

Pathologic Findings

Adenomatoid tumors are usually located subserosally in the cornual myometrium. They are typically small, measuring 0.5–1 cm in diameter, but some are larger and giant adenomatoid tumors have been reported. Adenomatoid tumors are round and rubbery and are often thought to be leiomyomas. The cut surfaces are gray or tan and may have a spongy appearance due to the presence of uniform small cysts.

Microscopically, adenomatoid tumors tend to be circumscribed, although rare diffuse variants have been described. They consist of tubules and cords of varying size and shape that are lined by flat or cuboidal epithelial cells (Fig. 13.46A). Collagen, elastic tissue, and smooth muscle surround the epithelial elements. The smooth muscle may so predominate that the tumor appears at first glance to be a leiomyoma. The cuboidal epithelial cells have cytologically bland, eccentric, round nuclei and abundant pale cytoplasm (Fig. 13.46B). The cytoplasm is often vacuolated, sometimes to the extent that some tumor cells resemble signet-ring cells. The growth of the epithelial cells between smooth muscle bundles and the presence of signet-ring-like cells may raise the suspicion of metastatic adenocarcinoma. Nuclear atypia, however, is absent or minimal, mitotic figures are infrequent, and stains for mucin are negative. When the cells lining the tubules are flattened, an adenomatoid tumor may resemble a hemangioma. However, the lumens do not contain blood, and immunostains for such vascular markers as factor VIII-related antigen and CD 31 are negative. Ultrastructural and immunohistochemical studies reveal that the epithelial cells in adenomatoid tumors have a mesothelial phenotype. Immunostains are positive for cytokeratin (Fig. 13.46C) and vimentin and for such mesothelial cell-associated antigens as thrombomodulin and HBME-1. Stains for adenocarcinoma-associated antigens such as CD 15, CEA, B72.3, and Ber-EP4 are usually negative, although variable positivity for the latter has been reported in adenomatoid tumors of the uterus.

Inflammatory Myofibroblastic Tumor

Inflammatory myofibroblastic tumor (IMT), also known as *inflammatory pseudotumor*, is a benign but potentially locally aggressive proliferation of myofibroblasts.[109,239] Grossly, the tumors range up to 12 cm in maximum diameter. They are firm or soft, and the cut surfaces are tan or white and often mucoid. Microscopically, the myofibroblasts are spindle shaped or stellate and have pale eosinophilic cytoplasm. Their nuclei are granular or vesicular and they may have prominent nucleoli. Mitotic activity is variable, but the mitotic index is generally less than 10/10 HPF and atypical mitotic figures are not present. The background is frequently edematous, and lymphocytes and plasma cells are scattered among the myofibroblasts. Immunohistochemical stains for smooth muscle actin or desmin typically are positive, although staining may be focal. Staining for specific markers of smooth muscle differentiation such as caldesmon is absent. Recent reports indicate that IMT may show cytoplasmic staining for ALK-1, a useful diagnostic feature.

IMT occurs in premenopausal women and may arise in children. The presentation is with symptoms related to the presence of a mass, such as pain or pressure, but some patients have constitutional symptoms including fever, weight loss, and fatigue. IMT is a benign lesion that does not metastasize. Recurrences of uterine IMT have not been reported, but there is a local recurrence rate of about 15% in patients with extrauterine IMT. IMT were initially considered to be inflammatory pseudotumors, but the documentation of the clonal nature of some IMT and the demonstration of chromosomal rearrangements involving the ALK locus region indicate that it may be more appropriate to view them as true neoplasms.[165,281]

Homologous and Heterologous Sarcoma

Most tumors in this category are high-grade sarcomas that resemble the mesenchymal component of a mixed müllerian tumor. They consist of round or spindled cells with variable amounts of cytoplasm and pleomorphic atypical nuclei. Mitotic figures are usually numerous. They differ from endometrial stromal sarcomas in that the tumor cells exhibit no clear resemblance to endometrial stromal cells. Pure *heterologous sarcomas* occasionally arise in the uterus. Rhabdomyosarcoma (Fig. 13.47) is the most common of these,[40,126,133,218,271] but chondrosarcoma,[44] osteosarcoma,[66,74,83] liposarcoma,[16] and tumors containing mixtures of heterologous elements also occur. Neoplasms resembling more ambiguous types of sarcomas such as malignant fibrous histiocytoma and malignant rhabdoid tumor have also been reported in the uterus. Histologically benign heterotopic bone, cartilage, and fat are occasionally found in the uterus, and rare benign tumors contain one or more of these elements.[22,244,295,315] They should not be mistaken for *heterologous sarcomas* or for an MMT.

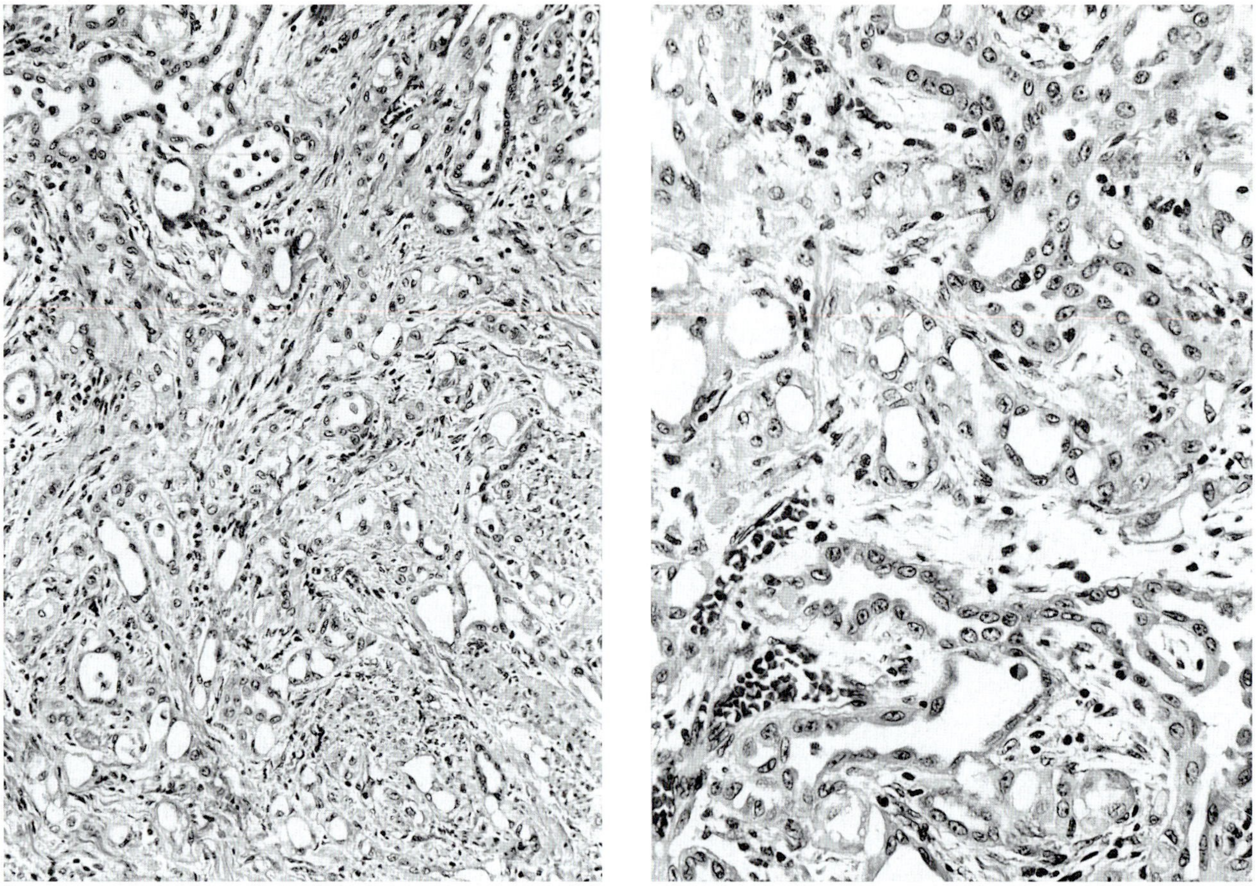

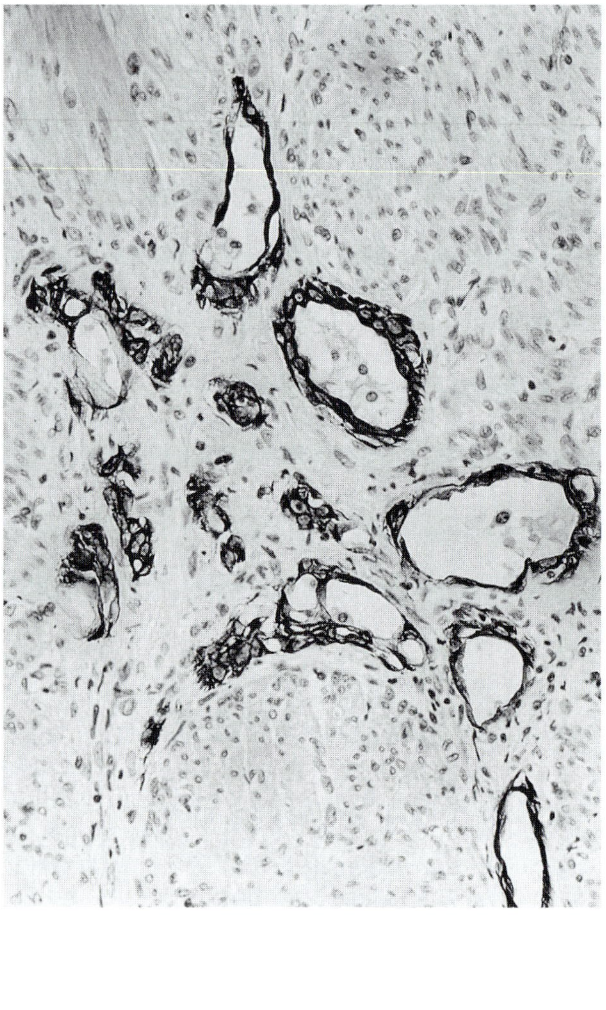

Fig. 13.46. Adenomatoid tumor. Tubules and microcystic spaces grow within the myometrium (**A**). The tubules and microcysts are lined by cuboidal or flattened mesothelial cells that have cytologically bland nuclei (**B**). An immunohistochemical stain for cytokeratin highlights the mesothelial cells (**C**).

Primitive Neuroectodermal Tumor

Rarely, a *primitive neuroectodermal tumor* (*PNET*) develops in the uterus.[68,99,130,276] PNET can occur at any age, but most are found in postmenopausal women. The usual clinical presentation is with abnormal vaginal bleeding. PNET is a soft, fleshy, gray or white polypoid mass that originates in the endometrium and invades the myometrium. Microscopically, it is composed of small cells with round to oval hyperchromatic nuclei and scanty cytoplasm (Fig. 13.48). Cellular areas merge with fibrillary foci of glial differentiation within which ganglion cells may be present. Rosettes, Homer–Wright pseudorosettes, and perivascular ependymal-type rosettes may be present. Immunostains are generally positive for one or more neural or neuroendocrine markers, such as neuron-specific enolase (NSE), glial fibrillary acidic protein (GFAP), chromogranin, or S-100 protein. Electron microscopic studies have revealed neural processes containing filaments and microtubules and, in some examples, neurosecretory granules. Too few patients have been studied to define the clinical behavior and most appropriate treatment for PNET of the uterus. Women with stage I neoplasms can be cured, but more advanced tumors generally are fatal. Foci of primitive neuroectodermal differentiation can be present in a mixed müllerian tumor, and a diag-

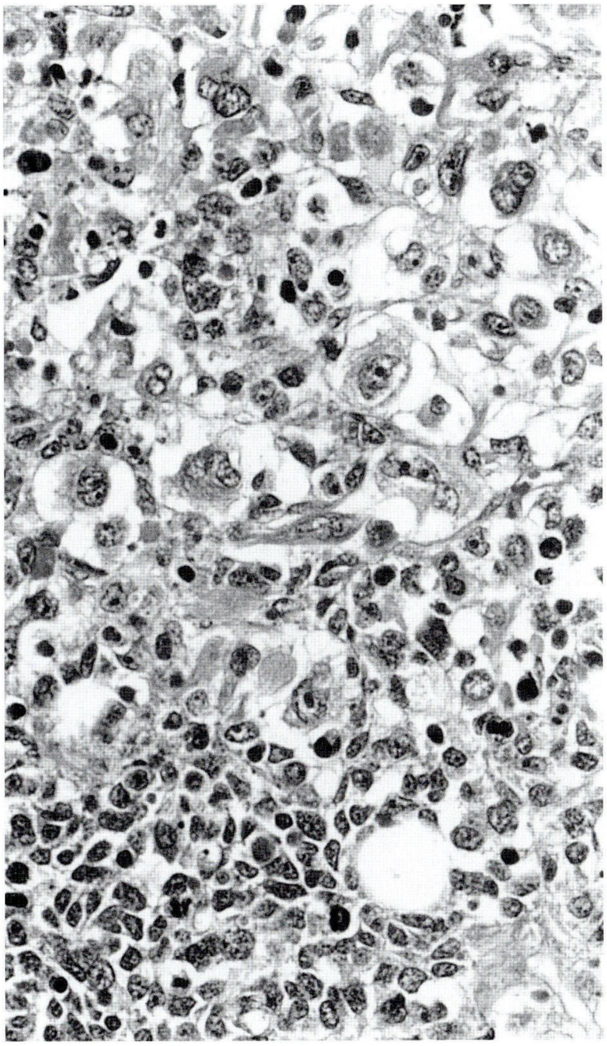

Fig. 13.47. Rhabdomyosarcoma of the uterus. The tumor consists of small round cells with scanty cytoplasm, round to polygonal cells with abundant eosinophilic cytoplasm, and spindled or strap-shaped cells with fibrillar eosinophilic cytoplasm. Immunohistochemical stains for muscle-specific actin, desmin, and myogenin were positive in these cells.

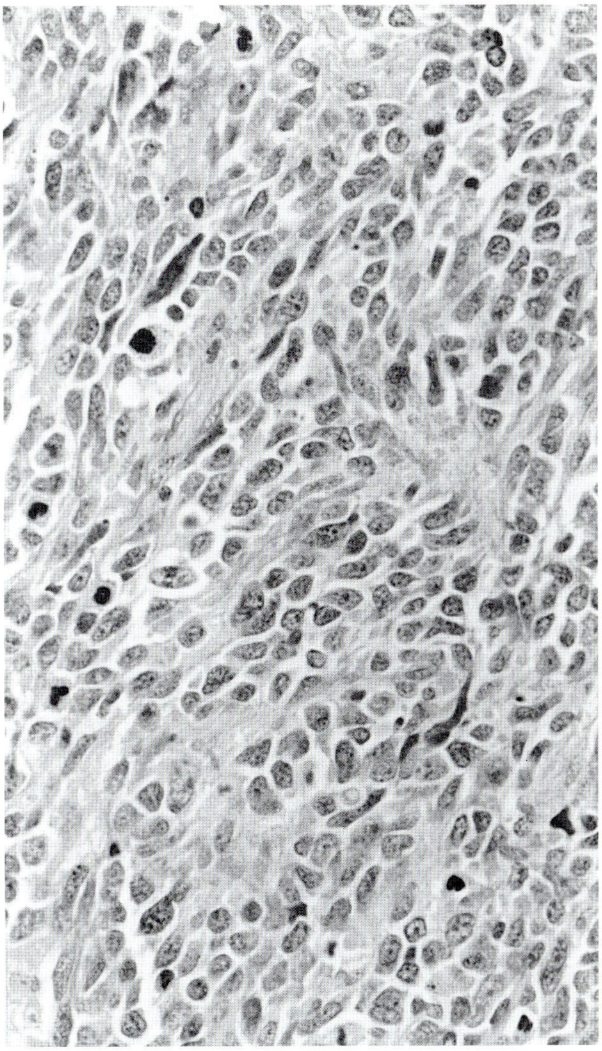

Fig. 13.48. Primitive neuroectodermal tumor of the uterus. The tumor cells are small and round or oval, and there is eosinophilic, fibrillar material in the background.

nosis of PNET is only appropriate when malignant epithelial elements are absent.

Vascular Tumors

Hemangiomas of the uterus, like those at other sites, are composed of neoplastic vessels lined by flat or cuboidal endothelial cells (Fig. 13.49). The endothelial cells have bland nuclei and mitotic figures are rare or, most typically, absent. Uterine hemangiomas can be subclassified as capillary, cavernous, or venous, depending on the appearance of the vessels.[171,308] There are no clinical differences between the subtypes. Capillary hemangiomas of the cervix are the most common vascular tumors of the uterus. Hemangiomas of the corpus are uncommon, and they vary considerably in size. Large hemangiomas can extend through the full thickness of the myometrium and can result in severe bleeding that requires a hysterectomy. Arteriovenous malformations can occur in the uterus.[95,173] They are differentiated from venous hemangiomas by the presence of thick-walled vessels of both arterial and venous types. The histologic distinction between a hemangioma and a vascular malformation can be difficult, but it is not critical because their clinical features are similar. A few examples of angiosarcoma of the uterus have been reported.[192,255,311] Angiosarcoma is a large, hemorrhagic, and often extensively necrotic tumor that grows in the myometrium. It consists of anastomosing vascular channels that are lined by atypical cuboidal or "tombstone"-shaped endothelial cells. Many mitotic figures are usually present. Some high-grade angiosarcomas consist partly or completely of solid sheets of difficult-to-recognize epithelioid endothelial cells.[287] When these cells predominate, the nature of the tumor can be determined by identifying characteristic foci of vascular growth, often at the periphery of the tumor, and by finding positive immunohistochemical stains for markers of vascular differentiation such as factor VIII-related antigen or CD 31. Angiosarcoma extensively invades and replaces the myometrium and has a poor prognosis.

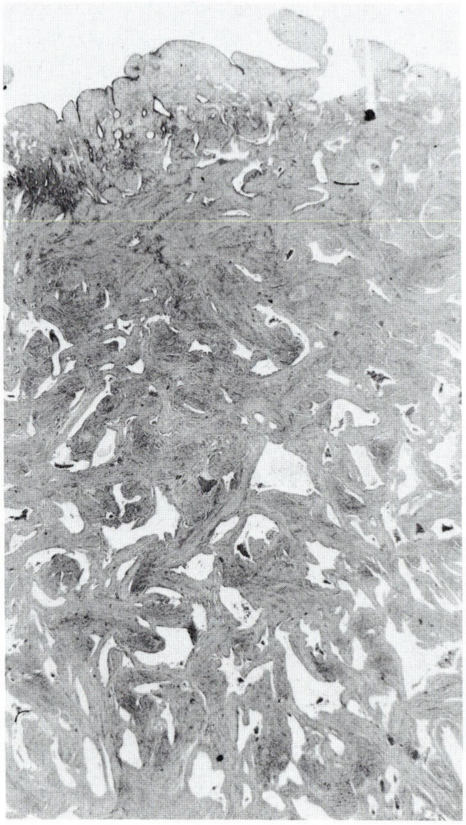

Fig. 13.49. Hemangioma. The tumor is composed of dilated vascular spaces that extend throughout the myometrium.

In the past, a few uterine tumors have been reported as hemangiopericytomas. Most of these appear to have been endometrial stromal nodules or low-grade endometrial stromal sarcomas that were misdiagnosed as hemangiopericytomas. Whether true hemangiopericytomas occur in the uterus is unclear, but if they do, they are certainly very rare. Whenever a diagnosis of hemangiopericytoma of the uterus is considered, the possibility that the tumor is an endometrial stromal tumor must be excluded.

Lymphoma

Lymphoma rarely occurs with initial signs or symptoms suggestive of a uterine tumor, but when it does, the cervix is involved three times more often than is the endometrium.[123] Most patients are older than 20 years and present with an abdominal or pelvic mass, abnormal vaginal bleeding, a vaginal discharge, or pelvic discomfort. Lymphoma involving the uterus can be staged using the FIGO system for gynecologic malignancies or by the lymphoma-staging classification; the latter appears to correlate most closely with the clinical evolution. Diffuse large cell lymphomas of B-cell type are most common.[8,300] An 80–90% survival rate has been reported for women with localized (Ann Arbor stage IE) lymphomas of the uterus and vagina.[123,280,300] The differential diagnosis includes a leiomyoma with a heavy lymphocytic infiltrate and an inflammatory lymphoma-like lesion (pseudolymphoma). Rare leiomyomas contain a heavy lymphocytic infiltrate; however, these are circumscribed tumors in which there are recognizable areas of residual smooth muscle tumor.[94] Additionally, the lymphocytic infiltrate consists of a mixture of cell types. Inflammatory "pseudolymphomas" mainly involve the cervical or endometrial surface or are just beneath it, whereas lymphoma is larger and more deeply situated.[317] Inflammatory processes contain a heterogeneous population of lymphoid cells in contrast to the more monomorphic population seen in most lymphomas, and they are polyclonal.

Uterine involvement as an initial manifestation of leukemia is rare, but a few cases have been reported.[123,147]

References

1. Abell MR (1971) Papillary adenofibroma of the uterine cervix. Am J Obstet Gynecol 110:990–993
2. Abrams J, Talcott J, Corson JM (1989) Pulmonary metastases in patients with low-grade endometrial stromal sarcoma. Clinicopathologic findings with immunohistochemical characterization. Am J Surg Pathol 13:133–140
3. Abu-Rustum NR, Curtin JP, Burt M, Jones WB (1997) Regression of uterine low-grade smooth-muscle tumors metastatic to the lung after oophorectomy. Obstet Gynecol 89:850–852
4. Adamson GD (1992) Treatment of uterine fibroids: current findings with gonadotropin-releasing hormone agonists. Am J Obstet Gynecol 166:746–751
5. Adany R, Fodor F, Molnar P, Ablin R, Muszbek L (1990) Increased density of histiocytes in uterine leiomyomas. Int J Gynecol Pathol 9(2):137–144

5a. Agoff SN, Grieco VS, Garcia R, Gown AM (2001) Immunohistochemical distinction of endometrial stromal sarcoma and cellular leiomyoma. Appl Immunohistochem Molecul Morphol 9(2):164–169

6. Andersen J (1998) Factors in fibroid growth. Baillieres Clin Obstet Gynaecol 12(2):225–243
7. Andrade LA, Derchain SFM, Vial JS, Alvarenga M (1992) Müllerian adenosarcoma of the uterus in adolescents. Int J Gynecol Obstet 38:119–123
8. Aozasa K, Saeki K, Ohsawa M, Horiuchi K, Mishima K, Tsujimoto M (1993) Malignant lymphoma of the uterus. Report of seven cases with immunohistochemical study. Cancer (Phila) 72(6): 1959–1964
9. Aterman K, Fraser GM, Lea RH (1977) Disseminated peritoneal leiomyomatosis. Virchows Arch [A] 374:13–26
10. Atkins K, Bell S, Kempson R, Hendrickson M (2001) Epithelioid smooth muscle neoplasms of the uterus. Mod Pathol 14(1):132A
11. Atkins K, Bell S, Kempson R, Hendrickson M (2001) Myxoid smooth muscle neoplasms of the uterus. Mod Pathol 14(1):132A
12. Azziz R (1989) Adenomyosis: current perspectives. Obstet Gynecol Clin North Am 16(1):221–235
13. Baiocchi G, Kavanagh JJ, Wharton JT (1990) Endometrioid stromal sarcomas arising from ovarian and extraovarian endometriosis: report of two cases and review of the literature. Gynecol Oncol 36:147–151
14. Baker RJ, Hildebrandt RH, Rouse RV, Hendrickson MR, Longacre TA (1999) Inhibin and CD99 (MIC2) expression in uterine stromal neoplasms with sex-cord-like elements. Hum Pathol 30(6):671–679
15. Baker TR, Piver MS, Lele SB, Tsukada Y (1988) Stage I uterine adenosarcoma: a report of six cases. J Surg Oncol 37:128–132
16. Bapat K, Brustein S (1989) Uterine sarcoma with liposarcomatous differentiation: report of a case and review of the literature. Int J Gynaecol Obstet 28:71–75
17. Barter JF, Smith EB, Szpak CA, Hinshaw W, Clarke-Pearson DL, Creasman WT (1985) Leiomyosarcoma of the uterus: clinicopathologic study of 21 cases. Gynecol Oncol 21:220–227
18. Bekkers RL, Willemsen WN, Schijf CP, Massuger LF, Bulten J, Merkus JM (1999) Leiomyomatosis peritonealis disseminata: does malignant transformation occur? A literature review. Gynecol Oncol 75(1):158–163
19. Bell SW, Kempson RL, Hendrickson MR (1994) Problematic uterine smooth muscle neoplasms: a clinicopathologic study of 213 cases. Am J Surg Pathol 18:535–558
20. Berchuck A, Rubin SC, Hoskins WJ, Saigo PE, Pierce VK, Lewis JL Jr (1988) Treatment of uterine leiomyosarcoma. Obstet Gynecol 71:845–850
21. Berchuck A, Rubin SC, Hoskins WJ, Saigo PE, Pierce VK, Lewis JL Jr (1990) Treatment of endometrial stromal tumors. Gynecol Oncol 36:60–65
22. Bhatia NN, Hoshiko MG (1982) Uterine osseous metaplasia. Obstet Gynecol 60:256–259
23. Binder SW, Nieberg RK, Cheng L, Al-Jitawi S (1991) Histologic and immunohistochemical analysis of nine endometrial stromal tumors: an unexpected high frequency of keratin protein positivity. Int J Gynecol Pathol 10:191–197
24. Blom R, Guerrieri C (1999) Adenosarcoma of the uterus: a clinicopathologic, DNA flow cytometric, p53 and mdm-2 analysis of 11 cases. Int J Gynecol Cancer 9:37–43
25. Blom R, Guerrieri C, Stal O, Malmstrom H, Simonsen E (1998) Leiomyosarcoma of the uterus: a clinicopathologic, DNA flow cytometric, p53, and mdm-2 analysis of 49 cases. Gynecol Oncol 68:54–61
26. Blom R, Malmstrom H, Guerrieri C (1999) Endometrial stromal sarcoma of the uterus: a clinicopathologic, DNA flow cytometric, p53, and mdm-2 analysis of 17 cases. Int J Gynecol Cancer 9: 98–104
27. Bradley LD, Falcone T, Magen AB (2000) Radiographic imaging techniques for the diagnosis of

abnormal uterine bleeding. Obstet Gynecol Clin North Am 27(2):245–276
28. Brescia RJ, Tazelaar HD, Hobbs J, Miller AW (1989) Intravascular lipoleiomyomatosis: a report of two cases. Hum Pathol 20:252–256
29. Brittingham J, Liaw D, Liddell R, McHugh M, McCue P, McHugh KM (1997) Comparative analysis of smooth muscle isoactin gene expression in normal and neoplastic tissues. Pathobiology 65(3):113–122
30. Brooks JJ, Wells GB, Yeh IT, LiVolsi VA (1992) Bizarre epithelioid lipoleiomyoma of the uterus. Int J Gynecol Pathol 11(2):144–149
31. Brown DC, Theaker JM, Banks PM, Gatter KC, Mason DY (1987) Cytokeratin expression in smooth muscle and smooth muscle tumours. Histopathology (Oxf) 11:477–486
32. Burns B, Curry RH, Bell MEA (1979) Morphologic features of prognostic significance in uterine smooth muscle tumors: a review of 84 cases. Am J Obstet Gynecol 135:109–114
33. Chang KL, Crabtree GS, Lim-Tan SK, Kempson RL, Hendrickson MR (1990) Primary uterine endometrial stromal neoplasms. A clinicopathologic study of 117 cases. Am J Surg Pathol 14:415–438
34. Chang KL, Crabtree GS, Lim-Tan SK, Kempson RL, Hendrickson MR (1993) Primary extrauterine endometrial stromal neoplasms: a clinicopathologic study of 20 cases and a review of the literature. Int J Gynecol Pathol 12:282–296
35. Chang V, Aikawa M, Druet R (1977) Uterine leiomyoblastoma: ultrastructural and cytological studies. Cancer (Phila) 39:1563–1569
36. Chauveinc L, Deniaud E, Plancher C, Sastre X, Amsani F et al (1999) Uterine sarcomas: the Curie Institut experience. Prognosis factors and adjuvant treatments. Gynecol Oncol 72:232–237
37. Chen KT (1984) Myxoid leiomyosarcoma of the uterus. Int J Gynecol Pathol 3:389–392
38. Chen KT (1999) Uterine leiomyohibernoma. Int J Gynecol Pathol 18(1):96–97
39. Cheung ANY, Ng WF, Chung LP, Khoo US (1996) Mixed low grade and high grade endometrial stromal sarcoma of uterus: differences on immunohistochemistry and chromosome in situ hybridisation. J Clin Pathol 49(7):604–607
40. Chiarle R, Godio L, Fusi D, Soldati T, Palestro G (1997) Pure alveolar rhabdomyosarcoma of the corpus uteri: description of a case with increased serum level of CA-125. Gynecol Oncol 66:320–323
41. Cho KR, Woodruff JD, Epstein JI (1989) Leiomyoma of the uterus with multiple extrauterine smooth muscle tumors: a case report suggesting multifocal origin. Hum Pathol 20:80–83
42. Christopherson WM, Williamson EO, Gray LA (1972) Leiomyosarcoma of the uterus. Cancer (Phila) 29:1512–1517
43. Chu PG, Arber DA (2000) Paraffin-section detection of CD10 in 505 nonhematopoietic neoplasms; frequent expression in renal cell carcinoma and endometrial stromal sarcoma. Am J Clin Pathol 113(3):374–382
44. Clement PB (1978) Chondrosarcoma of the uterus: report of a case and review of the literature. Hum Pathol 9:726–732
45. Clement PB (1988) Intravenous leiomyomatosis of the uterus. Pathol Annu 23(pt 2):153–183
46. Clement PB (1989) Müllerian adenosarcomas of the uterus with sarcomatous overgrowth. A clinicopathological analysis of 10 cases. Am J Surg Pathol 13:28–38
47. Clement PB (2000) The pathology of uterine smooth muscle tumors and mixed endometrial stromal-smooth muscle tumors: a selective review with emphasis on recent advances. Int J Gynecol Pathol 19(1):39–55
48. Clement PB, Oliva E, Young RH (1996) Müllerian adenosarcoma of the uterine corpus associated with tamoxifen therapy: a report of six cases and a review of tamoxifen-associated endometrial lesions. Int J Gynecol Pathol 15:222–229
49. Clement PB, Scully RE (1974) Müllerian adenosarcoma of the uterus. A clinicopathologic analysis of ten cases of a distinctive type of müllerian mixed tumor. Cancer (Phila) 34:1138–1149
50. Clement PB, Scully RE (1976) Uterine tumors resembling ovarian sex-cord tumors. A clinicopathologic analysis of 14 cases. Am J Clin Pathol 66: 512–525
51. Clement PB, Scully RE (1989) Müllerian adenosarcomas of the uterus with sex cord-like elements. A clinicopathologic analysis of eight cases. Am J Clin Pathol 91:664–672
52. Clement PB, Scully RE (1990) Müllerian adenofibroma of the uterus with invasion of myometrium and pelvic veins. Int J Gynecol Pathol 9:363–371
53. Clement PB, Scully RE (1990) Müllerian adenosarcoma of the uterus: a clinicopathologic analysis of 100 cases with a review of the literature. Hum Pathol 21:363–381
54. Clement PB, Scully RE (1992) Endometrial stromal sarcomas of the uterus with extensive glandular differentiation: a report of three cases that caused problems in differential diagnosis. Int J Gynecol Pathol 11:163–173
55. Clement PB, Young RH, Scully RE (1988) Intravenous leiomyomatosis of the uterus. A clinicopathological analysis of 16 cases with unusual histologic features. Am J Surg Pathol 12:932–945
56. Clement PB, Young RH, Scully RE (1992) Diffuse, perinodular, and other patterns of hydropic degeneration within and adjacent to uterine leiomyomas. Problems in differential diagnosis. Am J Surg Pathol 16:26–32
57. Coad JE, Sulaiman RA, Das K, Staley N (1997) Perinodular hydropic degeneration of a uterine leiomyoma: a diagnostic challenge. Hum Pathol 28(2):249–251
58. Cohen D, Mazur MT, Jozefczyk MA, Badawy SZA (1994) Hyalinization and cellular changes in uterine leiomyomata after gonadotropin releasing hormone agonist therapy. J Reprod Med 39:377–380
59. Colgan TJ, Pendergast S, LeBlanc M (1993) The

histopathology of uterine leiomyomas following treatment with gonadotropin-releasing hormone analogues. Hum Pathol 24:1073–1077
60. Cooper MM, Guillem J, Dalton J, Marboe CC, Corwin S, Todd GJ, et al (1992) Recurrent intravenous leiomyomatosis with cardiac extension. Ann Thorac Surg 53:139–141
61. Covens AL, Nisker JA, Chapman WB, Allen HH (1987) Uterine sarcoma: an analysis of 74 cases. Am J Obstet Gynecol 156:370–374
62. Cramer SF, Horiszny J, Patel A, Sigrist S (1996) The relation of fibrous degeneration to menopausal status in small uterine leiomyomas with evidence for postmenopausal origin of seedling myomas. Mod Pathol 9:774–780
63. Cramer SF, Patel A (1990) The frequency of uterine leiomyomas. Am J Clin Pathol 94:435–438
64. Crow J, Gardner RL, McSweeney G, Shaw RW (1995) Morphological changes in uterine leiomyomas treated by GnRH agonist goserelin. Int J Gynecol Pathol 14:235–242
65. Crow J, Wilkins M, Howe S, More L, Helliwell P (1991) Mast cells in the female genital tract. Int J Gynecol Pathol 10(3):230–237
66. Crum CP, Rogers BH, Anderson W (1980) Osteosarcoma of the uterus: case report and review of the literature. Gynecol Oncol 9:256–268
67. Darby AJ, Papadaki L, Beilby JOW (1975) An unusual leiomyosarcoma of the uterus containing osteoclast-like giant cells. Cancer (Phila) 36:495–504
68. Daya D, Lukka H, Clement PB (1992) Primitive neuroectodermal tumors of the uterus: a report of four cases. Hum Pathol 23:1120–1129
69. Daya DA, Scully RE (1988) Sarcoma botryoides of the uterine cervix in young women: a clinicopathological study of 13 cases. Gynecol Oncol 29: 290–304
70. De Fusco PA, Gaffey TA, Malkasian GD Jr, Long HJ, Cha SS (1989) Endometrial stromal sarcoma: review of Mayo Clinic experience, 1945–1980. Gynecol Oncol 35:8–14
71. Delahunt B, Eble JN, King D, Bethwaite PB, Nacey JN, Thornton A (2000) Immunohistochemical evidence for mesothelial origin of paratesticular adenomatoid tumour. Histopathology (Oxf) 36(2):109–115
72. Demopoulos RI, Jones KY, Mittal KR, Vamvakas EC (1997) Histology of leiomyomata in patients treated with leuprolide acetate. Int J Gynecol Pathol 16:131–137
73. Devaney K, Tavassoli FA (1991) Immunohistochemistry as a diagnostic aid in the interpretation of unusual mesenchymal tumors of the uterus. Mod Pathol 4:225–231
74. DeYoung B, Bitterman P, Lack EE (1992) Primary osteosarcoma of the uterus: report of a case with immunohistochemical study. Mod Pathol 5:212–215
75. Dharkar DD, Kraft JR, Gangadharam D (1981) Uterine lipomas. Arch Pathol Lab Med 105:43–45
76. Downes KA, Hart WR (1997) Bizarre leiomyomas of the uterus: a comprehensive pathologic study of 24 cases with long-term follow-up. Am J Surg Pathol 21(11):1261–1270
77. Downes KA, Hart WR (1999) Bizarre uterine leiomyomas: Ki-67 activity and DNA ploidy. Mod Pathol 12:116A
78. Dreyer L, Simson IW, Sevenster CB, Dittrich OC (1985) Leiomyomatosis peritonealis disseminata. A report of two cases and a review of the literature. Br J Obstet Gynaecol 92(8):856–861
79. Due W, Pickartz H (1989) Immunohistologic detection of estrogen and progesterone receptors in disseminated peritoneal leiomyomatosis. Int J Gynecol Pathol 8:46–53
80. Eddy GL, Mazur MT (1997) Endolymphatic stromal myosis associated with tamoxifen use. Gynecol Oncol 64:262–264
81. el-Naggar AK, Abdul-Karim FW, Silva EG, McLemore D, Garnsey L (1991) Uterine stromal neoplasms: a clinicopathologic and DNA flow cytometric correlation. Hum Pathol 22:897–903
82. Eldar-Geva T, Healy DL (1998) Other medical management of uterine fibroids. Baillieres Clin Obstet Gynaecol 12(2):269–288
83. Emoto M, Iwasaki H, Kawarabayshi T, Egami D, Yoshitake H, Kikuchi M, et al (1994) Primary osteosarcoma of the uterus: report of a case with immunohistochemical analysis. Gynecol Oncol 54: 385–388
84. Evans ATI, Symmonds RE, Gaffey TA (1981) Recurrent pelvic intravenous leiomyomatosis. Obstet Gynecol 57:260–264
85. Evans HL (1982) Endometrial stromal sarcoma and poorly differentiated endometrial sarcoma. Cancer (Phila) 50:2170–2182
86. Evans HL, Chawla SP, Simpson C, Finn KP (1988) Smooth muscle neoplasms of the uterus other than ordinary leiomyoma. A study of 46 cases, with emphasis on diagnostic criteria and prognostic factors. Cancer (Phila) 62:2239–2247
87. Eyden BP, Hale RJ, Richmond I, Buckley CH (1992) Cytoskeletal filaments in the smooth muscle cells of uterine leiomyomata and myometrium: an ultrastructural and immunohistochemical analysis. Virchows Arch A Pathol Anat Hispathol 420:51–58
88. Fanburg-Smith JC, Miettinen M (1999) Angiomatoid "malignant" fibrous histiocytoma: a clinicopathologic study of 158 cases and further exploration of the myoid phenotype. Hum Pathol 30(11): 1336–1343
89. Farhood AI, Abrams J (1991) Immunohistochemistry of endometrial stromal sarcoma. Hum Pathol 22:224–230
90. Fechner RE (1968) Atypical leiomyomas and synthetic progestogen therapy. Am J Clin Pathol 49: 697–703
91. Fehmian C, Jones J, Kress Y, Abadi M (1997) Adenosarcoma of the uterus with extensive smooth muscle differentiation: Ultrastructural study and review of the literature. Ultrastruct Pathol 21(1): 73–79
92. Fekete PS, Vellios F (1984) The clinical and histo-

logic spectrum of endometrial stromal neoplasms: a report of 41 cases. Int J Gynecol Pathol 3:198–212
93. Ferrer F, Sabater S, Farrus B, Guedea F, Rovirosa A, Anglada L, et al (1999) Impact of radiotherapy on local control and survival in uterine sarcomas: a retrospective study from the Grup Oncologic Catala-Occita. Int J Radiat Oncol Biol Phys 44(1): 47–52
94. Ferry JA, Harris NL, Scully RE (1989) Uterine leiomyomas with lymphoid infiltration simulating lymphoma: a report of seven cases. Int J Gynecol Pathol 8:263–270
95. Fleming H, Ostor AG, Pickel H, Fortune DW (1989) Arteriovenous malformations of the uterus. Obstet Gynecol 73:209–214
96. Fleming WP, Peters WA, Kumar NB, Morley GW (1984) Autopsy findings in patients with uterine sarcoma. Gynecol Oncol 19:168–172
97. Fornelli A, Pasquinelli G, Eusebi V (1999) Leiomyoma of the uterus showing skeletal muscle differentiation: a case report. Hum Pathol 30(3):356–359
98. Fox H, Harilal KR, Youell A (1979) Mullerian adenosarcoma of the uterine body: a report of nine cases. Histopathology (Oxf) 3:167–180
99. Fraggetta F, Magro G, Vasquez E (1997) Primitive neuroectodermal tumour of the uterus with focal cartilaginous differentiation. Histopathology (Oxf) 30(5):483–485
100. Franquemont DW, Frierson HF Jr, Mills SE (1991) An immunohistochemical study of normal endometrial stroma and endometrial stromal neoplasms. Evidence for smooth muscle differentiation. Am J Surg Pathol 15:861–870
101. Fukunaga M, Endo Y, Ushigome S, Ishikawa E (1995) Atypical polypoid adenomyomas of the uterus. Histopathology (Oxf) 27:35–42
102. Fukunaga M, Ishihara A, Ushigome S (1998) Extrauterine low-grade endometrial stromal sarcoma: report of three cases. Pathol Int 48(4):297–302
103. Fukunaga M, Ushigome S (1998) Dissecting leiomyoma of the uterus with extrauterine extension. Histopathology (Oxf) 32(2):160–164
104. Gadducci A, Landoni F, Sartori E, Zola P, Maggino T, Lissoni A, et al (1996) Uterine leiomyosarcoma: analysis of treatment failures and survival. Gynecol Oncol 62:25–32
105. Gadducci A, Sartori E, Landoni F, Zola P, Maggino T, Urgesi A, et al (1996) Endometrial stromal sarcoma: analysis of treatment failures and survival. Gynecol Oncol 63:247–253
106. Gal AA, Brooks JJ, Pietra GG (1989) Leiomyomatous neoplasms of the lung: a clinical, histologic, and immunohistochemical study. Mod Pathol 2:209–216
107. Gard GB, Mulvany NJ, Quinn MA (1999) Management of uterine leiomyosarcoma in Australia. Aust N Z J Obstet Gynaecol 39(1):93–98
108. Gilks CB, Clement PB, Hart WR, Young RH (2000) Uterine adenomyomas excluding atypical polypoid adenomyomas and adenomyomas of endocervical type: a clinicopathologic study of 30 cases of an underemphasized lesion that may cause diagnostic problems with brief consideration of adenomyomas of other female genital tract sites. Int J Gynecol Pathol 19(3):195–205
109. Gilks CB, Taylor GP, Clement PB (1987) Inflammatory pseudotumor of the uterus. Int J Gynecol Pathol 6:275–286
110. Gisser SD, Young I (1977) Neurilemoma-like uterine myomas: an ultrastructural reaffirmation of their non-Schwannian nature. Am J Obstet Gynecol 129:389–392
111. Gloor E (1979) Mullerian adenosarcoma of the uterus. Clinicopathologic report of five cases. Am J Surg Pathol 3:203–209
112. Goff BA, Rice LW, Fleischhacker D, Muntz HG, Falkenberry SS, Nikrui N, et al (1993) Uterine leiomyosarcoma and endometrial stromal sarcoma: lymph node metastases and sites of recurrence. Gynecol Oncol 50:105–109
113. Goldberg MF, Hurt WG, Frable WJ (1977) Leiomyomatosis peritonealis disseminata: report of a case and review of the literature. Obstet Gynecol 49:46s–52s
114. Goldblum JR, Clement PB, Hart WR (1995) Adenomyosis with sparse glands: A potential mimic of low-grade endometrial stromal sarcoma. Am J Clin Pathol 103:218–223
115. Gollard R, Kosty M, Bordin G, Wax A, Lacey C (1995) Two unusual presentations of müllerian adenosarcoma: case reports, literature review, and treatment considerations. Gynecol Oncol 59(3):412–422
116. Gown AM, Boyd HC, Chang Y, Ferguson M, Reichler B, Tippens D (1988) Smooth muscle cells can express cytokeratins of "simple" epithelium. Immunocytochemical and biochemical studies in vitro and in vivo. Am J Pathol 132:223–232
117. Grayson W, Fourie J, Tiltman AJ (1998) Xanthomatous leiomyosarcoma of the uterine cervix. Int J Gynecol Pathol 17:89–90
118. Grignon DJ, Carey MR, Kirk ME, Robinson ML (1987) Diffuse uterine leiomyomatosis: a case study with pregnancy complicated by intrapartum hemorrhage. Obstet Gynecol 69:477–480
119. Gutmann JN, Thornton KL, Diamond MP, Carcangiu ML (1994) Evaluation of leuprolide acetate treatment on histopathology of uterine myomata. Fertil Steril 61:622–626
120. Hales HA, Peterson CM, Jones KP, Quinn JD (1992) Leiomyomatosis peritonealis disseminata treated with a gonadotropin-releasing hormone agonist. Am J Obstet Gynecol 167:515–516
121. Han HS, Park IA, Kim SH, Lee HP (1998) The clear cell variant of epithelioid intravenous leiomyomatosis of the uterus: report of a case. Pathol Int 48(11):892–896
122. Han K, Lee W, Harris CP, Simsiman RC, Lee K, Kang C, et al (1994) Comparison of chromosome aberrations in leiomyoma and leiomyosarcoma us-

ing FISH on archival tissues. Cancer Genet Cytogenet 74(1):19–24
123. Harris NL, Scully RE (1984) Malignant lymphoma and granulocytic sarcoma of the uterus and vagina. A clinicopathologic analysis of 27 cases. Cancer (Phila) 53:2530–2545
124. Hart WR (1997) Problematic uterine smooth muscle neoplasms. Am J Surg Pathol 21(2):252–255
125. Hart WR, Billman JK Jr (1978) A reassessment of uterine neoplasms originally diagnosed as leiomyosarcomas. Cancer 41:1902–1910
126. Hart WR, Craig JR (1978) Rhabdomyosarcomas of the uterus. Am J Clin Pathol 70:217–223
127. Hart WR, Yoonessi M (1977) Endometrial stromatosis of the uterus. Obstet Gynecol 49:393–403
128. Hashimoto K, Azuma C, Kamura T, Nobunaga T, Kanai T, Sawada M, et al (1995) Clonal determination of uterine leiomyomas by analyzing differential inactivation of the X-chromosome-linked phosphoglycerokinase gene. Gynecol Obstet Invest 40:204–208
129. Hempling RE, Piver MS, Baker TR (1995) Impact on progression-free survival of adjuvant cyclophosphamide, vincristine, doxorubicin (adriamycin), and dacarbazine (CYVADIC) chemotherapy for stage I uterine sarcoma. A prospective trial. Am J Clin Oncol 18(4):282–286
130. Hendrickson MR, Scheithauer BW (1986) Primitive neuroectodermal tumor of the endometrium: report of two cases, one with electron microscopic observations. Int J Gynecol Pathol 5:249–259
131. Hilsenbeck SG, Allred DC (1992) Improved methods of estimating mitotic activity in solid tumors. Hum Pathol 23(6):601–602
132. Hirschfield L, Kahn LB, Chen S, Winkler B, Rosenberg S (1986) Müllerian adenosarcoma with ovarian sex cord-like differentiation. A light- and electron-microscopic study. Cancer (Phila) 57:1197–1200
133. Holcomb K, Francis M, Ruiz J, Abulafia O, Matthews RP, Lee YC (1999) Pleomorphic rhabdomyosarcoma of the uterus in a postmenopausal woman with elevated serum CA 125. Gynecol Oncol 74(3):499–501
134. Honore LH (1978) Uterine fibrolipoleiomyoma: report of a case with discussion of histogenesis. Am J Obstet Gynecol 132:635–636
135. Horie Y, Ikawa S, Kadowaki K, Minagawa Y, Kigawa J, Terakawa N (1995) Lipoadenofibroma of the uterine corpus: report of a new variant of adenofibroma (benign müllerian mixed tumor). Arch Pathol Lab Med 119:274–276
136. Hornback N, Omura G, Major F (1986) Observations on the use of adjuvant radiation therapy in patients with stage I and II uterine sarcoma. Int J Radiat Oncol Biol Phys 12(12):2127–30
137. Horstmann JP, Pietra GG, Harman JA, Cole NG, Grinspan S (1977) Spontaneous regression of pulmonary leiomyomas during pregnancy. Cancer (Phila) 39:314–321
138. Hyde KE, Geisinger KR, Marshall RB, Jones TL (1989) The clear-cell variant of uterine epithelioid leiomyoma. An immunohistologic and ultrastructural study. Arch Pathol Lab Med 113:551–553
139. Ito H, Sasaki N, Miyagawa K, Tahara E (1986) Bizarre leiomyoblastoma of the cervix uteri. Immunohistochemical and ultrastructural study. Acta Pathol Jpn 36:1737–1745
140. Jautzke G, Muller-Ruchholtz E, Thalmann U (1996) Immunohistological detection of estrogen and progesterone receptors in multiple and well differentiated leiomyomatous lung tumors in women with uterine leiomyomas (so-called benign metastasizing leiomyomas). A report on 5 cases. Pathol Res Pract 192:215–223
141. Jones MW, Norris HJ (1995) Clinicopathologic study of 28 uterine leiomyosarcomas with metastasis. Int J Gynecol Pathol 14(3):243–249
142. Kahanpaa KV, Wahlstrom T, Grohn P, Heinonen E, Nieminen U, Widholm O (1986) Sarcomas of the uterus: a clinicopathologic study of 119 patients. Obstet Gynecol 67(3):417–424
143. Kaku T, Silverberg SG, Major FJ, Miller A, Fetter B, Brady MF (1992) Adenosarcoma of the uterus: A Gynecologic Oncology Group clinicopathologic study of 31 cases. Int J Gynecol Pathol 11:75–88
144. Kalir T, Goldstein M, Dottino P, Brodman M, Gordon R, Deligdisch L, et al (1998) Morphometric and electron-microscopic analyses of the effects of gonadotropin-releasing hormone agonists on uterine leiomyomas. Arch Pathol Lab Med 122(5):442–446
145. Kaminski PF, Tavassoli FA (1984) Plexiform tumorlet: a clinical and pathologic study of 15 cases with ultrastructural observations. Int J Gynecol Pathol 3:124–134
146. Kantelip B, Cloup N, Dechelotte P (1986) Uterine tumor resembling ovarian sex cord tumors: report of a case with ultrastructural study. Hum Pathol 17:91–93
147. Kapadia SB, Krause JR, Kanbour AI, Hartsock RJ (1978) Granulocytic sarcoma of the uterus. Cancer (Phila) 41:687–691
148. Karpuz V, Joris F, Letovanec N, Branchmanski F, Kapanci Y (1998) Metastizing low-grade clear cell leiomyosarcoma of the uterus. Pathol Int 48(1):82–85
149. Katz L, Merino MJ, Sakamoto H, Schwartz PE (1987) Endometrial stromal sarcoma: a clinicopathologic study of 11 cases with determination of estrogen and progestin receptor levels in three tumors. Gynecol Oncol 26:87–97
150. Kawaguchi K, Fujii S, Konishi I, Nanbu Y, Nonogaki H, Mori T (1989) Mitotic activity in uterine leiomyomas during the menstrual cycle. Am J Obstet Gynecol 160:637–641
151. Kempson RL, Hendrickson MR (2000) Smooth muscle, endometrial stromal, and mixed Mullerian tumors of the uterus. Mod Pathol 13(3):328–342
152. Kerner H, Lichtig C (1993) Müllerian adenosarcoma presenting as cervical polyps: a report of seven cases and review of the literature. Obstet Gynecol 81:655–659

153. King ME, Dickersin GR, Scully RE (1982) Myxoid leiomyosarcoma of the uterus: a report of six cases. Am J Surg Pathol 6:589–598
154. Kjerulff KH, Langenberg P, Seidman JD, Stolley PD, Guzinski GM (1996) Uterine leiomyomas. Racial differences in severity, symptoms and age at diagnosis. J Reprod Med 41(7):483–490
155. Kondi-Paphitis A, Smyrniotis B, Liapis A, Kontoyanni A, Deligeorgi H (1998) Stromal sarcoma arising on endometriosis. A clinicopathological and immunohistochemical study of 4 cases. Eur J Gynaecol Oncol 19(6):588–590
155a. Koontz JI, Soreng AL, Nucci M, Kuo FC, Pauwels P, Van den BH et al (2001) Frequent fusion of the JAZF1 and JJAZ1 genes in endometrial stromal tumors. Proc Natl Acad Sci USA 98(11):6348–6353
156. Krishnamurthy S, Jungbluth AA, Busam KJ, Rosai J (1998) Uterine tumors resembling ovarian sex-cord tumors have an immunophenotype consistent with true sex-cord differentiation. Am J Surg Pathol 22(9):1078–1082
157. Kunzel KE, Mills NZ, Muderspach LI, d'Ablaing G III (1993) Myxoid leiomyosarcoma of the uterus. Gynecol Oncol 48:277–280
158. Kurman RJ, Norris HJ (1976) Mesenchymal tumors of the uterus. VI. Epithelioid smooth muscle tumors including leiomyoblastoma and clear cell leiomyoma: a clinical and pathological analysis of 26 cases. Cancer (Phila) 37:1853–1865
159. Lack EE, Bitterman P, Sundeen JT (1991) Müllerian adenosarcoma of the uterus with pure angiosarcoma: case report. Hum Pathol 22:1289–1291
160. Lai FM, Wong FW, Allen PW (1991) Diffuse uterine leiomyomatosis with hemorrhage. Arch Pathol Lab Med 115:834–837
161. Langlois PL (1970) The size of the normal uterus. J Reprod Med 4:220–228
162. Larson B, Silfversward C, Nilsson B, Pettersson F (1990) Endometrial stromal sarcoma of the uterus. A clinical and histopathological study. The Radiumhemmet series 1936–1981. Eur J Obstet Gynecol Reprod Biol 35:239–249
163. Larson B, Silfversward C, Nilsson B, Pettersson F (1990) Prognostic factors in uterine leiomyosarcoma. A clinical and histopathological study of 143 cases. The Radiumhemmet series 1936–1981. Acta Oncol 29:185–191
164. Lavin P, Hajdu SI, Foote FW (1987) Gastric and extragastric leiomyoblastomas. Cancer (Phila) 29: 305–311
165. Lawrence B, Perez-Atayde A, Hibbard MK, Rubin BP, Dal Cin P, Pinkus JL, et al (2000) TPM3–ALK and TPM4–ALK oncogenes in inflammatory myofibroblastic tumors. Am J Pathol 157(2):377–384
166. Leibsohn S, d'Ablaing G, Mischell DR Jr, Schlaerth JB (1990) Leiomyosarcoma in a series of hysterectomies performed for presumed uterine leiomyomas. Am J Obstet Gynecol 162:968–974
167. Levenback C, Rubin SC, McCormack PM, Hoskins WJ, Atkinson EN, Lewis JL Jr (1992) Resection of pulmonary metastases from uterine sarcomas. Gynecol Oncol 45:202–205
168. LevGur M, Abadi MA, Tucker A (2000) Adenomyosis: symptoms, histology, and pregnancy terminations. Obstet Gynecol 95(5):688–691
169. Lillemoe TJ, Perrone T, Norris HJ, Dehner LP (1991) Myogenous phenotype of epithelial-like areas in endometrial stromal sarcomas. Arch Pathol Lab Med 115:215–219
170. Longacre TA, Chung MH, Rouse RV, Hendrickson MR (1996) Atypical polypoid adenomyofibromas (atypical polypoid adenomyomas) of the uterus: a clinicopathologic study of 55 cases. Am J Surg Pathol 20:1–20
171. Lotgering FK, Pijpers L, van Eijck J, Wallenburg HC (1989) Pregnancy in a patient with diffuse cavernous hemangioma of the uterus. Am J Obstet Gynecol 160:628–630
172. Lumsden MA, Wallace EM (1998) Clinical presentation of uterine fibroids. Baillieres Clin Obstet Gynaecol 12(2):177–195
173. Majmudar B, Ghanee N, Horowitz IR, Graham D (1998) Uterine arteriovenous malformation necessitating hysterectomy with bilateral salpingo-oophorectomy in a young pregnant patient. Arch Pathol Lab Med 122(9):842–845
174. Major FJ, Blessing JA, Silverberg SG, Morrow CP, Creasman WT, Currie JL, et al (1993) Prognostic factors in early-stage uterine sarcoma: a Gynecologic Oncology Group study. Cancer (Phila) (Suppl) 71: 1702–1709
175. Malmstrom H, Schmidt H, Persson PG, Carstensen J, Nordenskjold B, Simonsen E (1992) Flow cytometric analysis of uterine sarcoma: ploidy and S-phase rate as prognostic indicators. Gynecol Oncol 44(2):172–177
176. Maluf HM, Gersell DJ (1994) Uterine leiomyomas with high content of mast cells. Arch Pathol Lab Med 118:712–714
177. Mansi JL, Ramachandra S, Wiltshaw E, Fisher C (1990) Endometrial stromal sarcomas. Gynecol Oncol 36:113–118
178. Marchese MJ, Liskow AS, Crum CP, McCaffrey RM, Frick HC (1984) Uterine sarcomas: a clinicopathologic study, 1965–1981. Gynecol Oncol 18:299–312
179. Marshall RJ, Braye SG, Jones DB (1986) Leiomyosarcoma of the uterus with giant cells resembling osteoclasts. Int J Gynecol Pathol 5:260–268
180. Martin-Reay D, Christ M, La Pata R (1991) Uterine leiomyoma with skeletal muscle differentiation. Report of a case. Am J Clin Pathol 96(3):344–347
181. Mashal RD, Fejzo ML, Friedman AJ, Mitchner N, Nowak RA, Rein MS, et al (1994) Analysis of androgen receptor DNA reveals the independent clonal origins of uterine leiomyomata and the secondary nature of cytogenetic aberrations in the development of leiomyomata. Genes Chromosomes Cancer 11(1):1–6
182. Mayerhofer K, Obermair A, Windbichler G, Petru

E, Kaider A, Hefler L, et al (1999) Leiomyosarcoma of the uterus: a clinicopathologic multicenter study of 71 cases. Gynecol Oncol 74(2):196–201
183. Mazur MT, Kraus FT (1980) Histogenesis of morphologic variations in tumors of the uterine wall. Am J Surg Pathol 4:59–74
184. Mazur MT, Priest JB (1986) Clear cell leiomyoma (leiomyoblastoma) of the uterus: ultrastructural observations. Ultrastruct Pathol 10:249–255
185. McCluggage WG, Alderdice JM, Walsh MY (1999) Polypoid uterine lesions mimicking endometrial stromal sarcoma. J Clin Pathol 52(7):543–546
185a. McCluggage WG, Surnathi VP, Maxwell P (2001) CD10 is a sensitive and diagnostically useful immunohistochemical marker of normal endometrial stroma and of endometrial stromal neoplasms. Histopathology 39(3):273–278
186. Melilli GA, Di Vagno G, Greco P, Vimercati A, Loizzi V, Putignano G, et al (1999) Endometrial stromal sarcoma: a clinicopathologic study. Eur J Gynaecol Oncol 20(1):33–34
187. Mesia AF, Demopoulos RI (2000) Effects of leuprolide acetate on low-grade endometrial stromal sarcoma. Am J Obstet Gynecol 182(5):1140–1141
188. Mesia AF, Williams FS, Yan ZQ, Mittal K (1998) Aborted leiomyosarcoma after treatment with leuprolide acetate. Obstet Gynecol 92(4 pt 2):664–666
189. Meyer WR, Mayer AR, Diamond MP, Carcangiu ML, Schwartz PE, DeCherney AH (1990) Unsuspected leiomyosarcoma: treatment with a gonadotropin-releasing hormone analogue. Obstet Gynecol 75(3 pt 2):529–532
190. Michalas S, Creatsas G, Deligeoroglou E, Markaki S (1994) High-grade endometrial stromal sarcoma in a 16-year-old girl. Gynecol Oncol 54:95–98
191. Miller KN, McClure SP (1992) Papillary adenofibroma of the uterus: report of a case involved by adenocarcinoma and review of the literature. Am J Clin Pathol 97:806–809
192. Milne DS, Hinshaw K, Malcolm AJ, Hilton P (1990) Primary angiosarcoma of the uterus: a case report. Histopathology (Oxf) 16:203–205
193. Minassian SS, Frangipane W, Polin JI, Ellis M (1986) Leiomyomatosis peritonealis disseminata. A case report and literature review. J Reprod Med 31:997–1000
194. Morrow C, Curtin J (1998) Synopsis of gynecologic oncology. Churchill Livingstone, New York
195. Mourits MJE, Hollema H, Willemse PHB, Devries EGE, Aalders JG, VanderZee AGJ (1998) Adenosarcoma of the uterus following tamoxifen treatment for breast cancer. Int J Gynecol Cancer 8:168–171
196. Mulvany NJ, Östör AG, Ross I (1995) Diffuse leiomyomatosis of the uterus. Histopathology (Oxf) 27:175–179
197. Mulvany NJ, Slavin JL, Ostor AG, Fortune DW (1994) Intravenous leiomyomatosis of the uterus: a clinicopathologic study of 22 cases. Int J Gynecol Pathol 13:1–9
198. Myles JL, Hart WR (1985) Apoplectic leiomyomas of the uterus. A clinicopathologic study of five distinctive hemorrhagic leiomyomas associated with oral contraceptive usage. Am J Surg Pathol 9:798–805
199. Nogales FF, Matilla A, Carrascal E (1978) Leiomyomatosis peritonealis disseminata: an ultrastructural study. Am J Clin Pathol 699:452–457
200. Nogales FF, Navarro N, Martinez de Victoria JM, Contreras F, Redondo C, Herraiz MA, et al (1987) Uterine intravascular leiomyomatosis: an update and report of seven cases. Int J Gynecol Pathol 6:331–339
201. Nola M, Babic D, Ilic J, Marusic M, Uzarevic B, Petrovecki M et al (1996) Prognostic parameters for survival of patients with malignant mesenchymal tumors of the uterus. Cancer (Phila) 78(12): 2543–2550
202. Nordal RR, Kristensen GB, Kaern J, Stenwig AE, Pettersen EO, Trope CG (1996) The prognostic significance of surgery, tumor size, malignancy grade, menopausal status, and DNA ploidy in endometrial stromal sarcoma. Gynecol Oncol 62:254–259
203. Nordal RR, Kristensen GB, Kaern J, Stenwig AE, Pettersen EO, Tropé CG (1995) The prognostic significance of stage, tumor size, cellular atypia and DNA ploidy in uterine leiomyosarcoma. Acta Oncol 34:797–802
204. Norris HJ, Hilliard GD, Irey NS (1988) Hemorrhagic cellular leiomyomas ("apoplectic leiomyoma") of the uterus associated with pregnancy and oral contraceptives. Int J Gynecol Pathol 7:212–224
205. Norris HJ, Parmley T (1975) Mesenchymal tumors of the uterus. V. Intravenous leiomyomatosis. A clinical and pathologic study of 14 cases. Cancer (Phila) 36:2164–2178
206. Norris HJ, Taylor HB (1966) Mesenchymal tumors of the uterus. I. A clinical and pathologic study of 53 endometrial stromal tumors. Cancer (Phila) 19:755–766
206a. Nucci MR, O'Connell JT, Huettner PC, Cviko A, Sun D, Quade BJ (2001) h-Caldesmon expression effectively distinguishes endometrial stromal tumors from uterine smooth muscle tumors. Am J Surg Pathol 25(4):455–463
207. Nunez-Alonso C, Battifora HA (1979) Plexiform tumors of the uterus: ultrastructural study. Cancer (Phila.) 44:1707–1714
208. O'Connor DM, Norris HJ (1990) Mitotically active leiomyomas of the uterus. Hum Pathol 21:223–227
209. O'Leary TJ, Steffes MW (1996) Can you count on the mitotic index? Hum Pathol 27:147–151
210. Oda Y, Nakanishi I, Tateiwa T (1984) Intramural müllerian adenosarcoma of the uterus with adenomyosis. Arch Pathol Lab Med 108(10):798–801
211. Olah KS, Dunn JA, Gee H (1992) Leiomyosarcomas have a poorer prognosis than mixed mesodermal tumours when adjusting for known prognostic factors: the result of a retrospective study of 423 cases of uterine sarcoma. Br J Obstet Gynaecol 99(7): 590–594

212. Oliva E, Clement PB, Young RH, Scully RE (1998) Mixed endometrial stromal and smooth muscle tumors of the uterus—a clinicopathologic study of 15 cases. Am J Surg Pathol 22:997–1005
213. Oliva E, Nielsen PG, Clement PB, Young RH, Scully RE (1997) Epithelioid smooth muscle tumors of the uterus: a clinicopathologic study of 80 cases. Mod Pathol 10:107A
214. Oliva E, Young RH, Clement PB, Bhan AK, Scully RE (1995) Cellular benign mesenchymal tumors of the uterus: a comparative morphologic and immunohistochemical analysis of 33 highly cellular leiomyomas and six endometrial stromal nodules, two frequently confused tumors. Am J Surg Pathol 19:757–768
215. Oliva E, Young RH, Clement PB, Scully RE (1999) Myxoid and fibrous endometrial stromal tumors of the uterus: a report of 10 cases. Int J Gynecol Pathol 18(4):310–319
216. Omura GA, Blessing JA, Major F, Lifshitz S, Ehrlich CE, Mangan C, et al (1985) A randomized clinical trial of adjuvant adriamycin in uterine sarcomas: a Gynecologic Oncology Group study. J Clin Oncol 3:1240–1245
217. Omura G, Major F, Blessing J, Sedlacek T, Thigpen J, Creasman W, et al (1983) A randomized study of adriamycin with and without dimethyl triazenoimidazole carboxamide in advanced uterine sarcomas. Cancer (Phila) 52(4):626–632
218. Ordi J, Stamatakos MD, Tavassoli FA (1997) Pure pleomorphic rhabdomyosarcomas of the uterus. Int J Gynecol Pathol 16:369–377
219. Orii A, Mori A, Zhai YL, Toki T, Nikaido T, Fujii S (1998) Mast cells in smooth muscle tumors of the uterus. Int J Gynecol Pathol 17(4):336–342
220. Ostor AG, Fortune DW (1980) Benign and low grade variants of mixed mullerian tumour of the uterus. Histopathology (Oxf) 4:369–382
221. Pang LC (1998) Endometrial stromal sarcoma with sex cord-like differentiation associated with tamoxifen therapy. South Med J 91(6):592–594
222. Parker WH, Shi Fu Y, Berek JS (1994) Uterine sarcoma in patients operated on for presumed leiomyoma and rapidly growing leiomyoma. Obstet Gynecol 83:414–418
223. Pautier P, Genestie C, Rey A, Morice P, Roche B, Lhommé C, et al (2000) Analysis of clinicopathologic prognostic factors for 157 uterine sarcomas and evaluation of a grading score validated for soft tissue sarcoma. Cancer (Phila) 88(6):1425–1431
224. Peacock G, Archer S (1989) Myxoid leiomyosarcoma of the uterus: case report and review of the literature. Am J Obstet Gynecol 160:1515–1518
225. Pedeutour F, Quade BJ, Sornberger K, Tallini G, Ligon AH, Weremowicz S, et al (2000) Dysregulation of HMGIC in a uterine lipoleiomyoma with a complex rearrangement including chromosomes 7, 12, and 14. Genes Chromosomes Cancer 27(2):209–215
226. Perrone T, Dehner LP (1988) Prognostically favorable "mitotically active" smooth-muscle tumors of the uterus. A clinicopathologic study of ten cases. Am J Surg Pathol 12:1–8
227. Peters WA III, Howard DR, Andersen WA, Figge DC (1992) Deoxyribonucleic acid analysis by flow cytometry of uterine leiomyosarcomas and smooth muscle tumors of uncertain malignant potential. Am J Obstet Gynecol 166:1646–1654
228. Peters WA III, Howard DR, Andersen WA, Figge DC (1994) Uterine smooth-muscle tumors of uncertain malignant potential. Obstet Gynecol 83:1015–1020
229. Pieslor PC, Orenstein JM, Hogan DL, Breslow A (1979) Ultrastructure of myofibroblasts and decidualized cells in leiomyomatosis peritonealis disseminata. Am J Clin Pathol 72:875–882
230. Piver MS, Rutledge FN, Copeland L, Webster K, Blumenson L, Suh O (1984) Uterine endolymphatic stromal myosis: a collaborative study. Obstet Gynecol 64:173–178
231. Pounder DJ (1982) Fatty tumors of the uterus. J Clin Pathol 35:1380–1383
232. Prakash S, Scully RE (1964) Sarcoma-like pseudopregnancy changes in uterine leiomyomas. Report of a case resulting from prolonged norethindrone therapy. Obstet Gynecol 24:106–110
233. Prayson RA, Goldblum JR, Hart WR (1997) Epithelioid smooth-muscle tumors of the uterus—a clinicopathologic study of 18 patients. Am J Surg Pathol 21(4):383–391
234. Prayson RA, Hart WR (1992) Mitotically active leiomyomas of the uterus. Am J Clin Pathol 97: 14–20
235. Prichard J, Lowenstein M, Silverman I, Brennan J (1986) *Streptococcus milleri* pyomyoma simulating infective endocarditis. Obstet Gynecol 68;46S–49S
236. Quade BJ (1995) Pathology, cytogenetics and molecular biology of uterine leiomyomas and other smooth muscle lesions. Curr Opin Obstet Gynecol 7(1):35–42
237. Quade BJ, McLachlin CM, Soto-Wright V, Zuckerman J, Mutter GL, Morton CC (1997) Disseminated peritoneal leiomyomatosis—clonality analysis by X chromosome inactivation and cytogenetics of a clinically benign smooth muscle proliferation. Am J Pathol 150(6):2153–2166
238. Quade BJ, Pinto AP, Howard DR, Peters WA III, Crum CP (1999) Frequent loss of heterozygosity fo chromosome 10 in uterine leiomyosarcoma in contrast to leiomyoma. Am J Pathol 154(3):945–950
239. Rabban J, Wei MQ, Tavassoli FA (2001) Inflammatory myofibroblastic tumors of the uterus: a benign mimic of myxoid leiomyosarcoma. Am J Surg Pathol (Submitted)
240. Regidor PA, Schmidt M, Callies R, Kato K, Schindler AE (1995) Estrogen and progesterone receptor content of GnRH analogue pretreated and untreated uterine leiomyomata. Eur J Obstet Gynecol Reprod Biol 63:69–73
241. Reich O, Regauer S, Urdl W, Lahousen M, Winter R (2000) Expression of oestrogen and progesterone

receptors in low-grade endometrial stromal sarcomas. Br J Cancer 82(5):1030–1034
242. Rizeq MN, Van de Rijn M, Hendrickson MR, Rouse RV (1994) A comparative immunohistochemical study of uterine smooth muscle neoplasms with emphasis on the epithelioid variant. Hum Pathol 25:671–677
243. Rose PG, Piver MS, Tsukada Y, Lau T (1989) Patterns of metastasis in uterine sarcoma. An autopsy study. Cancer (Phila) 63:935–938
244. Roth E, Taylor HB (1966) Heterotopic cartilage in the uterus. Obstet Gynecol 27:838–844
245. Roth LM, Reed RJ (1999) Dissecting leiomyomas of the uterus other than cotyledonoid dissecting leiomyomas: a report of eight cases. Am J Surg Pathol 23(9):1032–1039
246. Roth LM, Reed RJ (2000) Cotyledonoid leiomyoma of the uterus: report of a case. Int J Gynecol Pathol 19(3):272–275
247. Roth LM, Reed RJ, Sternberg WH (1996) Cotyledonoid dissecting leiomyoma of the uterus—the Sternberg tumor. Am J Surg Pathol 20(12):1455–1461
248. Rotter AJ, Lundell CJ (1991) MR of intravenous leiomyomatosis of the uterus extending into the inferior vena cava. J Comput Assist Tomogr 15:690–693
248a. Rush DS, Tan JY, Baergen RN, Soslow RA (2001) h-Caldesmon, a novel smooth muscle-specific antibody, distinguishes between cellular leiomyoma and endometrial stromal sarcoma. Am J Surg Pathol 25(2):253–258
249. Rutgers JL, Spong CY, Sinow R, Heiner J (1995) Leuprolide acetate treatment and myoma arterial size. Obstet Gynecol 86:386–388
250. Rywlin AM, Recher L, Benson J (1964) Clear-cell leiomyoma of the uterus: report of two cases of a previously undescribed entity. Cancer (Phila) 17: 100–104
251. Sabini G, Chumas JC, Mann WJ (1992) Steroid hormone receptors in endometrial stromal sarcomas. A biochemical and immunohistochemical study. Am J Clin Pathol 97:381–386
252. Sahin AA, Silva EG, Landon G, Ordóñez NG, Gershenson DM (1989) Endometrial tissue in myometrial vessels not associated with menstruation. Int J Gynecol Pathol 8:139–146
253. Saksela E, Lampinen V, Precope BJ (1974) Malignant mesenchymal tumors of the uterine corpus. Am J Obstet Gynecol 120:452–460
254. Schammel DP, Silver SA, Tavassoli FA (1998) Combined endometrial stromal/smooth muscle neoplasms of the uterus: a clinicopathological study of 38 cases. Mod Pathol 12(2):124A
255. Schammel DP, Tavassoli FA (1998) Uterine angiosarcomas—a morphologic and immunohistochemical study of four cases. Am J Surg Pathol 22(2):246–250
256. Schilder JM, Hurd WW, Roth LM, Sutton GP (1999) Hormonal treatment of an endometrial stromal nodule followed by local excision. Obstet Gynecol 93:805–807
257. Schmid C, Beham A, Kratochvil P (1991) Hematopoesis in a degenerating leiomyoma. Arch Obstet Gynecol 248:81
258. Schneider D, Halperin R, Segal M, Maymon R, Bukovsky I (1995) Myxoid leiomyosarcoma of the uterus with unusual malignant histologic pattern—a case report. Gynecol Oncol 59:156–158
259. Schwartz LB, Diamond MP, Schwartz PE (1993) Leiomyosarcomas: clinical presentation. Am J Obstet Gynecol 168:180–183
260. Scribner DR Jr, Walker JL (1998) Low-grade endometrial stromal sarcoma preoperative treatment with Depo-Lupron and Megace. Gynecol Oncol 71:458–460
261. Scully RE, Bonfiglio TA, Kurman RJ, Silverberg SG, Wilkinson EJ (1994) World Health Organization international histological classification of tumours: histological typing of female genital tract tumours, 2nd Ed. Springer, Berlin
262. Scully R (1992) Pathology of leiomyomas. Semin Reprod Endocrinol 10(4):325–331
263. Seidman JD, Kjerulff KH (1996) Pathologic findings from the Maryland Women's Health Study: practice patterns in the diagnosis of adenomyosis. Int J Gynecol Pathol 15:217–221
264. Seidman JD, Thomas RM (1993) Multiple plexiform tumorlets of the uterus. Arch Pathol Lab Med 117:1255–1256
265. Seidman JD, Wasserman CS, Aye LM, MacKoul PJ, O'Leary TJ (1999) Cluster of uterine mullerian adenosarcoma in the Washington, DC metropolitan area with high incidence of sarcomatous overgrowth. Am J Surg Pathol 23(7):809–814
266. Seidman JD, Yetter RA, Papadimitriou JC (1992) Epithelioid component of uterine leiomyosarcoma simulating metastatic carcinoma. Arch Pathol Lab Med 116:287–290
267. Seltzer VL, Levine A, Spiegal G, Rosenfeld D, Coffey EL (1990) Adenofibroma of the uterus: multiple recurrences following wide local excision. Gynecol Oncol 37:427–431
268. Sener AB, Seckin NC, Ozmen S, Gokmen O, Dogu N, Ekici E (1996) The effects of hormone replacement therapy on uterine fibroids in postmenopausal women. Fertil Steril 65(2):354–357
269. Shaw RW (1998) Gonadotrophin hormone-releasing hormone analogue treatment of fibroids. Baillieres Clin Obstet Gynaecol 12(2):245–268
270. Shih IM, Kurman RJ (1998) Epithelioid trophoblastic tumor—a neoplasm distinct from choriocarcinoma and placental site trophoblastic tumor simulating carcinoma. Am J Surg Pathol 22:1393–1403
271. Siegal GP, Taylor LL III, Nelson KG, Reddick RL, Frazelle M, Siegfried JM, et al (1983) Characterization of a pure heterologous sarcoma of the uterus: rhabdomyosarcoma of the corpus. Int J Gynecol Pathol 2:303–315

272. Sieinski W (1989) Lipomatous neometaplasia of the uterus. Report of 11 cases with discussion of histogenesis and pathogenesis. Int J Gynecol Pathol 8:357–363
273. Silva EG, Tornos C, Ordóñez NG, Morris M (1995) Uterine leiomyosarcoma with clear cell areas. Int J Gynecol Pathol 14:174–178
274. Silverberg SG, Kurman RJ (1992) Tumors of the uterine corpus and gestational trophoblastic disease. Armed Forces Institute of Pathology, Washington, DC
275. Sinkre P, Miller DS, Milchgrub S, Hameed A (2000) Adenomyofibroma of the endometrium with skeletal muscle differentiation. Int J Gynecol Pathol 19(3):280–283
276. Sorensen JB, Schultze HR, Madsen EL, Holund B (1998) Primitive neuroectodermal tumor (PNET) of the uterine cavity. Eur J Obstet Gynecol Reprod Biol 76(2):181–184
277. Sornberger KS, Weremowicz S, Williams AJ, Quade BJ, Ligon AH, Pedeutour F, et al (1999) Expression of HMGIY in three uterine leiomyomata with complex rearrangements of chromosome 6. Cancer Genet Cytogenet 114(1):9–16
278. Sreenan JJ, Prayson RA, Biscotti CV, Thornton MH, Easley KA, Hart WR (1996) Histopathologic findings in 107 uterine leiomyomas treated with leuprolide acetate compared with 126 controls. Am J Surg Pathol 20(4):427–432
279. Stovall TG, Ling FW, Henry LC, Woodruff MR (1991) A randomized trial evaluating leuprolide acetate before hysterectomy as treatment for leiomyomas. Am J Obstet Gynecol 164:1420–1423
280. Stroh EL, Besa PC, Cox JD, Fuller LM, Cabanillas FF (1995) Treatment of patients with lymphomas of the uterus or cervix with combination chemotherapy and radiation therapy. Cancer (Phila) 75:2392–2399
281. Su LD, Atayde-Perez A, Sheldon S, Fletcher JA, Weiss SW (1998) Inflammatory myofibroblastic tumor: cytogenetic evidence supporting clonal origin. Mod Pathol 11:364–368
282. Suginami H, Kaura R, Ochi H, Matsuura S (1990) Intravenous leiomyomatosis with cardiac extension: successful surgical management and histopathologic study. Obstet Gynecol 76:527–529
283. Sutton G, Blessing JA, Malfetano JH (1996) Ifosfamide and doxorubicin in the treatment of advanced leiomyosarcomas of the uterus: a Gynecologic Oncology Group study. Gynecol Oncol 62: 226–229
284. Sutton G, Blessing JA, Park R, DiSaia PJ, Rosenshein N (1996) Ifosfamide treatment of recurrent or metastatic endometrial stromal sarcomas previously unexposed to chemotherapy: a study of the Gynecologic Oncology Group. Obstet Gynecol 87: 747–750
285. Swisher EM, Gown AM, Skelly M, Ek M, Tamimi HK, Cain JM, et al (1996) The expression of epidermal growth factor receptor, HER-2/Neu, p53, and Ki-67 antigen in uterine malignant mixed mesodermal tumors and adenosarcoma. Gynecol Oncol 60:81–88
286. Taina E, Maenpäa J, Erkkola R, Ikkala J, Söderström O, Viitanen A (1989) Endometrial stromal sarcoma: a report of nine cases. Gynecol Oncol 32:156–162
287. Tallini G, Price FV, Carcangiu ML (1993) Epithelioid angiosarcoma arising in uterine leiomyomas. Am J Clin Pathol 100:514–518
288. Tang CK, Toker C, Ances IG (1979) Stromomyoma of the uterus. Cancer (Phila) 43:308–316
289. Tavassoli FA, Norris HJ (1981) Mesenchymal tumors of the uterus. VII. A clinicopathological study of 60 endometrial stromal nodules. Histopathology (Oxf) 5:1–10
290. Tavassoli FA, Norris HJ (1982) Peritoneal leiomyomatosis (leiomyomatosis peritonealis disseminata): a clinicopathologic study of 20 cases with ultrastructural observations. Int J Gynecol Pathol 1:59–74
291. Thatcher SS, Woodruff JD (1982) Uterine stromatosis: a report of 33 cases. Obstet Gynecol 59: 428–434
292. Tietze L, Guenther K, Hoerbe A, Pawlik C, Klosterhalfen B, Handt S, et al (2000) Benign metastasizing leiomyoma: a cytogenetically balanced but clonal disease. Hum Pathol 31(1):126–128
293. Tiltman AJ (1985) The effect of progestins on the mitotic activity of uterine fibromyomas. Int J Gynecol Pathol 4:89–96
294. Timmis AD, Smallpeice C, Davies AC, Macarthur AM, Gishen P, Jackson G (1980) Intracardiac spread of intravenous leiomyomatosis with successful surgical excision. N Engl J Med 303:1043–1044
295. TornÄ A, Jou P, Pagano R, Sanchez I, Ordi J, Vanrell JA (1996) Endometrial ossification successfully treated by hysteroscopic resection. Eur J Obstet Gynecol Reprod Biol 66(1):75–77
296. Tresukosol DR, Kudelka AP, Malpica A, Varma DGK, Edwards CL, Kavanagh JJ (1995) Leuprolide acetate and intravascular leiomyomatosis. Obstet Gynecol 86:688–692
297. Tsushima K, Stanhope CR, Gaffey TA, Lieber MM (1988) Uterine leiomyosarcomas and benign smooth muscle tumors: usefulness of nuclear DNA patterns studied by flow cytometry. Mayo Clin Proc 63:248–255
298. Upadhyaya NB, Doody MC, Googe PB (1990) Histopathological changes in leiomyomata treated with leuprolide acetate. Fertil Steril 54:811–814
299. Van Diest PJ, Baak JP, Matze-Cok P, Wisse-Brekelmans EC, van Galen CM, Kurver PH, et al (1992) Reproducibility of mitosis counting in 2,469 breast cancer specimens: results from the Multicenter Morphometric Mammary Carcinoma Project. Hum Pathol 23(6):603–607
300. Vang R, Medeiros LJ, Ha CS, Deavers M (2000) Non-Hodgkin's lymphomas involving the uterus: a

clinicopathologic analysis of 26 cases. Mod Pathol 13(1):19–28
301. Vardi JR, Tovell HMM (1980) Leiomyosarcoma of the uterus: clinicopathologic study. Obstet Gynecol 56:428–434
302. Vellios F, Ng AB, Reagen JW (1973) Papillary adenofibroma of the uterus: a benign mesodermal mixed tumor of mullerian origin. Am J Clin Pathol 60:543–551
303. Viville B, Charnock-Jones DS, Sharkey AM, Wetzka B, Smith SK (1997) Distribution of the A and B forms of the progesterone receptor messenger ribonucleic acid and protein in uterine leiomyomata and adjacent myometrium. Hum Reprod 12(4): 815–822
304. Vollenhoven B (1998) Introduction: the epidemiology of uterine leiomyomas. Baillieres Clin Obstet Gynaecol 12(2):169–176
305. Volpe R, Canzonieri V, Gloghini A, Carbone A (1992) "Lipoleiomyoma with metaplastic cartilage" (benign mesenchymoma) of the uterine cervix. Pathol Res Pract 188(6):799–801
306. Vu K, Greenspan DL, Wu TC, Zacur HA, Kurman RJ (1998) Cellular proliferation, estrogen receptor, progesterone receptor, and bcl-2 expression in GnRH agonist-treated uterine leiomyomas. Hum Pathol 29(4):359–363
307. Watanabe K, Hiraki H, Ohishi M, Mashiko K, Saginoya H, Suzuki T (1996) Uterine leiomyosarcoma with osteoclast-like giant cells: histopathological and cytological observations. Pathol Int 46(9): 656–660
308. Weissman A, Talmon R, Jakobi P (1993) Cavernous hemangioma of the uterus in a pregnant woman. Obstet Gynecol 81:825–827
309. West CP (1998) Hysterectomy and myomectomy by laparotomy. Baillieres Clin Obstet Gynaecol 12(2): 317–335
310. Wheelock JB, Krebs HB, Schneider V, Goplerud DR (1985) Uterine sarcoma: analysis of prognostic variables in 71 cases. Am J Obstet Gynecol 151:1016–1022
311. Witkin GB, Askin FB, Geratz JD, Reddick RL (1987) Angiosarcoma of the uterus: a light microscopic, immunohistochemical, and ultrastructural study. Int J Gynecol Pathol 6:176–184
312. Wolff M, Silva F, Kaye G (1979) Pulmonary metastases (with admixed epithelial elements) from smooth muscle neoplasms: report of nine cases, including three males. Am J Surg Pathol 3:325–342
313. Wolfson AH, Wolfson DJ, Sittler SY, Breton L, Markoe AM, Schwade JG, et al (1994) A multivariate analysis of clinicopathologic factors for predicting outcome in uterine sarcomas. Gynecol Oncol 52:56–62
314. Wood C, Maher P (1998) Endoscopic treatment of uterine fibroids. Baillieres Clin Obstet Gynaecol 12(2):289–316
315. Yamadori I, Kobayashi S, Ogino T, Ohmori M, Tanaka H, Jimbo T (1993) Uterine leiomyoma with a focus of fatty and cartilaginous differentiation. Acta Obstet Gynecol Scand 72:307–309
316. Yoonessi M, Hart WR (1977) Endometrial stromal sarcomas. Cancer (Phila) 40:898–906
317. Young RH, Harris NL, Scully RE (1985) Lymphoma-like lesions of the lower female genital tract: a report of 16 cases. Int J Gynecol Pathol 4:289–299
318. Young RH, Prat J, Scully RE (1984) Endometrioid stromal sarcomas of the ovary. A clinicopatholgic analysis of 23 cases. Cancer (Phila) 53:1143–1155
319. Young RH, Scully RE (1984) Placental-site trophoblastic tumor: current status. Clin Obstet Gynecol 27:248–258
320. Young RH, Silva EG, Scully RE (1991) Ovarian and juxtaovarian adenomatoid tumors: a report of six cases. Int J Gynecol Pathol 10:364–372
321. Young RH, Treger T, Scully RE (1986) Atypical polypoid adenomyoma of the uterus. A report of 27 cases. Am J Clin Pathol 86:139–145
322. Youngs LA, Taylor HB (1967) Adenomatoid tumors of the uterus and fallopian tube. Am J Clin Pathol 48:537–545
323. Zaloudek CJ, Norris HJ (1981) Adenofibroma and adenosarcoma of the uterus: a clinicopathologic study of 35 cases. Cancer (Phila) 48:354–366
324. Zamecnik M, Michal M (1998) Endometrial stromal nodule with retiform sex-cord-like differentiation. Pathol Res Pract 194:449–453

14

Diseases of the Fallopian Tube

James E. Wheeler, M.D.

Anatomy

The normal fallopian tube extends from the area of its corresponding ovary anteriorly and medially to its terminus in the posterosuperior aspect of the uterine fundus. In an adult during the reproductive years, its length is usually between 9 and 11 cm. The tube at the ovarian end opens to the peritoneal cavity and is composed of about 25 irregular finger-like extensions of the tube, the fimbriae. The fimbriae attach to the expanded end of the tube, the infundibulum, which is about 1 cm long and 1 cm in diameter. The infundibulum lies within a few millimeters of the superolateral or tubal end of the ovary. It narrows gradually to about 4 mm in diameter and merges medially with the ampullary portion of the tube, which extends about 6 cm, passing anteriorly as it passes around the ovary. At a point characterized by relative thickening of the muscular wall, the isthmic portion begins and extends some 2 cm to the uterus. Within the myometrium, the tube extends as a 1-cm-long intramural segment until it joins the extension of the endometrial cavity at the uterotubal junction. Throughout its extrauterine course, the tube lies in a peritoneal fold along the superior margin of the broad ligament, the mesosalpinx.

The arterial blood supply has a dual origin. A tubal branch of the uterine artery passes in the mesosalpinx laterally from the cornu of the uterus to anastomose with tubal branches of the ovarian artery. Venous drainage parallels the arterial supply via anastomosing tubal branches of uterine and ovarian veins, also located in the mesosalpinx. Tubal lymphatics pass laterally, accompanying the ovarian vessels. Thence, on the right side, lymph drains into nodes in the area of the right renal vein and the inferior vena cava, whereas on the left side, lymph drains into nodes lying between the left ovarian vein and the left renal vein. Lymph also drains into presacral and common ililac nodes. It is apparent that lymphatic spread of tubal malignancy may reach extrapelvic sites early in its dissemination.[86,87]

The nerve supply of the tube is both sympathetic and parasympathetic. Sympathetic fibers from T10 through L2 synapse in the celiac, aortic, renal, inferior mesenteric, cervicovaginal, and possibly presacral plexuses. Postsynaptic fibers pass into the myosalpinx, where they provide adrenergic innervation to the smooth muscle. The fact that isthmic and ampullary tubal muscle is innervated via presacral and ovarian plexuses, respectively, provides a possible neural explanation for differential myosalpingeal activity and formation of a physiologic sphincter. Sensory pain fibers pass along with the sympathetic nerves to the spinal cord at the level of T10–T12. Parasympathetic fibers from the vagus nerve supply the extrauterine tube via postganglionic fibers from the ovarian plexus, whereas the intramural portion is innervated via S2–S4 parasympathetic fibers synapsing in the pelvic plexuses. Unique connections are formed between autonomic nerve fibers and subepithelial stromal cells of the mucosa.[178]

Histology

A mucosal membrane, a wall of smooth muscle, and a serosal coat make up the three histologic layers of the tube. The serosa is lined by flattened mesothelial cells. Beneath the mesothelium lies a small amount of connective tissue containing a few collagen fibers and blood vessels. The tubal muscularis generally has two layers: an outer longitudinal layer and an inner circular layer. At the uterine end, beginning in the intramural tube and extending laterally about 2 cm, there is, in addition, an inner longitudinal layer. The outer longitudinal layer is easily overlooked, as it is composed of inconspicuous bundles of smooth muscle interspersed with loose connective tissue containing numerous small blood vessels. The circular layer forms the major muscle mass of the tube. Its thickness varies, being about 0.5 mm in the isthmus and only about 0.1 mm in the ampulla.

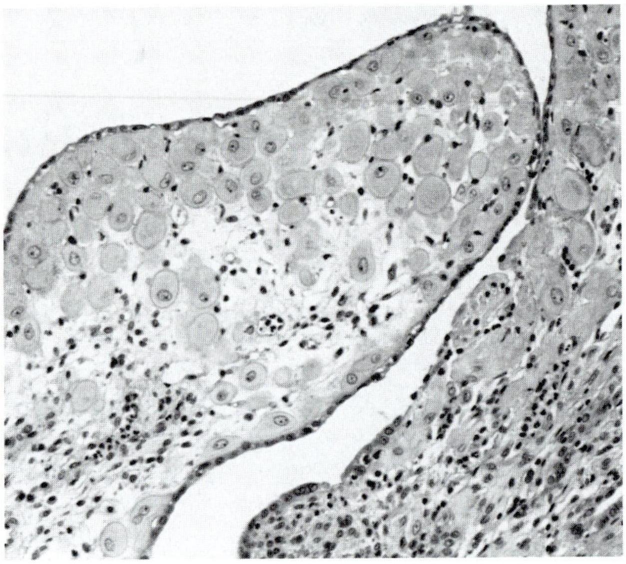

Fig. 14.1. Decidual reaction in tubal mucosa. The endosalpingeal folds are expanded by oval decidualized stromal cells characterized by well-defined cytoplasmic membranes.

The mucosal layer lies directly on the muscularis. It consists of a luminal epithelial lining and a scanty underlying lamina propria containing vessels and spindly or angular cells. Although these stromal cells seem sparse, they are the cells that lead to focally recognizable decidua in 5%–12% of postpartum tubes (Fig. 14.1) and may be seen in 80% of tubes removed for ectopic pregnancy.[64] The mucosa increases significantly in its gross structural complexity as the lumen enlarges from the uterine to the ovarian end. The interstitial and intramural portions each contain about five or six blunt plicae, or folds. In the isthmus, the plicae increase in height to more nearly occupy the larger lumen. A dozen or more plicae, some with secondary folds, are present. In the ampulla, the plicae are frondlike and delicate, and both secondary and tertiary branches may be appreciated. The infundibular plical pattern is similar.

The epithelial layer of the mucosa is composed of at least three histological cell types: ciliated, secretory, and intercalary. About 20%–30% of the cells contain prominent cilia, and about 55%–65% are secretory (Fig. 14.2). Although some investigators have found the ciliated cells in humans to be apparently randomly and equally distributed throughout the isthmic, ampullary,and fimbriated portions, others have found ciliated cells more numerous and preferentially located at the apical portions of the plicae, especially in the fimbriae and ampulla. Ciliated cells in the isthmus are less frequent[48] and occur in short strands. Ciliated cells are even scantier in the intramural tubal segment. The ciliated cell itself is columnar and approximately 20–30 μm long. Electron microscopic study reveals typical ciliary basal bodies and rootlets. The nucleus is oval to round, about 8–10 μm in greatest extent, and may lie parallel or perpendicular to the long axis of the cell. The chromatin pattern is moderately granular. A distinct but small nucleolus is present. The secretory cell also is columnar, approximately the same height as the ciliated cell but often narrower (Fig. 14.2). Its nucleus is ovoid and perpendicular to the long axis of the cell. The chromatin pattern may be somewhat denser than that of the ciliated cell, but its nucleolus is similar. The intercalary, or peg, cell is a columnar cell that appears to be occupied mainly by a thin, dark-staining nucleus. It is likely a morphologic variant of the secretory cell.

In addition to the three epithelial cell types described, scattered lymphocytes may be seen located basally above the basement membrane. Immunohistological analysis of these lymphocytes indicates a preponderance of the T-cytotoxic/suppressor subtype, consistent with formation of mucosal-associated lymphoid tissue (MALT).[118]

The wolffian or mesonephric duct develops in close proximity to the fallopian tube, and remnants from it normally persist throughout adult life. These remnants consist of 10–15 mesonephric tubules lying in the mesovarium. The tubules are lined by low columnar or cuboidal epithelium containing ciliated and nonciliated cells. There is only a thin, if any, muscular coat.[31] The tubules connect with the

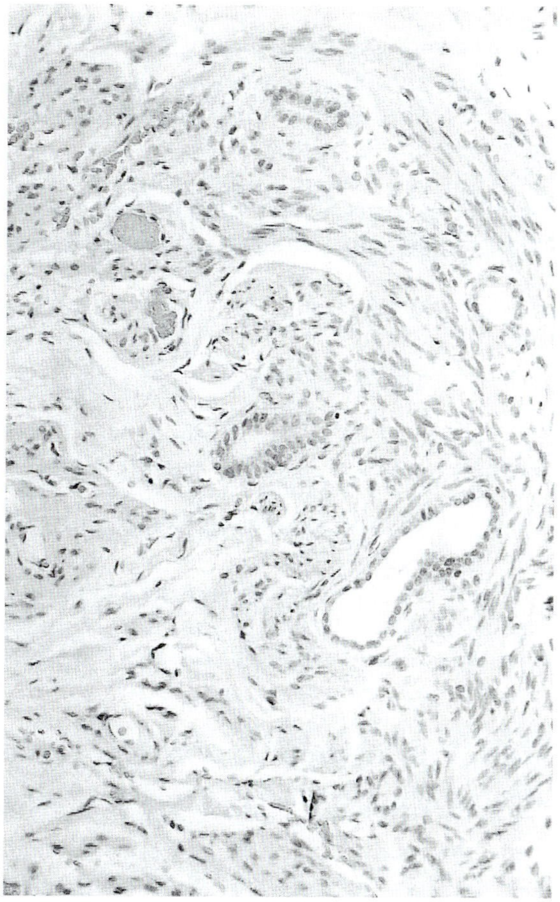

Fig. 14.3. Mesonephric duct remnants. These embryologic rests are commonly found on routine cross sections. Note small tubal lumens in the center lined by low cuboidal cells. The surrounding smooth muscle is characteristic.

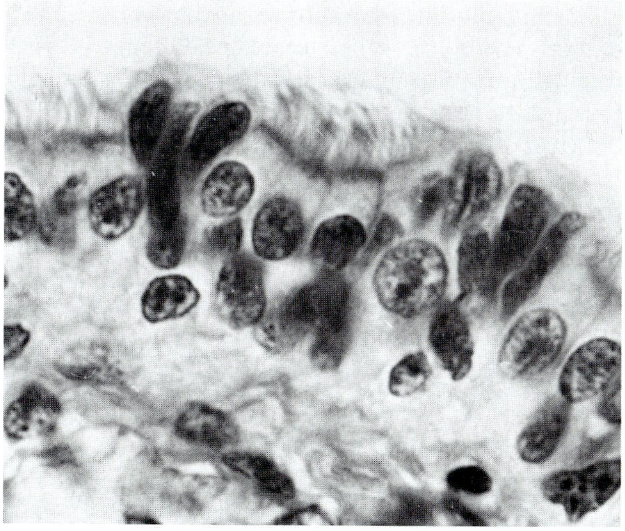

Fig. 14.2. Tubal epithelium. Ciliated cells are numerous. Secretory cells with columnar, somewhat compressed nuclei protrude above the level of the ciliated cells. Note vacuolated apical cytoplasm of secretory cells.

mesonephric duct, which runs parallel to the fallopian tube in the mesosalpinx. The duct is lined by nonciliated cuboidal or columnar cells surrounded by a relatively thick layer of inner longitudinal and outer circular smooth muscle. It is commonly seen on routine histological cross sections of tube lying outside the tubal muscularis (Fig. 14.3).

Physiology with Morphologic Correlation

The morphologic characteristics of the tubal epithelium change during life. Ciliated cells appear during early fetal development and persist until the postmenopausal years. At this time, as circulating estrogen levels drop, the cilia are gradually lost. Estrogen therapy in postmenopausal women, however, restores both the cilia and the ability to transport particulate matter. The demonstration of a specific estradiol receptor in the human tube suggests that there is a direct action of estrogen on ciliogenesis. The characteristics of the tubal epithelium change during the course of the menstrual cycle. Early in the cycle the cells are low, and the secretory cells appear relatively inactive. As ovulation approaches, probably under the influence of an increasing amount of estrogen, the secretory cells become prominent and actually project beyond the ciliated cells (see Fig. 14.2). There is a discharge of periodic acid–Schiff (PAS)-positive material, probably glycogen, into the tubal lumen.[58] Changes in cilial maturity and repeated ciliation and deciliation of a minor degree have been documented during the menstrual cycle.[48,170] Other cyclic changes in tubal physiology occur.[80]

The cilia and tubal muscularis play a dominant role in tubal function at ovulation. The cilia beat in synchronized waves in the direction of the uterus. During the course of ovum pickup, there appears to be a realignment of fimbriae in their relationship to the ovary itself. A distinct fimbria, the fimbria ovarica, runs from the tubal ostium to one pole of the ovary. It is thought that, at the time of ovulation, the muscle of the fimbria ovarica contracts, pulling the tube in the direction of the rupturing follicle. At the same time, some muscular elements in the paraovarian tissue contract, pulling the ovary toward the tubal ostium. This realignment of fimbriae over the rupturing follicle has been observed in several laboratory species, but for technical reasons it has not yet been satisfactorily evaluated in the human. Once the ovum is released from its follicle, surrounded by an entourage of sticky cumulus cells, it adheres to the cilia of the fimbriated end of the tube, and is transported along the surface by the ciliary action.[163] The ovum is retained within the tube for approximately 3 days, after which it is delivered into the uterus. In Kartagener's syndrome, where cilia are scanty and structurally and functionally defective, fertility is impaired, but not abolished[67]; this raises the likelihood that muscular contraction is more important than previously considered. The effect of adrenergic innervation or prostaglandins on muscle function and ova transport is not yet well defined.

Spermatozoa are transported upward through the uterus into the fallopian tube. The mechanisms by which they traverse the uterotubal junction and tubal isthmus in the face of a ciliary beat in a downward direction is still not understood. It is known, however, that spermatozoa in the human can reach the tube within minutes after they are placed in the vagina. It is likely that the fertilizing spermatozoon is already present in the fallopian tube at the time the ovum arrives there.[174]

The environment provided within the tubal lumen is of special importance in reproductive function. The fallopian tube does provide a temporary milieu for spermatozoa, the ovum, and finally the fertilized, cleaving zygote during its initial development. The secretory cells certainly must play a role in the provision of suitable conditions for the processes that occur within the tubal lumen. Fluid formation in the tube appears to be driven by transepithelial secretion of chloride ions.[50] The salient components of oviductal fluid include metabolic substrates, the most important of which are lactate, pyruvate, and bicarbonate, which appears in tubal fluid as a result of carbonic anhydrase in the tubal epithelium, and electrolytes, including calcium. Tubal fluid also contains trypsin inhibitors, which may influence the fertilization process, and a genital tract isoamylase. The bicarbonate ion is in part responsible for dispersion of cells that surround the ovum. On reaching the level of the zona pellucida (a protein–mucopolysaccharide layer immediately surrounding the egg), the spermatozoon is able to penetrate by virtue of the presence of a trypsin-like enzyme in its head. Trypsin inhibitors appear in high concentration both before and after ovulation, but for a matter of hours after ovulation, they are at their lowest concentration. Some investigators have speculated that trypsin inhibitors control the fertilization process so that aged ova that are in the fallopian tube in the presence of a high concentration of inhibitors are not fertilized. Be that as it may, the 3-day residence in the fallopian tube apparently serves a useful function in several experimental mammals. When zygotes are removed prematurely from the tube and placed in the uterus, implantation is less likely.

Most of the work on tubal physiology has focused on its role in reproduction, and only scanty information is available on the tubal immune system and its role in infection.[20] The immunoglobulin IgG is present in tubal fluid. Both subclasses of immunoglobulin A, IgA_1 and IgA_2, are formed by a scanty population of subepithelial lymphocytes and plasma cells[94] with the secretory component contributed by the epithelial cells.[118] CD 8+ and CD 4+ T cells and macrophages are also identified.[180] Primates vaccinated with sperm antigens may mount a antibody response in tubal fluid.[92]

Congenital Anomalies

Structural congenital anomalies of the fallopian tube are rare and may be simulated by inflammatory processes or torsion. Tubes associated with uterine abnormalities such as a rudimentary uterine horn or bicornuate uterus may be hypoplastic or partially atretic. Bilateral absence of the ampullary muscularis has been reported. Infertility patients who were exposed in utero to diethylstilbestrol (DES) may have shortened, sacculated, and convoluted fallopian tubes despite normal salpingograms. The fimbriae are described as constricted and the os as pinpoint. No detailed pathologic studies are available. A mouse model of DES exposure produces tubal changes more reminiscent of salpingitis isthmica nodosa. Apparent congenital absence of a segment of the tube has been reported,[90] as has tubal duplication and accessory tubes.[17] Tubes may be absent in phenotypic females in rare cases.

Torsion, Prolapse, and Intussusception

Among the various anatomic displacements of the tube, *torsion* is the most common. The usual predisposing factor is cystic enlargement of the ipsilateral ovary. A benign ovarian cyst or tumor is present in 65%–80% of patients, and a malignant ovarian tumor is present in 5%–15%. Paraovarian cysts also are associated with torsion. Tubal enlargement secondary to hydrosalpinx or pyosalpinx, or previous gynecologic surgery, especially sterilization,[21] are additional causes, but torsion may occur in the absence of apparent adnexal disease.[16] The typical patient is in the reproductive years, occasionally pregnant, and complains of the sudden onset of lower abdominal pain. At operation, the adnexa on one side is twisted, usually once or twice. Venous outflow is compromised early, and the resulting congestion may lead to arterial compression. The adnexa often is swollen and edematous, with hemorrhagic infarction and gangrene. If surgical intervention is prompt, the tube may be preserved. Undiagnosed torsion in an infant or adult may result in resorption and total disappearance of the infarcted adnexa or in calcification of the necrotic tissue.[63]

Tubal *prolapse* into the vagina may occur rarely as a complication of vaginal or abdominal hysterectomy.[138] (See Chapter 4, Diseases of the Vagina.) Clinically this is characterized by vaginal discharge, beginning a few days to several years after vaginal hysterectomy. On examination, an excresence is seen in the vaginal vault, suggestive of granulation tissue or carcinoma. Fimbriae may be apparent grossly. Severe acute and chronic inflammation is present microscopically, and pseudogland formation by the tubal epithelium may mimic adenocarcinoma. *Intussusception* of the tube has been reported once. A paraovarian cyst was engulfed by the end of the tube and pulled the fimbriated end into the ampulla. Simple eversion and cystectomy permitted tubal salvage.

Metaplasia

The tubal epithelium may undergo metaplastic changes without apparent reason. The metaplastic cells may be squamous, transitional, or mucinous, resembling endocervical epithelium.[51,152] *Mucinous metaplasia* may be associated with Peutz–Jeghers syndrome and may also accompany chronic inflammation. There may be *oncocytic metaplasia* with marked cytoplasmic eosinophilia on routine H&E staining (Fig 14.4). When associated with chronic salpingitis and papillary changes, occasionally it is interpreted as a benign papilloma.[145] Studies delineating the usual extent of epithelial variability demonstrate that focal nuclear crowding and tufting are frequent and normal (Fig. 14.5), but mitoses occur infrequently.

Psammoma bodies are an occasional finding in chronic salpingitis associated with IgG antibodies to *Chlamydia*[111] but may be seen in otherwise normal-appearing epithelium (Fig. 14.6). Accumulation of lipofuscin, accompanied by scanty iron pigment, in macrophages in the lamina propria has been reported as pigmentosis tubae[71] and may be associated with endometriosis[153] (see later under "Pseudoxanthomatous Salpingitis").

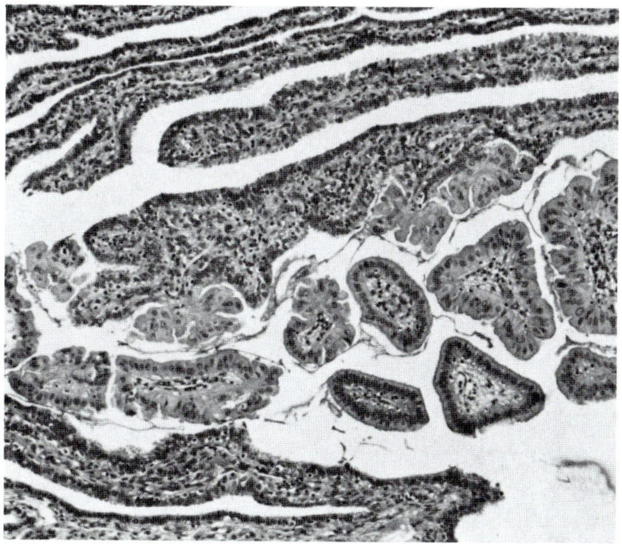

Fig. 14.4. Benign oncocytic (pink cell) metaplasia. Nuclear atypia and cell crowding in the absence of papillary formations and mitoses should not be confused with early carcinoma.

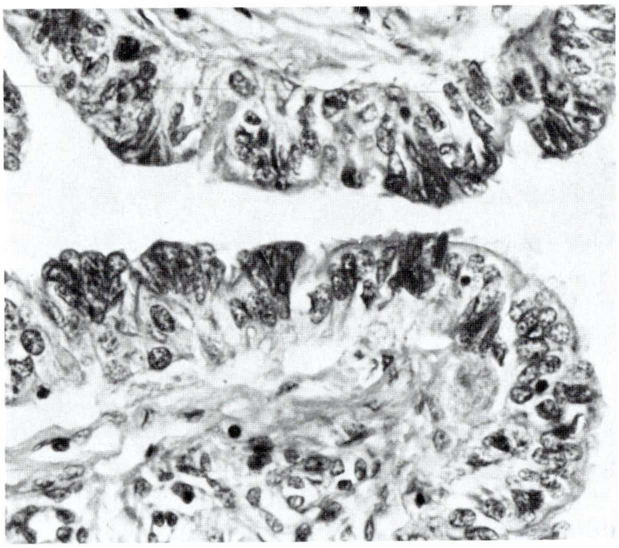

Fig. 14.5. Tubal epithelium. Crowding of nuclei and tufting of epithelial cells is a normal variant.

Endometriosis and Endosalpingiosis

Endometrial-type tissue may involve the tubal lumen, wall, or serosa. Heterotopic endometrium may entirely replace normal tubal epithelium, with luminal occlusion.[75] Endosalpingiosis is the ectopic location of tubal-type epithelium involving peritoneal surfaces. Both *endometriosis* and *endosalpingiosis* are discussed in detail in Chapter 17, Diseases of the Peritoneum.

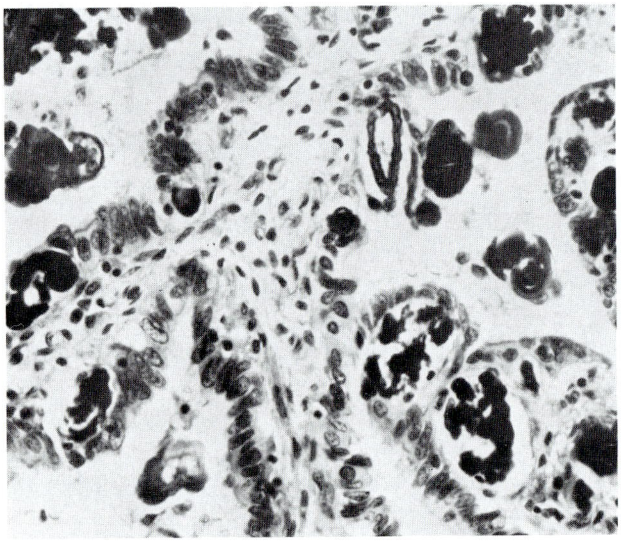

Fig. 14.6. Psammoma bodies in tubal epithelium. These calcific bodies may be found in chronic salpingitis or in relatively normal epithelium containing only rare lymphocytes.

Salpingitis

Salpingitis may be divided into three major types: *acute*, *chronic*, and *granulomatous*.

Acute Salpingitis

Acute salpingitis is a purulent inflammatory process usually secondary to the passage of bacteria from the uterine cavity into the tubal lumen.[113] It is not clear if organisms are carried upward by sperm or trichomonads as vectors or whether some form of passive transport is in effect.[83] Although *Neisseria gonorrhoeae* and *Chlamydia trachomatis* have been considered the most common causative organisms, meticulous bacteriologic studies indicate that most are polymicrobial and that anaerobic bacteria, especially *Bacteroides* species and peptostreptococci, frequently are present, as well as aerobes such as *Escherichia coli*. The presence in some of these women of serum antibodies against gonococcal pili, however, suggests that gonococci may initiate the process, only to be supplanted by anaerobes.

Elegant in vitro studies by Ward and others[172] have clarified the likely initial steps in gonococcal infection, and the molecular mechanisms involved have been reviewed.[24] *N. gonorrhoeae* perfused through the lumen of cultured whole tubes attach only to nonciliated cells. Within 3 hours, microvilli from the cells appear to embrace the gonococci and adhere to them. The bacteria then penetrate both the cells and intercellular junctions, with cell lysis and sloughing. Adjacent ciliated cells are also destroyed but are not invaded directly. Gonococcal lipopolysaccharide and gonococcal-induced tumor necrosis factor (TNF-alpha) may cause much of the epithelial damage,[114] and the degree of pathogenicity likely depends on the bacterial as well as the host genome.[10] After cell lysis, the bacteria penetrate the subepithelial connective tissue. In vivo, this process is considerably modified by the host response. A brisk diapedesis of granulocytes occurs from capillaries into the mucosa and lumen, and there is vascular engorgement and edema of all tubal layers (Fig. 14.7).

In severe cases, transudation of plasma proteins results in a fibrinous exudate on the serosal surface, which reddens because of vascular dilatation. As the lumen fills with granulocytes and cellular debris and as the tube distends, pus may be seen dripping from the fimbriated end in patients undergoing laparoscopy. The cell necrosis, distension of the tube, and focal peritonitis lead to abdominal and pelvic pain. The gonococcus gains access to the tube most readily at the time of menstruation. This situation corresponds to the typical clinical presentation in

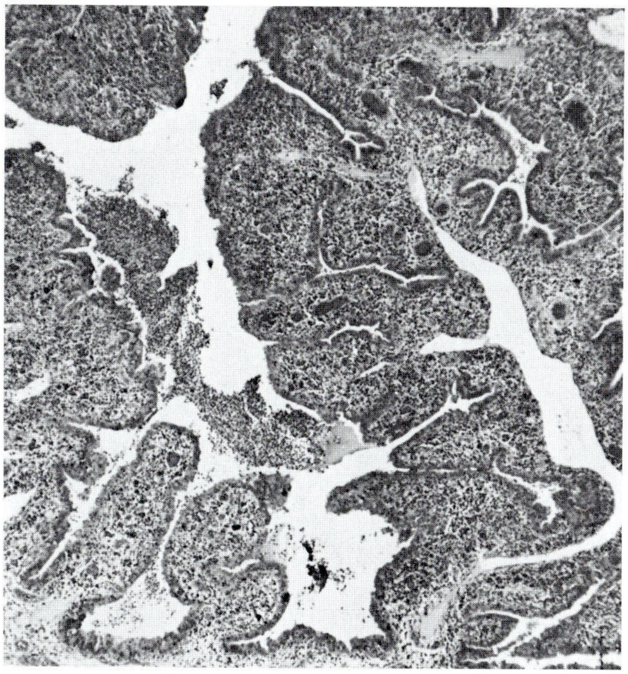

Fig. 14.7. Acute and chronic salpingitis. Plicae are broadened and blunted. Numerous granulocytes, lymphocytes, and plasma cells are present in the mucosa; many granulocytes are present in the lumen.

which the onset of acute pain occurs a few days after menses. The onset of nongonococcal, nonchlamydial acute salpingitis is not, however, clearly related to the recent onset of menses.[161] Over time, repeated infections result in recurrent symptoms as well as the anatomic changes of chronic salpingitis, discussed next. Acute bacterial salpingitis after tubal ligation is not rare, but may be milder than that occurring in nonligated tubes.[1] Although *N. gonorrhoeae* spreads via the epithelial surface and thus causes mucosal changes, other bacteria, such as streptococci, tend to spread into the tube by vascular or lymphatic channels; this results in acute inflammation of the tubal wall, with relative sparing of the mucosa.

Initial reports implicated the intrauterine contraceptive device in the etiology of salpingitis and pelvic inflammatory disease. However, newer information eliminating methodologic problems of control groups, ascertainment bias, and confounding factors indicate that any increased risk of infection in a stable monogamous sexual situation may be limited to a few weeks after insertion.[55,98,166,177] Vaginal douching may be a risk factor for acute pelvic inflammatory disease.[149]

Mycoplasmas have been reported in both acute salpingitis and tuboovarian abscess, although some studies sugggest that *Mycoplasma hominis* is not an important cause of salpingitis or infertility. Laparoscopically obtained pretreatment cultures from grossly infected tubes occasionally reveal *M. hominis*. Tubes examined histologically have shown a moderate infiltration with chronic inflammatory cells, some neutrophils, and focal epithelial ulceration. *Ureaplasma urealyticum* also may be responsible for acute salpingitis.

Chlamydia trachomatis is cultured frequently from the cervix, uterus, and fallopian tubes in women with acute salpingitis.[91,110] The histologic appearance of tubes removed during the acute or subacute phase of chlamydial salpingitis is virtually identical to that caused by the gonococcus. There is an initial transmural and mucosal infiltration of polymorphonuclear leukocytes with an intraluminal exudate. Subsequently, there is a lymphoplasmacytic response with variable numbers of residual granulocytes.[175] Antibodies to chlamydia antigen stain round circumnuclear vacuoles containing granular particles in epithelial cells. On occasion, the lymphofollicular response may be so florid as to suggest lymphoma.[171] Long-term tubal damage may be inferred by the finding of distorted tubal folds, areas of mucosal deciliation, and infertility in women with circulating antichlamydial antibodies, which occurs whether or not there is a history of overt acute salpingitis.[25,128] Indeed, the frequency of tubal damage appears similar to that caused by the gonococcus. There is a close association with chronic endometritis, and therefore patients with a diagnosis of chronic endometritis should be evaluated carefully for asymptomatic salpingitis (see Chapter 10, Benign Diseases of the Endometrium).

Coxsackie viruses B5 and ECHO6 have been recovered from tubes with acute salpingitis, but no histologic data are available. Herpes simplex infection involved the mucosa of a prolapsed tube, causing cytologic atypia of the epithelium.[110]

An asymptomatic form of acute salpingitis is seen in tubes removed during postpartum ligation. Beginning about 5 hours after delivery and present up to 7–10 days later, a small or moderate number of acute or mixed acute and chronic inflammatory cells are found in the mucosa or lumen of 10% or more of specimens. Attempts to culture aerobic or anaerobic bacteria have been almost uniformly unsuccessful. The process may be regarded as secondary to the trauma of delivery or intrauterine tissue necrosis.

Chronic Salpingitis

When acute salpingitis resolves, residual disease may be found in the fallopian tube. With acute in-

a

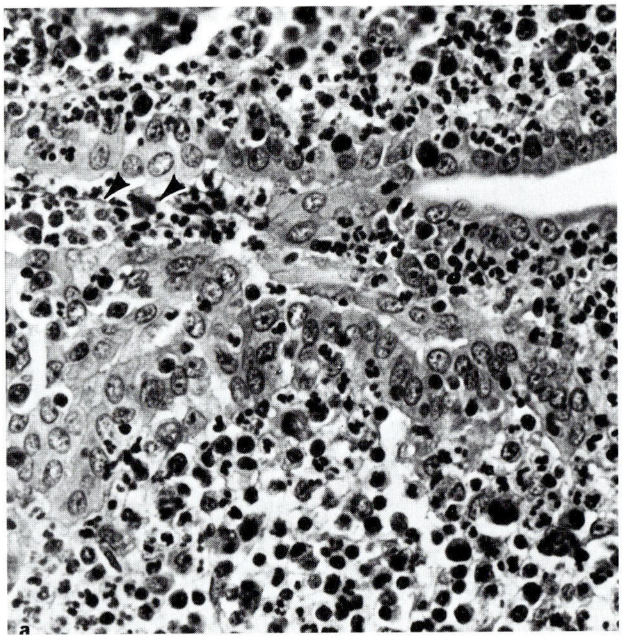

b

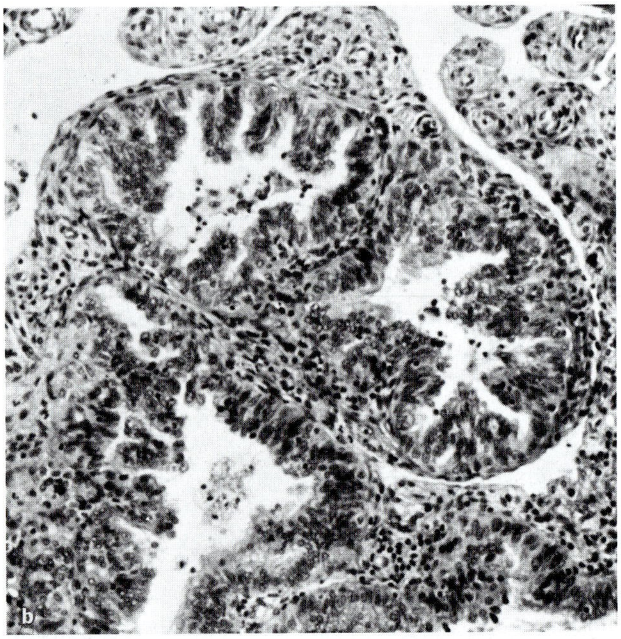

Fig. 14.8. a: **Acute and chronic salpingitis.** Plicae are distended with polymorphonuclear leukocytes, histiocytes, lymphocytes, and plasma cells. Fibrin strands lie in lumen at left (*arrowheads*). Note approximation of plicae and suggestion of early adhesion at center. **b**: **Chronic salpingitis.** Papillary tufts of reactive epithelial cells are prominent, but mitoses are absent. A few lymphocytes may be seen in the stroma; this should not be confused with carcinoma.

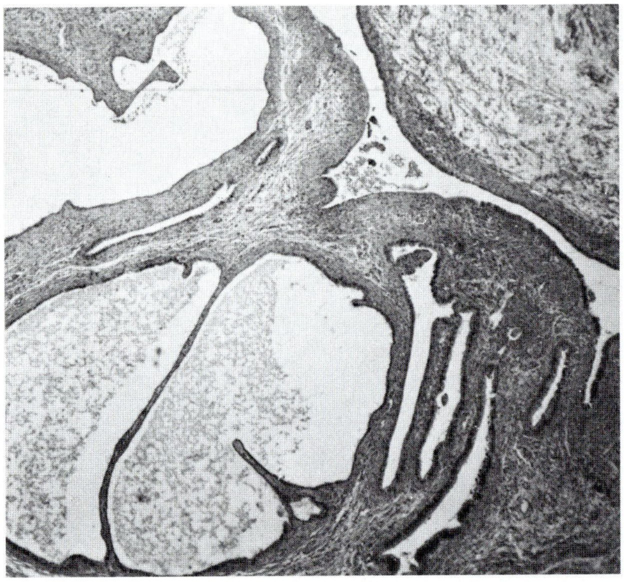

Fig. 14.9. Salpingitis follicularis. There is agglutination of plicae with formation of dilated glandlike spaces between them.

flammation, the mucosal plicae, secondary to surface fibrin deposition, adhere to one another (Fig. 14.8a,b). Healing and organization then lead to permanent bridging between folds. In the classic case, this results in follicular salpingitis (Fig. 14.9). In a primate model of chlamydial salpingitis, repeated episodes of inflammation are associated with accumulation of CD 8 T cells and tubal scarring.[168] In chronic salpingitis plicae may retain much of their size and shape, but plasma cells, lymphocytes, or both are still present in the mucosa. Often the height of the folds appears reduced, or their intricate pattern, so prominent in the ampulla and infundibulum, is subtly altered. The mucosa may become hyperplastic, forming cribriform pseudoglands which, accompanied by modest nuclear atypia with or without loss of polarity and invaginations of epithelium into the tubal muscularis, can simulate malignancy.[32] Fibrinous adhesions develop between the serosa and surrounding peritoneal surfaces that, unless routinely sought, are easily overlooked. Peritoneal inflammation may be widespread and thin, violin-string adhesions may form between liver and diaphragm. Agglutination of acutely inflamed fimbriae may be focal or massive. If it is severe enough, the bases of the fimbriae may coalesce in the center, with the fimbriae radiating outward like daisy petals, or the tips of the fimbriae may adhere, blocking the lumen and causing a blunted end, the so-called clubbed tube (Fig. 14.10).

The proximity of the ovary to the fimbriae allows multiple tuboovarian adhesions to form, with occlusion of the tubal ostium. The ovary itself may then become more directly involved, and a tuboovarian abscess may result (Fig. 14.11). If the fimbriae close before the ovary is seriously involved, the inflamed, dilated tube forms a pyosalpinx full of

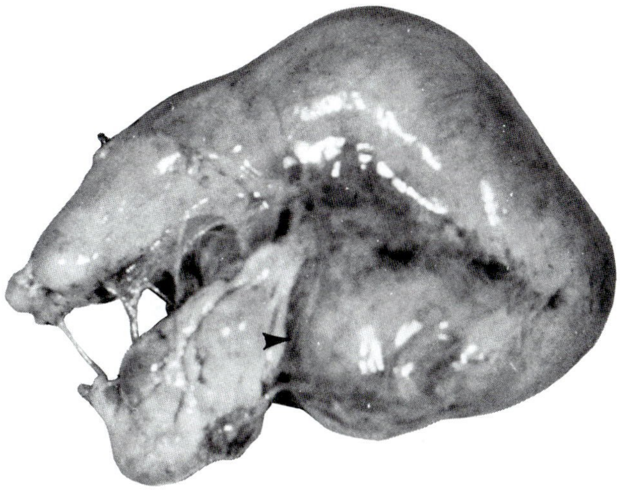

Fig. 14.10. Chronic salpingitis. Multiple, thin, fibrous adherences are present between tube and ovary and between ampulla and infundibulum. Distal portion of tube (*arrowhead*) has clubbed appearance because of obliteration of tubal ostium.

acute and chronic inflammatory cells. As the inflammation subsides, the acute and most of the chronic inflammatory cells gradually disappear, and the patient is left with either a severely scarred tube or a hydrosalpinx.

Both aerobic and anaerobic cultures of any tuboovarian abscess should be obtained in the operating room or laboratory. Prior treatment with antibiotics possibly may eliminate culturable organisms, but with careful technique, anaerobes are isolated in 63%–100% of cases. *E. coli*, *Bacteriodes fragilis*, *Bacterioides* species, *Peptostreptococcus*, *Peptococcus*, and aerobic streptococci are the most commonly found organisms; typically, infection is polymicrobial. *Pasteurella multocida* also has been isolated as a causative agent in a patient with a tuboovarian abscess.[144] Fungi, including *Blastomyces dermatitidis*, are cultured only rarely from tuboovarian abscesses and may be secondary to hematogenous spread. Tubal coccidioidomycosis also may be found secondary to disseminated disease. Malacoplakia only rarely involves the tube.

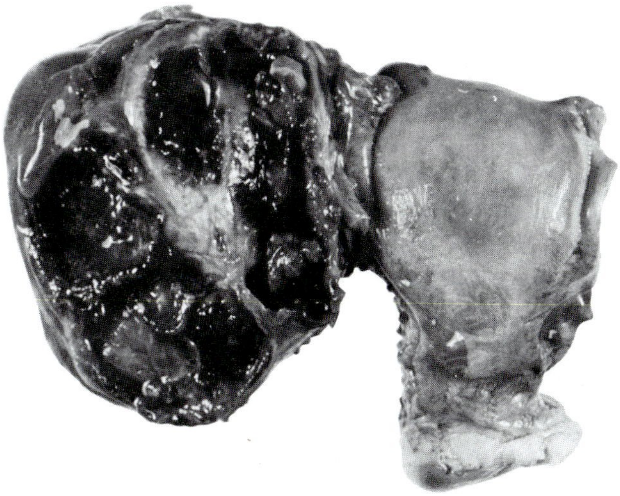

Fig. 14.11. Tuboovarian abscess. Posterior view shows bisected tuboovarian abscess involving entire left adnexa. Tube and ovary have been largely destroyed and replaced by a multiloculated mass containing foul-smelling pus.

Hydrosalpinx is one of the complications of salpingitis. It is characterized by obliteration of the fimbriated end and dilation of the tube, usually the ampullary and infundibular portions. If the ovary is first involved by tuboovarian adhesions, the ovary may be compressed by the dilated tube. The dilated tube may resemble the chemist's retort, and the wall is generally whitish, thin, and translucent, with occasional fibrous adhesions on its surface (Fig. 14.12). The tube usually contains clear serous fluid with an electrolyte composition similar to serum but

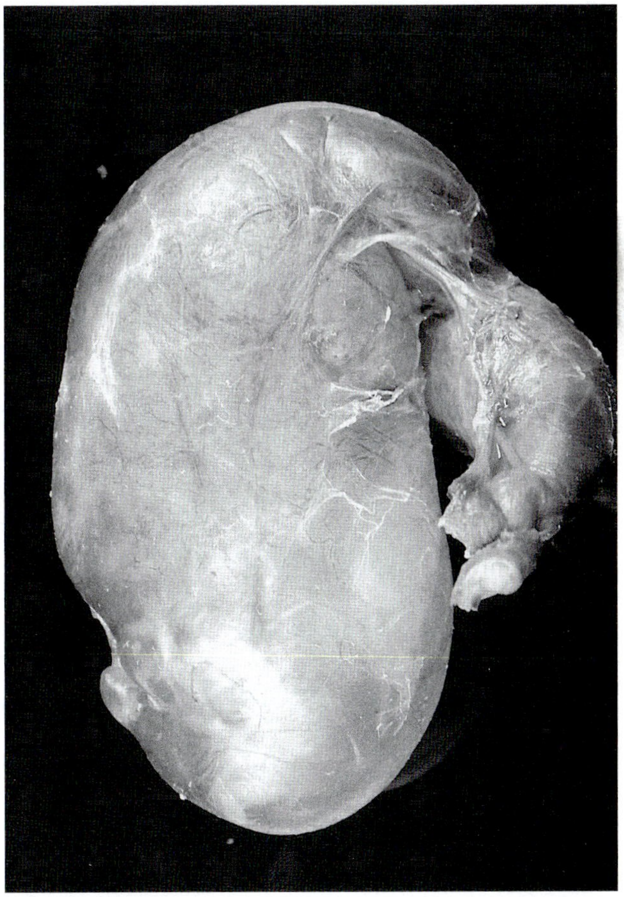

Fig. 14.12. Hydrosalpinx. The tube is markedly dilated in the ampullary portion. The fimbriae are obliterated; the wall is thickened but translucent.

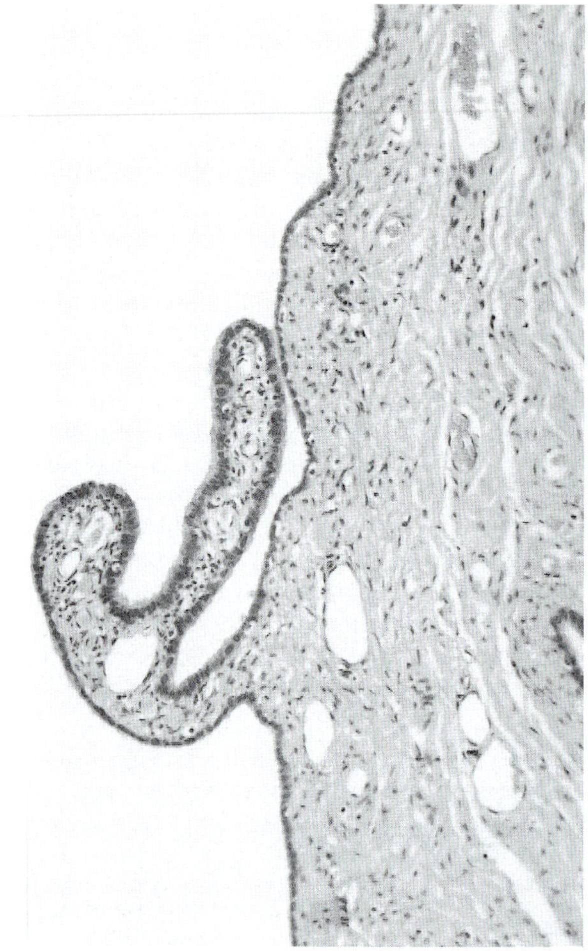

Fig. 14.13. Hydrosalpinx. Although most of the luminal epithelium is cuboidal or flattened, occasional plicae may remain with a normal epithelial surface.

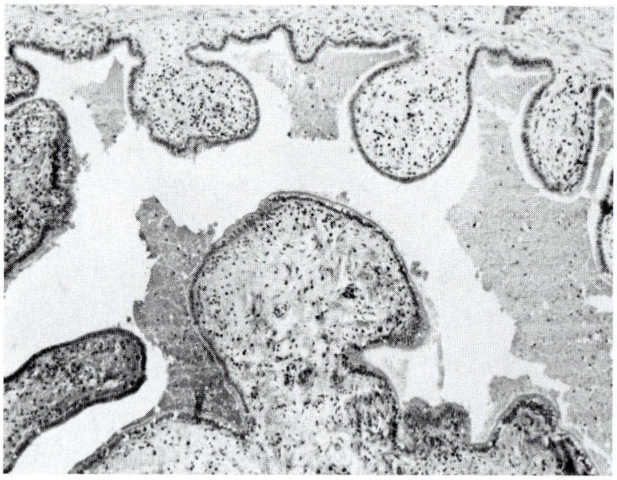

Fig. 14.14. Chronic salpingitis. Transitional stage between chronic salpingitis and hydrosalpinx. Marked blunting of plicae; only a scanty residual lymphocytic infiltrate is present.

with a low protein content.[41] Because a luminal communication usually can be demonstrated between dilated and nondilated portions of the tube, the etiology of the dilatation is obscure, but it may result in part from a sphincter-like action of isthmic muscularis. The muscle wall is either thin and atrophic or replaced by collagenous connective tissue. Most of the epithelial lining consists of low cuboidal cells, but an occasional plica may persist, with surprisingly intact columnar epithelium with histologically normal ciliated and secretory cells corresponding morphologically with the menstrual phase (Fig. 14.13). The persistence of healthy-appearing plicae is consistent with selective damage of the tubal folds, resulting in uneven scarring and plical disappearance (Fig. 14.14). The results of salpingoneostomy for infertility decrease with increasing degrees of mucosal damage.[169] A few lymphocytes may be found in the wall of the hydrosalpinx but are more commonly absent. Recovery of tubal function, even with expert surgery, is unlikely, and there is a possibility of tubal torsion with subsequent hemorrhagic infarction. The observation in 1991 that discharge of fluid from a hydrosalpinx might interfere with embryo implantation in assisted reproduction[106] has been confirmed by several additional studies of the relation between hydrosalpinx and in vitro fertilization success.[27,37] It appears that the hydrosalpinx may have to be large enough to be visible on ultrasound to affect pregnancy rates,[45] and it must be emphasized that fimbrial closure (clubbed tube) alone does not constitute a hydrosalpinx.[18] Because tubes are now being removed before attempted in vitro fertilization,[159] it is clear that the pathologist examining them must document the degree of dilatation and comment on mucosal abnormalities as well as peritubal adhesions.

Granulomatous Salpingitis

Granulomatous inflammation of the fallopian tube may result from infection by a number of different organisms or be induced by a variety of noninfectious processes. The histologic identification of one or more granulomas calls for immediate communication between pathologist and clinician to determine the likely etiology.

Tuberculous Salpingitis

Mycobacterium tuberculosis historically has been the predominant etiologic agent of granulomatous salpingitis. The frequency of *tuberculous salpingitis* in women studied for tubal causes of infertility ranges from much less than 1% in the United States to nearly 40% in India[127]; 10%–20% of women who die of tuberculosis have tubal involvement.[147] Primary infection of the genitalia, as by coitus with a partner with genitourinary tuberculosis, is extremely rare. Secondary spread, usually from a primary pulmonary infection, is the usual route of infection. For reasons still unknown, the blood-borne organism preferentially lodges in the tubes rather than the other parts of the female genital tract. The primary pulmonary lesion may not be radiologically evident, but extrapulmonary involvement of the peritoneum, kidneys, or other sites may be present. Lymphatic spread from primary intestinal tuberculosis or direct spread from bladder or gastrointestinal tract may occur. Although the earliest pathologic lesions are microscopic, with advancing disease the tube increases in diameter and may become nodular, mimicking salpingitis isthmica nodosa. In the more common adhesive form of the disease, multiple dense adhesions may form between the tube and ovary, and the fimbriae and ostium may be obliterated.[66] Frequently, the ostium remains patent and some investigators, in fact, regard the presence of an identifiable ostium and fimbriae in a grossly diseased tube as characteristic of tuberculous salpingitis.[147] With the exudative form of disease, progressive distension mimics bacterial pyosalpinx. Hematosalpinx, hydrosalpinx, tuboovarian masses, or a frozen pelvis may be found late in the disease process.[127] In either form, serosal tubercles may be present.

The earliest microscopic lesions are mucosal, with a typical granulomatous reaction of epithelioid cells and lymphocytes arranged in a nodular configuration. Giant cells often are seen, and central caseation, focal or massive, may be present. Immunosuppressive therapy may modify cellular immunity to a point where granulomas fail to form, and with this clinical information, the mere finding of acute and chronic inflammatory cells should lead to consideration of staining for acid-fast organisms. From the mucosa, extension to the muscularis and serosa may occur. As the tubercles enlarge, they may erode through the mucosa and discharge their contents into the tubal lumen (Fig. 14.15). The mucosal inflammatory reaction leads to progressive scarring, with plical distortion and conglutination. Large caseous nodules may form and coalesce, eventually filling the dilated tube. Calcification may occur in areas of fibrosis. Because tubercles may not be present in a given section, the presence of caseation, fibrosis, or calcification in a tube may be the only histologic finding pointing to the necessity for more thorough study. The presence of severe mucosal atypicality in tuberculous salpingitis and confusion with adenocarcinoma have been stressed by numerous authors, but similar atypia may be found in any chronic salpingitis[32] (see Fig. 14.8b).

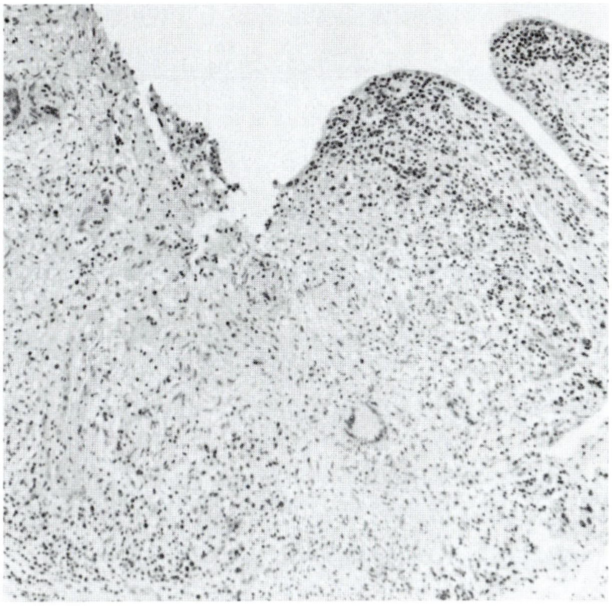

Fig. 14.15. Tuberculous salpingitis. Confluent focally necrotizing granulomas occupy most of the endosalpinx except on the *far right.* There is focal ulceration of the epithelial surface, illustrating a possible mechanism whereby *Mycobacterium tuberculosis* could reach the tubal lumen and seed the endometrial cavity.

Complications of tuberculous salpingitis are several. Alteration in function is the rule. Sterility is almost universal because of the common bilaterality of the disease. Rarely, successful pregnancies occur, but ectopic tubal nidation is likely in the event that fertilization is successful.[147] Pelvic pain, sterility, and menstrual irregularities are the most common complaints. Because of repeated seeding of the endometrium from the infected tubes, mycobacterial culture and the histologic finding of endometrial granulomas on curettage are diagnostically useful (see Chapter 10, Benign Diseases of the Endometrium). Laparoscopy may cause bowel perforation in cases of extensive pelvic and peritoneal tuberculosis.

Actinomycosis

Actinomycotic infections of the tube may occur, many of them associated with intrauterine contraceptive devices (IUDs) (see Chapter 10, Benign Diseases of the Endometrium).[47] There is good evidence that actinomycetes, probably of gastrointestinal origin, are intermittently a part of the indigenous female genital tract flora.[133] Grossly, a large fibrous mass is present that often includes the ovary. The mass may appear to be a dilated tube or may be more obviously inflammatory, being bound down to pelvic structures with adhesions or fistula formation. Pus is present in the shaggy-walled cavities within the tube. Anaerobic culture is necessary to permit growth of *Actinomyces israelii*. Microscopically, numerous histiocytes, plasma cells, and lymphocytes are present in the abscess wall, and gram-positive, filamentous clumps, and sulfur granules may be recognized in the pus. Complications in unrecognized cases include dissemination to the liver and lung.

Parasitic Salpingitis

Pinworm

The pinworm, *Enterobius vermicularis*, may migrate up the female genital tract, embed in the tube, and cause an inflammatory reaction. The tube may be involved with the ovary in what appears to be a tuboovarian abscess, or a fibrous nodular area may be present. Acute and chronic inflammatory cells may be found together with eosinophils, Charcot–Leyden crystals, and portions of gravid female worm. Ova may be released into the tissue, where they provoke a granulomatous reaction. The ova may be identified by their size (about 20×50 μm) and ovoid asymmetric shape, but they may be obscured by calcification of granulomas. The ova may be widely disseminated in the peritoneum in the absence of histologic tubal involvement, and the fibrous granulomas may simulate metastatic carcinoma.

Schistosomiasis

Although tubal bilharziasis probably is one of the most common causes of granulomatous salpingitis worldwide, it is rare in the United States. In Africa, reported tubal infections occur in as many as 20% of unselected women at autopsy. The ova of *Schistosoma haematobium* are most common, but *Schistosoma mansoni* eggs may be present in some women. If granulomas are present and there is a suspicion of schistosomiasis, sodium hydroxide digestion of the remaining tubal tissue may reveal ova. Gross findings appear to be related to fibrosis surrounding the ova, producing a nodular or fibrotic tube. Ectopic pregnancy in an infected tube may precipitate its removal, but the granulomas themselves may not always cause sufficient damage to account for abnormal nidation.

Other Parasites

Where the condition is common, hydatid disease secondary to *Echinococcus granulosus* infection may involve the female genital tract, including the adnexae. Cysticercosis also has been described in the tube.[2]

Sarcoid

Sarcoidosis of the tube is rarely reported[19] and appears to accompany disseminated disease. Histologically, noncaseating granulomas may be seen in the mucosa. Culture, special stains, and clinical information are necessary to exclude other granulomatous diseases.

Crohn's Disease

Crohn's disease of the ileum, colon, or appendix may secondarily involve the tube and ovary to produce a granulomatous salpingo-oophoritis. Noncaseating granulomas may involve the entire thickness of the tubal muscularis as well as the mucosa. The epithelium may react with severe cellular atypia (Fig. 14.16). Fistulas from bowel to tube also may occur.

Pseudoxanthomatous Salpingitis (Pigmentosis Tubae)

Rare cases are reported in patients with pelvic endometriosis[57,71,153] in whom the tubes may be grossly swollen and clubbed or edematous with dra-

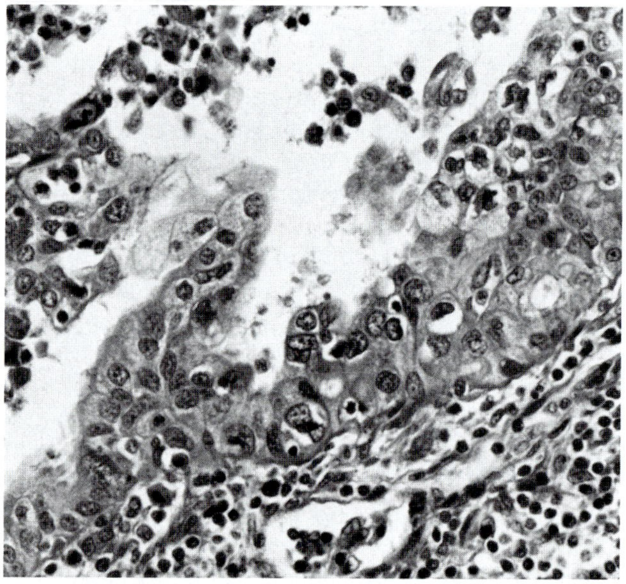

Fig. 14.16. Granulomatous salpingitis secondary to Crohn's disease. Underlying granulomas are not visible here, but severe chronic inflammation is present (*lower right*). Epithelium is piled up and has marked nuclear atypia. This change should not be confused with carcinoma in situ.

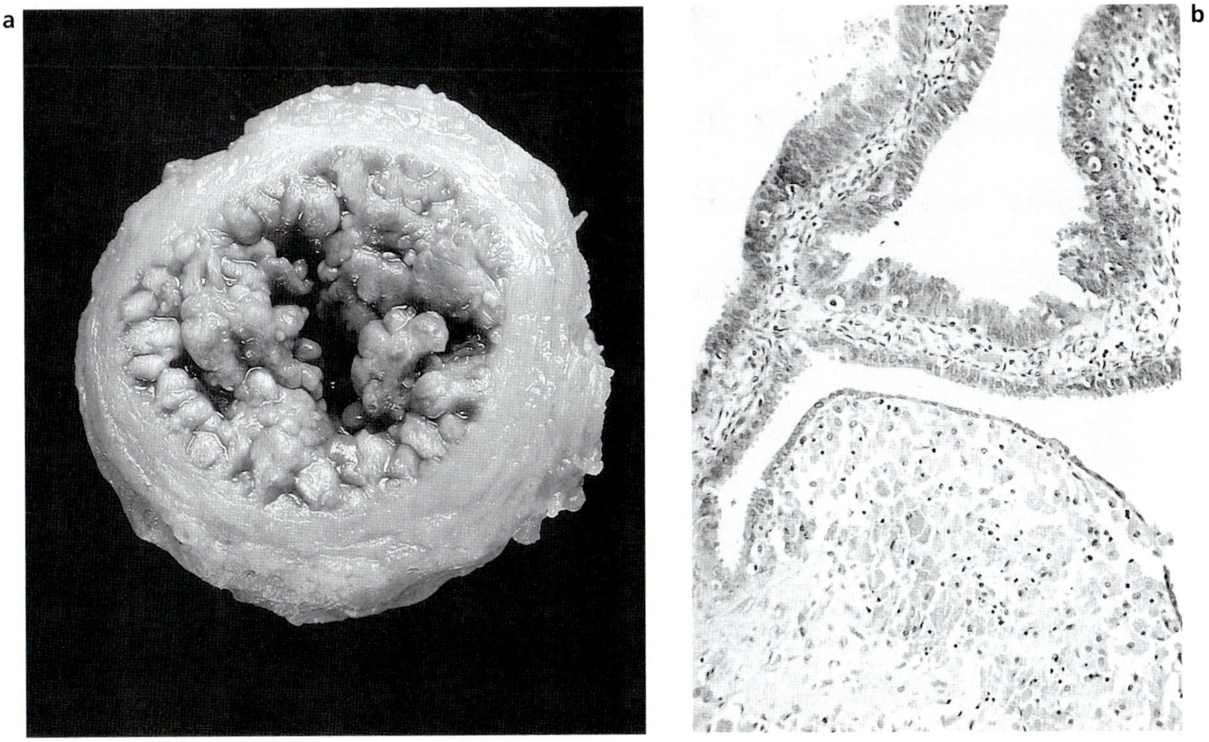

Fig. 14.17. Xanthogranulomatous salpingitis (pigmentosis tubae). a: The tubal cross section reveals golden-brown to chocolate-brown discoloration of the swollen plicae. b: The endosalpingeal fold (*bottom*) is swollen with foamy macrophages containing iron pigment.

matically dark brown polypoid mucosal surfaces (Fig 14.17a). The plicae are distended with lipofusion-laden and foamy macrophages with some hemosiderin (Fig 14.17b).[120] A mixed chronic inflammatory infiltrate with or without giant cells also may be seen. Despite the association with endometriosis this process also might result from salpingitis with associated bleeding.[35,153]

Foreign Body

Foreign material may be introduced into the tube in the course of gynecologic investigation, especially hysterosalpingography. Lubricant jelly, mineral oil, and starch and talc powder may cause a lipoid or granulomatous salpingitis. An intense phagocytic reaction to introduced lipid material causes accumulation of subepithelial foamy histiocytes. If the patient has received a blood substitute containing polyvinylpyrrolidone (PVP), this foreign material may be ingested by macrophages and deposited in many organs, including the tube. These histiocytes simulate signet-ring cell carcinoma, with mucicarmine-positive vacuolated cytoplasm. An appropriate history and a negative PAS stain should clarify the benign nature of the lesion. Talc may cause mucosal or serosal granulomas. Examination of all granulomas or foreign body reactions under polarized light is useful in the recognition of these processes. Other disease processes in the tube, such as leprosy or amyloidosis, are so infrequent that they are of little clinical or pathologic significance.

Giant cell arteritis involving the tube has been reported in postmenopausal women and may be part of a generalized process or an incidental finding.[15]

Salpingitis Isthmica Nodosa

Salpingitis isthmica nodosa (*SIN*) consists of one or more outpouchings or diverticula of tubal epithelium in the isthmic region. Involvement is often bilateral, and usually is accompanied by nodular hyperplasia of the surrounding muscularis.

The etiology is unknown. The disease is found in women between the ages of 25 and 60 years (average age at diagnosis is 30 years). Because the lesion is almost unknown before puberty, is not found congenitally, and may be progressive,[112] attention has focused on possible causes, especially postinflammatory distortion and an adenomyosis-like process. In some locales most, if not all, cases of SIN are associated with chronic salpingitis.[93] Evidence for a noninflammatory adenomyosis-like origin, at least in this country, is more convincing. The usual localization of nodularity is in the isthmic portion of the tube or immediately adjacent ampulla, unlike the usual picture in inflammatory salpingitis, where the ampulla is diffusely involved. When salpingitis isthmica nodosa is associated with inflammatory salpingitis, such as pyosalpinx and hydrosalpinx, the inflammatory process is contralateral nearly as often as it is ipsilateral. Although a few lymphocytes are found in the peridiverticular stroma, scarring usually is absent. Moderate or large numbers of endometrial-like stromal cells accompany the diverticula in more than half the patients. As in uterine adenomyosis, the presence of glands appears to stimulate muscular growth, with subsequent mural thickening. Unilateral tubal involvement often is accompanied by uterine adenomyosis on the same side.

The external gross appearance is of one or more nodular swellings in the isthmus to 1–2 cm in diameter. The serosa is smooth. On section, the tissue is firm, and careful inspection may disclose some of the dilated diverticula. Microscopically, the diverticula appear on cross section as dispersed glands of tubal epithelium surrounded by broad bands of muscularis (Fig. 14.18). Diverticula may closely approach the serosal surface but do not normally connect with it. Endometrial-like stromal cells lying beneath the epithelial outpouchings may be abundant, sparse, or absent. If both glands and stroma are present, a diagnosis of tubal endometriosis may be considered. Because the underlying configuration is diverticular rather than glandular and the condition is not clearly related to pelvic endometriosis, it seems best to continue using the term salpingitis isthmica nodosa until the etiology is better understood.

The most serious clinical and pathologic complications of salpingitis isthmica nodosa are infertility and the strong association with ectopic pregnancy.[64,132] Inflammatory tubal disease may be associated with it ipsilaterally or contralaterally. A rare complication that we have seen is rupture of a deep diverticulum through the serosa, with subsequent mild intraabdominal bleeding and pelvic pain.

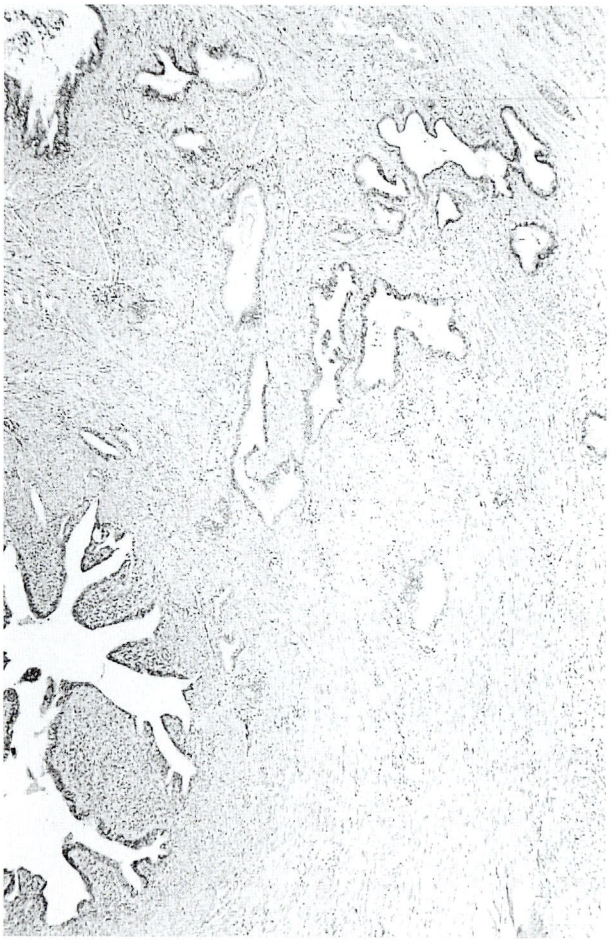

Fig. 14.18. Salpingitis isthmica nodosa. Tubal lumen is partially visible at *lower left.* Cross-sectioned diverticula in the thickened wall are widely separated by broad bands of smooth muscle.

Ectopic Pregnancy

An *ectopic pregnancy* occurs when the developing blastocyst implants at a site other than in the endometrium of the fundus or lower uterine segment. Because more than 95% of ectopic pregnancies occur in the fallopian tube, the terms ectopic pregnancy and tubal pregnancy are nearly synonymous. However, implantation on both tubal fimbriae and ovary, in the abdominal cavity, in the uterine interstitium (intramural pregnancy) or cornu, in the cervix,[21] or in the retroperitoneum also may occur, in descending order of frequency. Hepatic, diaphragmatic, and splenic pregnancy are all extremely rare.[43] Within the tube, most ectopic pregnancies are found in the ampulla (75%–80%), with about 10%–15% isthmic and 5% at the fimbriae.[21]

Right-sided ectopic pregnancies comprise 52%–57% of all tubal pregnancies.[21,22] Epidemiologic studies note an incidence of ectopic pregnancy increasing from about 1% to 2% during the past 25 years.[103] Ectopic pregnancies may be bilateral; in one series the frequency was approximately 1 in 500.

Simultaneous ectopic and intrauterine implantations, so-called heterotopic or combined pregnancy, used to occur in 1 in 10,000 to 30,000 pregnancies, but with in vitro fertilization programs, the incidence approaches 1%, no doubt related to an increased incidence of tubal disease.[109]

Etiology

The mechanisms responsible for ectopic pregnancy are largely unknown, although any disease process that alters the normal tubal anatomy seems to increase the frequency. Although delay in entering the uterine cavity may predispose the blastocyst to tubal nidation, experimentally delayed conceptuses in rabbit, guinea pig, and mouse oviducts degenerate and fail to implant. However, ectopic pregnancy is reported uncommonly in nonhuman primates. A history of previous pelvic inflammatory disease is the single most common antecedent factor in 35%–45% of patients,[22] and the risk of ectopic pregnancy increases sevenfold after acute salpingitis. A decline in chlamydial infection rates in one community was followed promptly by a decline in the rate of ectopic pregnancy.[52] As many as 88% of carefully studied tubes with an ectopic pregnancy also will show chronic salpingitis.[64]

Salpingitis isthmica nodosa,[132] previous pelvic surgery,[22] genital tuberculosis, a history of prenatal DES exposure, and vaginal douching also appear as ectopic risk factors. Although IUDs have been identified in some studies as an independent risk factor for tubal or ovarian ectopic pregnancy,[108,125,140] in general it appears that ectopic rates are lower than in the general population, possibly because of the selected population using the device.[166,177] The proportion of pregnancies that are ectopic in IUD users is quite high because of the efficacy of prevention of intrauterine pregnancy. Electively induced abortion does not appear to increase the frequency of ectopic pregnancy[154] unless there is postabortal infection. Tubal ectopic pregnancy after tubal sterilization may occur subsequent to tuboperitoneal fistula formation,[157] and repeat ectopic pregnancy on the same or opposite side is common (9%) after one ectopic pregnancy. The increasing use of linear salpingostomy for the removal of an unruptured ectopic pregnancy, especially when only one tube is patent, poses the highest known risk for a repeat ectopic pregnancy (20%) but is tolerated because of the 50%–60% chance for intrauterine pregnancy. Ectopic pregnancy after hysterectomy is rare. Abnormalities in the embryo may possibly lead to an increased tendency toward tubal implantation.[26]

Clinical Features

Although many women with an ectopic pregnancy still present with tubal rupture and hemorrhagic shock, because of the increasing frequency, clinicians consider any complaint of pelvic pain with or without menstrual irregularity as possible indication of an ectopic pregnancy. Quantitative, sensitive serum human chorionic gonadotropin (hCG) assays and ultrasonography to identify a gestational sac are subsequently performed.[103] Early diagnosis and operation result either in salpingostomy with conceptus removal or salpingectomy for an unruptured ectopic pregnancy. Trophoblastic tissue and villi may persist after salpingostomy and conceptus removal[104] and may implant elsewhere, forming nodules on pelvic and omental surfaces.[49] Tissue remaining may retain its viability and form an ectopic-like tubal mass with a persistent hCG titer, requiring reoperation, or may become implanted on pelvic or uterine serosal surfaces.[29] Single-dose methotrexate treatment for early ectopic pregnancy has superceded surgery in many cases, but patients require careful follow-up to detect the 10% who fail treatment, or instances of late rupture.[59,102,103]

Pathologic Findings

The unruptured tubal pregnancy is characterized grossly by a somewhat irregular sausage-like dilatation of the tube, with a bluish discoloration caused by hematosalpinx (Fig. 14.19). Chorionic villi usually are found in the blood-filled and dilated tubal lumen and, in 75% of cases, appear viable. Nearly two-thirds of cases contain a grossly or microscopically identifiable embryo, and multiple pregnancies may occur. Implantation is deeper and more apt to be associated with a viable pregnancy when the placentation occurs on the mesosalpingeal side of the tube, as compared with the antimesosalpingeal side.[84] The extravillous intermediate trophoblast of the conceptus penetrates deep in the tubal wall and into tubal blood vessels. Perhaps because of the limited ability of the endosalpingeal stroma to undergo decidualization, and analogous to a placenta increta, the chorionic villi then invade first muscularis and then serosa.[130] Another major difference with uterine implantation is the failure of tubal trophoblast to differentiate into chorion frondosum and chorion laeve.[139] Vascular changes in midsized tubal arteries adjacent to ectopic pregnancies are similar to those found in the vessels near uterine implantations, with invasion by intermediate trophoblast, proliferation of the vascular intima, and accumulation of foam cells in the intima. Chronic salpingitis is found adjacent to the ectopic pregnancy in nearly half the patients, with a reported range of 29%–88%.[64] Ultrastructural studies may demonstrate decreased or absent areas of ciliation in the mucosa adjacent to the ectopic pregnancy. The tubal wall should be examined micro-

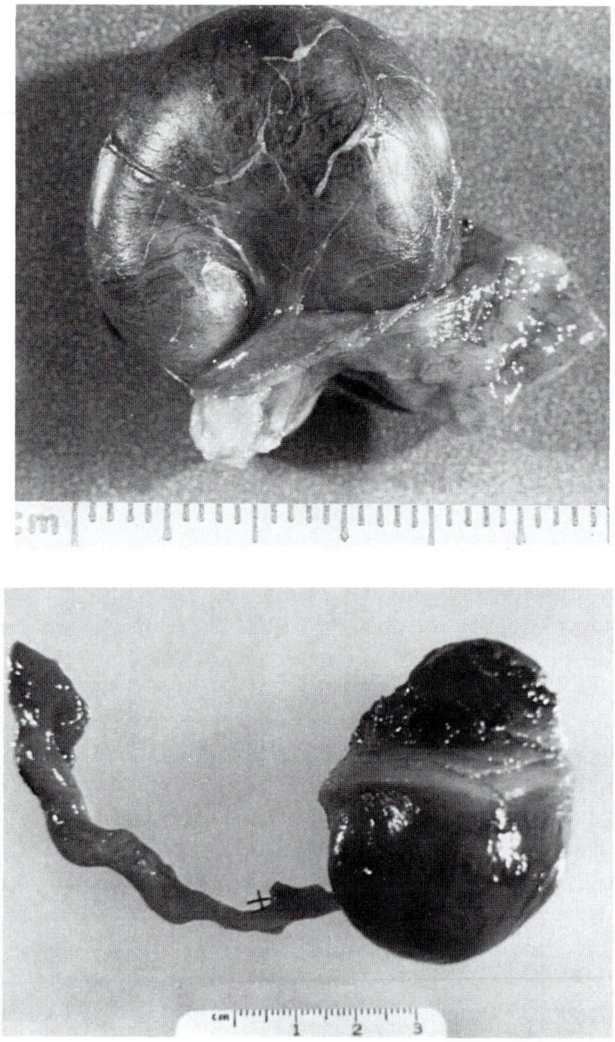

Fig. 14.19. Unruptured ectopic pregnancy. *Top*: Tubal pregnancy. A resected, kinked portion of tube is expanded by the growing pregnancy. Intraluminal blood imparts a bluish discoloration. The thin fibrous peritubal adhesions suggest previous salpingitis. *Bottom*: Cornual pregnancy. The attached tube is normal, but the resected uterine cornu is expanded by the hemorrhagic mass of a nonviable ectopic pregnancy.

scopically for the diverticula of salpingitis isthmica nodosa.

The pathology of extratubal ectopic pregnancy varies according to the site. Cornual or interstitial pregnancies may expand up to about 12 weeks, when rupture may lacerate one of the uterine arteries as well as the entire side of the uterus. Cervical ectopic pregnancy presents much as an incomplete abortion with bleeding. Because of the fibrous cervical tissue underlying placental implantation, control of bleeding may be difficult. Ovarian pregnancy is clinically similar to tubal pregnancy, including frequent preoperative rupture. More than half the patients in one series had a history of previous reproductive tract disease or infertility,[65] and 17%–25% had an IUD in place.[130] Macroscopic examination typically reveals a hemorrhagic mass replacing the ovary. The pathologic criteria for ovarian pregnancy proposed by Spiegelberg[155] are (1) the tube must be intact and separate from the ovary, (2) the gestational sac must occupy the normal position of the ovary, (3) the gestational sac must be connected to the uterus by the uteroovarian ligament, and (4) ovarian tissue must be demonstrated within the wall of the sac. Pathologic documentation of ovarian tissue within the pregnancy may be difficult or impossible if treatment consists of conservative resection or if the pregnancy has extensively replaced the ovarian tissue.

The epithelial changes described by Arias–Stella (see Chapter 9, Anatomy and Histology of the Uterine Corpus) may be found in the endometrial glands of at least 60% of women with ectopic pregnancy. In addition, similar changes of nuclear atypia and cytoplasmic clearing occasionally may be found in carefully studied tubes[116] (Fig. 14.20). In one case, there was clear cell hyperplasia.[167]

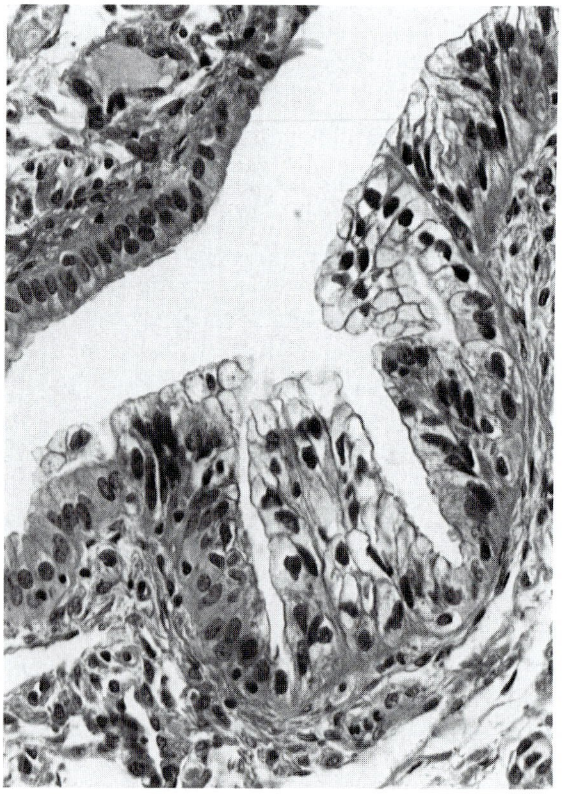

Fig. 14.20. Arias–Stella reaction in tubal epithelium. Note the focally clear epithelial cell cytoplasm, with nuclear enlargement and hyperchromatism.

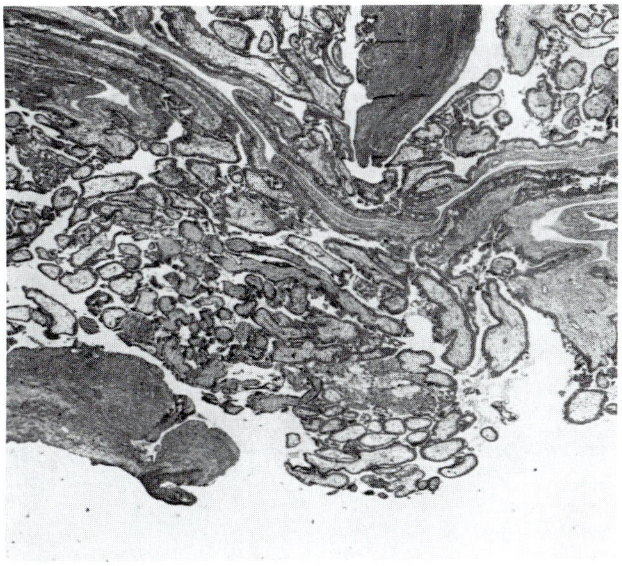

Fig. 14.21. Ruptured tubal pregnancy. After penetration of the tubal musculature by the trophoblastic cells of the ectopic pregnancy, the muscle wall (*top center* and *bottom left*) weakens and ruptures, with extrusion of chorionic villi.

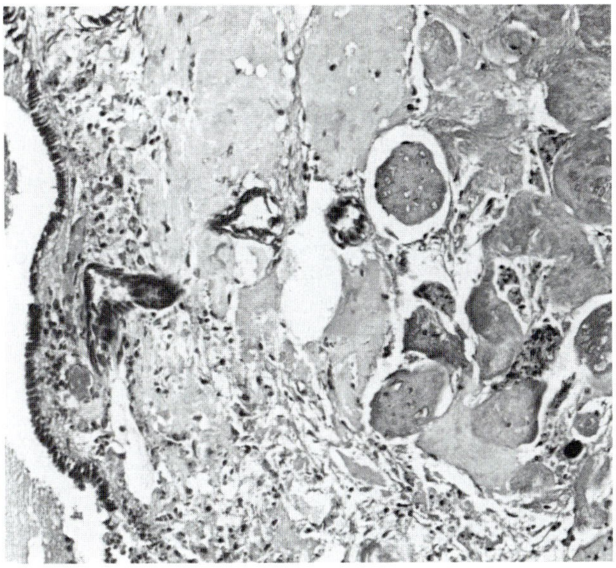

Fig. 14.23. Chronic ectopic pregnancy. Proteinaceous fluid is present in the distorted tubal lumen on the left. Fibrotic chorionic villi replacing the normal tubal architecture are present on the *right*.

Sequelae

The natural history of tubal ectopic pregnancy includes spontaneous expulsion from the fimbriated end—tubal abortion—as well as embryonal death and involution of the conceptus. Typically, however, continued growth of the trophoblast leads to increasing dilatation and weakening of the muscularis, with rupture about the eighth week (Fig. 14.21). About 25% of tubal pregnancies have ruptured by the time of diagnosis, but attempts to predict which ectopic will rupture have not proven fruitful.[54] Because hemorrhage may be massive, it is a major cause of maternal mortality. A few tubal pregnancies have proceeded to term with fetal viability. Peritoneal irritation and formation of dense intestinal adhesions is likely to occur in these patients.

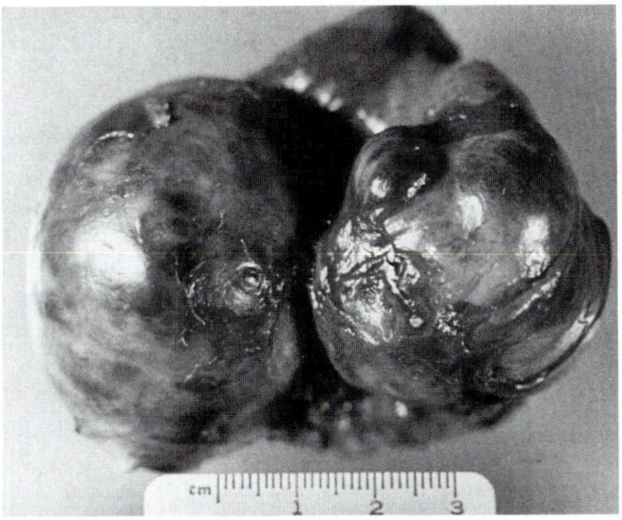

Fig. 14.22. Chronic ectopic pregnancy. This irregularly lobulated mass grossly simulated an ovarian neoplasm.

Some tubal pregnancies form a chronic inflammatory mass that, with involution of trophoblast and reestablishment of the menstrual cycle, may present problems in differential diagnosis. The convoluted, blood-filled tube, often with involved ipsilateral ovary, may simulate tumor[75] or an endometriotic mass (Fig. 14.22). Extensive microscopic sampling of a so-called chronic ectopic pregnancy may be required to demonstrate a few ghost villi (Fig. 14.23). In more advanced pregnancy, death of the fetus with retention in the extrauterine location may be followed by calcification of the fetus (lithopedion) or both membranes and fetus (lithokelyphopedion). The mass formed may be discovered only incidentally decades later.[79]

Infertility

Most of the diseases discussed in this chapter may result in sufficient anatomic distortion to cause tubal infertility. In contrast, purely physiologic tubal dysfunction is not well defined but may be illustrated by the immotile cilia of Kartagener's syndrome that may lead to reduced fertility: only 3 of 12 women in one series succeeded in becoming pregnant.[3] Peritubal adhesions secondary to endometriosis, prior pelvic inflammatory disease, or appendicitis may interfere with normal tubal motility and ovum pickup. Adhesion lysis may be curative. Multiple fimbrial adhesions secondary to gonococcal or other inflammatory tubal disease may be treated by operative lysis and surgical eversion of tubal mucosa. Obliterative fibrosis, possibly secondary to inflammation within the uterus, or polyp formation at the uterine tubal ostium may lead to obstruction at the uterotubal junction.[56,97] Resection of the obstruction and microsurgical anastomosis or tubal reimplantation may result in patency rates of about 80%–85% and term pregnancy rates of 50% to nearly 80%. Although tubal surgery for infertility has been criticized for lack of convincing evidence of effectiveness, untreated complete bilateral tubal obstruction offers no expectation of spontaneous cure, and surgery offers some hope of pregnancy. Typically, tubal patency rates are approximately double the rates for intrauterine pregnancy, and ectopic pregnancy is an ever-present risk.

Tubal patency is commonly assessed by hysterosalpingography, using radiopaque dye or intrauterine dye injection with tubal monitoring via laparoscopy (chromopertubation). Cannulation of the tube with a falloposcope of minute diameter and a 0.3-mm lens affords an opportunity to visually assess patency, luminal adhesions, and the state of the epithelial surface.[85]

Contraception by interference with tubal function involves procedures designed to damage the tube by caustic chemicals, electrocautery, or surgical removal of a segment of the tube, or to obstruct it by placement of a clip. Intrauterine placement of quinacrine hydrochloride pellets for sterilization leads to necrosis of intramural endosalpingeal mucosa. The associated inflammation and progressive submucosal fibrosis leads to luminal narrowing or obliteration with a dose-dependant success rate.[53,115,119] Tubal resection should be confirmed by histologic demonstration of a cross section of tube including the entire tubal lumen. Despite these procedures, spontaneous reanastomosis or fistula formation (Fig. 14.24) may occur in approximately 1% of all patients and may lead to fertilization and ectopic or intrauterine pregnancy. Failure rates may be higher in training programs in which clips and rings are more apt to be misapplied.[158] Ectopic pregnancy rates after bipolar electrocoagulation are higher than with other sterilization methods unless multiple sites are coagulated, and may occur 5 or 10 years after the procedure.[134,135] To identify the cause of failure of tubal sterilization procedures, careful gross examination of the specimen, occasionally specimen salpingography, longitudinal orientation of the tubal segment in paraffin, and meticulous sectioning techniques may be necessary. Fistula formation at suture and excision sites appears to be the most common cause of failure after segmental resection. Up to 70% of pregnancies after electrocoagulation are ectopic. There are a number of other rare complications of tubal sterilization,[33] which do not appear to include menstrual abnormalities.[133a]

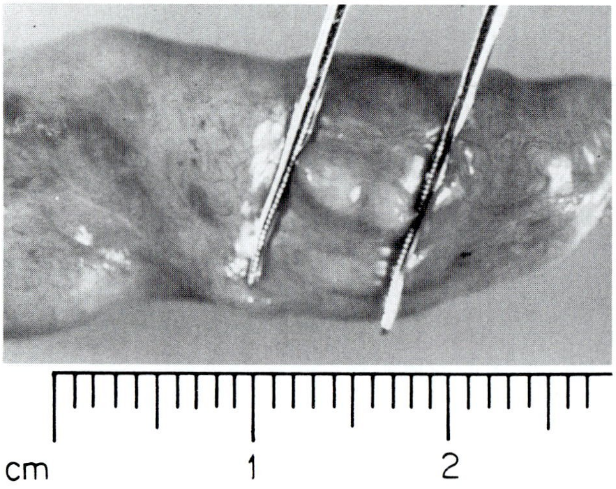

Fig. 14.24. Postligation tubal fistula. This proximal tubal segment was removed simultaneously with an ectopic pregnancy on the opposite side. Slight pressure on the forceps has caused the endosalpingeal mucosa to pout out through a 2- to 3-mm fistulous opening, with the lumen represented by a small dimple in the center.

The success of surgical reanastomosis in reestablishing a patent lumen varies with the extent of the initial procedure and the skill of the surgeon but is reported to be as high as 80%. Only 25%–40% of the patients, however, will subsequently become pregnant, and even with careful classification of the degree of tubal disease it is difficult to predict which patient will achieve term pregnancy.[107] The frequency of ectopic pregnancy after reanastomosis is increased; this may be caused by residual fibrosis after the original ligation or endosalpingeal distortion, which may mimic salpingitis isthmica nodosa. Scanning electron microscopic examination of tubal epithelium within 0.5 cm of the area of ligation shows loss of cilia.[100]

The American Fertility Society has proposed schemes for the classification of adhesions, tubal occlusions, tubal pregnancies, and müllerian anomalies.[8] The use of standardized nomenclature should make it easier to judge the efficacy of different treatment modalities.

Benign Neoplasms

Both benign and malignant tumors of the fallopian tube are uncommon. They are frequently mistaken for lesions of chronic salpingitis or pyosalpinx, both preoperatively and during the operative procedure itself. *Benign tumors* are most often of mesodermal origin and usually are small enough to be incidental findings at laparotomy.

Inclusion Cysts and Walthard Nests

The tubal serosa, by invagination, may give rise to a number of benign *inclusion cysts*. The simplest is a 1- to 2-mm unilocular cyst lying directly beneath the serosal surface lined by one or more layers of mesothelial cells, a mesothelial inclusion cyst. By a process of metaplasia, these cysts may become filled with polygonal epithelial-like cells to form a *Walthard nest*. On gross examination, a 1- to 2-mm yellowish-white nodule lies beneath the serosa. The cells of the Walthard nest often fully occupy it. Their nuclei are irregularly ovoid, and a longitudinal nuclear groove gives them a coffee-bean appearance (Fig. 14.25). Both mesothelial inclusion cysts and Walthard nests are common incidental findings of no clinical importance.

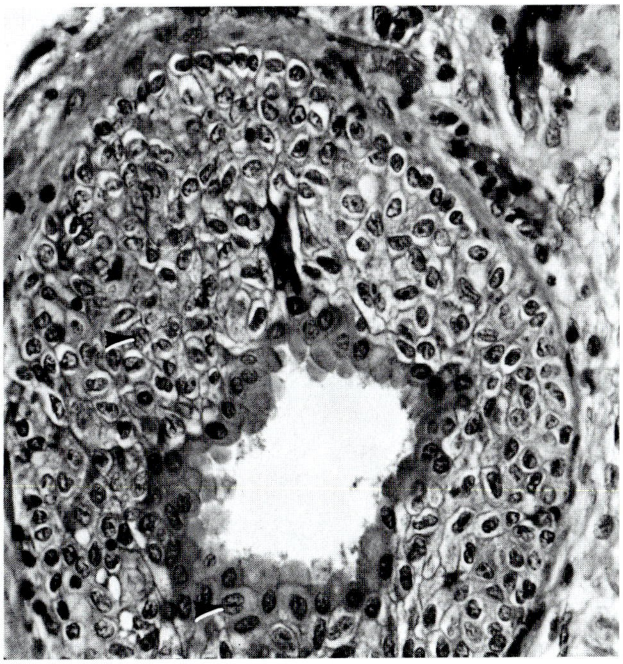

Fig. 14.25. Walthard nest. The most central epithelial cells have undergone columnar metaplasia. Nuclear grooves are visible (*arrowheads*) in other epithelial cells as dark lines in the long axis of ovoid nuclei. Note the serosal surface at *upper left*.

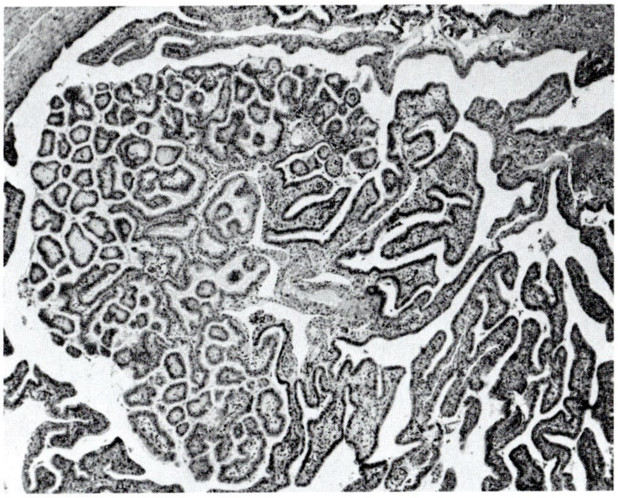

Fig. 14.26. Epithelial papilloma. Single layer of uniform cells lines a delicately branched papillary core.

Epithelial Papilloma

Epithelial papillomas or polyps are rare.[62,82] They are composed of a delicate, branching stromal stalk lined by a single layer of nonciliated columnar or oncocytic cells with regular nuclei (Fig. 14.26). Whether these lesions have malignant potential is unknown. Because papillary proliferations may accompany salpingitis (see Fig. 14.8b), a diagnosis of a papilloma in the presence of inflammation or plical distortion secondary to previous inflammation may not be warranted. The so-called metaplastic papillary tumor of the tube associated with pregnancy[14,145] in some cases appears to represent a papillary oncocytic metaplastic process rather than a true neoplasm. Rare cases of borderline (low malignant potential) papillary serous and endometrioid tumors of the tube have been reported.[6] In one case there was no evidence of disease 6 years after conservative surgery.[181]

Leiomyoma and Adenomyoma

Tumors of smooth muscle origin, chiefly *leiomyomas*, may originate from the tubal muscularis, from smooth muscle of the broad ligament, or from walls of blood vessels in either location. Compared with the frequency of uterine leiomyomas, tubal leiomyomas are quite uncommon. Microscopically, they are similar to those found in the uterus, and

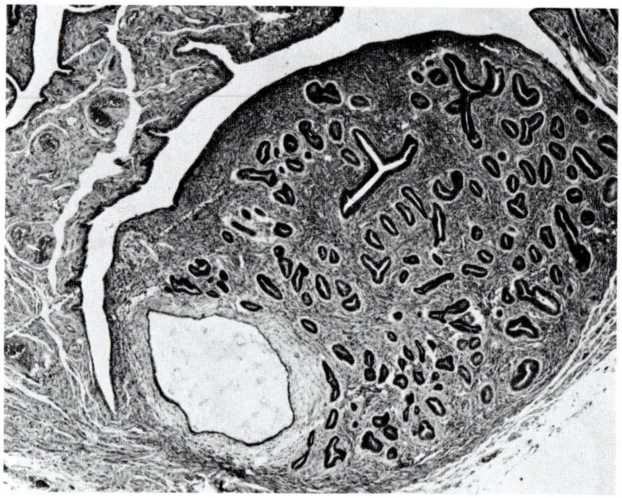

Fig. 14.27. Adenomyoma. A nodule of mixed simple glands and smooth muscle fibers protrudes into the tubal lumen.

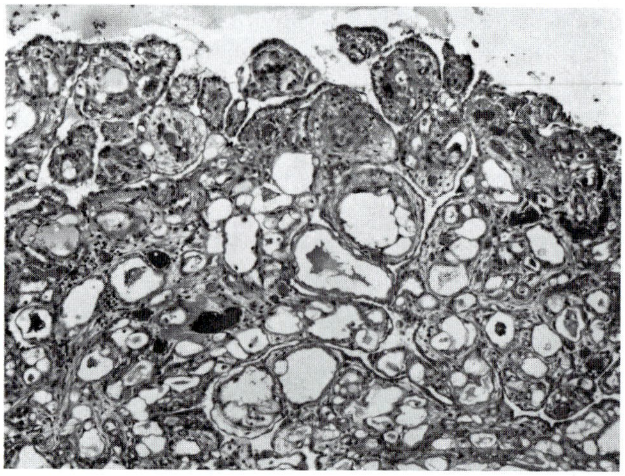

Fig. 14.28. Adenomatoid tumor (benign mesothelioma). Multiple connections with serosal surface are seen at *top*.

they can undergo similar degenerative changes. Rarely, benign glands and smooth muscle may be so intimately involved in a tumor that a true *adenomyoma* is produced (Fig. 14.27).

Adenomatoid Tumor

Adenomatoid tumor (*benign mesothelioma*) is the most frequent type of benign tubal tumor. Previously reported lymphangiomas probably represent examples of this entity. They are usually only 1–2 cm in diameter, appearing as a nodular swelling beneath the tubal serosa, and are yellow or whitish gray on section. They are rarely bilateral. Similar lesions may be found in the uterus, cul-de-sac, or ovary (see Chapter 13, Mesenchymal Tumors of the Uterus, and Chapter 21, Nonspecific Tumors of the Ovary, Including Mesenchymal Tumors and Malignant Lymphoma). Their origin is presumed to be from the cells of the serosal mesothelium. A fortuitous section may demonstrate a connection between serosa and tumor (Fig. 14.28), but usually the serosa covers the lesion.

Microscopically, multiple, small, slitlike or ovoid spaces are lined by a single layer of low cuboidal or flattened epithelial-like cells. The tumor may be large enough to displace the tubal lumen eccentrically and may grow into the supporting stroma of the luminal folds in an infiltrating manner. On frozen section the pathologist must differentiate the adenomatoid tumor from an infiltrating adenocarcinoma. Histochemical studies have shown hyaluronidase-digestible, alcian blue-positive material in the cells and spaces. No significant glycogen or intracellular mucin is present, as might be found in a tumor of müllerian origin. Electron microscopic and immunocytochemical studies support a mesothelial origin for these lesions. Microvilli project from the cell surfaces. Bundles of tonofilaments are present and occasionally are attached to desmosomes. Desmosomes are numerous between cells but are absent along the basal lamina on which the cells lie. These features are not characteristic of endothelial or müllerian epithelium but are seen in benign as well as in malignant mesotheliomas. Clinically, they are asymptomatic, and rarely, if ever, do they recur after adequate excision.

Other Benign Mesenchymal and Mixed Epithelial–Mesenchymal Tumors

These tumors are rare. *Hemangioma*, *lipoma*, *chondroma*, *angiomyofibroblastoma*, *angiomyolipoma*, *adenofibroma*, *cystadenofibroma*, and *neural tumors* have been reported. Their microscopic appearance is identical to that of similar tumors appearing elsewhere in the body.

Teratoma

Tubal teratomas are rare. Clinically, a patient with a tubal teratoma usually is nulliparous and in the fourth decade. Grossly, the tumors are located most frequently in the lumen, often attached by a pedicle to the inner tubal wall. They may, however, be intramural or attached to the serosa. On section, they are more often cystic than solid and may be small (1–2 cm in diameter) or large (10–20 cm in diameter). As with their ovarian counterparts, ectodermal, mesodermal, and endodermal tissues are represented by well-differentiated mature elements. Rare teratomas consisting entirely of mature thyroid tissue have been described in the tube of women without clinical hyperthyroidism. An isolated nodule of pancreatic tissue has been found beneath the tubal mucosa of one patient. Only rare cases of histologically immature tubal teratoma have been described.[101] Although ovarian teratomas appear to originate in abnormally developing ova, tissue containing ova is rarely found within tubal mucosa.

Malignant Neoplasms

Carcinoma In Situ

Carcinoma in situ (CIS) of the tube is diagnosed accurately only when the epithelial cells of the endosalpingeal lining form papillae with cytologically malignant mitotically active nuclei (Fig. 14.29). CIS may be seen adjacent to invasive tumor in carefully studied cases of tubal carcinoma or in cases of malignant mixed mesodermal tumor, and should not be confused with endosalpingeal seeding from primary ovarian carcinoma (see Fig. 14.35, later in this chapter). Some authors[129] have illustrated cases in which tubal epithelium showed nuclear crowding and atypia and termed the change *CIS*. It is clear that carefully studied tubes demonstrate similar changes in 18% of routinely accessioned salpingectomy specimens and even more frequent mucosal hyperplasia[117,179] (see Fig. 14.5). Although the lesions are more common in tubes with salpingitis (see Fig. 14.16), 14% of otherwise normal tubes show changes consisting of nuclear crowding and stratification, loss of polarity, and nuclear atypia. Mitoses are sparse. Frequently, changes are present in only one or two of many sections. Papillary formation with bridging reminiscent of some forms of mammary papillomatosis may occur. An oncocytic "pink cell" metaplasia with cytoplasmic acidophilia occasionally is present (see Fig. 14.4). Startling epithelial changes that mimic early papillary adenocarcinoma may be produced by accidental exposure of the specimen to heat.

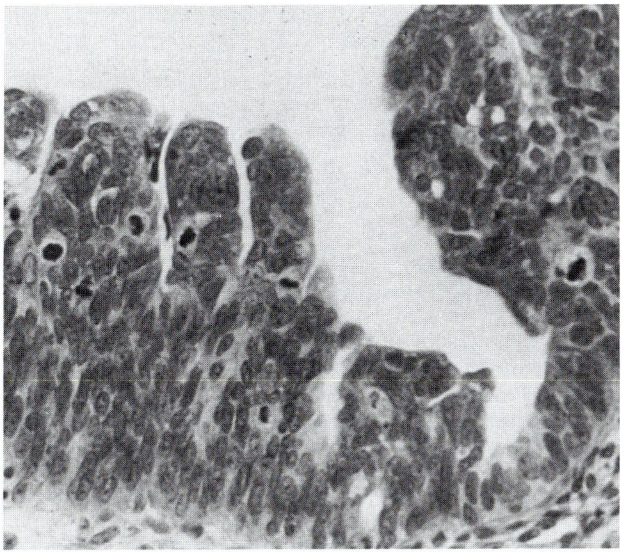

Fig. 14.29. Carcinoma in situ. The epithelial cells have lost their polarity and are growing in papillae without stromal cores. Nuclei are hyperchromatic, large, and irregular, and mitoses are numerous. The basement membrane is intact.

Invasive Adenocarcinoma

Primary adenocarcinoma of the tube is uncommon. Only 0.2%–0.5% of primary female genital malignancies are tubal, a prevalence of about 3.6 per million women per year.[13] Some tubal primaries with disseminated disease involving the ovaries are surely misclassified as ovarian in origin.[176] Although some patients with tubal carcinoma harbor a *BRCA1* germline mutation,[182] the implications for prophylactic surgery are not yet clear. Comparative genomic hybridization of tumor DNA reveals a rather consistent DNA gain in chromosome arm 3q, but there are numerous other chromosomal losses and gains.[72,131] There is prominent overexpression of p53 on immunohistochemical staining of most tumors, and less common overexpression of c-erbB-2.[34,96] p53 immunoreactivity has not proven helpful in predicting clinical behavior,[68] and the presence of estrogen and progesterone receptors in tumor tissue does not correlate with survival.[143]

Unfortunately, primary tubal carcinoma is rarely found in the in situ stage. The typical patient is usually in her sixth or seventh decade and is rarely younger than 35 years.[13,69] About 30% of patients are nulliparous, but no case-control studies have yet been done to confirm if this is significant.[126] The classic signs and symptoms of invasive tubal carcinoma include vaginal bleeding, clear or serosanguinous vaginal discharge (hydrops tubae profluens), pelvic pain, and a pelvic mass. The diagnosis is rarely made before operation, but occasionally positive cytology associated with negative endometrial curettage will suggest the correct location of the neoplasm.[105] Tubal carcinoma may occur as a part of multifocal upper genital tract malignancy.[6,141]

Grossly, the tube usually is swollen secondary to advanced intraluminal growth. Hydrosalpinx or tuboovarian abscess is ruled out only after the speci-

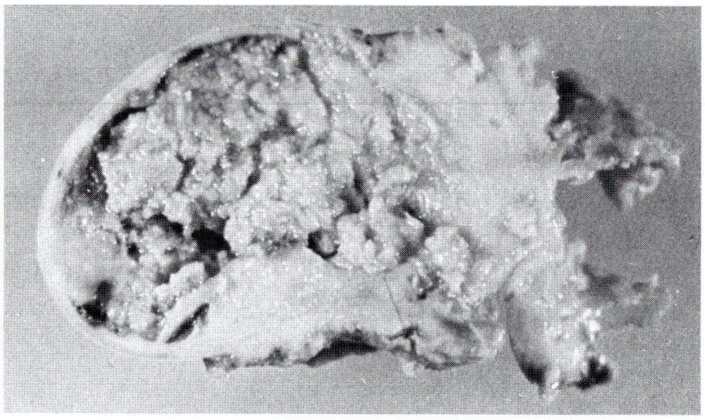

Fig. 14.30. Primary tubal adenocarcinoma. Tube is dilated and filled by papillary and solid tumor, which penetrates the muscularis along the lower margin of the specimen.

men is opened. The lumen usually is filled and dilated by papillary or solid and necrotic tumor (Fig. 14.30). The fimbriated end is closed in about half the cases. A detailed protocol for examination of a tube with carcinoma has been developed by the Cancer Committee of the College of American Pathologists that includes obtaining pertinent historical information as well as gross and microscopic data.[150] Bilateral involvement frequently occurs, but the reason for this is unknown. A common carcinogenic stimulus could cause simultaneous development of tumor in both tubes, or retrograde lymphatic spread after blockage by advanced tubal carcinoma of one side could lead to contralateral metastatic deposits. Subsequent growth might then mimic a second primary tumor. The fact that bilateral tubal carcinoma is present in some 7% of stage 0–II lesions but may be seen in as many as 30% of stage III and IV tumors suggests that metastatic spread in advanced lesions is an important cause of bilaterality.[148]

Microscopically, tubal neoplasms may be classified as epithelial, mixed epithelial–mesenchymal, or mesenchymal (Table 14.1). The majority of tumors are histologically similar to serous adenocarcinomas of the ovary. They are composed of fine branching papillae covered by one or more layers of epithelium with enlarged pleomorphic hyperchromatic nuclei with both increased and abnormal mitoses (Figs. 14.31 and 14.32). In poorly differentiated areas, the tumor may grow in solid sheets of cells with small or large foci of necrosis. Abrupt transitions from normal to neoplastic epithelium may be found. Attempts to grade tumor pattern or degree of nuclear atypia have proved to be of limited prognostic value.

Although serous histology is most common in the tube, comprising 70% of cases in one recent series, endometrioid and transitional cell types[89] each makes up about another 10%.[6] Mucinous carcinomas may be of borderline histology or in situ.[152] Synchronous mucinous primaries have been described in the tube and endocervix.[77] Endometrioid carcinoma may resemble that of the ovary, with or without focal squamous differentiation, or may have an unusual histologic appearance with microtubule formation suggestive of an adnexal tumor of probable wolffian origin.[42,123] Rare endometrioid tumors have a prominent spindle cell component, which may suggest sex cord stromal tumor, malignant mixed mesodermal tumor, or adnexal wolffian tumor. The spindle cells may be diffuse or whorled, or may palisade.[164,165] Primary squamous,[31] adenosquamous, clear cell, hepatoid,[9] small cell,[9] lymphoepithelioma-like,[6] giant cell,[6] and glassy cell[70] carcinomas are rarely seen.

Table 14.1. Tumors of the fallopian tube (WHO classification)

Epithelial tumors
Benign
Adenoma
Papilloma
Metaplastic papillary tumor
Other
Of borderline malignancy
Malignant
Carcinoma in situ
Serous carcinoma
Mucinous carcinoma
Endometrioid carcinoma
Clear cell carcinoma
Transitional cell carcinoma
Squamous cell carcinoma
Undifferentiated and other
Mixed epithelial-mesenchymal tumors
Benign
Adenofibroma
Adenomyoma
Adenomatoid
Other
Malignant
Adenosarcoma
Mesodermal (müllerian) mixed tumor
Homologous (carcinosarcoma)
Heterologous
Mesenchymal tumors
Benign
Leiomyoma
Adenomatoid
Others
Malignant
Leiomyosarcoma
Others

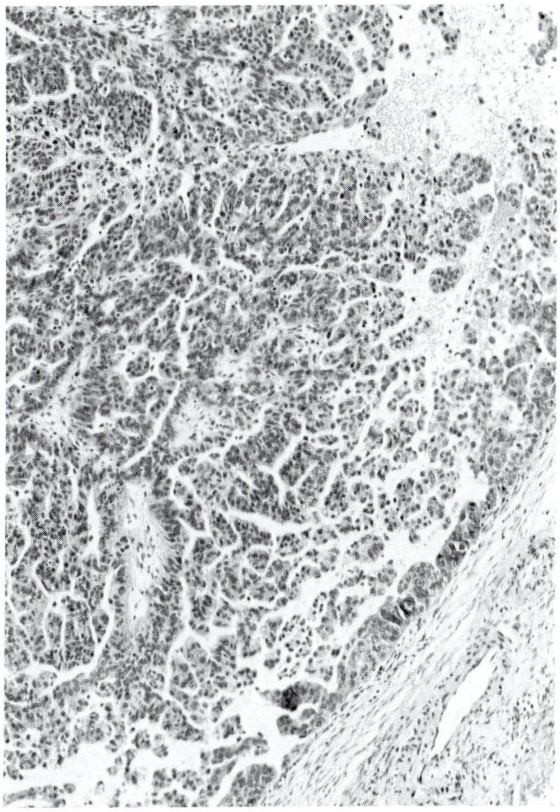

Fig. 14.31. Primary tubal serous carcinoma. The tumor is characterized by a delicate fibrovascular branching core supporting proliferating atypical epithelial cells. Invasion is present in adjacent areas of the wall.

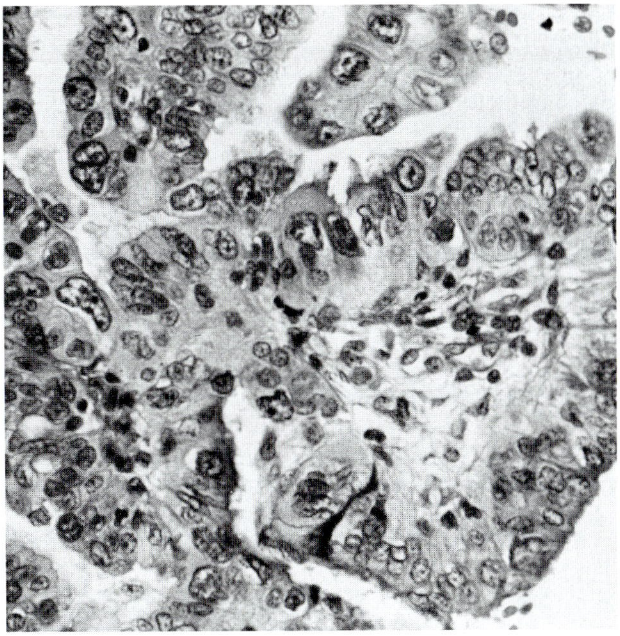

Fig. 14.32. Tubal serous adenocarcinoma. The tumor cells covering the fibrovascular core (*center*) have lost their nuclear polarity. Their nuclei are large, irregular, and hyperchromatic.

A number of staging schemes have been proposed based on operative or operative combined with pathologic findings.[7,148] In 1991 the Gynecology Oncology (GOG) Committee of the International Federation of Gynecology and Obstetrics (FIGO) adopted a staging system for tubal carcinoma based on that for ovarian carcinoma[39] (Table 14.2). Since then, modification has been suggested to account for such features as tumor without extension into the lamina propria (proposed IA-0), or tumor lacking invasion of the muscularis (IA-1).[6] These subcategories appear to separate patients who will do well from those with a guarded prognosis. Tumor at the fimbriated end, with ready access to the peritoneal cavity, may also warrant individual staging.[5] Tumor spreads via the lymphatics to paraaortic and pelvic nodes, and may be present when it appears that the tumor is limited to the tube.[46,86,87] Once tumor spreads to the serosa, 5-year survival drops to only one patient in six (Table 14.3), and even 5-year survival is not synonymous with cure.[141,148]

Current treatment by total abdominal hysterectomy and bilateral salpingo-oophorectomy with or without adjuvant radiation or chemotherapy usually fails because of transperitoneal spread. Aggressive cytoreduction and chemotherapy in advanced disease may yield complete responses for more than 3 years.[121] Postoperative radiation is no longer favored.[13] The CA-125 antigenic determinant found in ovarian carcinoma also is characteristic of tubal adenocarcinomas, and its serum level may prove useful in patient follow-up.[13,137,162] Recent series suggest that 5-year survival rates greater than 60% may be achieved with early-stage disease (stage I), whereas with more advanced disease survival is about 20%.[13,69,142] The value of second-look laparotomy for tubal cancer is unclear.[38] As do other gynecologic cancers, tubal carcinoma may cause a variety of paraneoplastic syndromes.[36,73]

Sarcomas and Mixed Epithelial–Mesenchymal Tumors

Sarcomas of the tube may be classified as pure or mixed (see Table 14.1). Neoplasms containing a mixture of sarcoma with cytologically benign epithelial elements are designated adenosarcoma, whereas those with a mixture of sarcoma and cytologically malignant epithelial areas are designated *malignant mesodermal mixed tumor* (*MMMT*). Pure sarcomas may be histologically subtyped if sufficient differentiation is present. Leiomyosarcomas[78] are per-

Table 14.2. International Federation of Gynecologists and Obstetricians (FIGO) fallopian tube tumor staging

Stage 0	Carcinoma in situ (limited to tubal mucosa)
Stage I	Growth limited to fallopian tubes
Stage IA	Growth limited to one tube with extension into submucosa and/or muscularis but not penetrating serosal surface; no ascites
Stage IB	Growth limited to both tubes with extension into submucosa and/or muscularis but not penetrating serosal surface; no ascites
Stage IC	Tumor either Stage IA or Stage IB but with extension through or onto tubal serosa or with ascites containing malignant cells or with positive peritoneal washings
Stage II	Growth involving one or more fallopian tubes with pelvic extension
Stage IIA	Extension and/or metastases to uterus and/or ovaries
Stage IIB	Extension to other pelvic tissues
Stage IIC	Tumor either Stage IIA or IIB and with ascites containing malignant cells or with positive peritoneal washings
Stage III	Tumor involving one or both fallopian tubes with peritoneal implants outside pelvis and/or positive retroperitoneal or inguinal nodes. Superficial live metastasis equals stage III. Tumor appears limited to true pelvis but with histologically proved malignant extension to small bowel or omentum
Stage IIIA	Tumor grossly limited to true pelvis with negative nodes but with histologically confirmed microscopic seeding of abdominal peritoneal surfaces
Stage IIIB	Tumor involving one or both tubes with histologically confirmed implants of abdominal peritoneal surfaces, none exceeding 2 cm in diameter. Lymph nodes are negative
Stage IIIC	Abdominal implants >2 cm in diameter and/or positive retroperitoneal or inguinal nodes
Stage IV	Growth involving one or both fallopian tubes with distant metastases. If pleural effusion is present, cytological fluid must be positive for malignant cells to be Stage IV. Parenchymal liver metastasis equals Stage IV

Note: Staging for fallopian tube carcinoma is by the surgical pathological system. Operative findings designating stage are determined before tumor debulking.

haps the most common type and may arise from the tube or broad ligament. Chondrosarcoma, malignant fibrous histiocytoma, and embryonal rhabdomyosarcoma have been described.

Primary stromal sarcoma[30] and adenosarcoma (Fig 14.33) arising in the tube are rare. The few dozen patients reported with tubal MMMT are nearly all postmenopausal, with a mean age of 58.[76] They may have watery or bloody vaginal discharge and abdominal pain with signs of peritoneal spread. Grossly, the tumors distend the tube, and by the time of discovery 85% have a pelvic mass with spread to adjacent pelvic and abdominal structures. The ovary must be identified clearly to rule out an origin in that organ. The grossly dilated tube when opened reveals a shaggy mucosal surface with areas of necrosis and hemorrhage (Fig. 14.34). Microscopically distinct sarcomatous and carcinomatous areas should be identifiable. Malignant squamous or glandular foci (or both) lie in an atypical mitotically active spindle cell background of sarcoma. In about half the cases, the sarcoma may consist only of malignant elements homologous to the tube, such as smooth muscle or stromal cells (for which the term *carcinosarcoma* was formerly used), but commonly there are foci of malignant cartilage, osteosarcoma, or rhabdomyosarcoma. Areas of mucosal carcinoma in situ may be apparent adjacent to the main tumor mass.[28] The histology of metastases from MMMTs of the female genital tract is typically carcinoma, but sarcoma and mixtures have been described.[156] The major differential diagnostic pitfall is a poorly differentiated carcinoma with spindle cell metaplasia. Life expectancy usually is measured in months, but surgery and chemotherapy may lead to longer remission.[28,76]

Table 14.3. Staging and survival in adenocarcinoma of the fallopian tube

Stage	*No. of patients*	*5-Year survival (%)*
0	8	87.5
I	41	73
II	33	37
III	52	29
IV	17	12

After Baekelandt et al.[13]

Metastatic Tumors

Metastatic tumors involving the tube usually are secondary to spread from carcinomas of the ovary or

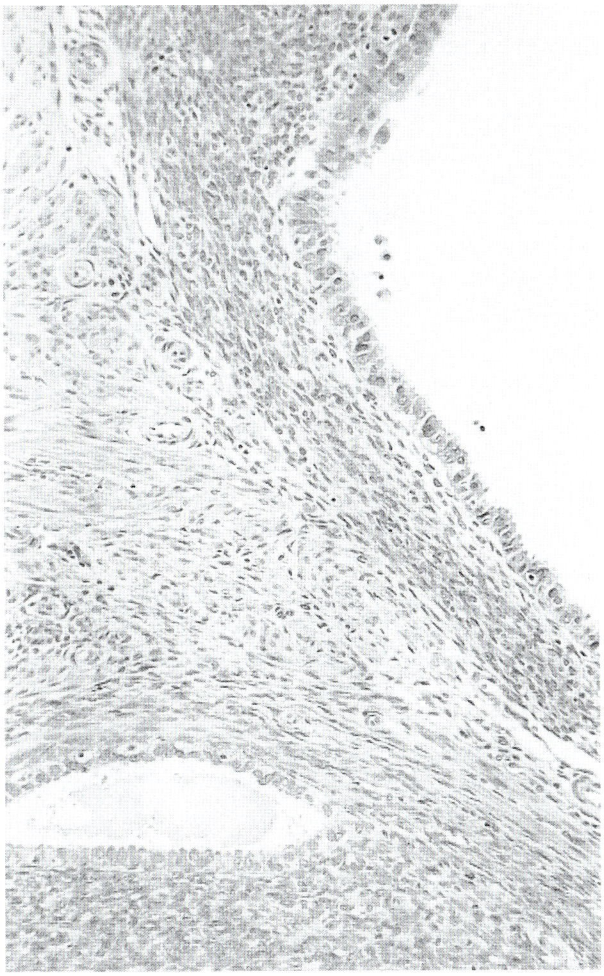

Fig. 14.33. Adenosarcoma. Benign-appearing glands (*right and bottom*) are admixed with hypercellular stroma that is closely applied to glands. (Case courtesy of Dr. S.R. Paik, Poughkeepsie, NY.)

endometrium. Peritoneal spread involves the serosal surface, whereas lymphatic metastases from adjacent primary sites may involve the mucosa or muscularis as well. Low-grade stromal sarcoma may extend to involve the tubes and ovaries. Spread takes place by the extension of wormlike tongues of tumor along tubal lymphatics. Blood-borne metastases from breast carcinomas or other extrapelvic tumors also may occur. On occasion, squamous carcinoma of the uterine cervix may spread in an in situ manner to involve the endometrial cavity, tubes, and even the ovarian surface.[136] The presence of a large ovarian primary tumor coupled with tumor in the lumen of the fallopian tube and tumor in the endometrial cavity suggests that the tubal lumen may serve as a conduit for tumor spread. Careful study of the tubes removed at surgery for primary ovarian carcinoma reveals that luminal groups of tumor cells may implant onto endosalpingeal surfaces and

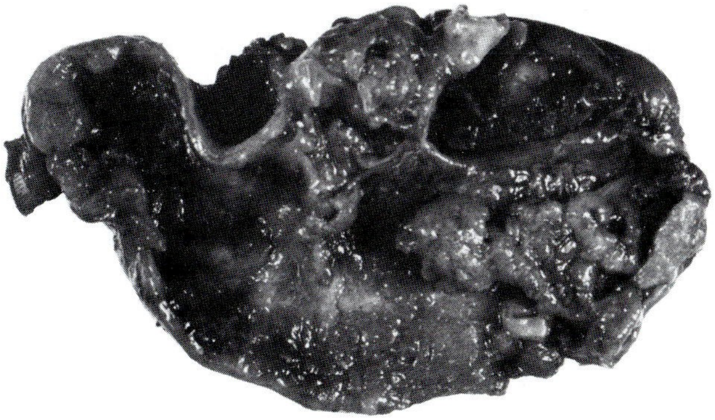

Fig. 14.34. Primary malignant mixed mesodermal tumor. Dilated tube has been opened to illustrate the irregular intraluminal projections and a shaggy, irregular mucosal surface.

simulate CIS or early primary tubal carcinoma (Fig. 14.35). Because of frequent secondary involvement of the tubes, Hu and colleagues suggested that the following criteria be used to determine primary tubal carcinoma: grossly, the main tumor is in the

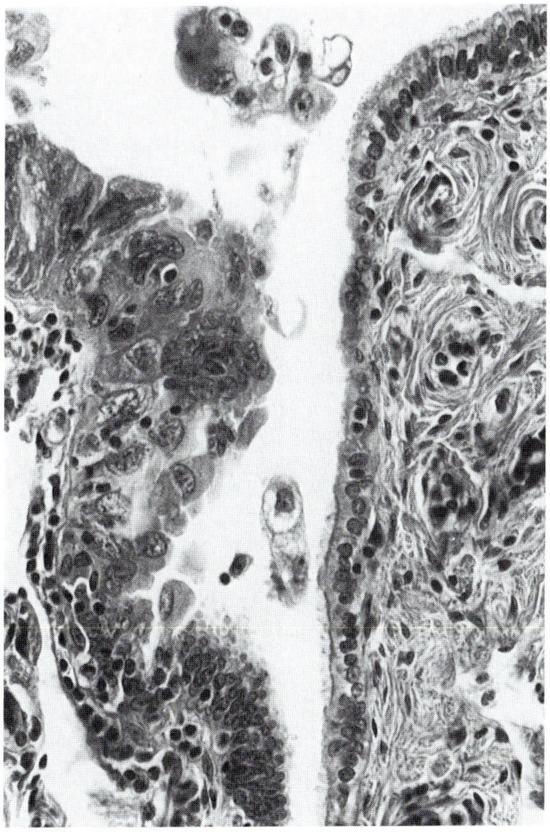

Fig. 14.35. Tubal implantation of ovarian carcinoma. Two clusters of malignant cells from an ipsilateral ovarian carcinoma lie free in the tubal lumen, and on the *left*, carcinoma has implanted and begun to spread over the mucosal surface.

tube; microscopically, the mucosa is involved and shows a papillary pattern; if the tubal wall is extensively involved, a transition between benign and malignant tubal epithelium should be found.[75] When both tube and ovary are intimately involved by a mass of tumor, the assumption of an ovarian primary tumor may not always be correct. However, because the current surgical and chemotherapeutic treatment for epithelial malignancies of tube and ovary are the same, the distinction is academic.

Lymphoma

Tubal involvement by *lymphoma* is rare and is associated almost invariably with simultaneous involvement of the ipsilateral ovary.[151] Undifferentiated carcinoma must be ruled out with appropriate immunohistochemical stains.

Trophoblastic Lesions

Trophoblastic tubal lesions are exceedingly uncommon. Patients have risk factors for ectopic pregnancy such as prior salpingitis and tubal occlusion.[122] Hydatidiform moles usually occur as isolated growths but may be associated with intrauterine pregnancy. Clinically, perhaps 1 in 5000 ectopic pregnancies will prove to be a mole. The histologic appearance may be that of a complete or a partial mole with clear evidence of trophoblastic proliferation in addition to hydropic swelling of the villi.[122] Choriocarcinoma rarely may arise in the tube. Clinically, the patient is believed to have an ectopic pregnancy. At operation, a large and hemorrhagic, fleshy mass may have largely destroyed the tube. Histologically, the malignant trophoblastic proliferation is similar to that of uterine choriocarcinomas. Response to modern chemotherapy in general has been excellent. Lesions of intermediate trophoblast, both placental site nodule[124] and placental site trophoblastic tumor,[160] are rare (see Chapter 24, Gestational Trophoblastic Disease and Related Lesions).

Paratubal Tumors and Cysts

Adrenal Rests

Adrenal cortical rests, if a careful search is made, may be found in the broad ligament in more than 20% of women. They lie adjacent to the ovarian vein and just beneath the peritoneum. Grossly, they appear as yellow nodules or disks, but they may be obscured by fat. Medullary tissue is absent, but microscopically all three cortical layers are recognizable. This accessory tissue may hypertrophy secondary to adrenal destruction or may, rarely, give rise to a functional or nonfunctional cortical adenoma.[146,173]

Nests of cells morphologically similar to ovarian hilus cells have been described in the midportion of the tube. In the absence of Reinke crystals, close association with nonmyelinated nerve fibers, or histochemical studies, it is difficult to exclude the possibility of an adrenal rest. Hilus cell nests with Reinke crystals may be seen, however, in fimbrial stroma. These may be the cells responsible for the only case reported of tubal Sertoli–Leydig cell tumor.

Adnexal Tumor of Probable Wolffian Origin

A small group of distinctive tumors is described as located either within the leaves of the broad ligament, the mesosalpinx, or in the ovarian hilus.[44,81] (These tumors are also described and illustrated in Chapter 21, Nonspecific Tumors of the Ovary, Including Mesenchymal Tumors and Malignant Lymphoma.) Briefly, patients range in age from 29 to 58 years. Either they have abdominal pain and a palpable mass or the tumor is discovered as an incidental finding. The lesions measure from 1.3 to 12 cm in greatest dimension and are lobulated, with gross encapsulation. On section, the consistency may be rubbery or friable, and cysts or calcification may be present.

The microscopic picture varies widely. Solid masses of epithelial cells may be present, or tubular areas may be found similar to a well-differentiated Sertoli–Leydig tumor of the ovary (Pick's tubular adenoma). A sievelike pattern reminiscent of benign tubal mesotheliomas also may be seen. Microscopically, the capsule often is breached by tongues of tumor. Ultrastructural analysis[81] and immunohistochemical positivity for cytokeratin and inhibin[44] support a mesonephric, specifically rete ovarii origin, but a sex cord–stromal origin cannnot be excluded. Although most of these tumors behave in a benign fashion, multiple local recurrences[23] and fatal metastases may occur. The differential diagnosis includes the recently described variant of tubal endometrioid carcinoma.[42]

Other Paraovarian Tumors

Other **solid paraovarian tumors** are most often leiomyomas. Sarcomas and malignant primary epithelial lesions are rare. The rare broad ligament adenocarcinomas reported tend to be in women in the reproductive years and are typically low-grade serous lesions.[11,12] Overdiagnosis of low malignant potential (borderline) serous tumors as carcinoma should be avoided.[40] Distinction of a borderline tumor from an invasive serous carcinoma is based on the absence of stromal invasion, using the same criteria that are applied to ovarian serous neoplasms (see Chapter 18, Surface Epithelial Tumors of the Ovary). The majority of broad ligament and paraovarian epithelial tumors are serous neoplasms of low malignant potential. The patients range in age from 13 to 76 years (mean, 32–43 years) and present with a pelvic mass with or without ascites or pain.[4,11] At operation there is no involvement of the ovary. Paraovarian cystadenofibromas are occasional, usually incidental findings. Papillary cystadenoma of the broad ligament may be associated with von Hippel–Lindau disease.[88] Extraovarian Brenner tumors, mesosalpingeal choriocarcinoma, broad ligament pheochromocytoma, extraskeletal Ewing's sarcoma, thecoma and mesovarial ependymoma are among the rare tumors reported adjacent to the tube and ovary.

Paratubal Cysts

Paratubal cysts may arise from mesonephric (wolffian) structures, from paramesonephric (müllerian) structures, or from mesothelial inclusions. Differentiation may be difficult because of compression and atrophy of the lining cells; paramesonephric cysts are lined by epithelium containing numerous ciliated cells. Such cysts also may have papillary infoldings similar to endosalpingeal folds. Mesonephric cysts contain only a few or no ciliated cells and may have a more prominent muscular coat. Ultrastructurally, mesonephric epithelial cells tend to have an inapparent Golgi apparatus, moderate rough endoplasmic reticulum (RER), numerous lysosomes, and minimal glycogen. Paramesonephric epithelial cells tend to have a prominent Golgi apparatus and RER, prominent glycogen, and only rare lysosomes.[60]

The hydatid of Morgagni is by far the most common paramesonephric cyst. Grossly, it is found dangling from one of the fimbriae. It is ovoid or round, 2–10 mm in diameter, and contains clear serous fluid surrounded by a thin translucent wall. Microscopically, it is lined by ciliated and nonciliated cells and may have small epithelial-covered plicae projecting into the lumen. A careful study of paraovarian cysts revealed that 86% of those more than 3 cm in diameter were mesothelial, 14% were paramesonephric, and none was mesonephric.[61]

References

1. Abbuhl SB, Muskin EB, Shofer FS (1997) Pelvic inflammatory disease in patients with bilateral tubal ligation. Am J Emerg Med 15:271–274
2. Abraham JL, Spore WW, Benirschke K (1982) Cysticercosis of the fallopian tube: histology and microanalysis. Hum Pathol 13:665–670
3. Afzelius BA, Eliasson R (1983) Male and female infertility problems in the immotile-cilia syndrome. Eur J Respir Dis 64(suppl 127):144
4. Altaras MM, Jaffe R, Corduba M, et al (1990) Primary paraovarian cystadenocarcinoma: clinical and management aspects and literature review. Gynecol Oncol 38:268–272
5. Alvarado-Cabrero I, Navani SS, Young RH, et al (1997) Tumors of the fimbriated end of the fallopian tube: a clinicopathologic analysis of 20 cases, including nine carcinomas. Int J Gynecol Pathol 16:189–196
6. Alvarado-Cabrero I, Young RH, Vamvakas EC, et al (1999) Carcinoma of the fallopian tube: a clinicopathologic study of 105 cases with observations on staging and prognostic factors. Gynecol Oncol 72:367–379
7. American College of Obstetricians and Gynecologists Committee on Terminology (1972) In: Hughes EC (ed) Obstetric–gynecologic terminology, with section on neonatology and glossary of congenital anomalies. Davis, Philadelphia, p 157
8. American Fertility Society (1988) The American Fertility Society classifications of adnexal adhesions, distal tubal occlusion, tubal occlusion secondary to tubal ligation, tubal pregnancies, Müllerian anomalies and intrauterine adhesions. Fertil Steril 49:944–955
9. Aoyama T, Mizuno T, Andoh K, et al (1996) Alphafetoprotein-producing (hepatoid) carcinoma of the fallopian tube. Gynecol Oncol 63:261–266
10. Arvidson CG, Kirkpatrick R, Witcamp MT, et al (1999) *Neisseria gonorrhoeae* mutants altered in toxicity to human fallopian tubes and molecular characterization of the genetic locus involved. Infect Immun 67:643–652
11. Aslani M, Ahn G-H, Scully RE (1988) Serous papillary cystadenoma of borderline malignancy of broad ligament. Int J Gynecol Pathol 7:131–138
12. Aslani M, Scully RE (1989) Primary carcinoma of the broad ligament: Report of four cases and review of the literature. Cancer (Phila) 64:1540–1545
13. Baekelandt M, Nesbakken AJ, Kristensen GB, Trope, CG, Abeler AM (2000) Carcinoma of the fallopian tube. Clinicopathologic study of 151 patients treated at The Norwegian Radium Hospital. Cancer (Phila) 89:2076–2084
14. Bartnik J, Powell WS, Moriber-Katz S, et al (1989) Metaplastic papillary tumor of the fallopian tube. Case report, immunohistochemical features and review of the literature. Arch Pathol Lab Med 113:545–547
15. Bell DA, Mondschein M, Scully RE (1986) Giant cell arteritis of the female genital tract. A report of three cases. Am J Surg Pathol 10:696–701
16. Bernardus RE, Van der Slikke JW, Roex AJM, Dijkhuizen GH, Stolk JG (1984) Torsion of the fallopian tube: some considerations on its etiology. Obstet Gynecol 64:675

17. Beyth Y, Kopolovic J (1982) Accessory tubes: a possible contributing factor in infertility. Fertil Steril 38:382–383
18. Bloechle M (1999) What is a hydrosalpinx? A plea for the use of a proper terminology in scientific discussion. Hum Reprod 14:578
19. Boakye K, Omalu B, Thomas L (1997) Fallopian tube and pulmonary sarcoidosis. A case report. J Reprod Med 42:533–555
20. Brandtzaeg P (1997) Mucosal immunity in the female genital tract. J Reprod Immunol 36:23–50
21. Breen JL (1970) A 21-year survey of 654 ectopic pregnancies. Am J Obstet Gynecol 106:1004–1019
22. Brenner PF, Roy S, Mishell DR Jr (1980) Ectopic pregnancy. A study of 300 consecutive surgically treated cases. JAMA 243:673–676
23. Brescia RJ, Cardoso de Almeida PC, Fuller AF Jr, Dickersin GR, Robboy SJ (1985) Female adnexal tumor of probable wolffian origin with multiple recurrences over 16 years. Cancer (Phila) 56:1456–1461
24. Britigan BE, Cohen MS, Sparling PF (1985) Gonococcal infection: A model of molecular pathogenesis. N Engl J Med 312:1683–1694
25. Brunham RC, Maclean IW, Binns B, Peeling RW (1985) *Chlamydia trachomatis*: its role in tubal infertility. J Infect Dis 152:1275–1282
26. Busch DH, Benirschke K (1974) Cytogenetic studies of ectopic pregnancies. Virch Arch [Cell Pathol] 16:319–330
27. Camus E, Poncelet C, Goffinet F, et al (1999) Pregnancy rates after in vitro fertilization in cases of tubal infertility with and without hydrosalpinx: a meta-analysis of published comparative studies. Hum Reprod 14:1243–1249
28. Carlson JA, Ackerman BL, Wheeler JE (1993) Malignant mixed müllerian tumor of the fallopian tube. Cancer (Phila) 71:187–192
29. Cataldo NA, Nicholson M, Bihrle D (1990) Uterine serosal trophoblastic implant after linear salpingostomy for ectopic pregnancy at laparotomy. Obstet Gynecol 76:523–525
30. Chang KL, Crabtree GS, Lim-Tan SK, et al (1993) Primary extrauterine endometrial stromal neoplasms: a clinicopathologic study of 20 cases and a review of the literature. Int J Gynecol Pathol 12: 282–296
31. Cheung AN, So KF, Ngan HYS, Wong LC (1994) Primary squamous carcinoma of the fallopian tube. Int J Gynecol Pathol 13:92–95
32. Cheung AN, Young RH, Scully RE (1994) Pseudocarcinomatous hyperplasia of the fallopian tube associated with salpingitis. Am J Surg Pathol 18: 1125–1130
33. Chi I-C, Potts M, Wilkens L (1986) Rare events associated with tubal sterilization: an international experience. Obstet Gynecol Surv 41:7–19
34. Chung TK, Cheung TH, To KF, et al (2000) Overexpression of p53 and HER-2/neu and c-myc in primary fallopian tube carcinoma. Gynecol Obstet Invest 49:47–51
35. Clement PB, Young RH, Scully RE (1988) Necrotic pseudoxanthomatous nodules of ovary and peritoneum in endometriosis. Am J Surg Pathol 12: 390–397
36. Clement PB, Young RH, Scully RE (1991) Clinical syndromes associated with tumors of the female genital tract. Semin Diagn Pathol 8:204–233
37. Cohen MA, Lindheim SR, Sauer MV (1999) Hydrosalpinges adversely affect implantation in donor oocyte cycles. Hum Reprod 14:1087–1089
38. Cormio G, Gabriele A, Maneo A, et al (1997) Second-look laparotomy in the management of fallopian tube carcinoma. Acta Obstet Gynecol Scand 76:369–372
39. Creasman WT (1992) Revision in classification by International Federation of Gynecology and Obstetrics [Letter]. Am J Obstet Gynecol 167:857–858
40. d'Ablaing G, Klatt EC, DiRocco G, Hibbard LT (1983) Broad ligament serous tumor of low malignant potential. Int J Gynecol Pathol 2:93–99
41. David A, Garcia C-R, Czernobilsky B (1969) Human hydrosalpinx. Histologic study and chemical composition of fluid. Am J Obstet Gynecol 105:400–411
42. Daya D, Young RH, Scully RE (1992) Endometrioid carcinoma of the fallopian tube resembling an adnexal tumor of probable wolffian origin: a report of six cases. Int J Gynecol Pathol 11:122–130
43. Delabrousse E, Site O, Le Mouel A, et al (1999) Intrahepatic pregnancy: sonography and CT findings. AJR Am J Roentgenol 173:1377–1378
44. Devouassoux-Shisheboran M, Silver SA, Tavassoli FA (1999) Wolffian adnexal tumor, so-called female adnexal tumor of probable wolffian origin (FATWO): immunohistochemical evidence in support of a wolffian origin. Hum Pathol 30:856–863
45. de Wit W, Gowrising CJ, Kuik DJ, et al (1998) Only hydrosalpinges visible on ultrasound are associated with reduced implantation and pregnancy rates after in vitro fertilization. Hum Reprod 13:1696–1701
46. di Re E, Grosso G, Raspagliesi F, et al (1996) Fallopian tube cancer: incidence and role of lymphatic spread. Gynecol Oncol 62:199–202
47. Dische FE, Burt JM, Davison NJH, Puntambekar S (1974) Tuboovarian actinomycosis associated with intrauterine contraceptive devices. J Obstet Gynaecol Br Commonw 81:724–729
48. Donnez J, Casanas-Roux F, Caprasse J, Ferin J, Thomas K (1985) Cyclic changes in ciliation, cell height, and mitotic activity in human tubal epithelium during reproductive life. Fertil Steril 43:554–559
49. Doss BJ, Jacques SM, Qureshi F, et al (1998) Extratubal secondary trophoblastic implants: clinicopathologic correlation and review of the literature. Hum Pathol 29:184–187
50. Downing SJ, Maguiness SD, Watson A, et al (1997) Electrophysiological basis of human fallopian tubal fluid formation. J Reprod Fertil 111:29–34
51. Egan AJ, Russell P (1996) Transitional cell (urothelial) cell metaplasia of the fallopian tube mucosa:

morphological assessment of three cases. Int J Gynecol Pathol 15:72–76
52. Egger M, Low N, Smith GD (1998) Screening for chlamydial infections and the risk of ectopic pregnancy in a county in Sweden: ecological analysis. Br Med J 316:1776–1780
53. El-Kady AA, Mansy MM, Nagib HS, et al (1991) Histopathologic changes in the cornual portion of the fallopian tube following a single transcervical insertion of quinacrine hydrochloride pellets. Adv Contracep 7:1–9
54. Falcone T, Mascha EJ, Goldberg JM, et al (1998) A study of risk factors for ruptured tubal ectopic pregnancy. J Womens Health 7:459–463
55. Farley TMM, Rosenberg MJ, Rowe PJ, et al (1992) Intrauterine devices and pelvic inflammatory disease: an international perspective. Lancet 339:785–788
56. Fortier KJ, Haney AF (1985) The pathologic spectrum of uterotubal junction obstruction. Obstet Gynecol 65:93–98
57. Franco V, Florena AM, Guarneri G, et al (1990) Xanthogranulomatous salpingitis. Case report and review of the literature. Acta Eur Fertil 21:197–199
58. Fredricsson B (1969) Histochemistry of the oviduct. In: Hafez ESE, Blandau RJ (eds) The mammalian oviduct. University of Chicago Press, Chicago
59. Fylstra DL (1998) Tubal pregnancy: a review of current diagnosis and treatment. Obstet Gynecol Surv 53:320–326
60. Gardner GH, Greene RR, Peckham BM (1948) Normal and cystic structures of broad ligament. Am J Obstet Gynecol 55:917–939
61. Genadry R, Parmley T, Woodruff JD (1977) The origin and clinical behavior of the parovarian tumor. Am J Obstet Gynecol 129:873–880
62. Gisser SD (1986) Obstructing fallopian tube papilloma. Int J Gynecol Pathol 5:179–182
63. Gold MA, Schmidt RR, Parks, N, et al (1997) Bilateral absence of the ovaries and distal fallopian tubes. A case report. J Reprod Med 42:375–377
64. Green LK, Kott ML (1989) Histopathologic findings in ectopic tubal pregnancy. Int J Gynecol Pathol 8:255–262
65. Grimes HG, Nosal RA, Gallagher JC (1983) Ovarian pregnancy: a series of 24 cases. Obstet Gynecol 61:174–180
66. Haines M (1958) Tuberculous salpingitis as seen by the pathologist and the surgeon. Am J Obstet Gynecol 75:472–481
67. Halbert SA, Patton DL, Zarutskie PW, et al (1997) Function and structure of cilia in the fallopian tube of an infertile woman with Kartagener's syndrome. Hum Reprod 12:55–58
68. Hellstrom AC, Blegen H, Malee M, et al (2000) Recurrent fallopian tube carcinoma: TP53 mutation and clinical course. Int J Gynecol Pathol 19:145–151
69. Hellstrom AC, Silfersward C, Nilsson B, Pettersson F (1994) Carcinoma of the fallopian tube. A clinical and histopathologic review. The Radiumhemmet series. Int J Gynecol Cancer 4:395–400
70. Herbold DR, Axelrod JH, Bobowski SJ, et al (1988) Glassy cell carcinoma of the fallopian tube. A case report. Int J Gynecol Pathol 7:384–390
71. Herrera GA, Reimann BEF, Greenberg HL, Miles PA (1983) Pigmentosis tubae, a new entity: light and electron microscopic study. Obstet Gynecol 61: 80S–83S
72. Heselmeyer K, Hellstrom A-C, Blegen H, et al (1998) Primary carcinoma of the fallopian tube: comparative genomic hybridization reveals high genetic instability and a specific, recurring pattern of chromosomal aberrations. Int J Gynecol Pathol 17:245–254
73. Hetzel DJ, Stanhope CR, O'Neill BP, et al (1990) Gynecologic cancer in patients with subacute cerebellar degeneration predicted by anti-Purkinje cell antibodies and limited in metastatic volume. Mayo Clin Proc 65:1558–1563
74. Hoda SA, Huvos AG (1993) Struma salpingis associated with struma ovarii. Am J Surg Pathol 17: 1187–1189
75. Hu CY, Taymor ML, Hertig AT (1950) Primary carcinoma of the fallopian tube. Am J Obstet Gynecol 59:58–67
76. Imachi M, Tsukamoto N, Shigematsu T, et al (1992) Malignant mixed Müllerian tumor of the fallopian tube: report of two cases and review of literature. Gynecol Oncol 47:114–124
77. Jackson-York GL, Ramzy I (1992) Synchronous papillary mucinous adenocarcinoma of the endocervix and fallopian tubes. Int J Gynecol Pathol 11:63–67
78. Jacoby AF, Fuller AF Jr, Thor AD, Muntz HG (1993) Primary leiomyosarcoma of the fallopian tube. Gynecol Oncol 51:404–407
79. Jacques SM, Qureshi F, Ramirez NC, et al (1997) Retained trophoblastic tissue in fallopian tubes: a consequence of unsuspected ectopic pregnancies. Int J Gynecol Pathol 16:219–224
80. Jansen RPS (1984) Endocrine response in the fallopian tube. Endocrin Rev 5:525
81. Kariminejad MH, Scully RE (1973) Female adnexal tumor of probable wolffian origin. Cancer (Phila) 31:671–677
82. Keeney GL, Thrasher TV (1988) Metaplastic papillary tumor of the fallopian tube: a case report with ultrastructure. Int J Gynecol Pathol 7:86–92
83. Keith LG, Berger GS, Edelman DA, et al (1984) On the causation of pelvic inflammatory disease. Am J Obstet Gynecol 149:215–224
84. Kemp B, Kertschanska S, Handt S, et al (1999) Different placentation patterns in viable compared with nonviable tubal pregnancy suggest a divergent clinical management. Am J Obstet Gynecol 181: 615–620
85. Kerin JF, Williams DB, San Roman GA, et al (1992) Falloposcopic classification and treatment of fallopian tube lumen disease. Fertil Steril 57:731–741

86. Klein M, Rosen AC, Lahousen M, et al (1994) Lymphogenous metastasis in the primary carcinoma of the fallopian tube. Gynecol Oncol 55:336–338
87. Klein M, Rosen AC, Lahousen M, et al (1999) Lymphadenectomy in primary carcinoma of the fallopian tube. Cancer Lett 147:63–66
88. Korn WT, Schatzki SC, DiSciullo AJ, et al (1990) Papillary cystadenoma of the broad ligament in Von Hippel–Lindau disease. Am J Obstet Gynecol 163:596–598
89. Koshiyama M, Konishi I, Yoshida M, et al (1994) Transitional cell carcinoma of the fallopian tube: a light and electron microscopic study. Int J Gynecol Pathol 13:175–180
90. Kozlowski D, Luciano AA (1995) Bilateral atresia of the proximal ampullary segment of the fallopian tubes. J Am Assoc Gynecol Laparosc 3:99–101
91. Kristensen GS, Bollerup AC, Lind K, et al (1985) Infections with *Neisseria gonorrhoeae* and *Chlamydia trachomatis* in women with acute salpingitis. Genitourin Med 61:179
92. Kurth BE, Weston C, Reddi PP, et al (1997) Oviductal antibody response to a defined recombinant sperm antigen in macques. Biol Reprod 57:981–989
93. Kutluay L, Viedan K, Turan C, et al (1994) Tubal histopathology in ectopic pregnancies. Eur J Obstet Gynecol Reprod Biol 57:91–94
94. Kutteh WH, Hatch KD, Blackwell RE, et al (1988) Secretory immune system of the female reproductive tract: I. Immunoglobulin and secretory component-containing cells. Obstet Gynecol 71:56–60
95. Kuzela DC, Speers WC (1985) Heterotopic endometrium of the fallopian tube. Fertil Steril 44: 552–553
96. Lacy MQ, Hartmann LC, Keeney GL, et al (1995) c-erbB-2 and p53 expression in fallopian tube carcinoma. Cancer (Phila) 75:2891–2896
97. Lee A, Ying YK, Novy MJ (1997) Hysteroscopy, hystersalpingography and tubal ostial polyps in infertility patients. J Reprod Med 42:337–341
98. Lee NC, Rubin GL, Borucki R (1988) The intrauterine device and pelvic inflammatory disease revisited: new results from the Women's Health Study. Obstet Gynecol 72:1–6
99. Lefrancq T, Orain I, Michalak S, et al (1999) Herpetic salpingitis and fallopian tube prolapse. Histopathology (Oxf) 34:548–550
100. Li J, Chen X, Zhou J (1996) Ultrastructural study on the epithelium of ligated fallopian tubes in women of reproductive age. Anat Anz 178:317–320
101. Li S, Zimmerman RL, LiVolsi VA (1999) Mixed malignant germ cell tumor of the fallopian tube. Int J Gynecol Pathol 18:183–185
102. Lipscomb GH, Bran D, McCord ML, et al (1998) Analysis of three hundred fifteen ectopic pregnancies treated with single-dose methotrexate. Am J Obstet Gynecol 178:1354–1358
103. Lipscomb GH, Stovall TG, Ling FW (2000) Nonsurgical treatment of ectopic pregnancy. N Engl J Med 343:1325–1329
104. Lundorff P, Hahlin M, Sjoblom P, et al (1991) Persistent trophoblast after conservative treatment of tubal pregnancy: prediction and detection. Obstet Gynecol 77:129–133
105. Luzzatto R, Sisson G, Luzzatto L, et al (1996) Psammoma bodies and cells from in situ fallopian tube carcinoma in endometrial smears: a case report. Acta Cytol 40:295–298
106. Mansour RT, Aboulghar MA, Serour GI, et al (1991) Fluid accumulation of the uterine cavity before embryo transfer: a possible hindrance for implantation. J In Vitro Fert Embryo Transf 8:157–159
107. Marana R, Rizzi M, Muzii L, et al (1995) Correlation between the American Fertility Society classifications of adnexal adhesions and distal tubal occlusion, salpingoscopy, and reproductive outcome in tubal surgery. Fertil Steril 64:924–929
108. Marchbanks PA, Annegers JF, Coulam CB, et al (1988) Risk factors for ectopic pregnancy. A population-based study. JAMA 259:1823–1827
109. Marcus SF, Macnamee M, Brinsden P (1995) Heterotopic pregnancies after in-vitro fertilization and embryo transfer. Hum Reprod 10:1232–1236
110. Mårdh P-A, Ripa T, Svensson L, Westrom L (1977) *Chlamydia trachomatis* infection in patients with acute salpingitis. N Engl J Med 296:1377–1379
111. Martin DC, Khare VK, Miller BE (1995) Association of *Chlamydia trachomatis* immunoglobulin gamma titers with dystrophic peritoneal calcification, psammoma bodies, adhesions, and hydrosalpinges. Fertil Steril 63:39–44
112. McComb PF, Rowe TC (1989) Salpingitis isthmica nodosa: evidence it is a progressive disease. Fertil Steril 51:542–545
113. McCormack WM (1994) Pelvic inflammatory disease. N Engl J Med 330:115–119
114. McGee ZA, Jensen RL, Clemens CM, et al (1999) Gonococcal infection of fallopian tube mucosa in organ culture: relationship of mucosal tissue TNF-alpha concentration to sloughing of ciliated cells. Sex Transm Dis 26:160–165
115. Merchant RN, Prabhu SR, Kessel E (1995) Clinicopathologic study of fallopian tube closure after single trancervical insertion of quinicrine pellets. Int J Fertil Menopaus Stud 40:47–54
116. Milchgrub S, Sandstad J (1991) Arias-Stella reaction in fallopian tube epithelium. A light and electron microscopic study with a review of the literature. Am J Clin Pathol 95:892–895
117. Moore SW, Enterline HT (1975) Significance of proliferative epithelial lesions of the uterine tube. Obstet Gynecol 45:385–390
118. Morris H, Emms H, Visser T, et al (1986) Lymphoid tissue of the normal fallopian tube—a form of mucosal-associated lymphoid tissue (MALT)? Int J Gynecol Pathol 5:11–22
119. Mumford SD, Kellel E (1992) Sterilization needs in the 1990s: the case for quinacrine nonsurgical female sterilization. Am J Obstet Gynecol 167:1203–1207

120. Munichor M, Kerner H, Cohen H, et al (1997) The lipofuscin-iron association in pigmentosis tubae. Ultrastruct Pathol 21:273–280
121. Muntz HG, Tarraza HM, Goff BA, et al (1991) Combination chemotherapy in advanced adenocarcinoma of the fallopian tube. Gynecol Oncol 40:268–273
122. Muto MG, Lage JM, Berkowitz RS, et al (1991) Gestational trophoblastic disease of the fallopian tube. J Reprod Med 36:57–60
123. Navani SS, Alvarado-Cabrero I, Young RH, et al (1996) Endometrial carcinoma of the fallopian tube: a clinicopathologic analysis of 26 cases. Gynecol Oncol 63:371–378
124. Nayar R, Snell J, Silverberg SG, et al (1996) Placental site nodule occurring in a fallopian tube. Hum Pathol 27:1243–1245
125. Nordenskjold F, Ahlgren M (1991) Risk factors in ectopic pregnancy. Results of a population-based case-control study. Acta Obstet Gynecol Scand 70: 575–579
126. Nordin AJ (1994) Primary carcinoma of the fallopian tube: a 20-year literature review. Obstet Gynecol Surv 49:349–361
127. Parikh FR, Nadkarni SG, Kamat SA, et al (1997) Genital tuberculosis: a major pelvic factor causing infertility in Indian women. Fertil Steril 67:497–500
128. Patton DL, Moore DE, Spadoni LR, et al (1989) A comparison of the fallopian tube's response to overt and silent salpingitis. Obstet Gynecol 73:622–630
129. Pauerstein CJ (1974) The fallopian tube: a reappraisal. Lea & Febiger, Philadelphia
130. Pauerstein CJ, Croxatto HB, Eddy CA, et al (1986) Anatomy and pathology of tubal pregnancy. Obstet Gynecol 67:301–308
131. Pere H, Tapper J, Seppala M, et al (1998) Genomic alterations in fallopian tube carcinoma: comparison to serous uterine and ovarian carcinomas reveals similarity suggesting likeness in molecular pathogenesis. Cancer Res 58:4274–4276
132. Persaud V (1970) Etiology of tubal ectopic pregnancy. Radiologic and pathologic studies. Obstet Gynecol 36:257–263
133. Persson E, Holmberg K (1984) A longitudinal study of *Actinomyces israelii* in the female genital tract. Acta Obstet Gynecol Scand 63:207–216

133a. Peterson HB, Jeng G, Folger SG, et al (2000) The risk of menstrual abnormalities after tubal sterilization. N Engl J Med 343:1681–1687

134. Peterson HB, Xia Z, Hughes JM, et al (1997) The risk of ectopic pregnancy after tubal sterization. U.S. Collaborative Review of Sterilization Working Group. N Engl J Med 336:762–767
135. Peterson HB, Xia Z, Wilcox LS, et al (1999) Pregnancy after tubal sterilization with bipolar electrocoagulation. U.S. Collaborative Review of Sterilization Working Group. Obstet Gynecol 94:163–167
136. Pins MR, Young RH, Crum CP, et al (1997) Cervical squamous cell carcinoma in situ with intraepithelial extension to the upper genital tract and invasion of tubes and ovaries: report of a case with human papilloma virus analysis. Int J Gynecol Pathol 16:272–278
137. Puls LE, Davey DD, DePriest PD, et al (1993) Immunohistochemical staining for CA-125 in fallopian tube carcinomas. Gynecol Oncol 48:360–363
138. Ramin SM, Ramin KD, Hemsel DL (1999) Fallopian tube prolapse after hysterectomy. South Med J 92:963–966
139. Randall S, Buckley CH, Fox H (1987) Placentation in the fallopian tube. Int J Gynecol Pathol 6:132–139
140. Raziel A, Golan A, Pansky M, et al (1990) Ovarian pregnancy: a report of twenty cases in one institution. Am J Obstet Gynecol 163:1182–1185
141. Rose PG, Piver MS, Tsukada Y (1990) Fallopian tube cancer. The Roswell Park experience. Cancer (Phila) 66:2661–2667
142. Rosen AC, Klein M, Hafner E, et al (1999) Management and prognosis of primary fallopian tube carcinoma. Austrian Cooperative Study Group for Fallopian Tube Carcinoma. Gynecol Obstet Invest 47:45–51
143. Rosen AC, Reiner A, Klein M, et al (1994) Prognostic factors in primary fallopian tube carcinoma. Austrian Cooperative Study Group for Fallopian Tube Carcinoma. Gynecol Oncol 53:307–313
144. Rowe R, Mikuta J (1992) Cat-scratch salpingitis [Letter]. N Engl J Med 327:1395–1396
145. Saffos RO, Rhatigan RM, Scully RE (1980) Metaplastic papillary tumor of the fallopian tube—a distinctive lesion of pregnancy. Am J Clin Pathol 74:232–236
146. Sasano H, Sato S, Yajima A, et al (1997) Adrenal rest tumor of the broad ligament: case report with immunohistochemical study of steroidogenic enzymes. Pathol Int 47:493–496
147. Schaefer G (1970) Tuberculosis of the female genital tract. Clin Obstet Gynecol 13:965–998
148. Schiller HM, Silverberg SC (1971) Staging and prognosis in primary carcinoma of the fallopian tube. Cancer (Phila) 28:389–395
149. Scholes D, Daling JR, Stergachis A, et al (1993) Vaginal douching as a risk factor for acute pelvic inflammatory disease. Obstet Gynecol 81:601–606
150. Scully RE, Henson DE, Nielsen ML, et al (1999) Protocol for the examination of specimens from patients with carcinoma of the fallopain tube. A basis for checklists. Arch Pathol Lab Med 123:33–38
151. Scully RE, Young RH, Clement PB (1998) Tumors of the ovary, maldeveloped gonads, fallopian tube, and broad ligament. In: Atlas of tumor pathology, series 3, fasc 23. Armed Forces Institute of Pathology, Washington, DC, p 481
152. Seidman JD (1994) Mucinous lesions of the fallopian tube. A report of seven cases. Am J Surg Pathol 18:1205–1212
153. Seidman JD, Oberer S, Bitterman P, et al (1993) Pathogenesis of pseudoxanthomatous salpingiosis. Mod Pathol 6:53–55

154. Skjeldestad FE, Gargiullo PM, Kendrick JS, et al (1997) Multiple induced abortions as risk factor for ectopic pregnancy: a prospective study. Acta Obstet Gynecol Scand 76:691–696
155. Spiegelberg O (1878) Zur Kasuistik der Ovarialschwanagenschaft. Arch Gynakol 13:73
156. Sreenan JJ, Hart WR (1995) Carcinosarcomas of the female genital tract. A pathologic study of 29 metastatic tumors: further evidence for the dominant role of the epithelial component and the conversion theory of histogenesis. Am J Surg Pathol 19:666–674
157. Stock RJ, Nelson KJ (1984) Ectopic pregnancy subsequent to sterilization: histologic evaluation and clinical implications. Fertil Steril 42:211–215
158. Stovall TG, Ling FW, O'Kelley KR, et al (1990) Gross and histologic examination of tubal ligation failures in a residency training program. Obstet Gynecol 76:461–465
159. Strandell A, Lindhard A, Waldenstrom U, et al (1999) Hydrosalpinx and IVF outcome: a prospective, randomized multicentre trial in Scandinavia on salpingectomy prior to IVF. Hum Reprod 14:2762–2769
160. Su YN, Cheng WF, Chen CA, et al (1999) Pregnancy with primary tubal placental site trophoblastic tumor—a case report and literature review. Gynecol Oncol 73:322–325
161. Sweet RL, Blankfort-Doyle M, Robbie MO, Schacter J (1986) The occurrence of chlamydial and gonococcal salpingitis during the menstrual cycle. JAMA 255:2062–2064
162. Takeshima N, Hirai Y, Yamauchi K, et al (1997) Clinical usefulness of endometrial aspiraton cytology and CA-125 in the detection of fallopian tube carcinoma. Acta Cytol 41:1445–1450
163. Talbot P, Geiske C, Knoll M (1999) Oocyte pickup by the mammalian oviduct. Mol Biol Cell 10:5–8
164. Tornos C, Silva EG, McCabe KM, et al (1992) The spindle cell variant of endometrioid carcinoma. Mod Pathol 5:69A
165. Tornos C, Silva EG, Ordonez NG, et al (1995) Endometrioid carcinoma of the ovary with a prominent spindle-cell component, a source of diagnostic confusion. A report of 14 cases. Am J Surg Pathol 19:1343–1353
166. Treiman K, Liskin L (1988) IUDs—a new look. Popul Rep Ser B 16(5):1–31
167. Tziortziotis DV, Bouros AC, Ziogas VS, et al (1997) Clear cell hyperplasia of the fallopian tube epithelium associated with ectopic pregnancy: report of a case. Int J Gynecol Pathol 16:79–80
168. Van Voorhis WC, Barrett LK, Sweeney YT, et al (1997) Repeated *Chlamydia trachomatis* infection of *Macaca nemistrina* fallopian tubes produces a Th1-like cytokine response associated with fibrosis and scarring. Infect Immun 65:2175–2182
169. Vasquez G, Boeckx W, Brosens I (1995) Prospective study of tubal mucosal lesions and fertility in hydrosalpinges. Hum Reprod 10:1075–1078
170. Verhege HG, Bareither ML, Jaffe RC, Akbar M (1979) Cyclic changes in ciliation, secretion and cell height of the oviductal epithelium in women. Am J Anat 156:505–521
171. Wallace TM, Hart WR (1991) Acute chlamydial salpingitis with ascites and adnexal mass simulating a malignant neoplasm. Int J Gynecol Pathol 10:394–401
172. Ward ME, Watt PJ, Robertson JN (1974) The human fallopian tube: a laboratory model for gonococcal infection. J Infect Dis 129:650–659
173. Wild RA, Albert RD, Zaino RJ, et al (1988) Virilizing paraovarian tumors: a consequence of Nelson's syndrome? Obstet Gynecol 71:1053–1056
174. Williams M, Hill CJ, Scudamore I, et al (1993) Sperm numbers and distribution within the human fallopian tube around ovulation. Hum Reprod 8:2019–2026
175. Winkler B, Reumann W, Mitao M, et al (1985) Immunoperoxidase localization of chlamydial antigens in acute salpingitis. Am J Obstet Gynecol 152: 275–278
176. Woolas R, Jacobs I, Prys Davies A, et al (1994) What is the true incidence of primary fallopian tube carcinoma? Int J Gynecol Cancer 4:384–388
177. World Health Organization (1987) Mechanism of action, safety, and efficacy of intrauterine devices. WHO Technical Report Series 753. WHO, Geneva
178. Yamazaki K, Eyden BP (1998) Gap junctions and nerve terminals among stromal cells in human fallopian tube ampullary mucosa. J Submicrosc Cytol Pathol 30:399–408
179. Yanai-Inbar I, Siriaunkgul S, Silverberg SG (1995) Mucosal epithelial proliferation of the fallopian tube: a particular association with ovarian serous tumor of low malignant potential? Int J Gynecol Pathol 14:107–113
180. Yeaman GR, White HD, Howell A, et al (1998) The mucosal immune system in the human female reproductive tract: potential insights into the heterosexual transmission of HIV. AIDS Res Hum Retroviruses 14(suppl):S57–S62
181. Zheng W, Wolf S, Kramer EE, et al (1996) Borderline papillary serous tumour of the fallopian tube. Am J Surg Pathol 20:30–35
182. Zweemer RP, van Diest PJ, Verheijen RH, et al (2000) Molecular evidence linking primary cancer of the fallopian tube to BRCA1 germline mutations. Gynecol Oncol 76:45–50

15

Anatomy and Histology of the Ovary

Philip B. Clement, M.D.

This chapter considers the normal macroscopic and microscopic morphology of the human ovary and its hormonal function. Ultrastructural features are considered in detail elsewhere.[21] Because the anatomy and function of the ovary vary considerably at different stages in a woman's life, these aspects are considered during adulthood, childhood, and after the menopause.

The Ovary in Adulthood

Gross Anatomy

The ovaries are paired pelvic organs that lie on either side of the uterus close to the lateral pelvic wall, behind the broad ligament and anterior to the rectum. Each ovary is attached along its anterior (hilar) margin by a double fold of peritoneum, the mesovarium, to the posterior aspect of the broad ligament. Each ovary is also attached at its medial pole to the ipsilateral uterine cornu by the ovarian (utero-ovarian) ligament, and from the superior aspect of its lateral pole to the lateral pelvic wall by the infundibulopelvic (suspensory) ligament. The location of the ovary posterior to the broad ligament and a similar relationship of the ovarian ligament to the ipsilateral fallopian tube aid in the determination of the laterality of a salpingo-oophorectomy specimen.

Adult ovaries are ovoid, approximately 3.0–5 cm by 1.5–3.0 cm by 0.6–1.5 cm, and weigh 5–8 g. Their size and weight, however, vary considerably depending on their content of follicular derivatives. Their pink-white exterior in early reproductive life is usually smooth (Fig. 15.1), but becomes increasingly convoluted thereafter. Thin-walled, fluid-filled cystic follicles and bright yellow corpora lutea may be partially visible from the external aspect. Three poorly defined zones are discernible on the sectioned surface: an outer cortex, an inner medulla, and the hilus. Follicular structures (cystic follicles, corpora lutea, corpora albicantia) are usually visible in the cortex and medulla (Fig. 15.2).

Blood Vessels

The ovarian artery, a branch of the aorta, courses along the infundibulopelvic ligament and the mesovarial border of the ovary where it anastomoses with the ovarian branch of the uterine artery. Approximately 10 arterial branches from this arcade penetrate the ovarian hilus and course through the medulla, becoming markedly coiled and branched.[14,113] These helicine arteries have longitudinal ridges of intimal smooth muscle.[14] At the corticomedullary junction, the medullary arteries and arterioles form a plexus from which smaller, straight cortical arterioles arise and penetrate the cortex in a radial fashion. These cortical arterioles branch and anastomose, forming sets of interconnecting vascular arcades that give rise to dense capillary networks within the theca layers of the ovarian follicles (Fig. 15.3).[113]

The veins within the ovary accompany the arteries and become large and tortuous in the medulla. The veins join together in the hilus, forming a plexus that drains into the ovarian veins[14,113]; the latter traverse the mesovarium and course along the in-

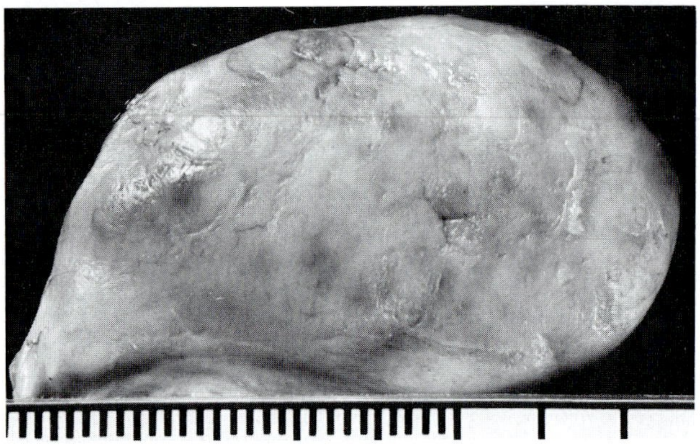

Fig. 15.1. Normal adult ovary from a 25-year-old woman. Except for occasional fibrous adhesions, the external surface is smooth and white.

fundibulopelvic ligament. The left and right ovarian veins drain into the left renal vein and the inferior vena cava, respectively.

Lymphatics

Ovarian lymphatics originate predominantly within the theca layers of the follicles. The granulosa layer of a maturing follicle is devoid of lymphatics in contrast to its counterpart within the corpus luteum, which possesses a rich supply of lymphatics.[106] The lymphatics, independent of blood vessels, traverse the ovarian stroma to drain into larger trunks that form a plexus at the hilus. Within the hilus, the lymphatics and blood vessels converge, with the former coiled around veins in a helicoid fashion.[106] Four to eight efferent channels enter the mesovarium, where they converge to form the subovarian plexus that is joined by branches from the fallopian tube and uterine fundus. Leaving the plexus, the drainage trunks diminish in number and size, passing along the free border of the infundibulopelvic ligament enmeshed with the ovarian veins. From there they accompany the ovarian vessels, juxtaposed to the psoas muscle, and drain into the upper paraaortic lymph nodes at the level of the lower pole of the kidney.[36,106] Accessory channels can bypass the subovarian plexus, passing through the broad ligament to the internal iliac, external iliac, and interaortic lymph nodes, or via the round ligament to the iliac and inguinal lymph nodes.[36,106] When the pelvic and paraaortic lymph nodes are extensively replaced by tumor, retrograde lymphatic flow may provide a rare route of tumor spread to the ovaries.

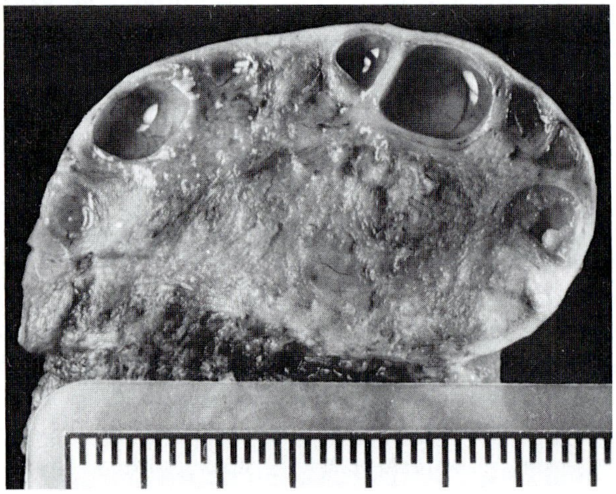

Fig. 15.2. Normal adult ovary (*cut surface*). Occasional cystic follicles are present in the cortex.

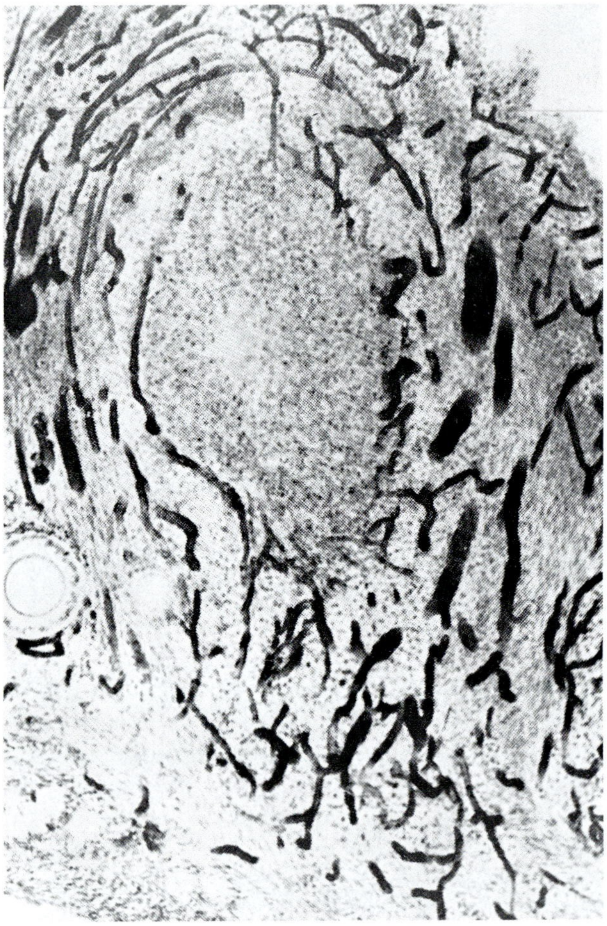

Fig. 15.3. Perifollicular capillary network. Ovarian vessels were injected with colored gelatin before sectioning. (Reprinted by permission of Leeson and Leeson (1970) Histology. Philadelphia, Saunders.)

Nerves

The nerve supply of the ovary arises from a sympathetic plexus that is enmeshed with the ovarian vessels in the infundibulopelvic ligament.[59] Nerve fibers, which are predominantly nonmyelinated, accompany the ovarian artery, entering the ovary at the hilus. Delicate terminal fibers, many surrounding small arteries and arterioles, penetrate the medulla and cortex to terminate as plexuses surrounding the follicules.[59,100] Adrenergic nerve fibers and terminals have been shown to be in close contact with smooth muscle cells in the cortical stroma and theca externa. Ovarian sympathetic innervation may play a role in follicular maturation, follicular rupture, or both.[7,59,91] In addition, catecholamines can stimulate progesterone production by the ovarian follicles and androgen production by the ovarian stroma in vitro.[35]

Surface Epithelium

The *ovarian surface epithelium* consists of a single, focally pseudostratified layer of modified mesothelial cells. The cells vary from flat to cuboidal to columnar, and several types may be seen in different areas of the same ovary (Fig. 15.4). The surface cells are separated from the underlying stroma by a distinct basement membrane. In oophorectomy specimens, the epithelium is almost always denuded as a result of handling by the surgeon and pathologist, as well as drying artifact as a result of delayed fixation. Preserved epithelium is usually confined to sulci and areas protected by surface adhesions. Surface epithelium within these crevices may lose its connection with the surface, giving rise to surface epithelial inclusion glands and cysts (see Chapter 16, Nonneoplastic Lesions of the Ovary).

Histochemical studies have demonstrated glycogen, as well as acid and neutral mucopolysaccharides, within surface epithelial cells.[13,81] Unlike extraovarian mesothelial cells, surface epithelial cells of the ovary have 17-beta-hydroxysteroid dehydrogenase activity.[13] The surface epithelial cells are immunoreactive for cytokeratin, Ber-EP4, desmoplakin, vimentin, transforming growth factor-alpha, and receptors for estrogen, progesterone, and epidermal growth factor receptors, but not desmin.[11,27–29,57,61,72,89,116] Several antigens associated with ovarian tumors of surface epithelial origin have been demonstrated with variable frequency, including CA125,[66,96,98] CA19-9 (CA 19-9),[20] and MH99,[23] but not carcinoembryonic antigen.[20,98]

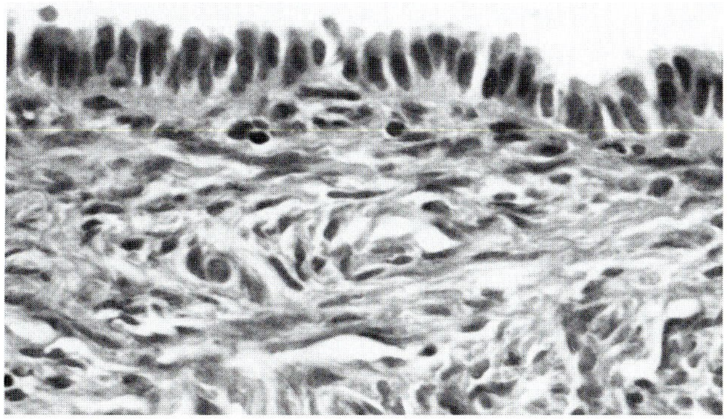

Fig. 15.4. Ovarian surface epithelium. A single layer of columnar cells overlies the ovarian stroma.

Stroma

Histology

Because the cortical and medullary stroma is continuous, similar in appearance, and varies in volume from one individual to another, the boundary between these two zones is poorly defined and arbitrary. The spindle-shaped stromal cells, which have scant cytoplasm and resemble fibroblasts, are typically arranged in whorls or a storiform pattern (Fig. 15.5a) within a dense reticulum network (Fig. 15.5b) and a variable amount of collagen, which is most abundant in the superficial cortex. Although the latter has been sometimes erroneously designated the tunica albuginea, it lacks the densely collagenous, almost acellular appearance and sharp delineation of this layer in the testis. Fine droplets of cytoplasmic lipid within the stromal cells may be appreciable with special stains, especially in the late reproductive and postmenopausal age groups.[38] The stromal cells are immunoreactive for vimentin, actin, and desmin,[11,28,29,71,89,124] as well as for estrogen, progesterone, and testosterone receptors.[4] In many women of late-reproductive and postmenopausal age, there is a decrease in stromal volume and cellularity, with an increase in collagen.

A variety of other cells may be found within the ovarian stroma, most of which are probably derived from the spindle-shaped stromal cells:

1. Luteinized stromal cells are found singly or in small nests at a distance from the follicles, most often in the medulla. They are polygonal with abundant eosinophilic to vacuolated cytoplasm containing variable amounts of lipid, a central round nucleus, and a prominent nucleolus. The cytoplasm is immunoreactive for inhibin[103] and occasionally testosterone.[92] Luteinized stromal cells increase during pregnancy and after the menopause, probably as a result of elevated levels of circulating gonadotropins during these periods.[16,38] In one autopsy study,[16] diligent searching found luteinized stromal cells in 13% of women under the age of 55

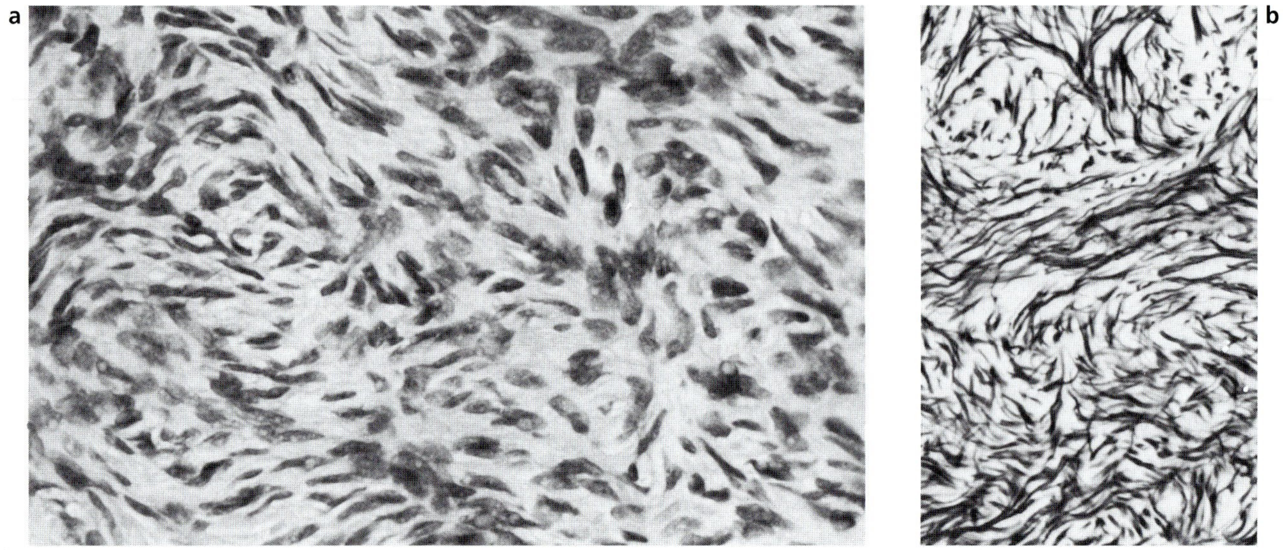

Fig. 15.5. Ovarian stroma. a: Plump, fibroblastic cells are arranged in whorls. **b:** Dense pericellular reticulum pattern is evident (reticulin stain).

years and in one-third of women over that age; the frequency of their detection increased with increasing degrees of stromal proliferation. More exhaustive sampling might indicate that luteinized stromal cells are a normal finding in the ovary, particularly in later life.[16] In this age group, the presence of luteinized cells is not usually associated with clinical evidence of an endocrine disturbance. In some older women, but more often in younger patients, more striking degrees of stromal luteinization (stromal hyperthecosis) are frequently associated with androgenic or estrogenic manifestations or both (see Chapter 16, Nonneoplastic Lesions of the Ovary).

2. Enzymatically active stromal cells (EASC) are characterized by their oxidative and other enzymatic activity.[38,76,93,122] Some EASC correspond to luteinized stromal cells, but most cannot be distinguished from neighboring, nonreactive stromal cells in routine histologic preparations.[122] They are typically found in the medulla and increase in number with age, occurring in more than 80% of postmenopausal women.[122]
3. Decidual cells, representing focal decidual transformation of the ovarian stroma in response to elevated progesterone levels, are found in almost every ovary examined at term. Similar cells are also occasionally found in nonpregnant women (see Chapter 16, Nonneoplastic Lesions of the Ovary).[10,12,49,58,128]
4. Endometrial stromal-type cells (stromal endometriosis, "ovarian stromatosis") (see Chapter 17, Diseases of the Peritoneum).
5. Smooth muscle cells have been demonstrated within the ovarian stroma in otherwise normal ovaries but also in certain pathologic conditions (see Chapter 16).[121] Smooth muscle cells have also been identified on ultrastructural examination within the normal theca externa of the follicles.[99]
6. Fat cells (see Chapter 16).
7. Stromal Leydig cells (see Chapter 16).

Rare cells of neuroendocrine or APUD (amino precursor uptake and decarboxylation) type, which may be of stromal origin, have been demonstrated within the ovarian stroma in approximately 6% of normal women in one study.[53] The cells occur in small groups in the corticomedullary–stromal junction and exhibit argyrophilia and argentaffinity. Their clinical significance and hormonal function, if any, are unknown.

Hormone Synthesis

Numerous studies have demonstrated the steroidogenic potential and the gonadotropin responsiveness of the ovarian stroma in both premenopausal and postmenopausal women.[19,32,46,64,65,75,79,84,87,134] In vitro incubation of ovarian stromal tissue indicates that it secretes androstenedione, as well as smaller quantities of testosterone and dehydroepiandrosterone.[115] In vitro production of these androgens is enhanced by human chorionic gonadotropin (hCG), pituitary gonadotropins, and insulin, consistent with the presence of receptors for these hormones within the stromal cells.[9,92,93] To what extent the ovarian stroma contributes to the androgen pool in normal premenopausal women is unknown; it is likely the source of small amounts of testosterone.

Primordial Follicles

Approximately 400,000 *primordial follicles* are present at birth. Subsequently, their numbers continue to decrease progressively by atresia and folliculogenesis until their eventual disappearance. In women of reproductive age, the primordial follicles are irregularly distributed throughout a narrow band in the superficial cortex. They consist of a primary oocyte, 40–70 μm in diameter, surrounded by a single layer of flattened, mitotically inactive, granulosa cells resting on a thin basal lamina (Fig. 15.6). Rare primordial (and maturing) follicles contain multiple

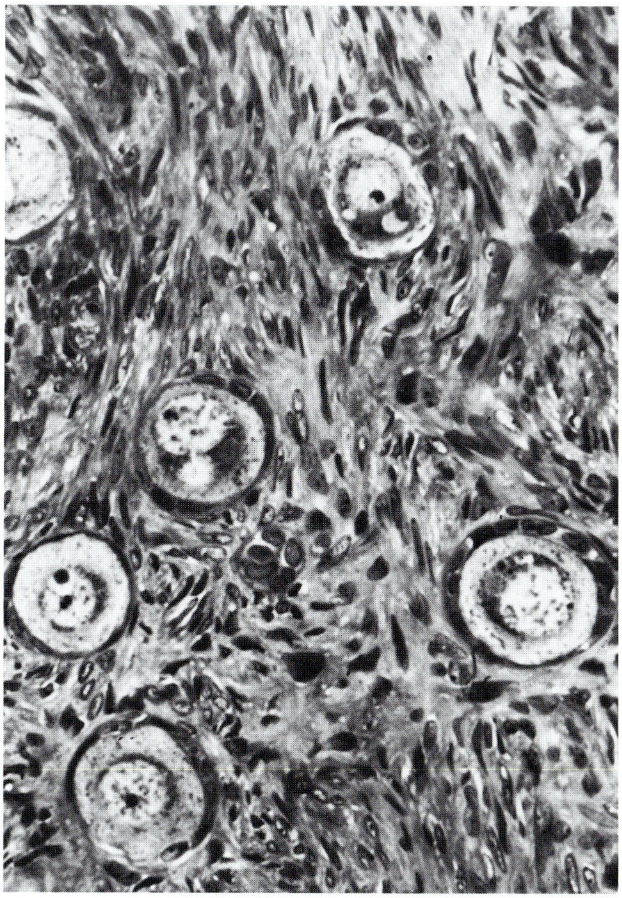

Fig. 15.6. Primoridal follicles within ovarian cortex. The primary oocytes are surrounded by a single layer of flattened granulosa cells. Note perinuclear crescentic zones (Balbiani's vitelline body) in the cytoplasm of several of the oocytes. (Reprinted by permission of Baca and Zamboni, ref. 6.)

oocytes, particularly in individuals less than 20 years of age.[43] The large spherical nucleus of the oocyte has finely granular, uniformly dispersed chromatin and one or more dense, threadlike nucleoli[6]; rare oocytes have multiple nuclei.[43,77] Within the cytoplasm of the oocyte is a paranuclear, eosinophilic, crescentic zone representing a complex of interelated organelles ("Balbiani's vitelline body") (Fig. 15.6).[51,52] Within the vitelline body is a dark spot, the centrosome, surrounded by a halo, which in turn is flanked by darker, periodic acid–Schiff- (PAS-) positive, granular zones rich in mitochondria.[51,52] The cytoplasm of the oocyte lacks the abundant glycogen and the high alkaline phosphatase activity characteristic of the primordial germ cells and the oogonia of the embryonic gonad.

Maturing Follicles

Folliculogenesis

Folliculogenesis refers to the continuous process occurring throughout reproductive life whereby cohorts of primordial follicles undergo maturation during each menstrual cycle. Follicular maturation begins during the luteal phase and continues throughout the follicular phase of the next cycle. Each month usually only one developing follicle is dominant, achieving complete maturation and release of the oocyte (ovulation). The other developing follicles undergo atresia (see "Atretic Follicles"). Folliculogenesis and atresia also occur prenatally, throughout childhood, and during pregnancy, although maturing follicles rarely reach the preovulatory follicle stage during these periods.[31,44,78,94]

The first morphologic evidence of follicular maturation is enlargement of the oocyte and alteration of the granulosa cells from flat to cuboidal or columnar (*primary follicle*). The granulosa cells proliferate, forming three to five concentric layers around the oocyte (*secondary* or *preantral follicle*) (Fig. 15.7). Preantral follicles measure from 50 to 400 μm in diameter; as they increase in size, they migrate into the deeper cortex and medulla. Simultaneously, the surrounding ovarian stromal cells become specialized into several layers of theca interna cells and an outer, poorly defined layer of theca externa cells. Secretion of mucopolysaccharide-rich fluid by the granulosa cells results in their separation by fluid-filled clefts. The latter eventually coalesce to form a single large cavity or antrum lined by several layers of granulosa cells (*tertiary*, *antral*, or *vesicular follicle*) (Fig. 15.8). As the follicle enlarges because of continued fluid secretion into the antrum, the oocyte reaches its definitive size and an eccentric position at one pole of the follicle. At this site the

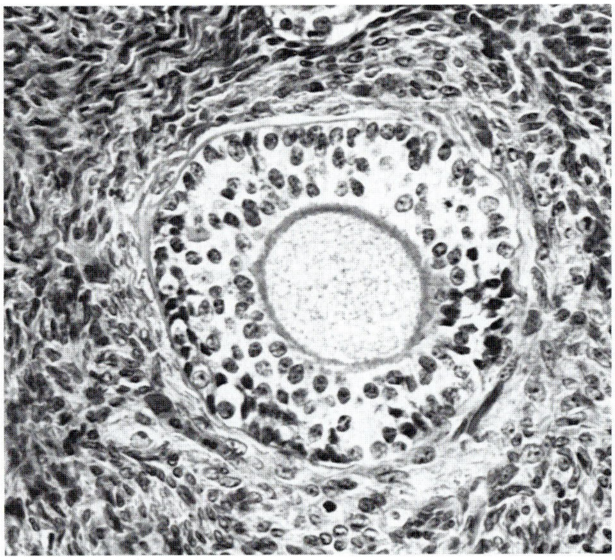

Fig. 15.7. Preantral follicle. Several layers of granulosa cells surround the oocyte. A theca interna layer is not yet apparent.

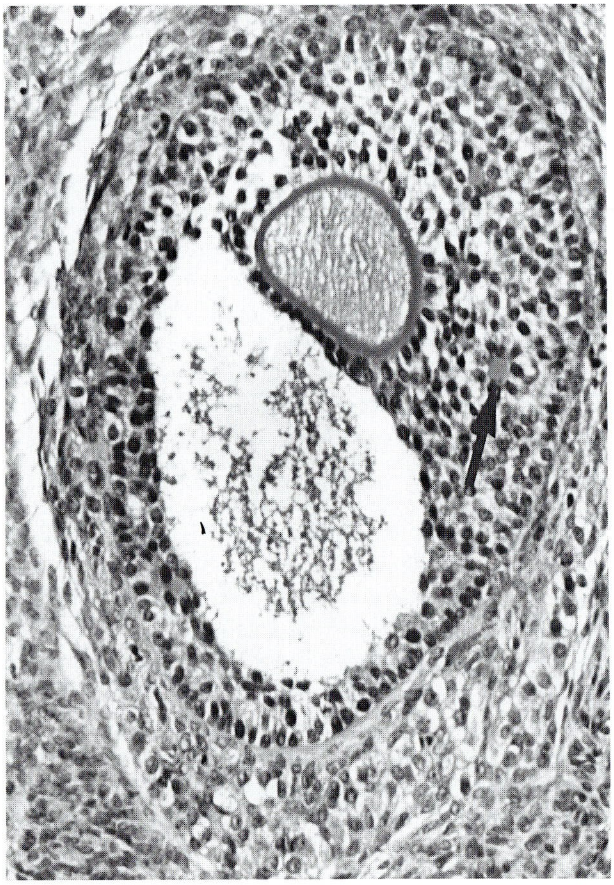

Fig. 15.8. Antral follicle. Note Call–Exner body (*arrow*) within the granulosa layer. A well-developed theca interna layer is now visible.

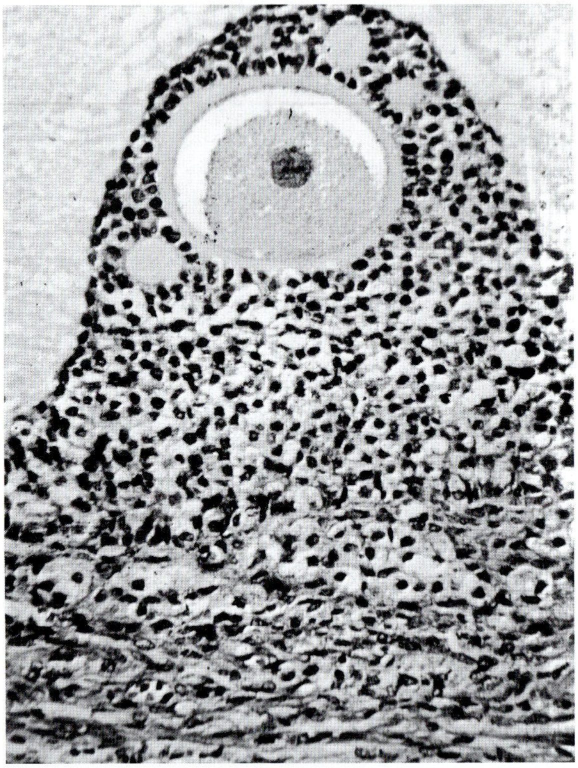

Fig. 15.9. Graafian follicle with antrum (*top*). Notice the cumulus oophorus containing the oocyte with its surrounding zona pellucida. Three Call–Exner bodies are present near the oocyte.

granulosa cells proliferate to form the cumulus oophorus, which contains the oocyte and protrudes into the antrum (*mature* or *graafian follicle*) (Fig. 15.9).

Ovulation

During each cycle, usually less than four mature follicles in each ovary reach a diameter of 4–5 mm by the middle to late luteal phase; one of them will become the preovulatory follicle of the next cycle.[86] Late in follicular growth, the oocyte, its surrounding zona pellucida, and a single layer of radially disposed, columnar granulosa cells, the corona radiata, detach from the cumulus oophorus and float in the antral fluid. The preovulatory follicle shortly before ovulation reaches a diameter of 15–25 mm[7,86]; it partially protrudes from the ovarian surface at a point that represents the eventual rupture point, or stigma. The surface epithelial and stromal cells in this area become attenuated and degenerate, changes that may be secondary to local ischemia and release of proteolytic enzymes and prostaglandins.[7] The preovulatory follicle then ruptures, possibly aided by contraction of the perifollicular smooth muscle cells, with liberation of the follicular fluid, the oocyte, and its corona radiata into the peritoneal cavity. Following ovulation, the stigma is occluded by a mass of coagulated follicular fluid, fibrin, blood, and granulosa and connective tissue cells.[7] The specific components of the maturing follicle are considered in more detail.

Oocyte and Zona Pellucida

As the oocyte matures it triples in size. When the oocyte of the preantral follicle is 80 μm in diameter, it is encased by an eosinophilic, PAS-positive, homogeneous, acellular layer, the zona pellucida (Fig. 15.7). Its formation is usually attributed to the granulosa cells, but the oocyte may also play a role. At the end of its development, the zona pellucida is a 20- to 25-μm-thick membrane (Figs. 15.8 and 15.9) consisting of fine filamentous material of medium electron density[6] rich in acid mucopolysaccharides and glycoprotein.[39]

During the early stages of follicular growth, the oocyte nucleus has an appearance similar to that seen in the primordial follicle. Shortly before ovulation, the oocyte within the preovulatory follicle enters telophase of the first meiotic division. Chromosomal reduction occurs by migration of one-half the oocyte chromosomes into a portion of the oocyte cytoplasm that separates from the cell as the first polar body. The latter lies within the perivitelline space between the plasma membrane of the oocyte and the inner aspect of the zona pellucida. After completion of the first meiotic division, the oocyte is now referred to as the secondary oocyte. Immediately after expulsion of the first polar body, the secondary oocyte enters the second meiotic division, arresting at metaphase until fertilization occurs.

Granulosa Cells

Granulosa cells within maturing and mature follicles are polyhedral and measure 5–7 μm in diameter; those resting on the basement membrane are often columnar. Granulosa cells have pale scanty cytoplasm, indistinct cell borders, and small, round to oval, hyperchromatic nuclei, which typically lack nuclear grooves (Fig. 15.10a).[140] Mitotic figures are usually numerous in maturing follicles but decrease in number immediately before ovulation. Until the onset of luteinization several hours before ovulation, cytoplasmic lipid is absent or sparse, as are the histochemical patterns of steroidogenesis. The cytoplasm of granulosa cells of primary, secondary, and mature follicles is immunoreactive for cytokeratin, vimentin, desmoplakin, and inhibin.[11,28,89,103]

Granulosa cells typically surround small cavities, Call–Exner bodies (see Figs. 15.8 and 15.9), that represent a distinctive feature of normal and neoplastic granulosa cells. Call–Exner bodies are delimited from the granulosa cells by a basal lamina and typically contain an eosinophilic, PAS-positive, filamentous material consisting of basal lamina.[14,39] Unlike the theca layers, the granulosa layer of maturing follicles is avascular and devoid of a reticulum framework (Fig. 15.10b).

Theca Cells

Theca cells differentiate continuously from the stromal cells at the periphery of developing follicles

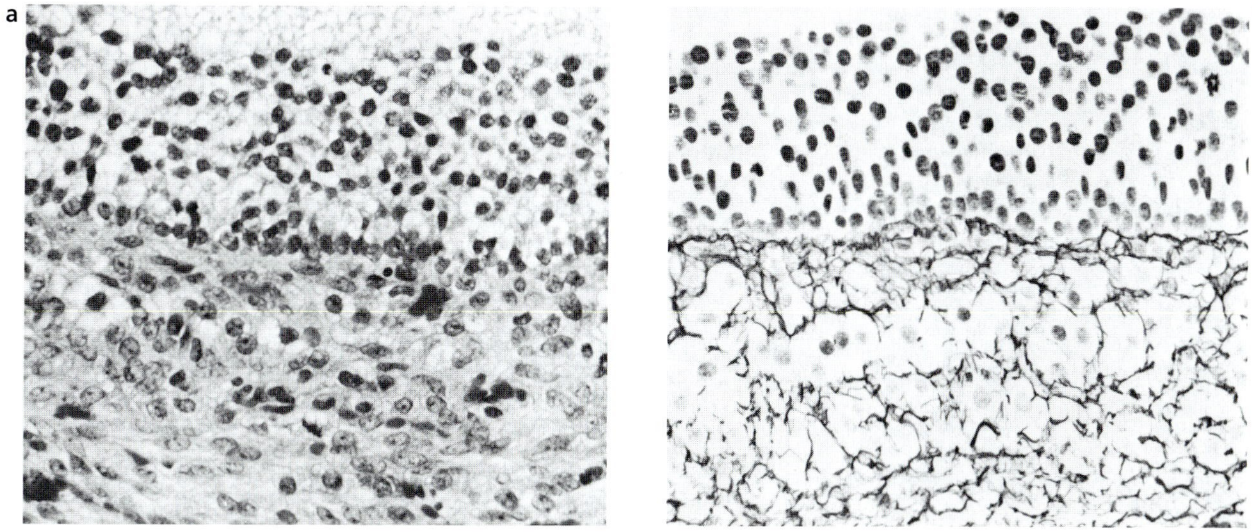

Fig. 15.10. Lining of mature follicle. a: The granulosa layer is surrounded by an outer layer of luteinized theca interna cells. **b**: A reticulin stain reveals a reticulum network in the theca interna layer but an absence of reticulum in the granulosa layer.

from fetal life to the termination of the menopause. The thecal component of the antral follicle is characterized by a well-developed theca interna and a less well defined theca externa.

The theca interna layer is three or four cells thick and lies external to the granulosa layer, from which it is separated by a basement membrane. Unlike the granulosa cells of developing and mature follicles, the theca interna cells typically have a luteinized or partially luteinized appearance and have steroidogenic histochemical patterns.[30,38,63] Luteinization of the theca interna of maturing follicles is particularly prominent during pregnancy. The round to polygonal luteinized theca cells are 12–20 μm in diameter and have abundant, eosinophilic to vacuolated cytoplasm containing variable amounts of lipid. A central, round, vesicular nucleus typically contains a single, prominent nucleolus (see Figs. 15.8–15.10). Theca cells are immunoreactive for inhibin[103] and vimentin but not cytokeratin.[11] Mitotic figures are typically present within the theca cells of maturing follicles and may be numerous. The theca interna layer contains a rich vascular plexus consisting of dilated capillaries, as well as a dense reticulum that surrounds each cell (Fig. 15.10b). Tangential sections through the luteinized theca interna may result in seemingly isolated nodules of luteinized theca cells, which are misinterpreted occasionally as foci of stromal luteinization.

The theca externa is a poorly defined layer of variable thickness that surrounds the theca interna and merges almost imperceptibly with the adjacent ovarian stroma. It is composed of plump, spindle stromal cells (which lack steroidogenic histochemical features), as well as circumferential collagen bundles, blood vessels, and lymphatics.[42] Some of the spindle cells are immunoreactive for actin.[29] The spindle cells are typically highly mitotic and may be misinterpreted as tumor cells, such as those of a fibrosarcoma, particularly when only the theca externa edge of the follicle is seen in a microscopic section (Fig. 15.11).

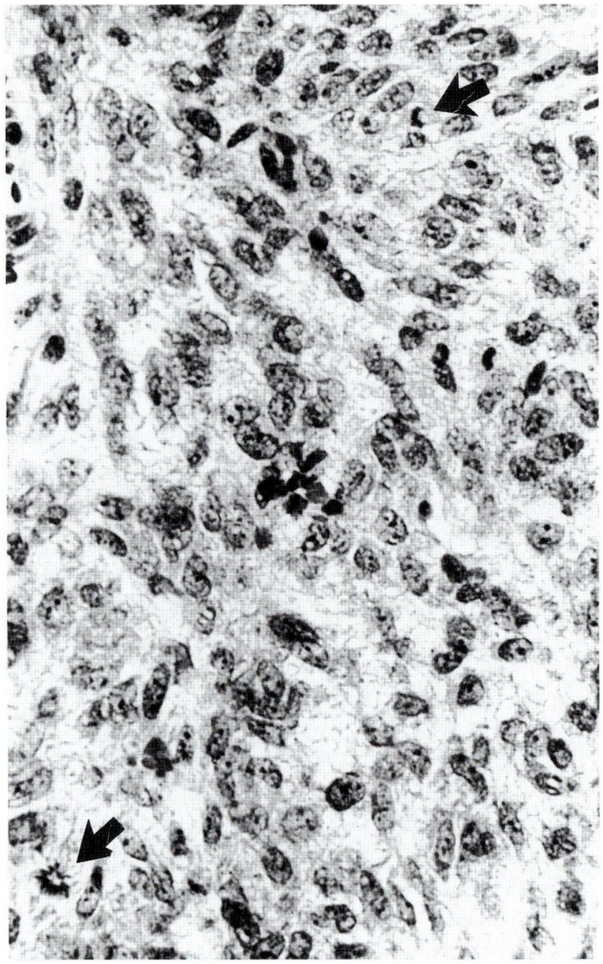

Fig. 15.11. Theca externa of maturing follicle. Notice the plump oval to spindle cells with mitotic figures (*arrows*).

Hormone Synthesis

Only the later stages of follicular maturation are under gonadotropin control. As a small antral follicle develops into a preovulatory follicle, the sequence of endocrine events within its antral fluid differs from most, if not all, other antral follicles.[82,83] Early in its development, follicle-stimulating hormone (FSH) receptors and intrafollicular FSH increase, accompanied by a rise in estradiol (E_2) receptors within the granulosa cells of the preovulatory follicle.[37,82,83,125] E_2 levels within the follicle and serum peak during the mid- to late-follicular phase, when plasma FSH falls to a basal level.[37,82,83] At this stage the follicle is self-sustaining, continuing to mature under the influence of intrafollicular FSH and E_2.[84] During the late follicular phase, plasma luteinizing hormone (LH) and LH receptors become apparent within the granulosa cells of the preovulatory follicle but not of other follicles.[125] In contrast, LH receptors are present within the theca cells of all follicles throughout the follicular phase.[125]

Although circulating E_2 is likely derived from both the granulosa cells and the LH-stimulated theca cells, intrafollicular E_2 is derived almost exclusively from the granulosa cells by FSH-dependent aromatization of theca-derived androgen.[84,85] Aromatase activity is highest in the preovulatory follicle, thereby maintaining a high E_2:androstenedione ratio.[54,82,83] In contrast, other follicles that will undergo atresia are FSH and aromatase deficient and have high androgen:estrogen ratios within their fluid. Granulosa and theca LH receptors increase gradually throughout follicular development, possibly under the control of FSH, reaching peak concentrations just before ovulation.[37,82,83] Simultaneously, high estrogen levels initiate a preovulatory surge of plasma LH,[102,142] which induces luteinization of the granulosa cells, an increase in intrafollicular progesterone (P) concentration, and a small preovulatory rise in circulating P.[40,82,83] The rising plasma P and peaking estrogen levels further augment the LH surge, initiate a smaller increase in FSH, and trigger ovulation. Ovulation occurs 36–38 hours after the onset of the LH surge, 24–36 hours after the estradiol peak, and 10–12 hours after the LH peak.[40]

The ovarian follicles also produce nonsteroidal hormones. Inhibin, a glycoprotein synthesized by the granulosa cells, is secreted into the follicular fluid and ovarian venous effluent in amounts that correlate with steroid levels.[40,131,132] Although inhibin secretion is predominantly under the control of LH,[80] it reduces, by negative feedback, FSH secretion from the hypothalamic–pituitary unit. Also secreted by granulosa cells is müllerian-inhibiting substance.[34] High concentrations of prorenin are present within the fluid of mature follicles[123]; their granulosa, theca, and stromal cells are immunoreactive for renin and angiotensin II.[101] The function of the renin-angiotensin system within the ovary is largely unknown.

Corpus Luteum of Menstruation

Dating the Corpus Luteum

After ovulation on the 14th day of the typical 28-day menstrual cycle, and in the absence of fertilization,

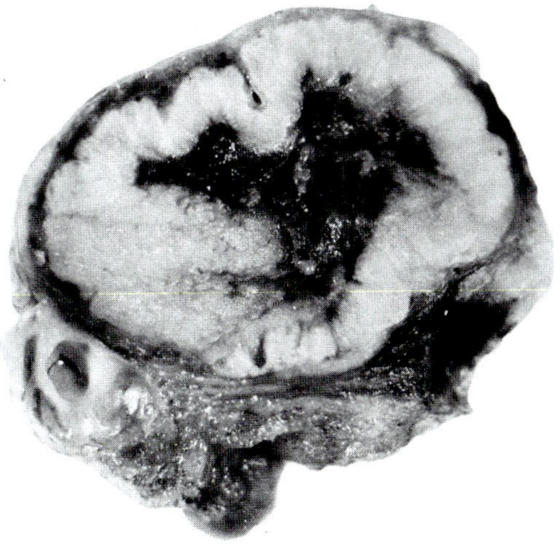

Fig. 15.12. Mature corpus luteum of menstruation. A yellow convoluted border surrounds a central hemorrhagic coagulum.

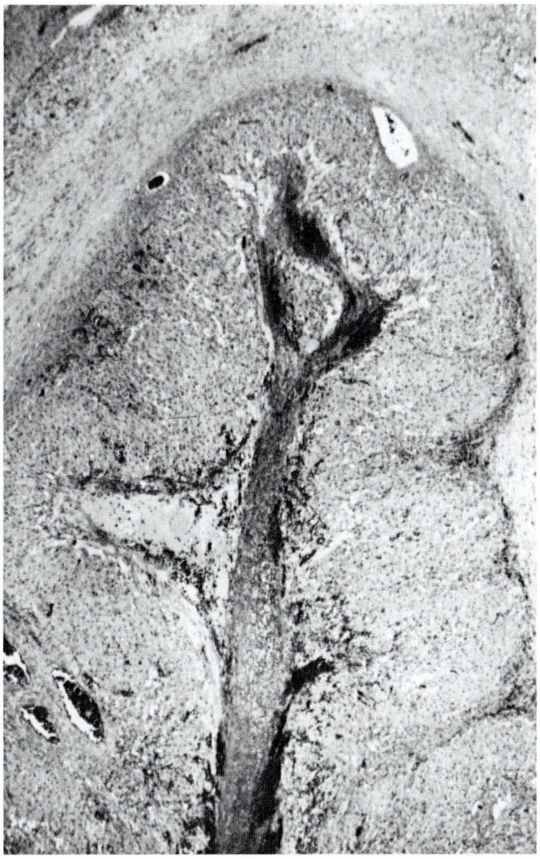

Fig. 15.13. Mature corpus luteum of menstruation. Festooned lining composed of granulosa–lutein cells surrounds a central cavity.

the collapsed ovulatory follicle becomes the *corpus luteum of menstruation* (*CLM*), a 1.5- to 2.0-cm, round structure with a festooned contour; a center filled with a gray, focally hemorrhagic coagulum; and a color that changes during the luteal phase from brown to orange-yellow as it acquires more lipid (Figs. 15.12 and 15.13). Occasionally, the CLM is cystic, but this feature is more characteristic of the corpus luteum of pregnancy (see following). If the cyst exceeds 3 cm, the structure is designated a corpus luteum cyst, and if smaller, a cystic corpus luteum.

Histology

The luteinized granulosa cells of the mature CLM are 30- to 35-μm polygonal cells with abundant, pale eosinophilic cytoplasm that contain numerous small lipid droplets[42] and a spherical nucleus with one or two large nucleoli (Figs. 15.14 and 15.15).[42] The histochemical pattern of these cells varies with the age of the CLM but generally is typical of steroidogenic cells.[30,38,141] The cytoplasm of luteinized granulosa cells immunoreacts for inhibin[103] and vimentin, but

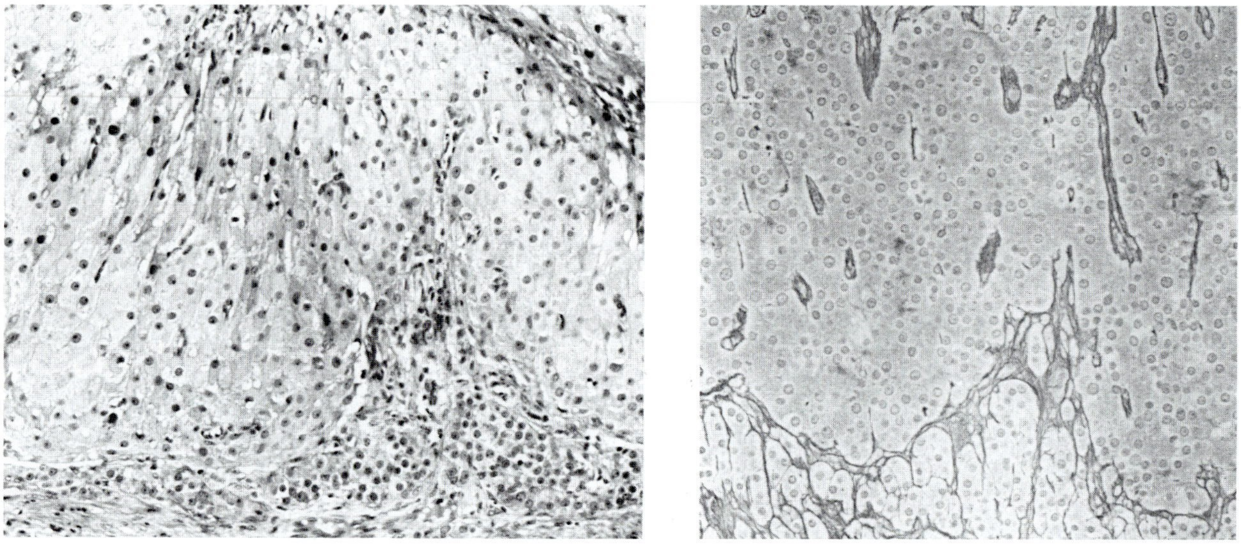

Fig. 15.14. Mature corpus luteum of menstruation. a: The lining is composed of a thick layer of large granulosa–lutein cells and an outer, thinner layer of smaller theca–lutein cells. **b**: A reticulin stain shows a dense reticulum network in the theca interna and a beginning reticulum network, predominantly perivascular, within the granulosa–lutein layer.

in contrast to granulosa cells of maturing and mature follicles, contains little or no cytokeratin.[28]

The theca interna forms an irregular outer layer of the CLM several cells in thickness and ensheathes the vascular septa that extend into the center of the structure (Figs. 15.14 and 15.15).[42] When these septa are cut in cross section, triangular-shaped wedges of theca cells appear in the sulci of the convoluted, thick granulosa lutein layer. In all but the earliest stages of the CLM, the theca lutein cells are approximately half the size of granulosa lutein cells; they contain a round to oval nucleus with a single prominent nucleolus. Their cytoplasm, which is less abundant and stains more deeply than that of the granulosa lutein cells, contains lipid droplets that are usually larger than those in granulosa lutein cells. Theca interna cells of the mature CLM are immunoreactive for inhibin.[103]

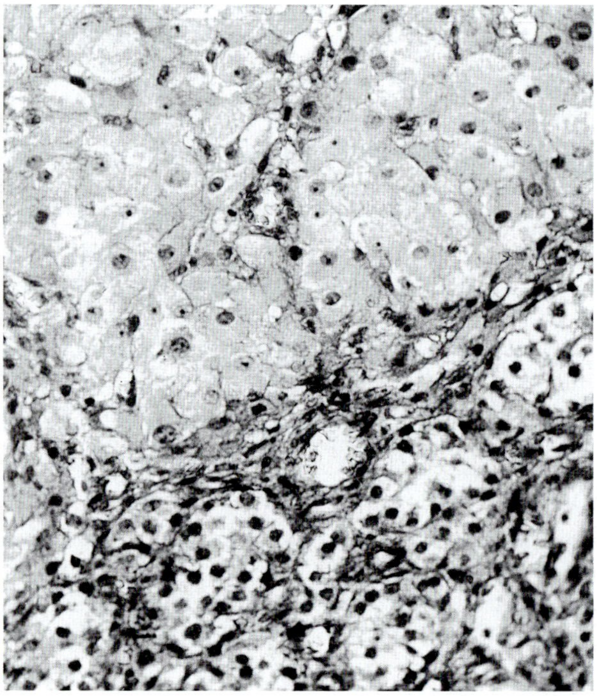

Fig. 15.15. Corpus luteum of menstruation. Notice the large luteinized granulosa cells (*top*) and the nests of luteinized theca interna cells (*bottom*).

During the maturation of the CLM, capillaries from the theca interna penetrate the granulosa layer and reach the central cavity. Fibroblasts that accompany the vessels form an increasingly dense reticulum within the granulosa layer and the inner fibrous layer that lines the central cavity (Fig. 15.14b).

If fertilization does not occur, involutional changes begin on postovulatory day 8 or 9.[24] The granulosa lutein cells decrease in size, their nuclei become pyknotic, and they accumulate abundant cytoplasmic lipid (Fig. 15.16). There is a progressive infiltration of T lymphocytes (mostly CD8+, a minority of which express perforin) and cells of monocyte/macrophage lineage.[48] There is a decrease in histochemical staining of enzymes associated with steroid biosynthesis and an increase in hydrolytic enzymes.[30] The cells eventually undergo dissolution and are phagocytosed.[1] During a period of several months, progressive fibrosis and shrinkage of the

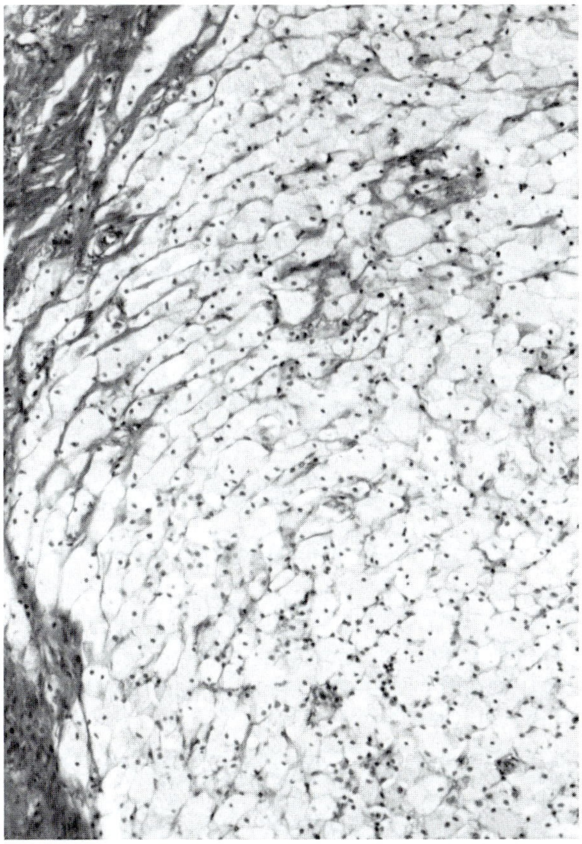

Fig. 15.16. Degenerating corpus luteum of menstruation. Granulosa–lutein cells have pyknotic nuclei and abundant cytoplasmic lipid.

corpus luteum occur, with conversion to a corpus albicans.[81]

Hormone Synthesis

The formation and function of the CLM are under the control of LH, reflected by the numerous LH receptors within the granulosa lutein cells.[40] FSH receptors have also been identified in the early corpus luteum, although the role of FSH in luteal function is unknown.[125] Although P is the major steroid hormone formed in vivo and in vitro by the CLM, it also synthesizes, both in vitro and in vivo, E_1 and E_2, as well as androgens, predominantly androstenedione.[74] In vitro P and estrogen synthesis is stimulated by both hCG and LH.[114]

After ovulation, LH, FSH, and E_2 levels fall, but the LH concentration is sufficient to maintain the CLM, producing a midluteal peak in P and E_2 concentration. If fertilization does not occur, the increased levels of P and estrogen result in a fall of LH and FSH to basal levels via a negative feedback mechanism, with a marked decline in P and E_2 synthesis after the 22nd day of the cycle.[17,37,40,110] These changes are accompanied by morphologic involution of the CLM and the onset of menses. Luteolysis appears to be estrogen related, possibly secondary to an estrogen-induced reduction in LH receptors or by enhancement of the luteolytic action of prostaglandins synthesized by the CLM.[40,135] A nonsteroidal LH receptor-binding inhibitor, which increases in concentration during the luteal phase, may also play a role.[40] Epidermal growth factor receptors have also been identified within the CLM, but their physiologic significance is unknown.[5]

Corpus Luteum of Pregnancy

Gross Appearance

On gross inspection, the *corpus luteum of pregnancy* (*CLP*) may be indistinguishable from the CLM, but it is usually larger and bright yellow in contrast to the orange-yellow of the late CLM.[50] The larger size, which may account for up to half the ovarian volume, primarily results from the presence of a central cystic cavity filled with fluid or a coagulum composed of fibrin and blood (Fig. 15.17).[95,128,136] When the cavity is large, typically in the first trimester, the wall of the CLP may lose its convolutions, becoming stretched and attenuated to the extent that it may consist focally of only the inner fibrous layer.[95] Obliteration of the cavity usually begins by the fifth month of gestation and is typically completed by term. The CLP thus gradually decreases in size, and

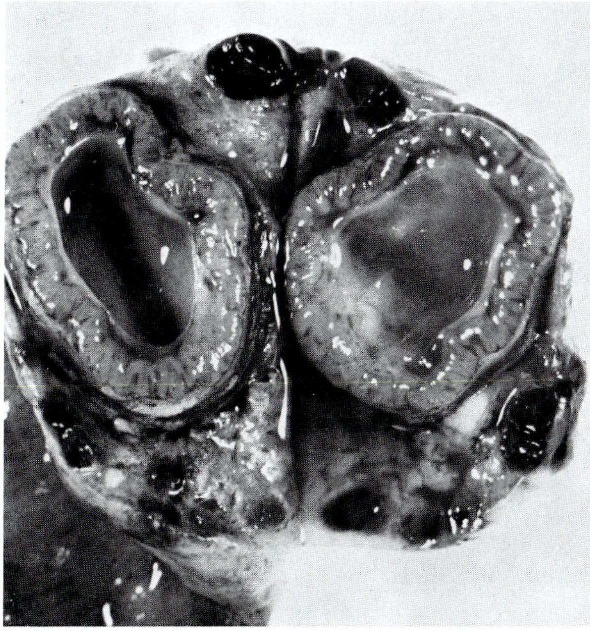

Fig. 15.17. Cystic corpus luteum of pregnancy. Note the convoluted lining, which was yellow.

by the last trimester is not conspicuous. During the puerperium, the CLP involutes and converts to a corpus albicans.

Histology

Granulosa Cells

The first morphologic evidence within the corpus luteum that conception has occurred is the absence of the regressive changes that normally appear in the CLM on the eighth or ninth days. Instead, the granulosa lutein cells enlarge, reaching their maximum size of 50–60 μm by 8–9 weeks gestation. The cells become round or polyhedral and contain abundant eosinophilic cytoplasm, round to oval vesicular nuclei, and one or two prominent nucleoli (Fig. 15.18a); typically, they have polyploid levels of DNA.[127]

The granulosa cells of the early CLP have cytoplasmic vacuoles that are initially minute but eventually increase in size to occupy almost the entire cell, often with displacement and flattening of the nucleus (Fig. 15.18a). The vacuoles tend to diminish in number and size as gestation progresses and typically disappear after the fourth month.[95] Fine, diffusely scattered, cytoplasmic lipid droplets are also commonly seen within the cells, particularly in early CLP. With increasing age of the CLP, the droplets become fewer and larger.[95]

Eosinophilic colloid or hyaline droplets appear within the granulosa cells of a CLP as early as 15 days after ovulation and are almost diagnostic of pregnancy, but these rarely occur within a CLM.[95] They initially appear as small, round or irregular, often multiple droplets but eventually enlarge, possibly by fusion of smaller droplets, into one or several large bodies that may fill the entire cell (Fig. 15.18a). The droplets become more numerous as gestation progresses,[136] although by term their numbers decrease as they undergo calcification, a process that continues into the puerperium (Fig. 15.18b).[95,136] It is likely that these calcified bodies eventually are resorbed, as they are not a feature of corpora albicantia.[95]

a

b

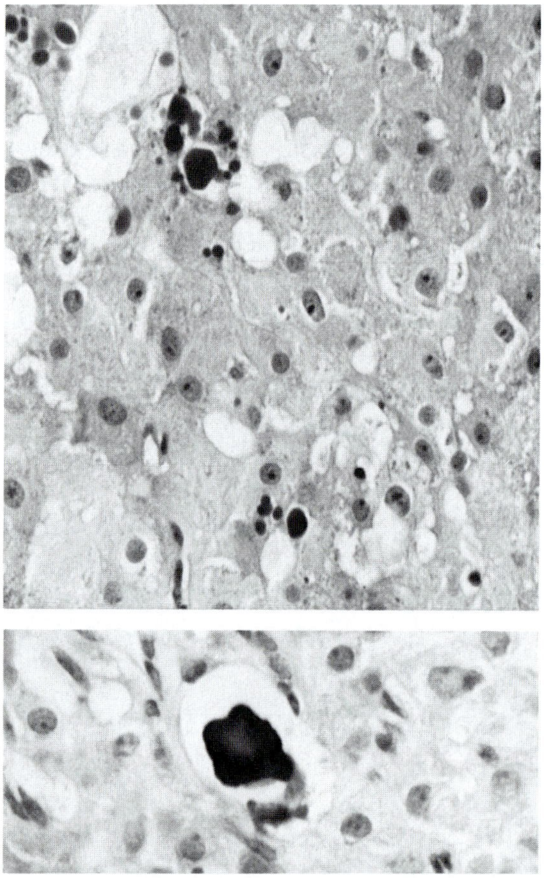

Fig. 15.18. Corpus luteum of pregnancy. a: Note granulosa–lutein cells with large irregular vacuoles and numerous, variably sized, darkly staining hyaline bodies. b: Focal calcification within a late corpus luteum of pregnancy.

Theca Cells

The theca interna is thickest in the early CLP, when it resembles its counterpart in the CLM. In the CLP, the theca cells are polyhedral or round and approximately one-fourth the size of the granulosa–lutein cells. Their cytoplasm is darker and more granular than that of the granulosa cells and is typically nonvacuolated. Their nuclei are central, round, and more hyperchromatic than those of the granulosa cells; one or two prominent nucleoli are usually present. The characteristic colloid inclusions seen within the granulosa cells are absent or very rare within the theca cells.[95] After the fourth month, the theca interna and its septa become thinner as the theca cells become smaller and fewer in number. Their nuclei become darker, more irregular, and oblong to spindle shaped, resembling fibroblasts.[136] By term, the theca interna layer has almost completely disappeared.[95] The theca externa layer may be more edematous and vascular than that of the CLM[95] or, in other examples, inapparent.[136]

Connective Tissue

As in the mature CLM, the central cystic cavity is typically lined by a layer of fibrous tissue, composed of variable numbers of fibroblasts, collagen, reticulin fibers, and blood vessels.[95] Its thickness is highly variable, not only within the same CLP, but also from one CLP to another and from one phase of pregnancy to another.[136] As gestation advances, the central cyst or coagulum is eventually obliterated by connective tissue, which may be focally hyalinized and calcified.[94]

Reticulin staining reveals a pattern similar to that of the mature CLM, that is, a dense pattern within the theca interna and inner fibrous layer and a sparser framework within the granulosa layer.[95] In the early CLP, many, often large, vessels are present in the theca externa and interna, which give origin to smaller vessels that penetrate the granulosa and inner fibrous layers. In the late CLP, the vessels develop sclerotic walls with luminal narrowing or obliteration.[95,136] The amount of connective tissue around the vessels increases in proportion to the decreasing vascularization and regression of the theca interna layer.[136]

Hormone Synthesis

Following fertilization, placental hCG stimulates P production by the granulosa–lutein cells. P concentration within the postovulatory corpus luteum increases sixfold, whereas the E_2 level drops to 10% of that within the preovulatory follicle.[82,83] HCG alone cannot maintain P secretion from the CLP for more than a few days, and the regulation of P secretion beyond that time is unknown.[25] P production by the CLP begins to decline by the end of the second month of gestation as the production of P is largely assumed by the placenta. However, in vivo and in vitro studies indicate that the CLP continues to produce P throughout the remainder of gestation, albeit in reduced amounts, consistent with the maintenance of its structural integrity until term.[2,45,74,90,139] It is not known if the P derived from the CLP has a biologic role during this period or is redundant because of the massive P production by the placenta. There is a rapid decline in function during the puerperium, reflecting falling hCG levels during this period.

Relaxin, a polypeptide hormone, is another substance produced during gestation and the puerperium by the CLP, probably under the control of hCG.[109,119,137,138] The concentration of relaxin in ovarian vein plasma during pregnancy correlates with P levels. The placenta and uterus have also been suggested as additional, but less important, sources for this hormone. Its reported actions include cervical dilatation and softening, inhibition of uterine contractions, and relaxation of the pubic symphysis and other pelvic joints.[109,119,137,138] Immunoreactivity for renin and angiotensin II, similar to that noted within the preovulatory follicle (see foregoing), has been demonstrated with the CLP,[101] consistent with the observation that prorenin, likely of ovarian origin, increases 10 fold in pregnant women soon after conception.[123]

Corpus Albicans

The regressing CLM is invaded by connective tissue that gradually converts it to a scar, the *corpus albicans*. The degenerating corpus luteum and the young corpus albicans may contain macrophages laden with ceroid and hemosiderin pigment.[111] The mature corpus albicans is well circumscribed, has convoluted borders, and is composed almost entirely of densely packed collagen fibers with occasional admixed fibroblasts (Fig. 15.19). Occasional corpora albicantia are focally calcified or cystic. Most are eventually resorbed and replaced by ovarian stroma,[62] although corpora albicantia often persist in the ovarian medulla of postmenopausal women.

Atretic Follicles

Histology

Of the original 400,000 primordial follicles present at birth, approximately 400 mature to ovulation. The remaining 99.9% undergo *atresia*, which begins be-

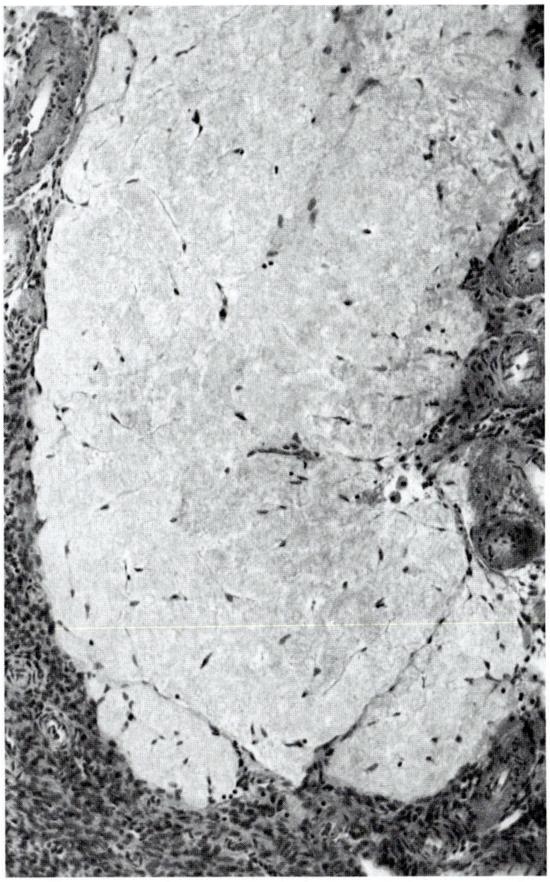

Fig. 15.19. Corpus albicans. Occasional fibroblasts are scattered throughout dense fibrous tissue.

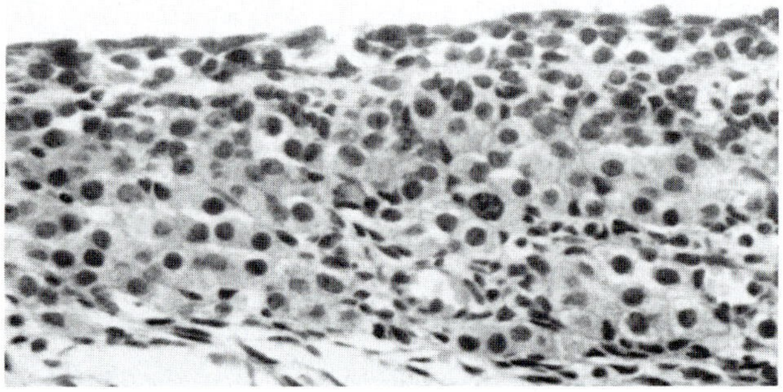

Fig. 15.20. Lining of atretic cystic follicle. The inner layer, composed of small granulosa cells, is thin and partially exfoliated. The outer, thicker theca interna layer exhibits prominent luteinization.

fore birth and continues throughout reproductive life, but is most intense immediately after birth and during puberty and pregnancy.[18,31,44,78,95] The factors that initiate atresia and determine which follicles will ultimately undergo atresia are unknown.

The atretic process varies with the stage of follicular maturation that has been reached (Figs. 15.20–15.23). Atresia of early follicles (primordial and preantral) begins with degeneration of the oocyte. Degeneration of the granulosa cells soon follows and the follicle completely disappears. In contrast, atresia of follicles that have reached the antral stage of development is more complex and variable, but ultimately leads to obliterative atresia and the formation of a scar, the corpus fibrosum (corpus atreticum).[14] The earliest evidence of this process is a decrease in mitotic activity and in the number of granulosa cells, resulting in a thinning and focal exfoliation of the granulosa layer. Some follicles may persist for an indefinite period of time (even for several years after the menopause) as atretic cystic follicles or follicular cysts (Fig. 15.20). Eventually, atretic follicles are invaded by vascular connective tissue that fills the central cavity (Fig. 15.21). The oocyte may persist for an indefinite period of time but eventually degenerates.[14] Concurrent with these

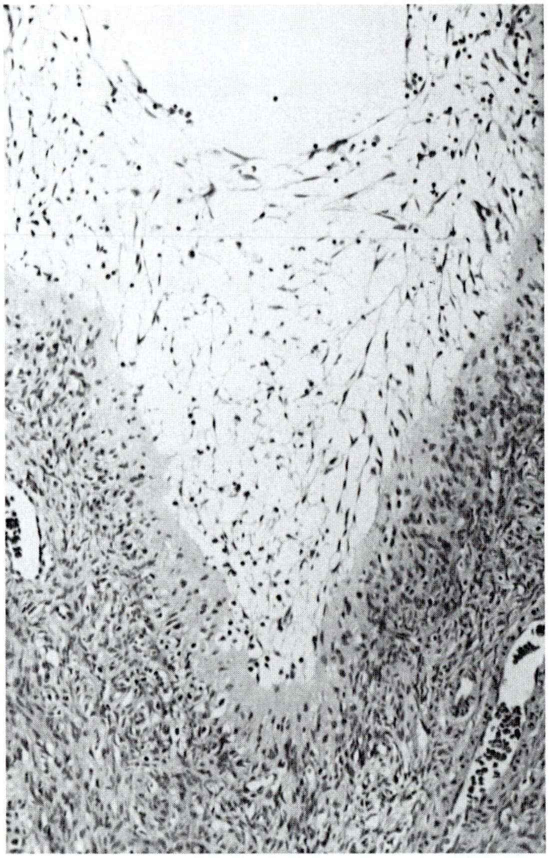

Fig. 15.21. Atretic cystic follicle undergoing obliterative atresia. Loose connective tissue is replacing the central cavity. The wavy basement membrane (glassy membrane) is thickened and hyalinized.

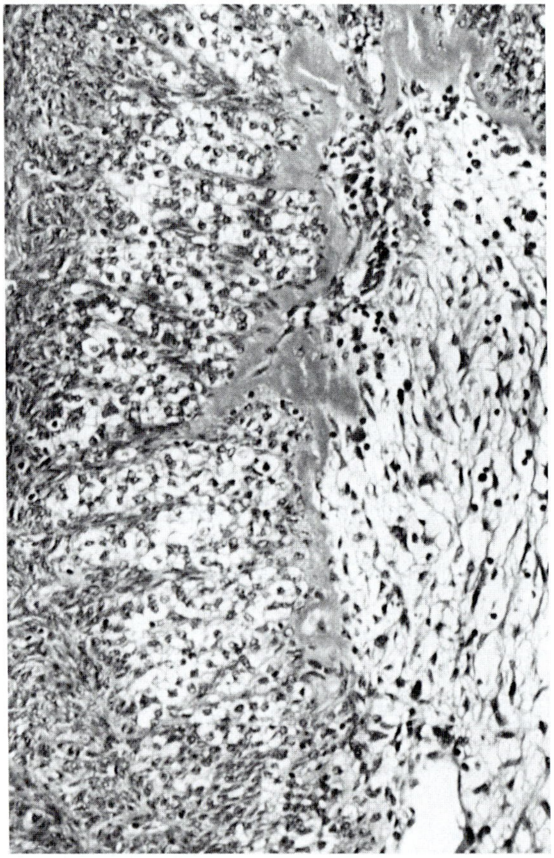

Fig. 15.22. Late stage of obliterative atresia. The thickened basement membrane separates the central fibrous tissue from the prominent luteinized theca interna layer.

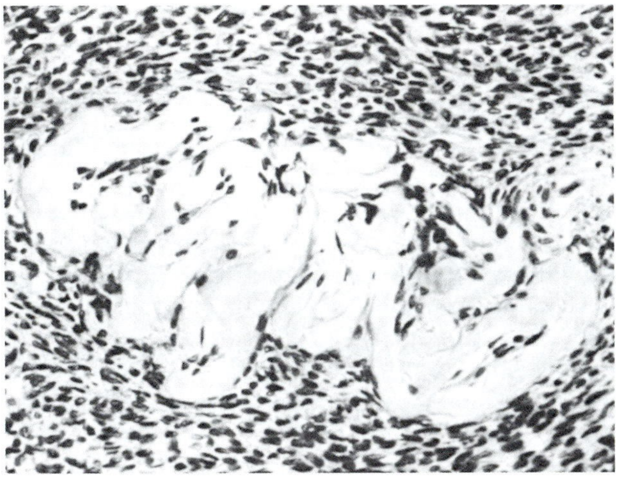

Fig. 15.23. **Corpus fibrosum.** The structure consists of a wavy hyalinized band.

changes, the basement membrane between the granulosa and theca interna layers becomes transformed into a thick, wavy, eosinophilic, hyalinized band (Figs. 15.21 and 15.22). The theca interna typically persists, often with prominent luteinization, until the late stages of atresia, at which time cords and nests of theca cells become surrounded by connective tissue (Fig. 15.22). Continued shrinkage and hyalinization produces the corpus fibrosum, a small scar consisting of a wavy strand of hyaline tissue (Fig. 15.23). Like corpora albicantia, most corpora fibrosa are resorbed.

Luteinization of both theca and granulosa layers is particularly striking in atretic follicles during infancy and childhood and pregnancy[95]; these cells are immunoreactive for inhibin.[103] Microscopic, often multifocal, proliferations of granulosa cells, potentially mimicking small granulosa cell tumors, are occasionally encountered within the centers of atretic follicles, most commonly during pregnancy (see Chapter 16, Nonneoplastic Lesions of the Ovary).[22]

Hormone Synthesis

In contrast to that of preovulatory follicles, the microenvironment of follicles undergoing atresia is predominantly androgenic, with high concentrations of intrafollicular androstenedione and low concentrations of FSH and E_2.[15,82,83,86,97] As noted, these follicles are deficient in granulosa cells, and the residual granulosa cells do not respond to FSH in vitro[86]; both FSH and LH receptors are lower than in nonatretic follicles.[125] Oocytes from atretic follicles are unable to complete the first meiotic division.[86] It is likely that an androgenic intrafollicular milieu is the major factor that halts follicular growth and initiates follicular atresia.

Hilus Cells

Histology

Ovarian hilus cells (*hilar Leydig cells*) are morphologically identical to testicular Leydig cells except for having a female chromatin pattern. Hilus cells are present during fetal life but are not identified in childhood. They reappear at the time of puberty and are demonstrable in virtually all postmenopausal women.[129,130] Their number and location can vary greatly, but they are more numerous during pregnancy, in parous women, with increasing age after the menopause, and with increasing degrees of ovarian stromal proliferation and stromal luteinization.[16] Hilus cell hyperplasia is discussed in Chapter 16, Nonneoplastic Lesions of the Ovary.

Hilus cell aggregates of variable size and shape are typically found in the ovarian hilus and adjacent mesovarium (Fig. 15.24). They are more numerous in the lateral and medial poles of the hilus and near

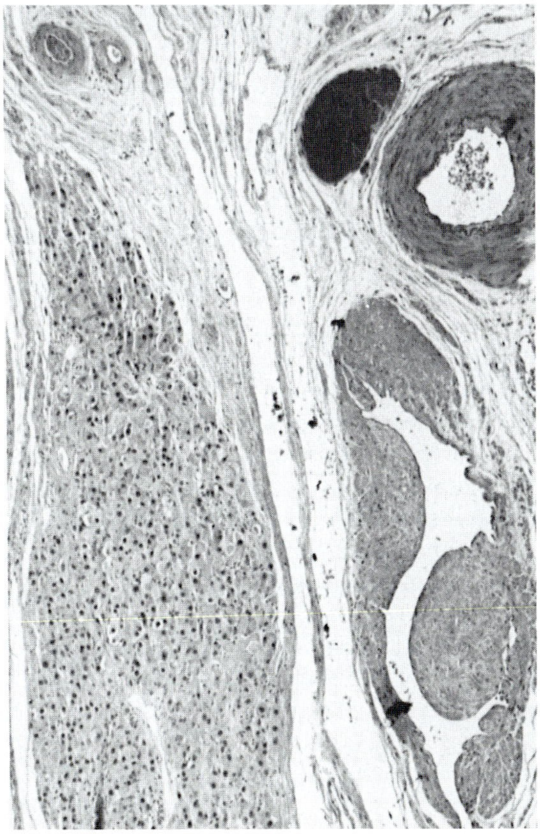

Fig. 15.24. **Hilus cells.** A nest of hilus cells lies adjacent to large vessels within the ovarian hilus.

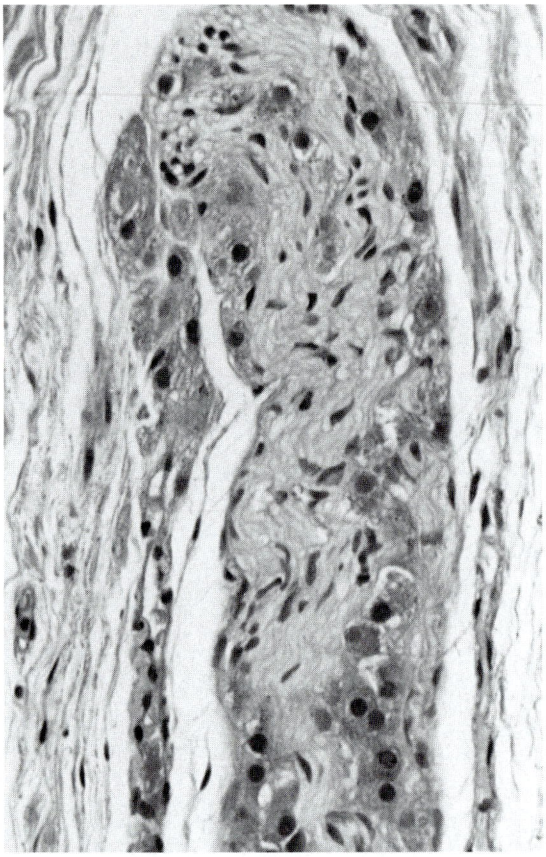

Fig. 15.25. Hilus cells. The cells ensheathe and lie within a nonmedullated nerve.

the junction of the ovarian ligament with the ovary, typically lying close to the junction of the hilus with the medullary stroma; they occasionally surround the rete ovarii.[129] The hilus cells characteristically ensheathe, or less commonly lie within, nonmedullated nerves (Fig. 15.25), and are frequently juxtaposed to large hilar venous and lymphatic sinusoids, occasionally forming nodular protrusions into their lumina.[129] Nests of hilus cells may also be seen within the ovarian stroma near the hilus, a finding probably resulting from irregularities in the junction between the hilus and medulla, and rarely, as previously noted, within the ovarian stroma away from the hilus (stromal Leydig cells) (see Chapter 16). Ectopic hilus cells may also be rarely encountered in the perisalpinx and fimbrial endosalpinx.[56]

Hilus cell nests are unencapsulated, typically lying within loose connective tissue, or rarely ovarian-type stroma, within the hilus.[143] The cells are 15–25 μm in diameter; are round to oval, and less commonly elongated; and contain abundant eosinophilic cytoplasm and a spherical vesicular nucleus, which contains one or two prominent nucleoli (Fig. 15.26). Rare multinucleated cells may be seen; those found incidentally in normal postmenopausal women do not exhibit mitotic activity in contrast to hyperplastic or neoplastic hilus cells.

Hilus cells contain specific crystals of Reinke, which are homogenous, eosinophilic, nonrefractile, rod-shaped structures, 10–35 μm long, with blunt to tapered ends (Fig. 15.26, inset). The crystals typically lie in a parallel or stacked arrangement within a cell, and often are surrounded by a clear halo; occasionally, they appear to extend through or overlie cell membranes. The crystals are typically unevenly distributed and present in only a minority of cells; frequently they are not identified.[60] Their visualization may be facilitated by the use of Masson's trichrome and iron hematoxylin methods, which stain them magenta and black, respectively. Additionally, the cystals exhibit yellow fluoresence when viewed by ultraviolet light in hematoxylin and eosin-stained sections.[120] Spherical or ellipsoidal, eosinophilic hyaline structures, which probably represent precursors of crystals, can be identified in hilus cells, often in greater numbers than crystals. Elongated erythrocytes com-

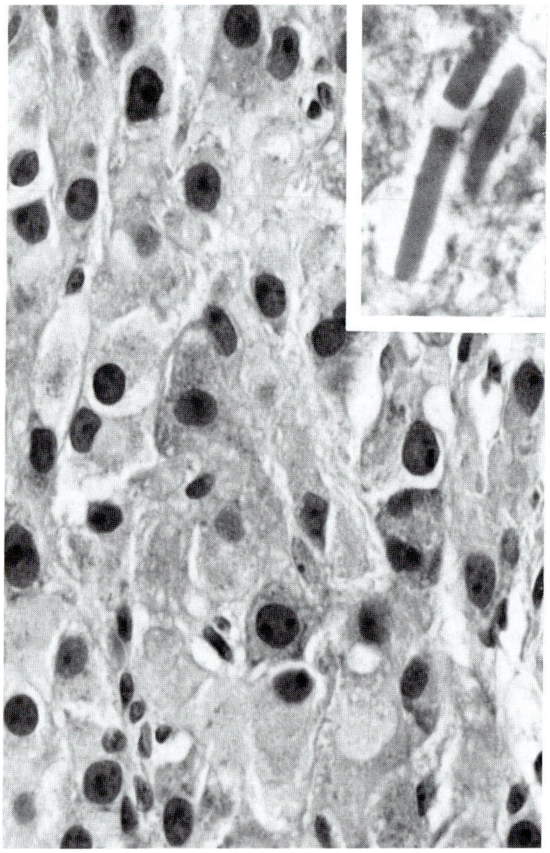

Fig. 15.26. Hilus cells. Note lipochrome pigment granules and Reinke crystals (*inset*).

pressed within capillaries should not be confused with crystals or their precursors.

The cytoplasm of hilus cells may also contain perinuclear eosinophilic granules, peripheral lipid vacuoles, and golden-brown lipochrome pigment (Fig. 15.26). Normal Leydig cells are immunoreactive for inhibin[103] and relaxin-like factor.[8] Typically admixed with the hilus cells are delicate collagen fibrils and fibroblasts and cells intermediate in appearance between the two cell types.[70] The hilus cells and intermediate cells have neural attachments, including true synaptic connections, suggesting that these cells may arise from hilar fibroblasts, possibly under the inductive influence of hilar nerves.[70] Hilus cells should be distinguished from encapsulated adrenocortical rests (see Chapter 16, Nonneoplastic Lesions of the Ovary).

Hormone Synthesis

The light and electron microscopic appearance and enzyme content of hilus cells are those of steroid hormone-producing cells, although to what extent hilus cells contribute to the steroid hormone pool in normal females is unknown.[81,122] In vitro incubation studies indicate that the major steroid produced by ovarian hilus cells is androstenedione and that it is produced in an amount higher than that secreted by the ovarian stroma.[33] Lesser amounts of E_2 and P are also produced in vitro. Hilus cells are responsive in vivo to both exogenous and endogenous hCG stimulation, as manifested by increase in cell size, mitotic activity, and cell number.[130]

Rete Ovarii

The *rete ovarii*, the ovarian analogue of the rete testis, which is present in the hilus of all ovaries, consists of a network of anastomosing branching tubules with intraluminal polypoid projections, lined by an epithelium that varies from flat to cuboidal to columnar (Fig. 15.27). Solid cords of similar cells may also be seen. The rete is surrounded by a cuff of spindle cell stroma morphologically similar to, but discontinuous from, the ovarian stroma. The rete epithelium is immunoreactive for cytokeratin, vimentin, and desmoplakin, as well as low levels of estrogen and progesterone receptors.[11,28,68] The rete lies adjacent to and may communicate with mesonephric tubules within the mesovarium.[41] The rete epithelium may undergo transitional metaplasia.[118] Occasional hilar cysts originate from the rete (see Chapter 16), and small tumor-like proliferations of the rete have been referred to as rete adenomas.[41]

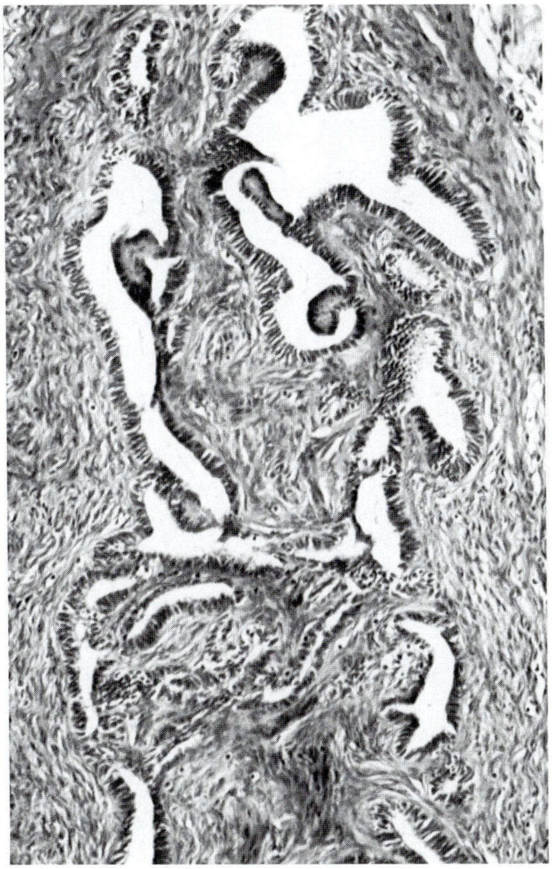

Fig. 15.27. Rete ovarii. Clefts and tubules, some with intraluminal papillae, are lined by a single layer of columnar epithelial cells.

The Ovary in Childhood

Gross Anatomy

The *newborn ovary* is a tan, elongated, and flat structure that lies above the true pelvis. It may have a lobulated appearance with irregular edges (Fig. 15.28).[108] Its approximate dimensions are 1.3 cm by 0.5 cm by 0.3 cm, and its weight is less than 0.3 g.[108,133] The ovary enlarges, increases in weight 30 fold, and changes in shape throughout infancy and childhood, and at puberty has the size and shape of an adult ovary and lies within the true pelvis.[108,133] The ovary may contain prominent cystic follicles, particularly during the first few months of life and around the time of puberty, an appearance that should not be misinterpreted as polycystic ovary disease (Fig. 15.29).

Histology

At the time of birth, the ovarian cortex is filled with approximately 400,000 closely packed primordial

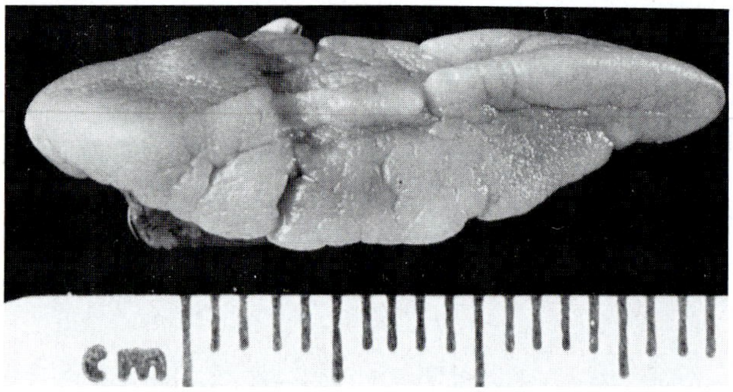

Fig. 15.28. Ovary of newborn. Note elongated shape and irregular edges.

follicles (Figs. 15.30 and 15.31). Some primordial follicles contain two or rarely a greater number of oocytes.[77,133] The oocyte is in meiotic prophase at the time of birth, entering an interphase period until preovulatory follicular maturation or degeneration during atresia. Follicle-derived structures resembling small sex cord tumors with annular tubules or, if germ cells are present, gonadoblastomas, may occur in normal ovaries from fetuses and children; they are probably a result of aberrent folliculogenesis.[67,77,117] Follicular maturation and atresia occur prenatally and throughout childhood, becoming more prominent after the age of 6.[26,55,88,97,105,133] Deceleration or arrest of folliculogenesis may occur in prepubertal patients with chronic illnesses, Down's syndrome, and in those exposed to cytotoxic drugs or irradiation.[105] Follicular maturation is identical to that occurring in premenopausal adult subjects except that it does not proceed beyond antral follicles measuring 5 mm in diameter. Because ovulation does not occur, corpora lutea and corpora albicantia are absent in the prepubertal ovary, and all maturing follicles undergo atresia in a manner identical to that occurring in adults. Prominent luteinization of the theca interna layer may also be seen in this age group.[69] By puberty, atresia has depleted more than 90% of

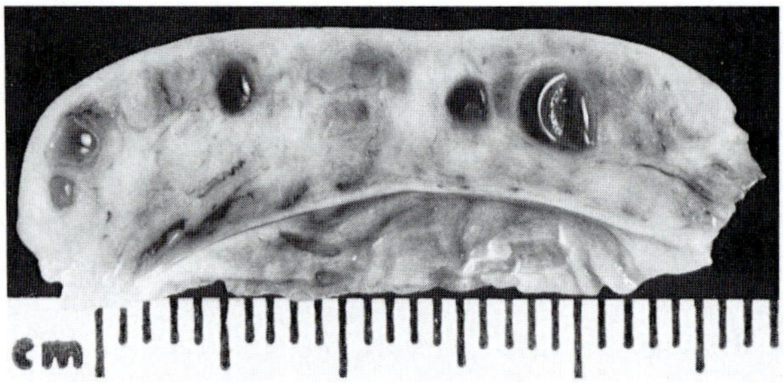

Fig. 15.29. Ovary of 14-year-old girl (*cut surface*). Note multiple cystic follicles within cortex.

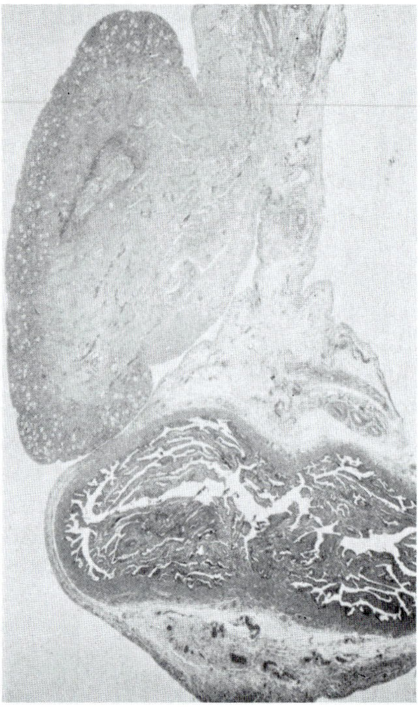

Fig. 15.30. Ovary and fallopian tube of newborn in cross section. Ovarian cortex is packed with primordial follicles.

the approximately 400,000 primordial follicles that were present at birth. This depletion and the concomitant increase in the amount of ovarian stroma results in the more sparse distribution of the primordial follicles in the pubertal girl and young adult compared to that in childhood.

Adolescent prepubertal ovaries, in addition to prominent cystic follicles with luteinization of the theca interna, may exhibit focal fibrosis of the superficial cortex, further enhancing their resemblance to the ovaries of polycystic ovary disease.[88] This sclerocystic appearance is consistent with the conclusion that such changes are not specific for polycystic ovary disease but are a reflection of chronic anovulation (see Chapter 16). As previously noted, hilus cells are demonstrable during fetal life but are not seen during infancy and childhood, reappearing at puberty.

Hormone Synthesis

Levels of gonadotropins and sex steroids, largely of placental origin, decline rapidly during the first few days of life. As a result, a rise in FSH and LH levels, paralleled by an elevation in follicle-derived estradiol (E_2), begins on the fifth day.[73] All three hormones reach peak levels at 3 to 4 months of age and then decline to low levels by the age of 2 years because of increasing sensitivity of the hypothala-

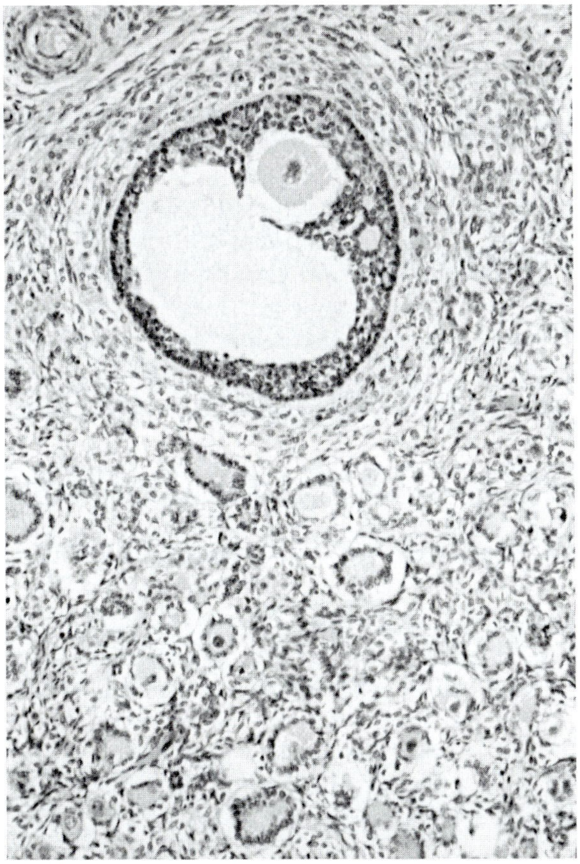

Fig. 15.31. Ovary of newborn. Note closely packed primordial follicles and antral follicle.

mic–pituitary unit to negative feedback by E_2. Low levels of gonadotropins are maintained until 6 to 8 years of age but are sufficient to maintain the growing ovary and stimulate continuous follicular development and atresia.[73,104] Only minimal quantities of E_2 are produced during this period. The onset of adrenal androgen secretion (adrenarche) at the age of 6 or 7 years usually precedes and may promote activation of the hypothalamic gonadostat.[73] As a result, there is a reduction in hypothalamic–pituitary sensitivity to negative feedback by estrogen, and FSH and LH levels progressively increase until menarche. These hormones stimulate the increased production of follicular estrogens that are responsible for the development of secondary sexual characteristics at puberty.

The Ovary in the Menopause

Gross Anatomy

After the menopause, the ovaries typically shrink to a size approximately one-half their size during the reproductive era. Their size varies considerably, however, depending on their content of ovarian stromal cells and the number of unresorbed corpora albicantia. Most postmenopausal ovaries have a shrunken, gyriform, external appearance (Fig. 15.32) but some have a smooth surface. The sectioned surface is usually firm and predominantly solid, although occasional cysts several millimeters in diameter (inclusion cysts) may be visible within the cortex. Small white scars (corpora albicantia) are typically present within the medulla. Thick-walled blood vessels may be appreciable within the medulla and hilus.

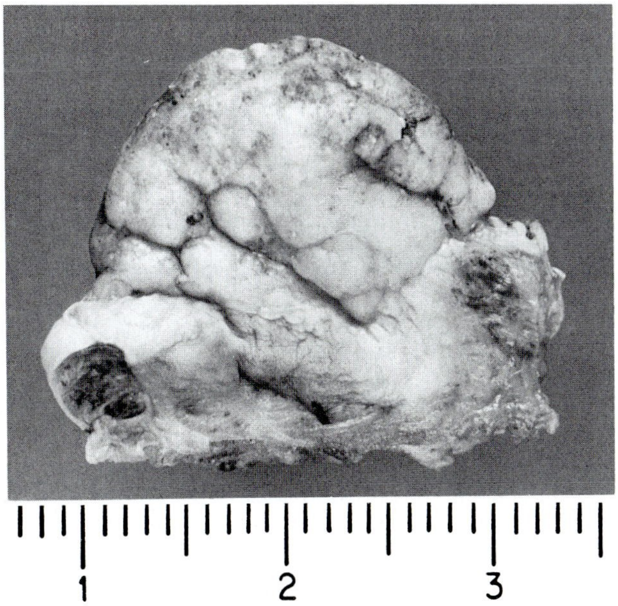

Fig. 15.32. Ovary of postmenopausal woman. Note the markedly irregular cortical surface.

Histology

The characteristic feature of the postmenopausal ovary is the absence of primordial follicles, and consequently, an absence of maturing follicles, corpora lutea, and atretic follicles. Occasional primordial follicles, however, may persist for several years after cessation of menses, accounting for sporadic ovulation and follicle cyst formation accompanied by postmenopausal bleeding. After this period, the only follicle-derived structures typically encountered are occasional unresorbed corpora fibrosa and corpora albicantia, the latter typically within the medulla (Figure 15.33).

Although the ovarian stroma typically increases in volume from the fourth to the seventh decades,[126] the ovarian stroma in postmenopausal women has a wide spectrum of appearances.[16,76,126] At one extreme there is stromal atrophy manifested by a thin

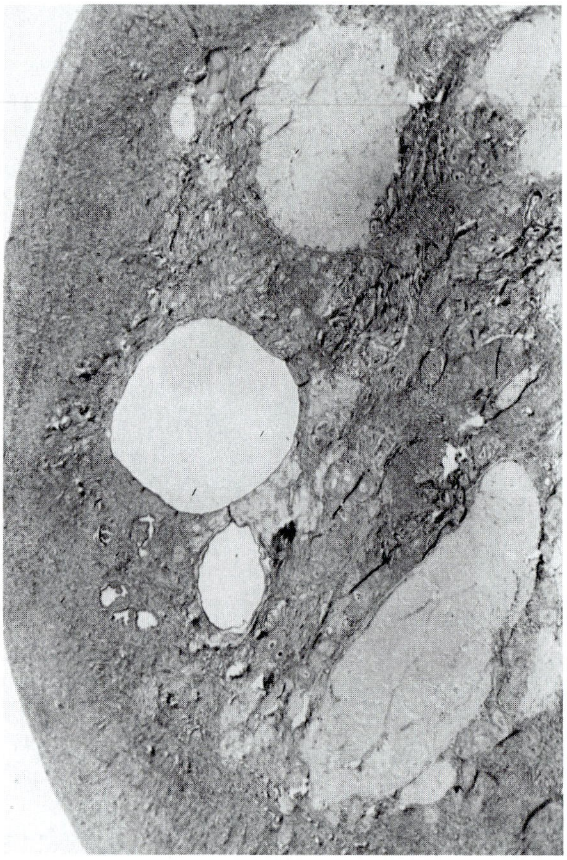

Fig. 15.33. Ovary of postmenopausal woman. Note the thin cortex devoid of follicular structures. Two inclusion cysts are present at the corticomedullary junction. Multiple corpora albicantia occupy the medulla.

cortex and mimimal amounts of medullary stroma (Fig. 15.33). In these subjects, the stroma becomes less cellular because of an increase in intercellular collagen, and its cells have smaller, darker, more inactive appearing nuclei (Fig. 15.34). At the other extreme, there is marked stromal proliferation warranting the designation "stromal hyperplasia" to connote a pathologic process (see Chapter 16). Most postmenopausal subjects, however, exhibit varying degrees of nodular or diffuse proliferation of cortical and medullary stromal cells that lie between these two extremes, making the normal quantity of ovarian stroma difficult to define. Ovarian stromal changes that can be considered normal aging phenomena include occasional luteinized stromal cells, broad irregular areas of cortical fibrosis or fibromatous nodules,[16] cortical "granulomas," spherical, cloudlike, hyaline scars, and surface papillary stromal proliferations (see Chapter 16). Less commonly, focal decidual transformation of the ovarian stroma may be seen in otherwise normal ovaries from postmenopausal subjects (see Chapter 16).

Other common changes within the ovaries of postmenopausal women include surface epithelial inclusion glands and cysts within the cortex and mild degrees of hilus cell hyperplasia (see Chapter 16). After the menopause, the medullary blood vessels exhibit a greater tortuosity, appearing more numerous and closely packed as a result of parenchymal atrophy, and should not be mistaken for a hemangioma on microscopic examination. Many of these vessels may be calcified or have thickened walls and narrowed lumens as a result of mural deposition of a hyaline, amyloid-like material.

Hormone Synthesis

With cessation of follicular activity at the time of the menopause, the ovarian stroma becomes, together with the adrenal glands, the major source of androgens. Testosterone and androstenedione are the major androgens secreted by the ovarian stroma in postmenopausal women.[3,19,33,64,65,75,79,107,134] Approximately 80% of the circulating levels of androstenedione in postmenopausal women, however, is of adrenal origin.[19] Despite a cessation of follicu-

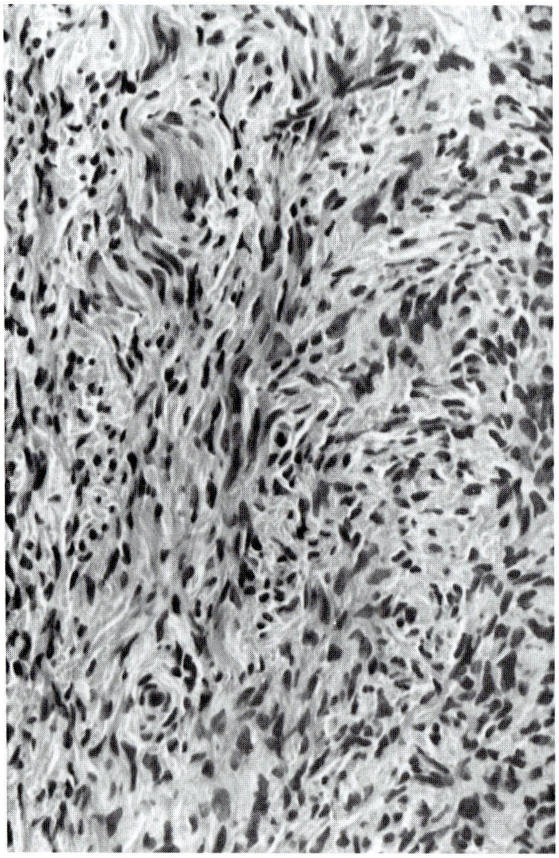

Fig. 15.34. Ovarian stroma in postmenopausal woman. Note the spindle-shaped cells with thin, darkly staining nuclei and abundant intercellular collagen.

lar synthesis of E_2 in postmenopausal subjects, small amounts of this hormone are present in the circulation, probably derived from the adrenal glands, by peripheral conversion of E_1,[19,112] and from the ovarian stroma itself.[3,75] E_1, however, becomes the major circulating estrogen after the menopause.

Estrone in postmenopausal women is derived predominantly from the peripheral aromatization of androstenedione that occurs in fat, muscle, liver, kidney, brain, and adrenals.[19,47,75] Increased aromatization in postmenopausal women, probably a result of high endogenous LH levels in this population, leads to an increase in the production of E_1 over that in premenopausal women; aromatization is also higher in obese subjects. In some postmenopausal women, sufficient estrogen may be elaborated by this mechanism to prevent the clinical manifestations of estrogen withdrawal and to play a role in the genesis of endometrial carcinoma.[19,126] Indeed, an association between the degree of stromal proliferation and postmenopausal endometrial adenocarcinoma has been found.[126] The variations that exist in the ovarian steroid hormone output from one postmenopausal woman to another may correspond to similar variations in the morphologic appearance of the stroma in this age group, although no correlative functional and structural studies have been performed.

References

1. Adams EC, Hertig AT (1969) Studies on the human corpus luteum. I. Observations on the ultrastructure of development and regression of the luteal cells during the menstrual cycle. J Cell Biol 41: 696–715
2. Adams EC, Hertig AT (1969) Studies on the human corpus luteum. II. Observations on the ultrastructure of luteal cells during pregnancy. J Cell Biol 41:716–735
3. Aiman J, Fornery JP, Parker R Jr (1986) Secretion of androgens and estrogens by normal and neoplastic ovaries in postmenopausal women. Obstet Gynecol 68:1–5
4. Al-Timimi A, Buckley CH, Fox H (1985) An immunohistochemical study of the incidence and significance of sex steroid hormone binding sites in normal and neoplastic human ovarian tissue. Int J Gynecol Pathol 4:24–41
5. Ayyagari RR, Khan-Dawood FS (1987) Human corpus luteum: presence of epidermal growth factor receptors and binding characteristics. Am J Obstet Gynecol 156:942–946
6. Baca M, Zamboni L (1967) The fine structure of the human follicular oocyte. J Ultrastruct Res 19:354–381
7. Balboni GC (1983) Structural changes: ovulation and luteal phase. In: Serra GB (ed) The ovary. Raven Press, New York, pp 123–141
8. Bamberger A-M, Ivell R, Balvers M, Kelp B, Bamberger CM, Riethdorf L, Löning T (1999) Relaxin-like factor (RLF): a new specific marker for Leydig cells in the ovary. Int J Gynecol Pathol 18:163–168
9. Barbieri RL, Makris A, Randall RW, et al (1986) Insulin stimulates androgen accumulation in incubations of ovarian stroma obtained from women with hyperandrogenism. J Clin Endocrinol Metab 62:904–910
10. Bassis ML (1956) Pseudodeciduosis. Am J Obstet Gynecol 72:1029–1037
11. Benjamin E, Law S, Bobrow LG (1987) Intermediate filaments cytokeratin and vimentin in ovarian sex cord-stromal tumours with correlative studies in adult and fetal ovaries. J Pathol 152:253–263
12. Bersch W, Alexy E, Heuser HP, Staemmler HJ (1973) Ectopic decidua formation in the ovary (so-called deciduoma). Virchows Arch A (Pathol Anat) 360:173–177
13. Blaustein A, Lee H (1979) Surface cells of the ovary and pelvic peritoneum: a histochemical and ultrastuctural comparison. Gynecol Oncol 8:34–43
14. Bloom W, Fawcett DW (1975) A textbook of histology. 10th Ed. Saunders, Philadelphia
15. Bomsel-Helmreich O, Gougeon A, Thebault A et al (1979) Healthy and atretic human follicles in the preovulatory phase: differences in evolution of follicular morphology and steroid content of follicular fluid. J Clin Endocrinol Metab 48:686–694
16. Boss, JH, Scully RE, Wegner KH, Cohen RB (1965) Structural variations in the adult ovary: clinical significance. Obstet Gynecol 25:747–763
17. Centola GM (1983) Structural changes: follicular development and hormonal requirements. In: Serra GB (ed) The ovary. Raven Press, New York, pp 95–111
18. Centola GM (1983) Structural changes: atresia. In: Serra GB (ed) The ovary. Raven Press, New York, pp 113–122
19. Chang RJ, Judd HL (1981) The ovary after menopause. Clin Obstet Gynaecol 24:181–191
20. Charpin C, Bhan AK, Zurawski VR Jr, Scully RE (1982) Carcinoembryonic antigen (CEA) and carbohydrate determinant 19–9 (CA 19–9) localization in 121 primary and metastatic ovarian tumors: an immunohistochemical study with the use of monoclonal antibodies. Int J Gynecol Pathol 1:231–245
21. Clement PB (1997) Histology of the ovary. In: Sternberg SS (ed) Histology for pathologists, 2nd Ed. Lippincott-Raven, New York, pp 929–959
22. Clement PB, Young RH, Scully RE (1988) Ovarian granulosa cell proliferations of pregnancy: a report of nine cases. Hum Pathol 19:657–662
23. Cordon-Cardo C, Mattes MJ, Melamed MR, et al (1985) Immunopathologic analysis of a panel of mouse monoclonal antibodies reacting with human ovarian carcinomas and other human tumors. Int J Gynecol Pathol 4:121–130

24. Corner GW Jr (1956) The histological dating of the human corpus luteum of menstruation. Am J Anat 98:377–401
25. Crowley WF (1986) Progesterone antagonism. N Engl J Med 315:1607–1608
26. Curtis EM (1962) Normal ovarian histology in infancy and childhood. Obstet Gynecol 19:444–454
27. Czernobilsky B, Moll R, Franke WW, et al (1984) Intermediate filaments of normal and neoplastic tissues of the female genital tract with emphasis on problems of differential tumor diagnosis. Pathol Res Pract 179:31–37
28. Czernobilsky B, Moll R, Levy R, Franke WW (1985) Co-expression of cytokeratin and vimentin filaments in mesothelial, granulosa and rete ovarii cells of the human ovary. Eur J Cell Biol 37:175–190
29. Czernobilsky B, Shezen E, Lifschitz-Mercer B, et al (1989) Alpha smooth muscle actin (alpha-SM actin) in normal human ovaries, in ovarian stromal hyperplasia and in ovarian neoplasms. Virchows Arch [B] 57:55–61
30. Deane HW, Lobel BL, Romney SL (1962) Enzymic histochemistry of normal human ovaries of the menstrual cycle, pregnancy, and the early puerperium. Am J Obstet Gynecol 83:281–294
31. Dekel N, David MP, Yedwab GA, Kraicer PF (1977) Follicular development during late pregnancy. Int J Fertil 22:24–29
32. Dennefors BL, Janson PO, Knutsson F, Hamberger L (1980) Steroid production and responsiveness to gonadotropin in isolated stromal tissue of human postmenopausal ovaries. Am J Obstet Gynecol 136: 997–1002
33. Dennefors BL, Janson PO, Hamberger L, Knutsson F (1982) Hilus cells from human postmenopausal ovaries: gonadotrophin sensitivity, steroid and cyclic AMP production. Acta Obstet Gynecol Scand 61:413–416
34. Donahoe PK, Cate RL, MacLaughlin DT, et al (1987) Mullerian inhibiting substance: gene structure and mechanism of action of a fetal regressor. Recent Prog Horm Res 43:431–67
35. Dyer CA, Erickson GF (1985) Norepinephrine amplifies human chorionic gonadotropin-stimulated androgen biosynthesis by ovarian theca-interstitial cells. Endocrinology 116:1645–1652
36. Eichner E, Bove ER (1954) In vivo studies on the lymphatic drainage of the human ovary. Obstet Gynecol 3:287–297
37. Erickson GF (1978) Normal ovarian function. Clin Obstet Gynecol 21:31–52
38. Feinberg R, Cohen RB (1965) A comparative histochemical study of the ovarian stromal lipid band, stromal theca cell, and normal ovarian follicular apparatus. Am J Obstet Gynecol 92:958–969
39. Ferenczy A, Richart RM (1974) Female reproductive system: dynamics of scan and transmission electron microscopy. Wiley, New York
40. Futterweit W (1985) Polycystic ovarian disease. Clinical perspectives in obstetrics and gynecology. Springer-Verlag, New York
41. Gardner GH, Greene RR, Peckham B (1957) Tumors of the broad ligament. Am J Obstet Gynecol 73:536–555
42. Gillim SW, Christensen AK, McLennan CE (1969) Fine structure of the human menstrual corpus luteum at its stage of maximum secretory activity. Am J Anat 126:409–428
43. Gougeon A (1981) Frequent occurrence of multiovular follicles and multinuclear oocytes in the adult human ovary. Fertil Steril 35:417–422
44. Govan ADT (1970) Ovarian follicular activity in late pregnancy. J Endocrinol 48:235–241
45. Green JA, Garcilazo JA, Maqueo M (1967) Ultrastructure of the human ovary. II. The luteal cell at term. Am J Obstet Gynecol 99:855–863
46. Greenblatt RB, Colle ML, Mahesh VB (1976) Ovarian and adrenal steroid production in the postmenopausal woman. Obstet Gynecol 47:383–387
47. Grodin JM, Siiteri PK, MacDonald PC (1973) Source of estrogen production in postmenopausal women. J Clin Endocrinol Metab 36:207–214
48. Hameed A, Fox WM, Kurman RJ, Hruban RH, Podack ER (1995) Perforin expression in human cell-mediated luteolysis. Int J Gynecol Pathol 14:151–157
49. Herr JC, Heidger PM Jr, Scott JR et al (1978) Decidual cells in the human ovary at term. I. Incidence, gross anatomy and ultrastructural features of merocrine secretion. Am J Anat 152:7–28
50. Hertig AT (1964) Gestational hyperplasia of endometrium. A morphologic correlation of ova, endometrium, and corpora lutea during early pregnancy. Lab Invest 13:1153–1191
51. Hertig AT (1968) The primary human oocyte: some observations on the fine structure of Balbiani's vitelline body and the origin of the annulate lamellae. Am J Anat 122:107–138
52. Hertig AT, Adams EC (1967) Studies on the human oocyte and its follicle. I. Ultrastructural and histochemical observations on the primordial follicle stage. J Cell Biol 34:647–675
53. Hidvegi D, Cibils LA, Sorensen K, Hidvegi I (1982) Ultrastructural and histochemical observations of neuroendocrine granules in nonneoplastic ovaries. Am J Obstet Gynecol 143:590–594
54. Hillier SG (1987) Intrafollicular paracrine function of ovarian androgen. J Steroid Biochem 27:351–357
55. Himelstein-Braw R, Byskov AG, Peters H, Faber M (1976) Follicular atresia in the infant human ovary. J Reprod Fertil 46:55–59
56. Honoré LH, O'Hara KE (1979) Ovarian hilus cell heterotopia. Obstet Gynecol 53:461–464
57. Isola J, Kallioniemi O, Korte J, et al (1990) Steroid receptors and Ki-67 reactivity in ovarian cancer and in normal ovary: correlation with DNA flow cytometry, biochemical receptor assay, and patient survival. J Pathol 162:295–301
58. Israel SL, Rubenstone A, Meranze DR (1954) The

ovary at term. I. Decidua-like reaction and surface cell proliferation. Obstet Gynecol 3:399–407

59. Jacobowitz D, Wallach EE (1967) Histochemical and chemical studies of the autonomic innervation of the ovary. Endocrinology 81:1132–1139
60. Janko AB, Sandberg EC (1970) Histochemical evidence for the protein nature of the Reinke crystalloid. Obstet Gynecol 35:493–503
61. Jindal SK, Snoey DM, Lobb DK, Dorrington JH (1994) Transforming growth factor alpha localization and role in surface epithelium of normal human ovaries and in ovarian carcinoma lines. Gynecol Oncol 53:17–23
62. Joel RV, Foraker AG (1960) Fate of the corpus albicans: a morphologic approach. Am J Obstet Gynecol 80:314–316
63. Jones GES, Goldberg B, Woodruff JD (1968) Histochemistry as a guide for interpretation of cell function. Am J Obstet Gynecol 100:76–83
64. Judd HL, Judd GE, Lucas WE, Yen SSC (1974) Endocrine function of the postmenopausal ovary: concentration of androgens and estrogens in ovarian and peripheral vein blood. J Clin Endocrinol Metab 39:1020–1024
65. Judd HL, Lucas WE, Yen SSC (1974) Effect of oophorecomy on circulating testosterone and androstenedione levels in patients with endometrial carcinoma. Am J Obstet Gynecol 118:793–798
66. Kabawat SE, Bast RC Jr, Bhan AK, et al (1983) Tissue distribution of coelomic-epithelium-related antigen recognized by the monoclonal antibody OC125. Int J Gynecol Pathol 2:275–285
67. Kedzia H (1983) Gonadoblastoma: structures and background of development. Am J Obstet Gynecol 147:81–85
68. Khan MS, Dodson AR, Heatley MK (1999) Ki-67, oestrogen receptor, and progesterone receptor proteins in the human rete ovarii and in endometriosis. J Clin Pathol 52:517–520
69. Kraus FT, Neubecker RD (1962) Luteinization of the ovarian theca in infants and children. Am J Clin Pathol 37:389–397
70. Laffargue P, Benkoel L, Laffargue F, et al (1978) Ultrastructural and enzyme histochemical study of ovarian hilar cells in women and their relationships with sympathetic nerves. Hum Pathol 9:649–659
71. Lastarria D, Sachdev RK, Babury RA, et al (1990) Immunohistochemical analysis for desmin in normal and neoplastic ovarian stromal tissue. Arch Pathol Lab Med 114:502–505
72. Latza U, Niedobitek G, Schwarting R, Nekarda H, Stein H (1990) Ber-EP4: new monoclonal antibody which distinguishes epithelia from mesothelia. J Clin Pathol 43:213–219
73. Lee PA (1983) Ovarian function from conception to puberty: physiology and disorders. In: Serra GB (ed) The ovary. Raven Press, New York, pp 177–189
74. LeMaire WJ, Rice BF, Savard K (1968) Steroid hormone formation in the human ovary: V. Synthesis of progesterone in vitro in corpora lutea during the reproductive cycle. J Clin Endocrinol Metab 28: 1249–1256
75. Longcope C, Hunter R, Franz C (1980) Steroid secretion by the postmenopausal ovary. Am J Obstet Gynecol 138:564–568
76. Loubet R, Loubet A, Leboutet M-J (1984) The ovarian stroma after the menopause: activity and ageing. In: de Brux J, Gautray J-P (eds) Clinical pathology of the ovary. MTP Press, Boston, pp 119–141
77. Manivel JC, Dehner LP, Burke B (1988) Ovarian tumorlike structures, biovular follicles, and binucleated oocytes in children: their frequency and possible pathologic significance. Pediatr Pathol 8: 283–292
78. Maqueo M, Goldzieher JW (1966) Hormone-induced alterations of ovarian morphology. Fertil Steril 17:676–683
79. Mattingly RF, Huang WY (1969) Steroidogenesis of the menopause and postmenopausal ovary. Am J Obstet Gynecol 103:679–693
80. McLachlan RI, Cohen NL, Vale WW, et al (1989) The importance of luteinizing hormone in the control of inhibin and progesterone secretion by the human corpus luteum. J Clin Endocrinol Metab 68:1078–1085
81. McKay DG, Pinkerton JHM, Hertig AT, Danziger S (1961) The adult human ovary: a histochemical study. Obstet Gynecol 18:13–39
82. McNatty KP (1978) Follicular determinants of corpus luteum function in the human ovary. In: Channing CP, Marsh JM, Sadler WA (eds) Ovarian follicular and corpus luteum function. Advances in experimental medicine and Biology, vol 112. Plenum Press, New York, pp 465–477
83. McNatty KP (1978) Cyclic changes in antral fluid hormone concentrations in humans. Clin Endocrinol Metab 7:577–600
84. McNatty KP, Makris A, DeGrazia C, et al (1979) The production of progesterone, androgens, and estrogens by granulosa cells, thecal tissue, and stromal tissue from human ovaries in vitro. J Clin Endocrinol Metab 49:687–699
85. McNatty KP, Makris A, DeGrazia C, et al (1979) The production of progesterone, androgens, and estrogens by human granulosa cells in vitro and in vivo. J Steroid Biochem 11:775–799
86. McNatty KP, Smith DM, Makris A, et al (1979) The microenvironment of the human antral follicle: interrelationships among the steroid levels in antral fluid, the population of granulosa cells, and the status of the oocyte in vivo and in vitro. J Clin Endocrinol Metab 49:851–860
87. McNatty KP, Smith DM, Makris A, et al (1980) The intraovarian sites of androgen and estrogen formation in women with normal and hyperandrogenic ovaries as judged by in vitro experiments. J Clin Endocrinol Metab 50:755–763
88. Merrill JA (1963) The morphology of the prepubertal ovary: relationship to the polycystic ovary syndrome. South Med J 56:225–231

89. Miettinen M, Lehto V, Virtanen I (1983) Expression of intermediate filaments in normal ovaries and ovarian epithelial, sex cord-stromal, and germinal tumors. Int J Gynecol Pathol 2:64–71
90. Mikhail G, Allen WM (1967) Ovarian function in human pregnancy. Am J Obstet Gynecol 99: 308–312
91. Mohsin S (1979) The sympathetic innervation of the mammalian ovary. A review of pharmacological and histochemical studies. Clin Exp Pharmacol Physiol 6:335–354
92. Nagamani M, Hannigan EV, Van Dinh T, Stuart CA (1988) Hyperinsulinemia and stromal luteinization of the ovaries in postmenopausal women with endometrial cancer. J Clin Endocrinol Metab 67: 144–148
93. Nakano R, Shima K, Yamoto M, et al (1989) Binding sites for gonadotropins in human postmenopausal ovaries. Obstet Gynecol 73:196–200
94. Nelson WW, Greene RR (1953) The human ovary in pregnancy. Int Abstracts Surg 97:1–23
95. Nelson WW, Greene RR (1958) Some observations on the histology of the human ovary during pregnancy. Am J Obstet Gynecol 76:66–89
96. Neunteufel W, Breitenecker G (1989) Tissue expression of CA 125 in benign and malignant lesions of ovary and fallopian tube: a comparison with CA 19–9 and CEA. Gynecol Oncol 32:297–302
97. Nicosia SV (1983) Morphological changes of the human ovary throughout life. In: Serra GB (ed) The ovary. Raven Press, New York, pp 57–81
98. Nouwen EJ, Hendrix PG, Eerdekens MW, De Broe ME (1987) Tumor markers in the human ovary and its neoplasms. A comparative immunohistochemical study. Am J Pathol 126:230–242
99. Okamura H, Virutamasen P, Wright KH, Wallach EE (1972) Ovarian smooth muscle in the human being, rabbit, and cat. Am J Obstet Gynecol 112: 183–191
100. Owman C, Rosengren E, Sjoberg N (1967) Adrenergic innervation of the human female reproductive organs: a histochemical and chemical investigation. Obstet Gynecol 30:763–773
101. Palumbo A, Jones C, Lightman A, et al (1989) Immunohistochemical localization of renin and angiotensin II in human ovaries. Am J Obstet Gynecol 160:8–14
102. Pauerstein CJ, Eddy CA, Croxatto HD, et al (1978) Temporal relationships of estrogen, progesterone, and luteinizing hormone levels to ovulation in women and infrahuman primates. Am J Obstet Gynecol 130:876–886
103. Pelkey TJ, Frierson HF Jr, Mills SE, Stoler MH (1998) The diagnostic utility of inhibin staining in ovarian neoplasms. Int J Gynecol Pathol 17:97–105
104. Pennington GW (1974) The reproductive endocrinology of childhood and adolescence. Clin Obstet Gynaecol 1:509–531
105. Peters H, Himelstein-Braw R, Faber M (1976) The normal development of the ovary in childhood. Acta Endocrinol 82:617–630
106. Plentl AA, Friedman EA (1971) Lymphatic system of the female genitalia. Saunders, Philadelphia
107. Plotz EJ, Wiener M, Stein AA, Hahn BD (1967) Enzymatic activities related to steroidogenesis in postmenopausal ovaries of patients with and without endometrial carcinoma. Am J Obstet Gynecol 99: 182–197
108. Pryse-Davies J (1974) The development, structure and function of the female pelvic organs in childhood. Clin Obstet Gynaecol 1:483–508
109. Quagliarello J, Goldsmith L, Steinetz B, et al (1980) Induction of relaxin secretion in nonpregnant women by human chorionic gonadotropin. J Clin Endocrinol Metab 51:74–77
110. Rao CV (1982) Receptors for gonadotropins in human ovaries. In: Recent advances in fertility research, part A: Developments in reproductive endocrinology. Alan R Liss, New York pp 123–135
111. Reagan JW (1950) Ceroid pigment in the human ovary. Am J Obstet Gynecol 59:433–436
112. Reed MJ, Beranek PA, Ghilchik MW, James VHT (1985) Conversion of estrone to estradiol and estradiol to estrone in postmenopausal women. Obstet Gynecol 66:361–365
113. Reeves G (1971) Specific stroma in the cortex and medulla of the ovary. Cell types and vascular supply in relation to follicular apparatus and ovulation. Obstet Gynecol 37:832–844
114. Rice BF, Hammerstein J, Savard K (1964) Steroid hormone formation in the human ovary. II. Action of gonadotropins in vitro in the corpus luteum. J Clin Endocrinol 24:606–615
115. Rice BF, Savard K (1966) Steroid hormone formation in the human ovary: IV. Ovarian stromal compartment; formation of radioactive steroids from acetate-1-^{14}C and action of gonadotropins. J Clin Endocrinol 26:593–609
116. Rodriguez GC, Berchuk A, Whitaker RS, et al (1991) Epidermal growth factor receptor expression in normal ovarian epithelium and ovarian cancer. II. Relationship between receptor expression and response to epidermal growth factor. Am J Obstet Gynecol 164:745–750
117. Safneck JR, DeSa DJ (1986) Structures mimicking sex cord-stromal tumours and gonadoblastomas in the ovaries of normal infants and children. Histopathology (Oxf) 10:909–920
118. Sauromo H (1954) Development, occurrence, function, and pathology of the rete ovarii. Acta Obstet Gynecol Scand Suppl 33:29–66
119. Schmidt CL, Black VH, Sarosi P, Weiss G (1986) Progesterone and relaxin secretion in relation to the ultrastructure of human luteal cells in culture: effects of human chorionic gonadotropin. Am J Obstet Gynecol 155:1209–1219
120. Schmidt WA (1986) Eosin-induced fluorescence of Reinke crystals. Int J Gynecol Pathol 5:88–89

121. Scully RE (1981) Smooth-muscle differentiation in genital tract disorders [Editorial]. Arch Pathol Lab Med 105:505–507
122. Scully RE, Cohen RB (1964) Oxidative-enzyme activity in normal and pathologic human ovaries. Obstet Gynecol 24:667–681
123. Sealey JE, Glorioso N, Itskovitz J, Laragh JH (1986) Prorenin as a reproductive hormone. New form of the renin system. Am J Med 81:1041–1046
124. Shaw JA, Dabbs DJ, Geisinger KR (1992) Sclerosing stromal tumor of the ovary: an ultrastructural and immunohistochemical analysis with histogenetic considerations. Ultrastruct Pathol 16:363–377
125. Shima K, Kitayama S, Nakano R (1987) Gonadotropin binding sites in human ovarian follicles and corpora lutea during the menstrual cycle. Obstet Gynecol 69:800–806
126. Snowden JA, Harkin PJR, Thornton JG, Wells M (1989) Morphometric assessment of ovarian stromal proliferation: a clinicopathological study. Histopathology (Oxf) 14:369–379
127. Stangel JJ, Richart RM, Okagaki T, Cottral G (1970) Nuclear DNA content of luteinized cells of the human ovary. Am J Obstet Gynecol 108:543–549
128. Starup J, Visfeldt J (1974) Ovarian morphology in early and late human pregnancy. Acta Obstet Gynecol Scand 53:211–218
129. Sternberg WH (1949) The morphology, androgenic function, hyperplasia, and tumors of the human ovarian hilus cells. Am J Pathol 25:493–521
130. Sternberg WH, Segaloff A, Gaskill CJ (1953) Influence of chorionic gonadotropin on human ovarian hilus cells (Leydig-like cells). J Clin Endocrinol Metab 13:139–153
131. Tanabe K, Gagliano P, Channing CP, et al (1983) Levels of inhibin-F activity and steroids in human follicular fluid from normal women and women with polycystic ovarian disease. J Clin Endocrinol Metab 57:24–31
132. Tsonis CG, Messinis IE, Templeton AA, et al (1988) Gonadotropic stimulation of inhibin secretion by the human ovary during the follicular and early luteal phase of the cycle. J Clin Endocrinol Metab 66:915–921
133. Valdes-Dapena MA (1967) The normal ovary of childhood. Ann NY Acad Sci 142:597–613
134. Vermeulen A (1976) The hormonal activity of the postmenopausal ovary. J Clin Endocrinol Metab 42:247–253
135. Vijayakumar R, Walters WAW (1987) Ovarian stromal and luteal tissue prostaglandins, 17-beta-estradiol, and progesterone in relation to the phases of the menstrual cycle in women. Am J Obstet Gynecol 156:947–951
136. Visfeldt J, Starup J (1974) Dating of the human corpus luteum of menstruation using histological parameters. Acta Pathol Microbiol Scand A 82:137–144
137. Weiss G, O'Byrne EM, Steinetz BG (1976) Relaxin: a product of the human corpus luteum of pregnancy. Science 194:948–949
138. Weiss G, O'Byrne EM, Hochman JA, Goldsmith LT, Rifkin I, Steinetz BG (1977) Secretion of progesterone and relaxin by the human corpus luteum at midpregnancy and at term. Obstet Gynecol 50:679–681
139. Weiss G, Rifkin I (1975) Progesterone and estrogen secretion by puerperal human ovaries. Obstet Gynecol 46:557–559
140. White RF, Hertig AT, Rock J, Adams E (1951) Histological and histochemical observations on the corpus luteum of human pregnancy with special reference to corpora lutea associated with early normal and abnormal ova. Contrib Embryol 34:55–74
141. Wiley CA, Esterly JR (1976) Observations on the human corpus luteum: histochemical changes during development and involution. Am J Obstet Gynecol 125:514–519
142. Yussman MA, Taymor ML (1970) Serum levels of follicle stimulating hormone and luteinizing hormone and of plasma progesterone related to ovulation by corpus luteum biopsy. J Clin Endocrinol 30:396–399
143. Zhang J, Young RH, Arseneau J, Scully RE (1982) Ovarian stromal tumors containing lutein or Leydig cells (luteinized thecomas and stromal Leydig cell tumors): a clinicopathological analysis of fifty cases. Int J Gynecol Pathol 1:270–285

16

Nonneoplastic Lesions of the Ovary

Philip B. Clement, M.D.

Nonneoplastic lesions of the ovary frequently form a pelvic mass and often are associated with abnormal hormonal manifestations, thus potentially mimicking an ovarian neoplasm on clinical examination, at operation, or on pathologic examination. Many occur in the reproductive years and may be associated with infertility. Their proper recognition is, therefore, important to allow appropriate, usually conservative therapy, thereby avoiding unnecessary oophorectomy.

Congenital Lesions

Absent Ovary

In phenotypic females, *absence of both ovaries* usually is associated with an abnormal karyotype and a syndrome of gonadal dysgenesis (see Chapter 1, Embryology of the Female Genital Tract and Disorders of Abnormal Sexual Development). In such cases, bilateral streak gonads or a unilateral streak gonad and a contralateral intraabdominal testis are usually found. However, rare cases of truly agonadal individuals have been reported, usually with a karyotype that is 46XY, but rarely, 46XX.[245] Rare patients with ataxia telangiectasia have had no evidence of ovarian tissue at laparotomy.[33]

Rarely, one ovary may be absent in an otherwise normal woman, usually representing an incidental finding at operation or postmortem examination. Associated findings frequently include agenesis or malformation of the ipsilateral fallopian tube, round ligament, kidney, or ureter, alone or in various combinations.[39,339] The differential diagnosis includes (1) ectopic ovary, which may lie at the level of the liver, close to the kidney, within the omentum,[245] or within an inguinal hernia,[37] and (2) adnexal torsion with atrophy or autoamputation.

Lobulated, Accessory, and Supernumerary Ovary

Examples of *lobulated*, *accessory*, and *supernumerary ovary* are among the rarest of gynecologic abnormalities. A lobulated ovary is a normally situated ovary divided by one or several fissures into two or more lobes. The lobes may be completely separate or connected by fibrous tissue or ovarian stroma; rarely both ovaries may be affected. A closely related anomaly is an accessory ovary, a structure containing normal ovarian tissue located in the vicinity of a normal, eutopic ovary with which it has a direct or ligamentous attachment. A supernumerary ovary is a similar structure but located at some distance from, and not connected to, a eutopic ovary.[69,112,161] It may be pelvic, attached to the uterus, bladder, or pelvic walls, or retroperitoneal, within the omentum, periaortic area, or mesentery. In most cases, the accessory or supernumerary ovary is less than 1 cm in size, and smaller examples may go unrecognized at operation or autopsy; they are multiple and bilateral in some cases.[112] The ectopic ovarian tissue possesses the functional potential, as evidenced by persistent menses after bilateral oophorectomy, as well as the pathologic potential of normal ovaries.[120,199] The presence of a supernumerary ovary therefore is one histogenetic mechanism for ovarian-type tumors in extraovarian sites. This derivation is even more likely for nonepithelial tumors, such as a granulosa-theca tumors within the broad ligament,[104] which are unlikely to have a mesothelial or secondary müllerian origin (see Chapter 17, Diseases of the Peritoneum).

Lobulated and accessory ovary are closely related embryonically. The former results from lobulation of the ovarian anlage, whereas the latter presumably develops from a slightly separated part of the otherwise normally developing and migrating ovarian anlage. Pathogenetic theories for supernumerary ovary include aberrent migration of part of the gonadal ridge after incorporation of the germ cells or, alternatively, arrest of some of the migrating germ cells in an ectopic location with inductive transformation of the surrounding tissue into ovarian stroma. As many as one-third of patients with lobulated ovaries, accessory ovary, and supernumerary ovary have other congenital genitourinary abnormalities.

Adrenal Cortical Rests

Although accessory adrenal cortical tissue frequently is observed within the wall of the fallopian tube and the broad ligament, it is an extremely rare finding in the ovary.[307] The adrenal rests are typically yellow, spherical, encapsulated nodules several millimeters in size (Fig. 16.1). Adrenal cortical ectopia in these sites can be explained by the close proximity of the anlage of the adrenal cortex to the gonadal ridge during embryonic development. Ovarian adrenal cortical rests may be the origin of occasional steroid cell tumors of the ovary that resemble adrenal cortical tissue in both their histologic appearance and endocrine manifestations.

Uterus-Like Ovarian Mass

The seven reported examples of a *uterus-like ovarian mass* have occurred in adult women (18–49 years of age) and were characterized by a central cavity lined by endometrial tissue and a thick wall of smooth muscle.[242] Additional findings have included an elevated CA-125 level (two cases), an associated breast carcinoma (two cases), and a contiguous endometrioid adenocarcinoma (one case). Although the lesion can be explained on the basis of an ovarian endometriotic cyst with smooth muscle metaplasia of its stromal component (endomyometriosis; see Chapter 17, Diseases of the Peritoneum), in some cases it may may be caused by a congenital malformation of the ipsilateral müllerian

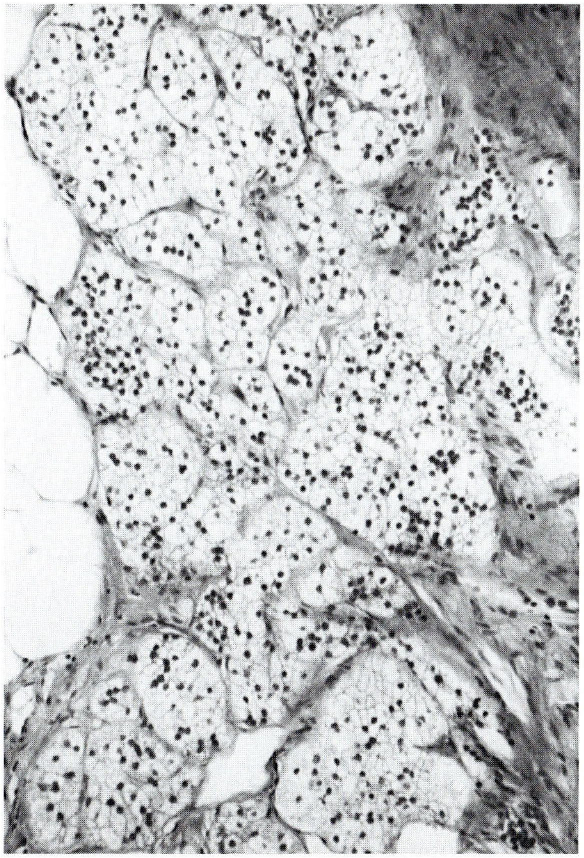

Fig. 16.1. **Adrenal cortical rest within mesovarium.** Nests of cells with foamy cytoplasm are separated by a scanty fibrous stroma.

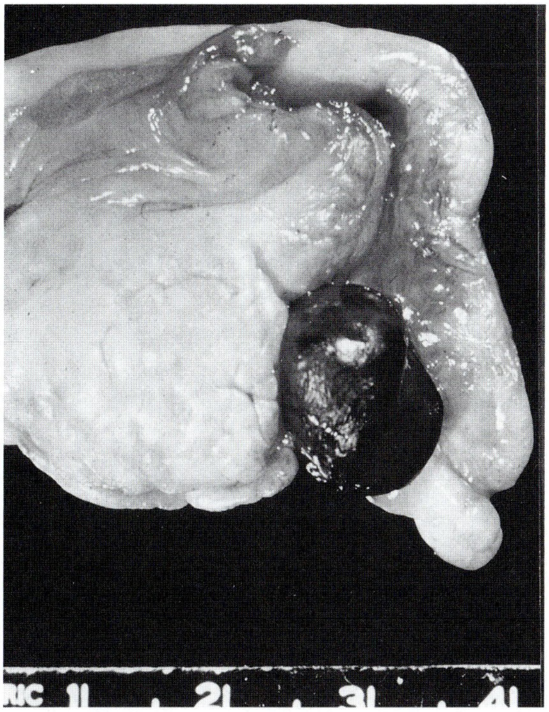

Fig. 16.2. **Splenic–gonadal fusion.** A nodule of splenic tissue is contiguous with the surface of the ovary.

duct,[264] an origin supported by the presence of congenital abnormalities of the urinary tract in two of the reported cases. In several other cases, however, residual ovarian parenchyma was identified at the periphery of the mass.

Splenic–Gonadal Fusion

Splenic–gonadal fusion (Fig. 16.2) is an extremely rare anomaly resulting from fusion of the anlage of both organs during embryonic development. The male/female ratio is 9:1. Three examples have been described in newborn female infants, two of which were associated with partially undescended ovaries, as well as other, multiple, congenital anomalies.[254] All three cases were of the continuous type in which a cordlike structure connected the spleen to the left ovary or surrounding structures. In one of these cases, several intraovarian splenic nodules were found. A case of discontinuous splenic–gonadal fusion has been reported in a 19-year-old woman with no other apparent congenital abnormalities.[198] In an additional case, a 44-year-old woman had a septate uterus and a cluster of splenic nodules surrounding the otherwise normal left ovary; multiple adhesions made it difficult to ascertain if a splenic–ovarian cord was present.[8] The differential diagnosis in the discontinuous cases is with traumatic splenosis. Affected women usually have a history of trauma, and at laparotomy, splenic nodules are widely dispersed throughout the peritoneal cavity (see Chapter 17, Disease of the Peritoneum).

Infections

Common Bacterial Infections

Pelvic inflammatory disease (PID) of bacterial origin accounts for most ovarian infections in the western world. Although some studies have indicated that the presence of an intrauterine device (IUD) increases the risk of infection, other studies have shown that when the number of sexual partners are controlled for, IUDs do not increase the risk of PID.[145] Ovarian involvement by PID is almost always secondary to salpingitis and typically takes the form of a tuboovarian abscess (Fig. 16.3), which usually is bilateral. The typical clinical manifestations are abdominal or pelvic pain, and, less often, fever, vaginal discharge or bleeding, and urinary symptoms.[165] An

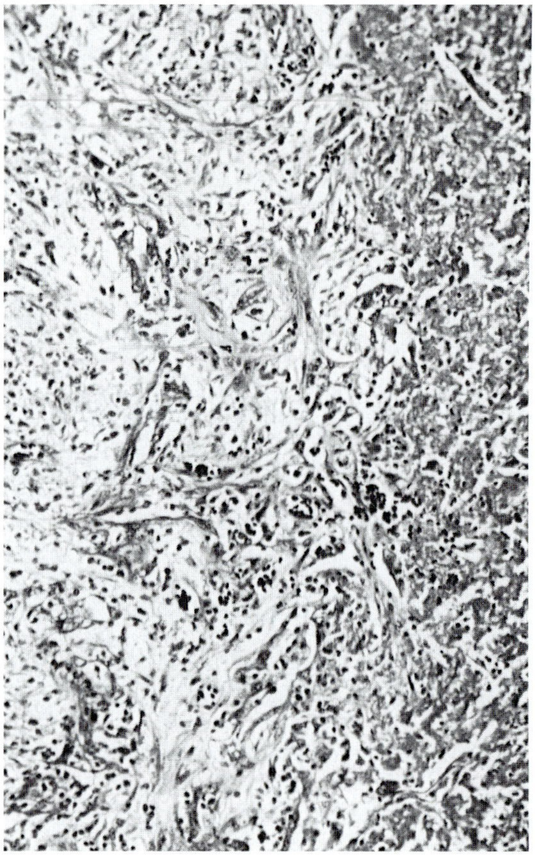

Fig. 16.3. **Tuboovarian abscess.** Lining consists of inflammatory debris with subjacent granulation tissue.

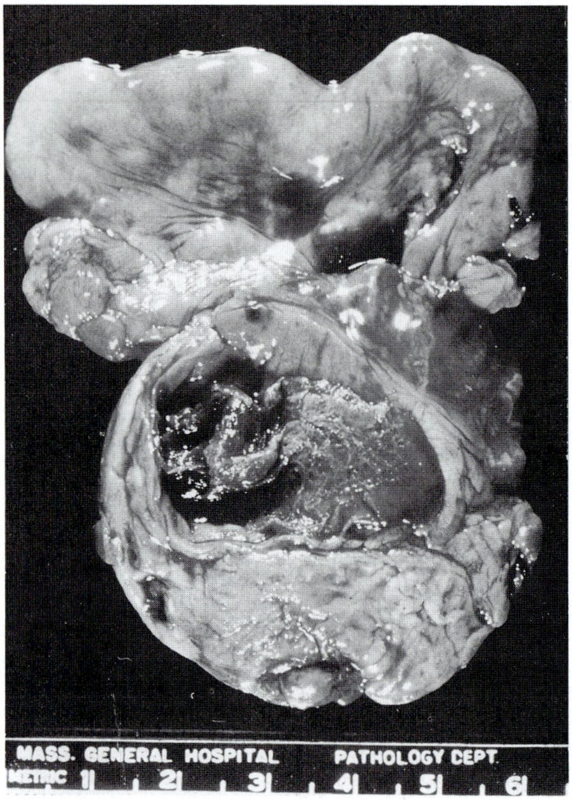

Fig. 16.4. **Ovarian abscess, sectioned surface.** Note the normal fallopian tube.

adnexal mass is palpable, demonstrable with imaging techniques or visible at laparoscopy. A history of an acute infectious episode is present in only one-third to one-half of patients, suggesting that subclinical infections are common.[165] A mixed flora with a preponderance of anaerobic organisms is typically recovered from the contents of the abscess.[82,165] With resolution, the only sequelae may be tuboovarian fibrous adhesions, but occasionally a healed abscess becomes a cyst.

A unilateral or bilateral ovarian abscess without tubal involvement is much rarer than a tuboovarian abscess. The former usually is secondary to direct or lymphatic spread of organisms from a nongynecologic pelvic inflammatory process, such as diverticulitis, appendicitis, inflammatory bowel disease, or postoperative pelvic infection.[325] Rarely, an ovarian abscess is the result of a blood-borne infection. The external ovarian surface in such cases often is unremarkable, and the process may not be apparent until the organ is sectioned (Fig. 16.4). Uncommonly, rupture of an ovarian or tuboovarian abscess leads to secondary peritonitis or, rarely, fistulas involving the colon, bladder, or vagina.[53,290]

Milder, chronic, or recurrent forms of ovarian involvement by PID may take the form of a chronic perioophoritis, with periovarian and tuboovarian adhesions. Sclerocystic ovarian changes have been described in such cases.[255] Rarely, a chronic ovarian abscess may result in a solid tumor-like mass, variably designated ovarian xanthogranuloma, xanthogranulomatous oophoritis, or inflammatory pseudotumor.[240] The involved ovary in such cases is replaced by a solid, yellow, lobulated mass characterized microscopically by foamy histiocytes admixed with multinucleated giant cells, plasma cells, fibroblasts, neutrophils, foci of necrosis, and fibrosis (Fig. 16.5). Several additional examples of pseudotumorous xanthogranulomatous inflammation with a more diffuse involvement of the adnexa have been described.[162]

Rare Bacterial Infections

Actinomycosis

Pelvic actinomyces infection is uncommon and usually represents a complication of an IUD, although most cases of IUD-related PID are nonactinomycotic.[147,165,213,280] Almost 85% of cases have occurred

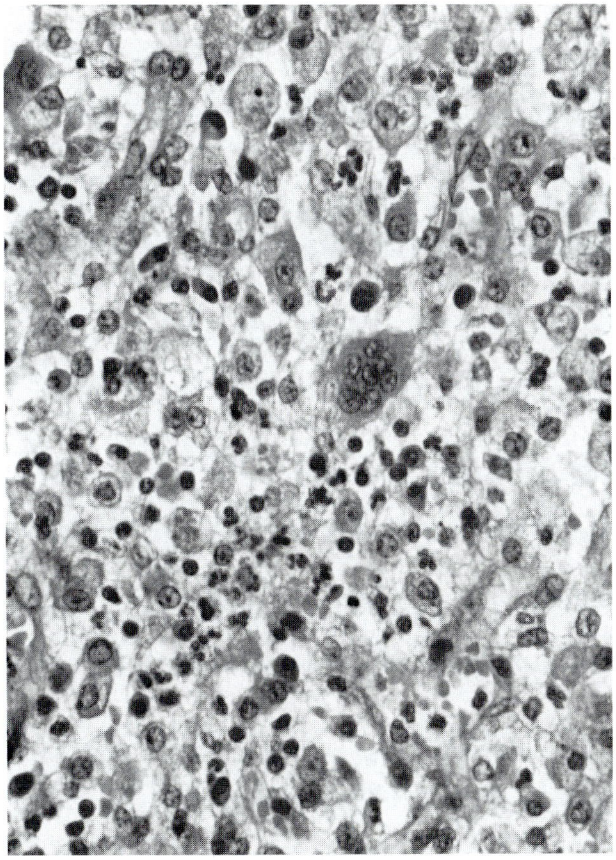

Fig. 16.5. Xanthogranuloma of ovary. Inflammatory reaction consists predominantly of foamy histiocytes, some of which are multinucleated. (Reprinted by permission of Pace et al., ref. 240.)

in women who have had an IUD in place for 3 or more years,[280] and the infection may be more common in women using plastic, rather than copper, IUDs.[147] There is a high likelihood of subsequent sterility.[280]

The adnexal involvement usually is unilateral, with destructive, often multiple, abscesses involving the ovary (Fig. 16.6) and fallopian tube (see Chapter 14, Diseases of the Fallopian Tube). Rarely, the characteristic actinomycotic (sulfur) granules are grossly visible within the abscess cavities. Microscopic examination typically reveals a nonspecific inflammatory response composed predominantly of neutrophils and foamy histiocytes sometimes admixed with lymphocytes and plasma cells. A specific diagnosis can be made only by finding the sulfur granules within the inflammatory exudate, but numerous blocks may be necessary to find them. The granules are composed of circumscribed rounded masses of basophilic, gram-positive, argyrophilic bacteria growing as branching filaments with a characteristic radial or palisading pattern at the periphery of the granule (Fig. 16.7). A fluorescent antibody stain may

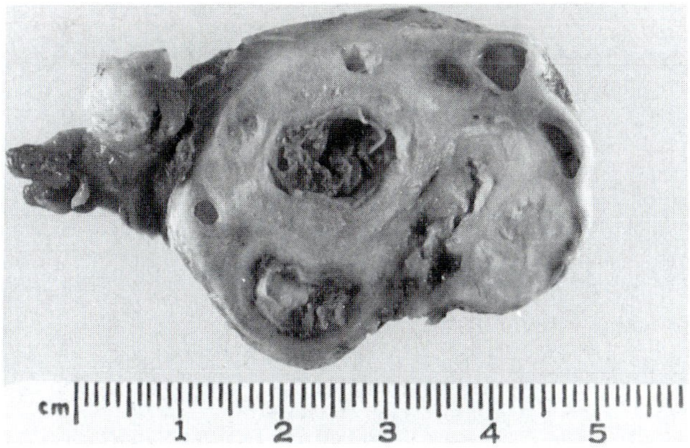

Fig. 16.6. Actinomycosis of ovary. The ovary is enlarged by many confluent abscesses. (Reprinted by permission of Schmidt et al., ref. 280.)

facilitate their detection.[249] A diagnosis of actinomycosis may be made before salpingo-oophorectomy in some cases by finding the granules within endometrial curettings or cervico-vaginal smears. In one study, almost 90% of patients with actinomyces demonstrated by the latter method were found to have a tubo-ovarian abscess.[42,147]

Tuberculosis

Tuberculous oophoritis is uncommon and usually secondary to tuberculous salpingitis (see Chapter 14, Diseases of the Fallopian Tube). The tubes are almost always involved in tuberculosis of the female genital tract, but the ovarian parenchyma is affected in only 10% of cases.[232] Unilateral or bilateral adnexal masses, in some cases accompanied by an elevated CA-125 level, may clinically simulate an ovarian tumor.[204] On macroscopic inspection, the ovaries are typically adherent to the tubal ampullae. Grossly visible caseation is rare. On histologic examination, the tuberculosis is typically confined to the cortex. In cases in which the ovary is enlarged, granulomas on the adjacent peritoneum may simulate metastatic ovarian cancer at operation.[232,306]

Malacoplakia

Of approximately 25 reported cases of gynecologic malacoplakia, only 3 have involved the ovary.[46,153] Friable, yellow, focally hemorrhagic and necrotic masses involve one or both ovaries and the ipsilateral fallopian tube. In one case, the process also involved contiguous portions of small and large bowel, simulating a malignant ovarian tumor at operation.[153] Histologic examination reveals the typical features of malacoplakia. Organisms (*Es-*

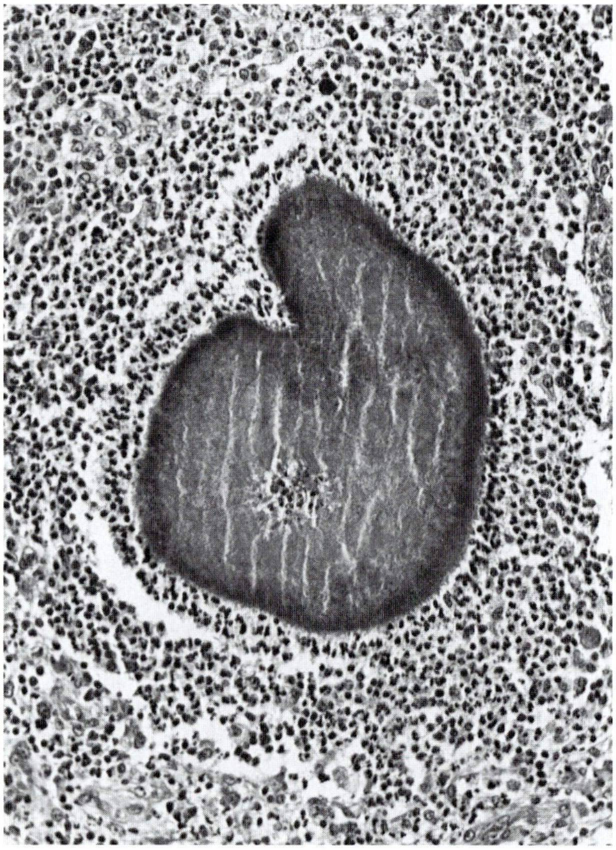

Fig. 16.7. Actinomycosis of ovary. A colony of actinomyces (sulfur granule) is surrounded by a purulent exudate. (Reprinted by permission of the Armed Forces Institute of Pathology, Neg. No. 74-13508.)

cherichia coli and *Enterococcus faecalis*) were demonstrated by culture in only one of the cases.[153]

Leprosy

Although *leprosy* rarely involves the female genital tract, the ovary is the most commonly involved gynecologic site.[35] In one well-documented case, microscopic examination of the grossly normal ovaries revealed numerous vacuolated histiocytes within the ovarian stroma that contained *Mycobacterium leprae*. In chronic forms of leprous oophoritis, a chronic inflammatory cell infiltrate and fibrosis are seen, and bacilli usually are demonstrable.

Syphilis

For unknown reasons, *syphilitic involvement* of the ovary is very rare. Luetic oophoritis has been described in congenital, secondary, and tertiary forms of the disease. The pathology of these various stages is similar to those in extraovarian sites.

Parasitic Infections

Parasitic infestations of the ovary are extremely rare in most parts of the world. Ovarian schistosomiasis, however, is common in endemic areas; the fallopian tube is typically also involved.[180] Patients usually have lower abdominal pain, a pelvic mass, and occasionally irregular menses and infertility. The typical operative findings are an enlarged tube and ovary, numerous adhesions, and scattered peritoneal nodules that may simulate the implants of a malignant tumor. On histologic examination, granulomas, often containing eosinophils, surround schistosoma ova. Dense fibrosis frequently is seen in the later stages of the disease.

Ovarian involvement by *Enterobius vermicularis* usually is an incidental operative finding on the external surface, or, rarely, within the ovary.[150,194] In several cases, there has been simultaneous involvement of the pelvic peritoneum, simulating a metastatic tumor. The granulomas, which may undergo caseation and contain eosinophils, surround the adult female worms and ova.[194] The worms probably reach the peritoneal cavity by migration from the perineum through the lumen of the genital tract.

Rare cases of ovarian echinococcosis have been described.[116] In one of them, a typical hydatid cyst 12 cm in diameter involved the ovary.

Viral Infections

Oophoritis secondary to cytomegalovirus (CMV) can occur as an incidental finding in surgical or autopsy specimens in immunosuppressed patients, usually as part of a generalized infection.[305,330] On macroscopic examination, the ovaries are usually of normal size but contain foci of superficial cortical hemorrhagic necrosis several millimeters in size.[305] Microscopic examination reveals foci of coagulative necrosis, with variable numbers of neutrophils, nuclear debris, and hemorrhage, as well as lymphocytes, plasma cells, and vascular dilatation in the surrounding stroma. Ovarian stromal and endothelial cells, even at a distance from the necrotic foci, contain typical intranuclear and occasional intracytoplasmic inclusion bodies (Fig. 16.8). Immunohistochemical staining for CMV may facilitate the diagnosis in some cases,[330] and intranuclear and intracytoplasmic herpes-type viral particles have been found on ultrastructural examination.

Mumps oophoritis as a clinical entity occurs much less commonly than mumps orchitis; clinical evidence of the lesion occurs in 5% of females with mumps. The pathology of the acute stage has not

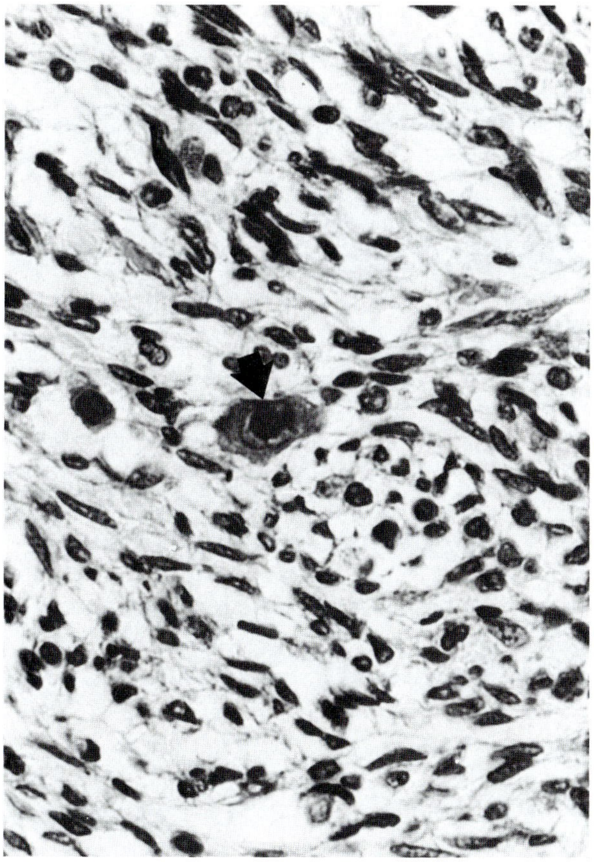

Fig. 16.8. Cytomegalovirus infection of ovary. Ovarian stromal cell contains an intranuclear inclusion (*arrow*). (Reprinted by permission of Subietas et al., ref. 305.)

been well described. It is postulated that germ cell depletion secondary to mumps oophoritis may result in premature menopause and possibly an increased risk of ovarian cancer.[6,68,210]

In view of the frequency of human papillomavirus (HPV) infection in the lower female genital tract, it is perhaps surprising that histologically documented examples of HPV infection of the ovary have not been described. Lai et al., however, recently have found HPV-16 or HPV-18 DNA sequences by the polymerase chain reaction (PCR) in 5 of 10 histologically normal ovaries.[163]

Fungal Infections

Fungal infections of the ovary are extremely rare, even in patients with disseminated mycoses. Three examples of tuboovarian abscess, caused by *Blastomyces dermatitidis,* have been reported.[84,115,215] In one case the abscesses were bilateral and associated with miliary nodules involving the pelvic peritoneum. In two of the cases the abscesses were probably secondary to hematogenous spread from the lungs, while in the third case the infection was sexually transmitted.

Seven of 11 patients with coccidioidomycosis of the upper female genital tract had tuboovarian and peritoneal involvement; 2 of the 7 had concomitant coccidioidal endometritis.[43] One case of tuboovarian abscess caused by *Aspergillus* has been reported in an IUD user.[156] Rupture of the abscess led to generalized peritonitis.

Noninfectious Inflammatory Disorders

A variety of noninfectious, typically granulomatous, inflammatory disorders may involve the ovary. In addition, granulomas may be seen rarely in autoimmune oophoritis.

Foreign Body Granulomas

A variety of foreign materials may evoke a *granulomatous reaction* on the ovarian and extraovarian peritoneal surfaces, potentially mimicking a malignant tumor at operation. Examples include suture material,[192] lipid material used in hysterosalpingographic contrast material, crystalline material such as talc,[211] and keratin (Fig. 16.9) from cystic teratomas and the squamous elements of endometrial and ovarian endometrioid adenocarcinomas (peritoneal and ovarian keratin granulomas are discussed in more detail in Chapter 17, Diseases of the Peritoneum). A foreign body reaction also occurs in response to starch granules from surgical gloves,[229,243] starch-containing douche fluid,[124] and lubricants.[277] Rarely, the starch granulomas are of the tuberculoid type, with or without caseous necrosis, and mimic tuberculosis on microscopic examination.[229] Granulomatous oophoritis is occasionally a response to bowel contents that reach the ovary via a coloovarian fistula.[23,106,185] Foreign body-type granulomas containing brown to black carbon pigment have been described in the ovary secondary to laser or electrocautery treatment (Fig. 16.10).[309]

Necrobiotic (Palisading) Granulomas

Necrobiotic granulomas have been encountered in the ovary, usually as an incidental microscopic finding.[5,122,149,192,309,332] In most cases, there is a history of an operation or cauterization involving the same ovary months to years earlier. The granulomas can be multiple and occasionally bilateral. A central zone of fibrinoid necrosis or hyalinization is

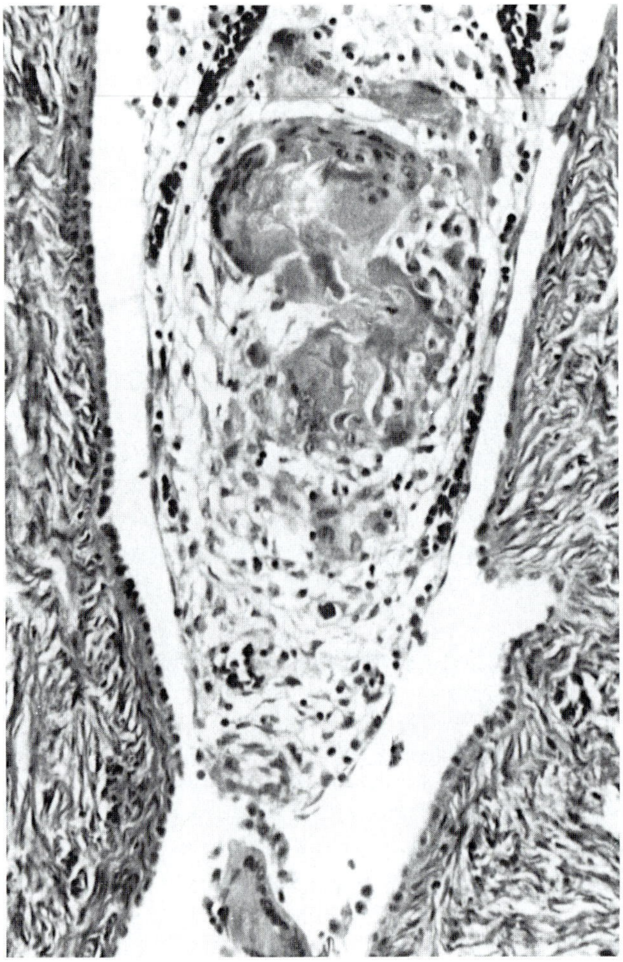

Fig. 16.9. Foreign body reaction to keratin implants on ovarian serosal surface. There was a coexistent endometrial adenocanthoma confined to the uterus.

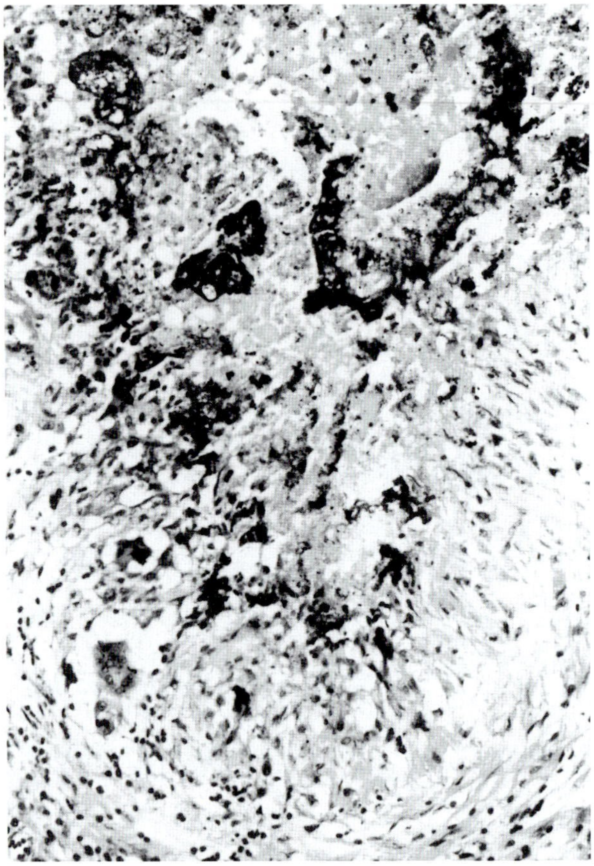

Fig. 16.10. Postcautery carbon pigment granuloma in ovary. Note black carbon pigment, some of which is in foreign-body type giant cells. Palisading histiocytes are seen at the *bottom* and *bottom right*

usually surrounded by palisading, sometimes multinucleated, histiocytes and variable numbers of other inflammatory cells including lymphocytes, plasma cells, and eosinophils; a fibrous pseudocapsule forms in some of the cases (Fig. 16.11). Brown to black carbon pigment (as already noted) is typically present in multinucleated giant cells in postcautery palisading granulomas.[309] The differential diagnosis of palisading granulomas includes the other ovarian granulomas discussed in this chapter, as well as necrotic pseudoxanthomatous nodules of endometriosis (see Chapter 17, Diseases of the Peritoneum).

Granulomas Secondary to Systemic Diseases

Four cases of ovarian involvement by sarcoidosis have been reported.[326] The sarcoid granulomas were an incidental microscopic finding in each case. In the three cases reported in detail, the patients had systemic sarcoidosis, as well as involvement of other gynecologic sites or paraaortic lymph nodes. The finding of sarcoid-like granulomas in the ovary should alert the pathologist to the possibility of a rare dysgerminoma with a granulomatous reaction sufficiently extensive to obscure the malignant tumor cells. Crohn's disease is another rare cause of granulomatous oophoritis, usually caused by direct extension of the inflammatory process from the bowel.[334] The ipsilateral fallopian tube is also involved in most cases. Although not strictly granulomatous, mucicarminophilic histiocytosis can occasionally involve the ovary (see Chapter 17).

Cortical Granulomas

Cortical granulomas are common, incidental, microscopic findings within the ovarian cortex. The granulomas are spherical, well circumscribed, 100–500

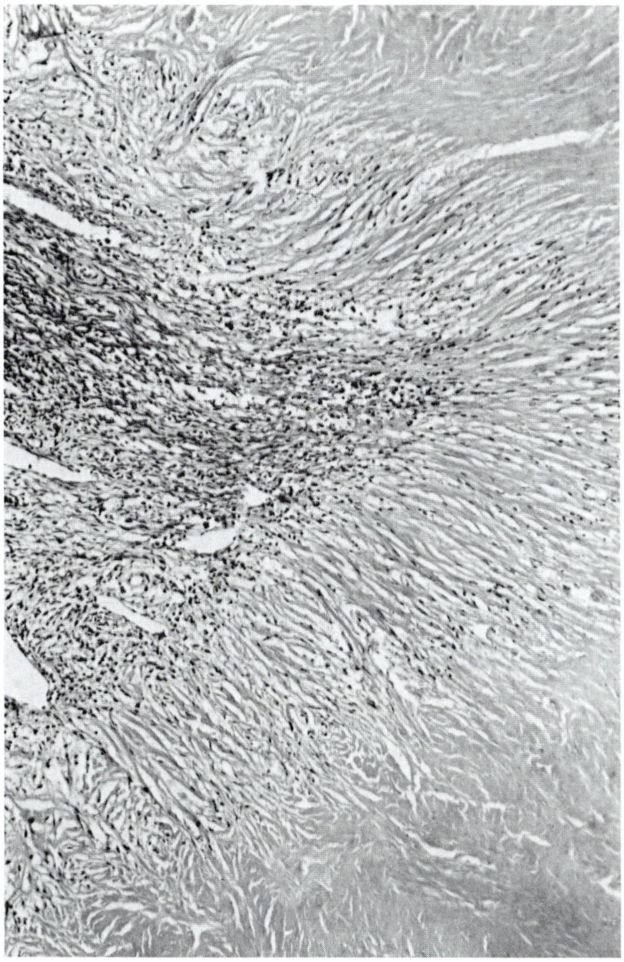

Fig. 16.11. Isolated palisading granuloma of ovary. (Reprinted by permission of Herbold et al., ref. 122.)

μm in diameter, and are composed of spindle cells, epithelioid cells, lymphocytes, and, in some, multinucleated giant cells; occasional anisotropic fat crystals also may be seen (Fig. 16.12a).[36,131,132,211] Hughesdon suggested that the granulomas become fibrotic with time, accounting for at least some of the spherical, cloudlike, hyaline scars commonly encountered in the cortical stroma of postmenopausal women.[131,132] These scars resemble corpora fibrosa but usually are distinguishable from the latter by their more superficial location within the cortex, greater cellularity, weaker eosinophilia, and the presence of a reticulin framework (Fig. 16.12b).[132] It also has been suggested that hyaline scars may represent foci of atrophic endometrial stromatosis, luteinized stromal cells, or ectopic decidua.[131,132]

The frequency of cortical granulomas appears to be related to age. They are not usually encountered before the age of 30 years, but Hughesdon found active lesions in 40% of women over the age of 40 years; the number of lesions per cross section of ovary increased in successive decades.[132] The clinical significance, if any, of cortical granulomas is unknown. Possible associations with ovarian stromal hyperplasia, endometrial carcinoma, or both have been suggested but not demonstrated consistently.

Surface Proliferative Lesions

Surface Epithelial Inclusion Glands and Cysts

Surface epithelial inclusion (*SEI*) *glands* and their cystic counterparts, *SEI cysts*, arise from cortical invaginations of the ovarian surface epithelium that have lost their connection with the surface. SEI glands and cysts can be found in ovaries from females of all ages, including fetuses, infants, and adolescents.[30,32] With advancing age their frequency increases to the extent that they are common in the late-reproductive and postmenopausal age groups.

SEI cysts may be visible on gross inspection of the ovary, although most SEI glands and cysts are appreciable only on microscopic examination; cysts greater than 1 cm in diameter are designated a cystadenoma (see Chapter 18, Surface Epithelial Tumors of the Ovary). SEI glands and cysts are usually multiple, scattered singly or in small clusters throughout the superficial cortex (Fig. 16.13); less commonly, they extend into the deeper cortical or medullary stroma. They are typically lined by a single layer of columnar cells that in postmenopausal patients is often ciliated, mimicking tubal (endosalpingeal) epithelium. Psammoma bodies may be seen within the cysts and the adjacent stroma (Fig. 16.13) and, rarely, within cervicovaginal Papanicolaou smears.[178] Similar glands, with or without associated psammoma bodies, encountered on the ovarian surface, within periovarian adhesions, and elsewhere on the peritoneum and in the omentum, are designated *endosalpingiosis* (see Chapter 17, Diseases of the Peritoneum).

Less commonly the lining of the glands and cysts consists of other müllerian cell types (endometrioid, mucinous) or nonspecific, flat, cuboidal, or columnar cells. One case of apocrine metaplasia within a SEI cyst has been reported.[7] An Arias–Stella-like reaction has been described within SEI glands in pregnant patients.[32] One study found that hyperplastic and metaplastic changes within SEI glands are more common in women with polycystic ovarian disease or endometrial carcinoma, suggesting a possible hormonal basis for these changes.[260] A rare pseudoneoplastic alteration in SEI glands is a striking vacuolar, presumably hydropic, cytoplasmic change of

a

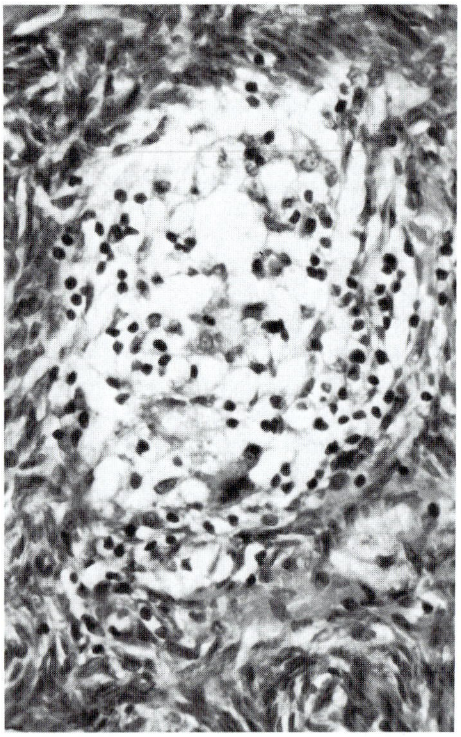

b

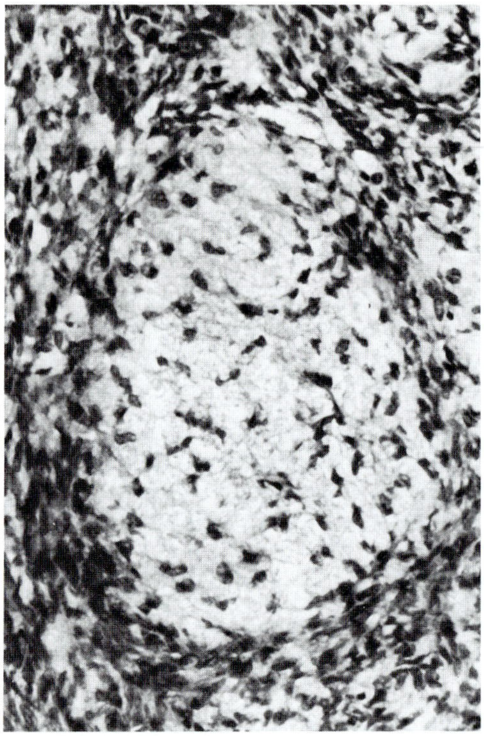

Fig. 16.12. a: **Cortical granuloma.** Circumscribed collection of lymphocytes, spindle cells, and occasional multinucleated giant cells lie within the ovarian stroma.

b: **Hyaline scar.** The circumscribed nodule consists of collagen and spindle cells.

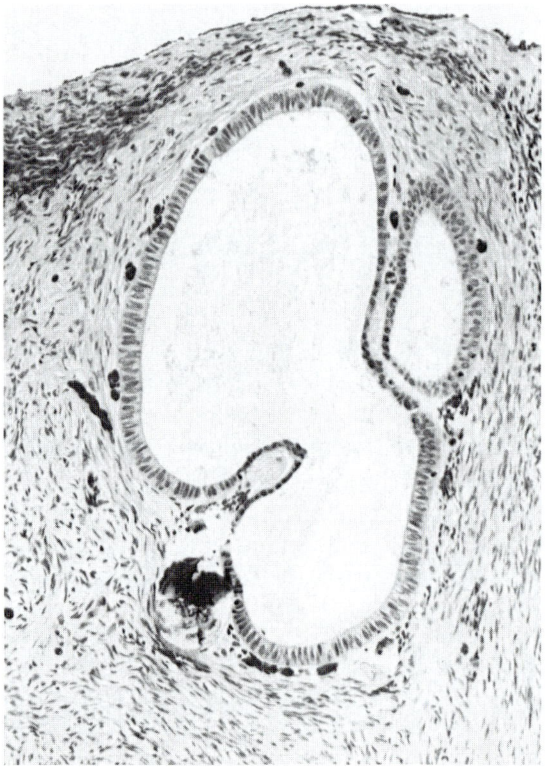

Fig. 16.13. Epithelial inclusion cyst. Cyst beneath ovarian surface epithelium is lined by a single layer of columnar cells. A psammoma body is present within the adjacent stroma.

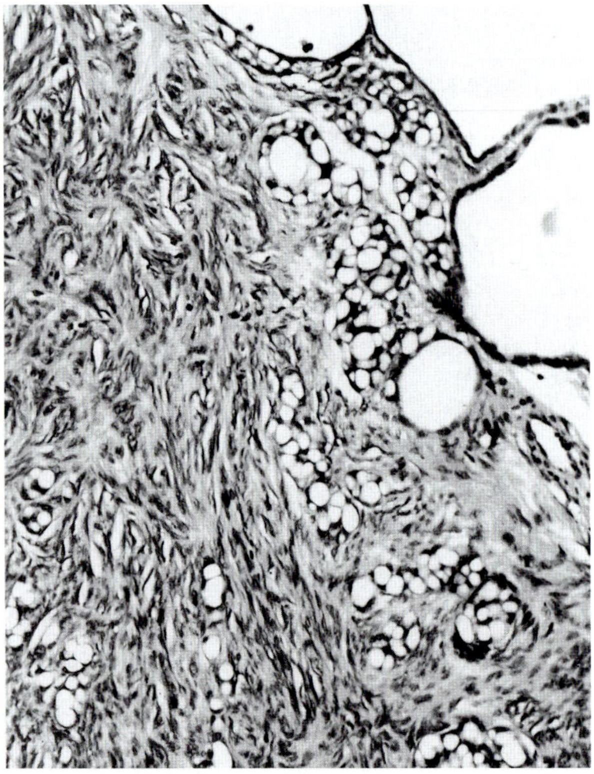

Fig. 16.14. Vacuolar change within surface epithelial inclusion glands. The lining cells exhibit hydropic change, simulating signet-ring cells. Similar cells form solid nests within the ovarian stroma.

the lining cells. In such cases, abundant clear cytoplasm displaces the nucleus, potentially mimicking signet-ring cell carcinoma, especially when the cells proliferate to form solid nests (Fig. 16.14). Awareness of this phenomenon, additional sectioning (if necessary) to demonstrate a relation to inclusion glands, and negative staining for mucin facilitate the diagnosis.

SEI glands and cysts are likely the site of origin for most common epithelial tumors of the ovary. Several studies have found that patients with ovarian carcinoma have an increased number of SEI cysts (or surface epithelial invaginations, their precursors) in the contralateral ovary compared to controls.[205,312] Additional support for this hypothesis is provided by the occasional presence of dysplastic changes within their linings[285] as well as immunoreactivity for a variety of ovarian epithelial tumor markers, including CA-125, CA-19-9, CEA, human chorionic gonadotropin (hCG), placental lactogen, alpha-2 glycoprotein, beta-1 glycoprotein, placental alkaline phosphatase, human milk fat globule protein, and p53.[31,51,61,72,134,141,234,235]

SEI cysts are distinguished from cystadenomas by their smaller size (see earlier). The differential diagnosis also includes other unilocular ovarian cysts.

Mesothelial Proliferations

Proliferation of mesothelial cells on the ovarian surface, within periovarian fibrous adhesions, or elsewhere on the pelvic peritoneum is usually a response to pelvic inflammation but also occurs in response to ovarian tumors and endometriosis. Florid examples may be associated with complex glandular and papillary proliferations of mesothelial cells that may exhibit mild to moderate atypia (Fig. 16.15). Such a process may simulate stromal invasion in a borderline ovarian tumor or simulate a metastatic carcinoma, primary serous surface carcinoma, or malignant mesothelioma. This subject is discussed in more detail in Chapter 17.

Surface Stromal Proliferations

Nodular, polypoid, and papillary stromal projections from the ovarian surface are a common incidental microscopic finding in women of late-reproductive and postmenopausal age. These projections are composed of ovarian stroma exhibiting varying degrees of hyalinization covered by a single layer of surface epithelium (Fig. 16.16). Detachment of these structures may give rise to "collagen balls" occasionally found in peritoneal washings.[335] Surface

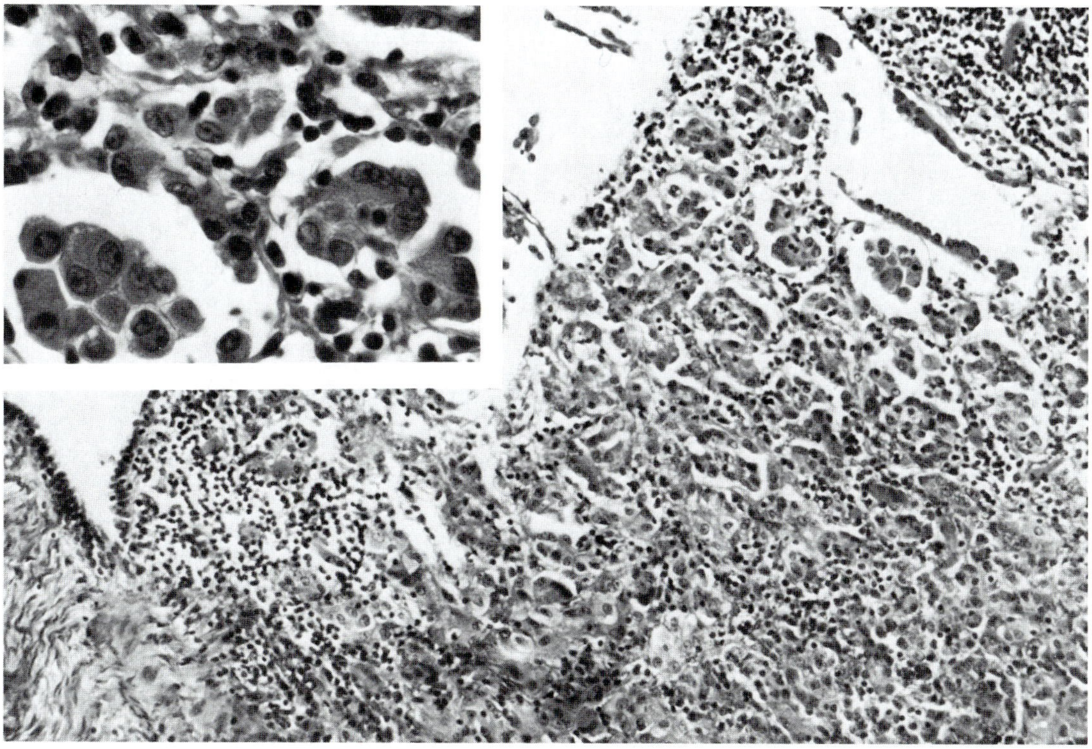

Fig. 16.15. Mesothelial proliferation on ovarian surface. Mesothelial cells, growing in papillary pattern, are admixed with lymphocytes. The mesothelial cells exhibit mild nuclear pleomorphism and multinucleation (*inset*).

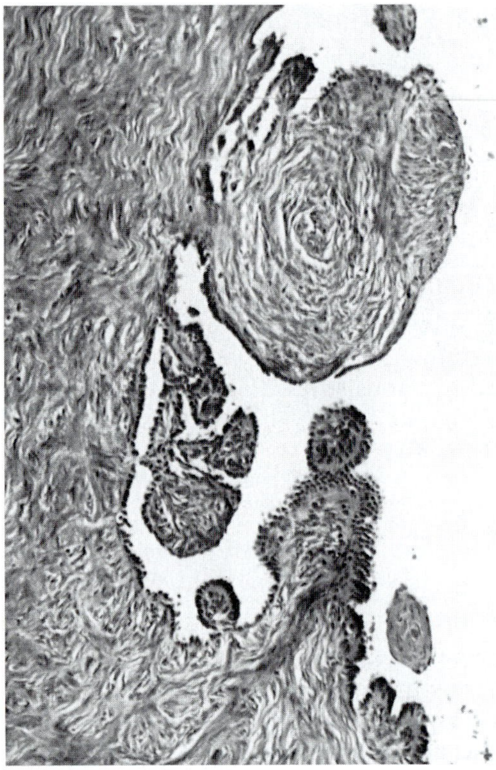

Fig. 16.16. Ovarian surface stromal proliferation. Papillary and nodular stromal proliferation involves ovarian surface.

stromal proliferations are typically 1–3 mm in maximal dimension and do not exceed 1 cm, the arbitrary dividing line between this type of proliferation and a serous surface papilloma.

Nonneoplastic Lesions of the Follicular and Stromal Elements

This section describes the wide spectrum of nonneoplastic lesions that arise from the ovarian follicles and stroma. Many of them are secondary to ovarian stimulation by pituitary or chorionic gonadotropins and may be associated with excessive production of estrogens, androgens, or both. Although most nonneoplastic proliferations of Leydig cells are not of stromal origin, these lesions are most conveniently discussed in this section.

Solitary Follicle Cysts

Solitary (or occasionally a few) *cysts of follicular origin* should be distinguished from disorders characterized by multiple, bilateral follicular cysts, which are discussed under a separate heading.

Clinical Features

Solitary follicle cysts (FCs) are most common in nonpregnant women of reproductive age, particularly around the menarche and menopause. FCs may also occur during fetal life,[196] in newborns,[74,169,328] throughout childhood,[169] and rarely after the onset of the menopause.[304] Solitary or multiple FCs can be a component of the McCune–Albright syndrome (polyostotic fibrous dysplasia, cutaneous melanin pigmentation, and endocrine organ hyperactivity), as discussed later, and postpubertal women with cystic fibrosis may be predisposed to the development of solitary FCs.[288] Corpus luteum cysts (CLCs) usually occur during the reproductive era but rarely are found in neonates[201] or follow sporadic ovulation in a postmenopausal woman.

The proportion of FCs and CLCs associated with clinical manifestations is unknown because many are incidentally discovered by pelvic ultrasononography, laparoscopy, or laparotomy. Patients with clinically evident FCs and CLCs typically have either a palpable adnexal mass or manifestations related to increased estrogen production that may include isosexual precocity or pseudoprecocity,[59,212,304] menstrual disturbances including amenorrhea and postmenopausal bleeding, or endometrial hyperplasia. A CLC is the most common finding in the ovarian remnant syndrome (see page 715). An uncommon clinical presentation of FCs and CLCs is rupture, which may cause abdominal pain, hemoperitoneum,[114] and rarely exsanguination. Rupture is more likely to occur in patients receiving anticoagulant therapy[166] or in those with bleeding diatheses.[324] Additionally, FCs occurring in utero or during the neonatal period may be complicated by adnexal torsion, as well as hemorrhage and rupture; most regress during the first 4 months of life.

Gross Findings

Solitary follicle cysts (FCs) and corpus luteum cysts (CLCs) are thin walled and unilocular, ranging from 3 to 8 cm in diameter, although larger examples occur rarely (Fig. 16.17), especially during pregnancy and the puerperium (see following). They usually have smooth surfaces and thin walls. CLCs are characterized by the presence of a convoluted yellow lining (Fig. 16.18). The contents of FCs and CLCs vary from serous or serosanguinous fluid to clotted blood.

Microscopic Findings

FCs are lined by an inner layer of granulosa cells that may be focally denuded and an outer layer of theca interna cells (Fig. 16.19a). The cells in either

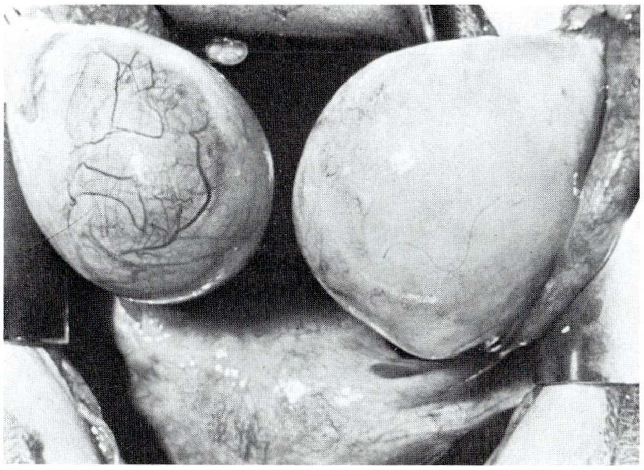

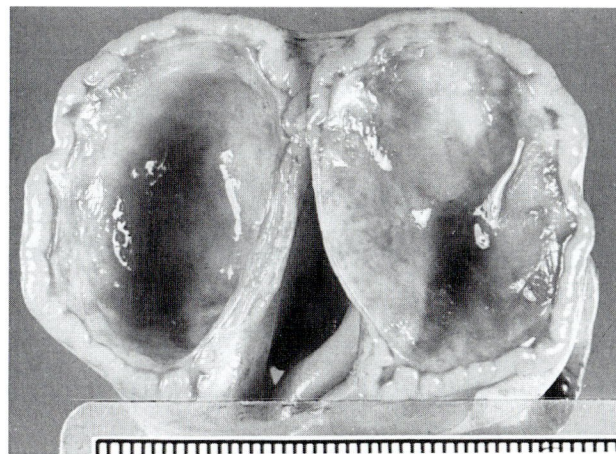

Fig. 16.17. Solitary follicle cyst within each ovary. (Reprinted by permission of The New England Journal of Medicine, 292:199–203, 1975)

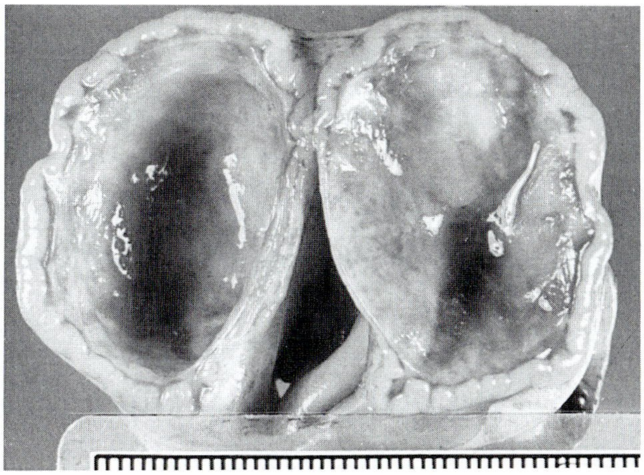

Fig. 16.18. Corpus luteum cyst. Note the convoluted lining, which was yellow.

layer may be luteinized. Distinction between the two layers can be facilitated by a reticulin stain, which reveals dense reticulum surrounding the theca cells but sparse or absent reticulum in the granulosa layer (Fig. 16.19b). CLCs exhibit a convoluted lining composed of large luteinized granulosa cells and an outer layer of smaller luteinized theca interna cells, with a prominent inner layer of connective tissue (Fig. 16.20). CLCs associated with pregnancy typically have characteristic hyaline bodies and calcific foci within the granulosa cells (Fig. 16.20, inset). Focal infarction of a CLC, possibly secondary to inadequate hCG production, has been encountered in association with tubal pregnancy. Involution of FCs and CLCs usually leads to the formation of corpora fibrosa and corpora albicantia, respectively; rarely, the latter may be cystic.

A rare type of solitary FC, designated "large solitary luteinized follicle cyst of pregnancy and the puerperium" with distinctive clinical and pathologic features, occurs during pregnancy and the puerperium and is presumably related to hCG stimula-

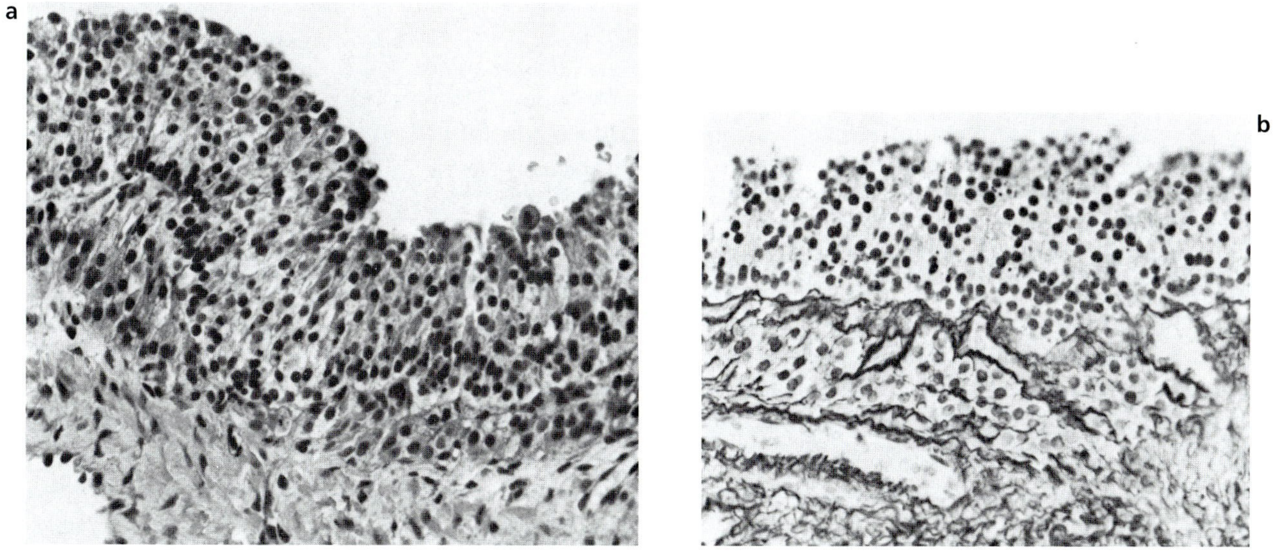

Fig. 16.19. Follicle cyst. **a**: Lining consists of an inner layer of granulosa cells and an outer layer of theca interna cells. **b**: Distinction between the two layers is enhanced with a reticulin stain, showing a reticulum network within the theca interna layer and an absence of reticulin within the granulosa layer. (Reprinted by permission of Clement (1985) In: Roth, Czernobilsky (eds). Contemporary Issues in Surgical Pathology, Vol 6. Churchill Livingstone, New York.)

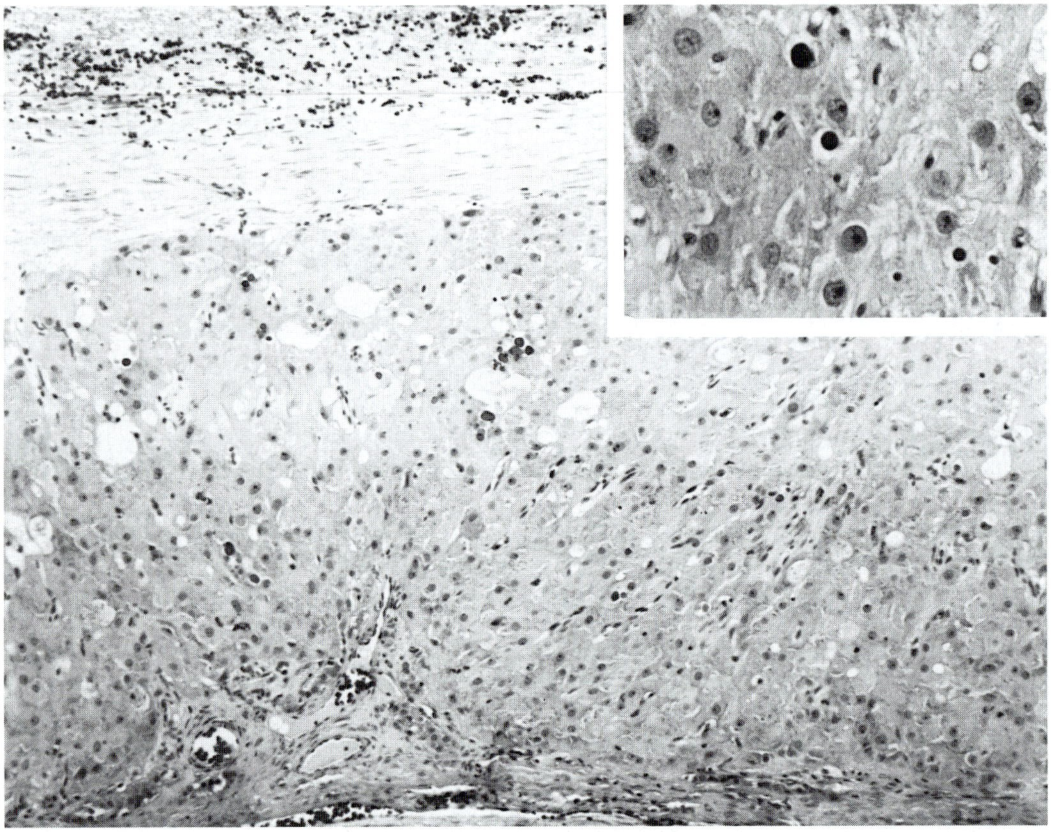

Fig. 16.20. Corpus luteum cyst of pregnancy. The cyst has an inner lining of connective tissue and an outer layer of large luteinized granulosa cells, some of which contain hyaline bodies (*inset*).

tion.[54,118] Patients present with a palpable adnexal mass (most commonly at the first postpartum visit) or are found to have a unilateral ovarian cyst at cesarean section. No endocrine disturbances have been reported to date. On gross inspection, the cyst resembles a typical FC except for its large size (median diameter, 25 cm). On microscopic examination, the cyst is lined by one to many layers of luteinized granulosa and theca cells that are usually indistinguishable. Nests of luteinized cells may be embedded within the fibrous tissue of the cyst wall. The cells have abundant vacuolated to eosinophilic cytoplasm, vary considerably in size and shape, and in all the reported cases have exhibited focal marked nuclear pleomorphism and hyperchromasia; mitotic figures have been absent (Fig. 16.21a,b).

Pathogenesis

The pathogenesis of some FCs is probably related to abnormalities in the release of anterior pituitary gonadotropins, such as a failure of the normal preovulatory luteinizing hormone surge. FCs occurring in females with abnormalities in gonadotropin release can be multiple, bilateral, recurrent, and in some cases are accompanied by corpora lutea and the possibility of pregnancy.[212] Other FCs appear to be autonomous and do not recur following removal. Girls with the McCune–Albright syndrome and precocious puberty secondary to a FC may have elevated gonadotropin levels, whereas in others with this syndrome the FCs appears to be mediated by a gonadotropin-independent mechanism.[59,71,329] Treatment with low-dose phasic oral contraceptives,[44] gonadotropin-releasing hormone analogues,[24] and tamoxifen[58] may also stimulate the development of FCs.

Clinical Behavior and Treatment

Most cases of FC and CLC regress spontaneously within 2 months; observation of small (<6 cm) ovarian cysts in women of reproductive age is justifiable for this period. Regression in some cases can be accelerated by administration of a high-dose, combined estrogen–progestogen preparation. FCs associated with isosexual pseudoprecocity can sometimes be treated by cyst puncture; others may require surgical removal. Persistence of a cyst suggests

a

b

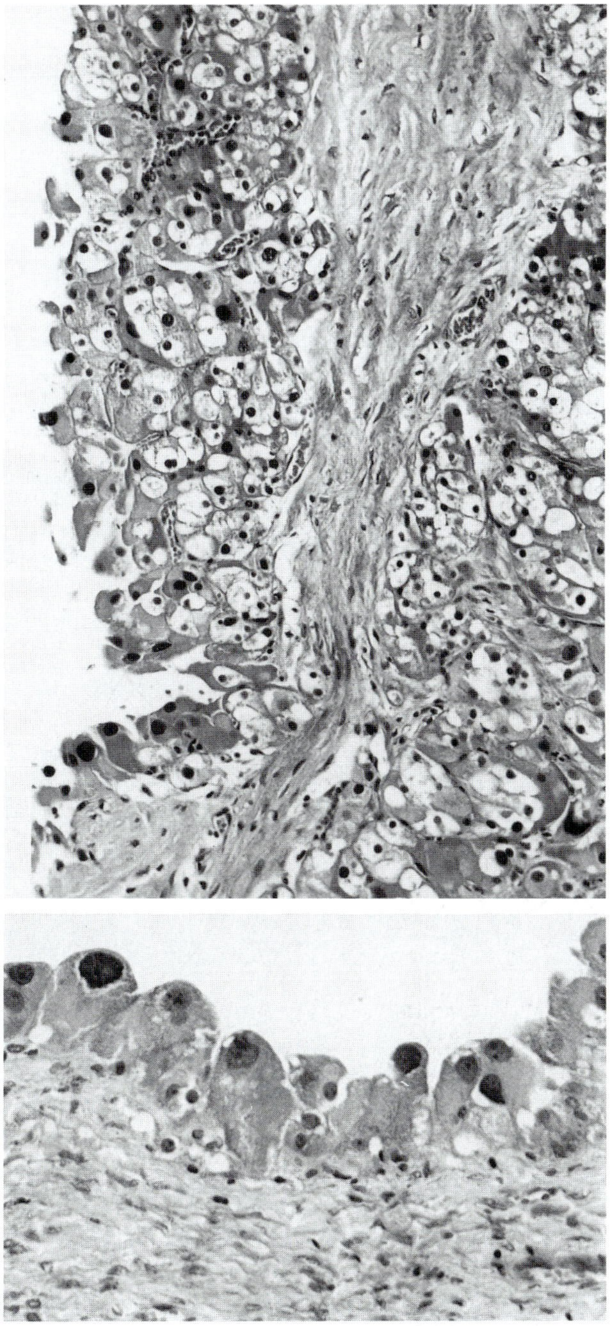

Fig. 16.21. Large solitary luteinized follicle cyst of pregnancy and puerperium. a: Luteinized cells with abundant (eosinophilic) to clear cytoplasm line cyst (*left*) and lie within its fibrous wall (*right*). Note focal nuclear atypicality. **b**: Higher-power view of lining cells showing marked nuclear hyperchromasia and atypicality. (Fig. 21a reprinted with permission from Clement et al. (1989) Nontrophoblastic pathology of the female genital tract and peritoneum associated with pregnancy. Semin Diagn Pathol 6:372–406.)[57]

that it is neoplastic, and in these cases laparotomy or laparoscopy is necessary.

Differential Diagnosis of Solitary Follicle Cysts

Solitary cysts of follicular origin should be distinguished on microscopic examination from other solitary unilocular ovarian cysts. Cysts otherwise identical to FCs and CLCs but less than 3.0 cm in diameter are generally regarded as physiologic, that is, cystic follicles and cystic corpora lutea, respectively. A simple cyst is of unknown origin because its lining has disappeared, was destroyed by rubbing or dessication after its removal, or because the lining consists of a thin layer of nonspecific epithelial-like cells. Additional sections may reveal theca lutein cells in its wall or foci of serous, endometrioid, or another type of epithelial lining allowing a more specific diagnosis. Even a rare cystic struma ovarii may be misdiagnosed as a simple cyst if inconspicuous follicles in its wall are overlooked or not sampled.

Cysts of surface epithelial origin that are usually small, incidental microscopic findings are designated inclusion cysts. Otherwise similar cysts measuring more than 1 cm are considered neoplastic and designated serous, endometrioid, or mucinous cystadenoma depending on the nature of their lining (see Chapter 18, Surface Epithelial Tumors of the Ovary). Epidermoid cysts are those lined exclusively by mature squamous epithelium and are considered either monodermal teratomas or of surface epithelial origin.[231,337] The finding of Walthard nests in the walls of some of these cysts favor the latter origin in at least some cases.[337] Endometriotic cysts are readily distinguishable by their characteristic lining of endometrial epithelium and stroma and pigmented histiocytes within their walls (see Chapter 17, Diseases of the Peritoneum). Solitary FCs should also be distinguished from those of rete origin that are located within the hilus (see page 716).[271]

Differentiating large FCs from unilocular cystic granulosa cell tumors of either the adult or juvenile type (see Chapter 19, Sex Cord–Stromal, Steroid Cell, and Other Ovarian Tumors with Endocrine, Paraendocrine, and Paraneoplastic Manifestations) may be difficult, especially if such a tumor has an orderly arrangement of granulosa and theca cells in its wall. Cystic granulosa cell tumors, however, are usually considerably larger than FCs, and the two cell types usually have a more disorderly pattern that may include obvious penetration of the cyst wall. In contrast to the large solitary luteinized FC of pregnancy, cystic granulosa cells tumors rarely have cells with bizarre nuclei.

Hyperreactio Luteinalis

Hyperreactio luteinalis (*HL*) is characterized by bilateral ovarian enlargement caused by the presence of multiple luteinized follicle cysts secondary to hCG stimulation.[121,208,319]

Clinical Features

Hyperreactio luteinalis most commonly occurs with disorders resulting in high levels of hCG, such as hydatidiform moles, choriocarcinoma, fetal hydrops (usually secondary to Rh sensitization but rarely of nonimmunologic type),[119] and multiple gestations. Sixty percent of cases unassociated with gestational trophoblastic disease (GTD), however, have accompanied a singleton pregnancy.[319] The frequency of HL in women with GTD ranges from 10% to 50% depending on whether it is detected by clinical examination or sonography.[275] The presence of HL in these patients may indicate an increased risk for persistent or metastatic GTD (see Chapter 24, Gestational Trophoblastic Disease and Related Lesions).[155,208] Rarely, HL has been preceded by the polycystic ovary syndrome.[25]

HL can be detected as a pelvic mass during any trimester, at cesarean section, or rarely during the puerperium. Symptoms are usually absent, but hemorrhage into the cysts may cause abdominal pain. Rarely, the involved ovary undergoes torsion or rupture, sometimes with intraabdominal bleeding, which can be fatal. In contrast to patients with the ovarian hyperstimulation syndrome (see following), ascites is rare.[319] In patients with HL accompanying GTD, HL is detected at the time of the diagnostic curettage or during the postoperative follow-up period.[250] In approximately 15% of cases unassociated with trophoblastic disease, there has been virilization of the patient but not the female infant.[25,121] Plasma testosterone levels have been elevated in these patients as well as nonvirilized patients with trophoblastic disorders, with the levels proportional to the degree of ovarian enlargement.

Pathological Findings

On macroscopic examination, multiple, usually bilateral, thin-walled cysts cause moderate to massive ovarian enlargement (up to 35 cm) (Fig. 16.22). The cysts are filled with clear or hemorrhagic fluid. Microscopic examination reveals FCs with prominent luteinization of the theca interna cells and, in some cases, the granulosa cells (Fig. 16.23). Occasionally, the latter have bizarre nuclei. There is usually marked edema of the theca layer and the intervening stroma; the latter frequently contains luteinized stromal cells.

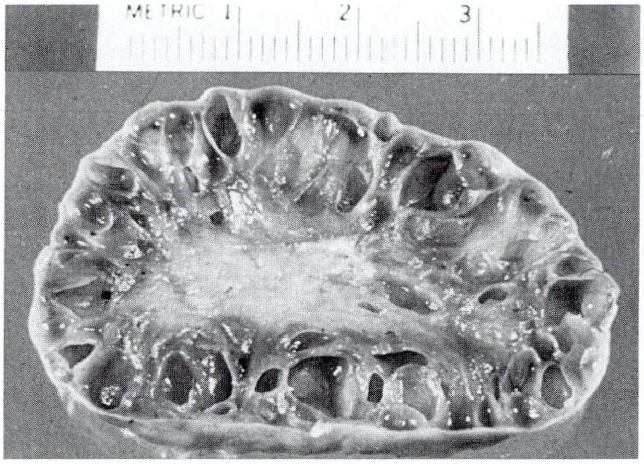

Fig. 16.22. Hyperreactio luteinalis. Multiple thin-walled follicle cysts are present within the cortex. (Courtesy of Dr. R.E. Scully. Reprinted by permission of Clement (1985) In: Roth, Czernobilsky (eds). Contemporary Issues in Surgical Pathology, Vol 6. Churchill Livingstone, New York.)

Pathogenesis

Because HL occasionally occurs in patients with otherwise normal pregnancies and normal hCG levels, and because HL does not occur in all women with high hCG levels, factors other than the latter likely play a role in the pathogenesis of HL. An increased ovarian sensitivity to hCG in patients with the disorder has been suggested.[38] One study found elevated levels of other hormones, specifically progesterone, prolactin, and estradiol, in patients with HL and GTD, possibly implicating these hormones in the pathogenesis or maintenance of HL.[239]

Clinical Behavior and Treatment

The cysts of HL typically involute during the puerperium, but occasionally regression is incomplete until 6 months postpartum. In exceptional cases, the cysts regress spontaneously during pregnancy. In cases associated with trophoblastic disease, gradual regression typically occurs 2–12 weeks after uterine evacuation, but occasionally the cysts persist for months or even enlarge after the hCG level has returned to normal.[208,250] Operative treatment of HL is needed only to remove infarcted tissue, control hemorrhage, or reduce ovarian size to diminish androgen production in virilized patients. Rarely, HL recurs in subsequent pregnancies.

Differential Diagnosis

Lack of knowledge of the gross appearance of the enlarged ovaries of hyperreactio luteinalis and their resultant misinterpretation as cystic ovarian tumors occasionally leads to an unwarranted bilateral

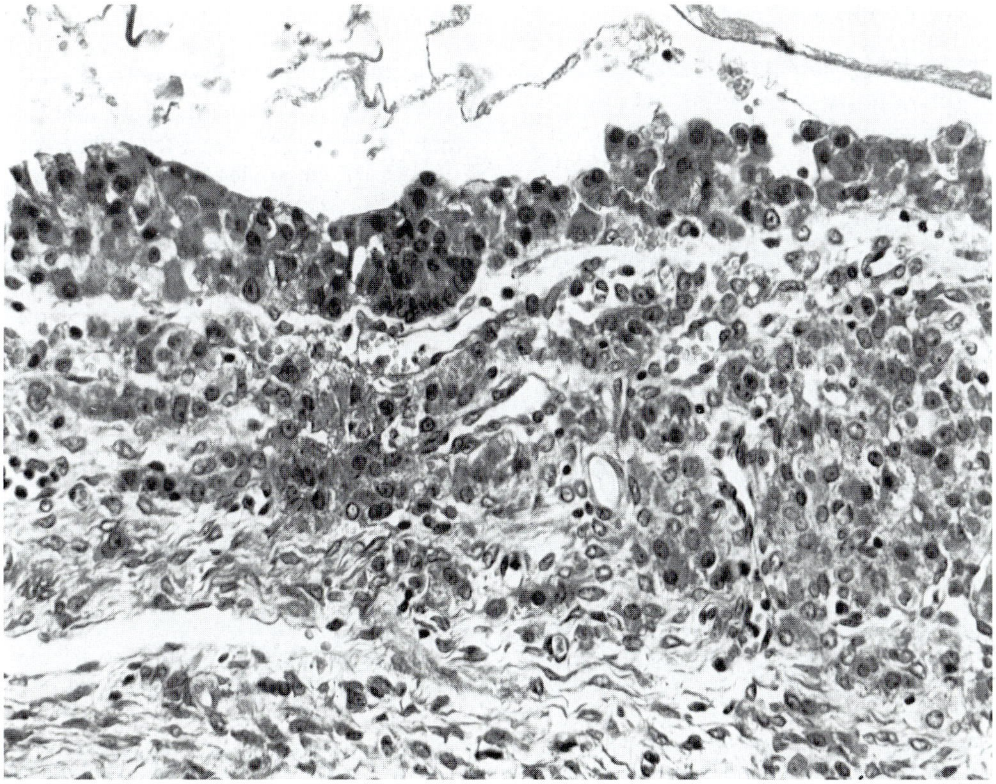

Fig. 16.23. Hyperreactio luteinalis. The cyst lining consists of granulosa and theca layers, both of which exhibit marked luteinization. (Reprinted by permission of Clement (1985) In: Roth, Czernobilsky (eds). Contemporary Issues in Surgical Pathology, Vol 6. Churchill Livingstone, New York.)

oophorectomy. If doubt exists, a frozen section examination of the cyst wall should solve the problem. Rarely, pregnancy luteomas coexist with HL, heightening the suspicion of a neoplastic process on gross examination.

Ovarian Hyperstimulation Syndrome

An iatrogenic form of HL, the *ovarian hyperstimulation syndrome* (*OHS*), occurs in a variable proportion of women undergoing ovulation induction, typically after the administration of follicle-stimulating hormone (FSH) followed by hCG, or rarely clomiphene alone.[97,117,191,314] The frequency of OHS has varied widely in the literature, although it has been suggested that some degree of the syndrome exists in all patients undergoing ovulation induction.[110] Mild OHS has been documented ultrasonographically in as many as 65% of such women.[191] OHS occurs only after ovulation, is more severe in patients who conceive, and is particularly prone to occur if the ovaries were polycystic before the institution of therapy. Several cases of spontaneous OHS unassociated with ovulation induction have been reported.[2,268] Three such patients, one with antecedent polycystic ovarian disease, had otherwise normal pregnancies[2]; one nonpregnant patient with spontaneous OHS had severe hypothyroidism.[268] Careful selection of patients and regulation of drug dosage by monitoring estrogen levels and ovarian size have reduced the frequency of OHS.

In severe cases, the ovaries become massively enlarged, and ascites, sometimes with hydrothorax (acute Meigs' syndrome) develops as a result of increased serosal permeability. Elevation of serum estrogens, progesterone, and testosterone typically occurs.[117] Hemoconcentration with secondary oliguria and thromboembolic phenomena is a life-threatening complication. High plasma levels of renin, aldosterone, and antidiuretic hormone may occur.[117] Patients usually respond to conservative therapy, such as cyst aspiration under ultrasonic guidance, and the cysts usually regress within 6 weeks. Operative intervention is only necessary in the rare instance of cyst torsion or rupture. Histologic examination of the ovaries reveals changes identical to those seen in HL, with the additional finding of one or more corpora lutea.

Rare Disorders Characterized by Multiple Follicle Cysts

Depending on the method of detection, as many as 75% of girls with juvenile hypothyroidism have multicystic ovaries.[171,262] Rarely, the ovarian enlargement may be the presenting sign leading to a diagnosis of hypothyroidism. The clinical features, in addition to ovarian enlargement and manifestations of hypothyroidism, include varying degrees of sexual precocity in more than half the patients and galactorrhea. The sexual precocity and galactorrhea appear to be caused by increased secretion of pituitary gonadotropins and prolactin, respectively. A similar clinical picture can occur rarely in adults. Histologic examination, which has been performed in only a few cases, has revealed FCs, some with luteinization of the theca interna layer. In two cases, a depletion of primordial follicles was also noted. Treatment with thyroxin has resulted in regression of the hypothyroidism, the ovarian cysts, and sexual precocity, and a decline in the elevated gonadotropin and prolactin levels.

Multiple, bilateral FCs associated with estradiol production have been described in infants born before the 30th week of gestation.[286] The cysts, which are secondary to elevated levels of FSH and luteinizing hormone (LH), appear at a postconception age that slightly precedes the expected time of delivery. It is postulated that marked prematurity is associated with relative insensitivity of the hypothalamus and anterior pituitary to negative feedback by estradiol.

Congenital deficiency of 17-hydroxylase, an enzyme required for both cortisol and estrogen synthesis, results in low estrogen levels and secondarily elevated levels of FSH and LH.[52,310] The rare patients with this disorder have congenital adrenal hyperplasia, hypokalemia, hypertension, primary amenorrhea, absence of sexual maturation, and ovarian enlargement due to multiple, bilateral FCs. A late onset of the disorder can mimic idiopathic hirsutism or polycystic ovary syndrome (PCOS).

Polycystic Ovary Syndrome

Polycystic ovary syndrome (*PCOS*) is an idiopathic disorder characterized by inappropriate gonadotropin secretion, chronic anovulation, hyperandrogenism, increased peripheral conversion of androgens to estrogens, and sclerocystic ovaries. Many patients also have abnormal glucose tolerance and hyperinsulinemia. The current clinical spectrum of PCOS is broader than that initially defined by Stein and Leventhal in 1935 (as the Stein–Leventhal syndrome), and as is discussed here, PCOS may be the result of multiple potential etiologies and be associated with variable clinical presentations.[310] Some patients with PCOS have the HAIR-AN syndrome of hyperandrogenism (HA), insulin resistance (IR), and acanthosis nigricans (AN), a syndrome discussed after the section on stromal hyperthecosis, a closely related disorder that overlaps both clinically and pathologically with PCOS.

Clinical Features

PCOS has been estimated to affect 5%–10% of the female population,[154] making it the most common endocrinopathy in women of reproductive age.[100] The affected women are typically in their third decade with a history of dysfunctional uterine bleeding related to anovulatory cycles and typically of peripubertal onset, or less commonly, secondary amenorrhea, as well as subfertility or infertility; 80% exhibit evidence of hyperandrogenism, usually in the form of hirsutism, and about half the patients are obese.[99,100,310] The skin may be involved by severe acne or acanthosis niricans (see HAIR-AN syndrome).[100] Hyperinsulinemia, insulin resistance, and impaired glucose tolerance are present in the majority of patients, particularly in those who are obese, although these features may not appear until later in life.[48] Frank virilization (clitoromegaly, deep voice, temporal baldness, male habitus) is rare, and if of sudden onset, suggests stromal hyperthecosis or a virilizing ovarian tumor rather than PCOS. The ovaries may or may not be palpably enlarged. Pelvic ultrasonography may help in establishing the diagnosis, as discussed below. Patients with PCOS have an increased risk for cardiovascular disease secondary to obesity, impaired glucose tolerance, and in some cases, hypertension and dyslipidemias.[11]

Current studies indicate that PCOS has a strong familial component and may be the most common endocrinopathy causing familial hirsutism, observations suggesting a genetic basis for PCOS in some patients. In one study of familial PCOS, approximately half the sisters of patients with PCOS were similarly affected, consistent with a autosomal dominant mode of inheritance. Other studies have suggested an X-linked transmission.[99] Genetic aspects of PCOS have been recently reviewed by Legro.[168]

Manifestations of unopposed estrogenic stimulation that occur in a significant proportion of patients include endometrial hyperplasia or, in approximately 1% of patients, endometrial carcinoma. The tumors typically occur in obese patients under the age of 40; conversely, up to one-quarter of patients with endometrial carcinoma under 40 have PCOS.[99] The tumors are almost always grade 1 endometrioid adenocarcinomas that are confined to the endometrium or invade the myometrium superficially.[64,86,101,256,257] The carcinomas are rarely, if ever, fatal, and many are reversible with progesterone therapy or by ovulation induction (see Chapter 11, Precursor Lesions of Endometrial Carcinoma, and Chapter 12, Endometrial Carcinoma). A wide variety of extrauterine tumors have also been described in patients with PCOS, but their association is probably coincidental.[64] One recent study, however, has found a 2.5-fold-increased risk of epithelial ovarian cancer in women with PCOS.[278]

Hyperprolactinemia is present in approximately 25% and galactorrhea in 13% of patients with PCOS.[98,99] Some hyperprolactinemic patients have pituitary adenomas, and therefore tomographic scanning of the sella may be necessary.[98,99]

Gross Findings

Both ovaries, or rarely, only one, are typically rounded and two to five times normal size; the ovarian volume can be three times that of control subjects.[177] Occasionally, however, the ovaries may be of normal size. Superficial cortical cysts are usually visible beneath the white ovarian surface. Examination of the sectioned ovarian surface reveals a thickened, white, capsule-like superficial cortex and numerous subjacent cysts, typically of similar size and usually less than 1 cm in diameter (Fig. 16.24). There is usually a central zone of stroma with only rare or no stigmata of ovulation (corpora lutea or albicantia).

Removal of ovarian tissue in PCOS is becoming increasingly uncommon as detection of the ovarian findings can be made by ultrasound examination. Polycystic ovaries are defined ultrasonographically by the presence of a peripheral array of many (at least eight) small cystic follicles (2–8 mm), and an increased ovarian stroma relative to the number of follicles.[310] The typical gross or ultrasonographic ovarian morphology, however, is unnecessary to make the diagnosis of PCOS, and in the absence of the typical clinical findings, is not diagnostic of the syndrome (see Differential Diagnosis).[310]

Microscopic Findings

The superficial cortex is fibrotic and hypocellular, resembling a capsule (Fig. 16.25), and may contain prominent thick-walled blood vessels.[133] Tongues of similarly fibrotic stroma may extend from the superficial cortex into the deeper cortex and medulla. The cysts are atretic cystic follicles and have an inner lining of several layers of nonluteinized, focally exfoliated granulosa cells. There is a prominent outer layer of luteinized theca interna cells (Fig. 16.26), giving rise to the term *follicular hyperthecosis*, but other studies have found that cystic follicles in women with PCOS differ from those in normal women only in their increased number.[177] Maturing follicles up to midantral stage and atretic follicles exhibiting prominent luteinization of the theca interna may be twice as numerous as in normal ovaries.[99,133] Primordial follicles are normal in number and appearance.[133] As noted, stigmata of prior ovulation are typically absent, but corpora lutea have been described in as many as 30% of otherwise typical cases of PCOS.[133] The deeper cortical and medullary stroma may have as much as a fivefold increase in volume. The stroma contains luteinized stromal cells in 80% of cases and, less commonly, foci of smooth muscle.[133] Nests of ovarian hilus (Leydig) cells may be more numerous in patients with PCOS than in age-matched controls.

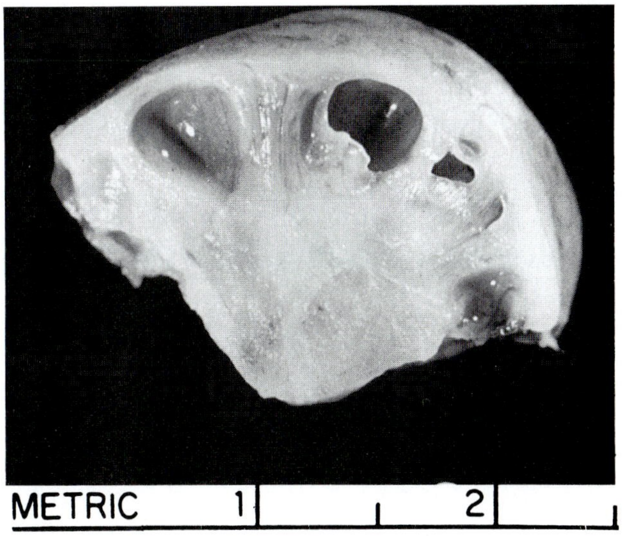

Fig. 16.24. Polycystic ovary disease. Superficial cortical fibrosis and multiple cystic follicles are present. (Courtesy of Dr. R.E. Scully. Reprinted by permission of Clement (1985) In: Roth, Czernobilsky (eds). Contemporary Issues in Surgical Pathology, Vol 6. Churchill Livingstone, New York.)

Pathophysiology

The pathophyiology of PCOS is complex, and the initiating factor(s) is (are) not yet completely understood.[310] A cardinal finding is a tonic elevation of the serum level of LH and an exaggerated response of LH to gonadotropin-releasing hormone.[99]

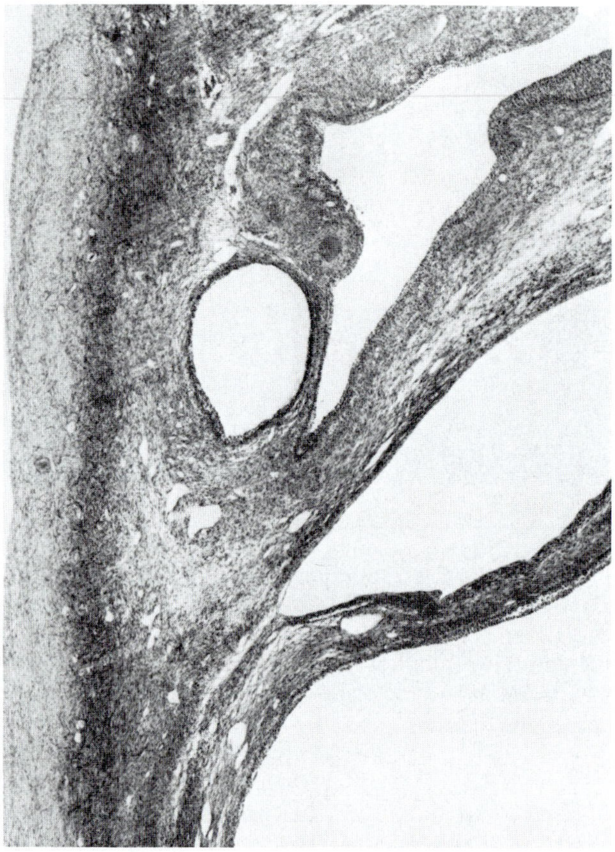

Fig. 16.25. Polycystic ovary disease. Multiple cystic follicles lie beneath the superficially fibrotic cortex. (Reprinted by permission of Clement (1985) In: Roth, Czernobilsky (eds). Contemporary Issues in Surgical Pathology, Vol 6. Churchill Livingstone, New York.)

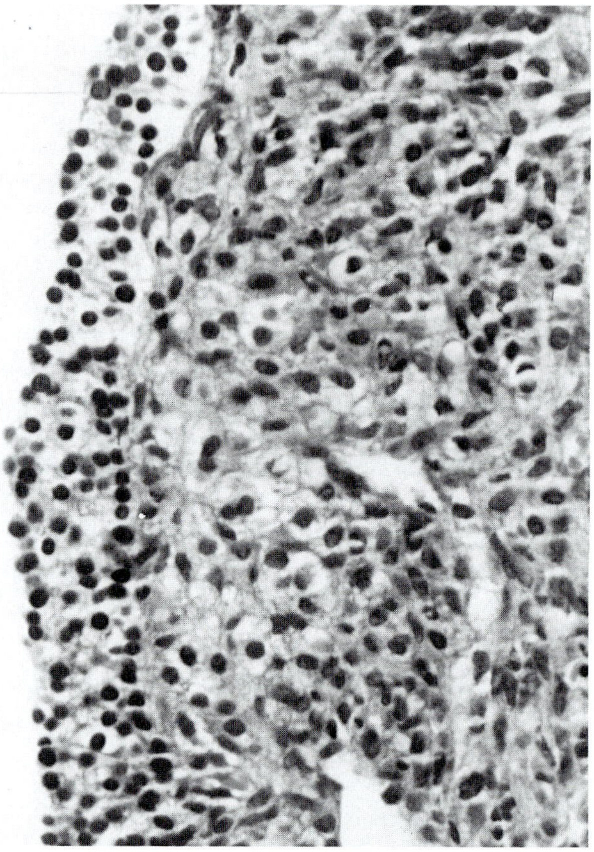

Fig. 16.26. Polycystic ovary disease. A cystic follicle is lined by nonluteinized granulosa cells and an outer, thicker layer of luteinized theca interna cells. (Reprinted by permission of Clement (1985) In: Roth, Czernobilsky (eds). Contemporary Issues in Surgical Pathology, Vol 6. Churchill Livingstone, New York.)

LH stimulates the follicular theca interna cells to produce androstenedione, which is converted peripherally, primarily within adipose tissue, to estrone (E_1), and to a lesser extent, testosterone. More importantly, ovarian follicular production of testosterone is also increased, leading to the small increases in serum testosterone concentrations that are present in PCOS. Estradiol (E_2) levels remain normal or low normal, resulting in an elevated E_1/E_2 ratio.[99] Elevated E_1 levels, and in some patients an increased secretion of inhibin, a nonsteroidal peptide produced by granulosa cells,[308] inhibit secretion of FSH. An elevated LH:FSH ratio is thus a characteristic finding in PCOS. Ovarian estrogen production in PCOS is markedly diminished, probably a result of inactivity of the FSH-dependent aromatase system within the granulosa cells.[99,195] Inadequate intrafollicular estrogen synthesis, increased intrafollicular androgens, and an elevated LH:FSH ratio result in cessation of follicle growth at the midantral stage, anovulation, and sclerocystic ovaries.

A number of interlinked factors potentially play a role in initiating or perpetuating PCOS. According to Taylor,[310] "there are correlations between gonadotropin secretion, insulin secretion, and androgen secretion across the spectum of patients with PCOS such that it remains impossible to determine the primary etiologic factor in the vast majority of patients."

Obesity

As the conversion of androstenedione to E_1 occurs predominantly in adipose tissue, the extent of the conversion correlates with the amount of adipose tissue.[20,99] Similarly, weight reduction in obese women is associated with a reduction in serum androgen and estrone levels.[20] Hyperestronemia, and as discussed later, hyperinsulinemia, are therefore two obesity-related factors that may play a role in the pathogenesis of PCOS.

ADRENAL ANDROGEN EXCESS

The adrenal contribution to the androgen pool is increased in half the patients with PCOS, as manifested by an elevated level of cortisol, the adrenal androgen dehydroepiandrosterone sulfate (DHES), and abnormal adrenal androgen responses to ACTH and metapyrone.[13,99,172,173,175,202,263] The increased adrenal androgens can lead to hyperestronemia and consequently an elevated LH:FSH ratio. Dexamethasone treatment can correct the abnormal LH:FSH ratio in some patients with PCOS, resulting in resumption of ovulation. Although some investigators believe that the adrenal abnormalities (which may include late-onset congenital adrenal hyperplasia) are a primary disturbance, others have concluded that they are secondary to the hormonal milieu of PCOS.[45,78]

HYPERINSULINEMIA

Insulin resistance and hyperinsulinemia are present in most obese and nonobese women with PCOS, although these features tend to be more severe in the former group.[48,49,226,316] In one study, glucose intolerance, impaired glucose tolerance, or type 2 diabetes mellitis were found in 40%, 31%, and 7.5% of patients, respectively, with PCOS.[77] Despite peripheral insulin resistance, ovarian tissues remain responsive to insulin in women with PCOS. Insulin appears to amplify LH action, enhancing production of estradiol and progesterone from the follicular granulosa cells and possibly contributing to the arrest of follicle growth.[94] As discussed later (see HAIR-AN syndrome), insulin and insulin-like growth factor stimulate proliferation of ovarian stromal cells and their production of androgen. Hyperinsulinemia thus can increase circulating androgen levels (and by peripheral conversion, estrone) in patients with PCOS. The resultant hyperandrogenism may in turn increase insulin resistance. Recently, it has been shown that in obese women with PCOS, decreasing serum insulin concentrations with metformin reduces ovarian cytochrome P-450-c-17-alpha activity and ameliorates but does not abolish hyperandrogenism.[227]

HYPERPROLACTINEMIA

The hyperprolactinemia occasionally present in PCOS may be caused by a pituitary adenoma, but in other cases may be related to a hyperplasia of prolactin secreting cells induced by the hyperestronemia in these patients.[99,100] The hyperprolactinemia, either through a direct effect on gonadotropin-secreting cells or indirectly through other mechanisms, may cause an elevated LFH:FSH ratio. Prolactin also may increase DHES secretion from the adrenal gland. In some patients, treatment with bromocriptine reverses hyperprolactinemia, lowers androgen levels, and may restore ovulatory cycles.

Differential Diagnosis

PCOS is a clinicopathologic syndrome, and the finding of polycystic ovaries with little or no evidence of prior ovulation in wedge biopsy specimens does not warrant the diagnosis per se in the absence of the usual clinical findings. Polycystic ovaries that resemble those of PCOS are seen occasionally in prepubertal children and in otherwise normal girls during the first few years after the onset of puberty. Similarly, ultrasonographic studies have revealed that ovulating women with minor evidence of hyperandrogenism, but without menstrual irregularity, can have polycystic ovaries similar to those of patients with overt clinical manifestations except that the ovaries also contain corpora lutea and albicantia.[252] Thus, the boundary between the clinical syndrome of PCOS and normality is not clear cut.

Although PCOS does not cause a problem in differential diagnosis with a neoplasm for the pathologist, the clinical manifestations may suggest the possibility of an androgenic or estrogenic ovarian tumor, particularly in the exceptional cases in which the disease coexists with a nonfunctioning ovarian neoplasm.[14] In some cases, in which the associated ovarian tumor is capable of function, such as a Sertoli–Leydig cell tumor, it may be difficult to determine which lesion was responsible for the endocrine manifestations.

The differential diagnosis includes a wide variety of other disorders that result in abnormal gonadotropin release, chronic anovulation, and sclerocystic ovaries. Sclerocystic ovaries are a nonspecific morphologic expression of chronic anovulation in the premenopausal patient and can accompany (1) adrenal lesions, such as Cushing's syndrome, congenital adrenal hyperplasia (most commonly 21-hydroxylase or 11-beta-hydroxylase deficiency), and virilizing adrenal tumors; (2) primary hypothalamic–pituitary disorders; and (3) ovarian lesions that produce excessive quantities of estrogens or androgens, including sex cord–stromal tumors, steroid cell tumors, and nonneoplastic lesions such as Leydig cell hyperplasia and stromal hyperthecosis. As previously noted, the latter overlaps both clinically and pathologically with PCOS, and the two disorders may represent opposite poles of a single disease spectrum. Sclerocystic ovaries have also been described in patients with autoimmune oophoritis,[15] after long-term use of oral contraceptives,[251,273] in association with periovarian adhesions,[255] and after long-term androgen therapy in female to male transsexuals.[241] An association between a PCOS-like syndrome and the use of the antiepileptic drug valproate has been found.[137]

Stromal Hyperplasia and Stromal Hyperthecosis

Stromal hyperplasia (*SH*) is characterized by varying degrees of proliferation of the ovarian stromal cells. *Stromal hyperthecosis* (*HT*) refers to the presence of luteinized cells within the stroma at a distance from the follicles; it is usually accompanied by at least a moderate degree of SH.

Clinical Features

The clinical manifestations are variable. Moderate to severe SH is most commonly encountered in women in their sixth and seventh decades and has been documented in more than one-third of autopsied patients in this age group.[36,294] Similar degrees of SH are found less commonly in patients in the eighth decade (18% of patients in one study[36]), suggesting that it may be a reversible process. A strong negative association with parity was found in one study.[294] SH of moderate to severe degree may be found in women with disorders associated with androgenic or estrogenic manifestations including endometrial carcinoma, obesity, hypertension, and glucose intolerance.

HT is most frequent in patients in the sixth to ninth decades. Some familial cases of HT have been reported,[140] and one case of HT has been described in a patient with acromegaly.[219] The process has been documented in one-third of autopsied patients over the age of 55, and exhaustive microscopic sampling may reveal that rare luteinized stromal cells are even more common in this age group (see Chapter 15, Anatomy and Histology of the Ovary).[36] In postmenopausal women, HT is usually mild and of doubtful clinical significance.

Clinically florid examples of HT are more common in patients in the younger reproductive age group, although rare cases occur in adolescents and postmenopausal patients.[40,167,179,236] The findings include marked virilization, obesity, hypertension, hyperinsulinemia, and decreased glucose tolerance. In addition, a small subset of women with HT (or occasionally PCOS) have the HAIR-AN syndrome (see following). The clinical picture of HT typically evolves gradually but occasionally there is an abrupt onset, potentially suggesting the presence of an androgenic tumor, especially if the process is unilateral and associated with ovarian enlargement. Less commonly, the clinical findings are more characteristic of PCOS. In some patients with HT, especially postmenopausal women, estrogenic findings predominate and may include endometrial hyperplasia or even well-differentiated adenocarcinoma.[148,179,217,276,294] Conversely, women with endometrial hyperplasia or carcinoma in some studies have had a high frequency of HT on microscopic examination of their ovaries.[217,276] HT-related virilization has been present in two cases of placental site trophoblastic tumor, and in one case it was the presenting manifestation of the tumor.[218,224]

Gross Findings

SH and HT are almost invariably bilateral, and the ovaries range from normal size to 7 cm in maximum dimension, thus potentially mimicking an ovarian neoplasm.[36,179] The sectioned surfaces are usually

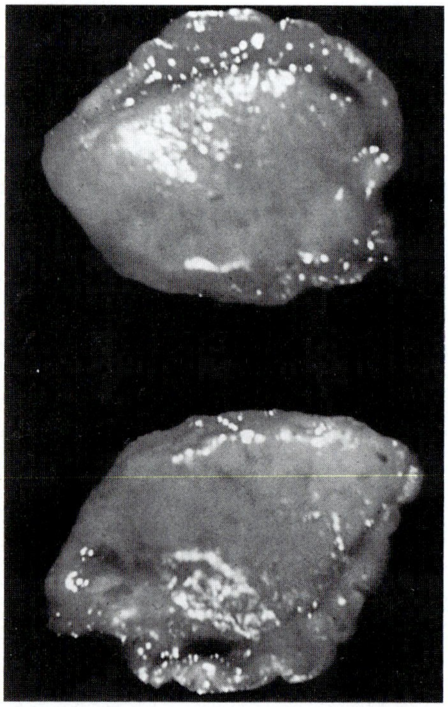

Fig. 16.27. Stromal hyperplasia and hyperthecosis. The ovaries are involved by a solid, homogeneous proliferation that had a yellow color in the unfixed state. (Courtesy of R.E. Scully, M.D., Boston, MA.)

solid, firm, homogenous, and white to yellow (Fig. 16.27).[36,219] In cases of nodular hyperthecosis, multiple yellow nodules may be appreciable.[167] In premenopausal women, sclerocystic changes similar to those seen in PCOS may also be present.[133,220] HT rarely coexists with a neoplasm, usually a stromal luteoma, which may also have hormone-secreting potential.

Microscopic Findings

In both SH and HT, a variable degree of nodular or diffuse cortical and medullary proliferation of ovarian stromal cells is present (Fig. 16.28). A mild degree of SH cannot be reliably distinguished from the normal appearance (see Chapter 15).[36] Follicular derivatives may lie within the hyperplastic stroma but may be rare or absent in advanced cases. The stromal cells in SH are plumper than normal postmenopausal ovarian stromal cells, and have oval to fusiform, vesicular nuclei, and, frequently, cytoplasmic lipid. The luteinized stromal cells of HT are more common in the medulla but may also be present in the cortex. They appear as single cells, small nests, or nodules of polygonal cells with abundant eosinophilic to vacuolated cytoplasm containing variable amounts of lipid (Fig. 16.29).[36] The round nucleus of the luteinized cells typically has a central small nucleolus. As noted, in premenopausal women including those with the HAIR-AN syndrome, sclerocystic changes characteristic of PCOS are also commonly present. In cases of HT accompanying the HAIR-AN syndrome (see following), edema and fibrosis of the ovarian stroma, rather than SH, are frequently a prominent change.[188]

Other ovarian findings occasionally encountered in HT include an increased number of atretic follicles,[236] small stromal nodules of metaplastic smooth muscle,[283] hilus cell hyperplasia,[36,301] hilus cell tumors,[265,301] stromal luteomas,[282] and thecomas.[340] SH in the absence of HT has also been associated with thecomas.[266,340] Some cases of HT may be associated with massive ovarian edema.

Histochemical analyses have shown that nonluteinized and luteinized stromal cells, and cells

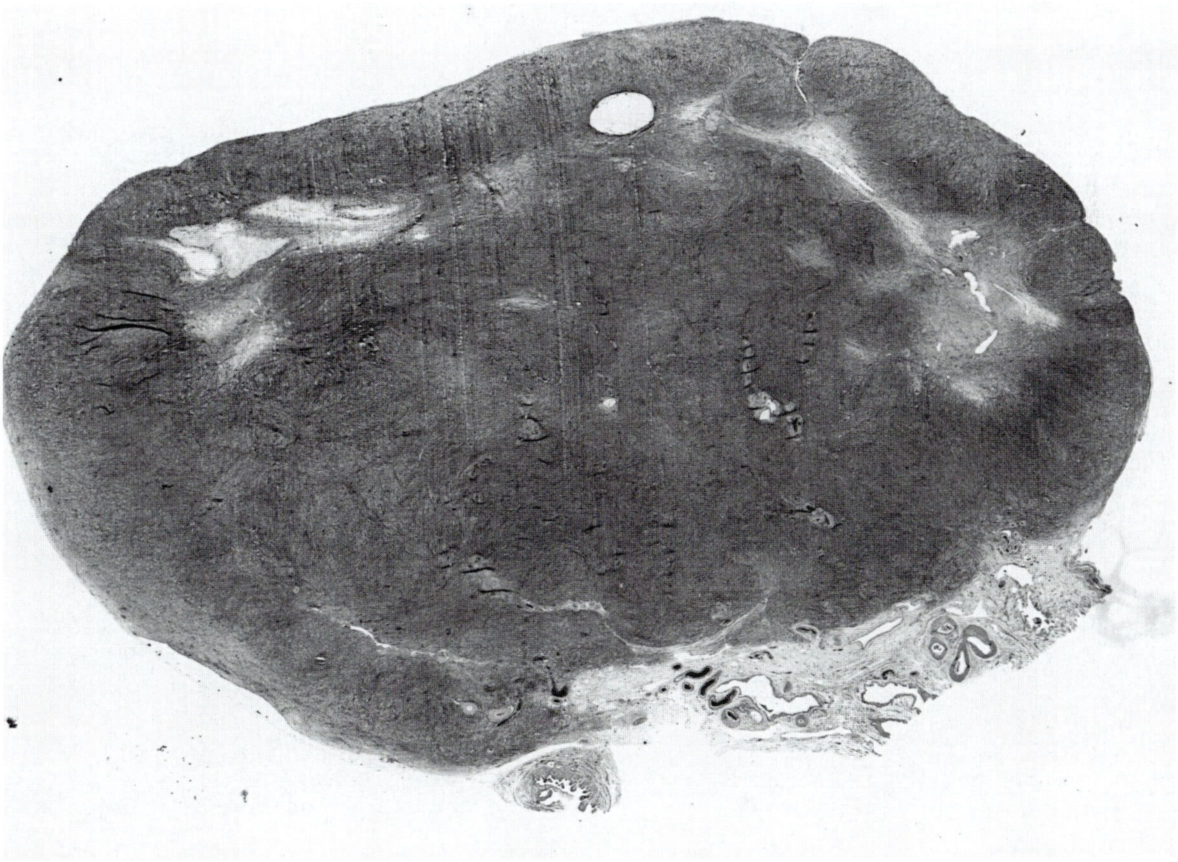

Fig. 16.28. Stromal hyperplasia. A diffuse proliferation of ovarian stromal cells within the cortex and medulla is seen. (Reprinted by permission of Clement (1985) In: Roth, Czernobilsky (eds). Contemporary Issues in Surgical Pathology, Vol 6. Churchill Livingstone, New York.)

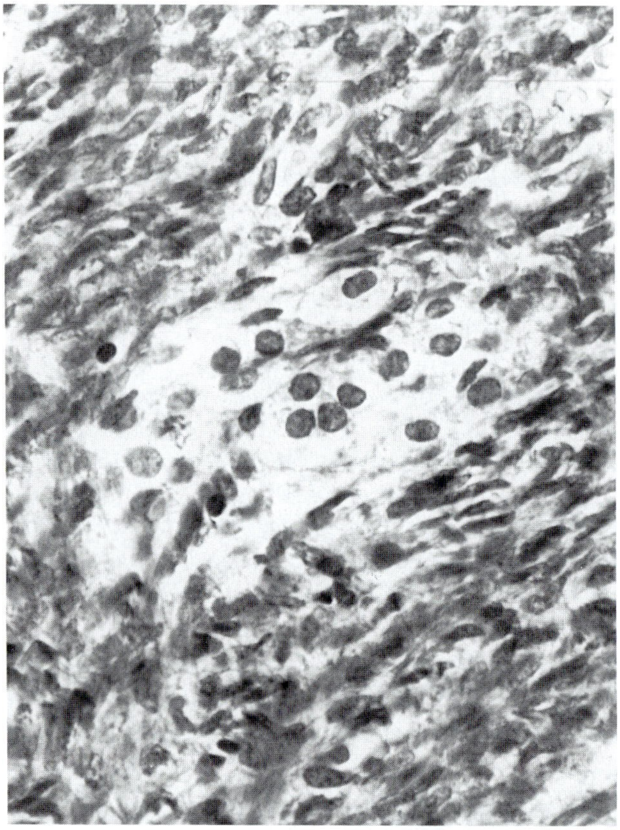

Fig. 16.29. Stromal hyperthecosis. A nest of luteinized stromal cells is present within the ovarian stroma. (Reprinted by permission of Clement (1985) In: Roth, Czernobilsky (eds). Contemporary Issues in Surgical Pathology, Vol 6. Churchill Livingstone, New York.)

transitional in appearance between the two, have oxidative activity important in steroid hormone production.[284] The luteinized cells were immunoreactive for cytochrome P-450-17-alpha, which catalyzes androgen synthesis, in approximately 50% of the cases of SH in one series.[276] Luteinized stromal cells are also immunoreactive for testosterone, estradiol, follicle-stimulating hormone (FSH), and inhibin.[179,217,247]

Pathophysiology

In vitro and in vivo studies have shown that ovaries with SH secrete more androstenedione, estrone, and estradiol than normal ovaries.[73,176] Similar studies using ovarian tissue from patients with HT[222] as well as in vivo studies in these patients have shown, respectively, markedly increased production rates and serum levels of ovarian testosterone, dihydrotestosterone, and androstenedione, usually in the male range.[85,179,219] As already noted, immunohistochemical staining for various enzymes involved in the conversion of cholesterol to steroid hormones in cases of HT has been consistent with androgen synthesis not only in the luteinized stromal cells characteristic of the disorder but also in the adjacent spindle-shaped stromal cells. Also, the demonstration of aromatase more frequently in the theca lutein cells of cystic follicles in young women with HT than in the luteinized stromal cells suggests a predominant role of the latter in the androgen overproduction of this disorder.[128] As in PCOS, the predominant estrogen in patients with SH and HT is estrone, derived predominantly from peripheral aromatization of ovarian androgens, resulting in an increased estrone/estradiol ratio.[219,276]

Unlike patients with PCOS, most premenopausal patients with HT have normal gonadotropin levels.[140,219] That gonadotropins may play a role in SH and HT, however, is suggested by (1) elevated LH levels in occasional premenopausal women with HT and most postmenopausal patients with SH and HT; (2) immunoreactivity for FSH and LH receptors within ovarian stromal cells[225]; (3) in vitro incubation studies showing that FSH and LH stimulate proliferation of the ovarian stroma of pre- and postmenopausal women[294]; (3) studies showing that androgen production by the ovarian stromal cells in patients with and without HT is enhanced by LH[17,73,222]; (4) the often prominent stromal luteinization during pregnancy; (5) cases of symptomatic HT complicating pregnancy and trophoblastic disease[218,224]; and (6) the increase in pituitary amphophils in some cases of severe HT.[179] As noted, insulin resistance and hyperinsulinemia occur in as many as 90% of patients with HT and likely play a role in the pathogenesis of the stromal luteinization in these patients (see HAIR-AN syndrome).[223]

Differential Diagnosis

In contrast to a fibroma, SH is almost always bilateral and is characterized by cells with smaller nuclei, scanty collagen, and nodules that commonly coalesce. The lesion is distinguished from a low-grade endometrioid stromal sarcoma by the spindle shape of its cells and by an absence of mitotic figures and regularly distributed arterioles.

The differential diagnosis of HT includes other nonneoplastic and neoplastic solid proliferations of luteinized cells, most of which are also virilizing. The nonneoplastic category includes pregnancy luteoma and Leydig cell hyperplasia (discussed elsewhere in this chapter) and the neoplasms include luteinized thecoma and steroid cell tumors (see Chapter 19, Sex Cord–Stromal, Steroid Cell, and Other Ovarian Tumors with Endocrine Paraendocrine, and Paraneoplastic Manifestations). These neoplasms, in contrast to HT, are almost always unilateral and typically form distinct tumors or nodules appreciable on gross examination. Luteinized stromal cells, histologically similar to those present in HT, may also be encountered within the nonneoplastic stroma of a variety of benign and malignant ovarian tumors, including primary surface epithelial and germ cell tumors as well as metastatic tumors, that is, "tumors with functioning stroma" (see Chapter 19).

Clinical Behavior and Treatment

In contrast to patients with PCOS, those with HT usually exhibit little or no response to clomiphene treatment and often only a transient response to wedge resection.[140,220] Many patients require bilateral oophorectomy to halt progressive virilization. Such treatment may also result in disappearance of hypertension and abnormalities in glucose tolerance.[40] More recently, successful treatment of HT has been achieved with gonadotropin-releasing hormone (GnRH) agonists.[297]

HAIR-AN Syndrome

In addition to the common occurrence of insulin resistance and hyperinsulinemia in patients with HT, some patients with HT have the *HAIR-AN syndrome*, a syndrome estimated to occur in as many as 5% of all women with hyperandrogenism.[12,18,79,183] The syndrome consists of *hyperandrogenism* (*HA*), typically of early, sometimes premenarcheal, onset; *insulin resistance* (*IR*); and *acanthosis nigricans* (*AN*).[18] Striking degrees of masculinization are present in some patients with the HAIR-AN syndrome and may be disproportionate to the degree of hyperandrogenism.[79] Some patients have a normal glucose tolerance whereas others have symptomatc diabetes.[142]

The syndrome has been most frequently described in patients with PCOS, although it appears likely that most, if not all, such patients also have HT.[79,188] Unusual histologic findings in patients with HT and the HAIR-AN syndrome have included prominent follicular atresia, large numbers of degenerating oocytes, medullary stromal fibrosis, and numerous small nests of granulosa cells forming Call–Exner bodies.[183] Dermoid cysts and stromal luteoma have been rarely described in patients with the HAIR-AN syndrome in association with HT, sclerocystic ovaries, or both.

The typical laboratory findings include hyperinsulinemia and increased production rates and elevated serum levels of testosterone and androstendione.[79,105] In some patients, the severity of the insulin resistance is proportional to the testosterone elevation. Proposed mechanisms of insulin resistance have included a decreased number or functional capacity of insulin receptors, which may be associated with obesity, or in other cases, genetic alterations in the structure of the receptors (type A); antiinsulin receptor antibodies that decrease insulin receptor affinity for insulin and which are often associated with autoimmune diseases (type B); and postreceptor defects in insulin action or clearance (type C).[16,19,88,91,142,206,207,311]

Several studies have demonstrated that (1) there is a 50 to 250 fold increase in testosterone production from the ovarian stroma in women with the syndrome compared to normal ovaries[195]; (2) in some women with hyperandrogenism and insulin resistance, a glucose load can produce an acute rise in cirulating androgens[292]; (3) insulin can stimulate the accumulation of androstenedione and testosterone in cultures of ovarian stromal cells in women with and without hyperandrogenism[17,18,222]; and (4) insulin and insulin-like growth factor I receptors are present in the ovarian stromal cells, the insulin-like growth factor possibly mediating the androgenic effects of insulin.[217,221,253] Additionally, insulin may enhance LH secretion from the pituitary and act synergistically with LH in stimulating the ovarian stromal cells.

On the basis of these and other findings, it has been postulated that the primary defect in the HAIR-AN syndrome is insulin resistance leading to hyperinsulinemia and the other findings in the syndrome. Thus, any cause of insulin resistance leading to hyperinsulinemia can produce the HAIR-AN syndrome. The hyperandrogenism itself may increase the severity of the insulin resistance, and thus a self-perpetuating cycle that increases in severity may result.[18] The acanthosis nigricans is probably an epiphenomenon secondary to the hyperandrogenism, hyperinsulinemia, or both.

Bilateral oophorectomy in patients with the HAIR-AN syndrome decreases hyperandrogenism but usually does not ameliorate insulin resistance.[183,223] Gonadotropin suppression with oral contraceptives has been successful in decreasing ovarian androgen production in some patients. Marked improvement of acanthosis nigricans may follow correction of the hyperandrogenism.

Massive Edema and Ovarian Fibromatosis

Tumor-like enlargement of one, or occasionally, both ovaries secondary to an accumulation of edema fluid within the ovarian stroma is referred to as *massive ovarian edema*. Approximately 80 cases of this disorder have been reported.[144,230,267,338] A rarer lesion designated *ovarian fibromatosis*,[338] characterized by diffuse ovarian fibrosis, is closely related to massive edema and is therefore considered in this section.

Clinical Features

Patients with massive edema are typically young, with a mean age of 21 years (range, 6–37 years) and have abdominal or pelvic pain, menstrual irregularities, and abdominal distension. The pain may be of several years duration or have a sudden onset and mimic the pain of acute appendicitis. Androgenic manifestations are present in approximately 20% of patients and are nearly always associated with the presence of luteinized stromal cells. Of these, two-thirds are masculinized and the rest exhibit only hirsutism.[317,338] Serum testosterone has been elevated in some cases. Rare patients have had estrogenic manifestations, manifested by isosexual pseudoprecocity.[230,267] Pelvic examination typically reveals a palpable adnexal mass, which in 70% of cases has been right sided. Abdominal exploration reveals unilateral involvement in 90% of cases, and in approximately half the patients, partial or complete torsion of the involved ovary. In one patient, the contralateral ovary had a twisted pedicle and was infarcted. Intraperitoneal fluid is not usually present, although rare patients have had an associated Meigs' syndrome.

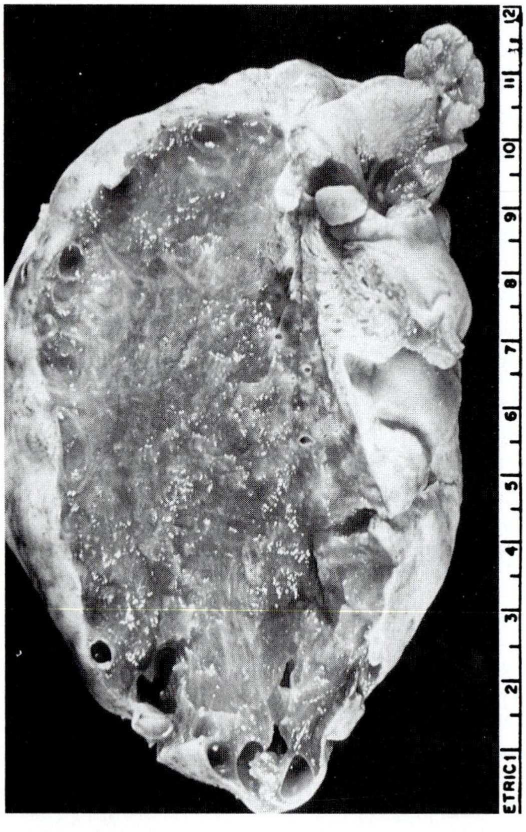

Fig. 16.30. Massive ovarian edema. The ovary is enlarged and markedly edematous. (Courtesy of Dr. R.E. Scully. Reprinted by permission of Clement (1985) In: Roth, Czernobilsky (eds). Contemporary Issues in Surgical Pathology, Vol 6. Churchill Livingstone, New York.)

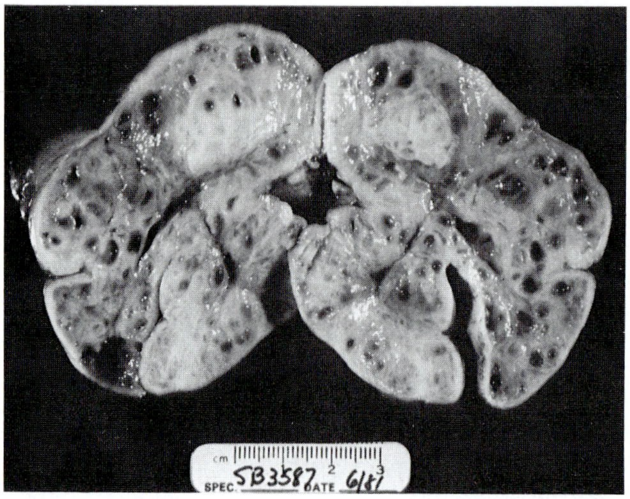

Fig. 16.31. Ovarian fibromatosis. The ovary is enlarged by a diffuse fibrous proliferation that surrounds multiple cystic follicles. (Courtesy of Young et al., ref. 337.)

Patients with ovarian fibromatosis have ranged in age from 13 to 39 years, with an average of 25 years.[338] Clinical manifestations include menstrual abnormalities or amenorrhea, abdominal pain, and rarely hirsutism or virilization. The majority of patients have a palpable adnexal mass. Occasionally, the ovarian enlargement is an incidental finding late in pregnancy or during cesarean section. In some cases, the involved ovary was found twisted on its pedicle at the time of operation. The endocrine manifestations, including, in several cases, infertility, disappear after oophorectomy, indicating that the lesion produces steroid hormones.

Gross Findings

The involved ovary in massive edema is enlarged, soft, and fluctuant, ranging from 5.5 to 35 cm in maximum dimension (mean, 11.5 cm). The heaviest ovary weighed 2400 g.[338] The ovary has a shiny, white, smooth exterior as a result of a white and fibrotic superficial cortex and a sectioned surface that is edematous or gelatinous and exudes watery fluid (Fig. 16.30). Occasional superficial FCs may be present. The ipsilateral fallopian tube may also be edematous.

In ovarian fibromatosis, there is usually complete or almost complete ovarian involvement by a fibromatous process.[338] In 20% of cases, the process is bilateral. The ovaries are 8–14 cm in maximum dimension with white and typically smooth or lobulated external surfaces. The cut surfaces are firm, white to gray, and solid except for the presence of cystic follicles in one-third of cases (Fig. 16.31).

Microscopic Findings

The striking finding on low magnification in massive edema is marked, diffuse, stromal edema that separates and sometimes involves the follicular structures but typically spares the superficial cortex (Fig. 16.32). The latter is usually thickened and fibrotic. Higher magnification reveals spindle-shaped ovarian stromal cells separated by abundant pale-staining fluid that focally may impart a microcystic appearance. In nonedematous areas, the stroma has the appearance of normal stroma, hyperplastic stroma, or ovarian fibromatosis.[338] In approximately 40% of cases, foci of luteinized cells are present (Fig. 16.33). Associated nonspecific findings include vascular and lymphatic dilatation within the ovary and occasionally the mesosalpinx, focal necrosis, extravasated erythrocytes, hemosiderin-laden macrophages, and mast cells.[267,338] The contralateral ovary is normal in more than 75% of cases; in the rest, it is enlarged and edematous, or is nonedematous but altered by stromal hyperthecosis or sclerocystic changes.

Ovarian fibromatosis is characterized by a fibromatoid proliferation of collagen-producing spindle cells that typically surrounds normal follicular structures and thickens the superficial cortex (Fig. 16.34).[338] In most cases of fibromatosis the process is diffuse but it may be localized, and occasionally it is confined to or predominantly involves the cortex ("cortical fibromatosis"). The process varies from moderately cellular fascicles of spindle cells with a focal storiform pattern to relatively acellular bands of dense collagen. Small foci of uninvolved ovarian stroma are usually present. In rare cases, luteinized cells are seen within the lesion or the adjacent non-fibrotic stroma. Minor foci of stromal edema and microscopic foci of sex cord elements within the fibromatous tissue, alone or in combination, have been encountered in occasional cases.[338]

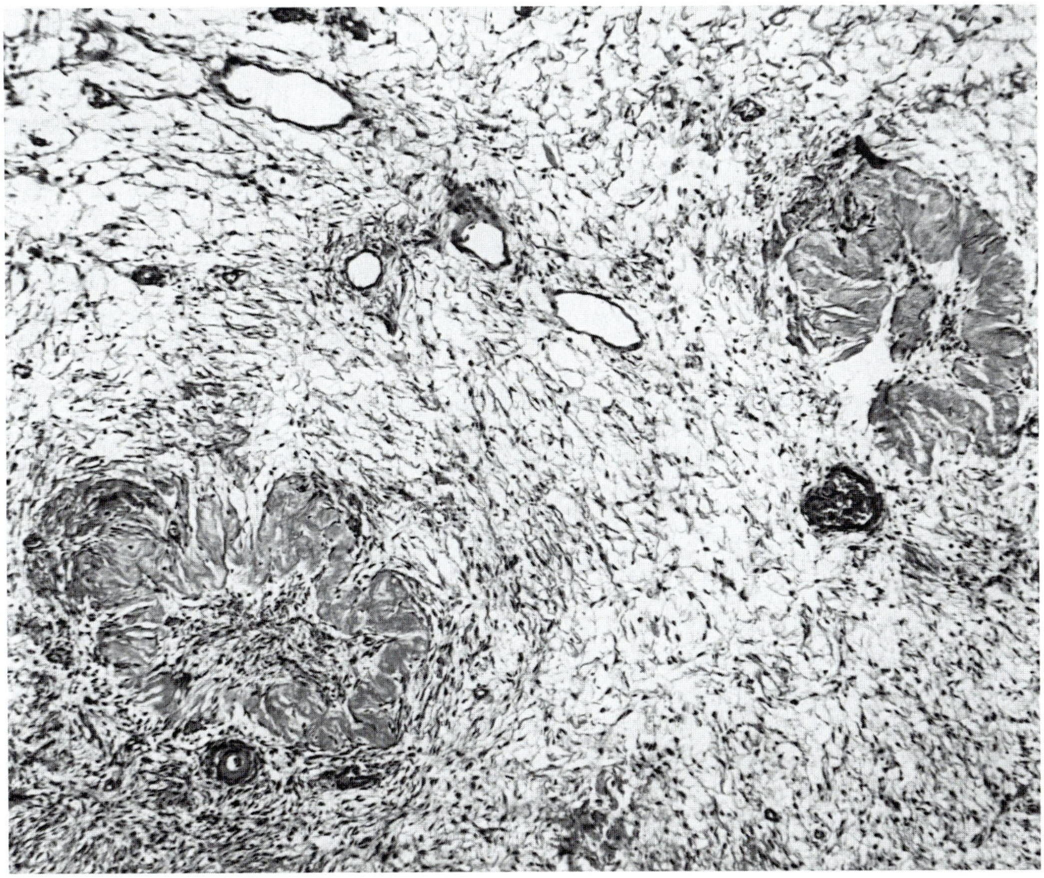

Fig. 16.32. Massive ovarian edema. The edematous ovarian stroma separates several corpora fibrosa. (Reprinted by permission of Clement (1985) In: Roth, Czernobilsky (eds). Contemporary Issues in Surgical Pathology, Vol 6. Churchill Livingstone, New York.)

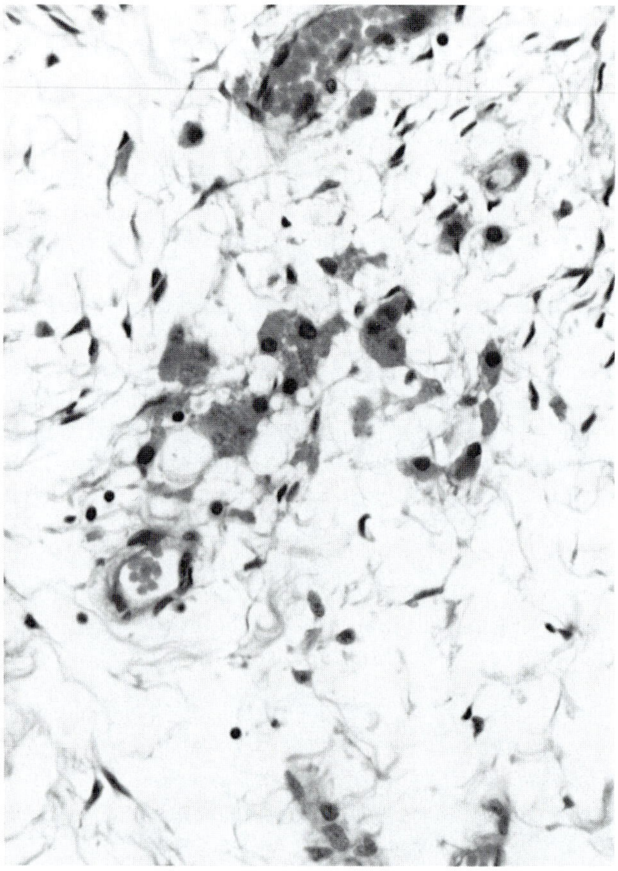

Fig. 16.33. Massive ovarian edema with luteinized stromal cells. (Reprinted by permission of Clement (1985) In: Roth, Czernobilsky (eds). Contemporary Issues in Surgical Pathology, Vol 6. Churchill Livingstone, New York.)

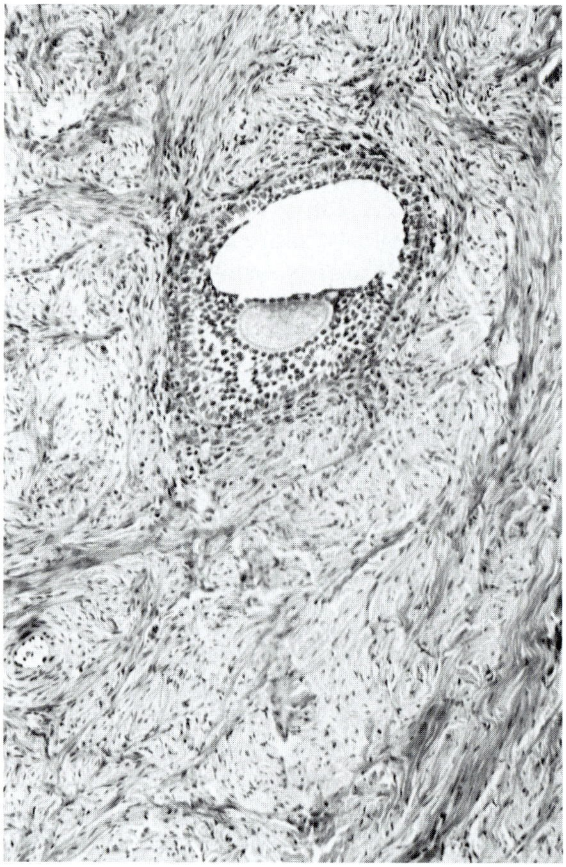

Fig. 16.34. Ovarian fibromatosis. Fibrotic ovarian stroma surrounds an antral follicle.

Pathogenesis

The pathogenesis of massive edema is thought to be intermittent torsion of the ovary on its pedicle, causing partial obstruction of venous and lymphatic drainage. Torsion is observed in half the cases of massive edema, and a few cases of massive edema have been reported in association with obstruction of ovarian lymphatics secondary to metastatic carcinoma within pelvic and paraaortic lymph nodes.[338] Luteinization of the ovarian stromal cells is considered a secondary phenomenon.[300]

In at least some cases, massive edema likely occurs in an ovary with an underlying stromal proliferation, either fibromatosis or stromal hyperthecosis, that enlarges the ovary, promoting torsion with subsequent edema.[338] This interpretation is supported by the clinical similarities and pathologic overlap between massive edema and ovarian fibromatosis. Young and Scully suggest that massive edema is simply ovarian fibromatosis following torsion and accumulation of edema fluid.[338] Similarly, some examples of massive edema in which luteinized stromal cells are present in the same ovary and in the contralateral, edematous or nonedematous ovary may represent cases of stromal hyperthecosis in which one or both ovaries have undergone torsion.

Rather than accepting that fibromatosis is a precursor of massive edema, Russell and Farnsworth[270] hypothesized that the fibromatoses described by Young and Scully represent the "burned-out" stage of a reactive fibroblastic proliferation that at one end of the spectrum is represented by massive edema and at the other by a variety of highly cellular fibroblastic tumor-like lesions.

Differential Diagnosis

The differential diagnosis of massive edema includes ovarian neoplasms that may exhibit an edematous or myxoid appearance, most commonly fibroma, but also sclerosing stromal tumor,[47] Krukenberg tumor, luteinized thecoma associated with sclerosing peritonitis, and the rare ovarian myxoma.[81] Recognition of massive edema is therefore of great importance to prevent unnecessary oophorectomy in a young female. Fibromatosis also may be confused with a fibroma, or if sex cord-like nests are prominent, a Brenner tumor.

Massive edema and fibromatosis are distinguished from a neoplasm by the presence of follicular derivatives visible on both macroscopic and microscopic examination. A neoplasm may be surrounded by a rim of normal ovarian tissue in contrast to massive edema and fibromatosis, which usually diffusely involve the ovarian tissue. Additionally, ovarian fibromas occur in an older age group and are hormonally inactive, and Krukenberg tumors, in contrast to massive edema and fibromatosis, are characterized by signet-ring cells. Finally, the sex cord-like nests in fibromatosis are distinguishable from those of a Brenner tumor in their number, shape, and cell type.

Clinical Behavior and Treatment

Although most of the reported patients with massive edema have been successfully treated by oophorectomy, the condition should be managed conservatively, especially if the patient is young, because there is a strong likelihood that the condition will resolve. After an intraoperative frozen section of a wedge biopsy to exclude a neoplasm, an ovarian suspension procedure should be performed, with fixation of the involved ovary.

Pregnancy Luteoma

Pregnancy luteoma is a distinctive, nonneoplastic lesion of pregnancy characterized by solid proliferations of luteinized cells resulting in tumor-like ovarian enlargement that regresses during the puerperium.[103,233,261,299,300]

Clinical Features

The patients are usually in their third or fourth decades, are multiparous in 80% of the cases, and a similar proportion are black. Most patients are asymptomatic, and the ovarian enlargement is discovered incidentally at cesarean section or postpartum tubal ligation. Rarely, a pelvic mass is palpable or obstructs the birth canal. In approximately 25% of cases, hirsutism or virilization appears or worsens during the latter half of pregnancy. Seventy percent of female infants born to virilized mothers are born with clitoromegaly and labial fusion. Plasma testosterone and other androgens may reach levels 70 times normal in virilized patients; increased values have also been demonstrated in nonvirilized patients.[216] Androgen levels in the infants may be increased but are usually lower than maternal levels or normal.[216] Regression of the luteomas usually begins within days after delivery and is complete within several weeks. Simultaneously, elevated androgen levels decrease rapidly, usually normalizing within 2 weeks postpartum. In rare cases, pregnancy luteomas occur in consecutive pregnancies. The diagnosis is made by excisional biopsy and frozen section examination of one nodule.

Gross Findings

Pregnancy luteomas are solid, fleshy, circumscribed, red to brown nodules ranging from microscopic up to 20 cm in diameter (median, 6.6 cm) (Fig. 16.35).[233] Hemorrhagic foci are common. The lesions are multiple in almost half the cases and bilateral in at least one-third. A separate corpus luteum of pregnancy may also be visible. Examination of the ovaries days to weeks postpartum reveals brown puckered scars.

Microscopic Findings

The lesions are composed of sharply circumscribed, rounded masses of cells (Fig. 16.36), that are also occasionally arranged in a trabecular or follicular pattern, the latter associated with spaces containing colloid-like material (Fig. 16.37a). The cells are intermediate in size between the luteinized granulosa cells and luteinized theca cells of adjacent follicles

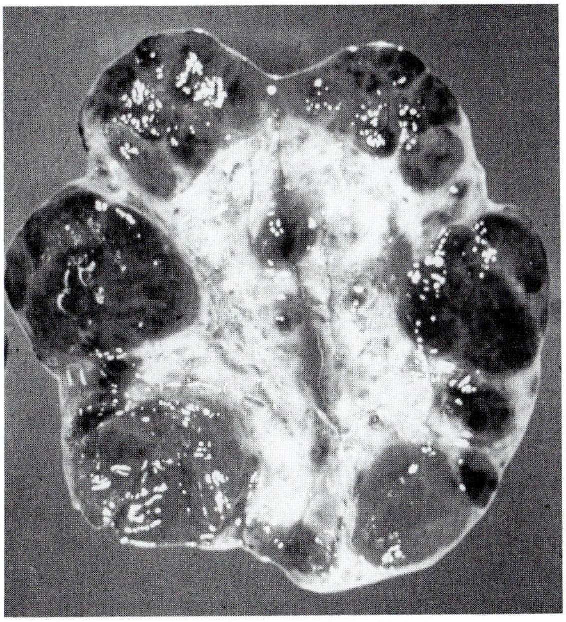

Fig. 16.35. Pregnancy luteoma. Multiple, solid, circumscribed, focally hemorrhagic nodules replace the normal parenchyma. [Reproduced by permission of Malinak and Miller (1965). Am J Obstet Gynecol 91:251–259.]

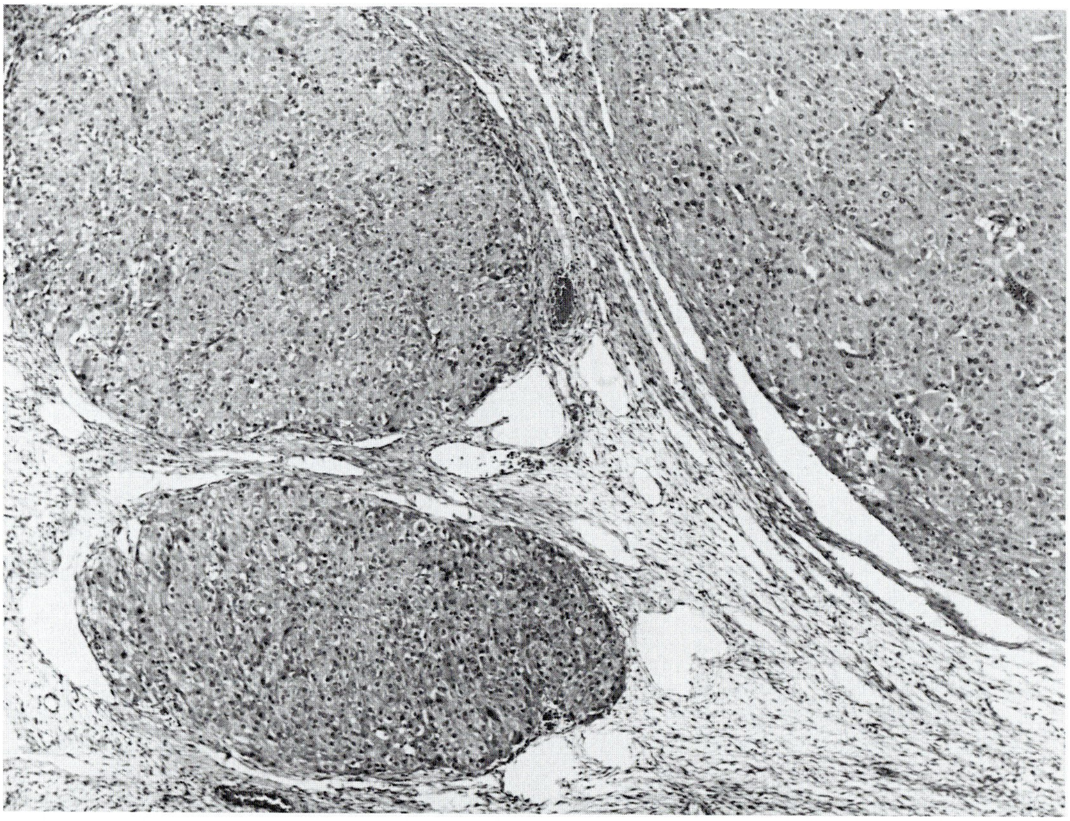

Fig. 16.36. Pregnancy luteoma. Three solid nodules of luteinized cells are present. (Reprinted by permission of Clement (1985) In: Roth, Czernobilsky (eds). Contemporary Issues in Surgical Pathology, Vol 6. Churchill Livingstone, New York.)

and have abundant eosinophilic cytoplasm that contains little or no stainable lipid and central nuclei (Fig. 16.37b). The nuclei may vary slightly in size and are hyperchromatic; nucleoli may be prominent. Mitotic figures may range up to 7 per 10 high-power fields, with an average of 2 or 3, and may be atypical.[233,299] Less common features include focal balloon-like cytoplasmic degeneration and colloid droplets similar to those seen in the corpus luteum of pregnancy. The stroma is scanty, and reticulin fibrils surround groups of cells. Examination of lesions removed postpartum shows shrunken aggregates of degenerating lipid-filled luteoma cells with pyknotic nuclei, infiltration by lymphocytes, and fibrosis.[300]

Pathogenesis

Pregnancy luteomas most likely arise from hCG-induced proliferations of luteinized ovarian stromal cells,[299] a conclusion favored by in vitro incubation studies that have shown that luteoma cells resemble ovarian stromal cells in their steroidogenic capacity. Some authors, however, have favored origin from luteinized follicular granulosa and theca cells.[233] The exclusive occurrence of the lesion in pregnancy suggests a role for hCG in its pathogenesis, and augmentation of steroidogenesis by pregnancy luteomas in response to hCG, both in vitro and in vivo, supports this interpretation. However, the rarity of pregnancy luteomas in association with gestational trophoblastic disease, which is typically accompanied by very high levels of hCG, and the almost exclusive recogition of the lesions during the third trimester when hCG levels are lower than earlier in pregnancy, indicate that hCG is not the only factor in their development. The occasional history of hirsutism, sometimes familial, antedating the pregnancy suggests that a preexistent endocrinopathy, such as stromal hyperthecosis or PCOS, may predispose to the development of the lesion in some patients.

Differential Diagnosis

When pregnancy luteomas are multiple, intraoperative inspection may suggest nodules of metastatic tumor. Such a diagnosis can usually be excluded by frozen section examination of one of the nodules, but the distinction may be difficult if the patient has

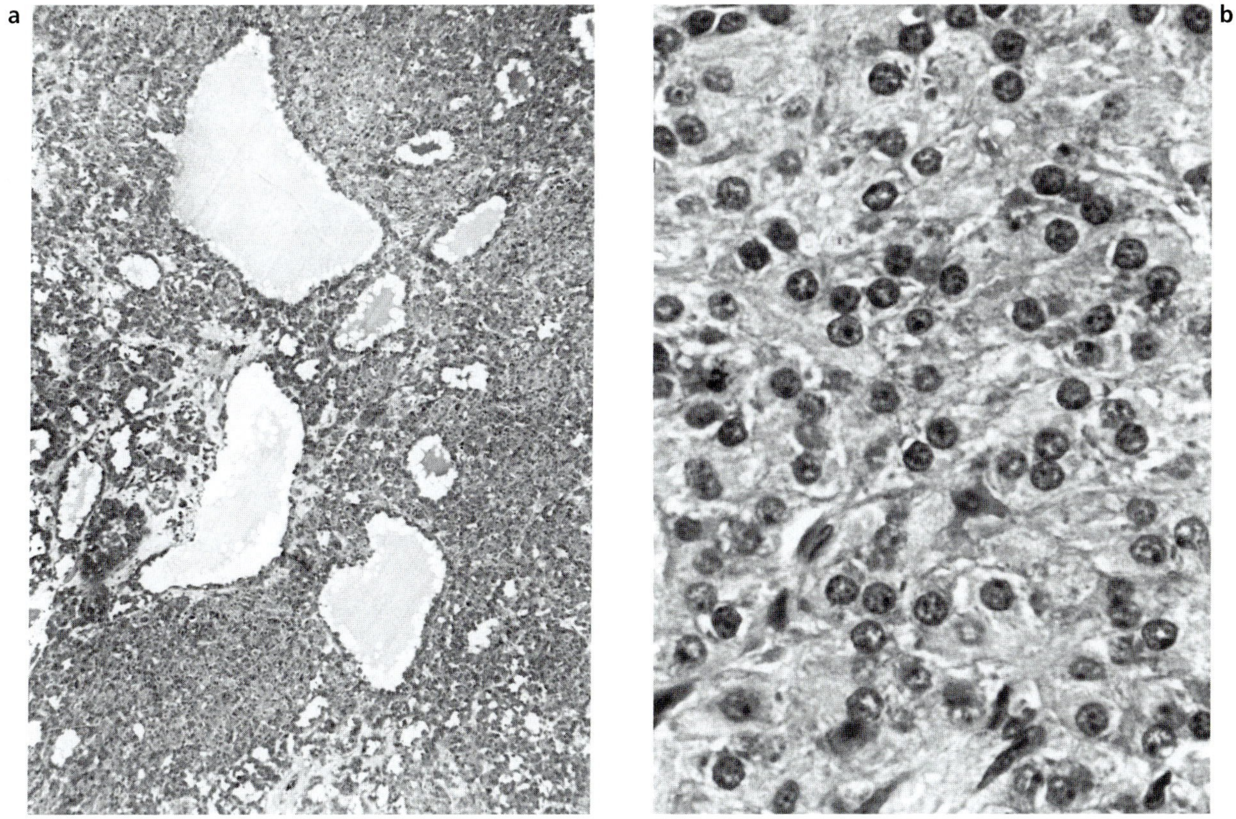

Fig. 16.37. Pregnancy luteoma. a: Follicular pattern. b: Solid growth pattern of polygonal luteinized cells.

a history or clinical evidence of an oxyphilic malignant tumor such as a malignant melanoma. When the luteoma is a single nodule, the microscopic differential diagnosis includes a number of lesions composed of luteinized cells occurring during pregnancy. However, the typical gross appearance of the pregnancy luteoma readily distinguishes it from a large solitary luteinized follicle cyst of pregnancy and puerperium, hyperreactio lueinalis, and corpus luteum of pregnancy. Solid primary neoplasms composed partially or entirely of luteinized cells such as granulosa tumors, thecomas, and steroid cell tumors may occur during pregnancy and enter the differential diagnosis. Such tumors are almost always unilateral and solitary compared to the more frequent bilaterality and multinodularity of the pregnancy luteoma. The partly luteinized group, that is, luteinized granulosa cell tumors and luteinized thecomas, contain typical nonluteinized foci and usually have denser reticulum patterns and more abundant intracellular lipid than seen in pregnancy luteoma. Entirely luteinized tumors belonging to the steroid cell category may closely resemble pregnancy luteoma histologically. Features favoring a steroid cell neoplasm include a dense reticulum pattern, intracellular lipid, lipochrome pigment, and in Leydig cell tumors, a hilar location and the presence of Reinke crystals (see Chapter 19). Differentiation of a solitary pregnancy luteoma from a lipid-poor steroid cell tumor may be impossible, but such a lesion in a pregnant woman is generally considered a pregnancy luteoma until proven otherwise.

Clinical Behavior and Treatment

Because the pregnancy luteoma is a benign, self-limited condition, no treatment is required.

Granulosa Cell Proliferations of Pregnancy

General and Pathologic Features

Granulosa cell proliferations that simulate small neoplasms have been encountered as incidental findings in the ovaries of pregnant women.[56] The older literature documented the presence of similar lesions in the ovaries of nonpregnant women,[193] and we have encountered them in the ovary of a newborn that also contained a corpus luteum. The lesions in pregnant women are usually multiple and lie within atretic follicles, which are typically enveloped by a thick layer of luteinized theca cells. The granulosa cells may be arranged in solid, insular,

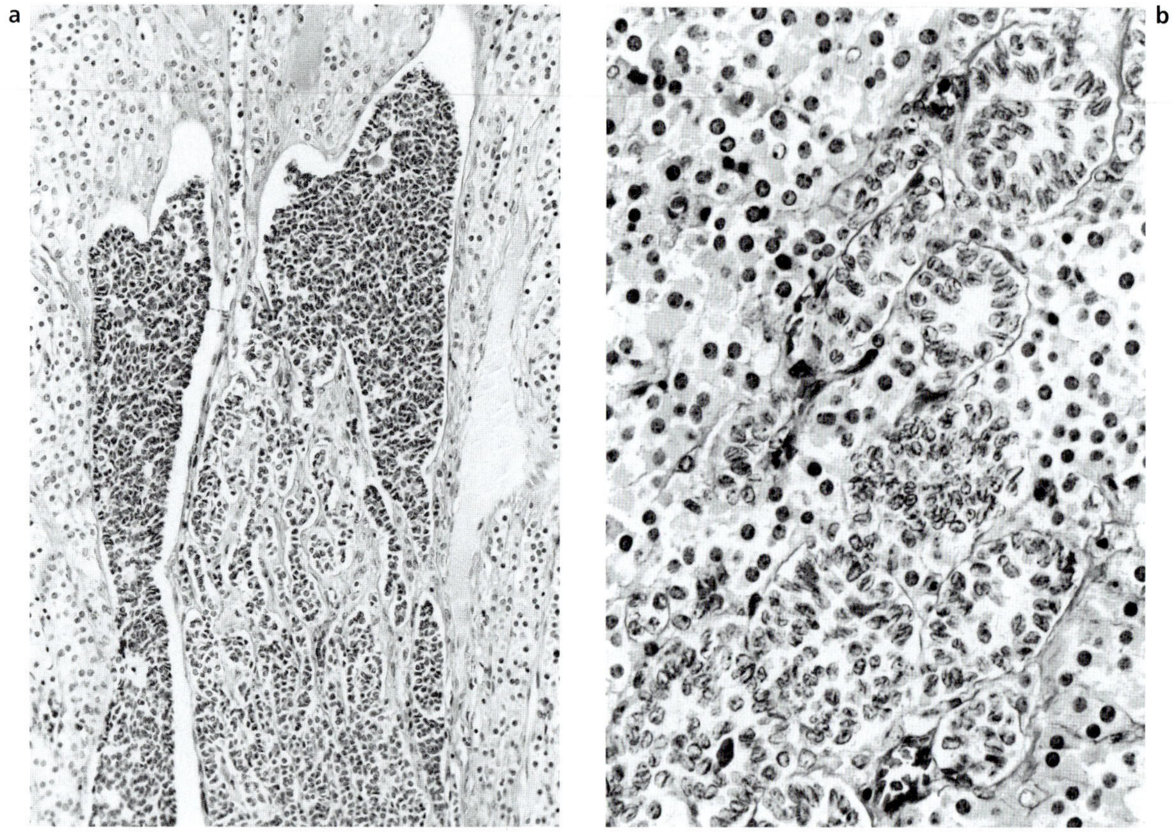

Fig. 16.38. Granulosa cell proliferations of pregnancy mimicking a small granulosa cell tumor. The proliferations are within the center of an atretic follicle, and are surrounded by the luteinized cells of the theca interna. **a**: The proliferating cells form sheets and cords. **b**: In a different case, the granulosa cells form small nests and contain nuclear grooves. [**a** is reprinted by permission of Clement PB (1993) Tumor-like lesions of the ovary associated with pregnancy. Int J Gynecol Pathol 12:105–115.]

microfollicular (Fig. 16.38), or trabecular patterns, mimicking similar patterns in clinically evident granulosa cell tumors. In one case, a solid tubular pattern was identical to that seen in some Sertoli cell tumors. The granulosa cells typically contain scanty cytoplasm and grooved nuclei resembling the cells of the adult-type granulosa cell tumor and in the case with a sertoliform pattern, the cells contained moderate amounts of finely vacuolated cytoplasm suggesting the presence of lipid. In one case, there were large nodules of luteinized granulosa cells with variably sized, round, nongrooved nuclei, resembling pregnancy luteomas except for their obvious origin in granulosa cells and the larger size of their cells.

Differential Diagnosis

The differential diagnosis in most of the cases is with a small granulosa or Sertoli cell tumor. Although similar proliferations have been previously interpreted as small tumors, the frequency of the lesions during pregnancy suggests an unusual nonneoplastic response to the hormonal milieu, possibly to the FSH-like property of hCG. The microscopic size of the lesions, their multifocality, and their confinement to atretic follicles support this interpretation.

Leydig Cell Hyperplasia

Leydig cells typically occur in the ovarian hilus, where they are also referred to as hilus cells, and can be found in virtually all adult ovaries, typically intermingled with nonmyelinated nerves (see Chapter 15). Rarely, Leydig cells occur in nonhilar locations, either within the ovarian stroma or in extraovarian sites, such as the lamina propria or adventitia of the fallopian tube.[129]

Hilar Leydig Cell Hyperplasia

Hilar Leydig cell hyperplasia is difficult to define because hilus cell nests are typically widely separated and cannot be quantitated adequately without sectioning both ovaries extensively. Also, hilus cell proliferation can occur physiologically as a result of elevated hCG or LH levels, such as during pregnancy and after the menopause (see Chapter 15). In such cases, the proliferation is often mild and generally not accompanied by a clinical endocrine disturbance, although such proliferations may account for at least some of the hirustism that is frequently observed during pregnancy (Fig. 16.39). Severe degrees of hyperplasia, often associated with virilization, may occur in both pregnant and nonpregnant women.[197,298,302] In some cases, elevated serum testosterone levels have been documented.[197] Hilus cell hyperplasia is characterized by an increased number of cells in a nodular or, less commonly, a diffuse arrangement, increased cell size, the presence of mitotic figures, cellular and nuclear pleomorphism, hyperchromasia, and multinucleation (Figs. 16.39 and 16.40).[302]

Hilar Leydig cell hyperplasia may be associated with other ovarian lesions, including stromal hyperplasia, stromal hyperthecosis, stromal Leydig cell hyperplasia, rete cysts (see "Miscellaneous Lesions"), and hilus cell neoplasia.[298,301] One case of hilus cell hyperplasia has been associated with the resistant ovary syndrome[197] and other cases have been associated with gonadal dysgenesis[139]; in both disorders, LH levels are elevated.

From a pathologic point of view, the distinction between a large hyperplastic nodule of hilus cells and a hilus cell tumor is arbitrary; we diagnose neoplasia when the nodule is more than 1 cm in diameter.

Leydig cells (containing Reinke crystals) rarely occur within the ovarian stroma, from which they are probably derived, usually representing a focal microscopic finding in ovaries exhibiting otherwise typical stromal hyperthecosis (Fig. 16.41).[34,301] In one such case, there was also bilateral hilar Leydig cell hyperplasia and bilateral hilar Leydig cell tumors.[301] Stromal Leydig cells are likely the origin of the rare Leydig cell tumors encountered within the ovarian stroma (see Chapter 19). Stromal Leydig cells have also been rarely encountered within the nonneoplastic stroma of a variety of ovarian neoplasms and cysts, including mucinous and serous cystadenomas, Brenner tumors, struma ovarii, and strumal carcinoid tumors.[272,300]

a b

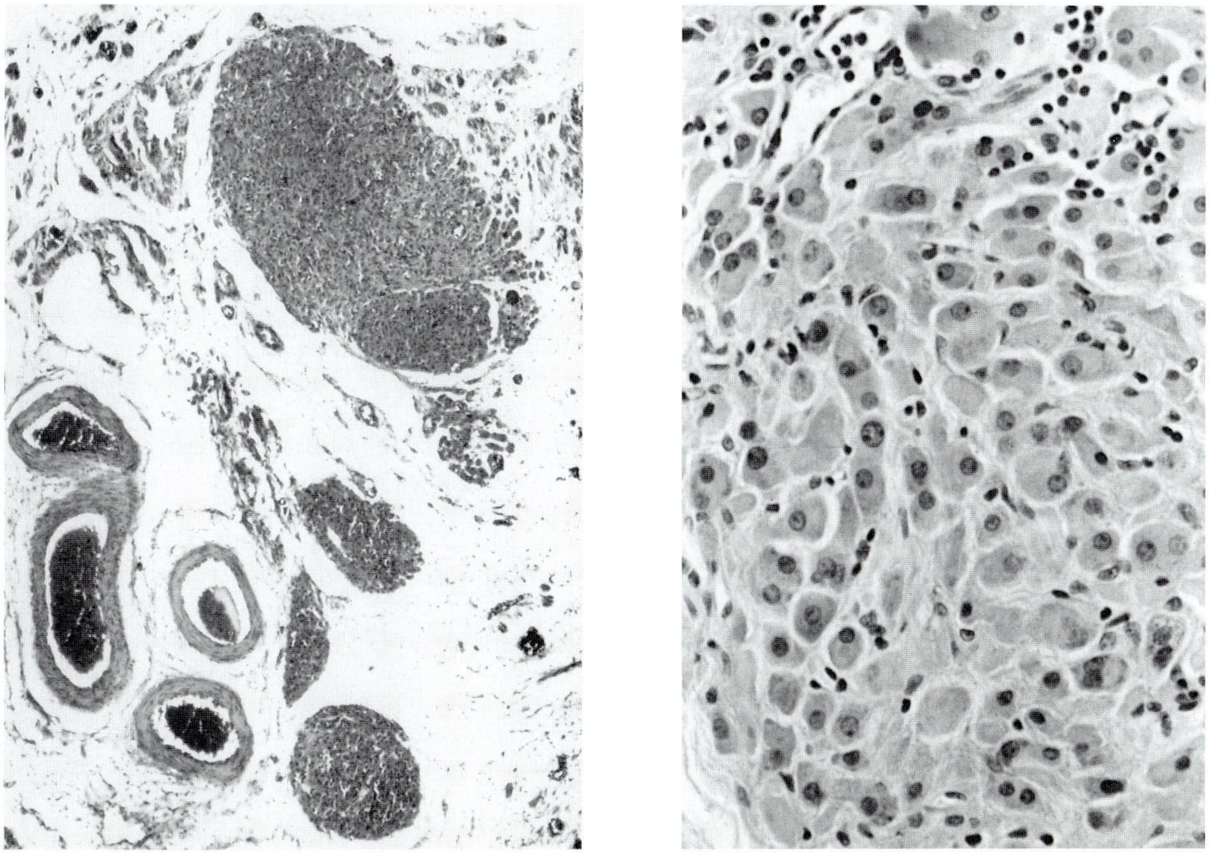

Fig. 16.39. Leydig cell hyperplasia. a: Nodular proliferation of hilar Leydig cells. **b**: There is mild nuclear pleomorphism, and occasional multinucleated cells are present. No crystals are seen in this field.

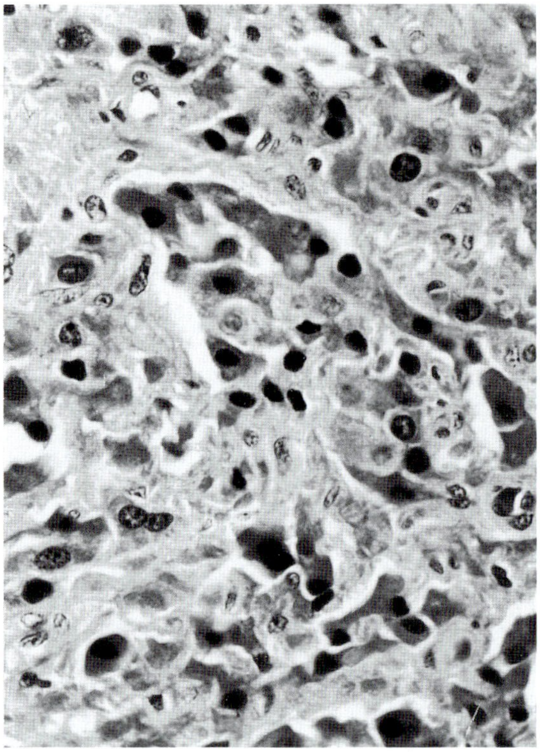

Fig. 16.40. Hilus cell hyperplasia in a postmenopausal woman. The hilus cells have bizarre shapes and abundant cytoplasm, which was eosinophilic. Some nuclei are enlarged and hyperchromatic.

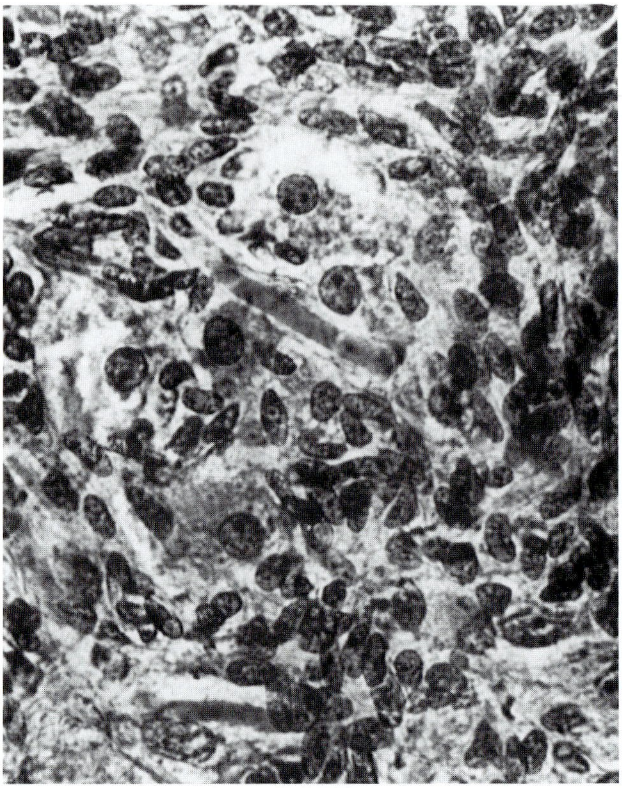

Fig. 16.41. Stromal Leydig cells. Occasional crystal-containing Leydig cells are present within the ovarian stroma. (Reprinted by permission of Sternberg and Roth, ref. 301.)

Ovarian Stromal Metaplasias Including Decidual Reaction

The ovarian stromal cell has the potential to differentiate, presumably by a process of metaplasia, into a variety of other mesenchymal cell types, most commonly decidua, but rarely smooth muscle, fat, and bone.

Ovarian Decidual Reaction

An ectopic decidual reaction may be encountered within the ovarian stroma as an isolated finding or as part of a more widespread decidual transformation of the subperitoneal pelvic mesenchyme (see Chapter 17, Diseases of the Peritoneum).[36] As in other sites of the secondary müllerian system, an *ovarian decidual reaction* usually represents a response of the indigenous stromal cells to the hormonal milieu of pregnancy. Ecopic decidua may be seen as early as the ninth week of gestation and is present in almost all ovaries at term. Less commonly, the decidua is associated with trophoblastic disease, in patients treated with progestagens, in the vicinity of a corpus luteum, and in association with hormonally active neoplastic and nonneoplastic lesions of the ovaries and adrenal glands.[36,237] Prior ovarian radiation may be a predisposing factor by increasing the sensitivity of the stromal cells to hormonal stimulation.[237] Foci of ectopic decidua occasionally may occur within the ovaries of pre- and postmenopausal women with no obvious cause.[237]

The decidual foci are usually seen only microscopically but in some cases may be visible on macroscopic examination as variably sized, soft, tan to hemorrhagic nodules or patches. The decidual cells typically occur singly, as small nodules, or confluent sheets in the superficial cortical stroma and the ovarian surface, often within periovarian adhesions (Fig. 16.42). The cells are indistinguishable from eutopic decidua on light microscopic and ultrastructural examination. Smooth muscle cells, probably derived from submesotheial fibroblasts or the ovarian stroma, may be admixed. A rich vascular network of distended capillaries and a sprinkling of lymphocytes are typically found within the decidual foci. Focal nuclear pleomorphism and hyperchromasia, sometimes in association with hemorrhagic necrosis, should not be misinterpreted as

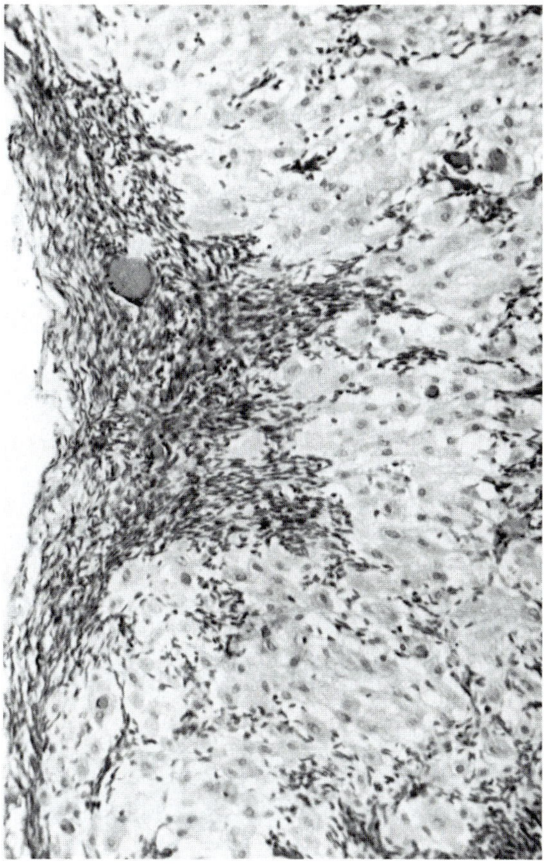

Fig. 16.42. **Ovarian decidual reaction.** Sheets of decidual cells replace the normal ovarian stroma.

evidence of a malignant tumor. Occasionally, ectopic decidual cells may have vacuoles and eccentric nuclei simulating signet-ring cells.[57] The bland appearance of most of the nuclei, the absence of mitotic figures, the PAS negativity of the vacuolar contents, and the association with pregnancy should facilitate the correct diagnosis. Ectopic decidua in postpartum patients may undergo hyalinization.

Rarer Ovarian Stromal Metaplasias and Calcification

Foci of metaplastic smooth muscle (Fig. 16.43a) may be rarely encountered in the ovarian stroma of otherwise normal ovaries, within hyperplastic ovarian stroma (as in stromal hyperthecosis or polycystic ovaries), or within the walls of nonneoplastic or neoplastic cysts.[133,283] Foci of mature fat have been described as a rare incidental histologic finding within the superficial ovarian stroma in obese women (Fig. 16.43b).[130] Heterotopic bone formation in the ovary in the absence of an ovarian neoplasm is also unusual, typically occurring within periovarian adhesions or the walls of endometriotic cysts but rarely within otherwise normal ovaries.[289]

In one case, extensive idiopathic calcification resulted in a stony hard consistency of both ovaries, which were of normal size.[55] Microscopic examination showed numerous spherical, laminated, calcific foci without accompanying epithelial cells (Fig. 16.44). This process must be distinguished from a

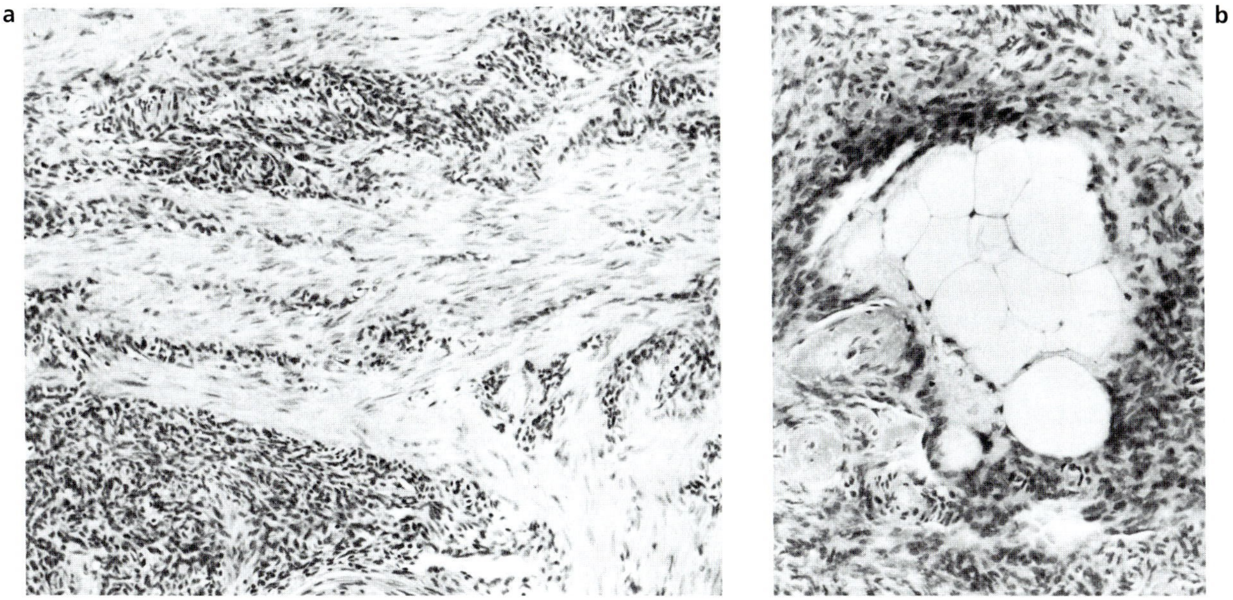

Fig. 16.43. **Ovarian stromal metaplasia.** **a**: Foci of smooth muscle are separated by ovarian stromal cells. **b**: A focus of adipose tissue lies within the ovarian stroma.

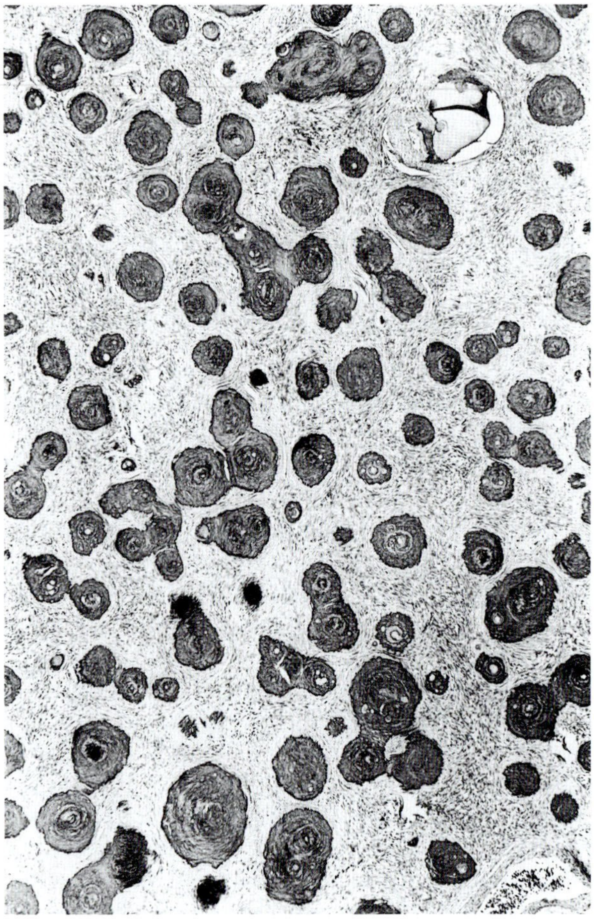

Fig. 16.44. Idiopathic ovarian calcification. Numerous spherical, laminated, calcific foci without accompanying epithelial cells occupy the ovarian stroma. Both ovaries were stony hard on gross examination.

serous borderline tumor or carcinoma with confluent psammoma bodies, in which at least occasional neoplastic epithelial cells should be identified, and from a "burned-out" gonadoblastoma replaced by laminated calcified masses. In the latter cases the patient almost always has evidence of abnormal gonadal development and Y-chromosome material in her karyotype, as well as residual typical gonadoblastoma in the same or contralateral gonad.

Disorders of Ovarian Failure

Premature ovarian failure (POF) or *premature menopause* is a result of a variety of disorders that lead to the onset of amenorrhea and infertility before the age of 35 years, or according to others, 40 years.[4,9,62,258,259,269,313] POF is uncommon, accounting for only 4–10% of patients with secondary amenorrhea.[269] The ovarian failure is usually permanent, but occasionally it is reversible, at least temporarily, as manifested by subsequent ovulation and even conception.[10,238,259]

Patients with POF typically have a 46XX karyotype, normal secondary sexual characteristics, and secondary amenorrhea, although rarely prepubertal ovarian failure causes primary amenorrhea or oligomenorrhea and incompletely developed secondary sexual features. POF, therefore, probably represents a continuum in which individuals may be affected at any age before the expected age of menopause.[259] In contrast to patients with POF, patients with gonadal dysgenesis (see Chapter 1, Embryology of the Female Genital Tract and Disorders of Abnormal Sexual Development) usually have an abnormal karyotype, streak gonads or abdominal testes, primary amenorrhea, ambiguous internal and external genitalia, and somatic abnormalities.

The absence or decline in follicular activity in patients with POF typically results in low serum estrogen levels, often accompanied by estrogen withdrawal symptoms. Because of the failure of negative feedback, the low estrogen levels lead to elevated levels of pituitary gonadotropins, a feature that differentiates POF from central causes of amenorrhea related to hypothalamic or pituitary dysfunction.

If the evaluation of a patient with hypergonadotropic POF is to include microscopic examination of ovarian tissue, the latter should be obtained by bilateral wedge biopsies at the time of laparotomy.[269] Although three histologic patterns have been recognized, specifically premature follicular depletion (true premature menopause), resistant ovary syndrome, and autoimmune oophoritis, it is not known with certainty if each represents a distinct disorder or a nonspecific morphologic manifestation of a number of different disorders.[269]

Premature Follicular Depletion

This disorder is characterized by ovaries that are typically small on gross inspection, resembling streak gonads. On microscopic examination, there is *premature follicular depletion*, with the ovaries resembling normal peri- or postmenopausal ovaries with complete, or nearly complete, absence of primordial and developing follicles (Fig. 16.45).[269] Follicles in varying stages of atresia and stigmata of prior ovulation are typically present, excluding a streak gonad.

Postulated pathogenetic mechanisms include a decreased number of ovarian germ cells at birth, acceleration of normal follicular atresia, or prepubertal or postpubertal destruction of germ cells. With respect to the latter, there is strong evidence, including

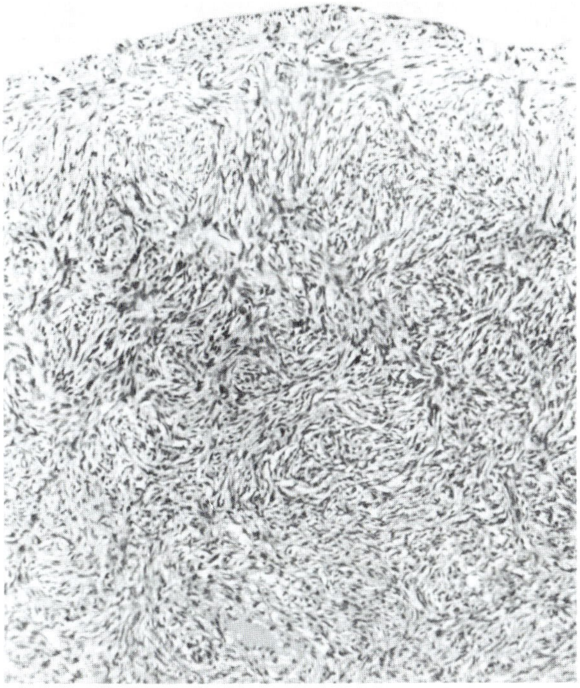

Fig. 16.45. Premature follicular depletion. No primordial or maturing follicles are present within the stroma.

the presence of antiovarian antibodies, autoimmune disorders, or both, implicating immune factors in a substantial proportion of women with POF. As some or all these cases likely represent an end stage of autoimmune oophoritis, they are considered further in that section (see page 712).[269] Additionally, postnatal destruction of germ cells may be caused by cytotoxic drugs or radiation (see "Changes Secondary to Cytotoxic Drugs and Radiation") and mumps oophoritis (see "Viral Infections"). Because mumps oophoritis is probably clinically occult in the majority of cases, it may be a more frequent cause of premature menopause, including familial cases, than is generally suspected.[6,210]

The occurrence of familial cases of POF, in a pattern consistent with an autosomal dominant mode of inheritance,[66,190] implicates genetic factors in some cases. Occasional patients with an otherwise typical presentation have had chromosomal abnormalities, usually 47XXX, pure or mosaic, but occasionally 45XO/46XX.[318] In some familial cases, the affected women were 46XX but had an interstitial deletion of the long arm of the X chromosome.[158] Some authors, however, exclude cases with chromosomal abnormalities from the category of POF so that it includes only "chromosomally competent" patients.

The presence of galactosemia in some patients with POF suggests that it may play a pathogenetic role. Approximately two-thirds of females with galactosemia in one study had POF.[146] In many such patients dietary treatment of galactosemia had been delayed. One galactosemic patient with POF had the pattern of the resistent ovary syndrome (see following) on ovarian biopsy, but in a series of galactosemic patients who were not biopsied, some patients had severely atrophic ovaries, suggesting premature follicular depletion.[83] Similarly, experimental studies indicate that galactose or its metabolites may interefere with normal prenatal oogenesis.

Depletion of primordial follicles has been described is several women with ataxia telangiectasia, which may be related to their severe immunosuppression or to their athymic state.[96,203] Athymic mice have been shown to have low neonatal gonadotropin levels, an abnormality that is believed to result in disorganized folliculogenesis and premature follicular depletion observed in these animals. The existence of a thymic–ovarian–pituitary–hypothalamic axis has also been suggested in human females.[96]

Resistant Ovary Syndrome

This rare syndrome, also known as Savage syndrome, is found in approximately 20% of patients with POF and characterized by primary or secondary amenorrhea, endogenous hypergonadotropinemia, and resistance to exogenous gonadotropins, often in massive doses.[152,170,187,269,295] The resistance to endogenous and exogenous gonadotropins may be relative or absolute, episodic or chronic.

The ovaries typically have a normal prepubertal or adult appearance on macroscopic inspection. Microscopic examination reveals an appropriate number of normal-appearing primordial follicles, but a complete, or nearly complete, absence of developing follicles. Atretic follicles and stigmata of prior ovulation may be present. In occasional patients, the space normally occupied by the ovum in some of the atretic follicles contains calcified material.[28,109] In another case, numerous abnormal preantral follicles were found that contained multiple nodules of basement membrane material.[187] A histologic pattern similar to that in the resistant ovary syndrome occurs in morbid obesity,[90] Cushing's syndrome,[135] and hypogonadotropic ovarian failure secondary to hypothalamic–pituitary dysfunction.

The pathogenesis of this disorder is not yet established, but a possible deficiency of FSH and LH receptors within the ovary, the presence of antibodies to these receptors, or a postreceptor defect have been postulated. An IgG-like substance that alters FSH receptors and thereby impairs binding of this hormone was present in the serum of several patients with associated myasthenia gravis.[83,159] In another patient with the resistent ovary syndrome, lupus erythematosus appeared while the ovarian failure was evolving, and a serum antibody specific for the FSH receptor was found.[187] In another study, circulating autoimmune antibodies to thyroglobulin and smooth muscle were found in some patients.[269] As noted earlier, one patient with the resistent ovary syndrome had galactosemia.[269]

Autoimmune Oophoritis

Clinical and Pathogenetic Features

Approximately 25 cases of *autoimmune oophoritis* have been documented pathologically.[15,29,65,95,108,174,186,269,287,336] The patients, who have ranged in age from 17 to 48 years (mean, 31), typically present with oligomenorrhea or amenorrhea, or symptoms relating to multiple follicular cysts, including pelvic pain, adnexal torsion, or estrogenic manifestations, such as abnormal bleeding, and in one case endometrial adenocarcinoma.[15,29,174] Most patients have steroid cell antibodies in their sera; Addison's disease, Hashimoto's thyroiditis, or both, have been additionally present in some cases.[15] The Addison's disease may arise at the same time or subsequent to the ovarian failure, and is associated at least in some cases with a lymphocytic adrenalitis. The steroid cell antibodies, which are rare in the general population, belong to a group of antibodies reactive with a range of antigens in steroid-producing cells. They are typically reactive against adrenal cortex, but in some cases also to theca interna, corpus luteum, thyroid epithelium and thyroglobulin, parathyroid cells, gastric parietal cells, and thymocytes, alone or in combination.[70,269,331] The antiovarian antibodies are cross reactive with antigens in the adrenal cortex, are cytotoxic to human granulosa cells in tissue culture, and have been localized by immunohistochemical methods to granulosa cells and oocytes.

There is also evidence supporting a role for cell-mediated immune mechanisms in the pathogenesis of autoimmune oophoritis: this includes clinical studies,[80] in vitro assays,[80] and experimental murine models.[136] Recent studies have shown expression of major histocompatibility class II antigens by granulosa cells in autoimmune oophoritis, a phenomenon inducible by interferon gamma, a product of activated T cells.[125] Additionally, there have been reports of occasional patients with POF, including some with documented autoimmune oophoritis, in whom menses and ovulation resumed after administration of corticosteroids.[67,87] All the foregoing observations suggest that a complex immune process with an interplay of humoral and cellular mechanisms is involved in the pathogenesis of autoimmune oophoritis.[287]

Autoimmune oophoritis is almost certainly more common than the small number of histologically documented cases would suggest. In two studies of women with POF who were not biopsied or in whom a biopsy revealed an afollicular pattern, two-thirds[246] and 90%[200] of patients, respectively, had some evidence of autoimmune phenomena with immunologic testing. In a third study, some women with POF had a decreased ratio of inducer/helper lymphocytes to suppressor/cytotoxic lymphocytes, as well as a decreased concentration of serum IgA, suggesting a mild suppression of immune competence.[96] Similarly, as many as one-half of patients with POF in some series have or subsequently develop one or more associated autoimmune disorders; an average figure calculated from the literature since 1980 is 20%.[160] Addison's disease or thyroid disease (Hashimoto's thyroiditis, Grave's disease) are the most common of these disorders, and are typically accompanied or preceded by the presence of steroid cell antibodies.[3,9,63] Conversely, as many as 25% of patients with idiopathic Addison's disease may have POF, the latter usually preceding the former by several, but occasionally many, years.[160] Other autoimmune diseases that occur less commonly in these patients include rheumatoid arthritis, hypoparathyroidism, myasthenia gravis, diabetes mellitus, atrophic gastritis, pernicious anemia, hemolytic anemia, idiopathic thrombocytopenia purpura, alopecia, vitiligo, and sicca syndrome.[9,63,80,331] POF occurs frequently in patients with two or more such diseases (polyglandular endocrinopathy).[160]

Additionally, a subgroup of patients with POF have chronic mucocutaneous candidiasis or chronic vaginal candidiasis, suggesting a defect in T-cell function, possibly secondary to circulating antibodies against T lymphocytes demonstrable in some of these patients.[189] Patients with these two types of candidiasis also frequently have anti-*Candida*, antithymocyte, and antiovarian antibodies, suggesting a shared antigen on these cells.[189]

A partial genetic basis is suggested by a family history of an autoimmune disease in 18% of patients in one study who had both POF and an autoimmune disease.[9] Similarly, a prevalence of certain HLA antigens has been found in some patients with autoimmune endocrine disease.[320]

The foregoing findings suggest that a substantial proportion of patients with the histologic pattern of premature follicular depletion likely represent an end stage of autoimmune oophoritis that is no longer recognizable on histologic examination.

Gross Findings

On gross examination, the ovaries may be small or normal in size, but in one-third of cases one or both are enlarged by multiple follicular cysts, potentially simulating cystic neoplasms.[15,29,174] The cysts are more common in the earlier phases of the disease and are likely caused by elevated gonadotropin levels.[29] Small ovaries presumably reflect a late- or end stage of the disorder, after complete destruction of the follicles.

Microscopic Findings

The cardinal feature of autoimmune oophoritis on microscopic examination is a folliculotropic lymphoid infiltrate that affects developing follicles with a theca layer, corpora lutea, and atretic follicles (Fig. 16.46). The intensity of the infiltrate increases with the degree of follicular maturation. The theca interna layer is typically more intensely infiltrated than the granulosa layer and may be focally destroyed; the granulosa layer may be focally disrupted with sloughing of its cells. The inflammatory infiltrate consists

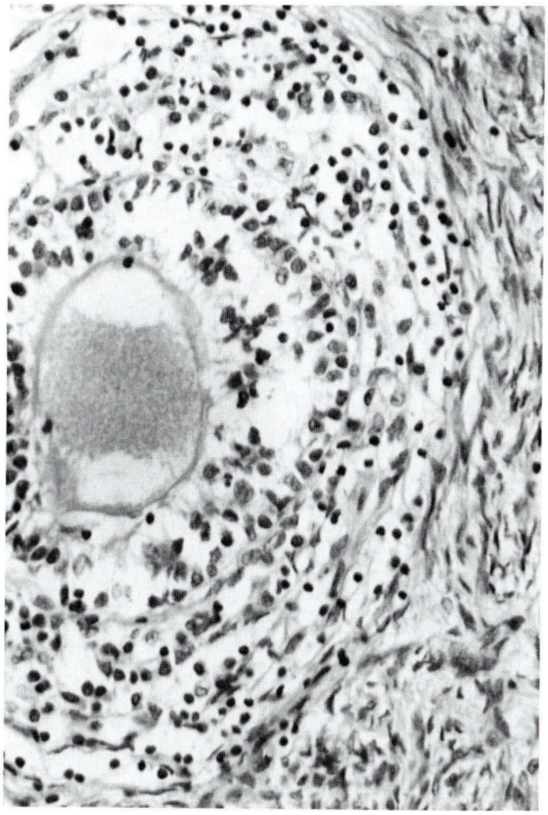

Fig. 16.46. Autoimmune oophoritis. A maturing follicle is infiltrated by mononuclear inflammatory cells.

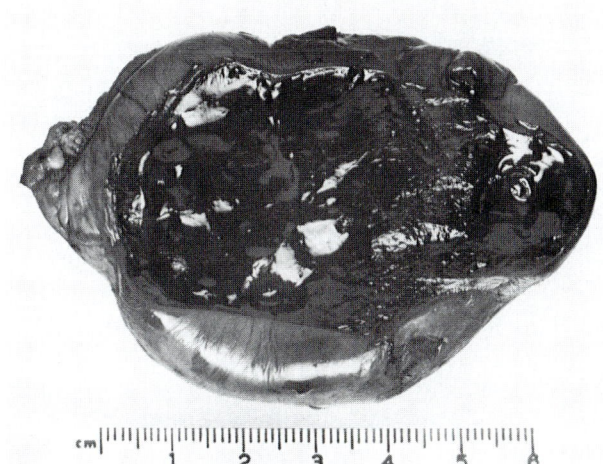

Fig. 16.47. Ovarian hemorrhage. Ovary from a patient being treated with anticoagulation therapy is replaced by a large hematoma.

predominantly of lymphocytes and plasma cells, but eosinophils, histiocytes, and, rarely, sarcoid-like granulomas are also present, and may predominate.[15] Primordial follicles are typically present but uninvolved. Additionally, perivascular and perineural lymphoid infiltrates may be found in the hilus, and in some such cases, there has been an absence of Leydig cells, suggesting destruction of the latter by the inflammatory process.[108,186] Nonspecific findings have included the presence of abnormal "dysplastic" follicles, follicle cysts (as noted earlier), and superficial cortical fibrosis.[15] Immunophenotyping of the inflammatory infiltrate has revealed, variously, B and T lymphocytes, polyclonal plasma cells, macrophages, and natural killer cells.[95,108,174,287]

Vascular Lesions

Ovarian Hemorrhage

Rupture of a normal corpus luteum or a corpus luteum cyst may occasionally result in *hemorrhage* and, rarely, *fatal hemoperitoneum*. Although hemorrhage may occur in otherwise normal women, it is observed more often in women receiving anticoagulant therapy (Fig. 16.47).[114] The right ovary is the source of the hemorrhage in almost two-thirds of patients, and the clinical manifestations frequently resemble acute appendicitis.[114]

Ovarian Torsion and Infarction

Ovarian or adnexal torsion is most frequently a complication of an underlying ovarian lesion, usually a nonneoplastic cyst, abscess, or benign tumor, but occasionally a malignant neoplasm.[123] Torsion of a normal ovary occurs rarely, especially in infants or children[281] but also in adults. Bilateral adnexal torsion, synchronous or asynchronous, has been reported.

The patients present with clinical findings similar to those of acute appendicitis or with recurrent episodes of abdominal pain; occasionally, an adnexal mass is palpable. Laparotomy reveals a swollen, hemorrhagic, and in some cases, infarcted, tuboovarian mass twisted on its pedicle. In rare cases the torsion and infarction may be asymptomatic,[26,27] and autoamputation can result in a mass, which is occasionally calcified, lying free in the peritoneal cavity or attached to adjacent structures. The differential diagnosis in such cases, as noted earlier (see "Congenital Lesions"), is with congenital unilateral absence of the ovary and tube.

It is crucial to examine thoroughly any hemorrhagic infarcted ovarian mass to exclude a neoplasm. A search should be made for viable foci at the periphery of the lesion, and the necrotic tissue should be scrutinized for shadows of neoplastic cells.

Ovarian Vein Thrombophlebitis

Ovarian vein thombosis or *thrombophlebitis* is an uncommon but potentially fatal disorder that most often occurs postpartum but may follow pelvic operations or pelvic trauma or complicate other pelvic disorders such as pelvic inflammatory disease.[41,76,151,214,333] Patients usually present with fever and lower abdominal pain and an abdominal mass, almost always on the right side. The clinical picture may simulate acute appendicitis or pyelonephritis. The marked right-sided predominance in the puerperal cases is explained on the basis of retrograde venous flow in the left ovarian vein during the puerperium, protecting that side from bacterial spread from the uterus.[214] Sonography, computed tomography, and magnetic resonance imaging studies may be useful in establishing the diagnosis preoperatively.

At operation, the involved ovarian vein is markedly enlarged and the thrombus usually extends to the inferior vena cava on the right or to the renal vein on the left. Rarely one or both of the latter structures are also be thrombosed. There is marked edema and inflammation of the surrounding retroperitoneal tissues. The ipsilateral ovary is usually congested but not infarcted, although asymptomatic bilateral ovarian infarction in a postpartum patient secondary to massive pelvic venous thrombosis has been reported. Some cases may be associated with the ovarian vein syndrome (see next section).

Rare Vascular Lesions

Giant cell arteritis can rarely involve the female genital tract, including the ovaries.[1,22,182] The patients are almost invariably postmenopausal, and some patients with ovarian involvement have had systemic manifestations, such as a history of polymyagia rheumatica or temporal arteritis, an elevated erythrocyte sedimentation rate (ESR), or both. Less commonly, the arteritis is an incidental microscopic finding in an asymptomatic patient. Treatment is probably unnecessary in this group of patients, but they should be followed carefully, including repeated determinations of the ESR.[22,182] Rare examples of *vasculitis of polyarteritis nodosa type* involving the ovaries or ovarian hilus have also been reported. Rarely, the finding is a reflection of systemic involvement, but usually polyarteritis in the female genital tract (typically the cervix) is an isolated finding without systemic manifestations on follow-up.[1,93,102]

A rare cause of retroperitoneal hemorrhage is rupture of an ovarian artery or vein, typically during pregnancy or the puerperium.[107] In some cases, the rupture represents a complication of an aneurysm of the ovarian artery.

Varicosities of the ovarian vein, almost always on the right side, may occur in pregnant or parous women and cause ipsilateral ureteric compression and pyelonephritis, constituting the so-called ovarian vein syndrome. Ovarian arteriovenous fistulas have been reported as a rare complication of gynecologic surgery.

Ovarian Pregnancy

In some series, up to 3% of all ectopic pregnancies have been ovarian.[113] The diagnosis of *ovarian pregnancy* should be restricted to cases in which there is no involvement of the fallopian tube. There is an increased frequency of ovarian pregnancy in patients with an intrauterine contraceptive device. The typical clinical presentation is severe pain with hemoperitoneum, and at laparotomy and on gross pathologic examination the enlarged hemorrhagic ovary may mimic a hemorrhagic neoplasm. In a minority of the cases, gross identification of an embryo is indicative of the diagnosis, and in other cases microscopic examination is diagnostic. Distinction between an ovarian pregnancy and the very rare examples of primary ovarian gestational trophoblastic disease (see Chapter 24, Gestational Trophoblastic Disease and Related Lesions) is made by applying criteria similar to those used in the uterus.

Ovarian Changes Secondary to Metabolic Diseases

Amyloidosis may rarely involve the ovaries, usually as an incidental microscopic finding in patients with systemic amyloidosis (Fig. 16.48).[60] There has been a single case of tumorous amyloidosis confined to the ovary that was associated with endometriosis in that site.[274]

Rare cases of ovarian enlargement secondary to involvement by systemic storage disorders (lipidoses, mucopolysaccharidoses) have been reported.[75,322] In such cases, the stored material is typically within macrophages, allowing histologic distinction from a steroid cell tumor or foci of fat within the ovarian stroma. An autopsy study in patients with diabetes mellitus revealed atrophic and fibrotic changes in the ovaries more frequently than in ovaries from control patients, although the differences were not statistically significant.[92]

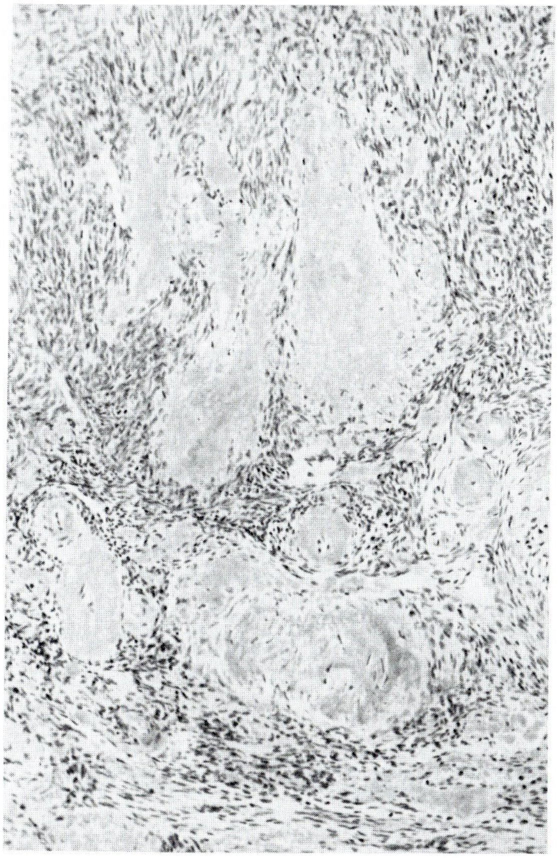

Fig. 16.48. Ovarian amyloidosis. Amyloid involves the ovarian stroma and vessels.

In contrast to frequent testicular involvement in hemochromatosis, in which hemosiderin is typically seen within walls of testicular blood vessels,[184] pathologic changes in the ovary secondary to this disorder appear to be rare or nonexistent.

Ovarian Changes Secondary to Cytotoxic Drugs and Radiation

Cytotoxic Drugs

Cytotoxic drugs may cause a variety of histologic changes in the ovaries of prepubertal and postpubertal patients, including focal or diffuse cortical fibrosis, impaired follicular maturation, and a reduction or depletion in follicle numbers.[126,127,157,181,209,228,321,323] Some studies have shown a direct correlation between the severity of these changes and the duration of the chemotherapy, the number of drugs, and malnourishment of the patients.[127,228] These morphologic findings are consistent with clinical observations of diminished ovarian endocrine function or ovarian failure in some of these patients.[21,50,209,279,291,321,327] The risk of ovarian failure appears to be greater in patients in whom treatment is begun after the age of 25.[21,279] In rare cases, the ovarian failure has reversed after cessation of the therapy.[291,321]

Radiation

The ovary is among the most radiosensitive of organs. Relatively low doses of *radiation* (500–600 R) to the ovaries cause complete or nearly complete disappearance of primordial and developing follicles, fibrosis of the ovarian stroma, and vascular sclerosis in more than 90% of patients (Fig. 16.49).[89,111,126] Follow-up studies of both children and adults who received pelvic radiation have shown that ovarian failure occurs in the majority of such patients.[126,303] The ovarian stroma appears to be more radioresistant than the follicles and may continue to secrete androgens after radiation.[138]

Miscellaneous Lesions

Ovarian Remnant Syndrome

Ectopic, accessory, and supernumerary ovary should be distinguished from examples of the *ovarian remnant syndrome* (*ORS*), which is also known as the

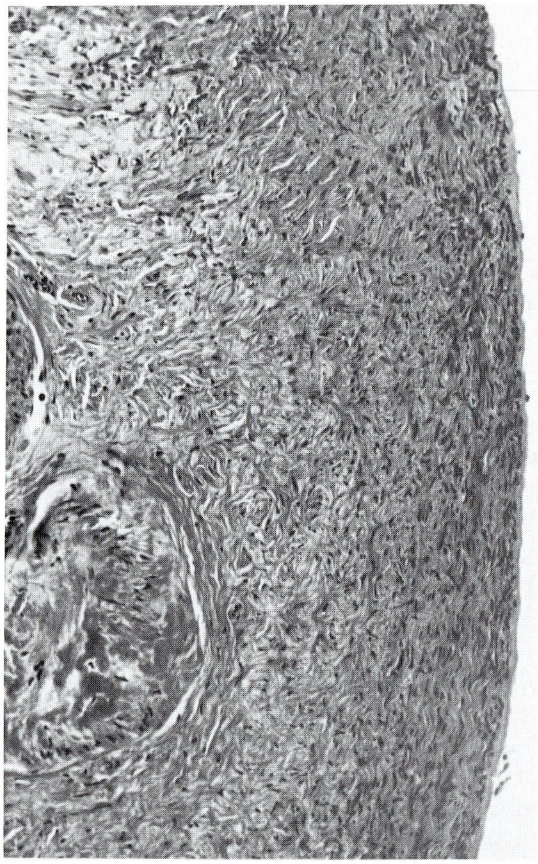

Fig. 16.49. Radiation changes. The ovarian stroma is fibrotic, and blood vessels are hyalinized.

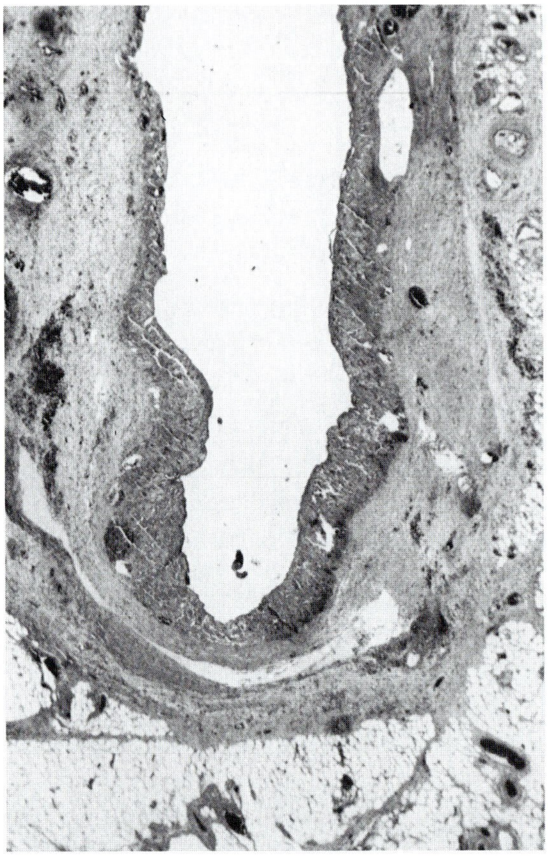

Fig. 16.50. Ovarian remnant syndrome. A corpus luteum cyst is surrounded by congested fibroadipose tissue.

ovarian implant syndrome.[143,164,244,248,296] The ORS should in turn be distinguished from the residual ovary syndrome, in which pelvic symptoms originate from ovaries preserved at the time of hysterectomy.[164] Patients with ORS have a history of a presumably total bilateral oophorectomy but present with findings related to the presence of residual ovarian tissue. The oophorectomy in such cases was often complicated by dense adhesions that are usually caused by endometriosis, pelvic inflammatory disease, a previous pelvic operation, inflammatory bowel disease, or combinations thereof. Clues to the diagnosis in patients who have had bilateral oophorectomy are premenopausal FSH and LH levels,[296] an absence of menopausal symptoms, and a lack of atrophic changes on cervicovaginal smears.

Within weeks to months, but occasionally years, after the oophorectomy, women with ORS usually present with chronic or cyclic pelvic pain and, in about half the cases, a palpable pelvic mass. Ultrasonography or computed tomographic (CT) scanning may aid preoperative detection of nonpalpable symptomatic remnants,[248] and stimulation of the residual ovarian tissue with clomiphene citrate therapy can facilitate their intraoperative localization.[143] Reoperation typically reveals a 3- to 4-cm cystic mass covered by dense adhesions on the pelvic side wall,[296] or less commonly, the mesentery[244]; bilateral ovarian remnants rarely have been encountered. Obstruction or compression of the ureter, the colon, the small intestine, or the bladder may occur.[244,248] Pathologic examination usually reveals one or several follicular or corpus luteum cysts within a remnant of ovarian tissue surrounded by chronically inflamed fibrous tissue (Fig. 16.50). Less common findings have included endometriosis, benign neoplasms, or normal ovarian tissue. Excision of the remnants may be difficult and require multiple operations.

Rete Cysts

Rete cysts are typically located in the ovarian hilus, and in one series, the cysts had a mean diameter of 8.7 cm (range, 1–24 cm).[271] Most are unilocular, although occasionally they are multilocular. Rete cysts typically are lined by a single layer of noncil-

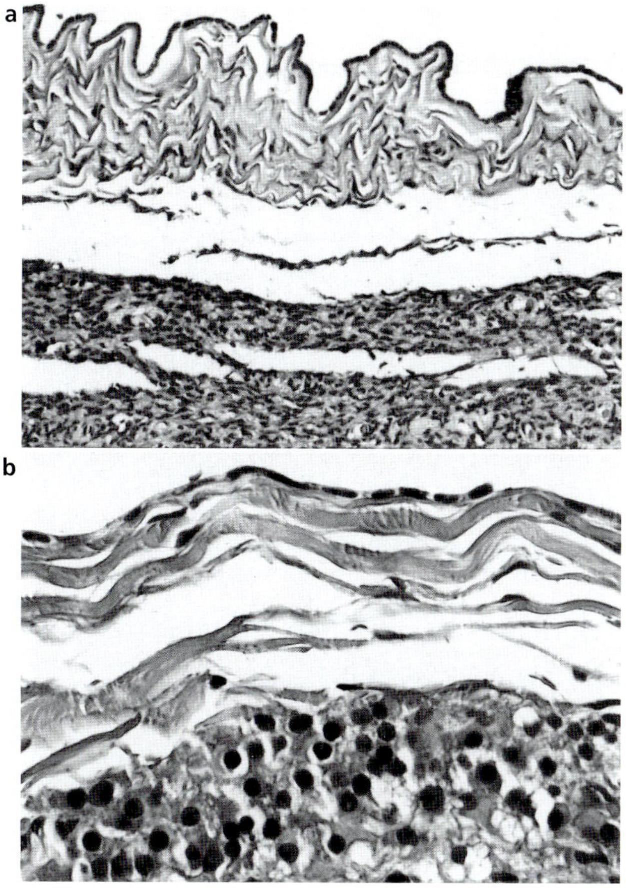

Fig. 16.51. Rete cyst. *Top*: The lining is composed of a single layer of flattened cells which line crevices. Note smooth muscle in wall. *Bottom*: Higher-power view of a different area of the cyst. Nests of Leydig cells are present in the wall.

iated epithelium that varies from flat to cuboidal to columnar. In addition to their hilar location, clues to the origin of the cysts are an irregular contour of their inner surface with small crevice-like outpouchings and a wall that often contains bundles of smooth muscle and hyperplastic hilus cells (Fig. 16.51).

Ectopic Tissues

Rare examples of *cholelithiasis of the ovary* have been a complication of laparoscopic cholecystectomy in which gallstones are released into the peritoneal cavity with implantation onto the surface of the ovary.[315]

A unique case of prostatic tissue within the ovary occurred in a 70-year-old woman who presented with ovarian enlargement.[293] The left ovary was enlarged by a hilar cystic dilatation related to a proliferation of mesonephric remnants. Within the wall of the cyst was a focus of prostatic tissue that was immunoreactive for prostate-specific antigen and prostatic acid phosphatase.

Artifacts and Normal Findings

The *granulosa cells of normal follicles* can be artifactually introduced into tissue spaces or vascular channels during sectioning (Fig. 16.52). This finding, especially when the displaced cells are shrunken or crushed, is occasionally misinterpreted as small cell carcinoma. Awareness of this artifact, the bland nuclear features of the cells, and their similarity to cells lining nearby follicles are helpful clues to the correct diagnosis. Granulosa cells that appear to be deposited on the surface of the ovary secondary to follicle rupture may be misinterpreted as mesothelial cells and when numerous may even suggest the possible diagnosis of a mesothelioma. Immunohistochemical staining for inhibin may be confirmatory of their presence in difficult cases.

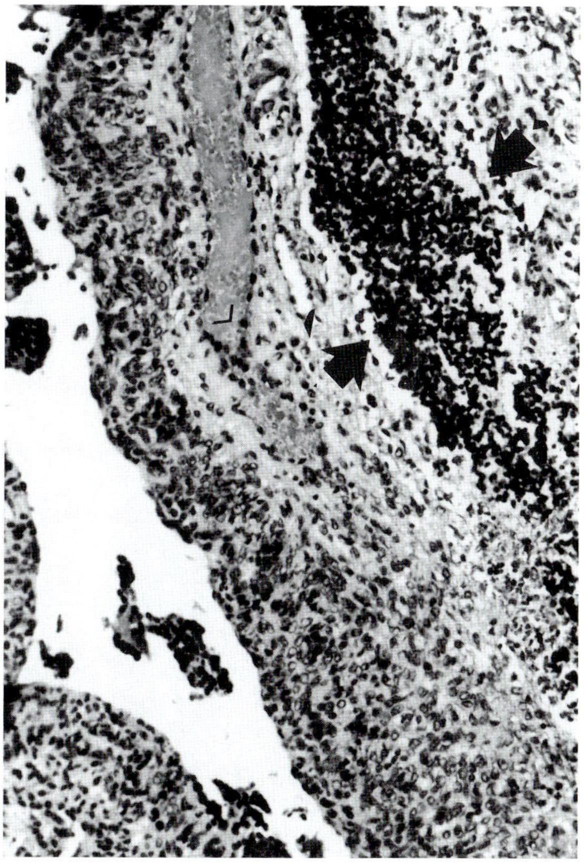

Fig. 16.52. Artifactual displacement of granulosa cells. Nests of granulosa cells (*between arrows*) occupy an artifactual space in the ovarian stroma. Note adjacent cystic follicle (*left*) with detached granulosa cells similar to those in the stroma.

Normal findings (see Chapter 15) that may be misinterpereted as neoplastic include the occasionally highly mitotic granulosa cells and the theca externa cells of the normal developing follicle (see Fig. 15.11). Similarly, the corpus luteum of late pregnancy and the puerperium may contain numerous calcific deposits; we have encountered one case in which their presence in a patient with a history of a serous borderline tumor was misinterpreted as recurrent tumor.

Lesions that can involve the ovary, but which are more appropriately discussed in Chapter 17 (Diseases of the Peritoneum), include mucicarminophilic histiocytosis and infarcted appendix epiploica.

References

1. Abu-Farsakh H, Mody D, Brown RW, Truong LD (1994) Isolated vasculitis involving the female genital tract: clinicopathologic spectrum and phenotyping of inflammatory cells. Mod Pathol 7:610–615
2. Abu-Louz SK, Ahmed AA, Swan RW (1997) Spontaneous ovarian hyperstimulation syndrome with pregnancy. Am J Obstet Gynecol 177:476–477
3. Ahonen P, Miettinen A, Perheentupa J (1987) Adrenal and steroidal cell antibodies in patients with autoimmune polyglandular disease type I and risk of adrenocortical and ovarian failure. J Clin Endocrinol Metab 64:494–500
4. Aiman J, Smentek C (1985) Premature ovarian failure. Obstet Gynecol 66:9–14
5. Al Dawoud A, Yates R, Foulis AK (1991) Postoperative necrotizing granulomas in the ovary. J Clin Pathol 44:524–525
6. Aleem FA (1981) Familial 46,XX gonadal dysgenesis. Fertil Steril 35:317–320
7. Allen C, Johnson S (1993) Apocrine metaplasia: a new type of mullerian metaplasia. J Clin Pathol 46: 569
8. Almenoff IA (1966) Splenic-gonadal fusion. N Y State J Med 66:1679–1691
9. Alper MM, Garner PR (1985) Premature ovarian failure: its relationship to autoimmune disease. Obstet Gynecol 66:27–30
10. Alper MM, Jolly EE, Garner PR (1986) Pregnancies after premature ovarian failure. Obstet Gynecol 67:59S–62S
11. Amowitz LL, Sobel BE (1999) Cardiovascular consequences of polycystic ovary syndrome. Endocrinol Metab Clin N Am 28:439–458
12. Annos T, Taymor ML (1981) Ovarian pathology associated with insulin resistance and acanthosis nigricans. Obstet Gynecol 58:662–664
13. Ayers JWT (1982) Differential response to adrenocorticotropin hormone stimulation in polycystic ovarian disease with high and low dehydroepiandrosterone sulfate levels. Fertil Steril 37:645–649
14. Babaknia A, Calfopoulos P, Jones HW (1976) The Stein-Leventhal syndrome and coincidental ovarian tumors. Obstet Gynecol 1976:47:223–224
15. Bannatyne P, Russell P, Shearman RP (1990) Autoimmune oophoritis: a clinicopathologic assessment of 12 case. Int J Gynecol Pathol 9:191–207
16. Bar RS, Muggeo M, Kahn CR, et al (1980) Characterization of insulin receptors in patients with the syndromes of insulin resistance and acanthosis nigricans. Diabetologia 18:209
17. Barbieri RL, Makris A, Randall RW, et al (1986) Insulin stimulates androgen accumulation in incubations of ovarian stroma obtained from women with hyperandrogenism. J Clin Endocrinol Metab 62:904–910
18. Barbieri RL, Ryan KJ (1983) Hyperandrogenism, insulin resistance, and acanthosis nigricans syndrome: a common endocrinopathy with distinct pathophysiologic features. Am J Obstet Gynecol 147:90–101
19. Barbieri Rl, Smith S, Ryan KJ (1988) The role of hyperinsulinemia in the pathogenesis of ovarian hyperandrogenism. Fertil Steril 50:197–212
20. Bates GW, Whitworth NS (1982) Effect of body weight reduction on plasma androgens in obese, infertile women. Fertil Steril 38:406–409
21. Beard MEJ, Conder JL, Clark VA (1984) Ovarian failure following cytotoxic therapy. NZ Med J 97:759–762
22. Bell DA, Mondschein M, Scully RE (1986) Giant cell arteritis of the female genital tract. A report of three cases. Am J Surg Pathol 10:696–701
23. Benirschke K, Bonin ML, Rost T (1984) Plant material in ovary following barium enema [Letter]. Arch Pathol Lab Med 108:359–360
24. Ben-Rafael Z, Bider D, Menashe Y, et al (1990) Follicular and luteal cysts after treatment with gonadotropin-releasing hormone analogue for in vitro fertilization. Fertil Steril 53:1091–1094
25. Berger NG, Repke JT, Woodruff JD (1984) Markedly elevated serum testosterone in pregnancy without fetal virilization. Obstet Gynecol 63:260–262
26. Best CL, Feldman DB, Sobenes JR, Sueldo CE (1991) Unexplained displacement of ipsilateral ovary and fallopian tube. Obstet Gynecol 78:558–560
27. Beyth Y, Bar-On E (1984) Tuboovarian autoamputation and infertility. Fertil Steril 42:932–934
28. Biberoglu KO, Damewood MD, Parmley T, Rock JA (1988) Insensitive ovary syndrome with a unique process of follicular degeneration. Fertil Steril 49:367–369
29. Biscotti CV, Hart WR, Lucas JG (1989) Cystic ovarian enlargement resulting from autoimmune oophoritis. Obstet Gynecol 74:492–495
30. Blaustein A (1981) Surface cells and inclusion cysts in fetal ovaries. Gynecol Oncol 12:222–233
31. Blaustein A, Kaganowicz A, Wells J (1982) Tumor markers in inclusion cysts of the ovary. Cancer (Phila) 49:722–726
32. Blaustein A, Kantius M, Kaganowicz A, et al (1982)

Inclusions in ovaries of females aged day 1–30 years. Int J Gynecol Pathol 1:145–153
33. Boder E, Sedgwick RP (1958) Ataxia-telangiectasia. A familial syndrome of progressive cerebellar ataxia, oculocutaneous telangiectasia and frequent pulmonary infection. Pediatrics 21:526–554
34. Bohm J, Roder-Weber M, Hofler H, Kolben M (1991) Bilateral stromal Leydig cell tumour of the ovary. Case report and literature review. Pathol Res Pract 187:348–352
35. Bonar BE, Rabson AS (1957) Gynecological aspects of leprosy. Obstet Gynecol 9:33–43
36. Boss, JH, Scully RE, Wegner KH, Cohen RB (1965) Structural variations in the adult ovary: clinical significance. Obstet Gynecol 25:747–763
37. Bradshaw KD, Carr BR (1986) Ovarian and tubal inguinal hernia. Obstet Gynecol 68:50S–51S
38. Bradshaw KD, Santos-Ramos R, Rawlins SC, et al (1986) Endocrine studies in a pregnancy complicated by ovarian theca lutein cysts and hyperreactio luteinalis. Obstet Gynecol 67:66S–69S
39. Bradley B, Gleicher N (1980) Grand multiparity associated with unilateral renal, ovarian, and mullerian agenesis. Mt Sinai J Med 47:418–422
40. Braithwaite SS, Erkman-Balis B, Avila TD (1978) Postmenopausal virilization due to ovarian stromal hyperthecosis. J Clin Endocrinol Metab 46:295–300
41. Brown CEL, Lowe TW, Cunningham FG, Weinreb JC (1986) Puerperal pelvic thrombophlebitis: impact on diagnosis and treatment using X-ray computed tomography and magnetic resonance imaging. Obstet Gynecol 68:789–794
42. Burkman R, Schlesselman S, McCaffrey L, et al (1982) The relationship of genital tract actinomycetes and the development of pelvic inflammatory disease. Am J Obstet Gynecol 143:585–589
43. Bylund DJ, Nanfro JJ, Marsh WL Jr (1986) Coccidioidomycosis of the female genital tract. Arch Pathol Lab Med 110:232–235
44. Caillouette JC, Koehler AL (1987) Phasic contraceptive pills and functional ovarian cysts. Am J Obstet Gynecol 156:1538–1542
45. Carmina E, Gonzalez F, Chang L, Lobi RA (1995) Reassessment of adrenal androgen secretion in women with polycystic ovary syndrome. Obstet Gynecol 85:971–976
46. Chalvardjian A, Picard L, Shaw R, et al (1980) Malacoplakia of the female genital tract. Am J Obstet Gynecol 138:391–394
47. Chalvardjian A, Scully RE (1973) Sclerosing stromal tumors of the ovary. Cancer (Phila) 31:664–670
48. Chang RJ, Katz SE (1999) Diagnosis of polycystic ovary syndrome. Endocrinol Metab Clin N Am 28:397–408
49. Chang RJ, Nakamura RM, Judd HL, Kaplan SA (1983) Insulin resistance in nonobese patients with polycystic ovarian disease. J Clin Endocrinol Metab 57:356–359
50. Chapman RM (1983) Gonadal injury resulting from chemotherapy. Am J Indust Med 4:149–161
51. Charpin C, Bhan AK, Zurawski VR Jr, Scully RE (1982) Carcinoembryonic antigen (CEA) and carbohydrate determinant 19–9 (CA 19–9) localization in 121 primary and metastatic ovarian tumors: an immunohistochemical study with the use of monoclonal antibodies. Int J Gynecol Pathol 1:231–245
52. Chrousos GP, Loriaux L, Mann DL, Cutler GB (1982) Late onset 21–hydroxylase deficiency mimicking idiopathic hirsutism or polycystic ovarian disease. Ann Intern Med 96:143–148
53. Claman P, Dover M, Saginur R, et al (1991) Spontaneous ovarian-to-vaginal fistula: A case report. Am J Obstet Gynecol 164:71–72
54. Clement PB, Scully RE (1980) Large solitary luteinized follicle cyst of pregnancy and puerperium. Am J Surg Pathol 4:431–438
55. Clement PB, Cooney TP (1992) Idiopathic multifocal calcification of the ovarian stroma. Arch Pathol Lab Med 116:204–205
56. Clement PB, Young RH, Scully RE (1988) Ovarian granulosa cell proliferations of pregnancy. A report of nine cases. Hum Pathol 19:657–662
57. Clement PB, Young RH, Scully RE (1989) Nontrophoblastic pathology of the female genital tract and peritoneum associated with pregnancy. Semin Diagn Pathol 6:372–406
58. Cohen I, Figer A, Tepper T, et al (1999) Ovarian overstimulation and cystic formation in premenopausal tamoxifen exposure: comparison between tamoxifen-treated and nontreated breast cancer patients. Gynecol Oncol 72:202–207
59. Comite F, Shawker TH, Pescovitz OH, et al (1984) Cyclical ovarian function resistent to treatment with an analogue of luteinizing hormone releasing hormone in McCune–Albright syndrome. N Engl J Med 311:1032–1036
60. Copeland W Jr, Hawley PC, Teteris NJ (1985) Gynecologic amyloidosis. Am J Obstet Gynecol 153: 555–556
61. Cordon-Cardo C, Mattes MJ, Melamed MR, et al (1985) Immunopathologic analysis of a panel of mouse monoclonal antibodies reacting with human ovarian carcinomas and other human tumors. Int J Gynecol Pathol 4:121–130
62. Coulam CB (1982) Premature gonadal failure. Fertil Steril 38:645–655
63. Coulam CB (1983) The prevalence of autoimmune disorders among patients with primary ovarian failure. Am J Reprod Immunol 4:63–66
64. Coulam CB, Annegers JF, Kranz JS (1983) Chronic anovulation syndrome and associated neoplasia. Obstet Gynecol 61:403–407
65. Coulam CB, Kempers RD, Randall RV (1981) Premature ovarian failure: evidence for autoimmune function. Fertil Steril 36:238–240
66. Coulam CB, Stringfellow S, Hoefnagel D (1983) Evidence for a genetic factor in the etiology of premature ovarian failure. Fertil Steril 40:693–695
67. Cowchock FS, McCabe JL, Montgomery BB (1988) Pregnancy after corticosteroid administration

in premature ovarian failure (polyglandular endocrinopathy syndrome). Am J Obstet Gynecol 158:118–119
68. Cramer DW, Welch WR, Cassells S, Scully RE (1983) Mumps, menarche, menopause, and ovarian cancer. Am J Obstet Gynecol 147:1–6
69. Cruikshank SH, Van Drie DM (1982) Supernumerary ovaries: update and review. Obstet Gynecol 60: 126–129
70. Damewood MD, Zacur HA, Hoffman GJ, Rock JA (1986) Circulating antiovarian antibodies in premature ovarian failure. Obstet Gynecol 68:850–854
71. D'Armiento M, Reda G, Camagna A, Tardella L (1983) McCune–Albright syndrome: evidence for autonomous multiendocrine function. J Pediatr 102:584–586
72. Deligdisch L, Einstein AJ, Guera D, Gil J (1995) Ovarian dysplasia in epithelial inclusion cysts. A morphometric approach using neural networks. Cancer (Phila) 76:1027–1034
73. Dennefors BL, Janson PO, Knutson F, Hamberger L (1980) Steroid production and responsiveness to gonadotropin in isolated stromal tissue of human postmenopausal ovaries. Am J Obstet Gynecol 136:997–1002
74. De Sa DJ (1975) Follicular ovarian cysts in stillbirths and neonates. Arch Dis Child 50:45–50
75. Dincsoy HP, Rolfes DB, McGraw CA, Schubert WK (1984) Cholesterol ester storage disease and mesenteric lipodystrophy. Am J Clin Pathol 81:263–269
76. Duff P, Gibbs RF (1983) Pelvic vein thrombophlebitis: diagnostic dilemma and therapeutic challenge. Obetet Gynecol Surv 38:365–373
77. Dunaif A (1999) Insulin action in the polycystic ovary syndrome. Endocrinol Metab Clin N Am 23: 341–359
78. Dunaif A, Futterweit W (1988) Polycystic ovary syndrome [Letter]. N Engl J Med 319:584
79. Dunaif A, Hoffman AR, Scully RE, et al (1985) Clinical, biochemical, and ovarian morphologic features in women with acanthosis nigricans and masculinization. Obstet Gynecol 66:545–552
80. Edmonds M, Lamki L, Killinger DW, Volpe R (1973) Autoimmune thyroiditis, adrenalitis and oophoritis. Am J Med 54:782–787
81. Eichhorn JH, Scully RE (1991) Ovarian myxoma: clinicopathologic and immunocytologic analysis of five cases and a review of the literature. Int J Gynecol Pathol 10:156–169
82. Eschenbach DA (1980) Epidemiology and diagnosis of acute pelvic inflammatory disease. Obstet Gynecol 55:142S–152S
83. Escobar ME, Cigorraga SB, Chiauzzi VA, et al (1982) Development of gonadotropin resistant ovary syndrome in myasthenia gravis: suggestion of similar autoimmune mechanisms. Acta Endocrinol 99:431–436
84. Farber ER, Leahy MS, Meadows TR (1968) Endometrial blastomycosis acquired by sexual contact. Obstet Gynecol 32:195–199
85. Farber M, Madanes A, O'Brian D, et al (1981) Asymmetric hyperthecosis ovarii. Obstet Gynecol 57: 521–525
86. Farhi DC, Nosanchuk J, Silverberg SG (1986) Endometrial adenocarcinoma in women under 25 years of age. Obstet Gynecol 68:741–745
87. Farid NR, Bear JC (1981) The human major histocompatibility complex and endocrine disease. Endocr Rev 2:50–86
88. Ferrannini E, Muggeo M, Navalesi R, Pilo A (1982) Impaired insulin degradation in a patient with insulin resistance and acanthosis nigricans. Am J Med 73:148–154
89. Fisher B, Cheung AYC (1984) Delayed effect of radiation therapy with or without chemotherapy on ovarian function in women with Hodgkin's disease. Acta Radiol Oncol 23:43–48
90. Fisher ER, Gregorio R, Stephan T, et al (1974) Ovarian changes in women with morbid obesity. Obstet Gynecol 44:839–844
91. Flier JS, Kahn CR, Roth J (1979) Receptors, antireceptor antibodies and mechanisms of insulin resistance. N Engl J Med 300:413–419
92. Fraley DS, Totten RS (1968) An autopsy study of endocrine organ changes in diabetes mellitus. Metabolism 17:896–900
93. Francke M, Mihaescu A, Chaubert P (1998) Isolated necrotizing arteritis of the female genital tract: a clinicopathologic and immunohistochemical study of 11 cases. Int J Gynecol Pathol 17:193–200
94. Granks S, Gilling-Smith C, Watson H, Willis D (1999) Insulin action in the normal and polycystic ovary. Endocrinol Metab Clin N Am 28:361–378
95. Friedman CI, Gurgen-Varol F, Lucas J, Neff J (1987) Persistent progesterone production associated with autoimmune oophoritis. J Reprod Med 32:293–296
96. Friedman CI, Neff J, Kim MH (1984) Immunologic parameters in premature follicular depletion: T and B lymphocytes, T-cell subpopulations, cutaneous reactivity, and serum immunoglobulin concentrations. Diagn Immunol 2:48–52
97. Friedman CI, Schmidt GE, Chang FE, Kim MH (1984) Severe ovarian hyperstimulation following follicular aspiration. Am J Obstet Gynecol 150:436–437
98. Futterweit W (1983) Pituitary tumors and polycystic ovarian disease. Obstet Gynecol 62:74S–79S
99. Futterweit W (1985) Polycystic ovarian disease. Clinical perspectives in obstetrics and gynecology. Springer, New York
100. Futterweit W (1999) Polycystic ovary syndrome: clinical perspectives and management. Obstet Gynecol Surv 54:403–413
101. Gallup DG, Stock RJ (1984) Adenocarcinoma of the endometrium in women 40 years of age or younger. Obstet Gynecol 64:417–419
102. Ganesan R, Ferryman SR, Meier L, Rollason TP (2000) Vasculitis of the female genital tract and its clinicopathologic correlation: a study of 46 cases with follow-up. Int J Gynecol Pathol 19:258–265

103. Garcia-Bunuel R, Berek JS, Woodruff JD (1975) Luteomas of pregnancy. Obstet Gynecol 45:407–414
104. Gardner GH, Greene RR, Peckham B (1957) Tumors of the broad ligament. Am J Obstet Gynecol 73:536–555
105. Gibson M, Schiff I, Tulchinsky D, Ryan KJ (1980) Characterization of hyperandrogenism with insulin-resistant diabetes type A. Fertil Steril 33: 501–505
106. Gilks CB, Clement PB (1987) Colo-ovarian fistula: a report of two cases. Obstet Gynecol 69:533–537
107. Ginsburg KA, Valdes C, Schnider G (1987) Spontaneous utero-ovarian vessel rupture during pregnancy: three case reports and a review of the literature. Obstet Gynecol 69:474–476
108. Gloor E, Hurlimann J (1984) Autoimmune oophoritis. Am J Clin Pathol 81:105–109
109. Gloor E, Juillard E. Curchod A, Legeret J (1982) Ovarian hypoplasia with follicular calcifications. Am J Clin Pathol 78:857–860
110. Golan A, Ron-El R, Herman A, et al (1989) Ovarian hyperstimulation syndrome: an update review. Obstet Gynecol Surv 44:430–440
111. Gronroos M, Klemi P, Piiroinen O, et al (1982) Ovarian function during and after curative intracavitary high dose-rate irradiation: steroidal output and morphology. Eur J Gynecol Reprod Biol 14: 13–21
112. Hahn-Pedersen J, Larsen PM (1984) Supernumerary ovary. Acta Obstet Gynecol Scand 63:365–366
113. Hallatt JG (1982) Primary ovarian pregnancy: a report of twenty-five cases. Am J Obstet Gynecol 143:55–60
114. Hallatt JG, Steele CH Jr, Snyder M (1984) Ruptured corpus luteum with hemoperitoneum: a study of 173 surgical cases. Am J Obstet Gynecol 149:5–9
115. Hamblen EC, Baker RD, Martin DS (1935) Blastomycosis of the female reproductive tract with report of a case. Am J Obstet Gynecol 30:345–356
116. Hangval H, Habibi H, Moshref A, Rahimi A (1979) Case report of an ovarian hydatid cyst. J Trop Med Hyg 82:34–35
117. Haning RV Jr, Strawn EY, Nolten WE (1985) Pathophysiology of the ovarian hyperstimulation syndrome. Obstet Gynecol 66:220–224
118. Harper SL, Tiltman AJ (1991) Non-neoplastic ovarian cysts with ectopic pregnancy. Int J Gynecol Pathol 10:372–379
119. Hatjis CG (1985) Nonimmunologic fetal hydrops associated with hyperreactio luteinalis. Obstet Gynecol 65:11S–13S
120. Heller DS, Harpaz N, Breakstone B (1990) Neoplasms arising in ectopic ovaries: a case of Brenner tumor in an accessory ovary. Int J Gynecol Pathol 9:185–189
121. Hensleigh PA, Woodruff JD (1978) Differential maternal-fetal response to androgenizing luteoma or hyperreactio luteinalis. Obstet Gynecol Surv 33:262–271
122. Herbold DR, Frable WJ, Kraus FT (1984) Isolated noninfectious granuloma of the ovary. Int J Gynecol Pathol 2:380–391
123. Hibbard LT (1985) Adnexal torsion. Am J Obstet Gynecol 152:456–461
124. Hidvegi D, Hidvegi I, Barrett J (1978) Douche-induced pelvic peritoneal starch granuloma. Obstet Gynecol 52:15S–18S
125. Hill JA, Welch WR, Faris HMP, Anderson DJ (1990) Indiction of class II major histocompatibility complex antigen expression in human granulosa cells by interferon gamma: a potential mechanism contributing to autoimmune ovarian failure. Am J Obstet Gynecol 162:534–540
126. Himelstein-Braw R, Peters H, Faber M (1977) Influence of irradiation and chemotherapy on the ovaries of children with abdominal tumours. Br J Cancer 36:269–275
127. Himelstein-Braw R, Peters H, Faber M (1978) Morphological study of the ovaries of leukaemic children. Br J Cancer 38:82–87
128. Hirakawa T, Thor AD, Osawa Y, Mason JI, Scully RE (1992) Stromal hyperthecosis of the ovary: immunohistochemical distribution of steroidogenic enzymes (Abstract). Mod Pathol 5:65a
129. Honoré LH, O'Hara KE (1979) Ovarian hilus cell heterotopia. Obstet Gynecol 53:461–464
130. Honoré LH, O'Hara KE (1980) Subcapsular adipocytic infiltration of the human ovary: a clinicopathological study of eight cases. Eur J Obstet Gynaecol Reprod Biol 10:13–20
131. Hughesdon PE (1972) The origin and development of benign stromatosis of the ovary. Br J Obstet Gynaecol 79:348–359
132. Hughesdon PE (1976) The endometrial identity of benign stromatosis of the ovary and its relation to other forms of endometriosis. J Pathol 119:201–209
133. Hughesdon PE (1982) Morphology and morphogenesis of the Stein-Leventhal ovary and of so-called "hyperthecosis." Obstet Gynecol Surv 37: 59–77
134. Hutson R, Ramsdale J, Wells M (1995) p53 protein expression in putative precursor lesions of epithelial ovarian cancer. Histopathology (Oxf) 27:367–371
135. Iannaccone A, Gabrilove JL, Sohval AR, Soffer LJ (1959) The ovaries in Cushing's syndrome. N Engl J Med 261:775–780
136. Ikeda H, Taguchi O, Takahashi T, et al (1988) L3T4 effector cells in multiple organ localized autoimmune disease in nude mice grafted with embronic rat thymus. J Exp Med 168:2397–2492
137. Isojärvi JIT, Laatikainen TJ, Pakarinen AJ, Juntunen KTS, Myllylä VV (1993) Polycystic ovaries and hyperandrogenism in women taking valproate for epilepsy. N Engl J Med 329:1383–1388
138. Janson PO, Jansson I, Skryten A, et al (1981) Ovarian endocrine function in young women undergoing radiotherapy for carcinoma of the cervix. Gynecol Oncol 11:218–223
139. Judd HL, Scully RE, Atkins L, Neer RM, Kliman B

(1970) Pure gonadal dysgenesis with progressive hirsutism. Demonstration of testosterone production by gonadal streaks. N Engl J Med 282:881–885
140. Judd HL, Scully RE, Herbst AL, et al (1973) Familial hyperthecosis: comparison of endocrinologic and histologic findings with polycystic ovarian disease. Am J Obstet Gynecol 117:976–982
141. Kabawat SE, Bast RC Jr, Bhan AK, et al (1983) Tissue distribution of a coelomic-epithelium-related antigen recognized by the monoclonal antibody OC125. Int J Gynecol Pathol 2:275–285
142. Kahn CR, Flier JS, Bar RS, et al (1976) The syndromes of insulin resistance and acanthosis nigricans: insulin-receptor disorders in man. N Engl J Med 294:739–745
143. Kaminski PF, Sorosky JI, Mandell MJ, et al (1990) Clomiphene citrate stimulation as an adjunct in locating ovarian tissue in ovarian remnant syndrome. Obstet Gynecol 76:924–926
144. Kanbour AI, Salazar H, Tobon H (1979) Massive ovarian edema. A nonneoplastic pelvic mass of young women. Arch Pathol Lab Med 103:42–45
145. Kaufman DW, Shapiro S, Rosenberg L, et al (1980) Intrauterine contraceptive device use and pelvic inflammatory disease. Am J Obstet Gynecol 136: 159–162
146. Kaufman FR, Kogut MD, Donnell GN, et al (1981) Hypergonadotropic hypogonadism in female patients with galactosemia. N Engl J Med 304: 994–998
147. Keebler C, Chatwani A, Schwartz R (1983) Actinomycosis infection associated with intrauterine contraceptive devices. Am J Obstet Gynecol 145:596–599
148. Kemmann E, Orenstein D, Smith C, et al (1980) Estrogenization in women with postmenopausal ovarian hyperthecosis. Int J Obstet Gynecol 18:188–191
149. Kernohan NM, Best PV, Jandial V, Kitchener HC (1991) Palisading granuloma of the ovary. Histopathology (Oxf) 19:279–280
150. Khan JS, Steele RJC, Stewart D (1981) *Enterobius vermicularis* infestation of the female genital tract causing generalized peritonitis. Case report. Br J Obstet Gynaecol 88:681–683
151. Khurana BK, Rao J, Friedman SA, Cho KC (1988) Computed tomographic features of puerperal ovarian vein thrombosis. Am J Obstet Gynecol 159: 905–908
152. Kim MH (1974) "Gonadotropin-resistant ovaries" syndrome in association with secondary amenorrhea. Am J Obstet Gynecol 120:257–263
153. Klempner LB, Giglio PG, Niebles A (1987) Malacoplakia of the ovary. Obstet Gynecol 69:537–540
154. Knochenhauer ES, Key TJ, Kahsar-Miller M, et al (1998) Prevalence of the polycystic ovary syndrome in unselected black and white women in the Southeastern United States: A prospective study. J Clin Endocrinol Metab 83:3078–3082
155. Kohorn EI (1983) Theca lutein ovarian cyst may be pathognomonic for trophoblastic neoplasia. Obstet Gynecol 62:80S–81S
156. Kostelnik FV, Fremount HN (1976) Mycotic tuboovarian abscess associated with the intrauterine device. Am J Obstet Gynecol 125:272–274
157. Kuhajda FP, Haupt HM, Moore GW, Hutchins GM (1982) Gonadal morphology in patients receiving chemotherapy for leukemia. Am J Med 72:759–767
158. Krauss CM, Turksoy N, Atkins L, et al (1987) Familial premature ovarian failure due to an interstitial deletion of the long arm of the X chromosome. N Engl J Med 317:125–131
159. Kuki S, Morgan RL, Tucci JR (1981) Myasthenia gravis and premature ovarian failure. Arch Intern Med 141:1230–1232
160. LaBarbera AR, Miller MM, Ober C, Rebar RW (1988) Autoimmune etiology in premature ovarian failure. Am J Reprod Immunol Microbiol 16:115–122
161. Lachman MF, Berman MM (1991) The ectopic ovary. A case report and review of the literature. Arch Pathol Lab Med 115:233–235
162. Ladefoged C, Lorentzen M (1988) Xanthogranulomatous inflammation of the female genital tract. Histopathology (Oxf) 13:541–551
163. Lai C, Hsueh S, Lin C, et al (1992) Human papillomavirus in benign and malignant ovarian and endometrial tissues. Int J Gynecol Pathol 11:210–215
164. Lafferty HW, Angioli R, Rudolph J, Penalver MA (1996) Ovarian remnant syndrome: Experience at Jackson Memorial Hospital, University of Miami, 1985 through 1993. Am J Obstet Gynecol 174:642–645
165. Landers DV, Sweet RL (1985) Current trends in the diagnosis and treatment of tuboovarian abscess. Am J Obstet Gynecol 151:1098–1110
166. Lee RA, Kazmier FJ (1977) Ovarian hematoma complicating anticoagulant therapy. Mayo Clin Proc 52:19–23
167. Leedman PJ, Bierre AR, Martin FIR (1989) Virilizing nodular ovarian stromal hyperthecosis, diabetes mellitus and insulin resistance in a postmenopausal woman. Case report. Br J Obstet Gynaecol 96:1095–1098
168. Legro RS (1999) Polycystic ovary syndrome. Phenotype to genotype. Endocrinol Metab Clin N Am 28:379–396
169. Liapi C, Evain-Brion D (1987) Diagnosis of ovarian follicular cysts from birth to puberty: a report of twenty cases. Acta Pediatr Scand 76:91–96
170. Lim HT, Meinders AE, de Haan LD, Bronkhorst FB (1984) Anovulation presumably due to the gonadotrophin-resistant ovary syndrome. Eur J Obstet Gynecol Reprod Biol 16:327–337
171. Lindsay AN, Voorhess ML, MacGillivray MH (1983) Multicystic ovaries in primary hypothyroidism. Obstet Gynecol 61:433
172. Lobo RA (1991) Hirsutism in polycystic ovary syndrome: current concepts. Clin Obstet Gynecol 34:817–826
173. Lobo RA, Goebelsmann U (1981) Evidence for reduced 3-beta-ol-hydroxysteroid dehydrogenase ac-

tivity in some hirsute women thought to have polycystic ovary syndrome. J Clin Endocrinol Metab 53:394–400
174. Lonsdale RN, Roberts PF, Trowell JE (1991) Autoimmune oophoritis associated with polycystic ovaries. Histopathology (Oxf) 19:77–81
175. Loughlin T, Cunningham S, Moore A, et al (1986) Adrenal abnormalities in polycystic ovary syndrome. J Clin Endocrinol Metab 62:142–147
176. Lucisano A, Russo N, Acampora MG, et al (1986) Ovarian and peripheral androgen and oestrogen levels in post-menopausal women: correlations with ovarian histology. Maturitas 8:57–65
177. Lunde O, Hoel PS, Sandvik L (1988) Ovarian morphology in patients with polycystic ovaries and in an age-matched reference material. Gynecol Obstet Invest 25:192–201
178. Luzzatto R, Brucker N (1981) Benign inclusion cysts of the ovary associated with psammoma bodies in vaginal smears. Acta Cytol 25:282–284
179. Madeido G, Tieu TM, Aiman J (1985) Atypical ovarian hyperthecosis in a virilized postmenopausal woman. Am J Clin Pathol 83:101–107
180. Mahmood K (1975) Granulomatous oophoritis due to *Schistosoma mansoni*. Am J Obstet Gynecol 123: 919–920
181. Marcello MF, Nuciforo G, Romeo R, et al (1990) Structural and ultrastructural study of the ovary in childhood leukemia after successful treatment. Cancer (Phila) 66:2099–2104
182. Marrogi AJ, Gersell DJ, Kraus FT (1991) Localized asymptomatic giant cell arteritis of the female genital tract. Int J Gynecol Pathol 10:51–58
183. Massachusetts General Hospital Case Records (1982) Case 25–1982. Ovarian stromal hyperthecosis. *Acanthosis nigricans*. N Engl J Med 306:1537–1544
184. Massachusetts General Hospital Case Records (1983) Case 25–1983. Hemochromatosis, involving liver and testes, with hypogonadotropic hypogonadism. N Engl J Med 308:1521–1529
185. Massachusetts General Hospital Case Records (1988) Case 13–1988. Diverticulitis, sigmoid colon, with colo-ovarian fistula formation and left ovarian abscess. N Engl J Med 318:835–842
186. Massachusetts General Hospital Case Records (1987) Case 46–1987. Autoimmune oophoritis with primary ovarian failure. N Engl J Med 317:1270–1278
187. Massachusetts General Hospital Case Records (1986) Case 46–1986. Resistant-ovary syndrome, with hyalinization of preantral follicles. N Engl J Med 315:1336–1344
188. Massachusetts General Hospital Case Records (1988) Case 22–1988. Ovarian stromal hyperthecosis, with virilization, insulin resistance, and acanthosis nigricans. N Engl J Med 318:1449–1457
189. Mathur S, Melchers JT III, Ades EW, et al (1980) Anti-ovarian and anti-lymphocyte antibodies in patients with chronic vaginal candidiasis. J Reprod Immunol 2:247–262
190. Mattison DR, Evans MI, Schwimmer WB, et al (1984) Familial premature ovarian failure. Am J Hum Genet 36:1341–1348
191. McArdle C, Seibel M, Hann LE, et al (1983) The diagnosis of ovarian hyperstimulation (OHS): the impact of ultrasound. Fertil Steril 39:464–467
192. McCluggage WG, Allen DC (1997) Ovarian granulomas: a report of 32 cases. J Clin Pathol 50:324–327
193. McKay DG, Hertig AT, Hickey WF (1953) The histogenesis of granulosa and theca cell tumors of the human ovary. Obstet Gynecol 1:125–136
194. McMahon JN, Connolly CE, Long SV, Meehan FB (1984) Enterobius granulomas of the uterus, ovary and pelvic peritoneum. Two case reports. Br J Obstet Gynaecol 91:289–290
195. McNatty KP, Smith DM, Makris A, et al (1980) The intraovarian sites of androgen and estrogen formation in women with normal and hyperandrogenic ovaries as judged by in vitro experiments. J Clin Endocrinol Metab 50:755–763
196. Meizner I, Levy A, Katz M, et al (1991) Fetal ovarian cysts: prenatal ultrasonographic detection and postnatal evaluation and treatment. Am J Obstet Gynecol 164:874–878
197. Meldrum DR, Frumar AM, Shamonki IM, et al (1980) Ovarian and adrenal steroidogenesis in a virilized patient with gonadotropin-resistant ovaries and hilus cell hyperplasia. Obstet Gynecol 56: 216–221
198. Meneses MF, Ostrowski ML (1989) Female splenic-gonadal fusion of the discontinuous type. Hum Pathol 20:486–488
199. Mercer LJ, Toub DB, Cibils LA (1987) Tumors originating in supernumerary ovaries. A report of two cases. J Reprod Med 32:932–934
200. Mignot MH, Schoemaker J, Kleingeld M, et al (1989) Premature ovarian failure. I: The association with autoimmunity. Eur J Obstet Gynecol Reprod Biol 30:59–66
201. Miles PA, Penney LL (1983) Corpus luteum formation in the fetus. Obstet Gynecol 61:525–529
202. Milewicz A, Silber D, Mielecki T (1983) The origin of androgen synthesis in polycystic ovary syndrome. Obstet Gynecol 62:601–604
203. Miller ME, Chatten J (1967) Ovarian changes in ataxia telangiectasia. Acta Paediatr Scand 56:559–561
204. Miranda P, Jacobs AJ, Roseff L (1996) Pelvic tuberculosis presenting as an asymptomatic pelvic mass with rising serum Ca-125 levels. A case report. J Reprod Med 41:273–275
205. Mittal KR, Zeleniuch-Jacquotte A, Cooper JL, Demopoulos RI (1993) Contralateral ovary in unilateral ovarian carcinoma: A search for preneoplastic lesions. Int J Gynecol Pathol 12:59–63
206. Moller DE, Flier JS (1988) Detection of an alteration in the insulin-receptor gene in a patient with insulin resistance, acanthosis nigricans, and the polycystic ovary syndrome (type A insulin resistance). N Engl J Med 319:1526–1529

207. Moller DE, Flier JS (1991) Insulin resistance—mechanisms, syndromes, and implications. N Engl J Med 325:938–948
208. Montz FJ, Schlaerth JB, Morrow CP (1988) The natural history of theca lutein cysts. Obstet Gynecol 72:247–251
209. Morgenfeld MC, Goldberg V, Parisier H, et al (1972) Ovarian lesions due to cytostatic agents during the treatment of Hodgkin's disease. Surg Gynecol Obstet 134:826–828
210. Morrison JC, Givens JR, Wiser WL, Fish SA (1975) Mumps oophoritis: a cause of premature menopause. Fertil Steril 26:655–659
211. Mostafa SAM, Bargeron CB, Flower RW, et al (1985) Foreign body granulomas in normal ovaries. Obstet Gynecol 66:701–702
212. Muechler EK, Florack AJ, Cary D, Kapakis M (1982) Isosexual precocious puberty with luteinized follicular cyst. NY State J Med 82:1353–1356
213. Muller-Holzner E, Ruth NR, Abfalter E, Schrocksnadel H, Dapunt O, Martin-Sances L, Nogales FF (1995) IUD-associated pelvic actinomycosis: a report of five cases. Int J Gynecol Pathol 14:70–74
214. Munslick RA, Gillanders LA (1981) A review of the syndrome of puerperal ovarian vein thrombophlebitis. Obstet Gynecol Surv 36:57–66
215. Murray JJ, Clark CA, Lands RH, Heim CR, Burnett LS (1985) Reactivation blastomycosis presenting as a tuboovarian abscess. Obstet Gynecol 64:828–830
216. Nagamani M, Gomez LG, Garza J (1982) In vivo steroid studies in luteoma of pregnancy. Obstet Gynecol 59:105S–111S
217. Nagamani M, Hannigan EV, Van Dinh T, Stuart CA (1988) Hyperinsulinemia and stromal luteinization of the ovaries in postmenopausal women with endometrial cancer. J Clin Endocrinol Metab 67:144–148
218. Nagamani H, Kaspar HG, Van Dinh T, et al (1990) Hyperthecosis of the ovaries in a woman with a placental site trophoblastic tumor. Obstet Gynecol 76:931–935
219. Nagamani M, Lingold JC, Gomez JR (1980) Hyperthecosis of the ovaries in acromegaly. Obstet Gynecol 56:258–262
220. Nagamani M, Lingold JC, Gomez JR, Garza JR (1981) Clinical and hormonal studies in hyperthecosis of the ovaries. Fertil Steril 36:326–332
221. Nagamani M, Stuart CA (1990) Specific binding sites for insulin-like growth factor I in the ovarian stroma of women with polycystic ovarian disease and stromal hyperthecosis. Am J Obstet Gynecol 163:1992–1997
222. Nagamani M, Stuart CA, Doherty MG (1992) Increased steroid production by the ovarian stromal tissue of postmenopausal women with endometrial cancer. J Clin Endocrinol Metab 74:172–176
223. Nagamani M, Van Dinh T, Kelver ME (1986) Hyperinsulinemia in hyperthecosis of the ovaries. Am J Obstet Gynecol 154:384–389
224. Nagelberg SB, Rosen SW (1985) Clinical and laboratory investigation of a virilized woman with placental-site trophoblastic tumor. Obstet Gynecol 65: 527–534
225. Nakano R, Shima K, Yamoto M, et al (1989) Binding sites for gonadotropins in human postmenopausal ovaries. Obstet Gynecol 73:196–200
226. Nestler JE, Clore JN, Blackard WG (1989) The central role of obesity (hyperinsulinemia) in the pathogenesis of the polycystic ovary syndrome. Am J Obstet Gynecol 161:1095–1097
227. Nestler JE, Jakubowicz DJ (1996) Decreases in ovarian cytochrome P450c-17-alpha activity and serum free testosterone after reduction of insulin secretion in polycystic ovary syndrome. N Engl J Med 335:617–623
228. Nicosia SV, Matus-Ridley M, Meadows AT (1985) Gonadal effects of cancer therapy in girls. Cancer (Phila) 55:2364–2372
229. Nissim F, Ashkenazy M, Borenstein R, Czernobilsky B (1981) Tuberculoid cornstarch granulomas with caseous necrosis. A diagnostic challenge. Arch Pathol Lab Med 105:86–88
230. Nogales FF, Martin-Sances L, Mendoza-Garcia E, et al (1996) Massive ovarian edema. Histopathology (Oxf) 28:229–234
231. Nogales FF, Silverberg SG (1976) Epidermoid cysts of the ovary: a report of five cases with histogenetic considerations and ultrastructural findings. Am J Obstet Gynecol 124:523–528
232. Nogales-Ortiz F, Taracon I, Nogales FF (1979) The pathology of female genital tract tuberculosis. Obstet Gynecol 53:422–428
233. Norris HJ, Taylor HB (1967) Nodular theca-lutein hyperplasia of pregnancy (so-called "pregnancy luteoma"). A clinical and pathologic study of 15 cases. Am J Clin Pathol 47:557–566
234. Nouwen EJ, Pollet DE, Schelstraete JB, et al (1985) Human placental alkaline phosphatase in benign and malignant ovarian neoplasia. Cancer Res 45:892–902
235. Nouwen EJ, Hendrix PG, Eerdekens MW, De Broe ME (1987) Tumor markers in the human ovary and its neoplasms. A comparative immunohistochemical study. Am J Pathol 126:230–242
236. Nuovo GJ (1989) Virilizing stromal thecosis of the ovary associated with multiple corpora atretica. Am J Clin Pathol 92:505–508
237. Ober WB, Grady HG, Schoenbucher AK (1957) Ectopic ovarian decidua without pregnancy. Am J Pathol 33:199–217
238. Ohsawa M, Wu M, Masahashi T, et al (1985) Cyclic therapy resulted in pregnancy in premature ovarian failure. Obstet Gynecol 66:64S–67S
239. Osathanondh R, Berkowitz RS, de Cholnoky C, et al (1986) Hormonal measurements in patients with theca lutein cysts and gestational trophoblastic disease. J Reprod Med 31:179–183
240. Pace EH, Voet EH, Melancon JT (1984) Xanthogranulomatous oophoritis: an inflammatory pseudotumor of the ovary. Int J Gynecol Pathol 3: 398–402

241. Pache TD, Chadha S, Goorens LJG, et al (1991) Ovarian morphology in long-term androgen-treated female to male transsexuals. A human model for the study of polycystic ovary syndrome? Histopathology (Oxf) 19:445–452
242. Pai SA, Desai SB, Borges AM (1998) Uterus-like masses of the ovary associated with breast cancer and raised serum CA 125. Am J Surg Pathol 22: 333–337
243. Paine CG, Smith P (1957) Starch granulomata. J Clin Pathol 10:51–55
244. Payan HM, Gilbert EF (1987) Mesenteric cyst-ovarian implant syndrome. Arch Pathol Lab Med 111: 282–284
245. Peer E, Peretz BA, Makler A, Paldi E (1981) Bilateral adnexal agenesis with an ectopic ovary: case report and review of the literature. Eur J Obstet Gynecol Reprod Biol 12:37–42
246. Pekonen F, Seigberg R, Makinen T, et al (1986) Immunological disturbances in patients with premature ovarian failure. Clin Endocrinol 25:1–6
247. Pelkey TJ, Frierson HF Jr, Mills SE, Stoler MH (1998) The diagnostic utility of inhibin staining in ovarian neoplasms. Int J Gynecol Pathol 17:97–105
248. Pettit PD, Lee RA (1988) Ovarian remnant syndrome: diagnostic dilemma and surgical challenge. Obstet Gynecol 71:580–583
249. Pine L, Curtis EM, Brown JM (1985) *Actinomyces* and the intrauterine contraceptive device: aspects of the fluorescent antibody stain. Am J Obstet Gynecol 152:287–290
250. Planner RS, Abell DA, Barbaro CA, Beischer NA (1982) Massive enlargement of the ovaries after evacuation of hydatidiform moles. Aust NZ J Obstet Gynaecol 22:96–100
251. Plate WP (1967) Ovarian changes after long-term oral contraception. Acta Endocrinol 55:71–77
252. Polson DW, Wadsworth J, Adams J, Franks S (1988) Polycystic ovaries—a common finding in normal women. Lancet ii:870–872
253. Poretsky L, Smith D, Seibel M, Pazionos A, Moses AC, Flier JS (1984) Specific insulin binding sites in human ovary. J Clin Endocrinol Metab 59:809–811
254. Putschar WGJ, Manion WC (1956) Splenic-gonadal fusion. Am J Pathol 32:15–33
255. Quan A, Charles D, Craig JM (1963) Histologic and functional consequences of periovarian adhesions. Obstet Gynecol 22:96–101
256. Ramzy I, Nisker JA (1979) Histologic study of ovaries from young women with endometrial adenocarcinoma. Am J Clin Pathol 71:253–256
257. Ravinsky E (1984) Ovarian hyperthecosis associated with pseudosarcomatous changes in the endometrial stroma. Am J Surg Pathol 8:939–943
258. Rebar RW (1982) Hypergonadotropic amenorrhea and premature ovarian failure. A review. J Reprod Med 27:179–186
259. Rebar RW, Erickson GF, Yen SSC (1982) Idiopathic premature ovarian failure: clinical and endocrine characteristics. Fertil Steril 37:35–41
260. Resta L, Scordari MD, Colucci GA, et al (1989) Morphological changes of the ovarian surface epithelium in ovarian polycystic disease or endometrial carcinoma and a control group. Eur J Gynaecol Oncol 10:39–41
261. Rice BF, Barclay DL, Sternberg WH (1969) Luteoma of pregnancy. Am J Obstet Gynecol 104: 871–878
262. Riddlesberger MM Jr, Kuhn JP, Munschauer RW (1981) The association of juvenile hypothyroidism and cystic ovaries. Radiology 139:77–80
263. Rodin A, Thakkar H, Taylor N, Clayton R (1994) Hyperandrogenism in polycystic ovary syndrome. Evidence of dysregulation of 11-beta-hydroxysteroid dehydrogenase. N Engl J Med 330:460–465
264. Rosai J (1982) Uterus-like mass replacing ovary [Letter]. Arch Pathol Lab Med 106:364–365
265. Roth LM, Sternberg WH (1973) Ovarian stromal tumors containing Leydig cells. II. Pure Leydig cell tumor, non-hilar type. Cancer (Phila) 32:952–960
266. Roth LM, Sternberg WH (1983) Partly luteinized theca cell tumor of the ovary. Cancer (Phila) 51:1697–1704
267. Roth LM, Deaton RL, Sternberg WH (1979) Massive ovarian edema. A clinicopathologic study of five cases including ultrastructural observations and review of the literature. Am J Surg Pathol 3:11–21
268. Rotmensch S, Scommenga A (1989) Spontaneous ovarian hyperstimulation syndrome associated with hypothyroidism. Am J Obstet Gynecol 160: 1220–1222
269. Russell P, Bannatyne P, Shearman RP, Fraser IS, Corbett P (1982) Premature hypergonadotropic ovarian failure: clinicopathological study of 19 cases. Int J Gynecol Pathol 1:185–201
270. Russell P, Farnsworth A (1997) Massive edema and fibromatosis. In: Russell P, Farnsworth A (authors) Surgical pathology of the ovaries. Churchill Livingstone, New York, pp 147–154
271. Rutgers JL, Scully RE (1988) Cysts (cystadenomas) and tumors of the rete ovarii. Int J Gynecol Pathol 7:330–342
272. Rutgers JL, Scully RE (1986) Functioning ovarian tumors with peripheral steroid cell proliferation: a report of twenty-four cases. Int J Gynecol Pathol 5:319–337
273. Ryan GM, Craig J, Reid DE (1964) Histology of the uterus and ovaries after long-term cyclic norethynodrel therapy. Am J Obstet Gynecol 90:715–725
274. Salomonowitz E (1980) Tumorformige Amyloidose des Ovars. Geburtsh Frauenheilkd 40:644–647
275. Santos-Ramos R, Forney JP, Schwarz BE (1980) Sonographic findings and clinical correlations in molar pregnancy. Obstet Gynecol 56:186–192
276. Sasano H, Fukunaga M, Rojas M, Silverberg SG (1989) Hyperthecosis of the ovary. Clinicopathologic study of 19 cases with immunohistochemical analysis of steroidogenic enzymes. Int J Gynecol Pathol 8:311–320
277. Saxen L, Kassinen A, Saxen E (1963) Peritoneal for-

eign-body reaction caused by condom emulsion. Lancet 1:1295–1296
278. Schildkraut J, Schwingl PJ, Bastos E, Evanoff A, Hughes C (1996) Epithelial ovarian cancer risk among women with polycystic ovary syndrome. Obstet Gynecol 88:554–559
279. Schilsky RL, Sherins RJ, Hubbard SM, et al (1981) Long-term follow-up of ovarian function in women treated with MOPP chemotherapy for Hodgkin's disease. Am J Med 71:552–556
280. Schmidt WA (1982) IUDs, inflammation, and infection: assessment after two decades of IUD use. Hum Pathol 13:878–881
281. Schultz LR, Newton WA Jr, Clatworthy HW Jr (1963) Torsion of previously normal tube and ovary in children. N Engl J Med 268:343–346
282. Scully RE (1964) Stromal luteoma of the ovary. Cancer (Phila) 17:769–778
283. Scully RE (1981) Smooth-muscle differentiation in genital tract disorders [Editorial]. Arch Pathol Lab Med 105:505–507
284. Scully RE, Cohen RB (1964) Oxidative-enzyme activity in normal and pathologic human ovaries. Obstet Gynecol 24:667–681
285. Scully RE (1986) Ovary. In: Henson DE, Albores-Saavedra J (eds) The pathology of incipient neoplasia. Saunders, Philadelphia, pp 279–293
286. Sedin G, Bergquist C, Lindgren PG (1985) Ovarian hyperstimulation syndrome in preterm infants. Pediatr Res 19:548–551
287. Sedmak DD, Hart WR, Tubbs RR (1987) Autoimmune oophoritis: a histopathologic study of involved ovaries with immunologic characterization of the mononuclear cell infiltrate. Int J Gynecol Pathol 6:73–81
288. Shawker TH, Hubbard VS, Reichert CM, Guerreiro de Matos OM (1983) Cystic ovaries in cystic fibrosis: an ultrasound and autopsy study. J Ultrasound Med 2:439–444
289. Shipton EA, Meares SD (1965) Heterotopic bone formation in the ovary. Aust N Z J Obstet Gynaecol 5:100–102
290. Simstein NL (1981) Colo-tubo-ovarian fistula as complication of pelvic inflammatory disease. South J Med 74:512–513
291. Siris ES, Leventhal BG, Vaitukaitis JL (1976) Effects of childhood leukemia and chemotherapy on puberty and reproductive function in girls. N Engl J Med 294:1143–1146
292. Smith S, Ravnikar VA, Barbieri RL (1987) Androgen and insulin response to an oral glucose challenge in hyperandrogenic women. Fertil Steril 48:72–77
293. Smith CET, Toplis PJ, Nogales FF (1999) Ovarian prostatic tissue originating from hilar mesonephric rests. Am J Surg Pathol 23:232–236
294. Snowden JA, Harkin PJR, Thornton JG, Wells M (1989) Morphometric assessment of ovarian stromal proliferation: a clinicopathological study. Histopathology (Oxf) 14:369
295. Starup J, Sele V, Henriksen B (1971) Amenorrhea associated with increased production of gonadotropins and a morphologically normal ovarian follicular apparatus. Acta Endocrinol 66:248–256
296. Steege JF (1987) Ovarian remnant syndrome. Obstet Gynecol 70:64–67
297. Steingold KA Judd HL, Nieberg RK, et al (1986) Treatment of severe androgen excess due to ovarian hyperthecosis with a long-acting gonadotropin-releasing hormone agonist. Am J Obstet Gynecol 154:1241–1248
298. Sternberg WH (1949) The morphology, androgenic function, hyperplasia, and tumours of the human ovarian hilus cells. Am J Pathol 25:493–521
299. Sternberg WH, Barclay DL (1966) Luteoma of pregnancy. Am J Obstet Gynecol 95:165–181
300. Sternberg WH, Dhurandhar HN (1977) Functional ovarian tumors of stromal and sex cord origin. Hum Pathol 8:565–582
301. Sternberg WH, Roth LM (1973) Ovarian stromal tumors containing Leydig cells. I. Stromal-Leydig cell tumor and non-neoplastic transformation of ovarian stroma to Leydig cells. Cancer (Phila) 32: 940–951
302. Sternberg WH, Segaloff A, Gaskill CJ (1953) Influence of chorionic gonadotropin on human ovarian hilus cells (Leydig-like cells). J Clin Endocrinol Metab 13:139–153
303. Stillman RJ, Schinfeld JS, Schiff I, et al (1981) Ovarian failure in long-term survivors of childhood malignancy. Am J Obstet Gynecol 139:62–66
304. Strickler RC, Kelly RW, Askin FB (1984) Postmenopausal ovarian follicle cyst: an unusual cause of estrogen excess. Int J Gynecol Pathol 3:318–322
305. Subietas A, Deppisch LM, Astarloa J (1977) Cytomegalovirus oophoritis: ovarian cortical necrosis. Hum Pathol 8:285–292
306. Sutherland AM (1982) Postmenopausal tuberculosis of the female genital tract. Obstet Gynecol 59:54s–57s
307. Symonds DA, Driscoll SG (1973) An adrenal cortical rest within the fetal ovary: report of a case. Am J Clin Pathol 60:562–564
308. Tanabe K, Gagliano P, Channing CP, et al (1983) Levels of inhibin-F activity and steroids in human follicular fluid from normal women and women with polycystic ovarian disease. J Clin Endocrinol Metab 57:24–31
309. Tatum ET, Beattie JF Jr, Bryson L (1996) Postoperative carbon pigment granuloma. A report of eight cases involving the ovary. Hum Pathol 27: 1008–1011
310. Taylor AE (1998) Polycystic ovary syndrome. Endocrinol Metab Clin N Am 27:877–902
311. Taylor SI, Dons RF, Hernandez E, et al (1982) Insulin resistance associated with androgen excess in women with autoantibodies to the insulin receptor. Ann Intern Med 97:851–855
312. Tressera F, Grases PJ, Labastida R, Ubeda A (1998) Histological features of the contralateral ovary in

patients with unilateral ovarian cancer: a case control study. Gynecol Oncol 71:437–441
313. Tulandi T, Kinch RAH (1981) Premature ovarian failure. Obstet Gynecol Surv 36:521–527
314. Tulandi T, McInnes RA, Arronet GH (1984) Ovarian hyperstimulation syndrome following ovulation induction with human menopausal gonadotropin. Int J Fertil 29:113–117
315. Tursi JP, Reddy UM, Huggins G (1993) Cholelithiasis of the ovary. Obstet Gynecol 82:653–654
316. Utiger RD (1996) Insulin and the polycystic ovary syndrome [Editorial]. N Engl J Med 335:657–658
317. Vasquez SB, Sotos JF, Kim MH (1982) Massive edema of the ovary and virilization. Obstet Gynecol 59:95s–99s
318. Villanueva AL, Rebar RW (1983) Triple-X syndrome and premature ovarian failure. Obstet Gynecol 62:70S–73S
319. Wajda KJ, Lucas JG, Marsh WL Jr (1989) Hyperreactio luteinalis. Benign disorder masquerading as an ovarian neoplasm. Arch Pathol Lab Med 113: 921–925
320. Walfish PG, Gottesman IS, Shewchuk AB, et al (1983) Association of premature ovarian failure with HLA antigens. Tissue Antigens 21:168–169
321. Warne GL, Fairley KF, Hobbs JB, Martin FIR (1973) Cyclophosphamide-induced ovarian failure. N Engl J Med 289:1159–1162
322. Wassman ER, Johnson K, Shapiro LJ, et al (1982) Postmortem findings in the Hurler-Scheie syndrome (mucopolysaccharidosis I-H/S). Birth Defects Orig Artic Ser 18(3B):13–18
323. Waxman JHX, Terry YA, Wrigley PFM, et al (1982) Gonadal function in Hodgkin's disease: long-term follow-up of chemotherapy. Br Med J 285:1612–1613
324. Weinstein D, Rabinowitz R, Malach D, et al (1983) Ovarian hemorrhage in women with Von Willebrand's disease. A report of two cases. J Reprod Med 28:500–502
325. Wetchler SJ, Dunn LJ (1985) Ovarian abscess. Report of a case and a review of the literature. Obstet Gynecol Surv 40:476–485
326. White A, Flaris N, Elmer D, et al (1990) Coexistence of mucinous cystadenoma of the ovary and ovarian sarcoidosis. Am J Obstet Gynecol 162:1284–1285
327. Whitehead E, Shalet SM, Blackledge G, et al (1983) The effect of combination chemotherapy on ovarian function in women treated for Hodgkin's disease. Cancer (Phila) 52:988–993
328. Widdowson DJ, Pilling DW, Cook RCM (1988) Neonatal ovarian cysts: therapeutic dilemma. Arch Dis Child 63:737–742
329. Wierman ME, Beardsworth DE, Mansfield MJ, et al (1985) Puberty without gonadotropins. A unique mechanism of sexual development. N Engl J Med 312:65–72
330. Williams DJ, Connor P, Ironside JW (1990) Premenopausal cytomegalovirus oophoritis. Histopathology (Oxf) 16:405–407
331. Williamson HO, Phansey SA, Mathur RS, et al (1980) Myasthenia gravis, premature menopause, and thyroid autoimmunity. Am J Obstet Gynecol 137:893–901
332. Wilson GE, Haboubi NY, McWilliam LJ, Hirsch PJ (1990) Postoperative necrotizing granulomata in the cervix and ovary [Letter]. J Clin Pathol 43: 1037–1038
333. Witlin AG, Sibai BM (1995) Postpartum ovarian vein thrombosis after vaginal delivery: a report of 11 cases. Obstet Gynecol 85:775–780
334. Wlodarski FM, Trainer TD (1975) Granulomatous oophoritis and salpingitis associated with Crohn's disease of the appendix. Am J Obstet Gynecol 122: 527–528
335. Wojcik EM, Naylor B (1992) "Collagen balls" in peritoneal washings. Acta Cytol 36:466–470
336. Wolfe CDA, Stirling RW (1988) Premature menopause associated with autoimmune oophoritis. Case report. Br J Obstet Gynaecol 95:63
337. Young RH, Prat J, Scully RE (1980) Epidermoid cyst of the ovary. A report of three cases with comments on histogenesis. Am J Clin Pathol 73:272–276
338. Young RH, Scully RE (1984) Fibromatosis and massive edema of the ovary, possibly related entities: a report of 14 cases of fibromatosis and 11 cases of massive edema. Int J Gynecol Pathol 3: 153–178
339. Zaitoon MM, Florentin H (1982) Crossed renal ectopia with unilateral agenesis of fallopian tube and ovary. J Urol 128:111
340. Zhang J, Young RH, Arseneau J, Scully RE (1982) Ovarian stromal tumors containing lutein or Leydig cells (luteinized thecomas and stromal Leydig cell tumors): a clinicopathological analysis of fifty cases. Int J Gynecol Pathol 1:270–285

17

Diseases of the Peritoneum

Philip B. Clement, M.D.

This chapter considers the wide range of nonneoplastic and neoplastic lesions that involve the peritoneum, and in some cases the retroperitoneal lymph nodes, of females. The first half of the chapter covers inflammatory lesions, tumor-like lesions (including mesothelial hyperplasia), mesothelial neoplasms, miscellaneous primary tumors, and metastatic tumors. The final half of the chapter is devoted to a large group of lesions that exhibit müllerian differentiation on microscopic examination and share a potential origin from the secondary müllerian system, the prototypical example of which is endometriosis.

Inflammatory Lesions

Acute Peritonitis

Acute diffuse peritonitis, characterized by a serosal fibrinopurulent exudate, is most commonly associated with a perforated viscus, and is usually bacterial or chemical (bile or gastric or pancreatic juice) in origin. The lipases in pancreatic juice typically produce fat necrosis. Spontaneous bacterial peritonitis occurs most often in children and in adults who are immunocompromised or have cirrhosis of the liver.[327,347] Rare infectious causes of acute peritonitis include *Candida*,[18] *Actinomycetes*, and amoebae.[164] Recurrent attacks of acute peritonitis are an almost constant feature of familial Mediterranean fever (recurrent polyserositis; periodic disease).[316] Localized acute peritonitis may be associated with infection (or infarction) of specific organs, as in pelvic inflammatory disease.

Granulomatous Peritonitis

A variety of infectious and noninfectious agents can cause *granulomatous peritonitis*. The peritoneum may be studded with nodules, which can mimic disseminated tumor at operation. The diagnosis rests on the histologic, and in some cases, microbiologic, identification of the causative agent.

Infectious

Tuberculous peritonitis, which is increasing in incidence, particularly among immunosuppressed patients, may be secondary to spread from a focus within the abdominopelvic cavity or be a manifestation of miliary spread.[17,133] The granulomas are characterized by caseous necrosis and Langhans type giant cells; mycobacteria may be demonstrated by acid-fast stains or immunofluorescence methods. Rarely, granulomatous peritonitis is a complication of fungal infections, including histoplasmosis,[266] coccidioidomycosis,[290] and cryptococcosis,[345] and parasitic infestations, including schistosomiasis,[28] oxyuriasis,[84,312] echinococcosis, ascariasis,[265] and strongyloidiasis.[191]

Noninfectious

Foreign material, typically recognizable on histologic examination, can elicit a granulomatous reaction on the peritoneum. Starch granules from surgical gloves,[74,143,151] douche fluid,[141] and lubricants[291] typically incite a granulomatous and fibrosing peritonitis; in occasional cases the inflammatory reaction may be of tuberculoid type with caseous necrosis.[231] The periodic acid–Schiff- (PAS) positive starch granules exhibit a characteristic Maltese-cross configuration under polarized light. Talc was once an important cause of granulomatous and fibrosing peritonitis because of its use as a lubricant on surgical gloves,[100] and talc-induced peritonitis has been described more recently in drug abusers.[48] Other iatrogenic causes of granulomatous peritonitis include cellulose and cotton fibers from surgical pads and drapes,[125,157,333] microcrystalline collagen hemostat (Avitene),[246] and oily materials such as hysterosalpingographic contrast medium, mineral oil, and paraffin.[202,233] The last three substances are associated with a lipogranulomatous reaction. In one recently described case, a foreign body reaction to Surgicel resulted in a pelvic mass that mimicked recurrent ovarian cancer.[93]

Contamination of the peritoneal cavity by bowel contents, including vegetable matter, food-derived starch,[87] and barium sulfate,[167] can produce a peritoneal foreign body reaction. Sebaceous material and keratin from ruptured dermoid cysts typically evoke an intense granulomatous, lipogranulomatous, and fibrosing peritoneal inflammatory reaction that may mimic a neoplasm at operation. Granulomatous inflammation to keratin derived from uterine and ovarian adenoacanthomas is discussed later in "Tumor-Like Lesions."

Spillage of amniotic fluid at cesarean section, with its content of vernix caseosa (keratin, squames, sebum, lanugo hair) and meconium (bile, pancreatic, and intestinal secretions), produces a granulomatous peritonitis.[121] Meconium peritonitis caused by bowel perforation in utero can also be a problem in newborn infants. In contrast to vernix caseosa peritonitis, calcification rather than granulomatous inflammation dominates the microscopic picture, which in some cases is associated with striking radiographic findings.[331] In boys, the process may involve the tunica vaginalis and result in a tumor-like scrotal mass.[112] Rare cases of meconium peritonitis are associated with disseminated intravascular spread of the meconium.[177] Chronic bile peritonitis may be associated with granulomatous inflammation and fibrosis; cholesterol crystals and bile pigment may be identifiable within giant cells.

Granulomatous peritonitis has also been described secondary to Crohn's disease,[85] sarcoidosis,[337,358] and Whipple's disease.[153] Necrotizing peritoneal granulomas have been recently described following diathermy ablation of endometriosis.[56] Necrotic pseudoxanthomatous nodules of endometriosis, which can resemble necrotic granulomas, are described on page 756.

Nongranulomatous Histiocytic Lesions

The peritoneum can be occasionally involved by *histiocytic infiltrates* rather than discrete granulomas. Ceroid- and lipid-rich histiocytes involving the peritoneum and omentum can be secondary to endometriosis[69] or can occur in association with a peritoneal decidual reaction.[351] Peritoneal lesions consisting of melanin-laden histiocytes have been referred to as peritoneal melanosis. The four reported cases of melanosis have all been associated with ovarian dermoid cysts; in two cases, the cysts had ruptured preoperatively.[288] At laparotomy, focal or diffuse, tan to black, peritoneal staining or similarly pigmented, tumor-like nodules are encountered within the pelvis and in the omentum. Some of the cysts within the ovarian tumors exhibit pigmentation of their contents and lining. On histologic examination, the ovarian and peritoneal pigmentation consists of melanin-laden histiocytes within a fibrous stroma. In at least three of the reported cases and in a fourth case we have encountered, gastric mucosa was prominent within an otherwise typical dermoid cyst. No obvious source for the pigment could be identified in any of the cases. These cases of benign peritoneal melanosis should obviously be distinguished from metastatic malignant melanoma, a distinction that is straightforward because of the bland nuclear features and absence of mitotic figures of the pigmented histiocytes.

Nonpigmented histiocytes can occasionally occur as nodular aggregates on the peritoneum that may appear as small grossly visible nodules at operation. We are aware of one such case from a patient with a granulosa cell tumor in which the histiocytes were initially misinterpreted microscopically as metastatic granulosa cell tumor. A recent report has described a diffuse histiocytic proliferation of the pelvic peritoneum associated with endocervicosis.[283] In these cases, the histiocytes should be distinguished from mesothelial cells, a distinction that can be aided by the different immunoreactivity of the two cell types.

Mucicarminophilic histiocytosis is characterized by histiocytes that contain polyvinylpyrrolidone (PVP), a substance that has been used as a blood substitute.[179] These cells can be found in many sites, both within and outside the female genital tract, including the ovary, the pelvic lymph nodes, and the omentum. The histiocytes have vacuolated basophilic to lavender cytoplasm and an eccentric nucleus, an appearance that may suggest the diagnosis of signet-ring cell adenocarcinoma (Fig. 17.1). The histiocytes are mucicarminophilic, but in contrast to neoplastic signet-ring cells, are PAS negative; a variety of other stains are also helpful in the differential diagnosis.[179]

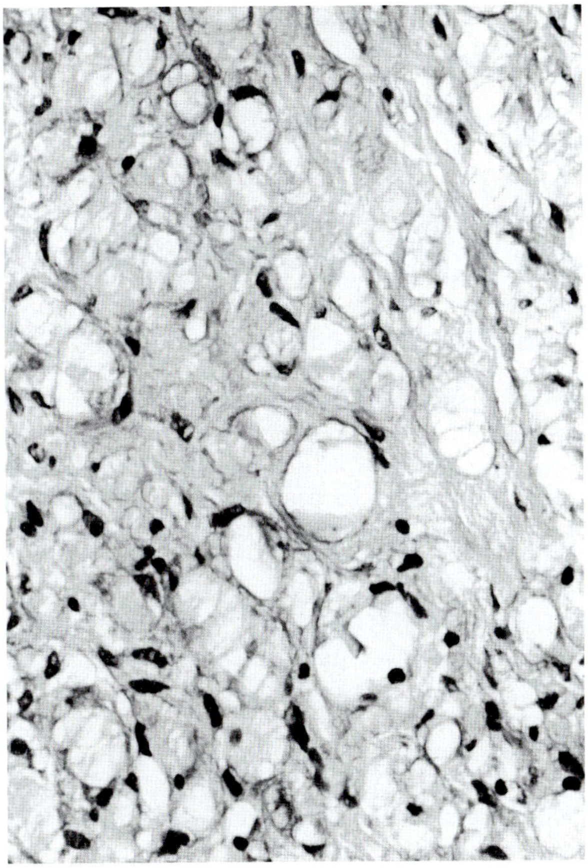

Fig. 17.1. Mucicarminophilic histiocytosis involving the ovary. Note multiple vacuolated histiocytes, some with a signet-ring-cell appearance.

Peritoneal collections of mucicarmine-positive histiocytes have also been described associated with topical administration of oxidized regenerated cellulose, a hemostatic agent.[172] The cytoplasm of these cells is PAS positive, diastase resistant, CD 68 positive, and S-100 and cytokeratin negative.

Peritoneal Fibrosis

Reactive *peritoneal fibrosis*, often accompanied by fibrous adhesions, is a common sequela of prior peritoneal inflammation and a frequent complication of a surgical procedure.[346] Some reactive peritoneal fibrous lesions may contain spindle cells that are immunoreactive for vimentin, smooth muscle actin, and cytokeratin, cells referred to as multipotential subserosal cells by Bolen et al.[30] Rarely, reactive fibrous proliferations of the peritoneum can form tumor-like nodules, in contrast to the more widespread peritoneal thickening of sclerosing peritonitis. In one case we have recently seen, three of these nodules, which we refer to as peritoneal fibrous nodules,[59] were found in the cul-de-sac in a woman with an ovarian mucinous cystadenocarcinoma. Similar nodules involved the serosal aspect of the tumor. The nodules were composed of moderately cellular fascicles of benign-appearing spindle cells resembling fibroblasts and myofibroblasts that contained occasional mitotic figures. Some of the spindle cells had the immunoprofile of the multipotential subserosal cells noted earlier.

Localized hyaline plaques are a common incidental finding on the splenic capsule and are probably related to splenic congestion.[344] Nonspecific fibrous thickening of the peritoneum has been described as a histologic finding in patients with hepatic cirrhosis and ascites.[38] The designation sclerosing peritonitis has been applied to a clinically significant, potentially fatal lesion that represents a reactive hyperplasia of the submesothelial mesenchymal cells to a variety of stimuli. The first description, by Concato, was that of pearly white thickening of the visceral peritoneum, either as discrete plaques or continuous sheets involving the hepatic, splenic, and diaphragmatic peritoneum. The process often encases the small bowel ("abdominal cocoon"), causing bowel obstruction. Sclerosing peritonitis occurs in an idiopathic form, which most frequently, but not invariably, affects adolescent girls in tropical countries.[94,111] Known causes include practolol therapy,[201] chronic ambulatory peritoneal dialysis,[32] the use of a peritoneovenous (LeVeen) shunt,[42] bacterial or mycobacterial infection, sarcoidosis,[232] the carcinoid syndrome, familial Mediterranean fever, and fibrogenic foreign materials as seen in drug users. Additionally, we have encountered six cases of sclerosing peritonitis associated with luteinized thecomas of the ovary (Fig. 17.2).[67]. Sclerosing peritonitis should be distinguished from the rarer "peritoneal encapsulation," a congenital malformation in which an accessory peritoneal membrane encases loops of small bowel in a saclike structure.[292,310] The latter condition is largely asymptomatic and is usually found incidentally at laparotomy or autopsy. Confusion arises when the two terms are used interchangeably or even together, as in "encapsulating peritonitis."

In occasional cases, it may be difficult to differentiate between markedly reactive peritoneal fibrosis and a desmoplastic mesothelioma lacking frankly sarcomatoid areas, particularly in a small biopsy specimen.[208] These tumors, however, are very rare in the peritoneal cavity, especially in women. Features favoring a diagnosis of mesothelioma include nuclear atypia, necrosis, organized patterns of collagen deposition (fascicular, storiform), and infiltration of adjacent tissues.[199,208]

Rare Types of Peritonitis

Eosinophilic peritonitis is seen rarely in cases of eosinophilic gastroenteritis and the hypereosinophilic syndrome.[3] Isolated cases of eosinophilic ascites have been associated with childhood atopy, peritoneal dialysis, vasculitis, lymphoma or metastatic carcinoma, and ruptured hydatid cysts.[3] Rare cases of peritonitis may be secondary to peritoneal involvement by collagen vascular diseases, includ-

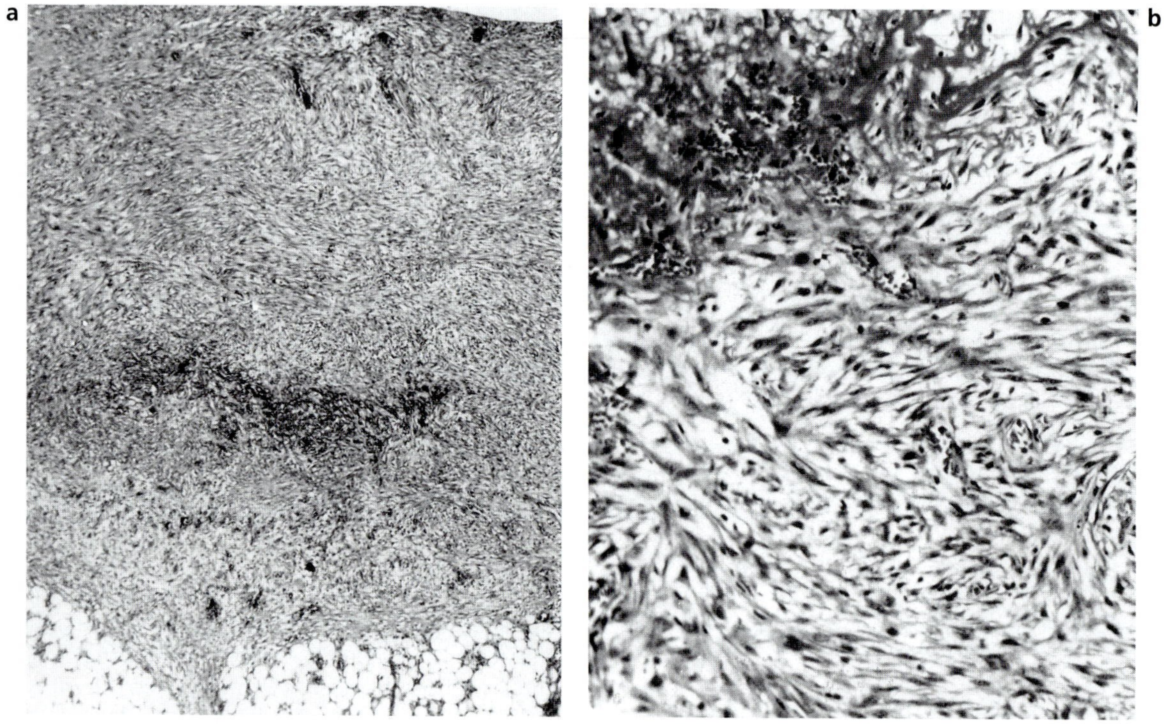

Fig. 17.2. Sclerosing peritonitis associated with bilateral luteinized thecomas of the ovary. **a**: Low-power view of omentum showing involvement of its surface by a layer of cellular fibrous tissue. **b**: Higher-power view showing fibrin (*top*), plump fibroblasts, and a sprinkling of chronic inflammatory cells.

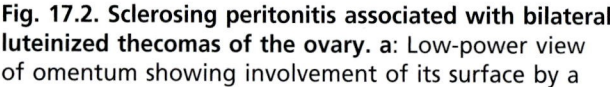

ing systemic lupus erythematosus[215] and Degos' disease.[196]

Tumor-Like Lesions

Mesothelial Hyperplasia

Hyperplasia of mesothelial cells is a common response to inflammation and chronic effusions (Figs. 17.3–17.5). Hyperplastic lesions may be noted at operation as solitary or multiple small nodules, but more commonly are incidental findings on microscopic examination.[91,114,137, 208,210] *Mesothelial hyperplasia* often involves the adnexal areas in cases of chronic salpingitis and endometriosis[171] and is occasionally encountered, particularly in the omentum, in association with ovarian tumors.[64] Mesothelial hyperplasia can also occur within the superficial ovarian stroma overlying a borderline epithelial tumor and in such cases can be misinterpreted as invasive tumor (Fig. 17.5).[64] Mesothelial hyperplasia may be confined to a hernia sac, and in such cases may be caused by trauma or incarceration.[278]

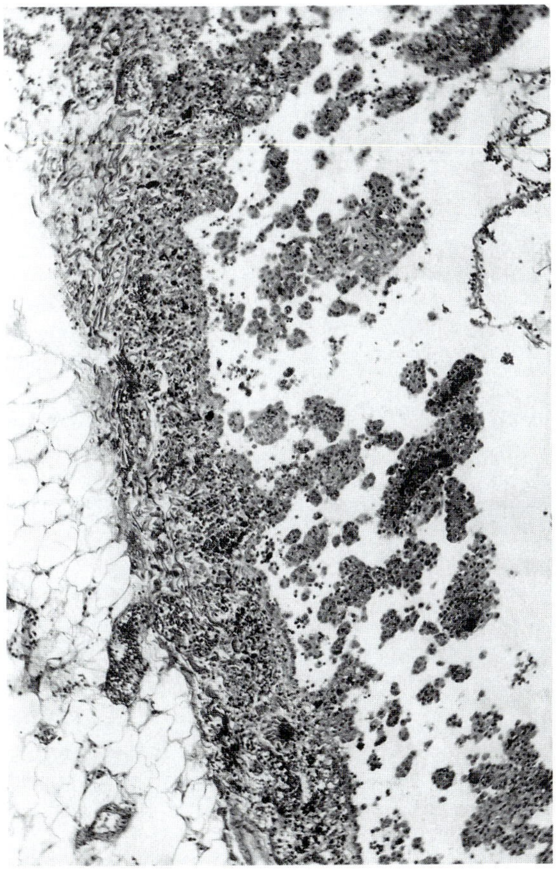

Fig. 17.3. Papillary mesothelial hyperplasia. (Reprinted by permission of Daya and McCaughey, ref. 90.)

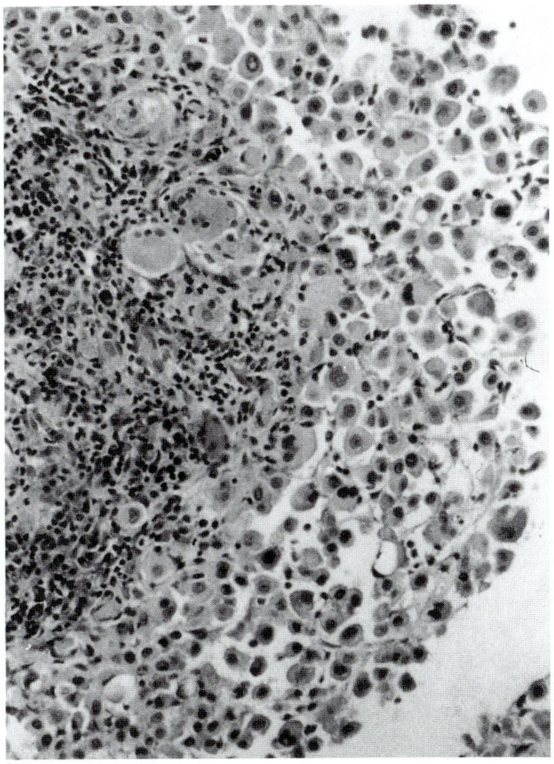

Fig. 17.4. Mesothelial hyperplasia with moderate nuclear atypia. (Reprinted by permission of Daya and McCaughey, ref. 90.)

Hyperplastic mesothelial cells occasionally are an incidental microscopic finding within pelvic and intraabdominal lymph nodes, and in such cases are usually associated with mesothelial hyperplasia of the peritoneum (Fig. 17.6).[68] The mesothelial cells may be misinterpreted as metastatic tumor, particularly in a woman with a known primary pelvic tumor. The appearance of the cells on routine stains suggests the correct diagnosis, and can be confirmed by histochemical and immunohistochemical staining (see following).

In florid examples, solid, trabecular, tubular, papillary, or tubulopapillary patterns (Figs. 17.3–17.5) and limited degrees of extension of the mesothelial cells into the underlying tissues may be seen. The cells are often focally disposed in linear, sometimes parallel, thin layers, separated by fibrin or fibrous tissue (Fig. 17.5). The mesothelial cells may have cytoplasmic vacuoles containing acid mucin (predominantly hyaluronic acid) or, less commonly, exhibit marked cytoplasmic clearing.[208] Mild to moderate nuclear pleomorphism (Fig. 17.4), mitotic figures, and occasional multinucleated cells may be seen. Psammoma bodies are encountered in occasional cases, and rarely, eosinophilic strap-shaped cells resembling rhabdomyoblasts have been described.[278]

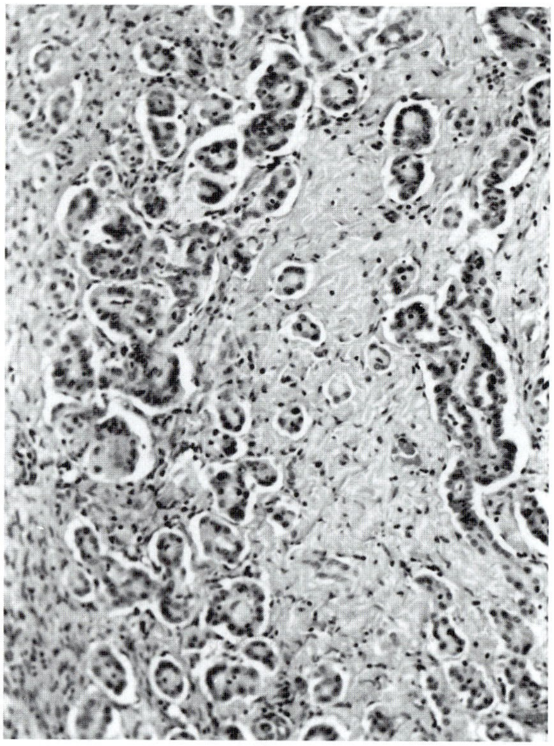

Fig. 17.5. Florid mesothelial hyperplasia in wall of borderline mucinous tumor of the ovary. The mesothelial proliferation was initially misdiagnosed as stromal invasion (Reprinted by permission of Clement and Young, ref. 64.)

The major differential diagnosis is with diffuse malignant mesothelioma (DMM). McCaughey and coworkers[91,208] have noted that the presence of grossly visible nodules, necrosis, conspicuous large cytoplasmic vacuoles, marked nuclear pleomorphism, and deep infiltration favor DMM over mesothelial hyperplasia. Some of these features, however, such as marked nuclear atypia, are not always present or may be present only focally within a DMM. Special techniques may facilitate the differential diagnosis. Immunoreactivity for p53[160] and intense cytoplasmic immunoreactivity for epithelial membrane antigen[140] are characteristic of the cells of DMM but not hyperplastic mesothelial cells. Morphometry has shown that reactive mesothelial cells generally have smaller nuclei that the cells of a DMM, and there are more nucleolar organizer regions in malignant mesothelial cells than in reactive ones.[11,140] Despite these differential features, in occasional cases the distinction between a hyperplastic and malignant mesothelial lesion may be difficult or impossible, particularly in a biopsy specimen. If the lesion in question is a DMM, follow-up usually reveals its nature within several months because of its typically rapid growth. In contrast, an atypical mesothelial proliferation occasionally persists for years without an apparent cause. An apparently benign, otherwise typical mesothelial proliferation, however, occasionally precedes the appearance of a DMM.[208,271] Some cases of "atypical mesothelial hyperplasia" evolving into DMM, however, likely represent DMM ab initio.[300]

The differential diagnosis of mesothelial hyperplasia also includes borderline serous tumors of primary peritoneal or ovarian origin. Grossly visible ovarian or peritoneal tumor, columnar cells with or without cilia, the presence of intracellular or extracellular neutral mucin, and numerous psammoma bodies all favor a serous tumor. Immunohistochemical markers for epithelial differentiation (see section on DMM) may also be of value in the differential diagnosis.

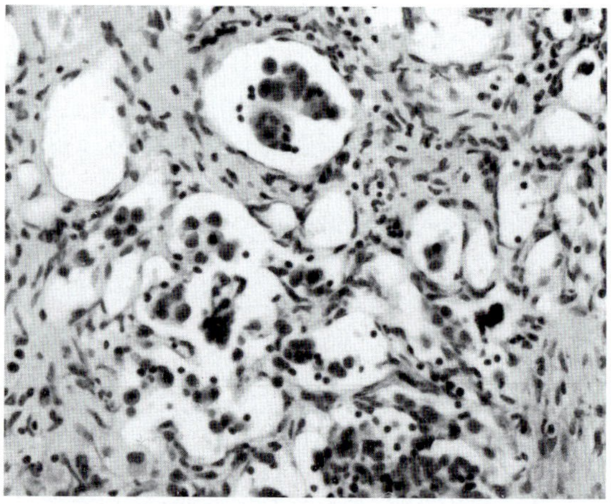

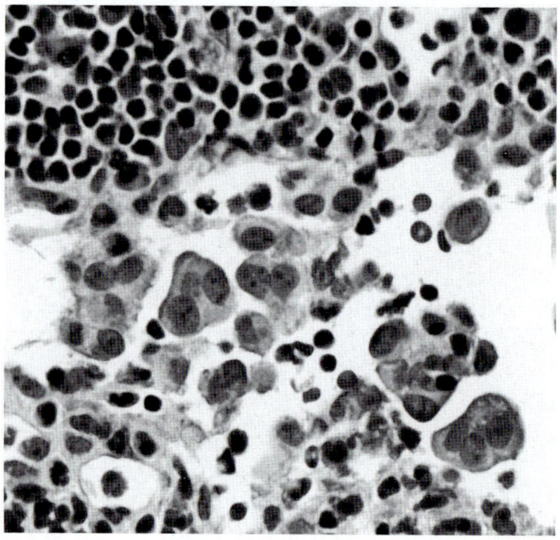

Fig. 17.6. Hyperplastic mesothelial cells within a pelvic lymph node. *Top*: Low magnification. *Bottom*: High-power magnification. Papillary clusters of mesothelial cells lie within capsular and subcapsular sinusoids.

Peritoneal Inclusion Cysts

Peritoneal inclusion cysts typically occur in the peritoneal cavity of women in the reproductive age group.[45,213,279,349] Rarely, they occur in males and in the pleural cavity.[219] Some are incidental findings at laparotomy in the form of single or multiple, small, thin-walled, translucent, unilocular cysts that may be attached or lie free in the peritoneal cavity. Occasionally, they may involve the round ligament simulating an inguinal hernia.[138] The cysts have a smooth lining, and contents that vary from yellow and watery to gelatinous. Microscopically, they are characterized by a single layer of flattened, benign-appearing mesothelial cells. Although most of these unilocular mesothelial cysts are probably reactive in origin, some of those located in the mesocolon, mesentery of the small intestine, retroperitoneum, and splenic capsule may be developmental.[279]

Multilocular peritoneal inclusion cysts (MPICs) may form large bulky masses (Fig. 17.7); these lesions have also been referred to as benign cystic mesotheliomas, inflammatory cysts of the peritoneum, or postoperative peritoneal cysts. MPICs are usually associated with clinical manifestations, most commonly lower abdominal pain, a palpable mass, or both. They are usually adherent to pelvic organs and may simulate a cystic ovarian tumor on clinical examination, at laparotomy,[213] or even on pathologic examination; the upper abdominal cavity, the retroperitoneum, or hernia sacs may also be involved.[279] Unlike the smaller unilocular cysts, the septa and walls of MPICs may contain considerable amounts of fibrous tissue. Their contents may resemble those of the unilocular cysts or be serosanguineous or bloody.

On microscopic examination, MPICs are typically lined by a single layer of flat to cuboidal, occasionally hobnail-shaped, mesothelial cells with generally bland nuclear features (Fig. 17.8), although a degree of reactive atypia is not infrequent. The lining cells occasionally form small papillae and cribriform patterns or undergo squamous metaplasia. In some cases, mural proliferations of typical or atypical mesothelial cells arranged singly, as gland-like structures or nests (Fig. 17.9),[213] or in patterns resembling those in adenomatoid tumors may be encountered. Occasional vacuolated mesothelial cells in the stroma may simulate signet-ring cells.[279] The septa typically consist of a loose, fibrovascular connective tissue with a sparse inflammatory infiltrate. In some cases, marked acute and chronic inflammation, abundant fibrin, broad bands of granulation and fibrous tissue, and evidence of recent and remote hemorrhage are present in the cyst walls.

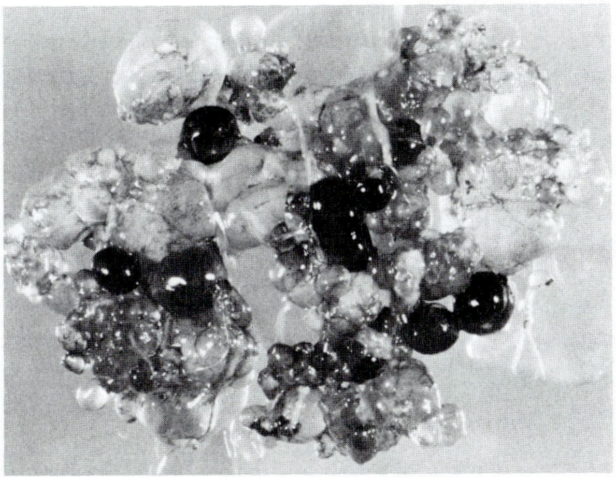

Fig. 17.7. Peritoneal inclusion cyst. Multilocular cystic masses consist of thin-walled cysts with a smooth lining. (Reprinted by permission of the Cleveland Clinic Foundation from Miles JM, Hart WR, McMahon JT (1986) Cystic mesothelioma of the peritoneum. Cleve Clin Q 53:109–114.)

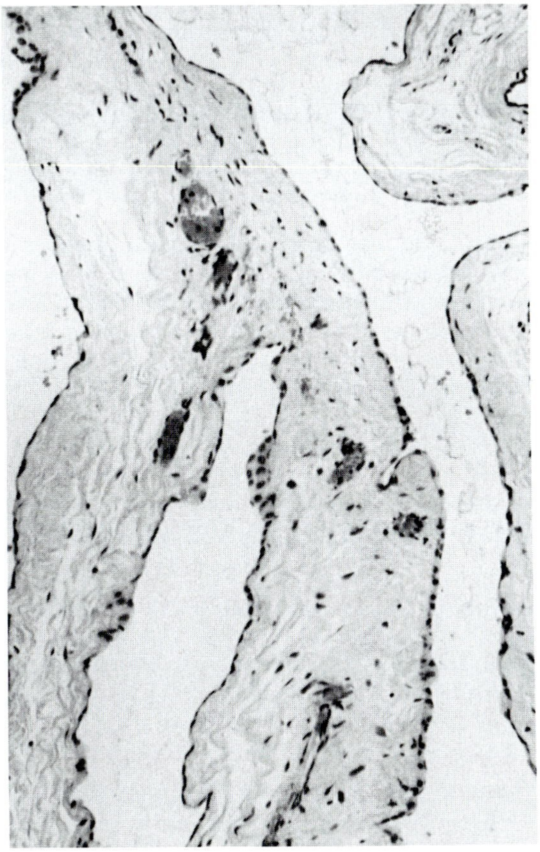

Fig. 17.8. Peritoneal inclusion cyst. Cystic spaces are lined by a single layer of flat mesothelial cells and are separated by thin fibrous septa.

a

b

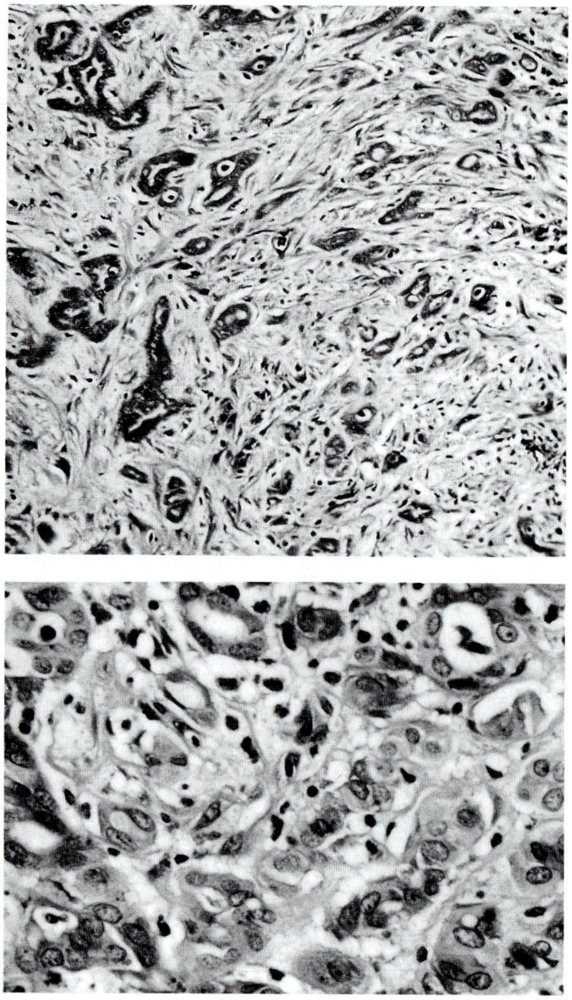

Fig. 17.9. Multiocular peritoneal inclusion cyst with mural mesothelial proliferation. **a**: Glandlike arrangements within a reactive fibrous stroma create an infiltrative pattern. **b**: Higher-power view showing benign-appearing mesothelial cells forming small nests, cords, and lining small tubules.

A history of a prior abdominal operation, pelvic inflammatory disease, endometriosis, or combinations thereof was present in 84% of patients in one series,[279] suggesting a role for inflammation in the pathogenesis of the cysts. An inflammatory pathogenesis is also supported by the occurrence of cases in which the dividing line between florid adhesions associated with inflammation and a MPIC may be difficult. With one exception, there has been no association with asbestos exposure. Follow-up examinations have not disclosed malignant behavior in cases that we consider MPICs, but in as many as one-half of these, the lesions have recurred from months to many years postoperatively.[279] It is likely, however, that at least some of these "recurrences" are the result of newly formed postoperative adhesions. For these reasons—although accepting that low-grade cystic mesotheliomas occur rarely (see page 738)—we prefer the designation multilocular peritoneal inclusion cyst to benign cystic mesothelioma for such lesions, until there is convincing evidence for their neoplastic nature.

Aside from the contentious problem of their distinction from "true" cystic mesotheliomas (see page 738), MPICs are confused most often with multilocular cystic lymphangiomas.[45] In contrast to MPICs, the latter typically occur in children, more frequently in boys. In addition, they are usually extrapelvic, being almost always localized to the mesentery of the small intestine, omentum, mesocolon, or retroperitoneum. Their contents may be chylous, and on histologic examination lymphoid aggregates and smooth muscle, which are rare findings in MPICs, are typically present within their walls. In problematic cases, immunohistochemical stains are useful in distinguishing endothelial from mesothelial cells. Another lesion that merits consideration in the differential diagnosis of MPICs is the rare multicystic adenomatoid tumor. In contrast to MPICs, the latter typically involve the myometrium, contain foci of typical adenomatoid tumor, and lack prominent numbers of inflammatory cells. A detailed discussion of other lesions in the differential diagnosis of MPICs has been presented elsewhere.[279]

Calcifying Fibrous Pseudotumor

The rare, presumably reactive lesion known as *calcifying fibrous pseudotumor* is typically an incidental finding involving the visceral peritoneum of the small bowel and stomach in adults.[176] The process, which can be misinterpreted intraoperatively as metastatic carcinoma, forms a well-circumscribed solid mass up to 2.0 cm in diameter that may have a gritty sectioned surface. Microscopic examination reveals dense hyalinized collagen often in concentric whorls, sparse benign-appearing fibroblasts, lymphocytes, and plasma cells (that may form perivascular aggregates), and numerous psammoma bodies.

Splenosis

Splenosis, which results from implantation of splenic tissue, is typically an incidental finding at laparotomy or autopsy months to years after splenectomy for traumatic splenic rupture.[46] A few to innumerable, red-blue, peritoneal nodules, ranging from punctate to 7 cm in diameter, are scattered widely thoughout the abdominal and, less commonly, the pelvic cavity. The intraoperative appearance may mimic endometriosis, benign or malignant vascular tumors, or metastatic cancer.

Trophoblastic Implants

Implants of trophoblast on the pelvic or omental peritoneum may complicate the operative treatment of tubal pregnancy.[47,270,329] The implants are more likely to occur in cases managed by laparoscopy (1.9% of cases) than those managed by laparotomy (0.6% of cases) and are more likely to occur after salpingotomy than salpingectomy. The clinical presentation in such cases includes an initial decline in the serum human chorionic gonadotropin (hCG) level after removal of the ectopic pregnancy, followed by a rising level, abdominal pain, and in some cases intraabdominal hemorrhage. Microscopic examination of the implants reveals viable trophoblastic tissue that may include chorionic villi.

Peritoneal Keratin Granulomas

Peritoneal granulomas that form in response to implants of keratin derived from neoplasms of the female reproductive tract may be confused with metastatic tumor.[53,174] The tumors are most commonly endometrioid carcinomas with squamous differentiation originating in the endometrium or ovary, or, rarely, squamous cell carcinomas of the cervix or atypical polypoid adenomyomas of the uterus. The granulomas consist of laminated deposits of keratin, sometimes with ghost squamous cells, surrounded by foreign body giant cells and fibrous tissue (see Fig. 16.10). Follow-up data on these patients suggest that the granulomas have no prognostic significance, although they should be thoroughly sampled by the gynecologist and carefully examined microscopically to exclude the presence of viable tumor. The differential diagnosis includes peritoneal granulomas in reponse to keratin derived from other sources, as discussed earlier in this chapter.

Infarcted Appendix Epiploica

Appendices epipolicae may undergo torsion and infarction.[104,343] Subsequent calcification can result in a hard tumor-like mass that may be found attached or loose in the peritoneal cavity. In the late stages, these structures are typically composed of layers of hyalinized connective tissue surrounding a central necrotic and calcified zone in which infarcted adipose tissue in usually recognizable.

Mesothelial Neoplasms

Solitary Fibrous Tumor

Although once referred to as fibrous mesotheliomas, these tumors are now designated *solitary fibrous tumors* and are believed to originate from submesothelial fibroblasts.[36] The clinical and pathologic features are similar to their much more common pleural counterparts, including immunoreactivity for CD 34 and lack of immunoreactivity for cytokeratin, an immunoprofile that is useful in distinguishing these tumors from desmoplastic mesotheliomas. Typical tumors are clinically benign. One peritoneal solitary fibrous tumor that was focally sarcomatous was clinically malignant.[116]

Adenomatoid Tumor

This benign tumor of mesothelial origin, *adenomatoid tumor*, rarely arises from extragenital peritoneum, such as the omentum or mesentery, but is much more commonly encountered within the fallopian tube and myometrium (see Chapter 13, Mesenchymal Tumors of the Uterus, and Chapter 14, Diseases of the Fallopian Tube), and, in the male, the epididymis.

Well-Differentiated Papillary Mesothelioma

Well-differentiated papillary mesotheliomas (*WDPMs*) of the peritoneum are uncommon lesions.[90,126] Eighty percent of the cases have occurred in women, who are usually of reproductive age; occasional patients are postmenopausal. WDPMs are usually an incidental finding at operation, but rare cases have been associated with abdominal pain or ascites. Occasional patients, including two who were sisters, have had possible exposure to asbestos.[90]

At laparotomy and on gross examination, WDPMs may be solitary but are usually multiple, and appear as gray to white, firm, papillary or nodular lesions measuring less than 2 cm in diameter. The omental and pelvic peritoneum are typically involved; several examples have also been encountered on the gastric, intestinal, or mesenteric peritoneum. Microscopic examination reveals fibrous papillae covered by a single layer of flattened to cuboidal mesothelial cells (Fig. 17.10) with occasional basal vacuoles; the nuclear features are bland, and mitotic figures are rare or absent. Uncommon patterns include tubulopapillary, adenomatoid-like, branching cords, or solid sheets.[128] The stroma of some tumors may be extensively fibrotic. Multinucleated stromal

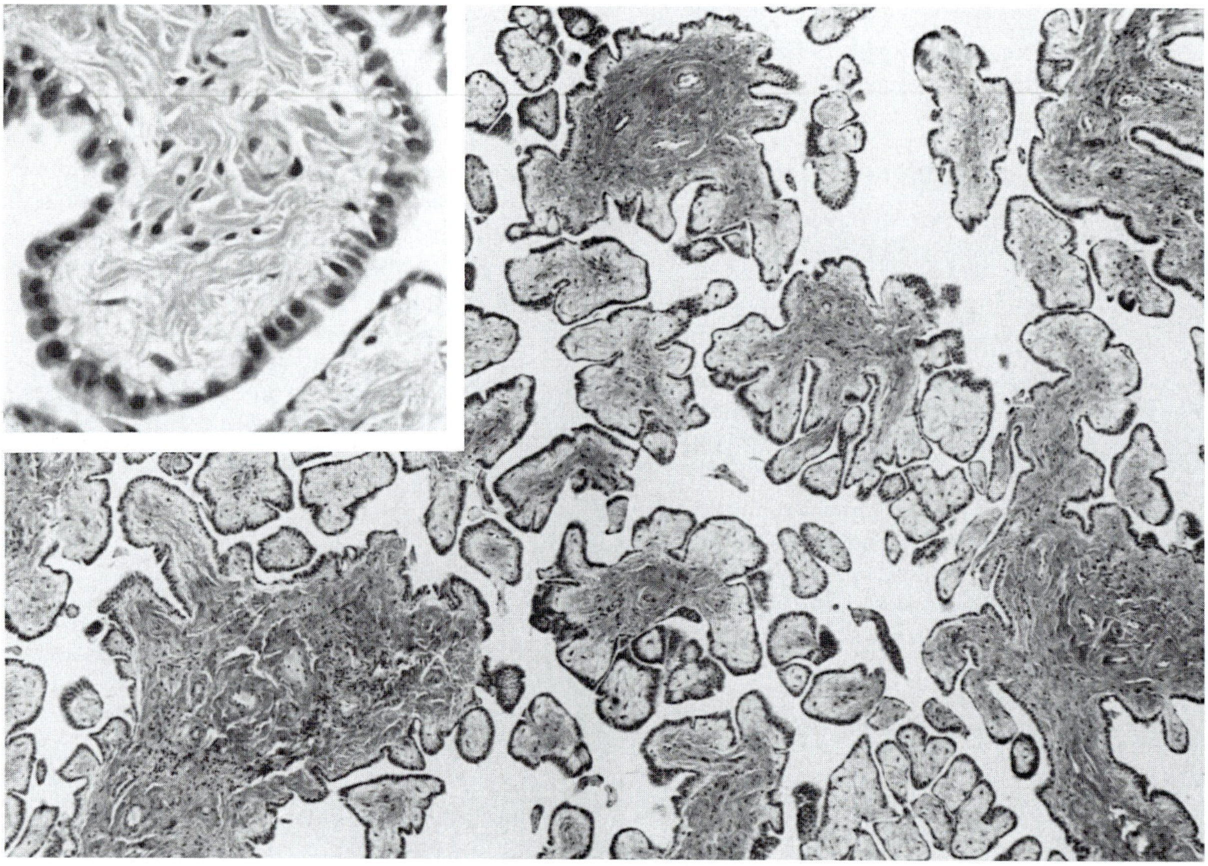

Fig. 17.10. Well-differentiated papillary mesothelioma. Fibrous papillae are lined by a single layer of uniform, flat to cuboidal, mesothelial cells (*inset*).

giant cells and psammoma bodies are encountered in occasional cases. When multiple lesions are present, they should each be sampled histologically as lesions with the appearance of a WDPM may rarely be associated with others that have the appearance of malignant mesothelioma and progressive disease.[126] The diagnosis of WDPM should be strictly reserved for tumors with bland nuclear features and no evidence of invasion.

With the exception of one case which appeared to evolve into a diffuse malignant mesothelioma, follow-up studies suggest that most WDPMs are benign. Occasional examples, however, have persisted for as many as 29 years.[90] Several patients with WDPM have died, although the adjuvant therapy used in such cases possibly was a contributory factor.[90]

Low-Grade Cystic Mesothelioma

Although we believe that most multilocular cystic mesothelial lesions are MPICs, we have seen very rare cases of what appear to be bona fide *multicystic mesotheliomas*. In contrast to MPICs, the cysts are lined, at least focally, by markedly atypical mesothelial cells (Fig. 17.11), and the tumors may contain areas of conventional malignant mesothelioma on histologic examination.[96]

Diffuse Malignant Mesothelioma

Clinical Features

Diffuse malignant mesotheliomas (DMMs) of the peritoneal cavity are much less common than similar tumors in the pleural cavity, and account for only 10%–20% of all mesotheliomas.[6,126,339] These tumors are particularly rare in women, in whom most malignant papillary neoplasms of the peritoneum are extraovarian papillary serous carcinomas (see "Lesions of the Secondary Müllerian System").

About two-thirds of the patients with DMM are male, usually middle aged or elderly; occasional peritoneal DMMs occur in young adults[162] or children. The patients typically present with nonspecific manifestations, including abdominal discomfort and distension, digestive disturbances, and weight

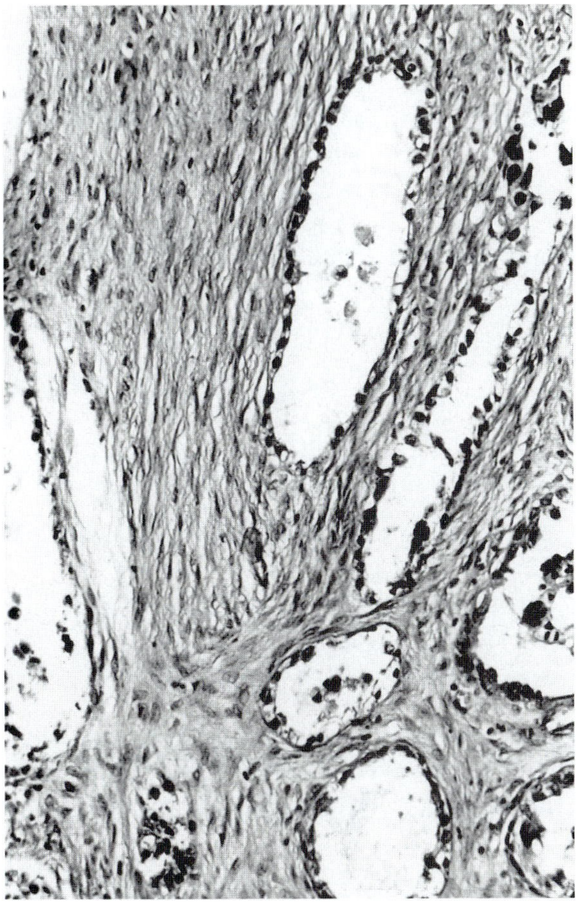

Fig. 17.11. Low-grade cystic mesothelioma. Small cysts are lined by mesothelial cells with hyperchromatic, pleomorphic nuclei. (Reprinted by permission of Thor et al., (1991) Pathology of the fallopian tube, broad ligament, peritoneum, and pelvic soft tissues. Hum Pathol 22:856–867.)

loss. Ascites is present in the majority of cases, and cytologic examination of the ascitic fluid may be diagnostic of DMM in some cases.[6] The diagnosis, however, usually requires laparotomy or laparoscopy and biopsy. Peritoneal DMMs may rarely present within a hernia or hydrocele sac,[6] as a retroperitoneal, umbilical, intestinal, or pelvic tumor, or as cervical or inguinal lymphadenopathy.[326] Rarely there is prominent ovarian involvement, the intraoperative appearance mimicking that of a primary ovarian tumor with peritoneal spread.[72]

More than 80% of the patients in one large series had a history of asbestos exposure, but most of them were identified because of an occupational exposure to asbestos. In contrast, two recent series of peritoneal DMMs in women found no association with a history of asbestos exposure.[126,339] Asbestos fibers, however, have been identified with special techniques in some of these women.[139] Aside from

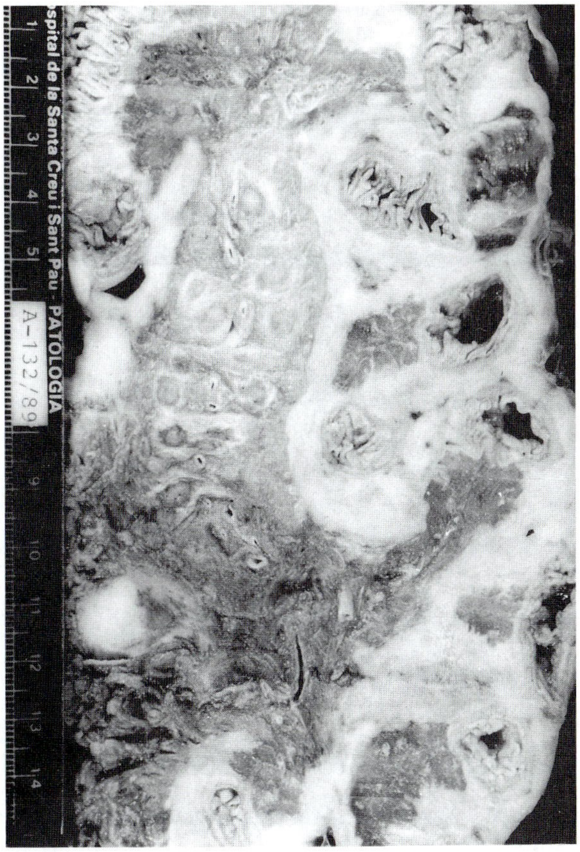

Fig. 17.12. Diffuse malignant mesothelioma encasing loops of bowel. (Courtesy of J. Prat, M.D., Barcelona, Spain.)

asbestos, radiation, chronic inflammation, organic chemicals, and nonasbestos mineral fibers may be etiologic agents in some cases.[80]

Most males with peritoneal DMMs reported in the literature survived less than 2 years after diagnosis, although there have been occasional long-term survivors. A recent study of peritoneal DMMs in women,[335] however, found that 40% of the patients survived longer than four years.

Pathologic Findings

At laparotomy, the visceral and parietal peritoneum are diffusely thickened or extensively involved by nodules and plaques. The viscera are often encased by tumor (Fig. 17.12) and may be invaded, although local invasion and metastases to lymph nodes, liver, lungs, and pleura are less frequent than in association with carcinomas with comparable degrees of peritoneal involvement. Significant degrees of invasion or metastatic involvement of abdominal viscera, however, may be encountered at autopsy, such as transmural invasion of bowel wall or massive re-

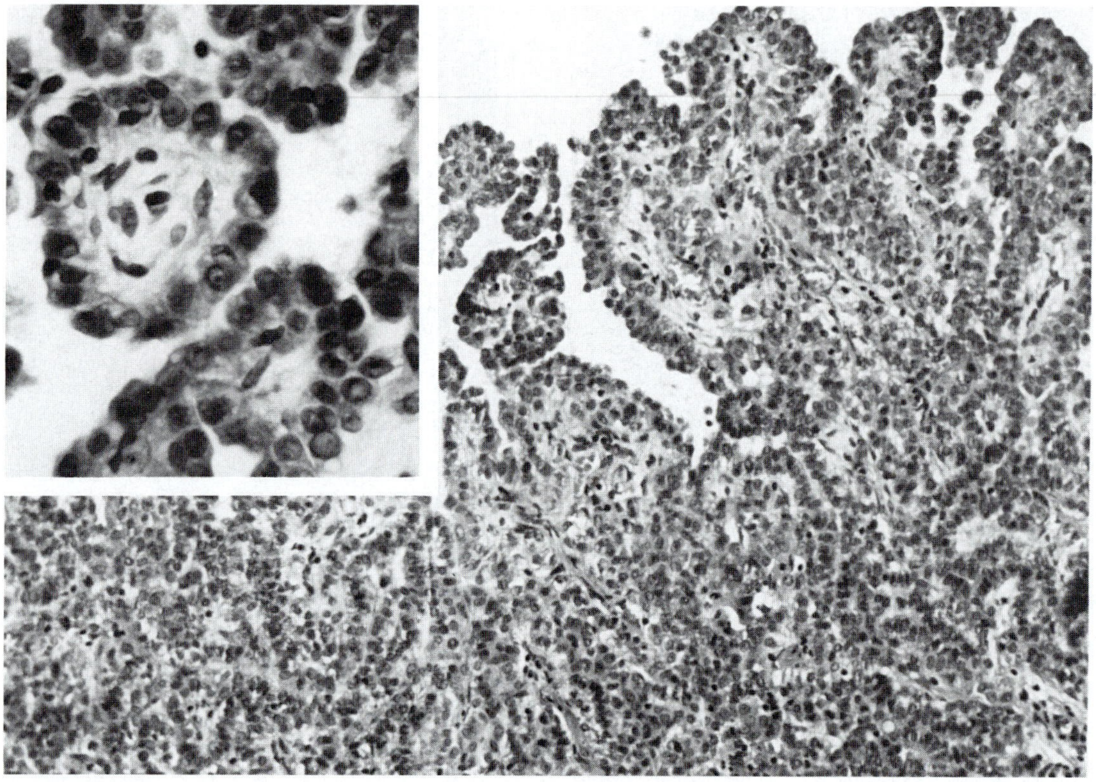

Fig. 17.13. Diffuse malignant mesothelioma. Atypical mesothelial cells (*inset*) are arranged in tubulopapillary and solid patterns.

placement of the pancreas. Some tumors incite a striking desmoplastic reaction. As noted earlier, rare peritoneal DMMs form localized solitary masses.

The typical histologic features (Figs. 17.13–17.15) are identical to DMMs involving the pleura. Most tumors are composed of epithelial cells arranged in tubulopapillary and solid patterns; areas of necrosis may be present. There is usually evidence of invasion of subperitoneal tissues, such as the omentum. As already noted, intraabdominal lymph nodes may be involved. The tumor cells usually retain some resemblance to mesothelial cells, with a cuboidal shape and eosinophilic cytoplasm. Usually there are mild to moderate degrees of nuclear atypicality and variably prominent nucleoli. Mitotic figures usually are present but are not numerous. Rare tumors with an exclusively solid pattern of polygonal cells with abundant eosinophilic cytoplasm and prominent nucleoli ("deciduoid" DMMs) (Fig. 17.16), with one exception, have arisen in the peritoneum.[304] Two-thirds of such tumors have occurred in females, some of whom were adolescents or young adults; deciduoid DMMs are usually rapidly fatal. Biphasic and sarcomatoid peritoneal DMMs occur, but are less common than their pleural counterparts. Occasional tumors contain a prominent inflammatory infiltrate, such as a dense lymphocytic infiltrate with lymphoid follicles, granulomas, or large numbers of foamy lipid-rich histiocytes.[175] The immunohistochemical (see next section) and ultrastructural features of peritoneal DMMs are similar to their pleural counterparts.

Differential Diagnosis

The differential diagnoses of DMM with atypical mesothelial hyperplasia (see "Mesothelial Hyperplasia") and of desmoplastic DMM versus reactive fibrosis (see "Peritoneal Fibrosis") have been previously discussed. Another frequently problematic lesion in the differential diagnosis is adenocarcinoma with diffuse peritoneal involvement, including metastatic adenocarcinomas (see "Metastatic Tumors") and adenocarcinomas of primary peritoneal origin (see "Lesions of the Secondary Müllerian System"). Features favoring a diagnosis of DMM include a prominent tubulopapillary pattern, polygonal cells with moderate amounts of eosinophilic cytoplasm, only mild to moderate nuclear atypia, a paucity of mitotic figures, and the presence of acid mucin (alcianophilic material) rather than neutral (PAS+) mucin.

DMMs usually lack immunoreactivity for a vari-

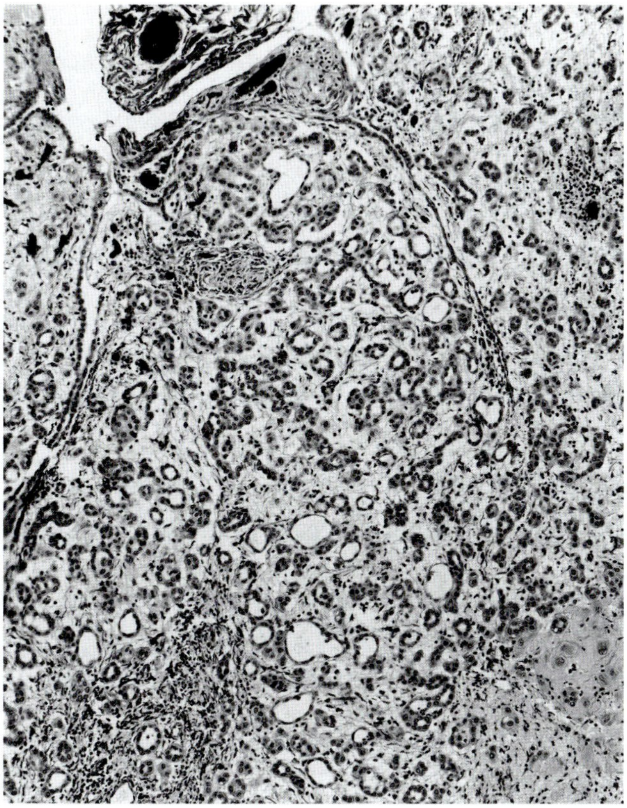

Fig. 17.14. Malignant mesothelioma. Tumor cells are arranged as small tubules, nests, and cords.

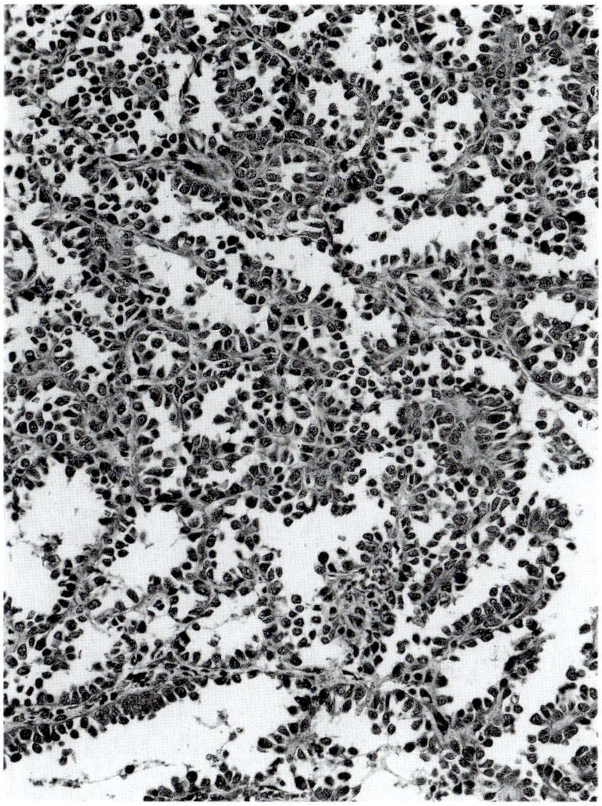

Fig. 17.15. Malignant mesothelioma. Tumors cells line irregular cystic and slitlike spaces.

ety of "epithelial" antigens, including carcinoembryonic antigen, B72.3, Leu-M1 (CD 15), MOC-31, CA 19-9, S-100 protein, Ber-EP4, and placental alkaline phosphatase.[31,209,240,241] Ordonez has found than B72.3, Leu-M1 (CD 15), MOC-31, and CA 19-9 are the most useful in the differential with primary peritoneal serous carcinoma.[33,240] Antigens that are usually present in epithelial DMMs but not in primary peritoneal serous carcinomas include cytokeratin 5/6, thrombomodulin, calretinin, and Wilms' tumor gene product.[240] However, no single immunohistochemical stain is diagnostic in the separation of peritoneal DMM from adenocarcinoma, and the results of a panel of antibodies should be interpreted in conjunction with the hematoxylin and eosin (H&E) and mucin stains.

"Deciduoid" peritoneal DMMs must be distinguished from an ectopic decidual reaction involving the peritoneum. Prominent nucleoli, often brisk mitotic activity, and cytokeratin immunoreactivity in the deciduoid tumors exclude an ectopic decidual reaction.

Lin et al. have reported peritoneal epithelioid hemangioendotheliomas or epithelioid angiosarcomas that have mimicked DMM.[190] Features that suggested the diagnosis of DMM in some of the cases included epithelioid cells in a tubulopapillary pattern and the presence of reactive or neoplastic spindle cells resulting in a focal biphasic pattern. Variable degrees of vascular differentiation and immunoreactivity of the neoplastic cells for endothelial antigens (and negative or weak cytokeratin staining) excluded the diagnosis of DMM.

Miscellaneous Primary Tumors

Intraabdominal Desmoplastic Small Round Cell Tumor

Clinical Features

This rare tumor (*desmoplastic small round cell tumor, DSRCT*) is of uncertain histogenesis, but it may ultimately prove to be a primitive tumor of mesothelial origin ("mesothelioblastoma").[122,237–239,242,355,362] Although most of the tumors are intraabdominal, similar tumors have also been described in the pleura and rarely at a distance from a mesothelium-lined surface (parotid gland, tentorium, hand). DSRCTs exhibit a reciprocal translocation [t(11;22) (p13;

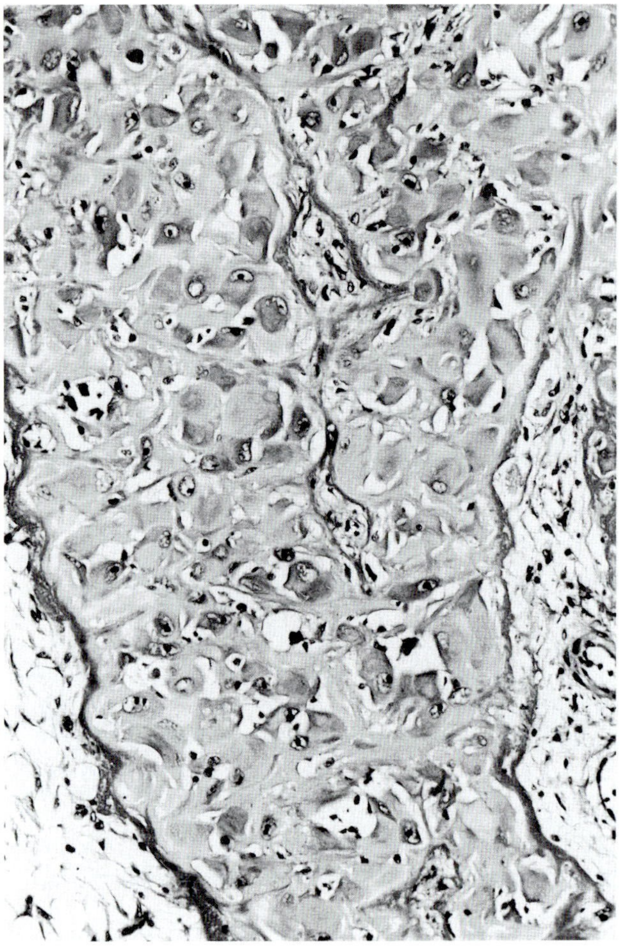

Fig. 17.16. Diffuse malignant mesothelioma of the peritoneum. The tumor had an exclusively solid growth pattern composed of cells with abundant cytoplasm that was eosinophilic.

q12)], resulting in fusion of the EWS1 gene on chromosome 22 and the Wilm's tumor suppressor gene (WT1) on chromosome 11 that appears to be unique for this tumor. This fusion results in the expression of the EWS/WT1 chimeric transcript detectable by reverse transcriptase polymerase chain reaction (PCR). The EWS/ERG fusion gene characteristic of Ewing's sarcoma/peripheral neuroectodermal tumors has been found in rare DSRCTs, suggesting some overlap between the two groups of tumors.

DSRCTs have a strong male predilection (M:F ratio, 4:1) and are most common in adolescents and young adults (range, 5–76 years) who usually have abdominal distension, pain, and a palpable abdominal, pelvic, or scrotal mass, sometimes in association with ascites. Some patients have had an elevated serum level of CA-125 or neuron-specific enolase. Laparotomy typically discloses variably sized but usually large, intraabdominal masses associated with smaller peritoneal "implants" of similar appearance. The tumor is sometimes confined to the pelvis, and prominent involvement of the tunica vaginalis or the ovaries may mimic a primary testicular or ovarian tumor.[362] The retroperitoneum is involved in some cases. One tumor appeared to originate within the liver.

After initial treatment (debulking and postoperative chemotherapy, irradiation, or both), there may be an initial response, but more than 90% of patients die of tumor progression. The bulk of the tumor tends to remain within the peritoneal cavity, although extraabdominal metastases occur in some patients.

Pathologic Findings

On gross examination, the tumors, which may reach 40 cm in maximal dimension, have smooth or bosselated outer surfaces and firm to hard, gray-white, focally myxoid and necrotic sectioned surfaces. Direct invasion of intraabdominal or pelvic viscera may occur.

Microscopic examination reveals sharply circumscribed aggregates of small epithelioid cells delimited by a cellular desmoplastic stroma (Fig. 17.17a). The aggregates vary from tiny clusters (or even single cells) to rounded or irregularly shaped islands. Other common features include rounded rosette-like or glandlike spaces, peripheral palisading of basaloid cells in some of the nests, and central necrosis with or without calcification. The tumor cells are typically uniform with scanty cytoplasm and indistinct cell borders (Fig. 17.17b), although tumor cells with eosinophilic cytoplasmic "inclusions" and an eccentric nucleus, resulting in a rhabdoid appearance, are frequently also present. Small to medium-sized, round, oval, or spindle-shaped hyperchromatic nuclei have clumped chromatin and nucleoli that are usually inapparent. Mitotic figures and single necrotic cells are numerous.

Architectural features noted in a minority of cases, which can occasionally predominate and lead to diagnostic problems, include tubules, glands (sometimes with luminal mucin), cysts, papillae, anastomosing trabeculae, cords of cells mimicking lobular breast carcinoma, adenoid cystic-like foci, and only a sparse desmoplastic stroma. Cytologic features noted in a minority of cases, which can occasionally predominate, include spindle cells, cells with abundant eosinophilic or clear cytoplasm, which may create a biphasic pattern (Fig. 17.18), signet-ring-like cells, and cells with marked nuclear pleomorphism.[238] Invasion of vascular spaces, especially lymphatics, is a common feature. Lymph nodes are occasionally involved by tumor.

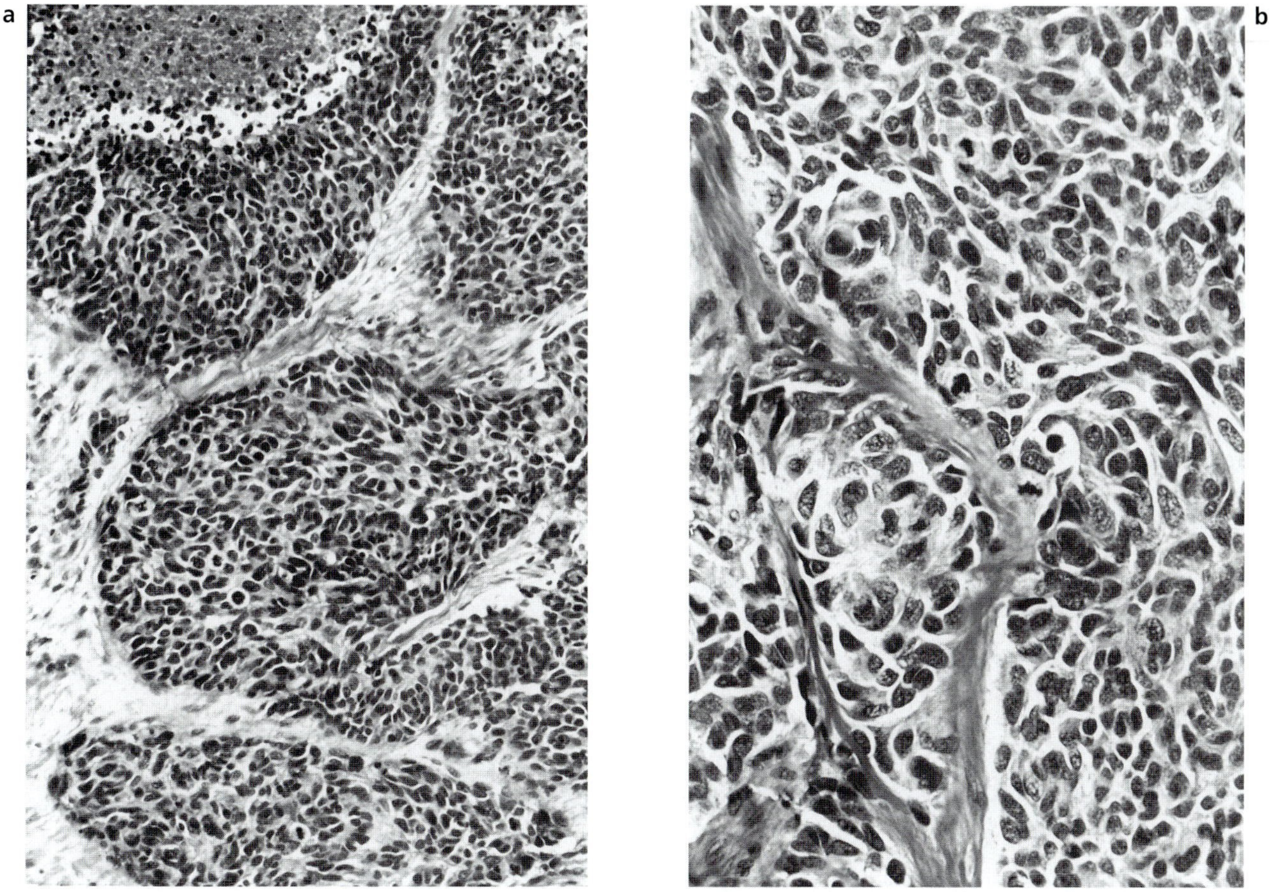

Fig. 17.17. Intraabdominal desmoplastic small round cell tumor. a: The cellular nests of tumor are sharply circumscribed and separated by a fibrous stroma. Focal necrosis of the tumor is seen in the *upper left*: **b**: The tumor cells have scant cytoplasm and malignant nuclear features.

Immunohistochemical and Ultrastructural Findings

The usual immunoreactivity for epithelial [low molecular weight cytokeratins, epithelial membrane antigen (EMA)], neural/neuroendocrine [neuron-specific enolase (NSE), CD57/Leu-7], and muscle (desmin) markers, as well as vimentin, suggests divergent differentiation. Desmin and vimentin immunoreactivity is typically paranuclear and globular and is particularly intense in the rhabdoid cells. Immunoreactivity for other antigens has been present in a variable proportion of cases, including Wilms' tumor protein (WT1), Leu-M1 (CD 15), S-100, B72.3, CA-125, MIC-2 protein, actin (MSA, SMA), desmoplakin, CD 99, MOC-31, NB84, Ber-EP4, chromogranin, and synaptophysin, but not HBA 71 (Ewing's sarcoma/PNET antigen). The stroma is typically immunoreactive for vimentin and muscle specific actin.

Ultrastructural variability suggests a range of differentiation. Cell junctions have varied from scant and primitive to more prominent ones including intermediate, desmosomal, and tight types. Paranuclear intermediate cytoplasmic filaments and basal lamina surrounding the nests of tumor have been prominent features in most of the cases.

Differential Diagnosis

The typical age of the patient, the absence of an extraoperitoneal primary tumor, the distribution of the tumor, and its typical microscopic features and immunoprofile facilitate the distinction from other malignant small cell tumors in most cases. Identification of the unique reciprocal translocation is diagnostic in problem cases.

Inflammatory Myofibroblastic Tumor

Day et al. reviewed the features of seven cases of abdominal "inflammatory pseudotumor,"[89] a lesion that has also been referred to as plasma cell granuloma or, more recently, *inflammatory myofibroblas-*

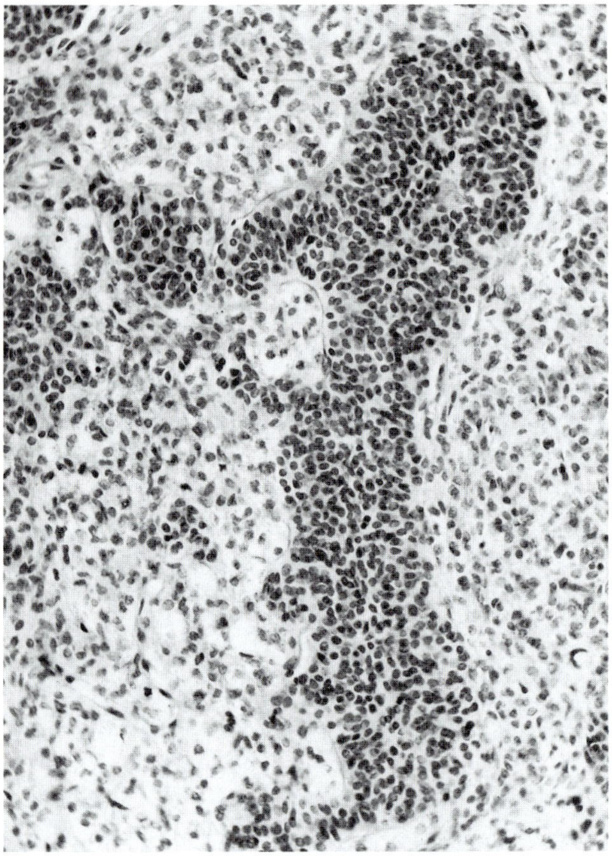

Fig. 17.18. Intraabdominal desmoplastic small round cell tumor. A nest of small cells is surrounded by cells with moderate amounts of pale cytoplasm.

tic tumor.[255] The abdominal lesions are typically encountered in patients younger than 20 years of age who present with a mass, fever, growth failure or weight loss, hypochromic anemia, thrombocytosis, and polyclonal hypergammaglobulinemia. Laparotomy typically reveals a solid mesenteric mass that on microscopic examination consists of myofibroblastic spindle cells, mature plasma cells, and small lymphocytes. All the patients have had an uneventful postoperative course with disappearance of the clinical manifestations.

Omental-Mesenteric Myxoid Hamartoma

The *omental-mesenteric myxoid hamartoma* designation was applied by Gonzalez-Crussi et al. to a lesion in infants characterized by multiple omental and mesenteric nodules composed of plump mesenchymal cells in a myxoid, vascularized stroma.[127] The diagnosis of the referring pathologists was usually that of some type of sarcoma, but the follow-up was uneventful. The lesions may be hamartomatous or a varient of inflammatory myofibroblastic tumor.

Metastatic Tumors

Peritoneal involvement by *metastatic tumor* is typically a result of seeding from a primary tumor arising within the abdomen or pelvis, most commonly the ovary. Peritoneal serous tumors in which the ovaries are normal or only minimally involved may arise directly from the peritoneum (see "Lesions of the Secondary Müllerian System") or rarely are metastatic from a serous papillary carcinoma of the endometrium or fallopian tube. Other tumors that may be associated with peritoneal seeding include carcinomas of the breast[2,214] and gastrointestinal tract, especially the colon and stomach, and the pancreas. In such cases, the metastatic tumor may take the form of signet-ring cells widely scattered in a fibrous stroma. Occasionally, the signet-ring cells can have relatively bland nuclear features, resulting in a deceptively benign appearance.

Pseudomyxoma Peritonei

Recent studies have indicated that *pseudomyxoma peritonei*, which refers to the presence of masses of jelly-like mucus in the pelvis and often the abdomen, is usually a result of peritoneal spread from a typically low-grade mucinous neoplasm, usually originating within the appendix or, less commonly, from a primary tumor elsewhere in the gastrointestinal tract.[257,273–276,363,365] Ovarian involvement is common in such cases and is discussed elsewhere (see Chapter 18, Surface Epithelial Tumors of the Ovary, and Chapter 22, Metastatic Tumors of the Ovary). Although controversial, rare cases of pseudomyxoma peritonei may be a result of peritoneal spread from an intestinal mucinous borderline tumor of the ovary, but such a diagnosis is tenable only if the appendix has been removed and completely sectioned for microscopic examination to exclude an appendiceal primary tumor.

Microscopic Findings

Extraovarian intraabdominal mucus may be of several types, all of which have been included in studies of pseudomyxoma peritonei, and there is no consensus as to how many of these types of intraabdominal mucus warrant the designation of pseudomyxoma peritonei: (1) free mucin in the abdominal cavity (mucinous ascites); (2) small or large deposits of mucin adherent to peritoneal surfaces, containing inflammatory and mesothelial cells and sometimes organizing capillaries and fibroblasts, but usually lacking neoplastic epithelial cells; and (3) masses composed of pools of mucin,

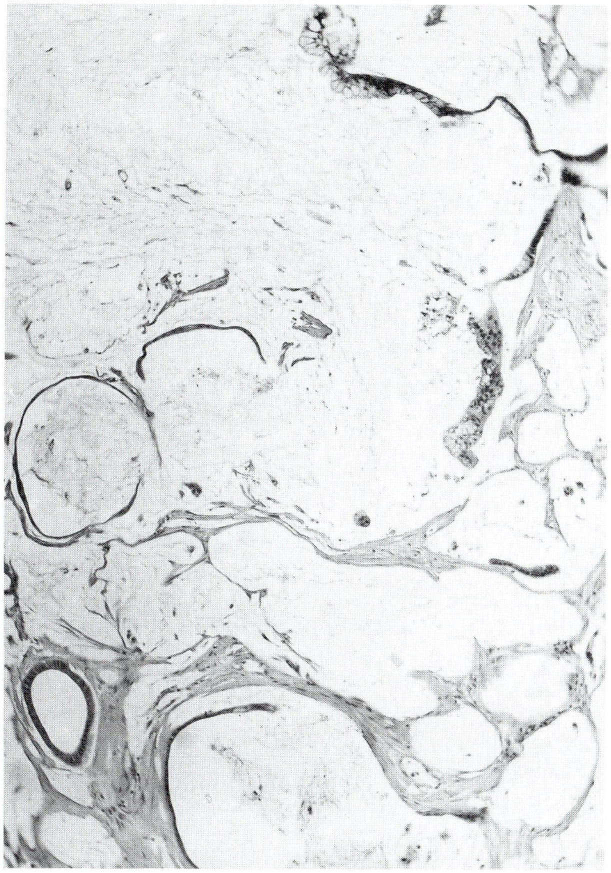

Fig. 17.19. Pseudomyxoma peritonei. Large pools of mucin are surrounded by hyalinized fibrous tissue.

which may or may not contain neoplastic cells, surrounded by dense collagenous tissue (dissecting mucin) (Fig. 17.19).

Prospective study of new cases of pseudomyxoma peritonei should include as extensive sampling of all the lesions as technically feasible in addition to further studies with special techniques such as immunohistochemistry and molecular biology. The appendix should be removed for complete histologic examination, even if its intraoperative appearance is normal. The term pseudomyxoma peritonei is most appropriately used only as a clinical and surgical designation and should not appear as a diagnosis in the pathology report. The latter should contain (1) an accurate appraisal of the appendiceal and, if present, the ovarian tumors as benign, borderline, or malignant, with a notation of the presence or absence of rupture; (2) assessment of the peritoneal lesions as mucinous ascites (free fluid in abdomen), organizing mucinous fluid, or mucin dissection with fibrosis; and (3) the presence or absence of neoplastic cells and whether they appear benign, atypical, or malignant.

Behavior

The typical peritoneal lesions of pseudomyxoma peritonei containing benign or atypical mucinous epithelium have a clinical course that is typically slowly progressive over a period of many years. Prayson et al. have found that patients in whom the peritoneal deposits are free of neoplastic epithelial cells have a more favorable prognosis than those with cell-containing deposits.[257] Conversely, Ronnett et al.[275,276] have shown that cases of pseudomyxoma arising from mucinous adenocarcinomas (usually of the appendix or large or small bowel) and with peritoneal deposits containing carcinomatous cells ("peritoneal mucinous carcinomatosis") are more likely to be associated with nodal and hepatic spread and have a much shorter survival than cases of pseudomyxoma characterized by only benign or atypical epithelium ("peritoneal adenomucinosis"). Tumors with intermediate features or in which the primary and metastatic tumor have discordant features (adenomucinous in the primary tumor, mucinous carcinomatosis in the metastases) behave more like mucinous carcinomatosis.

Lesions of the Secondary Müllerian System

These peritoneal lesions are characterized by müllerian differentiation on microscopic examination and share an origin from the so-called *secondary müllerian system*, that is, the pelvic and lower abdominal mesothelium and the subjacent mesenchyme of females.[185] The müllerian potential of this layer is consistent with its close embryonic relation to the müllerian ducts that arise by invagination of the coelomic epithelium. Displacement of coelomic epithelium and subcoelomic mesenchyme during embryonic development could account for the presence of identical lesions within pelvic and abdominal lymph nodes. The origin of many of these lesions, however, is not known with certainty, and other proposed histogenetic mechanisms are discussed where appropriate.

Lesions of the secondary müllerian system include those containing endometrioid, serous, and mucinous epithelium, simulating normal or neoplastic endometrial, tubal, and endocervical epithelium. The metaplastic potential of the pelvic peritoneum also includes differentiation toward cells of transitional (urothelial) type, exemplified most commonly by Walthard nests. Proliferation of the subjacent mesenchyme may accompany epithelial differentiation of the mesothelium or may give rise to a variety of pure mesenchymal lesions composed of endometrial stromal-type cells, decidua, or smooth muscle.

Endometriosis in Usual Sites

Endometriosis is defined as the presence of endometrial tissue outside the endometrium and myometrium. Usually both epithelium and stroma are seen, but occasionally the diagnosis of endometriosis can be made when only one component is present, as discussed next.

Etiology and Pathogenesis

Two theories have been proposed for the pathogenesis of endometriosis: (1) metastases of endometrial tissue to its ectopic location (metastatic theory); and (2) metaplastic development of endometrial tissue at the ectopic site (metaplastic theory). The metastatic theory explains the majority of cases, but a metaplastic origin likely accounts for ocasional cases in which metastatic spread of endometrial tissue is unlikely or impossible (see following).

Metastatic Theory

Sampson[289] proposed that endometriosis was caused by reflux of endometrial tissue through the fallopian tubes by a process of retrograde menstruation, with subsequent implantation and growth on peritoneal surfaces. Implantation of menstrual endometrium has also been proposed to explain endometriosis within surgical scars, on traumatized cervical and vaginal mucosa, and within perineal and vulvar scars following vaginal delivery. Passage of refluxed menstrual endometrium from the peritoneal cavity through diaphragmatic defects, diaphragmatic lymphatics, or both may explain pleural endometriosis.

Observations supporting the menstrual implantation hypothesis include the following: (1) endometriotic lesions are most common in areas closest to the tubal ostia and occur in a distribution that appears dependent on gravity and uterine postiion[155,159]; (2) retrograde menstruation through the fallopian tubes is a common physiologic process, occurring in 90% of menstruating women with patent tubes[29,135]; (3) endometriosis is more common in women with early menarche, heavy menstrual flow, long menstrual flow (>7 days), and frequent menses (cycle, <27 days); (4) menstrual endometrium is viable, capable of growth in tissue culture and after subcutaneous or intrapelvic injection[97]; (5) endometriosis is more frequent in females with congenital obstruction to menstrual flow[236]; and (6) endometriosis may follow uteropelvic or uteroabdominal wall fistulas in experimental animals and humans.

Although endometriosis in some scars may be a result of menstrual implantation, endometriosis within scars after uterine operations may be secondary to intraoperative implantation of endometrial tissue.[52,319] Supporting this theory is the greater frequency of scar endometriosis after abdominal hysterotomy than after cesarean section in some studies, consistent with the greater viability of transplanted early-pregnancy endometrium compared to late-pregnancy endometrium. Also, the occurrence of endometriosis within an episiotomy scar is much higher if uterine curettage is performed immediately after delivery than in patients without postdelivery curettage.[249]

The presence of endometriosis in distant sites (e.g., lungs, extremities, brain) is most easily explained by hematogenous spread from the uterus. Similarly, endometriosis within lymph nodes is likely a result of lymphatic spread. Evidence supporting the origin of endometriosis from lymphatic or hematogenous spread includes (1) the presence of normal endometrial tissue within endothelium-lined spaces as an incidental histologic finding within the myometrium, most often associated with adenomyosis; (2) the presence of intraluminal vascular involvement in rare endometriotic lesions; (3) the presence of intravascular or perivascular trophoblastic tissue and "decidua"* as an incidental microscopic finding within the lungs of pregnant patients[318]; (4) the occurrence of pulmonary endometriosis almost exclusively in women who have had prior uterine operations that could predispose to the embolization of endometrial tissue; (5) the experimental production of pulmonary endometriosis by intravenous injection of endometrial tissue in rabbits; and (6) the observations that tumor cells, blood, dye, and radiographic material can migrate from the pelvis to the umbilicus by retrograde lymphatic flow.

Metaplastic Theory

The origin of pelvic endometriosis by a process of metaplasia from the pelvic peritoneum is consistent with the putative müllerian potential of this tissue, which, as noted earlier, has been referred to as the secondary müllerian system.[185] Evidence for the metaplastic theory includes (1) the demonstration of endometriosis in subjects in whom metastasis of normally situated endometrium could not occur or

*By current criteria, these intrapulmonary foci of "decidua" would probably be interpreted as foci of intermediate trophoblast.

is highly unlikely, such as those with Turner's syndrome and pure gonadal dysgenesis who are amenorrheic and have hypoplastic uteri,[98,102,252] and in males; (2) the experimental induction of peritoneal endometriosis adjacent to millipore filters that contain endometrial tissue but that prevent cellular transfer; (3) the observation that autologous endometrial implants in rabbits degenerate but are associated with the subsequent development of endometriosis in adjacent tissues; and (4) the juxtaposition of endometriosis with other putative metaplastic lesions of the peritoneum, such as diffuse peritoneal leiomyomatosis.

Other Etiologic Factors

Endometriosis is an idiopathic disease in most patients, and the reason only a minority of females are affected despite the common occurrence of retrograde menstruation is unknown. Some potential etiologic factors have been discussed (congenital obstruction, iatrogenic implantation); others are summarized in the following section.

Genetic Factors Several studies concluded that the prevalence of endometriosis is greater in mothers and sisters of women with endometriosis than in the mothers and sisters of their husbands.[181,198,311] Lamb et al. calculated the overall risk for first-degree relatives to be 4.9%.[181] Genetic studies suggest a polygenic mode of inheritance (influenced by several different genes) or one that is multifactorial (a result of interaction between genetic and environmental factors). In opposition to the foregoing, Houston et al.[147] concluded that there were methodologic flaws in three of the studies[181,311] and that an inherited tendency to endometriosis has not yet been substantiated.

Hormonal Factors Because endometriosis occurs almost exclusively in women of reproductive age, hormonal factors may play an etiologic role. The rare examples of endometriosis in phenotypic females with gonadal dysgenesis and in males have usually been associated with the use of exogenous estrogens.[19,98,102,204,252,297,366] Also, it has been shown that maintenance of autologous peritoneal transplants of endometrium in monkeys requires either estradiol or progesterone or both. Similarly, smoking and exercise, which are inversely correlated with endogenous estrogen levels, appear to be protective factors for the development of endometriosis.

It has been suggested that the progestational milieu of pregnancy may inhibit the development of endometriosis. Many studies have indicated that endometriosis is more likely to occur in women who have delayed pregnancy and is less common in multiparous women.[268] Similarly, in some studies, patients with endometriosis are much less likely to have used oral contraceptives than similar patients without endometriosis.

Some studies have found an increased frequency of the luteinized unruptured follicle syndrome (LUFS) in patients with endometriosis. In normal women, the ruptured corpus luteum releases its progesterone-rich fluid into the peritoneal cavity. It has been postulated that this fluid may inhibit implantation and growth of refluxed endometrial fragments at the time of menstruation.[178] In patients with LUFS, a corpus luteum is formed, but rupture and fluid release do not occur, resulting in lowered luteal-phase levels of progesterone in the peritoneal fluid.[178] This local hormonal imbalance may be critical in allowing endometrial cells to implant on the peritoneum. Other studies, however, have shown no difference in the luteal-phase peritoneal fluid hormone values in women with and without endometriosis.

Immune Factors One study has demonstrated a reduced T-lymphocyte-mediated cytotoxicity to autologous endometrial cells and a decreased lymphocyte stimulation response to autologous endometrial antigens in patients with endometriosis.[320] The degree of depressed cellular immunity was directly proportional to the severity of the disease. The authors of this study suggested that certain cell-mediated immune mechanisms that may be operative in limiting the growth of endometriotic tissue may be impaired in patients with endometriosis. Other authors have suggested that the growth of endometriotic implants may be stimulated by activated macrophages.

Clinical Features

Epidemiologic Factors

The highest risk of the disease has traditionally been considered to be in the upper socioeconomic levels of developed societies, especially among women who delay pregnancy, although, according to Houston, these associations have not been proven statistically.[147] Although endometriosis was once considered to be more common in Caucasians, recent studies showing a similar frequency of the disease in Orientals and blacks cast doubt on this view.

The true prevalence of endometriosis is unknown as many patients are asymptomatic; estimates for the prevalence of the disease in women of reproductive age are 1%–7%,[15] 10%,[350] and 10%–15%.[216] Prevalence figures, however, have varied widely, depending on the population studied and the method of diagnosis (clinical, operative, or pathologic). Similarly, a study of the incidence rates of pelvic endometriosis in white females of reproductive age in Rochester, Minnesota (USA), found that the overall incidence of the disease more than doubled (from 108.8 to 246.9 cases per 100,000 person-years) as the definition of a case was extended from histologically confirmed cases to clinically and surgically diagnosed cases.[146]

More than 80% of affected patients are in the reproductive age group. In one study, the age-specific incidence rates increased in successive age groups through age 44 and then declined for women 45–49 years.[146] Less than 5% of cases occur in postmenopausal women, and in these patients the disease is frequently not diagnosed premenopausally.[168] Endometriosis can be clinically significant in this age group, with 20%–30% of affected patients requiring operative management.[168,260] In some postmenopausal patients with endometriosis, an association with obesity and endometrial carcinoma has been noted, suggesting that hyperestrinism may play a role, but in other series, a majority of patients have had no obvious exogenous or endogenous source of estrogen.[168] Almost 10% of patients with endometriosis are adolescents.[49] Endometriosis was found at laparoscopy in approximately 50% of teenage patients with dysmenorrhea or chronic pelvic pain in three studies.[49] In some studies, adolescents with endometriosis have a particularly high frequency of a congenital obstruction to menstrual flow.

Symptoms and Signs

The recurrent cyclic menstrual, inflammatory and fibrotic changes within endometriotic lesions are likely responsible for most of the symptomatology of endometriosis, although there is often no direct relationship between the extent of the disease and the severity of the symptoms.[49] One study, however, found that deeper implants were more likely to be associated with pain than superficial lesions.[77] Hormonal responsiveness of the lesions as judged histologically also does not correlate with symptoms, and microscopic examination of symptomatic endometriosis in postmenopausal patients typically reveals atrophic changes.[168] Age generally does not appear to affect disease severity in most studies.[147] An exception to the foregoing is one study in which women 26–52 years of age had less extensive disease than women 16–25 years of age.[268] A higher frequency of nulliparity in the younger women appeared to account for part of this difference.[147]

The typical symptoms that are attributed to pelvic endometriosis are acquired dysmenorrhea, lower abdominal, pelvic, and back pain, dyspareunia, irregular bleeding, and infertility. Infertility is present in up to 30% of women with endometriosis, although the putative association between mild endometriosis and infertility has recently been challenged.[44,325] The subject of endometriosis-related infertility has been reviewed elsewhere[132,216,325] and is not considered in detail here. Potential pathogenetic factors include tubal factors (adhesions, luminal obstruction), ovarian factors (anovulation, luteal-phase dysfunction, LUFS), immune factors (antiendometrial antibodies), peritoneal factors (increased prostaglandins, increased macrophages), and an increased risk of spontaneous abortion.

Pelvic examination may reveal tender nodules in the cul-de-sac and uterosacral ligments, tender, semifixed, cystic ovaries, and a fixed, retroverted uterus. The rectovaginal septum may also be tender and indurated. The endometriotic lesions frequently enlarge and become more painful during menses. The clinical manifestations also vary according to the site of the endometriosis, as is discussed later in this chapter. As the clinical manifestations of endometriosis are frequently nonspecific, vary widely between patients, and may be absent in a high proportion of patients, a definitive diagnosis requires direct visualization by laparoscopy (or laparotomy) and, ideally, biopsy.

Laparoscopic Findings

A number of recent studies have stressed that endometriotic foci, especially early ones, are frequently nonpigmented and may have a wide variety of laparoscopic appearances, including clear, white, and red lesions.[158,203,267,322,323] Sequential laparoscopic examinations indicate that nonpigmented endometriotic implants eventually evolve into the typical pigmented lesions.[158] Even in patients with laparoscopically typical disease, biopsy may yield only nondiagnostic tissue, and thus, in the opinion of some authors, diagnosis and treatment should not always depend on microscopic confirmation.[51] Laparoscopically detectable defects or "pockets" involving the pelvic peritoneum are frequently associated with, and likely caused by, endometriosis.[50,269] In one study, 80% of women with pelvic peritoneal defects had endometriosis,[50] and in another, the endometriotic foci were often located along the edges of the defects.[269] Conversely, 18%–28% of women with endometriosis in the two studies had peritoneal defects.

Serum Markers

Levels of CA-125 may be elevated in the serum and peritoneal fluid of patients with endometrio-

Sites

Common	*Less Common*	*Rare*
Ovaries	Large bowel, small bowel, appendix	Lungs, pleura
Uterine ligaments (uterosacral, round, broad)	Mucosa of cervix, vagina, and fallopian tubes	Soft tissues, breast
Rectovaginal septum	Skin (scars, umbilicus, vulva, perineum, inguinal region)	Bone
Cul-de-sac	Ureter, bladder, omentum, pelvic lymph nodes, inguinal (noncutaneous)	Upper abdominal peritoneum
Peritoneum of uterus, tubes, rectosigmoid, ureter, bladder		Stomach, pancreas, liver
		Kidney, urethra, prostate, paratesticular
		Sciatic nerve, subarachnoid space, brain

sis.[16,88,108] The concentrations of serum CA-125 correlate with both the severity and the clinical course of the disease. The serum test has low sensitivity, however, and is not appropriate for general screening purposes. In contrast, CA-125 levels have acceptable sensitivities and very high specificities in populations with a relatively high prevalence of the disease and are useful in monitoring response to treatment.

Antiendometrial antibodies have been found in up to 83% of women with laparoscopically confirmed endometriosis. In one study, the antibody titers in women who had had a good response to hormonal treatment were lower than in those with untreated endometriosis or in whom there had been a poor response to treatment, and in another study, sequential determination of antibody levels showed that they were lowered by hormonal treatment.

Effects of Pregnancy

Although rare cases of endometriosis undergo permanent regression during pregnancy, the ameliorative effect of pregnancy noted in many cases of endometriosis is only temporary.[207] The behavior of endometriosis during pregnancy is extremely variable among different patients and between one pregnancy and another in the same patient.[207] During pregnancy, visible endometriotic lesions frequently undergo initial enlargement, with occasional ulceration and bleeding, followed by shrinkage. In most sites, there is a decrease in the associated pain.

A rare complication of endometriosis during pregnancy is intrapartum or postpartum rupture of the lesion, most probably caused by a softening of the lesion secondary to stromal decidualization, pressure from the expanding uterus, or both. Rupture occurs most frequently in the ovaries or bowel, typically resulting in perforation and an acute abdomen. Rarely, hemoperitoneum, sometimes fatal, is caused by hemorrhage from decidualized endometriotic lesions at term.

Rare Complications

Massive, sometimes serosanguineous, ascites occurs in patients with pelvic endometriosis; a right pleural effusion is also present in one-third of such patients.[227] If one or both ovaries are involved, the operative findings may simulate those of an ovarian carcinoma. The pathogenesis of the ascites is not clear. Possible sources include production by endometriotic cysts, irritated peritoneal mesothelial cells, or the ovarian serosa (Meigs-like syndrome). Other rare complications include hemorrhage from an endometriotic focus and spontaneous rupture of ovarian endometriotic cysts, resulting in an acute abdomen.

Gross Features of Peritoneal and Ovarian Endometriosis

Depending on their duration and their superficial or deep location in relation to the peritoneal surface, endometriotic foci may appear as punctate, red, blue, brown, or white spots or patches with either a slightly raised or a puckered surface (Fig. 17.20). Ecchymotic or brown areas have sometimes been described as "powder burns." The endometriotic foci are frequently associated with dense fibrous adhesions. The lesions may form nodules or cysts or both. Rarely, endometriosis can take the form of polypoid masses that project from the serosal surfaces (Fig. 17.21), into the lumens of endometriotic cysts, or from the mucosa of the bowel or bladder. In some of these cases, there is a history of exogenous estrogen use and hyperplastic changes are found on microscopic examination.[82] This appearance, which we refer to as polypoid endometriosis, can simulate a malignant tumor on clinical, intraoperative, or pathologic examination.[82,225,299]

Endometriotic cysts (endometriomas) most commonly involve the ovaries, where they can partially or almost completely replace the normal tissue; bilateral involvement occurs in one-third to one-half of the cases.[99] The cysts rarely exceed 15 cm in diameter; larger examples are more likely to harbor a

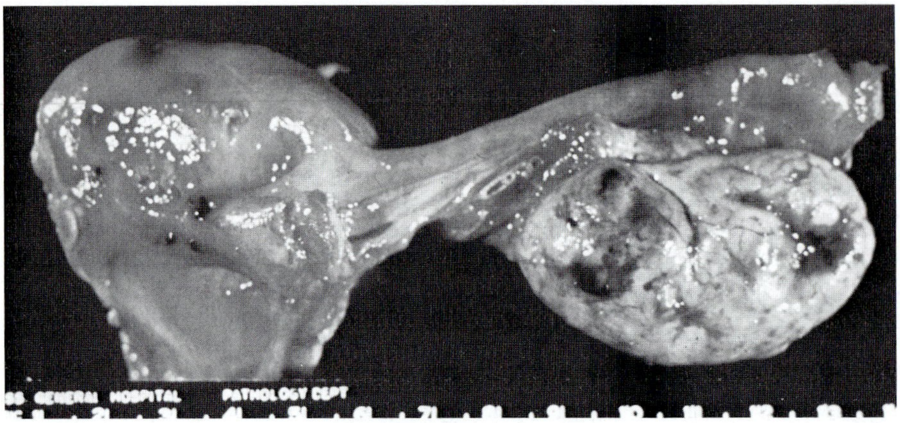

Fig. 17.20. Endometriosis of uterine serosa and ovary. Multiple, hemorrhagic lesions involve the serosal surfaces. (Courtesy of R.E. Scully, M.D., Boston, MA.)

neoplasm. Endometriotic cysts are commonly covered by dense fibrous adhesions, which may result in fixation to adjacent structures. The cyst walls are usually thick and fibrotic, with a smooth or shaggy, brown to yellow lining (Fig. 17.22). The cyst contents typically consist of altered, semifluid or inspissated, chocolate-colored material; rarely, the cyst is filled with watery fluid. Any solid areas in the cyst wall or intraluminal polypoid projections should be sampled histologically to exclude a neoplasm originating in the cyst (see page 767).

Typical Microscopic Findings

The typical appearance in reproductive age women, in whom the disease is usually diagnosed, is of one or more glands lined by endometrioid epithelium, surrounded by a mantle of densely packed small fusiform cells with scanty cytoplasm and bland cytology, typical of nonneoplastic endometrial stromal cells (Figs 17.23–17.25). Small blood vessels, which may be engorged, are present and sometimes draw attention to the lesion on low-power examination. When seen in the ovary, the most common site encountered by the surgical pathologist, endometriosis varies from simple to microscopically dilated glands (Fig. 17.26) to grossly recognizable endometriotic cysts. This spectrum is seen at extraovarian sites, although striking cysts are less common to rare, depending on the site. Endometriosis may occur anywhere in the ovary but is most common in the cortex. Sometimes it is very superficial and may occur on the surface as small nodules, irregularly shaped aggregates, or even have a plaque-like configuration (Fig. 17.26). Surface endometriosis is typically associated with fibrous tissue and inflammatory cells and, if prominent and of sig-

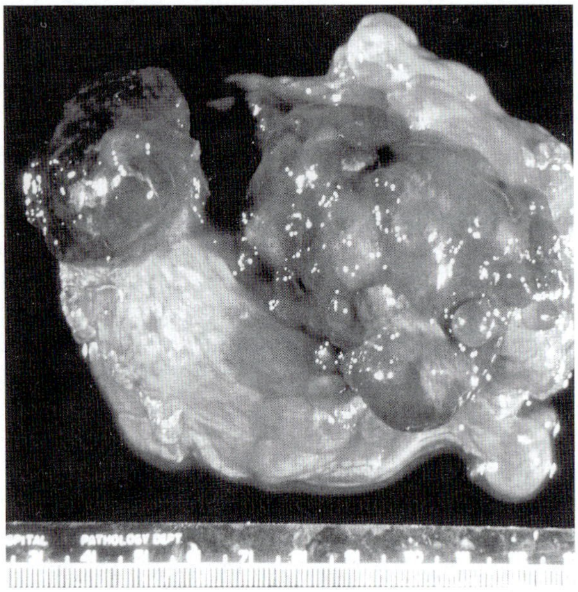

Fig. 17.21. Polypoid endometriosis. Polypoid tumor-like masses involve the pelvic peritoneum.

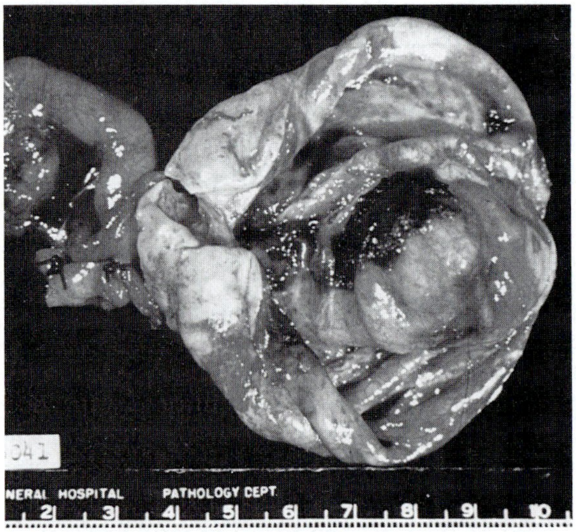

Fig. 17.22. Endometriotic cyst of ovary. The cyst has been opened to reveal a focally hemorrhagic lining. (Courtesy of R.E. Scully, M.D., Boston, MA.)

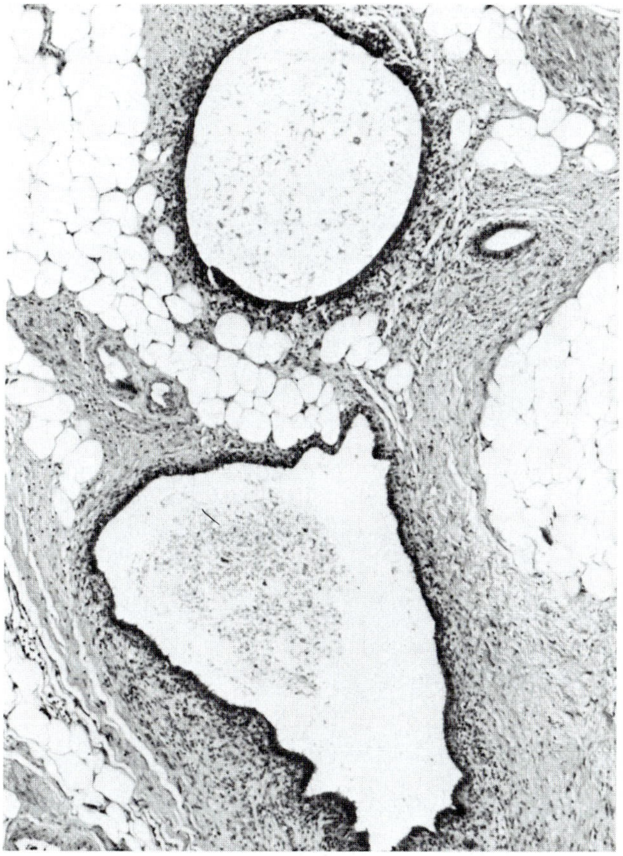

Fig. 17.23. Endometriosis of cul-de-sac. Cystic endometrial glands with a cuff of endometrial stroma are surrounded by fibrous and adipose tissue.

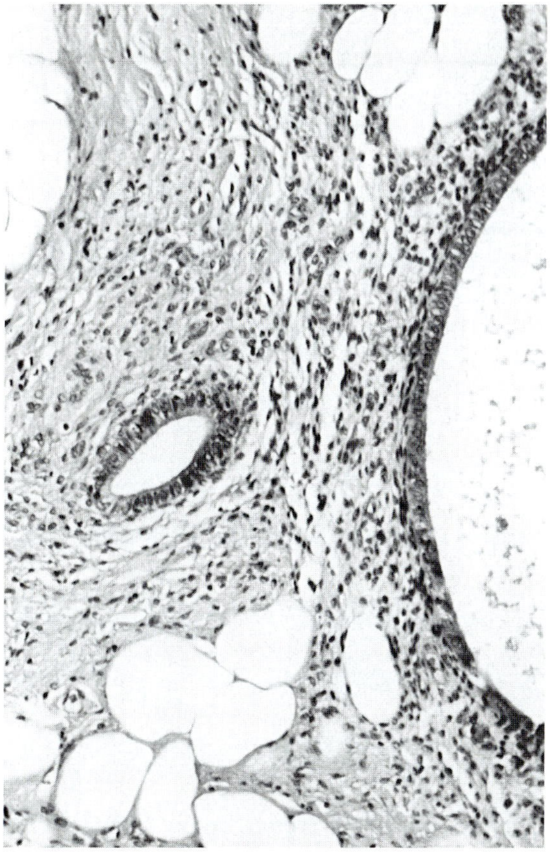

Fig. 17.24. Endometriosis of cul-de-sac (higher magnification of Fig. 17.23). Endometriotic glands are lined by inactive epithelium and surrounded by a thin rim of endometrial stroma.

nificant duration, there may be conspicuous adhesions. Glands, which can sometimes be cystic, may hang off the surface of the ovary, tethered to it by the associated stroma and fibrous tissue. Endometriotic glands in the cortex of the ovaries of perimenopausal or postmenopausal women, or glands that are atrophic for any reason, may be mistaken for inclusion glands and cysts if the often subtle, sometimes barely perceptible, cuffs of stroma are overlooked or obscured by hemorrhage (see Fig. 17.26).

The appearance of endometriotic tissue varies with the extent of its response to the normal hormonal fluctuations of the menstrual cycle and the duration of the process. When the appearances of simultaneous samples of eutopic endometrium and endometriotic foci from reproductive age women are compared, cyclic changes are seen in the endometriosis in 44%–80% of the cases, with considerable variability in glandular morphology.[36,218,361] When more than one endometriotic focus is examined in the same patient, the appearance of the specimens does not differ significantly from one to another.[25] In most postmenopausal patients, the endometriotic tissue is atrophic with glands, that are occasionally cystic, lined by flattened epithelial cells surrounded by a dense fibrotic stroma with sometimes a barely perceptible tendency for the stroma to be more cellular close to the gland, a feature that may be a diagnostic clue; the appearance is similar to that of simple or cystic atrophy of the endometrium (Fig. 17.27).[168] In a minority of cases, however, the endometriotic tissue has an active appearance, with or without the metaplastic and hyperplastic changes that are more commonly present in premenopausal women.

At the time of menstruation, hemorrhage may occur within the stroma and glandular lumens of endometriotic foci, as well as a secondary inflammatory response consisting predominantly of a diffuse infiltration of histiocytes. The histiocytes typically convert the extravasated red blood cells into glycolipid and granular brown pigment, becoming so-called pseudoxanthoma cells (Figs. 17.28 and 17.29) that can replace most or all the endometriotic stroma.[58,69] Most of the pigment is hemofuscin, and hemosiderin is typ-

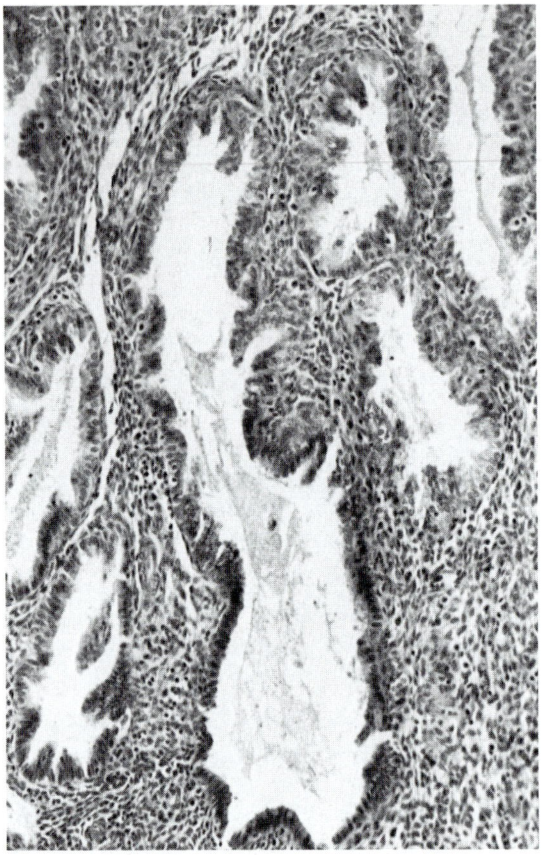

Fig. 17.25. Irregular secretory changes within a focus of endometriosis. The progestational response is less pronounced in the glandular epithelium at the bottom of the figure.

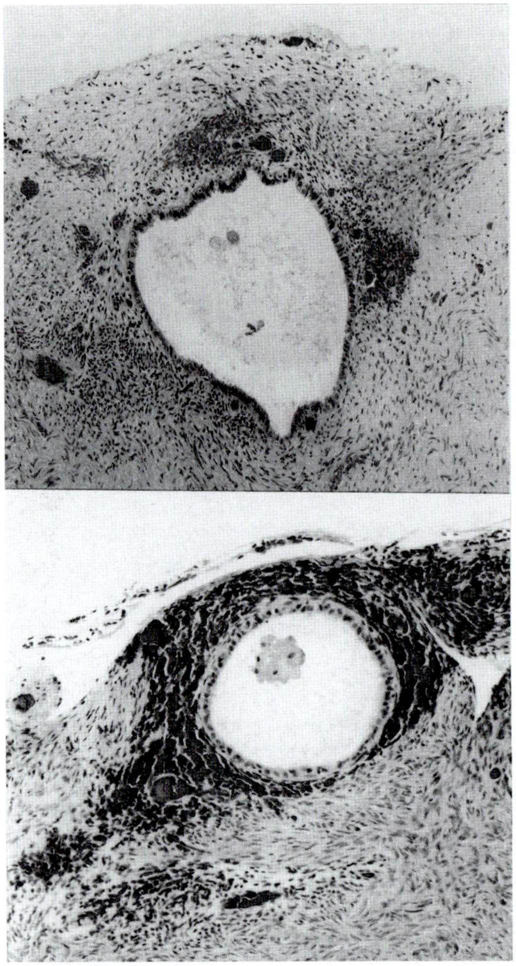

Fig. 17.26. Subtle endometriosis involving the ovarian surface. *Top*: The periglandular endometriotic stroma is only focal and less cellular than usual. *Bottom*: The periglandular endometriotic stroma is obscured by hemorrhage. In both examples, failure to recognize the endometriotic stroma could result in the diagnosis of endometriosis being missed and the endometriotic glands being misinterpreted as epithelial inclusion glands.

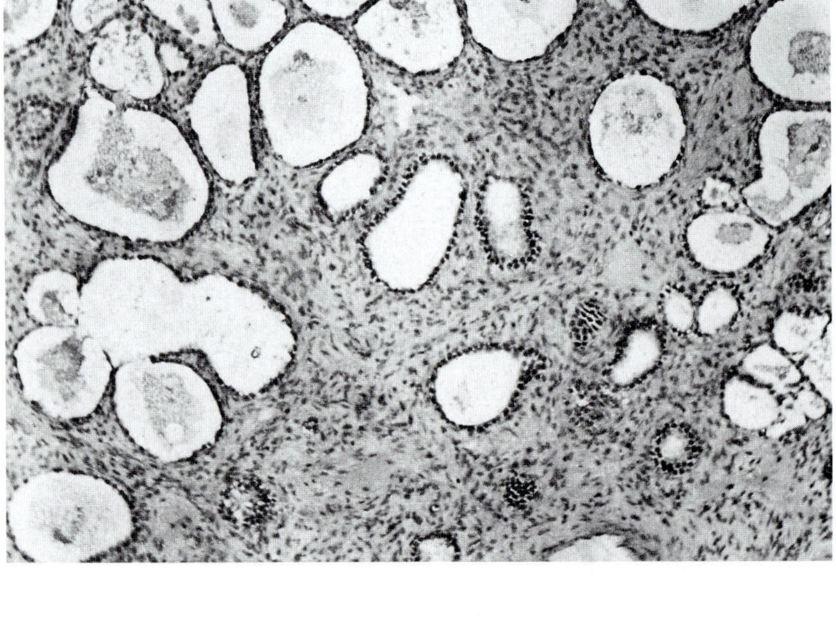

Fig. 17.27. Endometriosis in a postmenopausal woman. The glands are cystic, atrophic, and separated by a fibrous stroma. (Reprinted by permission of Clement, ref. 58.)

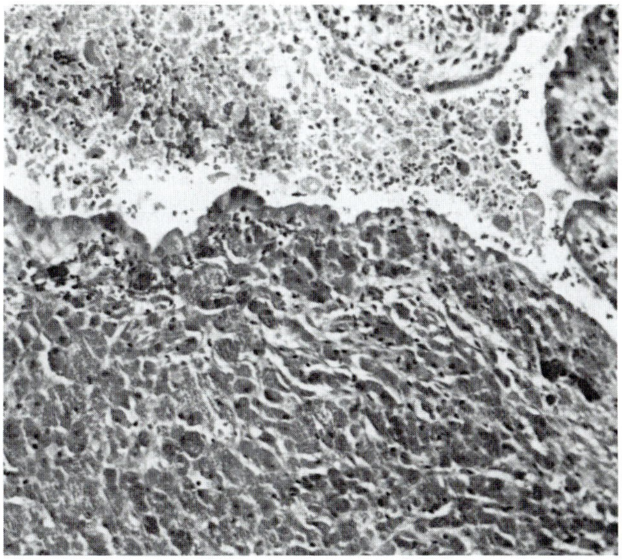

Fig. 17.28. Lining of ovarian endometriotic cyst. The lining consists of endometrial surface epithelium and numerous pigment-laden histiocytes within the subjacent stroma. Menstrual debris is present within the cyst lumen.

ically present to a much lesser extent.[58,69] The amount of pigment in an endometriotic lesion appears to increase with its age, and early lesions are frequently nonpigmented.[158] Variable numbers of lymphocytes and smaller numbers of other inflammatory cells may be present. Large numbers of neutrophils with microabscess formation should raise the possibility of secondary bacterial infection.[192,295]

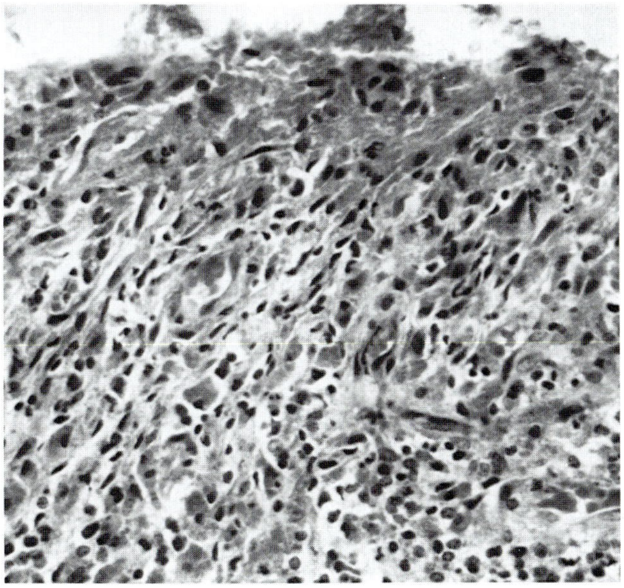

Fig. 17.29. Lining of ovarian endometriotic cyst. In this field, the lining consists only of fibrotic granulation tissue and pigment-laden histiocytes (presumptive endometriosis).

As already mentioned, a common manifestation of ovarian endometriosis is striking cystification resulting in an endometriotic cyst. The epithelial and stromal lining of an endometriotic cyst frequently becomes attenuated, and the former may be reduced to a single layer of cuboidal cells that may retain some endometrial characteristics but which are often devoid of specific features. In such circumstances, recognition of the cyst as endometriotic may only be possible if a rim of subjacent endometrial stroma persists. Commonly, the cyst lining of endometrial epithelium and stroma is totally lost, and replaced by granulation tissue, dense fibrous tissue containing fibroblasts with particularly small nuclei, and variable numbers of pseudoxanthoma cells (presumptive endometriosis) (Fig. 17.29). In some "old" endometriotic cysts, ossification, calcification, and old luminal blood clot can produce striking gross and microscopic appearances.[307] The epithelial cells lining endometriotic cysts are often focally large and cuboidal with abundant eosinophilic cytoplasm and large atypical nuclei (Fig. 17.30).[58,80,301] The significance of such nuclear atypia is unclear. Although it may be reactive, cells with these features may merge with clear cell ade-

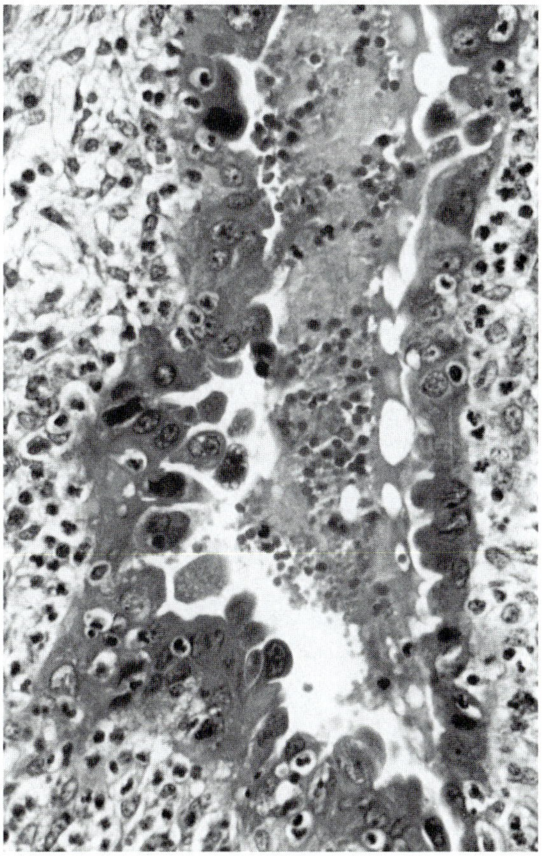

Fig. 17.30. Lining of ovarian endometriotic cyst. The surface epithelial cells show striking nuclear atypia.

nocarcinomas and endocervical-like mucinous borderline tumors.[285,286] When this atypia is an isolated finding in an endometriotic cyst, however, the follow-up is typically uneventful.[301]

Endometriosis that involves smooth muscle in the uterine ligaments or the walls of hollow viscera differs significantly in its appearance from that of endometriosis in the ovaries and the peritoneal surfaces. In the former, there is typically a striking proliferation of the indigenous smooth muscle, often resulting in a firm, solid, tumor-like mass.[58,299] The appearance is similar to that of adenomyosis with secondary striking myometrial hypertrophy.

Unusual Microscopic Findings

Metaplastic Glandular Changes

Metaplastic changes similar to those occurring in eutopic endometrial glands have been described in endometriotic glands.[118] These changes include ciliated,[80,184,185] eosinophilic,[118] hobnail,[80] and, rarely, squamous (Fig. 17.31a) and mucinous metaplasia (Fig. 17.31b); the latter may be characterized by the presence of endocervical-type cells or, less often, goblet cells.[364] In one study of ovarian endometriosis,[118] there was a significant association between the presence of metaplasia in the endometriosis and a synchronous ovarian epithelial cancer. Additionally, all four endocervical-like mucinous borderline tumors (EMBLTs) in the same study were associated with foci of ovarian endometriosis that exhibited both mucinous metaplasia and hyperplasia. In some cases of endometriosis, the distinction between papillary mucinous metaplasia and an early EMBLT may be arbitrary.

Unusual Hormonal Changes

Endometriotic tissue usually exhibits striking progestational changes (Fig. 17.32) during pregnancy or progestin therapy. In such cases, examination reveals a decidual reaction with atrophy of the endometrial glands, which are small and lined by cuboidal or flattened epithelial cells (Fig. 17.32a). In pregnancy the glands can rarely exhibit an Arias–Stella reaction (Fig. 17.32b), optically clear nuclei, or both.[223,315] Necrosis of the decidual cells, foci of marked stromal edema, and infiltration by lymphocytes are additional findings in patients receiving progestational agents. Inactive or atrophic changes similar to those that are seen typically in the endometriotic foci of postmenopausal patients may be present in premenopausal patients treated with oral contraceptives, danazol, antiprogesterone steroids (gestrinone), and some progestins.[76,78,230] Additionally, endometriotic foci often disappear or are replaced by fibrous tissue after danazol therapy.

a

b

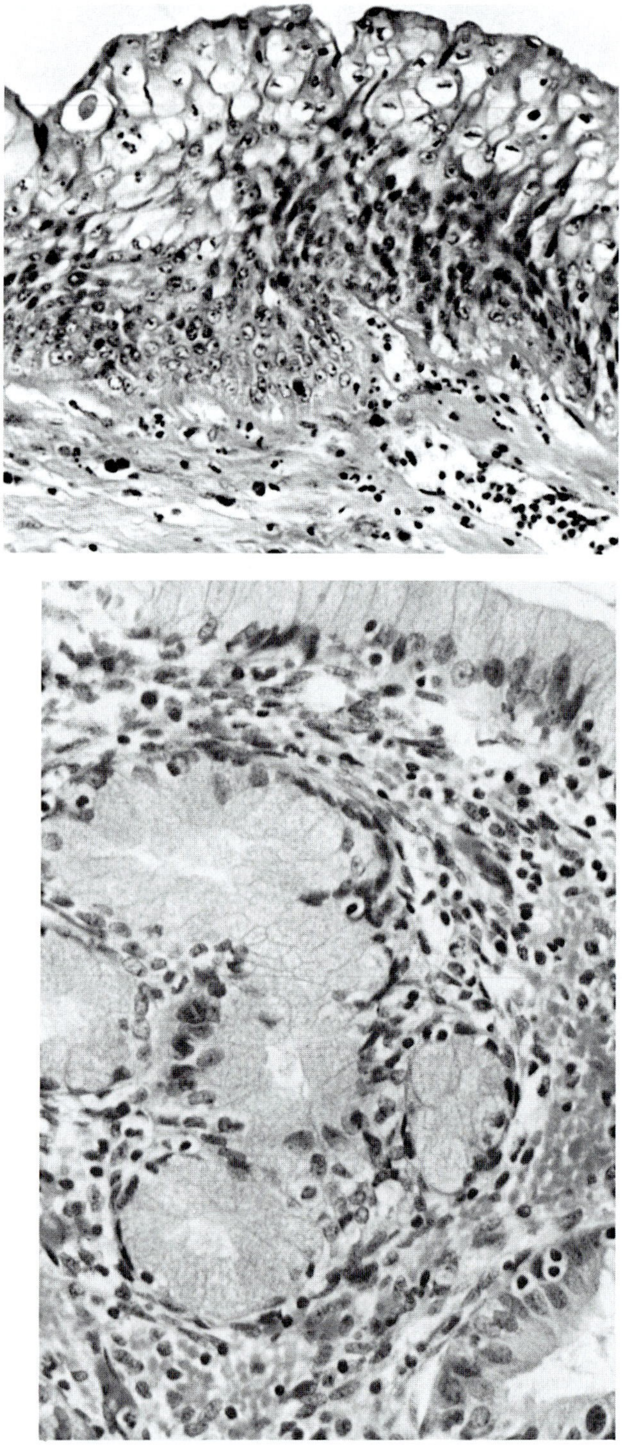

Fig. 17.31. Glandular metaplasia in endometriosis. a: Squamous metaplasia in the lining of an endometriotic cyst. **b**: Mucinous metaplasia of endometriotic glands.

Hyperplastic Glandular Changes

A variety of hyperplastic and atypically hyperplastic changes similar to those occurring in the endometrium have been described in endometriotic

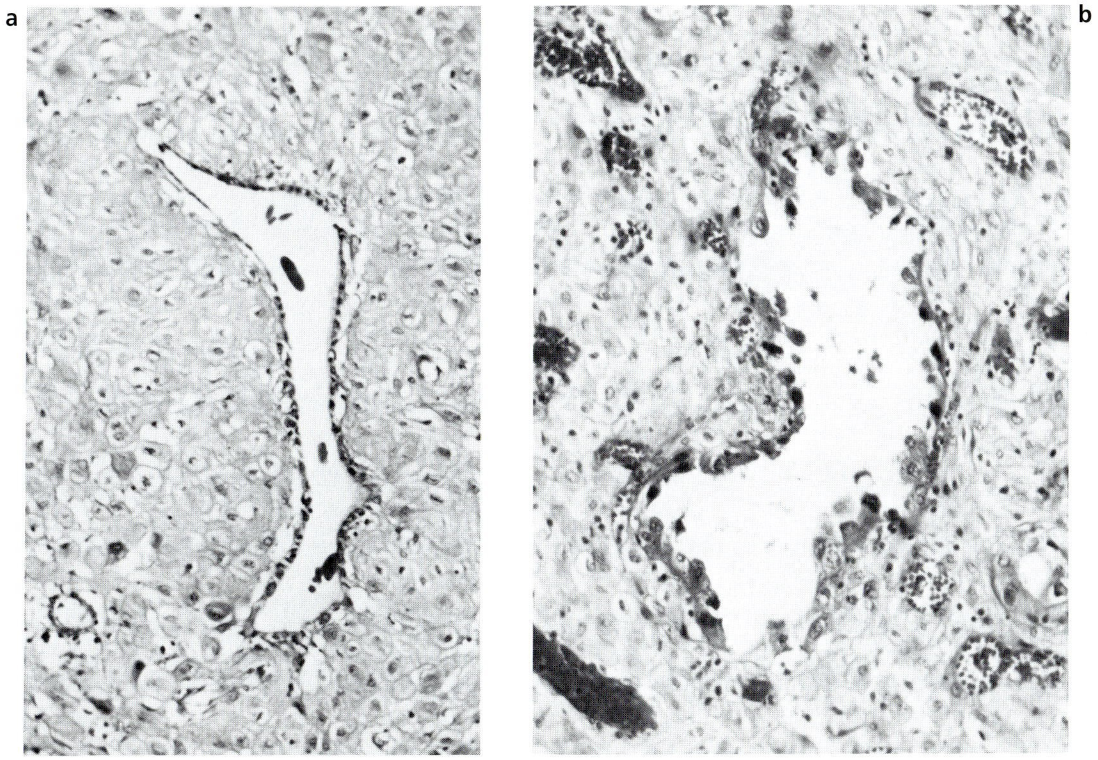

Fig. 17.32. Pregnancy-induced changes within endometriosis. a: The endometriosis gland is atrophic, and the stroma exhibits marked decidual transformation. b: The endometriotic gland exhibits an Arias–Stella reaction. The stroma is decidualized.

glands, sometimes related to an endogenous or exogenous estrogenic stimulus (Fig. 17.33)[80,82,117,163,289,359] or tamoxifen therapy.[37,294] Hyperplastic changes are particularly common in cases of polypoid endometriosis.[82] It is logical to conclude that such atypical changes have a malignant potential similar to those in the endometrium, and indeed, rare cases of hyperplastic endometriosis have preceded the development of an adenocarcinoma in the same area or have coexisted with carcinoma in the same specimen (Fig. 17.33; see also Fig. 17.50, later in this chapter).[180]

Stromal Changes

The endometriotic stroma may also undergo metaplasia, typically smooth muscle metaplasia, which is encountered most often within the walls of ovarian endometriotic cysts but occasionally elsewhere.[22,259,262,298] Extensive amounts of smooth muscle within the endometriotic stroma can result in "endomyometriosis" or uterus-like masses, which have been described within an obturator lymph node, the ovary, the small bowel, the broad ligament, and lumbosacral region, and in males, in the scrotum.[244,254,366] In some cases, a uterus-like mass in the region of the ovary may possibly represent a congenital malformation rather than an unusual manifestation of endometriosis.[277] Occasional cases of endometriosis can elicit a striking periglandular myxoid[60] (Fig. 17.34) or elastotic[66] response (Fig. 17.35), which in both situations can focally obliterate the endometriotic stroma. In one case, extensive myxoid change in endometriosis was misinterpreted at the time of frozen section as pseudomyxoma peritonei.[60]

Stromal Endometriosis

Rare cases of endometriosis are characterized by an absence or rarity of glands, so-called stromal endometriosis[66,71]; the same term was used in the older literature to refer to what is now designated low-grade endometrial stromal sarcoma. Stromal endometriosis is most commonly encountered in the ovary, where it is typically an incidental microscopic finding within the ovarian stroma ("benign stromatosis").[149] There is usually no associated pelvic endometriosis, and the process likely represents a metaplastic response of the ovarian stromal cells. A disproportionate number of cases of stromal endometriosis are seen within the superficial stroma of the uterine cervix (see page 759).[71] Rarely, endometriosis involving the pelvic peritoneum can take the form of multiple small nodules of en-

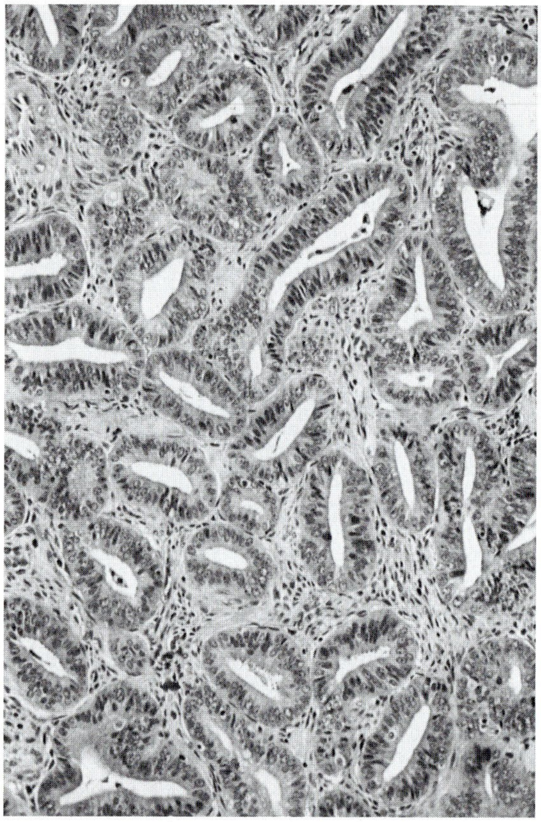

Fig. 17.33. Hyperplasia within endometriosis. Endometriotic glands exhibit architectural and cytologic atypia. Endometrioid carcinoma was found elsewhere in the specimen (see Fig. 17.50).

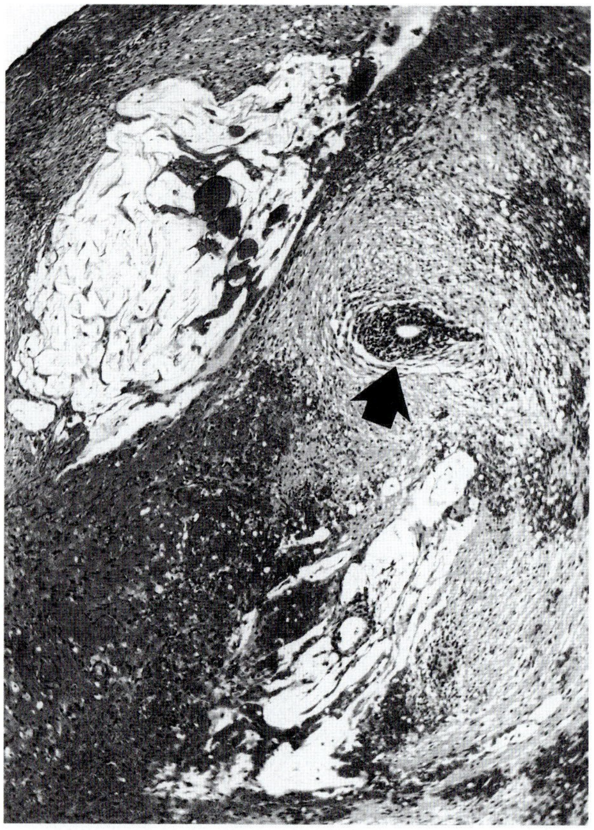

Fig. 17.34. Endometriosis with prominent myxoid stroma. A small endometriotic gland with a periglandular rim of endometriotic stroma (*arrow*) is surrounded by loose fibrous tissue and pools of acellular mucin. This appearance was misinterpreted as pseudomyxoma peritonei on frozen section examination.

dometriotic stroma in which endometriotic glands are absent or rare, a finding that we refer to as micronodular stromal endometriosis.[66] (Fig. 17.36).

Necrotic Pseudoxanthomatous Nodules

Occasionally ovarian and extraovarian endometriosis takes the form of "necrotic pseudoxanthomatous nodules," which typically occur in postmenopausal women.[69] Multiple nodules can be attached to the peritoneum or, less commonly, lie free in the peritoneal cavity. When associated with enlargement of one or both ovaries, the intraoperative findings can mimic those of carcinoma with peritoneal spread. The nodules are characterized by a central zone of necrosis surrounded by pseudoxanthoma cells, often in a palisaded arrangement, hyalinized fibrous tissue, or both (Fig. 17.37). Typical endometriotic glands and stroma are sparse or absent within the nodules and their immediate vicinity, but foci of recognizable endometriosis are usually present in the ovaries. The typical postmenopausal age group of the patient and the appearance of the nodules suggest that they represent end-stage or burned-out foci of endometriosis that should be distinguished from other necrotic peritoneal and ovarian granulomas, as well as necrotic tumor, on histologic examination.

Rare Miscellaneous Findings

Rare examples of endometriosis have been encountered in intimate association with foci of peritoneal leiomyomatosis,[144] glial implants of ovarian teratomas, and nodules of splenosis. Perineural[280] and vascular invasion can occur rarely in otherwise typical, benign endometriotic lesions, findings that may incorrectly suggest the diagnosis of malignancy.

Liesegang rings are eosinophilic, acellular, ringlike structures composed of periodic precipitation zones from colloidal solutions that are supersaturated in vitro or in vivo. They are typically encountered within necrotic, inflamed, or fibrotic tissues and have been found on microscopic examination within endometriotic cysts (Fig. 17.38). These structures have been confused with, and should be dis-

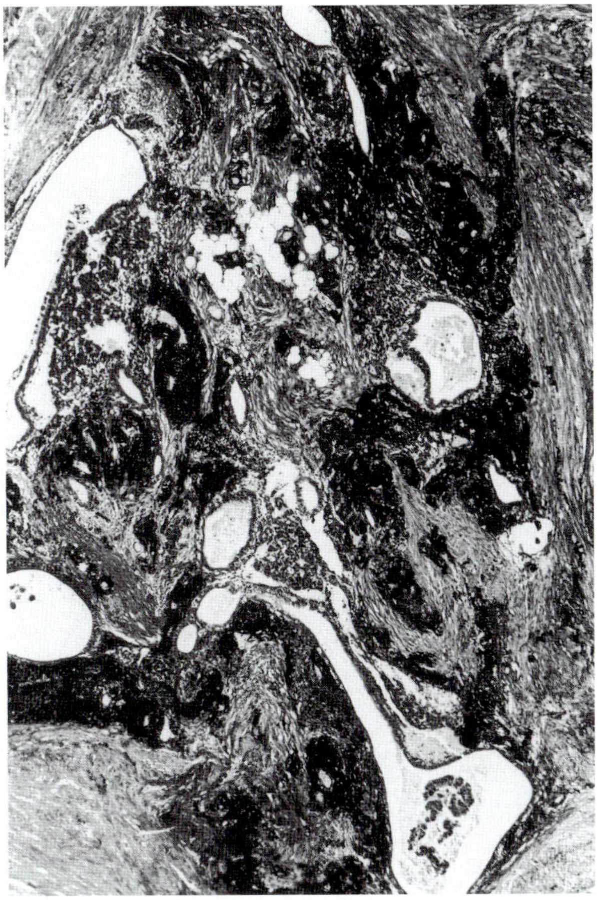

Fig. 17.35. Endometriosis with prominent elastotic stroma. Large masses of elastic tissue replace the normal endometriotic stroma. Elastic tissue stain.

tinguished from, parasites and foreign material on histologic examination.[70]

Microscopic examination of the fallopian tubes in patients with endometriosis has revealed nonspecific chronic salpingitis in as many as one-third of cases.[81] A less common lesion, so-called pseudoxanthomatous salpingitis or pseudoxanthomatous salpingiosis, characterized by infiltration of the tubal mucosa by pseudoxanthoma cells, is almost always been associated with pelvic endometriosis.[58,69,81,303]

Ultrastructural, Histochemical, and Steroid Receptor Studies

Endometriotic glands typically exhibit ultrastructural features that represent a response, but an incomplete one, to the prevailing hormonal milieu of the particular phase of the menstrual cycle. In contrast to eutopic endometrial glands, it is usually not possible to date the glands precisely within the secretory phase because of marked interglandular and intraglandular variability. Ultrastructural examination of endometriotic tissue following danazol treatment shows either arrest of the endometriotic glandular epithelium in the early proliferative phase or disorganization of the epithelial cells with atrophic changes.

Estrogen (ER) and progesterone receptors (PR) are present in endometriotic glands and stroma but usually in lower concentrations than in eutopic endometrium.[23,26,39,156] In a variable number of cases, one or both receptors are absent.[26] Moreover, the normal variation in the quantitity of both receptors exhibited by eutopic endometrium during the menstrual cycle is diminished or absent within foci of endometriosis.[24,188] Differences in receptor concentrations between eutopic endometrium and endometriotic epithelium in response to danazol have also been noted. No correlation has been found between receptor levels and severity of symptoms.

In summary, the findings of these studies are consistent with the incomplete and variable hormonal response of endometriotic foci observed on microscopic examination. They indicate a greater degree of autonomy of endometriotic tissue from the mechanisms controlling eutopic endometrium and may explain the failure of hormonal therapy in some patients.[217]

Differential Diagnosis

Endometriosis may also be accompanied by, and should be distinguished from, endosalpingiosis, which is characterized by glands lined by benign tubal-type epithelium, unassociated with endometrial stroma or the usual histiocytic inflammatory reaction of endometriosis (see "Endosalpingiosis"). A misdiagnosis of endosalpingiosis or, if in the ovary, an epithelial inclusion gland (see Chapter 16, Nonneoplastic Lesions of the Ovary) is likely when the endometriotic stroma is sparse or obscured by hemorrhage (see Fig. 17.26).

Necrotic pseudoxanthomatous nodules should be distinguished from other ovarian and peritoneal necrotic nodules, such as infectious granulomas and isolated palisading granulomas of the ovary (see Chapter 16), and as noted earlier, peritoneal granulomas related to diathermy.[56] Such lesions, in addition to having characteristic features, lack the numerous pseudoxanthoma cells that are typical of endometriotic lesions.

Rare low-grade endometrial stromal sarcomas (ESSs) contain numerous benign-appearing or atypical endometrial glands, to the extent that confusion with endometriosis may occur.[62] Indeed, it is likely that at least some cases referred to as aggressive endometriosis are examples of ESS with prominent glandular differentiation.[62] These tumors, however,

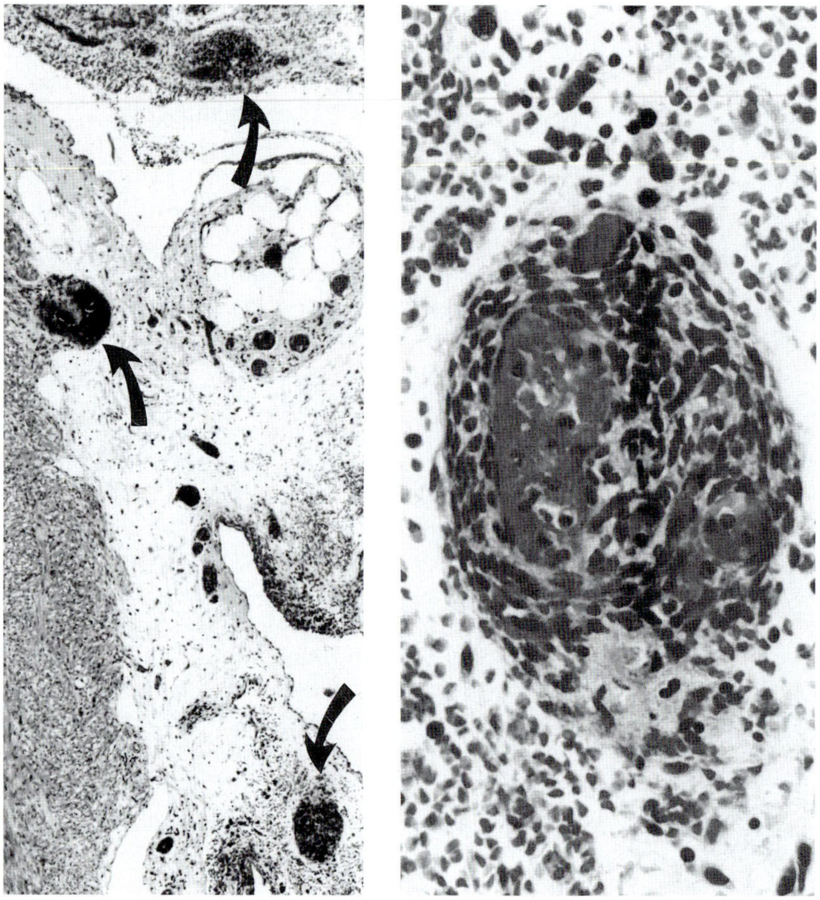

Fig. 17.36. Micronodular stromal endometriosis involving the appendiceal serosa. *Left*: Three stromal nodules are indicated by *arrows*. *Right*: High-power view of one nodule.

in contrast to typical endometriosis, contain foci of more typical ESS devoid of glands, and in some cases, prominent mitotic activity of the stromal cells, sex-cord-like elements, and prominent vascular invasion.

A diagnosis of adenosarcoma was initially considered in some cases of polypoid endometriosis. Adenosarcomas, in contrast to polypoid endometriosis, are characterized by a stromal component that usually exhibits dense periglandular cellularity, atypia (albeit mild in many cases), intraglandular papillae, and increased mitotic activity.

Cervical and Vaginal Endometriosis

Superficial *endometriosis of the uterine cervix* is more common than is generally appreciated.[13,71,120,234,342,353,357] It was documented in 2.4% of patients attending a colposcopic clinic in one study[342] but may occur in as many as 15% of patients who have had extensive cervical trauma, such as electocautery.[120] The prediliction for sites of trauma and the usual absence of associated pelvic endometriosis suggest implantation as the most likely pathogenetic mechanism. The condition may be an incidental finding in an asymptomatic patient or be associated with premenstrual or postcoital spotting or menorrhagia. The solitary or multiple lesions typically involve the ectocervix; endocervical lesions have been described only rarely.[357] The endometriotic foci appear as friable, ecchymotic streaks, patches, nodules, or cysts measuring from 1 mm to 2 cm in diameter. Rare lesions have been puckered secondary to fibrosis within the lesion, or papillary, simulating a carcinoma.[357] In patients who have had a recent cone biopsy or extensive cautery, the entire transformation zone may be involved.[154] Before menses, the lesions typically enlarge and change from bright red to blue; during menses they may rupture, leaving an irregular ulcer. Because a punch biopsy may yield nondiagnostic tissue due to the size of the lesion (which is frequently small), tissue crushing, and fragmentation, aspiration cytology may be useful in establishing the diagnosis.[342]

On histologic examination, the endometriotic fo-

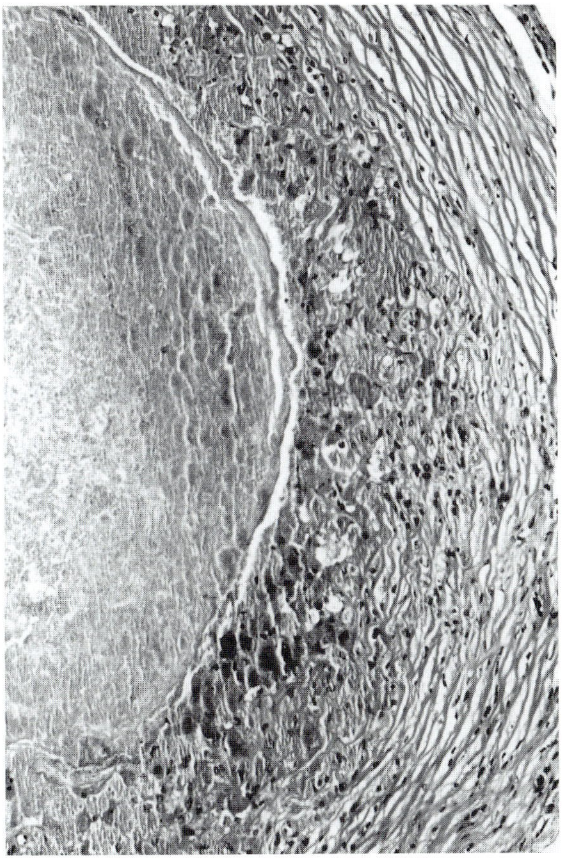

Fig. 17.37. Necrotic pseudoxanthomatous nodule of endometriosis. A central area of necrosis is surrounded by pseudoxanthoma cells and an outer zone of fibrous tissue.

cus is usually confined to the superficial lamina propria (Fig. 17.39). The diagnosis can be missed when the endometriotic stromal component is sparse or obscured by edema, hemorrhage, or inflammatory cells.[13] In such cases, the endometriotic glands, particularly when they show atypia or mitotic activity, can be misinterpreted as endocervical glandular dysplasia, adenocarcinoma in situ, or even invasive adenocarcinoma (Fig. 17.40). As previously noted, only endometrial stroma (stromal endometriosis) is found in occasional cases of superficial cervical endometriosis, even after serial sectioning (Fig. 17.41).[71]

In contrast to superficial cervical endometriosis, deep cervical endometriosis is usually an extension of cul-de-sac involvement in association with more widespread pelvic endometriosis. It may be palpable as deep, firm nodules or cysts in the posterior wall of the cervix.[120,334,357] The diagnosis is made by biopsy or pathologic examination of the hysterectomy specimen. The differential diagnosis in-

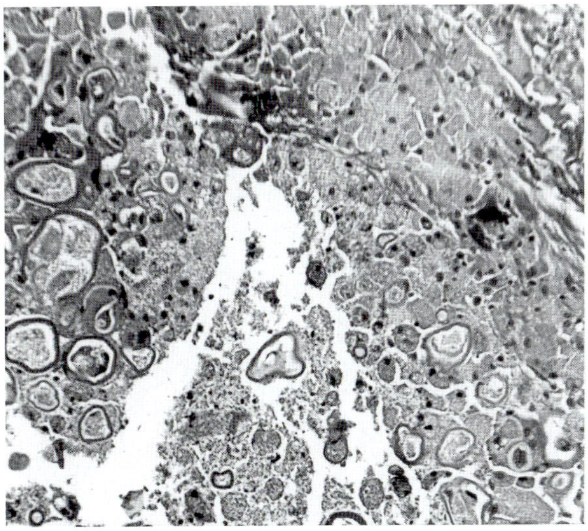

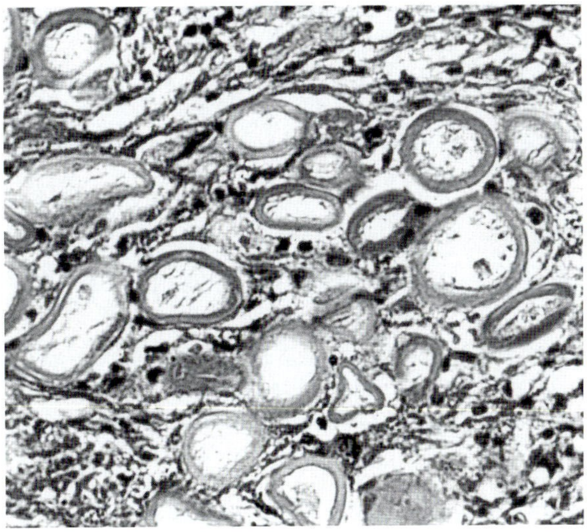

Fig. 17.38. Rare example of endometriosis. Liesang rings in an endometriotic cyst at low- and high-power magnifications.

cludes downgrowth of adenomyosis from the uterine corpus.

Superficial vaginal endometriosis, which typically involves the vault, is rarer than cervical endometriosis but is similar to the latter macroscopically, both in its predilection for involving sites of prior trauma and in its lack of associated pelvic endometriosis.[120] Deep vaginal endometriosis is more common, is typically associated with pelvic endometriosis, and appears as nodular or polypoid masses involving the posterior vaginal fornix.[120,234] The differential diagnosis of vaginal endometriosis, particularly of the superficial type, includes vaginal adenosis of the tuboendometrial variety; the latter, however, lacks endometrial stroma and the characteristic inflammatory response of endometriosis.

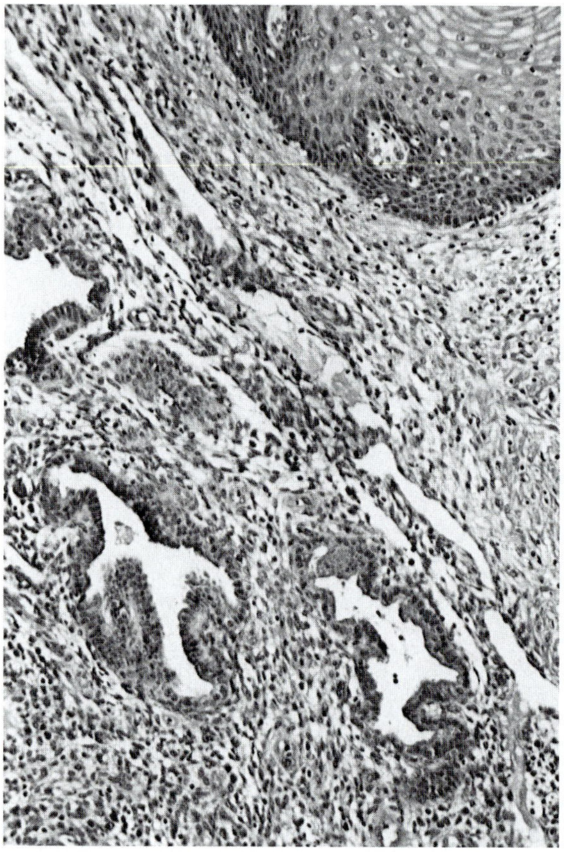

Fig. 17.39. Superficial cervical endometriosis. Endometrial glands (exhibiting secretory changes) and surrounding stroma lie beneath squamous epithelium.

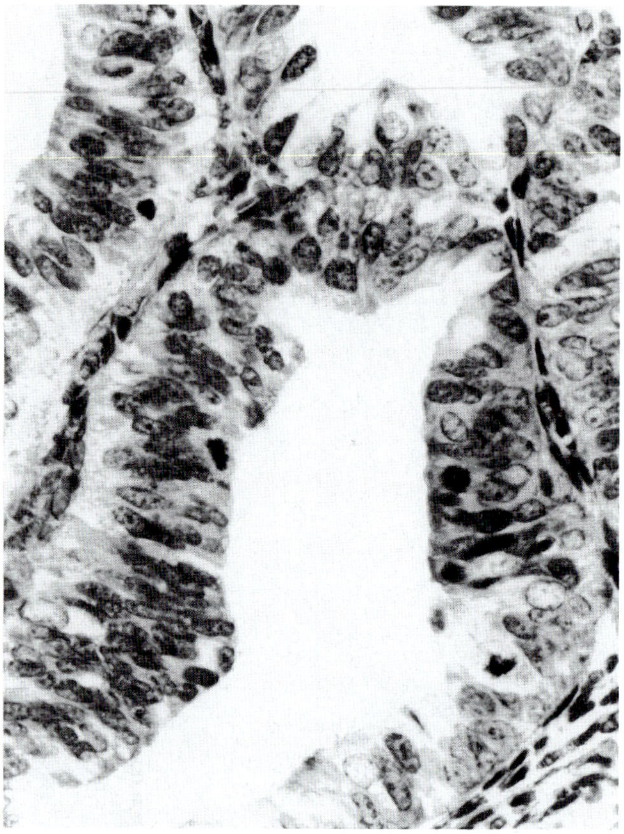

Fig. 17.40. Superficial endometriosis of the uterine cervix. The endometriotic glands show cellular stratification and mitotic figures. If the scanty endometriotic stroma (which is barely perceptible in the *lower right corner*) had not been appreciated, these glands may have been misinterpreted as endocervical glandular dysplasia or adenocarcinoma in situ. (Reproduced by permission of Baker et al., ref. 13.)

Endometriosis of the vulva is discussed in a subsequent section (see "Cutaneous Endometriosis").

Tubal Endometriosis

The term *endometriosis* has been applied to at least three different unrelated lesions of the fallopian tube. The most common type is *serosal or subserosal endometriosis*, typically associated with endometriosis elsewhere in the pelvis; the myosalpinx is usually not involved.[305]

Endometrial tissue may extend directly from the uterine cornu and replace the mucosa of the interstitial and isthmic portions of the tube in as many as 25% and 10% of women in the general population, respectively.[193,282] This finding is considered to represent a normal morphologic variation, although in some cases the ectopic endometrial tissue may give rise to intratubal polyps.[86] In occasional cases, the endometrial tissue may occlude the tubal lumen, that is, *intraluminal endometriosis* ("endometrial colonization") (Fig. 17.42); involvement may be bilateral.[55,92,113] Intraluminal endometriosis is typically unassociated with endometriosis elsewhere. The disorder accounts for 15%–20% of tubal-related infertility; it may also be associated with tubal pregnancy.

The third type of endometriosis involving the fallopian tube has been designated *postsalpingectomy endometriosis*. It occurs in the tip of the proximal tubal stump, typically 1 to 4 years following tubal ligation.[272,321] It is closely related to, and may be associated with, salpingitis isthmica nodosa. The lesion is analagous to uterine adenomyosis, consisting of endometrial glands and stroma extending from the endosalpinx into the myosalpinx and frequently to the serosal surface. Hysterosalpingography or India ink injection of the specimen may show tuboperitoneal fistulous tracts (Fig. 17.43); postligation pregnancies are a rare complication. Postsalpingectomy endometriosis has been documented in 20%–50% of tubes examined following ligation.

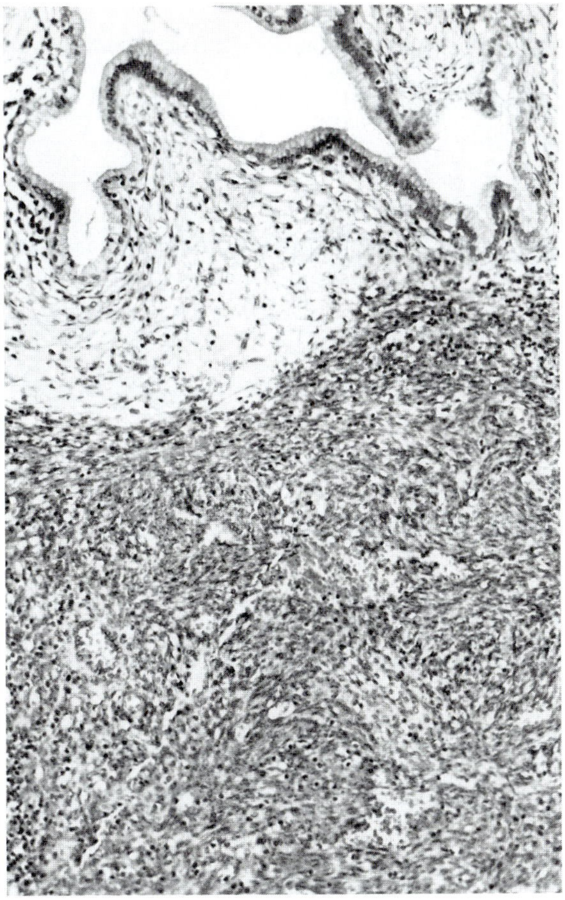

Fig. 17.41. Stromal endometriosis of uterine cervix. A cellular sheet of endometriotic stroma lies adjacent to an endocervical gland. (Reprinted by permission of Clement, ref. 58.)

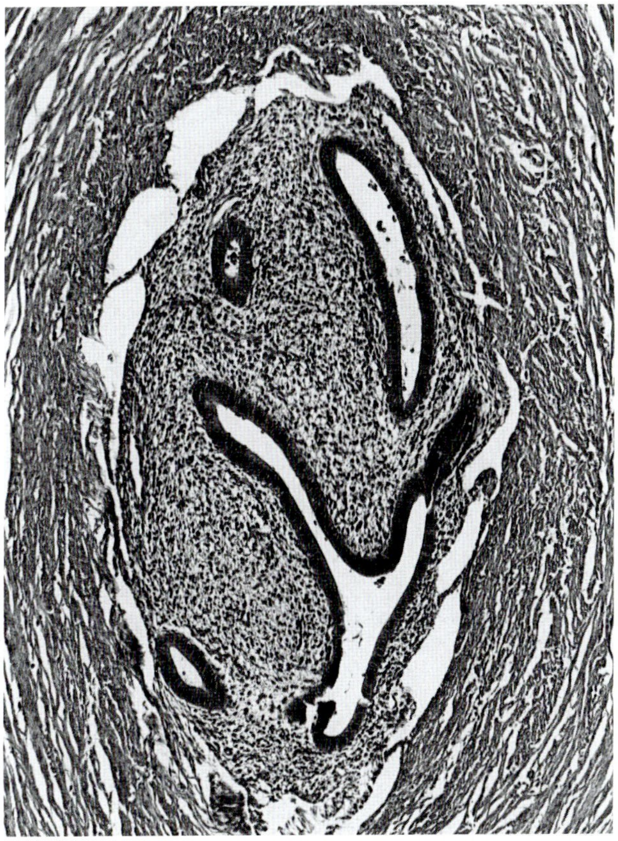

Fig. 17.42. Endometriosis (colonization) of the fallopian tube. The tubal lumen is occluded by endometrial glands and stroma. Spaces at the junction of endometrial tissue and myosalpinx represent dilated lymphatic channels.

The frequency of this complication is increased with the electrocautery method of ligation, with short proximal stumps, and with increasing postligation intervals.

Intestinal Endometriosis

Intestinal involvement has been documented in as many as 37% of patients with endometriosis undergoing laparotomy,[354] although the average frequency appears to be approximately 12%. In the majority of such cases, the involvement is confined to the serosa or subserosa and is unassociated with clinical manifestations referable to the intestinal tract. In contrast, from 0.7% to 2.5% of patients with endometriosis require bowel resection for symptomatic lesions.[258] In some series, as many as half the patients with symptomatic intestinal endometriosis have no extraintestinal involvement; the endometriotic nature of the intestinal lesions in such cases is more likely to be unrecognized preoperatively or at the time of laparotomy. Misdiagnosis is also common in postmenopausal patients because of a decreased index of suspicion, even though the intestine is one of the more common sites of clinically significant endometriosis in this age group.[168] As many as 7% of patients with symptomatic intestinal endometriosis are postmenopausal.

Intestinal sites of involvement include, in descending order of frequency, the rectum and sigmoid, the appendix, the terminal ileum, the cecum, and other parts of the large and small bowel, including Meckel's diverticulum.[58] In one large study,[258] 15% of patients had more than one site of involvement. The presenting symptoms include, alone or in combination, acute or chronic abdominal pain, diarrhea, constipation, hematochezia, and decrease in stool caliber. Although the frequent catamenial nature of the symptoms may suggest the correct diagnosis, the clinical presentation can mimic acute appendicitis, bowel obstruction due to adhesions or a hernia, a neoplasm, or even inflammatory bowel disease. En-

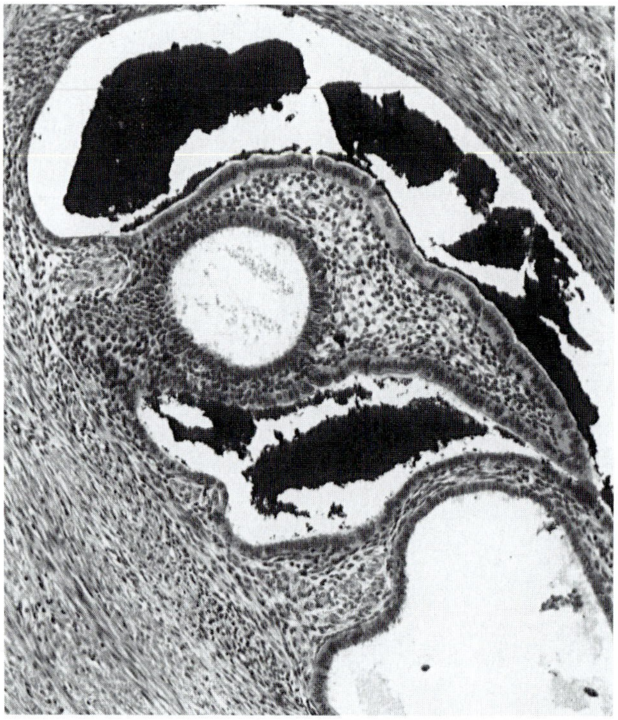

Fig. 17.43. Postsalpingectomy endometriosis of the fallopian tube. After removal, the lumen of the specimen has been injected with India ink. Endometrial glands and stroma are surrounded by smooth muscle of the myosalpinx. The lumens of the endometrial glands contain India ink. (From Rock JA, Parmley TH, King TM, Laufe LE, Su BC (1981) Endometriosis and the development of tuboperitoneal fistulas after tubal ligation. Fertil Steril 35:16. Reproduced by permission of the publisher, The American Fertility Society.)

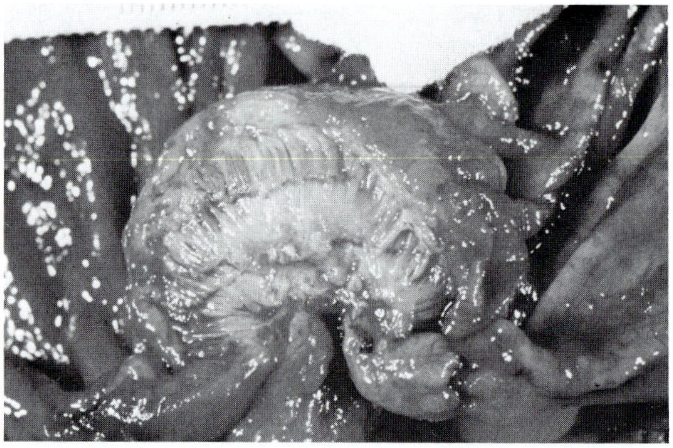

Fig. 17.44. Colonic endometriosis (cut surface). There is marked mural thickening and fibrosis. The serosal surface is retracted, and the overlying mucosa is intact. (Courtesy of R.D. Croom, M.D.)

doscopic and radiographic studies typically demonstrate an extramucosal stenosing lesion; endoscopic biopsies are usually of no diagnostic value.

Endometriosis of the rectosigmoid area is usually a solitary lesion, involving a segment several centimeters in length, whereas ileal involvement is frequently multifocal and may involve segments of bowel up to 45 cm in length.[58,103,194] On gross examination, the segment of bowel is indurated and often angulated by a poorly defined, usually noncircumferential mass; the serosal surface may be puckered and covered by adhesions. Sectioning typically reveals a firm, gray-white, solid, mural mass, the bulk of which represents markedly thickened muscularis propria; the latter often has a radiating fanlike appearance (Fig. 17.44). Small cystic spaces containing altered blood may be seen but are uncommon. In contrast to a primary adenocarcinoma, the overlying mucosa is usually intact, despite the high frequency of symptomatic bleeding in some series of patients. However, rare cases of polypoid endometriosis have involved the intestinal mucosa; such lesions can grossly mimic an adenocarcinoma.[82] On microscopic examination of typical intestinal endometriosis, islands of endometriotic tissue are typically scattered throughout the hyperplastic muscularis propria, with or without involvement of other layers (Fig. 17.45).

A complication of intestinal endometriosis is perforation, which is usually associated with pregnancy; a marked decidual reaction is typically seen with the endometriotic stroma in such cases. Other complications include volvulus, intussusception, acute appendicitis, appendiceal mucocoele, intramural hematoma, and the development of a malignant neoplasm.[35,182,225,359]

Urinary Tract Endometriosis

Urinary tract involvement has been documented at laparotomy in from 16% to 20% of patients with endometriosis.[268,354] In most of these cases, the endometriosis is found on the serosa of the urinary bladder or that overlying the ureter and is without local clinical manifestations. Similarly, high-volume intravenous urography has demonstrated subtle, clinically insignificant abnormalities in 15% of women with proven pelvic endometriosis before therapy. In contrast, only 0.5%–1% of patients with endometriosis have clinically significant urinary tract involvement; approximately 30% of such patients ultimately require nephrectomy for a hydronephrotic or nonfunctioning kidney. Most reported cases of urinary tract endometriosis have involved the urinary bladder or the ureters (with approximately equal frequency); the kidneys and the urethra are involved much less commonly. Urinary tract involvement is usually associated with endometriosis elsewhere in the pelvis, although the

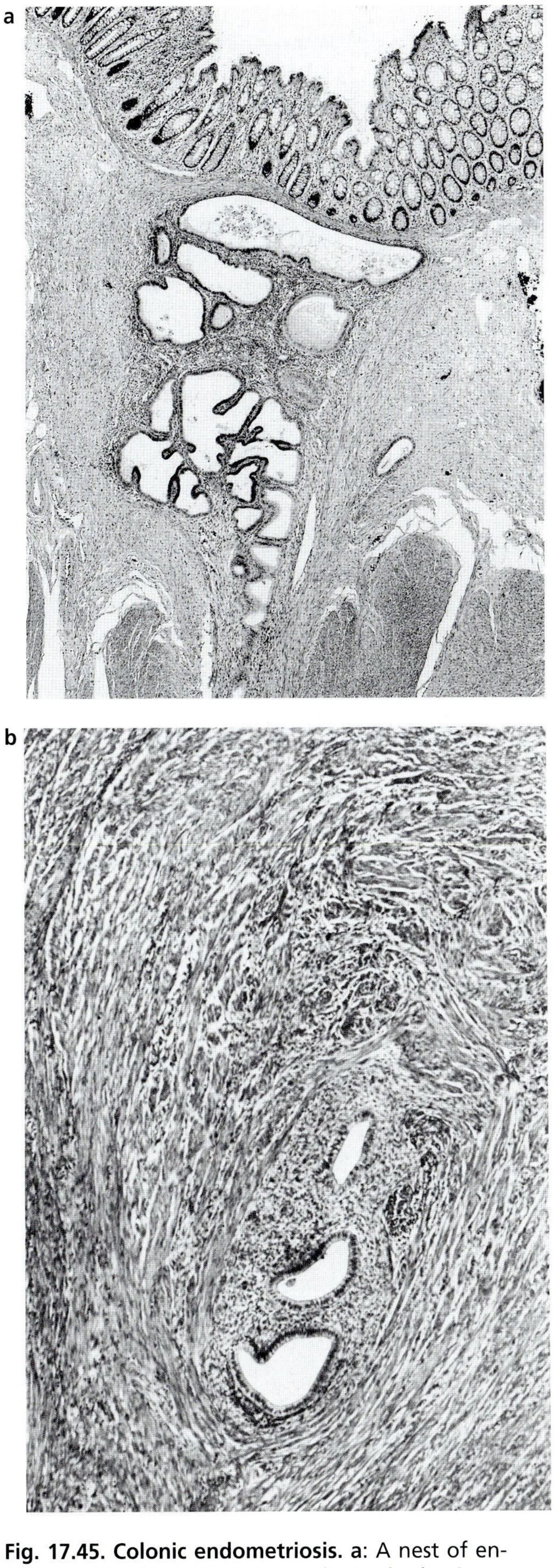

Fig. 17.45. **Colonic endometriosis.** a: A nest of endometriotic glands and stroma lie in the lamina propria. b: The endometriotic tissue within the muscularis is surrounded by hyperplastic smooth muscle.

symptoms relating to the urinary tract may be the initial or sole manifestations of the disease in such patients.[318] In some series, however, as many as half the patients with ureteral involvement have disease restricted to the ureter and the adjacent uterosacral ligament.[161] Patients with renal endometriosis typically do not have endometriosis elsewhere, suggesting an embolic, likely blood-borne, origin.

From one-third to one-half of the affected patients are over 40 years of age and almost 5% of the patients are postmenopausal, some of whom had received estrogen replacement therapy.[58,163] A preoperative diagnosis may be suspected by the catamenial nature of the symptoms, which include suprapubic or flank pain, frequency, urgency, dysuria, and hematuria; chills and fever secondary to a urinary tract infection have been the presenting symptoms in occasional cases. A tender suprapubic or flank mass may be palpable. Many patients, however, particularly those with ureteric involvement, have nonspecific manifestations or present with a silent obstructive uropathy, occasionally complicated by hypertension, renal failure (in cases of bilateral involvement), or both.[161,263,318] In patients with bladder involvement, urography may reveal a filling defect; a stricture in the lower ureter with hydroureter and hydronephrosis or a nonfunctioning kidney is the typical urographic finding in those with ureteral involvement. Endoscopy may confirm vesical or even ureteral involvement, and the lesions may exhibit catamenial enlargement, darkening, and bleeding. Endoscopy and biopsy, however, are often nondiagnostic.[318]

Symptomatic endometriosis of the bladder is almost always a result of mural involvement, and the lesions are typically located on the trigone, the floor of the bladder, or low on the posterior wall.[318] Involvement is rarely confined to the lateral walls, the dome, or the ureterovesical junction. Gross examination typically reveals a solitary, blue, red, gray, or brown multicystic mass that thickens the wall and sometimes projects into the bladder lumen (Fig. 17.46); the lesions have ranged from several millimeters to 14 cm in diameter. The mucosa is usually intact, but occasionally may be ulcerated and bleeding, particularly during menses. Histologic examination reveals fibrosis and proliferation of the muscularis around the foci of endometriosis; the lamina propria was also involved in 60% of the cases in one study.[318] Obstruction of both ureteric orifices, vesicolic fistula, and malignant transformation have been rare complications.

With rare exceptions, endometriosis of the ureter is confined to its lower one-third, usually involving a segment less than 2 cm in length that lies 2–5 cm from the ureterovesical junction; involvement has

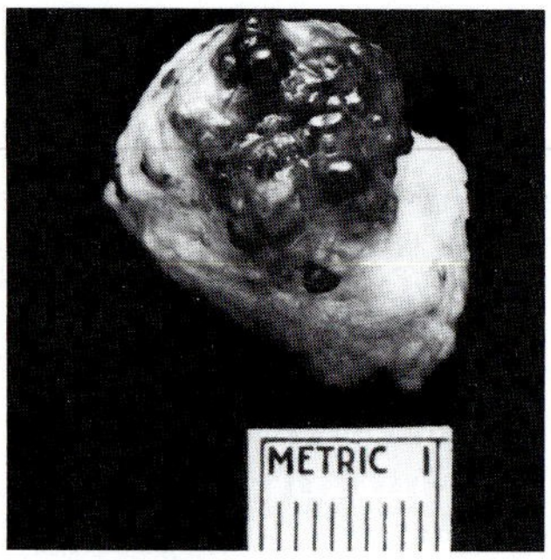

Fig. 17.46. Endometriosis of the bladder. The mucosal surface is replaced by a hemorrhagic, nodular lesion. (Reprinted by permission of Surgery, Gynecology & Obstetrics, ref. 512.)

been bilateral in approximately 10% of the cases.[197,318] Ureteral endometriosis has been traditionally divided into extrinsic and intrinsic forms, although this distinction has not been possible in many of the reported cases because the affected segment of ureter was not removed for microscopic examination. Also, it is likely that at least some intrinsic cases were initially of extrinsic type. In the latter, endometriosis of the uterosacral ligament or ureteral adventitia causes ureteral luminal narrowing by compression, fibrosis, or both; in some such cases, there is transmural scarring of the ureter. Intrinsic involvement is characterized by endometriotic tissue within a typically hyperplastic and fibrotic muscularis; in some cases, the lamina propria is also involved. Mucosal involvement rarely takes the form of a polypoid mass projecting into the lumen (Fig. 17.47).[163,225,318]

On gross examination, endometriosis of the kidney is typically a solitary, well-circumscribed, hemorrhagic, solid and cystic mass that focally replaces the renal parenchyma; the lesions in the 10 reported cases have measured from 1.5 cm to 13 cm in diameter.[58] In occasional cases, polypoid masses have projected into the renal pelvis. Foci of smooth muscle have been found admixed with the endometriotic tissue on microscopic examination in some of the cases.

Only two cases of urethral endometriosis have been described.[58] In one, a caruncle-like nodule projected from the urethral orifice in a 38-year-old woman with dysuria. In the other, a 24-year-old woman with dysuria and dyspareunia was found to have endometriosis in the wall of a large urethral diverticulum.[245]

Cutaneous Endometriosis

The majority of the reported cases of cutaneous endometriosis have occurred within surgical scars,[52,183,319,356] or rarely within needle tracts; the remainder are spontaneous. Both types are associated with pelvic endometriosis in only a minority of cases.[52,319] Because scar-related endometriosis typically occurs after operations on the uterus or fallopian tubes, the site most commonly involved is the lower abdominal wall; the umbilicus is involved less commonly. Similarly, most cases of endometriosis of the lower vagina, vulva, Bartholin's gland, perineum, and perianal region involve areas of obstetric or surgical trauma, most commonly episiotomy scars.[52,120,129,206,234,249,319] Scar-related cases occur less commonly after nongynecologic procedures, such as an appendectomy or inguinal hernia repair.[319] Spontaneous cutaneous endometriosis typically involves the umbilicus[220,319,332] and, less commonly, the inguinal[319] and perianal regions.[222]

The most common symptoms are those relating to a cutaneous mass or nodule that, in the scar-related cases, appears weeks to years following surgery; the average postoperative interval in one study

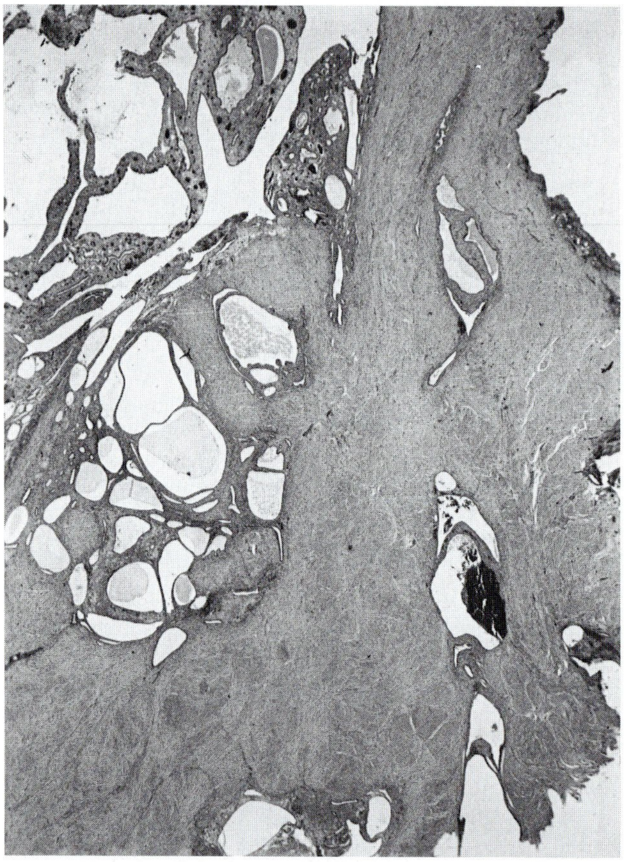

Fig. 17.47. Polypoid endometriosis of the ureter. The endometriosis involves the wall of the ureter and forms a polypoid mass projecting into its lumen (*top left*). (Reprinted by permission of Mostoufizadeh and Scully, ref. 225.)

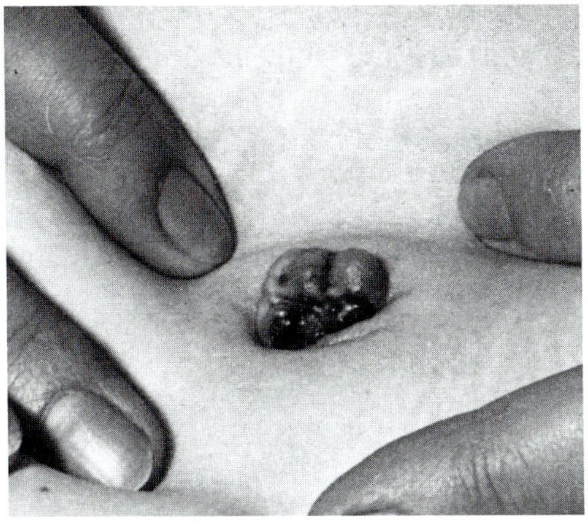

Fig. 17.48. Cutaneous endometriosis. A hemorrhagic, polypoid mass involves the umbilicus. (Reprinted by permission of Steck and Helwig, ref. 319.)

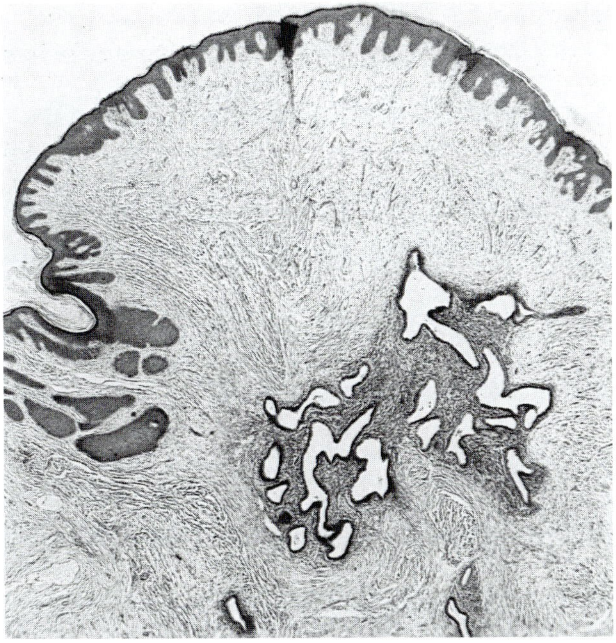

Fig. 17.49. Cutaneous endometriosis. Endometriotic foci are present within the dermis. (Reprinted by permission of Steck and Helwig, ref. 319.)

was 30 months.[319] A catamenial increase in size and tenderness, and occasionally bleeding from the lesion, suggest the diagnosis. Patients with perianal lesions may have involvement of the external sphincter producing anorectal pain and irritation simulating an anal fistula, abscess, or thrombosed hemorrhoid. Umbilical endometriosis may simulate an umbilical hernia on physical examination.[220] The lesions occasionally recur following excision.

On clinical examination, the lesions are firm, solitary nodules, varying up to 6 cm in diameter, and pink to brown to blue-black depending on the age of the lesion and the depth within the skin (Fig. 17.48). The cut surface of the scar-related lesions is typically gray-white, with or without focal areas of recent or old hemorrhage.[52] On microscopic examination, the endometriosis may involve the dermis (Fig. 17.49), the subcutis, or both[319] and, in occasional cases, underlying skeletal muscle.[142] There is typically no continuity between the cutaneous and peritoneal lesions in patients with associated pelvic endometriosis.

The association of abdominal scar-related endometriosis and episotomy scar-related endometriosis with uterine operations and episiotomies, respectively, suggests implantation of endometrial tissue as the most likely pathogenesis. The risk of implantation appears to be much higher after hysterotomy than after cesarean section or vaginal delivery, suggesting that the decidua of late pregnancy has a reduced ability to implant. When curettage is performed immediately after vaginal term delivery, however, the frequency of endometriosis in the episiotomy scar becomes much higher.[249] In nonpregnant patients, implantation of endometrium during endometrial curettage or spontaneous implantation of menstrual endometrium has also been implicated in occasional cases of scar-related endometriosis. Lymphatics have been demonstrated between the pelvis and umbilicus that may explain cases of spontaneous endometriosis in the latter site.

Inguinal Endometriosis

Noncutaneous *inguinal endometriosis*, secondary to involvement of the extraperitoneal portion of the round ligament, occurs in less than 1% of patients with endometriosis.[43,57,251] The usual presentation is that of a painful, typically right-sided, hernia-like inguinal mass, with catamenial exacerbation in some cases. In approximately one-third of the reported cases, an inguinal hernia was also present.[57] The lesion can impinge on the pubic tubercle and mimic arthritis, bursitis, or tendinitis.[251] Rarely, endometriosis in the inguinal region has also been described in inguinal or femoral hernia sacs or the canal of Nuck.[261,264] In one case of femoral hernial involvement, the adventitia of the femoral vein was involved and its lumen was thrombosed.[264]

Endometriosis of Lymph Nodes

Lymph node involvement by endometriosis is uncommon, and many examples reported as such, particularly in the older literature, are lymph nodes involved by benign müllerian (usually endosalpingiotic) glands devoid of an endometrial stromal component. The involved lymph nodes may be visibly or palpably enlarged at operation. On microscopic examination, in contrast to glandular inclusions, endometriotic foci are characterized by a more central location within the node, an endometrial stromal component, and the frequent presence of erythrocytes and pseudoxanthoma cells. Endosalpingiosis and endometriosis may coexist, however, in the same lymph node. As in other sites, decidual transformation of the endometriotic stroma has been encountered during pregnancy. As previously noted, one case of intranodal endomyometriosis has been reported.

Pleuropulmonary Endometriosis

Pathologically documented cases of endometriosis involving the lungs or pleura are rare. Some reported examples interpreted as *pulmonary endometriosis* have taken the form of microscopic foci of "decidua" found at autopsy in pregnant or recently pregnant women. Most such lesions would likely be interpreted by current criteria as foci of embolic intermediate trophoblast, although one case of bona fide deciduosis of the lung has been recently documented.[110] Many cases of purported pleuropulmonary endometriosis have been diagnosed solely on the basis of clinical manifestations or in conjunction with nonspecific histologic or cytologic findings. Coverage here is based on the 38 pathologically documented cases of thoracic endometriosis in the literature, 21 of which were pleural and 17 of which were parenchymal.[58,110]

The affected patients are usually in the reproductive age group, although rare patients are postmenopausal. The clinical manifestations of pleural endometriosis usually differ from those associated with parenchymal involvement. In the former, the characteristic presentation is one of recurrent catamenial shortness of breath related to catamenial pneumothorax, typically right sided. Less common presentations include recurrent right-sided, typically hemorrhagic effusions, hemoptysis, or catamenial pain. Chest X-rays usually reveal a pneumothorax, or occasionally, a hemothorax, pleural effusion, or a pleural lesion. Coexistent intraabdominal endometriosis has been demonstrated in approximately one-third of cases, although in another one-third of cases, its presence or absence was not confirmed. In contrast, patients with parenchymal endometriosis typically present with catamenial hemoptysis or blood-tinged cough; other patients are asymptomatic and the lesion is an incidental radiographic finding. Chest X-ray typically shows a nodule, infiltrates, or opacification of an entire lobe.[110] Only one patient has had documented peritoneal endometriosis, although in most patients the peritoneum has not been visualized. The majority of patients with parenchymal endometriosis have had prior uterine operations.

Pleural endometriosis is almost invariably confined to the right side; one case with bilateral involvement has been reported. The lesions are typically multiple, dark red or blue nodules or cysts on the diaphragmatic pleura; parietal, visceral, and pericardial pleural surfaces are also affected less commonly. Associated pathologic changes have included diaphragmatic fenestrations in 50% of the cases and occasionally pleural blebs. Parenchymal endometriotic lesions are typically solitary, tan to gray, focally hemorrhagic nodules or thin-walled cysts measuring up to 6 cm in diameter. Several lesions have been subpleural or have involved bronchial walls and lumina. Parenchymal lesions lack the almost exclusively right-sided location of pleural endometriosis; one case had a bilateral miliary distribution. In additional contrast to pleural lesions, associated diaphragmatic fenestrations have not been described.

The clinicopathologic differences between pleural and parenchymal endometriosis of the lung suggest that they differ in their histogenesis. The distribution of the parenchymal lesions and their strong association with prior uterine trauma strongly suggest an embolic origin. In contrast, most if not all pleural lesions are likely a result of passage of endometriotic tissue from the peritoneal cavity through diaphragmatic defects or diaphragmatic lymphatics, consistent with the right-sided predominance of both structures. The catamenial pneumothorax in these patients, and in those with catamenial pneumothorax unassociated with pleural endometriosis, may be related to the diaphragmatic defects that allow passage of air from the peritoneal into the pleural cavity. The escape of air from defects in the visceral pleura produced by the endometriotic lesions or from preexistent blebs is another possible explanation for the pneumothorax in these patients. It has been suggested that prostaglandins produced by eutopic endometrium or endometriotic tissue at the time of the menses may predispose to alveolar rupture.

Soft Tissue and Skeletal Endometriosis

Rarely, typical endometriomas have occurred in skeletal muscle or deep soft tissues in distant sites. The presentation is usually that of a mass associated with catamenial pain, tenderness, and enlargement. The involved sites have included the trapezius, extensor carpi radialis, thumb, biceps femoris, thigh, and the knee.[58,123,248] A unique endometrioma occurred in the breast of a patient with a 2-year history of catamenial bloody nipple discharge.[224] Rare pelvic endometriotic cysts have eroded lumbar vertebrae, causing catamenial lumbar pain.

Upper Abdominal Endometriosis

Endometriotic implants may occasionally occur on the omentum; omental endometriosis was only one-eighth as common as omental endosalpingiosis in one study.[368] Rarely, endometriotic implants may involve the peritoneal surfaces of the liver or diaphragm. As with pleural diaphragmatic involvement, implants on the peritoneal side of the diaphragm have occasionally been associated with diaphragmatic defects and catamenial pneumothorax. Rare endometriomas of the epigastrium, the tail of the pancreas,[130,200] and the liver parenchyma[109,281] have been reported.

Endometriosis of the Nervous System

Approximately 20 cases of endometriosis of the sciatic nerve sheath at the level of the sciatic notch have been described, typically associated with catamenial sciatica.[336] Some cases have been associated with a visible peritoneal evagination attached to the involved portion of the nerve ("pocket sign"). A case of subarachnoid endometriosis of the lumbar spinal cord caused catamenial radicular pain and recurrent subarachnoid hemorrhage.[195] In another case, a cerebral endometrioma was discovered in the parietal lobe of a patient who had a 3-year history of episodic headaches that culminated in a generalized seizure.[330]

Endometriosis in Males

Rare examples of endometriosis have been described in men receiving long-term estrogen therapy for prostatic carcinoma. With the exception of one case involving the abominal wall,[204] the sites of involvement have been confined to the genitourinary tract, specifically the urinary bladder, prostate, and paratesticular region.[19,58,297,366] The two paratesticular lesions were endomyometriotic in composition.

Neoplasms Arising from Endometriosis

A malignant tumor has been documented to arise in from 0.3% to 0.8% of cases of ovarian endometriosis, but the exact incidence of cancer originating in pelvic endometriosis is unknown because in many cases tumor arising in endometriosis may obliterate the latter or the endometriosis may not be sampled microscopically.[35,225] Approximately 75% of tumors complicating endometriosis arise within the ovary. The most common extraovarian site is the rectovaginal septum; less frequent sites include the vagina, colon and rectum,[359] urinary bladder, and other sites in the pelvis and abdomen. In some cases, there is a history of prolonged unopposed estrogen replacement therapy.[35,359] As previously noted, hyperplastic and metaplastic changes within endometriosis may precede or be found synchronously with the neoplasm. Tumors arising in endometriosis in unusual sites are more likely to be misdiagnosed than similar tumors arising in ovarian endometriosis, such as an endometrioid adenocarcinoma arising in colonic endometriosis being mistaken for a primary colonic adenocarcinoma, an error that could result in inappropriate staging and treatment.[359]

Endometrioid carcinoma (Fig. 17.50) is the most common tumor arising within endometriosis, accounting for almost 70% of such cases. Direct origin of endometrioid carcinoma from endometriotic tissue has been demonstrated in as many as 24% of cases in some series.[225] At least 90% of the carcinomas arising from extraovarian endometriosis have been of endometrioid type.[35,225] Rarely, endometrioid tumors arising in ovarian and extraovarian endometriosis may exhibit a benign or borderline adenofibromatous pattern.[299,359]

Clear cell carcinoma (Figs. 17.51 and 17.52) is the second most common tumor originating in endometriosis, accounting for approximately 14% of such cases. In some studies, the frequency of endometriosis coexisting with clear cell carcinoma of the ovary is even higher than with endometrioid carcinoma; pelvic endometriosis has been reported in 24%–49% of cases of ovarian clear cell carcinoma.[284,335] A few examples of clear cell carcinoma arising within extraovarian endometriosis have also been described.[4,142]

Rare epithelial tumors of other types arising from endometriosis include ovarian serous cystadenomas of low malignant potential,[359] benign and malignant mucinous tumors,[285,286,299] and squamous cell carcinomas.[187,228] Endometrioid stromal sarcomas (ESSs), malignant mesodermal mixed tumors, and adenosarcomas (Fig. 17.53) account for approximately 10% and 20% of tumors arising in ovarian and extraovarian endometriosis, respectively.[54,61,152,308,359,364] In one study, 60% of ESSs apparently arising within the ovary were associated with ovarian endometriosis.[364] Two examples of

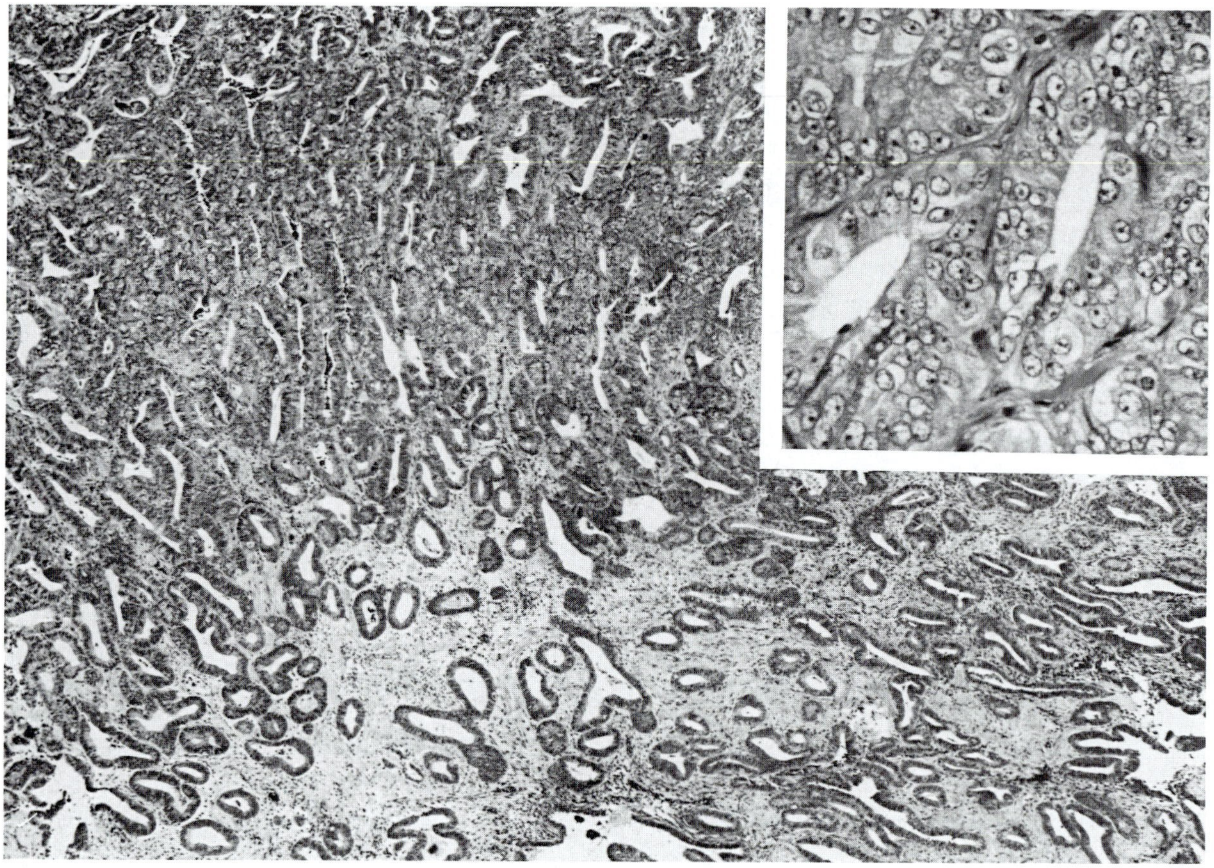

Fig. 17.50. Endometrioid carcinoma arising within endometriosis. Benign endometriotic glands and stroma merge with the carcinomatous glands. *Inset*: High-power view of carcinomatous glands.

yolk sac tumor have arisen in association with endometriosis,[182,287] and in one unique case, a sex cord tumor with annular tubules was intimately associated with endometriosis of the tubal serosa.[131]

Peritoneal Endometrioid Lesions Other Than Endometriosis

Benign glands lined by endometrial epithelium (but lacking endometrial stroma) with the peritoneal distribution of endosalpingiosis occasionally occur[185]; some may represent foci of endometriosis in which the stromal component has undergone atrophy. Benign endometrioid peritoneal "implants" lacking an endometrial stromal component have also been reported in association with a borderline ovarian endometrioid tumor.[284] The peritoneal lesions were interpreted as having arisen directly from the peritoneum.

A variety of extrauterine, extraovarian, pelvic, or retroperitoneal neoplasms of endometrioid type occur in the absence of demonstrable endometriosis. These tumors have generally been considered to arise directly from the mesothelium or submesothelial stroma. They have included endometrioid cystadenofibroma[134,243] and cystadenocarcinoma, endometrioid stromal sarcoma,[340] homologous and heterologous types of malignant mesodermal mixed tumor,[119,317] and mesodermal adenosarcoma.[71]

Endosalpingiosis

Clinical Findings

Endosalpingiosis typically refers to the presence of benign glands lined by tubal-type epithelium involving the peritoneum and subperitoneal tissues; the term may also be used to refer to similar glands within retroperitoneal lymph nodes (see "Benign Intranodal Glands of Müllerian Type"). This disorder occurs almost exclusively in females, typically during their reproductive years, with a mean age of 29.7 years in one study,[368] although occasional cases have been described in postmenopausal women. Endosalpingiosis is almost always an incidental finding either at the time of operation or more commonly on microscopic examination. Zinsser and

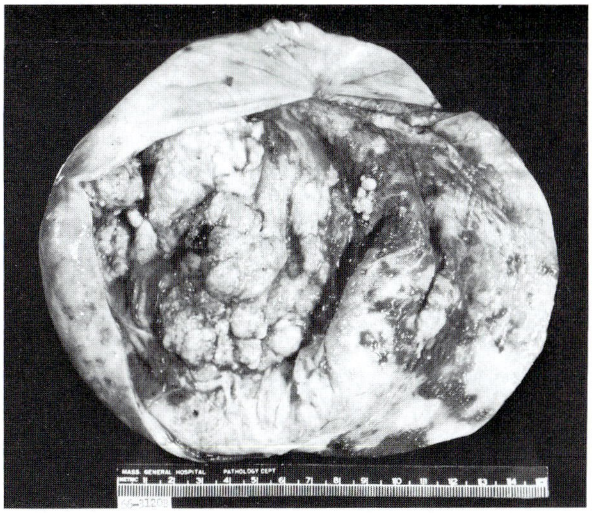

Fig. 17.51. Clear cell carcinoma arising within an endometriotic cyst. Fleshy pale tumor nodules protrude into the cyst lumen. (Reprinted by permission of Scully et al., ref. 299.)

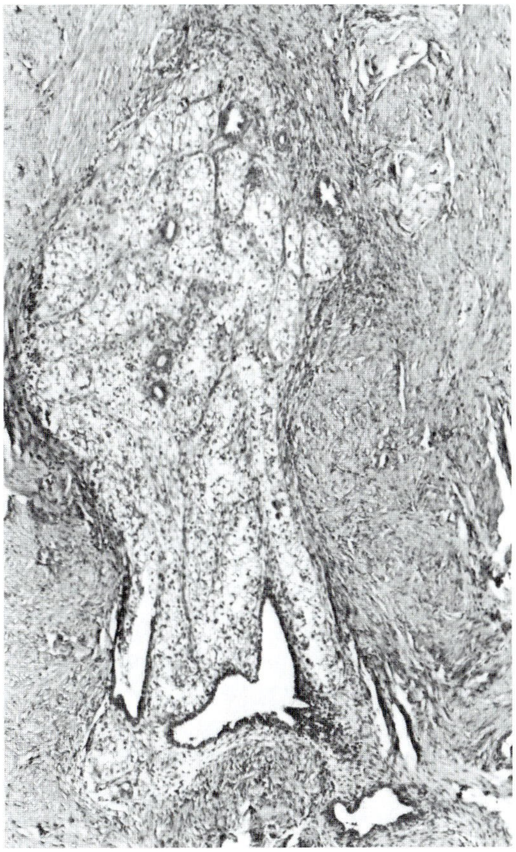

Fig. 17.52. Clear cell carcinoma arising within endometriosis. Benign endometriotic glands and stroma (*bottom*) merge with clear cell carcinoma. (Courtesy of A.B.P. Ng, M.D.)

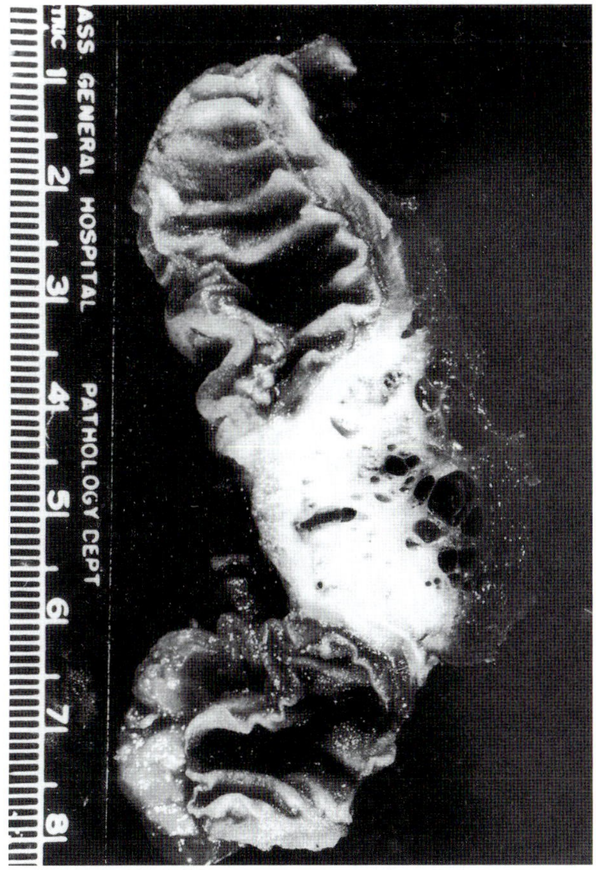

Fig. 17.53. Müllerian adenosarcoma arising in endometriosis of the small bowel. The sectioned surface is solid and cystic with focal hemorrhage. (Reprinted by permission of Yantiss et al., ref. 359).

Wheeler found endosalpingiosis in 12.5% of surgically removed omenta in a retrospective study, but this figure doubled when omenta were examined more thoroughly in a prospective study.[368] Endosalpingiosis may be detected as multiple fine pelvic calcifications on X-ray examination or as psammoma bodies within cul-de-sac fluid,[170] peritoneal washings,[309,313,314] the lumen of the fallopian tube, or cervical Papanicolaou smears.[169]

An origin from the secondary müllerian system is favored by most investigators, but the association of endosalpingiosis with chronic salpingitis implicates implantation of sloughed tubal epithelium as a possible histogenetic mechanism in some cases.[368] A similar association with serous tumors of borderline malignancy suggests that some endosalpingiotic foci may represent tumor implants that have undergone maturation.[212] Endosalpingiosis in the absence of residual tumor at the time of second-look laparotomy in patients with ovarian epithelial neoplasms does not justify additional treatment.[75]

Pathologic Findings

Endosalpingiosis is most commonly encountered on the pelvic peritoneum covering the uterus, fallopian tubes, ovaries, and cul-de-sac.[211,314] Less frequent sites include the pelvic parietal peritoneum, omentum,[211,368] bladder and bowel serosa,[41] paraaortic area,[306] and skin, including laparotomy scars. Endosalpingiosis is usually inapparent at the time of operation or on gross inspection of the involved tissues but may be visible as multiple, punctate (1–2 mm), white to yellow, opaque or translucent, fluid-filled cysts, which impart a vesicular or granular appearance to the involved surface; rarely larger cysts may be seen.[65] Rare examples of cystic endosalpingiosis have involved the wall of the uterus, resulting in grossly apparent transmural cysts.[65]

Microscopic examination reveals multiple, simple glands, often cystically dilated and lined by a single layer of epithelium resembling that of the normal fallopian tube (Figs. 17.54 and 17.55). The glands are frequently surrounded by a loose or dense connective tissue stroma that may contain a sparse mononuclear inflammatory cell infiltrate. The glands may exhibit irregular contours, crowding, and intraluminal stromal papillae. The three cell types of the normal fallopian tube epithelium are found in varying numbers: pale ciliated cells, secretory cells, and dark rodlike, intercalated or "peg" cells. The cells have prominent luminal margins, distinct borders, and basal nuclei. Focal cellular pseudostratification may be present. The nuclei have fine chromatin and delicate nuclear membranes and typically lack significant atypia or mitotic activity. Psammoma bodies are frequently present within the lumens or in the adjacent stroma, and, in occasional cases, numerous psammoma bodies are embedded in subserosal connective tissue. Endosalpingiotic glands can rarely extend into the underlying tissues, such as the wall of the appendix[41] or, as noted earlier, the uterus.[65] Staining with the PAS method reveals a basement membrane surrounding each gland and PAS-positive, diastase-resistant material in the apices of the lining cells and within the glandular lumens. Estrogen and progesterone receptors have been identified immunohistochemically within the cells.

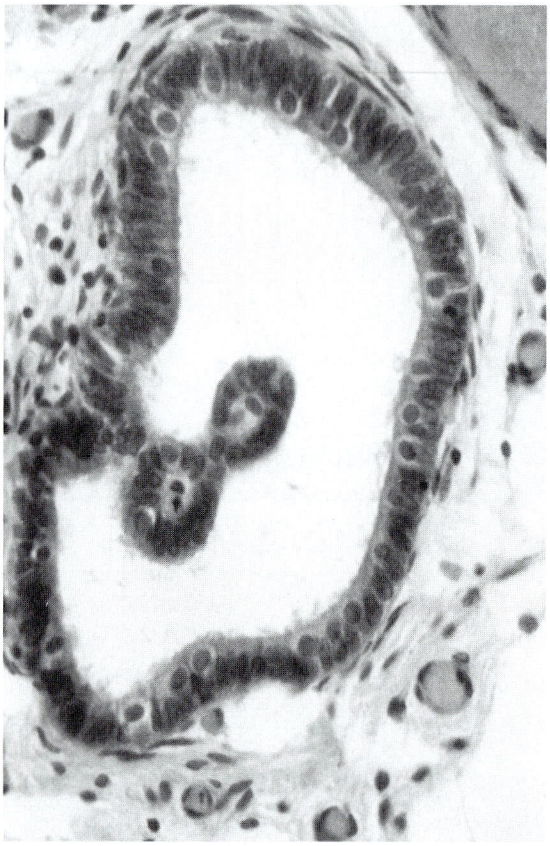

Fig. 17.55. Endosalpingiosis. A gland within the omentum is lined by benign endosalpingeal epithelium composed of multiple cell types.

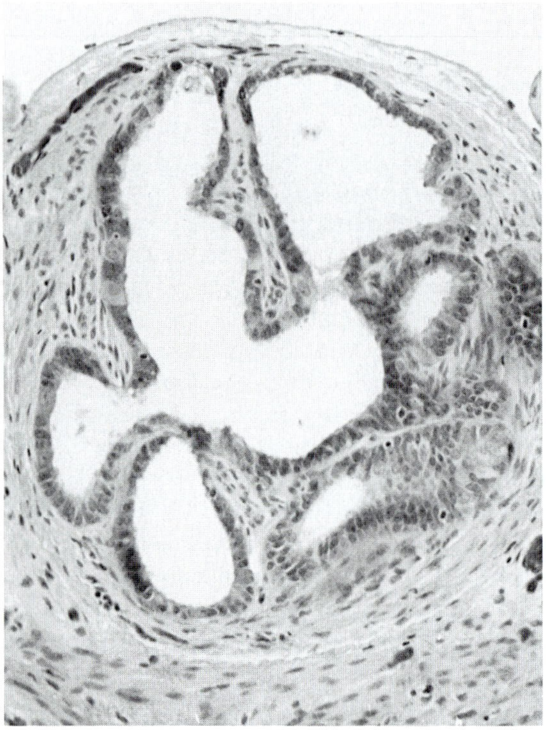

Fig. 17.54. Endosalpingiosis. Complex glandular structure lies beneath uterine serosa. Glands are lined by a single layer of benign endosalpingeal epithelium.

The term *atypical endosalpingiosis* has been applied to endosalpingiotic lesions in which there is cellular stratification, including cellular buds, cribriform patterns, and varying degrees of cellular atypia, occurring in the absence of a serous tumor of borderline malignancy. Such lesions merge histologically with peritoneal serous tumors of borderline malignancy (see next section). Bell and Scully use the latter term if the "lesions composed of tubal-type epithelium exhibit papillarity, tufting, or detachment of cell clusters . . . . even when they arise on a background of endosalpingiosis."[20] Endosalpingiotic glands should be differentiated from mesonephric remnants, which are common incidental microscopic findings in the region of the fallopian tube. Mesonephric tubules are typically located more deeply than endosalpingiosis and characteristically have a collar of smooth muscle under the epithelial lining, which is typically a single layer of nonciliated, low columnar to cuboidal cells.

Extraovarian Serous Tumors

The full spectrum of serous neoplasms arising within the ovary may also arise directly from the extraovarian peritoneum. These tumors are considered only briefly here because their clinicopathologic features closely resemble those of their ovarian counterparts. Primary peritoneal serous borderline tumors are usually associated with widespread extraovarian peritoneal involvement and normal-sized ovaries that are free of disease or which have serosal involvement similar to that involving the extraovarian peritoneum.[20,27] The most common presenting features in patients with these tumors, who are typically under the age of 35 years (range, 16–67), are infertility and chronic pelvic or abdominal pain. Many cases, however, are discovered incidentally at laparotomy for other conditions. At operation, focal or diffuse miliary granules, fibrous adhesions, or both involve the pelvic peritoneum and omentum and, less commonly, the abdominal peritoneum. Microscopic examination reveals superficial tumor that resembles noninvasive epithelial or desmoplastic implants of borderline serous tumors of ovarian origin. Coexistent endosalpingiosis has been found in 85% of cases.

Although most primary peritoneal serous carcinomas are high grade (see following paragraph), some have low-grade nuclear features and are distinguished from peritoneal serous borderline tumors by the presence of invasion. Low-grade peritoneal serous carcinomas (LGPSCs) resemble invasive implants of serous borderline tumors (Fig. 17.56)[348]; some may have a micropapillary pattern.[105] They lack high-grade nuclear atypia, invade tissue or lymphovascular spaces or both, and have appreciable solid epithelial proliferation. Peritoneal

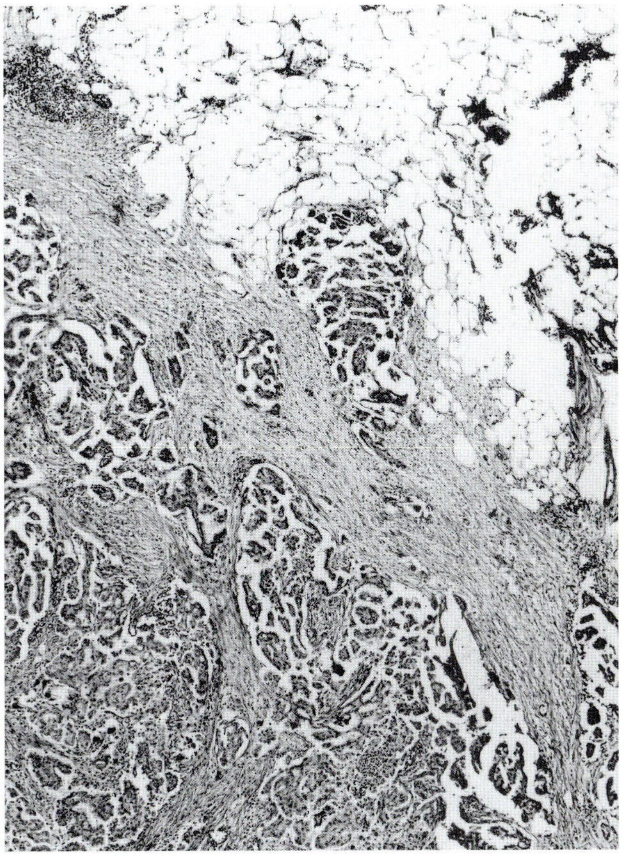

Fig. 17.56. Low-grade primary papillary serous carcinoma of the peritoneum. The tumor is infiltrating the omental fat.

psammocarcinomas[212,348] are a subtype of LGPSCs with psammoma bodies in most of the tumor nests and absent or rare solid epithelial proliferation (see Chapter 18, Surface Epithelial Tumors of the Ovary); lymphatic invasion is often conspicuous (Fig. 17.57). The average ages of patients in one study were 57 years (LGPSC of usual type) and 40 years (peritoneal psammocarcinomas).[348] Presenting features in both tumors are usually abdominal pain, mass, or both, but approximately 40% are incidental findings. Operative and gross findings vary from nodules to adhesions to a dominant mass. Short-term outcomes for LGPSCs and peritoneal psammocarcinomas are favorable, but follow-up is too limited in the reported cases to determine long-term outcomes. These tumors should be distinguished from peritoneal serous borderline tumors, which are very similar except for an absence of invasion. Adequate sampling is necessary to identify invasion, with highest yields of invasive foci in the omentum.

Typical *peritoneal serous carcinomas* have high-grade nuclear features and have been referred to

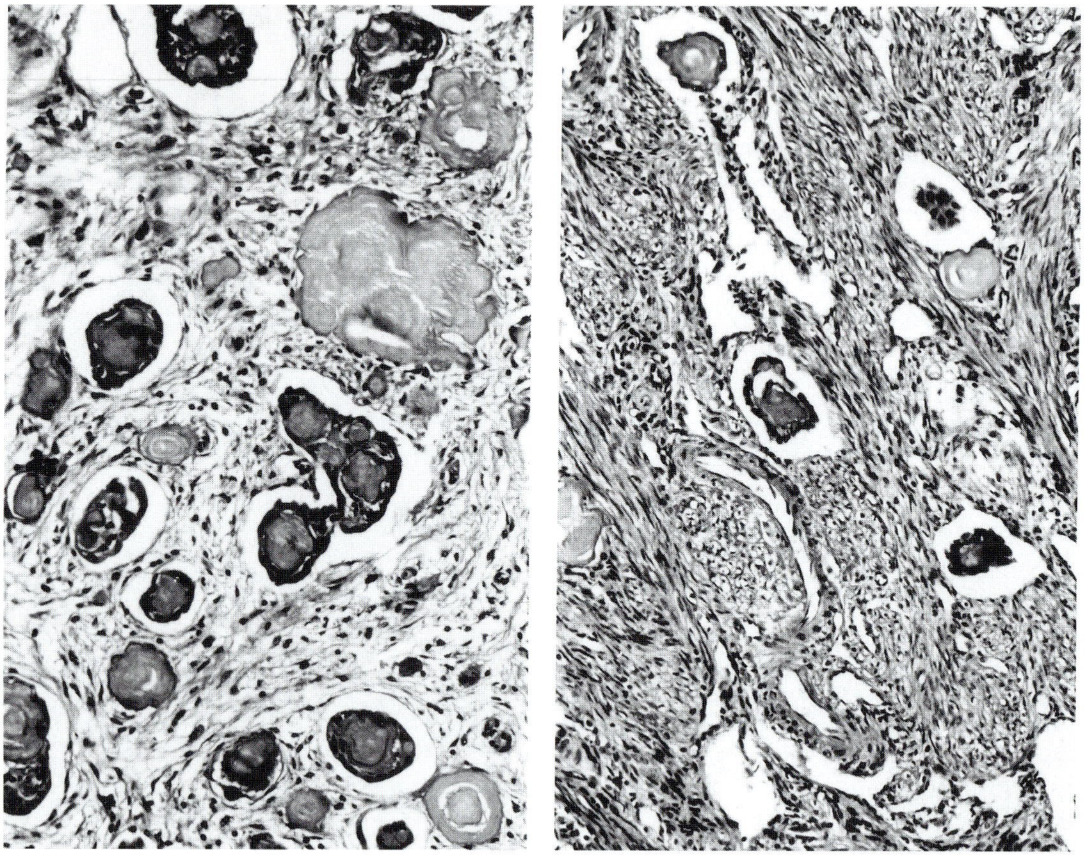

Fig. 17.57. Peritoneal psammocarcinoma. a: Numerous psammoma bodies, some of which are surrounded by a thin rim of neoplastic epithelial cells, lie within a demoplastic stroma. **b**: Tumor invades myometrial lymphatics. The patient was alive with no evidence of recurrent tumor 8 years after total abdominal hysterectomy and bilateral salpingo-oophorectomy. No adjuvant therapy was administered postoperatively.

as serous surface papillary carcinomas, serous papillary carcinomas of the peritoneum, or extra-ovarian peritoneal serous papillary carcinoma.[21,83,101,106,115,128,226,334,338,352] The typical intraoperative appearance of a primary peritoneal serous carcinoma, with widespread peritoneal tumor associated with ovaries of normal size, may mimic that of a diffuse malignant mesothelioma or peritoneal carcinomatosis associated with an unknown primary tumor. The ovaries are often involved by small surface "implants" but retain their normal size and shape. In some series, the patients have had an average age that is a decade older than patients with similar tumors of ovarian origin. Some tumors have occurred in women who had had bilateral oophorectomy performed as prophylactic treatment for familial ovarian cancer,[334] suggesting that some peritoneal serous carcinomas may be a phenotypic variant of familial ovarian cancer.[165]

Primary peritoneal serous carcinomas resemble their ovarian counterparts on microscopic and immunohistochemical examination; their distinction from malignant mesothelioma has been previously discussed. Criteria for their separation from primary ovarian serous carcinomas with peritoneal spread have been proposed by the Gynecologic Oncology Group: (1) both ovaries are either normal in size or enlarged by a benign process; (2) in the judgement of the surgeon and the pathologist, the bulk of the tumor is in the peritoneum and the extent of tumor involvement at one or more extraovarian sites is greater than on the surface of either ovary; (3) microscopic examination of the ovaries reveals no tumor, tumor confined to the surface epithelium with no evidence of cortical invasion, tumor involving the ovarian surface and the underlying cortical stroma but less than 5 mm in area, or tumor less than 5 mm in diameter within the ovarian substance, with or without surface involvement; and (4) the histologic and cytologic characteristics of the tumor are predominantly serous and similar or identical to those of ovarian serous papillary adenocarcinomas of any grade. In most series, these tumors have a prognosis similar to that of high-stage ovarian serous carcinomas with a similar volume of residual tumor and similar postoperative treatment.

Rare extraovarian serous tumors take the form of localized, typically cystic masses, usually within the broad ligament and less commonly within the retroperitoneum. Serous papillary cystadenomas and adenofibromas, serous borderline tumors, and serous carcinomas have been described in these sites.[8,9,341]

Endocervicosis

Benign glands of endocervical type involving the peritoneum, so-called *endocervicosis*, are rare, but examples involving the posterior uterine serosa, cul-de-sac, vaginal apex, outer wall of the uterine cervix, and the urinary bladder have been documented.[63,185,205,361a] In the last site, the lesions usually formed tumor-like masses that involved the posterior wall or posterior dome of the bladder in women of reproductive age. On microscopic examination, benign endocervical-type glands were located predominantly within the smooth muscle of the muscularis propria (Fig. 17.58).[63] In several cases, the infiltrative pattern of the glands, mild epithelial atypia, and a reactive periglandular stroma, alone or in combination, resulted in an initial misdiagnosis of well-differentiated adenocarcinoma.

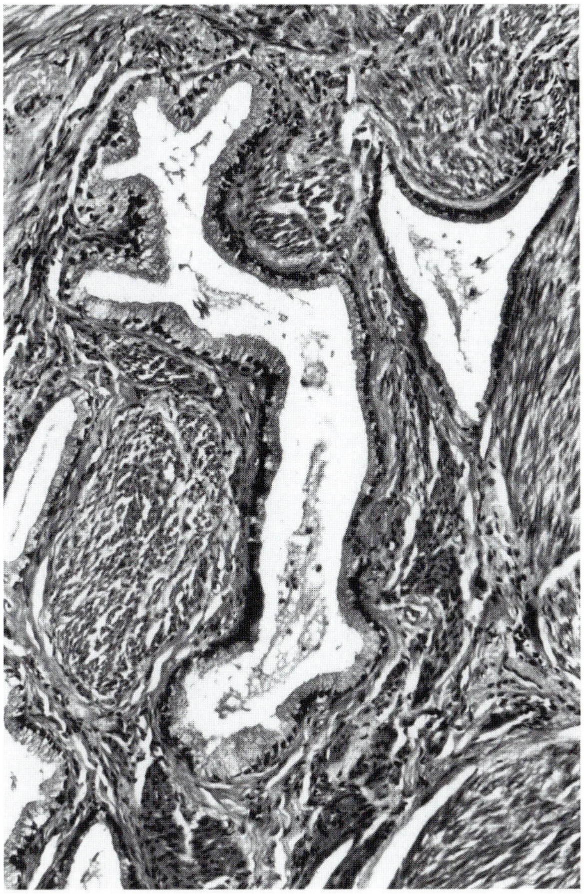

Fig. 17.58. Endocervicosis of urinary bladder. Benign endocervical-type glands lie within the muscularis propria.

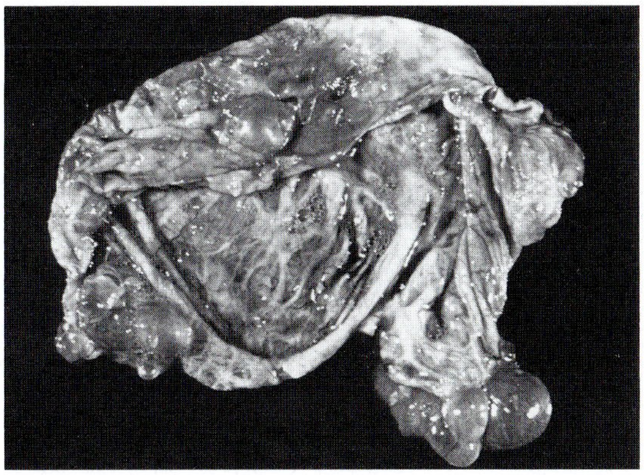

Fig. 17.59. Retroperitoneal mucinous tumor. The specimen has been opened to reveal multiple lobules with mucinous contents. (Courtesy of R.E. Scully, M.D., Boston, MA.)

Extraovarian Mucinous Tumors

Ovarian-type mucinous neoplasms, in the absence of a primary tumor within the ovary, have been described in extraovarian sites, typically in the retroperitoneum (Fig. 17.59)[14,95,185,189,247,250]; a single case has been described in the inguinal region.[324] These tumors form large cystic masses that on histologic examination resemble ovarian mucinous cystadenomas, borderline tumors, or cystadenocarcinomas (Fig. 17.60); some contain ovarian-type stroma in their walls. Although it is possible that some of these tumors originate within a supernumerary ovary, the great rarity of the latter, the absence of follicles or their derivatives within the ovarian-like stroma, and the rare occurrence of similar tumors in males strongly support a peritoneal origin. It has been recently suggested that, in some cases of pseudomyxoma peritonei associated with ovarian and appendiceal mucinous tumors, the peritoneal lesions may arise directly from the peritoneum as part of a multifocal neoplastic process.[302]

Peritoneal Transitional, Squamous, and Clear Cell Lesions

Nests of transitional (urothelial) epithelium referred to as Walthard nests are commonly present on the pelvic peritoneum in women of all ages, typically in-

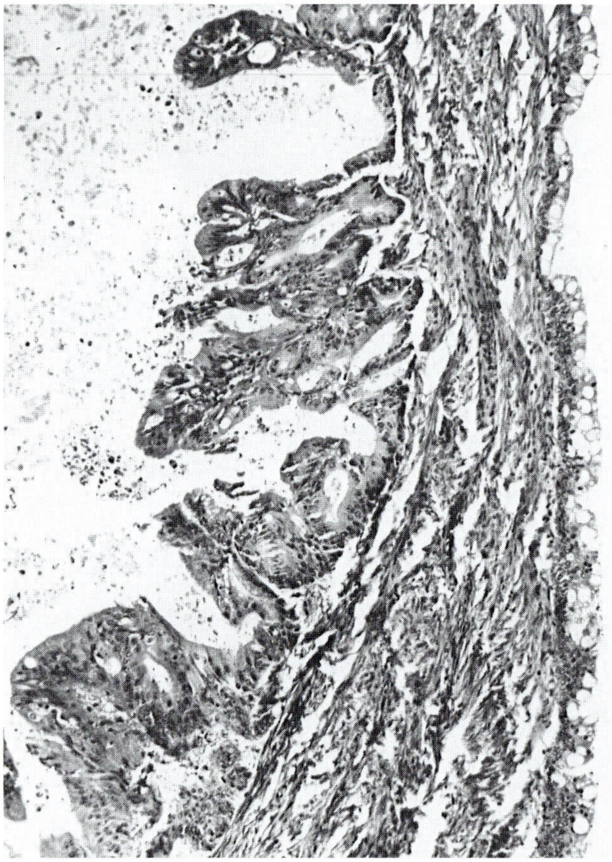

Fig. 17.60. Retroperitoneal mucinous cystadenocarcinoma. Cysts lined by papillary formations composed of atypical mucinous cells. (Reprinted by permission of The American College of Obstetricians and Gynecologists. Roth LM, Ehrlich CE (1977) Mucinous cystadenocarcinoma of the retroperitoneum. Obstet Gynecol 59:486–488.)

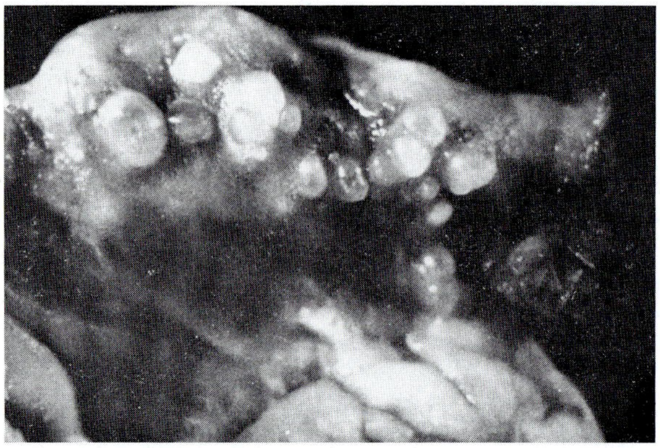

Fig. 17.61. Walthard nests. Multiple small cysts cover the serosa of fallopian tube and mesosalpinx. (From Teoh TB (1953) The structure and development of Walthard nests. J Pathol 66:433–439. Copyright 1953 by John Wiley & Sons, Ltd. Reprinted by permission of John Wiley & Sons, Ltd.)

volving the serosal surfaces of the fallopian tubes (Figs. 17.61 and 17.62), mesosalpinx, and mesovarium.[34,328] Walthard nests are uncommon on the ovarian surface but may be seen in the hilus, probably originating from the peritoneum of the mesovarium; they are most common on the tubal serosa (see Chapter 14, Diseases of the Fallopian Tube). Rare extraovarian Brenner tumors have been encountered, most commonly in the broad ligament.[136] In contrast to Walthard nests, squamous metaplasia of the peritoneum is rare; one such case has been described.[293] Two clear cell carcinomas of apparent peritoneal origin have been reported. One was a localized mass within the sigmoid mesocolon[107] whereas the other diffusely involved the peritoneum[186]; no endometriosis was identified in either case.

Ectopic Decidua

Clinical and Operative Findings

An ectopic decidual reaction similar to that seen in the lamina propria of the fallopian tube, cervix, and

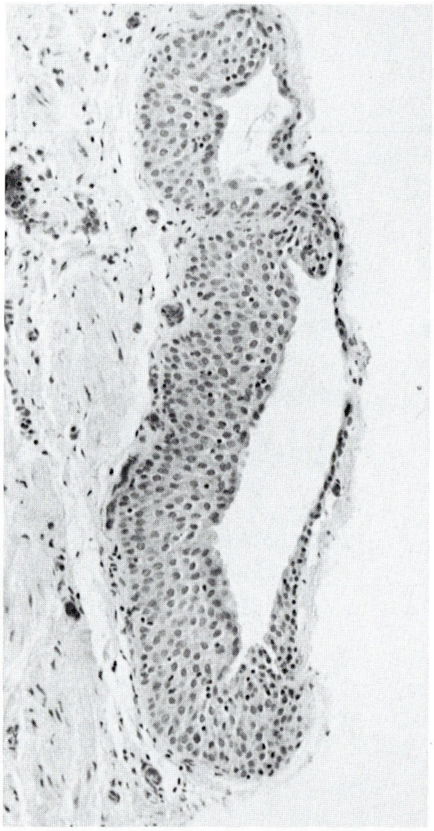

Fig. 17.62. Walthard nests on fallopian tube serosa. Nests with central cystic spaces are formed by benign transitional-type cells.

vagina may also be seen within the submesothelial stroma of the peritoneal cavity.[235,367] Frequent sites of *ectopic decidua* include the submesothelial stroma of the fallopian tubes, uterus and uterine ligaments, appendix and omentum, and within pelvic adhesions. Rare sites have included the serosal surfaces of the diaphragm, liver, spleen, and the renal pelvis.

Submesothelial decidua is typically an incidental microscopic finding, but florid lesions may be visible at the time of cesarean section or postpartum tubal ligation as multiple, gray to white, focally hemorrhagic nodules or plaques studding the peritoneal surfaces and simulating a malignant tumor. Several cases have been associated with massive, occasionally fatal, intraperitoneal hemorrhage during the third trimester, labor, or the puerperium. Other rare clinical presentations include abdominal pain, which may simulate that of appendicitis, and hydronephrosis and hematuria secondary to renal pelvic involvement.

Microscopic Findings

Microscopic examination discloses submesothelial decidual cells disposed individually or arranged in nodules or plaques (Fig. 17.63). Smooth muscle cells, probably derived from submesothelial myofibroblasts, may be admixed. The decidual foci are typically vascular and contain a sprinkling of lymphocytes. Focal hemorrhagic necrosis and varying degrees of nuclear pleomorphism and hyperchromasia of the decidual cells may suggest a tumor such as a deciduoid malignant mesothelioma,[304] but their bland appearance and mitotic inactivity militate against such a diagnosis. We have seen several cases of an omental decidual reaction in which most of the decidual cells exhibited striking vacuolization with basophilic mucin and an eccentric location of the nucleus. The appearance of the cells raised the possibility of metastatic signet-ring cell carcinoma, but in contrast to the cells of the latter, the vacuoles within the decidual cells contain acid rather than neutral mucin, and their cytoplasm lacks immunoreactivity for cytokeratin.

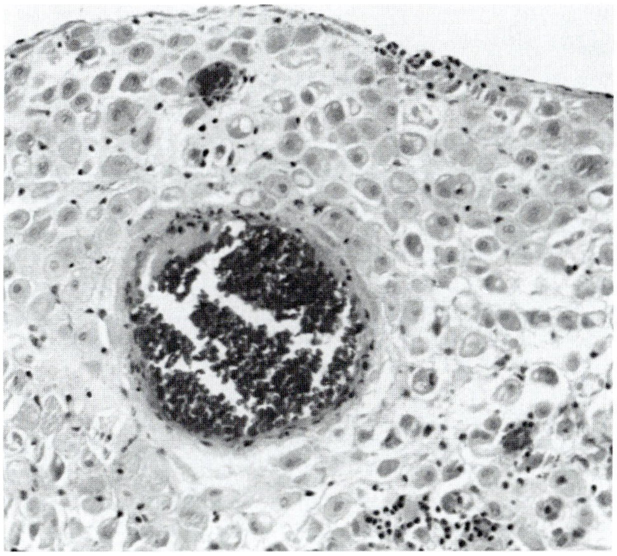

Fig. 17.63. Ectopic decidua beneath pelvic peritoneum. Note marked vascularity.

Leiomyomatosis

Disseminated peritoneal leiomyomatosis is a rare disorder characterized by the presence of multiple submesothelial nodules of cytologically benign smooth muscle, frequently associated with uterine leiomyomas and, rarely, ovarian leiomyomas. The nodules are generally considered to arise from multipotential submesothelial mesenchymal cells. This disorder is discussed elsewhere (see Chapter 13, Mesenchymal Tumors of the Uterus).

Benign Intranodal Glands of Müllerian Type

Clinical Features

Benign glands of müllerian type are most commonly encountered within the pelvic and paraaortic lymph nodes of females,[145,166,173,306] and less often in inguinal and femoral lymph nodes. Because these glands are almost always incidental microscopic findings in lymph nodes removed in cases of pelvic carcinoma, their reported frequency, which has varied from 2% to 41%, depends on the number of lymph nodes removed and the extent of the histologic sampling. Almost all the patients have been adults, although rare examples have been reported in children.[306] In males, the presence of similar glands has been recorded rarely within lymph nodes in the pelvis and abdomen[150] and mediastinum. Although typically without clinical or intraoperative manifestations, rare examples of lymph nodes containing müllerian-type glands have been associated with a false-positive lymphangiogram,[296] ureteral obstruction secondary to lymph node enlargement, or visible enlargement at the time of operation.

In a number of patients, intranodal glandular inclusions have been accompanied by endosalpingiosis of the peritoneum,[306] salpingitis isthmica nodosa, or acute and chronic salpingitis.[173,306] Other patients have had coexistent ovarian serous tumors, which have been benign, borderline tumors, or carcinomas.[296]

Pathologic Findings

On gross examination, the glands are usually not apparent, although rarely they are recognizable as cysts measuring up to a few millimeters in diameter. The glands are typically located in the periphery of the node, most commonly within its capsule or between the lymphoid follicles in the superficial cortex (Fig. 17.64); rarely, they lie free within the subcapsular sinuses.[173] In florid cases, they can be diffusely distributed throughout the lymph node. Intraglandular or periglandular psammoma bodies are commonly present. Intranodal glands may be surrounded by a thin rim of fibrous tissue or abut directly on the surrounding lymphoid cells.

The glands may be round and cystically dilated or exhibit an irregular contour as a result of infolding. They are most commonly lined by a single layer of cuboidal to columnar tubal-type epithelium, with an admixture of ciliated, secretory, and intercalated cell types (Fig. 17.65). With special stains, mucin can be demonstrated in the apical portion of the secretory cells and within the gland spaces.[166]

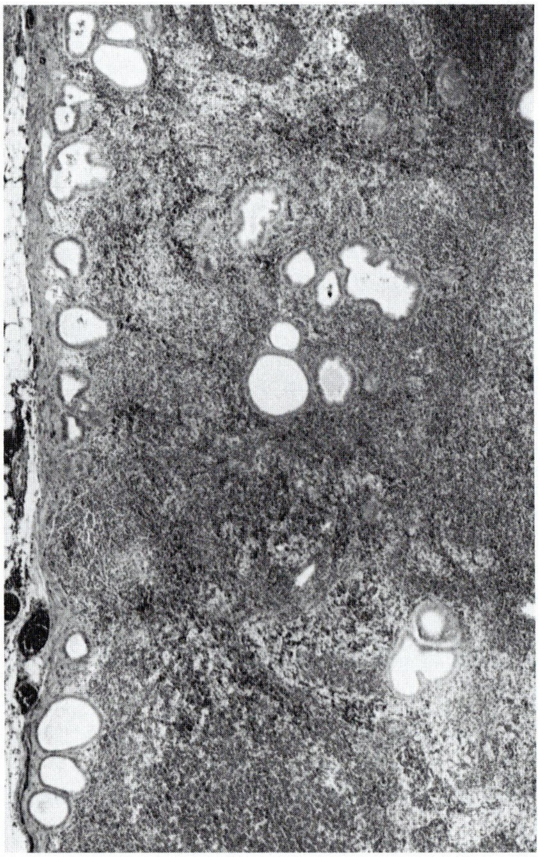

Fig. 17.64. Endosalpingiotic glands within pelvic lymph node. The glands are located within and immediately beneath the node capsule as well as deeper within the node.

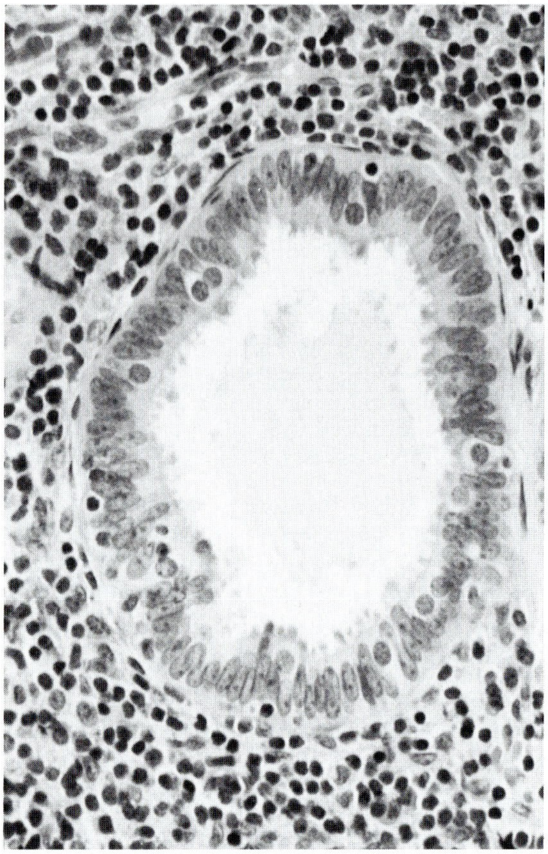

Fig. 17.65. Endosalpingiotic gland within pelvic lymph node. The gland is lined by benign cells of multiple types, including ciliated cells.

The cells have a benign appearance with regular, basally oriented or pseudostratified, oval to round nuclei, fine nuclear chromatin, and occasional small nucleoli; mitotic figures are typically absent. In rare cases, the cells can exhibit varying degress of atypia and stratification; the latter can produce an intraglandular cribriform pattern or luminal obliteration by sheets of cells (Fig. 17.66). These cases of atypical endosalpingiosis may rarely be the origin of intranodal serous neoplasms (see following).

Examples of intranodal glandular inclusions lined by benign endometrioid epithelium,[185] mucinous epithelium of endocervical[12] or goblet cell type, or metaplastic squamous epithelium[221] have been reported.

Differential Diagnosis

In most cases the distinction between glandular inclusions and metastatic adenocarcinoma is not difficult unless a primary ovarian serous tumor of low malignant potential is present, in which case the distinction may be difficult or impossible. Features favoring a benign diagnosis include a capsular or in-

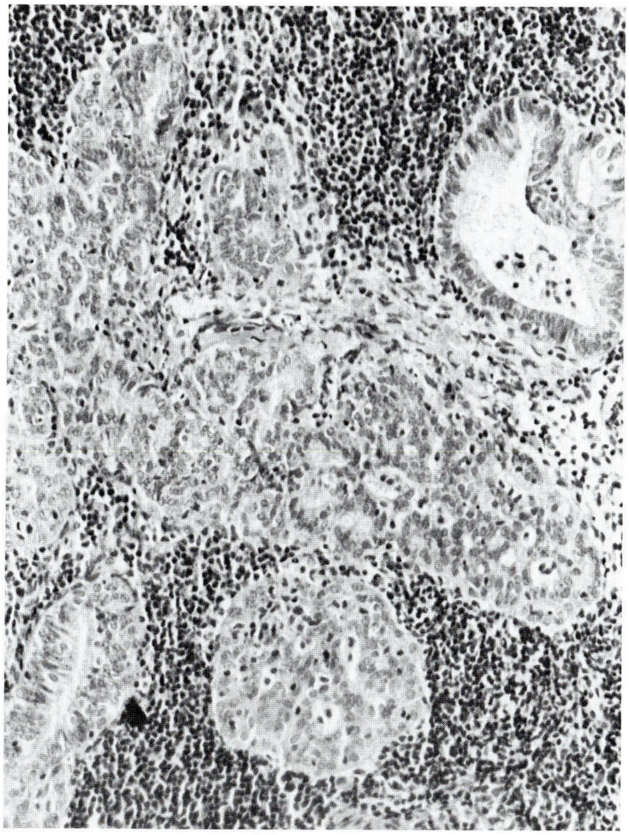

Fig. 17.66. Atypical endosalpingiotic glands within pelvic lymph node. Some of the glands exhibit luminal obliteration by cells growing in solid and cribriform patterns. (Reprinted by permission of Chen KTK (1981) Benign glandular inclusions of the peritoneum and periaortic lymph nodes. Diagn Gynecol Obstet 3:265–268.)

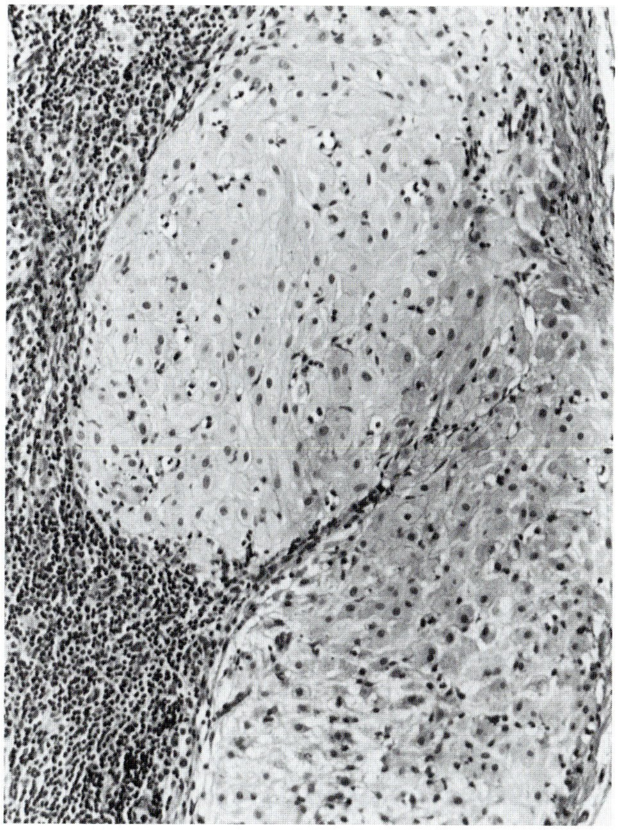

Fig. 17.67. Ectopic decidual within pelvic lymph node. The nodal architecture is focally replaced by sheets of decidualized cells. (Reprinted by permission of Mills, ref. 221.)

terfollicular location of the glands, lining cells of multiple types including ciliated forms, a lack of significant cellular atypia and mitotic activity, and an absence of a desmoplastic stromal reaction. Complicating the differential diagnosis is the very rare development of borderline or frankly malignant change in müllerian glandular inclusions in lymph nodes. This diagnosis is suggested in cases in which the intranodal neoplasm merges with foci of atypical endosalpingiosis. Intranodal nests of benign squamous epithelium should not be mistaken for metastatic squamous cell carcinoma. Features favoring a benign diagnosis include bland cytologic features, mitotic inactivity, and, in some cases, an origin within benign glands.

Intranodal Ectopic Decidua

Ectopic decidua unassociated with endometriosis has been described as a rare, incidental microscopic finding in paraaortic and pelvic lymph nodes, usually removed as part of a radical hysterectomy for carcinoma of the cervix in pregnant patients.[7,40,73,221,360,367] A subserosal ectopic decidual reaction may be present elsewhere in the pelvis. In some cases, the decidual tissue has been recognized on careful macroscopic examination as tiny, gray, subcapsular nodules. On microscopic examination, the decidual nests typically occupy the subcapsular sinus and superficial cortex (Fig. 17.67), although more central parts of the lymph node may also be involved. The cells appear benign, but may contain occasional bizarre, hyperchromatic nuclei, mimicking metastatic squamous cell carcinoma. The absence of mitotic activity, keratinization, and stromal desmoplasia facilitate the diagnosis. Metastatic squamous cell carcinoma, however, may be present in the same node.[73]

Intranodal Leiomyomatosis

Rare cases of lymph node involvement by mitotically inactive, cytologically benign smooth muscle

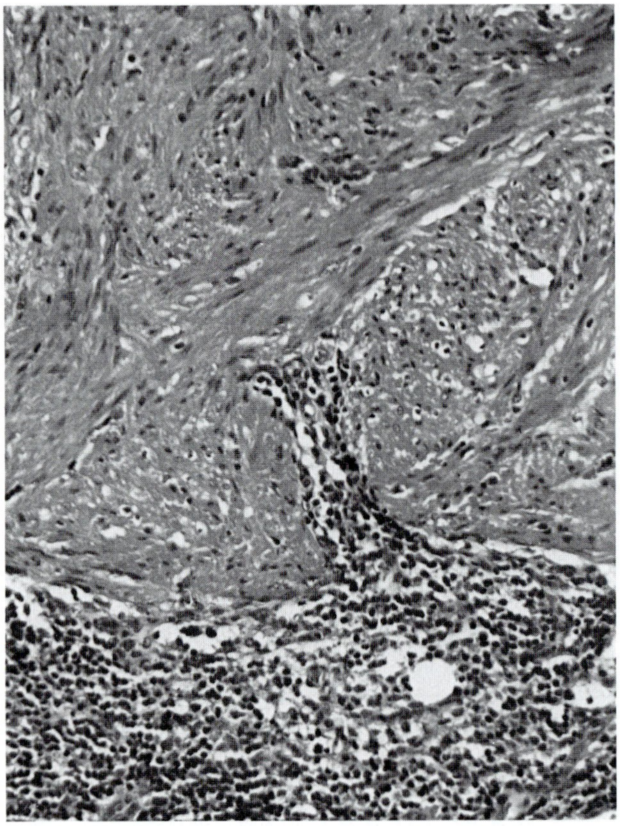

Fig. 17.68. Benign smooth muscle within pelvic lymph node. (Reprinted by permission of Abell and Littler, ref. 1.)

have been described (Fig. 17.68).[1,79,144,148] Most patients have had concurrent typical uterine leiomyomas or, less commonly, diffuse peritoneal leiomyomatosis[148] or similar nodules within the lungs.[79] In pregnant patients, the process may merge with intranodal decidua.[148] The finding in most cases likely is secondary to lymphatic spread from uterine leiomyomas ("benign metastasizing leiomyoma"; see Chapter 13, Mesenchymal Tumors of the Uterus), but in some cases the intranodal smooth muscle may arise from entrapped subcoelomic mesenchyme or myofibroblastic organization of intranodal decidua. The presence of benign-appearing smooth muscle in a lymph node should also bring into consideration the diagnosis of lymphangioleiomyomatosis. This disorder is usually, but not invariably, associated with pulmonary involvement. Benign intranodal smooth muscle should also be distinguished from metastatic well-differentiated leiomyosarcoma of uterine origin. Patients with the latter usually have a large uterine mass, and on histologic examination the intranodal tumor is cellular and exhibits evidence of cellular atypicality and mitotic activity.

References

1. Abell MR, Littler ER (1975) Benign metastasizing uterine leiomyoma. Multiple lymph nodal metastases. Cancer (Phila) 36:2206–2213
2. Abu-Rustum NR, Aghajanian CA, Venkatraman ES, Feroz F, Barakat RR (1997) Metastatic breast carcinoma to the abdomen and pelvis. Gynecol Oncol 66:41–44
3. Adams HW, Mainz DL (1977) Eosinophilic ascites. A case report and review of the literature. Digest Dis 22:40–42
4. Ahn GH, Scully RE (1991) Clear cell carcinoma of the inguinal region arising from endometriosis. Cancer (Phila) 67:116–120
5. Altaras MM, Aviram R, Cohen I et al (1991) Primary peritoneal papillary serous adenocarcinoma: clinical and management aspects. Gynecol Oncol 40:230–236
6. Asensio JA, Goldblatt P, Thomford NR (1990) Primary malignant peritoneal mesothelioma. A report of seven cases and a review of the literature. Arch Surg 125:1477–1481
7. Ashraf M, Boyd CB, Beresford WA (1984) Ectopic decidual reaction in para-aortic and pelvic lymph nodes in the presence of cervical squamous cell carcinoma during pregnancy. J Surg Oncol 26:6–8
8. Aslani M, Scully RE (1989) Primary carcinoma of the broad ligament. Report of four cases and review of the literature. Cancer (Phila) 64:1540–1545
9. Aslani M, Ahn G, Scully RE (1988) Serous papillary cystadenoma of borderline malignancy of broad ligament. Int J Gynecol Pathol 7:131–138
10. Attanoos R, Gibbs AR (1997) Pathology of malignant mesothelioma. Histopathology (Oxf) 30:403–418
11. Ayres JG, Crocker JG, Skilbeck NQ (1988) Differentiation of malignant from normal and reactive mesothelial cells by the argyrophil technique for nucleolar organiser region associated proteins. Thorax 43:366–370
12. Baird DB, Reddick RL (1991) Extraovarian mucinous metaplasia in a patient with bilateral mucinous borderline ovarian tumors: a case report. Int J Gynecol Pathol 10:96–103
13. Baker PM, Clement PB, Bell DA, Young RH (1999) Superficial endometriosis of the uterine cervix: a report of 20 cases of a process that may be confused with endocervical glandular dysplasia or adenocarcinoma in situ. Int J Gynecol Pathol 18:198–205
14. Banerjee R, Gough J (1988) Cystic mucinous tumours of the mesentery and retroperitoneum: Report of three cases. Histopathology (Oxf) 12:527–532
15. Barbieri RL (1990) Etiology and epidemiology of endometriosis. Am J Obstet Gynecol 162:565–567
16. Barbieri RL, Niloff JM, Bast RC Jr, et al (1986) Elevated serum concentrations of CA-125 in patients

with advanced endometriosis. Fertil Steril 45: 630–634
17. Bastani B, Shariatzadeh MR, Dehdashti F (1985) Tuberculous peritonitis. Report of 30 cases and review of the literature. Q J Med 56:549–557
18. Bayer AS, Blumenkrantz MJ, Montgomerie JZ, et al (1976) Candida peritonitis. Report of 22 cases and review of the English literature. Am J Med 61:832–840
19. Beckman EN, Leonard GL, Pintado SO, Sternberg WH (1985) Endometriosis of the prostate. Am J Surg Pathol 9:374–379
20. Bell DA, Scully RE (1990) Serous borderline tumors of the peritoneum. Am J Surg Pathol 14:230–239
21. Ben-Baruch G, Sivan E, Moran O, Rizel S, Menczer J, Seidman DS (1996) Primary peritoneal serous papillary carcinoma: a study of 25 cases and comparison with stage III-IV ovarian papillary serous carcinoma. Gynecol Oncol 60:393–396
22. Bergen S, Owen J, Snider WR, Lim YC (1981) Disseminated adenomyomas of the abdominal and pelvic cavities. Am Surg 47:232–235
23. Bergqvist A, Carlstrom K, Jeppsson S, Ljungberg O (1984) Histochemical localization of specific estrogen and progesterone binding in human endometrium and endometriotic tissue. A preliminary report. Acta Obstet Gynecol Scand (Suppl) 123:15–18
24. Bergqvist A, Jeppsson S, Ljungberg O (1985) Histochemical demonstration of estrogen and progesterone binding in endometriotic tissue and in uterine endometrium. J Histochem Cytochem 33:155–161
25. Bergqvist A, Ljungberg O, Myhre E (1984) Human endometrium and endometriotic tissue obtained simultaneously: a comparative histological study. Int J Gynecol Pathol 3:135–145
26. Bergqvist A, Rannevik G, Thorell J (1981) Estrogen and progesterone cytosol receptor concentration in endometriotic tissue and intrauterine endometrium. Acta Obstet Gynecol Scand (Suppl) 101: 53–58
27. Biscotti CV, Hart WR (1992) Peritoneal serous micropapillomatosis of low malignant potential (serous borderline tumors of the peritoneum). A clinicopathologic study of 17 cases. Am J Surg Pathol 16:467–475
28. Blumberg H, Srinivasan K, Parnes IH (1966) Peritoneal schistosomiasis simulating carcinoma. NY State J Med 66:758–761
29. Blumenkrantz MJ, Gallagher N, Bashore RA, Tenckhoff H (1981) Retrograde menstruation in women undergoing chronic peritoneal dialysis. Obstet Gynecol 57:667–670
30. Bolen JW, Hammar SP, McNutt MA (1986) Reactive and neoplastic serosal tissue. A light microscopic, ultrastructural and immunohistochemical study. Am J Surg Pathol 10:34–47
31. Bollinger DJ, Wick MR, Dehner LP, et al (1989) Peritoneal malignant mesothelioma versus serous papillary adenocarcinoma. A histochemical and immunohistochemical comparison. Am J Surg Pathol 13:659–670
32. Bradley JA, McWhinnie DL, Hamilton DNH, et al (1983) Sclerosing obstructive peritonitis after continuous ambulatory peritoneal dialysis. Lancet 2:113–114
33. Brainard JA, Goldblum JR (1998) An immunohistochemical analysis of the Wilms' tumor as a discriminator of peritoneal mesothelioma from primary peritoneal serous adenocarcinoma in women [abstract]. Mod Pathol 11:101A
34. Bransilver BR, Ferenczy A, Richart RM (1974) Brenner tumors and Walthard cell nests. Arch Pathol Lab Med 98:76–86
35. Brooks JJ, Wheeler JE (1977) Malignancy arising in extragonadal endometriosis. A case report and summary of the world literature. Cancer (Phila) 40:3065–3073
36. Brunnemann RG, Ro JY, Ordonez NG, Mooney J, EL-Naggar AK, Ayala AG (1999) Extrapleural solitary fibrous tumor: a clinicopathologic study of 24 cases. Mod Pathol 12:1034–1042
37. Buckley CH (1990) Tamoxifen and endometriosis. Case report. Br J Obstet Gynaecol 97:645–646
38. Buhac I, Jarmolych J (1978) Histology of the intestinal peritoneum in patients with cirrhosis of the liver and ascites. Dig Dis 23:417–422
39. Bur ME, Greene GL, Press MF (1987) Estrogen receptor localization in formalin-fixed, paraffin-embedded endometrium and endometriotic tissues. Int J Gynecol Pathol 6:140–151
40. Burnett RA, Millan D (1986) Decidual change in pelvic lymph nodes: a source of possible diagnostic error. Histopathology (Oxf) 10:1089–1092
41. Cajigas A, Axiotis CA (1990) Endosalpingiosis of the vermiform appendix. Int J Gynecol Pathol 9:291–295
42. Cambria RP, Shamberger RC (1984) Small bowel obstruction caused by the abdominal cocoon syndrome: possible association with the LeVeen shunt. Surgery (St. Louis) 95:501–503
43. Candiani GB, Vercellini P, Fedele L, et al (1991) Inguinal endometriosis: pathogenetic and clinical implications. Obstet Gynecol 78:191–194
44. Candiani GB, Vercellini P, Fedele L, et al (1991) Mild endometriosis and infertility: a critical review of epidemiologic data, diagnostic pitfalls, and classification limits. Obstet Gynecol Surv 46:374–381
45. Carpenter HA, Lancaster JR, Lee RA (1982) Multilocular cysts of the peritoneum. Mayo Clin Proc 57:634–638
46. Carr NJ, Turk EP (1992) The histological features of splenosis. Histopathology (Oxf) 21:549–553
47. Cartwright PS (1991) Peritoneal trophoblastic implants after surgical management of tubal pregnancy. J Reprod Med 36:523–524
48. Castelli MJ, Armin A, Husain A, et al (1985) Fibrosing peritonitis in a drug abuser. Arch Pathol Lab Med 109:767–769
49. Chatman DL, Ward AB (1982) Endometriosis in adolescents. J Reprod Med 27:156–160

50. Chatman DL, Zbella EA (1986) Pelvic peritoneal defects and endometriosis: further observations. Fertil Steril 46:711–714
51. Chatman DL, Zbella EA (1987) Biopsy in laparoscopically diagnosed endometriosis. J Reprod Med 32:855–857
52. Chatterjee SK (1980) Scar endometriosis: a clinicopathologic study of 17 cases. Obstet Gynecol 56:81–84
53. Chen KT, Kostich ND, Rosai J (1978) Peritoneal foreign body granulomas to keratin in uterine adenoacanthoma. Arch Pathol Lab Med 102:174–177
54. Chumas JC, Thanning L, Mann WJ (1986) Malignant mixed müllerian tumor arising in extragenital endometriosis: report of a case and review of the literature. Gynecol Oncol 23:227–233
55. Cioltei A, Tasca L, Titiriga L, Maakaron G, Calciu V (1979) Nodular salpingitis and tubal endometriosis. I. Comparative clinical study. Acta Eur Fertil 10:135–141
56. Clarke TJ, Simpson RHW (1990) Necrotizing granulomas of peritoneum following diathermy ablation of endometriosis. Histopathology (Oxf) 16: 400–402
57. Clausen I, Nielsen KT (1987) Endometriosis in the groin. Int J Gynaecol Obstet 25:469–471
58. Clement PB (1990) Pathology of endometriosis. Pathol Annu 25(1):245–295
59. Clement PB (1995) Reactive tumor-like lesions of the peritoneum [Editorial]. Am J Clin Pathol 103: 673–676
60. Clement PB, Granai CO, Young RH, Scully RE (1994) Endometriosis with myxoid change: a case simulating pseudomyxoma peritonei. Am J Surg Pathol 18:849–853
61. Clement PB, Scully RE (1978) Extrauterine mesodermal (müllerian) adenosarcoma. A clinicopathologic analysis of five cases. Am J Clin Pathol 69: 276–283
62. Clement PB, Scully RE (1992) Endometrial stromal sarcomas of the uterus with extensive endometrioid glandular differentiation. A report of three cases that caused problems in differential diagnosis. Int J Gynecol Pathol 11:163–173
63. Clement PB, Young RH (1992) Endocervicosis of the urinary bladder: A report of six cases of a benign müllerian lesion that may mimic adenocarcinoma. Am J Surg Pathol 16:533–542
64. Clement PB, Young RH (1993) Florid mesothelial hyperplasia associated with ovarian tumors: a possible source of error in tumor diagnosis and staging. Int J Gynecol Pathol 12:51–58
65. Clement PB, Young RH (1999) Tumor-like manifestations of florid cystic endosalpingiosis: a report of four cases including the first reported cases of mural endosalpingiosis of the uterus. Am J Surg Pathol 23:166–175
66. Clement PB, Young RH (2000) Two previously unemphasized features of endometriosis: micronodular stromal endometriosis and endometriosis with stromal elastosis. Int J Surg Pathol 8:223–227
67. Clement PB, Young RH, Hanna W, Scully RE (1993) Sclerosing peritonitis associated with luteinized thecomas of the ovary: a clinicopathological analysis of six cases. Am J Surg Pathol 18:1–13
68. Clement PB, Young RH, Oliva E, Sumner HW, Scully RE (1996) Hyperplastic mesothelial cells within abdominal lymph nodes: a mimic of metastatic ovarian carcinoma and serous borderline tumor. A report of two cases associated with ovarian neoplasms. Mod Pathol 9:879–886
69. Clement PB, Young RH, Scully RE (1988) Necrotic pseudoxanthomatous nodules of the ovary and peritoneum in endometriosis. Am J Surg Pathol 12:390–397
70. Clement PB, Young RH, Scully RE (1989) Liesegang rings in endometriosis. A report of three cases. Int J Gynecol Pathol 8:271–276
71. Clement PB, Young RH, Scully RE (1990) Stromal endometriosis of the uterine cervix. A variant of endometriosis that may simulate a sarcoma. Am J Surg Pathol 14:449–455
72. Clement PB, Young RH, Scully RE (1996) Malignant mesotheliomas presenting as ovarian masses. Am J Surg Pathol 20:1067–1080
73. Cobb CJ (1988) Ectopic decidua and metastatic squamous carcinoma: presentation in a single pelvic lymph node. J Surg Oncol 38:126–129
74. Coder DM, Olander GA (1972) Granulomatous peritonitis caused by starch glove powder. Arch Surg 105:83–86
75. Copeland LJ, Silva EG, Gershenson DM, et al (1988) The significance of müllerian inclusions found at second-look laparotomy in patients with epithelial ovarian neoplasms. Obstet Gynecol 71: 763–770
76. Cornillie FJ, Brosens A, Vasquez G, Riphagen I (1986) Histologic and ultrastructural changes in human endometriotic implants treated with the antiprogesterone steroid ethylnorgestrienone (gestrinone) during 2 months. Int J Gynecol Pathol 5: 95–109
77. Cornillie FJ, Oosterlynck D, Lauweryns JM, Koninckx PR (1990) Deeply infiltrating pelvic endometriosis: histology and clinical significance. Fertil Steril 53:978–983
78. Cornillie FJ, Puttemans P, Brosens IA (1987) Histology and ultrastructure of human endometriotic tissues treated with dydrogesterone (duphaston). Eur J Obstet Reprod Biol 26:39–55
79. Cramer SF, Meyer JS, Kraner JF, et al (1980) Metastasizing leiomyoma of the uterus. S-phase fraction, estrogen receptor, and ultrastructure. Cancer (Phila) 45:932–937
80. Czernobilsky B, Morris WJ (1979) A histologic study of ovarian endometriosis with emphasis on hyperplastic and atypical changes. Obstet Gynecol 53:318–323
81. Czernobilsky B, Silverstein A (1978) Salpingitis and ovarian endometriosis. Fertil Steril 30:45–49
82. Dadmanesh F, Young RH, Clement PB (1999) Poly-

poid endometriosis. A clinicopathologic analysis of 15 cases [abstract]. Mod Pathol 12:115A
83. Dalrymple JC, Bannatyne P, Russell P, et al (1989) Extraovarian peritoneal serous papillary carcinoma. A clinicopathologic study of 31 cases. Cancer (Phila) 64:110–115
84. Dalrymple JC, Hunter JC, Ferrier A, et al (1986) Disseminated intraperitoneal oxyuris granulomas. Aust NZ J Obstet Gynaecol 26:90–91
85. Daum F, Boley SJ, Cohen MI (1974) Miliary Crohn's disease. Gastroenterology 67:527–530
86. David MP, Ben-Zwi D, Langer L (1981) Tubal intramural polyps and their relationship to infertility. Fertil Steril 35:526–531
87. Davies JD, Ansell ID (1983) Food-starch granulomatous peritonitis. J Clin Pathol 36:435–438
88. Dawood MY, Khan-Dawood FS, Ramos J (1988) Plasma and peritoneal fluid levels of CA 125 in women with endometriosis. Am J Obstet Gynecol 159:1526–1531
89. Day DL, Sane S, Dehner LP (1986) Inflammatory pseudotumor of the mesentery and small intestine. Pediatr Radiol 16:210–215
90. Daya D, McCaughey WTE (1990) Well-differentiated papillary mesothelioma of the peritoneum. A clinicopathologic study of 22 cases. Cancer (Phila) 65:292–296
91. Daya D, McCaughey WTE (1991) Pathology of the peritoneum: a review of selected topics. Semin Diagn Pathol 8:277–289
92. De Brux J (1975) The contribution of pathological anatomy to the diagnosis and prognosis of different forms of tubal sterility. Acta Eur Fertil 6: 185–195
93. Deger RB, LiVolsi VA, Noumoff JS (1995) Foreign body reaction (gossypiboma) masking as recurrent ovarian cancer. Gynecol Oncol 56:94–96
94. Dehn TCB, Lucas MG, Wood RFM (1985) Idiopathic sclerosing peritonitis. Postgrad Med J 61:841–842
95. de Peralta MN, Delahoussaye PM, Tornos CS, Silva EG (1994) Benign retroperitoneal cysts of müllerian type: a clinicopathologic study of three cases and review of the literature. Int J Gynecol Pathol 13:273–278
96. DeStephano DB, Wesley JR, Heidelberger KP, Hutchison RJ, Blane CE, Coran AG (1985) Primitive cystic hepatic neoplasm of infancy with mesothelial differentiation: report of a case. Pediatr Pathol 4:291–302
97. D'Hooghe T, Bambra CS, Raeymaekers BM, De Jonge I, Lauweryns JM, Koninckx PR (1995) Intrapelvic injection of menstural endometrium causes endometriosis in baboons (*Papio cynocephalus* and *Papio anubis*). Am J Obstet Gynecol 173:125–134
98. Doty DW, Gruber JS, Wolf GC, Winslow RC (1980) 46 XY pure gonadal dysgenesis: report of 2 unusual cases. Obstet Gynecol 55:61S-63S
99. Egger H, Weigmann P (1982) Clinical and surgical aspects of ovarian endometriotic cysts. Arch Gynecol 233:37–45
100. Eiseman B, Seelig MG, Womack NA (1947) Talcum powder granuloma: a frequent and serious postoperative complication. Ann Surg 126:820–832
101. Eltabbakh GH, Werness BA, Piver S, Blumenson LE (1998) Prognostic factors in extraovarian primary peritoneal carcinoma. Gynecol Oncol 71:230–239
102. El-Mahgoub S, Yassen S (1980) A positive proof for the theory of coelomic metaplasia. Am J Obstet Gynecol 137:137–140
103. Elliott GB, Christensen RM, Elliott KA (1970) Invasive endometriosis of the intestine: report of 21 cases. Can J Surg 13:387–395
104. Elliott GB, Freigang B (1962) Aseptic necrosis, calcification and separation of appendices epiploicae. Ann Surg 155:501–505
105. Elmore LW, Sherman ME, Seidman JD, Kurman RJ (2000) p53 expression and mutational status of primary peritoneal micropapillary serous carcinoma [abstract]. Mod Pathol 13:124A
106. Eltabbakh GH, Werness BA, Piver S, Blumenson LE (1998) Prognostic factors in extraovarian primary peritoneal carcinoma. Gynecol Oncol 71: 230–239
107. Evans H, Yates WA, Palmer WE, et al (1990) Clear cell carcinoma of the sigmoid mesocolon: a tumor of the secondary müllerian system. Am J Obstet Gynecol 162:161–163
108. Fedele L, Vercellini P, Arcaini L, et al (1988) CA 125 in serum, peritoneal fluid, active lesions, and endometrium of patients with endometriosis. Am J Obstet Gynecol 158:166–170
109. Finkel L, Marchevsky A, Cohen B (1986) Endometrial cyst of the liver. Am J Gastroenterol 81: 576–578
110. Flieder DB, Moran CA, Travis WD, Koss MN, Mark EJ (1998) Pleuro-pulmonary endometriosis and pulmonary ectopic deciduosis: a clinicopathologic and immunohistochemical study of 10 cases with emphasis on diagnostic pitfalls. Hum Pathol 29:1495–1503
111. Foo KT, Ng KC, Rauff A, et al (1978) Unusual small intestinal obstruction in adolescent girls: the abdominal cocoon. Br J Surg 65:427–430
112. Forouhar F (1982) Meconium peritonitis. Pathology, evolution, and diagnosis. Am J Clin Pathol 78:208–213
113. Fortier KJ, Haney AF (1985) The pathologic spectrum of uterotubal junction obstruction. Obstet Gynecol 65:93–98
114. Foyle A, Al-Jabi M, McCaughey WTE (1981) Papillary peritoneal tumors in women. Am J Surg Pathol 5:241–249
115. Fromm G, Gershenson DM, Silva EG (1990) Papillary serous carcinoma of the peritoneum. Obstet Gynecol 75:89–95
116. Fukunaga M, Naganuma H, Ushigome S, Endo Y, Ishikawa E (1996) Malignant solitary fibrous tumour of the peritoneum. Histopathology (Oxf) 28:463–466
117. Fukunaga M, Nomura K, Ishikawa E, Ushigome S

(1997) Ovarian atypical endometriosis: Its close association with malignant epithelial tumors. Histopathology (Oxf) 30:249–255

118. Fukunaga M, Ushigome S (1998) Epithelial metaplastic changes in ovarian endometriosis. Mod Pathol 11:784–788
119. Garde JR, Jones MA, McAfee R, Tarraza HM (1991) Extragenital malignant mixed müllerian tumor: review of the literature. Gynecol Oncol 43:186–190
120. Gardner HL (1966) Cervical and vaginal endometriosis. Clin Obstet Gynecol 9:358–372
121. George E, Leyser S, Zimmer HL, et al (1995) Vernix caseosa peritonitis: an infrequent complication of cesarean section with distinctive histopathologic features. Am J Clin Pathol 103:681–684
122. Gerald W, Ladanyi M, de Alava E, et al (1997) Clinical, pathological and molecular spectrum of desmoplastic small round cell tumor based on a review of 100 cases [abstract]. Mod Pathol 10:10A
123. Giangarra C, Gallo G, Newman R, Dorfman H (1987) Endometriosis in the biceps femoris. J Bone Joint Surg 69A:290–292
124. Gilks CB, Bell DA, Scully RE (1990) Serous psammocarcinoma of the ovary and peritoneum. Int J Gynecol Pathol 9:110–121
125. Godleski JJ, Gabriel KL (1981) Peritoneal responses to implanted fabrics used in operating rooms. Surgery (St Louis) 90:828–834
126. Goldblum, J, Hart WR (1995) Localized and diffuse mesotheliomas of the genital tract and peritoneum in women. A clinicopathological study of nineteen true mesothelial neoplasms, other than adenomatoid tumors, multicystic mesotheliomas and localized fibrous tumors. Am J Surg Pathol 19:1124–1137
127. Gonzalez-Crussi F, deMello DE, Sotelo-Avila C (1983) Omental-mesenteric myxoid hamartomas. Am J Surg Pathol 7:567–578
128. Gooneratne S, Sassone M, Blaustein A, et al (1982) Serous surface papillary carcinoma of the ovary: a clinicopathologic study of 16 cases. Int J Gynecol Pathol 1:258–269
129. Gordon PH, Schottler JL, Balcos EG, Goldberg SM (1976) Perianal endometrioma. Report of five cases. Dis Colon Rectum 19:260–265
130. Goswami AK, Sharma SK, Tandon SP, et al (1986) Pancreatic endometriosis presenting as a hypovascular renal mass. J Urol 135:112–113
131. Griffith LM, Carcangiu M (1991) Sex cord tumor with annular tubules associated with endometriosis of the fallopian tube. Am J Clin Pathol 96:259–262
132. Guzick DS (1989) Clinical epidemiology of endometriosis and infertility. Obstet Gynecol Clin N Am 16:43–59
133. Haddad FS, Ghossain A, Sawaya E, et al (1987) Abdominal tuberculosis. Dis Colon Rectum 30:724–735
134. Hafiz MA, Toker C (1986) Multicentric ovarian and extraovarian cystadenofibroma. Obstet Gynecol 68:94S-98S
135. Halme J, Hammond MG, Hulka JF, et al (1984) Retrograde menstruation in healthy women and in patients with endometriosis. Obstet Gynecol 64:151–154
136. Hampton HL, Huffman HT, Meeks GR (1992) Extraovarian Brenner tumor. Obstet Gynecol 79:844–846
137. Hansen RM, Caya JG, Clowry LJ Jr, et al (1984) Benign mesothelial proliferation with effusion. Clinicopathologic entity that may mimic malignancy. Am J Med 77:887–892
138. Harper GB Jr, Awbrey BJ, Thomas CG Jr, et al (1986) Mesothelial cysts of the round ligament simulating inguinal hernia. Report of four cases and review of the literature. Am J Surg 151:515–517
139. Heller DS, Gordon RE, Clement PB, Turnnir R, Katz N (1999) Presence of asbestos in peritoneal mesotheliomas in women. Int J Gynecol Cancer 9:452–455
140. Henderson DW, Shilkin KB, Whitaker D (1998) Reactive mesothelial hyperplasia vs. mesothelioma, including mesothelioma in situ. Am J Clin Pathol 110:397–404
141. Hidvegi D, Hidvegi I, Barrett J (1978) Douche-induced pelvic peritoneal starch granuloma. Obstet Gynecol 52:15S-18S
142. Hitti IF, Glasberg SS, Lubicz S (1990) Clear cell carcinoma arising in extraovarian endometriosis: report of three cases and review of the literature. Gynecol Oncol 39:314–320
143. Holmes EC, Eggleston JC (1972) Starch granulomatous peritonitis. Surgery (St Louis) 71:85–90
144. Horie A, Ishii N, Matsumoto M, et al (1984) Leiomyomatosis in the pelvic lymph node and peritoneum. Acta Pathol Jpn 34:813–819
145. Horn L-C, Bilek K (1995) Frequency and histogenesis of pelvine retroperitoneal lymph node inclusions of the female genital tract. An immunohistochemical study of 34 cases. Path Res Pract 191:991–996
146. Houston DE, Noller KL, Melton J, et al (1987) Incidence of pelvic endometriosis in Rochester, Minnesota, 1970–1979. Am J Epidemiol 125:959–969
147. Houston DE, Noller KL, Melton J III, Selwyn BJ (1988) The epidemiology of pelvic endometriosis. Clin Obstet Gynecol 31:787–800
148. Hsu YK, Rosenshein NB, Parmley TH, et al (1981) Leiomyomatosis in pelvic lymph nodes. Obstet Gynecol 57:91S-93S
149. Hughesdon PE (1976) The endometrial identity of benign stromatosis of the ovary and its relation to other forms of endometriosis. J Pathol 119:201–209
150. Huntrakoon M (1985) Benign glandular inclusions in the abdominal lymph nodes of a man. Hum Pathol 16:644–646
151. Ignatius JA, Hartmann WH (1972) The glove starch peritonitis syndrome. Ann Surg 175:338–397
152. Irvin W, Pelkey T, Rice L, Andersen W (1998) Endometrial stromal sarcoma of the vulva arising in extraovarian endometriosis: a case report and literature review. Gynecol Oncol 71:313–316

153. Isenberg JI, Gilbert SB, Pitcher JL (1971) Ascites with peritoneal involvement in Whipple's disease. Gastroenterology 60:305–310
154. Ismail SM (1991) Cone biopsy causes cervical endometriosis and tubo-endometrioid metaplasia. Histopathology (Oxf) 18:107–114
155. Ishimaru T, Masuzaki H (1991) Peritoneal endometriosis: endometrial tissue implantation as its primary etiologic mechanism. Am J Obstet Gynecol 165:210–214
156. Janne O, Kauppila A, Kokko E, et al (1981) Estrogen and progestin receptors in endometriosis lesions: comparison with endometrial tissue. Am J Obstet Gynecol 141:562–566
157. Janoff K, Wayne R, Huntwork B, et al (1984) Foreign body reactions secondary to cellulose lint fibers. Am J Surg 147:598–600
158. Jansen RPS, Russell P (1986) Nonpigmented endometriosis: clinical, laparoscopic, and pathologic definition. Am J Obstet Gynecol 155:1154–1159
159. Jenkins S, Olive DL, Haney AF (1986) Endometriosis: pathogenetic implications of the anatomic distribution. Obstet Gynecol 67:335–338
160. Kafiri G, Thomas DM, SHepherd NA, et al (1992) p53 expression is common in malignant mesotheliomas. Histopathology (Oxf) 21:331–334
161. Kane C, Drouin P (1985) Obstructive uropathy associated with endometriosis. Am J Obstet Gynecol 151:207–211
162. Kane MJ, Chahinian AP, Holland JF (1990) Malignant mesothelioma in young adults. Cancer (Phila) 65:1449–1455
163. Kapadia SB, Russak RR, O'Donnell WF, et al (1984) Postmenopausal ureteral endometriosis with atypical adenomatous hyperplasia following hysterectomy, bilateral oophorectomy, and long-term estrogen therapy. Obstet Gynecol 64:60S-63S
164. Kapoor OP, Nathwani BN, Joshi VR (1972) Amoebic peritonitis. A study of 73 cases. J Trop Med Hyg 75:11–15
165. Karlan BY, Baldwin RL, Lopez-Luevanos E, et al (1999) Peritoneal serous papillary carcinoma, a phenotypic variation of familial ovarian cancer: Implications for ovarian cancer screening. Am J Obstet Gynecol 180:917–928
166. Karp LA, Czernobilsky B (1969) Glandular inclusions in pelvic and abdominal para-aortic lymph nodes. Am J Clin Pathol 52:212–218
167. Kay S (1954) Tissue reaction to barium sulfate contrast medium. Arch Pathol 57:279–284
168. Kempers RD, Dockerty MB, Hunt AB, et al (1960) Significant postmenopausal endometriosis. Surg Gynecol Obstet 111:348–356
169. Kern SB (1991) Prevalence of psammoma bodies in Papanicolaou-stained cervicovaginal smears. Acta Cytol 35:81–88
170. Kern WH (1969) Benign papillary structures with psammoma bodies in culdocentesis fluid. Acta Cytol 13:178–180
171. Kerner H, Gaton E, Czernobilsky B (1981) Unusual ovarian, tubal and pelvic mesothelial inclusions in patients with endometriosis. Histopathology (Oxf) 5:277–282
172. Kershisnik MM, Ro JY, Cannon GH, Ordonez NG, Ayala AG, Silva EG (1994) Histiocytic reaction in pelvic peritoneum associated with oxidized regenerated cellulose. Am J Clin Pathol 103:27–31
173. Kheir SM, Mann WJ, Wilkerson JA (1981) Glandular inclusions in lymph nodes. The problem of extensive involvement and relationship to salpingitis. Am J Surg Pathol 5:353–359
174. Kim K, Scully RE (1990) Peritoneal keratin granulomas with carcinomas of endometrium and ovary and atypical polypoid adenomyoma of endometrium. Am J Surg Pathol 14:925–932
175. Kitazawa M, Kaneko H, Toshima M, et al (1984) Malignant peritoneal mesothelioma with massive foamy cells. Acta Pathol Jpn 34:687–692
176. Kocova L, Michal M, Sulc M, Zamecnik A (1997) Calcifying fibrous pseudotumor of visceral peritoneum. Histopathology (Oxf) 31:182–184
177. Kolker SE, Ferrell LD, Bollen AW, Ursell PC (1999) Disseminated intravascular meconium in a newborn with meconium peritonitis. Hum Pathol 30: 592–594
178. Koninckx PR, Ide P, Vandenbroucke W, Brosens IA (1980) New aspects of the pathophysiology of endometriosis and associated infertility. J Reprod Med 24:257–260
179. Kuo T, Hsueh S (1984) Mucicarminophilic histiocytosis. A polyvinylpyrrolidone (PVP) storage disease simulating signet-ring cell carcinoma. Am J Surg Pathol 8:419–428
180. LaGrenade A, Silverberg SG (1988) Ovarian tumors associated with atypical endometriosis. Hum Pathol 19:1080–1084
181. Lamb K, Hoffmann RG, Nichols TR (1986) Family trait analysis: a case-control study of 43 women with endometriosis and their best friends. Am J Obstet Gynecol 154:596–601
182. Lankerani MR, Aubrey RW, Reid JD (1982) Endometriosis of the colon with mixed "germ cell" tumor. Am J Clin Pathol 78:555–559
183. Lauchlan SC (1965) Two types of müllerian epithelium in an abdominal scar. Am J Obstet Gynecol 93:89–90
184. Lauchlan SC (1966) The cytology of endometriosis. Am J Obstet Gynecol 94:533–535
185. Lauchlan SC (1972) The secondary müllerian system. Obstet Gynecol Surv 27:133–146
186. Lee KR, Verma U, Belinson J (1991) Primary clear cell carcinoma of the peritoneum. Gynecol Oncol 41:259–262
187. Lele SB, Piver S, Barlow JJ, et al (1978) Squamous cell carcinoma arising in ovarian endometriosis. Gynecol Oncol 6:290–293
188. Lessey BA, Metzger DA, Haney AF, McCarty KS Jr (1989) Immunohistochemical analysis of estrogen and progesterone receptors in endometriosis: comparison with normal endometrium during the men-

strual cycle and the effect of medical therapy. Fertil Steril 51:409–415
189. Lee I, Ching K, Pang M, Ho T (1996) Two cases of primary retroperitoneal mucinous cystadenocarcinoma. Gynecol Oncol 63:145–150
190. Lin BT-Y, Colby T, Gown AM, et al (1996) Malignant vascular tumors of the serous membranes mimicking mesothelioma. A report of 14 cases. Am J Surg Pathol 20:1431–1439
191. Lintermans JP (1975) Fatal peritonitis, an unusual complication of *Strongyloides stercoralis* infestation. Clin Pediatr 14:974–975
192. Lipscomb GH, Ling FW, Photopulos GJ (1991) Ovarian abscess arising within an endometrioma. Obstet Gynecol 78:951–954
193. Lisa JR, Gioia JD, Rubin IC (1954) Observations on the interstitial portion of the fallopian tube. Surg Gynecol Obstet 99:159–169
194. LiVolsi VA, Perzin KH (1974) Endometriosis of the small intestine, producing intestinal obstruction or simulating neoplasm. Am J Dig Dis 19:100–108
195. Lombardo L, Mateos JH, Barroeta FF (1968) Subarachnoid hemorrhage due to endometriosis of the spinal canal. Neurology 18:423–426
196. Lomholt G, Hjorth N, Fischermann K (1968) Lethal peritonitis from Degos' disease (malign and atrophic papulosis). Acta Chir Scand 134:495–501
197. Lucero SP, Wise HA, Kirsh G, et al (1988) Ureteric obstruction secondary to endometriosis: report of three cases with review of the literature. Br J Urol 61:201–204
198. Malinak LR, Buttram VC, Elias S, Simpson JL (1980) Heritable aspects of endometriosis. II. Clinical characteristics of familial endometriosis. Am J Obstet Gynecol 137:332–337
199. Mangano WE, Cagle PT, Churg A, Vollmer RT, Roggli VL (1998) The diagnosis of desmoplastic malignant mesothelioma and its distinction from fibrous pleurisy. A histologic and immunohistochemical analysis of 31 cases including p53 immunostaining. Am J Clin Pathol 110:191–199
200. Marchevsky AM, Zimmerman MJ, Aufses AH Jr, Weiss H (1984) Endometrial cyst of the pancreas. Gastroenterology 86:1589–1591
201. Marshall AJ, Baddeley H, Barritt DW, et al (1977) Practolol peritonitis. A study of 16 cases and a survey of small bowel function in patients taking beta adrenergic blockers. Q J Med 46:135–149
202. Marshall SF, Forse RA (1952) Peritoneal adhesions: report of a case of paraffinoma. Surg Clin North Am 32:903–908
203. Martin DC, Hubert GD, Vander Zwaag R, El-Zeky FA (1989) Laparoscopic appearances of peritoneal endometriosis. Fertil Steril 51:63–67
204. Martin JD Jr, Hauck AE (1985) Endometriosis in the male. Am Surg 51:426–430
205. Martinka M, Allaire C, Clement PB (1999) Endocervicosis presenting as a painful vaginal mass: a case report. Int J Gynecol Pathol 18:274–276
206. Matseoane S, Harris T, Moscowitz E (1987) Isolated endometriosis in a Bartholin gland. NY State J Med 87:575–576
207. McArthur JW, Ulfelder H (1965) The effect of pregnancy upon endometriosis. Obstet Gynecol Surv 20:709–733
208. McCaughey WTE, Al-Jabi M (1986) Differentiation of serosal hyperplasia and neoplasia in biopsies. Pathol Annu 21(1):271–292
209. McCaughey WTE, Colby TV, Battifora H, et al (1991) Diagnosis of diffuse malignant mesothelioma: experience of a US/Canadian mesothelioma panel. Mod Pathol 4:342–353
210. McCaughey WTE, Kannerstein M, Churg J (1985) Tumors and pseudotumors of the serous membranes. Atlas of tumor pathology, ser 2, fasc 20. Armed Forces Institute of Pathology, Washington, DC
211. McCaughey WTE, Schryer MJP, Lin X, et al (1986) Extraovarian pelvic serous tumor with marked calcification. Arch Pathol Lab Med 110:78–80
212. McCaughey WTE, Kirk ME, Lester W, et al (1984) Peritoneal epithelial lesions associated with proliferative serous tumours of the ovary. Histopathology (Oxf) 8:195–208
213. McFadden DE, Clement PB (1986) Peritoneal inclusion cysts with mural mesothelial proliferation. A clinicopathological analysis of six cases. Am J Surg Pathol 10:844–854
214. Merino MJ, Livolsi VA (1981) Signet ring carcinoma of the female breast: a clinicopathologic analysis of 24 cases. Cancer (Phila) 48:1830–1837
215. Metzger AL, Coyne M, Lee S, et al (1974) In vivo LE cell formation in peritonitis due to systemic lupus erythematosus. J Rheumatol 1:130–133
216. Metzger DA, Haney AF (1988) Endometriosis: etiology and pathophysiology of infertility. Clin Obstet Gynecol 31:801–812
217. Metzger DA, Lessey BA, Soper JT, et al (1991) Hormone-resistant endometriosis following total abdominal hysterectomy and bilateral salpingo-oophorectomy: correlation with histology and steroid receptor content. Obstet Gynecol 78:946–950
218. Metzger DA, Olive DL, Haney AF (1988) Limited hormonal responsiveness of ectopic endometrium: histologic correlation with intrauterine endometrium. Hum Pathol 19:1417–1424
219. Michael H, Sutton G, Roth LM (1987) Ovarian carcinoma with extracellular mucin production: reassessment of "pseudomyxoma ovarii et peritonei." Int J Gynecol Pathol 6:298–312
220. Michowitz M, Baratz M, Stavorovsky M (1983) Endometriosis of the umbilicus. Dermatologica (Basel) 167:326–330
221. Mills SE (1983) Decidua and squamous metaplasia in abdominopelvic lymph nodes. Int J Gynecol Pathol 2:209–215
222. Minvielle UL, de la Cruz JV (1968) Endometriosis of the anal canal: presentation of a case. Dis Col Rect 11:32–35

223. Moller NE (1959) The Arias–Stella phenomenon in endometriosis. Acta Obstet Gynecol Scand 38:271–274
224. Moloshok AA, Ivanko AI (1984) Endometriosis of the breast (an observation). Vopr Onkol 30:88–89
225. Mostoufizadeh M, Scully RE (1980) Malignant tumors arising in endometriosis. Clin Obstet Gynecol 23:951–963
226. Mulhollan TJ, Silva EG, Tornos C, Guerrieri C, Fromm G, Gershenson D (1994) Ovarian involvement by serous surface papillary carcinoma. Int J Gynecol Pathol 13:120–126
227. Muneyyirci-Delale O, Neil G, Serur E, Gordon D, Maiman M, Sedlis A (1998) Endometriosis with massive ascites. Obstet Gynecol 69:42–46
228. Naresh KN, Ahuja VK, Rao CR, et al (1991) Squamous cell carcinoma arising in endometriosis of the ovary. J Clin Pathol 44:958–959
229. Nazeer T, Ro JY, Tornos C, Ordonez NG, Ayala AG (1996) Endocervical type glands in urinary bladder: a clinicopathologic study of six cases. Hum Pathol 27:816–820
230. Nisolle-Pochet M, Casanas-Roux F, Donnez J (1988) Histologic study of ovarian endometriosis after hormonal therapy. Fertil Steril 49:423
231. Nissim F, Ashkenazy M, Borenstein R, et al (1981) Tuberculoid cornstarch granulomas with caseous necrosis. Arch Pathol Lab Med 105:86–88
232. Ngo Y, Messing B, Marteau P, et al (1992) Peritoneal sarcoidosis: an unrecognized cause of sclerosing peritonitis. Dig Dis Sci 37:1776–1780
233. Norris JC, Davison TC (1934) Peritoneal reaction to liquid petrolatum. JAMA 103:1846–1847
234. Novak ER, Hoge AF (1958) Endometriosis of the lower genital tract. Obstet Gynecol 12:687–693
235. Ober WB, Grady HG, Schoenbucher AK (1957) Ectopic ovarian decidua without pregnancy. Am J Pathol 33:199–214
236. Olive DL, Henderson DY (1987) Endometriosis and müllerian anomalies. Obstet Gynecol 69:412–415
237. Ordi J, de Alava E, Torné A, et al (1998) Intraabdominal desmoplastic small round cell tumor with EWS/ERG fusion transcript. Am J Surg Pathol 22:1026–1032
238. Ordonez NG (1998) Desmoplastic small round cell tumor. I: A histopathologic study of 39 cases with emphasis on unusual histologic patterns. Am J Surg Pathol 22:1303–1313
239. Ordonez NG (1998) Desmoplastic small round cell tumor. II: An ultrastructural and immunohistochemical study with emphasis on new histochemical markers. Am J Surg Pathol 22:1303–1313
240. Ordonez NG (1998) Role of immunohistochemistry in distinguishing epithelial peritoneal mesotheliomas from peritoneal and ovarian serous carcinomas. Am J Surg Pathol 22:1203–1204
241. Ordonez NG (1999) The immunohistochemical diagnosis of epithelial mesothelioma. Hum Pathol 30:313–323
242. Ordonez NG, Zirkin R, Bloom RE (1989) Malignant small-cell epithelial tumor of the peritoneum coexpressing mesenchymal-type intermediate filaments. Am J Surg Pathol 13:413–421
243. Ortega I, Nogales F, Gonzalez-Campora R, et al (1982) Extragenital endometrioid cystadenofibroma. Acta Obstet Gynecol Scand 61:283–284
244. Pai SA, Desai SB, Borges AM (1998) Uterus-like masses of the ovary associated with breast cancer and raised serum CA 125. Am J Surg Pathol 22:333–337
245. Palagiri A (1978) Urethral diverticulum with endometriosis. Urology 11:271–272
246. Park SA, Giannattasio C, Tancer ML (1981) Foreign body reaction to the intraperitoneal use of avitene. Obstet Gynecol 58:664–668
247. Park U, Han KC, Chang HK, Huh MH (1991) A primary mucinous cystadenocarcinoma of the retroperitoneum. Gynecol Oncol 42:64–67
248. Patel VC, Samuels H, Abeles E, Hirjibehedin PE (1982) Endometriosis of the knee. A case report. Clin Orthop 171:140–144
249. Paull T, Tedeschi LG (1972) Perineal endometriosis at the site of episiotomy scar. Obstet Gynecol 40:28–34
250. Pearl ML, Valea F, Chumas J, Chalas E (1996) Primary retroperitoneal mucinous cystadenocarcinoma of low malignant potential: a case report and literature review. Gynecol Oncol 61:150–152
251. Pellegrini VD Jr, Pasternak HS, Macaulay WP (1981) Endometrioma of the pubis: a differential in the diagnosis of hip pain. A report of two cases. J Bone Joint Surg 63A:1333–1334
252. Peress MR, Sosnowski JR, Mathur RS, Williamson HO (1982) Pelvic endometriosis and Turner's syndrome. Am J Obstet Gynecol 144:474–476
253. Perrotta PL, Ginsburg FW, Siderides CI, Parkash V (1998) Liesegang rings and endometriosis. Int J Gynecol Pathol 17:358–362
254. Peterson CJ, Strickler JG, Gonzalez R, Dehner LP (1990) Uterus-like mass of the small intestine. Heterotopia or monodermal teratoma? Am J Surg Pathol 14:390–394
255. Pettinato G, Manivel JC, De Rosa N, Dehner LP (1990) Inflammatory myofibroblastic tumor (plasma cell granuloma). Clinicopathologic study of 20 cases with immunohistochemical and ultrastructural observations. Am J Clin Pathol 94:538–546
256. Prade M, Spatz A, Bentley R, Duvillard P, Bognel C, Robboy SJ (1995) Borderline and malignant serous tumor arising in pelvic lymph nodes: evidence of origin in benign glandular inclusions. Int J Gynecol Pathol 14:87–91
257. Prayson RA, Hart WR, Petras RE (1994) Pseudomyxoma peritonei. A clinicopathologic study of 19 cases with emphasis on site of origin and nature of associated ovarian tumors. Am J Surg Pathol 18:591–603

258. Prystowsky JB, Stryker SJ, Ujiki GT, Poticha SM (1988) Gastrointestinal endometriosis. Incidence and indications for resection. Arch Surg 123:855–858
259. Pueblitz-Peredo S, Luevano-Flores E, Rincon-Taracena R, Ochoa-Carrillo FJ (1985) Uteruslike mass of the ovary: endomyometriosis or congenital malformation? A case with a discussion of histogenesis. Arch Pathol Lab Med 109:361–364
260. Punnonen R, Klemi PJ, Nikkanen V (1980) Postmenopausal endometriosis. Eur J Obstet Gynecol Reprod Biol 11:195–200
261. Quagliarello J, Coppa G, Bigelow B (1985) Isolated endometriosis in an inguinal hernia. Am J Obstet Gynecol 152:688–689
262. Rahilly MA, Al-Nafusi A (1991) Uterus-like mass of the ovary associated with endometrioid carcinoma. Histopathology (Oxf) 18:549–551
263. Ray J, Conger M, Ireland K (1985) Ureteral obstruction in postmenopausal woman with endometriosis. Urology 26:577–578
264. Recalde AL, Majmudar B (1977) Endometriosis involving the femoral vein. South Med J 70:69–74
265. Reddy CRRM, Venkateswar Rao D, Sarma ENB, et al (1975) Granulomatous peritonitis due to *Ascaris lumbricoides* and its ova. J Trop Med Hyg 78:146–149
266. Reddy P, Gorelick DF, Brasher CA, et al (1970) Progressive disseminated histoplasmosis as seen in adults. Am J Med 48:629–636
267. Redwine DB (1987) Age-related evolution in color appearance of endometriosis. Fertil Steril 48:1062–1063
268. Redwine DB (1987) The distribution of endometriosis in the pelvis by age groups and fertility. Fertil Steril 47:173–175
269. Redwine DB (1989) Peritoneal pockets and endometriosis. Confirmation of an important relationship, with further observations. J Reprod Med 34:270–272
270. Reich H, De Caprio J, McGlynn F, et al (1989) Peritoneal trophoblastic tissue implants after laparoscopic treatment of tubal ectopic pregnancy. Fertil Steril 52:337
271. Riddell RH, Goodman MJ, Moossa AR (1981) Peritoneal malignant mesothelioma in a patient with recurrent peritonitis. Cancer (Phila) 48:134–139
272. Rock JA, Parmley TH, King TM, et al (1981) Endometriosis and the development of tuboperitoneal fistulas after tubal ligation. Fertil Steril 35:16–20
273. Ronnett BM, Kurman RJ, Zahn CM, Shmookler BM, Jablonski KA, Kass ME, Sugarbaker PH (1995) Pseudomyxoma peritonei in women: a clinicopathologic analysis of 30 cases with emphasis on site of origin, prognosis, and relationship to ovarian mucinous tumors of low malignant potential. Hum Pathol 56:509–524
274. Ronnett BM, Shmookler BM, Sugarbaker PH, Kurman RJ (1997) Pseudomyxoma peritonei: new concepts in diagnosis, origin, nomenclature, and relationship to mucinous borderline (low malignant potential) tumors of the ovary. Anat Pathol 2:198–226
275. Ronnett BM, Zahn CM, Kurman RJ, Kass ME, Sugarbaker PH, Shmookler BM (1995) Disseminated peritoneal adenomucinosis and peritoneal mucinous carcinomatosis. Am J Surg Pathol 19:1390–1408
276. Rosai J (1982) Uteruslike mass replacing ovary [Letter] Arch Pathol Lab Med 106:364
277. Rosai J, Dehner LP (1975) Nodular mesothelial hyperplasia in hernia sacs. A benign reactive condition stimulating a neoplastic process. Cancer (Phila) 35:165–175
278. Ross MJ, Welch WR, Scully RE (1989) Multilocular peritoneal inclusion cysts (so-called cystic mesotheliomas). Cancer (Phila) 64:1336–1346
279. Roth LM (1973) Endometriosis with perineural involvement. Am J Clin Pathol 59:807–809
280. Rovati V, Faleschini E, Vercellini P, et al (1990) Endometrioma of the liver. Am J Obstet Gynecol 163:1490–1492
281. Rubin IC, Lisa JR, Trinidad S (1956) Further observations on ectopic endometrium of the fallopian tube. Surg Gynecol Obstet 103:469–474
282. Ruffolo R, Suster S (1993) Diffuse histiocytic proliferation mimicking mesothelial hyperplasia in endocervicosis of the female pelvic peritoneum. Int J Surg Pathol 1:101–106
283. Russell P (1979) The pathological assessment of ovarian neoplasms. II. The proliferating 'epithelial' tumours. Pathology 11:251–282
284. Rutgers JL, Scully RE (1988) Ovarian müllerian mucinous papillary cystadenomas of borderline malignancy. A clinicopathological analysis. Cancer (Phila) 61:340–348
285. Rutgers JL, Scully RE (1988) Ovarian mixed-epithelial papillary cystadenomas of borderline malignancy of mullerian type. A clinicopathological analysis. Cancer (Phila.) 61:546–554
286. Rutgers JL, Young RH, Scully RE (1987) Ovarian yolk sac tumor arising from an endometrioid carcinoma. Hum Pathol 18:1296–1299
287. Sahin AA, Ro JY, Chen J, Ayala AG (1990) Spindle cell nodule and peptic ulcer arising in a fully developed gastric wall in a mature cystic teratoma. Arch Pathol Lab Med 114:529–531
288. Sainz de la Cuesta R, Eichhorn JH, Rice LW, Fuller AF, Nikrui N, Goff BA (1996) Histologic transformation of benign endometriosis to early epithelial ovarian cancer. Gynecol Oncol 60:238–244
289. Sampson JA (1927) Peritoneal endometriosis due to the menstrual dissemination of endometrial tissue into the peritoneal cavity. Am J Obstet Gynecol 14:422–469
290. Saw EC, Shields SJ, Comer TP, et al (1974) Granulomatous peritonitis due to coccidioides immitis. Arch Surg 108:369–371
291. Saxen L, Kassinen A, Saxen E (1963) Peritoneal foreign-body reaction caused by condom emulsion. Lancet 1:1295–1296

292. Sayfan J, Adam YG, Reif R (1979) Peritoneal encapsulation in childhood. Case report, embryologic analysis, and review of literature. Am J Surg 138:725–727
293. Schatz JE, Colgan TJ (1991) Squamous metaplasia of the peritoneum. Arch Pathol Lab Med 115:397–398
294. Schlesinger C, Silverberg SG (1999) Tamoxifen-associated polyps (basalomas) arising in multiple endometriotic foci: a case report and review of the literature. Gynecol Oncol 73:305–311
295. Schmidt CL, Demopoulos RI, Weiss G (1981) Infected endometriotic cysts: clinical characterization and pathogenesis. Fertil Steril 36:27–30
296. Schneider V, Walsh JW, Goplerud DR (1980) Benign glandular inclusions in para-aortic lymph nodes: a cause for false positive lymphangiography. Am J Obstet Gynecol 138:350–352
297. Schrodt GR, Alcorn MO, Ibanez J (1980) Endometriosis of the male urinary system: a case report. J Urol 124:722–723
298. Scully RE (1981) Smooth-muscle differentiation in genital tract disorders [Editorial]. Arch Pathol Lab Med 105:505–507
299. Scully RE, Richardson GS, Barlow JF (1966) The development of malignancy in endometriosis. Clin Obstet Gynecol 9:384–411
300. Scurry J, Duggan MA (1999) Malignant mesothelioma eight years after a diagnosis of atypical mesothelial hyperplasia. J Clin Pathol 52:535–537
301. Seidman JD (1996) Prognostic importance of hyperplasia and atypia in endometriosis. Int J Gynecol Pathol 15:1–9
302. Seidman JD, Elsayed AM, Sobin LH, Tavassoli FA (1993) Association of mucinous tumors of the ovary and appendix. A clinicopathologic study of 25 cases. Am J Surg Pathol 17:22–34
303. Seidman JD, Oberer S, Bitterman P, Aisner SC (1993) Pathogenesis of pseudoxanthomatous salpingiosis. Mod Pathol 6:53–55
304. Shanks JH, Harris M, Banerjee SS, et al (2000) Mesotheliomas with deciduoid morphology. A morphologic spectrum and a variation not confined to young females. Am J Surg Pathol 24:285–294
305. Sheldon RS, Wilson RB, Dockerty MB (1967) Serosal endometriosis of fallopian tubes. Am J Obstet Gynecol 99:882–884
306. Shen SC, Bansal M, Purrazzella R, et al (1983) Benign glandular inclusions in lymph nodes, endosalpingiosis, and salpingitis isthmica nodosa in a young girl with clear cell adenocarcinoma of the cervix. Am J Surg Pathol 7:293–300
307. Shipton EA, Meares SD (1965) Heterotopic bone formation in the ovary. Aust N Z J Obstet Gynaecol 5:100–102
308. Shiraki M, Otis CN, Powell JL (1991) Endometrial stromal sarcoma arising from ovarian and extraovarian endometriosis: report of two cases and review of the literature. Surg Pathol 4:333–343
309. Sidaway MK, Silverberg SG (1987) Endosalpingiosis in female peritoneal washings: a diagnostic pitfall. Int J Gynecol Pathol 6:340–346
310. Sieck JO, Cowgill R, Larkworthy W (1983) Peritoneal encapsulation and abdominal cocoon. Case report and review of the literature. Gastroenterology 84:1597–1601
311. Simpson JL, Elias S, Malinak LR, Buttram VC (1980) Heritable aspects of endometriosis. I. Genetic studies. Am J Obstet Gynecol 137:327–331
312. Sjövall A, Åkerman M (1968) Peritoneal granulomas in women due to the presence of enterobius S. oxyuris vermicularis. Acta Obstet Gynecol Scand 47:361–372
313. Sneige N, Fanning CV (1992) Peritoneal washing cytology in women: diagnostic pitfalls and clues for correct diagnosis. Diagn Cytopathol 8:632–642
314. Sneige M, Fernandez T, Copeland LJ, et al (1986) Müllerian inclusions in peritoneal washings. Acta Cytol 30:271–276
315. Sobel HJ, Marquet E, Schwarz R, Mazur MT (1984) Optically clear endometrial nuclei. Ultrastruct Pathol 6:229–231
316. Sohar E, Gafni J, Pras M, et al (1967) Familial Mediterranean fever. A survey of 470 cases and review of the literature. Am J Med 43:227–253
317. Solis OG, Bui HX, Malfetano JH, Ross JS (1991) Extragenital primary mixed malignant mesodermal tumor. Gynecol Oncol 43:182–185
318. Stanley KE, Utz DC, Dockerty MB (1965) Clinically significant endometriosis of the urinary tract. Surg Gynecol Obstet 120:491–498
319. Steck WD, Helwig EB (1966) Cutaneous endometriosis. Clin Obstet Gynecol 9:373–383
320. Steele RW, Dmowski WP, Marmer DJ (1984) Immunologic aspects of human endometriosis. Am J Reprod Immunol 6:33–36
321. Stock RJ (1982) Postsalpingectomy endometriosis: a reassessment. Obstet Gynecol 60: 560–570
322. Stripling MC, Martin DC, Chatman DL, et al (1988) Subtle appearance of pelvic endometriosis. Fertil Steril 49:427–431
323. Stripling MC, Martin DC, Poston WM (1988) Does endometriosis have a typical appearance? J Reprod Med 33:879–884
324. Sun CJ, Toker C, Masi JD, et al (1979) Primary low grade adenocarcinoma occurring in the inguinal region. Cancer (Phila) 44:340–345
325. Surrey ES, Halme J (1989) Endometriosis as a cause of infertility. Obstet Gynecol Clin N Am 16:79–91
326. Sussman J, Rosai J (1990) Lymph node metastasis as the initial manifestation of malignant mesothelioma. Report of six cases. Am J Surg Pathol 14: 818–828
327. Targan SR, Chow AW, Guze LB (1977) Role of anaerobic bacteria in spontaneous peritonitis of cirrhosis. Report of two cases and review of the literature. Am J Med 62:397–403
328. Teoh TB (1953) The structure and development of Walthard nests. J Pathol 66:433–439
329. Thatcher SS, Grainger DA, True LD, DeCherney AH

(1989) Pelvic trophoblastic implants after laparoscopic removal of a tubal pregnancy. Obstet Gynecol 74:514–515
330. Thibodeau LL, Prioleau GR, Manuelidis EE, et al (1987) Cerebral endometriosis. J Neurosurg 66: 609–610
331. Tibboel D, Gaillard JLJ, Molenaar JC (1986) The importance of mesenteric vascular insufficiency in meconium peritonitis. Hum Pathol 17:411–416
332. Tidman MJ, MacDonald DM (1988) Cutaneous endometriosis: a histopathologic study. J Am Acad Dermatol 18:373–377
333. Tinker MA, Burdman D, Deysine M, et al (1974) Granulomatous peritonitis due to cellulose fibers from disposable surgical fabrics. Ann Surg 180: 831–835
334. Tobacman JK, Tucker MA, Kase R, Greene MH, Costa J, Fraumeni JF Jr (1982) Intra-abdominal carcinomatosis after prophylactic oophorectomy in ovarian-cancer-prone families. Lancet 2:795–797
335. Toki T, Fujii S, Silverberg SG (1996) A clinicopathologic study of the association of endometriosis and carcinoma of the ovary using a scoring system. Int J Gynecol Cancer 6:68–75
336. Torkelson SJ, Lee RA, Hildahl DB (1988) Endometriosis of the sciatic nerve: a report of two cases and a review of the literature. Obstet Gynecol 71:473
337. Trimble EL, Saigo PE, Freeberg GW, Rubin SC, Hoskins WJ (1991) Peritoneal sarcoidosis and elevated CA 125. Obstet Gynecol 78:976–977
338. Truong LD, Maccato ML, Awalt H, et al (1990) Serous surface carcinoma of the peritoneum: a clinicopathologic study of 22 cases. Hum Pathol 21:99–110
339. Turrnir R, Kerrigan SAJ, Clement PB, Young RH, Churg A Diffuse malignant epithelial mesotheliomas of the peritoneum in women. A clinicopathologic study of 25 cases. Cancer (in press)
340. Ulbright TM, Kraus FT (1981) Endometrial stromal tumors of extra-uterine tissue. Am J Clin Pathol 76:371–377
341. Ulbright TM, Morley DJ, Roth LM, et al (1983) Papillary serous carcinoma of the retroperitoneum. Am J Clin Pathol 79:633–637
342. Veiga-Ferreira MM, Leiman G, Dunbar F, Margolius KA (1987) Cervical endometriosis: facilitated diagnosis by fine needle aspiration cytologic testing. Am J Obstet Gynecol 157:849–856
343. Vuong PN, Guyot H, Moulin G, et al (1990) Pseudotumoral organization of a twisted epiploic fringe or `hard-boiled egg' in the peritoneal cavity. Arch Pathol Lab Med 114:531–533
344. Wanless IR, Bernier V (1983) Fibrous thickening of the splenic capsule. Arch Pathol Lab Med 107: 595–599
345. Watson NE Jr, Johnson AH (1973) Cryptococcal peritonitis. South Med J 66:387–388
346. Weibel MA, Majno G (1973) Peritoneal adhesions and their relation to abdominal surgery. Am J Surg 126:345–353
347. Weinstein MP, Iannini PB, Stratton CW, et al (1978) Spontaneous bacterial peritonitis. A review of 28 cases with emphasis on improved survival and factors influencing prognosis. Am J Med 64:592–598
348. Weir M, Bell DA, Young RH (1998) Grade 1 peritoneal serous carcinomas. A report of 14 cases and comparison with 7 peritoneal serous psammocarcinomas and 19 peritoneal serous borderline tumors. Am J Surg Pathol 22:849–862
349. Weiss SW, Tavassoli FA (1988) Multicystic mesothelioma: an analysis of pathologic findings and biologic behavior in 37 cases. Am J Surg Pathol 12:737–746
350. Wheeler JM (1989) Epidemiology of endometriosis-associated infertility. J Reprod Med 34:41–46
351. White J, Chan Y-F (1994) Lipofuscinosis peritonei associated with pregancy-related ectopic decidua. Histopathology (Oxf) 25:83–85
352. Wick MR, Mills SE, Dehner LP, et al (1989) Serous papillary carcinomas arising from the peritoneum and ovaries. A clinicopathologic and immunohistochemical comparison. Int J Gynecol Pathol 8:179–188
353. Williams GA (1969) Endometriosis of the cervix uteri: a common disease. Am J Obstet Gynecol 80: 734–741
354. Williams TJ, Pratt JH (1977) Endometriosis in 1,000 consecutive celiotomies: incidence and management. Am J Obstet Gynecol 129:245–250
355. Wolf AN, Ladanyi M, Paull G, Blaugrund JE, Westra WH (1999) The expanding clinical spectrum of desmoplastic small round-cell tumor: a report of two cases with molecular confirmation. Hum Pathol 30:430–435
356. Wolf GC, Singh KB (1989) Cesarean scar endometriosis: a review. Obstet Gynecol Surv 44:89–95
357. Wolfe SA, Mackles A, Greene HJ (1961) Endometriosis of the cervix. Am J Obstet Gynecol 81: 111–123
358. Wong M, Rosen SW (1962) Ascites in sarcoidosis due to peritoneal involvement. Ann Intern Med 57:277–280
359. Yantiss RK, Clement PB, Young RH (2000) Neoplastic and pre-neoplastic changes in gastrointestinal endometriosis: A study of 17 cases. Am J Surg Pathol 24:513–524
360. Yoonessi M, Satchindanand SK, Ortinez CG, et al (1982) Benign glandular elements and decidual reaction in retroperitoneal lymph nodes. J Surg Oncol 19:81–86
361. Young RH, Clement PB (1996) Müllerianosis of the urinary bladder. Mod Pathol 9:731–737
361a. Young RH, Clement PB (2000) Endocervicosis involving the uterine cervix: A report of four cases of a benign process that may be confused with deeply

invasive endocervical adenocarcinoma. Int J Gynecol Pathol 19:322–328

362. Young RH, Eichhorn JH, Dickersin GR, Scully RE (1992) Ovarian involvement by the intra-abdominal desmoplastic small round cell tumor with divergent differentiation: a report of three cases. Hum Pathol 23:454–464
363. Young RH, Gilks CB, Scully RE (1991) Mucinous tumors of the appendix associated with mucinous tumors of the ovary and pseudomyxoma peritonei. A clinicopathological analysis of 22 cases supporting an origin in the appendix. Am J Surg Pathol 15:415–429
364. Young RH, Prat J, Scully RE (1984) Endometrioid stromal sarcomas of the ovary. A clinicopathologic analysis of 23 cases. Cancer (Phila) 53:1143–1155
365. Young RH, Rosenberg AE, Clement PB (1997) Mucin deposits presenting within inguinal hernia sacs: a presenting finding of low grade mucinous cystic tumors of the appendix. A report of two cases and review of the literature. Mod Pathol 10:1228–1232
366. Young RH, Scully RE (1986) Testicular and paratesticular tumors and tumor-like lesions of ovarian common epithelial and müllerian types. A report of four cases and review of the literature. Am J Clin Pathol 86:146–152
367. Zaytsev P, Taxy JB (1987) Pregnancy-associated ectopic decidua. Am J Surg Pathol 11:526–530
368. Zinsser KR, Wheeler JE (1982) Endosalpingiosis in the omentum. A study of autopsy and surgical material. Am J Surg Pathol 6:109–117

18

Surface Epithelial Tumors of the Ovary

Jeffrey D. Seidman, M.D., Peter Russell, M.D., and Robert J. Kurman, M.D.

Epidemiology

Geographic Distribution, Incidence, and Mortality

Worldwide, ovarian cancer is the sixth most common cancer in women.[50] In most Western countries, ovarian carcinoma is the fifth most common malignancy and ranks fourth in cancer mortality. In the Western hemisphere, it accounts for 4% of cancer in women and is the most frequent cause of death from gynecologic cancer.[50] In U.S. women, ovarian cancer accounts for 5% of cancer deaths.[148] It is estimated that in the United States in 2000 there will be 23,100 new ovarian cancer cases and 14,000 deaths.[148] Approximately 1.4% of American women will develop ovarian cancer in their lifetime. In general, the disease is more common in industrialized countries where parity is lower, but there are notable exceptions, such as Japan, which has a low parity and low rate of ovarian cancer. The lifetime risk varies widely, from 0.45% in Japan to 1.7% in Sweden. Annual incidence rates of ovarian cancer range from less than 5 per 100,000 women in Gambia, Brazil, Thailand, Algeria, and India, to greater than 13 per 100,000 in the UK, United States, Germany, Norway, Denmark, and Sweden.[50] Migration studies have shown that ovarian cancer rates approach those of the place of immigration rather than the place of emigration, suggesting a significant environmental component to ovarian cancer risk.[23,373]

Age and Genetic Factors

Ovarian cancer rates increase exponentially with *age*. In the United States, the annual risk steadily increases from less than 3 per 100,000 in women under age 30 and plateaus at 54 per 100,000 in the 75-

to 79-year-old group.[473] The mean age of women with ovarian cancer is about 60 years.

Genetic factors are important in ovarian cancer risk. Hereditary ovarian cancer is responsible for approximately 10% of cases due to the markedly increased risk conferred by the *BRCA1* and *BRCA2* tumor suppressor genes (see "Molecular Basis of Hereditary Predisposition to Ovarian Cancer," later in this chapter). Notably, the increased frequency of ovarian cancer in relatives of women with ovarian cancer is not paralleled by an increase among relatives of women with "borderline" ovarian tumors.[374] White women have higher rates than blacks; in the United States, African-American women have a rate two-thirds that of caucasian women.[50,315] Ovarian cancer rates vary among different ethnic groups. For example, in Israel, Jewish women have a risk eightfold that of non-Jewish women.[23]

Reproductive Factors: Risk Factors and Protective Factors

Evidence suggests that *reproductive factors* are important in ovarian cancer risk. Established protective factors include increasing parity and oral contraceptive use.[323] Some but not all studies have demonstrated that early menarche and late menopause are significant risk factors.[50] Although it is well established that increased parity is associated with decreased ovarian cancer risk worldwide,[23] it is not clear whether this reflects a protective effect of pregnancy or a hazardous effect of infertility.[373] It is also unclear whether the alleged increase in risk associated with fertility drugs simply reflects the risk of infertility itself.[23] High socioeconomic status is associated with an increased ovarian cancer risk; this is believed to be a result of lower fertility rates in these women. The protective effect of increased parity and oral contraceptive use is strongest for nonmucinous tumors; the risk of mucinous ovarian tumors alone is not significantly reduced.[331] Surgically induced protective factors against ovarian cancer include hysterectomy, tubal ligation, and oophorectomy. The mechanism for risk reduction with hysterectomy and tubal ligation is unclear.

In addition to the risk factors just noted, several other risk factors have been studied, but any associations with ovarian cancer risk are inconclusive; these include age at birth of first child, hormone replacement therapy (HRT), breastfeeding, weight, diet, talc, smoking, certain types of viral infections in childhood, and ionizing radiation.[23] A recent meta-analysis of HRT and ovarian cancer risk showed a slightly elevated risk with ever-use of HRT (odds ratio of 1.15) that was of marginal statistical significance.[135]

Screening and Prevention

An effective *cancer screening test* that is cost-effective and feasible on a population scale should have some of the following attributes: (1) the disease must be sufficiently common; (2) the organ must be accessible for screening; (3) the precursor lesions of the cancer must be defined; and (4) early diagnosis must have demonstrable survival benefit. Regrettably, ovarian cancer at most has only one of these features. The excellent prognosis of patients with stage I disease and the poor outcome of advanced-stage disease suggests but does not prove a significant survival benefit of early diagnosis. Ovarian cancer is uncommon, the ovaries are relatively inaccessible, and the precursor lesions are largely unknown. Therefore, development of a screening test for ovarian cancer will be difficult. Among more than 50,000 women screened with ultrasound, most in conjunction with serum CA 125 levels, fewer than one cancer per thousand women screened was identified.[462a]

Few data are available regarding *prevention of ovarian cancer*. Preventive measures that could be recommended on a population-wide basis, such as diet modification and cessation of smoking, have an unclear relationship to ovarian cancer risk. Prophylactic oophorectomy is often performed in patients at high risk of ovarian cancer. Unfortunately, subsequent to the removal of benign ovaries, a few of these women develop primary peritoneal serous carcinomas at rates from 1.9%[314] to 10.7%[112] after varying follow-up periods; this would suggest a multifocal, multiclonal origin of ovarian-type serous carcinomas in these women in contrast to the suspected clonal origin of typical ovarian carcinomas. In fact, there is molecular evidence that patients with *BRCA1* mutations may develop polyclonal peritoneal serous carcinomas, even before oophorectomy, based on loss of heterozygosity and X-chromosome inactivation study of the androgen receptor gene locus.[112,376] Alternatively, it has been suggested that apparent primary peritoneal carcinomas in these women may represent metastases from occult microscopic primary ovarian carcinomas that were overlooked in the oophorectomy specimens.[462a]

Etiology and Pathogenesis

Surface epithelial tumors of the ovary display a wide variety of histologic types, and for purposes of understanding their pathogenesis they need to be considered individually by cell type. One useful way of considering the pathogenesis of ovarian carcinoma is by dividing them into those that appear to develop de novo (serous carcinomas) and those that appear to develop from benign and atypical proliferative precursor lesions (mucinous, endometrioid, and clear cell carcinomas). Although most investigators believe serous carcinomas develop de novo, there is a reasonable alternative hypothesis. The difference between serous and nonserous tumors may reflect the rapidity of the adenoma–carcinoma sequence rather than a qualitative difference in the pathogenesis. Specifically, it can be argued that the adenoma–carcinoma sequence for serous tumors is variable but, on average, shorter than that for mucinous, endometrioid, and clear cell tumors; this would explain the relative uniformity of serous carcinomas and the relatively infrequent presence of neoplastic precursor lesions. High-grade carcinomas, rather than developing de novo, simply obliterate the precursor lesions because of rapid growth.

Approximately three-quarters of serous carcinomas at the time of diagnosis are high grade and widely disseminated throughout the peritoneum (FIGO [Internal Federation of Gynecology and Obstetrics] stage II and III) with the largest volume of the tumor outside the ovary. Some data support the view that these tumors arise directly from the surface epithelium or from inclusion cysts and less frequently from benign serous cystadenomas. Evidence for this is derived from three different types of studies: (1) examination of uninvolved contralateral ovaries from patients with carcinoma confined to one ovary; (2) examination of ovaries removed prophylactically from women with a strong family history of ovarian and/or breast carcinoma or with known *BRCA1* or *BRCA2* mutations; and (3) examination of the surface epithelium and inclusions adjacent to ovarian carcinomas. Although all these studies are to some extent biased and flawed because of their retrospective nature and design, some tentative conclusions can be drawn. A range of surface lesions from those with very subtle abnormalities to those displaying marked cytologic atypia have been described. These findings and the relative infrequency of associated benign and atypical proliferative serous tumors (as compared to the high frequency in mucinous and endometrioid neoplasms) suggest that the majority of invasive serous carcinomas may be derived from the surface epithelium or inclusions. As already noted, a rapid adenoma–carcinoma sequence for serous tumors could also explain these observations. Because of the inaccessibility of the ovaries to close monitoring, as compared to the cervix or endometrium, the likelihood of ever identifying a precursor lesion whose natural history can be clinically followed is very low.

In contrast to the usual type of serous carcinoma, a relatively unusual type of low-grade serous carcinoma termed micropapillary serous carcinoma (MPSC) is commonly associated with atypical proliferative (borderline) serous tumors (APST). In fact, the noninvasive form of this tumor is associated with APST in approximately 90% of cases. Because transitions of APSTs to MPSCs are frequently observed and because small foci of micropapillary architecture are not uncommon in APSTs, it appears likely that MPSCs are derived from them. This mechanism would suggest a prolonged adenoma–carcinoma sequence in this subtype of serous tumors, in contrast to the de novo origin or the rapid adenoma–carcinoma sequence in typical serous carcinomas.

Molecular studies aimed at clarifying the pathogenesis of serous tumors have been limited but thus far have consistently demonstrated different molecular alterations in cystadenomas, APSTs, and frankly invasive serous carcinomas, supporting the conclusion that the majority of typical serous carcinomas do not develop from cystadenomas and APSTs. For example, although *p53* mutations are found in approximately 50%–60% of invasive serous carcinomas, and loss of heterozygosity (LOH) is common in these tumors, *p53* mutations and LOH of the *p53* locus are extremely uncommon in adenomas and APSTs. Alternatively, it could be argued that *p53* mutation is a relatively late event in the transformation of a cystadenoma to a carcinoma. Finally, although several molecular studies of advanced-stage serous carcinomas have shown that they are clonal, there have been no studies of ovarian carcinomas with minimal spread and therefore the possibility of multifocal development cannot be entirely excluded. In particular, the clonality of stage IB tumors to determine whether the right and left ovarian tumors are independent would be important. Thus, the available evidence is most consistent with serous carcinoma arising de novo from the surface epithelium or surface epithelial inclusions in the majority of cases. MPSC, a relatively uncommon low-grade carcinoma that arises from APST, does not arise de novo.

In contrast to their serous counterparts, mucinous, endometrioid, and clear cell carcinomas more convincingly appear to develop from benign counterparts that include mucinous cystadenomas, endometriotic cysts, and endometrioid adenofibromas. Mucinous, endometrioid, and clear cell carcinomas frequently display benign-appearing areas that probably reflect the precursor lesion, in contrast to serous carcinomas that uncommonly display benign-appearing areas. Hyperplasia and atypical hyperplasia in endometriosis and atypical proliferative (borderline) mucinous and endometrioid tumors are also frequently found in association with their benign and frankly malignant counterparts, suggesting a pathway of carcinogenesis similar to the adenoma–carcinoma sequence in colon cancer. Several lines of evidence support this view, including data on intratumoral heterogeneity, the high proportion of stage I cases, and K-*ras* mutational analyses. The finding of foci of intraepithelial carcinoma merging with areas of atypical proliferative mucinous tumors (APMT), also supports this view of ovarian mucinous carcinogenesis. Approximately two-thirds of mucinous carcinomas contain areas of APMT or intraepithelial carcinoma.[330] Although it appears certain that virtually all mucinous carcinomas follow this pattern of carcinogenesis, the same cannot be said for all endometrioid carcinomas because some of them, particularly the poorly differentiated ones, are morphologically very similar to serous carcinomas and at times can show the same widespread dissemination as serous carcinoma at diagnosis.

Molecular biologic studies of mucinous tumors have confirmed the morphologic findings by demonstrating similar frequencies of K-*ras* mutations in APMTs and carcinomas and have also shown similar K-*ras* mutations in adenomas, APMTs, and mucinous carcinomas. Similarly, molecular studies of endometriotic cysts have shown that many of them are monoclonal and have also demonstrated LOH at the same genetic loci in both endometrioid carcinomas and in endometriosis adjacent to the tumor.

An understanding of the pathogenesis of ovarian cancer has important implications for ovarian cancer screening. Most "ovarian cancers" are serous carcinomas of the usual type. As these tumors develop from the surface epithelium or epithelial inclusions that progress through a rapid adenoma–carcinoma sequence and can be relatively small even when they are widely disseminated, both vaginal ultrasound and serum CA-125 lack sufficient sensitivity and, for that matter, specificity to detect serous carcinomas at a curable stage. In fact, screening studies using these modalities merely identify functional cysts and cystadenomas and have not been successful in identifying carcinomas at a frequency sufficiently high enough to warrant implementation in the general population. In contrast, only a small proportion of ovarian carcinomas are mucinous and endometrioid tumors. These tumors appear to grow slowly from benign cystadenomas that become quite large before undergoing malignant transformation. As a result, most patients with these tumors are diagnosed with large pelvic masses on pelvic examination without the need of ultrasound before the neoplasms have undergone malignant transformation. This sequence of events with delayed transformation and dissemination accounts for the high proportion of well-differentiated and FIGO stage I cases among mucinous and endometrioid carcinomas as compared to serous carcinomas, which are typically poorly differentiated and disseminate early in their natural history.

Putative Histopathologic Precursor Lesions

Despite the accumulating evidence of the pathogenesis just described, it is widely acknowledged that the *precursors of ovarian carcinoma* are for the most part uncertain.[124,377] The candidates for precursors of ovarian carcinoma include epithelial dysplasia of the surface epithelium or germinal inclusions, a benign proliferative lesion such as endometriosis, and benign neoplasms, that is, cystadenomas and cystadenofibromas. Alternatively, carcinomas could arise directly from the surface epithelium without an intermediate precursor lesion.[33] It is conceivable that all these mechanisms account for ovarian carcinomas. The important questions include what proportion of ovarian carcinomas, and what cell types, are accounted for by each of these mechanisms. As already discussed, serous carcinomas either arise de novo from the surface epithelium or inclusions or arise from adenomas and undergo a rapid adenoma–carcinoma sequence. Many mucinous, endometrioid, and clear cell carcinomas clearly arise from preexisting benign lesions.

The study of precursors of ovarian carcinoma is difficult because the ovaries are not readily accessible for screening and ovarian carcinomas are often large and present in advanced stage, obliterating or rendering unrecognizable any precursor lesion that may have been present. Furthermore, identification of a putative precursor lesion within an ovary generally involves removal of that ovary and hence the natural history of the lesion cannot be observed. Limited data have been recently reported in a few studies on ovaries removed prophylactically from high-risk women and normal-appearing ovaries contralateral to stage I carcinomas.

Surface Epithelial Dysplasia

Investigators have studied ovarian surface epithelium in the vicinity of carcinomas in an attempt to define the putative entity of *ovarian dysplasia* and have reported atypical cellular and nuclear features that appear more frequently in ovarian surface epithelium near carcinomas in comparison to distant from carcinomas and in control ovaries. These data are difficult to interpret because the studies were not blinded and the criteria developed were not tested on an independent set of cases.[95,152,317] For example, in one of these studies, the criteria that were used to diagnose the dysplasia that was subsequently "confirmed" by nuclear texture analysis were never defined at the outset.[96] Furthermore, atypical ovarian surface epithelium adjacent to a carcinoma could represent an intraepithelial component or intraepithelial extension of the tumor rather than a precursor,[263] as suggested by molecular evidence from one study.[488] Some investigators have reported that, although not identifiable by light microscopy, subtle nuclear changes identified by image analysis are detectable in the surface epithelium of ovaries prophylactically removed from high-risk women in comparison to controls.[461] In contrast, another group of investigators[394] examined high-risk ovaries under oil immersion and found only subtle atypical features that were not significantly more common in cases than controls.

A recent study examining the surface epithelium and germinal epithelial inclusions in ovaries prophylactically removed from high-risk women found no increased expression of *p53*, c-*erbB*-2, or the proliferation marker Ki-67 compared to controls.[462]

Germinal Epithelial Inclusions

Simple glands and cysts lined by a single layer of tubal-type epithelium, termed *surface epithelial, cortical*, or *germinal inclusions*, frequently are present in the superficial ovarian cortex, particularly in older women. They arise when invaginations of the ovarian cortex lined by surface epithelium lose their connection to the surface, and are not related to ovulation.[378] Although ovarian carcinomas are generally acknowledged to arise from the surface epithelium, observations on small ovarian epithelial neoplasms, particularly the cystic forms, indicate that they more frequently arise within germinal inclusions.[124,377–380] Dysplasia may theoretically occur within these inclusions,[94] but whether dysplasia in the inclusion is an intermediate lesion in the progression from benign to malignant is unknown.

Similarly, epithelial proliferations within such inclusions occur but their natural history is unknown. Tubal metaplasia and several ovarian carcinoma markers including CA-125, CA-19-9, placental-like alkaline phosphatase, and human milk fat globule protein are more commonly identified in these inclusions in comparison to the ovarian surface epithelium.[378] Some studies on prophylactic oophorectomy specimens in high-risk women and normal-appearing ovaries contralateral to stage I carcinomas have shown a higher number of these cortical inclusions in comparison to controls,[263,461] but others have not confirmed these findings.[394,441] Some studies have also evaluated cortical invaginations and surface papillomatosis and found them to be more common in cancer-prone ovaries than in controls,[441] but again, these findings have not been confirmed by other investigators.[461]

Endometriosis

Although the precursors of ovarian carcinoma are for the most part unknown, *endometriosis* is the best documented precursor of ovarian carcinoma. Endometriosis is common, found in 7%–20% of women, and the risk of malignant transformation in an individual patient is negligible. Nonetheless, endometriosis may be a precursor for as many as 21% of ovarian cancers. Endometriosis is acknowledged to be the precursor of at least some endometrioid and clear cell carcinomas and, rarely, serous carcinomas. Premalignant lesions of many sites share common clinical and pathologic features,[385] some of which are displayed by endometriosis.

Endometriosis is the most plausible and recognizable morphologic precursor of ovarian carcinomas. Atypical endometrial hyperplasia in the uterus is a well-defined precursor of endometrial adenocarcinoma (see Chapter 11, Precancerous Lesions of Endometrial Carcinomas), and changes similar to this lesion are occasionally observed in endometriosis.[386] In addition, atypical changes are also seen in endometriosis in the vicinity of endometrioid adenocarcinomas of the ovary, which, on occasion, displays the full morphologic spectrum of neoplastic progression, that is, endometriosis without atypia, with atypical hyperplasia, and well-differentiated endometrioid adenocarcinoma.[102,130,254,360] Limited data suggest that atypical hyperplasia in endometriosis is associated with an increased risk of neoplastic transformation.[386] Further support for the premalignant potential of endometriosis comes from DNA ploidy and molecular biologic studies. One study identified DNA aneuploidy in severely atypical epithelial cells lining endometriotic cysts.[22] Loss of heterozygosity on chromosomes 9p, 11q, and/or 22q was found in 28% of 40 cases of endometriosis.[181] In another series, a monoclonal X-inactivation pattern in 3 of 5 endometriotic cysts was identified.[284] In a series of 11 endometriotic cysts, all cases showed monoclonal methylation patterns of the androgen receptor gene locus.[182] It is thus apparent that a significant proportion of endometriotic lesions are clonal and thus neoplastic, and therefore have the potential to undergo further genetic changes and malignant transformation.

On average, approximately 6% of all ovarian carcinomas are associated with endometriosis in that ovary, and 9% of all ovarian carcinomas are associated with extraovarian endometriosis. In large series in which endometriosis was specifically sought,

12%–21% of ovarian cancer patients had endometriosis.[182,355,439] These figures could be an overestimate because the association of endometriosis with carcinoma could be coincidental in some cases. On the other hand, these figures may be an underestimate because carcinomas often overgrow and obliterate precursor lesions. It is important to note that endometriosis is a common disorder and therefore the risk of an individual with endometriosis of developing ovarian carcinoma is extremely low. The relative proportion of endometrioid and clear cell carcinomas that are associated with endometriosis is much higher than that for serous and mucinous carcinomas, supporting endometriosis as a precursor of the endometrioid and clear cell subtypes of ovarian cancer; the association with serous and mucinous carcinomas is more likely to be coincidental.

Further evidence that endometriosis is a precursor of ovarian carcinoma is provided by a Swedish study of more than 20,000 women hospitalized with endometriosis. After a mean follow-up of 11.4 years, the overall cancer risk was 1.2 in comparison to the control population. The highest risk was for ovarian cancer with a relative risk of 1.9 [95% confidence interval (CI), 1.3–2.8]. Patients with a long-standing history of endometriosis (10 years or longer) had a relative risk of 4.2 (95% CI, 2.0–7.7).[51]

Benign and Atypical Proliferative Neoplasms

It well recognized that benign neoplasms of many sites undergo malignant transformation at varying frequencies, and the ovaries appear to be no exception. However, this is speculative and based on circumstantial evidence. The natural history of benign tumors usually cannot be observed because they are generally completely removed for diagnosis. Whether benign ovarian neoplasms undergo malignant transformation at any appreciable frequency is unknown.[124,377,379] Ovarian carcinomas are often heterogeneous, and morphologically benign areas often are present within carcinomas.[322,488] However, there is only circumstantial evidence that ovarian cystadenomas may undergo malignant transformation.[124,377] Benign-appearing epithelium has been identified at different frequencies in carcinomas of the various epithelial types: 74% for mucinous, 46% for endometrioid, 39% for clear cell, and 15% for serous carcinomas.[378] Furthermore, benign-appearing epithelium was generally found in younger women than those without identifiable benign-appearing epithelium.[378] Although some data suggest that benign-appearing epithelium in an ovarian carcinoma may reflect a well-differentiated portion of the neoplasm rather than a precursor,[488] the findings of other investigators do not support this conclusion.[469] It is well documented that carcinomas, particularly those metastatic to the ovaries, may have morphologically benign-appearing components (see Chapter 22, Metastatic Tumors of the Ovary); this is an example of another situation in which *morphologically* benign epithelium can be, in fact, malignant. The progressive increase in mean age of women with benign, atypical proliferative, and malignant ovarian epithelial tumors is also suggestive of progression but is circumstantial as well.[377] Other evidence suggesting progression of benign to malignant is the increased frequency of benign epithelial ovarian neoplasms in first- and second-degree relatives of ovarian cancer patients.[378]

Molecular biology has provided additional information involving the potential of benign ovarian neoplasms to progress to carcinoma. Molecular studies on morphologically benign and malignant components of the same neoplasms are limited and have not yet answered the important question of the nature of the benign-appearing components of carcinomas.[469,488] However, there appear to be significant differences between serous and mucinous tumors that provide some insight into their pathogenesis. The presence of K-*ras* mutations in benign, atypical proliferative, and malignant ovarian mucinous neoplasms supports an important role for this gene in ovarian mucinous carcinogenesis[82,244] and suggests a neoplastic progression from benign to proliferative to malignant,[57] as already discussed. In contrast, most studies on the spectrum of serous ovarian neoplasms suggest that they are molecularly distinct and do not support a progression from benign to malignant. For example, atypical proliferative serous tumors lack *p53* mutations while serous carcinomas often harbor *p53* mutations.[217,229,488] However, a specific low-grade variant of serous carcinoma, designated micropapillary serous carcinoma (MPSC) (see "Serous Tumors," following), displays features that strongly suggest an origin in a preexisting atypical proliferative serous tumor. MPSC displays a distinctive pattern of *p53* immunostaining but lacks *p53* mutation, suggesting increased expression of wild-type *p53* protein.[189]

Hormonal Factors: The "Incessant Ovulation" and Gonadotropin Hypotheses

The most commonly cited hormonal mechanism for the etiology of ovarian cancer is the *incessant ovulation hypothesis*.[119] It was hypothesized that ovulation repeatedly traumatizes the ovarian surface epithelium and thus stimulates proliferation, creating a milieu that predisposes the actively proliferating epithelium to malignant transformation. This hypothesis is supported by epidemiologic observations that indicate a direct correlation between the number of ovulations, that is, the length of the reproductive years uninterrupted by pregnancies or oral contraceptive use, and the risk of ovarian cancer (see "Epidemiology," earlier, and Chapter 27, Epidemiology). However, the degree of protection conferred by factors such as oral contraceptive use are incompletely explained.[23,323]

Factors that reduce the number of ovulations reduce ovarian cancer risk at varying and disproportionate amounts.[279] In addition, proponents of the incessant ovulation theory believe that ovulation results in the formation of surface epithelial inclusion cysts, the site at which the majority of ovarian carcinomas arise (see "Putative Histopathologic Precursor Lesions"), but there is strong evidence that this is not an important mechanism in humans.[378] Among this evidence, the presence of inclusions in fetal ovaries[44] and their increased occurrence in hypoovulatory states such as polycystic ovary syndrome are the most convincing.[378] Even if the incessant ovulation hypothesis is correct, it could not possibly contribute to explaining extraovarian carcinogenesis of homologous neoplasms, that is serous carcinomas of the peritoneum, which are epidemiologically, clinically, and pathologically essentially identical to ovarian serous carcinomas.

The *gonadotropin hypothesis,* which is less favored than the incessant ovulation hypothesis, proposes that high levels of circulating gonadotropins increase the risk of ovarian cancer, either directly by altering estrogen levels or via mechanisms that cause primary ovarian failure.[77] Although the gonadotropin levels associated with pregnancy and oral contraceptive use are consistent with this hypothesis, it has been argued that the age distribution of ovarian cancer is inconsistent with it.[23] One prospective study was unable to correlate serum gonadotropin levels with ovarian cancer risk.[279]

Angiogenesis

An important aspect of carcinogenesis is *neoangiogenesis.* Solid neoplasms require a blood supply to maintain their viability and growth in both the primary as well as metastatic sites. This requirement may be of considerable clinical importance, as some evidence suggests that antagonists of angiogenesis can retard or inhibit tumor growth and thus may prove to be an effective therapy for some cancers.[458] A recent study showed that certain antiangiogenic agents inhibited growth of ovarian cancer in athymic mice.[475] Neovascularization is histologically apparent in most malignant tumors and is manifested by areas with prominent capillary networks. This microvasculature may play an important role in metastasis by providing access to the circulation. The degree of angiogenesis in a variety of malignant tumors has been correlated with clinical behavior.[213] Assessment of the degree of angiogenesis in tumors involves the labor-intensive process of counting vessels, and further work is needed to establish uniform methods for counting, and reproducibility of the data. This evaluation is facilitated by the use of immunohistochemical markers to highlight the endothelial cell layer.

Angiogenesis in nonneoplastic and neoplastic ovarian conditions has been recently reviewed.[2] Ovarian carcinomas have been shown to have higher microvessel density (MVD) than benign ovarian neoplasms,[52,86] but some authors have found no difference in MVD in atypical proliferative tumors versus carcinomas.[295] Angiogenesis in ovarian carcinomas has been reported by some investigators to correlate directly with stage and grade and inversely with survival,[86,169] but others have found no such correlations.[3,295,375] Microvessel counts in omental metastases have been correlated with survival.[3]

A variety of growth factors that are important for angiogenesis have been identified.[127] Vascular endothelial growth factor (VEGF) is a dimeric glycoprotein related to platelet-derived growth factor. Certain subtypes of VEGF have been found to be significantly overexpressed in ovarian carcinomas as compared to normal ovaries and benign ovarian neoplasms.[127,409] VEGF has been identified in normal and neoplastic ovaries and in the ascites of ovarian cancer patients.[291] Antibodies to VEGF have been shown to inhibit the development of ascites and the growth of ovarian carcinoma cell lines in immunodeficient mice.[409] VEGF is more commonly overexpressed in endometriosis compared to normal endometrium, suggesting a mechanism for endometriosis-derived carcinomas.[253a] Gonadotropins at elevated levels have also been found to induce angiogenesis of ovarian carcinomas implanted in mice.[372]

Tumor–Host Cell Interactions

Tumor-infiltrating lymphocytes have been studied in benign and malignant ovarian epithelial tumors. Significant phenotypic and functional differences were observed between lymphocytes infiltrating ovarian carcinomas as compared to atypical proliferative ovarian tumors.[449] Carcinomas contained more activated T lymphocytes and more CD 4+ lymphocytes as compared to atypical proliferative tumors; both benign and malignant tumors contained similar proportions of natural killer cells.[449] Some soluble factors such as various cytokines are released by tumor-infiltrating lymphocytes as well as by tumor cells and may play an important role in tumor progression.[257] Antigen-presenting dendritic cells are present in ovarian carcinomas; one study correlated the number of dendritic cells present with prognosis.[112a] Ovarian carcinomas often express c-*fms*, which encodes the receptor for macrophage colony-stimulating factor, a cytokine important in the control of macrophage behavior.[66]

Angiogenesis may be related to host inflammatory cell infiltrates. Ovarian tumors release factors that are chemotactic for monocytes, and the numerous cell products secreted by macrophages include angiogenic promotors and inhibitors. Macrophages may play an important role in angiogenesis of ovarian neoplasms.[296]

Ovarian stromal cells, which are nonneoplastic, are often a conspicuous component of primary ovarian neoplasms. These cells are often enzymatically active and occasionally account for clinically detected hormonal effects. Luteinized stromal cells, or steroid cells, are seen in 14% of mucinous cystadenomas, but rarely in other ovarian epithelial tumors, and usually express adrenal 4-binding protein, the transcription factor of steroidogenesis.[177] (see Chapter 19, Sex Cord–Stromal, Steroid Cell, and Other Ovarian Tumors with Endocrine, Paraendocrine, and Paraneoplastic Manifestations).

Cellular and Molecular Biology

Cell growth and division are integral elements of neoplasia. Normal and neoplastic cells progress through phases of the cell division cycle, which includes DNA replication and repair phases and checkpoints, and also undergo programmed cell death. Cancer is a derangement of this process, and is the final outcome of the replication of cells with unrepaired DNA abnormalities.[340] More specifically, mutations, deletions, methylation, and other DNA abnormalities that involve oncogenes and tumor suppressor genes are critical components of the DNA damage that characterize the stages of neoplastic progression. At present, a number of genetic abnormalities have been identified in ovarian carcinoma but few studies have correlated these changes with specific histologic types. Because the pathobiology of ovarian carcinoma is highly cell type specific, the molecular biologic data thus far have made a limited contribution to our understanding of ovarian carcinogenesis. Nonetheless, oncogenes and tumor suppressor genes can be used as targets for novel types of therapy.[26]

Cell Cycle Regulation

The cell cycle is tightly regulated by a large number of genes and their respective proteins in a complex interrelated series of events. Neoplastic cells manifest deregulated growth, division, and senescence by a variety of mechanisms. Proto-oncogenes are normal cellular growth control genes that, when mutated, amplified, or overexpressed, facilitate malignant behavior and are then designated oncogenes. Oncogenes exert their growth-promoting effects through several pathways that often include growth factors and their cell-surface receptors. Oncogenes that have been studied extensively in ovarian cancer include c-*erbB-2* (*HER2/neu*), c-*erbB-1* (EGFR), c-*myc*, and K-*ras*. Tumor suppressor genes normally inhibit cell growth through a variety of growth regulatory pathways, and when mutated lose this inhibitory effect, thus promoting cell growth. Important tumor suppressor genes in ovarian cancer include *p53*, *BRCA1*, and *BRCA2*. The cell cycle is also influenced by epigenetic mechanisms, that is, those that do not relate to specific gene sequences but rather to overall DNA and chromosome structure. Epigenetic mechanisms of cell cycle control that have been studied in ovarian cancer include telomerase activity and DNA methylation.

Oncogenes and Growth Factor Receptors

The most widely studied proto-oncogene in ovarian cancer is c-*erbB-2* or *HER2/neu*. This gene, located on chromosome 17q, encodes a tyrosine kinase growth factor receptor, designated p185, that is closely related to the epidermal growth factor (EGF) receptor. Its amplification and overexpression lead to increased cellular proliferation as a result of the growth-promoting effects of growth factor receptors as part of the cell signal pathway. Efforts to identify a direct ligand for the receptor have not been successful, suggesting a nonconventional receptor function. Evidence indicates that c-*erbB-2* may have evolved as a shared receptor subunit of a group of related growth factors in the EGF family and that it acts as a shared coreceptor for multiple growth factors rather than one specific ligand; thus, it is believed to be a "master coordinator of a signaling network."[205] The c-*erbB-2* gene is amplified or overexpressed in approximately 42% of ovarian carcinomas, but thus far no consistent prognostic effect of *HER2/neu* overexpression has been observed.[171,184,342,401] One study suggested an association of HER2 overexpression with resistance to chemotherapy.[255]

The EGF receptor (EGFR), which is encoded by the c-*erbB-1* gene, has been identified by immunohistochemistry in 46%–100% of ovarian carcinomas,[38,413,415] and a correlation between tyrosine kinase growth factor receptor p185 and EGFR has been observed in ovarian carcinomas.[178] EGF itself is also found in a similarly high proportion of ovarian carcinomas.[415] EGF-related proteins have been identified in benign and malignant ovarian epithelial neoplasms,[282] and a high-affinity EGF-binding site has been identified in several ovarian cancer cell lines.[371] Other growth factors that have been studied in ovarian carcinomas include insulin-like growth factor 2 (IGF-2), transcripts of which have been detected in the majority of ovarian cancers,[485] vascular endothelial growth factor,[409] basic fibroblast growth factor, midkine, and pleiotropin.[275]

The *ras* gene family (H-*ras*, N-*ras*, K(Ki)-*ras*) encodes a group of proteins with GTPase activity, designated p21-*ras*, that are involved in normal receptor signal transduction pathways. *Ras* mutation abolishes GTPase activity and results in constitutive stimulation of the pathway.[114] K-*ras* mutations are present in ovarian carcinoma cell lines[172] and in 10%–25% of ovarian carcinomas.[435,472] Immunoreactive p21-*ras* is found in about half of ovarian carcinomas.[172] However, when classified according to cell type, K-*ras* mutations are present most often in mucinous neoplasms in comparison to serous neoplasms,[57,82,114,244] and evidence suggests that K-*ras* mutations are closely related to the development of a mucinous phenotype in ovarian tumors.[80] A correlation of mutation with prognosis has been observed by some[370] but not by others.[472] K-*ras* mutation has been identified in the majority of atypical proliferative mucinous tumors and in about one-third of atypical proliferative serous tumors.[264] K-*ras* mutation has also been observed in serous cystadenomas and Brenner tumors.[80] K-*ras* mutation in ovarian epithelial tumors is closely correlated with overexpression of the farnesyltransferase beta subunit gene; the enzyme coded by this gene plays an important role in the posttranslational processing of *ras*.[430]

The *c-myc* gene, which encodes a DNA-binding protein that acts as a transcription factor and thereby plays a role in cell proliferation, is amplified and overexpressed in some ovarian cancers[20,28,366] but is not related to stage, grade, or survival.[432] *C-fos* and *c-jun* are related transcription factors that, along with *c-myc*, are linked in a pathway with transforming growth factor-alpha (TGFA) and the EGF receptor. High mRNA levels for TGFA and *c-jun* were found in 30% and 38%, respectively, of ovarian carcinomas in one study,[28] and another series found immunoreactive TGFA in 64% of ovarian carcinomas.[415] In the former series of 47 ovarian carcinomas, 2 were found to have rearrangements of the EGF receptor gene.[28]

The beta catenin gene located on chromosome 3p encodes a protein that plays a role in stimulation of transcription factors as well as in cell–cell adhesion. This gene is mutated in 16% of endometrioid carcinomas of the ovary but is rarely mutated in other cell types of ovarian carcinoma.[298,471] Interestingly, β-catenin is also mutated in some endometrial adenocarcinomas of the uterine corpus,[471] suggesting some similarities in the mechanisms of carcinogenesis in these different but histologically related neoplasms. Other cell cycle regulators that have been found to be upregulated in ovarian cancers include $p34^{cdc2}$ protein kinase, which controls mitotic division,[25] and *c-met*, a tyrosine kinase growth factor receptor.[173]

Tumor Suppressor Genes

Tumor suppressor genes normally downregulate the cell cycle and act as cell cycle checkpoints. When a tumor suppressor gene is mutated, it loses its inhibitory effect on proliferation and thus contributes to abnormal proliferation. Of the various tumor suppressor genes, *p53*, *BRCA1*, and *BRCA2* have been those most extensively studied in ovarian cancer. The retinoblastoma tumor suppressor gene, which is mutated in several different types of carcinomas, has been found to be normal in the majority of ovarian cancers.[147a,202,364] The *BRCA* genes are discussed later (see "Molecular Basis of Hereditary Predisposition to Ovarian Cancer"). Mutation of the *p53* tumor suppressor gene located on the short arm of chromosome 17 is the most frequent genetic abnormality found in human cancer. The protein product of the *p53* gene is a transcription factor that is activated in response to DNA damage. *p53* induces the transcription of $p21^{WAF1/Cip1}$ a cyclin-dependent kinase inhibitor, which arrests DNA synthesis and thus leads to cell cycle arrest in response to DNA damage.[117] The p53 gene is mutated in approximately 50%–60% of ovarian cancers.[39,175,212,262,290,435] Immunoperoxidase staining for the p53 protein correlates positively with missense mutation but not nonsense or splicing mutations or deletions.[218] Positive immunostaining occurs because of the long cellular half-life of mutated p53 protein compared to wild-type p53 protein, which is not detected by immunohistochemistry. Immunoperoxidase staining for p53 protein has been found in approximately 50% of ovarian carcinomas.[11,47,203,246] Some studies have shown a correlation with increasing stage[12,39,137,160,212,392,435] and grade,[12,47,460] suggesting that mutation of *p53* in ovarian carcinogenesis is a relatively late event. *p53* mutation has also been correlated with stage.[285] Data on whether *p53* status provides prognostic information independent of stage are conflicting. Atypical proliferative tumors of serous and mucinous types only very rarely have *p53* mutations.[465]

Multiple different cyclins, cyclin-dependent kinases (CDK), and their inhibitors are also an important aspect of cell cycle regulation. The expression of some of these proteins and their respective genes has been evaluated in ovarian cancers.[128,339a,418] Mutations of WAF1/Cip1 also occur in ovarian carcinomas, and immunostaining for p21, the protein product of this gene, which is a CDK inhibitor, has been reported.[240] Although expression of p21 is regulated by p53, investigators have found no correlation between p21 and p53 immunohistochemical staining.[74,463] Ki-67 staining increases with increasing stage of ovarian cancer[160] and correlates with p53 staining.[164]

Because mutations of p53 are so diverse, the finding of the identical mutation in tumors at different sites has been interpreted as evidence of clonality. Mutational analyses of p53 in disseminated ovarian carcinomas suggest a unifocal clonal origin of these tumors.[179,265] Studies of less-advanced cases need to be done before these findings can be considered definitive evidence of clonality.

The p53 protein is strongly immunogenic. Serum antibodies to p53 are found in about 17% of all cancer patients and in 22% of ovarian cancer patients.[408] Antibodies against the p53 protein have also been detected in the ascitic fluid of women with ovarian carcinoma.[10]

Apoptosis and the *bcl-2* Family of Genes

Apoptosis, an evolutionarily conserved physiologic process that culminates in cell death, so-called programmed cell death or cell suicide, is distinct from necrosis and appears to be controlled by multiple genes.[436] Normal cellular and tissue growth, as well as neoplasia, depend on a delicate balance between cell proliferation and apoptosis. The proliferative features of malignancy can be a result of deregulated cell growth or inhibition of apoptosis and often involve both processes.[239] *p53* is involved in the regulation of apoptosis via its interactions with the proapoptotic genes *bax* and *bcl-x$_S$* and the antiapoptotic genes *bcl-2* and *bcl-x$_L$*. A recent study found that the regulation of these genes differs in normal ovaries as compared to ovarian neoplasms.[247] Paradoxically, some studies have found lower expression of antiapoptotic genes in ovarian serous carcinomas as compared to benign serous tumors, suggesting an alternative function of these genes.[67,457] One study has correlated chemosensitivity of ovarian cancer with apoptosis-related variables,[368] which is consistent with the finding that some chemotherapeutic agents such as cisplatin and paclitaxel induce cell death by the induction of apoptosis.[436,453]

Metallothioneins are low molecular weight proteins that protect cells against apoptosis induced by oxidative stress. In a study of mucinous ovarian tumors, metallothionein expression was found to be significantly higher in carcinomas than in benign tumors.[429]

DNA Methylation

In vertebrates, the dinucleotide doublet, CpG, is methylated at the 5 position on the cytosine ring in 60%–90% of its locations. DNA methylation appears to be essential in embryogenesis and represses gene transcription.[43] One of the most consistent findings in human cancers is changes in genomic methylation, which may contribute to neoplasia by altering growth control gene expression.[69] Patterns of DNA methylation are heritable, tissue specific, and are altered during embryologic development. Altered DNA methylation has been identified in ovarian carcinomas but not in benign tumors.[69] Hypermethylation of promoter regions of both the *BRCA1* tumor suppressor gene and the *hMLH1* mismatch repair gene appears to be an alternative mechanism of gene inactivation (see "Molecular Basis of Hereditary Predisposition to Ovarian Cancer").[115,116] The short arm of chromosome 17, where the *p53* gene is located, contains a hot spot for hypermethylation in many human malignancies including ovarian carcinoma.[309]

Telomerase

Telomeres are repetitive nucleotide sequences and associated proteins located at the distal ends of chromosomes. With every cell division, each chromosome loses a portion of its distal end, and thus progresive telomere shortening has been associated with cellular senescence and aging. It has been proposed that telomeric shortening is a mitotic clock, and a sufficiently short telomere signals cellular senescence. The enzyme telomerase reverses telomeric shortening and is required for a cell to be immortalized. Telomerase activity has been detected in virtually all human cancers as well as most immortal cells and germline cells.[53,476] Telomerase activity has been found in 85% of all tumors examined as compared to 4% of normal tissues.[53] Telomerase activity has been detected in 92%–96% of ovarian carcinomas[274,476] and has also been identified in ovarian carcinoma cell lines and in ascitic fluid containing ovarian carcinoma cells.[76] In the latter study, it was noted that telomerase was detected after telomeres had become very short. These investigators proposed that tumor cells lose telomeric DNA until a critically short telomere length is reached, after which proliferation is possible only in those cells that can maintain functional chromosome ends, for example, via telomerase.[76] A recent study found evidence that upregulation of hTERT (human telomerase catalytic subunit) may be important in ovarian carcinoma development.[221]

Molecular Basis of Hereditary Predisposition to Ovarian Cancer

There are three hereditary syndromes that predispose to ovarian cancer: the *breast–ovarian cancer syndrome* caused by mutations in the tumor suppressor genes *BRCA1* and *BRCA2*, *Lynch syndrome II*, and *hereditary site-specific ovarian cancer*. All three syndromes are transmitted in an autosomal dominant fashion.[241]

Breast–Ovarian Cancer Susceptibility Genes

Approximately 10% of women with ovarian cancer are carriers of a breast/ovarian cancer susceptibility gene. The proportion of cases of ovarian cancer resulting from such a gene decreases with age and is estimated to be 14% for women diagnosed in the fourth decade, dropping to 7% for women diagnosed in the sixth decade. Gene carriers have a greater than 15-fold risk of ovarian cancer compared to noncarriers.[72] The lifetime risk for ovarian cancer in the general population is 1.3%, whereas estimates for gene carriers range from 10% to 60%.[242] *BRCA1* and *BRCA2* together have been estimated to account for 95% of breast–ovarian cancer families.[123]

Both *BRCA1* and *BRCA2* are transmitted in an autosomal dominant fashion. Certain ethnic groups have high rates of specific mutations of these genes.[238,416] The large number of mutations described makes genetic testing and patient counseling complex, and at present there is no consensus on the proper clinical implementation of testing. Clinical implementation in the general population will require data on cost-effectiveness and influence on mortality, as well as a variety of psychosocial issues. At present, these data are limited.

BRCA1

The *BRCA1* tumor suppressor gene on chromosome 17q was cloned in 1994.[260] It encodes a protein composed of 1863 amino acids that is believed to play a role in repair of DNA damage.[125] More than 200 different mutations have been identified in this gene in women with hereditary breast/ovarian cancer susceptibility.[341] Eighty-six percent of mutations in the gene are predicted to result in a truncated protein.[390] Evidence suggests that the majority of breast–ovarian cancer families are linked to mutations of this gene, with estimates of 80–90%[75,123]; however, this figure is not constant worldwide. For example, a report from Amsterdam indicates that in only 36% of ovarian cancer families was ovarian cancer attributable to *BRCA1* mutation.[493] The proportion of ovarian cancers in the general population attributable to this gene is estimated to be 5.9% for women in the third decade or younger and steadily declines with increasing age, dropping to 1.8% in the seventh decade.[122] It has been estimated that, by age 70, 32.5–44% of carriers will develop ovarian cancer,[121,122] although others express more uncertainty about the lifetime risk, with estimates from 20% to 60%.[242]

The *BRCA1* gene has been studied in sporadic ovarian cancers. The evidence suggests that *BRCA1* mutation is not critical for ovarian carcinogenesis. In one study, only 1 of 12 ovarian cancers showed *BRCA1* mutation.[131] In another study, 42% of sporadic ovarian carcinomas had loss of heterozygosity for *BRCA1* and 31% of the tumors with LOH had hypermethylated promoter regions.[116] One study showed reduced *BRCA1* expression in sporadic ovarian carcinomas.[489]

BRCA2

The *BRCA2* tumor suppressor gene on chromosome 13q is a larger gene than *BRCA1* and is also associated with high rates of breast and ovarian cancer.[145] It has been estimated that this gene is linked to 15% of breast–ovarian cancer families.[123] The risk of ovarian cancer in gene carriers is estimated to be 0.5% by age 50 and 27% by age 70.[123] Others estimate the lifetime risk of ovarian cancer as 10%–20%.[242]

Lynch Syndrome II

Lynch syndrome II is a subtype of hereditary nonpolyposis colon cancer (HNPCC) that is associated with an increased risk of ovarian cancer (Lynch syndrome I is not associated with extracolonic tumors). The relative risk of ovarian cancer in these family members is 3.5. Families with HNPCC are heterogeneous with respect to the different sites of extracolonic cancers seen at elevated rates in these families. Certain families account for most of the excess of ovarian cancers as well as endometrial and upper urologic cancers, but whether these families are genetically distinct is unknown.[248,455]

Germline mutations of mismatch repair (MMR) genes have been demonstrated in individuals with

HNPCC. This genetic abnormality is manifested by widespread genomic instability, or a hypermutable state, which provides the background for an accelerated accumulation of mutations.[248]

The genomic instability in patients with HNPCC is characterized by changes in the length of tandem repeat segments in microsatellites, a class of short repetetive DNA sequences in noncoding regions, and reflects the molecular phenotype of a loss of normal function of a MMR gene. The variation in length of these sequences is referred to as microsatellite instability (MSI), and this type of genetic abnormality has been identified in the DNA of all the tumor types that occur in HNPCC patients, including ovarian carcinoma.[248] Some sporadic tumors with MSI display somatic mutations in MMR genes but many do not.[248] An alternative mechanism for inactivation of the *hMLH1* MMR gene, recently identified in sporadic colonic and endometrial cancers, involves hypermethylation of the promoter region of the gene with subsequent loss of expression of the protein.[115,165,467]

Site-Specific Ovarian Cancer

Limited data are available on the site-specific ovarian cancer syndrome, the least common of the three hereditary cancer syndromes characterized by an increased risk of ovarian cancer. Findings from one group of investigators suggested that most families with this syndrome are linked to mutation in the *BRCA1* gene.[134,411]

Clinicopathologic Features of Familial Ovarian Cancers

Ovarian cancer in women with familial ovarian cancer occurs at a younger age than sporadic ovarian cancer. For BRCA-associated ovarian cancer, the age at diagnosis is about 50 years, and for Lynch syndrome II, 40 years. The stage distribution is similar to sporadic cases. Histologically, the tumors are usually papillary serous carcinomas with similar features to sporadic tumors,[41] but others have found that familial ovarian cancers tend to be more poorly differentiated.[464] Nonserous histology is very uncommon. The prognosis for BRCA-associated familial cases appears to be somewhat better than for sporadic cases.[49,352] It has been suggested that the favorable prognosis of young women with ovarian cancer is a result of the high frequency of *BRCA1* mutations in this group;[352] however, the alleged favorable prognosis of young women with ovarian "carcinoma" could result from the inclusion of atypical proliferative ("borderline") tumors, which is officially a subset of carcinoma, because these tumors occur more often in younger women. Molecular studies of familial ovarian cancers suggest a higher than expected proportion of ovarian tumors showing overexpression of *HER2/neu*.[16] One group studied nine loci for loss of heterozygosity (LOH) in multiple tumor sites from 12 familial ovarian cancers and found an identical pattern of LOH for at least one locus in each case, thus favoring a unifocal origin of disease.[132]

Cytogenetic and Chromosomal Abnormalities

Changes associated with neoplastic progression occur at specific nucleotide sites within DNA that can be localized by sequencing. However, certain aspects of these changes can also be recognized at the cytogenetic level by methods that detect gross chromosomal changes such as deletions, translocations, inversions, and gene amplification.[300]

Karyotypic analyses of ovarian carcinomas have shown complex *chromosomal abnormalities*, particularly of chromosomes 1, 3, 7, 11,[133] 6, 8, 17, and X.[103] Allelic loss of the region of chromosome 17p containing the *p53* gene frequently occurs in ovarian carcinoma. Loss of heterozygosity studies have demonstrated allelic deletions on chromosome 17p near the *p53* locus in ovarian serous carcinomas[106] as well as primary peritoneal ("serous surface") carcinomas.[324] One study found LOH, possibly involving the entirety of chromosome 17, in serous tumors more frequently than in endometrioid and mucinous tumors.[308] In addition, other loci on chromosome 17[132,153,306] as well as sites on chromosomes 4, 6, 7, 8, 12, 13, 16, and 19 have shown allelic losses.[70,132,202,332,369] Allelic loss at the Peutz–Jeghers locus on chromosome 19p was recently reported in 24% of ovarian carcinomas.[451] Loss of chromosome 12, a well-established abnormality in ovarian germ cell tumors, is also found frequently in ovarian carcinomas.[433] Atypical proliferative (borderline) ovarian tumors, predominantly of the serous type, have shown allelic losses on chromosomes 1, 2, 3, 5, 6, 7, 17, and X,[70,103,153,332] and trisomy 12 has been reported in a high proportion of cases.[211,304] LOH is occasionally found in benign ovarian epithelial neoplasms.[362] Loss of heterozygosity and X-inactivation studies have also supported the unifocal clonal origin of advanced ovarian carcinomas.[233,443]

Cell–Cell and Cell–Extracellular Matrix Interactions

The extracellular matrix (ECM) is an inconspicuous tissue component on light microscopy. However, on a molecular level, the ECM is a highly complex structure with a backbone of collagen and rich in macromolecules including glycoproteins, proteoglycans, and glycosaminoglycans. A wide variety of cell–matrix interactions are modulated in part by cell-surface receptors that are specific for matrix elements. Cell–matrix interactions were first elucidated in embryologic studies and found to be crucial for cell division, differentiation, migration, and morphogenesis[301]; these are now suspected to be pivotal in the processes that mediate tumor cell invasion and metastasis.[235,301]

The stroma of neoplasms contains components of the normal ECM, which includes several types of collagens, elastic fibers, laminin, entactin, fibronectin, glycoproteins, glycosaminoglycans, and proteoglycans. Most of the matrix within tumors is newly secreted and may be of dual origin, from the host and the neoplasm.[249] Structural ECM components such as collagens are produced by ovarian cancers.[192] Normal and neoplastic cells have cell-surface receptors that are specific for components of the ECM and thus modulate their interactions.

Cell–Extracellular Matrix Interactions

Cancer cells overexpress matrix-degrading enzymes that are believed to be important in the processes of invasion and metastasis.[333] Some of these proteinases have dual functions, serving as activators of angiogenic and growth factors.[448] The major extracellular proteinases involved in this process are the serine proteases and the metalloproteinases; the latter group includes several types of collagenase.[18] Evaluation of collagenase mRNA and immunoreactivity for the enzyme in ovarian neoplasms, particularly type IV collagenase, has demonstrated their presence in both benign and malignant ovarian tumors, with ovarian carcinomas showing collagenase in primary as well as metastatic sites. Of note, several groups have demonstrated that the enzymes are present in the host's nonneoplastic stromal cells within carcinomas to a greater extent than the neoplastic epithelial cells,[4,18] suggesting that the stromal cells play an important role in the modulation of the extracellular matrix within neoplasms.

The 72-kDa type IV collagenase, MMP-2, is expressed in higher levels in ovarian carcinomas as compared to benign tumors, and is inversely correlated with basement membrane integrity.[100] Several serine proteases have also been found to be overexpressed in ovarian carcinomas.[167,431,448] Hyaluronidase is another matrix-degrading enzyme that has been studied in ovarian cancer. This enzyme digests hyaluronan and has been demonstrated in normal ovaries as well as ovarian cancer.[426] Cathepsin B, which can degrade laminin, fibronectin, and type IV collagen, has been found to be increased in ovarian carcinomas compared to normal ovaries.[154] Protein kinase C may play a role in the migration of ovarian carcinoma cells through ECM, and there is evidence that this role is independent of the production of proteolytic enzymes.[422]

Cell–Cell Interactions

Cell–cell interactions are modulated in part by the extracellular matrix and may contribute to the particular metastatic patterns of neoplasms.[249,487] Cell adhesion molecules that are important in these interactions include integrins, cadherins, the immunoglobulin supergene family, selectins, and CD 44.[310] Of particular relevance to the dissemination of ovarian cancer is the ECM component hyaluronan (hyaluronic acid, hyaluronate) and its major cell-surface receptor, CD 44, especially the CD 44H isoform.[14] CD 44 is a member of a group of cell adhesion molecules referred to as cell membrane-associated proteoglycans that generally function as receptors for ECM components. CD 44 isoforms are upregulated in most carcinomas.[215] Hyaluronan is a glycosaminoglycan that is composed of an unbranched chain of repeating disaccharide units. It is highly hydrophilic, said to be one of the most water-loving molecules in nature,[490] and plays an important role in tissue hydration, cell–cell adhesion, and cell migration.[209]

An important step in the dissemination of ovarian cancer is the adherence of tumor cells to the peritoneal surface. Recent evidence suggests that this adhesion is mediated in part by CD 44. Ovarian cancer cell lines, freshly isolated ovarian cancer cells, and ovarian carcinoma cells in tissue sections express CD 44.[59,88,232] A complex pattern of CD 44 splice variants has been observed in ovarian carcinomas.[58] CD 44-mediated binding of ovarian cancer cells to mesothelium in vitro has been found to result from hyaluronan associated with the surface of mesothelial cells. In addition, CD 44 expression is associated more strongly with tumor cells from peritoneal implants in contrast to tumor cells from ascites, suggesting the importance of CD 44 in peritoneal implantation.[59,474] Evidence suggests that tumor cells stimulate host mesothelial cells or fibroblasts to synthesize and secrete large amounts of hyaluronan.[474] Subsequent in vivo experiments in mice have demonstrated the inhibition of peritoneal implantation of ovarian cancer cells by antibodies to CD 44.[414] Mesothelial cells in vitro display a pericellular matrix containing hyaluronan that is largely eliminated by hyaluronidase treatment. Hyaluronidase treatment also reduces the binding of ovarian cancer cell lines to mesothelial cells.[232] Elevated hyaluronan levels in the stroma of ovarian carcinomas have been found to correlate with high grade, high stage, and residual tumor, but not with CD 44 expression, suggesting that hyaluronan may contribute to the aggressive behavior of ovarian carcinoma by multiple mechanisms.[13]

Cell adhesion molecules such as integrins and cadherins have been studied in ovarian cancer. Integrins serve as cell-surface receptors for other adhesion molecules including osteopontin, vitronectin, and laminin. Ovarian cancer cell lines express several species of integrins,[59] and β-1 integrin may play a role in the adhesion of ovarian cancer cells to mesothelial cells.[232] Several integrins as well as their ligands osteopontin, vitronectin, and laminin have been evaluated in ovarian carcinoma cell lines and tumor tissues; significant differences between normal ovary and carcinomas, benign and malignant neoplasms, and primary and metastatic sites have been found.[62,234,403,438]

E (epithelial)-cadherin is present in normal ovarian surface epithelium and, to a greater degree, in the epithelium lining cortical invaginations and epithelial inclusions.[243] Reduced levels of E-cadherin have been associated with invasion and metastasis in many tumors,[147] and ovarian carcinomas have lower levels than benign ovarian epithelial tumors.[87] E-cadherins have been identified in serous, mucinous, and endometrioid ovarian carcinomas, but N (neural)-cadherin, although present in serous and endometrioid carcinomas, is absent in mucinous tumors.[405] E-cadherin is present in primary ovarian carcinomas but reduced in metastatic sites. The catenins, ligands of E-cadherin, are present in normal ovary and benign neoplasms but reduced in carcinomas.[15,90]

Steroid Hormones and Receptors

The *steroid hormones estrogen and progesterone* bind to specific receptors in the nucleus. Once bound, the hormone–receptor complex undergoes a conformational change that allows the complex to bind to glucocorticoid regulatory elements of the DNA and activate transcription. Estrogen receptors (ER) and progesterone receptors (PR) are expressed in approximately half of ovarian carcinomas and are also present in ovarian cancer cell lines.[136] Androgen receptors are present in the majority of ovarian carcinomas. Of note, specific, high-affinity binding sites for tamoxifen have been observed in ovarian neoplasms.[27] Ovarian carcinomas contain a higher quantity of ER than either normal ovary or benign ovarian tumors. Recent data indicate that there are two homologous estrogen receptors, ER-α and ER-β, and that mRNA for ER-β is found predominantly in normal ovaries and benign ovarian neoplasms, whereas mRNA encoding ER-α is found predominantly in ovarian carcinomas.[321] One recent study suggests that ER-α is present in the majority of ovarian carcinomas with the exception of clear cell carcinomas.[127a] There are conflicting data on the relationship of steroid receptor status and prognosis. Many studies claiming prognostic significance have not demonstrated that receptor status is a prognostic factor independent of other well-documented factors such as stage. Similar studies on androgen receptor status have reached the same conclusion.[325]

Elevated plasma levels of a variety of steroid hormones including estrogens, progestins, and androgens have been observed in ovarian cancer patients, and some studies have correlated these levels with tumor burden. These data and other evidence, which include elevated hormone levels in the ovarian vein draining the affected ovary, suggest that some ovarian cancers produce these hormones. Confounding factors in these studies, however, include variation in the levels of serum proteins, such as sex hormone-binding globulin, that bind the steroid hormones. Decreased levels of luteinizing hormone (LH) and follicle-stimulating hormone (FSH) have been observed in postmenopausal ovarian cancer patients.[325]

Aromatase, an enzyme complex that catalyzes the conversion of androgens to estrone, plays an important role in the pathogenesis of estrogen-dependent cancers such as breast cancer. Aromatase activity has been demonstrated in the majority of ovarian carcinomas and has been localized to the stromal cells. In contrast, benign epithelial ovarian tumors do not display aromatase activity. Intratumoral aromatase is more common in serous than in mucinous carcinomas. Evidence suggests that aromatase activity of ovarian stromal cells has a different pathogenesis from the hormonal activities displayed by luteinized or enzymatically active ovarian stromal cells, which are frequently observed in the stroma of ovarian neoplasms.[365]

Prognostic Factors

The literature is replete with studies of putative prognostic factors, but unfortunately most of these studies are of limited value.[155] First, nearly all of them are retrospective and therefore are subject to a variety of biases that result in data accrual and analysis which lack the blinded and randomized design necessary for rigorous study of a possible prognostic factor. Second, many of the studies are small and lack the statistical power to demonstrate prognostic utility even if it exists for the particular factor under study. Third, the sheer number of different factors examined ensures that, by chance, roughly 5% of them will appear to show prognostic utility at the $p < 0.05$ level. Fourth, many studies do not account for previously well-established prognostic factors in their analyses. Finally, many prognostic studies are uninterpretable because of the failure to separate the data on atypical proliferative ("borderline" or "low malignant potential") tumors versus invasive carcinomas.[163]

It has been recognized that, even if a certain factor is of independent significance, the temporal order in which prognostic data are received is important. Specifically, stage is generally known before the results of DNA flow cytometry, and therefore the important questions become (1) does flow cytometry add prognostic data beyond that already provided by stage? and (2) are these data worth the cost?[163]

The only universally accepted prognostic factors for patients with ovarian cancer are FIGO stage and, in advanced-stage patients, volume of residual disease. Other factors that may be important but about which there is continued debate include patient age, histopathologic grade, and DNA ploidy. Many other putative prognostic factors have been reported, but the data are still considered preliminary. For all major cell types of ovarian carcinoma, histologic subtype is not an independent prognostic factor when stage is taken into account, with the possible exception of stage III clear cell carcinoma.[126,163,303,417] Nonetheless, because of the distinctly different stage distributions of the various histologic types, there are differences in the overall prognosis for each type.

Stage

The International Federation of Gynecology and Obstetrics (FIGO) has standardized the staging of gynecologic cancers. The latest version of the staging system for ovarian cancer is shown in Table 18.1.[303] FIGO stage is so powerful a predictor of prognosis in ovarian cancer that most other putative prognostic factors are of little importance in comparison to stage.[163]

Table 18.1. Carcinoma of the ovary: FIGO nomenclature (Rio de Janeiro 1988)

Stage I		Growth limited to the ovaries
	Ia	Growth limited to one ovary; no ascites present containing malignant cells. No tumor on the external surface; capsule intact
	Ib	Growth limited to both ovaries; no ascites present containing malignant cells. No tumor on the external surfaces; capsules intact
	Ic[a]	Tumor either stage Ia or Ib, but with tumor on surface of one or both ovaries, or with capsule ruptured, or with ascites present containing malignant cells, or with positive peritoneal washings
Stage II		Growth involving one or both ovaries with pelvic extension
	IIa	Extension and/or metastases to the uterus and/or tubes
	IIb	Extension to other pelvic tissues
	IIc[a]	Tumor either stage IIa or IIb, but with tumor on surface of one or both ovaries; or with capsule(s) ruptured; or with ascites present containing malignant cells or with positive peritoneal washings
Stage III		Tumor involving one or both ovaries with histologically confirmed peritoneal implants outside the pelvis and/or positive retroperitoneal or inguinal nodes. Superficial liver metastases equals stage III. Tumor is limited to the true pelvis, but with histologically proven malignant extension to small bowel or omentum
	IIIa	Tumor grossly limited to the true pelvis, with negative nodes, but with histologically confirmed microscopic seeding of abdominal peritoneal surfaces, or histologic-proven extension to small bowel or mesentery
	IIIb	Tumor of one or both ovaries with histologically confirmed implants, peritoneal metastasis of abdominal peritoneal surfaces, none exceeding 2 cm in diameter; nodes are negative
	IIIc	Peritoneal metastasis beyond the pelvis >2 cm in diameter and/or positive retroperitoneal or inguinal nodes
Stage IV		Growth involving one or both ovaries with distant metastases. If pleural effusion is present, there must be positive cytology to allot a case to stage IV; parenchymal liver metastasis equals stage IV

[a]To evaluate the impact on prognosis of the different criteria for allotting cases to stage Ic or IIc; it would be of value to know if rupture of the capsule was spontaneous, or caused by the surgeon; and if the source of malignant cells detected was peritoneal washings, or ascites. From Pecorelli et al.[303]

Standard surgical procedures for staging have evolved during the past two decades. In the early 1980s, it became apparent that approximately one-third of ovarian cancer patients with apparent stage I disease (confined to the ovaries) were staged higher at subsequent complete staging laparotomy.[477] The extent of surgical exploration and tissue sampling are currently quite thorough when performed by a gynecologic oncologist, but suboptimal staging often still occurs when performed by nonspecialists.[126,163] Survival rates for the lower stages gradually improved in the 1970s and 1980s[305] as occult advanced-stage tumors were detected and properly categorized.

Staging takes both surgical and pathologic findings into account; hence the term surgicopathologic stage. Stage can usually be deduced solely from the histopathologic and cytologic findings. However, evidence suggests that dense adhesions of an apparent stage I tumor that require sharp dissection, leaving a raw area following dissection, or when dissection results in tumor rupture, are associated with a prognosis similar to that of a more advanced-stage tumor. In fact, it is common practice to reassign densely adherent stage I tumors to stage II or III.[297]

The stage distribution of ovarian cancer varies by histologic type. The highest proportion of FIGO stage I cases is found among mucinous and clear cell carcinomas, both of which are stage I in approximately 50% of cases. Endometrioid carcinomas are stage I in 43% of cases,[36] and only 16% of serous carcinomas are diagnosed in stage I.[305]

Five-year survival rates by stage, including substages, are shown in Table 18.2. These data are from a total of more than 15,000 patients from three sources: the FIGO annual report,[305] the Commission on Cancer of the Americal College of Surgeons (CCACS),[281] and the National Cancer Data Base.[299] These data show similar survival rates, with the exception of a notably better survival for stage I in the CCACS review; this could be due to the inclusion of "borderline" tumors, as the separation or exclusion of such cases was not specifically stated,[281] or to a lower frequency of understaged cases in this group. In fact, the latter is probably the correct explanation because recent data show that well-staged FIGO stage I ovarian cancer patients have a survival rate of approximately 90% or better.[163]

Table 18.2. Five-year survival (%) of patients with ovarian carcinoma

Stage	*FIGO*	*CCACS*	*NCDB*
I	78	89	85
Ia	84	92	
Ib	79	85	
Ic	73	82	
II	59	57	60
IIa	65	67	
IIb	54	56	
IIc	61	51	
III	22	24	27
IIIa	52	39	
IIIb	29	26	
IIIc	18	17	
IV	14	12	16

From International Federation of Gynecology and Obstetrics (FIGO),[305] Commission on Cancer of the American College of Surgeons (CCACS),[281] and the National Cancer Data Base (NCDB).[299]

Stage I ovarian cancer is confined to the ovaries and peritoneal fluid or washings. Tumor cells in peritoneal washings or in ascitic fluid warrant a stage of IC. Ovarian surface involvement by tumor is also considered to reflect stage IC disease. Ovarian surface involvement has not been precisely defined. We consider ovarian surface involvement to be present only when tumor cells are exposed to the peritoneal cavity. Thus, only two scenarios qualify for surface involvement: (1) exophytic papillary tumor on the surface of the ovary or on the outer surface of a cystic neoplasm replacing the ovary, and (2) an intracystic tumor in which carcinoma has invaded through the full thickness of the cyst wall such that tumor cells are exposed to the peritoneal cavity. Women with FIGO stage I ovarian carcinomas, if staged by current meticulous procedures by a gynecological oncologist, have an excellent prognosis. Stage I patients with grade I tumors have a 5-year survival of more than 90%, as do patients in stages IA and IB. Poor prognostic factors in stage I include grade 3 histology and IC substage, both of which are associated with substantially poorer survival rates.[7,98,450] Although it is possible that the IC substage based on malignant cells in ascites or peritoneal washings is the first evidence of true metastatic ability, these cells may merely be exfoliated. Most stage IB cases are serous and probably reflect independent primary tumors, although occasional examples displaying small foci of tumor on the surface of a normal-sized ovary with a large contralateral primary tumor are obviously metastatic.

Stage II ovarian cancer is a small and heterogeneous group, comprising 10% of ovarian cancers.[303] It is defined as extension or metastasis to extraovarian pelvic organs, most commonly the fallopian tubes and pelvic peritoneum. As such, it includes examples of direct extension to the tubes and pelvic sidewall, as well as metastatic seeding of the pelvic peritoneum, and therefore may include tumors with a wide range of prognoses, ranging from curable tumors that have directly extended to adjacent organs but not yet metastasized to tumors that have seeded the pelvic peritoneum by metastasis and therefore have a poor prognosis. Although stage II is subclassified into three substages, these substages do not clearly separate direct extension from metastasis, and therefore there is room for substantial improvement in this classification. Unfortunately, stage II is uncommon, and therefore retrospective studies are the only type of studies likely to provide clues to more prognostically useful substages.

Ovarian cancer most commonly presents in stage III, comprising 51% of cases.[303] These tumors characteristically spread along peritoneal surfaces, involving both pelvic and abdominal peritoneum including the omentum, surfaces of the small and large bowel, mesentery, paracolic gutters, undersurface of the diaphragm, and peritoneal surfaces of the liver and spleen. Metastases to retroperitoneal lymph nodes commonly occur and to inguinal lymph nodes less commonly, indicating stage IIIC even in the absence of peritoneal metastases, a rare occurrence.

Stage IV includes patients with parenchymal liver metastases and extraabdominal metastases. Thirteen percent of patients present in stage IV.[303] Among these, liver and lungs/pleurae are the most common metastatic sites. In one large series, at presentation 15% of ovarian cancer patients had pulmonary metastases and an additional 30% developed pulmonary metastases after a mean of 9.3 months.[197] During the course of the disease, one-third of all ovarian cancer patients have pleural effusions, and three-quarters of these contain malignant cells on cytopathologic examination. Among patients with pulmonary involvement, malignant pleural effusion is three times as common as solid parenchymal lung metastasis.[197] Splenic parenchymal metastases occur on occasion[224] and may necessitate splenectomy. Although there are no specific guidelines for changing the stage based on splenic parenchymal metastasis, we consider these stage IV because they are analogous to liver parenchymal metastasis. Brain metastases are present in 0.1% of patients at presentation, are eventually clinically diagnosed in 0.6% of patients, and are found in 0.9% of patients at autopsy. In 6% of patients diagnosed during life, CNS involvement is clinically manifested as carcinomatous meningitis. Among patients who develop brain parenchymal involvement after diagnosis, the median time after diagnosis is 29 months.[89,159,225,231,252,318]

Cytopathology

The cytopathologic examination of ovarian epithelial neoplasms generally involves two types of specimens: fine-needle aspirates (FNA) of ovarian cysts and peritoneal fluids (obtained by peritoneal washing or by removal of ascitic fluid). Intraoperative smears of specimens can also be useful adjuncts to or replacements for frozen section examination. Once disseminated, ovarian cancers may also be examined in FNA specimens or effusions from sites of distant metastasis.

Fine-Needle Aspiration of Ovarian Cysts

Although several studies have shown that 90% of ovarian cysts can be accurately diagnosed by FNA,[393] a recent study reported an unacceptably high false-positive rate of 73%; the false-negative rate in this study was 12%.[166] The most important factor in the accuracy of FNA is the ability to retrieve diagnostic cells. Unsatisfactory specimens from ovarian cyst aspirates are found in 18–70% of cases.[42]

Most cysts in premenopausal women are functional. FNA may be useful in patients who appear to have inoperable ovarian cancer or who cannot undergo surgery for other reasons. The alleged risk of disseminating cells by FNA from early-stage disease has not been substantiated.

FNA specimens from most carcinomas are cellular and contain cytologically malignant cells, but accurate subclassification is often difficult and may be impossible solely on the basis of cytologic material. Cell block material can be of assistance in this regard. Features useful in subclassification of epithelial neoplasms include psammoma bodies and papillary structures, which suggest serous differentiation, elongated cells and focal squamous features, which suggest endometrioid differentiation, cells with abundant clear, frothy cytoplasm and prominent enlarged nucleoli, which suggest clear cell differentiation, and columnar cells with large cytoplasmic vacuoles containing basophilic cytoplasmic mucin, which suggest mucinous differentiation. FNA specimens from serous carcinomas are usually very cellular and display malignant cells, singly and in clusters, with nuclear enlargement, hyperchromasia, irregular chromatin clumping, and prominent nucleoli. Occasional bizarre mononuclear tumor giant cells are regularly seen.

Mucinous carcinomas yield viscous mucus and high cellularity with single cells, clusters, and syncytial fragments displaying pleomorphism, multinucleation, coarse chromatin, prominent nucleoli, and vacuolated cytoplasm.[97] Exclusion of metastatic mucinous carcinoma is generally not possible in cytologic material. Cytologic material from endometrioid carcinomas resembles that from serous carcinomas but with scanty, more granular cytoplasm, nuclear crowding, and microacini. Squamous differentiation or hemosiderin-laden macrophages may be present. Clear cell carcinomas display cells with abundant pale vacuolated cytoplasm. Hyaline cytoplasmic inclusions may be present. Nuclear features often include pleomorphism and macronucleoli. Metastatic tumors such as renal cell carcinoma may need to be considered, but this is a rare occurrence.[97]

Atypical proliferative epithelial tumors of all types may display a degree of cytologic atypia that overlaps with invasive well-differentiated carcinoma, and therefore this distinction requires tissue examination in all cases. Nonetheless, preoperative FNA can be of some value in surgical planning, although in our experience this is not commonly performed.

FNA of benign epithelial neoplasms usually produces a paucicellular specimen. Most of the material consists of macrophages and lymphocytes with few epithelial cells.[42] The background is generally clean, unless torsion or necrosis has occurred. Benign serous tumors may display cohesive sheets of uniform cells with round to oval nuclei, moderate amounts of cytoplasm with well-defined cell borders, and occasionally cilia. The nuclei have finely granular chromatin and small nucleoli. Cystadenofibromas also may display spindled stromal cells without atypia. Mucinous cystadenomas display tall columnar cells with basal nuclei without atypia and occasionally signet-ring cells.[97]

Peritoneal Fluid Cytology

Cytologic samples of peritoneal fluid are routinely obtained during staging procedures for ovarian cancer. These findings are important in substaging early (FIGO I and II) ovarian cancer; malignant cells in peritoneal washings or ascites warrant assignment of tumors to stage IC or IIC. Cytology is more sensitive in detecting ovarian carcinoma in ascites than in peritoneal washes, as well as in patients with peritoneal metastases measuring greater than 0.5 cm. Cytologic examination of ascitic fluid in women with advanced-stage ovarian carcinoma often displays numerous large hypervacuolated adenocarcinoma cells in papillary groups and singly.[278] The cytologic features of the carcinoma cells generally resemble those in FNA specimens (see foregoing) but may be more degenerate, depending on cellular viability. In 3%–10% of patients, a positive peritoneal cytology is the only indicator of extraovarian disease.[393] Peritoneal cytology and histology are concordant in 87% of patients with ovarian cancer.[492] The prognosis of patients with stage IC ovarian cancer based on positive peritoneal cytology is poorer than for stages IA and IB. In addition, patients with stage III disease with positive cytology have a poorer prognosis than stage III patients with negative cytology.[492]

The main component of benign peritoneal washings is mesothelial cells arranged singly and in sheets. In Papanicolaou stains, mesothelial cells appear as round or polygonal cells with dense, cyanophilic cytoplasm and centrally placed, round nuclei with smooth contours and finely granular chromatin. Degenerate and reactive mesothelial cells often display fine or coarse cytoplasmic vacuolation and a lightly stained perinuclear zone.[393]

The presence of epithelial cells in peritoneal fluid samples from patients with "borderline" (atypical proliferative) epithelial ovarian tumors has been highlighted in the past as a problematic area of cytopathology. This problem no longer exists because accurate subclassification of these neoplasms into benign and malignant types (see serous and mucinous tumor sections) renders the peritoneal fluid cytology specimens in most of these patients who have benign tumors of no importance. The small proportion of patients who have bona fide carcinomas (patients with micropapillary serous carcinoma (MPSCs) or atypical proliferative serous tumor (APSTs) with invasive implants) can be substaged on the basis of the presence or absence of epithelial cells resembling the primary ovarian tumor in the cytology specimens.

The most important pitfall in the examination of peritoneal cytology specimens in women involves benign epithelial proliferations. Women with or without cancer can have endometriosis or endosalpingiosis involving peritoneal surfaces. These lesions often shed epithelial fragments into peritoneal washings or ascites if present; in addition, benign fallopian tubal epithelium, particularly if salpingitis is present, and benign eutopic endometrial tissue via expulsion through the fallopian tubes may also be shed into the fluid.[393] Therefore, it is important to be aware of the cytologic appearances of these entities and not to ovardiagnose cancer in women without neoplasms or to assign to a higher stage women with ovarian cancer based solely on the presence of epithelium in the peritoneal fluid.[42,399] If the cells in the fluid are not obviously malignant, comparison and correlation of the cytologic features of the epithelium in the fluid with those of the tissue sections are essential in arriving at the correct diagnosis. It is also important to be aware of the cytologic abnormalities that may be caused by intraperitoneal chemotherapy, as they may mimic malignancy.[42]

Grade

Many studies have shown that *grade* appears to be an important prognostic factor for ovarian carcinoma, despite the fact that there is no uniform grading system currently in use, that most studies do not indicate what grading system was used, and that grade is among the most poorly reproducible observations among pathologists. The consistent findings of the prognostic value of grade despite these limitations suggests that either grade is an extremely important prognostic factor or that there is an obscure statistical reason that inflates the apparent prognostic importance of grade. We favor the latter interpretation because any three-grade system can arguably be shown to be statistically significantly related to prognosis by virtue of skewed data because of very small groups of patients with extreme prognoses at the morphologically highly reproducible extremes of low and high grade.

Recently, a three-grade system was developed and tested in a series of 461 patients with epithelial ovarian cancer. The grading system was modified from several breast cancer grading systems that include three variables to be scored and then summed: architectural grade, nuclear grade, and mitotic count. The investigators claimed that the system was prognostically useful in early stage (I and II) and advanced stage (III and IV) patients. Unfortunately, the individual stages were not separately analyzed, and therefore whether grade is a prognostic factor independent of stage was not adequately tested. In fact, these authors did find a positive correlation of grade and stage, suggesting that the apparent prognostic importance of grade was indeed confounded by stage. In addition, analysis of their findings revealed highly significant correlations among the three components of grade ($p = 0.003$ or lower for all possible paired comparisons), indicating that they are not independent (i.e., they are dependent on one another) and that, perhaps, a single factor such as nuclear grade alone would suffice.[396,397] Efforts to confirm this proposed grading system suffer from similar limitations particularly regarding stratification by stage.[252a]

At present, grading of ovarian carcinoma is clinically important only for stage I patients because chemotherapy is witheld for low-grade tumors in view of their outstanding prognosis when untreated.[120] Most proposed grading systems are three-grade systems and are unlikely to be reproducible. Because the decision to treat or not to treat is a binary one, we believe that criteria should be developed to classify ovarian carcinomas into low-grade and high grade, with chemotherapy witheld for low grade stage I cases.

Other Prognostic Factors

Volume of residual disease is an important prognostic factor in most studies; this is supported by the demonstrated value of cytoreductive surgery, both primary and secondary, in prolonging survival and progression-free interval. Data are conflicting on tumor rupture and capsular penetration. Although either of these findings warrants reassigning of an otherwise stage I or II tumor to IC or IIC, the prognostic value of these features is unclear.

Serum levels of CA-125 correlate with volume of disease. CA-125 levels in most studies are not independent factors in multivariate analyses. Although high preoperative CA-125 levels may predict unresectability and poor survival, postoperative CA-125 levels appear to be more prognostic. Some investigators believe that although CA-125 levels may be useful in predicting group outcomes they lack the power to guide individual treatment decisions.[297]

The prognostic utility of DNA flow and image cytometry is controversial. Many of the published data are conflicting. In addition, there are significant interlaboratory reproducibility problems as well as many other methodologic and interpretive issues. Image cytometry is very labor intensive. At present, these techniques remain investigational.

Patient age is difficult to evaluate as a prognostic factor. A number of studies addressing the age distribution of ovarian cancer do not separate the survival data on "borderline tumors" from invasive carcinomas, and because borderline tumors are much more common in younger women in the third to fifth decades, these data are difficult to interpret.[316,473] Among women under 40 years of age, in whom invasive ovarian carcinoma is rare, prognostic differences among subgroups appear to be largely explained by higher proportions of "borderline" tumors in the younger groups;[251,334] stage for stage, the survival rates are similar to those in older women.[105] Nonetheless, it does appear that younger women (i.e., age 40–50) with invasive ovarian cancer on average do have a slightly more favorable stage distribution and thus a better prognosis, although the difference is small.[303] Other studies have shown that stage-for-stage survival rates are better for younger than older women.[245] It has been observed that older women with ovarian cancer are treated less aggressively than younger women; in the Surveillance Epidemiology End Results (SEER) database, more than 40% of women older than 85 years did not receive definitive treatment.[328]

Treatment

Surgery

Initial surgical management of ovarian cancer includes staging, which is aimed at defining the extent of disease, and debulking, which is aimed at reducing tumor burden. Staging is performed through a vertical incision to allow assessment of the upper abdomen. Aspiration of ascites and washings of the pelvis as well as the paracolic gutters and surface of the diaphragm are obtained. In addition to removing the primary tumor intact, total abdominal hysterectomy and bilateral salpingo-oophorectomy, omentectomy, random peritoneal biopsies including the diaphragm, and paraaortic and often pelvic lymph node sampling are essential.[297]

Comprehensive staging is generally sufficient surgical treatment for patients in stages I and II. Patients with advanced-stage disease often require debulking or cytoreductive surgery as well. The rationale for cytoreductive surgery despite the incurability of nearly all these women includes the following: improved patient comfort; reduction in adverse metabolic consequences due to tumor, including enhanced ability to maintain nutrition; enhanced ability to tolerate chemotherapy; and enhanced responsiveness of residual tumor to chemotherapy.[297] Aggressive primary cytoreductive surgery has a low morbidity and mortality rate and is supported by an improved survival rate in multiple studies. Many patients with bulky disease cannot be optimally cytoreduced at primary surgery. It has been found that two to three cycles of chemotherapy followed by interval debulking significantly increases the proportion of patients who can be successfully cytoreduced. Secondary cytoreductive surgery (i.e., after recurrence) has similar advantages and is also supported by evidence of a survival benefit.[297]

Chemotherapy

The survival for patients with stage IA and IB, grade I tumors is 90% or better, and there is no demonstrable benefit for adjuvant chemotherapy. For early-stage ovarian cancer with poor prognostic features (FIGO IA and IB grades 2 and 3; FIGO IC and II), it is not clear whether adjuvant chemotherapy is superior to no treatment. Management options for this group include platinum-based chemotherapy, paclitaxel-based chemotherapy, or no treatment.

Patients with advanced-stage (FIGO III and IV) disease generally benefit from platinum- or paclitaxel-based chemotherapy. Cisplatin-based chemotherapy has resulted in a significant improvement in response rate, response duration, and time to progression; however, the effect on overall survival, although significant, is small. Long-term survival (>5 years) can be achieved with platinum-based combination chemotherapy in more than 20% of patients with stage III ovarian cancer with small-volume residual disease. At present, a platinum compound in combination with paclitaxel is the best first-line chemotherapy of advanced-stage ovarian cancer.[307]

As in early-stage disease, second-look laparotomy has no demonstrated effect on survival in an advanced stage. The survival of patients who recur after a complete remission is poor. In recurrent ovarian cancer, platinum and paclitaxel can be of value. Paclitaxel is active in a significant proportion of patients whose tumors are platinum resistant.

Other Therapeutic Modalities

Radiation, intraperitoneal chemotherapy, and hormonal therapy, although not standard therapy, may be alternatives in specific clinical situations, particularly for patients who cannot tolerate surgery or withstand the adverse effects of systemic chemotherapy.

Pathology of Ovarian Epithelial Neoplasms

The approximate distribution of ovarian surface epithelial tumors is shown in Table 18.3. Ovarian epithelial tumors comprise about half of all ovarian tumors, accounting for about 40% of benign tumors and 86% of malignant tumors.[214]

Serous Tumors

The classification of serous neoplasms of the ovary presented in this chapter, unlike the WHO classification,[381] categorizes the proliferative noninvasive epithelial ovarian neoplasms as "atypical proliferative" tumors rather than "borderline" or of "low malignant potential." The borderline category of ovarian epithelial tumors was officially introduced in the early 1970s to describe a group of tumors that did not display overtly malignant features but which occasionally appeared to behave in a malignant fashion. These tumors were distinguished from frankly invasive serous carcinomas by the absence of destructive infiltrative growth or stromal invasion.[176,389] Thus, their behavior appeared to be intermediate between benign cystadenomas and frank serous carcinomas. The FIGO committee charged with the development of the classification that was subsequently adopted by the WHO stated that this "intermediate" group may be composed of several different types of tumors but that the differences could not be discerned.[176] The classification was therefore viewed as provisional, but with its continued use over the past three decades, the "borderline" category has become firmly entrenched and is now regarded as a specific entity.

Although it has been recognized for many years

Table 18.3. Approximate distribution of surface epithelial tumors (% of all ovarian epithelial tumors)

	Benign	*Atypical proliferative ("borderline")*	*Carcinoma*	*Total*
Serous	30.7	5.5	16.5	52.7
Mucinous	23.7	3.8	3.6	31.1
Endometrioid	—[a]	0.4	5.7	6.1
Clear cell	—[a]	0.2	2.4	2.6
Transitional	3.1	0.1	0[b]	3.2
Undifferentiated	—	—	2.1	2.1
Mixed	0.5	0.1	1.8	2.4
Totals	57.5	9.9	32.6	100

[a]Less than 0.5%.
[b]This percentage is inaccurate because older studies did not include this category.
Data are derived from the following series: refs. 55, 190, 214, 299, 303, 354, 355, 444.
The totals do not exactly equal 100% as a result of rounding and lack of comparable data in some studies.

that the category includes a heterogeneous group of tumors, it is only recent studies that have clearly documented the biologic spectrum encompassed by the borderline category. Some borderline tumors more closely resemble their benign counterparts and others more closely resemble malignant tumors. The latter tumors are more likely to pursue a progressive clinical course or behave as low-grade carcinomas. Thus, some experts classify the highly proliferative upper end of the spectrum of borderline or "atypical proliferative" tumors as low-grade carcinomas ("micropapillary serous carcinomas") whereas other experts prefer to retain the borderline category but designate these tumors as borderline tumors with "micropapillary architecture."

Using the former approach to classification, which those authors of this chapter who live above the equator prefer, noninvasive serous tumors with a papillary architecture in which papillae display a hierarchical branching pattern are termed atypical proliferative serous tumors (APST) whereas those displaying a more complex papillary architecture characterized by delicate micropapillae are classified as micropapillary serous carcinomas (MPSC). Thus, the intermediate behavior of tumors in the borderline group results from the inclusion of a wide range of neoplasms, some benign, some approaching biologic malignancy, and some crossing the line, thereby creating the illusion of intermediate behavior. With the subdivision of the borderline group into benign and malignant tumors as preferred by some experts, the need for a borderline category disappears. Those who prefer to retain the borderline or atypical proliferative category as an intermediate group maintain that tumors at the upper end of the spectrum of atypical proliferation (i.e., MPSCs, also termed serous borderline tumors with a micropapillary pattern) are more likely to have extraovarian manifestations and those, in turn, are more likely to be invasive, but that a dichotomous classification into benign and malignant is not warranted.

The experts who prefer to retain the borderline category of ovarian tumors cite recurrences and deaths in an unpredictable minority of patients.[194,383] These investigators maintain that, in at least some cases, peritoneal implants reflect spread from the ovarian tumors, that microinvasion indicates transformation to bonafide carcinoma, and that some associated lymph node lesions represent metastases.

The literature demonstrates that assessment of the prognosis of APST and MPSC requires evaluation of the peritoneal implants that often accompany serous ovarian tumors. For a tumor classification to have clinical utility, it should categorize tumors in a way that the terms used in the classification correlate with clinical behavior. The classification presented in this chapter is based on that principle. This plan is another departure from the WHO classification, as the WHO classification requires that ovarian tumors be classified solely on the basis of the appearance of the primary tumor regardless of the appearance of the peritoneal lesions. However, studies over the past 20 years[139,388] have shown that classifying implants as invasive or noninvasive plays a critical role in determining prognosis. Patients whose tumors are associated with noninvasive implants have a 10-year survival that is close to 100%. In contrast, patients whose tumors are associated with invasive implants have a mortality rate of 34% after more than 7 years of follow-up. The difference in survival for patients with invasive versus noninvasive implants is highly significant and supports the subclassification of implants for purposes of clinical management.

Serous Cystadenomas and Adenofibromas

Benign serous tumors include *cystadenomas, adenofibromas, cystadenofibromas,* and *surface papillomas.* These tumors are common, accounting for about 25% of all benign ovarian neoplasms and 58% of all ovarian serous tumors. The peak incidence is in the fourth and fifth decades, and the median age is 41 years.[187] The symptoms and signs are nonspecific and most commonly include pelvic pain, discomfort, or an asymptomatic pelvic mass discovered on routine examination. Bilaterality rates are variable, depending on both the thoroughness with which an apparently uninvolved ovary is examined as well as the threshold for diagnosis of a small serous neoplasm. Accordingly, 12–23% of cystadenomas are bilateral.

Cystadenomas are composed of cysts filled with clear watery (serous) fluid or thin mucoid material. Occasionally, they contain thick mucus-like material more typical of mucinous neoplasms. The external surfaces of the cysts are smooth and glistening, often with a prominent vascular pattern. Occasionally, small papillary excrescences are found on the external surface of the cyst. The tumors may be unilocular or multilocular and vary in size up to 30 cm, with a median of 9 cm.[187] The lining of the cyst is either entirely flat or may have a varying number of coarse papillary projections (Fig. 18.1). Such papillary excrescences rarely cover the entire inner surface of the cyst. Cystadenofibromas are solid neoplasms composed of tough, rubbery tissue with interspersed glandular spaces.

Normal-sized ovaries often have small papillary projections with a fibrotic stromal component resembling a microscopic adenofibroma or cystadenofibroma arising from the surface; furthermore, simple germinal or cortical inclusions may become cystically dilated. Therefore, it has been suggested that serous neoplasms be diagnosed only if the lesion is greater than 1 cm in diameter.[383] This designation is obviously arbitrary and therefore is unlikely to distinguish true examples of neoplastic growth from simple serous cysts (Fig. 18.2) or nonneoplastic hyperplasias of the ovarian cortex.

There is a broad spectrum of epithelial proliferation in benign serous tumors that is manifested by

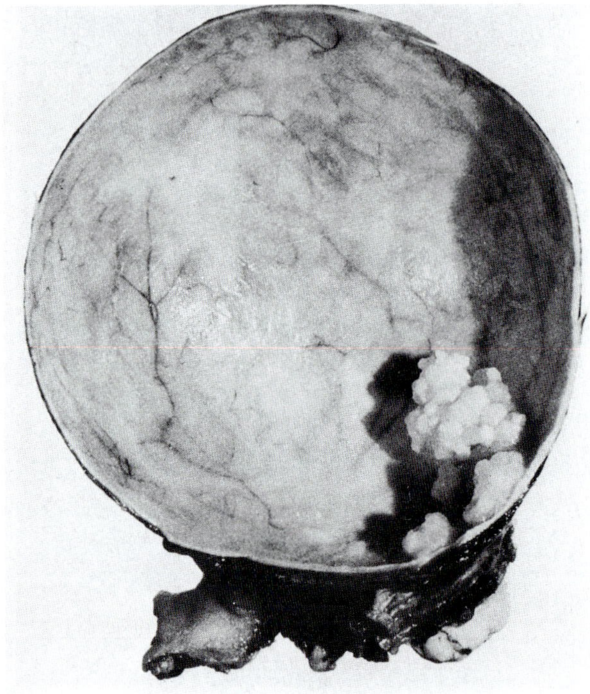

Fig. 18.1. Serous cystadenoma. A small papillary component is present in the lumen of a unilocular cyst.

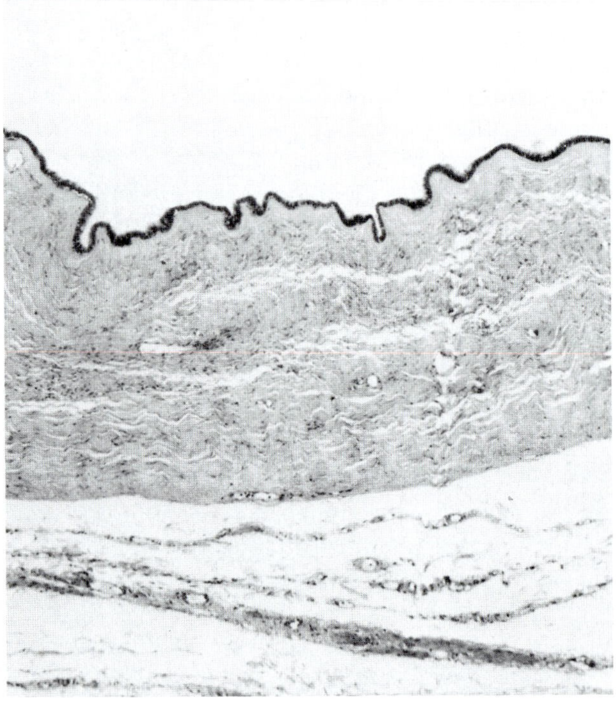

Fig. 18.2. Serous cyst. A simple cyst is lined by a single layer of epithelium overlying a fibrotic wall.

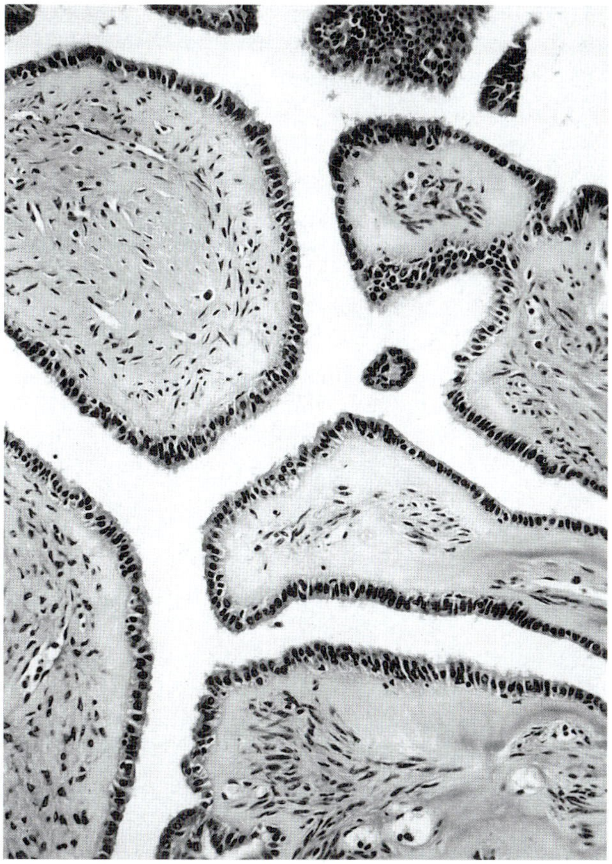

Fig. 18.3. **Serous cystadenoma.** Papillary processes are lined by a single layer of tubal-type columnar epithelium with cilia.

variation in the prominence and complexity of the papillae, from a simple, single layer and blunt papillae (Fig. 18.3) to focal epithelial stratification and detachment of cell clusters approaching the degree of proliferation seen in APSTs. Identification of these features in 10% of the histologic material is the boundary between benign and APST, but this is equally an arbitrary and artificial division in an otherwise smooth morphologic continuum. Cystadenomas are generally lined by a single layer of flattened to cuboidal cells with uniform basal nuclei. In addition, the epithelial cells can be pseudostratified and tubal in type, with the characteristic elongated (secretory cell) or rounded (ciliated cell) nuclei. Although the cells often produce mucin that is secreted into the cystic spaces, they do not contain the basophilic cytoplasmic vacuoles characteristic of mucinous neoplasms. In large cysts, the epithelium often becomes attenuated because of the pressure exerted by the cyst contents. Mitoses and atypia are generally absent. Psammoma bodies are present in the stroma in 15% of cystadenomas.

The stroma of benign serous tumors can resemble normal ovarian stroma but is generally more fibrous. Edema is sometimes present. When the stroma is highly cellular and fibrous, the tumor can be designated as an "adenofibroma" (Figs. 18.4 and 18.5). Pseudoxanthoma cells with granular light brown cytoplasmic pigment beneath the epithelium can be seen.

A variety of benign cysts may occur in and around the ovary and broad ligament and may simulate serous cystadenomas both grossly and microscopically. Functional ovarian cysts may have a denuded or attenuated lining. Similarly, an endometriotic cyst on occasion will mimic a serous cystadenoma if it lacks hemorrhage and endometriotic stroma is inconspicuous. Broad ligament cysts, such as hydatid cysts of Morgagni (tubal diverticulosis), mesonephric cysts, and mesothelial (peritoneal) cysts often mimic a serous cystadenoma. Any of these cysts, if large, may adhere to or compress the ovary, thus suggesting an ovarian origin. Mesonephric cysts are lined by cuboidal cells and are usually surrounded by concentric smooth muscle bundles. Peritoneal cysts are very common and are lined by mesothelial cells. Rarely, benign

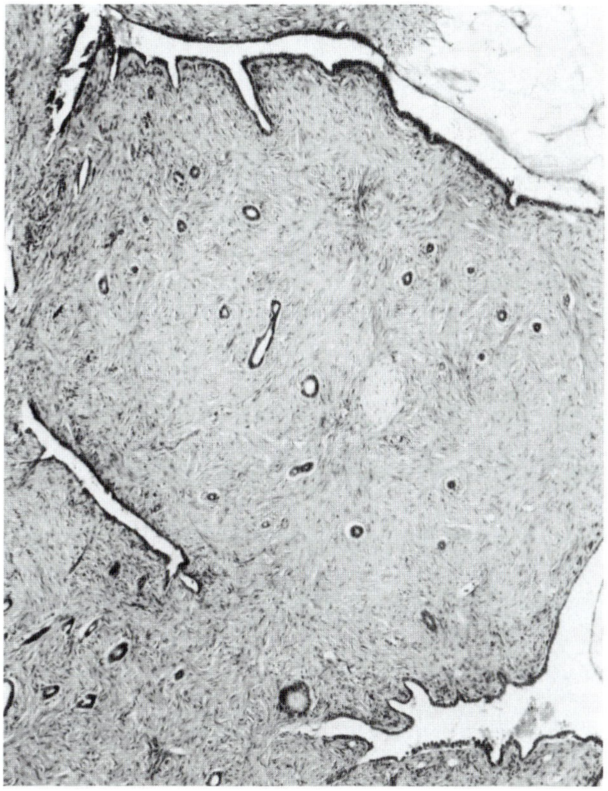

Fig. 18.4. **Serous adenofibroma.** Glands and clefts are lined by a single epithelial layer within a dense fibrous stroma.

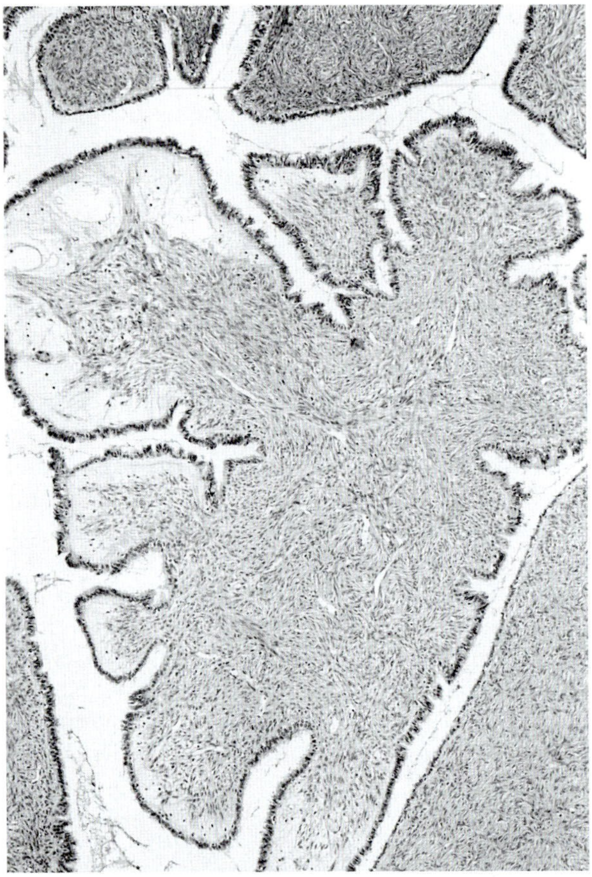

Fig. 18.5. Serous cystadenofibroma. Broad papillae with cellular fibrous stroma and lined by a single layer of epithelium project into the lumen of a cyst.

cystic teratomas may mimic serous cystadenomas, particularly the cystic variant of struma ovarii.[425] Patients with von Hippel–Lindau syndrome may develop a characteristic benign paraovarian cyst that resembles serous cystadenoma.[138]

Because serous cystadenomas are benign, unilateral salpingo-oophorectomy or ovarian cystectomy is adequate treatment. Recurrence is extremely rare and reflects either incomplete resection or a new primary tumor.

Atypical Proliferative ("Borderline") Serous Tumors

APSTs comprise about 10% of ovarian serous neoplasms and 56% of atypical proliferative ovarian tumors.

Clinical Findings

The clinical features of patients with APSTs are similar to those for serous cystadenomas, except that the mean patient age is slightly older for APSTs as compared to cystadenomas.

Operative Findings

Thirty-seven percent of atypical proliferative serous tumors are bilateral. Exophytic papillae reflecting ovarian surface involvement are common and are more often found in patients who also have peritoneal implants.[384]

APSTs are often associated with serous-type lesions involving the peritoneum. Endosalpingiosis or benign glandular inclusions are found in 40% of patients.[253] Likewise, papillary serous-type proliferations, so-called noninvasive implants (see "Associated Peritoneal Lesions"), that may resemble the ovarian tumor are found on peritoneal surfaces and are manifested as either small granular lesions or as fibrous plaques. At present, because of the current thorough staging procedures, 40% of APSTs are associated with peritoneal implants, in contrast to an average of 25% in the pre-1980 literature; among the 40% with implants, 31% are noninvasive and 9% are invasive.[388]

Gross Findings

APSTs have gross features similar to cystadenomas but tend to have finer, more friable, and more exuberant papillary projections (Fig. 18.6). Papillae are nearly always present on the internal surfaces of the cyst and are present on the external surfaces in as

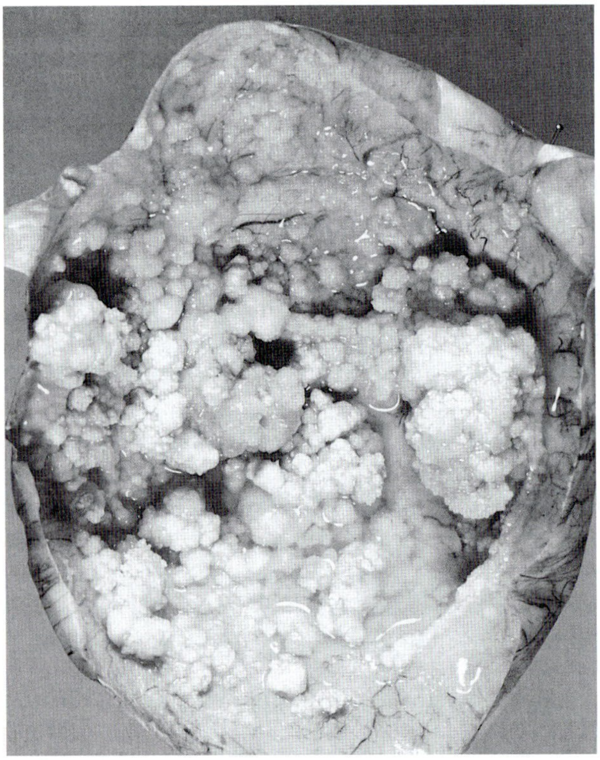

Fig. 18.6. Atypical proliferative serous tumor. The tumor is characterized by an intracystic proliferation of broad, soft papillary excrescences.

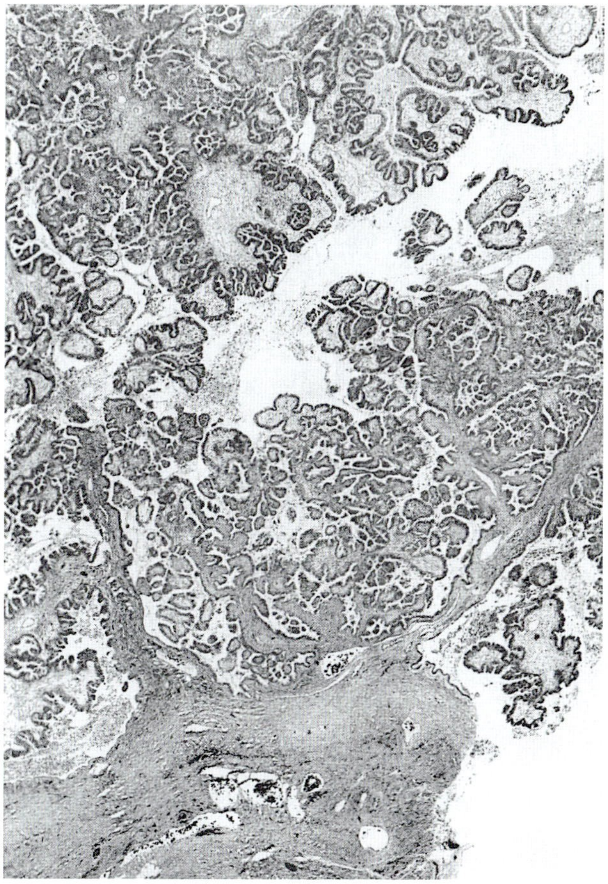

Fig. 18.7. Atypical proliferative serous tumor. Low-magnification view showing a hierarchical branching pattern with thick papillae giving rise to intermediate-sized papillae and then to small detached cell clusters.

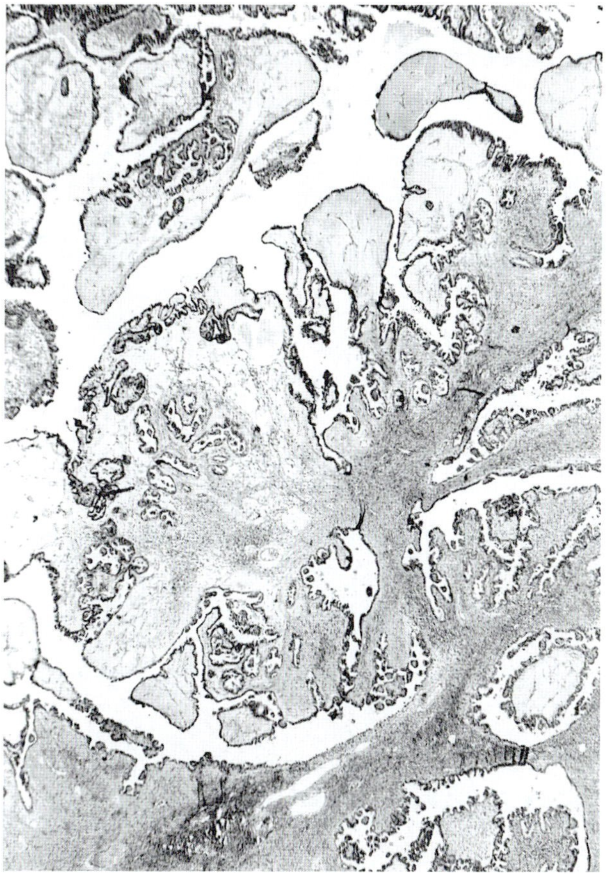

Fig. 18.8. Atypical proliferative serous tumor. Glands within the broad stromal cores of the larger papillae reflect tangential sectioning through a highly complex papillary surface and do not indicate invasion.

many as 70% of cases.[253] The adenofibromatous variant of APST is uncommon and grossly resembles its nonatypical counterpart.

Microscopic Findings

APSTs display extensive epithelial stratification and tufting and detachment of cell clusters in addition to hierarchical branching with successively smaller papillae emanating from the larger, more centrally located papillae (Figs. 18.7 and 18.8). The two most easily quantifiable proliferative changes in these tumors are epithelial stratification and the extent of tufting or budding with detachment of cells from the surface (Figs. 18.9–18.11). It has been recommended that a serous neoplasm should display stratification and budding in at least 10% of the available material to qualify as an APST.[353] Focal areas of fusion of the epithelial buds creates a roman bridge or cribriform pattern. Similarly, foci of nonhierarchical branching with fine elongated micropapillae emanating directly from large central papillae are seen not infrequently (Fig. 18.12). The cribriform and micropapillary patterns, when present in a 5-mm or greater area of confluent growth, warrant classification as micropapillary serous carcinoma (see "Malignant Serous Tumors").

The cells in APSTs show features of epithelial and mesothelial differentiation. Ciliated cells resembling those in the fallopian tube are present in about one-third of tumors (Fig. 18.13). Hobnail-type cells may be present (Fig. 18.14) and, not infrequently, the epithelium becomes attenuated and resembles mesothelium (Fig. 18.15). In addition, cells with abundant eosinophilic cytoplasm and rounded nuclei resembling mesothelial cells are also present, particularly on the tips of the papillae (Fig. 18.16). Very rarely, squamous morules are found. The nuclei of APSTs resemble those in cystadenomas but tend to display slightly more atypia. Nuclei are basally located and tend to be ovoid or rounded. The chromatin is usually fine but nucleoli are sometimes prominent (Fig. 18.17). Mitoses are not common and rarely exceed 4 per 10 high-power fields. Psammoma bodies are present in up to half of APSTs. Oc-

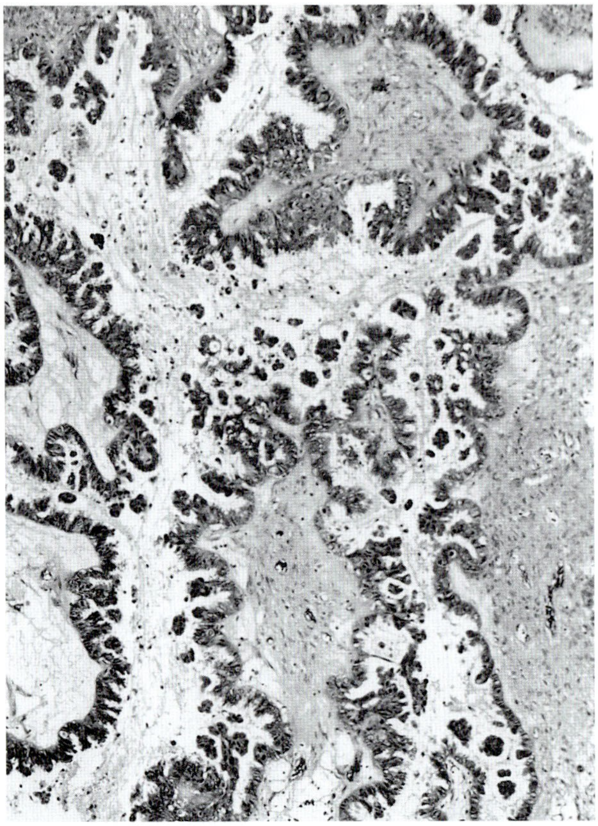

Fig. 18.9. Atypical proliferative serous tumor. Detachment of small cell clusters directly overlying stratified areas of the lining epithelium is one of the hallmarks of this tumor.

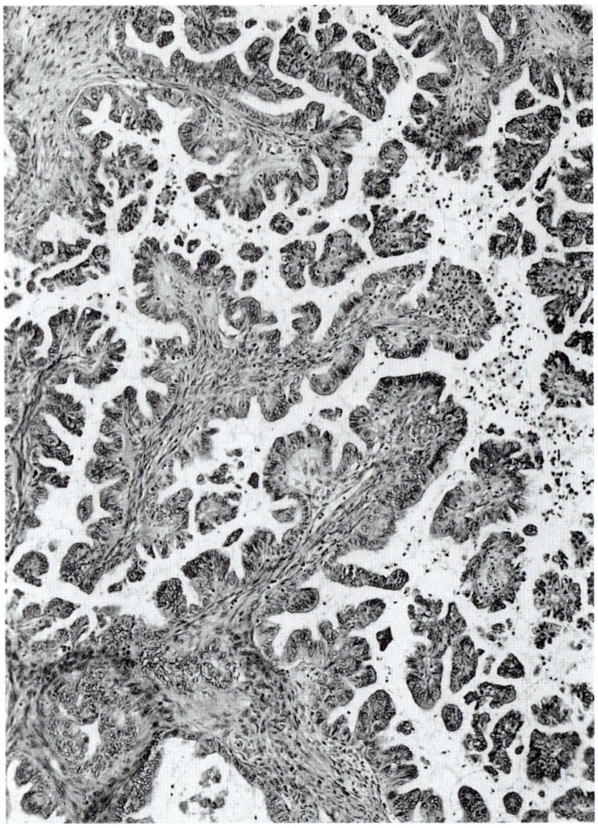

Fig. 18.10. Atypical proliferative serous tumor (APST). The stroma of this APST is cellular and closely resembles normal ovarian stroma. Note hierarchical branching pattern.

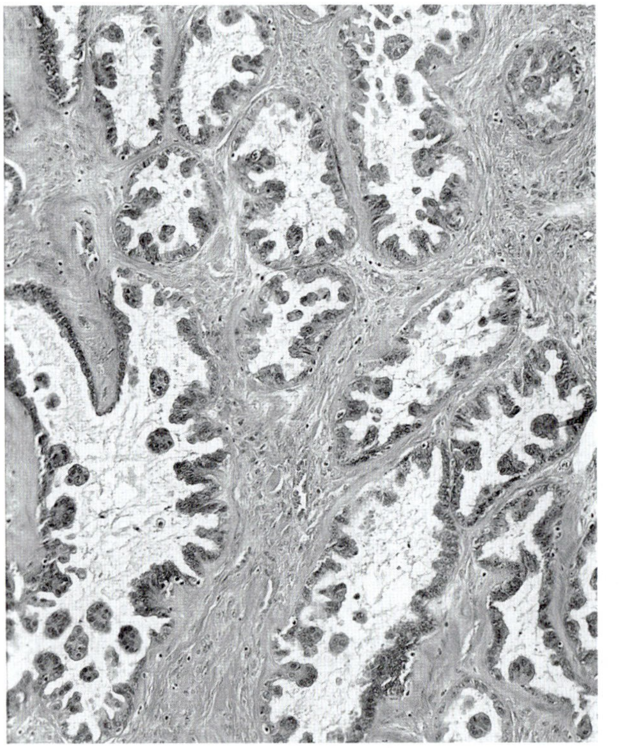

Fig. 18.11. Atypical proliferative serous tumor. This is the atypical proliferative counterpart of the serous adenofibroma. The epithelium is similar to that in ordinary APSTs, but the stroma is densely fibrous and the tumor is not cystic.

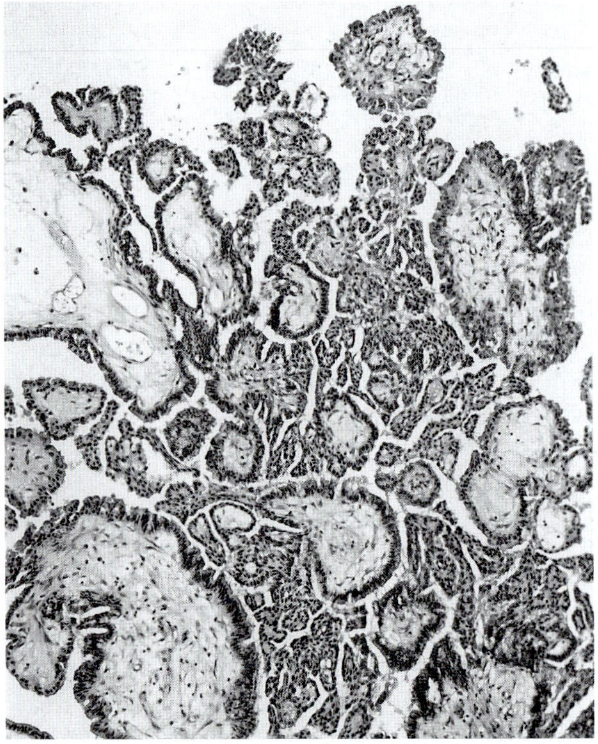

Fig. 18.12. Atypical proliferative serous tumor. Fusion of elongated micropapillae is present in an area measuring less than 5 mm in diameter. The tumor therefore does not meet the size requirement of a micropapillary serous carcinoma.

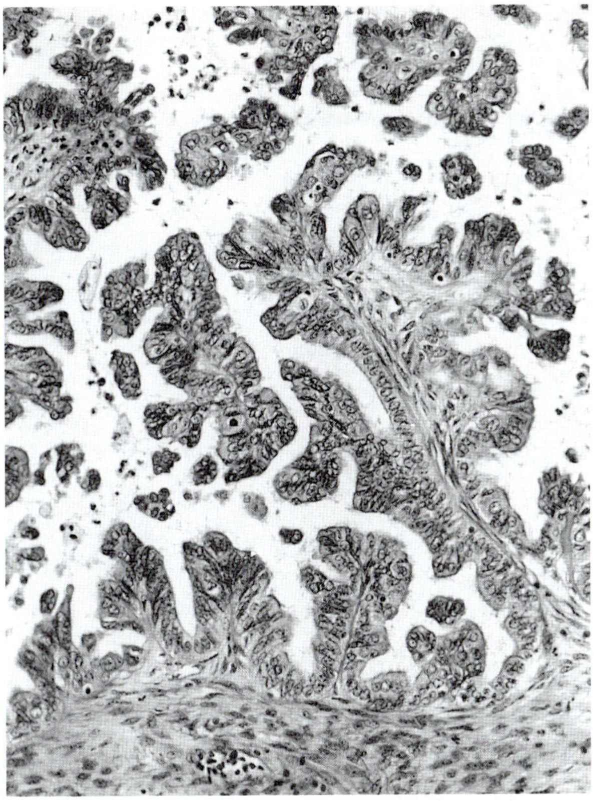

Fig. 18.13. Atypical proliferative serous tumor. The epithelium resembles tubal epithelium with some ciliated cells. A mild degree of cytologic atypia is present. The same features are present in the "detached" cell clusters.

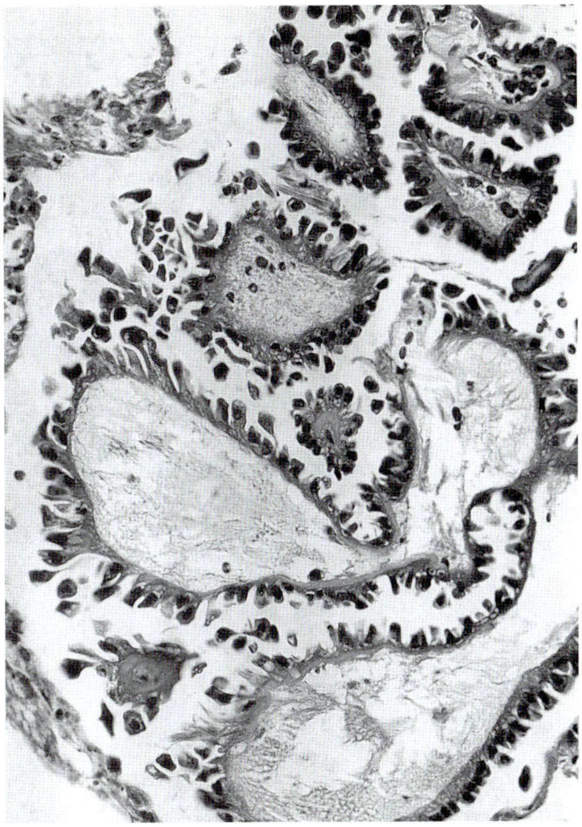

Fig. 18.14. Atypical proliferative serous tumor. The epithelium occasionally shows a hobnail-like pattern resembling that seen in some clear cell neoplasms.

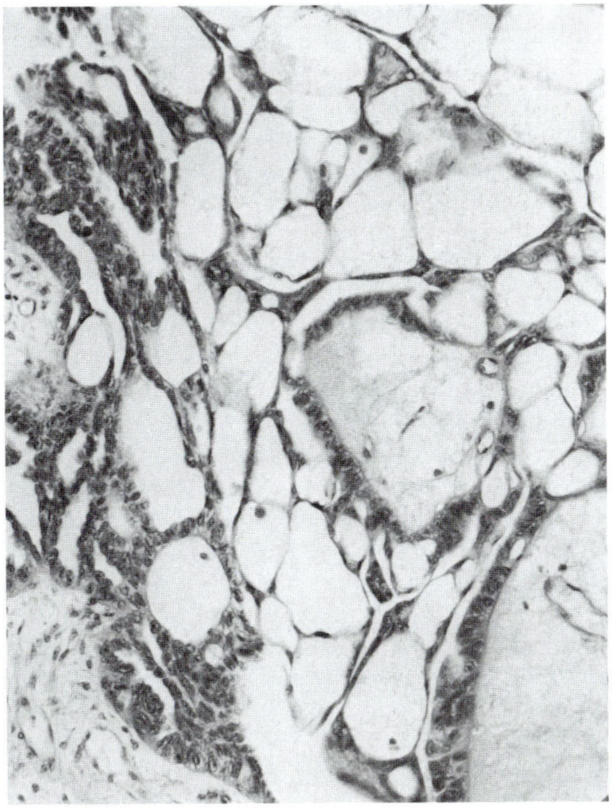

Fig. 18.15. Atypical proliferative serous tumor. There is attenuation of the epithelium creating a mesothelial-like appearance.

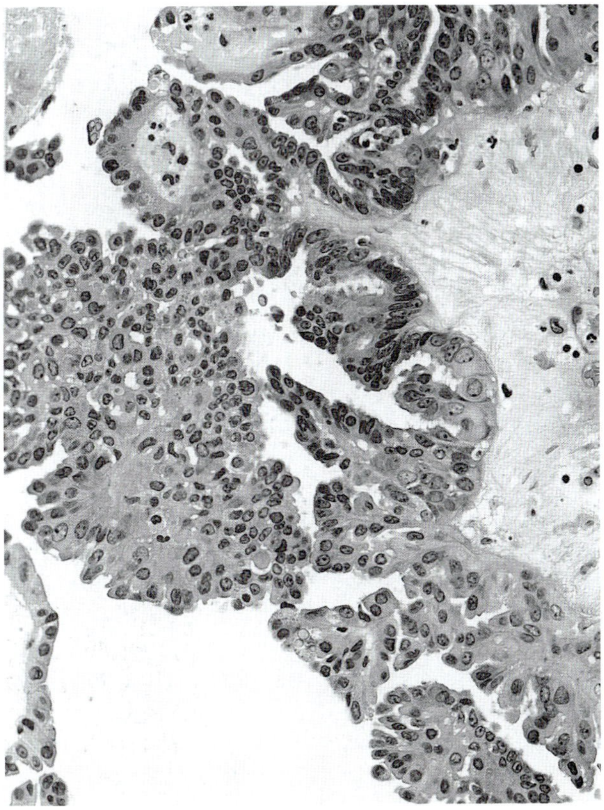

Fig. 18.16. Atypical proliferative serous tumor. Rounded cells in large clusters at the tips of the papillae resemble mesothelial cells.

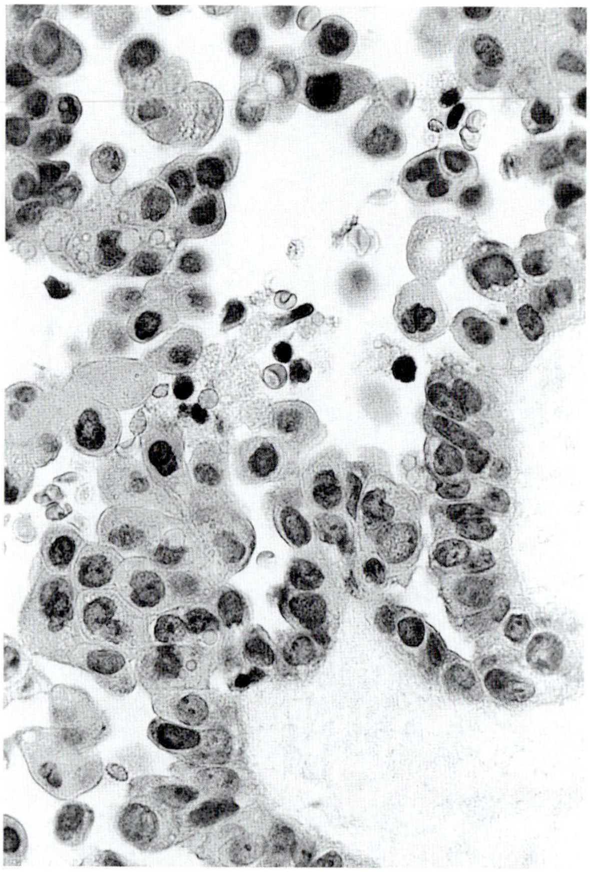

Fig. 18.17. Atypical proliferative serous tumor. The cells have a mesothelial-like appearance. Nuclei show mild to moderate pleomorphism, prominent nucleoli, and mild hyperchromasia.

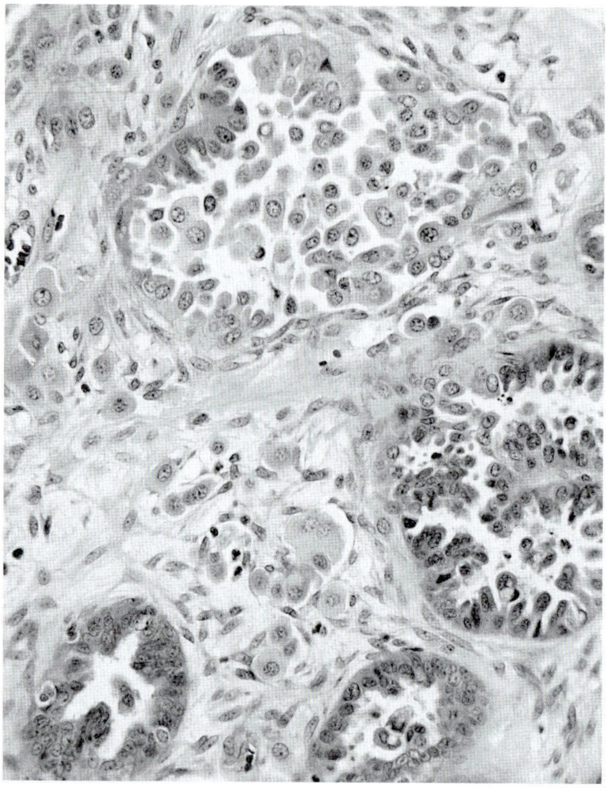

Fig. 18.18. Atypical proliferative serous tumor with microinvasion. Rounded cells with abundant cytoplasm appear to project into the stroma from the surface which displays a proliferation of cells with similar cytologic features. The cells are similar to those in Fig. 18.17.

casionally, foci resembling noninvasive desmoplastic peritoneal implants (see "Associated Peritoneal Lesions") are found on the surfaces of the ovarian tumor; this phenomenon has been referred to as autoimplantation.

Stromal Invasion APSTs, because of their complex papillary patterns, often display stromal invaginations that must be distinguished from stromal invasion as occurs in bona fide invasive carcinoma.

Microinvasion Two distinct types of lesions have been designated as microinvasion in APSTs. The more common type is characterized by isolated cells with abundant eosinophilic cytoplasm that appear to be budding from the epithelium into the superficial stromal cores of the papillae (Fig. 18.18). The true nature of these clusters of eosinophilic cells is not clear. In most cases, they do not evoke a host stromal response, and they bear no resemblance to invasive carcinoma. The second type of "microinvasion" occurs less commonly. This lesion is characterized by a haphazard infiltrative pattern of small nests of cells forming micropapillae, often surrounded by a clear space and associated with an identifiable stromal response (i.e., desmoplasia). Occasionally, the nests display a cribriform pattern. This second pattern of invasion resembles primary ovarian invasive well-differentiated serous carcinomas as well as the peritoneal lesions that have been designated invasive implants.

The second type of microinvasion appears to be a manifestation of true invasive carcinoma. In either case, the "invasion" is limited in extent and should occupy a total area of no more than 10 mm^2, with no single focus exceeding 3 mm, to qualify for the diagnosis.[31] When a careful search is made, 10% of APSTs contain microinvasion; however microinvasion has been specifically noted in only 1.3% of reported APSTs.[388] Interestingly, a high proportion of APSTs diagnosed during pregnancy show microinvasion.[269] The survival of 94 patients followed for a mean of 7.4 years was 100% (Table 18.4).[388] Thus, it is likely that microinvasion is frequently overlooked with no adverse affect on outcome. The majority of published cases display the first pattern; the clinical behavior associated with the second pat-

Table 18.4. Follow-up of 94 patients with serous "borderline" tumors (SBT) displaying microinvasion

Series	*No. of cases*	*Last known status*
Katzenstein[191]	7	NED, approximately 11 year
Tavassoli[434]	18	NED, 17 patients, mean 3.8 year DOD, 1 patient, 0.1 year
Bell[31]	21	NED, 17 patients, mean 5.2 year[a]
Lage[222]	2	NR
Casey[63]	2	NED, 12.9 and 16.2 year
Hanselaar[158]	9	NED, mean 4.5 year
Tan[428]	2	NED, 2 and 11 year[b]
Nayar[277]	7	NED, mean 10.6 year
Kennedy[195]	4	NED, 2.25, 9.1, 10.9, 13 year
Burks[54]	2[c]	AWD (1 recurred), 1 NR
Seidman[387]	4	NED, mean 8.8 year (6.6–14 year)
Sykes[421]	3	NED, mean 1.9 year
Mooney[269]	8	NED, 0.2–21 year
Silva[400]	3	NED, 1 patient, >15 year AWD, 2 patients, >7 year
Eichorn[109]	9[c]	NED, mean approximately 6 year
Total	101	94 patients, mean 6.7 years 7 patients NR

NED, no evidence of disease; DOD, dead of disease; NR, not reported; AWD, alive with disease.
Adequate sampling not documented.
[a]One patient developed a contralateral ovarian SBT after 2.8 years and was alive and well 6 months later.
[b]In the latter case, tumor "recurred" in a lymph node at 7 year, and the patient was NED 4 years later.
[c]Two cases were MPSCs.
From Seidman and Kurman,[388] with permission.

tern of microinvasion is based on a small number of cases. Although more data are needed, particularly about the second pattern, from the standpoint of prognosis and patient management, microinvasion at present appears to have no clinical relevance.

Associated Peritoneal Lesions: Endosalpingiosis and "Implants" The peritoneum in patients with APSTs often contains serous epithelial proliferations displaying a wide range of proliferative changes: benign glands designated endosalpingiosis; papillary epithelial proliferations, sometimes with stromal desmoplasia, designated "noninvasive implants"; and invasive carcinoma, also designated "invasive implants." Useful features that distinguish invasive from noninvasive desmoplastic implants are summarized in Table 18.5. It is important to note that some patients have both invasive and noninvasive implants; in addition, endosalpingiosis often coexists with both types of implant.

Endosalpingiosis Endosalpingiosis, or benign glandular inclusions, may involve the peritoneal surfaces in patients with or without benign or malignant serous ovarian tumors (see Chapter 17, Diseases of the Peritoneum). These glands typically are lined by simple columnar epithelium, often displaying tubal-type differentiation. The epithelium may display minor degrees of cytologic atypia and form simple papillary structures (Figs. 18.19 and 18.20); psammoma bodies are sometimes present and may persist after degeneration of the associated epithelial structures. Mitotic figures are absent.

Noninvasive Peritoneal Implants Among women with APSTs, 31% have peritoneal epithelial lesions that display a degree of proliferation beyond that usually seen in endosalpingiosis but which lack features of invasion. These lesions have been designated noninvasive implants and have two morphologic forms: epithelial and desmoplastic. Some patients have both types of noninvasive implants; patients with desmoplastic implants usually also have epithelial implants.

Epithelial implants are papillary and resemble the ovarian APST. The cores of the papillae have fibrovascular support, and the epithelial cells resemble those in endosalpingiosis. Thus, mild atypia is

Table 18.5. Morphologic features distinguishing invasive from noninvasive peritoneal implants

		Noninvasive implants	
Feature	*Invasive implants*	*Desmoplastic*	*Epithelial*
Growth pattern	Haphazard infiltration High ratio of epithelium to stroma	Orderly arrangement Low ratio of epithelium to stroma	Exophytic or in submesothelial invaginations beneath the peritoneal surface
Epithelial component	Small rounded nests containing serous and mesothelial-type cells with high nuclear: cytoplasmic ratio, surrounded by a clear space Endophytic micropapillae displaying a confluent pattern Exophytic micropapillae resembling MPSC of the ovary	Irregular glandlike structures lined by one or two layers of nondescript epithelial and mesothelial-type cells, often with abundant eosinophilic cytoplasm The lining epithelial cells of the glandlike structures often appear to merge with the surrounding stromal cells	Papillary structures with thick papillae displaying a hierarchical branching pattern similar to primary ovarian APST
Stromal component	Loose or dense fibrous tissue	Granulation tissue appearance frequently	No stromal reaction
Psammoma bodies	Generally infrequent and sparse, but may at times be extensive	Frequent and can be extensive	Frequent
Cytologic atypia	Generally mild to moderate	Mild to moderate, rarely marked	Mild to moderate
Inflammation	Generally minimal	Frequent and occasionally marked; fibrinopurulent exudate may be present	Minimal

MPSC, micropapillary serous carcinoma; APST, atypical proliferative serous tumor.

often present, but mitoses are usually absent (Figs. 18.21–18.23). Calcification, usually in the form of psammoma bodies, is common and may be extensive (Fig. 18.23).

Desmoplastic implants are plaquelike lesions with fibrosis that entraps glandlike structures. The glandlike structures bear little resemblance to the ovarian serous tumor and usually have features of a benign reactive mesothelial proliferation. Both epithelial and desmoplastic implants are often associated with abundant psammoma bodies and usually appear "tacked on" to the peritoneal surface. Occasionally, a peritoneal lesion is entirely calcified or fibrotic; these should not be considered implants if an epithelial component is absent.

The characteristic architectural feature of the desmoplastic noninvasive implant is a plaquelike thickening overlying peritoneal surfaces (Fig. 18.24), which may extend into the septae that separate omental lobules (Fig. 18.25) and create an appearance that under low power may suggest invasion.[35,387] They display an exuberant fibroblastic proliferation that engulfs glandlike or papillary structures lined by epithelial cells with minimal and occasionally more marked cytologic atypia. The fibroblastic proliferation often has a granulation tissue-like appearance characterized by edematous fascicles of plump fibroblasts, often with interspersed small vascular channels (Figs. 18.26–18.28). A helpful feature in distinguishing a desmoplastic noninvasive implant from an invasive implant is that the fibroblastic reaction associated with the noninvasive implant is generally much more extensive than the glandlike proliferation, which tends to be sparse; this creates an appearance suggestive of sclerosing peritonitis with florid reactive mesothelial proliferation. In contrast, the ratio of epithelium to stroma is much higher in the invasive implant. It should be noted that there is little direct evidence that the epithelial-like structures in noninvasive implants are derived from the ovarian tumor, and some of these lesions might, in fact, be mesothelial in origin. At times, the glandlike structures are more crowded, but the proliferation lacks the haphazard infiltrative pattern of carcinoma. Typically, the cells forming the glandlike structures merge with the sur-

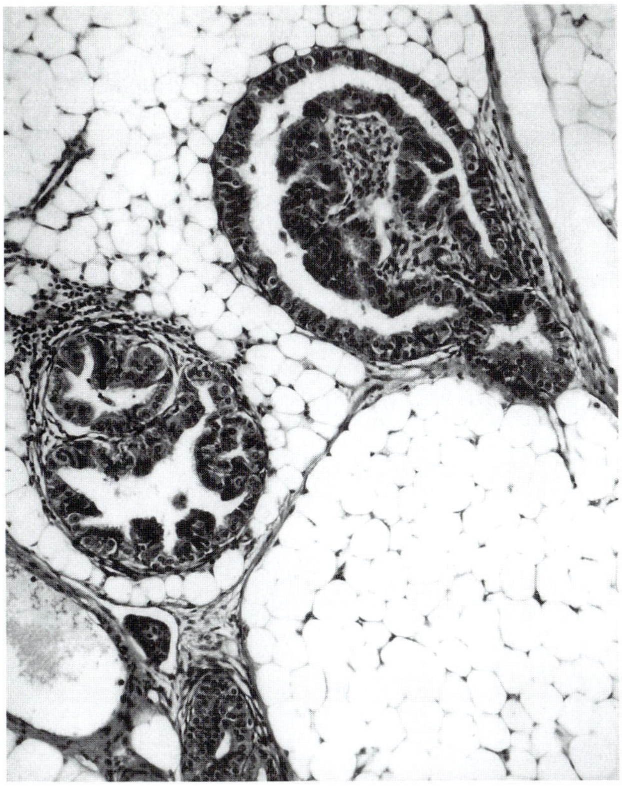

Fig. 18.19. Endosalpingiosis. Glands within the omentum are lined by a single layer of tubal-type epithelium with a few simple papillary projections.

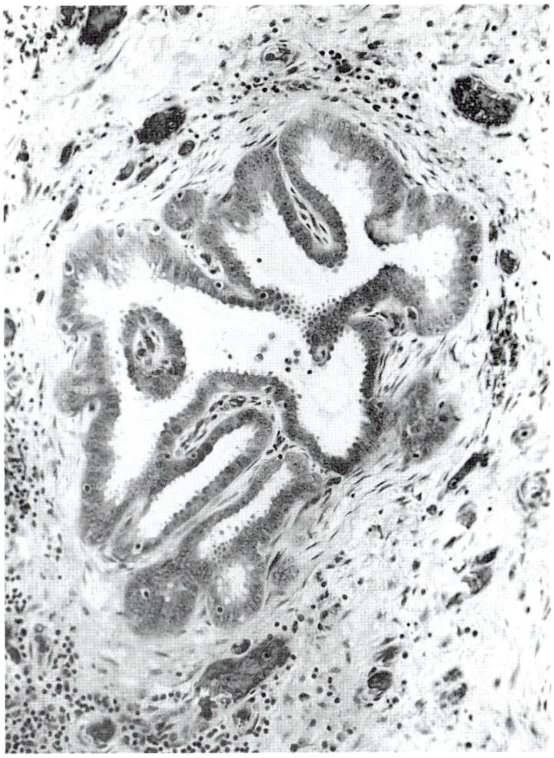

Fig. 18.20. Endosalpingiosis. Glands within a peritoneal fibrous adhesion are lined by a single layer of tubal-type epithelium with simple papillary projections containing delicate fibrovascular support.

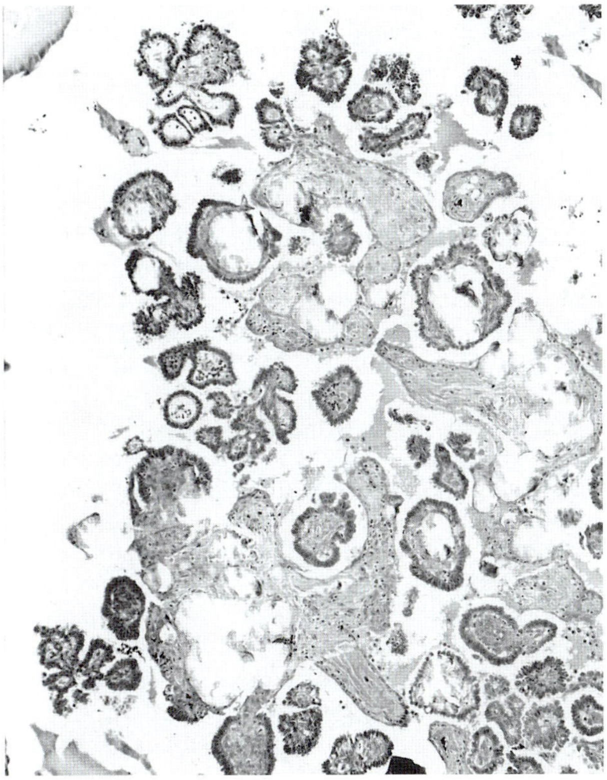

Fig. 18.21. Noninvasive peritoneal implant, epithelial type. Multiple small papillae on the surface of the peritoneum.

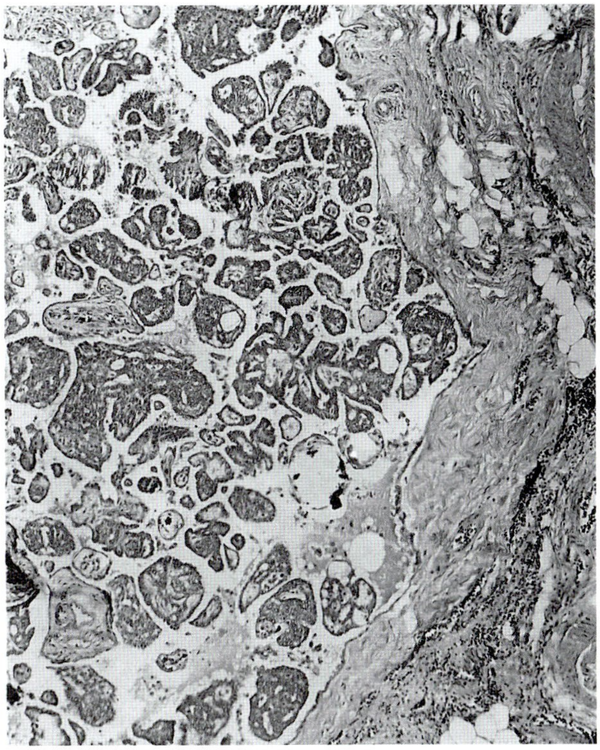

Fig. 18.22. Noninvasive peritoneal implant, epithelial type. A papillary serous proliferation resembling the ovarian APST is present on the surface of the peritoneum without invading underlying tissue.

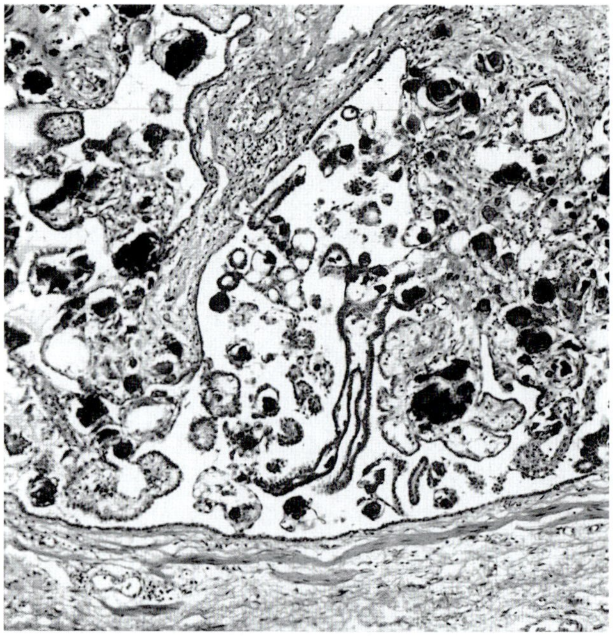

Fig. 18.23. Noninvasive peritoneal implant, epithelial type. Abundant psammoma bodies are present in this papillary serous proliferation within folds of the peritoneum without invasion of underlying tissue.

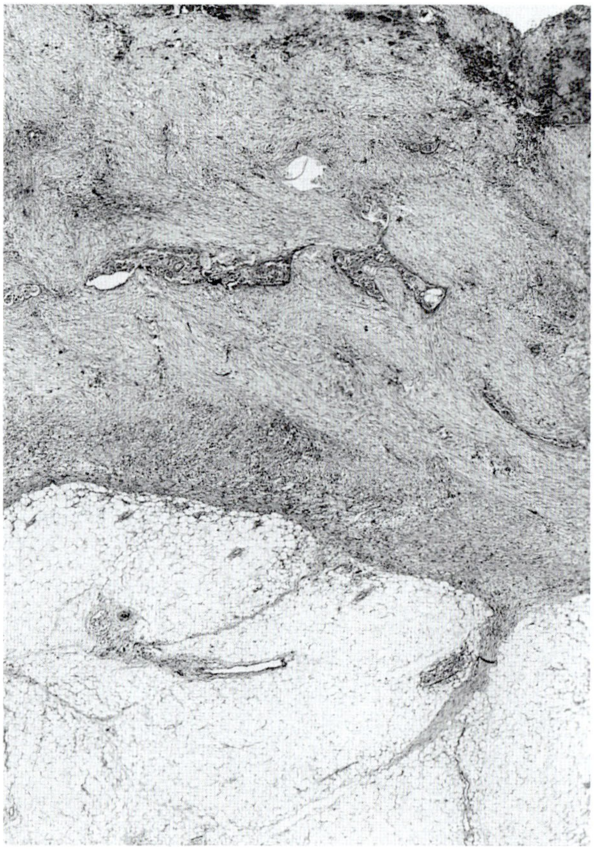

Fig. 18.24. Noninvasive peritoneal implant, desmoplastic type. Plaquelike thickening of cellular fibroblastic tissue with entrapped epithelial-like structures overlying omental fat.

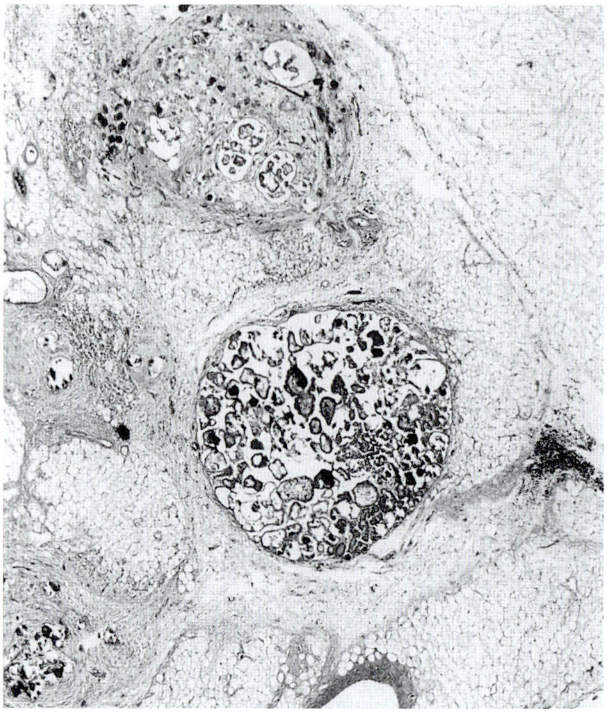

Fig. 18.25. Noninvasive peritoneal implant, desmoplastic and epithelial type. In *upper and left parts of field*, small papillary structures are surrounded by fibrous tissue. In *center*, a rounded well-circumscribed area contains small papillary structures without associated fibrosis. Note the preservation of omental fat lobules.

rounding fibroblasts, which surround the glands in a concentric fashion, making distinction between the two cell populations difficult at times; again, this is suggestive of a reactive mesothelial proliferation (Figs. 18.29 and 18.30). A chronic inflammatory response is nearly always present, and in 20% of cases, an acute inflammatory exudate overlies the implant. Mitotic figures are usually absent, and psammoma bodies are present in more than 90% of cases.

Invasive Peritoneal Implants The characteristic architectural feature of an invasive implant is a haphazard infiltrative growth pattern (Figs. 18.31–18.33). A confluent or cribriform glandular pattern may be present. An exophytic micropapillary pattern, as described later (see "Micropapillary Serous Carcinoma"), also qualifies for the designation of invasive implant (Fig. 18.34), but more often micropapillae are nonbranched, embedded in fibrous stroma, and surrounded by a clear space or cleft (Figs. 18.32, 18.35–18.37). Sometimes micropapillae are present within glands and may fuse with one another to create a weblike appearance (Fig. 18.38). Invasive implants often display only mild cytologic

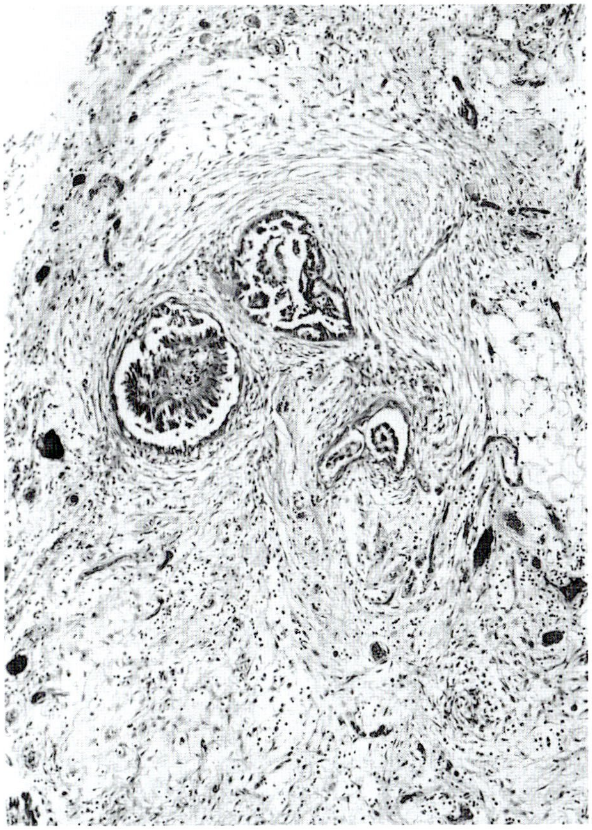

Fig. 18.26. Noninvasive peritoneal implant, desmoplastic type. The stroma engulfs glandlike structures that may display papillary projections into the spaces. There is a mild chronic inflammatory infiltrate in the stroma.

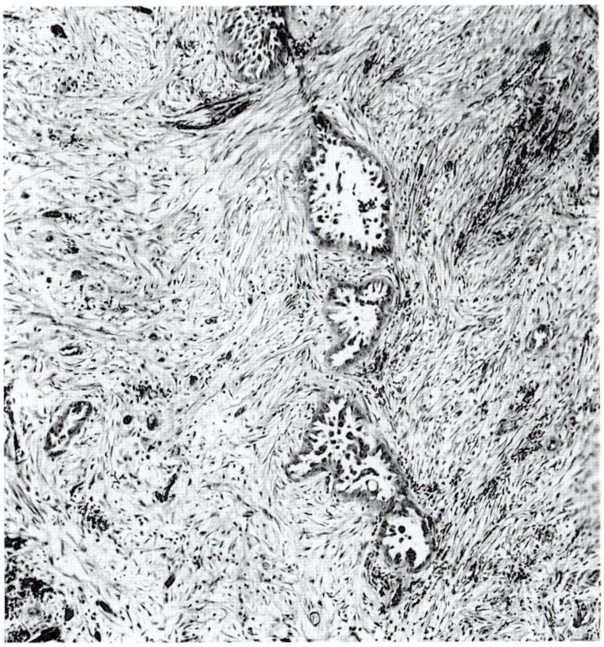

Fig. 18.27. Noninvasive peritoneal implant, desmoplastic type. Edematous, moderately cellular fibroblastic proliferation resembling granulation tissue engulfs glandlike structures.

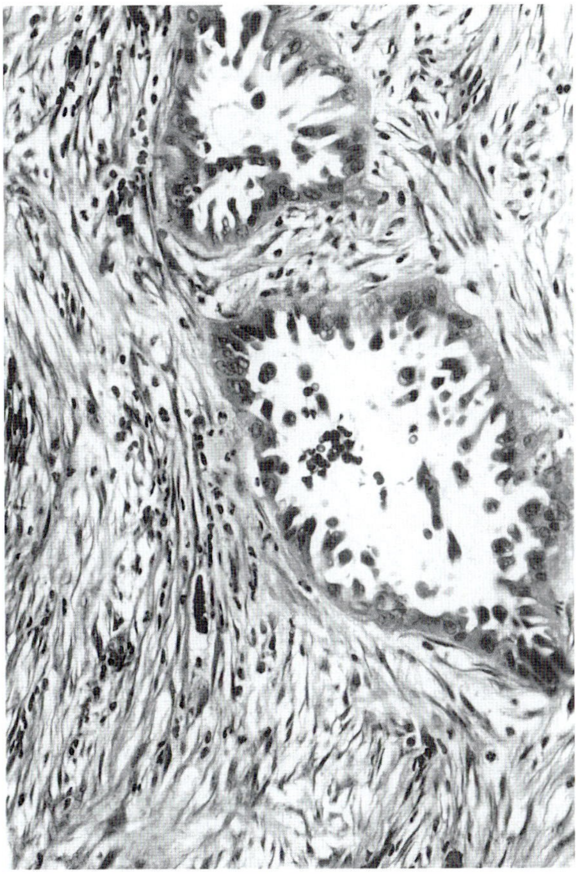

Fig. 18.28. Noninvasive peritoneal implant, desmoplastic type. Entrapped glandlike structures are lined by columnar epithelium with minimal cytologic atypia. Many cells have a hobnail-like appearance.

atypia, but occasionally atypia is moderate and rarely marked (Fig. 18.39). Mitotic figures are occasionally present.

The distinction of desmoplastic implants from invasive implants (carcinoma) may be very difficult at times but is important because it is this feature that is the best predictor of outcome for tumors with extraovarian disease. In the past, criteria for the diagnosis of invasive implants have been difficult to apply and controversial. For example, it has been stated that to qualify as invasive, an implant must clearly display invasion of underlying normal tissue, but in many cases peritoneal biopsies obtained during surgical staging procedures are small and devoid of underlying normal tissue. Controversy over what constitutes the appropriate criteria for the diagnosis of an invasive implant is illustrated by the debate over the significance of individual cells with abundant eosinophilic cytoplasm within the stroma. Most investigators state that this is a feature commonly seen in noninvasive implants[35,387] whereas

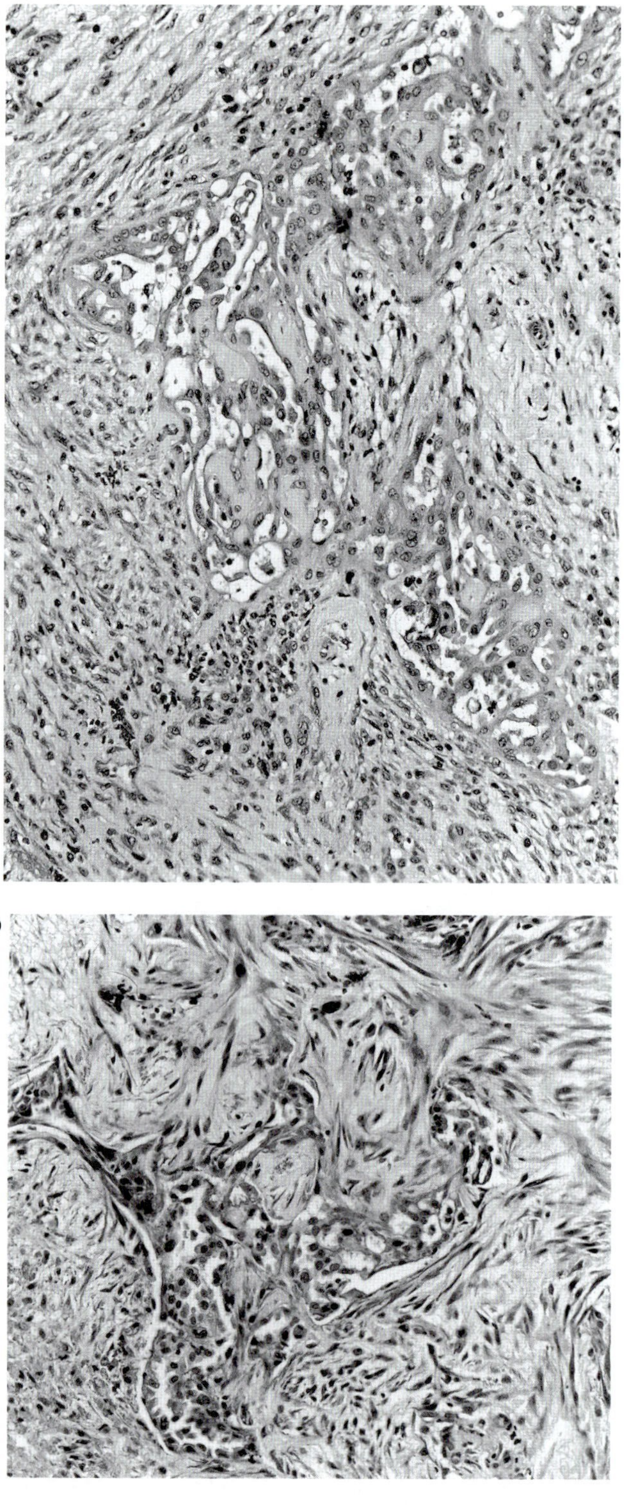

Fig. 18.29. Noninvasive peritoneal implant, desmoplastic type. a: The epithelium appears to merge with the surrounding stroma, which has a granulation tissue-like appearance. b: The cells lining the glandlike structures merge with the surrounding fibroblasts, an appearance resembling a florid reactive mesothelial proliferation.

others dispute this, claiming that this feature is diagnostic of an invasive implant.[141]

A recent study in which implants designated as invasive were associated with a 65% recurrence rate compared with a recurrence rate of 14% for implants designated as noninvasive[37] confirmed that the presence of individual cells within the stroma was not helpful in separating invasive from noninvasive implants. Furthermore, it was found that most invasive implants could be identified in the absence of overt invasion of underlying normal tissue and yet still accurately predict poor outcome. Features that were found to be useful in diagnosing invasive implants were the presence of solid nests and glandlike structures haphazardly or radially infiltrating the stroma that either displayed a micropapillary or cribriform architecture or a confluent growth pattern or were surrounded by a clear space or cleft.[37] Some have observed that the epithelial structures extend into the surrounding tis-

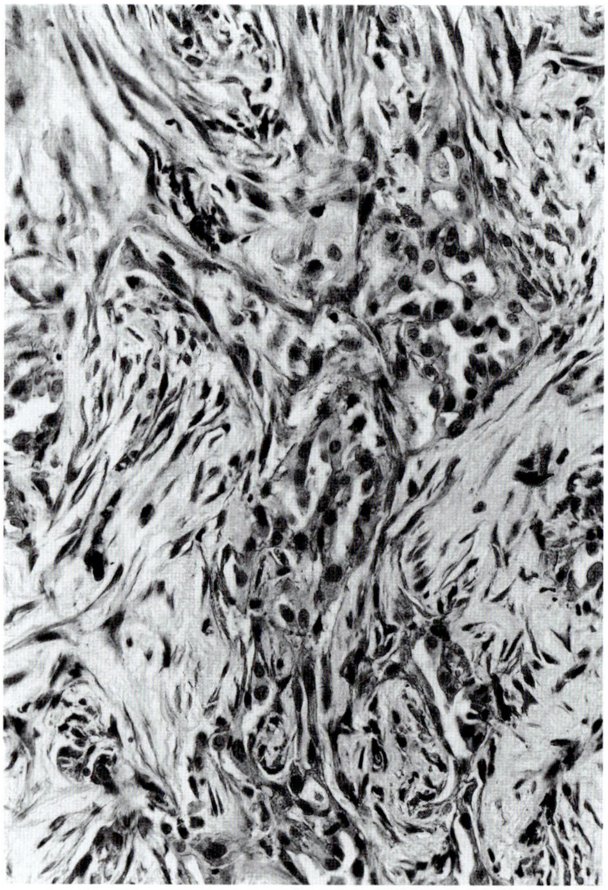

Fig. 18.30. Noninvasive peritoneal implant, desmoplastic type. The cells lining the glandlike structures merge with the surrounding fibroblasts, making distinction between the two cell types difficult. Note the minimal cytologic atypia in the cells lining the glandlike structures.

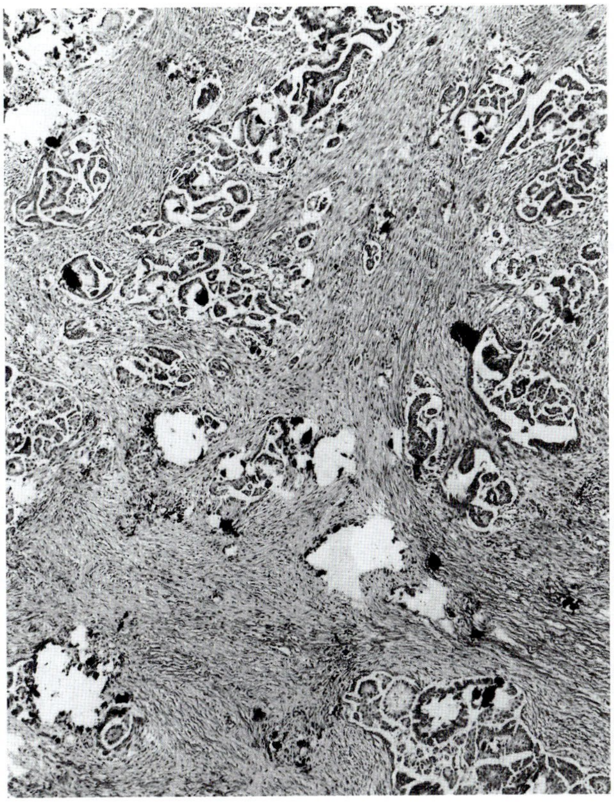

Fig. 18.31. Invasive peritoneal implant. A haphazard infiltrative pattern of predominantly small papillae invading cellular fibrous tissue.

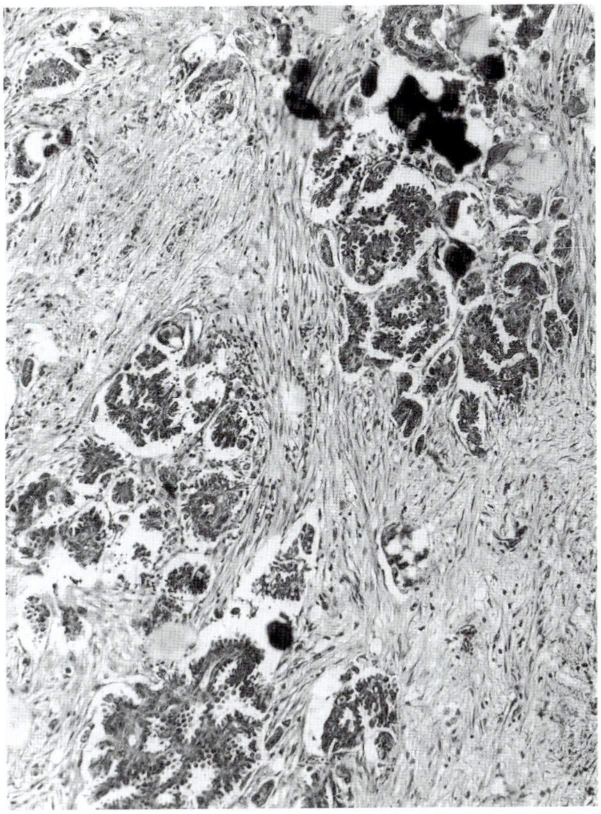

Fig. 18.32. Invasive peritoneal implant. Micropapillae invading fibrous tissue. Note the spaces surrounding most of the papillae.

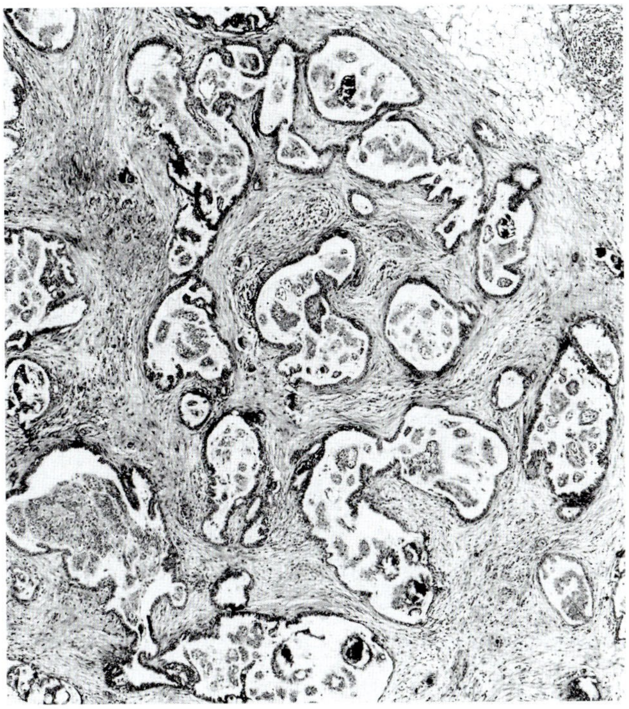

Fig. 18.33. Invasive peritoneal implant. Each gland contains micropapillary structures. The haphazard infiltrative pattern is best appreciated from low magnification by noting the haphazard infiltrative relationship of the glands to one another.

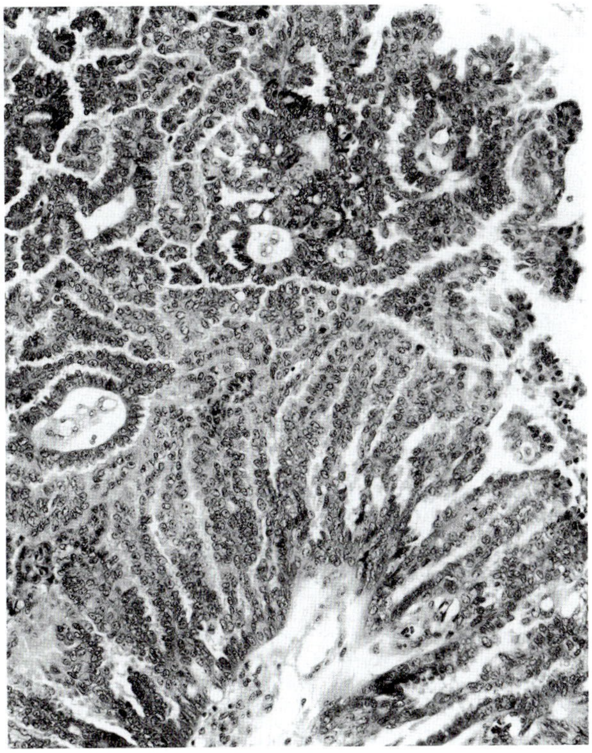

Fig. 18.34. Invasive peritoneal implant. An exophytic micropapillary pattern with fusion and bridging of the micropapillae warrants a diagnosis of invasive implant.

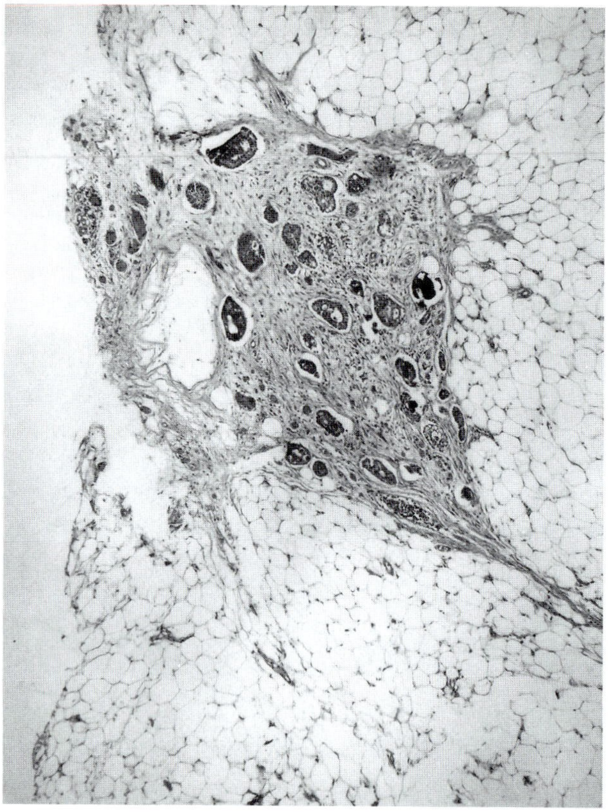

Fig. 18.35. **Invasive peritoneal implant.** Invasion of omental fat by micropapillae surrounded by a space.

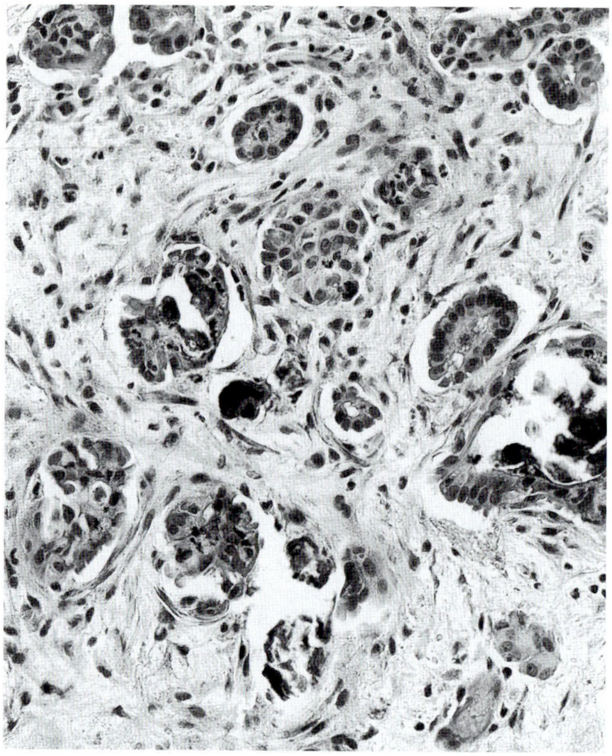

Fig. 18.36. Invasive peritoneal implant. Haphazard infiltrative pattern of micropapillae. Each papillary structure is surrounded by a space.

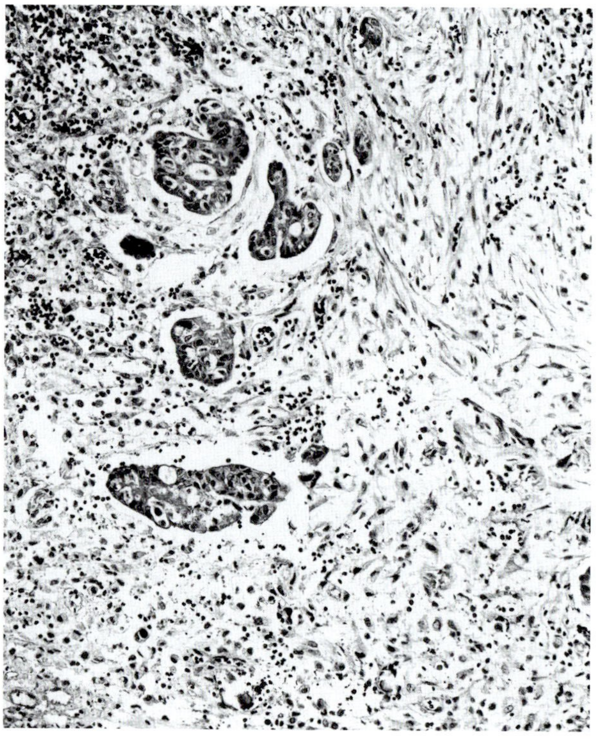

Fig. 18.37. Invasive peritoneal implant. When an infiltrative pattern is not apparent, the presence of spaces around the papillae is a very useful feature of invasion.

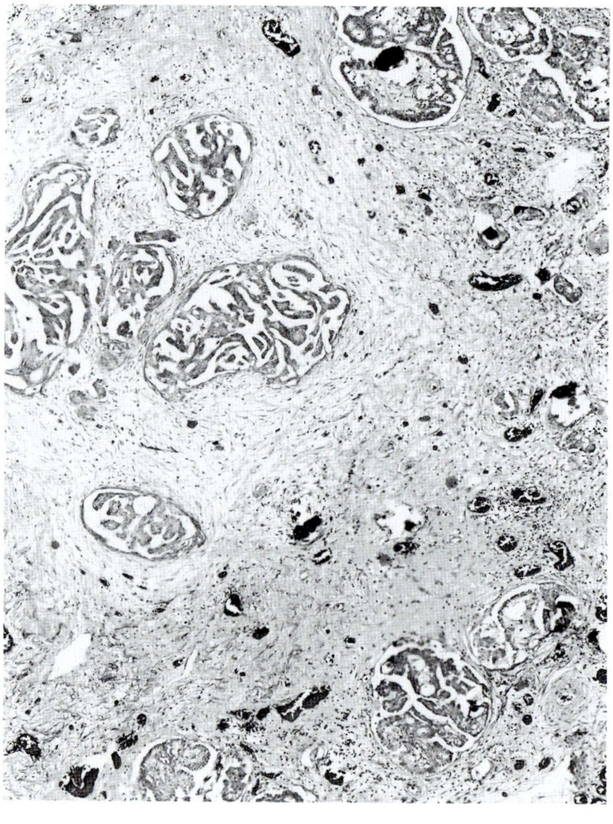

Fig. 18.38. Invasive peritoneal implant. The invading glands occasionally contain micropapillae that may fuse with one another, creating a weblike confluent pattern.

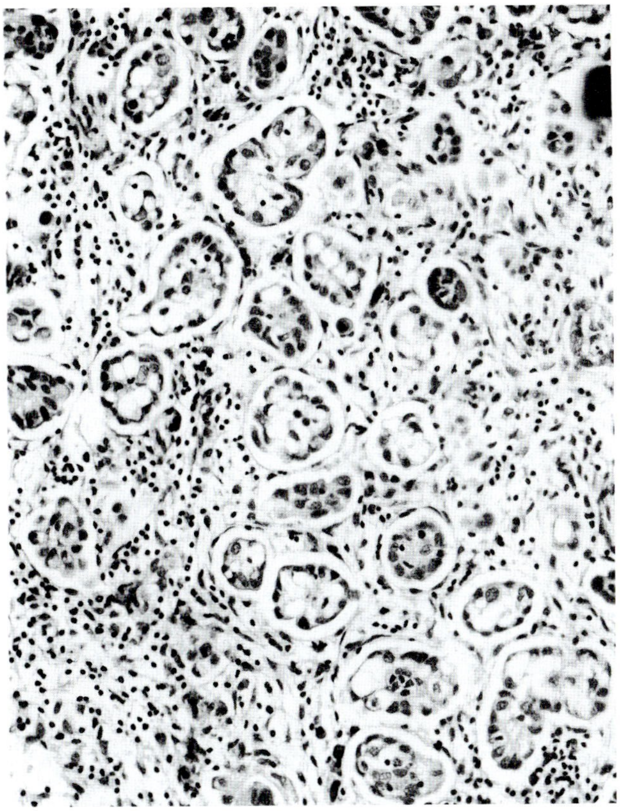

Fig. 18.39. Invasive peritoneal implant. Mild to moderate cytologic atypia is present in the glands. The stroma displays a chronic inflammatory infiltrate.

sues marginally ahead of the desmoplastic response in an invasive implant, in contrast to the lack of this feature in noninvasive desmoplastic implants.

Pathogenesis of Peritoneal Implants The pathogenesis of the peritoneal lesions associated with APSTs is unknown. Molecular data are conflicting in resolving whether these lesions are independent primary peritoneal lesions, as suggested by one study showing a different X-inactivation pattern of the primary ovarian tumor and the peritoneal implants,[237] or arise from exfoliation or detachment from the ovarian tumor with subsequent attachment to the peritoneal surface, as suggested by another study showing concordance between the primary tumor and the peritoneal implants for LOH at three loci on chromosome 17p13.[486] As noninvasive epithelial implants to some degree resemble the ovarian tumors, these are the ones most likely to arise by the detachment–implantation mechanism, although evidence for this is only circumstantial.[384] In contrast, noninvasive desmoplastic implants more closely resemble a reactive mesothelial process and, in our view, are likely to be independent of the primary ovarian tumor. Invasive implants are rare, and bonafide invasive implants most likely reflect peritoneal metastases of MPSCs (micropapillary serous carcinoma) or inadequately sampled invasive serous carcinomas but also could be independent primary peritoneal serous carcinomas. A recent report notes that calcified fallopian tube mucosal lesions designated "salpingoliths" resemble noninvasive epithelial implants and are found more often in the tubes of patients with peritoneal implants as compared to those without impalnts.[388a]

Lymph Nodes Lymph node involvement has been reported in approximately 63 cases of APSTs.[388] Putative lymph node "metastases" of APSTs can be divided into two types. Excluded from consideration is endosalpingiosis involving lymph nodes, which are nonneoplastic glandular inclusions of müllerian type and occur in pelvic lymph nodes of 5%–14% of unselected women and in 45%–65% of women with borderline ovarian tumors.[73,270] One of the two types of metastatic lymph node lesions that has been associated with APSTs is characterized by individual cells and clusters of cells with abundant eosinophilic cyto-

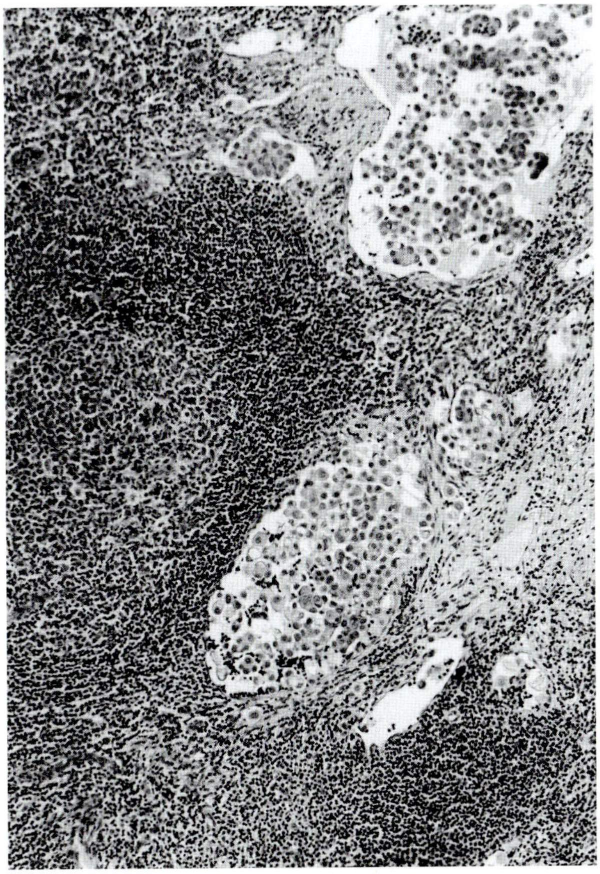

Fig. 18.40. Lymph node "involvement" by atypical proliferative serous tumor. The subcapsular sinus of this lymph node is filled with isolated cells and cell clusters.

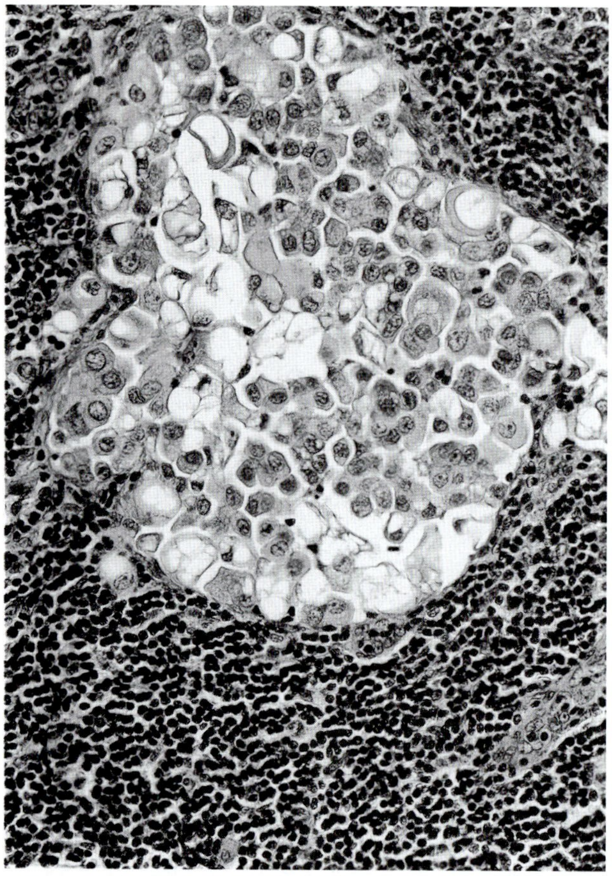

Fig. 18.41. Lymph node "involvement" by atypical proliferative serous tumor. The clusters of cells in the subcapsular sinus have abundant eosinophilic cytoplasm and nuclear grooves and folds resembling reactive mesothelial cells. Compare to Fig. 18.17.

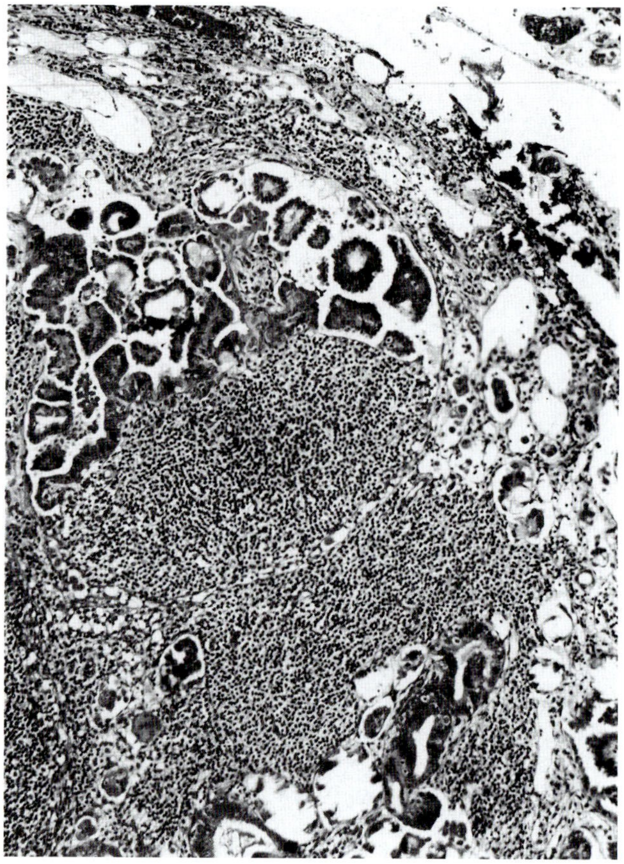

Fig. 18.42. Lymph node "involvement" by atypical proliferative serous tumor (APST). Papillary structures resembling the ovarian APST are filling the subcapsular sinus.

plasm in the sinuses, predominantly subcapsular sinuses (Figs. 18.40 and 18.41). The nature of these cells is unclear, but a recent study suggested that they may be mesothelial in origin. Similar cells are nearly always present on the surface of primary APSTs and are often present in the stroma of noninvasive desmoplastic implants. It is plausible that these cells exfoliate and are filtered from the peritoneal fluid by regional lymph nodes, so-called deportation.

The second type of lymph node lesion is characterized by glandular inclusions and papillary serous structures, usually just beneath the capsule of the lymph node, that resemble the ovarian APST (Figs. 18.42 and 18.43). The majority of these papillary serous lesions are also associated with endosalpingiosis in the same lymph node. The observation of papillary proliferations arising within endosalpingiosis, and the rare reports of APSTs and carcinomas arising within lymph nodes from endosalpingiosis, suggest an independent origin of this second type of lymph node lesion.[388] Identification of lymph node metastases of APSTs has been cited as evidence of malignant potential for APSTs (borderline tumors). However, this conclusion is not supported by the data because the survival rate of 43 reported patients with lymph node metastases is 98% after a mean follow-up of 6.5 years (Table 18.6).[388]

Immunohistochemistry

Limited data on the immunohistochemistry of APSTs indicate that they are positive for CK 7 and OC-125. About half of cases are positive for Leu M1. Focal positivity for CK 20 is seen in a small minority of cases. Most cases express estrogen[1] and progesterone receptors.[60] They are also positive for other epithelial markers including epithelial membrane antigen (EMA) and other cytokeratins.

Differential Diagnosis

Most papillary neoplasms in the ovary that are not serous cystadenomas or APSTs are obviously malignant; these are discussed later (see "Differential Di-

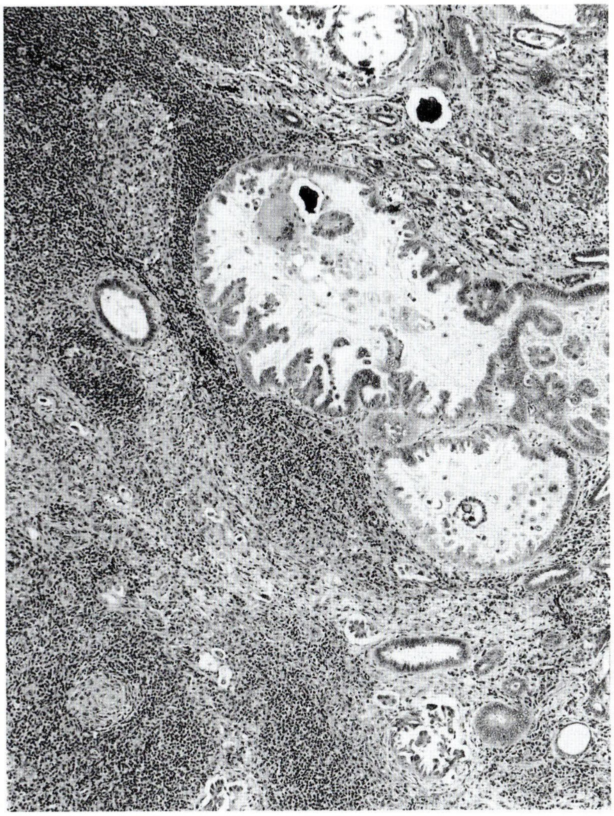

Fig. 18.43. Lymph node "involvement" by atypical proliferative serous tumor. Endosalpingiosis, or benign müllerian glandular inclusions, is closely associated with a papillary proliferation resembling the ovarian APST. (Photograph courtesy of Chris Clark, M.D., Acworth, GA.)

agnosis of Malignant Serous Tumors"). Benign epithelial neoplasms that may display a papillary pattern resembling APST include atypical proliferative müllerian (endocervical-like type) mucinous tumor and atypical proliferative endometrioid tumor. These tumors are discussed in their respective sections.

The distinction of a serous cystadenoma from an APST is not of major importance because both lesions are biologically benign. More importantly, the distinction of an MPSC from an APST separates benign from a malignant neoplasm and is critical. A 5-mm confluent area of micropapillary growth is required for a diagnosis of MPSC (see "Malignant Serous Tumors").

Intraoperative Consultation Ovarian epithelial tumors are often heterogeneous, and carcinomas may have benign-appearing areas resembling a cystadenoma or an APST. It should therefore come as no surprise that approximately 20%–30% of ovarian epithelial tumors diagnosed as atypical proliferative ("borderline") at the time of frozen section examination prove to be carcinomas on further sampling.[339,445] Accordingly, it is important that the surgeon perform a thorough exploration when the frozen section is diagnosed as an APST. Because only 15% of unilateral tumors are associated with extraovarian disease, formal staging is not necessary for a unilateral ovarian tumor unless suspicious peritoneal lesions are found. In contrast, 56% of bilateral tumors are associated with extraovarian disease, and therefore staging in this setting is advisable.[384] Pathologists should be aware that exploration and staging are different procedures. Exploration is a careful and thorough examination of peritoneal surfaces with minimal additional morbidity, whereas staging entails hysterectomy, bilateral salpingo-oophorectomy, omentectomy, peritoneal biopsies, lymph node sampling, and peritoneal washings of the pelvis, paracolic gutters, and hemidiaphragms, with greater attendant morbidity.

Clinical Behavior and Treatment

The disease-specific survival rate of patients with APSTs confined to the ovaries after a mean of approximately 6.7 years, based on more than 2,000 reported cases, exceeds 99.5%.[388] As indicated earlier, survival of 94 reported patients who had tumors that showed "microinvasion" was 100%, and survival of 43 reported patients with "lymph node involvement" was 98%.[388] In six prospective randomized trials including approximately 373 patients with serous borderline tumors followed for a mean of 6.7 years, the survival was 100% (Table 18.7). The behavior of APSTs with extraovarian disease is based on the type of implants that are present. The survival rate of patients with APSTs with noninvasive implants is 95%–100% after a mean follow-up of 7.4 years.[109,387,388] Recurrences and deaths reported in the literature are poorly documented in the majority of cases. When carefully documented, most deaths are either treatment related or are the result of complications from adhesions and bowel obstruction rather than carcinoma.[220] Finally, in a literature review of more than 18,000 borderline tumors, we were unable to identify a single well-documented case of an APST with noninvasive peritoneal implants whose primary ovarian tumor had been adequately sampled to exclude invasion (one section per centimeter of maximum tumor diameter) that had progressed to documented invasive carcinoma[388] (one such case was recently reported[229a]) although it is conceivable that a noninvasive peritoneal implant can undergo malignant transformation on rare occasion. Among 30 cases that reportedly progressed to invasive carcinoma, only one recent case was documented to have

Table 18.6. Lymph node "involvement" by serous "borderline" tumors (SBT) at disease presentation

Series	*No. of patients*	*Node group*	*Last known status*
Ehrmann[108]	2	Paraaortic	NR
Farhi[118]	2	Pelvic	NR
Tavassoli[434]	1	Pelvic	NED, 2.5 years
Bell[31]	1	Paraaortic	LFU
Gershenson[140]	3	Paraaortic	NR
Rice[327]	3	Pelvic or paraaortic	NED, 1.9, 5.8, 10.8 years
Massad[250]	1	Pelvic	NED, 3.75 years
Leake[228]	7[a]	Pelvic and/or paraaortic	NED, 6 patients, mean 4.6 years; 4 recurrences; 1 death due to "bowel obstruction with persistent disease"
Sutton[420]	5[b]	Pelvic/paraaortic	NED, mean 2.7 years
Segal[384]	2	NR	NR
Shiraki[398]	1	Pelvic, paraaortic	NED, 0.5 years
Piura[313]	1	Paraaortic	NED, presumably for mean follow-up of 5.4 years
Goldman[146]	1	Supraclavicular	NED, >3.0 years
Tan[428]	4	Paraaortic	NED, 5 years
		Omental	NED, 9 years
		Iliac	NED, 2 years
		External iliac	NED, 7 years
Di Re[104]	9	5 pelvic, 2 para-aortic, 2 pelvic and paraaortic	NED, mean 8.5 years
Abu-Jawdeh[1]	1	Paraaortic	NR
Kennedy[c 195]	1	NR	NED, 13.3 years
Burks[54]	1[d]	Paraaortic	NR
Seidman[387]	4	Pelvic and/or paraaortic	NED, mean 9.7 years (6.25–13 years)
Sykes[421]	3	Pelvic	NR
Mooney[269]	1	Supraclavicular	NED, 21.75 years
Weir[459]	2	NR	NED, 0.9–6.4 years
Gershenson[141]	2	Pelvic, peripheral	NR
Gershenson[142]	2	Pelvic, peripheral	NR
Rota[343]	3	2 pelvic, 1 pelvic and paraaortic	NED, 6.5, 8.5, 10.9 years
Total	63		43 patients, mean 6.5 years

NR, not reported; LFU, lost to follow-up; NED, no evidence of disease.
[a]One of the seven cases was a seromucinous tumor.
[b]Approximate.
[c]Case also reported in ref. 384; case not repeated in table.
[d]This was an MPSC associated with invasive peritoneal implants.
From Seidman and Kurman,[388] with permission.

been adequately sampled for pathologic examination (Table 18.8).[229a,388]

In general, the noninvasive serous tumors associated with invasive implants are MPSCs, not APSTs. Some experts suggest that this could be equally well explained by thinking of MPSC as the upper end of the spectrum of APST rather than a low-grade carcinoma. Based on a literature review of 467 noninvasive serous tumors that included both invasive and noninvasive implants, the survival rate for patients with in-

Table 18.7. Prospective randomized trials of serous "borderline" tumors (SBT)

Series	No. of SBTs	FIGO stage	No. of deaths	No. of tumor deaths	Mean/median follow-up (years)
Creasman[78]	40[a]	I	0	0	3.0
Barnhill[24]	146	I	0	0	3.5
Young[478]	30[b]	I/II	2	0	>6.0
Trope[442]	114[c]	I/II	0	0	12.25
Klaassen[204]	14[b]	II	0	0	8.0
Sutton[420]	29[d]	III	1	0	2.6
Totals	373		3	0	6.7

[a]The single tumor death in this study occurred in a patient with a 34-cm mucinous tumor, for which 3 slides were examined; the total number of SBTs is corrected due to a typographical error in the published report (H.J. Norris, MD, personal communication, 1999).
[b]Study included borderline tumors of all types: the number of SBTs was estimated to be 59% of all borderline tumors.
[c]Excludes "nonrandomized controls."
[d]Excludes 1 patient with 0.3 months of follow-up.
From Seidman and Kurman,[388] with permission.

vasive implants was 66% after a mean follow-up of 7.4 years, compared to 95% for patients with noninvasive implants (Table 18.9); the difference was highly significant ($p < 0.0001$).[388] The finding of invasive implants in association with an APST is very unusual; this is probably a result of inadequate sampling and reflects foci of occult invasion in the primary tumor.

Malignant Serous Tumors

Micropapillary Serous Carcinoma

In 1979, Russell described a noninvasive serous tumor with morphology that closely approached the degree of proliferation displayed by low-grade carcinomas, but lacked invasion, and therefore fulfilled the WHO

Table 18.8. Serous "borderline" tumors with noninvasive implants reportedly progressing to invasive carcinoma

Series	No. of patients	Time to progression	Last known status
Michael[258]	1[b]	7 years	AWD, 11 years
Bell[a 32]	2[b]	7 years	AWD, 11.8 years
		7.5 years	DOD, 9.5 years, with lung metastases
Demirel[99]	1[b]	2 years	NED, 6 years
Kennedy[195]	1[b]	4.75 years	DOD, 8.6 years
Seidman[387]	2[c]	2.8 years	DOD, 3.5 years
		5.5 years	AWD, 8.25 years
Burks[54]	1[b]	2.8 years	AWD, 11.7 years
Sykes[421]	3[b]	3.5, 5, 14 years	DOD, 2 patients
			AWD, 1 patient, 8.5 years
Weir[459]	2[d]	2.3 years	NED, 3.9 years
		2.8 years	AWD, 3.3 years
Gershenson[142]	14[b]	7.1 years (median)	DOD, 6 patients
Lee[229a]	3[e]	4, 6, and 9 years	NED, 8 years
			AWD, DOD, 8 years and 10 years

AWD, alive with disease; DOD, dead of disease; NED, no evidence of disease.
[a]Primary peritoneal tumors.
[b]Adequate sampling not documented.
[c]Both cases documented to have been inadequately sampled.
[d]One case documented to have been inadequately sampled.
[e]One case was adequately sampled.
Modified from Seidman and Kurman,[388] with permission.

Table 18.9. Mortality in advanced-stage serous "borderline" tumors (SBT): invasive versus noninvasive implants

First author	*Total stage II and III patients*	*Noninvasive implants deaths/ total*	*Invasive implants deaths/ total*	*Follow-up, mean or median months (Range)*
Russell[352a]	12	1/6	3/6	101 (24–264)
McCaughey[253]	21	2/15	4/6	39 (12–84)
Friedlander[126a]	10	0/6	1/4	36 (7–84)
Kliman[207]	10	1/8	0/2	66 (32–120)
Michael[258]	12	0/5	1/7	88 (12–180)
Bell[35]	56	3/50	5[a]/6	72 (NR)
Bell[32]	28[b]	1/28	0/0	96 (12–167)
Snider[403a]	3	0/2	0/1	47 (12–87)
De Nictolis[100a]	19	0/10	4/9	64 (12–168)
Casey[63]	4	0/3	1/1	108 (45–185)
Tan[428]	5	0/4	0/1	76 (24–132)
Di Re[104]	7	0/7	0/0	72 (18–213)
Kennedy[195]	26	1/25	0/1	102 (23–204)
Demirel[99]	11	0/11	0/0	79 (24–156)
Burks[54]	7	0/3	2/4	70 (38–140)
Seidman[387]	65	1/52	6/13	100 (17–171)
Darai[87a]	2	0/2	0/0	44 (12–96)
Kuoppala[216]	2	0/2	0/0	139 (NR)
Sykes[421]	15[c]	1/13	0/2	54 (12–160)
Weir[459]	14[b]	0/14	0/0	37 (8–88)
Gershenson[141,142]	112[d]	6/73	6/39	119 (NR)
Eichorn[109]	26	0/24	2/2	93 (6–222)
Totals	467	17/363 (4.7%)	35/104 (34%)	Mean, 89 months $p < 0.0001$

Mortality for invasive versus noninvasive implants: $p < 0.0001$.
When possible, the following cases were excluded: patients with less than 1 year of uneventful follow-up; patients with unknown types of implants; patients without implants (ie, advanced stage cases based on positive nodes); nontumor deaths are censored.
NR, not reported.
[a]Four deaths were originally reported[35] and 1 additional death was reported later.[109]
[b]Primary peritoneal SBTs.
[c]Excluding cases previously reported.[207]
[d]Combined data from two studies[141,142] which included data from one earlier study.[140]
From Seidman and Kurman,[388] with permission.

criteria for serous borderline tumor. He designated these tumors as "grade IV proliferating serous tumors" and reported that they were more prone to be associated with peritoneal implants and that the degree of proliferation in the implants was similar to that of the primary ovarian tumor.[354,356] This pattern was also recognized by others around the same time,[191] but despite numerous studies of ovarian borderline tumors or tumors of low malignant potential in the ensuing two decades,[388] very few data on this variant were published until 1996, when two series appeared,[54,387] followed by a third in 1999.[109] At this time, some investigators observed that these tumors, despite no apparent evidence of invasion, behaved like low-grade carcinomas in contrast to the other tumors in this group, and therefore proposed that they be designated *micropapillary serous carcinomas*[54,387] or serous borderline tumors with a micropapillary pattern.[109]

Because the published data on MPSC are limited to only a few large studies, many of the data describing the clinical presentation, behavior, and treatment of this tumor are preliminary. MPSCs that do not display destructive infiltrative growth are considered "noninvasive" for purposes of this discussion, although it is conceivable that the complex exophytic micropapillary pattern may be a form of invasion. This distinction may be of academic interest only because the neoplastic cells on the surface of the ovarian tumor have direct access to the peritoneal cavity and may exfoliate and implant on peritoneal surfaces, thus ac-

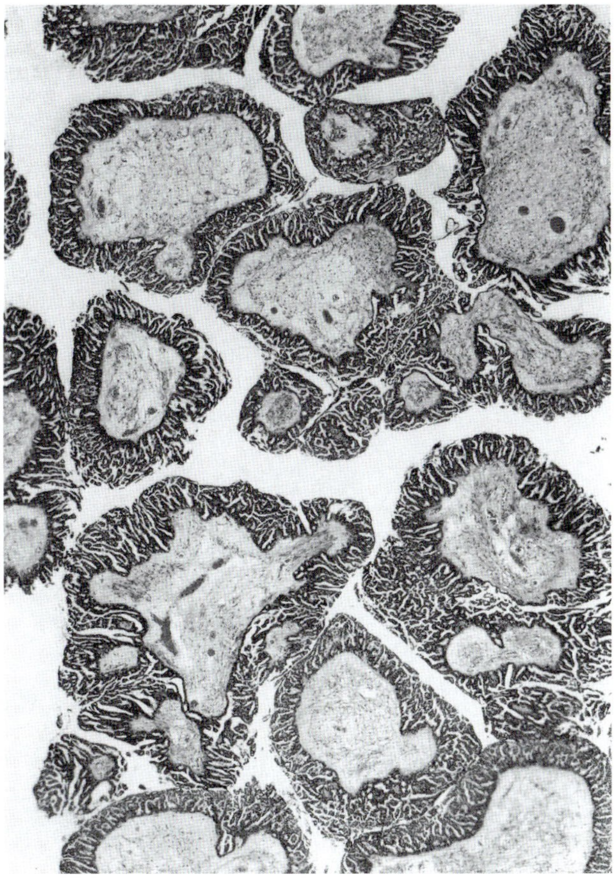

Fig. 18.44. Micropapillary serous carcinoma, noninvasive type. The "medusa" pattern characterized by an extensive proliferation of thin elongated micropapillae arising from thick centrally located papillae, with extensive fusion and confluence of the micropapillae. Invasion into the underlying stromal cores is not present.

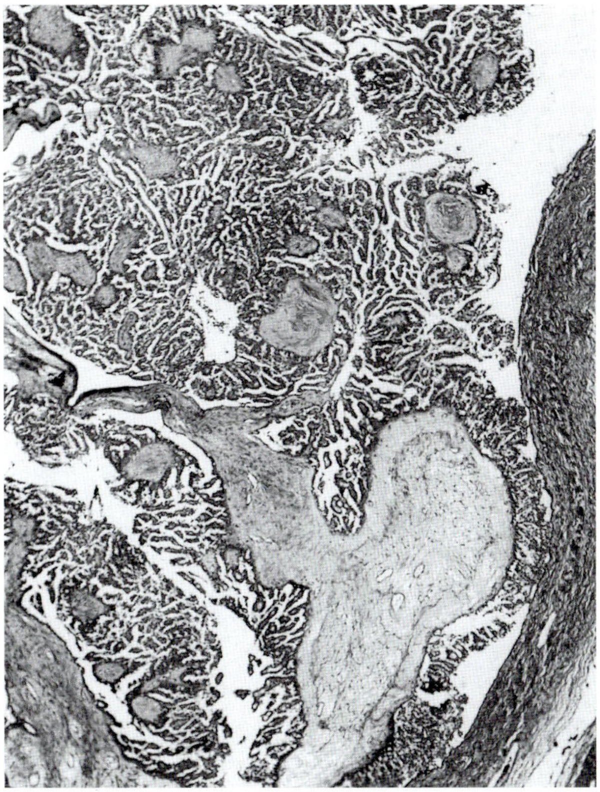

Fig. 18.45. Micropapillary serous carcinoma, noninvasive type. Marked proliferation of micropapillae creates a filigree pattern.

counting for the strong association of this pattern with so-called invasive implants (metastatic carcinoma). When areas of obvious stromal invasion exceeding the criteria for microinvasion (see earlier) are present, the neoplasm is interpreted as the invasive form of MPSC.

Clinical Findings The mean age of patients with the noninvasive form of MPSC is 43 years. The most common presentation is an asymptomatic pelvic mass, but abdominal pain, fullness, or distension are common symptoms in advanced-stage cases.

Operative Findings Sixty-four percent of tumors are bilateral. Forty-five percent of patients are stage I, 18.1 are stage II, and 37.1 are stage III.[54,109,146a]

Gross Findings The mean tumor size is 8.5 cm. Surface involvement is present in 54% of cases. As these tumors are very well differentiated, they tend to have a more papillary and cystic gross appearance resembling APSTs, and little if any necrosis, in contrast to many typical serous carcinomas that often have solid areas and extensive necrosis.

Microscopic Findings Noninvasive MPSC is a proliferating serous neoplasm that displays a high degree of epithelial proliferation and complexity but is morphologically intraepithelial because diagnostic features of invasion are not present; perhaps it is an in situ carcinoma. Some experts believe that the association with invasive carcinoma and high mortality rate warrant classification of this variant as a well-differentiated papillary serous carcinoma, thus the designation MPSC. In either case, this variant displays a characteristic pattern of papillary branching (Figs. 18.44–18.47). The distal papillary branches are thin and delicate with minimal fibrovascular support, and emanate abruptly from thick, more centrally located papillae without intervening branches of successive intermediate sizes, unlike the hierarchical branching pattern of APSTs. The papillae often fuse to form a cribriform pattern or a roman bridgelike pattern on the surfaces of the

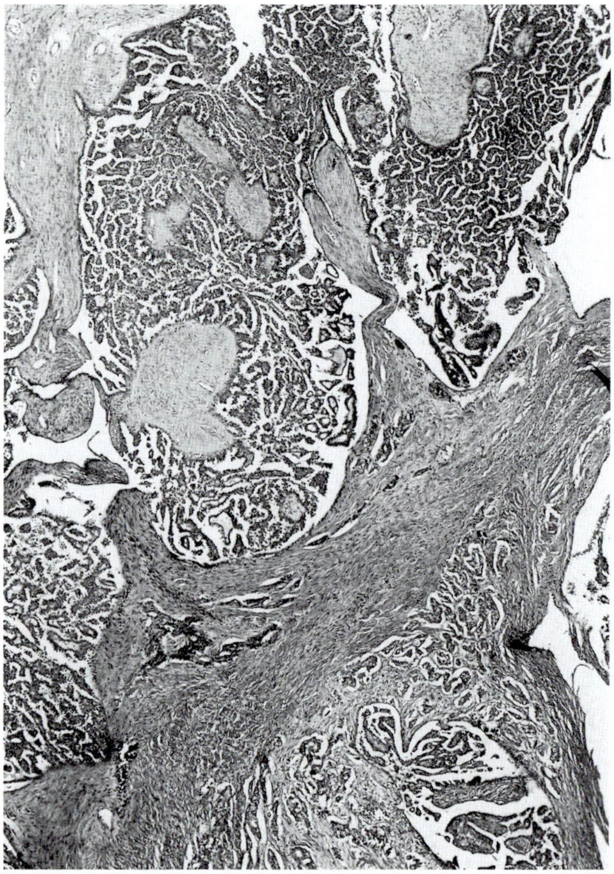

Fig. 18.46. Micropapillary serous carcinoma, invasive type. Noninvasive micropapillary pattern is present at *upper left*, and stromal invasion characterized by micropapillae infiltrating the stroma in a haphazard pattern is present at *lower right.*

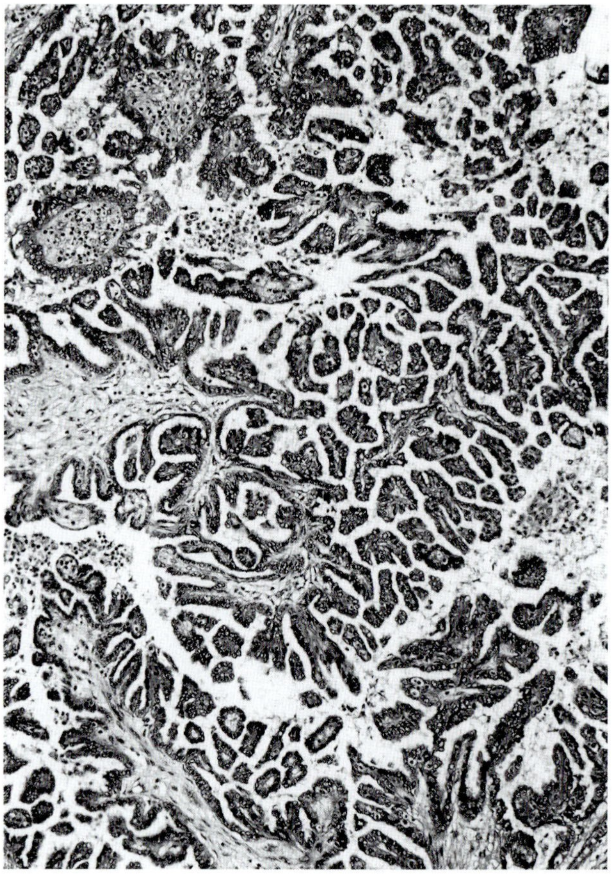

Fig. 18.47. Micropapillary serous carcinoma, noninvasive type. Although micropapillary serous carcinomas typically display very little if any fibrovascular stromal support within the distal papillae, in this case stromal support is conspicuous.

large papillae (Fig. 18.48). Because micropapillary and cribriform areas may be focally present in APSTs, an area 5 mm in diameter of a confluent micropapillary pattern is required for the designation of MPSC; anything less than this, in the absence of other features of invasion, should be classified as an APST (Fig. 18.49). Extensive sampling of the ovarian tumor may be necessary to resolve difficult cases. MPSC displays no apparent invasion of the stromal cores of the papillae. Invasion occurring in MPSC is recognized by a haphazard infiltrative growth composed of solid nests or complex glandlike structures displaying micropapillae or a confluent pattern. The nests, glands, and glandlike structures are often surrounded by a clear space or cleft. Psammoma bodies may be numerous in either the MPSC or invasive areas.

MPSCs with or without invasion display similar cytologic features. Cells tend to be rounded with scant cytoplasm, and there is mild or moderate nuclear atypia, often with prominent small nucleoli (Figs. 18.50 and 18.51). It should be noted that these cytologic features differ from APST. The cells in the latter tend to be columnar, are often ciliated, and have less nuclear atypia. Mitotic activity tends to be low. Severe nuclear atypia warrants a designation of a conventional serous carcinoma, even in the absence of overt invasion (Fig. 18.52). This latter pattern is very uncommon; when this pattern is present, further sampling of the tumor generally reveals obvious invasion.

The peritoneal implants associated with MPSC are frequently invasive (i.e., carcinoma). Among 44 reported cases of advanced-stage noninvasive MPSC, 24 (55%) of the implants were invasive[54,109,146a,387] in comparison to 6% of the implants associated with APSTs.[387]

Immunohistochemistry There are few published data on the immunohistochemistry of MPSC. These tumors should be positive for EMA and cytokeratin 7, as are the other serous ovarian epithelial neoplasms.

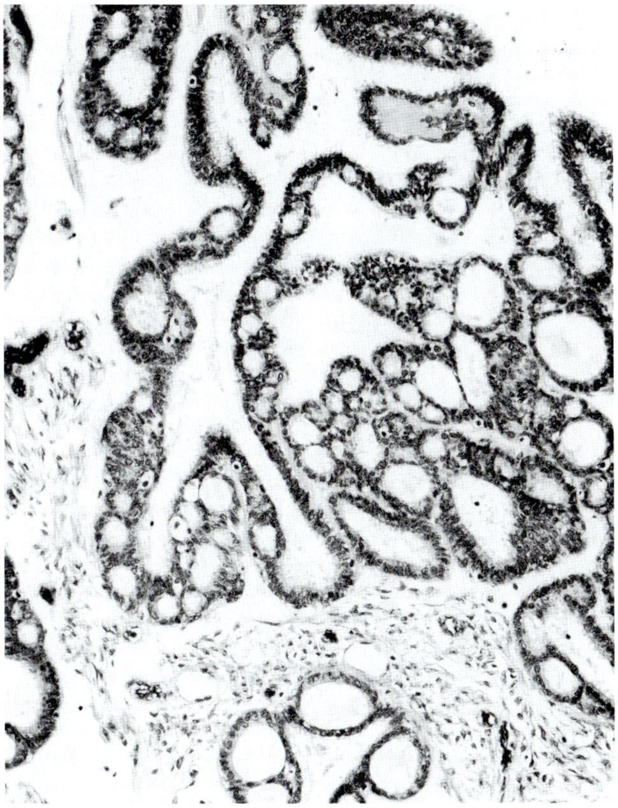

Fig. 18.48. Micropapillary serous carcinoma, noninvasive type. A surface cribriform pattern created by fusion of micropapillae is present on the surface of the larger papillae.

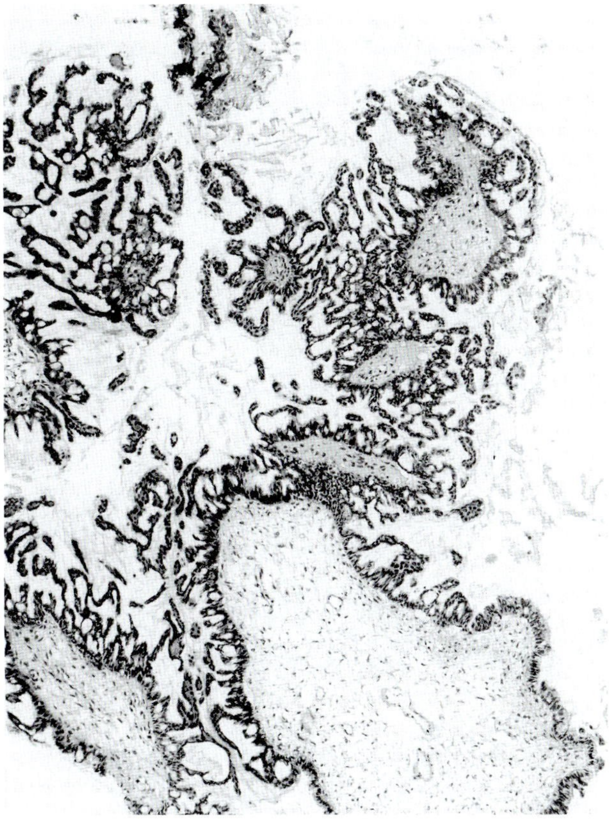

Fig. 18.49. Micropapillary serous carcinoma, noninvasive type. The micropapillary pattern is present at *upper left.* Most of the tumor had an APST pattern, part of which appears at *lower right.* These patterns are commonly intermixed. The tumor had greater than 5 mm of confluent micropapillary architecture and therefore qualified for the diagnosis of micropapillary serous carcinoma.

Differential Diagnosis A 5-mm-diameter area of confluent micropapillary architecture distinguishes this tumor from APSTs, which often have scattered small foci of a micropapillary pattern. High-grade malignant nuclear features, even in the presence of the typical micropapillary patterns, warrant a diagnosis of ordinary papillary serous carcinoma. The distinguishing morphologic features of serous neoplasms, including the invasive and noninvasive variants of MPSC, are shown in Table 18.10.

Clinical Behavior and Treatment Despite the apparent absence of destructive infiltrative growth in the noninvasive variant of MPSC, the limited available data indicate that it behaves as a low-grade serous carcinoma. Stage I MPSC appear to be cured by adnexectomy alone, although only a small number of stage I tumors have been reported. Based on relatively limited data from three studies, the 5- and 10-year survival rates for patients with advanced-stage MPSC are approximately 84% and 58%, respectively.[54,109,387] Documented recurrences of invasive carcinoma have been reported in 35.1% of advanced-stage MPSCs. One invasive recurrence from an inadequately sampled primary ovarian MPSC that was reportedly stage I (but for which slides of the omentum were not reviewed by the authors) has been reported.[109] Insufficient data are available on the invasive variant of MPSC to comment on their behavior.

Psammocarcinoma

Psammocarcinoma is a very rare variant of serous neoplasm that appears to arise as often in the peritoneum as in the ovaries.[144,459] Psammocarcinoma has been defined by some investigators as a serous neoplasm displaying (1) destructive invasion, (2) no more than moderate nuclear atypia, (3) no areas of solid epithelial proliferation except for occasional nests no more than 15 cells in diameter, and (4) at least 75% of papillae or nests associated with or completely replaced by psammoma bodies.[144] We

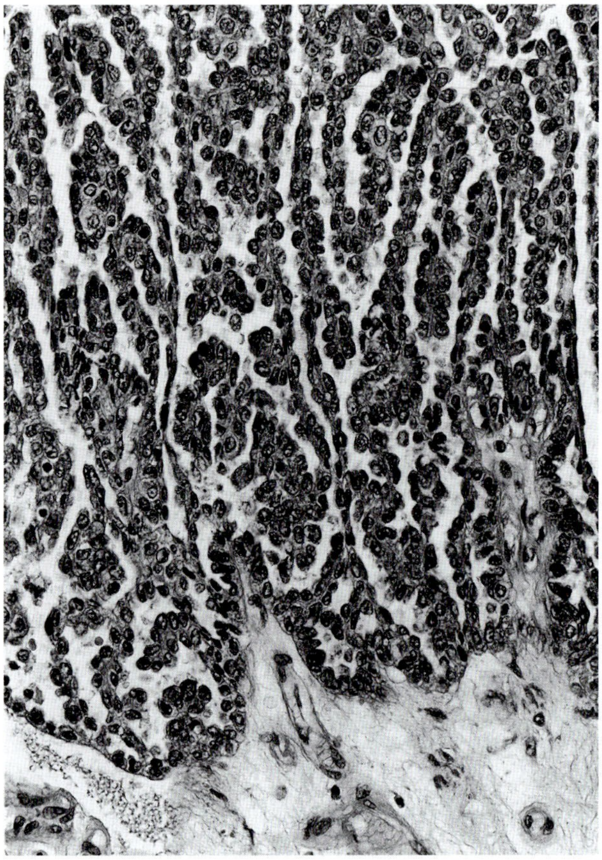

Fig. 18.50. Micropapillary serous carcinoma, noninvasive type. In contrast to APSTs, cells are rounded instead of columnar and have a higher nuclear:cytoplasmic ratio. Nuclear atypia is minimal but greater than that in APSTs. Small but prominent nucleoli are present.

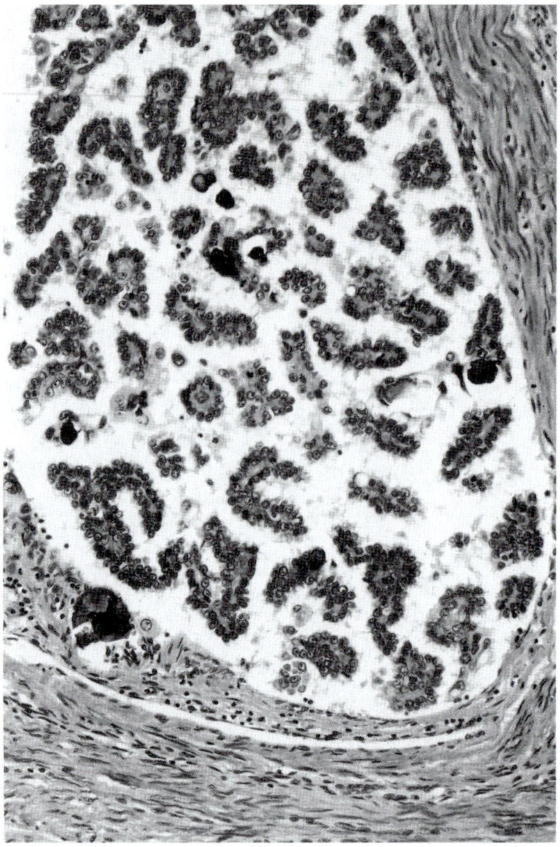

Fig. 18.51. Micropapillary serous carcinoma in a vascular/lymphatic space in the myometrium. The ovarian tumor showed no evidence of invasion. It is conceivable that malignant cells exfoliate into the peritoneal cavity and gain access to lymphatic channels.

believe that this definition describes a group of lesions with limited malignant potential, as they lack a significant proliferative epithelial component. Based on this definition, a review of 18 reported cases indicates that the mean mitotic rate is 1 mitotic figure (MF) per 10 high-power fields (HPF), and although all tumors were stage III at presentation, there has been only 1 death, yielding a survival rate of 94%. If the diagnosis is used at all, we recommend that it be applied to tumors that have a clear-cut epithelial component that predominates over the presence of abundant psammoma bodies.

In the reports describing psammocarcinoma as defined by at least 75% of papillae or nests replaced by psammoma bodies and lack of solid epithelial proliferation, the mean age of 8 reported patients with ovarian psammocarcinoma was 59 and that of 10 peritoneal psammocarcinomas was 50 years. The most common presenting symptoms and signs for ovarian tumors included abdominal or pelvic pain and pelvic mass and, for peritoneal tumors, a pelvic mass. All 8 ovarian psammocarcinomas have involved the peritoneum; the bowel wall and myometrium are sometimes involved, and 1 case had positive lymph nodes. All have been FIGO stage III. Peritoneal psammocarcinomas have invaded the myometrium from the serosal surface in 3 of 10 cases and may also involve omentum, fallopian tubes, and broad ligament.

The mean size of ovarian psammocarcinoma is 11 cm. They may be solid, cystic, or mixed. Peritoneal psammocarcinoma may occur as a dominant extraovarian mass 4–19 cm in diameter or as multiple small nodules ranging from several millimeters to 2.5 cm. The characteristic low-power appearance is dominated by a myriad of psammoma bodies, which may fuse with one another, with a sparse epithelial component (Fig. 18.53). The psammoma bodies are usually surrounded by a single layer of low columnar epithelium that displays mild or moderate atypia and rare mitotic figures. Peritoneal tumor deposits may appear noninvasive or invasive.

a

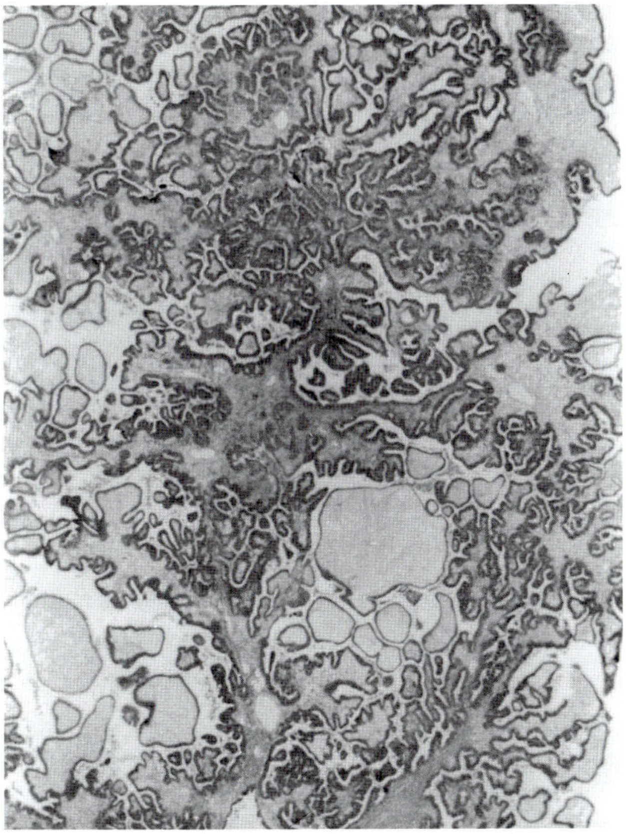

b

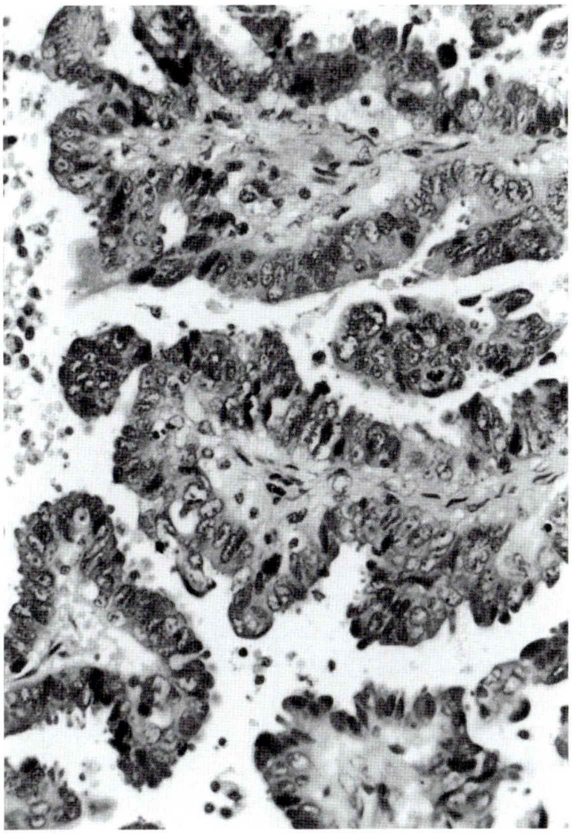

Fig. 18.52. Noninvasive serous carcinoma. a: A papillary serous neoplasm with no obvious evidence of invasion. **b**: Although by WHO criteria this tumor qualifies as "borderline" because it lacks stromal invasion, we diagnose these tumors as "carcinoma" in view of the high-grade nuclear atypia and abundant mitotic activity.

Among all patients with follow-up reported in the two series, including both ovarian and peritoneal primary tumors, there have been three recurrences and one tumor death.

Serous Carcinoma

Clinical Findings *Serous carcinoma* is the most common type of ovarian cancer and accounts for approximately 50% of malignant ovarian neoplasms. The peak age group is 45–65 years and the mean age is 57 years. Inasmuch as 70%–84% of patients present in advanced stage (FIGO stage II or higher) with tumor disseminated throughout the abdominal and pelvic cavities,[299,305] common presenting symptoms are abdominal pain and distension caused by ascites or bulky abdominal tumor. Gastrointestinal symptoms are also common. Other symptoms may include urinary frequency, dysuria, and vaginal bleeding. Stage I tumors usually present as an asymptomatic mass on a routine pelvic examination.[297]

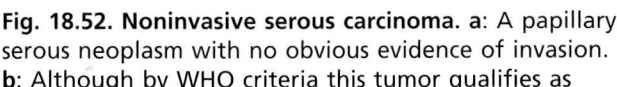

Table 18.10. Distinguishing morphologic features of serous ovarian neoplasms

Diagnosis	*Atypia*	*Stratification and detachment*	*Micropapillary pattern*	*Stromal invasion*
Serous cystadenoma	Absent, or present in <10%	Absent, or present in <10%	Absent	Absent
APST	Present in >10%	Present in >10%	May be present, <5 mm of confluence	Absent
MPSC, noninvasive	Present	Usually present	Present, >5 mm of confluence	Absent
MPSC, invasive	Present	Usually present	Present	Present
Serous carcinoma	Present	May be present	May be present	Present

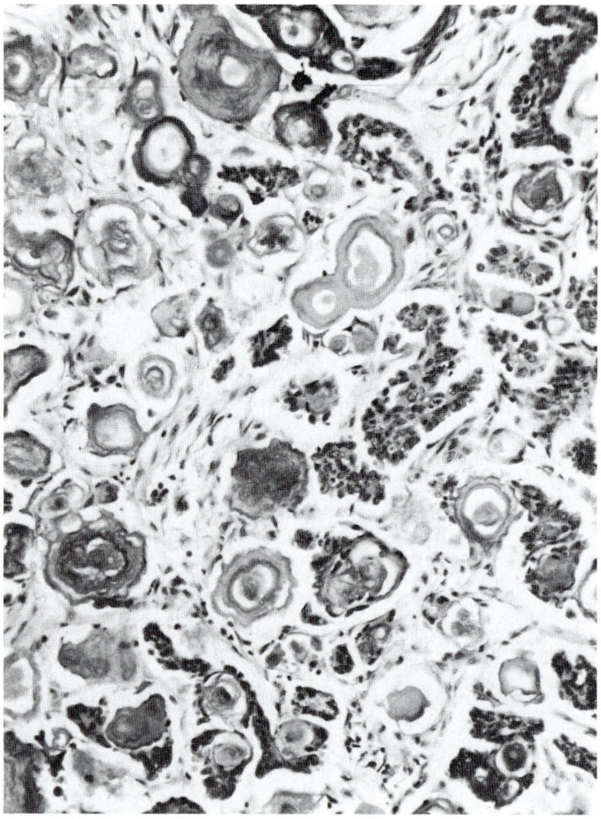

Fig. 18.53. Psammocarcinoma. Psammoma bodies are prominent in this variant of well-differentiated papillary serous carcinoma.

Serum levels of CA-125 are elevated in about 90% of patients. Serum levels of inhibin are elevated in 18% of postmenopausal patients and fall after tumor removal.[162] Neither CA-125 nor inhibin is sufficiently specific for population-based screening.

Operative Findings Two-thirds of cases involve both ovaries. For stage I cases, about 40% are bilateral. Nearly all advanced-stage ovarian carcinomas spread along peritoneal surfaces, including the pelvic peritoneum (stage II), the surfaces of the bowel, and other abdominal organs (stage III). Both pelvic and abdominal spread can be by direct extension or metastasis. For example, direct extension to the rectosigmoid, broad ligament, or uterus can occur by contiguous growth, or exfoliation of malignant cells can result in seeding of the peritoneal surfaces of the bowel or pelvic peritoneum. Tumor rupture preoperatively or intraoperatively may occur and warrants assignment of a stage I or II tumor to stage IC or IIC, respectively. Assessment of the character of the external surface is an important component of staging for tumors that are confined to the ovaries; this is best done by the surgeon but should also be evaluated by the pathologist. Grossly exophytic papillary tumor on the surface of an ovarian neoplasm that is confined to the ovaries warrants a stage of IC. Intracystic neoplasms without gross or microscopic tumor on the external surfaces do not qualify for surface involvement unless tumor cells invade through the full thickness of the cyst wall and are thus exposed to the peritoneal cavity. Dense adhesions to pelvic structures or bowel are reassigned to FIGO stage II or III (see earlier, "Stage").

Patients with stage III disease usually have omental involvement which, in advanced cases, is manifested by a solid tumorous mass ("omental cake"). Pelvic and paraaortic lymph node metastases are found frequently, with a direct relationship to the extent of disease. Rarely, inguinal lymph nodes contain metastatic tumor. Patients with tumors that appear to be stage I have lymph node metastases in 4%–14% of cases; the corresponding figures for stages II, III, and IV are 36%, 41%–68%, and 88%, respectively. Liver metastases usually manifest as studding of the peritoneal surface of the liver. Parenchymal liver metastases are rarely present, and very rarely, splenic metastases are found, necessitating splenectomy.

In 8%–12.5% of women with advanced-stage papillary serous carcinoma, the ovaries are small and display predominantly surface involvement.[351,355] These findings warrant a diagnosis of primary peritoneal serous carcinoma (see "Differential Diagnosis"; and Chapter 17, Diseases of the Peritoneum). On very rare occasions, typical serous carcinomas arise in extraperitoneal loca-

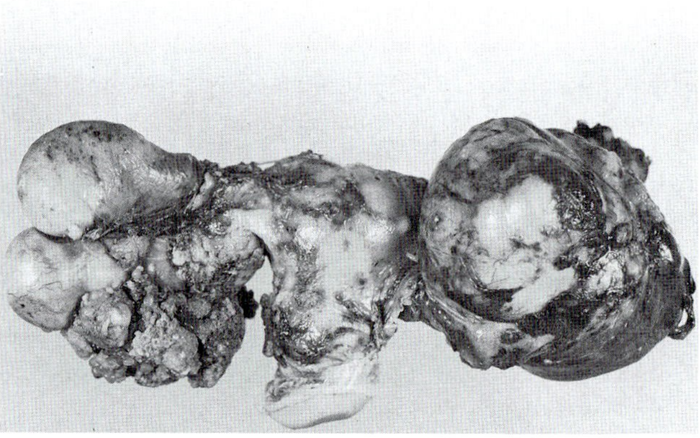

Fig. 18.54. Serous carcinoma. Bilateral ovaries are involved by papillary serous carcinoma. A surface papillary component is present on the inferior aspect of the right ovarian tumor (*left side* of photo).

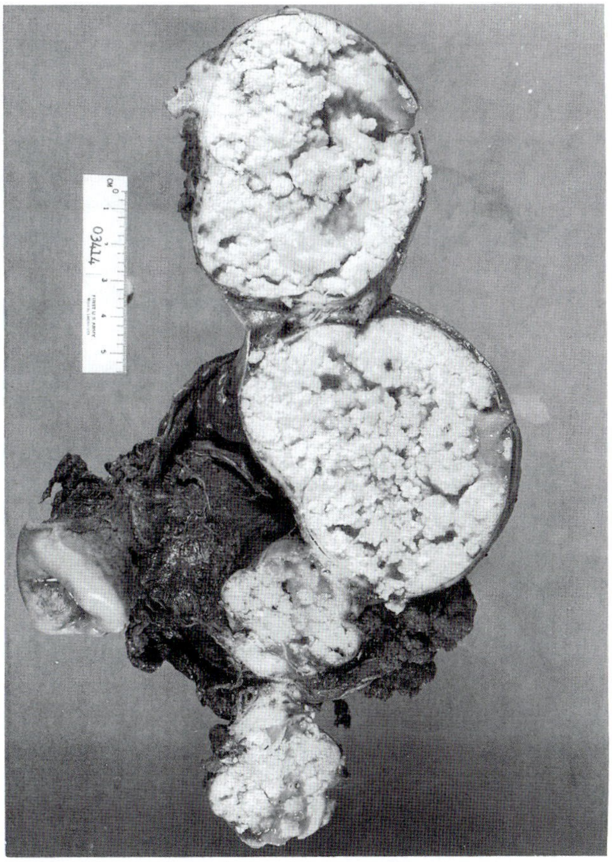

Fig. 18.55. Serous carcinoma. Cut section of a cystic tumor shows intracystic papillations.

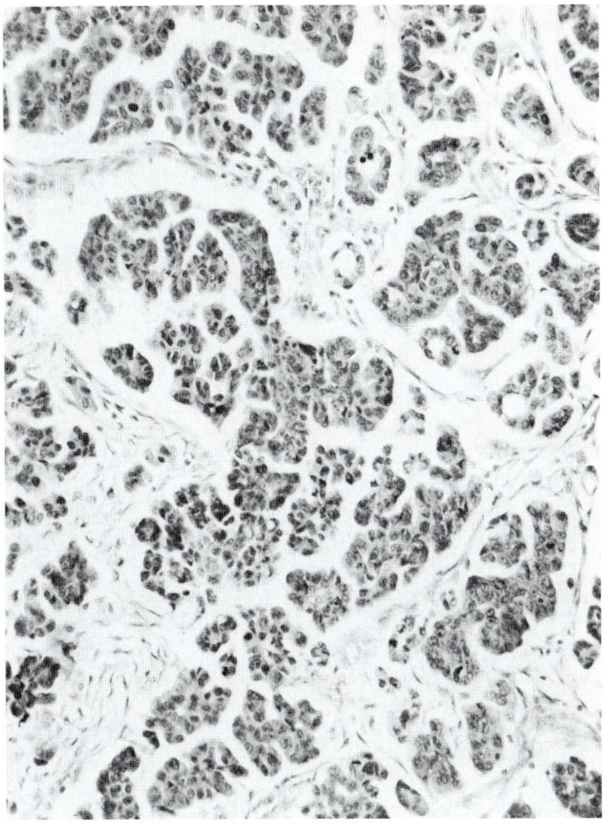

Fig. 18.56. Serous carcinoma. Complex invasive papillary pattern. The cells display grade 1 nuclear atypia. This tumor qualifies as an invasive micropapillary serous carcinoma.

tions including pelvic or retroperitoneal lymph nodes, within the leaves of the broad ligament, in the retroperitoneum, or in the endocervix. More commonly, serous carcinomas arise in the endometrium (see Chapter 12, Endometrial Carcinoma).

Gross Findings Serous carcinomas range from microscopic to about 20 cm in diameter. They are typically multilocular and cystic, with soft, friable papillae, filling the cyst cavities and containing serous, turbid, or bloody fluid. The external surfaces may be smooth or bosselated and sometimes display surface papillae (Figs. 18.54 and 18.55). Tumors are often solid, pink to gray with less obvious papillae, and may be soft or firm depending on the character of the tumor stroma. Hemorrhage and necrosis are often present. Omental metastases are characterized by firm nodules of variable size with white or gray cut surfaces, which may coalesce into an omental cake. Grossly normal omenta are found to contain microscopic tumor in 22% of cases.[412]

Microscopic Findings Well-differentiated serous carcinomas are discussed under "MPSC." Typical serous carcinomas display complex papillary (Fig. 18.56) and solid patterns and marked nuclear atypia. A frequently encountered and quite characteristic pattern is a lacelike or labyrinthine pattern (Figs. 18.57 and 18.58). This pattern may be focal but often predominates, and is characterized by extensive bridging and coalescence of papillae resulting in slitlike spaces between the papillae. Areas of solid growth are common (Fig. 18.59). Other patterns include retiform arrangements of slitlike spaces and glandular patterns. An uncommon pattern that is occasionally seen in well-differentiated serous carcinomas is characterized by broad papillae invading the stroma in lymphatic-like spaces (Fig. 18.60). A glandular pattern is not necessarily diagnostic of endometrioid differentiation, and the distinction of a high-grade endometrioid carcinoma from a serous carcinoma may be difficult. Secretory change can occur but, as the cell shape is usually not altered by this process, should not be confused with secretory endometrioid or clear cell carcinoma. Intracytoplasmic mucinous inclusions may be present.[289] The cells

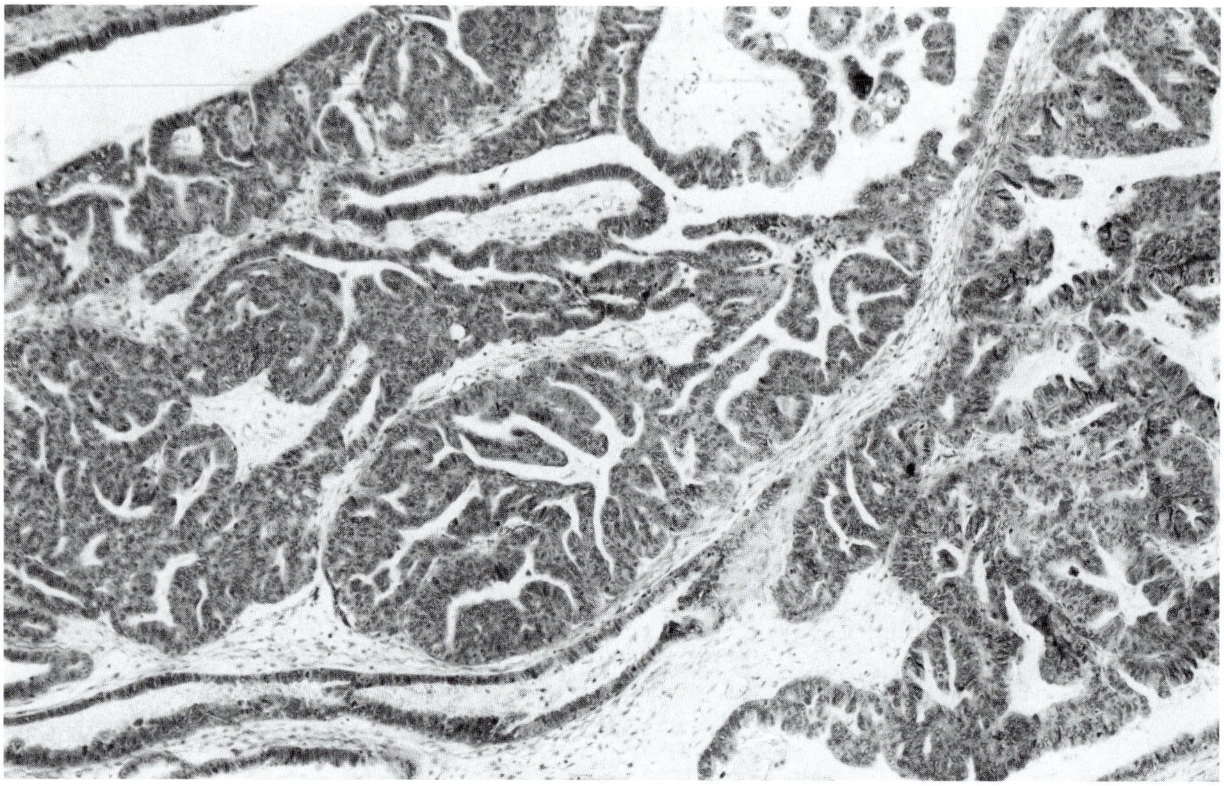

Fig. 18.57. Serous carcinoma. Lacelike pattern.

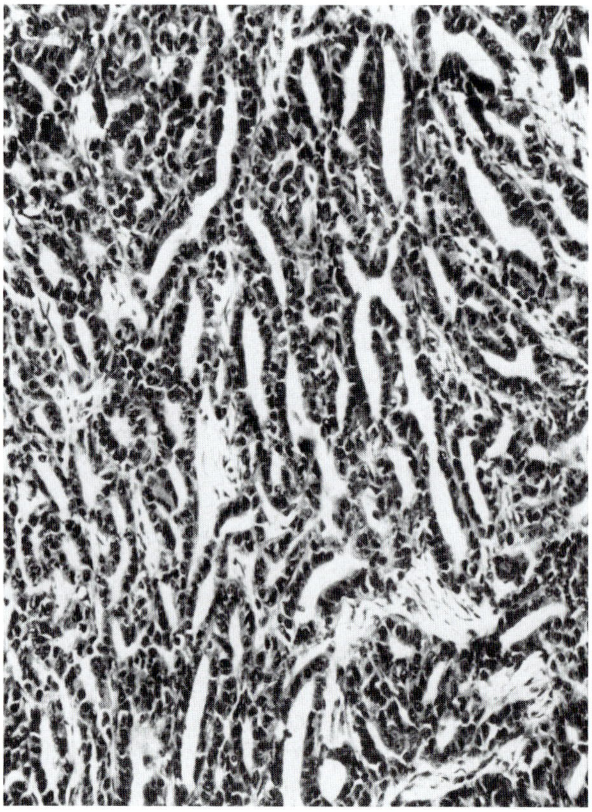

Fig. 18.58. Serous carcinoma. A labyrinthine, slitlike glandular pattern.

may be small and uniform with grade 2 nuclear atypia but more often are large, pleomorphic, and display obviously malignant cytologic features (Fig. 18.61).

Serous carcinomas that display extensive solid areas are usually composed of uniform sheets of cells with high-grade nuclear atypia and may display isolated bizarre mononuclear giant cells or syncytial-like aggregates. Signet ring cells may rarely be present.[68a] Mitoses, including abnormal mitoses, are usually numerous and necrosis is often pronounced. Areas with grade 2 nuclei often merge with areas of grade 3 nuclei. Nuclear grade is subjective and not very reproducible; we therefore designate these tumors as "high grade." Usually there are focal areas with papillary architecture that permit the diagnosis of a serous carcinoma as opposed to an undifferentiated carcinoma. Psammoma bodies are present in 25% of cases. A completely solid carcinoma without any evidence of glands or papillae warrants a designation of undifferentiated carcinoma (see "Undifferentiated Carcinoma").

Microscopic tumors, so-called early de novo ovarian carcinoma, are usually unilateral and may be multifocal. In one series, they measured up to 7 mm in diameter.[33] Early de novo ovarian carcinoma involves the ovarian surface or superficial cortex; these are usually high-grade serous carcinomas (Fig. 18.62).

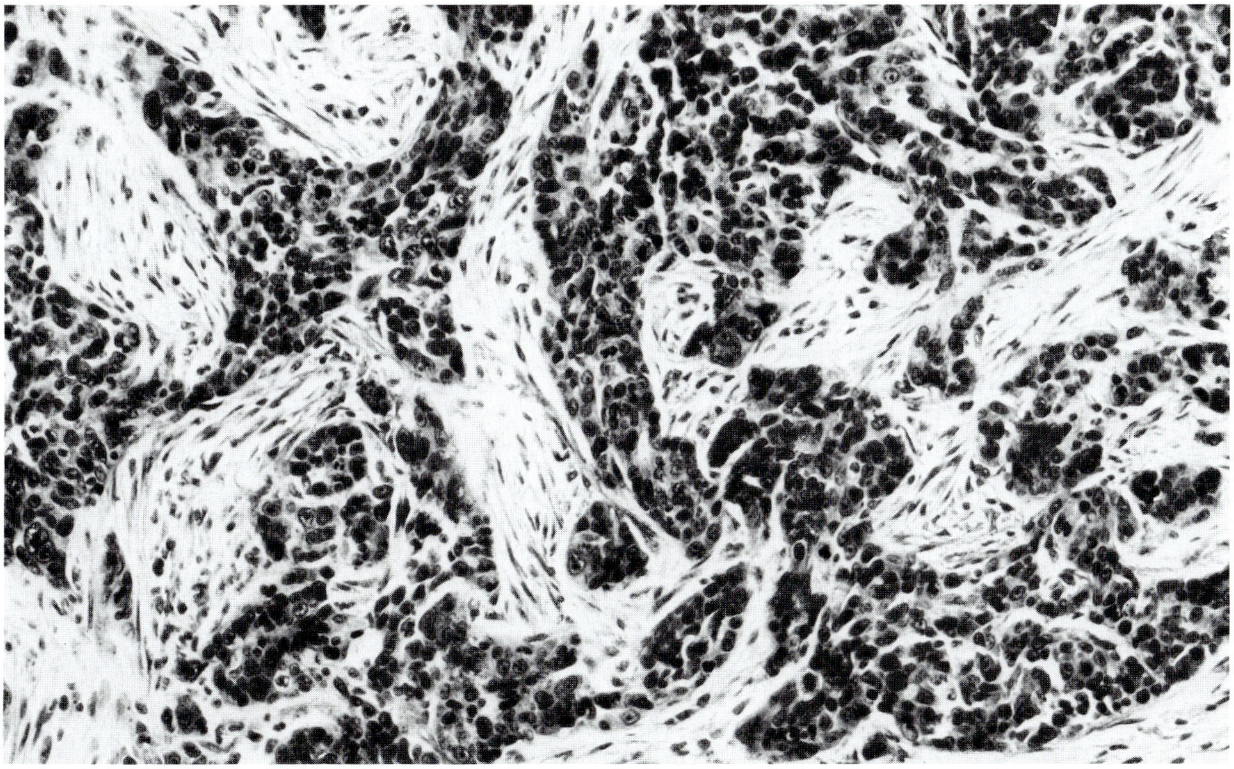

Fig. 18.59. Serous carcinoma. Solid pattern with sheets of small to moderate-size cells with scanty cytoplasm and a high nuclear:cytoplasmic ratio.

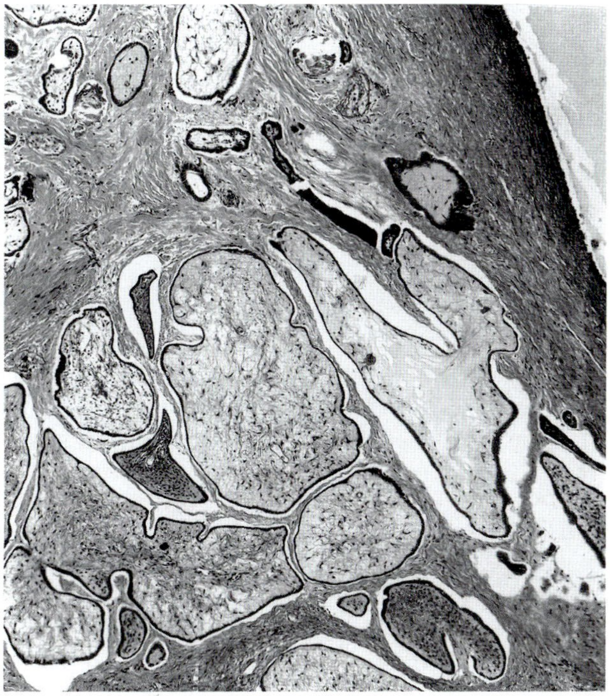

Fig. 18.60. Serous carcinoma. An uncommon pattern of invasion in well-differentiated serous carcinomas is characterized by broad papillae invading the stroma. It is not clear whether the spaces surrounding the papillae represent retraction artifact, destruction of tissue by enzymes secreted from the tumor, or lymphatic channels.

Immunohistochemistry Serous carcinomas have been extensively evaluated by immunohistochemistry.* Based on a compilation of data from these studies, the following immunoprofile for serous carcinoma emerges (proportion of tumors showing positive staining): epithelial membrane antigen (EMA), 100%; CAM 5.2, 100%; cytokeratin 7, 100%; cytokeratin 20, 34%; vimentin, 45%; B72.3 (antibody to tumor-associated glycoprotein 72), 92%; carcinoembryonic antigen (CEA), 19%; OC-125, 91%; gross cystic disease fluid protein-15 (GCDFP-15), 2%, S-100, 30%. The CK7/20 panel shows CK 7+/CK 20− in the majority of serous and endometrioid ovarian carcinomas; the remainder are CK 7+/CK 20+.[40,236,273,452] Inhibin, a valuable marker of sex cord–stromal tumors, is rarely positive in serous carcinomas (see Chapter 19). Occasional serous carcinomas are positive for thyroglobulin.[193]

Differential Diagnosis When faced with a neoplasm in the ovary, particularly when bilateral, the pathologist should always consider the possibility of metastatic tumor to the ovary. Although metastatic carcinomas to the ovary most often mimic mucinous or endometrioid ovarian carcinomas, metastases may display a wide variety of patterns (see Chapter 22, Metastatic Tumors of the Ovary).

---

*40,46,85,157,183,193,198,210,223,236,266,268,273,280, 293,391,437,452,456,468.

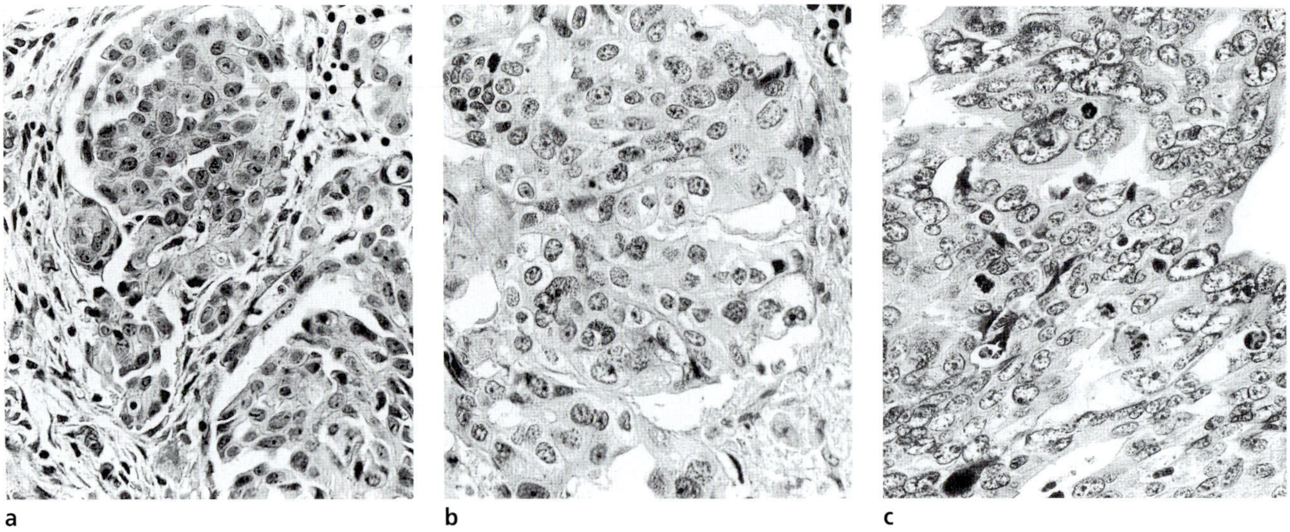

Fig. 18.61. **Serous carcinoma.** a: Grade 1 cytologic atypia shows relatively small cells with a uniform nuclear chromatin distribution, prominent small nucleoli, and abundant cytoplasm. **b**: Grade 2 cytologic atypia shows larger nuclei compared to grade 1, with a greater degree of chromatin clumping. **c**: Grade 3 cytologic atypia shows marked cellular and nuclear enlargement, marked nuclear pleomorphism, and occasional bizarre nuclear forms. There is a high nuclear:cytoplasmic ratio and scattered enlarged nucleoli.

Serous carcinomas may invade the fallopian tubes, and on occasion, the distinction of an ovarian from a primary tubal carcinoma may be difficult (see Chapter 22, Metastatic Tumors of the Ovary). Meticulous dissection of the fallopian tube, which is nearly always dilated and filled with tumor when primary, can be of value. Microscopically, the presence of carcinoma in situ in uninvolved tubal epithelium is also helpful.

Approximately 8%–12.5% of patients with apparent advanced-stage serous carcinoma have normal-sized or slightly enlarged ovaries with only surface involvement; these are classified as primary peritoneal serous carcinomas. The criteria for distinguishing ovarian carcinoma from primary peritoneal carcinoma are arbitrary. From a practical standpoint the distinction is not critical because the behavior and treatment are similar. Nonetheless, the

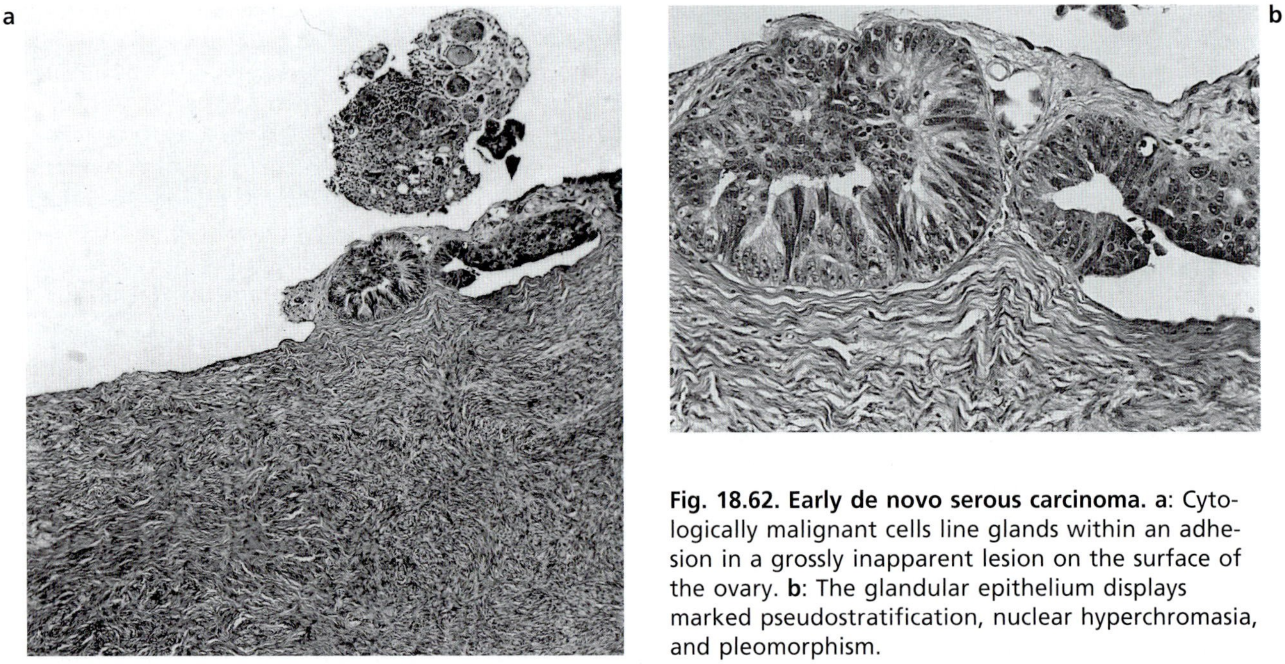

Fig. 18.62. Early de novo serous carcinoma. a: Cytologically malignant cells line glands within an adhesion in a grossly inapparent lesion on the surface of the ovary. **b**: The glandular epithelium displays marked pseudostratification, nuclear hyperchromasia, and pleomorphism.

following criteria for this distinction have been proposed by the Gynecologic Onocology Group (GOG): (1) both ovaries must be either physiologically normal in size or enlarged by a benign process; (2) the involvement in the extraovarian sites must be greater than the involvement on the surface of either ovary; (3) microscopically, the tumor in the ovary must be one of the following: (a) nonexistent; (b) confined to the ovarian surface epithelium with no evidence of cortical invasion; (c) involving ovarian surface epithelium and/or underlying cortical stroma but with no tumor nodule measuring greater than 5 × 5 mm; and (4) the histological and cytological characteristics of the tumor must be predominantly of the serous type that is similar or identical to ovarian serous papillary adenocarcinoma, any grade.[45]

The uterus is removed as part of the staging procedure for ovarian and peritoneal serous carcinomas. When the tumor appears to be primary peritoneal, the pathologist should meticulously examine the endometrium both grossly and microscopically. Serous carcinoma of the endometrium, and its putative precursor, endometrial intraepithelial carcinoma, can disseminate throughout the peritoneum even when microscopic and lacking myometrial invasion (see Chapter 12, Endometrial Carcinoma). It is possible that a small proportion of apparent primary peritoneal serous carcinomas reflect disseminated endometrial serous carcinomas with an inapparent or occult primary endometrial tumor.[406,466]

Primary ovarian epithelial tumors of nonserous types may occasionally mimic serous carcinoma, typically clear cell and endometrioid carcinomas; this is not surprising as ovarian carcinomas may display mixed cell types (see "Mixed Epithelial Tumors," following), and secretory change may be present in otherwise typical serous carcinomas. More importantly, malignant germ cell tumors, particularly embryonal carcinoma and yolk sac tumor, often have solid and papillary patterns, respectively, which may mimic serous carcinoma. The age of the patient is an important clue to their diagnosis, as these malignant germ cell tumors usually occur in much younger patients. Immunohistochemistry utilizing antibodies against alpha fetoprotein (AFP), which reliably stains yolk sac tumors, can be very useful in this distinction (see Chapter 20, Germ Cell Tumors of the Ovary). Clinical correlation with serum levels of AFP may also be of value. On occasion, distinction of serous carcinoma from the retiform variant of Sertoli–Leydig cell tumor is difficult. Positive inhibin and negative EMA staining in the latter tumors, as well as the younger age of these patients, are useful features (see Chapter 19).

Ovarian carcinoma is often considered in the differential diagnosis of a metastatic adenocarcinoma of unknown primary site in women. Of particular value in this differential diagnosis is the panel of CK7 and CK20, as the CK7/CK20 profiles of carcinomas of a variety of sites have been studied and tabulated.[452] The CK7/CK20 profiles of endometrioid and serous ovarian carcinomas, the two most common types of ovarian carcinoma, which together account for 68% of all ovarian carcinomas, are similar. The antibody to CA-125, designated OC-125, is not as useful, as it is often positive in endometrial and nongynecologic carcinomas and has been reported in breast, colon, lung, and pancreatic carcinomas.[46] In addition, pancreatic carcinoma is often CK7 positive and CK20 negative, making distinction of ovarian from pancreatic carcinoma difficult. When breast cancer is in the differential diagnosis, GCDFP-15 is often useful as it is frequently positive in breast carcinomas and is nearly always negative in ovarian carcinomas.

Clinical Behavior and Treatment The survival rates for ovarian carcinomas, of which the majority are serous, are shown in Table 18.2 (see earlier in this chapter). As discussed earlier, stage I patients who have been carefully staged have a 5-year survival rate that exceeds 90%. Survival for stages III and IV is generally very poor. Some of the older literature overestimates the survival rate for stage III patients because of the inclusion of "borderline" tumors. Stage II tumors are uncommon (8% of serous carcinomas[303]) and represent an intermediate group that, depending on other factors including completeness of surgical removal and substage, can have widely varying survival and cure rates. Early de novo carcinoma, despite its small size, is associated with recurrence and death in about one-third of cases, usually with widespread peritoneal disease.

Mucinous Tumors

An understanding of the current status of *mucinous ovarian tumors* from the standpoint of their classification and behavior must start with a brief review of the evolution of ovarian tumor classification over the past half century as well as a survey of recent clinicopathologic studies performed during the past 10 years. With the acceptance, at the beginning of the twentieth century, of the view that classification of ovarian "cancer" should be based on histologic principles, investigators devised classifications of surface epithelial tumors based on cell type. For the mucinous tumors, classifications utilized from the 1940s through the 1960s generally divided them into three categories: pseudomucinous cystadenoma, pseudomucinous carcinoma, and pseudomyxoma ovarii et peritonei. At that time there was considerable controversy as to whether these latter tumors, which typically displayed a bland histologic appearance but often resulted in the death of the patient, should be classified as benign or malignant.[161]

In the early 1970s, FIGO and WHO introduced a radically different classification in which tumors of surface epithelial origin were not only classified according to cell type but also were subdivided into benign, frankly malignant, or "of borderline malignancy" or "low malignant potential".[176, 389] This tripartite categorization, with the category of borderline malignancy at its core, was conceived in an effort to reconcile the disparate behavior and histologic appearance of a certain group of serous tumors. It had been recognized that a group of "noninvasive" serous tumors with minimal cytologic atypia associated with "implants" outside the ovary behaved in a relatively innocuous fashion even when inadequately treated compared to advanced-stage, frankly invasive serous carcinoma. In an effort to construct a uniform classification, it was reasoned that this tripartite categorization could be extended to all the histologic subtypes of surface epithelial tumors. The behavior of mucinous ovarian tumors associated with pseudomyxoma peritonei, which often proved to be malignant despite a bland histologic appearance, was interpreted as yet another example of borderline malignancy. Accordingly, mucinous ovarian tumors associated with *pseudomyxoma peritonei (PMP)* were placed in the borderline category.

In the ensuing years, it was found that the long-term survival for *mucinous borderline tumors (MBTs)* confined to the ovary was close to 100% whereas survival for advanced-stage MBTs was 40%–50%. Thus, the only MBTs that displayed malignant behavior were those that were advanced stage. A recent review[330] showed that about 85% of all reported advanced-stage MBTs were associated with PMP.* Furthermore, when carefully analyzed virtually all these can be shown to be secondary tumors from a mucinous cystadenoma of the appendix that ruptured and presumably discharged mucinous epithelium into the peritoneal cavity.[336] This epithelium is capable of implanting on peritoneal surfaces and producing copious amounts of mucin. Bona fide primary ovarian MBTs that have ruptured before or at the time of surgery have never been reported to have recurred or resulted in the development of PMP. Thus, most investigators believe that PMP is a condition associated with certain gastrointestinal neoplasms but not with primary ovarian mucinous tumors, although some believe that the ovaries are capable of producing this condition on rare occasion. Concomitant mucinous neoplasms of the ovary and appendix in the absence of PMP may occur very rarely and probably represent independent primary tumors.

Other studies have shown that metastatic carcinomas from the upper gastrointestinal tract, notably the pancreas, biliary tract, and occasionally from the cervix, can display a beguilingly innocous appearance in the ovary such that they are easily mistaken for ovarian MBTs. Furthermore, the ovarian tumors in these cases are typically much larger than the primary carcinoma, thus heightening the resemblance to a primary ovarian tumor. Thus, ovarian MBTs are a heterogeneous group of neoplasms. The majority are benign proliferative tumors confined to the ovary. The minority that are "advanced stage" are either secondary tumors from a ruptured mucinous adenoma of the appendix associated with PMP or are metastatic carcinomas from a primary site in the upper gastrointestinal tract or cervix that masquerade as advanced-stage MBTs. Thus, when properly diagnosed, ovarian MBTs are benign tumors that rarely if ever involve extraovarian sites. From this discussion it should be clear that the need for a category of borderline mucinous tumors no longer exists, and accordingly, in this chapter, the term "atypical proliferative" replaces "borderline" or "low malignant potential." Cystadenomas with increased proliferative activity and varying degrees of cytologic atypia are classified as *atypical proliferative mucinous tumors (APMTs)*. Although it has been suggested that APMTs with more than three layers of epithelial stratification and/or marked cytologic atypia qualify as intraepithelial carcinoma, epithelial stratification is difficult to quantify and is unlikely to be reproducible. Therefore, we consider only those tumors with marked cytologic atypia to represent APMT with intraepithelial carcinoma. APMTs with clear-cut foci of invasion measuring less than 5 mm in diameter are designated APMT with microinvasion.

Benign Mucinous Tumors

Mucinous cystadenomas and *adenofibromas* comprise 41% of all benign ovarian epithelial neoplasms and 76% of ovarian mucinous neoplasms. *Benign mucinous neoplasms* occur most often in the third to sixth decades with a mean age of about 43 years.[230] Small tumors are often found incidentally whereas large tumors present as an obvious pelvic or abdominal mass.

Bilaterality is uncommon, occurring in 2%–5%

*63,65,151,185,207,216,250,276,283,356,358,402,421.

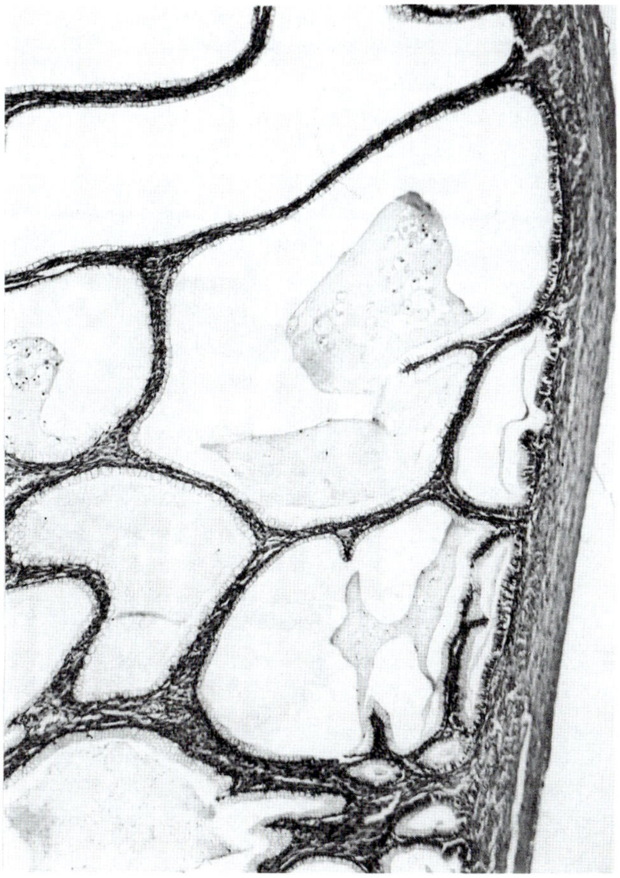

Fig. 18.63. Mucinous cystadenoma. Back-to-back cysts are lined by a single layer of mucinous epithelium.

of cases. Mucinous cystadenomas are typically large multiloculated cystic tumors that measure up to 50 cm in diameter. Locules are usually small and multiple but are variable in number; rarely, mucinous adenomas are large simple cysts with no loculations. These are the largest ovarian tumors on record; mucinous cystadenomas measuring 25–30 cm in diameter are not unusual. Tumors weighing more than 100 kg have been reported. The outer cyst wall is usually thick with a smooth opaque surface. The cysts contain thick tenacious gelatinous material that is usually pale yellow but may be turbid, brown, and more watery when associated with areas of infarction. Fibrous stroma is usually inconspicuous, but when it is abundant, these tumors are termed mucinous adenofibromas. Mucinous adenofibromas vary from 1 to 23 cm in diameter with a mean of 7 cm, and are predominantly solid with small cysts on sectioning and without surface involvement.[29]

Microscopically, mucinous cystadenomas are lined by a single layer of uniform tall columnar cells with clear or basophilic cytoplasm and small basal hyperchromatic nuclei. Goblet cells are almost always present and indicate gastrointestinal-type differentiation (Figs. 18.63–18.65). Rarely, endocervical-type mucinous epithelium predominates, usually associated with a papillary architecture (Fig. 18.66). Not infrequently, the cyst is lined by nondescript tall columnar epithelium more typical of gastric antral-type epithelium. The intestinal-type tumors are usually glandular and cystic. Simple mucinous cysts have thick, collagenous, acellular outer walls, sometimes with dystrophic calcification. More complex cystadenomas have multiple locules that may be of similar or widely varying size, some of which display a peripheral arrangement of small acini or "daughter cysts" that may create a pseudoinvasive pattern. These areas may exhibit cryptlike epithelial structures with mitoses at the bases of the crypts and also often display reduced intracytoplasmic mucin.

The complexity of glandular and papillary arrangements may be quite florid, and the presence or absence of invasion is often difficult to assess. Accumulation of mucin within the cysts causes at-

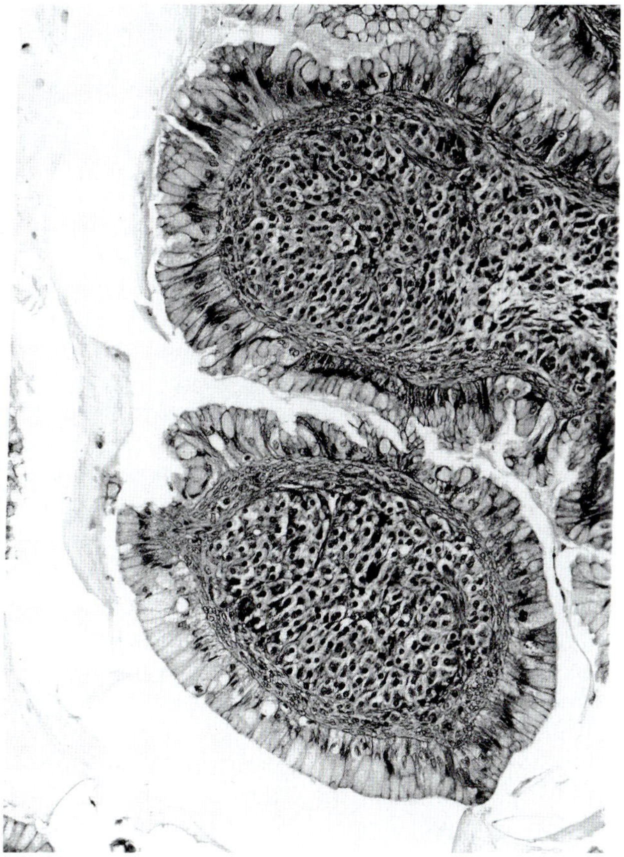

Fig. 18.64. Mucinous cystadenoma. The epithelium contains prominent vacuoles containing mucin. Luteinized stromal cells lie immediately beneath the epithelium, which is a relatively uncommon finding.

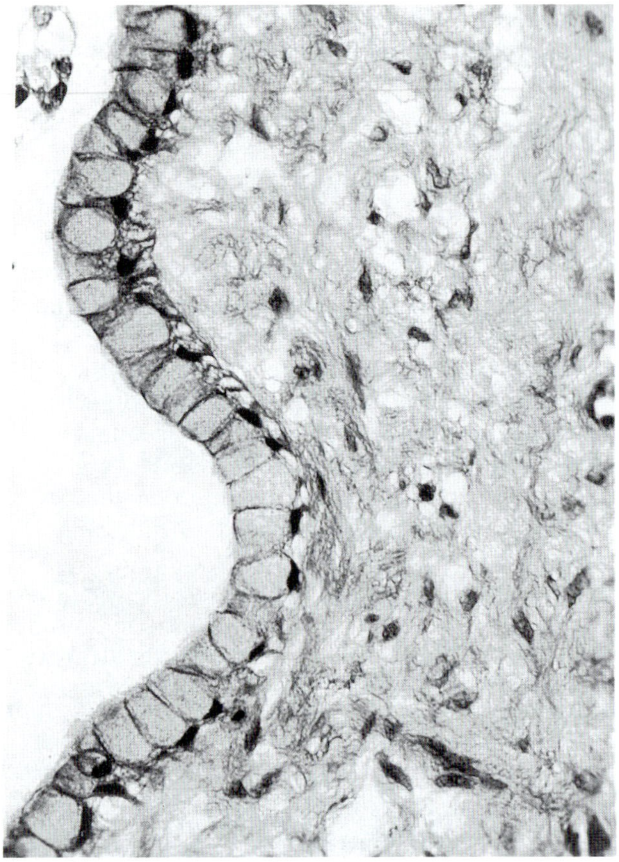

Fig. 18.65. Mucinous cystadenoma. Goblet cells resembling gastrointestinal epithelium are prominent.

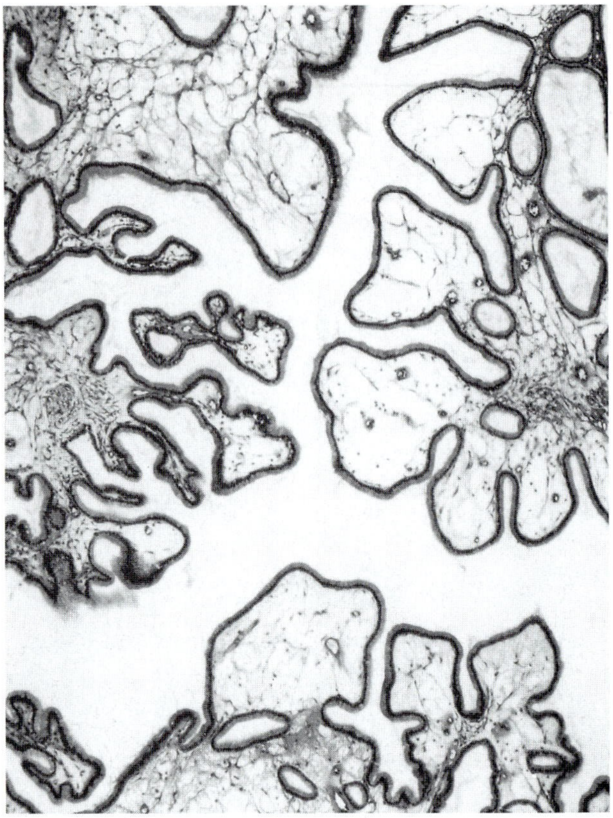

Fig. 18.66. Mucinous cystadenoma, müllerian (endocervical-like) type. This tumor is also referred to as a seromucinous cystadenoma. Coarse papillae are lined by a single layer of tall columnar mucinous epithelium of endocervical type.

tenuation of the epithelium, which may lead to leakage of mucin into the stroma; the latter can also be caused by infarction. The mucin in the stroma may elicit no stromal reaction, an acute or chronic inflammatory response with numerous muciphages, or a foreign body-type reaction. Extensive dissection of mucin through the tumor stroma is designated pseudomyxoma ovarii. The presence of mucin lakes in the stroma does not alter the diagnosis of mucinous cystadenoma but must be considered carefully in conjunction with the clinical and operative findings because extensive dissection of paucicellular mucin in the stroma is a characteristic morphologic feature of mucinous ovarian tumors associated with PMP, a condition that is nearly always of gastrointestinal origin (see "Mucinous Tumors Associated with Pseudomyxoma Peritonei"; and Chapter 22, Metastatic Tumors of the Ovary).

The stroma of mucinous cystadenomas is fibrocollagenous and the cellularity is variable but rarely approaches the high cellularity of the stroma of serous tumors. Stromal cellularity is often increased immediately surrounding the epithelium, and in this zone, luteinized stromal cells are occasionally seen (see Fig. 18.64). Mucinous adenofibromas contain dense fibrous stroma with scattered mucinous glands (Fig. 18.67).

Immunohistochemical studies have shown that mucinous cystadenomas are positive for keratins AE1, AE3 and CAM 5.2, and 40% are positive for vimentin.[101] About half of cases are positive for CEA.[21] Approximately a third of cases have argyrophil cells (demonstrated by positive Grimelius stain)[21] that are positive for serotonin,[363] ACTH, gastrin, and usually positive for somatostatin.[5]

Atypical Proliferative (Borderline) Mucinous Tumors, Gastrointestinal Type

Clinical Findings

These tumors comprise about 38% of "borderline" tumors and 12% of mucinous ovarian neoplasms. The clinical features associated with APMTs are similar to those for mucinous cystadenomas. The age distribution of patients with these tumors peaks in the fifth and sixth decades.[64,151,330,354]

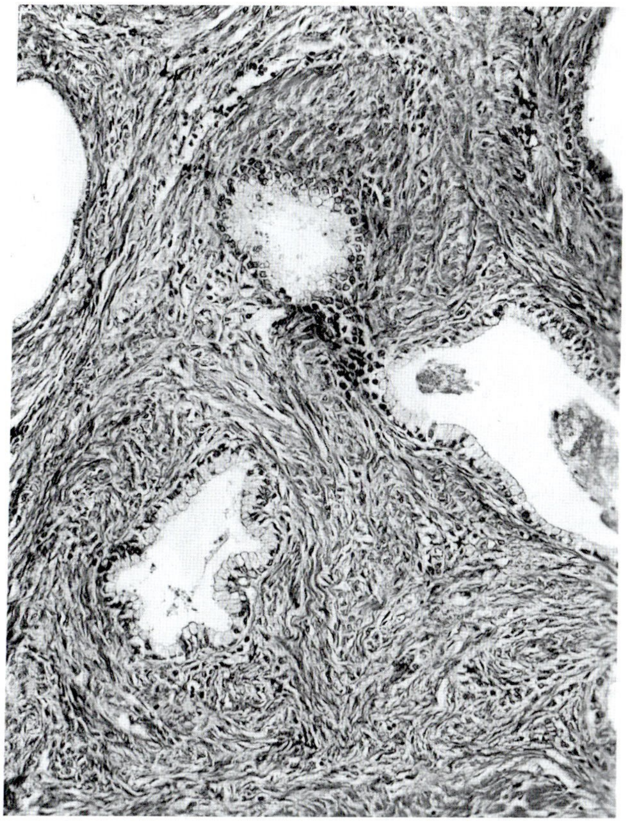

Fig. 18.67. Mucinous adenofibroma. A prominent dense fibrous stroma contains benign mucinous glands.

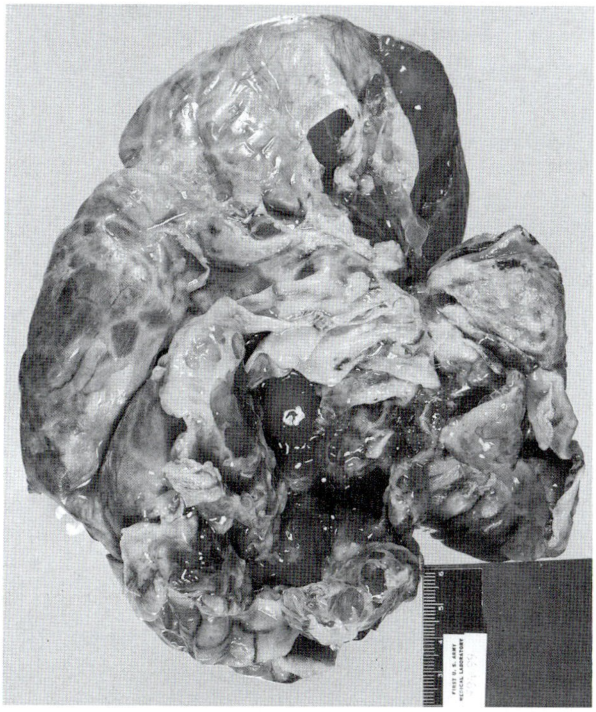

Fig. 18.68. Atypical proliferative mucinous tumor. A multiloculated, cystic gross appearance similar to that of mucinous cystadenomas is characteristic.

Operative Findings

APMTs are bilateral in up to 6% of cases.[151,330] Like mucinous cystadenomas, APMTs are often very large neoplasms and may be adherent to other pelvic or abdominal organs. However, these tumors are noninvasive and therefore adherence to adjacent organs is not an ominous feature.

Gross Findings

The characteristic gross features of APMT are identical to those of mucinous cystadenomas (Fig. 18.68). This is not surprising because APMTs arise in preexisting mucinous cystadenomas (see following and also preceding pathogenesis section).

Microscopic Findings

APMT of gastrointestinal type is characterized by cytologic atypia and epithelial stratification of mucinous epithelium that is otherwise similar to that of gastrointestinal-type mucinous cystadenomas (Figs. 18.69 and 18.70). At least 10% of the neoplasm should display these features to be included in the

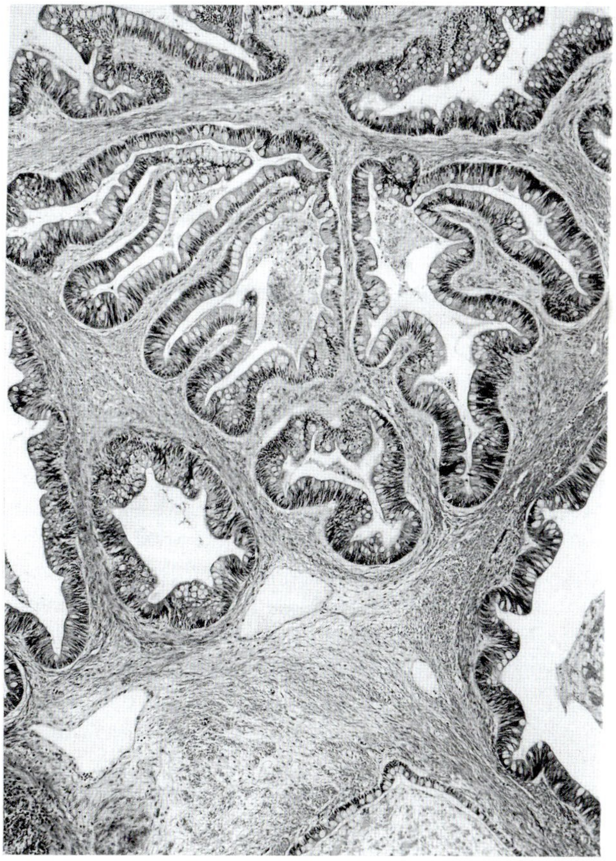

Fig. 18.69. Atypical proliferative mucinous tumor. Crowded branched glands are lined by gastrointestinal-type epithelium.

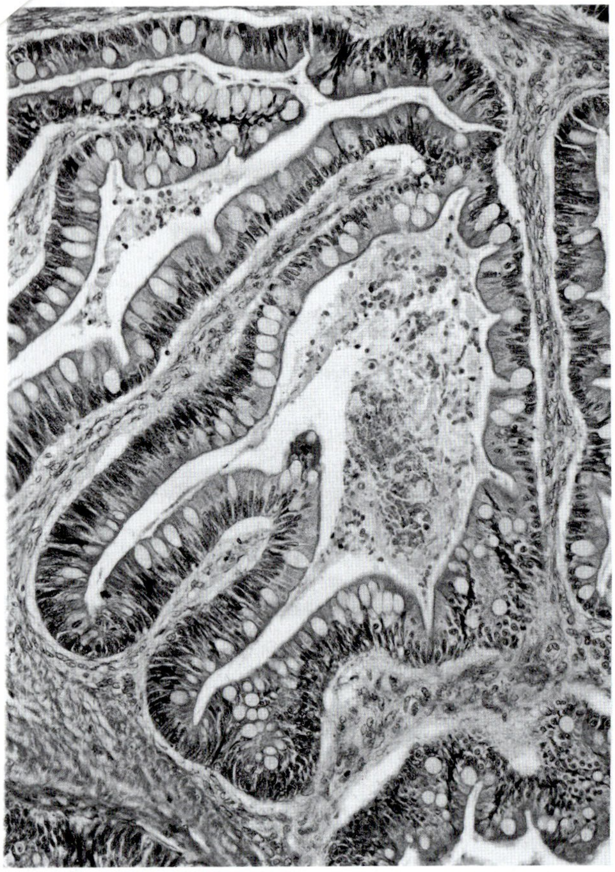

Fig. 18.70. Atypical proliferative mucinous tumor. The epithelium contains numerous goblet cells. There is nuclear stratification.

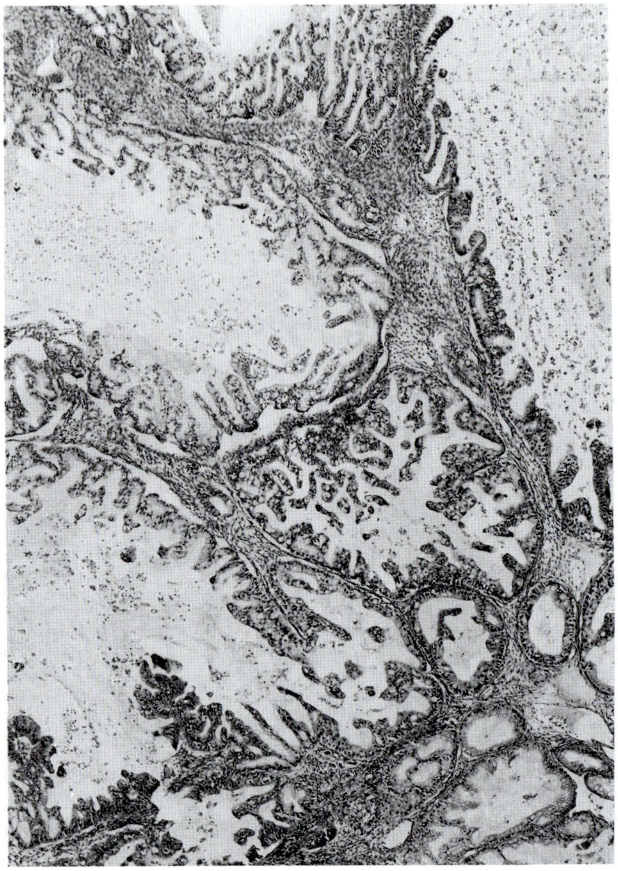

Fig. 18.71. Atypical proliferative mucinous tumor. Cystically dilated glands contain intraluminal papillary tufts with focal areas of fusion of the papillae.

APMT category.[353] Stromal invasion is absent. The epithelial stratification is often manifested by intraluminal papillary tufts of varying size that lack fibrovascular support (Figs. 18.71–18.74). A villoglandular architecture is occasionally present. Although the older literature suggests that epithelial stratification greater than three cell layers conveys a worse prognosis,[161] these data have not been substantiated, and furthermore the degree and extent of epithelial stratification may not be reproducible. The glands are often crowded and may be back to back (Fig. 18.75). Foci of a true cribriform pattern characterized by absence of fibrovascular support between adjacent glands may occur but must be confined within cysts to qualify as an APMT. Nests or masses of epithelium displaying a cribriform pattern within the stroma reflect invasion and depending on the size of these foci qualify as microinvasive (less than 5 mm) or frank carcinoma (see following). Cytologic atypia and mitotic activity are variable (Fig. 18.76). Marked cytologic atypia qualifies for the diagnosis of intraepithelial carcinoma (see following) and should prompt further sampling for areas of invasion.

Immunohistochemistry

APMTs are positive for keratins including AE1, AE3, and CAM 5.2, and 70% are positive for vimentin.[101] Nearly all tumors are positive for CEA, CK7, and CK18, and the majority also stain for HAM-56 and CK20.[337] Estrogen receptors are not present.[1] The majority (60%–86%) have argyrophil (Grimelius-positive) cells[21,358] that nearly always stain for serotonin and gastrin and often are positive for ACTH, somatostatin, pancreatic polypeptide, chromogranin, and neuron-specific enolase.[5,363]

Differential Diagnosis

The most important differential diagnostic consideration when evaluating a mucinous neoplasm in the ovary is whether the tumor is primary in the

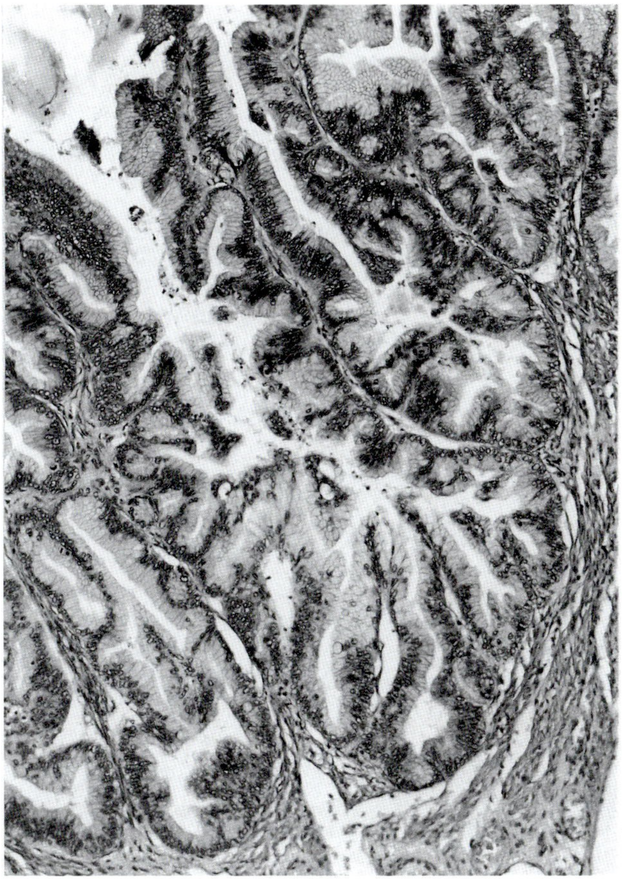

Fig. 18.72. Atypical proliferative mucinous tumor. Markedly crowded complex glands. (Courtesy of Brigitte M. Ronnett, M.D., Baltimore, MD.)

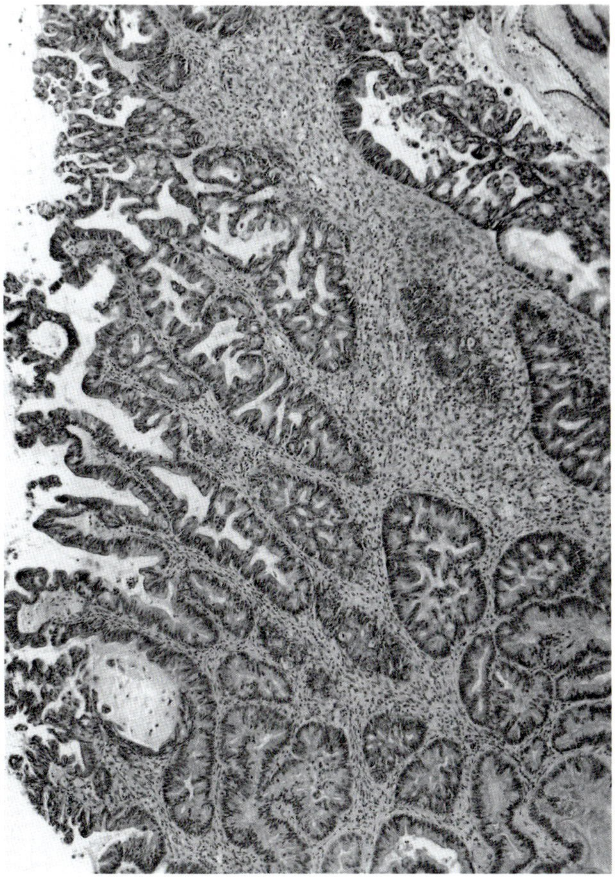

Fig. 18.73. Atypical proliferative mucinous tumor. Fusion of papillary tufts creates foci of an intraglandular cribriform pattern. This pattern when confined to glandular lumens is not indicative of invasion.

ovary or metastatic. If primary, an APMT must be distinguished from invasive carcinoma (see "Mucinous Carcinoma"). Features suggestive of metastatic ovarian involvement include bilaterality, and if bilateral, size less than 10 cm, ovarian surface involvement, extensive pseudomyxoma ovarii, and certain patterns of haphazard, nodular infiltrative growth.

It is important to be aware that mucinous epithelial proliferations can occur in association with other benign or low-grade malignant tumor types, most commonly transitional cell (Brenner), teratomas, and Sertoli–Leydig cell tumors (SLCT). Mucinous epithelium in these tumors usually is a minor component; however, at times the mucinous component can form the dominant mass. For example, a mucinous epithelial element in a benign cystic teratoma may be the predominant component and appear to be a mucinous neoplasm, and only after extensive sampling is another teratomatous element discovered. Similarly, heterologous gastrointestinal-type mucinous epithelium, found in 20% of Sertoli–Leydig cell tumors, may occasionally form the dominant part of the tumor. The intimate admixture of endocervical-type mucinous and transitional epithelium in the "metaplastic Brenner tumor" (see "Transitional Cell Tumors") suggests that the association of transitional cell and mucinous neoplasms is also based on overgrowth of a mucinous element in the former. On very rare occasions, the mucinous element of a teratoma, transitional cell tumor, or SLCT may appear atypical or may undergo malignant transformation.

Clinical Behavior and Treatment

APMTs are benign, with survival rates of 98–99% based on literature reviews including approximately 900 patients[330,402] (Table 18.11). Very rare reports of aggressive behavior most likely reflect inadequate sampling with failure to detect occult invasion, or the ovarian tumor may be a metastasis from an occult primary source elsewhere. Although the litera-

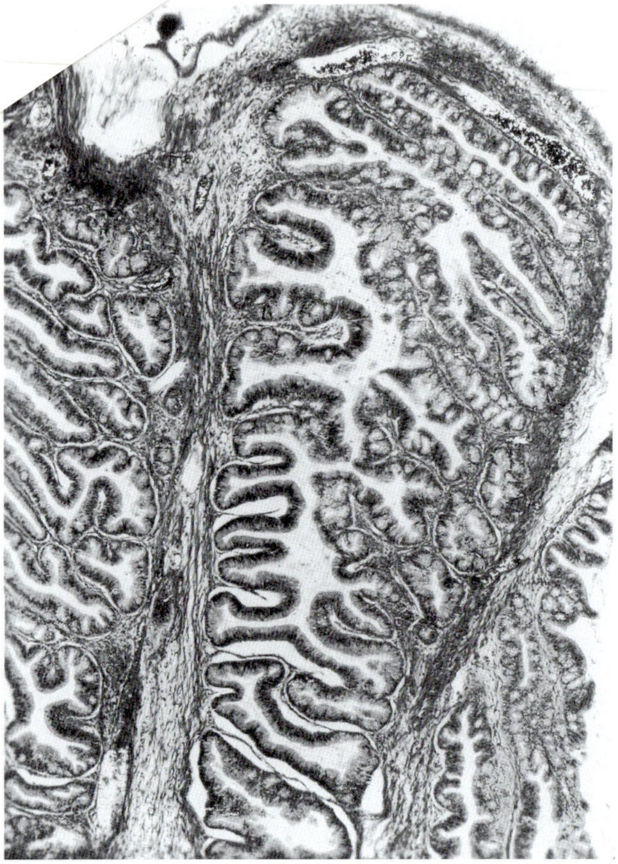

Fig. 18.74. Atypical proliferative mucinous tumor. There is prominent papillary infolding, but the glands do not display a confluent pattern.

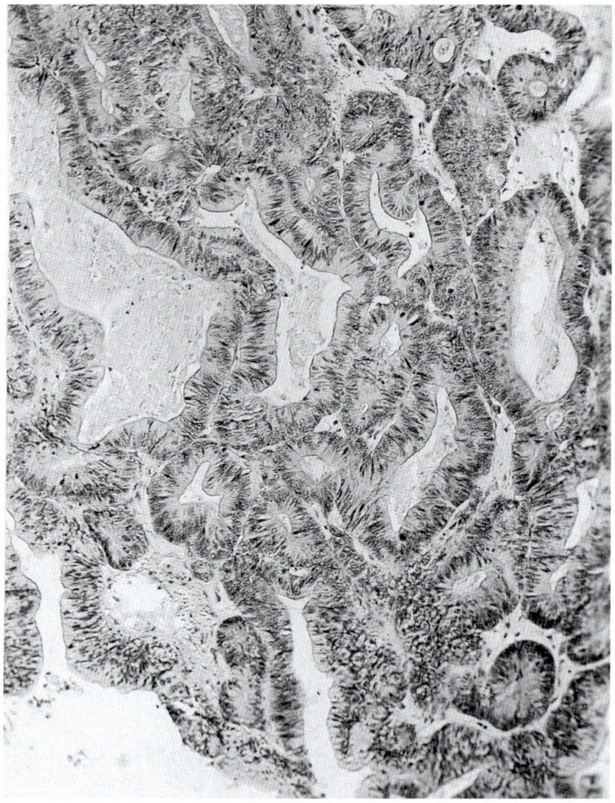

Fig. 18.75. Atypical proliferative mucinous tumor. Back-to-back glandular crowding is prominent.

ture suggests that the survival of patients with advanced stage MBTs is only 54%, it is now clear that bona fide advanced-stage MBT rarely if ever occurs. Eighty-five percent of women who have been reported to have advanced-stage MBTs present with the syndrome of pseudomyxoma peritonei, a condition that is not of ovarian origin[330]; (see "Pseudomyxoma Peritonei").

APMT, Endocervical-Like (Seromucinous) Type, and Atypical Proliferative Tumors of Mixed Epithelial Type

Fifteen percent of ovarian APMTs are of the müllerian, endocervical-like type, also referred to as seromucinous to reflect the combination of serous and mucinous features. The mean patient age is 34; 77% are stage I, and 40% are bilateral. In the largest reported series,[358] the 23% of patients who had stage

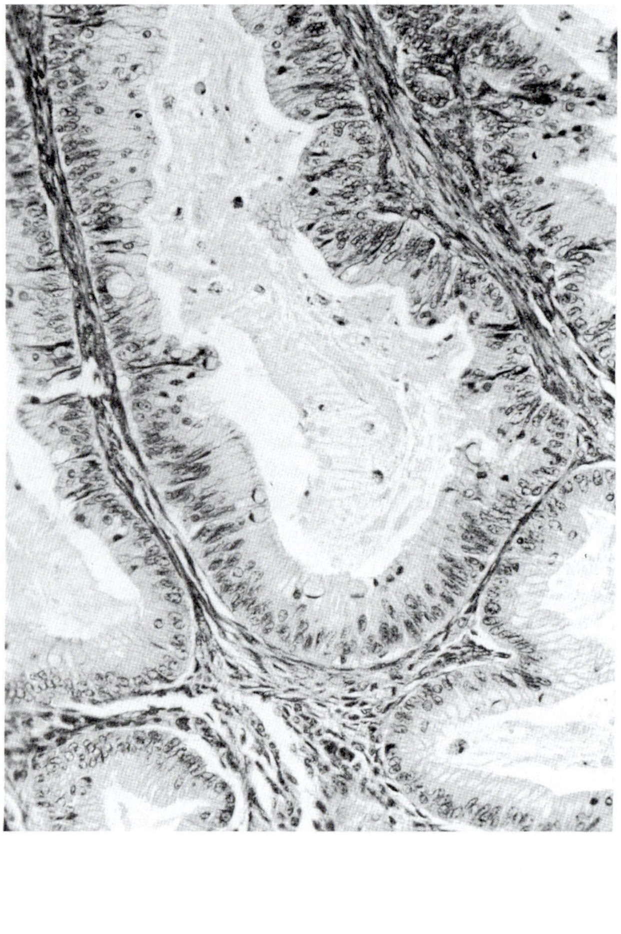

Fig. 18.76. Atypical proliferative mucinous tumor. Epithelial stratification and mild to moderate cytologic atypia are present.

Table 18.11. Review of studies reporting survival of patients with stage I mucinous borderline tumors (MBTs) and MBTs with intraepithelial (noninvasive) mucinous carcinomas

Series	*No. of MBTs*	*No. of disease-related deaths*	*No. of intraepithelial carcinomas*	*No. of disease-related deaths*
Hart[161]	87	1[a]	12	1[a]
Chaitin[64]	21	2	—[b]	—[b]
Sumithran[419]	41	0	12	3
Watkin[454]	19	0	16	1
de Nictolis[101]	32	0	15	0
Guerrieri[151]	48	0	18	1
Siriaunkgul[402]	32	0	12	0
Hoerl[168]	0	—	15	0
Lee[230]	47[c]	0	74[d]	2[e]
Riopel[330]	44	0	11	0
Totals	371	3 (0.8%)	185	8 (4.31%)

[a]Does not include two patients who died of disease but were acknowledged by the investigators to have had tumors that were inadequately sampled.
[b]Deaths not reported by stage for 19 noninvasive carcinomas.
[c]Excludes two cases which were classified as stage IC based on the superficial organizing type of pseudomyxoma peritonei.
[d]Includes 5 cases which had both carcinoma in situ and microinvasion.
[e]Both cases were incompletely staged.
Modified with permission from Riopel MA, et al, ref. 333.

II and III disease did not have PMP, suggesting that the peritoneal implants associated with this type of APMT are more akin to those seen with APSTs. This finding is also consistent with the papillary architecture of these tumors, a feature that closely resembles the architecture of serous tumors and is quite dissimilar to the architecture of intestinal-type mucinous neoplasms. The mean tumor size is 8 cm.

The microscopic architectural features as noted earlier are similar to APSTs, with a hierarchical branching pattern, stratification, tufting, and detachment of cell clusters (Figs. 18.77–18.79). A prominent acute inflammatory infiltrate is nearly always present, at least focally (Fig. 18.80). The epithelium is tall columnar and mucinous, resembling endocervical epithelium. Cells with cilia can be found in a third of cases, reflecting serous-type differentiation (Fig. 18.81). Atypia is usually minimal. Cells with slightly larger and rounded nuclei containing densely eosinophilic cytoplasm, particularly at the tips of the papillae, are present in nearly all cases. A small component (less than 10%) of other müllerian epithelial cell type differentiation, for example endometrioid, is common. There is a strong association with endometriosis, which is present in 30% of patients; in two-thirds of these patients, the neoplasm has been observed to arise directly from the atypical epithelial component of an endometriotic cyst.[358] Immunoperoxidase studies show these

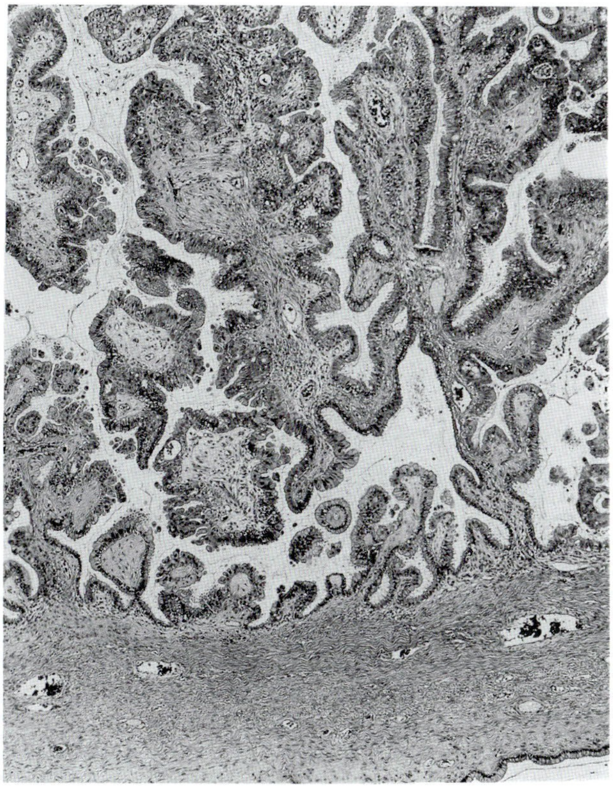

Fig. 18.77. Atypical proliferative mucinous tumor, endocervical-like or seromucinous type. The hierarchical branching pattern is characterized by large thick papillae giving rise to papillae of successively smaller sizes.

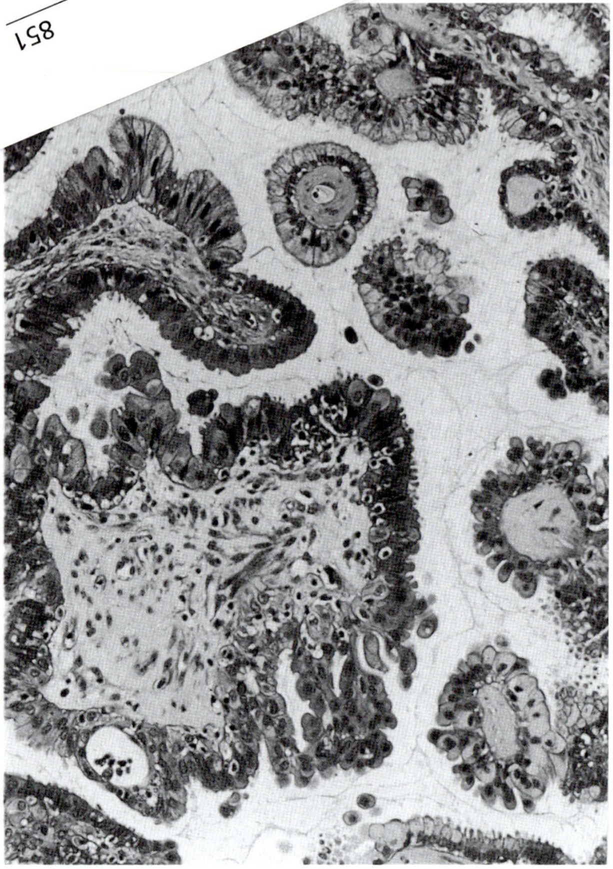

Fig. 18.78. Atypical proliferative mucinous tumor, endocervical-like or seromucinous type. The combination of a papillary architecture and cells containing mucin is characteristic.

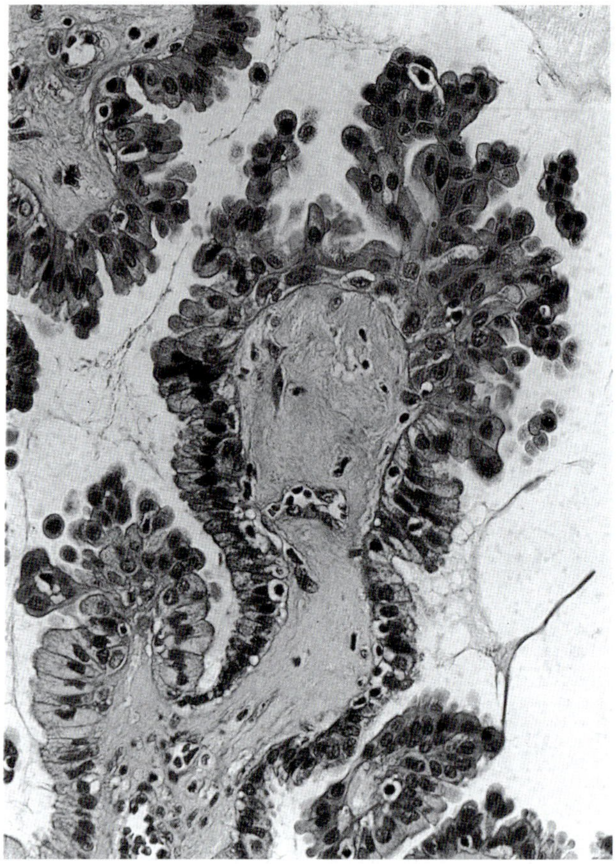

Fig. 18.79. Atypical proliferative mucinous tumor, endocervical-like or seromucinous type. Mucinous cells and polygonal cells with eosinophilic cytoplasm are present. The latter cells are typically found in APSTs.

tumors are positive for estrogen receptors[1] and epithelial markers. After a short mean follow-up of 3.7 years, all patients were alive and well, but two who underwent unilateral salpingo-oophorectomy developed contralateral APMTs, which most likely reflect new primary tumors.

The authors of the largest series of these tumors also reported a series of 36 patients with a closely related tumor classified as "mixed epithelial papillary cystadenoma of borderline malignancy of müllerian type".[359] The distinguishing feature of these tumors from the APMTs of müllerian type is the presence of a significant component (at least 10%) of endometrioid, serous, or squamous differentiation in addition to müllerian mucinous differentiation. Many of the clinical and pathologic features of this tumor closely resemble those of the APMT of müllerian type, including the mean patient age of 35 years, bilaterality rate of 22%, presence of an acute inflammatory infiltrate in 86% of cases, and endometriosis in 53% of cases with three-quarters of the latter displaying atypical endometriosis in the ipsilateral ovary. These features indicate a close relationship between this tumor and APMT of müllerian type. All the mixed epithelial tumors were stage I, and 3 patients reportedly had pelvic recurrences, but there were no tumor deaths after 4.8 years of follow-up. It is likely that an apparent recurrence of this type of tumor reflects a new primary tumor developing in endometriosis.

APMT with Intraepithelial Carcinoma

The term *atypical proliferative mucinous tumor with intraepithelial carcinoma* is relatively new and has been employed to describe a subset of atypical mucinous neoplasms that display extensive epithelial stratification (greater than three cell layers) (Fig. 18.82), or marked cytologic atypia (Figs. 18.83–18.85), which are characteristic features of invasive carcinoma in many sites; in these cases, however, unequivocal stromal invasion cannot be demonstrated. Because epithelial stratification is difficult

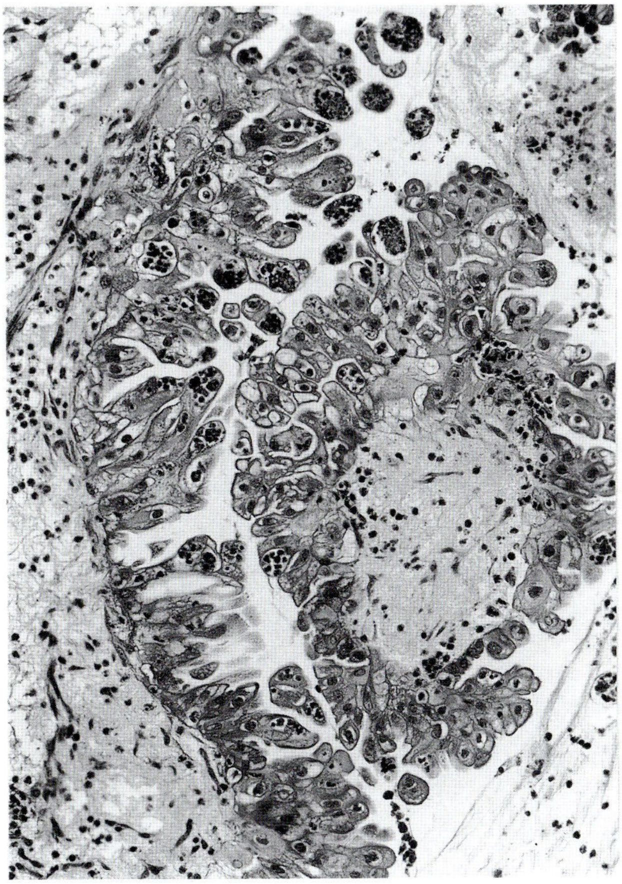

Fig. 18.80. Atypical proliferative mucinous tumor, endocervical-like or seromucinous type. Microabscesses containing neutrophils in the epithelium on the surface of papillae are characteristic.

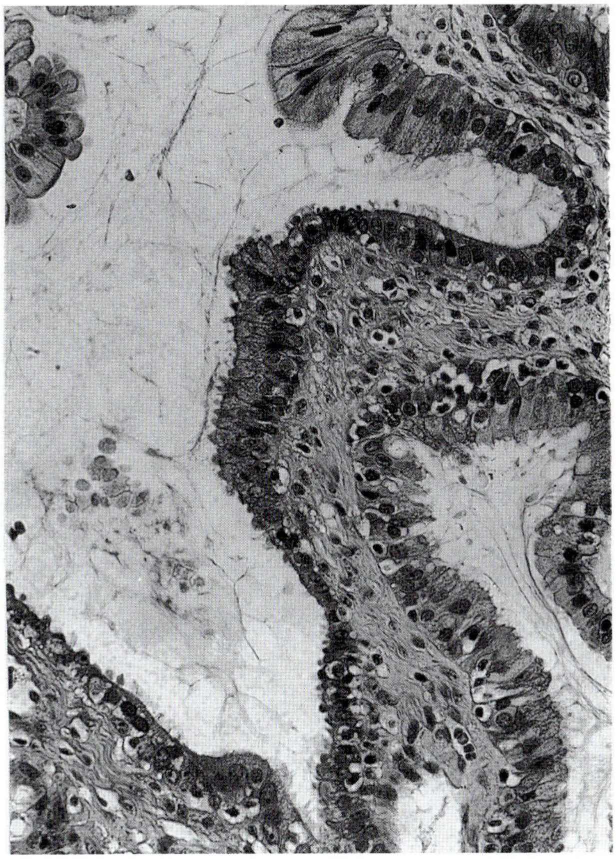

Fig. 18.81. Atypical proliferative mucinous tumor, endocervical-like or seromucinous type. In addition to cytoplasmic mucin, many cells display cilia at their apical borders.

to quantify and may not be reproducible, we reserve the diagnosis of APMT with intraepithelial carcinoma for those tumors displaying areas of high-grade nuclear atypia. APMT with intraepithelial carcinoma has been considered by some to reflect the morphologic upper end of the spectrum of proliferation of APMT, or as intraglandular, or in situ, mucinous carcinoma. APMT with intraepithelial carcinoma comprises approximately one-quarter of all mucinous neoplasms in the atypical proliferative and invasive carcinoma groups combined.[64,151,330] The survival of patients with intraepithelial carcinoma exceeds 95% following salpingo-oophorectomy and for all practical purposes is the same as that of APMTs (see Table 18.11).[330]

APMT with Microinvasion

To qualify as APMT with microinvasion, no single invasive area should exceed 5 mm in diameter (Fig. 18.86). Multiple foci of invasion are permitted.[330] Some authors have proposed a 3-mm criterion as the maximum size of the invasive area to qualify for this diagnosis. In most cases, microinvasion measures less than 2 mm.[199] Further studies are needed to quantitatively define microinvasion. Stromal invasion in mucinous neoplasms is described later (see "Mucinous Carcinomas"). Limited data on microinvasion in APMTs indicate a survival of 100%, based on 42 patients (34 intestinal type, 6 müllerian type, 2 mixed) followed for a mean of about 6 years.[168,199,230,277,330]

Mucinous Tumors Associated with Pseudomyxoma Peritonei

Historically, the term pseudomyxoma peritonei (PMP) referred to the gross appearance of mucinous ascites associated with a mucinous tumor of the appendix, colon, or ovary. The literature on PMP before the 1990s is very difficult to evaluate for several reasons. First, PMP has never been a specific histopathologic diagnosis, but rather an operative/gross description. Second, much of the literature on this entity lacks descriptive data on the histology of the lesion. Third, PMP in women often involves the ovaries, and, until recently, it had not been clear whether the primary site was in the appendix, ovary, or both in such women. Some investigators have also proposed that the primary site may be the colon. Another problem plaguing the diagnosis of PMP is the subclassification, by some authors, of cases into those with and without epithelial cells. These problems have recently been addressed.

Some investigators have proposed that the clinical presentation and gross appearance of PMP encompass two distinct histopathologic entities: peritoneal mucinous carcinomatosis (PMCA), which is histologically a high-grade metastatic adenocarcinoma usually from the appendix or colon with a high early mortality rate; and disseminated peritoneal adenomucinosis (DPAM), which is an indolent proliferation of morphologically benign or minimally atypical neoplastic ("adenomatous") mucinous epithelium nearly always derived from a ruptured mucinous neoplasm of the appendix. The mucinous epithelium released from the appendiceal neoplasm implants on peritoneal surfaces and is capable of producing copious amounts of mucin that persistently reaccumulates in the form of mucinous ascites. The mucinous epithelium has little capacity to invade tissue, but the mucin that accumulates in the peritoneal cavity is an irritant which induces fibrosis and dense adhesions. Patients with this entity usually have prolonged survival, but eventually many succumb from bowel obstruction. Although most cases of PMP can be reliably classified into DPAM or PMCA, approximately 12% display discordant or intermediate histologic features and, on average, have a prognosis intermediate between the two major groups.[338]

The term DPAM is less than optimal because it fails to communicate the ability of this tumor to produce serious complications and death, albeit over a

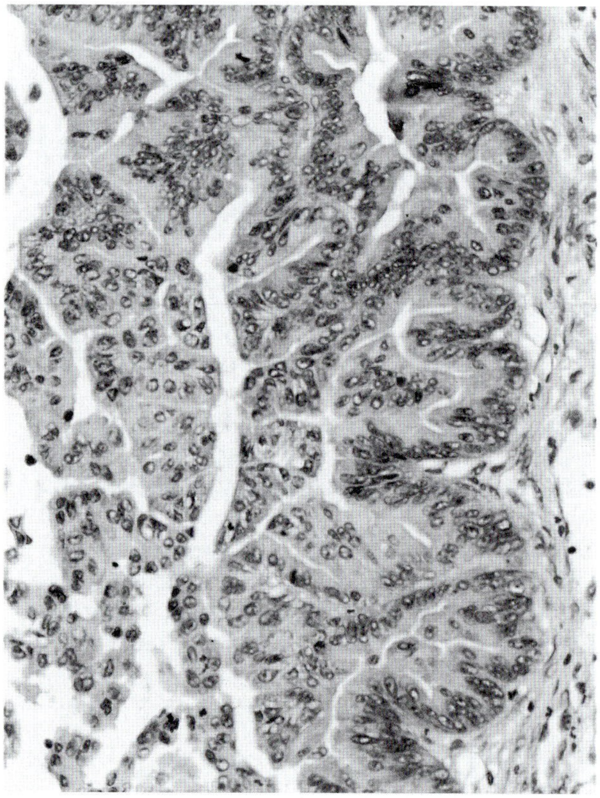

Fig. 18.82. Atypical proliferative mucinous tumor with extensive epithelial stratification. In the older literature, this tumor would qualify as a mucinous carcinoma based on stratification exceeding three cell layers. Currently, this is regarded as an APMT. Some authors would accept this as an example of APMT with intraepithelial carcinoma, although others prefer to restrict the designation of APMT with intraepithelial carcinoma to those displaying cytologically malignant features (see Figs 18.83–18.85). (Courtesy of Brigitte M. Ronnett, M.D., Baltimore, MD.)

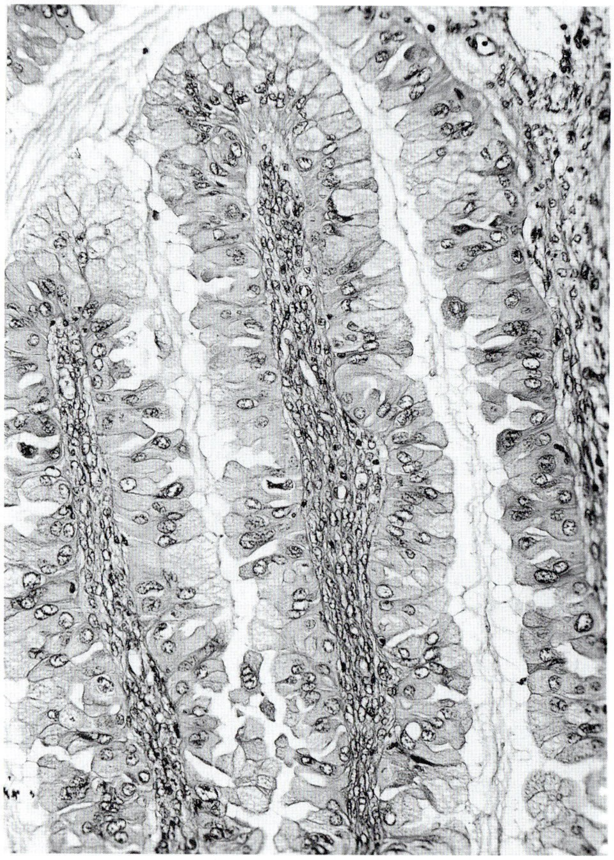

Fig. 18.83. Atypical proliferative mucinous tumor with intraepithelial carcinoma. Marked cytologic atypia and loss of polarity.

prolonged period, and in only a minority of patients. As defined earlier, DPAM describes a condition in which the majority of patients survive for long periods if all lesions are surgically removed. In some patients in whom this has been done, as well as in those who have been inadequately treated, the tumor can lead to extensive adhesions with attendant bowel obstruction and may be fatal. The development of bonafide invasive carcinoma, however, is extremely rare. On the other hand, mucinous neoplasms of the appendix that implant on the peritoneum as PMP are classified as carcinomas by some expert gastrointestinal pathologists, even if they display no significant cytologic atypia.[61] We favor the view that these tumors are not true carcinomas. This is a very low grade, clinically indolent neoplastic process that needs to be distinguished from the clinically aggressive peritoneal mucinous carcinomatosis rather than lumped together under the rubric PMP. The term PMP should be restricted to the description of the clinical entity and should not be used as a pathologic term.[337a]

Only 39% of patients with pseudomyoma peritonei in the largest series reported are women, and of these, 44% have ovarian involvement by a mucinous neoplasm.[338] It is now generally accepted that ovarian involvement in women with PMP is secondary; PMP is nearly always of gastrointestinal origin, usually from a mucinous adenoma of the vermiform appendix.[320,338] Mucinous ovarian tumors that are associated with pseudomyxoma peritonei are typically classified as borderline because tumor is present throughout the peritoneal cavity. As noted, these tumors are not ovarian in origin but are derived from appendiceal mucinous cystadenomas. Finally, it should be noted that most of the mucinous ovarian tumors associated with pseudomyxoma peritonei demonstrate gross and microscopic features that are distinctive from those of primary ovarian MBTs (see following). We prefer to refer to the ovarian tumors in these cases descriptively as "ovarian involvement by DPAM from an appendiceal mucinous neoplasm"; they are identical to the appendiceal mucinous neoplasms from which they are derived.

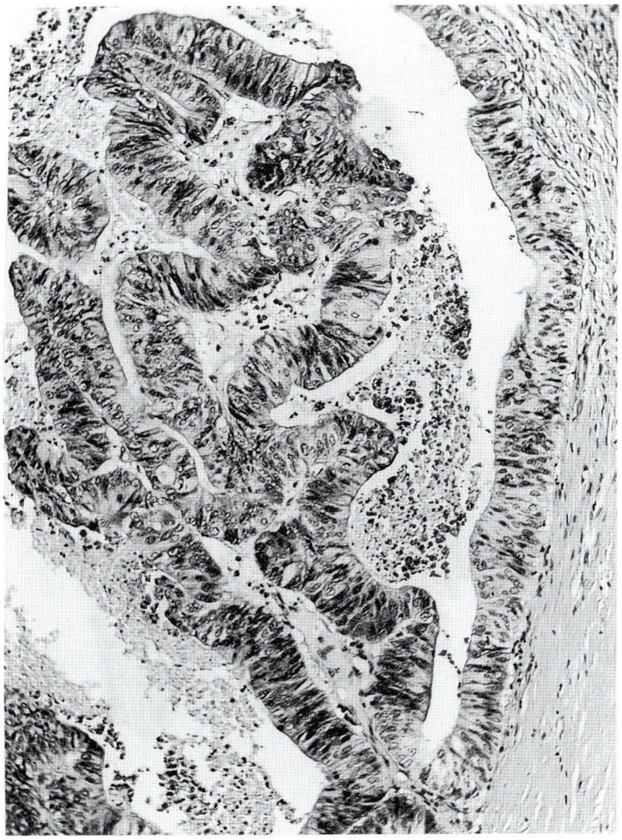

Fig. 18.84. Atypical proliferative mucinous tumor with intraepithelial carcinoma. Extensive epithelial stratification and marked cytologic atypia manifest as nuclear hyperchromasia and chromatin clumping warrant a designation of intraepithelial carcinoma.

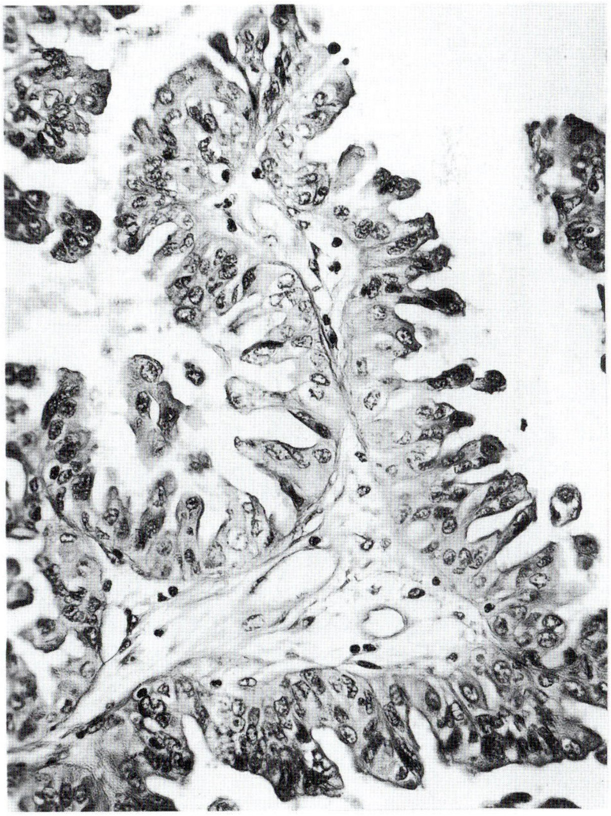

Fig. 18.85. Atypical proliferative mucinous tumor with intraepithelial carcinoma. Cytologically malignant nuclear features warrant a designation of intraepithelial carcinoma.

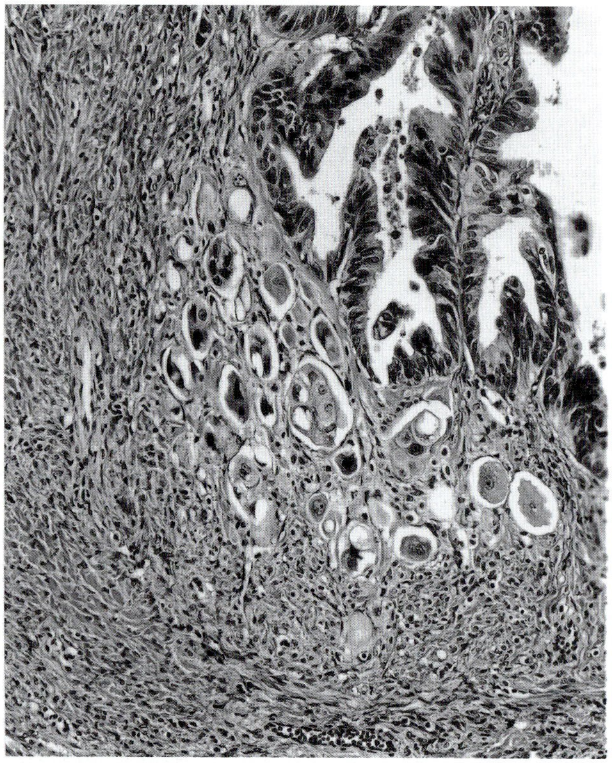

Fig. 18.86. Atypical proliferative mucinous tumor with microinvasion. Atypical mucinous epithelial cells are budding singly and in small nests into the stroma of an APMT.

Clinical Findings

Mean patient age is 44 years, with two-thirds of patients presenting in the fourth and fifth decades. Presenting clinical symptoms are often dominated by the effects of mucinous ascites, including abdominal distension and abdominal pain.

Operative Findings

Mucinous ovarian tumors associated with pseudomyxoma peritonei are bilateral in 80% of cases with a mean diameter of 7 cm. When unilateral, there is a right-sided predominance. These findings contrast with primary ovarian APMTs, which are almost invariably unilateral, large (mean diameter greater than 15 cm), stage I, and are equally distributed in the right and left ovaries. Mucinous ascites or mucoid nodules scattered throughout the peritoneal surfaces are characteristic.

Gross Findings

Ovaries involved by DPAM are often cystic and usually display mucoid surfaces, surface nodules, or implants. Metastatic mucinous carcinomas (PMCA) in the ovaries appear similar but are more often solid.[336] In 75% of patients with pseudomyxoma peritonei, there is gross or microscopic evidence of rupture of the appendiceal tumor. Gastrointestinal perforations can be very small, can heal, and can be overlooked as a result of inadequate sampling by the pathologist; these are the best explanations for most of the remaining 25% of apparently unruptured appendices. It is also possible that there can be chronic leakage of mucus from a small perforation that repeatedly heals and reruptures. In contrast, rupture of bona fide stage I primary ovarian MBTs is not associated with recurrence or the development of pseudomyxoma peritonei.

Microscopic Findings

The majority of tumors associated with PMP display mucoid nodules or implants involving the ovarian surface; in 20% of cases, the involvement is confined to the surface. Surface and superficial or deep cortical involvement is seen in more than 50% of cases, and about 25% are confined to the ovarian stroma.

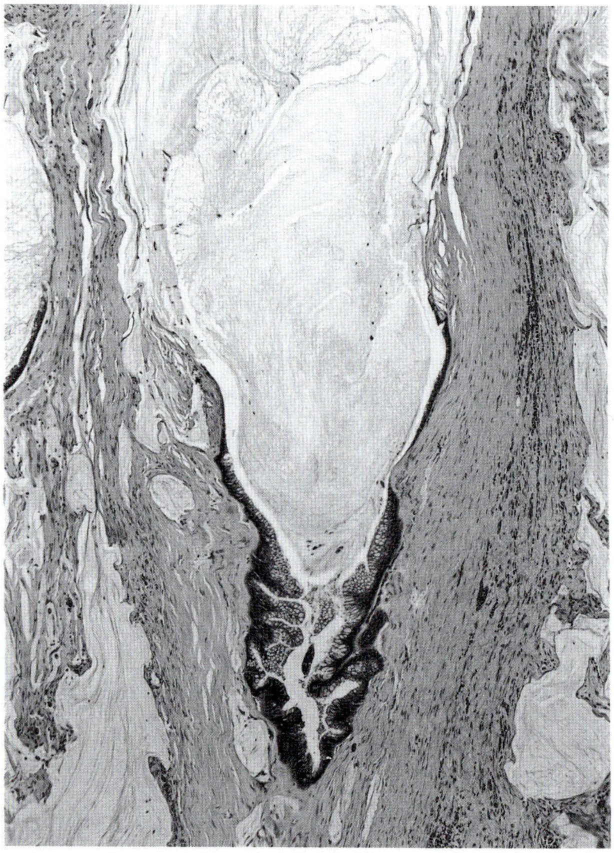

Fig. 18.87. Ovarian tumor in disseminated peritoneal adenomucinosis. There is dissection of large acellular pools of mucin through the ovarian stroma. A large mucinous gland is distended with mucin and has ruptured, creating this appearance. (Courtesy of Brigitte M. Ronnett, M.D., Baltimore, MD.)

Pseudomyxoma ovarii, an appearance characterized by dissection of acellular lakes of mucin through the ovarian stroma, is present in two-thirds of cases and is usually multifocal or extensive. Although this lesion generally does not invade organs in the usual sense, the mucin does dissect through tissue. One might speculate that enzymes in the mucin allow for dissection through tissue.

The ovarian tumors associated with mucinous tumors that are disseminated throughout the peritoneum are of two types. Tumors composed of pools of mucin with scanty simple or focally proliferative mucinous epithelium displaying minimal cytologic atypia and rare mitotic figures have been designated disseminated peritoneal adenomucinosis (DPAM) along with the abdominal disease. Additional morphologic features that are characteristically seen in these secondary ovarian lesions include strips of mucinous epithelium floating in mucin pools, often with a hypersecretory or "hypermucinous" appearance (Figs. 18.87–18.89). The latter is defined as mucinous epithelium containing mucin with a basally located nucleus resembling gastric foveolar-type epithelium. There is loss of the apical portion of the cell such that there is direct continuity of the intracellular with extracellular mucin[336] (also see Fig. 18.94, later in this chapter); these are nearly always associated with appendiceal adenomas lacking significant atypia. The ovarian mucinous proliferation closely resembles the peritoneal mucinous lesions as well as the appendiceal adenoma.

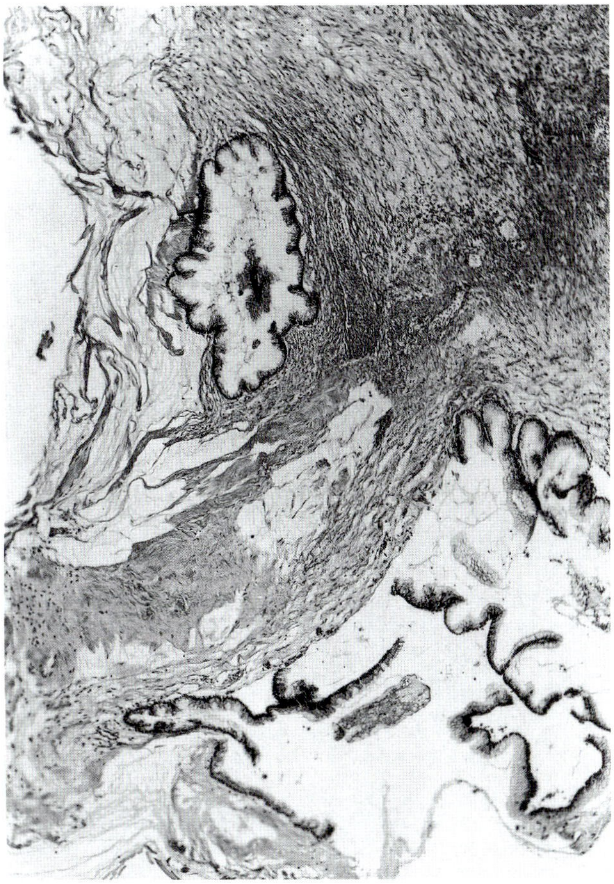

Fig. 18.88. Ovarian tumor in disseminated peritoneal adenomucinosis. Glands and strips of mucinous epithelium float in large pools of mucin within the ovarian stroma.

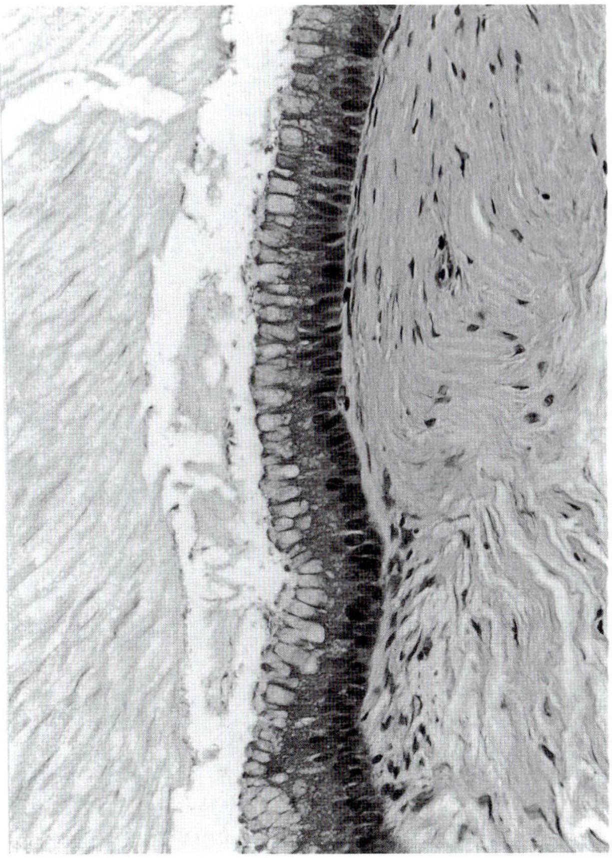

Fig. 18.89. Ovarian tumor in disseminated peritoneal adenomucinosis. Mucinous epithelium with very minimal cytologic atypia produces abundant mucin. (Courtesy of Brigitte M. Ronnett, M.D., Baltimore, MD.)

In the past, ovarian mucinous tumors characterized by epithelial proliferation and moderate to marked atypia or signet-ring cells, significant mitotic activity, and obvious stromal invasion were often included in the category of PMP because of the abundant extracellular mucin production. However, because they contain overtly histologically malignant epithelium, are associated with gastrointestinal carcinomas, and have a poor prognosis, they are not diagnosed as PMP but rather as metastatic mucinous carcinomas. They are the ovarian manifestation of PMCA and are virtually always metastatic.[336] Because

Table 18.12. Distinguishing features of disseminated peritoneal adenomucinosis (DPAM) and peritoneal mucinous carcinomatosis (PMCA)

Feature	*DPAM*	*PMCA*
Primary site	Appendix	Appendix, colon, small intestine
Primary diagnosis	Mucinous adenoma	Mucinous adenocarcinoma
Surgical appearance	Mucinous ascites with characteristic distribution[a]	Carcinomatosis with invasive implants
Peritoneal tumor		
Cellularity	Scant	Moderate to abundant
Morphology	Abundant extracellular mucin containing simple to focally proliferative mucinous epithelium	Moderate to abundant extracellular mucin containing extensively proliferative mucinous epithelium or mucinous glands, clusters of cells, or individual cells consistent with carcinoma
Cytologic atypia	Minimal	Moderate to marked
Mitotic activity	Rare	Infrequent to abundant
Lymph node involvement	Rare	Frequent
Parenchymal organ involvement	Rare (except ovary)	Frequent

[a]The distribution is characterized by superficial noninvasive involvement of the omentum, undersurface of the diaphragm, pelvis, right retrohepatic space, left abdominal gutter, and ligament of Treitz, with sparing of the peritoneal surfaces of the bowel.
Modified with permission from Ronnett et al, ref. 338.

these tumors display obvious cytologically malignant features, they are rarely confused with ovarian APMTs (see Chapter 22, Metastatic Tumors of the Ovary). The cytologic examination of peritoneal washings can assist in the distinction of DPAM and PMCA.[178a]

IMMUNOHISTOCHEMISTRY

Immunohistochemical and molecular biologic studies have provided supportive evidence that the bland-appearing mucinous tumors associated with PMP involving the ovaries are secondarily derived

Table 18.13. Distinguishing features of ovarian mucinous tumors in disseminated peritoneal adenomucinosis (DPAM) and peritoneal mucinous carcinomatosis (PMCA) and primary ovarian atypical proliferative mucinous tumors (APMT)

Feature	*Mucinous ovarian tumors in DPAM and PMCA*	*Primary ovarian APMT*
Size (mean)	7 cm	19 cm
Laterality		
Bilateral	80%	7%
Unilateral	20%	93%
	Right >> left	Right = left
Gross		
Mucinous nodules	90%	0%
Multiloculated cyst	10%	100%
Rupture	7%	3%
Location of tumor		
Surface ± cortical stroma	37%	0%
Surface + stroma	40%	3%
Stroma only	23%	97%
Pseudomyxoma ovarii	Often prominent	Infrequent
Cytologic atypia	Adenoma-associated: minimal Carcinoma-associated: moderate to marked	Variable
Associated appendiceal or intestinal tumor	Very frequent (some cases obliterated or not sampled)	Rare
Prognosis (5-year survival)	Adenoma-associated: 75% Carcinoma-associated: <10%	99%

Modified with permission from Ronnett et al., ref. 337a.

from the associated appendiceal mucinous tumor. The immunohistochemical profile of these tumors is similar to the associated appendiceal mucinous adenoma with concordance between the two sites in the majority of cases. Specifically, these tumors display diffusely positive staining for CK20 and negative staining for CK7. In contrast, primary ovarian APMTs are all diffusely positive for CK7. In addition, they are often also positive for CK20, but the distribution of positivity is often patchy, in contrast to PMP cases in which CK20 staining is strong and diffuse.[337] Data from most molecular biologic studies that have addressed the issue have also supported the appendiceal origin of the ovarian tumors associated with PMP.[71,81] For example, in a series of 16 well-characterized cases of PMP, identical K-*ras* mutations were demonstrated in the ovarian and appendiceal neoplasms. A discordant pattern of allelic loss was demonstrated in a few cases, characterized by loss of heterozygosity in the ovarian tumor and not in the appendiceal adenoma; this most likely reflects the acquisition of additional genetic alterations as a part of tumor progression.[423]

Differential Diagnosis

The distinguishing morphologic features of DPAM and PMCA are shown in Table 18.12. As the mucinous tumors in the ovary of patients with PMP usually reflect secondary involvement, they must be distinguished from primary ovarian mucinous neoplasms. The distinguishing features of primary versus metastatic mucinous tumors in the ovary are compared above (see "APMT"), below (see "Mucinous Carcinomas"), in Table 18.13,[337a] and in Chapter 22 (Metastatic Tumors of the Ovary).

Clinical Behavior and Treatment

The behavior of mucinous tumors that are disseminated throughout the peritoneal cavity depends on tumor morphology. Cases designated DPAM are nearly always associated with appendiceal mucinous adenomas and constitute the classic description of pseudomyxoma peritonei found in the older literature, in which the behavior is characterized as slowly progressive, with reaccumulation of mucinous ascites, and compatible with prolonged survival if treated symptomatically by periodic evacuation of the ascites. The 5- and 10-year survival rates are 75% and 68%, respectively.[337b,338] In contrast, those cases characterized by morphologic features of carcinoma, designated PMCA, are metastatic mucin-secreting carcinomas from the appendix or colon and are associated with an aggressive clinical course; more 90% of patients die within 3 years. The latter group, by morphology and behavior, are high-grade carcinomas. It is clear, therefore, that the term pseudomyxoma peritonei, although useful as an operative and gross description, lacks sufficient specificity for use as a histologic diagnosis.[337a,338]

Mucinous Tumors with Mural Nodules

Mucinous neoplasms have been reported to contain mural nodules that display a wide variety of histologic features. A classification of mural nodules that includes six categories has been proposed,[19] but because only a few more than 50 cases have been reported, we prefer classifying them as either benign or malignant. Benign mural nodules may appear sarcoma-like or have features of leiomyoma. Sarcoma-like mural nodules range up to 6 cm in diameter and are composed of pleomorphic cells with bizarre nuclei, spindle cells, epulis-type giant cells, variably increased mitotic activity (often in the range of 5–10 MF/10 HPF including atypical mitotic figures), and acute and chronic inflammation (Fig. 18.90).

Malignant mural nodules usually occur in the wall of an APMT or a mucinous carcinoma. These lesions range up to 12 cm in diameter, and usually have the

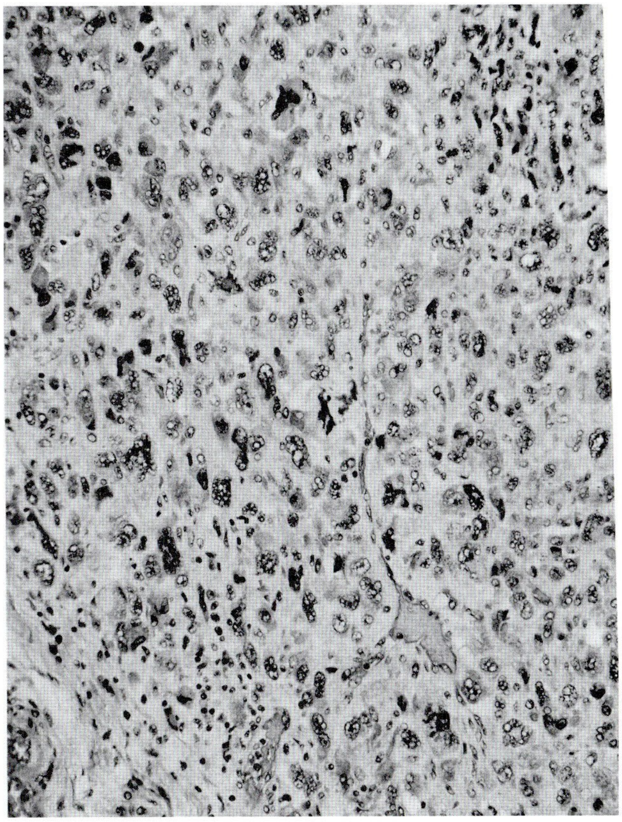

Fig. 18.90. Atypical proliferative mucinous tumor (not shown) **with sarcoma-like mural nodule.** The sarcoma-like mural nodule contains scattered giant cells with multilobated nuclei displaying marked atypia and abundant eosinophilic cytoplasm.

appearance of anaplastic carcinoma or sarcoma. Solid sheets of large rounded epithelial or spindle cells with high-grade nuclear atypia, and often with abundant eosinophilic cytoplasm, are characteristic.[383] Mucinous tumors with malignant mural nodules are probably best classified as variants of mucinous carcinoma or carcinosarcomas. Mural nodules of carcinoma or carcinosarcoma usually stain strongly for cytokeratins. Sarcoma-like mural nodules may stain focally for cytokeratins, but the clinical importance of this finding is unclear.[383] Limited data are available on the behavior of mucinous neoplasms with mural nodules. Benign mural nodules have not been reported to recur. Malignant mural nodules are fatal in 50% of cases.[19] Because of the markedly atypical histologic features that may be seen in mural nodules currently classified as benign and the limited number of cases reported, the data on their behavior should be regarded as preliminary.

Mucinous Carcinoma

After exclusion of metastatic tumors to the ovaries, primary ovarian *mucinous carcinomas* are uncommon and in fact are much less common than metastatic mucinous carcinomas.[330] Because of the limitations of the published data, as already discussed, clinical and pathologic features including proportion of ovarian neoplasms, bilaterality rates, and stage distribution are variable and may be unreliable. Mucinous carcinomas appear to comprise approximately 3.6% of ovarian epithelial neoplasms, 12% of ovarian mucinous neoplasms, and 11% of ovarian carcinomas, although these are probably overestimates because some of the studies from which these data are derived (see Table 18.3) were published before the recognition of the variety of patterns of metastatic mucinous carcinomas in the ovaries.

Clinical Findings

Mucinous carcinomas occur in women in the fourth to seventh decades; the mean age is 53 years. The clinical presentation is similar to that of benign mucinous neoplasms, inasmuch as the majority of cases are stage I. Therefore, these patients do not generally present with signs and symptoms of abdominal carcinomatosis as do the majority of women with serous ovarian carcinomas. Rather, as these tumors can be quite large, the clinical presentation is generally that of a large pelvic or abdominal mass and abdominal distension.

Operative Findings

Approximately 63% of patients with mucinous carcinoma have FIGO stage I disease. Nearly all stage I cases have unilateral ovarian involvement.[168] If microinvasive tumors are excluded from the carcinoma category, this figure drops to approximately 58%.[64,151,168,200,230,330] The proportion of stage I cases varies widely among studies,[454] a finding that reflects variation in criteria as well as the difficulty of distinguishing intraepithelial carcinoma from invasive carcinoma. Nearly all intraepithelial carcinomas have been stage I, but in one study there were several advanced-stage cases.[454] Ascites may occur, but the gelatinous, mucinous ascites characteristic of pseudomyxoma peritonei does not occur in association with primary ovarian mucinous tumors (see "Pseudomyxoma Peritonei").

Gross Findings

As mucinous carcinomas arise from atypical proliferative mucinous neoplasms, their gross appearance is similar. Mucinous carcinomas are typically large, cystic, and multiloculated. Solid areas and intracystic nodules are more common in carcinomas than in cystadenomas and APMTs. Rarely, the tumor is predominantly solid.

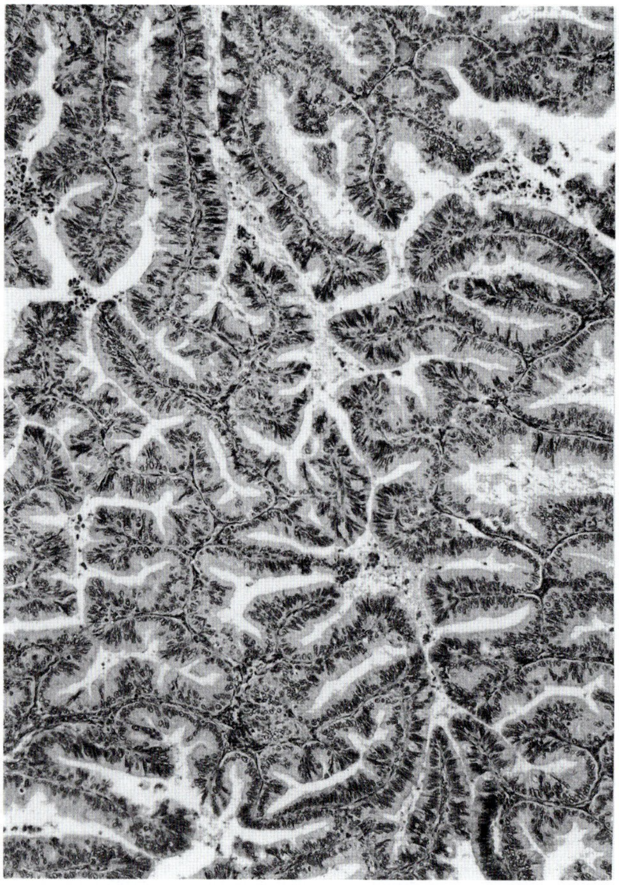

Fig. 18.91. Mucinous carcinoma, well-differentiated. Confluent glandular and papillary growth with loss of most of the intervening stromal support.

MICROSCOPIC FINDINGS

Invasive mucinous carcinomas resemble APMTs but display unequivocal stromal invasion measuring more than 5 mm. Stromal invasion in primary ovarian mucinous neoplasms is characterized by three different patterns: (1) a confluent glandular growth with crowded glands that merge together without intervening stroma (Fig. 18.91) and back-to-back cribriform glands with well-defined, sharply etched rounded spaces (Fig. 18.92); (2) clusters of single cells with abundant eosinophilic cytoplasm surrounded by clear spaces (see Fig. 18.86); and (3) glands of varying sizes infiltrating the stroma in a haphazard pattern (Figs. 18.93–18.95). A nodular pattern with glands and nests of tumor in a nodular arrangement surrounded by normal ovarian stroma is strongly suggestive of metastatic disease (Fig. 18.96).

Cytologic atypia is usually marked and characterized by an increased nuclear/cytoplasm ratio, irregularly clumped chromatin, and prominent nucleoli. The cytoplasm is scant and eosinophilic with irregular borders and occasional mucin droplets. Stratification is usually prominent but exceeds three cell layers in fewer than 50% of cases.[330] Necrosis is often present. Mitotic figures are usually prominent, with more than 5 per 10 high-power fields in most cases. Although there are few data on grading, most mucinous carcinomas are well differentiated.

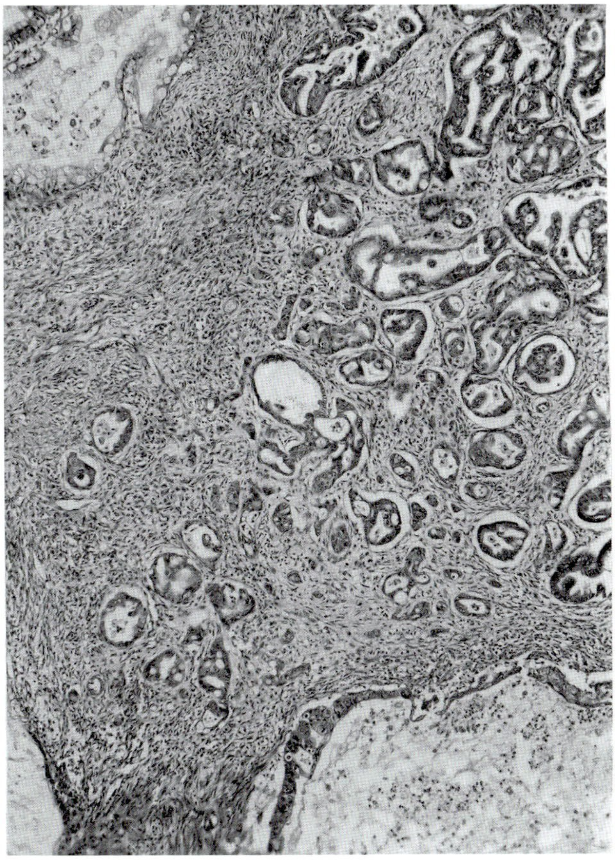

Fig. 18.93. Mucinous carcinoma, well-differentiated. Haphazard infiltrative pattern of mucinous glands of varying size and shape.

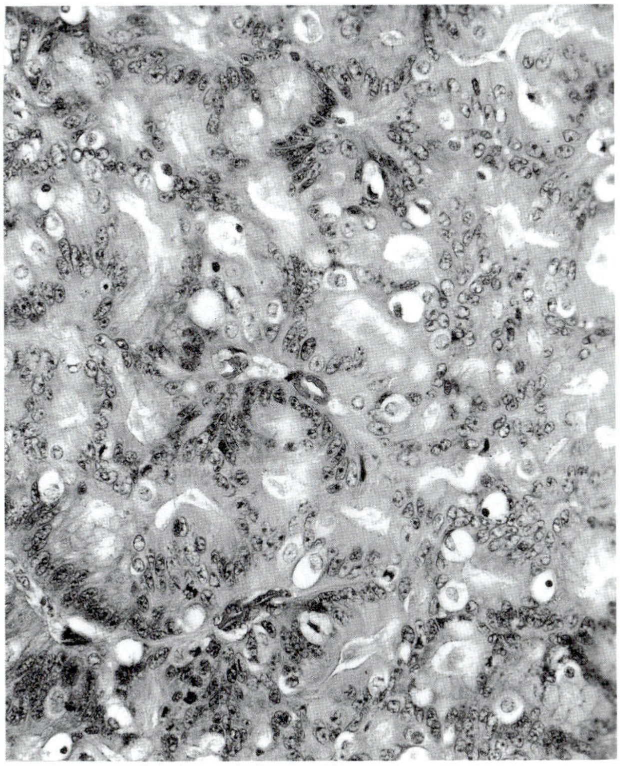

Fig. 18.92. Mucinous carcinoma, well to moderately differentiated. Confluent cribriform pattern with loss of intervening stroma.

IMMUNOHISTOCHEMISTRY

Mucinous carcinomas are positive for epithelial membrane antigen and cytokeratins, including AE1, AE3, and CAM 5.2; approximately half are positive for vimentin.[101] Positivity for other antibodies is as follows: CEA, 80%; B72.3, 88%; CK 7, 93%; CK 20, 69%; OC-125, 33%.[40,46,157,183,198,210,223,236,273,280,335,391,437,456] CK 18 and HAM-56 are usually positive. GCDFP-15 is usually negative.[268] Seventeen to 30% of cases contain Grimelius-positive argyrophil cells that are usually positive for serotonin and gastrin and are occasionally positive for somatostatin, pancreatic polypeptide, neurotensin, and chromogranin.[5,363] Fewer than 10% of tumors with argyrophil cells are positive for neuron-specific enolase.[363]

DIFFERENTIAL DIAGNOSIS

Before making a diagnosis of mucinous carcinoma of the ovary, it is imperative to exclude metastatic

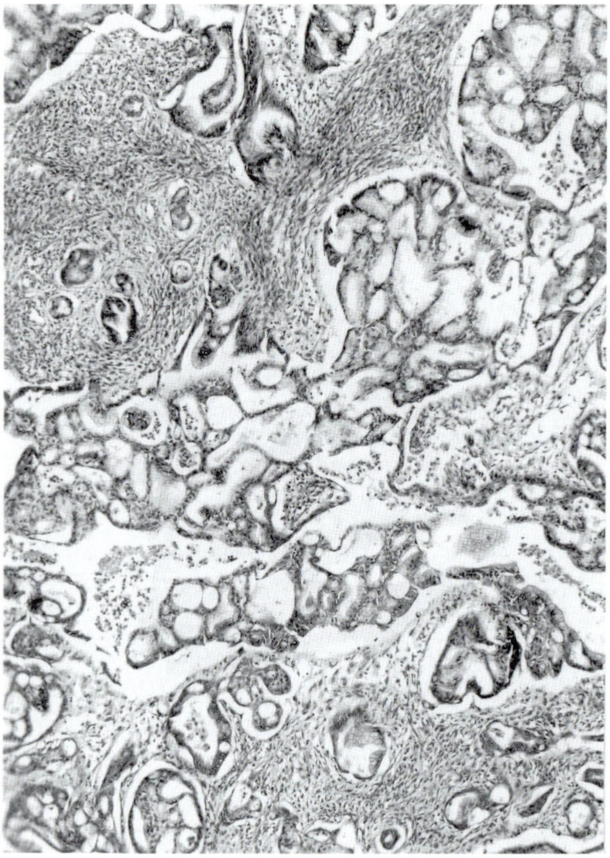

Fig. 18.94. Mucinous carcinoma, well-differentiated. Haphazard infiltrative growth of isolated glands and glands with a cribriform pattern.

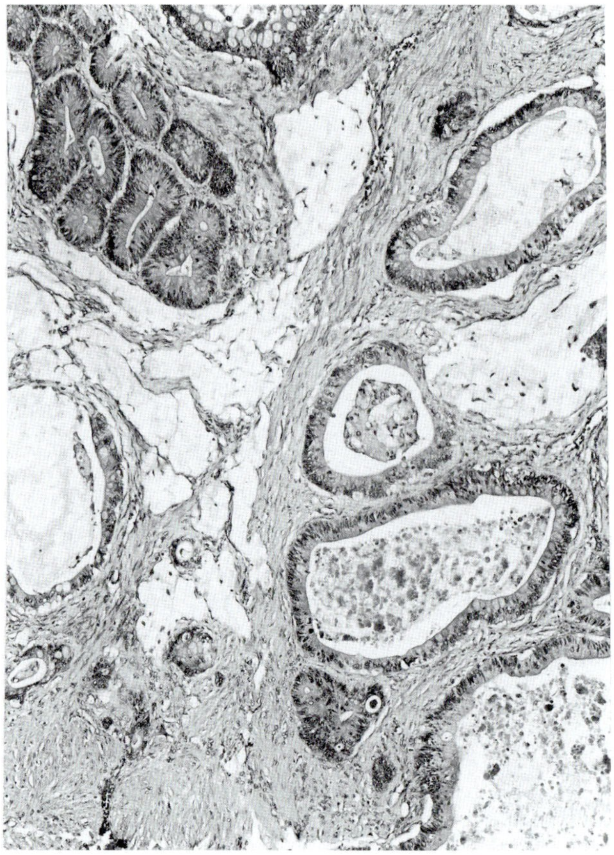

Fig. 18.95. Mucinous carcinoma, well-differentiated. Mucin has been discharged from some glands and is dissecting through the stroma. This simulates disseminated peritoneal adenomucinosis (DPAM), but the epithelium in this case is malignant.

mucinous carcinoma (see Chapter 22, Metastatic Tumors of the Ovary). Mucinous adenocarcinomas of the pancreas, biliary tract, colon, appendix, and cervix can mimic ovarian mucinous tumors.[91,226,335,479] The morphologic features of primary versus metastatic mucinous neoplasms in the ovary were detailed earlier (see "Pseudomyxoma peritonei" and "APMTs"; also see Chapter 22, Metastatic Tumors of the Ovary). Cytokeratins 7 and 20 are useful markers in the differential diagnosis with colonic carcinomas. Colonic tumors are usually (90%) negative for CK 7 and nearly always positive for CK 20.[337]

The distinction of APMT from mucinous carcinoma can be difficult. Stromal invasion must be identified to diagnose mucinous carcinoma; the various patterns of stromal invasion were discussed under "Microscopic Findings." If cytologically malignant features are present but unequivocal stromal invasion cannot be confidently identified, a diagnosis of APMT with intraepithelial carcinoma is warranted.

Rare examples of malignant tumors with a mucinous component that can be confused with ovarian mucinous carcinoma include the hypercalcemic type of small cell carcinoma and mucinous (goblet cell) carcinoid tumors; the latter tumor may rarely be primary[19a] but more commonly is metastatic from the gastrointestinal tract, usually the appendix. Twelve percent of hypercalcemic small cell carcinomas contain a neoplastic mucinous epithelial element.[480]

Clinical Behavior and Treatment

The overall prognosis of patients with mucinous carcinoma is better than that for serous carcinoma because a high proportion of patients present in stage I. Nonetheless, despite the differing clinical and pathologic features of ovarian serous and mucinous carcinomas, their behavior when stratified by stage is similar. Recurrence and mortality in stage I mucinous carcinoma occurs in 8%–12% of cases,[64,151,168,200,303,330] similar to well-staged stage I serous carcinomas. Advanced-stage mucinous carcinoma (FIGO III and IV) is uniformly fatal, as is serous carcinoma

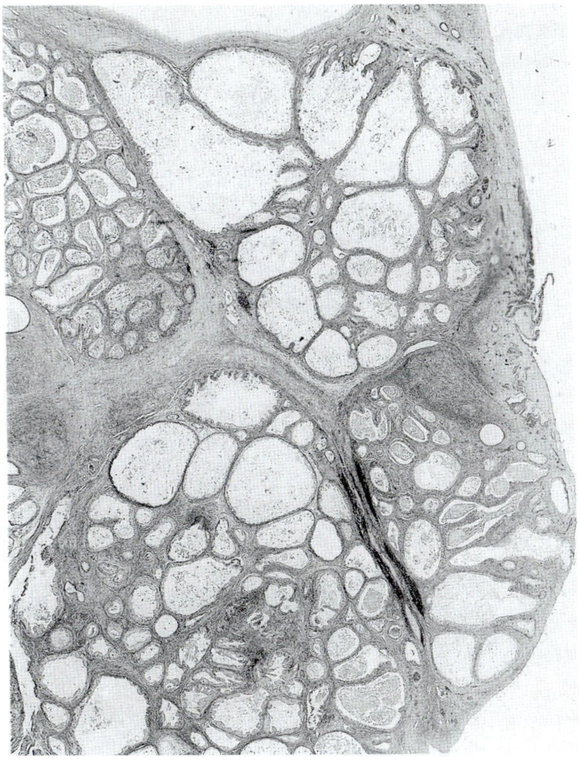

Fig. 18.96. Metastatic mucinous carcinoma. A nodular pattern of invasion is characteristic of metastatic adenocarcinoma to the ovary. This example of metastatic pancreatic carcinoma displays nodules of tumor composed of well-formed glands and aggregates of irregularly infiltrative glands surrounded by ovarian stroma. (Courtesy Brigitte M. Ronnett, M.D., Baltimore, MD.)

of advanced stage. Limited data are available on FIGO stage II tumors as only 10% of patients are in stage II. Similarly, few data are available on high-grade stage I mucinous carcinomas. Occult advanced-stage mucinous carcinoma is rare compared to serous carcinoma.[227]

Endometrioid Tumors

Most *endometrioid ovarian neoplasms* are carcinomas. Endometrioid adenofibromas and atypical proliferative endometrioid tumors are very uncommon, comprising less than 1% of ovarian epithelial neoplasms. Endometrioid carcinomas were first described in detail in 1964, but had previously been recognized as resembling tumors of the endometrium and were designated endometrial-like carcinomas in 1954. Molecular biologic studies have shown that endometrioid ovarian carcinomas have similarities with and differences from their uterine counterparts. For example, expression of the *p53* gene product, and allelic loss on 17q, are both significantly more common in the ovarian tumors than in the uterine tumors.[56] In contrast, both uterine and ovarian endometrioid carcinomas occasionally exhibit mutation of the β-catenin gene (see "Cellular and Molecular Biology").

Endometrioid Adenofibromas

Endometrioid adenofibromas are uncommon and are usually unilateral. The median age of women with these tumors is 57 years. The mean diameter is about 10 cm, and 17% are bilateral.[188] The external surface is smooth and the cut surface is densely fibrous, often with intermixed cystic areas creating a honecomb appearance similar to a serous cystadenofibroma (Fig. 18.97). The cysts contain clear or yellowish fluid. Microscopically, the dominant pattern is that of an adenofibroma or cystadenofibroma. The epithelial elements are arranged in branching tubular glands and cysts and usually resemble those of proliferative endometrium (Figs. 18.98 and 18.99). The epithelium lining the glands is tall and columnar with oval nuclei containing coarse chromatin and small nucleoli; the cytoplasm is basophilic to amphophilic. Sometimes, the nuclei

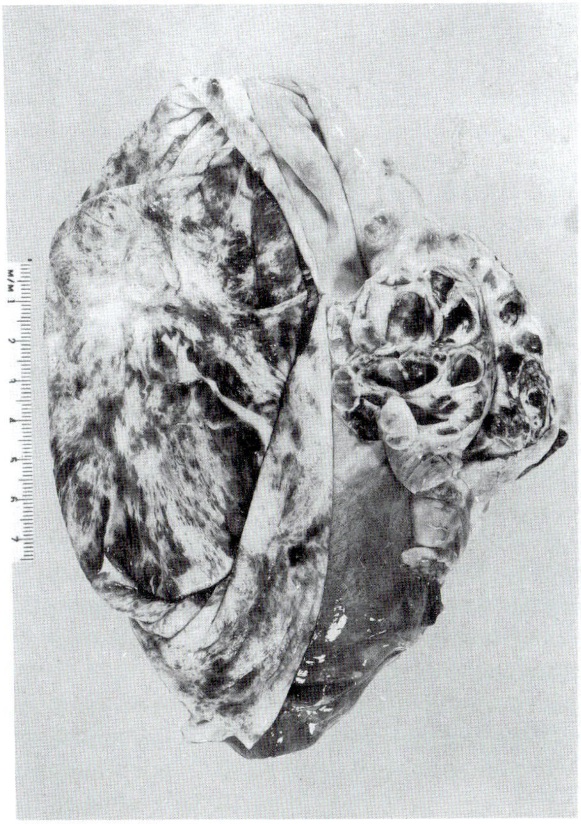

Fig. 18.97. Endometrioid adenofibroma. The tumor is predominantly cystic and can also be referred to as endometrioid cystadenofibroma.

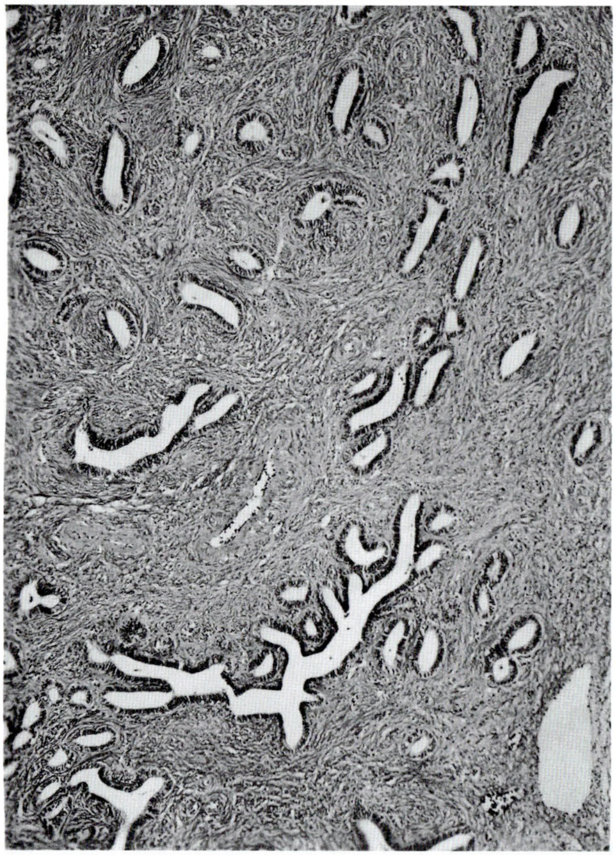

Fig. 18.98. Endometrioid adenofibroma. Proliferative-type endometrioid glands are widely dispersed in a dense fibrotic stroma.

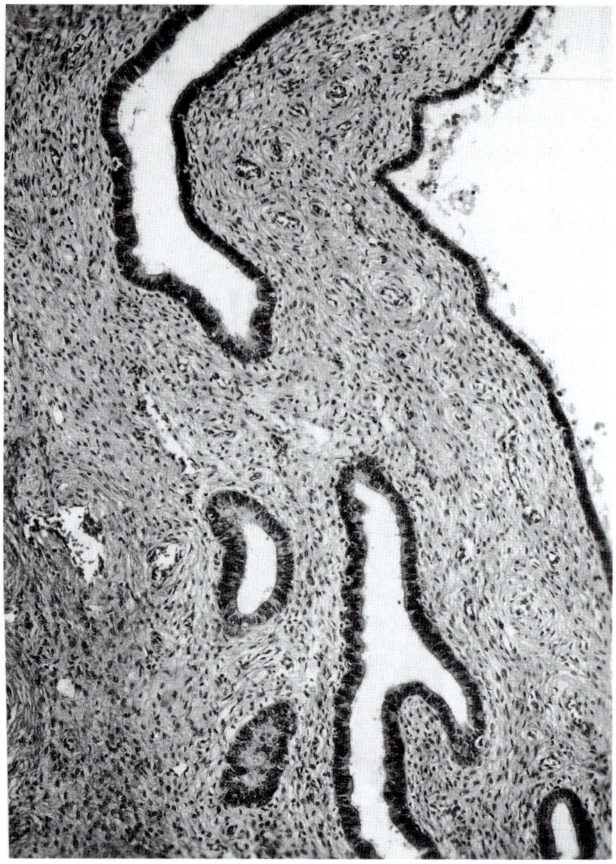

Fig. 18.99. Endometrioid adenofibroma. A single layer of tall columnar epithelial cells is present in a mildly cellular stroma.

resemble those of atrophic or inactive endometrium, with uniform, elongated dark nuclei and scanty cytoplasm. Mitoses are variable but usually rare. Secretory changes and focal squamous differentiation may be present. The stroma is usually densely fibrotic; focal areas may resemble ovarian cortex. Occasional endometrioid adenofibromas are associated with endometriosis. These tumors are benign, although rarely they may recur.

Atypical Proliferative Endometrioid Tumors (APET)

There is a spectrum of epithelial proliferation, glandular crowding, and cytologic atypia in *benign endometrioid neoplasms* ranging from mild atypia, mild glandular crowding, and epithelial stratification slightly beyond that seen in typical endometrioid adenofibromas to confluent epithelial proliferation lacking stromal support in areas up to 5 mm in diameter resembling atypical hyperplasia and well-differentiated adenocarcinoma of the endometrium. A variety of terms have been employed for these tumors, including proliferating or proliferative endometrioid tumor, atypical endometrioid adenofibroma, endometrioid tumor of borderline or low malignant potential, and atypical proliferative endometrioid tumor.[34,36,404] The criteria for these diagnoses have differed among these series. Because the behavior of all these tumors has been benign, we prefer to combine these groups and refer to them as *atypical proliferative endometrioid tumors* (APET).

Among three series, there were 96 patients with a mean patient age of 50 years. Five patients (5%) had bilateral tumors, and all but one were confined to the ovaries; one had a colonic "implant".[404] The mean tumor size was about 8 cm. The characteristic gross appearance is solid and cystic; the cyst fluid is usually hemorrhagic, brown or green. A few patients have had endometriosis and some have also had endometrial hyperplasia.

The two characteristic microscopic architectural appearances of APET are adenofibromatous and glandular/papillary. The glandular/papillary proliferation can show varying degrees of glandular complexity and crowding (Figs. 18.100 and 18.101). An underlying adenofibroma is often present. When the glandular proliferation becomes confluent, this is considered evidence of invasion by some experts but could also reasonably be considered examples of the upper end of the spectrum of atypical proliferative tumors, or APET with intraepithelial carcinoma, as other experts prefer. A confluent epithelial proliferation that exceeds 5 mm in diameter warrants a diagnosis of carcinoma according to one group.[36] The glands show crowding and mild or moderate cytologic atypia and epithelial stratification (Fig. 18.102); tufting and bridging may be present. Severe cytologic atypia warrants a diagnosis of intraepithelial carcinoma (Fig. 18.103).[36] Squamous metaplasia is present in up to half of cases (Figs. 18.104 and 18.105). The stroma is usually cellular with periglandular cuffing characterized by increased stromal cellularity around the glandular elements; however, these areas lack the stromal mitoses and atypia of adenosarcoma. Necrosis is common and is often confined to gland lumens or cysts. The single case with a colonic implant most likely represents an independent lesion arising in endometriosis.[286] All reported cases have had a benign behavior after a mean follow-up period of approximately 5 years.

Criteria for microinvasion in APETs differ among investigators. In two series, microinvasion was characterized by a haphazard infiltrative pattern in the stroma of epithelial cells, glands, and nests with cytologically malignant features. Among the five APETs with microinvasion reported in these series, all patients were alive and well 0.3–11 years postoperatively (mean, 5.3 years).[34,404] Different criteria employed by another group required one or more foci of confluent glandular growth, each measuring less than 5 mm, for a designation of APET with microinvasion[36] (Fig. 18.106). The five cases in that series had limited follow-up; all were alive but only two were known to be free of disease at 2 years of follow-up.[36] In summary, microinvasion, intraepithelial carcinoma, and confluence of glandular growth when limited in extent are atypical mor-

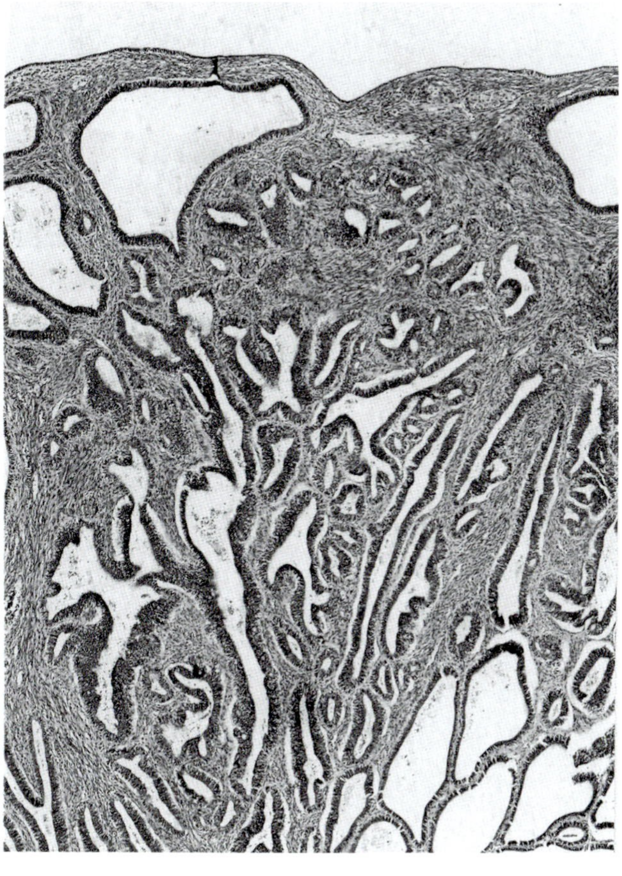

Fig. 18.100. Atypical proliferative endometrioid tumor (APET). This degree of gland crowding is the lower end of the spectrum of APETs and is similar to the degree of crowding seen in complex endometrial hyperplasia.

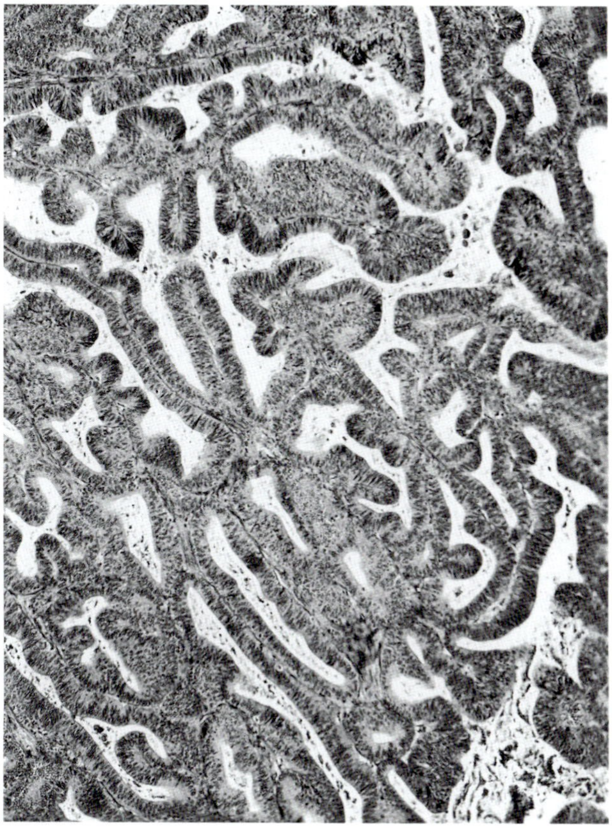

Fig. 18.101. Atypical proliferative endometrioid tumor. Back-to-back glands create a confluent pattern measuring less than 5 mm in diameter.

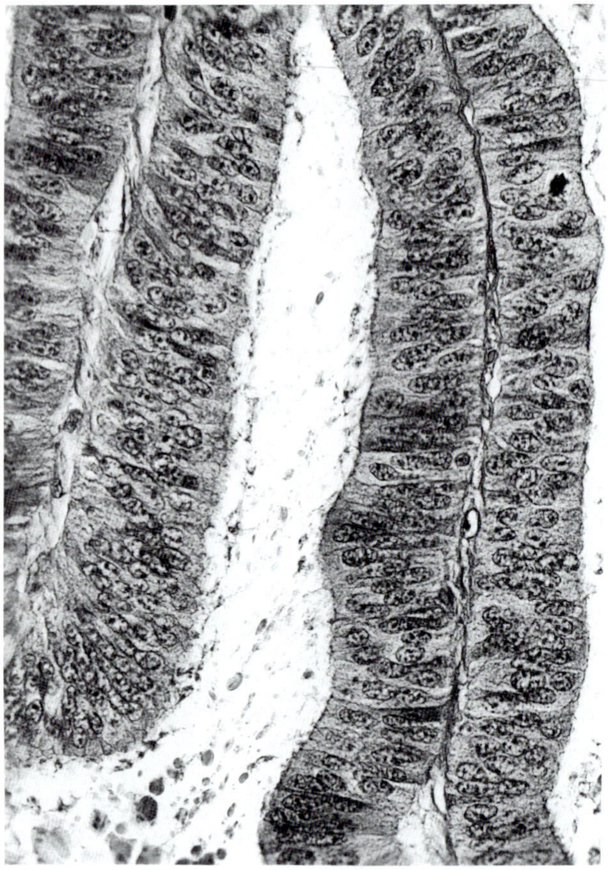

Fig. 18.102. Atypical proliferative endometrioid tumor. The cytologic features are characterized by nuclear rounding, coarsening of the chromatin, and stratification, similar to atypical endometrial hyperplasia. A mitotic figure is present in *upper right.*

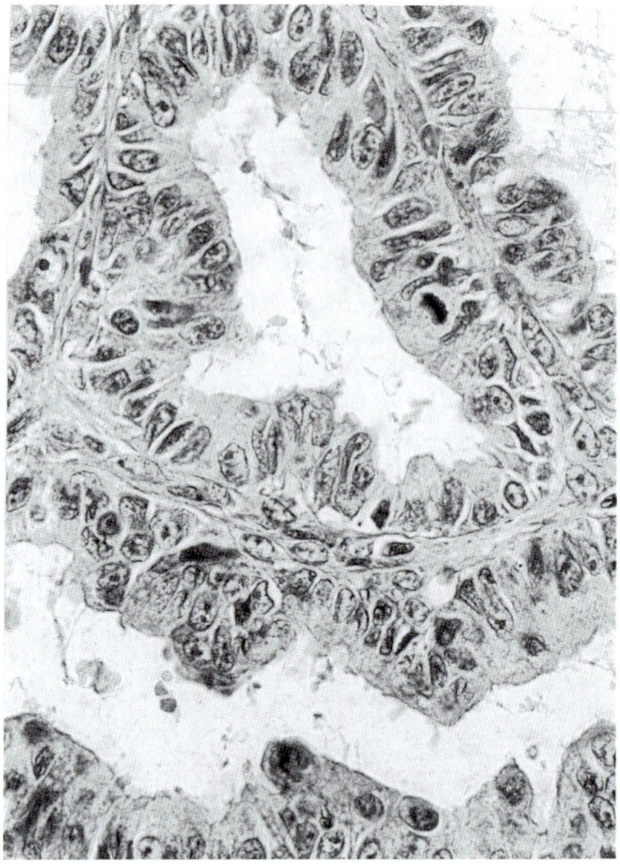

Fig. 18.103. Atypical proliferative endometrioid tumor with intraepithelial carcinoma. High-grade cytologic features and lack of invasion warrant a designation of intraepithelial carcinoma. (Reprinted by permission, ref. 36.)

phologic features and appear to be biologically benign, but only a few cases have been reported and clinical follow-up data are limited.

Endometrioid Adenocarcinoma

Endometrioid carcinomas comprise 5.7% of ovarian surface epithelial neoplasms, 17.5% of ovarian carcinomas, and 93% of endometrioid ovarian neoplasms.

Clinical Findings

These tumors are most common in the fifth and sixth decades, and the mean patient age is 56 years. The most common symptoms are abdominal distension and pelvic or abdominal pain. Abnormal vaginal bleeding is also frequent; this is, in part, related to the association of endometrioid ovarian carcinoma with endometrial hyperplasia and carcinoma (see following).[84] Most patients have an adnexal mass on pelvic examination. Another clinical association of significant interest is breast cancer. In a 1970 series, 7% of patients with endometrioid ovarian carcinoma also had breast cancer.[84]

Operative Findings

Tumor size ranges from 12 to 20 cm with a mean of about 15 cm. The stage distribution differs significantly from serous carcinoma. A high proportion of endometrioid carcinomas are diagnosed in stage I, 43% in a review of 874 cases from 19 series.[36] In the FIGO database, 52% of patients are diagnosed in stage I or II.[303] About 13% of early stage (FIGO I–II) cases are bilateral. Endometriosis, which may be extraovarian, in the ipsilateral or contralateral ovary, or within the tumor itself, is found in 15%–20% of patients.

Gross Findings

Endometrioid carcinomas have a smooth outer surface. On cut section, they are solid and cystic, with the cysts containing friable soft masses and bloody

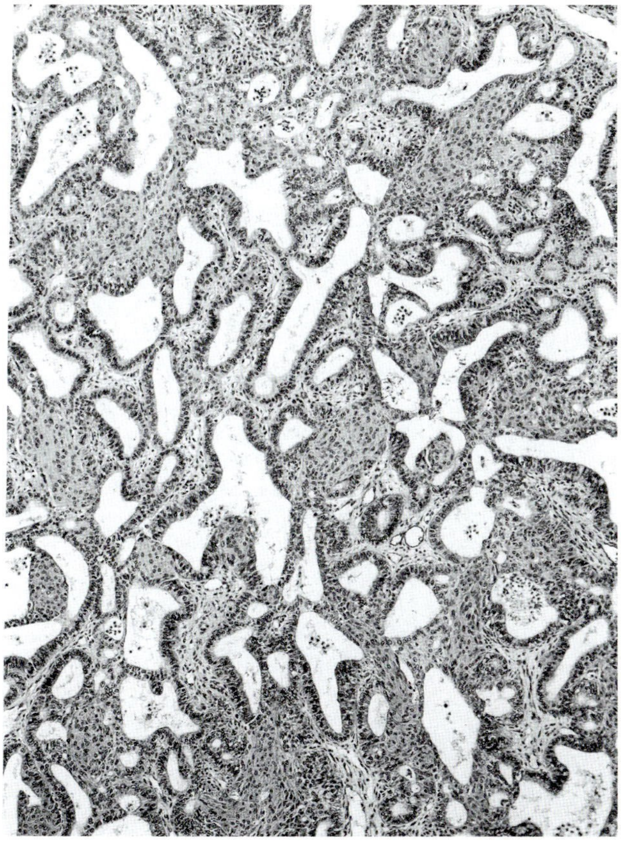

Fig. 18.104. Atypical proliferative endometrioid tumor. Squamous morules within glands.

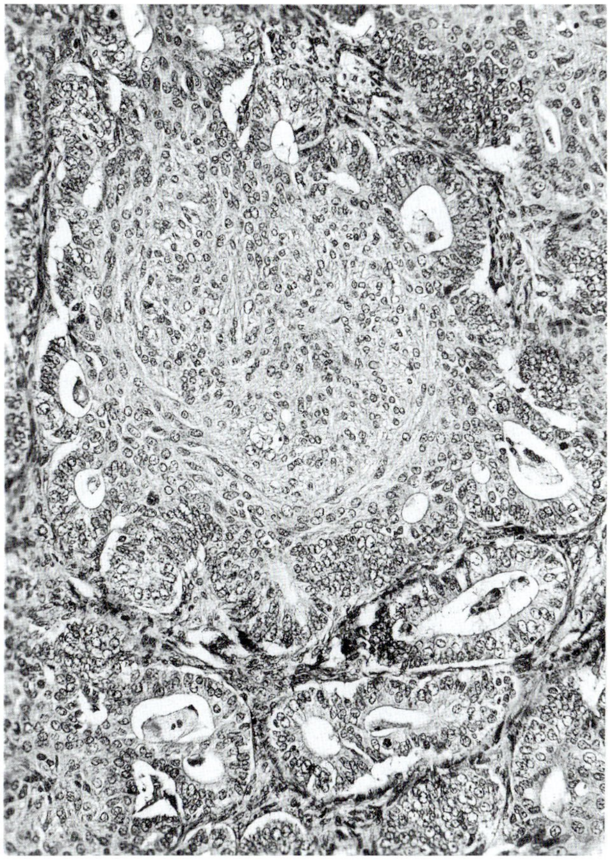

Fig. 18.105. Atypical proliferative endometrioid tumor. A squamous morule in the *center* displays a similar degree of nuclear atypia as the endometrioid glands.

fluid (Fig. 18.107). Cysts occasionally contain mucus or greenish fluid. Less commonly, the tumor is solid with extensive hemorrhage and necrosis. Tumors arising in endometriosis may display gross findings of an endometriotic cyst containing chocolate-colored fluid, with a solid nodule in the wall reflecting the focus of malignant transformation.

Microscopic Findings

Destructive infiltrative growth is definitional of ovarian carcinoma. Some authors also interpret a confluent glandular epithelial proliferation exceeding 5 mm as a pattern of invasion, which corresponds to a pattern of stromal invasion for tumors in the uterine corpus[36] (see Chapter 12, Endometrial Carcinoma).

Well-differentiated endometrioid adenocarcinoma accounts for the majority of cases and is characterized by a confluent or cribriform proliferation of glands (Fig. 18.108) lined by tall stratified columnar epithelium with sharp luminal margins (Fig. 18.109). A villoglandular growth pattern also occurs (Fig. 18.110). Mitotic figures are commonly seen. Squamous differentiation is present in up to 50% of cases (Figs. 18.108 and 18.109). Degeneration of squamous cells may induce a foreign body-type giant cell reaction in the stroma. Focal secretory changes are seen in up to one-third of cases (Fig. 18.111); this may result from an endogenous or exogenous progestin effect or may occur in the absence of hormonal stimulation. Areas of APET are commonly associated with endometrioid carcinoma.[36] Luteinized stromal cells are seen in 12% of cases.[84] Moderately and poorly differentiated endometrioid carcinomas show solid growth and complex glandular and microglandular patterns. Nuclear pleomorphism and mitotic activity are marked, and necrosis and hemorrhage are often prominent.

Approximately one-third of ovarian carcinomas classified as endometrioid based on the predominant epithelial component are mixed with other epithelial types.[219] A clear cell component is present in 20% and a papillary serous component is seen in 10% of cases.[84]

In addition to pure endometrioid carcinoma, which is the most common, several of the variants of endometrioid carcinoma of the uterine corpus also occur in the ovary; these include endometrioid car-

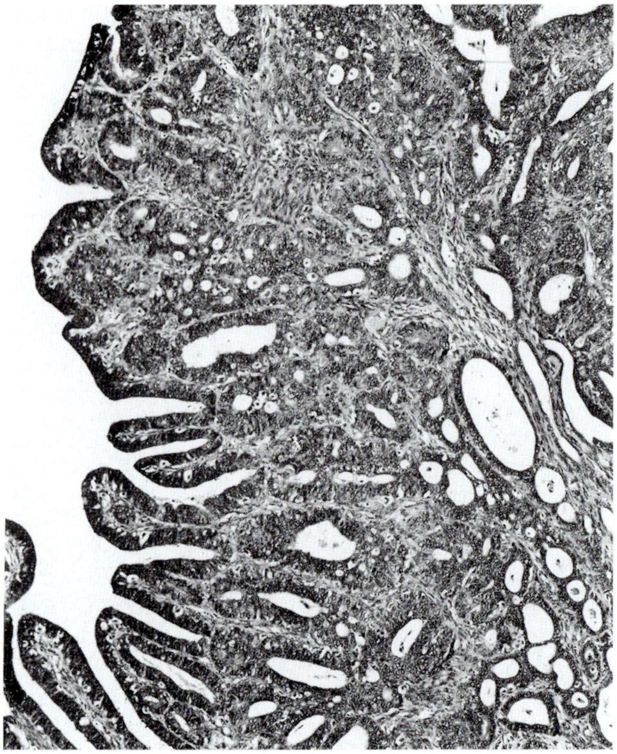

Fig. 18.106. Atypical proliferative endometrioid tumor with microinvasion. A villoglandular-type papillary pattern on the surface reflects an APET. A well-differentiated carcinoma characterized by a confluent glandular pattern arises from it. The confluent glandular pattern measured less than 5 mm and therefore qualified for microinvasion.

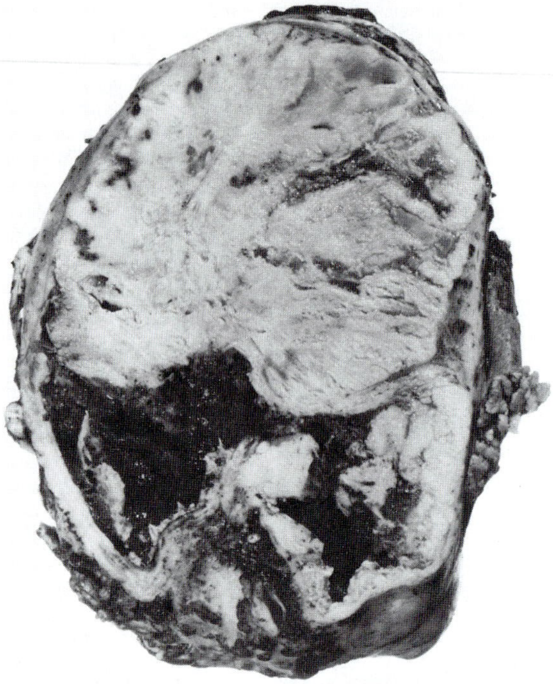

Fig. 18.107. Endometrioid carcinoma. A large solid nodule protrudes into a cyst, which contains altered blood

cinoma with squamous differentiation and secretory and ciliated variants. Other variant microscopic patterns of endometrioid ovarian carcinoma have been described. One variant has been designated sertoliform endometrioid carcinoma or endometrioid carcinoma resembling sex cord–stromal tumor by different authors. These tumors are characterized by a predominant pattern resembling a sex cord–stromal tumor, usually Sertoli–Leydig type, characterized by small tubular glands lined by cuboidal or low columnar epithelium, creating a resemblance to well-differentiated Sertoli cell tumor (Pick's tubular adenoma). Anastomosing solid tubules are often present[482] (Fig. 18.112). Moderately cellular fibrous stroma resembling the spindle cell component of stromal tumors may also be present. In a few cases, large islands of cells with round nuclei and scanty cytoplasm may mimic a granulosa cell tumor, but nuclear grooves are absent (Fig. 18.113). In nearly all these cases, foci of typical endometrioid carcinoma can be identified. In addition, transitional areas with mixed features are sometimes present. Among 30 patients in three series, 87% were FIGO stage I.[292,349,482]

Endometrioid carcinomas occasionally contain a prominent spindle cell component.[440] Other rare

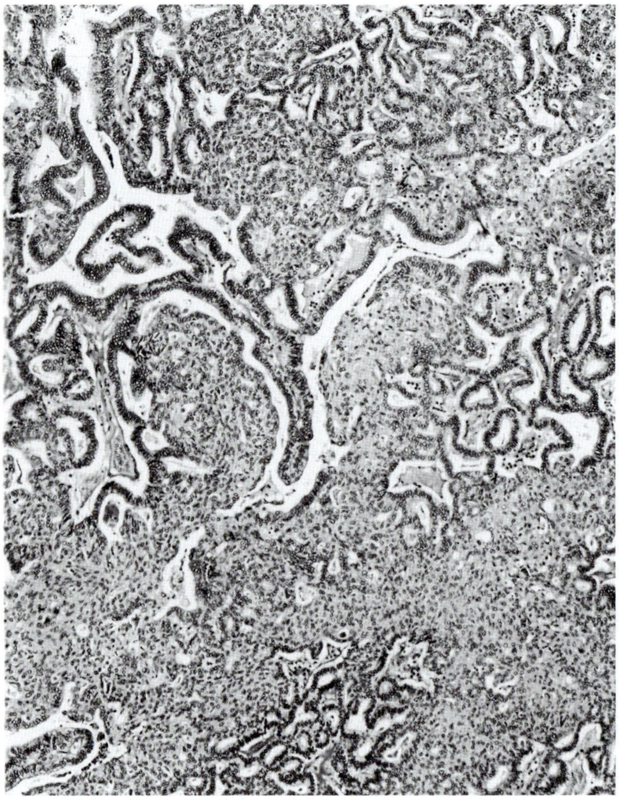

Fig. 18.108. Endometrioid carcinoma, well-differentiated. A confluent glandular pattern with extensive squamous differentiation.

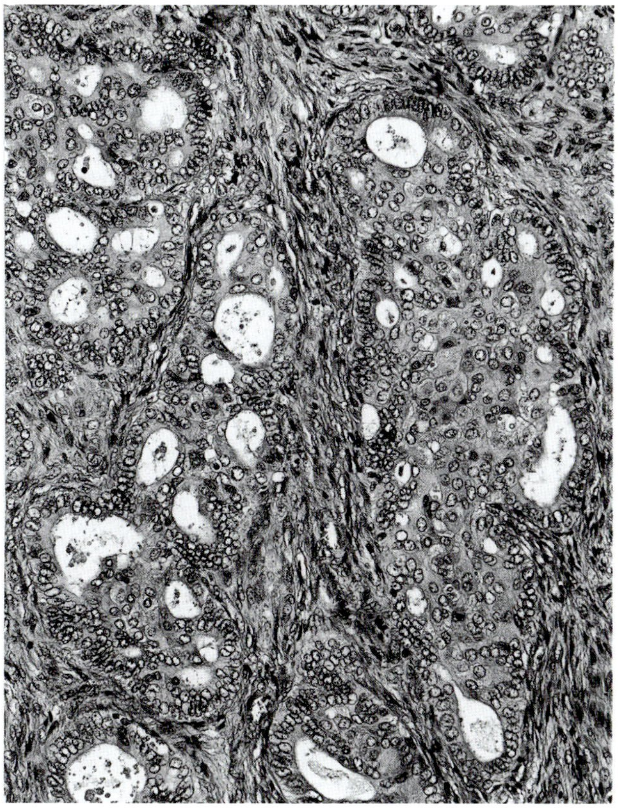

Fig. 18.109. Endometrioid carcinoma. Cribriform glandular growth with sharp luminal margins and squamous differentiation. (Reprinted by permission, ref. 36.)

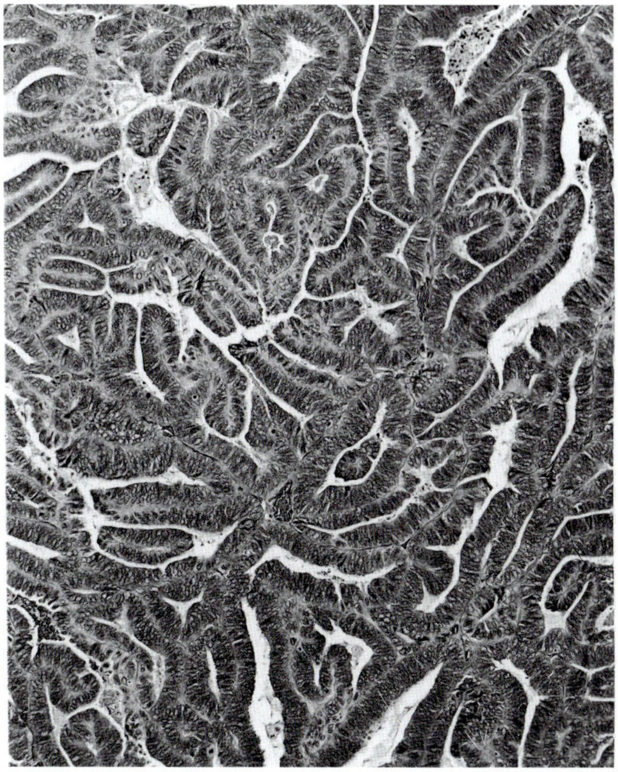

Fig. 18.110. Endometrioid carcinoma. A confluent villoglandular pattern is present. (Reprinted by permission, ref. 36.)

variants include oxyphilic endometrioid carcinoma[312] and a ciliated cell variant.[110]

Peritoneal keratin granulomas may be found in women with endometrioid ovarian carcinomas as a result of rupture of the neoplasm. The keratin within the metaplastic squamous component of these tumors incites a foreign body-type reaction. Follow-up of a limited number of these patients reveals that these lesions have no prognostic significance and therefore should not be considered evidence of advanced-stage disease.[201,286]

Immunohistochemistry

Endometrioid carcinomas stain strongly with epithelial markers, including keratins (CK 7, 97%; CK 20, 13% positive) and epithelial membrane antigen (EMA). Positivity for other markers are as follows: vimentin, 31%; B72.3, 86%; CEA, 30%; OC-125, 76%.[40,46,85,92,157,183,198,210,236,266,273,280,391,437,452] The immunohistochemical profiles of typical endometrioid carcinomas and sertoliform endometrioid carcinomas appear to be identical.[6,150,292,349] Forty-five percent of endometrioid carcinomas contain argyrophil cells; these cells rarely contain peptide hormones.[446]

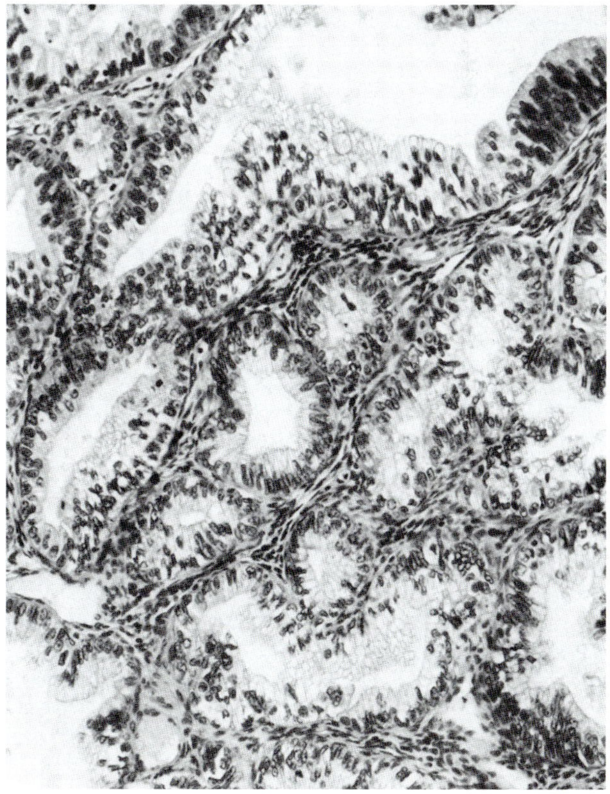

Fig. 18.111. Endometrioid carcinoma. Supranuclear vacuoles reflect secretory change in this well-differentiated endometrioid carcinoma.

Differential Diagnosis

The sertoliform or sex cord-like variant of endometrioid carcinoma creates the most problems in the differential diagnosis; this has important therapeutic and prognostic implications because sex cord–stromal tumors are usually benign and require no therapy if confined to the ovaries, whereas carcinomas usually require chemotherapy and have a worse prognosis. The age of the patient is helpful as the mean age of patients with Sertoli–Leydig cell tumors (SLCT) is 25 years, whereas women with endometrioid carcinoma are usually peri- or postmenopausal. In addition, hormonal manifestations such as virilization are often associated with sex cord–stromal tumors and generally not with endometrioid carcinomas. The retiform variant of SLCT, which occurs in adolescent girls, can closely simulate endometrioid or serous carcinoma, but this pattern is usually only focal. In most cases of sertoliform endometrioid carcinoma, extensive sampling of the tumor discloses areas of typical endometrioid carcinoma. Other helpful features include squamous metaplasia, which does not occur in sex cord–stromal tumors, an adenofibromatous component, which is typical of endometrioid carcinoma, and prominent luminal mucin, which occurs in endometrioid carcinomas.[482]

Although sex cord–stromal tumors often stain with keratins, they are almost always negative for EMA.[6,329] In addition, inhibin is a very useful marker that is positive in most granulosa and Sertoli–Leydig cell tumors, and nearly always negative in ovarian epithelial tumors, although inhibin may be positive in the nonneoplastic stromal cells within the tumor. Other epithelial markers including neuron-specific enolase, OM-1, and B72.3 are negative in granulosa and most Sertoli–Leydig cell tumors and positive in the majority of endometrioid carcinomas.[6] Occasionally, a prominent spindle cell component in an endometrioid carcinoma creates an appearance resembling a sex cord–stromal tumor, an adnexal tumor of wolffian origin, or a carcinosarcoma.[440] The spindle cells are generally uniform and have nuclear features resembling the glandular component. In most cases, the spindle cells merge imperceptibly with the glands. The spindle cells in the spindle cell variant of endometrioid carcinoma are strongly positive for keratins and EMA.[440]

Another common problem in the differential diagnosis of endometrioid carcinoma is metastatic

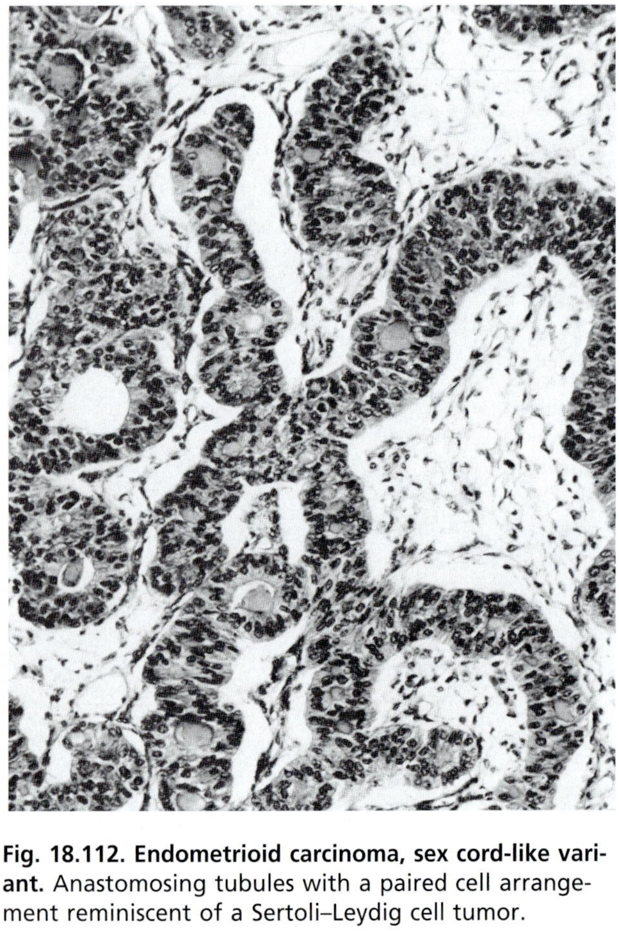

Fig. 18.112. Endometrioid carcinoma, sex cord-like variant. Anastomosing tubules with a paired cell arrangement reminiscent of a Sertoli–Leydig cell tumor.

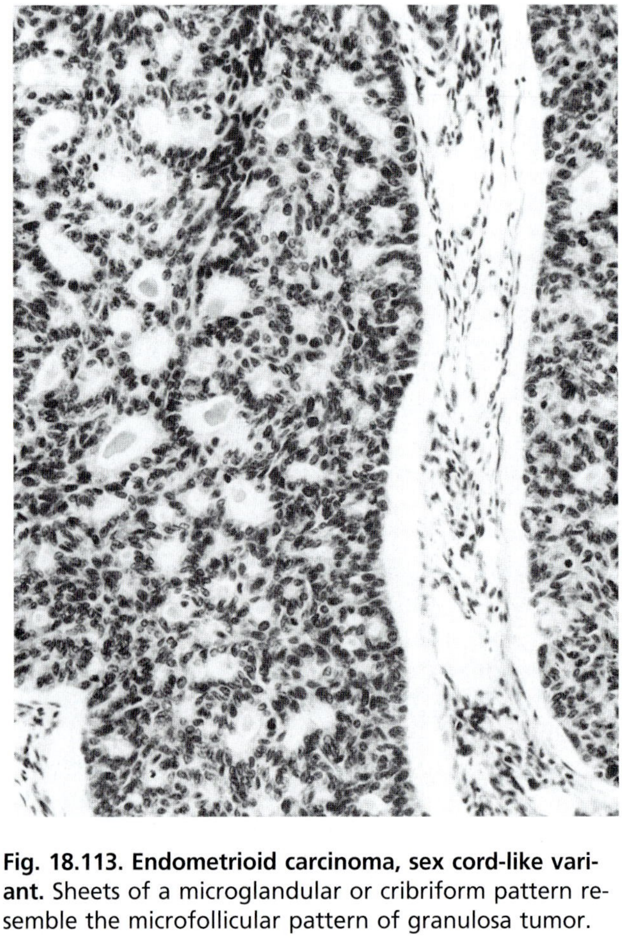

Fig. 18.113. Endometrioid carcinoma, sex cord-like variant. Sheets of a microglandular or cribriform pattern resemble the microfollicular pattern of granulosa tumor.

adenocarcinoma, particularly metastatic adenocarcinoma from the colon. Colonic metastases to the ovaries are often cystic and grossly mimic primary ovarian neoplasms. Useful features in the distinction are a characteristic "garland" pattern characterized by cysts lined by cytologically malignant tall columnar cells with bridging and cribriforming, in addition to bilaterality and surface involvement.[91,226] Although extensive "dirty necrosis" has also been cited as a feature of metastatic colonic carcinoma, this type of necrosis, characterized by abundant basophilic karyorrhectic nuclear debris intermixed with eosinophilic necrotic material, often in a geographic or zonal distribution, is often seen in primary ovarian carcinomas and therefore is of limited value.[92] The immunoperoxidase panel of CK7/20 can be of value in the distinction of primary ovarian versus metastatic colonic carcinoma.

Clinical Behavior and Treatment

It has often been stated that endometrioid carcinomas of the ovary have a better prognosis than typical serous carcinomas of the ovary. However, this is largely if not completely because of the high proportion of cases presenting in stage I. When stratified by stage, essentially all subtypes of ovarian carcinoma have a similar prognosis.[303] The apparent favorable prognosis may also be due, in part, to a high proportion of grade I cases, although data on the influence of grade on prognosis are less clear (see "Prognostic Factors"). Treatment for endometrioid carcinoma is generally the same as that for other ovarian carcinomas. However, progestational agents, antiestrogens, tamoxifen, and other hormonal therapies have been used with limited success in previously treated endometrioid carcinomas; 10%–15% response rates have been reported. There may be a correlation between the presence of steroid hormone receptors in tumor tissue and response rates, but data are limited.[297] Hormonal therapy may be an option for treatment of recurrence in patients who have failed or cannot tolerate chemotherapy or surgery.

Endometrioid Carcinoma Associated with Uterine Endometrial Carcinoma

Approximately 14% of women with endometrioid ovarian carcinoma also have endometrial cancer of the uterine corpus.[84,149,206,208,254] Endometrial hyperplasia is also commonly present. As both tumors are often well-differentiated endometrioid adenocarcinomas, they usually resemble each other, and excluding the possibility that the ovarian tumor is metastatic can be a problem; usually this can be determined on the basis of a careful evaluation of the clinicopathologic features. If the uterine endometrial tumor is low grade with no or only inner-half myometrial invasion, its metastatic potential is very low and the ovarian tumor can confidently be regarded as independent. If the endometrial tumor is high grade or deeply myoinvasive, the features of the ovarian tumors come into play. Bilaterality and a multinodular pattern, as well as other patterns characteristic of metastatic disease (see Chapter 22, Metastatic Tumors of the Ovary), indicate metastatic tumor.[447] Close association of the ovarian tumors with either an underlying adenofibroma or endometriosis can also provide evidence that the ovarian tumor is independent.

Follow-up of patients considered to have independent primary tumors also supports their independence, because most of these patients survive without recurrence, a finding compatible with stage I endometrial and ovarian carcinomas but not with a stage III endometrial cancer.[111,302,319,447]

Molecular studies can be of value in difficult cases. One group found selective loss of heterozygosity at two loci in only one of the two tumor sites in 8 of 13 cases, supporting the interpretation that these 8 cases were independent primary tumors.[113] Another useful approach is examination of the pattern of X-chromosome inactivation, or mutations in the K-*ras* and *p53* genes; 2 of 5 cases studied had different findings, indicating independent primaries.[129]

Endometrioid Carcinoma Arising in Endometriosis

On average, 15%–20% of endometrioid carcinomas of the ovary are associated with endometriosis, which may occur within the tumor, the ipsilateral or contralateral ovary, or elsewhere. The frequency can be as high as 42%.[130] In only a small minority of cases, however, can direct continuity from endometriosis to atypical hyperplasia to carcinoma be demonstrated.[272] This connection is most commonly seen in the lining of an endometriotic cyst, which may contain a thickening of the cyst wall or a solid nodule protruding into the cyst. The mean age of women with endometrioid carcinoma associated with endometriosis is 5–10 years younger than when unassociated with endometriosis.[130,272,360] Tumors associated with endometriosis, and particularly those arising in an endometriotic cyst, are usually well differentiated and stage I, and therefore the prognosis is excellent.[439] On rare occasions, a limited atypical epithelial proliferation in an endometriotic cyst raises the differential diagnosis of atypical hyperplasia similar to the type seen in the uterine corpus versus well-differentiated endometrioid adenocarcinoma. In such cases, criteria for this distinction have been modified from those used in the uterine corpus.[386]

Clear Cell Tumors

The müllerian nature of *clear cell tumors of the ovary*, previously thought to be of mesonephric origin and referred to as mesonephroma, is supported by the close association with endometriosis, their frequent admixure with endometrioid carcinoma, the occurrence of identical tumors in the endometrium, and their origin in vaginal adenosis in DES-exposed women.[383] Most clear cell neoplasms of the ovaries are carcinomas; *clear cell adenofibromas* and *atypical proliferative clear cell neoplasms* are rare.

Clear Cell Adenofibromas

Among approximately 12 reported cases of benign clear cell tumors, the mean age is 45 years.[30,188,348] One case was bilateral. The median diameter was 12 cm. The tumors display a smooth lobulated external surface, and the cut surfaces have a fine honeycomb appearance with minute cysts embedded in firm rubbery stroma ("parvilocular"). The cyst fluid is clear. Microscopically, the tumor is characterized by tubular glands lined by one or two layers of peglike or hobnail cells that bulge into the lumen (Fig. 18.114). The cytoplasm is either scanty, often in the hobnail cells, or abundant clear, granular, or eosinophilic in the large polyhedral cells. Nuclear atypia and mitotic activity are minimal. The stroma is compact and fibrocollagenous (Fig. 18.115). The apical cell borders and lumens often contain mucin. The cytoplasm usually contains glycogen. The clinical behavior is benign.

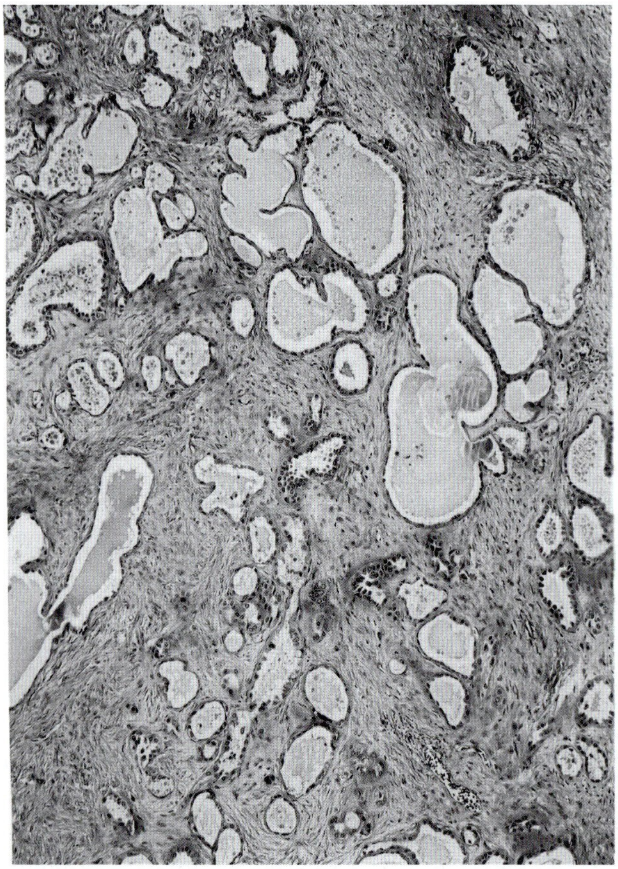

Fig. 18.114. Clear cell adenofibroma. Glands and tubules, some dilated and filled with pale eosinophilic secretions, are embedded in a dense fibrous stroma. The glands are only slightly crowded and lack a haphazard infiltrative pattern.

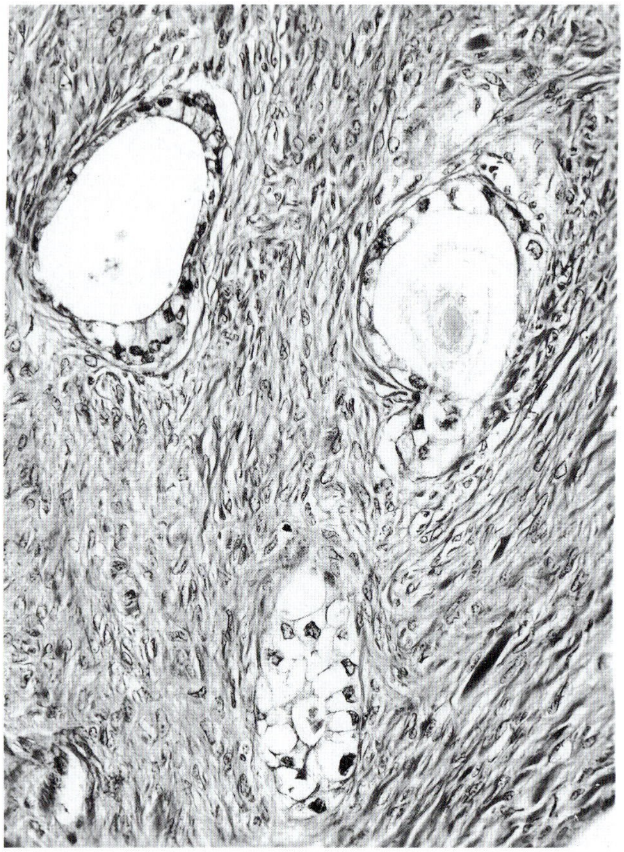

Fig. 18.115. Clear cell adenofibroma. Glands lined by epithelium with clear cytoplasm and minimal cytologic atypia are embedded in a fibrous stroma.

Atypical Proliferative Clear Cell Tumors (APCCT)

Among approximately 30 cases of *APCCT* (clear cell adenofibroma of borderline malignancy or low malignant potential) in the literature,[30,348,354] the mean age is 60–70 years. The mean tumor diameter is about 15 cm. The gross appearance is similar to that of the clear cell adenofibroma, but in addition there are softer and fleshier areas (Fig. 18.116). Microscopically, the architecture is similar to the clear cell adenofibroma. The tumor has greater epithelial proliferation and atypia than the adenofibroma and lacks stromal invasion (Fig. 18.117). The cell types lining the glands and cystic spaces are similar to those in

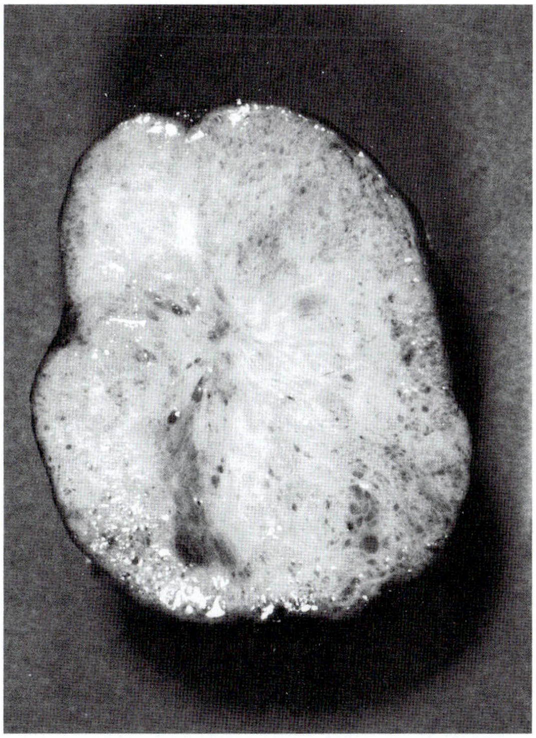

Fig. 18.116. Atypical proliferative clear cell tumor. Solid neoplasm displays a honeycomb pattern on cut surface.

benign tumors but display significant nuclear atypia with coarse chromatin clumping, prominent nucleoli, and mitotic activity up to 3 MF/10 HPF. The epithelium often displays stratification and budding; true papillary structures are uncommon (Fig. 18.118). Small solid nests of clear cells may be present and can raise the possibility of stromal invasion.

Peritoneal "implants" as occur in the more common atypical proliferative serous tumor have not been described with APCCTs. Among the limited reported cases, there is one alleged recurrence[30] and no tumor deaths. Accordingly, we prefer the term atypical proliferative clear cell tumor for these neoplasms.

Clear Cell Carcinomas

Clear cell carcinomas comprise 2.4% of ovarian epithelial neoplasms and 7.4% of ovarian carcinomas.

Clinical Findings

The mean age of patients with clear cell carcinoma is 57 years. Symptoms usually relate to a pelvic or abdominal mass. Interestingly, clear cell carcinoma is the most common epithelial ovarian neoplasm to be associated with paraneoplastic hypercalcemia (see Chapter 19).

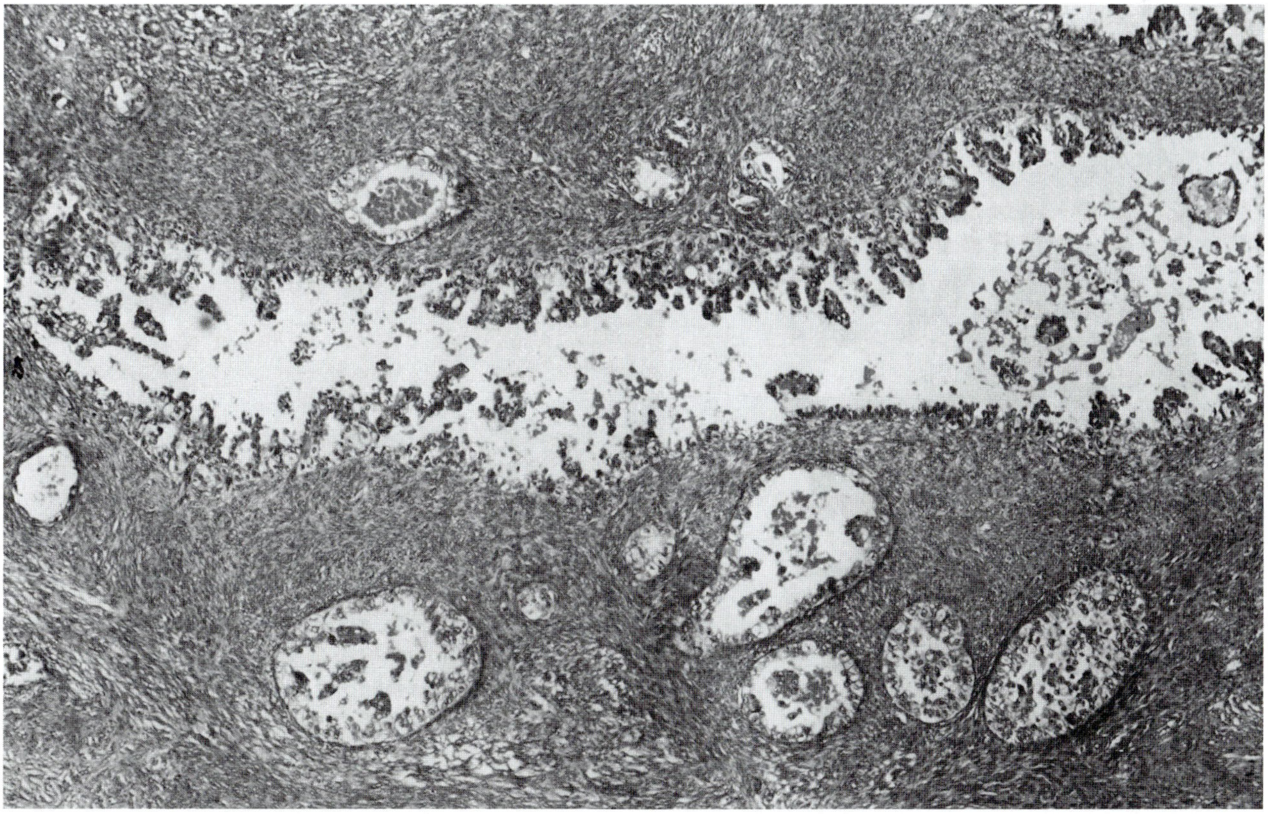

Fig. 18.117. Atypical proliferative clear cell tumor. Tubules are lined by epithelium displaying stratification, micropapillae with budding, and mild cytologic atypia. There is no stromal invasion.

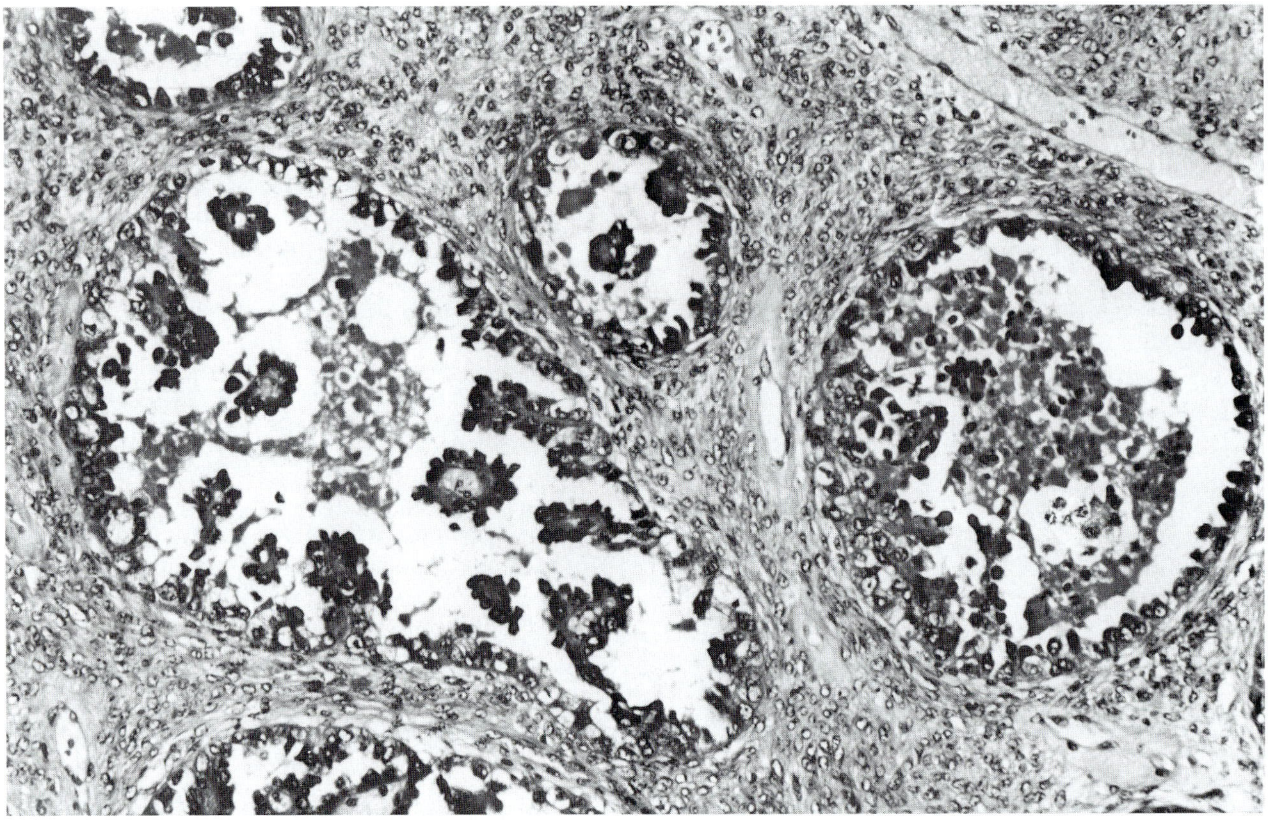

Fig. 18.118. Atypical proliferative clear cell tumor. Tubules are lined by cells with a hobnail pattern, epithelial stratification, and mild cytologic atypia.

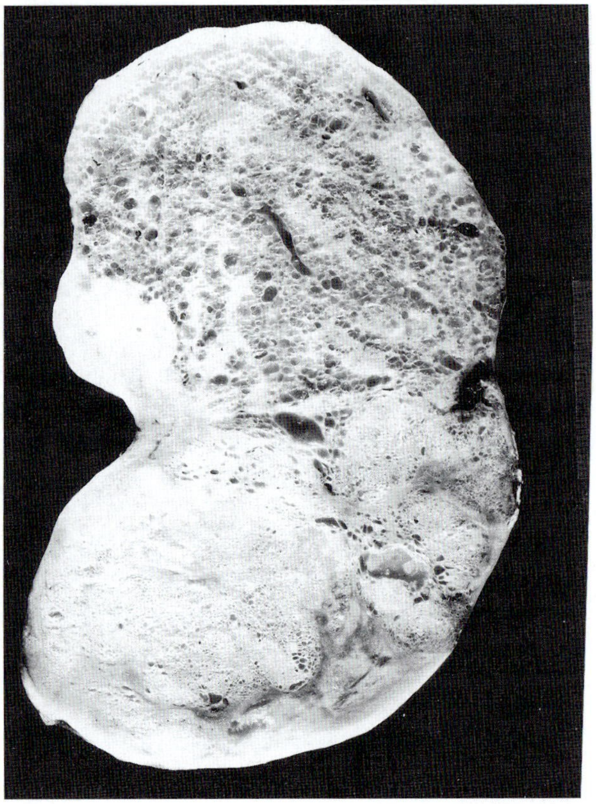

Fig. 18.119. Clear cell carcinoma. Solid neoplasm with a honeycomb cut surface resembles its benign and atypical proliferative counterparts.

Operative Findings

As the relationship with endometriosis is strongest for clear cell carcinoma among all types of ovarian carcinoma, endometriotic implants are commonly present in close proximity to the tumor or elsewhere in the pelvis or abdomen. Approximately half of patients present in FIGO stage I and 15% in stage II.[303] Four percent of stage I cases are bilateral.

Gross Findings

Tumors range up to 30 cm in diameter with a mean of about 15 cm. Although they may be solid and fibrous with a honeycomb cut surface resembling benign and atypical proliferative clear cell tumors (Fig. 18.119), more commonly the cut surfaces reveal a thick-walled unilocular cyst with multiple yellow-beige fleshy nodules protruding into the lumen, or a multiloculated cystic mass with cysts containing watery or mucinous fluid. Tumors arising in endometriosis may display features of an endometri-

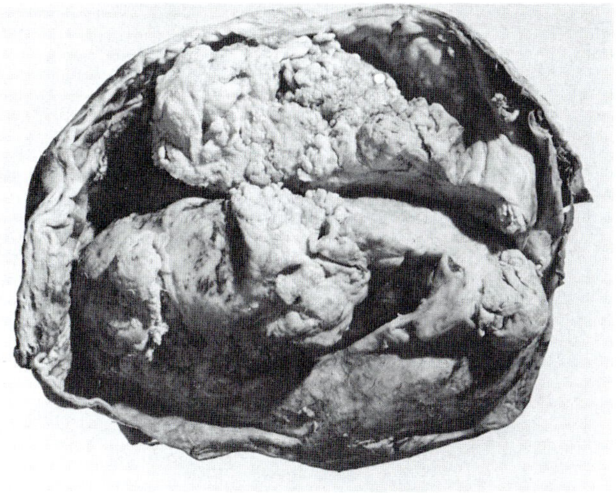

Fig. 18.120. Clear cell carcinoma. Unilocular cystic neoplasm with large nodules protruding into the lumen.

otic cyst, which typically contains chocolate-brown fluid, and a thickened, polypoid, or nodular area in the wall reflecting the area of malignant transformation (Fig. 18.120).

Microscopic Findings

Clear cell carcinomas display several different patterns, which often occur together.[83,219,287,382] The most common patterns are solid and tubulopapillary. The solid pattern is characterized by sheets of polyhedral cells with abundant clear cytoplasm separated by delicate fibrovascular septae or dense hyalinized fibrotic stroma (Fig. 18.121). The tubulopapillary pattern is characterized by papillae with varying degrees of complexity (Fig. 18.122). The fibrovascular cores of the papillae are often hyalinized. In fact, the hyalinized and homogeneous eosinophilic stromal fibrosis is a very characteristic feature of this tumor and is found in almost all cases. This hyaline stroma probably reflects basement membrane-type matrix production. One report suggested that papillary areas and areas with high-grade nuclear features most often display this matrix in comparison to areas displaying the other architectural patterns and grade 1 nuclear features.[259] Complex tubules and cysts may be intermixed with the papillae, creating a tubulocystic pat-

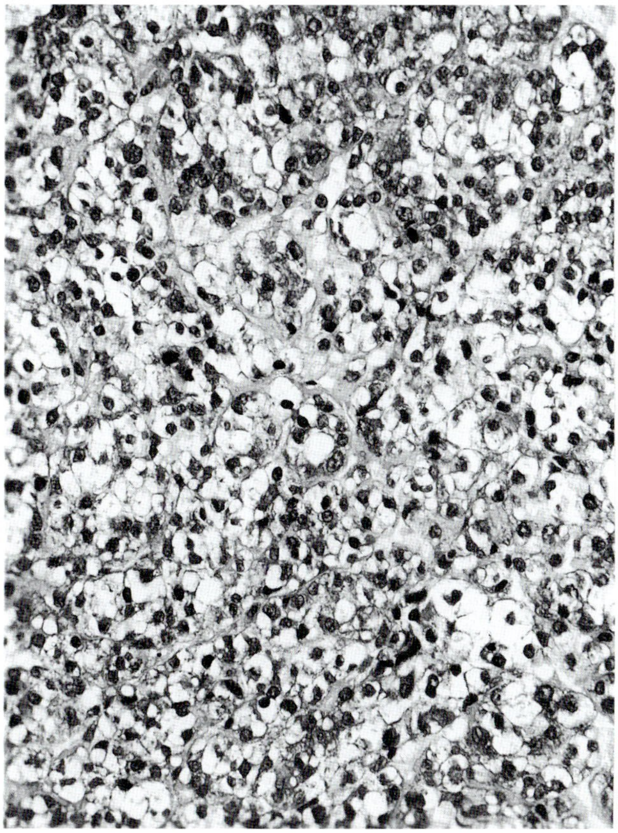

Fig. 18.121. Clear cell carcinoma. Solid sheets of cells with clear cytoplasm.

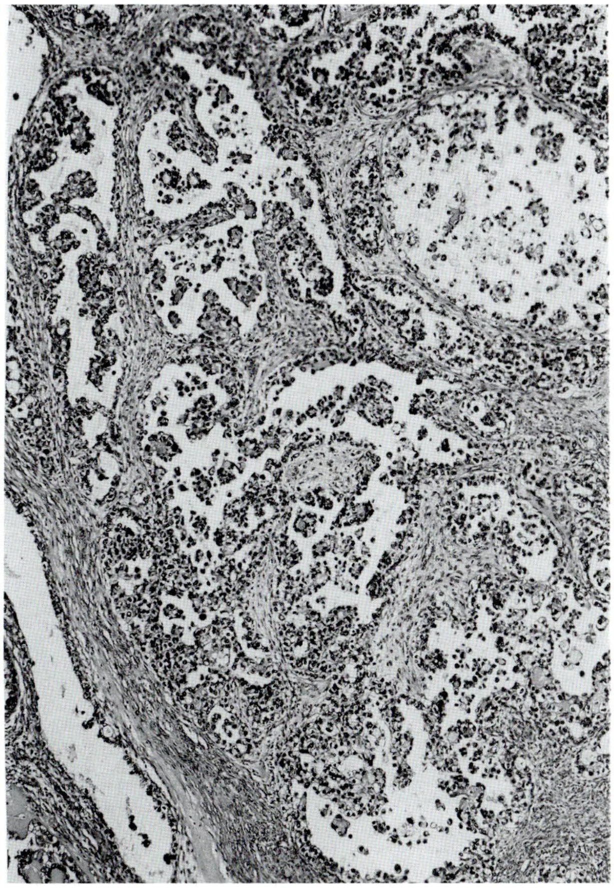

Fig. 18.122. Clear cell carcinoma. A complex tubulopapillary pattern.

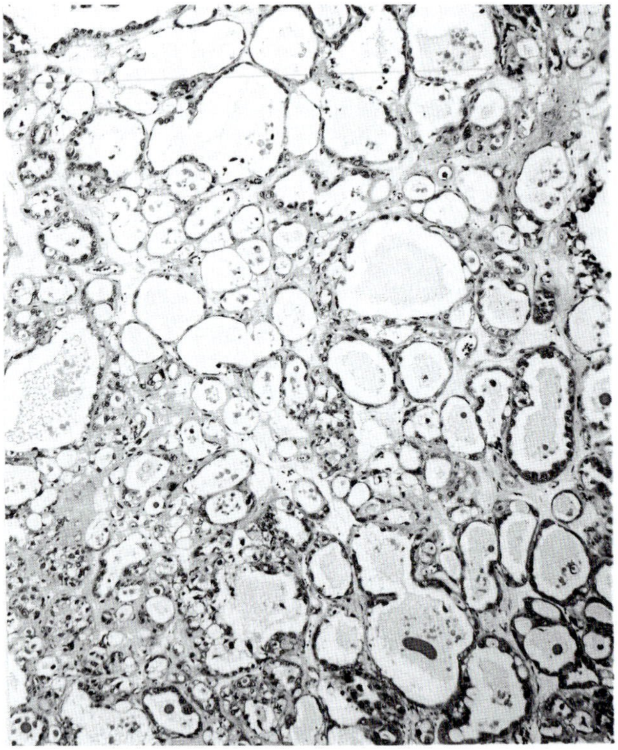

Fig. 18.123. Clear cell carcinoma. The tubulocystic pattern. The tubules are lined by flattened epithelial cells that appear deceptively bland.

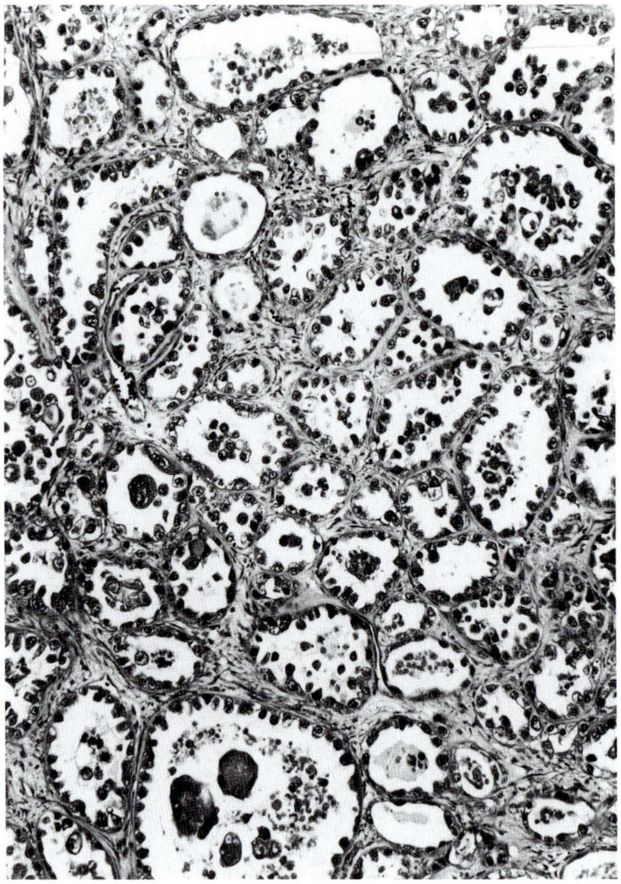

Fig. 18.124. Clear cell carcinoma. The tubulocystic pattern. Most of the cells lining the tubules are hobnail shaped.

tern (Figs. 18.123 and 18.124). The cell borders are usually prominent, and the nuclei vary from small and rounded or angular (Fig. 18.125) to large and pleomorphic with large prominent nucleoli (Figs. 18.126 and 18.127). The cytoplasm is filled with glycogen. In addition, intracytoplasmic mucinous inclusions may be present.[289] In the tubulopapillary pattern, the cells are often columnar with a hobnail appearance, with the nucleus protruding from the papillae, gland, or cyst into the lumen (Figs. 18.124 and 18.126). Occasionally, the epithelium lining the glands and cysts is flattened. A less common appearance of the cytoplasm is granular and eosinophilic. When this cytologic feature is diffuse, the term oxyphilic clear cell carcinoma is appropriate[484] (Fig. 18.128). The majority of clear cell carcinomas contain eosinophilic or hyaline cytoplasmic globules that are PAS positive[8] (Fig. 18.129). Mitotic activity is often prominent. Necrosis, hemorrhage, and stromal lymphocytic infiltrates are variable. Luteinized stromal cells and microcalcifications are occasionally present.

On average, 30%–35% of ovarian clear cell carcinomas are associated with endometriosis, either in the involved ovary or elsewhere in the pelvis or abdomen. These figures vary widely, and several studies have observed 50% or greater associated with endometriosis.[130,267,382,439] When carefully sought, the majority of ovarian clear cell carcinomas are associated with endometriosis, and one-third of cases can be convincingly demonstrated to have arisen within endometriosis, usually an endometriotic cyst.[174,272]

Immunohistochemistry

Like other ovarian carcinomas, clear cell carcinomas stain strongly and diffusely for epithelial markers including keratins, epithelial membrane antigen, Leu M1, Ber-Ep4, and B72.3.[46,157,183,198,210,266,280,285a,437,449a] Alpha fetoprotein (AFP) is rarely positive. CEA is positive in 63% of cases, and OC-125 is positive in 72%. The hyalinized stroma is usually immunoreactive for type IV collagen and laminin, indicating it is composed of basement membrane-like material.[259]

Differential Diagnosis

Germ cell tumors, including yolk sac (endodermal sinus) tumor, dysgerminoma, and rarely struma ovarii, are important to consider in the differential diagnosis of a clear cell neoplasm in the ovary. Clinical information including young age for yolk sac tumors and dysgerminomas and elevated serum AFP levels in women with yolk sac tumors can be helpful. Morphologically, the papillary structures of clear cell carcinomas are more complex and have hyalinized cores, thus differing from the festoon pattern of yolk sac tumors. In addition, yolk sac tumors display a variety of features not seen in clear cell carcinoma, including the characteristic Schiller–Duvall (glomeruloid) bodies as well as other patterns (see Chapter 20, Germ Cell Tumors of the Ovary). Negative immunoperoxidase stain for AFP is an important feature in excluding yolk sac tumor. The combination of positive LeuM1 and negative AFP appears to be a good discriminator of clear cell carcinoma from yolk sac tumor.[491] Positivity for EMA and strong diffuse positivity for cytokeratins help exclude dysgerminoma.[383] The solid pattern of clear cell carcinoma can resemble dysgerminoma, but the latter may be distinguished by the presence of stromal chronic inflammation, granulomas, and occasionally by the presence of syncytiotrophoblastic giant cells. Extensive sampling of a germ cell tumor often reveals other germ cell components that can assist in diagnosis. Rarely, struma ovarii will mimic benign or malignant clear cell tumors.[424,425]

Although hyaline globules are commonly found in clear cell carcinomas, these are nonspecific. They are described as a characteristic feature of yolk sac tumor, but also occur in the majority of carcinosarcomas, and in a small minority of endometrioid, serous, and mucinous ovarian neoplasms.[8]

Endometrioid carcinomas with secretory changes can mimic clear cell carcinoma. When the cells are tall columnar with sub- or supranuclear vacuoles resembling early secretory endometrium, the tumor is classified as secretory variant of endometrioid carcinoma. When the clear cell changes are more extensive and the cells become more cuboidal, the distinction is more difficult, and inasmuch as endometrioid and clear cell ovarian carcinomas are often intermixed, the distinction may be of only academic interest. Rarely, a metaplastic squamous component of an endometrioid carci-

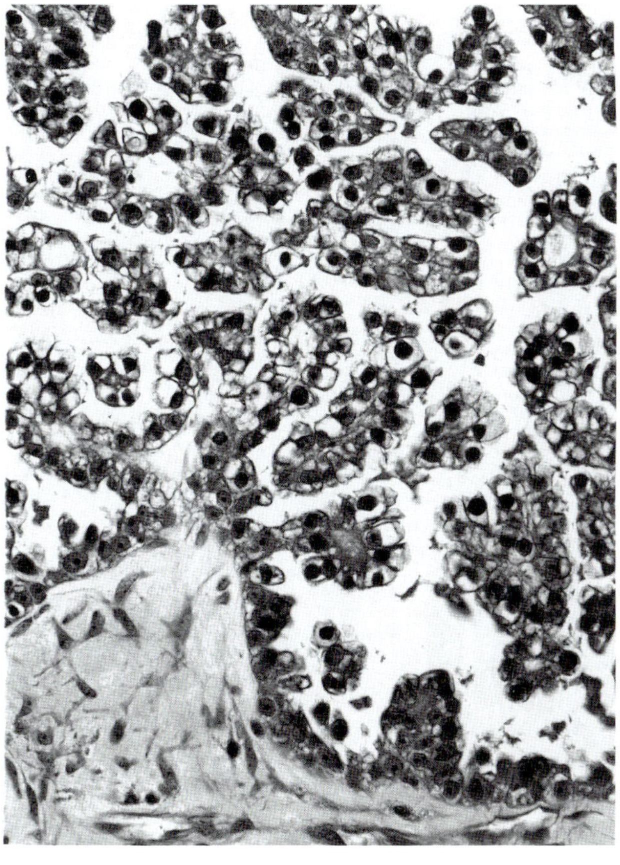

Fig. 18.125. Clear cell carcinoma. Papillary pattern with epithelium displaying prominent cell borders and small, rounded hyperchromatic nuclei.

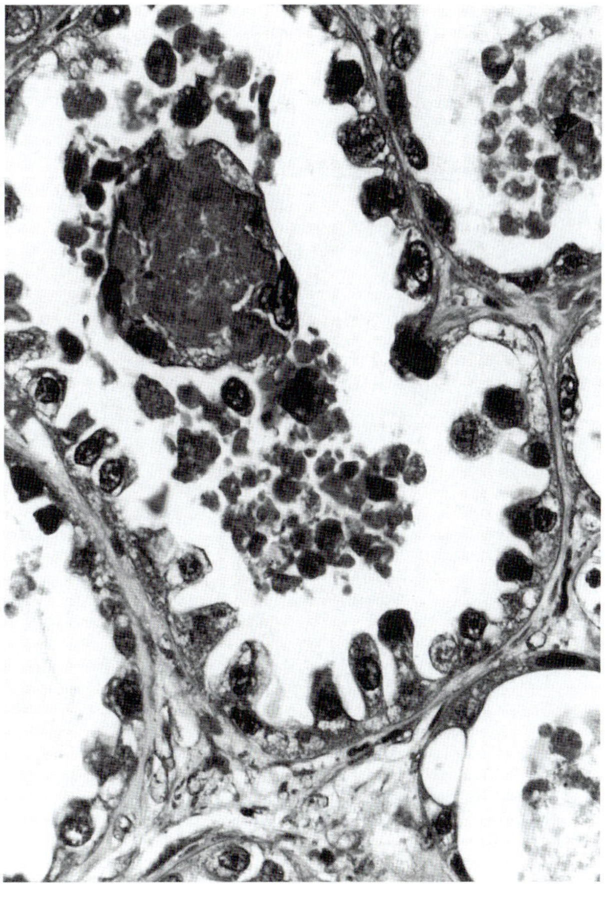

Fig. 18.126. Clear cell carcinoma. Hobnail cells with large, pleomorphic and hyperchromatic nuclei.

noma in which the squamous cells contain abundant glycogen can be confused with clear cell carcinoma. Steroid cell (lipid cell) tumors of the ovary can have prominent areas of clear cytoplasm. Benign or low-grade nuclear features, a delicate fibrovascular stroma, small size, and confinement within the ovarian stroma are features of a steroid cell tumor that help to distinguish it from clear cell carcinoma. Metastatic clear cell neoplasms to the ovaries are very rare (see Chapter 22).

Clinical Behavior and Treatment

There are conflicting data on the behavior of clear cell carcinoma of the ovary. In some studies, the prognosis appears similar to that for other ovarian carcinomas,[79,180] but in others, the prognosis is said to be worse.[196,288,303,383,427] In two series in which analyses were stratified by stage, clear cell carcinoma had a significantly worse prognosis than serous carcinoma only in stage III, based on a total of 81 stage III patients with clear cell carcinoma in these studies.[303,417] In summary, when controlled for stage, survival of women with clear cell carcinoma may be slightly lower than that of patients with serous carcinoma, but in most studies a rigorous comparison to a control group of non-clear cell carcinomas, stratified by stage, has not been made. It is possible that survival analyses are confounded by the possibility that clear cell carcinomas tend to be of higher histologic grade more often than other epithelial cell types. However, there are insufficient reproducible data correlating grade with prognosis of ovarian carcinomas at present to confirm this.

The treatment for clear cell carcinoma is similar to that of other epithelial cell types of ovarian carcinoma. Of note, one large series found that women with clear cell carcinoma treated with platinum-based chemotherapy were at significantly increased risk of thromboembolic complications compared to those with non-clear cell carcinomas, with a corresponding negative impact on survival.[326]

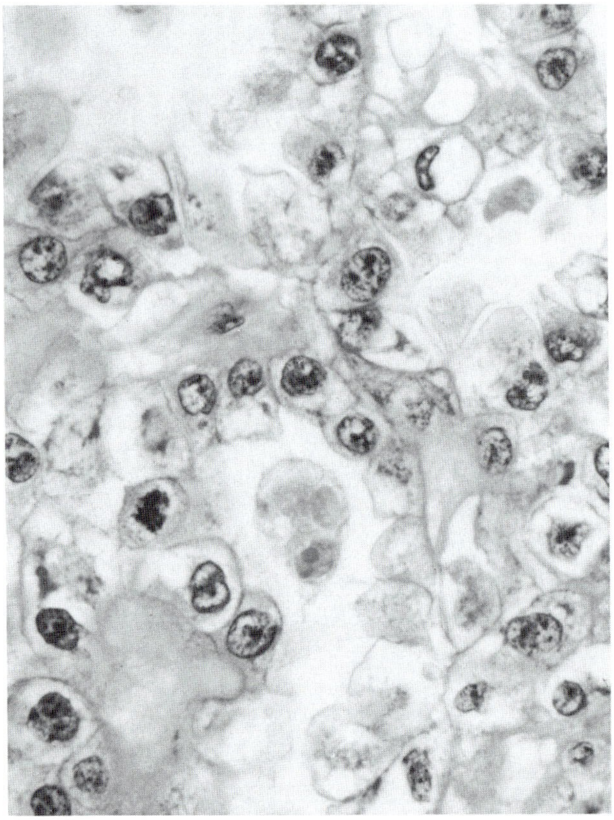

Fig. 18.127. Clear cell carcinoma. Large cells with clear cytoplasm and vesicular, pleomorphic nuclei with large prominent nucleoli.

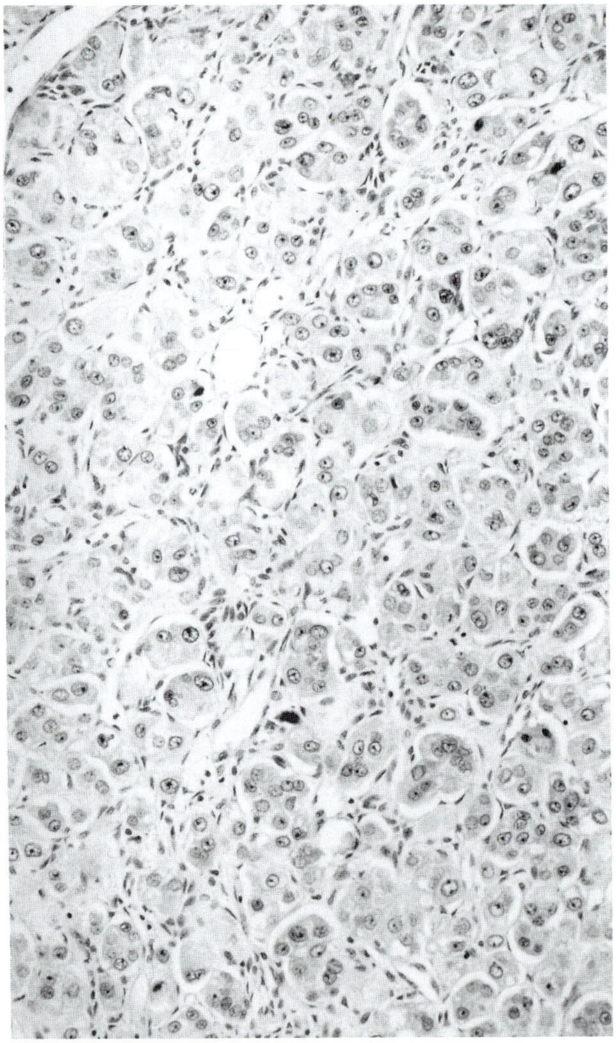

Fig. 18.128. Clear cell carcinoma. Oxyphilic variant displaying an organoid pattern of large cells displaying abundant eosinophilic granular cytoplasm.

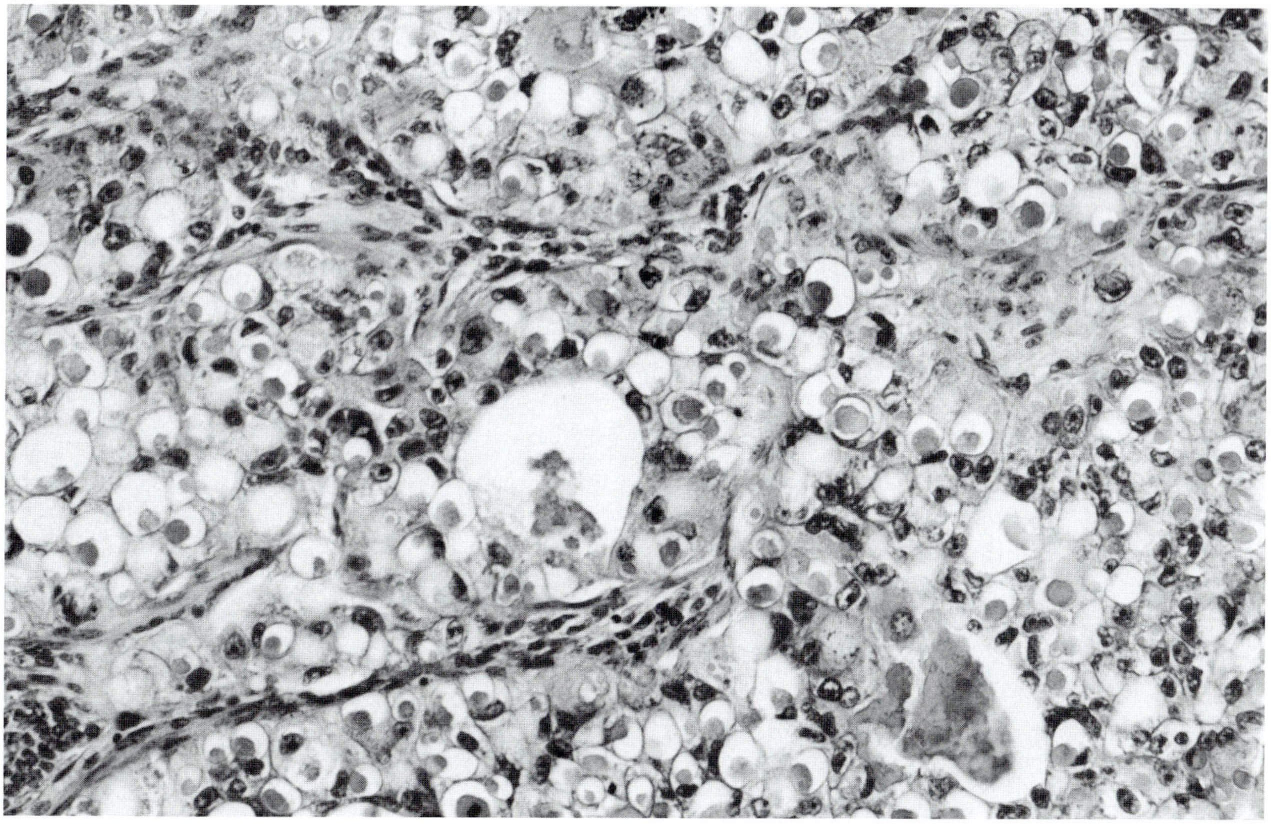

Fig. 18.129. Clear cell carcinoma. Cytoplasmic vacuoles contain homogeneous eosinophilic globules creating a "targetoid" appearance.

Transitional Cell (Brenner) Tumors

The term preferred by WHO for this group of tumors is transitional cell; however, the term Brenner tumor, based on one of the earliest descriptions of the tumor by Brenner, remains firmly entrenched in the literature and remains an approved term for some variants in this tumor group. *Transitional cell tumors* comprise 3.2% of ovarian epithelial neoplasms. Nearly all these are benign Brenner tumors; atypical proliferative and malignant forms are very uncommon. The transitional epithelial cell type, characterized by a relatively uniform population of stratified cells with ovoid nuclei displaying nuclear grooves, is named because of its resemblance to urothelium. Although a few studies have shown immunohistochemical and ultrastructural similarities to native urothelium,[344,347,395] at present the resemblance is considered to be predominantly morphologic.[407] The same type of epithelium is characteristic of Walthard nests, which commonly occur beneath the peritoneal surfaces of the superior and posterior aspects of the fallopian tubes, ovarian hilus, and elsewhere in the broad ligament and are thought to represent a metaplastic change of the mesothelium. Because transitional cell tumors nearly always arise within the ovary, an origin in Walthard nests is unlikely.

Benign Transitional Cell Tumors

Benign transitional cell tumors comprise approximately 3.1% of ovarian epithelial neoplasms. The mean patient age is 50 years. The tumors are common incidental findings and are often microscopic in size. Therefore, the presenting symptoms are often unrelated to the ovarian tumor.[107] Most tumors are 2 cm or smaller, but occasionally they are large and may exceed 10 cm. Most tumors are well circumscribed, firm, and rubbery, with a smooth or slightly bosselated serosal surface. The cut surfaces are typically solid and fibrous, usually gray, white, or yellow, and may be whorled or lobulated; occasionally a cystic component is present. Calcification is sometimes seen. Small tumors can usually be seen to be arising in the ovarian cortex.

Microscopically, the characteristic feature is sharply demarcated epithelial nests in a dense fibrous stroma (Figs. 18.130 and 18.131). The epithelial cells are relatively uniform in size with

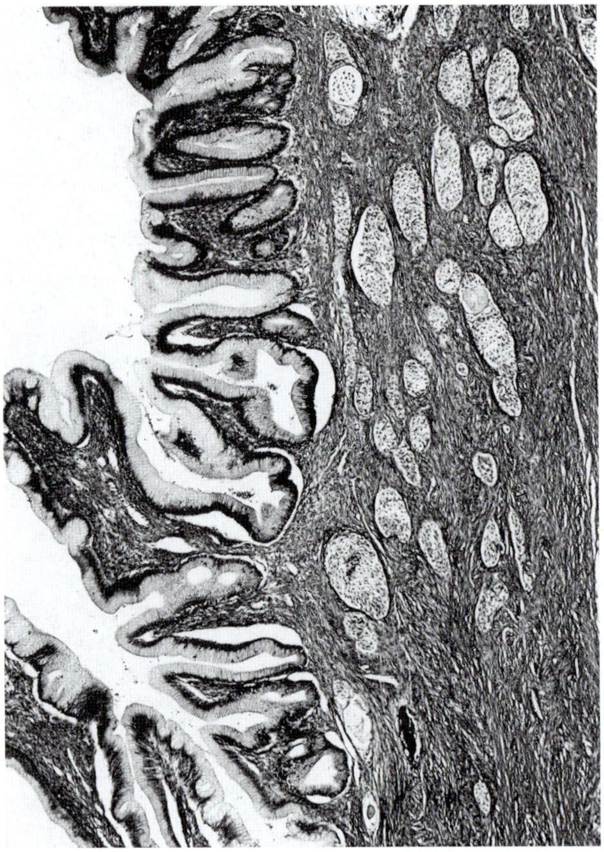

Fig. 18.130. Benign transitional cell (Brenner) tumor with mucinous cystadenoma. On the *right side*, nests of transitional-type cells are distributed in a fibrous stroma. On the *left side*, a benign mucinous cystadenoma is present.

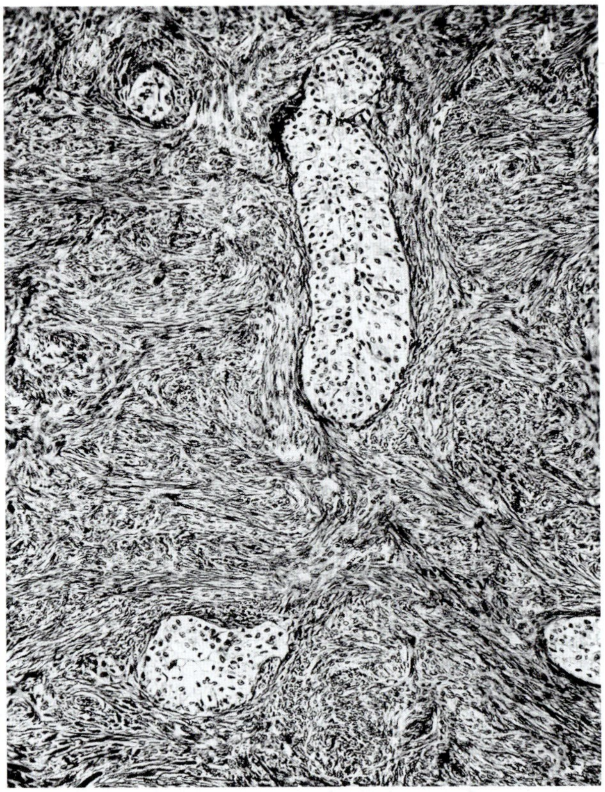

Fig. 18.131. Benign transitional cell (Brenner) tumor. Sharply demarcated epithelial nests are embedded in a dense fibrous stroma.

prominent cell borders and pale to eosinophilic cytoplasm. The nuclei are oval, often with small nucleoli, and longitudinal grooves are usually present (Fig. 18.132). Atypia and mitotic activity are generally not present. The nests often become cystic and contain eosinophilic debris or mucin. Occasionally, metaplastic endocervical-like mucinous epithelium lines the cystic nests; some investigators have termed these tumors "metaplastic Brenner tumor".[346] The metaplastic mucinous component may occasionally form the dominant part of the tumor and may account for the association of Brenner tumors with mucinous cystadenomas (Fig. 18.130). The stroma varies from closely resembling ovarian cortical stroma to densely fibrous. Hyalinized areas are common, and dystrophic calcification is present in 50% of cases, often in the hyalinized areas. The stroma is occasionally luteinized. Rare examples of epidermoid cyst of the ovary may represent cystic variants of Brenner tumor.[481] Histochemical stains indicate that the cells contain glycogen, and mucin is present at the luminal borders and in the luminal contents. By immunoperoxidase stains, the epithelial nests typically stain strongly for epithelial markers including keratins and EMA. CK7 is typically positive and CK20 negative. CEA and CA19-9 are positive in the majority of cases,[407] and chromogranin and neuron-specific enolase are typically positive.[361] Stains for steroidogenic enzymes are usually negative.[367] The clinical behavior is benign.

Atypical Proliferative Transitional Cell Tumors

These uncommon neoplasms, also termed proliferating or borderline transitional cell or Brenner tumor, or transitional cell or Brenner tumor of low malignant potential, present in patients whose mean age is 59 years. They are always unilateral and confined to the ovary. The tumors are larger than their benign counterparts and are usually cystic and measure 10–28 cm with a mean diameter of 18 cm. Friable papillary or polypoid masses project into the cyst lumens, and there is usually a benign Brenner component with a more solid and fibrous cut sur-

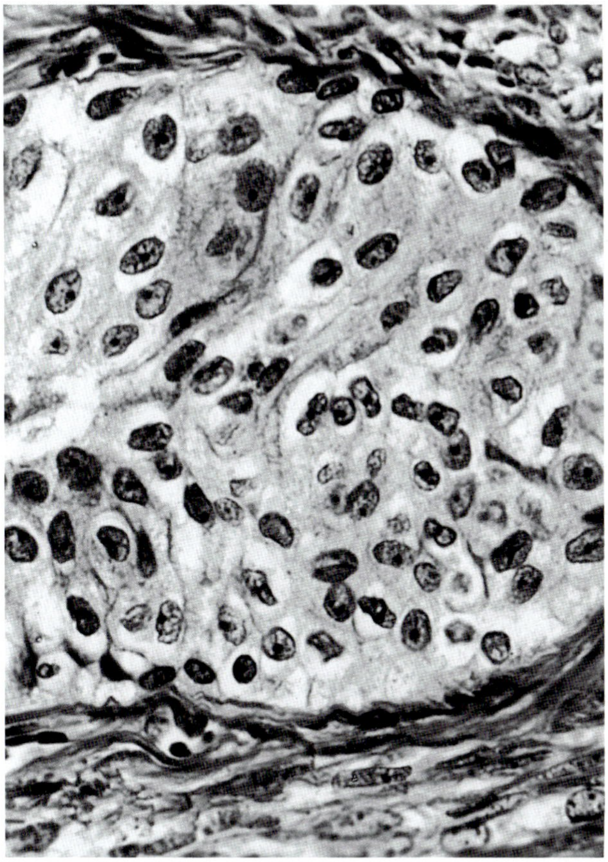

Fig. 18.132. Benign transitional cell (Brenner) tumor. Transitional-like epithelial cells display ovoid nuclei with longitudinal grooves. Some nuclei have prominent nucleoli.

face. Microscopically, the intracystic papillary component is composed of transitional-type epithelium resembling low-grade noninvasive papillary transitional cell neoplasms of the urinary tract (Fig. 18.133). Mucinous metaplasia may be present in the epithelium lining the papillae. Underneath the papillae and within the wall there may be solid sheets of transitional epithelium with little intervening stroma (Fig. 18.134). Nearly all cases display areas of benign transitional cell neoplasm, and occasionally the proliferating component can be seen to be arising directly from the benign component.

The cytologic features are similar to those in benign transitional cell tumors, but occasionally significant atypia and mitotic activity are present. Some authors have separately classified "proliferative" and "low malignant potential" transitional cell tumors, the former characterized by a resemblance to grade 1–2 urothelial papillary transitional cell carcinoma and the latter displaying high-grade nuclear atypia resembling grade 3 urothelial papillary transitional cell carcinoma or in situ squamous cell carcinoma.[346] In all cases, stromal invasion is absent. Benign and atypical proliferative Brenner tumors usually contain carcinoembryonic antigen.[395] Among more than 50 reported cases of atypical proliferative transitional cell tumors, there has been 1 local recurrence and no convincing evidence of malignant behavior.[156,261,346,350,470] Accordingly, we prefer the term "atypical proliferative transitional cell (Brenner) tumor."

Malignant Transitional Cell Tumors

Malignant transitional cell tumors are difficult to define clinicopathologically for several reasons. First, published data are very limited. Second, large databases including the FIGO annual report and the SEER database do not separately classify ovarian transitional cell carcinomas; in addition, malignant Brenner tumor is erroneously classified by SEER in a miscellaneous category for noncarcinomas.[315] Third, papillary serous carcinomas not infrequently have focal areas that display features resembling transitional cell carcinoma. In fact, at present, many

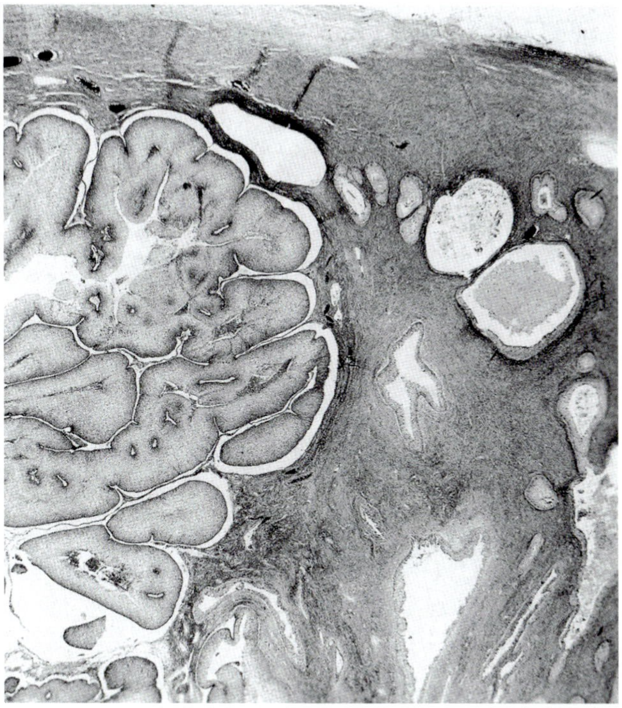

Fig. 18.133. Atypical proliferative transitional cell (Brenner) tumor. On the *left side*, there is a papillary proliferation of transitional-type epithelium resembling a low-grade papillary transitional cell carcinoma of the urinary tract. On the *right*, there are several benign transitional cell nests, some of which are cystically dilated. (Reprinted by permission from Colgan TJ, Norris HJ. Int J Gynecol Pathol 1983;1:367–382.)

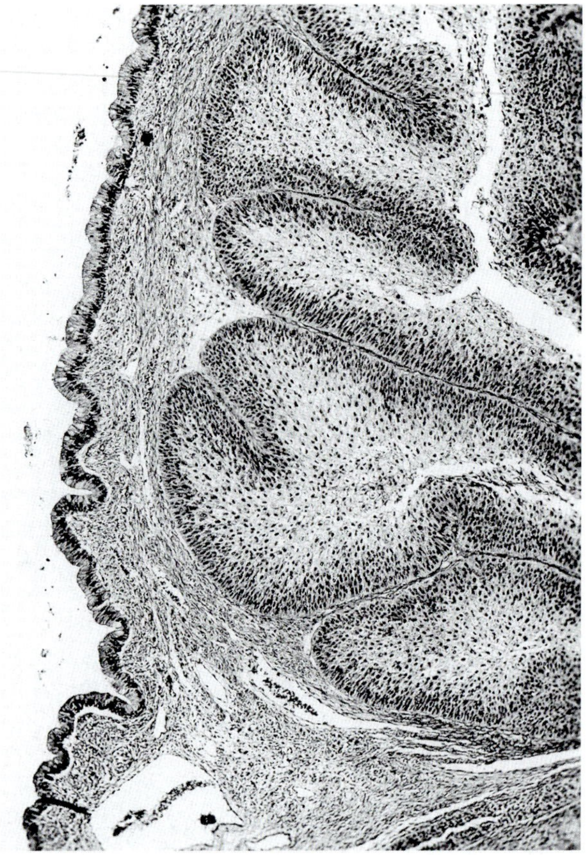

Fig. 18.134. Atypical proliferative transitional cell (Brenner) tumor. Within the wall of a cyst, the base of a papillary transitional cell proliferation displays undulating borders and a solid epithelial proliferation. On the *left side*, a mucinous cystadenoma is lined by a single layer of benign mucinous epithelium.

experts believe that most tumors classified as ovarian transitional cell carcinomas (TCC) are serous carcinomas with a pseudopapillary pattern and that genuine TCC of the ovary is very rare.

Approximately 10%–15% of advanced-stage ovarian carcinomas contain a transitional cell component;[143] some authors have found that a transitional cell pattern predominates in 22% of advanced-stage ovarian carcinomas.[170] Some investigators have defined two clinicopathologic types: malignant Brenner tumor, in which a benign or atypical proliferative Brenner component is identified, and transitional cell carcinoma (TCC), in which no benign or atypical proliferative Brenner component is identified.[17]

Clinical Findings

The clinical presentation is nonspecific and is similar to those of the more common cell types of ovarian cancer; thus, pelvic or abdominal pain and a mass are common. Malignant Brenner tumors occur at a mean age of 63 years,[17,156,261,345,470] whereas TCCs present at a median age of about 55 years.[17,143]

Operative Findings

The size of malignant Brenner tumors ranges up to 25 cm with a mean diameter of 14 cm. Among stage I tumors, 16% are bilateral. The stage distribution is as follows: stage I, 64%; stage II, 12%; stage III, 18%; stage IV, 6%.[17,156,261,345,470] In contrast, 69% of transitional cell carcinomas present in advanced stage.[17] The median size is 13 cm.

Gross Findings

The gross appearance is typically solid and cystic. The cysts may exhibit polypoid, friable mural nodules, and the cyst fluid is watery or mucinous. Hemorrhage and necrosis may be prominent, and half have foci of gritty calcification. In the malignant Brenner tumor, the benign Brenner component may be identifiable as a solid fibrous nodule within a cyst wall. Serous carcinomas that have a minor transitional cell component have the gross features of papillary serous carcinoma (see "Malignant Serous Tumors").

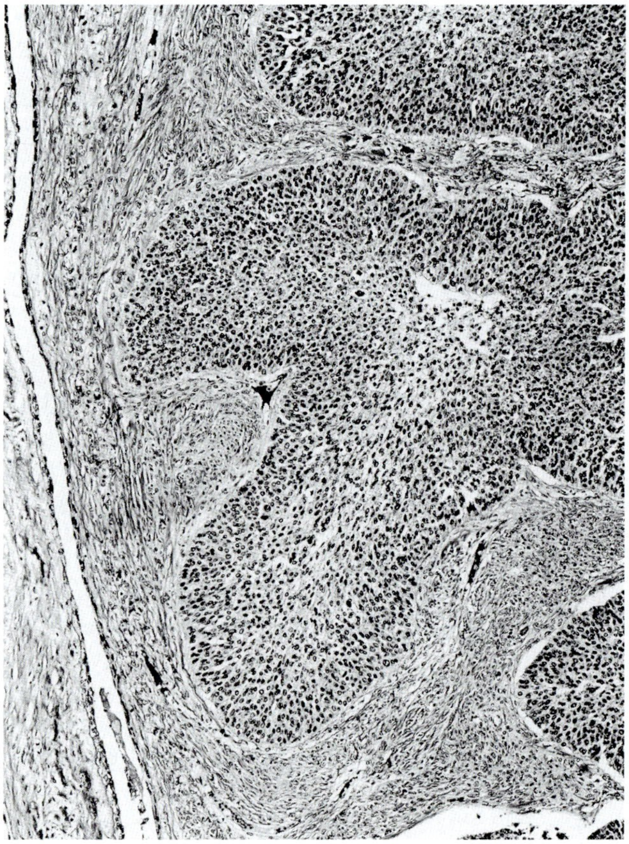

Fig. 18.135. Transitional cell carcinoma. Cyst wall with stratified transitional-type epithelium

Microscopic Findings

The histologic patterns of TCC are often mixed with other types of carcinoma, most often serous. Approximately 10% of ovarian carcinomas containing the TCC pattern are said to be pure.[143] More than 50% of the tumor should display the patterns of TCC for a diagnosis of TCC. A diagnosis of malignant Brenner tumor is warranted when a benign or atypical proliferative Brenner component is identified.

The characteristic microscopic feature is thick, blunt, and often elongated papillary folds with fibrovascular cores, lined by transitional-type epithelium resembling urothelium. The papillae often appear to arise from a cyst wall with a similar lining of stratified and atypical transitional cells (Figs. 18.135 and 18.136). Foci of squamous or glandular differentiation are common. Stromal invasion is present, characterized by haphazard infiltrative growth of epithelium at the base of the papillae into the cyst wall or extensive areas of solid epithelial proliferation with scant or no fibrovascular support.

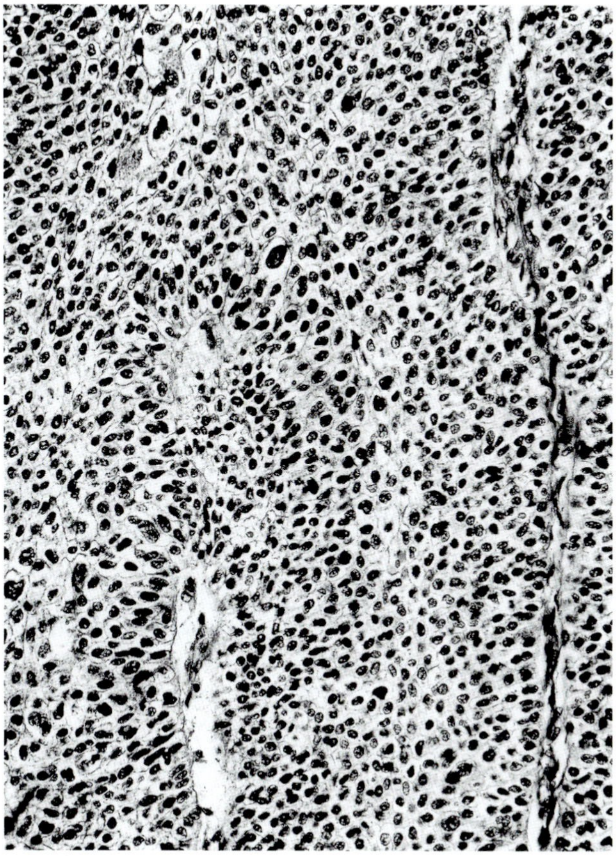

Fig. 18.136. Transitional cell carcinoma. Fibrovascular cores reflect the papillary pattern of this tumor. The papillae are thick and lined by transitional type epithelium with severe cytologic atypia, manifested by pleomorphism and hyperchromasia.

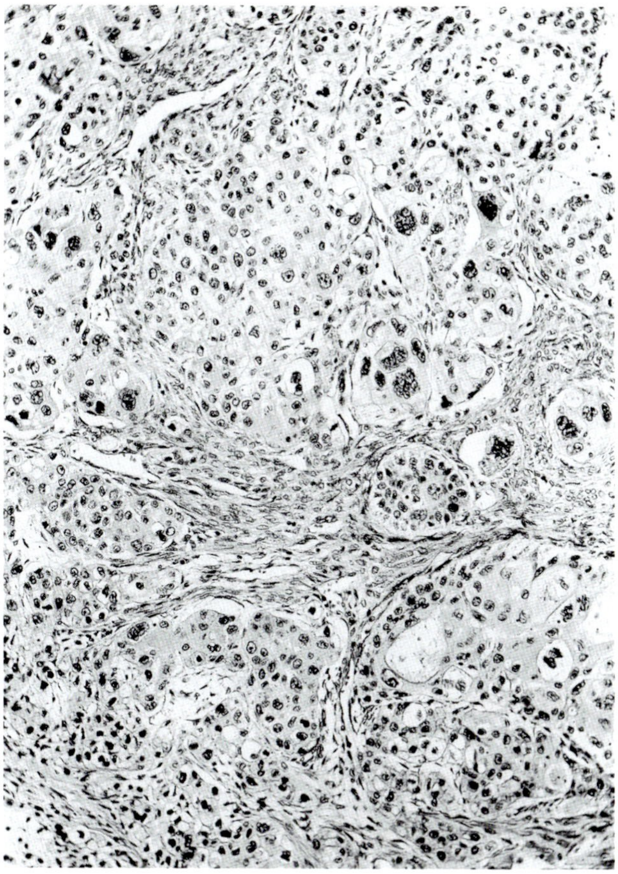

Fig. 18.137. Malignant Brenner tumor. This is the less common pattern of malignant transitional cell tumor, characterized by a haphazard infiltrative pattern of crowded transitional cell nests with marked nuclear atypia including some bizarre nuclei. (Reprinted by permission from Miles PA, Norris HJ, Cancer 1972;30:174–186.[261])

A less common architectural pattern is characterized by solid areas resembling benign Brenner tumor, but the epithelial nests have a disorderly growth pattern that appears invasive and is sometimes associated with stromal desmoplasia[347] (Fig. 18.137). Cytologic atypia is usually prominent and corresponds to grade 2 or 3 papillary transitional cell carcinoma of the urinary tract. High-grade pleomorphic nuclear features and bizarre giant cells may occur, further supporting the opinion that these tumors are transitional-like variants of papillary serous carcinoma. Mitotic activity is prominent. Stromal inflammation, necrosis, and dystrophic calcification are often present. Benign or atypical proliferative Brenner components are required for the diagnosis of a malignant Brenner tumor and are absent in TCCs. In addition, malignant Brenner tumors, like their benign counterparts, often have prominent stromal calcification, in contrast to TCCs in which calcification is uncommon.[17]

Immunohistochemistry

Very limited immunohistochemical data are available on malignant Brenner tumors and TCCs. They are positive for keratins, in particular CK7, and negative for CK20, in contrast to TCCs of the urinary tract, which are usually CK7 and CK20 positive. A minority of ovarian TCCs are positive for CEA and CA19-9.[294,407]

Differential Diagnosis

TCCs must be distinguished from metastatic TCC from the urinary tract, which is usually done clinically; urinary tract TCCs that metastasize to the ovaries generally do so late in their evolution and therefore are generally large, deeply invasive, and thus clinically evident.

The presence or absence of a benign or atypical proliferative Brenner component distinguishes a TCC from a malignant Brenner tumor, as just discussed. Poorly differentiated papillary serous carcinomas may have transitional-like areas in up to 22% of cases. The appearance of thick, blunt papillae of transitional cell differentiation contrasts with the papillae of serous carcinoma, which are generally thinner.

Clinical Behavior and Treatment

Limited data indicate that ovarian TCC is more aggressive than malignant Brenner tumor, as is suggested by the tendency for TCC to present in more advanced stage, with most malignant Brenner tumors presenting in stage I.[17] However, it is not clear that the behavior is different when stratified by stage. The apparent behavioral difference may arguably be a result of obliteration of a recognizable benign Brenner component by the more rapidly growing, clinically aggressive tumors, rendering their classification as TCC only because a benign component can no longer be identified. Alternatively, TCC may simply reflect a variant of papillary serous carcinoma; this is supported by many similar clinical and pathologic features between these two types of ovarian carcinoma, and an immunophenotype that resembles papillary serous carcinoma of the ovary rather than TCC of the urinary tract.[294]

Limited data suggest that advanced-stage TCCs are more chemosensitive to platinum-containing chemotherapeutic regimens in comparison to advanced-stage serous carcinomas;[143] however, other investigators have not confirmed these findings.[170]

Squamous Cell Carcinoma

Pure invasive *squamous cell carcinoma* is very rare. In a series of 18 cases, endometriosis was found in 7 cases, and no underlying lesion was found in 11 cases.[311] Invasive squamous cell carcinoma in the ovary is most commonly caused by malignant transformation of a mature cystic teratoma; in such cases, the tumor is classified as being not of surface epithelial origin but rather of germ cell origin (see Chapter 20, Germ Cell Tumors of the Ovary). Rarely, metastatic disease from the uterine cervix is the source of squamous cell carcinoma in the ovary, and very rarely in situ squamous cell carcinoma of the cervix spreads intraepithelially by unknown mechanisms into the endometrium, fallopian tubes, and may involve the ovaries.

Transitional cell tumors often display focal squamous differentiation and on very rare occasion are the site of origin of an invasive squamous cell carcinoma. Rare reports of in situ squamous cell carcinoma of the ovary not arising in a teratoma probably represent atypical proliferative transitional cell tumors (see "Atypical Proliferative Transitional Cell Tumors," earlier). Rarely, an endometrioid carcinoma with a prominent metaplastic squamous component mimics a pure squamous cell carcinoma. Generous sampling will disclose diagnostic features in most cases.

Most patients with primary ovarian squamous cell carcinoma are in advanced stage and die within 1 year; this appears to be a significantly worse prognosis compared to squamous cell carcinoma arising in a mature cystic teratoma.[311]

Mixed Epithelial Tumors

The presence of two epithelial cell types in an ovarian epithelial neoplasm, each comprising at least 10% of the tumor, warrants a designation of a *mixed epithelial tumor*. Nonetheless, as mixed epithelial tumors are by necessity a heterogeneous group, it is more convenient and of no significant clinical import to ignore the minor components and classify tumors based solely on the predominant component, unless of course the minor component is malignant in an otherwise benign tumor or is of a higher grade than the remainder of the tumor. As the prognosis for all cell types is essentially the same when stratified by stage, it is preferable to designate tumors based on the predominant component.

Serous and endometrioid differentiation often occur together. In particular, poorly differentiated serous and endometrioid carcinomas often display

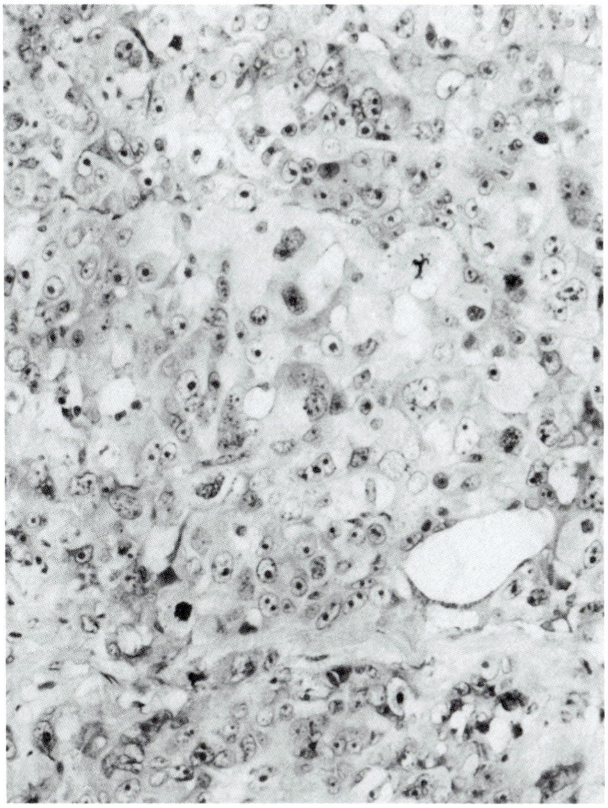

Fig. 18.138. Undifferentiated carcinoma. Large anaplastic cells with abundant pale cytoplasm, large prominent nucleoli, and a high mitotic rate, including an abnormal mitotic figure.

overlapping features, and at times assignment to one or the other group is arbitrary and varies among observers. Similarly, endometrioid and clear cell differentiation are often mixed in these carcinomas. Mucinous differentiation is commonly observed in benign transitional cell neoplasms. Among atypical proliferative tumors, the most common mixed type is seromucinous, also called müllerian mucinous, or endocervical-like type atypical proliferative ("borderline") tumor. Furthermore, the combination of papillary (serous) architectural features and mucinous cytologic features in these tumors is often mixed with other cell types (see "Atypical Proliferative Mucinous Tumors").

Undifferentiated Carcinomas

Undifferentiated carcinomas show no readily identifiable features of any of the cell types of ovarian surface epithelial neoplasms. Therefore, any element of glands, papillae, or psammoma bodies removes a tumor from this category. There are three types of primary ovarian undifferentiated carcinoma, referred to as follows: undifferentiated carcinoma, the hypercalcemic type of small cell carcinoma, and the pulmonary type of small cell carcinoma. When strict pathologic criteria are employed for these diagnoses, all three types are very uncommon. In all cases when this diagnosis is considered, it is very important to exclude metastatic tumor, particularly from the lungs.

Although data are limited, undifferentiated carcinoma appears to be more common than the small cell types, both of which are very rare. However, the small cell type of undifferentiated carcinoma associated with hypercalcemia is the most common type of undifferentiated carcinoma in women under 40 years of age. For the usual type of undifferentiated carcinoma, the mean age at presentation is 60 years; 78% of patients present in stages III and IV. Tumors are composed of solid sheets of large pleomorphic cells with high-grade nuclear features and usually with abundant cytoplasm that is often eosinophilic (Figs. 18.138 and 18.139). Immunoperoxidase stains for epithelial markers (EMA, CAM 5.2, B72.3) are positive. In nearly all cases, CK7 is positive and CK20 is negative; 21% stain for CEA and 79% for OC-125.[46,157,210,266,280,437,456] Overall, 22% of patients survive 5 years, but only 14% of stage III and IV patients survive 5 years. Surprisingly, more than 90% of stage I patients survive 5 years. Although overall survival is worse than that for serous carcinoma, when stratified by stage they do not have a significantly worse prognosis.[303]

Undifferentiated small cell carcinoma associated with hypercalcemia is a distinctive neoplasm and is described in detail in Chapter 19 (Sex Cord–Stromal, Steroid Cell, and Other Ovarian Tumors with Endocrine, Paraendocrine, and Paraneoplastic Manifestations). Undifferentiated small cell carcinoma, pulmonary type, is extremely rare and is described in Chapter 21 (Nonspecific Tumors of the Ovary, Including Mesenchymal Tumors and Malignant Lymphoma).

Malignant Mixed Mesodermal Tumor (Carcinosarcoma) (MMMT)

MMMTs comprise less than 1% of ovarian neoplasms. There are more than 300 cases in the literature.[357] The mean age of patients with this tumor is about 60 years; over 85% present in advanced stage. The tumors are typically large, ranging from 15 to 20 cm in diameter. The morphology is similar to its uterine counterpart (see Chapter 12, Endometrial Carcinoma). The characteristic microscopic feature is an intimate admixture of malignant

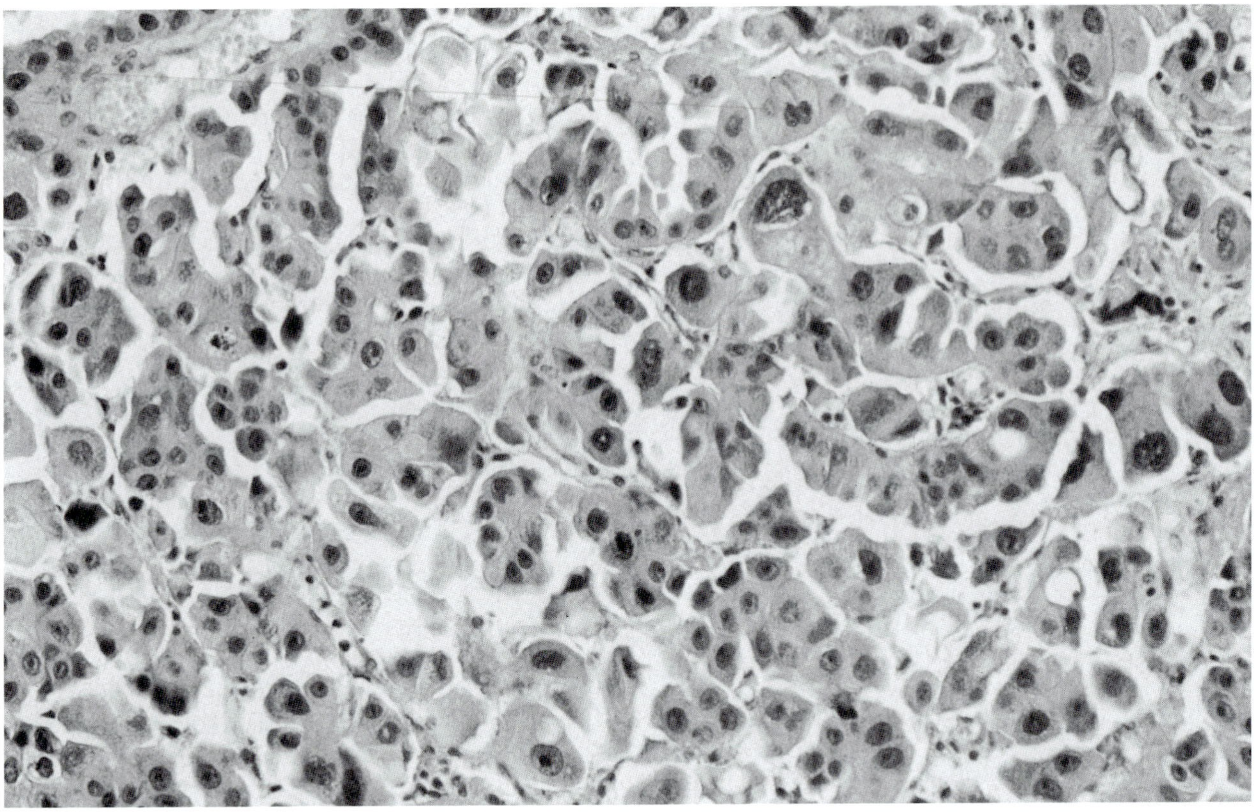

Fig. 18.139. Undifferentiated carcinoma. Pleomorphic giant cells with abundant eosinophilic cytoplasm, and malignant nuclear features with some bizarre nuclear forms.

epithelial and stromal elements. The malignant epithelial element is most commonly a high-grade serous or endometrioid carcinoma but can be of any of the surface epithelial cell types of ovarian tumors. The stromal component usually contains sheets of hyperchromatic rounded to spindled cells with marked nuclear atypia and a high mitotic rate (Fig. 18.140). Heterologous elements, most commonly cartilage, osteoid, and rhabdomyoblasts, are commonly found and, as in the uterine counterpart, their frequency depends on the diligence with which the search is conducted (Fig. 18.141).

An occasionally problematic situation is a tumor that is otherwise a typical carcinoma but in which a small focus of malignant stroma is identified. Although there are few published data on such tumors, they are classified as MMMTs. Immunohistochemical stains for epithelial markers are often positive in the sarcomatous component, and their behavior and patterns of spread are similar to high-grade carcinomas.[410] These observations suggest that these tumors should be classified as metaplastic carcinomas like their uterine counterpart[256] (see Chapter 12, Endometrial Carcinoma). Immunohistochemistry for skeletal muscle markers such as desmin can be used to help identify heterologous rhabdomyoblasts. MMMTs are aggressive, rapidly fatal tumors with a median survival of approximately 1 year.[9,48,93,271,357,410] The presence of heterologous elements does not influence prognosis.

Sarcomas

Although primary pure or mixed sarcomas of the ovary are very uncommon, they constitute a heterogeneous group with four different types of neoplasms: *endometrioid stromal sarcoma, adenosarcoma, sarcoma arising in a mature teratoma,* and *miscellaneous soft tissue sarcomas.* Carcinosarcomas (MMMTs) were already discussed (see "Malignant Mixed Mesodermal Tumors"). All these tumors are extremely rare. Sarcomas arising in teratomas are classified as germ cell tumors with secondary malignant transformation (see Chapter 20, Germ Cell Tumors of the Ovary). Miscellaneous soft tissue sarcomas rarely arise in the ovary. Their pathologic features are not significantly different from those of their soft tissue counterparts.

Endometrioid Stromal Sarcoma (ESS)

ESS is an extremely rare primary ovarian neoplasm that is morphologically identical to its uterine counterpart (see Chapter 13, Mesenchymal Tumors of the Uterus). Among approximately 27 reported cases,[68,483] 63% have been closely associated with endometriosis from which the tumor may have arisen. The mean patient age is 52 years; more than 70% present in advanced stage (FIGO II–III). Mean tumor size is 10 cm. Because primary uterine ESS is often slow growing and prone to late recurrence, it is important to consider the possibility of metastatic tumor from a uterine primary, even if the patient has had a hysterectomy in the remote past. Ovarian sex cord–stromal tumors with a predominant spindle cell component, including cellular fibroma, thecoma, and poorly differentiated Sertoli–Leydig cell tumor, are also important differential diagnostic considerations. The behavior appears to parallel that of advanced-stage uterine ESS, although data are limited.[68]

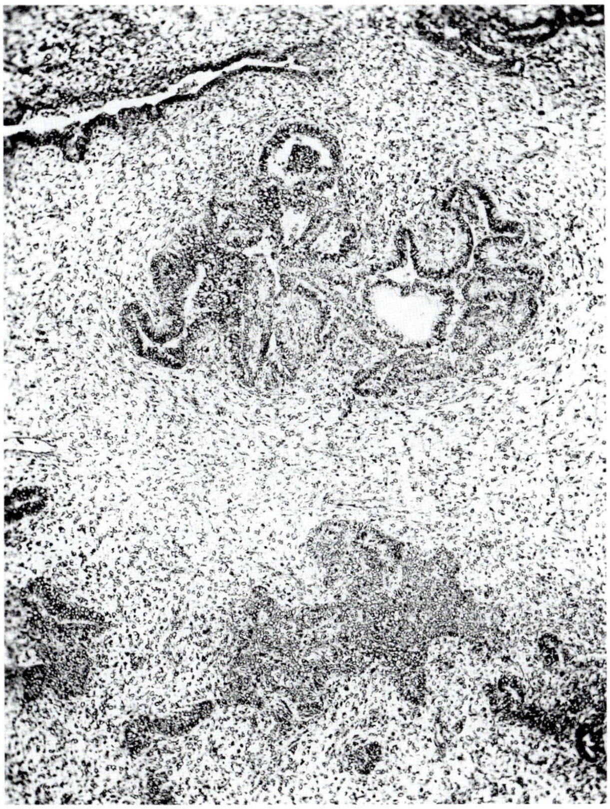

Fig. 18.140. Malignant mixed mesodermal tumor (carcinosarcoma). An intimate admixture of malignant glands and a malignant spindle cell stroma resembles its uterine counterpart.

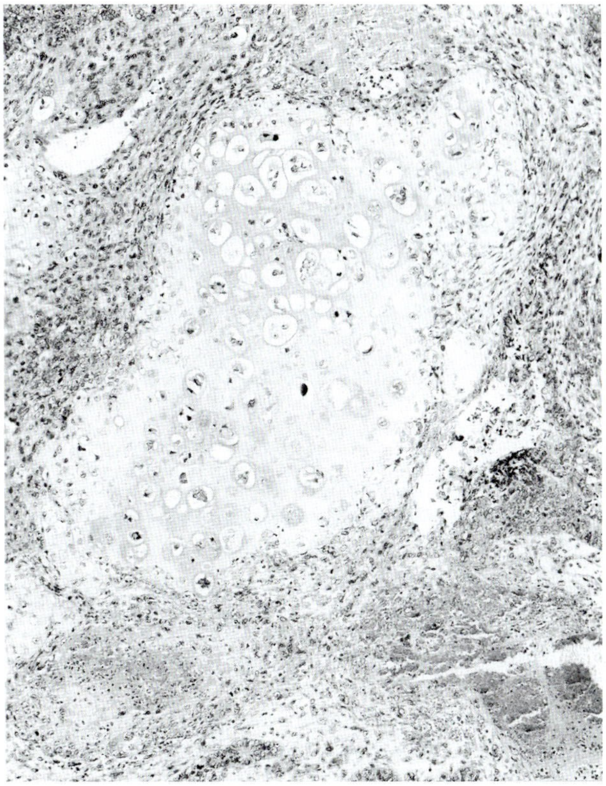

Fig. 18.141. Malignant mixed mesodermal tumor (carcinosarcoma) (MMMT). Heterologous cartilage is present in this example of MMMT.

Müllerian Adenosarcoma

Müllerian adenosarcoma of the ovary is very rare. It is morphologically identical to its uterine counterpart (see Chapter 13, Mesenchymal Tumors of the Uterus). In a series of five cases,[186] the mean patient age was 46, and the median tumor size was more than 15 cm; two were stage I and three were stages II and III. The characteristic microscopic feature is periglandular stromal condensation with atypia and mitotic activity in these hypercellular areas of stroma. The mitotic rate usually exceeds 5 MF/10 HPF. After limited follow-up with a mean of 3.4 years, two patients were alive with disease, two were alive and well, and one had died of unrelated causes.

Acknowledgments. Richard Roden, Ph.D., and Brigitte Ronnette, M.D., are thanked for critical evaluation of selected portions of this chapter.

References

1. Abu-Jawdeh GM, Jacobs TW, Niloff J, et al (1996) Estrogen receptor expression is a common feature

of ovarian borderline tumors. Gynecol Oncol 60: 301–307
2. Abulafia O, Sherer DM (2000) Angiogenesis of the ovary. Am J Obstet Gynecol 182:240–246
3. Abulafia O, Triest WE, Sherer DM (1997) Angiogenesis in primary and metastatic epithelial ovarian carcinoma. Am J Obstet Gynecol 177:541–547
4. Afzal S, Lalani E-N, Poulsom R, et al (1998) MT1-MMP and MMP-2 mRNA expression in human ovarian tumors: possible implications for the role of desmoplastic fibroblasts. Hum Pathol 29:155–165
5. Aguirre P, Scully RE, Dayal Y, et al (1984) Mucinous tumors of the ovary with argyrophil cells: an immunohistochemical analysis. Am J Surg Pathol 8:345–356
6. Aguirre P, Thor AD, Scully RE (1989) Ovarian endometrioid carcinomas resembling sex cord-stromal tumors: an immunohistochemical study. Int J Gynecol Pathol 8:364–373
7. Ahmed FY, Wiltshaw E, A'Hern RP, et al (1996) Natural history and prognosis of untreated stage I epithelial ovarian carcinoma. J Clin Oncol 14: 2968–2975
8. Al-Nafussi AI, Hughes DE, Williams ARW (1993) Hyaline globules in ovarian tumors. Histopathology (Oxf) 23:563–566
9. Andersen WA, Young DE, Peters WA, et al (1989) Platinum-based combination chemotherapy for malignant mixed mesodermal tumors of the ovary. Gynecol Oncol 32:319–322
10. Angelopoulou K, Diamandis EP (1997) Detection of TP53 tumour suppressor gene product and p53 auto-antibodies in the ascites of women with ovarian cancer. Eur J Cancer 33:115–121
11. Anreder MB, Freeman SM, Merogi A, et al (1999) P53, c-erbB2, and PCNA status in benign, proliferative, and malignant ovarian surface epithelial neoplasms: a study of 75 cases. Arch Pathol Lab Med 123:310–316
12. Anttila MA, Ji H, Juhola MT, et al (1999) The prognostic significance of p53 expression quantitated by computerized image analysis in epithelial ovarian cancer. Int J Gynecol Pathol 18:42–51
13. Anttila MA, Tammi RH, Tammi MI, et al (2000) High levels of stromal hyaluronan predict poor disease outcome in epithelial ovarian cancer. Cancer Res 60:150–155
14. Aruffo A, Stamenkovic I, Melnick M, et al (1990) CD44 is the principal cell surface receptor for hyaluronate. Cell 61:1303–1313
15. Auersperg N, Pan J, Grove BD, et al (1999) E-cadherin induces mesenchymal-to-epithelial transition in human ovarian surface epithelium. Proc Natl Acad Sci USA 96:6249–6254
16. Auranen A, Grenman S, Klemi P-J (1997) Immunohistochemically detected p53 and HER-2/neu expression and nuclear DNA content in familial epithelial ovarian carcinomas. Cancer (Phila) 79:2147–2153
17. Austin RM, Norris HJ (1987) Malignant Brenner tumors and transitional cell carcinoma of the ovary. Int J Gynecol Pathol 6:29–39
18. Autio-Harmainen H, Karttunen T, Hurskainen T, et al (1993) Expression of 72 kilodalton type IV collagenase (gelatinase A) in benign and malignant ovarian tumors. Lab Invest 69:312–321
19. Baergen RN, Rutgers JL (1994) Mural nodules in common epithelial tumors of the ovary. Int J Gynecol Pathol 13:62–72
19a. Baker PM, Oliva E, Young RH, et al (2001) Ovarian mucinous carcinoids including some with a carcinomatous component: a report of 17 cases. Am J Surg Pathol 25:557–568
20. Baker VV, Borst MP, Dixon D, et al (1990) *c-myc* amplification in ovarian cancer. Gynecol Oncol 38:340–342
21. Ball NJ, Robertson I, Duggan MA, et al (1990) Intestinal differentiation in ovarian mucinous tumours. Virch Arch A Pathol Anat 417:197–201
22. Ballouk F, Ross JS, Wolf BC (1994) Ovarian endometriotic cysts: an analysis of cytologic atypia and DNA ploidy patterns. Am J Clin Pathol 102: 415–419
23. Banks E, Beral V, Reeves G (1997) The epidemiology of epithelial ovarian cancer: a review. Int J Gynecol Cancer 7:425–438
24. Barnhill DR, Kurman RJ, Brady MF, et al (1995) Preliminary analysis of the behavior of stage I ovarian serous tumors of low malignant potential: a Gynecologic Oncology Group study. J Clin Oncol 13:2752–2756
25. Barrette BA, Srivatsa PJ, Cliby WA, et al (1997) Overexpression of $p34^{cdc2}$ protein kinase in epithelial ovarian carcinoma. Mayo Clin Proc 72:925–929
26. Bast RC Jr, Yu Y, Xu F-J, et al (2000) Molecular approaches to management of epithelial ovarian cancer. Int J Gynecol Cancer 10 (suppl 1):2–7
27. Batra S, Iosif CS (1996) Elevated concentrations of antiestrogen binding sites in membrane fractions of human ovarian tumors. Gynecol Oncol 60: 228–232
28. Bauknecht T, Angel P, Kohler M, et al (1993) Gene structure and expression analysis of the epidermal growth factor receptor, transforming growth factor-alpha, myc, jun, and metallothionein in human ovarian carcinomas: classification of malignant phenotypes. Cancer (Phila) 71:419–429
29. Bell DA (1991) Mucinous adenofibromas of the ovary: a report of 10 cases. Am J Surg Pathol 15: 227–232
30. Bell DA, Scully RE (1985) Benign and borderline clear cell adenofibromas of the ovary. Cancer (Phila) 56:2911–2931
31. Bell DA, Scully RE (1990) Ovarian serous borderline tumors with stromal microinvasion: a report of 21 cases. Hum Pathol 21:397–403
32. Bell DA, Scully RE (1990) Serous borderline tumors of the peritoneum. Am J Surg Pathol 14: 230–239

33. Bell DA, Scully RE (1994) Early de novo ovarian carcinoma: a study of fourteen cases. Cancer (Phila) 73:1859–1864
34. Bell DA, Scully RE (1985) Atypical and borderline endometrioid adenofibromas of the ovary: a report of 27 cases. Am J Surg Pathol 9:205–214
35. Bell DA, Weinstock MA, Scully RE (1988) Peritoneal implants of ovarian serous borderline tumors: histologic features and prognosis. Cancer (Phila) 62:2212–2222
36. Bell KA, Kurman RJ (2000) A clinicopathologic analysis of atypical proliferative (borderline) tumors and well differentiated endometrioid adenocarcinomas of the ovary. Am J Surg Pathol 24(11):1465–1479
37. Bell KA, Sedhev AES, Kurman RJ (2001) Refined diagnostic criteria for implants associated with ovarian atypical proliferative serous tumors (borderline) and micropapillary serous carcinomas. Am J Surg Pathol 25:419–432
38. Berchuck A, Rodriguez GC, Kamel A, et al (1991) Epidermal growth factor expression in normal ovarian epithelium and ovarian cancer. I. Correlation of receptor expression with prognostic factors in patients with ovarian cancer. Am J Obstet Gynecol 164:669–674
39. Berchuck A, Kohler MF, Marks JR, et al (1994) The p53 tumor suppressor gene frequently is altered in gynecologic cancers. Am J Obstet Gynecol 170:246–252
40. Berezowski K, Stastny JF, Kornstein MJ (1996) Cytokeratins 7 and 20 and carcinoembryonic antigen in ovarian and colonic carcinoma. Mod Pathol 9:426–429
41. Bewtra C, Watson P, Conway T, et al (1992) Hereditary ovarian cancer: a clinicopathological study. Int J Gynecol Pathol 11:180–187
42. Bibbo M, van Hoeven KH, Fitzpatrick BT (1997) Peritoneal washings and ovary. In: Bibbo M (ed) Comprehensive cytopathology, 2nd Ed. Saunders, Philadelphia, pp 315–323
43. Bird A (1992) The essentials of DNA methylation. Cell 70:5–8
44. Blaustein A (1981) Surface cells and inclusion cysts in fetal ovaries. Gynecol Oncol 12:222–233
45. Bloss JD, Liao S-Y, Buller RE, et al (1993) Extraovarian peritoneal serous papillary carcinoma: a case-control retrospective comparison to papillary adenocarcinoma of the ovary. Gynecol Oncol 50:347–351
46. Boerman OC, van Niekerk CC, Makkink K, et al (1991) Comparative immunohistochemical study of four monoclonal antibodies directed against ovarian carcinoma-associated antigens. Int J Gynecol Pathol 10:15–25
47. Bosari S, Viale G, Radaelli U, et al (1993) p53 accumulation in ovarian carcinomas and prognostic implications. Hum Pathol 24:1175–1179
48. Boucher D, Tetu B (1994) Morphologic prognostic factors of malignant mixed mullerian tumors of the ovary: a clinicopathologic study of 15 cases. Int J Gynecol Pathol 13:22–28
49. Boyd J, Sonoda Y, Federici MG, et al (2000) Clinicopathologic features of BRCA-linked and sporadic ovarian cancer. JAMA 283:2260–2265
50. Boyle P, Maisonneuve P, Autier P (1998) Towards cancer control in women. J Epidemiol Biostat 3:137–168
51. Brinton LA, Gridley G, Persson I, et al (1997) Cancer risk after a hospital discharge diagnosis of endometriosis. Am J Obstet Gynecol 176:572–579
52. Brustmann H, Riss P, Naude S (1997) The relevance of angiogenesis in benign and malignant epithelial tumors of the ovary: a quantitative histologic study. Gynecol Oncol 67:20–26
53. Burger AM, Bibby MC, Double JA (1997) Telomerase activity in normal and malignant mammalian tissues: feasability of telomerase as a target for cancer chemotherapy. Br J Cancer 75:516–522
54. Burks RT, Sherman ME, Kurman RJ (1996) Micropapillary serous carcinoma of the ovary: a distinctive low grade carcinoma related to serous borderline tumors. Am J Surg Pathol 20:1319–1330
55. Buttini M, Nicklin JL, Crandon A (1997) Low malignant potential ovarian tumours: a review of 175 consecutive cases. Aust NZJ Obstet Gynaecol 37: 100–103
56. Caduff RF, Svoboda-Newman SM, Bartos RE, et al (1998) Comparative analysis of histologic homologues of endometrial and ovarian carcinomas. Am J Surg Pathol 22:319–326
57. Caduff RF, Svoboda-Newman SM, Ferguson AW, et al (1999) Comparison of mutations of Ki-RAS and p53 immunoreactivity in borderline and malignant epithelial ovarian tumors. Am J Surg Pathol 23:323–328
58. Cannistra SA, Abu-Jawdeh G, Niloff J, et al (1995) CD44 variant expression is a common feature of epithelial ovarian cancer: lack of association with standard prognostic factors. J Clin Oncol 13:1912–1921
59. Cannistra SA, Kansas GS, Niloff J, et al (1993) Binding of ovarian cancer cells to peritoneal mesothelium *in vitro* is partly mediated by CD44H. Cancer Res 53:3830–3838
60. Carano KS, Soslow RA (1997) Immunophenotypic analysis of ovarian and testicular mullerian papillary serous tumors. Mod Pathol 10:414–420
61. Carr NJ, McCarthy WF, Sobin LH (1995) Epithelial noncarcinoid tumors and tumor-like lesions of the appendix: a clinicopathologic study of 184 patients with a multivariate analysis of prognostic factors. Cancer (Phila) 75:757–768
62. Carreiras F, Denoux Y, Staedel C, et al (1996) Expression and localization of αv integrins and their ligand vitronectin in normal ovarian epithelium and in ovarian carcinoma. Gynecol Oncol 62:260–267
63. Casey A, Bell D, Lage J, et al (1993) Epithelial ovarian tumors of borderline malignancy: long-term follow-up. Gynecol Oncol 50:316–322
64. Chaitin BA, Gershenson DM, Evans HL (1985)

Mucinous tumors of the ovary: a clinicopathologic study of 70 cases. Cancer (Phila) 55:1958–1962
65. Chambers JT, Merino MJ, Kohorn EI, et al (1988) Borderline ovarian tumors. Am J Obstet Gynecol 159:1088–1094
66. Chambers SK, Wang Y, Gertz RE, et al (1995) Macrophage colony-stimulating factor mediates invasion of ovarian cancer cells through urokinase. Cancer Res 55:1578–1585
67. Chan W-Y, Cheung K-K, Schorge JO, et al (2000) Bcl-2 and p53 protein expression, apoptosis, and p53 mutation in human epithelial ovarian cancers. Am J Pathol 156:409–417
68. Chang KL, Crabtree GS, Lim-Tan SK, et al (1993) Primary extrauterine endometrial stromal neoplasms: a clinicopathologic study of 20 cases and a review of the literature. Int J Gynecol Pathol 12:282–296
68a. Che M, Tornos C, Deavers MT, et al (2001) Ovarian mixed-epithelial carcinomas with a microcystic pattern and signet-ring cells. Int J Gynecol Pathol 20:323–328
69. Cheng P, Schmutte C, Cofer KF, et al (1997) Alterations in DNA methylation are early, but not initial, events in ovarian tumorigenesis. Br J Cancer 75:396–402
70. Cheng PC, Gosewehr JA, Kim TM, et al (1996) Potential role of the inactivated X chromosome in ovarian epithelial tumor development. J Natl Cancer Inst 88:510–518
71. Chuaqui RF, Zhuang Z, Emmert-Buck MR, et al (1996) Genetic analysis of synchronous mucinous tumors of the ovary and appendix. Hum Pathol 27:165–171
72. Claus EB, Schildkraut JM, Thompson WD, et al (1996) The genetic attributable risk of breast and ovarian cancer. Cancer (Phila) 77:2318–2324
73. Copeland LJ, Silva EG, Gershenson DM, et al (1988) The significance of müllerian inclusions found at second-look laparotomy in patients with epithelial ovarian neoplasms. Obstet Gynecol 71:763–770
74. Costa MJ, Hansen CL, Walls JE, et al (1999) Immunohistochemical markers of cell cycle control applied to ovarian and primary peritoneal surface epithelial neoplasms: p21 WAF1/CIP1 predicts survival and good response to platinum-based chemotherapy. Hum Pathol 30:640–647
75. Couch FJ, Garber J, Kiousis S, et al (1995) Genetic analysis of eight breast-ovarian cancer families with suspected BRCA1 mutations. J Natl Cancer Inst 17:9–14
76. Counter CM, Hirte HW, Bacchetti S, et al (1994) Telomerase activity in human ovarian carcinoma. Proc Natl Acad Sci USA 91:2900–2904
77. Cramer DW, Welch WR (1983) Determinants of ovarian cancer risk: II. Inferences regarding pathogenesis. J Natl Cancer Inst 71:717–721
78. Creasman WT, Park R, Norris H, et al (1982) Stage I borderline ovarian tumors. Obstet Gynecol 59: 93–96
79. Crozier MA, Copeland LJ, Silva EG, et al (1989) Clear cell carcinoma of the ovary: a study of 59 cases. Gynecol Oncol 35:199–203
80. Cuatrecasas M, Erill N, Musulen E, et al (1998) K-*ras* mutations in nonmucinous ovarian epithelial tumors: a molecular analysis and clinicopathologic study of 144 patients. Cancer (Phila) 82:1088–1095
81. Cuatrecasas M, Matias-Guiu X, Prat J (1996) Synchronous mucinous tumors of the appendix and the ovary associated with pseudomyxoma peritonei: a clinicopathologic study of six cases with comparative analysis of c-Ki-*ras* mutations. Am J Surg Pathol 20:739–746
82. Cuatrecasas M, Villanueva A, Matias-Guiu X, et al (1997) K-ras mutations in mucinous ovarian tumors: a clinicopathologic and molecular study of 95 cases. Cancer (Phila) 79:1581–1586
83. Czernobilsky B, Silverman B, Enterline HT (1970) Clear cell carcinoma of the ovary: a clinicopathologic analysis of pure and mixed forms and comparison with endometrioid carcinoma. Cancer (Phila) 25:762–772.
84. Czernobilsky B, Silverman BB, Mikuta JJ (1970) Endometrioid carcinoma of the ovary: a clinicopathologic study of 75 cases. Cancer (Phila) 26: 1141–1152
85. Dabbs DJ, Sturtz K, Zaino RJ (1996) The immunohistochemical discrimination of endometrioid adenocarcinomas. Hum Pathol 27:172–177
86. Darai E, Bringuier A-F, Walker-Combrouze F, et al (1998) CD31 expression in benign, borderline, and malignant epithelial ovarian tumors: an immunohistochemical and serological analysis. Gynecol Oncol 71:122–127
87. Darai E, Scoazec J-Y, Walker-Combrouze F, et al (1997) Expression of cadherins in benign, borderline, and malignant ovarian epithelial tumors: a clinicopathologic study of 60 cases. Hum Pathol 28:922–928
87a. Darai E, Teboul J, Walker F, et al (1996) Epithelial ovarian carcinoma of low malignant potential. Eur J Obstet Gynecol Reprod Biol 66:141–145
88. Darai E, Walker-Combrouze F, Fauconnier A, et al (1998) Analysis of CD44 expression in serous and mucinous borderline tumors of the ovary: comparison with cystadenomas and overt carcinomas. Histopathology (Oxf) 32:151–159
89. Dauplat J, Nieberg RK, Hacker NF (1987) Central nervous system metastases in epithelial ovarian carcinoma. Cancer (Phila) 60:2559–2562
90. Davies BR, Wordsley SD, Ponder BAJ (1998) Expression of E-cadherin, α-catenin and β-catenin in normal ovarian surface epithelium and epithelial ovarian cancers. Histopathology (Oxf) 32:69–80
91. Daya D, Nazerali L, Frank GL (1992) Metastatic ovarian carcinoma of large intestinal origin simulating primary ovarian carcinoma: a clinicopathologic study of 25 cases. Am J Clin Pathol 97:751–758

92. DeCostanzo DC, Elias JM, Chumas JC (1997) Necrosis in 84 ovarian carcinomas: a morphologic study of primary versus metastatic colonic carcinoma with a selective immunohistochemical analysis of cytokeratin subtypes and carcinoembryonic antigen. Int J Gynecol Pathol 16:245–249
93. Dehner LP, Norris HJ, Taylor HB (1971) Carcinosarcomas and mixed mesodermal tumors of the ovary. Cancer (Phila) 27:207–216
94. Deligdisch L, Einstein AJ, Guera D, et al (1995) Ovarian dysplasia in epithelial inclusion cysts: a morphometric approach using neural networks. Cancer (Phila) 76:1027–1034
95. Deligdisch L, Gil J (1989) Characterization of ovarian dysplasia by interactive morphometry. Cancer (Phila) 63:748–755
96. Deligdisch L, Miranda C, Barba J, et al (1993) Ovarian dysplasia: nuclear texture analysis. Cancer (Phila) 72:3253–3257
97. DeMay RM (1996) The art and science of cytopathology: aspiration cytology. ASCP Press, Chicago, pp 1163–1165
98. Dembo AJ, Davy M, Stenwig AE, et al (1990) Prognostic factors in patients with stage I epithelial ovarian cancer. Obstet Gynecol 75:263–273
99. Demirel D, Laucirica R, Fishman A, et al (1996) Ovarian tumors of low malignant potential: correlation of DNA index and S-phase fraction with histopathologic grade and clinical outcome. Cancer (Phila) 77:1494–1500
100. de Nictolis M, Garbisa S, Lucarini G, et al (1996) 72-Kilodalton type IV collagenase, type IV collagen, and Ki-67 antigen in serous tumors of the ovary: a clinicopathologic, immunohistochemical, and serological study. Int J Gynecol Pathol 15:102–109
100a. de Nictolis M, Montironi R, Tommasoni S, et al (1992) Serous borderline tumors of the ovary: a clinicopathologic, immunohistochemical, and quantitative study of 44 cases. Cancer 70:152–160
101. de Nictolis M, Montironi R, Tommasoni S, et al (1994) Benign, borderline, and well-differentiated malignant intestinal mucinous tumors of the ovary: a clinicopathologic, histochemical, immunohistochemical, and nuclear quantitiative study of 57 cases. Int J Gynecol Pathol 13:10–21
102. DePriest PD, Banks ER, Powell DE, et al (1992) Endometrioid carcinoma of the ovary and endometriosis: the association in postmenopausal women. Gynecol Oncol 47:71–75
103. Diebold J, Deisenhofer I, Baretton GB, et al (1996) Interphase cytogenetic analysis of serous ovarian tumors of low malignant potential: comparison with serous cystadenomas and invasive serous carcinomas. Lab Invest 75:473–485
104. Di Re F, Paladini D, Fontanelli R, et al (1994) Surgical staging for epithelial ovarian tumors of low malignant potential. Int J Gynecol Cancer 4:310–314
105. Duska LR, Chang Y, Flynn CE, et al (1999) Epithelial ovarian carcinoma in the reproductive age group. Cancer (Phila) 85:2623–2629
106. Eccles DM, Brett L, Lessells A, et al (1992) Overexpression of the p53 protein and allele loss at 17p13 in ovarian carcinomas. Br J Cancer 65:40–44
107. Ehrlich CE, Roth LM (1971) The Brenner tumor: a clinicopathologic study of 57 cases. Cancer (Phila) 27:332–342
108. Ehrmann RL, Federschneider JM, Knapp RC (1980) Distinguishing lymph node metastases from benign glandular inclusions in low-grade ovarian carcinoma. Am J Obstet Gynecol 136:737–746
109. Eichorn JH, Bell DA, Young RH, et al (1999) Ovarian serous borderline tumors with micropapillary and cribriform patterns: a study of 40 cases and comparison with 44 cases without these patterns. Am J Surg Pathol 23:397–409
110. Eichhorn JH, Scully RE (1996) Endometrioid ciliated-cell tumors of the ovary: a report of five cases. Int J Gynecol Pathol 15:248–256
111. Eifel P, Hendrickson M, Ross J, et al (1982) Simultaneous presentation of carcinoma involving the ovary and the uterine corpus. Cancer (Phila) 50:163–170
112. Eisen A, Weber BL (1998) Primary peritoneal carcinoma can have multifocal origins: implications for prophylactic oophorectomy. J Natl Cancer Inst 90:797–799
112a. Eisenthal A, Polyvkin N, Bramante-Schreiber L, et al (2001) Expression of dendritic cells in ovarian tumors correlates with clinical outcome in patients with ovarian cancer. Hum Pathol 32:803–807
113. Emmert-Buck MR, Chuaqui R, Zhuang Z, et al (1997) Molecular analysis of synchronous uterine and ovarian endometrioid tumors. Int Gynecol Pathol 16:143–148
114. Enomoto T, Weghorst CM, Inoue M, et al (1991) K-*ras* activation occurs frequently in mucinous adenocarcinomas and rarely in other common epithelial tumors of the human ovary. Am J Pathol 139:777–785
115. Esteller M, Catasus L, Matias-Guiu X, et al (1999) HMLH1 promoter hypermethylation is an early event in human endometrial tumorigenesis. Am J Pathol 155:1767–1772
116. Esteller M, Silva JM, Dominguez G, et al (2000) Promoter hypermethylation and BRCA1 inactivation in sporadic breast and ovarian tumors. J Natl Cancer Inst 92:564–569
117. Facher EA, Becich MJ, Deka A, et al (1997) Associations between human cancer and two polymorphisms occurring together in the $p21^{Waf1/Cip1}$ cyclin-dependent kinase inhibitor gene. Cancer (Phila) 79:2424–2429
118. Farhi DC, Silverberg SG (1982) Pseudometastases in female genital cancer. Pathol Ann 17(part I): 47–76
119. Fathalla MF (1971) Incessant ovulation—a factor in ovarian neoplasia? Lancet 2:163

120. Finn CB, Dunn J, Buxton EJ, et al (1993) Can we predict a high risk group in stage I epithelial ovarian cancer? Int J Gynecol Cancer 3:226–230
121. Ford D, Easton DF, Bishop DT, et al (1994) Risks of cancer in BRCA1-mutation carriers. Lancet 343:692–695
122. Ford D, Easton DF, Peto J (1995) Estimates of the gene frequency of BRCA1 and its contribution to breast and ovarian cancer incidence. Am J Hum Genet 57:1457–1462
123. Ford D, Easton DF, Stratton M, et al (1998) Genetic heterogeneity and penetrance analysis of the BRCA1 and BRCA2 genes in breast cancer families. Am J Hum Genet 62:676–689
124. Fox H (1993) Pathology of early malignant change in the ovary. Int J Gynecol Pathol 12:153–155
125. Frank TS (1999) Laboratory determination of hereditary susceptibility to breast and ovarian cancer. Arch Pathol Lab Med 123:1023–1026
126. Friedlander ML (1998) Prognostic factors in ovarian cancer. Semin Oncol 25:305–314
126a. Friedlander ML, Russell P, Taylor IW, et al (1984) Influence of cellular DNA content on survival in advanced ovarian cancer. Cancer Res 44:397–400
127. Fujimoto J, Sakaguchi H, Hirose R, et al (1998) Biologic implications of the expression of vascular endothelial growth factor subtypes in ovarian carcinoma. Cancer (Phila) 83:2528–2533
127a. Fujimura M, Hidaka T, Kataoka K, et al (2001) Abscence of estrogen receptor-alpha expression in human ovarian clear cell adenocarcinoma compared with ovarian serous, endometroid, and mucinous adenocarcinoma. Am J Surg Pathol 25:667–672
128. Fujita M, Enomoto T, Haba T, et al (1997) Alteration of p16 and p15 genes in common epithelial ovarian tumors. Int J Cancer 74:148–155
129. Fujita M, Enomoto T, Wada H, et al (1996) Application of clonal analysis: differential diagnosis for synchronous primary ovarian and endometrial cancers and metastatic cancer. Am J Clin Pathol 105:350–359
130. Fukunaga M, Nomura K, Ishikawa E, et al (1997) Ovarian atypical endometriosis: its close association with malignant epithelial tumours. Histopathology (Oxf) 30:249–255
131. Futreal PA, Liu Q, Shattuck-Eidens D, et al (1994) BRCA1 mutations in primary breast and ovarian carcinomas. Science 266:120–122
132. Gallion HH, Guarino DA, DePriest PD, et al (1996) Evidence for a unifocal origin in familial ovarian cancer. Am J Obstet Gynecol 174:1102–1108
133. Gallion HH, Powell DE, Smith LW, et al (1990) Chromosome abnormalities in human epithelial ovarian malignancies. Gynecol Oncol 38:473–477
134. Gallion HH, Smith SA (1994) Hereditary ovarian carcinoma. Semin Surg Oncol 10:249–254
135. Garg PP, Kerlikowske K, Subak L, et al (1998) Hormone replacement therapy and the risk of epithelial ovarian carcinoma: a meta-analysis. Obstet Gynecol 92:472–479
136. Geisinger KR, Kute TE, Pettenati MJ, et al (1989) Characterization of a human ovarian carcinoma cell line with estrogen and progesterone receptors. Cancer (Phila) 63:280–288
137. Geisler JP, Geisler HE, Wiemann MC, et al (1997) Quantification of p53 in epithelial ovarian cancer. Gynecol Oncol 66:435–438
138. Gersell DJ, King TC (1988) Papillary cystadenoma of the mesosalpinx in von Hippel–Lindau disease. Am J Surg Pathol 12:145–149
139. Gershenson DM (1999) Contemporary treatment of borderline ovarian tumors. Cancer Invest 19: 206–210
140. Gershenson DM, Silva EG (1990) Serous ovarian tumors of low malignant potential with peritoneal implants. Cancer (Phila) 65:578–585
141. Gershenson DM, Silva EG, Levy L, et al (1998) Ovarian serous borderline tumors with invasive peritoneal implants. Cancer (Phila) 82:1096–1103
142. Gershenson DM, Silva EG, Tortolero-Luna G, et al (1998) Serous borderline tumors of the ovary with noninvasive peritoneal implants. Cancer (Phila) 83:2157–2163
143. Gershenson DM, Silva EG, Mitchell MF, et al (1993) Transitional cell carcinoma of the ovary: a matched control study of advanced-stage patients treated with cisplatin-based chemotherapy. Am J Obstet Gynecol 168:1178–1187
144. Gilks CB, Bell DA, Scully RE (1990) Serous psammocarcinoma of the ovary and peritoneum. Int J Gynecol Pathol 9:110–121
145. Goldgar DE, Neuhausen SL, Steele L, et al (1995) A 45-year follow-up of kindred 107 and the search for BRCA2. Monogr Natl Cancer Inst 17:15–19
146. Goldman TL, Chalas E, Chumas J, et al (1993) Management of borderline tumors of the ovary. South Med J 86:423–425
146a. Goldstein NS, Ceniza N (2000) Ovarian micropapillary serous borderline tumors: clinicopathologic features and outcome of seven surgically staged patients. Am J Clin Pathol 114:380–386
147. Gould VE, Gould KA (1999) E-cadherin as a tumor differentiation marker and as architectural determinant [Editorial] Human Pathol 30:1273–1275
147a. Gras E, Pons C, Machin P, et al (2001) Loss of heterozygosity at the RB-1 locus and pRB immunostaining in epithelial ovarian tumors: a molecular, immunohistochemical, and clinicopathologic study. Int J Gynecol Pathol 20:335–340
148. Greenlee RT, Murray T, Bolden S, et al (2000) Cancer statistics, 2000. CA Cancer J Clin 50:7–33
149. Grosso G, Raspagliesi F, Baiocchi G, et al (1998) Endometrioid carcinoma of the ovary: a retrospective analysis of 106 cases. Tumori 84:552–557
150. Guerrieri C, Franlund B, Malmstrom H, et al (1998) Ovarian endometrioid carcinomas simulating sex cord-stromal tumors: a study using inhibin and cytokeratin 7. Int J Gynecol Pathol 17: 266–271

151. Guerrieri C, Hogberg T, Wingren S, et al (1994) Mucinous borderline and malignant tumors of the ovary: a clinicopathologic and DNA ploidy study of 92 cases. Cancer (Phila) 74:2329–2340
152. Gusberg SB, Deligdisch L (1984) Ovarian dysplasia: a study of identical twins. Cancer (Phila) 54:1–4
153. Haas CJ, Diebold J, Hirschmann A, et al (1999) Microsatellite analysis in serous tumors of the ovary. Int J Gynecol Pathol 18:158–162
154. Haczynska H, Gerber J, Osada J, et al (1997) The activities and subcellular localization of cathepsin B and cysteine proteinase inhibitors in human ovarian carcinoma. Acta Biochim Pol 44:113–120
155. Hall PA, Going JJ (1999) Predicting the future: a critical appraisal of cancer prognosis studies. Histopathology (Oxf) 35:489–494
156. Hallgrimsson J, Scully RE (1972) Borderline and malignant Brenner tumours of the ovary: a report of 15 cases. Acta Path Microbiol Scand A 80(suppl 233):56–66
157. Hammond RH, Bates TD, Clarke DG, et al (1991) The immunoperoxidase localization of tumour markers in ovarian cancer: the value of CEA, EMA, cytokeratin and DD9. Br J Obstet Gynaecol 98:73–83
158. Hanselaar AGJM, Vooijs GP, Mayall B, et al (1993) Epithelial markers to detect occult microinvasion in serous ovarian tumors. Int J Gynecol Pathol 12:20–27
159. Hardy JR, Harvey VJ (1989) Cerebral metastases in patients with ovarian cancer treated with chemotherapy. Gynecol Oncol 33:296–300
160. Harlozinska A, Bar JK, Sedlaczek P, et al (1996) Expression of p53 protein and Ki-67 reactivity in ovarian neoplasms: correlation with histopathology. Am J Clin Pathol 105:334–340
161. Hart WR, Norris HJ (1973) Borderline and malignant mucinous tumors of the ovary: histologic criteria and clinical behavior. Cancer (Phila) 31: 1031–1045
162. Healy DL, Burger HG, Mamers P, et al (1993) Elevated serum inhibin concentrations in postmenopausal women with ovarian tumors. N Engl J Med 329:1539–1542
163. Hendrickson MR, Longacre TA, Kempson RL (1993) Clinicopathology of malignant surface epithelial neoplasms of the ovary. In: Hendrickson MR (ed) Surface epithelial neoplasms of the ovary. Hanley & Belfus, Philadelphia, pp 367–410
164. Henriksen R, Strang P, Wilander E, et al (1994) p53 expression in epithelial ovarian neoplasms: relationship to clinical and pathological parameters, Ki-67 expression and flow cytometry. Gynecol Oncol 53:301–306
165. Herman JG, Umar A, Polyak K, et al (1998) Incidence and functional consequences of hMLH1 promoter hypermethylation in colorectal carcinoma. Proc Natl Acad Sci USA 95:6870–6875
166. Higgins RV, Matkins JF, Marroum M-C (1999) Comparison of fine-needle aspiration cytologic findings of ovarian cysts with ovarian histologic findings. Am J Obstet Gynecol 180:550–553
167. Hirahara F, Miyagi E, Nagashima Y, et al (1998) Differential expression of trypsin in human ovarian carcinomas and low-malignant-potential tumors. Gynecol Oncol 68:162–165
168. Hoerl HD, Hart WR (1998) Primary ovarian mucinous cystadenocarcinomas: a clinicopathologic study of 49 cases with long-term follow-up. Am J Surg Pathol 22:1449–1462
169. Hollingsworth HC, Kohn EC, Steinberg SM, et al (1995) Tumor angiogenesis in advanced stage ovarian carcinoma. Am J Pathol 147:33–41
170. Hollingsworth HC, Steinberg SM, Silverberg SG, et al (1996) Advanced stage transitional cell carcinoma of the ovary. Hum Pathol 27:1267–1272
171. Huettner PC, Carney WP, Naber SP, et al (1992) *neu* oncogene expression in ovarian tumors: a quantitative study. Mod Pathol 5:250–256
172. Hung W-C, Chai C-Y, Huang J-S, et al (1996) Expression of cyclin D1 and c-Ki-*ras* gene product in human epithelial ovarian tumors. Hum Pathol 27:1324–1328
173. Huntsman D, Resau JH, Klineberg E, et al (1999) Comparison of c-*met* expression in ovarian epithelial tumors and normal epithelia of the female reproductive tract by quantitative laser scan microscopy. Am J Pathol 155:343–348
174. Imachi M, Tsukamoto N, Shimamoto T, et al (1991) Clear cell carcinoma of the ovary: a clinicopathologic analysis of 34 cases. Int J Gynecol Cancer 1:113–119
175. Inoue M, Fujita M, Enomoto T, et al (1994) Immunohistochemical analysis of p53 in gynecologic tumors. Am J Clin Pathol 102:665–670
176. International Federation of Gynecology and Obstetrics (1971) Classification and staging of malignant tumors in the female pelvis. Acta Obstet Gynecol Scand 50:1–7
177. Ishikura H, Sasano H (1998) Histopathologic and immunohistochemical study of steroidogenic cells in the stroma of ovarian tumors. Int J Gynecol Pathol 17:261–265
178. Ito K, Sasano H, Ozawa N, et al (1992) Immunolocalization of epidermal growth factor receptor and c-erbB-2 oncogene product in human ovarian carcinoma. Int J Gynecol Pathol 11:253–257
178a. Jackson SL, Fleming RA, Loggie BW, et al (2001) Gelatinous ascites: a cytohistologic study of pseudomyxoma peritonei in 67 patients. Modern Pathol 14:664–671
179. Jacobs IJ, Kohler MF, Wiseman RW, et al (1992) Clonal origin of epithelial ovarian carcinomas: analysis by loss of heterozygosity, p53 mutation, and X-chromosome inactivation. J Natl Cancer Inst 84:1793–1798
180. Jenison EL, Montag AG, Griffiths CT, et al (1989) Clear cell adenocarcinoma of the ovary: a clinical analysis and comparison with serous carcinoma. Gynecol Oncol 32:65–71

181. Jiang X, Hitchcock A, Bryan EJ, et al (1996) Microsatellite analysis of endometriosis reveals loss of heterozygosity at candidate ovarian tumor suppressor gene loci. Cancer Res 56:3534–3539
182. Jimbo H, Hitomi Y, Yoshikawa H, et al (1997) Evidence for monoclonal expansion of epithelial cells in ovarian endometrial cysts. Am J Pathol 150:1173–1178
183. Kabawat SE, Bast RC, Bhan AK, et al (1983) Tissue distribution of a coelomic-epithelium-related antigen recognized by the monoclonal antibody OC125. Int J Gynecol Pathol 2:275–285
184. Kacinski BM, Mayer AG, King BL, et al (1992) *NEU* protein overexpression in benign, borderline, and malignant ovarian neoplasms. Gynecol Oncol 44:245–253
185. Kaern J, Trope C, Kristensen G, et al (1993) DNA ploidy: the most important prognostic factor in patients with borderline tumors of the ovary. Int J Gynecol Cancer 3:349–358
186. Kao GF, Norris HJ (1978) Benign and low grade variants of mixed mesodermal tumor (adenosarcoma) of the ovary and adnexal region. Cancer (Phila) 42:1314–1324
187. Kao GF, Norris HJ (1978) Cystadenofibromas of the ovary with epithelial atypia. Am J Surg Pathol 2:357–363
188. Kao GF, Norris HJ (1979) Unusual cystadenofibromas: endometrioid, mucinous, and clear cell types. Obstet Gynecol 54:729–736.
189. Katabuchi H, Tashiro H, Cho KR, et al (1998) Micropapillary serous carcinoma of the ovary: an immunohistochemical and mutational analysis of p53. Int J Gynecol Pathol 17:54–60
190. Katsube Y, Berg JW, Silverberg SG (1982) Epidemiologic pathology of ovarian tumors: a histopathologic review of primary ovarian neoplasms diagnosed in the Denver Standard Metropolitan Statistical Area, 1 July–31 December 1969 and 1 July–31 December 1979. Int J Gynecol Pathol 1:3–16
191. Katzenstein AA, Mazur MT, Morgan TE, et al (1978) Proliferative serous tumors of the ovary: histologic features and prognosis. Am J Surg Pathol 2:339–355
192. Kauppila S, Saarela J, Stenback F, et al (1996) Expression of mRNAs for type I and type III procollagens in serous ovarian cystadenomas and cystadenocarcinomas. Am J Pathol 148:539–548
193. Keen CE, Szakacs S, Okon E, et al (1999) CA125 and thyroglobulin staining in papillary carcinomas of thyroid and ovarian origin is not completely specific for site of origin. Histopathology (Oxf) 34:113–117
194. Kempson RL, Hendrickson MR (2000) Ovarian serous borderline tumors: the citadel defended [Editorial]. Hum Pathol 31:525–526
195. Kennedy AW, Hart WR (1996) Ovarian papillary serous tumors of low malignant potential (serous borderline tumors): a long term follow-up study, including patients with microinvasion, lymph node metastasis, and transformation to invasive serous carcinoma. Cancer (Phila) 78:278–286
196. Kennedy AW, Markman M, Biscotti CV, et al (1999) Survival probability in ovarian clear cell adenocarcinoma. Gynecol Oncol 74:108–114
197. Kerr VE, Cadman E (1985) Pulmonary metastases in ovarian cancer: analysis of 357 patients. Cancer (Phila) 56:1209–1213
198. Khalifa MA, Sesterhenn IA (1990) Tumor markers of epithelial ovarian neoplasms. Int J Gynecol Pathol 9:217–230
199. Khunamornpong S, Russell P, Dalrymple JC (1999) Proliferating (LMP) mucinous tumors of the ovaries with microinvasion: morphologic assessment of 13 cases. Int J Gynecol Pathol 18:238–246
200. Kikkawa F, Kawai M, Tamakoshi K, et al (1996) Mucinous carcinoma of the ovary: clinicopathologic analysis. Oncology (Basel) 53:303–307
201. Kim K-R, Scully RE (1990) Peritoneal keratin granulomas with carcinomas of the endometrium and ovary and atypical polypoid adenomyoma of the endometrium: a clinicopathological analysis of 22 cases. Am J Surg Pathol 14:925–932
202. Kim TM, Benedict WF, Xu H-J, et al (1994) Loss of heterozygosity on chromosome 13 is common only in the biologically more aggressive subtypes of ovarian epithelial tumors and is associated with normal retinoblastoma gene expression. Cancer Res 54:605–609
203. Kiyokawa T (1994) Alteration of p53 in ovarian cancer: its occurrence and maintenance in tumor progression. Int J Gynecol Pathol 13:311–318
204. Klaassen D, Shelley W, Starreveld A, et al (1988) Early stage ovarian cancer: a randomized clinical trial comparing whole abdominal radiotherapy, melphalan, and intraperitoneal chromic phosphate: a National Cancer Institute of Canada Clinical Trials Group report. J Clin Oncol 6:1254–1263
205. Klapper LN, Glathe S, Vaisman N, et al (1999) The ErbB-2/HER2 oncoprotein of human carcinomas may function solely as a shared coreceptor for multiple stroma-derived growth factors. Proc Natl Acad Sci USA 96:4995–5000
206. Klemi PJ, Gronroos M (1979) Endometrioid carcinoma of the ovary: a clinicopathologic, histochemical, and electron microscopic study. Obstet Gynecol 53:572–579
207. Kliman L, Rome RM, Fortune DW (1986) Low malignant potential tumors of the ovary: a study of 76 cases. Obstet Gynecol 68:338–344
208. Kline RC, Wharton JT, Atkinson EN, et al (1990) Endometrioid carcinoma of the ovary: retrospective review of 145 cases. Gynecol Oncol 39:337–346
209. Knudson W (1996) Tumor-associated hyaluronan: providing an extracellular matrix that facilitates invasion. Am J Pathol 148:1721–1726
210. Koelma IA, Nap M, van Steenis GJ, et al (1988) Tumor markers for ovarian cancer: a comparative

immunohistochemical and immunocytochemical study of two commercial monoclonal antibodies (OV632 and OC125). Am J Clin Pathol 90:391–396
211. Kohlberger PD, Kieback DG, Mian C, et al (1997) Numerical chromosomal aberrations in borderline, benign, and malignant epithelial tumors of the ovary: correlation with p53 protein overexpression and Ki-67. J Soc Gynecol Invest 4:262–264
212. Kohler MF, Kerns BM, Humphrey PA, et al (1993) Mutation and overexpression of p53 in early-stage epithelial ovarian cancer. Obstet Gynecol 81:643–650
213. Kohn EC (1997) Angiogenesis in ovarian carcinoma: a formidable biomarker. Cancer (Phila) 80:2219–2221
214. Koonings PP, Campbell K, Mishell DR Jr, et al (1989) Relative frequency of primary ovarian neoplasms: a 10-year review. Obstet Gynecol 74:921–926
215. Koukoulis GK, Patriarca C, Gould VE (1998) Editorial: adhesion molecules and tumor metastasis. Hum Pathol 29:889–892
216. Kuoppala T, Heinola M, Aine R, et al (1996) Serous and mucinous borderline tumors of the ovary: a clinicopathologic and DNA ploidy study of 102 cases. Int J Gynecol Cancer 6:302–308
217. Kupryjanczyk J, Bell DA, Dimeo D, et al (1995) p53 gene analysis of ovarian borderline tumors and stage I carcinomas. Hum Pathol 26:387–392
218. Kupryjanczyk J, Thor AD, Beauchamp R, et al (1993) p53 mutations and protein accumulation in human ovarian cancer. Proc Natl Acad Sci USA 90:4961–4965
219. Kurman RJ, Craig JM (1972) Endometrioid and clear cell carcinoma of the ovary. Cancer (Phila) 29:1653–1664
220. Kurman RJ, Trimble CL (1993) The behavior of serous tumors of low malignant potential: are they ever malignant? Int J Gynecol Pathol 12:120–127
221. Kyo S, Kanaya T, Takakura M, et al (1999) Expression of human telomerase subunits in ovarian malignant, borderline and benign tumors. Int J Cancer 80:804–809
222. Lage JM, Weinberg DS, Huettner PC, Mark SD (1992) Flow cytometric analysis of nuclear DNA content in ovarian tumors: association of ploidy with tumor type, histologic grade, and clinical stage. Cancer (Phila) 69:2668–2675
223. Lagendijk JH, Mullink H, van Diest PJ, et al (1998) Tracing the origin of adenocarcinomas with unknown primary using immunohistochemistry: differential diagnosis between colonic and ovarian carcinomas as primary sites. Hum Pathol 29:491–497
224. Lam KY, Tang V (2000) Metastatic tumors to the spleen: a 25-year clinicopathologic study. Arch Pathol Lab Med 124:526–530
225. Larson DM, Copeland LJ, Moser RP, et al (1986) Central nervous system metastases in epithelial ovarian carcinoma. Obstet Gynecol 68:746–750
226. Lash RH, Hart WR (1987) Intestinal adenocarcinoma metastatic to the ovaries: a clinicopathologic evaluation of 22 cases. Am J Surg Pathol 11: 114–121.
227. Le T, Krepart GV, Lotocki RJ, et al (1999) Clinically apparent early stage invasive epithelial ovarian carcinoma: should all be treated similarly? Gynecol Oncol 74:252–254
228. Leake JF, Rader JS, Woodruff JD, Rosenshein NB (1991) Retroperitoneal lymphatic involvement with epithelial ovarian tumors of low malignant potential. Gynecol Oncol 42:124–130
229. Lee J-H, Kang Y-S, Park S-Y, et al (1995) P53 mutation in epithelial ovarian carcinoma and borderline ovarian tumor. Cancer Genet Cytogenet 85:43–50
229a. Lee KR, Castrillon DH, Nucci M (2001) Pathologic findings in eight cases of ovarian serous borderline tumors, three with foci of serous carcinoma, that preceded death or morbidity from invasive carcinoma. Int J Gynecol Pathol 20:329–334
230. Lee KR, Scully RE (2000) Mucinous tumors of the ovary: a clinicopathologic study of 196 borderline tumors (of intestinal type) and carcinomas, including an evaluation of 11 cases with 'pseudomyxoma peritonei.' Am J Surg Pathol 24:1447–1464
231. LeRoux PD, Berger MS, Elliott JP, et al (1991) Cerebral metastases from ovarian carcinoma. Cancer (Phila) 67:2194–2199
232. Lessan K, Aguiar DJ, Oegema T, et al (1999) CD44 and $\beta 1$ integrin mediate ovarian carcinoma cell adhesion to peritoneal mesothelial cells. Am J Pathol 154:1525–1537
233. Li S, Han H, Resnik E, et al (1993) Advanced ovarian carcinoma: molecular evidence of unifocal origin. Gynecol Oncol 51:21–25
234. Liapis H, Adler LM, Wick MR, et al (1997) Expression of $\alpha_v \beta_3$ integrin is less frequent in ovarian epithelial tumors of low malignant potential in contrast to ovarian carcinomas. Hum Pathol 28:443–449
235. Liotta LA (1986) Tumor invasion and metastases: role of the extracellular matrix. Cancer Res 46:1–7
236. Loy TS, Calaluce RD, Keeney GL (1996) Cytokeratin immunostaining in differentiating primary ovarian carcinoma from metastatic colonic adenocarcinoma. Mod Pathol 9:1040–1044
237. Lu KH, Bell DA, Welch WR, et al (1998) Evidence for the multifocal origin of bilateral and advanced human serous borderline ovarian tumors. Cancer Res 58:2328–2330
238. Lu KH, Cramer DW, Muto MG, et al (1999) A population-based study of BRCA1 and BRCA2 mutations in Jewish women with epithelial ovarian cancer. Obstet Gynecol 93:34–37
239. Lu Q-L, Abel P, Foster CS, et al (1996) Bcl-2: role in epithelial differentiation and oncogenesis. Hum Pathol 27:102–110
240. Lukas J, Groshen S, Saffari B, et al (1997) WAF1/Cip1 gene polymorphism and expression in

carcinomas of the breast, ovary, and endometrium. Am J Pathol 150:167–175

241. Lynch HT, Watson P, Bewtra C, et al (1991) Hereditary ovarian cancer: heterogeneity in age at diagnosis. Cancer (Phila) 67:1460–1466
242. Lynch HT, Watson P, Tinley S, et al (1999) An update on DNA-based BRCA1/BRCA2 genetic counseling in hereditary breast cancer. Cancer Genet Cytogenet 109:91–98
243. Maines-Bandiera S, Auersperg N (1997) Increased E-cadherin expression in ovarian surface epithelium: an early step in metaplasia and dysplasia? Int J Gynecol Pathol 16:250–255
244. Mandai M, Konishi I, Kuroda H (1998) Heterogeneous distribution of K-*ras*-mutated epithelia in mucinous ovarian tumors with special reference to histopathology. Hum Pathol 28:34–40
245. Markman M, Lewis JL, Saigo P, et al (1993) Impact of age on survival of patients with ovarian cancer. Gynecol Oncol 49:236–239
246. Marks JR, Davidoff AM, Kerns BJ, et al (1991) Overexpression and mutation of p53 in epithelial ovarian cancer. Cancer Res 51:2979–2984
247. Marone M, Scambia G, Mozzetti S, et al (1998) Bcl-2, bax, bcl-x_L and bcl-x_S expression in normal and neoplastic ovarian tissues. Clin Cancer Res 4:517–521
248. Marra G, Boland CR (1995) Hereditary nonpolyposis colorectal cancer: the syndrome, the genes, and historical perspectives. J Natl Cancer Inst 87:14–25
249. Martinez-Hernandez A (1988) Editorial: The extracellular matrix and neoplasia. Lab Invest 58:609–612
250. Massad L, Hunter V, Szpak C, et al (1991) Epithelial ovarian tumors of low malignant potential. Obstet Gynecol 78:1027–1032
251. Massi D, Susini T, Savino L, et al (1996) Epithelial ovarian tumors in the reproductive age group: age is not an independent prognostic factor. Cancer (Phila) 77:1131–1136
252. Mayer RJ, Berkowitz RS, Griffiths CT (1978) Central nervous system involvement by ovarian carcinoma: a complication of prolonged survival with metastatic disease. Cancer (Phila) 41:776–783
252a. Mayr D, Diebold J (2000) Grading of ovarian carcinomas. Int J Gynecol Pathol 19:348–353
253. McCaughey WTE, Kirk ME, Lester W, et al (1984) Peritoneal epithelial lesions associated with proliferative serous tumors of the ovary. Histopathology (Oxf) 8:195–208
253a. McLaren J (2000) Vascular endothelial growth factor and endometriotic angiogenesis. Hum Reprod Update 6:45–55
254. McMeekin DS, Burger RA, Manetta A, et al (1995) Endometrioid adenocarcinoma of the ovary and its relationship to endometriosis. Gynecol Oncol 59:81–86
255. Meden H, Marx D, Roegglen T, et al (1998) Overexpression of the oncogene c-erbB-2 (HER2/neu) and response to chemotherapy in patients with ovarian cancer. Int J Gynecol Pathol 17:61–65
256. Meis JM, Lawrence WD (1990) The immunohistochemical profile of malignant mixed mullerian tumor: overlap with endometrial adenocarcinoma. Am J Clin Pathol 94:1–7
257. Merogi AJ, Marrogi AJ, Ramesh R, et al (1997) Tumor-host interaction: analysis of cytokines, growth factors, and tumor-infiltrating lymphocytes in ovarian carcinomas. Hum Pathol 28:321–331
258. Michael H, Roth LM (1986) Invasive and noninvasive implants in ovarian serous tumors of low malignant potential. Cancer (Phila) 57:1240–1247
259. Mikami Y, Hata S, Melamed J, et al (1999) Basement membrane material in ovarian clear cell carcinoma: correlation with growth pattern and nuclear grade. Int J Gynecol Pathol 18:52–57
260. Miki Y, Swensen J, Shattuck-Eidens D, et al (1994) A strong candidate for the breast and ovarian cancer susceptibility gene BRCA1. Science 266:66–71
261. Miles PA, Norris HJ (1972) Proliferative and malignant Brenner tumors of the ovary. Cancer (Phila) 30:174–186
262. Milner BJ, Allan LA, Eccles DM, et al (1993) p53 mutation is a common genetic event in ovarian carcinoma. Cancer Res 53:2128–2132
263. Mittal KR, Zeleniuch-Jacquotte A, Cooper JL, et al (1993) Contralateral ovary in unilateral ovarian carcinoma: a search for preneoplastic lesions. Int J Gynecol Pathol 12:59–63
264. Mok SC, Bell DA, Knapp RC, et al (1993) Mutation of K-*ras* protooncogene in human ovarian epithelial tumors of borderline malignancy. Cancer Res 53:1489–1492
265. Mok C-H, Tsao S-W, Knapp RC, et al (1992) Unifocal origin of advanced human epithelial ovarian cancers. Cancer Res 52:5119–5122
266. Moll R, Pitz S, Levy R, et al (1991) Complexity of expression of intermediate filament proteins, including glial filament protein, in endometrial and ovarian adenocarcinomas. Hum Pathol 22:989–1001
267. Montag AG, Jenison EL, Griffiths CT, et al (1989) Ovarian clear cell carcinoma: a clinicopathologic analysis of 44 cases. Int J Gynecol Pathol 8:85–96
268. Monteagudo C, Merino MJ, LaPorte N, et al (1991) Value of gross cystic disease fluid protein-15 in distinguishing metastatic breast carcinomas among poorly differentiated neoplasms involving the ovary. Hum Pathol 22:368–372
269. Mooney J, Silva EG, Tornos C, et al (1997) Unusual features of serous neoplasms of low malignant potential during pregnancy. Gynecol Oncol 65:30–35
270. Moore WF, Bentley RC, Berchuck A, et al (2000) Some müllerian inclusion cysts in lymph nodes may sometimes be metastases from serous borderline tumors of the ovary. Am J Surg Pathol 24:710–718

271. Morrow CP, d'Ablaing G, Brady LW, et al (1984) A clinical and pathologic study of 30 cases of malignant mixed mullerian epithelial and mesenchymal ovarian tumors: a Gynecologic Oncology Group Study. Gynecol Oncol 18:278–292
272. Mostoufizadeh M, Scully RE (1980) Malignant tumors arising in endometriosis. Clin Obstet Gynecol 23:951–963
273. Multhaupt HAB, Arenas-Elliott CP, Warhol MJ (1999) Comparison of glycoprotein expression between ovarian and colon adenocarcinomas. Arch Pathol Lab Med 123:909–916
274. Murakami J, Nagai N, Ohama K, et al (1997) Telomerase activity in ovarian tumors. Cancer (Phila) 80:1085–1092
275. Nakanishi T, Kadomatsu K, Okamoto T, et al (1997) Expression of midkine and pleiotropin in ovarian tumors. Obstet Gynecol 90:285–290
276. Nakashima N, Nagasaka T, Oiwa N, et al (1990) Ovarian epithelial tumors of borderline malignancy in Japan. Gynecol Oncol 38:90–98
277. Nayar R, Siriaunkgul S, Robbins KM, et al (1996) Microinvasion in low malignant potential tumors of the ovary. Hum Pathol 27:521–527
278. Naylor B (1997) Pleural, peritoneal, and pericardial fluids. In: Bibbo M (ed) Comprehensive cytopathology, 2nd Ed. Saunders, Philadelphia, pp. 551–621
279. Ness RB, Cottreau C (1999) Possible role of ovarian epithelial inflammation in ovarian cancer. J Natl Cancer Inst 91:1459–1467
280. Neunteufel W, Breitenecker G (1989) Tissue expression of CA 125 in benign and malignant lesions of ovary and fallopian tube: a comparison with CA 19-9 and CEA. Gynecol Oncol 32:297–302
281. Nguyen HN, Averette HE, Hoskins, W, et al (1993) National Survey of ovarian carcinoma VI: critical assessment of current International Federation of Gynecology and Obstetrics staging system. Cancer (Phila) 72:3007–3011
282. Niikura H, Sasano H, Sato S, et al (1997) Expression of epidermal growth factor-related proteins and epidermal growth factor receptor in common epithelial ovarian tumors. Int J Gynecol Pathol 16:60–68
283. Nikrui N (1981) Survey of clinical behavior of patients with borderline epithelial tumors of the ovary. Gynecol Oncol 12:107–119
284. Nilbert M, Pejovic T, Mandahl N, et al (1995) Monoclonal origin of endometriotic cysts. Int J Gynecol Cancer 5:61–63
285. Niwa K, Itoh M, Murase T, et al (1994) Alteration of p53 gene in ovarian carcinoma: clinicopathological correlation and prognostic significance. Br J Cancer 70:1191–1197
285a. Nolan LP, Heatley MK (2001) The value of immunocytochemisty in distinguishing between clear cell carcinoma of the kidney and ovary. Int J Gynecol Pathol 20:155–159
286. Norris HJ (1993) Proliferative endometrioid tumors and endometrioid tumors of low malignant potential of the ovary. Int J Gynecol Pathol 12: 134–140
287. Norris HJ, Robinowitz M (1971) Ovarian adenocarcinoma of mesonephric type. Cancer (Phila) 28:1074–1081
288. O'Brien ME, Schofield JB, Tan S, et al (1993) Clear cell epithelial ovarian cancer (mesonephroid): bad prognosis only in early stages. Gynecol Oncol 49:250–254
289. O'Donnell M, Al-Nafussi AI (1995) Intracytoplasmic lumina and mucinous inclusions in ovarian carcinomas. Histopathology (Oxf) 26:181–184
290. Okamoto A, Sameshima Y, Yokoyama S, et al (1991) Frequent allelic losses and mutations of the p53 gene in human ovarian cancer. Cancer Res 51:5171–5176
291. Olson TA, Mohanraj D, Carson LF, et al (1994) Vascular permeability factor gene expression in normal and neoplastic human ovaries. Cancer Res 54:276–280
292. Ordi J, Schammel DP, Rasekh L, et al (1999) Sertoliform endometrioid carcinomas of the ovary: a clinicopathologic and immunohistochemical study of 13 cases. Mod Pathol 12:933–940
293. Ordonez NG (1998) Role of immunohistochemistry in distinguishing epithelial peritoneal mesotheliomas from peritoneal and ovarian serous carcinomas. Am J Surg Pathol 22:1203–1214
294. Ordonez NG (2000) Transitional cell carcinomas of the ovary and bladder are immunophenotypically different. Histopathology (Oxf) 36:433–438
295. Orre M, Lotfi-Miri M, Mamers P, et al (1998) Increased microvessel density in mucinous compared with malignant serous and benign tumors of the ovary. Br J Cancer 77:2204–2209
296. Orre M, Rogers PAW (1999) Macrophages and microvessel density in tumors of the ovary. Gynecol Oncol 73:47–50
297. Ozols RF, Rubin SC, Thomas G, et al (1997) Epithelial ovarian cancer. In: Hoskins WJ, Perez CA, Young RC (eds) Principles and practice of gynecological oncology, 2nd Ed. Lippincott-Raven, Philadelphia, pp 919–986
298. Palacios J, Gamallo C (1998) Mutations in the β-catenin gene (CTNNB1) in endometrioid ovarian carcinomas. Cancer Res 58:1344–1347
299. Partridge EE, Phillips JL, Menck HR (1996) The National Cancer Data Base report on ovarian cancer treatment in United States hospitals. Cancer (Phila) 78:2236–2246
300. Pathak S (1992) Cytogenetics of epithelial malignant lesions. Cancer (Phila) 70:1660–1670
301. Pauli BU, Knudson W (1998) Tumor invasion: a consequence of destructive and compositional matrix alterations. Hum Pathol 19:628–639
302. Pearl ML, Johnston CM, Frank TS, et al (1993) Synchronous dual primary ovarian and endometrial carcinomas. Int J Gynecol Obstet 43:305–312
303. Pecorelli S (ed) (1998) FIGO annual report on the

results of treatment in gynaecological cancer, vol 23. J Epidemiol Biostat 3:1–168
304. Pejovic T, Iosif CS, Mitelman F, et al (1996) Karyotypic characteristics of borderline malignant tumors of the ovary: trisomy 12, trisomy 7, and r(1) as nonrandom features. Cancer Genet Cytogenet 92:95–98
305. Pettersson F (ed) (1994) Annual report on the results of treatment in gynecological cancer, vol 22. International Federation of Gynecology and Obstetrics, Stockholm
306. Phillips NJ, Ziegler MR, Radford DM, et al (1996) Allelic deletion on chromosome 17p13.3 in early ovarian cancer. Cancer Res 56:606–611
307. Piccart MJ, Bertelsen K, James K, et al (2000) Randomized intergroup trial of cisplatin-paclitaxel versus cisplatin-cyclophosphamide in women with advanced epithelial ovarian cancer: three-year results. J Natl Cancer Inst 92:699–708
308. Pieretti M, Powell DE, Gallion HH, et al (1995) Genetic alterations on chromosome 17 distinguish different types of epithelial ovarian tumors. Hum Pathol 26:393–397
309. Pieretti M, Powell DE, Gallion HH, et al (1995) Hypermethylation of a chromosome 17 "hot spot" is a common event in ovarian cancer. Hum Pathol 26:398–401
310. Pignatelli M, Vessey CJ (1994) Adhesion molecules: novel molecular tools in tumor pathology. Hum Pathol 25:849–856
311. Pins MR, Young RH, Daly WJ, et al (1996) Primary squamous cell carcinoma of the ovary: a report of 37 cases. Am J Surg Pathol 20:823–833
312. Pitman MB, Young RH, Clement PB, et al (1994) Endometrioid carcinoma of the ovary and endometrium, oxyphilic cell type: a report of nine cases. Int J Gynecol Pathol 13:290–301
313. Piura B, Dgani R, Blickstein I, et al (1992) Epithelial ovarian tumors of borderline malignancy: a study of 50 cases. Int J Gynecol Cancer 2:189–197
314. Piver MS, Jishi MF, Tsukuda Y, et al (1993) Primary peritoneal carcinoma after prophylactic oophorectomy in women with a family history of ovarian cancer: a report of the Gilda Radner familial ovarian cancer registry. Cancer (Phila) 71:2751–2755
315. Platz CE, Benda JA (1995) Female genital tract cancer. Cancer (Phila) 75:270–294
316. Plaxe SC, Braly PS, Freddo JL, et al (1993) Profiles of women age 30–39 and age less than 30 with epithelial ovarian cancer. Obstet Gynecol 81:651–654
317. Plaxe SC, Deligdisch L, Dottino PR, et al (1990) Ovarian intraepithelial neoplasia in patients with stage I ovarian carcinoma. Gynecol Oncol 38:367–372
318. Plaxe SC, Dottino PR, Lipsztein R, et al (1990) Clinical features and treatment outcome of patients with epithelial carcinoma of the ovary metastatic to the central nervous system. Obstet Gynecol 75:278–281
319. Prat J, Matias-Guiu X, Barreto J (1991) Simultaneous carcinoma involving the endometrium and the ovary: a clinicopathologic, immunohistochemical, and DNA flow cytometric study of 18 cases. Cancer (Phila) 68:2455–2459
320. Prayson RA, Hart WR, Petras RE (1994) Pseudomyxoma peritonei: a clinicopathologic study of 19 cases with emphasis on site of origin and nature of associated ovarian tumors. Am J Surg Pathol 18:591–603
321. Pujol P, Rey J-M, Nirde P, et al (1998) Differential expression of estrogen receptor-α and β messenger RNAs as a potential marker of ovarian carcinogenesis. Cancer Res 58:5367–5373
322. Puls LE, Powell DE, DePriest PD, et al (1992) Transition from benign to malignant epithelium in mucinous and serous ovarian cystadenocarcinoma. Gynecol Oncol 47:53–57
323. Purdie D, Bain CJ, Siskind V, et al (1999) Hormone replacement therapy and risk of epithelial ovarian cancer. Br J Cancer 81:559–563
324. Quezado MM, Moskaluk CA, Bryant B, et al (1999) Incidence of loss of heterozygosity of p53 and BRCA1 loci in serous surface carcinoma. Hum Pathol 30:203–207
325. Rao BR, Slotman BJ (1991) Endocrine factors in common epithelial ovarian cancer. Endocr Rev 12:14–26
326. Recio FO, Piver MS, Hempling RE, et al (1996) Lack of improved survival plus increase in thromboembolic complications in patients with clear cell carcinoma of the ovary treated with platinum versus nonplatinum-based chemotherapy. Cancer (Phila) 78:2157–2163
327. Rice LW, Berkowitz RS, Mark SD, et al (1990) Epithelial ovarian tumors of borderline malignancy. Gynecol Oncol 39:195–198
328. Ries LAG (1993) Ovarian cancer: survival and treatment differences by age. Cancer (Phila) 71: 524–529
329. Riopel MA, Perlman EJ, Seidman JD, et al (1998) Inhibin and epithelial membrane antigen immunohistochemistry assist in the diagnosis of sex cord-stromal tumors and provide clues to the histogenesis of hypercalcemic small cell carcinomas. Int J Gynecol Pathol 17:46–53
330. Riopel MA, Ronnett BM, Kurman RJ (1999) Evaluation of diagnostic criteria and behavior of ovarian intestinal-type mucinous tumors: atypical proliferative (borderline) tumors, and intraepithelial, microinvasive, invasive, and metastatic carcinomas. Am J Surg Pathol 23:617–635
331. Risch HA, Marrett LD, Jain M, et al (1996) Differences in risk factors for epithelial ovarian cancer by histologic type: results of a case-control study. Am J Epidemiol 144:363–372
332. Rodabaugh KJ, Blanchard G, Welch WR, et al (1995) Detailed deletion mapping of chromosome

6q in borderline epithelial ovarian tumors. Cancer Res 55:2169–2172

333. Rodgers W (1999) Editorial: Matrix metalloproteinases and carcinogenesis. Hum Pathol 30:363–364

334. Rodriguez M, Nguyen HN, Averette HE, et al (1994) National survey of ovarian carcinoma XII: epithelial ovarian malignancies in women less than or equal to 25 years of age. Cancer (Phila) 73:1245–1250

335. Ronnett BM, Kurman RJ, Shmookler BM, et al (1997) The morphologic spectrum of ovarian metastases of appendiceal adenocarcinomas: a clinicopathologic and immunohistochemical analysis of tumors often misinterpreted as primary ovarian tumors or metastatic tumors from other gastrointestinal sites. Am J Surg Pathol 21:1144–1155

336. Ronnett BM, Kurman RJ, Zahn CM, et al (1995) Pseudomyxoma peritonei in women: a clinicopathologic analysis of 30 cases with emphasis on site of origin, prognosis, and relationship to ovarian mucinous tumors of low malignant potential. Hum Pathol 26:509–524

337. Ronnett BM, Shmookler BM, Diener-West M, et al (1997) Immunohistochemical evidence supporting the appendiceal origin of pseudomyxoma peritonei in women. Int J Gynecol Pathol 16:1–9

337a. Ronnett BM, Shmookler BM, Sugarbaker PH, et al (1997) Pseudomyxoma peritonei: new concepts in diagnosis, origin, nomenclature, and relationship to mucinous borderline (low malignant potential) tumors of the ovary. Anat Pathol 2:197–226

337b. Ronnett BM, Yan H, Kurman RJ, et al (2001) Patients with pseudomyxoma peritonei associated with disseminated peritoneal adenomucinosis have a significantly more favorable prognosis than patients with peritoneal mucinous carcinomatosis. Cancer 92:85–91

338. Ronnett BM, Zahn CM, Kurman RJ, et al (1995) Disseminated peritoneal adenomucinosis and peritoneal mucinous carcinomatosis: a clinicopathologic analysis of 109 cases with emphasis on distinguishing pathologic features, site of origin, prognosis, and relationship to "pseudomyxoma peritonei." Am J Surg Pathol 19:1390–1408

339. Rose PG, Rubin RB, Nelson BE, et al (1994) Accuracy of frozen-section (intraoperative consultation) diagnosis of ovarian tumors. Am J Obstet Gynecol 171:823–826

339a. Rosenberg E, Demopoulos RI, Zelenuich-Jacquotte A, et al (2001) Expression of cell cycle regulators $p57^{KIP2}$, cyclin D1, and cyclin E in epithelial ovarian tumors and survival. Hum Pathol 32:808–813

340. Ross DW (1998) Introduction to oncogenes and molecular cancer medicine. Springer, New York

341. Ross DW (1997) BRCA1:genetic testing and hereditary breast and ovarian cancer. Arch Pathol Lab Med 121:754–755

342. Ross JS, Yang F, Kallakury BVS, et al (1999) HER-2/neu oncogene amplification by fluorescence in situ hybridization in epithelial tumors of the ovary. Am J Clin Pathol 111:311–316

343. Rota SM, Zanetta G, Ieda N, et al (1999) Clinical relevance of retroperitoneal involvement from epithelial ovarian tumors of borderline malignancy. Int J Gynecol Cancer 9:477–480

344. Roth LM (1974) The Brenner tumor and the Walthard cell nest: an electron microscopic study. Lab Investig 31:15–23

345. Roth LM, Czernobilsky B (1985) Ovarian Brenner tumors: II. Malignant. Cancer (Phila) 56:592–601

346. Roth LM, Dallenbach-Hellweg G, Czernobilsky B (1985) Ovarian Brenner tumors: I. Metaplastic, proliferating, and of low malignant potential. Cancer (Phila) 56:582–591

347. Roth LM, Gersell DJ, Ulbright TM (1993) Ovarian Brenner tumors and transitional cell carcinoma: recent developments. Int J Gynecol Pathol 12:128–133

348. Roth LM, Langley FA, Fox H, et al (1984) Ovarian clear cell adenofibromatous tumors: benign, of low malignant potential, and associated with invasive clear cell carcinoma. Cancer (Phila) 53: 1156–1163

349. Roth LM, Liban E, Czernobilsky B (1982) Ovarian endometrioid tumors mimicking Sertoli and Sertoli-Leydig cell tumors: sertoliform variant of endometrioid carcinoma. Cancer (Phila) 50:1322–1331

350. Roth LM, Sternberg WH (1971) Proliferating Brenner tumors. Cancer (Phila) 27:687–693

351. Rothacker D, Mobius G (1995) Varieties of serous surface papillary carcinoma of the peritoneum in Northern Germany: a thirty-year autopsy study. Int J Gynecol Pathol 14:310–318

352. Rubin SC, Benjamin I, Behbakht K, et al (1996) Clinical and pathological features of ovarian cancer in women with germ line mutations of BRCA1. N Engl J Med 335:1413–1416

352a. Russell P (1984) Borderline epithelial tumors of the ovary: a conceptual dilemma. Clin Obstet Gynecol 1984;11:259–277

353. Russell P (1994) Surface epithelial-stromal tumors of the ovary. In: Kurman RJ (ed) Blaustein's pathology of the female genital tract, 4th Ed. Springer, New York, pp. 705–782

354. Russell P (1979) The pathological assessment of ovarian neoplasms. II. The 'proliferating' epithelial tumours. Pathology 11:251–282

355. Russell P (1979) The pathological assessment of ovarian neoplasms. III: The malignant 'epithelial' tumours. Pathology 11:493–532

356. Russell P, Merkur H (1979) Proliferating ovarian "epithelial" tumours: a clinico-pathological analysis of 144 cases. Aust NZJ Obstet Gynaecol 19: 45–51

357. Russell P, Farnsworth A (1997) Mullerian mesenchymal tumors. In: Russell P, Farnsworth A (eds) Surgical pathology of the ovaries, 2nd Ed. Churchill Livingstone, New York, pp 319–333

358. Rutgers JL, Scully RE (1988) Ovarian müllerian mucinous papillary cystadenomas of borderline malignancy: a clinicopathologic analysis. Cancer (Phila) 61:340–348
359. Rutgers JL, Scully RE (1988) Ovarian mixed-epithelial papillary cystadenomas of borderline malignancy of mullerian type: a clinicopathologic analysis. Cancer (Phila) 61:546–554
360. Sainz de la Cuesta R, Eichhorn JH, Rice LW, et al (1996) Histologic transformation of benign endometriosis to early epithelial ovarian cancer. Gynecol Oncol 60:238–244
361. Santini D, Gelli MC, Mazzoleni G, et al (1989) Brenner tumor of the ovary: a correlative histologic, histochemical, immunohistochemical, and ultrastructural investigation. Hum Pathol 20:787–795
362. Saretzki G, Hoffmann U, Rohlke P, et al (1997) Identification of allelic losses in benign, borderline, and invasive epithelial ovarian tumors and correlation with clinical outcome. Cancer (Phila) 80:1241–1249
363. Sasaki E, Sasano N, Kimura N, et al (1989) Demonstration of neuroendocrine cells in ovarian mucinous tumors. Int J Gynecol Pathol 8:189–200
364. Sasano H, Comerford J, Silverberg SG, et al (1990) An analysis of abnormalities of the retinoblastoma gene in human ovarian and endometrial carcinoma. Cancer (Phila) 66:2150–2154
365. Sasano H, Harada N (1998) Intratumoral aromatase in human breast, endometrial, and ovarian malignancies. Endocr Rev 19:593–607
366. Sasano H, Nagura H, Silverberg SG (1992) Immunolocalization of c-myc oncoprotein in mucinous and serous adenocarcinomas of the ovary. Hum Pathol 23:491–495
367. Sasano H, Wargotz ES, Silverberg SG, et al (1989) Brenner tumor of the ovary: immunoanalysis of steroidogenic enzymes in 23 cases. Hum Pathol 20:1103–1107
368. Sato S, Kigawa J, Minagawa Y, et al (1999) Chemosensitivity and p53-dependent apoptosis in epithelial ovarian carcinoma. Cancer (Phila) 86: 1307–1313
369. Sato T, Saito H, Morita R, et al (1991) Allelotype of human ovarian cancer. Cancer Res 51:5118–5122
370. Scambia G, Masciullo V, Benedetti Panici P, et al (1997) Prognostic significance of ras/p21 alterations in human ovarian cancer. Br J Cancer 75: 1547–1553
371. Scambia G, Benedetti Panici P, Battaglia F, et al (1991) Presence of epidermal growth factor (EGF) receptor and proliferative response to EGF in six human ovarian carcinoma cell lines. Int J Gynecol Cancer 1:253–258
372. Schiffenbauer YS, Abramovitch R, Meir G, et al (1997) Loss of ovarian function promotes angiogenesis in human ovarian carcinoma. Proc Natl Acad Sci USA 94:13203–13208
373. Schiffman MH, Brinton LA (1994) Epidemiology. In: Kurman RJ (ed) Blaustein's pathology of the female genital tract, 4th Ed. Springer, New York, pp 1199–1223
374. Schildkraut JM, Thompson WD (1988) Familial ovarian cancer: a population-based case-control study. Am J Epidemiol 128:456–466
375. Schoell WMJ, Pieber D, Reich O, et al (1997) Tumor angiogenesis as a prognostic factor in ovarian carcinoma: quantification of endothelial immunoreactivity by image analysis. Cancer (Phila) 80:2257–2262
376. Schorge JO, Muto MG, Welch WR, et al (1998) Molecular evidence for multifocal papillary serous carcinoma of the peritoneum in patients with germline BRCA1 mutations. J Natl Cancer Inst 90:841–845
377. Scully RE (1993) Ovary. In: Henson DE, Albores-Saavedra J (eds) Pathology of incipient neoplasia, 2nd Ed. Saunders, Philadelphia, pp 283–300
378. Scully RE (1995) Pathology of ovarian cancer precursors. J Cell Biochem Suppl 23:208–218
379. Scully RE (1995) Early de novo ovarian cancer and cancer developing in benign ovarian lesions. Int J Gynecol Obstet Suppl 49:S9–S15
380. Scully RE (1977) Ovarian tumors: a review. Am J Pathol 87:686–720
381. Scully RE (1999) Histological typing of ovarian tumors. World Health Organization International Histological Classification of Tumors, 2nd Ed. Springer, New York
382. Scully RE, Barlow JF (1967) "Mesonephroma" of ovary: tumor of mullerian nature related to the endometrioid carcinoma. Cancer (Phila) 20:1405–1417
383. Scully RE, Young RH, Clement PB (1998) Tumors of the ovary, maldeveloped gonads, fallopian tube and broad ligament. In: Atlas of tumor pathology, ser 3, fasc 23. Armed Forces Institute of Pathology, Washington, DC
384. Segal GH, Hart WR (1992) Ovarian serous tumors of low malignant potential (serous borderline tumors): the relationship of exophytic surface tumor to peritoneal "implants." Am J Surg Pathol 16: 577–583
385. Seidman JD, Berman JJ (1993) Premalignant nonepithelial lesions: a biological classification. Mod Pathol 6:544–554
386. Seidman JD (1996) Prognostic importance of hyperplasia and atypia in endometriosis. Int J Gynecol Pathol 15:1–9
387. Seidman JD, Kurman RJ (1996) Subclassification of serous borderline tumors of the ovary into benign and malignant types: a clinicopathologic study of 65 advanced stage cases. Am J Surg Pathol 20:1331–1345
388. Seidman JD, Kurman RJ (2000) Ovarian serous borderline tumors: a critical review of the literature with emphasis on prognostic indicators. Hum Pathol 31:539–557
388a. Seidman JD, Sherman ME, Bell KA, et al (2002) Salpingitis, salpingoliths and serous tumors of

the ovaries: is there a connection? Int J Gynecol Pathol, in press
389. Serov SF, Scully RE, Sobin LH (1973) Histologic typing of ovarian tumors. In: International histological classification and staging of tumors, 9. World Health Organization, Geneva
390. Shattuck-Eidens D, McClure M, Simard J, et al (1995) A collaborative survey of 80 mutations in the BRCA1 breast and ovarian cancer susceptibility gene: implications for presymptomatic testing and screening. JAMA 273:535–541
391. Sheahan K, O'Brien MJ, Burke B, et al (1990) Differential reactivities of carcinoembryonic antigen (CEA) and CEA-related monoclonal and polyclonal antibodies in common epithelial malignancies. Am J Clin Pathol 94:157–164
392. Sheridan E, Silcocks P, Smith J, et al (1994) p53 mutation in a series of epithelial ovarian cancers from the U.K., and its prognostic significance. Eur J Cancer 30A: 1701–1704
393. Sherman ME (1994) Cytopathology. In: Kurman RJ (ed) Blaustein's pathology of the female genital tract, 4th Ed. Springer, New York, pp 1097–1130
394. Sherman ME, Lee JS, Burks RT, et al (1999) Histopathologic features of ovaries at increased risk for carcinoma: a case-control analysis. Int J Gynecol Pathol 18:151–157
395. Shevchuk MM, Fenoglio CM, Richart RM (1980) Histogenesis of Brenner tumors. II: Histochemistry and CEA. Cancer (Phila) 46:2617–2622
396. Shimizu Y, Kamoi S, Amada S, et al (1998) Toward the development of a universal grading system for ovarian epithelial carcinoma. I. Prognostic significance of histopathologic features: problems involved in the architectural grading system. Gynecol Oncol 70:2–12
397. Shimizu Y, Kamoi S, Amada S, et al (1998) Toward the development of a universal grading system for ovarian epithelial carcinoma: testing of a proposed system in a series of 461 patients with uniform treatment and follow-up. Cancer (Phila) 82:893–901
398. Shiraki M, Otis CN, Donovan JT, Powell JL (1992) Ovarian serous borderline epithelial tumors with multiple retroperitoneal nodal involvement: metastasis or malignant transformation of epithelial glandular inclusions? Gynecol Oncol 46:255–258
399. Sidawy MK, Silverberg SG (1987) Endosalpingiosis in female peritoneal washings: a diagnostic pitfall. Int J Gynecol Pathol 6:340–346
400. Silva EG, Tornos C, Zhuang Z, Merino MJ, Gershenson DM (1998) Tumor recurrence in stage I ovarian serous neoplasms of low malignant potential. Int J Gynecol Pathol 17:1–6
401. Singleton TP, Perrone T, Oakley G, et al (1994) Activation of c-erbB-2 and prognosis in ovarian carcinoma: comparison with histologic type, grade, and stage. Cancer (Phila) 73:1460–1466
402. Siriaungkul S, Robbins KM, McGowan L, et al (1995) Ovarian mucinous tumors of low malignant potential: a clinicopathologic study of 54 tumors of intestinal and mullerian type. Int J Gynecol Pathol 14:198–208
403. Skubitz APN, Bast RC Jr, Wayner EA, et al (1996) Expression of $\alpha 6$ and $\beta 4$ integrins in serous ovarian carcinoma correlates with expression of the basement membrane protein laminin. Am J Pathol 148:1445–1461
403a. Snider DD, Stuart GCE, Nation JG, et al (1991) Evaluation of surgical staging in stage I low malignant potential ovarian tumors. Gynecol Oncol 40:129–132
404. Snyder RR, Norris HJ, Tavassoli FA (1988) Endometrioid proliferative and low malignant potential tumors of the ovary: a clinicopathologic study of 46 cases. Am J Surg Pathol 12:661–671
405. Soler AP, Knudsen KA, Tecson-Miguel A, et al (1997) Expression of E-cadherin and N-cadherin in surface epithelial-stromal tumors of the ovary distinguishes mucinous from serous and endometrioid tumors. Hum Pathol 28:734–739
406. Soslow RA, Pirog E, Isaacson C (2000) Endometrial intraepithelial carcinoma with associated peritoneal carcinomatosis. Am J Surg Pathol 24: 726–732
407. Soslow RA, Rouse RV, Hendrickson MR, et al (1996) Transitional cell neoplasms of the ovary and urinary bladder: a comparative immunohistochemical analysis. Int J Gynecol Pathol 15:257–265
408. Soussi T (2000) p53 antibodies in the sera of patients with various types of cancer: a review. Cancer Res 60:1777–1788
409. Sowter HM, Corps AN, Evans AL, et al (1997) Expression and localization of the vascular endothelial growth factor family in ovarian epithelial tumors. Lab Invest 77:607–614
410. Sreenan JJ, Hart WR (1995) Carcinosarcomas of the female genital tract: a pathologic study of 29 metastatic tumors: further evidence for the dominant role of the epithelial component and the conversion theory of histogenesis. Am J Surg Pathol 19:666–674
411. Steichen-Gersdorf E, Gallion HH, Ford D, et al (1994) Familial site-specific ovarian cancer is linked to BRCA1 on 17q12-21. Am J Hum Genet 55:870–875
412. Steinberg JJ, Demopoulos RI, Bigelow B (1986) The evaluation of the omentum in ovarian cancer. Gynecol Oncol 24:327–330
413. Stewart CJR, Owens OJ, Richmond JA, et al (1992) Expression of epidermal growth factor receptor in normal ovary and in ovarian tumors. Int J Gynecol Pathol 11:266–272
414. Strobel T, Swanson L, Cannistra SA (1997) *In vivo* inhibition of CD44 limits intraabdominal spread of a human ovarian cancer xenograft in nude mice: a novel role for CD44 in the process of peritoneal implantation. Cancer Res 57:1228–1232
415. Stromberg K, Johnson GR, O'Connor DM, et al

(1994) Frequent immunohistochemical detection of EGF supergene family members in ovarian carcinogenesis. Int J Gynecol Pathol 13:342–347
416. Struewing JP, Hartge P, Wacholder S, et al (1997) The risk of cancer associated with specific mutations of BRCA1 and BRCA2 among Ashkenazi Jews. N Engl J Med 336:1401–1408
417. Sugiyama T, Kamura T, Kigawa J, et al (2000) Clinical characteristics of clear cell carcinoma of the ovary: a distinct histologic type with poor prognosis and resistance to platinum-based chemotherapy. Cancer (Phila) 88:2584–2589
418. Sui L, Tokuda M, Ohno M, et al (1999) The concurrent expression of $p27^{kip1}$ and cyclin D1 in epithelial ovarian tumors. Gynecol Oncol 73:202–209
419. Sumithran E, Susil BJ, Looi LM (1988) The prognostic significance of grading in borderline mucinous tumors of the ovary. Hum Pathol 19:15–18
420. Sutton GP, Bundy BN, Omura GA, et al (1991) Stage III ovarian tumors of low malignant potential treated with cisplatin combination therapy (a Gynecologic Oncology Group study). Gynecol Oncol 41:230–233
421. Sykes PH, Quinn MA, Rome RM (1997) Ovarian tumors of low malignant potential: a retrospective study of 234 patients. Int J Gynecol Cancer 7:218–226
422. Szaniawska B, Gawrychowski K, Janik P (1998) The effects of protein kinase C inhibitors on invasion of human ovary cancer cells. Neoplasma 45:7–11
423. Szych C, Staebler A, Connolly DC, et al (1999) Molecular genetic evidence supporting the clonality and appendiceal origin of pseudomyxoma peritonei in women. Am J Pathol 154:1849–1855
424. Szyfelbein WM, Young RH, Scully RE (1995) Struma ovarii simulating ovarian tumors of other types: a report of 30 cases. Am J Surg Pathol 19: 21–29
425. Szyfelbein WM, Young RH, Scully RE (1994) Cystic struma ovarii: a frequently unrecognized tumor: a report of 20 cases. Am J Surg Pathol 18: 785–788
426. Tamakoshi K, Kikkawa F, Maeda O, et al (1997) Hyaluronidase activity in gynaecological cancer tissues with different metastatic forms. Br J Cancer 15:1807–1811
427. Tammela J, Geisler JP, Eskew PN Jr, et al (1998) Clear cell carcinoma of the ovary: poor prognosis compared to serous carcinoma. Eur J Gynaecol Oncol 19:438–440
428. Tan LK, Flynn SD, Carcangiu ML (1994) Ovarian serous borderline tumors with lymph node involvement: clinicopathologic and DNA content study of seven cases and review of the literature. Am J Surg Pathol 18:904–912
429. Tan Y, Sinniah R, Bay B-H, et al (1999) Expression of metallothionein and nuclear size in discrimination of malignancy in mucinous ovarian tumors. Int J Gynecol Pathol 18:344–350
430. Tanimoto H, Mehta KD, Parmley TH, et al (1997) Expression of the farnesyltransferase β-subunit gene in human ovarian carcinoma: correlation to K-ras mutation. Gynecol Oncol 66:308–312
431. Tanimoto H, Yan Y, Clarke J, et al (1997) Hepsin, a cell surface serine protease identified in hepatoma cells, is overexpressed in ovarian cancer. Cancer Res 57:2884–2887
432. Tanner B, Hengstler JG, Luch A, et al (1998) c-myc mRNA expression in epithelial ovarian carcinomas in relation to estrogen receptor status, metastatic spread, survival time, FIGO stage, and histologic grade and type. Int J Gynecol Pathol 17:66–74
433. Tanyi J, Tory K, Amo-Takyi BK, et al (1998) Frequent loss of chromosome 12 in human epithelial ovarian tumors: a chromosomal in situ hybridization study. Int J Gynecol Pathol 17:106–112
434. Tavassoli FA (1988) Serous tumor of low malignant potential with early stromal invasion (serous LMP with microinvasion). Mod Pathol 1:407–414
435. Teneriello MG, Ebina M, Linnoila RI, et al (1993) p53 and Ki-*ras* gene mutations in epithelial ovarian neoplasms. Cancer Res 53:3103–3108
436. Thompson CB (1995) Apoptosis in the pathogenesis and treatment of disease. Science 267:1456–1462
437. Thor A, Gorstein F, Ohuchi N, et al (1986) Tumor-associated glycoprotein (TAG-72) in ovarian carcinomas defined by monoclonal antibody B72.3. J Natl Cancer Inst 76:995–1006
438. Tiniakos DG, Yu H, Liapis H (1998) Osteopontin expression in ovarian carcinomas and tumors of low malignant potential (LMP). Hum Pathol 29: 1250–1254
439. Toki T, Fujii S, Silverberg SG (1996) A clinicopathologic study on the association of endometriosis and carcinoma of the ovary using a scoring system. Int J Gynecol Cancer 6:68–75
440. Tornos C, Silva EG, Ordonez NG, et al (1995) Endometrioid carcinoma of the ovary with a prominent spindle-cell component, a source of diagnostic confusion: a report of 14 cases. Am J Surg Pathol 19:1343–1353
441. Tresserra F, Grases PJ, Labastida R, et al (1998) Histological features of the contralateral ovary in patients with unilateral ovarian cancer: a case control study. Gynecol Oncol 71:437–441
442. Trope C, Kaern J, Vergote IB, et al (1993) Are borderline tumors of the ovary overtreated both surgically and systemically? A review of four prospective randomized trials including 253 patients with borderline tumors. Gynecol Oncol 51:236–243
443. Tsao S-W, Mok C-H, Knapp RC, et al (1993) Molecular genetic evidence of a unifocal origin for human serous ovarian carcinomas. Gynecol Oncol 48:5–10
444. Tuncer ZS, Gunalp S, Aksu T, et al (1998) Benign epithelial ovarian tumors. Eur J Gynaecol Oncol 19:391–393

445. Twaalfhoven FCM, Peters AAW, Trimbos JB, et al (1991) The accuracy of frozen section diagnosis of ovarian tumors. Gynecol Oncol 41:189–192
446. Ueda G, Yamasaki M, Inoue M, et al (1984) Argyrophil cells in the endometrioid carcinoma of the ovary. Cancer (Phila) 54:1569–1573
447. Ulbright TM, Roth LM (1985) Metastatic and independent cancers of the endometrium and ovary: a clinicopathologic study of 34 cases. Hum Pathol 16:28–34
448. Underwood LJ, Tanimoto H, Wang Y, et al (1999) Cloning of tumor-associated differentially expressed gene-14, a novel serine protease overexpressed by ovarian carcinoma. Cancer Res 59: 4435–4439
449. Vaccarello L, Kanbour A, Kanbour-Shakir A, et al (1993) Tumor-infiltrating lymphocytes from ovarian tumors of low malignant potential. Int J Gynecol Pathol 12:41–50
449a. Vang R, Whitaker BP, Farhood AI, et al (2001) Immunohistochemical analysis of clear cell carcinoma of the gynecologic tract. Int J Gynecol Pathol 20:252–259
450. Vergote IB, Kaern J, Abeler VM, et al (1993) Analysis of prognostic factors in stage I epithelial ovarian carcinoma: importance of degree of differentiation and deoxyribonucleic acid ploidy in predicting relapse. Am J Obstet Gynecol 169:40–52
451. Wang Z-J, Churchman M, Campbell IG, et al (1999) Allele loss and mutation screen at the Peutz–Jeghers (LKB1) locus (19p13.3) in sporadic ovarian tumours. Br J Cancer 80:70–72
452. Wang NP, Zee S, Zarbo RJ, et al (1995) Coordinate expression of cytokeratins 7 and 20 defines unique subsets of carcinomas. Appl Immunohistochem 3:99–107
453. Wang T-H, Wang H-S, Soong Y-K (2000) Paclitaxel-induced cell death: where the cell cycle and apoptosis come together. Cancer (Phila) 88:2619–2628
454. Watkin WG, Silva EG, Gershenson DM (1992) Mucinous carcinoma of the ovary: pathologic prognostic factors. Cancer (Phila) 69:208–212
455. Watson P, Lynch HT (1993) Extracolonic cancer in hereditary nonpolyposis colorectal cancer. Cancer (Phila) 71:677–685
456. Wauters CCAP, Smedts F, Gerrits LGM, et al (1995) Keratins 7 and 20 as diagnostic markers of carcinomas metastatic to the ovary. Hum Pathol 26:852–855
457. Wehrli BM, Krajewski S, Gascoyne RD, et al (1998) Immunohistochemical analysis of bcl-2, bax, mcl-1, and bcl-X expression in ovarian surface epithelial tumors. Int J Gynecol Pathol 17: 255–260
458. Weidner N (1995) Intratumor microvessel density as a prognostic factor in cancer. Am J Pathol 147:9–19
459. Weir MM, Bell DA, Young RH (1998) Grade 1 peritoneal serous carcinomas: a report of 14 cases and comparison with 7 peritoneal serous psammocarcinomas and 19 peritoneal serous borderline tumors. Am J Surg Pathol 22:849–862
460. Wen W-H, Reles A, Runnebaum IB, et al (1999) P53 mutations and expression in ovarian cancers: correlation with overall survival. Int J Gynecol Pathol 18:29–41
461. Werness BA, Afify AM, Bielat KL, et al (1999) Altered surface and cyst epithelium of ovaries removed prophylactically from women with a family history of ovarian cancer. Hum Pathol 30:151–157
462. Werness BA, Afify AM, Eltabbakh GH, et al (1999) P53, c-erbB, and Ki-67 expression in ovaries removed prophylactically from women with a family history of ovarian cancer. Int J Gynecol Pathol 18:338–343
462a. Werness BA, Eltabbakh GH (2001) Familial ovarian cancer and early ovarian cancer: biologic, pathologic, and clinical features. Int J Gynecol Pathol 2001;20:48–63
463. Werness BA, Jobe JS, DiCioccio RA, et al (1997) Expression of the p53 induced tumor suppressor $p21^{waf1/cip1}$ in ovarian carcinomas: correlation with p53 and Ki-67 immunohistochemistry. Int J Gynecol Pathol 16:149–155
464. Werness BA, Ramus SJ, Whittemore AS, et al (2000) Histopathology of familial ovarian tumors in women from families with and without germline BRCA1 mutations. Hum Pathol 31:1420–1424
465. Wertheim I, Muto MG, Welch WR, et al (1994) P53 gene mutation in human borderline epithelial ovarian tumors. J Natl Cancer Inst 86:1549–1551
466. Wheeler DT, Bell KA, Kurman RJ, et al (2000) Minimal uterine serous carcinoma: diagnosis and clinicopathologic correlation. Am J Surg Pathol 24:797–806
467. Wheeler JMD, Beck NE, Kim HC, et al (1999) Mechanisms of inactivation of mismatch repair genes in human colorectal cancer cell lines: the predominant role of hMLH1. Proc Natl Acad Sci 96:10296–10301
468. Wick MR, Lillemoe TJ, Copland GT, et al (1989) Gross cystic disease fluid protein-15 as a marker for breast cancer: immunohistochemical analysis of 690 human neoplasms and comparison with alpha-lactalbumin. Hum Pathol 20:281–287
469. Wolf NG, Abdul-Karim FW, Schork NJ, et al (1996) Origins of heterogeneous ovarian carcinomas: a molecular cytogenetic analysis of histologically benign, low malignant potential, and fully malignant components. Am J Pathol 149: 511–520
470. Woodruff JD, Dietrick D, Genadry R, et al (1981) Proliferative and malignant Brenner tumors: review of 47 cases. Am J Obstet Gynecol 141:118–125
471. Wright K, Wilson P, Morland S, et al (1999) β-catenin mutation and expression analysis in ovarian cancer: exon 3 mutations and nuclear translocation in 16% of endometrioid tumors. Int J Cancer 82:625–629

472. Yaginuma Y, Yamashita K, Kuzumaki N, et al (1992) ras oncogene product p21 expression and prognosis of human ovarian tumors. Gynecol Oncol 46:45–50
473. Yancik R (1993) Ovarian cancer: age contrasts in incidence, histology, disease stage at diagnosis, and mortality. Cancer (Phila) 71:517–523
474. Yeo T-K, Nagy JA, Yeo K-T, et al (1996) Increased hyaluronan at sites of attachment to mesentery by CD44-positive mouse ovarian and breast tumor cells. Am J Pathol 148:1733–1740
475. Yokoyama Y, Dhanabal M, Griffioen AW, et al (2000) Synergy between angiostatin and endostatin: inhibition of ovarian cancer growth. Cancer Res 60:2190–2196
476. Yokoyama Y, Takahashi Y, Shinohara A, et al (1998) Telomerase activity in the female reproductive tract and neoplasms. Gynecol Oncol 68:145–149
477. Young RC, Decker DG, Wharton JT, et al (1983) Staging laparotomy in early ovarian cancer. JAMA 250:3072–3076
478. Young RC, Walton LA, Ellenberg SS, et al (1990) Adjuvant therapy in stage I and stage II epithelial ovarian cancer: results of two prospective randomized trials. N Engl J Med 322:1021–1027
479. Young RH, Hart WR (1989) Metastases from carcinomas of the pancreas simulating primary mucinous tumors of the ovary: a report of seven cases. Am J Surg Pathol 13:748–756
480. Young RH, Oliva E, Scully RE (1994) Small cell carcinoma of the ovary, hypercalcemic type: a clinicopathological analysis of 150 cases. Am J Surg Pathol 18:1102–1116
481. Young RH, Prat J, Scully RE (1980) Epidermoid cyst of the ovary: a report of three cases with comments on histogenesis. Am J Clin Pathol 73:272–276
482. Young RH, Prat J, Scully RE (1982) Ovarian endometrioid carcinomas resembling sex cord-stromal tumors: a clinicopathological analysis of 13 cases. Am J Surg Pathol 6:513–522
483. Young RH, Prat J, Scully RE (1984) Endometrioid stromal sarcomas of the ovary: a clinicopathologic analysis of 23 cases. Cancer (Phila) 53:1143–1155
484. Young RH, Scully RE (1987) Oxyphilic clear cell carcinoma of the ovary: a report of nine cases. Am J Surg Pathol 11:661–667
485. Yun K, Fukumoto M, Jinno Y (1996) Monoallelic expression of the insulin-like growth factor-2 gene in ovarian cancer. Am J Pathol 148:1081–1087
486. Zanotti KM, Hart WR, Kennedy AW, et al (1999) Allelic imbalance on chromosome 17p13 in borderline (low malignant potential) epithelial ovarian tumors. Int J Gynecol Pathol 18:247–253
487. Zetter BR (1990) The cellular basis of site-specific tumor metastasis. N Engl J Med 322:605–612
488. Zheng J, Benedict WF, Xu H-J, et al (1995) Genetic disparity between morphologically benign cysts contiguous to ovarian carcinomas and solitary cystadenomas. J Natl Cancer Inst 87:1146–1153
489. Zheng W, Luo F, Lu JJ, et al (2000) Reduction of BRCA1 expression in sporadic ovarian cancer. Gynecol Oncol 76:294–300
490. Ziegler J (1996) Hyaluronan seeps into cancer treatment trials. J Natl Cancer Inst 88:397–399
491. Zirker TA, Silva EG, Morris M, et al (1989) Immunohistochemical differentiation of clear cell carcinoma of the female genital tract and endodermal sinus tumor with the use of alpha-fetoprotein and Leu M1. Am J Clin Pathol 91:511–514
492. Zuna RE, Behrens A (1996) Peritoneal washing cytology in gynecologic cancers: long-term follow-up of 355 patients. J Natl Cancer Inst 88:980–987
493. Zweemer RP, Verheijen RHM, Gille JJP, et al (1998) Clinical and genetic evaluation of thirty ovarian cancer families. Am J Obstet Gynecol 178:85–90

19

Sex Cord–Stromal, Steroid Cell, and Other Ovarian Tumors with Endocrine, Paraendocrine, and Paraneoplastic Manifestations

Robert H. Young, M.D., F.R.C. PATH.
and Robert E. Scully, M.D.

Sex Cord–Stromal Tumors

This category of ovarian neoplasms includes all those that contain granulosa cells, theca cells, and their luteinized derivatives: Sertoli cells, Leydig cells, and fibroblasts of gonadal stromal origin, singly or in various combinations and in varying degrees of differentiation.[122,156] The generic terms that have been applied most widely to these tumors reflect differing views of gonadal embryology. Those who believe that all these cell types are derived from the "specialized stroma" of the genital ridge have proposed the term gonadal stromal tumors for these neoplasms.[90] In contrast, others, recognizing that many embryologists favor the participation of coelomic and mesonephric epithelium in the formation of the sex cords, which are the proximal precursors of granulosa cells and Sertoli cells, favor the term *sex cord–stromal tumors*, and it is now the most widely accepted designation.[122]

In the developing testis, the sex cords are clearly distinguishable by the fifth week of embryonic life as slender columns of primitive Sertoli cells, but similar cords, at least in the sense of thin columns, are not encountered in the developing ovary; instead, packets of small pregranulosa cells enveloping germ cells become evident later in embryonic life. For that reason, the term *sex cords* has been criticized as inaccurate to describe the progenitors of granulosa cells. Nevertheless, the long-established usage of this designation by embryologists and the lack of a better term justify its retention. The term sex cord–stromal tumors has the advantage of acknowledging the presence of neoplasms in this general category of derivatives of either or both the sex cords and the stroma. The components derived from the sex cords (granulosa and Sertoli cells) typically are arranged in epithelial configurations, whereas those derived from the stroma have the appearance of cellular gonadal stroma or its specialized derivatives, the theca and Leydig cells.

Most *sex cord–stromal tumors* (*granulosa–stromal cell tumors*) are composed of ovarian cell types but some (*Sertoli–stromal cell tumors*) contain cells of only testicular type; occasionally cells and patterns of growth characteristic of both gonads are present in single tumors (*gynandroblastomas*). When the neoplastic cells are immature and their appearance is intermediate between those of testicular and ovarian cell types, or when the architectural patterns of the tumor are not specific for either the testis or ovary, it may be impossible to determine whether the tumor belongs in the granulosa–stromal or Sertoli–stromal cell category; in such cases the term sex cord–stromal tumor, unclassified is used. The classification of sex cord–stromal tumors used in this chapter is presented in Table 19.1. Sex cord–stromal tumors account for approximately 8% of all ovarian tumors, with fibromas, which are very exceptionally associated with endocrine manifestations, accounting for approximately half the cases. Most of the other tumors in this category are *granulosa cell tumors*, which are neoplasms of a low grade of malignancy.

Granulosa–Stromal Cell Tumors

This category includes all ovarian tumors composed of granulosa cells, theca cells, and fibroblasts, singly or in any combination and in varying degrees of differentiation. *Granulosa cell tumors* that occur typically in middle-aged and older women differ in several important respects from those that usually arise in children and young adults and these two subtypes, which are referred to as adult and juvenile granulosa cell tumors, are discussed separately. Tumors in the thecoma–fibroma group are composed exclusively or almost exclusively of theca cells, fi-

Table 19.1. Classification of sex cord–stromal tumors

Granulosa–stromal cell tumors
- A. Granulosa cell tumor
  - i. Adult type
  - ii. Juvenile type
- B. Tumors in the thecoma-fibroma group
  - i. Thecoma
    - a. Typical
    - b. Luteinized
  - ii. Fibroma-fibrosarcoma
    - a. Fibroma
    - b. Cellular fibroma
    - c. Fibrosarcoma
  - iii. Stromal tumors with minor sex cord elements
  - iv. Sclerosing stromal tumor
  - v. Signet-ring stromal tumor
  - vi. Unclassified

Sertoli–stromal cell tumors
- A. Sertoli cell tumor
- B. Leydig cell tumor
- C. Sertoli–Leydig cell tumors
  - i. Well differentiated
  - ii. Of intermediate differentiation
  - iii. Poorly differentiated
  - iv. With heterologous elements
  - v. Retiform
  - vi. Mixed

Gynandroblastoma

Sex cord tumor with annular tubules

Unclassified

broblasts of ovarian stromal origin, or both. The presence of occasional small nests of granulosa cells or occasional tubules lined by Sertoli cells does not exclude tumors from this category; such tumors have been referred to as fibromas or thecomas with minor sex cord elements.[156]

Adult Granulosa Cell Tumor

Clinical Features

Adult granulosa cell tumors account for approximately 1%–2% of all ovarian tumors and 95% of all granulosa cell tumors. They occur more often in postmenopausal than premenopausal women, with a peak incidence between 50 and 55 years of age.[14,90,127,129] They are the most common estrogenic ovarian tumors clinically, but the precise proportion of adult granulosa cell tumors that secrete hormones is difficult to establish because a specimen of endometrium to evaluate the effects of estrogenic stimulation often is unavailable. The typical endometrial alteration associated with functioning tumors in this category is simple hyperplasia, usually exhibiting some degree of precancerous atypicality. Carcinoma of the endometrium, which almost always is well differentiated, has been reported in from slightly less than 5% to slightly more than 25% of the cases; the wide variation in these figures is attributable, at least in part, to differing views of the dividing line between complex atypical hyperplasia and grade 1 adenocarcinoma. If strict criteria for the diagnosis of carcinoma are used and if all patients with a granulosa cell tumor, not only those who have had an endometrial curettage or hysterectomy, are considered, the best estimate for the frequency of associated endometrial carcinoma is under 5%.[129]

The endometrial changes associated with adult granulosa cell tumors are manifested clinically in women in the reproductive age group by metropathia hemorrhagica, which is characterized by irregular, excessive uterine bleeding, but amenorrhea, lasting from months to years, may precede the abnormal bleeding or may be the only hormonal manifestation at the time of presentation. Postmenopausal bleeding is the most common endocrine symptom in older women, in whom carcinoma of the endometrium is encountered about twice as often as in younger patients. Occasionally, swelling and tenderness of the breasts are prominent symptoms. Elevated levels of estrogens have been reported in the blood and urine, and vaginal cytologic smears typically show increased maturation of squamous epithelial cells. Alterations resembling those seen in a secretory endometrium have been observed rarely in association with granulosa cell tumors, suggesting the possibility of a significant production of progesterone[152] as well as estrogen by the neoplasm.

Rarely, androgenic changes are the sole endocrine manifestation of an adult granulosa cell tumor.[85,91] Most of the patients have been frankly virilized but some have been only hirsute. The tumors may be solid or solid and cystic. The cysts typically are thin walled and may be single or multiple, resembling serous cystadenomas. Because granulosa cell tumors in general are composed exclusively of thin-walled cysts in only about 3% of the cases, the almost 50% frequency of a cystic gross appearance of tumors associated with androgenic manifestations is of great interest. From another standpoint, 17% of granulosa cell tumors composed of thin-walled cysts seen in consultation by one of us (R.E.S.) have been androgenic in contrast to only 1.5% of solid or solid and cystic granulosa cell tumors.[85] The nature of the association of androgen production with the formation of thin-walled cysts remains an enigma.

Gross Findings

Adult granulosa cell tumors vary in size from those that are too small to be felt on pelvic examination (10%–15%)[40] to very large masses that distend the abdomen; the average diameter is approximately 12 cm. At operation the tumor may appear predominantly solid or predominantly cystic, and is unilateral in more than 95% of the cases. Sectioning a solid tumor reveals a gray-white or yellow color, depending on its lipid content, and a soft or firm consistency, depending on its relative content of neoplastic cells and fibrothecomatous stroma. Hemorrhage, which may be massive, is common. Most characteristically, however, the tumor is predominantly cystic, with numerous compartments that are typically filled with fluid or clotted blood and separated by solid tissue (Fig. 19.1). An interesting clinical corollary of the hemorrhage in both solid and solid and cystic granulosa cell tumors is the presentation, in 10%–12% of these, with an acute abdominal disorder caused by rupture and hemoperitoneum.[12–14,129] The occasional tumor that is a multilocular or unilocular cyst (Fig. 19.2) typically has a smooth lining.

Microscopic Findings

Microscopic examination of an adult granulosa cell tumor reveals only granulosa cells or, more often, an additional component of theca cells, fibroblasts, or both; in some cases, the latter cell types predominate. The granulosa cells grow in a wide variety of patterns, which are commonly admixed (Figs.

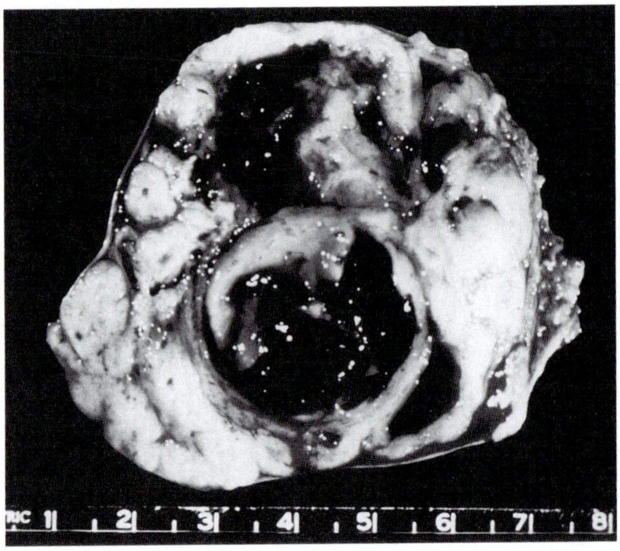

Fig. 19.1. Granulosa cell tumor. The sectioned surface of the neoplasm is solid and cystic with the cysts containing clotted blood. (Reprinted by permission from Young RH, Scully RE (1992) Ovarian sex cord–stromal tumors. Recent progress. Int J Gynecol Pathol 1:101.)

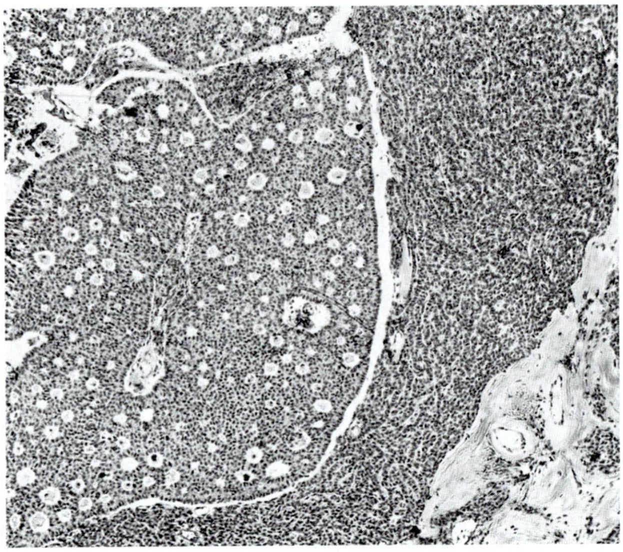

Fig. 19.3. Granulosa cell tumor. Microfollicular pattern (*left*); watered-silk pattern (*right*). (Reprinted by permission from Morris L McL, Scully RE (1958) Endocrine Pathology of the Ovary. St. Louis, Mosby.)

19.3–19.9). The better-differentiated tumors typically have microfollicular, macrofollicular, insular, trabecular, solid-tubular, and rarely hollow-tubular patterns (Figs. 19.3–19.6). The microfollicular pattern is characterized by the presence of numerous small cavities simulating the Call–Exner bodies of the developing graafian follicle (Figs. 19.4 and 19.10). These cavities may contain eosinophilic fluid and often one or a few degenerating nuclei (Fig. 19.10), hyalinized basement membrane material, or rarely basophilic fluid. The microfollicles are separated typically by well-differentiated granulosa cells that contain scanty cytoplasm and pale, angular or oval, often grooved nuclei (Fig. 19.11) arranged haphazardly in relation to one another and to the follicles (Fig. 19.4). The macrofollicular pattern of the granulosa cell tumor (Fig. 19.5) is characterized by cysts lined by well-differentiated granulosa cells, beneath which theca cells usually are present.

The trabecular (Fig. 19.6) and insular forms of granulosa cell tumors are characterized by bands and islands of granulosa cells separated by a fibromatous or thecomatous stroma. In the solid tubular pattern, the tubules may be uniformly cellular or contain peripheral nuclei and central masses of cytoplasm; occasionally a few hollow tubules or glandlike structures are encountered. The various tubular patterns encountered in granulosa cell tumors are indistinguishable from those of well-differentiated Sertoli cell tumors; their presence is ignored as a diagnostic criterion unless they account for a significant portions of the tumor (10% or more); in such cases, a diagnosis of mixed granulosa cell and Sertoli cell tumor, or gynandroblastoma, is warranted. The less well differentiated forms of granulosa cell tumor typically have a watered-silk (moiré silk) (Fig. 19.3), gyriform (Fig. 19.7), or diffuse (sarcomatoid)

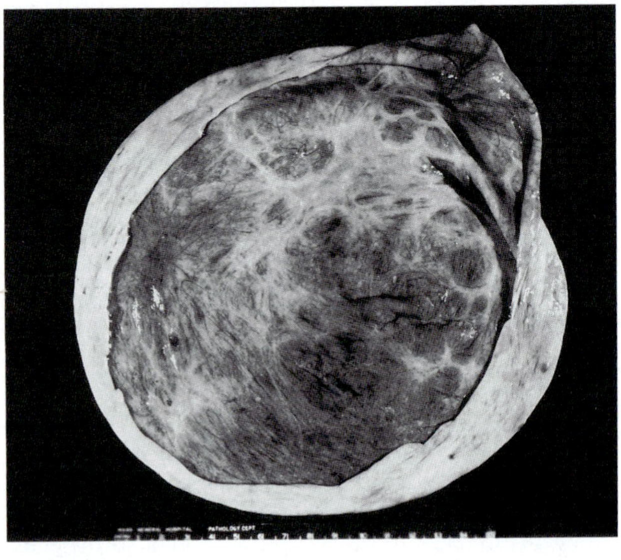

Fig. 19.2. Granulosa cell tumor. The neoplasm is a unilocular cyst with a smooth inner lining. (Reprinted by permission of Nakashima et al, ref. 85.)

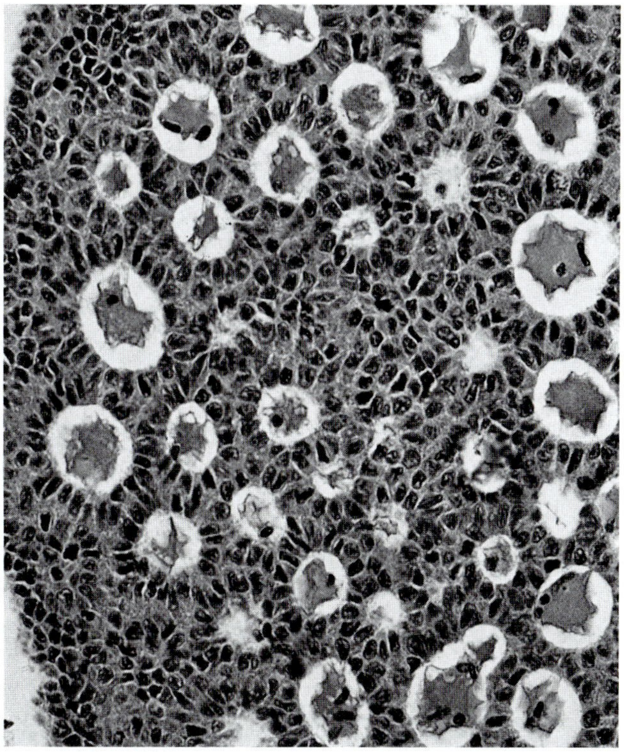

Fig . 19.4. Granulosa cell tumor, microfollicular pattern. Call–Exner bodies are surrounded by granulosa cells with angular nuclei in a haphazard arrangement. (Reprinted by permission of Scully and Morris (1957) Functioning ovarian tumors. In: Meigs LV, Sturgis SH (eds). Progress in Gynecology, Vol. 3 New York, Grune & Stratton, pp 20–34.)

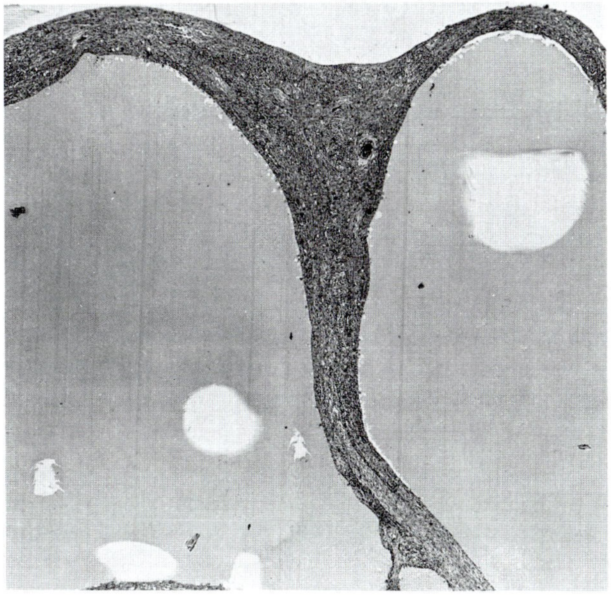

Fig . 19.5. Granulosa cell tumor, macrofollicular pattern. (Reprinted by permission from Case Records of the Massachusetts General Hospital (Case 89-1961). N Engl J Med 265:1213, 1961.)

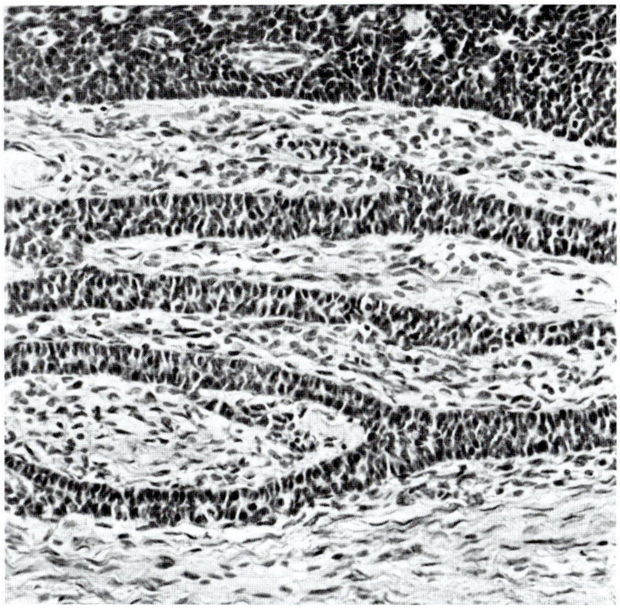

Fig. 19.6. Granulosa cell tumor, trabecular pattern. (Reprinted by permission of Serov SF, Scully RE, Sobin LH (1973) International Histological Classification of Tumours, No. 9. Histological Typing of Ovarian Tumours. Geneva, World Health Organization.

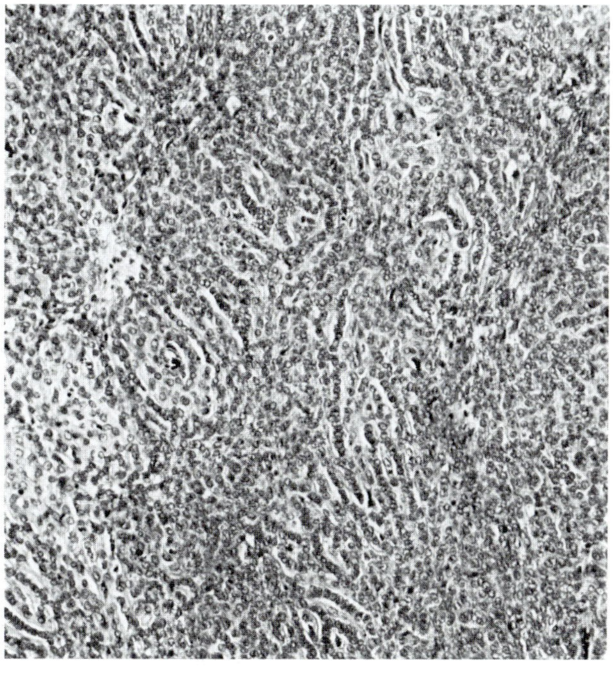

Fig. 19.7. Granulosa cell tumor, gyriform pattern.

pattern (Fig. 19.8), alone or in combination. The first two patterns are manifested by undulating or zigzag rows of granulosa cells, generally in single file, whereas the diffuse pattern is characterized by a monotonous cellular growth. In some granulosa cell tumors, the neoplastic cells contain abundant dense or vacuolated cytoplasm (Fig. 19.12), approaching, to varying degrees, the appearance of the granulosa cells of the corpus luteum; in such cases the term luteinized granulosa cell tumor is appropriate.[152] Very rarely a granulosa cell tumor undergoes sarcomatous transformation[133] or transforms into an anaplastic carcinoma.[122] One granulosa cell tumor was intimately associated with a mucinous cystic tumor.[106]

The nuclear features of a granulosa cell tumor are characteristic, and although the diagnosis usually is apparent, or at least suggested, on the basis of low-power features, the diagnosis must be confirmed by appropriate supportive cytologic features on high power, specifically pale, relatively uniform nuclei, at least some of which contain nuclear grooves (Fig. 19.9). The prominence of the latter varies from one neoplasm to the next. Sometimes they are seen in virtually every nucleus, whereas in other cases they are seen only occasionally. In cases of the latter type the characteristic nuclear pallor is still usually seen. An exception to the characteristic nuclear features just described is seen in approximately 2% of granulosa cell tumors that contain bizarre, enlarged hyperchromatic nuclei, including multinucleated forms[157] (Fig. 19.13). Cells with these nuclear features typically are a focal finding but rarely are conspicuous and may overshadow more characteristic foci, which can be overlooked if not carefully sought. The mitotic rate in granulosa cell tumors is variable but usually not pronounced. If numerous mitoses are found, the diagnosis of granulosa cell tumor should be made with caution although it is acceptable if other features are compatible with the diagnosis and lesions in the differential diagnosis have been carefully excluded.

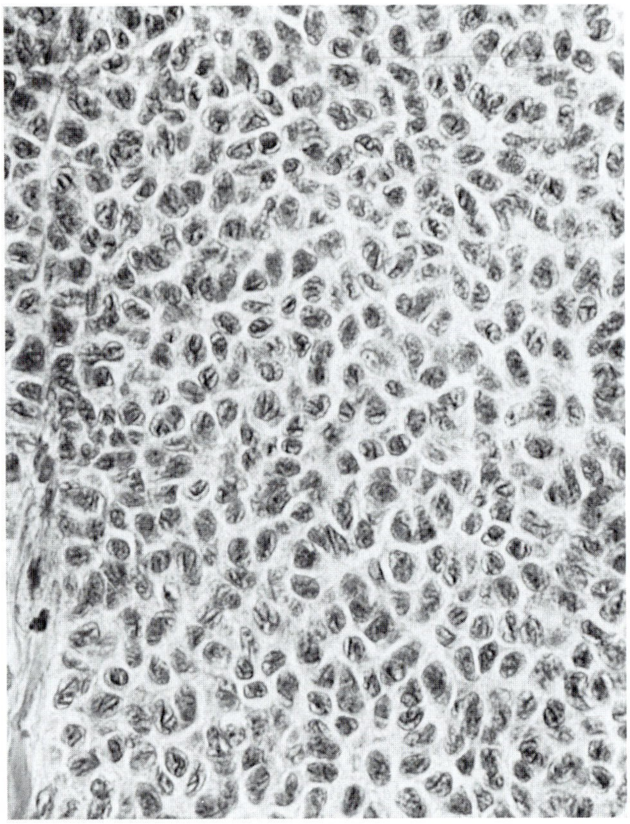

Fig. 19.9. Granulosa cell tumor. The nuclei are pale and have prominent grooves. (Reprinted by permission of Young RH, Scully RE (1985) Ovarian sex cord-stromal and steroid cell tumors. In: Roth LM, Czernobilsky B (eds) Tumors and tumor-like conditions of the ovary. Contemporary Issues in Surgical Pathology, Vol. 6. New York, Churchill Livingstone.)

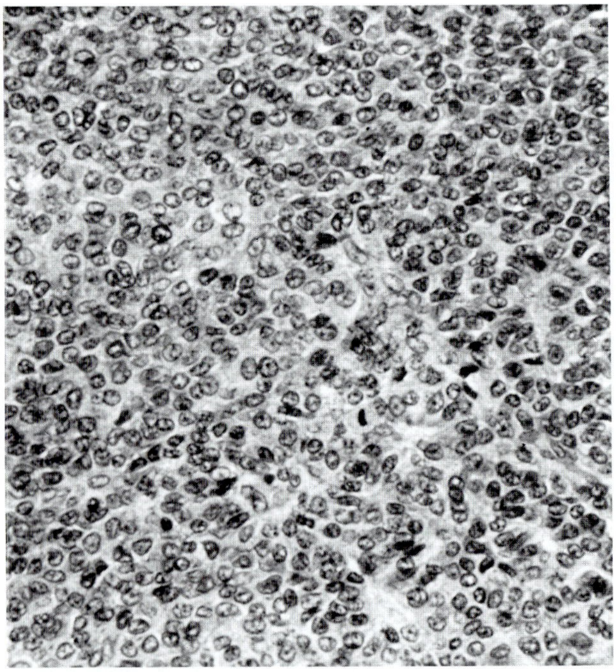

Fig. 19.8. Granulosa cell tumor, diffuse pattern. The nuclei are pale and oval. (Reprinted by permission from Case Records of the Massachusetts General Hospital (Case 45292). N Engl J Med 261:146, 1959.)

The prominence and nature of the stromal component in granulosa cell tumors vary considerably. In some cases, usually those with a diffuse pattern, it is essentially absent. In tumors in which the granulosa cells form nests or trabeculae the stroma is usually conspicuous and composed of fibroblasts and theca cells that contain appreciable to abundant eosinophilic or vacuolated lipid-rich cytoplasm. Rarely,

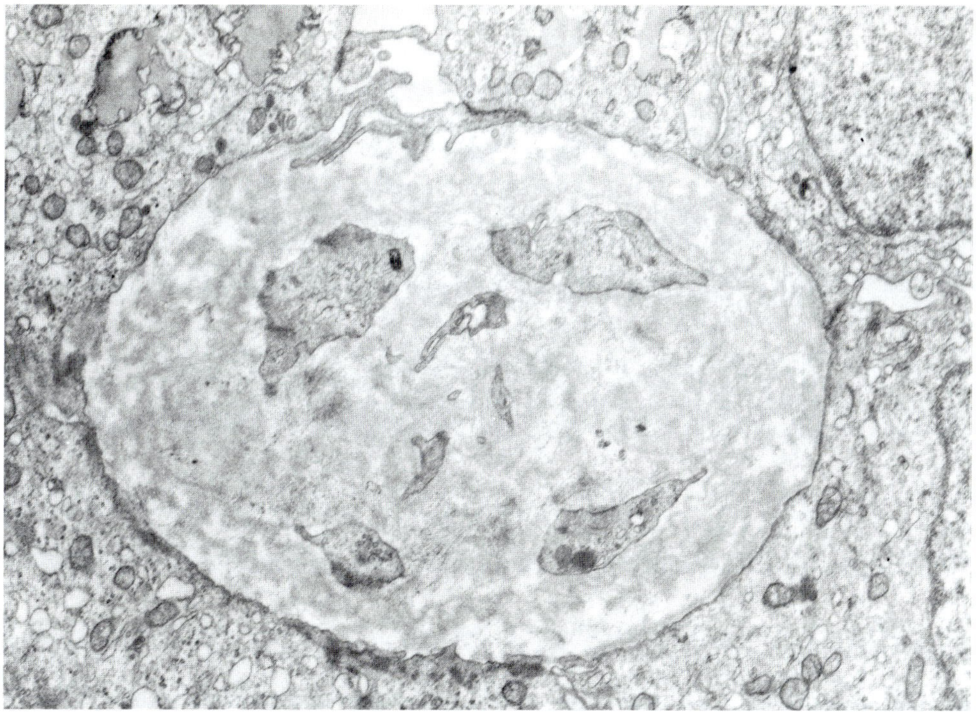

Fig. 19.10. Granulosa cell tumor. A Call–Exner body contains cellular fragments and amorphous debris. The surrounding cells show prominent microvilli and junctional complexes. ×12,000. (Reprinted by permission of Gondos and Monroe. Obstet Gynecol 38:683–689, 1971.)

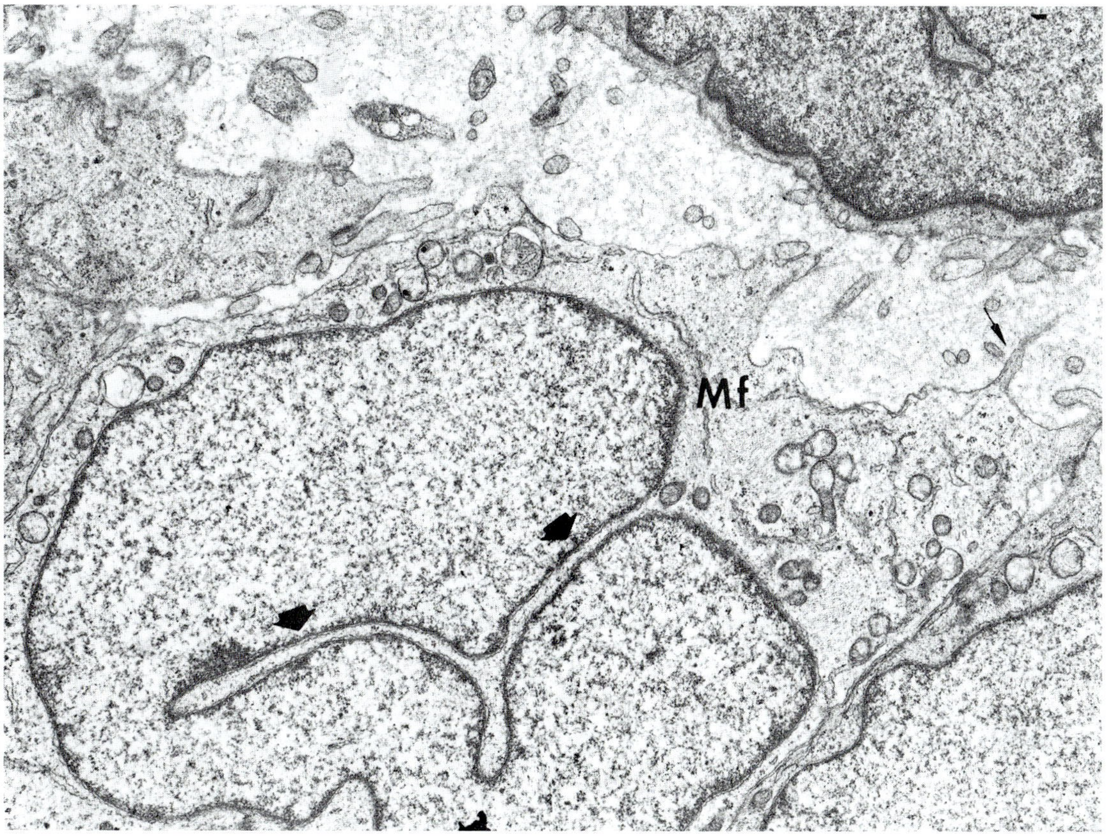

Fig. 19.11. Granulosa cell tumor. The deep indentation of the nuclear membranes (*large arrows*) corresponds to the nuclear wrinkling on light microscopic examination. The sparse cytoplasm contains clusters of small mitochondria and numerous microfibrils (*Mf*). The plasma membrane has hairlike microvillous processes (*small arrow*) projecting into the intercellular space. (×8000.) (Courtesy of Dr. A. Ferenczy, Montreal, Canada.)

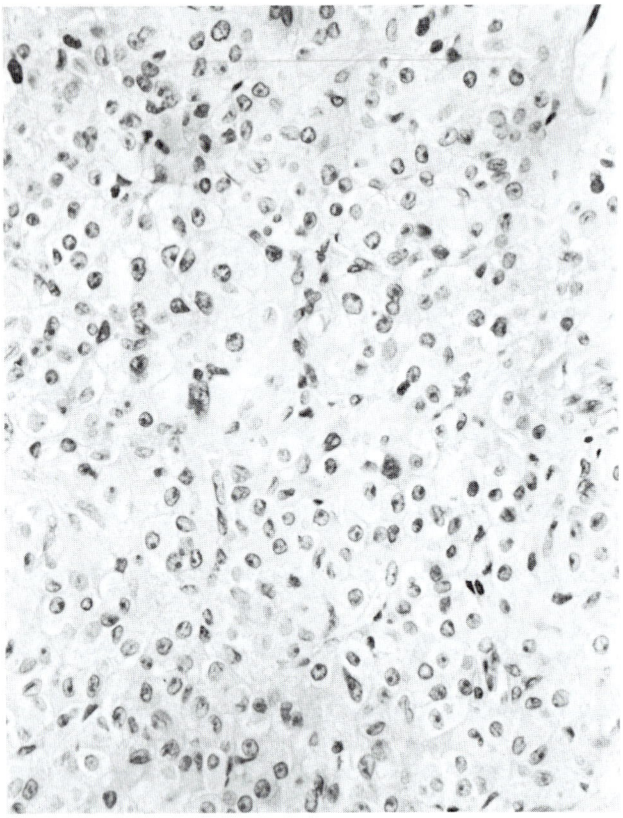

Fig. 19.12. Granulosa cell tumor, luteinized. The tumor cells have abundant cytoplasm.

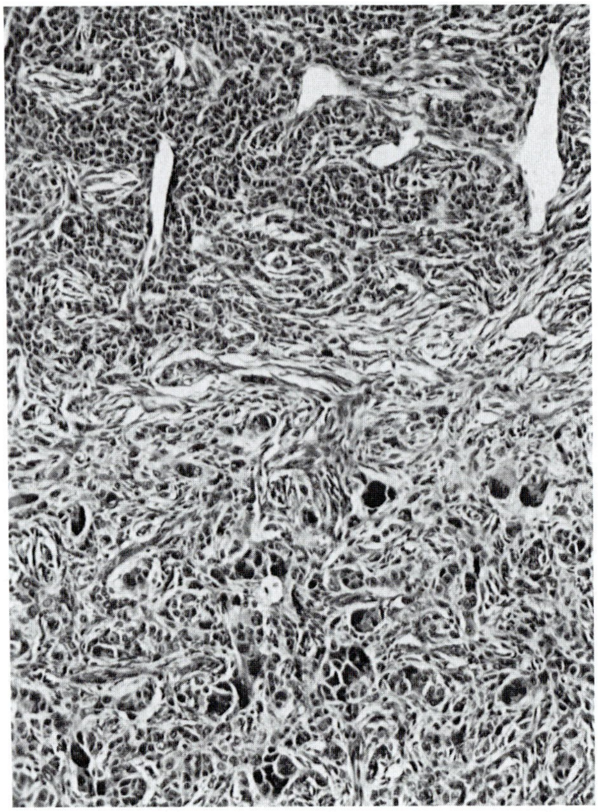

Fig. 19.13. Granulosa cell tumor. The tumor (*top*) is adjacent to area with bizarre nuclei (*bottom*). (Reprinted by permission of Young and Scully, ref. 157.)

crystals of Reinke are present in the lutein-type cells, enabling them to be specifically identified as Leydig cells.[4] Another recently recognized rare component of the stromal compartment of granulosa cell tumors is hepatic-type cells[4,89] (Fig. 19.14). These cells are typically larger and have denser eosinophilic cytoplasm than lutein or Leydig cells. Bile pigment has been detected in canaliculi between some of the hepatic-type cells in three cases. The hepatic-type cells have been immunoreactive for epithelial membrane antigen (EMA), carcinoembryonic antigen (CEA), which stained canaliculi between the cells, and CAM 5. In contrast to lutein or Leydig cells, the hepatic-type cells are negative for inhibin.[4]

The presence of theca cells in varying quantities in most granulosa cell tumors has led to the occasional usage of the term granulosa–theca cell tumor. Although this designation accurately describes the cellular content of many of these neoplasms, the term granulosa cell tumor is more widely accepted for tumors containing both cell types. One reason for this preference is the probability that the presence of theca cells in some cases reflects a response of the ovarian stroma to the growth of granulosa cells rather than the coexistence of a second neoplastic cell component. Evidence favoring such an interpretation includes the nonspecific presence of theca-like cells in a variety of ovarian tumors, both benign and malignant and both primary and metastatic, and the observation that theca cells usually are absent in granulosa cell tumors that have extended beyond the ovary.[41] It is possible, however, that some tumors in which the theca cell element is prominent or even greatly preponderant are truly mixed neoplasms. The theca cells in granulosa cell tumors may resemble theca externa or theca interna cells and may be luteinized. In some tumors, particularly those with a diffuse pattern, differentiation of granulosa and theca cells with routine staining may be difficult or impossible. In such cases a reticulum stain may be helpful. Just as in a developing graafian follicle, so in a granulosa cell tumor the fibrils typically invest theca cells individually. In contrast, the granulosa cell layer of a follicle contains no fibrils, and in a granulosa cell tumor the reticulum usually is sparse, being typically confined to perivascular zones (Fig. 19.15). In occasional tumors an intermediate pattern of fibril distribution is present, and the reticulum stain is not useful in the differentiation of the two cell types.

The presence of blood-filled cysts in many granulosa cell tumors results in the frequent presence in the tumors of related changes that are nonspecific but in the context of other typical features of granulosa cell tumors are at the same time quite characteristic. For example, the cysts often are lined by fibrous tissue associated with evidence of old and recent hemorrhage that is sometimes conspicuous.

Several histochemical reactions that are characteristic of steroid hormone-producing cells, particularly those that demonstrate various types of lipid content or oxidative enzyme activity, usually are positive in the theca cells and negative or only weakly positive in the granulosa cells of a tumor containing both cell types.[70,72,124] This finding, as well as ultrastructural observations, have led some observers to conclude that the theca cell component of granulosa cell tumors produces the hormones responsible for estrogenic manifestations. Additional evidence in favor of this conclusion is the observation that granulosa cell tumors that recur outside ovarian tissue and lack theca cells typically are not obviously estrogenic. In some cases, however, histochemical and other evidence has suggested a role for the granulosa cells in estrogen secretion. Likewise, Kurman et al.[72] have demonstrated immunohistochemically the presence of a variety of steroid hormones in granulosa cells; whether these findings reflect production, storage, or binding of these hormones, however, has not been established. Possibly the theca cells in granulosa cell tumors produce androgens, and aromatase in the granulosa cells converts these hormones to estrogens according to the two-cell theory of estrogen production by the normal graafian follicle.[7,37]

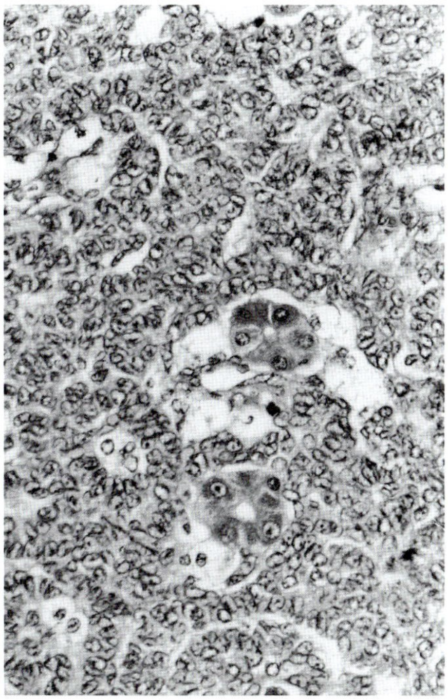

Fig. 19.14. Granulosa cell tumor with hepatic-like cells. The liver-like cells are forming small acini. (Reprinted by permission of Ahmed et al., ref. 4.)

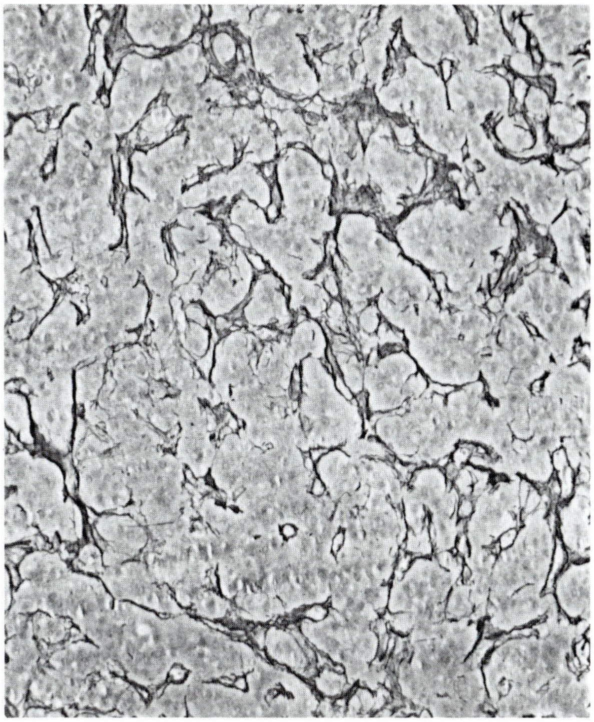

Fig. 19.15. Granulosa cell tumor (reticulum stain.) Reticulum surrounds aggregates of granulosa cells. Contrast with Fig. 19.23.

Differential Diagnosis

The misinterpretation of an undifferentiated carcinoma as an adult granulosa cell tumor (AGCT) with a diffuse pattern is one of the most frequent errors in ovarian tumor pathology. If the clinical course of the patient is atypically malignant for an AGCT, the possibility of such a misdiagnosis must be considered. The single best criterion for distinguishing these two tumors is the appearance of the nuclei, which are typically uniform, pale, and often grooved in the AGCT (see Figs. 19.8 and 19.9) and are hyperchromatic, usually of unequal size and shape, and rarely grooved in undifferentiated carcinomas; atypical mitotic figures often are found in the latter as well. Other features helpful in the differential diagnosis are summarized in Table 19.2. The highly malignant small cell carcinoma, which usually is associated with hypercalcemia,[34] also may be misdiagnosed as an AGCT. The differential features of these tumors are pre-

Table 19.2. Granulosa cell tumor versus undifferentiated carcinoma and poorly differentiated adenocarcinoma

Granulosa cell tumor	*Carcinoma*
Bilateral, less than 5%	Bilateral, more than 25%
Stage I in 90% of cases	Stage III or IV in most cases
Nuclei round to angular, pale and commonly grooved[a]	Nuclei hyperchromatic, often bizarre with atypical mitoses
Mucin occasionally in follicles, (mainly in juvenile type)	Intracellular droplets or extracellular pools of mucin, psammoma bodies or glands may be present
Good prognosis	Poor prognosis
Indolent course, when clinically malignant[b]	Rapid course

[a]Exception: dark, ungrooved nuclei of juvenile granulosa cell tumor.
[b]Exception: rare juvenile granulosa cell tumors.

sented in Table 19.3. The most helpful features are the much higher mitotic rate of the small cell carcinoma and the lack in that tumor of the typical cytologic features of the AGCT. A diffuse AGCT occasionally is confused with a primary endometrioid stromal sarcoma or metastatic endometrial stromal sarcoma of the ovary but a variety of features, including the frequent high stage and bilaterality of the latter tumors, the characteristic pattern of growth in extraovarian sites of spread, their typical content of numerous arterioles, and their rich reticulum content aid in this differential diagnosis. In this, as in other problems in the diagnosis of granulosa cell and other sex cord–stromal tumors, extensive sampling of the specimen often is helpful as is an appreciation of the rarity of bilaterality and extraovarian spread at presentation in cases of sex cord–stromal tumors.

AGCTs may be difficult to distinguish from pure stromal tumors such as cellular thecomas, fibromas, and fibrosarcomas. Reticulum stains may show abundant intercellular fibrils in these tumors, unlike the scant reticulum of AGCTs. In some cases the pattern of fibrils is intermediate between an AGCT and a typical thecoma, and in such cases, the differential diagnosis may be difficult or impossible. The almost exclusive spindle cell nature of the cells in fibromas and fibrosarcomas is rarely seen in an AGCT.

Occasionally, the distinction of a unilocular or multilocular macrofollicular AGCT from one or more follicular cysts may be troublesome; this is particularly likely if the patient is pregnant, or in the puerperium, because a large solitary luteinized follicle cyst of pregnancy and the puerperium is indistinguishable grossly from a unilocular cystic AGCT. The large luteinized cells of the former, some of which contain large bizarre nuclei, differ from those of a unilocular AGCT, which are rarely uniformly luteinized and rarely contain bizarre nuclei.

Endometrioid carcinomas occasionally are misdiagnosed as AGCT when the former have small

Table 19.3. Granulosa cell tumors (GCTs) versus small cell carcinoma

Juvenile GCT	*Adult GCT*	*Small cell carcinoma*
Mostly before 30 years	All ages, but mostly postmenopausal	Always premenopausal
Rarely malignant	Occasionally malignant, often with protracted course	Highly malignant
No hypercalcemia	No hypercalcemia	Hypercalcemia common
Usually estrogenic	Usually estrogenic	Never estrogenic
Thecomatous component common	Fibrothecomatous component common	Stroma scanty and non specific
Cytoplasm usually abundant	Cytoplasm usually scanty	Cytoplasm usually scanty, but may be abundant
Nuclei dark, ungrooved, and often pleomorphic	Nuclei pale and often grooved	Nuclei dark, uniform, and ungrooved
Mitoses usually numerous	Mitoses variable	Mitoses numerous

acini imparting a microfollicular pattern. In addition, some endometrioid carcinomas have an insular pattern that on low power may suggest the diagnosis of an insular AGCT. In most of these cases the cytologic features in an endometrioid carcinoma differ from those of an AGCT, although there are rare cases in which the former tumors have pale nuclei that on cytologic grounds are consistent with a diagnosis of AGCT. In our experience a combination of at least focal cytologic differences, and the presence in endometrioid tumors that are well sampled of other foci incompatible with the diagnosis of an AGCT, such as squamous foci, establish the diagnosis.

The rare AGCT in which the cells are extensively luteinized (see Fig. 19.12) may superficially resemble a steroid cell tumor. The focal presence of areas with the architectural and cytologic features of an AGCT usually facilitates the diagnosis in these cases. AGCTs should be distinguished from the small proliferations of granulosa cells within atretic follicles that are typically an incidental finding within the ovaries of pregnant women. Another rare problem in differential diagnosis is distinction between a granulosa cell tumor, usually a luteinized one, and an epithelioid smooth muscle tumor. The latter diagnosis does not tend to be considered as quickly, not unreasonably, when examining an ovarian tumor as it does when evaluating a uterine one. This is an area in which immunohistochemistry, specifically desmin staining, may play a major role.

It is important to distinguish the Call–Exner bodies of AGCTs from the acini of carcinoid (Table 19.4) and from the hyaline bodies that are seen in gonadoblastomas and sex cord tumors with annular tubules. The acini of carcinoids often contain dense eosinophilic secretion that is sometimes calcified; the latter is not a feature of the AGCT. The nuclei of carcinoids, which have coarse chromatin, contrast with the pale nuclei of the AGCT. The hyaline bodies of gonadoblastomas and sex cord tumors with annular tubules typically are larger than Call–Exner bodies. Sometimes the hyaline bodies can be observed to be continuous with hyaline thickenings of the basement membrane along the periphery of the tumor cell nests; these bodies also undergo calcification. The AGCT may be confused with two types of metastatic tumors, metastatic malignant melanoma and metastatic breast carcinoma (see Chapter 22, Metastatic Tumors of the Ovary). Metastatic melanomas may have cells with scant cytoplasm that grow diffusely, imparting a low-power appearance that may closely mimic that of an AGCT. Patterns of growth incompatible with a diagnosis of AGCT usually are found when a tumor is thoroughly sampled, and the finding of melanin pigment or immunohistochemical stains may be helpful in problematic cases. Metastatic breast carcinoma sometimes also has a diffuse growth of cells with scant cytoplasm, particularly in cases of lobular carcinoma. The history often is helpful in these cases because breast carcinoma rarely presents with an ovarian metastasis. In cases in which a breast cancer is not known in the patient, it is only the presence of focal patterns more suggestive of breast cancer than a granulosa cell tumor and a lack of the typical cytologic features of granulosa cell tumor that will alert the pathologist to the possible correct diagnosis. In both this situation and that of metastatic melanoma, the ovarian metastatic tumors are much more frequently bilateral than is the AGCT. Immunohistochemical staining for gross cystic disease fluid protein 15, S-100, and HMB45 can be helpful in the distinction of metastatic breast carcinoma and metastatic malignant melanoma from the adult granulosa cell tumor.

Table 19.4. Granulosa cell tumor versus carcinoid

Granulosa cell tumor	*Insular carcinoid*
Variety of patterns	Islands, round acini, solid tubules and ribbons
Call–Exner bodies, ill-defined, with watery to dense eosinophilic content, occasionally pyknotic nuclei	Acini sharply outlined with dense content, sometimes calcified
Nuclei round to angular, pale, often grooved, haphazardly oriented	Nuclei round with coarse chromatin and regular orientation
Thecomatous stroma common, at least focally	Fibromatous or hyalinized stroma, may be focally luteinized
Usually uninodular and almost always unilateral; no teratomatous elements	Often multinodular and almost always bilateral if metastatic; always unilateral and usually associated with other teratomatous elements if primary
Cells nonargentaffin; may contain fine argyrophilic granules	Cells usually argentaffin: almost always argyrophilic

Clinical Behavior and Treatment

After the removal of a granulosa cell tumor, the manifestations of hyperestrinism typically regress. If the uterus has been conserved in a young woman, estrogen withdrawal bleeding usually occurs in 1 or 2 days and regular menses ensue shortly thereafter. Granulosa cell tumors of all patterns have a malignant potential, with a capacity to extend beyond the ovary or recur after apparently successful removal. Spread is largely within the pelvis and lower abdomen; distant metastases are rare but have been reported in many sites. Although recurrences may appear within 5 years, they often are not evident until a much longer postoperative interval has elapsed, and numerous cases have been reported in which the tumor has reappeared two or even three or more decades after the initial therapy. The 10-year survival figures that have been recorded in the literature have varied widely from less than 60% to more than 90%, and progressive declines in survival have been documented after longer follow-up periods.[12–15,129]

The optimal treatment of a granulosa cell tumor in menopausal or postmenopausal women is total hysterectomy with bilateral salpingo-oophorectomy. In younger women in whom the preservation of fertility is an important consideration, however, removal of only the ovary and the adjacent fallopian tube is justifiable if spread beyond the ovary is not demonstrable and examination of the contralateral ovary shows no suggestion of involvement. Recurrence usually is fatal, but some recurrent tumors have been treated successfully by reoperation, radiation therapy, or a combination of these. Too little information is available on the chemotherapy of granulosa cell tumors to evaluate the comparative merits of various agents, but several of them have been used with varying degrees of success.

Ninety percent of granulosa cell tumors are stage I and these tumors have a considerably better prognosis than higher-stage tumors, as shown by an 86% versus a 49% relative survival at 10 years, respectively, in one large series and a 96% versus a 26% survival in another.[14] Rupture also adversely affects the outlook, with an 86% relative 25-year survival of patients with intact stage I tumors compared with only 60% survival of those with ruptured tumors that are otherwise in the same stage.[14]

The size of granulosa cell tumors also has been related to their prognosis. In one series all the patients with tumors 5 cm or less in diameter survived 10 years but only 57% of those with tumors 6–15 cm in diameter and 53% of those with even larger tumors survived for that period of time.[45] Another investigation reported a 73% crude overall survival of patients with tumors less than 5 cm in diameter, a 63% survival of those with tumors between 5 and 15 cm, and a 34% survival of those with a tumor greater than 15 cm in diameter.[129] In a final series, stage I tumors 5 cm or less in diameter were associated with a 100% relative 10-year survival in contrast to a 92% survival of patients with larger stage I tumors.[14] The last series is the only one in which the survival rate was corrected for stage, and on that basis the improvement in prognosis for the smaller stage I tumors was not statistically significant. Therefore, a relationship between tumor size and prognosis independent of stage has not been clearly established. Attempts to correlate the histologic pattern and the degrees of nuclear atypia and mitotic activity with prognosis have met with varying success; most investigators have been unable to show a prognostic importance for pattern alone in granulosa cell tumors.[14,90,127,129]

The degree of nuclear atypicality within granulosa cell tumors has been correlated with their prognosis. In one study, the 5-year survival of patients whose tumors showed no atypia was 92% compared with 80% for those with slight atypicality and 30% for those with moderate atypicality.[129] In another study there was an 80% relative 25-year survival in cases with grade 1 nuclear atypicality in contrast to only a 60% survival in those with grade 2 atypia.[14] In both of these studies, nuclear atypicality was the most reliable prognostic index in cases of stage I tumors; for higher-stage tumors nuclear atypicality and mitotic rate were of similar significance. With regard to the relation of nuclear atypicality to prognosis, it should be noted that assessment of its degree is somewhat subjective. Also, as noted earlier, approximately 2% of granulosa cell tumors contain mononucleate and multinucleate cells with large, bizarre, hyperchromatic nuclei (see Fig. 19.13), the presence of which has not been shown to worsen the prognosis. These nuclear changes, which resemble those seen in the uterine leiomyoma with bizarre nuclei, also are encountered in occasional Sertoli–Leydig cell tumors and thecomas and probably are degenerative. In a study of 8 granulosa cell tumors, 7 Sertoli–Leydig cell tumors and 2 thecomas with bizarre nuclei, follow-up was obtained on 11 patients, all of whom were alive without evidence of disease 3–21 years postoperatively.[157]

The mitotic activity of granulosa cell tumors also has been correlated with their prognosis. In one study there was a 70% 10-year survival associated with tumors that had 2 or fewer mitotic figures (MF) per 10 high-power fields (HPF) compared with only a 37% survival for those with 3 or more.[129] In another investigation,[90] tumors with many mitotic figures were associated with a worse prognosis than those with few, but most of the tumors with high mitotic rates also were at a higher stage than those with low mitotic rates, and differences in mitotic rate did not have a statistically significant effect on the prognosis of stage I tumors.

Juvenile Granulosa Cell Tumor

Clinical Features

Somewhat less than 5% of granulosa cell tumors are diagnosed before the age of normal puberty. The great majority of these tumors as well as many granulosa cell tumors in young adults differ histologically from adult granulosa cell tumors (Table 19.5), and the designation juvenile has been selected for such tumors because 97% of them occur in the first three decades.[150] Approximately 80% of *juvenile granulosa cell tumors* (*JGCTs*) occurring in children result in isosexual precocity, accounting for 10% of cases of that syndrome in the female. More common forms of isosexual precocity are those of central origin, with premature release of gondadotropins from the anterior pituitary gland and those resulting from apparently autonomous formation of one or more follicle cysts. The precocity caused by granulosa cell tumors is more specifically designated pseudoprecocity because there is no associated ovulation or progesterone production, precluding the possibility of pregnancy, which exists, in contrast, in cases of true sexual precocity. Typically, pseudoprecocity is heralded by development of the breasts, followed by the appearance of pubic and axillary hair, stimulation and enlargement of the external and internal secondary sex organs, irregular uterine bleeding, and a whitish vaginal discharge, believed to originate in the stimulated endocervical glands. Somatic and skeletal development typically are accelerated as well. Androgenic manifestations such as clitoromegaly occasionally occur.[150]

Table 19.5. Adult versus juvenile granulosa cell tumor (GCT)

Adult GCT	*Juvenile GCT*
Less than 1% prepubertal	50% prepubertal
Usual after 30 years	Rare after 30 years
Mature follicles and Call–Exner bodies common	Immature follicles with mucin content Call–Exner bodies rare
Nuclei pale, angular, commonly grooved	Nuclei darker, round, rarely grooved
Luteinization infrequent	Luteinization frequent

When it occurs after puberty the JGCT usually presents with abdominal pain or swelling, sometimes associated with menstrual irregularities or amenorrhea. Approximately 6% of all the patients present with acute abdominal symptoms because of rupture of the tumor and hemoperitoneum. An interesting clinical association of the JGCT has been its association with Ollier's disease (enchondromatosis) in some patients and with Maffucci's syndrome (enchondromatosis and hemangiomatosis) in a few others.[150] The JGCT is bilateral in only about 2% of the cases.[150] It appears ruptured at operation in approximately 10% of the cases, and ascites is present in a similar percentage. Spread beyond the ovary is unusual; in our series only 2% of the tumors were stage II; rare tumors are stage III.[150] The diameter of the tumor has ranged from 3.0 to 32.0 cm, with an average of 12.5 cm. Because of a usual moderate to large size of the tumor, an adnexal mass is almost always detectable clinically. Rarely, however, a mass has not been palpable preoperatively even on bimanual rectal examination.

Gross Findings

The range of gross appearances of the JGCT is similar to that of an adult form. Like the latter, the single most common presentation is as a solid and cystic neoplasm in which the cysts may contain hemorrhagic fluid (Fig. 19.16). Uniformly solid and uniformly cystic neoplasms also are encountered; the latter may be multilocular or, rarely, unilocular. The solid component typically is yellow-tan or gray, and occasionally exhibits extensive necrosis, hemorrhage, or both.

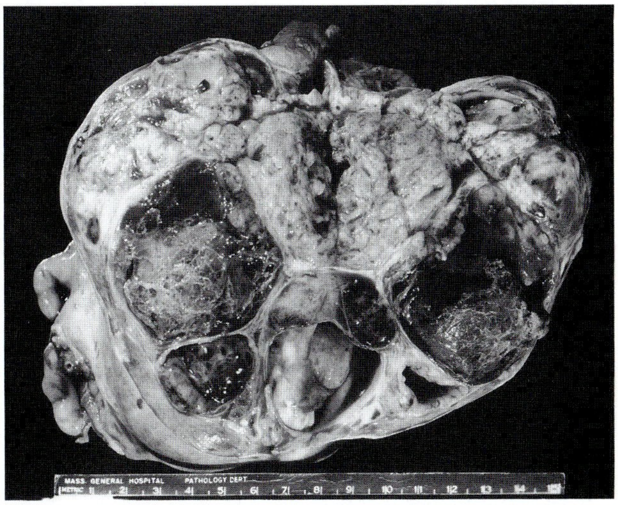

Fig. 19.16. Juvenile granulosa cell tumor. The sectioned surface of the neoplasm is solid and cystic. Clotted blood is present in most of the cysts.

Microscopic Findings

Microscopic examination typically reveals a solid cellular neoplasm, with focal follicle formation (Figs. 19.17 and 19.18), but the tumor also may be uniformly solid or uniformly follicular. In the solid areas the neoplastic cells may be arranged diffusely or divided into nodules by fibrous septa; occasionally, small clusters of tumor cells are present in a fibrous stroma. In the solid foci the granulosa cells usually predominate, but often there is an admixture of theca cells and in some areas the latter may predominate. Occasionally, the granulosa cells and theca cells are admixed in a haphazard fashion; in such cases reticulum stains may aid in their differentiation. Foci resembling typical thecoma with hyaline bands are encountered rarely, but usually are minor in extent. Rarely, areas of sclerosis and calcification are seen.

The follicles usually vary in size and shape (Fig. 19.17) but may be regular and round to oval (Fig. 19.18). They generally do not reach the large size of the follicles in the macrofollicular form of the AGCT.

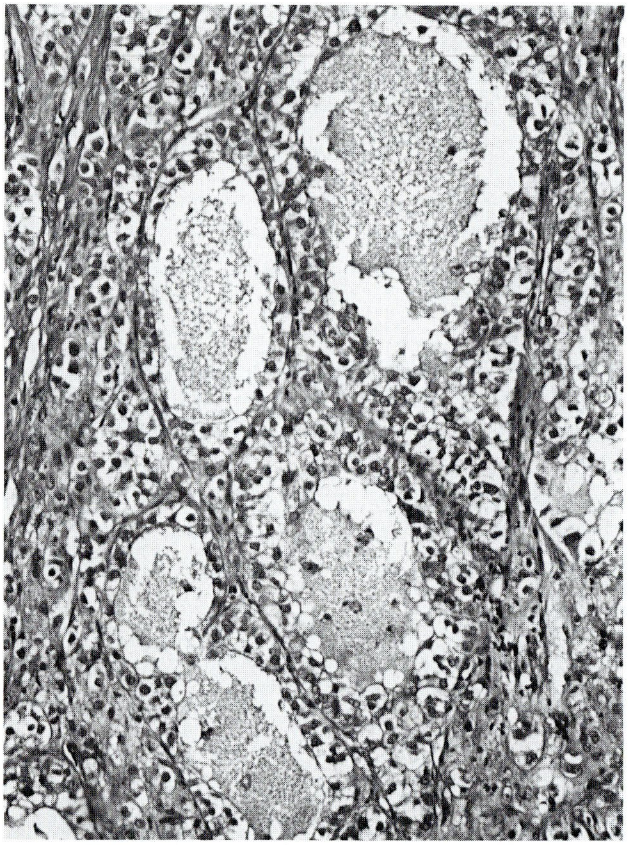

Fig. 19.18. Juvenile granulosa cell tumor. Round to oval follicles lined by cells with abundant pale cytoplasm enclose secretion that was basophilic. (Reprinted by permission from Young RH, Scully RE (1982) Ovarian sex cord–stromal tumors. Recent progress. Int J Gynecol Pathol 1:101.)

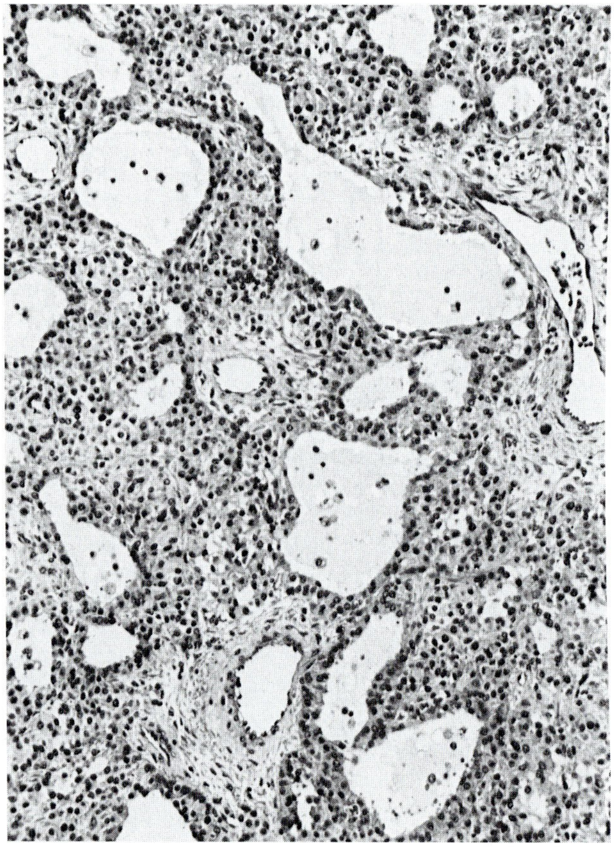

Fig. 19.17. Juvenile granulosa cell tumor. Follicles of varying sizes and shapes are separated by cellular areas. (Reprinted by permission of Young et al., ref. 150.)

Their lumens contain eosinophilic or basophilic secretion, which stains with mucicarmine in approximately two-thirds of the cases. Granulosa cells of varying layers of thickness line the follicles and occasionally are surrounded by mantles of theca cells. More often, however, the granulosa cells lining the follicles blend into the intervening diffusely cellular areas. Rarely, the lining cells resemble hobnail cells.

The two characteristic cytologic features of the neoplastic granulosa cells that distinguish them from those of the AGCT are their generally rounded, hyperchromatic nuclei, which lack grooves in most cases, and their frequent abundant content of eosinophilic (luteinized) cytoplasm (Fig. 19.19). The theca cell element of the tumors usually is also luteinized, and lipid stains typically disclose moderate to large amounts of fat within the cytoplasm of both cellular components. The theca cells are more often spindle shaped than the granulosa cells and, like the latter, usually contain hyperchromatic

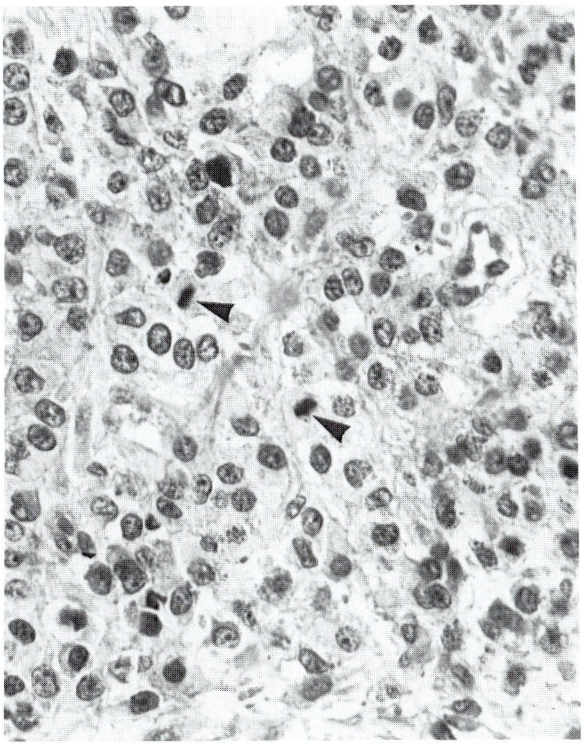

Fig. 19.19. Juvenile granulosa cell tumor. The cells have abundant cytoplasm; their nuclei are hyperchromatic, lack grooves, and exhibit mitotic activity (arrows). (Reprinted by permission of Young and Scully (1985) Ovarian sex cord–stromal and steroid cell tumors. In: Roth LM, Czernobilsky B (eds) Tumors and Tumor-like Conditions of the Ovary. Contemporary Issues in Surgical Pathology, Vol. 6. Churchill Livingstone, New York.)

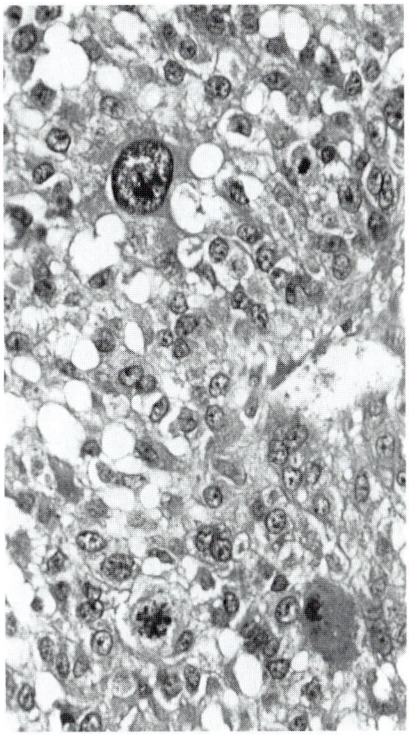

Fig. 19.20. Juvenile granulosa cell tumor. Marked nuclear atypicality and an abnormal mitotic figure are visible. This tumor was clinically malignant. (Reprinted by permission from Young RH, Scully RE (1982) Ovarian sex cord–stromal tumors. Recent progress. Int J Gynecol Pathol 1:101.)

nuclei. In rare JGCTs small foci more characteristic of the AGCT are encountered.

Nuclear atypicality in JGCTs varies from minimal to marked. In approximately 13% of the cases severe degrees are present (Fig. 19.20). The mitotic rate also varies greatly but is generally higher than that seen in AGCTs. In our series the average count was 7 MF/10 HPF and in the series[150] from the Armed Forces Institute of Pathology[164] it was 5.5 MF/10 HPF.

There are very rare neoplasms that we designate anaplastic juvenile granulosa cell tumor. In contrast to conventional neoplasms with striking nuclear atypia but which still have an orderly architecture, these neoplasms have zones with a sheetlike growth that when viewed in isolation are not recognizable as juvenile granulosa cell tumor and indeed, in some instances, resemble undifferentiated carcinoma. A diagnosis of anaplastic juvenile granulosa cell tumor can only be made when thorough sampling discloses characteristic features of that neoplasm in the form of the typical follicles.

Differential Diagnosis

The differential diagnosis of the JGCT includes the AGCT and a wide variety of other neoplasms. The follicles of the JGCT are more irregular in size and shape than those of an AGCT, and its cells are more extensively luteinized with nuclei that are typically round and more hyperchromatic and lack nuclear grooves (see Table 19.5). The mucicarminophilic, often basophilic follicular content in the JGCT also differs from the eosinophilic fluid often accompanied by degenerating nuclei or basement membrane material that is usually present in the microfollicles of AGCTs.

The JGCT often is misdiagnosed as a malignant germ cell tumor. The latter are more common in young females than the JGCT and may be associated with human chorionic gonadotropin- (hCG-) induced isosexual pseudoprecocity. The nuclei of the JGCT are not as primitive appearing as those of either a yolk sac tumor or an embryonal carcinoma and the follicular pattern of the JGCT is not a feature of either germ cell tumor, although the cysts of the polyvesicular variant of yolk sac tumor can superficially resemble the follicles of a JGCT in rare cases. Immunohistochemical demonstration of hCG in embryonal carcinomas and of alpha fetoprotein in yolk sac tumors may be helpful in difficult cases.

The JGCT is sometimes misinterpreted as a thecoma because of the occasional absence or rarity of follicles, the typically abundant cytoplasm of the neoplastic cells, and the occasional predominance of theca cells. Thorough sampling to demonstrate follicles and the performance of reticulum stains to establish the granulosa cell nature of at least some of the tumor cells are important diagnostically. Also, thecomas rarely exhibit significant mitotic activity, rarely occur before 30 years of age, and are exceptionally rare in children. A focally diffuse pattern in a luteinized JGCT may suggest the diagnosis of a steroid (lipid) cell tumor, but the uniformity of the pattern and cytologic features of the latter tumor would be unusual for a JGCT, which almost always contains more diagnostic areas. The pregnancy luteoma rarely contains rounded follicle-like spaces and may suggest a luteinized JGCT but, like the steroid cell tumor, its cells are uniform in appearance, and it is multiple and bilateral in one-half and one-third of the cases, respectively.

The common epithelial tumors with which a JGCT may be confused are clear cell, undifferentiated, and transitional cell carcinomas. The tubulocystic variant of the clear cell carcinoma is rarely suggested when follicles in a JGCT are lined by cells resembling hobnail cells, and JGCTs with high-grade nuclear atypia may suggest an undifferentiated carcinoma. Transitional cell carcinoma is mimicked in rare cases in which a cystic JGCT contains pseudopapillae lined by uniform granulosa cells. The young age of the patient and the presence of follicles and of focal areas typical of a JGCT should help indicate the correct diagnosis in these cases.

The JGCT may be confused with a small cell carcinoma of hypercalcemic type (see Table 19.3) because both neoplasms contain follicles and both are characteristically found in young patients. In the typical case of small cell carcinoma the presence of cells with scanty cytoplasm is in marked contrast to the JGCT, in which the tumors almost without exception have cells with appreciable to abundant cytoplasm. The follicles in the small cell carcinoma rarely contain the basophilic secretion that is seen in many JGCTs. Although the JGCT characteristically has easily found mitotic figures, mitoses are in general much more numerous in the small cell carcinoma. Particular difficulty may be caused by cases of small cell carcinoma in which the tumor cells have abundant eosinophilic cytoplasm. The tumors usually can be distinguished even in these cases because the small cell carcinomas have a much more disorderly growth than seen in the JGCT. Additionally, the large cells seen in cases of small cell carcinoma often have a rather distinctive dense, globular cytoplasm, a feature only occasionally seen in the JGCT.

The only metastatic tumor that we have seen confused with a JGCT is metastatic malignant melanoma, because some malignant melanomas, like many metastatic tumors, contain follicle-like spaces and this metastatic tumor frequently has cells with abundant eosinophilic cytoplasm. The result may be a striking simulation of the solid and follicular pattern of a JGCT. It is helpful clinically that metastatic malignant melanoma is very rare in the first two decades, when approximately 80% of JGCTs are encountered. The clinical history, of course, is helpful in many cases but as the history of malignant melanoma may be remote, or the primary tumor may have regressed, the possibility of malignant melanoma should be considered when entertaining the diagnosis of JGCT in a patient over 20 years of age. The likelihood of this diagnosis will be heightened if the ovarian tumor is bilateral. Other features of metastatic melanoma discussed in Chapter 22 also may be helpful.

Clinical Behavior and Treatment

Although the JGCT usually appears less well differentiated than the adult type, follow-up to date indicates a high cure rate. In contrast to AGCTs, which often recur late, all the clinically malignant juvenile tumors have reappeared within 3 years and several have had a rapid course.[150]

In our series, the feature of greatest prognostic significance was the stage of the tumor.[150] Only 2 of the 80 stage I tumors for which follow-up information was available were clinically malignant. Rupture did not have an adverse effect on prognosis. Two of the 10 stage IC tumors were malignant; in 1 of them, malignant cells were present on cytologic examination of the ascitic fluid. All 3 stage II tumors were fatal. Although both the mitotic rate and the degree of nuclear atypicality correlated with the prognosis when tumors of all stages were considered, no such correlation was evident when only stage I tumors were evaluated. In conclusion, despite the frequent presence of disquieting features such as severe nuclear atypicality and very high mitotic rates, a JGCT that is confined to the ovary appears to have an excellent prognosis.

In view of the rarity of bilateral ovarian involvement, and their excellent prognosis, a stage 1A JGCT can be treated by a unilateral salpingo-oophorectomy. Little experience has accumulated on the role of radiation therapy and chemotherapy in the management of persistent or recurrent tumor, but isolated examples of the efficacy of these modes of therapy have been recorded.

The comments just made on behavior, prognosis, and therapy do not apply to the rare cases that we designate anaplastic juvenile granulosa cell tumor, which are highly malignant in our experience.

Thecoma

Thecomas can be divided into typical and luteinized forms.[10,49,61,114,167] The typical thecoma is composed of swollen lipid-laden stromal cells resembling theca cells; varying numbers of fibroblasts usually are present as well. Although differing criteria for the microscopic separation of thecoma and fibroma have resulted in varying estimates of the frequency of these tumors, thecomas are approximately one-third as common as granulosa cell tumors if one includes in the former category only those tumors containing moderate to abundant lipid or those tumors associated with evidence of estrogen secretion. The thecoma occurs at an older average age than the granulosa cell tumor, being very rare before puberty and uncommon before the age of 30 years. In one large series 84% of the patients were postmenopausal, with a mean age of 59 years; only 10% of the patients were under 30 years of age.[15] In the same series 60% of the postmenopausal women presented because of uterine bleeding and 21% of the patients had endometrial carcinoma.

Thecomas range in size from small, impalpable tumors to large, solid masses, most of which are 5–10 cm in diameter. Sectioning typically discloses a solid yellow mass (Fig. 19.21), but in some cases the tumor is white with only focal tinges of yellow; cystic change and foci of hemorrhage and necrosis occur occasionally. Microscopic examination reveals masses of cells, most of which are ill defined and oval or rounded; the cytoplasm usually is abundant, pale, and vacuolated, containing moderate to abundant amounts of lipid (Fig. 19.22). In occasional cellular thecomas the cytoplasm is less conspicuous. The nuclei vary from round to spindle shaped and exhibit little or no atypia; mitoses are absent or infrequent. Hyaline plaques often are conspicuous (Fig. 19.22). In thecomas, in contrast to granulosa cell tumors, reticulum fibrils typically surround individual tumor cells (Fig. 19.23).

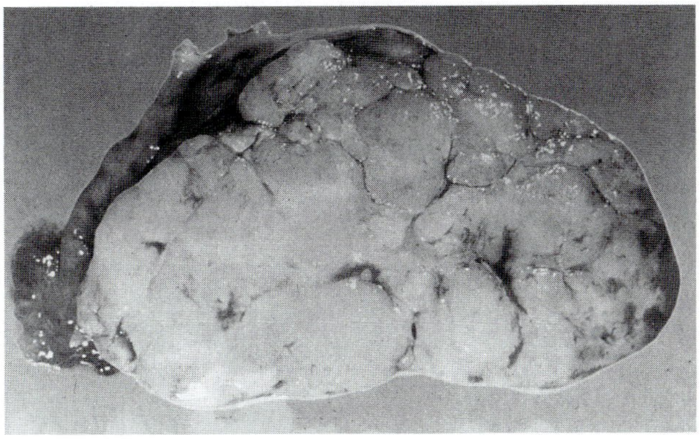

Fig. 19.21. Thecoma. The sectioned surface of the neoplasm is uniformly solid and lobulated. The tumor was yellow in the fresh state.

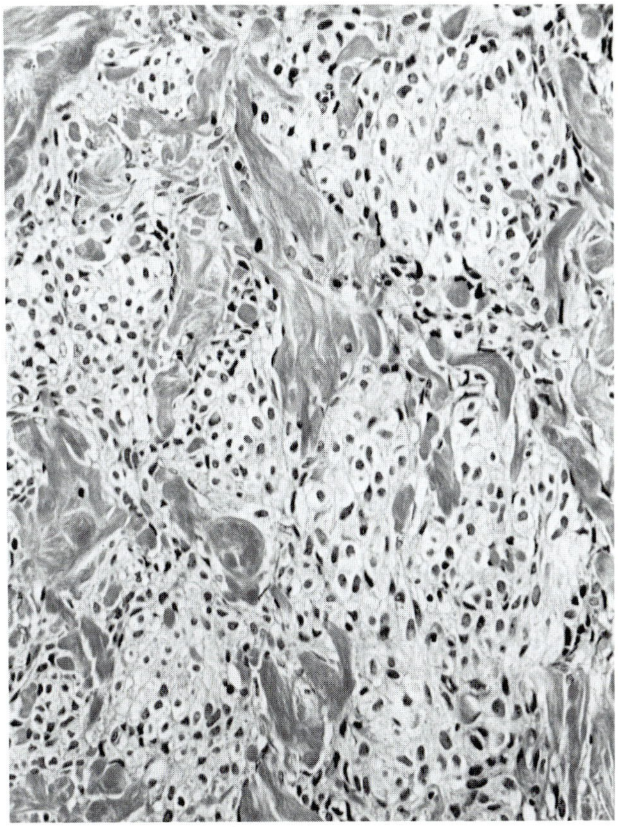

Fig. 19.22. Thecoma. The tumor cells have abundant pale cytoplasm. Hyaline plaques are conspicuous. (Reprinted by permission from Young RH, Scully RE (1984) Ovarian sex cord–stromal tumors: Recent advances and current status. Clin Obstet Gynecol 11:93.)

Typical thecomas are unilateral in 97% of the cases and are almost never malignant. A number of tumors have been reported as "malignant thecomas," but some of these tumors are better interpreted as endocrinologically inactive fibrosarcomas or diffuse granulosa cell tumors.[148] In cases in which the preservation of fertility is important, a thecoma can be treated adequately by oophorectomy. Total hysterectomy with bilateral salpingo-oophorectomy is indicated, however, in most patients who are menopausal or postmenopausal.

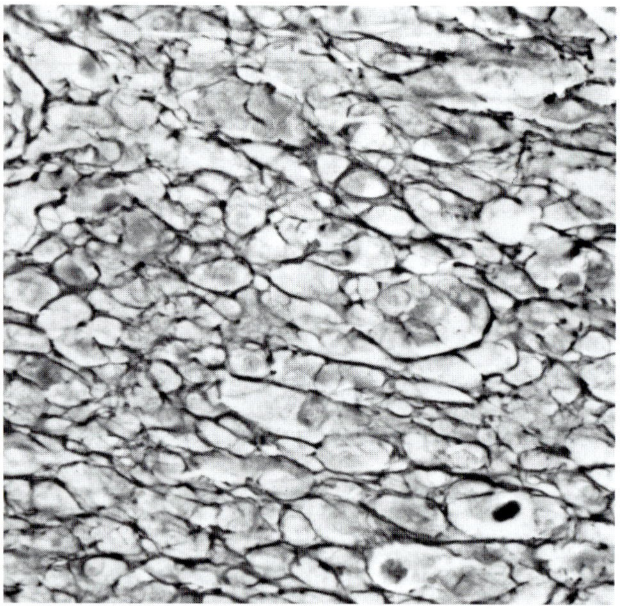

Fig. 19.23. Thecoma (reticulum stain). Contrast with reticulum pattern of granulosa cell tumor in Fig. 19.15. (Reprinted by permission from Serov SF, Scully RE, Sobin LH (1973) International Histological Classification of Tumours, No. 9. Histological Typing of Ovarian Tumours. World Health Organization, Geneva.)

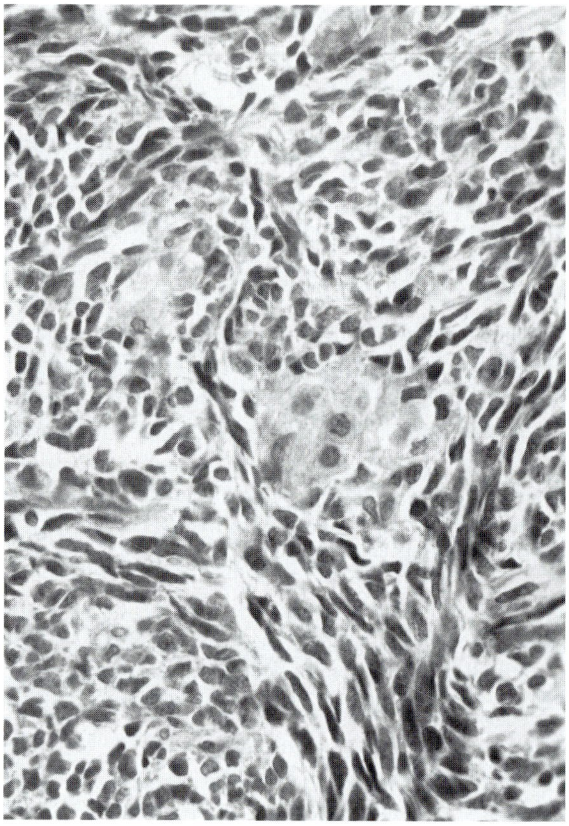

Fig. 19.24. Luteinized thecoma. Luteinized cells are present within a fibromatous background. (Reprinted by permission of Young and Scully, ref. 156.)

Tumors that are predominantly fibromatous or thecomatous but also contain collections of steroid-type cells resembling luteinized theca and luteinized stromal cells have been called luteinized thecomas (Fig. 19.24). In our series of 46 cases of these tumors, half of them were estrogenic, 39% were nonfunctioning, and 11% were androgenic.[167] Two of the four patients with tumors of this type described by Roth and Sternberg[114] also were virilized. This relatively high frequency of masculinization contrasts with its great rarity in association with nonluteinized thecomas. Luteinized thecomas also occur in a younger age group than typical thecomas; although they are most frequent in postmenopausal women, 30% of them have occurred in patients under 30 years of age. When, on rare occasions, crystals of Reinke are identified in the steroid-type cells (Fig. 19.25),[120] the term stromal-Leydig cell tumor is appropriate.[16,97,131,167] Approximately half these tumors have been virilizing.

A rare subtype of luteinized thecoma with distinctive features is that associated with potentially fatal sclerosing peritonitis.[26] Almost 20 cases of this neoplasm have now been reported. In contrast to typical thecomas and luteinized thecomas of the usual type, this lesion is often bilateral and may enlarge the ovary irregularly, instead of forming a discrete mass, suggesting a hyperplastic rather than neoplastic process in some cases (Fig. 19.26). Microscopic examination discloses a process with densely cellular areas and less cellular areas in which edema with microcystic change is often con-

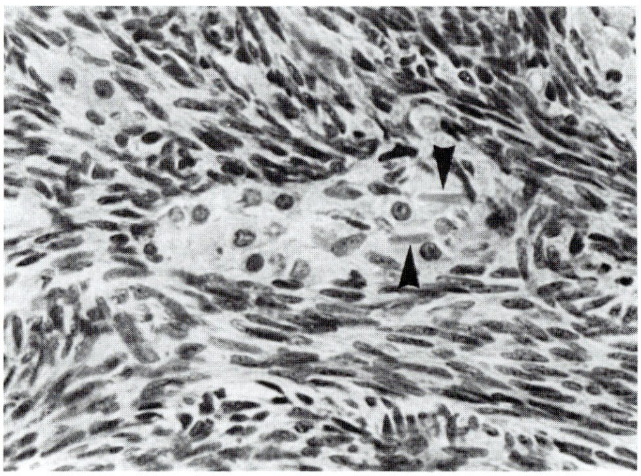

Fig. 19.25. Stromal–Leydig cell tumor. Crystalloids of Reinke (*arrowheads*) are present within steroid type cells. (Reprinted by permission of Scully, ref. 120.)

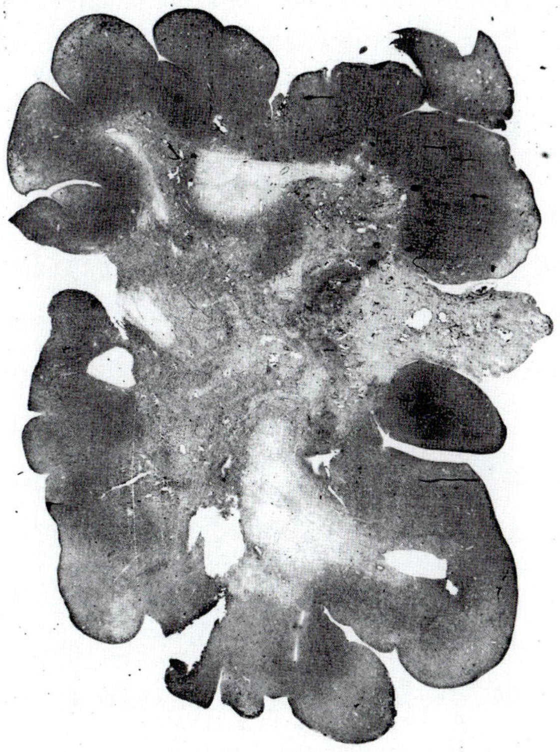

Fig. 19.26. Luteinized thecoma of type associated with sclerosing peritonitis. The ovarian cortex has a striking polypoid configuration (Reprinted by permission of Clement et al., ref. 26.)

spicuous (Fig. 19.27). Lutein cells are present but are smaller and less easy to recognize that those in the usual luteinized thecoma. Another unusual aspect of this neoplasm is the brisk mitotic activity present in many cases despite the lack of evidence that the lesion has the potential to metastasize. The pathogenesis of the sclerosing peritonitis in these cases remains a mystery.

Fibroma

This tumor, which is composed of spindle cells forming variable amounts of collagen, accounts for 4% of all ovarian tumors. *Fibroma* occurs at all ages, but is most frequent during middle age, with an average age of 48 years[36]; fewer than 10% of the cases are encountered under the age of 30 years. The fibroma is rarely associated with steroid hormone production but may be accompanied by two unusual clinical syndromes, Meigs' syndrome,[80] and the basal cell nevus syndrome (Gorlin's syndrome).[50] The former, which complicates about 1% of ovarian fibromas, is defined as ascites and pleural effusion accompanying a fibrous ovarian tumor, usually a fibroma, and disappearing after the removal of the tumor. Ascites alone is present in association with 10%–15% of ovarian fibromas larger than 10 cm in diameter.[116] The most widely accepted explanation of Meigs' syndrome is seepage of fluid from the tumor through its serosal surface into the peritoneal

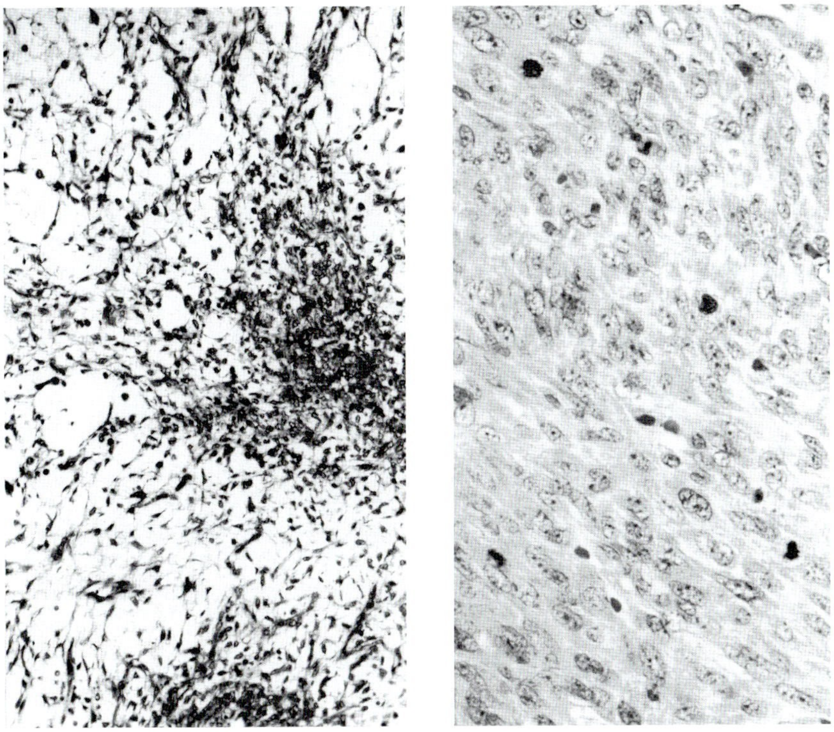

Fig. 19.27. Luteinized thecoma of type associated with sclerosing peritonitis. Edema with microcystic change is conspicuous on the *left* and mitotic activity on the *right*. (Reprinted by permission of Clement et al., ref. 26.)

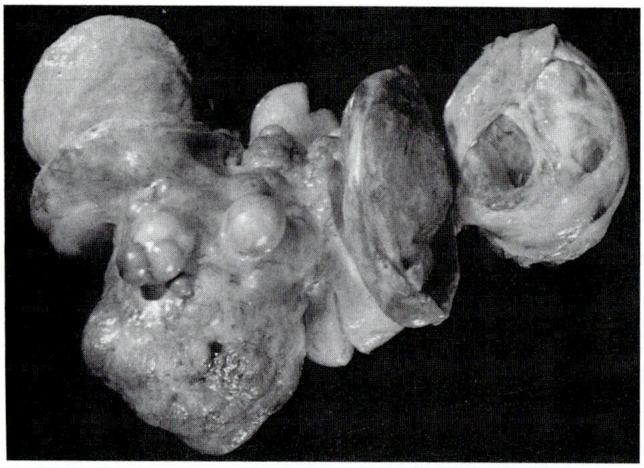

Fig. 19.28. Multinodular fibroma. The tumor is partly sectioned. The patient had basal cell nevus syndrome. (Reprinted by permission from Case Records of the Massachusetts General Hospital (Case 14-1976).)

cavity, with subsequent passage into one or both pleural cavities either via lymphatics or through a communication between the abdominal and pleural cavity, such as the foramen of Bochdalek.

The hereditary basal cell nevus syndrome is characterized by one or more of the following findings: basal cell carcinomas appearing early in life, keratocysts of the jaw, calcification of the dura, mesenteric cysts, and other less common abnormalities,[50] as well as ovarian fibromas, which typically are bilateral, multinodular, and calcified (Fig. 19.28). A case of fibrosarcoma of the ovary in a child with the basal cell nevus syndrome has been reported.[68]

Fibromas range in size from microscopic to very large. Very small tumors are not uncommon, and their occurrence probably accounts for the high frequency of such tumors in some series of ovarian neoplasms. For statistical purposes a fibromatous nodule less than 3 cm in diameter should not be considered a true neoplasm.

Sectioning of fibromas typically reveals hard, flat, chalky-white surfaces that have a whorled appearance. Areas of edema, occasionally with cyst formation, are relatively common (Fig. 19.29). Focal or diffuse calcification and bilaterality are each observed in fewer than 10% of the cases but, as already mentioned, these features are characteristic of the fibromas associated with the basal cell nevus syndrome. Microscopic examination reveals intersecting bundles of spindle cells producing collagen; a storiform pattern often is encountered (Figs. 19.30 and 19.31). The presence of bands of hyalinized fibrous tissue is not uncommon. Many tumors show varying degrees of intercellular edema (Fig. 19.32), which may have

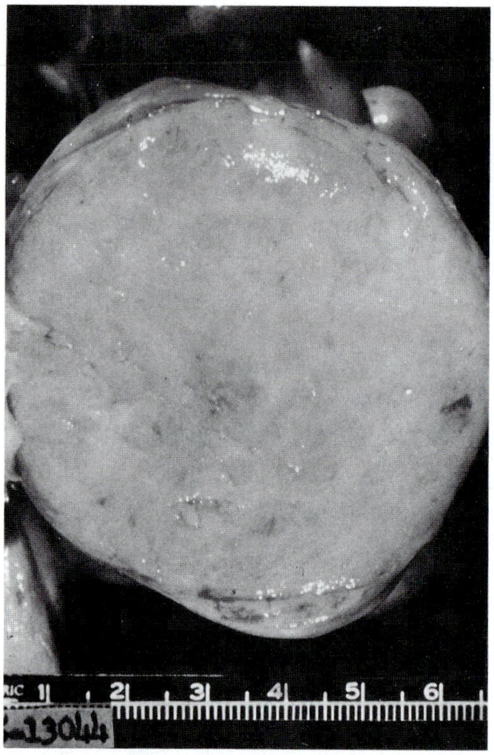

Fig. 19.29. Fibroma. The sectioned surface of the neoplasm is solid. In the fresh state the neoplasm was white and slightly edematous.

a myxoid appearance, and immunohistochemical findings provide some support that the ovarian myxoma may be variant of a stromal tumor.[30] However, the World Health Organization classifies myxomas under the miscellaneous category of ovarian tumors, and these are considered elsewhere in this volume. The cytoplasm of the neoplastic cells of fibromas may contain small quantities of lipid. In rare tumors the cytoplasm contains small red granules reminiscent of hyaline bodies, probably representing a degenerative phenomenon. As previously mentioned, an occasional fibroma contains a minor component of sex cord elements (Fig. 19.33).

The fibroma must be distinguished from several nonneoplastic ovarian processes, specifically massive edema, fibromatosis, and stromal hyperplasia. The first two disorders usually are unilateral but may be bilateral and are characterized by proliferation of ovarian stromal cells with marked intercellular edema and the production of abundant dense collagen, respectively. Unlike fibromas, which almost always displace follicles, corpora lutea, and corpora albicantia, massive edema and fibromatosis encompass these structures. Stromal hyperplasia, in contrast to the ovarian fibroma, is bilateral and is characterized by a multinodular or diffuse

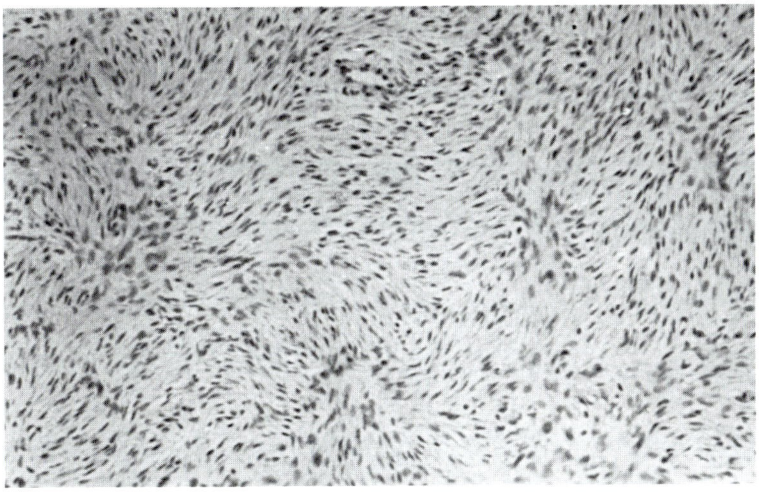

Fig. 19.30. Fibroma. The tumor has a storiform pattern.

proliferation of closely packed, small stromal cells with minimal collagen formation.

Ovarian fibromas are almost always benign, but cellular forms containing an average of 1–3 MF/10 HPF and showing no more than slight nuclear atypicality are of low malignant potential (Fig. 19.34), occasionally recurring, particularly if they are adherent or have ruptured.[104] Very rarely, fibromas without any atypical features are associated with peritoneal implants. Tumors with an average of 4 or more MF/10 HPF and significant nuclear atypicality are almost always associated with a malignant course and warrant the designation fibrosarcoma.[24,104]

Sclerosing Stromal Tumor

This tumor differs from the fibroma and the thecoma both clinically and pathologically. Although the latter tumors are uncommon in the first three decades, more than 80% of *sclerosing stromal tumors* have been encountered during the second and third decades, with an average age at diagnosis of

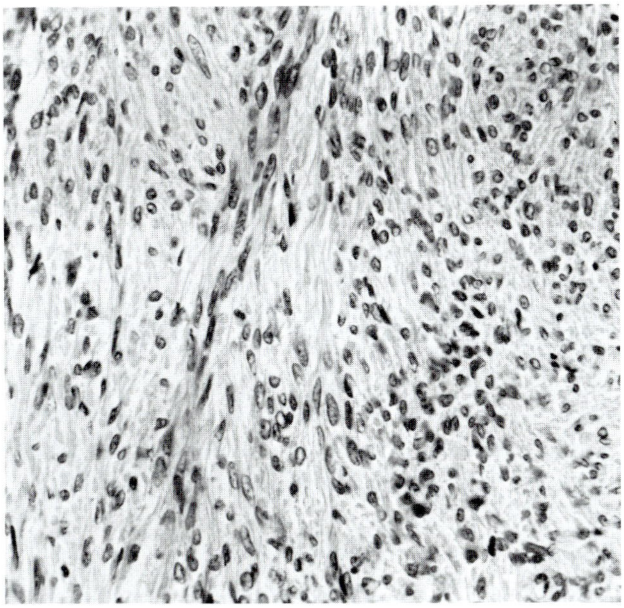

Fig. 19.31. Fibroma. The cells have small, spindle-shaped nuclei lacking atypia or mitotic activity. (Reprinted by permission from Serov SF, Scully RE, Sobin LH (1973) International Histological Classification of Tumours, No. 9. Histological Typing of Ovarian Tumours. World Health Organization, Geneva.)

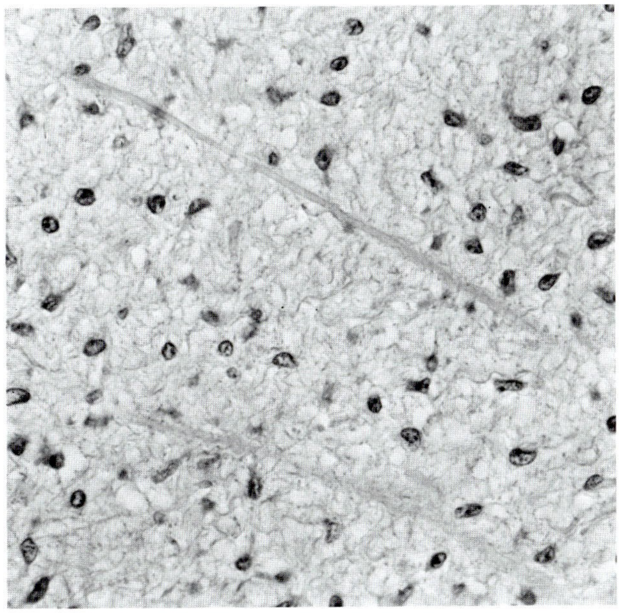

Fig. 19.32. Edematous fibroma. (Reprinted by permission from Serov SF, Scully RE, Sobin LH (1973) International Histological Classification of Tumours, No. 9. Histological Typing of Ovarian Tumours. World Health Organization, Geneva.)

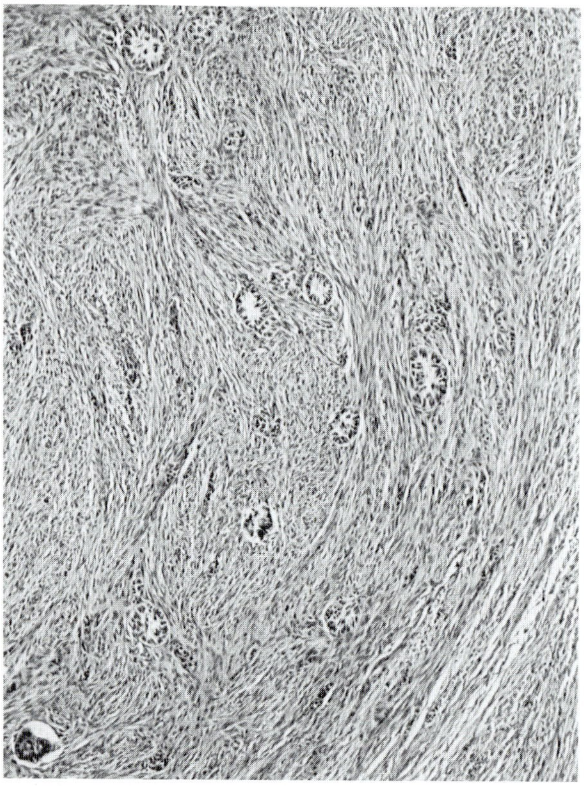

Fig. 19.33. **Fibroma with minor sex cord elements.** Sertoliform tubules are scattered within a fibromatous tumor. (Reprinted by permission of Young and Scully, ref. 156.)

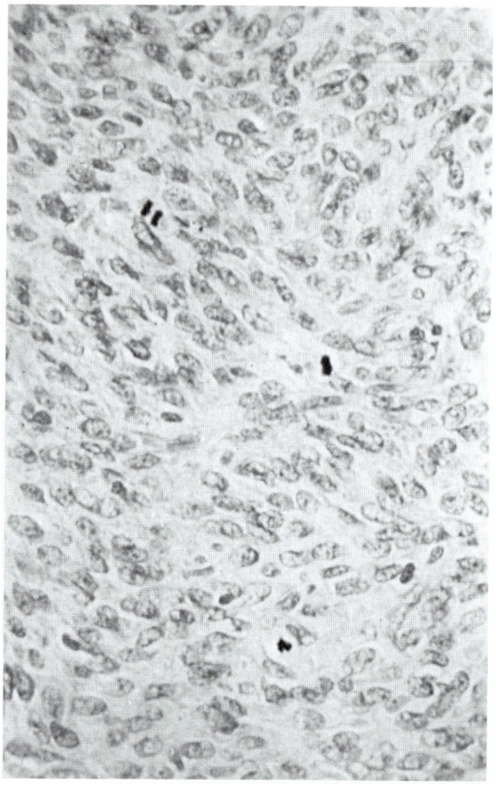

Fig. 19.34. **Cellular fibroma.** Note mitotic figures.

27 years. In contrast to the thecoma, the sclerosing stromal tumor has been associated with evidence of estrogen or androgen secretion, or both in only a few cases.[167] All sclerosing stromal tumors encountered to date have been benign.

Gross examination typically reveals a unilateral, discrete, sharply demarcated mass; the neoplasm is rarely bilateral.[62] Its sectioned surface is solid and white but often shows areas of edema and cyst formation and foci of yellow discoloration (Fig. 19.35). A rare specimen presents as a unilocular cyst. Microscopic examination discloses a number of distinctive features: a pseudolobular pattern (Fig. 19.36), in which cellular nodules are separated by less cellular areas of densely collagenous or edematous connective tissue; sclerosis within the nodules; prominent thin-walled vessels in some of the nodules (Fig. 19.37); and a disorganized admixture of fibroblasts and rounded, vacuolated cells within the nodules (Fig. 19.38). Occasionally, the vacuolated cells have a signet cell appearance, creating some confusion with the signet cells of a Krukenberg tumor, but the former cells contain lipid instead of mucin. The lipid-laden cells appear to be inactive or weakly active lutein cells; in the rare functioning tumors, the lutein cells resemble more closely those encountered in a luteinized thecoma. Although overlap exists between fibromas, thecomas, sclerosing stromal tumors, and even steroid cell tumors, the presence of various distinctive features of these four tumors, which are presented in Table 19.6, almost always allows a specific diagnosis.

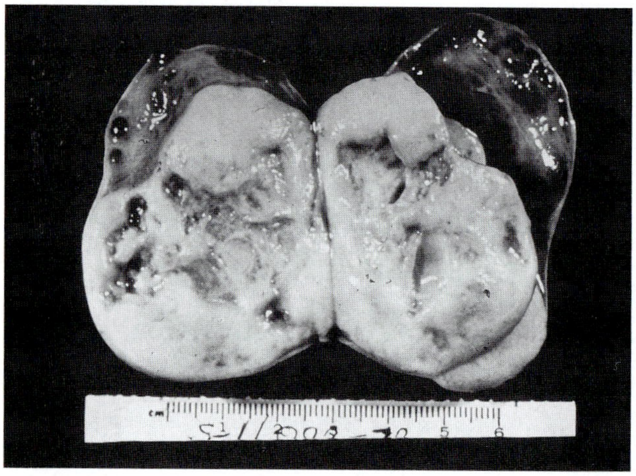

Fig. 19.35. **Sclerosing stromal tumor.** The sectioned surface of the neoplasm is solid and cystic. The solid tissue was white to focally tan.

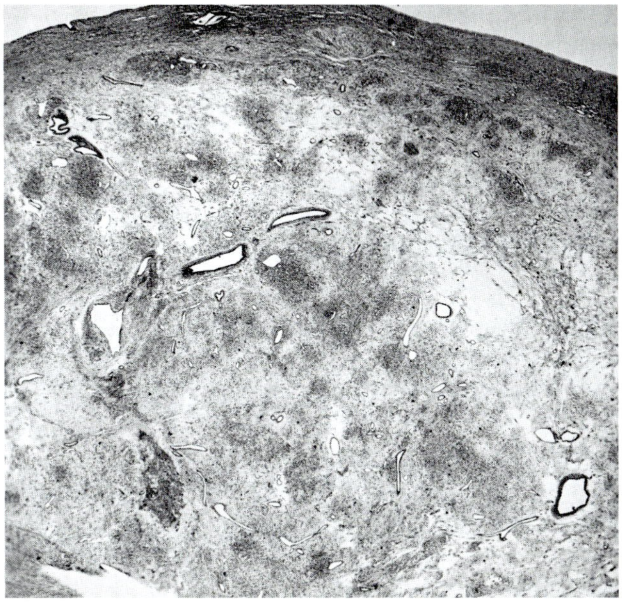

Fig. 19.36. Sclerosing stromal tumor. Cellular pseudolobules are separated by edematous hypocellular tumor. (Reprinted by permission of Chalvardjian and Scully, ref. 23.)

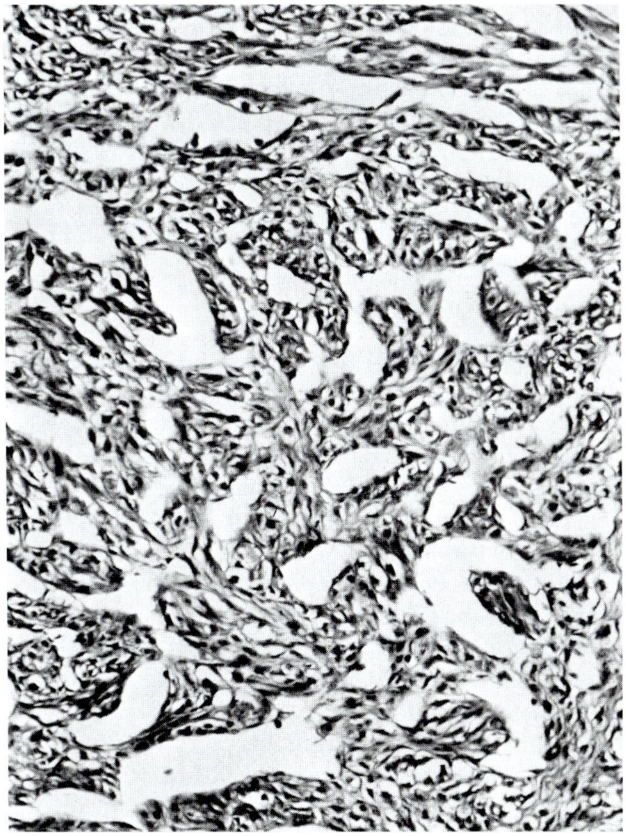

Fig. 19.37. Sclerosing stromal tumor. Pseudolobule is richly vascularized. (Reprinted by permission of Chalvardjian and Scully, ref. 23.)

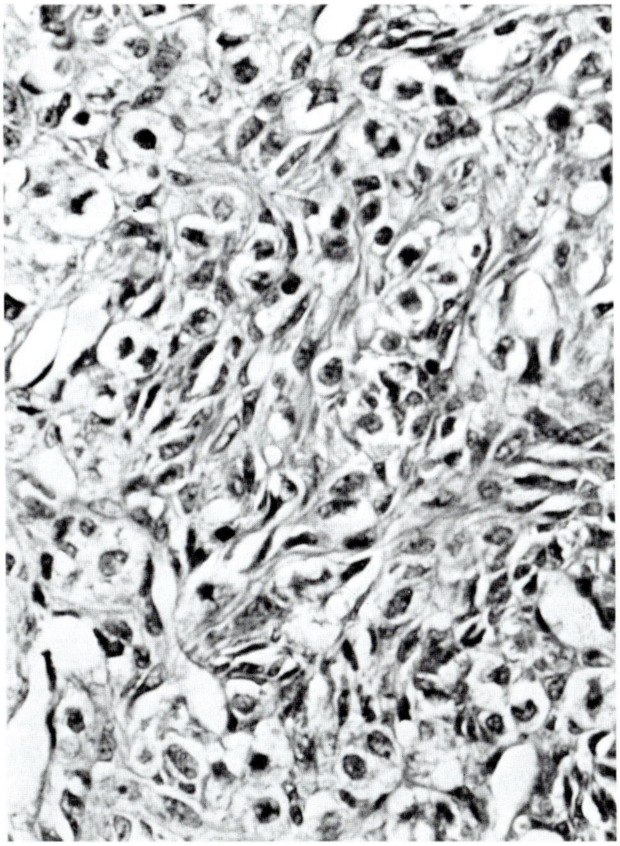

Fig. 19.38. Sclerosing stromal tumor. Spindle cells are mixed with large rounded vacuolated cells. (Reprinted by permission of Chalvardjian and Scully, ref. 23.)

Signet-Ring Stromal Tumor

In 1976, Ramzy[107] described an unusual ovarian tumor from a 28-year-old woman, which he designated *signet-ring stromal tumor*. Five examples have now been described, all in adults and all nonfunctioning and all benign.[35] There are no noteworthy gross features. On microscopic examination spindle cells are diffusely distributed and merge imperceptibly with rounded cells containing eccentric nuclei and single large vacuoles resembling signet-ring cells (Fig. 19.39). These cells may be diffusely scattered or focally distributed. Stains for lipid and mucin are negative. Electron microscopic examination has shown that in some cases the vacuoles result from generalized edema of the cytoplasmic matrix, in others from swelling of mitochondria, and in still others from cytoplasmic pseudoinclusions of edematous extracellular matrix.[35] Negative staining for mucin excludes a Krukenberg tumor, the most realistic and impor-

Table 19.6. Sclerosing versus other stromal tumors and steroid cell tumors

	Sclerosing stromal tumor	*Fibroma*	*Thecoma*	*Steroid cell tumor*
Age	80% under 30 years	10% under 30 years	Average age, 63 years	25% under 30 years
Function	Almost always absent	Absent	Typically estrogenic[a]	Typically androgenic
Gross variegation	Yes	No	No	No
Pseudolobulation	Yes	Rare	Rare	No
Prominent ectatic vessels	Yes	Rare	Rare	Rare
Two cell types	Yes	No	Only in luteinized form	No
Hyaline plaques	No	Common	Common	No
Behavior	Benign	Almost always benign	Almost always benign	Sometimes malignant

[a]Luteinized form androgenic in 11% of cases.

tant lesion in the differential diagnosis. The signet-ring stromal tumor lacks the pseudolobulation, lipid-rich cells, and prominent vascularity of the sclerosing stromal tumor.

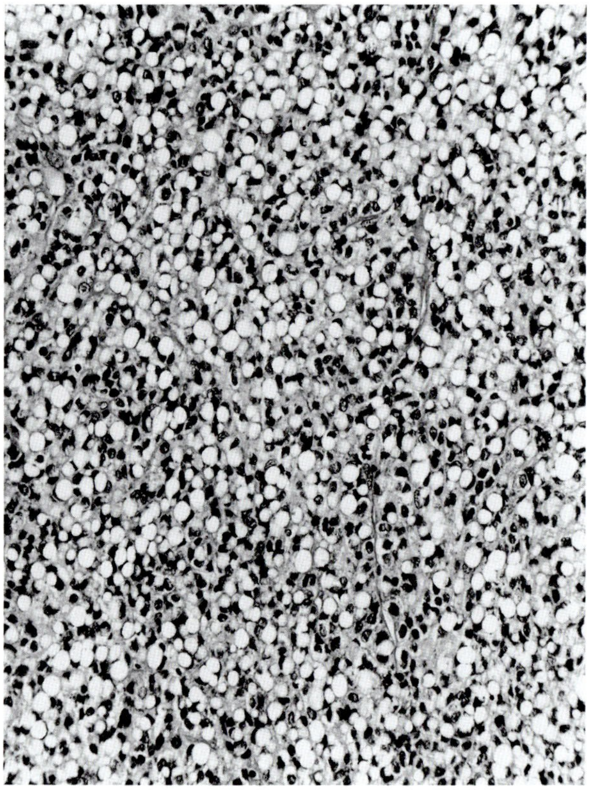

Fig. 19.39. Signet-ring stromal tumor.

Unclassified Tumors

Rare tumors in the intermediate zone between fibromas and thecomas are impossible to classify more specifically. Such tumors are made up of cells having some but not all the features of theca cells, containing small to moderate amounts of lipid, and being associated with equivocal evidence of estrogen secretion. Such tumors should be diagnosed as "tumor in the fibroma–thecoma category, unclassified," and often a descriptive notation is warranted to remark on the particular features of a given case.

Sertoli–Stromal Cell Tumors (Androblastomas)

Sertoli–stromal cell tumors contain Sertoli cells, Leydig cells, fibroblasts, or all these cells, in varying proportions and varying degrees of differentiation. Because the less well differentiated neoplasms within this category may recapitulate the development of the testis, the terms androblastomas and arrhenoblastomas have been used as synonyms. However, the connotation of masculinization associated with the latter designations is misleading because many tumors in this category have no endocrine manifestations and a few are estrogenic or progestagenic. Nevertheless, *androblastoma* is an approved alternative term for these tumors. Other tumors within this group are pure Sertoli cell tumors, pure Leydig cell tumors, and stromal-Leydig cell tumors; the latter already have been mentioned in the discussion of luteinized thecomas, and pure Leydig cell tumors are considered in the section on steroid cell tumors.

Sertoli Cell Tumors

Sertoli cell tumors account for approximately 4% of Sertoli–stromal cell tumors.[137,139,159] They are characterized by a predominant pattern of hollow (Fig. 19.40) or solid tubules (Figs. 19.41 and 19.42), usually dispersed within a fibrous stroma that contains no Leydig cells or very few of them. When the Sertoli cells contain abundant cytoplasmic lipid (Figs. 19.41 and 19.42), the term lipid-rich Sertoli cell tumor is appropriate. Occasional Sertoli cell tumors have cells with abundant eosinophilic cytoplasm.[43] Seven Sertoli cell tumors, most or all of which appear to have been of the lipid-rich type, have resulted in isosexual pseudoprecocity. Two of these tumors were from patients with Peutz–Jeghers syndrome.[128,159] One Sertoli cell tumor was associated with progesterone as well as estrogen production.[141] All the Sertoli cell tumors reported to date have been

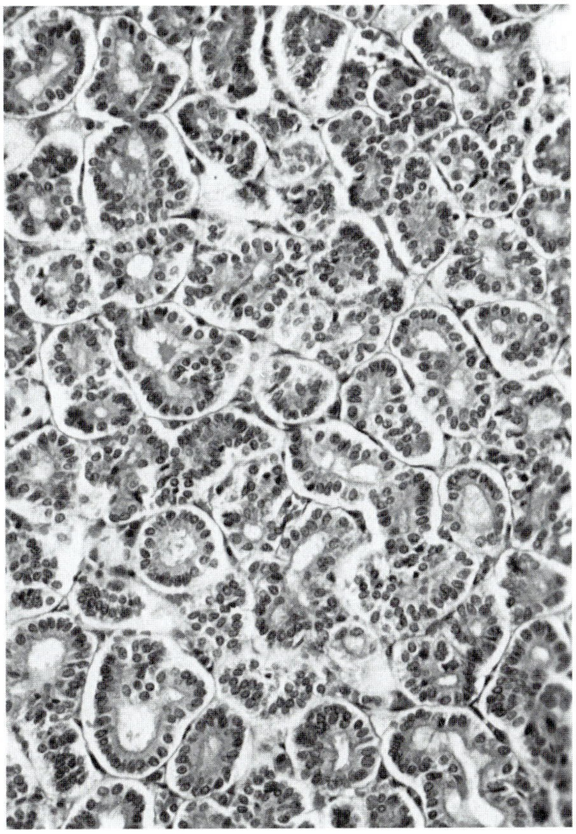

Fig. 19.40. Sertoli cell tumor. Closely packed hollow tubules lined by well-differentiated cuboidal to columnar epithelial cells. (Reprinted by permission of Young and Scully, ref. 159.)

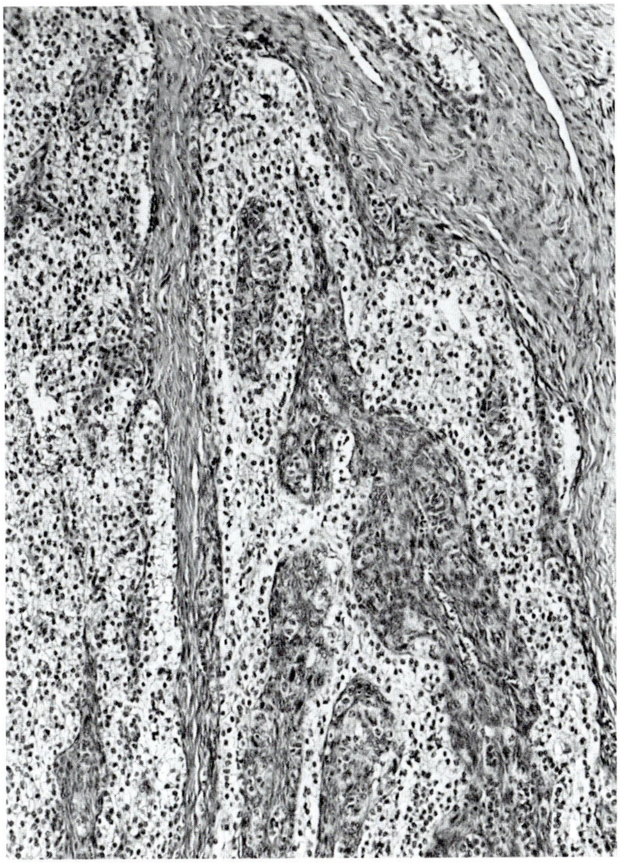

Fig. 19.41. Sertoli cell tumor, lipid rich. Reprinted by permission from Serov SF, Scully RE, Sobin LH (1973) International Histological Classification of Tumours, No. 9. Histological Typing of Ovarian Tumours. World Health Organization, Geneva.

unilateral and stage I. They have averaged approximately 9 cm in diameter and typically formed lobulated, solid, yellow or brown masses. Microscopic examination may show a focal solid pattern as well as definitional tubules. There is little if any nuclear atypia or mitotic activity, and the prognosis is excellent. A few tumors exhibit moderate degrees of nuclear atypicality, and exceptionally there is a malignant appearance with metastases.[103,159]

Sertoli–Leydig Cell Tumors

Sertoli–Leydig cell tumors account for less than 0.5% of all ovarian tumors.[111,165] They have been divided into six subtypes: well differentiated, of intermediate differentiation, poorly differentiated, with heterologous elements, retiform, and mixed. Sertoli–Leydig cell tumors occur in all age groups but are encountered most often in young women. In our series of more than 200 cases, the average age was 25 years;

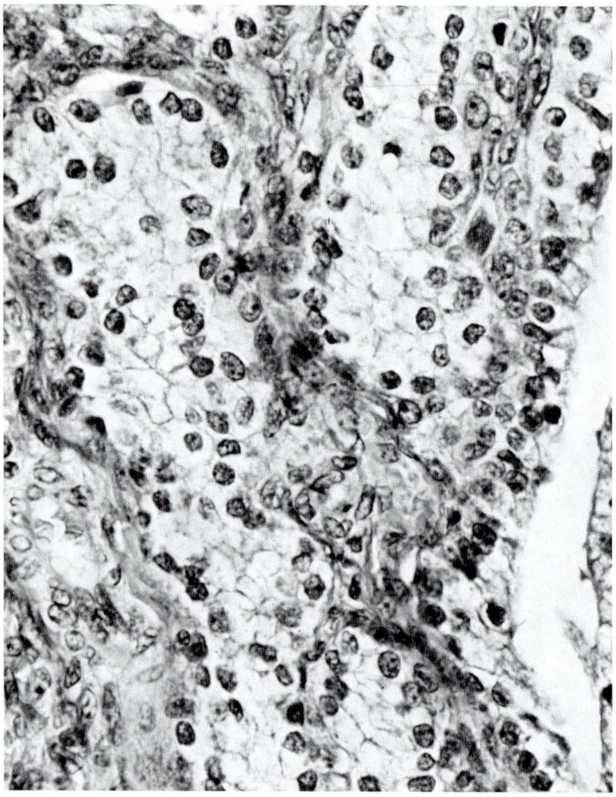

Fig. 19.42. Sertoli cell tumor, lipid rich. Reprinted by permission from Serov SF, Scully RE, Sobin LH (1973) International Histological Classification of Tumours, No. 9. Histological Typing of Ovarian Tumours. World Health Organization, Geneva.

75% of the patients were 30 years of age or younger and only 9.5% were over 50 years of age.[162] The average age in the two other large series was 24 and 24.5 years.[111,165] The well-differentiated tumors[161] occur on an average a decade later, and retiform tumors[158] a decade earlier, than other Sertoli–Leydig cell tumors. Tumors with a retiform pattern are more common in the first decade than any other subtype.

Clinical Features

Although the most striking mode of presentation of Sertoli–Leydig cell tumors is virilization, it develops in only about one-third of the cases.[162] In such cases a patient who has been having normal menstrual periods typically begins to have oligomenorrhea, followed within a few months by amenorrhea. There is a concomitant loss of female secondary sex characteristics, with atrophy of the breasts and disappearance of normal bodily contours. Progressive masculinization is heralded by acne, with hirsutism, temporal balding, deepening of the voice, and enlargement of the clitoris following in its wake. There was no significant difference in the frequency of androgenic manifestations among the various subtypes in our series except that it was lower with tumors containing heterologous elements and lowest with tumors having a prominent retiform component.[162] The androgen secretion by the tumor also may result in erythrocytosis.

Plasma levels of testosterone, androstenedione, and other androgens, alone or in combination, may be elevated in patients with Sertoli–Leydig cell tumors. The urinary 17-ketosteroid values usually are normal or only slightly raised, although occasionally a high level has been recorded. These findings are in contrast to those associated with virilizing adrenal tumors, which often are accompanied by high urinary levels of 17-ketosteroids.[160] The values for plasma androgens and urinary 17-ketosteroids are not reliable, however, in the differentiation of ovarian and adrenal virilizing tumors because the latter often are associated with elevated testosterone and normal urinary 17-ketosteroid levels.[5] Also, tests involving attempted stimulation by tropic hormones and suppression by gonadal and adrenocortical steroids have not proved decisive in differentiating these tumors. Approximately 20 Sertoli–Leydig cell tumors associated with elevated plasma levels of alpha-fetoprotein have been reported,[11,47] but values as high as those accompanying yolk sac tumors are rare.

Approximately 50% of patients with Sertoli–Leydig cell tumors have no endocrine manifestations and usually complain of abdominal swelling or pain. Occasional tumors have been associated with various estrogenic syndromes, including irregular menses, menorrhagia, or menometrorrhagia in women in the reproductive age group and postmenopausal bleeding in older women.[162] No well-documented case of a Sertoli–Leydig cell tumor associated with isosexual precocity has been reported.

At laparotomy almost all Sertoli–Leydig cell tumors are unilateral; in our series only 1.5% were bilateral. Rare tumors are asynchronously bilateral. The tumors are stage Ia in about 80% of the cases; in 12% the tumor has either ruptured or involved the external surface of the ovary and in 4% ascites is present. Only about 2.5% of the tumors have spread beyond the ovary, usually within the pelvis and rarely into the upper abdomen. All the well-differentiated tumors in our series were stage Ia; the poorly differentiated tumors more often were ruptured or presented at a higher stage than the tumors of intermediate differentiation.[162]

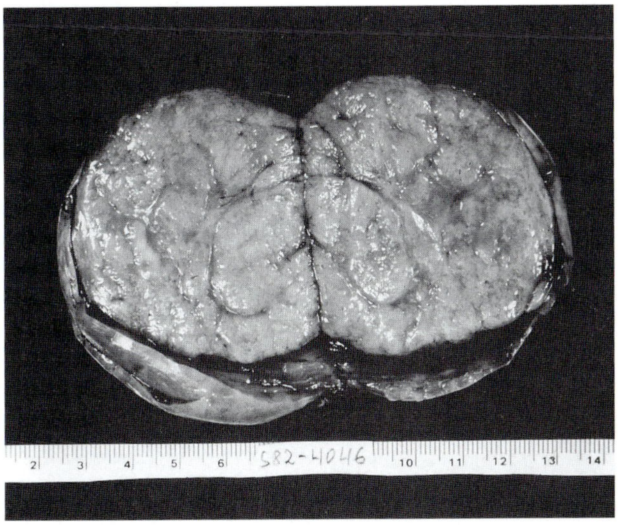

Fig. 19.43. Sertoli–Leydig cell tumor. The sectioned surface of the neoplasm is solid and lobulated. The neoplasm was yellow in the fresh state.

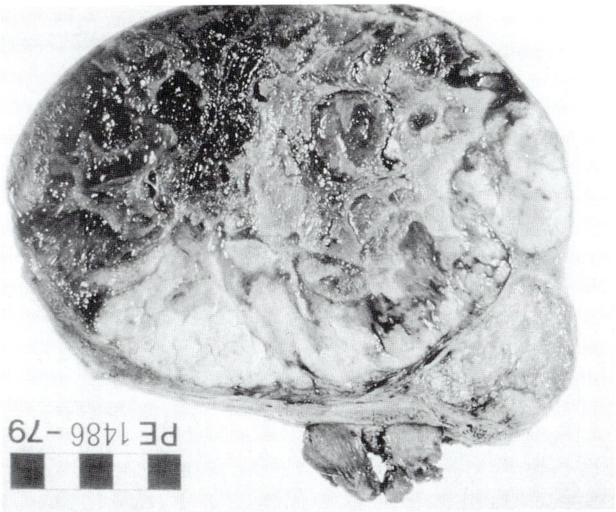

Fig. 19.44. Sertoli–Leydig cell tumor with mesenchymal heterologous elements. The sectioned surface of the tumor exhibits extensive areas of hemorrhage and necrosis. (Reproduced by permission of Prat et al., ref. 105.)

Pathologic Findings

Sertoli–Leydig cell tumors vary as greatly in their gross appearance as granulosa cell tumors, and these neoplasms cannot be distinguished on gross examination alone. There are, however, a few general differences. Sertoli–Leydig cell tumors contain blood-filled cysts less often than granulosa cell tumors and, unlike the latter, almost never have the appearance of a unilocular thin-walled cyst. Sertoli–Leydig cell tumors vary in size from microscopic to huge masses but most are between 5 and 15 (average, 13.5) cm in diameter (Fig. 19.43). Poorly differentiated tumors including those with mesenchymal heterologous elements tend to be larger than those of better differentiation and contain areas of hemorrhage and necrosis more frequently (Fig. 19.44). Tumors with heterologous or retiform components are cystic more often than tumors without these elements. The heterologous tumors occasionally simulate mucinous cystic tumors on gross examination (Fig. 19.45), and retiform tumors may contain large, edematous papillae, resembling serous papillary tumors (Fig. 19.46).

Well-Differentiated Sertoli–Leydig Cell Tumor

These tumors are characterized by a predominantly tubular pattern (Fig. 19.47).[161] On low-power examination a nodular architecture often is conspicuous, with fibrous bands separating lobules composed of hollow or less often solid tubules; in some tumors tubules of both types are present. The hollow tubules typically are round to oval and small, but may be cystically dilated, and some of them resemble the tubular glands of a well-differentiated endometrioid adenocarcinoma. The lumens usually are devoid of conspicuous secretion but in some cases eosinophilic fluid, which is occasionally mucicarminophilic, is present. The solid tubules typically are elongated but may be round or oval and

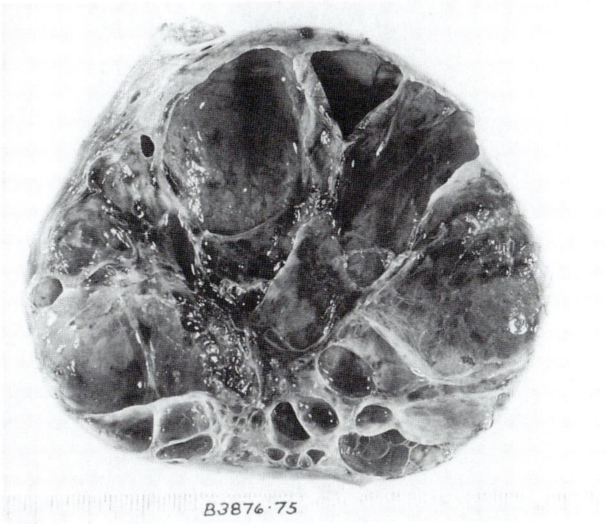

Fig. 19.45. Sertoli–Leydig cell tumor with mucinous heterologous elements. The sectioned surface of the tumor displays a multiloculated cystic neoplasm. (Reproduced by permission of Young et al., ref. 155.)

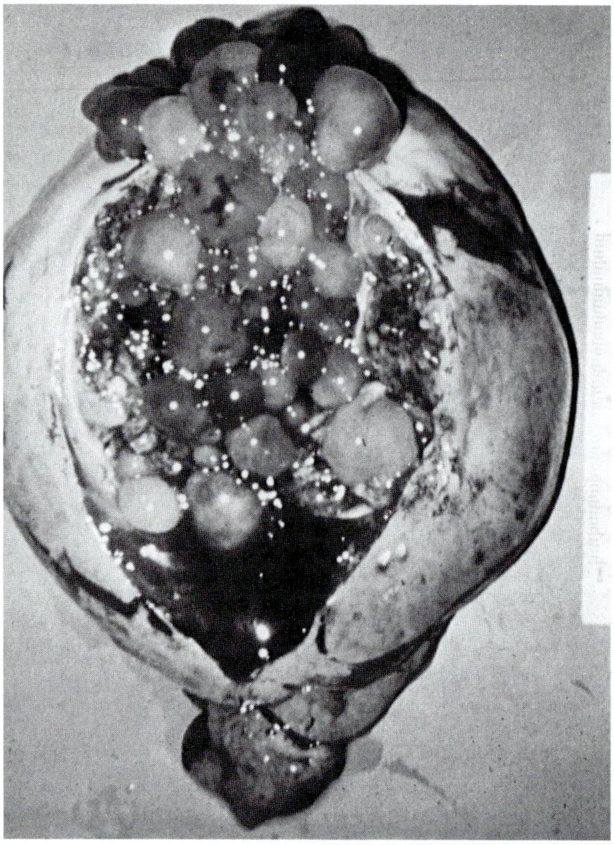

Fig. 19.46. Sertoli–Leydig cell tumor with retiform pattern. Edematous polypoid structures project into lumen of cystic neoplasm. (Reprinted by permission of Young and Scully, ref. 158.)

occasionally resemble prepubertal or atrophic testicular tubules. The tubules contain cuboidal to columnar epithelial cells with round or oblong nuclei without prominent nucleoli. Nuclear atypicality usually is absent or minimal, and mitotic figures are rare. The cells lining the hollow tubules and filling the solid tubules typically contain moderate amounts of dense cytoplasm, but in some cases varying numbers of them have abundant pale cytoplasm rich in lipid. The stromal component consists of bands of mature fibrous tissue containing variable but usually conspicuous numbers of Leydig cells. These cells may contain abundant lipochrome pigment; in our series crystals of Reinke were identified in some of the Leydig cells in approximately 20% of the cases (Fig. 19.48).

Sertoli–Leydig Cell Tumors of Intermediate and Poor Differentiation

These tumors form a continuum characterized by a variety of patterns and combinations of cell types. Some tumors exhibit intermediate differentiation in some areas and poor differentiation in others and, less commonly, tumors of intermediate differentiation contain well-differentiated foci. Either the Sertoli cells or Leydig cells or both may exhibit varying degrees of immaturity. In the tumors of intermediate differentiation, immature Sertoli cells with small, round, oval, or angular nuclei are arranged typically in poorly defined masses, often creating a lobulated appearance on low power (Fig. 19.49); solid and hollow tubules (Fig. 19.50), nests, thin cords resembling the sex cords of the embryonic testis (Fig. 19.51), and broad columns of Sertoli cells (Fig. 19.52) often are present. Cysts containing eosinophilic secretion may create a thyroid-like appearance, and follicle-like spaces are encountered rarely. The Sertoli cells, or the Leydig cells, may have bizarre nuclei similar to those seen in some granulosa cell tumors.[157] The Sertoli cell aggregates are separated by a stromal component that ranges from fibromatous to densely cellular to edematous and typically contain clusters of well-differentiated Leydig cells. Occasionally, part or all of the stromal

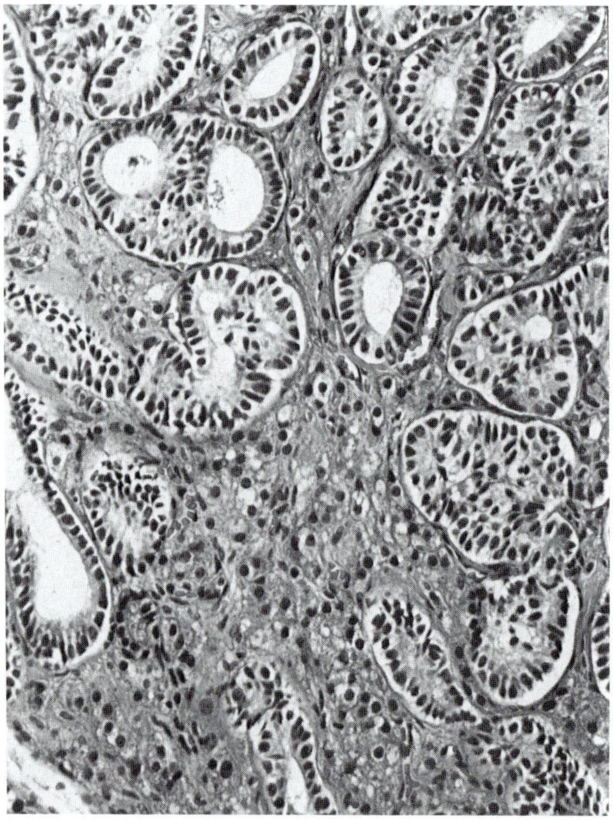

Fig. 19.47. Sertoli–Leydig cell tumor, well differentiated. Hollow tubules are separated by Leydig cells in intervening stroma. (Reprinted by permission of Young and Scully, ref. 161.)

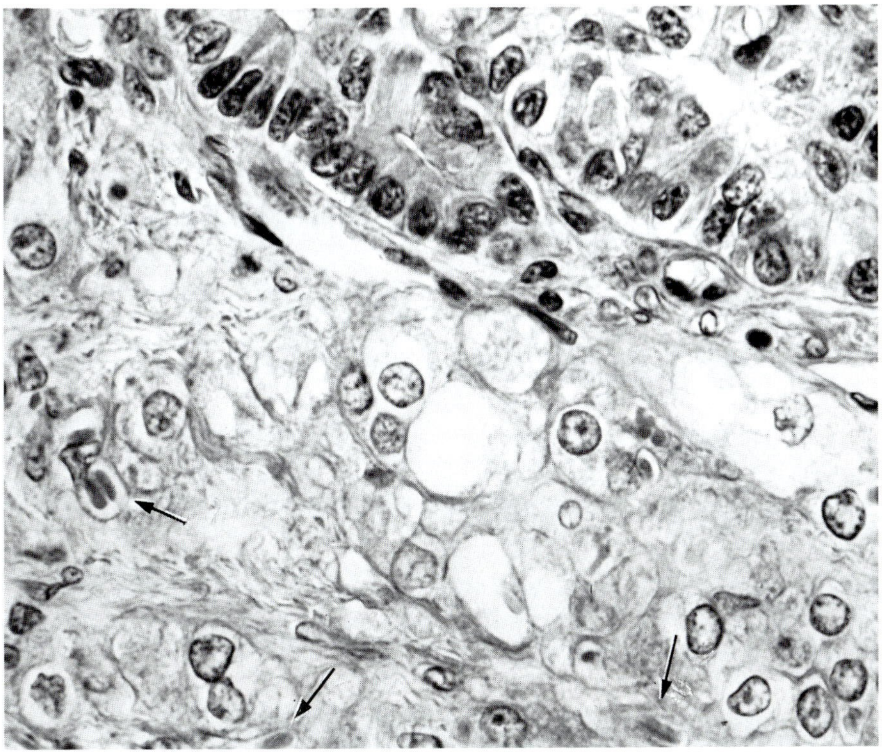

Fig. 19.48. Sertoli–Leydig cell tumor, well differentiated. *Arrows* point to crystals of Reinke.

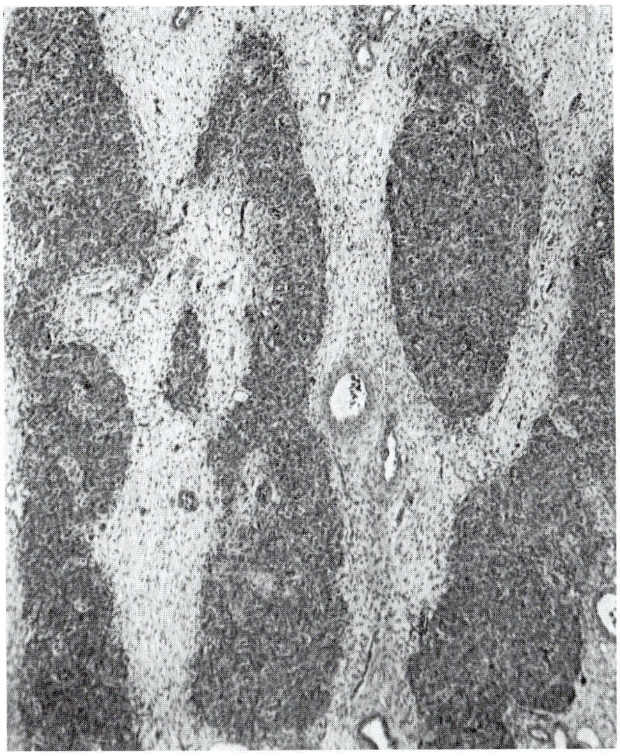

Fig. 19.49. Sertoli–Leydig cell tumor of intermediate differentiation. Cellular lobules are intersected by slightly edematous stromal component. (Reprinted by permission of Young and Scully, ref. 162.)

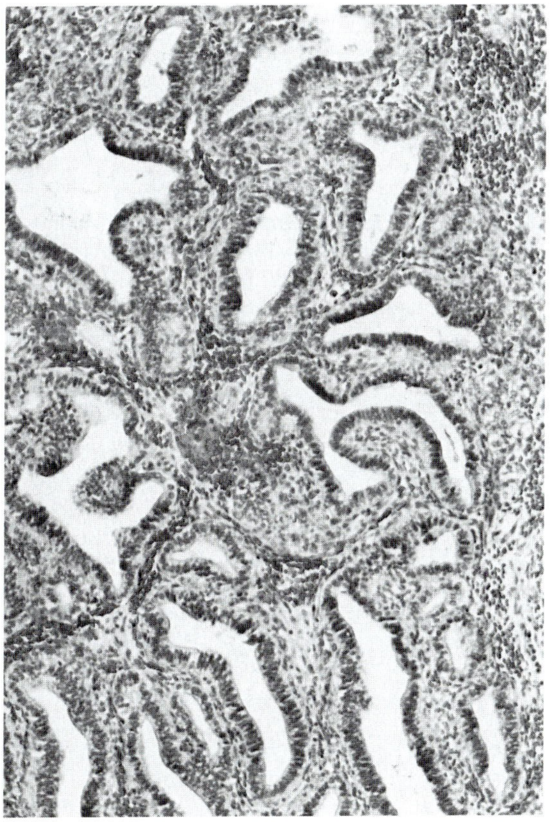

Fig. 19.50. Sertoli–Leydig cell tumor of intermediate differentiation. The tubules in this neoplasm resemble those of an endometrioid tumor.

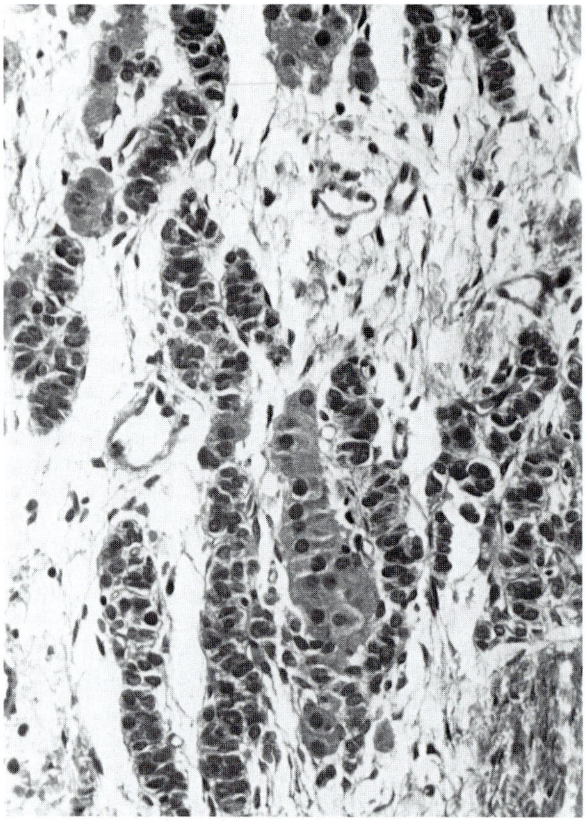

Fig. 19.51. Sertoli–Leydig cell tumor of intermediate differentiation. Cords of immature Sertoli cells and clusters of Leydig cells with abundant cytoplasm. (Reprinted by permission of Young and Scully, ref. 158.)

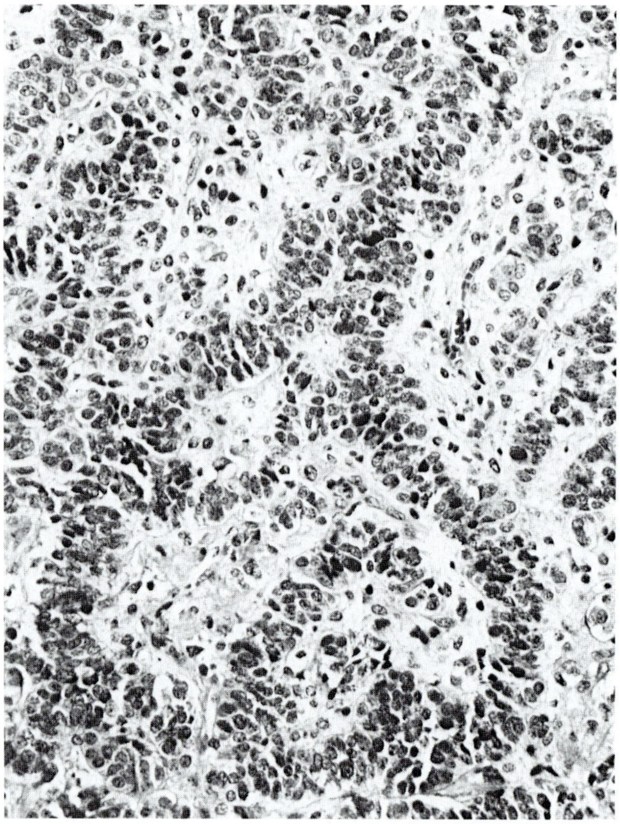

Fig. 19.52. Sertoli–Leydig cell tumor of intermediate differentiation. Anastomosing columns of immature Sertoli cells. (Reprinted by permission of Young and Scully, ref. 162.)

component is made up of immature, cellular mesenchymal tissue resembling a nonspecific sarcoma. The Sertoli and Leydig cell elements, singly or together, may contain varying and sometimes large amounts of lipid in the form of small or large droplets (Fig. 19.53). Poorly differentiated Sertoli–Leydig cell tumors originally were classified as sarcomatoid because, aside from the presence of specifically diagnostic elements, they resemble fibrosarcomas (Fig. 19.54); however, they often have a diffuse pattern that is not clearly recognizable as that of a fibrosarcoma.

Retiform Sertoli–Leydig Cell Tumor

Fifteen percent of Sertoli–Leydig cell tumors are composed, usually partially but occasionally entirely, of tubular structures arranged in a pattern resembling that of the rete testis.[112,134,158] So far a retiform pattern has been encountered only in tumors that are otherwise intermediate, poorly differentiated, or heterologous. Microscopic examination reveals a network of irregularly branching, elongated, narrow, often slitlike tubules and cysts into which papillae or polypoid structures may project (Fig. 19.55). The tubules and cysts may contain eosinophilic secretion; they are lined by epithelial cells that exhibit varying degrees of stratification and nuclear atypicality. The papillae and polyps are of three types: most commonly they are small and rounded or blunt, often containing hyalinized cores (Fig. 19.56); sometimes they are large and bulbous, containing edematous cores. Finally, in some cases they are delicate and branch extensively and may be lined by stratified cells, simulating the papillae of a serous tumor of borderline or invasive type (Fig. 19.57). A common finding in the retiform Sertoli–Leydig cell tumor is the presence of columns or ribbons of immature Sertoli cells. The stroma within a retiform area may be hyalinized or edematous, moderately cellular, or densely cellular and immature.

Heterologous Sertoli–Leydig Cell Tumor

Heterologous elements occur in approximately 20% of Sertoli–Leydig cell tumors, most of which are

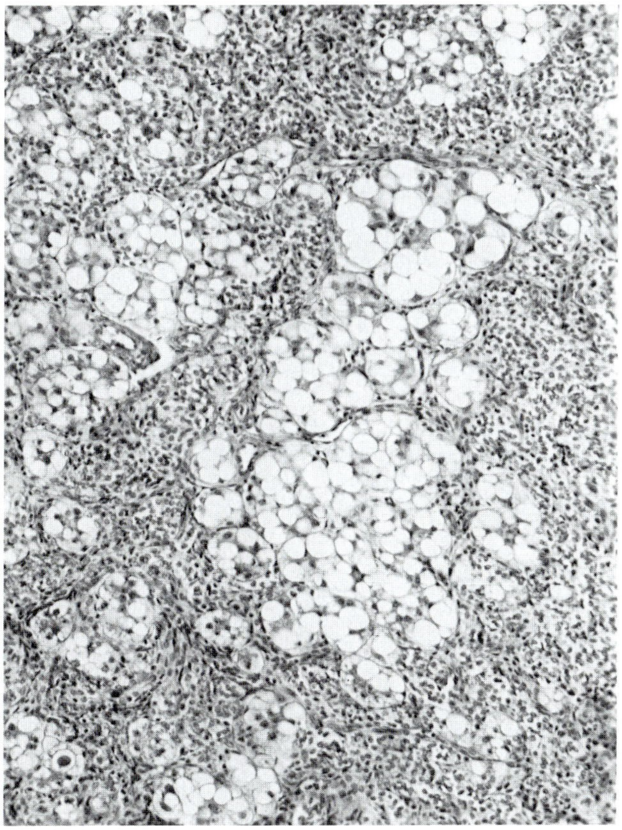

Fig. 19.53. Sertoli–Leydig cell tumor of intermediate differentiation. Nests of Leydig cells with large lipid vacuoles. (Reprinted by permission of Young and Scully, ref. 162.)

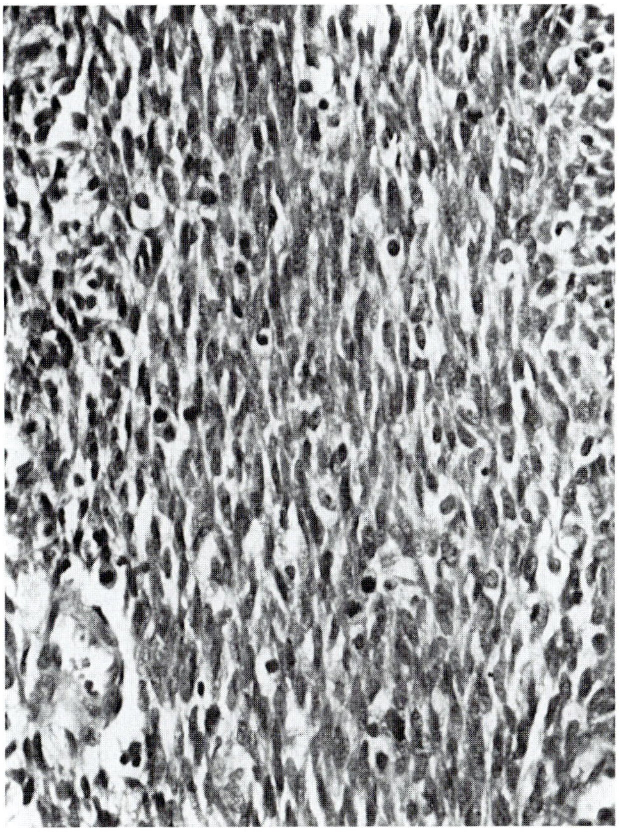

Fig. 19.54. Sertoli–Leydig cell tumor, poorly differentiated. The tumor cells are spindle shaped and exhibit nuclear atypia and mitotic activity. ×400. (Reprinted by permission of Young and Scully, ref. 162.)

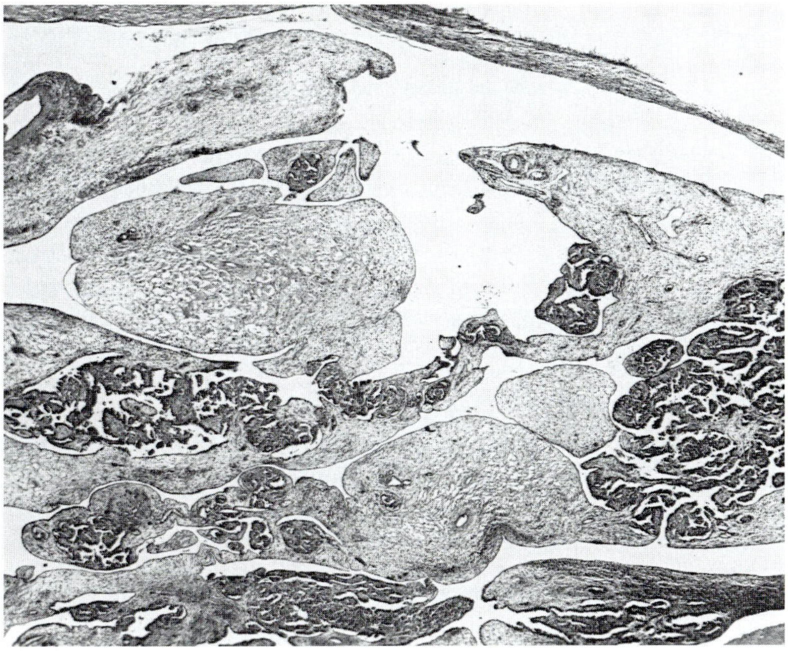

Fig. 19.55. Sertoli–Leydig cell tumor with retiform pattern. Large edematous polypoid structures and many small papillae. (Reprinted by permission of Young and Scully, ref. 158.)

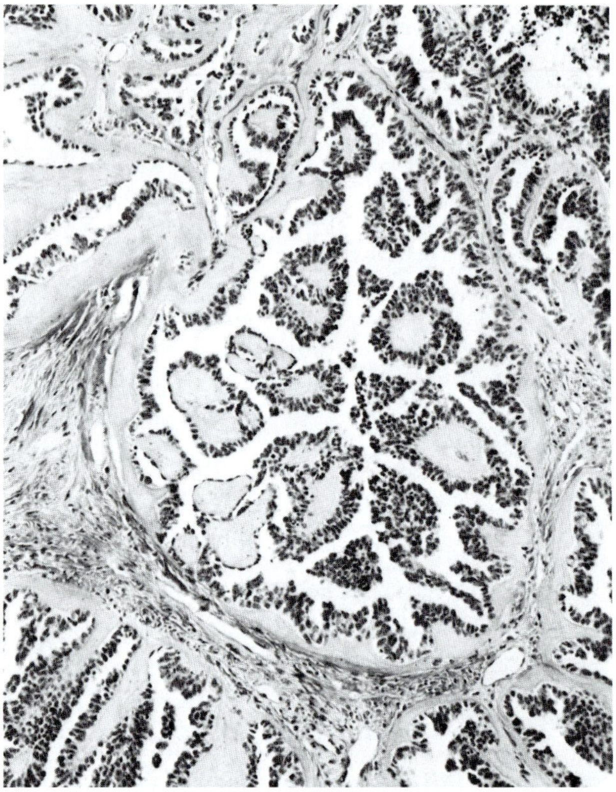

Fig. 19.56. Sertoli–Leydig cell tumor with retiform pattern. The papillae have prominent hyalinized cores and are lined by stratified epithelial cells. (Reprinted by permission of Young and Scully (1985) Ovarian sex cord-stromal and steroid cell tumors. In: Roth LM, Czernobilsky B (eds) Tumors and Tumor-like Conditions of the Ovary. Contemporary Issues in Surgical Pathology, Vol. 6. Churchill Livingstone, New York.)

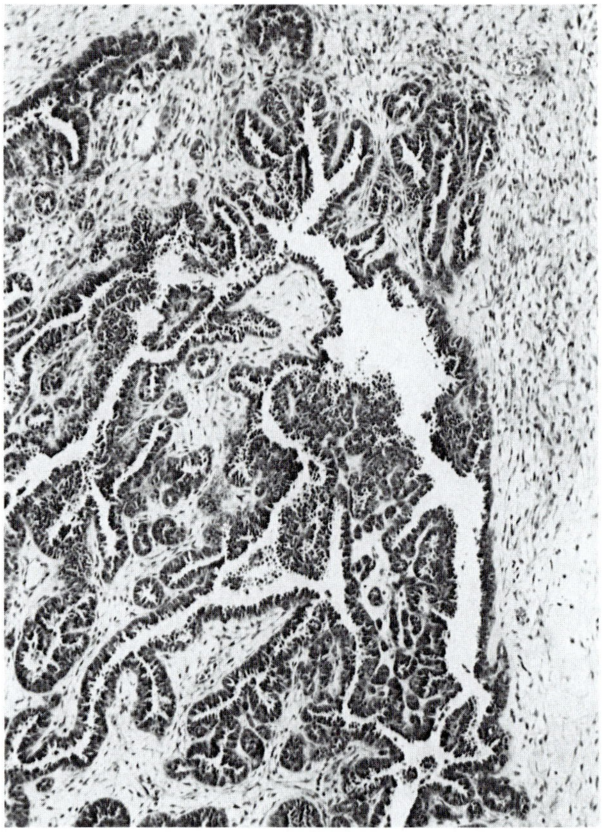

Fig. 19.57. Sertoli–Leydig cell tumor with retiform pattern. A complex papillary pattern simulates a serous papillary adenocarcinoma.

otherwise of intermediate differentiation, but some of which are poorly differentiated.[105,155] In our series of more than 200 tumors, 18% contained glands and cysts lined by moderately to well-differentiated gastric-type or intestinal-type epithelium (Fig. 19.58). The intestinal-type epithelium at times may contain goblet cells, argentaffin cells, and rarely Paneth cells. Sixteen percent of heterologous Sertoli–Leydig cell tumors had one or a few microscopic foci of carcinoid tumor (Fig. 19.59).[147,155] Stromal heterologous elements, encountered in 5% of all Sertoli–Leydig cell tumors,[105] include islands of cartilage arising on a sarcomatous background, areas of embryonal rhabdomyosarcoma, or both (Fig. 19.60). We also have seen one heterologous tumor that contained cells resembling hepatocytes,[154] one containing retinal tissue, and another with neuroblastoma, in a recurrent tumor.[105] Despite the variety of unexpected tissues in heterologous Sertoli–Leydig cell tumors, it appears unlikely that such neoplasms are of germ cell origin[108] inasmuch as neither Sertoli nor Leydig cells have ever been identified in gonadal tumors clearly recognizable as teratomas.

Differential Diagnosis

Because of their many patterns, Sertoli–stromal cell tumors often are difficult to differentiate from tumors outside the sex cord–stromal category as well as from granulosa cell tumors. The small hollow tubular structures, solid tubular aggregates, and cords that occasionally are seen in endometrioid carcinomas may closely mimic structures characteristically encountered in Sertoli and Sertoli–Leydig cell tumors. Endometrioid carcinomas also may contain luteinized stromal cells that resemble Leydig cells, creating an even greater problem in differentiation. At least some of the glands of endometrioid carcinomas, however, usually are larger than the tubules of Sertoli–Leydig cell tumors and are lined by epithelium that is less well differentiated. In addition, mucin secretion, areas of squamous differentiation that range from nests of uniform immature spindle-

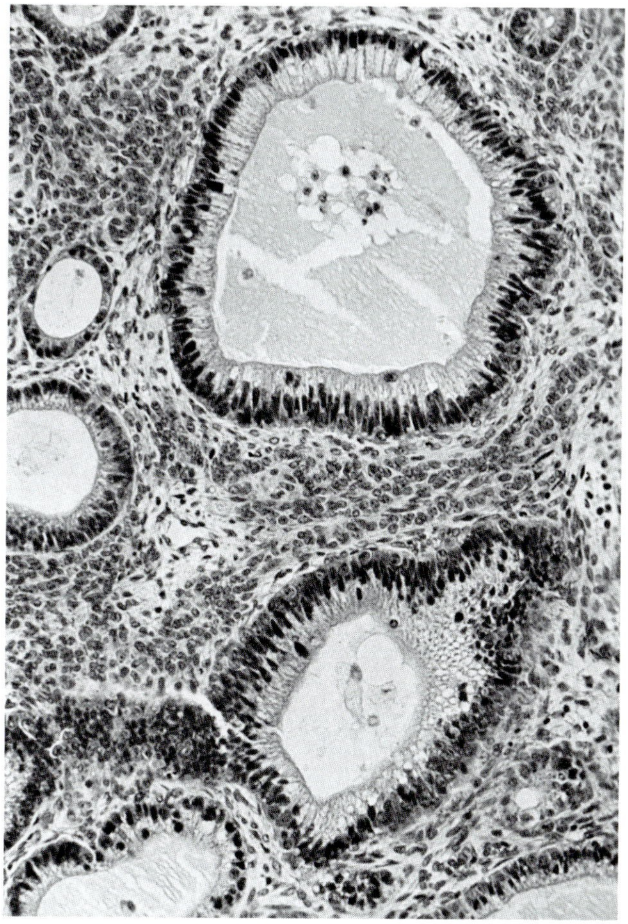

Fig. 19.58. Sertoli–Leydig cell tumor with heterologous elements. Mucinous glands are separated by intermediate form of tumor. (Reprinted by permission from Serov SF, Scully RE, Sobin LH (1973) International Histological Classification of Tumours, No. 9. Histological Typing of Ovarian Tumours. World Health Organization, Geneva.)

shaped epithelial cells to morules to keratinizing foci, and an adenofibromatous component of common epithelial type are present in most endometrioid carcinomas, facilitating their diagnosis. Clinical features, such as the usual older age of the patient and the absence of androgenic manifestations, support the diagnosis of endometrioid carcinoma, but it must be emphasized that endometrioid carcinomas occasionally have a functioning stroma, which sometimes is manifested clinically by estrogenic changes and rarely by virilization. Immunohistochemical staining for epithelial membrane antigen (and other antigens, see later) may be helpful in difficult cases because it is almost always positive in cases of endometrioid carcinoma and only rarely focally positive in a few cells within a Sertoli–Leydig cell tumor.[2] Sertoli–Leydig cell tumors may be simulated by primary or metastatic endometrioid stromal sarcomas. Criteria that are applicable in the differential diagnosis of these tumors with granulosa cell tumors also are helpful in this situation.

The tubular Krukenberg tumor (see Chapter 22, Metastatic Tumors of the Ovary) may mimic a Sertoli–Leydig cell tumor especially if luteinization of the stroma is present; further confusion arises in the rare case in which the former tumor is associated with virilization. Tubular Krukenberg tumors have been reported to be bilateral, however, in 50% of the cases and contain markedly atypical cells, including signet-ring cells that contain mucin, easily demonstrable by special stains.

Carcinoid tumors, especially those of the trabecular type, may be confused with Sertoli–Leydig cell tumors of intermediate differentiation. The ribbons of the former, however, are longer, thicker, and more uniformly distributed than the sex cordlike formations of the latter. Also, rare carcinoid tumors with a solid tubular pattern can be difficult to distinguish from well-differentiated Sertoli cell tumors. Examination of the stroma of carcinoid tumors may be helpful in the differential diagnosis. It is typically

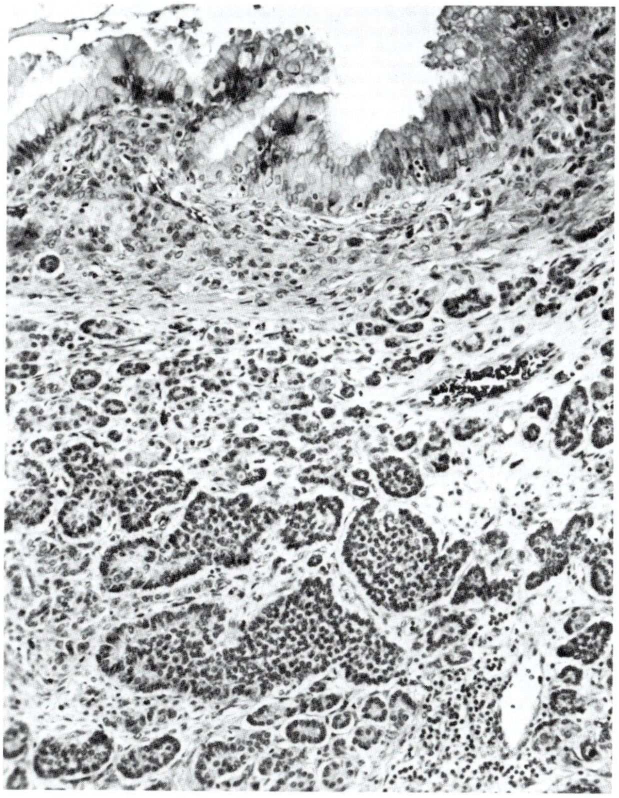

Fig. 19.59. Sertoli–Leydig cell tumor with heterologous elements. Insular carcinoid adjacent to mucinous epithelium.

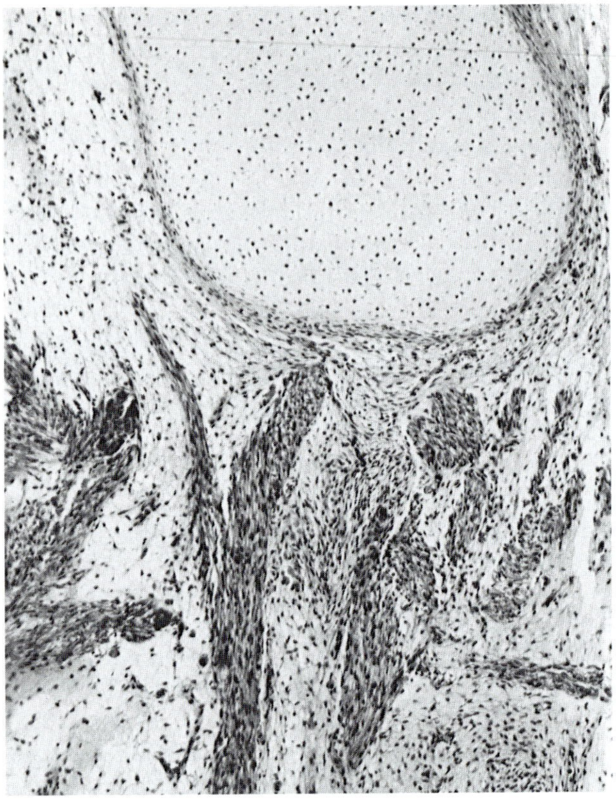

Fig. 19.60. Sertoli–Leydig cell tumor with heterologous elements. Nodule of fetal type cartilage and bundles of strap cells. (Reprinted by permission of Prat et al., ref. 105.)

less cellular and more fibromatous than that of Sertoli–Leydig cell tumors and does not contain Leydig cells. The most specific diagnostic criterion is the presence of argyrophil granules in almost all carcinoid tumors and of argentaffin granules in many of them; in contrast, only heterologous Sertoli–Leydig cell tumors with glands and cysts lined by gastrointestinal-type epithelium contain such granules. Finally, primary carcinoid tumors are associated with teratomatous elements in 70% of the cases, and metastatic carcinoids are almost always bilateral and usually are associated with an obvious primary tumor of the intestine and metastases elsewhere in the abdomen (see Chapter 22).

The tubules seen in ovarian wolffian tumors (see Chapter 21, Nonspecific Tumors of the Ovary, Including Mesenchymal Tumors and Malignant Lymphoma) may be indistinguishable from those seen in Sertoli and Sertoli–Leydig cell tumors but are virtually always accompanied by other patterns that exclude the diagnosis of a sex cord–stromal tumor.

The retiform variant of Sertoli–Leydig cell tumor causes specific problems in differential diagnosis. The most common misdiagnosis is yolk sac tumor, which is suggested clinically by the young age of the patient and pathologically by the presence of papillae within cystic spaces. The occurrence of androgenic manifestations with about one-quarter of cases of retiform Sertoli–Leydig cell tumor, however, contrasts with the rare occurrence of such changes in cases of yolk sac tumor, attributable to a functioning stroma. On gross examination, the retiform tumors generally appear less malignant than yolk sac tumors, and microscopic examination reveals less primitive-appearing cells. The presence of other distinctive patterns of either tumor and positive immunohistochemical staining for alpha-fetoprotein in the yolk sac tumor almost always facilitate the diagnosis.

A greater problem in the differential diagnosis of retiform Sertoli–Leydig cell tumors arises because of their characteristic papillary patterns and the frequent presence of cellular stratification particularly if those features predominate. Under such circumstances, a misdiagnosis of a serous cystadenoma of borderline malignancy or a serous or endometrioid carcinoma occasionally is made. A variety of clinical and pathologic features, including the young age of the patient, the association with virilization, and the presence of other more easily recognizable patterns of Sertoli–Leydig cell tumor, are helpful clues to the correct diagnosis. Finally, the juxtaposition of epithelial and immature mesenchymal elements in some retiform tumors has caused confusion with a malignant mesodermal mixed tumor, but the features already outlined also serve to exclude the latter diagnosis.

Because occasional sex cord–stromal tumors have a morphologic appearance intermediate between granulosa cell tumors and Sertoli–Leydig cell tumors or exhibit features of both tumors, it is sometimes difficult to decide whether a given tumor should be placed in the granulosa, Sertoli–Leydig cell, or mixed category. Major criteria that help to differentiate granulosa cell tumors and Sertoli–Leydig cell tumors are listed in Table 19.7.

Clinical Behavior and Treatment

After the removal of a virilizing Sertoli–Leydig cell tumor, normal menses characteristically resume in about 4 weeks. The excessive hair usually diminishes to some extent. Clitoromegaly and deepening of the voice are less apt to regress. The prognosis in cases of Sertoli–Leydig cell tumor is closely related to their stage and degree of differentiation. The rare tumors that present in an advanced stage have a poor prognosis, with a mortality rate of 100% in our series of cases.[162] The survival rates of patients with stage I

Table 19.7. Adult granulosa cell tumor versus Sertoli–Leydig cell tumor

Granulosa cell tumor	*Sertoli–Leydig cell tumor*
All age groups, mostly postmenopausal	Mainly young women
Usually estrogenic, rarely androgenic	Usually androgenic, occasionally estrogenic
Microfollicular, macrofollicular, trabecular, insular and diffuse patterns	Hollow or solid tubules, cords, diffuse patterns
Granulosa cells usually mature with pale, often grooved nuclei	Sertoli cells often immature
Fibrothecomatous component common	Fibromatous component uncommon; mesenchyme often immature and cellular, or edematous
Steroid-type cells (lutein cells) usually not prominent and uncommonly clustered	Steroid-type cells (Leydig cells) tend to cluster; rarely contain crystals of Reinke
Heterologous elements absent	Heterologous elements in 20% of cases
Retiform elements absent	Retiform elements in 15% of cases

tumors correlate with the degree of differentiation. In our series none of the well-differentiated tumors, 11% of those of intermediate differentiation, 59% of the poorly differentiated tumors, and 19% of those with heterologous elements were clinically malignant. The homologous component of the tumor was poorly differentiated in all eight clinically malignant tumors in the heterologous category, and in seven of these the heterologous elements included skeletal muscle, cartilage, or both.

Earlier studies in the literature failed to establish a relation between the degree of differentiation of Sertoli–Leydig cell tumors and their prognosis, but later investigations have supported the findings in our series. The only clinically malignant tumor in the series of Roth et al.[111] was poorly differentiated, and 4 of the 20 poorly differentiated tumors reported by Zaloudek and Norris[165] were malignant in contrast to only 1 of the 44 tumors of intermediate differentiation and none of the 7 well-differentiated tumors. In our series there also was evidence that the presence of a retiform pattern had an adverse effect on the prognosis; 25% of stage I tumors of intermediate differentiation with a retiform component were malignant as opposed to 10% of those with no retiform component.[162] It is noteworthy that the only stage III tumor of intermediate differentiation in our series had an almost completely retiform pattern, and we have seen an additional Sertoli–Leydig cell tumor with a predominantly retiform pattern that was stage III. Rupture also adversely affected the outcome of stage I tumors. Thirty percent of the tumors of intermediate differentiation that had ruptured were clinically malignant, in contrast to only 7% of those that were intact; in the poorly differentiated category 86% of the ruptured tumors were malignant compared with 45% of those that had not ruptured.

In contrast to granulosa cell tumors, which often recur many years after primary therapy, Sertoli–Leydig cell tumors typically reappear relatively early. Sixty-six percent of the malignant tumors in our series recurred within 1 year and only 6.6% recurred after 5 years. The recurrent tumor usually is confined to the pelvis and abdomen, but distant metastases to the lung, scalp, and supraclavicular lymph nodes have been reported. Three of the patients in our series had parenchymal liver metastases.

The treatment of a patient with Sertoli–Leydig cell tumor depends on her age, the stage of her tumor, the presence or absence of rupture, and the degree of differentiation. In young women the low frequency of bilaterality justifies the performance of a unilateral salpingo-oophorectomy if the tumor is stage IA and preservation of fertility is desired. More aggressive surgical therapy and adjuvant therapy are indicated for advanced-stage tumors. Adjuvant therapy also may be advisable for stage I tumors that are poorly differentiated, contain mesenchymal heterologous elements, or are ruptured tumors of intermediate differentiation. Radiation therapy, combination chemotherapy, or both seem to have been of benefit in occasional reported cases.[106,162]

Other Types of Sex Cord–Stromal Tumors

Gynandroblastoma

Gynandroblastoma, an extremely rare tumor,[5] has been greatly overdiagnosed. Because small foci of ovarian cell types often are encountered in well-sampled, otherwise typical Sertoli–Leydig cell tumors and conversely, testicular cell types are demonstrable focally in occasional granulosa–stromal cell tumors, the diagnosis of gynandroblastoma should

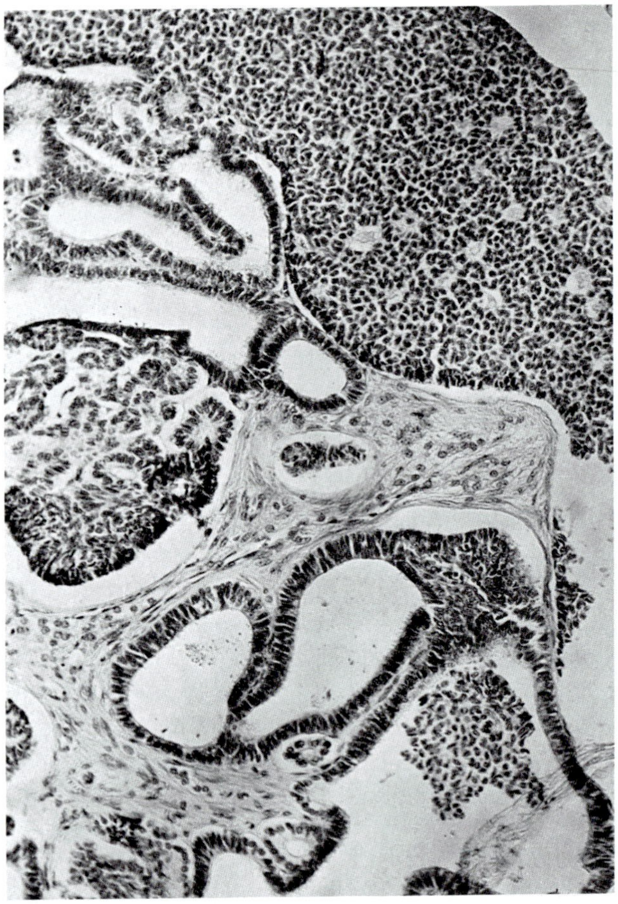

Fig. 19.61. Gynandroblastoma. (Reprinted by permission from Scully RE (1962) Androgenic lesions of the ovary. In: Grady HG, Smith DE (eds). The Ovary, International Academy of Pathology Monograph No. 3. Lippincott Williams & Wilkins, Baltimore.)

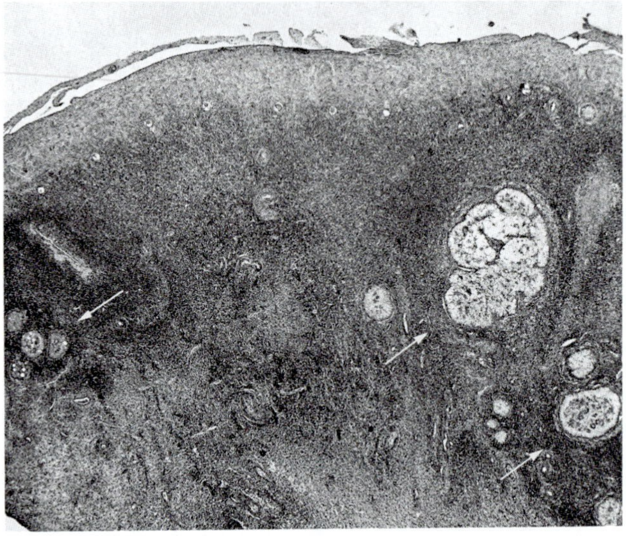

Fig. 19.62. Sex cord tumor with annular tubules. Multicentric foci are present within ovary from patient with Peutz–Jeghers syndrome. (Reprinted by permission of Scully, ref. 121.)

be restricted to the very rare tumors that contain significant components of both forms of neoplasia (Fig. 19.61). According to our criteria, the minor component should account for at least 10% of a tumor in the sex cord–stromal category to warrant a diagnosis of gynandroblastoma. The nature of the hormones secreted by a sex cord–stromal tumor should not, of course, determine its morphologic diagnosis in view of the proven capacity of tumors of testicular cell types to secrete estrogens and of those of ovarian cell types to produce androgens.

Sex Cord Tumor with Annular Tubules

The *sex cord tumor with annular tubules* (Figs. 19.62–19.65), has been established as a distinctive entity.[121,163] It is characterized basically by the presence of simple and complex annular tubules (Figs. 19.63 and 19.65). The simple tubules have the shape

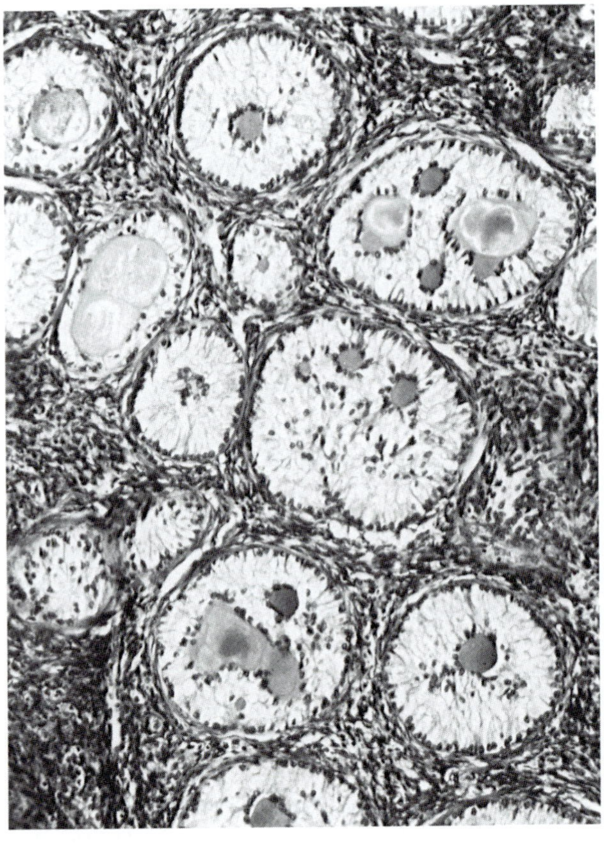

Fig. 19.63. Sex cord tumor with annular tubules. Simple and complex annular tubules encircle hyaline material.

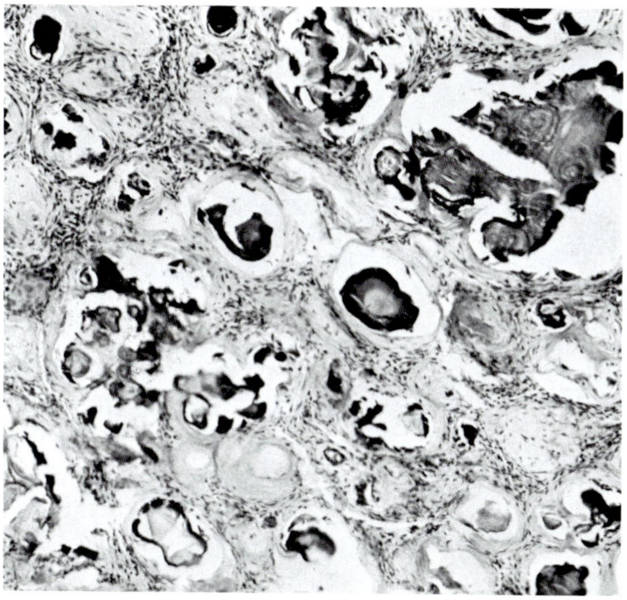

Fig. 19.64. Sex cord tumor with annular tubules. Extensive calcification of the epithelial nests has occurred in this tumor from a patient with Peutz–Jeghers syndrome.

of a ring, with the nucleus oriented peripherally and around a central hyalinized body composed of basement membrane material; an intervening anuclear cytoplasmic zone forms the major component of the ring. The much more numerous complex tubules are rounded structures made up of intercommunicating rings revolving around multiple hyaline bodies. Tumors containing annular tubules have been interpreted as Sertoli cell tumors by some observers[137] and granulosa cell tumors by others,[53] but the pattern of growth has features intermediate between these two tumors and focal differentiation into both typical Sertoli cell tumor with elongated tubules and typical granulosa cell tumor with Call–Exner bodies is seen in some of the cases. Sertoli-type cells have been identified ultrastructurally by the demonstration of Charcot–Bottcher filament bundles (Fig. 19.66,[137] which are considered specific cytoplasmic inclusions of Sertoli cells. A study of small tumors of this type suggests an origin in the ovarian cortex from the granulosa cells of follicles. Other evidence of such an origin is the well-known tubular differentiation of follicles that occurs in the canine ovary and the occasional observation of tubular differentiation in graafian follicles during pregnancy.

Sex cord tumors with annular tubules vary both clinically and pathologically, depending on whether the patient has Puetz–Jeghers syndrome[163] (mucocutaneous melanin pigmentation, gastrointestinal hamartomatous polyposis, and occasionally carcinomas of the gastric intestinal tract and adenoma malignum of the cervix) (Table 19.8). Almost all female patients with this syndrome whose ovaries have been examined microscopically have had sex cord tumorlets with annular tubules, which have been multifocal (see Fig. 19.62) and bilateral in at least two-thirds of the cases; the largest reported lesion in a patient with this syndrome was 3 cm in diameter. Focal calcification has been seen in more than half the cases (see Fig. 19.64). In almost all the patients the lesions have been incidental findings in ovaries removed for other reasons. All the tumorlets associated with Peutz–Jeghers syndrome have been benign, warranting conservative treatment.

In patients without Peutz–Jeghers syndrome (see Fig. 19.65), in contrast, the tumors are almost always unilateral and usually form palpable masses. Transitions to typical granulosa cell tumor are much more common than in tumorlets associated with Peutz–Jeghers syndrome. Forty percent of the patients have had manifestations of estrogen secretion; progesterone secretion, as evidenced by a decidual change of the endometrium, is relatively common. At least one-fifth of the tumors have been clinically malignant, with a characteristic spread via the

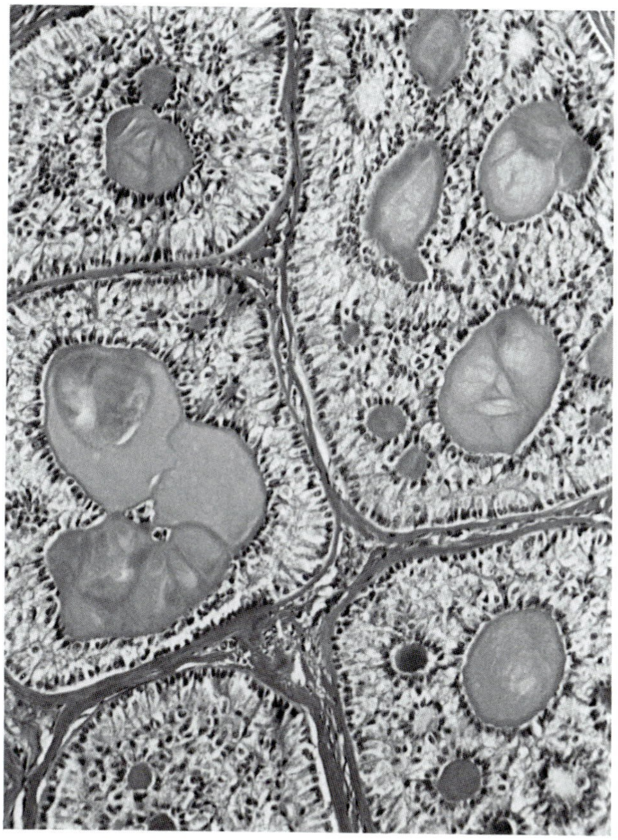

Fig. 19.65. Sex cord tumor with annular tubules. There was no evidence of Peutz–Jeghers syndrome in the patient with this neoplasm.

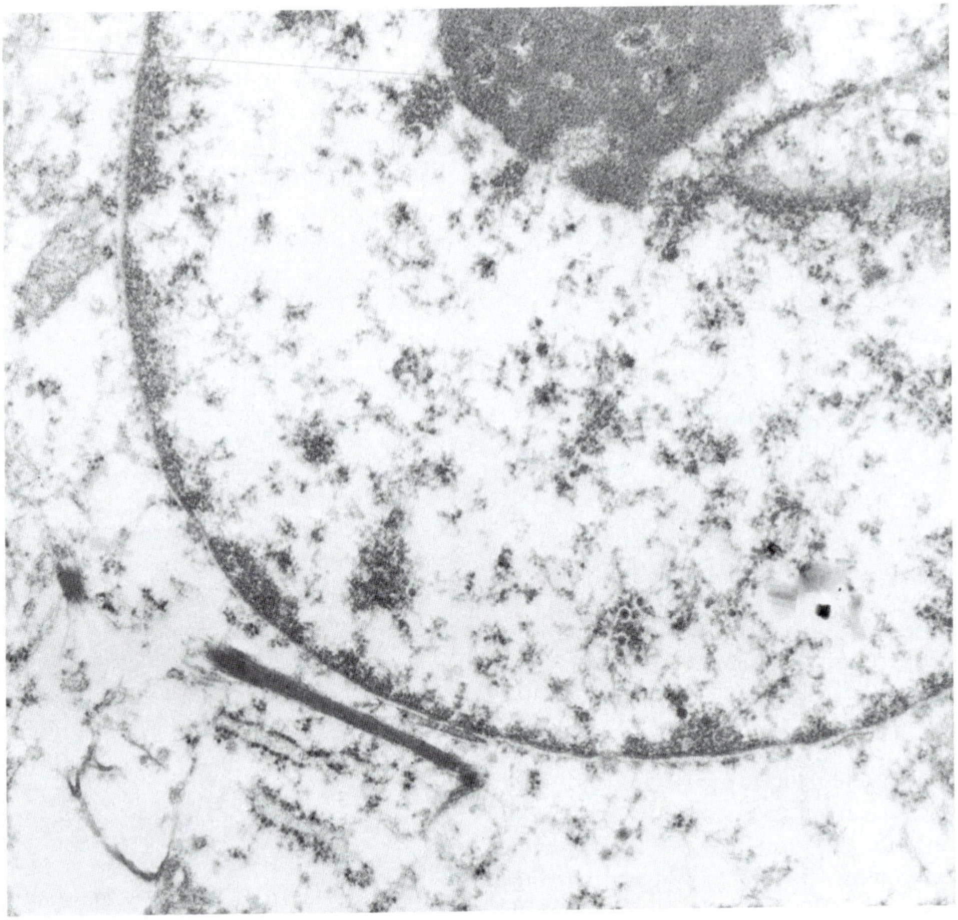

Fig. 19.66. Charcot–Bottcher filament in characteristic paranuclear location. ×27,300. (Reprinted by permission of Tavassoli and Norris, ref. 137.)

lymphatic system. Recurrences often are late. In one remarkable case multiple recurrences occurred, mostly within regional and distal lymph nodes, over a period of 24 years, with each recurrent tumor removed surgically. In that case the tumor produced large amounts of müllerian-inhibiting substance as well as progesterone, both of which were found useful as tumor markers in the serum in monitoring the course of the patient.[52]

Table 19.8. Sex cord tumor with annular tubules with and without Peutz–Jeghers syndrome

	With	*Without*
Bilateral	62%	5%
Grossly visible	27%	75%
Size	3 cm or less	Usually large
Multifocal	82%	6%
Calcification	62%	12%
Clinically malignant	0	20%[a]
Adenoma malignum cervix	15%	4%

[a]Only grossly visible tumors used in this evaluation.

Four other ovarian tumors from girls with Peutz–Jeghers syndrome have caused sexual precocity. Two of them, occurring in sisters, had the features of Sertoli cell tumors with lipid storage,[128] whereas the other two had microscopic findings that were unique in our experience, including diffuse areas, tubular differentiation, microcysts, and papillae, and the presence of two distinctive cell types, one containing abundant eosinophilic cytoplasm and the other scanty cytoplasm (Figs. 19.67 and 19.68).[149] All four tumors appeared to be clinically benign. The occurrence of these unusual neoplasms in association with Peutz–Jeghers syndrome suggested an association.

Sex Cord–Stromal Tumors, Unclassified

Sex cord–stromal tumors, unclassified, is a poorly defined group of tumors that accounts for less than 10% of those in the sex cord–stromal category. This group includes neoplasms in which a predominant

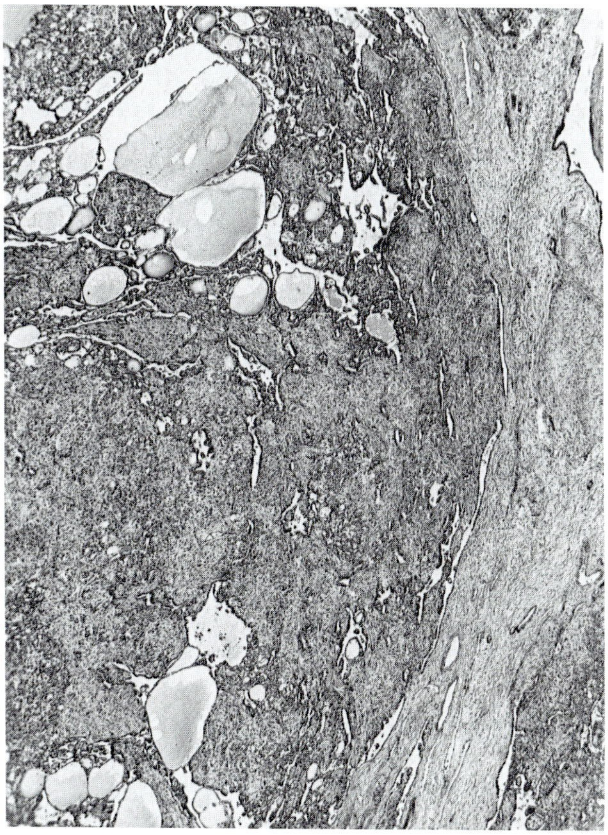

Fig. 19.67. Ovarian sex cord tumor from patient with sexual precocity and Peutz–Jeghers syndrome. Solid areas are interrupted by cysts of varying sizes. (Reprinted by permission of Young et al., ref. 149.)

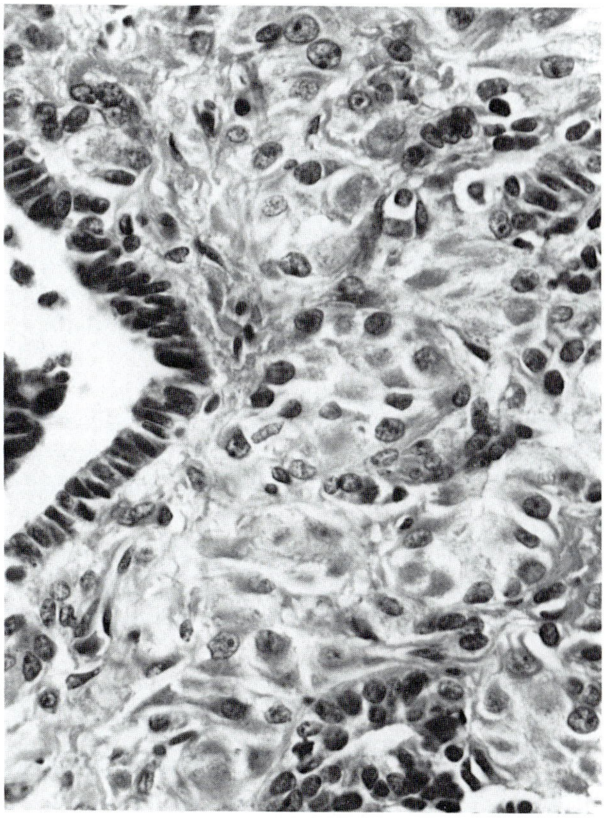

Fig. 19.68. Ovarian sex cord tumor from patient with sexual precocity and Peutz–Jeghers syndrome. Tubules are separated by cells with abundant cytoplasm and vesicular nuclei. (Reprinted by permission of Young et al., ref. 149.)

pattern of testicular or ovarian differentiation is not clearly recognizable. The boundary lines between these tumors and those of both ovarian and testicular cell types are vague because interpretations of intermediate patterns of growth and closely similar cell types inevitably are subjective.

Talerman and his associates[135] have described a group of sex cord–stromal tumors containing diffuse fibrothecomatous and/or granulosa celllike proliferation as well as areas of tubular differentiation in most of the cases. These authors have interpreted these tumors, which differ in appearance from usual forms of Sertoli–Leydig cell tumor, as diffuse nonlobular androblastomas, but in our opinion it is more appropriate to place them in the unclassified sex cord–stromal category.

Sex Cord–Stromal Tumors During Pregnancy

Sex cord–stromal tumors may be particularly difficult to subclassify when they occur in pregnant patients[151] because of alterations of their usual clinical and pathologic features. Their diagnosis is rarely suggested clinically because estrogenic manifestations are not recognizable during pregnancy, and androgenic manifestations are rare, possibly because of the ability of the placenta to aromatize androgens to estrogens. Indeed, virilization of a pregnant patient is much more likely to be caused by a nonneoplastic lesion such as the pregnancy luteoma or hyperreactio luteinalis or by a tumor with functioning stroma than a sex cord–stromal tumor. In one study, 17% of 36 sex cord–stromal tumors that were removed during pregnancy were placed in the unclassified group, and many of those which were classified in the granulosa cell or Sertoli–Leydig cell category had large areas with an indifferent appearance.[151] The features that led to difficulty in classification were the presence of prominent intercellular edema, increased luteinization in the granulosa cell tumors, and marked degrees of Leydig cell maturation in one-third of the Sertoli–Leydig cell tumors. All these changes, which were most common in tumors removed during the third trimester, tended to obscure the underlying architecture. The behavior of sex cord–stromal tumors during pregnancy appeared to be similar to that of tumors of similar type unassociated with pregnancy on the basis of limited follow-up of the 36 cases.

Immunohistochemistry of Sex Cord–Stromal Tumors

Kurman and his associates[70–72] have demonstrated immunohistochemically a variety of steroid hormones, including estrogens, androgens, and progesterone in the granulosa, theca, Sertoli, and Leydig cells of sex cord–stromal tumors. It is not clear, however, whether their presence reflects secretion or binding of these hormones to cellular receptors. Sasano and others[117,118] have used antibodies to demonstrate immunohistochemically many of the enzymes that are involved in the conversion of cholesterol to various steroid hormones, helping to pinpoint their site of origin in the cells of sex cord–stromal tumors.

Immunohistochemical techniques occasionally are of help in the differential diagnosis of sex cord–stromal tumors, particularly in their distinction from epithelial–stromal cancers.[2,31,109] Although both granulosa cells and Sertoli cells initially were thought to be positive for vimentin and negative for keratin, it has since been demonstrated that both cell types in neoplasms are commonly positive for various cytokeratins. Epithelial membrane antigen, however, can be demonstrated in the great majority of the epithelial cancers, but it has not been shown to be stainable in granulosa cell tumors and is present immunohistochemically in only rare cells in Sertoli–stromal cell tumors.[2] Cytokeratin 7 is usually positive in surface epithelial carcinomas and negative in sex cord–stromal tumors.[51] S-100 protein can be demonstrated immunohistochemically in approximately one-third of both adult and juvenile granulosa cell tumors but has not yet been demonstrated in the small number of Sertoli–stromal cell tumors studied.[2]

The most recently intensively studied marker in this area of investigation is inhibin.[29,44,65,77,109,110,132,168] Inhibin has been found to be typically immunoreactive in sex cord–stromal tumors of diverse types and is typically negative, or at most weakly positive, in tumors that are not sex cord–stromal tumors. Accordingly, it can play an important role in confirming or, in some cases, establishing the diagnosis of a tumor of sex cord-stromal type. A combination of positive staining for inhibin and negative staining for epithelial membrane antigen is particularly supportive of placement of a tumor in the sex cord–stromal category.[109] Positive staining for desmin may aid in establishing the diagnosis of an epithelioid smooth muscle tumor of the ovary, a rare lesion but one which may enter into the differential diagnosis of a sex cord tumor, particularly a granulosa cell tumor as mentioned earlier. Calretinin may stain Sertoli cells (personal observations) and is not reliable in distinguishing Sertoli tubules from mesothelial tubules

One sex cord tumor with annular tubules has been shown to be positive immunohistochemically for müllerian-inhibiting substance[52]; its presence has not been tested for as yet in other types of ovarian tumors.

The argyrophil cells of mucinous and carcinoid components of heterologous Sertoli–Leydig cell tumors have reacted for serotonin and one or more polypeptide hormones on immunohistochemical examination.[123] In one Sertoli–Leydig cell tumor associated with elevated levels of alpha-fetoprotein in the serum, immunohistochemical staining for this antigen was localized in cells resembling liver cells within the tumor[154]; in other cases, there was staining of the Sertoli–Leydig cell component of the neoplasm.[47]

Steroid Cell Tumors

The terms *lipid cell tumor* and *lipoid cell tumor* have been applied to ovarian neoplasms composed entirely of cells resembling typical steroid hormone-secreting cells, that is, lutein cells, Leydig cells, and adrenal cortical cells.[138] These terms are nonspecific and inaccurate, however, because as many as 25% of tumors in this category contain little or no lipid. Several years ago one of us proposed the term *steroid cell tumors* for these neoplasms, because it reflects both the morphologic features of the neoplastic cells and their propensity to secrete steroid hormones.[122] These tumors, which account for approximately 0.1% of ovarian tumors, have been subdivided into two subtypes according to their cell of origin and a third subtype whose specific cell lineage is unknown (Table 19.9). The features of the various subtypes of steroid cell tumors are contrasted in Table 19.10.

Stromal Luteoma

The *stromal luteoma* accounts for approximately 25% of steroid cell tumors. This designation is ap-

Table 19.9. Steroid cell tumors

Stromal luteoma
Leydig cell tumors
Hilus cell tumor
Leydig cell tumor, nonhilar type
Steroid cell tumor, not otherwise specified

Table 19.10. Clinical and pathologic features of steroid cell tumors

	Stromal luteoma	*C+ hilus cell tumor*	*C− hilus cell tumor*	*Steroid cell tumor nos*
No. of cases	25	12	9	63
Age range, years (mean)	28–74 (58)	32–75 (57)	34–82 (61)	2–80 (43)
Virilization/hirsutism	12%	83%	33%	52%
Estrogenic manifestations	60%	0	44%	8%
Duration of androgenic manifestations	1.5–5 years	2–20 years	1–24 years	0.5–30 years
Cushing's syndrome	0	0	0	6%
Diameter, cm (mean)	1.3	2.4	1.8	8.4
Stromal hyperthecosis	92%	42%	67%	23%

C, Reinke crystal; NOS, not otherwise specified.
From Paraskevas and Scully (1989), ref. 98.

plied to small steroid cell tumors that lie within the ovarian stroma (Fig. 19.69) and therefore are presumed to arise from it. Such an origin is supported by the capacity of the ovarian stroma to differentiate into lutein cells in the nonneoplastic disorder designated *stromal hyperthecosis*.[131] Adrenal rest cells and Leydig cells, the other possible sources of tumors of this type, on the other hand, have been identified within the ovarian stroma on only extremely rare occasions. The diagnosis of stromal luteoma is supported in approximately 90% of the cases by the finding of stromal hyperthecosis elsewhere in the same or contralateral ovary. In some cases of the latter disorders, the nests of lutein cells may form nodules (nodular hyperthecosis). The dividing line between a large hyperthecotic nodule and a stromal luteoma is arbitrary; we reserve the former designation for large nodular foci of microscopic size and the latter for nodules that are grossly visible.

Stromal luteomas are almost always less than 3 cm in diameter and, with rare exceptions, are unilateral.[55] They are well circumscribed, solid, and usually gray-white or yellow, but one-third of them have red or brown areas.

Microscopic examination of a stromal luteoma reveals a more or less rounded nodule of cells of lutein type that generally contain relatively little lipid. Intracytoplasmic lipochrome pigment may be conspicuous. The nuclei are small and round with a single prominent nucleolus. Mitoses generally are rare. The cells may be arranged diffusely or in small nests or cords and are more or less completely surrounded by ovarian stroma. One confusing feature, seen in about 20% of the cases, is focal degeneration, with the formation of irregular spaces that may simulate glands or vessels (Fig. 19.70). These spaces may contain, or be surrounded by, lipid-laden cells and chronic inflammatory cells and may be associated with fibrosis. In some cases they contain red blood cells. Some steroid cell tumors in the "not otherwise specified" category may be overgrown stromal luteomas, but the specific diagnosis cannot be made with certainty when the tumor is no longer confined to the ovarian stroma.

Eighty percent of stromal luteomas occur in

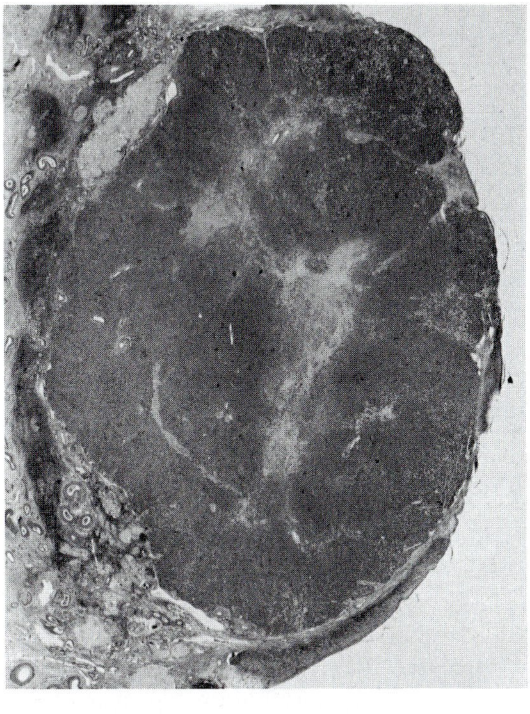

Fig. 19.69. Stromal luteoma. The tumor is partly surrounded by ovarian stroma.

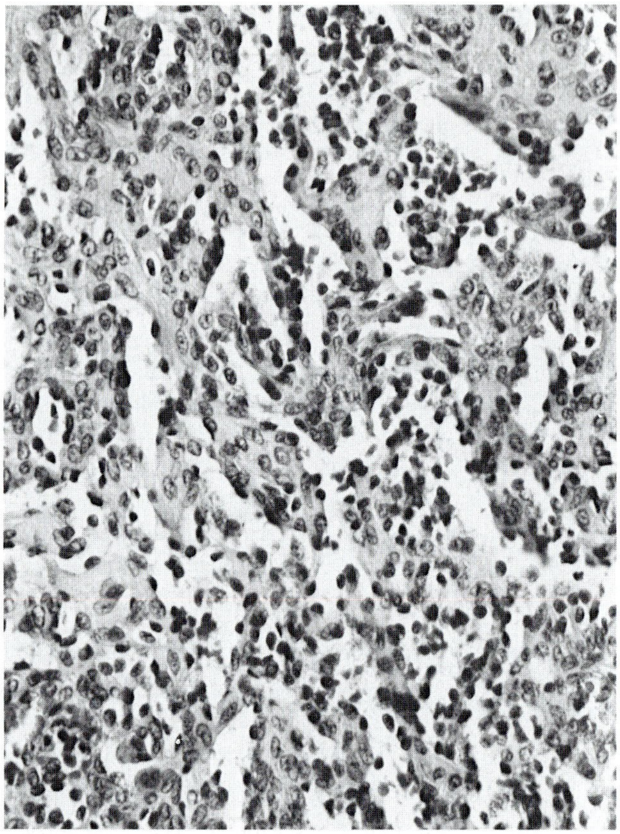

Fig. 19.70. Stromal luteoma. Degenerative changes have produced irregular spaces.

postmenopausal women.[55] The initial symptom in 60% of patients is abnormal vaginal bleeding probably related to hyperestrinism, although whether the tumor secretes estrogen directly or secretes an androgen that is converted peripherally to an estrogen is unknown. Androgenic manifestations are present in only 12% of the cases. This profile of hormonal function is the opposite of that associated with other categories of steroid cell tumor, which usually are androgenic and only occasionally estrogenic. Underlying stromal hyperthecosis may contribute to the clinical picture in some cases, particularly those in which there is a long history of hormonal disturbance. Stromal luteomas are benign.

Leydig Cell Tumors

A *Leydig cell nature of a steroid cell tumor* (Figs. 19.71–19.74) can be proved only by the identification of the more or less specific crystals of Reinke in the cytoplasm of the neoplastic cells on either light microscopic (Fig. 19.73) or electron microscopic (Fig. 19.74) examination. Because only 35%–40% of Leydig cell tumors of the testis contain crys-

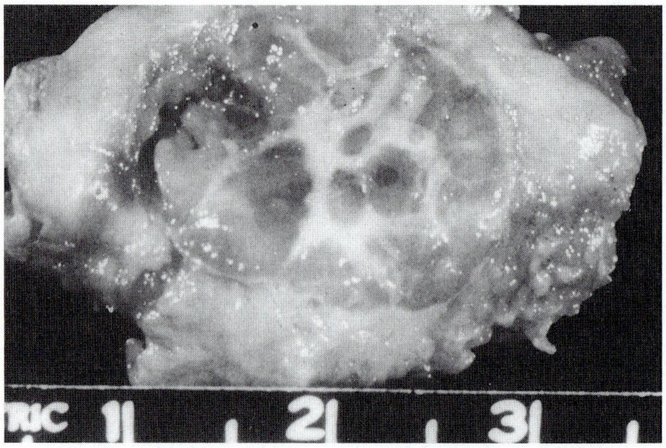

Fig. 19.71. Hilus cell tumor. A dark mass lobulated by septa occupies the center of the sectioned surface of the ovary. (Reprinted by permission of Scully RE (1979) Tumors of the Ovary and Maldeveloped Gonads. In: Atlas of Tumor Pathology, 2nd series, Fascicle No. 16, Armed Forces Institute of Pathology, Washington DC.)

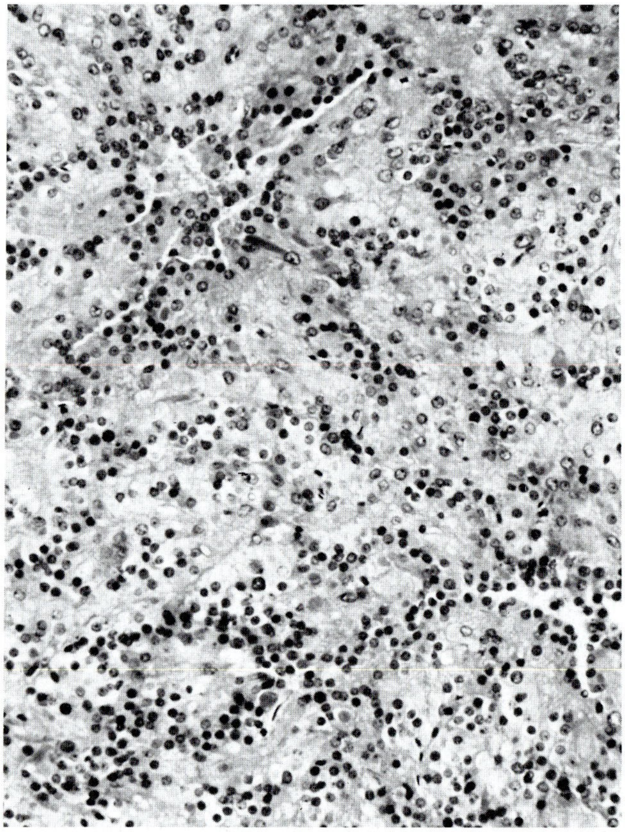

Fig. 19.72. Hilus cell tumor. (Reprinted by permission of Scully RE (1979) Tumors of the Ovary and Maldeveloped Gonads. In: Atlas of Tumor Pathology, 2nd series, Fascicle No. 16, Armed Forces Institute of Pathology, Washington DC.)

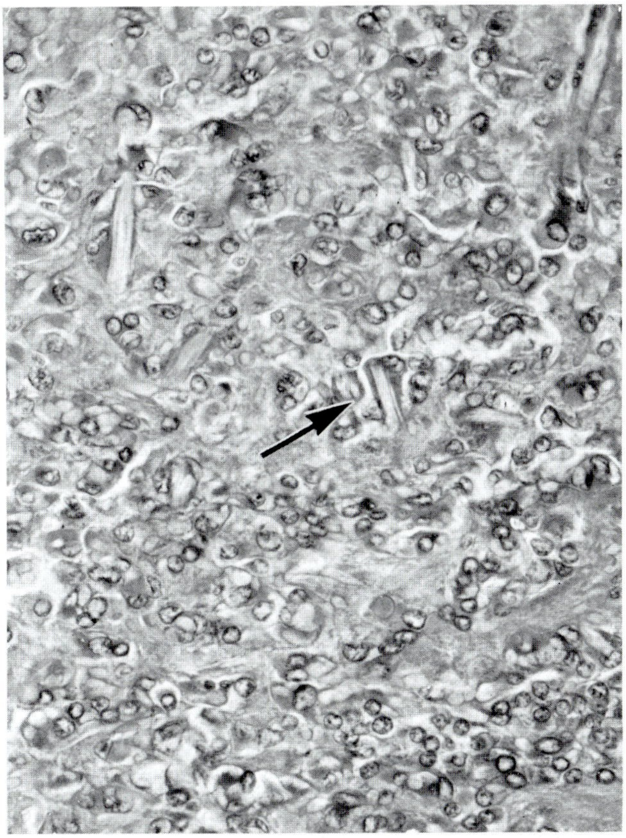

Fig. 19.73. **Hilus cell tumor.** *Arrow* points to crystals of Reinke (Reprinted by permission from Morris L McL, Scully RE (1958) Endocrine Pathology of the Ovary. Mosby, St. Louis.)

tals of Reinke on light microscopic examination and Leydig cells cannot be differentiated from lutein cells or adrenal cortical cells in the absence of these inclusions, it is probable that a number of unclassified steroid cell tumors are Leydig cell tumors that cannot be identified specifically as such.

Ovarian Leydig cell tumors have been divided into two subtypes by Roth and Sternberg,[113] the hilus cell tumor and the Leydig cell tumor, nonhilar type. The former, which are much more common, originate in the ovarian hilus from hilar Leydig cells, which have been identified in 80%–85% of adult ovaries, usually lying in relation to nonmedullated nerve fibers.[130] Hilus cell tumors, which account for approximately 20% of steroid cell tumors,[98] occur at an average age of 58 years and cause hirsutism or virilization in three-quarters of the cases; they are rarely associated with estrogenic manifestations. The androgenic changes typically have a less abrupt onset and are milder than those associated with Sertoli–Leydig cell tumors. They sometimes have been present for many years. The urinary 17-ketosteroid levels usually are normal or only slightly elevated because these tumors produce predominantly the potent androgen, testosterone, which is not a 17-ketosteroid, instead of the weaker androgens androstenedione and dehydroepiandrosterone, elevations of which are typically associated with high values of urinary 17-ketosteroids. Hilus cell tumors occasionally are palpable preoperatively. They are rarely bilateral.[32] There is no convincing example of malignant Leydig cell tumor in the literature.

Hilus cell tumors usually are reddish brown to yellow, are centered in the hilar region, and rarely are large (see Fig. 19.71) (mean diameter, 2.4 cm). Microscopic examination typically reveals a circumscribed mass of steroid cells with abundant eosinophilic cytoplasm and little intracellular lipid; cytoplasmic lipochrome pigment may be abundant. The cells usually are distributed diffusely but occasionally their nuclei cluster and are separated by nucleus-free eosinophilic zones (see Fig. 19.72); this pattern is highly suggestive of a hilus cell tumor even in the absence of crystals of Reinke. In some tumors

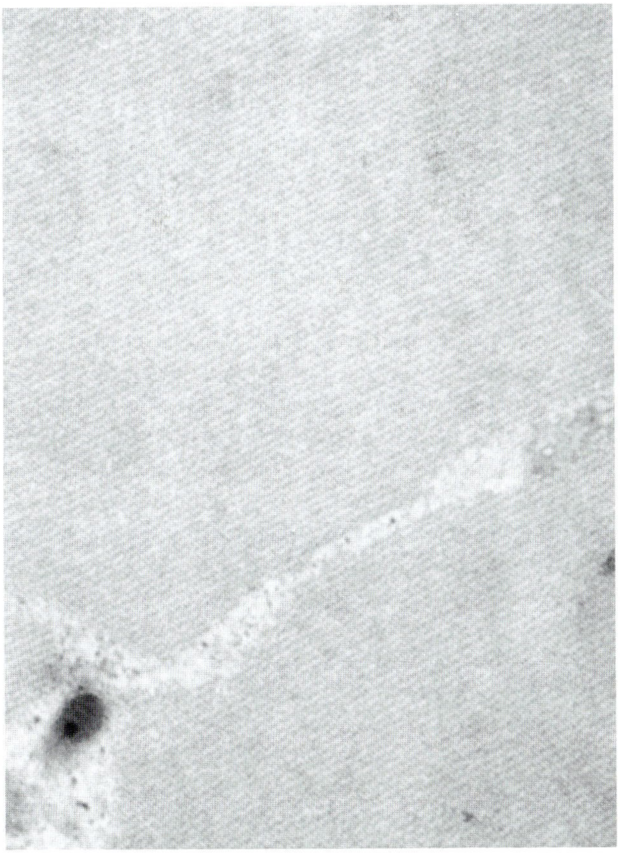

Fig. 19.74. **Hilus cell tumor.** Reinke crystal is composed of protein-containing, tightly apposed 300 Å wide hexagonal microtubular units. (Courtesy of Dr. A. Ferenczy, Montreal, Canada.)

the presence of a prominent fibrous stroma imparts a nodular appearance. An unusual feature in one-third of the cases is fibrinoid replacement of the walls of moderate-sized vessels unaccompanied by inflammatory cell infiltration.[98] Degenerative spaces similar to those seen in stromal luteomas may be present. The tumor cells typically contain abundant granular eosinophilic cytoplasm; occasional cells have spongy cytoplasm, indicating the presence of lipid. Cytoplasmic lipochrome pigment, which usually is sparse, is present in most cases. The typically round nuclei often are hyperchromatic and contain single small nucleoli, there may be slight to moderate variation in nuclear size and shape, and occasionally bizarre nuclei and multinucleated cells are encountered. Rare mitotic figures occasionally are present. Pseudoinclusions of cytoplasm into the nucleus may be seen. Elongated eosinophilic Reinke crystals of varying sizes are present in varying numbers in the cytoplasm (see Fig. 19.73) or sometimes in the nucleus, but often are found only after prolonged search.

The diagnosis of hilus cell tumor is favored if a crystal-free steroid cell tumor located in the hilus has a background of hilus cell hyperplasia, is associated with nonmedullated nerve fibers, has fibrinoid necrosis of blood vessel walls, or shows nuclear clustering with intervening nucleus-free zones. On electron microscopic examination, crystals of Reinke typically are needle shaped when cut longitudinally and hexagonal when cut in cross section (see Fig. 19.74). The interior of the crystal has a cross-hatched appearance. Intracytoplasmic eosinophilic spheres, which may be crystal precursors, also are typically present but are not specific for hilus cell tumors. Stromal hyperthecosis, hilus cell hyperplasia, or both are associated findings in occasional cases. The Leydig cell tumor of nonhilar type is thought to arise directly from ovarian stromal cells. Only four examples of this tumor have been reported[113] and, except for their location, their clinical and pathologic features have not differed from those of hilus cell tumors. An ovarian stromal cell derivation of these tumors is supported by the very rare finding of Leydig cells containing crystals in the steroid cell nests of ovaries that otherwise have the typical appearance of stromal hyperthecosis. In some cases in which a Leydig cell tumor is in equal contact with ovarian stroma and hilar stroma, it may be impossible to determine whether it is of the hilar or nonhilar type.

Steroid Cell Tumor, Not Otherwise Specified

Steroid cell tumors, not otherwise specified (NOS), which account for approximately 60% of steroid cell tumors, in all probability are large stromal luteomas or Leydig cell tumors but because they lack crystals of Reinke and their topographic features have been obliterated, they cannot be identified specifically as either type of tumor. These tumors occur at any age but typically at a younger age (mean, 43 years) than other types of steroid cell tumor, and in contrast to the latter occasionally occur before puberty.[54] Steroid cell tumors NOS are associated with androgenic changes, which may be of many years duration, in approximately half the cases, estrogenic changes including rare examples of isosexual pseudoprecocity in approximately 10% of the cases, and occasionally progestagenic changes. Five tumors have secreted cortisol and caused Cushing's syndrome,[122,160] and occasional others have been accompanied by elevated cortisol levels in the absence of clinical manifestations of the syndrome; one secreted aldosterone. Rare tumors have been associated with hypercalcemia, erythrocytosis, or ascites. The remaining cases have not been accompanied by endocrine or paraendocrine manifestations. Hormone studies performed in patients with androgenic changes, Cushing's syndrome, or both typically show elevated urinary levels of 17-ketosteroids and 17-hydroxycorticosteroids as well as increased serum levels of testosterone and androstenedione. The tumors that resulted in Cushing's syndrome were associated with elevated levels of free cortisol in the blood or urine.

Gross Findings

The tumors typically are solid and well circumscribed (Fig. 19.75), occasionally are lobulated, and have a mean diameter of 8.4 cm; only about 5% of

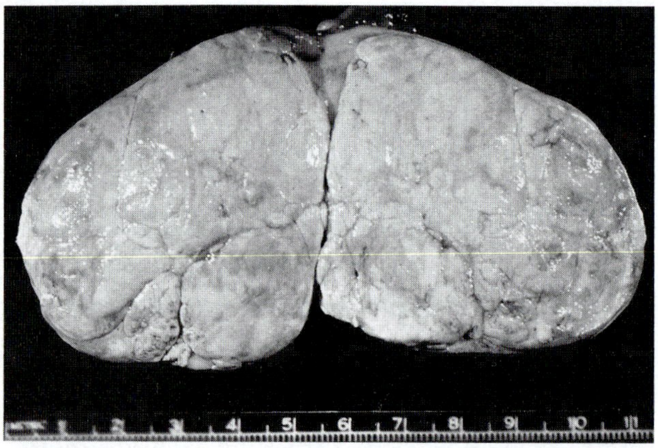

Fig. 19.75. Sertoid cell tumor, not otherwise specified. The sectioned surface of the tumor is uniformly solid and focally lobulated. The neoplasm was bright orange in the fresh state and was from a young girl who was virilized.

them are bilateral.[54] The sectioned surfaces typically are yellow or orange if large amounts of intracytoplasmic lipid are present, red to brown if the cells are lipid poor, or dark brown to black if large quantities of intracytoplasmic lipochrome pigment are present. Necrosis, hemorrhage, and cystic degeneration occasionally are observed.

Microscopic Findings

On microscopic examination, the cells typically are arranged diffusely (Fig. 19.76), but occasionally they grow in large aggregates, small nests (Fig. 19.77), irregular clusters, thin cords, or columns. The stroma is inconspicuous in most cases but in approximately 15% of them it is relatively prominent. A minor fibromatous component may be seen, indicating, as suggested by Hughesdon,[61] that steroid cell tumors may be completely luteinized thecomas. Rarely the stroma is edematous or myxoid, with tumor cells loosely dispersed within it and, exceptionally, it exhibits calcification and even psammoma body formation. Necrosis and hemorrhage may be prominent, particularly in tumors that have significant cytologic atypia.

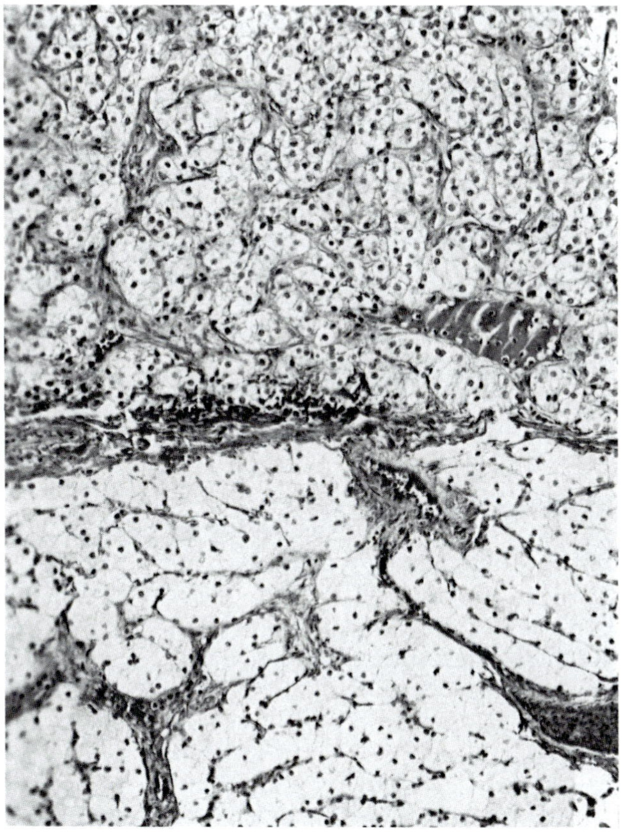

Fig. 19.76. Steroid cell tumor, not otherwise specified. Cells at the *bottom* have abundant pale cytoplasm whereas those at the *top* have less abundant cytoplasm. (Reprinted by permission of Young RH, Scully RE (1985). Ovarian sex cord-stromal and steroid cell tumors. In: Roth LM, Czernobilsky B (eds) Tumors and Tumor-like Conditions of the Ovary. Contemporary Issues in Surgical Pathology, Vol. 6. Churchill Livingstone, New York.)

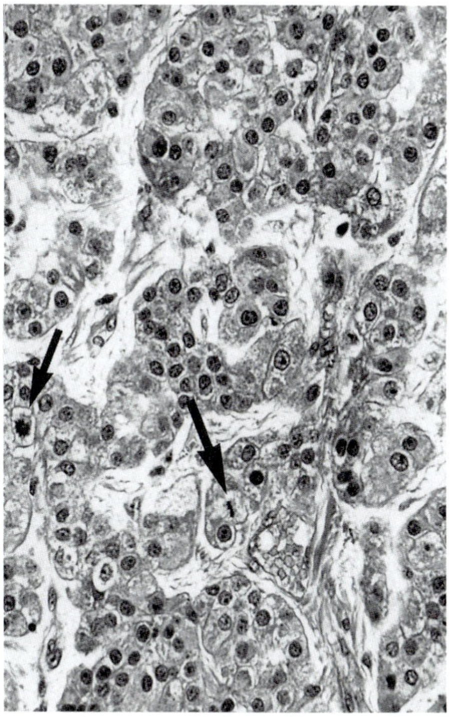

Fig. 19.77. Steroid cell tumor, not otherwise specified. This tumor, which was from a patient with Cushing's syndrome, exhibited prominent mitotic activity (*arrows*). (Reprinted by permission from Clement PB, Young RH, Scully RE (1991) Clinical syndromes associated with tumors of the female genital tract. Semin Diagn Pathol 8:204–233.)

The polygonal to rounded tumor cells have distinct cell borders, central nuclei, and moderate to abundant amounts of cytoplasm that varies from eosinophilic and granular (lipid free or lipid poor) to vacuolated and spongy (lipid rich) (see Figs. 19.76 and 19.77); lipid was present in 75% of the tumors in one series.[54] Steroid cell tumors NOS have lipid-rich cytoplasm more often than other subtypes of steroid cell tumor. Rarely, cells with large fat droplets have a signet-ring appearance. Intracytoplasmic lipochrome pigment has been found in 40% of the cases. In 60% of the cases in the largest published series, nuclear atypia was absent or slight, and mitotic activity was low (less than 2 MF/10 HPFs).[54] In the remaining cases, grade 1 to 3 nuclear atypia, usually associated with an increase in mitotic activity (up to 15 MFs/10 HPFs), was present (Fig. 19.77).

As already mentioned, tumors in this category are thought to arise from the ovarian stroma or hilus cells. The striking resemblance of many of these tumors to adrenal cortical tumors has suggested, however, the possibility that some of them arise from adrenal cortical rests, but such rests are extremely rare within the ovary. However, in a few patients with steroid cell tumors the responses of elevated levels of urinary 17-ketosteroids and 17-hydroxycorticosteroids to adrenocorticotropic hormone (ACTH) stimulation and dexamethasone suppression have been more suggestive of an origin from cells of adrenal cortical than gonadal type, but such responses are not diagnostic. The strongest evidence that rare steroid cell tumors arise from adrenal cortical rests is their association with Cushing's syndrome. Despite this, the confinement of these tumors to the ovary on gross and microscopic examination strongly supports an atypical production of adrenal cortical hormones by gonadal cells rather an ectopic adrenal cortical tumor.

Clinical Behavior and Treatment

In 20% of the cases, extraovarian spread of tumor is present at the time of operation; three of the patients with Cushing's disease (Fig. 19.77) had extensive intraabdominal spread of tumor.[160] In the two largest series in the literature, the proportion of tumors that were clinically malignant was 25% and 43%[54,138]; rare tumors have recurred as many as 19 years postoperatively. Patients with clinically malignant tumors were on average 16 years older than patients with benign tumors in one series; no malignant steroid cell tumors have been reported in patients in the first two decades.

The best pathologic correlates with malignant behavior in one series[54] were 2 or more MF/10 HPFs (92% malignant); necrosis (86% malignant); a diameter of (7 cm (78% malignant); hemorrhage (77% malignant); and grade 2 or 3 nuclear atypia (64% malignant); occasional tumors that appear cytologically benign, however, may be malignant. The metastatic tumor appears similar to the primary tumor in some cases but more poorly differentiated in others.

Differential Diagnosis of Steroid Cell Tumors

Stromal luteomas and Leydig cell tumors usually do not pose great diagnostic difficulty for the pathologist because of their characteristic locations and obvious composition of steroid-type cells, which contain crystals of Reinke in the Leydig cell tumor. The extensive formation of spaces in occasional tumors in these categories, however, may cause confusion with an adenocarcinoma and more often with a vascular tumor. Awareness of this degenerative phenomenon and its association with cellular debris, inflammatory cell infiltration, and fibrosis, as well as the finding of typical areas elsewhere in the specimen, particularly at the periphery, should facilitate the diagnosis.

Steroid cell tumors in the NOS category vary more widely in appearance than the stromal luteoma and Leydig cell tumor both architecturally and cytologically and are accordingly the cause of greater diagnostic difficulty. The tumors that may enter the differential diagnosis include extensively luteinized granulosa cell tumors and thecomas, lipid-rich Sertoli cell tumors, clear cell carcinomas, particularly those of the oxyphilic type, rare oxyphilic endometrioid carcinomas, hepatoid yolk sac tumors and hepatoid carcinomas, endocrine tumors such as oxyphilic struma ovarii, pituitary-type tumors and paragangliomas (pheochromocytoma), metastatic renal cell carcinomas, adrenocortical carcinomas, hepatocellular carcinomas, other metastatic tumors with oxyphilic appearance, and primary and metastatic melanomas.

The presence of characteristic nonluteinized cells in both luteinized granulosa cell tumors and thecomas, as well as the typical cytologic features and patterns of these neoplasms, and the finding of abundant reticulum in thecomas are of help in the identification of these tumors. The recognition of areas with a solid tubular pattern helps distinguish a usually estrogenic lipid-rich Sertoli cell tumor with a predominant diffuse pattern from a typically androgenic steroid cell tumor. In contrast to steroid cell tumors, the clear cells of clear cell carcinomas and metastatic renal cell carcinomas have glycogen-rich cytoplasm and eccentric nuclei. Also, the presence of tubular, glandular, and papillary patterns, which are inconsistent with a steroid cell tumor, generally facilitate the differential diagnosis. Radiologic studies to rule out a renal cell carcinoma may be additionally helpful.

Oxyphilic clear cell carcinomas and endometrioid carcinomas, and hepatoid yolk sac tumors and hepatoid carcinomas are all characterized by neoplastic cells with abundant eosinophilic cytoplasm. The first two tumors generally exhibit epithelial patterns, may contain glandular lumens, and are almost always accompanied by more easily recognized patterns. The oxyphilic clear cell carcinoma is almost always accompanied by a variable component of clear and hobnail cells not seen in steroid cell tumors. The hepatoid tumors also have epithelial patterns and may contain glandular lumens; they are characterized by immunohistochemical staining for alpha-fetoprotein. We are not aware of any cases of adrenocortical carcinoma that have presented in the form of a metastatic mass involving the ovary, but the possibility exists. Primary and metastatic melanomas can simulate steroid cell tumors if amelanotic, and if they are pigmented the pigment granules may be confused with the lipochrome granules of a steroid cell tumor. Melanomas generally have more malignant nuclear features than steroid cell tumors. Special staining, including staining for S-100 protein and HMB-45, may be helpful in difficult cases. An association with other teratomatous elements and the presence of colloid and immunohistochemical staining for thyroglobulin should enable one to distinguish an oxyphil struma from a steroid cell tumor NOS.

A rare pituitary-type tumor containing cells with abundant eosinophilic cytoplasm that arose in a wall of a dermoid cyst secreted ACTH and caused Cushing's syndrome.[9] Such a tumor might be confused with a steroid cell tumor. In that case, immunohistochemical staining for ACTH and several other pituitary hormones was positive. In one case we have seen of pheochromocytoma of the ovary, immunohistochemical staining of the tumor cells for chromogranin was helpful in establishing that diagnosis over steroid cell tumor. Electron microscopic examination of most of the neoplasms that simulate steroid cell tumors should disclose strikingly different features. Finally, the presence or absence of endocrine manifestations and their nature may be important clinical clues to the diagnosis.

Pregnancy luteomas, which are hyperplastic nodules composed of lutein cells that develop during pregnancy, may form large masses that resemble steroid cell tumors grossly and microscopically (see Chapter 16, Nonneoplastic Lesions of the Ovary). As with the latter, they also may be virilizing (in about one-quarter of the cases). Unlike steroid cell tumors, however, approximately one-third of pregnancy luteomas are bilateral and approximately one-half are multiple. Microscopic examination reveals masses of cells with abundant eosinophilic cytoplasm containing little or no lipid; mitotic figures may be numerous, sometimes up to 2 or 3/10 HPF. In contrast, a steroid cell tumor with minimal cytologic atypia that resembles a pregnancy luteoma usually contains only rare mitotic figures. Although it may be impossible to distinguish a lipid-poor or lipid-free steroid cell tumor from a solitary pregnancy luteoma, a lesion encountered during the third trimester of pregnancy is presumed to be a solitary pregnancy luteoma unless clear-cut evidence indicates otherwise.

Other Ovarian Tumors with Endocrine Function

Ovarian Tumors with Functioning Stroma

A wide variety of ovarian tumors other than those in the sex cord–stromal and steroid cell categories may be hormonally active as a result of steroid hormone production by stromal cells within or adjacent to the tumor (Figs 19.78–19.81). These tumors, which have been designated *ovarian tumors with functioning stroma*,[122] may be benign or malignant and, if in the latter category, primary or metastatic. Almost every ovarian tumor has been reported to be associated with steroid hormone production but, as discussed next, this phenomenon is seen much more often with some neoplasms than others.

Ovarian tumors with functioning stroma are associated infrequently with overt endocrine manifestations but commonly accompanied by subclinical elevations of steroid hormone values.[122] The stromal cells responsible for the hormone secretion in ovarian tumors with functioning stroma typically resemble lutein or Leydig cells and have been referred to as luteinized stromal cells. These cells almost al-

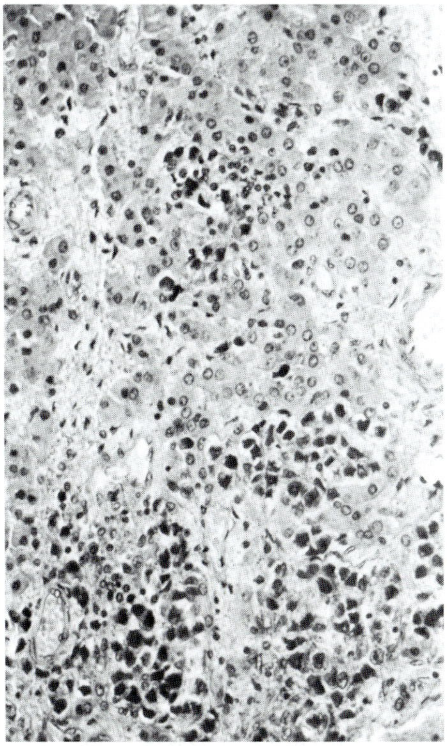

Fig. 19.78. Dysgerminoma with syncytiotrophoblast cells. Degenerating dysgerminoma cells are separated by steroid-type cells with pale nuclei and abundant dense cytoplasm in the peripheral portion of the tumor.

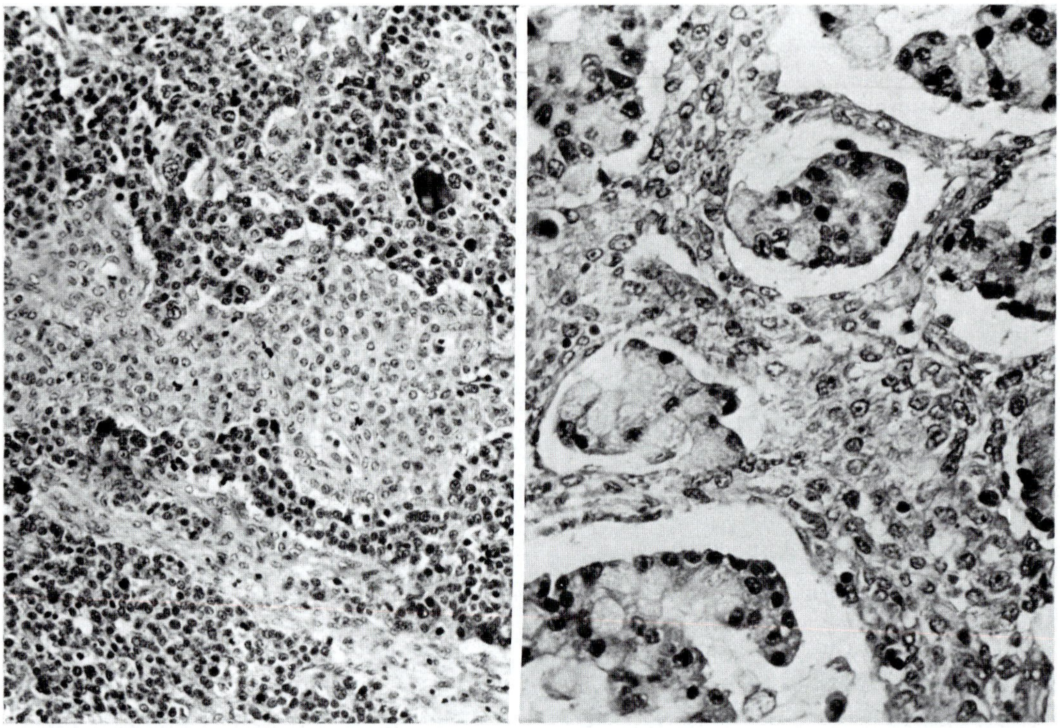

Fig. 19.79. Krukenberg tumor with luteinization of stroma. *Left*: Cords of carcinoma cells are separated by masses of luteinized cells. *Right*: Clusters of mucin-filled cells are separated by luteinized stromal cells. This tumor was associated with virilization and decidual change of the endometrium. (Reprinted by permission of Scully and Richardson, ref. 123.)

ways lie within the tumor singly, diffusely, or in clusters (Figs. 19.78–19.80), but rarely they are mainly distributed just outside the tumor, sometimes forming a peripheral band (Fig 19.81).[115] Exceptionally, crystals of Reinke can be identified in the lutein-like cells, warranting their interpretation as Leydig cells. It must be emphasized, however, that steroid-type cells may be prominent in the absence of clinical evidence of hormone overproduction and, conversely, evidence of function may exist in the absence of fully developed cells of steroid type. Ovarian tumors with functioning stroma can be divided into three major categories. In the first two categories, germ cell tumors that contain syncytiotrophoblast cells and tumors in pregnant patients, the luteinized stromal cells probably develop as a result of stimulation by hCG. The cause of the stromal alteration in the third (idiopathic) group, which accounts for most of the cases, is unclear, but ectopic production of hCG or some other stromal stimulant by the neoplastic cells may be responsible.

Germ Cell Tumors Containing Syncytiotrophoblast Cells

Two dysgerminomas with syncytiotrophoblast cells have been associated with luteinization of the stroma (Fig. 19.78) and endocrine manifestations; one was accompanied by isosexual precocity and the other by postpubertal virilization.[122,144]

Germ cell tumors that produce hCG, including *dysgerminomas with syncytiotrophoblast giant cells*,[166] *choriocarcinomas*, *embryonal carcinomas*, and *polyembryomas* and *mixed primitive germ cell tumors*, also may cause manifestations of steroid hormone secretion as a result of hCG stimulation of the ovary contralateral to the tumor to form luteinized follicles that secrete steroid hormones.[122]

Tumors with Functioning Stroma Occurring During Pregnancy

Although it is logical to speculate that ovarian tumors with functioning stroma in pregnant patients may secrete estrogens, this possibility has not been investigated by hormone assay, and clinical manifestations of estrogen excess are not expected to be present during gestation. In contrast, more than 20 examples of virilization caused by *ovarian tumors with functioning stroma during pregnancy* have been reported. These tumors were mostly Krukenberg tumors or mucinous cystic tumors, but a few have been Brenner tumors or isolated other tumor types. The onset of the virilization in these patients has

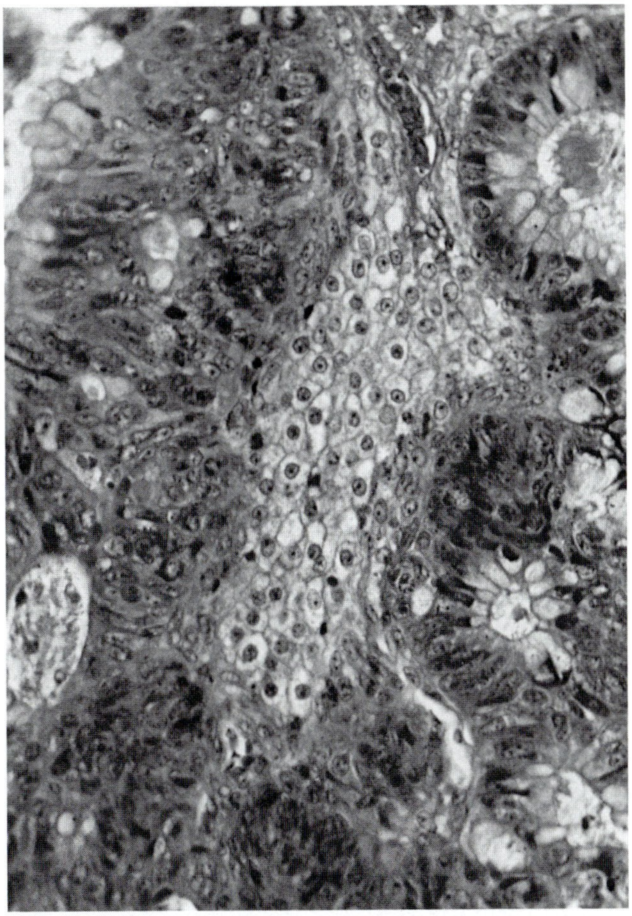

Fig. 19.80. **Metastatic adenocarcinoma from colon.** The neoplastic glands are separated by vacuolated luteinized stromal cells. (Reprinted by permission of Scully and Richardson, ref. 125.)

ranged from the third to the ninth month of gestation. Female offspring may be virilized.

Idiopathic Group

Although ovarian tumors with functioning stroma in the first two categories are encountered in young girls, patients with tumors in the *idiopathic group* usually are postmenopausal, reflecting the higher prevalence of ovarian tumors, both primary and metastatic, and possibly the higher levels of circulating luteinizing hormone in this age group. A wide variety of ovarian tumors has been associated with an idiopathic functioning stroma but its frequency has varied from one type of neoplasm to another.

Mucinous tumors often contain functioning stroma, occasionally resulting in either estrogenic or androgenic manifestations. Brenner tumors have been accompanied by endometrial hyperplasia in 10%–16% of the cases and occasionally are virilizing.[122] Rare cases of endometrioid carcinoma have

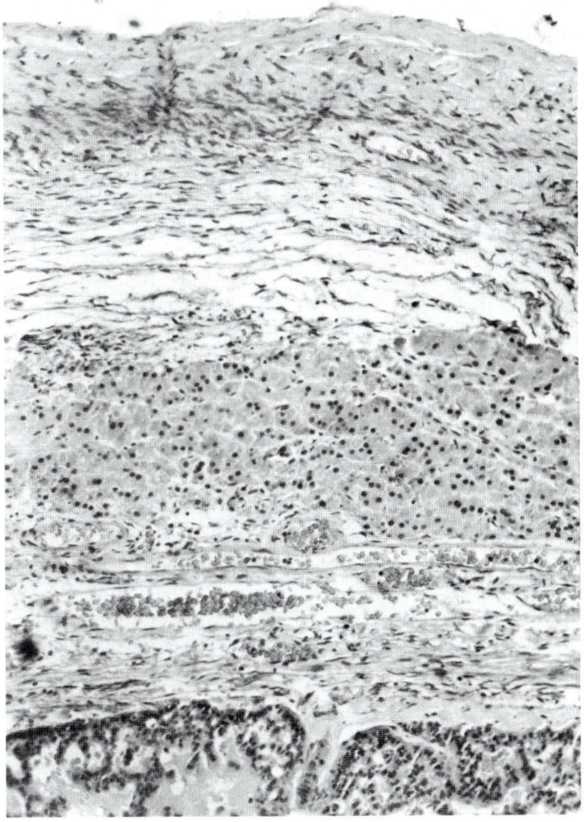

Fig. 19.81. **Strumal carcinoid.** There is a peripheral band of steroid-type cells.

been reported to be associated with endometrial hyperplasia in postmenopausal women, and in one case virilization and breast secretion developed.[122] We have seen a well-differentiated endometrioid carcinoma from a patient with an elevated serum testosterone level and the recent development of hirsutism. Serous and clear cell tumors have been accompanied only exceptionally by hormone manifestations. Germ cell tumors of various types lacking trophoblastic cells have been associated rarely with stromal luteinization and evidence of steroid hormone secretion in the absence of pregnancy. The germ cell tumors within the idiopathic category that have been accompanied by androgenic or estrogenic manifestations have included a variety of subtypes such as dermoid cyst, struma ovarii, carcinoid tumors, embryonal carcinoma, and yolk sac tumor. The steroid cells that are stimulated in cases of germ cell tumor are peripheral (see Fig. 19.81) rather than within the tumor in many, if not most, of the cases. The lesions associated with peripheral steroid cell formation in the series of Rutgers and Scully[115] describing this phenomenon were struma ovarii (nine cases), strumal or trabecular carcinoids (four cases), rete cysts (four cases), mucinous cystadenomas (three cases), dermoid cysts (two cases), and single examples of dysgerminoma with syncytiotrophoblast giant cells and metastatic carcinoid. In three of the cases, all strumas, a yellow color was appreciated grossly at the periphery or on the surface of the tumor.

The steroid cells that develop adjacent to ovarian tumors rather than within them are of three types: lutein cells within adjacent ovarian stroma, Leydig cells within ovarian stroma, and hilus cells, which are present only along the hilar border of the tumor. The number of cases in each of these three categories in the series of Rutgers and Scully[115] were 14, 2, and 8, respectively. The tumors with hilus cell hyperplasia were typically large with an average greatest diameter of 18 cm. The lutein cells and stromal Leydig cells were located predominantly or exclusively in the cortex or medulla peripheral to the tumor and were arranged singly and in nests forming a discontinuous band up to 2 mm in thickness. The hilus cells were arranged singly and in small nests forming discontinuous bands in the walls of the cysts in which they arose. Lutein cell formation is accompanied most often by estrogenic manifestations, whereas stromal Leydig cell formation and hilar Leydig cell hyperplasia are associated most often with androgenic changes.

Metastatic carcinomas that contain mucinous cells, such as primary mucinous tumors of the ovary, frequently are associated with luteinization of the stroma (see Figs. 19.79 and 19.80) and in a significant proportion of cases with clinical evidence of elevated steroid hormone levels. Scully and Richardson[125] found clinical evidence of excess estrogens as manifested by irregular premenopausal bleeding or postmenopausal bleeding in one-quarter of patients with metastatic adenocarcinoma from the large intestine and stomach. Occasional Krukenberg tumors from nonpregnant patients have been associated with virilization (see Fig. 19.77).[122] Other metastatic tumors are associated much less often with stromal luteinization. One postmenopausal woman was virilized as a result of luteinization caused by bilateral metastatic lobular carcinoma of the breast.[22] One metastatic colonic carcinoid was associated with peripheral stromal luteinization.[115] Finally, in one case of malignant lymphoma stromal luteinization was associated with secondary amenorrhea.[82]

Ovarian Tumors with Thyroid Hyperfunction

Although strumas and strumal carcinoids of the ovary have been demonstrated by immunohistochemical staining to contain thyroglobulin, triiodothyronine, and thyroxine and, therefore, probably produce thyroid hormones at subclinical levels in many cases, clinical evidence suggestive of *hyperthyroidism* is present in only 25% of the cases, and florid thyrotoxicosis in only about 5%. Factors that make it difficult to determine accurately the frequency of hyperthyroidism in patients with struma ovarii include variable criteria for the amount of thyroid tissue required for a diagnosis of struma, the observation that approximately one-sixth of patients with struma ovarii have concomitant enlargement of the thyroid gland, and a lack of confirmation of the hyperthyroidism by modern laboratory tests in most of the reported cases.

In some patients with clinical or laboratory evidence of hyperthyroidism, the preoperative diagnosis of hyperfunctioning struma ovarii has been established by high iodine uptake in the pelvis with low radioiodine uptake in the neck.[19] Other cases of struma-associated hyperthyroidism have not been recognized until the symptoms regressed after removal of an ovarian tumor. In some of these cases, a prior thyroidectomy had had no effect on the hyperthyroidism. Occasionally, oophorectomy for struma may precipitate compensatory enlargement of the thyroid gland, increased uptake of radioactive iodine by the thyroid gland, or an episode of thyrotoxicosis. Similarly, torsion of an ovary containing a struma precipitated striking hyperthyroxinemia in a pregnant patient.[122] Occasional strumal carcinoids (see Chapter 20, Germ Cell Tumors of the Ovary) have been accompanied by evidence of hypersecretion of thyroid hormone in the form of postoperative thyroid storm or hypothyroidism, and thyroglobulin has been demonstrated in the colloid within tumors of this type.

Ovarian Tumors Associated with the Carcinoid Syndrome

Of the four major categories of primary carcinoid tumor of the ovary (see Chapter 20), insular, trabecular, strumal, and mucinous, one-third of the insular tumors and a single example of strumal carcinoid have been associated with the *carcinoid syndrome*.[122] One patient with the syndrome also had elevated serum levels of calcitonin.[126] Metastatic carcinoids involving the ovary are associated with the carcinoid syndrome in almost half the cases. The volume of the carcinoid is an important factor determining the presence or absence of the syndrome in cases of primary carcinoids. The syndrome is present in about two-thirds of the cases when the tumor is large.[122] One 74-year-old woman had the carcinoid syndrome attributable to an ovarian tumor that resembled an atypical carcinoid with areas of neuroendocrine (oat cell) carcinoma.[18] That patient also was virilized and had Cushing's syndrome. Although no immunohistochemical staining was performed, the authors concluded that the tumor was elaborating both serotonin and ACTH. The carcinoid syndrome typically occurs in the absence of hepatic or other metastases in cases of ovarian carcinoid, because the hormonal effluent of the tumor enters the systemic circulation directly, bypassing the portal venous system and avoiding inactivation in the liver. The carcinoid syndrome caused by a primary ovarian carcinoid, therefore, is usually curable if the tumor is confined to the ovary and irreversible damage to cardiac valves has not occurred.

Ovarian Tumors Associated with Zollinger–Ellison Syndrome

Eleven mucinous tumors (two cystadenomas, five borderline tumors, and four cystadenocarcinomas) have caused the *Zollinger–Ellison syndrome* with disappearance of the syndrome after removal of the tumor.[17,48] Most of the tumors were large, with a mean diameter of 21.5 cm. Gastrin-containing cells were identified immunohistochemically within the cyst lining in all cases in which staining was performed (Fig. 19.82), and gastrin was demonstrated within the cyst fluid in about half of them.

The association between ovarian mucinous tumors and Zollinger–Ellison syndrome is consistent with the frequent finding of neuroendocrine intestinal-type cells within mucinous tumors. A number of studies have shown that all categories of mucinous tumors (benign, borderline, and malignant) commonly contain argyrophil and hormone-immunoreactive cells, although in most of the studies, these cells have been found most frequently in mucinous borderline tumors.[1] The argyrophilic cells often are immunoreactive for serotonin and a variety of polypeptide hormones. The most commonly identified of the latter have been corticotropin, gastrin, somatostatin, glucagon, secretion, and pancreatic polypeptide; in many cases, the tumors have been immunoreactive for multiple hormones.

Ovarian Tumors with Paraendocrine Disorders

A variety of *paraendocrine disorders* have been described in association with numerous types of ovarian tumor, some manifested by signs and symptoms of a well-known endocrine disease and others by subclinical laboratory abnormalities, indicating ectopic production of hormones or hormone-like substances by the tumor cells. In some of these cases the hormone being produced has been identified whereas in others, such as in cases of hypercal-

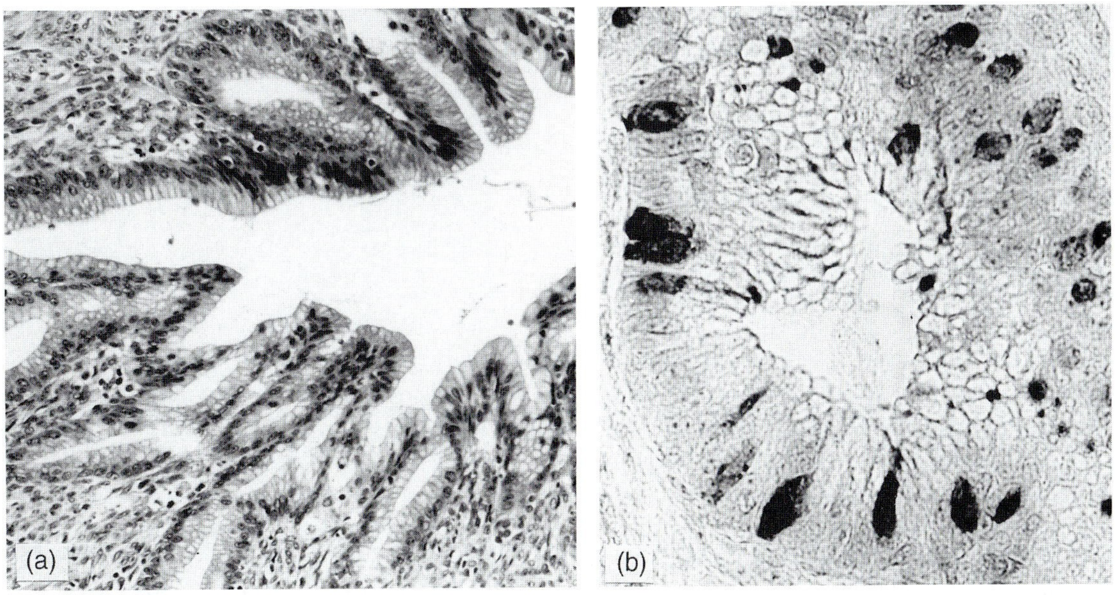

Fig. 19.82. Mucinous cystic tumor of borderline malignancy that was associated with the Zollinger–Ellison syndrome. *In the right panel* (*b*), some of the neoplastic cells are immunoreactive for gastrin. (Reprinted by permission from Clement PB, Young RH, Scully RE (1991) Clinical syndromes associated with tumors of the female genital tract. Semin Diagn Pathol 8:204–233.)

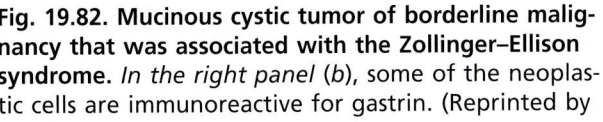

cemia, the mechanism of the disorder remains unclear. In all the cases included within this category of neoplasms, successful therapy of the tumor has led to disappearance of the paraendocrine state.

Hypercalcemia, Including Small Cell Carcinoma

Slightly more than 100 ovarian tumors have been reported to be associated with *paraendocrine hypercalcemia*.[153] The tumors have not been accompanied by recognizable clinical manifestations of hypercalcemia in most of the cases. About 60% of the tumors have been a distinctive type of small cell carcinoma; almost half the remainder have been clear cell carcinomas with serous carcinomas, squamous cell carcinoma arising in a dermoid cyst, dysgerminoma, and miscellaneous other neoplasms each accounting for about one quarter of the remainder.

The mechanism of the hypercalcemia associated with ovarian cancers is unknown. Attempts to demonstrate parathormone (PTH) within the tumor cells have been unsuccessful with rare exceptions, and in several cases in which PTH has been measured in the serum, the level was normal. Recent evidence has implicated PTH-related peptide (PTHRP) which has been elevated in the serum[56,142] or detected by radioimmunoassay in some cases[46]; three tumors (one a small cell carcinoma) were immunoreactive for PTHRP.[20,142] Because of the binding of PTHRP to a receptor common for PTH and PTHRP, the secretion of PTHRP by a neoplasm may produce the biochemical features of hyperparathyroidism. In one case the patient also had abnormally high serum concentrations of 1,25-dihydroxyvitamin D (1,25-DHD) and increased intestinal calcium absorption.[56] Tumor removal was followed by normalization of the serum calcium, PTHRP, and 1,25-DHD levels, suggesting an intestinal contribution to the maintenance of the hypercalcemia in this patient.

The small cell carcinoma of hypercalcemic type (see Figs. 19.72 and 19.73).is the most common form of undifferentiated carcinoma of the ovary in females under 40 years of age and has been accompanied by elevated levels of calcium in 66% of the cases in which it has been measured. The age of the patients has ranged from 14 months to 44 (average, 24) years. The presenting symptoms usually are abdominal pain and swelling.

At laparotomy almost all the tumors have been unilateral; spread beyond the ovary is usual. Gross examination reveals fleshy white to pale tan masses, often containing large areas of hemorrhage and necrosis (Fig. 19.83). The most common microscopic appearance is a diffuse arrangement of closely packed epithelial cells interrupted focally in most cases by distinctive follicle-like structures containing eosinophilic fluid (Fig. 19.84). The neoplastic cells typically have scanty cytoplasm and small nu-

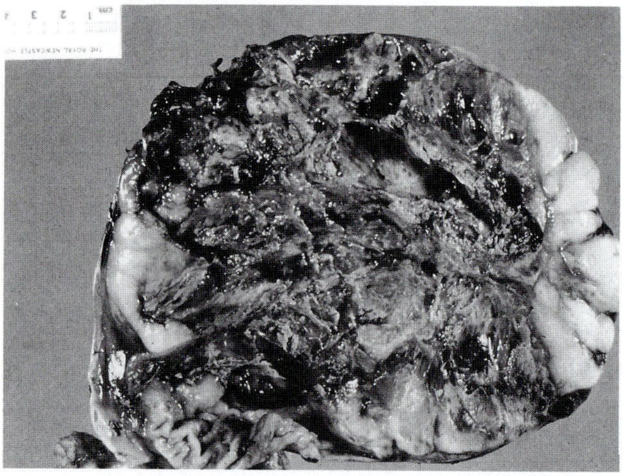

Fig. 19.83. Small cell carcinoma, hypercalcemic type. The sectioned surface of the neoplasm exhibits massive hemorrhage and necrosis. Viable lobulated tumor that was creamy white is still visible at the periphery.

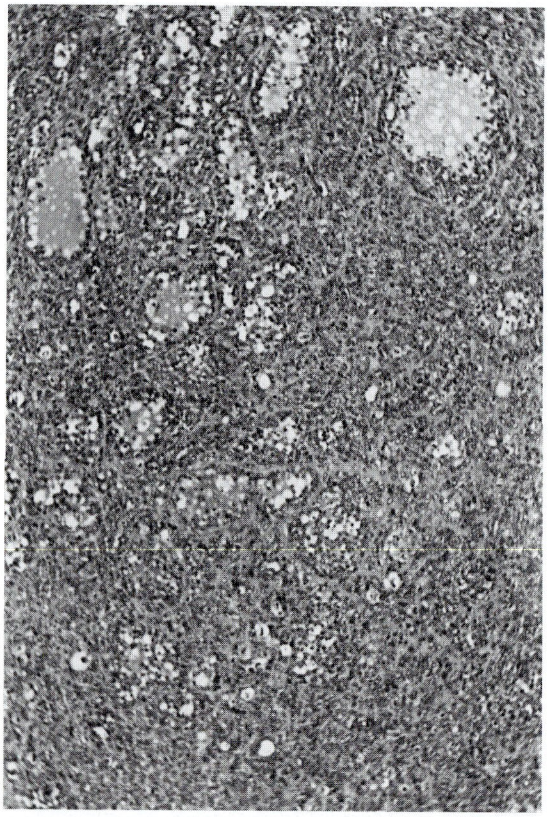

Fig. 19.84. Small cell carcinoma. Many small follicles are present within an otherwise densely cellular neoplasm.

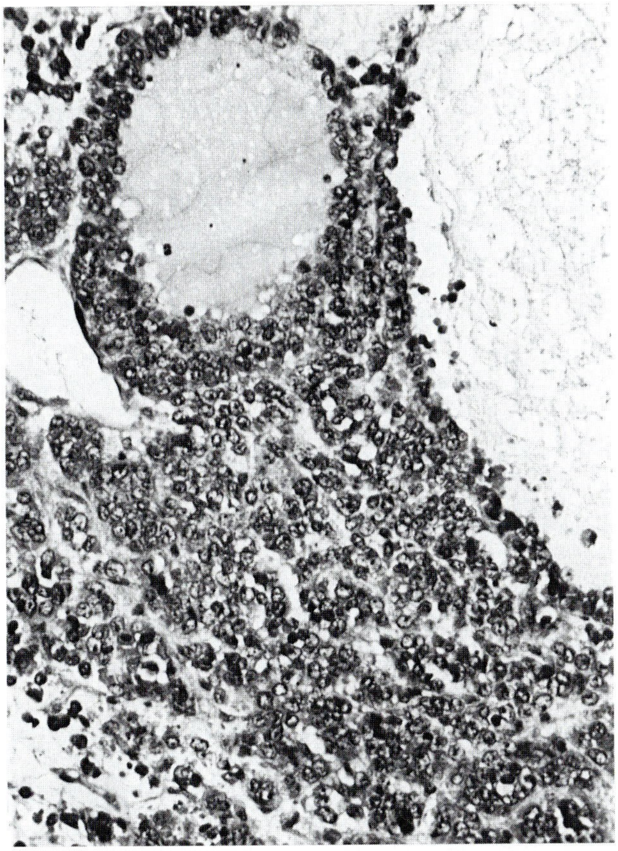

Fig. 19.85. **Small cell carcinoma.** Follicle-like structures lined by and surrounded by small cells with scanty cytoplasm and hyperchromatic nuclei.

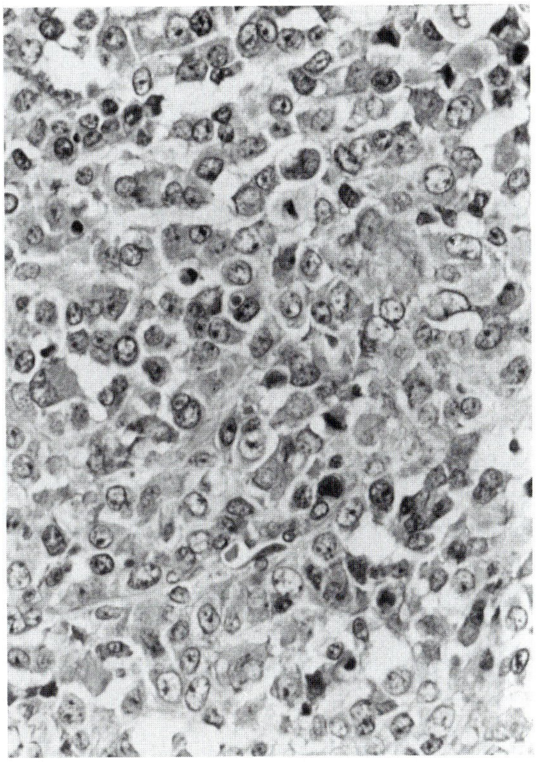

Fig. 19.86. **Small cell carcinoma.** Focal area is composed of large cells with abundant dense cytoplasm.

clei that typically contain single small nucleoli; mitotic figures are numerous (Fig. 19.85). The tumor cells also grow in nests, cords, and irregular groups. In many tumors large cells with abundant eosinophilic cytoplasm resembling lutein cells to varying extent have been present focally (Fig. 19.86); rarely, these cells predominate. In about 10% of the cases occasional glands lined by mature mucinous epithelium, signet cells, or highly atypical cells containing mucin are present. The stroma is generally relatively scanty and consists of nonspecific fibrous tissue.

Special staining and immunohistochemical[3] and ultrastructural[78] examination have not revealed any features that identify the specific cell type of this epithelial tumor; dense-core granules have been absent in most cases. Flow cytometry on paraffin-embedded material typically shows that the cells are diploid.[39] The age distribution and the characteristic presence of uniform small cells and follicle formation suggest a sex cord derivation, but transitions to recognizable forms of sex cord tumors have not been observed.

The small cell carcinoma often is confused with a granulosa cell tumor of either adult or juvenile type. The features of these three types of tumor are contrasted in Table 19.3 (earlier in this chapter). Diffuse small cell carcinomas also may resemble malignant lymphomas, particularly on low-power examination, but adequate sampling reveals patterns of growth that indicate the epithelial nature of the tumor; also, the cytologic features of the neoplastic cells are incompatible with any form of malignant lymphoma. Exceptionally, the differential diagnosis of a small cell carcinoma includes other small cell malignant tumors of the ovary, including several metastatic tumors such as metastatic melanoma and metastatic small cell sarcomas (see Chapter 22, Metastatic Tumors of the Ovary). The small cell carcinoma has a poor prognosis even when stage I, and no form of adjuvant therapy is of proven benefit.

Cushing's Syndrome

Five cases of clinically typical and biochemically documented *Cushing's syndrome* have been caused by cortisol production by a steroid cell tumor. Most of the tumors occurred in adults and had metastasized within the abdomen at the time of presentation and had atypical cytologic features. Rarely, primary ovarian tumors other than those of steroid cell type have been associated with Cushing's syndrome, probably in most cases on the basis of ectopic production of corticotropin or corticotropin-releasing factor.

These cases have included bilateral endometrioid adenocarcinoma,[33] a poorly differentiated adenocarcinoma,[99] a malignant Sertoli cell tumor,[88] a trabecular carcinoid (in which the tumor cells were immunoreactive for corticotropin),[122] and a tumor that resembled an atypical carcinoid and small cell carcinoma of the lung.[18] Finally, two cases have been described in which anterior pituitary tissue within a dermoid cyst caused Cushing's syndrome. In one of these cases, it was not clear whether the pituitary tissue was neoplastic or hyperplastic, but in the other case there was a chromophobe adenoma in which the neoplastic cells were immunoreactive for corticotropin.[27]

Human Chorionic Gonadotropin Secretion

Ectopic hCG production was reported by Civantos and Rywlin[25] in three women with serous papillary or mucinous adenocarcinomas of the ovary. All the patients had elevated urinary hCG level. Each tumor contained poorly differentiated areas with cells resembling syncytiotrophoblast cells; these cells were positive for hCG on immunofluorescence. In one case the contralateral ovary contained numerous lutein cells, and a decidual reaction was present in the endometrium; that patient had vaginal bleeding but no endocrine effects were present in the others. Oliva et al.[94] described two poorly differentiated surface epithelial carcinomas with a choriocarcinomatous component that occurred in patients with elevated serum hCG levels. The choriocarcinoma appeared grossly as a necrotic, hemorrhagic, circumscribed, brown nodule. Matias-Guiu and Prat[76] conducted the most extensive immunohistochemical investigation of hCG in ovarian tumors, using single polyclonal antibodies to the whole hormone and its beta subunit and four monoclonal antibodies to the whole hormone, its beta subunit, and two regions of the carboxyl terminal of the beta subunit. Correlating positive staining results with the presence or absence of an "active" stroma of the tumor (luteinization and/or "condensation"), these authors found that the epithelial cells of 41% of the tumors with active stroma reacted with the polyclonal antibodies and 62% with the monoclonal antibodies; the corresponding figures for the epithelial cells of the tumor with an inactive stroma were 14% and 37%, respectively.

Hypoglycemia

Six ovarian neoplasms have been associated with *hypoglycemia*: a serous cystadenocarcinoma, a dysgerminoma, a fibroma, a malignant schwannoma, a strumal carcinoid and a carcinoid tumor with a mixed insular and trabecular pattern.[8,84,122] In the case of the malignant schwannoma, insulin and proinsulin were recovered from the tumor tissue and the cells of the carcinoid tumor were immunoreactive for insulin. The patient with the insular-trabecular carcinoid tumor also had a parathyroid adenoma and pituitary hyperplasia.

Renin and Aldosterone Secretion

Three cases of hypertension related to hormone secretion by an ovarian tumor have been reported; two of the patients also had Gorlin's syndrome. In 8 cases, the hypertension was associated with a renin-secreting tumor, hyperreninism, and secondary hyperaldosteronism.[6,67] In 3 cases, an *aldosterone-secreting ovarian tumor* resulted in primary hyperaldosteronism associated with low or normal plasma renin levels.[63,69,140] Elevated aldosterone levels were present in a 12th case (but plasma renin levels were not measured),[122] and in the 13th case, reported in 1966, neither renin nor aldosterone levels were determined.[122] In 4 cases, the tumor also elaborated steroid hormones, as manifested by isosexual pseudoprecocity in 2 cases and elevated serum levels of estradiol and testosterone in 2.[122] Eight of the ovarian tumors were interpreted as sex cord–stromal tumors and 2 as steroid cell tumors. Three tumors in the first category were well-differentiated Sertoli cell tumors, whereas the other 4 had an appearance that was too nonspecific or poorly differentiated to subclassify. One of these last 4 tumors occurred in a woman with Peutz–Jeghers syndrome and was benign, whereas the other 3 were clinically malignant and 2 were fatal. One of the "steroid cell" tumors occurred in a 7-year-old girl and had a prominent follicular pattern, more in keeping with a diagnosis of JGCT. The final 2 tumors were a leiomyosarcoma and a mucinous adenocarcinoma. Immunohistochemical staining in 5 of the sex cord–stromal tumors and the leiomyosarcoma showed cells containing immunoreactive renin or prorenin.[122]

Prolactin Secretion

Two ovarian dermoid cysts have been associated with the elaboration of prolactin.[64,96] The patients were both in the reproductive age group. In one

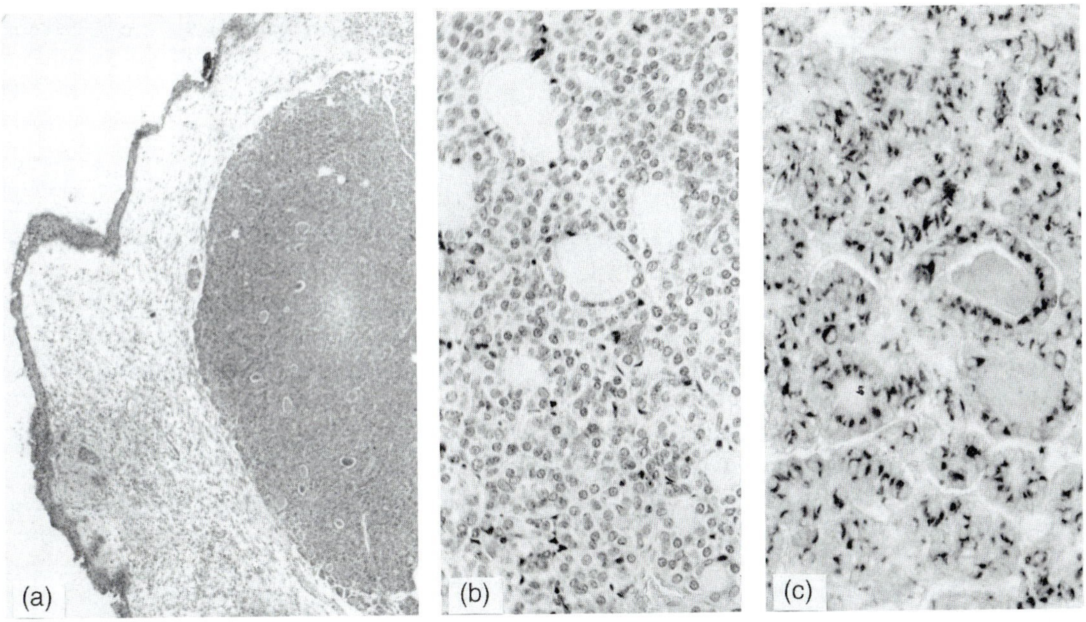

Fig. 19.87. Prolactinoma within ovarian dermoid cyst. **a**: A nodule of tumor is present beneath the squamous epithelial lining of the dermoid cyst. **b**: The tumor is composed of epithelial cells with scanty cytoplasm and small round uniform nuclei, some of which surround lumens filled with colloid-like material. **c**: Most of the tumor cells are strongly immunoreactive for prolactin. (Reprinted by permission from Clement PB, Young RH, Scully RE (1991) Clinical syndromes associated with tumors of the female genital tract. Semin Diagn Pathol 8:204–233.)

case, the dermoid cyst contained a 2.5-cm tumor composed of small rounded nests of epithelial cells, some of which surrounded lumens filled with colloid-like material (Fig. 19.87). The cells had scanty cytoplasm and small, round, uniform, mitotically inactive nuclei. Most of the tumor cells were strongly immunoreactive for prolactin (Fig. 19.87). In the other case, pathologic examination of an otherwise typical dermoid cyst disclosed a 1-mm focus of pituitary tissue composed of large polygonal cells with abundant eosinophilic cytoplasm that was immunoreactive for prolactin. In one patient with gonadoblastoma[57] a prolactin gradiant was present between the vein draining the tumor and peripheral veins, although the patient did not have hyperperlactonemia. Cells within the gonadoblastoma that resembled Sertoli cells were immunoreactive for prolactin.

Ovarian Tumors Associated with Paraneoplastic Syndromes

Nervous System Disorders

Ovarian cancer of surface epithelial type is one of the malignant tumors most often associated with *nervous system disorders*. The tumor is occasionally occult.[75] A variety of lesions affecting both the gray matter and white matter of the cerebrum, cerebellum, and spinal cord, the peripheral nerves, and the myoneural junction, accompanied by myasthenia gravis, may occur.[143] Paraneoplastic subacute cerebellar degeneration (SCD) is one of the most common lesions, with ovarian cancer accounting for from 16% to 47% of the cases.[101] The cerebellar manifestations usually antedate recognition of the cancer, and typically there is no improvement after removal of the tumor. In one case manifestations of the cerebellar degeneration partially regressed after plasmapheresis.[27] The pathogenesis of SCD in these cases appears to be related to the presence of circulating anti-Purkinje cell antibodies that have been shown to react with antigens in the tumor. The presence of such antibodies appears to be much more common in patients with SCD and gynecologic or breast cancer than in patients with SCD and other types of carcinoma. Limbic encephalitis and necrotizing myelopathy have also rarely been associated with ovarian carcinoma.[122]

Connective Tissue Disorders

The connective tissue disorder most commonly associated with ovarian cancer is *dermatomyositis*. In one study of 10 patients with dermatomyositis or polymyositis and a malignant tumor of the female genital tract, 5 had ovarian cancer.[145] The tumors are most commonly high-grade, high-stage serous carcinomas,[83] but there is 1 case of dysgerminoma and 1 of leiomyoma associated with dermatomyositis.[122] The onset of the dermatomyositis generally precedes recognition of the tumor, which usually becomes evident within 2 years. Medsger and his associates[79] described 6 patients with ovarian carcinoma in whom polyarthritis and palmar fasciitis preceded the diagnosis of carcinoma by 5–25 months. The arthritic symptoms were similar to those of rheumatoid arthritis. Four of the ovarian tumors were endometrioid carcinomas, 1 a serous carcinoma, and 1 an undifferentiated carcinoma. Occasional patients have had hypertrophic pulmonary osteoarthropathy, rheumatoid arthritis, scleroderma, systemic lupus erythematosus, or the shoulder–hand syndrome.

Cutaneous Disorders

Acanthosis nigricans occurs in some, typically young, women in association with polycystic ovary disease (POD), stromal hyperthecosis, or combinations thereof,[38] representing a component of the so-called HAIR-AN syndrome (hyperandrogenemia, insulin resistance, and acanthosis nigricans). Four cases of so-called malignant acanthosis nigricans have been cases of ovarian carcinoma.[122] The sign of Leser–Trelat, the sudden onset and rapid increase in size of numerous seborrheic keratoses in association with an occult cancer, considered by some a variant of "malignant" acanthosis nigricans, has been associated with ovarian cancer in one case.[58] Rarely, ovarian carcinomas have occurred in patients with the Torre–Muir syndrome or Sweet's syndrome.[87] Cutaneous melanosis has occurred with a strumal carcinoid[8]; the tumor cells were immunoreactive for alpha-melanocyte-stimulating hormone.

Nephrotic Syndrome

In cases of the *nephrotic syndrome*, 5%–10% have a paraneoplastic background, although the causative tumors in such cases are located only rarely in the female genital tract. Hoyt and Hamilton[59] described a 65-year-old woman who was found to have the nephrotic syndrome 8 months before the detection of a stage IV poorly differentiated serous carcinoma of the ovary. A renal biopsy showed membranous glomerulopathy. The proteinuria markedly diminished after debulking of the tumor, and after 10 months of combination chemotherapy the proteinuria had disappeared and there was no evidence of tumor at a second-look laparotomy.

Hematologic Disorders

Approximately 30 ovarian tumors have been reported to be associated with autoimmune hemolytic anemia, which is usually Coombs positive.[122] Most of these tumors have been dermoid cysts,[100] but occasional examples of carcinoma and a single case of granulosa cell tumor also have been reported.[122] In the last case, the patient also had splenic angiomas. In many cases corticosteroid therapy, splenectomy, or both have resulted in little or no improvement, but removal of the ovarian tumor has produced a rapid remission of the hemolytic disorder. Payne and coworkers[100] have listed several mechanisms proposed to explain the relation of the dermoid cyst to the anemia: (1) liberation by the tumor of a substance that alters the surface of red cells, making them antigenic to the host, (2) stimulation of production of an antibody that cross-reacts with the red cells by an antigen in the wall or lumen of the cyst, and (3) direct production of a red cell antibody by the tumor. Support for the last theory is provided by the finding of immunoglobulin in the cyst fluid in several cases.

Ovarian tumors are commonly associated with laboratory evidence of disseminated intravascular coagulation (DIC), but clinical manifestations of this disorder are uncommon. Ovarian tumors also have been associated with migratory thrombophlebitis (Trousseau's syndrome). Nonbacterial thrombotic endocarditis also has been recorded as a complication of ovarian cancer, as has microangiopathic hemolytic anemia.[122] Excluding cases of mild erythrocytosis that may accompany androgenic ovarian tumors, paraneoplastic erythrocytosis is associated only rarely with ovarian tumors.[122] Examples of erythropoetin-secreting ovarian tumors have included a dermoid cyst and a steroid cell tumor.[122] Other hematologic abnormalities that have been described rarely in association with ovarian tumors include nonthrombocytopenic purpura (mucinous cystadenoma), granulocytosis (clear cell carcinoma), thrombocytosis (serous carcinoma), thrombocytopenia (hemangioma, adenofibroma), and pancytopenia (granulosa cell tumor).[122]

Miscellaneous Rare Conditions

One ovarian example of *inappropriate antidiuresis syndrome* has been reported in association with a serous carcinoma that had a component of small cell carcinoma of pulmonary type.[136] Electron microscopic examination of the tumor disclosed neuroendocrine granules, and the neoplastic cells were also immunoreactive for antidiuretic hormone.

A small number of patients with ovarian tumors, usually with high-stage serous carcinomas but rarely with low-stage endometrioid carcinomas, have had hyperamylasemia.[95] Monitoring the serum amylase level may be a marker of tumor progression and response to therapy in such cases. Rarely, patients with ovarian cancer have had a clinical presentation that has mimicked that of acute pancreatitis.[92] In one unusual case a patient with pseudo-Meigs' syndrome had a pleural infusion rich in amylase that disappeared after removal of a serous tumor or borderline malignancy, which had ruptured preoperatively.[32] Six patients with poorly differentiated surface epithelial carcinomas[22a] have had uveal melanocytic lesions as may be seen with other visceral cancers. Microscopic examination of the eyes from these patients who undergo progressive blurring and loss of vision shows bilateral diffuse proliferation of melanocytes throughout the uvueal tracts with involvement of the sclerae in some instances.[22a,74] Rarely pyrexia is a presenting manifestation of a patient with ovarian carcinoma.[119] One of the two cases in this category was classified as a clear cell carcinoma, and the other was not classified as to specific cell type.

References

1. Aguirre P, Scully RE, Delellis RA (1986) Ovarian heterologous Sertoli–Leydig cell tumors with gastrointestinal-type epithelium. An immunohistochemical analysis. Arch Pathol Lab Med 110:528–533
2. Aguirre P, Thor AD, Scully RE (1989) Ovarian endometrioid carcinomas resembling sex cord-stromal tumors: an immunohistological study. Int J Gynecol Pathol 8:364–373
3. Aguirre P, Thor AD, Scully RE (1989) Ovarian small cell carcinoma: histogenetic considerations based on immunohistochemical and other findings. Am J Clin Pathol 92:140–149
4. Ahmed E, Young RH, Scully RE (1999) Adult granulosa cell tumor of the ovary with foci of hepatic cell differentiation. A report of four cases and comparison with two cases of granulosa cell tumor with Leydig cells. Am J Surg Pathol 23:1089–1093
5. Anderson MC, Rees DA (1975) Gynandroblastoma of the ovary. Br J Obstet Gynaecol 82:68–73
6. Anderson PW, Macaulay L, Do YS, et al (1989) Extrarenal renin-secreting tumors: Insights into hypertension and ovarian renin production. Medicine (Baltim) 68:257–268
7. Armstrong DT, Papkoff H (1976) Stimulation of aromatization by endogenous and exogenous androgens in ovaries of hypophysectomized rats in vivo by FSH. Endocrinology 99:1144–1151
8. Ashton MA (1995) Strumal carcinoid of the ovary associated with hyperinsulinemic hypoglycemia and cutaneous melanosis. Histopathology (Oxf) 27: 463–467
9. Axiotis CA, Lippes HA, Merino MJ, deLanerolle NC, Stewart AF, Kinder B (1987) Corticotroph cell pituitary adenoma within an ovarian teratoma. A new cause of Cushing's syndrome. Am J Surg Pathol 11: 218–224
10. Banner EA, Dockerty MB (1945) Theca cell tumors of the ovary. A clinical and pathological study of twenty-three cases (including thirteen new cases) with a review. Surg Gynecol Obstet 81:234–242
11. Benfield GFA, Tapper-Jones L, Stout TV (1982) Androblastoma and raised serum alpha-fetoprotein with familial multinodular goitre. Case report. Br J Obstet Gynaecol 89:323–326
12. Bjorkholm E (1980) Granulosa cell tumors: a comparison of survival in patients and matched controls. Am J Obstet Gynecol 138:329–331
13. Bjorkholm E, Pettersson F (1980) Granulosa-cell and theca-cell tumors. The clinical picture and long term outcome for the Radiumhemmet series. Acta Obstet Gynecol Scand 59:361–365
14. Bjorkholm E, Silfversward C (1981) Prognostic factors in granulosa cell tumors. Gynecol Oncol 11: 261–274
15. Bjorkholm E, Silfversward C (1980) Theca-cell tumors. Clinical features and prognosis. Acta Radiol Oncol Radiat Phys Biol 19:241–244
16. Bohm J, Roder-Weber M, Hofler H (1991) Bilateral stromal Leydig cell tumor of the ovary. Case report and literature review. Path Res Pract 187:348–352
17. Boixeda D, Roman AL, Pascasio JM, et al (1990) Zollinger-Ellison syndrome due to gastrin-secreting ovarian cystadenocarcinoma. Case report. Acta Chir Scand 156:409–410
18. Brown H, Lane M (1965) Cushing's and malignant carcinoid syndromes from ovarian neoplasm. Arch Intern Med 115:490–494
19. Brown WW, Shetty KR, Rosenfeld PS (1973) Hyperthyroidism due to struma ovarii: demonstration by radioiodine scan. Acta Endocrinol 73:266–272
20. Burton PBJ, Knight DE, Quirke P, et al (1990) Parathyroid hormone related peptide in ovarian carcinoma. J Clin Pathol 43:784
21. Callen JP (1986) Dermatomyositis and female malignancy. J Surg Oncol 32:121–124
22. Caron P, Roche H, Gorguet B, Martel P, Bennet A, Carton M (1990) Mammary ovarian metastases with stroma cell hyperplasia and postmenopausal virilization. Cancer (Phila) 66:1221–1224

22a. Chahud F, Young RH, Remulla JF, et al (2001) Bilateral diffuse uveal melanocytic proliferation associated with extraocular cancers. Am J Surg Pathol 25:212–218

23. Chalvardjian A, Scully RE (1973) Sclerosing stromal tumors of the ovary. Cancer (Phila) 31:664–670
24. Christman JE, Ballon SC (1990) Ovarian fibrosarcoma associated with Maffucci's syndrome. Gynecol Oncol 37:290–291
25. Civantos F, Rywlin AM (1972) Carcinomas with trophoblastic differentiation and secretion of chroionic gonadotrophins. Cancer (Phila) 29:789–798
26. Clement PB, Young RH, Hanna W, Scully RE (1994) Sclerosing peritonitis associated with luteinized thecomas of the ovary. A clinicopathological analysis of six cases. Am J Surg Pathol 18:1–13
27. Cocconi G, Ceci G, Juvarra G, et al (1985) Successful treatment of subacute cerebellar degeneration in ovarian carcinoma with plasmapheresis. A case report. Cancer (Phila) 56:2318–1320
28. Cohen PR, Kohn SR, Kurzrock R (1991) Association of sebaceous gland tumors and internal malignancy: the Muir-Torre syndrome. Am J Med 90: 606–613
29. Costa MJ, Ames PF, Walls J, Roth LM (1997) Inhibin immunohistochemistry applied to ovarian neoplasms: a novel, effective, diagnostic tool. Hum Pathol 281:247–254
30. Costa MJ, Morris R, DeRose PB, Cohen C (1993) Histologic and immunohistochemical evidence for considering ovarian myxoma as a variant of the thecoma-fibroma group of ovarian stromal tumors. Arch Pathol Lab Med 117:802–808
31. Costa MJ, Morris RJ, Wilson R, Judd R (1992) Utility of immunohistochemistry in distinguishing ovarian Sertoli-stromal cell tumors from carcinosarcomas. Hum Pathol 23:787–797
32. Cramer SF, Bruns DE (1979) Amylase-producing ovarian neoplasm with pseudo-Meigs' syndrome and elevated pleural amylase. Cancer (Phila) 44: 1715–1721
33. Crawford SM, Pyrah RD, Ismail SM (1994) Cushing's syndrome associated with recurrent endometrioid adenocarcinoma of the ovary. J Clin Pathol 47:766–768
34. Dickersin GR, Kline IW, Scully RE (1982) Small cell carcinoma of the ovary with hypercalcemia. A report of eleven cases. Cancer (Phila) 49:188–197
35. Dickersin GR, Young RH, Scully RE (1995) Signet-ring stromal and related tumors of the ovary. Ultrastruct Pathol 19:401–419
36. Dockerty MB, Masson JC (1944) Ovarian fibromas: A clinical and pathologic study of two hundred and eighty-three cases. Am J Obstet Gynecol 47:741–752
37. Dorrington JH, Moon YS, Armstrong DT (1975) Estradiol-17β biosynthesis in cultured granulosa cells from hypophysectomized immature rats: stimulation by FSH. Endocrinology 97:1328–1331
38. Dunaif A, Hoffman AR, Scully RE, et al (1985) Clinical, biochemical, and ovarian morphologic features in women with acanthosis nigricans and masculinization. Obstet Gynecol 66:545–552
39. Eichhorn JH, Bell DA, Young RH, et al (1992) DNA content and proliferative activity in ovarian small cell carcinomas of the hypercalcemic type. Implications for diagnosis, prognosis and histogenesis. Am J Clin Pathol 98:579–586
40. Fathalla MF (1967) The occurrence of granulosa and theca tumors in clinically normal ovaries. A study of 25 cases. J Obstet Gynaecol Br Commonw 74:279–282
41. Fathalla MF (1968) The role of the ovarian stroma in hormone production by ovarian tumors. J Obstet Gynaecol Br Commonw 75:78–83
42. Fathizadeh A, Medenica MM, Soltani K, et al (1982) Aggressive keratoacanthoma and internal malignant neoplasm. Arch Dermatol 118:112–114
43. Ferry JA, Young RH, Engel G, Scully RE (1994) Oxyphilic Sertoli cell tumor of the ovary: a report of three cases, two in patients with the Peutz-Jeghers syndrome. Int J Gynecol Pathol 13:259–266
44. Flemming P, Wellmann A, Maschek HJ et al (1995) Monoclonal antibodies against inhibin represents key markers of adult granulosa cell tumors of the ovary even in their metastases. Am J Surg Pathol 19:927–933
45. Fox H, Agrawal K, Langley FA (1975) A clinicopathological study of 92 cases of granulosa cell tumor of the ovary with special reference to the factors influencing prognosis. Cancer (Phila) 35:231–241
46. Fujino T, Watanabe T, Yamaguchi K, et al (1992) The development of hypercalcemia in a patient with an ovarian tumor producing parathyroid hormone-related protein. Cancer (Phila) 70:2845–2850
47. Gagnon S, Tetu B, Silva EG, McCaughey WTE (1989) Frequency of a-fetoprotein production by Sertoli-Leydig cell tumors of the ovary: an immunohistochemical study of eight cases. Mod Pathol 2: 63–67
48. Garcia-Villaneuva M, Figuerola NB, del Arbol LR, Ortiz MJH (1990) Zollinger–Ellison syndrome due to a borderline mucinous cystadenoma of the ovary. Obstet Gynecol 75:549–551
49. Geist SH, Gaines JA (1938) Theca cell tumors. Am J Obstet Gynecol 35:39–51
50. Gorlin RJ (1987) Nevoid basal-cell carcinoma syndrome. Medicine (Baltim) 66:98–113
51. Guerrieri C, Frånlund B, Malmström H, Boeryd B (1998) Ovarian endometrioid carcinomas simulating sex cord-stromal tumors: a study using inhibin and cytokeratin 7. Int J Gynecol Pathol 17:266–271
52. Gustafson ML, Lee MM, Scully RE, et al (1992) Müllerian inhibiting substance as a marker for ovarian sex-cord tumor. N Engl J Med 326:466–471
53. Hart WR, Kumar N, Crissman JD (1980) Ovarian neoplasms resembling sex cord tumors with annular tubules. Cancer (Phila) 45:2352–2363
54. Hayes MC, Scully RE (1987) Ovarian steroid cell

tumor (not otherwise specified): a clinicopathological analysis of 63 cases. Am J Surg Pathol 11:835–845
55. Hayes MC, Scully RE (1987) Stromal luteoma of the ovary: a clinico-pathological analysis of 25 cases. Int J Gynecol Pathol 6:313–321
56. Hoekman K, Tjandra Y, Papapoulos SE (1991) The role of 1,25-dihydroxyvitamin D in the maintenance of hypercalcemia in a patient with an ovarian carcinoma producing parathyroid hormone-related protein. Cancer (Phila) 68:642–647
57. Hoffman WH, Gala RR, Kovacs K, Subramanian MG (1987) Ectopic prolactin secretion from a gonadoblastoma. Cancer (Phila) 60:2690–2695
58. Holguin T, Padilla RS, Ampuero F (1986) Ovarian adenocarcinoma presenting with the sign of Leser–Trelat. Gynecol Oncol 25:128–132
59. Hoyt RE, Hamilton JF (1987) Ovarian cancer associated with the nephrotic syndrome. Obstet Gynecol 70:513–514
60. Hughesdon PE (1958) Thecal and allied reactions in epithelial ovarian tumours. J Obstet Gynaecol Br Commonw 65:702–709
61. Hughesdon PE (1983) Lipid cell thecomas of the ovary. Histopathology (Oxf) 7:681–692
62. Ismail SM, Walker SM (1990) Bilateral virilizing sclerosing stromal tumours of the ovary in a pregnant woman with Gorlin's syndrome: implications for pathogenesis of ovarian stromal neoplasms. Histopathology (Oxf) 17:159–163
63. Jackson B, Valentine R, Wagner G (1986) Primary aldosteronism due to a malignant ovarian tumour. Aust NZ J Med 16:69–71
64. Kallenberg GA, Pesce CM, Norman B, Ratner RE, Silverberg SG (1990) Ectopic hyperprolactinemia resulting from an ovarian teratoma. JAMA 263: 2472–2474
65. Kommoss F, Oliva E, Bhan AK, Young RH, Scully RE (1998) Inhibin expression in ovarian tumors and tumor-like lesions: an immunohistochemical study. Mod Pathol 11:656–664
66. Konishi I, Fujii S, Ishikawa Y, Suzuki A, Okamura H, Mori T (1986) Ovarian fibroma with Leydig cell hyperplasia of the adjacent stroma: a light and electron microscopic study. Int J Gynecol Pathol 5:170–178
67. Korzets A, Nouriel H, Steiner Z, et al (1986) Resistant hypertension associated with a renin-producing ovarian Sertoli cell tumor. Am J Clin Pathol 85:242–247
68. Kraemer BB, Silva EG, Sneige N (1984) Fibrosarcoma of the ovary. A new component in the nevoid basal-cell carcinoma syndrome. Am J Surg Pathol 8:231–236
69. Kulkarni JN, Mistry RC, Kamat MR, Chinoy R, Lotlikar RG (1990) Autonomous aldosterone-secreting ovarian tumor. Gynecol Oncol 37:284–289
70. Kurman RJ, Andrade D, Goebelsmann U, Taylor CR (1978) An immunohistochemical study of steroid localization in Sertoli–Leydig tumors of the ovary and testis. Cancer (Phila) 42:1772–1783
71. Kurman RJ, Ganjei P, Nadjii M (1984) Contributions of immunocytochemistry to the diagnosis and study of ovarian neoplasms. Int J Gynecol Pathol 3:3–26
72. Kurman RJ, Goebelsmann U, Taylor CR (1979) Steroid localization in granulosa–theca tumors of the ovary. Cancer (Phila) 43:2377–2384
73. Lack EE, Perez-Atayde AR, Murthy ASK, Goldstein DP, Crigler JF, Vawter GF (1981) Granulosa theca cell tumors in premenarchal girls. A clinical and pathologic study of ten cases. Cancer (Phila) 48: 1846–1854
74. Margo CE, Pavan PR, Gendelman D, Gragoudas E (1987) Bilateral melanocytic uveal tumors associated with systemic non-ocular malignancy. Malignant melanomas or benign paraneoplastic syndrome? Retina 7:137–141
75. Mason WP, Dalman J, Curtin MP, Posner JB (1997) Normalization of the tumor marker CA-125 after oophorectomy in a patient with paraneoplastic cerebellar degeneration without detectable cancer. Gynecol Oncol 65:1558–1563
76. Matias-Guiu X, Prat J (1990) Ovarian tumors with functioning stroma. An immunohistochemical study of 100 cases with human chorionic gonadotropin monoclonal and polyclonal antibodies. Cancer (Phila) 65:2001–2005
77. McCluggage WG, Maxwell P, Sloan JM (1997) Immunohistochemical staining of ovarian granulosa cell tumors with monoclonal antibodies against inhibin. Hum Pathol 28:1034–1038
78. McMahon JT, Hart WR (1988) Ultrastructural analysis of small cell carcinomas of the ovary. Am J Clin Pathol 90:523–529
79. Medsger TA, Dixon JA, Garwood VF (1982) Palmar fasciitis and polyarthritis associated with ovarian carcinoma. Ann Intern Med 96:424–431
80. Meigs JV (1954) Fibroma of the ovary with ascites and hydrothorax. Meigs' syndrome. Am J Obstet Gynecol 67:962–987
81. Miettinen M, Talerman A, Wahlstrom T, Astengo-Osuna C, Virtanen I (1988) Cellular differentiation in ovarian sex-cord-stromal and germ-cell tumors studied with antibodies to intermediate filament proteins. Am J Surg Pathol 9:640–651
82. Mittal KR, Blechman A, Greco MA, Alfonso F, Demopoulos R (1992) Lymphoma of ovary with stromal luteinization, presenting as secondary amenorrhea. Gynecol Oncol 45:69–75
83. Mordel N, Margalioth EJ, Harats N, et al (1988) Concurrence of ovarian cancer and dermatomyositis. A report of two cases and literature review. J Reprod Med 33:649–655
84. Morgello S, Schwartz E, Horwith M, et al (1988) Ectopic insulin production by a primary ovarian carcinoid. Cancer (Phila) 61:800–805
85. Nakashima N, Young RH, Scully RE (1984) An-

drogenic granulosa cell tumors of the ovary. A clinicopathological analysis of seventeen cases and review of the literature. Arch Pathol Lab Med 108: 786–791
86. Napoli VM, Wallach H (1976) Pancytopenia associated with a granulosa-cell tumor of the ovary. Report of a case. Am J Clin Pathol 65:344–350
87. Nguyen KQ, Hurst CG, Pierson DL, et al (1983) Sweet's syndrome and ovarian carcinoma. Cutis 32: 152–154
88. Nichols J, Warren JC, Mantz FA (1962) ACTH-like excretion from carcinoma of the ovary. JAMA 182: 713–718
89. Nogales FF, Concha A, Plata C, Ruiz-Avila I (1993) Granulosa cell tumor of the ovary with diffuse true hepatic differentiation simulating stromal luteinization. Am J Surg Pathol 17:85–90
90. Norris HJ, Taylor HB (1968) Prognosis of granulosa-theca tumors of the ovary. Cancer (Phila) 21:255–263
91. Norris HJ, Taylor HB (1969) Virilization associated with cystic granulosa tumors. Obstet Gynecol 34: 629–635
92. Norwood SH, Torma MJ, Fontanelle LJ (1981) Hyperamylasemia due to poorly differentiated adenosquamous carcinoma of the ovary. Arch Surg 116: 225–226
93. Nussbaum SR, Gas R, Arnold A (1990) Hypercalcemia and ectopic secretion of parathyroid hormone by an ovarian carcinoma with rearrangement of the gene for parathyroid hormone. N Engl J Med 323:1324–1328
94. Oliva E, Andrada E, Pezzica E, Prat J (1993) Ovarian carcinomas with choriocarcinomatous differentiation. Cancer (Phila) 72:2441–2446
95. O'Riordan T, Gaffney E, Tormey V, Daly P (1990) Hyperamylasemia associated with progression of a serous surface papillary carcinoma. Gynecol Oncol 36:432–434
96. Palmer PE, Bogojavlensky S, Bhan AK, Scully RE (1990) Prolactinoma in wall of ovarian dermoid cyst with hyperprolactinemia. Obstet Gynecol 75: 540–543
97. Paoletti M, Pridjian G, Okagaki T, Talerman A (1987) A stromal Leydig cell tumor of the ovary occurring in a pregnant 15-year-old girl. Ultrastructural findings. Cancer (Phila) 60:2806–2810
98. Paraskevas M, Scully RE (1989) Hilus cell tumor of the ovary. A clinicopathological analysis of 12 Reinke crystal-positive and 9 crystal-negative cases. Int J Gynecol Pathol 8:299–310
99. Parsons V, Rigby R (1958) Cushing's syndrome associated with adenocarcinoma of the ovary. Lancet 2:992–994
100. Payne D, Muss HB, Homesley HD, Jobson VW, Baird FG (1981) Autoimmune hemolytic anemia and ovarian dermoid cysts: case report and review of the literature. Cancer (Phila) 48:721–724
101. Peterson K, Rosenblum MK, Kotanides H, Posner MP (1992) Paraneoplastic cerebellar degeneration. I. A clinical analysis of 55 anti-Yo antibody-positive patients. Neurology 42:1931–1937
102. Pelkey TJ, Frierson HF, Mills SE, Stoler MH (1998) The diagnostic utility of inhibin staining in ovarian neoplasms. Int J Gynecol Pathol 17:97–105
103. Phadke DM, Weisenberg E, Engel G, Rhone DP (1999) Malignant Sertoli cell tumor of the ovary metastatic of the lung mimicking neuroendocrine carcinoma: report of a case. Ann Diagn Pathol 3: 213–219
104. Prat J, Scully RE (1981) Cellular fibromas and fibrosarcomas of the ovary: a comparative clinicopathologic analysis of seventeen cases. Cancer (Phila) 47:2663–2670
105. Prat J, Young RH, Scully RE (1982) Ovarian Sertoli-Leydig cell tumors with heterologous elements. (ii) cartilage and skeletal muscle: a clinicopathologic analysis of twelve cases. Cancer (Phila) 50: 2465–2475
106. Price A, Russell P, Elliott P, Bannatyne P (1990) Composite mucinous and granulosa-cell tumor of ovary: case report of a unique neoplasm. Int J Gynecol Pathol 9:372–378
107. Ramzy I (1976) Signet-ring stromal tumor of ovary. Histochemical, light, and electron microscopic study. Cancer (Phila) 38:166–172
108. Reddick RL, Walton LA (1982) Sertoli-Leydig cell tumor of the ovary with teratomatous differentiation. Cancer (Phila) 50:1171–1176
109. Riopel MA, Perlman EJ, Seidman JD et al (1998) Inhibin and epithelial membrane antigen immunohistochemistry assist in the diagnosis of sex cord-stromal tumors and provide clues to the histogenesis of hypercalcemic small cell carcinomas. Int J Gynecol Pathol 17:46–53
110. Rishi M, Howard LN, Bratthauer GL, Tavassoli FA (1997) Use of monoclonal antibodies against human inhibin as a marker for sex cord-stromal tumors of the ovary. Am J Surg Pathol 19:927–933
111. Roth LM, Anderson MC, Govan ADT, Langley FA, Gowing NFC, Woodcock AS (1981) Sertoli-Leydig cell tumors. A clinicopathologic study of 34 cases. Cancer (Phila) 48:187
112. Roth LM, Slayton RE, Brady LW, Blesdsing JA, Johnson G (1985) Retiform differentiation in ovarian Sertoli–Leydig cell tumors. A clinicopathologic study of six cases from a gynecologic oncology study group. Cancer (Phila) 55:1093–1098
113. Roth LM, Sternberg WH (1973) Ovarian stromal tumors containing Leydig cells. II. Pure Leydig cell tumor, non-hilar type. Cancer (Phila) 32:952–960
114. Roth LM, Sternberg WH (1983) Partly luteinized theca cell tumor of the ovary. Cancer (Phila) 51: 1697–1704
115. Rutgers J, Scully RE (1986) Functioning ovarian tumors with peripheral steroid cell proliferation: a report of twenty-four cases. Int J Gynecol Pathol 5:319–337
116. Samanth KK, Black WC (1970) Benign ovarian

stromal tumors associated with free peritoneal fluid. Am J Obstet Gynecol 107:538–545

117. Sasano H, Sasano N (1989) What's new in the localization of sex steroids in the human ovary and its tumors? Pathol Res Pract 185:942–948
118. Sasano H, Okamoto M, Mason JI, et al (1989) Immunohistochemical studies of steroidogenic enzymes (aromatase, 17–hydroxylase and cholesterol side-chain cleavage cytochromes P-450) in sex cord-stromal tumors of the ovary. Hum Pathol 20: 452–457
119. Schofield PM, Kirsop BA, Reginald P, Harington M (1985) Ovarian carcinoma presenting as pyrexia of unknown origin. Postgrad Med J61:177–178
120. Scully RE (1953) An unusual ovarian tumor containing Leydig cells but associated with endometrial hyperplasia, in a postmenopausal woman. J Clin Endocrinol Metab 13:1254–1263
121. Scully RE (1970) Sex cord tumor with annular tubules. A distinctive ovarian tumor of the Peutz–Jeghers syndrome. Cancer (Phila) 25:1107–1121
122. Scully RE, Young RE, Clement PB (1998) Tumors of the ovary, maldeveloped gonads, fallopian tube, and broad ligament. In: Atlas of tumor pathology, 3rd series, fasc 23. Armed Forces Institute of Pathology, Washington, DC
123. Scully RE, Aguirre P, DeLellis RA (1984) Argyrophilia, serotonin, and peptide hormones in the female genital tract and its tumors. Int J Gynecol Pathol 3:51–70
124. Scully RE, Cohen RB (1964) Oxidative-enzyme activity in normal and pathologic human ovaries. Obstet Gynecol 24:667–681
125. Scully RE, Richardson GS (1961) Luteinization of the stroma of metastatic cancer involving the ovary and its endocrine significance. Cancer (Phila) 14:827–840
126. Sens MA, Levenson TB, Metcalf JS (1982) A case of metastatic carcinoid arising in an ovarian teratoma. Case report with autopsy findings and review of the literature. Cancer (Phila) 49:2541–2546
127. Sjostedt S, Wahlen T (1961) Prognosis of granulosa cell tumors. Acta Obstet Gynecol Scand 40:1–26
128. Solh HM, Azoury RS, Najjar SS (1983) Peutz–Jeghers syndrome associated with precocious puberty. J Pediatr 103:593–595
129. Stenwig JT, Hazekamp JT, Beecham JB (1979) Granulosa cell tumors of the ovary. A clinicopathological study of 118 cases with long-term follow-up. Gynecol Oncol 7:136–152
130. Sternberg WH (1949) The morphology, endocrine function, hyperplasia and tumors of the human ovarian hilus cells. Am J Pathol 25:493–511
131. Sternberg WH, Roth LM (1973) Ovarian stromal tumors containing Leydig cells. 1. Stromal-Leydig cell tumor and non-neoplastic transformation of ovarian stroma to Leydig cells. Cancer (Phila) 32: 940–951
132. Stewart CJR, Jeffers MD, Kennedy A (1997). Diagnostic value of inhibin immunoreactivity in ovarian gonadal stromal tumours and their histological mimics. Histopathology (Oxf) 31:67–74
133. Susil BJ, Sumithran E (1987) Sarcomatous change in granulosa cell tumor. Hum Pathol 18:397–399
134. Talerman A (1987) Ovarian Sertoli-Leydig cell tumor (androblastoma) with retiform pattern: a clinicopathologic study. Cancer (Phila) 60:3056–3064
135. Talerman A, Hughesdon PE, Anderson MC (1982) Diffuse nonlobular ovarian androblastoma usually associated with feminization. Int J Gynecol Pathol 1:155–171
136. Taskin M, Barker B, Calanog A, Jormark S (1996) Syndrome of inappropriate antidiuresis in ovarian serous carcinoma with neuroendocrine differentiation. Gynecol Oncol 62:400–404
137. Tavassoli FA, Norris HJ (1980) Sertoli tumors of the ovary. A clinicopathologic study of 28 cases with ultrastructural observations. Cancer (Phila) 46:2282–2297
138. Taylor HB, Norris HJ (1967) Lipid cell tumors of the ovary. Cancer (Phila) 20:1953–1962
139. Teilum G (1958) Classification of testicular and ovarian androblastoma and Sertoli cell tumors. Cancer (Phila) 11:769–782
140. Todesco S, Terribile V, Borsatti A, et al (1975) Primary aldosteronism due to a malignant ovarian tumor. J Clin Endocrinol Metab 41:809–819
141. Tracy SL, Askin FB, Reddick RL, Jackson B, Kurman RJ (1985) Progesterone secreting Sertoli cell tumor of the ovary. Gynecol Oncol 22:85–96
142. Tsunematsu R, Saito T, Iguchi H, Fukuda T, Tsukamoto N (2000) Hypercalcemia due to parathyroid hormone-related protein produced by primary ovarian clear cell adenocarcinoma: case report. Gynecol Oncol 76:218–222
143. Tyler HR (1974) Paraneoplastic syndromes of nerve, muscle, and neuromuscular junction. Ann NY Acad Sci 230:348–357
144. Ueda G, Nobuaki H, Hayakawa K, et al (1972) Clinical histochemical and biochemical studies of an ovarian dysgerminoma with trophoblasts and Leydig cells. Am J Obstet Gynecol 114:748–754
145. Verducci MA, Malkasian GD, Friedman SJ, Winkelmann RK (1984) Gynecologic carcinoma associated with dermatomyositis-polymyositis. Obstet Gynecol 64:695–698
146. von dem Borne AEGK, van Oers RHJ, Wiersinga WM, et al (1990) Complete remission of autoimmune thrombocytopenia after extirpation of a benign adenofibroma of the ovary. Br J Rheumatol 74:119–120
147. Waxman M, Damjanov I, Alpert L, Sardinsky T (1981) Composite mucinous ovarian neoplasms associated with Sertoli-Leydig and carcinoid tumors. Cancer (Phila) 47:2044–2052
148. Waxman M, Vuletin JC, Urcuyo R, Belling CG (1979) Ovarian low-grade stromal sarcoma with thecomatous features. A critical reappraisal of the so-called "malignant thecoma." Cancer (Phila) 44: 2206–2217

149. Young RH, Dickersin GR, Scully RE (1983) A distinctive ovarian sex cord–stromal tumor causing sexual precocity in the Peutz–Jeghers syndrome. Am J Surg Pathol 7:233–243
150. Young RH, Dickersin GR, Scully RE (1984) Juvenile granulosa cell tumor of the ovary. A clinicopathologic analysis of 125 cases. Am J Surg Pathol 8:575–596
151. Young RH, Dudley AG, Scully RE (1984) Granulosa cell, Sertoli-Leydig cell and unclassified sex cord-stromal tumors associated with pregnancy. A clinicopathological analysis of thirty-six cases. Gynecol Oncol 18:181–205
152. Young RH, Oliva E, Scully RE (1994) Lutenized adult granulosa cell tumors of the ovary: a report of four cases. Int J Gynecol Pathol 13:302–310
153. Young RH, Oliva E, Scully RE (1994) Small cell carcinoma of the ovary, hypercalcemia type. A clinicopathological analysis of 150 cases. Am J Surg Pathol 18:1102–1116
154. Young RH, Perez-Atayde AR, Scully RE (1984) Ovarian Sertoli-Leydig cell tumor with retiform and heterologous components. Report of a case with hepatocytic differentiation and elevated serum alpha-fetoprotein. Am J Surg Pathol 8:709–718
155. Young RH, Prat J, Scully RE (1982) Ovarian Sertoli-Leydig cell tumors with heterologous elements. (i) Gastrointestinal epithelium and carcinoid: a clinicopathologic analysis of thirty-six cases. Cancer (Phila) 50:2448–2456
156. Young RH, Scully RE (1983) Ovarian stromal tumors with minor sex cord elements: a report of seven cases. Int J Gynecol Pathol 2:227–234
157. Young RH, Scully RE (1983) Ovarian sex cord-stromal tumors with bizarre nuclei. A clinicopathologic analysis of seventeen cases. Int J Gynecol Pathol 1:325–335
158. Young RH, Scully RE (1983) Ovarian Sertoli-Leydig cell tumors with a retiform pattern: a problem in histopathologic diagnosis. A report of 25 cases. Am J Surg Pathol 7:755–771
159. Young RH, Scully RE (1984) Ovarian Sertoli cell tumors. A report of ten cases. Int J Gynecol Pathol 2:349–363
160. Young RH, Scully RE (1987) Ovarian steroid cell tumors associated with Cushing's syndrome. A report of three cases. Int J Gynecol Pathol 6:40–48
161. Young RH, Scully RE (1984) Well-differentiated ovarian Sertoli–Leydig cell tumors. A clinicopathological analysis of 23 cases. Int J Gynecol Pathol 3:277–290
162. Young RH, Scully RE (1985) Ovarian Sertoli-Leydig cell tumors. A clinicopathological analysis of 207 cases. Am J Surg Pathol 9:543–569
163. Young RH, Welch WR, Dickersin GR, Scully RE (1982) Ovarian sex cord tumor with annular tubules: review of 74 cases including 27 with Peutz–Jeghers syndrome and 4 with adenoma malignum of the cervix. Cancer (Phila) 50:1384–1402
164. Zaloudek C, Norris HJ (1982) Granulosa tumors of the ovary in children. A clinical and pathologic study of 32 cases. Am J Surg Pathol 6:503–512
165. Zaloudek C, Norris HJ (1984) Sertoli-Leydig tumors of the ovary. A clinicopathologic study of 64 intermediate and poorly differentiated neoplasms. Am J Surg Pathol 8:405–418
166. Zaloudek CJ, Tavassoli FA, Norris HJ (1981) Dysgerminoma with syncytiotrophoblastic giant cells. A histologically and clinically distinctive subtype of dysgerminoma. Am J Surg Pathol 5:361–367
167. Zhang J, Young RH, Arseneau J, Scully RE (1982) Ovarian stromal tumors containing lutein or Leydig cells (luteinized thecomas and stromal Leydig cell tumors). A clinicopathological analysis of fifty cases. Int J Gynecol Pathol 1:270–285
168. Zheng W, Sung CJ, Hanna I, et al (1997) α and β subunits of inhibin/activin as sex cord-stromal differentiation markers. Int J Gynecol Pathol 16:263–271

20

Germ Cell Tumors of the Ovary

Aleksander Talerman, M.D., Ph.D., F.R.C. Path.

Germ cell tumors are composed of a number of histologically different tumor types derived from the primitive germ cells of the embryonic gonad. The concept of germ cell tumors as a specific group of gonadal neoplasms has evolved in the last five decades. It is based on (1) the common histogenesis of these neoplasms, (2) the relatively frequent presence of histologically different neoplastic elements within the same tumor, (3) the presence of histologically similar neoplasms in extragonadal locations along the line of migration of the primitive germ cells from the wall of the yolk sac to the gonadal ridge,[214] and (4) the remarkable homology between the various tumors in the male and the female. In no other group of gonadal neoplasms is this homology better illustrated. Although the strong morphologic resemblance between the testicular seminoma and its ovarian counterpart, the dysgerminoma, was noted soon after these neoplasms were first described, for a long time there was no agreement as to their histogenesis. Nevertheless, these were the first neoplasms to become accepted as originating from germ cells. It was not until the studies by Teilum[194,195] on the homology of ovarian and testicular neoplasms, the studies by Friedman and Moore[46] and Dixon and Moore[40] on testicular tumors, and those by Friedman[45] on related extragonadal neoplasms that the germ cell origin of other neoplasms belonging to this group was suggested. These views were supported by the embryologic studies of Witschi[214] and Gillman,[53] and later by the experimental work of Stevens[167–169] and Pierce et al.[132,134] on germ cell tumors in rodents.

Although occasional unusual neoplasms composed of germ cells and sex cord derivatives had been noted previously, it was not until Scully's detailed description of gonadoblastoma[153] that these neoplasms were recognized. More recently, another neoplasm composed of germ cells and sex cord derivatives, the mixed germ cell–sex cord–stromal tumor, has been described in detail.[174,175] This chapter, therefore, is devoted not only to neoplasms of germ cell origin but also to those composed of germ cells and sex cord derivatives.

Histogenesis

The histogenesis and interrelationships of the various types of germ cell neoplasms, as suggested by Teilum,[198] are shown in Fig. 20.1. According to Teilum,[198] dysgerminoma (seminoma) is a primitive germ cell neoplasm that has not acquired the potential for further differentiation. Embryonal carcinoma is regarded as a conceptual as well as a morphologic entity and represents a germ cell neoplasm composed of multipotential cells that are capable of further differentiation. This process can take place in an embryonal or somatic direction, resulting in teratomatous neoplasms showing various degrees of maturity, or in an extraembryonal direction along either of two pathways: vitelline, differentiating toward yolk sac (endodermal sinus) tumor, or trophoblastic, differentiating toward a choriocarcinoma. The process of differentiation is dynamic and, therefore, the resulting neoplasms may be composed of different elements showing various stages of development. According to this view,[198] dysgerminoma is considered incapable of further differentiation, but immunocytochemical evidence indicates that some seminoma or dysgerminoma cells can differentiate into embryonal carcinoma and further. Although the great majority of seminoma or dysgerminoma cells are cytokeratin negative, whereas embryonal carcinoma, yolk sac tumor, and choriocarcinoma are composed entirely of cytokeratin-positive cells,[100,101] some seminomas and dysgerminomas contain cytokeratin-positive cells.[100] The intimate admixture of dysgerminoma cells with other neoplastic germ cell elements seen in some germ cell tumors also supports this view.[68]

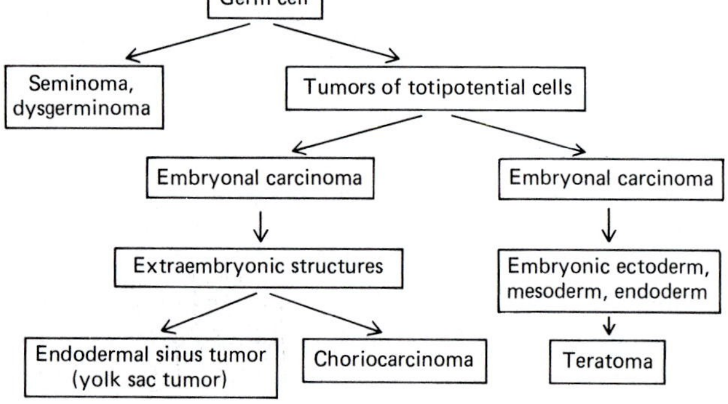

Fig. 20.1. Histogenesis and interrelationship of tumors of germ cell origin. (Modified from Teilum, ref. 198.)

Classification

A number of classifications of germ cell neoplasms of the ovary have been proposed over the years, each one becoming progressively more detailed. Some years ago, a panel of pathologists was established under the auspices of the World Health Organization (WHO) to formulate a histologic classification of ovarian neoplasms to be used throughout the world. This classification[157] divides the germ cell tumors into a number of groups and also includes neoplasms composed of germ cells and sex cord–stromal derivatives. Recently, the WHO classification of ovarian neoplasms has been modified based on advances in our understanding of the pathology of ovarian neoplasms that have taken place during the past two decades (Table 20.1).[156]

There are several changes in the new classification. The main change is the use of the term yolk sac tumor instead of the more specific term endodermal sinus tumor. The latter term is retained as a synonym. The yolk sac tumor category has been expanded to include the polyvesicular vitelline, hepatoid, and glandular subtypes, which unlike other patterns of differentiation in yolk sac tumors can occur in pure form and thus pose diagnostic problems. The new classification also expands the category of teratoma, especially the group of monodermal teratomas, to include some newly described entities. The tumors composed of germ cells and the sex cord–stromal derivatives are divided into two categories, gonadoblastoma and mixed germ cell–sex cord–stromal tumor; each of these is subclassified to include those tumors associated with dysgerminoma or other germ cell tumors.

Cytogenetic Aspects

Most ovarian germ cell tumors are mature cystic teratomas that are diploid, have a normal 46,XX karyotype, and have been considered to originate from germ cells after the first meiotic division[86]; thus, these are unlike testicular germ cell tumors, which are nearly always malignant, aneuploid, have a higher than normal chromosome complement,[10] and are considered to originate before the first meiotic division. Recent studies[108,119] using new and more advanced banding techniques have demonstrated diverse modes of origin of mature cystic teratoma. Although most ovarian mature cystic teratomas originate from germ cells after the first meiotic division, it has been demonstrated conclusively that some originate before this event.[108,119]

Table 20.1. WHO classification of germ cell tumors of the ovary

Germ cell tumors
Dysgerminoma
Variant—with syncytiotrophoblastic cells
Yolk sac tumor (endodermal sinus tumor)
Variants
Polyvesicular vitelline tumor
Hepatoid
Glandular
Embryonal carcinoma
Polyembryoma
Choriocarcinoma
Teratomas
Immature
Mature
Solid
Cystic (dermoid cyst)
With secondary tumor formation (specify type)
Fetiform (homunculus)
Monodermal and highly specialized
Struma ovarii
Variant—with thyroid tumor (specify type)
Carcinoid
Insular
Trabecular
Strumal carcinoid
Mucinous carcinoid
Neuroectodermal tumors
Sebaceous tumors
Others
Mixed (specify type)
Mixed forms (tumors composed of two or more of the above pure types)
Tumors composed of germ cells and sex cord–stromal derivatives
Gonadoblastoma
Variant—with dysgerminoma or other germ cell tumor
Germ cell–sex cord–stromal tumor
Variant—with dysgerminoma or other germ cell tumor

WHO, World Health Organization.

This distinction also applies to immature ovarian teratomas, which tend to be aneuploid, resembling their testicular counterparts. The demonstration of a small isochromosome, i(12p), as a specific abnormality and therefore a possible chromosomal marker for testicular germ cell tumors, especially seminoma,[11] has been extended to some ovarian germ cell neoplasms. The presence of this chromosome has been noted in two dysgerminomas.[12] Neither mature cystic teratoma,[119] immature cystic teratoma,[74] or mixed germ cell tumors and their metastases[52] have demonstrated this abnormality.

Clinical and Pathologic Features of Germ Cell Tumors

Germ cell tumors constitute the second largest group of ovarian neoplasms after the surface epithelial stromal tumors and comprise approximately 20% of all ovarian neoplasms observed in Europe and North America. In countries in Asia and Africa where the prevalence of surface epithelial stromal tumors is much lower, germ cell tumors constitute a much larger proportion of ovarian neoplasms. Germ cell tumors are encountered at all ages from infancy to old age but are seen most frequently from the first to the sixth decades. They also have been observed during fetal life. In children and adolescents, more than 60% of ovarian neoplasms are of germ cell origin and one-third are malignant.[111] In adults, the great majority of germ cell tumors (95%) are benign and consist of mature cystic teratomas (dermoid cysts).

Dysgerminoma

General Features

Although the term *dysgerminoma* was first introduced by Meyer[99] in 1931, ovarian neoplasms showing this histologic pattern had been recognized earlier. Chenot[30] in 1911 was the first to note their occurrence and their similarity to the testicular seminoma described some years earlier.[31] In view of the strong resemblance to their testicular counterparts, the tumor was named ovarian seminoma by Masson,[96] and this became the most popular term until its replacement by dysgerminoma. It is still widely used in the French literature. The term disgerminoma, as originally suggested by Meyer,[99] and which later became dysgerminoma, has over the years gained almost universal acceptance.

Histogenesis

Dysgerminoma is composed entirely of germ cells that show morphologic, including ultrastructural,[88] and histochemical[91] similarity to primordial germ cells. The cells of dysgerminoma are considered to be in an early and sexually indifferent stage of differentiation; they have been believed to be arrested at a developmental stage at which they have not yet gained the ability for further differentiation.[198] However, there is now evidence that occasional cells may acquire this ability and differentiate to embryonal carcinoma and further.[100] These cells are hormonally inert. An origin from the primordial germ cells that migrate to the ovary during early embryogenesis from their site of origin in the wall of the yolk sac[214] is the most widely accepted view of the histogenesis of dysgerminoma. It is supported by the occurrence of homologous neoplasms in the testis (seminoma) and along the route of migration of the primordial germ cells from the wall of the yolk sac to the primitive gonad, in the mediastinum, retroperitoneum, posterior abdominal wall, and parapineal and sacrococcygeal regions.

The presence of sex chromatin bodies (Barr bodies) in the cells of dysgerminoma is a matter of controversy. Sex chromatin bodies were said by some investigators[200] to be present in the cells of a number of dysgerminomas, whereas others[9] could not identify them. The latter view is more in accordance with an origin from the primordial germ cells. The finding of twice the amount of DNA in the nuclei of dysgerminoma cells as compared with the nuclei of lymphocytes in all the cases studied[9,79] further supports the origin from primordial germ cells, which have the same amount of DNA in their nuclei (twice the amount present in normal diploid cells).

Genetic Aspects

When Meyer[99] described dysgerminoma, he observed that the tumor frequently occurred in hermaphrodites, pseudohermaphrodites, and patients with underdeveloped or malformed genitalia. In fact, 27 of 48 cases collected by Meyer[99] occurred in sexually abnormal patients, and this relationship was strongly emphasized. It is considered that most of these reports described patients with gonadal dysgenesis and dysgerminoma that had originated from a gonadoblastoma. Although subsequent authors supported Meyer's contention about the very close association between dysgerminoma and developmental and sexual abnormalities, later reports suggested that it is not as close as had been postulated. These later reports stated that most patients with dysgerminoma were normally developed females without any sexual abnormalities.[9,22]

Most patients with dysgerminoma do not exhibit any menstrual abnormalities and are either capable of bearing or have actually borne children.[9,22] In a number of cases, the diagnosis has been made during pregnancy.[9,22] A number of patients have become pregnant and have had normal offspring after therapy.[9,22] Most recent reports emphasize the occurrence of dysgerminoma in normal female patients[9,22] and some have even cast doubt on the relationship with developmental and sexual abnormalities.[9]

The common association of dysgerminoma with gonadoblastoma, a tumor that nearly always occurs in patients with dysgenetic gonads,[147,148,154] indicates that there is a relationship between dysgerminoma and genetic and somatosexual abnormalities (see Chapter 1, Embryology of the Female Genital Tract and Disorders of Abnormal Sexual Development).

Endocrine Aspects

In the great majority of cases, dysgerminoma is not associated with endocrine manifestations. Occasional cases have been described in which the tumor was associated with elevated urinary chorionic gonadotropins, positive pregnancy tests, or signs of precocious puberty, and these manifestations have disappeared after tumor excision. Although in these cases the tumor has been said to be a pure dysgerminoma, the possibility of admixture with choriocarcinomatous elements that have not been detected, perhaps because of inadequate sampling, is the most likely explanation.

The presence of choriocarcinoma in association with dysgerminoma is not frequent, but most of the reported series contain cases of this type.[123,146] Occasional cases of pure dysgerminoma, containing multinucleated syncytiotrophoblastic giant cells but lacking cytotrophoblastic elements, have been noted to be associated with gonadotropin production. Although some cases of dysgerminoma showing these histologic appearances were recognized previously, evidence of gonadotropin production by the syncytiotrophoblastic giant cells was obtained more recently. This evidence provides another possible explanation, apart from the presence of true choriocarcinomatous elements, for the occasional presence of endocrine activity in cases of dysgerminoma. However, there remains a small group of cases in which, despite a careful search, trophoblastic elements have not been found. In some of these cases, the dysgerminoma has been associated with an increase in luteinized stromal or Leydig-like cells and it is likely that these cells may be responsible for the feminizing side effects. These cells may be found within the stroma of the tumor, within the uninvolved ovarian stroma either in the vicinity of the tumor, or located at the periphery of the ovary.[144] These cells also may be responsible for the virilizing side effects observed in occasional cases of dysgerminoma. Dysgerminoma associated with evidence of virilization is found mostly in association with gonadoblastoma in patients with pure or mixed gonadal dysgenesis.

Prevalence

Dysgerminoma is an uncommon tumor, accounting for 1–2% of primary ovarian neoplasms and 3–5% of ovarian malignancies.[102,146] Although until 1950 only 427 cases had been recorded in the literature,[102] more than twice as many cases have been reported since, and dysgerminoma is considered the most common malignant ovarian germ cell neoplasm occurring in pure form. The exact prevalence of dysgerminoma in different parts of the world is not known, because most cancer registry reports do not differentiate between the various types of ovarian neoplasms. In some countries there are considerable regional variations. Although most reports emanate from Europe and North America, dysgerminoma has been encountered in all parts of the world and in all races.

Clinical Features

The tumor may occur at any age from infancy to old age; the reported cases range between the ages of 7 months and 70 years[102] but most cases occur in adolescence and early adult life.[9,22,59,102] Dysgerminoma occurs not infrequently before puberty but is very rare after menopause. Most cases occur in the second and third decades; nearly half the patients are under 20 years of age and 80% are under 30 years.[9,22,59,102] Therefore, dysgerminoma is one of the most common malignant ovarian neoplasms of childhood, adolescence, and early adult life.[9,22,59,102,111]

Pure dysgerminoma has been reported in siblings[190] as well as in a mother and daughter.[66] The symptomatology of dysgerminoma is not distinctive and is similar to that observed in patients with other solid ovarian neoplasms.[9,22,59,102] The duration of symptoms is usually short; despite this, the tumor is often large, indicating a rapid growth.[22] The most common presenting symptoms are abdominal enlargement and presence of a mass in the lower abdomen, sometimes associated with abdominal pain that may be caused by torsion. Loss of weight may also be an accompanying symptom. In a number of cases, the tumor has been found incidentally; in these cases, the tumor is usually small. Sometimes the tumor may be detected during pregnancy.[9] In such cases, it may be discovered as an incidental finding or may be obstructing labor.

Dysgerminoma is one of the two most common ovarian neoplasms observed in pregnancy, the other being serous cystadenoma. Dysgerminoma occurring during pregnancy shows rapid growth. The relatively common finding of dysgerminoma in pregnant patients is nonspecific and relates to the age of the patients. Dysgerminoma may also be discovered incidentally in patients investigated for primary amenorrhea; in these cases it is not infrequently associated with gonadoblastoma.[147,148,154,212] Occasionally, menstrual and endocrine abnormalities may be the presenting symptom, but this finding tends to be more common in patients with dysgerminoma combined with other neoplastic germ cell elements, especially choriocarcinoma. In children, precocious sexual development may occur.[144] Dysgerminoma has also been encountered in a patient with triple-X syndrome.[72]

Gross Findings

Dysgerminoma usually is unilateral. It tends to occur more often in the right ovary,[102] which is affected in approximately 50% of cases, whereas the left is affected in 33–35% and bilateral involvement occurs in 10–17%.[9,59,102] Bilateral involvement has been reported more frequently in some series[123,190] and less frequently in others.[9,22] A much higher frequency of bilateral tumors is observed in patients with dysgerminoma associated with gonadoblastoma, the dysgerminoma arising from and overgrowing the gonadoblastoma.[147,148,154] Thus, inclusion of such cases tends to increase the prevalence of bilaterality.

Pure dysgerminomas are solid tumors that are round, oval, or lobulated, with a smooth, gray-white, slightly glistening fibrous capsule. They vary in size from a few centimeters in diameter to large masses measuring 50 cm across,[9] that fill the pelvic and abdominal cavities. Tumors weighing more than 5 kg have been described.[102] Compressed ovarian tissue may be seen surrounding small tumors, but in large tumors it is not discernible. The capsule is usually intact but may be ruptured, especially in large tumors, which may lead to the formation of adhesions between the tumor and the surrounding structures. The consistency of dysgerminoma varies from firm and rubbery in small and medium-sized tumors to soft in the large ones. On cut surface (Fig. 20.2), the tumor is solid and varies from gray-pink to light tan. Red, brown, or yellow discoloration caused by hemorrhage or necrosis is also seen, especially in large tumors; this may sometimes lead to the formation of small cysts, but cystic areas are seen only occasionally in pure dysgerminoma. The presence of cystic areas suggests the possibility that other neoplastic elements may be present, most likely teratoma. In view of the important therapeutic and prognostic implications concerning the presence of other neoplastic germ cell elements, extensive and judicious sampling of different parts of the tumor, especially of the less typical areas, is strongly recommended.

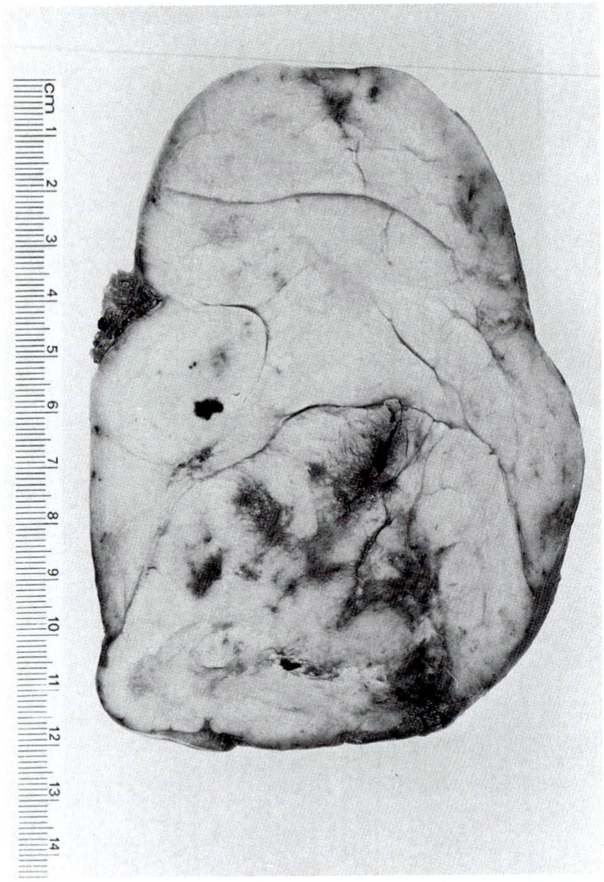

Fig. 20.2. Dysgerminoma. The cut surface is solid. There is some lobulation. Focally hemorrhage is present.

Microscopic Findings

Dysgerminoma exhibits a distinctive histologic appearance. It is histologically identical to classic seminoma of the testis. It is composed of aggregates, islands, or strands of large uniform cells surrounded by varying amounts of connective tissue stroma containing lymphocytes (Figs. 20.3 and 20.4). The cells are large and measure from 15 to 25 micrometers (μm) across. They are oval or round and usually have distinguishable cytoplasmic borders (Fig. 20.5). In well-fixed material, the cell boundaries are well-defined. The cells contain an ample amount of pale, slightly granular eosinophilic or clear cytoplasm.

The centrally located vesicular nucleus is large, occupying nearly half the cell. The nucleus is oval or round, has a sharp nuclear membrane with unevenly dispersed finely granular chromatin, and contains usually one, but sometimes two, prominent eosinophilic nucleoli. Some variation in the size of the cells and nuclei and in the amount of nuclear chromatin is usually seen. Large or giant mononucleate tumor cells, which in all other respects resemble typical dysgerminoma cells, may be seen (Fig. 20.6). Mitotic activity is almost always detectable (Figs. 20.5 and 20.6) and may vary from slight to brisk. This difference in mitotic activity may be observed not only in different tumors but also in different parts of the same tumor.

The cytoplasm of the tumor cells contains glycogen, which is removed by diastase digestion. The glycogen can be demonstrated with the periodic acid–Schiff (PAS) reaction, and this can be used as an aid in diagnosis. The amount of glycogen in tumor cells is variable, and glycogen is lost from the cytoplasm on prolonged fixation in formalin. In view of this, the PAS reaction may vary from strong to very weak. Most dysgerminoma cells do not show positive immunocytochemical staining for cytokeratin, although occasional cells may show a positive reaction.[100,101] In view of this, immunocytochemical staining for cytokeratin provides a useful diagnostic test that distinguishes between dysgerminoma and embryonal carcinoma or endodermal sinus tumor, which show a uniformly positive staining reaction for cytokeratin.[100,101]

Lipid can be demonstrated in the cytoplasm of the tumor cells in frozen tissue. The cells of dysgerminoma, like the primordial germ cells, show a positive alkaline phosphatase reaction beneath the cytoplasmic rim[91] and, in general, show similar his-

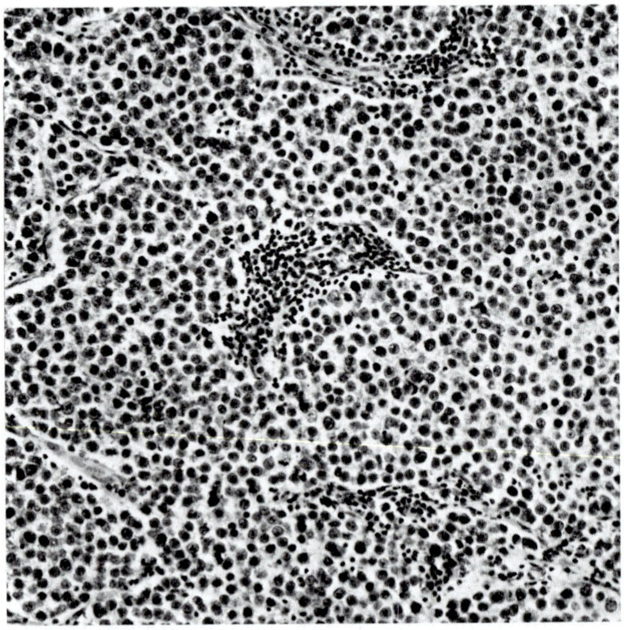

Fig. 20.3. Dysgerminoma. The tumor is composed of large aggregates of uniform cells surrounded by delicate strands of connective tissue containing lymphocytes.

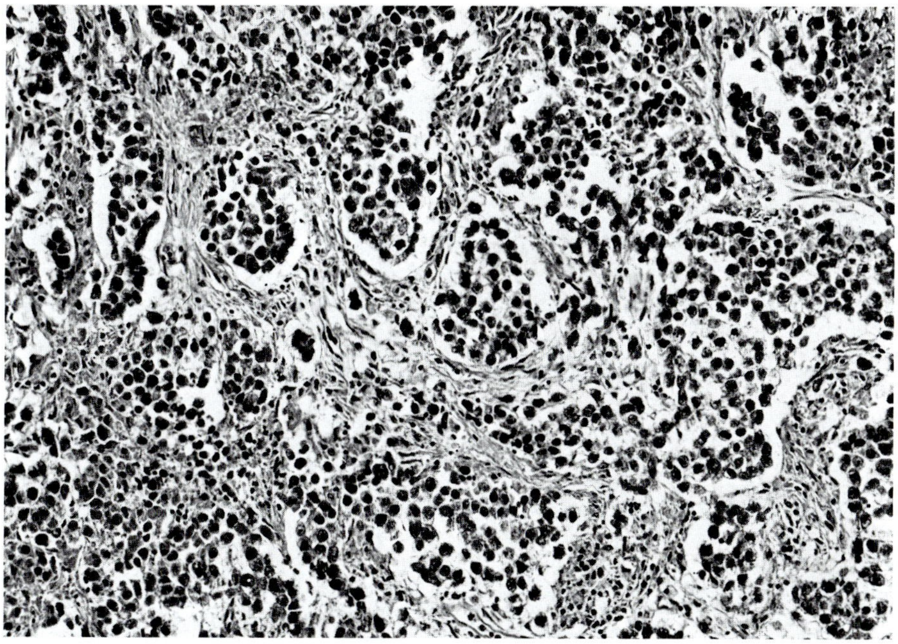

Fig. 20.4. Dysgerminoma. The tumor is composed of islands of tumor cells surrounded by connective tissue stroma containing lymphocytes.

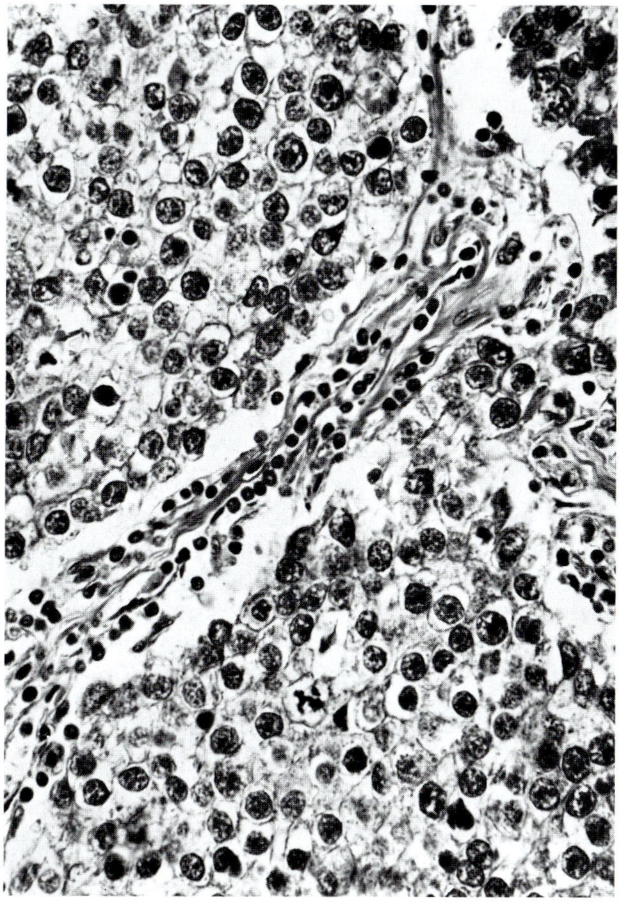

Fig. 20.5. Dysgerminoma. Nests of dysgerminoma cells surrounded by a connective tissue septum infiltrated by lymphocytes. An abnormal mitosis is seen just below the *center*.

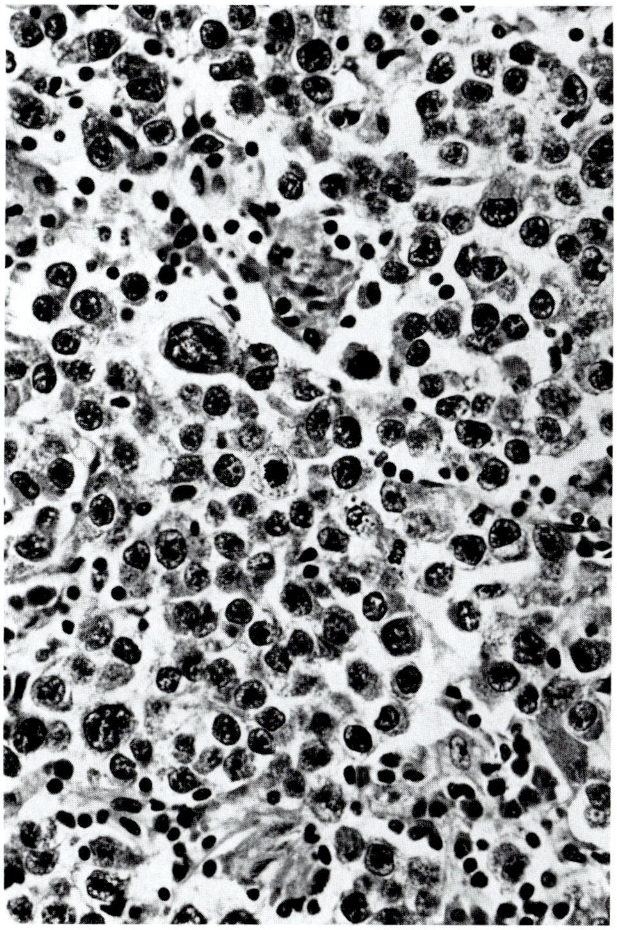

Fig. 20.6. Dysgerminoma. There is slight variation in size of the cells, a large uninucleate cell and a mitosis are seen in the *center*.

tochemical reactions to those of primordial germ cells. An increased amount of DNA, double the amount present in normal somatic cells, has been observed in the nuclei of dysgerminoma using densitometry[9] and more sophisticated methods of DNA measurement.[79]

The stroma that surrounds the tumor cells is almost always infiltrated by lymphocytes. The lymphocytic infiltration may vary from slight to marked (Fig. 20.7). Occasionally, lymphoid follicles containing germinal centers may be seen. Plasma cells and eosinophils are not infrequently seen within the connective tissue stroma. Granulomatous reaction is also not infrequently seen; this manifests itself as collections of histiocytes surrounded by lymphocytes, plasma cells, and occasional giant cells of both the Langhans and foreign body types (Fig. 20.8). The lymphoreticular cell infiltrate recently has been studied immunocytochemically, and most of the cells were found to consist of T cells and macrophages. There were relatively few B cells, natural killer cells, and other types of lymphoreticular cells.[39] Similar findings were observed in testicular seminoma.[17]

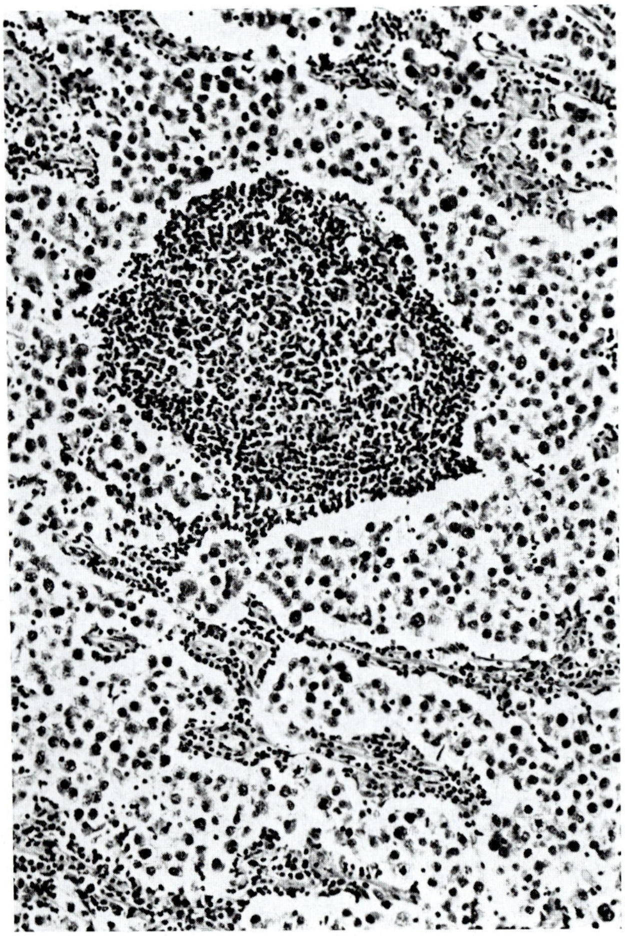

Fig. 20.7. Dysgerminoma. A large collection of lymphocytes and fine connective tissue septa surround the tumor cells.

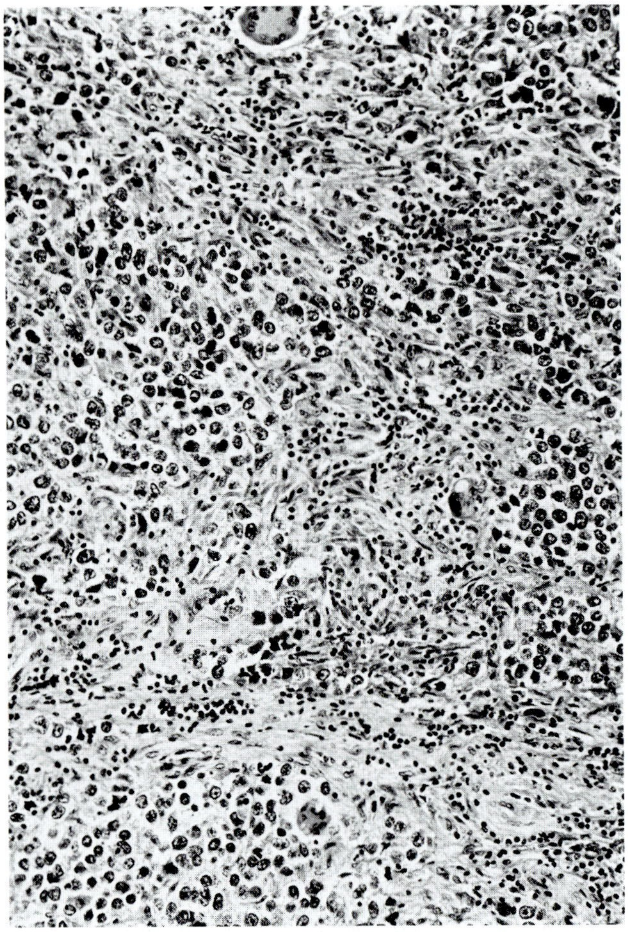

Fig. 20.8. Dysgerminoma. A granulomatous reaction with foreign body and Langhans giant cells present.

The connective tissue stroma shows considerable variation in its appearance. Depending on the amount of stroma, the tumor cells form large aggregates, smaller nests, islands, cords, or strands. The stroma varies from a fine, delicate fibrovascular network that can be loose and edematous to densely hyalinized. Occasionally, the amount of stroma may be very large, and this leads to wide separation of the nests of tumor cells (see Fig. 20.4). In some cases hyalinization may be so marked that tumor cells are detected with difficulty. At the opposite end of the spectrum, there are tumors that are cellular and contain only an imperceptible amount of stroma. There may be considerable variation in the amount of stroma in various parts of the same tumor.

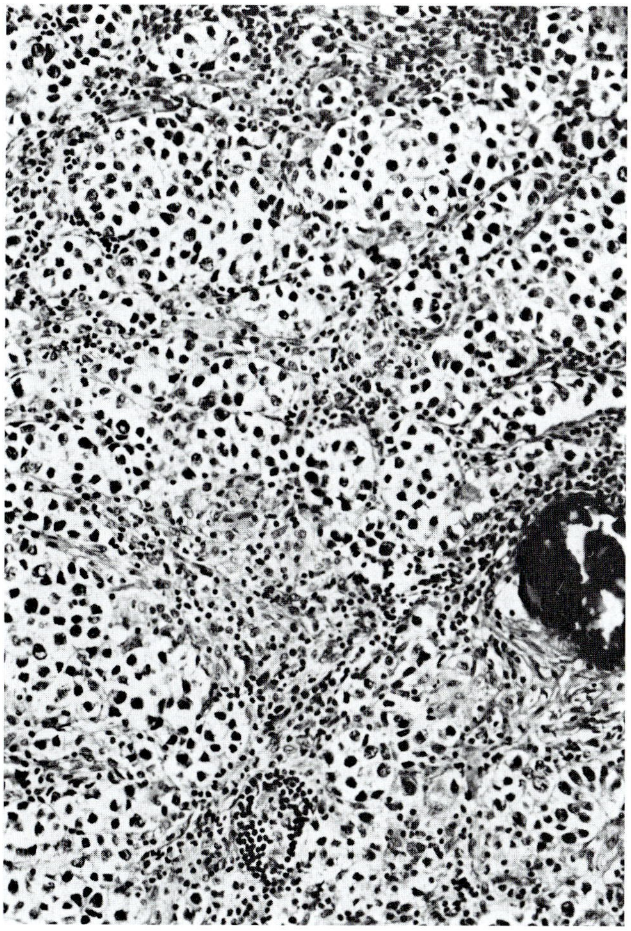

Fig. 20.9. Dysgerminoma. A large calcified concretion is present. Nests of gonadoblastoma were found in other parts of the tumor.

Foci of necrosis and hemorrhage are frequently found and may be of considerable size in large tumors or in tumors affected by torsion. Small foci of hyalinization may also be present, but large hyalinized areas sometimes observed in testicular seminoma are uncommon. Calcification is only occasionally seen in dysgerminoma. It occurs as small untidy spots or flecks of calcified material that are found in association with necrosis, hemorrhage, fibrosis, or hyalinization. Occasionally, relatively large, round, or ovoid calcified bodies are found, which may indicate the presence of a burnt-out gonadoblastoma[154] (Fig. 20.9). In 6%–8% of dysgerminomas, there are individual or collections of syncytiotrophoblastic giant cells that produce human chorionic gonadotropin (hCG). The presence of these cells is associated with elevation of serum hCG levels; hCG can also be demonstrated in tissue sections by immunoperoxidase techniques.

The syncytiotrophoblastic giant cells may form large syncytial masses resembling the syncytiotrophoblast of a choriocarcinoma, but they differ from the latter because there is no cytotrophoblast (Fig. 20.10). The syncytiotrophoblastic cells must also be differentiated from foreign body and Langhans' giant cells and from mononucleate and multinucleate tumor giant cells, which are seen in some dysgerminomas. There is no evidence that dysgerminomas containing syncytiotrophoblastic giant cells are associated with a worse prognosis.[219] The serum hCG level can be monitored as a tumor marker in the same way as in patients with gestational trophoblastic disease (see Chapter 24, Gestational Trophoblastic Disease and Related Lesions) or with mixed germ cell tumors containing choriocarcinoma. The serum hCG levels in these cases are much lower compared with dysgerminoma admixed with typical choriocarcinoma.

Pure dysgerminoma is not associated with elevated levels of serum alpha fetoprotein (AFP).[189] The presence of elevated levels of AFP is an indication of presence of other neoplastic germ cell elements, virtually always yolk sac tumor (YST), either within the primary tumor or its metastases.

Immunocytochemical staining for placenta-specific alkaline phosphatase (PLAP) has been used less extensively in ovarian dysgerminoma as compared to testicular seminoma,[68] but when applied PLAP stains dysgerminoma cells in the same

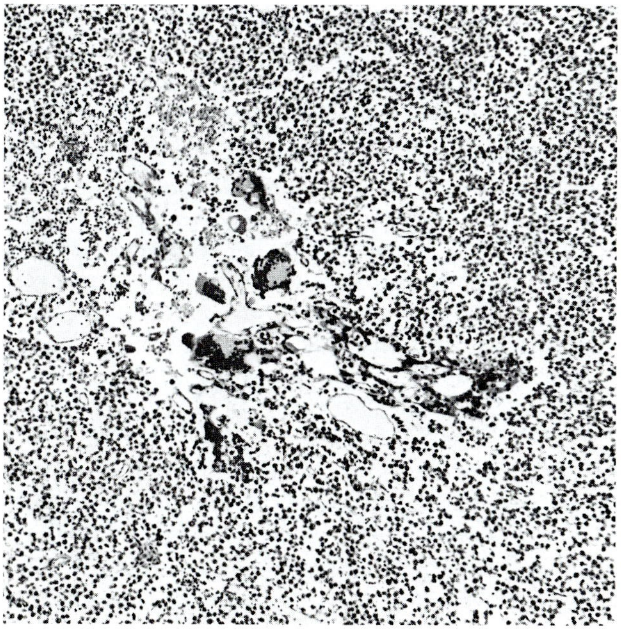

Fig. 20.10. Dysgerminoma. Collections of giant cells form large syncytial masses resembling syncytiotrophoblast.

way as testicular seminoma cells, showing membrane-bound staining in most cells.[141] As PLAP also stains positively the tumor cells in other malignant germ cell tumors, it cannot be used to differentiate dysgerminoma from other malignant germ cell neoplasms.[68] It may be useful in differentiating dysgerminoma from nongerm cell malignancies that occasionally may resemble it such as clear cell carcinoma, malignant lymphoma, and granulosa cell tumor. Dysgerminoma cells stain positively with the C-kit product.[205] This reaction is not very useful for the diagnosis of dysgerminoma, however, because the C-kit product stains a great variety of cells.

The cells of dysgerminoma, when studied with the electron microscope,[88] have been found to resemble closely the cells of testicular seminoma[128] and germ cell neoplasms in other locations showing a similar histologic pattern, as well as normal maturing germ cells in the ovary. Slight ultrastructural differences have been noted between individual germ cells present within a tumor, as well as between those present in the different tumors studied. It is likely that some of these differences are related to the degree of differentiation and maturity of the tumor cells.

Dysgerminoma may be associated with other neoplastic germ cell elements. Recent studies indicate a greater frequency of these mixed tumors[83,123] as compared with earlier reports.[102] This finding is a result of a more detailed examination of the tumors and a better recognition of the fact that germ cell tumors may be composed of histologically different neoplastic elements occurring in combination. For example, dysgerminoma may be combined with teratoma, yolk sac tumor, embryonal carcinoma, and choriocarcinoma. Some tumors may contain all these neoplastic germ cell elements. The association of dysgerminoma with gonadoblastoma is frequent, occurring in 50% of cases of gonadoblastoma.[154] Histologically, the other neoplastic germ cell elements may be intimately admixed with the dysgerminoma or may be found adjacent to the dysgerminoma and separated from it by a fibrous septum.

Clinical Behavior

Dysgerminoma is a malignant neoplasm capable of metastatic and local spread. Despite its less aggressive behavior and its marked radiosensitivity as compared with other malignant germ cell neoplasms, the malignant potential of dysgerminoma should not be minimized. Dysgerminoma is a rapidly growing neoplasm, but metastatic spread does not occur early in the course of the disease (although it is not possible to predict this in individual cases). When the tumor is small and freely mobile, its capsule is usually intact, but large tumors may be adherent to the surrounding structures or may rupture. Rupture may occur either spontaneously or at operation; this leads to spillage of the tumor contents and peritoneal implantation, causing serious consequences. Penetration of the ovarian surface by the tumor and formation of adhesions to surrounding structures may lead to direct extension by the tumor.

Metastatic spread occurs via the lymphatic system; the lymph nodes in the vicinity of the common iliac arteries and the terminal part of the abdominal aorta are first affected. Occasionally, there may be marked enlargement of these lymph nodes, with formation of large masses. Usually the enlargement is slight to moderate and can be detected by lymphangiography, computerized tomography (CT) scanning, or magnetic resonance imaging (MRI). In view of the superior results and fewer side effects with the last two methods, the use of lymphangiography, in this context, has been virtually abandoned in the developed countries. From the abdominal lymph nodes, the tumor spreads to the mediastinal and supraclavicular lymph nodes. Hematogenous spread to distant organs occurs later, and any organ may be affected, although involvement of the liver, lungs, and bones tends to be most common.[9,22,102] In cases of pure dysgerminoma, the metastases usually present a similar histologic appearance to the primary tumor, but occasionally tumors composed of pure dysgerminoma may be associated with metastases composed of other neoplastic germ cell elements. This metastatic pattern is observed much more commonly in combined tumors. It has been suggested that cellular tumors with small amounts of stroma, slight lymphocytic infiltration, and associated with cellular atypia and high mitotic activity tend to be more aggressive.[9] However, in view of the inconstancy of these findings, that is, marked histologic variations within the same tumor and its radiosensitivity and chemosensitivity, there is at present no good evidence that the behavior of an individual tumor can be assessed from its histologic appearance.[22] The presence of other neoplastic germ cell elements, however, has an adverse effect on prognosis.[9,22,83,123]

Dysgerminoma, similar to its testicular counterpart, the classic seminoma, is associated with elevated levels of serum lactic dehydrogenase (LDH) and its isoenzyme-1 (LDH-1). These substances can be used as tumor markers.[47,152] There is a good correlation between the volume of tumor tissue present and the serum levels of the enzymes. It has been shown that patients with testicular seminoma have elevated levels of serum placental alkaline phosphatase (Regan isoenzyme) (PLAP), but so far serum PLAP has not come into use as a tumor marker. On the other hand, because PLAP produces very distinctive membranous staining of dysgerminoma cells, it can be used immunocytochemically to confirm the diagnosis of dysgerminoma.[68]

The prognosis of patients with pure dysgerminoma is now considered to be very favorable. Although earlier reports indicated that the prognosis was poor and that the 5-year survival was only 27%,[102] more recent studies have reported a much better prognosis for pure dysgerminoma, with a 5-year survival of 75%–90%.[22,50,59,122,201] At the same time, the 5-year survival of patients with unilateral encapsulated dysgerminoma has been reported as greater than 90%,[9,22,50,122,201] although patients who were treated by unilateral salpingo-oophorectomy had 18%–52% recurrence rates. The recurrences were treated successfully with radiation therapy. Unfavorable prognostic features include presence of metastases at the time of diagnosis, presence of adhesions, spread into adjacent structures, bilaterality, and large size of the tumor.[59,123] It should be noted that even when these features are present many patients have been cured with radiotherapy or chemotherapy. Some investigators have considered patients younger than 20 years[123] as well as patients older than 40 years[123] to have a worse prognosis. More recent studies, however, do not regard age as an important prognostic factor.[9,22,50,122]

Eighty percent of recurrences occur in the first 2 years after diagnosis,[123] and it has been reported that more than 75% occur in the first year. In a few cases, recurrences occurred many years after excision of the original tumor, but this is very rare.

Treatment

Dysgerminoma, like its testicular counterpart the classic seminoma, is a highly radiosensitive tumor. It also responds very well to the combination chemotherapy of *cis*-diamino platinum, etopoxide (VP16), and bleomycin (BEP), which has been very successful in treatment of other malignant germ cell tumors. Until recently patients with bilateral or disseminated dysgerminoma, as well as patients with unilateral encapsulated tumors no longer desirous of having children, were treated by hysterectomy and bilateral salpingo-oophorectomy followed by radiation therapy to the abdominal and, in some centers, to the mediastinal lymph nodes. Nowadays, instead of radiation therapy such patients are treated with three to four cycles of combination chemotherapy with very good results.

For young women with unilateral encapsulated pure dysgerminoma, two different therapeutic approaches have been advocated. One consists of unilateral oophorectomy, or salpingo-oophorectomy, and careful follow-up of the patient. At one time wedge biopsy of the contralateral ovary was also advocated, but it has been abandoned because of the risk of damage to the ovary and decreased fertility. The second approach advocates similar surgical therapy, but to decrease and prevent metastases and recurrences, chemotherapy or radiotherapy is administered. The advantages of the first approach are that fertility is preserved and there are no genetic hazards associated with administration of chemotherapy or radiotherapy. Although the second approach tends to decrease the risk of metastases and recurrences,[22,190] this risk is not very serious especially because the metastases or recurrences can be treated successfully by combination chemotherapy if they develop.[9,22,50,122]

The conservative approach to the therapy of unilateral encapsulated dysgerminoma is recommended, but each individual case should be considered on its merits. It should be noted that before this mode of treatment can be considered, the opposite ovary must be normal, there should be no evidence of spread of the tumor in the abdominal cavity, and the abdominal and pelvic lymph nodes must be free from metastases on inspection, CT scanning, and MRI. In addition, the patient must be chromatin positive and have a normal female 46,XX karyotype.

In patients with widely disseminated metastases, administration of three to four cycles of combination chemotherapy composed of *cis*-diamino platinum, etopoxide (VP16), and bleomycin combination (BEP) has been successful in eradicating the disease.[50,122] The treatment of patients with dysgerminoma occurring in dysgenetic gonads must be hysterectomy and bilateral salpingo-gonadectomy in view of the high risk of development of bilateral neoplasms in these patients.[48] Furthermore, their gonads are hormonally and functionally inactive (see Chapter 1, Embryology of the Female Genital Tract and Disorders of Abnormal Sexual Development). Therefore, determination of the karyotype of all patients with dysgerminoma, especially those with evidence of virilization or developmental and menstrual abnormalities, is recommended. This is important in prepubertal patients, because these patients lack other signs of abnormal function, such as primary amenorrhea, virilization, and absence of normal sexual development. Following adnexectomy, patients are given hormone replacement therapy. Adequate treatment in these cases prevents development of a tumor in the opposite gonad.[48]

Yolk Sac Tumor

Histogenesis

Yolk sac tumor is a malignant germ cell neoplasm that is thought to arise from the undifferentiated and multipotential embryonal carcinoma by selective differentiation toward yolk sac or vitelline structures, in the same way as nongestational choriocarcinoma differentiates toward trophoblastic structures. The recognition and classification of yolk sac (endodermal sinus) tumor as a specific entity stems from the studies of Teilum, extending over nearly three decades.[195–197] The concepts regarding the histogenesis of this neoplasm that Teilum proposed have been supported by the experimental studies of the neoplastic rodent yolk sac by Pierce et al.[134]

In 1939, Schiller[150] described an ovarian neoplasm composed of clear and hobnail cells with a pattern that he designated a mesonephroma because of the presence of structures resembling immature glomeruli. Other investigators[71] were unable to demonstrate the mesonephric origin of this tumor and considered it an endothelioma of the ovary, as suggested earlier.[151] In 1946, Teilum[195] demonstrated that the tumor described as mesonephroma[150] included two distinct neoplasms with different histogenesis, histologic pattern, age distribution, and clinical behavior. One of these tumors was highly malignant, occurred in young patients, was homologous with certain testicular neoplasms, and was of germ cell origin.[195] The other tumor was less aggressive, occurred in older women, and ultimately was shown by Scully to be of müllerian-type origin. He designated this neoplasm *clear cell carcinoma*.

In addition to the terms mesonephroma and endothelioma, yolk sac tumors have been designated as embryonal carcinoma because of certain similarities to the embryonal carcinoma of the testis.[40] Although embryonal carcinoma showing the histologic pattern resembling the typical embryonal carcinoma of the testis[40] is seen occasionally in ovarian tumors,[82] most ovarian tumors of this type show a distinctive pattern with differentiation toward yolk sac or vitelline structures[197,198] and should be termed yolk sac tumor.

The term yolk sac tumor is more inclusive than the original term endodermal sinus tumor. Ovarian yolk sac tumor differs from the undifferentiated embryonal carcinoma[40] and resembles closely the yolk sac tumor of both infantile and adult testes.[177,197,198] It is now generally accepted that the term embryonal carcinoma should be used only to designate ovarian neoplasms showing the typical histologic pattern of the embryonal carcinoma as described in testicular tumors.[40,82] It is notable that most true ovarian embryonal carcinomas are combined with yolk sac tumor. The not infrequent combination of yolk sac tumor elements in ovarian tumors with other neoplastic germ cell elements[83,188] is one of the arguments in favor of the germ cell origin of this neoplasm. Yolk sac tumor, either pure or combined with other neoplastic germ cell elements, has been encountered in extragonadal locations where germ cell tumors are known to occur, in the mediastinum, the sacrococcygeal region, the pineal gland, and the vagina.

Alpha-fetoprotein (AFP), an alpha$_1$-globulin, was first identified as a specific constituent of normal human fetal serum by Bergstrand and Czar[19] in 1956. In the human embryo, serum AFP peaks at approximately 3000 mg/l at about 12–13 weeks of gestation. The level then decreases slowly until birth, when it is approximately 55 mg/l. After birth, AFP disappears rapidly from the serum, and 3 weeks after full-term delivery, it can be detected only in very small amounts (0–15 ng/ml) by radioimmunoassay or sensitive enzyme immunoassays. The sites of AFP synthesis in the human fetus and in other mammalian species have been studied by Gitlin et al.,[54] who demonstrated that during fetal life AFP is produced by the yolk sac, liver, and upper gastrointestinal tract. They also demonstrated that AFP synthesis commences in the yolk sac. In recent years there has been considerable interest in the histologic aspects of germ cell neoplasms associated with elevated serum AFP, and it has been demonstrated that germ cell tumors in patients with elevated serum AFP either are composed entirely of or contain yolk sac tumor elements.[110,189] Table 20.2 shows the results of preoperative serum AFP determinations in patients with ovarian germ cell tumors. Elevation of serum AFP has not been observed in patients with pure dysgerminoma or seminoma of the testis,[189] mature cystic teratoma of the ovary,[189] or pure gonadoblastoma.[189] Slight elevations of serum AFP have been noted in occasional cases of immature teratoma of the ovary; this is most likely caused by neuroepithelium, related to the neural tube defects associated with elevations of serum AFP in pregnancy.

Apart from yolk sac tumor, elevated levels of serum AFP are seen in patients with hepatoid carcinoma of the ovary and occasional Sertoli–Leydig cell tumors, especially those showing a retiform pattern.[180,184,217] Slightly elevated levels of serum AFP up to 60 ng/ml (upper limit of normal serum AFP, 20 ng/ml) have been observed in some cases of embryonal carcinoma of the testis.[189] Using immuno-

Table 20.2. Serum AFP in patients with ovarian germ cell tumors measured by radioimmunoassay[a]

	No. of cases	*Serum AFP*
Mixed germ cell tumors containing EST	39	Elevated
Pure EST	23	Elevated
Pure dysgerminoma	25	Normal
Dysgerminoma with syncytiotrophoblastic giant cells	4	Normal
Teratoma (immature and mature)	12	Normal
Teratoma (immature and mature) with dysgerminoma	8	Normal
Mature cystic teratoma (dermoid cyst)	15	Normal

[a]Unpublished data.
AFP, alpha-fetoprotein; EST, endodermal sinus tumor.

fluorescent and immunoperoxidase techniques, AFP has been identified in the cells of yolk sac tumor and embryonal carcinoma of the ovary,[68,82] and in the eosinophilic, PAS-positive, diastase-resistant globules present both inside and outside the tumor cells. Large amounts of AFP have been extracted from tumor tissue in yolk sac tumors of the ovary and testis.[188] The results of these studies indicate that yolk sac tumor elements are associated with AFP synthesis.

In view of the fact that normal yolk sac in the human and other mammalian species has been shown to be associated with AFP synthesis,[56] it is reasonable to assume that the selective synthesis of AFP by yolk sac tumors provides further support to the view that yolk sac tumor develops as a result of differentiation of primitive malignant germ cell elements in the direction of yolk sac or vitelline structures.[68,81,183,189] The immunocytochemical localization of AFP in embryonal carcinoma and in areas of yolk sac tumor showing no morphologic evidence of yolk sac differentiation suggests that the biochemical manifestations of yolk sac differentiation, such as AFP synthesis, precede morphologic differentiation.[68,82]

Prevalence

Although originally yolk sac tumor was considered very rare, it is being diagnosed with much greater frequency nowadays and is the second most common malignant ovarian germ cell neoplasm after dysgerminoma. Yolk sac tumor often occurs in pure form, but it is also a frequent component of mixed malignant germ cell tumors. More than 350 cases have been reported.[51,81,188] It is one of the most common malignant ovarian neoplasms of childhood, adolescence, and early adult life.[68]

Although most reports discuss Caucasians, yolk sac tumor has been encountered in other races.[51,68,81] The reported age distribution of patients with yolk sac tumor ranges from 16 months to 46 years, but most patients have been under 30 years of age.[51,68,81] Yolk sac tumor is encountered most frequently in the second and third decades, followed by first and fourth, and is rare in women in the fifth decade. Yolk sac tumor of the ovary has been encountered in occasional postmenopausal patients. As ovarian surface epithelial–stromal tumor associated with yolk sac tumor occurs in elderly patients,[98,107,145] it is possible that such cases were examples of this entity. Although the histogenesis of the yolk sac component of these tumors is uncertain, the likely explanation is that it originates from the surface epithelium by a process of neoplastic differentiation or transformation and therefore the histogenesis is totally different from that of germ cell neoplasms.[98,145]

Clinical Features

The symptomatology of yolk sac tumor is nonspecific. Most patients have symptoms of abdominal enlargement and pain and present with a lower abdominal or pelvic mass.[51,68,81] Occasionally, the symptoms are acute and severe and may lead to the diagnosis of acute appendicitis or a ruptured ectopic pregnancy; this usually is caused by torsion of the tumor. A number of cases have been encountered during pregnancy.[68,81] The presence of yolk sac tumor is not associated with endocrine symptoms, although endocrine symptoms may be present if the tumor is combined with choriocarcinoma.[68,81] Such neoplasms are classified as mixed germ cell tumors. On clinical examination, a tumor mass is usually palpable and is frequently of considerable size.[51,68,81] Increased levels of AFP are found in sera of patients with yolk sac tumor,[51,110,188] and this is considered a useful diagnostic test for the presence of yolk sac tumor elements in the primary tumor, its metastases, and recurrences.[188,189]

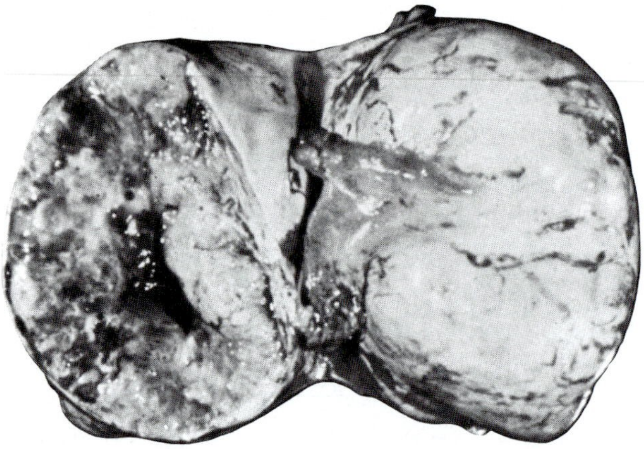

Fig. 20.11. Yolk sac tumor. The tumor is oval shaped, encapsulated, with a central area of cystic degeneration. (Courtesy of R.E. Scully, M.D., Boston, MA.)

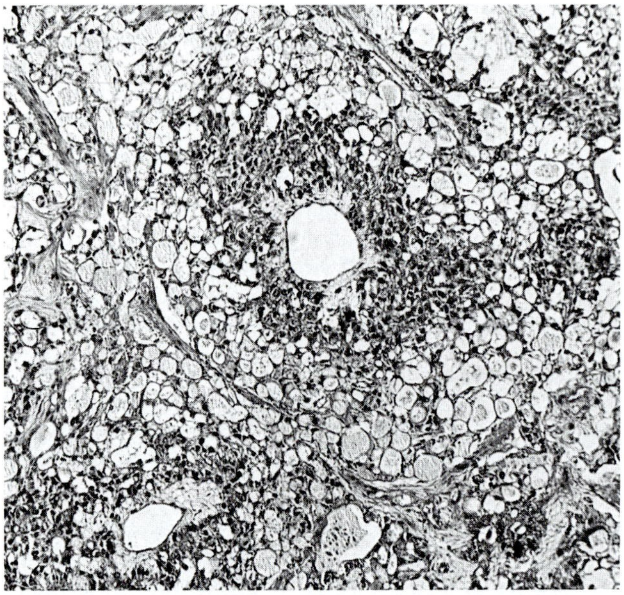

Fig. 20.12. Yolk sac tumor, microcystic pattern. A labyrinthine structure composed of tumor cells radiating around a blood vessel resembling a perivascular formation is seen in the *center*.

Gross Findings

Yolk sac tumors are almost always unilateral.[51,68,81,188] Bilaterality typically is a manifestation of metastatic spread. Yolk sac tumor shows a certain predilection for the right ovary.[68,81] The tumor is usually large, varying in size from 3 to 30 cm in diameter, with most tumors measuring more than 10 cm.[68,81,188] It frequently weighs more than 500 g; tumors weighing 5 kg have been recorded. The tumors are usually encapsulated, round, oval, or globular; firm, smooth, or somewhat lobulated; and gray-yellow, with areas of hemorrhage and cystic or gelatinous changes (Fig. 20.11). The tumor may form adhesions to the surrounding structures and invade them. On sectioning, yolk sac tumors are mainly solid, but cystic spaces frequently are present. The fluid present in the cysts also may be gelatinous. Necrosis and hemorrhage and the presence of other neoplastic germ cell elements, especially teratoma, may alter the appearance of the tumor.

Microscopic Findings

Yolk sac tumors exhibit a wide range of histologic patterns that differ considerably from each other and, although all the different patterns are frequently observed in the same tumor, one or two may predominate. The following histologic patterns may be observed in yolk sac tumor: (1) microcystic, (2) endodermal sinus, (3) solid, (4) alveolar-glandular, (5) polyvesicular vitelline, (6) myxomatous, (7) papillary, (8) macrocystic, (9) hepatoid, and (10) glandular or primitive endodermal (intestinal).

The polyvesicular vitelline, the hepatoid, and the primitive endodermal (intestinal) patterns tend to occur in pure form, unassociated with other yolk sac tumor elements forming a yolk sac tumor exhibiting a single histologic pattern. Although such tumors are rare, they pose considerable diagnostic difficulties, and because of this they have been classified as specific subtypes of yolk sac tumor in the revised WHO classification of ovarian neoplasms[156] (see Table 20.1).

The first five histologic patterns were described by Teilum.[198] Microcystic (Fig. 20.12) and myxomatous (Fig. 20.13) patterns are composed of a loose vacuolated network with small cystic spaces or microcysts forming a honeycomb pattern. The microcysts are lined by flat, pleomorphic, mesothelial-like cells with large hyperchromatic or vesicular nuclei that show brisk mitotic activity. There is usually some variation in the size of the cysts (Fig. 20.12). In the underlying capillary spaces, hematopoiesis may be seen. The vacuolated network may contain pale, PAS-positive, mucinous material forming small lakes or precipitates as well as small, round, brightly eosinophilic, PAS-positive, diastase-resistant globules or droplets. These globules are also found within the cytoplasm of the tumor cells (Fig. 20.14). Areas composed of fine, loose myxomatous tissue containing alveolar spaces (Fig. 20.15), occasional gland-like structures lined by cuboidal epithelium (Fig. 20.16), and small cellular aggregates, often merging with the microcystic or other patterns, are also present (Fig. 20.17). The loose myxomatous pattern was considered to be analogous to the magma reticulare or the extraembryonic mesoderm of the exocoelom,

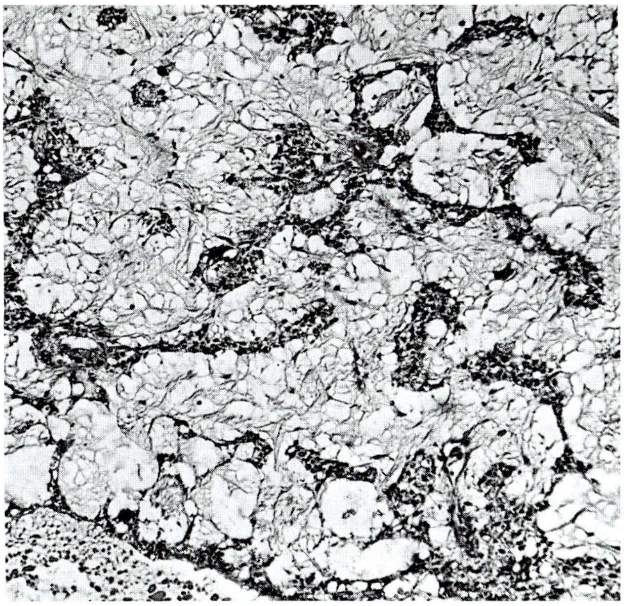

Fig. 20.13. Yolk sac tumor, myxomatous pattern. Small collections of epithelial-like cells forming strands or glandlike structures are seen within myxomatous tissue.

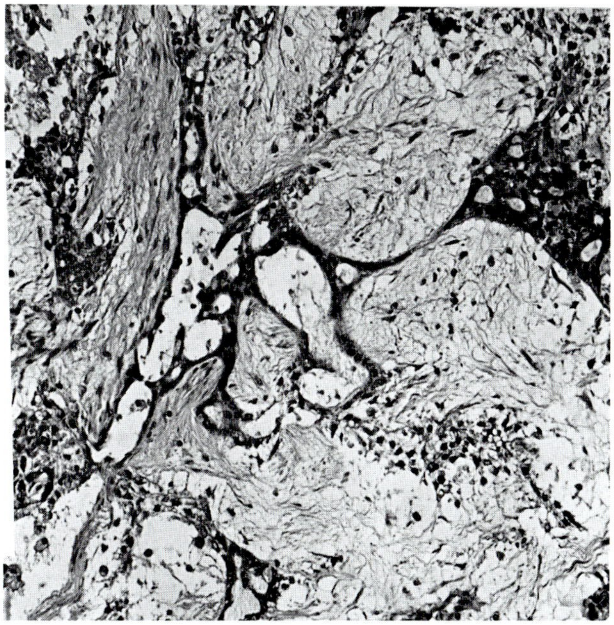

Fig. 20.15. Yolk sac tumor. The tumor is composed of myxomatous tissue containing glandular and alveolar spaces and channels.

and the presence of this pattern led to the recognition of the mesoblastic nature of this tumor.[196]

These two histologic patterns should be considered as separate principal patterns. Endodermal sinus pattern (Fig. 20.18) is composed of perivascular formations, consisting of a narrow band of connective tissue with a capillary blood vessel in the center and lined by a layer of cuboidal or low columnar embryonal epithelial-like cells. The cells have large, slightly vesicular nuclei, prominent nucleoli, and show mitotic activity. The surrounding capsular sinusoid space is lined by a single layer of flat

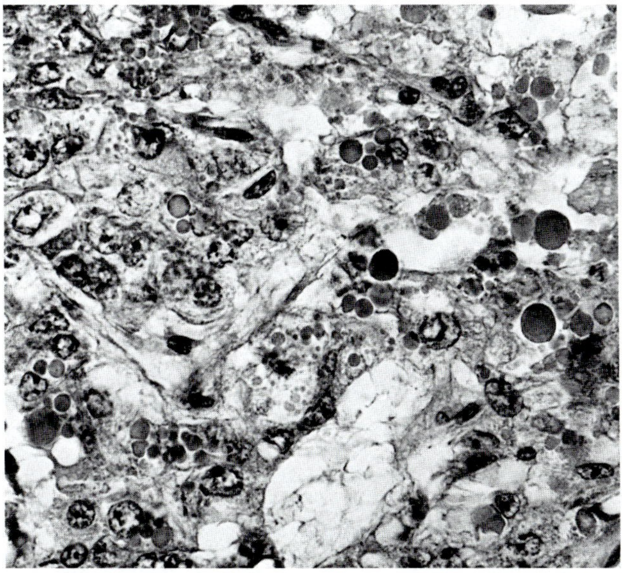

Fig. 20.14. Yolk sac tumor. Numerous round hyaline globules are present both inside and outside the cells. Larger precipitates of this material are seen at the *upper right.*

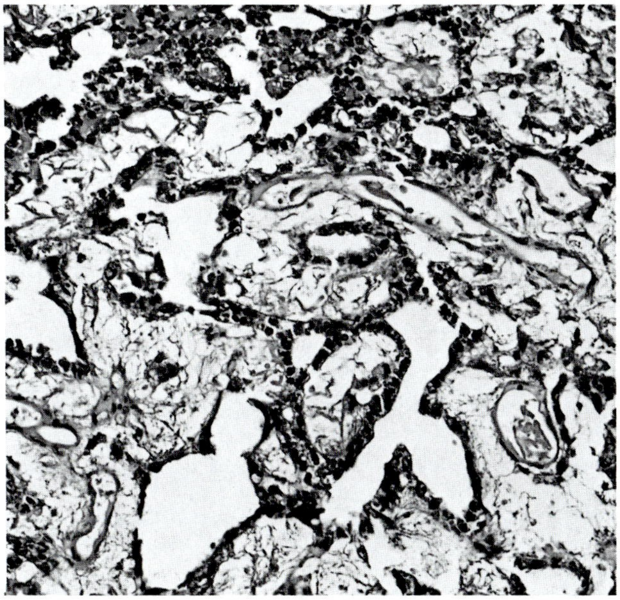

Fig. 20.16. Endodermal sinus tumor, glandulas-alveolar and myxomatous pattern. Numerous cavities and channels are present. Note hyaline material at *top left.*

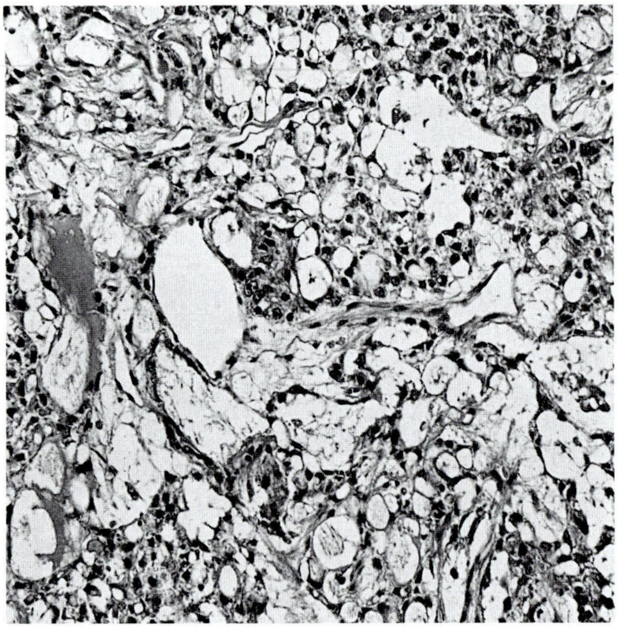

Fig. 20.17. Yolk sac tumor. Small cellular aggregates, microcysts, and myxomatous tissue are present. Mucinous material also is seen.

cells with prominent hyperchromatic nuclei. These characteristic perivascular formations are said to recapitulate the so-called endodermal sinuses[197,198] that, although not conspicuous in the human placenta, are well-defined embryologic structures in the rat placenta. These structures are also known as sinuses of Duval, Schiller–Duval bodies, or glomerulus-like structures and resemble superficially immature renal glomeruli. When sectioned longitudinally, the perivascular structures consist of a central connective tissue core containing a longitudinal vessel surrounded by epithelial-like cells that often form small papillary formations projecting into the surrounding capsular sinusoid space.

The presence of these perivascular formations or Schiller–Duval bodies can be considered diagnostic of yolk sac tumor, but in some tumors they may be poorly represented, somewhat atypical, or absent. Although the tumor should always be examined carefully and searched to identify these structures, their absence does not preclude the diagnosis, if the appearances of the tumor are typical in all other respects. Apart from the presence of the perivascular structures, this pattern consists of a complicated labyrinth of communicating cavities and channels. In addition, there are papillary processes and blood vessels surrounded by narrow connective tissue cores and epithelial-like cells radiating into the surrounding stroma, resembling the typical perivascular formations but differing from them by the absence of the sinusoid space (see Fig. 20.12).

The solid pattern (Fig. 20.19) is composed of aggregates of small epithelial-like polygonal cells with clear cytoplasm and large vesicular or pyknotic nuclei with prominent nucleoli and exhibits brisk mi-

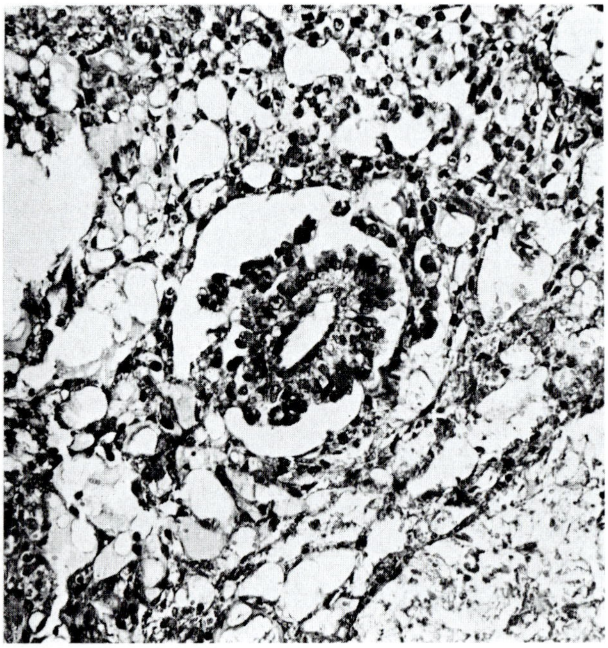

Fig. 20.18. Yolk sac tumor. A typical perivascular formation (Schiller–Duval body) is illustrated.

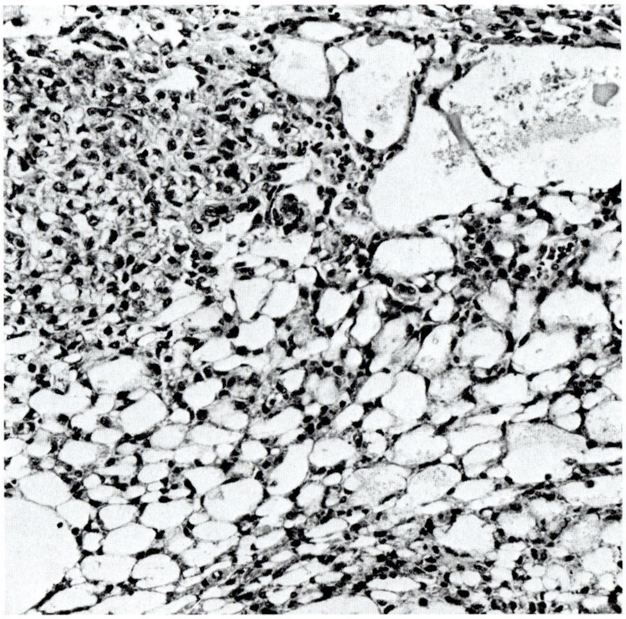

Fig. 20.19. Yolk sac tumor, solid and microcystic patterns. Some larger cysts (macrocysts) are seen at *top right*.

totic activity. The tumor cells in the solid aggregates may resemble dysgerminoma cells, but they usually show greater cellular and nuclear pleomorphism and presence of at least occasional microcysts (Fig. 20.19). The presence of the latter helps to differentiate between these two entities. The presence of other patterns of yolk sac tumor is also helpful in this respect, as is diffuse or focal staining for AFP and uniformly positive staining for cytokeratin, which are observed in yolk sac tumor and not in dysgerminoma.

The alveolar-glandular pattern (Figs. 20.16 and 20.20) is composed of alveolar, glandlike, or larger cystic spaces and cavities lined by flat or cuboidal epithelial-like cells with large, prominent nuclei and surrounded by myxomatous stroma or cellular aggregates. Some of these spaces may be lined by more than one layer of cells, and sometimes the lining cells form small papillary projections protruding into the lumen. The layer of cells lining these spaces may be continuous with the lining of the perivascular sinusoid spaces.[197] Glandlike formations lined by columnar or cuboidal epithelial-like cells may be seen and in some tumors may be prominent and may form bizarre patterns (see Fig. 20.15).

The polyvesicular vitelline pattern[198] is composed of numerous cysts or vesicles surrounded by compact connective tissue stroma (Figs. 20.21 and 20.22). The vesicles are lined partly by columnar or cuboidal epithelial cells, frequently showing basal or paraluminal vacuolation, and partly by flat mesothelial-like cells (Fig. 20.22). The individual vesicles or cysts vary in size and shape. The wall of the cyst may show a constriction dividing the part lined by the mesothelial cells from that lined by the

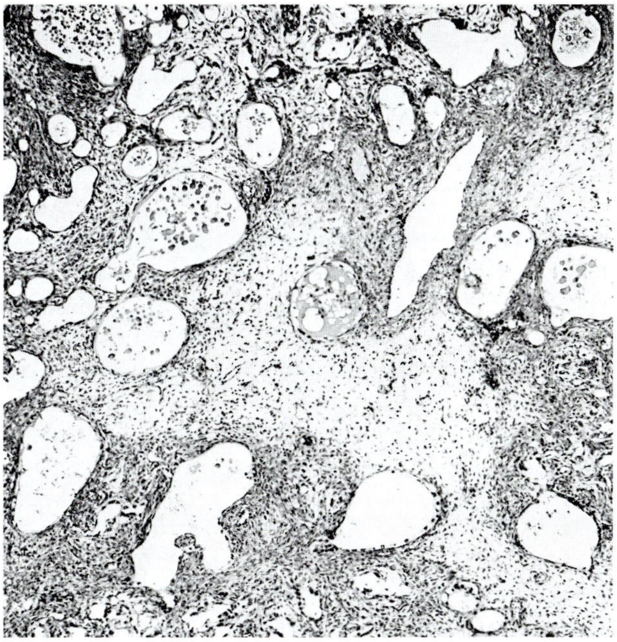

Fig. 20.21. Yolk sac tumor, polyvesicular vitelline pattern. The tumor is composed of numerous small vesicles surrounded by connective tissue.

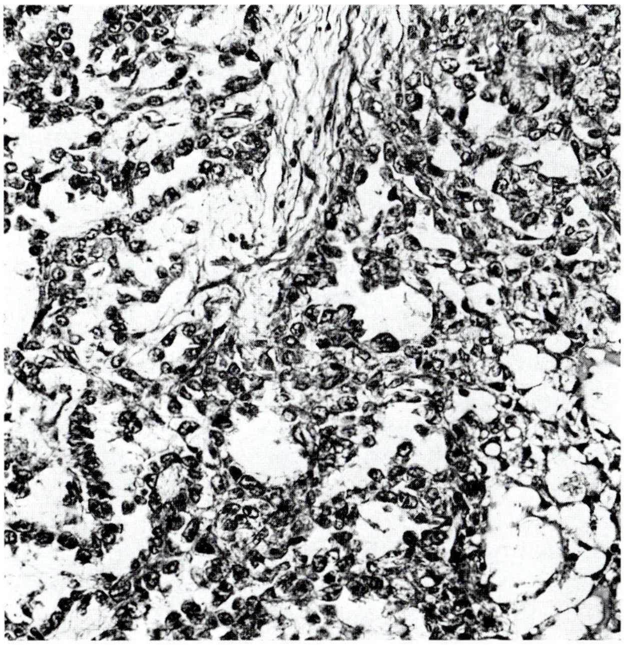

Fig. 20.20. Yolk sac tumor, glandular alveolar pattern. Note the alveoli lined by epithelial-like cells (*left* and *center*).

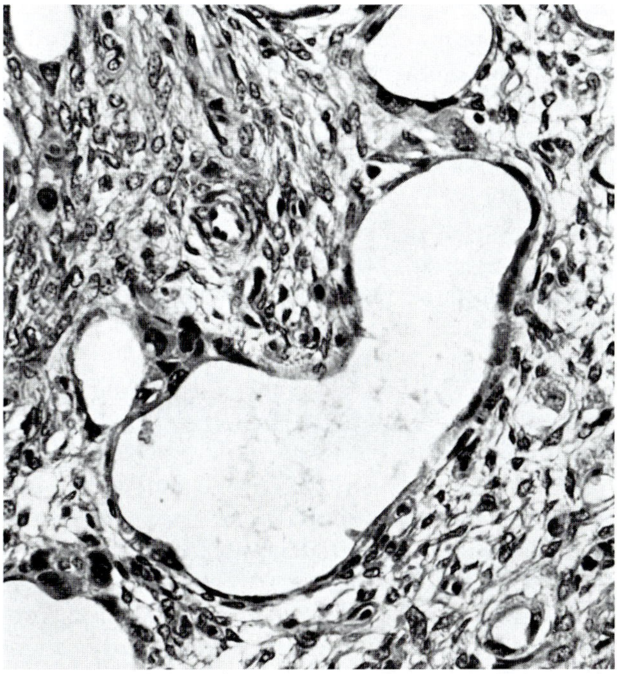

Fig. 20.22. Yolk sac tumor, polyvesicular vitelline pattern. A typical vesicle is surrounded by cellular stroma.

columnar or cuboidal epithelium (Fig. 20.22). This division was considered to reflect the embryologic conversion of the primary yolk sac into the secondary yolk sac.[198] Occasionally, the whole tumor may exhibit the polyvesicular vitelline pattern; such tumors have been designated as polyvesicular vitelline tumors.[198]

The eosinophilic, hyaline droplets may be present either within the tumor cells or outside them; they may be numerous and prominent in some tumors (see Fig. 20.14). The droplets may be observed in tumors exhibiting all the histologic patterns described, and their identification is a helpful diagnostic feature. However, their presence is not diagnostic of yolk sac tumor because they are observed in many malignant, often poorly differentiated neoplasms. The droplets are considered to be secreted by the tumor cells and accumulate within the cytoplasm. As the amount of secretion increases, the cell becomes distended and ruptures, discharging its contents into the surrounding tissue. Recently, the significance of these globules in yolk sac tumor has been enhanced further by demonstrating with immunofluorescent and immunoperoxidase techniques that some contain AFP.[68,81,160] Other globules may contain alpha$_1$-antitrypsin and other plasma proteins such as transferrin.[68,160,204]

The presence of hyaline, PAS-positive material forming bands or connective tissue cores surrounded by tumor cells is not an infrequent finding in yolk sac tumor; in some tumors, it may be a prominent feature, with the tumor cells resting on and surrounding the bands of hyaline material (Fig. 20.23). There may be an increased amount of the eosinophilic, PAS-positive globules described here in the vicinity of the hyaline bands, suggesting a relationship between them and a possibility of common origin.[198] The hyaline, PAS-positive material in yolk sac tumor has been found to be similar to the hyaline material produced by mouse teratocarcinoma during its conversion to the ascitic form, and this is considered to be a strong argument in favor of the yolk sac origin of the tumor.[129,130,134] When examined with the electron microscope, the cells of yolk sac tumor resemble those of the normal human yolk sac.[58,68,106]

In addition to the five histologic patterns already described, five additional patterns merit consideration as specific patterns. The myxomatous pattern (see Fig. 20.13), which Teilum[198] combined with the microcystic, may be observed on its own or may predominate. The papillary pattern (Fig. 20.23) is composed of papillary structures consisting of connective tissue cores lined by epithelial-like cells showing a considerable degree of cellular and nuclear pleomorphism and mitotic activity. The connective tissue may show variable hyalinization (Fig. 20.24). This pattern may be the predominant pattern within a tumor. The macrocystic pattern is observed when yolk sac tumor exhibits larger cysts in contrast to microcysts or alveolar spaces. In some tumors, this pattern may predominate.

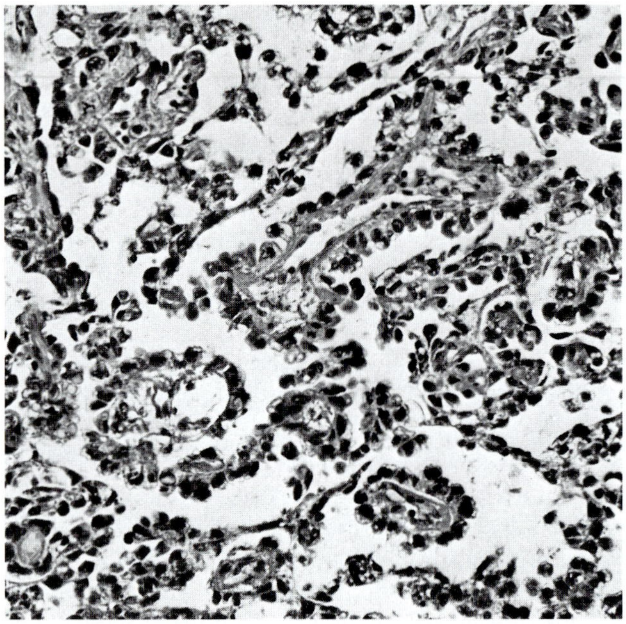

Fig. 20.23. Yolk sac tumor, papillary pattern. The papillae are composed of hyaline material lined by tumor cells.

The hepatoid pattern is composed of cells with eosinophilic, uniform, or granular cytoplasm, showing a solid pattern and considerable resemblance to hepatocytes. This pattern was considered by Teilum[198] as a variant of the solid pattern. Although such collections of hepatocyte-like cells are not infrequently observed in yolk sac tumors, tumors composed entirely or predominantly of such cells have been designated as hepatoid yolk sac tumors[135] or yolk sac tumors with hepatoid pattern (Figs. 20.25 and 20.26). These tumors are admixed only infrequently with other histologic patterns of yolk sac tumor or other neoplastic germ cell elements, and this, together with the rarity of the tumor, may cause diagnostic problems. The presence of a solid ovarian tumor composed of hepatocyte-like cells surrounded by connective tissue and forming solid aggregates, cords, or clusters and associated with elevated serum AFP in a young patient would strongly favor a diagnosis of yolk sac tumor with a hepatoid pattern.

The glandular or primitive endodermal (intestinal) pattern, in which the tumor is composed en-

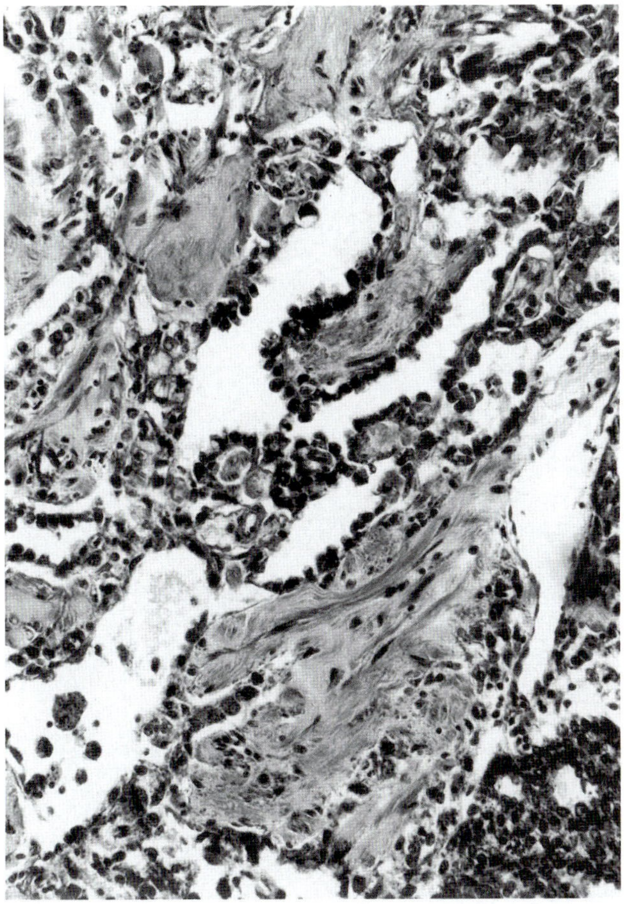

Fig. 20.24. **Yolk sac tumor, papillary pattern.** Broad papillae are composed of fibrous tissue with only slight hyalinization.

tirely of primitive endodermal glands, is encountered occasionally[34] (Fig. 20.27). This pattern has been designated as glandular (intestinal) yolk sac tumor. The tumor in these cases is composed of nests or collections of primitive endodermal glands surrounded by connective tissue, which varies from loose and edematous to dense and hyalinized. The degree of differentiation varies from primitive to relatively well differentiated. The glands may contain inspissated secretion within the lumen, and the tumor may resemble a mucin-secreting adenocarcinoma. Ultrastructurally, the nuclei are large and show prominent nucleolonema, whereas the cytoplasm contains many ribosomes, rough endoplasmic reticulum, and mitochondria. Dense amorphous intracellular material is also present. Yolk sac tumors showing this pattern have been associated with very high levels of serum AFP.[34]

The presence of primitive endodermal glandular tissue, lobular or nestlike pattern, and high levels of serum AFP differentiate this type of yolk sac tumor from mucinous tumors of the ovary. A variant of this pattern composed of primitive glands of various sizes lined by tall columnar or cuboid cells with basophilic or clear cytoplasm containing subnuclear vacuoles resembling secretory endometrial carcinoma, so-called endometrioid variant (Fig. 20.28), has been described.[33] This variant may be seen in pure form, showing a pronounced glandular or villoglandular pattern, or may be composed of glands surrounded by fibrous or densely cellular stroma.[33] Elevated levels of serum AFP and immunocytochemical demonstration of AFP within the tumor cells confirm the diagnosis of yolk sac tumor.

Occasionally, yolk sac tumor may exhibit a greater degree of cellular and nuclear pleomorphism with some giant cells, usually mononucleated, but sometimes multinucleated. This picture may be seen in association with the solid, papillary, and glandular-alveolar patterns. The pleomorphic cells show variable immunocytochemical staining for AFP, and the absence of hCG confirms that the

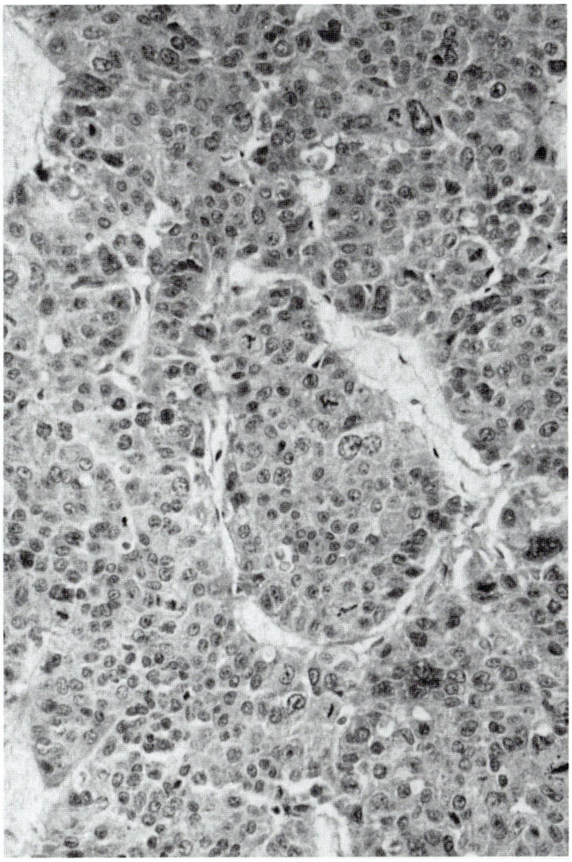

Fig. 20.25. **Yolk sac tumor, hepatoid pattern.** The tumor is composed of solid aggregates or cords of polygonal cells with even or granular eosinophilic cytoplasm resembling hepatocytes. Note brisk mitotic activity.

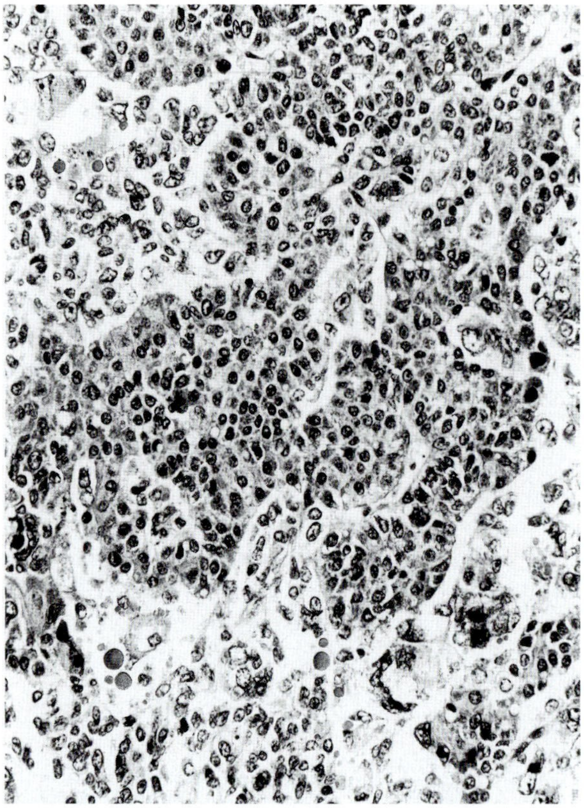

Fig. 20.26. Yolk sac tumor, hepatoid pattern. The appearances are more primitive and less orderly than in Fig. 20.25.

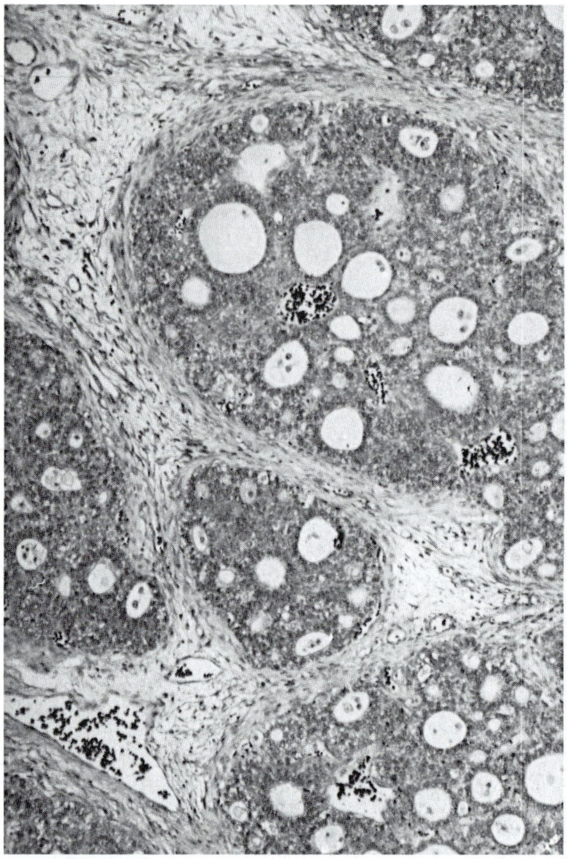

Fig. 20.27. Yolk sac tumor, endodermal (intestinal) pattern. The tumor is composed of nests of primitive endodermal cells forming glands or solid aggregates, which are surrounded by connective tissue.

giant cells are not trophoblastic in origin but are part of a yolk sac tumor.

Differential Diagnosis

Yolk sac tumor may be confused with clear cell carcinoma, embryonal carcinoma, and dysgerminoma. The clear cell tumors of the ovary show more regular tubular patterns, lack the honeycomb network composed of microcysts, and have papillary frond-like projections that are often lined by clear or hobnail cells. The typical perivascular formations, endodermal sinuses, or Schiller–Duval bodies present in yolk sac tumor are absent. The epithelial cells lining the tubules are cuboidal with clear cytoplasm or are hobnail with nuclei bulging into the lumen. Areas composed of large polygonal cells with clear cytoplasm and small, dark, uniform, centrally situated nuclei resembling those of renal carcinoma are present. Because these cells line cystic spaces, they frequently proliferate in a papillary fashion or form solid aggregates. When the clear cell carcinoma is composed entirely of tubules or spaces, confusion may arise with the polyvesicular vitelline pattern. However, the epithelial lining is usually composed of the projecting hobnail cells and not of the two types of epithelia seen in the vesicles forming the polyvesicular vitelline pattern. The cystic spaces are more tubular and less vesicle like. The clear cell tumors occur also in other parts of the female genital tract, usually occurring in older patients.

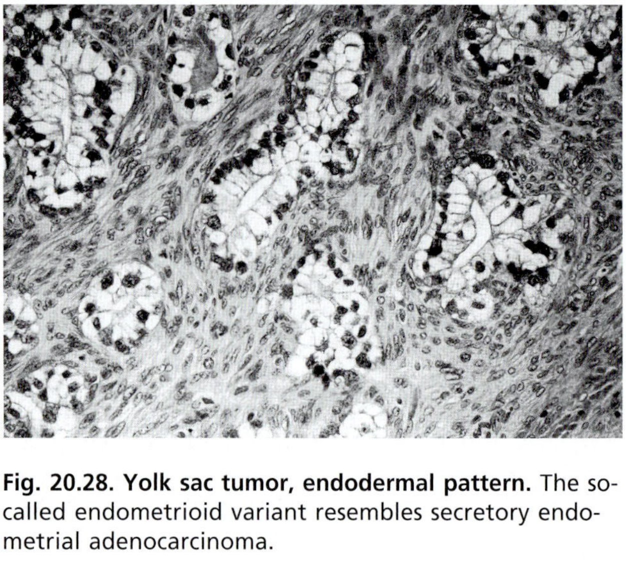

Fig. 20.28. Yolk sac tumor, endodermal pattern. The so-called endometrioid variant resembles secretory endometrial adenocarcinoma.

The embryonal carcinoma, which is uncommon in the ovary,[82,188,197] lacks the specific patterns observed in the yolk sac tumor. In its undifferentiated form, it is composed of aggregates of primitive embryonal cells. The tumor cells are frequently larger than those seen in the solid cellular aggregates in yolk sac tumor. The cytoplasm is more granular, there is more marked cellular and nuclear pleomorphism, and the nucleoli are more prominent. Even when the tumor is somewhat better differentiated, with the embryonal cells forming cords, tubules, or papillae and lining clefts or spaces, it still lacks the typical patterns associated with yolk sac tumor.

The cells of yolk sac tumor are uniformly cytokeratin positive.[100,101] The presence of this feature as well as positive staining for AFP differentiates between yolk sac tumor showing solid pattern and dysgerminoma, with which it may be confused and which shows only occasional cytokeratin-positive cells. The cells of dysgerminoma are usually more uniform, lack microcysts, and are usually associated with lymphocytic and granulomatous reactions.

Yolk sac tumor, because of its cystic pattern and the presence of numerous small blood vessels, has been confused with vascular tumors, but careful examination reveals that the pattern is more cystic and the absence of a true vascular pattern is confirmed by reticulum stains. It should be pointed out in this context that yolk sac tumor elements are sometimes intimately associated with immature vascular tissue in some mixed germ cell tumors and that this may also contribute to the diagnostic problem. The presence of positive immunocytochemical staining for vimentin, CD 31, CD 34, and factor VIII further confirms the presence of vascular tissue, whereas positive staining for cytokeratin favors yolk sac tumor. Confusion may arise occasionally, with some Sertoli–Leydig cell tumors showing a retiform pattern.[180,217] The presence of more marked cellular and nuclear pleomorphism, brisk mitotic activity, the presence of other histologic patterns observed in yolk sac tumor, and their absence in Sertoli–Leydig cell tumors aid in the differential diagnosis.

Occasionally, confusion may arise with juvenile granulosa cell tumor when it presents with small vesicle-like collections of cells surrounded by connective tissue stroma that simulate the vesicles seen in polyvesicular vitelline yolk sac tumor. Presence of solid nests typical of juvenile granulosa cell tumor, absence of the various patterns of yolk sac tumor, absence of immunocytochemical staining for AFP, and a lack of elevated levels of serum AFP indicate that the tumor is a juvenile granulosa cell tumor. Presence of positive alpha inhibin further confirms the diagnosis of the latter.

Clinical Behavior

Yolk sac tumor of the ovary is a highly malignant neoplasm, metastasizing early and invading the surrounding structures and organs. Local invasion and intracoelomic spread frequently lead to extensive involvement of the abdominal cavity by tumor deposits. Yolk sac tumor metastasizes first via the lymphatic system to the paraaortic and common iliac lymph nodes and then to the mediastinal and supraclavicular lymph nodes. Hematogenous spread occurs later, with metastases found in the lungs, liver, and other organs. The tumor is aggressive locally, and spread beyond the ovary is observed in a number of patients at the time of operation.[51,68,81,188] Recurrences in the pelvis are frequent, even when the tumor and the affected adnexa have been excised completely.[68,81,188] Such recurrences usually appear within a few weeks or months after excision of the primary tumor.

Treatment

Until the advent of efficacious combination chemotherapy, the treatment of patients with yolk sac tumor was disappointing. The treatment was primarily surgical,[81,197] because yolk sac tumor is not sensitive to radiation therapy. Extensive surgery was not justified as it did not improve prognosis.[81,197] The small number of long-term survivors in the past were mainly patients with tumors confined to the ovary, most of whom were treated by unilateral adnexectomy.[81,197] In recent years, there has been marked improvement in prognosis with conservative surgery (unilateral salpingo-oophorectomy) and adjuvant multiagent combination chemotherapy.[50,122,188] The combination chemotherapy originally used was dactinomycin, vincristine, and cyclophosphamide or dactinomycin, 5-fluorouracil, and cyclophosphamide. Although this therapy proved to be effective in many cases, the number of tumors that recurred was still high.

The introduction of a combination of *cis*-platinum, bleomycin, and vinblastine, which has now been superseded by *cis*-platinum, etopoxide (VP 16), and bleomycin (BEP) in combination, has been found to be much more effective and has produced remissions in patients with advanced-stage disease and in patients in whom other combinations of multiagent chemotherapy have failed.[50,122] This combination chemotherapy has revolutionized the treatment of patients with yolk sac tumor. Complete cure for all stages is now more than 80%.[50,122] The occasional cases of pure hepatoid and glandular (primitive intestinal) yolk sac tumor show a less satisfactory response to combination chemotherapy and are therefore associated with a poorer prognosis.[33,34,135] It is of interest that the only tumor that was diploid in a series of 20 yolk sac tumors was a tumor of the pure glandular (primitive intestinal) type whereas all the other tumors were aneuploid.[79]

Serum AFP determination is a useful diagnostic test in patients with yolk sac tumor. It is also of value in monitoring the results of therapy and for early detection of metastases and recurrences. It should be noted, however, that a normal result may not always indicate the absence of active disease but only the absence of the tumor element associated with AFP synthesis. Preoperatively, if the tumor contains yolk sac tumor elements, the AFP can be detected in the serum. AFP levels fall postoperatively and, if there are no metastases, reach normal levels within 4–6 weeks, depending on the preoperative serum AFP level. The use of serial serum AFP estimations for diagnosis, monitoring of therapy, and early detection of metastases and recurrences in patients with tumors containing yolk sac tumor elements is of considerable value in management and highly recommended.

It has been shown by Gitlin and Pericelli[55] that, apart from AFP, normal human yolk sac synthesizes a number of other proteins, and their presence has been demonstrated by immunofluorescence within yolk sac tumor.[160,204] One of these proteins, alpha$_1$-antitrypsin, has been studied serially together with AFP in sera of a number of patients with yolk sac tumor.[187,204] Although it was found to be capable of monitoring disease activity, it was shown to be inferior to AFP in this respect.[187]

Human chorionic gonadotropin (hCG) and its beta subunit (beta-hCG) have been found to be normal in patients with yolk sac tumor. Carcinoembryonic antigen (CEA) has also been studied in patients with germ cell neoplasms and has been found to be of no value as a tumor marker in this group of patients.[191] Estrogen and progesterone receptors are not detected in yolk sac tumors.[78]

Embryonal Carcinoma

The term *embryonal carcinoma* in this text includes only ovarian neoplasms showing histologic appearances resembling those observed in embryonal carcinomas occurring in the testis of adults. Dixon and Moore[40] consider embryonal carcinoma as both a morphologic and a conceptual entity, and this interpretation is being followed. Embryonal carcinoma is considered to be the least differentiated form of germ cell tumor, which may differentiate either toward somatic structures (teratomatous tumors of various degrees of differentiation) or toward extraembryonal structures, forming yolk sac or vitelline structures (yolk sac tumor) or trophoblastic structures (choriocarcinoma) (see Fig. 20.1). Although ovarian embryonal carcinoma[68,82] shows similar appearances and is considered to be homologous with its testicular counterpart, it is uncommon as a component of mixed germ cell tumors and rare as a pure entity. However, tumors showing this histologic pattern are relatively frequent in the testis. The reason for this difference is unknown.

Ovarian embryonal carcinoma is usually combined with other neoplastic germ cell elements, most frequently yolk sac tumor, and forms a part of a mixed germ cell tumor.[68,83,188] Embryonal carcinoma occasionally has been observed in association with gonadoblastoma.[154,176,181]

Clinical Features

The age incidence, clinical presentation, and findings of embryonal carcinoma are similar to those observed in patients with other malignant germ cell neoplasms, such as yolk sac tumor, immature teratoma, and dysgerminoma, with the tumor occurring in children and young adults.[68,82,188]

Embryonal carcinoma may produce AFP, even when it is not combined with yolk sac tumor (YST), but the serum AFP levels in such cases are only slightly elevated. When embryonal carcinoma contains syncytiotrophoblastic giant cells, as is often the case, or is combined with choriocarcinoma, it produces hCG and is associated with endocrine manifestations, such as isosexual precocious puberty in children and abnormal vaginal bleeding in adults.[82] A positive pregnancy test is found in almost all such patients.

Gross Findings

Because embryonal carcinoma usually is a component of mixed germ cell tumors, the appearances of the tumor vary according to the type and amount of the different components present. On sectioning, the embryonal carcinomatous component is solid, gray-white, and slightly granular, with foci of necrosis and hemorrhage in the larger tumors (Fig. 20.29).

Microscopic Findings

In its most primitive and undifferentiated form, embryonal carcinoma is composed of solid aggregates of epithelial-like, medium to large, polygonal or ovoid cells containing an ample amount of somewhat pale eosinophilic granular cytoplasm, with poorly defined cytoplasmic borders, frequently forming a syncytial arrangement (Fig. 20.30). The cells have a large, prominent, centrally situated, and somewhat irregular vesicular or hyperchromatic nucleus with a fine nuclear membrane and frequently

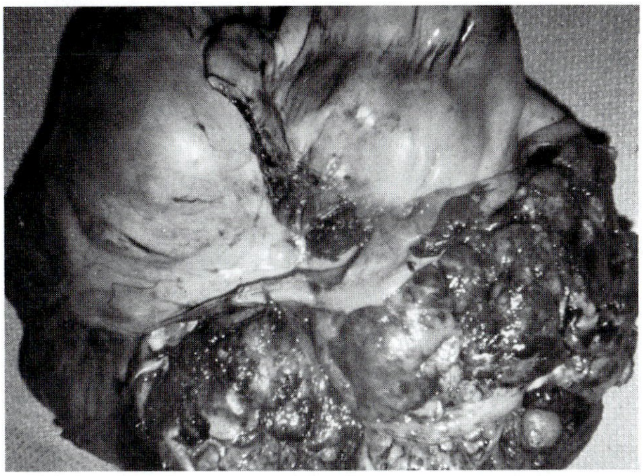

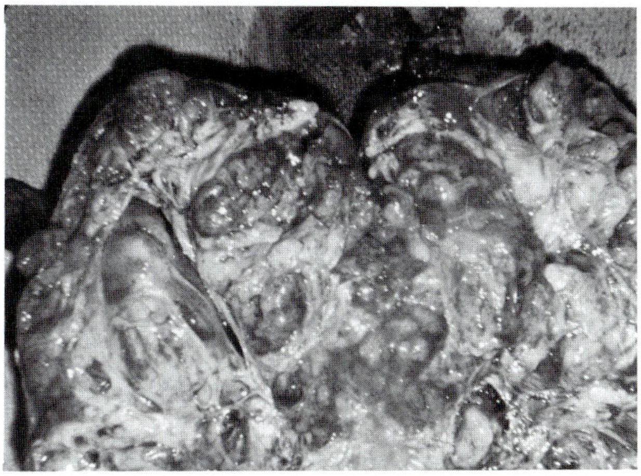

Fig. 20.29. Embryonal carcinoma. A large lobular mass is partially encapsulated.

more than one nucleolus. Mitotic activity is usually brisk, and abnormal mitoses are frequently seen. Cellular and nuclear pleomorphism is usually marked. Giant cells and multinucleated cells may be seen.

In the slightly better differentiated tumors, the cells, apart from forming solid areas, also tend to line clefts and spaces and form papillae (Fig. 20.31). The cells appear more epithelial than those of the more undifferentiated type, being more cuboidal or columnar in shape (Fig. 20.31). Although there is a suggestion of glandular differentiation, true gland formation is absent. The papillae are composed of solid collections of cells or may contain a cystic space or a small vessel surrounded by tumor cells. They must be differentiated from perivascular formations observed in yolk sac tumor. Very primitive mesenchymal tissue may be present in conjunction with the epithelial-like component. Syncytiotrophoblastic giant cells immediately adjacent to aggregates of embryonal carcinoma cells or lying isolated in the stroma are found very frequently. Foci of necrosis and hemorrhage are frequently seen.

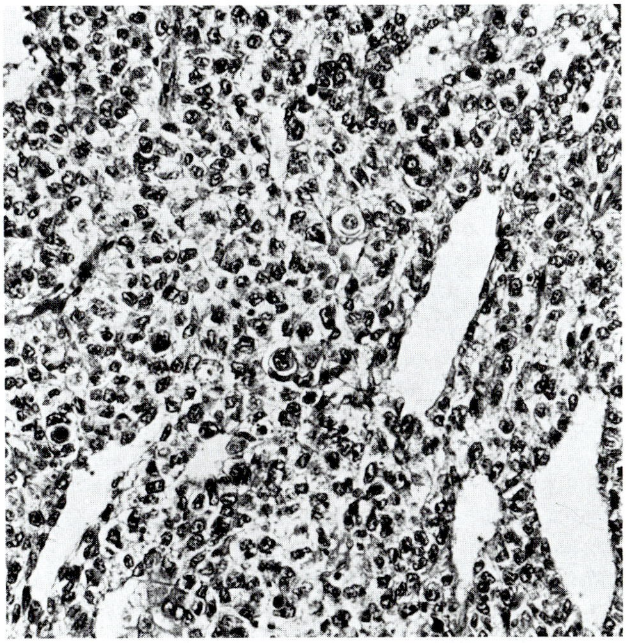

Fig. 20.30. Embryonal carcinoma. The tumor displays a solid pattern. The tumor was admixed with teratoma and endodermal sinus tumor.

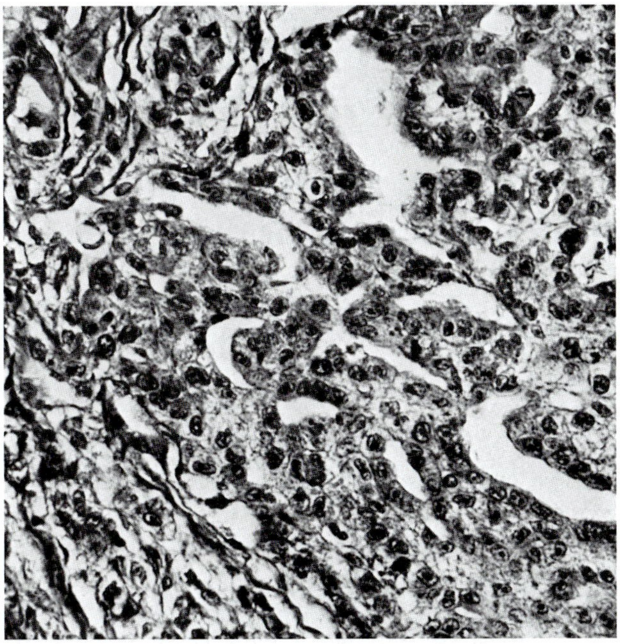

Fig. 20.31. Embryonal carcinoma. The tumor forms clefts and spaces. (Reprinted with permission from The American College of Obstetricians and Gynecologists. Obstetrics and Gynecology 43:138, 1974.)

Differential Diagnosis

Embryonal carcinoma may be present in the form of small solid aggregates or pseudoglandular or cleft-like formations surrounded by better-differentiated malignant teratomatous elements showing somatic differentiation. It may coexist with other neoplastic germ cell elements, such as yolk sac tumor, immature or mature teratoma, choriocarcinoma, polyembryoma, or dysgerminoma. Differentiation from dysgerminoma is important because of a totally different prognosis and response to treatment. It is usually the solid primitive type of embryonal carcinoma that is more likely to be confused with dysgerminoma, but the presence of clefts, alveoli, or cell-lined spaces militates against the diagnosis of dysgerminoma.

The cells of embryonal carcinoma are usually larger and show much more marked cellular and nuclear pleomorphism. Mitotic activity is usually more prominent, and bizarre mitoses are more frequent. The nuclear membrane is less sharp and the nuclei are more irregular, larger, and usually contain more than one dark hyperchromatic nucleolus, in contrast with the rounded, prominent, usually single, and frequently eosinophilic nucleolus of dysgerminoma. The presence of connective tissue stroma infiltrated by lymphocytes and at times a granulomatous reaction is a prominent feature of dysgerminoma. These features usually are absent in embryonal carcinoma. Cells of embryonal carcinoma stain positively for cytokeratin, whereas most dysgerminoma cells are negative. In addition, some embryonal carcinoma cells show positive staining for AFP, whereas dysgerminoma cells are invariably negative. Most embryonal carcinoma cells stain positively for CD 30 whereas only occasional dysgerminoma cells are CD 30 positive. Therefore immunocytochemical localization of cytokeratin, CD 30, and AFP provides a useful method for differentiating between these two neoplasms.

Clinical Behavior and Treatment

Embryonal carcinoma of the ovary is a highly malignant neoplasm. It is aggressive locally, spreads extensively in the abdominal cavity, and metastasizes early. The metastatic spread is similar to that observed with other germ cell neoplasms, taking place first via the lymphatic system and later by hematogenous spread. The primary treatment of embryonal carcinoma is surgical. Because the tumors are usually unilateral, conservative treatment is advocated if the tumor is localized to the ovary. Embryonal carcinoma is not radiosensitive. Prognosis in the past has been unfavorable, but introduction of the various forms of combination chemotherapy effective in the treatment of malignant germ cell tumors has led to marked improvement, resulting in a complete cure in most patients. The response to combination chemotherapy using bleomycin, vinblastine, and cisplatin or, preferably, cisplatin, etopoxide (VP 16), and bleomycin[50,122] is similar to that observed in patients with embryonal carcinoma of the testis.

Polyembryoma

General Features

Polyembryoma is a rare ovarian germ cell neoplasm composed of numerous embryoid bodies resembling morphologically normal presomite embryos. Similar homologous neoplasms occur more frequently in the human testis,[16,43] although pure polyembryoma is very rare. Less than a dozen cases of ovarian polyembryoma have been recorded.[16,75,172] In all these cases the polyembryoma was associated with other neoplastic germ cell elements, mainly immature or mature teratoma.[16,75,161,172] All these tumors occurred in young patients or in patients in the reproductive age group[16,75,161,172]; the oldest patient was 38 years old.[161] The clinical findings are similar to those observed in patients with other malignant germ cell neoplasms of the ovary.

Histogenesis

There are conflicting views of the origin of embryoid bodies. It has been suggested that they arise by parthenogenic development from primitive germ cells present in a malignant teratoma.[94,127,161] Other investigators question this view as well as the entire concept that embryoid bodies bear a close similarity to early human embryos because embryoid bodies never appear to develop beyond the 18-day stage.[16] They consider that embryoid bodies probably develop transiently by bizarre differentiation, possibly in response to local release of organizers in malignant teratomas of the gonads.

Another view that has been advanced accepts the morphologic similarities between the early embryo and the embryoid bodies but disputes their parthenogenic origin.[43,130,168] It maintains that embryoid bodies are formed after initiation of teratogenesis, most likely from multipotential malignant embryonal cells present in a tumor and not directly from germ cells.[169] This concept is supported by the observations of the development of embryoid bodies from undifferentiated embryonal cells in strain 129 mice. The tumor, a teratoma that had been serially transplanted for many years, was considered to be devoid of germ cells.[130,168] These findings are in accordance with the view that embryoid bodies probably persist only transiently within the tumor, and while new embryoid bodies are being formed others lose their identity and their multipotential cells undergo further differentiation.[43] Although the origin and development of embryoid bodies are still a matter of dispute, the view that they originate from multipotential malignant embryonal cells, which is supported by experimental observations,[130,168] is most favored at present.

Gross Findings

Polyembryoma is usually unilateral. Macroscopically, the tumor resembles other malignant germ cell tumors, varying in size from relatively small (9.5 cm in longest diameter)[16] to tumors filling almost the whole abdominal cavity and invading the surrounding structures.[161] The tumor is usually solid and contains hemorrhagic and necrotic areas.

Microscopic Findings

Polyembryoma is composed of numerous embryoid bodies, and the better-differentiated ones are composed of an embryonic disk, amniotic cavity, and yolk sac surrounded by primitive extraembryonic mesenchyme (Fig. 20.32). Sometimes trophoblastic differentiation may be seen in the vicinity of the embryoid body. When the embryoid bodies are less well formed, they are composed of a medullary plate and amnion associated with a blastocystic space or with extraembryonic mesenchyme. They may have two or more amniotic cavities and share a single yolk sac cavity or vice versa. There may be a considerable disproportion between the two cavities, and the cavities may be malformed. There may be considerable variation in size between the different embryoid bodies; some may be more primitive and others appear to be better developed.

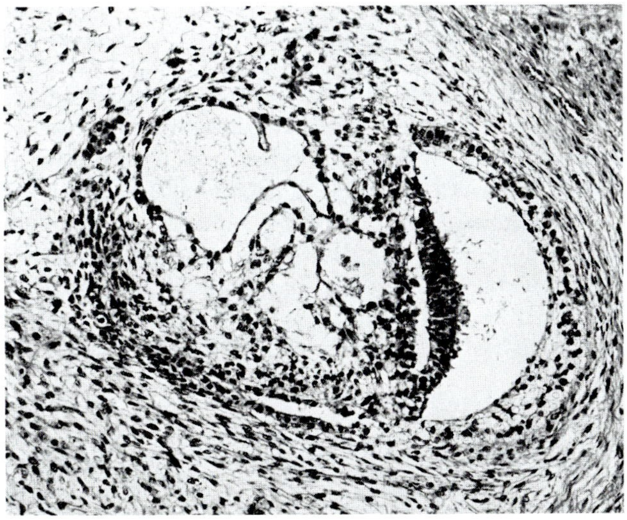

Fig. 20.32. Polyembryoma. Embryoid body shows amniotic cavity (*right*), embryonic disk (*center*), and atypical yolk sac (*left*).

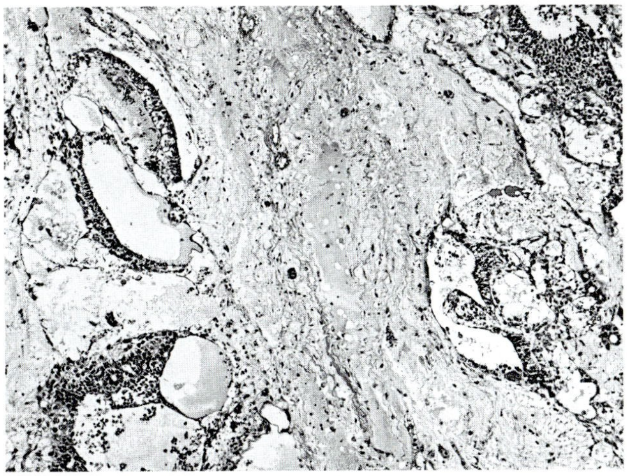

Fig. 20.33. Polyembryoma. Embryoid bodies show bizarre appearances.

Some embryoid bodies may be malformed and show bizarre appearances (Fig. 20.33). None of the embryoid bodies appear to have developed beyond the 18-day stage. The embryonic disk of a typical embryoid body is lined on one side by cuboidal epithelial cells of uniform size, resembling endoderm, and on the other by tall columnar epithelium, resembling ectoderm. The latter merges with low cuboidal epithelium lining the rest of the cavity, which resembles the amnion. The cavity resembling the yolk sac is on the opposite side of the embryonic disk from the amnion (Fig. 20.32). The embryoid bodies are surrounded by extraembryonic mesenchyme, which is composed of either closely or more loosely packed spindle-shaped cells of regular appearance (Fig. 20.32) and showing occasional mitotic figures. Loose myxomatous areas may be present (Fig. 20.33).

Occasionally, embryoid bodies in earlier developmental stages, mainly the blastocyst and morula stage, form numerous round or oval structures. In some tumors this pattern may predominate, although occasional fully developed embryoid bodies may be seen.[75] Teratomatous structures in various stages of differentiation are frequently seen interspersed among the embryoid bodies. In one reported case,[16] hCG and human placental lactogen were demonstrated within syncytiotrophoblastic cells that were present in the vicinity of the embryoid bodies. Cytotrophoblastic cells were not identified in this tumor. In another reported case, there was elevation of serum AFP and hCG. AFP was demonstrated by immunoperoxidase within the cells lining the yolk sac cavities and hCG within the syncytiotrophoblastic giant cells that were present in the vicinity of the embryoid bodies.[172]

Clinical Behavior and Treatment

Polyembryoma is a highly malignant germ cell neoplasm. In most cases, it has been associated with invasion of adjacent structures and extensive metastases, which were mainly confined to the abdominal cavity.[161]

The primary treatment of polyembryoma is surgical, and because the tumor is usually unilateral unless there is spread beyond the ovary, excision of the tumor and the adjoining adnexa is the treatment of choice. The tumor is not sensitive to radiotherapy, but responds to the combination chemotherapy used in treatment of malignant germ cell tumors.[50,172]

One patient with a relatively small mobile tumor, absence of capsular penetration, and no evidence of metastases survived more than 5 years.[16] Another patient was alive and free of disease for more than 12 years after excision of the affected adnexa and excision of intraabdominal metastases composed of grade 1 immature teratoma.[75] A third patient was well and disease free 6 months after diagnosis.[172] Before the introduction of effective combination chemotherapy, most patients with polyembryoma died of their disease.

Choriocarcinoma

General Features

Pure *ovarian choriocarcinoma* of germ cell origin is a rare neoplasm,[67,68,209] and even the presence of choriocarcinomatous elements admixed with other neoplastic germ cell elements is uncommon. In most cases, the tumor is admixed with other neoplastic germ cell elements, and their presence is diagnostic of nongestational choriocarcinoma, except for the remote possibility of the tumor being a gestational choriocarcinoma metastatic to an ovarian germ cell tumor. The presence of other neoplastic germ cell elements is a particularly helpful diagnostic feature in postmenarchal patients in whom exclusion of gestational origin of the tumor may be difficult. In view of this, nongestational choriocarcinoma may be diagnosed with confidence in postmenarchal patients and not only in young children, as had been considered earlier. At least 50 cases of ovarian germ cell tumors containing choriocarcinoma have been reported.[67,95,209] The tumor occurs in children and young adults. Its occurrence in children has been emphasized; in some series, 50% of cases occurred in children who had not reached puberty.[95] This high frequency in children may stem from the reluctance of making the diagnosis in adults.

Histogenesis

Choriocarcinoma of the ovary may originate in three different ways: (1) as a primary gestational choriocarcinoma associated with ovarian pregnancy, (2) as metastatic choriocarcinoma from a primary gestational choriocarcinoma arising in other parts of the genital tract, mainly the uterus, and (3) as a germ cell tumor differentiating in the direction of trophoblastic structures, usually admixed with other neoplastic germ cell elements. In each case it is important to ascertain the mode of origin of the tumor because this has important therapeutic and prognostic implications. Alternatively, choriocarcinoma of the ovary may be divided into two broad groups: (1) gestational choriocarcinoma encompassing the first two groups mentioned and (2) nongestational choriocarcinoma, a germ cell tumor differentiating toward trophoblastic structures. As this chapter is concerned solely with germ cell tumors, only the nongestational choriocarcinoma is discussed here.

Clinical Features

The clinical findings in patients with ovarian nongestational choriocarcinoma are similar to those observed in patients with other malignant ovarian germ cell neoplasms, except that they may be modified by the endocrine activity of the tumor, which secretes hCG. This effect is particularly noticeable in prepubertal children who show evidence of isosexual precocious puberty, with mammary development, growth of pubic and axillary hair, and uterine bleeding. Adult patients may have signs of ectopic pregnancy. Because the nongestational choriocarcinoma, resembling its gestational counterpart, is associated with increased production of hCG, determination of urinary or plasma hCG is a useful diagnostic test. Serum hCG, or preferably beta-hCG levels are also useful in monitoring the response to therapy, as well as in detecting metastases and recurrences containing choriocarcinomatous tissue. It should be noted that normal levels of hCG do not exclude the presence of metastases or recurrences composed of other neoplastic germ cell elements. Table 20.3 shows the results of preoperative serum hCG and beta-hCG determinations in patients with ovarian germ cell tumors.

Gross Findings

The tumor typically is large, unilateral, solid, gray-white, and hemorrhagic. Necrosis may be evident. Because most of these tumors are composed of a combination of neoplastic germ cell elements, the appearances tend to vary according to the elements present in the tumor.

Table 20.3. Serum hCG and beta-hCG in ovarian germ cell tumors measured by radioimmunoassay[a]

	No. of cases	*Serum hCG*
Mixed germ cell tumors containing choriocarcinoma	8	Elevated
Mixed germ cell tumors containing EST	26	Normal
Pure EST	15	Normal
Pure dysgerminoma	18	Normal
Dysgerminoma with syncytiotrophoblastic giant cells	3	Elevated
Teratoma (immature and mature)	8	Normal
Teratoma (immature and mature) and dysgerminoma	7	Normal
Mature cystic teratoma (dermoid cyst)	11	Normal

[a]Unpublished data.
hCG, human chorionic gonadotropin; EST, endodermal sinus tumor.

Microscopic Findings

Choriocarcinoma is composed of two types of cells, cytotrophoblast and syncytiotrophoblast (Fig. 20.34). The cytotrophoblast is composed of medium-sized polygonal, round, or oval cells with clear cytoplasm and sharp borders. Some cells have centrally situated, small, round, and hyperchromatic nuclei whereas others have larger vesicular nuclei containing nucleoli and showing brisk mitotic activity. The syncytiotrophoblast is composed of large basophilic, vacuolated cells with irregular outlines, and although frequently elongated they may vary in shape. These cells contain multiple hyperchromatic nuclei, varying in shape and size. The cytotrophoblastic cells are usually disposed centrally within a tumor mass and are partly or completely surrounded by irregular collections or layers of the syncytiotrophoblastic cells (Fig. 20.34).

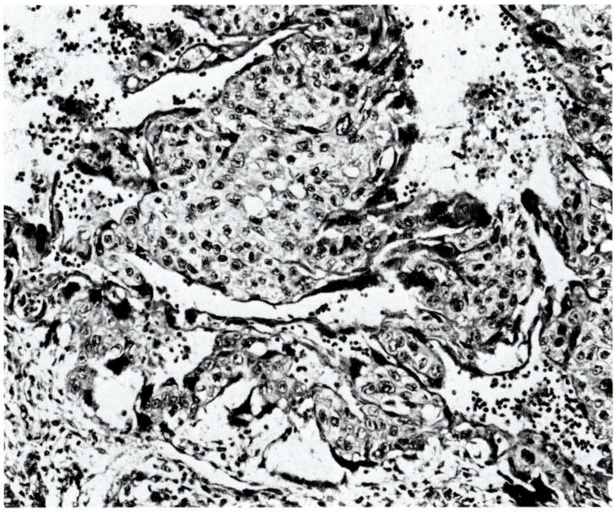

Fig. 20.34. Choriocarcinoma. Cytotrophoblast composed of medium-sized cells is situated centrally; syncytiotrophoblast composed of very large multinucleated cells is situated peripherally.

There is a considerable variation in the pattern and in the ratio of the two components in different parts of the same tumor and in different tumors. The tumor cells form solid aggregates, nearly always associated with hemorrhage and necrosis. At times the tumor is limited to the periphery of the hemorrhagic mass. When the tumor is combined with other germ cell elements, the choriocarcinoma may form small nodules associated with hemorrhage and surrounded by other germ cell elements. The presence of other germ cell elements within the tumor is a frequent finding. As choriocarcinoma is often affected by hemorrhage, a careful search may be necessary to demonstrate the presence of choriocarcinomatous elements.

The cytotrophoblast is the more primitive element, and the syncytiotrophoblast is formed from it either directly or indirectly. The syncytiotrophoblast is the differentiated, nondividing, hormone-secreting component. These findings are supported by electron microscopic and immunohistochemical studies.[131,133] Immunocytochemical staining for hCG or beta-hCG provides a useful confirmatory diagnostic method. Although intermediate trophoblastic cells may be seen occasionally in nongestational choriocarcinomas, ovarian tumors composed of intermediate trophoblast have not been reported to date. A mixed germ cell tumor with a predominant component suggestive of intermediate trophoblast has been seen by the author, suggesting that such tumors may occur.

Clinical Behavior and Treatment

Nongestational choriocarcinoma of the ovary is a highly malignant germ cell neoplasm. It invades adjacent structures, spreads widely throughout the abdominal cavity, and metastasizes via the lymphatics and the blood vessels. Although gestational choriocarcinoma tends to spread primarily via the bloodstream, nongestational choriocarcinoma shows lymphatic and intraabdominal spread as well as hematogenous spread. Sometimes the hematogenous spread may be less marked.

Until the introduction of effective combination chemotherapy, the prognosis of patients with choriocarcinoma was distinctly unfavorable but was somewhat better than of patients with yolk sac tumor. The treatment has been revolutionized by the introduction of combination chemotherapy containing cisplatin with marked improvement in prognosis and survival. Cisplatin, etopoxide (VP 16), and bleomycin currently is the most favored combination.[50,122]

Teratoma

The origin of *teratomas* has been a matter of interest, speculation, and dispute for centuries. The parthenogenic theory, which suggests an origin from the primordial germ cell, is now the most widely accepted. Two other theories, one suggesting an origin from blastomeres segregated at an early stage of embryonic development and the second suggesting an origin from embryonal rests, have few adherents nowadays. Support for the germ cell theory has come from the anatomic distribution of the tumors, which occur along the line of migration of the primordial germ cells from the yolk sac to the primitive gonad, and from the fact that the tumors occur most commonly during the years of reproductive activity. Support also comes from animal experiments in which cystic teratomas can be produced only during the period of reproductive activity of the gonad, as in roosters injected with zinc and copper salts,[14,28] and from the nuclear sexing and karyotyping of teratomas. It has been shown that cells of ovarian teratomas are always chromatin positive, unlike the cells of testicular teratomas, which may be chromatin negative, chromatin positive, or mixed. The karyotypes of all mature ovarian teratomas studied have been found to be 46,XX.[87,137]

Further support for the germ cell theory of origin has come from the work of Linder et al.[87] They studied the histogenesis of mature cystic teratoma of the ovary using both cytogenetic techniques and the electrophoretic variants of four enzymes in normal as well as in tumor cells. They demonstrated that these tumors are of germ cell origin and arise from a single germ cell after the first meiotic division.[86,87] Recent studies using more advanced cytogenetic techniques further confirm these observations. Although most mature cystic teratomas arise in this manner, some arise before the first meiotic division.[108,119] The classification of ovarian teratomas is shown in Table 20.1. Briefly, they are divided into three main groups: (1) immature teratomas, (2) mature teratomas, and (3) monodermal and highly specialized teratomas. Most cases (99%) are mature cystic teratomas also known as dermoids or dermoid cysts.

Immature Teratoma

Immature teratomas are composed of tissues derived from the three germ layers—ectoderm, mesoderm, and endoderm—and, in contrast to the much more common mature teratoma, they contain immature or embryonal structures. Mature tissues are frequently present and sometimes may predominate. In these cases, the tumor should be differentiated from a mature teratoma with malignant transformation. The presence of immature or embryonal elements as opposed to the neoplastic transformation of mature tissues differentiates between these two types of neoplasm.

Clinical Features

The immature teratoma of the ovary is an uncommon tumor, comprising less than 1% of teratomas of the ovary.[25,29,93,215] In contrast with the mature cystic teratoma, which is encountered most frequently during the reproductive years but occurs at all ages, the immature teratoma has a specific age incidence, occurring most commonly in the first two decades of life and being almost unknown after the menopause.[25,26,93,215] In view of this, teratomas occurring in childhood, adolescence, and early adult life should always be examined carefully and thoroughly sampled.

The tumor is usually asymptomatic until it reaches a considerable size. It tends to grow rapidly and may manifest itself as a pelvic or lower abdominal mass. It may cause pressure symptoms, abdominal heaviness, or dull pain, or it may undergo torsion, causing acute abdominal pain.

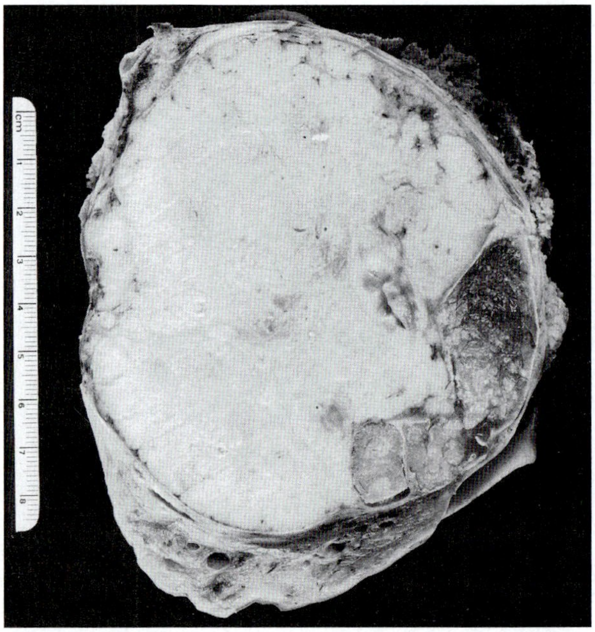

Fig. 20.35. Immature teratoma. A large lobulated, firm, solid tumor with focal areas of mature adipose tissue (*right*). Most of the tumor consisted of grade 3 immature teratoma.

Gross Findings

The tumor is usually unilateral,[25,26,29,62,215] but may coexist with a mature cystic teratoma in the opposite ovary,[213] as is seen in at least 10–15% of cases. Immature teratomas are usually large, with the reported range from 9 to 28 cm in the largest dimension.[26] They may form a round, oval, or lobulated soft or firm mass (Fig. 20.35). The tumor is often prone to perforate its capsule, which is not always well defined.[26,213] It tends to form adhesions to the surrounding structures and to invade locally.[26] The tumor is predominantly solid (Fig.20.35) but frequently contains cystic structures.[25,26,29,62,93,213] Occasionally, it may be predominantly cystic, with solid areas present in the cyst wall.[26] The cut surface is usually variegated, trabeculated, and lobulated, varying in color from gray (Fig. 20.35) to dark brown. Occasionally, foci of cartilage or bone may be recognizable and hair may be present. The cystic areas are usually filled with serous or mucinous fluid, colloid, or fatty material.

Microscopic Findings

The tumor is composed of a variety of immature and mature tissues derived from the three germ layers. Occasionally, the tumor may be composed of a small number of tissues, although usually derivatives of all the three germ layers are present. Ectoderm is usually represented by neural tissue. Glia, ganglion cells, neuroblastic tissue (Fig. 20.36), neuroepithelium, nerve trunks, and ocular structures are often represented. Skin elements (Fig. 20.36), including pilosebaceous units, sweat glands, and hair, are not infrequently present. Mesodermal elements include fibrous connective tissue, cartilage (Fig. 20.36), bone, muscle, usually smooth but occasionally striated, lymphoid tissue, and undifferentiated embryonic mesenchyme. Endodermal elements are usually represented by tubules lined by columnar, sometimes ciliated, epithelium. Occasionally, gastrointestinal or renal epithelium (Fig. 20.37) may be present.

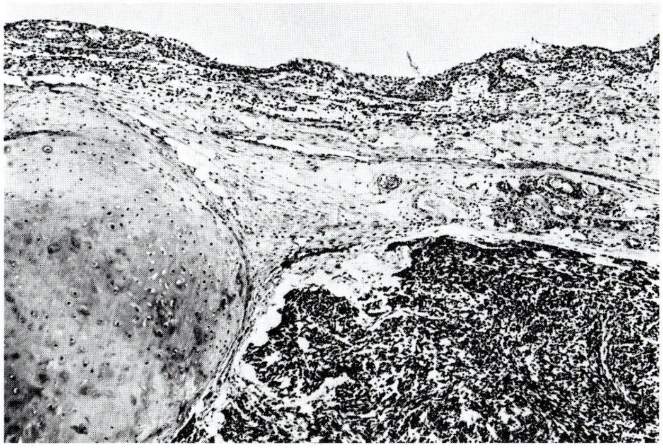

Fig. 20.36. Immature teratoma. Both solid and cystic areas are shown. The tumor was mainly composed of neuroblastic tissue (*right*). Note the squamous epithelium, adnexal glands, and cartilage.

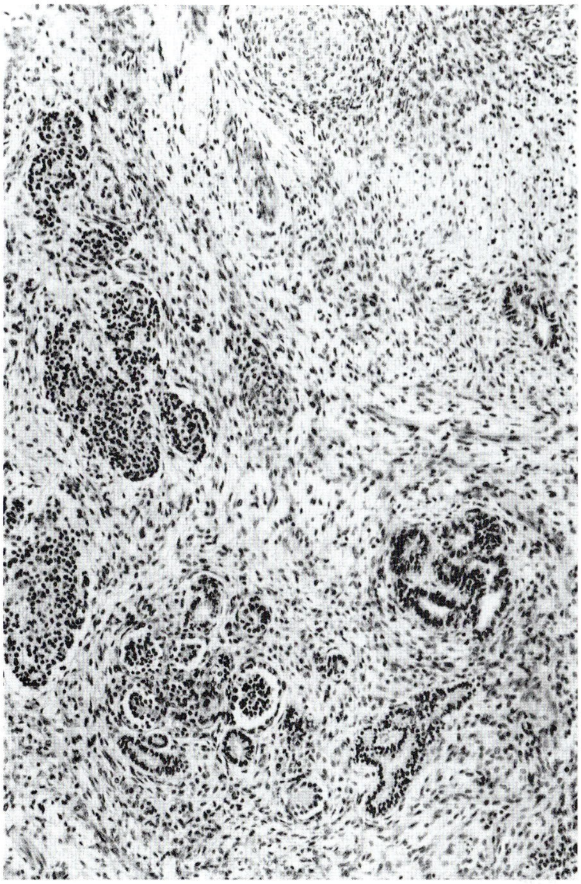

Fig. 20.37. Immature teratoma. The tumor contains embryonal renal tissue, glomeruli and blastema, and immature connective and neural tissue.

All these tissues, which may be in stages of maturity varying from embryonic to mature, are scattered haphazardly throughout the tumor (Fig. 20.37) and so differ from the orderly organoid arrangement seen in a mature teratoma. In cases in which the tumor is composed mainly of mature tissues, differentiation from mature teratoma may be difficult, and patients have been diagnosed as having a benign lesion only to return within a short time with recurrence. In a number of such cases, review of the material taken from the original tumor has revealed immature elements. Therefore, careful examination and thorough sampling of the tumor are strongly recommended. Immature teratoma may be combined with other neoplastic germ cell elements, such as yolk sac tumor, dysgerminoma, embryonal carcinoma, choriocarcinoma, and polyembryoma. It can therefore form a part of a malignant germ cell tumor composed of two or more neoplastic germ cell elements (mixed germ cell tumor). Immature teratoma has been reported to develop from the germ cell element of gonadoblastoma and mixed germ cell–sex cord–stromal tumor.

Differential Diagnosis

Immature teratoma must be differentiated from the malignant mixed müllerian (mesodermal) tumor, which although occurring most frequently in the uterus, also occurs in the ovary. Malignant mixed müllerian (mesodermal) tumor is composed of derivatives of müllerian mesoderm, a primitive structure that gives rise to both the stroma and the epithelium of the endometrium. The monodermal origin of malignant mixed müllerian (mesodermal) tumor distinguishes it from teratoma. Malignant mixed müllerian (mesodermal) tumor occurs most frequently in postmenopausal women between the ages of 50 and 70 years and, unlike immature teratoma, occurs only occasionally in younger patients.

The tumor is composed of sarcomatous and carcinomatous tissue. The carcinoma is invariably an adenocarcinoma, squamous cell carcinoma, or adenosquamous carcinoma, and the sarcomatous elements may be composed of a wide variety of tissues, including leiomyosarcoma, chondrosarcoma, rhabdomyosarcoma, fibrosarcoma, undifferentiated sarcomatous tissue, and myxomatous tissue. Derivatives of the three germ layers are absent in malignant mixed müllerian (mesodermal) tumor; neuroectodermal derivatives, prominent in solid immature teratoma, are seen only exceptionally. Malignant mixed müllerian (mesodermal) tumor does not exhibit the great variety of tissues present in teratoma, and the tissues present in malignant mixed müllerian (mesodermal) tumor generally form more typical sarcomatous or carcinomatous patterns (see Chapter 13, Mesenchymal Tumors of Uterus).

Clinical Behavior and Treatment

Immature teratoma is a malignant neoplasm that usually grows rapidly, penetrates its capsule, and forms adhesions to the surrounding structures. It spreads throughout the peritoneal cavity by implantation. It metastasizes first to the retroperitoneal, paraaortic, and more distant lymph nodes and later to the lungs, liver, and other organs. Peritoneal implants and metastases are not infrequently present at operation for the removal of the primary tumor.[26,213] Excision of the tumor is often followed by a local recurrence within a few weeks or months. Recurrences usually occur within the first year after the primary treatment.[26] Rupture of the tumor with spillage of the contents during operation is not infrequent, but because of the satisfactory response of the tumor to combination chemotherapy the favorable prognosis is not affected. The metastases and peritoneal implants may be composed of different tissues, and thus their teratomatous nature is readily apparent, but they may also be composed of a single tissue. The histologic appearances of the metastases and of the peritoneal implants may or may not reflect the appearances of the primary tumor.

In the past prognosis was poor, with less than 20% of patients surviving 5 years after the operation.[29,93] Better results have been claimed in cases in which the only immature element was neurogenic.[93,215] It has been noted that there is a good correlation between the histologic appearances of the tumor and prognosis.[25,62,112,114] Very immature and poorly differentiated tumors have been found to be associated with worse prognosis, whereas a more favorable outcome has been observed in patients with more mature and better differentiated tumors.[62,112,213] A recent study of immature teratoma in children showed that less mature tumors were more likely to be associated with YST.[62]

A histologic grading has been proposed and it is of value for predicting prognosis and planning treatment. This grading is based on the relative amounts of immature and mature tissues, the degree of differentiation, and the mitotic activity within the immature components. The most common immature element present and the one that is evaluated most often in grading is primitive neuroepithelium, but other immature tissues present must also be evaluated. The grading is as follows:

Grade 0	All tissues mature; no mitotic activity
Grade 1	Minor foci of abnormally cellular or immature tissue mixed with mature elements; slight mitotic activity
Grade 2	Moderate quantities of immature tissue mixed with mature elements; moderate mitotic activity
Grade 3	Large quantities of highly immature tissue present; high mitotic activity

This grading system has been widely accepted and its use is strongly recommended. Recently, O'Connor and Norris[114] proposed that immature teratomas should be divided into two grades, those with a slight degree of immaturity (grade 1), which are not treated with combination chemotherapy, and those with a more marked degree of immaturity (grades 2 and 3), which are treated. It was demonstrated that although there was considerable inter- and intraobserver disagreement when a large series of immature teratomas were being graded into three grades, this was markedly decreased when a two-grade system was used. The study further confirmed the good correlation between the grade of the tumor and its behavior.

The recommended treatment for patients with grade 1 (low grade) immature teratoma confined to one ovary is unilateral salpingo-oophorectomy and careful follow-up. This treatment is curative in nearly all cases.[25,122] For grade 2 and 3 (high grade) tumors, adjuvant chemotherapy is administered following surgery, resulting in complete cure in the majority of patients.[25] More extensive surgery is necessary if the tumor extends beyond the ovary. Current combination therapy is either vincristine, dactinomycin, and cyclophosphamide (VAC), vinblastine, bleomycin, and cisplatin (VBP), or cisplatin, etopoxide (VP 16), and bleomycin (BEP) regimens. Therapy with VAC has been the treatment of choice[112] because the results obtained were considered to be similar to those with VBP or BEP regimens and the latter are more toxic. There is evidence that the recurrence rate with BEP is less than with VAC regimen, and for patients with metastatic disease the cisplatin-containing regimens are the treatment of choice, especially as the more recently introduced BEP regimen is less toxic than the VBP.[25,50,122]

In a recent large collaborative study of immature teratoma in children, the authors[62] have demonstrated that pure immature teratomas in this population are associated with very good prognosis. There is no correlation between age and tumor grade and recurrences occur almost exclusively in children whose tumor contains foci of YST. The authors[62] concluded that grading of immature teratoma in children is of little value.

Mature Solid Teratoma

General Features

Mature solid teratoma is an uncommon ovarian teratoma. The age incidence is similar to that of immature solid teratoma, the tumor occurring mainly in children and young adults.[124,215] Most solid ovarian teratomas are composed at least partly of immature tissues and therefore are considered to be malignant. The occasional cases of solid ovarian teratoma composed entirely of mature tissues have usually been included in this group and thus misinterpreted as malignant. At the same time, this practice has improved the survival statistics, which were generally very poor in patients with immature ovarian teratoma. Mature solid teratoma is composed entirely of mature tissues derived from the three germ layers. Rigid diagnostic criteria must be used, and the examination and sampling of the tumor must be thorough, because inclusion of cases with immature elements completely changes the prognosis of this neoplasm, which otherwise is excellent.[124,213,215] Neurogenic elements, which are among the most common tissues present in this tumor, often pose diagnostic problems because they may not be recognized as mature. As the presence of immature neural elements immediately excludes the tumor from this group, it is very important to recognize the mature tissue as such, as by definition only tumors composed entirely of mature tissues may be diagnosed as mature solid teratoma.

Gross Findings

The tumors are usually large, do not exhibit any specific features, and show similar appearance to most solid teratomas, which are composed of immature tissues. They grow slowly in comparison with immature solid teratoma, but because they are usually discovered after they have reached a considerable size, this feature is of little help in diagnosis. In all reported cases of mature solid teratoma, the tumor has been unilateral.[124,213,215]

Microscopic Findings

The tumor is composed of a variety of tissues derived from the three germ layers and arranged in an orderly manner resembling the much more common mature cystic teratoma, except that the neoplasm is solid or at least predominantly solid. The tumor is composed entirely of mature tissues (Figs. 20.38 and 20.39). Sometimes neurogenic elements may predominate (Fig. 20.39). Occasionally, mature solid teratoma may be associated with peritoneal implants composed entirely of mature glial tissue (gliomatosis) (Fig. 20.40). Despite extensive peritoneal disease and irrespective of the mode of therapy employed, the prognosis is excellent.[138] Presence of peritoneal implants composed entirely of mature glial tissue occasionally may be observed in patients with immature solid teratoma and with mature cystic teratoma. The presence of these implants does not affect the prognosis.[62,104,138]

Clinical Behavior and Treatment

Because the tumor is unilateral, oophorectomy or unilateral adnexectomy is the treatment of choice, resulting in a complete cure.[124,213,215]

Mature Cystic Teratoma

General Features

Mature cystic teratoma of the ovary, or *dermoid cyst*, has been known since antiquity. The tumor is composed of well-differentiated derivatives of the three germ layers—ectoderm, mesoderm, and endoderm—with ectodermal elements predominating. In its pure form, mature cystic teratoma is always benign, but occasionally it may undergo malignant change

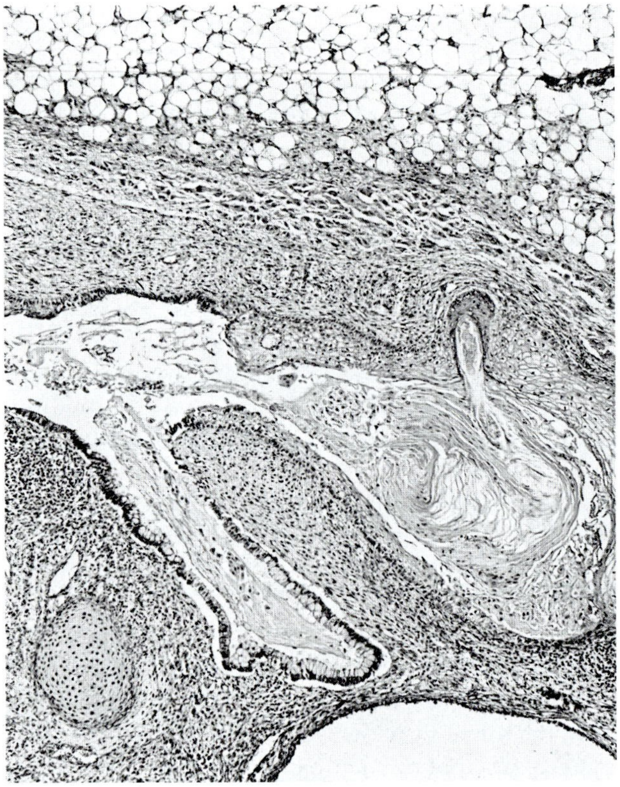

Fig. 20.38. **Mature solid teratoma.** The tumor is composed of squamous and glandular epithelium, adipose and fibrous tissue, and cartilage.

in one of its elements. It may also form a part of a germ cell neoplasm composed of a number of different neoplastic germ cell elements (mixed germ cell tumor).

Clinical Features

Mature cystic teratoma is the most common type of ovarian teratoma and the most common type of ovarian germ cell neoplasm. It occurs relatively frequently and comprises approximately 20% of all ovarian neoplasms.[126] Mature cystic teratoma occurs most commonly during the reproductive years, but, unlike other germ cell tumors of the ovary, it has a wider age distribution and may be encountered at any age from infancy to old age.[13,29,126] In some series, more than 25% of cases have been observed in postmenopausal women.[92] It has also been encountered in newborns. Mature cystic teratoma is often discovered as an incidental finding on physical examination, radiologic examination, or during abdominal surgery performed for other indications.

When symptoms are present, they usually manifest as abdominal pain (47.6%), abdominal mass or swelling (15.4%), and abnormal uterine bleeding (15.1%).[126] The abdominal pain is usually constant, slight, or moderate but, in a number of cases, may be severe and acute because of torsion or rupture of the tumor; this tends to occur more commonly when the tumor is large. In children and young adults the tumors tend to be more easily mobile and therefore are more frequently affected by torsion. The abnormal uterine bleeding and its relief after excision of the tumor suggests hormone synthesis by the tumor, but histologic examination has failed to reveal any explanation for the endocrine function.[92] Slightly decreased fertility has been observed in patients with mature cystic teratoma, but in most cases there is no satisfactory explanation. In 10% of cases, the tumor is diagnosed during pregnancy.[13,29] Mature cystic teratoma has been diagnosed radiologically because of the presence of teeth, bone, and cartilage[92,126] (Fig. 20.41).

Gross Findings

Mature cystic teratoma does not have a predilection for either ovary; 8–15% of cases are bilateral.[126] The

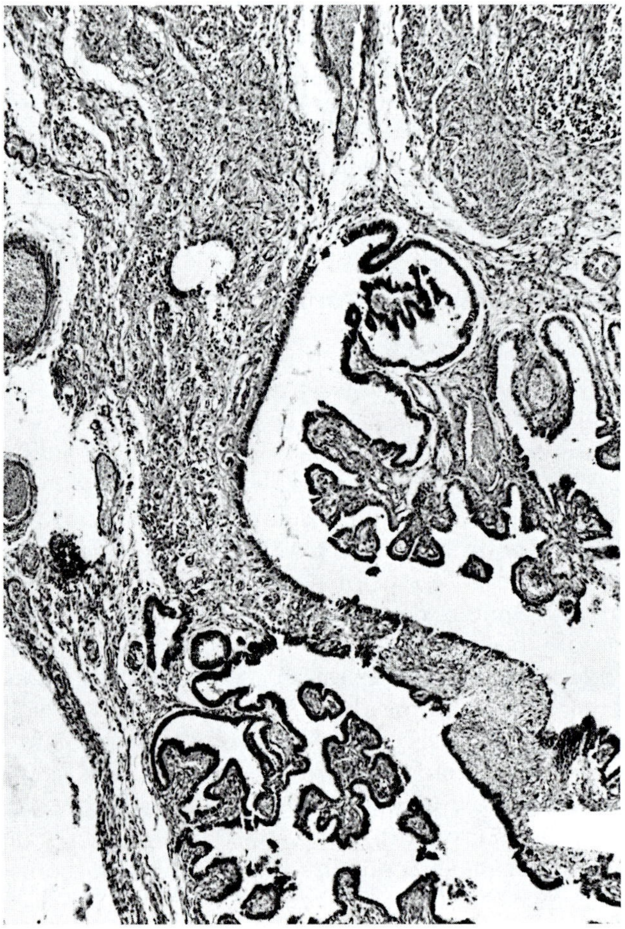

Fig. 20.39. **Mature solid teratoma.** The tumor is composed of mature neural tissue and choroid plexus.

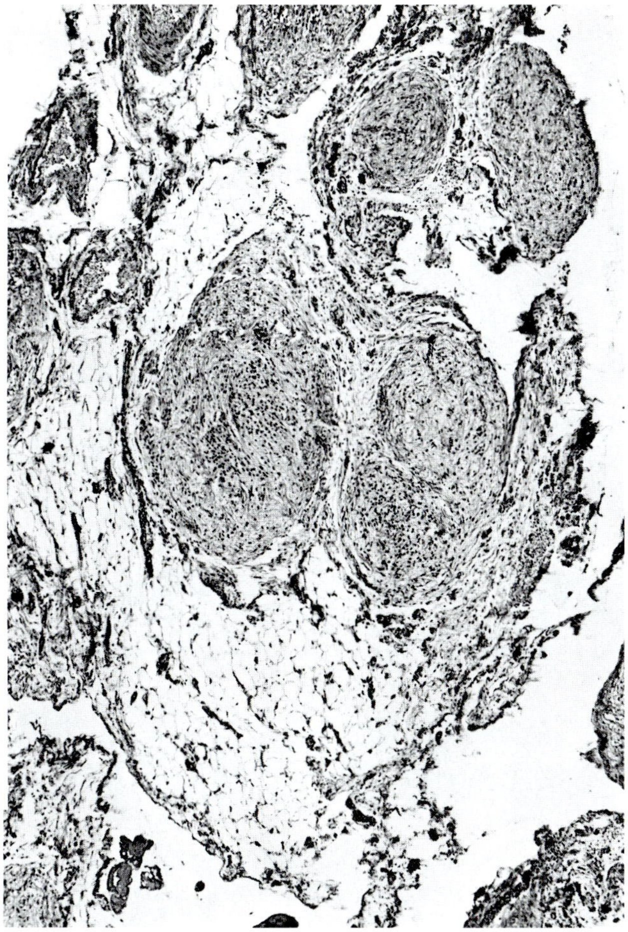

Fig. 20.40. **Mature solid teratoma.** Mature glial implants on omentum.

tumor varies in size from very small (0.5 cm across) to large (measuring more than 40 cm) and weighing several kilograms. Approximately 60% of mature cystic teratomas measure from 5 to 10 cm across, and more than 90% measure less than 15 cm across.[126] The tumor is round, oval, or globular, with a smooth, gray-white, glistening surface (Fig. 20.41). It is usually freely mobile but occasionally may form adhesions to the surrounding structures, especially if there has been leakage of the contents. On palpation, the tumor is soft and fluctuant, with firm or hard areas; this is usually observed immediately after its removal, because at room temperature the tumor tends to solidify. The contents of the tumor are liquid at temperatures above 34°C and become solid at temperatures below 25°C.[23] The cut surface of the tumor reveals a cavity filled with fatty material and hair surrounded by a firm capsule of varying thickness. The fatty material is similar to normal sebum. The tumor is usually unilocular but may be multilocular. Several tumors may be present in the same ovary.

Arising from the cyst wall and projecting into the cavity is a protuberance that may vary in size from a small nodule to a rounded elevated mass. It is usually single but may be multiple. It is frequently solid but may be partly cystic. This protuberance has been variously termed dermoid mamilla, dermoid protuberance, Rokitansky protuberance, embryonic node, or dermoid nipple. The hair present in the tumor arises from this protuberance, and when bone or teeth are present they tend to be located within this area, which is composed of a variety of different tissues and is one of the sites that should always

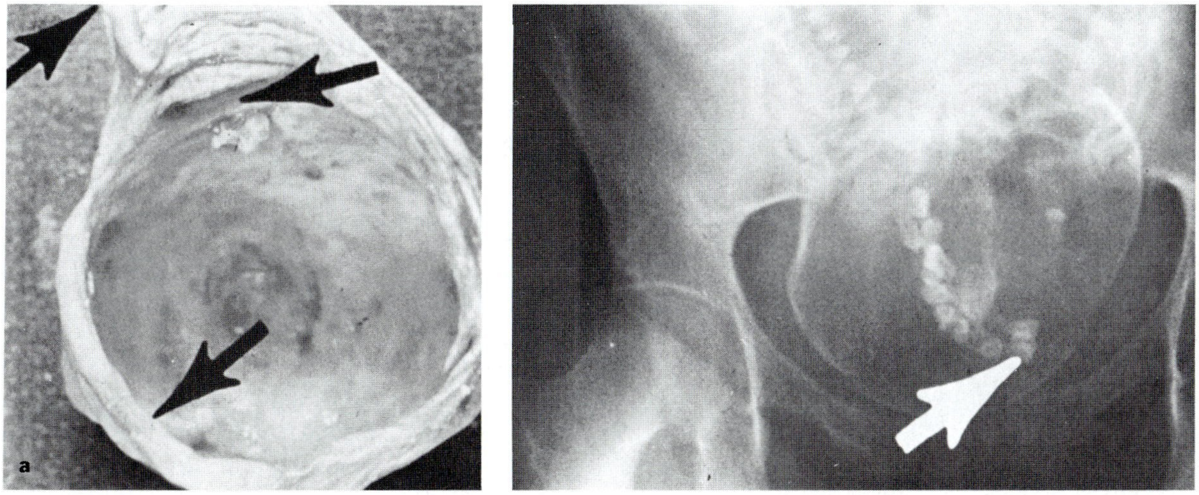

Fig. 20.41. **Mature cystic teratoma.** *Left*: Well-encapsulated spherical cystic mass. *Arrows* point to teeth. *Right*: Tumor produced dystocia and was diagnosed by pelvimetry. A row of teeth is seen at *arrow tip*. (Courtesy of A. Blaustein, M.D.)

be carefully sampled. Mature cystic teratomas contain macroscopically recognizable and well-formed teeth in 31% of cases.[23] Phalanges, long and other bones, parts of the rib cage, loops of intestine, and even fetus-like structures are occasionally encountered.[1,211]

Microscopic Findings

The outer side of the cyst wall is composed of ovarian stroma that may often be hyalinized, making its recognition difficult. The cavity of the cyst is lined mainly by skin, and in small tumors cutaneous structures may form the entire lining. The skin is composed of keratinized squamous epithelium (Figs. 20.42 and 20.43) and usually contains abundant sebaceous and sweat glands (Fig. 20.42). Hair and other dermal appendages are usually present. Occasionally, the cyst wall may be lined by bronchial or gastrointestinal epithelium or epithelium of columnar or cuboidal type. The squamous epithelium may be present only in the region of the dermoid protuberance. Sometimes there may be loss of the lining epithelium caused by desquamation, and this may be associated with a foreign body giant cell reaction. The latter may be seen in other parts of the tumor as a reaction to the contents of the tumor. Foreign body giant cell reaction may also be seen when the contents of the tumor are spilled, leading to the formation of adhesions.

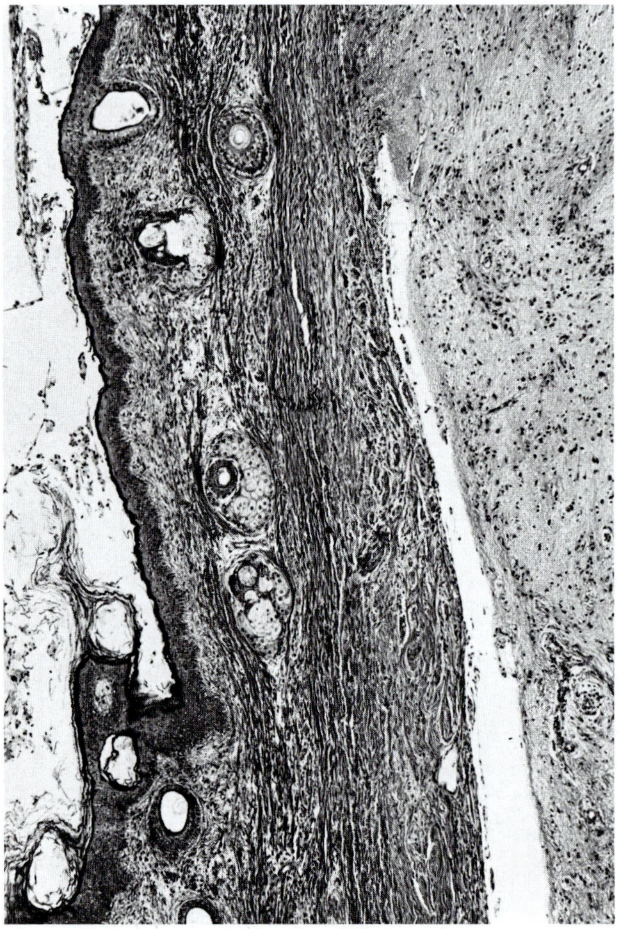

Fig. 20.42. Mature cystic teratoma. The lining of the cyst is composed of skin with its appendages. Mature neural tissue is seen beneath the cutaneous structures.

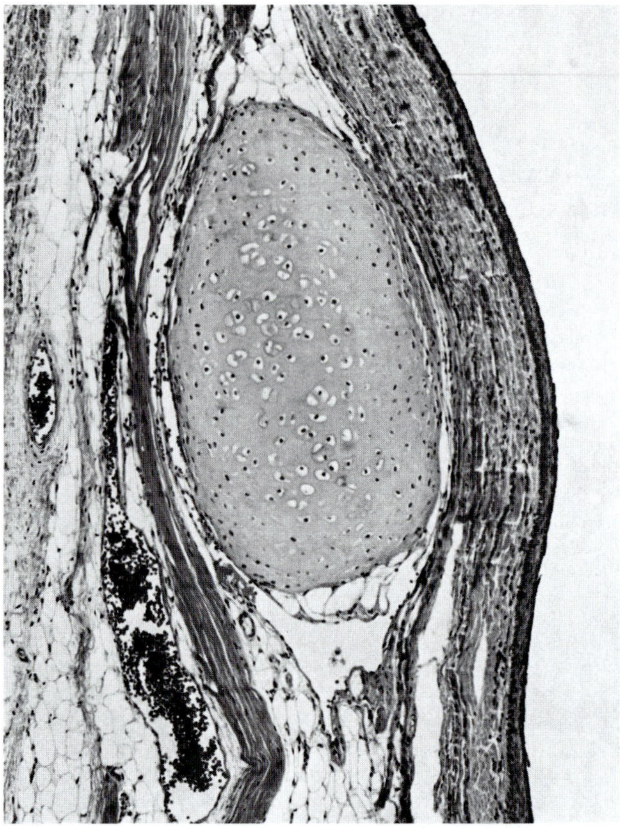

Fig. 20.43. Mature cystic teratoma. The tumor is lined by squamous epithelium and contains cartilage, muscle, and fatty tissue.

The area around the dermoid protuberance may contain a large variety of tissues derived from the three germ layers. Ectodermal tissue, represented by squamous epithelium and other skin derivatives, is usually most abundant. Brain tissue, glia, neural tissue, retina, choroid plexus, and ganglia may also be encountered. Mesodermal tissue is represented by bone, cartilage (Fig. 20.43), smooth muscle, and fibrous and fatty tissue. Endodermal tissue is represented by gastrointestinal and bronchial epithelium and glands, thyroid, and salivary gland tissue. In a careful study of 100 cases, ectodermal structures were found in 100%, mesodermal in 93%, and endodermal in 71% of cases.[23] The various tissues present in mature cystic teratoma show an orderly organoid arrangement forming cutaneous, bronchial, and gastrointestinal tissues, as well as bone and other structures. Although these tissues may be scattered diffusely, they do not exhibit the disorderly haphazard arrangement that is observed in immature teratoma.

With the exception of thyroid tissue, the presence of endocrine tissue of other types is distinctly uncommon in mature cystic teratoma, but pituitary, adrenal, and parathyroid tissue have been documented. Occasionally functioning endocrine tissue, forming an adenoma, may be found in a mature cystic teratoma. Mature cystic teratoma must be differentiated from the rare cases of fetus in fetu, considered most likely to be caused by an inclusion of a monozygotic diamniotic twin. Fetus in fetu can be distinguished from a teratoma by its location in the retroperitoneal space, presence of vertebral organization with formation of limb buds, and a well-developed organ system. Fetus in fetu shows better organization than the most differentiated teratomas. Like mature cystic teratoma, fetus in fetu is a benign lesion.

Clinical Behavior

Mature cystic teratoma of the ovary may be associated with various complications. In view of the fact that in many of these cases the condition is amenable to cure, their recognition is of considerable importance. These complications include (1) torsion, (2) rupture, (3) infection, (4) hemolytic anemia, and (5) development of malignancy.

Torsion is the most frequent complication,[13,29,116,126] occurring in 16.1% of cases in one large series.[126] This complication tends to be more common during pregnancy and puerperium.[92,126] Mature cystic teratoma is said to comprise from 22% to 40% of ovarian tumors in pregnancy, and from 0.8% to 12.8% of reported cases of mature cystic teratoma have occurred during pregnancy.[29,126] The fact that these tumors, when they occur during pregnancy, are more liable to be associated with torsion is of considerable importance. Torsion is also more common in children and younger patients.[116,126] The patients usually have severe acute abdominal pain, and the condition is an acute abdominal emergency. Excision of the affected ovary or salpingo-oophorectomy is the treatment of choice.

Torsion tends to predispose to rupture of the tumor. Rupture of mature cystic teratoma is an uncommon complication, occurring in approximately 1% of cases.[92,126] It is much more common during pregnancy and may manifest itself during labor.[92,126] The immediate result of the rupture may be shock or hemorrhage, especially during pregnancy or labor, but the prognosis even in these cases is usually favorable. Rupture of the tumor into the peritoneal cavity may be followed by chemical peritonitis caused by the spillage of the contents of the tumor. It produces a marked granulomatous reaction and leads to the formation of dense adhesions throughout the peritoneal cavity. Rupture of the tumor occasionally may be followed by the development of glial implants on the peritoneum. This condition occurs when the tumor contains mature neuroglial elements, and spillage leads to deposition of numerous small nodules composed of mature glia in the peritoneal cavity. Despite the wide dissemination of these deposits throughout the peritoneal cavity, the prognosis is favorable, and simple surgical excision of the primary tumor is considered to be adequate therapy.[138] Mature cystic teratoma may rupture not only into the peritoneal cavity but also into adjacent organs, usually the bladder or the rectum. More than 30 such cases have been reported.[35] Infection is an uncommon complication and occurs in approximately 1% of cases.[92] The infecting organism is usually a coliform, but *Salmonella* infection causing typhoid fever has also been reported.[63]

Autoimmune hemolytic anemia has been noted occasionally in patients with teratoma of the ovary, mainly mature cystic teratoma. Excision of the tumor in these cases resulted in the disappearance of the anemia and a complete cure.[20,37,121] Nineteen cases of mature cystic teratoma and 7 other cystic ovarian tumors associated with this complication have been reported.[20,121] The patients have symptoms and signs of progressive anemia, which may be moderate or severe; it is accompanied by reticulocytosis, spherocytosis, and increased osmotic fragility. Normoblasts may be present in the peripheral blood. The indirect serum bilirubin is elevated, and the direct antiglobulin test (Coombs' test) is positive, indicating the presence of autoantibodies that react with the patient's red blood cells. The platelets are normal in number. The spleen may be palpable but is only slightly enlarged. Steroids are only transiently effective in treating the disease, and splenectomy has no effect on the progress of the disease.[20,121] Excision of the ovarian tumor leads to the permanent disappearance of the anemia.[20,37,121] The following possible pathogenetic mechanisms have been suggested[20]:

1. Presence in the tumor of substances that are antigenically different from the host and that stimulate the production by the host of antibodies, which cross-react with the patients own red blood cells

2. Antibody production by the tumor directed specifically against the host's red blood cells resembling the graft-versus-host reaction
3. Coating of red blood cells with products secreted by the tumor, resulting in changed red blood cell antigenicity

In view of this, pelvic and radiologic examination is indicated in a young woman with autoimmune hemolytic anemia that does not respond to steroid treatment, as it may help to detect an ovarian teratoma and prevent an unnecessary splenectomy.[121]

Treatment

The treatment of choice for an uncomplicated mature cystic teratoma in young patients is excision of the cyst with conservation of part of the ovary if possible. This treatment usually results in a complete cure. Local recurrences after conservative treatment for mature cystic teratoma are uncommon and occur in less than 1% of cases.

Mature Cystic Teratoma (Dermoid Cyst) with Malignant Transformation

General Features

Malignant transformation is an uncommon complication of mature cystic teratoma. It occurs in approximately 2% of cases,[13,80,92,125,166] although in one report the frequency was almost 4%.[117] The age of patients with this complication as reported in the literature ranges from 19 to 88 years,[125] but this tumor usually is observed in postmenopausal patients.[80,92,117,125,166]

Clinically, this tumor cannot be readily differentiated from an uncomplicated mature cystic teratoma or other ovarian tumor, although evidence of its rapid growth, pain, loss of weight, and other systemic symptoms suggest the presence of a malignant tumor. Sometimes, the tumor may be found as an incidental observation. We have encountered, at autopsy, a large mature cystic teratoma containing a squamous cell carcinoma (Fig. 20.44) in a 56-year-old woman.

Gross Findings

The tumor is frequently larger than an average mature cystic teratoma[29,80,166]; it may exhibit a more solid appearance, but differentiation cannot be made on gross examination. Malignant transformation in mature cystic teratoma tends to occur in patients with unilateral tumors.[125,126]

Microscopic Findings

The tumor exhibits malignant transformation in one of its constituent tissues, most frequently squamous epithelium (see Fig. 20.44), with formation of a typical squamous cell carcinoma.[29,80,117,125,166] Any of the tissues present in a mature cystic teratoma may undergo malignant transformation, and a variety of malignant tumors have been reported, including carcinoid tumor, thyroid carcinoma, basal cell carcinoma (Fig. 20.45), adenocarcinoma of the intestinal epithelium (Fig. 20.46), malignant melanoma, leiomyosarcoma, chondrosarcoma, and hemangiosarcoma.[125,206] The malignant element invades other parts of the tumor and its wall (Fig. 20.45), which it tends to perforate. Invariably, only one tissue element becomes malignant, and the presence of many different malignant elements indicates that the tumor is an immature teratoma and not a mature cystic teratoma that has undergone malignant transformation.

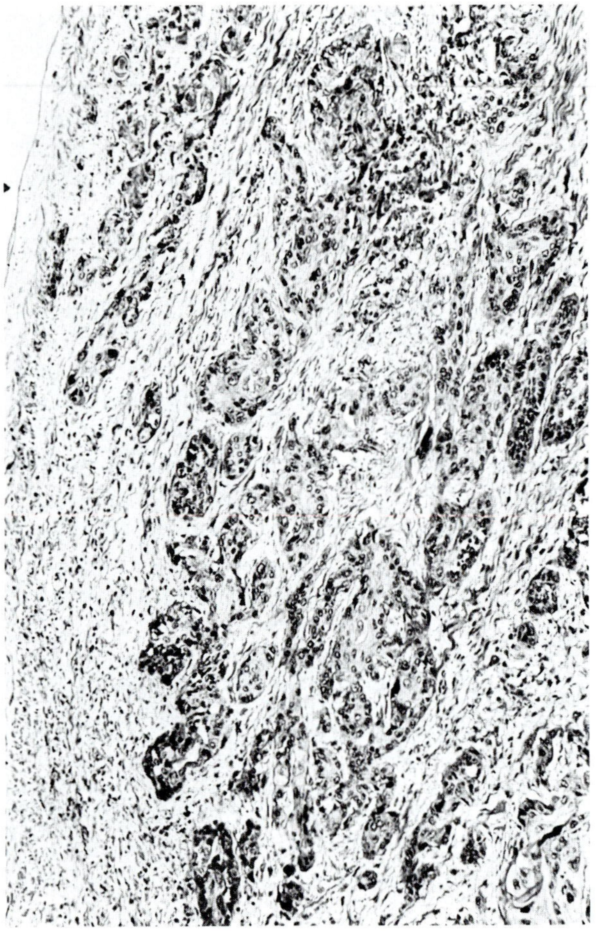

Fig. 20.44. Squamous cell carcinoma arising in a mature cystic teratoma. Surface of the ovary is seen at *top left*.

Clinical Behavior and Treatment

The mode of spread of the malignant tumor differs from that observed in other tumors of germ cell ori-

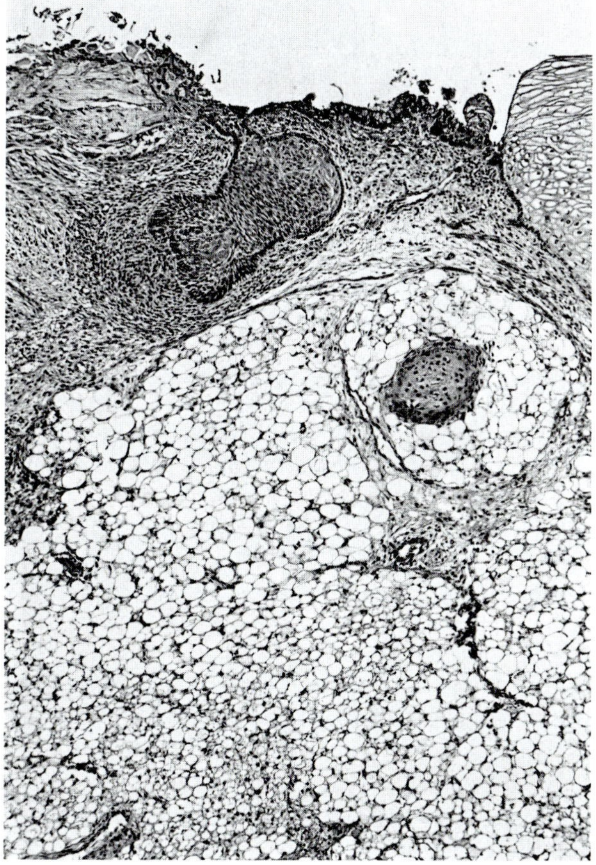

Fig. 20.45. Basal cell carcinoma arising in a mature cystic teratoma.

gin. The tumor spreads by direct invasion and peritoneal implantation and generally does not metastasize to the lymph nodes.[80,125] Extensive local invasion and absence of lymph node involvement usually is observed at laparotomy.[117,166] Hematogenous dissemination is uncommon.

The prognosis of patients with mature cystic teratoma with malignant transformation is unfavorable[80,117,125,166]; only 15%–30.8% of patients are 5-year survivors.[80,125] Better prognosis has been reported when the malignant element is a squamous cell carcinoma confined to the ovary and is excised without spillage of the contents. In such cases, the reported 5-year survival is 63%.[125] Although previous reports have indicated that there have been no 5-year survivors when the malignant element was an adenocarcinoma or a sarcoma, Ueda et al.[206] reported a case of a patient with an adenocarcinoma arising in a mature cystic teratoma who has survived for more than 15 years. The authors also cite a number of other cases, but include thyroid and sebaceous carcinomas, which are usually considered as separate entities. The present author has seen a patient with an intestinal-type adenocarcinoma arising in a mature cystic teratoma (Fig. 20.46) who has survived for more than 5 years. The outlook with this type of neoplasm may not be as dismal as previously believed, especially if there is no evidence of metastases at presentation.

Treatment is hysterectomy and bilateral adnexectomy.[80,166] Because the tumors are usually unilateral, in cases where there is no penetration of the capsule and no involvement of the adjacent structures, a more conservative surgical procedure may be just as effective. However, because malignant transformation of a mature cystic teratoma almost always occurs in postmenopausal women, total abdominal hysterectomy and bilateral salpingo-oophorectomy is the treatment of choice. If the tumor has spread beyond the confines of the ovary and there is involvement of the adjacent structures, a more radical procedure with resection of the tumor and the involved structures or viscera is advo-

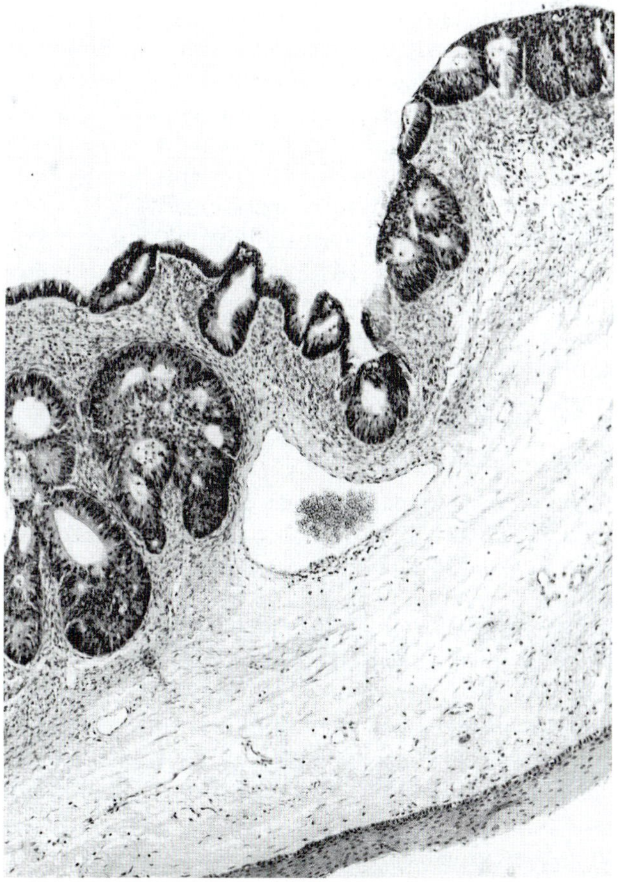

Fig. 20.46. Intestinal adenocarcinoma arising in a mature cystic teratoma.

cated.[117] Response to radiation and chemotherapy is unsatisfactory.[80,117]

Struma Ovarii

General Features

Thyroid tissue is a relatively frequent constituent of mature cystic teratoma and has been demonstrated in 5%–20% of cases. *Struma ovarii* is considered a one-sided development of a teratoma, in which the thyroid tissue has overgrown all other tissues, or one in which only the thyroid tissue has developed. The term struma ovarii should be reserved for tumors composed either entirely or predominantly of thyroid tissue.

Clinical Features

Struma ovarii is uncommon; it comprises 2.7% of ovarian teratomas. The age distribution of patients with struma ovarii is generally the same as that of patients with mature cystic teratoma and ranges from 6 to 74 years. Most patients are in the reproductive years.[105,216] There are usually no specific symptoms; the clinical findings are similar to those observed in patients with mature cystic teratoma. The only differences are that in some cases struma ovarii is associated with enlargement of the thyroid gland, and in other cases there is clinical evidence that the struma ovarii is responsible for the development of thyrotoxicosis, although this has not been confirmed preoperatively by laboratory tests.[105,162,216] Some cases of thyrotoxicosis have been associated with struma ovarii, which has also shown evidence of thyroid hyperactivity. The ectopic thyroid tissue present within struma ovarii, therefore, may be the subject of the same physiologic and pathologic changes as the thyroid gland.[162]

Gross Findings

Struma ovarii is usually unilateral[105,216] but is often associated with mature cystic teratoma and rarely with a cystadenoma in the contralateral ovary.[105,216] In some cases, the teratoma present in the contralateral ovary contained thyroid tissue.

Struma ovarii varies in size but usually measures less than 10 cm in diameter. The surface is usually smooth and, before sectioning, the tumor shows similar appearances to mature cystic teratoma. Occasionally, adhesions may be present. The cut surface of the tumor may be composed entirely of light tan, glistening thyroid tissue (Fig. 20.47). Hemorrhage, necrosis, and foci of fibrosis may be present. Solid tumors with small amounts of colloid appear less glistening and more fleshy.

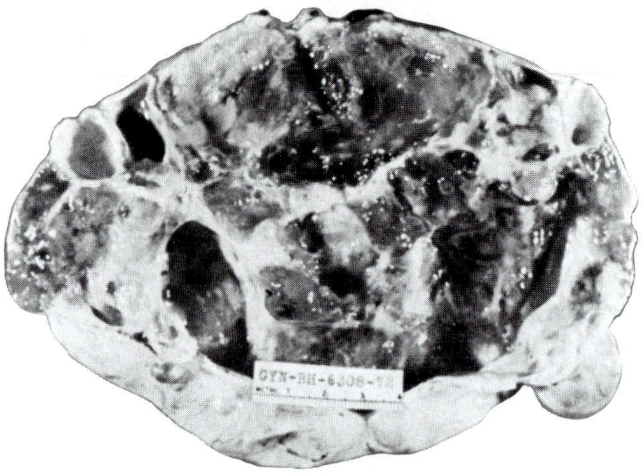

Fig. 20.47. Struma ovarii. The cut surface shows compartments of amber-colored thyroid tissue separated by thick fibrous septae. (Courtesy of B. Bigelow, M.D., New York, NY.)

Microscopic Findings

The tumor is composed of mature thyroid tissue consisting of acini of various sizes, lined by a single layer of columnar or flattened epithelium (Fig. 20.48). The acini contain eosinophilic, PAS-positive colloid. The intensity of the staining may vary. There may be a considerable variation in the size of the acini, which may be large, containing a large amount of colloid, or may be small. Thyroglobulin can be identified in the epithelial cells by immunohistochemistry. Occasionally, the lining of the acini may be columnar, containing small papillary projections not unlike those seen in hyperactive thyroid gland. Sometimes the appearances may resemble a nodular adenomatous goiter. Adenoma-like lesions may also be observed. Struma ovarii showing appearances suggestive of Hashimoto's thyroiditis has also been reported.[41]

Clinical Behavior and Treatment

Most cases of struma ovarii are benign and can be treated by excision of the ovary or by unilateral salpingo-oophorectomy. In a small number of cases, there are complications, the most important being the development of malignancy and the presence of ascites or ascites associated with pleural effusion producing a pseudo-Meigs' syndrome.[70] Ascites may be found in 17% of cases of struma ovarii, and its presence does not indicate that the tumor is malignant.[162] The cause of the ascites and pleural effusion has not been fully elucidated. In most reported cases, excision of the tumor led to complete remission.

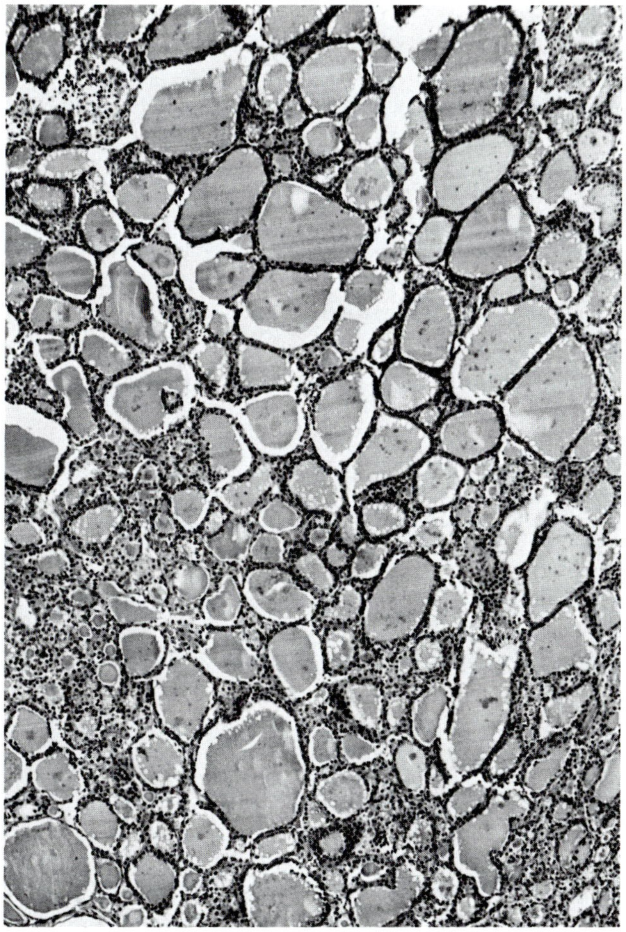

Fig. 20.48. Struma ovarii. The tumor is composed of normal thyroid tissue.

Malignant change in struma ovarii is uncommon. In a number of reported cases, the diagnosis was based on the histology of the tumor, and there were no metastases or other features of malignancy. The diagnosis of malignancy is difficult in such cases; this applies mainly to the tumors showing a follicular pattern, as papillary carcinomas occurring in struma ovarii are much easier to diagnose. The tumor must be extensively sampled. The criteria for malignancy in struma ovarii are the same as those for thyroid tumors.

A number of reported cases of malignant struma ovarii were examples of strumal carcinoid. Only 17 of 45 reported cases of malignant struma ovarii were associated with metastases.[57,105,216] Malignant struma ovarii often shows a follicular pattern, but papillary carcinoma is not infrequent. We have encountered a 26-year-old patient with a mature cystic teratoma containing thyroid tissue and a typical well-differentiated papillary adenocarcinoma of the thyroid (Fig. 20.49), which was associated with metastases in the para-aortic lymph nodes. The patient was well and symptom free 5 years after excision of the tumor followed by laparotomy and dissection of the paraaortic lymph nodes, as well as a course of radiation therapy. There was no evidence of metastases elsewhere. In three other cases of papillary carcinoma developing in struma ovarii known to the author, the patients were cured by excision of the affected adnexa, although in a fourth case the patient died of extensive metastatic disease. In two cases of follicular carcinoma arising in struma ovarii known to the author the patients were cured by excision of the affected adnexa, whereas in two other cases the patients succumbed to extensive metastatic disease.

Malignant struma ovarii may involve the peritoneum. The tumor deposits, which are composed of malignant thyroid tissue, should not be confused with deposits of benign thyroid tissue representing peritoneal spread of nonmalignant struma ovarii (see following discussion of benign strumosis). Occasionally, the distinction between these entities

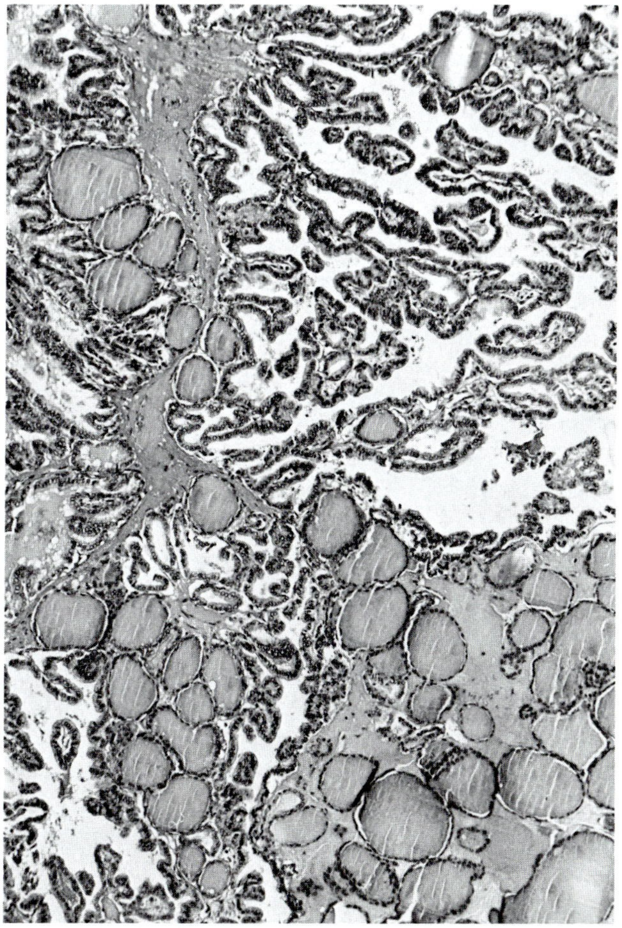

Fig. 20.49. Papillary thyroid carcinoma in mature cystic teratoma.

may pose considerable difficulties, especially when the malignant neoplasm is of the well-differentiated follicular type. Other routes of spread are via the lymphatics to the paraaortic and other lymph nodes and via the bloodstream to the lungs and bones. The prognosis in cases unassociated with metastases is generally good, but when metastases are present, it is less favorable. Treatment consists of surgery and administration of radioactive iodine (^{131}I) and other agents used in the treatment of thyroid malignancy, including radiation therapy.

Occasionally, struma ovarii may be associated with extraovarian extension caused either by rupture of the tumor or by local spread. In such cases, the peritoneal cavity contains tumor deposits, which may be numerous and are composed of mature thyroid tissue. The condition is benign and is termed benign strumosis. It is only rarely associated with untoward side effects, which are mainly caused by the formation of adhesions. Benign strumosis may be treated by excision of the tumor deposits or by administration of radioactive iodine (^{131}I).

Carcinoid

Carcinoid tumors of the ovary may be primary or metastatic. Primary carcinoids are subdivided into four categories: (1) insular or islet, (2) trabecular, (3) mucinous, and (4) mixed (composed of any combination of the three pure types). The latter are uncommon and often associated with a mature cystic teratoma. Of the metastatic carcinoids, the insular carcinoid tumor is the most common, followed by the trabecular and mucinous types. The metastatic carcinoid tumors of the ovary are discussed in Chapter 22, Metastatic Tumors of the Ovary.

Insular or Islet Carcinoid

General Features

Insular carcinoid tumor, considered to be of midgut derivation, is the most common type of primary ovarian carcinoid tumor. It usually arises in association with gastrointestinal or respiratory epithelium present in a mature cystic teratoma. It may also be observed within a solid teratoma, a mucinous tumor, in association with a Sertoli–Leydig cell tumor,[218] or may occur in a pure form.[140,179] The latter is considered to arise either as a one-sided development of a teratoma or from enterochromaffin cells present within the ovary. The former is much more likely. Approximately 40% of ovarian insular carcinoids occur in pure form; the remaining 60% are combined.[179]

Clinical Features

More than 80 cases of primary ovarian insular carcinoid tumors have been reported.[36,140] The author is aware of an even greater number of unreported cases. The age of patients ranges from 31 to 83 years, but most patients are either postmenopausal or perimenopausal.[36,140] One-third of the reported cases have been associated with the typical carcinoid syndrome, despite the absence of metastases.[36,140] This is in contrast to intestinal carcinoids, which are associated with the syndrome only when there is metastatic spread to the liver. The reason for this difference is that the blood flow from the ovary goes directly into the systemic circulation and does not pass through the liver, which inactivates the serotonin produced by the tumor. The presence or absence of symptoms of carcinoid syndrome is also dependent on the number of secreting tumor cells.

Functioning ovarian carcinoid tumors, with only one exception, have all measured approximately 10 cm in diameter, whereas intestinal carcinoids are usually smaller. Thus, there is a good correlation between the size of the tumor and the presence of carcinoid syndrome. The excision of the tumor is associated with rapid remission of the symptoms, disappearance of 5-hydroxyindole acetic acid (5-HIAA) from the urine,[140] and marked decrease of serum serotonin. Determination of serum serotonin and urinary 5-HIAA may be used to monitor disease activity and response to therapy. If the tumor is nonfunctioning, there is no specific presentation.

Gross Findings

The tumor shows similar appearances to those of mature cystic teratoma within which it is usually found. The same applies if the tumor is associated with a solid teratoma or a mucinous tumor. If the carcinoid is not associated with other tissue elements, the tumor is solid. The carcinoid may vary in size from microscopic to 20 cm in longest diameter and is solid and homogeneous (Fig. 20.50). Its color may vary from light brown to yellow or pale gray. Primary ovarian carcinoids practically always are unilateral, although they may be associated with a mature cystic teratoma in the contralateral ovary.

Microscopic Findings

The primary ovarian insular carcinoid usually shows the typical appearance associated with midgut carcinoids.[140] The tumor is composed of collections of small acini and solid nests of uniform polygonal cells with ample amounts of cytoplasm and round or oval, centrally located hyperchromatic nuclei (Fig. 20.51). Mitotic activity is low. The cy-

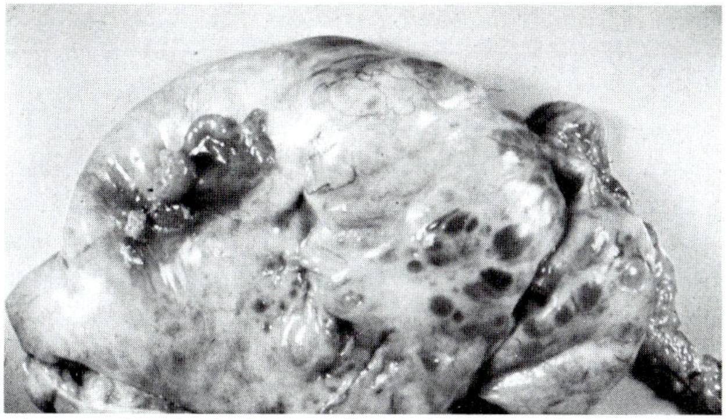

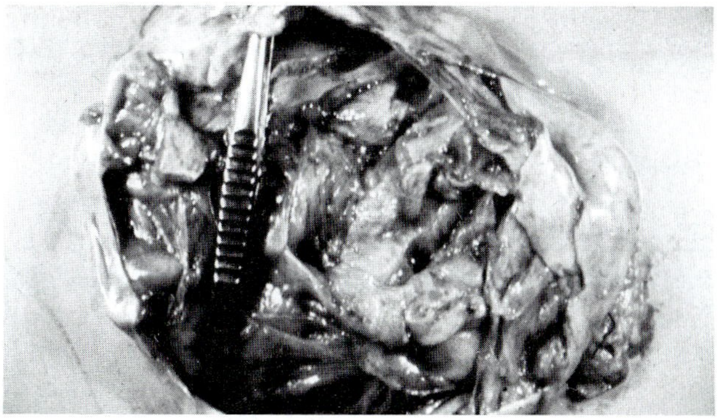

Fig. 20.50. Primary insular carcinoid. *Left*: The tumor is oval shaped and encapsulated. *Right*: The cut surface is yellow to brown and largely cystic. (Courtesy of B. Bigelow, M.D., New York, NY.)

toplasm is basophilic or amphophilic and may contain red, brown, or orange argentaffin (Fig. 20.52) or argyrophil granules, which are demonstrated in the majority of cases of primary ovarian carcinoids.[140] Ultrastructurally, the cells of the ovarian insular carcinoid show similar appearances to those of insular carcinoid tumors from other locations[179] and show abundant neurosecretory granules, which exhibit marked variation in size and shape, being round, oval, or elongated.

Serotonin may be demonstrated within the cytoplasm of the tumor cells by immunoperoxidase techniques.[164] Demonstration of positive chromogranin A staining immunocytochemically further supports the diagnosis and has become the method of choice to confirm the diagnosis. Occasionally, other neurohormonal polypeptides may also be demonstrated within the cytoplasm of the tumor cells, but their finding is much less frequent than in trabecular or strumal carcinoids.[164] The connective

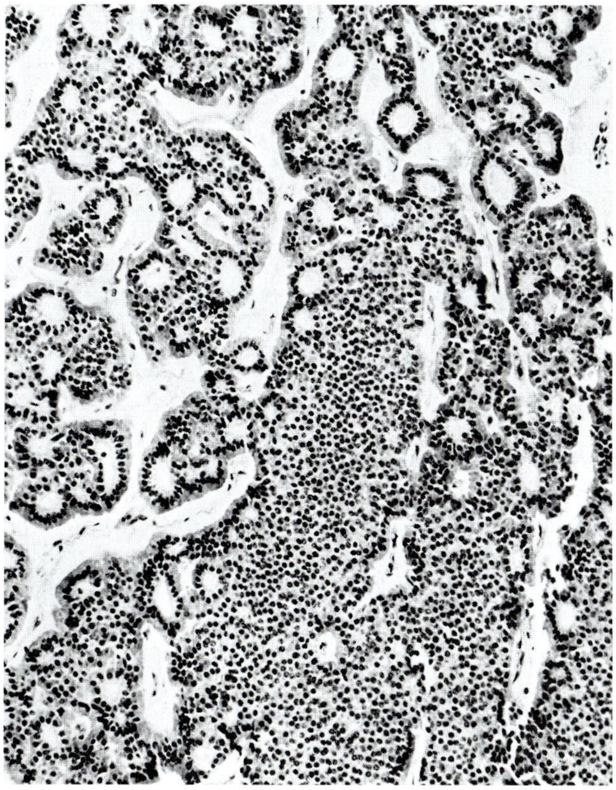

Fig. 20.51. Primary insular ovarian carcinoid. The typical solid and acinar patterns of midgut carcinoid are shown.

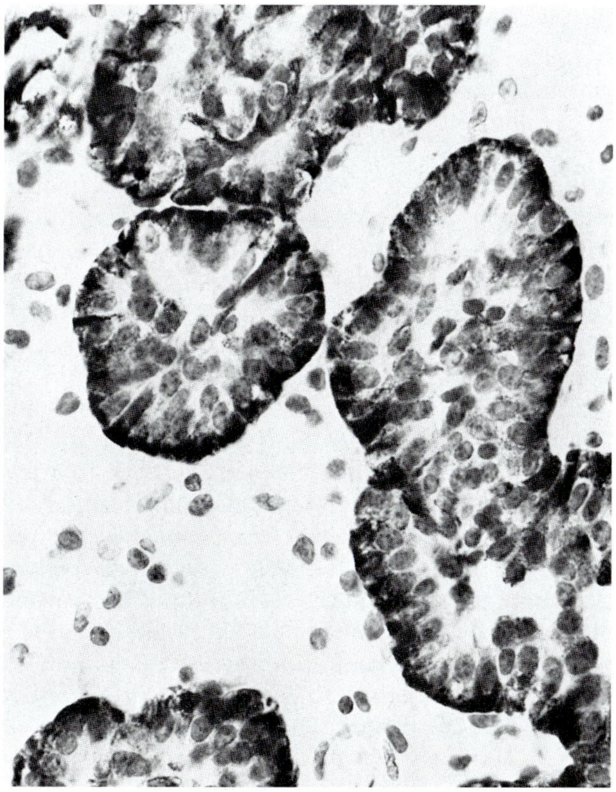

Fig. 20.52. Ovarian insular carcinoid. The tumor cells contain numerous argentaffin granules stained *black*.

tissue surrounding the tumor nests is frequently dense and hyalinized as a result of the fibrogenic effect of the serotonin produced by the tumor.

Differential Diagnosis

Primary insular carcinoid of the ovary must be differentiated from metastatic insular carcinoid of the ovary, which is usually of gastrointestinal origin. Metastatic carcinoid nearly always affects both ovaries,[141] unlike primary ovarian carcinoid, which is unilateral.[140] Macroscopically, the metastatic carcinoid is composed of tumor nodules, whereas primary ovarian carcinoid forms a single homogeneous mass. Presence of other teratomatous elements associated with an ovarian carcinoid, confirms that it is primary.[140,179]

Primary ovarian carcinoid sometimes may be confused with Brenner tumor, but the appearances of the cell nests and the grooved coffee-bean nuclei of the cells of Brenner tumor are against the diagnosis of a carcinoid, whereas the typical small acinar pattern and the presence of argyrophil- and argentaffin-positive cells, as well as positive chromogranin A staining, are in favor of a carcinoid. Confusion with granulosa cell tumor may also arise because Call–Exner bodies may be mistaken for carcinoid acini, but the cells of the carcinoid tumor usually show an acinar pattern and contain more cytoplasm and argentaffin granules.[140] Cystic areas that may be present in a granulosa cell tumor are nearly always absent in a carcinoid.

Occasionally, ovarian carcinoid may be confused with a Krukenberg tumor, but the latter is usually bilateral and larger. The cells of Krukenberg tumor tend to merge with the stroma, are larger, and show greater pleomorphism, a signet-ring appearance, and more brisk mitotic activity. An acinar pattern is less evident. Demonstration of argyrophil and argentaffin granules, which can be detected in most ovarian carcinoids and are often abundant, confirms the diagnosis. Although these granules may be observed in some cells in Krukenberg tumors, they are much more numerous in ovarian carcinoids and are best identified immunocytochemically with chromogranin A stains; this is the most widely used method to demonstrate them at the present time. These granules can also be demonstrated with the aid of the electron microscope, manifesting themselves as numerous pleomorphic membrane-bound neurosecretory granules present within the cytoplasm.[140,158,179]

Clinical Behavior and Treatment

Although insular carcinoid tumors of the ovary are considered to be malignant, they are slow growing and only occasionally are associated with metastases. Metastases has been observed in 11 patients, 7 of whom died with metastatic disease[36,140]; this includes 6 patients with metastatic disease from a series of 9 cases of insular carcinoid tumors of the ovary collected over 40 years by Davis et al.[36] This series suggested that metastatic disease may be more frequent than generally reported. Although the malignant potential of insular carcinoid should not be minimized, it is considered that the series of Davis et al[36] was somewhat selective as regards its content of metastasizing tumors.

In occasional patients, features of carcinoid syndrome, such as tricuspid incompetence resulting in right-sided heart failure, may progress after the excision of the tumor and lead to the death of the patient, as has been observed in two cases.[140] In most patients with the carcinoid syndrome, the symptoms and signs of the syndrome observed preoperatively disappear or regress during the postoperative period.[140] Because nearly all patients with this tumor are postmenopausal or perimenopausal, bilateral salpingo-oophorectomy and hysterectomy is the treatment of choice. Surgical excision of foci of extraovarian spread or of metastases if present is indicated. The tumor does not respond to radiation therapy, and there is at present little experience with chemotherapy. Estimation of serum serotonin and 5-HIAA in the urine may be used to monitor the progress of the disease.

Trabecular Carcinoid

General Features

Trabecular carcinoid includes carcinoid tumors of hindgut or foregut derivation. Primary trabecular or ribbon carcinoid usually arises in association with teratomatous elements,[142] but in a later study of four cases of trabecular carcinoid, two tumors were pure and not associated with teratomatous elements.[182]

Clinical Features

Trabecular carcinoid is rare; fewer than 25 cases have been reported. The age varies from 24 to 74 years, with most patients being postmenopausal.[36,142,182] Trabecular carcinoid is a slowly growing neoplasm that can reach a large size. None of the known cases have been associated with the carcinoid syndrome. In three patients whose urine was examined immediately after the operation, 5-HIAA was normal.[142]

Gross Findings

The appearance of trabecular carcinoid depends on whether the tumor is associated with teratomatous elements. When associated with teratoma, the ap-

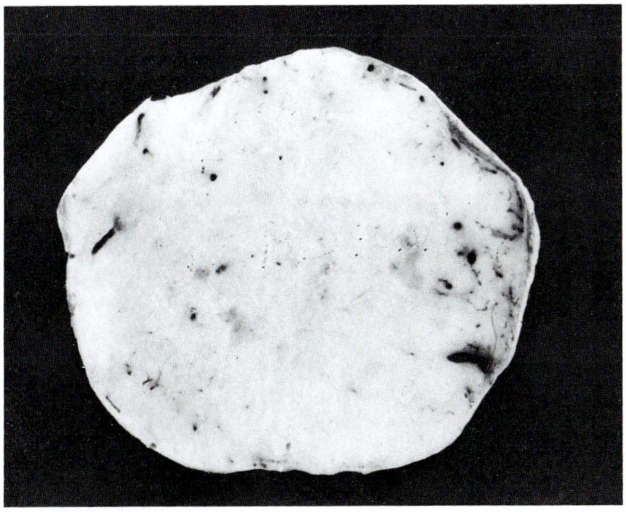

Fig. 20.53. Pure trabecular carcinoid tumor of the ovary. The cut surface is solid, uniform, and yellow. The outer surface is smooth.

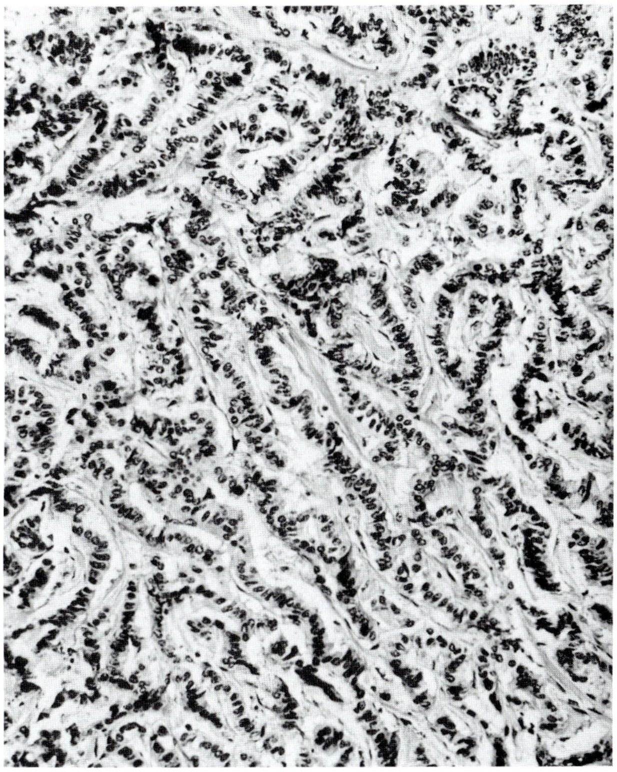

Fig. 20.54. Trabecular carcinoid. The tumor is composed of long ramifying cords of tumor cells surrounded by dense fibrous stroma.

pearance is similar to that of a mature cystic teratoma. When the tumor is pure, it is a solid, firm to hard, round or oval mass with a smooth outline and tan to yellow on cross section (Fig. 20.53). The tumors have always been unilateral[142,182] but occasionally have been associated with mature cystic teratoma in the opposite ovary.[142] In the reported cases, the tumors measured from 4 to 25 cm in the longest diameter.[142,182]

Microscopic Findings

The tumor is composed of long, usually wavy ribbons, cords, or parallel trabeculae surrounded by fibromatous connective tissue stroma that is usually dense (Fig. 20.54). The ribbons, cords, or trabeculae are composed of cells that form usually one but sometimes two cell layers (Fig. 20.54). The nuclei are elongated or ovoid and contain finely dispersed chromatin. The cytoplasm is abundant and often contains orange to red-brown granules, which usually stain with argyrophil and argentaffin stains. Ultrastructurally, the neurosecretory granules are round or oval and show slight variation in size,[158,185] thus differing from those seen in insular carcinoids. Immunocytochemistry is positive for chromogranin A and demonstrates a much wider range of neurohormonal polypeptides than insular carcinoids; these include serotonin, pancreatic polypeptide, glucagon, enkephalin, gastrin, vasoactive intestinal polypeptide, and calcitonin.[164]

Differential Diagnosis

Primary trabecular carcinoid must be distinguished from metastatic trabecular carcinoid, which is usually bilateral and frequently associated with metastases elsewhere. The presence of teratomatous elements, which are found frequently in the primary lesion, helps to distinguish the primary from a metastatic lesion. Trabecular carcinoid sometimes may exhibit an insular pattern in foci, but unless this is a major component the tumor need not be classified as a mixed carcinoid.

The presence of thyroid follicles indicates that the tumor is a struma ovarii and carcinoid (strumal carcinoid), and their presence must be excluded before a diagnosis of trabecular carcinoid is made. Occasionally, trabecular carcinoid must be distinguished from a Sertoli–Leydig cell tumor showing a cordlike pattern. In contrast to a Sertoli–Leydig tumor, trabecular carcinoid lacks tubules. The presence of argyrophil and argentaffin granules, positive chromogranin A staining, and neurosecretory granules ultrastructurally confirm the diagnosis of carcinoid.

Clinical Behavior and Treatment

The prognosis of patients with trabecular carcinoid of the ovary is favorable because these tumors are not associated with metastases.[36,142,182] In one case, a peritoneal implant was found 2 years after bilateral salpingo-oophorectomy and hysterectomy.[142]

The optimal treatment is the excision of the affected adnexa, which results in a complete cure, but follow-up of the patient is advisable.

Mucinous Carcinoid (Goblet Cell Carcinoid)

General Features

Mucinous carcinoid is a variant of carcinoid tumor that has been encountered mainly in the vermiform appendix[76,170,210] and occasionally has been observed in the ovary.[3,179] However, it should be noted that at least some of the tumors described as primary Krukenberg tumors of the ovary may have been examples of this entity. A number of cases of mucinous carcinoid tumor metastatic to the ovary have been reported, and several more are known to the author.

Clinical Features

The age of patients ranges from 14 to 74 years. Mucinous carcinoid is usually observed in pure form but may be seen in association with mature cystic teratoma. The tumor is unilateral but may be associated with metastases in the contralateral ovary.[3,115,179]

Gross Findings

Macroscopically, the tumor is usually of considerable size, ranging from 4 to 30 cm, and most of the tumors have been more than 8 cm in the longest diameter. The tumor is gray-yellow, firm, and usually solid but may contain cystic areas.[3,115,179] Similar appearances are encountered when the tumor forms part of a mature cystic teratoma.

Microscopic Findings

Microscopically, mucinous carcinoid is composed of numerous small glands or acini with very small lumens lined by uniform columnar or cuboid epithelium. The cells contain small round or oval nuclei or appear as goblet cells distended with mucin (Fig. 20.55). Some cells may be disrupted by excessive distension with mucin, which may result in the formation of small pools of mucin within the glands or even in the obliteration of the gland with pools of mucinous material within the connective tissue (Fig. 20.56). The glands are surrounded by connective tissue, which may vary from loose and edematous to dense fibrous or hyalinized. Some of the glands or acini may be larger and occasionally may be cystic (Fig. 20.56); this represents the typical or classical pattern of mucinous carcinoid. In some areas the tumor cells tend to invade the surrounding connective tissue, often assuming signet-ring appearance. The tumor cells may form large solid aggregates and show a less uniform appearance and more atypical features, with large hyperchromatic nuclei and brisk mitotic activity.

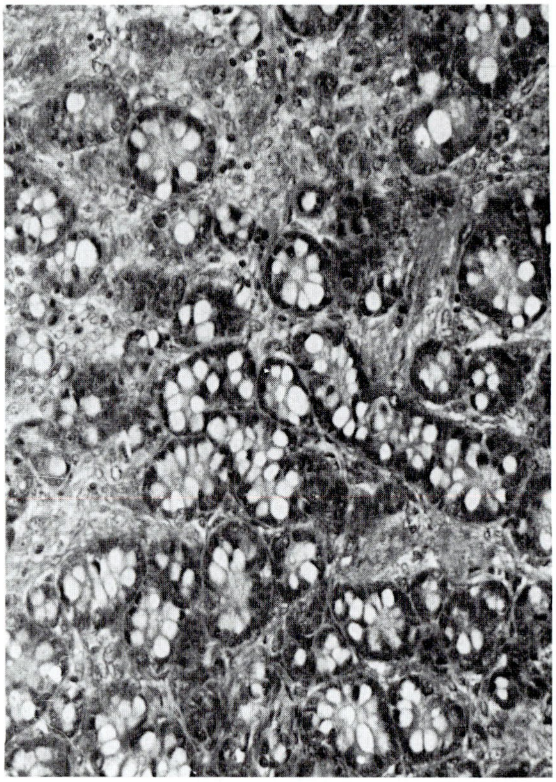

Fig. 20.55. Mucinous carcinoid tumor. The tumor is composed of numerous small glands and acini with imperceptible or very small lumens. Numerous goblet cells distended with mucin are present.

In some tumors, such appearances may predominate. This second pattern resembles Krukenberg tumor and is described as atypical or Krukenberg tumor-like pattern. Sometimes mucinous carcinoid showing either the typical or atypical pattern or both merges with intestinal-like adenocarcinoma showing numerous neuroendocrine cells (Fig. 20.57); this is regarded as a third pattern present in this tumor. Some mucinous carcinoids may be admixed with other types of carcinoid tumor, such as insular or trabecular, forming a mixed carcinoid tumor. Thus, primary ovarian mucinous carcinoid tumors can be divided into these four histologic types. In a recent study of 17 mucinous carcinoid tumors, 6 were of the typical type, 4 of the atypical or Krukenberg tumor-like type, 5 were admixed with intestinal-like adenocarcinoma, and 2 were of the mixed type.[115] The cytoplasm of the tumor cells may exhibit orange-red granules and may even be bright red. Argyrophil

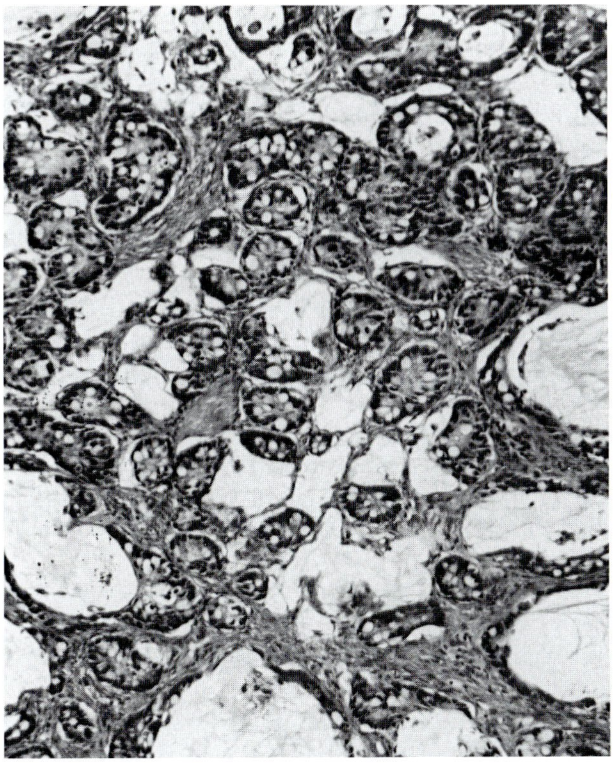

Fig. 20.56. Mucinous carcinoid tumor. The tumor is composed of small glands and acini. Many acini are disrupted by excessive distension with mucin, resulting in the formation of pools of mucin within the surrounding connective tissue. Larger glands distended with mucin also are present.

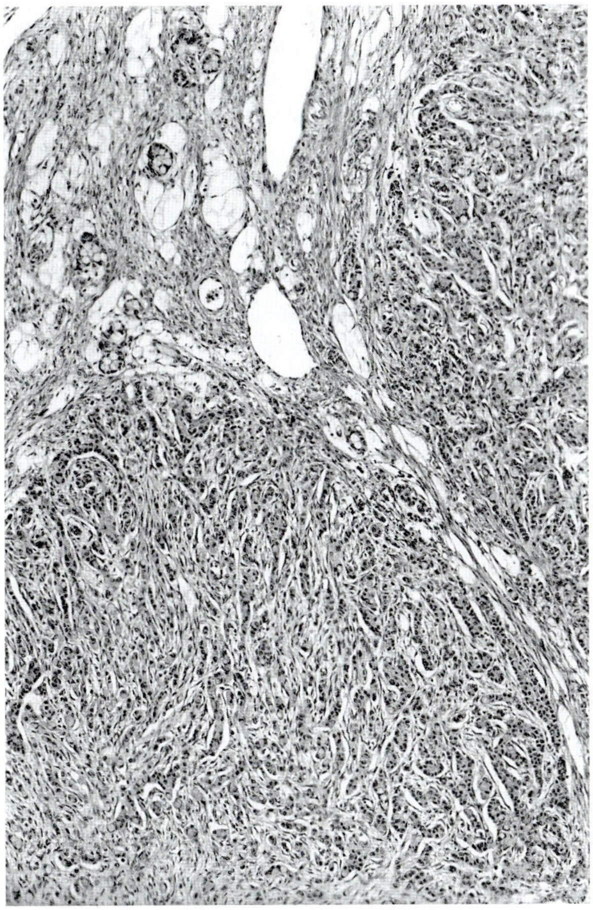

Fig. 20.57. Mucinous carcinoid tumor. Classical pattern (*top left*) associated with the atypical pattern.

and argentaffin granules are always present and, in some tumors, may be abundant.[3,115,179]

Ultrastructurally, neurosecretory granules are present in some cells and absent in others. The tumor cells may contain both neurosecretory granules and mucinous material. The neuroendocrine nature of the tumor cells is further confirmed using immunocytochemical stains. The tumor cells react positively with chromogranin A. Using immunocytochemical techniques, some of the tumor cells have been shown to contain serotonin and gastrin, and these substances may be present within the same tumor cell. Other neurohormonal polypeptides such as pancreatic polypeptide and prolactin also have been detected in the tumor cells, but the range is narrower than that observed in trabecular carcinoids. CEA and low molecular weight cytokeratin also can be demonstrated within the cytoplasm of the tumor cells.

Differential Diagnosis

Primary mucinous carcinoid tumor of the ovary must be differentiated from its metastatic counterpart. The latter, in common with other types of carcinoid metastatic to the ovary, is nearly always bilateral and instead of forming a single tumor mass shows scattered tumor deposits involving ovarian tissue. Depending on their size, these deposits may form tumor nodules observed macroscopically or may be detectable only microscopically. Histologically, they may have appearances indistinguishable from the primary tumor.

Mucinous carcinoid must be distinguished from mucinous tumors of the ovary, especially when the carcinoid tumor is composed of large acini, shows increased mucin production, and exhibits a pleomorphic pattern. Occasionally, confusion may arise with well-differentiated endometrioid tumors of the ovary, which may resemble mucinous tumors.

Mucinous carcinoid must be distinguished from a Krukenberg tumor. The differentiation between these two entities may be difficult, especially if the mucinous carcinoid assumes a predominantly Krukenberg-like pattern or if the Krukenberg tumor contains numerous argentaffin and argyrophil granules. The presence of these granules as well as of the neurosecretory granules observed ultrastructurally cannot be used for differentiation between these two entities. Involvement of both ovaries and the presence of primary extraovarian signet-ring or mucinous adenocarcinoma are indicative of Krukenberg tumor.

Clinical Behavior and Treatment

Primary mucinous carcinoid of the ovary behaves in a slightly more aggressive manner than other types of primary ovarian carcinoid tumors,[3,115,179] similar to the behavior of mucinous carcinoid tumors of the vermiform appendix.[76,170,210] The tumor tends to spread mainly via the lymphatics, and metastases may be present at the time of initial laparotomy. Patients who do not exhibit metastatic disease at the time of diagnosis have very much better prognosis compared with those who have metastases, however small, at the time of diagnosis.[3,115,179] In a recent series of 17 patients,[115] follow-up was available in 13 cases. Eleven patients were alive without recurrence for periods of 28–168 months, 2 patients with mucinous carcinoid of the atypical type died of widespread disease within 2 years of diagnosis, and all 6 patients with mucinous carcinoid of the typical or classical type had tumors confined to the ovary and all were well and disease free after excision of the tumor.[115]

The treatment is surgical, depending on the extent of the disease, but in postmenopausal women, patients with involvement of the contralateral ovary, and patients who do not want children, hysterectomy, bilateral salpingo-oophorectomy, and omentectomy, as well as excision of all the tumor deposits present, are indicated. Paraaortic lymph node dissection may be necessary because metastatic tumor deposits may be present. Surgery may be followed by combination chemotherapy, including 5-fluorouracil, although the efficacy of this mode of therapy is not proven. Radiation therapy does not appear to be effective. Premenopausal patients with tumors localized to the ovary may be treated by unilateral salpingo-oophorectomy with careful follow-up.

Strumal Carcinoid

General Features

Strumal carcinoid is an uncommon ovarian tumor composed of thyroid tissue intimately admixed with carcinoid tumor, showing a ribbon-like or cordlike pattern. Other teratomatous elements are also present in most of the tumors.[139] Tumors showing the histologic pattern of struma ovarii, merging imperceptibly with carcinoid tumor exhibiting the ribbon-like pattern observed in hindgut carcinoids, were usually interpreted as a carcinoma developing in a struma ovarii, although the resemblance to a carcinoid tumor has been noted in some cases.[57]

Clinical Features

More than 60 cases have been reported,[139,163] and there are probably as many unreported cases. The age distribution is similar to struma ovarii, ranging from 21 to 77 years.[139,163] The tumor is usually not associated with any specific clinical findings. In one reported case, it was associated with virilization. Like hindgut carcinoids and unlike the primary ovarian insular carcinoid, strumal carcinoid is not as a rule associated with the carcinoid syndrome,[139,163] although this association has been described in a single case.[207]

Gross Findings

Macroscopically, this tumor, if pure, may be similar to struma ovarii or carcinoid. If the tumor is a part of a teratoma, it manifests as a yellow nodule within the teratoma.[139,163]

Microscopic Findings

Microscopically, the strumal carcinoid is composed of thyroid follicles containing colloid that merge with ribbons of neoplastic cells usually set in dense fibrous tissue stroma similar to the trabecular carcinoid (Figs. 20.58 and 20.59). The thyroid follicles are often small in size at the junction between the two types of tissue. The carcinoid is usually composed of long, winding or straight ribbons of columnar cells with elongated hyperchromatic nuclei (Fig. 20.59). It may also be composed of small islands of tumor cells surrounded by dense fibrous tissue stroma (Fig. 20.58). Slight mitotic activity is present in the carcinoid part of the lesion.

Argyrophil and argentaffin granules are identified in the carcinoid cells,[139,163,165] as well as in some cells lining the thyroid follicles both histochemically and immunohistochemically. Ultrastructural examination demonstrates neurosecretory granules in the carcinoid component and in some of the thyroid follicular cells.[163,165] In two tumors, amyloid deposits were identified and were verified both histochemically and ultrastructurally.[7,38]

Some investigators consider that strumal carcinoid is a carcinoid tumor and that the thyroid tissue only resembles thyroid.[61] Other investigators have conclusively demonstrated thyroglobulin within the thyroid component of the tumor, thus indicating its thyroid nature.[139,163] It is, therefore, considered that in verified cases of strumal carci-

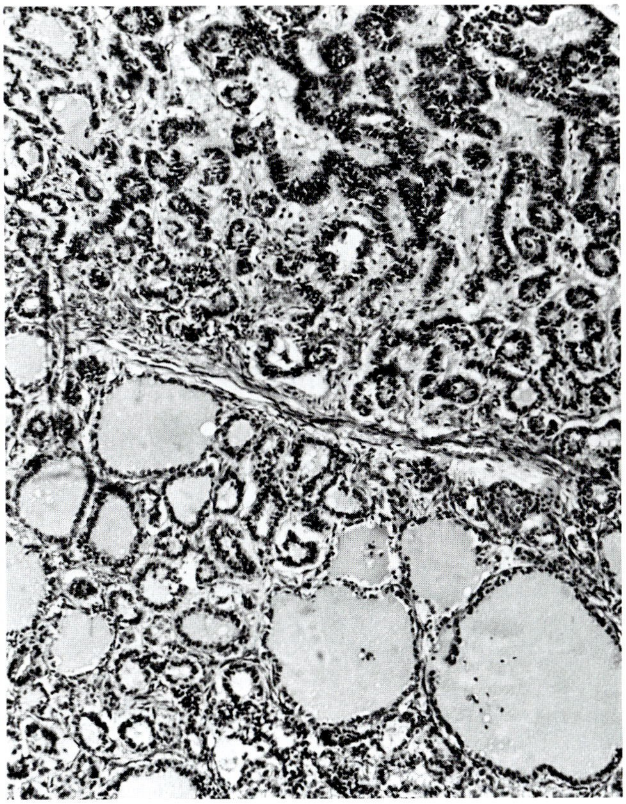

Fig. 20.58. Struma ovarii and carcinoid. The carcinoid forms long narrow cords and ribbons (*top*), merging with thyroid follicles (*bottom*).

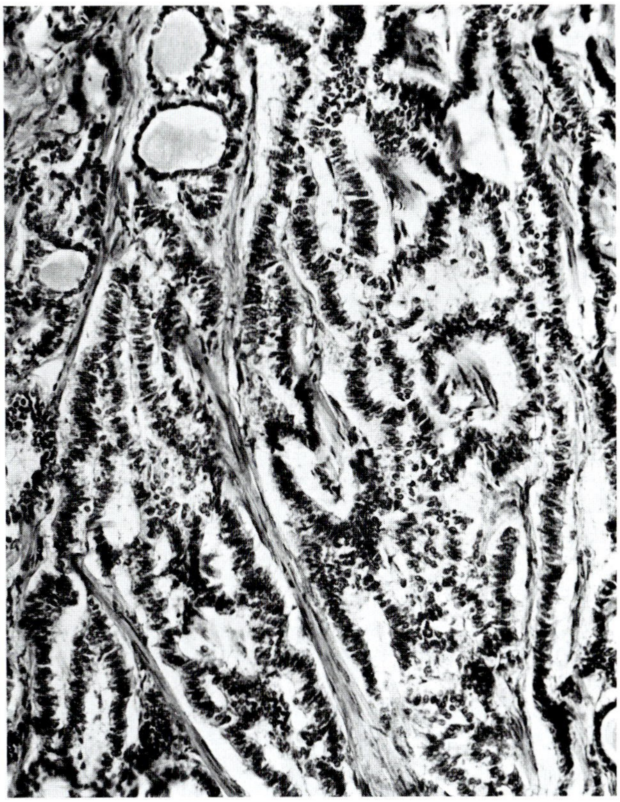

Fig. 20.59. Struma ovarii and carcinoid. The carcinoid is composed of columnar or cuboidal epithelial cells forming narrow winding cords and ribbons. Thyroid follicles also are seen.

noid the tumor consists of thyroid tissue intimately admixed with a carcinoid. Strumal carcinoid should be distinguished from carcinoma of the thyroid arising in struma ovarii, with which it has often been confused. The latter has the typical appearances observed in carcinoma of the thyroid and usually exhibits the follicular or papillary pattern.

Clinical Behavior and Treatment

Strumal carcinoid only once has been associated with metastases, and even in this case the patient was apparently cured by a combination of surgery and radiation therapy.[216] All other cases have followed a benign course.[139,163]

Monodermal Teratomas with Neuroectodermal Differentiation

During the past decade, both malignant[2,77] and benign[202,208] *monodermal teratomas with neuroectodermal differentiation* have been described. The benign tumors consist of a cyst lined entirely by mature glial tissue[208] or by ependymal tissue.[202] The former has been described as a neurogenic cyst. It is important to recognize the benign nature of such tumors. The fact that the tumor is composed of mature neural tissue distinguishes it from its malignant counterparts. The malignant tumors can be divided into malignant neuroectodermal tumor[2] and ependymoma.[77]

Malignant Neuroectodermal Tumor

Aguirre and Scully[2] described five ovarian tumors occurring in patients in the second decade that showed pure *neuroectodermal differentiation* characterized by histologic patterns resembling those of glioblastoma, medulloblastoma, and neuroblastoma present alone or in combination. Small foci of more mature glia or ependyma, as well as small foci of mature teratoma, may also be seen in these tumors. Although tumors of this type may be confused with other ovarian tumors composed of small cells, special stains for neural tissue and immunocytochemical stains for glial fibrillary acidic protein (GFAP) and neurofilaments are helpful in reaching the correct diagnosis. The tumors thus far reported occurred in patients in the second decade; they pursue an aggressive course, and the prognosis is poor.[2]

Ependymoma

Four cases of pure *ovarian ependymoma* representing one-sided development of a teratoma have been reported.[77] The patients were all in the third and fourth decades and presented with abdominal pain and a palpable abdominal mass. Three patients had intraabdominal metastases, and in one case the tumor was confined to the ovary.

The tumors were cystic, containing fleshy mural nodules or papillary processes arising from the cyst wall. Microscopically, they showed typical features of ependymoma arising in the central nervous system (Fig. 20.60). Perivascular pseudorosettes, consisting of a blood vessel surrounded by tumor cells with long radiating processes and antipodally arranged nuclei characteristic of ependymoma, were prominent. Central lumen (Homer Wright) rosettes were also seen (Fig. 20.60). Mitotic activity varied from 1 to 3 mitotic figures (MF) per 10 high-power fields (HPF). Special stains for neural tissue and for GFAP are helpful in confirming the diagnosis.[77]

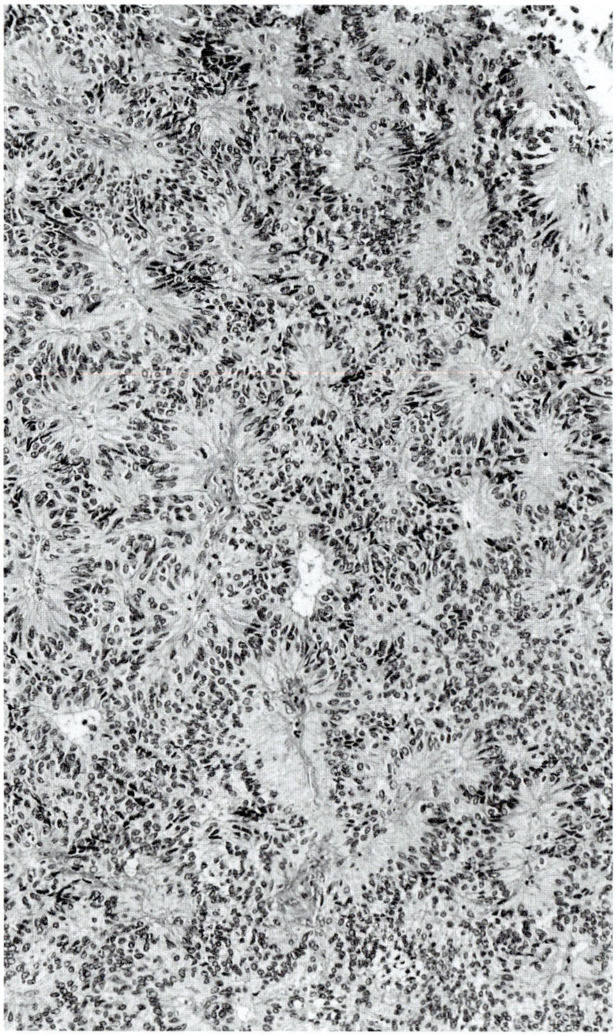

Fig. 20.60. Monodermal teratoma with ependymona. Homer Wright rosettes and perivascular pseudorosettes are present.

The prognosis of patients with this tumor is much more favorable than that of those with malignant neuroectodermal tumor; despite the presence of metastases on presentation in three of the four patients, only one of them succumbed to the disease.[77]

Monodermal Teratoma Composed of Vascular Tissue

Another type of *monodermal teratoma* is represented by neoplasms composed entirely or predominantly of *immature vascular tissue*. These occur in children and young adults, and the patients present with symptoms and signs suggestive of an ovarian tumor. The tumors may vary in size and are smooth, soft, solid, and gray-pink but may be hemorrhagic. Microscopically they consist of collections of small vascular spaces lined by immature endothelial cells and surrounded by connective tissue, which varies from loose and edematous to dense and fibrous. The lining of the vascular spaces may be multilayered and the endothelial cells may form small projections bulging into the lumen. Small collections of endothelial cells, some forming abortive lumina and some devoid of a lumen, are also seen within the connective tissue and may predominate (Fig. 20.61).

The endothelial cells show a considerable degree of cellular and nuclear pleomorphism, and mitotic activity is usually evident. Occasionally hematopoietic activity may be seen within some of the vascular spaces. When these tumors contain small teratomatous foci their nature is more readily apparent, but when they occur in pure form, especially when the endothelial cells form a more solid pattern with fewer obvious vascular spaces (Fig. 20.61), the nature of the lesion is more difficult to recognize. Occasionally these tumors may be composed of immature pericytes and resemble a hemangiopericytoma. Further sectioning of the tumor, which may reveal a more typical vascular pattern, and immunocytochemical stains for CD 31 and CD 34 as well as for factor VIII may be helpful in reaching the correct diagnosis. This distinction is important because monodermal teratomas composed of immature vascular tissue or with a predominant vascular component behave on the whole in a less aggressive manner compared with high-grade immature teratomas and hemangioendothelial sarcomas of the ovary, with which they tend to be confused. As in most immature teratomas, the grade of the tumor is an important prognostic feature.

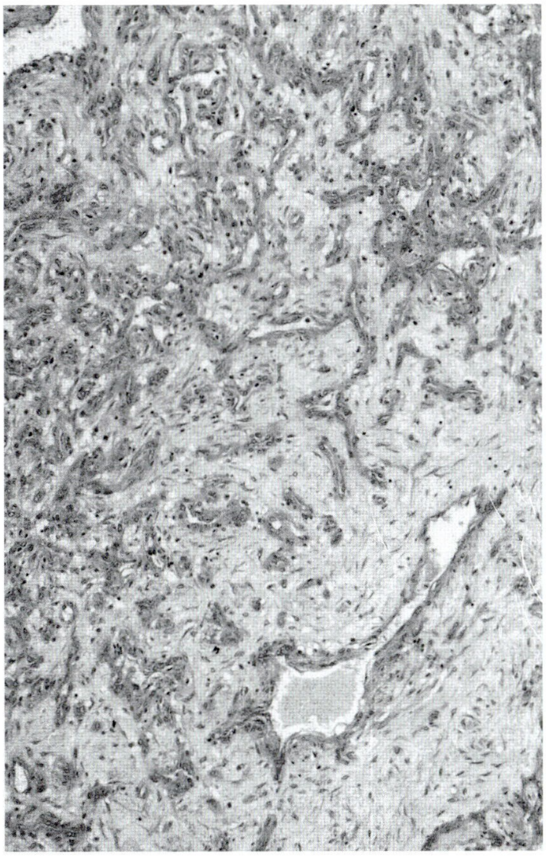

Fig. 20.61. Monodermal teratoma with vascular differentiation. The tumor is composed of immature vessels, including some forming cordlike structures either with small inconspicuous lumina, or devoid of a lumen.

Monodermal Teratoma with Sebaceous Differentiation

Sebaceous tumors showing one-sided development of a teratoma or arising in mature cystic teratomas are rare, and until a recent report describing five such tumors[32] only three cases had been recorded in the literature. Review of these eight cases shows an age range from 31 to 79 years at presentation, but most patients were older than 49 years. All presented with lower abdominal enlargement. The ovarian tumors found at laparotomy were all large, ranging from 10 to 35 cm. Three of the patients were found to have a mature cystic teratoma in the contralateral ovary. The tumors were mainly cystic. Partly solid yellow and tan masses protruded into the cysts. The latter contained necrotic or cheesy material.[32]

Microscopically, the tumors consisted of five cases of sebaceous adenomas, two cases of basal cell carcinomas with sebaceous differentiation, and a single sebaceous carcinoma.[32] The adenomas were all composed of nodules or lobules of proliferating normal sebaceous cells showing various degrees of maturity, with mature cells predominating. The basal cell carcinomas with sebaceous differentiation were composed of masses or nests of malignant basal cells containing collections of mature sebaceous cells. The sebaceous carcinoma was composed of sebaceous cells showing marked cellular and nuclear pleomorphism growing in an infiltrative pattern. The cells comprising the tumors had the typical appearance of sebaceous cells. Lipid stains were strongly positive in all the tumors, confirming the diagnosis.[32]

The patients were treated either by excision of the affected adnexa or by hysterectomy and bilateral salpingo-oophorectomy. The outcome was favorable; only one tumor was known to have recurred. The tumor, a basal cell carcinoma with sebaceous differentiation, recurred in the pelvis; further follow-up was not available. All the other patients were well and disease free for periods ranging from 1.5 to 6 years postoperatively.[32] One patient had, in addition to the sebaceous adenoma, a squamous cell carcinoma arising in the same ovary and died as a result of disseminated disease 1 year after the diagnosis. The patient with sebaceous carcinoma was well and disease free 6 years after diagnosis.[32]

Other Types of Monodermal Teratoma

Mucinous tumors of the ovary usually are described with surface epithelial–stromal neoplasms and are considered to be derived from the surface epithelium of the ovary; they are generally not regarded as germ cell neoplasms. However, there is undoubtedly a considerable number of cases in which the tumor is of germ cell origin, forming a *monodermal teratomatous neoplasm* in which the mucinous element (of intestinal derivation) developed in a pure form or has overgrown all the other tissues in the same manner that the thyroid tissue in a pure struma ovarii has developed in a pure form or has overgrown all the other tissues. The presence of occasional teratomatous tumors composed mainly of mucinous (intestinal-type) epithelium of endodermal derivation and only a small amount of other tumor elements, as well as a 5% association of mature cystic teratoma with mucinous cystadenoma, lends strong support to this mode of origin for at least some mucinous tumors.

Mucinous epithelium resembling intestinal epithelium has been observed in association with struma ovarii and with strumal carcinoid. In these cases, it was the only other tissue element present. The mucinous epithelium frequently contains goblet cells and so shows greater resemblance to intestinal than to endocervical epithelium. In 21% of cases, the epithelium lining mucinous tumors of the ovary contains argyrophil and argentaffin granules. In a number of cases, Paneth cells are also present. These findings are considered to be a strong argument in favor of the derivation of at least some mucinous ovarian tumors from intestinal-type epithelium and their teratomatous (germ cell) origin. It is possible that studies of the type undertaken by Linder et al.[87] using both chromosomal and isoenzyme techniques, may help to clarify the origin of mucinous tumors of the ovary and confirm that some of these are of germ cell origin. Mucinous tumors of the ovary are discussed fully with tumors of surface epithelial–stromal derivation (see Chapter 18, Surface Epithelial Tumors of the Ovary).

Other rare examples of monodermal teratomatous neoplasms observed in the ovary include the epidermoid cyst, which is lined by epidermis without appendages, the melanotic tumor, resembling the retinal anlage tumor,[73] and the possible benign cystic counterpart of the latter.[6] Monodermal teratomatous origin of some malignant connective tissue tumors is difficult to prove because of the occurrence of connective tissue neoplasms derived from normal ovarian tissue. Monodermal teratomatous origin of tumors derived from ectodermal or endodermal tissues is more easily acceptable, and there may be as yet undescribed tumors of this type.

Mixed Germ Cell Tumors

Mixed germ cell tumors are tumors composed of more than one neoplastic germ cell element, such as dysgerminoma combined with teratoma, yolk sac tumor, choriocarcinoma, embryonal carcinoma, or polyembryoma, as well as any other possible combination of these tumor types. This group includes only neoplasms composed entirely of neoplastic germ cell elements and does not include gonadoblastoma and mixed germ cell–sex cord–stromal tumor, which in addition to germ cells contain sex cord–stromal derivatives as an integral component. The relatively frequent finding of different neoplastic germ cell elements in gonadal tumors of germ cell origin is considered to be a strong argument in favor of the common histogenesis of this group of neoplasms. The various tumor elements present in these tumors may be intimately admixed or may form separate areas adjacent to each other and separated by fibrous septa.

Although many ovarian tumors belonging to this group are classified according to the predominant element present, it is emphasized that when these tumors are examined all areas of varying appearance should be sampled carefully and thoroughly analyzed. All the neoplastic germ cell elements observed within the tumor, however small, should be reported and described and, if possible, their relative size estimated. The importance of this practice is by no means only academic, because the behavior and treatment of neoplasms belonging to this group vary considerably, and the presence of a small area composed of a more malignant element may alter the therapeutic approach and the prognosis, especially in children.[62]

Although the presence of very small foci of YST or high-grade immature teratoma may not alter the behavior of a mixed germ cell tumor largely composed of less aggressive components, the presence of larger amounts of more malignant elements within a tumor is usually associated with a more aggressive behavior. Before the introduction of effective combination chemotherapy, it was associated with an unsatisfactory response to therapy and poor prognosis.[9,83,190] However, it should be noted that the clinical course in most patients with tumors composed of yolk sac tumor associated with dysgerminoma or other germ cell elements usually does not differ materially from that observed in patients with pure yolk sac tumor.[50,122] The different response to treatment and the different behavior of some cases of dysgerminoma described in the past may have been a result of the presence of other germ cell elements that were not identified. Although in the past mixed germ cell tumors were considered to be uncommon, they tend to figure quite frequently in more recent reports, probably because of more careful and extensive examination of the tumors.

Clinical and Pathologic Features of Tumors Composed of Germ Cells and Sex Cord–Stromal Derivatives

Gonadoblastoma

General Features

In 1953, Scully[153] described two patients with a distinctive gonadal tumor, which he designated *gonadoblastoma*. The tumor was composed of germ cells and sex cord-stromal derivatives, resembling immature granulosa, and Sertoli cells. One of the tumors also contained stromal elements indistinguishable from lutein or Leydig cells. Both tumors occurred in phenotypic females who showed abnormal sexual development. The older patient, who was postpubertal, showed virilization, and it was considered that the tumor was capable of steroid hormone secretion. The tumors were located at the site of normal ovaries, but normal ovarian tissue was not discernible and the exact nature of the gonads in which the tumors had originated could not be determined. Both patients had bilateral tumors that were partly overgrown by dysgerminoma. It was subsequently demonstrated that both patients were chromatin negative. The tumor was designated gonadoblastoma because it appeared to recapitulate the development of the gonads and because it occurred in individuals with abnormal sexual development and in gonads, the nature of which could not be determined.[154]

The neoplastic nature of gonadoblastoma has been questioned because some lesions are very small and may undergo complete regression by hyalinization and calcification. Furthermore, when malignancy supervenes, it manifests itself as germ cell neoplasia despite the fact that gonadoblastoma is composed of two or three different cell types. When the tumor has metastasized, gonadoblastoma as such has never been observed in the metastases. Nevertheless, gonadoblastoma shows exactly the same pattern in the very small lesions as in the large ones, including mitotic activity in the germ cell element and early overgrowth by dysgerminoma. The association with dysgerminoma is seen in 50% of cases and with other more malignant germ cell neoplasms in an additional 10%.[154] In view of this, the concept that gonadoblastoma represents an in situ germ cell malignancy is considered to be fully justified.

Genetic Aspects

Gonadoblastoma occurs almost entirely in patients with pure or mixed gonadal dysgenesis or in male pseudohermaphrodites (see Chapter 1, Embryology of the Female Genital Tract and Disorders of Abnormal Sexual Development). Occasional patients are of short stature and may have other stigmata of Turner's syndrome.[147,159] Most patients are chromatin negative; this has been observed in 89% of cases.[154] Nearly all patients with gonadoblastoma whose karyotype was recorded (96%) were found to have a Y chromosome.[147] Eight patients had 46,XX karyotype,[18,42,103,113,192] and 4 of these were fertile.[18,42,103,192] One patient had a 45,X/46,XX mosaicism.[120] The most frequently encountered karyotype was 46,XY, which was seen in half the cases; this was followed by 45,X/46,XY mosaicism, which was seen in a quarter of the cases. The remainder showed many different forms of mosaicism.[147] Six patients had morphologic abnormalities of the Y chromosome. Of 25 patients with gonadal dysgenesis and dysgerminoma, 24 had a Y chromosome. The karyotype was 46,XY in 60%, followed by 45,X/46,XY in 24%. The remainder showed various forms of mosaicism.[147] One patient had 45,X monosomy and Turner syndrome. All other patients with features of Turner syndrome had various forms of mosaicism containing a Y chromosome.

The similarity between the distribution of the karyotypes in the gonadoblastoma group and the patients with dysgerminoma and gonadal dysgenesis is striking, and 62% of the former group and 45% of the latter had clitoral hypertrophy.[147] Gonadal dysgenesis and dysgerminoma has been reported in a female with a 46,XX karyotype who had no evidence of Y chromosomal DNA material as studied by sophisticated karyotypic techniques.[85] Gonadoblastoma was not detected in the affected gonad, but the authors[85] suggested that it was probably overgrown by the dysgerminoma. This finding indicates that gonadoblastoma and gonadal dysgenesis may occur in patients who do not have Y chromosome DNA.

Family history of gonadal dysgenesis has been noted in at least 10 reports of patients with gonadoblastoma.[4,5,24,173] Evidence of gonadal dysgenesis affecting three generations of the family of a patient with gonadoblastoma was obtained in two instances.[4,15] Gonadoblastoma has been reported in one pair of twins[44] and in four pairs of siblings.[4,5,24,173] All these patients had 46,XY karyotype. It has been postulated that the mode of inheritance is either an X-linked recessive gene or an autosomal sex-linked mutant gene.[15,147,148]

Endocrine Aspects

The association of gonadoblastoma with certain endocrine abnormalities was noted in one of the two cases first reported.[153] In view of the fact that gonadoblastoma occurs almost entirely in patients with gonadal dysgenesis, the defective gonadal development present in these patients should not be confused with the presence of endocrine effects that are associated with the tumor and are not a result of the abnormal gonadal development. Although the virilization produced by the tumor may regress after the excision of the tumor, there is no further gonadal development and the gonadal abnormalities remain. Although the exact source of the steroid hormone production was not originally known, the interstitial cells resembling Leydig or lutein cells were considered to be the most likely source of the androgens.[153] Further observations have shown that the presence of Leydig or lutein-like cells is not always associated with the presence of virilization, although they are encountered more frequently in tumors from virilized phenotypic female patients than in those from nonvirilized patients. The possibility that the tumor may secrete estrogens, as evidenced by complaints of hot flushes and other menopausal symptoms after the excision of the tumor, has also been noted.[154] Originally, the evidence of hormone secretion was mainly clinical, usually evidenced by virilization occurring after puberty and manifesting itself as masculine body contour, hirsutism, and clitoromegaly. Slight elevation of the urinary 17-ketosteroid excretion was noted in some cases. The gonadotropins, when estimated, were usually elevated.

In recent years it has been shown that gonadoblastoma is capable of producing testosterone and estrogens from progesterone in vitro.[5,143] Evidence of testosterone secretion in vivo in patients with gonadal dysgenesis has been presented.[69] Androgen and estrogen formation from progesterone in vitro has been demonstrated in a streak gonad that did not contain any Leydig and lutein cells microscopically, but from the description it may have contained a small burned-out gonadoblastoma.[89] Although in vitro testosterone formation has been ascribed to the Leydig or lutein-like cells present in gonadoblastoma,[143] the demonstration of steroid production by a streak gonad that did not contain Leydig or lutein cells indicates that the stromal tissue also has the capability of steroid synthesis.[89]

Despite all these advances in the study and understanding of the hormonal aspects of gonadoblastoma and dysgenetic gonads, considerable problems remain, the most important being why some patients become virilized and others do not. Although there is a relationship between the virilization of patients with gonadoblastoma and the presence of Leydig or lutein-like cells, this relationship is not constant. It may be that the reason is quantitative and that the amount of the steroid secretion may be inadequate to produce virilization because of a small cell mass. Another possible reason is that the steroid metabolic pathways may be different and that gonadoblastoma may produce different steroid hormones or different quantities of various steroid hormones. Some of these hormones may be metabolically nonfunctioning and therefore unassociated with endocrine side effects, whereas the metabolically active steroids may be associated with evidence and visible signs of endocrine activity.

Clinical Features

The exact prevalence of gonadoblastoma is not known. Although more than 200 cases have been reported, it is considered to be uncommon. Gonadoblastoma is usually seen in young patients, occurring most frequently in the second and somewhat less frequently in the third and first decades, in that order. With a few exceptions all the reported cases occurred in patients under 30 years of age. Gonadoblastoma is much more common in phenotypic females than in phenotypic males, the ratio being 4:1.[154] Patients with gonadoblastoma usually have primary amenorrhea, virilization, or developmental abnormalities of the genitalia (see Chapter 1, Embryology of the Female Genital Tract and Disorders of Abnormal Sexual Development). The discovery of gonadoblastoma is made in the course of investigations of these conditions. Another mode of presentation is the presence of a gonadal tumor. The gonadoblastoma forms part of the tumor in these cases and is discovered on histologic examination. Most patients with gonadoblastoma (80%) are phenotypic females, and the remainder are phenotypic males with cryptorchidism, hypospadias, and female internal secondary sex organs. Among the phenotypic females, 60% are virilized and the remainder are normal in appearance.[154]

Most of the phenotypic female patients exhibit abnormal genital development, and breast development is often diminished even among the nonvirilized females. Although primary amenorrhea is a common presenting symptom among phenotypic females with gonadoblastoma, a few patients have episodes of spontaneous cyclical bleeding, but in most of these patients the episodes are sporadic and the bleeding scanty; occasional patients menstruate normally.[154] The virilization present in phenotypic female patients with gonadoblastoma usually does not regress after excision of the tumor, although this has been seen in occasional cases, and in a few additional cases there was partial regression.

Although most patients have gonadal dysgenesis, gonadoblastoma has been described in patients who have had normal pregnancies. One patient had two normal pregnancies after the excision of a dysgerminoma containing a small focus of gonadoblastoma. The patient was chromatin positive and had a 46,XX karyotype[18] Normal pregnancies have also been documented in a patient with a normal female 46,XX karyotype and gonadoblastoma occurring in a normal ovary[103] in a true hermaphrodite with bilateral ovotestes, gonadoblastomas, and dysgerminomas,[192] and in a normal 46,XX female with one normal ovary and the other gonad overgrown by a large dysgerminoma originating in a gonadoblastoma.[42]

Gonadoblastoma has been observed in seven true hermaphrodites, four of whom had 46,XX karyotype[90,192] and the other three 46,XY.[118,171] It was also seen in five males with normally descended testes,[64,181] some of whom fathered children subsequent to the excision of the testis bearing the lesion.

Gross Findings

Gonadoblastoma has been found more often in the right gonad than in the left and has been bilateral in 38% of cases.[154] Recent reports suggest an even higher frequency of bilateral involvement. Although many tumors are recognized on gross examination, in a number of cases the lesion is detected only on histologic examination; this may be the case with bilateral tumors, only one of which may be recognized macroscopically. In most cases, the gonad of origin is indeterminate because it is overgrown by the tumor. When the nature of the gonad can be identified, it is usually a streak or a testis. The contralateral gonad in these cases may be a streak or a testis, and the former is more likely to harbor a gonadoblastoma.[154] Occasionally gonadoblastoma has been found in otherwise normal ovaries.[103,109,136] A number of such cases are known to the author.

Pure gonadoblastoma varies in size from a microscopic lesion to 8 cm in diameter, with most tumors measuring a few centimeters. When gonadoblastoma becomes overgrown by dysgerminoma (Fig. 20.62) or other malignant germ cell elements, much larger tumors may be observed.[154,176] The macroscopic appearance of the tumor varies to some extent according to the presence of hyalinization and calcification, as well as overgrowth by dysgerminoma.

Gonadoblastoma is a solid tumor and presents a smooth or slightly lobulated surface. It varies from soft and fleshy to firm and hard. It is speckled with calcific granules and may be almost completely calcified. Calcification has been recognized on gross examination in 45% of cases, and in more than 20% it has been detected radiologically.[154] The tumor varies in color from gray or yellow to brown, and on cross section it appears to be somewhat granular.

Although the external sex organs in patients with gonadoblastoma present a wide variety of appearances ranging from normal to completely ambiguous, the secondary internal sex organs consist almost always of a uterus, which is hypoplastic in most cases, and two or occasionally one normal fallopian tube; this is also seen in the phenotypic males. Male secondary internal sex organs, such as the epididymis, vas deferens, and prostate, are found occasionally in the virilized phenotypic females and are always found in the phenotypic male pseudohermaphrodites.[154]

Microscopic Findings

Gonadoblastoma is composed of collections of cellular nests surrounded by connective tissue stroma (Fig. 20.63). The nests are solid, usually small, and oval or round but occasionally may be larger and

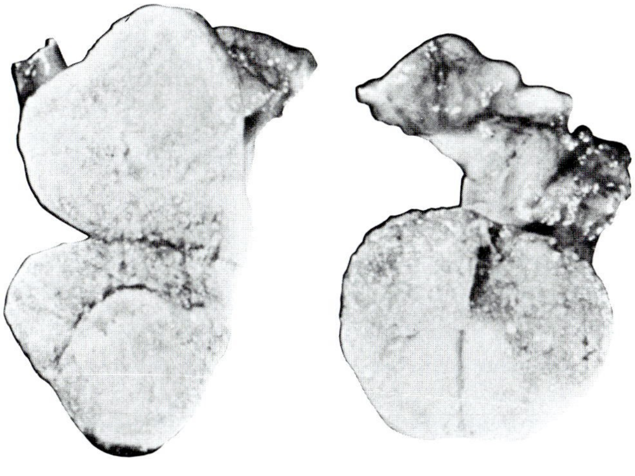

Fig. 20.62. Gonadoblastoma with dysgerminoma. The outer surface is smooth, the cut surface solid, granular, and yellow-brown in color. (Courtesy of R.E. Scully, M.D., Boston, MA.)

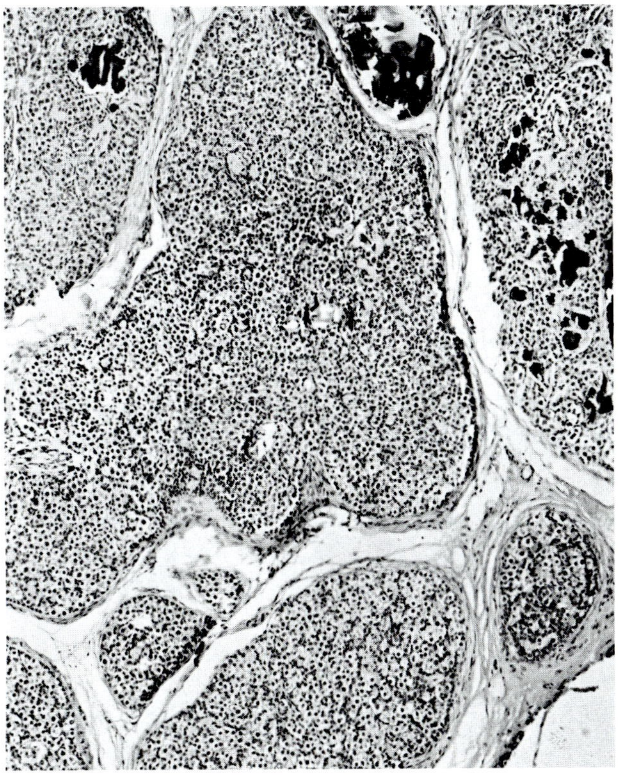

Fig. 20.63. Gonadoblastoma. Cellular nests surrounded by connective tissue stroma. Note foci of calcification (*heavy black areas*).

elongated. The cellular nests contain a mixture of germ cells and sex cord derivatives resembling immature Sertoli and granulosa cells (Fig. 20.64). The germ cells are large and round, with pale or slightly granular cytoplasm and large round vesicular nuclei, often with prominent nucleoli showing histologic and ultrastructural appearances and histochemical reactions similar to the germ cells of dysgerminoma or seminoma.

The germ cells show mitotic activity, which may be marked in some cases. They are intimately admixed with immature Sertoli and granulosa cells, which are smaller and epithelial like. The latter are round or oval and have dark, oval or slightly elongated carrot-shaped nuclei. Mitotic activity is not seen in these cells. The immature Sertoli and granulosa cells are arranged within the cell nests in three typical patterns (Fig. 20.64): (1) along the periphery of the nests in a coronal pattern, (2) surrounding individual or collections of germ cells in the same way as the follicular epithelium surrounds the ovum of the primary follicle, or (3) surrounding small round spaces containing amorphous hyaline, eosinophilic, and PAS-positive material that resemble Call–Exner bodies.

The connective tissue stroma surrounding the cellular nests frequently contains collections of cells indistinguishable from Leydig cells or luteinized stromal cells (Fig. 20.65). There is considerable variation in the number of these cells from case to case; in some cases they are numerous, in others they are identified with difficulty, or may be absent.

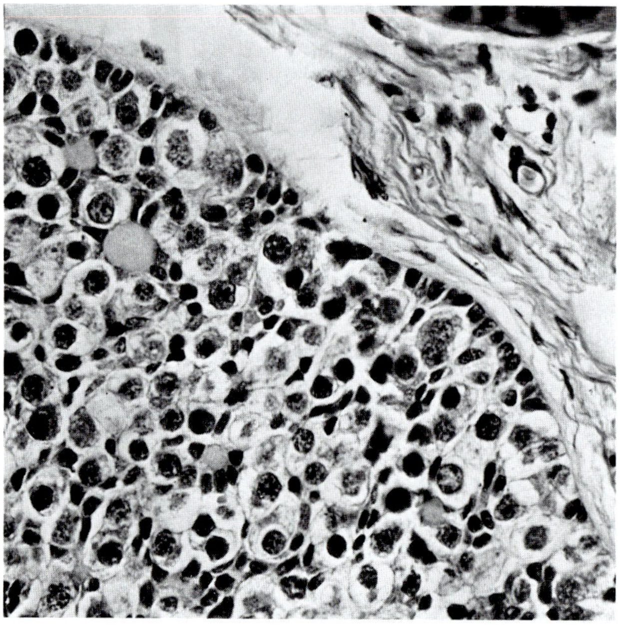

Fig. 20.64. Gonadoblastoma. A nest composed of large germ cells is intimately admixed with smaller sex cord derivatives. Hyaline Call–Exner-like bodies also are seen.

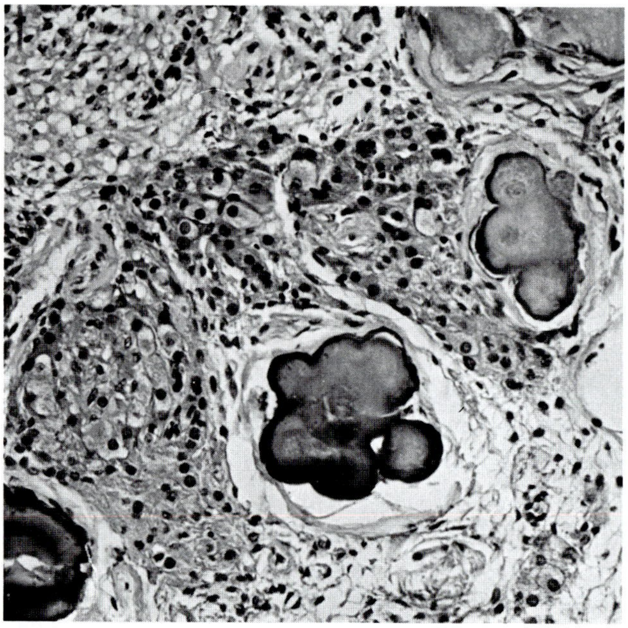

Fig. 20.65. Gonadoblastoma. Calcified nest is surrounded by connective tissue containing numerous Leydig or lutein-like cells. Same case as in Fig. 20.62.

Although in many cases the cells are indistinguishable from Leydig cells and may contain lipochrome granules, Reinke crystals, which are specifically diagnostic of Leydig cells, have never been identified in their cytoplasm. The Leydig or lutein-like cells are identified in 66% of cases, and they are present nearly twice as frequently in older patients as in those 15 years of age or younger.[154] The presence of Leydig or lutein-like cells is not necessary for the diagnosis of gonadoblastoma. The connective tissue stroma surrounding the cellular nests may be scanty or abundant, and may vary from dense and hyalinized to cellular, resembling ovarian stroma. These latter appearances are more common in tumors that either have arisen in, or are suspected to originate in, a gonadal streak.[154] Occasionally, the stroma may be loose and edematous.

The basic composition of gonadoblastoma, consisting of the two cell types present within the cellular nests and with the Leydig or lutein-like cells present in the stroma, has been confirmed by electron microscopy.[49,65,89] Although there is agreement concerning the nature of the germ cells, the nature of the sex cord–stromal cells is in dispute. They are considered by some to be Sertoli cells or granulosa cells or their precursors,[89] whereas others consider them to be primitive sex cord–stromal cells and are unable to differentiate them further.[154,178] The latter view is more widely accepted. The nature of the amorphous, hyaline, eosinophilic material forming Call–Exner-like bodies also was a matter of dispute. It was considered to be either of basement membrane origin[65,89] or composed of fibrillar material formed by the stromal cells before they undergo fragmentation and cell death. The former view is supported by most investigators.

The basic histologic appearance of gonadoblastoma may be altered by three processes: hyalinization, calcification, and overgrowth by dysgerminoma.[154] Hyalinization takes place by coalescence of the hyaline Call–Exner-like bodies within the nests and of the basement membrane-like band of similar material present around the nests. The hyaline material replaces the tumor cells, and the whole nest may be replaced. Calcification is a common feature (Figs. 20.63 and 20.65) and is seen microscopically in 81% of cases; it usually begins in the Call–Exner-like bodies with formation of small calcific spherules that are frequently laminated, resembling psammoma bodies (Fig. 20.65). The process continues with enlargement and fusion of the calcified bodies and calcification of the hyalinized material, resulting in formation of a calcified mass embracing the whole nest. The process may extend to the stroma, which may also undergo hyalinization and calcification. In such cases, tumor cells become very scarce or absent, and the presence of smooth, rounded, calcified masses may be the only evidence that gonadoblastoma was present (see Fig. 20.9). Although this finding is not considered to be diagnostic of gonadoblastoma, and has been called a burned-out gonadoblastoma,[154] it is a strong argument in favor of the diagnosis and indicates that a careful search should be made for more viable areas of the tumor.

Gonadoblastoma is frequently overgrown by dysgerminoma (Figs. 20.66 and 20.67), as is seen in 50% of cases.[154] The overgrowth may vary from the presence of a small collection of malignant germ cells in the stroma outside the gonadoblastoma nests to massive overgrowth of the whole tumor, in which occasional nests of gonadoblastoma may be seen. The dysgerminoma in these cases shows the typical appearances of pure dysgerminoma or seminoma, histologically, histochemically, and ultrastructurally. It should be noted that when gonadoblastoma becomes overgrown by dysgerminoma, the germ cell component present within the gonadoblastoma nests shows marked proliferative activity and overgrows the sex cord elements (Figs. 20.66 and 20.67). When gonadoblastoma undergoes regressive changes, they manifest first as a decrease in germ cells. Gonadoblastoma may also be associated with and overgrown by other more malignant germ cell neoplasms, such as immature teratoma, yolk sac tumor, embryonal carcinoma, and choriocarcinoma, as occurs in 10% of cases.[154,178] A gonadoblastoma overgrown by dysgerminoma and

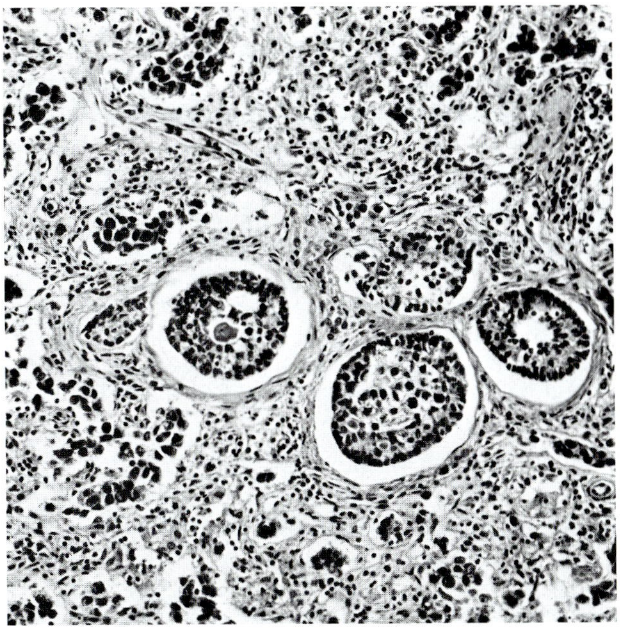

Fig. 20.66. Gonadoblastoma nests surrounded by dysgerminoma. (Reprinted with permission from The American College of Obstetricians and Gynecologists. Obstetrics and Gynecology 38:416, 1971.)

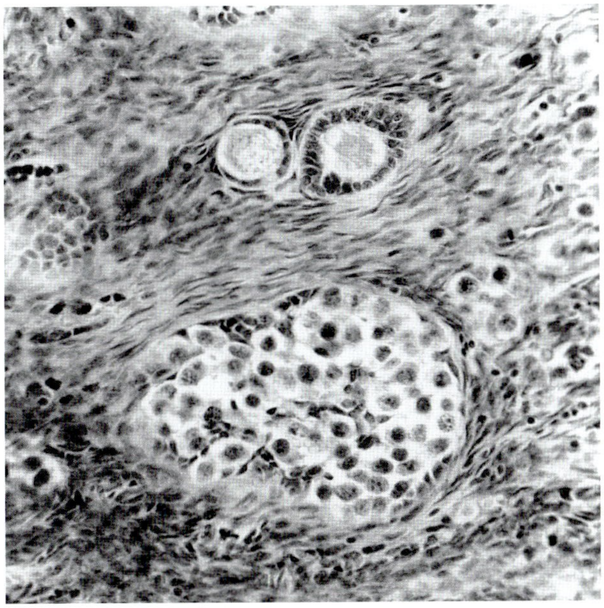

Fig. 20.67. Gonadoblastoma arising in a normal ovary. Elsewhere the tumor was overgrown by dysgerminoma. The patient had a normal female 46,XX karyotype.

containing a proliferation of sex cord element resembling a Sertoli cell tumor and occurring in a dysgenetic gonad of a 19-year-old phenotypic female with 46,XY karyotype has been reported.[109] Therefore, it is possible that Sertoli cell tumors may occur in association with gonadoblastoma, but this is considered to be unique.

Although it has been postulated that gonadoblastoma may coexist with mixed germ cell–sex cord–stromal tumor, the only case describing such an association[21] was in reality a typical gonadoblastoma and not a combined tumor.

Differential Diagnosis

Gonadoblastoma, because of its distinctive histologic appearance and its cellular composition, cannot be easily confused with any of the well-recognized gonadal neoplasms. The gonadal tumors with which confusion may arise are all newly recognized entities and may be related to it. Gonadoblastoma may be confused with the mixed germ cell–sex cord–stromal tumor,[174,175] which shares with gonadoblastoma the unique distinction of being composed of germ cells and sex cord–stromal derivatives. The mixed germ cell–sex cord–stromal tumor shows less uniform appearance, absence of nestlike pattern, absence of calcification and hyalinization, a more pronounced proliferative activity involving also the sex cord–stromal derivatives, the tendency to occur in normal gonads, and other genetic, endocrine, and somatic differences. The other lesion resembling gonadoblastoma is the ovarian sex cord tumor with annular tubules,[155] which is frequently found in patients with Peutz–Jeghers syndrome. This lesion, which is also frequently bilateral, is composed of tubules lined by Sertoli and granulosa-like cells, contains similar round, eosinophilic, and hyaline Call–Exner-like bodies, and tends to calcify in the same manner as gonadoblastoma. The basic difference from gonadoblastoma is the absence of germ cells (see Chapter 19, Sex Cord–Stromal, Steroid Cell, and Other Ovarian Tumors with Endocrine, Paraendocrine, and Paraneoplastic Manifestations).

Clinical Behavior and Treatment

The prognosis of patients with pure gonadoblastoma is excellent, provided the tumor and the contralateral gonad, which may be harboring a macroscopically undetectable gonadoblastoma, are excised. When gonadoblastoma is associated with dysgerminoma, the prognosis is still very good. Metastases tend to occur later and more infrequently than in dysgerminoma arising de novo. All patients with gonadoblastoma and dysgerminoma with known follow-up, including the occasional cases with metastases,[60,149] are alive and well after treatment, with the exception of two patients who died of disseminated dysgerminoma.[60,199] The prognosis is different when gonadoblastoma is associated with more malignant germ cell neoplasms, such as embryonal carcinoma, yolk sac tumor, choriocarcinoma, and immature teratoma. In the past, none of these patients survived longer than 18 months.[176] More recently, the administration of combination chemotherapy used successfully in the treatment of malignant germ cell tumors has markedly improved this dismal prognosis, which with adequate treatment is now favorable.

Because gonadoblastoma occurs almost entirely in patients with dysgenetic gonads, which are not capable of normal function and because the gonadoblastoma may act as a source from which malignant germ cell neoplasms may originate,[147] there is general agreement that excision of the gonads is the treatment of choice.[148,154,178] This consensus applies not only to a contralateral gonad that appears to be abnormal but also, in most cases, to a normal-appearing gonad. There is no complete agreement regarding whether the uterus should be excised together with the gonads. It has been considered that for psychologic reasons it should be left in situ so that periodic bleeding simulating menstruation can take place on estrogen-progesterone substitution therapy. However, because estrogen administration is associated with a risk of development of endometrial carcinoma, excision of the uterus together with the gonads has been advocated.[148]

Mixed Germ Cell–Sex Cord–Stromal Tumor

General Features

The descriptive term *mixed germ cell–sex cord–stromal tumor* originally was intended to embrace all the tumors composed of these cell types, including the gonadoblastoma. In view of the fact that the latter term is now so well established, the term mixed germ cell–sex cord–stromal tumor should be reserved for tumors composed of these cell types that exhibit distinctive histologic appearances differing from those of gonadoblastoma.[174,175] This term is preferable to Pflügerome[27] or epithelioma Pflügerien[97] because the latter terms imply a possible origin from Pflüger's tubes (germ cell clusters in a granulosa cell envelope that are formed during gonadal embryogenesis and may persist into infancy). Because there is no good evidence for this mode of origin and there is some doubt as to the formation of Pflüger's tubes during human embryogenesis, the term Pflügerome is not considered to be satisfactory. The term mixed germ cell tumor[64] is unsatisfactory because it implies a tumor composed of a mixture of different types of neoplastic germ cell elements without the presence of sex cord–stromal elements, and this term is used in this context in the classification of ovarian tumors proposed by the WHO ovarian tumor panel.[156,157]

Genetic Aspects

Nearly all female patients with this neoplasm have had genotype and karyotype determinations and have been found chromatin positive and to have the normal female chromosome complement of 46,XX. All the patients with this tumor showed normal somatosexual development. Therefore, there is no evidence that patients with this tumor have chromosomal abnormalities or gonadal dysgenesis.

Endocrine Aspects

Most patients with mixed germ cell–sex cord–stromal tumor do not exhibit any endocrine abnormalities as observed clinically. In most cases, tests of hormonal function have not been performed preoperatively. In cases in which tests have been performed postoperatively, function has been found to be normal. In one case, the patient, an 8-year-old girl, exhibited signs of precocious pseudopuberty manifesting as mammary development and menstrual bleeding for 3 years before the discovery of a large ovarian tumor.[186] There was an increased urinary estrogen excretion. After excision of the ovarian tumor, the uterine bleeding ceased and the urinary estrogens became normal.[186]

Isosexual precocious pseudopuberty has been seen in nine other patients in the first decade, including four infants under 1 year of age, who exhibited mammary development and vaginal bleeding. The urinary estrogens were elevated, and vaginal smears showed estrogen effect. After the excision of the tumor, there was a complete return to normality. There was no evidence of virilization in any of the patients. These findings indicate that female patients with this neoplasm either do not have any associated endocrine abnormalities or, if these are present, that they are manifested as feminization. One of the patients, who had a mixed germ cell–sex cord–stromal tumor excised at the age of 10 years,[174] has developed normally and commenced menstruating at the age of 15 years. She was well and disease free 12 years after excision of the tumor.

Clinical Features

These neoplasms are rare, and only a few adequately documented cases have been recorded, although it is likely that some cases may not have been recognized and have been classified with tumors of germ cell origin or with sex cord–stromal tumors. This concept is supported by the fact that because this neoplasm has been recognized as a specific entity, additional well-documented and so far unreported cases have been encountered. Tumors of this type have been observed more frequently in normal phenotypic female patients but have also been encountered in normal adult males. Most of the known cases in females were encountered in children in the first decade. More than a dozen cases occurred in infants under 1 year of age.[175,178] In three cases, the tumor occurred in women aged 26, 31, and 43 years, respectively, who had normal pregnancies. In the ovary, the tumor is most common in the first decade, followed by the second and third, and is uncommon thereafter. Therefore, the age distribution of patients with this neoplasm differs from that of patients with gonadoblastoma.[178]

Gross Findings

The tumors encountered have been relatively large (Fig. 20.68), varying from 7.5 to 18 cm in diameter and weighing from 100 to 1050 g. The tumor was found to be unilateral in all except two patients, and the contralateral gonad has always been described as a normal ovary. In some cases in which excision or biopsy was performed, this was confirmed on microscopic examination.

The tumor is usually round or oval, firm in consistency, and surrounded by a smooth, slightly glistening gray or gray-yellow capsule. In most cases the tumor is solid[174,175] (Fig. 20.68), but in some cases it is partly cystic.[186] The cut surface of the tumor is uniformly gray, pink, or yellow to pale brown. Neither calcified areas nor foci of necrosis have been observed on gross examination. The fallopian tubes and the uterus have always been found to be normal. There have been no abnormalities affecting the external genitalia.

Microscopic Findings

The tumor is composed of germ cells and sex cord derivatives, intimately admixed with each other. The tumor cells form three different histologic patterns.[174,175,178,186] One is composed of long, narrow ramifying cords or trabeculae (Fig. 20.69), which in places expand to form wider columns and larger round or oval cellular aggregates surrounded by connective tissue stroma (Fig. 20.70). The second consists of tubular structures devoid of a lumen and surrounded by a fine connective tissue network (Figs. 20.71 and 20.72). In some places, the tubular pattern is less obvious, and the tumor forms small

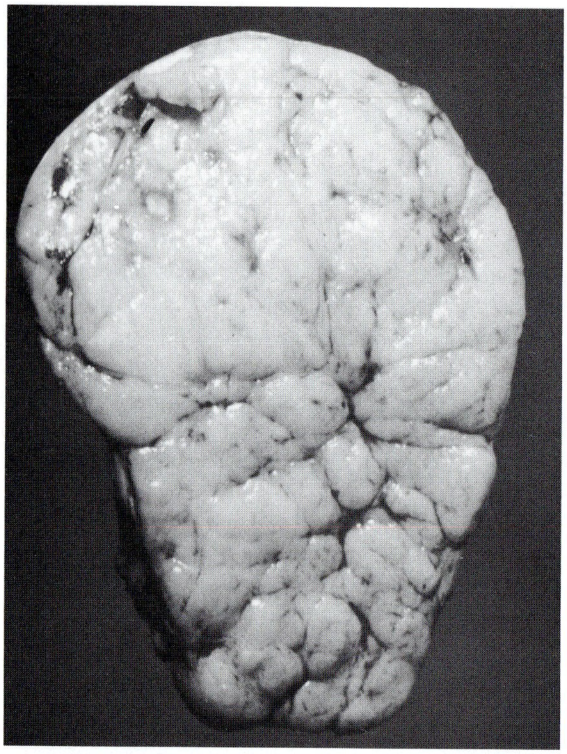

Fig. 20.68. Mixed germ cell–sex cord–stromal tumor. The tumor is large, and the external surface is lobulated. The cut surface is solid, bulging, uniform, and gray-yellow. (Courtesy H.W. Oechler, M.D.)

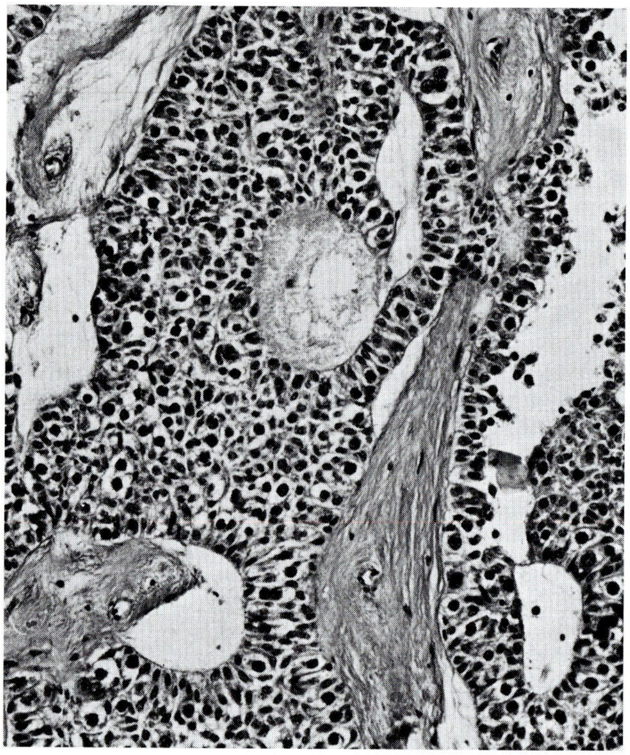

Fig. 20.70. Mixed germ cell–sex cord–stromal tumor. The neoplasm is composed of large cellular aggregates and more slender cords. Note the hyaline connective tissue stroma.

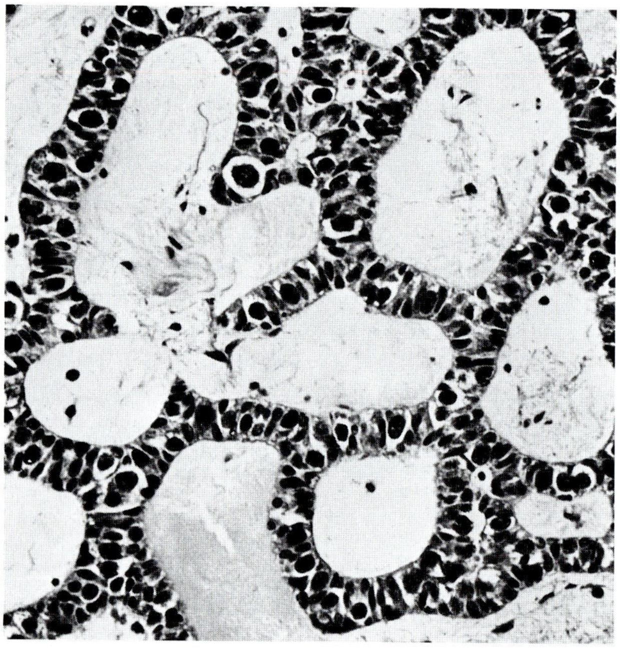

Fig. 20.69. Mixed germ cell–sex cord–stromal tumor. The neoplasm is composed of long ramifying cords. Note the large germ cells and smaller sex cord derivatives and the loose connective tissue stroma.

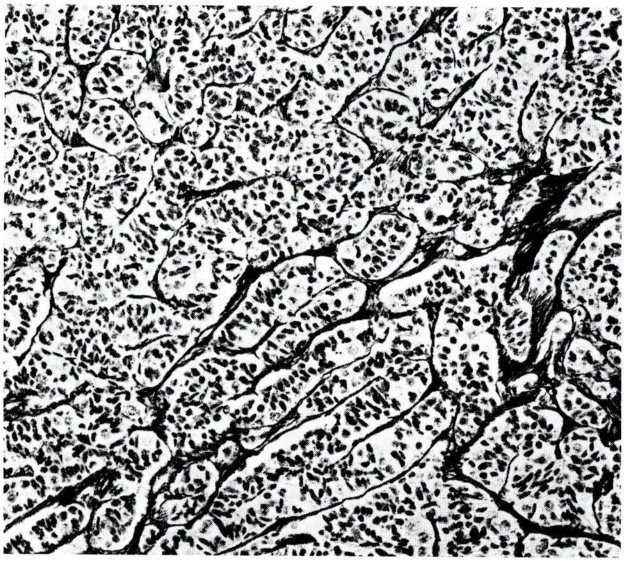

Fig. 20.71. Mixed germ cell–sex cord–stromal tumor. The neoplasm is composed of solid tubules surrounded by fine connective tissue septa. (Reprinted with permission from The American College of Obstetricians and Gynecologists. Obstetrics and Gynecology 40:473, 1972.)

clusters or larger round or oval cellular masses surrounded by connective tissue stroma. The latter varies in amount and appearance and tends to be more abundant in tumors showing mainly the cordlike or trabecular pattern (Fig. 20.69), whereas the tubular variety tends to be more cellular and contains less connective tissue (Figs. 20.71 and 20.72). The stroma may vary from loose and edematous (Fig. 20.69) to dense fibrous and hyalinized (Fig. 20.70). The former is seen more often where the cordlike pattern is most prominent, whereas the latter surrounds the larger cellular aggregates.

The third pattern consists of scattered collections of germ cells surrounded by sex cord elements that may be very abundant. The germ cells admixed with sex cord derivatives may also be scattered individually and in small groups within connective tissue stroma. Sometimes there may be a suggestion of an insular pattern with islands of various sizes surrounded by fine fibrovascular stroma coalescing and forming aggregates (Fig. 20.73), or occasionally being separated by large amounts of connective tissue and forming a more pronounced insular pattern. Admixture with all these patterns is often seen. The typical nestlike pattern present in gonadoblastoma is not observed. In only one case were a few small collections of Leydig or lutein-like cells observed,[174] but in all the remaining cases these cells were not identified.

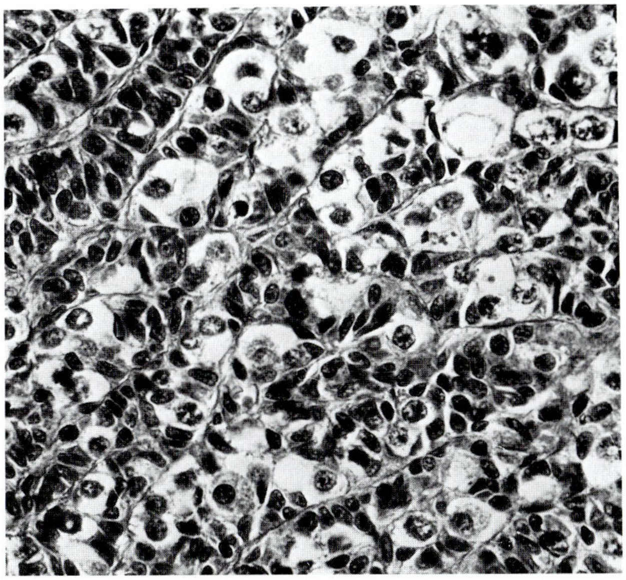

Fig. 20.72. Mixed germ cell–sex cord–stromal tumor. The tubular pattern is illustrated. Note large germ cells surrounded by sex cord–stromal cells. (Reprinted with permission from The American College of Obstetricians and Gynecologists. Obstetrics and Gynecology 40:473, 1972.)

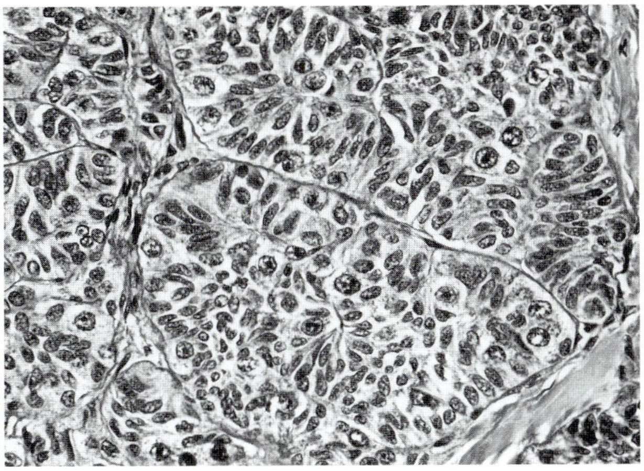

Fig. 20.73. Mixed germ cell–sex cord–stromal tumor. There is a suggestion of an insular pattern. The tumor islands are surrounded by fine fibrovascular connective tissue.

The two cellular elements present in the tumor, the germ cells and the sex cord derivatives, are intimately admixed. The sex cord derivatives are arranged peripherally in a single file, forming long rows at the periphery of the cords (Figs. 20.69 and 20.74), or peripherally lining the tubular structures (Fig. 20.72) as well as surrounding individual or groups of germ cells within the small clusters or larger aggregates. The germ cells resemble those observed in dysgerminoma and gonadoblastoma in all respects, including histochemical reactions. In some cases, a number of the germ cells present in this tumor appear more mature than the germ cells observed in gonadoblastoma or dysgerminoma and tend to resemble primordial germ cells. In view of this, it is possible that they may represent a later stage in the maturation of the germ cell than that seen in gonadoblastoma or dysgerminoma. The germ cells show brisk mitotic activity (Fig. 20.74). The sex cord derivatives generally tend to resemble Sertoli cells more than granulosa cells. They show variable degrees of mitotic activity.

The tumor does not show hyalinization, calcification, or the regressive changes observed in gonadoblastoma and appears to be actively proliferative. There is some variation in the cellular content in some parts of the tumor; in some areas there is a preponderance of germ cells, whereas in others the sex cord derivatives predominate. However, the intimate admixture of these two cell types is seen everywhere. Most tumors show a solid pattern, although occasional small clefts lined by sex cord elements may be present. In some tumors cystic spaces of varying size either lined by sex cord de-

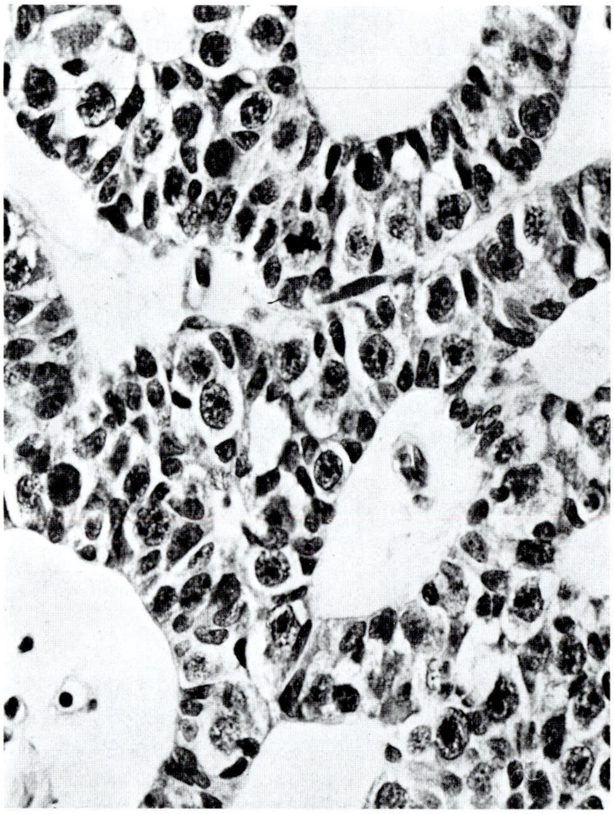

Fig. 20.74. Mixed germ cell–sex cord–stromal tumor. The cordlike pattern is shown. Tripolar mitosis is seen above *center*.

rivatives or flattened epithelial-like cells or devoid of lining may be observed[186,193,203]; they closely resemble the cystic spaces observed in some retiform Sertoli–Leydig cell tumors[180,184,217] or cystic sex cord–stromal tumors. In occasional tumors, this pattern may be pronounced and may suggest that the tumor contains epithelial cells in addition to germ cells and sex cord derivatives.[193] It is considered that these cells are in fact sex cord derivatives and that the tumor in common with some sex cord tumors exhibits a retiform or cystic pattern or both.

Normal ovarian tissue as evidenced by the presence of normal ovarian stroma and at least some primordial follicles has been identified in all cases, including a case in which it could not be identified in the original sections available.[174] In a number of cases, graafian follicles also are present.[175,186] In other cases, tumor deposits are found very close to the surface of the ovary, obliterating primordial and graafian follicles.

Differential Diagnosis

Histologically, this tumor is most likely to be confused with gonadoblastoma. In contrast to gonadoblastoma, this tumor lacks the typical nestlike pattern, has greater proliferative activity of both the germ cell and sex cord component, and lacks calcification, hyalinization, and in most cases Leydig or lutein-like cells. Macroscopically, the tumors are larger. The gonad of origin is a normal ovary, and there is no evidence of gonadal dysgenesis or any somatosexual abnormalities. The patients are chromatin positive and have a normal female 46,XX karyotype. There is no evidence of virilization, and if there are signs of abnormal endocrine activity, they manifest themselves as feminization.

Occasionally, if the germ cells are relatively scanty, the tumor may be confused with the sex cord–stromal tumors of the ovary, but the presence of germ cells should alert the observer to the true identity of the tumor. If the sex cord derivatives are few in number, are missed, or are disregarded, the tumor may be included with the germ cell tumors, but the presence of sex cord elements intimately admixed with the germ cells should indicate its true identity. The presence of prominent clefts and cystic spaces, especially when the latter contain papillary projections, may cause confusion with Sertoli–Leydig cell tumors showing the retiform pattern or even with serous papillary tumors. The presence of germ cells admixed with sex cord derivatives indicates that the tumor is a mixed germ cell–sex cord–stromal tumor.

Clinical Behavior and Treatment

The prognosis of patients with mixed germ cell–sex cord–stromal tumor of the ovary occurring in pure form is favorable. In the great majority of known cases when the tumor was confined to the ovary and not associated with other malignant neoplastic germ cell elements, there has been no recurrence or metastases after excision of the affected adnexa. The patients are well and disease free for periods varying from 1 to 15 years.[178] Accordingly, after a unilateral salpingo-oophorectomy, careful examination of the abdomen and a biopsy of the contralateral ovary are recommended. After this procedure, the patient should have chromosome studies. If the karyotype is 46,XX and if no other abnormalities are detected, further therapy is not necessary, although careful long-term follow-up is essential.

One well-documented case of metastasizing mixed germ cell–sex cord–stromal tumor occurring in an 8-year-old girl has been reported.[84] The metastases were found in the paraaortic lymph nodes and in the peritoneal cavity. The patient was well and disease free 2 years after excision of the affected adnexa, paraaortic lymphadenectomy, excision of peritoneal metastases, and a course of cisplatin-based combination chemotherapy.[84] Another case of metastasizing mixed germ cell–sex cord–stromal tumor showing an unusual pattern resembling the sex cord tumor with annular tubules (SCTAT) occurring in a 30-year-old woman has been reported.[8] Three years after excision of a right-sided ovarian tumor, a large tumor mass was noted in the region of the uterine fundus. The mass and a number of peritoneal implants were excised together with the uterus and the left ovary. The primary and the metastatic tumors showed identical appearances. The left ovary was normal. The patient was well and disease free 1 year after excision of the metastases and administration of combination chemotherapy.[8]

In three patients in their twenties, one in her early thirties, and one in her early forties, the mixed germ cell–sex cord–stromal tumor was associated with dysgerminoma. There was no evidence of metastases. The patients are well and disease free from 2 to 7 years after one-sided adnexectomy and radiation therapy.

In four children aged 5–16 years, the tumor was overgrown by other malignant germ cell elements, including choriocarcinoma and yolk sac tumor. In three of these cases, the tumor metastasized and resulted in the death of the patient. The metastases were composed of the malignant germ cell elements. One patient treated with *cis*-platinum-based chemotherapy was alive and well 5 years later. When the tumor is associated with malignant germ cell elements, the patient should be treated with the appropriate combination chemotherapy used in treatment of nondysgerminomatous malignant germ cell tumors.

When the tumor is encountered in postmenarchal women, there is an increased possibility that the tumor may not present in pure form but is associated with other neoplastic germ cell elements. In such cases, in addition to excision of the affected adnexa appropriate therapy to treat the neoplastic germ cell elements present is recommended.

References

1. Abbot TM, Herman WJ Jr, Scully RE (1984) Ovarian fetiform teratoma (homunculus) in a 9-year-old girl. Int J Gynecol Pathol 2:392
2. Aguirre P, Scully RE (1982) Malignant neuroectodermal tumor of the ovary: a distinctive form of monodermal teratoma. Report of five cases. Am J Surg Pathol 6:283
3. Alenghat E, Okagaki T, Talerman A (1986) Primary mucinous carcinoid tumor of the ovary. Cancer (Phila) 58:777
4. Allard S, Cadotte M, Boivin Y (1972) Dysgenesie gonadique pure familiale et gonadoblastome. Union Med Can 101:448–452
5. Anderson CT Jr, Carlson IH (1975) Elevated plasma testosterone and gonadal tumors in two 46XY "sisters." Arch Pathol 99:360
6. Anderson MC, McDicken IW (1971) Melanotic cyst of the ovary. J Obstet Gynaecol Br Commonw 78: 1047
7. Arhelger RB, Kelly B (1974) Strumal carcinoid. Report of a case with electron microscopical observations. Arch Pathol 97:323
8. Arroyo JG, Harris W, Laden SA (1998) Recurrent mixed germ cell-sex cord-stromal tumor of the ovary in an adult. Int J Gynecol Pathol 17:281
9. Asadourian LA, Taylor HB (1969) Dysgerminoma. An analysis of 105 cases. Obstet Gynecol 33:370
10. Atkin NB (1973) High chromosome numbers of seminomata and malignant teratomata of the testis: a review of data on 103 tumors. Br J Cancer 28:275
11. Atkin NB, Baker MC (1983) i(12p): specific chromosomal marker in seminoma and malignant teratoma of the testis? Cancer Genet Cytogenet 10:199
12. Atkin NB, Baker MC (1987) Abnormal chromosomes including small metacentrics in 14 ovarian cancers. Cancer Genet Cytogenet 26:355
13. Ayhan A, Bukulmez O, Genc C, Kuramursel BS, Ayhan A (2000) Mature cystic teratomas of the ovary. A case series from one institution over 34 years. Eur J Obstet Gynecol 88:153
14. Bagg HJ (1936) Experimental production of teratoma testis in a fowl. Am J Cancer 26:69
15. Bartlett DJ, Grant JK, Pugh MA, Aherne W (1968) A familial feminizing syndrome. A family showing intersex characteristics with XY chromosomes in three female members. J Obstet Gynaecol Br Commonw 75:199
16. Beck JS, Fulmer HF, Lee ST (1969) Solid malignant ovarian teratoma with "embryoid bodies" and trophoblastic differentiation. J Pathol 99:67
17. Bell DA, Flotte TJ, Bhan AK (1987) Immunohistochemical characterization of seminoma and its inflammatory infiltrate. Hum Pathol 18:511
18. Bergher de Bacalao E, Dominguez I (1969) Unilateral gonadoblastoma in a pregnant woman. Am J Obstet Gynecol 105:1279
19. Bergstrand CG, Czar B (1956) Demonstration of a new protein fraction in serum from human fetus. Scand J Lab Invest 8:174
20. Bernstein D, Naor S, Rikover M, Manahem H (1974) Hemolytic anemia related to ovarian tumor. Obstet Gynecol 43:276
21. Bhatena D, Haning RV Jr, Shapiro S, Hafez GR (1985) Coexistence of a gonadoblastoma and mixed germ cell–sex cord stroma tumor. Pathol Res Pract 180:203
22. Bjorkholm E, Lundell M, Gyftodimos A, Silversward C (1990) Dysgerminoma. The Radiumhemmet series 1927–1984. Cancer (Phila) 65:38
23. Blackwell WJ, Dockerty MB, Masson JC, Mussey

RD (1946) Dermoid cysts of the ovary: clinical and pathological significance. Am J Obstet Gynecol 51: 151
24. Boczkowski K, Teter J, Sternadel Z (1972) Sibship occurrence of XY gonadal dysgenesis with dysgerminoma. Am J Obstet Gynecol 113:952
25. Bonazzi C, Peccatori F, Colombo N, Lucchini V, Cantu MG, Mangioni C (1994) Pure ovarian immature teratoma, a unique and curable disease: 10 years experience of 32 prospectively treated patients. Obstet Gynecol 84:598
26. Breen JL, Neubecker RD (1967) Ovarian malignancy in children with special reference to the germ cell tumors. Ann NY Acad Sci 142:658
27. Cabanne F (1971) Gonadoblastomes et tumeurs de l'ebauche gonadique. Ann Anat Pathol (Paris) 16:387
28. Carleton RL, Friedman NB, Bomze EJ (1953) Experimental teratomas of testis. Cancer (Phila) 6:464
29. Caruso PA, Marsh MR, Minkowitz S, Karten G (1971) An intense clinicopathologic study of 305 teratomas of the ovary. Cancer (Phila) 27:343
30. Chenot M (1911) Contribution ê l'etude des epitheliomas primitifs de l'ovaire. Thesis, Sorbonne, Paris
31. Chevassu M (1906) Tumeurs du Testicule. Thesis, Steinhall, Paris
32. Chumas JC, Scully RE (1991) Sebaceous tumors arising in ovarian dermoid cysts. Int J Gynecol Pathol 10:356
33. Clement PB, Young RH, Scully RE (1987) Endometrioid-like variant of ovarian yolk sac tumor. A clinicopathological analysis of eight cases. Am J Surg Pathol 11:767
34. Cohen MB, Friend DS, Molnar JJ, Talerman A (1987) Gonadal endodermal sinus (yolk sac) tumor with pure intestinal differentiation; a new histologic type. Pathol Res Pract 182:609
35. Dandia SD (1967) Rectovesical fistula following an ovarian dermoid with recurrent vesical calculus. A case report. J Urol 97:85
36. Davis KP, Hartmann LK, Keeney GL, Shapiro H (1996) Primary ovarian carcinoid tumors. Gynecol Oncol 61:259
37. Dawson MA, Wilimer T, Yarbro JW (1971) Hemolytic anemia associated with an ovarian tumor. Am J Med 50:552
38. Dayal Y, Tashjian AH Jr, Wolfe HJ (1979) Immunocytochemical localization of calcitonin-producing cells in a strumal carcinoid with amyloid stroma. Cancer (Phila) 43:1331
39. Dietl J, Horny HP, Ruck P, Kaiserling E (1993) Dysgerminoma of the ovary. An immunohistochemical study of tumor-infiltrating lymphoreticular cells and tumor cells. Cancer (Phila) 71:2562
40. Dixon FJ, Moore RA (1952) Tumors of the male sex organs. Atlas of tumor pathology, sect VIII, fasc 31b, 32. Armed Forces Institute of Pathology, Washington, DC
41. Erez SE, Richart RM, Shettles LB (1965) Hashimoto's disease in a benign cystic teratoma of the ovary. Am J Obstet Gynecol 92:273
42. Erhan Y, Toprak AS, Ozdemir N, Tiras B (1992) Gonadoblastoma and fertility. J Clin Pathol 45:828
43. Evans RW (1957) Developmental stages of embryo-like bodies in teratoma testis. J Clin Pathol 10:321
44. Frazier SD, Bashore RA, Mosier HD (1964) Gonadoblastoma associated with pure gonadal dysgenesis in monozygous twins. J Pediatr 64:740
45. Friedman NB (1951) The comparative morphogenesis of extragenital and gonadal teratoid tumors. Cancer (Phila) 4:265
46. Friedman NB, Moore RA (1946) Tumors of the testis. A report of 922 cases. Mil Surg 99:573
47. Fujii S, Konishi I, Suzuki A, Okamura H, Okazaki T, Mori T (1985) Analysis of serum lactic dehydrogenase levels and its isoenzymes in ovarian dysgerminoma. Gynecol Oncol 22:65
48. Galager HS, Lewis RP (1973) Sequential gonadoblastoma and choriocarcinoma. Obstet Gynecol 41: 123
49. Garvin AJ, Pratt-Thomas HR, Spector M, Spicer SS, Williamson HO (1976) Gonadoblastoma: histologic ultrastructural and histochemical observations in five cases. Am J Obstet Gynecol 125:459
50. Gershenson DM (1993) Update on malignant ovarian germ cell tumors. Cancer (Phila) 71:1581
51. Gershenson DM, Del Junco G, Herson J, Rutledge FN (1983) Endodermal sinus tumor of the ovary. The M.D. Anderson experience. Obstet Gynecol 61: 194
52. Gibas Z, Talerman A, Faruqi S, Carlson J, Noumoff J (1993) Cytogenetic analysis of an immature teratoma of the ovary and its metastasis. Int J Gynecol Pathol 12:276
53. Gillman J (1948) The development of the gonads in man with consideration of the role of fetal endocrines and the histogenesis of ovarian tumors. Contrib Embryol 32:83
54. Gitlin D, Boesman M (1967) Sites of serum alpha-fetoprotein synthesis in the human and in the rat. J Clin Invest 46:1010
55. Gitlin D, Pericelli A (1970) Synthesis of serum albumin, prealbumin, alpha-fetoprotein, alpha-1-antitrypsin and transferrin by the human yolk sac. Nature (Lond) 228:995
56. Gitlin D, Pericelli A, Gitlin G (1972) Synthesis of alpha-fetoprotein by liver, yolk sac and gastrointestinal tract of the human conceptus. Cancer Res 32: 979
57. Gonzalez-Angulo A, Kaufman R, Braungardt CD, Chapman FC, Hinshaw AJ (1963) Adenocarcinoma of thyroid arising in struma ovarii (malignant struma ovarii). Report of two cases and review of the literature. Obstet Gynecol 21: 567
58. Gonzalez-Crussi F, Roth LM (1976) The human yolk sac and yolk sac carcinoma. Hum Pathol 7:675
59. Gordon A, Lipton D, Woodruff JD (1981) Dysgerminoma: a review of 158 cases from the Emil Novak Ovarian Tumor Registry. Obstet Gynecol 58: 497
60. Hart WR, Burkons DM (1979) Germ cell neoplasms arising in gonadoblastomas. Cancer (Phila) 34:669

61. Hart WR, Regezi JA (1978) Strumal carcinoid of the ovary. Ultrastructural observations and long-term follow-up study. Am J Clin Pathol 69:356
62. Heifetz SA, Cushing B, Giller R, et al (1998) Immature teratomas in children: Pathologic considerations. Am J Surg Pathol 22:1115
63. Hingorani V, Narula RK, Bhalla S (1963) *Salmonella typhi* infection in an ovarian dermoid. Report of a case. Obstet Gynecol 22:118
64. Hughesdon PE, Kumarasamy T (1970) Mixed germ cell tumors (gonadoblastomas) in normal and dysgenetic gonads. Virch Arch [Pathol Anat] 349:258
65. Ishida T, Tagatz GE, Okagaki T (1976) Gonadoblastoma. Ultrastructural evidence of testicular origin. Cancer (Phila) 37:1770
66. Jackson SM (1967) Ovarian dysgerminoma. Br J Radiol 40:459
67. Jacobs AJ, Newland JR, Green RK (1982) Pure choriocarcinoma of the ovary. Obstet Gynecol Surv 37:603
68. Jacobsen GK, Talerman A (1989) Atlas of germ cell tumors. Munksgaard, Copenhagen
69. Judd HL, Scully RE, Atkins L, Neer RM, Kliman B (1970) Pure gonadal dysgenesis with progressive hirsutism. N Engl J Med 282:881
70. Kawahara H (1963) Struma ovarii with ascites and hydrothorax. Am J Obstet Gynecol 85:85
71. Kazancigil TR, Laquer W, Ladewig P (1940) Papilloendothelioma of the ovary; report of three cases and discussion of Schiller's "mesonephroma ovarii." Am J Cancer 40:199
72. Kemp B, Hauptmann S, Schroder W, Amo-Takyi B, Leeners B, Rath W (1995) Dysgerminoma of the ovary in a patient with triple-X syndrome. Int J Obstet Gynecol 50:51
73. King ME, Mouradian JA, Micha JP, Chaganti RSK, Allen SL (1985) Immature teratoma of the ovary with predominant malignant retinal anlage tumor. A parthenogenetically derived tumor. Am J Surg Pathol 9:221
74. King ME, DiGiovanni LM, Yung JF, Clarke-Pearson DL (1990) Immature teratoma of the ovary grade 3, with karyotype analysis. Int J Gynecol Pathol 9:178
75. King ME, Hubbell MJ, Talerman A (1991) Mixed germ cell tumor of the ovary with prominent polyembryoma component. Int J Gynecol Pathol 10: 88
76. Klein HZ (1974) Mucinous carcinoid tumor of the vermiform appendix. Cancer (Phila) 33: 770
77. Kleiman GM, Young RH, Scully RE (1984) Ependymoma of the ovary: report of three cases. Hum Pathol 15:632
78. Kommoss F, Franklin WA, Talerman A (1989) Estrogen and progesterone receptors in endodermal sinus (yolk sac) tumor. Evaluation of immunocytochemical and biochemical methods. J Reprod Med 34:943
79. Kommoss F, Bibbo M, Talerman A (1990) Nuclear deoxyribonucleic acid content (ploidy) of endodermal sinus (yolk sac) tumor. Lab Invest 62:223
80. Krumerman MS, Chung A (1977) Squamous carcinoma arising in benign cystic teratoma of the ovary. Cancer (Phila) 39:1237
81. Kurman RJ, Norris HJ (1976) Endodermal sinus tumor of the ovary. A clinical and pathological analysis of 71 cases. Cancer (Phila) 38:2404
82. Kurman RJ, Norris HJ (1976) Embryonal carcinoma of the ovary. A clinicopathologic entity distinct from endodermal sinus tumor resembling embryonal carcinoma of the adult testis. Cancer (Phila) 38:2420
83. Kurman RJ, Norris HJ (1976) Malignant mixed germ cell tumors of the ovary. A clinical and pathological analysis of 30 cases. Obstet Gynecol 48:579
84. Lacson AG, Gillis DA, Shawwa A (1988) Malignant mixed germ cell–sex cord stromal tumors of the ovary associated with isosexual precocious puberty. Cancer (Phila) 61:2122
85. Letterie GS, Page DC (1995) Dysgerminoma and gonadal dysgenesis in 46,XX female with no evidence of Y chromosomal DNA. Gynecol Oncol 57: 423
86. Linder D, Power J (1970) Further evidence for postmeiotic origin of teratomas in the human female. Ann Hum Genet 34:21
87. Linder D, McCaw BK, Hecht F (1975) Parthenogenic origin of benign ovarian teratoma. N Engl J Med 292:63
88. Lynn JA, Varon HH, Kingsley WB, Martin JH (1967) Ultrastructure and biochemical studies of estrogen-secreting capacity of a "non-functional" ovarian neoplasm (dysgerminoma). Am J Pathol 51: 639
89. Mackay AM, Pattigrew N, Symington T, Neville AM (1974) Tumors of dysgenetic gonads (gonadoblastoma). Ultrastructural and steroidogenic aspects. Cancer (Phila) 34:1108
90. McDonough PG, Byrd JR, Tho PT, Otken L (1976) Gonadoblastoma in a true hermaphrodite with 46XX karyotype. Obstet Gynecol 47:355
91. McKay DG, Hertig AT, Adams EC, Danziger S (1953) Histochemical observations on the germ cells of human embryos. Anat Rec 117:201
92. Malkasian GD Jr, Dockerty MB, Symmonds RE (1967) Benign cystic teratomas. Obstet Gynecol 29: 719
93. Malkasian GD Jr, Symmonds RE, Dockerty MB (1965) Malignant ovarian teratomas. Report of 31 cases. Obstet Gynecol 25:810
94. Marin-Padilla M (1965) Origin, nature and significance of the "embryoids" of human teratomas. Virchows Arch [Pathol Anat] 340:105
95. Marrubini G (1949) Primary chorionepithelioma of the ovary. Report of two cases. Acta Obstet Gynecol Scand 28:251
96. Masson P (1912) Seminomes ovariennes. Bull Soc Anat (Paris) 87:402
97. Masson P (1923) Epitheliomas pflugeriens. In: Diagnostics de Laboratoire. Les Tumeurs. Maloine, Paris
98. Mazur MT, Talbot WH Jr, Talerman A (1988) Endodermal sinus tumor and mucinous cystadenofi-

broma of the ovary. Occurrence in an 82-year-old woman. Cancer (Phila) 62:2011
99. Meyer R (1931) The pathology of some special ovarian tumors and their relation to sex characteristics. Am J Obstet Gynecol 22:697
100. Miettinen M, Virtanen I, Talerman A (1985) Intermediate filament proteins in human testis and testicular germ-cell tumors. Am J Pathol 120:402
101. Miettinen M, Talerman A, Wahlstrom T, Astengo-Osuna C, Virtanen I (1985) Cellular differentiation in ovarian sex cord-stromal and germ-cell tumors studied with antibodies to intermediate-filament proteins. Am J Surg Pathol 9:640
102. Mueller CW, Topkins P, Lapp WA (1950) Dysgerminoma of the ovary. An analysis of 427 cases. Am J Obstet Gynecol 60:153
103. Nakashima M, Nagasaka T, Fukata S, Oiwa N, Nara Y, Fukatsu T, Takeuchi J (1989) Ovarian gonadoblastoma with dysgerminoma in a woman with two normal children. Hum Pathol 20:814
104. Nielsen SNJ, Scheithauer BW, Gaffey TA (1985) Gliomatosis peritonei. Cancer (Phila) 56:2499
105. Nieminen I, Von Numers C, Widholm O (1964) Struma ovarii. Acta Obstet Gynecol Scand 42:399
106. Nogales FF Jr, Silverberg SG, Bloustein PA, Martinez-Hernandez A, Pierce GB (1977) Yolk sac carcinoma (endodermal sinus tumor). Ultrastructure and histogenesis of gonadal and extragonadal tumors in comparison with normal human yolk sac. Cancer (Phila) 39:1462
107. Nogales FF, Bergeron C, Carvia RE, Alvaro T, Fulwood HR (1996) Ovarian endometrioid tumors with yolk sac tumor component, an unusual form of ovarian neoplasm. Analysis of six cases. Am J Surg Pathol 20:1056
108. Nomura K, Ohama K, Okamoto E, Fujiwara A (1983) Cytogenetic studies of multiple ovarian dermoid cysts in a single host. Acta Obstet Gynecol Jpn 35:1938
109. Nomura K, Matsui T, Aizawa S (1999) Gonadoblastoma with proliferation resembling Sertoli cell tumor. Int J Gynecol Pathol 18:91
110. Norgaard-Pedersen B, Albrechtsen R, Teilum G (1975) Serum alpha-fetoprotein as a marker for endodermal sinus tumor (yolk sac tumor), or a vitelline component of teratocarcinoma. Acta Pathol Microbiol Scand (A) 83:573
111. Norris HJ, Jensen RD (1972) Relative frequency of ovarian neoplasms in children and adolescents. Cancer (Phila) 30:713
112. Norris HJ, Zirkin HJ, Benson WL (1976) Immature (malignant) teratoma of the ovary. A clinical and pathologic study of 58 cases. Cancer (Phila) 37:2359
113. Obata NH, Nakashima N, Kawai M, Kikkawa F, Mamba S, Tomoda Y (1995) Gonadoblastoma with dysgerminoma in one ovary and gonadoblastoma with dysgerminoma and yolk sac tumor in the contralateral ovary in a girl with 46,XX karyotype. Gynecol Oncol 58:124
114. O'Connor DM, Norris HJ (1994) The influence of grade on the outcome of stage I ovarian immature (malignant) teratomas and the reproducibility of grading. Int J Gynecol Pathol 13:283
115. Oliva E, Baker PM, Talerman A, Young RH, Scully RE (2000) Primary mucinous carcinoid tumors of the ovary: a report of 17 cases with emphasis on their histologic spectrum. Mod Pathol 13:129A
116. Pantoja E, Noy MA, Axtmayer RW, Colon FE, Pelegrina I (1975) Ovarian dermoids and their complications. Comprehensive historical review. Obstet Gynecol Surv 30:1
117. Pantoja E, Rodriguez-Ibanez I, Axtmayer RW, Noy MA, Pelegrina I (1975) Complications of dermoid tumors of the ovary. Obstet Gynecol 45:89
118. Park IJ, Pyeatte JC, Jones HW, Woodruff JD (1972) Gonadoblastoma in a true hermaphrodite with 46XY genotype. Obstet Gynecol 40:466
119. Parrington JM, West LF, Povey S (1984) The origin of ovarian teratomas. J Med Genet 21:4
120. Patel SK, Prentice SA (1972) Gonadoblastoma: distinctive ovarian tumor. Arch Pathol 94:165
121. Payne D, Muss HB, Homesley HD, Jobson VM, Baird FG (1981) Autoimmune hemolytic anemia and ovarian dermoid cysts. Case report and review of the literature. Cancer (Phila) 48:721
122. Peccatori F, Bonazzi C, Chiari F, Landoni F, Colombo N, Mangioni C (1995) Surgical management of malignant ovarian germ cell tumors: 10 years' experience with 129 patients. Obstet Gynecol 86:367
123. Pedowitz P, Felmus LB, Grayzel DM (1955) Dysgerminoma of the ovary. Prognosis and treatment. Am J Obstet Gynecol 70:1284
124. Peterson WF (1956) Solid histologically benign teratomas of the ovary. A report of four cases and review of the literature. Am J Obstet Gynecol 72:1094
125. Peterson WF (1957) Malignant degeneration of benign cystic teratomas of the ovary: a collective review of the literature. Obstet Gynecol Surv 12:793
126. Peterson WF, Prevost EC, Edmunds FT, Huntley JM Jr, Morris FK (1955) Benign cystic teratomas of the ovary. A clinicostatistical study of 1007 cases with review of the literature. Am J Obstet Gynecol 70:368
127. Peyron A (1939) Faits nouveaux relatifs ê l'origine et ê l'histogenese des embryomes. Bull Assoc Fr Cancer 28:658
128. Pierce GB Jr (1966) Ultrastructure of human testicular tumors. Cancer (Phila) 19:1963
129. Pierce GB Jr, Dixon FJ (1959) Testicular teratomas. 1. Demonstration of teratogenesis by metamorphosis of multipotential cells. Cancer (Phila) 12:573
130. Pierce GB Jr, Dixon FJ (1959) Testicular teratomas. 2. Teratocarcinoma as ascitic tumor. Cancer (Phila) 12:584
131. Pierce GB Jr, Midgley AR (1963) The origin and function of human syncytiotrophoblastic giant cells. Am J Pathol 43:153
132. Pierce GB Jr, Verney EL (1961) An in vitro and in

vivo study of differentiation in teratocarcinomas. Cancer (Phila) 14:1017
133. Pierce GB Jr, Midgley AR, Beals TF (1962) An ultrastructural study of differentiation and maturation of trophoblast of the monkey. Lab Invest 13: 451
134. Pierce GB Jr, Midgley AR, Sri Ram J, Feldman JD (1964) Parietal yolk sac carcinoma. Clue to the histogenesis of Reichert's membrane of the mouse embryo. Am J Pathol 41:549
135. Prat J, Bhan AK, Dickersin GR, Robboy SJ, Scully RE (1982) Hepatoid yolk sac tumor of the ovary (endodermal sinus tumor with hepatoid differentiation). A light microscopic ultrastructural and immunohistochemical study of seven cases. Cancer (Phila) 50:2355
136. Pratt-Thomas HR, Cooper JM (1976) Gonadoblastoma with tubal pregnancy. Am J Clin Pathol 65: 121
137. Rashad MH, Fathalla MF, Kerr MC (1966) Sex chromatin and chromosome analysis in ovarian teratomas. Am J Obstet Gynecol 96:461
138. Robboy SJ, Scully RE (1970) Ovarian teratoma with glial implants on the peritoneum. An analysis of 12 cases. Hum Pathol 1:643
139. Robboy SJ, Scully RE (1980) Strumal carcinoid of the ovary. An analysis of 50 cases of a distinctive tumor composed of thyroid tissue and carcinoid. Cancer (Phila) 46:2019
140. Robboy SJ, Norris HJ, Scully RE (1975) Insular carcinoid primary in the ovary: a clinicopathologic analysis of 48 cases. Cancer (Phila) 36:404
141. Robboy SJ, Scully RE, Norris HJ (1974) Carcinoid metastatic to the ovary. A clinicopathologic analysis of 35 cases. Cancer (Phila) 33:798
142. Robboy SJ, Scully RE, Norris HJ (1977) Primary trabecular carcinoid of the ovary. Obstet Gynecol 49:202
143. Rose LI, Underwood RH, Williams GH, Pincus GS (1974) Pure gonadal dysgenesis. Studies of in vitro androgen metabolism. Am J Med 57:957
144. Rutgers JL, Scully RE (1986) Functioning ovarian tumors with peripheral steroid cell proliferation. A report of 24 cases. Int J Gynecol Pathol 5: 319
145. Rutgers JL, Young RH, Scully RE (1987) Ovarian yolk sac tumor arising from endometrioid carcinoma. Hum Pathol 18:1296
146. Santesson L (1947) Clinical and pathological survey of ovarian tumours treated at the Radiumhemmet. 1. Dysgerminoma. Acta Radiol (Stockh) 28:643
147. Schellhas HF (1974) Malignant potential of the dysgenetic gonad. Part 1. Obstet Gynecol 44:298
148. Schellhas HF (1974) Malignant potential of the dysgenetic gonad. Part 2. Obstet Gynecol 44:455
149. Schellhas HF, Trujillo JM, Rutledge FN, Cork A (1971) Germ cell tumors associated with XY gonadal dysgenesis. Am J Obstet Gynecol 109:1197
150. Schiller W (1939) Mesonephroma ovarii. Am J Cancer 35:1
151. Schmitz EF (1925) Malignant endothelioma of perithelioma type in the ovary. Am J Obstet Gynecol 9:247
152. Schwartz PE, Morris JM (1988) Serum lactic dehydrogenase. A tumor marker for dysgerminoma. Obstet Gynecol 72:511
153. Scully RE (1953) Gonadoblastoma. A gonadal tumor related to dysgerminoma (seminoma) and capable of sex hormone production. Cancer (Phila) 6: 455
154. Scully RE (1970) Gonadoblastoma. Cancer (Phila) 25:1340
155. Scully RE (1970) Sex cord tumor with annular tubules. A distinctive ovarian tumor of the Peutz–Jeghers syndrome. Cancer (Phila) 25:1107
156. Scully RE (1999) Histological typing of ovarian tumours, 2nd Ed. World Health Organization histological classification of tumours. Springer, Heidelberg
157. Serov SF, Scully RE, Sobin LH (1973) Histological typing of ovarian tumors. International histological classification of tumors, no 9. World Health Organization, Geneva
158. Serratoni FT, Robboy SJ (1975) Ultrastructure of primary and metastatic ovarian carcinoids: analysis of 11 cases. Cancer (Phila) 36:157
159. Shah KD, Kaffe S, Gilbert F, Dolgin S, Gertner M (1988) Unilateral microscopic gonadoblastoma in a prepubertal Turner mosaic with Y chromosome material identified by restriction fragment analysis. Am J Clin Pathol 90:622
160. Shirai T, Itoh T, Yoshiki T, Noro T, Tomino Y, Hayasaka T (1976) Immunofluorescent demonstration of alpha-fetoprotein, and other plasma proteins in yolk sac tumor. Cancer (Phila) 38:1661
161. Simard LC (1957) Polyembryonic embryoma of the ovary of parthenogenetic origin. Cancer (Phila) 10: 215
162. Smith FG (1946) Pathology and physiology of struma ovarii. Arch Surg 53:603
163. Snyder RR, Tavassoli FA (1986) Ovarian strumal carcinoid: Immunohistochemical, ultrastructural, and clinicopathologic observations. Int J Gynecol Pathol 5:187
164. Sporrong B, Falkmer S, Robboy SJ, et al (1982) Neurohormonal peptides in ovarian carcinoids. An immunohistochemical study of 81 primary carcinoids and of intraovarian metastases from six midgut carcinoids. Cancer (Phila) 49:68
165. Stagno PA, Petras RE, Hart WR (1987) Strumal carcinoids of the ovary. An immunohistologic and ultrastructural study. Arch Pathol Lab Med 111:440
166. Stamp GWH, McConnell EM (1983) Malignancy arising in cystic ovarian teratomas. Br J Obstet Gynecol 90:671
167. Stevens LC (1959) Embryology of testicular teratomas in strain 129 mice. J Natl Cancer Inst 23:1249
168. Stevens LC (1960) Embryonic potency of embryoid bodies derived from a transplantable testicular teratoma of the mouse. Dev Biol 2:285
169. Stevens LC (1962) The biology of teratomas in-

cluding evidence indicating their origin from primordial germ cells. Ann Biol 1:585
170. Subbuswamy SG, Gibbs NM, Ross CF, Morson BC (1974) Goblet cell carcinoid of the appendix. Cancer (Phila) 34:338
171. Szokol M, Kondrai G, Papp Z (1977) Gonadal malignancy and 46 XY karyotype in a true hermaphrodite. Obstet Gynecol 49:358
172. Takeda A, Ishizuka T, Goto T, et al (1982) Polyembryoma of ovary producing alpha-fetoprotein and HCG. Immunoperoxidase and electron microscopic study. Cancer (Phila) 49:1878
173. Talerman A (1971) Gonadoblastoma and dysgerminoma in two siblings with dysgenetic gonads. Obstet Gynecol 38:416
174. Talerman A (1972) A distinctive gonadal neoplasm related to gonadoblastoma. Cancer (Phila) 30:1219
175. Talerman A (1972) A mixed germ cell-sex cord stroma tumor in a normal female infant. Obstet Gynecol 40:473
176. Talerman A (1974) Gonadoblastoma associated with embryonal carcinoma. Obstet Gynecol 43:138
177. Talerman A (1975) The incidence of yolk sac tumor (endodermal sinus tumor) elements in germ cell tumors of the testis in adults. Cancer (Phila) 36:211
178. Talerman A (1980) The pathology of gonadal neoplasms composed of germ cells and sex cord stroma derivatives. Pathol Res Pract 170:24
179. Talerman A (1984) Carcinoid tumors of the ovary. J Cancer Res Clin Oncol 107:125
180. Talerman A (1987) Ovarian Sertoli–Leydig cell tumor (androblastoma) with retiform pattern. A clinicopathologic study. Cancer (Phila) 60:3056
181. Talerman A, Delemarre JFM (1975) Gonadoblastoma associated with embryonal carcinoma in an anatomically normal male. J Urol 113:355
182. Talerman A, Evans MI (1982) Primary trabecular carcinoid tumor of the ovary. Cancer (Phila) 50: 1407
183. Talerman A, Haije WG (1974) Alpha-fetoprotein and germ cell tumors. A possible role of yolk sac tumor in production of alpha-fetoprotein. Cancer (Phila) 34:1722
184. Talerman A, Haije WG (1985) Ovarian Sertoli cell tumor with retiform and heterologous elements. Am J Surg Pathol 9:459
185. Talerman A, Okagaki T (1985) Ultrastructural features of primary trabecular carcinoid tumor of the ovary. Int J Gynecol Pathol 4:153
186. Talerman A, van der Harten JJ (1977) A mixed germ cell-sex cord stroma tumor of the ovary associated with isosexual precocious puberty in a normal female child. Cancer (Phila) 40:889
187. Talerman A, Haije WG, Baggerman L (1977) Alpha-1-antitrypsin (AAT) and alpha-foetoprotein (AFP) in sera of patients with germ cell neoplasms. Value as tumor markers in patients with endodermal sinus tumour (yolk sac tumour). Int J Cancer 19:741
188. Talerman A, Haije WG, Baggerman L (1978) Serum alpha-fetoprotein in diagnosis and management of endodermal sinus (yolk sac) tumor and mixed germ cell tumor of the ovary. Cancer (Phila) 41:272
189. Talerman A, Haije WG, Baggerman L (1980) Serum alpha-fetoprotein (AFP) in patients with germ cell tumors of the gonads and extragonadal sites. Correlation between endodermal sinus (yolk sac) tumor and raised serum AFP. Cancer (Phila) 46:340
190. Talerman A, Huyzinga WT, Kuipers T (1973) Dysgerminoma. Clinicopathologic study of 22 cases. Obstet Gynecol 41:137
191. Talerman A, van der Pompe WB, Haije WG, Baggerman L, Boekestein-Tjahjadi HM (1977) Alphafetoprotein and carcinoembryonic antigen in germ cell neoplasms. Br J Cancer 35:288
192. Talerman A, Verp M, Senekjian E, Gilewski T, Vogelzang N (1990) True hermaphrodite with normal female 46,XX karyotype, bilateral gonadoblastomas and dysgerminomas and normal pregnancy. Cancer (Phila) 66:2668
193. Tavassoli FA (1983) A combined germ cell-gonadal stromal-epithelial tumor of the ovary. Am J Surg Pathol 7:73
194. Teilum G (1944) Homologous tumours in ovary and testis: contribution to classification of gonadal tumours. Acta Obstet Gynecol Scand 24:480
195. Teilum G (1946) Gonocytoma; homologous ovarian and testicular tumours. 1. With discussion of "mesonephroma ovarii" (Schiller: Am J Cancer 1939). Acta Pathol Microbiol Scand 23:242
196. Teilum G (1950) "mesonephroma ovarii" (Schiller) extraembryonic mesoblastoma of germ cell origin in ovary and testis. Acta Pathol Microbiol Scand 27:249
197. Teilum G (1959) Endodermal sinus tumors of the ovary and testis. Comparative morphogenesis of the so-called mesonephroma ovarii (Schiller) and extraembryonic (yolk sac-allantoic) structures of the rat's placenta. Cancer (Phila) 12:1092
198. Teilum G (1965) Classification of endodermal sinus tumour (mesoblastoma vitellinum) and so-called embryonal carcinoma of the ovary. Acta Pathol Microbiol Scand 64:407
199. Teter J (1970) Prognosis, malignancy and curability of the germ cell tumor occurring in dysgenetic gonads. Am J Obstet Gynecol 108:894
200. Theiss EA, Ashley DJB, Mostofi FK (1959) Nuclear sex of testicular tumors and some related ovarian and extragonadal neoplasms. Cancer (Phila) 13:323
201. Thomas GM, Dembo AJ, Hacker NE, DePetrillo AD (1987) Current therapy for dysgerminoma of the ovary. Obstet Gynecol 70:268
202. Tiltman AJ (1985) Ependymal cyst of the ovary. South Afr Med J 68:424
203. Tokuoka S, Aoki Y, Yokoyama T, Ishii T (1985) A mixed germ cell-sex cord stromal tumor of the ovary with retiform tubular structure. A case report. Int J Gynecol Pathol 4:161
204. Tsuchida Y, Kaneko M, Yokomori K, et al (1978) Alpha-fetoprotein, prealbumin, albumin, alpha-1-antitrypsin, and transferrin as diagnostic and ther-

apeutic markers for endodermal sinus tumors. J Pediatr Surg 13:25
205. Tsuura Y, Hiraki H, Watanabe K, et al (1996) Preferential localization of C-kit product in tissue mast cells, basal cells of skin, epithelial cells of breast, small cell lung carcinoma and seminoma/dysgerminoma in the human. Immunohistochemical study on formalin-fixed paraffin-embedded tissues. Virchows Arch 424:135
206. Ueda G, Fujita M, Ogawa H, Sawada M, Inoue M, Tanizawa O (1993) Adenocarcinoma in a benign cystic teratoma of the ovary. Report of a case with a long survival period. Gynecol Oncol 48:259
207. Ulbright TM, Roth LM, Erlich CE (1982) Ovarian strumal carcinoid. An immunocytochemical and ultrastructural study of two cases. Am J Clin Pathol 77:622
208. Ulirsch RC, Goldman RL (1982) An unusual teratoma of the ovary: neurogenic cyst with lactating breast tissue. Obstet Gynecol 60:400
209. Vance RP, Geisinger KR (1985) Pure nongestational choriocarcinoma of the ovary. Report of a case. Cancer (Phila) 56:2321
210. Warkel RL, Cooper PH, Helwig EB (1978) Adenocarcinoid, a mucin-producing carcinoid of the appendix. Cancer (Phila) 42:2781
211. Weldon-Linne CM, Rushovich AM (1983) Benign ovarian cystic teratomas with homunculi. Obstet Gynecol 61:88S
212. Williamson HO, Underwood PB Jr, Kreutner A Jr, Rogers JF, Mathur RS, Pratt-Thomas HR (1976) Gonadoblastoma: Clinicopathologic correlation in six patients. Am J Obstet Gynecol 126:579
213. Wisniewski M, Deppisch LM (1973) Solid teratomas of the ovary. Cancer (Phila) 32:440
214. Witschi E (1948) Migration of the germ cells of human embryos from the yolk sac to the primitive gonadal folds. Contrib Embryol 32:69
215. Woodruff JD, Protos P, Peterson WF (1968) Ovarian teratomas. Relationship of histologic and ontogenic factors to prognosis. Am J Obstet Gynecol 102:702
216. Woodruff JD, Rauh JT, Markley RL (1966) Ovarian struma. Obstet Gynecol 27:194
217. Young RH, Scully RE (1983) Ovarian Sertoli–Leydig cell tumors with a retiform pattern. A problem in histopathologic diagnosis. A report of 25 cases. Am J Surg Pathol 7:755
218. Young RH, Prat J, Scully RE (1982) Ovarian Sertoli–Leydig cell tumors with heterologous elements (1) gastrointestinal epithelium and carcinoid: A clinicopathologic analysis of thirty six cases. Cancer (Phila) 50:2448
219. Zaloudek C, Tavassoli FA, Norris HJ (1981) Dysgerminoma with syncytiotrophoblastic giant cells. A histologically and clinically distinctive subtype of dysgerminoma. Am J Surg Pathol 5:361

21

Nonspecific Tumors of the Ovary, Including Mesenchymal Tumors and Malignant Lymphoma

Aleksander Talerman, M.D., Ph.D., F.R.C. Path.

The tumors discussed in this chapter comprise a heterogeneous group of neoplasms that are not specific to the ovary. They are uncommon in this location, occurring much more frequently in other parts of the body. Consequently, whenever they are encountered in the ovary, these tumors pose difficult problems in diagnosis, histogenesis, behavior, and therapy for the pathologist and clinician. These neoplasms must be differentiated from primary ovarian neoplasms containing mesenchymal tissue, as well as from metastatic and disseminated neoplasms affecting the ovary. Thus, mesenchymal neoplasms nonspecific to the ovary must be differentiated primarily from teratomatous neoplasms containing large amounts of mature or immature mesenchymal elements and from the malignant mixed müllerian (mesodermal) tumors (MMMT), composed of different malignant connective tissue elements in addition to their malignant epithelial components. In contrast, the primary malignant lymphomas must be differentiated from the more common disseminated malignant lymphoma and leukemia, which not infrequently affect the ovary.

These two different groups of neoplasms—the connective tissue neoplasms nonspecific to the ovary and malignant lymphoma of the ovary—are discussed separately, although included under the same heading, because of their different nature, behavior, and histogenesis. In addition, the adenomatoid tumor, which is of mesothelial origin, the ovarian tumor of probable wolffian origin, ovarian neoplasms of neural origin, hepatoid carcinoma of the ovary, small cell carcinoma of the ovary with pulmonary differentiation, and tumors of salivary gland type are included.

Mesenchymal Tumors Nonspecific to the Ovary

Mesenchymal neoplasms nonspecific to the ovary include all primary ovarian neoplasms of connective tissue origin found in the ovary that are nonspecific to it but are considered to originate from ovarian tissue, and not of teratomatous or surface epithelial–stromal (müllerian) origin. However, this mode of origin cannot be excluded in a number of cases. The neoplasms discussed here are composed of a single neoplastic mesenchymal element, either benign or malignant, in contrast to teratomatous or malignant mixed müllerian tumors, which usually are composed of a number of tissue elements.

Some issues of classification and histogenesis may not be reconcilable in view of the possibility of one-sided differentiation of a teratoma or of a malignant mixed müllerian tumor of the ovary. Thus, although some of these neoplasms can be shown to originate directly from ovarian tissue, a considerable number of cases are of indeterminate histogenesis and origin. Mesenchymal neoplasms nonspecific to the ovary can be benign or malignant, and are classified on the basis of the tissue of origin.

Tumors of Fibrous Tissue Origin

Fibroma

Fibroma is the most common ovarian neoplasm of connective tissue origin and constitutes 3%–5% of ovarian neoplasms. An even higher frequency occurs when fibrosed thecomas are included in this category.

The histogenesis of ovarian fibroma is controversial. The neoplasm most likely arises from mesenchymal cells of the ovarian stroma, which differentiate in the fibroblastic direction. Some investigators postulate that it arises from a fibrosed thecoma or a Brenner tumor, whereas others believe that it originates from the connective tissue within the ovary, primarily within the ovarian cortex or in the walls of blood and lymphatic vessels. Although it can be difficult or even impossible to differentiate between fibroma and fibrosed thecoma, it is worthwhile to make the attempt.

Ovarian fibroma is bilateral in 4%–8% of patients, and in 10% of patients, the tumors are multiple.[15] Ovarian fibroma usually is encountered in meno-pausal and postmenopausal women but is seen at all ages. It is rare in children: fewer than 10 examples have been reported.[7,9,29,37]

Clinically, patients with ovarian fibroma frequently are asymptomatic, mainly because of the tumor's small size. When symptoms do occur, they manifest with abdominal enlargement, urinary symptoms, and abdominal pain. Acute pain is associated with torsion of the tumor. Ascites is a relatively common associated finding and is seen in 50% of cases of fibromas measuring more than 5 cm in diameter. Ascites and hydrothorax (Meigs' syndrome) are seen in 1%–3% of cases.[15,44] Excision of the tumor results in resolution of the ascites and hydrothorax. In one case[46] the tumor was associated with hypoglycemia, which resolved after excision of the fibroma. An increased frequency of ovarian fibroma has been noted in women with hereditary basal cell nevus (Gorlin) syndrome.[9,37] In these women, the fibroma usually is bilateral[9,37,60] and may become malignant[37] or recur.[60]

Macroscopically, the tumors vary from small round nodules 1–2 cm in diameter to large masses weighing up to 13 kg. The tumor usually forms a round or oval solid mass that is gray-white and firm in consistency. It sometimes may be bosselated or lobulated, but usually the external surface is smooth. The cut surface is uniformly white or gray-white, with a whorled pattern similar to that observed in leiomyoma. In large tumors, foci of hemorrhage or necrosis, sometimes resulting in cyst formation, may be seen.

Microscopically, the tumor is composed of short spindle-shaped cells having narrow or ovoid spindle-shaped nuclei. Mitotic activity is absent or very low. The cells form bundles frequently intersected by hyalinized tissue. Hyalinization and myxomatous change frequently are present. Calcification, edema, hemorrhage, and necrosis also may be seen. Fat is absent except in necrotic areas.

The absence of fat differentiates a fibroma from a thecoma, but it cannot distinguish between a fibroma and a completely fibrosed thecoma. Thus, these two entities cannot always be distinguished satisfactorily. Massive edema of the ovary[33,77] and fibromatosis, which may be related to massive edema and usually affects the entire ovary, may resemble an edematous fibroma and must be differentiated from it (see Chapter 16, Nonneoplastic Lesions of the Ovary). Cellular fibroma of the ovary must be differentiated from fibrosarcoma. Although in well-differentiated examples of the latter the distinction may be difficult, the presence of mitotic activity tends to be the best distinguishing feature, and the presence of more than 4 mitoses (MF)/10 high-power fields (HPF) places the tumor in the fibrosarcoma category.[37,57,67]

Fibroma of the ovary is a benign neoplasm, and the treatment of choice is excision of the affected ovary; this results in resolution of all symptoms. In the occasional patient, ovarian fibroma may be associated with implants in the peritoneum.[41] The presence of these implants should not be taken as evidence of malignancy. The prognosis in these, as in other cases of ovarian fibroma, is excellent.

Fibrosarcoma

Primary fibrosarcoma of the ovary is uncommon.[37,57,67] In a series of 283 ovarian tumors of fibrous tissue origin, there were 4 primary fibrosarcomas.[15] Although some fibrosarcomas of the ovary may have been classified as malignant thecomas and as spindle-cell sarcomas, fully documented tumors of this type are uncommon, although they occur more frequently than do other pure primary sarcomas of the ovary. Fibrosarcoma usually is seen in menopausal and postmenopausal patients.[47,57,67] This tumor may arise de novo from ovarian stroma or may originate as a result of malignant change in a preexistent fibroma. Occasional cases have been observed in children. In 1 case, the tumor was associated with nevoid basal cell carcinoma syndrome.[37]

Macroscopically, fibrosarcoma of the ovary resembles ovarian fibroma, but the tumor usually is larger and is more likely to be associated with hemorrhage and necrosis.[47,57] Microscopically, ovarian fibrosarcoma shows typical appearances of fibrosarcoma seen in other locations and usually shows marked cellular pleomorphism and brisk mitotic activity.[47,57] The prognosis is generally poor, the tumor metastasizing early via the bloodstream to the lungs. Occasionally, the course of the disease is more protracted, with patients surviving up to 9 years from time of diagnosis.[37,47] Tumors showing less marked mitotic activity tend to be less aggressive.[37,57] The treatment is excision of the affected adnexa and excision of any intraabdominal metastases. Chemotherapy is used in treatment of fibrosarcoma when distant metastases are present.

Myxoma

Primary *myxoma* of the ovary is a very rare neoplasm: only 16 cases have been reported in the literature.[8,17,67] The patients were aged 14–45 years and in each case had an adnexal mass; the other adnexa was normal.[8,17,67] Macroscopically, the tumors measured from 5 to 22 cm in the greatest dimension.[17,67] They were encapsulated, gray-white, and soft; on cut section, they were found to be partly cystic. Solid areas were slimy and mucinous, whereas the cystic spaces contained a viscous, glassy, gelatinous material.

Microscopically, the tumors showed typical appearances of myxoma as seen in other locations. They were composed of loose myxomatous stroma within which there were scattered stellate or spindle-shaped cells, some of which contained hyperchromatic nuclei. There was no nuclear pleomorphism and mitotic activity was absent. The tumors varied from poorly vascularized, containing only a few capillary blood vessels and showing absence of plexiform vessels, to tumors with prominent capillary vessels within the tumor, and larger vessels with muscular walls at its periphery. The myxomatous stroma stained positively with alcian blue stain and contained a network of fine reticulum fibers. Stains for fat were negative. In some areas, fibrosis was present. There were no other connective tissue elements, and the tumors had a homogeneous appearance.

Myxoma is immunoreactive for vimentin and focally for actin, but negative for desmin, cytokeratins, vascular markers, S-100, and neurofilaments.[17] Most myxomas originate within connective tissue, and the origin of the tumor is still a matter of dispute. The histogenesis of ovarian myxomas is unknown.

Although myxoma is a benign neoplasm, because of its viscous nature it is difficult to excise completely and recurrences are not uncommon unless the entire adnexa bearing the tumor is excised. All the patients treated by unilateral adnexectomy and for whom there is follow-up information are free of disease after 1–13 years.[17]

Myxoma must be differentiated from fibroma with myxoid degeneration, which contains normal fibrous tissue in some areas. Ovarian myxoma must be distinguished from massive edema of the ovary (see Chapter 16, Nonneoplastic Lesions of the Ovary).[33,77] The patients with massive edema usually are younger, and the lesion shows entrapment of follicular derivatives, which is not observed in ovarian myxoma. More importantly, myxoma must be differentiated from myxomatous liposarcoma, which contains fat, is more vascularized, and shows lipoblasts at least in some areas. It also must be differentiated from mucinous cystadenomas and carcinomas, either primary or metastatic, which contain epithelial cells, show absence of stellate and spindle-shaped cells, and may show glandular differentiation. The epithelial tumor cells are cytokeratin positive.

Myxoma also should be distinguished from embryonal rhabdomyosarcoma. The latter tumor shows less of a uniform appearance, displays greater cellular and nuclear pleomorphism, and contains rhabdomyoblasts. In addition, embryonal rhabdomyosarcoma shows positive immunocytochemical staining for sarcomeric actin filaments and desmin. Ultrastructurally, Z-band formation, glycogen granules, and thick filament ribosomal complexes are observed.

Tumors of Muscle Origin

Leiomyoma

Primary leiomyoma of the ovary is uncommon.[34,58,67] Approximately 50 cases are on record, but it is likely that many cases are not reported, especially when the tumor is small and is discovered incidentally. More than a dozen unreported cases are known to the author.

Primary ovarian leiomyoma probably originates from smooth muscle present in the walls of blood vessels in the cortical stroma, in the corpus luteum, and in the ovarian ligaments at their point of attachment to the ovary; its precise histogenesis is uncertain, however. This tumor usually is found in menopausal and postmenopausal women but sometimes occurs in young women. The age of patients ranges from 20 to 65 years.[58,67] Clinically, many patients are asymptomatic, and the tumor is discovered incidentally. When symptoms are present, they are related to the presence of an adnexal mass, often accompanied by abdominal swelling and abdominal pain. The latter may be acute because of torsion. Ascites is rare, and hydrothorax has not been reported. The uterus usually contains leiomyomas.

Ovarian leiomyoma is unilateral, although a single case of large bilateral ovarian leiomyomas occuring in a 21-year-old woman has been reported.[34] Macroscopically the tumors are solid, firm, round or oval masses having a smooth surface. On cut section they have a white or gray-white solid whorled surface. Hemorrhage and necrosis may be evident, altering the appearance. Cyst formation caused by necrosis may occur, and calcification also may be present.

Microscopically, the tumor shows typical appearances of a leiomyoma, as observed in the uterus, the tumor being composed of smooth muscle cells that are uniformly spindle shaped or elongated and contain elongated blunt-ended or cigar-shaped nuclei. Palisading of the nuclei may be present and may be prominent. Mitotic activity is absent or very low, and cellular and nuclear pleomorphism is not a feature. The tumor cells form bundles intersected by fibrous septa that may be wide and show marked hyalinization. Other degenerative changes seen in uterine leiomyomas also may be present. Occasionally a leiomyoma may show an epithelioid pattern, which may cause some diagnostic problems. Connective tissue stains and immunocytochemical stains for vimentin, smooth muscle actin and desmin confirm the leiomyomatous nature of the tumor. In four tumors that I have studied, this was further confirmed ultrastructurally.

A well-documented case of a large ovarian lipoleiomyoma occurring in a 63-year-old woman has been reported.[48] The tumor replaced nearly the entire ovary. The adipose tissue was found replacing and dissecting the smooth muscle within the tumor. There was no associated uterine leiomyomatosis.[48]

Primary ovarian leiomyoma must be differentiated from pedunculated subserosal (parasitic) uterine leiomyoma, which has lost its attachment and instead has become attached to the ovary, from which it draws its blood supply. Leiomyoma also must be differentiated from ovarian fibroma as the latter is much more common. There is a tendency to diagnose leiomyoma as a fibroma, but a careful examination of the tumor supported by histochemical and immunocytochemical stains would prevent this. The treatment is excision of the affected adnexa.

Leiomyosarcoma

Primary leiomyosarcoma of the ovary is very rare; fewer than 20 cases have been reported. These tumors usually are found in postmenopausal women, but may be seen in younger women.[1,58] The tumors usually are large and solid, and patients have symptoms and signs related to the presence of an abdominal or pelvic mass. The tumors are gray-yellow, soft, fleshy, and frequently associated with hemorrhage and necrosis.

Microscopically, they differ from a leiomyoma by the presence of mitotic activity and cellular and nuclear pleomorphism (Figs. 21.1 and 21.2). In well-differentiated tumors, the mitotic activity may be the only distinguishing feature from a cellular leiomyoma and is considered to be far more important in this respect than cellular and nuclear pleomorphism.

Occasional ovarian leiomyosarcomas may be of the myxoid or epithelioid type. It is important to recognize these unusual variants, which are similar to their counterparts in the uterus. Primary leiomyosarcoma of the ovary metastasizes via the bloodstream; the prognosis is generally unfavorable, although the use of combination chemotherapy may improve it. Primary leiomyosarcoma of the ovary must be distinguished from MMMT's containing a prominent leiomyosarcomatous component. Primary leiomyosarcoma also should be distinguished from immature teratoma with a prominent leiomymatous tissue component. It also must be distinguished from metastatic leiomyosarcoma of uterine or other origin, as well as from poorly differentiated sarcomas and carcinosarcomas, both primary and metastatic to the ovary.

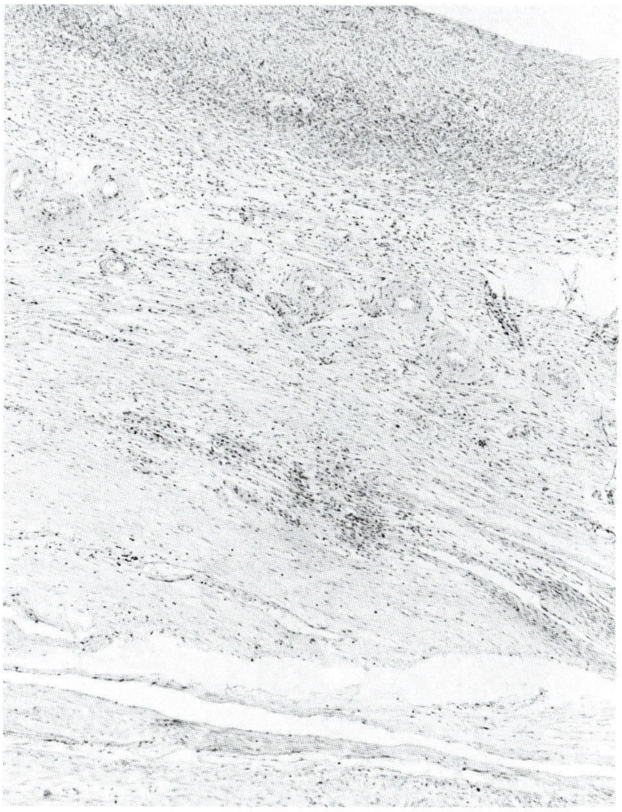

Fig. 21.1. Primary ovarian leiomyosarcoma. The tumor is seen beneath normal ovarian cortex (*top*).

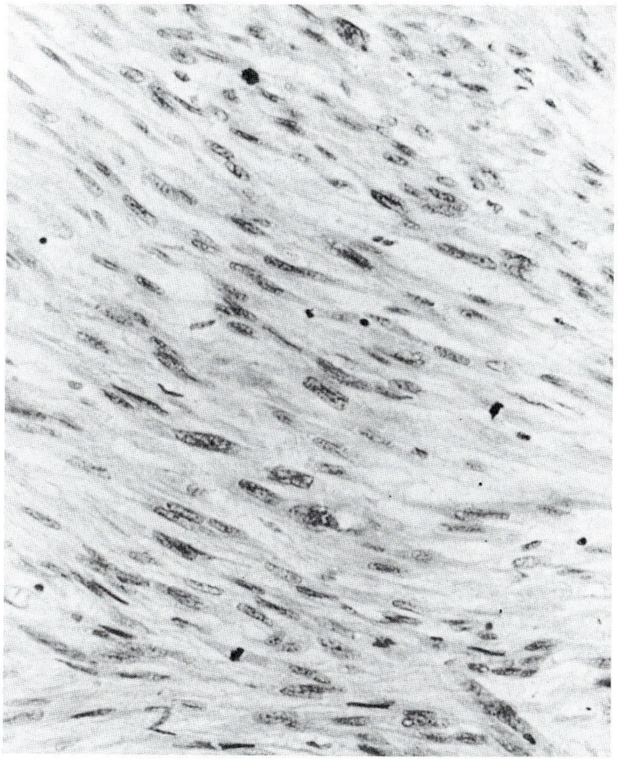

Fig. 21.2. Primary ovarian leiomyosarcoma. Higher magnification of tumor shown in Fig. 21.1. Note brisk mitotic activity and cellular and nuclear pleomorphism.

Rhabdomyoma

No well-documented case of *ovarian rhabdomyoma* has been recorded.

Rhabdomyosarcoma

Primary rhabdomyosarcoma of the ovary is uncommon. Nearly 30 well-documented cases have been reported in the literature, and 9 unreported cases are known to the author. A careful review of the literature shows that some cases, such as the frequently quoted case reported by Sandison,[64] were not pure rhabdomyosarcomas but rather examples of MMMT or teratomas with a marked rhabdomyoblastic component. Therefore, before a diagnosis of primary ovarian rhabdomyosarcoma can be made, the tumor must be sampled carefully and extensively to exclude the presence of other neoplastic elements, the presence of which would preclude a diagnosis of a pure rhabdomyosarcoma of the ovary.

The histogenesis of primary rhabdomyosarcoma of the ovary is uncertain. These tumors may originate from the connective tissue of the ovary, as a one-sided development of a teratoma, as a result of malignant transformation of a mature cystic teratoma with the malignant element overgrowing the tumor, or as a one-sided development of a MMMT.

The age of patients with ovarian rhabdomyosarcoma ranges from 2.5 to 84 years. The small number of cases makes it impossible to state whether there is a predilection for any particular age group, but, as with rhabdomyosarcomas occurring in other locations, the pleomorphic type occurs in older patients, whereas the embryonal and alveolar types occur in young women.[11] Patients with ovarian rhabdomyosarcoma usually have symptoms associated with the presence of a large, usually rapidly growing, abdominal mass, often associated with hemorrhagic ascites. Metastases frequently are seen at presentation.

Macroscopically, the tumors are unilateral, but metastatic involvement of the contralateral ovary may be present and should be differentiated from bilateral involvement. The tumors usually are large, exceeding 10 cm in diameter. They are solid, soft, fleshy, and gray-pink to yellow-tan, with areas of hemorrhage and necrosis that may be prominent.

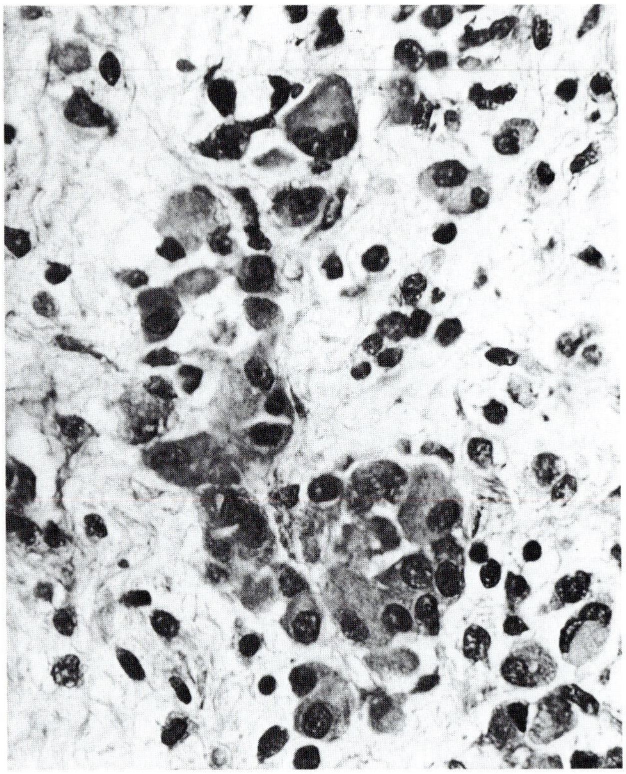

Fig. 21.4. Primary rhabdomyosarcoma of ovary of embryonal type. The tumor is composed of primitive rhabdomyoblasts with ample amount of bright eosinophilic cytoplasm and eccentric nuclei.

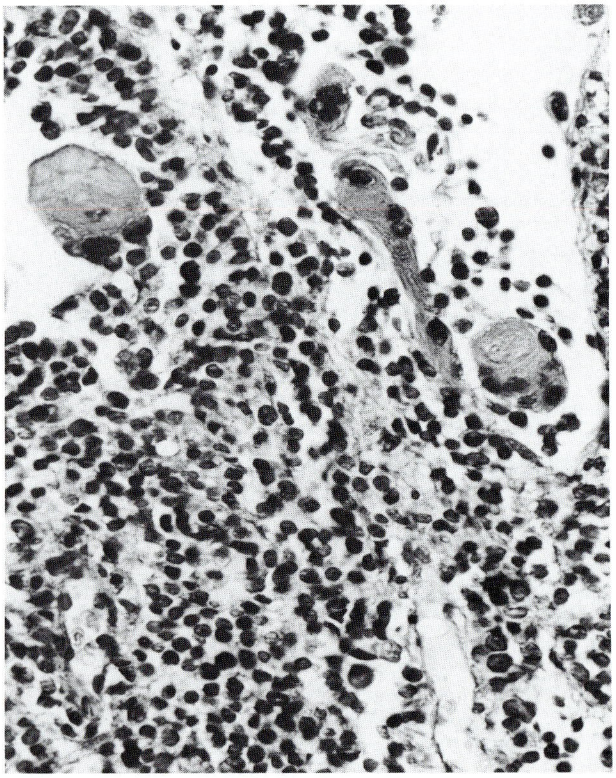

Fig. 21.3. Primary rhabdomyosarcoma of ovary in embryonal type. Most tumor cells are of small round type, but occasional large rhabdomyoblasts, some exhibiting cross-striations, are seen.

Microscopically, the tumors are composed entirely of rhabdomyoblasts, either of the embryonal type (Figs. 21.3 and 21.4) admixed with the alveolar (Fig. 21.5) or botryoid types, or of the pleomorphic type. Tumors composed of the former types occur in children and young adults, whereas those of the pleomorphic type are observed in older women. Although the diagnosis of pleomorphic rhabdomyosarcoma should not present undue difficulty, because of the presence of at least some typical rhabdomyoblasts showing cross-striation, the diagnosis of embryonal rhabdomyosarcoma is much more difficult because the tumor cells are poorly differentiated, making rhabdomyoblastic differentiation discernible only with difficulty. Furthermore, it is necessary to recognize the distinctive alveolar (Fig. 21.5) or botryoid patterns, which may not be easy.

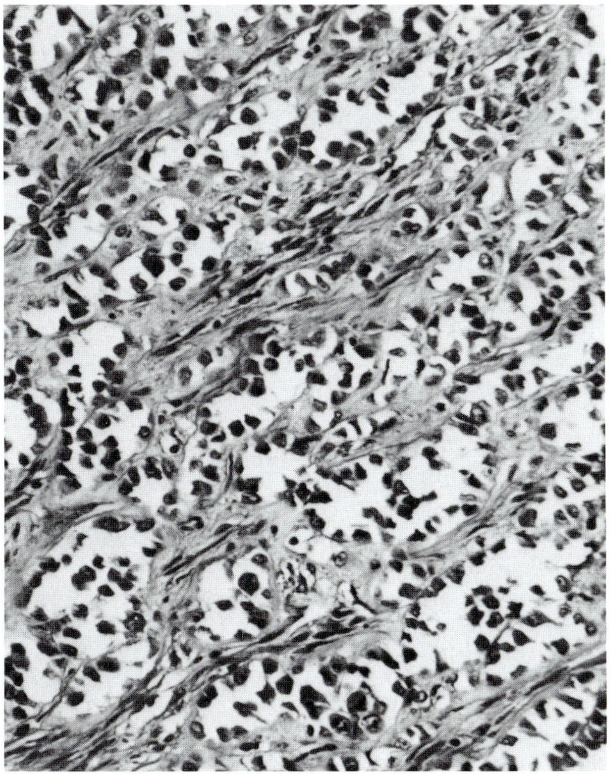

Fig. 21.5. Primary rhabdomyosarcoma of the ovary. The tumor has a pronounced alveolar pattern.

The embryonal rhabdomyosarcoma is composed of rhabdomyoblasts in various stages of differentiation (Figs. 21.3 and 21.4) and is composed at least partly of collections of small round cells having a narrow rim of cytoplasm (Fig. 21.3) that are poorly differentiated. Therefore, the lesion is difficult to distinguish from poorly differentiated small cell carcinoma, malignant lymphoma, or even neuroblastoma or leukemia.[53,55,67] Among the small round cells are scattered occasional better-differentiated cells with bright eosinophilic cytoplasm and eccentric nuclei (see Fig. 21.4).

Occasionally, large, more typical rhabdomyoblasts are seen. The presence of cross-striations is not necessary for diagnosis, but the cells comprising the tumor may be well enough differentiated to exhibit cross-striations (see Fig. 21.3). Demonstration of Z bands or their precursors by electron microscopy is helpful in making the diagnosis. Immunocytochemical demonstration of myoglobin, desmin, and especially sarcomere-specific actin are helpful in this respect. The tumor is frequently affected by edema, hemorrhage, and necrosis, making the diagnosis even more difficult. Therefore, thorough examination and sampling of the tumor are essential to make the correct diagnosis. The tumor may be more common than has been hitherto believed, but because of its poor differentiation, it may have been either assigned to the group of undifferentiated ovarian tumors or misdiagnosed. In some cases, the tumor infiltrated the bone marrow and was originally diagnosed as leukemia. It is therefore emphasized that embryonal rhabdomyosarcoma must be considered in the differential diagnosis of undifferentiated small round cell tumor of the ovary in a young patient. The presence of other neoplastic elements always must be excluded when making this diagnosis.

The importance of making the correct diagnosis is not only academic but practical, in view of the advances that have been made in the therapy of embryonal rhabdomyosarcoma during the past two decades. In the past, the prognosis was poor, and in most reported cases, the patients died of extensive metastatic disease within 1 year of diagnosis. Recently, patients with embryonal rhabdomyosarcoma, some of whom had metastases, are well and disease free after surgery, chemotherapy, and radiotherapy. The combination chemotherapy advocated in such patients consists of dactinomycin, vincristine, and cyclophosphamide. The addition of methotrexate with folinic acid rescue and doxorubicin to this combination also may be of value.

Myofibroblastoma

A well-documented case of an *ovarian myofibroblastoma* has been reported recently.[61] A 22-year-old woman who was involved in an automobile accident was found to have an enlarged right ovary but refused laparotomy. Over the next 3 years the mass gradually increased in size, and laparotomy was performed. A $9 \times 8.5 \times 6$ cm, right-sided ovarian tumor weighing 215 g and adherent to the right fallopian tube and omentum was found and excised. The tumor was solid, white-tan, and on sectioning revealed whorled areas and focal calcification. Microscopically, it was composed of uniform bland-looking spindle cells arranged haphazardly in fascicles separated by bands of hyalinazed collagen. In some areas there was increased vascularity. There was no atypia or mitotic activity. The tumor cells showed vimentin, smooth muscle actin, and muscle-specific actin positivity. There was no immunoreactivity with desmin and cytokeratin. The patient was well and disease free 21 months after treatment.[61] Myofibroblastoma is a benign lesion, and complete excision results in cure.

Tumors of Vascular and Lymphatic Origin

Hemangioma

Hemangioma is found only occasionally in the ovary; the number of well-documented cases does not exceed 50. Although some cases may not have been recognized or recorded, all investigators consider ovarian hemangioma uncommon.[38,73] This is somewhat surprising, as the ovary has a very rich and complex vasculature.

The origin of ovarian hemangioma in common with hemangioma in general is a matter of controversy; it is considered either a hamartomatous malformation or a true neoplasm. It is likely that both modes of origin are responsible for their formation. The reported age of patients with ovarian hemangioma ranges from 4 months to 63 years[38,73] and does not show a predominance in any decade. In most patients, ovarian hemangioma has been noted as an incidental finding at operation or autopsy.[73] In a few cases, the lesion was large and the patient had abdominal enlargement because of the presence of an ovarian mass[24,42,43] or had acute abdominal pain associated with torsion of the tumor.[42,69] In some cases, there was ascites.[24,43,66] The lesions usually are unilateral, although in four patients they were bilateral.[73] Ovarian hemangiomas have been noted in patients with generalized hemangiomatosis[38] and in patients with hemangiomas in other parts of the genital tract.[38,73] One patient with bilateral ovarian hemangiomas and diffuse abdominopelvic hemangiomatosis had thrombocytopenia. The platelet count returned to normal after excision of the affected ovaries.[38]

Macroscopically, the lesions are small, red or purple, round or oval nodules, measuring from a few millimeters to 1.5 cm in diameter. Larger lesions also have been encountered measuring up to 11.5 cm in the longest diameter.[24,42] On cut section, they usually are spongy and show a honeycomb appearance. Although they have been found in different parts of the ovary, the medulla and the hilar region appear to be the most common sites.[73]

Microscopically, ovarian hemangioma is of the cavernous or mixed capillary-cavernous type. It consists of collections of vascular spaces, which may vary in size but usually are small, lined by a single layer of endothelial cells, and usually contain red blood cells in their lumen (Fig. 21.6). Occasionally, thrombosis may be seen. A small amount of connective tissue may be present within the lesion. In a few reported cases, the hemangioma was associated with the presence of lutein cells in the stroma of the lesion. In one such case, there was evidence of hormonal function.[66] In a recent case, a patient with capillary hemangioma presenting as an adnexal mass had elevated serum CA-125 and massive ascites.[24] Excision of the affected adnexa resulted in a complete cure.

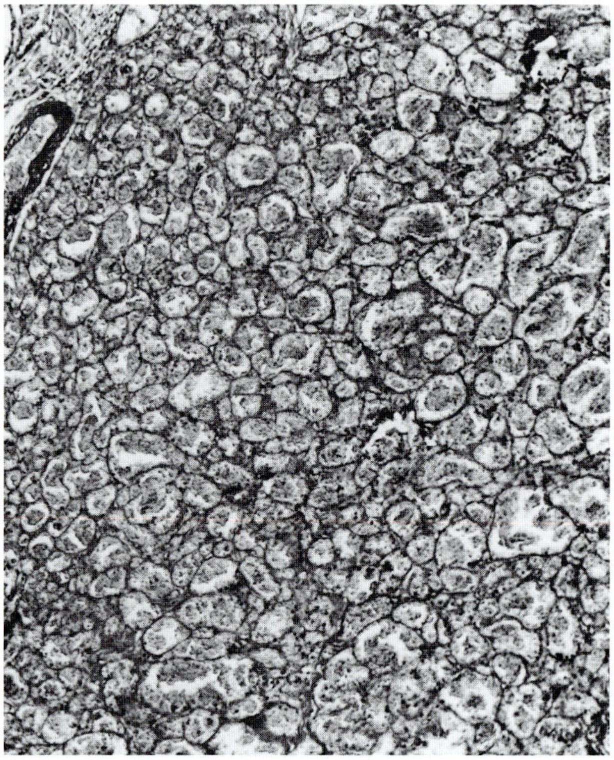

Fig. 21.6. Hemangioma of the ovary. The tumor is composed of numerous small vascular spaces lined by a single layer of endothelial cells. Elastic van Gieson.

Hemangioma must be differentiated from proliferations of dilated blood vessels, frequently seen in the hilar region of the ovary. Although a very small hemangioma may not be easily distinguished from such vascular proliferations, the hemangioma usually forms a nodule or a small mass. The presence of a circumscribed nodule composed of vascular spaces tends to distinguish hemangioma from vascular proliferations, which usually are smaller and more diffuse. The presence of numerous blood cells within the vascular spaces and the absence of pale eosinophilic homogeneous material usually distinguish hemangioma from the less common lymphangioma. Hemangioma also must be distinguished from teratoma with a prominent vascular component. In such cases, careful sampling will detect other teratomatous elements, the presence of which distinguishes the lesion from a hemangioma.

The treatment of choice is oophorectomy or adnexectomy, which results in a complete cure.

Hemangioendothelial Sarcoma (Hemangioendothelioma, Hemangiosarcoma, Angiosarcoma)

Hemangioendothelial sarcoma is a very rare ovarian neoplasm; fewer than 25 cases have been recorded.[52,67] Five unreported cases have been seen by me. In some reported cases the hemangioendothelial sarcoma had arisen within a mature cystic teratoma, or may have been associated with an immature teratoma. Such cases are considered as germ cell tumors and are excluded from consideration here. The age of the patients with hemangioendothelial sarcoma varies from 19 to 77 years. The tumor usually is unilateral, but bilateral tumors have been recorded. Bilaterality must be differentiated from metastatic spread to the contralateral ovary, which was seen in one personally observed case. The histogenesis of the tumor is uncertain. It may originate from the vascular tissue present in the ovary, as a one-sided development of a teratoma, or from a teratoma in which the vascular component has overgrown the other parts of the tumor. Patients usually have symptoms related to the presence of a lower abdominal mass, which may be associated with torsion and rupture of the tumor and hemorrhage.

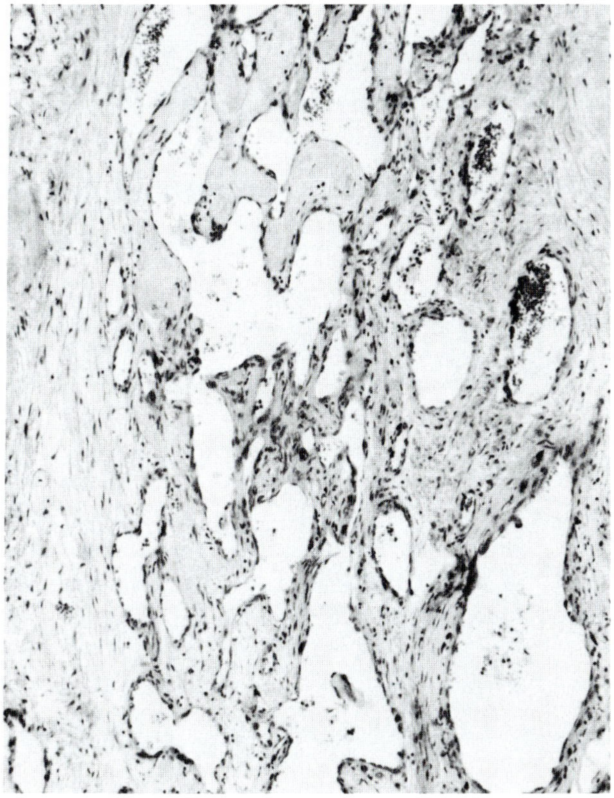

Fig. 21.7. Primary hemangioendothelial sarcoma of ovary. The tumor is composed of vascular spaces surrounded by connective tissue.

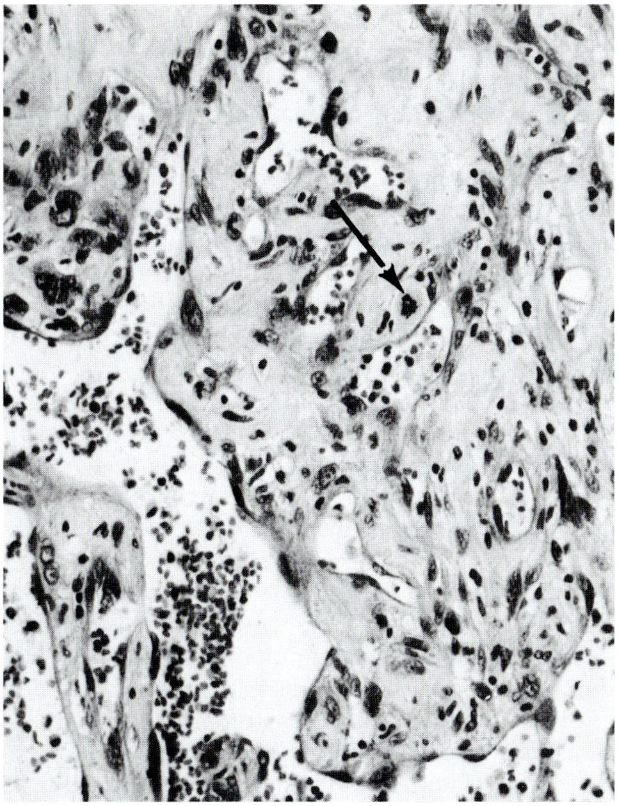

Fig. 21.8. Primary hemangioendothelial sarcoma of ovary. Note the large endothelial cells lining vascular spaces. Large abnormal mitosis is seen to right of center (*arrow*).

Macroscopically, the tumors usually are large, blue-brown, hemorrhagic, soft, and friable. They may be confined to the ovary but often are associated with invasion of the surrounding structures.

Microscopically, they are composed of vascular spaces of varying size and appearance, lined by endothelial cells that usually are large, showing atypical appearance, bizarre nuclei, and mitotic activity (Figs. 21.7 and 21.8). In some areas, the tumor may contain a considerable amount of connective tissue interspersed between the vascular spaces (Fig. 21.7). Some tumors are composed of small closely packed spaces lined by atypical cells with a suggestion of a solid pattern.

Hemangioendothelial sarcoma of the ovary must be distinguished from immature teratomatous neoplasms with a prominent vascular component. The presence of other neoplastic germ cell elements distinguishes teratoma from primary hemangioendothelial sarcoma. It also must be distinguished from the occasional lymphangiosarcoma, which is composed of lymphatics and not of blood vessels, as well as from malignant hemangiopericytoma, which is composed of a proliferation of pericytes and shows a different histologic pattern. Hemangioendothelial sarcoma can be distinguished from hemangiopericytoma with the help of reticulum stains. Immunocytochemical stains for CD 31 and CD 34 are useful in confirming the diagnosis of hemangioendothelial sarcoma when the tumor is poorly differentiated, especially when showing a solid pattern.

The tumor invades locally and metastasizes via the bloodstream. Prognosis is poor, especially in patients who have metastases at the time of presentation. When the tumor is confined to the ovary, the prognosis is better and a few survivors have been reported. The tumor has not responded to combination chemotherapy regimens.

Lymphangioma

Lymphangioma of the ovary is very rare, with fewer than 15 documented cases reported. I have seen 2 cases. In both cases, the tumor was small and was found incidentally. The tumor is usually unilateral but bilateral lesions have been reported. In the latter cases, it is possible that the lesions were malformations and not tumors. Macroscopically, the tumor is small with a smooth, gray surface. On cut section, it is yellow, honeycombed, and composed of numerous small cystic spaces exuding clear yellow fluid.

Microscopically, lymphangioma of the ovary is composed of closely packed, thin-walled vascular spaces lined by flattened endothelial cells and containing pale homogeneous eosinophilic fluid. Lymphocytes may be seen within the vascular spaces. The histogenesis is a matter of controversy. Some investigators consider these lesions as malformations and some as neoplasms. Both modes of histogenesis are likely.

Lymphangioma is differentiated from a teratoma with a prominent vascular component by the absence of other germ cell elements. Lymphangioma also must be distinguished from hemangioma and an adenomatoid tumor that contains thin-walled, vessel-like spaces. In contrast to hemangioma, lymphangioma does not contain blood cells in the vascular spaces. The adenomatoid tumor has solid areas, and the cells lining the vessel-like spaces stain positively with periodic acid–Schiff (PAS) and alcian blue stains as well as show positive staining for low molecular weight cytokeratin.

Lymphangiosarcoma

Only one case of *lymphangiosarcoma of the ovary* has been reported.[62] The tumor, which measured 15 cm in diameter, was found in a 31-year-old woman who had symptoms of a rapidly enlarging abdominal mass. The tumor was composed of proliferating, closely packed lymphatic vessels that, in one area, showed cytologic atypia. There was extensive necrosis and hemorrhage. The patient died 1 year after diagnosis of extensive metastatic disease. Recently it has been suggested that this tumor may have been an example of hemangioendothelial sarcoma.[52]

Hemangiopericytoma

A single case of *hemangiopericytoma of the ovary* has been reported.[36] Histologically, the tumor resembled hemangiopericytoma in other locations. The excision of the affected adnexa resulted in a complete cure.

Tumors of Cartilage Origin

Chondroma

Only a few reports of *ovarian chondroma* are available, and documentation in most cases is unsatisfac-

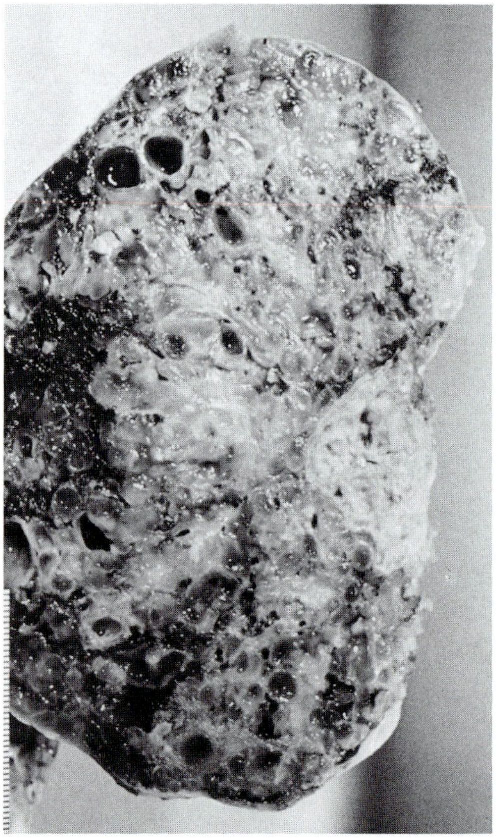

Fig. 21.9. Primary ovarian chondrosarcoma. The tumor is large, solid, hard, and gray-white.

tory. One well-documented case considered to originate from the ovarian stroma has been reported.[54] The tumor, which measured 4 × 3 × 3 cm and was composed entirely of mature cartilage, was found incidentally. Although chondroma may originate from the connective tissue of the ovary by a process of metaplasia, it is more likely that most ovarian tumors described as chondroma were either fibromas showing cartilaginous metaplasia or teratomas having a prominent cartilaginous component.

Chondrosarcoma

A single example of pure *chondrosarcoma of the ovary* has been reported[74] (Fig. 21.9). A 61-year-old woman had an abdominal mass that, on extensive microscopic examination, proved to be a pure, well-differentiated chondrosarcoma (Figs. 21.10 and 21.11). The patient was well and disease free 6 years after one-sided adnexectomy. The histogenesis of this tumor is uncertain, but the age of the patient and the histologic appearances of the tumor point to an origin in a dermoid cyst with malignant transformation and overgrowth by the malignant cartilaginous component.[74] A well-documented case of mature cystic teratoma (dermoid cyst) with malignant transformation of the cartilaginous element has been reported; the patient died of extensive metastatic disease.[13]

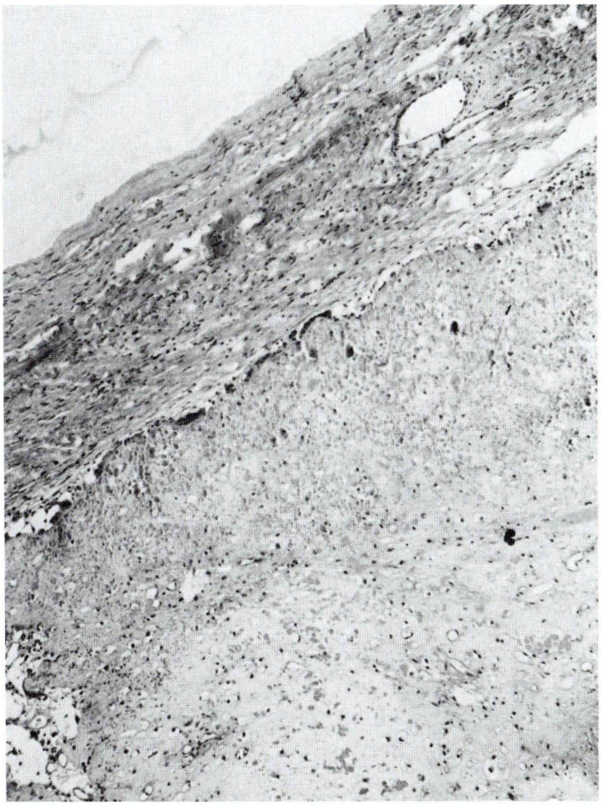

Fig. 21.10. Primary ovarian chondrosarcoma. Tumor is seen beneath normal ovarian cortex.

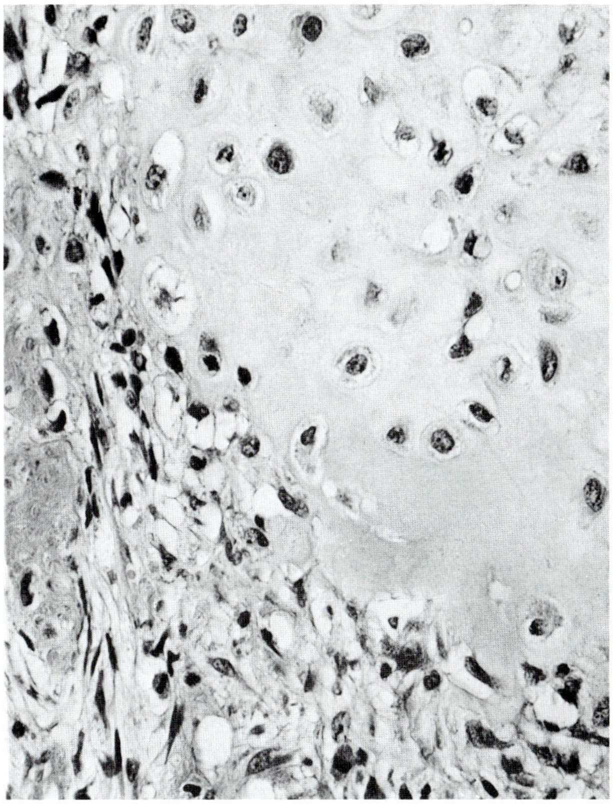

Fig. 21.11. Primary ovarian chondrosarcoma. Higher magnification shows well-differentiated tumor.

Tumors of Bone Origin

Osteoma

Few documented examples of *osteoma* occurring in the ovary exist. Although an origin from ovarian stroma is possible, most such lesions probably were examples of osseous metaplasia occurring in fibromas or leiomyomas, or possibly examples of metaplasia or heterotopia and not neoplasia occurring in the connective tissue of the ovary. The lesions usually are small, but may be large and are histologically composed of dense cortical bone.

Osteosarcoma

Four cases of pure *osteosarcoma of the ovary* have been reported.[27,28,67] The age of patients ranged from 24 to 47 years. In all cases the tumor was associated with extensive metastastic disease. None of the patients survived more than 8 months. In one case metastatic tumor deposits affecting the abdominal cavity were excised at operation, and the patient was treated with triple chemotherapy consisting of cyclophosphamide, mitomycin C, and bleomycin.[28] The tumor recurred, and cisplatin and doxorubicin were added to the chemotherapeutic regimen. Inspite of this, the tumor progressed and the patient died 8 months after diagnosis.

Histologically, the tumors showed typical appearances of osteosarcoma occurring in the skeleton. Although it was believed that the tumors originated directly from ovarian stroma, their histogenesis is uncertain. Occasional cases of osteosarcoma originating in ovarian teratoma have been recorded,[72] but such cases should not be confused with pure ovarian osteosarcoma or with cases of MMMT with a prominent osteosarcomatous component.

Giant Cell Tumor of the Ovary

A single case of *giant cell tumor of the ovary* histologically indistinguishable from a giant cell tumor of bone has been reported.[40] The tumor was found incidentally in an ovary of a 31-year-old woman. It was composed of small ovoid or spindle-shaped stromal cells admixed with multinucleated giant cells, many of which contained between 50 and 100 small hyperchromatic nuclei. In places, there was brisk mitotic activity. The patient was well and disease free 4.5 years after excision of the affected adnexa.

Tumors of Neural Tissue Origin

Ovarian tumors originating from neural tissue are rare. The presenting symptoms usually are related to the presence of an intraabdominal mass. The tumors are solid and usually are small. The histogenesis is uncertain and probably is similar to that of other mesenchymal tumors of the ovary.

Neurofibroma

Two cases of *neurofibroma of the ovary* have been reported in patients with generalized neurofibromatosis (von Recklinghausen's disease),[26,70] one as an incidental finding.[70] Histologically, the tumors resembled neurofibroma occurring elsewhere.

Neurofibrosarcoma

One case of *neurofibrosarcoma* occurring in a 38-year-old woman with generalized neurofibromatosis (von Recklinghausen's disease) has been described.[16] The tumor was an incidental finding and had replaced the ovary. It was solid, and histologically showed the typical appearance of a neurofibrosarcoma with a moderate degree of nuclear pleomorphism and mitotic activity. There was no evidence of metastases, and the patient was well and disease free 1 year after diagnosis.[16]

Neurilemmoma

Three cases of *ovarian neurilemmoma (schwannoma)* have been reported.[45,49] In one case, the tumor was large.[49] The tumors were solid, and the patients were well and disease free after the excision of the tumor. Histologically, the tumors resembled neurilemmoma occurring in other locations.

Malignant Neurilemmoma

One case of *malignant neurilemmoma (schwannoma) of the ovary* has been reported.[71] The affected patient, a 71-year-old, nulliparous woman, was admitted for evaluation of lower abdominal enlargement and pain. There were no stigmata of generalized neurofibromatosis. At laparotomy, a 15-cm, firm, somewhat hemorrhagic tumor was found arising from the left ovary. There were numerous tumor deposits involving the peritoneal cavity. A debulking procedure was performed, and the ovarian tumor was excised together with the omentum. Histologic and ultrastructural examinations revealed that the tumor was a malignant neurilemmoma. After surgery the patient was treated with combination chemotherapy consisting of doxorubicin and cyclophosphamide, but the disease progressed and she died 5 months after surgery of extensive intraabdominal metastatic disease.[71]

Ganglioneuroma

A single case of *ovarian ganglioneuroma* occurring in a 4-year-old girl has been reported.[67] The child had abdominal enlargement. The tumor was solid, weighing 200 g, and replaced nearly the whole ovary. Histologically, the tumor was composed of well-differentiated ganglion cells. There was a recurrence after the excision of the tumor. True ganglioneuroma must be differentiated from teratomas showing prominence of ganglion cells and from proliferations of ganglion cells occasionally seen in the hilar region of the ovary; the latter are nonneoplastic and probably hamartomatous in nature.

Pheochromocytoma

A single case of *ovarian pheochromocytoma* has been reported in a 15-year-old girl.[21] The patient had hypertension, convulsions, and a large, left-sided abdominal tumor mass. The tumor had undergone torsion and weighed 970 g. It was solid, and microscopic examination showed typical appearances of pheochromocytoma. Epinephrine and norepinephrine were extracted from tumor tissue. The symptoms disappeared after excision of the tumor, and the patient was well and disease free 15 months after the operation.[21] Two additional cases were mentioned by Scully et al.,[67] but no further details were provided.

Primitive Neuroectodermal Tumors

These tumors are described in Chapter 20, Germ Cell Tumors of the Ovary.

Tumors of Adipose Tissue Origin

There are no well-documented cases of *tumors of adipose tissue origin in the ovary*. Some reports relating to the presence of both benign and malignant neoplasms composed of adipose tissue in the ovary exist, but they are not well substantiated. Collections of adipose cells forming islands of fatty tissue that are not encapsulated are seen occasionally within ovarian tissue and are attributed to metaplasia of connective tissue of the ovary. These collections have been described as *adipose prosoplasia*. Benign adipose tissue seen in the ovary may be part of a teratoma with a prominent adipose tissue component. Malignant adipose tissue may be part of a MMMT with a prominent liposarcomatous component, or it may represent metastases from a liposarcoma occurring at another location.

Tumors of Mesothelial Origin

Adenomatoid Tumor

The *adenomatoid tumor*, which in the female is found most frequently in the fallopian tubes and broad ligament and occasionally in the uterus near the serosal surface, is found only rarely in the ovary (see Chapter 13, Mesenchymal Tumors of the Uterus, and Chapter 14, Diseases of the Fallopian Tube). Although its histogenesis was long disputed, it is now considered to be of mesothelial origin, as is supported by morphologic, histochemical, and ultrastructural observations. Adenomatoid tumor is benign and, therefore, is considered a benign mesothelioma.

Ten cases of ovarian adenomatoid tumor have been recorded, most of which occurred in patients in the third and fourth decades.[67,79] The lesions, which are small, round or oval, and 0.5–3 cm in diameter, usually are found in the hilus of the ovary as incidental findings. In two cases the tumors were larger, measuring 6 and 8 cm in the longest diameter, respectively, and were symptomatic.

Histologically, the tumors show similar appearances to adenomatoid tumors occurring in other locations and are composed of clefts and spaces lined by cuboidal, low columnar, or flattened epithelial-like cells (Fig. 21.12) and of solid aggregates of similar cells surrounded by connective tissue that varies from loose and edematous to dense and hyalinized. The epithelial-like cells may exhibit marked vacuolation. They exhibit positive staining with alcian blue, which is digestible with hyaluronidase, and similarly staining material is present in the clefts and spaces. Occasionally, the cells may show weak PAS staining. The tumor cells show strong positive staining with low molecular weight cytokeratin. Ultrastructural observations support the mesothelial origin of this lesion and show an abundance of microvilli, bundles of cytoplasmic filaments, tight junctional complexes, and intercellular spaces. The lesion is benign, and its excision results in a complete cure.

Adenomatoid tumor may be confused with yolk sac tumor (YST) because the clefts and spaces may resemble the microcystic pattern of YST, but the

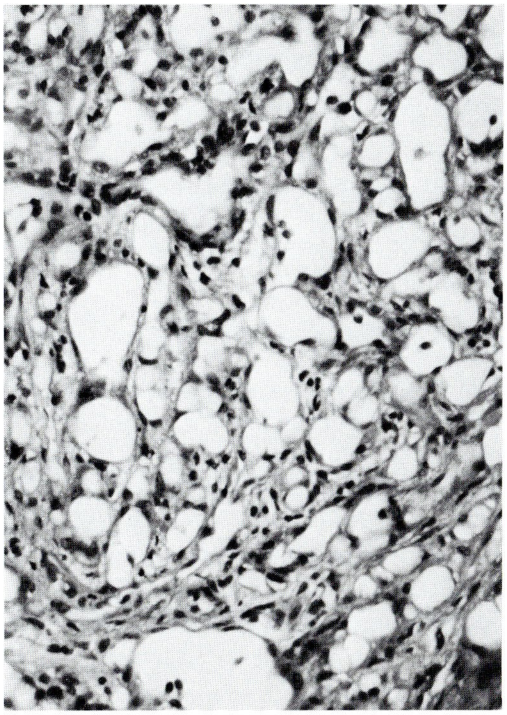

Fig. 21.12. Adenomatoid tumor. The tumor has numerous clefts and spaces lined by a single layer of flattened epithelial-like or low cuboid cells.

nuclear appearances are totally different. The nuclei of adenomatoid tumor are bland and generally small and flattened, differing from the larger round and ovoid vesicular nuclei of YST, which exhibit brisk mitotic activity. The absence of other patterns associated with YST helps to distinguish adenomatoid tumor from YST. Confusion with lymphangioma may arise, and I have seen an adenomatoid tumor diagnosed as lymphangioma and vice versa. Immunocytochemical studies can be helpful in differentiating between these two entities. Lymphangioma is low molecular weight cytokeratin negative, whereas adenomatoid tumor is strongly positive. Vascular markers such as factor VIII, CD 34, and CD 31 show negative reactions with adenomatoid tumor and positive staining with lymphangioma.

Peritoneal Mesothelioma

Occasionally, *peritoneal mesothelioma* may involve the surface of the ovary (see Chapter 17, Diseases of the Peritoneum). When the tumor affects the ovary, confusion with primary ovarian neoplasms or benign conditions may occur.[75] The involvement of the ovary may be very extensive, and the presentation is that of a primary ovarian neoplasm. In one series of nine malignant peritoneal mesotheliomas presenting as ovarian masses, two tumors were considered as primary ovarian malignant mesotheliomas because the tumors were confined to the ovary.[12,67] The histologic pattern, ultrastructural and immunohistochemical observations, and behavior and distribution of the lesion are helpful in making the correct diagnosis.[6,12,67,75] Most patients with malignant peritoneal mesothelioma are middle-aged or elderly adults, and the tumor shows a considerable male predominance. Very rarely, it may occur in children.[75]

Other Mesenchymal Tumors

Other *mesenchymal tumors* occurring in the ovary include the *sclerosing stromal tumor of the ovary* described in detail in Chapter 19 (Sex Cord–Stromal, Steroid Cell, and Other Ovarian Tumors with Endocrine, Paraendocrine, and Paraneoplastic Manifestations). Tumors of teratomatous origin containing mesenchymal tissue are described in Chapter 20, Germ Cell Tumors of the Ovary, and MMMTs, carcinosarcomas, endometrial stromal sarcomas, and adenosarcoma are discussed in Chapter 18, Surface Epithelial Tumors of the Ovary.

Undifferentiated Sarcomas

Some ovarian tumors are poorly differentiated, and although a diagnosis of sarcoma can be made, the tumor does not exhibit further differentiation beyond showing its mesenchymal origin. Careful and extensive histologic examination in such cases is helpful and may result in finding better-differentiated areas, which will yield a more accurate diagnosis. Immunocytochemical investigations may be very helpful in detecting accurately the tissue of origin and should be undertaken in all such cases. In some cases, a more precise diagnosis cannot be made despite very extensive investigations.

Tumors of Hematopoietic Origin

Malignant Lymphoma

Malignant lymphoma affecting the ovary can be divided into two types: primary malignant lymphoma of the ovary, and disseminated malignant lymphoma affecting the ovary.

Primary malignant lymphoma of the ovary is rare and, in turn, can be divided further into two categories: (1) first manifestation of generalized malignant lymphoma and (2) localized extranodal malignant lymphoma. *Disseminated malignant lymphoma* is far more common than the primary type. It too can be divided into two categories: (1) the ovarian tumor being either the initial or predominant presenting manifestation of the disease and (2) ovarian involvement occurring during the course of the disseminated disease, only discovered histologically after surgery or autopsy.

One specific type of malignant lymphoma, Burkitt's lymphoma, frequently affects the ovary, the second most common site after the jaws. The ovary may be the site of primary disease as well as of disseminated disease, and the manifestations of Burkitt's lymphoma may accord with any of the specific types described for both primary and disseminated disease. Patients with primary disease localized to the ovary and with disseminated disease discovered only by histologic examination at surgery or autopsy are uncommon. Consequently, Burkitt's lymphoma is the most common malignant lymphoma in which involvement of the ovary manifests itself clinically and is an important feature of the disease.

Other hematopoietic neoplasms affecting the ovary, such as leukemia, myelomatosis, or plasmacytoma, also can be classified in a manner similar to malignant lymphoma. It should be noted, however, that their primary manifestation in the ovary is rare, even when compared with primary malignant lymphoma, which is itself very uncommon.

Primary Extranodal Malignant Lymphoma of the Ovary

Before the diagnosis of *primary extranodal malignant lymphoma* can be made, the presence of lymph node as well as blood and bone marrow involvement by the disease must be carefully excluded, and the involvement of the affected organ must be the first manifestation of the disease. This distinction is of considerable importance, because there is now good evidence that primary extranodal malignant lymphoma tends to run a less aggressive course than does malignant lymphoma affecting the lymph nodes. Although primary extranodal malignant lymphoma is not uncommon, the ovary is an infrequent site, and fewer than 70 well-documented cases have been reported.[22,23,50,56]

The diagnosis of primary malignant lymphoma of the ovary can be made only if, in addition to the general criteria for the diagnosis of extranodal malignant lymphoma mentioned earlier, the tumor is confined to the ovary at the time of diagnosis. If, in addition to the ovarian involvement, only the lymph nodes immediately draining the ovary are affected or if local spread from the ovary to the adjacent structures is present, this should not preclude the diagnosis. Primary malignant lymphoma of the ovary shows a wide age range but tends to occur more frequently before menopause. The most common symptoms are abdominal enlargement or abdominal pain. Primary malignant lymphoma of the ovary also has been noted as an incidental finding. On examination, ovarian enlargement is nearly always present and often is bilateral. The tumors range in size from 3.5 to 27 cm.[22,23,50,56] They usually are soft, white to gray-white, with a lobulated or nodular external surface, and solid and white to gray-pink on cut section, with evidence of hemorrhage and necrosis.

Microscopically, the ovarian tissue is replaced almost completely by a diffuse proliferation of malignant lymphoma cells forming a diffuse pattern, although occasionally a nodular (follicular) pattern, which may be pure or associated with the diffuse pattern, also is seen.[50,56] Normal ovarian structures, for example, corpora lutea and corpora albicantia, sometimes are present and are surrounded by the neoplastic cells, which may invade them.[22,23,50,56] Acute inflammatory cells, plasma cells, and normal lymphocytes may be admixed with the tumor cells, causing diagnostic difficulties. The malignant lymphoma usually is of a poorly differentiated type and may be difficult to classify (Fig. 21.13). It usually is of the lymphoblastic or histiocytic type or the large cleaved or noncleaved type. Using recent nomenclature, most tumors are classified as of the diffuse large cell type, or diffuse mixed large and small cell type, and the great majority are B-cell tumors.[22,50]

Malignant lymphoma of the ovary must be distinguished from other small round all tumors composed of diffuse or nodular proliferations of small uniform tumor cells. Malignant lymphoma, especially of the lymphoblastic or poorly differentiated lymphocytic (small cell and large cell cleaved) types, must be distinguished from poorly differentiated metastatic carcinoma, most frequently of mammary origin. The carcinoma cells tend to be less uniform, show usually less marked mitotic activity, may be associated with evidence of fibroblastic reaction, and in places may exhibit an attempt at acinar formation. Malignant lymphoma also must be distinguished from primary or metastatic small (oat) cell carcinoma (see following).

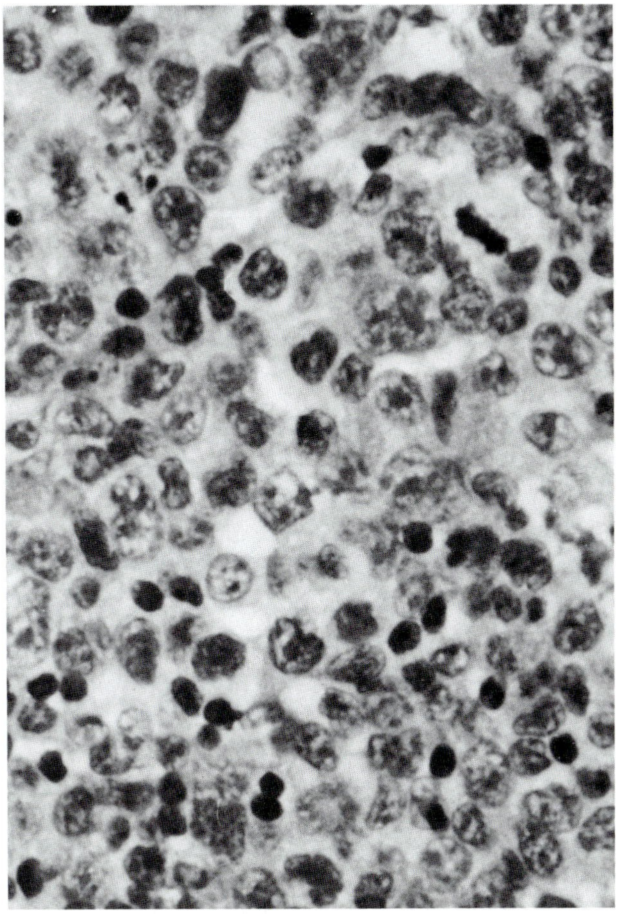

Fig. 21.13. Primary malignant lymphoma of ovary, poorly differentiated type. Note brisk mitotic activity and infiltration by inflammatory cells.

The presence of positive immunocytochemical staining for leukocyte common antigen (LCA) distinguishes malignant lymphoma from neoplasms that are not composed of lymphoreticular cells and is the most valuable diagnostic aid in this context. Further immunocytochemical typing with large panels of antibodies for light and heavy chains, and various B- and T-marker antibodies, are recommended in LCA-positive cases. Molecular studies, including gene rearrangement, also can be performed if fresh frozen tissue is available.

Histochemical demonstration of mucin and positive immunocytochemical staining for cytokeratin, which indicate carcinoma, also are helpful in distinguishing between these two entities. The presence of occasional, better-differentiated rhabdomyoblasts and of rosette formation helps to distinguish embryonal rhabdomyosarcoma and metastatic neuroblastoma, respectively, from malignant lymphoma. Further confirmation is provided by immunocytochemical studies demonstrating the presence of muscle and neural markers, respectively. Malignant lymphoma also must be distinguished from ovarian involvement by leukemia, and in such cases, blood and bone marrow studies obviously are helpful. The presence of red granular staining in the cytoplasm of the tumor cells when using naphthol-AS-D-chloroacetate esterase (Leder's stain) distinguishes malignant lymphoma cells, which do not stain by this method, from myeloid series cells, which stain positively. Immunocytochemical stains for myeloid series markers are also useful in this respect.

Malignant lymphoma also must be distinguished from granulosa cell tumors showing diffuse pattern, but other patterns seen in granulosa cell tumor may be evident, at least in some parts of the tumor. Mitotic activity is less brisk in granulosa cell tumor, and the cellular and nuclear appearances are different. Positive immunocytochemical staining for LCA and negative staining for inhibin further confirms the diagnosis of malignant lymphoma. Malignant lymphoma of the histiocytic (large cell noncleaved) type, which sometimes contains normal lymphocytes, must be distinguished from dysgerminoma. The dysgerminoma cells are more uniform in size and appearance and usually contain larger amounts of cytoplasm, which tends to be clear or pale and granular. The cytoplasm typically contains abundant glycogen, which stains positively with PAS stain and is removed by diastase digestion. The nuclei of dysgerminoma cells are more uniform and do not display the marked variation in shape and size seen in the nuclei of the malignant lymphoma cells. Negative membranous staining of the tumor cells for placenta-specific alkaline phosphatase (PLAP) and positive staining for LCA and other markers of malignant lymphoma confirms the diagnosis of malignant lymphoma in such cases.

The course of the disease of patients with primary malignant lymphoma of the ovary is variable. Although generalized disease develops in most patients within a few months of the excision of the ovarian neoplasm, in some patients generalized disease does not develop for years. An occasional patient does not show any further involvement, and in some patients the only further involvement is enlargement of paraaortic and parailiac lymph nodes, the lymph nodes that provide lymphatic drainage of the ovary. Although some patients in whom generalized disease develops might not have been examined carefully enough to detect the presence of further disease, on presentation there is little doubt that in some patients with malignant lymphoma confined to the ovary generalized disease will develop within a few months. Unfortunately, at present it is not possible to determine which patients will and which will not develop generalized disease. Therefore, all patients should be staged properly and given adequate therapy, which should include radiation to the regional lymph nodes and the most efficacious combination chemotherapy. Occasional cases have been reported[22,23,50,56] in which patients were well and disease free for periods of 2–5 years after initial treatment; some further unreported cases are known as well.

Hodgkin's Disease Localized to the Ovary

Two cases of *Hodgkin's disease* localized to the ovary have been reported.[4,39] In both cases, the tumor was unilateral. Microscopically, the ovary was replaced by a malignant cellular infiltrate consisting of lymphocytes, eosinophils, plasma cells, atypical histiocytic cells, and typical Sternberg–Reed cells. Fibrosis and necrosis also were evident. Both patients were well and disease free for periods of 2 and 6 years after diagnosis. Although it is difficult to draw any conclusions from only two cases, it appears that Hodgkin's disease, when localized to the ovary, has a better prognosis than does primary non-Hodgkin's lymphoma of the ovary.

Disseminated Malignant Lymphoma Affecting the Ovary

As mentioned earlier, this entity must be divided into two categories: (1) the ovarian tumor being either the initial or predominant presenting manifestation of the disease and (2) ovarian involvement occurring during the course of the disease and being noted at surgery or autopsy, either grossly or microscopically.

The first type of *disseminated malignant tumor* is uncommon, although it is more common than primary malignant lymphoma of the ovary, with more than 100 examples recorded.[22,23,50] The second type is common and is becoming even more so because of the longer survival of patients with malignant lymphoma as a result of recent therapy.

The age of patients in whom ovarian involvement is the presenting sign of malignant lymphoma ranges from childhood to old age, but most are 20–50 years of age.[22,23,50] The symptoms in these patients are largely similar to those observed in patients with primary malignant lymphoma of the ovary, the most common being abdominal enlargement, often associated with abdominal pain. In contrast to women with primary malignant lymphoma of the ovary, these patients frequently complain of malaise, weight loss, pallor, and fatigue. On physical examination, in addition to the finding of an adnexal mass, which is frequently bilateral, lymph node enlargement may be noted, either widespread or localized. There may be enlargement of the spleen and the liver. The blood count may show anemia. A leukemic blood picture or pancytopenia may be observed.

The macroscopic and microscopic appearances of the ovarian tumor are similar to those described in cases of malignant lymphoma localized to the ovary. The malignant lymphoma usually is of a poorly differentiated B-cell type, either lymphoblastic, poorly differentiated lymphocytic, or reticulum cell sarcoma, or of large or small cleaved or noncleaved type, or diffuse large cell, or diffuse mixed large and small cell type.[50]

It is extremely uncommon for generalized Hodgkin's disease to present in this manner. The course of the disease and the prognosis are similar to those observed in patients with generalized non-Hodgkin's malignant lymphoma of the poorly differentiated cell type, which are, at best, very guarded despite recent advances in treatment of these conditions. Ovarian involvement is observed nowadays in up to 50% of cases of disseminated malignant lymphoma examined at autopsy, but it occurs rarely in patients with disseminated Hodgkin's disease. Patients with malignant lymphoma live longer with the disease because of the improved therapy, which contributes to the wider dissemination once response to therapy is lost. In such cases, the lymphoma affects many sites that did not become affected in the past, when patients died earlier, with the disease involving mainly the lymphoreticular system. The involvement of the ovaries usually is bilateral, and the ovaries may be of normal size or only slightly enlarged. Microscopically, extensive infiltration by malignant lymphoma cells usually is present, but sometimes the infiltration may be slight. These patients should be treated according to the most effective current protocols used for treating patients with disseminated malignant lymphoma.

Burkitt's Lymphoma

Burkitt's lymphoma is a specific type of malignant lymphoma showing a typical age prevalence, clinical and histologic picture, and specific geographic distribution. It is observed primarily in East and West Africa south of the Sahara desert and in Papua and New Guinea,[5] which are considered the endemic areas where the tumor is common. The tumor also occurs sporadically outside the endemic areas.[50]

Burkitt's lymphoma is a poorly differentiated malignant lymphoma, showing multicentric or multifocal origin. Clinically, it is seen affecting the jaw, ovary, orbit, kidney, thyroid, testis, and other sites, with involvement of the lymph nodes a minor feature. Frequent ovarian involvement by the disease was first noted in West Africa and also was found in the East African cases. Relatively frequent involvement of the ovary also is observed in cases from outside the endemic areas.[50]

Abdominal pain and swelling caused by ovarian enlargement represent the principal symptoms in 38% of patients with Burkitt's lymphoma. Burkitt's lymphoma occurs mainly in children, with a peak incidence at 4–7 years. Young adults also are affected. Occasionally, the tumor is localized to the ovary without involvement of other sites. Macroscopically, ovarian involvement by Burkitt's lymphoma usually is bilateral. The ovarian tumors are large, white, and solid with a slightly lobulated surface and on cut section have a solid, white, firm surface that can be altered by the presence of necrosis and hemorrhage.

Microscopically, the ovary is completely or nearly completely replaced by proliferation of primitive lymphoreticular cells (Figs. 21.14 and 21.15) that appear round, oval, or indented with a narrow rim of basophilic cytoplasm, exhibiting strong pyroninophilia. The nuclei are large, prominent, and usually round but sometimes oval or reniform (Fig. 21.15). The nuclear membrane is sharp and well defined, and the chromatin is coarse, containing a few small nucleoli. Mitotic activity is brisk. The cytoplasm of the tumor cells contains numerous small vacuoles that contain lipid material; this is more obvious in imprint preparations from the tumor, a procedure that should al-

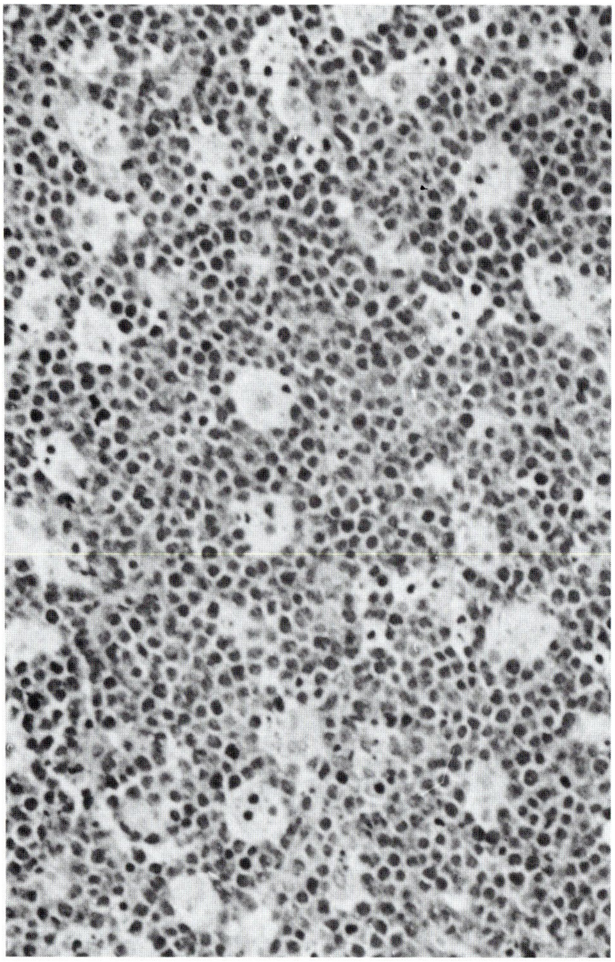

Fig. 21.14. Burkitt's lymphoma affecting ovary. The tumor has a typical starry-sky appearance.

ways be undertaken because it provides a very good diagnostic aid. Interspersed among the tumor cells are numerous nonneoplastic macrophages (histiocytes) containing phagocytosed material that stains positively with PAS and lipid stains. It is the presence of these macrophages scattered between the tumor cells that gives the tumor its typical starry-sky appearance (Fig. 21.14). It should be noted that this starry-sky appearance is not pathognomonic of Burkitt's lymphoma and may be observed in other types of poorly differentiated neoplasms. The histologic appearance of the cells and the histochemical reactions mentioned earlier are the main features leading to the diagnosis of Burkitt's lymphoma.

Burkitt's lymphoma progresses quickly and, in the absence of therapy, is rapidly fatal. It responds dramatically to chemotherapy with antimetabolites and alkylating agents, leading to long remissions, and to complete cure in approximately 20% of cases. Radiotherapy can be used in conjunction with chemotherapy. The behavior of the tumor and its response to therapy are similar, whether it is encountered in the endemic or nonendemic areas.[81]

Involvement of the Ovary by Leukemia

Ovarian involvement by leukemia as seen at autopsy is common and is observed in 30%–50% of cases. Recent reports indicate more frequent involvement than earlier studies, which may result from longer containment of the disease by chemotherapy and radiotherapy, such as that observed in malignant lymphoma of the non-Hodgkin's type.

Lymphocytic and Granulocytic Leukemia

Occasionally, the ovary has been found to be the site of a relapse of *childhood acute lymphocytic leukemia,*

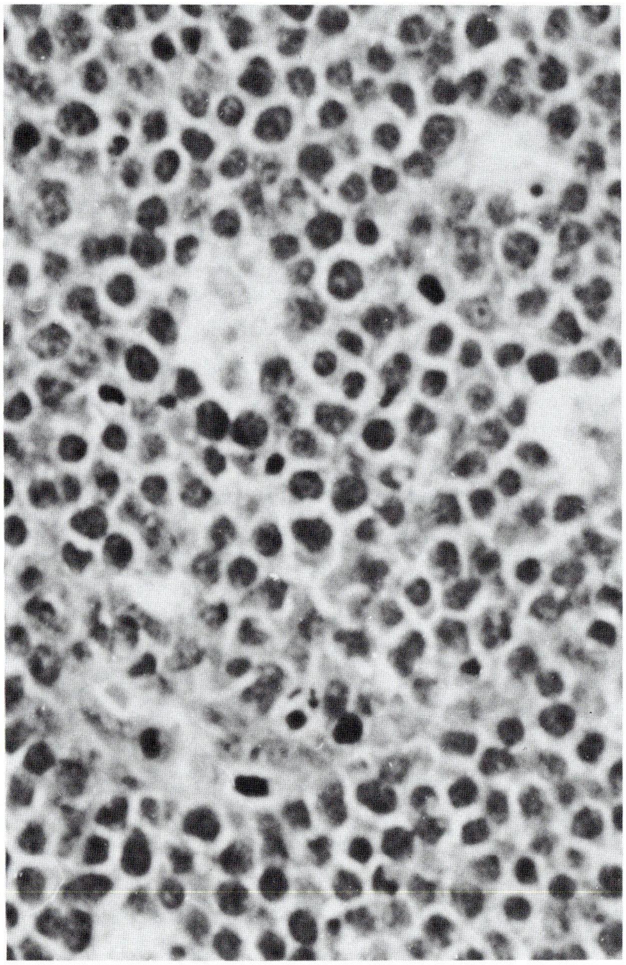

Fig. 21.15. Burkitt's lymphoma affecting ovary. Higher magnification of tumor shown in Fig. 21.14.

although this course of events is by far not as common as in the case of the testes.[10] At times, ovarian enlargement may be the first sign of *granulocytic leukemia*, the ovarian tumor being designated *ovarian granulocytic sarcoma* or *chloroma*, the latter term a result of the green color of the tumor mass. Such cases usually are observed in children[2,51,67] but occasionally are seen in adults. On examination, the peripheral blood or the bone marrow usually shows evidence of leukemia. Occasionally, the presence of an ovarian mass precedes the leukemia by a number of months.[2,51,59] The tumors frequently are bilateral, although one tumor may be larger than the other.

Microscopically, the tumor may resemble malignant lymphoma, especially if it is composed of early and primitive hematopoietic cells (Figs. 21.16 and 21.17). The presence of myeloblasts and better-differentiated cells (Fig. 21.17) that may be seen in places is helpful in making the diagnosis. The application of naphthol-AS-D-chloroacetate esterase (Leder's) stain and positive immunocytochemical staining for myeloid series markers confirm the diagnosis. Electron microscopy also is helpful in making the diagnosis.

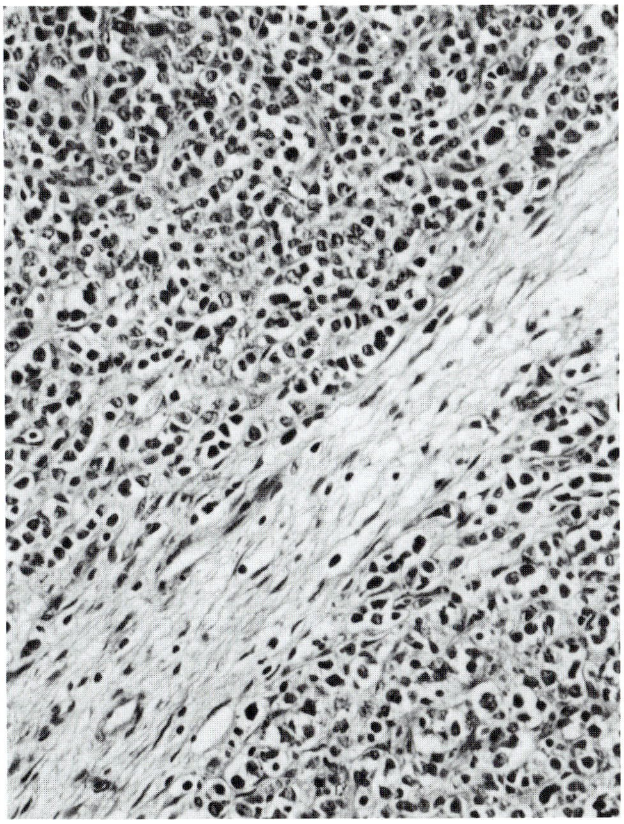

Fig. 21.16. Myelocytic sarcoma of ovary. Tumor is composed of collections of small round cells separated by bands of unaffected connective tissue.

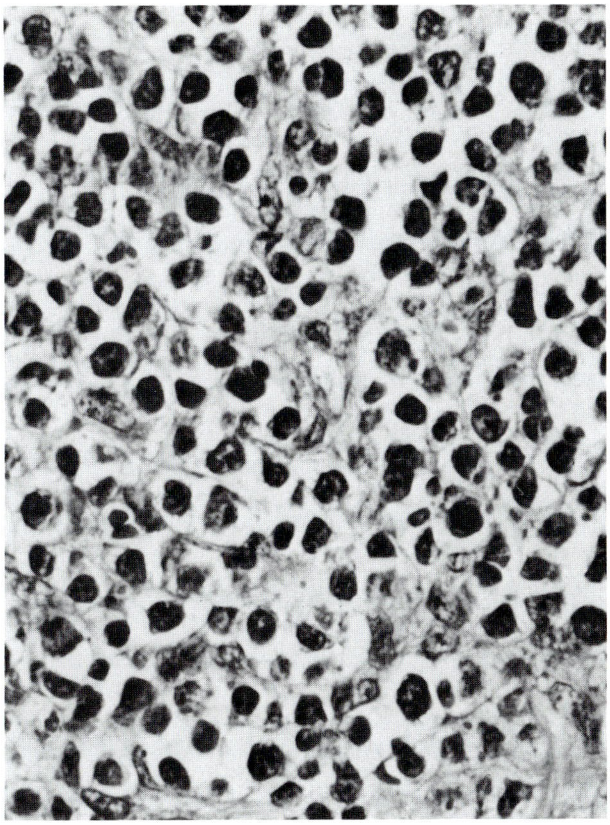

Fig. 21.17. Myelocytic sarcoma of ovary. Tumor is composed of primitive myeloid series cells. In places, slightly better differentiation indicates the myelocytic nature of the lesion.

The prognosis is generally poor, but some patients survive a few years. The treatment of choice in patients with granulocytic sarcoma is the combination chemotherapy used in patients with acute or subacute myelocytic leukemia.

Plasma Cell Dyscrasia

Involvement of the ovary by malignant disorders of plasma cells is very rare. The disorder can manifest either as involvement of the ovary by *multiple myeloma*, usually observed at autopsy, although one case in a 44-year-old living woman has been reported,[3] or rarely as a *primary extranodal plasmacytoma* similar to primary malignant lymphoma of the ovary. One such case, which I observed, occurred in a 35-year-old woman, who had a painful lower abdominal mass. The tumor was unilateral, solid, firm, and gray-white. It measured 15 × 12 × 9 cm and showed ovarian tissue replaced by diffuse proliferation of plasma cells, including many immature forms. There was no evidence of biochemical abnormalities, including monoclonal gammopathy, and no evidence of bone or bone marrow involvement. The patient was well and disease free 9 months after the operation, when she was lost to follow-up. A few similar cases have been reported in the literature.[14,25,67]

Plasmacytoma must be differentiated from malignant lymphoma affecting the ovary as well as from granulocytic sarcoma. The appearance of the tumor cells, aided by special stains such as methyl green-pyronin, immunocytochemical staining for light and heavy chains, and B-cell antibodies as well as electron microscopy are helpful in differentiating these lesions. Biochemical studies including electrophoresis, full blood, and radiologic examinations are necessary to differentiate between the disseminated disease and primary plasmacytoma. Because of the rarity of primary plasmacytoma of the ovary, it is possible only to speculate about the prognosis, but in common with extramedullary plasmacytoma found in other locations, it probably is better than in cases of multiple myeloma. The treatment of choice is excision of the lesion and careful follow-up of the patient. Chemotherapy used in cases of multiple myeloma may be administered prophylactically.

Ovarian Tumor of Probable Wolffian Origin

In the original report describing tumors of this type,[35] all the tumors were located within the leaves of the broad ligament or were attached to it or to the fallopian tube; this also applied to subsequent reports dealing with this entity. Subsequently, 12 *ovarian tumors of probable wolffian origin* were reported,[30,76] indicating that tumors of this type also occur in the ovary. The age of the patients ranged from 28 to 79 years. Five patients had abdominal enlargement, and in the remaining 7 patients, the tumor was found on physical examination.[30,76] At laparotomy, all the tumors were found to be unilateral. In 11 patients, they were confined to the ovary, and in the remaining patient, there were metastatic deposits in the abdominal cavity. In the latter case, the tumor contained foci of undifferentiated carcinoma.[76] The tumors range in size from 2 to 20 cm in the largest diameter. They are smooth and often lobulated and are either solid or solid and cystic. The cysts vary in size and may range up to 11 cm.[76]

Microscopically, the tumor is composed of relatively uniform epithelial cells that line cysts and tubules, sometimes forming a sievelike pattern (Fig. 21.18). The tumor cells also may form closely packed tubules (Fig. 21.19), grow in a diffuse pattern, or fill tubules or tubular spaces. They have uniform round or oval nuclei, and there is low mitotic activity. The tumor cells do not contain mucin but occasionally may contain glycogen. The amount of intervening connective tissue varies from imperceptible to considerable, forming fibrous bands separating the islands of tumor cells and producing a lobular pattern.[76] In two patients in whom the tumors were associated with aggressive behavior, there was brisk mitotic activity with 10 or more mitoses (MF)/10 high-power fields (HPF), and in one of the these patients, there was nuclear pleomorphism.

Two patients have subsequently developed metastases.[76] Eight patients were known to be alive and disease free from 1 to 15 years postoperatively, and one was lost to follow-up,[76] indicating that in most cases the tumor is not associated with an aggressive course. It is also of note that there is a good correlation between the mitotic activity and the behavior of this neoplasm. Ovarian tumor of probable wolffian origin may be confused with sex cord–stromal tumors, especially various types of Sertoli–

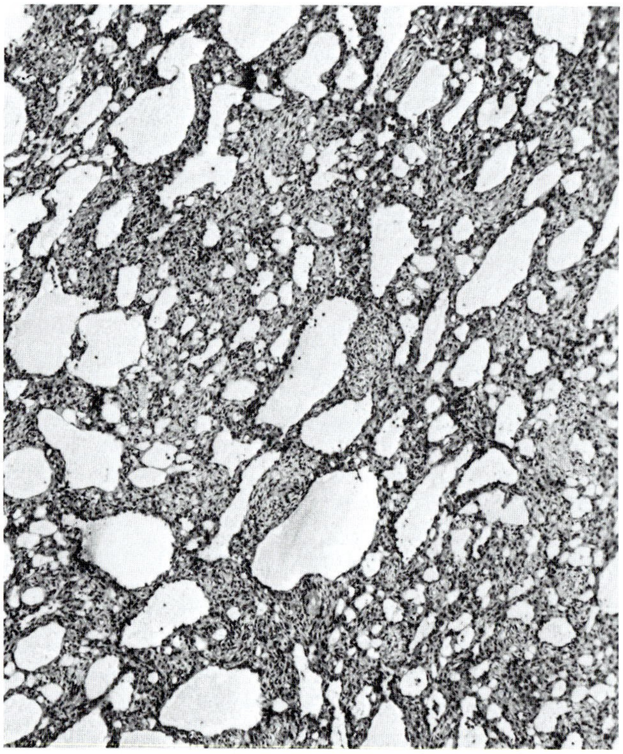

Fig. 21.18. Ovarian tumor of probable wolffian origin. The tumor shows a sievelike pattern. The tumor cells line clefts and spaces and form solid aggregates. (Reprinted by permission of Young and Scully, ref. 76.)

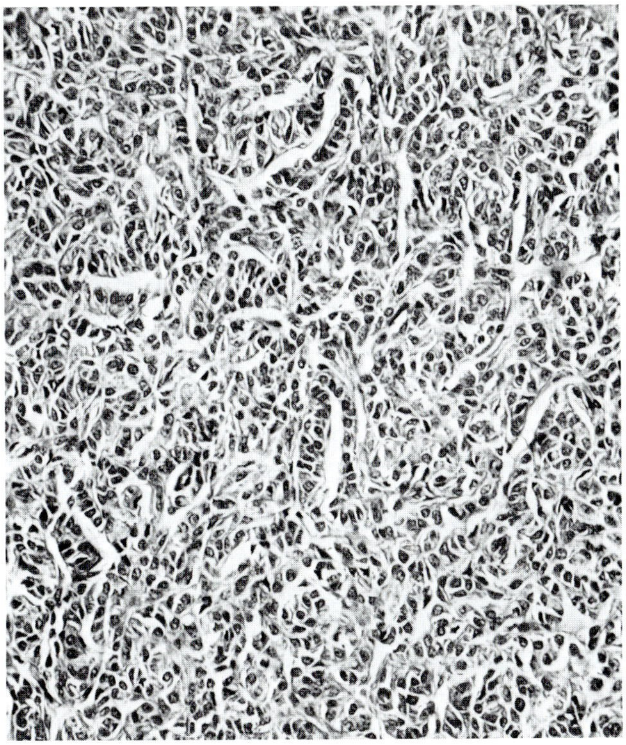

Fig. 21.19. Ovarian tumor of probable wolffian origin. The tumor is composed of closely packed tubules with compressed lumens and is lined by cuboid epithelial cells. (Reprinted by permission of Young and Scully, ref. 76.)

Leydig cell tumors and surface epithelial–stromal tumors from which it must be differentiated (see Chapter 19, Sex Cord–Stromal, Steroid Cell, and Other Ovarian Tumors with Endocrine, Paraendocrine, and Paraneoplastic Manifestations). The presence of the typical features of this tumor described here and the absence of the various patterns observed in Sertoli–Leydig cell tumors differentiate it from the latter. The tumor of probable wolffian origin is distinguished from the various surface epithelial–stromal tumors of the ovary by the absence of cellular and nuclear pleomorphism, a papillary pattern, and intraluminal and intracellular mucin.

Tumors of Uncertain Histogenesis

Hepatoid Carcinoma of the Ovary

In 1987, Ishikura and Scully[31] described five cases of ovarian carcinoma with hepatoid features, three of them primary and two probably primary. The age of the patients ranged from 42 to 78 years and thus differed considerably from patients with yolk sac tumor with a hepatoid pattern, which is invariably seen in children, adolescents, and young women. The age range, as well as the histologic appearances of the tumors, showed considerable similarity to gastric carcinomas with hepatic features described some years earlier.[32]

Unlike yolk sac tumor with a hepatoid pattern, which may be pure, mixed with other yolk sac tumor patterns, or combined with other germ cell tumors, *hepatoid carcinoma of the ovary* occurs in pure form, although occasionally it is associated with serous adenocarcinoma or other types of ovarian surface epithelial–stromal tumors.[67,68] Hepatoid carcinoma of the ovary,[31] like yolk sac tumor with hepatoid pattern and gastric adenocarcinoma with hepatoid features,[32] is associated with alpha–fetoprotein (AFP) secretion, and AFP can be demonstrated within the tumor cells by immunohistochemical techniques. In two cases known to the author, high levels of serum AFP were noted, and serum AFP was used to monitor the disease activity.

Clinically, patients present with symptoms and signs related to the presence of an adnexal mass. Abdominal enlargement, which may be associated with pain, malaise, and weight loss, is the main presenting sign.[31]

Hepatoid carcinomas of the ovary are large and are associated with metastatic tumor deposits within the abdominal cavity (stage III) in most cases.[31] Histologically, the tumor shows a close resemblance to hepatocellular carcinoma, and is composed of solid sheets or aggregates of uniform cells with moderate or abundant eosinophilic cytoplasm, distinct cell borders, and centrally located nuclei with prominent nucleoli (Fig. 21.20).[31] Mitotic activity generally is brisk, and abnormal forms are seen. In some parts of the tumor there may be a considerable degree of nuclear pleomorphism, and multinucleated giant cells may be seen.[31] PAS-positive diastase-resistant hyaline globules may be seen, and glycogen can be demonstrated within the cytoplasm of the tumor cells. Histologic patterns seen in germ cell tumors or surface epithelial–stromal tumors are not detectable when the tumor is seen in pure form.[31,67]

Immunohistochemical studies demonstrate the presence of AFP in a considerable number of tumor cells. In addition, the tumor cells are immunoreactive for albumin, alpha$_1$-antitrypsin, and alpha$_1$-antichymotrypsin. Focal positive immunostaining for carcinoembryonic antigen (CEA) also is seen.[31]

Hepatoid carcinoma of the ovary is a highly malignant neoplasm.[31,67] Most patients present with disseminated disease and die of the disease within

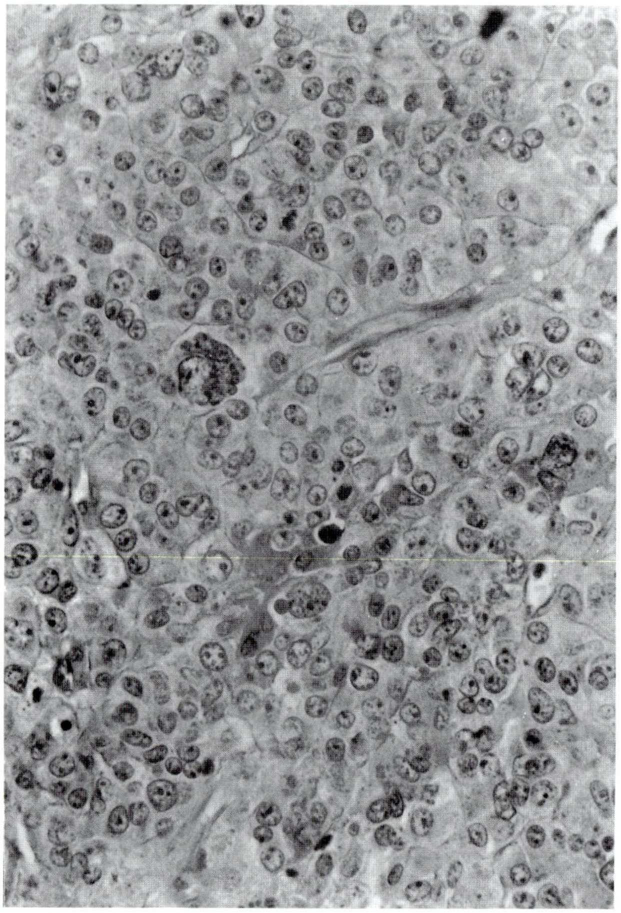

Fig. 21.20. Hepatoid carcinoma of the ovary. Note the close resemblance to hepatocellular carcinoma. Occasional giant cells help to differentiate this tumor from yolk sac tumor with hepatoid pattern. (Courtesy of R.E. Scully, M.D., Boston, MA.)

a few years of diagnosis. One patient was well and disease free for 2 years after pelvic irradiation.[31] One patient was alive with evidence of disease 2 years after surgery and combination chemotherapy. She was treated with Taxol and for some time responded to treatment, as evidenced by some decrease in the highly elevated serum AFP level. She then relapsed and died of extensive disease.

The histogenesis of hepatoid carcinoma of the ovary has not been established. Unlike yolk sac tumor with hepatoid pattern, it is not of germ cell origin, as it occurs in older patients, is not associated with other neoplastic germ cell elements, and is not found in patients with gonadal dysgenesis. Because of the age distribution and the occasional association with ovarian surface epithelial–stromal tumors, it is likely that it is a metaplastic tumor and represents a variant of a surface epithelial–stromal tumor.[31,67,68]

Hepatoid carcinoma of the ovary must be distinguished from yolk sac tumor with hepatoid pattern. It can be distinguished clinically by its occurrence in older, usually postmenopausal patients, and by its presentation in a more advanced clinical stage, usually in stage III. Histologically, hepatoid carcinoma shows a greater degree of nuclear pleomorphism, and tumor giant cells are much more frequently seen.

Demonstration of positive immunocytochemical staining for AFP in the tumor cells and elevated levels of serum AFP differentiate hepatoid carcinoma from other ovarian tumors such as undifferentiated adenocarcinomas, endometrioid adenocarcinomas with marked squamous differentiation, and steroid cell tumors.[31] Primary hepatoid carcinoma of the ovary also must be differentiated from primary hepatocellular carcinoma, metastatic to the ovary. Although the latter is uncommon, this possibility must be carefully excluded before the diagnosis of primary hepatoid carcinoma of the ovary is made.

Primary Ovarian Small Cell Carcinoma with Pulmonary Differentiation

Eichhorn et al.[18] have reported 11 primary ovarian tumors that resembled small cell carcinoma of the lung and differed both clinically and histologically from primary small cell carcinoma of the ovary, usually associated with hypercalcemia.[80] The age of the patients ranged from 28 to 85 years.[18] Most patients presented with abdominal enlargement. Six of the tumors were unilateral, and 5 were bilateral. Spread beyond the ovary was noted in 7 tumors. None of the patients had distant metastases at presentation.[18] The tumors measured from 4.5 to 26 cm in the greatest dimension; they were mostly solid with a variable minor cystic component.[18]

Histologically, the tumor was composed of small to medium-sized round to spindle-shaped cells with scanty cytoplasm, hyperchromatic nuclei, and inconspicuous nucleoli forming sheets, large aggregates, and closely packed nests (Fig. 21.21). Sometimes an insular or a trabecular pattern was seen.[18] In four tumors a component of endometrioid carcinoma was present, one tumor showed focal squamous differentiation, two tumors were associated with Brenner tumor, and one contained a cyst lined by atypical mucinous cells.[18] In two of six tumors, argyrophil granules were demonstrated. In nine cases immunocytochemical studies were performed that demonstrated positive staining for cytokeratin in six cases, for epithelial membrane antigen (EMA) in five, for neuron-specific enolase (NSE) in seven, for chromogranin in two, and for Leu-7 in a single

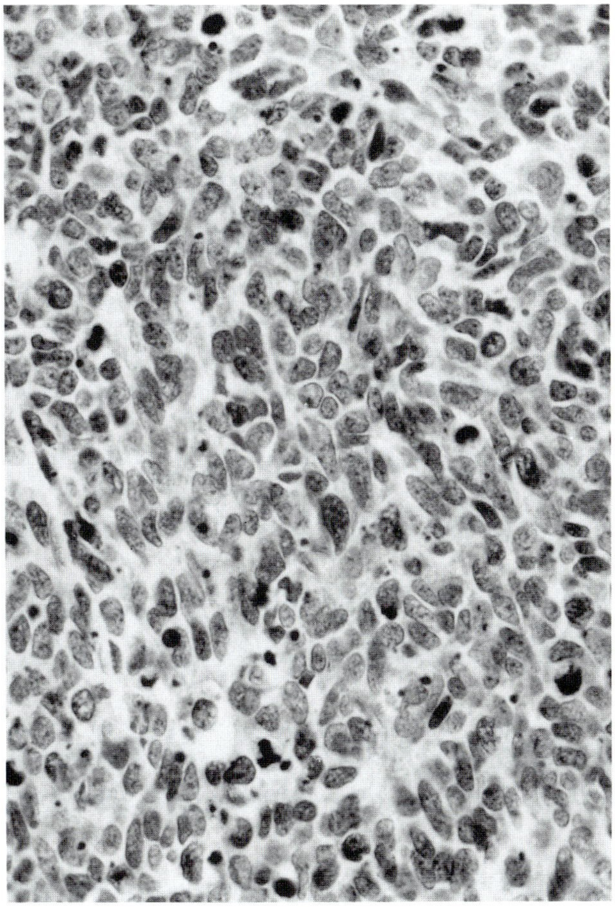

Fig. 21.21. Small cell carcinoma of the ovary with pulmonary differentiation. Note the ovoid and spindle shape of the nuclei, the finely dispersed chromatin, and inconspicuous nucleoli. (Courtesy of R.E. Scully, M.D., Boston, MA.)

case. All nine tumors were vimentin negative.[18] Flow cytometric studies performed on eight tumors showed that five tumors were aneuploid and three were diploid.[18]

The tumors were aggressive, and of the nine patients with known follow-up, five died of the disease 1–13 months after diagnosis, one died after an unknown interval, and two had recurrent disease 6 and 8 months after surgery. One patient was alive without evidence of disease 7.5 years after surgery.[18] Five of the patients with stage III tumors and two with stage I tumors were treated with combination chemotherapy, which included cisplatin in all cases and doxorubicin in most cases; one of these treated patients is the 7.5-year survivor.[18] Aggressive treatment with agents effective in treating small cell pulmonary carcinoma appears to be the treatment of choice.

Primary ovarian small cell carcinoma with pulmonary differentiation must be distinguished from *pulmonary small cell carcinoma metastatic to the ovary*, which shows both clinical and pathologic differences.[78] It also must be differentiated from primary ovarian small cell carcinoma, usually associated with hypercalcemia[67,80] (see Chapter 19, Sex Cord–Stromal, Steroid Cell, and Other Ovarian Tumors with Endocrine, Paraendocrine, and Paraneoplastic Manifestations). The patients with primary ovarian small cell carcinoma with pulmonary differentiation are older. The tumor is seen either in perimenopausal or postmenopausal women.[18,67] Hypercalcemia is absent. The tumors are bilateral in 45% of cases, whereas in the hypercalcemic type, this is seen only rarely (1% of cases).[18]

Histologically, the cells of primary ovarian small cell carcinoma with pulmonary differentiation differ from those of the hypercalcemic type in having finely dispersed chromatin and inconspicuous nucleoli, whereas the latter is composed of cells with nuclei showing clumped chromatin and prominent nucleoli, as well as showing the presence of larger cells with abundant eosinophilic cytoplasm in 40% of cases.[18] Folliculoid spaces are always seen in the hypercalcemic type and are virtually absent in the pulmonary type of small cell carcinoma.[18] Endometrioid and Brenner tumor components are present in more than half the small cell carcinomas with pulmonary differentiation and are absent in the hypercalcemic type. The former also tend to be more frequently aneuploid.[81]

Although the histogenesis of the primary ovarian small cell carcinoma with pulmonary differentiation has not been established, the frequent association with endometrioid and Brenner tumors points toward a surface epithelial–stromal origin, as is supported further by the age range of the patients.[18]

Neuroendocrine Carcinoma of Non-Small Cell Type

Eight ovarian tumors composed of solid sheets, nests, cords, trabeculae, or solid islands of cells showing *neuroendocrine differentiation* have been reported.[20,67] All these tumors were associated with a surface epithelial–stromal component, which in seven cases was of the mucinous and in the remaining case of the endometrioid type. The age of the patients ranged from 22 to 77 years. Most of the tumors were stage I, but in spite of this the prognosis was poor in common with neuroendocrine tumors occurring in other sites.

Histologically, the neuroendocrine component of the tumor consisted of solid islands or cords of medium to large epithelial cells with variable amount of cytoplasm and large nuclei, some of which had prominent nucleoli. Mitotic activity was variable. The cellular islands and cords were surrounded only by a small amount of connective tissue. Argyrophil granules were invariably present in the cytoplasm of the tumor cells, and immunocytochemical stains were strongly positive for chromogranin and serotonin. Other neurohormonal polypeptides were also detected in some of the tumors.[20]

The neuroendocrine component of the tumor may resemble insular carcinoid tumor of the ovary, but the cells are usually larger and show much greater degree of cellular and nuclear pleomorphism. The presence of the surface epithelial–stromal component also helps to differentiate between these two entities. The distinction between them is very important because the prognosis of patients with neuroendocrine carcinoma is by far worse than that of patients with carcinoid tumors. The size of the tumor cells and the strong positive immunocytochemical reactions distinguish this tumor from the ovarian carcinoma of the small cell pulmonary type. The presence of the surface epithelial–stromal component confirming the ovarian origin differentiates this tumor from metastatic small cell tumors to the ovary.[20]

Adenoid Cystic and Polymorphous Low-Grade Adenocarcinoma (PLGA)

Ovarian tumors resembling *adenoid cystic and polymorphous low-grade adenocarcinoma (PLGA)* of the salivary gland type are rare, but a series of eight tumors with a predominant or entire such pattern has been reported.[19] Most of the tumors also exhibited a minor component of surface epithelial–stromal neoplasia. The latter were of various histologic types and, although most were poorly differentiated, they included a case in which this component was of the serous borderline type.[19,67]

The affected patients were elderly; nearly all were in the seventh or eighth decade. Most of the tumors were associated with extensive metastatic disease and the prognosis was poor, except for one case where the tumor was in pure form and another case in which the associated surface epithelial–stromal component was of the serous borderline type.

Histologically the tumors resemble adenoid cystic carcinoma or PLGA (Fig. 21.22). The tumor cells resemble myoepithelial cells, although this has not been confirmed immunocytochemically because in the majority of cases the cells did not stain positively for actin and S-100 protein.[19,67] As this sometimes is seen in PLGA, the importance of the negative findings may not be very significant. Histogenetically, these tumors are probably of surface epithelial–stromal origin, because they are usually associated with a surface epithelial–stromal component.

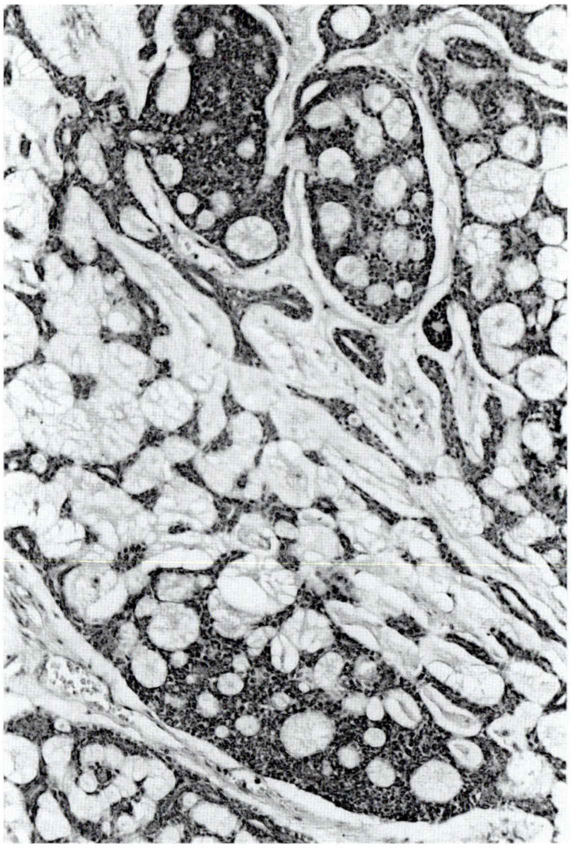

Fig. 21.22. Ovarian carcinoma resembling adenoid cystic carcinoma. (Courtesy of R.E. Scully, M.D., Boston, MA.)

Basaloid Carcinomas

Six ovarian tumors showing *basaloid* or *ameloblastomatous* features have been reported.[19,67] The age distribution was wide, ranging from 19 to 65 years. Most of the tumors were confined to the ovary (stage IA), and the prognosis was excellent after excision of the tumor, although some of the follow-up periods were relatively short, varying from 19 to 71 months.

Histologically, the tumors showed either basaloid or ameloblastomatous pattern. Several of them showed focal squamous and glandular differentiation, and one showed a minor component of endometrioid adenocarcinoma.[19,67] The histogenesis of this neoplasm is uncertain but surface epithelial–-stromal origin appears to be most likely.

Nephroblastoma (Wilms' Tumor)

A single case of *ovarian nephroblastoma* occurring in a 56-year-old woman has been reported.[65] The patient was treated by excision of the affected adnexa followed by radiotherapy and chemotherapy. She was well and disease free 9 years after diagnosis. The tumor showed typical features of well-differentiated nephroblastoma with glomeruloid formations, small tubules, and prominent blastema. There were no other neoplastic elements.[65] Although the tumor was described as a primary ovarian nephroblastoma, its histogenetic origin is uncertain. It is considered that one-sided development of a teratoma, or a teratoma overgrown by its nephroblastomatous component, is the likely origin of this tumor.

Nephroblastoma differentiation is seen in a number of ovarian teratomas and has not been seen in association with other ovarian neoplasms, providing support for this contention. Occasionally retiform Sertoli–Leydig cell tumors, because of the presence of tubules and papillary pattern resembling glomeruloid formations, have been misdiagnosed as ovarian nephroblastomas. Careful sectioning and examination of the tumor for the presence of other patterns associated with Sertoli–Leydig cell tumors and absence of renal blastema are helpful in differentiating between these two entities. Demonstration of positive inhibin staining using immunocytochemistry further supports the diagnosis of Sertoli–Leydig cell tumor.

Carcinoma of Rete Ovarii

Cysts and cystadenomas of *rete ovarii* are uncommon, although probably more common than it is realized. Only one well-documented case of *adenocarcinoma of rete ovarii* occurring in a 52-year-old woman with abdominal enlargement and ascites has been reported.[63] The patient had bilateral, partly solid and partly cystic tumors without specific macroscopic features. The tumor showed a predominant pattern of branching tubules and cysts containing simple papillae with fibrovascular or hyalinized cores. Some cysts contained eosinophilic material. Focally the tumor showed a solid tubular pattern. The cells lining the tubules and papillae were cuboidal, nonciliated, and atypical. Focally, they were multilayered and stratified. There was brisk mitotic activity.[63]

Adenocarcinoma of rete ovarii can only be diagnosed if the tumor has hilar location and is composed of collections of slitlike retiform tubules and cysts containing papillae lined by cells similar to those of normal rete ovarii.[63,67] Confusion may occur with retiform Sertoli–Leydig cell tumor, but the latter is likely to show other patterns of Sertoli–Leydig cell tumor and positive staining for inhibin. Some serous papillary adenocarcinomas may also resemble adenocarcinoma of the rete ovarii, but they tend to be found in cortical location, generally do not show the fine slitlike papillae, and exhibit much greater nuclear pleomorphism.

References

1. Balaton A, Vaury P, Imbert MC, Mussy MA (1987) Primary leiomyosarcoma of the ovary. A histological and immunocytochemical study. Gynecol Oncol 28:116–120
2. Ballon SC, Donaldson RC, Berman ML, Swanson GA, Byron RL (1978) Myeloblastoma (granulocytic sarcoma) of the ovary. Arch Pathol Lab Med 102:474
3. Bambirra EA, Miranda D, Magalhaes GMC (1982) Plasma cell myeloma simulating Krukenberg's tumor. South Med J 75:511
4. Bare WW, McCloskey JF (1961) Primary Hodgkin's disease of the ovary. Obstet Gynecol 17:447
5. Berard C, O'Conor GT, Thomas LB, Torloni H (1969) Histopathological classification of Burkitt's tumour. Bull WHO 40:601
6. Bollinger DJ, Wick MR, Dehner LP, Mills SE, Swanson PE, Clark RE (1989) Peritoneal malignant mesothelioma versus serous papillary adenocarcinoma. A histochemical and immunohistochemical comparison. Am J Surg Pathol 13:659
7. Bower JF, Erikson ER (1967) Bilateral ovarian fibromas in a 5 year old. Am J Obstet Gynecol 99:880
8. Brady K, Page DV, Benn LE, de las Morenas A, O'Brien M (1987) Ovarian myxoma. Am J Obstet Gynecol 156:1240
9. Burket RL, Rauh JL (1976) Gorlin's syndrome. Ovarian fibromas at adolescence. Obstet Gynecol 47:43S
10. Cecalupo AJ, Frankel LS, Sullivan MP (1982) Pelvic and ovarian extramedullary leukemic relapse in young girls. A report of four cases and review of the literature. Cancer (Phila) 50:587
11. Chan YF, Leung CS, Ma L (1989) Primary embryonal rhabdomyosarcoma of the ovary in a 4-year-old girl. Histopathology (Oxf) 15:211
12. Clement PB, Young RH, Scully RE (1996) Malignant mesotheliomas presenting as ovarian masses: a report of nine cases, including two primary ovarian mesotheliomas. Am J Surg Pathol 20:1067
13. Climie AR, Heath LP (1968) Malignant degeneration of benign cystic teratoma of the ovary. Review of the literature and report of a chondrosarcoma and a carcinoid tumor. Cancer (Phila) 22:824
14. Cook HT, Boylston AW (1988) Plasmacytoma of the ovary. Gynecol Oncol 29:378
15. Dockerty MB, Masson JC (1944) Ovarian fibromas: a clinical and pathologic study of two hundred eighty three cases. Am J Obstet Gynecol 47:741
16. Dover H (1950) Neurofibrosarcoma of the ovary, associated with neurofibromatosis. Can Med Assoc J 63:488

17. Eichhorn JH, Scully RE (1991) Ovarian myxoma. Clinicopathologic and immunocytologic analysis of five cases and a review of the literature. Int J Gynecol Pathol 10:156
18. Eichhorn JH, Young RH, Scully RE (1992) Primary ovarian small cell carcinoma of pulmonary type. A clinicopathologic, immunohistologic and flow cytometric analysis of 11 cases. Am J Surg Pathol 16:926
19. Eichhorn JH, Scully RE (1995) "Adenoid cystic" and basaloid carcinomas of the ovary: evidence for a surface epithelial lineage. A report of 12 cases. Mod Pathol 8:731
20. Eichhorn JH, Lawrence WD, Young RH, Scully RE (1996) Ovarian neuroendocrine carcinomas of non-small cell type associated with surface epithelial adenocarcinomas. A study of five cases and review of the literature. Int J Gynecol Pathol 15:303
21. Fawcett FJ, Kimbell NKB (1971) Phaeochromocytoma of the ovary. J Obset Gynaecol Br Commonw 78:458
22. Ferry JA, Young RH (1991) Malignant lymphoma, pseudolymphoma and hematopoietic disorders of the female genital tract. Pathol Annu 26:227
23. Fox H, Langley FA, Govan ADT, Hill AS, Bennett MM (1988) Malignant lymphoma presenting as an ovarian tumor. A clinicopathologic analysis of 34 cases. Br J Obstet Gynecol 95:386
24. Gehrig PA, Fowler WC Jr, Liniger RA (2000) Ovarian capillary hemangioma presenting as adnexal mass with massive ascites and elevated CA-125. Gynecol Oncol 76:130
25. Hautzer NW (1984) Primary plasmacytoma of the ovary. Gynecol Oncol 18:115
26. Hegg CA, Flint A (1990) Neurofibroma of the ovary. Gynecol Oncol 37:437
27. Hines JF, Compton DM, Stacy CC, Potter ME (1990) Pure primary osteosarcoma of the ovary presenting as an extensively calcified adnexal mass: a case report and review of the literature. Gynecol Oncol 39: 259
28. Hirakawa T, Tsuneyoshi M, Enjoji M, Shigyo R (1988) Ovarian sarcoma with histologic features of telangiectatic osteosarcoma of bone. Am J Surg Pathol 12:567
29. Howell CG, Rogers DA, Gable DS, Falls GD (1990) Bilateral ovarian fibromas in children. J Pediatr Surg 25:690
30. Hughesdon PE (1982) Ovarian tumors of wolffian or allied nature. Their place in ovarian oncology. J Clin Pathol 35:526
31. Ishikura H, Scully RE (1987) Hepatoid carcinoma of the ovary. A newly described tumor. Cancer (Phila) 60:2775
32. Ishikura H, Kirimoto K, Shamoto M, et al (1986) Hepatoid adenocarcinomas of the stomach. An analysis of seven cases. Cancer (Phila) 58:119
33. Kalstone CE, Jaffe RB, Abell MR (1969) Massive edema of the ovary simulating fibroma. Obstet Gynecol 34:564
34. Kandalaft PL, Esteban JM (1992) Bilateral massive ovarian leiomyomata in a young woman. A case report with review of the literature. Mod Pathol 5:586
35. Kariminejad MH, Scully RE (1973) Female adnexal tumor of probable wolffian origin. Cancer (Phila) 31:671
36. Kawauchi S, Fukuda T, Amada S, Kaku T, Nakano H, Tsuneyoshi M (1996) Hemangiopericytoma of the ovary. A case report. Int J Surg Pathol 4:115
37. Kraemer BB, Silva EG, Sneige N (1984) Fibrosarcoma of the ovary. A new component in the nevoid basal-cell carcinoma syndrome. Am J Surg Pathol 8:231
38. Lawhead RA, Copeland LJ, Edwards CL (1985) Bilateral ovarian hemangiomas associated with diffuse abdominopelvic hemangiomatosis. Obstet Gynecol 65:597
39. Long JP, Patchefsky AS (1971) Primary Hodgkin's disease of the ovary. Obstet Gynecol 38:680
40. Lorentzen M (1980) Giant cell tumor of the ovary. Virchows Arch [Pathol Anat] 388:113
41. Lyday RO (1952) Fibroma of the ovary with abdominal implants. Am J Surg 84:737
42. Mann LS, Metrick S (1961) Hemangioma of the ovary. Report of a case. J Int Coll Surg 36:500
43. McBurney RC, Trumbull M (1955) Hemangioma of the ovary with ascites. Miss Doct 32:271
44. Meigs JV (1954) Fibroma of the ovary with ascites and hydrothorax. Meigs' syndrome. Am J Obstet Gynecol 67:962
45. Meyer R (1943) Nerve tumors of the female genitals and pelvis. Arch Pathol 36:437
46. Michael CA (1966) Pelvic fibroma causing recurrent attacks of hypoglycaemia in a post-menopausal patient. Proc R Soc Med 59:835
47. Miles PA, Kiley KC, Mena H (1985) Giant fibrosarcoma of the ovary. Int J Gynecol Pathol 4:83
48. Mira JL (1991) Lipoleiomyoma of the ovary. Report of a case and review of the English literature. Int J Gynecol Pathol 10:198
49. Mishura VI (1963) Report of large benign tumor—report of three cases. Vopr Onkol 9:103
50. Monterosso V, Jaffe ES, Merino MJ, Medeiros LJ (1993). Malignant lymphomas involving the ovary. A clinicopathologic analysis of 39 cases. Am J Surg Pathol 17:154
51. Morgan ER, Labotka RJ, Gonzalez-Crussi F, Wiederhold M, Sherman JO (1981) Ovarian granulocytic sarcoma as a primary manifestation of acute infantile myelomonocytic leukemia. Cancer (Phila) 48:1819
52. Nielsen GP, Young RH, Prat J, Scully RE (1997) Primary angiosarcoma of the ovary. A report of seven cases and review of the literature. Int J Gynecol Pathol 16:378
53. Nielsen GP, Young RH, Rosenberg AE, Oliva E, Prat J, Scully RE (1998) Primary ovarian rhabdomyosarcoma. A report of 13 cases. Int J Gynecol Pathol 17:113
54. Nogales FF (1982) Primary chondroma of the ovary. Histopathology (Oxf) 6:376
55. Nunez C, Abboud SL, Lemon NC, Kemp JA (1983)

Ovarian rhabdomyosarcoma presenting as leukemia. Case report. Cancer (Phila) 52:297
56. Paladugu RR, Bearman RM, Rappaport H (1980) Malignant lymphoma with primary manifestation in the gonad. A clinicopathologic study of 38 patients. Cancer (Phila) 45:561
57. Prat J, Scully RE (1981) Cellular fibromas and fibrosarcomas of the ovary. A comparative clinicopathologic analysis of seventeen cases. Cancer (Phila) 47:2663
58. Prayson RS, Hart WR (1992) Primary smooth muscle tumors of the ovary. A clinicopathologic study of four leiomyomas and two mitotically active leiomyomas. Arch Pathol Lab Med 116:1068
59. Pressler H, Horny HP, Wolf A, Kaiserling E (1992) Isolated granulocytic sarcoma of the ovary: histologic electron microscopic and immunohistochemical findings. Int J Gynecol Pathol 11:68
60. Raggio M, Kaplan AL, Harberg JF (1983) Recurrent ovarian fibromas with basal cell nevus syndrome (Gorlin syndrome). Obstet Gynecol 61:95S
61. Rhoades CP, McMahon JT, Goldblum JR (1999) Myofibroblastoma of the ovary. Mod Pathol 12:907
62. Rice M, Pearson B, Treadwell WB (1943) Malignant lymphangioma of the ovary. Am J Obstet Gynecol 45:884
63. Rutgers JL, Scully RE (1988) Cysts (cystadenomas) and tumors of the rete ovarii. Int J Gynecol Pathol 7:330
64. Sandison AT (1955) Rhabdomyosarcoma of the ovary. J Pathol Bacteriol 70:433
65. Sahin A, Benda JA (1998) Primary ovarian Wilms' tumor. Cancer (Phila) 61:1460
66. Savargaonkar PR, Wells S, Graham I, Buckley CH (1994) Ovarian hemangiomas and stromal luteinization. Histopathology (Oxf) 25:185
67. Scully RE, Young RH, Clement PB (1998) Tumors of the ovary, maldeveloped gonads, Fallopian tube, and broad ligament, vol 23, 3rd ser. Armed Forces Institute of Pathology, Washington, DC
68. Scurry JP, Brown RW, Jobling T (1996) Combined ovarian serous papillary and hepatoid carcinoma. Gynecol Oncol 63:138
69. Shaeffer MD, Cancelmo JJ (1939) Cavernous hemangioma of the ovary in a girl twelve years of age. Am J Obstet Gynecol 38:722
70. Smith FR (1931) Neurofibroma of the ovary associated with Recklinghausen's disease. Am J Cancer 15:859
71. Stone GC, Bell DA, Fuller A, Dickersin GR, Scully RE (1986) Malignant Schwannoma of the ovary. Report of a case. Cancer (Phila) 58:1575
72. Stowe LM, Watt JY (1952) Osteogenic sarcoma of the ovary. Am J Obstet Gynecol 64:422
73. Talerman A (1967) Hemangiomas of the ovary and the uterine cervix. Obstet Gynecol 30:108
74. Talerman A, Auerbach WM, Van Meurs AJ (1981) Primary chondrosarcoma of the ovary. Histopathology (Oxf) 5:319
75. Talerman A, Montero JR, Chilcote RR, Okagaki T (1985) Diffuse malignant peritoneal mesothelioma in a 13-year-old girl. Am J Surg Pathol 9:73
76. Young RH, Scully RE (1983) Ovarian tumors of probable wolffian origin. A report of 11 cases. Am J Surg Pathol 7:125
77. Young RH, Scully RE (1984) Fibromatosis and massive edema of the ovary, possibly related entities. A report of 14 cases of fibromatosis and 11 cases of massive edema. Int J Gynecol Pathol 3:153
78. Young RH, Scully RE (1985) Ovarian metastases from cancer of the lung. Problems in interpretation. A report of seven cases. Gynecol Oncol 21:337
79. Young RH, Silva EG, Scully RE (1991) Ovarian and juxtaovarian adenomatoid tumors: a report of six cases. Int J Gynecol Pathol 10:364
80. Young RH, Oliva E, Scully RE (1994) Small cell carcinoma of the ovary, hypercalcemic type. A clinicopathologic analysis of 150 cases. Am J Surg Pathol 18:1102
81. Ziegler JL (1977) Treatment results of 54 American patients with Burkitt's lymphoma are similar to the African experience. N Engl J Med 297:75

22

Metastatic Tumors of the Ovary

Robert H. Young, M.D., F.R.C. Path., and
Robert E. Scully, M.D.

Metastatic tumors are an important group of ovarian neoplasms because the misinterpretation of those cases encountered as surgical pathology specimens may have important adverse consequences for the patient. Tumors may metastasize to the ovary from numerous organs and tissues outside the female genital tract, but neoplasms arising in the intestines, stomach, and breast, and hematopoietic tumors (rare examples of which are also primary in the ovary), are the most common forms encountered by the pathologist. Hematopoietic tumors are discussed in Chapter 21 (Nonspecific Tumors of the Ovary, Including Mesenchymal Tumors and Malignant Lymphoma), and are not considered further here. Tumors that extend to the ovary directly from adjacent organs or tissues (secondary tumors) are also considered here; determination of the origin of the tumor in such cases may be impossible when both ovarian and extraovarian involvement is extensive.

Recognition of the metastatic nature of an ovarian tumor depends on several factors: (1) an awareness of the frequency with which metastases occur and simulate a variety of primary tumors; (2) a detailed clinical history; (3) a thorough clinical and operative search by the surgeon for a primary tumor outside the ovary and for other sites of tumor spread; (4) a careful evaluation of the gross and routine microscopic features of the ovarian tumor by the pathologist; and (5) judicious use of conventional special stains and immunohistochemistry.

It is surprising how often the diagnosis of a metastatic tumor is missed by the pathologist because the existence of a present or prior tumor in another organ is either not known or, if known, disregarded.[116,119] The surgical and pathologic findings from previous operations should be reviewed if there is any possibility that they could be related to the ovarian tumor being evaluated. In some cases a search for an extraovarian primary tumor must be conducted postoperatively on the basis of the suspicion of the pathologist that the ovarian tumor is metastatic. Even if an extraovarian primary tumor is not detected, a diagnosis of ovarian metastasis must be strongly considered if the distribution of the metastatic disease is atypical for primary ovarian cancer or if pathologic examination is highly suggestive of metastasis. For example, the presence of pulmonary or hepatic metastases in the absence of extensive peritoneal spread would be unusual for an ovarian cancer, but not for certain other tumors that are prone to metastasize to the ovary. The mere presence of tumor outside the ovaries should lead to the serious consideration of a metastasis in certain situations. For example, if a well-differentiated ovarian mucinous tumor is associated with extensive mucinous adenocarcinoma in the omentum and on the peritoneal surfaces, the possibility of spread to the ovary from, for example, the pancreas or biliary tract should be entertained. Additionally, certain tumors, such as Sertoli cell tumors or primary carcinoid tumors, which are almost always benign, should be diagnosed with caution in cases in which there also is extraovarian tumor. In cases of these types the putative Sertoli cell tumor may prove to be a metastatic tumor that is mimicking it, for example, a tubular Krukenberg tumor, and the carcinoid tumor probably is metastatic rather than primary in the ovary. It also must be emphasized that an association of an ovarian tumor with clinical or pathologic evidence of excess estrogens, androgens, or progesterone does not exclude the diagnosis of a metastatic tumor, which may have a functioning stroma (see Chapter 19, Sex Cord–Stromal, Steroid Cell, and Other Ovarian Tumors with Endocrine, Paraendocrine, and Paraneoplastic Manifestations).

For a variety of reasons it is difficult to establish accurately the frequency of metastatic tumors among all ovarian tumors from the available literature. Some studies have been based on autopsy findings, others on surgical specimens, and still others on both. In addition, some series have included clinically silent metastases such as breast carcinoma found in prophylactic or therapeutic oophorectomy specimens and small metastases detected incidentally during operations for gastric or intestinal carcinoma. In contrast, other series have been restricted to metastatic tumors that presented clinically as pelvic or abdominal masses. Finally, some investigations have included as metastases ovarian carcinomas associated with uterine cancers of similar histologic type, whereas in many cases the ovarian tumors are independent primary tumors.

The frequency of metastases to the ovary also varies from one country to another because of wide differences in the prevalence of the various cancers that are associated with high rates of ovarian spread. For example, metastatic carcinoma was reported to account for approximately 40% of all ovarian cancers in one series from Japan, where gastric carcinoma is common, but for fewer than 3% in a series from Uganda, where this form of cancer is relatively rare.[47] The frequency of metastases also has varied greatly in series in which differences in the prevalence of the primary tumors do not adequately explain the discrepant results. Such variations may be related, in part, to the frequency and thoroughness of microscopic examination of the ovaries, because gross inspection may not reveal evidence of involvement in one-third to one-half the cases. The figure for the frequency of ovarian metastases that is most meaningful to the surgeon is one that expresses the probability that an ovarian neoplasm found on exploration of a pelvic or abdominal mass is metastatic; this figure is of the order of 5%–10%.[77,107]

The age distribution of patients with ovarian metastases depends to a great extent on that of the corresponding primary tumors, but for each of the most common types (intestinal, gastric, and breast) the average age of patients with ovarian involvement is significantly lower than that of those without ovarian spread suggesting that the richly vascularized ovaries of young women are more receptive to metastases than are those of older patients.

Tumors spread to the ovary by several routes.[46] Direct spread is an important pathway for carcinomas of the fallopian tube and uterus, for mesotheliomas, and for occasional colonic carcinomas and retroperitoneal sarcomas. A second mechanism of spread of genital tract carcinomas is through the lumen of the fallopian tube and onto the surface of the ovary; this route is taken most often by carcinomas of the uterine corpus.[17] Spread from more distant sites is mainly via blood vessels and lymphatics. The frequent association of ovarian metastases with other blood-borne metastases, the common finding of tumor within ovarian blood vessels on microscopic examination in cases of metastasis, and the higher frequency of ovarian metastases in young patients are consistent with the important role of hematogenous spread. Retrograde flow within lymphatics is an unlikely route of spread except in the presence of extensive involvement of the lymph nodes draining the ovaries. Such a mechanism of spread also seems inconsistent with the sporadic reports of prolonged survival after a primary tumor and its apparently solitary ovarian metastatic tumor have been removed. Finally, transcoelomic dissemination with surface implantation is an important route by which intraabdominal cancers spread to the ovary, as is supported by the common association of ovarian involvement with generalized peritoneal spread. The pathologist often encounters foci of metastatic carcinoma on the surface of the ovary, or superficially located within the cortex in these cases, supporting implantation as the mechanism. It is possible that ovulation, by creating a defect in the ovarian surface, provides a portal of entry for cancer cells floating in the peritoneal cavity in premenopausal patients.

The gross features of tumors metastatic to the ovary vary greatly and may resemble those of a variety of primary ovarian tumors. Because of the relatively high frequency with which metastases are bilateral (Fig. 22.1) (two-thirds to three-quarters of the cases), the possibility of metastasis should be considered particularly in evaluating bilateral tumors other than serous and undifferentiated carcinomas, which also are commonly bilateral. Endometrioid

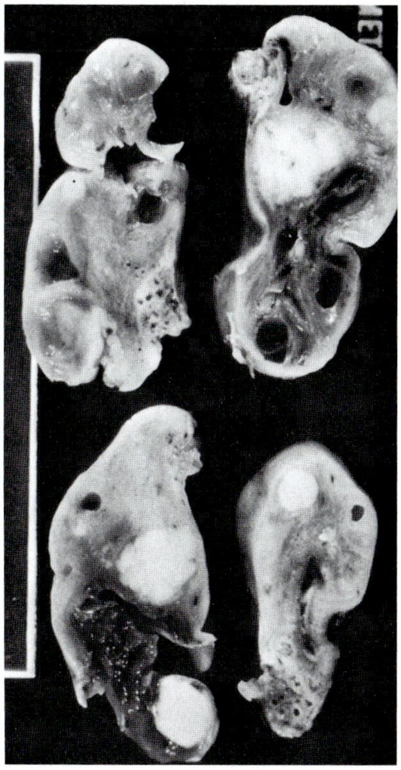

Fig. 22.1. Metastatic carcinoma from the breast. Multiple nodules are seen on the sectioned surfaces of both ovaries.

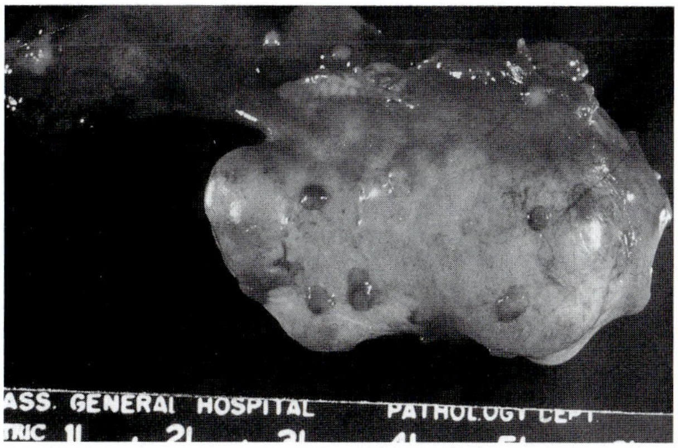

Fig. 22.2. Metastatic carcinoma from the breast. Several discrete nodules of tumor are present on the external aspect of the ovary. (Reproduced by permission of ref. 135.)

and mucinous carcinomas, in contrast, are bilateral in less than 15% of the cases, and bilateral tumors with endometrioid-like and mucinous features merit more serious consideration for possibly being metastatic.[135] Although metastatic tumors often are bilateral, many metastatic tumors are unilateral and, if the microscopic features of a tumor suggest metastasis, unilaterality should not be considered a significant argument against it. In general, almost 10% of bilateral ovarian cancers presenting as adnexal masses prove to be metastatic on careful evaluation. Two other gross findings that are suggestive, but not pathognomonic, of metastasis in cases with certain microscopic appearances (see following) are the presence of multiple nodules (Fig. 22.1) and the location of nodules on the surface of the ovary (Fig. 22.2), sometimes without significant involvement of the underlying parenchyma. Conversely, a gross feature of some metastastic tumors, which should not be regarded as establishing the primary nature of the tumor, is the presence of cysts, which often are large and occasionally thin walled, despite the absence of cysts in the primary neoplasm (Fig. 22.3).

The microscopic appearance of a metastatic tumor obviously varies with the appearance of the primary neoplasm. In addition to the presence of specific features of various primary tumors, the presence of implants on the surface of the ovary (Fig. 22.4), and growth in the form of multiple nodules (Fig. 22.5), suggests metastasis in many cases. This distribution of disease may be seen with serous

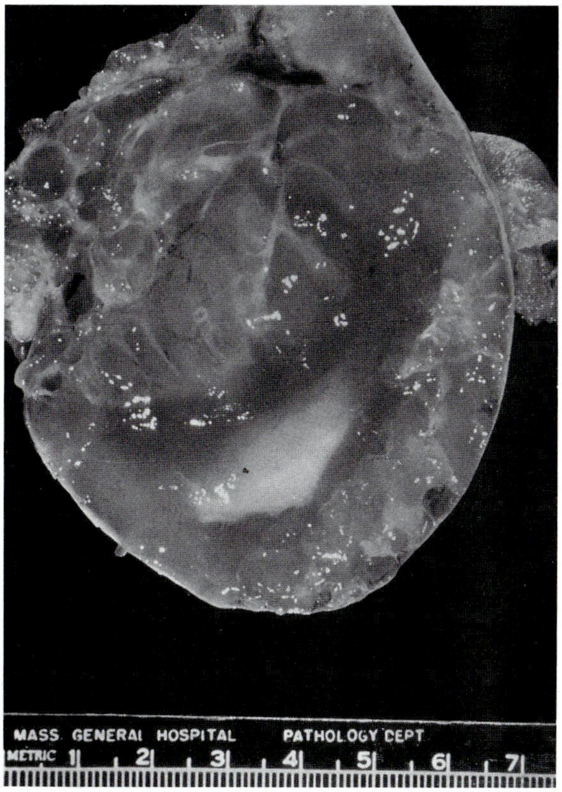

Fig. 22.3. Metastatic carcinoma from the cecum. The tumor is indistinguishable on gross examination from a primary mucinous cystic tumor of the ovary. (Reproduced by permission of ref. 135.)

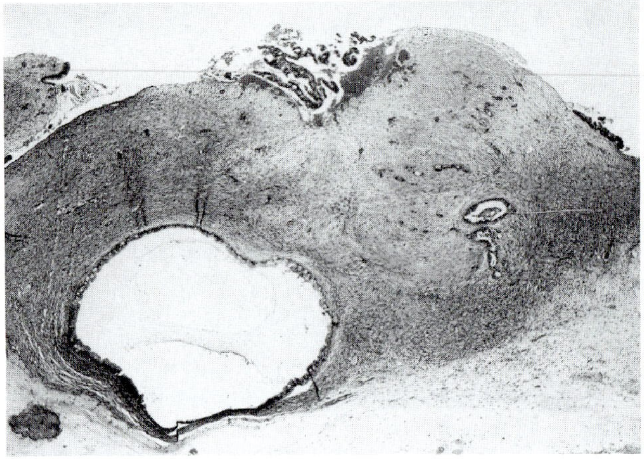

Fig. 22.4. Metastatic carcinoma from the pancreas. Tumor is present on the external aspect of the specimen (*top center*) and is associated with an underlying desmoplastic stromal reaction in the superficial cortex. One neoplastic gland has become cystic in the deeper portion of the ovary (*lower left*). (Reproduced by permission of ref. 135.)

carcinomas, particularly those of so-called surface type, and some undifferentiated carcinomas and has no weight in cases with those microscopic features, but does in cases of mucinous and endometrioid-

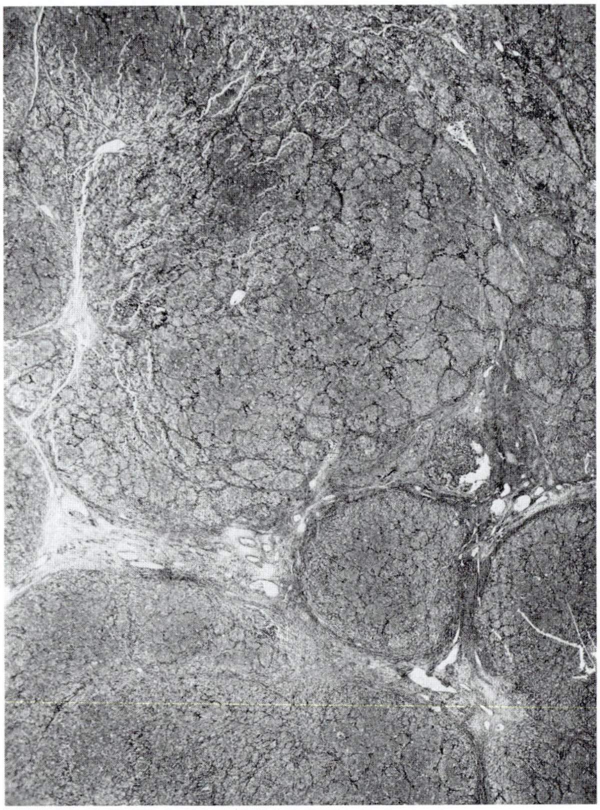

Fig. 22.5. Metastatic carcinoma from the lung. The tumor is growing in the form of multiple nodules.

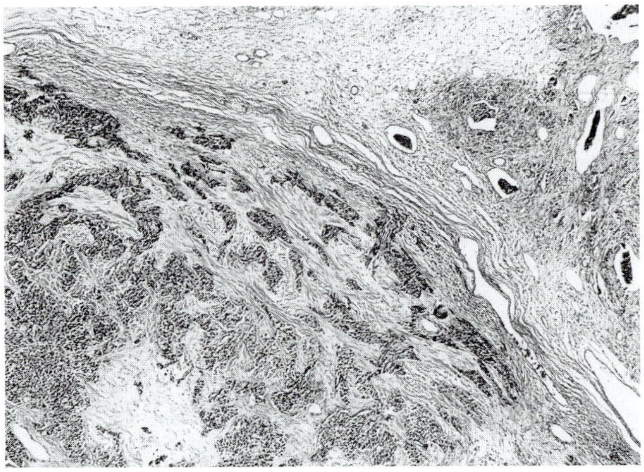

Fig. 22.6. Metastatic carcinoma from the breast. Vascular channels at the periphery of the tumor (*upper right*) contain metastatic tumor. (Reproduced by permission of ref. 135.)

like morphology as well as in cases with any of a diverse number of unusual microscopic appearances. The surface implants typically are focal, often projecting above the surface of the adjacent cortex, and characteristically are embedded in desmoplastic or hyalinized fibrous tissue (Fig. 22.4). The presence of surface implants in cases of metastasis sometimes correlates with the presence of excrescences on the external surface of the ovary that may be detected on careful gross inspection. Lymphatic or blood vessel invasion strongly suggest metastasis (Fig. 22.6). A confusing microscopic feature of some metastatic tumors is the presence of cysts, some of which simulate follicles (Fig. 22.7). These follicle-like spaces may be encountered in a variety of metastatic tumors including gastric and intestinal carcinomas, carcinoids, small cell carcinomas from various

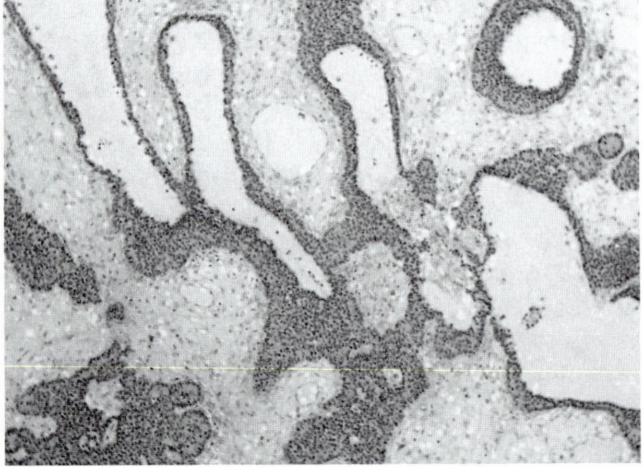

Fig. 22.7. Metastatic small cell carcinoma from the cervix. The tumor contains many follicle-like spaces.

sites (Fig. 22.7), and malignant melanomas.[135] A wide variety of other patterns and cell types in metastatic tumors suggest diverse possible primary sites, as discussed in detail elsewhere.[135] Immunohistochemistry, selectively applied according to the routine microscopic features, may aid in certain cases but is uncommonly diagnostic on its own. We have personally found it most helpful in occasional cases of amelanotic malignant melanoma when staining for S-100 protein and HMB-45 has been present. Even after the most thorough evaluation, it is sometimes impossible for the pathologist to be definitive whether a neoplasm is primary or metastatic but on the basis of the morphology may suggest the most likely possible extra-ovarian primary sites to direct clinical evaluation.

Female Genital Tract Tumors

Tubal Carcinoma

The ovary is involved secondarily in approximately 13% of *tubal carcinomas*, usually by direct extension, sometimes via tuboovarian inflammatory adhesions, and at other times by surface implantation on the ipsilateral or contralateral ovary.[94] In some cases, there is clinical or pathologic evidence of salpingitis and salpingo-oophoritis, but often it is unclear whether the inflammatory process preceded or followed the development of the carcinoma. If the involvement of the tube and the ovary is extensive, the primary site of the tumor may not be established with certainty; the term tuboovarian carcinoma has been suggested for these cases. Green and Scully[34] encountered six such tumors in an investigation of 24 carcinomas initially considered to be of tubal origin. The tuboovarian carcinomas formed solid or cystic masses; at least one of the cystic tumors appeared to have developed in a postinflammatory tuboovarian cyst.

Because most tubal carcinomas closely resemble serous, endometrioid, or undifferentiated carcinomas of the ovary, microscopic examination often fails to establish whether a carcinoma involving both organs is primary in one or the other unless the tumor is grossly clearly centered in one of them. Because of the great rarity of primary mucinous and clear cell carcinomas of the fallopian tube, a tumor of either of these cell types involving both organs usually is considered primary in the ovary. It should be emphasized that surface growth within the tube may be seen as a result of implantation from an ovarian carcinoma and does not necessarily indicate a tubal primary.

Endometrial Carcinoma

Ovarian involvement in cases in which a diagnosis of *endometrial carcinoma* has been made has been reported in 34%–40% of autopsy cases,[5,10] and 5%–15% of hysterectomy and bilateral salpingo-oophorectomy specimens (see Chapter 12, Endometrial Carcinoma). Conversely, in approximately one-third of the cases in which a diagnosis of endometrioid carcinoma of the ovary has been made, an endometrial carcinoma also has been found. When the uterine corpus and the ovary are both involved by carcinomas, the question arises whether both cancers are primary or one is metastatic from the other.[28,105,142] If the endometrial carcinoma extends deeply into the myometrium with lymphatic or vascular invasion, if tumor is present in the lumen of the fallopian tube, or if tumor is on the ovarian surface or within its lymphatics or blood vessels, it is usually reasonable to conclude that the ovarian involvement is secondary. On the other hand, if lymphatic or hematogenous spread is absent, if the corpus carcinoma is small and limited to the endometrium or superficial myometrium, if it arises on a background of atypical hyperplasia, and if there is a centrally located ovarian tumor, sometimes arising on a background of endometriosis, the tumors probably are independent primaries. Criteria that are helpful in the determination of primary versus metastatic concomitant ovarian and endometrial carcinomas are presented in Table 22.1. Although the ovarian and uterine tumors are of the endometrioid type in most cases, occasionally they are similar but of other cell types, and rarely the histologic type of tumor is different in the two organs.[28]

In some cases of combined involvement it is impossible to establish the site of origin even after consideration of the features just described. In our experience and that of most series, most synchronous ovarian and corpus carcinomas are independent primary tumors; in one study, however, the ovarian tumors were interpreted as metastatic from the corpus in most of the cases,[105] and other valid cases of metastasis are reported in the literature.[85] An independent–primary explanation for most concomitant ovarian and corpus carcinomas is supported by the survival rates associated with this combination of tumors, which have generally been high. These results would be surprising if either the ovarian or corpus carcinoma was metastatic in most of the cases.

Rarely, ovarian spread from an adenocarcinoma of the uterine corpus with squamous differentiation takes the form of deposits of keratin or degenerated mature squamous cells associated with a foreign body giant cell response on the serosal surface of one or both ovaries.[13,52] If no viable-appearing tu-

Table 22.1. Criteria for interpretation of nature of concomitant uterine corpus and ovarian carcinomas

Corpus primary ovarian metastasis	*Ovarian primary corpus metastasis*	*Ovarian primary corpus primary*	*Ovarian metastasis corpus metastasis*	*Uncertain primary*
Direct extension to ovary from large corpus tumor	Direct extension to corpus from large ovarian primary	No direct extension of either tumor	Usually no direct extension of tumors	Massive involvement of both organs or conflicting findings listed in first four columns
Deep myometrial invasion from endometrium	Myometrial invasion from serosal surface	Myometrial invasion usually absent or superficial	Tumor characteristically in endometrial stroma. Myometrial invasion may be present	
Lymphatic or blood vessel invasion in corpus, ovary, or both	Lymphatic or blood vessel invasion in corpus, ovary, or both	No lymphatic or blood vessel invasion	Lymphatic or blood vessel invasion frequent in ovary and corpus	
Atypical hyperplasia of endometrium frequent	Atypical hyperplasia of endometrium usually absent	Atypical hyperplasia of endometrium frequent	Atypical hyperplasia of endometrium absent	
Tumor present in fallopian tube	Tumor present on peritoneal surfaces and sometimes in fallopian tube	Usually both tumors confined to primary sites or have spread minimally	Tumor usually evident outside female genital tract	
Tumor predominant on surface of ovary	Tumor predominant within ovary	Tumor predominant within ovary and endometrium	Ovarian tumor usually bilateral—ovarian surface involvement frequent	
Usually no endometriosis in ovary	Endometriosis sometimes present in ovary	Endometriosis sometimes present in ovary	Endometriosis absent	
Histological types uniform and consistent with corpus primary	Histological types uniform and consistent with ovarian primary	Histological types uniform or dissimilar	Type of tumor inconsistent with or unusual for either organ	

mor cells can be identified in these deposits on careful sampling, this finding does not appear to worsen the prognosis even when the granulomas are also found elsewhere on the peritoneum.

Cervical Carcinoma

Ovarian spread of *cervical carcinomas* of all types generally has been considered rare. There has been considerable recent interest in this topic, however, stimulated in part by observations suggesting that it is more common in cases of adenocarcinoma than in cases of squamous cell carcinoma, and raising the question of whether ovarian conservation is justified in patients with cervical adenocarcinoma. In addition, occasional patients with cervical carcinomas of diverse types have had clinically significant ovarian metastases.[125]

One of the most detailed studies of ovarian spread of cervical carcinoma is that of Tabata et al.[101] In their autopsy series, ovarian metastases were detected in 104 of 597 (17%) cases of squamous cell carcinoma and in 22 of 77 (28.6%) cases of adenocarcinoma. The frequency of ovarian metastases of squamous cell carcinoma at autopsy in their series is much higher than the 3% frequency in the prior literature. Ovarian metastases discovered during life are much rarer. In their series of 318 patients with stage IA cervical carcinoma treated by hysterectomy with ovarian preservation, Tabata et al.[101] found no examples of subsequent ovarian metastasis during follow-up periods that exceeded 5 years in more than half the cases. In cases of stage IB, II, and III carcinoma in their series, there were no ovarian metastases in 278 cases of squamous cell carcinoma in contrast to 6 ovarian metastases of 48 (12.5%) cases of adenocarcinoma. In another series there were 3 cases of microscopic ovarian metastasis in 185 cases of stage IIB cervical carcinoma[103]; in the same series, there were no metastases in 335 cases of stage IB disease, 71 cases of stage IIA disease, and 6 cases of stage IIIB disease; 1 of the ovarian metastases was from a squamous cell carcinoma (0.2% of all squamous cell carcinomas) whereas 2 were adenocarcinomas (5.5% of these tumors). The cervical carcinomas in these 3 cases had invaded the uterine corpus and vascular spaces. Tabata et al.[101] also found that ovarian metastasis was much more common when a cervical carcinoma had invaded the uterine corpus.

There are only eight well-documented examples of clinically significant ovarian metastases from invasive squamous cell carcinomas of the cervix.[70,125] The youngest patient was 30 years old and the oldest 59 years. The ovarian and cervical tumors were discovered at essentially the same time in three of the patients. In four others, the ovarian metastases occurred 18 months to 10 years after the cervical primary tumor had been treated. In the eighth case the cervical tumor was not discovered until autopsy 7 months after the patient had been treated for a squamous cell carcinoma involving the left ovary. The cervical tumor in that case was invasive only to 3.8 mm, whereas in the other cases there appears to have been deep infiltration of the cervical wall with frequent extrauterine extension of the neoplasm.[125] The ovarian tumors, 2 of which were bilateral, ranged from 5 to 17 cm in greatest dimension. Four of the 10 tumors in these patients were solid, 3 solid and cystic, and 3 cystic. Microscopic examination has shown the typical features of squamous cell carcinoma except that many of the tumors had striking cystification within the squamous nests. In one case, a cervical squamous cell carcinoma that was invasive to only 1.2 mm extended in an in situ manner to involve the endometrium and involved the surface and inclusion glands and cysts within one ovary, tumor cells presumably having spread there via the tubal lumen.[125] In a final remarkable case, a cervical squamous cell carcinoma in situ was associated with contiguous spread to the endometrium, fallopian tubes, and ovaries, extensively replacing the endometrial and tubal epithelium and focally invading the wall of the tubes and parenchyma of both ovaries (Fig. 22.8).[79]

The differential diagnosis in cases of metastatic squamous cell carcinoma from the cervix with primary squamous cell carcinoma of the ovary usually has been aided by the knowledge of the presence of a cervical tumor, but in the one case in which the cervical tumor was not detected until autopsy and some of the others, there were major problems in diagnosis.[125] Before the diagnosis of primary squamous cell carcinoma of the ovary is made, the possibility of spread of a cervical tumor, even one that is occult, should be considered. As most squamous cell carcinomas of the ovary arise on the background of a preexistent neoplasm such as a dermoid or endometriotic cyst, thorough sampling to identify such a component may be crucial in determining the primary nature of the neoplasm. Although the evidence strongly points to the ovarian tumors being metastatic when both organs have been involved by squamous cell carcinoma, the rare association of squamous cell carcinoma of the ovary with squamous cell carcinoma in situ of the cervix leaves open the possibility of independent primary neoplasms in some cases.

In a series from the Armed Forces Institute of Pathology, 10% of mucinous adenocarcinomas of the cervix were reported to metastasize to the ovary,[50] and occasional other examples have been reported in detail[136] or included in series of metastatic mucinous carcinomas in the ovary.[86] When a cervical mucinous adenocarcinoma and an ovarian mucinous adenocarcinoma coexist, however, particular difficulty may be encountered in deciding whether they are independent primary tumors[57] or metastatic from one organ to the other,[78] although the general features of metastatic spread to the ovary often help. Two adenosquamous carcinomas and two glassy cell carcinomas with ovarian metastases have been reported.[125] Both metastatic adenosquamous carcinomas were discovered at the same time as the cervical primary tumors. The ovarian tumors were bilateral in both cases, and the cervical tumors were deeply invasive with extracervical extension, findings facilitating the diagnosis in these cases. In one of the cases of glassy cell carcinoma the ovarian involvement was a microscopic finding; in the other the ovarian involvement was grossly evident but the ovary was not enlarged.

Four cases have been reported in detail in which cervical small cell carcinomas or mixed tumors with a component of adenocarcinoma and small cell carcinoma or poorly differentiated carcinoid have been associated with ovarian metastases. In each of these four cases, the ovarian spread was manifest clinically.[125] In one, the patient had evidence of the carcinoid syndrome. The four patients were from 23 to 34 years of age. The cervical tumors and ovarian tumors were synchronous findings in two of them. In

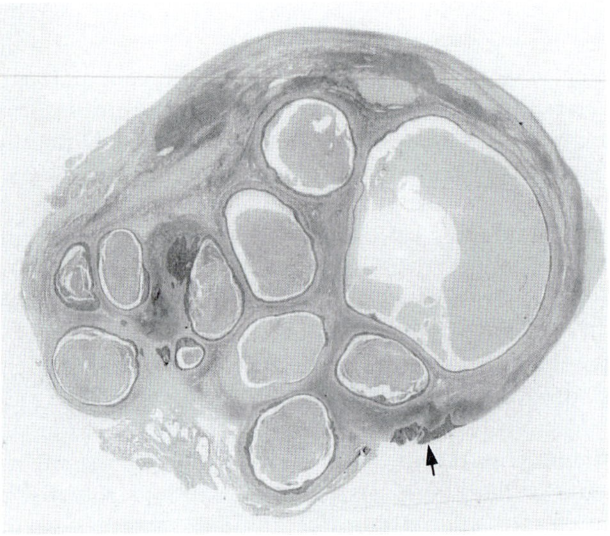

Fig. 22.8. Metastatic squamous cell carcinoma from the cervix. The whole-mount photomicrograph shows the normal-sized ovary containing cystic nests of squamous cell carcinoma. Surface involvement is focally present (*arrow*). In this case the cervical neoplasia was all in situ; there was contiguous spread of the in situ carcinoma to the ovarian surface, and then apparent growth into the underlying parenchyma. (Reproduced by permission of ref. 79.)

the other two, the ovarian tumors were discovered 10 months and 3 years after the cervical tumors. In one final case, a cervical transitional cell carcinoma metastasized to the ovary and was detected before the cervical tumor, which was not discovered until pathologic examination.[125] The ovarian metastatic tumor in this case was a large cystic mass that was indistinguishable microscopically from a primary transitional cell carcinoma of the ovary but was associated with prominent vascular space invasion, suggesting its metastatic nature.

Other Uterine Tumors

Endometrial stromal sarcomas metastasize to the ovary more frequently than *leiomyosarcomas*. In a series of 11 uterine sarcomas that metastasized to the ovary (none of which were autopsy findings), 8 were endometrial stromal sarcomas and 3 leiomyosarcomas.[139] The patients with endometrial stromal sarcomas ranged from 33 to 79 (average, 50) years of age; 5 of them were less than 50 years old. The ovarian metastases accounted for the clinical presentation in 3 of the patients. In 2 patients, the primary uterine tumors were not discovered until 7 months and 10 months after bilateral ovarian tumors had been resected. In 4 of the other cases the ovarian and uterine tumors were found synchronously, and in the remaining 2 the ovarian metastases occurred 4 to 9 years after the uterine neoplasms had been discovered. The ovarian tumors were bilateral in 6 cases and ranged up to 17 cm in greatest dimension. These tumors usually are solid (Fig. 22.9) or solid and cystic, but rarely are they cystic.

The major problem with the interpretation of these tumors on microscopic examination is that, when growing in the ovary, the tongue-like pattern of infiltration characteristic of this neoplasm often is inconspicuous. Other problems result from the presence in some of the tumors of large fibromatous areas that may contain hyaline plaques, a finding that may cause diagnostic problems. Yu et al.[141] described the case of a 24-year-old woman with an ovarian metastatic endometrial–stromal sarcoma that was misinterpreted initially as a thecoma for this reason. In other cases, the ovarian tumors have a diffuse pattern (Fig. 22.10) and in areas their characteristic content of small arteries resembling the spiral arteries of the endometrium is inconspicuous, resulting in a resemblance to a diffuse granulosa cell tumor. Confusion with sex cord–stromal tumors may be heightened by the occasional presence of areas of sex cord-like differentiation in metastatic endometrial stromal sarcomas. However, high-power examination does not show the typical nuclear features of granulosa cell tumors and careful examination usually shows, at least focally, the typical vascular pattern of endometrial stromal tumors

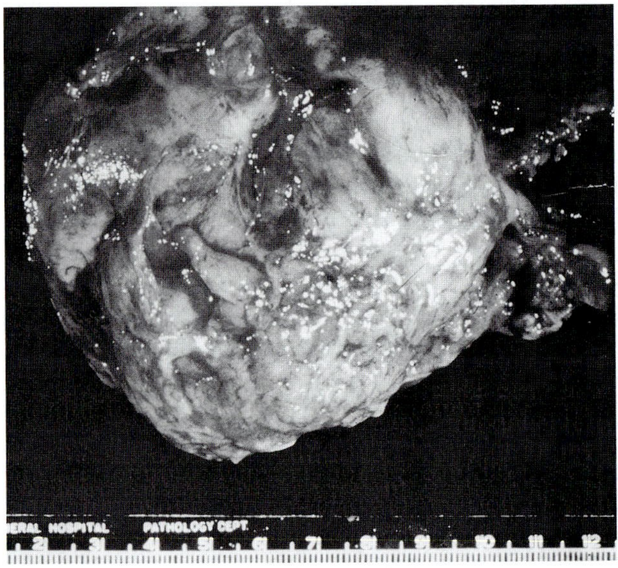

Figure 22.9. Metastatic endometrial stromal sarcoma from the uterus. Several wormlike foci of tumor are visible.

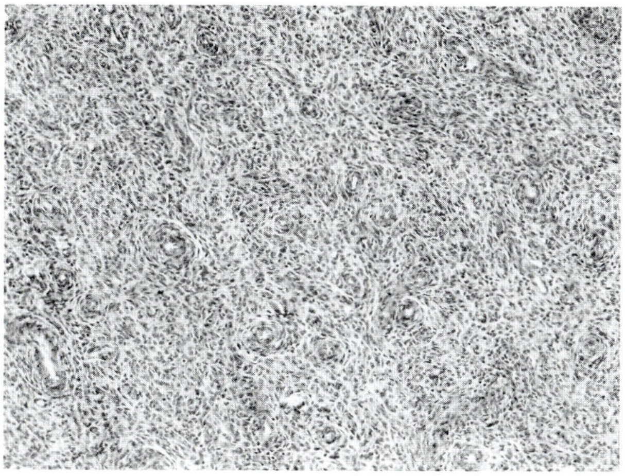

Fig. 22.10. Metastatic endometrial stromal sarcoma from the uterus. The tumor has a diffuse pattern. Note the presence of many characteristic small arterioles.

(Fig. 22.10). Reticulum stains often are helpful in the differential diagnosis showing individual cell investment by fibrils in the endometrial stromal sarcoma and only small amounts, mainly perivascular, in the granulosa cell tumor. Bilaterality also is far more common in the former than the latter as is the presence of extraovarian tumor, examination of which often shows the distinctive growth pattern of endometrial stromal sarcoma.

Metastatic endometrial stromal sarcomas in the ovary must be distinguished from primary endometrioid stromal sarcomas.[132] An association of the tumor with endometriosis is evidence of an ovarian origin; bilaterality favors metastasis. When both organs are involved, it is possible that the tumors may be independent primary tumors in some instances.

Leiomyosarcomas of the uterus with ovarian metastases probably are more common than the rare reports in the literature suggest, particularly in patients with widespread disease. The three leiomyosarcomas with ovarian metastases in our series occurred in patients 35, 44, and 49 years of age.[139] In the first patient a large ovarian metastatic tumor became symptomatic 14 months after hysterectomy. In the second patient, the ovarian metastatic tumor was in the setting of widespread disease. In the third case the ovarian involvement was only microscopic. Ovarian spread of malignant mixed müllerian tumors is common but not a diagnostic problem. Ovarian involvement in cases of müllerian adenosarcoma of the uterus is uncommon and in some cases may be an independent primary.

Gestational choriocarcinoma of the uterus may spread to the ovary, but in the light of known uterine disease is not a diagnostic problem.[3,74] If such an ovarian tumor in a woman of childbearing age is not clearly metastatic from a uterine or tubal choriocarcinoma, thorough sampling may be needed to demonstrate the presence or absence of teratomatous elements. If such elements are not found, it may be difficult or impossible to differentiate between a primary choriocarcinoma of the ovary of either gestational or germ cell origin and a metastatic tumor from a choriocarcinoma of the uterus that has regressed. Invasive hydatidiform mole also has been documented to spread to the ovary, and at least two placental site trophoblastic tumors have spread through the uterine wall to involve an ovary.[1]

Vulvar and Vaginal Tumors

Vulvar and vaginal carcinomas rarely exhibit ovarian spread. Occasional *vaginal clear cell adenocarcinomas* have metastasized to the ovary, in most cases associated with extensive pelvic spread.

Extragenital Tract Tumors

Breast Carcinoma

Ovarian involvement is seen at autopsy in about 10% of cases of *breast cancer*. The metastases are bilateral in approximately 80% of the cases and in approximately two-thirds of all cases, autopsy[109] and surgical combined.[31] Most surgical pathologic experience with ovarian metastases of mammary carcinoma has resulted from examination of ovaries removed to decrease the estrogen level in patients with known spread of the tumor.[56,82,84] In such cases, ovarian involvement has been reported in up to half the cases but is often only a microscopic finding.

It is unusual for metastatic carcinoma of the breast to produce signs or symptoms of an ovarian tumor, and only rarely is the ovarian metastasis evident before the primary tumor is detected.[31,107,122] In a series of 79 ovarian metastases presenting as pelvic or abdominal masses, Johansson[48] found 11 (14%) to be of mammary origin. The ovarian involvement was discovered before diagnosis of the primary tumor in only 1 case; in the remaining 10 cases in that series the ovarian tumors became evident clinically at subsequent intervals ranging from less than 1 year to 16 years. Death occurred within 1 year of the detection of ovarian involvement in all but 1 of the 11 patients. In contrast, Osborne and Pitts[73] recorded a mean survival of more than 20 months after the diagnosis of metastasis in therapeutic oophorectomy specimens. In one large series breast metastases accounted for almost 40% of all metastases, being slightly more common than gastrointestinal tract metastases.[31] However, 22 of the 59 cases of breast metastasis were autopsy findings and 28 were incidental findings in therapeutic oophorectomy specimens. In 4 of the remaining 9 cases, the ovarian metastases were incidental findings during an operation for another indication; in the remaining 5 patients, however, the ovarian metastases caused a mass of sufficient size to be the clinical indication for operation. The ovarian metastatic tumor was detected before the breast cancer in only 1 case. This patient presented with hepatic and ovarian tumors, and her primary breast cancer was not identified until 15 months later. The median interval between the diagnosis of breast cancer and the ovarian metastasis was 11.5 months and was related to the stage of the breast cancer. The median survival after the diagnosis of ovarian metastasis was 16 months. One patient with metastatic breast carcinoma in the ovaries presented 10 years after initial treatment of the breast cancer, as a result of virilization caused by stromal luteinization associated with the ovarian metastasis.[11] Although ovarian metastases of breast cancer usually are accompanied by other foci of abdominal spread, isolated ovarian metastases occasionally are encountered. In one series the metastasis was limited to the ovary in 8 of 59 cases.[31] Lobular carcinomas, including those of signet-ring cell type, spread to the ovary more frequently than those of ductal type; in an autopsy study 36% of the former metastasized to the ovaries in contrast to only 2.6% of the latter.[38]

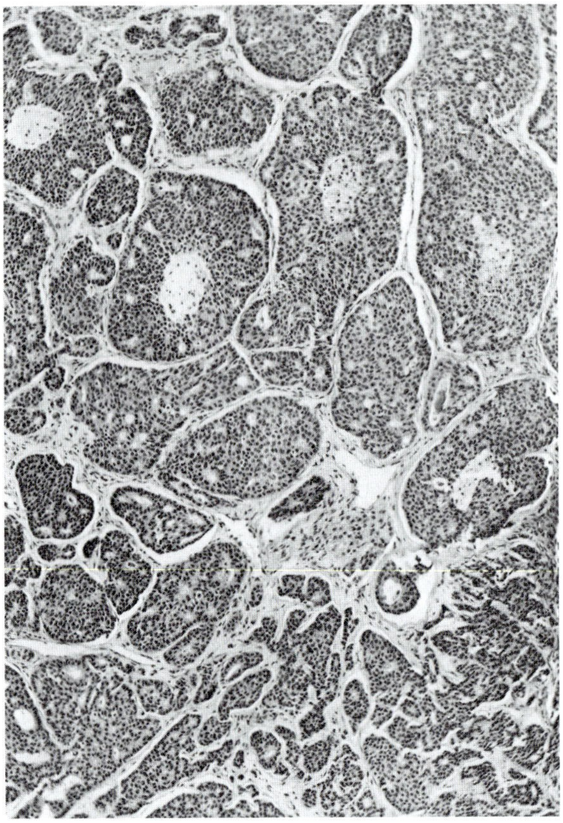

Fig. 22.11. Metastatic ductal carcinoma from the breast. A cribriform pattern is present.

Gross Findings

On gross examination, the visibly involved ovaries often have irregular, nodular surfaces and typically contain firm or gritty, white nodules of various sizes (see Fig. 22.1). When the organ is replaced by tumor, it is transformed into a smooth-surfaced or bosselated mass; exceptionally, it contains cysts and very rarely it is entirely cystic. When all cases are considered tumors larger than 5 cm are uncommon, accounting for only 15% of the cases in one large study.[31]

Microscopic Findings

Microscopic examination reveals the same variety of patterns and cell types that are observed in primary breast carcinomas (Figs. 22.11–22.13). In early examples, small cords and clusters of cells may be found in the ovarian cortex. In premenopausal women, small deposits often are situated in the highly vascular theca interna of a graafian follicle or in the granulosa or theca layer of a corpus luteum. In larger metastatic foci a pattern of tubular glands and nests similar to that of ductal carcinoma is common (Fig. 22.11), as is an Indian-file pattern such as that of lobular carcinoma (Fig. 22.12); such patterns were seen in 42% and 32% of the cases, respectively, in one series.[31] A pure cribriform pattern is infrequent but focal cribriform areas are relatively common. In approximately 10% of the cases, there is a diffuse pattern and occasionally the tumor cells grow as single cells or in clusters.[31] Rarely, papillae are seen. Admixtures of these various patterns may be seen. Signet cells usually are not a conspicuous feature of metastatic breast carcinoma unless the primary tumor is of the relatively uncommon signet-ring type but, rarely, the features of a metastatic breast cancer are those of a typical Krukenberg tumor,[61] as described below; 1.8% of Krukenberg tumors in one series were of breast origin.[118] The stroma of the tumor varies from sparse to abundant; it rarely shows luteinization, no examples being found in one series of 59 cases,[31] in contrast to the stroma of metastatic carcinomas of intestinal origin. Rare tumors with a Krukenberg pattern have been associated with luteinization and evidence of

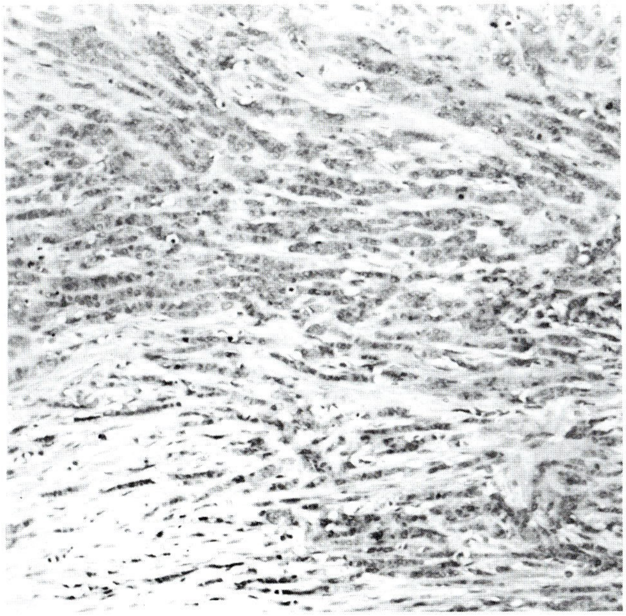

Fig. 22.12. **Metastatic lobular carcinoma from the breast.** An Indian-file pattern is present.

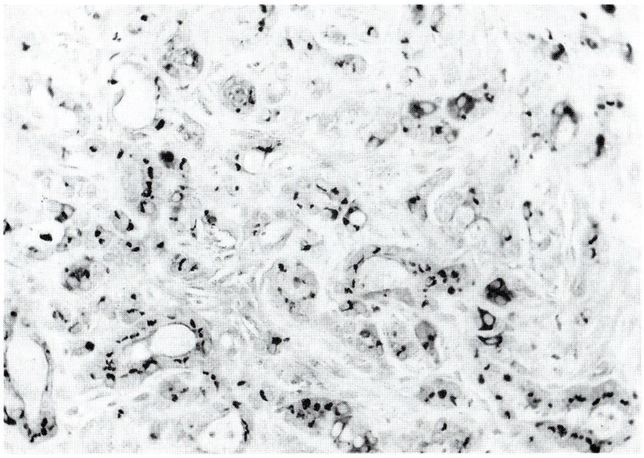

Fig. 22.14. **Metastatic ductal carcinoma from the breast.** A section of the tumor has been stained by the immunohistochemical technique for gross cystic disease fluid protein-15 and is strongly positive.

virilization. Lymphatic invasion was seen in 15% of the cases in one series.[31]

Differential Diagnosis

The differential diagnosis of metastatic breast carcinoma may be difficult, particularly if the primary tumor is remote, or not apparent, or if its existence is not known by the pathologist. Rare, predominantly glandular, tumors may resemble surface epithelial tumors, particularly those of endometrioid type, and the insular pattern may mimic a carcinoid tumor. Exceptionally, a tumor with a diffuse pattern or one with an Indian-file arrangement of the cells simulates a lymphoma or granulocytic sarcoma (chloroma). Metastatic breast carcinomas also have been misinterpreted as granulosa cell tumors (see Fig. 22.13). The growth patterns and characteristics of the neoplastic cells and the clinical features, however, almost always permit their distinction from these and other tumors, but this is occasionally difficult on the evaluation of routinely stained sections alone. It should be remembered that patients with breast cancer have an increased frequency of ovarian carcinoma,[19] and rarely ovarian carcinoma metastasizes to the breast. Staining of an ovarian neoplasm immunohistochemically for gross cystic disease fluid protein-15 (GCDFP-15) may be helpful in distinguishing a metastasis from the breast (Fig. 22.14) from a primary ovarian carcinoma.[68] In one study, 11 of 14 cases (71%) of ovarian metastatic tumors from the breast exhibited strong cytoplasmic staining, usually in a paranuclear pattern; in contrast, 7 ovarian metastases of other tumors and 32 primary ovarian carcinomas failed to stain.[115] Finally, in cases of ovarian involvement by the intraabdominal desmoplastic small round cell tumor,[123] the diagnosis of metastatic breast cancer may be suggested in areas. However, these patients usually are in their teens, when breast cancer is rare, and other more characteristic foci of the tumor and the typical immunohistochemical profile of the former tumor facilitate the interpretation. We have seen one case in which this tumor involved the breast, confusing the picture, but the breast involvement suggested metastasis and the tumor exhibited the characteristic immunohistochemical staining of the desmoplastic small round cell tumor.

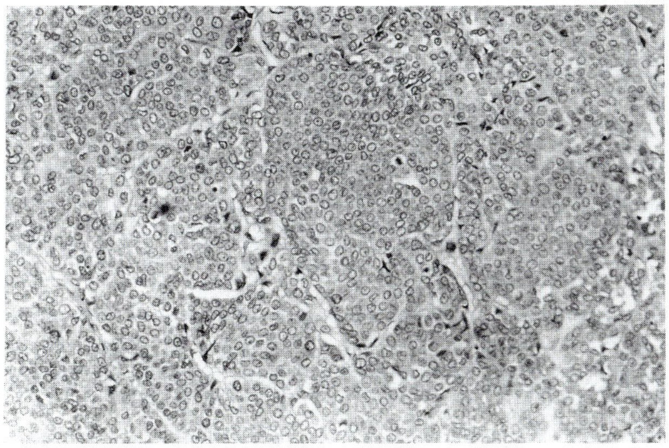

Fig. 22.13. **Metastatic lobular carcinoma from the breast.** An insular growth of small cells with pale nuclei superficially resembles an insular granulosa cell tumor.

Carcinoma of the Stomach, Including Krukenberg Tumor

The great majority of metastatic gastric carcinomas to the ovary are *Krukenberg tumors*,[25,37,42,117] which are defined as tumors characterized entirely or prominently by the presence of mucin-filled signet-ring cells, typically lying within a cellular stroma derived from the ovarian stroma. The source of Krukenberg tumors in 70%–100% of the reported cases is a gastric carcinoma, usually arising in the pylorus. Carcinomas of the large intestine, appendix, and breast are the next most common primary sites; the gallbladder, biliary tract, pancreas, cervix, and urinary bladder are rare sources of these tumors. Saphir[92] demonstrated in an autopsy study that signet-ring cell carcinomas of various organs are associated more often with ovarian metastasis than carcinomas of other histologic types by a ratio of about 4:1. More recent studies have supported his observation; gastric signet-ring cell carcinomas metastasize to the ovary in 41% of the cases whereas intestinal-type carcinomas of the stomach do so in only 17%[35]; signet-ring cell carcinoma of the colon also metastasizes to the ovaries more frequently than does the usual colonic adenocarcinoma.[4]

The frequency of the Krukenberg tumor varies with that of gastric carcinoma in the population analyzed. At the Radiumhemmett, 39% of ovarian metastases presenting as ovarian tumors were of gastric origin, although not specified to be of the Krukenberg type.[48] In a similar series, Krukenberg tumors of gastric origin accounted for approximately 30% of clinically apparent ovarian metastases.[93] In countries such as Japan, with a high prevalence of gastric carcinoma and a low prevalence of primary ovarian carcinoma, the Krukenberg tumor accounts for a large proportion of all ovarian cancers.[118] The average age of patients with Krukenberg tumors is about 45 years. From one-quarter to almost one-half the patients have been under 40 years, and only slightly more than 10% of them have been over 60 years of age. This age distribution is related in part to the disproportionate frequency of gastric signet-ring cell carcinomas in young women as well as the greater vascularity of the ovary in young women. In one study, 10% of women 35 years or younger with this tumor had ovarian metastases at presentation.[104] Almost 90% of patients with Krukenberg tumors have symptoms related to ovarian involvement, the most common of which are abdominal pain and swelling; occasionally, there is abnormal uterine bleeding and rarely overt signs of excess hormone production such as virilization (see Chapter 19, Sex Cord–Stromal, Steroid Cell, and Other Ovarian Tumors with Endocrine, Paraendocrine, and Paraneoplastic Manifestations). The remainder of the patients have gastrointestinal or miscellaneous symptoms or are asymptomatic. A history of prior carcinoma of the stomach or, rarely, another organ can be obtained in 20%–30% of the cases.[37,48] The interval between the diagnosis of a gastric carcinoma and the subsequent discovery of ovarian involvement usually is 6 months or less,[48] but periods as long as 12 years have been reported.[37] In most cases, the diagnosis of the gastric carcinoma is made preoperatively, during the operation for the ovarian metastasis, or within a few months thereafter. Often, the primary tumor is too small to be detected at operation,[42] and radiographic examination of the upper gastrointestinal tract also may fail to reveal evidence of a tumor even after the diagnosis of Krukenberg tumor has been established. Rarely, the gastric carcinoma may not be detected until 5 or more years after discovery of the ovarian metastatic tumor.

Almost all the patients die within a year of the diagnosis of ovarian metastasis, with an average duration of 7 months from diagnosis to death,[37] but a rare patient has survived, apparently free of tumor, for as long as 6 years after gastrectomy and bilateral oophorectomy.[42] Such a result, even though exceptional, justifies removal of both the stomach and the ovarian metastases for possible cure in cases in which the tumor appears limited to those organs. It also is prudent for the surgeon to remove the ovaries routinely in menopausal and postmenopausal women who have a gastric resection for carcinoma so as to prevent the later complication of ovarian metastasis and avoid another operation.

Almost all tumors with microscopic features of the Krukenberg tumor are metastatic, but very rare examples may be primary. Joshi[49] accepted as primary 18 reported cases, including 11 in which autopsy examination revealed no evidence of an extraovarian source, and 7 in which the patient survived for 5–13 years after the removal of the ovarian tumor. These tumors occurred in patients ranging in age from 16 to 61 years, with an average of 38 years. Although a primary Krukenberg tumor probably exists, one should exercise considerable caution before making such a diagnosis or accepting reported cases as valid. Primary carcinomas, particularly those arising in the breast and stomach, may be very small, requiring exhaustive sectioning to detect them, despite the presence of metastases in some cases. It is possible that tiny primary tumors were missed in these or other organs in the reported autopsied cases of "primary" Krukenberg tumors. Ulbright and Roth[106] cited a case observed by Kraus

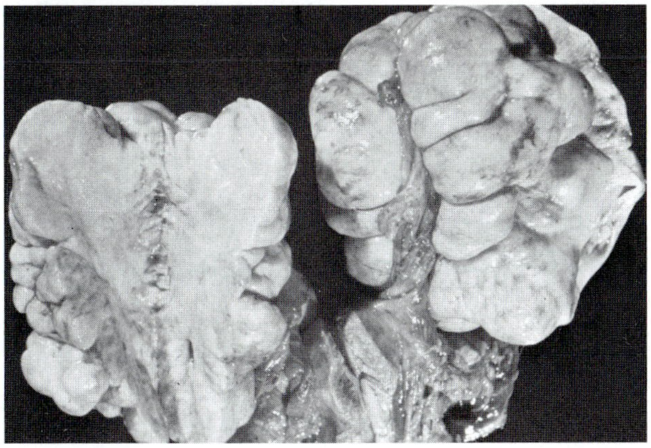

Fig. 22.15. Krukenberg tumor. Bilateral bosselated masses are composed of solid white tissue.

in which a primary tumor in the stomach was detected only after microscopic sections prepared from 200 blocks had been examined. Also, it is well known that mammary and gastric carcinomas may remain silent for many years. We have seen one case of a Krukenberg tumor in which a primary gastric carcinoma did not become apparent until 5.5 years after the ovarian tumor had been removed. Thus, clinical dormancy of the primary tumor probably accounts for some of the cases of Krukenberg tu-

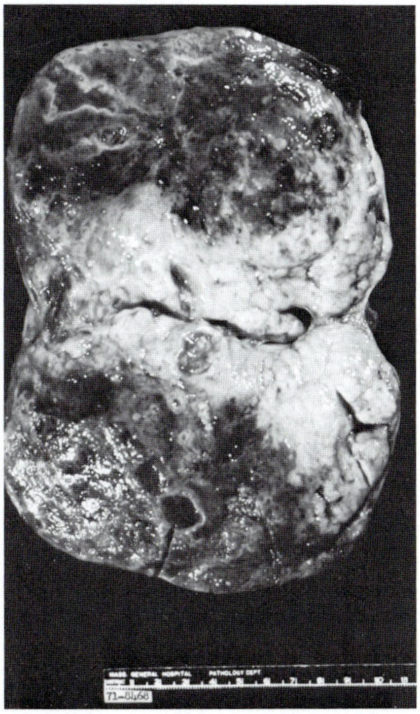

Fig. 22.16. Krukenberg tumor. There is extensive hemorrhagic necrosis.

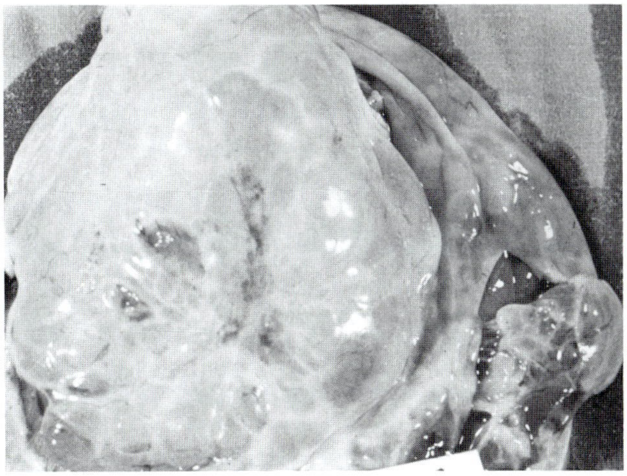

Fig. 22.17. Metastatic carcinoma from the stomach. Multiloculated cystic neoplasm simulates a mucinous cystadenoma.

mor with long survival. As poorly differentiated primary mucinous carcinoids of the ovary may have extensive foci of signet-ring cell proliferation, it is possible that some of the "primary Krukenberg" tumors in the literature may be in that category.

Gross Findings

Krukenberg tumors typically form rounded or reniform, firm, white masses that may be bosselated and may attain a large size. The sectioned surfaces usually are yellow or white (Fig. 22.15) but areas of purple, red, or brown discoloration and extensive hemorrhage also are encountered (Fig. 22.16). The consistency is characteristically firm but fleshy, gelatinous, or spongy areas are common. Occasionally, the gross presentation is atypical with large, thin-walled cysts containing mucinous or watery fluid, separated by relatively small amounts of solid tissue. Both ovaries are involved in 80% or more of the cases. The occasional metastatic gastric carcinoma that is not a Krukenberg tumor may be predominantly solid or predominantly cystic (Fig. 22.17).

Microscopic Findings

Microscopic examination of a Krukenberg tumor reveals mucin-laden, signet-ring cells strewn individually and in small clusters within a cellular ovarian stroma (Figs. 22.18 and 22.19); occasionally the stroma has a storiform pattern. Frequent variations from the classical appearance include small glands, a prominent tubular architecture (Fig. 22.20), mucin-poor tumor cells in trabeculae, and large masses, abundant collagen formation, marked stromal edema (Fig. 22.21), and cell-free pools of mucin in the stroma. Occasionally, small or large cysts

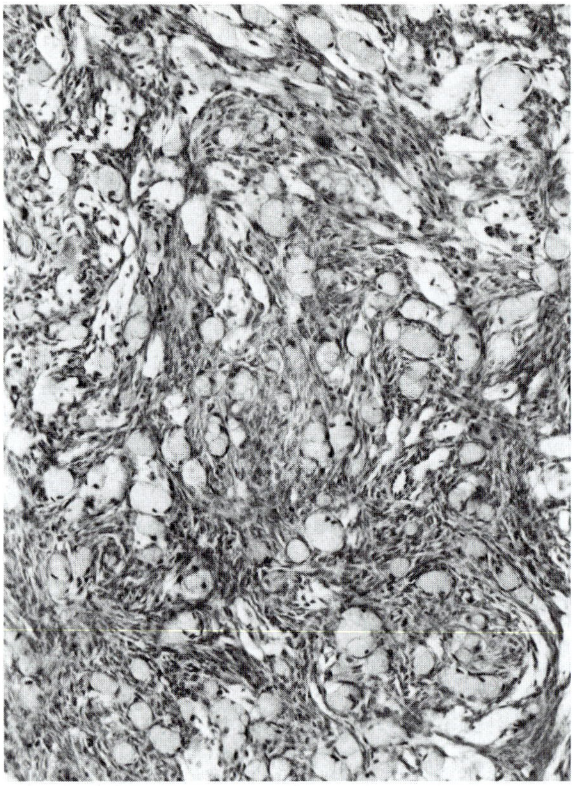

Fig. 22.18. Krukenberg tumor. Numerous signet-ring cells are present within a cellular stroma.

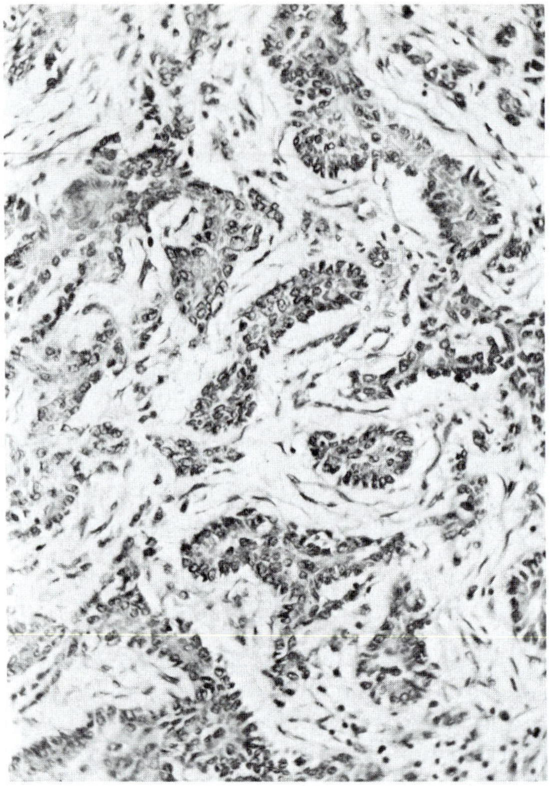

Fig. 22.20. Tubular Krukenberg tumor. The tubules simulate those of a Sertoli–Lydig cell tumor. Signet-ring cells are not evident in this illustration.

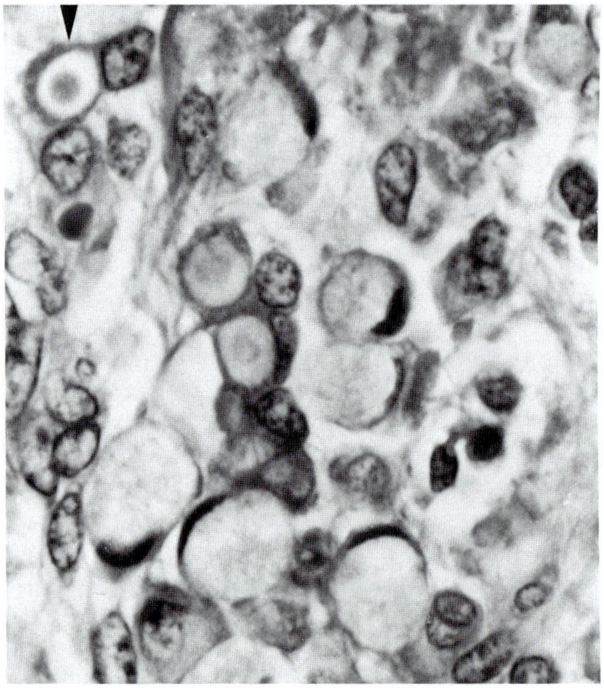

Fig. 22.19. Krukenberg tumor. Signet-ring cells with eccentric nuclei and abundant pale cytoplasm. In one cell a droplet of mucin with a targetoid appearance is present (*arrow*). (Reprinted by permission of Scully RE (1979) Tumors of the ovary and maldeveloped gonads. In: Atlas of Tumor Pathology, second series, fascicle 16. Armed Forces Institute of Pathology, Washington, DC.)

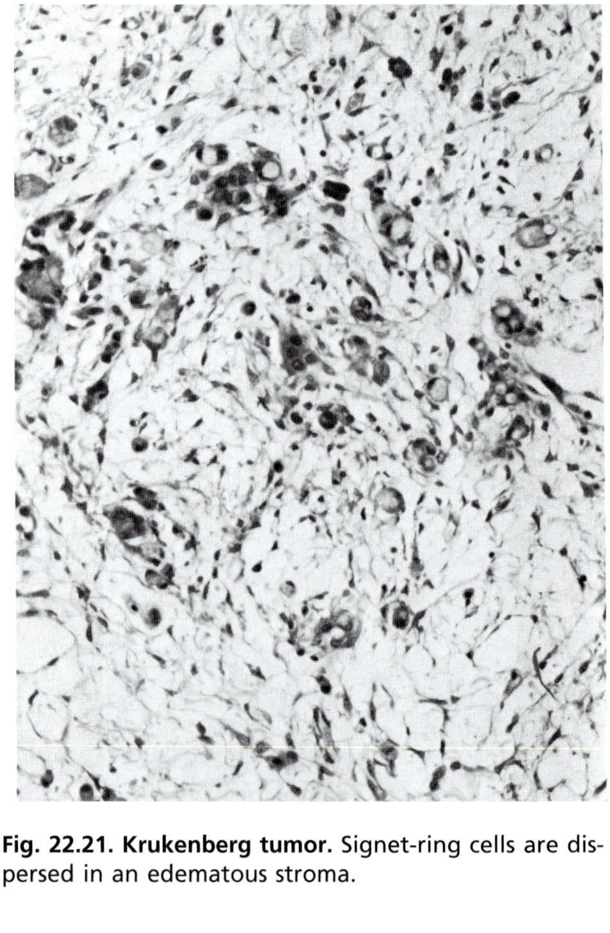

Fig. 22.21. Krukenberg tumor. Signet-ring cells are dispersed in an edematous stroma.

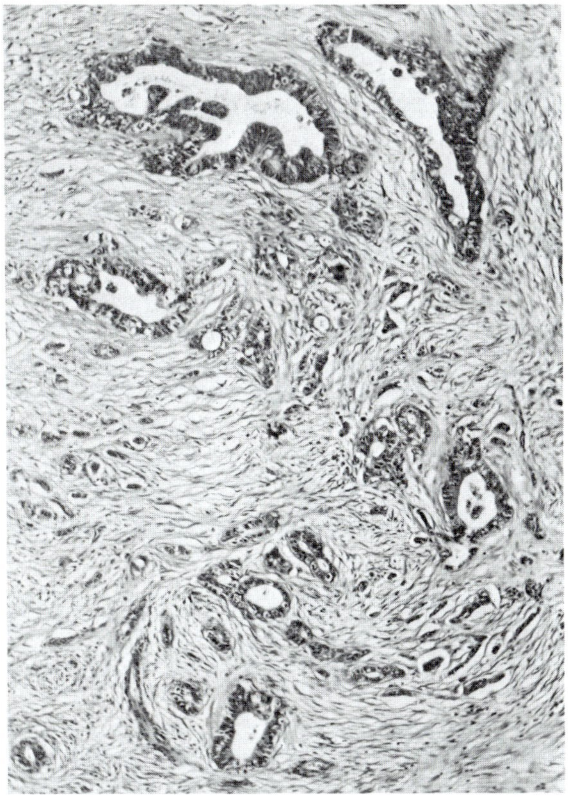

Fig. 22.22. Metastatic carcinoma from the stomach. Glands of varying sizes and shapes and small clusters of tumor cells lie in a fibrous stroma.

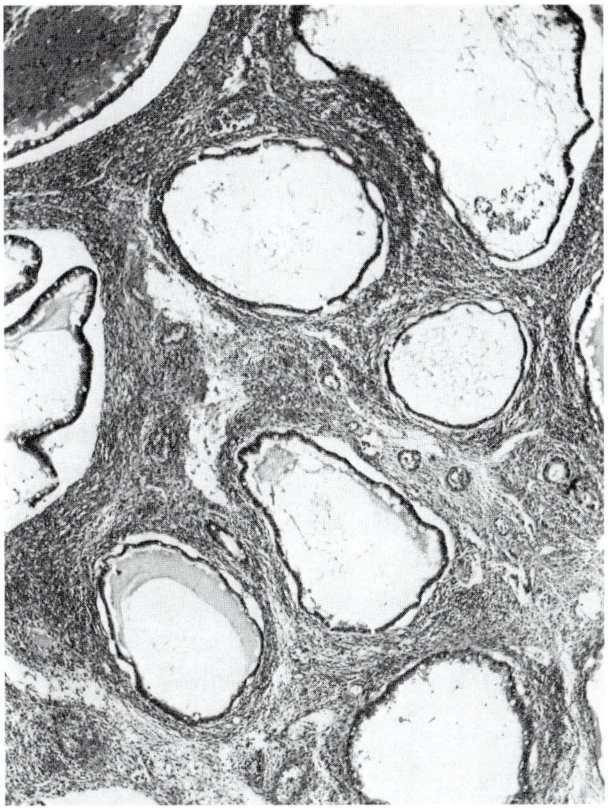

Fig. 22.23. Metastatic carcinoma from the stomach. Cystic glands are separated by stroma lacking tumor cells. Same case as shown in Fig. 22.22. ×50.

lined by minimally atypical-appearing mucinous epithelium forms a conspicuous component of the tumor, with more characteristic areas lying between the cysts. The cytoplasm of the signet-ring cells occasionally is granular and eosinophilic rather than pale and vacuolated; the cytoplasm sometimes has a bull's-eye appearance, containing a large vacuole with a central eosinophilic body (Fig. 22.19). As with metastases in general, blood vessel and lymphatic invasion is common. Lutein cells occasionally are present in the stroma, particularly if the patient is pregnant (see Chapter 19). Although most metastatic gastric carcinomas to the ovary have the characteristics of a Krukenberg tumor, occasional examples do not and may be composed of glands of intestinal type in varying degrees of differentiation (Fig. 22.22) that occasionally are cystically dilated (Fig. 22.23), as well as sheets and irregular aggregates of poorly differentiated carcinoma cells.

Differential Diagnosis

The Krukenberg tumor may resemble a fibroma or any other type of solid ovarian tumor on gross examination. Its appearance also occasionally may be deceptive on frozen section or low-power examination[68] (Fig. 22.24) but should be readily diagnosable on high-power microscopic examination, especially with the aid of mucin stains. A frequent misdiagnosis is a Sertoli–Leydig cell tumor, particularly when a prominent tubular component and luteinization of the stroma are encountered in a Krukenberg tumor[9]; signet-ring cells, however, are not a feature of Sertoli–Leydig cell tumors except for occasional tumors of heterologous type (see Chapter 19). The sclerosing stromal tumor may contain cells resembling signet cells as well as a proliferating fibroblastic component, but such cells contain lipid rather than mucin. The rare signet-ring stromal tumor also may enter the differential diagnosis (see Chapter 19), but the signet-ring cells in that tumor also fail to react with mucin stains.

In clear cell carcinomas, the clear cells contain glycogen; mucin, when present, is typically luminal and extracellular. In rare cases portions of the tumor contain signet-ring cells but the presence of other characteristic features of this tumor permit its identification. Primary mucinous tumors may contain signet-ring cells but rarely in great number, and

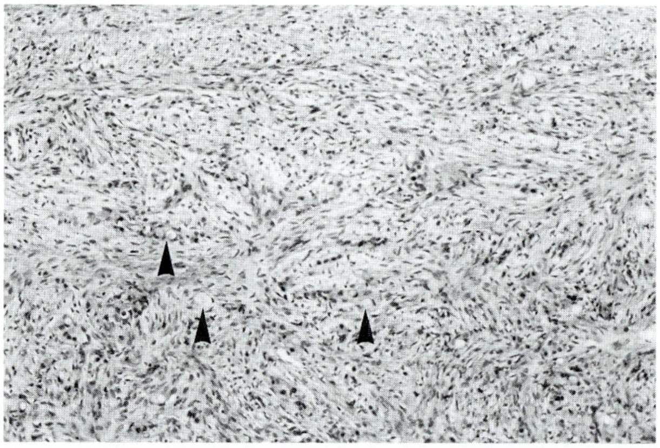

Fig. 22.24. Krukenberg tumor. At this magnification the appearance is similar to that of an ovarian fibroma, but occasional signet-ring cells are evident on careful inspection (*arrows*). (Reproduced by permission of ref. 135.)

confusion with a Krukenberg tumor is rarely a realistic problem. Mucinous carcinoid tumors that contain large numbers of signet-ring cells are distinguished from Krukenberg tumors by their additional component of carcinoid, the presence of which can be confirmed by special stains. These tumors are discussed further in the section on metastatic carcinoid tumor. Finally, the rare nonneoplastic lesion, mucicarminophilic histiocytosis,[53] which is caused by injection of substances containing polyvinylpyrrolidine, is characterized by signet-ring-like cells and may involve numerous tissues and organs including the ovaries. Although these cells are stained by mucicarmine, they are periodic acid–Schiff (PAS) negative.

Intestinal Carcinoma

Most metastatic ovarian tumors of intestinal origin are from the large intestine, with occasional examples of small intestinal derivation.[48,76] Three of the small number of clear cell adenocarcinomas of the intestine that spread to the ovaries were primary in the small intestine.[128] Ovarian metastases from intestinal carcinomas have been reported to be less common than those from gastric carcinomas at autopsy, 14% versus 38%, respectively,[92] but when malignant ovarian tumors encountered at the time of operation are evaluated, metastases from intestinal carcinomas are almost five times as frequent as those from gastric carcinomas.[2,7,48,66,93,112,114] Lash and Hart[55] have estimated that up to 45% of large intestinal metastases to the ovary are thought clinically to be primary ovarian tumors and many are misinterpreted as such on pathologic examination, even when there is a known intestinal cancer.

Approximately 4% of women with intestinal cancer have ovarian metastases at some time during the course of their disease,[7,33] but in one study this figure was as high as 10% when the ovaries were cut into 2-mm slices.[33] Four of the six metastatic ovarian tumors in that series of 58 cases were not recognized on gross examination. Metastasis from the large intestine to the ovary is seen relatively more frequently when this cancer occurs in women under 40 years of age (in 18–27% of the patients in this age group).[80]

From a clinical point of view, patients with this type of metastatic carcinoma fall into three categories: (1) patients who present with an intestinal carcinoma (50%–75% of the cases), which antedates diagnosis of the ovarian tumor by as much as 3 years in 90% of the cases, (2) patients in whom ovarian involvement is found unexpectedly during an operation for resection of an intestinal carcinoma, and (3) patients whose initial manifestations are those of an ovarian tumor (3%–20% of the cases). Ovarian metastases have been found in up to 8% of patients who have bilateral prophylactic oophorectomy because of intestinal carcinoma.[62] It has been estimated that routine preoperative barium X-ray examination of the large intestine in women suspected of having an ovarian tumor would be positive for carcinoma in approximately 1 or 2 of 1000 cases. In one study, 77% of the intestinal primary tumors were in the rectum or sigmoid colon, 5% in the descending colon, 9% in the ascending colon, and 9% in the cecum.[55] Occasional patients with an intestinal metastasis have endocrine symptoms because of the presence of luteinized stromal cells in the ovarian tumor with resultant hormone production.

Webb et al.[112] reported a 5-year survival of 5% after treatment of ovarian metastases from gastrointestinal carcinomas. Routine removal of the ovaries in menopausal and postmenopausal women having intestinal resections for carcinoma is indicated to prevent the later development of symptoms of ovarian metastasis and avoid another operation, which has been necessary in up to 7% of these patients.[7] There is no evidence, however, that prophylactic oophorectomy enhances the overall survival rate.

Gross Findings

Metastatic ovarian carcinomas of intestinal origin, which are bilateral in approximately 60% of the cases, may form solid masses (Fig. 22.25), but are more often predominantly cystic (Figs. 22.3 and 22.6); frequently they are large, with a median largest dimension in one series of 11 cm,[55] and may simulate closely primary carcinomas of the ovary

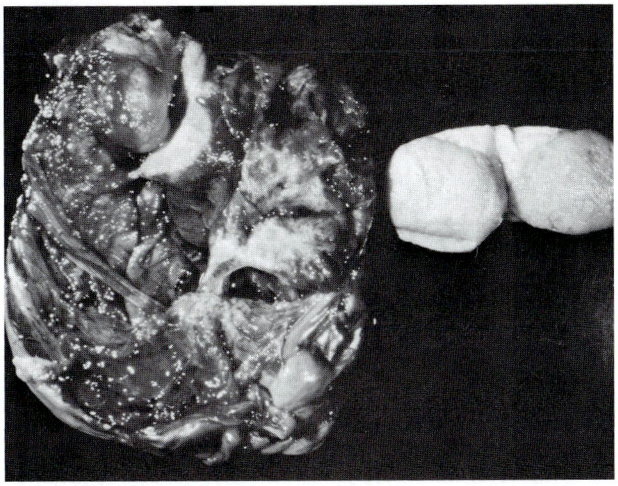

Fig. 22.25. **Metastatic carcinoma from the colon.** The smaller tumor is solid and buff-colored. The larger tumor is cystic with extensive hemorrhage and necrosis. (Reprinted by permission of Scully RE (1979) Tumors of the ovary and maldeveloped gonads. In: Atlas of Tumor Pathology, second series, fascicle 16. Armed Forces Institute of Pathology, Washington, DC.)

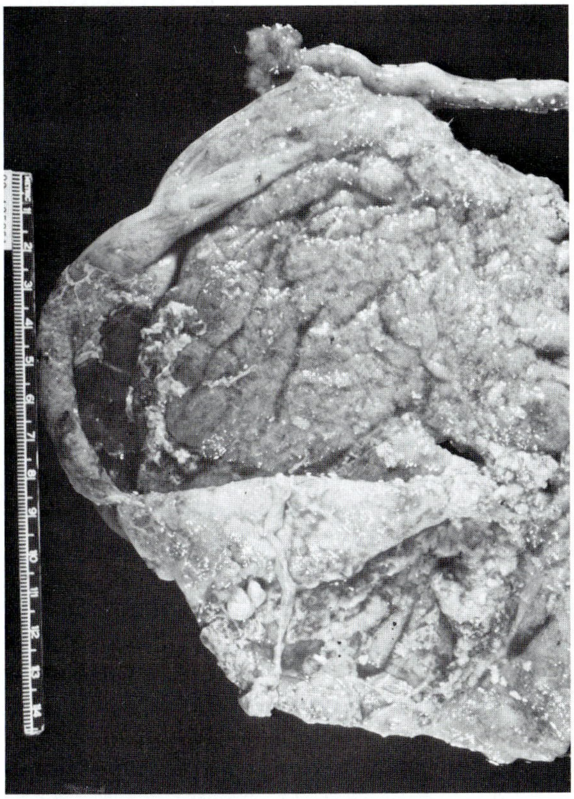

Fig. 22.26. **Cystic metastatic carcinoma from the colon.** The cyst is lined by shaggy necrotic tumor tissue.

(see Fig. 22.3). They may be much larger than the small primary tumor in the intestine. Sectioning typically reveals friable or mushy yellow, red, or gray tissue with cystic compartments that contain necrotic tumor (Fig. 22.26), mucinous or clear fluid, or fresh or old blood. Approximately 10% of the tumors rupture spontaneously during pelvic examination or removal. An occasional example is composed of multiple, thin-walled cysts filled with mucinous or clear fluid (see Fig. 22.3).

Microscopic Findings

The neoplastic cells characteristically grow in patterns similar to those of primary intestinal carcinomas of usual type (Figs. 22.27 and 22.28), typically forming small or large glands with a frequent cribriform pattern; mucin-containing cells including goblet cells may be scattered among mucin-free cells, the latter usually predominating or being the exclusive cell type. Glands and cysts lined by well-differentiated mucin-rich cells may be a prominent component of the tumor (Fig. 22.29) and rarely the tumor has the pattern of colloid carcinoma. Necrosis is common and often extensive, forming striking eosinophilic masses containing nuclear debris within the lumens (see Fig. 22.26); this feature, referred to as dirty necrosis, was present in all the cases in one series.[55] Two other features of the tumor, the frequent disposition of glands in a ring at the edge of the necrotic material (likened to a garland) and focal segmental necrosis of the glandular

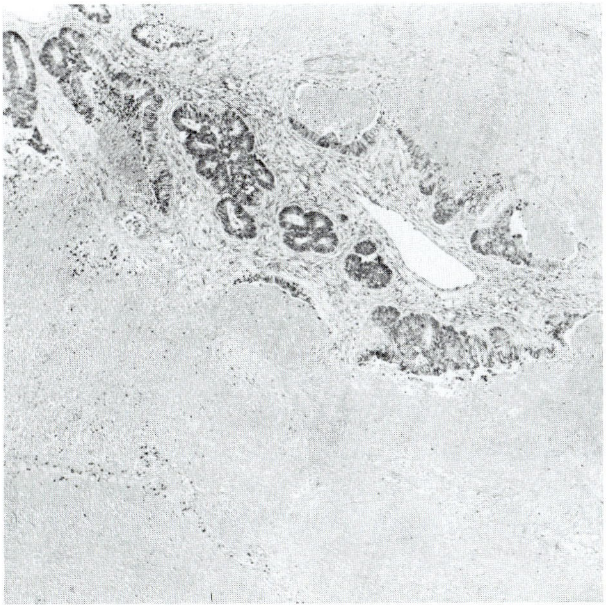

Fig. 22.27. **Metastatic carcinoma from the colon.** There is extensive necrosis.

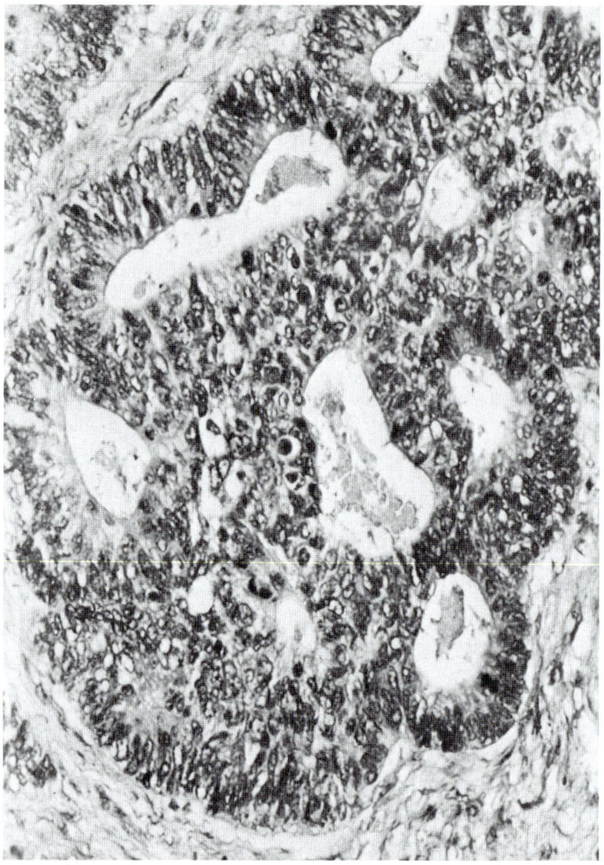

Fig. 22.28. Metastatic carcinoma from the colon. The shape of the glands suggests an endometrioid adenocarcinoma but they are lined by more poorly differentiated stratified epithelial cells than usually seen in gland-forming endometrioid tumors.

epithelium, were emphasized by Lash and Hart.[55] The stroma varies from negligible to abundant; it may be desmoplastic, edematous, or mucoid, but often resembles ovarian stroma, containing cells re-

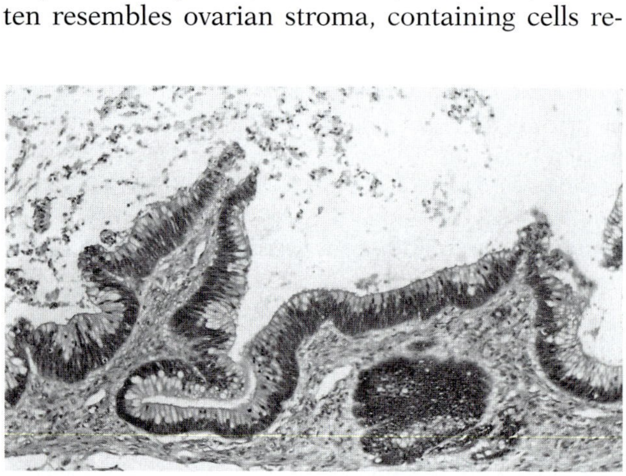

Fig. 22.29. Metastatic carcinoma from the colon. The mucinous epithelium in this illustration is indistinguishable from that of a primary mucinous borderline tumor. (Reproduced by permission of ref. 135.)

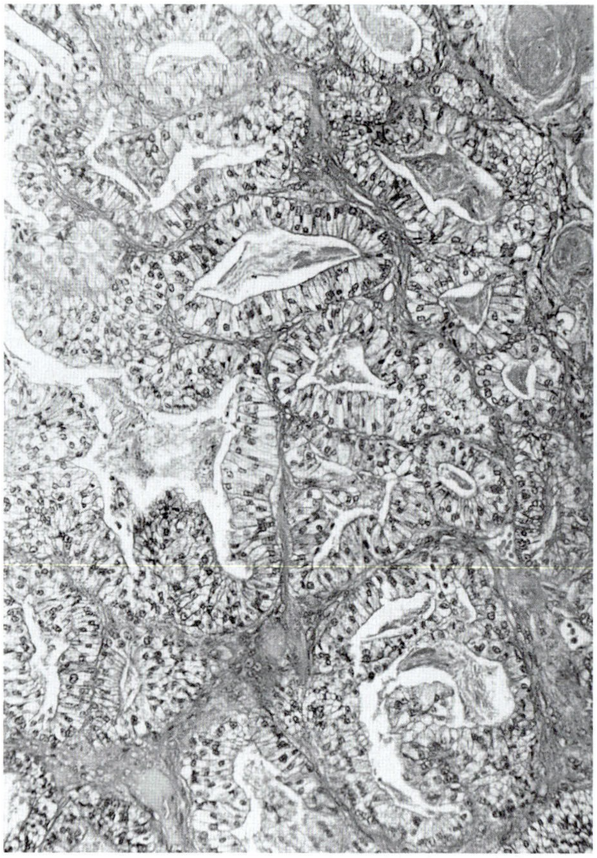

Fig. 22.30. Metastatic carcinoma, clear cell type, from the small intestine. Note the conspicuous clear cytoplasm.

sembling theca externa cells or theca-lutein cells in one-quarter to one-third of the cases.[55,107]

The tumors metastatic from intestinal clear cell adenocarcinomas have a glandular pattern architecturally similar to that of the usual intestinal adenocarcinoma metastatic in the ovary, including dirty necrosis.[128] In a few of them, a colloid-like secretion has been conspicuous. These tumors, however, differ in the conspicuous clear cytoplasm of the tumor cells (Fig. 22.30). In some instances the clarity is subnuclear, imparting a resemblance to the secretory variant of endometrioid carcinoma, but in most the closest resemblance is to clear cell adenocarcinoma.

Signet-ring cell carcinomas of the colon may form typical Krukenberg tumors; 5.4% of the latter originated in the sigmoid colon in one large series.[118] Three cases of intestinal small cell carcinoma with ovarian metastases have been reported.[27]

Differential Diagnosis

In one series, more than two-thirds of the cases of metastatic intestinal carcinoma were misinterpreted initially as primary ovarian adenocarcinomas.[107] The most difficult tumors to exclude on microscopic examination are primary endometrioid and mucinous adenocarcinomas.[22,55] In the series of 22 metastatic intestinal cancers described by Lash and Hart,[55] 19 mimicked endometrioid carcinoma, 2 mucinous carcinoma, and 1 a mixed endometrioid and mucinous carcinoma. Aside from clinical clues, gross features may be helpful in the differential diagnosis. The usual bilaterality of metastatic intestinal carcinomas contrasts with the less than 15% frequency of bilateral involvement in cases of primary endometrioid and mucinous carcinomas. A confusing gross feature of metastatic intestinal carcinomas is the presence of solid masses and cysts lined by necrotic debris and thin-walled cysts with smooth linings. These cysts occasionally are so numerous as to suggest a primary benign or borderline mucinous cystic tumor (see Fig. 22.3). Endometrioid adenocarcinomas often are cystic but the cysts are sometimes filled with chocolate material, the presence of which is generally related to a background of endometriosis, and a more homogeneous, less often necrotic, solid component usually is present.

With regard to the microscopic differential diagnosis of metastatic intestinal adenocarcinoma and endometrioid adenocarcinoma, the glands of the former typically are lined by more poorly differentiated cells with greater degrees of nuclear hyperchromatism and loss of polarity (see Fig. 22.28) than those of endometrioid adenocarcinomas with similar degrees of glandular differentiation. In addition, extensive confluent necrosis is common in metastatic intestinal carcinomas (see Fig. 22.27), being present in 50% of the tumors in the series of Lash and Hart,[55] but uncommon in gland-forming endometrioid carcinomas. A similar comment pertains to so-called dirty necrosis within gland lumens, but it should be emphasized that this and the other features correctly emphasized by Lash and Hart[55] as typical of metastatic intestinal carcinoma, such as focal segmental necrosis of glandular lining epithelium, may be seen in some cases of endometrioid carcinoma.[23] Foci of squamous differentiation are frequent in endometrioid carcinomas, but extremely rare in intestinal carcinomas, and an adjacent or background adenofibromatous component or endometriosis strongly favors endometrioid carcinoma. The features just summarized and the general features of metastatic tumors to the ovaries in general, as well as, of course, clinical findings, aid in the uncommon problem of differentiating a metastatic clear cell adenocarcinoma from the intestines from a primary secretory endometrioid adenocarcinoma or clear cell adenocarcinoma.

In cases in which the differential is between a metastatic intestinal adenocarcinoma and primary mucinous adenocarcinoma, the frequent presence of glands and cysts lined by endocervical-type mucinous cells with basal nuclei favors a primary ovarian mucinous carcinoma over a metastasis, although, as already mentioned, differentiated glands and cysts are encountered in some metastatic intestinal carcinomas. Although goblet cells are encountered more commonly in primary mucinous carcinomas, they also may be seen in metastatic mucinous tumors. Other typical features of metastatic disease in the ovary already discussed are helpful in many cases but in occasional cases it may be impossible to make a differential diagnosis of metastatic versus primary mucinous adenocarcinoma on the basis of examination of the ovarian tumor alone. As emphasized by Lash and Hart,[55] the differential diagnosis of metastatic intestinal adenocarcinoma is most commonly with an endometrioid, as opposed to mucinous, carcinoma. Metastatic mucinous carcinomas are more characteristically from the pancreas although they can be from diverse sites. In one series eight metastatic mucinous adenocarcinomas were from the pancreas, six from the colon and rectum, three from the endocervix, two from the stomach, one possibly from the appendix, and one from the esophagus.[86] Other primary sites of metastatic mucinous carcinomas include the gallbladder and even urachus (see below).

In the occasional cases in which consideration of these criteria for the distinction of a primary endometrioid or mucinous carcinoma from a metastatic carcinoma of the large intestine do not yield a confident diagnosis, additional evidence may be obtained, particularly in the case of nonmucinous lesions, by the use of immunohistochemical staining for CA-125, cytokeratin (CK) 7, CK 20, HAM 56, and CEA.[6,14,15,18,20,30,59,60,66,67,77,83,110,111] Positive staining for CEA and CK 20 is typical of metastatic intestinal adenocarcinomas in the ovary but unusual in nonmucinous primary ovarian carcinomas such as endometrioid carcinoma. In contrast, although not specific, positive staining for CA-125, CK 7, and HAM 56 is much more typical of a primary as opposed to metastatic carcinoma in the ovary.

Tumors of the Appendix

Ovarian metastases from appendiceal tumors may be seen in cases of frankly invasive adenocarcinomas of the usual intestinal and, typical mucinous types,[88] as well as colloid and signet-ring cell carcinomas, and carcinoids. Almost all the latter are of the mucinous (goblet cell) type (adenocarcinoids). Finally, ovarian involvement is common in cases of low-grade mucinous epithelial tumors of the appendix that microscopically resemble borderline mucinous tumors of the ovary and often have the gross features of a so-called mucocele.

The largest proportion of cases of spread of tumor from the appendix to ovary are in the last category,[81,89,126] but some interpret the ovarian tumor in such cases as an independent primary tumor,[95] and the relation between the ovarian and mucinous tumors in these cases, in which pseudomyxoma peritonei is typically present, has been controversial. The appendiceal and ovarian tumors are usually synchronous. Laparotomy typically discloses cystic ovarian tumors that are often bilateral, average about 16 cm in diameter, and usually are multilocular (Fig. 22.31). The appendix is usually dilated, often covered with mucus, and there is typically abundant intraabdominal mucus. The ovarian and appendiceal tumors are typically similar, having histologic features similar to those of mucinous cystadenomas (Fig. 22.32) and cystic tumors of borderline malignancy. In many of the ovarian tumors, mucin dissects into the ovarian stroma (pseudomyxoma ovarii), and the mucinous cells typically are taller than those seen in ovarian mucinous tumors encountered in women without pseudomyxoma peritonei. The typical synchronous presentation of the ovarian and appendiceal tumors, their histologic similarity, the frequent bilaterality of the ovarian tumors, and the predominance of right-sided ovarian involvement in unilateral cases favors spread to the ovary. An argument against this is the failure to detect rupture of the appendiceal tumor in many of the cases. However, the site of rupture of an appendiceal tumor of this type may be very small and require extensive sectioning to demonstrate; such examinations have not been performed in most of the cases in which a site of rupture has not been identified. Additionally, in some cases a rupture site heals over and is represented only by fibrosis in the appendiceal wall. Another argument against independent primary tumors in the appendix and ovary is the infrequency of their coexistence in the absence of pseudomyxoma peritonei.

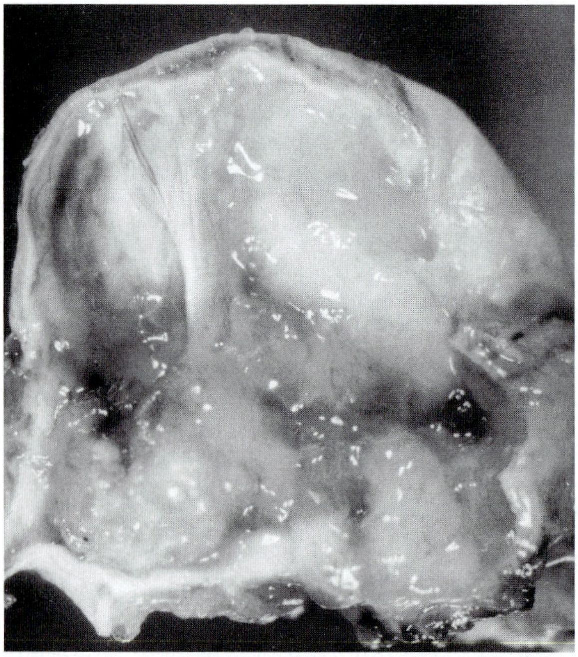

Fig. 22.31. Mucinous cystic tumor of ovary in patient with borderline mucinous cystadenoma of appendix. The thin-walled cyst is filled with jelly-like material. (Reproduced by permission of ref. 126.)

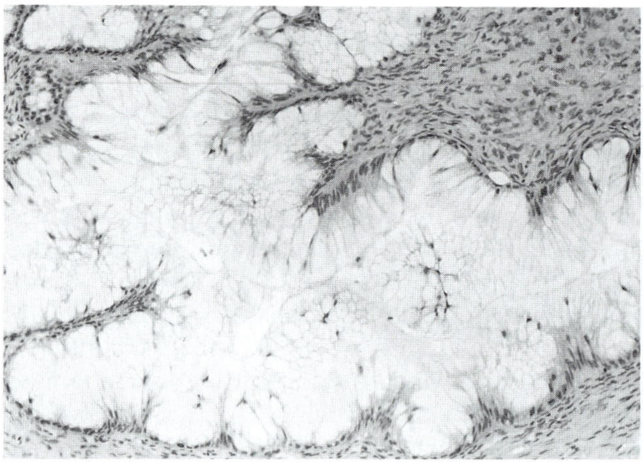

Fig. 22.32. Mucinous cystic tumor of ovary in patient with borderline mucinous cystadenoma of appendix. The tumor is characterized by tall, stratified mucinous cells with minimal atypia.

Seidman and his associates[95] reviewed 25 cases of coexistent ovarian and appendiceal lesions and presented the following evidence for an independent primary origin of the tumors. In 6 of their cases, the tumors coexisted in the absence of pseudomyxoma peritonei; in 13 cases, the tumor in one organ appeared to be of a different degree of malignancy than that in the other organ; and in two-thirds of the cases there was a lack of complete concordance of immunocytochemical staining of the ovarian and appendiceal tumors for four antigens.

There have been several other immunohistochemical studies investigating the association of synchronous appendiceal and ovarian mucinous tumors. Guerrieri et al.[36] examined 10 cases, all associated with pseudomyxoma peritonei, and found 6 of them to be negative for cytokeratin 7 at both sites on immunohistochemical staining, supporting an appendiceal origin. However, in the other 4 cases, both sites were cytokeratin 7 positive, leaving the possibility that at least some of the tumors may have originated in the ovary or were examples of cytokeratin 7-positive appendiceal primaries. Ronnett et al.[90] did a similar study with a panel of antibodies including cytokeratins 7, 18, and 20 as well as HAM-56 and CEA. The majority of cases with pseudomyxoma peritonei (10/14) showed an identical pattern in the appendiceal and ovarian tumors of negative staining for cytokeratin 7 and HAM-56 and positivity for cytokeratins 18–20 and CEA, supporting a primary appendiceal tumor.

Molecular studies have examined clonality in synchronous ovarian and mucinous tumors by looking at mutations in K-*ras* and loss of heterozygosity (LOH) at multiple genetic loci. Chuaqui et al.[16] studied LOH at three loci in 12 cases with synchronous tumors. Three of the cases showed an identical mutation pattern between the appendix and ovary suggesting a common origin, but an additional 3 showed different mutation patterns between the appendix and ovary, raising the possibility that a subset may represent independent primary tumors. The remaining 6 cases were negative for mutations at any of the three loci studied. The differing results may be complicated by the morphologic heterogeneity of the cases studied.

Szych et al.[100] studied 16 cases with the typical picture of pseudomyxoma peritoneii and morphologically similar synchronous ovarian and appendiceal mucinous tumors. They found all to have identical K-*ras* mutations in the ovarian and appendiceal tumors, suggesting a common origin, and demonstrated additional mutations in the ovarian tumor in 5 cases, likely related to tumor progression following spread to the ovary. Cuatrecasas et al.[18] had similar findings, with 5 of 6 cases showing identical c-Ki-*ras* mutations in the appendiceal and ovarian tumors. The weight of evidence, both conventional gross and microscopic as well as immunohistochemical and molecular, in our opinion, favors spread of the low-grade mucinous cystic tumors of the appendix to the ovaries in these cases.

Irrespective of the relation of the ovarian and appendiceal tumors in these cases, it is important from the practical point of view for the pathologist to carefully examine specimens of peritoneal mucin in these cases for mucinous epithelial cells because the prognosis appears to be better in their absence. The epithelium in the peritoneal mucin in these cases is typically in the form of glands and cysts lined by epithelium with atypia that equates to that seen in mucinous borderline tumors of the ovary. It has not had the degree of atypia seen in cases of frank mucinous carcinoma with peritoneal spread, although the clinical picture in the latter may also be that of pseudomyxoma peritonei.[91]

Ovarian spread has occurred in 18 cases of mucinous carcinoid.[12,41,45,64] In 13 of the cases the ovarian metastatic tumor was found at presentation, and in 11 of these cases the patient presented with an ovarian mass; in 3 cases the ovary was the only known site of metastasis. In 5 patients, ovarian spread occurred after disease-free intervals of 6 months to 8 years. In cases of metastatic mucinous carcinoid, the distinction from a primary mucinous carcinoid may be difficult, and criteria similar to those discussed next are helpful in the differential diagnosis. Only very rare pure carcinoids of the appendix have been reported to spread to the ovary.[43]

For the most part, the interest in ovarian disease in cases of appendiceal neoplasms has centered on the foregoing issues of low-grade mucinous cystic tumors and mucinous carcinoid tumors. However, recently Ronnett and colleagues[88] have emphasized that conventional invasive appendiceal adenocarcinomas of various types may be associated with striking ovarian spread with a tendency for the primary appendiceal nature of the disease in these cases to be overlooked, the ovarian tumors sometimes being considered primaries, or metastatic from sites other than the appendix. In her series of 20 cases, the ovarian tumors were bilateral in 16 cases and were similar histologically to the associated appendiceal tumor in every case. Some of the ovarian tumors had signet-ring cell, glandular, and goblet cell features that suggested metastasis from a gastric adenocarcinoma; those that were well-differentiated mucinous adenocarcinomas often suggested a possible primary in the pancreas or biliary tract; and the remainder, being of intestinal type, suggested a primary intestinal adenocarcinoma. As is the usual situation with intestinal-type adenocarcinomas metastatic to the ovary in general, the latter catergory of cases were sometimes mistaken for primary ovarian endometrioid carcinoma. The conventional clinical, gross, and microscopic features of metastatic spread to the ovary in general already summarized, as well as the immunohistochemical features already mentioned, in combination, should faciliate the establishment of the correct diagnosis in these cases.

Carcinoid Tumors

Carcinoid tumors account for approximately 2% of metastases that form ovarian masses, and a similar percentage of small intestinal carcinoids greater than 1 cm in diameter spread to the ovary. Although most metastatic carcinoids are of small intestinal origin, rarely the primary tumor originates in the appendix (in this case mucinous carcinoids as just noted), colon, stomach, pancreas, or lung.[8,87,107,131,137] In the largest series of carcinoids metastatic to the ovary, the age of the 35 patients ranged from 21 to 82 years, with a median of 57 years; almost all were older than 40 years.[87] Ten of the tumors in that series were not diagnosed until autopsy. Forty percent of the women whose metastases were discovered at operation had preoperative manifestations of the carcinoid syndrome. Some of them also had signs and symptoms referable to intestinal or ovarian involvement. Extraovarian metastases were found in at least 90% of the cases, a figure that contrasts with the rarity of similar spread of primary ovarian carcinoids. The primary site usually was in the ileum, but the cecum, jejunum, appendix, and pancreas were sources in occasional cases.[87] One-third of the patients died within 1 year and three-fourths of them within 5 years after unilateral or bilateral salpingo-oophorectomy, which was accompanied by a hysterectomy and an intestinal operation in some of the cases. Six of the 25 patients, however, were asymptomatic for a median period of 5 years postoperatively; all 4 patients with the carcinoid syndrome had postoperative relief, 2 for periods of more than 3 years after the removal of the ovarian tumors.

In view of the occasional complications of ovarian metastasis, menopausal or postmenopausal patients with gastrointestinal carcinoids should have a bilateral oophorectomy even in the absence of obvious ovarian involvement to prevent the subsequent growth of occult metastases or the appearance of new metastases. Whenever bilateral ovarian carcinoids are detected, a careful search for an extraovarian primary tumor should be instituted. Both the metastases and the primary tumor, if found, should be excised whenever feasible. In a young woman with a unilateral neoplasm, careful examination of the intestine and its mesentery and other organs for a primary tumor, biopsy of the opposite ovary if enlarged, a thorough search for teratomatous elements in the tumor, and postoperative radiologic studies and measurement of 5-hydroxyindole acetic acid in the urine may be necessary before a determination of the primary or metastatic nature of the tumor and selection of appropriate therapy is made. Because the primary tumor in the intestine may be very small, it may not be detected by radiologic studies for a year or more after the diagnosis of the ovarian metastasis.

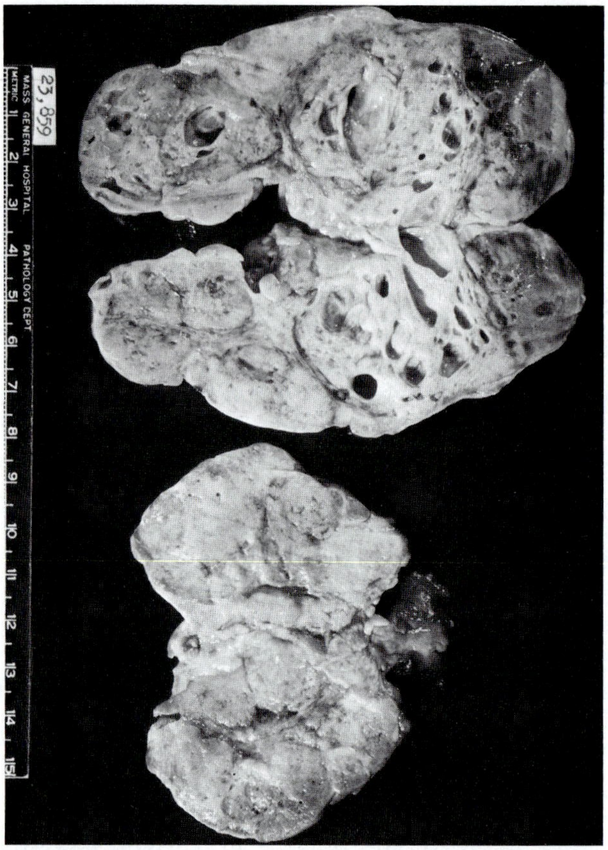

Fig. 22.33. Metastatic carcinoid. The larger tumor contains multiple cysts simulating a cystadenofibroma. (Reprinted by permission of Scully RE (1979) Tumors of the ovary and maldeveloped gonads. In: Atlas of Tumor of Pathology, second series, fascicle 16. Armed Forces Institute of Pathology, Washington, DC.)

Gross Findings

Metastatic carcinoids may be large and typically are predominantly solid, with smooth or bosselated surfaces (Fig. 22.33). Sectioning reveals single or confluent firm, white or yellow nodules, which may resemble ovarian fibromas or thecomas; cysts of varying size (Fig. 22.34) occasionally are present and typically are filled with clear, watery fluid, resulting in a gross appearance similar to that of a cystadenofibroma (Fig. 22.33); focal necrosis and hemorrhage may occur (Fig. 22.34). Most of these tumors are bilateral in contrast to primary ovarian carcinoids, which are almost always unilateral.

Microscopic Findings

The microscopic features of metastatic carcinoids are similar to those of primary ovarian carcinoids except that teratomatous elements are not encountered, multinodularity often is prominent, and vascular invasion occasionally is observed. An insular pattern is most common (Figs. 22.35 and 22.36) but trabecular, mixed, and rarely solid tubular patterns (Fig. 22.37) also are encountered. Acini, which typically are uniformly small and round, are common

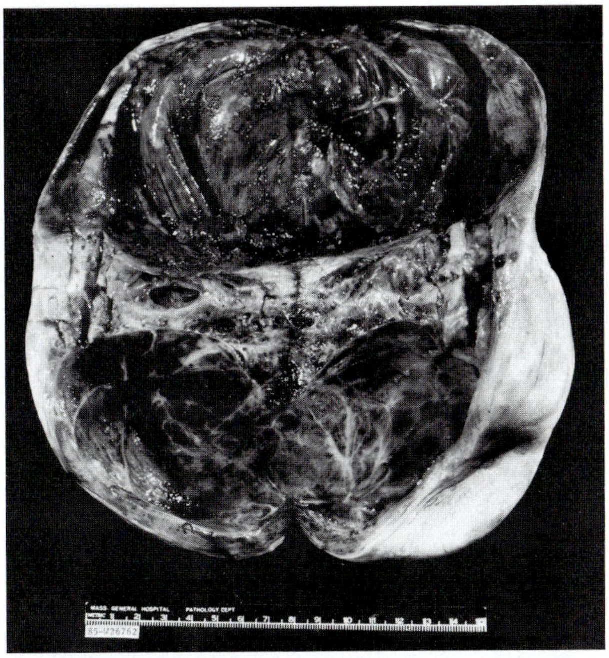

Fig. 22.34. Metastatic carcinoid. The tumor is predominantly cystic with extensive hemorrhage.

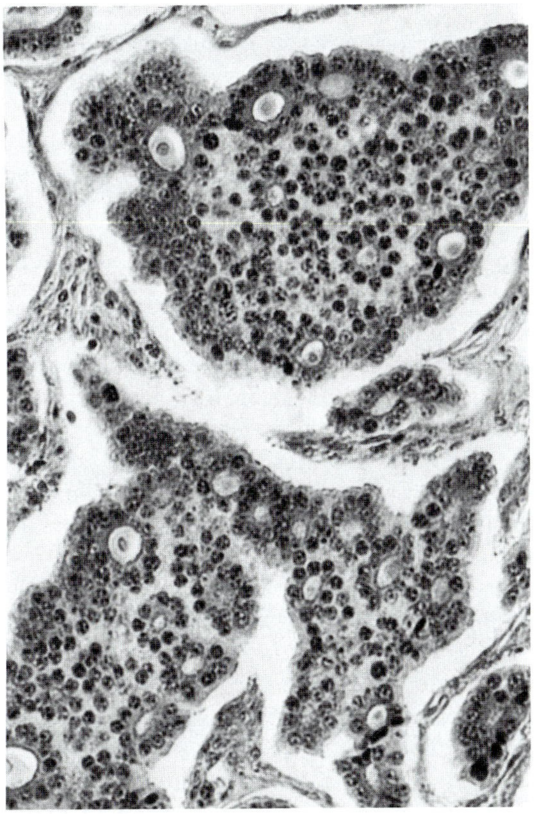

Fig. 22.35. Metastatic insular carcinoid. The gland lumens have smooth, rounded outlines; the nuclei are round with evenly distributed, coarse chromatin.

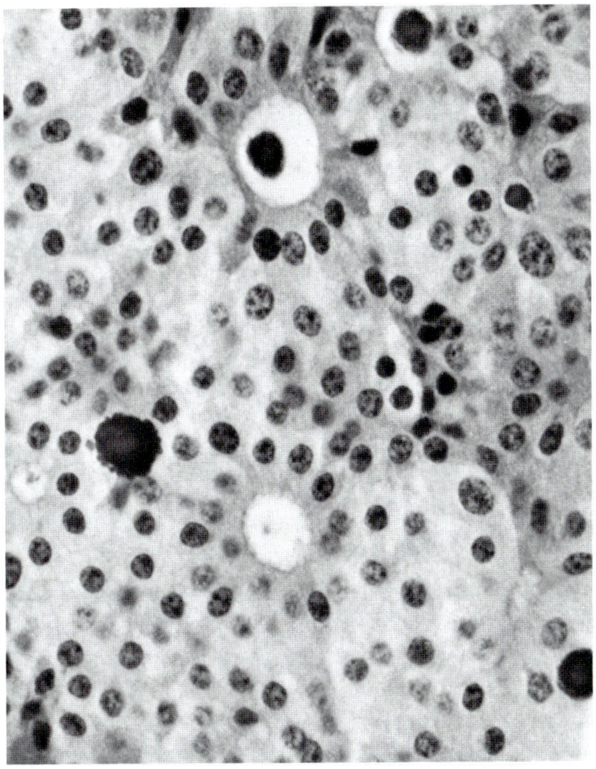

Fig. 22.36. Metastatic insular carcinoid. Several lumens contain dark calcified secretion.

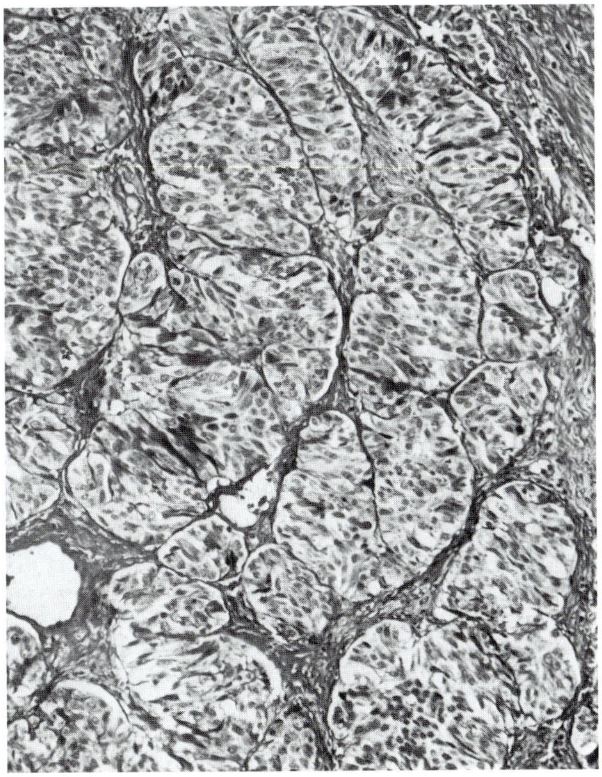

Fig. 22.37. Metastatic carcinoid. A solid tubular pattern simulates a Sertoli cell tumor.

(Fig. 22.35); they often contain a homogeneous eosinophilic secretion that may undergo calcification (Fig. 22.36), sometimes in the form of psammoma bodies. Large glands and cysts lined by one or a few layers of neoplastic cells sometimes are seen (Fig. 22.38). With rare exceptions the carcinoid is the only ovarian metastatic tumor that elicits an extensive stromal proliferation which closely resembles an ovarian fibroma; occasionally this stroma becomes extensively hyalinized (Fig. 22.39). Metastatic carcinoids of mucinous (goblet cell) type, which are almost always of appendiceal origin, have rounded nests containing goblet cells and argentaffin or argyrophil cells are present (Fig. 22.40). These tumors also may have foci resembling a Krukenberg tumor as well as cystic glands filled with mucin.

Differential Diagnosis

Metastatic carcinoids may be confused with a number of tumors other than primary carcinoid tumors, including granulosa cell tumors, Sertoli or Sertoli–Leydig cell tumors, Brenner tumors, adenofibromas and cystadenofibromas, whether benign or borderline, and adenocarcinomas of various types. The microfollicular granulosa cell tumor often is confused with a metastatic carcinoid. The Call–Exner body of the granulosa cell tumor may resemble the acinus of the carcinoid when it is filled with eosinophilic dense basement membrane material, but it often differs by containing watery, eosinophilic fluid and shrunken nuclei in its lumen. Examination of the neoplastic cells is the most helpful clue to the correct diagnosis. The cells of a microfollicular granulosa cell tumor usually have scanty cytoplasm and ovoid, angular, or round nuclei that typically are pale and grooved. The cells typically are haphazardly oriented with respect to one another and the cavities of the Call–Exner bodies.

In contrast, the cells of carcinoid tumors characteristically have round nuclei with coarse chromatin, and their cytoplasm often contains prominent red or red-brown argentaffin granules. The sex cord-like formations of Sertoli–Leydig cell tumors may resemble the ribbons of the trabecular carcinoid but the latter usually are longer and thicker and have a more orderly architecture. The tubules of Sertoli or Sertoli–Leydig cell tumors may simulate the acini of insular carcinoids. Further confusion may be caused by the presence of a carcinoid component, which

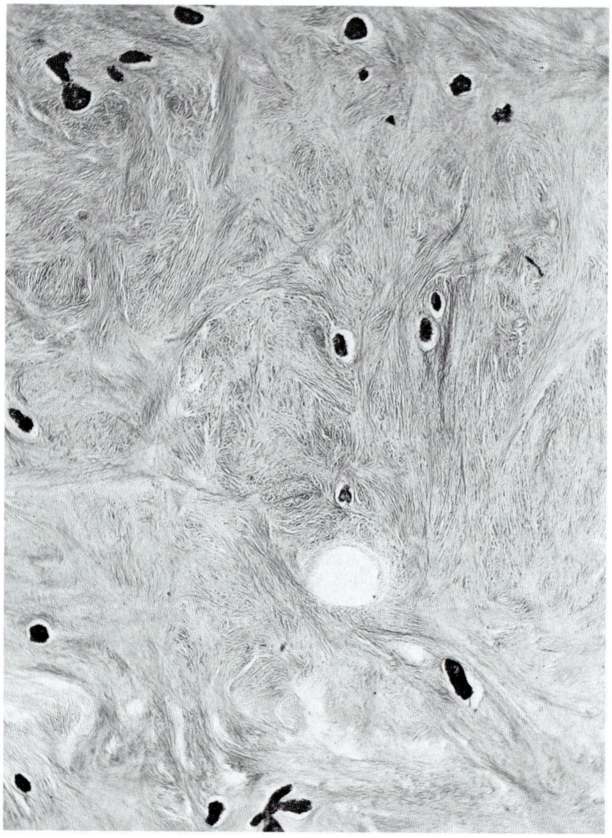

Fig. 22.39. Metastatic carcinoid. There is abundant hyalinized stroma.

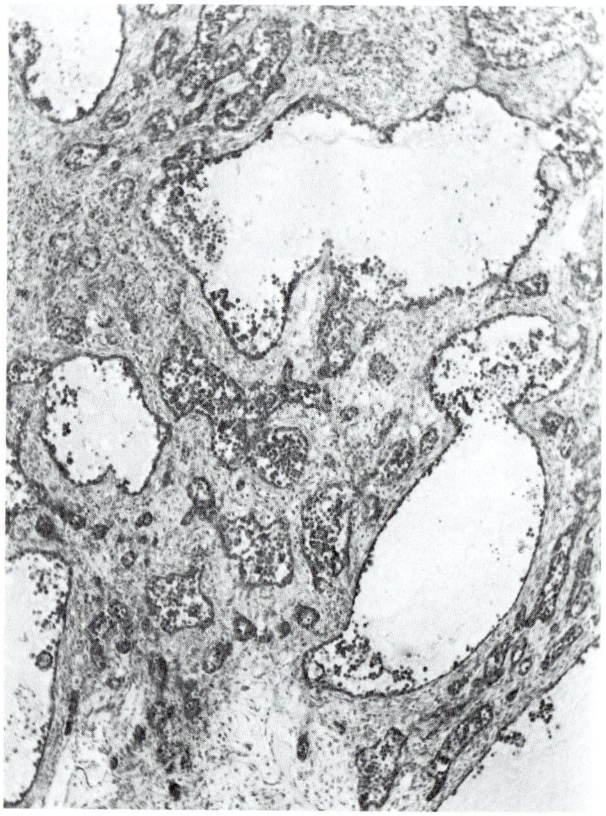

Fig. 22.38. Metastatic carcinoid. Cysts are lined by one or a few layers of neoplastic cells.

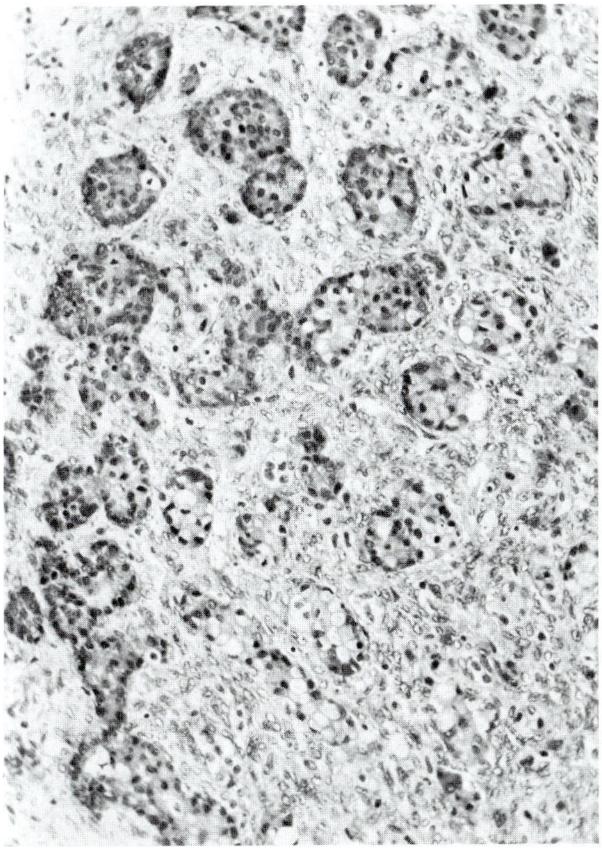

Fig. 22.40. Metastatic mucinous carcinoid. Nests containing cells with dense cytoplasm, which contained argentaffin granules and signet-ring cells.

typically is minor in extent, in a Sertoli–Leydig cell tumor with heterologous elements. The presence of other distinctive patterns of Sertoli–Leydig cell tumor and attention to the characteristic cytologic features of carcinoid cells, however, should enable one to make the correct diagnosis.

The fibromatous stroma of a Brenner tumor often is indistinguishable from that of a carcinoid but the epithelial nests of the former contain cells of urothelial type with oval, pale, grooved nuclei rather than cells with the characteristic features of carcinoid tumors. Benign and malignant adenofibromatous tumors and endometrioid adenocarcinomas containing small tubules and acini are generally readily distinguished from carcinoids by recognition of the differing patterns and cytologic features of these tumors. As mentioned earlier, a metastatic breast carcinoma with a prominent insular pattern may simulate a carcinoid tumor (see Fig. 22.11). Rarely, an adenocarcinoma of the pancreas with a microglandular pattern metastasizes to the ovary and, in the absence of a known pancreatic primary tumor, prompts an initial diagnosis of probable metastatic carcinoid. If the diagnosis of a carcinoid tumor is difficult, more thorough sampling, histochemical staining for argentaffin and argyrophil granules, immunohistochemical staining for chromogranin, neuron-specific enolase, peptide hormones, and serotonin, and electron microscopy for dense-core granules should resolve the differential diagnosis. It must be emphasized, however, that some of the other tumors already mentioned on occasion may contain scattered cells that stain for these substances and contain dense-core granules.

Metastatic mucinous carcinoids may contain foci of adenocarcinoma and be difficult to distinguish from pure metastatic adenocarcinomas unless the characteristic pattern of the mucinous carcinoid is recognized and the presence of argentaffin or argyrophil cells is confirmed by special staining. Adenocarcinomas of the stomach, intestine, and ovary may contain scattered argentaffin or argyrophil cells, and the diagnosis of mucinous carcinoid should be reserved for cases in which the distinctive pattern of that tumor is present. Distinction of a metastatic mucinous carcinoid from the rare primary mucinous carcinoid of the ovary may be difficult and depends on knowledge of the distribution of disease and the presence or absence of teratomatous elements; bilaterality and extraovarian spread strongly favor a metastasis.

Tumors of the Pancreas

Spread of pancreatic carcinoma to the ovary was considered uncommon until relatively recently, but recent experience indicates that it is more common than was previously thought and that it has almost certainly been responsible for the miscategorization of some metastatic tumors in the ovary as primary mucinous carcinoma and even sometimes as mucinous borderline tumors. Seven pancreatic adenocarcinomas that spread to the ovary and mimicked primary mucinous tumors of the ovary were reported in detail in 1989.[127] The patients were 29 to 87 (average, 63) years of age. The ovarian and pancreatic tumors were discovered synchronously in five patients. In two patients, the pancreatic tumor preceded the ovarian tumor by 9 months and 8.5 years, respectively. The clinical presentation simulated that of primary ovarian carcinoma in four patients. The ovarian tumors were typically large, cystic, and multiloculated (Fig. 22.41); six of them were bilateral and the status of the contralateral ovary was not known in the remaining case. Subsequently, pancreatic primaries accounted for 7 of 82 nongenital cancers that spread to the ovary in one large se-

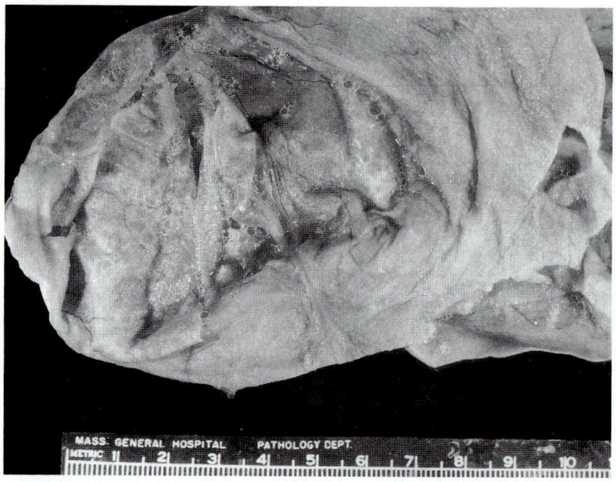

Fig. 22.41. Metastatic carcinoma from the pancreas. The multiloculated cystic ovarian tumor is indistinguishable from a primary mucinous cystic tumor.

ries,[78] and in another recent series of metastatic mucinous carcinomas the single greatest number of cases, 8, originated in the pancreas.[86]

Microscopic examination in these cases shows varying degrees of differentiation, but usually foci resemble mucinous cystadenoma (Fig. 22.42), mucinous cystic tumor of borderline malignancy, and moderated or well-differentiated mucinous cystadenocarcinoma (Fig. 22.43). The pancreatic tumors are usually typical ductal adenocarcinomas cases but may be mucinous cystadenocarcinomas. A number of features are helpful in distinguishing between a primary and metastatic mucinous tumor in these

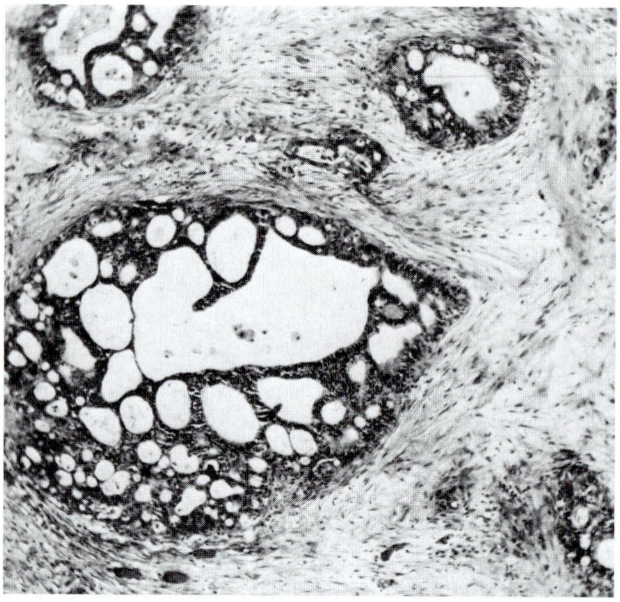

Fig. 22.43. Metastatic carcinoma from the pancreas. There is a prominent cribriform pattern.

cases. The usual bilaterality of the ovarian tumors strongly favors metastasis. A helpful finding in many cases is the presence of desmoplastic implants of carcinoma on the ovarian surface and in the superficial ovarian cortex. The clinical findings often aid and the frequent presence of abdominal spread is most consistent with spread to the ovary in cases of bilateral ovarian mucinous carcinomas. We have seen two adenocarcinomas of the pancreas with microglandular features that had ovarian metastases (Fig. 22.44), one of which accounted for the clinical

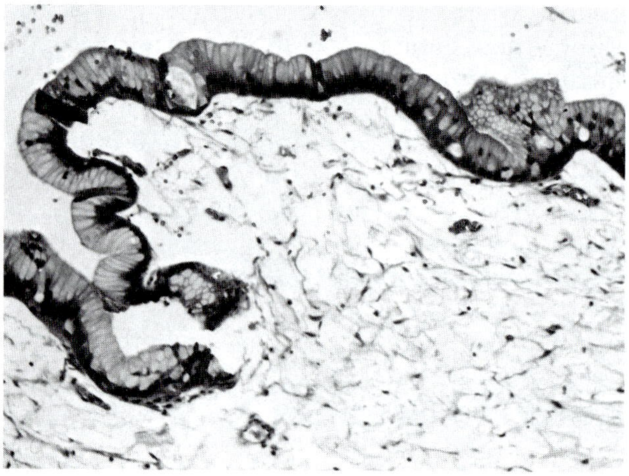

Fig. 22.42. Metastatic carcinoma from the pancreas. Cysts lined by only slightly atypical mucinous epithelium were a prominent component of this neoplasm. Same neoplasm as that in Fig. 22.43.

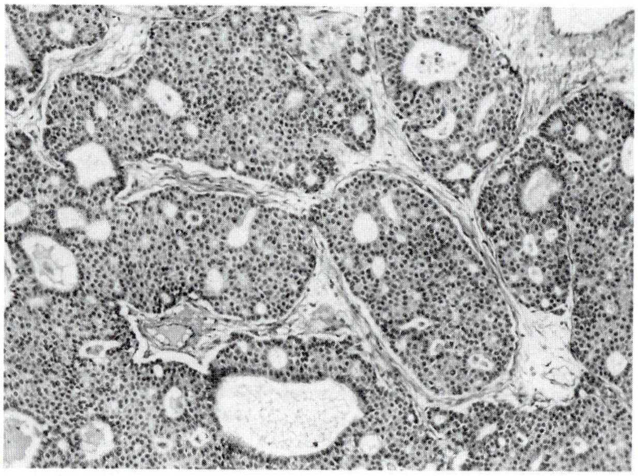

Fig. 22.44. Metastatic microadenocarcinoma from the pancreas. Islands of tumor cells contain numerous small acini. The tumor mimics a carcinoid tumor. (Reproduced by permission of ref. 135.)

presentation. These tumors, as already noted, may mimic a carcinoid tumor, primary or metastatic, but are negative with silver stains. Most series of Krukenberg tumors do not contain any of pancreatic origin, but 6% of these tumors in one series were primary in the pancreas.[118] A probable example of islet cell carcinoma metastatic to the ovaries has been reported.[113]

Tumors of the Gallbladder and Bile Ducts

Ovarian metastases of biliary tumors occasionally are clinically significant. Seven such cases have recently been reported.[54,138] The patients ranged from 33 to 72 (average, 55) years of age. In one case the ovarian tumor was discovered 5 weeks before a gallbladder carcinoma was detected; in four cases the gallbladder tumors and ovarian metastases were discovered simultaneously, and in two cases the ovarian metastases were recognized 1 and 2 years after the biliary tumors, respectively. The ovarian tumors were bilateral in six cases, and in one case the metastatic tumor was a large multiloculated cystic tumor, simulating a primary mucinous tumor of the ovary, and in another case the ovarian tumors were "cystic masses."[54] The remaining neoplasms were uniformly or predominantly solid, usually had lobulated external surfaces, and often were multinodular on section. The ovarian tumors in three of these cases posed problems in differential diagnosis. One of them closely simulated an endometrioid carcinoma; the neoplasm that simulated a mucinous tumor grossly also simulated one on microscopic examination (Fig. 22.45); and, finally, one neoplasm initially raised the question of a Sertoli–Leydig cell tumor. The general features of metastatic involvement of the ovaries were helpful in the evaluation of these cases.

Tumors of the Liver

Spread of hepatocellular carcinoma to the ovary is even rarer than that of pancreatic and biliary tumors, but four clinically important cases recently have been reported.[124] The patients ranged from 31 to 67 (average, 43) years of age. One patient had bilateral ovarian tumors discovered at the same time as the liver tumor. In another patient, the liver tumor was discovered by radiologic investigation after bilateral ovarian tumors had been removed. In the other two cases unilateral ovarian tumors were discovered 3 and 7 months, respectively, after the liver tumors had been detected.

The ovarian neoplasms ranged from 4 to 11 cm in diameter and three of them were solid (Fig. 22.46). Microscopic examination has shown features characteristic of hepatocellular carcinoma (Fig. 22.47) except for one case, in which cysts were prominent. The major differential diagnosis in these cases involves both primary and metastatic hepatoid tumors of the ovary.[124] In most cases of hepatoid

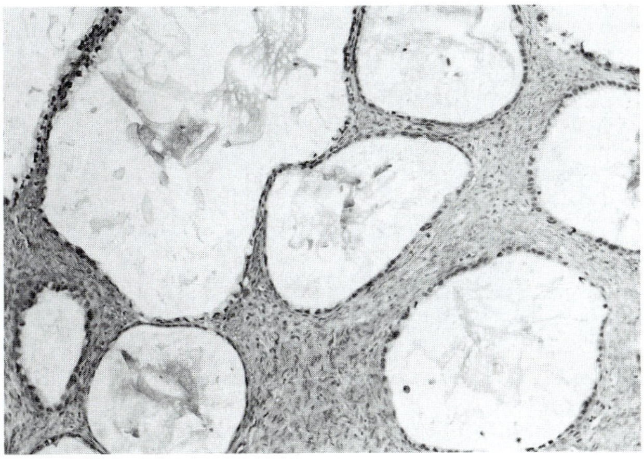

Fig. 22.45. Metastatic carcinoma from the gallbladder. In this field there are many cystically dilated glands lined by slightly atypical epithelium, imparting a resemblance to a cystadenoma of the ovary. (Reproduced by permission of ref. 135.)

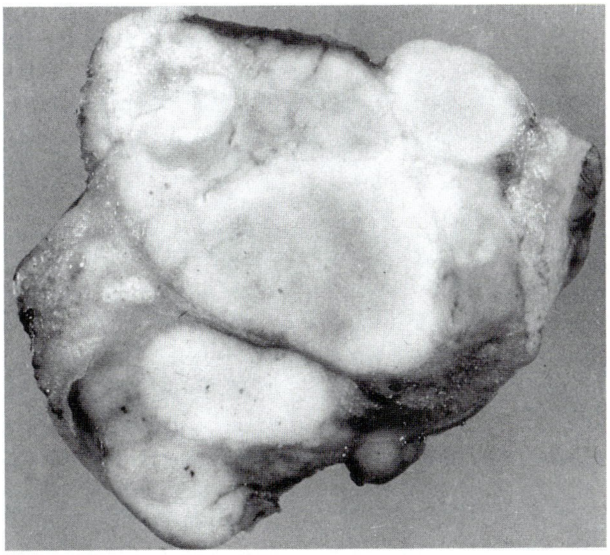

Fig. 22.46. Metastatic hepatocellular carcinoma. Multiple nodules are visible on the sectioned surface of a tumor that was yellow-green in the fresh state. (Reproduced by permission of ref. 124.)

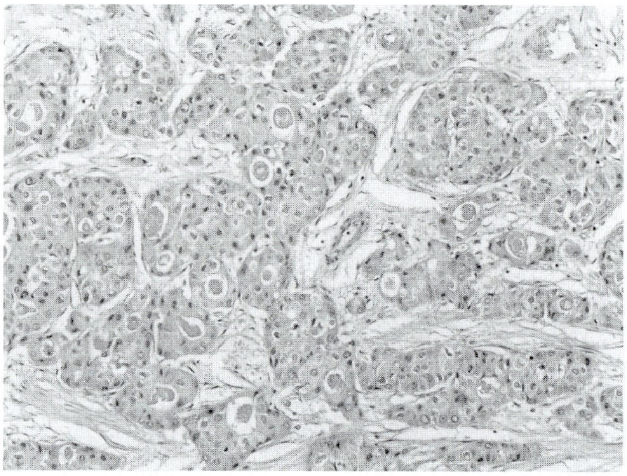

Fig. 22.47. **Metastatic hepatocellular carcinoma.** Tumor cells with abundant cytoplasm are arranged in trabeculae punctuated by occasional small glands.

yolk sac tumor, the finding of foci of more typical yolk sac neoplasia or of other germ cell elements exclude the diagnosis of metastatic hepatocellular carcinoma and the young age of the patient will argue against the latter diagnosis. In a postmenopausal patient the differential diagnosis involves hepatoid carcinoma rather than a hepatoid yolk sac tumor. In this situation, bilaterality and other characteristic findings of metastatic spread to the ovary may be helpful in indicating the metastatic nature of the tumor. Hepatoid carcinomas may arise outside the ovary, for example, in the stomach and lung, and may metastasize to the ovary. There is one report in the literature of a cholangiocarcinoma that metastasized to the ovaries,[51] and we have seen an additional example. A hepatoblastoma that occurred in a 19-year-old woman and was associated with bilateral ovarian metastases at presentation has recently been reported.[35]

Renal Tumors

Renal cell carcinoma rarely spreads to the ovary, with only 11 cases of clinically detectable ovarian metastatic tumors reported in detail.[98,108,129] In 6 of the cases, the ovarian tumor was discovered first, leading to the initial misdiagnosis of primary ovarian clear cell carcinoma in 3 cases. The renal tumors usually were detected within a short period of time in these patients, but in 1 the renal primary was not detected until 8 years later. In the other 4 cases the ovarian tumor was detected 5 months to 14 years after the renal tumors had been removed. The ovarian tumors, 3 of which were bilateral, were usually large (average, 12.5 cm in greatest dimension), and were either solid or solid and cystic (Fig. 22.48), with one cystic tumor being unilocular and containing a 2.5-cm solid nodule in one area. The solid components of the tumors were either uniformly or focally yellow. With one possible exception the renal tumors were well-differentiated clear cell adenocarcinomas; microscopic examination showed a relatively uniform picture of diffuse sheets of clear cells or tubules lined by similar cells and containing eosinophilic material or blood (Fig. 22.49); a prominent sinusoidal vascular pattern was almost always present. It is helpful from the aspect of the differential diagnosis that primary clear cell carcinomas of the ovary have a tubulocystic and papillary component, or both, hobnail cells, and intraluminal mucin in the greater majority of cases. Hobnail cells and conspicuous mucin production, in contrast, are exceptional in renal cell carcinomas. In addition, the typical sinusoidal vascular framework of renal cell carcinoma is not a feature of ovarian clear cell carcinoma. In cases of pure clear cell carcinoma of the ovary without hobnail cells or mucin secretion, radiologic evaluation of the kidney may be necessary to exclude a renal cell carcinoma. Renal transitional cell tumors rarely spread to the ovary,[24,71] but in one case a patient with a renal pelvic tumor of this type had an ovarian metastasis at the time of presentation.[44]

Ovarian metastases from Wilms' tumor of the

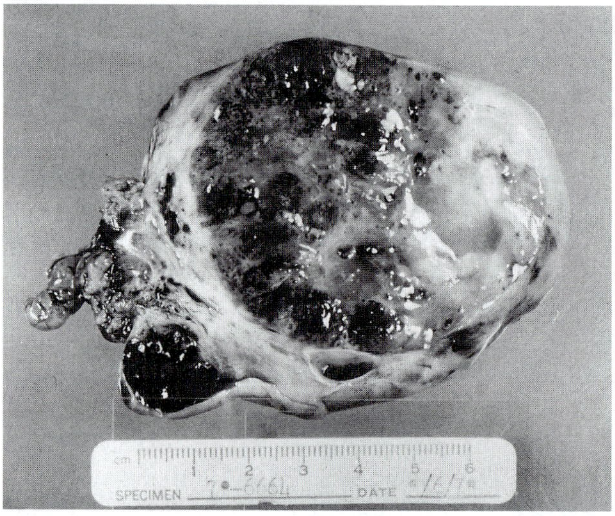

Fig. 22.48. **Metastatic renal cell carcinoma.** The tumor has a solid and cystic sectioned surface. (Reproduced by permission of Buller RE, et al. (1983) Renal-cell carcinoma metastatic to the ovary. A case report. J Reprod Med 28:217–220.)

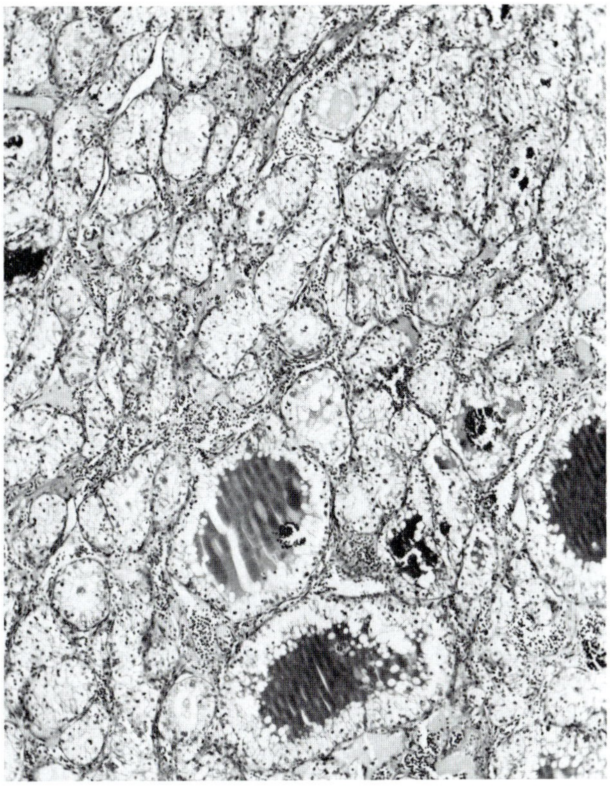

Fig. 22.49. Metastatic renal cell carcinoma, clear cell type. The primary tumor in this case was not diagnosed until 8 years after the removal of the metastasis.

kidney must be very rare as no examples are present in several large series of this neoplasm. In one remarkable case, a patient with a rhabdoid tumor of the kidney presented with an ovarian metastasis, initially misinterpreted as a granulosa cell tumor, the primary renal tumor being undiscovered until autopsy.[131]

Tumors of the Urinary Bladder, Ureter, and Urethra

Tumors from these sites uncommonly metastasize to the ovaries. Three signet-ring cell carcinomas metastatic from the bladder have had the appearance of a Krukenberg tumor.[140] In one of them the ovarian tumor was an autopsy finding and in another the ovarian involvement was an incidental finding on microscopic examination. In the third case the ovarian metastatic tumor, which was symptomatic, was not discovered until 7 years after the primary bladder tumor had been resected. We have seen two cases of urachal adenocarcinoma that formed metastatic mucinous cystic tumors in the ovary and in one case led to the initial misinterpretation of a primary mucinous tumor of the ovary.[121] Only isolated examples of ovarian metastasis of ureteral or urethral cancer have been reported in the literature.[140]

In many cases of possible transitional cell carcinoma metastatic to the ovary, it is difficult to distinguish between a metastatic tumor and a borderline or malignant Brenner tumor or independent primary transitional cell carcinoma of the ovary.[97,140] In almost all borderline or malignant Brenner tumors, however, foci of typical benign Brenner tumor also can be found and the presence of associated benign mucinous elements also favors the diagnosis of a Brenner tumor. The extent of invasion of the primary extraovarian tumor, and the general features of metastatic involvement of the ovary, all have to be considered in the evaluation of these cases. The metastatic transitional cell carcinoma in the series of Ulbright et al.[107] was cystic, exemplifying the great propensity of ovarian metastases from various sites to undergo cystic change.

Adrenal Gland Tumors

Neuroblastoma spreads to the ovary more frequently than other tumors of the adrenal gland. From 25% to 50% of females with neuroblastoma have ovarian involvement at autopsy.[65] Clinically significant metastases during life are rare. In one reported case there was bilateral ovarian involvement at presentation[86] and in two others ovarian metastatic tumor caused the clinical presentation.[99,131] Rarely neuroblastoma is primary in the ovary, and such tumors must be distinguished from metastatic neuroblastomas. The unilaterality of the primary tumors, their occasional association with a teratoma, and the absence of a known primary tumor elsewhere are helpful in the differential diagnosis in individual cases. The prominent fibrillary background of neuroblastoma and the presence of pseudorosettes should aid in the distinction of metastatic neuroblastoma from other metastatic small cell tumors; immunohistochemical staining also may help in a case in which routine stains are not diagnostic.

Adrenal cortical carcinomas metastasize to the ovary rarely even at autopsy. We are not aware of a case in which an ovarian metastatic tumor from the adrenal cortex was the presenting manifestation of the disease. Pheochromocytomas spread to the ovary even less commonly; a review of the literature has failed to disclose a documented case.

Malignant Melanoma

Autopsies of patients who died of *malignant melanoma* have revealed ovarian involvement in 18% of the cases; 95% of these tumors were bilateral.[21] Most of them have originated in the skin, but occasional examples have arisen in the choroid or elsewhere. Occasionally ovarian involvement is clinically symptomatic, as exemplified by many of the cases in two relatively large series of melanomas metastatic to the ovary.[29,134] In the first, ovarian tumors were discovered during life in 7 of the 10 patients.[29] The patients ranged from 29 to 55 (average, 38) years of age and had symptoms attributable to the ovarian metastases. Five of them had a known history of malignant melanoma, and most of them also had extraovarian metastases as well. The tumors were bilateral in 3 of the 7 cases and had an average diameter of 11.4 cm. In the second study,[134] none of the tumors were autopsy findings. The 20 patients ranged from 21 to 60 (average, 37.5) years of age and typically presented because of abdominal swelling or pain. In 75% of the cases there was a history of removal of a cutaneous malignant melanoma or "pigmented lesion." The history of melanoma was more than 5 years previously (7–13 years) in 3 patients. Laparotomy disclosed unilateral ovarian tumors in 11 cases and bilateral tumors in 9.

Approximately 50% of the patients also had metastatic tumor outside the ovary, usually within the pelvis and upper abdomen. The ovarian tumors averaged 10.5 cm in diameter; only 30% of them were noted to be black or brown (Fig. 22.50). On low-power examination, a feature suggesting the metastatic nature in a number of the cases was growth of the tumor in the form of multiple nodules. The

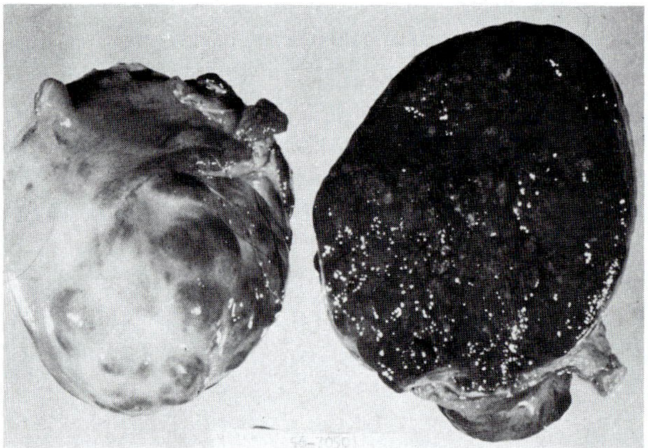

Fig. 22.50. Metastatic malignant melanoma. The tumor has a bosselated external surface; the sectioned surface is *black.*

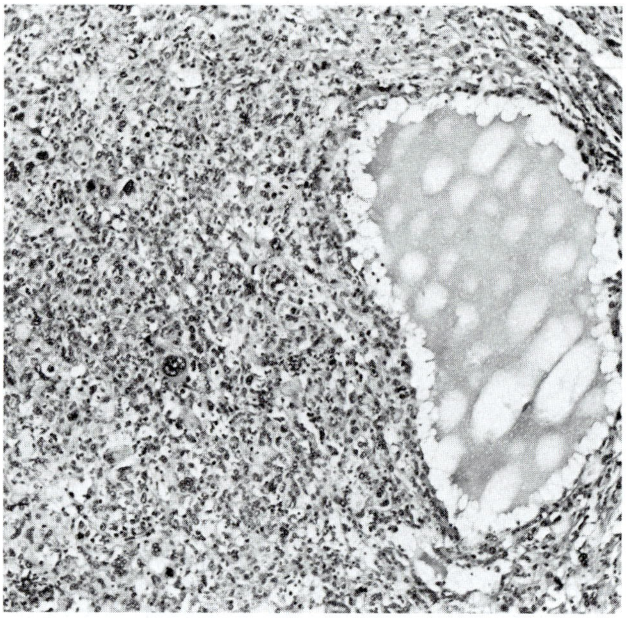

Fig. 22.51. Metastatic malignant melanoma. A follicle-like space is present adjacent to sheets of cells exhibiting conspicuous nuclear atypicality.

most common microscopic appearance in one series was the presence of large cells with abundant eosinophilic cytoplasm.[134] Occasional tumors were characterized by small cells with scanty cytoplasm, and in five tumors spindle cells were present. In the other series, small cells with scanty cytoplasm predominated in most of the cases, often suggesting a sex cord–stromal tumor.[43] Metastatic melanoma may mimic closely a juvenile granulosa cell tumor[77] because of the presence of cells with abundant eosinophilic cytoplasm and follicle-like spaces, which are seen in approximately 40% of the cases[134] (Fig. 22.51). A helpful diagnostic feature of many metastatic melanomas is the presence of discrete rounded aggregates with a nevoid appearance (Fig. 22.52). In our series of metastatic melanomas, prominent nucleoli were seen in 65% of the cases and cytoplasmic pseudoinclusions in many nuclei in 25%.[134] The presence of melanin pigment is an obvious clue to the nature of the tumor in these cases, but melanin was inconspicuous or absent in approximately half the cases in the two series just summarized.[29,134]

Metastatic melanoma must be distinguished from the rare primary melanoma that usually arises in the wall of a dermoid cyst, and sometimes is accompanied by junctional activity beneath the squamous lining of the cyst or is associated with another teratomatous component such as a struma ovarii. Because recognition of teratomatous elements is im-

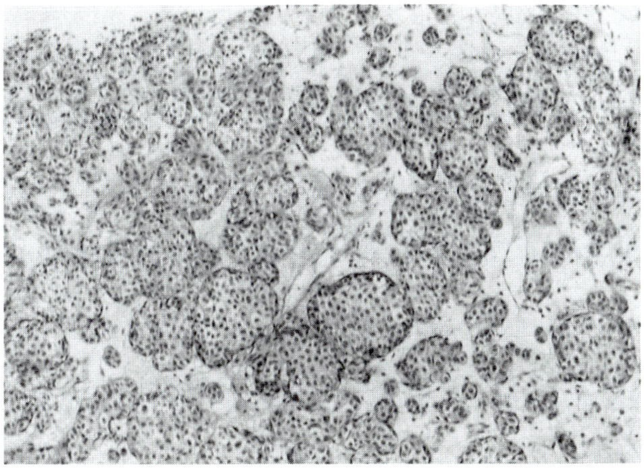

Fig. 22.52. Metastatic malignant melanoma. Nests of cells have a nevoid appearance.

portant in establishing the primary nature of a melanoma, the pathologist should sample the specimen extensively. In cases of apparently pure ovarian melanoma without obvious evidence of a primary tumor elsewhere, a meticulous search for an occult primary tumor should be conducted. If there is no evidence of a primary tumor elsewhere, it is possible that a primary cutaneous melanoma that has regressed was the source of the ovarian tumor. In these cases, bilaterality or growth of the ovarian tumor in the form of multiple nodules strongly suggests metastasis even in the absence of a known primary tumor. In some cases, removal of a primary melanoma may be remote and possibly not considered relevant by the patient or known by the clinician.

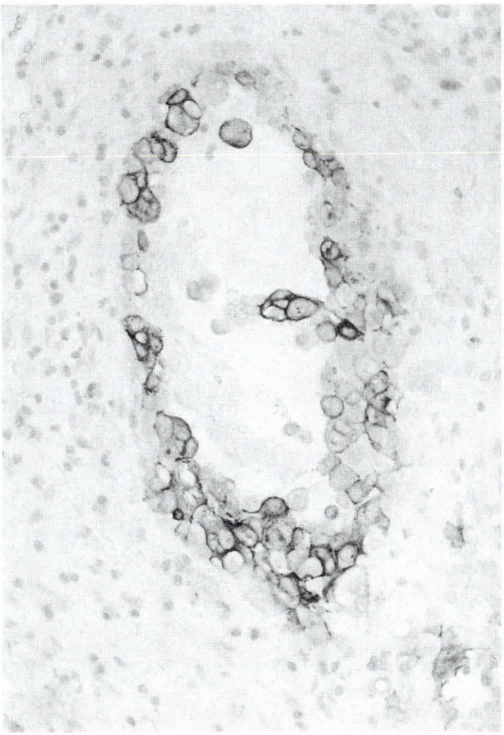

Fig. 22.53. Metastatic malignant melanoma. The cells surrounding a follicle-like space are positive for HMB-45. (Reproduced by permission of ref. 135.)

Metastatic melanoma, particularly if it is amelanotic, may resemble closely a lipid-poor steroid cell tumor or, if it is found during pregnancy, a pregnancy luteoma. Melanin can be misinterpreted as lipochrome pigment, the presence of which may be a feature of steroid cell tumors and impart a dark green-brown or almost black color to the neoplastic tissue. The presence of follicle-like spaces in metastatic melanomas (see Fig. 22.51) has resulted in their confusion with small cell carcinomas of the hypercalcemic type as well as juvenile granulosa cell tumors. The diagnosis of metastatic melanoma to the ovary may be confirmed in problem cases by the immunohistochemical demonstration of S-100 protein and HMB-45 (Fig. 22.53) and negative staining for keratin and other antigens characteristic of other neoplasms that may be in the differential diagnosis.

Pulmonary and Mediastinal Tumors

Only approximately 5% of women with lung cancer have ovarian metastases at autopsy, and the surgical pathologist uncommonly encounters an ovarian tumor of this type.[63,69] Exceptionally, an ovarian metastatic tumor either precedes the discovery of a pulmonary tumor or is found simultaneously.[137] In our series of seven cases of pulmonary tumors metastatic to the ovary, the ovarian tumors were discovered first in three cases, the ovarian and pulmonary tumors were synchronous in three cases, and in the final case the ovarian tumor was found less than 1 year after the pulmonary tumor.[137] In the first category a pulmonary neoplasm was detected 2, 4, or 26 months after the ovarian metastasis. The seven patients ranged from 26 to 66 (average, 42) years of age. Four of them were heavy smokers and one had scleroderma with diffuse interstitial pulmonary fibrosis. Six patients had symptoms referable to the presence of an ovarian mass. The ovarian metastasis was not associated with other foci of intraabdominal spread in any of the cases, indicating the propensity for isolated ovarian spread of neoplasms to occur occasionally. Only one of the ovarian tumors was bilateral. On microscopic examination, three tumors were small cell undifferentiated carcinomas, two large cell undifferentiated carcinomas, one a poorly differentiated adenocarcinoma, and one an atypical spindle cell carcinoid. In our experience since the time of publication of our paper on this subject, the small cell carcinoma has been the most commonly encountered type. An additional case of large cell carcinoma was associated with bilateral ovarian metastases and rupture with intraabdominal hemorrage.[69]

When a patient has a pulmonary and ovarian neoplasm, it can be difficult to decide which tumor is primary. When the histologic features are typical of a lung carcinoma (Figs. 22.54 and 22.55), a pulmonary origin can be assumed with rare exceptions. Small cell carcinomas of pulmonary type may be primary in the ovary, but there is typically no pulmonary involvement in such cases facilitating the diagnosis of an ovarian primary. The focal presence of a surface epithelial tumor is also sometimes helpful in excluding a metastasis. In the absence of such a finding and in the presence of tumor in the lung, it may be impossible to decide whether an ovarian small cell carcinoma of pulmonary type is primary or metastatic.

Metastatic small cell carcinomas in the ovary may originate in sites other than the lung.[27] Three such tumors were primary in the mediastinum, apparently of thymic origin, and had ovarian metastases at the time of presentation.[27] One neuroblastoma primary in the posterior mediastinum metastasized to the ovary.[131] Thymomas have involved the ovary rarely.[120]

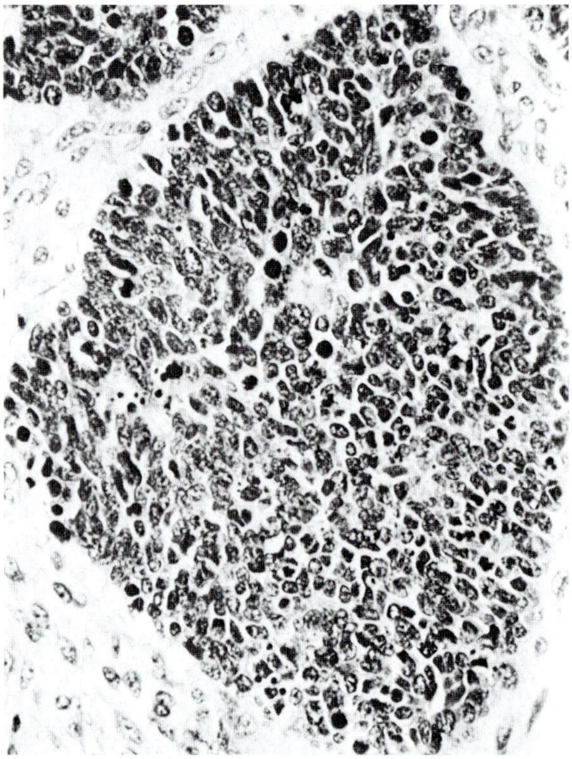

Fig. 22.54. Metastatic small cell carcinoma from the lung. (Reprinted by permission of ref. 137.)

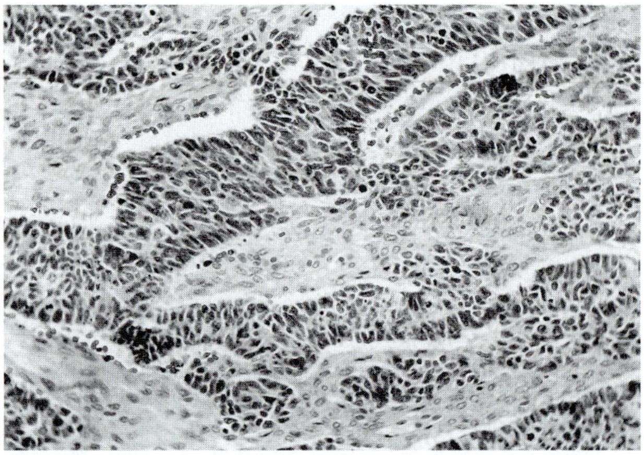

Fig. 22.55. Metastatic small cell carcinoma from the lung. The tumor cells are growing in trabeculae.

Extragenital Sarcomas

Extragenital sarcomas, whether from the viscera or the soft tissues, uncommonly metastasize to the ovary except in late stages of the disease. Eleven rhabdomyosarcomas metastatic to the ovary (Fig. 22.56) have been reported in patients 6 to 27 years of age.[133] Six tumors were alveolar rhabdomyosarcomas, three embryonal, one mixed embryonal, and alveolar rhabdomyosarcoma, and one of unstated subtype. In most of the cases, the ovarian spread was a late manifestation of disease. The ovarian tumors were symptomatic in only two patients, in whom the ovarian involvement was detected within a few weeks of discovery of a soft tissue mass by the patient. The ovarian tumors were bilateral in two cases. In cases of embryonal rhabdomyosarcoma metastatic to the ovary, the diagnosis of rhabdomyosarcoma usually is evident because of the presence of strap cells, and the tumor must be distinguished from a primary embryonal rhabdomyosarcoma, which is the most common subtype of primary malignant striated muscle tumor of the ovary. Because a primary alveolar rhabdomyosarcoma of the ovary has not, to the best of our knowledge, been reported, metastatic alveolar rhabdomyosarcoma more commonly raises the question of other primary and metastatic small cell tumors of the ovary in young women. Two other cases in which the ovary was involved by rhabdomyosarcoma have occurred in patients with a clinical picture that simulated acute leukemia.[39]

In our study of 21 metastatic sarcomas, other than rhabdomyosarcoma, 10 were extragenital and

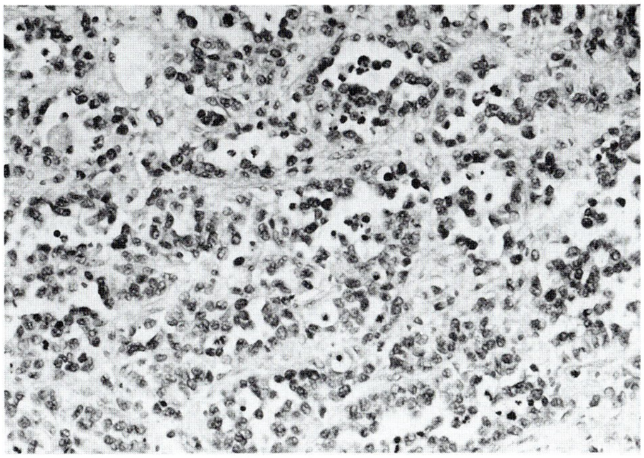

Fig. 22.56. Metastatic alveolar rhabdomyosarcoma. (Reproduced by permission of ref. 135.)

all of them were clinically significant.[139] These tumors included three leiomyosarcomas, one primary in the stomach and two in the small intestine, and single examples of retrovesical leiomyosarcoma, fibrosarcoma of the anterior abdominal wall, sarcoma of the mesentery of smooth muscle or neural type, hemangiosarcoma probably primary in the heart, osteosarcoma of the maxilla, chondrosarcoma of the rib, and Ewing's sarcoma of a pubic bone. Rare other cases of hemangiosarcoma that metastasized to the ovaries have been documented as have a few cases of Ewing's sarcoma. The only tumor in our series that caused major difficulty in diagnosis was a primary epithelioid leiomyosarcoma of the stomach; a unilateral ovarian metastasis accounted for the clinical presentation. The primary tumor was not discovered until 4 months later.

Ovarian Involvement by Peritoneal Tumors

Although ovarian involvement in cases of malignant mesothelioma and malignant serous tumors of the peritoneum is secondary in most of the cases, this subject is generally not included in discussions of secondary tumors of the ovary because the ovarian involvement is only one part of widespread peritoneal disease. It should be noted, however, that in a recent series of peritoneal mesotheliomas ovarian involvement was common[32] and indeed was the focus of another report that included seven cases of peritoneal malignant mesothelioma which presented clinically as "ovarian cancer."[14] The differential diagnosis in these cases is primarily with an ovarian surface epithelial carcinoma, particularly serous carcinoma. Although there is some overlap, in typical cases the tubulopapillary and diffuse patterns of mesothelioma, and the characteristic cuboidal to rounded cell type with abundant eosinophilic cytoplasm, produce a picture that is distinctly different from that of serous carcinoma. Psammoma bodies, although occasionally seen in mesotheliomas, are rarely numerous and if present in significant number their presence strongly favors a serous neoplasm. Histochemical and immunohistochemical stains may aid in this differential. Special stains in serous tumors frequently reveal apical or luminal neutral mucin and one or more antigens that are usually absent in mesothelioma including TAG-72, S-100, Leu-M1, PLAP, CEA, and Ber-EP4.14 Criteria for the differential diagnosis of peritoneal serous neoplasia and serous neoplasms of the ovary with peritoneal spread are beyond the scope of this chapter and are covered elsewhere in this volume.

One recently described peritoneal tumor that may have ovarian manifestations as a major component of the clinical presentation and present as "ovarian cancer" is the intraabdominal desmoplastic small round cell tumor with divergent differentiation (see Chapter 17, Diseases of the Peritoneum). A few examples of this tumor with ovarian involvement at presentation have been described in teenagers and one in a 22-year-old.[123,143] In some cases the ovarian tumor initially was thought to be the primary neoplasm. In all the cases there was extensive extraovarian tumor at the time of presentation. The ovarian involvement is usually bilateral. Microscopic examination of the ovarian tumors shows nodules composed predominantly of small cells with hyperchromatic nuclei and scanty cytoplasm surrounded by a prominent desmoplastic stroma (Fig. 22.57). The neoplasms exhibit the characteristic im-

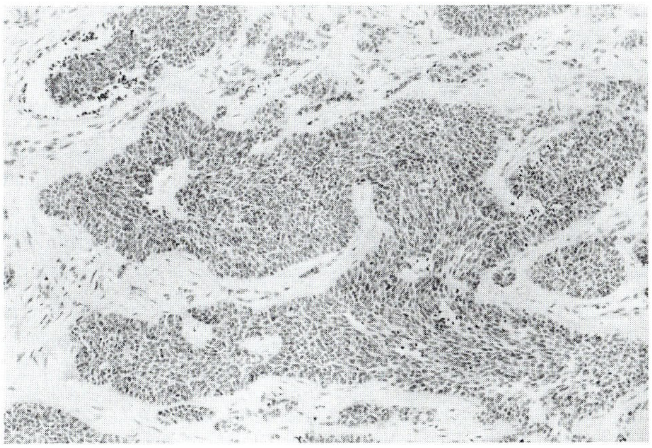

Fig. 22.57. Ovarian involvement by intraabdominal desmoplastic small round cell tumor. Nests of small cells with scanty cytoplasm are embedded in a desmoplastic stroma.

munohistochemical staining profile, with many of the tumor cells staining for cytokeratin, epithelial membrane antigen, desmin, and vimentin. The differential diagnosis in these cases is extensive and includes a number of small cell tumors that may involve the ovary, either primarily or secondarily in young females, as presented in detail elsewhere,[141] and whose features are considered elsewhere in this volume.

Miscellaneous Rare Ovarian Metastases

Metastases to the ovary other than those already discussed are of great rarity and generally only of relevance to autopsy pathology. Carcinomas of the thyroid only exceptionally spread to the ovary; rare examples of spread at autopsy in cases of follicular, medullary, and anaplastic carcinoma are mentioned in the literature. We are not aware of a documented case of ovarian spread of papillary carcinoma. There is only one case in which ovarian spread of thyroid carcinoma is documented to have caused some diagnostic difficulty.[130] In that case, a 29-year-old woman had a 17-cm right ovarian tumor 12 years after undergoing a partial thyroidectomy for follicular carcinoma. The tumor also had spread to the brain and one adrenal gland by the time the ovarian tumor was discovered. Initial consideration was given to the diagnosis of a malignant struma ovarii in this case because of the interval since the thyroid tumor and also because it was only the existence of the ovarian tumor that prompted review of the thyroid neoplasm and its reinterpretation as carcinoma, a diagnosis not made initially.

A review of the literature on parathyroid carcinoma has not disclosed any examples of ovarian metastasis. Rare examples of head and neck carcinoma metastatic to the ovary are documented,[72] and we have seen one case in which the primary tumor was an undifferentiated carcinoma of the ethmoid sinus. Salivary gland tumors also spread to the ovary with extreme rarity. We have seen a case of a young woman who had an adenoid cystic carcinoma of the parotid gland excised at the age of 12 years followed by local recurrence, lung metastasis, and bilateral symptomatic ovarian metastases 11 years after presentation. Longacre and colleagues[58] described a case of a 30-year-old woman with an adenoid cystic carcinoma of the submandibular gland who had a 10-cm left ovarian metastasis, followed by smaller tumor in the opposite ovary 10 years later. These cases emphasize that a history of neoplasia of any type, even relatively remote, may be relevant in the evaluation of an unusual ovarian tumor. Esophageal cancer rarely spread to the ovary. In one report "gonadal" spread is mentioned in 2 of 73 patients who came to autopsy.[102] A case of metastatic esophageal adenocarcinoma to the ovary is briefly mentioned in one series.[86]

There are only two reports to our knowledge in which ovarian spread of tumors of the central nervous system and cranium is mentioned. One was a case of metastatic meningioma[69] and the other was a metastatic medulloblastoma in a 4-year-old girl, in whose ovary "a cleft near the hilum was full of tumor cells."[75] Tumors of the skin, other than malignant melanoma, rarely spread to the ovary; clinically significant spread of Merkel cell tumor is documented.[27] One chordoma has metastasized to the ovary.[144] Rarely a metastatic tumor involves an ovary that contains a primary ovarian neoplasm; two of these metastatic tumors that were of gastric origin and involved dermoid cysts,[118] one was a breast carcinoma and another a cystosarcoma phyllodes, both metastatic to a Brenner tumor.[40,96] Additionally, we have seen one Krukenberg tumor of gastric origin in an ovary containing a granulosa cell tumor and another involving an ovarian fibroma.

References

1. Abdul-Hafeez M, Akhtar M, Aqeel HS Ba, Kidess EA (1987) Placental site trophoblastic tumor: Report of a case with review of literature. Ann Saudi Med 7:340–344
2. Abu-Rustum NR, Barakat RR, Curtin JP (1997) Ovarian and uterine disease in women with colorectal cancer. Gynecol Oncol 89:85–87
3. Acosta-Sison H (1958) The relative frequency of various anatomic sites as the point of first metastasis in 32 cases of chorionepithelioma. Am J Obstet Gynecol 75:1149–1152
4. Amorn Y, Knight WA (1978) Primary linitis plastica of the colon: report of two cases and review of the literature. Cancer (Phila) 41:2420–2425
5. Beck RP, Latour JPA (1963) Necropsy reports on 36 cases of endometrial carcinoma. Am J Obstet Gynecol 85:307–311
6. Berezowski K, Stastny JF, Kornstein MJ (1996) Cytokeratins 7 and 20 and carcinoembryonic antigen in ovarian and colonic carcinoma. Mod Pathol 9: 426–429
7. Birnkrant A, Sampson J, Sugarbaker PH (1986) Ovarian metastasis from colorectal cancer. Dis Colon Rectum 29:767–771
8. Brown BL, Scharifker DA, Gordon R, Deppe GG, Cohen CJ (1980) Bronchial carcinoid tumor with ovarian metastasis. A light microscopic and ultrastructural study. Cancer (Phila) 46:543–546

9. Bullon A, Arseneau J, Prat J, Young RH, Scully RE (1981) Tubular Krukenberg tumor. A problem in histopathologic diagnosis. Am J Surg Pathol 5: 225–232
10. Bunker ML (1959) The terminal findings in endometrial carcinoma. Am J Obstet Gynecol 77:530–538
11. Caron P, Roche H, Gorguet B, Martel P, Bennet A, Carton M (1990) Mammary ovarian metastases with stromal cell hyperplasia and postmenopausal virilization. Cancer (Phila) 66:1221–1224
12. Chen KTK (1990) Appendiceal adenocarcinoid with ovarian metastasis. Gynecol Oncol 38:286–288
13. Chen KTK, Kostich ND, Rosai J (1978) Peritoneal foreign body granulomas to keratin in uterine adenoacanthoma. Arch Pathol Lab Med 102:174–177
14. Clement PB, Young RH, Scully RE (1996) Malignant mesotheliomas presenting as ovarian masses. A report of nine cases, including two primary ovarian mesotheliomas. Am J Surg Pathol 20:1067–1080.
15. Cheung ANY, Chiu P-M, Khoo U-S (1997) Is immunostaining with HAM56 antibody useful in identifying ovarian origin of metastatic adenocarcinomas? Hum Pathol 28:91–94
16. Chuaqui RF, Zhuang Z, Emmert-Buck, MR, Bryant BR, Nogales F, Tavassoli FA, Merino MJ (1996) Genetic analysis of synchronous mucinous tumors of the ovary and appendix. Hum Pathol 27:165–171
17. Creasman WT, Lukeman J (1972) Role of the fallopian tube in dissemination of malignant cells in corpus cancer. Cancer (Phila) 20:456–457
18. Cuatrecasas M, Matias-Guiu X, Prat J (1996) Synchronous mucinous tumors of the appendix and the ovary associated with pseudomyxoma peritonei: a clinicopathologic study of six cases with comparative analysis of c-Ki-*ras* mutations. Am J Surg Pathol 20:739–746
19. Curtin JP, Barakat RR, Hoskins WJ (1994) Ovarian disease in women with breast cancer. Obstet Gynecol 84:449–452.
20. Dabbs DJ, Sturtz K, Zaino RJ (1996) The immunohistochemical discrimination of endometrioid adenocarcinomas. Hum Pathol 27:172–177
21. Das Gupta T, Brasfield R (1964) Metastatic melanoma: a clinicopathological study. Cancer (Phila) 17:1323–1339
22. Daya D, Nazerali L, Frank GL (1992) Metastatic ovarian carcinoma of large intestinal origin simulating primary ovarian carcinoma. A clinicopathologic study of 25 cases. Am J Clin Pathol 97:751–758
23. DeCostanzo DC, Elias JM, Chumas JC (1997) Necrosis in 84 ovarian carcinomas: a morphologic study of primary versus metastatic colonic cancer with a selective immunohistochemical analysis of cytokeratin subtypes and carcinoembryonic antigen. Int J Gynecol Pathol 16:245–249
24. Demopoulos RI, Touger L, Dubin N (1987) Secondary ovarian carcinoma: a clinical and pathological evaluation. Int J Gynecol Pathol 6:166–175
25. Diddle AW (1955) Krukenberg tumors: Diagnostic problem. Cancer (Phila) 8:1026–1034
26. Duarte I, Llanos O (1981) Patterns of metastases in intestinal and diffuse types of carcinoma of the stomach. Hum Pathol 12:237–242
27. Eichhorn JH, Young RH, Scully RE (1993) Nonpulmonary small cell carcinomas of extragenital origin metastatic to the ovary: a report of seven cases. Cancer (Phila) 71:177–186
28. Eifel P, Hendrickson M, Ross J, Ballon S, Martinez A, Kempson R (1982) Simultaneous presentation of carcinoma involving the ovary and the uterine corpus. Cancer (Phila) 50:163–170
29. Fitzgibbons PL, Martin SE, Simmons TJ (1987) Malignant melanoma metastatic to the ovary. Am J Surg Pathol 11:959–964
30. Fowler LJ, Maygarden SJ, Novotny DB (1994) Human alveolar macrophage-56 and carcinoembryonic antigen monoclonal antibodies in the differential diagnosis between primary ovarian and metastatic gastrointestinal carcinomas. Hum Pathol 25:666–670
31. Gagnon Y, Tetu B (1989) Ovarian metastases of breast carcinoma. A clinicopathologic study of 59 cases. Cancer (Phila) 64:892–898
32. Goldblum J, Hart WR. (1995) Localized and diffuse mesotheliomas of the genital tract and peritoneum in women. A clinicopathological study of nineteen true mesothelial neoplasms, other than adenomatoid tumors, multicystic mesotheliomas and localized fibrous tumors. Am J Surg Pathol 19:1124–1137
33. Graffner HOL, Alm POA, Oscarson JEA (1983) Prophylactic oophorectomy in colorectal carcinoma. Am J Surg 146:233–235
34. Green TH Jr, Scully RE (1962) Tumors of the fallopian tube. Clin Obstet Gynecol 5:886–906
35. Green LK, Silva EG (1989) Hepatoblastoma in an adult with metastasis to the ovaries. Am J Clin Pathol 92:110–115
36. Guerrieri C, Frånlund B, Fristedt S, Gillooley JF, Boeryd B (1997) Mucinous tumors of the vermiform appendix and ovary, and pseudomyxoma peritonei: histogenetic implications of cytokeratin 7 expression. Hum Pathol 28:1039–1045
37. Hale RW (1968) Krukenberg tumor of the ovaries. A review of 81 records. Obstet Gynecol 32:221–225
38. Harris M, Howell A, Chrissohou M, Swindell RIC, Hudson M, Sellwood RA (1984) A comparison of the metastatic pattern of infiltrating lobular carcinoma and infiltrating duct carcinoma of the breast. Br J Cancer 50:23–30
39. Hayashi Y, Kikuchi F, Oka T, et al (1988) Rhabdomyosarcoma with bone marrow metastasis simulating acute leukemia. Report of two cases. Acta Pathol Jpn 38:789–798
40. Hines JR, Gordon RT, Widger C, et al (1976) Cystosarcoma phyllodes metastatic to a Brenner tumor of the ovary. Arch Surg 111:299–300
41. Hirschfield LS, Kahn LB, Winkler B, Bochner RZ,

Gibstein AA (1985) Adenocarcinoid of the appendix presenting as bilateral Krukenberg's tumor of the ovaries. Immunohistochemical and ultrastructural studies and literature review. Arch Pathol Lab Med 109:930–933
42. Holtz F, Hart WR (1982) Krukenberg tumors of the ovary. A clinicopathologic analysis of 27 cases. Cancer (Phila) 50:2438–2447
43. Hopping RA, Dockerty MB, Masson JC (1942) Carcinoid tumor of the appendix. Report of a case in which extensive intra-abdominal metastases occurred, including involvement of the right ovary. Arch Surg 45:613–622
44. Hsiu J-G, Kemp GM, Singer GA, Rawls WH, Siddiky MA (1991) Transitional cell carcinoma of the renal pelvis with ovarian metastasis. Gynecol Oncol 41:178–181
45. Ikeda E, Tsutsumi Y, Yoshida H, Yanagi K (1991) Goblet cell carcinoid of the vermiform appendix with ovarian metastasis mimicking mucinous cystadenocarcinomas. Acta Pathol Jpn 41:455–460
46. Israel SL, Helsel EV, Hausman DH (1965) The challenge of metastatic ovarian carcinoma. Am J Obstet Gynecol 93:1094–1101
47. James PD, Taylor CW, Templeton AC (1973) Tumors of the female genitalia. In: Templeton AC (ed) Tumours in a tropical country. Springer, New York
48. Johansson H (1960) Clinical aspects of metastatic ovarian cancer of extragenital origin. Acta Obstet Gynecol Scand 39:681–697
49. Joshi VV (1968) Primary Krukenberg tumor of ovary. Review of literature and case report. Cancer (Phila) 22:1199–1207
50. Kaminski PF, Norris HJ (1984) Coexistence of ovarian neoplasms and endocervical adenocarcinoma. Obstet Gynecol 64:553–556
51. Karsh J (1951) Secondary malignant disease of the ovaries. A study of 72 autopsies. Am J Obstet Gynecol 61:154–160
52. Kim K-R, Scully RE (1990) Peritoneal keratin granulomas with carcinomas of endometrium and ovary and atypical polypoid adenomyoma of endometrium. A clinicopathological analysis of 22 cases. Am J Surg Pathol 14:925–932
53. Kuo T-T, Hsueh S (1984) Mucicarminophilic histiocytosis. A polyvinylpyrrolidone (PVP) storage disease simulating signet-ring cell carcinoma. Am J Surg Pathol 8:419–428
54. Lashgari M, Behmaram B, Hoffman JS, Garcia J (1992) Primary biliary carcinoma with metastasis to the ovary. Gynecol Oncol 47:272–274
55. Lash RH, Hart WR (1987) Intestinal adenocarcinomas metastatic to the ovaries. A clinicopathological evaluation of 22 cases. Am J Surg Pathol 11: 114–121
56. Lee YN, Hori JM (1971) Significance of ovarian metastases in therapeutic oophorectomy for advanced breast cancer. Cancer (Phila) 27:1374–1378
57. LiVolsi VA, Merino MJ, Schwartz PE (1983) Coexistent endocervical adenocarcinoma and mucinous adenocarcinoma of ovary: a clinicopathological study of four cases. Int J Gynecol Pathol 1:391–402
58. Longacre TA, O'Hanlan K, Hendrickson MR (1996) Adenoid cystic carcinoma of the submandibular gland with symptomatic ovarian metastases. Int J Gynecol Pathol 15:349–355
59. Loy TS, Calaluce RD, Kenney GL (1996) Cytokeratin immunostaining in differentiating primary ovarian carcinoma from metastatic colonic adenocarcinoma. Mod Pathol 9:1040–1044
60. Loy TS, Quesenberry JT, Sharp SC (1992) Distribution of CA 125 in adenocarcinomas. An immunohistochemical study of 481 cases. Am J Clin Pathol 98:175–179
61. Lumb G, Mackenzie DH (1959) The incidence of metastases in adrenal glands and ovaries removed for carcinoma of the breast. Cancer (Phila) 12:521–526
62. MacKeigan JM, Ferguson JA (1979) Prophylactic oophorectomy and colorectal cancer in premenopausal patients. Dis Colon Rectum 22:401–405
63. Mazur MT, Hsueh S, Gersell DJ (1984) Metastases to the female genital tract. Analysis of 325 cases. Cancer (Phila) 53:1978–1984
64. Merino MJ, Edmonds P, LiVolsi V (1985) Appendiceal carcinoma metastatic to the ovaries and mimicking primary ovarian tumors. Int J Gynecol Pathol 4:110–120
65. Meyer WH, Yu GW, Milvenan ES, Jeffs RD, Kaizer H, Leventhal BG (1979) Ovarian involvement in neuroblastoma. Med Pediatr Oncol 7:49–54
66. Miller BE, Pittman B, Wan JY, Fleming M (1997) Colon cancer with metastasis to the ovary at time of initial diagnosis. Gynecol Oncol 66:368–371
67. Miettinen M (1996) Keratin 20: immunohistochemical marker for gastrointestinal, urothelial, and Merkel cell carcinomas. Mod Pathol 8:384–388
68. Monteagudo C, Merino MJ, Laporte N, Neumann RD (1991) Value of gross cystic disease fluid protein-15 in distinguishing metastatic breast carcinomas among poorly differentiated neoplasms involving the ovary. Hum Pathol 22:368–372
69. Nelson BE, Carcangiu ML, Chambers JT (1992) Intraabdominal hemorrhage with pulmonary large cell carcinoma metastatic to the ovary. Gynecol Oncol 47:377–381
70. Nguyen L, Brewer CA, DiSaia PJ (1998) Ovarian metastasis of Stage 1B1 squamous cell cancer of the cervix after radical parametrectomy and oophoropexy. Gynecol Oncol 68:198–200
71. Oliva E, Musulen E, Prat J, Young RH (1993) Transitional cell carcinoma of the renal pelvis with symptomatic ovarian metastases. Int J Surg Pathol 2:231–236
72. Orr JW, Grizzle WE, Huddleston JF (1982) Squamous cell carcinoma metastatic to placenta and ovary. Obstet Gynecol 59:81S—83S
73. Osborne MP, Pitts RM (1961) Therapeutic oophorectomy for advanced breast cancer. The significance of metastases to the ovary and of ovarian cor-

tical stromal hyperplasia. Cancer (Phila) 14:126–130
74. Park WLH, Lees JC (1950) Choriocarcinoma. A general review, with an analysis of five hundred and sixteen cases. Arch Pathol 49:205–241
75. Paterson E (1961) Distant metastases from medulloblastoma of the cerebellum. Brain 84:301–330
76. Patsner B (1990) Jejunal adenocarcinoma manifested as an adnexal mass. South Med J 83:1493–1494
77. Pavelic ZP, Pavelic L, Pavelic K, Peacock JS (1991) Utility of anti-carcinoembryonic antigen monoclonal antibodies for differentiating ovarian adenocarcinomas from gastrointestinal metastasis to the ovary. Gynecol Oncol 40:112–117
78. Petru E, Pickel H, Heydarfadai M, Lahousen M, Haas J, Schaider H, Tamussino K (1992) Nongenital cancers metastatic to the ovary. Gynecol Oncol 44:83–86
79. Pins MR, Young RH, Crum CP, Leach IH, Scully RE (1997) Cervical squamous carcinoma in situ with superficial extension to corpus and tubes and invasion of tubes and ovaries. Int J Gynecol Pathol 16:272–278
80. Pitluk H, Poticha SM (1983) Carcinoma of the colon and rectum in patients less than 40 years of age. Surg Gynecol Obstet 157:335–337
81. Prayson RA, Hart WR, Petras RE (1994) Pseudomyxoma peritonei. A clinicopathologic study of 19 cases with emphasis on site of origin and nature of associated ovarian tumors. Am J Surg Pathol 18: 591–603
82. Puga FJ, Gibbs CP, Williams TJ (1973) Castrating operations associated with metastatic lesions of the breast. Obstet Gynecol 41:713–719
83. Ramaekeres F, van Niekerk C, Poels L, et al (1990) Use of monoclonal antibodies to keratin 7 in the differential diagnosis of adenocarcinomas. Am J Pathol 136:641–655
84. Resta L, De Benedictis G, Colucci GA, Cimmino A, Borraccino V, Milillo F (1989) Secondary tumors of the ovary. II: Breast carcinoma. J Exp Clin Cancer Res 8:147–151
85. Resta L, De Benedictis G, Colucci GA, Napoli A, Borraccino V, Milillo F (1989) Secondary tumors of the ovary. I: Tumors of the female genital tract. J Exp Clin Cancer Res 8:87–94
86. Riopel MA, Ronnett BM, Kurman RJ (1999) Evaluation of diagnostic criteria and behavior of ovarian intestinal-type mucinous tumors. Atypical proliferative (borderline) tumors and intraepithelial, microinvasive, invasive, and metastatic carcinomas. Am J Surg Pathol 23:617–635
87. Robboy SJ, Scully RE, Norris HJ (1974) Carcinoid metastatic to the ovary. A clinicopathologic analysis of 35 cases. Cancer (Phila) 33:798–811
88. Ronnett BM, Kurman RJ, Shmookler BM, Sugarbaker PH, Young RH (1997) The morphologic spectrum of ovarian metastases of appendical adenocarcinomas. A clinicopathologic and immunohistochemical analysis of tumors often misinterpreted as primary ovarian tumors or metastatic tumors from other gastrointestinal sites. Am J Surg Pathol 2:1144–1155
89. Ronnett BM, Kurman RJ, Zahn CM, Shmookler BM, Jablonski KA, Kass ME (1995) Pseudomyxoma peritonei in women. A clinicopathologic analysis of 30 cases with emphasis on site of origin, prognosis, and relationship to ovarian mucinous tumors of low malignant potential. Hum Pathol 26:509–524
90. Ronnett BM, Shmookler BM, Diener-West M, Sugarbaker PH, Kurman RJ (1997) Immunohistochemical evidence supporting the appendiceal origin of pseudomyxoma peritonei in women. Int J Gynecol Pathol 16:1–9
91. Ronnett BM, Zahn CM, Kurman RJ, Kass ME, Sugarbaker PH, Shmookler BM (1995) Disseminated peritoneal adenomucinosis and peritoneal mucinous carcinomatosis: a clinicopathologic analysis of 109 cases with emphasis on distinguishing pathologic features, site of origin, prognosis, and relationship to "pseudomyxoma peritonei". Am J Surg Pathol 19:1390–1408
92. Saphir O (1951) Signet-ring cell carcinoma. Mil Surg 109:360–369
93. Scully RE, Richardson GS (1961) Luteinization of the stroma of metastatic cancer involving the ovary and its endocrine significance. Cancer (Phila) 14: 827–840
94. Sedlis A (1961) Primary carcinoma of the fallopian tube. Obstet Gynecol Surv 16:209–226
95. Seidman JD, Elsayed AM, Sobin LH, Tavassoli FA (1993) Association of mucinous tumors of the ovary and appendix. A clinicopathologic study of 25 cases. Am J Surg Pathol 17:22–34
96. Smale L (1980) Metastatic breast adenocarcinoma to Brenner tumors. Gynecol Oncol 9:251–253
97. Soslow RA, Rouse RV, Hendrickson MR, Silva EG, Longacre TA (1996) Transitional cell neoplasms of the ovary and urinary bladder: a comparative immunohistochemical analysis. Int J Gynecol Pathol 15:257–265
98. Spencer JR, Eriksen B, Garnett JE (1993) Metastatic renal tumor presenting as ovarian clear cell carcinoma. Urology 41:582–584
99. Sty JR, Kun LE, Casper JT (1980) Bone scintigraphy in neuroblastoma with ovarian metastasis. Wis Med J 79:28–29
100. Szych C, Staebler A, Connolly DC, Wu R, Cho KR, Ronnett BM (1999) Molecular genetic evidence supporting the clonality and appendiceal origin of pseudomyxoma peritonei in women. Am J Pathol 154:1849–1855
101. Tabata M, Ichinoe K, Sakuragi N, Shina Y, Yamaguchi T, Mabuchi Y (1987) Incidence of ovarian metastasis in patients with cancer of the uterine cervix. Gynecol Oncol 28:255–261
102. Takita H, Vincent RG, Caicedo V, Gutierrez AC (1977) Squamous cell carcinoma of the esophagus: a study of 153 cases. J Surg Oncol 9:547–554

103. Toki N, Tsukamoto N, Kaku T, et al (1991) Microscopic ovarian metastasis of the uterine cervical cancer. Gynecol Oncol 41:46–51
104. Tso PL, Bringaze WL III, Dauterive AH, Correa P, Cohn I Jr (1987) Gastric carcinoma in the young. Cancer (Phila) 59:1362–1365
105. Ulbright TM, Roth LM (1985) Metastatic and independent cancers of the endometrium and ovary: a clinicopathologic study of 34 cases. Hum Pathol 16:28–34
106. Ulbright TM, Roth LM (1985) Secondary tumors of the ovary. In: Roth LM, Czernobilsky B (eds) Tumors and tumor-like conditions of the ovary. Contemporary issues in surgical pathology, no. 6. Churchill-Livingstone, New York, pp 129–152
107. Ulbright TM, Roth LM, Stehman FB (1984) Secondary ovarian neoplasia. A clinicopathologic study of 35 cases. Cancer (Phila) 53:1164–1174
108. Vara A, Madrigal B, Veiga M, Diaz A, Garcia J, Calvo J (1998) Bilateral ovarian metastases from renal clear cell carcinoma. Acta Oncol (Stockh) 37:379–380
109. Viadana E, Bross IDJ, Pickren JW (1973) An autopsy study of some routes of dissemination of cancer of the breast. Br J Cancer 27:336–340
110. Wang NP, Zee S, Zarbo RJ, Bacchi CE, Gown AM (1995) Coordinate expression of cytokeratins 7 and 20 defines unique subsets of carcinomas. Apol Immunohistochem 3:99–107
111. Wauters CCAP, Smedts F, Gerrits LGM, Bosman FT, Ramaekers FCS (1995) Keratins 7 and 20 as diagnostic markers of carcinomas metastatic to the ovary. Hum Pathol 26:852–855
112. Webb MJ, Decker DG, Mussey E (1975) Cancer metastatic to the ovary. Factors influencing survival. Obstet Gynecol 45:391–396
113. Weitberg AB, Weitzman SA (1983) Metastatic islet cell carcinoma: a potentially treatable cause of "carcinoma of unknown origin." CA Cancer J Clin 33: 167–171
114. Wheelock MC, Putong P (1959) Ovarian metastases from adenocarcinomas of colon and rectum. Obstet Gynecol 14:291–295
115. Wick MR, Lillemoe TJ, Copland GT, Swanson PE, Manivel JC, Kiang DT (1989) Gross cystic disease fluid protein-15 as a marker for breast cancer: immunohistochemical analysis of 690 human neoplasms and comparison with alphalactalbumin. Hum Pathol 20:281–287
116. Woodruff JD, Murthy YS, Bhaskar TN, Bordbar F, Tseng S-S (1970) Metastatic ovarian tumors. Am J Obstet Gynecol 107:202–209
117. Woodruff JD, Novak ER (1960) The Krukenberg tumor. Study of 48 cases from the Ovarian Tumor Registry. Obstet Gynecol 15:351–360
118. Yakushiji M, Tazaki T, Nishimura H, Kato T (1987) Krukenberg tumors of the ovary: a clinicopathologic analysis of 112 cases. Acta Obstet Gynaecol Jpn 39:479–485
119. Yazigi R, Sandstad J (1989) Ovarian involvement in extragenital cancer. Gynecol Oncol 34:84–87
120. Yoshida A, Shigematsu T, Mori H, Yoshida H, Fukunishi R (1981) Non-invasive thymoma with widespread blood-borne metastasis. Virchows Arch (Path Anat) 390:121–126
121. Young RH (1995) Urachal adenocarcinoma metastatic to the ovary simulating primary mucinous cystadenocarcinoma of the ovary: report of a case. Virchows Arch 426:529–532
122. Young RH, Carey RW, Robboy SJ (1981) Breast carcinoma masquerading as a primary ovarian neoplasm. Cancer (Phila) 48:210–212
123. Young RH, Eichhorn JH, Dickersin GR, Scully RE (1992) Ovarian involvement by the intra-abdominal desmoplastic small round cell tumor with divergent differentiation. A report of three cases. Hum Pathol 23:454–464
124. Young RH, Gersell DJ, Clement PB, Scully RE (1992) Hepatocellular carcinoma metastatic to the ovary: a report of three cases discovered during life with discussion of the differential diagnosis of hepatoid tumors of the ovary. Hum Pathol 23:574–580
125. Young RH, Gersell DJ, Roth LM, Scully RE (1993) Ovarian metastases from cervical carcinomas other than pure adenocarcinomas: A report of 12 cases. Cancer (Phila) 71:407–418
126. Young RH, Gilks CB, Scully RE (1991) Mucinous tumors of the appendix associated with mucinous tumors of the ovary and pseudomyxoma peritonei: a clinicopathological analysis of 22 cases supporting an origin in the appendix. Am J Surg Pathol 15: 415–429
127. Young RH, Hart WR (1989) Metastases from carcinomas of the pancreas simulating primary mucinous tumors of the ovary: a report of seven cases. Am J Surg Pathol 13:748–756
128. Young RH, Hart WR (1998) Metastatic intestinal carcinomas simulating primary ovarian clear cell carcinoma and secretory endometrioid carcinoma. A clinicopathologic and immunohistochemical study of five cases. Am J Surg Pathol 22:805–815
129. Young RH, Hart WR (1992) Renal cell carcinoma metastatic to the ovary: a report of three cases emphasizing possible confusion with ovarian clear cell adenocarcinoma. Int J Gynecol Pathol 11:96–104
130. Young RH, Jackson A, Wells M (1994) Ovarian metastasis from thyroid carcinoma twelve years after partial thyroidectomy mimicking struma ovarii. Report of a case. Int J Gynecol Pathol 13:181–185
131. Young RH, Kozakewich HPW, Scully RE (1993) Metastatic ovarian tumors in children: a report of 14 cases and review of the literature. Int J Gynecol Pathol 12:8–19
132. Young RH, Prat J, Scully RE (1984) Endometrial stromal sarcomas of the ovary. A clinicopathologic analysis of 23 cases. Cancer (Phila) 53:1143–1155
133. Young RH, Scully RE (1989) Alveolar rhabdomyosarcoma metastatic to the ovary. A report of two

cases and discussion of the differential diagnosis of small cell malignant tumors of the ovary. Cancer (Phila) 64:899–904
134. Young RH, Scully RE (1991) Malignant melanoma metastatic to the ovary: a clinicopathologic analysis of 20 cases. Am J Surg Pathol 15:849–860
135. Young RH, Scully RE (1991) Metastatic tumors in the ovary: a problem-oriented approach and review of the recent literature. Semin Diagn Pathol 8:250–276
136. Young RH, Scully RE (1988) Mucinous tumors of the ovary associated with mucinous adenocarcinomas of the cervix. A clinicopathological analysis of 16 cases. Int J Gynecol Pathol 7:99–111
137. Young RH, Scully RE (1985) Ovarian metastases from cancer of the lung: problems in interpretation—a report of seven cases. Gynecol Oncol 21:337–350
138. Young RH, Scully RE (1990) Ovarian metastases from carcinoma of the gallbladder and extrahepatic bile ducts simulating primary tumors of the ovary: a report of six cases. Int J Gynecol Pathol 9:60–72
139. Young RH, Scully RE (1990) Sarcomas metastatic to the ovary. A report of 21 cases. Int J Gynecol Pathol 9:231–252
140. Young RH, Scully RE (1988) Urothelial and ovarian carcinomas of identical cell types: problems in interpretation. A report of three cases and review of the literature. Int J Gynecol Pathol 7:197–211
141. Yu TJ, Iwasaki I, Horie H, Tamaru J, Takahashi A (1986) Endolymphatic stromal myosis of the uterus with metastasis to ovary and recurrence in vagina. Acta Pathol Jpn 36:301–308
142. Zaino RJ, Unger ER, Whitney C (1984) Synchronous carcinomas of the uterine corpus and ovary. Gynecol Oncol 19:329–335
143. Zaloudek C, Miller TR, Stern JL (1995) Desmoplastic small cell tumor of the ovary: a unique polyphenotypic tumor with an unfavorable prognosis. Int J Gynecol Oncol 14:260–265
144. Zukerberg LR, Young RH (1990) Chordoma metastatic to the ovary: report of a case. Arch Path Lab Med 114:208–210

23

Diseases of the Placenta

Deborah J. Gersell, M.D., and Frederick T. Kraus, M.D.

The placenta is crucial for fetal growth and survival, performing the most important functions of many somatic organs before birth. Thus, pathologic processes interfering with placental function may result in abnormalities of fetal growth or development, malformations, or stillbirth, and there is increasing recognition that some long-term (especially neurologic) disabilities can be traced to injury occurring before birth. It is the purpose of this chapter to describe clinically important placental lesions and to emphasize the context in which these lesions are directly or indirectly important to the fetus, the mother, or both.

Normal Anatomy and Development

The monograph by Boyd and Hamilton[76] provides a detailed description and exquisite illustrations of the various stages of human implantation. The ovum is fertilized in the fallopian tube and develops rapidly, reaching the endometrial cavity as a blastocyst. At this stage, the outer cell layer of the blastocyst has differentiated into trophoblast, and there are only a few cells in the inner cell mass from which the embryo will ultimately be derived. The trophoblast attaches to and penetrates the endometrium on the 6th to 7th postovulatory day, and by the 10th to 11th postovulatory day, the blastocyst is totally embedded in endometrial stroma that has reestablished continuity over the penetration defect. The trophoblast grows rapidly and circumferentially, invading maternal blood vessels. Blood-filled spaces (lacunae) separate the trophoblast into trabecular columns (Fig. 23.1), with an outer syncytiotrophoblastic layer oriented radially around central solid cores of cytotrophoblast. As the extraembryonic mesenchyme penetrates the cytotrophoblastic cores, small blood vessels form within it, and these eventually connect with each other and with those in the body stalk (allantois), establishing the fetoplacental

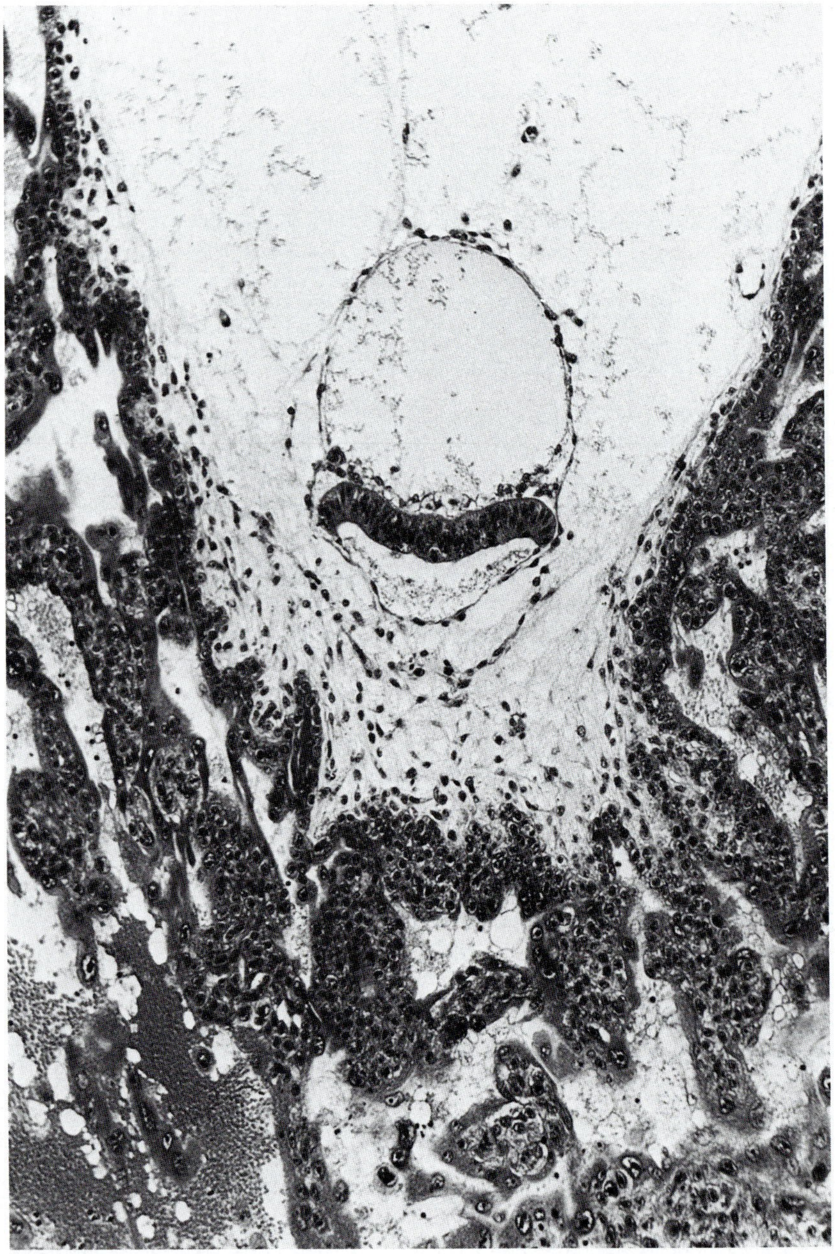

Fig. 23.1. Implantation at 13 days. Trophoblast has differentiated into inner (cytotrophoblast) and outer (syncytiotrophoblast) layers. Focally, the cytotrophoblast has proliferated to form projections, the forerunners of the primary villi. The germ disk is located near the center. (Reprinted courtesy of Department of Embryology, Davis Division, Carnegie Institute of Washington.)

circulation by early in the 5th week. Solid trophoblastic aggregates remain at the periphery of the stem villi, anchoring them to the basal plate (Fig. 23.2) and forming a complete shell that continues to grow and expand the intervillous space (Fig. 23.3).

Successful implantation requires a series of complex, coordinated interactions between maternal tissue and trophoblast. The trophoblast consists of several morphologically and functionally distinct cell types, each with characteristic anatomic distribution. The great majority of cytotrophoblastic and syncytiotrophoblastic cells are located on chorionic villi (villous trophoblast). Cytotrophoblast (CT), the germinative, mitotically active component of trophoblast, is present as a layer of uniform cells with single, round–oval nuclei, clear cytoplasm, and distinct cell borders directly overlying the stromal core of the villus. The syncytiotrophoblast (ST) overlies the cytotrophoblast and is the terminally differentiated component of trophoblast responsible for transport functions and hormone production. Its abundant, often vacuolated cytoplasm is amphophilic with multiple small dark nuclei and a distinct brush border. Intermediate trophoblast (IT) is a constituent of villous trophoblast, primarily in the anchoring cell columns, but is most prevalent in extravillous sites including the fetal membranes (chorion laeve) and implantation site.[309] Subpopulations of IT in different locations [villous, implantation site, and membranous ("chorionic")] are morphologically and immunohistochemically distinct.[525–527,612] IT nuclei are irregular and hyperchromatic with coarsely granular chromatin, and most cells are mononucleate, although bi-, tri-, and multinucleate forms occur. IT cells may be round, polyhedral, or spindle shaped with abundant eosinophilic, amphophilic, or clear cytoplasm. The cytologic features are generally sufficient to distinguish IT,[592] but the intermingling of intermediate trophoblast and decidua at the implantation site is so intimate that it may be difficult to characterize any particular cell as maternal or fetal by conventional light microscopy. When findings are equivocal (as in some abortion specimens), immunohistochemical stains for keratin help distinguish IT (keratin positive) from decidua (keratin negative).[122,123]

The intermediate trophoblast that infiltrates the decidua and myometrium at the implantation site is responsible for remarkable physiologic structural modifications in the spiral arteries essential to in-

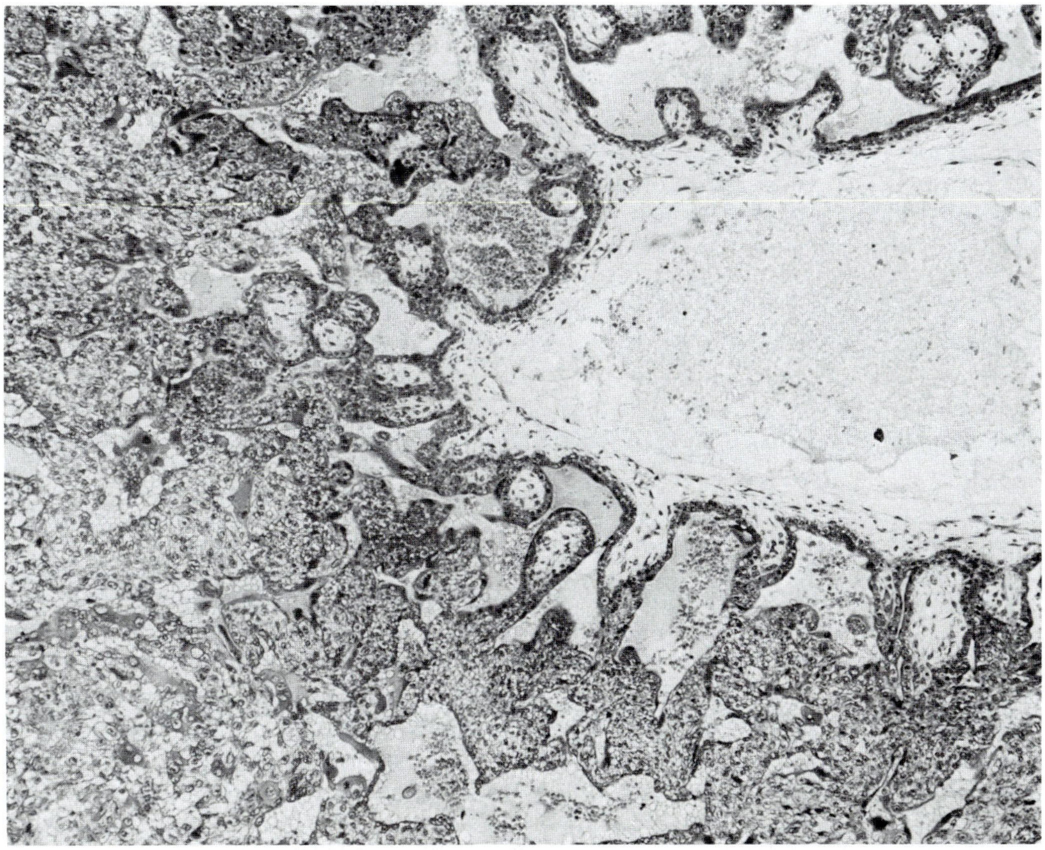

Fig. 23.2. Secondary villi. Solid cytotrophoblastic cores are penetrated by mesenchyme.

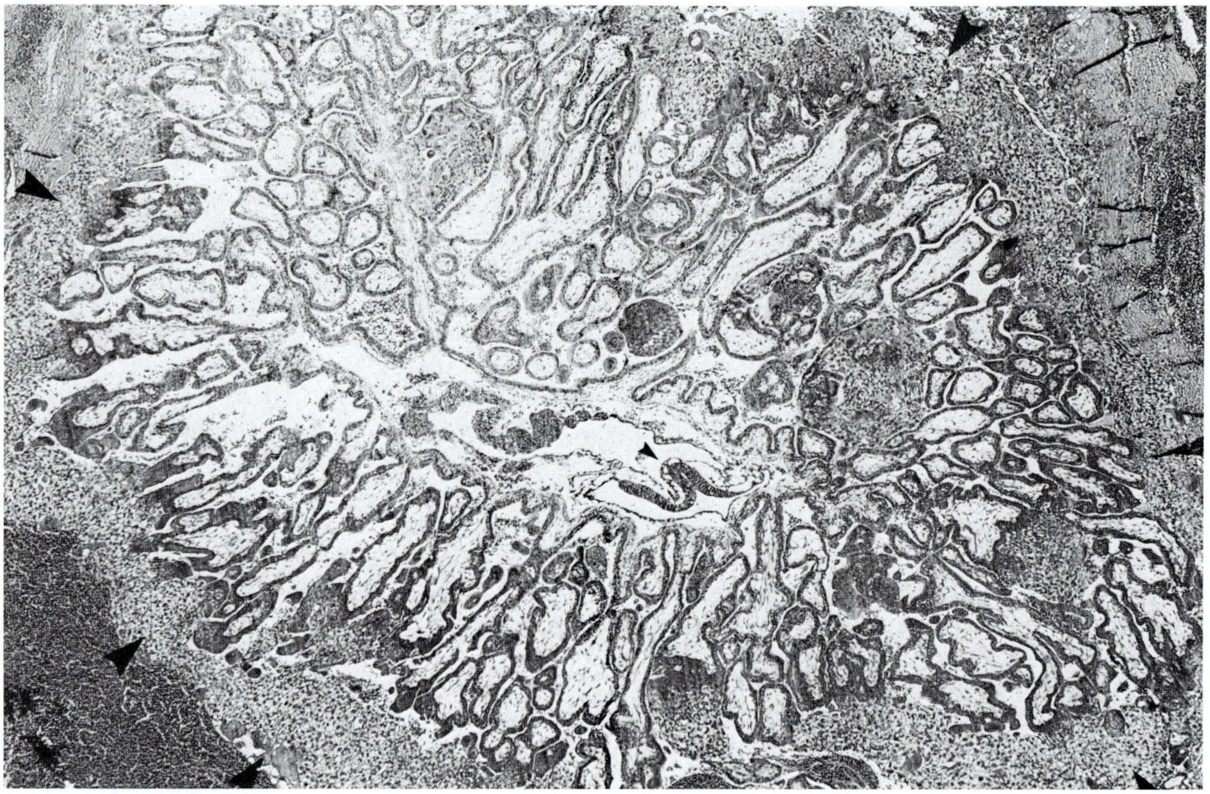

Fig. 23.3. Cytotrophoblastic shell. Complete cytotrophoblastic shell (*large arrows*) surrounds the entire conceptus. Portions of the germ disk and yolk sac are present at center (*small arrow*).

crease blood flow to the implantation site. In the early weeks of pregnancy, IT invades the decidual segments of the spiral arteries,[137,309,464,465,466] and with fibrinoid material composed of a complex of fibrin, plasma constituents, and proteinaceous substances produced by the trophoblast, it replaces the endothelium and the muscular and elastic tissue of the media (Fig. 23.4). Between 14 and 20 weeks of pregnancy, endovascular IT extends from the decidual segments into the myometrial segments of the spiral arteries, and the latter are similarly remodeled. As detailed by Pijnenborg, adaptation of the myometrial segments of the spiral arteries by migrating IT may be necessary before endovascular trophoblastic migration can occur.[423] The spiral arteries altered by this process undergo progressive distension, eventuating in large funnel-shaped channels that augment blood flow from 100 ml/min in the nonpregnant uterus to more than 500 ml/min in the uterus at term.

The trophoblast is also responsible for the production of a number of protein and steroid hormones. The ratio and distribution of pregnancy-specific and pregnancy-associated hormones changes during development suggesting a link between hormone biosynthesis and trophoblastic differentiation.[244,309,310,496,578] In normal placentas, hormones are most widely distributed in the syncytiotrophoblast, and none of these hormones is localized in the cytotrophoblast. The intermediate trophoblast produces a considerable amount of human placental lactogen (hPL) throughout pregnancy as well as a small amount of human chorionic gonadotrophin (hCG) early in gestation. Although there is a marked diminution of hCG in both syncytiotrophoblast and intermediate trophoblast after the first trimester, hPL increases during the second and third trimesters. The normal pattern of trophoblastic hormone expression may be altered in abnormal gestations.[144,300]

As it grows and enlarges, the chorion undergoes gross structural modifications. Initially, villi surround the entire chorionic cavity, but as the chorion prolapses into the endometrial cavity, the villi on the embryonic aspect of the chorion continue to proliferate, forming the definitive placenta (chorion frondosum) while the villi oriented toward the uterine cavity undergo progressive atrophy to form the smooth chorion (chorion laeve) or fetal membranes. Remnants of these atrophic villi are still apparent in sections of extraplacental membranes in the mature placenta (Fig. 23.5). A departure from this orderly process of villous growth and atrophy is

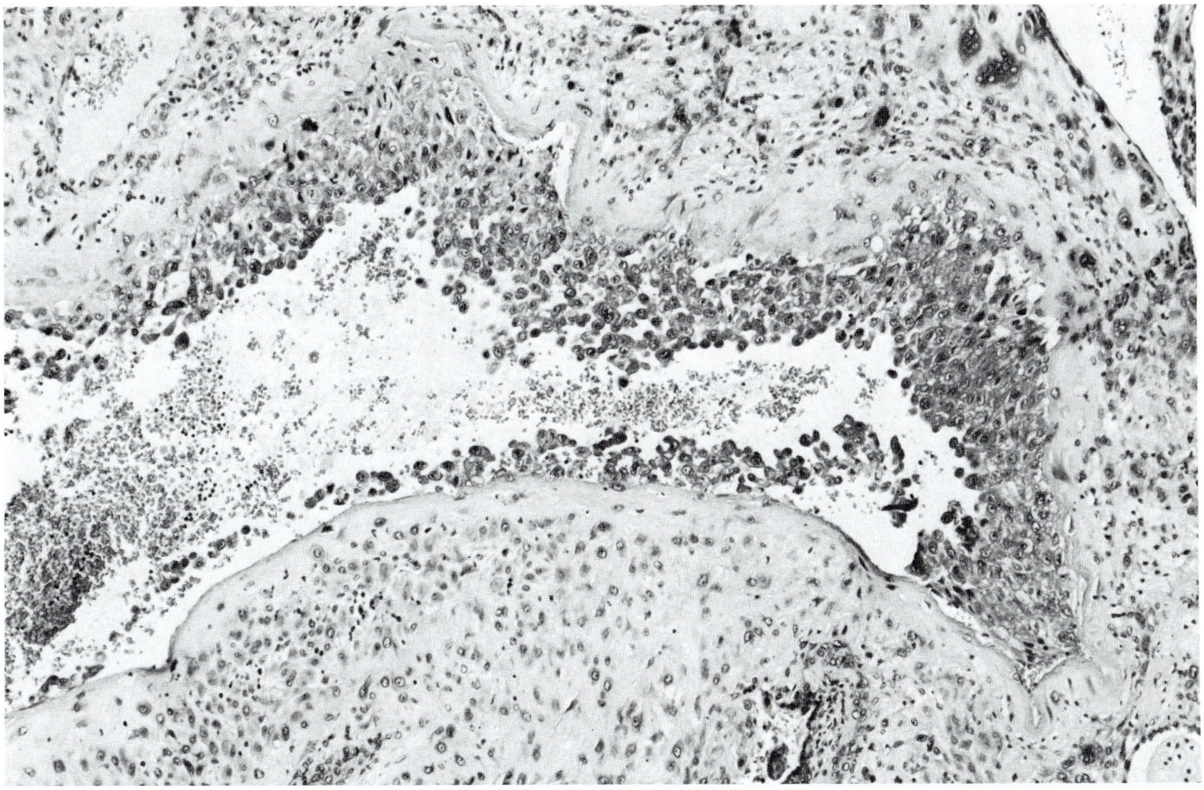

Fig. 23.4. Normal physiologic changes in a spiral artery. Replacement of maternal endothelium and destruction of the media by intermediate trophoblast and fibrinoid deposits result in marked vascular dilatation.

thought to result in some of the aberrant placental shapes described later. Continued growth and enlargement of the chorion results in eventual obliteration of the uterine cavity through fusion of the decidua capsularis and the decidua vera of the opposite uterine wall, usually around 20 weeks. In time, the chorionic cavity is obliterated by progressive expansion of the amnion.

Septae, appearing at about 3 months, are irregular folds of the basal plate drawn into the intervillous space by the relatively slow growth of the anchoring villi. The septae partition the maternal surface incompletely and irregularly into 15 to 20 divisions that have no physiologic significance. Islands of intermediate trophoblast (previously referred to as "X" cells) in the septae may be prominent.

Villous structure changes dramatically over the course of a normal gestation reflecting placental growth, development and maturation. Five villous types have been detailed in the work of Kaufmann and others.[51] *Mesenchymal villi* are a primitive, transient stage in villous development. The loose stroma of mesenchymal villi is abundant with numerous Hofbauer cells, central small vessels, and an orderly surface bilayer of CT and ST. Mesenchymal villi predominate in early pregnancy but may be found in small numbers even at term.[494] According to Kaufmann, mesenchymal villi begin to develop into *immature intermediate villi* around 7–8 weeks. Immature intermediate villi are defined by abundant loose reticular stroma with empty channels containing Hofbauer cells, features that may lead to erroneous interpretation as villous edema. Immature intermediate villi predominate through the second trimester, but small clusters persist in the center of lobules at term (normally 0–5% volumetrically). Immature intermediate villi are gradually transformed into *stem villi* as their vessels acquire a distinct muscular media and progressively prominent adventitia and fibrous stroma. Stem villi comprise 20%–25% of villi in a normal term placenta, with the highest concentration centrally beneath the chorionic plate. Stem villi support the villous tree and transport blood but do not participate significantly in oxygen or nutrient exchange. The stem villi divide progressively, and some insert into the basal plate, anchoring the placenta to the uterus. The aggregate of villi derived from a primary stem villus defines the fetal cotyledon. The subunit referred to as a lobule is composed of villous parenchyma derived from a single secondary stem villus.

Beginning in the last trimester, newly formed

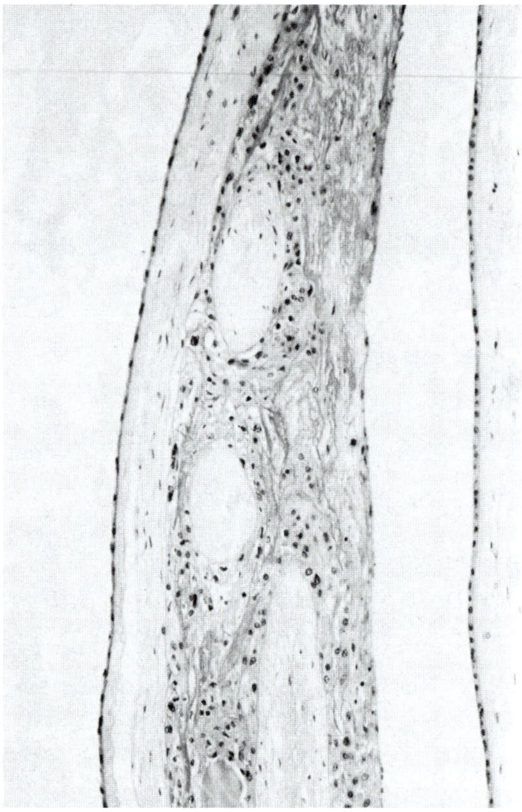

Fig. 23.5. Chorion laeve. Remnants of atrophic villi in the fetal membranes of a normal term gestation.

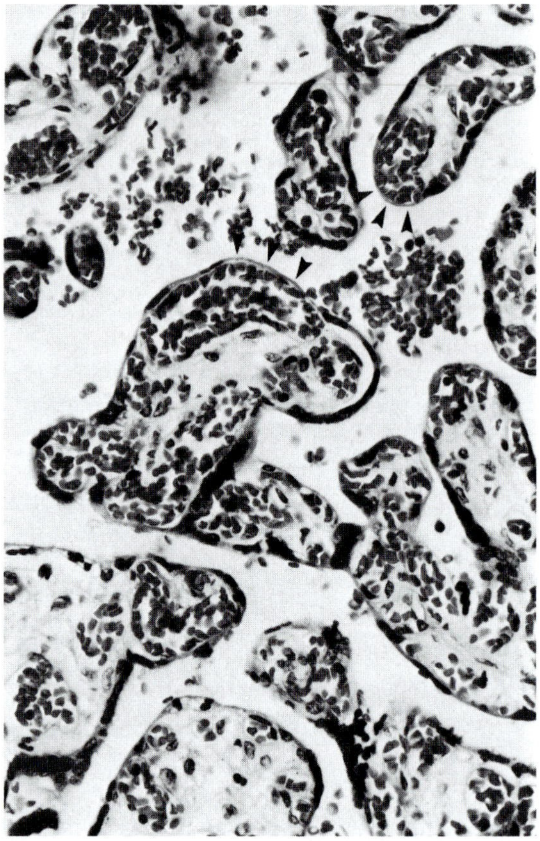

Fig. 23.6. Third-trimester terminal villi, vasculosyncytial membranes. Syncytiotrophoblastic nuclei aggregate to form knots. Fetal capillaries protrude beneath and fuse with the syncytiotrophoblast to form vasculosyncytial membranes (*arrows*).

mesenchymal villi transform into *mature intermediate villi*. Mature intermediate villi are long and slender with roughly the same diameter as terminal villi and numerous small vessels and capillaries, comprising less than 50% of the villus. Roughly one-fourth of the villous volume at term is made up of mature intermediate villi. *Terminal villi* are the final ramifications of the villous tree produced along the surfaces of mature intermediate villi during the third trimester. Terminal villi have sinusoidally dilated capillaries (occupying more than 50% of the villous stroma) that bulge beneath and fuse with the overlying attenuated syncytiotrophoblast forming vasculosyncytial membranes (Fig. 23.6). In these areas, the maternal and fetal circulations are most closely approximated and most gas and nutrient exchange occurs. Normally, terminal villi make up more than 35% of the villous volume at term.

With villous maturation, the barrier between maternal and fetal circulations is reduced by thinning of syncytiotrophoblast, diminution in cytotrophoblast, decrease in mean villous diameter, and apposition of fetal capillaries to the villous surface. The factors that normally control villous maturation are not understood, but considerable evidence suggests that the maturational rate is altered in pathologic states. The villi in any placenta are not completely homogeneous. The peripheral villi and those beneath the chorionic plate tend to be smaller with more collagenous stroma and a thicker trophoblastic basement membrane, and the villi located centrally in the fetal lobule are less mature than those at the periphery. These regional differences, probably related to maternal blood flow, should always be considered when judging placental maturity, which is best assessed in standardized sections from central placental zones.[198]

Circulation

Maternal blood is delivered to the intervillous space through spiral arterial inlets in the basal plate. Maternal blood flows toward the chorionic plate, disperses laterally, percolates around the villi, and exits through venous outlets in the placental floor. The precise anatomic relationship between the maternal arterial inlets in the basal plate and the fetal placental lobules is a matter of debate. Deoxygenated fetal blood reaches the placenta through the two umbilical arteries that branch and divide until they ultimately terminate in the complex anastomosing capillary network of the terminal villi. At this interface, gas and nutrient exchange occurs across the vasculosyncytial membranes (capillary endothelium, fused endothelial and trophoblastic basement membranes, and attenuated trophoblastic cytoplasm). Oxygenated and fortified blood returns via venous tributaries to the umbilical vein.

Abnormal Placentation

Anomalous Shapes

Occasionally, the placenta may deviate from its usual round or oval discoid shape. The pathogenesis of shape variation is not completely understood, but these anomalies probably reflect a failure or disturbance in the pattern of orderly villous atrophy and proliferation that generally results in a single round or oval placental disk with transition to fetal membranes at the disk edge.

One of the most common shape variations is the *accessory* or *succenturiate lobe*, a condition in which usually one but occasionally multiple discrete masses of placental tissue are separated from the main placenta (Fig. 23.7). The accessory lobe may be attached to the main disk by a narrow isthmus of placental tissue or separated from it by fetal membranes. The umbilical cord generally inserts into the main placental mass, and the fetal vessels supplying the accessory lobe traverse membranes unsupported by underlying villous parenchyma. If these large intramembranous vessels are traumatized during delivery, severe fetal hemorrhage may result. Thrombosis of membranous vessels may be associated with fetal thromboembolic events (Fig. 23.8).[444] Occasionally, an accessory lobe presents as placenta previa or is retained in utero after delivery, resulting in postpartum bleeding or infection. Succenturiate lobes have a tendency to infarct but otherwise show no specific histologic changes. The reported frequency of the accessory lobe is variable; Fox estimates that it occurs in about 3% of placentas.[174]

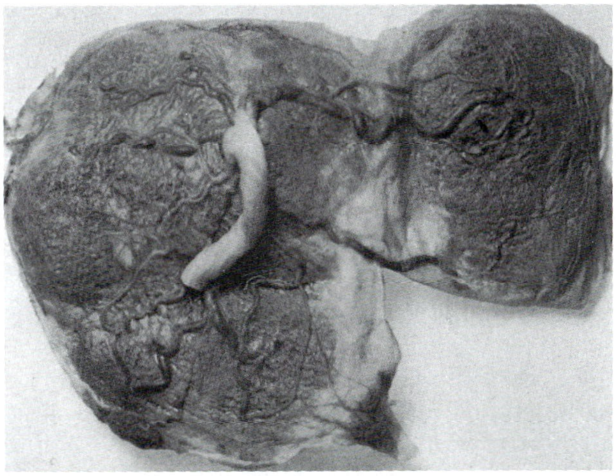

Fig. 23.7. Accessory (succenturiate) lobe. Discrete mass of placental tissue separated from the main placental mass by fetal membranes. Fetal vessels supplying the accessory lobe must traverse unsupported membranes.

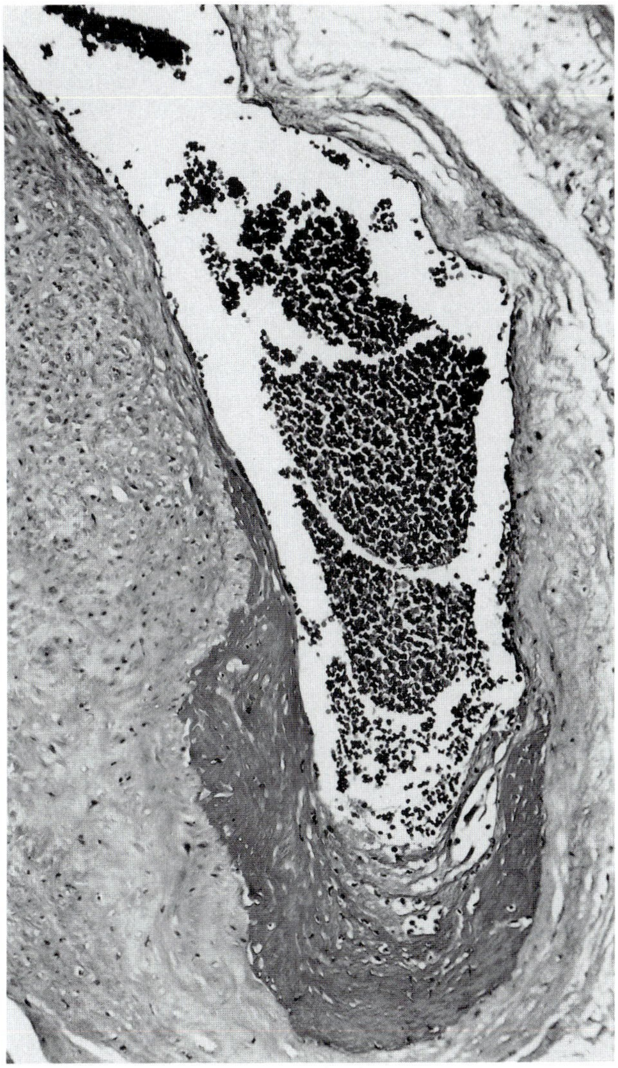

Fig. 23.8. Membranous vessel supplying succenturiate lobe. This large membranous vessel supplying a succenturiate lobe contains a mural thrombus.

The *bilobate* or *bipartite placenta* is a specific variant in which two equally sized placental lobes are separated by fetal membranes or connected by a narrow isthmus of placental tissue. The umbilical cord usually inserts centrally between the lobes into the placental bridge or membranes. The clinical significance of this abnormality has not been extensively studied. Fujikura et al. noted a significant association between bilobate placenta and multiparity, advanced maternal age, and a history of infertility. They also found a higher frequency of first-trimester bleeding, placenta previa, and undue placental adherence requiring manual extraction in association with this condition.[188]

A variety of other anomalous shapes occur, but these are very uncommon and rarely encountered. The *multilobate placenta* consists of three or more lobes of roughly equal size. *Placenta membranacea* is a large, thin placenta in which functional chorionic villi cover the entire gestational sac. In this condition, the differential atrophy of the chorion laeve and proliferation of the chorion frondosum does not occur, leaving most or all the membranes covered by chorionic villi. The placental parenchyma may vary in thickness, but only exceptionally is there a dominant area resembling a placental disk. Placenta membranacea occurs commonly in animal species but is extremely rare in humans. The few reported cases have been complicated by antepartum bleeding and abnormal placental adherence, undoubtedly relating to the obligate placenta previa that accompanies this form of placentation. Nearly all cases are associated with preterm delivery, and the fetal mortality rate is high.[219,249] The annular or cylindrical *ring-shaped placenta* is also very rare. In *fenestrate placenta*, there is focal absence of villous parenchyma resulting in either a through-and-through hole or the chorionic plate may remain intact over the parenchymal defect.

Extrachorial Placentae

Extrachorial placentation is a common gross structural deviation in which the chorionic plate of the placenta is smaller than its basal plate. The chorionic plate does not extend to the placental margin as in a normal placenta, but undergoes transition to fetal membranes central to the disk edge, leaving a rim of bare placental tissue (extrachorial portion) extending beyond the limits of the chorionic plate (Fig. 23.9).

Etiology and Pathogenesis

The many theories attempting to explain the etiology and pathogenesis of extrachorial placentation have been summarized by Scott.[504] Recently, recurrent marginal hemorrhages resulting in circumvallation have been documented on serial ultrasound images, providing evidence that recurrent hemorrhage at the disk margin elevates and displaces the membrane insertion site centrally.[58,395] This condition may represent the pathologic correlate of recurrent and persistent maternal bleeding throughout pregnancy (chronic abruption).

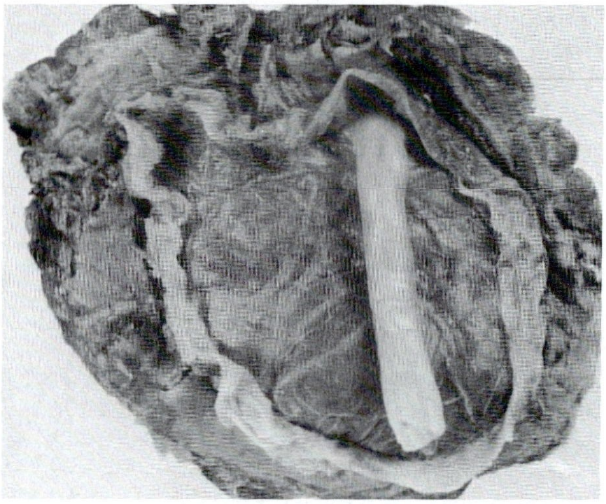

Fig. 23.9. Extrachorial placenta. The fetal membranes do not extend to the peripheral margin of the placenta, leaving a ring of placental tissue extending beyond the chorionic plate.

Pathology

There are two types of extrachorial placenta, *circummarginate* and *circumvallate*, categorized on the basis of the nature of the transition from the chorionic plate to the fetal membranes. In circumvallate placentas, the marginal membrane ring is reflected centrally, folded, and rolled back upon itself (Fig. 23.10). Variable amounts of fibrin and recent and old blood clot are consistently found at the margin in the reflected membrane fold, and compressed old clot and hemosiderin deposits are common behind the membranes. In circummarginate placentas, the transition from the chorionic plate to the membranes is flat without reflection or prominent accumulation of old blood. In both types of extrachorial placentation, fetal vessels appear to terminate at the margin of the chorionic plate (Fig. 23.11) but actually continue their course peripherally in the deeper villous tissue. These two forms of extrachorial placentas may be partial or complete (circumferential) and may occur in combination.

Clinical Behavior

Estimates of the frequency of extrachorial placentation vary widely (presumably because the terms are not used uniformly), but it is more common in

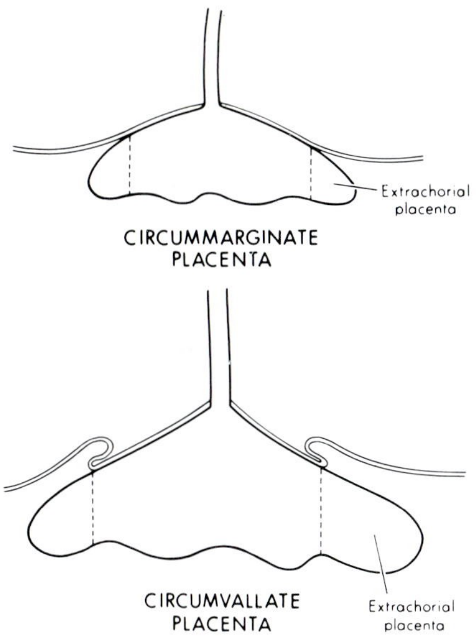

Fig. 23.10. Extrachorial placenta. Diagram comparing the rolled membrane ring in the circumvallate placenta to the flat transition in the circummarginate placenta. (After Fox H (1997) Pathology of the placenta, 2nd Ed. Saunders, Philadelphia, p 55.)

multigravidas.[56,182,597] Most investigators agree that circummarginate placentation has no clinical significance. An increased frequency of antepartum bleeding, preterm labor and delivery, fetal hypoxia, low birth weight, and perinatal mortality has been associated with circumvallate placentation.[56,182,316,395,471,504,618] Circumvallate placentation may recur in successive pregnancies.[605]

Placenta Accreta, Increta, Percreta

Placenta accreta, increta, percreta are defined clinically as abnormal adherence of the placenta to the

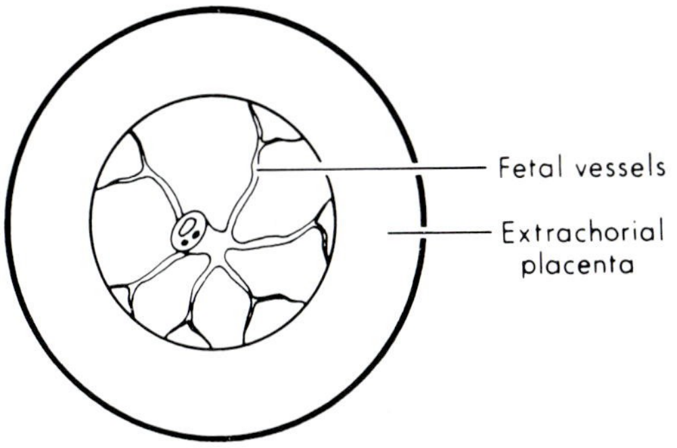

Fig. 23.11. Diagram of an extrachorial placenta, fetal side. Vessels appear to terminate at the margin of the chorionic plate but actually continue peripherally in the extrachorial portion. (After Fox H. Pathology of the Placenta. Second edition. Saunders, Philadelphia, 1997:55.)

uterine wall so that separation does not occur after delivery of the newborn. The degree of abnormal adherence/invasion is variable; placental villi may adhere to (*placenta accreta*), invade into (*placenta increta*), or penetrate through (*placenta percreta*) the myometrium. The condition may be total (involving the entire placenta), partial (involving one or more cotyledons), or focal (involving isolated foci of the placenta).

Etiology

The pathologic basis of this condition is partial or complete absence of the decidua, which normally separates the placenta from the myometrium during gestation and allows the placenta to separate after delivery of the newborn.[257] Deficient endometrial decidualization may be associated with abnormal placental adherence in nonfundic (cornual, tubal, cervical) implantation or in scarred endometrium [over leiomyomas; cesarean section (C-section) scars]. Alternatively, it has been suggested that abnormal trophoblastic invasion (in addition to, or rather than deficient decidualization) may be an important factor in the pathogenesis of abnormally adherent placentas.[522]

Clinical Features

The true frequency of placenta accreta is difficult to determine. Reported figures have varied widely from 1 in 1,667 to 1 in 70,000 pregnancies.[78] Fox emphasized the particular tendency for placenta accreta to occur in multigravid and obstetrically elderly women.[180] A number of predisposing factors have been linked to this condition, the two most significant being placenta previa and previous cesarean section (Fig. 23.12).[248,258,345,351] In some reports, as many as 64% of patients with placenta accreta have associated placenta previa,[78] and many placenta previa accretas occur in cesarean section scars.[370,559] In some cases, only that portion of the placenta implanted over the lower uterine segment or cesarean section scar has been abnormally adherent.[577] Other risk factors include a history of prior uterine curettage or uterine infection that may result in scarring,[197] previous manual removal of the placenta indicating abnormal adherence in a prior pregnancy, and nonfundic implantation (cornual, cervical, over leiomyomas, or in a rudimentary horn). The common endpoint in all these conditions is presumably a deficiency in or absence of the decidua. In only a small percentage (less than 10%) of cases are no risk factors identified.

Pathology

Microscopically, the cardinal feature is partial or complete absence of the decidua basalis, which may

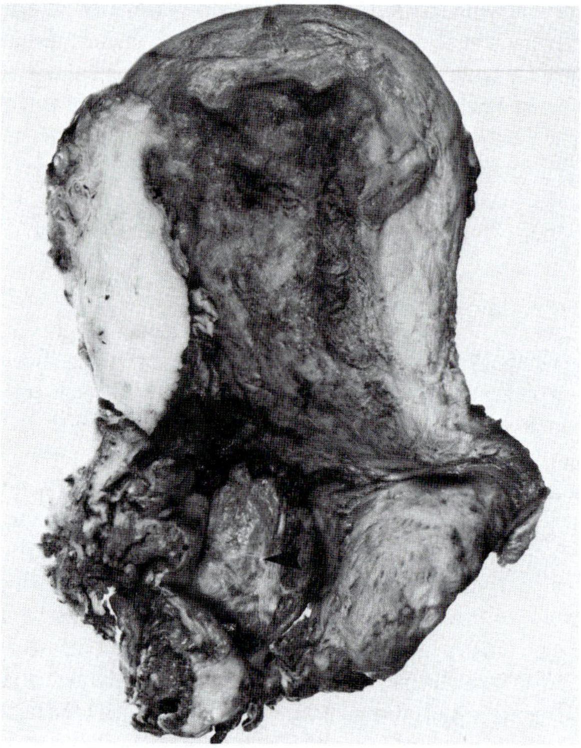

Fig. 23.12. Placenta percreta. Placenta penetrating the serosa at the site of three previous cesarean sections (*lower left* portion of the specimen). A portion of the chorionic plate is indicated by the *arrowhead*.

be replaced by loose connective tissue.[350] The decidua parietalis may be normal but is commonly absent or deficient as well. Placental villi adhere directly to or invade the myometrium (Fig. 23.13) often partially separated from focally hyalinized myometrial smooth muscle cells by a layer of fibrin. Abnormalities in the uteroplacental vasculature have been reported.[63,289] The diagnosis is often made in a hysterectomy specimen, but evaluation is difficult, because both placenta and uterus are frequently markedly disrupted by attempts to remove the adherent placenta at the time of delivery. Gross fragmentation, especially in a low-lying placenta or one requiring manual removal, should prompt a careful evaluation for placenta accreta, and any hysterectomy performed for postpartum bleeding requires a similar search. On occasion, microscopic examination will show a thin layer of myometrial fibers adherent to the maternal surface of the placenta, representing a focal form of accreta,[261] which occurs more frequently after manual removal and after preterm birth, especially in association with the vascular changes of preeclampsia. Occasionally the diagnosis can be established in a postpartum curettage when the sample includes villi in direct connection with myometrium. This finding may call attention to the potential for further bleeding or infection if all the placental tissue is not removed.

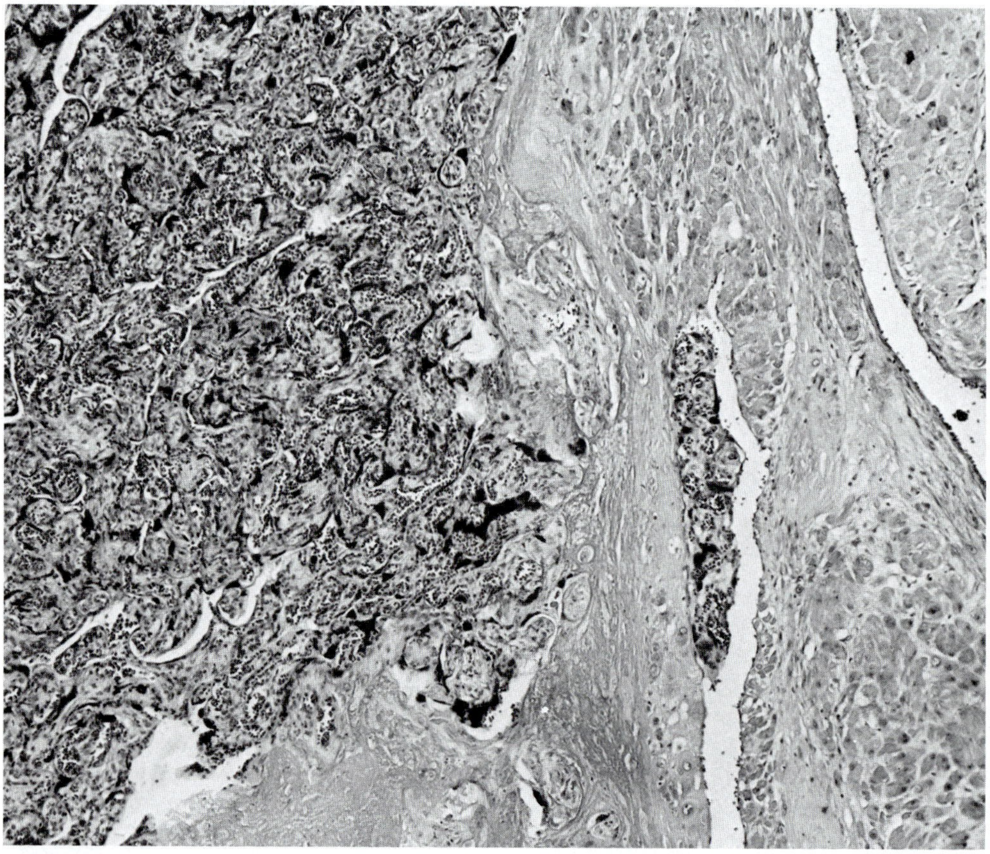

Fig. 23.13. Placenta accreta. Chronic villi adherent to myometrium without intervening decidua.

Clinical Behavior and Treatment

Placenta accreta is compatible with normal fetal growth and development and usually is not suspected until the placenta fails to separate in the third stage of labor. Postpartum bleeding is often life threatening, requiring immediate hysterectomy, or bleeding may be delayed, for which curettage is appropriate. More recently, selected cases have been managed expectantly, leaving the retained placenta in situ with or without systemic administration of methotrexate.[323] Some patients have had subsequent normal pregnancies with vaginal delivery. Antepartum bleeding and premature labor, also common, are caused by the high frequency of associated placenta previa. Uterine rupture may occur at any stage of pregnancy or during labor.[74,128,559] Maternal mortality is now uncommon, and fetal death occurs in about 1% of cases, usually in association with uterine rupture or severe antepartum bleeding.

Multiple Pregnancy

Pathologists are frequently asked to examine placentas of multiple pregnancies. Multiple gestations are common, even more so with assisted reproductive techniques, and they are associated with a disproportionate share of complications. Multiple gestations have higher rates of fetal morbidity, mortality, low birth weight, anomalous development, and malformation than singletons. Careful pathologic examination of the placenta can provide important insight into problems peculiar to multiples, and pathologists must be aware of the special considerations required in the examination of placentas from multiple births. A number of excellent and detailed accounts describing various aspects of multiple pregnancy are recommended to supplement the abbreviated coverage of the subject presented here.[33,52–54]

Twin Gestation

Twins may arise from the fertilization of two separate ova (dizygous or fraternal twins) or from the division of a single fertilized ovum (monozygous or identical twins). Monozygous twins are usually genetically and phenotypically identical, although there are rare examples of genetic and phenotypic discordance (monovular dispermic/monozygous heterokaryotic twins).[33,223,266] Dizygotic twins are no more similar genetically than other singleton siblings.

The frequency of monozygous twinning is relatively constant worldwide (about 3.5 in 1000 pregnancies), but there are marked geographic differences in total twinning rate, reflecting the predisposition for polyovulation in certain populations and families. Twins occur in about 1 in 80 Caucasian pregnancies in the United States, and about one-third of these are monozygotic.

Placentas in twin gestations are either monochorionic or dichorionic. All dizygous twins have dichorionic placentas (diamnionic-dichorionic, DiDi). In double ovulation, each blastocyst generates a placenta; if these implant in close proximity, varying degrees of fusion may result (DiDi fused), but otherwise, they are entirely separate. Monozygous twins may show any type of placentation depending on when division occurs (Fig. 23.14). If the single

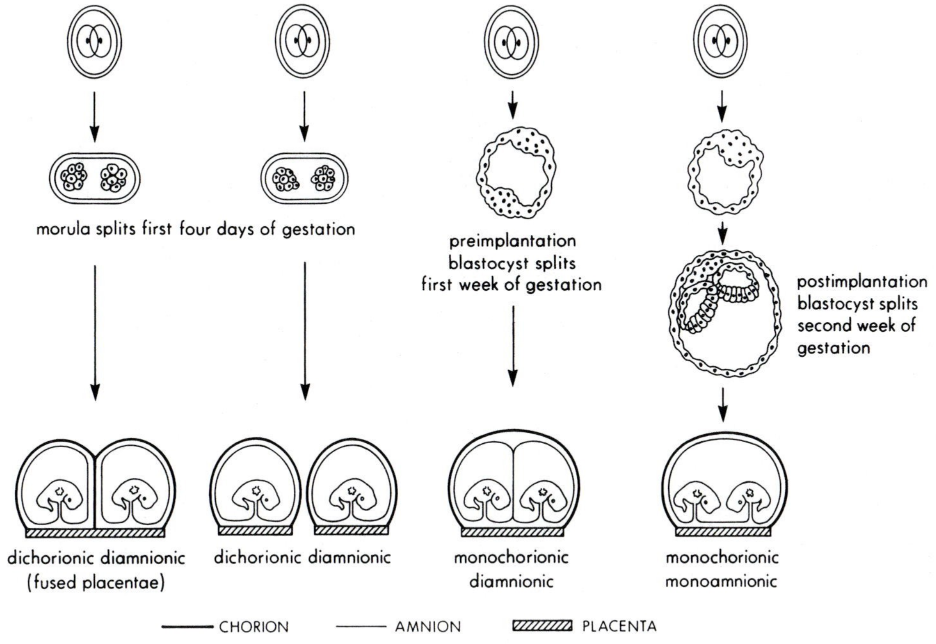

Fig. 23.14. Diagrammatic representation of placentation of monozygous twins. (After Fox H. (1997) Pathology of the Placenta. Second edition. Saunders, Philadelphia, p. 80.)

fertilized ovum divides very early, before differentiation of the chorion (first 2 or 3 days), the situation is analogous to dizygous twinning. If splitting occurs in the blastocyst stage, after formation of the chorion but before formation of the amnion (3rd to 8th day after fertilization), there will be a single placenta with two amnionic sacs (diamnionic-monochorionic, DiMo). A split after formation of the amnion, between the 8th and 13th days, will result in one placenta and one amnionic cavity (monoamnionic-monochorionic, MoMo), and later splitting, in conjoined twins. All twins with monochorionic placentas, therefore, are monozygous. Twins with dichorionic placentas, however, may be either dizygous or monozygous. Obviously, different fetal sex establishes a dizygous relation, but further investigation (blood group analysis, HLA typing, DNA analysis) may be required if determination zygosity is necessary in like-sex dichorionic twins. The frequencies of different placentation types in 250 consecutive twin deliveries summarized in Table 23.1 is reflective of the literature in general.[48] Overall, about 20% of twins with dichorionic placentas are monozygous.

Establishment of placentation type is important because it has a significant relationship to perinatal morbidity and mortality, which is much higher in twins than in singleton pregnancies. Many factors contribute to the increased morbidity/mortality in multiples, most importantly the premature onset of labor and delivery. Placentation type is also significant. Twins with monochorionic placentas have a much higher perinatal mortality than those with dichorionic placentas. Monoamnionic placentation is associated with highest fetal mortality rate (33–70%), presumably because of the high frequency of cord complications in twins that share an amnionic cavity.[33,52,416,575,601]

Pathologic examination should establish the type of placentation. Two entirely separate placentas are obviously dichorionic, each requiring routine examination. Practically speaking, the principal task for the pathologist is to distinguish a diamnionic-monochorionic placenta from a diamnionic-dichorionic fused placenta, and this can usually be reliably accomplished on gross exam. The septum in dichorionic fused placentas is thick and opaque because of the presence of chorionic tissue between the two amnionic layers. In contrast, the septum in a diamnionic monochorionic placenta is thin and translucent, composed of only two directly apposed layers of amnion. Histologic examination of the membranous septum confirms the gross impression (Figs. 23.15 and 23.16); this is most easily accomplished in a section of rolled septal membranes, although identical information may be obtained from a section of the T-zone where the septum meets the fetal surface. The latter method is useful in cases in which the septal membranes have been torn or otherwise distorted and cannot be rolled, but is technically more difficult, especially in monochorionic placentas (see Chapter 28, Gross Description, Processing, and Reporting of Gynecologic and Obstetric Specimens). The distribution of the fetal vessels on the chorionic plate is also helpful in distinguishing DiDi fused from DiMo placentas. In di-

Table 23.1. Frequency of different types of placentation in 250 consecutive twin deliveries

77 Monochorionic (31%)	*173 Dichorionic (69%) by blood group analysis*
3 MoMo (1%)	33 Monozygotic (13%)
74 DiMo (30%)	140 Dizygotic (56%)

From Benirschke and Driscoll.[48]

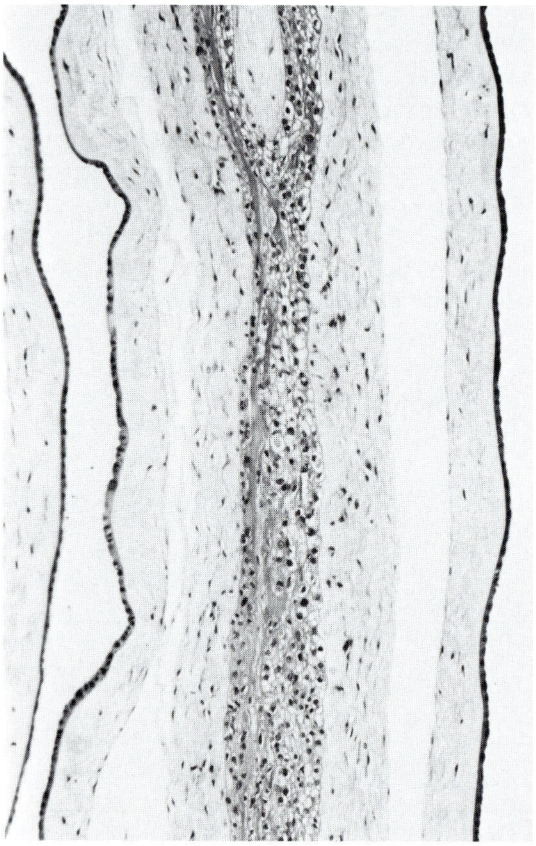

Fig. 23.15. Diamnionic-dichorionic (DiDi) fused twin placenta. Histologic section of the septal membranes shows an intervening central layer of chorion between two amnions.

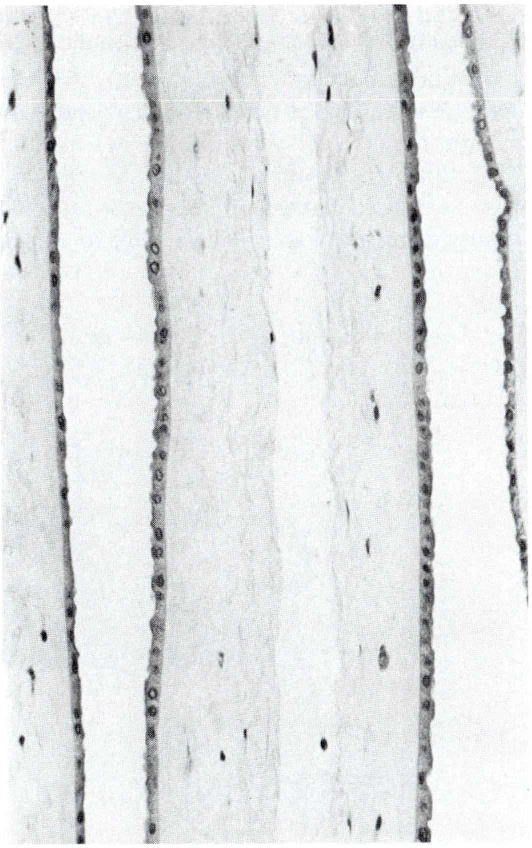

Fig. 23.16. **Diamnionic-monochorionic (DiMo) twin placenta.** Septal membranes are composed of two directly apposed amnions without intervening chorionic tissue.

chorionic placentas, fetal chorionic vessels approach, but do not cross, the area of fusion (Fig. 23.17). In diamnionic-monochorionic placentas, the two vascular districts are generally imperceptibly merged, and portions of the placenta are shared by both fetuses (Fig. 23.18). The position of the membranous septum in the DiMo placenta does not necessarily conform to the vascular equator.

An important feature of monochorionic placentas is the presence of vascular communications between the two fetal circulations. It is generally agreed that some form of vascular communication occurs in essentially all monochorionic placentas, although the size and location of anastomotic vessels varies. Some anastomoses occur between the large vessels on the chorionic plate. The majority of superficial anastomoses are between arteries; vein-to-vein anastomoses are much less common. Of greater physiologic significance are the arteriovenous anastomoses that occur between capillaries deep within shared villous parenchyma. Although arteriovenous anastomoses are very common, their physiologic importance varies markedly depending

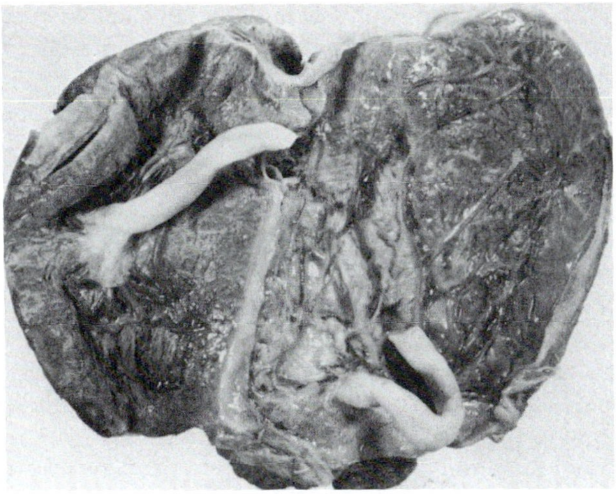

Fig. 23.17. **DiDi fused twin placenta.** The two placental masses are fused but discrete. Fetal vessels do not approach or cross the area of fusion.

on their size, number, and the overall balance of blood flow. Arteriovenous anastomoses may be modified by communication between large superficial branches of the same vessels. Vascular communications in DiDi fused placentas are absent with rare exceptions.[89,319,442,462]

Stripping the amnion from the fetal surface of the placenta facilitates the study of chorionic plate vessels. Large vessel anastomoses are easily identified grossly and can be highlighted by the injection of milk, colored dye, or air. The size (diameter) and type (arteries cross over veins) of anastomosis should be recorded. Arteriovenous (A-V) anastomoses are physiologically more important but more difficult to identify because they involve capillaries and cannot be directly visualized. Potential sites of

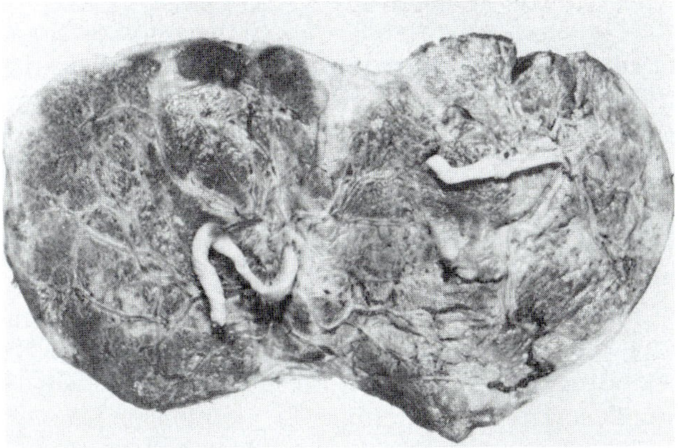

Fig. 23.18. **DiMo twin placenta.** Intimate intermingling of the two vascular districts with anastomosis of superficial vessels.

A-V anastomoses can be suspected when an unpaired artery from one twin penetrates the chorionic plate in close proximity to an unpaired vein from the co-twin. A simple method to confirm the presence of an A-V anastomosis is to inject any colored substance (milk, dye) into a vessel supplying a suspected anastomosis and document its return to the co-twin. This procedure can be repeated at multiple sites in an attempt to document the number of anastomoses.[33,462] The injection of air is particularly effective (also very quick and easy) because by displacing blood it renders the shared placental district pale, allowing estimation of its volume.[33] It should be emphasized that injection studies are merely qualitative and do not necessarily reflect the physiologic significance of the anastomoses in vivo. Nevertheless, their documentation is essential if anastomoses are to be invoked as a cause of discordant fetal growth (see following). Areas of villous disruption will compromise any injection technique.

Complications of Multiple Pregnancy

Twin–Twin Transfusion Syndrome

Etiology

A major cause of perinatal mortality in monochorionic twins is the *twin–twin transfusion* syndrome. Schatz proposed the now widely accepted view that the twin–twin transfusion syndrome results occurs when there is unbalanced flow of blood from one twin (the donor) to its co-twin (recipient) through arteriovenous anastomoses deep within shared placental lobules (the "third circulation").[557]

Pathology

Typically, the twin–twin transfusion syndrome is clinically manifest in the second trimester with acute hydramnios and growth discrepancy between the twins. Chronic unidirectional diversion of blood results in relative deprivation and growth retardation of the donor as compared to the larger recipient. Hydramnios, usually in the recipient, may be sufficient to cause maternal discomfort or respiratory compromise. The donor twin frequently exhibits oligohydramnios and decreased movement, and is sometimes referred to as the "stuck twin."

Postnatally, there is a marked discrepancy in the size and appearance of the infants and their corresponding placental territories. The donor twin is smaller, pale, and anemic; the recipient is heavier, edematous, plethoric, and polycythemic. Either twin may be hydropic. Classically, there is marked discordance in the size and weight of the fetal organs, the organs of the recipient being larger and heavier than those of the donor. The recipient's heart especially is comparatively enlarged, and there is myocardial hypertrophy involving all chambers as well as increased smooth muscle mass in the media of the pulmonary and systemic arteries and arterioles. The donor heart is usually subnormal in size, and arterial muscle mass is decreased. Glomeruli are enlarged, up to twice normal size, in the recipient twin, and they are either normal or reduced in size in the donor.[382]

The placental territories of the donor and recipient twins may also be discordant.[1,5,109,484] The donor's placental territory may be large, bulky, and pale, reflecting fetal anemia. (Fig. 23.19). The villi

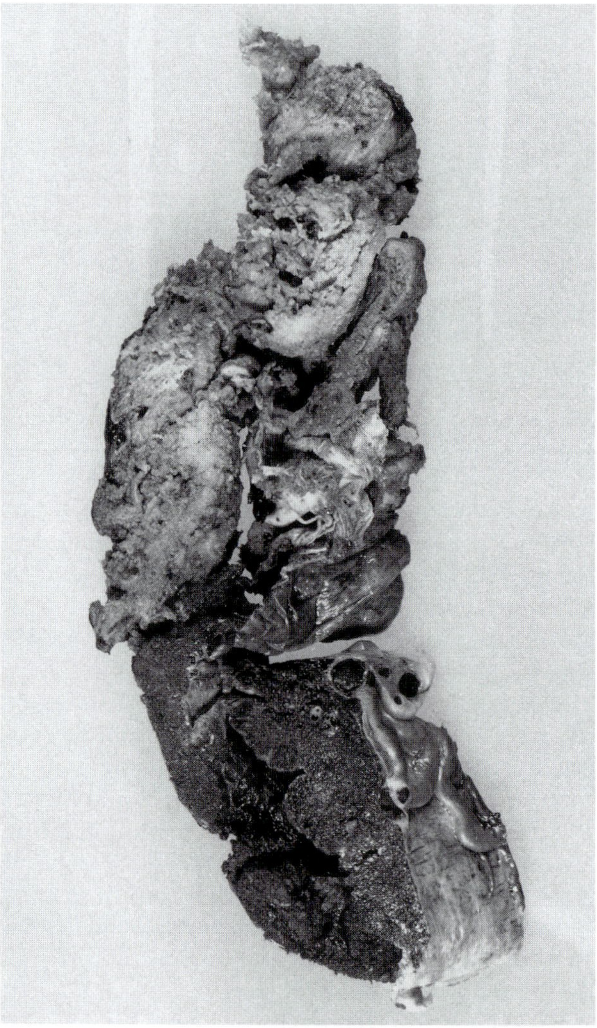

Fig. 23.19. Placenta, twin–twin transfusion syndrome. The donor portion (*top*) of this twin gestation complicated by the twin-twin transfusion syndrome is pale in comparison to the congested, darker recipient portion (*bottom*). Only a portion of the donor's placental territory, which was approximately three times the size of the recipient's territory, is included in this photograph.

are large and edematous with numerous Hofbauer cells and small capillaries containing nucleated red blood cells (Fig. 23.20). Amnion nodosum may be found when there is associated oligohydramnios. The recipient's placental territory is generally smaller, firm, and deep red. The villi are appropriately mature with dilated and intensely congested vessels (Fig. 23.20).

The clinical definition of the twin–twin transfusion syndrome is imprecise.[117] Hematologic (hemoglobin concentration difference greater than 5 g/100 ml) and anatomic (weight difference of 15%–20%) criteria are considered definitive by some.[71,329,442] The diagnosis is complicated because monochorionic twins may show asymmetric growth for reasons other than a chronic twin–twin transfusion (maternal, fetal, umbilical cord, or placental factors).[156,260] Furthermore, plethora of one twin and anemia of the other do not always signify a chronic twin–twin transfusion but may instead reflect acute shifts of blood through large superficial anastomoses (often occurring at the time of delivery) or fetomaternal hemorrhage. Either or both of the latter phenomena may be superimposed on a chronic intrauterine transfusion, further complicating an already complex clinical situation.[41]

The difficulty in establishing a uniform, clear definition of the twin–twin transfusion syndrome explains, in part, the great discrepancy, in its reported frequency which varies from 15% to 30% of monochorionic gestations.[442,557] Whatever the true frequency, the twin–twin transfusion syndrome does not occur as often as would be anticipated given the universal presence of vascular communications in monochorionic twin pregnancies. Interestingly, the twin–twin transfusion syndrome is not a significant cause of fetal mortality in monoamnionic twins.[601]

Clinical Behavior and Treatment

The consequences of the twin–twin transfusion syndrome are grave. Mortality rates are as high as 70%–100%, depending on the gestational age at diagnosis and delivery.[38,215,511] When the condition develops in the second trimester, it is usually associated with preterm labor and either death of one or both fetuses (if delivered before viability) or sig-

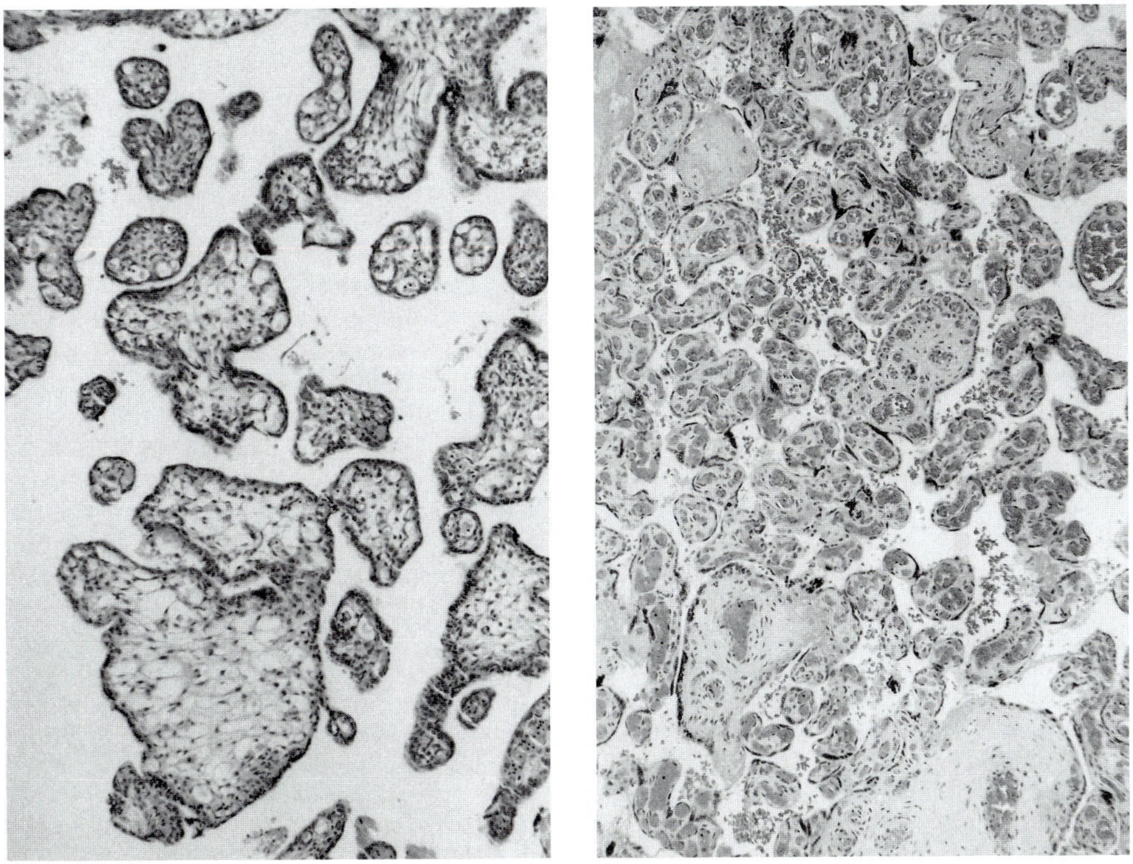

Fig. 23.20. Twin–twin transfusion, 32 weeks. In these photomicrographs taken at the same power for comparison, the donor villi (*left*) are large, relatively immature, and edematous, and the fetal capillaries contain numerous red blood cell precursors. The recipient villi (*right*) are more mature and congested.

nificant morbidity (if the neonates survive). Both twins are at great risk. The recipient twin is subject to cardiac failure, hemolytic jaundice, kernicterus, and thrombosis caused by hemoconcentration. The donor twin may be severely anemic or hypoglycemic.

If one twin dies in utero and the transfusion ceases, the situation may resolve itself. Alternatively, the surviving twin (usually the recipient) may exsanguinate acutely into the suddenly relaxed circulatory system of the dead co-twin (usually the donor).[44,327] In this event, the expected color/weight relationships between the twins may be paradoxically reversed. Multiorgan necrotic lesions (hydranencephaly, porencephaly, intestinal atresia, aplasia cutis) may occur in either or both twins[40,91,117,154,245,246,274,565,615] and have been attributed to the altered hemodynamics and transitory cardiovascular compromise associated with complex placental vascular connections.

Management options are limited and frequently unsuccessful. Serial amniocenteses, maternal digoxin treatment, intrauterine ligation of one umbilical cord, and selected feticide have been attempted in severe cases.[34,146,329] Successful outcome has been reported in a few cases of severe twin–twin transfusion syndrome following YAG laser ablation of vascular communications[127] or inadvertent puncture of vessels.[588] Doppler studies may be helpful in evaluating the results of intervention in the twin–twin transfusion syndrome.[162,201,433]

Acardia

Acardiac fetuses (*chorangiopagus parasiticus*, *CAPP*) occur in about 1% of monozygous twin gestations. The acardius is a bizarre and grossly malformed fetus attached to the placenta by an umbilical cord usually containing a single artery and vein (Fig. 23.21). These fetuses differ greatly in size, gross appearance, and degree of organogenesis; some are amorphous, shapeless masses, others exhibit rudimentary trunk and limb (usually lower) development, and rarely they are remarkably well developed. Regardless of the degree of development and organogenesis, all acardiac fetuses lack a functioning heart; their circulation is accomplished entirely by the co-twin (the "pump" twin).[73,204,399,510,606] Blood from the normal twin reaches the acardius through a large artery–artery anastomosis, flows through the acardius in reverse course, and returns to the pump twin via a large vein–vein anastomosis. These vascular anastomoses occur at the level of the umbilical cord or chorionic plate. The acardiac has no placental parenchymal vascular connections and is therefore more akin to a conjoined twin than a twin–twin transfusion. The pump twin is at risk for cardiovascular overload and preterm delivery. Intervention strategies similar to those utilized in the twin–twin transfusion syndrome have been attempted in this setting as well.

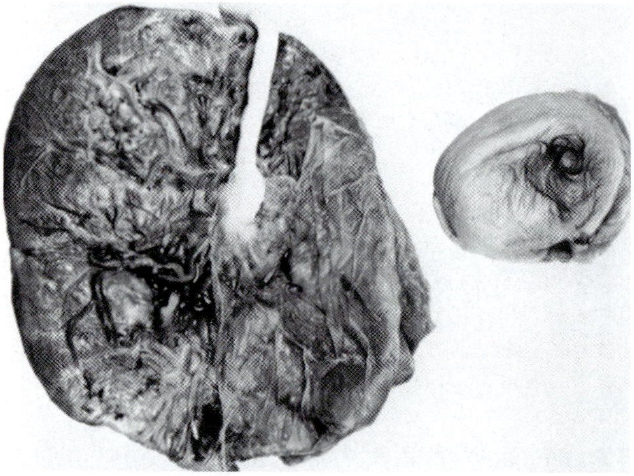

Fig. 23.21. Acardiac fetus.

There are two main theories of pathogenesis: (1) the reversed circulation is responsible for regression or resorption of a previously formed heart in the acardiac, or (2) the anomaly results from primary agenesis of the heart, the acardiac fetus surviving only when maintained by very specific vascular anastomoses with a normal co-twin. When karyotyped, the acardius and its co-twin have been isosexual. Chromosomal abnormalities have been documented in some acardiacs, all of whom have been associated with a genotypically normal co-twin.[21,124]

Fetus Papyraceus

Careful monitoring indicates that many twin pregnancies are converted to singleton pregnancies. The pathologic findings vary depending on the time of fetal death and the length of intrauterine retention.[33] When a twin dies early in gestation (first trimester), it may be completely undetectable when delivered at term, or a flattened mass of sclerotic placenta with a collapsed sac may be the only residue. *Fetus papyraceus* results from intrauterine death of a twin, usually in the second trimester. The dead fetus shrinks and is compressed against the membranes, eventually resembling amorphous necrotic tissue (Fig. 23.22). Undoubtedly, many are overlooked. Fetus papyracei occur in both monochorionic and dichorionic placentation.

Higher Multiple Births

The same principles of zygosity and placentation apply to *triplet*, *quadruplet*, and other *higher multiple births*. For example, triplets may be trizygotic, dizy-

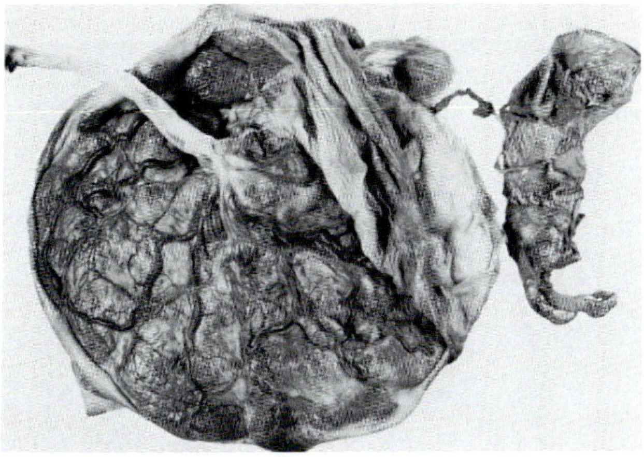

Fig. 23.22. Fetus papyraceus. Necrotic, compressed twin.

gotic, or monozygotic. Trizygotic triplets have trichorionic-triamnionic placentation but may be separate or variably fused. Dizygotic triplets may be dichorionic or trichorionic. Monozygotic triplets may be monochorionic, dichorionic, or trichorionic.

Placental Inflammation and Intrauterine Infections

Placental inflammatory infiltrates, a very common histologic finding, are variable in character and pattern of involvement. Different patterns of inflammation are associated with different routes of infection and, in general, with different causative organisms. Ascending infections in which microorganisms, usually bacteria, ascend into the uterus from the vagina or cervix produce an acute inflammatory reaction in the fetal membranes (*chorioamnionitis*), umbilical cord (*funisitis*), and ultimately within the fetus itself. Less often an inflammatory infiltrate, usually chronic, is found in the villous parenchyma (*villitis*) rather than the fetal membranes. This pattern of inflammation is the histologic hallmark of hematogenous infection whereby infectious agents reach the placenta through the maternal blood. The microorganisms that reach the placenta in this manner are often viruses, but also include some bacteria and protozoa. Passage through an infected birth canal is an important mode of fetal infection, but the placenta is not involved in this circumstance.

The consequences of intrauterine infection include abortion, stillbirth, preterm birth, fetal malformation, active postnatal infection, and long-term sequelae, frequently neurologic. At worst, affected children may be severely handicapped, mentally retarded, blind, or deaf. The social, financial, and emotional burden posed by the support of these children is enormous.

Ascending Infection and Chorioamnionitis

Chorioamnionitis is by far the most common form of placental inflammation in humans. Histologic chorioamnionitis reportedly occurs in about 4% of otherwise uncomplicated term births. Its frequency is inversely proportional to gestational age, emphasizing the strong association between chorioamnionitis and preterm birth (PTB). Chorioamnionitis is increased in black women.[389,394,474] Coitus has been implicated in increasing the frequency and severity of ascending infection,[380,391] and the role of the incompetent cervix has been stressed by Russell.[476]

Etiology and Pathogenesis

It is now generally accepted that chorioamnionitis is caused by infection. Microorganisms, usually bacteria, have been cultured from fetal membranes, amnionic fluid, cord blood, and fetal tissues in a high percentage of cases, and chorioamnionitis can be produced experimentally in animals by the intraamniotic injection of bacteria but not by sterile exogenous irritants.[321,340,412] The ascent of bacteria from the vagina or cervix into the uterus causing chorioamnionitis may either preceed or follow membrane rupture.[378,392] There is a consistent and well-documented relationship between chorioamnionitis and membrane rupture; the longer that membranes have been ruptured, the greater the likelihood that chorioamnionitis will occur.[108,205] This sequence of events, membrane rupture followed by chorioamnionitis, occurs commonly at term, and in these circumstances the threat of infection is universally recognized.

Chorioamnionitis, however, frequently precedes membrane rupture, causing premature rupture of membranes (PROM) and/or preterm labor (PTL), explaining the strong association between chorioamnionitis and preterm birth.[210,211,352,390,391,414] The bacteria most commonly identified in women with spontaneous preterm labor and intact membranes are low-virulence vaginal and enteric organisms, *Ureaplasma urealiticum*, *Mycoplasma hominis*, *Gardnerella vaginalis*, peptostreptococci, and *Bacterioides* species.[145,240,338,435,524] Rarely, nongenital organisms such as *Capnocytophaga* are found in association with PTL and chorioamnionitis.[149,256] Vaginal organisms appear to ascend into the uterus in the choriodecidual space and then broach the chorion and amnion in some cases to reach the amnionic fluid and ultimately the fetus itself. Although it is unclear when bacteria ascend from the vagina, recent evidence suggests that intrauterine infection may occur quite early in pregnancy, remaining undetected for months until eventuating in preterm labor or membrane rupture.[210]

Data accumulating from experimental and human studies are clarifying how bacterial infection and chorioamnionitis result in spontaneous preterm delivery. The inflammatory response to bacterial invasion results in the production of cytokines [principally IL-1, IL-6, and tumor necrosis factor (TNF)] that initiate prostaglandin synthesis, resulting in uterine contractions.[26,98,210,213,252,341,549] Certain bacterial species commonly associated with chorioamnionitis are high in phospholipase A_2, which releases the prostaglandin precursor arachidonic acid from membrane phospholipids.[15,16,414] The inflammatory response also results in increased synthesis of metalloproteases that are thought to remodel and soften cervical collagen and to degrade the extracellular matrix of the fetal membranes, leading to membrane rupture.[414]

Pathology

In most cases of chorioamnionitis, the placenta and fetal membranes are macroscopically normal. Occasionally, the membranes may be opaque, friable, or foul smelling in cases of particularly severe, longstanding bacterial infection. In rare instances of *Candida* infection, tiny white foci of colonization 2–3 mm in size may be seen, especially on the amniotic surface of the umbilical cord.[437,500,587,602]

Histologically, there is evidence of maternal and usually fetal response to amniotic infection.[61,66,67,252] The maternal reaction is manifested by an accumulation of neutrophils in the decidua that migrate progressively through the chorion, amnion, and into the amnionic fluid in response to chemotactic factors released by the infecting agent or inflammatory cells in the fetal membranes or amniotic cavity (Fig. 23.23). Various terms, including membranous deciduitis, membranous chorionitis, and membranous chorioamnionitis, have been applied to these stages in the progression of the inflammatory response (Fig. 23.24). Frequently, the membranous inflammatory response is most intense at the site of membrane rupture. Maternal neutrophils also migrate out of the intervillous space of the placenta and accumulate immediately beneath the chorionic plate (Fig. 23.25). In some cases, this may be the first evidence of amniotic infection and is best demonstrated in thin regions of the chorionic plate without significant subchorionic fibrin deposition. With time these neutrophils are thought to migrate across

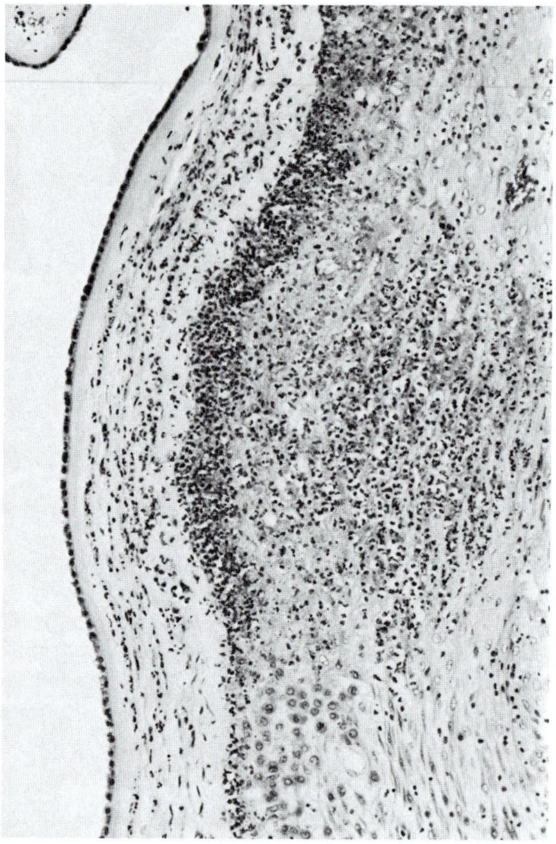

Fig. 23.23. Ascending infection, fetal membranes. Maternal neutrophils migrate from decidual vessels progressively through the chorion and amnion toward the source of infection in the amnionic cavity.

the chorionic plate toward an infection in the amniotic cavity. The time course of the inflammatory reaction in ascending infection is poorly defined.

Depending on the gestational age and status of the fetal immune system, the fetus may also respond to amniotic infection. A fetal leukocytic response is often absent in gestations less than 19–20 weeks and in fetuses less than 500 g and will not occur when infection occurs after fetal death. The fetal reaction is manifested by the migration of fetal neutrophils from umbilical and chorionic plate vessels into Wharton's jelly or the chorionic plate. The migration of inflammatory cells is crescent shaped, oriented toward the source of infection in the amniotic cavity (Figs. 23.26–23.28). Umbilical cord inflammation may be segmental, sometimes identified in only one of multiple sections.

Amniotic infection, then, is a unique situation in which two individuals, mother and fetus, respond to the same infectious stimulus. The traditional view that the majority of leukocytes participating in this process are maternal is based on the lack of fetal blood vessels in the fetal membranes and early sex chromatin analysis of the inflammatory cells in the amnionic exudate.[66] More recent studies utilizing fluorescence in situ hybridization have demonstrated that the majority of neutrophils in amnionic fluid and fetal lung in some cases of chorioamnionitis are fetal rather than maternal,[491,505] raising questions regarding the relative contributions of the maternal and fetal immune systems to the overall inflammatory response in chorioamnionitis.

The acute inflammatory infiltrate in chorioamnionitis is characteristically confined to the fetal membranes and umbilical cord. Villous tissue is not involved unless fetal septicemia results secondarily in villitis. The character of the inflammatory infiltrate is usually not specific enough to identify a particular offending agent. In fact, it is relatively unusual to find bacteria in histologic sections even when they have been demonstrated on smears of the amnion. Notable exceptions to this include infections with group B β-hemolytic streptococci in which colonies of the organism are frequently found

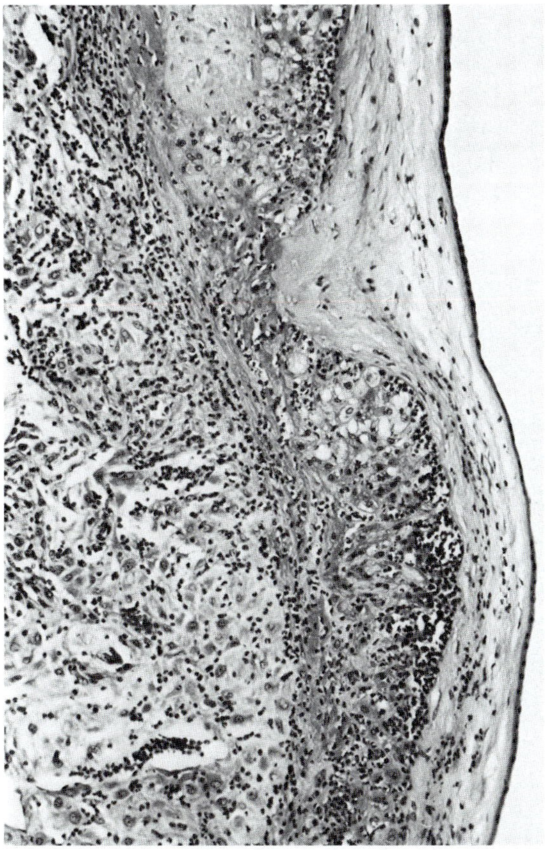

Fig. 23.24. Ascending infection, fetal membranes. The progression of the inflammatory response is illustrated. Neutrophilic infiltration confined to the decidua and chorion (*top*) has extended into the amnion as well (*bottom*).

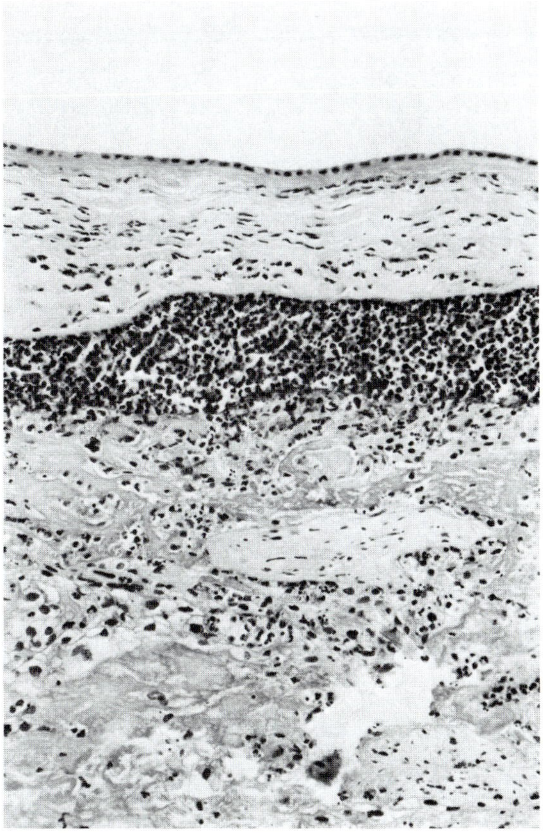

Fig. 23.25. Ascending infection, chorionic plate. Maternal neutrophils migrate out of the intervillous space to accumulate beneath the chorionic plate.

without difficulty even in the absence of histologic evidence of chorioamnionitis (Fig. 23.29).[67] *Fusobacterium* species may be visible on conventional hematoxylin and eosin (H&E) stains as long (at least 15 μm), faintly basophilic wavy organisms usually associated with very severe inflammation and often necrosis of the membranes. *Fusobacterium* may be demonstrated with silver stains but is only faintly gram negative on Brown and Hopps stain.[15,16,155,239] Yeast and hyphal forms of *Candida* may also be identified on conventional H&E stains, characteristically in small, superficial, crescentic microabscesses under the amniotic surface of the umbilical cord (Fig. 23.30).[242,342,437,500,587,602] The rarity of ascending candidal infection is surprising in view of the frequency with which it is found in the vagina. Natural defenses against *Candida* and other organisms in amnionic fluid may help control their spread.[27,31,495,571]

Clinical Significance

Although there are maternal hazards associated with chorioamnionitis (maternal sepsis), the princi-

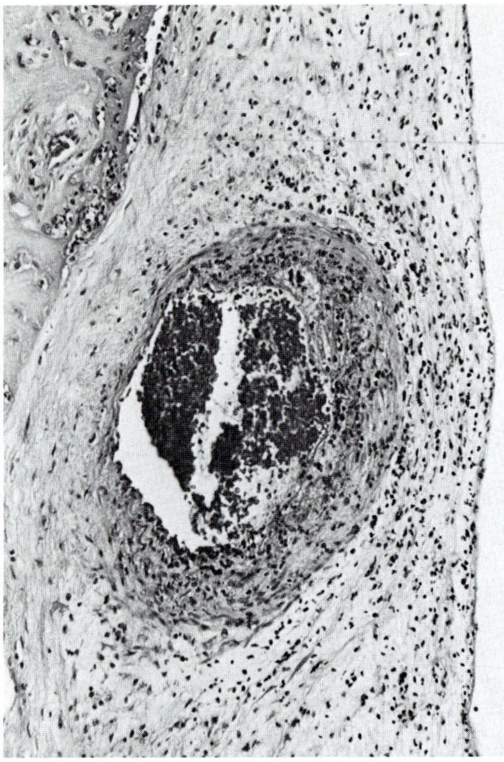

Fig. 23.26. Ascending infection, chorionic plate. Fetal neutrophils migrate through large fetal vessels of the chorionic plate. Orientation toward the source of infection in the amnionic cavity results in crescentic pattern.

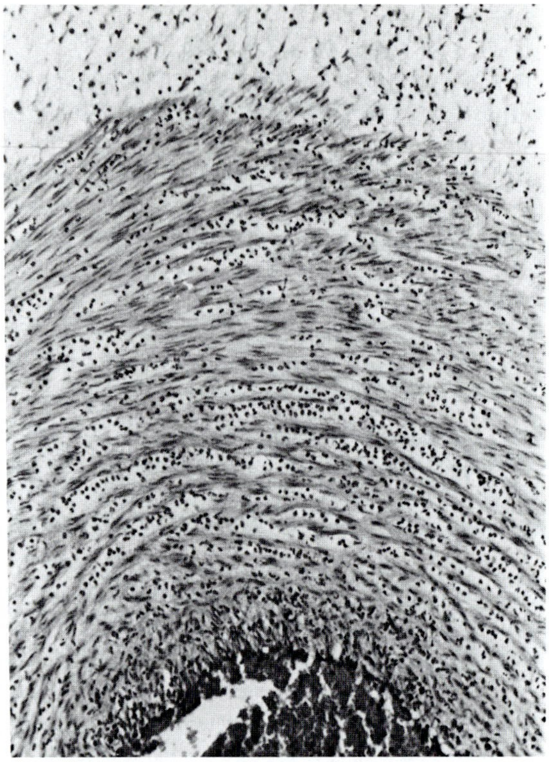

Fig. 23.28. Ascending infection, umbilical cord. Migration of fetal leukocytes from the umbilical vein.

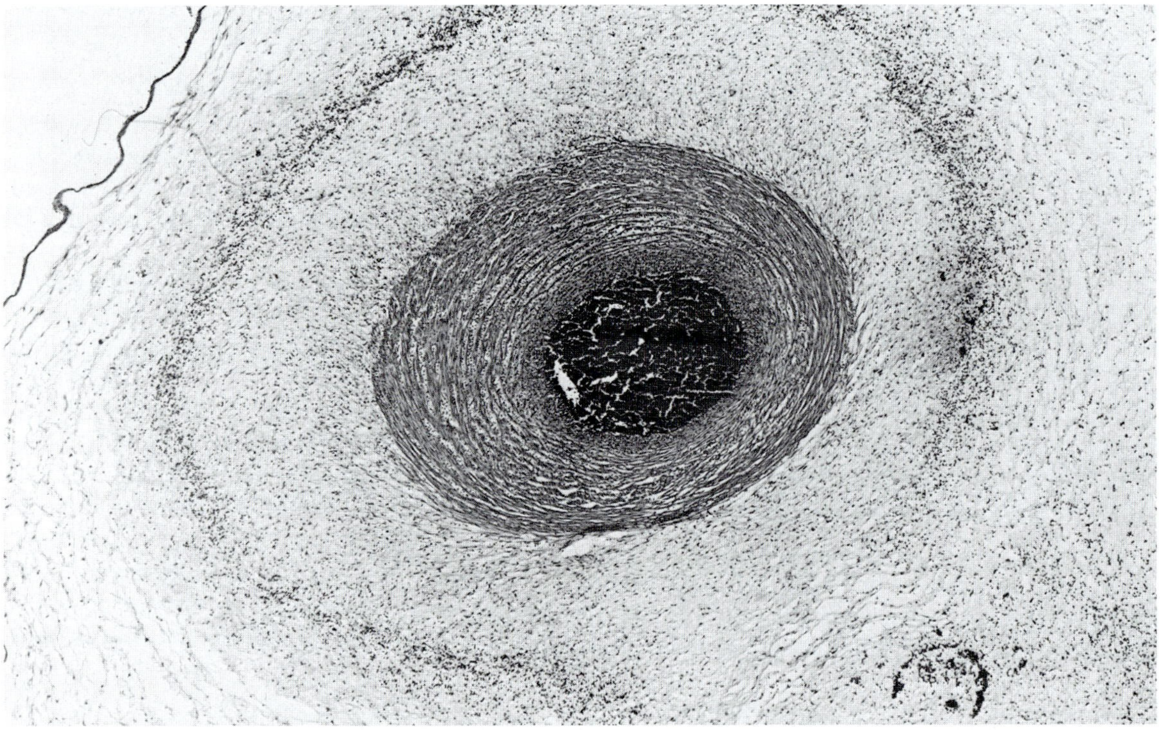

Fig. 23.27. Subacute necrotizing funisitis. Prominent crescentic band of necrotic leukocytes is accompanied by continued migration of neutrophils from the umbilical vein. This pattern of inflammation is thought to result from prolonged low-grade amnionic infection.

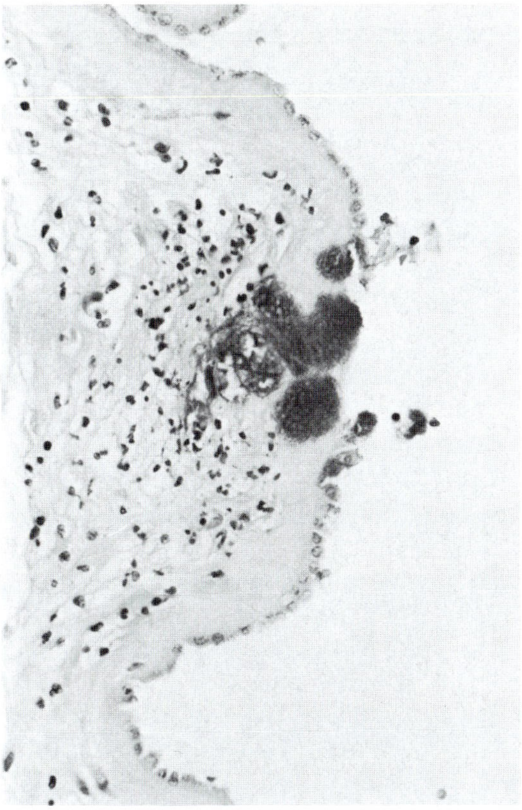

Fig. 23.29. **Ascending infection.** Colonies of group B β-hemolytic streptococci in amnion.

pal clinical impact of chorioamnionitis is its potential adverse affects on the fetus.

Preterm Birth

It is estimated that approximately 70% of perinatal mortality and nearly half of long-term neurologic morbidity can be attributed to *preterm birth* (*PTB*).[211] Multiple factors contribute to PTB, but chorioamnionitis is associated in a high percentage of cases.[203,210] Intrauterine infection as a cause of PTB is usually asymptomatic until labor begins or the membranes rupture prematurely, and therefore early diagnosis is difficult. Many recent strategies have been aimed at the identification of women at risk (measurement of fibronectin and cytokines in cervical/vaginal secretions, serum concentration of cytokines, c-reative protein, and ferritin, ultrasonographic assessment for short cervix, and assessment for bacterial vaginosis) and the development of therapeutic interventions targeting infection and the inflammatory response to reduce spontaneous preterm delivery and its associated mortality and long-term morbidity.[210]

Traditional thinking has attributed many of the neonatal complications of PTB associated with chorioamnionitis to prematurity, not to infection per se. Evidence is accumulating that many pathologic lesions predictive of long-term morbidity (periventricular leucomalacia, intraventricular hemorrhage, bronchopulmonary dysplasia) may be initiated in utero through exposure to the infectious process. Most data would not implicate infectious organisms as a direct cause of tissue damage but rather inflammatory mediators such as cytokines (maternal and fetal) or coagulation abnormalities in the genesis of fetal lesions, especially white matter damage predictive of cerebral palsy.[116,159,214,222,227,613,614] Altered umbilical vascular reactivity associated with inflammation may also contribute to fetal morbidity.[251,488]

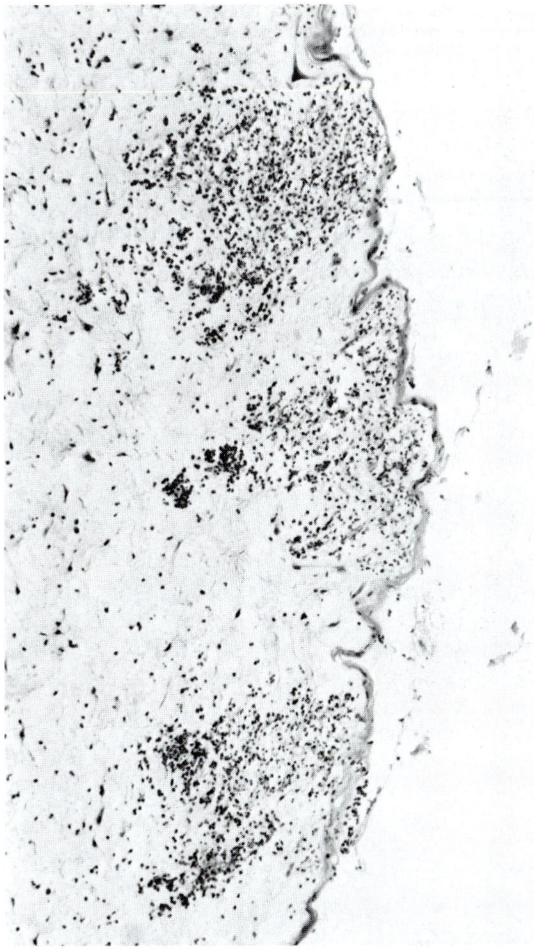

Fig. 23.30. ***Candida* infection of umbilical cord.** Small candidal microabscesses beneath the amnion of the umbilical cord. Gomori methenamine silver stain showed yeast and hyphal forms.

Neonatal Infection

Infants whose placentas show chorioamnionitis are at increased risk to develop sepsis and die in the neonatal period. Although neither mother nor neonate is overtly ill in most cases of chorioamnionitis, *neonatal infection* is an important cause of perinatal death, and most serious neonatal infections are associated with chorioamnionitis.[297,379,381,435,476,620] Fetal outcome is determined by a number of factors including gestational age and causative organism. Group B β-hemolytic streptococcus, *Escherichia coli*, and *Hemophilus influenzae* are the most common causes of significant neonatal infection.[210,475] The magnitude of the risk of neonatal infection has been correlated with the severity of the inflammatory reaction.[145,286,297,387,584,620] Naeye noted that placental villous edema (Fig. 23.31) correlated with morbidity and mortality in neonates with chorioamnionitis.[393]

Chorioamnionitis implies that the fetus has been exposed to infection but not necessarily that the fetus is infected. The exposed fetus may be infected through the fetal skin, eyes, nose, or ear canals or by aspiration or swallowing of infected amniotic fluid. Inspired (Fig. 23.32) or swallowed amniotic elements including neutrophils and amniotic debris in the fetal bronchoalveolar tree and gastrointestinal tract often accompany chorioamnionitis and may result in bronchopneumonia, gastritis, ileitis, or gastrointestinal perforation with peritonitis. Hematogenous spread of organisms from infected amniotic fluid directly into the fetal circulation via the superficial chorionic vessels is another possible route of fetal infection.

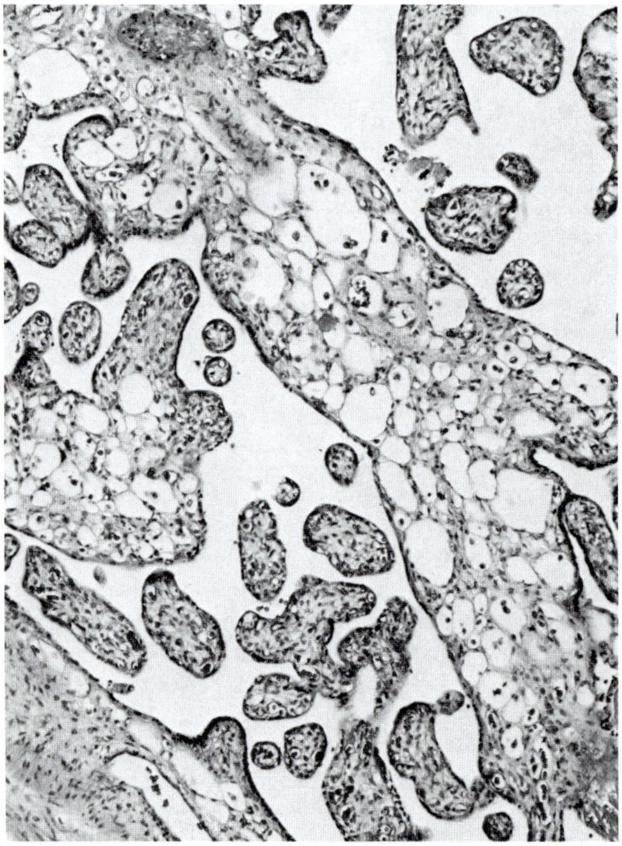

Fig. 23.31. Villous edema. Open spaces are delimited by attenuated strands of stromal cell cytoplasm. When associated with chorioamnionitis, fetal morbidity and mortality is more likely.

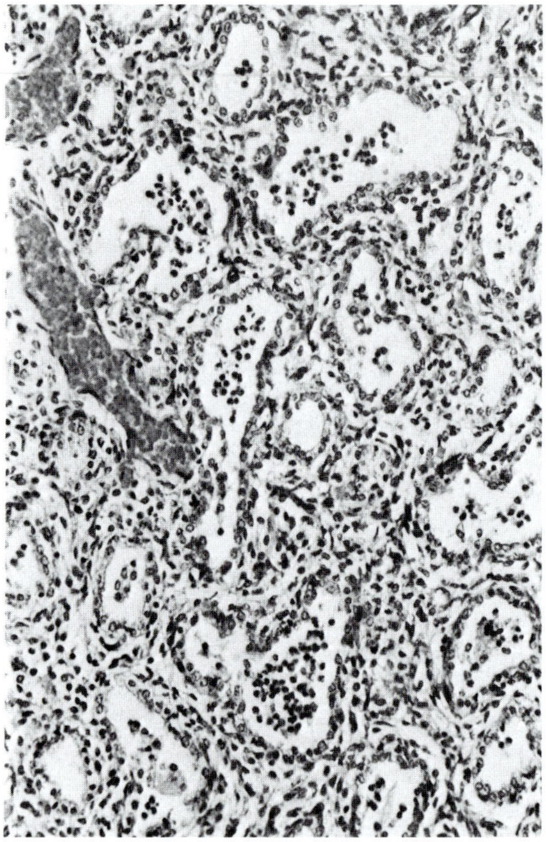

Fig. 23.32. Chorioamnionitis, fetal lung. Neutrophils aspirated from amnionic fluid and/or produced by fetus are accumulated in the fetal bronchoalveolar tree.

Chronic Chorioamnionitis

Rarely, an inflammatory infiltrate occurring in the same distribution as acute chorioamnionitis is composed of chronic inflammatory cells.[199,200,262] Typically, small mature lymphocytes predominate, but plasma cells, histiocytes, and rarely large lymphoid cells and immunoblasts are admixed. In some cases, the chronic inflammatory cells may be accompanied by a minor component of neutrophils, which may be either entirely distinct from or intimately admixed with the chronic inflammatory component. The inflammatory infiltrate in chronic chorioamnionitis is commonly focal and typically concentrated in the free fetal membranes, although involvement of the chorionic plate may occur. Rarely, the large fetal vessel of the chorionic plate and umbilical cord may show a chronic inflammatory infiltrate as well. Chronic chorioamnionitis is often accompanied by villitis and occasionally by chronic or subacute necrotizing funisitis. Rarely, chronic chorioamnionitis occurs in association with rubella, herpes simplex, *Treponema pallidum*, or *Toxoplasma gondii* infection, although a specific infectious etiology is not identified in most cases.

Hematogenous Infections

Etiology

In hematogenous infections, infectious agents reach the placenta through the maternal blood. In contrast to chorioamnionitis, a local infection, placental involvement in hematogenous infection is just one manifestation of maternal systemic disease. Infectious agents reaching the placenta in this way include viruses, some bacteria, and parasites. The histologic hallmark of hematogenous infection is villitis, inflammation of the villous parenchyma. It has been suggested that villitis may also result from local spread of an endometrial infection or reflect a noninfectious immunologic process, a host-versus-graft reaction (see following).

Pathology

Villitis is almost always discovered incidentally on microscopic examination. Typically, there is neither clinical suspicion of nor gross pathologic clue to the underlying inflammatory process. Only rarely are necrotic foci identified grossly, but commonly there are associated but nonspecific abnormalities such as placental enlargement or pallor.

The essential feature common to all villitides is an inflammatory infiltrate in the villi, but its character and the nature of associated changes are highly variable from case to case.[12,181,199,281,445] The inflammatory infiltrate is usually chronic, composed of lymphocytes, histiocytes, and plasma cells in variable proportion, but occasionally it may be granulomatous, and rarely neutrophils predominate. Usually the inflammatory infiltrate is accompanied by necrosis and destruction of the villous stroma and vessels, but rarely it may infiltrate passively without appreciable alteration in villous landmarks. Dystrophic calcification, stromal hemosiderin deposition, and/or complete stromal fibrosis may be prominent in some cases. The inflammatory cells are generally concentrated within the villi, but may also extend into the surrounding perivillous or intervillous space, a feature commonly associated with syncytiotrophoblastic necrosis, intervillous fibrin deposition, and agglutination of contiguous inflamed villi. Rarely, the intervillous component (intervillositis) may be pure or predominate.[147,259]

Inflamed villi are usually randomly distributed but in some cases may be concentrated in the basal regions of the placenta juxtaposed to the decidua or septae. The degree of villous involvement varies greatly from case to case and may be graded semiquantitatively (very mild, mild, moderate, severe) as outlined by Russell,[478] Knox and Fox,[295] or Redline.[445] Villitis is often a very focal process that may be overlooked unless an adequate number of sections is examined. Knox and Fox found that examination of four blocks of placental parenchyma was adequate for detection of all but a "tiny minority" of cases.[295]

The villitides often exhibit all degrees of active inflammation, resolution, and repair, an evolutionary process that is responsible, in part, for the histologic variability from case to case.[18] Rarely, the morphologic features may suggest a causative agent, although differences between the morphologic manifestations of the various infectious villitides are quite subtle. An infectious etiology is identified by any means [conventional histology, culture, electron microscopy (EM), immunohistochemistry] in only a very small percentage of cases. The majority (≥95%) of chronic villitides are of unknown etiology (villitis of unknown etiology, or VUE).

Specific Infectious Villitides

Cytomegalovirus (CMV)

Grossly, the placenta may be normal, small (in cases of fetal growth retardation), or large and edematous (when associated with fetal anemia). Histologically, the villi may exhibit any or all of a wide spectrum of changes related in part to gestational age.[55,65,281,365,372] A plasmacytic villous infiltrate and stromal hemosiderin, often deposited around the remnants of occluded vessels, are characteristic features (Figs. 23.33–23.36). Villous histiocytes and stromal cells are usually increased, and foci of stromal necrosis, calcification, and fibrosis may be found. The diagnostic cytopathic viral changes, large eosinophilic intranuclear and smaller basophilic cytoplasmic inclusions, may be found in endothelial cells, Hofbauer cells, or trophoblast (Fig. 23.37). They are most numerous and easily found in early, severe infections; as gestation proceeds, viral inclusions are typically scarce. When inclusions are not visualized on conventional H&E stains, CMV

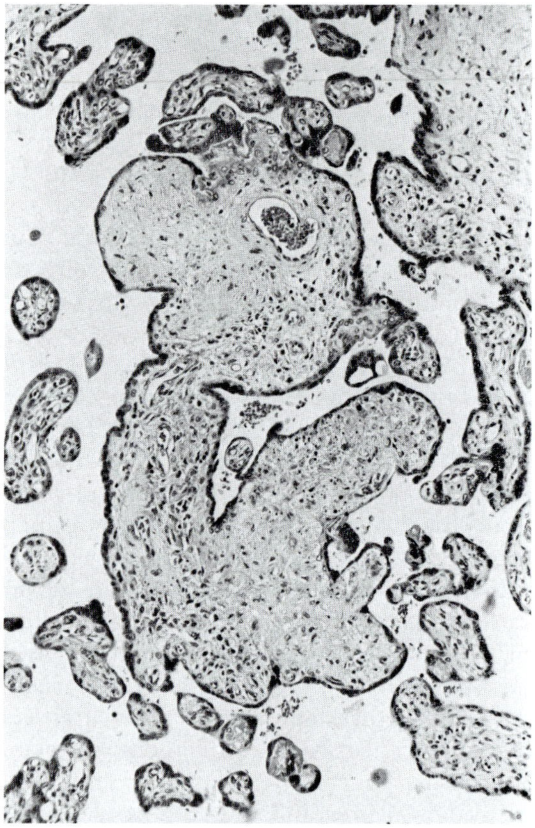

Fig. 23.33. Cytomegalovirus (CMV) villitis. Lymphoplasmacytic villous infiltrate and focal villous necrosis.

infection may be confirmed by immunohistochemistry, polymerase chain reaction (PCR), or in situ hybridization.[375,411,483]

CMV is the commonest identified infectious cause of villitis. The prevalence of congenital infection ranges from 0.2% to 2.2% of all live births. The natural history of cytomegalovirus infection in pregnancy is complex and not completely understood.[544,546–548] Epidemiologic data indicate that (1) transmission to the baby may occur in utero, at birth, or postnatally; (2) intrauterine infection may result from either primary or recurrent maternal infection, the latter despite substantial humoral immunity; (3) congenital infection may be symptomatic at birth (hepatosplenomegaly, microcephaly, petechiae), but in most infants is subclinical; (4) late complications, including mental retardation, chorioretinitis, seizures, and especially neurosensory hearing loss, are most common among the survivors of symptomatic congenital infection but may also occur later in children with no clinical manifestations at birth; and (5) congenital infections resulting from reactivation of latent virus are less likely to produce fetal damage and late sequelae than those resulting from primary maternal infections. Cytomegaloviruses readily infect the fetus and newborn, causing both acute infection and chronic subtle disease that may not be manifest for months or years. At the present time, CMV is the most commonly recognized infectious cause of developmental impairments. Some authors have found a "fairly good"correlation between the severity of placental lesions and the clinical outcome.[65]

Rubella

Congenital rubella infection is now rare due to the effectiveness of immunization programs. The placental findings have been well documented during previous rubella epidemics, mainly in first- and second-trimester abortions[152,410,576] but in a few term placentas as well.[48,194,410] Placental tissue examined shortly after an acute maternal infection often shows necrotizing villitis and vasculitis of variable severity and extent. Necrotic trophoblast associated with perivillous fibrin and acute inflammation may be prominent. Endothelial necrosis, often associated with fragmentation of fetal red cells, is a characteristic finding. Eosinophilic cytoplasmic viral inclusions may be found in endothelial cells, Hof-

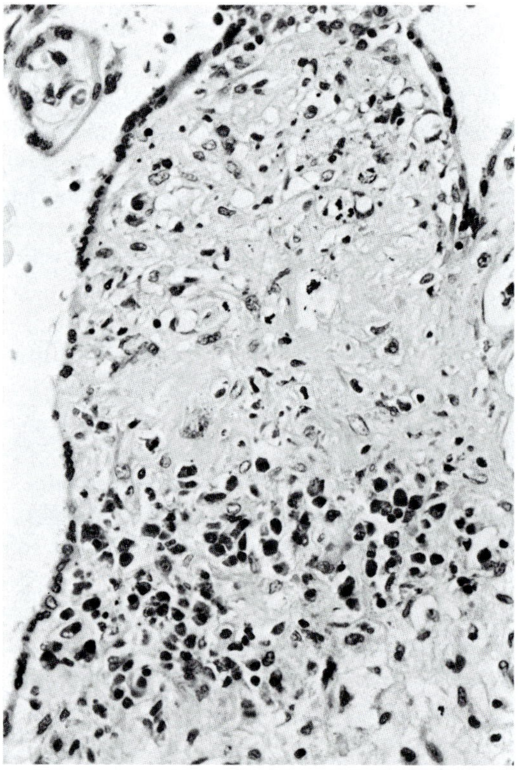

Fig. 23.34. CMV villitis. Plasmacytic villous inflammatory infiltrate is associated with focal necrosis and fibrosis (*top*).

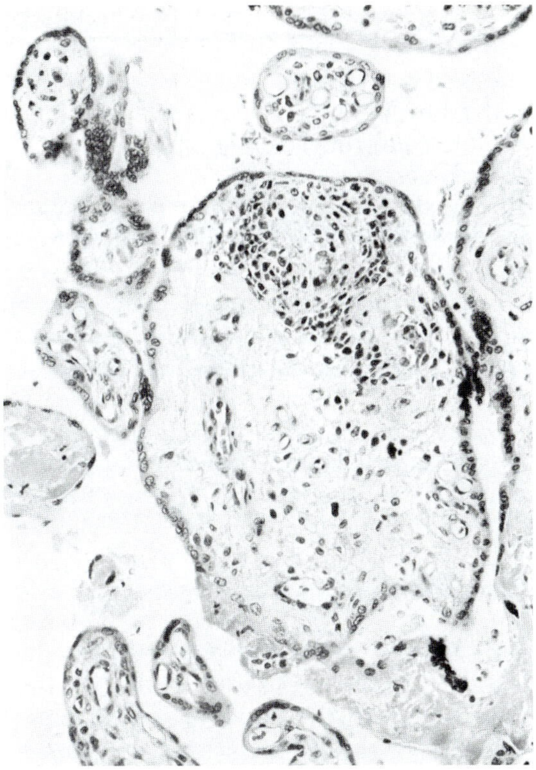

Fig. 23.35. CMV villitis. Segmental vasculitis.

bauer cells, villous stromal cells, trophoblast, and decidua.[410] A mild, focal chronic inflammatory infiltrate occurs infrequently in the membranes and cord.[194] Placentas delivered and examined long after acute maternal illness are often very small, showing only scattered, shrunken, avascular villi. In some cases, these remote lesions coexist with more acute changes. Some placentas from which rubella virus has been isolated show no inflammatory changes or other morphologic abnormalities.[410]

The consequences of rubella infection during pregnancy include spontaneous abortion, fetal death, intrauterine growth retardation, congenital malformations, active neonatal infection, and delayed manifestations including deafness and mental retardation.[388] Survivors of congenital rubella infection can also suffer from late sequelae including panencephalitis[580,595] and diabetes mellitus.[167,265,348] Infection during the first trimester appears to present the greatest risk to the fetus.[281]

Herpes Simplex Virus

Disseminated herpes simplex virus infection is an important cause of devastating disease and death in the newborn. Intrapartum infection of the fetus is the most common,[545] although histologic evidence of both ascending[11,67,234,254] and transplacental dissemination[67,498,609] has been described. Villous necrosis and agglutination, lymphocytic villitis, and fibrinoid necrosis of villous vessels have been documented in the rare cases of hematogenous infection. Acute necrotizing and chronic lymphoplasmacytic chorioamnionitis, amnionic viral inclusions, and funisitis have been described in cases of ascending infection. An increased frequency of spontaneous abortion and congenital malformations have been reported in patients with primary infection in the first 20 weeks of pregnancy.[165,228,366,396–398,540,545]

Varicella Zoster

Varicella infection in pregnancy is uncommon in the United States because the majority of women of childbearing age (95%) are immune. In congenital infection, the placenta may show small, grossly visible necrotic foci and villous necrosis, vascular occlusion, lymphoplasmacytic infiltrates, and granulomas with giant cells microscopically.[438,463] Viral inclusions have been reported in villi and decidua. The spectrum of fetal manifestations is wide, ranging from completely asymptomatic babies to those

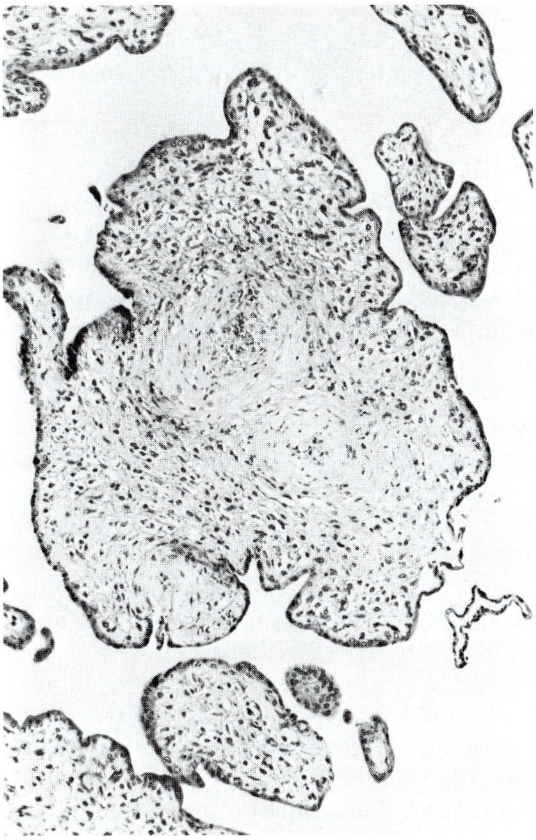

Fig. 23.36. CMV villitis. Villi show remnants of hyalinized, obliterated vessels.

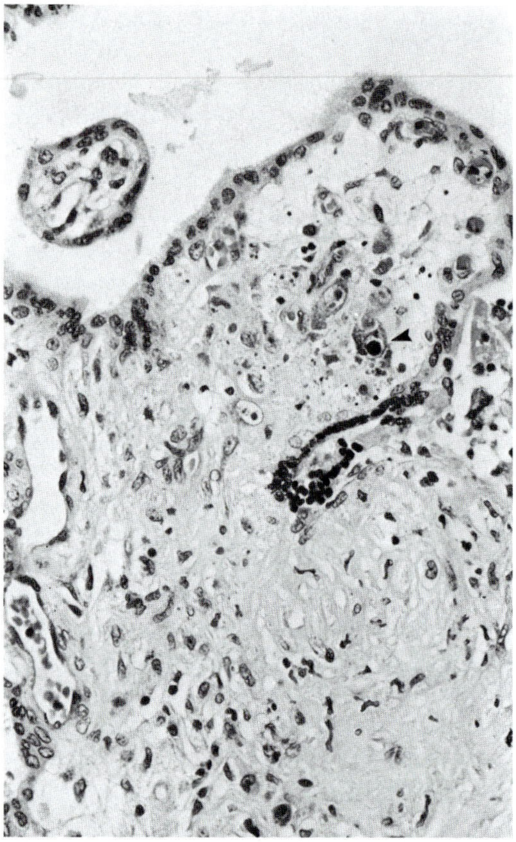

Fig. 23.37. CMV villitis, infection. Typical CMV intranuclear inclusion (*arrow*) associated with focal villous necrosis.

with perinatal varicella/zoster or full-blown embryopathy, the latter occurring in less than 5% of fetuses infected in the first trimester. Reactivation of maternal zoster during pregnancy does not appear to be associated with severe fetal sequelae.

Parvovirus B19

Parvovirus B19 has only recently been added to the growing list of viruses that may cross the placenta and result in fetal infection, morbidity, and death.[22,96,183,434,490,528] Human parvovirus B19 is the agent of "fifth disease," or erythema infectiosum, a mild, acute, exanthematous disease of children. In adults, most infections are asymptomatic, although self-limited polyarthropathy is common, especially in women, and aplastic crises occur in individuals with chronic hemolytic anemias.[96] Parvovirus B19 preferentially infects actively replicating cells, especially erythroblasts, which are then destroyed. To date, the most commonly recognized consequences of fetal parvovirus infection are nonimmune hydrops, which may resolve spontaneously,[514] and abortion. Most abortions occur between the 10th and 28th weeks of pregnancy, but the risk of fetal loss is low, estimated to be less than 10%.[96,290,501] Neonatal anemia has also been observed in a few infants infected in the third trimester,[107,528] and malformations reminiscent of ocular rubella embryopathy have been reported only very rarely.[231,596]

Grossly, the placenta is typically large, pale, and friable, reflecting fetal anemia. Microscopically, there is a uniform pattern of relative villous immaturity and edema. Erythroblasts, some containing diagnostic intranuclear eosinophilic inclusions with peripheral chromatin condensation, are present in the villous vessels (Fig. 23.38).[95,183,293,369,528] In situ hybridization and immunohistochemistry are somewhat more sensitive than conventional microscopy in identifying infected cells,[428,501] or PCR may be used to confirm the diagnosis.[160,212,514] Unlike most other congenital hematogenous infections, there is no villous inflammation in parvovirus infection.

Human Immunodeficiency Virus

Human immunodeficiency virus (HIV) may be transmitted to the fetus transplacentally, at the time of delivery, or after birth (through breastfeeding).[68,417,469,482,543,552] In utero transmission can be

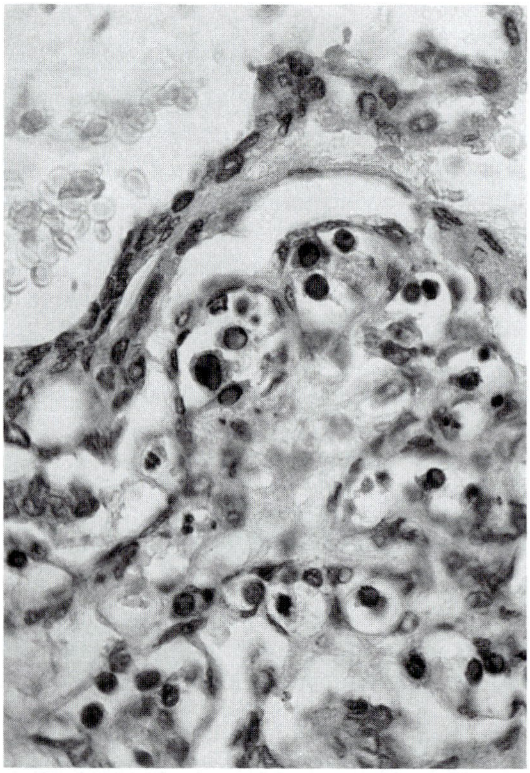

Fig. 23.38. Parvovirus infection. Erythroblasts in the villous capillaries show central nuclear eosinophilic inclusions with peripheral chromatin condensation.

confirmed by the detection of virus in infants by PCR or coculture within 48 hours of birth. Several factors (maternal, fetal, obstetric, and virologic) affect maternal–infant viral transmission, and timing of transmission may determine the subsequent course of infection in the infant. Antiretroviral therapy with zidovudine given to the mother before and during delivery and to the infant after delivery has reduced vertical transmission substantially.[470,542]

No histopathologic lesions directly attributable to HIV have been described in the placenta.[99,263] Specifically, there have been no reports of villitis. Placentas from seropositive mothers have demonstrated an increased incidence of chorioamnionitis.[99,263,339] In some studies, seropositive mothers have been more likely to deliver prematurely and to produce infants with relatively low birth weights.[360,482] Immunohistochemical studies, in situ hybridization, and PCR of placentas from HIV-seropositive pregnancies have demonstrate variable expression of HIV antigens in amnion,[264,543] trophoblast,[99,325] and macrophages,[264,325,337,339] and ultrastructurally, retrovirus-like particles have been detected in syncytiotrophoblast, villous fibroblasts, and fetal endothelial cells.[263] The immunohistochemical demonstration of HIV antigens does not correlate perfectly with culture status,[339] and neither immunohistochemical localization of HIV antigen nor recovery of HIV in placental cell culture predicts fetal HIV infection.[339]

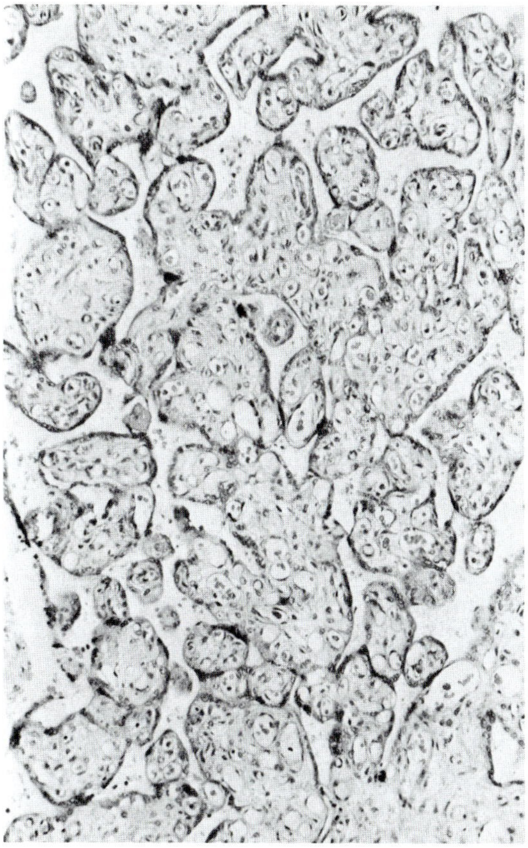

Fig. 23.39. Congenital syphilis at term in a liveborn infant. Note large, immature branching villi.

Other Viruses

Pathologic findings in the few placentas with documented infection by other viruses, such as vaccinia, variola, Coxsackie B, and hepatitis B virus, have been detailed by Fox,[175,181] Blanc,[65,67] Kaplan,[281] and Altshuler and Russell.[18] The effects of many of the most common viruses (enteroviruses, adenoviruses, influenza viruses) are not well known.[192,556]

Treponema pallidum

Congenital syphilis as a major cause of abortion and stillbirth declined after the discovery of penicillin, but has reemerged as a significant problem, especially in large urban centers.[57,97,344] Grossly, infected placentas tend to be large and bulky. Histologically, the villi are large and relatively immature but not markedly edematous (Fig. 23.39). The villous stroma is cellular as a result the prominence of Hofbauer cells, and a lymphoplasmacytic villous infiltrate with subtrophoblastic neutrophils and microabscesses may be seen focally. Rarely, the inflammatory reaction has granulomatous features. Subendothelial and perivascular fibrosis resulting in luminal narrowing, recanalization, or occlusion of villous vessels (Figs. 23.40 and 23.41) is particularly characteristic. Marked decidual plasmacytic vasculitis and a chronic inflammatory infiltrate in the fetal membranes and umbilical cord have been noted in some cases.[45,196,436,479,590] Necrotizing funisitis, a lesion characterized by perivascular necrotic bands containing inflammatory debris, is a frequent finding but is neither universal in nor specific for congenital syphilis (Fig. 23.42).[113,166]

The histologic changes in the placenta and umbilical cord are not diagnostic but are highly suggestive, especially when accompanied by fetal lesions (pneumonia alba, pancreatic fibrosis, cirrhosis, osteitis). Definitive diagnosis depends on identification of spirochetes, often most easily demonstrated in the umbilical cord (whether inflamed or not)[499] by silver stains (Dieterle, Warthin–Starry, Steiner), immunofluorescence, immunohistochemistry, or PCR.[196] Transplacental transmission of circulating spirochetes may occur at any time during pregnancy,[67,229] but morphologic expression of infection in the placenta and fetus seems to depend on gestational age and the magnitude of the inflammatory response.[537]

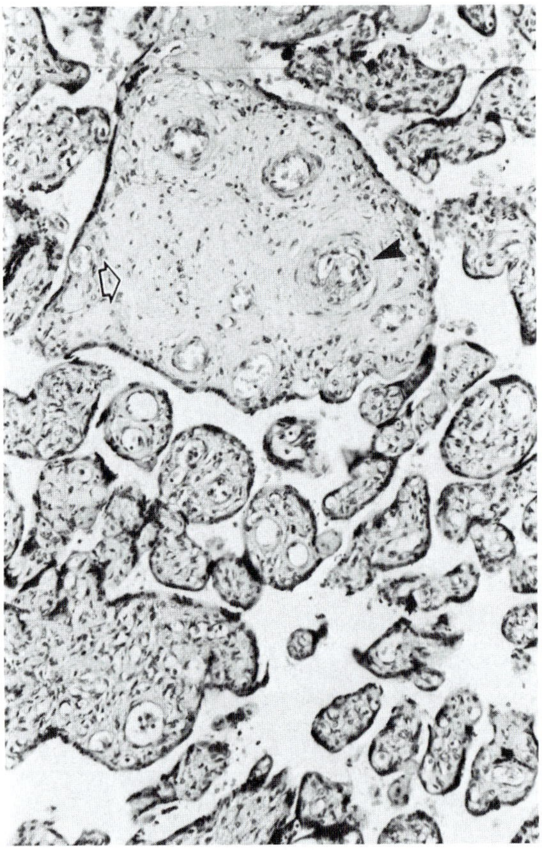

Fig. 23.40. Congenital syphilis at term in a liveborn infant. Perivascular and subendothelial fibrosis results in partial (*black arrow*) and complete (*open arrow*) vascular obliteration in a stem villus.

Listeria monocytogenes

In the villitis caused by *Listeria monocytogenes*, neutrophils predominate, unlike most other villitides, which feature lymphocytes, histiocytes, and plasma cells. Typically, scattered villi exhibit a rim of neutrophils localized between the trophoblast and villous stroma (Fig. 23.43). Other more diffusely inflamed villi are commonly enmeshed in a perivillous inflammatory infiltrate and fibrin, which, when extensive, may result in villous necrosis and abscesses.[550] On occasion, the inflammatory process may include palisaded histiocytes and multinucleated giant cells.[153,292,413,506,611] The placenta is usually grossly normal but may contain minute yellow-white necrotic foci or, rarely, larger abscesses or infarcts near the maternal surface.[550] The amniotic fluid is frequently meconium stained.

Almost invariably, the villitis in *Listeria* infection is accompanied by chorioamnionitis, and funisitis is also a common finding.[67,153,611] Amnionic "plaques" composed of disordered amnionic cells with granular cytoplasm (caused by accumulation of bacteria) with or without an acute inflammatory reaction have been described.[413] Given the coexistence of villitis (usually a marker of transplacental infection) and chorioamnionitis (indicative of ascending infection), it is unclear by which route(s) congenital *Listeria* infection is acquired.[533]

Listeria monocytogenes is a small, gram-positive motile bacillus with rounded ends. It may be demonstrated with Brown–Hopps, Warthin–Starry, or Dieterle stains but is often difficult to identify in either placental or fetal lesions. Recently, immunohistochemical stains have been utilized to establish the diagnosis definitively[413,506] and to exclude other infections (*Campylobacter* spp.,[106,349] *E. coli, H. influenzae, Francisella tularesis*, streptococci, *Brucella abortus, Chlamydia psittaci*[253]) that produce similar histologic findings.

Listeria monocytogenes is a significant cause of intrauterine infection, spontaneous abortion, prematurity, and neonatal sepsis, morbidity, and death.[23,92,226,243,422,443.619] Perinatal listeriosis takes one of two forms. In the "early type," congenital in-

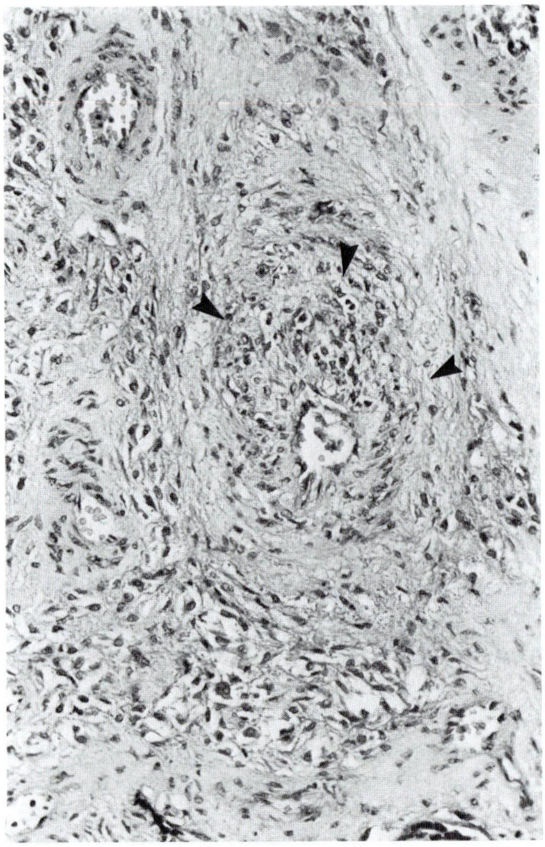

Fig. 23.41. Congenital syphilis at term in a liveborn infant. Stem villus with a lymphohistiocytic infiltrate and vasculitis. *Arrows* indicate vessel infiltrated by lymphocytes.

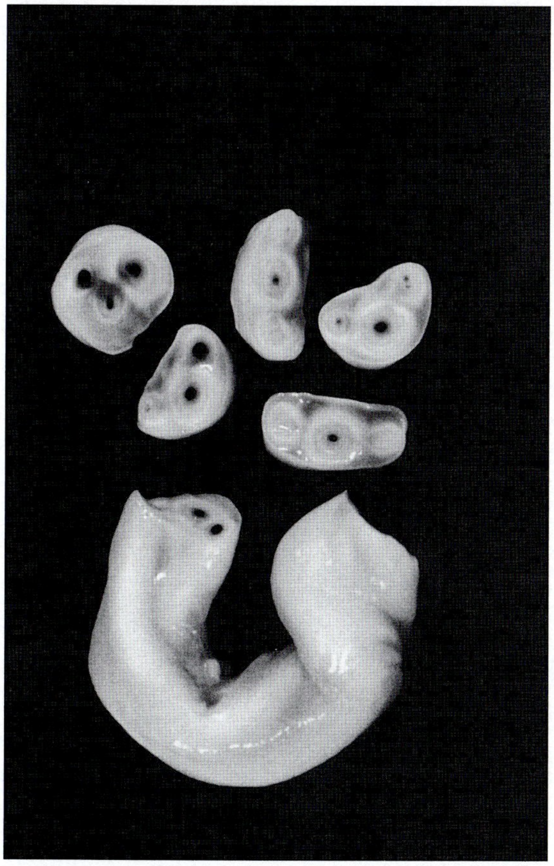

Fig. 23.42. **Necrotizing funisitis.** Perivascular necrotic bands are well seen in cross section.

fection results in devastating neonatal sepsis (granulomatosis infantiseptica) in which microabscesses similar to those in the placenta are disseminated in fetal organs.[509] Nonimmune fetal hydrops rarely complicates congenital listeriosis. Diagnosis by amniocentesis[421] and antibiotic treatment during pregnancy has resulted in successful pregnancy outcome.[112] The "late type" of perinatal listeriosis, presumably acquired during birth, presents as meningitis in the second or third week of life.

The most common mode of maternal infection is thought to be from ingestion of contaminated food, often a milk product. Cervical colonization has been documented, but its role in habitual abortion is controversial.[217,322,441] *Listeria monocytogenes* usually does not cause serious disease in the normal adult, although gravidas may experience a flu-like syndrome and fever. The particular predisposition for significant listerial infection in pregnant women and the fetus appears to be related to local factors at the maternofetal interface that compromise an effective immune response, including a deficiency in T cells and macrophages and properties of decidual cells themselves which prevent macrophage functions crucial for defense against *Listeria*.[447–449]

Toxoplasma gondii

The placenta infected with *Toxoplasma gondii* may be grossly normal but is commonly large and edematous, resembling the hydropic placenta of the anemic fetus.[10,32] Microscopically, the changes are highly variable, ranging from a subtle low-grade lymphocytic villous infiltrate to a destructive process associated with necrosis or fibrosis. True granulomas with central necrosis, palisaded histiocytes, and Langerhans giant cells may predominate in some cases (Fig. 23.44).[158,427] Nodular accumulations of histiocytes beneath the trophoblast or extending into the intervillous space have been described.[158,193] Decidual plasmacytic infiltrates and vasculitis,[193] villous nucleated RBCs, "hemorrhagic endovasculitis," thrombosis and calcification of chorionic vessels, and chronic inflammatory infiltrates in the fetal membranes and umbilical cord have been reported in congenital toxoplasmosis.[158,191,402]

The organism, when identified, is usually in the encysted form and may be found in the fetal

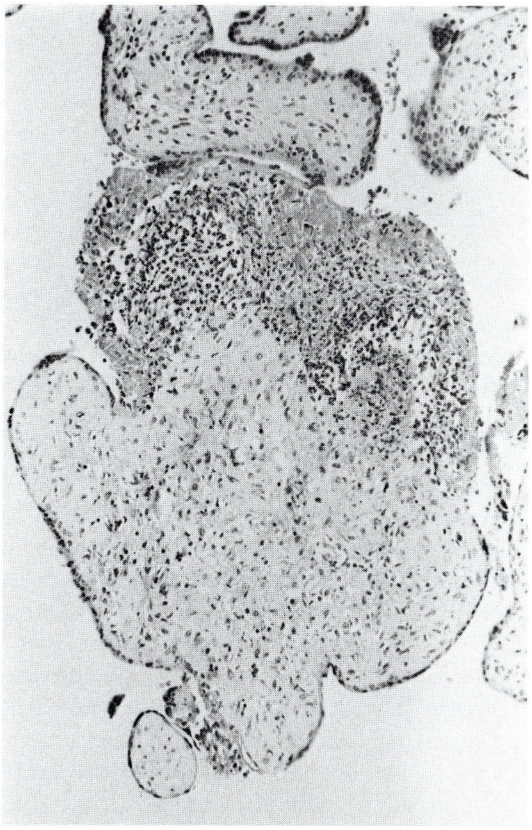

Fig. 23.43. **Congenital listeriosis.** Subtrophoblastic acute villitis with necrosis.

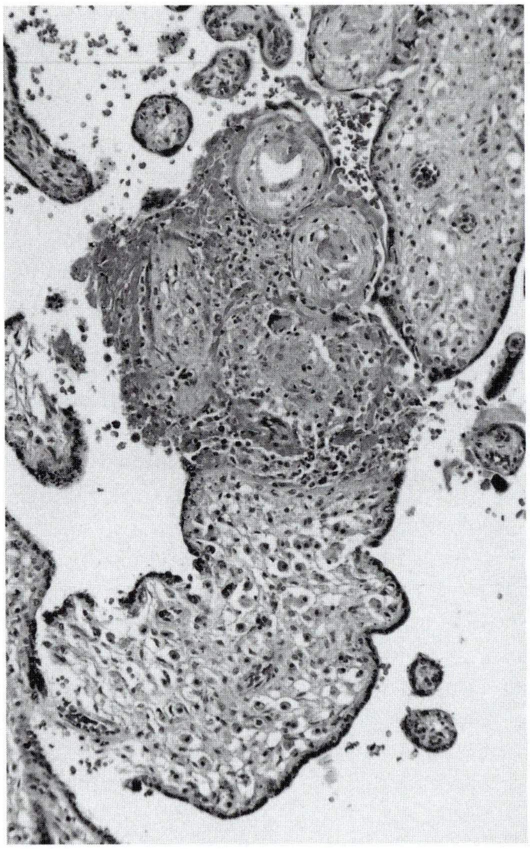

Fig. 23.44. Toxoplasma villitis. Villous necrosis and granulomatous inflammation.

membranes, chorionic plate, umbilical cord, or villi.[39,158,208] *Toxoplasma* cysts are typically unassociated with inflammation,[10,158] but once ruptured, the tachyzoites incite an intense inflammatory reaction and necrosis.[427] Identification of tachyzoites, very difficult on H&E stains, is aided by immunohistochemistry, immunofluorescence, or PCR.[582]

Congenital infection appears to result mainly from primary maternal infection acquired early in pregnancy, usually by the ingestion of oocytes in undercooked meat or by contact with cat feces.[184] During the parasitemic stage of maternal infection, the organism is transmitted to the placenta and fetus. The risk of fetal infection in these circumstances is about 50%. The likelihood of fetal transmission increases with gestational age, although the severity of infection is greatest when the infection is acquired in the first trimester.[129,241] The clinical spectrum of fetal involvement ranges from severe damage to the central nervous system and eyes to completely asymptomatic infection, recognized only by the development of chorioretinitis after months or years of follow-up.[129,299,604] Prenatal diagnosis (via fetal blood sampling, culture)[130,168,169] and antibiotic treatment seem to reduce the frequency of congenital infection.[111,115,129,202,241,604] In the presence of maternal antibodies from past infections, fetal lesions, with rare exception, do not occur.[70,129,320,555]

Other Organisms

Hematogenous dissemination of other organisms to the placenta occurs but is uncommon. The placental lesions associated with hematogenous spread of pyogenic and enteric bacteria, *Francisella tularesis, Brucella, Campylobacter, Mycobacterium tuberculosis,* and *Mycobacterium leprae,* are detailed in the treatises by Fox[175] and Blanc.[67] Recurrent villitis has been described in association with nonsyphilitic spirochetes.[2,446] Massive chronic intervillositis may occur in malaria.[409,591] Rarely, fungi reach the placenta hematogenously.[363]

Villitis of Unknown Etiology

Although catastrophic fetoplacental infections caused by the hematogenously acquired "TORCH" agents have been well documented, they are infrequent. Far more commonly, a focal chronic villitis for which no etiology can be established is discovered incidentally in sections of the placenta (*villitis of unknown etiology, VUE*). Estimates of the frequency of this phenomenon vary. Russell identified VUE in 7.6% of 7500 consecutively examined singleton placentas.[477] Knox and Fox reported a frequency of 13.6% in 1000 randomly selected patients,[295] and even higher frequencies have been reported.[312,489] Differences in the reported frequency may reflect true regional variation, differences in the studied populations, the extent of tissue sampling, or diagnostic criteria, but by any estimate VUE is a common lesion. Histologically, the villitis may exhibit any of the morphologic features previously described,[478] and the histologic characteristics of the villitis do not seem to be related to clinical presentation or neonatal outcome.[450,478] The intensity of the inflammation in the majority of VUE cases (75%–85%) is either very mild or mild.[295,478] Massive chronic intervillositis may represent an unusual variant of VUE.[147,259]

When VUE is found in the placenta, the infant is generally unaffected, although Russell and others have stressed that VUE is associated with intrauterine growth retardation and an increased perinatal mortality rate.[9,295,312,450,477] The severity of the villitis seems to correlate directly with these complications.[295,408,472,478] When fatal, VUE is usually massive, suggesting that impaired placental function may be the mechanism of injury. VUE has a considerable tendency to recur,[313,450,477,478,480] and total reproductive failure is reportedly increased in patients with recurrent VUE. The morphologic features of villitis in recurrent VUE tend to be consistent but often with an increase in the proportion of inflamed villi and earlier onset.[450]

The histologic similarity between VUE and the well-known infectious villitides suggests that VUE may be the result of chronic infection, although a causative agent has not been identified and fetuses show no evidence of infection. Alternatively, consideration has been given to the possibility that VUE may be an expression of an abnormal immune reaction culminating in rejection of the fetal allograft.[312,313,315,450] Humoral (complement-fixing immune complexes and a deficiency of blocking factors) and cellular mechanisms have been proposed but not well delineated. These theories are not mutually exclusive; an unrecognized pathogen, for example, could be the initial stimulus culminating in a host-versus-graft reaction. Utilizing interphase cytogenetics, it has been demonstrated that many of the inflammatory cells in chronic villitis are maternal.[452] Macrophages and T lymphocytes predominate, and mononuclear cells expressing HLA-DR have been present in a high percentage of cases.[7,218,315,452] B lymphocytes have not been observed.

Circulatory Disorders

The placenta is a vascular organ with a dual blood supply, and the integrity of both fetal and maternal circulations is essential to placental function. Many of the most clinically significant lesions in the placenta are the cause or consequence of maternal or fetal vascular compromise.

Thrombi and *hematomas* in the vessels and spaces in and around the placenta cause both fetal and maternal injury in proportion to their size and extent and according to location. Whether there is injury to the mother or fetus or both depends on how the circulation of each is affected. Individual lesions should be measured, and when extensive, the percent of placental involvement should be estimated. There is, however, no absolute "cutoff" beyond which a bad outcome is inevitable or below which a good outcome is assured. The functional status of the uninvolved parenchyma is an important element in this equation. Thus, even a relatively small lesion in a compromised placenta may have greater clinical significance than a larger lesion in an otherwise normal placenta.

Maternal Circulation

Incomplete Physiologic Change in Spiral Arteries and Acute Atherosis

When the normal physiologic changes in the spiral arteries of the maternal decidua (see Fig. 23.4) do not evolve properly, arterial smooth muscle persists, the lumina fail to expand, and uteroplacental blood flow is relatively low. The usual effect on the pregnant woman is the syndrome of *preeclampsia*, also called *pregnancy-induced hypertension* (*PIH*), and *toxemia of pregnancy* (see following). The spiral arteries develop a distinctive lesion, *acute atherosis*, characterized by necrosis with dense eosinophilia of the vessel wall and large foamy lipid-filled cells. The lumens may become partly or completely occluded by thrombus. The subsequent chronic placental ischemia causes a reduction in the growth rate of both the fetus and the placenta. In more severe cases the placental villi develop abnormally, resulting in slender stem villi, reduced branching, and very tiny terminal villi, a pattern called *accelerated maturation*. The synctiotrophoblast nuclei cluster, forming trophoblastic knots. Localized areas of especially severe ischemia may become necrotic, forming *infarcts*.

Infarct

Etiology

An infarct in the placenta, as in any other organ, is an area of ischemic necrosis resulting from obstruction of its blood supply, the spiral arteries, by occlusion by thrombi, narrowing by mural thrombi, or complete blocking by a retroplacental hematoma.

Pathology

Infarcts are usually small and are most common at the placental margin. They are often triangular in shape with the base abutting the basal plate (Fig. 23.45). The gross appearance of a placental infarct changes with age. Fresh infarcts are very difficult to see; they differ little in color, but are firmer and drier than the surrounding normal placenta. They are more readily appreciated on palpation than visual inspection. With age, infarcts grow progressively firmer and change in color from red to brown, then tan, yellow, or white.

The histologic appearance of an infarct also changes with age. The earliest change microscopically is extreme narrowing or obliteration of the intervillous space (Fig. 23.46). In some infarcts, small amounts of fibrin may accumulate in the intervillous space. The villous vessels are dilated and con-

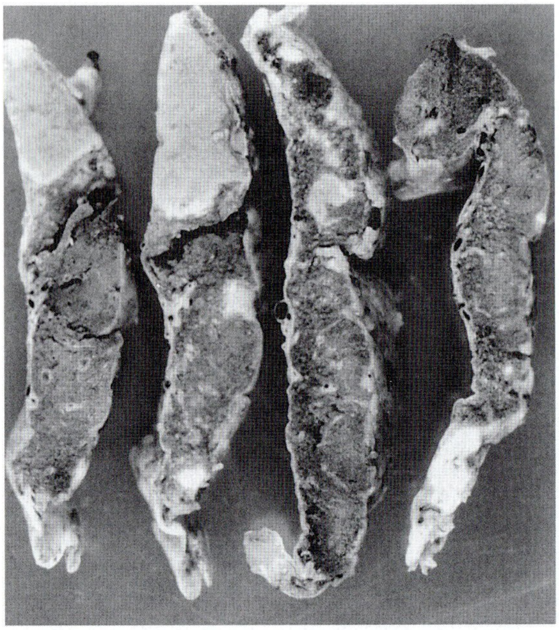

Fig. 23.45. Multiple placental infarcts at 25 weeks gestation. The mother had severe preeclampsia and the HELLP syndrome.

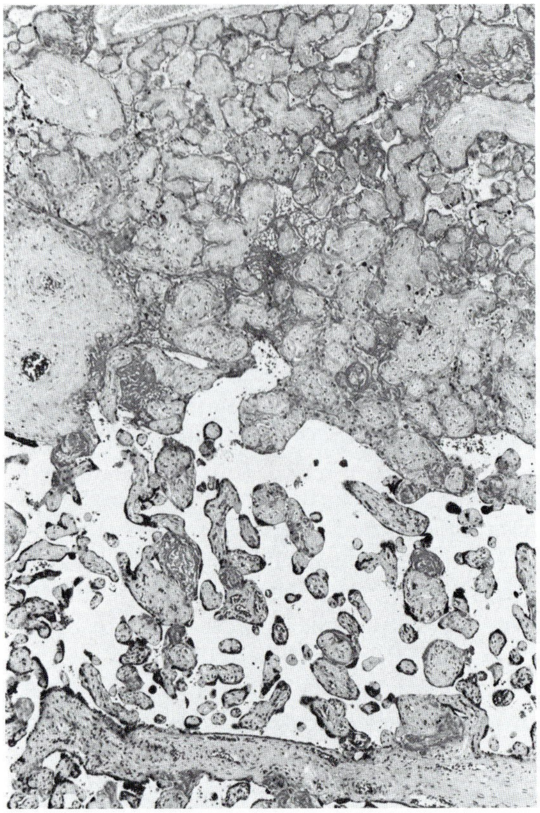

Fig. 23.46. Placental infarct (*top*). Aggregation of villi and obliteration of the intervillous space. Adjacent normal placenta is on the *bottom*.

gested, and trophoblastic nuclei cluster together forming trophoblastic "knots." The syncytiotrophoblast, vascular endothelium, and villous stroma undergo progressive necrosis until eventually the infarct consists of crowded, ghostlike remnants of necrotic villi (Fig. 23.47). The fetal stem arteries supplying the infarcted villi undergo fibromuscular sclerosis and, along with the villous capillaries, eventually disappear. There may be an acute inflammatory response at the margin of the infarct that does not actually involve the villous parenchyma and is generally mild. The mummified remnants of infarcted villi in the placenta are not removed by macrophages or replaced by fibrous tissue as occurs in other organs, and the scant amounts of fibrin between the villi, like all forms of clot in the intervillous space, do not become organized.

Clinical Behavior

Infarcts are common; they occur in about 25% of otherwise normal term placentas.[178] The finding of a small infarct in an otherwise normal placenta is of no clinical significance. Multiple or large (>3 cm) infarcts, central infarcts, or infarcts in the first or second trimester are indicative of significant, underlying maternal vascular disease, especially preeclampsia. In women with hypertension (preeclampsia and essential hypertension), the frequency and extent of infarction are increased in proportion to the severity of the underlying maternal disease.[178] Extensive placental infarction has also been documented in thrombophilic states.[28,142,288,444]

Extensive placental infarction is associated with fetal hypoxia, intrauterine growth retardation, and fetal death in utero.[178] These ill effects on the fetus are probably not simply the result of the destruction of villous tissue but are the result of the superimposition of infarction on a placenta already compromised by a pathologically altered maternal vascular tree and low uteroplacental blood flow.

Spiral Artery Thrombosis

Recurrent pregnancy loss related to acute atherosis, placental ischemia, and infarcts is a well-recognized complication in women with scleroderma,[148] systemic lupus erythematosis,[3,77,135,403] and the related circulating antiphospholipid antibody (lupus anticoagulant) syndrome.[138,163,407,485] The same problem occurs with other maternal coagulation disorders such as deficiencies of protein C, protein S, and antithrombin III,[305] and the factor V Leiden and methylenetetrahydrofolate reductase gene mutations.[28,142,288] Some patients have experienced mul-

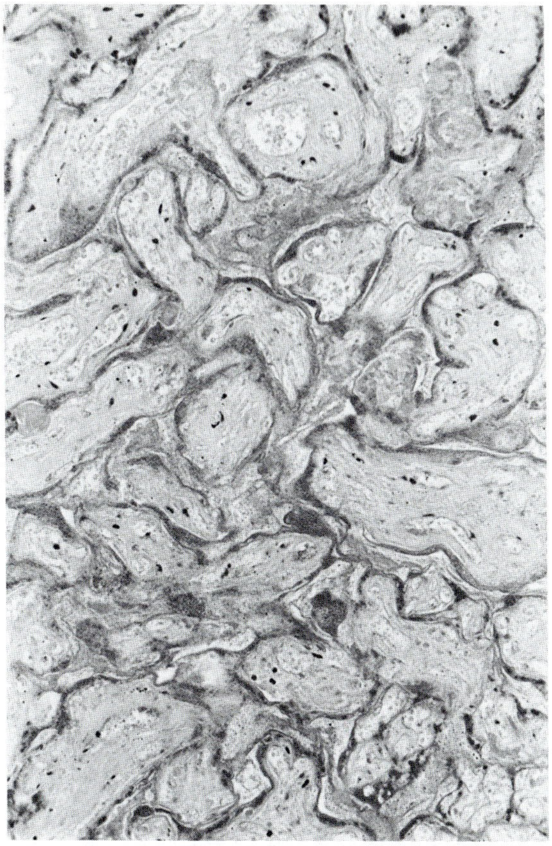

Fig. 23.47. Placental infarct. The villi in this old infarct are ghostlike. A perivillous eosinophilic rim is all that remains of the completely necrotic trophoblast.

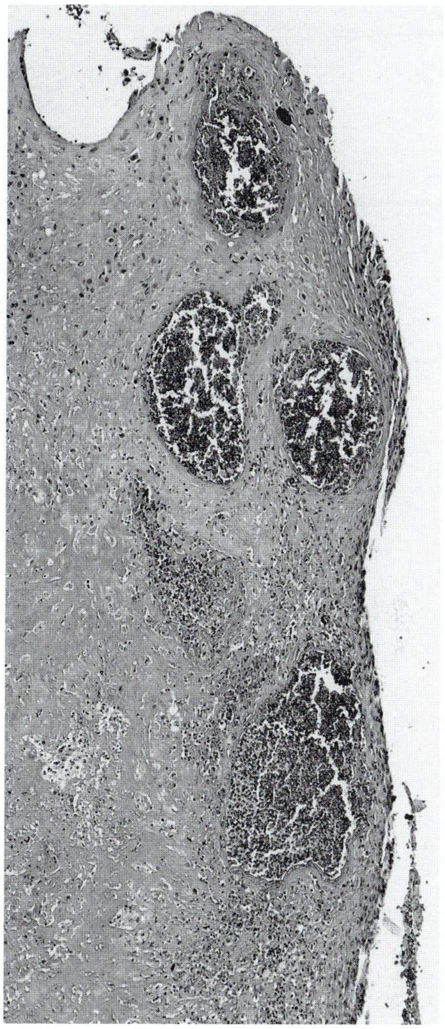

Fig. 23.48. Spiral artery thrombosis. The spiral arteries show thrombi in various stages of development in this patient with lupus anticoagulant.

tiple abortions occurring late in the second or early in the third trimesters, and some have had unexplained intrauterine growth retardation in previous gestations. In these conditions, both acute and organizing thrombi may occur in spiral arteries (Fig. 23.48), and infarcts are common.[444] Thrombi may also occur in the fetal circulation, evident in the placenta as fetal artery thrombosis or in the newborn as castrophic large vessel thrombi.[303,508,523]

Maternal Floor Infarct and Perivillous Fibrin Deposit

These two lesions have many similar features, differing mainly in distribution and size. *Maternal floor infarct* is a disorder characterized by heavy deposition of fibrin in the region of the basal villi immediately adjacent to the decidua basalis. The fibrin extends into the intervillous space where it envelops the basal villi, which become avascular and sclerotic (Fig. 23.49). It is not an infarct, and is most directly distinguished from a placental infarct by the fact that the affected villi are widely separated by the fibrin, whereas the villi in infarcts are typically crowded together. Grossly, the maternal surface of the placenta is thickened, firm, and yellow. The lesion is often but not always diffuse.

The reported frequency of maternal floor infarction ranges from 0.09% to 5%.[25,384] The entity has been associated with a high rate of fetal mortality (17%–40%) and intrauterine growth retardation (51%). The pathophysiologic basis for the lesion is unclear. An occasional patient has had a coagulopathy,[28] but most have not been tested. Maternal floor infarction frequently recurs in successive pregnancies,[25,104] and there is evidence that it develops rapidly. Diagnosis of the lesion and anticipation of recurrence have prompted careful monitoring and intervention with successful pregnancy outcome in some cases.

Perivillous fibrin deposits are a regular finding in the normal term placenta. Fibrin routinely deposits

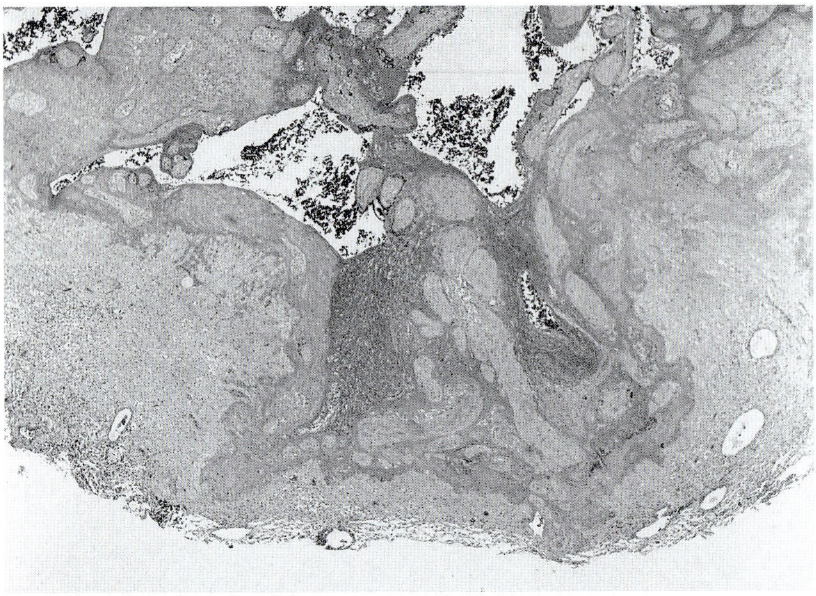

Fig. 23.49. Maternal floor infarct. Fibrin deposits surround the basal villi. This was the fifth consecutive intrauterine fetal death (IUFD). The mother's antithrombin III level was low.

around stem villi, being grossly visible as lacelike strands. Trophoblastic apoptosis resulting in fibrin deposits which may then reepithelialize on the villous surface has been proposed as the mechanism for the apparently normal, generally small, fibrin deposits confined to scattered clumps of villi.[404]

Massive perivillous fibrin deposition refers to very large, macroscopically visible accumulations of perivillous fibrin that appear hard and waxy, pale tan or gray, and may range from one or two to several centimeters in size (Fig. 23.50). This deposition represents a pathologic process in which large groups of villi become encased in wide bands of dense fibrin-like material. As seen microscopically, the villous stroma becomes sclerotic, villous capillaries and the synctiotrophoblast layer disappear, and mononuclear cytotrophoblast or intermediate trophoblastic cells survive and migrate into the fibrin matrix (Fig. 23.51). In significant contrast to an infarct, the villi are widely separated by the fibrin, and early acute necrosis of the villi does not occur. Even in older lesions, the villous outlines including a few surviving stromal cells may remain.

The etiology of this condition is unknown, but it is thought to result from localized stasis and thrombosis of the maternal blood in the intervillous space. Several instances have occurred in association with maternal coagulopathy.[28,303,485] The fibrin deposition isolates the entrapped villi from their maternal blood supply, and they become nonfunctional. Fox has presented evidence that the process seems to require good maternal blood flow and is less frequent in the placentas of women with preeclampsia.[177] Fox found no adverse clinical effects, specifically no relationship between perivillous fibrin deposition and decreased fetal weight, fetal distress, or intrauterine fetal death.[177] Redline and Patterson observed that perivillous fibrin deposits that entrapped more than 20% of terminal villi in the central basal portion of the placenta, thought to be the primary region of gas and nutrient exchange, were significantly associated with intrauterine growth retarda-

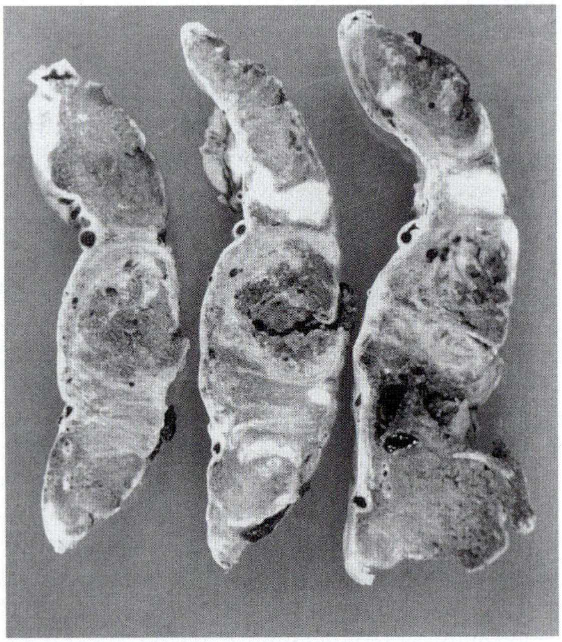

Fig. 23.50. Massive perivillous fibrin deposits. The mother's antithrombin III level (also her brother's and father's) was depressed, and she was heterozygous for the methylene tetrahydrofolate reductase gene mutation.

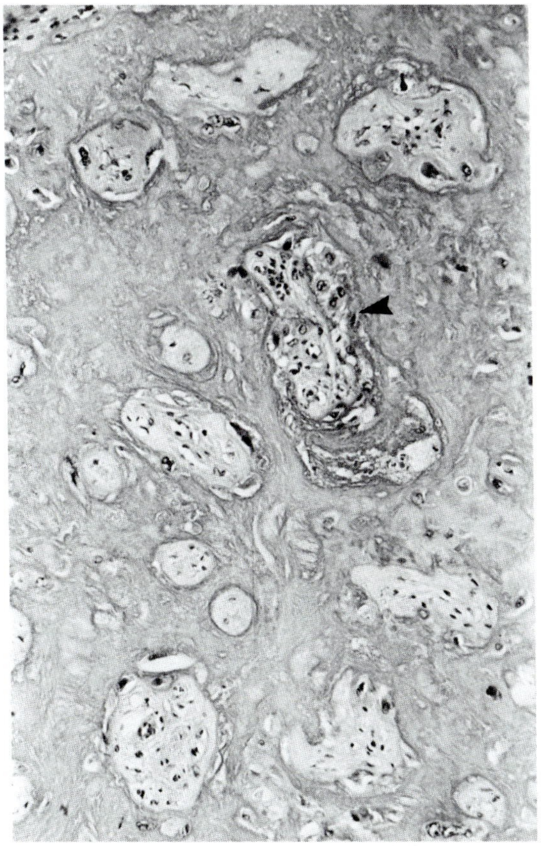

Fig. 23.51. Perivillous fibrin deposition. Villi are separated by and enmeshed in dense perivillous fibrin plaque. Intermediate trophoblast proliferates around villi (*arrow*) and extends into surrounding fibrin.

tion (IUGR) and low placental weight.[453] Although not as carefully localized or quantitated, Fuke et al. also found a significant relationship between massive intervillous fibrin deposition and IUGR.[189] It appears that massive perivillous fibrin deposition is clinically significant in proportion to its extent and location. Fibrin obliteration of large portions of the intervillous space in its prime exchange region (midbasal/central) is more likely to result in IUGR than smaller deposits at the periphery or beneath the chorionic plate. We have encountered three cases of massive perivillous fibrin deposits associated with maternal coagulopathies resulting in stillbirth, usually sudden, with little or no warning, as in the case of maternal floor infarct.[28]

Subchorionic Fibrin

Fibrin plaques and nodules are normally distributed beneath the chorionic plate of the term placenta. These pale gray or white amorphous old fibrin clots range in size from 2 or 3 cm in diameter and vary from 2 or 3 mm to about 1 cm in thickness. The pathogenesis is probably comparable to perivillous fibrin deposition, that is, thrombosis of maternal blood in the subchorionic space. Clot is deposited in layers, with amorphous fibrin just beneath the chorionic plate and the most recent layer of red cells enmeshed in fibrin adjacent to the circulating blood in the intervillous space. The amount of subchorionic fibrin and its distribution varies considerably, but in general it seems to increase with gestational age. These plaques do not appear to have any adverse effects on the placenta or the fetus. One study has linked the absence of subchorionic fibrin with markers of fetal hypoactivity.[386]

Massive Subchorial Thrombosis (Breus' Mole)

The massive *subchorial thrombohematoma* has been defined as coagulated blood, at least 1 cm in thickness, which separates the chorionic plate from the underlying villi over much of its area (Fig. 23.52).[513] These are generally relatively fresh, red thrombi that distort the chorionic plate and protrude as nodular or tuberous masses into the amnionic cavity. They may dissect into the chorionic plate or extend into the intervillous space, sometimes as far as the basal plate. Histologically, they consist of laminated thrombus devoid of villi.

A massive thrombohematoma in the subchorionic region is a rare event. The incidence of massive subchorial thrombohematoma was estimated to be 0.53 per 1000 deliveries in one large study.[513] The etiology and pathogenesis of the lesion are unknown. Early descriptions by Breus and others attributed the lesion to fetal demise, although the subsequent demonstration of massive subchorial thrombohematomas in mature placentas of liveborns refutes this view. Although smaller lesions may be innocuous, large hematomas may stimulate

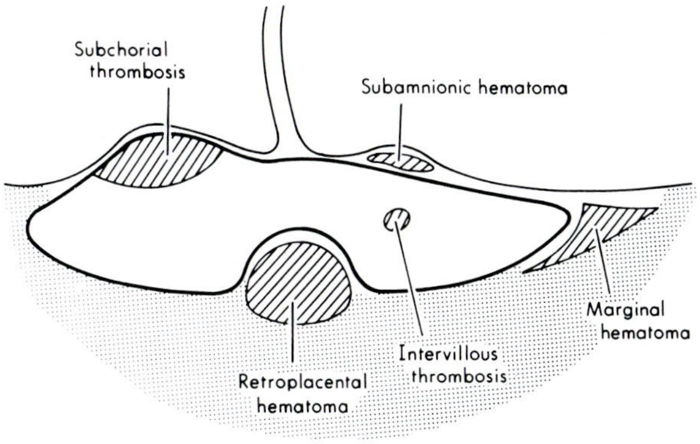

Fig. 23.52. Diagrammatic representation of various placental thrombi and hematomas. (After Fox H. (1997) Pathology of the Placenta. Second edition. Saunders, Philadelphia.)

onset of labor, or, if sufficiently large, cause severe perinatal injury or death of the fetus. Most authors agree that the thrombi are maternal in origin.

Intervillous Thrombus

Intervillous thrombi are round or oval blood clots that may occur anywhere in the intervillous space but are most common midway between the chorionic and basal plates. They begin as red, fluid, or semifluid blood (Kline's hemorrhage) and become progressively laminated and depigmented with age (Fig. 23.53). They may be single, although multiple lesions are common. Most are 1–3 cm in diameter. Early intervillous thrombohematomas should be distinguished from naturally occurring "holes" in the villous tissue at sites of maternal blood injection. Basilar intervillous thrombohematomas should be distinguished from intervillous extension of retroplacental thrombohematomas.

Microscopically, the thrombi consist of erythrocytes and fibrin, the proportion of fibrin increasing with the age of the lesion (Fig. 23.54). The villi are displaced to the margins of the clot. Nucleated red blood cells have been identified in these thrombi,[132,282] and more recent immunohistochemical studies have confirmed the presence of fetal hemoglobin containing RBCs,[282] although maternal erythrocytes seem to constitute the majority of the lesion.

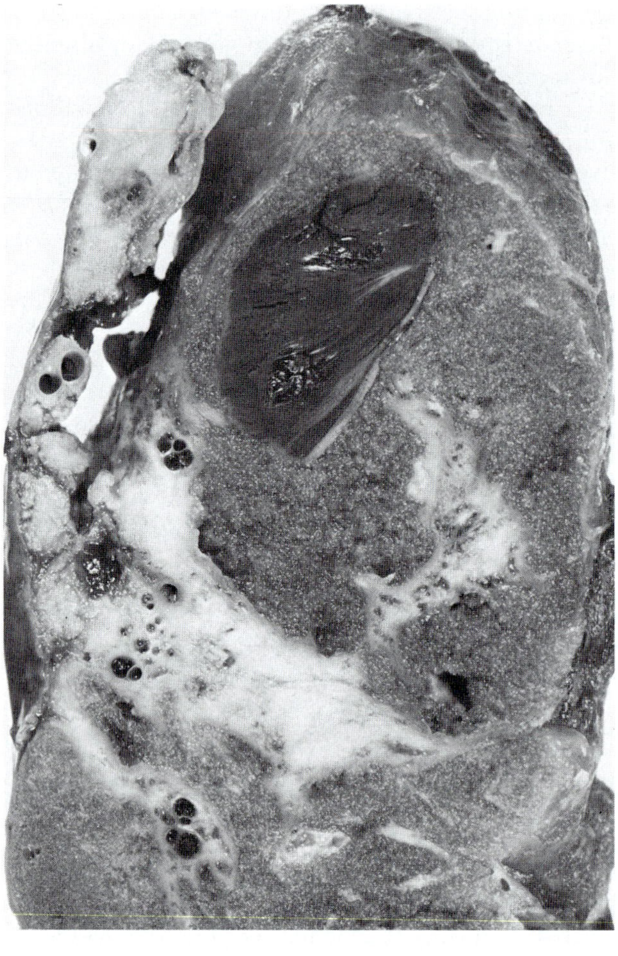

Fig. 23.53. Intervillous thrombus. Intervillous thrombi become laminated as they age.

An intervillous thrombus is significant in that it marks the site of hemorrhage from the fetal to the maternal circulation. Fetal bleeding into the intervillous space is thought to occur through rupture of the attenuated vasculosyncytial membrane. Factors cited as potential causes of villous damage resulting in fetomaternal hemorrhage include trauma, amniocentesis, and external version.[459] Small fetomaternal hemorrhages, as assessed by the Kleihauer–Betke technique, are relatively common in the third trimester of pregnancy, occurring in 15%–30% of pregnancies. There appears to be good correlation between the number of fetal cells in the maternal circulation and the number of intervillous thrombi.[132,600] The same relationship applies to other placental lesions, including retroplacental hematomas and infarcts.[600] Fetomaternal hemorrhage, when massive, may be a cause of severe fetal anemia or intrauterine fetal demise.[459]

Retroplacental Hematoma

Pathology

A *retroplacental hematoma* is a clot located between the basal plate of the placenta and the uterine wall (Fig. 23.55). The pathologic findings reflect a number of factors including its size, location, and duration. When confined by peripherally attached placenta, a retroplacental hematoma distorts and indents the overlying placental parenchyma, which is often infarcted (Fig. 23.56). This characteristic depression is easily recognized even in the absence of hematoma itself. Older retroplacental hematomas may be much more subtle, forming only a thin, inconspicuous layer of red-brown clot beneath an infarct. When retroplacental hematomas extend to the placental margin, the blood may be evacuated without causing any indentation. Very recent extensive placental separation is typically associated with little, if any, gross or histologic change in the placenta. These large hematomas generally result in immediate fetal distress, necessitating emergent delivery. The observation of a large fresh clot behind a "floating" detached placenta observed at the time of cesarean section may be the only objective sign of an acute retroplacental hemorrhage. Obstetricians should document this observation and submit the

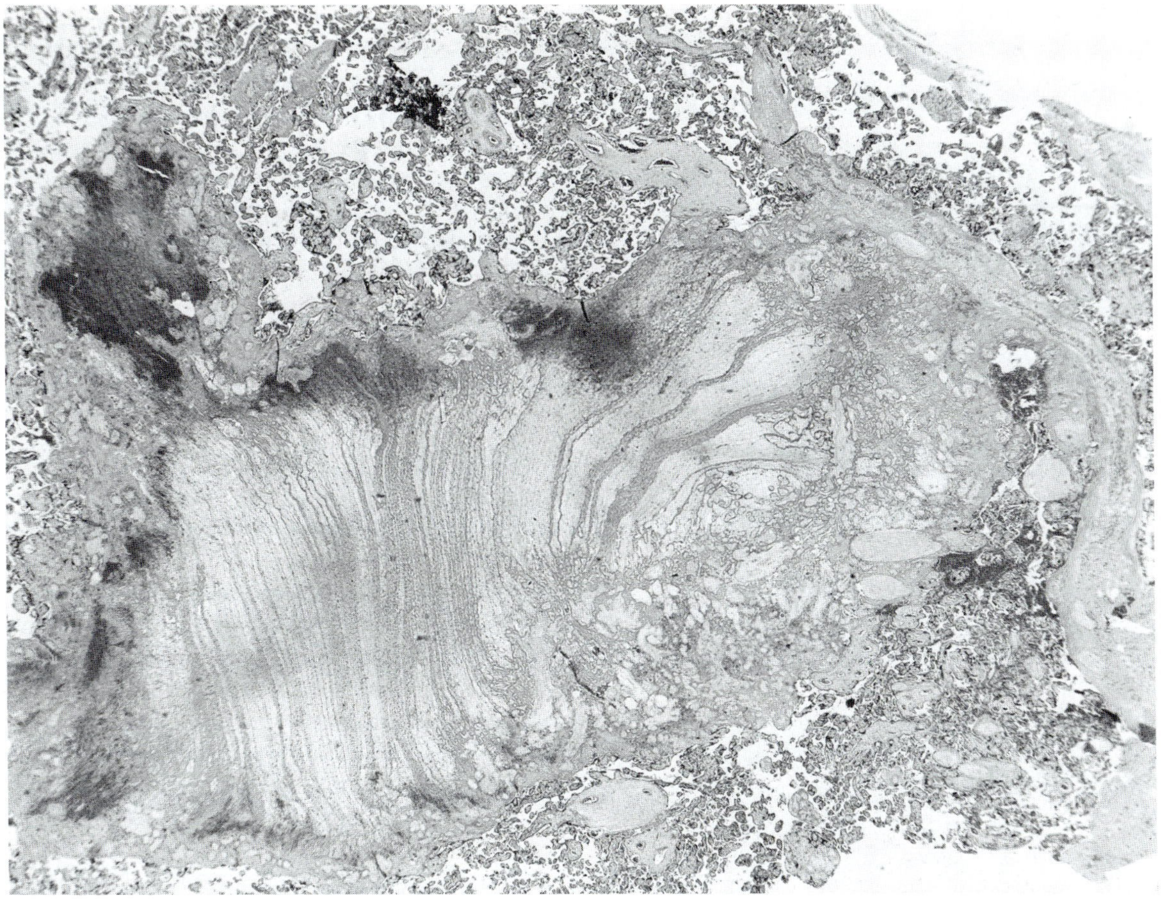

Fig. 23.54. Intervillous thrombus. Histologic appearance of laminated fibrin and erythrocytes in an intervillous thrombus.

clot along with the placenta when requesting pathologic examination.

Microscopically, retroplacental hematomas consist of red cells and fibrin, the proportion of fibrin increasing as the lesion ages and the red cells degenerate. The time course of these evolutionary changes is unknown. The basal plate decidua may be normal in instances of acute retroplacental hemorrhage, but there is usually patchy bland necrosis; this is to be expected after normal labor and vaginal delivery, but not in a placenta that has been delivered by cesarean section with no prior labor. An acute inflammatory infiltrate may occur in the decidua basalis adjacent to early clots, and hemosiderin deposits are often present in macrophages around older clots. Retroplacental hematomas are composed predominantly of maternal blood, but in some cases, there may be a significant fetal component as well.[90]

The infarcted placenta overlying the hematoma is microscopically identical to the infarcts just described. Blanc described a "divergent" infarction pattern characterized by necrotic villi widely separated by a markedly enlarged and congested intervillous space.[64] This pattern has been attributed to interruption of both venous and arterial circulations. Villous stromal hemorrhage may occur in placentas with clinically suspected abruption (Fig. 23.57).[367]

Etiology

The overall prevalence of retroplacental hematoma is reportedly about 4.5%, but it is increased threefold in women with preeclampsia.[301] Other factors associated with retroplacental hematoma include trauma, typically from automobile accidents, heavy cigarette smoking, acute chorioamnionitis,[118] cocaine abuse, and previous abruption.[283] Recent studies implicate maternal coagulopathies.[288,603] Rupture of a spiral artery weakened by the pathologic alterations that occur in preeclampsia is the usual explanation in patients with that condition. Alternative mechanisms include venous rupture following thrombosis of decidual arterioles and decid-

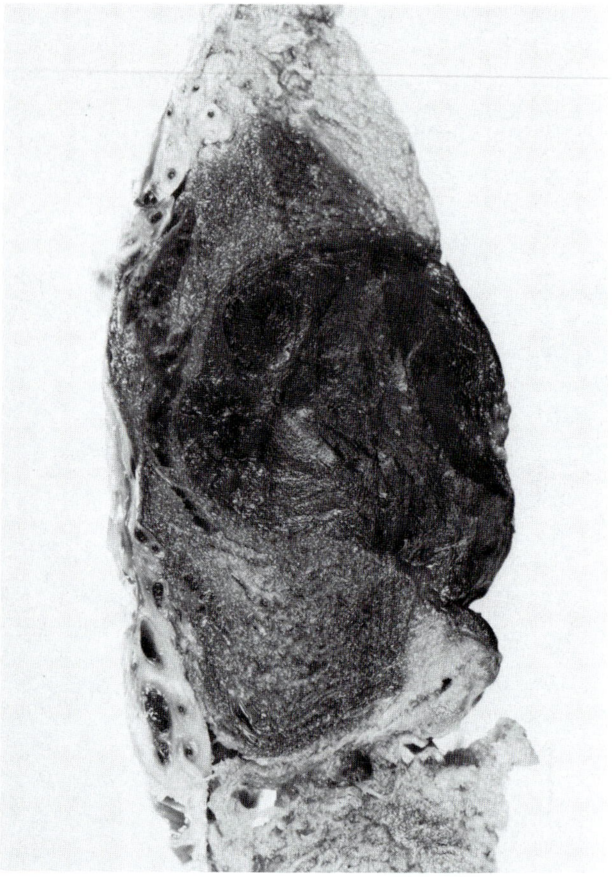

Fig. 23.55. Retroplacental hematoma. Characteristic compression and infarction of the placental parenchyma overlie a large retroplacental hematoma. The surrounding, lighter, normal placenta contrasts with the darker, infarcted tissue.

ual necrosis, venous outflow obstruction, or primary placental separation. A deficiency of folic acid and hyperhomocysteinemia have been proposed as factors predisposing to abnormal placental separation.[209,237,288]

Clinical Features

Retroplacental hematoma, the *pathologic* lesion, is related to but not synonymous with placental abruption (abruptio placentae), an acute *clinical* syndrome characterized by pain, uterine tetany, fetal distress, and sometimes a consumptive coagulopathy.[224] Clinical abruption occurs in about 11.5 of 1000 deliveries. It is associated with a 20%–40% fetal mortality rate and accounts for 10% of all stillbirths and 6% of maternal deaths. Although placental abruption and retroplacental hematoma share the same risk factors, only about one-third of patients with clinical abruption will have a retroplacental hematoma. Clinical abruption may not be associated with any discernible placental abnormality, especially if the entire placenta separates suddenly and completely. A retroplacental hematoma must have been present for some period of time to be recognizable as such. Because abruption is an acute clinical situation, it is not surprising that the associated placenta often lacks a recognizable hematoma. Conversely, small retroplacental hematomas are sometimes found in the absence of clinical signs or symptoms. In only about 35% of cases with retroplacental hematomas will abruption have been diagnosed clinically. Retroplacental hematomas in some instances probably occur in stages, resulting finally in the clinical syndrome of complete placental abruption.

The clinical significance of a retroplacental hematoma appears to be related primarily to its size. In separating a portion of the placenta from its maternal blood supply, the retroplacental hematoma is responsible for defunctionalizing the overlying placenta, which eventually will be recognizable as an infarct. The larger the infarct, the more likely it will exceed the functional reserve capability of the placenta, which may be already marginal in a background of chronic uteroplacental ischemia. A large hematoma may sometimes initiate the blood coagulation cascade in the mother, resulting in disseminated intravascular coagulation. In such cases abruption is also responsible for high maternal morbidity and mortality.

Marginal Hematoma

A *marginal hematoma* occurs where the lateral margin of the placental disk joins the fetal membranes (Fig. 23.52). Grossly, the marginal hematoma forms a crescent-shaped clot adherent to the lateral margin of the placenta. It may extend beneath the adjacent fetal membranes or for some distance onto the maternal aspect of the placenta, but in contrast to retroplacental hematoma, it does not cause depression of the basal plate or infarction of overlying villous parenchyma. On cut section, the clot is triangular in shape, the apex of the triangle being formed by the junction of the membranous and villous chorion.

Microscopically, a recent marginal clot may be accompanied by an acute inflammatory infiltrate and older clots by hemosiderin deposition. The clot usually lies entirely outside the placental disk but may occasionally involve the intervillous space. With this exception, the presence of a marginal hematoma has no effect on the adjacent villi.

Marginal hematomas are thought to result from rupture of uteroplacental veins at the margin of a low-lying placenta. The hematoma is found at the margin of the placenta closest to the site of mem-

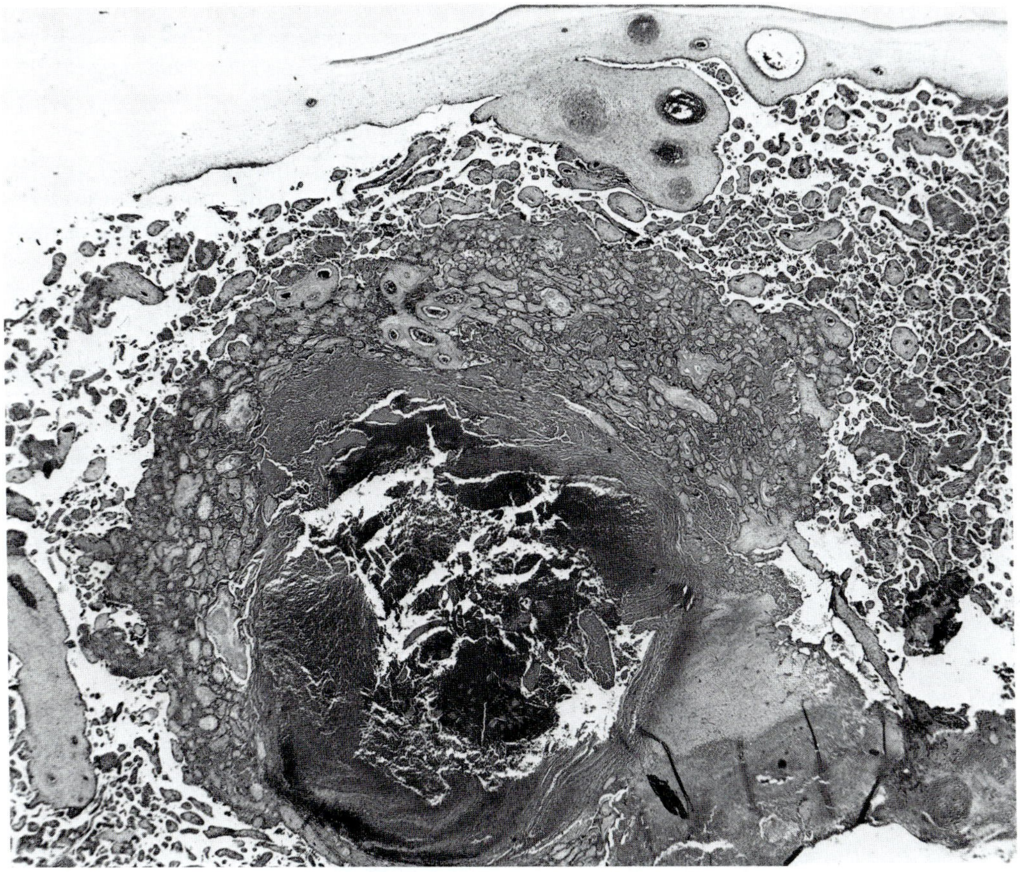

Fig. 23.56. Retroplacental hematoma. Histologic appearance of a retroplacental hematoma showing elevation of the basal plate and infarction of the adjacent placenta.

brane rupture, which is usually only a few centimeters from the placental margin. A marginal hematoma may be associated with antepartum maternal hemorrhage and in some cases may be followed by onset of labor, but it does not have any untoward direct affects on the fetus. Chronic marginal separation and thrombohematomas are common in circumvallation, and in this context retroplacental hematomas and abruption are also more frequent.

Fetal Circulation

Fetal blood is pumped through the umbilical arteries in the cord into placental stem vessels and smaller branches, eventually reaching the villous capillaries. Reoxygenated and fortified blood returns to the fetus through the umbilical vein. Clots may obstruct any part of this system from the largest vessels in the umbilical cord to the smallest villous capillaries. Clots in the largest vessels may significantly compromise the fetal circulation, leading to fetal death; clots in smaller vessels defunctionalize the portion of placenta distal to the clot. A clot in any part of the fetal vascular tree also implies a significant risk for clotting elsewhere in the fetus.

Fetal Vessel Thrombosis and Fetal Thrombotic Vasculopathy

Pathology

Thrombosed large chorionic plate vessels, arteries and veins, are often grossly abnormal: enlarged, distended, and hard. Occlusion of a large fetal artery on the chorionic plate or a smaller fetal stem artery results in degeneration and ultimately in the disappearance of the distal smaller vessels and capillaries. The pattern of clustered avascular villi downstream from an occluded vessel is called *fetal thrombotic vasculopathy* (*FTV*). Because many thrombi involve smaller vessels, the clusters of distal fibrotic avascular villi are often small, identifiable only microscopically. When a larger fetal vessel is obstructed, the downstream villous changes may be appreciated grossly as a well-delineated triangular area of pallor with its base on the maternal

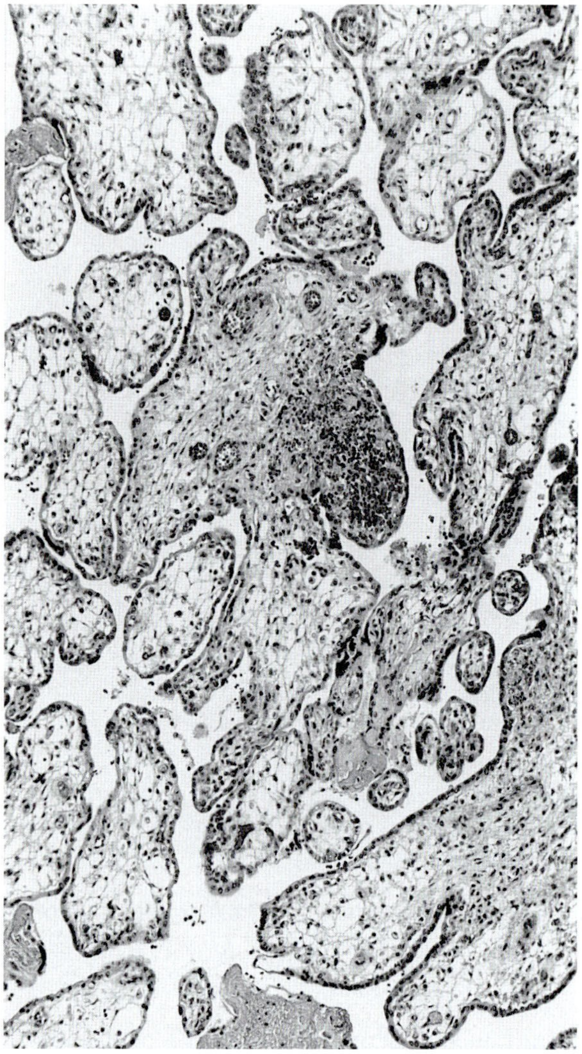

Fig. 23.57. Placenta with acute abruption. A circumvallate placenta with a large old marginal hematoma that extended beneath the placenta caused clinical features of abruption. Patchy villous edema and focal villous stromal hemorrhage is shown in the large central villus.

surface. Generally, these have the same consistency as the surrounding normal parenchyma (Fig. 23.58), although some older lesions in a term placenta may become firmer, gray or white, and well delimited. The extent of the villous lesions is easily underestimated on gross examination, and many lesions are very hard to see or invisible, even after fixation (Fig. 23.59).

Microscopically, the downstream villi are avascular with densely collagenized, hyalinized stroma, and the nuclei of the syncytiotrophoblast cells, which typically survive this injury, may cluster to form syncytial knots (Fig. 23.60).[304] The intervillous space is normally patent. The larger fetal stem vessels distal to the thrombus undergo septation (Fig. 23.61) and fibromuscular sclerosis characterized by medial hyperplasia and intimal proliferation with eventual luminal obliteration. The proximal thrombosed vessel(s) may or may not be apparent depending on the plane of sectioning, but the constellation of villous changes is specific enough to infer the nature of the pathologic process. It is impossible to distinguish between stem arteries and veins in histologic sections when they have been altered by thrombi. Nonocclusive forms of FTV in stem or surface vessels known as *fibrinous vasculosis*[502] and *intimal cushions*[119] refer to deposits of fibrin in the vascular wall that in time resemble organized re-epithelialized mural thrombi which bulge into the lumen and ultimately may calcify (Fig. 23.62).

Clinical Significance

Fetal thrombotic vasculopathy has been associated with IUGR, intrauterine fetal demise, nonimmune

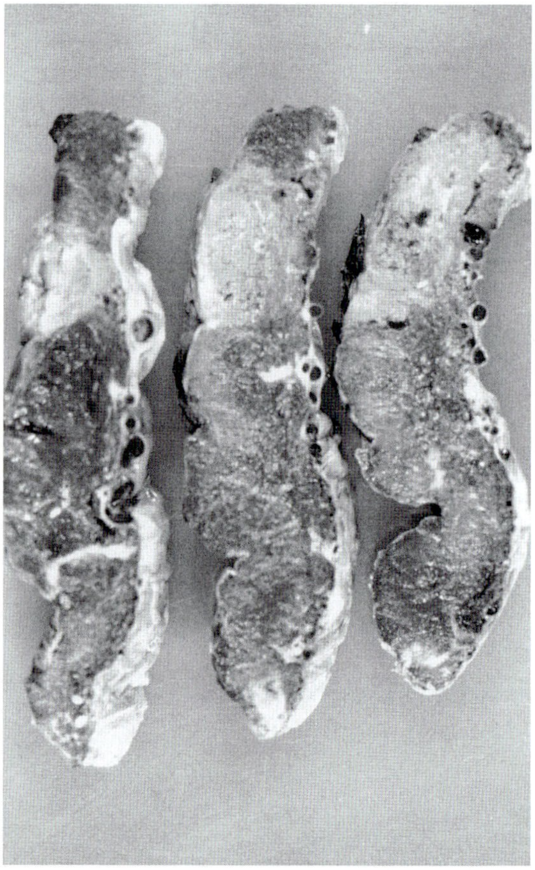

Fig. 23.58. Fetal thrombotic vasculopathy. The pale areas *on top* are composed of fibrotic avascular villi comparable to those shown in Fig. 23.59. The large surface vessel toward the *left* in the *left* slice contains a partly organized mural thrombus.

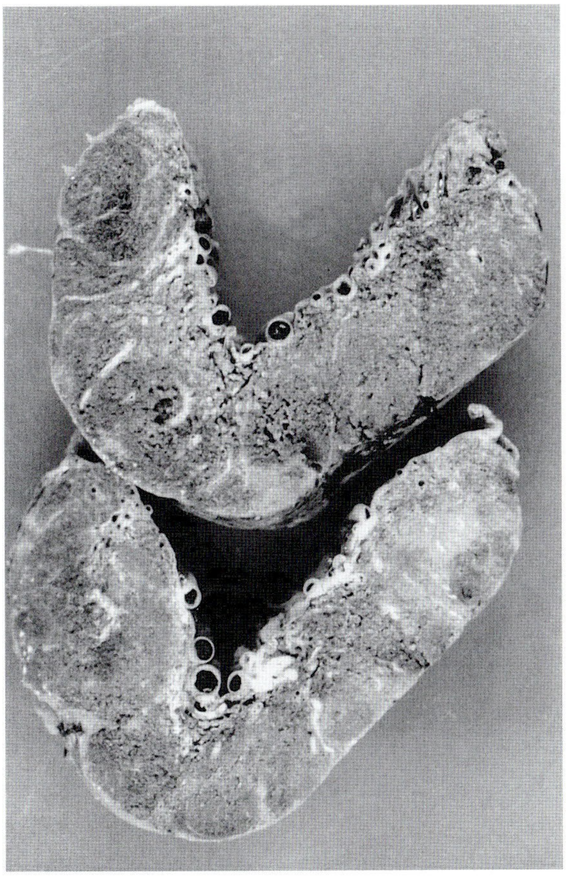

Fig. 23.59. Fetal thrombotic vasculopathy. Although very difficult to identify grossly, fetal thrombotic vasculopathy was found throughout this placenta. Cesarean section was done for fetal heartbeat irregularities. The newborn was flaccid at birth with established periventricular leukomalacia by ultrasound.

hydrops, acute and chronic fetal monitoring abnormalities, and thromboembolic disease.[444,451] The pathologic findings provide direct evidence of clot formation in the fetal circulation. The somatic circulation of the fetus is therefore also clearly at risk, and there is a significant association between FTV and thrombotic lesions in the newborn, of which neurologic injury has been the most important.[303,572] Somatic thrombi also occur in the lungs and kidneys,[303] and probably represent the basis for some instances of limb reduction defects[246] and myocardial infarct.[610] Massive FTV affecting about 50% of the placenta usually causes stillbirth.[170,303] Some relationship to inherited or transplacental coagulopathy appears likely.[302,303] Postnatal coagulation testing of 92 children with cerebral thromboembolism demonstrated that 38% had coagulopathies[131]; tests of another group of children with stroke showed that 23% were homozygous for the methylene tetrahydrofolate reductase gene mutation.[432] The finding of FTV in a placenta may be the earliest identifying sign of risk for stroke in children; studies to calculate the magnitude of this risk are needed before strategies for intervention can be developed. Adverse outcomes have not been identified in many babies with placentas showing FTV.

Hemorrhagic Endovasculitis (HEV)

The lesion described by Sander in 1980 as *hemorrhagic endovasculitis* (*HEV*)[492] is characterized by a constellation of histologic findings including villous endothelial and stromal necrosis, thrombi in various stages of organization, endothelial proliferation, luminal fibrotic strands (recanalization) of vessels, fragmentation and diapedesis of red cells, and villous stromal hemorrhage and hemosiderin deposition (Figs. 23.63 and 23.64). Associated placental findings have included umbilical cord abnormalities, meconium staining, VUE, and erythroblastosis.[493]

The reported prevalence of HEV is highly variable; Sander diagnosed the lesion in 19.5% of pla-

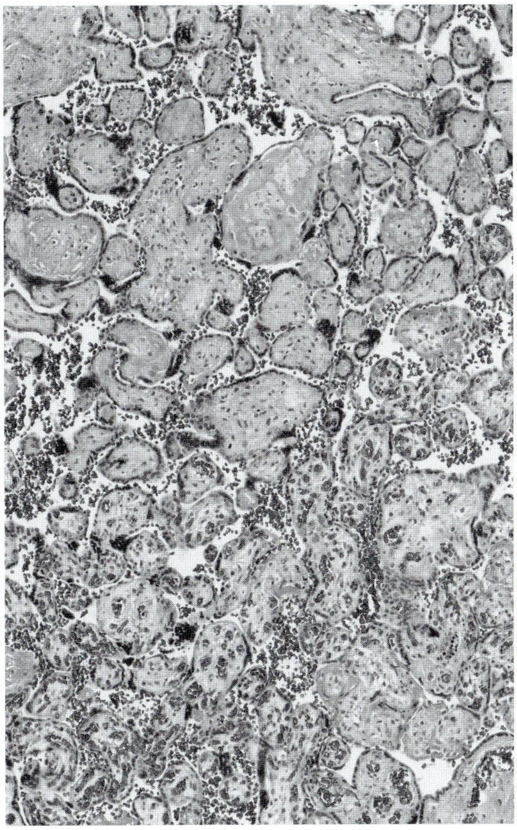

Fig. 23.60. Fetal thrombotic vasculopathy. The avascular villi (*upper*) reflect the changes associated with fetal artery thrombosis and contrast with the functional villi (*lower*) in this placenta from a liveborn baby.

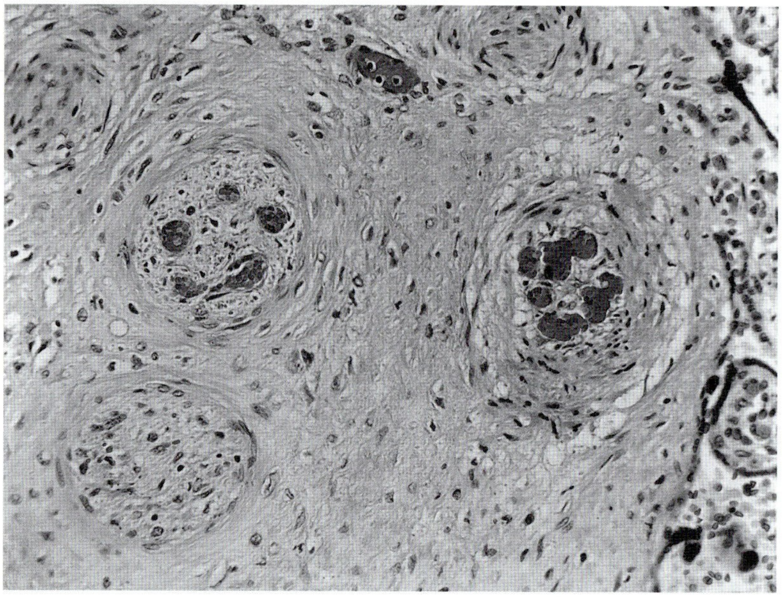

Fig. 23.61. Fetal thrombotic vasculopathy. Large vessels downstream from a thrombus undergo septation of the vascular lumen and then fibromuscular obliteration.

centas submitted to the Michigan Placental Tissue Registry, but Shen-Schwarz and others found it in only 0.67% of placentas from unselected pregnancies.[492,517] Clinically, the lesion has been significantly associated with stillbirth, intrauterine growth retardation, long-term developmental delay, maternal hypertension or preeclampsia, postterm gestation, and the presence of a nuchal cord during delivery.[493,517] HEV has recurred in successive pregnancies in some patients.[493]

The etiology and pathogenesis of HEV are controversial, but currently it is considered to represent a form of fetal thrombotic vasculopathy. Some believe that the villous changes in HEV are secondary to upstream venous thrombosis rather than the downstream reflection of arterial occlusion.[445] The finding of localized HEV adjacent to venous thrombi, its frequent association with nuchal cord, and the identification of an HEV-like lesion in human chorionic villous organ culture provide support for this hypothesis.[517,535] Because it is impossible to distinguish arteries from veins in placental sections, it may be difficult to resolve this issue. The sequence of regressive vascular changes in stillborns is identical,[171,195] although in intrauterine fetal demise, the vascular alterations are generalized in contrast to sharply demarcated focal involvement of the placenta in liveborns.

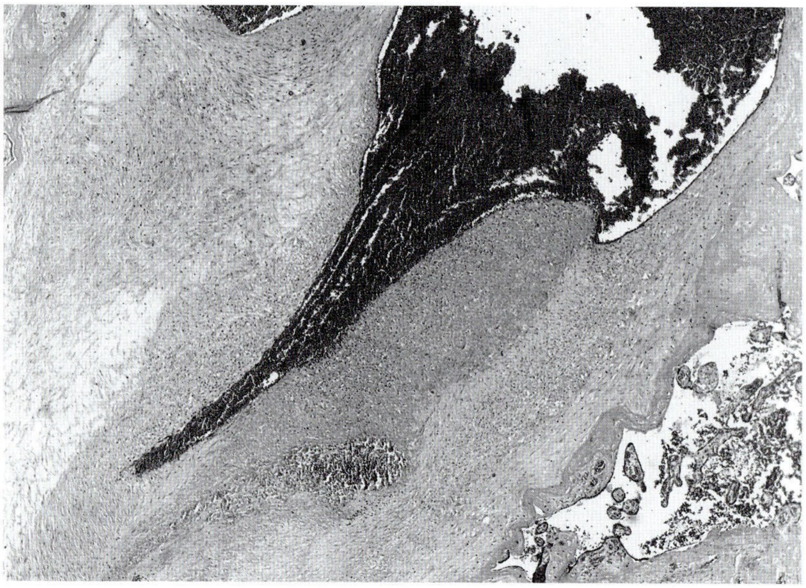

Fig. 23.62. Mural thrombus in large stem vessel. A mural thrombus is attached at center and the external media is calcified (*bottom, center*). This pattern has been illustrated as fibrinous vasculosis by Scott.[502]

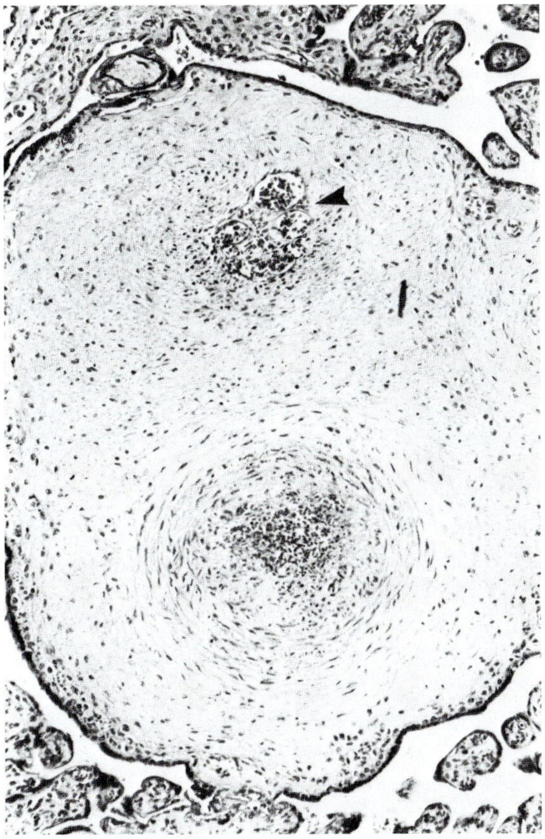

Fig. 23.63. Hemorrhagic endovasculitis. Thrombi in various stages of organization in vessels of stem villi. Recanalized channels (septation) are apparent (*arrow*). Extravasated red cells are noted around vessel at *bottom.*

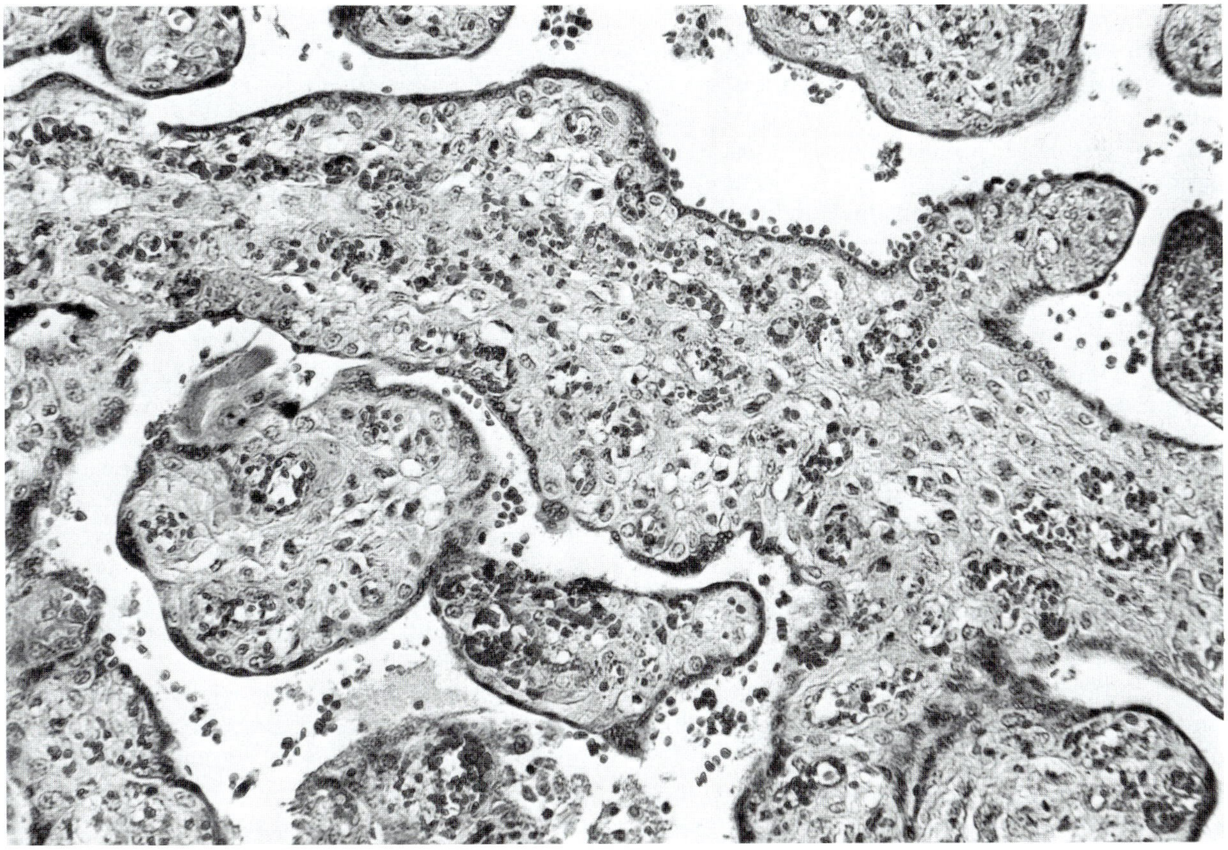

Fig. 23.64. Hemorrhagic endovasculitis. Fragmented red blood cells, many of which are extravasated, and nuclear debris are present in and around the capillaries of the terminal villi. This pattern is typical of more acute villous change upstream from a recent thrombus.

Villous Edema and Villous Stromal Hemorrhage

Chorionic villous swelling caused by abnormal accumulations of water occurs in three different contexts, each with distinct pathologic features. The first and most obvious form is the gross vesicular swelling of hydatidiform mole and certain other abnormal karyotypes. The second most common and also most controversial form of villous edema is a pattern in which both terminal and intermediate villi are expanded by many small reticular stromal spaces separated by strands of stromal cell cytoplasm, often in a patchy distribution. It is necessary, but often difficult, to separate this lesion from the appearance of immature intermediate villi as seen in premature placentas, which normally have this appearance.[50,51,173]

Naeye[387,393] described this pattern of villous edema in association with acute chorioamnionitis and abruption, a relationship not supported by other observers. Shen-Schwartz et al.[516] found villous edema associated significantly with fetal and neonatal death but not with chorioamnionitis. We have found occasional instances of villous edema together with both acute chorioamnionitis and abruption (see Fig. 23.57), but these placentas also had other significant problems, especially vascular thromboses. In a series of very low birth weight infants with cerebral palsy or other neurologic impairment, Redline et al. found severe villous edema and nonocclusive fetal vessel thrombi to be the most significant pathologic abnormalities.[455] A third category of villous edema occurs in both immune and nonimmune fetal hydrops. In this condition, virtually all terminal and stem villi are expanded by diffuse interstitial edema and enveloped by immature trophoblast including a persistent layer of cytotrophoblast. Some diabetic placentas may have a component of villous edema that is usually mild and inconspicuous.

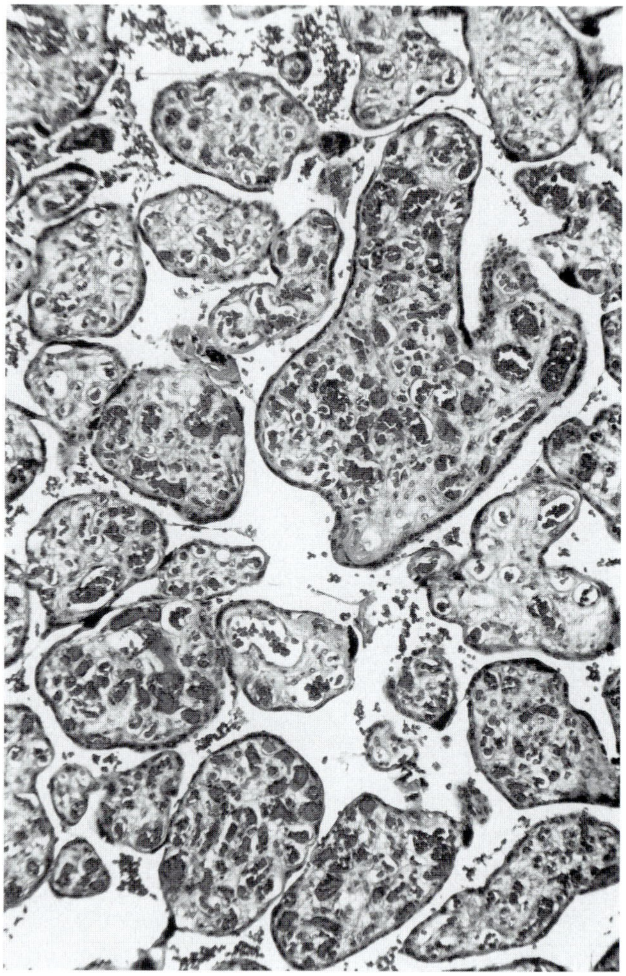

Fig. 23.65. Chorangiosis. Greatly increased numbers of villous capillaries in chorangiosis.

Chorangiosis

Chorangiosis refers to the occurrence of numerous enlarged, highly vascular villi throughout the placenta. The villous stroma is usually abundant and is diffusely interspersed with the numerous capillaries (Fig. 23.65). As defined by Altshuler,[13] there should be more than 10 terminal villi containing more than 10 capillaries per villus in 10 medium-power fields, occurring in multiple areas (at least three) of the placenta.

Chorangiosis appears to be a nonspecific change related to a variety of conditions including maternal diabetes, hypertension, infections, anomalies, intrauterine fetal death, and growth retardation.[13,541] Placentas with chorangiosis are often large for gestational age and exhibit delayed villous maturation. In one large study, chorangiosis occurred in 3% of 1614 deliveries and was associated with placental lesions including infarcts, chronic villitis, fetal artery thrombi, and spiral artery thrombi.[541] Altshuler et al. found chorangiosis in 5.5% of 1350 placentas of babies admitted to the neonatal intensive care unit; among 38- to 40-week gestations, 39% of infants with chorangiosis died, and 27% had major congenital malformations.[13]

The pathogenesis of chorangiosis is unknown. Chorangiosis is increased in placentas of gestations occurring at high altitude, suggesting that it may be an adaptive response to hypoxia. The central location of the capillaries might suggest the possibility of a shunt, comparable to hemangioma, which could become clinically significant if sufficient numbers of villi are affected. The finding of occasional villi with these features seems to have no clinical significance.

Subamnionic Hematoma

A subamnionic hematoma lies between the amnion and chorion on the fetal surface of the placenta (see Fig. 23.52). Very recent lesions often result from trauma to the chorionic veins during delivery, especially after excessive traction on the umbilical cord. Occasionally laceration of chorionic plate vessels during amniocentesis may lead to subamnionic hemorrhage, sometimes severe, and therefore chorionic vessels in the region of a subamnionic hemorrhage always deserve careful inspection. Older subamnionic fibrin clots, of unknown pathogenesis, form dome-shaped blisters and contain a mixture of brown-tinged fluid and fibrin.

The Placenta in Maternal Disorders

One of the commonest situations in which the pathologist is asked to evaluate the placenta is in the setting of underlying maternal disease. The goal is to define what if any effect such diseases have had on the placenta and fetus. Although a large number of studies have focused on these very issues, there is, unfortunately, a great deal of disagreement and direct contradiction about the nature and significance of the lesions described.

Preeclampsia (Pregnancy-Induced Hypertension) and Eclampsia

As a major cause of both maternal and fetal morbidity and mortality, *preeclampsia*, also known as *pregnancy-induced hypertension* (*PIH*), is the most important underlying maternal condition to complicate pregnancy. Preeclampsia is defined as the development of hypertension with proteinuria or generalized edema or both after 20 weeks of gestation. Eclampsia signifies the occurrence of convulsions in a patient with preeclampsia. Not every case of hypertension in pregnancy is preeclampsia. Recent classification schemes have categorized the hypertensive disorders of pregnancy to exclude early or preexisting hypertension and those lacking proteinuria.[120]

Pathology

No single lesion is invariably found in the placenta in preeclampsia, nor are there any absolutely specific abnormalities. In the great majority of cases, the placenta shows the effects of low uteroplacental flow. The placenta is smaller on average than the placenta from an uncomplicated pregnancy, and infarcts are more numerous, larger, and often centrally located.[598] The infarcts may be old or recent. Recent infarcts may be difficult to see grossly, but they are easily felt, being firmer than the surrounding noninfarcted placenta. The extent of infarction is directly proportional to the severity of the preeclampsia. Although extensive placental infarction is a cardinal sign of preeclampsia, it is neither specific for nor invariable in that condition. In preeclampsia, even relatively minor degrees of infarction may be associated with fetal compromise (growth retardation; fetal death in utero) reflecting underlying chronic uteroplacental ischemia and decreased reserve capacity. Retroplacental hematoma is also identified with undue frequency (12%–15%) in preeclamptic women; this is an added factor contributing to the increased frequency of infarction in these placentas.

The villi in preeclampsia show subtle but consistent microscopic changes reflecting placental ischemia including cytotrophoblastic proliferation, trophoblastic basement membrane thickening, small, inconspicuous fetal capillaries, and prominence of the villous stroma.[271,385] The villi show accelerated maturation and are often abnormally small, with increased syncytial knots ("Tenney–Parker" change) (Fig. 23.66).[385,570] Syncytial knotting occurs as a part of normal villous maturation, but syncytial knots on more than 30% of the villi (especially in the premature placenta) are indicative of perfusional compromise. Similar changes occur in villi cultured under conditions of low oxygen tension as well as in the placentas of animals with experimentally produced toxemia. These villous changes are focal with normal villi present in variable proportion. The uneven pattern of villous morphology results from normal blood flow through some spiral arteries and low/absent flow through others. It is important to assess these changes in areas remote from other abnormalities and in central portions of the placenta because uteroplacental flow is normally low at the periphery and beneath the chorionic plate.

Low uteroplacental flow and its effect on the placenta are attributable to pathologic abnormalities occurring in the spiral arteries of the placental bed in preeclampsia. These arteries differ from their normal counterparts in two important respects. First, the adaptive, physiologic remodeling that occurs normally in the vessels of the placental bed is decreased in degree and extent. In women with preeclampsia, the second wave of intravascular trophoblastic migration does not occur. The intramyometrial segments of the spiral arteries retain their musculoelastic media and do not dilate. Physiologic vascular changes that accompany normal implan-

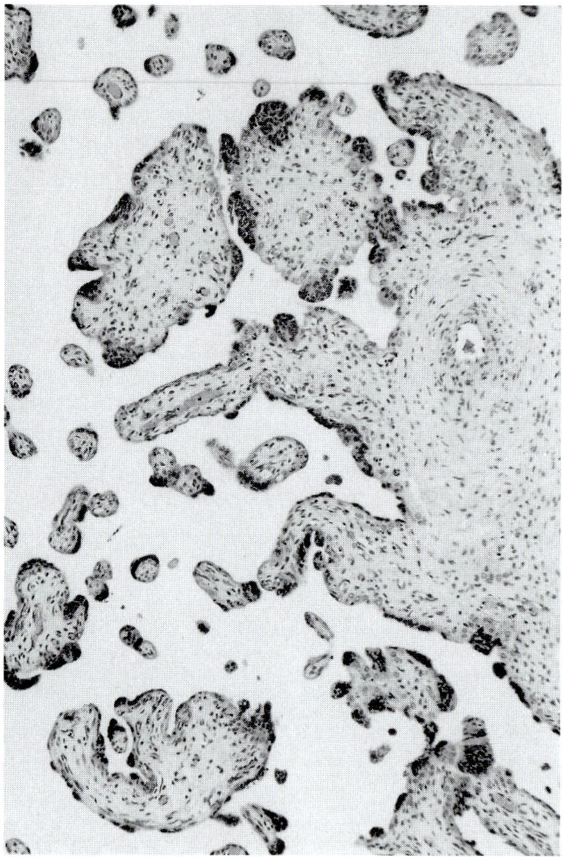

Fig. 23.66. Villi in preeclampsia. The villous changes in this placenta from a pregnancy complicated by severe preeclampsia at 17 weeks include markedly accelerated maturation and increased syncytial knots (Tenney–Parker change).

tation are, therefore, incomplete in women with preeclampsia. Physiologic remodeling of spiral arteries is also limited in other pathologic states, including some normotensive women with SGA babies.[8,134,518]

Second, the spiral arteries in women with preeclampsia exhibit an acute necrotizing arteriopathy (acute atherosis).[617] This lesion is characterized by fibrinoid necrosis of the vessel wall, accumulation of lipid-laden cells, and a perivascular mononuclear infiltrate (Fig. 23.67).[136] Spiral arteries altered by acute atherosis may be thrombosed; the infarcts and retroplacental hematomas so common in preeclamptics are thought to be the direct result of acute atherosis and related vascular changes.[79]

Acute atherosis is thought by some to be a specific feature of preeclampsia with a characteristic distribution. According to Robertson, acute atherosis is a lesion limited to vessels that have not been altered by the normal adaptive processes of implantation: the decidual segments of spiral arteries outside the placental bed, the basal arteries, and the myometrial segments of the spiral arteries in the placental bed that have not undergone physiologic adaptation.[464] Identical vascular alterations, however, have been described in placentas from pregnancies complicated by other hypertensive disorders, diabetes, systemic lupus erythematosus (SLE), and the antiphospholipid antibody syndrome.[3,4,138,291] The lesion has also been observed in the spiral arteries of the placental bed in normotensive women with intrauterine growth retardation.[80,134,287,518]

The examination of spiral arteries is desirable, but they are rarely obtained in random sections of the placenta. Spiral arteries can often be directly visualized in the normal placenta, usually toward the center of a cotyledon, but the pathologic alterations that occur in preeclampsia make them difficult or impossible to see. The decidua capsularis is frequently the best place to identify spiral arteries and their pathologic alterations. Alternatively, additional random sections of the basal plate may increase the odds of obtaining them. Even when spiral arteries are not identified, the status of the uteroplacental circulation can be inferred from placental weight, extent and size of infarcts, and villous morphology.

Redline and Patterson recently described increased amounts of abnormally proliferative, immature intermediate trophoblast (IT) in the decidua basalis of preeclamptics at all gestational ages.[454] They proposed that these changes, termed atypical implantation site, be considered characteristic of the preeclamptic placenta and theorized that the overabundant immature trophoblast might initiate the disease by triggering the maternal immune system leading to the vascular pathology.

A second and smaller group of patients with preeclampsia is more heterogeneous but seems to be linked by excessive placental size. This group includes patients with multiple gestations, very large placentas with abundant immature trophoblast (especially some diabetics), hydropic placentas, and hydatidiform moles.[503]

Etiology

Preeclampsia is a common disease and intensively studied, but it is still not completely understood. It is a disease unique to pregnancy, mediated by the placenta, and its pathophysiologic alterations regress completely after delivery. Reduced placental perfusion and relative placental ischemia play a central role and may be exacerbated by maternal diseases associated with vascular compromise (diabetes mellitus, hyper-

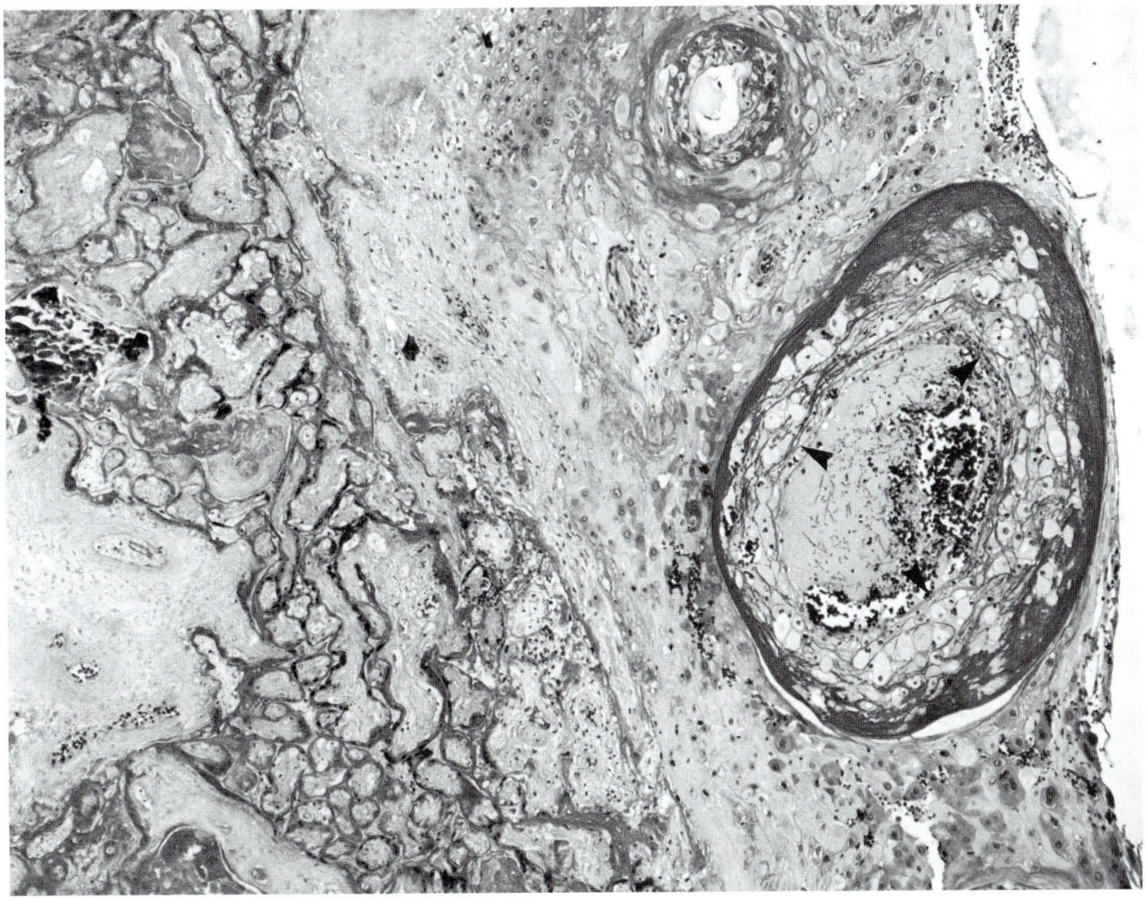

Fig. 23.67. Acute atherosis, preeclampsia. The spiral arteries are distorted by fibrinoid necrosis of the vessel wall and accumulation of lipid-containing macrophages (*arrows*). The largest artery is thrombosed, and there is infarction of the overlying placenta (*left*).

tension, collagen vascular disease) or excessive placental size.[81,82,141,330] Incomplete physiologic remodeling of the spiral arteries undoubtedly impedes uteroplacental blood flow,[621] and there is abundant evidence that endothelial dysfunction is the final common pathway. A review of current hypotheses relating to the pathogenesis of preeclampsia has been presented by Dekker and Sibai.[126] Severe early-onset preeclampsia is associated with a disproportionately high prevalence of maternal coagulopathies including factor V Leiden, activated protein C resistance, hyperhomocysteinemia, anticardiolipin antibodies, and protein S deficiency.[125,143,308,431,586]

Essential Hypertension

The pathology of the placenta in mothers with *preexisting essential hypertension* as an isolated problem has received little attention. A few studies have shown that morphologic changes in the placenta in this disease are qualitatively very similar to those found in preeclampsia. The similarities extend to the ultrastructural level, although the extent and degree of pathologic changes are less marked in placentas from cases of essential hypertension than in preeclampsia.[272] A maternal vascular abnormality termed hyperplastic arteriosclerosis, characterized by marked medial thickening of all coats of the vessel wall, intimal hyperplasia, and luminal narrowing, has been described in women with essential hypertension.[464,465,519] These changes are most conspicuous in the myometrial segments of the spiral arteries. When preeclampsia complicates essential hypertension there may be superimposition of acute atherosis on hyperplastic arteriosclerosis. The placental changes in cases of essential hypertension complicated by preeclampsia are less marked than those found in the placentas of previously normotensive women who develop preeclampsia of comparable severity.[272]

Immunologic Diseases: Systemic Lupus Erythematosis, Scleroderma, and Related Conditions

Placental abnormalities comparable to those in preeclampsia, including acute atherosis, infarcts, and other manifestations of reduced placental blood flow, are found in some[148,333,403] but not all[4] cases of collagen vascular disease. The presence of antiphospholipid antibodies appears to enhance the presence and severity of the morphologic abnormalities. Repeated abortion and stillbirth are common. Fetal thrombotic disease may also occur,[523,534,566] suggesting that the associated maternal coagulopathy can be transmitted in some cases. Placental lesions associated with significant fetal morbidity include thrombi in decidual and fetal stem vessels (see Fig. 23.48) and chronic villitis.[333,485] Fetomaternal alloimmune thrombocytopenia may predispose the fetus to intracranial hemorrhage antenatally, as shown by ultrasound.[521]

Acute Fatty Liver of Pregnancy and HELLP Syndrome

Both the HELLP syndrome (Hemolysis, Elevated Liver enzyme levels, Low Platelet count) and acute fatty liver of pregnancy (AFLP) occur during pregnancy as maternal diseases resembling preeclampsia complicated by liver malfunction.[294] The HELLP syndrome is more common and usually has a reasonably good prognosis under appropriate management.[529] AFLP, although rare, has a significant mortality rate. Although these conditions are recognized by maternal diseases, one very important cause of both is an inherited gene mutation expressed in the fetus that causes a deficiency of long-chain 3-hydroxyl-CoA dehydrogenase.[255] The infants have severe liver dysfunction and also may have severe cardiac and neuromuscular abnormalities. Appropriate early dietary management may reduce both morbidity and mortality.[255]

Diabetes Mellitus

Reports on the pathology of the placenta in diabetes mellitus are numerous but often contradictory. The inconsistency may be explained, in part, by the fact that the category of diabetic pregnant women is very heterogeneous. Diabetes established before pregnancy (overt diabetes) may be of variable severity, sometimes with superimposed vascular disease. Of women who become diabetic during pregnancy, the diabetes may persist (early diabetes) or regress (gestational diabetes) after pregnancy. Some nondiabetic women giving birth to infants resembling those born to women with established diabetes become diabetic later and, in retrospect, may be considered to have had prediabetes during pregnancy.

Placentas from diabetic women vary considerably. Many placentas are essentially normal, although in more than half, the placenta is large, thick, and heavier than normal controls of the same gestational age.[6,172,232,269] The umbilical cord is often increased in diameter, and there is an increased likelihood of finding a single umbilical artery (3%–5%) as compared with the general population (1%).[150,232]

Histologically, there are no specific features allowing absolute distinction of the diabetic placenta from any other. There are, however, a constellation of abnormalities that, when taken together, are fairly characteristic. Some degree of villous immaturity and mild edema is common. Cytotrophoblastic cells are numerous and may contain mitotic figures. The trophoblastic basement membrane often shows focal, marked thickening. Villous vascularity is variable, but chorangiosis is more common than in nondiabetics.[13,150] Fibrotic avascular villi (fetal thrombotic vasculopathy) is reportedly increased,[150] but in these observations the possibility of an associated coagulopathy was not considered. Fibrinoid necrosis, the deposition of fibrinoid material between the trophoblast and basement membrane, is unduly frequent in the placentas of diabetics.[268] When there is severe maternal vascular or renal disease, the placenta may be small with accelerated villous maturation and infarcts reflecting low uteroplacental flow. Many of the variations in diabetic placentas may reflect complications introduced by unrelated disease processes such as PIH, autoimmune disorders, or coagulopathies.

Driscoll has described two types of vascular lesions in the decidual vessels of diabetics: (1) arteriolar medial hypertrophy, hyalinization, and onion skinning; and (2) acute atherosis identical to that described in preeclamptic women.[150] The latter change has been reported both in diabetics with superimposed preeclampsia and in normotensive diabetic women.[291] Others have found no specific morphologic abnormalities in the maternal vessels.[424]

So far, there has been no good correlation between the presence or extent of the pathologic changes in the placenta and the well-documented increase in congenital malformations, neonatal morbidity, or macrosomia in the babies of diabetic mothers.[232,247,401,419]

Sickle-Cell Trait/Disease and Other Hemoglobinopathies

The placenta is a very sensitive detector of sickle cells.[72,187] In both sickle trait and homozygous (SS) disease, the maternal erythrocytes in the intervillous space undergo sickling, and can be identified on careful placental examination (Fig. 23.68). Neither clinical problems nor placental lesions are likely in uncomplicated sickle trait,[69] although maternal pyelonephritis, refractory anemia,[461] premature rupture of membranes, prematurity,[461] and increased perinatal mortality[425] have been reported rarely. Lethal maternal complications are rare.[415] We have seen an occasional instance of extensive placental infarction and postnatal morbidity in instances of sickle cell trait complicated by other hemoglobinopathies or maternal coagulopathies.

In contrast, pregnant patients with sickle cell disease experience increased maternal and fetal morbidity and mortality. Reported maternal complications include urinary tract infections, pneumonia, painful crises, and worsening anemia. Sickle cell disease is associated with a high rate of spontaneous abortion, stillbirth, premature delivery, and fetal growth retardation.[24,100,164,298,358,430] Meticulous obstetric care and close hematologic surveillance have resulted in a significant reduction in maternal and fetal mortality. Prophylactic transfusion reduces the frequency of painful maternal crises but does not appear to affect fetal outcome.[298]

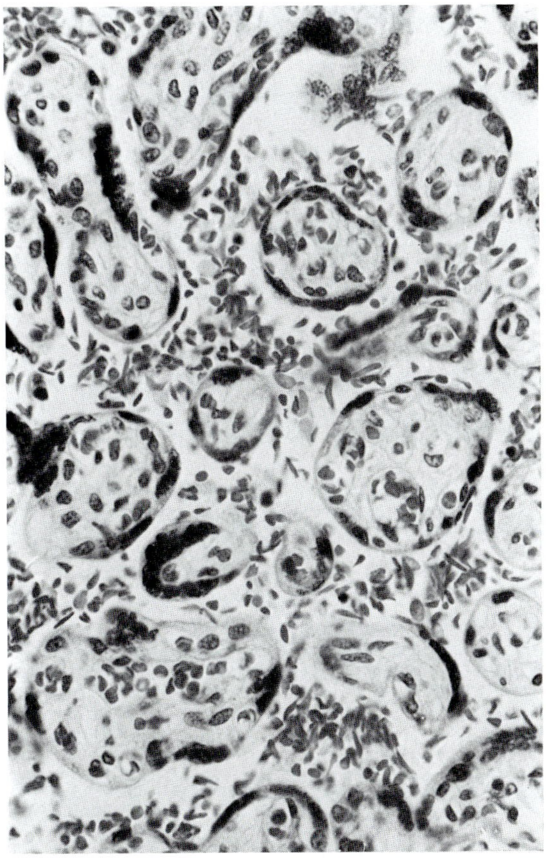

Fig. 23.68. Placenta from a patient with sickle-cell trait. Maternal erythrocytes in the intervillous space show marked sickling.

Small placentas with infarction may occur in SS disease and in combination with other hemoglobinopathies such as sickle-thalassemia and hemoglobin S-C disease.[298,430]

Maternofetal Disease

Maternofetal Rhesus (Rh) Incompatibility

Etiology

Maternofetal rhesus incompatibility occurs when maternal antibodies directed against Rh (D) antigens cross the placenta and destroy fetal red blood cells, resulting in severe fetal anemia and fetoplacental hydrops. This disease is no longer common, but before the advent of standard Rho-gam prophylaxis in the 1960s, maternofetal Rh incompatibility was a significant cause of fetal compromise. The placental changes in this condition are considered part of generalized fluid accumulation in the fetus (fetoplacental hydrops–hydrops fetalis). Anemia, decreased plasma oncotic pressure, and cardiac failure together are the pathophysiologic factors involved in the development of fetoplacental hydrops.

Pathology

Classically, the placenta is large, bulky, edematous, and strikingly pale (Fig. 23.69), although a proportion may be grossly normal.[599] Placental color is a reflection of fetal hemoglobin content. Placental pallor is associated with conditions of fetal blood loss or anemia. Intervillous thrombi are present in almost 50% of placentas and are often multiple. Septal cysts are more common in edematous placentas and are, therefore, frequently found in cases of maternofetal Rh incompatibility.

Histologically, the villi typically exhibit a combination of nonspecific but characteristic changes. There is a generalized delay in villous maturation, with clumps of markedly immature villi scattered throughout the placenta (Fig. 23.70). Mitotically active cytotrophoblastic cells are conspicuous, and the trophoblastic basement membrane is thickened (Fig. 23.71). The villous stroma is edematous and abundant, containing numerous Hofbauer cells. Nucleated red blood cells and erythroblasts are present within the fetal capillaries (Fig. 23.72). This finding reflects the fetal anemia and is, therefore, characteristic of but not specific for maternofetal Rh incompatibility. There is some evidence that pla-

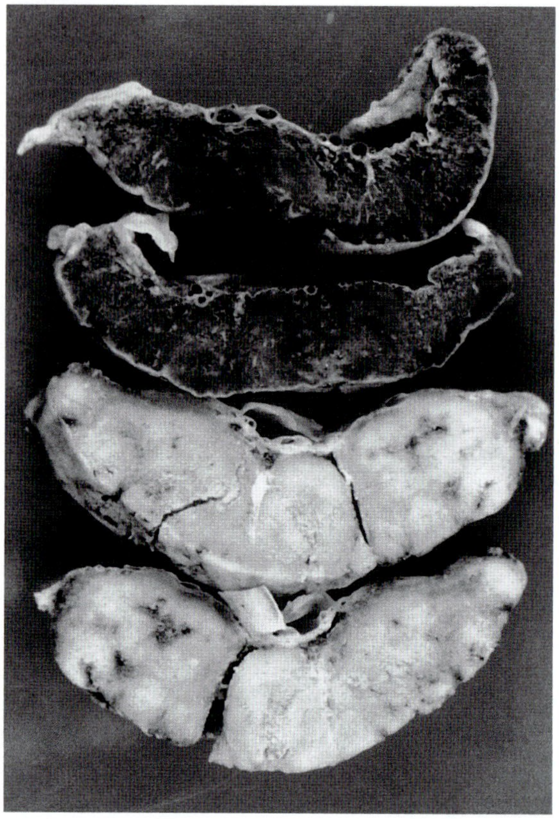

Fig. 23.69. **Maternofetal Rh incompatibility.** Both twins were anemic but with much greater severity in the twin whose placenta was large and pale (*lower slices*).

cental hyperplasia may contribute to the increased placental bulk[114,270] and reduction in the intervillous space.[20]

The constellation of gross and microscopic findings typical of maternofetal Rh incompatibility is a common end-stage picture of variable etiology. Now that Rh incompatibility is no longer common, other etiologic factors have assumed greater prominence. Other documented causes of fetoplacental hydrops include isoimmunization against other blood group antigens (ABO, Kell antigens), red cell enzyme defects, alpha-thalassemia, cardiac failure (malformations, endocardial fibroelastosis, large arteriovenous shunts, arrhythmias), hypoproteinemia (congenital nephrotic syndrome, defects in hepatic protein synthesis), congenital malformations (cystic adenomatoid malformation), congenital infections, fetal blood loss (fetomaternal hemorrhage), and other miscellaneous disorders (Gaucher's disease, sacrococcygeal teratoma).[151,161,332,334,373] It has been estimated that 1:4000 to 1:500 pregnancies are complicated by the latter disorders. When none of these immunologic or nonimmunologic causative factors is identified, the hydrops is considered to be idiopathic. Idiopathic fetoplacental hydrops has been reported to recur in successive pregnancies.

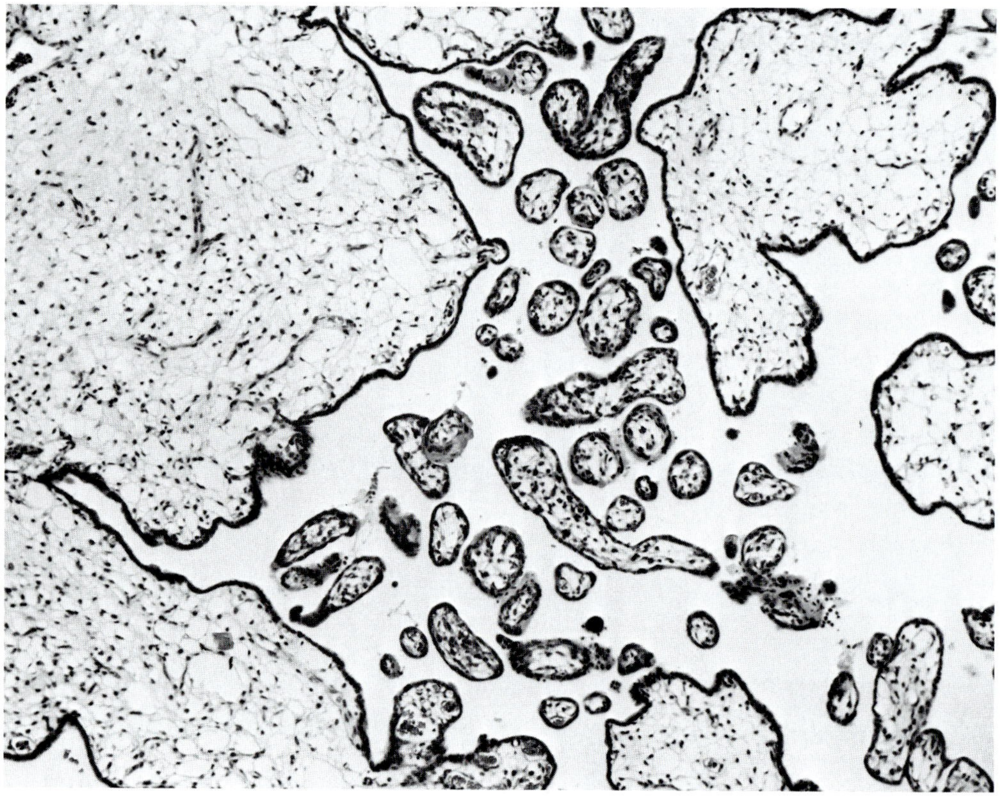

Fig. 23.70. Maternofetal Rh incompatibility, placenta at term. Pronounced variability in villous appearance is characterized by markedly immature (*large*) villi interspersed among normal, mature villi.

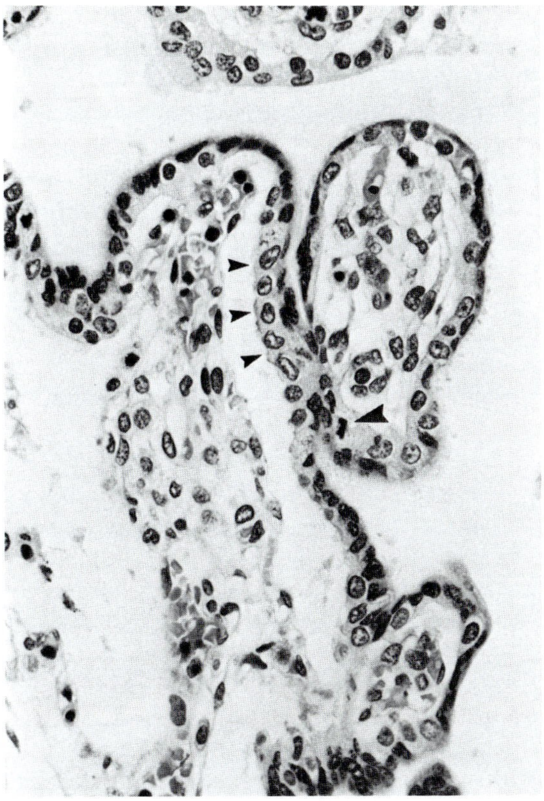

Fig. 23.71. Maternofetal Rh incompatibility, placenta at term. Immature villi with conspicuous cytotrophoblast (*small arrows*) show some mitotic activity (*large arrow*).

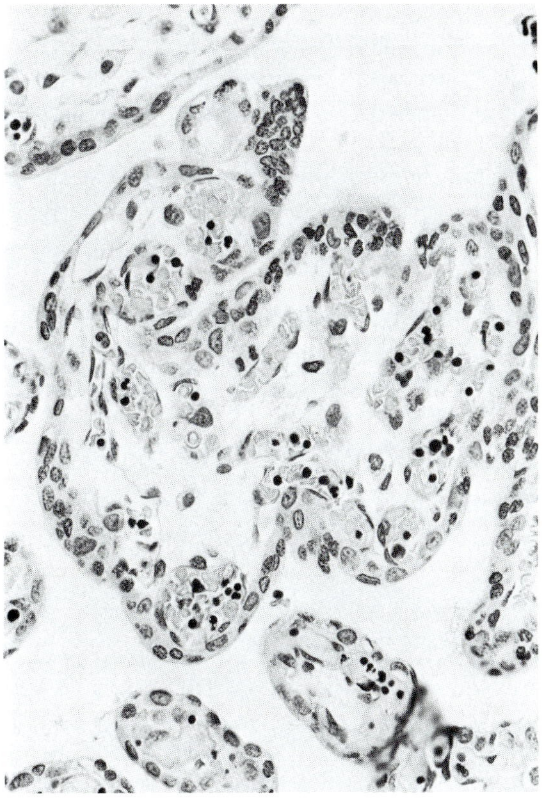

Fig. 23.72. Maternofetal Rh incompatibility, placenta at term. Fetal capillaries are filled with normoblasts and erythroblasts.

Increased Nucleated Red Blood Cells

Increased nucleated red blood cells (*nRBCs*) are a significant finding in the third-trimester placenta that should be noted. Only rare nRBCs are normal in placental sections after the first trimester. Excessive nRBCs are a consequence of fetal anemia and/or hypoxia, resulting in increased erythropoietin and release of nRBCs from the bone marrow. Accurate nRBCs counts can be established in cord blood, although identification of excessive nRBCs in placental sections may be the only means of detection in some circumstances (stillborns). The precise number of nRBCs that constitutes an "increase" in placental sections is not well defined. According to Redline, nRBCs in more than two fetal capillaries in a random 10× field indicates a mild increase; nRBCs in the majority of capillaries constitutes a marked increase.[445]

Storage Disorders

Placental abnormalities in some inherited metabolic storage diseases include vacuolar changes in trophoblastic stromal and Hofbauer cells.[267,539] Placentas from two infants with Gaucher's disease causing nonimmune fetal hydrops and stillbirth were found to have circulating Gaucher cells as well as immature erythroblasts in the fetal capillaries.[539] Refined enzymatic and other biochemical studies on snap-frozen placental tissue as well as genetic and ultrastructural studies are required to evaluate specific enzymatic defects.[272] Chorionic villus sampling for diagnosis requires careful advance coordination between clinicians and the specific laboratories that may be involved.

Fetal Membranes

The fetal membranes should be examined in their natural anatomic configuration after reconstructing the gestational sac as it exists in utero; this permits assessment of size, completeness, membrane insertion, and point of rupture. Some aspects of immediate clinical relevance (completeness and likelihood of intrauterine retention) should be addressed by the obstetrician at the time of delivery. The distance from the point of membrane rupture to the edge of the placental disk reflects the site of uterine implantation; the lower the implantation, the closer the membrane rupture site to the disk. A configuration indicative of low implantation should prompt consideration of associated conditions such as marginal hematoma or placenta accreta.

Squamous Metaplasia

Foci of *squamous metaplasia* are common on the amnionic surface of the fetal membranes and umbilical cord. Grossly, these foci are slightly elevated, sometimes targetoid, pearly-white macules that tend to be most numerous at the site of cord insertion (Fig. 23.73). Although they are generally very small, measuring no more than a few millimeters in diameter, rarely they may form larger plaques. Histologically, foci of squamous epithelium, with or without keratinization, have a sharp transition with the surrounding amnionic epithelium (Fig. 23.74). Squamous metaplasia has no clinical significance, but it is important to distinguish from amnion nodosum, which it superficially resembles.

Amnion Nodosum

Amnion nodosum is a rare condition in which the amnionic surface is studded with small (1–5 mm), irregular, yellowish elevated nodules (Fig. 23.75). These nodules are generally concentrated on the chorionic plate, particularly around the insertion of the umbilical cord, although they may occur anywhere on the amnionic surface. The nodules are composed of amorphous, eosinophilic material containing cells and hair fragments (Figs. 23.76 and 23.77). The amnionic epithelium may be totally or partially preserved or absent beneath the nodules, and a layer of amnionic epithelium is commonly present over their surfaces.

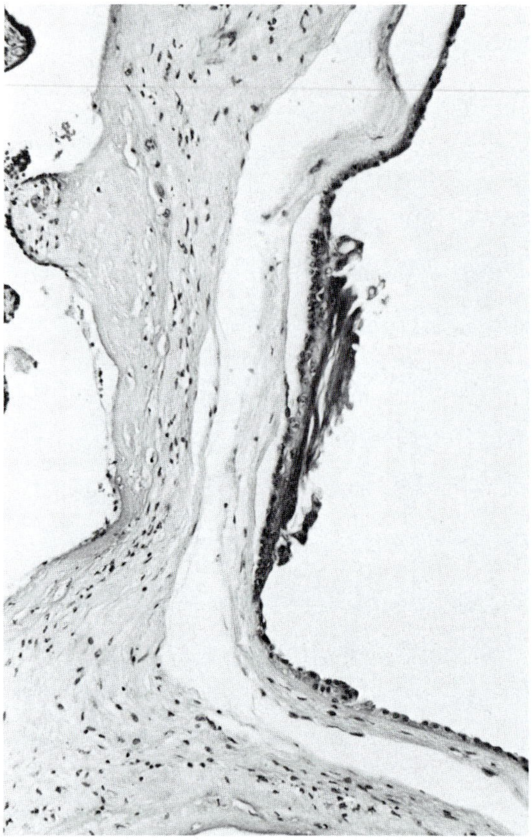

Fig. 23.74. Squamous metaplasia of amnion. Small focus of squamous metaplasia show keratinization.

Amnion nodosum is associated with oligohydramnios. The particulate debris and cellular elements from the fetal epidermis, oral cavity, urinary and gastrointestinal tracts, and the amnion itself are abnormally concentrated when amnionic fluid is

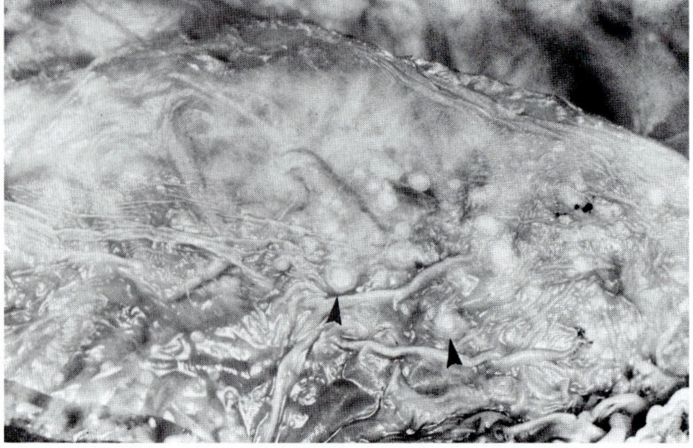

Fig. 23.73. Squamous metaplasia of amnion. Elevated white macules of squamous metaplasia (*arrows*).

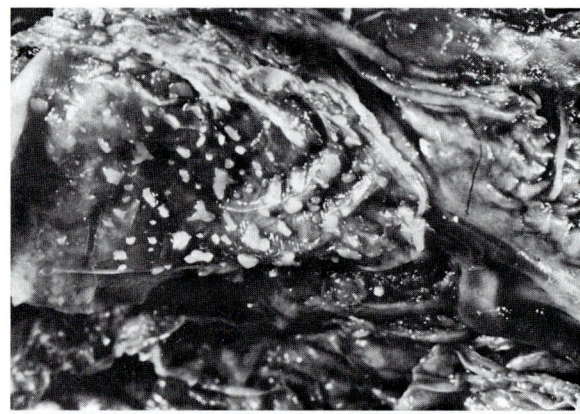

Fig. 23.75. Amnion nodosum. Elevated, irregular nodules on the fetal surface of the placenta.

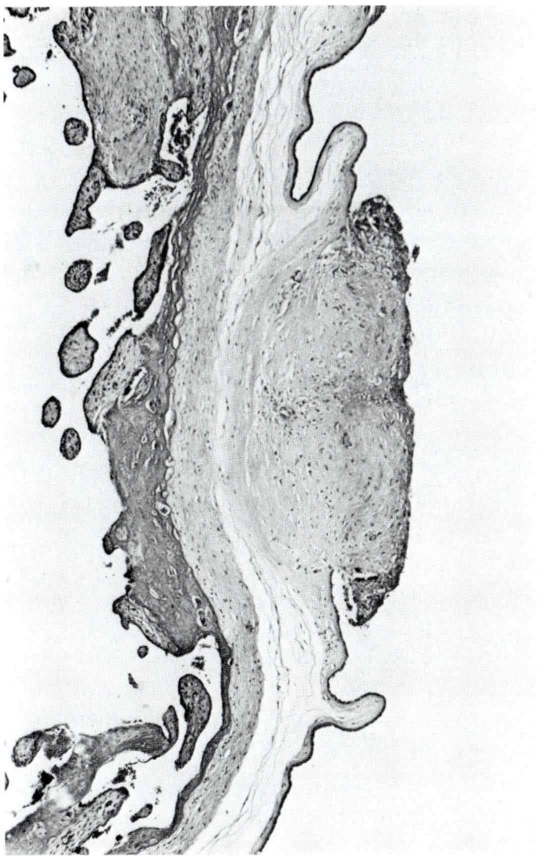

Fig. 23.76. Amnion nodosum. Nodular deposit on the amnionic surface of the placenta.

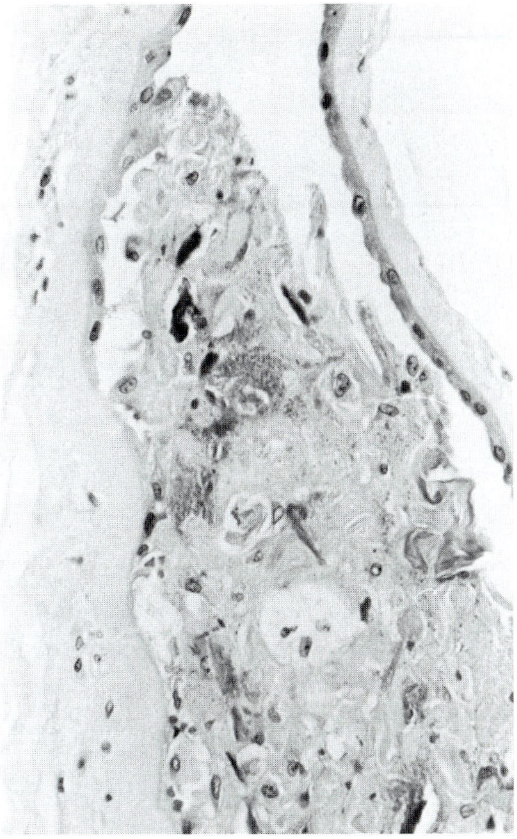

Fig. 23.77. Amnion nodosum. Nodular deposits are composed of degenerating cell fragments and hair embedded in amorphous granular material. Amnionic epithelium is preserved under a portion of this nodule.

scant and are deposited on the amnionic surface.[62] The cause of the oligohydramnios varies. In many cases, a fetal urinary tract abnormality (renal agenesis or urinary tract obstruction) is responsible for diminished fetal urine, resulting in decreased amnionic fluid. Oligohydramnios may occur in association with IUGR or the donor twin in the twin–twin transfusion syndrome. Long-standing amniorrhea is less likely to result in amnion nodosum than conditions resulting in decreased amnionic fluid production, presumably because in the former the cellular and particulate debris are lost along with the amnionic fluid. Amnion nodosum is a reliable indicator of oligohydramnios that should prompt an investigation for fetal abnormalities known to accompany it, including urinary tract anomalies and pulmonary hypoplasia.

Amnionic Bands

Amnionic bands, strings, and adhesions have been associated with a wide variety of fetal deformities. Amnionic fragmentation and shredding with separation of amnion and chorion and exposure of mesoblastic tissue results in the formation of thin fibrous strands that encircle fetal limbs, digits, neck, and umbilical cord causing characteristic constriction, amputation, and syndactyly (Fig. 23.78). Malformations are thought to result when a band interferes with the normal sequence of embryonic development. Some babies with characteristic amnionic band defects have additional structural anomalies, usually severe, including major limb deficiencies, body wall defects, open cranial defects, short umbilical cord and club feet, or internal defects in a number of organ systems.[59,230,235,236,317,328,354,507,553,583] The wide spectrum of anomalies in this condition has been variously referred to as the amnionic band syndrome, amniotic band disruption complex, early amnion rupture spectrum, limb–body–wall complex, and amnion adhesion malformation syndrome.

Gross identification of the bands and strings may be facilitated by submersion of the placenta in water. Microscopically, the bands usually consist of fi-

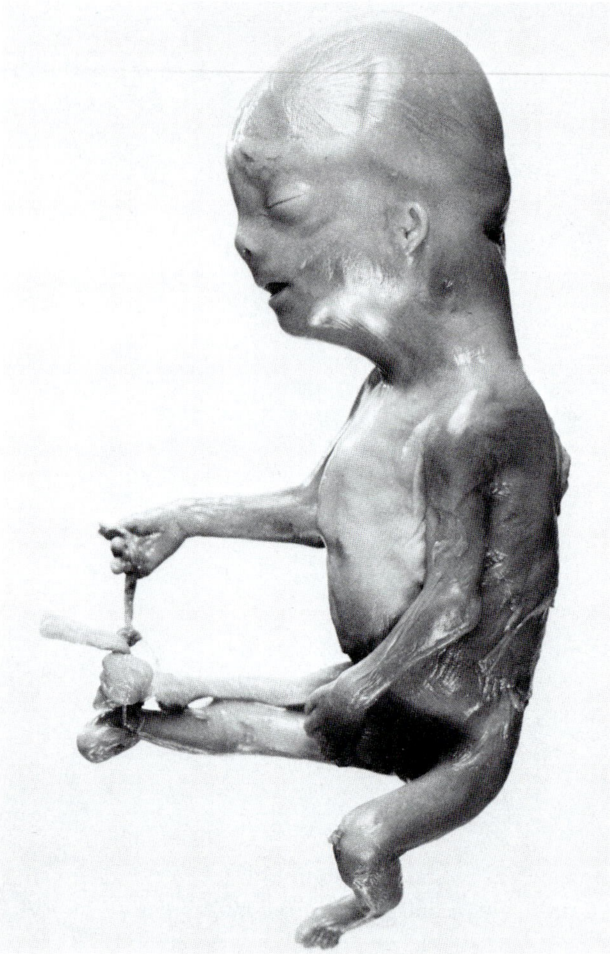

Fig. 23.78. Amnionic bands. Thin fibrous bands encircled and deformed the leg and digits of this fetus.

brous tissue, but occasionally amnionic epithelium is recognizable. Amnion is absent from the placental surface and the chorion is fibrotic. In cases associated with body wall or open cranial defects, amnion may be continuous with the fetal skin at the site of the defect. Broad adhesions may occur between the placenta and fetus.

Multiple theories have been proposed to explain the abnormalities in this syndrome. Torpin strongly espoused the concept that amnionic bands cause the structural defects.[579] The widely variable nature of the defects has been attributed to the timing of amnionic rupture; early rupture is thought to result in fetal compression, tethering, or swallowing of bands resulting in severe multisystem defects,[581] whereas constriction and amputation defects of limbs and digits have been attributed to amnionic rupture later in pregnancy.[238] Kalousek maintained that the extent of amnionic bands is as important as the developmental stage at which they occur in the determination of the pattern of fetal involvement.[280] The etiology of amnionic rupture is unknown; amnionic bands have been noted rarely after trauma, amniocentesis, and in women with connective tissue disorders.[30,317,361,458,616] Others have postulated that the amnionic bands are secondary and that the more severe fetal abnormalities are the result of vascular disruption or a primary embryologic defect.[35,368,583]

The recognition and correct diagnosis of amnion rupture and its consequences are important in counseling parents because the risk of recurrence is negligible. Unless accompanied by typical constriction/amputation lesions, major craniofacial or body wall defects may be difficult to diagnose. An important clue is the variety and asymmetry of the fetal defects, which are unlike the pattern of any heritable syndrome. No two cases are alike.

Meconium Stain

Fetal passage of meconium can often be suspected on gross examination by green or brown membrane staining. The gross appearance correlates roughly with the chronicity of meconium passage. Meconium passed shortly before delivery may be recognizable as such, or the membranes may be blue-green and slimy. With longer exposure the membranes become dark and edematous, eventually dull, muddy brown.

Microscopically, free meconium consists of amorphous green-brown material and anucleate squames. The amnionic epithelium exposed to meconium shows reactive changes, including heaping, stratification, and eventually nuclear pyknosis and necrosis. There may be marked edema of the spongy layer. With time, meconium is engulfed by macrophages in the amnion, chorion, and decidua (Fig. 23.79). The progression of meconium-induced changes in the membranes has been studied in vitro, but how closely these observations approximate events in vivo is unknown.[356] A rare finding in chronic meconium exposure is pigment-related necrosis of umbilical vascular smooth muscle cells.[14]

Meconium must be distinguished from hemosiderin, generally a larger, more refractile, yellowish crystalline granule. Iron stain is helpful when an ambiguous pigment is encountered. Membrane hemosiderin is believed to reflect remote bleeding episodes, chronic abruption, or hemolytic disease, and has been associated with preterm birth. Lipochrome and nonhemosiderin, nonmeconium pigments of unknown composition have been identified in a variety of diverse clinical situations. It has been hypothesized that these pigments may represent metabolites of remotely passed meconium.

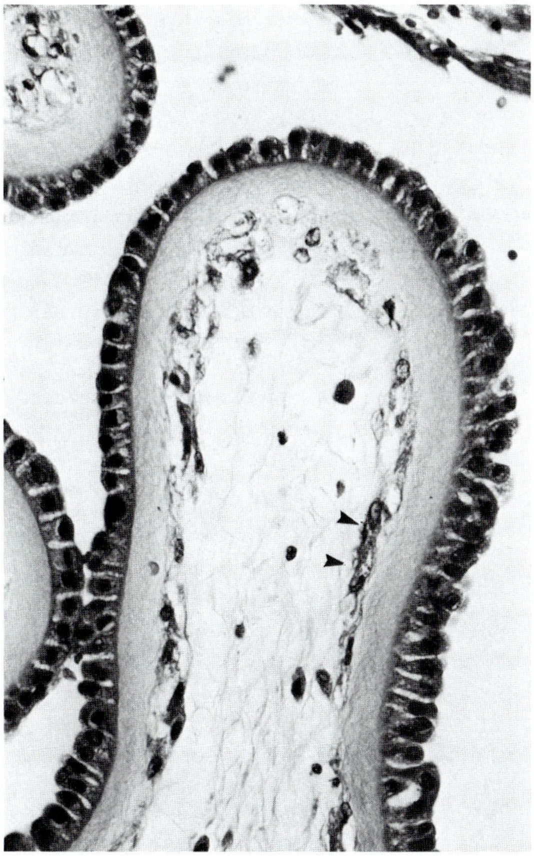

Fig. 23.79. Meconium stain. Accumulation of granular meconium pigment in the amnionic macrophages (*arrows*).

Many questions concerning the cause, effect, clinical significance, and pathologic expression of in utero meconium passage are, as yet, unresolved. In the majority of infants, meconium passage is a reflection of physiologic maturity, although in some, it appears to be associated with adverse stimuli. Meconium passage has been significantly associated with parameters of fetal distress including low Apgar scores, umbilical artery pH of 7.0 or less, respiratory distress, seizures in the first 24 hours, and need for delivery room resuscitation.[400,439,574,608] What is unclear is whether meconium passage is the cause or the result of fetal distress.

The extent to which meconium may produce injury or inflammation is also unclear, although direct meconium-induced injury to umbilical cord vessels[14] and amnionic epithelium has been described. Meconium has also been demonstrated to induce vasoconstriction, a potential cause of ischemia.[17,377,531] There is some evidence that meconium may interfer with surfactant function and, in high enough concentrations, have a direct toxic effect on type II pneumocytes, contributing to the meconium aspiration syndrome.[85,103] Meconium has also been shown to inhibit neutrophil function in vitro, perhaps relating to its association with chorioamnionitis.[102] Pathologic findings predict neither the causes nor the consequences of in utero meconium passage.

Gastroschisis

Gastroschisis is associated with an alteration in the amnionic epithelial cells characterized by extensive fine, uniform vacuolization[29] (Fig. 23.80). Ultrastructural studies confirm that the vacuoles contain lipid, but the origin of the lipid is obscure.[216] These amnionic changes have not been noted in cases of omphalocele.

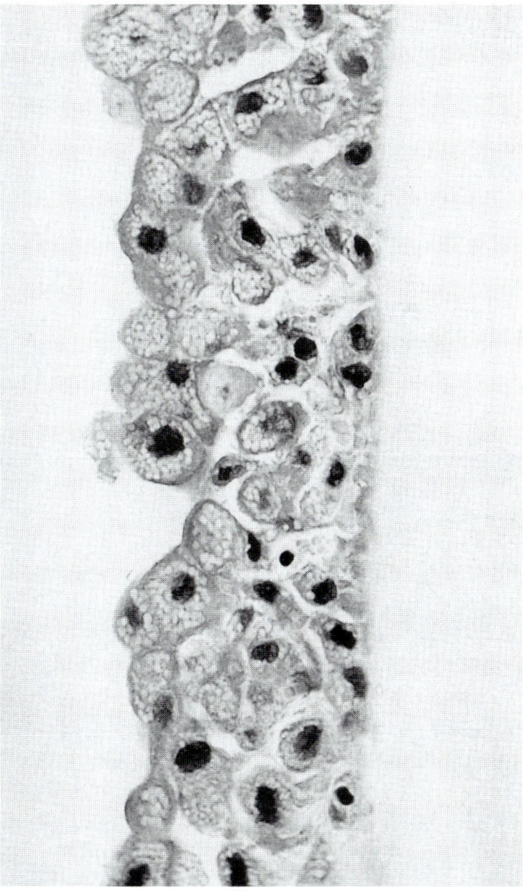

Fig. 23.80. Amnion, gastroschisis. The amnionic epithelium in this case of gastroschisis shows the typical fine vacuolation. The epithelial stratification is a result of meconium passage.

Umbilical Cord

The umbilical cord is an important lifeline between the fetus and placenta. It should be examined carefully along its entire length because clinically significant lesions are often focal.

Vestigial Remnants

The normal umbilical cord contains two arteries and one vein surrounded by Wharton's jelly, a loosely structured myxomatous tissue covered by a layer of amnion. No other vessels, specifically vasa vasorum, or lymphatics are found in the cord. Occasionally, vestigial remnants dating back to fusion of the yolk sac and body stalk may be apparent on microscopic examination. Traces of the omphalomesenteric duct that connects the fetal ileum and the yolk sac in the early embryo are infrequent. These remnants are usually discontinuous, located peripherally, and may be lined by either nondescript flat or columnar epithelium resembling intestinal epithelium (Fig. 23.81). Rarely, omphalomesenteric remnants show remarkable differentiation: gastric, small intestinal, or pancreatic. The remainder of the original yolk sac, a tiny, yellow-white nodule between the amnion and chorion, consists of amorphous, basophilic material histologically.

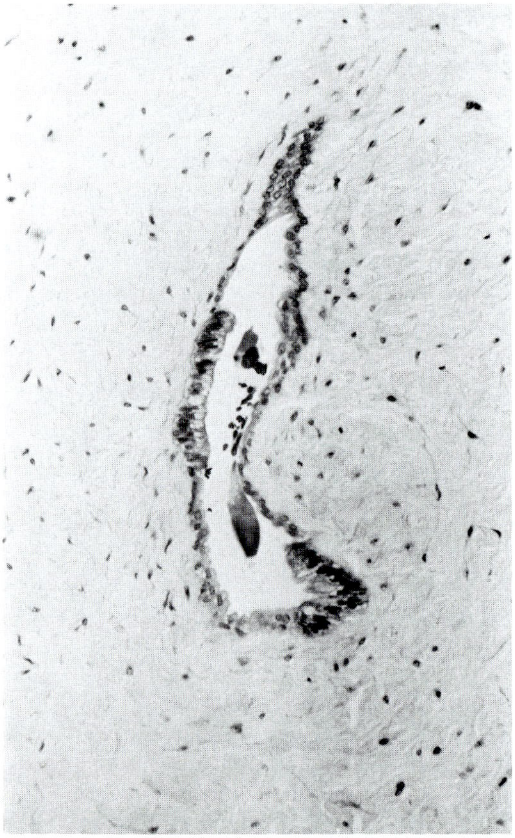

Fig. 23.81. Omphalomesenteric duct remnant, umbilical cord. This omphalomesenteric duct remnant is lined by columnar, mucin-containing epithelium.

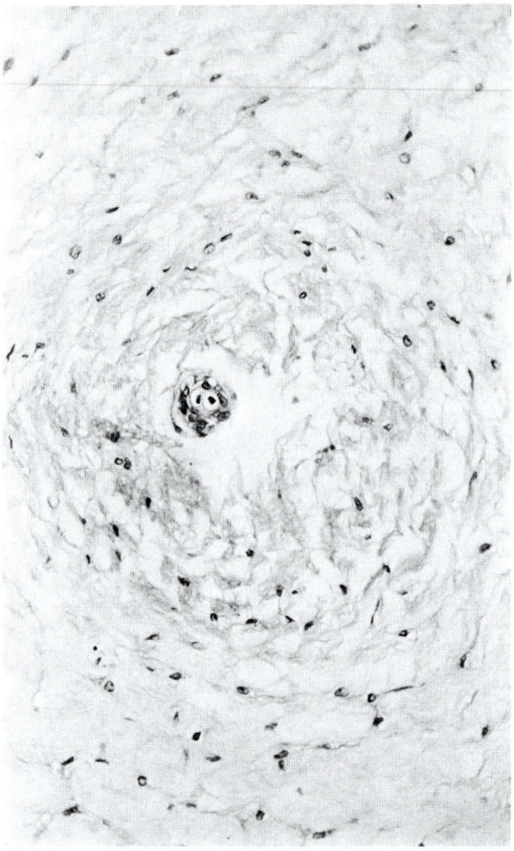

Fig. 23.82. Allantoic duct remnant, umbilical cord. Allantoic duct remnant is lined by transitional type cuboidal cells.

Remnants of the allantoic duct, the connection between the bladder via the urachus and rudimentary allantois, are more frequent. These are lined by flat or cuboidal cells, often reminiscent of transitional epithelium (Fig. 23.82), with or without a lumen. Allantoic duct remnants are usually located between the umbilical arteries.

Insertion

The site of cord insertion is variable, usually central or eccentric, but occasionally (about 7%), it is marginal (Battledore) or into the fetal membranes (*velamentous*). The significance of a marginal insertion is debated. Marginal insertion has been reported to occur with increased frequency in abortions, with malformed fetuses, and in association with neonatal asphyxia and premature labor, although Fox could not confirm any of the reported associations.[176]

Velamentous insertion is a common anomaly, occurring in about 1% of placentas. It is increased in multiple pregnancies, extrachorial placentas, and in cords with a single umbilical artery. Velamentous insertion is associated with an increased incidence of fetal anomalies (usually of deformation type), low birth weight, and intrapartum complications related to compression or trauma of membranous vessels.[157,364,467] Having lost their protective covering of Wharton's jelly and unsupported by underlying villous tissue, these vessels are vulnerable to injury or compression, especially when they traverse the cervical os (vasa previa). Thrombosis of membranous vessels may be associated with fetal thromboembolic events.[444] Membranous vessels are not limited to velamentously inserted cords but may arise aberrantly from marginally or even centrally inserted cords, and they regularly supply succenturiate lobes. The distance between cord insertion and the disk margin (the length of membranous vessels) provides one measure of the degree of their vulnerability. As a site of potentially clinically significant alterations, membranous vessels should be inspected carefully grossly and included in sections submitted for microscopic examination.

The mode of cord insertion is less variable than the site of insertion. Rarely, the cord may lose Wharton's jelly before insertion onto the placental surface (*furcate insertion*), leaving unsupported vessels subject to trauma and thrombosis. Alternatively, the cord may insert velamentously but retain Wharton's jelly until its vessels branch on the placental surface (*interposito velamentosa*).

Cord Length and Diameter

Umbilical cord length is an important parameter most accurately documented in the delivery room before cord segments are removed for other studies. When the cord is received in several segments, each should be measured, and the cord should be reconstructed as accurately as possible. Standards for cord length relative to gestational age have been established and should be considered in all cases.[357] The mean length at term is 55–60 cm. Extremes of cord length have been correlated with potentially adverse outcomes. Excessively long cords (≥80 cm) have been associated with encirclement around body parts, knots, torsion, prolapse, and partial or complete vascular occlusion. Abnormally short cords (≤40 cm) may predispose to intrauterine distress, neonatal asphyxia, cord rupture and hemorrhage, placental abruption, and uterine inversion.[43] Some consideration of relative as well as absolute cord length is appropriate. A long cord with extensive looping many function as a short cord; this obviously requires clinical assessment. Acordia, absence of the umbilical cord, is an anomaly usually identified in abortions or stillbirths in which the fetal umbilical region, often malformed, merges with the placenta.

Cord length reflects factors that influence its growth, mainly tensile forces related to fetal activity and intrauterine conditions affecting fetal movement.[353,355,362] Conditions restricting fetal mobility, such as amnionic bands and oligohydramnios, are often associated with short umbilical cords. Whether cord length as an indirect indicator of fetal activity can be correlated ultimately with antenatal neurologic development deserves additional study.[383]

Umbilical cord diameter is affected by the number of vessels and the amount of Wharton's jelly and its fluid content. A thin cord with decreased or absent Wharton's jelly is often a sign of fetal growth retardation. Cord edema, focal or diffuse, occurs inconsistently in a variety of clinical situations, especially diabetes, but often the cause is unknown. A cross-sectional area of 1.3 cm^2 has been arbitrarily defined as the threshold of significant cord edema.[110]

Single Umbilical Artery

Single umbilical artery (*SUA*) (Fig. 23.83) is a common and important abnormality associated with low birth weight and major congenital anomalies.[233,573] Vascularity should be assessed at least 3–5 cm from the placental insertion site because anastomosis of the umbilical arteries close to the placenta may lead to the false impression of single umbilical artery. Fixation aids in assessment of vascularity. The reported frequency of SUA varies depending on the population studied. In prospective studies of consecutive deliveries, the frequency of SUA is consistently somewhat less than 1%,[46,83,185] but it is considerably higher (2.5%–3.0%) in neonatal autopsies and spontaneous abortions.[233] SUA is more common in whites than in blacks or Asians, in babies of diabetic mothers, in chromosomal abnormalities (especially trisomies), in twins, and in velamentously inserted cords.[46,185,233,418,538]

There is a well-documented association between SUA and fetal malformations, but no particular organ or specific abnormality characterizes this association.[46,47,83,185,186,233,306,538] Any organ system may be involved, and malformations are frequently multiple. Congenital malformations are most nu-

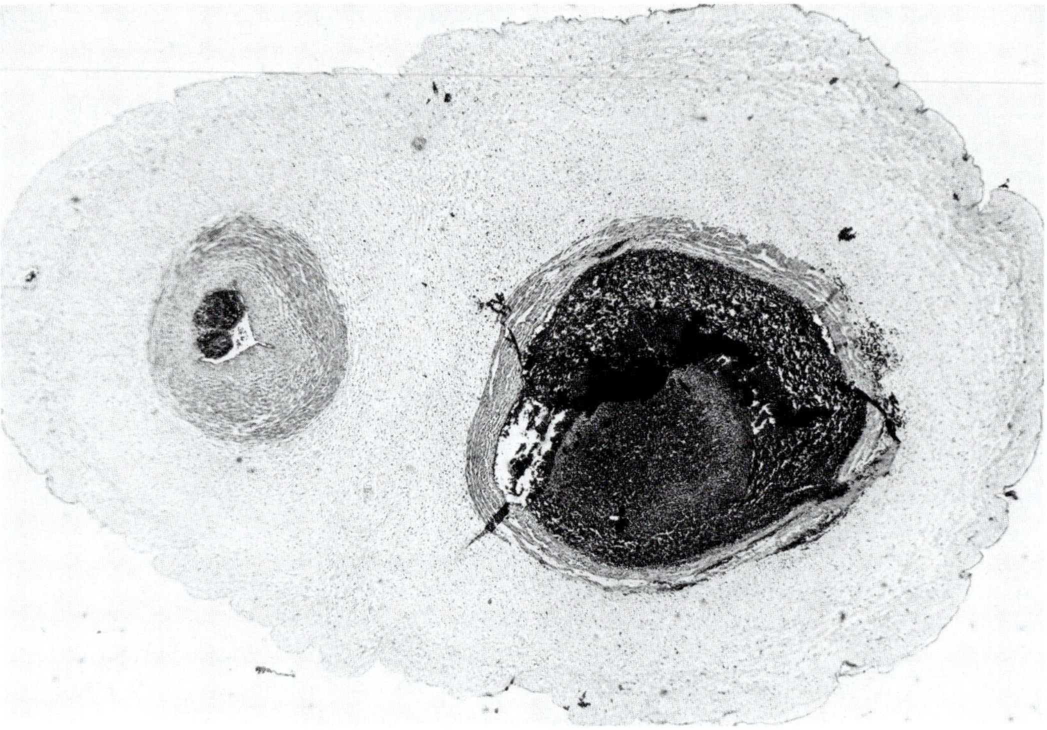

Fig. 23.83. Single umbilical artery. On *left*, umbilical cord.

merous and most severe in stillborn babies and those dying in the neonatal period.[83,84,185,186] Infants with SUA but no detectable malformations at birth who survive the neonatal period are unlikely to have a significant abnormality detected subsequently.[84,186] The perinatal mortality rate of infants with SUA is greatly increased (11%–41%), mainly by the associated major malformations, although otherwise normal infants with SUA experience an increased perinatal mortality rate as well.[83] SUA is associated with a tendency toward low birth weight even when infants with major malformations have been excluded from analysis.[83]

Whether SUA is caused primary aplasia or secondary atrophy is debatable. Histologic evidence of vascular remnants supports secondary atrophy in some cases (Figs. 23.84 and 23.85).[19] The higher incidence of SUA in early embryos as compared to fetuses provides circumstantial evidence that SUA may be an acquired defect. Whether SUA plays a role in the development of congenital malformations or is just another manifestation of them is a matter of conjecture.

Focal Lesions

Focal aberrations in the umbilical cord have important clinicopathologic associations. All cord lesions should be carefully assessed for evidence of functionally significant alterations in blood flow. Clinically significant circulatory compromise is usually accompanied by pathologic changes including thrombosis, edema, congestion, or hemorrhage.

Torsion and Stricture

The umbilical cord is normally spiraled, usually in a counterclockwise direction from the fetal end, with an average of 10 or 11 coils. Neonates with noncoiled or hypocoiled cords (below the 10th percentile) have a higher incidence of fetal distress, IUGR, meconium staining, karyotypic abnormalities, and perinatal mortality.[440,558] *Excessive torsion* may be associated with interruption of fetal blood flow and fetal death.[207] Excess torsion is more common in long cords and is most common at the fetal end of the cord where it is sometimes associated with stricture. *Strictures* are usually single, sharply defined, short segments most common at the fetal end of the cord with contraction of vessels, loss of Wharton's jelly, or fibrosis.[594] Associated venous congestion, edema, and thrombi provide evidence that the lesion is not a postmortem artifact.[225,560]

Knots

True *knots* (Fig. 23.86) occur in less than 1% of umbilical cords, often in an excessively long cord. They

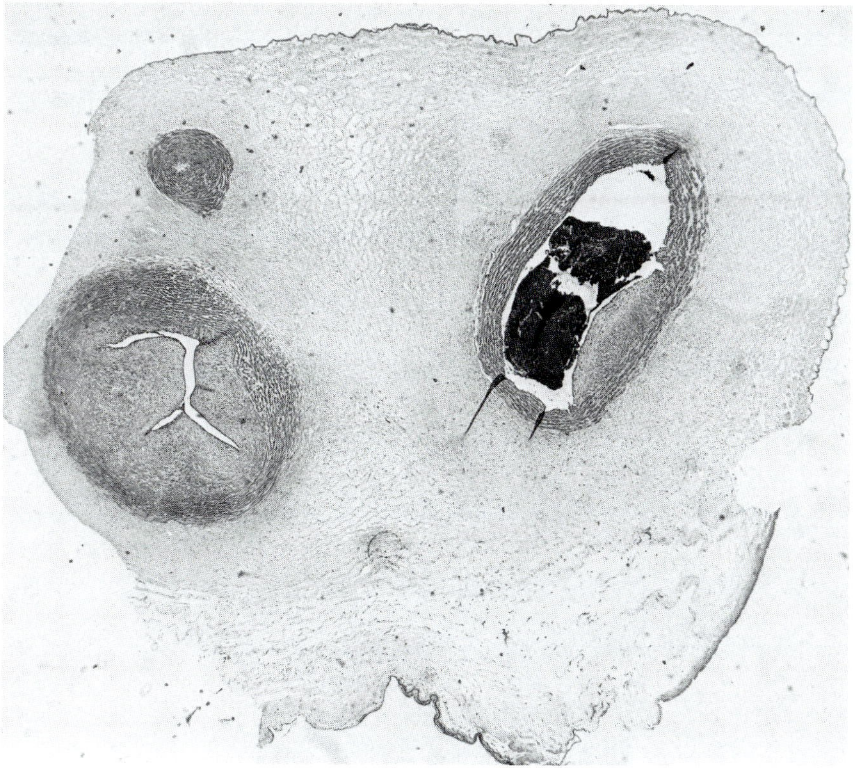

Fig. 23.84. This anomaly was found in conjunction with several congenital malformations in a fetus dying shortly after birth.

must be distinguished from false knots, which are merely focal accentuations of the vascular spiral, a varicosity, or excess Wharton's jelly. The majority of true knots are clinically insignificant, although overall they are associated with an increased perinatal mortality rate in the range of 8%–11%, presumably a result of obstruction of the fetal circulation (Fig. 23.87).[346] Either an acutely tightened or a long-standing tight knot may be responsible for intrauterine or intrapartum fetal death. Long-standing tight knots are evidenced by a definite groove and loss of Wharton's jelly at the site of the knot, changes that persist after the knot is untied. Acutely tightened knots may be associated signs of circulatory compromise including edema, congestion and vascular thrombi.

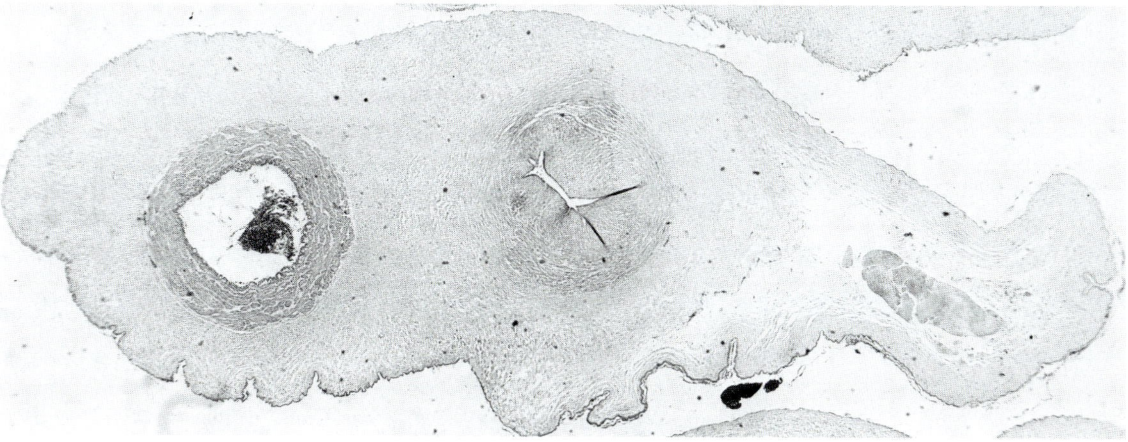

Fig. 23.85. Marked hypoplasia of one umbilical artery. Amorphous remnant of one umbilical artery (*right*).

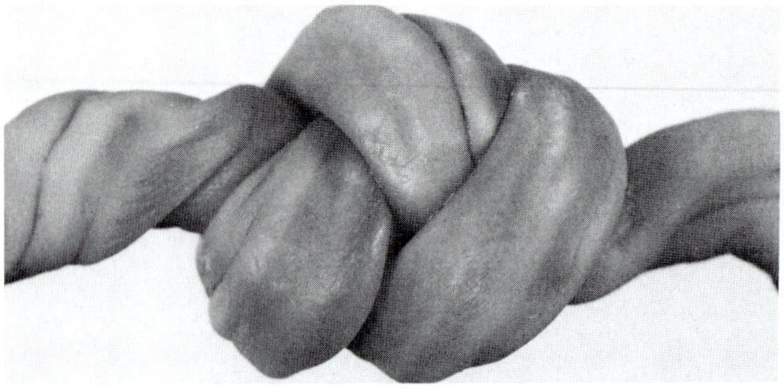

Fig. 23.86. True knot of umbilical cord. This true knot occurred in a normal liveborn infant.

Hematoma

Hematomas of the umbilical cord are a rare but clinically significant abnormality associated with a reported perinatal mortality rate of 40%–50%.[140,481,497] Most umbilical cord hematomas present as red-purple fusiform swellings, usually at the fetal end. They are generally confined to the cord but occasionally may rupture into the amnionic cavity. In some cases, the hemorrhage may be demonstrated to originate from the umbilical vein and, very rarely, from an umbilical artery. In the great majority of cases, an obvious source is not apparent. The etiology is unknown, but rupture of a varix, traumatic or mechanical damage, inflammation, or structural anomalies of the vessel wall have been proposed as possible mechanisms. Fetal death may be caused by blood loss or compression of fetal vessels with circulatory compromise. Small collections of fresh blood are often the result of cord blood sampling at the time of delivery.

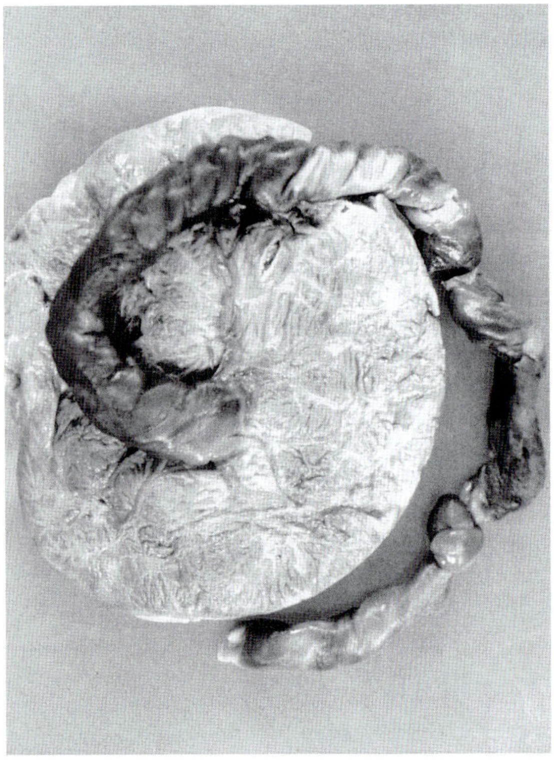

Fig. 23.87. Tight knot with congestion and edema in IUFD.

Ulceration/Absence of Wharton's Jelly

Linear *ulceration of Wharton's jelly* over the umbilical vessels has been associated with severe intraamniotic hemorrhage, profound fetal anemia, and fetal death in utero. Microscopically, the Wharton's jelly overlying the vessels is necrotic and replaced by amorphous debris. The vessels may show myonecrosis and aneurysmal dilatation (Fig. 23.88). These cord findings have been reported in conjunction with intestinal atresia.[42] Rarely, Wharton's jelly is completely absent around the arteries, an anomaly that has also been associated with fetal death in utero.[314]

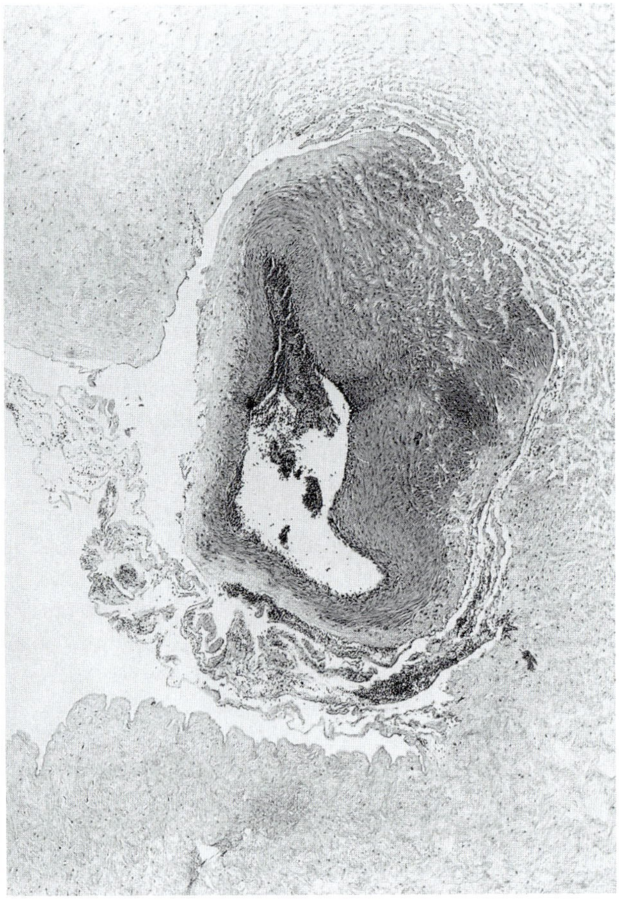

Fig. 23.88. Wharton's jelly, ulceration. Wharton's jelly is completely necrotic over the umbilical artery, which is markedly thinned and focally necrotic. This pregnancy was complicated by massive intraamnionic hemorrhage and fetal death in utero.

Common Clinical Syndromes of Pregnancy: Placental Pathologic Correlations

The clinical data provided with placentas that come to the pathologist will (or should) identify the clinical diagnosis or problem, but the difficulty faced by most pathologists is to decide what specific pathologic lesions are relevant to the clinical problem. This determination is not always easy. The terminology is often confusing, unfamiliar, or even misleading, and tissue reactions in the placenta may evolve in patterns that do not occur in other organs. Placental disease can affect both mother and fetus, but sometimes in different ways. The placental pathology report must satisfy both the obstetrician–perinatologist, whose first patient is the mother, and the pediatrician–neonatologist, who is preoccupied with the newborn. This section is intended to assist the pathologist by identifying which of the pathologic lesions described in this chapter are to be sought in placentas of infants born with some of the more common clinical syndromes or problems.

Clinical and Pathologic Chorioamnionitis

Chorioamnionitis is a *fetal* disease, identified in a *fetal* organ, the placenta. It is caused by the presence of bacteria growing in the fetal membranes and amnionic fluid. *Pathologic chorioamnionitis* is identified in the placenta by the finding of maternal neutrophils that have migrated from the decidual vessels toward the chorioamnionic interface in the membranes or from maternal blood in the intervillous space into the chorionic plate. It is this microscopically visible inflammatory response in the placenta that makes it possible to conclude that the fetus has been exposed to a potentially serious bacterial infection. Fetal neutrophils may invade the vessel wall of umbilical vessels in the cord or fetal vessels in the chorionic plate. The bacteria usually have little or no toxicity for the mother even when they injure or kill the fetus.

Standardized criteria for the *clinical diagnosis of chorioamnionitis* are based on signs and symptoms identified in the examination of the *mother*. These signs include maternal temperature elevation (at least 100.4°F), with or without additional features such as maternal tachycardia, fetal tachycardia, uterine tenderness, foul-smelling amnionic fluid, and maternal leukocytosis (more than 15,000 WBC/mm^3). Maternal fever and other symptoms that may occur when the *fetus* has chorioamnionitis are sometimes the result of an associated *maternal endometritis*, but all these problems very often have another cause; the mother has an infection somewhere and is responding to it, and the fetus is not affected.

The diagnosis of *clinical chorioamnionitis* is not supported by the demonstration of inflammatory changes of *pathologic chorioamnionitis* in the placenta in about 40% of cases. On the other hand, the mother is commonly asymptomatic in the presence of significant amnionic fluid infection. Finally, fetal illness does not occur in all cases in which pathologic chorioamnionitis is found in the placenta. Fetal illness depends on the pathogenicity of the organism and on the resistance of the fetus, which increases steadily as the fetus matures. Passive transfer of maternal antibodies may protect the fetus, as demonstrated best in most instances of group B streptococcal colonization of the maternal vagina. In the absence of maternal antibodies, chorioamnionitis caused by intraamnionic growth of this organism will often either kill or cause serious injury.

The injurious effects to the fetus associated with the finding of pathologic chorioamnionitis are caused by the products or effects of bacterial growth (toxins and cytokines) in the amnionic fluid, which is inhaled, swallowed, and absorbed by the fetus. Serious injury and stillbirth can occur in the absence of any symptoms in the mother, and, unfortunately, all too often they do just that.

Preterm Labor and Prematurity

Labor, whether at term or preterm, is initiated by prostaglandin release, which in turn is mediated by cytokines produced by either the decidua, amnion, or chorion.[98] The most common cause of preterm labor is bacterial infection involving the membranes, amnionic fluid, and adjacent decidua, identified pathologically as chorioamnionitis. The direct effect on the fetus, if any, depends on bacterial toxins and cytokines (especially IL-1, IL-6, and TNF-α) produced in the decidua and placenta in response to toxins or other products of bacterial growth.[443] The second most common cause of premature birth are decidual vasculopathies and their sequelae, including acute atherosis, decidual necrosis, retroplacental clots (abruption), and infarcts,[118] which may also cause prostaglandin release. The same cytokines can initiate labor resulting in preterm birth and probably also injure the fetus as well. The complications of preterm birth include hyaline membrane disease, periventricular leukomalacia, intraventricular hemorrhage, retinopathy, necrotizing enterocolitis, and death.

Intrauterine Growth Retardation (IUGR) and Infants Small for Gestational Age (SGA)

A newborn whose weight is below the tenth percentile may be considered small for gestational age. The expression IUGR indicates a reduction in the *rate of growth* as determined by two or more measurements of weight plotted on a normal growth curve. There are dozens of potential causes, including abnormal karyotypes, metabolic disorders, various congenital anomalies, and intrauterine infections. The more common relevant identifiable *placental lesions* include decidual vasculopathy, multiple infarcts, chronic retroplacental hematomas, large chorangiomas, fetal thrombotic vasculopathy, chronic intrauterine infections of the TORCH group, chronic villitis of unknown etiology, and multiple gestations.[486] A specific chromosomal anomaly involving the placenta but not the fetus called *confined placental mosaicism* merits greater attention, especially when no other explanation seems apparent.

Thrombophilia: Maternal, Paternal, and Fetal Coagulopathies

Pregnancy itself is a thrombophilic state: the maternal coagulation system balance is shifted toward clotting in normal pregnancy. The impact of other coagulopathies on both the pregnant mother and the fetus raises the risk for thromboembolic disease. Homozygosity for coagulation gene mutations and the occurrence of multiple different coagulopathies in the same patient increase both the frequency and severity of both maternal and fetal injury. Some acquired maternal coagulopathies, such as anticardiolipin antibodies, have been associated with thrombi in the fetal circulation. In the evaluation of potential gene mutations affecting the newborn, it is important to remember that both parents contribute to the fetal coagulation genome. Important correlations in clinical history include prior thromboembolic disease in either parent, repeated spontaneous abortions, intrauterine fetal death, prematurity, abruptions, and visceral thrombi in any organ.

The main thrombophilias are *deficiencies* of antithrombin III and proteins C and S; *gene mutations* for factor V Leiden, the prothrombin 20210 variant, and methylene tetrahydrofolate reductase; and *elevations* of homocysteine, factor VIII, and fibrinogen.[133,206,221,307,336,586] Placental lesions relevant to thrombophilias include fetal thrombotic vasculopathy, fetal vessel and umbilical cord thrombosis,[28,303] massive perivillous fibrin deposits, spiral artery thromboses, placental infarcts (especially multiple or large infarcts),[288,301,444] and retroplacental hematoma (abruption).[133,221,288,307] Relevant lesions that may occur in the fetus and newborn include intrauterine fetal death,[303,326] neonatal death with or without extensive or focal intravascular thrombi,[105,303,508,523] intrauterine growth retardation,[206,221,307] cerebral infarcts[296,303,324] and cerebral palsy,[131,432,572] recurrent spontaneous abortion,[142] renal vein thrombosis,[303] myocardial infarcts,[88,610] and some instances of limb reduction defect.[246] Because the occurrence together of multiple inherited or acquired coagulopathies appears to have the most serious impact and the location of a clot is a matter of chance, it should be no surprise that severe sublethal problems such as cerebral palsy are uncommon in the same family or that most of affected siblings become identified as "abortions" or "miscarriages."

Cerebral Palsy

Significant placental lesions associated with *cerebral palsy* as an isolated problem include chorioamnionitis[222,455] and fetal thrombotic vasculopathy.[302,572] Prematurity is a significant factor in periventricular leukomalacia. Significant placental lesions in very low birth weight infants studied by Redline et al. were severe villous edema and recent nonocclusive thrombi in fetal vessels of the chorionic plate. Autopsy studies on neonates and stillborns with short death-to-delivery intervals have shown that some central nervous system lesions are chronic and well-established prenatal events.[86,190,303,420,520] An important underlying factor in many cases has been the occurrence of parental coagulopathies. A clinical study of 46 infants of normal birth weight with spastic quadriplegic cerebral palsy found tight nuchal cord as the only significant potentially asphyxiating condition noted in the clinical history. Intrapartum difficulties during delivery occurred with equal frequency in cases and controls; unfortunately, the placentas were not evaluated.[406] Epidemiologic studies of large groups of infants with cerebral palsy have confirmed the etiologic importance of infection,[222] as well as cytokines and coagulation factors.[405] Sudden acute intrapartum anoxia as may occur with abruption and cord compression also causes brain injury, but usually as a part of severe multisystem organ failure affecting especially the lungs, kidneys, liver, and gastrointestinal tract.

Fetal and Placental Hydrops

Fetal hydrops means global severe edema of head, trunk, and extremities and serous effusions in all serous cavities. It is the end result of many fetal diseases that cause anemia, hypoproteinemia, and heart failure. Specific disease entities include hemolytic anemia caused by *Rhesus* isoimmunization; infections such as parvovirus, cytomegalic inclusion disease; congestive failure from congenital heart disease or circulatory overload, as in the recipient in the twin transfusion syndrome; and chromosomal anomalies, especially 45,XO karyotype.[331,332]

Fetal–Maternal Hemorrhage

Small amounts of fetal blood likely leak into the maternal circulation in nearly every pregnancy. Identifiable transplacental hemorrhage occurs in about 1 in 300 pregnancies and may be fatal in as many as 1 in 2000 pregnancies.[49] Bleeding severe enough to cause anemia is associated with nucleated red blood cells in the fetal circulation. Massive fetomaternal hemorrhage may result from severe abdominal trauma, but most often no specific event can be identified. Intraplacental hematomas, which consistently contain a component of fetal erythrocytes, appear to represent the locus of the bleeding.[282] In cases of chronic or episodic bleeding causing severe anemia or death, the placenta is enlarged, pale, and hydropic. Fetal red cells are demonstrable in the maternal blood by the Kleihauer–Bethke technique[49] or by flow cytometry[121] and may persist for as long as 2–3 weeks.

Abortion, Miscarriage, Stillbirth

Products of conception, either spontaneously passed or curetted from the uterus, are submitted for pathologic examination to confirm the presence of an intrauterine gestation and to exclude other problems, especially trophoblastic disease. This examination requires the identification of trophoblast, either in the form of placental villi or intermediate trophoblast infiltrating the decidua or myometrium at the implantation site. The presence of decidua or gestational endometrium alone does not constitute adequate documentation of intrauterine pregnancy because this change may be associated with ectopic pregnancy or hormonal manipulation. When trophoblastic elements are not found in initial sections, the entire specimen should be examined microscopically. If trophoblast is still not identified, the clinician should be alerted to the possibility of an ectopic gestation. It should be recognized that no combination of findings in the endometrium, including villi, can exclude an ectopic pregnancy because occasionally intrauterine and tubal pregnancies occur simultaneously.[607]

Villi, when present, may be normal or show characteristic pathologic changes known to be associated with fetal death in utero. A constellation of morphologic alterations in the villi begins about 6 hours after fetal death and is fully established within 2 weeks.[179,195,250] These changes include sclerosis and obliteration of fetal stem arteries and villous capillaries, progressive villous stromal fibrosis, increased numbers of syncytial knots and cytotrophoblastic cells, and thickening of the trophoblastic basement membrane (Fig. 23.89). Vascular changes in the placenta may be useful in establishing the time of death in stillborn fetuses.[195]

Approximately one-half of all human gestations abort, of which about half are actually recognized by the mother or her physician. Of clinically recognized pregnancies, those that abort can be divided into two significantly different groups, early and late, according to age of gestation. In general, the factors associated with early abortion are fetal, primarily chromosomal abnormalities. Late spontaneous abortion is more likely to be associated with

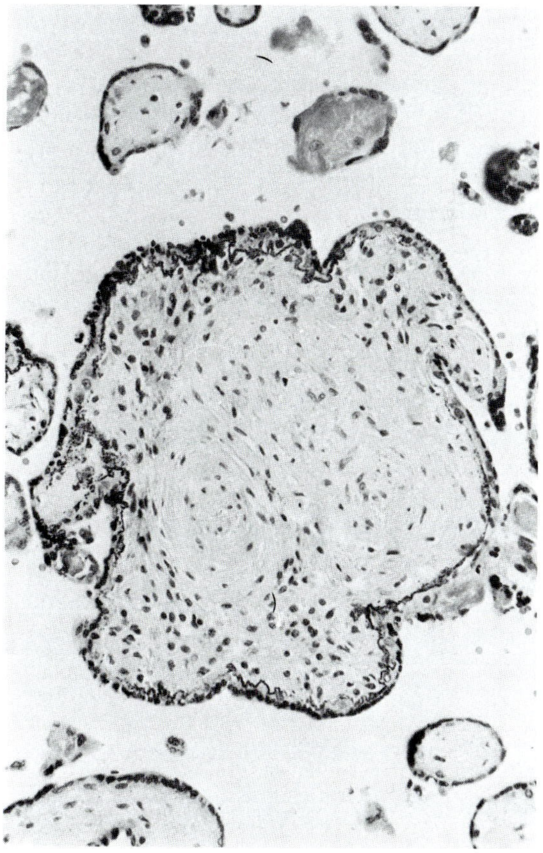

Fig. 23.89. Fetal death in utero. The villous alterations resulting from fetal death in utero include sclerosis and obliteration of the fetal vessels, stromal fibrosis, and prominence of the cytotrophoblast.

other causes, mainly maternal factors, such as infection, maternal disease, uterine anomalies, immunologic factors, nutrition, medication, and age.

Embryonic Stage (1 to 10 Menstrual Weeks)

More than half of early spontaneous abortions have demonstrable chromosomal anomalies, and most of those are eliminated in the embryonic period. Trisomies, triploidy, and monosomy X are most common (Table 23.2).[139]

Pathology

The chorionic cavity when present is frequently empty but should be examined for remnants of cord or embryo. The amnionic sac when present is often abnormally large and prematurely fused to the chorion (this occurs normally at 9 weeks developmental age). An embryo is often absent but when present frequently exhibits generalized abnormal development (growth disorganization). Morphologic recognition of embryonic growth disorganization points to a high probability of a chromosomal anomaly (Fig. 23.90).[276,277] Localized developmental defects (fusion defects in the face, ocular anomalies, limb bud deformities, neural tube defects, and cervical edema) are also commonly genetically determined. Many localized defects, however, have several causes and the risk of recurrence is related to the particular pathogenetic mechanisms.[276,277,278] Specific morphologic defects are often difficult to identify in the early embryo; they are more easily evaluated in the previable fetus (Figs. 23.91 and 23.92). The finding of a well-developed, normal embryo is important; this should suggest a maternal causative factor, some of which are treatable, although 20%–25% of morphologically normal embryos are karyotypically abnormal (usually triploid). Accurate assessment of embryonic development requires familiarity with normal developmental stages, which are amply illustrated in the comprehensive work of Kalousek et al.[279]

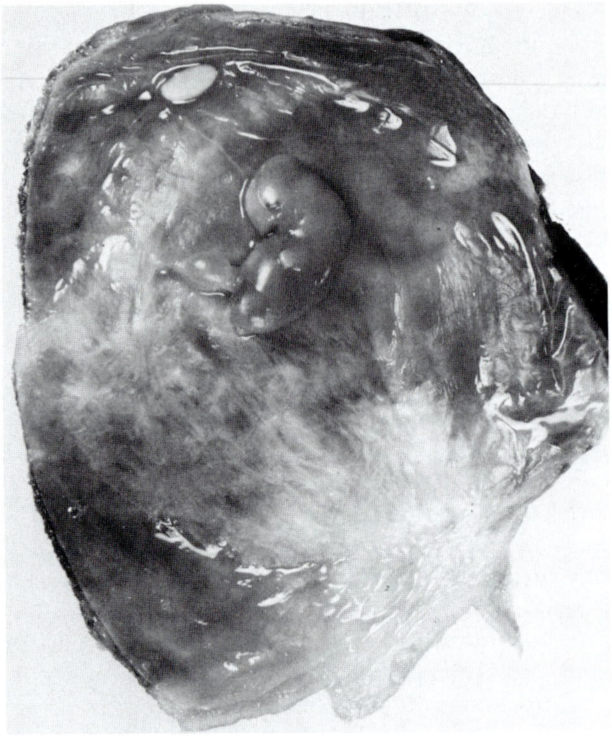

Fig. 23.90. Spontaneous abortion with intact amnion and deformed embryo. The bulbous, amorphous limb buds, distorted facial clefts, constricted body stalk (umbilical cord), and greatly distended amnion all suggest abnormal karyotype.

Table 23.2. Proportions of abnormal karyotypes in 1500 spontaneous abortions

Karyotype abnormality	*Approximate percentage*
Trisomies	52
Triploidy	20
XO	15
Tetraploidy	6
Translocation	4
Double trisomy	2
Mosaics	1

From data of Boue et al.[75]

The villi of abortions with abnormal karyotypes often appear abnormal, but the patterns are variable and nonspecific. Some dysmorphic features suggestive of chromosomal abnormality—villous enlargement with myxoid stroma, irregular villous outlines, multiple trophoblastic invaginations, large trophoblastic cells in the villous stroma, and trophoblastic hyperplasia—are common (Figs. 23.93 and 23.94) and may be more marked in karyotypically abnormal abortions, but are found in abortions with normal karyotypes as well.[75,284,456,457,585,593] The placental villi seem to react similarly to a spectrum of chromosomal and nonchromosomal factors. Morphologic changes in the villi seem, to a large degree, to be determined more by the time of embryonic or fetal death and the length of intrauterine retention than the specific nature of the insult.

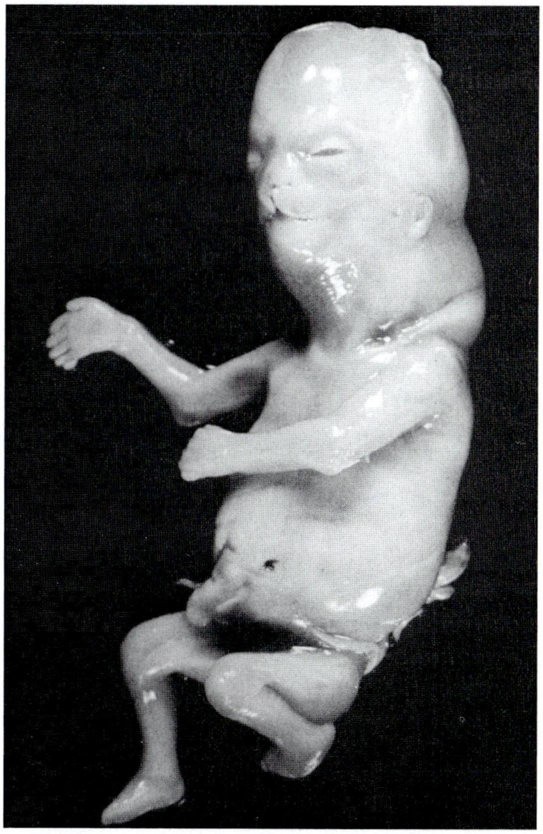

Fig. 23.91. Aborted 47,XX (trisomy 13) fetus. Note supernumerary digits, facial fusion defect, cervical swelling, low-set ears, and ventral hernia.

Complete and partial moles are the only morphologic entities with defined karyotype abnormalities that can be diagnosed with any degree of confidence (Fig. 23.95).[562–564] The diagnosis of trophoblastic disease, however, has become more difficult because of the practice of routine early sonography and curettage when there is no evidence of a fetus. Increasingly, the histologic distinction between complete hydatidiform mole, partial mole, and hydropic abortion has to be made before either form of mole has developed its most distinctive attributes. All three lesions have some degree of villous edema (hydrops) and trophoblastic hyperplasia at the early stage at which most hydropic abortions occur spontaneously (and when early moles may be curetted). The distinction is still possible, however. *Early complete moles* have a single population of enlarged villi with some persistence of stromal vessels, karyorrhexis of endothelial and stromal cells, primitive cellular stroma, focal but marked trophoblastic hyperplasia with atypia, and distinctively clubbed villous outlines.[285,343,359,371,515] They have a paternally derived diploid or tetraploid karyotype. *Early partial moles* characteristically have two populations of villi by size, scalloped villous margins, circumferential trophoblastic hyperplasia and some have trophoblastic invaginations, pseudoinclusions, and large dilated empty endothelial-lined stromal spaces.[101] They are typically triploid, with two sets of paternal chromosomes. Karyotyped triploid abortions show interesting differences based upon which parent contributed the extra set of chromosomes. Digynic triploidy results in small placentas without villous hydrops and a growth-retarded fetus with facial clefts and syndactyly of digits 3 and 4; diandric triploidy results in a larger placenta with vesicular change (partial hydatiform mole). *Hydropic abortions* have mildly swollen villi and only focal mild trophoblastic hyperplasia. The karyotype is variable. The distinction between diploid, triploid, and

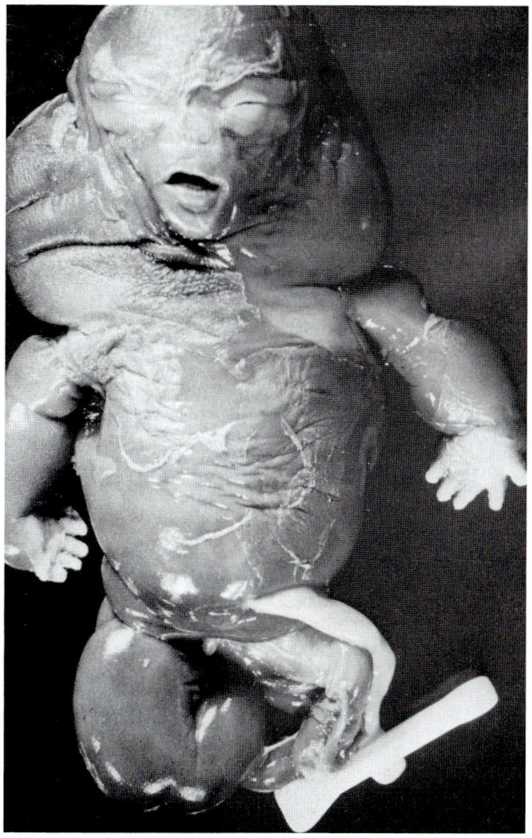

Fig. 23.92. Aborted 45,XO fetus. The large, symmetric cervical swellings and generalized edema are characteristic features. Cardiovascular anomalies are also common, as in Turner syndrome.

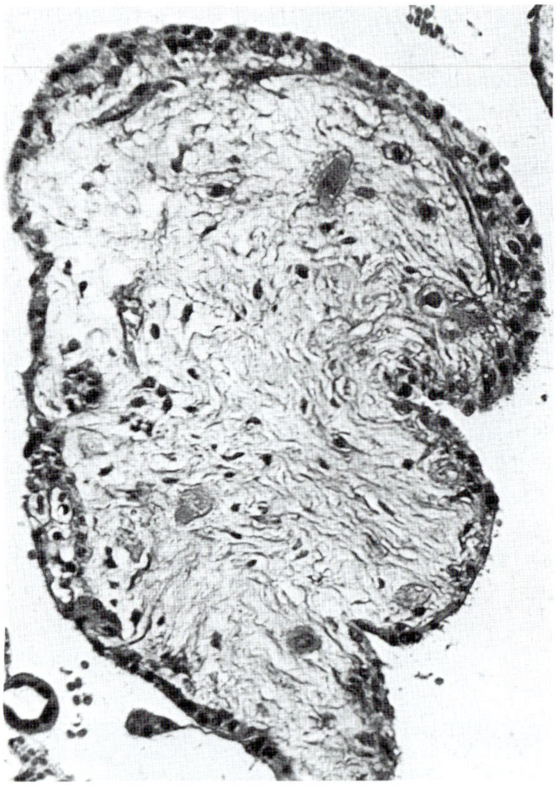

Fig. 23.93. Villus from D-trisomy spontaneous abortion. A few large, irregular cells resembling cytotrophoblast extend into the villous stroma at *top*, *center*, and *bottom center*.

tetraploid karyotypes can be made by flow cytometry[318] or image analysis.[284]

Some abnormalities, especially trisomies when they occur repeatedly, may reflect chromosomal anomalies in the parents. Karyotyping may be clinically very useful in the evaluation of couples distressed by repeated spontaneous abortion.[551] Balanced translocations are the most common parental karyotypic defects and may represent the basis for repeated abortion in such cases.[551] Although these are not currently treatable, they are of immense importance in genetic counseling as the prospects for future pregnancies are evaluated.

The role of immunologic rejection as a significant cause of abortion has received attention for some years; in fact, a satisfactory explanation of immunologic tolerance sufficient to allow the fetal autograft to survive until term delivery has been a major problem. The role of abnormal immune response in human infertility and of therapeutic interventions is not settled. Recent experimental studies in mice[376] suggest that local catabolism of tryptophan by 2,3-dioxygenase produced by the placenta suppresses maternal T-cell responses. An adjustment of the experimental model to provide adequate tryptophan results in more normal T-cell function, and the fetal placental site is rejected like any other allograft.

Rocklin et al.[468] identified a maternal immunoglobulin G (IgG) antibody in normal multigravid

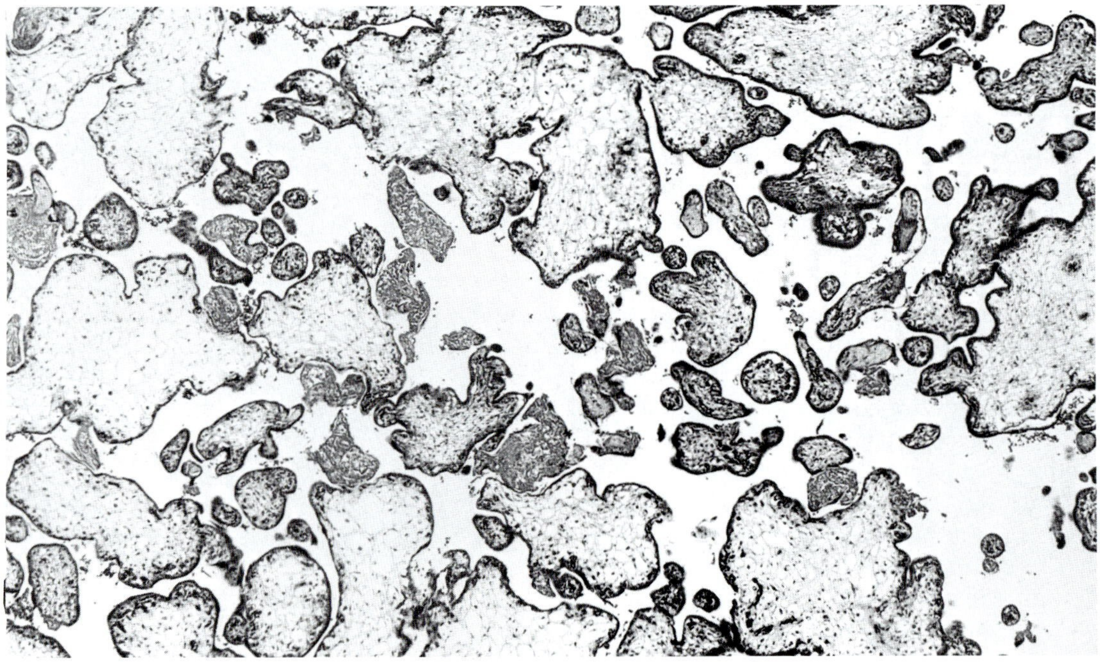

Fig. 23.94. Placenta, 45,XO. Immature, enlarged villi from a 45,XO spontaneous abortion similar to the fetus shown in Fig. 23.92, but of longer (26 weeks) gestation. Patchy clusters of larger immature villi with abundant stroma are not specific but suggestive of this and other abnormal placental genotypes, including trisomies.

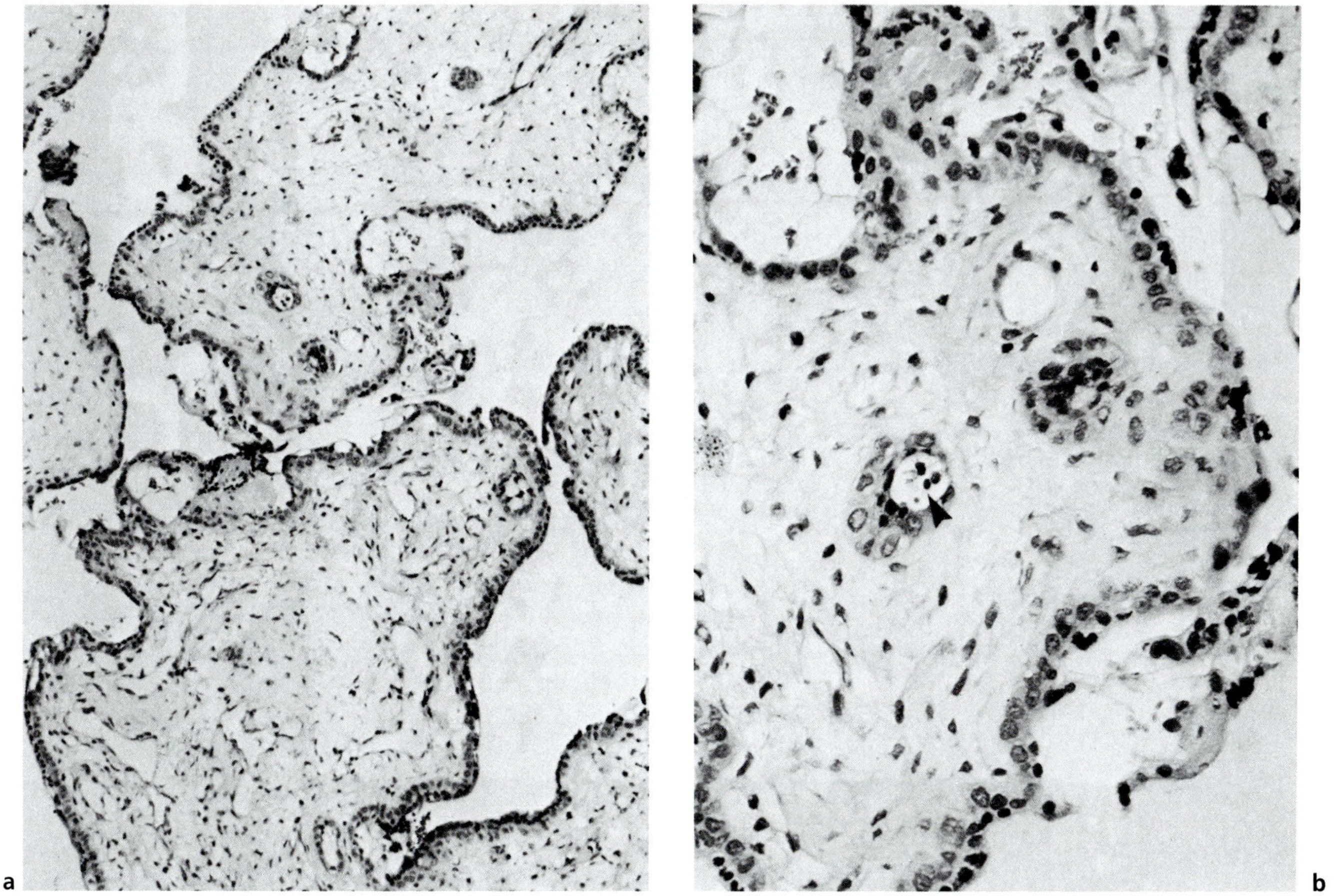

Fig. 23.95. Partial mole (69,XXY). a: Distinctive features are trophoblastic invaginations that appear circular in cross section (villous at *top center*), the scalloped, irregular margins, and empty endothelium-lined vascular sinusoids (villus at *bottom*). **b**: Higher magnification of trophoblastic invaginations. Note the peripheral, pale-staining, larger cytotrophoblast cells and the more central, darker, syncytiotrophoblast nuclei. The central space (*arrow*) communicates with the maternal intervillous space.

women that is absent in some women who experience repeated abortion. The presence of this serum blocking factor is believed to support the fetus and placenta as an allograft. Morphologic changes at the implantation site in these abortions have not been correlated with the immunologic findings. It would be interesting and very desirable to see if placental site trophoblast is altered or absent in women who experience this form of habitual abortion. The absence of vessel changes and intermediate trophoblast is another easily recognized pattern variation in some abortions, but clinical correlations with this deficit are lacking (Fig. 23.96).

Fetal Stage (10–20 Weeks)

Most late abortions are caused by infections, mainly bacterial invasion of the amnionic fluid represented histologically by acute chorioamnionitis. Midtrimester abortions are also caused by viral infections, toxoplasmosis, and other pathogens described elsewhere in this chapter. A second major category of late abortions includes women with immunologic abnormalities, including lupus anticoagulant, anticardiolipin antibodies, and antinuclear antibodies, and a third group is related to coagulopathies.

Intrauterine Fetal Death; Stillbirth

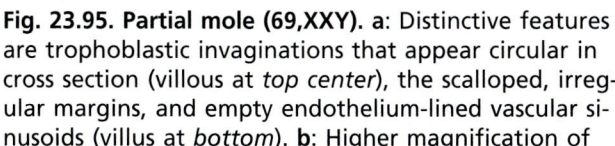

Most instances of *intrauterine fetal death* (*IUFD*) are caused by one or more of the placental conditions described in this chapter or by fetal malformations incompatible with life. A reasonable explanation for fetal death should be possible from examination of the fetal autopsy and placenta together in a significant percentage of cases, assuming a complete examination and the availability of specialized techniques such as cytogenetics. A very important category to evaluate when the fetus is normally formed and the placental findings seem trivial is

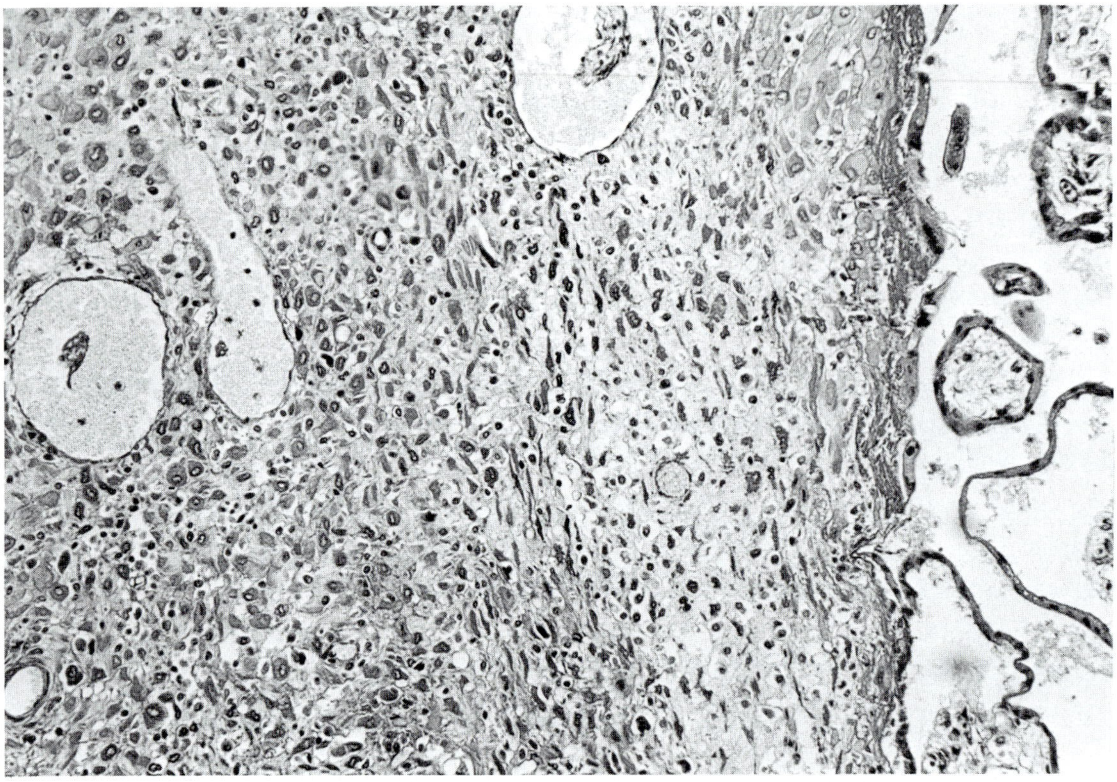

a

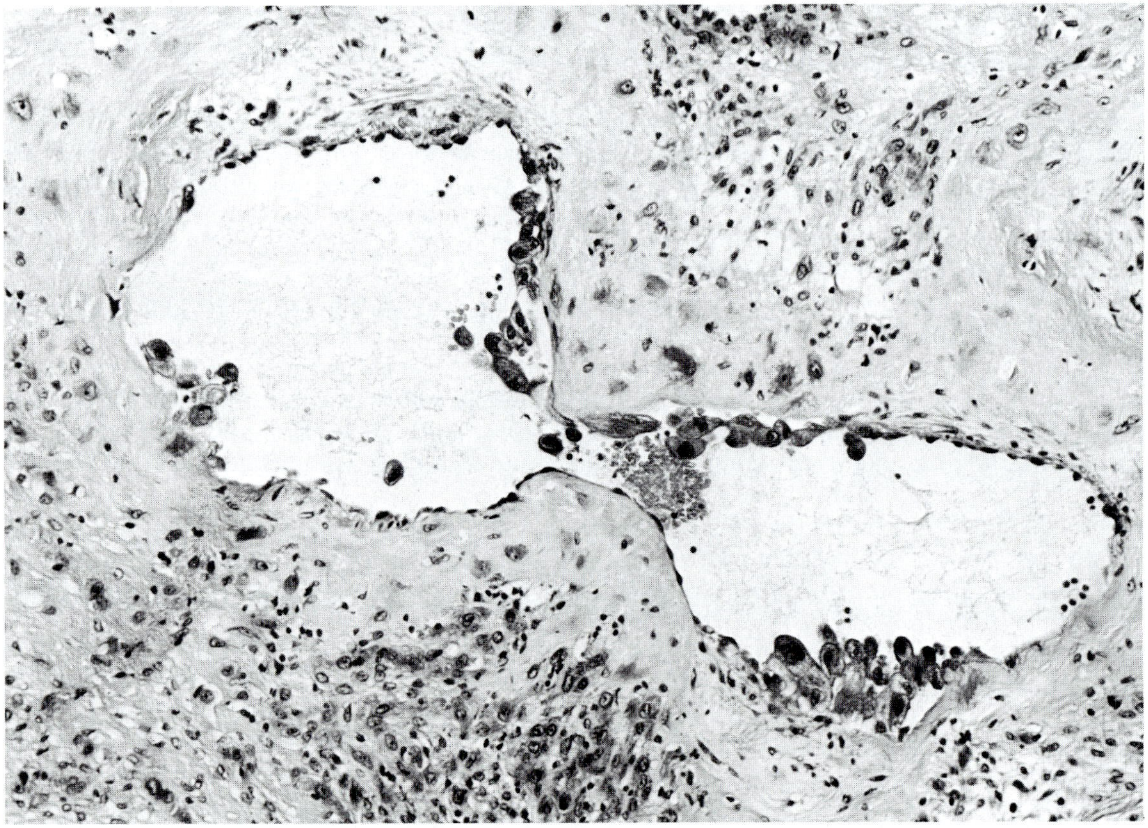

b

Fig. 23.96. a: **Implantation site of spontaneous abortion.** Placental site intermediate trophoblast cells are markedly deficient in size and numbers. **b**: Normal appearance of intermediate trophoblast at implantation site. Numerous trophoblast cells replace intima, infiltrate the wall of the large spiral artery at center, and cluster irregularly in the surrounding decidua, especially at *bottom center.*

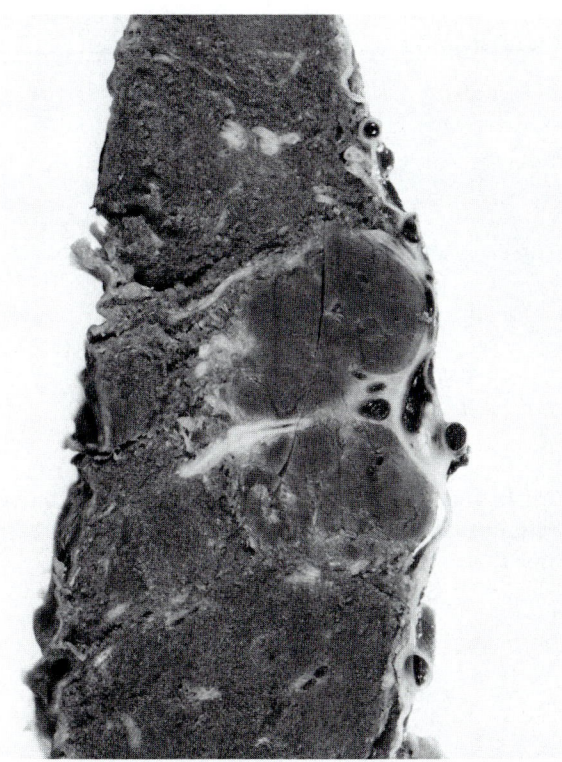

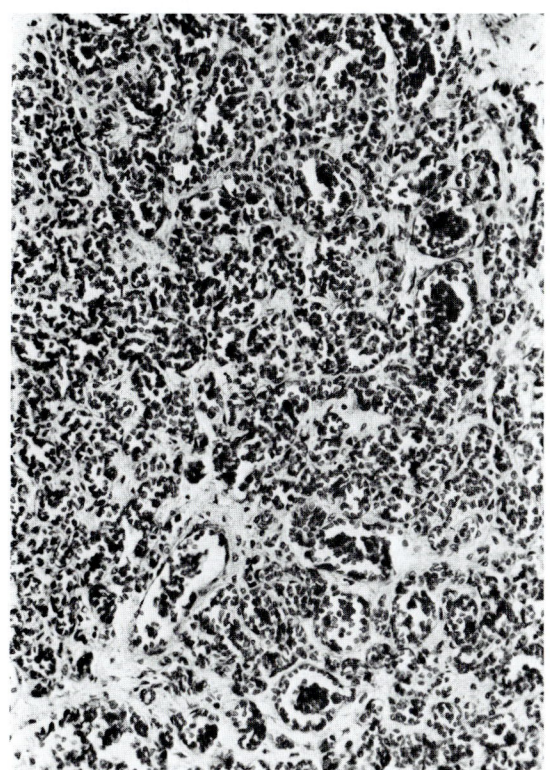

Fig. 23.97. **Placental hemangioma.** Firm, red hemangioma, well demarcated from the surrounding placental parenchyma.

confined placental mosaicism.[275] As this diagnosis requires fresh tissue from both the fetus and placenta for cell culture and karyotyping, the decision to employ it should be made as soon as possible before the placenta has been immersed in formalin.

Nontrophoblastic Tumors

Hemangioma (Chorangioma)

Placental hemangiomas (chorangiomas) occur in about 1% of carefully examined placentas.[589] They are usually small and entirely intraplacental and may be difficult to appreciate on gross examination, especially in the unfixed specimen. Large tumors distorting either the chorionic or basal plates of the placenta are rare, and exceptionally a chorangioma is attached to the placenta by a thin pedicle. Chorangiomas are usually solitary, but they may be multiple or, rarely, involve the placenta diffusely. Chorangiomas may be brown, yellow, tan, red, or white and are usually firm and well demarcated from the surrounding parenchyma (Fig. 23.97). Most chorangiomas are composed of numerous blood vessels, usually capillary but occasionally cavernous in type, supported by inconspicuous, loose stroma (Fig. 23.98). Occasionally, they are more cellular or show

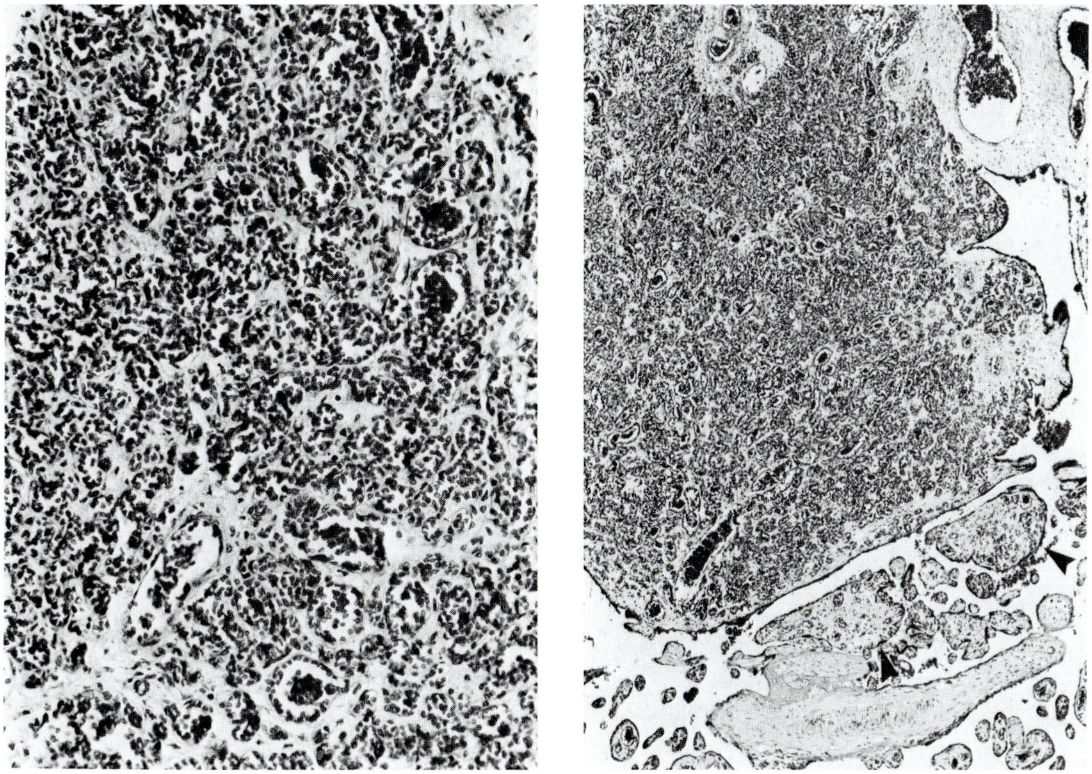

Fig. 23.98. **Placental hemangioma.** Numerous capillary-sized vessels are separated by inconspicuous stroma (*left*). Adjacent villi show telangiectatic change (*arrowheads, right*).

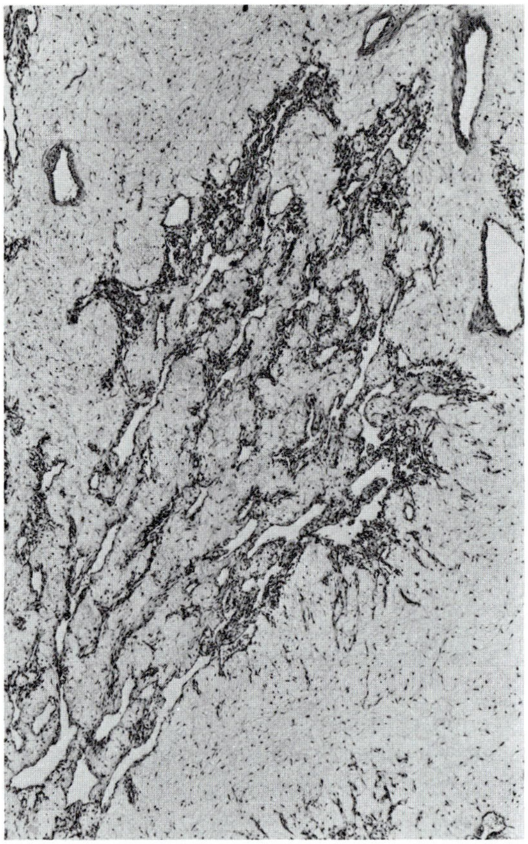

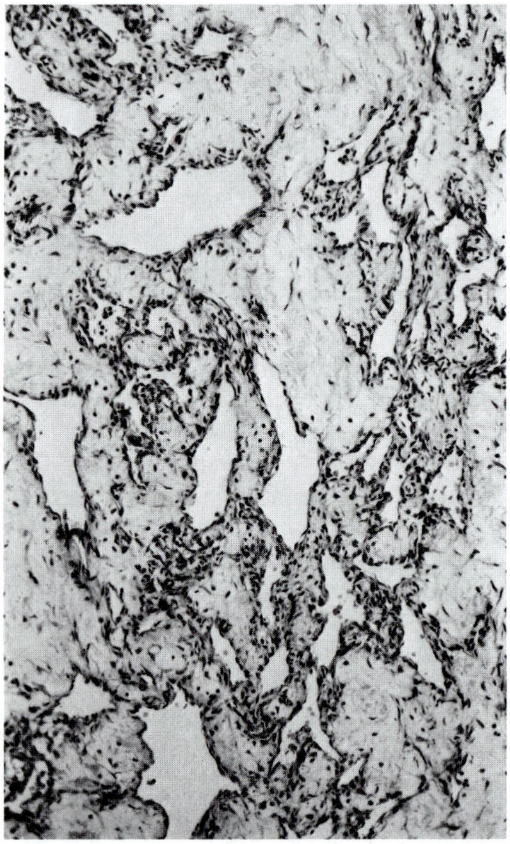

Fig. 23.99. **Hemangioma of umbilical cord.** Large, cavernous vessels suspended in abundant, myxoid stroma. *Top*: Low power. *Bottom*: High power.

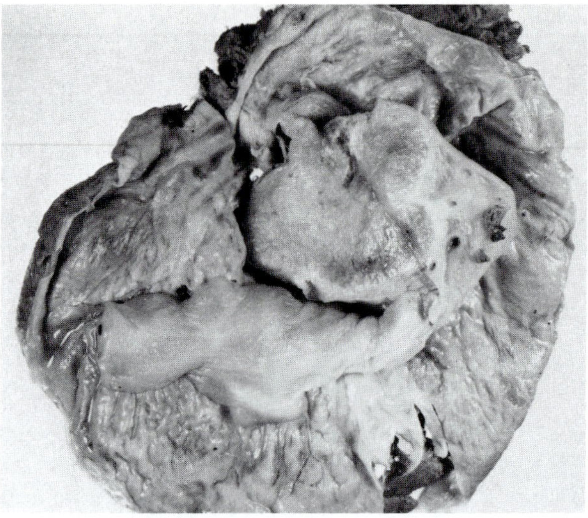

Fig. 23.100. Hemangioma of umbilical cord in a liveborn normal infant. Large hemangioma is located near cord insertion.

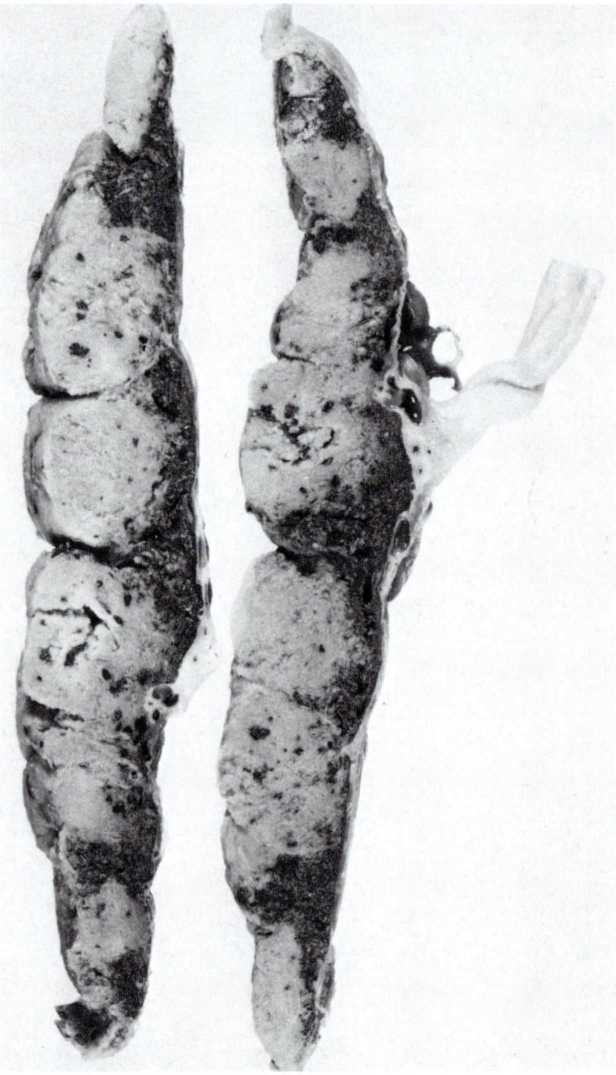

Fig. 23.101. Metastatic malignant melanoma of placenta. Dark areas represent metastatic deposits of malignant melanoma.

prominent myxoid change, hyalinization, necrosis, or calcification (Fig. 23.99). Mitotic figures and nuclear atypicality have been reported in some chorangiomas, but these have not behaved aggressively.[335] Localized groups of large telangiectatic villi are often identified adjacent to the dominant lesion (Fig. 23.98). Hemangiomas of identical gross and microscopic appearance occur occasionally in the umbilical cord (Fig. 23.100).[36]

Although the majority of chorangiomas are of no clinical significance, various complications have been reported, usually in association with large lesions.[87,93,512,532,589] Hydramnios and premature delivery, the latter apparently a consequence of the former, are the most significant. Fetal cardiomegaly, congestive heart failure, and hydrops have been attributed the increased workload in shunting blood through a large chorangioma. When significant amounts of blood are directed through the chorangioma away from functional villi, chronic hypoxia may lead to intrauterine growth retardation. A relationship between growth retardation and chorangioma size has been stressed.[374] Other fetal complications including anemia and thrombocytopenia may reflect sequestration or destruction of cellular elements as they traverse the chorangioma. Skin angiomas have been reported in a few babies with placental hemangiomas.

Teratoma

Placental teratomas are rare. The few tumors reported have been located between the amnion and chorion, usually on the placental surface, and rarely in the umbilical cord. Histologically, they have the usual features of a mature teratoma, and are distinguished from an acardiac fetus by the lack of an umbilical cord and disorganization of the component tissues.

Placental Metastases

Metastases to the placenta from either maternal or fetal neoplasms are very rare. Although carcinomas of the cervix and breast are the most frequently encountered malignancies in pregnant women, malignant melanoma (Fig. 23.101) is by far most common maternal tumor to metastasize to the placenta or spread to the fetus.[429,460,461] A variety of other maternal neoplasms metastatic to the placenta have been reported.[94,311,347,426]

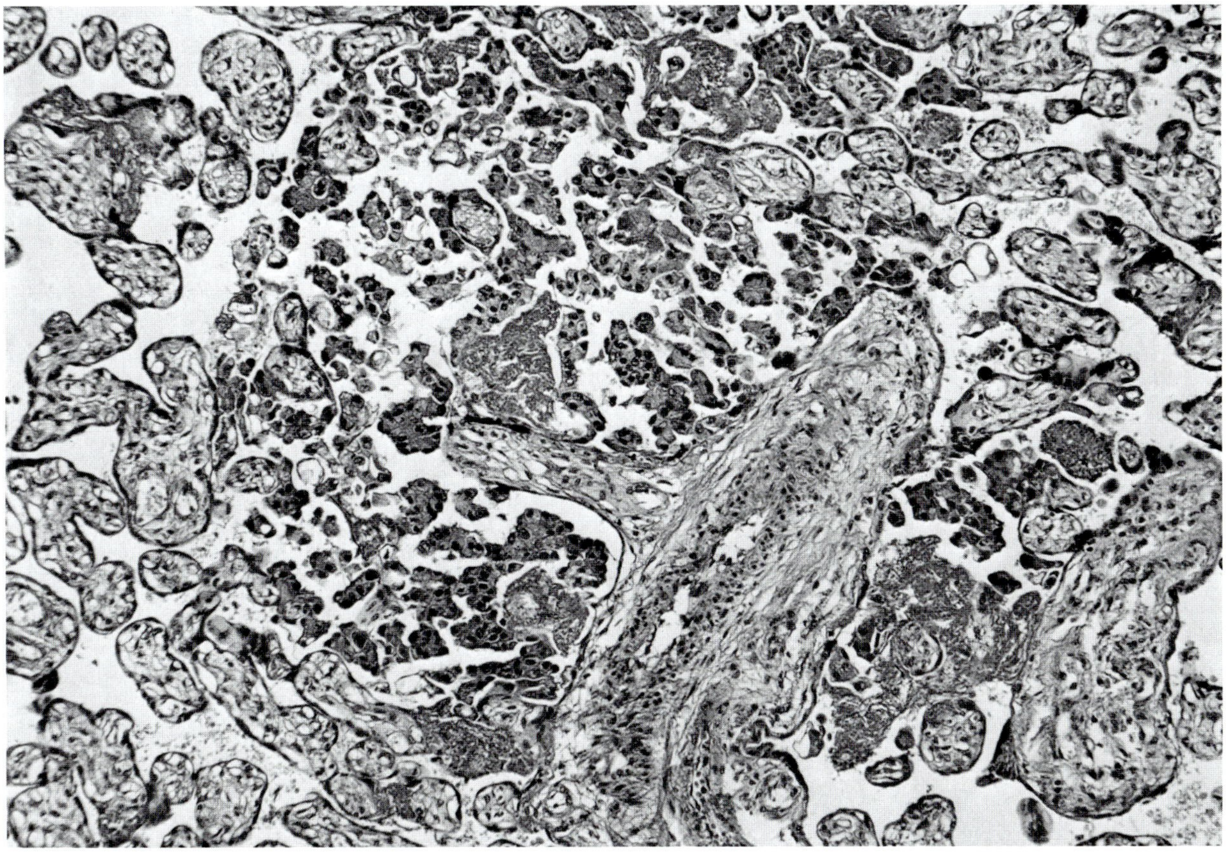

Fig. 23.102. Metastatic breast carcinoma of placenta. Metastatic breast carcinoma is confined to the intervillous space. There is no villous invasion.

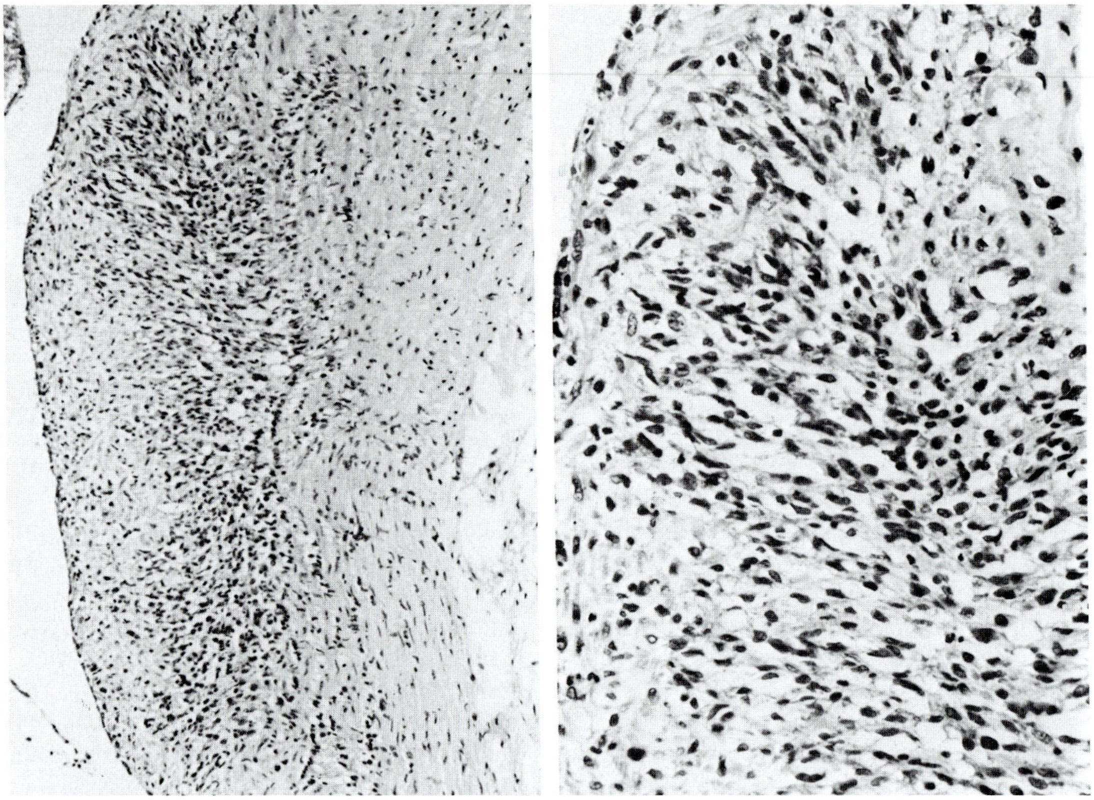

Fig. 23.103. Umbilical artery. Disseminated histiocytosis in subendothelial location. *Left*: Low power. *Right*: High power.

Placentas harboring metastases are usually normal on gross inspection, although on occasion metastatic tumor deposits may be apparent grossly. Tumor cells are usually confined to the intervillous space, and villous or fetal vascular invasion is very uncommon (Fig. 23.102).

Dissemination of a congenital fetal tumor to the placenta is also very rare. The few well-documented cases of placental metastasis from neuroblastoma have been pale and bulky, resembling the hydropic placentas of Rh incompatibility.[60,554] Clumps of neuroblastoma cells plugging villous vessels have been found microscopically. Rare cases of fetal leukemic involvement of the placenta and disseminated histiocytosis involving the vessels of the umbilical cord have been reported (Fig. 23.103).

References

1. Abraham JM (1967) Intrauterine feto-fetal transfusion syndrome. Clinical observations and speculations on pathogenesis. Clin Pediatr 6:405–410
2. Abramowsky C, Beyer-Patterson P, Cortinas E (1991) Nonsyphilitic spirochetosis in second-trimester fetuses. Pediatr Pathol 11:827–838
3. Abramowsky CR, Vegas ME, Swinehart G, Gyves MT (1980) Decidual vasculopathy of the placenta in lupus erythematosus. N Engl J Med 303:668–672
4. Ackerman J, Gonzolez EF, Gilbert-Barness E (1999) Immunologic studies of the placenta in maternal connective tissue disease. Pediatr Dev Pathol 2:19–24
5. Aherne W, Strong SJ, Corney G (1968) The structure of the placenta in the twin transfusion syndrome. Biol Neonate 12:121–135
6. Aladjem S (1967) Morphologic aspects of the placenta in gestational diabetes seen by phase-contrast microscopy. An anatomicroclinical correlation. Am J Obstet Gynecol 99:341–349
7. Altemani AM (1992) Immunohistochemical study of the inflammatory infiltrate in villitis of unknown etiology. A qualitative and quantitative analysis. Pathol Res Pract 188:303–309
8. Althabe O, LaBarrere C, Telenta M (1985) Maternal vascular lesions in placentae of small-for-gestational-age infants. Placenta 6:265–276
9. Althabe O, LaBarrere C (1985) Chronic villitis of unknown aetiology in placentae of idiopathic small for gestational age infants of normal and low ponderal index. Placenta 6:369–373
10. Altshuler G (1973) Toxoplasmosis as a cause of hydranencephaly. Am J Dis Child 125:251–252
11. Altshuler G (1974) Pathogenesis of congenital herpesvirus infection. Am J Dis Child 127:427–429

12. Altshuler G (1977) Placentitis, with a new light on and old torch. Obstet Gynecol Annu 6:197–221
13. Altshuler G (1984) Chorangiosis. Arch Pathol Lab Med 108:71–74
14. Altshuler G, Arizawa M, Molnar-Nadasdy G (1992) Meconium-induced umbilical cord vascular necrosis and ulceration: a potential link between placenta and poor pregnancy outcome. Obstet Gynecol 79:760–766
15. Altshuler G, Hyde S (1985) Fusobacteria: an important cause of chorioamnionitis. Arch Pathol Lab Med. 109:739–743.
16. Altshuler G, Hyde S. (1988) Clinicopathologic considerations of fusobacteria chorioamnionitis. Acta Obstet Gynecol Scand 67:513–517
17. Altshuler G, Hyde S (1989) Meconium-induced vasocontraction: a potential cause of cerebral and other fetal hypoperfusion and of poor pregnancy outcome. J Child Neurol 4:137–142
18. Altshuler G, Russell P (1975) The human placental villitides. A review of chronic intrauterine infection. Curr Top Pathol 60:63–112
19. Altshuler G, Tsang RC, Ermocilla R (1975) Single umbilical artery. Correlation of clinical status and umbilical cord histology. Am J Dis Child 129:697–700
20. Alvarez H, Sala MA, Benedetti WL (1972) Intervillous space reduction in the edematous placenta. Am J Obstet Gynecol 112:819–820
21. Amatuzio JC, Gorlin RJ (1981) Conjoined acardiac monsters. Arch Pathol 105:253–255
22. Anand A, Gray ES, Brown T, et al (1987) Human parvovirus infection in pregnancy and hydrops fetalis. N Engl J Med 316:183–186
23. Anderson GD (1975) Listeria monocytogenes septicemia in pregnancy. Obstet Gynecol 46:102–104
24. Anderson M, Went LN, MacIver JE, Dixon HG (1960) Sickle-cell disease in pregnancy. Lancet 2: 516–521
25. Andres RL, Kuyper W, Resnik R, et al (1990) The association of maternal floor infarction of the placenta with adverse perinatal outcome. Am J Obstet Gynecol 163:935–938
26. Andrews WW, Goldenberg RL, Hauth JC (1995) Preterm labor: emerging role of genital tract infections. Infect Agents Dis 4:196–211
27. Appelbaum PC, Shulman G, Chambers NL, et al (1980) Studies on the growth-inhibiting property of amniotic fluids from two United States population groups. Am J Obstet Gynecol 137:579–582
28. Arias F, Romero R, Joist H, Kraus FT (1998) Thrombophilia: A mechanism of disease in women with adverse pregnancy outcome and thrombotic lesions in the placenta. J Matern Fetal Med 7:277–286
29. Ariel IB, Landing BH (1985) A possibly distinctive vacuolar change of the amniotic epithelium associated with gastroschisis. Pediatr Pathol 2:283–289
30. Ashkenazy M, Borenstein R, Katz Z, Segal M (1982) Constriction of the umbilical cord by an amniotic band after midtrimester amniocentesis. Acta Obstet Gynecol Scand 61:89–91
31. Auger P, Marquis G, Dallaire L, et al (1980) Natural occurrence of a humoral response to *Candida* in human amniotic fluid. Am J Obstet Gynecol 136: 1075–1079
32. Bain AD, Bowie JH, Flint WF, et al (1956) Congenital toxoplasmosis simulating haemolytic disease of the newborn. J Obstet Gynaecol Br Emp 63: 826–832
33. Baldwin VJ. (1994) Pathology of multiple pregnancy. Springer, New York
34. Baldwin VJ, Wittmann BK (1990) Pathology of intragestational intervention in twin-to-twin transfusion syndrome. Pediatr Pathol 10:79–93
35. Bamforth JS (1993) Amnionic band sequence: Streeter hypothesis revisited. Birth Defects Orig Artic Ser 29:279–289
36. Barry FE, McCoy CP, Callahan WP Jr (1951) Hemangioma of the umbilical cord. Am J Obstet Gynecol 62:675–680
37. Batcup G, Tovey LAD, Longster G (1983) Fetomaternal blood group incompatibility studies in placental intervillous thrombosis. Placenta 4:449–454
38. Bebbington MW, Wittmann BK (1989) Fetal transfusion syndrome: antenatal factors predicting outcome. Am J Obstet Gynecol 160:913–915
39. Beckett RS, Flynn FJ (1953) Toxoplasmosis. Report of two new cases with a classification and with a demonstration of the organisms in the human placenta. N Engl J Med 249:345–350
40. Bejar R, Vigliocco G, Gramajo H, et al (1990) Antenatal origin of neurologic damage in new born infants. II. Multiple gestations. Am J Obstet Gynecol 162:1230–1236
41. Bendon RW, Siddiqi (1989) Clinical pathology conference: acute twin-to-twin in utero transfusion. Pediatr Pathol 9:591–598
42. Bendon RW, Tyson RW, Baldwin VJ, et al (1991) Umbilical cord ulceration and intestinal atresia: a new association? Am J Obstet Gynecol 164:582–586
43. Benirschke K (1994) Obstetrically important lesions of the umbilical cord. J Reprod Med 39:262–272
44. Benirschke K (1993) Intrauterine death of a twin: mechanisms, implications for surviving twin, and placental pathology. Semin Diagn Pathol 10:222–231
45. Benirschke K (1974) Syphilis—The placenta and the fetus. Am J Dis Child 128:142–143
46. Benirschke K, Bourne GL (1960) The incidence and prognostic implication of congenital absence of one umbilical artery. Am J Obstet Gynecol 79:251–254
47. Benirschke K, Brown WH (1955) A vascular anomaly of the umbilical cord: The absence of one umbilical artery in the umbilical cords of normal and abnormal fetuses. Obstet Gynecol 6:399–404
48. Benirschke K, Driscoll SG (1967) The pathology of the human placenta. Springer, New York
49. Benirschke K, Kaufmann P (2000) Pathology of the human placenta, 4th Ed. Springer, New York, pp 497–506

50. Benirschke K, Kaufmann P (2000) Pathology of the human placenta, 4th Ed. Springer, New York, pp 120, 432
51. Benirschke K, Kaufman P (1995) Pathology of the human placenta, 3rd Ed. Springer, New York, pp 116–150
52. Benirschke K, Kaufmann P (1995) Pathology of the human placenta, 3rd Ed. Springer, New York, pp 719–826
53. Benirschke K, Kim CK (1973) Multiple pregnancy (first of two parts). N Engl J Med 288:1276–1284
54. Benirschke K, Kim CK (1973) Multiple pregnancy (second of two parts). N Engl J Med 288:1329–1335
55. Benirschke K, Mendoza GR, Bazely PL (1974) Placental and fetal manifestations of cytomegalovirus infection. Virchows Arch [B Cell Pathol] 16:121–139
56. Benson RC, Fujikura T (1969) Circumvallate and circummarginate placenta. Obstet Gynecol 34:799–804
57. Berry MC, Dajani AS (1992) Resurgence of congenital syphilis. Infect Dis Clin N Am 6:19–29
58. Bey M, Dott A, Miller JM Jr (1991) The sonographic diagnosis of circumvallate placenta. Obstet Gynecol 78:515–516
59. Beyth Y, Perlman M, Ornoy A (1977) Amniogenic bands associated with facial dysplasia and paresis. J Reprod Med 18:83–86
60. Birner WF (1961) Neuroblastoma as a cause of antenatal death. Am J Obstet Gynecol 82:1388–1391
61. Blanc WA (1959) Amniotic infection syndrome. Pathogenesis, morphology, and significance in circumnatal mortality. Clin Obstet Gynaecol 2:705–734
62. Blanc WA (1961) Vernix granulomatosis of amnion ("amnion nodosum") in oligohydramnios. Lesion associated with urinary abnormalities, retention of dead fetuses, and prolonged leakage of amniotic fluid. NY State J Med 61:1492–1496
63. Blanc WA (1976) Pathology of placenta accreta. Verh Dtsch Ges Pathol 60:393–399
64. Blanc WA (1976) Circulatory lesions of the human placenta in abruptio. Verh Dtsch Ges Pathol 60: 386–392
65. Blanc WA (1978) Pathology of the placenta and cord in some viral infections. In: Hanshan JB, Dregeon JA (eds). Viral diseases of the fetus and newborn. Major problems in clinical pediatrics, vol 17. Saunders, Philadelphia
66. Blanc WA (1980) Pathology of the placenta and cord in ascending and in haematogenous infection. Excerpta Medica Ciba Found Symp 77:17–38
67. Blanc WA (1981) Pathology of the placenta, membranes, and umbilical cord in bacterial, fungal and viral infections in man. In: Naeye RL, Kissane JM, Kaufman N (eds) Perinatal diseases. International Academy of Pathology Monograph. Williams & Wilkins, Baltimore
68. Blanche S, Rouzioux C, Moscata M-LG, et al (1989) A prospective study of infants born to women seropositive for human immunodeficiency virus Type I. N Engl J Med 320:1643–1648
69. Blattner P, Dar H, Nitowsky HM (1977) Pregnancy outcome in women with sickle cell trait. JAMA 238:1392–1394
70. Blattner R (1964) Repeated congenital infection with *Toxoplasma gondii*. J Pediatr 64:452–455
71. Blickstein I (1990) The twin-twin transfusion syndrome. Obstet Gynecol 76:714–722
72. Bloomfield RD, Suarez JR, Malangit AC (1978) The placenta: A diagnostic tool in sickle cell disorders. J Natl Med Assoc 70:87–88
73. Boronow RC, West RH (1964) Monster acardius parasiticus. Am J Obstet Gynecol 88:233–237
74. Botha MC (1969) Spontaneous rupture of the uterus due to placenta percreta. S Afr Med J 43: 39–4l
75. Boue J, Phillipe E, Girond A, Boue A (1976) Phenotypic expression of lethal chromosomal anomalies in human abortuses. Teratology 14:3–20
76. Boyd JD, Hamilton WJ (1970) The human placenta. Heffer, Cambridge
77. Branch DW, Scott JR, Kochenour NK, Hershgold E (1985) Obstetric complications associated with the lupus anticoagulant. N Engl J Med 313:1322–1326
78. Breen JL, Neubecker R, Gregori CA, Franklin JE (1977) Placenta accreta, increta and percreta. Obstet Gynecol 49:43–47
79. Brosens I, Renaer M (1972) On the pathogenesis of placental infarcts in pre-eclampsia. J Obstet Gynaecol Br Commonw 79:794–799
80. Brosens I, Dixon HG, Robertson WB (1977) Fetal growth retardation and the arteries of the placental bed. Br J Obstet Gynaecol 84:656–663
81. Browne JC (1958) The uterine circulation in toxemia. Clin Obstet Gynaecol 1:341–348
82. Browne JC, Veall N (1953) The maternal placental blood flow in normotensive and hypertensive women. J Obstet Gynaecol Br Emp 60:141–147
83. Bryan EM, Kohler HG (1974) The missing umbilical artery. I. Prospective study based on a maternity unit. Arch Dis Child 49:844–852
84. Bryan EM, Kohler HG (1975) The missing umbilical artery. II. Paediatric follow-up. Arch Dis Child 50:714–718
85. Burgess AM, Hutchins GM (1996) Inflammation of the lungs, umbilical cord and placenta associated with meconium passage in utero. Review of 123 autopsied cases. Path Res Pract 192:1121–1128
86. Burke CJ, Tannenberg AE, Payton DJ (1997) Ischaemic cerebral injury, intrauterine growth retardation, and placental infarction. Dev Med Child Neurol 39:726–730
87. Burrows S, Gaines JL, Hughes FJ (1973) Giant chorioangioma. Am J Obstet Gynecol 115:579–580
88. Byard RW (1996) Idiopathic arterial calcifications

and unexpected infant death. Pediatr Pathol Lab Med 16:985–994
89. Cameron AH (1968) The Birmingham twin survey. Proc R Soc Med 61:229–234
90. Cardwell, MS (1987) Ultrasound diagnosis of abruptio placentae with fetomaternal hemorrhage. Am J Obstet Gynecol 157:358–359
91. Carlson NJ, Towers CV (1989) Multiple gestation complicated by the death of one fetus. Obstet Gynecol 73:685–689
92. Case records of the Massachusetts General Hospital (case 15-1997). (1997) N Engl J Med 336:1439–1446
93. Cash JB, Powell DE (1980) Placental chorioangioma. Presentation of a case with electron microscopic and immunochemical studies. Am J Surg Pathol 4:87–92
94. Catlin EA, Roberts JD, Erana R, et al (1999) Transplacental transmission of natural-killer-cell lymphoma. N Engl J Med 341:85–91
95. Caul EO, Usher MJ, Burton PA (1988) Intrauterine infection with human parvovirus B19: a light and electron microscopy study. J Med Virol 24:55–66
96. Centers for Disease Control (1989) Risks associated with human parvovirus B19 infection. MMWR 38:81–97
97. Centers for Disease Control (1988) Continuing increase in infectious syphilis-United States. MMWR 37:35–38
98. Challis JRG, Patel F, Pomini F (1999) Prostaglandin dehydrogenase and initiation of labor. J Perinat Med 27:26–34
99. Chandwani S, Greco MA, Mittal K, et al (1991) Pathology and human immunodeficiency virus expression in placentas of seropositive women. J Infect Dis 163:1134–1138
100. Charache S, Scott J, Niebyl J, Bonds D (1980) Management of sickle cell disease in pregnant patients. Obstet Gynecol 55:407–410
101. Chew SH, Ronnet B, Williams R, Kurman RJ, Perlman EJ (1998) Morphology and DNA content in evaluation of first trimester placentas for partial hydatidiform mole. Mod Pathol 11:102
102. Clark P, Duff P (1995) Inhibition of neutrophil oxidative burst and phagocytosis by meconium. Am J Obstet Gynecol 173:1301–1305
103. Cleary GM, Wiswell TE (1998) Meconium-stained amniotic fluid and the meconium aspiration syndrome. An update. Pediatr Clin North Amer 45:511–529
104. Clewell WH, Manchester DK (1983) Recurrent maternal floor infarction: a preventable cause of fetal death. Am J Obstet Gynecol 147:346–347
105. Cocker J, George SW, Yates PO (1965) Perinatal occlusion of the middle cerebral artery. Dev Med Child Neurol 7:235–243
106. Coid CR, Fox H (1983) Short review: Campylobacters as placental pathogens. Placenta 4:295–306
107. Committee on Infectious Diseases, American Academy of Pediatrics. (1990) Parvovirus, erythema infectiosum, and pregnancy. Pediatrics 85:131
108. Cooperman NR, Kasim M, Rajashekaraiah KR (1980) Clinical significance of amniotic fluid, amniotic membranes, and endometrial biopsy cultures at the time of cesarean section. Am J Obstet Gynecol 137:536–542
109. Corney G, Aherne W (1965) The placental transfusion syndrome in monozygous twins. Arch Dis Child 40:264–270
110. Coulter JBS, Scott JM, Jordan MM (1975) Oedema of the umbilical cord and respiratory distress in the newborn. Br J Obstet Gynaecol 82:453–459
111. Couvreur J, Desmonts G, Thulliez P (1988) Prophyllaxis of congenital toxoplasmosis. Effects of spiramycin on placental infection. J Antimicrob Chemother 22:193–200
112. Craig S, Permezel M, Doyle L et al (1996) Perinatal infection with *Listeria monocytogenes*. Aust NZ J Obstet Gynaecol 36:3:286–290
113. Craver RD, Baldwin V (1992) Necrotizing funisitis. Obstet Gynecol 79:64–70
114. Crawford JM (1959) A study of human placental growth with observations on the placenta in erythroblastosis foetalis. J Obstet Gynaecol Br Emp 66:885–896
115. Daffos F, Forestier F, Capella-Pavlovsky M et al (1988) Prenatal management of 746 pregnancies at risk for congenital toxoplasmosis. N Engl J Med 318:271–275
116. Damman O, Leviton A (1997) Maternal intrauterine infection, cytokines and brain damage in the preterm newborn. Pediatr Res 42:1–8
117. Danskin FH, Neilson JP (1989) Twin-to-twin transfusion syndrome: what are appropriate diagnostic criteria? Am J Obstet Gynecol 161:365–369
118. Darby MJ, Caritis SN, Shen-Schwarz S (1989) Placental abruption in the pre-term gestation: an association with chorioamnionitis. Obstet Gynecol 74:88–92
119. DaSa DJ (1973) Intimal cushions of foetal placental veins. J Pathol 110:347–352
120. Davey DA, MacGillivray I (1988) The classification and definition of the hypertensive disorders of pregnancy. Am J Obstet Gynecol 158:892–898
121. Davis BH, Olsen S, Bigelow NC, Chen JC (1998) Detection of fetal red cells in fetomaternal hemorrhage using a fetal hemoglobin monoclonal antibody by flow cytometry. Transfusion 38:749–756
122. Daya D, Sabet L (1991) The use of cytokeratin as a sensitive and reliable marker for trophoblastic tissue. Am J Clin Pathol 95:137–141
123. Daya D, Sabet L (1990) Can one make a diagnosis of intrauterine pregnancy in the absence of chorionic villi? Surg Pathol 3:205–210
124. Deacon JS, Machin GA, Martin JME, et al (1980) Investigation of acephalus. Am J Med Genet 5:85–99

125. Dekker GA, de Vries JIP, Doelitsch PM, et al (1995) Underlying disorders associated with severe early-onset preeclampsia. Am J Obstet Gynecol 173: 1042–1048
126. Dekker GA, Sibai BM (1998) Etiology and pathogenesis of preeclampsia: current concepts. Am J Obstet Gynecol 179:1359–1375
127. DeLia JE, Cruikshank DP, Keye WR (1990) Fetoscopic neodymium:Yag laser occlusion of placental vessels in severe twin-twin transfusion syndrome. Obstet Gynecol 75:1046–1053
128. deRoux SJ, Prendergast NC, Adsay NV (1999) Spontaneous uterine rupture with fatal hemoperitoneum due to placenta accreta percreta: a case report and review of the literature. Int J Gynecol Pathol 18:82–86
129. Desmonts G, Couvreur J (1974) Congenital toxoplasmosis. A prospective study of 378 pregnancies. N Engl J Med 290:1110–1116
130. Desmonts G, Forestier F, Thulliez PH, et al (1985) Prenatal diagnosis of congenital toxoplasmosis. Lancet 1:500–504
131. DeVeber C, Monagle P, Chan A, et al (1998) Prothrombotic disorders in infants and children with cerebral thromboembolism. Arch Neurol 55:1539–1543
132. Devi B, Jennison RF, Langley FA (1968) Significance of placental pathology in transplacental haemorrhage. J Clin Pathol 21:322–331
133. de Vries JIP, Dekker GA, Huigens PC, Jakobs C, Blomberg BME, van Geijn HP (1997) Hyperhomocysteinaemia and protein S deficiency in complicated pregnancies. Br J Obstet Gynaecol 104:1248–1254
134. DeWolf F, Brosens I, Renaer M (1980) Fetal growth retardation and the maternal arterial supply of the human placenta in the absence of sustained hypertension. Br J Obstet Gynaecol 87:678–685
135. DeWolf F, Carreras LO, Moerman P, et al (1982) Decidual vasculopathy and extensive placental infarction in a patient with repeated thromboembolic accidents, recurrent fetal loss, and a lupus anticoagulant. Am J Obstet Gynecol 142:829–834
136. DeWolf F, Robertson WB, Brosens I (1975) The ultrastructure of acute atherosis in hypertensive pregnancy. Am J Obstet Gynecol 123:164–174
137. DeWolf F, DeWolf-Peeters C, Brosens I, Robertson WB (1980) The human placental bed: electron microscopic study of trophoblastic invasion of spiral arteries. Am J Obstet Gynecol 137:58–70
138. DeWolf F, Carreras LO, Moerman P, et al (1982) Decidual vasculopathy and extensive placental infarction in a patient with repeated thromboembolic accidents, recurrent fetal loss, and a lupus anticoagulant. Am J Obstet Gynecol 142:829–834
139. Dimmick JE, Kalousek DK (1992) Developmental pathology of the embryo and fetus. Lippincott, Philadelphia
140. Dippel AL (1940) Hematomas of the umbilical cord. Surg Gynecol Obstet 70:51–57
141. Dixon HG, Browne JCM, Davey DA (1963) Choriodecidual and myometrial blood-flow. Lancet 2:369–373
142. Dizon-Townson DS, Meline L, Nelson L, Varner M, Ward K (1997) Fetal carriers of the factor V Leiden mutation are prone to miscarriage and placental infarction. Am J Obstet Gynecol 177:402–405
143. Dizon-Townson DS, Nelson LM, Easton K, Ward K (1996) The factor V Leiden mutation may predispose women to severe preeclampsia. Am J Obstet Gynecol 175:902–905
144. Dobashi K, Ajika K, Ohkawa T, et al (1984) Immunohistochemical localization of pregnancy-associated plasma protein A (PAPP-A) in placentae from normal and pre-eclamptic pregnancies. Placenta 5:205–212
145. Dong Y, St (1987) Clair PJ, Ramzy I, et al. A microbiologic and clinical study of placental inflammation at term. Obstet Gynecol 70:175–182
146. Donnenfeld AE, Glazerman LR, Cutillo DM, et al (1989) Fetal exsanguination following intrauterine angiographic assessment and selective termination of a hydrocephalic, monozygotic co-twin. Prenatal Diagn 9:301–308
147. Doss BJ, Greene MF, Hill J, Heffner LJ, Bieber FR, Genest DR (1995) Massive chronic intervillositis associated with recurrent abortions. Hum Pathol 26:1245–1251
148. Doss BJ, Jacques SM, Mayes MD, Qureshi F (1998) Maternal scleroderma: placenta findings and perinatal outcome. Hum Pathol 28:1524–1530
149. Douvier S, Neuwirth C, Filipuzzi L, Kisterman J-P (1999) Chorioamnionitis with intact membranes caused by *Capnocytophaga sputigena*. Eur J Obstet Gynecol Reprod Biol 83:109–112
150. Driscoll SG (1965) The pathology of pregnancy complicated by diabetes mellitus. Med Clin North Am 49:1053–1067
151. Driscoll SG (1966) Current concepts. Hydrops fetalis. N Engl J Med 275:1432–1434
152. Driscoll SG (1969) Histopathology of gestational rubella. Am J Dis Child 118:49–53
153. Driscoll SG, Gorbach A, Feldman D (1962) Congenital listeriosis: diagnosis from placental studies. Obstet Gynecol 20:216–220
154. Dudley DKL, D'Alton ME (1986) Single fetal death in twin gestation. Semin Perinatol 10:65–72
155. Easterling TR, Garite TJ (1985) Fusobacterium: anaerobic occult amnionitis and premature labor. Obstet Gynecol 66:825–828
156. Eberle AM, Levesque D, Vintzileos AM, Egan JF, Tsapanos V, Salafia CM (1993) Placental pathology in discordant twins. Am J Obstet Gynecol 169:931–935
157. Eddleman KA, Lockwood CJ, Berkowitz GS, Lapinski RH, Berkowitz RL (1992) Clinical significance and sonographic diagnosis of velamentous umbilical cord insertion. Am J Perinatol 9:123–126
158. Elliott WG (1970) Placental toxoplasmosis: report of a case. Am J Clin Pathol 53:413–417

159. Eschenbach DA (1997) Amniotic fluid infection and cerebral palsy. Focus on the fetus. JAMA 278:247–248
160. Essary LR, Vnencak-Jones CL, Manning SS, et al (1998) Frequency of parvovirus B19 infection in nonimmune hydrops fetalis and utility of three diagnostic methods. Hum Pathol 29:696–701
161. Etches PC, Lemons JA (1979) Nonimmune hydrops fetalis: report of 22 cases including three siblings. Pediatrics 64:326–332
162. Farmakides G, Schulman H, Saldana LR, et al (1985) Surveillance of twin pregnancy with umbilical arterial velocimetry. Obstet Gynecol 153:789–792
163. Feinstein DI (1985) Lupus anticoagulant, thrombosis, and fetal loss. N Engl J Med 313:1348–1350
164. Fiakpui EZ, Moran EM (1973) Pregnancy in the sickle hemoglobinopathies. J Reprod Med 11:28–34
165. Florman AL, Gershon AA, Blackett PR, Nahmias AJ (1973) Intrauterine infection with herpes simplex virus. Resultant congenital malformations. JAMA 225:129–132
166. Fojaco RM, Hensley GT, Moskowitz L (1989) Congenital syphilis and necrotizing funisitis. JAMA 261:1788–1790
167. Forrest JM, Menser MA, Burgess JA (1971) High frequency of diabetes mellitus in young adults with congenital rubella. Lancet 2:332–334
168. Foulon W, Naessens A, Mahler T, et al (1990) Prenatal diagnosis of congenital toxoplasmosis. Obstet Gynecol 76:769–772
169. Foulon W, Naessens A, deCalte L, et al (1990) Detection of congenital toxoplasmosis by chorionic villus sampling and early amniocentesis. Am J Obstet Gynecol 163:1511–1513
170. Fox H (1966) Thrombosis of the foetal stem arteries in the human placenta. J Obstet Gynaecol Br Commonwealth 73:961–965
171. Fox H (1997) Pathology of the placenta, 2nd Ed. Saunders, Philadelphia, pp 237–241
172. Fox H (1997) Pathology of the placenta, 2nd Ed. Saunders, Philadelphia, pp 216–224
173. Fox H (1997) Pathology of the placenta, 2nd Ed. Saunders, Philadelphia, p 168
174. Fox H (1997) Pathology of the placenta, 2nd Ed. Saunders, Philadelphia, p 64
175. Fox H (1997) Pathology of the placenta, 2nd Ed. Saunders, Philadelphia, pp 294–343
176. Fox H (1997) Pathology of the placenta, 2nd Ed. Saunders, Philadelphia, pp 418–452
177. Fox H (1967) Perivillous fibrin deposition in the human placenta. Am J Obstet Gynecol 98:245–251
178. Fox H (1997) The significance of placental infarction in perinatal morbidity and mortality. Biol Neonate 11:87–105
179. Fox H (1968) Morphological changes in the human placenta following fetal death. J Obstet Gynaecol Br Commonw 75:839–843
180. Fox H (1972) Placenta accreta, 1945–1969. Obstet Gynecol 27:475–486
181. Fox H (1981) Placental involvement in maternal systemic infection. In: Rosenberg HS, Bernstein J (eds). Perspectives in pediatric pathology. Infectious diseases, vol 6. Masson, New York
182. Fox H, Sen DK (1972) Placenta extrachorialis. A clinico-pathologic study. J Obstet Gynaecol Br Commonw 79:32–35
183. Franciosi RA, Tattersall P (1988) Fetal infection with human parvovirus B19. Hum Pathol 19:489–491
184. Frenkel JK (1971) Toxoplasmosis. Mechanisms of infection, laboratory diagnosis and management. Curr Top Pathol 54:28–75
185. Froehlich LA, Fujikura T (1966) Significance of a single umbilical artery. Report from the collaborative study of cerebral palsy. Am J Obstet Gynecol 94:274–279
186. Froehlich LA, Fujikura T (1973) Follow-up of infants with single umbilical artery. Pediatrics 52:22–29
187. Fujikura T, Froehlich L (1968) Diagnosis of sickling by placental examination. Geographic differences in incidence. Am J Obstet Gynecol 100:1122–1124
188. Fujikura T, Benson RC, Driscoll SG (1970) The bipartite placenta and its clinical features. Am J Obstet Gynecol 107:1013–1017
189. Fuke Y, Aono T, Imai S, et al (1994) Clinical significance and treatment of massive intervillous fibrin deposition associated with recurrent fetal growth retardation. Gynecol Obstet Invest 38:5–9
190. Funsch C, Ozdoba C, Kuhn P, et al (1997) Perinatal ultrasonography and magnetic resonance imaging findings in congenital hydrocephalus associated with fetal intraventricular hemorrhage. Am J Obstet Gynecol 177:512–518
191. Garcia AGP (1968) Congenital toxoplasmosis in two successive sibs. Arch Dis Child 43:705–710
192. Garcia AGP, Basso NGDS, Fonseca MEF, et al (1991) Enterovirus associated placental morphology: a light, virological, electron microscopic and immunohistologic study. Placenta 12:533–547
193. Garcia AGP, Coutinho SG, Amendoeira MR, Assumpcao MR, Albano N (1983) Placental morphology of newborns at risk for congenital toxoplasmosis. J Trop Pediatr 29:95–103
194. Garcia AGP, Marques RLS, Lobato YY, et al (1985) Placental pathology in congenital rubella. Placenta 6:281–295
195. Genest DR (1992) Estimating the time of death in stillborn fetuses: II. Histologic evaluation of the placenta; a study of 71 stillborns. Obstet Gynecol 80:585–592
196. Genest DR, Choi-Hong SR, Tate JE, Qureshi F, Jacques SM, Crum C (1996) Diagnosis of congenital syphilis from placental examination: comparison of histopathology, Steiner stain, and polymerase chain reaction for *Treponema pallidum* DNA. Hum Pathol 27:366–372
197. Georgakopoulos P (1974) Placenta accreta following lysis of uterine synechiae (Asherman's syn-

drome). J Obstet Gynaecol Br Commonw 81:730–733
198. Gersell DJ (1998) ASCP survey on placental examination. Am J Clin Pathol 109:127–143
199. Gersell DJ (1993) Chronic villitis, chronic chorioamnionitis and maternal floor infarction. Semin Diagn Pathol 10:251–266
200. Gersell DJ, Phillips NJ, Beckerman K (1991) Chronic chorioamnonitis: A clinicopathologic study of 17 cases. Int J Gynecol Pathol 10:217–229
201. Gerson AG, Wallace DM, Bridgens NK, et al (1987) Duplex Doppler ultrasound in the evaluation of growth in twin pregnancies. Obstet Gynecol 70: 419–423
202. Ghidini A, Sirtori M, Spelta A, et al (1991) Results of a preventive program for toxoplasmosis. J Reprod Med 36:270–273
203. Gibbs RS, Romero R, Hillier SL, Eschenbach DA, Sweet RL (1992) A review of premature birth and subclinical infections. Am J Obstet Gynecol 166: 1515–1528
204. Gillim DL, Hendricks CH (1953) Holoacardius. Review of the literature and case report. Obstet Gynecol 2:647–653
205. Gilstrap LC III, Cunningham FG (1979) The bacterial pathogenesis of infection following cesarean section. Obstet Gynecol 53:545–549
206. Girling J, De Sweit M (1998) Inherited thrombophilia and pregnancy. Curr Opin Obstet Gynecol 10:135–144
207. Glanfield PA, Watson R (1986) Intrauterine death due to umbilical cord torsion. Arch Pathol Lab Med 110:357–358
208. Glasser L, Delta BG (1971) Congenital toxoplasmosis with placental infection in monozygous twins. Curr Top Pathol 54:28–75.
209. Goddijn-Wessel TAW, Wouters MGAJ, Vd Molen EF, et al (1996) Hyperhomocysteinemia: a risk factor for placental abruption and infarction. Eur J Obstet Gynecol Reprod Biol 66:21–29
210. Goldenberg RL, Hauth JC, Andrews WW (2000) Intrauterine infection and preterm delivery. N Engl J Med 342:1500–1507
211. Goldenberg RL, Rouse DJ (1998) Prevention of premature birth. N Engl J Med 339:313–320
212. Goldstein LJ, Strenger R, King TC, et al (1995) Retrospective diagnosis of sickle cell-hemoglobin C disease and parvovirus infection by molecular DNA analysis of postmortem tissue. Hum Pathol 26: 1375–1378
213. Gomez R, Ghezzi F, Romero R, Munoz H, Tolosa JE, Rojas I (1995) Premature labor and intraamniotic infection. Clinical aspects and role of the cytokines in diagnosis and pathophysiology. Clin Perinatol 22:281–342
214. Gomez R, Romero R, Ghezzi F, et al (1998) The fetal inflammatory response syndrome. Am J Obstet Gynecol 179:194–202
215. Gonsoulin W, Moise KJ, Kirshon B, et al (1990) Outcome of twin-twin transfusion diagnosed before 28 weeks of gestation. Obstet Gynecol 75:214–216
216. Grafe MR, Benirschke K (1990) Ultrastructural study of the amniotic epithelium in a case of gastroschisis. Pediatr Pathol 10:95–101
217. Gray ML (1960) Genital listeriosis as a cause of repeated abortion. Lancet 2:315–317156
218. Greco MA, Wieczorek R, Sachdev R, Kaplan C, Nuovo GJ, Demopoulos RI (1992) Phenotype of villous stromal cells in placentas with cytomegalovirus, syphilis, and nonspecific villitis. Am J Pathol 141:835–842
219. Greenberg JA, Sorem KA, Shifren JL, Riley LE (1991) Placenta membranacea with placenta increta: a case report and literature review. Obstet Gynecol 78:512–514
220. Greenberg P, Collins JD, Voet RL, Jariwala L (1982) Ewing's sarcoma metastatic to placenta. Placenta 3:191–196
221. Greer IA (1999) Thrombosis in pregnancy: maternal and fetal issues. Lancet 353:1258–1265
222. Grether JK, Nelson KB (1997) Maternal infection and cerebral palsy in infants of normal birth weight. JAMA 278:207–211
223. Gruenwald P (1970) Environmental influences on twins apparent at birth. Biol Neonate 15:79–93
224. Gruenwald P, Levin H, Yousem H (1968) Abruption and premature separation of the placenta. The clinical and the pathologic entity. Am J Obstet Gynecol 102:604–610
225. Hallak M, Pryde PG, Qureshi F, Johnson MP, et al (1994) Constriction of the umbilical cord leading to fetal death: a report of three cases. J Reprod Med 39:561–565
226. Halliday HL, Hirata T (1979) Perinatal listeriosis—a review of twelve patients. Am J Obstet Gynecol 133:405–410
227. Hallman M (1999) Cytokines, pulmonary surfactant and consequences of intrauterine infection. Biol Neonate 76:2–9
228. Hanshaw JB (1973) Herpes virus hominis infections in the fetus and the newborn. Am J Dis Child 126:546–555
229. Harter CA, Benirschke K (1976) Fetal syphilis in the first trimester. Am J Obstet Gynecol 124:705–711
230. Hartwig NG, Vermeij-Keers C, DeVries HE, et al (1989) Limb body wall malformation complex: an embryologic etiology? Hum Pathol 20:1071–1077
231. Hartwig NG, Vermeij-Keers C, Van Elsacker-Neile VE, Fleuren GF (1989) Embryonic malformations in a case of intrauterine parvovirus B19 infection. Teratology 39:295–302
232. Haust MD (1981) Maternal diabetes mellitus: effects on the fetus and placenta. In: Perinatal diseases. International Academy of Pathology monograph no. 22. Williams & Wilkins, Baltimore, pp 201–285
233. Heifetz SA (1984) Single umbilical artery: a statistical analysis of 237 autopsy cases and review of the literature. Perspect Pediatr Pathol 8:345–378
234. Heifetz SA, Baumann M (1994) Necrotizing funisitis and herpes simplex infection of placental and decidual issues: study of four cases. Hum Pathol 25:715–719

235. Herva R, Karkinen-Jaaskelainen M (1984) Amnionic adhesion malformation syndrome: fetal and placental pathology. Teratology 29:11–19
236. Herva R, Rapola J, Rosti J, Karlson H (1980) Cluster of severe amniotic adhesion malformations in Finland. Lancet 1:818–819
237. Hibbard BM, Jeffcoate TNA (1966) Abruptio placentae. Obstet Gynecol 27:155–167
238. Higginbottom MC, Jones KL, Hall BD, Smith DW (1979) The amniotic band disruption complex: timing of amniotic rupture and variable spectra of consequent defects. J Pediatr 95:544–549
239. Hill GB (1993) Investigating the source of amniotic fluid isolates of *Fusobacteria.* Clin Infect Dis 16: S423–424
240. Hillier SL, Martius J, Krohn M, et al (1988) A case-control study of chorioamnionic infection and histologic chorioamnionitis in prematurity. N Engl J Med 319:972–978
241. Hohlfeld P, Daffos F, Thulliez P, et al (1989) Fetal toxoplasmosis: outcome of pregnancy and infant follow-up after in utero treatment. J Pediatr 115: 765–769
242. Hood IC, Desa DJ, Whyte RK (1983) The inflammatory response in candidal chorioamnionitis. Hum Pathol 14:984–990
243. Hood M (1961) Listeriosis as an infection of pregnancy manifested in the newborn. Pediatrics 27: 390–396
244. Hoshina M, Boothby M, Hussa R, et al (1985) Linkage of human chorionic gonadotrophin and placental lactogen biosynthesis to trophoblast differentiation and tumorigenesis. Placenta 6:163–172
245. Hoyme HE, Higginbottom MC, Jones KL (1981) Vascular etiology of disruptive structural defects in monozygotic twins. Pediatr 67:288–291
246. Hoyme HE, Jones KL, Allen MIV, Saunders BS, Benirschke K (1982) Vascular pathogenesis of transverse limb reduction defects. J Pediatr 101: 839–843
247. Hubbell JP, Muirhead DM, Drorbaugh JE (1965) The newborn infant of the diabetic mother. Med Clin North Am 49:1035–1052
248. Hung TH, Shau WY, Hsieh CC, et al. (1999) Risk factors for placenta accreta. Obstet Gynecol 93: 545–550
249. Hurley VA, Beischer NA (1987) Placenta membranacea. Case reports. Br J Obstet Gynaecol 94: 798–802
250. Hustin J, Gaspard U (1977) Comparison of histological changes seen in placental tissue cultures and in placentae obtained after fetal death. Br J Obstet Gynaecol 84:210–215
251. Hyde S, Smotherman J, Moore JI, Altshuler G (1989) A model of bacterially induced umbilical vein spasm, relevant to fetal hypoperfusion. Obstet Gynecol 73:996–970
252. Hyde SR, Altshuler G (1999) Infectious disorders of the placenta. In: Lewis SH, Perrin E (eds) Pathology of the placenta, 2nd Ed. Churchill Livingstone, New York, pp 317–342
253. Hyde SR, Benirschke K (1997) Gestational psittacosis: case report and literature review. Mod Pathol 10:602–607
254. Hyde SR, Giacoia GP (1993) Congenital herpes infection: placental and umbilical cord findings. Obstet Gynecol 81:852–855
255. Ibdah JA, Bennett MJ, Rinaldo P, et al (1999) A fetal fatty acid oxydation disorder as a cause of liver disease in pregnant women. N Engl J Med 340: 1723–1731
256. Iralu JV, Roberts D, Kazanjian PH (1993) Chorioamnionitis caused by capnocytophaga: case report and review. Clin Infect Dis 17:457–461
257. Irving FL, Hertig AT (1937) A study of placenta accreta. Surg Gynecol Obstet 64:178
258. Iyasu S, Saftlas AK, Rowley DL et al (1993) The epidemiology of placenta previa in the United States, 1979 through 1987. Am J Obstet Gynecol 168:1424–1449
259. Jacques SM, Qureshi F (1993) Chronic intervillositis of the placenta. Arch Pathol Lab Med 117: 1032–1035
260. Jacques SM, Qureshi F (1994) Chronic villitis of unknown etiology in twin gestations. Ped Pathol 14: 575–584
261. Jacques SM, Qureshi F, Trent VS, Ramirez NC (1996) Placenta accreta: mild cases diagnosed by placental examination. Int J Gynecol Pathol 15:28–33
262. Jacques SM, Qureshi F (1998) Chronic chorioamnionitis: a clinicopathologic and immunohistochemical study. Hum Pathol 29:1457–1461
263. Jauniaux E, Nessmann C, Imbert C, et al (1988) Morphological aspects of the placenta in HIV pregnancies. Placenta 9:633–642
264. Jimenes E, Unger M, Eitelbach F, et al (1989) Demonstration of HIV-antigens in birth placentae and therapeutic abortions. Placenta 10:467
265. Johnson GM, Tudor RB (1970) Diabetes mellitus and congenital rubella infection. Am J Dis Child 120:453–455
266. Johnstone BH, Benirschke K (1975) Monozygotic twins discordant for urinary tract anomalies and presenting as hydramnios. Obstet Gynecol 47:610–615
267. Jones CJP, Lendon M, Chawner LE, Jauniauz E (1990) Ultrastructure of the human placenta in metabolic storage disease. Placenta 11:395–411
268. Jones CJP, Fox H (1976) Placental changes in gestational diabetes. An ultrastructural study. Obstet Gynecol 48:274–280
269. Jones CJP, Fox H (1976) An ultrastructural and ultrahistochemical study of the placenta of the diabetic woman. J Pathol 119:91–99
270. Jones CJP, Fox H (1978) An ultrastructural study of the placenta in materno-fetal Rhesus incompatibility. Virchows Arch [A Pathol Anat] 379:229–241
271. Jones CJP, Fox H (1980) An ultrastructural and ultrahistochemical study of the human placenta in maternal pre-eclampsia. Placenta 1:61–76
272. Jones CJP, Fox H (1981) An ultrastructural and

ultrahistochemical study of the human placenta in maternal essential hypertension. Placenta 2:193–204
273. Jones CJP, Lendon M, Chawner LE, Jauniauz E (1990) Ultrastructure of the human placenta in metabolic storage disease. Placenta 11:395–411
274. Jones KL, Benirschke K (1983) The developmental pathogenesis of structural defects: the contribution of monozygotic twins. Semin Perinatol 7:239–243
275. Kalousek DK, Barrett I (1994) Confined placental mosaicism and stillbirth. Pediatr Pathol 14:151–159
276. Kalousek DK (1987) Anatomic and chromosomal anomalies in specimens of early spontaneous abortion: seven years experience. Birth Defects 23:153–168
277. Kalousek DK (1991) Pathology of abortion. In: Kraus FT, Danjanov I, Kaufman N (eds) Pathology of reproductive failure. Williams & Wilkins, Baltimore, pp 228–256
278. Kalousek DK (1957) Pathology abortion. In: Gilbert-Barness E (ed) Potter's pathology of the fetus and infant. Mosby, St. Louis
279. Kalousek DK, Fitch N, Paradice (1990) Pathology of the human embryo and previable fetus. An atlas. Springer, New York
280. Kalousek DK, Bamforth S (1988) Amnion rupture sequence in previable fetuses. Am J Med Genet 31:63–73
281. Kaplan CG (1993) The placenta and viral infections. Semin Diagn Pathol 10:232–250
282. Kaplan C, Blanc WA, Elias J (1982) Identification of erythrocytes in intervillous thrombi. A study using immunoperoxidase identification of hemoglobins. Hum Pathol 13:554–557
283. Karegard M, Gennser G (1986) Incidence and recurrence rate of abruptio placentae in Sweden. Obstet Gynecol 67:523–528
284. Kaspar HG, Kraemer BB, Kraus FT (1998) DNA ploidy by image cytometry and karyotype analysis in spontaneous abortion. Hum Pathol 29:1013–1016
285. Keep D, Zaragoza MV, Hassold T, Redline RW (1996) Very early complete mole. Hum Pathol 27: 708–713
286. Keenan WJ, Steichen JJ, Mahmood K, Altshuler G (1977) Placental pathology compared with clinical outcome. Am J Dis Child 131:1224–1227
287. Khong TY (1991) Acute atherosis in pregnancies complicated by hypertension, small-for-gestational-age infants, and diabetes mellitus. Arch Pathol Lab Med 115:722–725
288. Khong TY (1999) The placenta in maternal hyperhomocysteinaemia. Br J Obstet Gynaecol 106: 2733–2738
289. Khong TY, Robertson WB (1987) Placenta creta and placenta praevia creta. Placenta 8:399–409
290. Kinney JS, Anderson LJ, Farrar J, et al (1988) Risk of adverse outcome after human parvovirus B19 infection. J Infect Dis 157:663–667
291. Kitzmiller JL, Watt N, Driscoll SG (1981) Decidual arteriopathy in hypertension and diabetes in pregnancy: immunofluorescent studies. Am J Obstet Gynecol 141:733–779
292. Klatt EC, Pavlova Z, Teberg AJ, Yonekura ML (1986) Epidemic perinatal listeriosis at autopsy. Hum Pathol 17:1278–1281
293. Knisely AS, O'Shea PA, McMillan P, Singer DB, Magid MA (1988) Electron microscopic identification of parvovirus virions in erythroid-line cells in fatal hydrops fetalis. Pediatr Pathol 8:163–170
294. Knox TA, Olans LB (1996) Liver disease in pregnancy. N Engl J Med 335:569–576
295. Knox WF, Fox H (1984) Villitis of unknown aetiology: Its incidence and significance in placentae from a British population. Placenta 5:395–402
296. Koelfen W, Freund M, Varnholt W (1995) Neonatal stroke involving the middle cerebral artery in term infants: clinical presentation, EEG and imaging studies, outcome. Dev Med Child Neurol 37: 204–212
297. Korbage de Araujo MC, Schultz R, Costa Vaz FA, et al (1994) A case-control study of histological chorioamnionitis and neonatal infection. Early Hum Dev 40:51–58
298. Koshy M, Burd L, Wallace D, et al (1988) Prophylactic red-cell transfusions in pregnant patients with sickle cell disease. N Engl J Med 319:1447–1452
299. Koskimiemi M, Lappalainen M, Hedman K (1989) Toxoplasmosis needs evaluation. Am J Dis Child 143:724–728
300. Kraemer BB, Kraus FT, Sheldon G (1985) Expression of pregnancy-specific proteins in maternal diabetes. An immunocytochemical study of placental bed biopsies and placental tissues. Lab Invest 52:37A
301. Kramer MS, Usher RH, Pollack R, Boyd M, Usher S (1997) Etiologic determinants of abruptio placentae. Obstet Gynecol 89:221–226
302. Kraus FT (1997) Cerebral palsy and thrombi in placental vessels of the fetus: insights from litigation. Hum Pathol 28:246–248
303. Kraus FT, Acheen VI (1999) Fetal thrombotic vasculopathy in the placenta: cerebral thrombi and infarcts, coagulopathies, and cerebral palsy. Hum Pathol 30:759–769
304. Kraus FT (1993) Placental thrombi and related problems. Semin Diagn Pathol 10:275–283
305. Kraus FT (1991) Role of the pathologist in evaluation of infertility: current practice and future developments. In: Kraus FT, Damjanov I, Kaufman N (eds) Pathology of reproductive failure. Williams & Wilkins, Baltimore p 339
306. Kristoffersen K (1969) The significance of absence of one umbilical artery. Acta Obstet Gynecol Scand 48:195–214
307. Kupferminc MJ, Eldor A, Steinman N, et al (1999) Increased frequency of genetic thrombophilia in women with complications of pregnancy. New Engl J Med 340:9–13

308. Kupferminc MJ, Fait C, Mauy A, et al. Severe preeclampsia and high frequency of genetic thrombophilia. Obstet Gynecol 2000;96:45–49
309. Kurman RJ, Main CS, Chen H-C (1984) Intermediate trophoblast: a distinctive form of trophoblast with specific morphological, biochemical and functional features. Placenta 5:349–370
310. Kurman RJ, Young RH, Norris HJ, et al (1984) Immunocytochemical localization of placental lactogen and chorionic gonadotropin in the normal placenta and trophoblastic tumors, with emphasis on intermediate trophoblast and the placental site trophoblastic tumor. Int J Gynecol Pathol 3:101–121
311. Kurtin PJ, Gaffey TA, Habermann TM (1992) Peripheral T-cell lymphoma involving the placenta. Cancer (Phila) 70:2963–2968
312. LaBarrere C, Althabe O, Telenta M (1982) Chronic villitis of unknown aetiology in placentae of idiopathic small for gestational age infants. Placenta 3:309–318
313. LaBarrere C, Althabe O (1987) Chronic villitis of unknown aetiology in recurrent intrauterine fetal growth retardation. Placenta 8:167–173
314. Labarrere C, Sebastiani M, Siminovich M, et al (1985) Absence of Wharton's jelly around the umbilical arteries: an unusual cause of perinatal mortality. Placenta 6:555–559
315. LaBarrere C, McIntyre JA, Faulk WP (1990) Immunohistologic evidence that villitis in human normal term placentas is an immunologic lesion. Am J Obstet Gynecol 162:515–522
316. Lademacher DS, Vermeulen RCW, Harten JJ, Arts NF (1981) Circumvallate placenta and congenital malformation. Lancet 1:732
317. Lage JM, VanMarter LJ, Bieber FR (1988) Questionable role of amniocentesis in the etiology of amniotic band formation. J Reprod Med 33:71–73
318. Lage JM, Mark SD, Roberts DJ, et al (1992) A flow cytometric study of 137 fresh hydropic placentas: correlation between types of hydatidiform moles and nuclear DNA ploidy. Obstet Gynecol 79:403–410
319. Lage JM, Vanmarter LJ, Mikhail E (1989) Vascular anastomoses in fused, dichorionic twin placentas resulting in twin transfusion syndrome. Placenta 10:55–59
320. Langer H (1963) Repeated congenital infection with *Toxoplasma gondii*. Obstet Gynecol 21:318–329
321. Lauweryns J, Bernat R, Lerut A, Detournay G (1973) Intrauterine pneumonia. An experimental study. Biol Neonate 22:301–318
322. Lawler FC, Wood WS, King S, Metzger W (1964) Listeria monocytogenes as a cause of fetal loss. Am J Obstet Gynecol 89:915–923
323. Legro RS, Price FV, Hill LM, Caritis SN (1994) Nonsurgical management of placenta percreta: a case report. Obstet Gynecol 83:847–849
324. Levy SR, Abroms IF, Marshall PC, Rosquete EE (1985) Seizures and cerebral infarctions in the full term newborn. Ann Neurol 17:366–370
325. Lewis SH, Reynolds-Kohler C, Fox HE, Nelson JA (1990) HIV-1 in trophoblastic and villous Hofbauer cells, and haematologic precursors in eight-week fetuses. Lancet 1:565–568
326. Lissak A, Sharon A, Fruchter A, et al (1999) Polymorphism for mutation of cytosine to thymine at location 677 in the methylenetetrahydrofolate reductase gene is associated with recurrent early fetal loss. Am J Obstet Gynecol 181:126–130
327. Liu S, Benirschke K, Scioscia AL, Maunino FL (1992) Intrauterine death in multiple gestation. Acta Genet Med Gemellol 41:5–26
328. Lockwood C, Ghidini A, Romero R, Hobbins JC (1989) Amniotic band syndrome: Reevaluation of its pathogenesis. Am J Obstet Gynecol 160:1030–1033
329. Lopriore E, Vandenbussche FP, Tiersma ES, de Beaufort AJ, de Leeuw JP (1995) Twin-to-twin transfusion syndrome: new perspectives. J Pediatr 127:675–680
330. Lunell NO, Nylund LE, Lewander R, et al (1982) Uteroplacental blood flow in pre-eclampsia measurements with indium-113m and a computer-linked gamma camera. Clin Exp Hyper-Hyper Preg B1(1), 105–117
331. Machin GA (1989) Hydrops revisited: literature review of 1414 cases published in the 1980's. Am J Med Genet 34:366–378
332. Machin GA (1981) Differential diagnosis of hydrops fetalis. Am J Med Genet 9:341–350
333. Magid MS, Kaplan C, Sammaritano LR, Peterson M, Druzin ML, Lockshin MD (1998) Placental pathology in systemic lupus erythematosis: A prospective study. Am J Obstet Gynecol 179:226–236
334. Maidman JE, Yeager C, Anderson V, et al (1980) Prenatal diagnosis and management of nonimmunologic hydrops fetalis. Obstet Gynecol 56:571–576
335. Majlessi HF, Wagner KM, Brooks JJ (1983) Atypical cellular chorangioma of the placenta. Int J Gynecol Pathol 1:403–408
336. Mandel H, Brenner B, Berant M, et (1996) al. Coexistence of hereditary homocystinuria and factor V Lieden: effect on thrombosis. N Engl J Med 334:763–768
337. Martin AE, Brady K, Smith SI, et al (1992) Immunohistochemical localization of human immunodeficiency virus p24 antigen in placental tissue. Hum Pathol 23:411–414
338. Martin DH, Koutsky L, Eschenbach DA, et al (1982) Prematurity and perinatal mortality in pregnancies complicated by maternal Chlamydia trachomatis infections. JAMA 247:1585–1588
339. Mattern CFT, Murray K, Jensen A, et al (1992) Localization of human immunodeficiency virus core antigen in term human placentas. Pediatrics 89: 207–209
340. Maudsley RF, Brix GA, Hinton NA, et al (1966) Placental inflammation and infection. A prospective

bacteriologic and histologic study. Am J Obstet Gynecol 95:648–659
341. Mazor M, Chaim W, Horowitz S, Romero R, Glezerman M (1994) The biomolecular mechanisms of preterm labor in women with intrauterine infection. Isr J Med Sci 30:317–322
342. Mazor M, Chaim W, Shinwell ES, Glezerman M (1993) Asymptomatic amniotic fluid invasion with *Candida albicans* in preterm premature rupture of membranes. Acta Obstet Gynecol Scand 72:52–54
343. McConnell HD, Carr DH (1975) Recent advances in the cytogenetic study of human spontaneous abortions. Obstet Gynecol 45:547–552
344. McIntosh K (1990) Congenital syphilis-breaking through the safety net. N Engl J Med 323:1339–1341
345. McKeogh RP, D'Errico E (1951) Placenta accreta: clinical manifestations and conservative management. N Engl J Med 245:159–165
346. McLennan H, Price E, Urbanska M, Craig N, Fraser M (1988) Umbilical cord knots and encirclements. Aust NZJ Obstet Gynaecol 28:116–119
347. Megurian-Bedoyan Z, Lamant L, Hoptner C, et al (1997) Anaplastic large cell lymphoma of maternal origin involving the placenta: case report and literature survey. Am J Surg Pathol 21:1236–1241
348. Menser MA, Forrest JM, Bransby RD (1978) Rubella infection and diabetes mellitus. Lancet 1: 57–60
349. Meyer A, Stallmach T, Goldengert D, Altwegg M (1997) Lethal maternal sepsis caused by *Campylobacter jejuni*: pathogen preserved in placenta and identified by molecular methods. Mod Pathol 10: 1253–1256
350. Meyer B (1955) Placenta accreta. An analysis based on an unusual case. Acta Obstet Gynecol Scand 34:189–201
351. Miller DA, Chollet JA, Goodwin TM (1997) Clinical risk factors for placenta previa-placenta accreta. Am J Obstet Gynecol 177:210–214
352. Miller JM, Pupkin MJ, Hill GB (1980) Bacterial colonization of amniotic fluid from intact fetal membranes. Am J Obstet Gynecol 136:796–804
353. Miller ME, Higginbottom M, Smith DW (1981) Short umbilical cord: Its origin and relevance. Pediatrics 67:618–621
354. Miller ME, Graham JM Jr, Higginbottom MC, Smith DW (1981) Compression-related defects from early amnion rupture: evidence for mechanical teratogenesis. J Pediatr 98:292–297
355. Miller ME, Jones MC, Smith DW (1982) Tension: the basis of umbilical cord growth. J Pediatr 101: 844
356. Miller PW, Coen RW, Benirschke K (1985) Dating the time interval from meconium passage to birth. Obstet Gynecol 66:459–462
357. Mills JL, Harley EE, Moessinger AC (1983) Standards for measuring umbilical cord length. Placenta 4:423–426
358. Milner PF, Jones BR, Dobler J (1980) Outcome of pregnancy in sickle cell anemia and sickle cell-hemoglobin C disease. An analysis of 181 pregnancies in 98 patients, and a review of the literature. Am J Obstet Gynecol 138:239–245
359. Minguillon C, Eiben B, Bahr-Porsch S, et al (1989) The predictive value of chorionic villus histology for identifying chromosomally normal and abnormal spontaneous abortions. Hum Genet 82:373–376
360. Minkoff H, Nanda D, Menez R, Fikrig S (1987) Pregnancies resulting in infants with acquired immunodeficiency syndrome or AIDS-related complex. Obstet Gynecol 69:285–287
361. Moessinger AC, Blanc WA, Byrne J, et al (1981) Amniotic band syndrome associated with amniocentesis. Am J Obstet Gynecol 141:588–591
362. Moessinger AC, Blanc WA, Marone PS, Polsen DC (1982) Umbilical cord length as an index of fetal activity: Experimental study and clinical implications. Pediatr Res 16:109–112
363. Molnar-Nadasdy G, Haesly I, Reed J, Altshuler G (1994) Placental cryptococcosis in a mother with systemic lupus erythematosus. Arch Pathol Lab Med 118:757–759
364. Monie IW (1965) Velamentous insertion of the cord in early pregnancy. Am J Obstet Gynecol 93:276–281
365. Monif GRG, Dische RM (1972) Viral placentitis in congenital cytomegalovirus infection. Am J Clin Pathol 58:445–449
366. Montgomery JR, Flanders RW, Yow MD (1973) Congenital anomalies and herpes virus infection. Am J Dis Child 126:364–366
367. Mooney EE, Shunnar AA, O'Regan M, Gillan JE (1994) Chorionic villous hemorrhage is associated with retroplacental hemorrhage. Br J Obstet Gynecol 101;965–969
368. Moreman P, Fryns JP, Vandenberghe K, Lauweryns JM (1992) Constrictive amniotic bands, amniotic adhesions and limb-body wall complex: discrete disruption sequences with pathogenetic overlap. Am J Med Genet 42:470–479
369. Morey AL, Keeling JW, Porter HJ, Fleming KA (1992) Clinical and histopathological features of parvovirus B19 infection in the human fetus. Fetal Neonat Med 99:566–574
370. Morison JE (1978) Placenta accreta: a clinicopathologic review of 67 cases. Obstet Gynecol Annu 7:107–123
371. Mosher R, Genest D (1998) Early complete hydatidiform mole. Prevalence, histopathology, and persistence. Mod Pathol 11:109
372. Mostoufi-Zadeh M, Driscoll SG, Biano SA, Kundsin RB (1984) Placental evidence of cytomegalovirus infection of the fetus and neonate. Arch Pathol Lab Med 108:403–406
373. Mostoufi-Zadeh M, Weiss LM, Driscoll SG (1985) Non-immune hydrops fetalis. A challenge in perinatal pathology. Hum Pathol 16:785–789
374. Mucitelli DR, Charles EZ, Kraus FT (1990) Chor-

angiomas of intermediate size and intrauterine growth retrdation. Pathol Res Pract 186:455–458
375. Muhlemann K, Miller RK, Metlay L, Menegus MA (1992) Cytomegalovirus infection of the human placenta: an immunocytochemical study. Hum Pathol 23:1234–1237
376. Munn DH, Zhou M, Attwood JT, et al (1998) Prevention of fetal rejection by tryptophan catabolism. Science 281:1191–1193
377. Naeye RL (1995) Can meconium in the amnionic fluid injure the fetal brain? Obstet Gynecol 86:720–724
378. Naeye RL (1975) Causes and consequences of chorioamnionitis. N Engl J Med 293:40–41
379. Naeye RL (1977) Causes of perinatal mortality in the U.S. Collaborative Perinatal Project. JAMA 238: 228–229
380. Naeye RL (1979) Coitus and associated amniotic-fluid infections. N Engl J Med 301:1198–1200
381. Naeye RL (1980) Factors in the mother/infant dyad that influence the development of infections before and after birth. Excerpta Med Ciba Found Symp 77:3–16
382. Naeye RL (1963) Human intrauterine parabiotic syndrome and its complications. N Engl J Med 268: 804–809
383. Naeye RL (1985) Umbilical cord length: clinical significance. J Pediatr 107:278–281
384. Naeye RL (1985) Maternal floor infarction. Hum Pathol 16:823–828
385. Naeye RL (1989) Pregnancy hypertension, placental evidence of low uteroplacental blood flow, and spontaneous premature delivery. Hum Pathol 20: 441–444
386. Naeye RL (1990) The clinical significance of absent subchorionic fibrin in the placenta. Am J Clin Pathol 94:196–198
387. Naeye RL Acute chorioamnionitis and the disorders that produce placental insufficiency. In: Kraus FT, Damjanov I, Kaufman N (eds) Pathology of reproductive failure. Williams & Wilkins, Baltimore, p 293
388. Naeye RL, Blanc W (1965) Pathogenesis of congenital rubella. JAMA 194:109–115
389. Naeye RL, Blanc WL (1970) Relation of poverty and race to antenatal infection. N Engl J Med 283:555–560
390. Naeye RL, Peters EC (1978) Amniotic fluid infections with intact membranes leading to perinatal death: a prospective study. Pediatrics 61:171–177
391. Naeye RL, Peters EC (1980) Causes and consequences of premature rupture of fetal membranes. Lancet 1:192–194
392. Naeye RL, Dellinger WS, Blanc WA (1971) Fetal and maternal features of antenatal bacterial infections. J Pediatr 79:733–739
393. Naeye RL, Maisels J, Lorenz RP, Botti JJ (1983) The clinical significance of placental villous edema. Pediatrics 71:588–594
394. Naeye RL, Tafari N, Judge D, et al (1977) Amniotic fluid infections in an African city. J Pediatr 90: 965–970
395. Naftolin F, Khudr G, Benirschke K, Hutchinson DL (1973) The syndrome of chronic abruptio placentae, hydrorrhea, and circumvallate placenta. Am J Obstet Gynecol 116:347–350
396. Nahmias AJ, Alford CA, Korones SB (1970) Infection of the newborn with herpes virus hominis. Adv Pediatr 17:185–226
397. Nahmias AJ, Josey WE, Naib ZM, et al (1971) Perinatal risk associated with maternal genital herpes simplex virus infection. Am J Obstet Gynecol 110: 825–837
398. Naib ZM, Nahmias AJ, Josey WE, Wheeler JH (1970) Association of maternal genital herpetic infection with spontaneous abortion. Obstet Gynecol 35:260–263
399. Napolitani FD, Schreiber I (1960) The acardiac monster. A review of the world literature and presentation of 2 cases. Am J Obstet Gynecol 80:582–589
400. Nathan L, Leveno KJ, Carmody TJ 3rd, Kelly MA, Sherman ML (1994) Meconium: a 1990's perspective on an old obstetric hazard. Obstet Gynecol 83:329–32
401. Navarrete VN, Torres IH, Rivera IR, et al (1967) Maternal carbohydrate disorder and congenital malformations. Diabetes 16:127–130
402. Navarro C, Blanc WA (1977) Chronic viral funisitis. J Pediatr 91:967–973
403. Nayar R, Lage JM (1996) Placental changes in a first trimester missed abortion in maternal systemic lupus erythematosis with antiphospholipid syndrome: a case report and review of the literature. Hum Pathol 27:201–206
404. Nelson DM (1996) Apoptotic changes occur in syncytiotrophoblast of human placental villi where fibrin type fibrinoid is deposited in discontinuities in the villous trophoblast. Placenta 17:387–391
405. Nelson KB, Dambrosia JM, Grether JK, Phillips TM (1998) Neonatal cytokines and coagulation factors in children with cerebral palsy. Ann Neurol 44: 665–675
406. Nelson KB, Grether KJ (1998) Potentially asphyxiating conditions and spastic cerebral palsy in infants of normal birth weight. Am J Obstet Gynecol 179;507–513
407. Nilsson IM, Astedt B, Hedner U, Berezin D (1975) Intrauterine death and circulating anticoagulant ("antithromboplastin"). Acta Med Scand 197:153–159
408. Nordenvall M, Sandstedt B (1990) Placental villitis and intrauterine growth retardation in a Swedish population. APMIS 98:19–24
409. Ordi J, Ismail MR, Ventura PJ, et al (1998) Massive chronic intervillositis of the placenta associated with malaria infection. Am J Surg Pathol 22: 1006–1011
410. Ornoy A, Segal S, Nishmi M, et al (1973) Fetal and placental pathology in gestational rubella. Am J Obstet Gynecol 116:949–956

411. Ozono K, Mushiake S, Takeshima T, Nakayama M (1997) Diagnosis of congenital cytomegalovirus infection by examination of placenta: application of polymerase chain reaction and in situ hybridization. Pediatr Pathol Lab Med 17:249–258
412. Pankuch GA, Applebaum PC, Lorenz RP, et al (1983) Placental microbiology in the diagnosis of chorioamnionitis. Abstracts of the annual meeting of American Society for Microbiology. American Society for Microbiology, Washington, DC, p 319
413. Parkash V, Morohi RA, Jorlin V, Cartun R, Rauch C, West AB (1998) Immunohistochemical reflection of *Listeria* antigens in the placenta in prenatal listeriosis. Int J Gynecol Pathol 17:343–350
414. Parry S, Strauss JF (1998) Premature rupture of the fetal membranes. N Engl J Med 338:663–670
415. Pastorek JG II, Seiler B (1985) Maternal death associated with sickle cell trait. Am J Obstet Gynecol 152:295–297
416. Pauls F (1969) Monoamniotic twin pregnancy: a review of the world literature and a report of two new cases. Can Med Assoc J 100:254–256
417. Peckham C, Gibbs D (1995) Mother-to-child transmission of the human immunodeficiency virus. N Engl J Med 333:298–302
418. Peckham CH, Yerushalmy J (1965) Aplasia of one umbilical artery: incidence by race and certain obstetric factors. Obstet Gynecol 26:359–366
419. Pedersen LM, Tygstrup I, Pedersen J (1964) Congenital malformations in newborn infants of diabetic women. Correlation with maternal diabetic vascular complications. Lancet 1:1124–1126
420. Petrikovsky BM, Schneider E, Smith-Leviton M, Gross B (1998) Cephalhematoma and caput succedaneum: do they always occur in labor? Am J Obstet Gynecol 179:906–908
421. Petrilli ES, D'Ablaing G, Ledger WJ (1980) *Listeria monocytogenes* chorioamnionitis: diagnosis by transabdominal amniocentesis. Obstet Gynecol 55s:5–8
422. Pezeshkian R, Fernando N, Carne CA, Simanowita MD (1984) Listeriosis in mother and fetus during the first trimester of pregnancy. Case report. Br J Obstet Gynaecol 91:85–86
423. Pijnenborg R, Bland JM, Robertson WB, Brosens I (1983) Uteroplacental arterial changes related to interstitial trophoblast migration in early human pregnancy. Placenta 4:397–414
424. Pinkerton JHM (1963) The placental bed arterioles in diabetes. Proc R Soc Med 56:1021–1022
425. Platt HS (1971) Effect of maternal sickle cell trait on perinatal mortality. Br Med J 4:334–336
426. Pollack RN, Sklarin NT, Rao S, Divon MY (1993) Metastatic placental lymphoma associated with maternal immunodeficiency virus infection. Obstet Gynecol 81:856–857
427. Popek EJ (1992) Granulomatous villitis due to toxoplasma gondii. Pediatr Pathol 12:281–288
428. Porter HJ, Khong TY, Evans MF, et al (1988) Parvovirus as a cause of hydrops fetalis: detection by in situ DNA hybridization. J Clin Pathol 41:381–383
429. Potter JF, Schoeneman M (1970) Metastasis of maternal cancer to the placenta and fetus. Cancer (Phila) 25:380–388
430. Powars DR, Sandhu M, Niland-Weiss J, et al (1986) Pregnancy in sickle cell disease. Obstet Gynecol 67: 217–228
431. Powers RW, Evans RW, Majors AK et al (1998) Plasma homocysteine concentration is increased in preecalmpsia and is associated with evidence of endothelial activation. Am J Obstet Gynecol 179:605–611
432. Prengler M, Sturt N, Flanagan M, et al (1998) The homozygous thermolabile variant of the methylenetetrahydrofolate reductase gene: a risk factor for cerebrovascular disease and stroke in childhood. Dev Med Child Neurol 40(suppl 79):10–11
433. Pretorius DH, Manchester D, Barkin S, et al (1988) Doppler ultrasound of twin transfusion syndrome. J Ultrasound Med 7:117–124
434. Public Health Laboratory Service Working Party on Fifth Disease (1990) Prospective study of human parvovirus (B19) infection in pregnancy. Br Med J 300:1166–1170
435. Quinn PA, Butany J, Taylor J, Hannah W (1987) Chorioamnionitis: its association with pregnancy outcome and microbial infection. Am J Obstet Gynecol 156:379–387
436. Qureshi F, Jacques SM, Reyes MP (1993) Placental histopathology in syphilis. Hum Pathol 24:779–784
437. Qureshi F, Jacques SM, Bendon RW, et al (1998) Candida funisitis: A clinicopathologic study of 32 cases. Pediatr Dev Pathol 1:118–124
438. Qureshi F, Jacques S (1996) Maternal varicella during pregnancy: correlation of maternal history and fetal outcome withplacental histopathology. Hum Pathol 27:191–195
439. Ramin KD, Leveno KJ, Kelly MA, Carmody TJ (1996) Amnionic fluid meconium: a fetal environmental hazard. Obstet Gynecol 87:181–184
440. Rana J, Ebert GA, Kappy KA (1995) Adverse perinatal outcome in patients with an abnormal umbilical coiling index. Obstet Gynecol 85:573–577
441. Rappaport F, Rabinovitz M, Toaff R, Krochik N (1960) Genital listeriosis as a cause of repeated abortion. Lancet 1:1273–1275
442. Rausen AR, Seki M, Strauss L (1965) Twin transfusion syndrome. A review of 19 cases studied at one institution. J Pediatr 66:613–628
443. Ray CG, Wedgwood RJ (1964) Neonatal listeriosis. Six case reports and a review of the literature. Pediatrics 34:378–392
444. Rayne SC, Kraus FT (1993) Placental thrombi and other vascular lesions. Classification, morphology, and clinical correlations. Pathol Res Pract 189:2–17
445. Redline RW (1999) Disorders of the placental parenchyma. In: Lewis SH, Perin E (eds) Pathology of the placenta. Churchill Livingstone, New York, pp 161–184
446. Redline RW (1996) Recurrent villitis of bacterial etiology. Pediatr Pathol Lab Med 16:995–1001

447. Redline RW (1988) Role of local immunosuppression in murine fetoplacental listeriosis. J Clin Invest 79:1234–1241
448. Redline RW (1988) Specific defects in the anti-listerial immune response in discrete regions of the murine uterus and placenta account for susceptibility to infection. J Immunol 140:3947–3955
449. Redline RW (1988) Defective anti-listerial responses in deciduoma of pseudopregnant mice. Am J Pathol 133:485–497
450. Redline RW, Abramowsky CR (1985) Clinical and pathologic aspects of recurrent placental villitis. Hum Pathol 16:727–731
451. Redline RW, Pappin A (1995) Fetal thrombotic vasculopathy: the clinical significance of extensive avascular villi. Hum Pathol 26:80–85
452. Redline R, Patterson R (1993) Villitis of unknown etiology is associated with major infiltration of fetal tissues by maternal cells. Am J Pathol 143:332–336
453. Redline RW, Patterson P (1994) Patterns of placental injury; correlation with gestational age, placental weight, and clinical diagnosis. Arch Pathol Lab Med 118:698–701
454. Redline RW, Patterson P (1995) Preeclampsia is associated with an excess of proliferative immature intermediate trophoblast. Hum Pathol 26:594–600
455. Redline RW, Wilson-Costello D, Borawski E, Fanaroff AA, Hack M (1998) Placental lesions associated with neurologic impairment and cerebral palsy in very low birth weight infants. Arch Pathol Lab Med 122:1091–1098
456. Redline RW, Zaragoza M, Hassold T (1999) Prevalence of developmental and inflammatory lesions in nonmolar first-trimester spontaneous abortions. Hum Pathol 30:93–100
457. Rehder H, Coerdt W, Eggers R, et al (1989) Is there a correlation between morphological and cytogenetic findings in placental tissue from early missed abortions. Hum Genet 82:337–385
458. Rehder H, Weitzel H (1978) Intrauterine amputations after amniocentesis. Lancet 1:382
459. Renaer M, Van de Putte I, Vermylen C (1976) Massive feto-maternal hemorrhage as a cause of perinatal mortality and morbidity. Eur J Obstet Gynecol Reprod Biol 6:125–140
460. Rewell RE, Whitehouse WL (1966) Malignant metastasis to the placenta from carcinoma of the breast. J Pathol 91:255–256
461. Rimer BA (1975) Sickle-cell trait and pregnancy: a review of a community hospital experience. Am J Obstet Gynecol 123:6–11
462. Robertson EG, Neer KJ (1983) Placental injection studies in twin gestation. Am J Obstet Gynecol 147:170–174
463. Robertson NJ, McKeever PA (1992) Fetal placental pathology in two cases of maternal varicella infection. Pediatr Pathol 12:545–550
464. Robertson WG (1976) Uteroplacental vasculature. J Clin Pathol (Suppl) 10:9–17
465. Robertson WB, Brosens I, Dixon G (1975) Uteroplacental vascular pathology. Eur J Obstet Gynecol Reprod Biol 5:47–65
466. Robertson WB, Khong TY, Brosen I, et al (1986) The placental bed biopsy: review from three European centers. Am J Obstet Gynecol 155:401–412
467. Robinson LK, Jones KL, Benirschke K (1983) The nature of structural defects associated with velamentous and marginal insertion of the umbilical cord. Am J Obstet Gynecol 146:191–193
468. Rocklin RE, Kitzmiller VL, Carpenter CB, et al (1976) Maternal-fetal relation. Absence of an immunologic blocking factor from the serum of women with chronic abortions. N Engl J Med 295: 1209–1213
469. Rogers MF, Ou C-Y, Rayfield M, et al (1989) Use of the polymerase chain reaction for early detection of the proviral sequences of human immunodeficiency virus in infants born to seropositive mothers. N Engl J Med 320:1649–1654
470. Rogers MF, Shafer N (1999) Reducing the risk of maternal-infant transmission of HIV by attacking the virus. N Engl J Med 341:441–443
471. Rolschau J (1978) Circumvallate placenta and intrauterine growth retardation. Acta Obstet Gynecol Scand 72:11–14
472. Rolschau J (1978) The significance of different forms of placentitis. Acta Obstet Gynecol Scand 72 (suppl):5–10
473. Romero R, Gomez R, Ghezzi F et al (1998) A fetal systemic inflammatory response is followed by the spontaneous onset of preterm parturition. Am J Obstet Gynecol 179:186–193
474. Ross SM, MacPherson T, Wallace J, et al (1978) Unsuccessful pregnancies—report on 200 perinatal postmortems. S Afr Med J 53:828–829
475. Rusin P, Adam RD, Petersen EA, et al (1991) *Haemophilus influenzae*: an important cause of maternal and neonatal infections. Obstet Gynecol 77: 92–96
476. Russell P (1979) Inflammatory lesions of the human placenta I. Am J Diagn Gynecol Obstet 1:127–137
477. Russell P (1979) Inflammatory lesions of the human placenta II. Villitis of unknown etiology in perspective. Am J Diagn Gynecol Obstet 1:339–346
478. Russell P (1980) Inflammatory lesions of the human placenta. III. The histopathology of villitis of unknown etiology. Placenta 1:227–244
479. Russell P, Altshuler G (1974) Placental abnormalities of congenital syphilis. A neglected aid to diagnosis. Am J Dis Child 128:160–163
480. Russell P, Atkinson K, Krishnan L (1980) Recurrent reproductive failure due to severe placental villitis of unknown etiology. J Reprod Med 24:93–98
481. Ruvinsky ED, Wiley TL, Morrison JC, Blake PG (1981) In utero diagnosis of umbilical cord hematoma by ultrasonography. Am J Obstet Gynecol 140:833–834
482. Ryder RW, Hassig SE, Behets F, et al (1989) Peri-

natal transmission of the human immunodeficiency virus type I to infants of seropositive women in Zaire. N Engl J Med 320:1637–1642
483. Sachdev R, Nuovo GJ, Kaplan C, Greco MA (1990) In situ hybridization for cytomegalovirus in chronic villitis. Pediatr Pathol 10:909–917
484. Sala MA, Matheus M (1989) Placental characteristics in twin transfusion syndrome. Arch Gynecol Obstet 246:51–56
485. Salafia CM, Parke A (1995) Placental pathology in the phospholipid antibody syndrome and systemic lupus erythematosis. Am J Obstet Gynecol 172:336
486. Salafia CM, Minior VK, Pezzullo JC, Popek EJ, Rosenkrantz TS, Vintzileos AM (1995) Intrauterine growth restriction in infants of less than thirty-two weeks gestation: Associated placental pathologic features. Am J Obstet Gynecol 173:1049–1057
487. Salafia CM, Cowchock FS (1997) Placental pathology and antiphospholipid antibodies: a descriptive study. Am J Perinatol 14:435–441
488. Salafia CM, Mangam HE, Weigl CA, et al (1989) Abnormal fetal heart rate patterns and placental inflammation. Am J Obstet Gynecol 160:140–147
489. Salafia CM, Silverman L, Herreva NE, et al (1988) Placental pathology at term associated with elevated midtrimester maternal serum alpha fetoprotein. Am J Obstet Gynecol 158:1064–1066
490. Samra JS, Obhrai MS, Constantine G (1989) Parvovirus infection in pregnancy. Obstet Gynecol 73:832–834
491. Sampson JE, Theve RP, Blatman RN, et al (1997) Fetal origin of amniotic fluid polymorphonuclear leukocytes. Am J Obstet Gynecol 176:77–81
492. Sander CH (1980) Hemorrhagic endovasculitis and hemorrhagic villitis of the placenta. Arch Pathol Lab Med 104:371–373
493. Sander CH, Kinnane L, Stevens NG, Echt R (1986) Haemorrhagic endovasculitis of the placenta: a review with clinical correlation. Placenta 7:551–574
494. Sands J, Dobbing J (1985) Continuing growth and development of the third-trimester human placenta. Placenta 6:13–22
495. Schlievert P, Johnson W, Galask RP (1976) Bacterial growth inhibition by amniotic fluid. VI. Evidence for a zinc-peptide antibacterial system. Am J Obstet Gynecol 125:906–910
496. Schindler A-M, Bordignon P, Bischop P (1984) Immunohistochemical localization of pregnancy-associated plasma protein A in decidua and trophoblast: comparison with human chorionic gonadotropin and fibrin. Placenta 5:227–236
497. Schreier R, Brown S (1962) Hematoma of the umbilical cord. Report of a case. Obstet Gynecol 20: 798–800
498. Schwartz DA, Caldwell E (1991) Herpes simplex virus infection of the placenta: The role of molecular pathology in the diagnosis of viral infection of placental-associated tissues. Arch Pathol Lab Med 115:1141–1144
499. Schwartz DA, Larsen SA, Beck-Sague C, Fears M, Rice RJ (1995) Pathology of the umbilical cord in congenital syphilis: analysis of 25 specimens using histochemistry and immunofluorescent antibody to *Treponema pallidum*. Hum Pathol 26:784–791
500. Schwartz DA, Reef S (1990) *Candida albicans* placentitis and funisitis: early diagnosis of congenital candidemia by histopathologic examination of umbilical cord vessels. Pediatr Infect Dis J 9:661–665
501. Schwarz TF, Nerlich A, Hottentrager B, et al (1991) Parvovirus B19 infection of the fetus. Histology and in situ hybridization. Am J Clin Pathol 96:121–126
502. Scott JM (1983) Fibrinous vasculosis in the human placenta. Placenta 4:87–100
503. Scott JS (1958) Pregnancy toxaemia associated with hydrops foetalis, hydatidiform mole and hydramnios. J Obstet Gynaecol Br Emp 65:689–701
504. Scott JS (1960) Placenta extrachorialis (placenta marginata and placenta circumvallata). A factor in antepartum hemorrhage. J Obstet Gynaecol Br Emp 67:904–918
505. Scott RJ, Peat D, Rhodes CA (1994) Investigation of the fetal pulmonary inflammatory reaction in chorioamnionitis, using an in situ Y chromosome marker. Pediatr Pathol 14:997–1003
506. Scully RE, Mark EJ, McNeely WF, Ebeling SH, Phillips LD (1997) Weekly clinicopathological exercises. N Engl J Med 336:1439–1446
507. Seidman JD, Abbondanzo SL, Watkin WG, et al (1989) Amniotic band syndrome. Arch Pathol Lab Med 113:891–897
508. Seligsohn U, Berger A, Abend M, et al (1984) Homozygous protein C deficiency manifested by massive venous thrombosis in the newborn. New Engl J Med 310:559–562
509. Sepp AH, Roy TE (1963) *Listeria monocytogenes* infections in metropolitan Toronto. Can Med Assoc J 88:549–561
510. Severn CB, Holyoke EA (1973) Human acardiac anomalies. Am J Obstet Gynecol 116:358–365
511. Shah DM, Chaffin D (1989) Perinatal outcome in very preterm births with twin-twin transfusion syndrome. Am J Obstet Gynecol 161:1111–1113
512. Shanklin DR (1999) Chorangioma and other tumors. In: Lewis SH, Perrin E (eds) Pathology of the placenta, 2nd Ed. Churchill Livingstone, New York
513. Shanklin DR, Scott JS (1975) Massive subchorial thrombohaematoma. (Breus' mole). Br J Obstet Gynaecol 82:476–487
514. Sheikh AU, Ernest JM, O'Shea M (1992) Long-term outcome in fetal hydrops from parvovirus B19 infection. Am J Obstet Gynecol 167:337–341
515. Sheikh SS, Lage JM (1998) Diagnosis of early complete hydatidiform mole. A study of 35 cases. Mod Pathol 11:115
516. Shen-Schwarz S, Ruchelli E, Brown D (1989) Villous oedema of the placenta; a clinicopathologic study. Placenta 10:297–307
517. Shen-Schwarz S, Macpherson TA, Mueller-Heubach E (1988) The clinical significance of hemorrhagic endovasculitis of the placenta Am J Obstet Gynecol 159:48–51

518. Sheppard BL, Bonnar J (1976) The ultrastructure of the arterial supply of the human placenta in pregnancy complicated by fetal growth retardation. Br J Obstet Gynaecol 83:948–959
519. Sheppard BL, Bonnar J (1980) Uteroplacental arteries and hypertensive pregnancy. In: Bonnar J, McGilliray I, Symonds E (eds) Pregnancy hypertension. MTP Press, Lancaster, pp 213–219
520. Sher MS, Belfar H, Martin J, Painter MJ (1991) Destructive brain lesions of presumed fetal onset: antepartum causes of cerebral palsy. Pediatrics 88: 898–906
521. Sherer DM, Anyaegbunam A, Onyeije C (1998) Antepartum fetal intracranial hemorrhage, predisposing factors and prenatal sonography: a review. Am J Perinatol 15:431–441
522. Sherer DM, Salafia CM, Minior VK, et al (1996) Placental basal plate myometrial fibers: clinical correlations of abnormally deep trophoblast invasion. Obstet Gynecol 87:444–449
523. Sheridan-Pereira M, Porreco RP, Hays T, Burke MS (1988) Neonatal aortic thrombosis associated with the lupus anticoagulant. Obstet Gynecol 71:1016–1018
524. Sherman DJ, Tovbin J, Lazarovich T, et al (1997) Chorioamnionitis caused by gram-negative bacteria as an etiologic factor in preterm birth. Eur J Clin Microbiol Infect Dis 16:417–423
525. Shih I-M, Kurman RJ (1999) Immunohistochemical localization of inhibin-α in the placenta and gestational trophoblastic lesions. Int J Gynecol Pathol 18:144–150
526. Shih I-M, Schnaar RL, Gearhart JD, Kurman RJ (1997) Distribution of cells bearing the HNK-1 epitope in the human placenta. Placenta 18:667–674
527. Shih I-M, Kurman RJ (1996) Expression of melanoma cell adhesion molecule in intermediate trophoblast. Lab Invest 75:377–388
528. Shmoys S, Kaplan C (1990) Parvovirus and pregnancy. Clin Obstet Gynecol 33:268–275
529. Sibai BM, Ramadan MK, Usta I, Salama M, Mercer BM, Friedman SA (1993) Maternal morbidity and mortality in 442 pregnancies with hemolysis. Am J Obstet Gynecol 169:1000–1006
530. Siedman JD, Abbondanzo SL, Watkin WG, Ragsdale B, Manz HJ (1989) Amnionic band syndrome: report of 2 cases and review of the literature. Arch Pathol Lab Med 113:891–897
531. Sienko A, Altshuler G (1999) Meconium-induced umbilical vascular necrosis in abortuses and fetuses: a histopathologic study for cytokines. Obstet Gynecol 94:415–420
532. Sieracki JC, Panke TW, Horvat BL, et al (1975) Chorioangiomas. Obstet Gynecol 46:155–159
533. Silver HM (1998) Listeriosis during pregnancy. Obstet Gynecol Surv 53:737–740
534. Silver RK, MacGregor SN, Pasternak JF, et al (1992) Fetal stroke associated with maternal cardiolipin antibodies. Obstet Gynecol 80:497–499
535. Silver MM, Yeger H, Lines LD (1988) Hemorrhagic endovasculitis-like lesion induced in placental organ culture. Hum Pathol 19:251–256
536. Silverstein AJ, Kanbour AI (1981) Repetitive idiopathic fetal hydrops. Obstet Gynecol (Suppl) 57: 18s–21s
537. Silverstein AM (1962) Congenital syphilis and the timing of immunogenesis in the human foetus. Nature (Lond) 194:196–197
538. Soma H (1979) Single umbilical artery with congenital malformations. Curr Top Pathol 66:159–173
539. Soma H, Yamada K, Osawa H, et al (2000) Identification of Gaucher cells in the chorionic villi in association with recurrent hydrops fetalis. Placenta 21:412–416
540. South MA, Tompkins WAF, Morris CR, Rawls WE (1969) Congenital malformation of the central nervous system associated with genital type (type 2) herpesvirus. J Pediatr 75:13–18
541. Spencer GD, Kraus FT (1992) Placental chorangiosis: a nonspecific marker of abnormal gestation (unpublished observations)
542. Sperling RS, Shapiro DE, Coombs RW, et al (1996) Maternal viral load, zidovudine treatment, and the risk of transmission of human immunodeficiency virus type 1 from mother to infant. N Engl J Med 335:1621–1629
543. Sprecher S, Soumenkoff G, Puissant F, Degueldre M (1986) Vertical transmission of HIV in 15-week fetus. Lancet 2:288
544. Stagno S, Whitley RJ (1985) Herpes virus infections of pregnancy. Part I. Cytomegalovirus and Epstein-Barr virus infections. N Engl J Med 313:1270–1274
545. Stagno S, Whitley RJ (1985) Herpes virus infections of pregnancy. Part II. Herpes simplex virus and varicella zoster infections. N Engl J Med 313:1327–1330
546. Stagno S, Pass RF, Dworsky ME, Alford CA (1983) Congenital and perinatal cytomegalovirus infections. Semin Pathol 7:31–42
547. Stagno S, Reynolds DW, Huang E-S, et al (1977) Congenital cytomegalovirus infection. Occurrence in an immune population. N Engl J Med 296:1254–1258
548. Stagno S, Pass RF, Dworsky ME, et al (1982) Congenital cytomegalovirus infection. The relative importance of primary and recurrent maternal infection. N Engl J Med 306:945–949
549. Stallmach T, Hebisch G, Joller-Jemelka HI, Orban P, Schwaller J, Engelmann M (1995) Cytokine production and visualized effects in the fetomaternal unit. Quantitative and topographic data on cytokines during intrauterine disease. Lab Invest 73: 384–392
550. Steele PE, Jacobs DS (1979) *Listeria monocytogenes* macroabscesses of placenta. Obstet Gynecol 53: 124–127
551. Stenchever MA, Parks KA, Daines TL, et al (1977) Cytogenetics of habitual abortion and other reproductive wastage. Am J Obstet Gynecol 127:143–150
552. Stiehm ER (1996) Newborn factors in maternal-

infant transmission of pediatric HIV infection. J Nutr 126:2632S–2636S
553. Stock RJ, Stock ME (1979) Congenital annular constrictions and intrauterine amputations revisited. Obstet Gynecol 53:592–598
554. Strauss L, Driscoll SG (1964) Congenital neuroblastoma involving the placenta. Pediatrics 34:23–31
555. Stray-Pedersen B, Lorentzen-Styr AM (1977) Uterine toxoplasma infections and repeated abortions. Am J Obstet Gynecol 128:716–721
556. Strong BS, Young SA (1995) Intrauterine coxsackie virus, group B type 1, infection: viral cultivation from amniotic fluid in the third trimester. Am J Perinatol 12:78–79
557. Strong SJ, Corney G (1967) The placenta in twin pregnancy. Pergamon Press, London, pp 1–13
558. Strong TH Jr, Elliott JP, Radin TG (1993) Non-coiled umbilical blood vessels: a new marker for the fetus at risk. Obstet Gynecol 81:409–411
559. Sumawong V, Nondasuta A, Thanapath S, Budthimedhee V (1966) Placenta accreta. A review of the literature and a summary of 10 cases. Obstet Gynecol 27:511–516
560. Sun Y, Arbuckle S, Hocking G, Billson V (1995) Umbilical cord stricture and intrauterine fetal death. Pediatr Pathol Lab Med 15:723–732
561. Sweet LK, Connerty HV (1941) Congenital melanoma. Report of a case in which antenatal metastasis occurred. Am J Dis Child 62:1029–1040
562. Szulman AE, Surti U (1978) The syndromes of hydatidiform mole. I. Cytogenetic and morphologic correlations. Am J Obstet Gynecol 131:665–671
563. Szulman AE, Surti U (1978) The syndromes of hydatidiform mole. II. Morphologic evolution of the complete and partial mole. Am J Obstet Gynecol 132:20–27
564. Szulman AE, Philippe E, Boue JG, Boue A (1981) Human tripoloidy: association with partial hydatidiform moles and non-molar conceptuses. Hum Pathol 12:1016–1021
565. Szymonowicz W, Preston H, Yu VYH (1986) The surviving monozygotic twin. Arch Dis Child 61: 454–458
566. Tabbutt S, Griswold WR, Ogino MT, et (1994) al. Multiple thromboses in a premature infant associated with maternal phospholipid antibody syndrome. J Perinatol 14:66–70
567. Teasdale F (1981) Histomorphometry of the placenta of the diabetic woman: class A diabetes mellitus. Placenta 2:241–252
568. Teasdale F (1983) Histomorphometry of the human placenta in class B diabetes mellitus. Placenta 4: 1–12
569. Teasdale F (1985) Histomorphometry of the human placenta in class C diabetes mellitus. Placenta 6: 69–82
570. Tenney B, Parker F (1940) The placenta in toxemia of pregnancy. Am J Obstet Gynecol 39:1000–1005
571. Thadepalli H, Appleman MD, Maidman JE, et al (1977) Antimicrobial effect of amniotic fluid against anaerobic bacteria. Am J Obstet Gynecol 127:250–254
572. Thorarensen O, Ryan S, Hunter J, Younkin DP (1997) Factor V Leiden 19 mutations: an unrecognized cause of hemiplegic cerebral palsy, neonatal stroke, and placental thrombosis. Ann Neurol 42:372–375
573. Thummala MR, Raju TN, Langenberg P (1998) Isolated single umbilical artery anomaly and the risk for congenital malformation: a meta analysis. J Pediatr Surg 33:580–585
574. Thureen PJ, Hall DM, Hoffenberg A, Tyson RW (1997) Fatal meconium aspiration in spite of appropriate perinatal airway management: pulmonary and placental evidence of prenatal disease. Am J Obstet Gynecol 176:967–975
575. Timmons JD, de Alvarez RR (1963) Monoamniotic twin pregnancy. Am J Obstet Gynecol 86:875–881
576. Tondury G, Smith DW (1966) Fetal rubella pathology. J Pediatr 68:867–879
577. Torbet TE, Tsoutsoplides GC (1968) Placenta praevia accreta: conservative management. J Obstet Gynaecol Br Commonw 75:737–740
578. Tornehave D, Chemnitz J, Teisner B, et al (1984) Immunohistochemical demonstration of pregnancy-associated plasma protein A (PAPP-A) in the syncytiotrophoblast of the normal placenta at different gestational ages. Placenta 5:427–432
579. Torpin R (1965) Amniochorionic mesoblastic fibrous strings and amnionic bands: associated contricting fetal malformations of fetal death. Am J Obstet Gynecol 91:65–75
580. Townsend JJ, Baringer JR, Wolinsky JS, et al (1975) Progressive rubella panencephalitis. N Engl J Med 292:990–993
581. Trasler DG, Walker BE, Fraser FC (1956) Congenital malformations produced by amnionic sac puncture. Science 124:439
582. Tsai MM, O'Leary TJ (1993) Identification of *Toxoplasma gondii* in formalin-fixed, paraffin-embedded tissue by polymerase chain reaction. Mod Pathol 6:185–188
583. Van Allen MI, Curry C, Gallagher L (1987) Limb body wall complex: I. Pathogenesis. Am J Med Genet 28:529–548
584. Van Hoeven KH, Anyaegbunam A, Hochster H, et al (1996) Clinical significance of increasing histologic severity of acute inflammation in the fetal membranes and umbilical cord. Pediatr Pathol Lab Med 16:731–744
585. Van Lijnschoten G, Arends JW, Leffers P, et al (1993) The value of histomorphological features of chorionic villi in early spontaneous abortion for the prediction of karyotype. Histopathology (Oxf) 22: 557–563
586. Van Pampus MG, Dekker GA, Wolf HA, et al (1999) High prevalence of hemostatic abnormalities in women with a history of preeclampsia. Am J Obstet Gynecol 180:1146–1150
587. Van Winter JT, Ney JA, Ogburn PL Jr, Johnson RV

(1994) Preterm labor and congenital candidiasis. A case report. J Reprod Med 39:987–990
588. Vetter K, Schneider KTM (1988) Iatrogenic remission of twin transfusion syndrome. Am J Obstet Gynecol 158:221
589. Wallenburg HCS (1971) Chorioangioma of the placenta. Obstet Gynecol Surv 26:411–425
590. Walter P, Blot P, Ivanoff B (1982) The placental lesions in congenital syphilis. A study of six cases. Virchows Arch A Pathol Anat 397:313–326
591. Walter PR, Garin Y, Blot P (1982) Placental pathologic changes in malaria. A histologic and ultrastructural study. Am J Pathol 109:330–342
592. Wan SK, Lam PWY, Pau MY, et al (1992) Multiclefted nculei. A helpful feature for identification of intermediate trophoblastic cells in uterine curetting specimens. Am J Surg Pathol 16:1226–1232
593. Warren CT, Kraus FT, Taysi K, et al (1990) Histologic-karyotypic correlations in spontaneous abortions. Mod Pathol 3:105A
594. Weber J (1963) Constriction of the umbilical cord as a cause of fetal death. Acta Obstet Gynecol Scand 42:259–268
595. Weil ML, Itabashi HH, Cremer NE, et al (1975) Chronic progressive panencephalitis due to rubella virus simulating subacute sclerosing panencephalitis. N Engl J Med 292:994–998
596. Weiland HT, Vermey-Keers C, Salimans MMM, et al (1987) Parvovirus B19 associated with fetal abnormality. Lancet 1:682–683
597. Wentworth P (1968) Circumvallate and circummarginate placentas. Am J Obstet Gynecol 102:44–47
598. Wentworth P (1967) Placental infarction and toxemia of pregnancy. Am J Obstet Gynecol 99:318–326
599. Wentworth P (1967) The placenta in cases of hemolytic disease of the newborn. Am J Obstet Gynecol 98:283–289
600. Wentworth P (1964) A placental lesion to account for feotal haemorrhage into the maternal circulation. J Obstet Gynaecol Br Commonw 71:379–387
601. Wharton B, Edwards JH, Cameron AH (1968) Monoamniotic twins. J Obstet Gynaecol Br Commonw 75:158–163
602. Whyte RK, Hussain Z, deSA D (1982) Antenatal infections with *Candida* species. Arch Dis Child 57: 528–535
603. Wiener-Meynagi Z, Ben-Schlomo I, Goldbeg Y, Shaler E (1998) Resistance to activated protein C and Leiden mutation: high prevalence of patients with abruptio placenta. Am J Obstet Gynecol 179: 1565–1567
604. Wilson CB, Remington JS (1980) What can be done to prevent congenital toxoplasmosis? Am J Obstet Gynecol 138:357–363
605. Wilson D, Paalman J (1967) Clinical significance of circumvallate placenta. Obstet Gynecol 29:774–778
606. Wilson EA (1972) Holoacardius. Obstet Gynecol 40:740–748
607. Winer AE, Bergman WD, Fields C (1957) Combined intra- and extrauterine pregnancy. Am J Obstet Gynecol 74:170–178
608. Wiswell TE, Bent RC (1993) Meconium staining and the meconium aspiration syndrome. Unresolved issues. Pediatr Clinic N Am 40:955–81
609. Witzleben CL, Driscoll SG (1965) Possible transplacental transmission of herpes simplex infection. Pediatrics 36:192–199
610. Wolf PL, Jones KL, Longway SR, Benirshke K, Bloor C (1985) Prenatal death from acute myocardial infarction and cardiac tamponade due to embolus from the placenta. Am Heart J 109:603–609
611. Yamazaki K, Price JT, Altshuler G (1977) A placental view of the diagnosis and pathogenesis of congenital listeriosis. Am J Obstet Gynecol 129: 703–705
612. Yeh I-T, O'Connor DM, Kurman RJ (1989) Vacuolated cytotrophoblast: a subpopulation of trophoblast in the chorion laeve. Placenta 10:429–438
613. Yoon BH, Jun JK, Romero R, et al (1997) Amniotic fluid inflammatory cytokines (interleukin-6, interleukin-1β, and tumor necrosis factor-α), neonatal brain white matter lesions, and cerebral palsy. Am J Obstet Gynecol 177:19–26
614. Yoon BH, Romero R, Kim CJ, et al (1997) High expression of tumor necrosis factor-α and interleukin-6 in periventricular leukomalacia. Am J Obstet Gynecol 177:406–411
615. Yoshioka H, Kadomoto Y, Mino M, et al (1979) Multicystic encephalomalacia in liveborn twin with a stillborn macerated co-twin. J Pediatr 95:798–800
616. Young ID, Lindenbaum RH, Thompson EM, Pembrey ME (1985) Amniotic bands in connective tissue disorders. Arch Dis Child 60:1061–1063
617. Zeek PM, Assali NS (1950) Vascular changes in the decidua associated with eclamptogenic toxemia of pregnancy. Am J Clin Pathol 20:1099–1109
618. Ziel H (1963) Circumvallate placenta, a cause of antepartum bleeding, premature delivery, and perinatal mortality. Obstet Gynecol 22:798–802
619. Zervoudakis IA, Cederqvist LL (1977) Effect of *Listeria monocytogenes* septicemia during pregnancy on the offspring. Am J Obstet Gynecol 129:465–467
620. Zhang J, Kraus FT, Aquino TI (1985) Chorioamnionitis: a comparative histologic, bacteriologic, and clinical study. Int J Gynecol Pathol 4:1–10
621. Zhou Y, Damsky CH, Fisher SJ (1997) Preeclampsia is associated with failure of human cytotrophoblasts to mimic a vascular adhesion phenotype. J Clin Invest 99:2152–2164

24

Gestational Trophoblastic Disease and Related Lesions

Ie-Ming Shih, M.D., Ph.D., Michael T. Mazur, M.D., and Robert J. Kurman, M.D.

Gestational trophoblastic disease (GTD) encompasses a heterogeneous group of lesions with specific clinical features, morphologic characteristics, and pathogenesis. The modified World Health Organization classification of GTD includes complete and partial hydatidiform mole, invasive mole, choriocarcinoma, placental site trophoblastic tumor, epithelioid trophoblastic tumor, exaggerated placental site, and placental site nodule. Some of these lesions are true neoplasms, whereas others represent abnormally formed placentas with a predisposition for neoplastic transformation of the trophoblast. Two entities, the exaggerated placental site and the placental site nodule, are included because they are trophoblastic lesions that must be distinguished from other entities with malignant potential. The literature on this subject is extensive and at times confusing because of inconsistencies in classification and terminology. In fact, the necessity of a morphologic classification has been questioned, because current management is largely medical and in the case of trophoblastic disease following a mole, treatment is often conducted in the absence of a histologic diagnosis. Thus, all trophoblastic lesions are frequently combined under the rubric of GTD without applying specific pathologic terms. Recent studies demonstrate profound differences in the etiology, morphology, and clinical behavior of various forms of the disease, however. These studies underscore the importance of a uniform histologic classification to facilitate standardized reporting of data and to ensure appropriate clinical management. Nonetheless, the term GTD has clinical utility, as the principles of human chorionic gonadotropin (hCG) monitoring in follow-up and the chemotherapy of metastatic or persistent disease are similar for all these entities.

This chapter discusses the clinical and pathologic features of each specific form of GTD as well as its clinical behavior, management, and treatment.

In addition, the morphologic and immunohistochemical features of the distinct subtypes of trophoblastic cells are reviewed because these have important implications for diagnosis. Recent studies have shed light on the molecular mechanisms of trophoblastic function, especially as it relates to trophoblastic disease, and this material is reviewed because it enhances our understanding of the biology of these entities.

Overview of Morphology and Biology of Trophoblast

The abnormal trophoblastic tissue in GTD recapitulates the trophoblast present in the early developing placenta and the implantation site. In normal placentation, the trophoblast growing in association with chorionic villi is referred to as *villous trophoblast*, whereas the trophoblast in all other locations is termed *extravillous trophoblast*. Three distinct types of trophoblastic cells have been recognized: *cytotrophoblast (CT)*, *syncytiotrophoblast (ST)*, and *intermediate trophoblast (IT)*. Villous trophoblast is composed, for the most part, of CT and ST with small amounts of IT. In contrast, extravillous trophoblast that infiltrates the decidua, myometrium, and spiral arteries of the placental site is composed of IT.

The CT or Langhans' cell is the germinative trophoblastic cell, whereas the ST is the highly differentiated cell that interfaces with the maternal circulation and produces most of the placental hormones. The IT is a distinct form of trophoblastic cell that shares some of the morphologic and functional features of both CT and ST. It has been referred to by several terms, including X-cell, interstitial (cyto)trophoblast, extravillous (cyto)trophoblast,[10] and "cytotrophoblast." The term *intermediate trophoblast* is preferred by pathologists because it more clearly reflects the morphologic and functional features, including hormone secretion, of this unique cell population, which is "intermediate" between cytotrophoblast and syncytiotrophoblast. Recent morphologic and immunohistochemical studies have shown that intermediate trophoblast is a heterogenous cell population that can be further categorized according to its anatomic location (Fig. 24.1). Accordingly, we have proposed that intermediate trophoblast extending from the trophoblastic column at the anchoring villi be designated "villous intermediate trophoblast," that in the placental site (or basal plate) "implantation site intermediate trophoblast," and that in the chorion laeve of the fetal membranes "chorionic-type intermediate trophoblast" (Fig. 24.1). The intermediate trophoblastic cells in the trophoblastic shell, trophoblastic islands, and placental septae appear to be equivalent to the implantation site intermediate trophoblastic cells.

Human trophoblast is derived from the trophoectoderm, the outermost layer of the blastocyst. Shortly after implantation (day 7–8), the trophoectoderm differentiates into a syncytiotrophoblastic mass at the implantation pole. Small intrasyncytial vacuoles then appear in the syncytiotrophoblastic mass and expand, becoming confluent and forming a system of lacunae that are separated by syncytiotrophoblastic trabeculae. At approximately day 12, the previllous mononucleate trophoblast from the primary chorionic plate invades the syncytiotrophoblastic trabeculae where, in the peripheral ends of the trabeculae, they join together and form the outermost layer of the trophoblast, the trophoblastic shell. After 2 weeks of gestation, the extraembryonic mesenchyme grows into the trabeculae, transforming them into the primary chorionic villi. The lacunae coalesce to form the intervillous space.

After the development of the chorionic villi, distinctive trophoblastic subpopulations can be recognized (see Fig. 24.1). The chorionic villus surface is lined by a continuous inner layer of cytotrophoblast and an outer layer of syncytiotrophoblast. Cytotrophoblast is the trophoblastic stem cell on the villous surface, demonstrating proliferative activity with a Ki-67 nuclear labeling index of approximately 30% in the first trimester. Cytotrophoblast, in early gestation, differentiates along two main pathways—villous and extravillous.[2,9,115,127,187] On the villous surface, cytotrophoblast fuses directly to form syncytiotrophoblast. The differentiation of cytotrophoblast into syncytiotrophoblast is accompanied by complete loss of proliferation activity.[140,189] As gestation progresses, the proliferative activity of cytotrophoblast decreases with an increase in the relative number of syncytiotrophoblast to cytotrophoblast. The nuclei of syncytiotrophoblast gradually become apoptotic, forming so-called syncytial knots, clusters of pyknotic nuclei with a small amount of cytoplasm, that are eventually extruded into the intervillous space. The second pathway of differentiation of cytotrophoblast occurs at the pole of the villi that make contact with the placental bed. These villi, the so-called anchoring villi, display a morphologic spectrum of differentiation where cytotrophoblast (CT) merges imperceptibly into intermediate trophoblast within these trophoblastic columns (see Fig. 24.1).

These intermediate trophoblastic cells in the trophoblastic columns are termed "villous intermediate trophoblast." The proliferative activity of villous intermediate trophoblast gradually decreases as the cells move away from the villi.[189] At the base of the

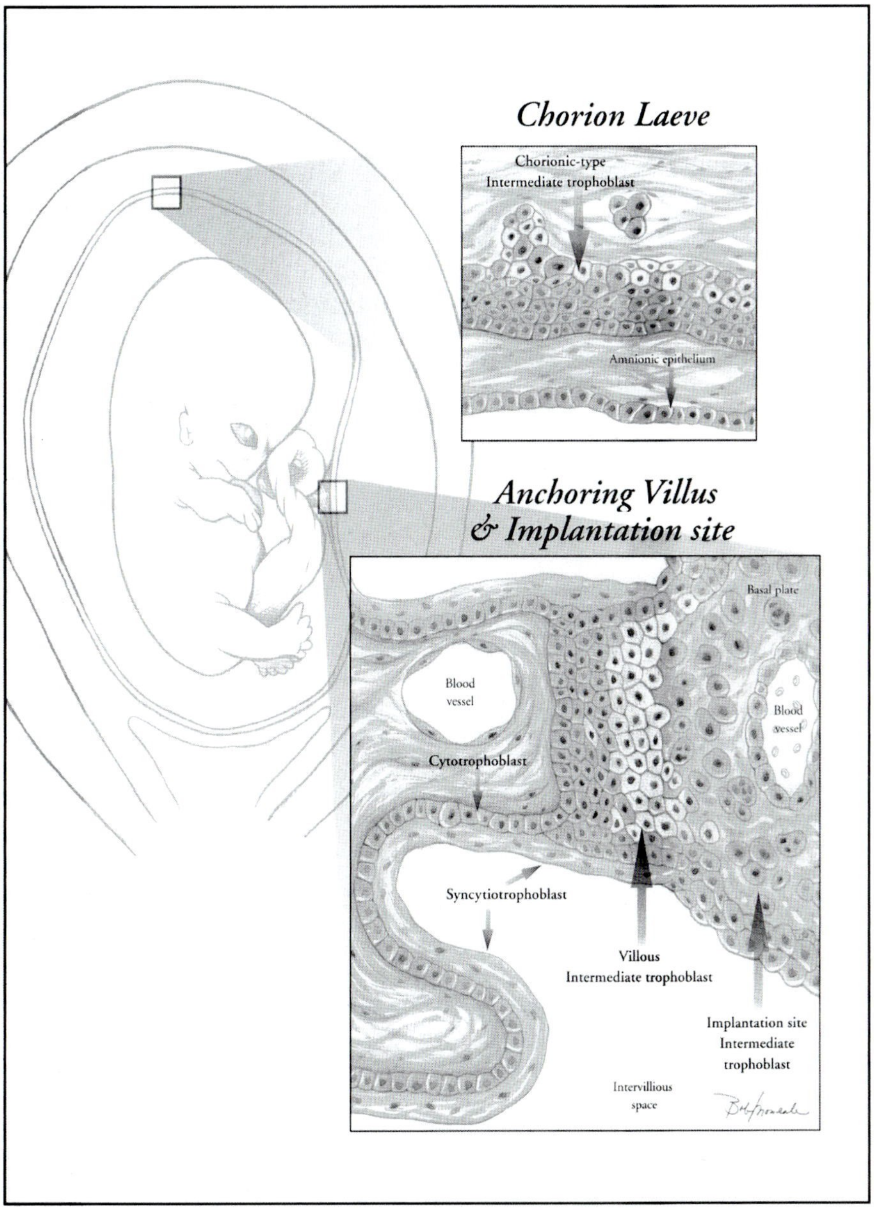

Fig. 24.1. Schematic representation of the trophoblastic subpopulations in the placenta and fetal membranes. (Reprinted by permission from Shih et al., ref. 194.)

trophoblastic column where it makes contact with the endometrium, intermediate trophoblast infiltrates the decidua and myometrium and invades and replaces the spiral arteries of the implantation site (basal plate) to establish the maternal–fetal circulation. This subpopulation of intermediate trophoblast in the implantation site is designated *implantation site intermediate trophoblast*.[194] Although these trophoblastic cells extensively infiltrate the placental bed, they do not demonstrate proliferative activity.[189] Some mononucleate implantation site intermediate trophoblastic cells fuse into multinucleated cells that are terminally differentiated. In contrast to anchoring villi, floating villi are not in contact with the placental bed. The trophoblast at the tips of these villi appears to be analogous to implantation site intermediate trophoblast. This cell population of trophoblast is associated with extensive deposition of extracellular matrix protein and fibrin, forming "balloon-like" structures that have been designated trophoblastic islands.[10] Like implantation site intermediate trophoblast, the trophoblastic cells in the trophoblastic islands are not proliferative. In contrast, the intermediate trophoblast away from implantation site (i.e., the chorion frondosum) differentiates into chorionic-type intermediate trophoblast. At around 20 weeks of gestation the expanding gestational sac obliterates the endometrial cavity and the chorion frondosum fuses with the decidua parietalis to form the chorion laeve (Fig. 24.2). As the surface area of the chorionic laeve increases toward term, the chorionic-type intermediate tro-

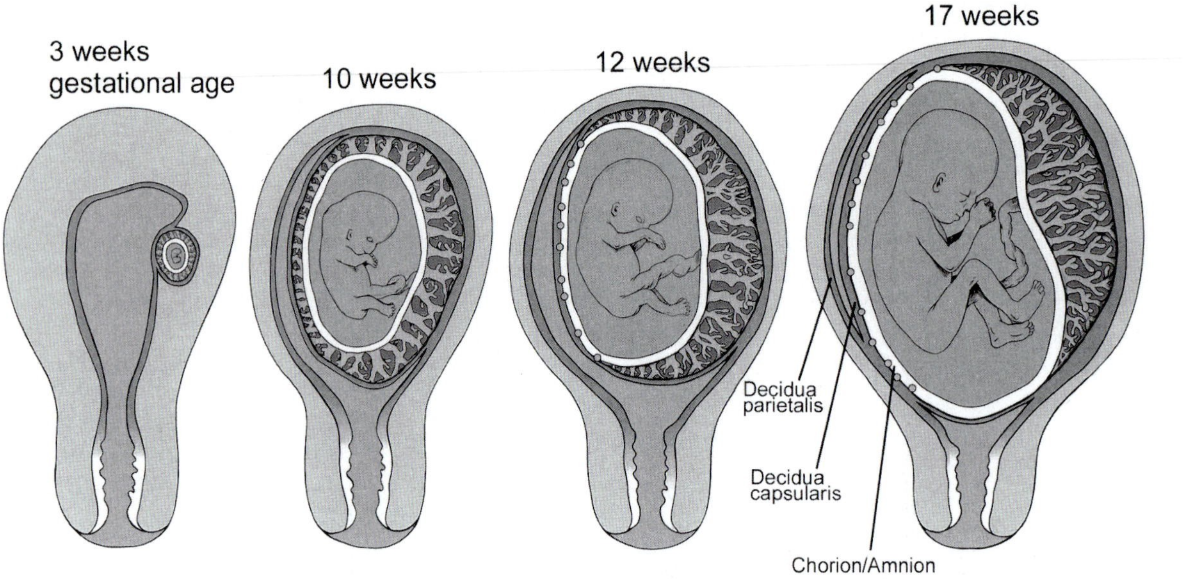

Fig. 24.2. Schematic representation of the formation of the chorion laeve. At *3 weeks of gestation*, the entire blastocyst is embedded in the endometrium at the implantation site and is surrounded by the trophoblastic shell. At *10 weeks*, the definitive placenta is established at the implantation site and the chorionic villi at the opposite pole begin to degenerate. At approximately *12 weeks*, the *amnion/chorion* at the opposite end of the placental site fuses with the *decidua capsularis*. The intervillous space is obliterated and the chorionic villi (the *small, round grayish structures*) degenerate. This process continues, and at approximately 17 weeks of gestation the uterine cavity begins to be obliterated as the amnion and chorion laeve become apposed to the endometrium on the opposite side of the uterine cavity. The chorion laeve, amnion, and underlying decidua constitute the fetal membranes. (Reprinted by permission from Shih et al., ref. 194.)

phoblast appears to proliferate throughout gestation, albeit at a low level.

Morphology of Trophoblast

Previllous trophoblast. By light microscopy, the previllous trophoblast is composed of mononucleate trophoblast and primitive syncytiotrophoblast that invade the endometrium. The dimorphic pattern of previllous trophoblast is reminiscent of the dimorphic pattern of trophoblast in choriocarcinoma, and it has been hypothesized that the morphologic appearance of choriocarcinoma is a recapitulation of the appearance of previllous trophoblast (Fig. 24.3). Unlike choriocarcinoma,

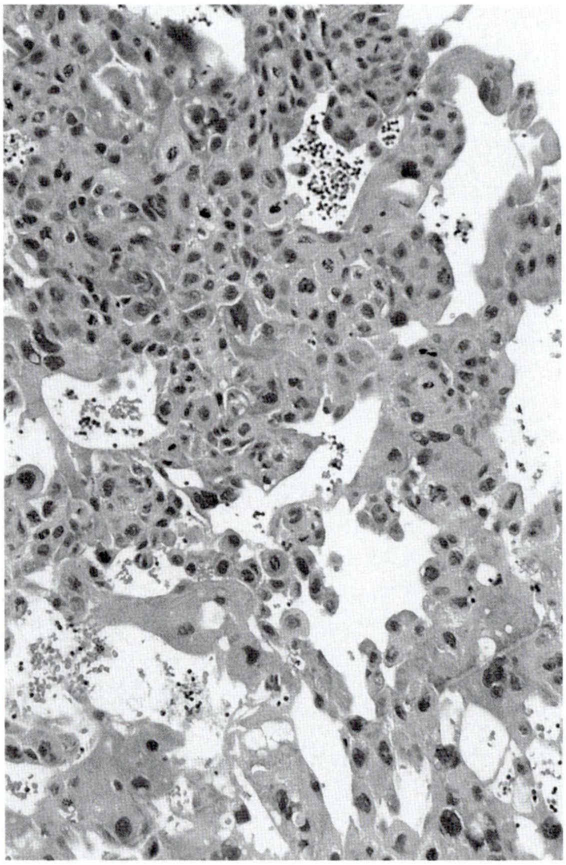

Fig. 24.3. Primitive trophoblast. In an early placenta, the trophoblast demonstrates a dimorphic pattern composed of mononucleate trophoblastic cells and syncytiotrophoblastic cells that resembles choriocarcinoma. The mononucleate trophoblastic cells, in contrast to those in choriocarcinoma, are smaller and uniform with less nuclear atypia. Unlike choriocarcinoma, the trophoblast does not invade and destroy adjacent tissue.

previllous trophoblastic cells are less pleomorphic and exhibit little cellular necrosis.

Cytotrophoblast. Following the development of villi, cytotrophoblastic cells are small primitive epithelial cells, uniform and polygonal to oval in shape (Fig. 24.4; Table 24.1). Cytotrophoblastic cells have a single nucleus, clear to granular cytoplasm, and well-defined cell borders (Fig. 24.4). Mitotic activity is evident.

Syncytiotrophoblast. Syncytiotrophoblast is composed of a large, multinucleate cellular mass with dense amphophilic cytoplasm containing multiple vacuoles that vary in size (Fig. 24.4). A distinct brush order often lines the cell membrane. The syncytiotrophoblastic nuclei are dark and often appear pyknotic. They do not show mitotic activity.

Villous intermediate trophoblast. Villous interme-

a
b
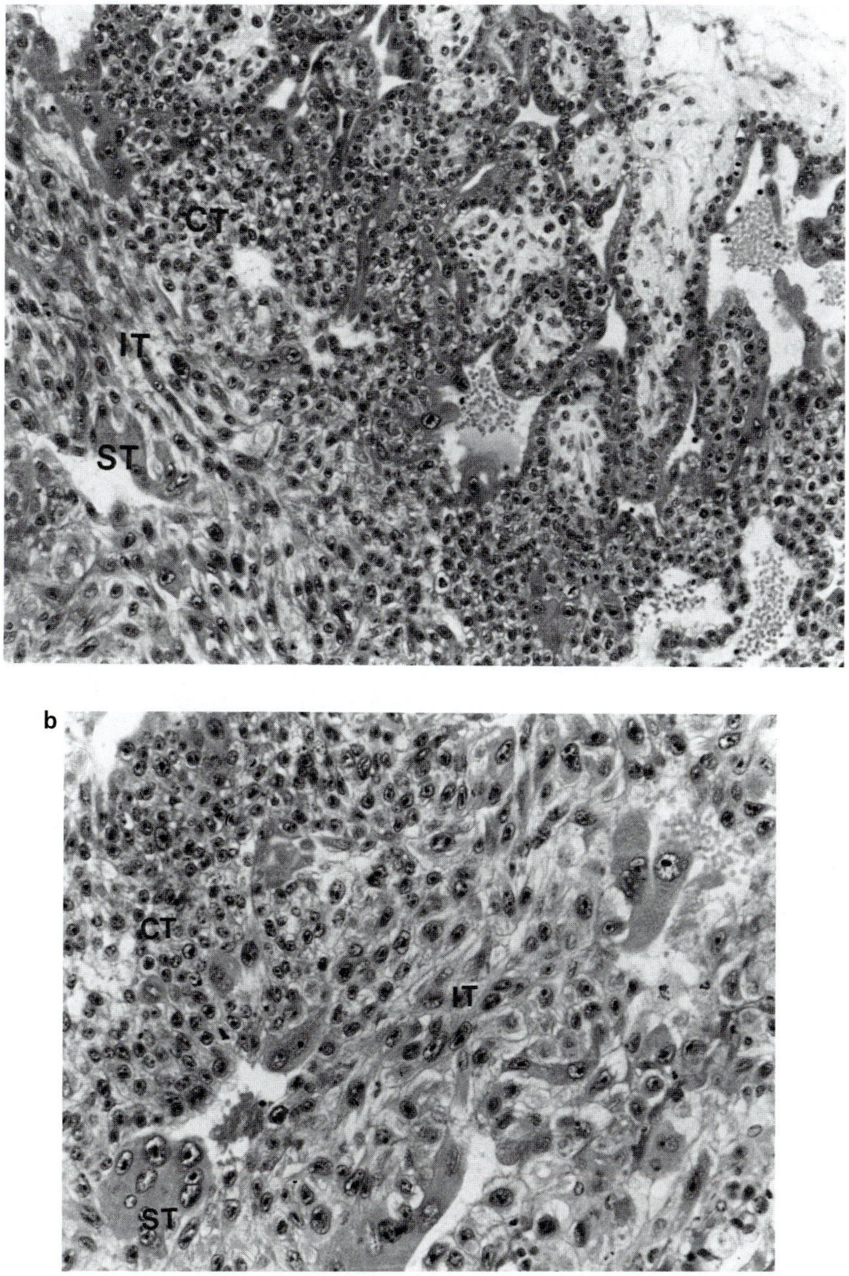

Fig. 24.4. Villous and extravillous trophoblast of a 16-day blastocyst. a: Cytotrophoblast (*CT*), intermediate trophoblast (*IT*), and syncytiotrophoblast (*ST*). **b**: Cytotrophoblast (*CT*) is characterized by small, unfiorm, mononucleate cells with distinct cell membranes, intermediate trophoblast (*IT*) by larger cells that are mononucleate but show greater pleomorphism, and syncytiotrophoblast (*ST*) by multinucleate giant cells with much larger nuclei.

Table 24.1. Morphologic and immunohistochemical features of trophoblastic cells throughout gestation

		Intermediate trophoblast (IT)			
	Cytotrophoblast	*Villous IT*	*Implantation site IT*	*Chorionic-type IT*	*Syncytiotrophoblast*
Morphology	Round, uniform, and small; scant, clear to granular cytoplasm; prominent cell borders	Polyhedral; abundant, eosinophilic to clear cytoplasm; prominent cell borders	Pleomorphic and large; abundant, eosinophilic cytoplasm; occasional multinucleated cells	Round to polyhedral, regular abundant eosinophilic and clear[a] cytoplasm	Linearly arranged multinucleated cells; abundant dense cytoplasm with multiple vacuoles and lacunae
Growth pattern	Cohesive	Cohesive	Infiltrating	Cohesive	Syncytial
Immunostaining					
Cytokeratin[b]	++++[c]	++++	++++	++++	++++
hCG	–	–	–; + in multinucleated IT	–	++/++++[d]
hPL	–	–/+	++++	++	++/++++[d]
Mel-CAM	–	–/++++[e]	++++	++	–
PLAP	–	–	+	+++	++++
HNK-1	–	++++	–	–	–
EMA	–	–	– (1st trimester); ++ (term)	+++	–
Inhibin-α	–	–	–/+ (1st trimester); ++ (term)	++	+++ (1st trimester); –/+ (term)
Ki-67 index[f]	25%–50%	>90%[g]	0	3%–10%	0

hCG, human chorionic gonadotropin; hPL, human placental lactogen; Mel-CAM, melanoma cell adhesion molecule (CD 146); EMA, epithelial membrane antigen; PLAP, placental alkaline phosphatase; HNK-1 is also known as Leu-7 and CD57.

[a]The chorionic-type IT with clear cytoplasm is more often positive for PLAP. In contrast, the cells with eosinophilic cytoplasm is more often positive for hPL and Mel-CAM.

[b]Trophoblast is positive for cytokeratins 7, 8, 18, 19, and AE1/AE3 cocktail, variable for cytokeratin 20, and negative for high molecular weight cytokeratin (antibody 903).

[c]++++ denotes semiquantitative scoring of proportion of cells showing a positive reaction; + = <25%; ++ = 25%–50%; +++ = >50%–75%; ++++ = >75%.

[d]The immunodistribution of hPL and hCG in syncytiotrophoblast is variable depending on gestational age. hCG decreases and hPL increases in intensity toward term.

[e]Mel-CAM immunointensity increases from the base to the tip of the trophoblastic column.

[f]The percentage of Ki-67-positive trophoblastic cells in 300 randomly selected trophoblastic cells.

[g]Ki-67 immunointensity decreases from the base to the tip of the trophoblastic column.

diate trophoblastic cells are mononucleate and larger than cytotrophoblast with pale cytoplasm and uniform round nuclei.

Implantation site intermediate trophoblast. Implantation site intermediate trophoblastic cells have a variable appearance that to some extent is dependent on their anatomic location (see Table 24.1). For example, implantation site intermediate trophoblastic cells in the endometrium are polygonal or round and contain abundant amphophilic cytoplasm closely resembling the decidualized stromal cells with which they are admixed. In contrast, implantation site intermediate trophoblastic cells in the myometrium are frequently spindle shaped and resemble the smooth muscle cells of the myometrium. Generally, the cytoplasm of implantation site intermediate trophoblastic cells is abundant and is eosino-philic to amphophilic. Scattered small vacuoles may be present in the cytoplasm of implantation site intermediate trophoblastic cells. The nuclei of implantation site intermediate trophoblastic cells have highly irregular outlines and hyperchromatic, coarsely granular chromatin. Often the nuclei are lobulated or show multiple deep nuclear clefts. Nucleoli are smaller and less prominent than those in cytotrophoblast. Cytoplasmic nuclear invaginations may be seen. Mono-nucleate implantation site intermediate trophoblastic cells occasionally fuse into multinucleated cells.

Implantation site intermediate trophoblastic cells infiltrate the decidua, surround glands, and invade the myometrium, dissecting between smooth muscle fibers without destroying them (see Table 24.1). These cells characteristically invade spiral arteries, replacing the smooth muscle of the vessel wall but leaving the overall structure intact. Eosinophilic fibrinoid material is often deposited around implantation site intermediate trophoblast. The material contains a variety of extracellular matrix proteins including adult-type and oncofetal fibronectin, type IV collagen, laminin, and a small amount of fibrin.[187] Implantation site intermediate trophoblastic cells are the predominant cellular population of the exaggerated placental site and the placental site trophoblastic tumor.

The intermediate trophoblastic cells in the trophoblastic islands are mononucleate, round and uniform in size, and contain rounded nuclei. They are embedded in an abundant, homogenous and eosinophilic fibrinoid matrix. In vitro studies suggest that the cell islands are derived from the floating cell columns, which are not anchored to the endometrium.[73,152] As a result, abundant extracellular matrix accumulates among the cells, replacing those in the center of the islands.

Chorionic-type intermediate trophoblast. Chorionic-type intermediate trophoblast is composed for the most part of relatively uniform cells with either eosinophilic or clear (glycogen-rich) cytoplasm arranged in a cohesive layer in the chorion laeve (see Table 24.1; Fig. 24.1). Most of the cells are smaller than implantation site intermediate trophoblast but larger than cytotrophoblast. Occasionally, the cells from nests or cords that extend into the underlying decidua. As with implantation site intermediate trophoblastic cells, some chorionic-type intermediate trophoblastic cells are multinucleated. Chorionic-type intermediate trophoblast is the cellular population found in placental site nodules and epithelioid trophoblastic tumors.[194]

Gene Expression and Immunohistochemical Features of Trophoblastic Subpopulations

Trophoblast-associated gene expression as detected by immunohistochemistry has great value in the diagnosis of GTD as well as in the study of the biology of trophoblast.[105] The β-subunit of human chorionic gonadotropin (hCG), human placental lactogen (hPL), placental alkaline phosphatase (PLAP), and cytokeratin are well-recognized markers of trophoblast. Recently, several other genes, although not specifically expressed in trophoblast, have been identified in human trophoblast. Antibodies against these markers, especially those that are commercially available and recognize the epitopes on formalin-fixed, paraffin-embedded tissue sections, have considerable value in the study and differential diagnosis of different types of GTD (Fig. 24.5).

All forms of trophoblastic subpopulations and gestational trophoblastic lesions react strongly for cytokeratin when broad-spectrum antibodies (for example, the AE1/AE3 antibody cocktail) are used. More specifically, trophoblast is positive for simple epithelium-type cytokeratins including cytokeratins 7, 8, 18, and 19. In contrast, trophoblast is variably positive for cytokeratin 20 and is rarely positive for high molecular weight cytokeratin that is normally expressed by stratified squamous epithelium.[191] Cytokeratin

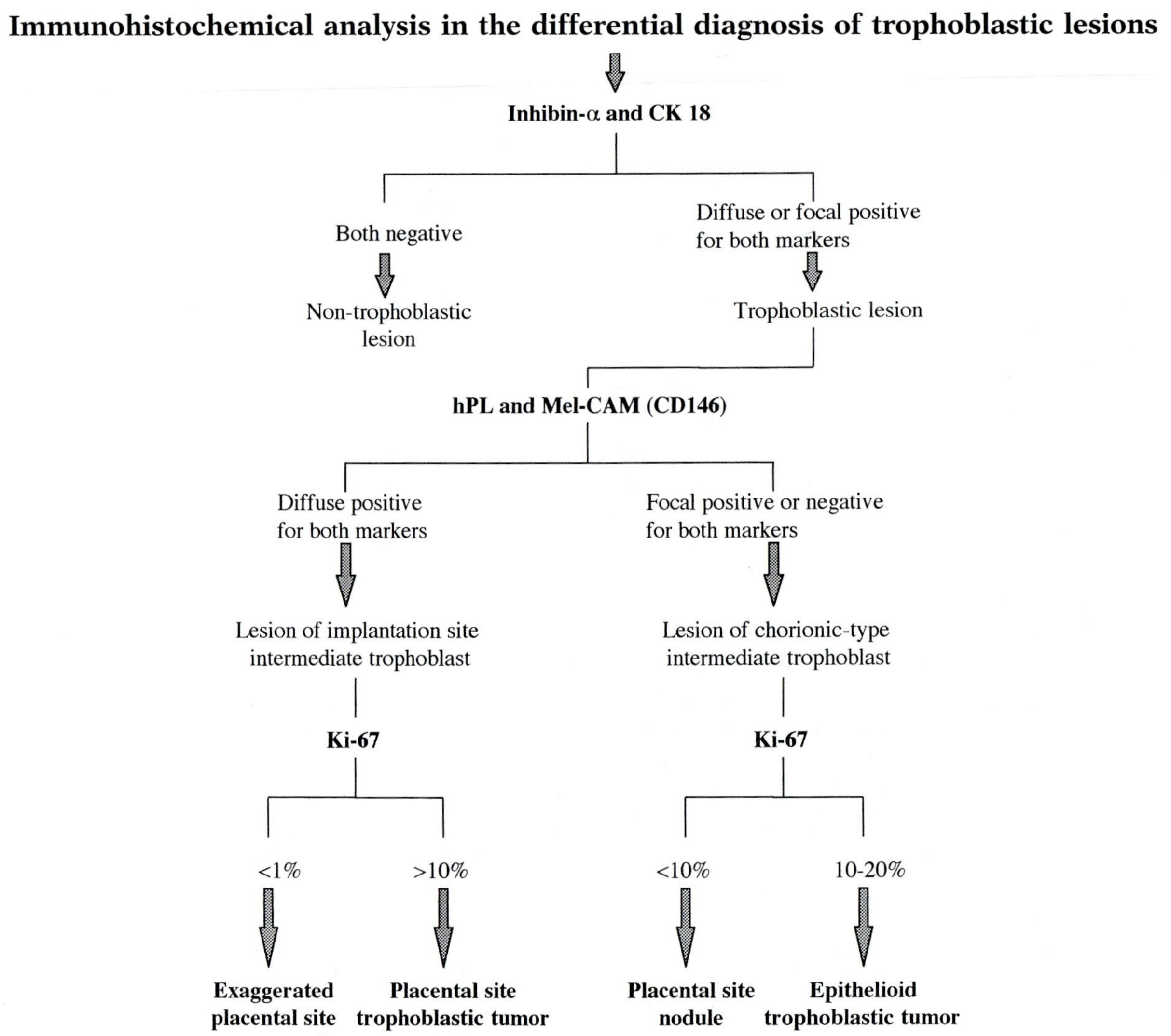

Fig. 24.5. Immunohistochemical analysis using antibodies against cytokeratin 18, inhibin-α, hPL, Mel-CAM (CD 146), and Ki-67 in the differential diagnosis of trophoblastic lesions.

immunostaining is especially useful for demonstrating the presence of implantation site intermediate trophoblastic cells at the placental site because these cells are always admixed with the other cell types. The intermediate trophoblastic cells that are positive for cytokeratin are easily identified amid nonreactive decidual cells and smooth muscle cells.[49,161] Myometrial smooth muscle cells can display punctate cytoplasmic cytokeratin immunoreactivity that is easily distinguished from the diffusely membrane staining of intermediate trophoblastic cells.

Before 10 weeks of gestation, cytotrophoblast is immunoreactive for the monoclonal antibody Ber-EP4, which reacts with two membrane antigens.[5] Cytotrophoblast is immunoreactive for a variety of antigens including leukemia inhibitory factor receptor,[184] epidermal growth factor receptor, P2Y6 purinergic receptor,[200] and a number of cell adhesion molecules including $\alpha_6\beta_4$ integrin and E-cadherin.[43,127] Unlike syncytiotrophoblast, cytotrophoblast fails to react with antibodies against a wide variety of steroid and pregnancy-associated hormones. Ki-67 proliferation-related antigen is highly expressed by cytotrophoblast (labeling index, 25%–50%), especially in the region forming the trophoblastic columns. These findings confirm that cytotrophoblast is a stem cell with a high level of proliferative activity and a limited functional role.

The differentiation of cytotrophoblast into syncytiotrophoblast is accompanied by dramatic changes in gene expression.[226] For example, syncytiotrophoblast expresses several pregnancy-associated hormones including hCG, hPL, estradiol, progesterone, placental growth hormone, pregnancy-specific β_1

glycoprotein, relaxins, and inhibin. The immunodistribution of some of these hormones in syncytiotrophoblast is variable depending on gestational age. For example, syncytiotrophoblast contains abundant hCG from at least 12 days of gestation until approximately 8–10 weeks, after which it diminishes. By 40 weeks it is present only focally. hPL is also localized in syncytiotrophoblast at 12 days but increases steadily thereafter. From late in the second trimester to term, hPL is diffusely distributed in the syncytiotrophoblast overlying the chorionic villi.[115] Inhibin-α exhibits the highest expression in the first trimester and gradually decreases in immunointensity through the third trimester (see Table 24.1).[190] Syncytiotrophoblast also expresses placental alkaline phosphatase, leukemia inhibitory factor receptor,[184] placental growth hormone,[1] epidermal growth factor receptor,[127] syndecan-1,[42,103] $p27^{kip1}$ (a negative regulator in cell cycle progression),[166] c-*fms* oncoprotein,[70] and syncytin.[145] Expression of syncytin has been shown to be involved in the fusion process of syncytiotrophoblast.[145] In contrast, several genes are downregulated in syncytiotrophoblast as compared with cytotrophoblast. For example, syncytiotrophoblast fails to express E-cadherin and Ki-67 nuclear antigen. These findings are concordant with the view that syncytiotrophoblast is terminally differentiated and that its major functions are hormone production and molecular transport across the villous surface.

Among the various populations of trophoblast, the pattern of gene expression is most complex in intermediate trophoblast and depends on the differentiation status and anatomic location of the intermediate trophoblastic cells, that is, the subpopulation of intermediate trophoblast (see Table 24.1). The villous intermediate trophoblast in the trophoblastic columns uniquely expresses the HNK-1 carbohydrate epitope on glycosphingolipids, which is not present in other subpopulations of trophoblastic cells.[193] The genes that are upregulated as villous intermediate trophoblast differentiates into implantation site intermediate trophoblast include 92-kDa and 72-kDa type IV collagenase, interstitial collagenase (matrix metalloproteinase 1),[146,169] plasminogen activator inhibitor 1 (PAI-1),[169] cell-surface proteoglycans, syndecan 1 and 4,[42] cyclin-dependent kinase inhibitors ($p57^{kip\text{-}2}$ and $p21^{WAF1/CIP1}$),[71] HLA-G,[141] melanoma cell adhesion molecule (Mel-CAM or CD146),[187] oncofetal fibronectin,[59] prolyl 4-hydroxylase,[219] insulin-like growth factor-II,[212] pleiotrophin,[182] c-*erbB-2* oncogene product,[152] $\alpha_5\beta_1$, $\alpha_1\beta_1$, and $\alpha_v\beta_3$ integrins,[20] inhibin-α,[190] human placental lactogen (hPL),[117] and pregnancy-associated major basic protein.[131] The genes that are downregulated during differentiation of villous to implantation site intermediate trophoblast are Ki-67 nuclear antigen, epidermal growth factor (EGF) receptor, $\alpha_6\beta_4$ integrin, and E-cadherin.[40] In terms of hormone production, implantation site intermediate trophoblast resembles syncytiotrophoblast. It contains abundant hPL, which appears as early as 12 days and reaches a peak at 11–15 weeks of gestation.[115] Inhibin-α is also immunolocalized in the implantation site intermediate trophoblast after 10 weeks of gestation. In contrast, hCG is present only focally in implantation site intermediate trophoblast, appearing as early as 12 days and remaining until 6 weeks, after which it disappears. The so-called multinucleated trophoblastic giant cells exhibit an identical immunostaining pattern to the mononucleate counterparts except the former are negative for pregnancy-associated major basic protein.[114] Accordingly, these giant cells should be designated "multinucleated intermediate trophoblastic cells" rather than syncytiotrophoblastic giant cells.[187]

The implantation site intermediate trophoblastic cells that invade the spiral arteries show the same staining pattern as those within the decidua and myometrium except that expression of neural cell adhesion molecule (NCAM),[21] E-cadherin, and β-catenin are upregulated and expression of pregnancy-associated major basic protein is downregulated.[21] Implantation site intermediate trophoblast in both the endometrium and myometrium expresses leukemia inhibitory factor receptor,[184] which interacts with leukemia inhibitory factor expressed by maternal decidual leukocytes. Although leukemia inhibitory factor plays an important role in implantation and placentation in several species, the paracrine role of leukemia inhibitory factor in the biology of human implantation site intermediate trophoblastic cells is not known.[184]

In contrast to implantation site intermediate trophoblast, chorionic-type intermediate trophoblast is diffusely positive for placental alkaline phosphatase but is only focally positive for several trophoblast-associated antigens including hPL, Mel-CAM (CD 146), and oncofetal fibronectin (see Table 24.1). Chorionic-type intermediate trophoblastic cells exhibit mild proliferative activity as indicated by an increased Ki-67 labeling index (3–10%) in contrast to the absence of Ki-67 labeling in implantation site intermediate trophoblast. Some of the chorionic-type intermediate trophoblastic cells express epithelial membrane antigen (EMA), which is rarely expressed in other types of trophoblastic cells.[228]

The immunophenotype of trophoblastic cells in gestational trophoblastic lesions is similar to their normal counterparts. In routine pathologic practice, cytokeratin 18, hPL, inhibin-α, Mel-CAM (CD 146), and Ki-67 are particularly useful markers in the diagnosis of trophoblastic lesions. An algorithm that assists in the differential diagnosis of trophoblastic lesions is shown in Fig. 24.5. The practical application of immunohistochemistry in the differential diagnosis of gestational trophoblastic lesions is discussed under the specific trophoblastic lesions.

Functional Aspects of Trophoblast

Trophoblast plays a crucial role in implantation and embryonic development.[43,122] The major functions of trophoblast are as follows. First, the villous trophoblast (syncytiotrophoblast and cytotrophoblast) provides a structural interface for molecular transport between the maternal and fetal compartments. Second, implantation site intermediate trophoblast establishes the fetomaternal circulation in the placental site. Third, syncytiotrophoblast secretes several pregnancy-associated hormones that are necessary for successful maintenance of the placenta and fetus. Finally, syncytiotrophoblast as well as chorionic-type intermediate trophoblast in the fetal membranes serve as an immunologic barrier that prevents allograft rejection of the fetus by the maternal immune system. Functional abnormalities of trophoblast may account for several common gestational disorders including failure of implantation, which leads to spontaneous abortion, preeclampsia, and intrauterine growth retardation. The function of specific trophoblastic subpopulations are discussed next.

Previllous Trophoblast

The *previllous syncytiotrophoblast* is responsible for the initial erosion of maternal tissues during the early stages of implantation. Subsequently, it appears that the previllous mononucleate trophoblastic cells are responsible for further invasion and expansion of the implantation site. At approximately 13 days of gestation, mesenchyme penetrates the trophoblastic mass and chorionic villi develop, thus forming the rudimentary structure of the definitive placenta.

Cytotrophoblast

Cytotrophoblast is the trophoblastic stem cell and is located on the villous surface. Cytotrophoblast expresses epidermal growth factor receptor (EGFR), which binds to EGF secreted by the decidua.[83] It has been postulated that by a paracrine mechanism EGFR and its ligand may provide persistent growth stimulation for cytotrophoblast. Cytotrophoblast differentiates along two main pathways. Along one pathway, cytotrophoblast continues to proliferate and fuses to form the overlying syncytiotrophoblast. This process results in expansion of the surface area of chorionic villi in the developing placenta. In the second pathway, cytotrophoblast differentiates into villous intermediate trophoblast in the trophoblastic columns and then into implantation site intermediate trophoblast in the placental site or chorionic-type intermediate trophoblast in the chorion laeve.

Syncytiotrophoblast

Syncytiotrophoblast is composed of terminally differentiated cells that synthesize and secrete a variety of pregnancy-associated hormones thought to be critical in the establishment and maintenance of pregnancy. Some of these secretory proteins may also have a paracrine function by regulating the local microenvironment of decidua cells, inflammatory cells, and smooth muscle cells at the placental site. In addition to its role as an endocrine organ, the syncytiotrophoblast is bathed in maternal blood and is responsible for the exchange for oxygen, nutrients, and a variety of metabolic products between the mother and fetus.

Villous Intermediate Trophoblast

Villous intermediate trophoblastic cells proliferate in the proximal portion of trophoblastic columns and serve as the source from which implantation site and chorionic-type intermediate trophoblast are derived. In addition, villous intermediate trophoblastic cells may play an important role in maintaining the structural integrity of the villi that anchor the placenta to the basal plate. HNK-1 carbohydrate moiety expressed on the surface of the villous intermediate trophoblast may contribute to the intercellular cohesion in the trophoblastic columns, which counteract the mechanical shearing forces resulting from fetal movements and the turbulence created by the pulsatile blood flow in the placental bed.[193]

Implantation Site Intermediate Trophoblast

The major function of *implantation site intermediate trophoblast* is to establish the maternofetal circulation by invading the spiral arteries in the basal plate during early pregnancy.[62] The mechanisms underlying trophoblastic invasion are similar to those involved in tumor cell invasion.[27,227] For example, proteases are responsible for matrix degradation and tissue remodeling, a prerequisite for trophoblastic migration and invasion. Loss of E-cadherin expression is closely associated with the infiltrative phenotype of implantation site intermediate trophoblast.[192] Expression of growth factors and their receptors constitutes a unique molecular mechanism regulating trophoblastic behavior and cell-to-cell communication (autocrine or paracrine), including cellular migration, proliferation and differentiation. Expression of cell adhesion molecules is important for trophoblastic migration in different extracellular substrates and for cross talk between trophoblastic cells and their microenvironment.

Unlike malignant tumors, the invasion of implantation site intermediate trophoblast is tightly regulated, confined spatially to the implantation site and limited temporally to early pregnancy.[62,80,81] While extensively infiltrating the endometrium of the basal plate, the implantation site intermediate trophoblast invades only the inner third of the myometrium in the first trimester, decreasing to less than 10% of the myometrium by term. although the molecular mechanisms underlying the control of trophoblastic invasion currently are unclear, the invasive process can be modulated by both the trophoblast and the local microenvironment.[24,81] Fusion of mononucleate implantation site intermediate trophoblastic cells into multinucleated cells leads to the loss of their invasive and migratory phenotype. Although multinucleated implantation site intermediate trophoblastic cells can be seen in trophoblastic neoplasms such as placental site trophoblastic tumor, they are more frequently encountered in the normal or exaggerated placental site, a morphologic feature helpful in distinguishing exaggerated placental site from placental site trophoblastic tumor.

The binding of $\alpha_5\beta_1$ integrin to fibronectin has been shown to restrain invasion of implantation site intermediate trophoblastic cells.[47] Recently, it has been demonstrated that Mel-CAM (CD 146) expressed by implantation site intermediate trophoblastic cells binds to its putative ligand on the surface of smooth muscle cells and that the Mel-CAM–ligand interaction confers a stationary phenotype on trophoblastic cells, limiting their invasion into the superficial portion of myometrium.[195]

Another feature that distinguishes nonneoplastic trophoblastic cells from tumor cells is their pattern of cellular proliferation. The differentiation of implantation site intermediate trophoblast is accompanied by a decrease in cellular proliferation, in contrast to the uncontrolled proliferation in malignant neoplasms. Indeed, implantation site intermediate trophoblastic cells are negative for Ki-67, a proliferative marker, and are positive for several proteins that are involved in the arrest of cell cycle progression including $p21^{WAF1/CIP}$[130] and $p57^{kip\text{-}2}$.[35] Accordingly, any proliferative activity (mitotic figures or Ki-67-positive trophoblastic cells) in the implantation site intermediate trophoblast should be considered abnormal and a neoplastic process must be considered.

Spiral arteries at the implantation site are the targets for invasion by implantation site intermediate trophoblast. The mechanisms that are responsible for the tropism of implantation site intermediate trophoblast to the spiral arteries and not to other structures is unclear; one postulate is that the *oxygen gradient* may be a guiding cue. The trophoblastic invasion into the vascular wall is associated with abundant deposition of extracellular matrix that eventually replaces the entire smooth muscle layer of spiral arteries, resulting in the transformation of the arteries to large-caliber and low-resistance vascular channels. This unique feature of vascular invasion is not only observed in the normal placental site but also in the placental site trophoblastic tumor. Implantation site intermediate trophoblast replaces the lining endothelial cells and undergoes an epithelial–endothelial transdifferentiation characterized by the acquisition of several endothelial markers including VCAM-1, VE-cadherin, and α_4 integrin,[237] and Mel-CAM (CD 146),[187] all of which are expressed by endothelial cells. Accordingly, the term trophoblast pseudovasculogenesis has been proposed to describe this unique differentiation pathway of implantation site intermediate trophoblast.[46,237]

Some of the implantation site intermediate trophoblastic cells that invade the spiral arteries migrate along the vascular wall in a retrograde fashion to reach the spiral arteries beyond the implantation site in the myometrium. The intravascular implantation site intermediate trophoblastic cells tend to form trophoblastic aggregates that act like valves or a sieve to control the blood flow in the trophoblast-modified spiral arteries. The process of aggregation is associated with the expression of NCAM and E-cadherin. These cell adhesion molecules may be responsible for the enhanced intercellular cohesion among cells in trophoblastic aggregates in the spiral arteries because NCAM and E-cadherin function as homotypic cell–cell adhesion molecules. This hypothesis has been supported by a recent study in which the E-cadherin gene was introduced into an E-cadherin negative implantation site intermediate trophoblastic cell line, IST-1, resulting in a stationary and cohesive phenotype of IST-1 cells in culture (Shih, unpublished).

Chorionic-Type Intermediate Trophoblast

The functional role of chorionic-type intermediate trophoblastic cells is unknown. Unlike the implantation site intermediate trophoblast, the chorionic-type intermediate trophoblast proliferates throughout gestation as the total surface area of fetal membrane increases. Chorionic-type intermediate trophoblast may contribute to the synthesis of extracellular matrix, which is required to maintain the tensile strength of the fetal membrane.[19] It is also possible that chorionic-type intermediate trophoblast acts as a biologic and mechanical barrier to the maternal immune system and is important for fetal allograft survival (see following).

Classification of Gestational Trophoblastic Disease

We have modified the current WHO classification of GTD[183] to include recently described entities (Table 24.2).[188] In the modified classification, GTD can be broadly divided into molar lesions and nonmolar lesions. The molar lesions include partial and complete hydatidiform moles and invasive moles. The nonmolar lesions include choriocarcinoma and lesions derived from implantation site intermediate trophoblast (exaggerated placental site and placental site trophoblastic tumor) and those from the chorionic-type intermediate trophoblast (placental site nodule and epithelioid trophoblastic tumor) (Fig. 24.6). In the past, exaggerated placental site and placental site nodule were classified as "unclassified GTD." Both lesions are benign and have distinct histogenesis and morphologic features that justify their separate designation. The modified classification also includes epithelioid trophoblastic tumor, which is a recently described trophoblastic neoplasm distinct from choriocarcinoma and placental site trophoblastic tumor.

Table 24.2. Modified World Health Organization classification of gestational trophoblastic disease

Molar lesions		
	Hydatidiform mole	
		Complete
		Partial
	Invasive mole	
Nonmolar lesions		
	Choriocarcinoma	
	Placental site trophoblastic tumor	
	Epithelioid trophoblastic tumor	
	Miscellaneous trophoblastic lesions	
		Exaggerated placental site
		Placental site nodule

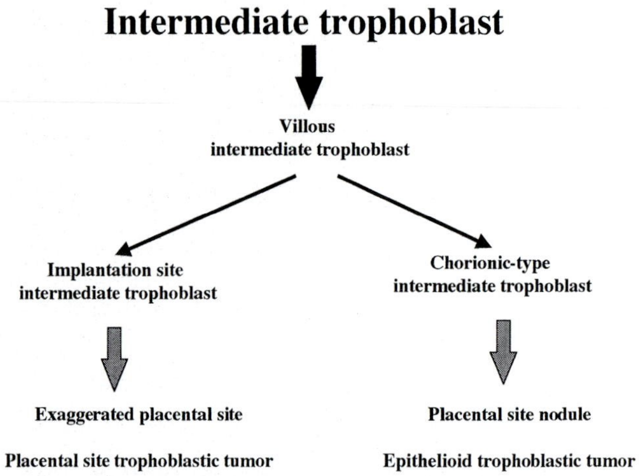

Fig. 24.6. Gestational trophoblastic disease (GTD) of placental site can be related to the different subpopulations of intermediate trophoblastic cells. Exaggerated placental site and placental site trophoblastic tumor are related to the differentiation of implantation site intermediate trophoblast whereas placental site nodule and epithelioid trophoblastic tumor are related to chorionic-type intermediate trophoblast.

General Features of Gestational Trophoblastic Disease

Epidemiology

The reported incidence of hydatidiform mole and choriocarcinoma varies widely throughout the world, being greatest in Asia, Africa, and Latin America and substantially lower in North America, Europe, and Australia.[17,41,75,82,86,107,163,201] The incidence rates are difficult to compare, however, because of limitations in the methodology of these studies.[17,82] Furthermore, some studies of incidence rates have used hospital-based rather than population-based figures, which probably result in overreporting.[82,163] There are no reported epideminologic data on incidence or geographic distribution for the more recently described placental site trophoblastic tumor and epithelioid trophoblastic tumor. Despite the various incidence rates documented, the overall incidence of GTD has been decreasing in recent years, especially in those geographic areas that have previously reported a higher incidence.[86,107]

The incidence rate for hydatidiform mole in the United States and Europe is approximately 1 in 1000 to 1 in 2000 pregnancies.[41,88,101,163] There is wide regional variation in the incidence of molar disease. In some other regions, especially Asia, the incidence can be as high as 1 in 500 pregnancies[17,82,108,201] and as low as 1 in 5000 pregnancies in other third-world countries such as Paraguay.[98,220] Based on recent studies, the estimated worldwide incidence of complete and partial mole is 1 per 1500–2000 pregnancies and 1 per 700 pregnancies, respectively.[101,163]

Choriocarcinoma occurs with a frequency of 1 in 20,000 to 1 in 40,000 pregnancies in the United States and Europe.[17,82,163] Estimates for incidence in Asia, Africa, and Latin America generally are higher, with incidence rates as high as 1 in 500–1000 pregnancies reported.[17,82,163] As with molar disease, there are marked regional variations in incidence rates. In Nigeria, choriocarcinoma is the third most common malignant tumor in women at one institution, ranking behind breast and cervical carcinoma. Thus, despite methodologic problems it appears that choriocarcinoma occurs at a substantially higher rate in developing countries than it does in North America and Europe. Previous studies found that 50% of choriocarcinomas were preceded by hydatidiform mole, 25% by abortion, 23% by a normal pregnancy, and 3% by an ectopic pregnancy.[129] Similar to hydatidiform moles, the overall incidence of choriocarcinoma in recent years has decreased dramatically as socioeconomic conditions improve.[86,107] These observations suggest that low socioeconomic conditions or dietary factors may contribute to the development of GTD.[13]

Gestational trophoblastic lesions are nearly always disorders of the reproductive years. Women who are sexually active are at risk for developing GTD, but the incidence is substantially higher in women before 20 and after 40 years.[13,163,164] In rare cases, GTD can develop in a postmenopausal woman with a long interval between the diagnosis of GTD and the antecedent pregnancy.[134,213] The absolute number of cases of mole or choriocarcinoma in women over 40 years is smaller because of their lower fertility. In contrast, maternal age has no effect on the risk of partial mole.[98] Neither paternal age nor race seems to affect the risk of developing a hydatidiform mole. Malignant sequelae for hydatidiform mole occur more frequently in older patients.[213] Although hydatidiform mole, choriocarcinoma, exaggerated placental site, and placental site nodule are nearly always confined to reproductive age women, placental site trophoblastic tumors and epithelioid trophoblastic tumors occur infrequently in postmenopausal women.

Several studies have revealed that a history of prior spontaneous abortions is more common in patients with hydatidiform mole and choriocarcinoma than with a normal pregnancy.[143] Furthermore, women who have had one hydatidiform mole are at increased risk of having another.[15,163] Conversely, term pregnancy and live births have a protective effect, with GTD less common in patients who are parous.[165] The protective effect appears to increase with an increased number of live births. A case-control study demonstrated that the risk factors for partial molar pregnancy include irregular cycles, only male infants among prior live births, and oral contraceptive use more than 4 years.[12] Compared to the influence of maternal age and antecedent obstetric history of molar disease, the evidence for a role of diet, ethnicity, endogenous estrogen levels, ABO blood group, and environment toxins is weaker.[163]

Cytogenetics

Cytogenetic studies of complete and partial hydatidiform mole show that *chromosomal abnormalities* play an important role in their development.[120] The karyotypic patterns of the two types of moles are considerably different. Most complete hydatidiform moles (>98%) have a normal DNA content or twice the normal DNA content. 46,XX is the most common karyotype[220] but both X chromosomes are androgenic, that is, of paternal origin (Fig. 24.7). This 46,XX karyotype results from duplication of a hap-

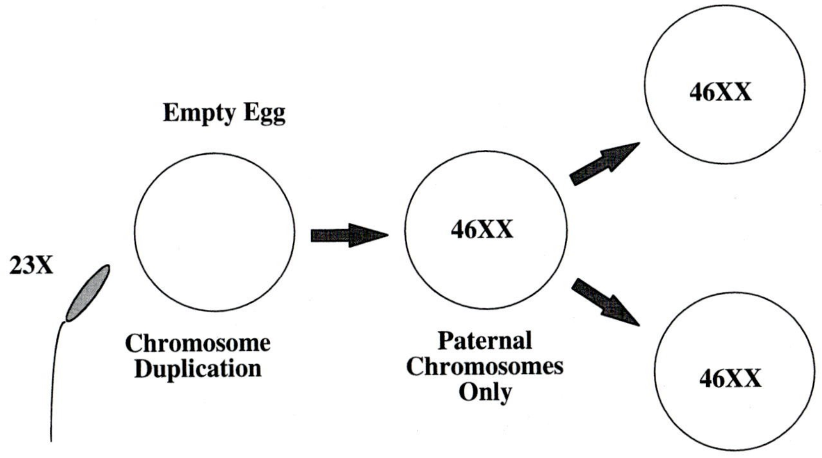

Fig. 24.7. Chromosomal origin of a complete hydatidiform mole. A single sperm fertilizes an empty egg. Reduplication of its 23,X set results in a completely homozygous diploid genome of 46,XX. A similar process follows fertilization of an empty egg by two sperms with two independently drawn sets of 23,X or 23,Y. Note that both karyotypes 46,XX and 46,XY can ensue.

loid sperm (23 chromosomes) pronucleus in an empty ovum that lacks functional maternal DNA. Duplication of a 23,Y sperm results in a nonviable 46,Y cell. A smaller proportion (3%–13%) of complete moles have a 46,XY chromosome complement, but in these moles, too, the chromosomes are androgenic. In this instance, the 46,XY-complete mole is believed to result from dispermy, that is, fertilization of an empty ovum by two sperm pronuclei, one with an X and the other with a Y chromosome. Accordingly, the complete mole, being paternally derived, constitutes a total allograft in the mother. On rare occasions, complete moles are triploid or aneuploid.

The karyotype of a partial mole is nearly always triploid (69 chromosomes) (Fig. 24.8) with a maternal chromosome complement. Conversely, not all triploid conceptuses demonstrate the histologic features of a partial mole. The percentage of partial moles among triploid conceptuses depends on the histologic criteria for the diagnosis and on the type of cytogenetic assays employed.[139,171] Rare examples of a partial mole with a 46,XX karyotype and an identifiable fetus,[98] as well as tetraploidy, aneuploidy, and haploidy, have been reported.[121] When triploidy is present in a partial mole, the chromosomal complement usually is 69,XXY or 69,XXX or, rarely, 69,XYY. These abnormal conceptuses result from the fertilization of an egg with a haploid set of chromosomes by either two sperms, each with a set of haploid chromosomes, or by a single sperm with a diploid genome of 46,XY.[100] This condition is known as diandric (paternally derived) triploidy in which two of the three haploid sets are of paternal origin. Diandric tripolids at early stages of development frequently show features of an early partial mole, but only a subgroup go on to develop the complete phenotype of a partial mole.[171] A conceptus with a diploid 46,XX maternal genome caused by failure of the first meiotic division and a haploid paternal set of chromosomes results in an abnormal, triploid (69,XXX or 69,XXY) fetus.[171] This event is referred to as a digynic (maternally derived) conceptus in which two of the three haploid sets are of maternal origin. There is no agreement as to the percentage of digynic triploids among all triploid placentas, but it is believed that digynic triploids generally do not present as a molar pregnancy.[98,139,171] In conclusion, most well-documented partial moles are (diandric) triploids, but not all triploid conceptuses are associated with partial moles. Partial molar pregnancies may have a grossly identifiable embryo or fetus with congenital anomalies.

Genetic studies of choriocarcinoma have shown that most choriocarcinomas are diploid[67] and that choriocarcinomas with aneuploidy may be associated with a poorer prognosis.[133] Several studies have demonstrated the androgenetic origin of choriocarcinoma following a complete hydatidiform mole.[48,63,180]

The cytogenetics of GTD other than molar pregnancy and choriocarcinoma, such as placental site trophoblastic tumor and epithelioid trophoblastic tumor, has not been as well studied because of the rarity of these neoplasms. However, new techniques such as fluorescence in situ hybridization, interphase cytogenetics, and polymorphism of oligonucleotide repeat sequences (microsatellites) have been recently performed on fixed tissue.[32,123,208,216] Although most GTD can be diagnosed by the pathologist on morphologic grounds alone, the application of these techniques may in the future play a role in diagnosis and management of GTD.[4,8,64,162] For ex-

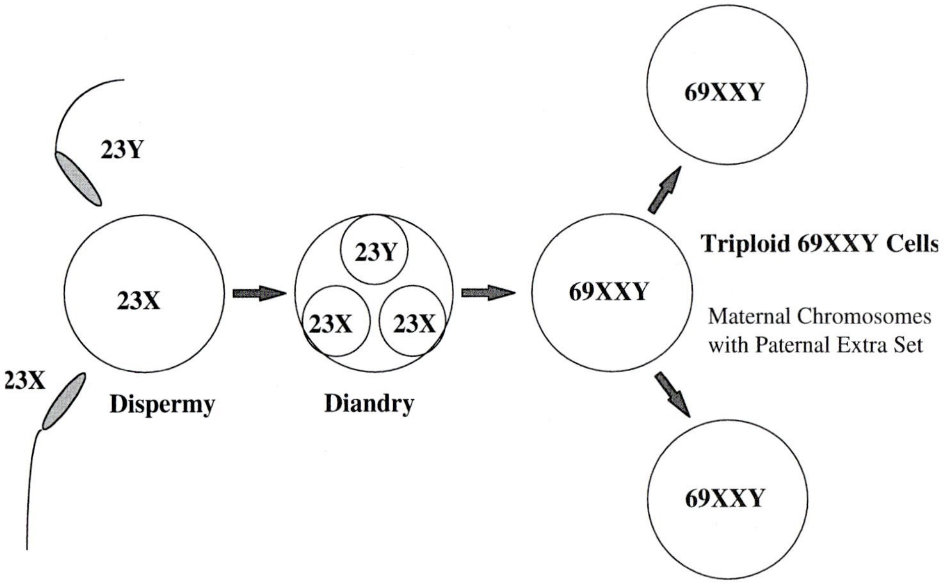

Fig. 24.8. Chromosomal origin of the triploid, partial hydatidiform mole. A normal egg with a 23,X haploid set is fertilized by two sperm that carry either sex chromosome, to give a total of 69 chromosomes with a sex configuration of XXY, XXX, or XYY. A similar result can be obtained by fertilization of a sperm carrying the unreduced paternal genome 46,XY (resulting sex complement, XXY only).

ample, microsatellite markers that differ in maternal or paternal origins have been used to confirm a complete mole.[123] Both fluorescence in situ hybridization using chromosome-specific markers and polymerase chain reaction using polymorphic markers have been employed to assist in differentiating a hydropic abortus from a partial mole and a partial mole from a complete mole.[8,32] Likewise, image DNA cytometric analysis and interphase cytogenetic analysis provide objective measurements that contribute to the differential diagnosis of complete mole, partial mole, and a hydropic abortion.[216]

Serum Markers

Treatment of GTD is based on determining, if possible, the specific histologic type of trophoblastic lesion, monitoring *serum human chorionic gonadotropin (hCG) titers*, and instituting chemotherapy when appropriate, hCG has proved to be an ideal marker for all forms of GTD, and measurement of serum hCG levels is an integral part of the management of this disease.[36,37]

hCG is produced mainly by syncytiotrophoblast,[117] and it is almost invariably detectable in the serum if trophoblastic tissue is present and when sensitive assays are used.[37] hCG is a glycoprotein composed of two polypeptide chains, alpha and beta, attached to a carbohydrate moiety. The configuration of hCG is similar to other gonadotropins, particularly luteinizing hormone (LH). The alpha-polypeptide chain in all these hormones is identical; it is the difference in the beta chain that gives the hormones their unique immunologic specificity and biologic function.[36] Accordingly, β-hCG is the most specific marker for GTD.

In normal pregnancy, β-hCG peaks to 50,000–100,000 mIU/ml at about 10 weeks gestation and decreases to 10,000–20,000 mIU/ml by 20 weeks, remaining at that level until term. Levels as high as 600,000 mIU/ml in early pregnancy have been reported. In molar gestations, β-hCG levels at diagnosis are variable, but most show a markedly elevated hCG titer, which is a useful diagnostic feature. Levels greater than 2 million mIU/ml have been reported. β-hCG titers are generally higher in complete as compared to partial moles.[45] In contrast to the high levels in hydatidiform moles and choriocarcinoma, β-hCG levels are much lower in placental site trophoblastic tumors and epithelioid trophoblastic tumors.[188] Nevertheless, β-hCG levels are very useful in monitoring patients with these tumors.

Recently, a β-core fragment of hCG in urine has been reported to be an even more sensitive marker, being detected in patients whose serum hCG levels are near or below the limit of detection.[173] Also recently, a sensitive radioimmunoassay (RIA) and immunoradiometric assay (IRMA) have been developed[36,37] that can measure serum β-hCG to a level of 0.5 mIU/ml. The assay can detect β-hCG production from as few as 1000 trophoblast cells, thus permitting follow-up to complete disappearance of trophoblastic tissue. Disappearance of β-hCG from the serum as measured by half-life shows two components, one with a half-life of 6 hours and a slower component with a half-life of about 30 hours.[36,37] Because heterophilic antibodies are known to interfere with the measurement of serum analytes, concurrent serum and urine testing for hCG should be used as routine policy in the diagnosis and follow-up of the patients with GTD.[177]

Staging and Prognostic Factors

Several systems including the modified International Federation of Gynecology and Obstetrics (FIGO) staging system, the World Health Organization (WHO) prognostic index score system, and the National Institute of Health (NIH) classification of metastatic GTD have been developed to predict prognosis and guide treatment.[202] The FIGO system uses an anatomic staging system (Table 24.3). Within each stage, patients with no risk factors are assigned to substage A, those with only one risk factor to substage B, and those with two risk factors to substage C.[52] The NIH classification is a clinical classification based on a variety of clinical features and serum hCG levels that segregates patients into good and poor prognosis (Table 24.4). The WHO scoring system divides patients into low-, intermediate-, and high-risk groups based on the total score of a variety of prognostic features (Table 24.5). All these systems have been shown to correlate with survival.[150,199] Of the three, the NIH clinical classification is the simplest to apply and is the best for identifying patients who are likely to fail therapy. Accordingly, the NIH system is currently preferred for determining initial therapy.[202] In addition to the diagnosis of choriocarcinoma, poor prognostic factors include metastatic disease at diagnosis, cerebral or hepatic metastases, symptoms for more than

Table 24.3. International Federation of Gynecology and Obstetrics (FIGO) staging of gestational trophoblastic disease

Stage	*Definition*
I	Confined to uterine corpus
II	Metastases to pelvis and vagina
III	Metastases to lung
IV	Distant metastases

Table 24.4. Clinical classification of malignant trophoblastic disease

Nonmetastatic GTD
Metastatic GTD
Good prognosis
Low hCG level (<40,000 mIU/ml serum β-hCG)
Symptoms present for less than 4 months
No brain or liver metastases
No prior chemotherapy
Pregnancy event is not term delivery (i.e., mole, ectopic, or spontaneous abortion)
Poor prognosis
High pretreatment hCG level (>40,000 mIU/ml serum β-hCG)
Symptoms present for more than 4 months
Brain or liver metastases
Prior chemotherapeutic failure
Antecedent term pregnancy

GTD, gestational trophoblastic disease; hCG, human chorionic gonadotropin.

4 months, failure of prior chemotherapy, and a pretreatment serum β-hCG titer of more than 100,000 mIU/ml.[128,149] More recently, the critical hCG level has been reduced to 40,000 mIU/ml by some investigators. Metastatic disease limited to the lungs or vagina is not a poor prognostic sign. In contrast, although it is difficult to assess precisely the prognostic significance of extrapulmonary metastases, patients with CNS metastases have an approximately 50% remission rate compared with involvement of other visceral organs.[58] Development of CNS metastases during the course of treatment confers an even worse prognosis.[58,129] Patients with hepatic metastases also have a poor prognosis, but multiagent chemotherapy appears to increase the survival rate. Choriocarcinoma diagnosed after a term gestation has a worse prognosis than choriocarcinoma diagnosed after a mole.

Pathogenesis of Gestational Trophoblastic Disease

The *pathogenesis of GTD* is largely unknown because few molecular studies have been performed.[174] This lack is in part due to the relative rarity of GTD and the absence of appropriate experimental models. The best-studied gestational trophoblastic lesion in hydatidiform mole and, to a lesser extent, the choriocarcinoma.

Development of a mole appears to be associated with an excess of paternal haploid set of chromosomes. The higher the ratio of paternal/maternal chromosomes, the greater the molar change. Complete moles show a 2:0 paternal/maternal ratio whereas partial moles show a 2:1 ratio. This hypothesis is supported by experimental evidence in a mouse model in which molecularly engineered mice that were either androgenetic or gynogenetic were created by microtransfer of male or female pronuclei into enucleated eggs.[207] Androgenetic embryos transplanted to a foster mother developed a bulky, hypertrophic placenta similar to complete moles in humans, whereas the gynogenetic embryos developed only a small placenta with a secondarily stunted embryo.

Table 24.5. World Health Organization scoring system based on prognostic factors[a]

	Score			
Prognostic factors	*0*	*1*	*2*	*4*
Age (years)	≤39	>39		
Antecedent pregnancy	Mole	Abortion	Term	
Interval[b]	4	4–6	7–12	>12
hCG (IU/L)	$<10^3$	10^3–10^4	10^4–10^5	$>10^5$
ABO groups (female × male)		O × A	B	
		A × O	AB	
Largest tumor (including uterine tumor)		3–5 cm	>5 cm	
Site of metastases		Spleen, kidney	GI tract, liver	Brain
No. of metastases identified		1–4	4–8	>8
Prior chemotherapy			Single drug	Two or more drugs

hCG, human chorionic gonadotropin; GI tract, gastrointestinal tract.
[a]The total score for a patient is obtained by adding the individual scores for each prognostic factor. Total score ≤ 4, low risk; 5–7, middle risk; and ≥8, high risk.
[b]Interval time (months) between end of antecedent pregnancy and start of chemotherapy.

Other than imprinted genes, several oncogenes and tumor suppressor genes have been studied in complete moles and choriocarcinoma. Synergistic upregulation of c-*myc*, c-*erb-*, c-*fms*, and *bcl-2* oncoproteins has been suggested in the pathogenesis of complete moles and choriocarcinomas.[70] Mutational analysis of K-*ras* and *p53* failed to show mutations in complete moles and choriocarcinomas,[28,70,185] although immunoreactivity of *p53* has occasionally been found in complete moles and choriocarcinomas.[71] The other genes that are potentially involved in development of choriocarcinomas include *DOC-2/hDab2*, a candidate tumor suppressor gene,[69] and a putative tumor suppressor gene(s) located in the chromosome 7p12-7q11.23,[135] and the *ras* GTPase-activating protein.[204]

Clinicopathologic Features, Behavior, and Treatment

Hydatidiform Mole

A *hydatidiform mole* is an abnormal placenta characterized by enlarged, edematous, and vesicular chorionic villi accompanied by a variable amount of proliferative trophoblast. It is subdivided into complete hydatidiform mole and partial hydatidiform mole based on morphologic, cytogenetic, and clinicopathologic features. Although typical complete and partial moles are easily distinguished on histologic examination, the routine use of ultrasound in pregnancy has led to the clinical diagnosis and evacuation of moles much earlier in gestation, often in the first trimester. As a result, the classical features of complete and partial moles that in the past were based on examination of specimens obtained in the second trimester are not as apparent, making the histopathologic diagnosis more difficult.

In addition, it has been recognized that a variety of other genetic abnormalities such as trisomy and monosomy may be associated with abnormal placentas that display minor degrees of hydropic change and trophoblastic proliferation but do not qualify as moles. Although recent studies have proposed new and expanded criteria for the diagnosis of these early moles and abnormal placentas, the criteria are subtle and difficult to reproduce, making the histologic diagnosis somewhat subjective. Furthermore, with the recognition that the genetic alterations that underlie these various lesions are distinctly different, one can legitimately question whether the diagnosis should be based on genetic as well as morphologic assessment. At present there are insufficient data to provide a definitive answer. Genetic analysis is costly, labor intensive, and is not available in most pathology laboratories. However, as these techniques become cheaper and more widespread, it is likely that genetic analysis will complement histopathologic evaluation in the diagnosis of difficult cases.

Complete Mole

Complete mole is characterized by hydropic swelling of the majority of villi and a variable degree of trophoblastic proliferation and atypia. Fetal tissue usually is not present. Most complete hydatidiform moles have a 46,XX karyotype. Early complete moles may lack hydropic swelling but trophoblastic proliferation and atypia are present.

Clinical Features

As already discussed, complete moles are being diagnosed now at an earlier gestational age than in the past (8.5–12 weeks versus 16–18 weeks) because of the routine use of sonography in pregnancy. Pelvic ultrasonic examination discloses a diagnostic "snowstorm" pattern. This pattern, especially when associated with a markedly elevated hCG level, is clinically diagnostic of molar pregnancy. Consequently, a complete mole now rarely presents with the classic signs and symptoms such as excessive uterine size, hyperemesis, theca lutein ovarian cysts, hyperthyroidism, or preeclampsia.[39,151,203] The majority of patients present with vaginal bleeding or are discovered by sonography. Although a presumptive diagnosis of an incomplete or missed abortion is usually made, serum β-hCG levels greater than 100,000 mIU/ml should prompt the physician to consider the diagnosis of molar pregnancy. In the past, excessive uterine enlargement for the gestational age occurred in approximately two-thirds of patients. Occasionally, the initial clinical manifestation is sudden passage of molar vesicles.

Preeclampsia (pregnancy-induced hypertension with edema and proteinuria) occurs in up to one-fourth of patients with complete mole. In contrast to nonmolar gestations in which preeclampsia occurs typically in the last trimester, in molar gestations preeclampsia occurs in the first trimester. Thus, early onset of preeclampsia, especially when coupled with excessive uterine enlargement, suggests the presence of a molar pregnancy. Additional clinical signs of molar pregnancy include hyperemesis gravidarum, occurring in a quarter of patients, and hyperthyroidism in 7%. Pulmonary embolization of trophoblast and massive ovarian enlargement caused by benign

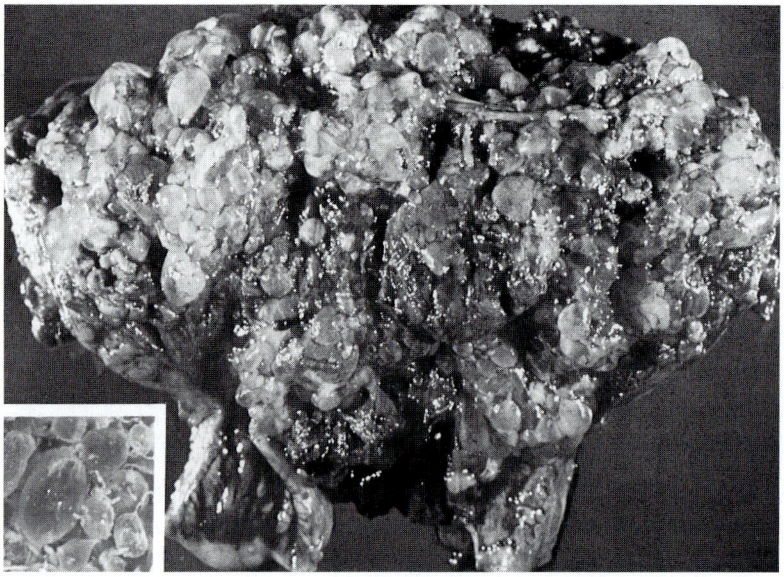

Fig. 24.9. Complete hydatidiform mole. Hysterectomy specimen shows an enlarged uterus with molar placental tissue protruding from the opened specimen. *Inset*: The hydropic villi range from a few millimeters to more than 1 cm in diameter.

theca lutein cysts (see Chapter 16, Nonneoplastic Lesions of the Ovary) are other possible clinical manifestations of a hydatidiform mole. With complete mole the hCG titer usually is markedly elevated.

Although these clinical signs and symptoms permit the diagnosis of a molar pregnancy before evacuation, the clinical presentation is quite variable. Up to 80% of cases are first diagnosed by histologic study of spontaneously passed or curetted tissue.[98]

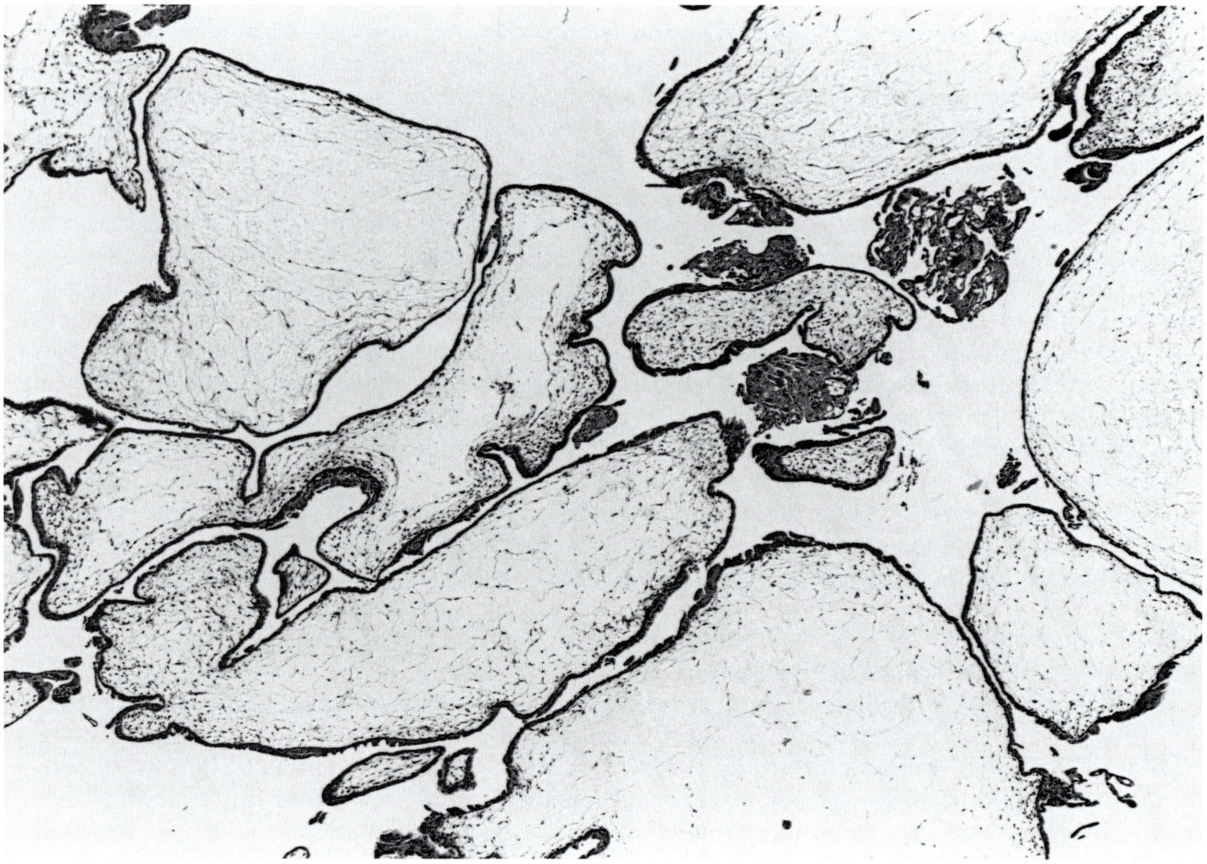

Fig. 24.10. Complete hydatidiform mole. Villi have extensive stromal edema with central cisterns. There is a minimal amount of proliferative trophoblast in this field.

Hydatidiform moles also can be found unexpectedly in elective abortion specimens of asymptomatic patients.[234] Hydatidiform mole may also occur in the fallopian tube and ovary.[205] A primary mole involving the adnexa should be discriminated from the hydropic change that is frequent in an aborting ectopic pregnancy and from invasive mole with extension into the broad ligament.

Gross Findings

In typical cases, massively enlarged, edematous villi give the characteristic grapelike appearance to the placenta (Fig. 24.9). However, the specimen volume of contemporary complete moles is significantly less than in the past,[151] and in very early complete moles hydropic change may be absent. In the typical mole, swollen villi may range from a few millimeters to as large as 3.0 cm in diameter but usually average about 1.5 cm. Rarely, fetal development may occur in complete mole. After suction curettage, molar villi may collapse and a large amount of bloody tissue may obscure the edematous villi, especially if a mole is extracted early in pregnancy when villous enlargement is less striking. In this instance, there may be no gross evidence of molar enlargement. Histologic evaluation of the tissue adherent to the gauze that collects suctioned uterine contents is necessary to establish the diagnosis. Immersing the gross tissue in saline or formalin can resuspend collapsed villi.[38]

Microscopic Findings

Complete moles have two key features: trophoblastic proliferation and villous edema. Many villi display central cistern formation characterized by a prominent central space that is entirely acellular (Fig. 24.10). A few smaller villi usually are present but these, too, are edematous. Previous studies reported that the villi of complete moles were avascular; however, using a CD 34 monoclonal antibody that identifies endothelial cells, a recent study not only identified numerous blood vessels in villi of complete moles but also found that the number of vessels was equivalent to those in normal placentas.[168]

All hydatidiform moles display some degree of trophoblastic proliferation on the villous surface. This trophoblastic proliferation in complete hydatidiform mole is circumferential around the villus. Columns and streamers of cells composed of a mixture of cytotrophoblast, syncytiotrophoblast, and villous intermediate trophoblast project randomly from the vil-

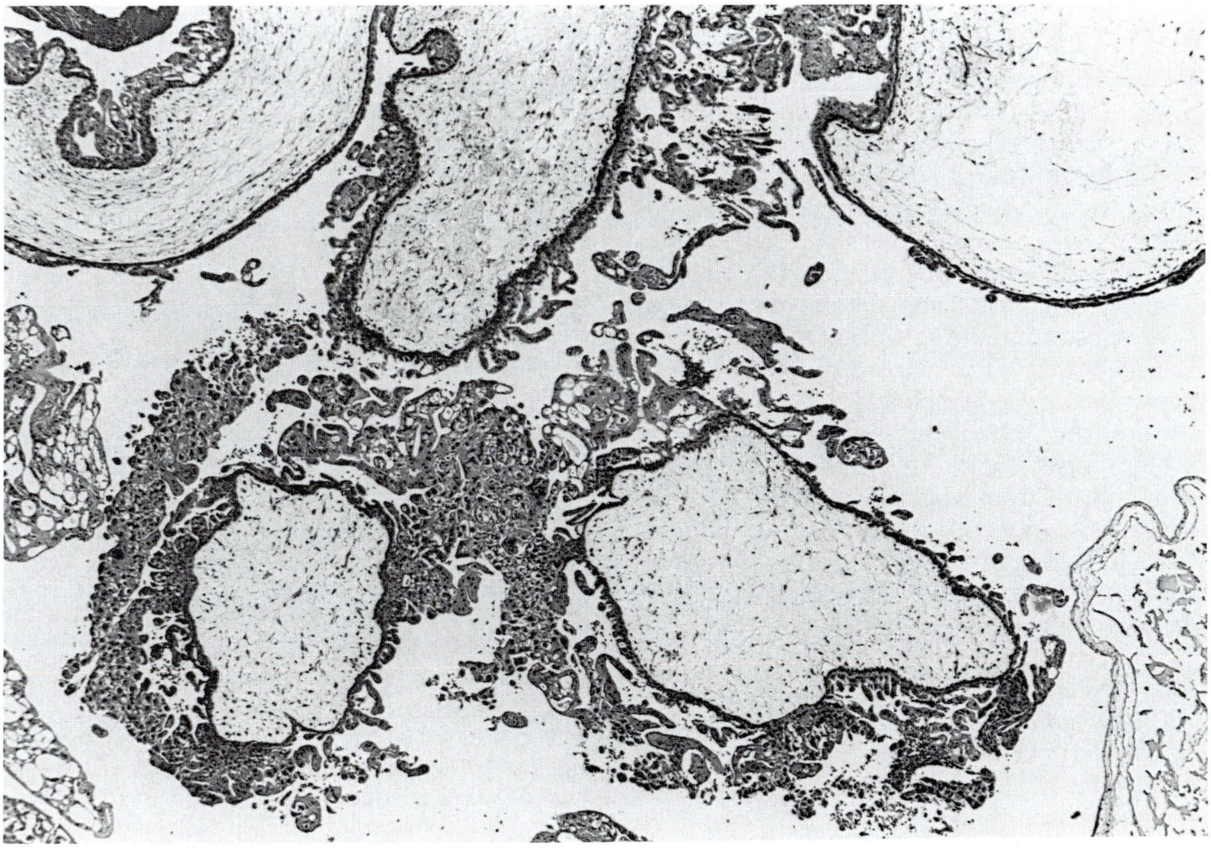

Fig. 24.11. Complete hydatidiform mole. Enlarged villi have a circumferential proliferation of trophoblast from the surface of several villi.

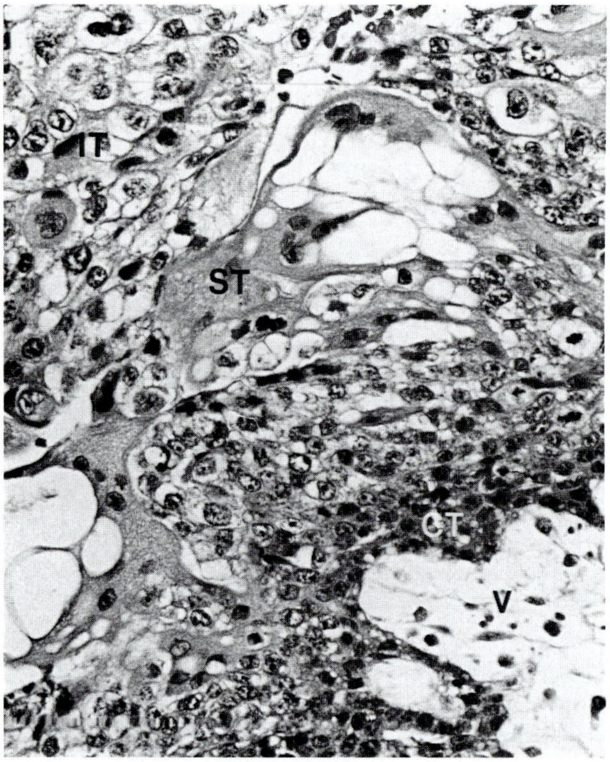

Fig. 24.12. Trophoblast in a complete mole. A mixture of cytotrophoblast (*CT*), intermediate trophoblast (*IT*), and syncytiotrophoblast (*ST*) grows from the surface of a villus (*V*).

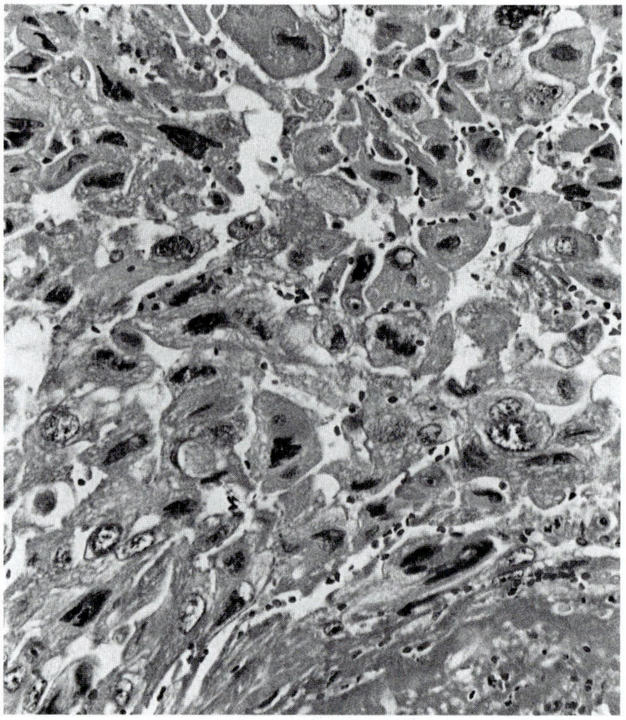

Fig. 24.13. Intermediate trophoblast in a complete hydatidiform mole. The mononucleate cells are pleomorphic with abundant amphophilic cytoplasm.

lous surface (Figs. 24.11 and 24.12). The amount of proliferative trophoblast in moles varies greatly. It may be marked, affecting most villi, or it may be subtle and only focally present, emphasizing the need for thorough sampling.[74] Large sheets of trophoblast including villous intermediate trophoblast that appear to be unattached to villi also may be present (Fig. 24.13); these may result from tangential sectioning or represent detached fragments of the trophoblast from the implantation site. Trophoblastic islands, structures seen in the normal early placentas, are rarely present in complete moles. The trophoblast of a complete mole always displays cytologic atypia. At times, it may be as marked as in choriocarcinoma (Fig. 24.14; see following).

Besides the trophoblastic hyperplasia on the villous surface, there is also a proliferation of implantation site intermediate trophoblastic cells in the placental site that morphologically resembles an exaggerated placental site.[189] As with the trophoblastic hyperplasia on the villous surface, the cells are more abundant and atypical than those encountered with an abortus and for that matter an exaggerated placental site. The immunostaining pattern for the markers of implantation site intermediate trophoblast is identical between the molar implanta-

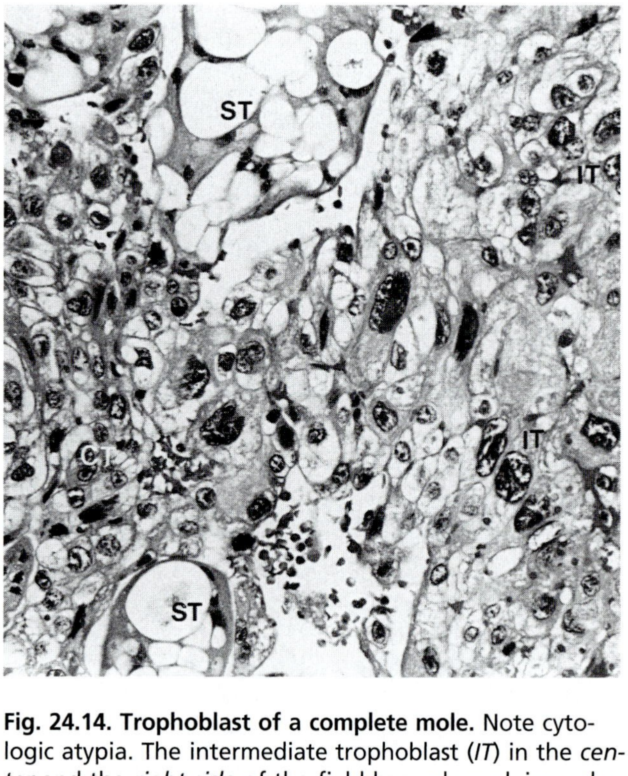

Fig. 24.14. Trophoblast of a complete mole. Note cytologic atypia. The intermediate trophoblast (*IT*) in the *center* and the *right side* of the field has enlarged, irregular nuclei. Cytotrophoblast (*CT*) is present on the left, and vacuolated syncytiotrophoblast (*ST*) is present in the *upper* and *lower* portions of the photo micrograph.

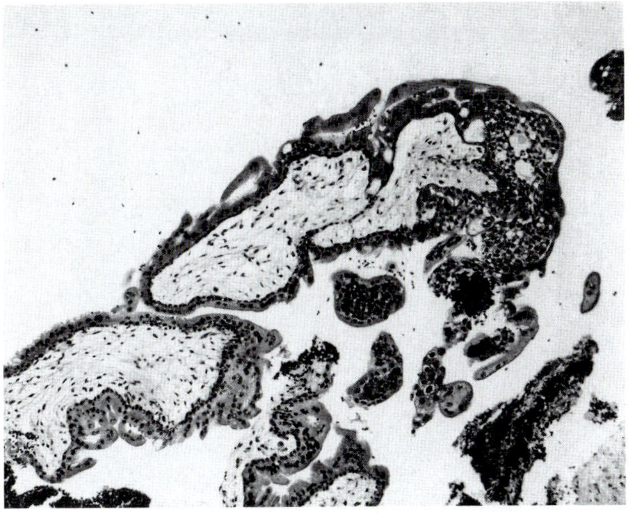

Fig. 24.15. An early complete hydatidiform mole. The villi are not particularly hydropic, and the trophoblastic hyperplasia and atypia are not marked. The circumferential proliferation of villous trophoblastic cells that project randomly from the villous surface is most characteristic.

tion site and an exaggerated placental site except the Ki-67 labeling index in a mole is 5.2% ± 4.0% compared to *no* Ki-67 labeling index in an nonmolar exaggerated placental site, suggesting that these two types of lesions are different despite their similar morphologic features.[147,189] Interestingly, as compared with the normal placentas, complete moles exhibit a higher level of apoptosis in cytotrophoblast, indicating a complex but delicate regulation of the cell population in complete moles.[167]

As noted previously, the typical morphologic features of a complete mole may be absent or very subtle in molar specimens evacuated in the first trimester (Fig. 24.15). These complete moles are referred to as "early complete moles." The histologic features of an early complete mole are (1) redundant bulbous terminal villi; (2) hypercellular villous stroma with primitive stellate cells and karyorrhexia; (3) a labyrinthine network of villous stromal canaliculi; (4) focal hyperplasia of cytotrophoblast and syncytiotrophoblast on both villi and the undersurface of the chorionic plate; and (5) atypical trophoblast lining the villi and in the implantation site.[106,151]

Differential Diagnosis

See following: "Partial Mode."

Behavior and Treatment

Between 2% and 12% of patients experience severe respiratory distress immediately after uterine evacuation of a hydatidiform mole.[112] This phenomenon usually is attributed to massive deportation of trophoblast to the lungs,[112] an exaggeration of a physiologic process occurring in normal pregnancy. Other factors, such as fluid overload, dilutional edema, preeclampsia, and hyperthyroidism may also contribute to the pathogenesis of the respiratory distress. The most serious complication after molar evacuation is persistent or metastatic GTD and the risk of developing choriocarcinoma.[39] Postmolar trophoblastic disease may represent a persistent mole in the uterine cavity or it may be an invasive mole or a choriocarcinoma. Persistent GTD occurs in approximately 17%–20% of women who have undergone evacuation and in 3%–5% of women who have undergone hysterectomy.[74] The risk of development of choriocarcinoma following a complete mole is about 2%–5% in the United States[39,57] and 13% in Japan.[136]

A number of clinical, morphologic, and immunohistochemical studies have tried to predict the prognosis of complete moles. In one study, age greater than 40 years, previous history of molar pregnancy, preevacuation hCG levels above 100,000 mIU/ml, uterine size greater than 20 weeks, and ovarian enlargement caused by theca lutein cysts[148] were important risk factors, but another study failed to confirm these findings.[153] In the past, some investigators argued that the degree of trophoblastic proliferation and atypia was useful in predicting prognosis, but more recent studies have found that grading of moles has no predictive value.[74,147] Similarly, DNA ploidy, chromosomal abnormalities, the presence of a Y chromosome, the Ki-67 labeling index, expression of oncogenes c-*erB-2* and *p53*, and a cyclin-dependent kinase inhibitor, $p21^{WAF1/CIP1}$, fail to consistently predict behavior.[22,29,30,31,33,102,217]

Apoptosis index has been recently proposed as a potentially useful prognostic marker of complete moles.[224] The apoptotic index of complete moles that spontaneously regressed was statistically higher than those that developed persistent GTD, but further studies are necessary to confirm this. Currently, follow-up with serial serum hCG titers using sensitive assays remains the mainstay of management.

Only 0.6%–1.5% of patients who have had a complete hydatidiform mole are at risk of having recurrent molar pregnancies.[15] After treatment with chemotherapy there is no increase in the risk of spontaneous abortion or congenital anomalies, and many patients subsequently have successful term pregnancies.[108]

A chest radiograph before treatment and 4 weeks later should be performed to exclude metastases. Following evacuation of a mole, careful hCG monitoring is mandatory because it is the most reliable and sensitive method for the early detection of persistent GTD.[78] The titers of β-hCG should fall to normal between 10 and 170 days after evacuation of a mole, and most patients will have normal titers by 60 days postevacuation. Persistent GTD after molar pregnancy is heralded by plateauing hCG titers for 2–4 weeks, rising hCG titers, persistent uterine disease such as abnormal bleeding, or evidence of metastases.[111] Initial therapy for persistent disease is usually methotrexate, dactinomycin, or a combination of the two.[129] Multiagent chemotherapy that includes etoposide (VP-16)[181] is used for the treatment of high-risk patients and for those who fail to respond to conventional forms of chemotherapy. The inclusion of etoposide in combination chemo-therapy, however, may increase the risk of secondary cancers.[178]

Partial Mole

A *partial hydatidiform mole* has an intimate admixture of two populations of villi, enlarged, edematous villi and normal-sized villi that may be fibrotic. Evidence of fetal development often is present in partial moles. Partial moles are usually the result of diandric triploidy; however, not all triploid conceptuses are partial moles.

Clinical Features

Partial moles usually present between the 9th and 34th weeks of pregnancy.[45,100] Patients with partial moles may have signs and symptoms similar to those seen in complete moles but usually this is less likely.[14,45,100] Uterine size is generally small for dates. Enlargement in excess of that expected for the gestational age is uncommon.[14] Frequently, patients with partial moles appear to have a missed abortion and vaginal bleeding is the main presenting symptom. Forty-two percent of patients with partial moles are at risk of preeclampsia, which tends to occur later than in complete mole but it can be equally severe.[100] Serum hCG levels often are in the low or normal range for gestational age.[14] Only a few patients with partial moles show markedly elevated hCG titers such as those seen with complete moles.[45]

Gross Findings

The volume of tissue is generally small, less than 100–200 ml. The villi may be grossly evident and recognizable as molar, yet are smaller than those found in a complete mole (Fig. 24.16). For early partial moles, these gross features may not be apparent. In some cases a fetus or fetal membranes is present (Fig. 24.17). When a fetus is found, it often shows gross congenital anomalies.

Microscopic Findings

Partial mole shows features in some villi that are similar to those seen in complete moles, but the molar change is focal (Fig. 24.18). By definition, there should be a mixture of edematous villi and small, relatively normal-sized villi.[45] Central cisterns are less conspicuous than in complete moles. Smaller villi usually show stromal fibrosis similar to that seen in missed abortions (Fig. 24.19). Trophoblastic hyperplasia is less marked than in complete mole. Generally it is focal and shows little, if any, atypia, consisting of small, haphazard tufts of trophoblast, often syncytiotrophoblast, emanating from the surface of some of the abnormal villi. Another feature commonly encountered in partial mole is a scalloped outline of the enlarged villi, yielding a pattern of trophoblastic invaginations into the villous stroma. When the invaginations do not show conti-

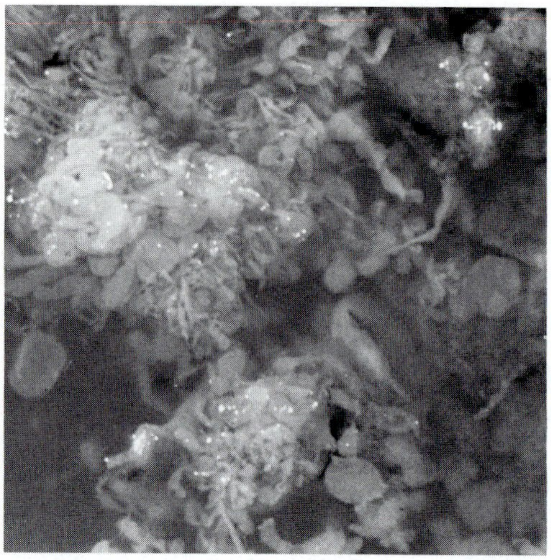

Fig. 24.16. Partial hydatidiform mole. Hydropic villi mixed with smaller villi.

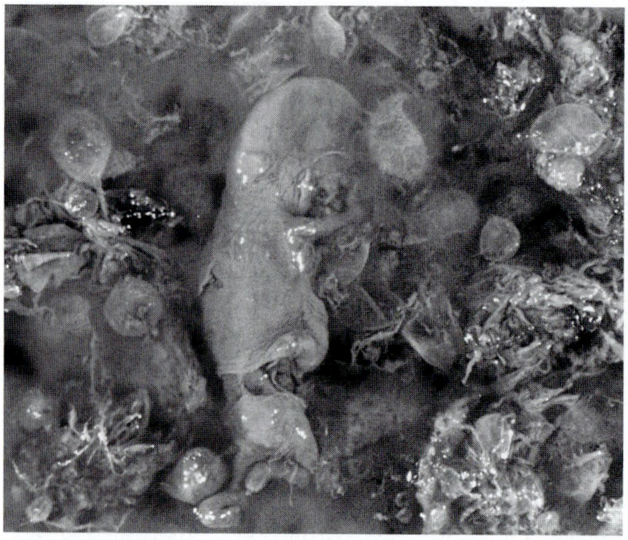

Fig. 24.17. Partial hydatidiform mole. A macerated fetus surrounded by villi with visible hydropic change. Often, the fetus in partial mole shows congenital abnormalities.

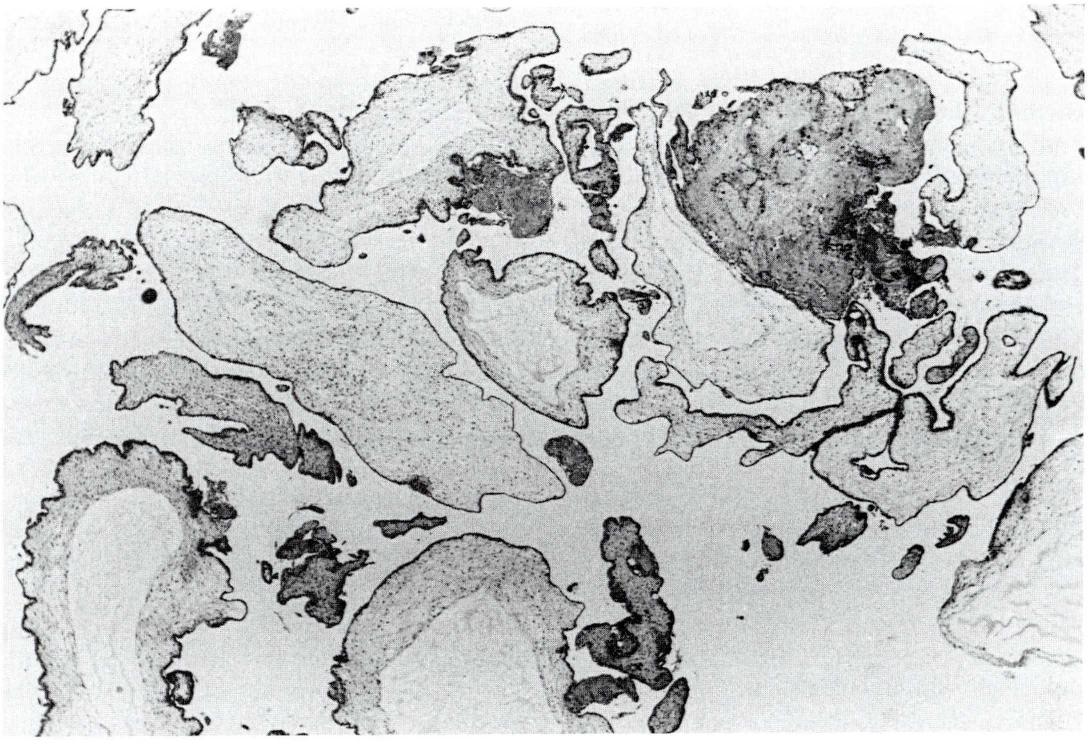

Fig. 24.18. Partial hydatidiform mole. A mixture of enlarged villi with cisterns and small, normal-sized and fibrotic villi. A small degenerating fetus was present elsewhere.

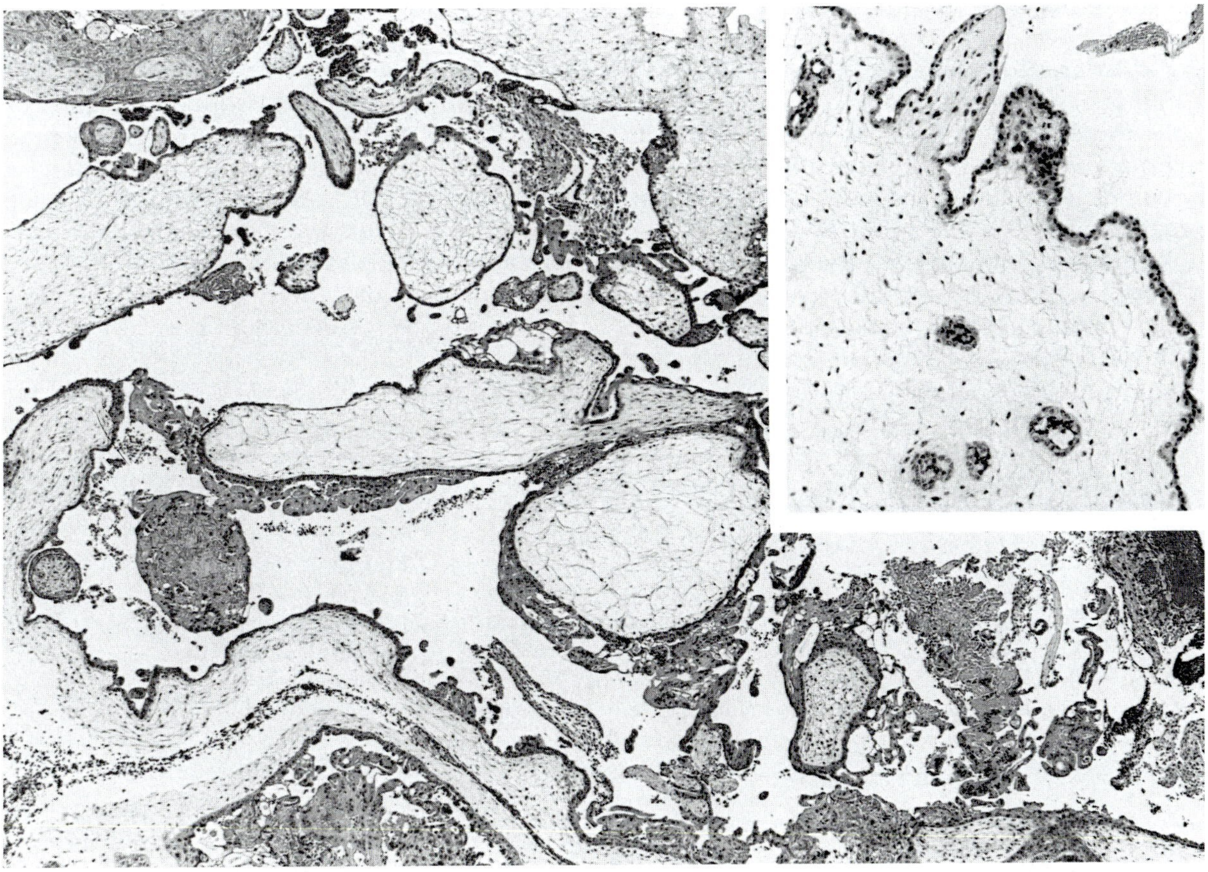

Fig. 24.19. Partial hydatidiform mole. Proliferative trophoblast projecting randomly from the villus surface. Normal-sized, fibrotic villi are present in the *left upper corner*. This specimen consisted of 50 ml of tissue. There was no evidence of a fetus. *Inset*: Scalloped villous surface with trophoblast infolding, forming inclusions.

nuity with the surface trophoblast, they appear as inclusions within the stroma (Fig. 24.19). Invaginations are not exclusive for partial moles and may, on occasion, be found in other conditions including complete mole and nonmolar hydropic abortus.

Partial moles with triploid are usually associated with the presence of a fetus or its amnion (see Fig. 24.17), in contrast to the absence of fetal structures in most complete moles. Fetal demise with subsequent degeneration of fetal structures may make identification of fetal tissue difficult. A subtle clue is the presence of a functioning villous circulation containing nucleated red cells, a feature that requires fetal development. In contrast, the embryo associated with a complete mole usually dies before organogenesis and, therefore, fetal structures are not present in the specimen and fetal erythrocytes are not present within placental vessels. One concern in the diagnosis of an apparent partial mole is that the specimen represents a twin gestation with a fetus and a complete mole. Such twin pregnancies may occur[119] but probably are an infrequent occurrence relative to singleton gestations of a partial mole.

Differential Diagnosis

Diagnosis of hydatidiform moles by histology and polidy analysis is compromised by overlap of morphologic criteria for complete mole, partial mole, and a nonmolar hydropic abortus. The diagnosis of complete versus partial moles is usually relatively straightforward but can be more difficult when an early complete hydatidiform mole is encountered. The pathologic features of partial as compared with complete moles are shown in Table 24.6. Evidence of a fetus or embryo strongly favors the diagnosis of partial mole, although the rare event of a twin gestation with one conceptus being a complete mole should be borne in mind.

Morphologic distinction of a hydatidiform mole from an abortus with abnormal villous morphology may be problematic, and there is a considerable degree of interobserver variance in making this distinction.[34,94,144] Spontaneous abortions often are associated with failure of development or early demise of the embryo, the so-called blighted ovum or hydropic abortus. These specimens show some villous edema with hydropic swelling, features shared with molar placentas. The hydropic abortus usually is a smaller specimen, however.[38] The villi in a hydropic abortus are enlarged only slightly and do not assume the large dimensions found in complete or partial moles (Fig. 24.20). Cisterns can be seen in nonmolar abortions but they are focally distributed. Hyperplasia of villous trophoblast is not evident in these cases. The proliferative trophoblast on the villous surface of early pregnancy also must be distinguished from the trophoblastic hyperplasia of molar pregnancy. The trophoblast proliferating from the villous surface of an abortus shows polar distribution characterized by proliferation of trophoblast at the distal end of the villus that implants into the basal plate. Similarly, villi with trophoblastic islands can be regarded as polarized villi that are also associated with a nonmolar abortus (Fig. 24.20). This directional orientation contrasts with the irregular or circumferential proliferation of molar trophoblast. In conclusion, partial moles display at least three of the following histologic features: two discrete populations of villi, circumferential mild trophoblastic hyperplasia, trophoblastic inclusions, prominent scalloping of villi, or cistern formation. In contrast, nontriploid abortus display at most two of the diag-

Table 24.6. Pathologic features and behavior of complete and partial moles

Feature	*Complete*	*Partial*
Karyotype	46,XX, 46,XY	Triploid
Embryo/fetus	Absent	Present
Villous outline	Round	Scalloped
Hydropic swelling	Marked; cisterns present	Less pronounced and focal
	All villi involved	Cisterns less prominent
	Circumferential	Villous fibrosis
Trophoblastic proliferation	Variable, may be marked	Focal and minimal
Trophoblastic atypia	Often present	Absent
Implantation site	Exaggerated[a]	Normal or occasionally exaggerated
p57 (kip2) staining	Negative or weakly positive	Diffusely positive
Behavior	10%–30% develop GTD	0.5%–4% develop GTD

[a]Exaggerated implantation site indicates an increase in the number and the extent in invasion of implantation site intermediate trophoblastic cells.

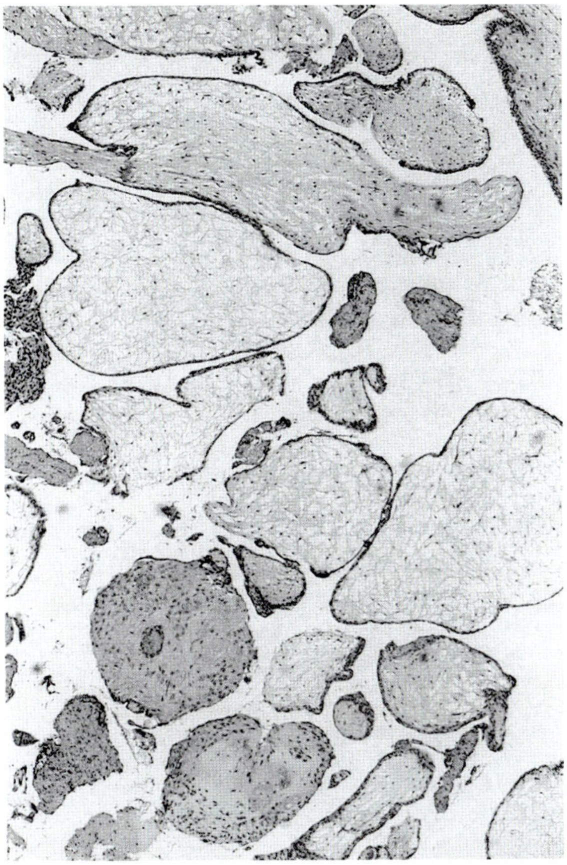

Fig. 24.20. Hydropic abortus. The villi are only slightly enlarged. They do not assume the large dimensions found in complete or partial moles. In addition, there is no trophoblastic hyperplasia in a hydropic abortus.

nostic features of partial moles.[34] If a specimen consists of only one or two cassettes of tissue with mild microscopic villous edema, it is most likely a hydropic abortus (M.T. Mazur, unpublished finding).

Immunohistochemical stains with the p57^{kip2} antibody can be helpful in the differential diagnosis of complete hydatidiform moles. Expression of p57^{kip2}, a maternally imprinted gene, is either absent or low in intermediate trophoblast in cases of complete moles in contrast to diffuse staining in partial moles and nonmolar placentas.[35] Finally, molecular genetic analysis including polymerase chain reaction (PCR) assay for polymorphic markers, fluorescence in situ hybridization (FISH), and flow cytometry from paraffin-embedded tissue may be helpful in classifying cases that do not clearly fall into the category of complete mole, partial mole, or nonmolar hydropic abortion based on morphologic features alone.[8,32,38,118,119,120]

When large aggregates of atypical or proliferating trophoblast are encountered without any villi, the differential diagnosis should include choriocarcinoma or placental site trophoblastic tumor. Care must be taken to be certain that sampling is adequate because villi may be sparse. The entire specimen should be processed. Limited examination of a uterine, vaginal, or pulmonary lesion may show only trophoblast, but deeper sectioning may reveal molar villi.

Behavior and Treatment

Recent studies have shown that partial moles are rarely followed by persistent or metastatic GTD with risk estimates ranging from 0.5% to 4%.[7,16,45,79,119,136,142,235] Misinterpretation of complete moles as partial moles is a major factor contributing to the overestimated frequency of persistent GTD after partial mole in previous studies.[14]

Invasive mole and metastatic pulmonary lesions have been reported in association with a partial mole.[136] A rare well-documented case of choriocarcinoma following a partial mole,[72] and as in situ choriocarcinoma arising in a partial mole have been reported.[89] The magnitude of the risk of repeated partial moles is not known, although repetitive partial moles do occur.[172]

Although the development of persistent GTD following a partial mole is uncommon, follow-up of patients after evacuation of a partial mole is warranted.

Invasive Mole

Invasive mole is a hydatidiform mole in which hydropic villi invade the myometrium or blood vessels or, more rarely, are deported to extrauterine sties.

Clinical Features

Invasive mole is a possible sequela of a hydatidiform mole, complete or partial. It is unusual for invasive mole to present primarily, although invasive mole may occur simultaneously with intracavitary molar pregnancy. Pathologic diagnosis requires demonstration of molar villi invading the myometrium or deported to extrauterine sites. When deportation occurs, invasive moles generally are found in the lungs, vagina, vulva, or broad ligament. The diagnosis usually is made on a hysterectomy specimen. However, invasive mole is rarely confirmed histologically because hysterectomy is rarely performed in patients with persistent hCG titers after removal of an intrauterine mole and because metastatic lesions of GTD usually are treated successfully with cytotoxic chemotherapy without biopsy.[210]

Gross Findings

In the uterus, invasive mole is an erosive, hemorrhagic lesion extending from the uterine cavity into

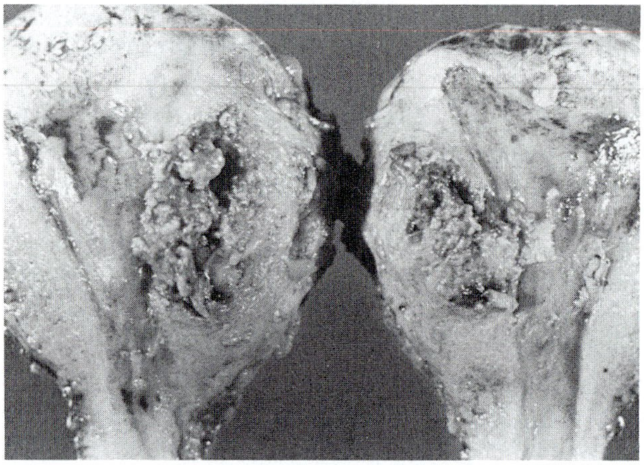

Fig. 24.21. Invasive mole. The lesion infiltrates deeply into the myometrium, forming a ragged, irregular mass.

the myometrium (Fig. 24.21). Invasion can range from superficial penetration to extension through the wall, with perforation or involvement of the broad ligament. Molar vesicles often are grossly apparent.

Microscopic Findings

Microscopically, the diagnostic feature is the presence of molar villi along with trophoblast in the myometrium or at an extrauterine site (Fig. 24.22). Trophoblastic proliferation with atypia accompanies the enlarged villi and is as variable as in noninvasive mole, ranging from slightly proliferative with minimal atypia to marked trophoblastic proliferation with extreme atypia (Fig. 24.23). Hydropic swelling tends not to be as marked as in noninvasive mole. Molar villi usually are no more than 4–5 mm in diameter. In metastatic sites, the diagnosis is based on the presence of villi. Careful searching may be necessary to identify villi within a lesion seemingly composed entirely of highly proliferative trophoblast. Lesions at distant sites usually are composed of molar villi confined within blood vessels without invasion into adjacent tissue. The molar villi at the extrauterine sites are the result of intravascular deportation.

Differential Diagnosis

Because the pathologic diagnosis of invasive moles requires identification of molar villi and trophoblast either within the myometrium or at an extrauterine site, few lesions enter into the differential. Recurettage of the endometrium after diagnosis of a mole may show proliferative trophoblast with villi but this does not represent an invasive mole unless myometrial invasion is found. If postmolar curettage yields only trophoblast, the diagnosis of invasive mole is not established. Two forms of placenta accreta, specifically placenta increta or percreta, represent normal placenta that has implanted without an intervening decidual layer and invaded myometrium. In contrast to invasive mole, however, the villi in accreta are not hydropic and the trophoblast does not show the proliferative activity found in a mole.

Invasive mole must be discriminated from choriocarcinoma. Both invasive mole and choriocarcinoma after a hydatidiform mole are manifested by a plateau or elevation in the hCG titer. Furthermore, both can give rise to secondary lesions. Consequently, it is often not possible clinically to distinguish between these lesions. A repeat curettage may yield more molar tissue, obvious choriocarcinoma, or scant fragments of trophoblast unaccompanied by villi but lacking unequivocal features of choriocarcinoma. In the latter instance, a diagnosis of atypical trophoblast is appropriate, accompanied by a description and the reasons why a diagnosis of residual mole or choriocarcinoma was not made. When more molar tissue is found, a diagnosis of persistent hydatidiform mole is made.

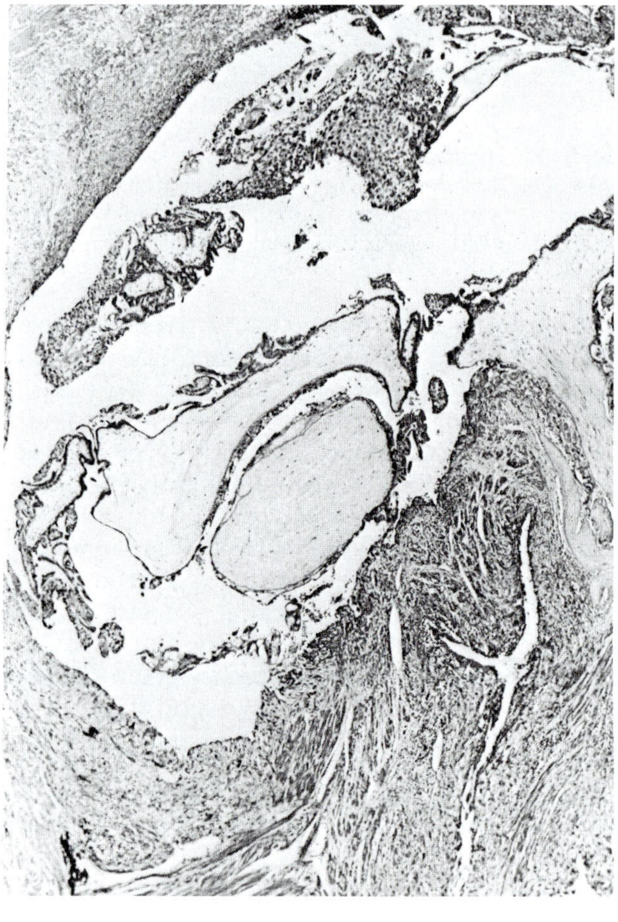

Fig. 24.22. Invasive mole. A hydropic villus within a large vein deep within the myometrium. Proliferative trophoblast accompanies the villi.

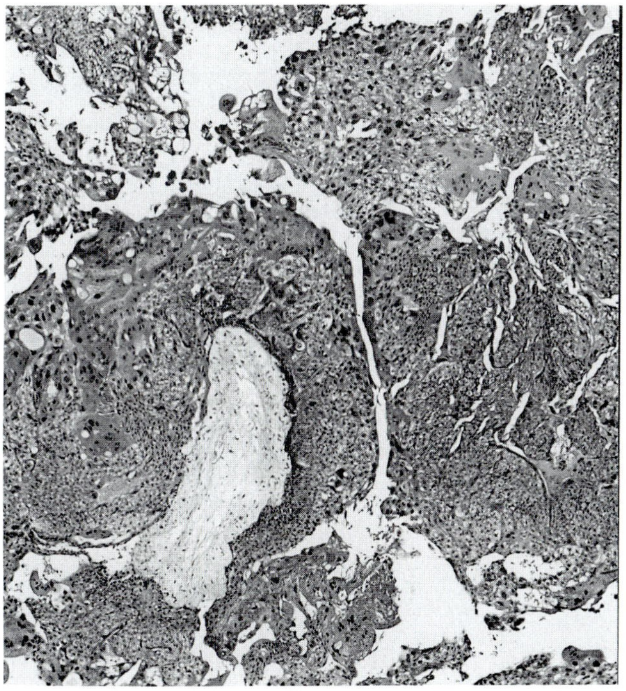

Fig. 24.23. Invasive mole. A single hydropic villus with marked trophoblastic hyperplasia is found in a biopsy of the uterine serosa. The lesion perforated the uterus and formed multiple hemorrhagic nodules on the serosa several months after abortion of a complete mole.

Behavior and Treatment

Invasive mole is the most common form of persistent or metastatic GTD after hydatidiform mole, occurring 6–10 times more frequently than choriocarcinoma.[210] In histologically verified cases the lesion most often is confined to the uterus, with distant spread occurring in 20%–40% of cases. Typically this involves the lungs, but the vagina, vulva, and broad ligament are also well recognized. Rare examples of spread t other sites such as the paraspinal soft tissue have been reported. Using modern chemotherapy, death from invasive mole is unusual[129]; most patients, even with distant spread, survive. The risk of progression to choriocarcinoma is no greater than that after complete mole.

Invasive mole is the clinical diagnosis given to many patients with extrauterine disease or abnormally persistent hCG titers after molar pregnancy and no residual hydatidiform mole within the uterine cavity.[129,210] In such instances, there is, however, a possibility that persistent hCG levels may be caused by choriocarcinoma. In these cases, the clinical term persistent GTD or gestational trophoblastic neoplasia[111] is used without attempting to discriminate between invasive mole and choriocarcinoma.

Choriocarcinoma

Gestational choriocarcinoma is a highly malignant epithelial tumor arising from the trophoblast of any type of gestational event, most often a hydatidiform mole. Choriocarcinoma is for all practical purposes limited to reproductive age women, but rare examples of choriocarcinoma in postmenopausal women have been reported.[53] It consists predominantly of a biphasic proliferation of mononucleate trophoblast and syncytiotrophoblast that morphologically recapitulates the primitive trophoblast of the previllous stage during placental development. Chorionic villi are not a component of this tumor.

Clinical Features

Theoretically, choriocarcinoma may arise in the trophoblast of the primitive blastocyst during implantation, but most cases of choriocarcinoma appear to follow a recognizable gestational event. Indeed, "in situ" choriocarcinoma can be found in a third-trimester placenta with a transition from normal-appearing cytotrophoblast to neoplastic cytotrophoblast. The more abnormal the pregnancy, the more likely that choriocarcinoma may supervene. Hertig and Mansell found an incidence of 1 in 160,000 normal gestations, 1 in 15,386 abortions, 1 in 5,333 ectopic pregnancies, and 1 in 40 molar pregnancies.[90] In that series, one-half of the cases of choriocarcinoma were preceded by hydatidiform mole, with 25% following abortion, 22.5% following normal pregnancy, and 2.5% following ectopic pregnancy.[90] Other studies have generally confirmed these figures.[129]

The signs and symptoms of choriocarcinomas are protean. Abnormal uterine bleeding is one of the most frequent presentations of choriocarcinoma, but uterine lesions may be restricted to the myometrium and remain asymptomatic. Not all patients have a demonstrable lesion in the uterus after an intrauterine gestation. Many examples of metastatic choriocarcinoma without a primary uterine tumor have been described.[138] It is highly likely that the neoplasm undergoes regression in the uterus. Although the majority of choriocarcinomas develop shortly after the preceding gestation (Table 24.7), long latency (>10 years) between the gestation and diagnosis can occur.[53] A rare case of choriocarcinoma has been reported in which an intervening normal pregnancy occurred 7 years before the diagnosis of choriocarcinoma.[208]

Sometimes, symptoms related to metastases are the first indication that a choriocarcinoma is present, and the lungs are the most frequent sites for metastasis.[126,138] Symptomatology related to hem-

Table 24.7. Clinical features of placental site trophoblastic tumor (PSTT), epithelioid trophoblastic tumor (ETT) and choriocarcinoma

Feature	*PSTT*	*ETT*	*Choriocarcinoma*
Clinical presentation	Missed abortion	Abnormal vaginal bleeding	Persistent GTD after hydatidiform mole
Last known pregnancy or GTD	Variable, can be remote	Variable, can be remote	Months
History of mole	5%–8%	14%	50%
Serum hCG	Low (<2,000 mIU/ml)	Low (<2,000 mIU/ml)	High (>10,000 mIU/ml)
Behavior	Self-limited, persistent, or aggressive	Self-limited, persistent, or aggressive	Aggressive if untreated
Response to chemotherapy	Variable	Variable	Good
Treatment	Surgery (hysterectomy)	Surgery (hysterectomy)	Chemotherapy

GTD, gestational trophoblastic disease; hCG, human chorionic gonadotropin.

orrhagic events in the central nervous system, liver, and gastrointestinal or urinary tracts also occurs. Thyrotoxicosis may occur in choriocarcinoma.[159]

Although rare, gestational choriocarcinoma may coexist with an intrauterine pregnancy, either as an incidental microscopic finding or a concurrent disease with the diagnosis of choriocarcinoma during pregnancy.[236] Gestational choriocarcinoma also may be primary in the fallopian tube, and in this instance, the tumor probably is a sequela to an ectopic pregnancy. This is a rare event, estimated to be 1 tubal choriocarcinoma for every 1.6 million intrauterine pregnancies.[130,154,160] These tumors usually cause symptoms suggesting an ectopic pregnancy or appear as an adnexal mass that mimics an ovarian tumor. Primary gestational choriocarcinoma of the ovary is difficult to document but does occur.[221]

Gross Findings

Uterine choriocarcinoma generally is a dark red, hemorrhagic mass with a shaggy, irregular surface and variable amounts of necrosis (Figs. 24.24 and 24.25). Occasionally, a lesion may lack significant hemorrhage and appear as a fleshy, tan-gray mass with necrosis. The size of uterine lesions varies greatly, ranging from tiny, microscopic foci to huge, necrotic tumors. Metastases beyond the uterus appear well circumscribed and hemorrhagic (Figs. 24.26 and 24.27).

Microscopic Findings

Choriocarcinoma is characterized by masses and sheets of trophoblastic cells that invade surrounding tissue and permeate vascular spaces (Figs. 24.28–24.31). Choriocarcinoma is generally not associated with chorionic villi, but the presence of chorionic villi in the specimen does not necessarily exclude the diagnosis because choriocarcinoma rarely may be found in a placenta.[236] Central hemorrhage and necrosis with viable tumor constituting only a thin peripheral rim is a characteristic feature.

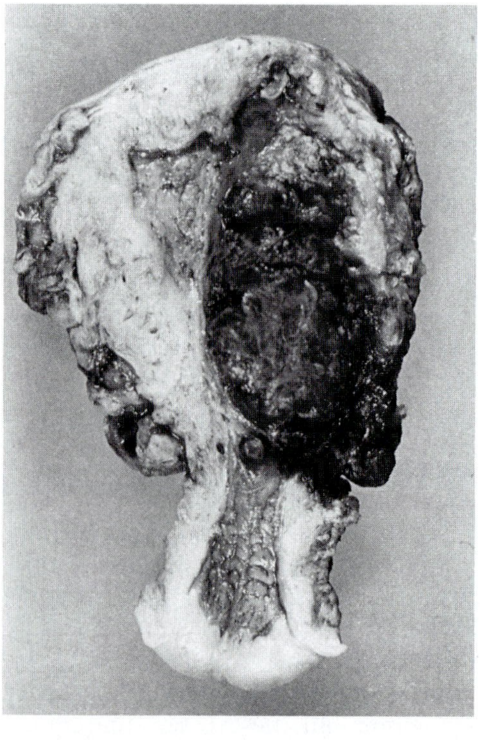

Fig. 24.24. Choriocarcinoma. The tumor forms a large, hemorrhagic mass that involves the endometrium and myometrium.

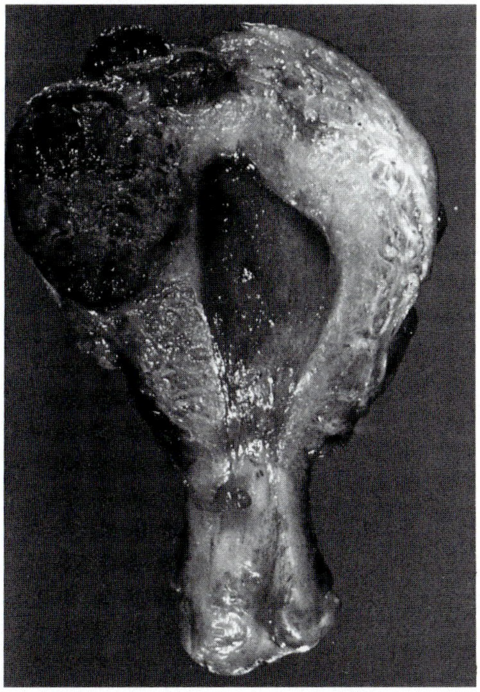

Fig. 24.25. **Choriocarcinoma.** The tumor forms a circumscribed mass within the myometrium that does not involve the endometrium. Lesions such as this may be asymptomatic because of their location.

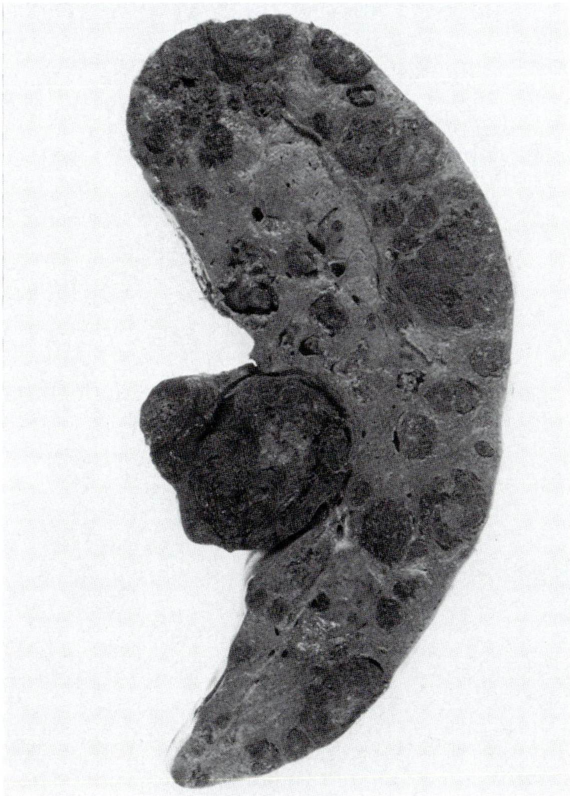

Fig. 24.26. Liver metastases from choriocarcinoma. Multiple, circumscribed, hemorrhagic masses are evident.

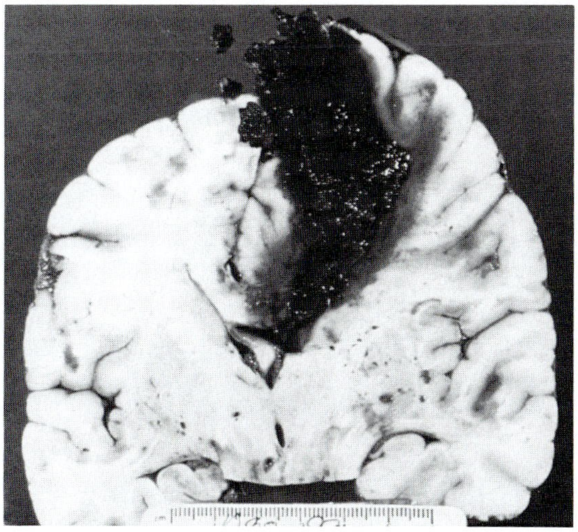

Fig. 24.27. Metastatic choriocarcinoma to the brain. Extensive hemorrhage caused death. At autopsy, the patient had metastases in multiple organs.

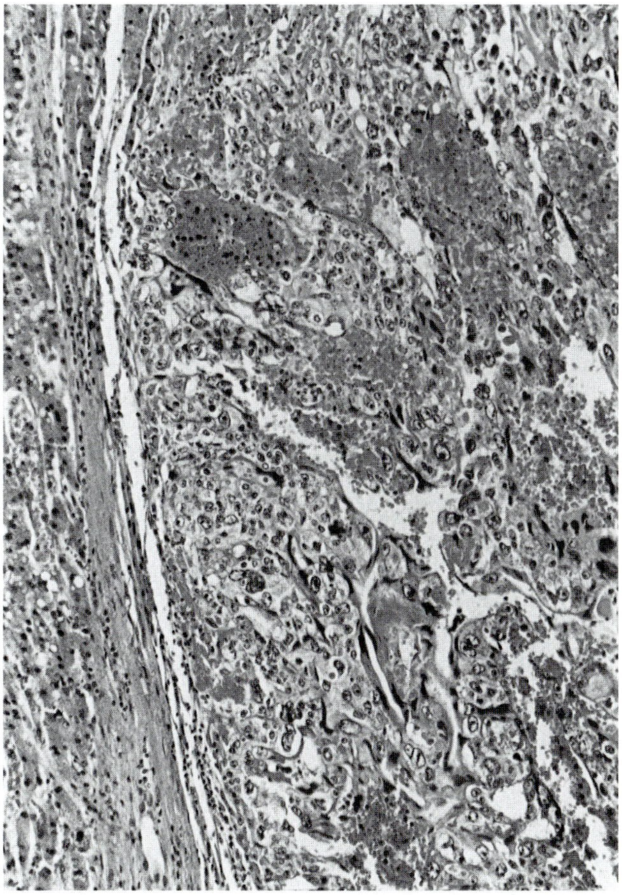

Fig. 24.28. Metastatic choriocarcinoma in the liver. Syncytiotrophoblast, cytotrophoblast, and intermediate trophoblast are present. On the *left*, the boundary with preserved liver is circumscribed.

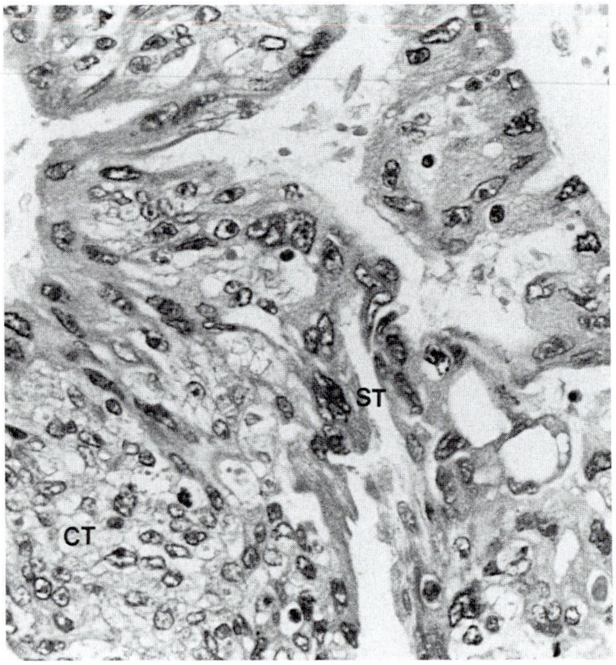

Fig. 24.29. Trophoblast in choriocarcinoma. Syncytiotrophoblast (*ST*) lining vascular spaces and capping cytotrophoblast (CT).

The interface with normal tissue, if preserved, is circumscribed and appears expansile (Fig. 24.28).

An intimate mixture of cytotrophoblast, intermediate trophoblast, and syncytiotrophoblast forms the cellular population of choriocarcinoma (Fig. 24.31). The cytotrophoblast and intermediate trophoblast (Fig. 24.30) tend to grow in clusters and sheets, separated by syncytiotrophoblast, forming the characteristic dimorphic growth pattern (Fig. 24.31). These patterns of growth recapitulate the relationship of the trophoblast to the maternal–placental circulation of the early implanting previllous blastocyst. A network of syncytiotrophoblast intimately admixed with cytotrophoblast and intermediate trophoblast comprises the plexiform pattern of trophoblast in many cases. The percentage of intermediate trophoblast in choriocarcinomas is highly variable, ranging from 1% to 90% of the mononucleate trophoblastic cellular population.[187] The intermediate trophoblastic cells in a choriocarcinoma tend to be larger with more abundant cytoplasm (Fig. 24.30); they are usually located adjacent to the cytotrophoblast, assuming a zonal pattern of differentiation from cytotrophoblast. Occasionally, choriocarcinoma appears predominately composed of cytotrophoblast and intermediate trophoblast, forming a monotonous and cohesive shear or mass with indistinct or attenuated syncytiotrophoblast (Fig. 24.32). This monomorphic variant may cause a problem in the differential diagnosis. Careful search for syncytiotrophoblast, deeper sectioning of the paraffin blocks, and immunostaining for β-hCG may reveal syncytiotrophoblast in focal areas. β-hCG staining can be very useful in demonstrating attenuated or indistinct syncytiotrophoblast.

There may be considerable cytologic atypia in the trophoblast with pleomorphic enlarged nuclei, abnormal mitotic figures, and bizarre cellular configurations. Nuclear chromatin is coarsely granular, with an uneven distribution, and multiple nucleoli may be present. Enlarged, multinucleated intermediate trophoblastic cells with two or several nuclei also occur, and they are distinguished from syncytiotrophoblast by their cytoplasm, which lacks the dense eosinophilia and vacuolization, and by positive Mel-CAM (CD 146) immunostaining*.[187] Choriocarcinoma can undergo sufficient necrosis so that

*Mel-CAM (CD 146) is a marker for implantation site intermediate trophoblast, and the Mel-CAM specific antibody is available on request to Dr. Shih (ishih@jhmi.edu).

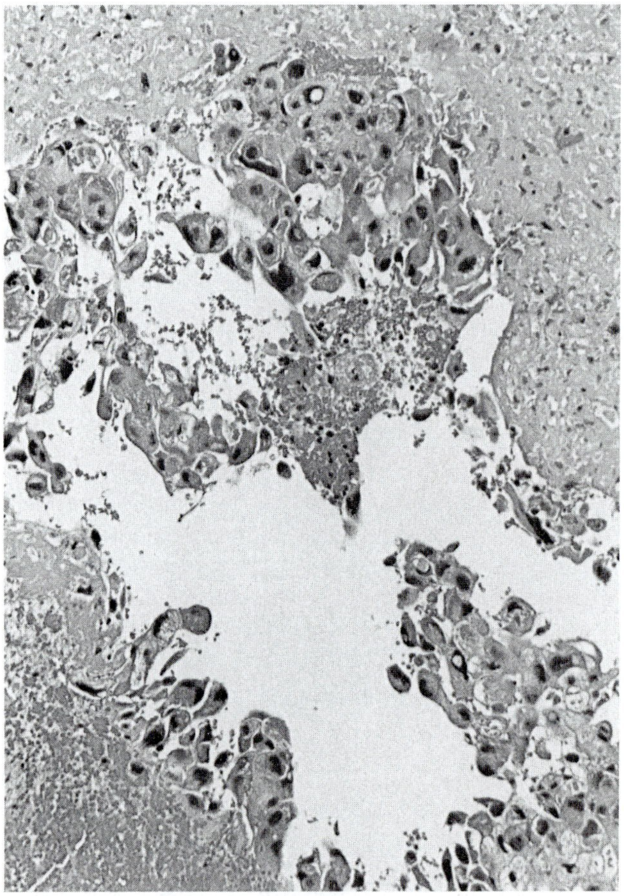

Fig. 24.30. Intermediate trophoblast in choriocarcinoma. Intermediate trophoblast can be found in choriocarcinoma and is composed of mononucleate and binucleate cells with amphophilic cytoplasm. In other areas, this tumor contains cytotrophoblast and syncytiotrophoblast.

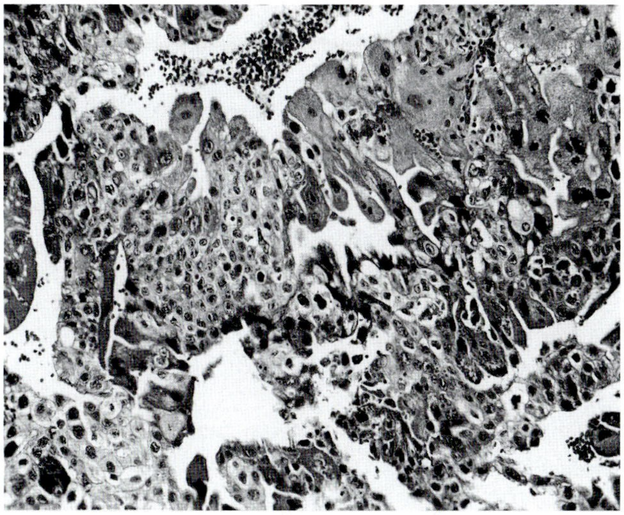

Fig. 24.31. Choriocarcinoma. Mononucleate trophoblast (cytotrophoblast and intermediate trophoblast) alternating with syncytiotrophoblast is most characteristic.

little or no viable tissue is present in a lesion. Diagnosis may require extensive sectioning to identify the typical pattern of choriocarcinoma. Generally, choriocarcinoma has no intrinsic vascular stroma, the tumor receiving its vascular supply by permeating and replacing host vessels. Infiltrative growth of normal tissues and blood vessels, however, can be observed in the periphery of a lesion.[138]

Ultrastructure

The fine structure of the trophoblastic cells of choriocarcinoma correlates with its functional and light microscopic features.[54] The neoplastic cells have features similar to trophoblast in the normally developing placenta and in hydatidiform mole. The most striking feature of cytotrophoblast is its simplicity, with electron-lucent cytoplasm containing numerous free cytoplasmic ribosomes and aggregates of particulate glycogen. Others organelles, including mitochondria, rough endoplasmic reticulum (RER), and Golgi complexes, are sparse. The nuclei have smooth, round to oval contours and contain a prominent nucleolus. The cells are joined by widely separated, well-formed desmosomes. The syncytiotrophoblast contrasts markedly with cytotrophoblast.[54] These highly developed epithelial cells have a complex cytoplasm and cell membrane structure. Thick bundles of tonofilaments are scattered throughout the cell. Syncytiotrophoblast is joined directly to cytotrophoblast by desmosomes. In addition to the multiple nuclei, syncytiotrophoblast demonstrate an electron-dense cytoplasm because of the presence of multiple organelles including RER and free cytoplasmic ribosomes, lipid droplets, vesicles, and lysosomes. The syncytiotrophoblastic cell surface is covered with many long microvilli. Infolding of the microvillous surface into the cytoplasm forms interconnecting lacunae and gives an appearance of multiple intracytoplasmic lumens when viewed in cross section. The syncytiotro-

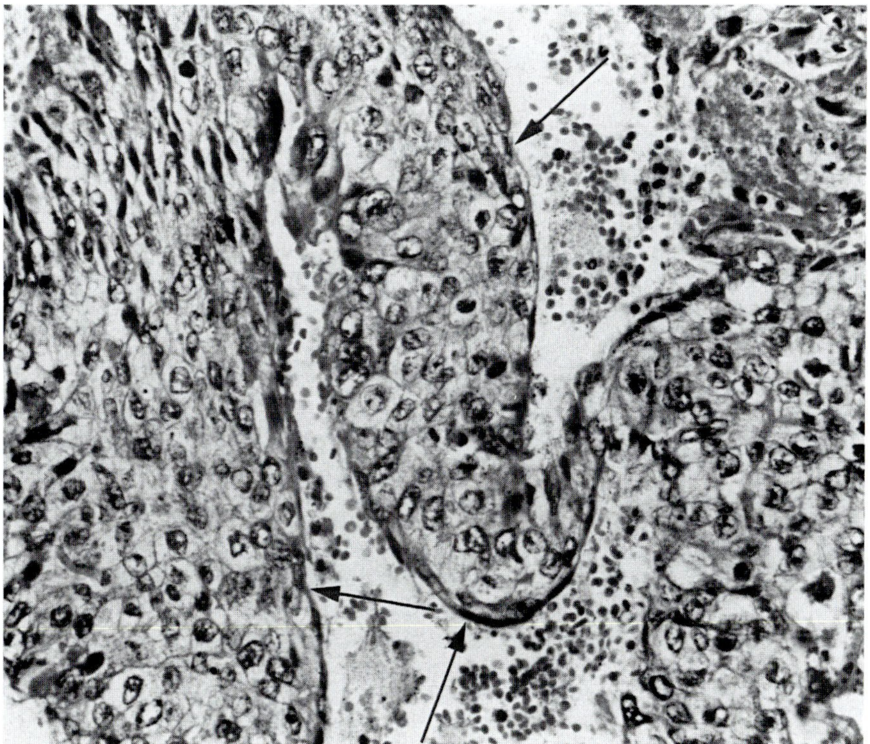

Fig. 24.32. Choriocarcinoma. Occasionally, choriocarcinoma appears predominately composed of cytotrophoblast and intermediate trophoblast with indistinct or attenuated syncytiotrophoblast (*arrows*) forming a monotonous and cohesive sheet or mass. This pattern may simulate a poorly differentiated carcinoma.

phoblastic nuclei tend to have highly irregular outlines and coarsely clumped chromatin.[54,137]

Differential Diagnosis

Choriocarcinoma must be distinguished from the normal trophoblast of early gestation, from molar pregnancies, from placental site trophoblastic tumor, and from other forms of epithelial malignancy. The differential diagnosis is primarily based on morphologic grounds. Occasionally, normal trophoblast of an early gestation is found in curettings without associated villi. In this circumstance, the trophoblast should be present only in small quantities. Normal trophoblast of an early gestation, although proliferative, does not show atypical features including the marked cellular enlargement and nuclear abnormalities found in choriocarcinoma. Most importantly, fragments of normal trophoblast in curettings do not show tumor necrosis or destructive invasion. Large amounts of trophoblast showing atypia should be viewed suspiciously for choriocarcinoma. If the diagnosis is in doubt, a chest radiograph and careful monitoring of β-hCG levels should resolve the problem. As a general rule, choriocarcinoma should not be diagnosed in the presence of villi. Proliferative trophoblast in association with villi usually indicates either an abortion or hydatidiform mole. The differential diagnosis of these lesions is discussed under "Hydatidiform Mole." Rarely, gestational choriocarcinoma arises within normally developing placenta, with the neoplasm intimately associated with well-formed, mature nonmolar villi (Fig. 24.33).[236]

Discriminating choriocarcinoma from other carcinomas either within the uterus or at other sites usually is not a problem. On occasion a biopsy of choriocarcinoma may show a few syncytiotrophoblastic cells, or the entire lesion is composed of mononucleate trophoblastic cells, a pattern that can mimic a poorly differentiated carcinoma (see Fig. 24.32).[138] When this differential diagnosis arises, the clinical history may reveal a previous molar pregnancy or another suspicious pregnancy event that can assist in the diagnosis. Serum hCG levels and immunohistochemical localization of hCG, hPL, and inhibin-α in syncytiotrophoblast can be useful.

Choriocarcinoma has been described as a primary tumor arising in a number of different sites besides the uterus and gonads. In women of reproductive age, however, pure choriocarcinoma that appears to be an extrauterine primary tumor probably represents gestational choriocarcinoma in which the index pregnancy is undetected. True primary choriocarcinoma at an unusual site may be an extragonadal germ cell tumor, or it may be derived from dedifferentiation of an ordinary carcinoma.[225] Primary somatic tumors of the gastrointestinal tract, bladder, breast, lung, or endometrium rarely show choriocarcinomatous differentiation, and these show transitions from ordinary carcinoma to the trophoblastic component. Because somatic tumors also may produce hCG without showing choriocarcinoma histology, the classic biphasic growth pattern should be present before rendering the diagnosis of choriocarcinoma.

The differential diagnosis of choriocarcinoma and placental site trophoblastic tumor and epithelioid tro-

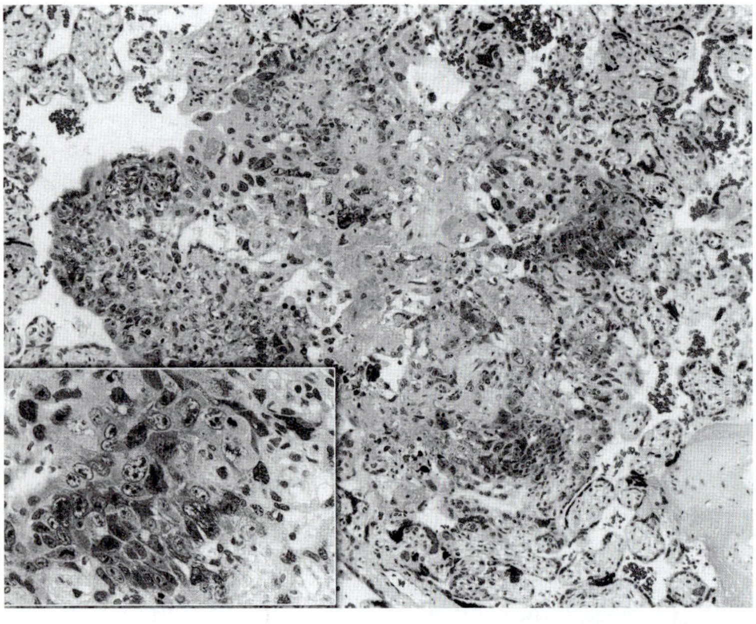

Fig. 24.33. Choriocarcinoma arising in a mature placenta. Malignant trophoblast arising from the surface of normally formed villi. Highly atypical cytotrophoblastic cells with irregular hyperchromatic nuclei are mixed with syncytiotrophoblast (*inset*).

phoblastic tumor are discussed in the following specific sections and summarized in Table 24.8.

Clinical Behavior and Treatment

Metastasis of choriocarcinoma most frequently occurs in lung, brain and liver, and the majority of therapeutic failures have liver and/or brain metastases.[138,222] High β-hCG level is a risk factor for predicting the occurrence of brain and liver metastases.[233] Kidney and abdomen, including intestinal tract, are the other common sites of spread, but almost any organ, including the skin, may be involved.[138] Lymph nodes contain tumor on occasion, often as tertiary metastatic lesions from other organs.[138] Vaginal involvement has been reported in 16–32% of patients.[138] There have been a few isolated reports of metastatic choriocarcinoma occurring in the mother and child of a term pregnancy.[66,236] In most cases, the infant is disease free, however.

Death from choriocarcinoma most commonly results from hemorrhage or pulmonary insufficiency.[138] Fatal hemorrhage usually occurs in the central nervous system or lungs, but intraperitoneal and gastrointestinal hemorrhage also can cause death.[138] Exsanguination may occur after biopsy of a vaginal metastasis. Pulmonary insufficiency can result from either a large tumor burden or the effects of irradiation and cytotoxic chemotherapy.[138] An interval of less than 4 months since the antecedent pregnancy, a pretreatment hCG level less than 40,000 mIU/ml, and absence of brain or liver metastases appear to be the significant predictors of a favorable outcome in postterm choriocarcinoma.[175]

In the past, gestational choriocarcinoma usually was fatal. Before cytotoxic chemotherapy was available, hysterectomy and, in some instances, irradiation were the only forms of treatment. The absolute 5-year survival for patients treated by hysterectomy alone was 32%. Survival rates have improved dramatically since the introduction of cytotoxic chemotherapy combined with accurate and sensitive assays for β-hCG to monitor the course of the disease. With the introduction of chemotherapy regimens, choriocarcinoma represents one of the few cancers that are potentially curable by chemotherapeutic agents alone.[128] The overall survival for choriocarcinoma at the present time approaches 100%.[77,97,181]

The principles of management of choriocarcinoma are similar to those for GTD after hydatidiform mole; β-hCG monitoring and chemotherapy are essential.[129] In following patients with hCG, a compulsory test for urinary hCG is important because of possible false-positive hCG concentrations in serum.[177] Hysterectomy can reduce hospitalization and the amount of chemotherapy needed to induce remission. Resection of pulmonary metastases may have therapeutic value in patients with persistent but limited pulmonary disease, if there is no evidence of tumor at other sites and the hCG titer is low.[104,211] Irradiation combined with chemotherapy will give a 50% remission rate for cerebral metastases,[223] but irradiation to other sites generally is not useful.[129] When a pure choriocarcinoma is present in the ovary, the principles of β-hCG monitoring and chemotherapy remain the same whether it is a gestational or germ cell neoplasm.[3]

Placental Site Trophoblastic Tumor

The *placental site trophoblastic tumor (PSTT)* is a relatively uncommon form of GTD composed of neoplastic implantation site intermediate trophoblastic cells. PSTT resembles the trophoblastic infiltration of the endometrium and myometrium of the placental site during early pregnancy. The neoplasm lacks the biphasic pattern seen in choriocarcinoma and the epithelial-like growth pattern of epithelioid trophoblastic tumor. The PSTT was originally termed atypical chorioepithelioma by Marchand in 1895,[132] but because of its rarity, it has been periodically rediscovered and renamed. Terms that have been used include atypical choriocarcinoma, syncytioma, chorioepitheliosis, and trophoblastic pseudotumor.[116] PSTT is generally benign but behaves in an aggressive fashion in approximately 15% of cases.[214,215]

Clinical Features

Patients usually are in the reproductive age group (19–62 years with an average of 30 years) and can present with either amenorrhea or abnormal bleeding, often accompanied by uterine enlargement,[55,76,116,231] and frequently are thought to be pregnant. When uterine enlargement ceases, the diagnosis of a missed abortion is made.[116] Serum levels of β-hCG are generally low. Rarely, PSTT is associated with virilization,[155] nephrotic syndrome,[50,232] and erythrocytosis.[18] In contrast to choriocarcinoma, which is preferentially associated with a complete mole, PSTT occurs most commonly following a normal pregnancy or nonmolar abortion, whereas in only 5%–8% of patients is there a clinical history of complete mole (Table 24.7).[114,179,183] Flow cytometric DNA analysis of six cases of PSTT revealed a diploid DNA stemline and one case that was tetraploid.[68,113] Interestingly, more than 85% of patients with PSTT have had a female antecedent gestation either by history or by genetic analysis, suggesting a role of the paternally derived X chromosome in the pathogenesis of PSTT.[65,110,124] Rare examples of primary tubal PSTT have been reported.[206] An apparently unique form of renal disease accompanied by the nephrotic syndrome has occurred in a few patients with PSTT.[55] Renal biopsies showed glomerular lesions with prominent eosinophilic deposits in the capillary lumens that stained for fibrinogen and IgM. This lesion has been found in 3 and possibly 4 of more than 90 patients with PSTT, suggesting that the lesion is specific and not fortuitous. Its pathogenesis in unknown. Nephrotic syndrome is not observed in association with other forms of GTD. The clinical features of PSTT as compared with choriocarcinoma and epithelioid trophoblastic tumor are shown in Table 24.7.

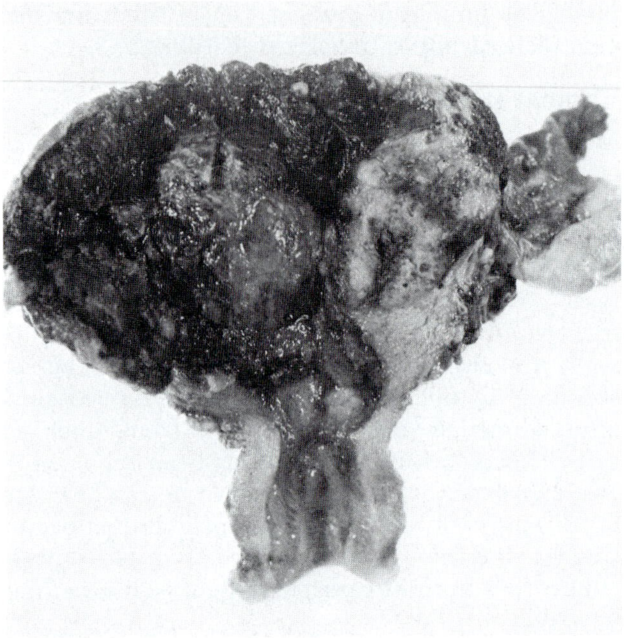

Fig. 24.34. Placental site trophoblastic tumor. Opened uterus showing a large, erosive tumor involving most of the fundus with invasion to the serosal surface. The uterus was perforated at curettage.

Gross Findings

Most of the tumors are well circumscribed. PSTTs may be polypoid, projecting into the uterine cavity, or may predominantly involve the myometrium (Fig. 24.34). The sectioned surface is soft and tan and contains only focal areas of hemorrhage or necrosis. Invasion frequently extends to the uterine serosa and, in rare instances, to the adnexal structures.

Microscopic Findings

The predominant cell type in PSTT is implantation site intermediate trophoblast.[115,117] The microscopic features of PSTT are summarized in Table 24.8. Most of the cellular population is monomorphic in contrast to the mixture of cell types in choriocarcinoma (Figs. 24.35–24.37). PSTT is composed of large, polygonal implantation site intermediate trophoblastic cells with irregular, hyperchromatic

Table 24.8. Pathologic features of placental site trophoblastic tumor (PSTT), epithelioid trophoblastic tumor (ETT), and choriocarcinoma

Feature	*PSTT*	*ETT*	*Choriocarcinoma*
Cellular population	Monomorphic; implantation site intermediate trophoblastic	Monomorphic; chorionic-type intermediate trophoblastic	Dimorphic; primitive previllous-type trophoblastic
Cell size and shape	Large and pleiomorphic	Small round and uniform	Irregular, highly variable
Cytoplasm	Abundant and eosinophilic	Eosinophilic or clear	Eosinophilic to purple
Growth pattern	Infiltrating single cells or confluent sheets	Epithelioid nests or cords or solid masses	Dimorphic; mononucleate trophoblast and syncytiotrophoblast
Margin	Infiltrating	Circumscribed; expansile	Circumscribed; expansile
Hemorrhage	Focal or haphazard	Usually present	Massive and central
Cellular necrosis	Usually absent	Extensive	Extensive
Calcification	Absent	Usually present	Absent
Vascular invasion	From periphery to lumen	Absent	From lumen to periphery
Fibrinoid change	Present	Present	Absent
Mitosis	Variable; 0–6/10 HPF	Variable; 1–10/10 HPF	High; 2–22/10 HPF
Associated chorionic villi	Absent	Absent	Absent

HPF, high-power fields (400×).

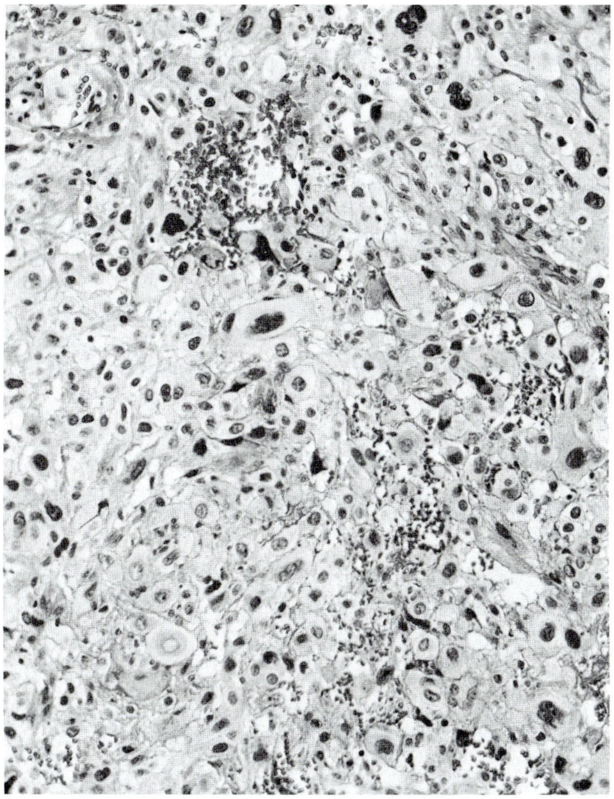

Fig. 24.35. **Placental site trophoblastic tumor.** Sheets of intermediate trophoblast characterized by large polyhedral cells with pleomorphic nuclei. (Reprinted by permission of Kurman et al., ref. 116.)

nuclei and dense eosinophilic to amphophilic cytoplasm with occasional vacuoles. Although most of the implantation site intermediate cells are polyhedral, many of them assume a spindle shape especially where they are closely apposed to myometrial cells (Fig. 24.38). PSTT also contains scattered multinucleated implantation site intermediate trophoblastic cells that can be mistaken for syncytiotrophoblast. The cells often aggregate into confluent sheets. At the periphery of the tumor, however, the trophoblastic cells invade singly or in cords and nests, characteristically separating individual muscle fibers and groups of fibers. Rarely, PSTT is composed almost entirely of single cells or small nests of cells without forming sheets or masses. The individual neoplastic cells extensively infiltrate the endomyometrium and penetrate the uterine wall deeply. Although some tumors appear to cause relatively little tissue destruction, others are associated with extensive necrosis, a microscopic feature that is often associated with malignant behavior (see following).

As in the normal placental site, abundant extracellular eosinophilic fibrinoid is present in the tumor. The neoplasm displays a characteristic form of vascular invasion in which blood vessel walls are extensively replaced by trophoblastic cells and fibrinoid material, as observed in the normal placental site (Figs. 24.39 and 24.40). Decidua or an Arias–Stella reaction may be present in the adjacent, uninvolved endometrium. Villi are almost never identified.

Rarely a PSTT shows histologic features of both choriocarcinoma and PSTT, and these are termed mixed choriocarcinoma and PSTT. Similarly, PSTT can also be associated with epithelioid trophoblastic tumor. These tumors display hybrid features of both PSTT and epithelioid trophoblastic tumor. The neoplasms have an infiltrative growth pattern as occurs in PSTT but are composed almost entirely of a monotonous population of mononucleate trophoblastic cells that form rounded nests and cords with a distinctly epithelioid growth pattern.[188] Too few of these mixed cases have been studied to determine their clinical behavior.

PSTT is immunoreactive to cytokeratin (AE1/AE3 cocktail and cytokeratin 18), epithelial membrane antigen (EMA), and inhibin-α.[190] For the tro-

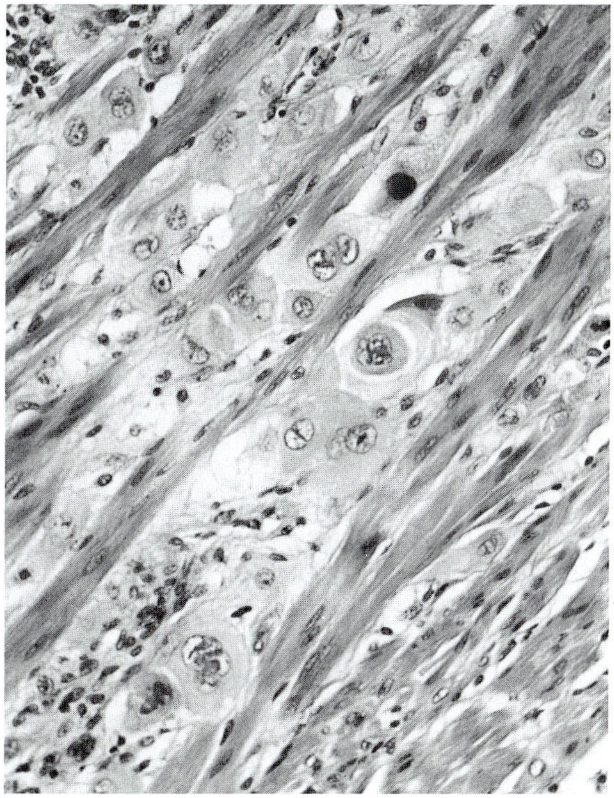

Fig. 24.36. **Placental site trophoblastic tumor.** The implantation site intermediate trophoblastic cells characteristically separate muscle bundles as they invade myometrium. (Reprinted by permission of Kurman et al., ref. 116.)

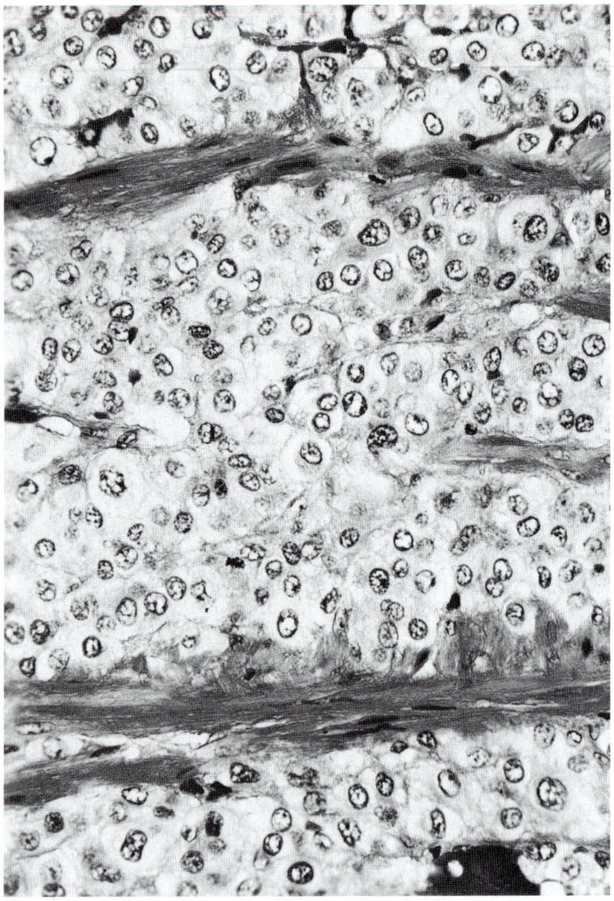

Fig. 24.37. Placental site trophoblastic tumor. Tumor is composed of a monomorphic population of intermediate trophoblast in contrast to the mixture of cytotrophoblast, syncytiotrophoblast, and intermediate trophoblast in choriocarcinoma.

phoblast-associated markers, PSTT is diffusely positive for hPL and Mel-CAM (CD 146), but rarely positive for hCG or PLAP, an immunophenotype characteristic of implantation site intermediate trophoblast (Table 24.9; see Fig. 24.5). Immunohistochemical analysis has shown that PSTT is associated with abnormal expression of cell cycle regulatory gene products including cyclins, cyclin-dependent kinases, and p53.[96]

Differential Diagnosis

The differential diagnosis of PSTT includes exaggerated placental site, choriocarcinoma, epithelioid trophoblastic tumor, and epithelioid smooth muscle tumor. The most difficult differential diagnosis is that of an exaggerated placental site. Both lesions are characterized by an exuberant infiltration of implantation site intermediate trophoblastic cells. The immunophenotype of both lesions is similar. The histologic features that favor the diagnosis of PSTT include confluent masses of trophoblastic cells, unequivocal mitotic figures, and absence of chorionic villi (see Table 24.8). In contrast, the exaggerated placental site is microscopic in size, lacks mitotic activity, is composed of intermediate trophoblastic cells separated by masses of hyaline, and usually is admixed with decidua and chorionic villi (Table 24.8). In addition, an exaggerated placental site contains larger numbers of multinucleated trophoblastic cells as compared to PSTT. Immunostaining for Ki-67, a proliferation marker, to determine the Ki-67 labeling index in the implantation site intermediate trophoblastic cells has been recently shown to be superior to the mitotic index as a diagnostic adjunct in the differential diagnosis of an exaggerated placental site versus a PSTT (see Fig. 24.5).[189] The Ki-67 labeling index in PSTT is significantly elevated

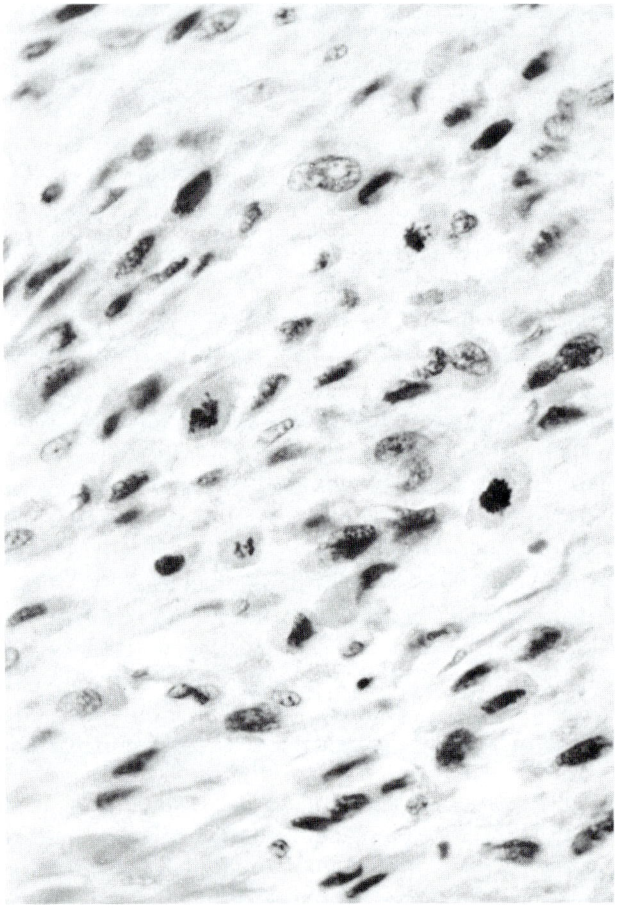

Fig. 24.38. Placental site trophoblastic tumor. Implantation site intermediate trophoblastic cells may assume a spindle shape and may, therefore, be confused with leiomyosarcoma. Four mitotic figures are in *center* of field. (Reprinted by permission from Kurman et al., ref. 116.)

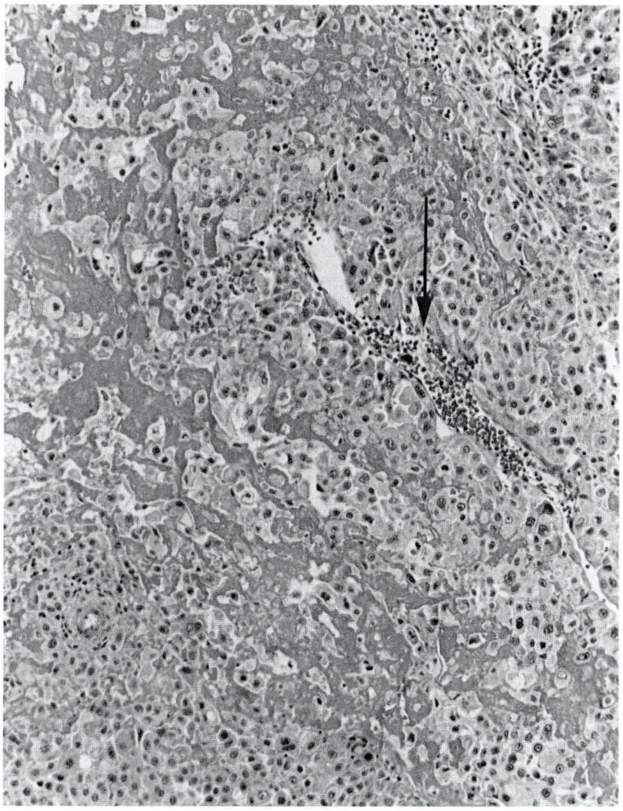

Fig. 24.39. Placental site trophoblastic tumor. Fibrin and implantation site intermediate trophoblast replace the wall of a uterine blood vessel. The vessel lumen (*arrow*) still contains red cells.

(14% ± 6.9%) in PSTT but is near zero in the normal and exaggerated implantation site.

A diagnosis of a PSTT should be strongly considered if the Ki-67 index in implantation site intermediate trophoblastic cells exceeds 5%. Although the Ki-67 index in a molar implantation site that is morphologically indistinguishable with exaggerated placental site can be 5% or slightly higher, the diagnosis of a PSTT versus a complete hydatidiform mole is not a problem. The Ki-67 labeling in the implantation site intermediate trophoblastic cells should be carefully assessed using stringent morphologic criteria because implantation site intermediate trophoblastic cells can closely resemble other cell types in the placental site. Many Ki-67 positive cells in the placental site or PSTT are natural killer cells and activated T lymphocytes that can be highly positive for Ki-67. A double-staining technique utilizing MIB-1 antibody to determine the Ki-67 proliferative index and Mel-CAM (CD 146) to identify implantation site intermediate trophoblastic cells has been shown to be very useful in distinguishing an exaggerated placental site from a PSTT†.[189] The labeling index for an exaggerated placental site is close to zero whereas the labeling index for PSTT is about 15%. In estimating the Ki-67 labeling index, the proximal portions of trophoblastic columns should not be counted because these normally contain proliferating trophoblastic cells and tangential sectioning of trophoblastic columns could lead to an erroneously high labeling index.

In contrast to the biphasic pattern of choriocarcinoma, PSTT is composed of a relatively monomorphic population of trophoblast. The multinucleated intermediate trophoblastic cells in PSTT should not be confused with syncytiotrophoblast in choriocar-

†The antibody specific for Mel-CAM (CD 146) is available on request to Dr. Shih (ishih@jhmi.edu).

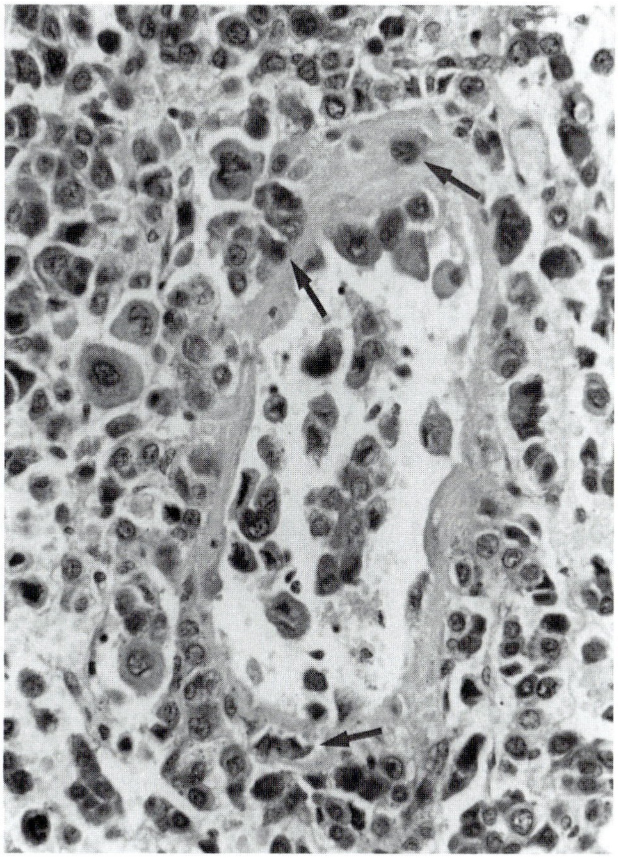

Fig. 24.40. Placental site trophoblastic tumor. Vascular invasion by implantation site intermediate trophoblast resembles that of the normal implantation site. The neoplastic cells surround and invade (*arrows*) a blood vessel, extending into the vascular lumen. The vessel wall has been replaced by fibrin. The tissue is immunostained for human placental lactogen (hPL), and all the neoplastic cells in this field contain hPL. (Reprinted by permission of Kurman et al., ref. 117.)

Table 24.9. Immunohistochemical marker profile of exaggerated placental site (EPS) placental site nodule (PSN), placental site trophoblastic tumor (PSTT), epithelioid trophoblastic tumor (ETT), and choriocarcinoma

	Lesions of implantation site IT		*Lesions of chorionic type IT*		
Markers	*EPS*	*PSTT*	*PSN*	*ETT*	*Choriocarcinoma*
hPL	+++	+++	−/+	−/+	+/+++
hCG	−	−	−/+	−/+	++/+++
Mel-CAM	+++	+++	−/+	−/+	+/+++
PLAP	−	−	++	++	−/+

IT, intermediate trophoblast; hPL, human placental lactogen; hCG, human chorionic gonadotropin; Mel-CAM, melanoma cell adhesion molecule (CD146); PLAP, placental alkaline phosphatase.

cinoma. In contrast to the interlacing pattern of elongated syncytiotrophoblast in choriocarcinoma, the multinucleated intermediate trophoblastic cells in PSTT are usually polygonal or round. Additionally, PSTT is diffusely positive for hPL but only focally positive for hCG, whereas the reverse staining pattern is seen in choriocarcinoma. Ki-67 labeling index in Mel-CAM (CD 146) defined intermediate trophoblastic cells is also helpful in the differential diagnosis of PSTT versus choriocarcinoma.[189] The Ki-67 index in intermediate trophoblastic cells of PSTT is 14% ± 6.9% and in choriocarcinoma is 69% ± 20% ($p < 0.001$).

The differential diagnosis of epithelioid smooth muscle tumor can at times present a problem because of the infiltrative pattern of PSTT within the myometrium. The distinctive pattern of vascular invasion and the deposition of fibrinoid material in PSTT are helpful morphologic clues. Positive staining for hPL, inhibin-α, and cytokeratin 18 and the negative staining for smooth muscle markers are helpful in this differential diagnosis (see Fig. 24.5).

Poorly differentiated carcinoma and metastatic melanoma can sometimes be confused with PSTT. The pattern of prominent blood vessel invasion, characteristic myometrial invasion (see Figs. 24.39 and 24.40) and extensive deposition of fibrinoid material are key diagnostic features of PSTT. Immunohistochemical stains for hPL, inhibin-α, and HMB-45 help to distinguish PSTT from poorly differentiated carcinoma and melanoma (see Fig. 24.5).

The differential diagnosis of the PSTT from epithelioid trophoblastic tumor is considered in the section describing the latter lesion.

Ultrastructure

Implantation site intermediate trophoblastic cells are large and have abundant cytoplasm.[11,54] When they are closely apposed, their cell outlines are polygonal, and they are joined by well-formed desmosomes. Free surfaces show microvilli that are less numerous and more blunt than the microvilli of syncytiotrophoblast. The cytoplasm of implantation site intermediate trophoblast is electron dense and contains numerous organelles, although lacking the overall complexity of syncytiotrophoblastic cytoplasm. Typically, moderate numbers of mitochondria, RER, and free ribosomes are present. Some cells contain vesicles of smooth endoplasmic reticulum, Golgi complexes, and pools of glycogen. One feature described in most of the reported cases is the presence of large bundles of paranuclear intermediate filaments that are apparently distinctive for implantation site intermediate trophoblast as compared with syncytiotrophoblast or cytotrophoblast.

Behavior and Treatment

PSTTs often invade through the myometrium to the serosa, and therefore perforation at the time of curettage may occur. Direct invasion into the broad ligament and ovary may occur.[55] Despite deep myometrial invasion, most cases of PSTT are self-limited,[11,55,116,176] and some patients have been cured by curettage alone. Approximately 10%–15% of PSTT are clinically malignant,[55,56,229] and patients have died despite intensive multiagent chemotherapy. The mortality rate in patients with PSTT is about 15–20%, which may be overestimated because benign cases generally are not reported.[93,116] The overtly malignant tumors have had widely disseminated metastases resembling choriocarcinoma in their distribution with lung, liver, abdominal cavity, and brain involved. Metastasis to other more unusual sites such as scalp has also been reported.[87] Metastases have the same histologic appearance as the primary tumor and may develop several years after the initial diagnosis; one fatal case recurred 5 years after hysterectomy.

Because these tumors are composed of neoplastic implantation site intermediate trophoblastic cells that contain only small amounts of β-hCG, serum levels of β-hCG are usually in the range of 1000–2000 mIL/ml. These levels are much lower than those in choriocarcinoma.[179] Despite the low level of serum β-hCG in patients with PSTT, it is the best available marker to monitor the course of the disease. It is important to emphasize that the disease may still progress even if β-hCG levels are low.[93] For those patients with undetectable or very low serum levels of β-hCG, the urinary β-core fragment of β-hCG may be a better method to monitor treatment.[173]

It is difficult to predict with certainty the behavior of PSTT[192] because it has been shown that there is no correlation between clinical outcome and DNA ploidy, histopathologic features, immunohistochemical features, B-hCG levels, and S-phase fraction.[60,67,68] In one study, the most significant adverse prognostic variable in 17 patients was an interval from the antecedent pregnancy that was greater than 2 years.[158] In our experience, malignant PSTTs as compared with benign cases generally are composed of larger masses and sheets of cells, many with clear instead of amphophilic cytoplasm. They have more extensive necrosis and higher mitotic activity. In general, PSTTs with a mitotic rate of 2 mitotic figures (MF) or less/10 high-power fields (HPF) have behaved in a benign fashion in contrast to PSTTs with more than 5 MF/10 HPF that develop recurrent disease.[60] However, a mean mitotic rate of less than 2 MF/10 HPF has been reported in some recurrent or fatal cases.[68,109,110] Abnormal mitotic figures can be found in benign or malignant tumors. Our preliminary findings suggest that the Ki-67 labeling index may be a reliable indicator of prognosis as the index is usually higher than 50% in malignant tumors in contrast to 14% in benign ones. In addition to the histologic features that predict outcome, Chang et al. have recently analyzed 91 cases of PSTT and concluded that FIGO stage is the most important prognostic factor.[26] In that study, the outcome of patients with FIGO stage I–II disease after hysterectomy was excellent, whereas those patients with FIGO stage III–IV diseases had a 30% survival.

The treatment of choice for patients whose disease is confined to the uterus is hysterectomy.[93] In some patients with localized PSTT who desire preservation of fertility, more conservative surgical therapy may be considered.[125] Curettage[124] and local excision (F. Montz, unpublished data) may be therapeutic, but if uterine disease persists, as evidenced by persistently elevated serum hCG levels, hysterectomy is indicated.[117] For patients with more extensive or metastatic disease, chemotherapy is indicated although the clinical outcome is variable.[26,50,51,55,61,76,91,99,109,157,209,214,215] Combination chemotherapy usually results in a high response rate and long-term remission even in patients with recurrent, metastatic PSTT, but only a few patients achieve a complete response.[26,50,99,170] Addition of platinum in the treatment regimens may be helpful in patients who have recurred or progressed after treatment with nonplatinum-containing regimens.[170] Radiation has been used to treat localized and isolated recurrences.[50] In conclusion, with the use of dose-intensive chemotherapy, imaging techniques to define disease spread, surgery for localized disease and the close surveillance with serologic measurement of the β-hCG level, most patients with PSTT can be cured.[93,214]

Epithelioid Trophoblastic Tumor

The term *epithelioid trophoblastic tumor* was introduced to describe an unusual type of trophoblastic tumor that is distinct from placental site trophoblastic tumor and choriocarcinoma with features resembling a carcinoma. The tumor was originally termed "atypical choriocarcinoma" and was described in the lungs of patients with antecedent choriocarcinoma following intensive chemotherapy.[104,137,138] Similar lesions referred to as "multiple nodules of intermediate trophoblast" were subsequently reported in the uteri of patients following evacuation of hydatidiform moles.[197] Subsequently, similar tumors were observed in the uterus of patients without history of antecedent GTD.[188] The relatively recent recognition of epithelioid trophoblastic tumor as a distinctive form of trophoblastic disease is in part due to its rarity and partly because many of the morphologic features of epithelioid trophoblastic tumor are more reminiscent of a carcinoma than of a trophoblastic tumor.[188]

Clinical Features

Based on published and unpublished data, the age of patients ranges from 15 to 48 (average, 36.1) years.[188] The antecedent gestational events include full-term deliveries (67%), spontaneous abortions (16%), and hydatidiform moles (16%). The interval between the preceding gestation and the diagnosis of epithelioid trophoblastic tumor has ranged from 1 to 18 (average, 6.2) years. Abnormal vaginal bleeding is the most common presenting symptom. Extrauterine epithelioid trophoblastic tumor without an identifiable trophoblastic lesion in the uterus has also been described.[84,188] The origin of the tumor in the three reported patients is not clear. It is well recognized that choriocarcinoma can develop after a long latent period without evidence of disease in the uterus[92]; thus, it is conceivable that extrauterine epithelioid trophoblastic tumors develop in a similar fashion. Serum β-hCG levels are nearly al-ways elevated at the time of diagnosis, although as with PSTTs the levels are generally low (<2,500 mIU/ml).[84,188]

Gross Findings

In one study, 30% of 14 epithelioid trophoblastic tumors were located in the uterine corpus, 50% in the lower uterine segment or endocervix, and the remaining 20% in extrauterine sites including the small bowel and lungs.[188] In cases in which a hysterectomy was performed, tumor size varied from 0.5 to 4.0 cm. All were solitary, discrete nodules that deeply invaded the cervix or myometrium. The cut surface was solid or cystic. Solid areas were typically tan to brown with varying amounts of hemorrhage and necrosis (Fig. 24.41).

Microscopic Findings

Epithelioid trophoblastic tumors are nodular and generally well circumscribed, although focal infiltrative features can be present at the periphery. The tumors are composed of a relatively uniform population of mononucleate trophoblastic cells typically arranged in nests and cords and masses of cells that are intimately associated with an eosinophilic, fibrillar, hyaline-like material and necrotic debris (Figs. 24.42–24.44). This hyaline-like material, which is composed of type IV collagen and fibronectin of oncofetal and adult types, is either located within the nests or surrounds them, coalescing to form large aggregates. This dense eosinophilic material and necrotic debris can simulate keratin. The extensive areas of necrosis that surround islands of viable tumor cells create a "geographic" pattern (Fig. 24.45). Typically, a small blood vessel is located within the center of tumor nests. Blood vessels within the tumor are preserved with occasional deposition of amorphous fibrinoid material in the wall. Focal calcification can sometimes be identified within the lesions. A lymphocytic infiltrate often surrounds the tumor.

Chorionic-type intermediate trophoblast is the predominate cell population in the epithelioid tro-

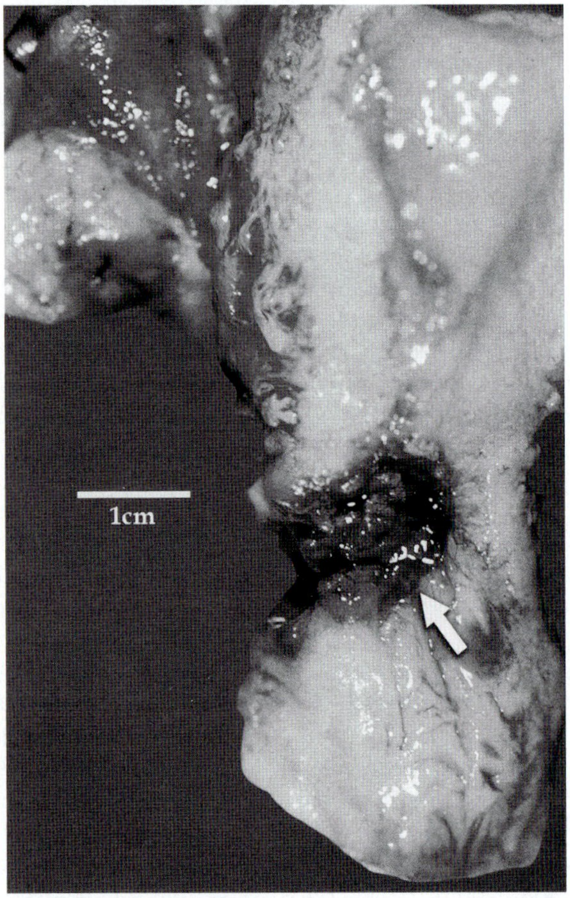

Fig. 24.41. Epithelioid trophoblastic tumor. The tumor is located in the endocervical canal. It is well circumscribed and ulcerated with hemorrhage and necrosis. (Reprinted by permission of Shih and Kurman, ref. 188.)

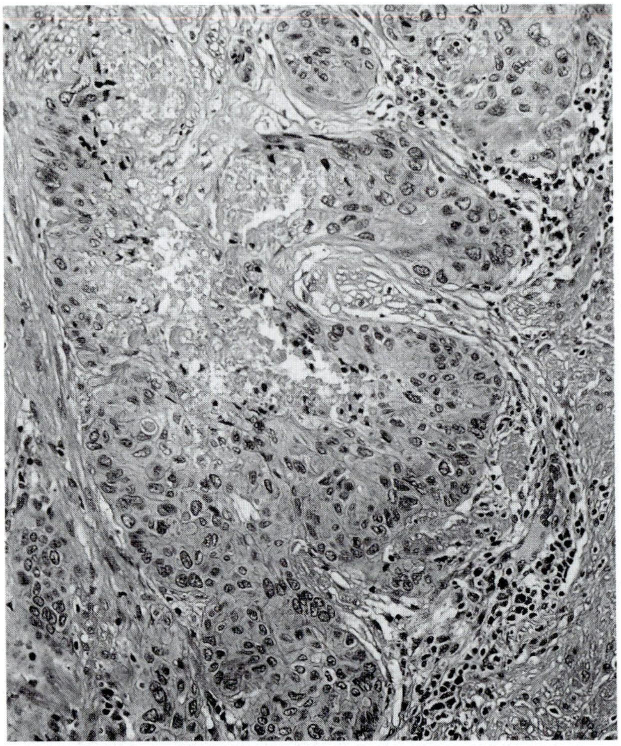

Fig. 24.42. Epithelioid trophoblastic tumor. Tumor in a hysterectomy specimen shows nests of atypical mononucleate trophoblastic cells. The tumor lacks the typical dimorphic pattern of choriocarcinoma.

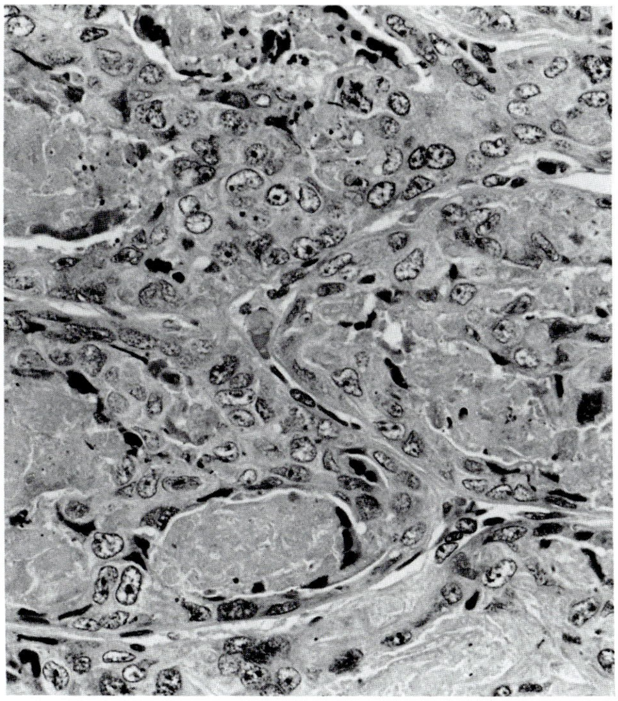

Fig. 24.43. **Epithelioid trophoblastic tumor.** Solitary lung metastasis after chemotherapy for typical dimorphic choriocarcinoma shows a rim of enlarged, mononucleate trophoblast surrounding dense eosinophilic debris.

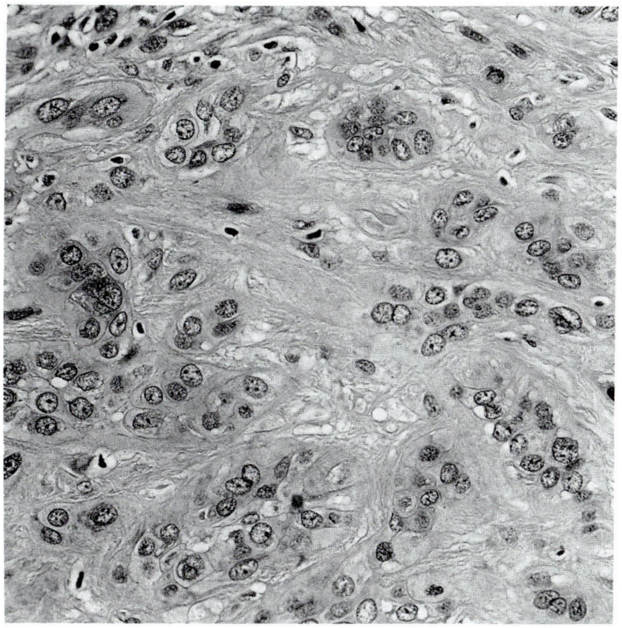

Fig. 24.44. **Epithelioid trophoblastic tumor.** Tumor in uterus shows infiltrating cords and nests of cells surrounded by dense hyaline material. Cells have single nuclei with vesicular chromatin and a moderate amount of finely granular cytoplasm.

phoblastic tumor.[188] These cells contain round, uniform nuclei and eosinophilic or clear (glycogen-rich) cytoplasm surrounded by a well-defined cell membrane. For the most part, the cells are larger than cytotrophoblastic cells but smaller than the implantation site intermediate trophoblastic cells. The tumor cell nuclei have finely dispersed chromatin and prominent or inconspicuous nucleoli. Ultrastructurally these cells are transitional between cytotrophoblast and syncytiotrophoblast but differ from the implantation site intermediate trophoblast.[137] Occasionally, larger cells resembling implantation site intermediate trophoblastic cells can be found among the smaller tumor cells or embedded in the extracellular hyaline matrix. The mitotic index varies from 0 to 9 mitoses per 10 high-power fields (×40) with an average of 2 mitoses per 10 high-power fields.[188] Apoptotic cells and apoptotic bodies are diffusely distributed throughout the tumor in most cases. Although most epithelioid trophoblastic tumors display a uniform architectural pattern, focal areas resembling placental site nodule, placen-

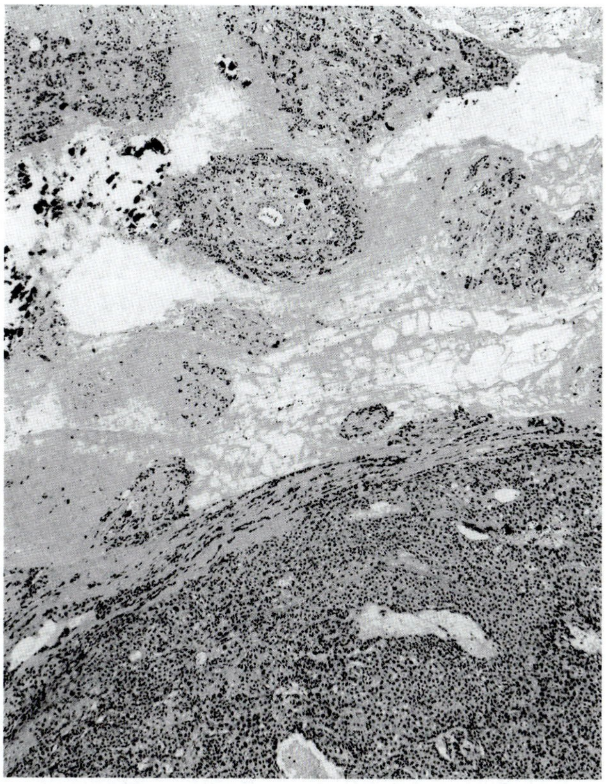

Fig. 24.45. **Epithelioid trophoblastic tumor.** Large areas of necrosis surround islands of tumor cells that encircle small blood vessels. In the *lower part of the field*, there is a solid sheet of tumor cells in which there are several large vessels. (Reprinted by permission of Shih and Kurman, ref. 188.)

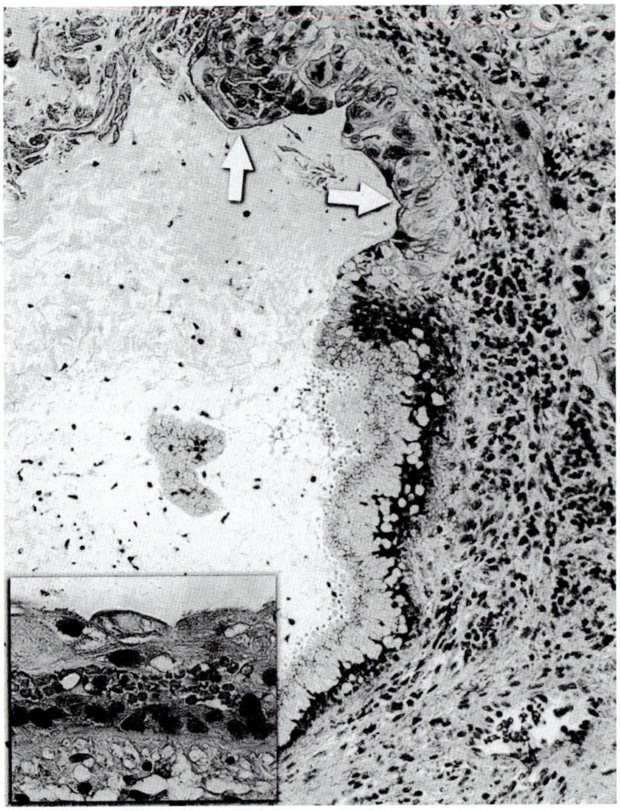

Fig. 24.46. Epithelioid trophoblastic tumor. An endocervical gland shows replacement of epithelium by epithelioid trophoblastic tumor with an abrupt transition between the tumor and the endocervical epithelium (arrows). *Inset*: High magnification of this area. The cells of the epithelioid trophoblastic tumor that replace the surface epithelium are larger and more pleomorphic than the squamous cells and are arranged parallel to the basement membrane. (Reprinted by permission of Shih and Kurman, ref. 188.)

tal site trophoblastic tumor, and choriocarcinoma can occasionally be identified within the tumor.

Epithelioid trophoblastic tumors located in the cervix sometimes appear to replace the surface endocervical epithelium (Fig. 24.46).[188] The tumor cells usually stratify into two or three layers and are larger than cervical squamous cells, with abundant eosinophilic cytoplasm and large hyperchromatic, pleomorphic nuclei.

The immunohistochemical features of the epithelioid trophoblastic tumor are similar to those of chorionic-type intermediate trophoblast. All the tumors are positive for cytokeratin (AE1/AE3 and cytokeratin 18), epithelial membrane antigen, E-cadherin, and epidermal growth factor receptor, consistent with their epithelial origin. In our experience, all epithelioid trophoblastic tumors are positive for inhibin-α, with the percentage of positive cells ranging from 20% to 80%. The "classic" trophoblastic markers including hPL, hCG, and Mel-CAM (CD 146) are only focally expressed (see Fig. 24.5). The immunophenotype of the epithelioid trophoblastic tumor contrasts with the placental site trophoblastic tumor, which is diffusely positive for Mel-CAM and hPL. The mean Ki-67 labeling index in epithelioid trophoblastic tumors is 17.7% ± 4.5% (mean ± standard deviation) with a range from 10% to 25%. The morphologic and immunohistochemical features of extrauterine epithelioid trophoblastic tumors are similar to those in the uterus.[84]

Differential Diagnosis

The differential diagnosis of epithelioid trophoblastic tumor includes placental site trophoblastic tumor, placental site nodule, choriocarcinoma, epithelioid smooth muscle tumor, and keratinizing squamous cell carcinoma of the cervix.[188] Epithelioid trophoblastic tumors exhibit a nodular growth pattern, and the border between the tumor and the myometrium is expansile. In contrast, the cells of placental site trophoblastic tumor infiltrate the myometrium by insinuating themselves between muscle bundles and fibers. In addition, the cells in epithelioid trophoblastic tumor are smaller than in placental site trophoblastic tumor and tend to grow in nests and cords, a pattern usually not observed in the placental site trophoblastic tumor. In epithelioid trophoblastic tumors, there is extensive geographic necrosis accompanied by dystrophic calcification, and the tumor cells are surrounded by fibrillar eosinophilic material instead of the more homogeneous fibrinoid material found in the placental site trophoblastic tumor. Blood vessels in epithelioid trophoblastic tumor are often surrounded by tumor cells, but vascular invasion is not a striking feature. In contrast, vascular invasion in a placental site trophoblastic tumor, like that seen at an implantation site, results in replacement of the smooth muscle of the walls of the vessels by hyaline-like material. Finally, immunostains can be useful in difficult cases. Figure 24.5 is a proposed algorithm for the differential diagnosis of epithelioid trophoblastic tumor. For example, hPL and Mel-CAM (CD 146) are diffusely positive in placental site trophoblastic tumor,[117,186] whereas staining for hPL and Mel-CAM (CD 146) is generally focal in epithelioid trophoblastic tumor.[188]

The distinction of an epithelioid trophoblastic tumor from a placental site nodule is usually not difficult because placental site nodules are microscopic lesions with sharply circumscribed borders.[194] Epithelioid trophoblastic tumors are larger and display substantial necrosis. The placental site nodule is much less cellular than epithelioid trophoblastic tumor. In addition, the lesional cells in a placental site nodule in contrast to an epithelioid trophoblastic tumor are bland and mitotic activity is low or absent. The Ki-67 index in epithelioid trophoblastic tumors is significantly higher (>10%) than in placental site nodules (<10%) (see Fig. 24.5).

As compared with choriocarcinoma, the cells in an epithelioid trophoblastic tumor are aggregated into nests and cords. In addition, epithelioid trophoblastic tumor is not associated with marked hemorrhage as is the case with choriocarcinoma. Immunostains for β-hCG can be helpful in the differential diagnosis. β-hCG immunostains highlight the dimorphic trophoblastic population of cells in choriocarcinoma with hCG-negative cytotrophoblast and intermediate trophoblast alternating with β-hCG-positive syncytiotrophoblast. In contrast, β-hCG-positive cells are randomly distributed as single mononucleate cells or small clusters of cells in epithelioid trophoblastic tumor.

Epithelioid smooth muscle tumors usually display areas composed of typical smooth muscle cells in addition to epithelioid areas. In addition, epithelioid smooth muscle tumors are positive for muscle markers including desmin and smooth muscle actin that are not expressed by epithelioid trophoblastic tumors. Conversely, epithelioid trophoblastic tumors are positive for cytokeratin 18 and inhibin-α, which are not detected in smooth muscle tumors.[188]

Distinction between an epithelioid trophoblastic tumor and a keratinizing squamous cell carcinoma of the cervix can be challenging. The differential diagnosis is particularly difficult because of the tendency of epithelioid trophoblastic tumor to grow in the lower uterine segment and cervix and involve the endocervical epithelium. In this situation, immunostains for inhibin-α and cytokeratin 18 are particularly helpful. Almost all epithelioid trophoblastic tumors are positive for inhibin-α and cytokeratin 18, whereas squamous cell carcinomas of the cervix are negative for these two markers.[188,190] Furthermore, unlike epithelioid trophoblastic tumor in which the Ki-67 labeling index is relatively low (10%–25%), cervical squamous cell carcinomas almost invariably have a very high Ki-67 labeling index (>50%) (see Fig. 24.5).

The morphologic distinction between a pulmonary epithelioid trophoblastic tumor and a primary squamous cell carcinoma of the lung can be extremely difficult, especially in a postmenopausal patient.[84,188] Useful clues that support the diagnosis of epithelioid trophoblastic tumor include (1) lack of cytoplasmic eosinophilia and intercellular bridges, which are frequently observed in differentiated squamous cell carcinoma; and (2) infiltration of alveolar spaces by highly atypical tumor cells and preservation of the alveolar septa, features not frequently seen in squamous cell carcinoma.[84] As in squamous cell carcinomas of the cervix, primary squamous cell carcinoma of the lung fails to react with antibodies to inhibin-α and cytokeratin 18.[194]

Behavior and Treatment

Experience with epithelioid trophoblastic tumor is limited because only 35 cases have been reported to date.[84,137,138,188,197] Generally, the behavior of epithelioid trophoblastic tumor is similar to that of placental site trophoblastic tumor. For the most part, epithelioid trophoblastic tumors behave in a benign fashion. Metastasis and death occur in approximately 25% and 10% of patients, respectively.[188] Because the number of tumors that have behaved in an aggressive fashion is small and follow-up for many cases has been short, we have been unable to identify any feature that predicts outcome.

Although serum β-hCG levels are variable and generally low in patients with epithelioid trophoblastic tumors, serum hCG levels have been used successfully to monitor treatment.[188] For those patients with undetectable or very low serum levels of hCG, urinary β-core fragment of hCG may be useful.[173] The available data suggest that, similar to placental site trophoblastic tumor, epithelioid trophoblastic tumor may not be responsive to the chemotherapeutic agents used in the treatment of other types of GTD.[188] Hysterectomy and lung resection have been used successfully.[84,188] The effectiveness of curettage and chemotherapy for the treatment of early lesions requires further evaluation.

Exaggerated Placental Site

This lesion is an exuberant infiltration of the myometrium by implantation site intermediate trophoblast. The distinction between a normal and *exaggerated placental site* is somewhat arbitrary as there are no reliable data quantifying the amount and extent of trophoblastic infiltration at different stages of normal gestation.[198] The lesion has been termed "syncytial endometritis" in the past, but this designation is no longer used because the process is neither inflammatory, confined to the endometrium, nor composed of syncytiotrophoblast.

The exaggerated placental site can occur in a normal pregnancy or an abortion from the first trimester. The incidence is approximately 1.6% of spontaneous and elective abortions from the first trimester, based on a review of the surgical pathology files at the Johns Hopkins Hospital.

The exaggerated placental site is characterized by an extensive infiltration of the endometrium and myometrium by intermediate trophoblastic cells, many of which are multinucleated (see Figs 24.47 to 24.49). Despite the massive infiltration by trophoblastic cells, the overall architecture of the placental site is not disturbed. Endometrial glands and spiral arteries may be completely engulfed by trophoblastic cells, but there is no necrosis. Similarly, the smooth muscle cells of the myometrium are separated by cords, nests, and individual trophoblastic cells that diffusely infiltrate the myometrium without producing necrosis (Fig. 24.47).[114,115] Cytologically, the trophoblastic cells in an exaggerated placental site are identical to the implantation site intermediate trophoblastic cells in the normal placental site. They contain abundant eosinophilic cytoplasm with hyperchromatic and irregular nuclei (Figs. 24.48 and 24.49). In many cases, there are profuse numbers of multinucleated implantation site intermediate trophoblastic cells (Fig. 24.49). Mitotic activity is absent. The associated placentas are morphologically unremarkable.

The trophoblastic cells in the exaggerated placental site display an immunophenotypic profile identical to that of the implantation site intermediate trophoblastic cells found in the normal placental site (see Tables 24.1 and 24.9). These cells are strongly positive for Mel-CAM (CD 146), prolyl 4-hydroxylase, oncofetal fibronectin, and hPL, moderately positive for EGFR and E-cadherin, and negative for Ber-EP4, EMA, HNK-1, and NCAM. These findings indicate that the differentiation of implantation site intermediate trophoblastic cells is unaltered in an exaggerated placental site and suggests that an exaggerated placental site is a normal variation of an implantation site. Despite the profuse infiltration of implantation site intermediate trophoblast in an exaggerated placental site, the Ki-67 indices of implantation site intermediate trophoblast are near zero.[189] Complete hydatidiform moles are always accompanied by exaggerated placental sites in which the implantation site intermediate trophoblastic cells are often more atypical and the Ki-

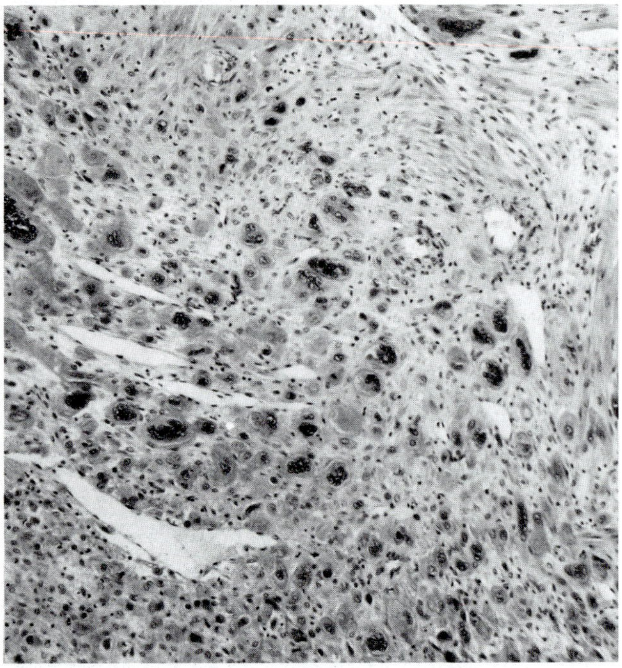

Fig. 24.48. Exaggerated placental site. Numerous mononucleate and multinucleated implantation site intermediate trophoblastic cells infiltrate decidua and myometrium. The trophoblastic cells are widely spaced, lacking confluent growth or necrosis.

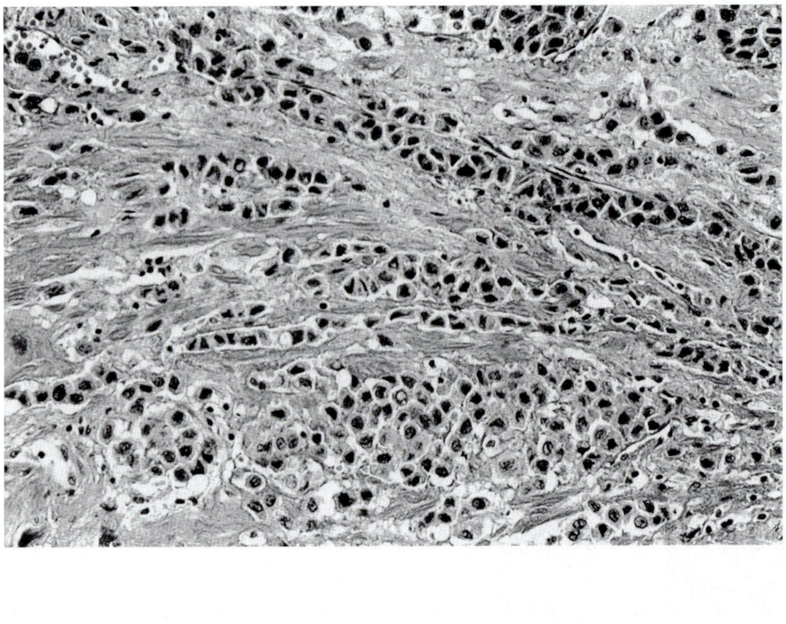

Fig. 24.47. Exaggerated placental site. The lesion is characterized by an increased amount of implantation site intermediate trophoblast exceeding that normally present in the implantation site.

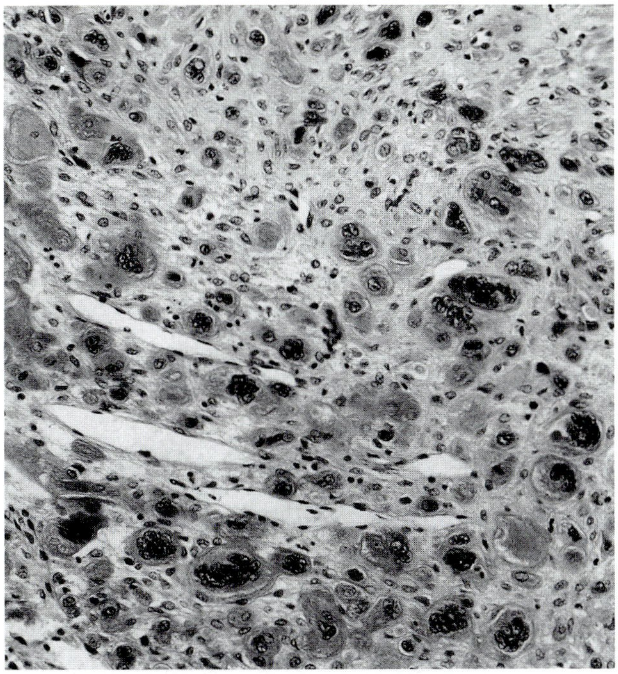

Fig. 24.49. Exaggerated placental site. Mixture of mononucleate and multinucleated implantation site intermediate trophoblastic cells in which the latter is more commonly seen in an exaggerated placental site rather than in a placental site trophoblastic tumor. The cells show no mitotic activity.

67 labeling index is higher (5%) than those in the exaggerated placental sites that are not associated with complete moles.[189]

The most important differential diagnosis of an exaggerated implantation site is placental site trophoblastic tumor, which is discussed in the section describing that entity. Occasionally, implantation site intermediate trophoblastic cells that infiltrate the myometrium may resemble the atypical smooth muscle cells found in symplastic leiomyomas. The presence of chorionic villi, the infiltrative growth pattern of the trophoblastic cells and positive cytokeratin and hPL stains support the diagnosis of an exaggerated implantation site.

Exaggerated placental site probably represents a physiologic process that resolves spontaneously after curettage. Exaggerated placental site that is not associated with a hydatidiform mole does not carry an increased risk of persistent GTD. No specific treatment or follow-up is required.

Placental Site Nodule

Placental site nodules are small, well-circumscribed nodular aggregates of chorionic-type intermediate trophoblastic cells that are embedded in a hyalinized stroma. Placental site nodules have been thought to represent a portion of uninvoluted placental site from remote gestations in the uterus. However, the constituent cells in placental site nodules are more closely related to the intermediate trophoblast of chorion laeve (chorionic-type intermediate trophoblast) than to the intermediate trophoblast of placental site (implantation site intermediate trophoblastic cells).[194] Based on morphologic and immunohistochemical studies, the placental site nodule appears to represent the benign counterpart of the epithelioid trophoblastic tumor.

Patients are in the reproductive age group. Placental site nodules are typically incidental findings in uterine curettings, cervical biopsies, and occasionally in hysterectomy specimens.[42,156,194] In one study, 40% of placental site nodules were present in the endocervix, 56% in the endometrium, and 4% in the fallopian tube.[194] The diagnosis of placental site nodule has been made in a variety of clinical settings, including evaluation of cervical intraepithelial neoplasm following an abnormal cervical smear (35%), dysmenorrhea and metromenorrhagia (30%), recurrent spontaneous abortion (5%), retained products of conception (5%), postcoital bleeding (2.5%), and infertility (2.5%).[194] Many patients have a prior history of therapeutic abortion and cesarean section. A significant number of patients have had a history of a tubal ligation.[25,95,194] The antecedent pregnancy has been reported to have been as little as 2 months to as much as 108 months before the diagnosis,[95,156,196,230] suggesting that these lesions can persist in the uterus for a long period of time.

Placental site nodules are small, ranging from 1 to 14 (average, 2.1) mm. Occasionally, multiple nodules are found. When grossly visible, placental site nodules appear as a yellow and tan nodule or plaque in the endometrium or superficial myometrium.

Microscopically, placental site nodules are small nodular lesions with rounded, well-circumscribed borders (see Figs. 24.50 to 24.53). The nodules are surrounded by a thin rim of chronic inflammatory cells and occasionally decidua cells. The nodules typically are composed of trophoblastic cells that resemble those found in the chorion laeve and therefore have been termed chorionic-type intermediate trophoblast (see Fig. 24.1). These cells occupy the central portion of the nodule and are surrounded by a hyalinized extracellular matrix that forms the outer border of the lesion (Figs. 24.50 and 24.51). The trophoblastic cells within the placental site nodule share several features with chorionic-type intermediate trophoblast in the chorion laeve of the fetal membranes (see Tables 24.1 and 24.9).[194] They vary in size; many have relatively small uniform nuclei and a few have

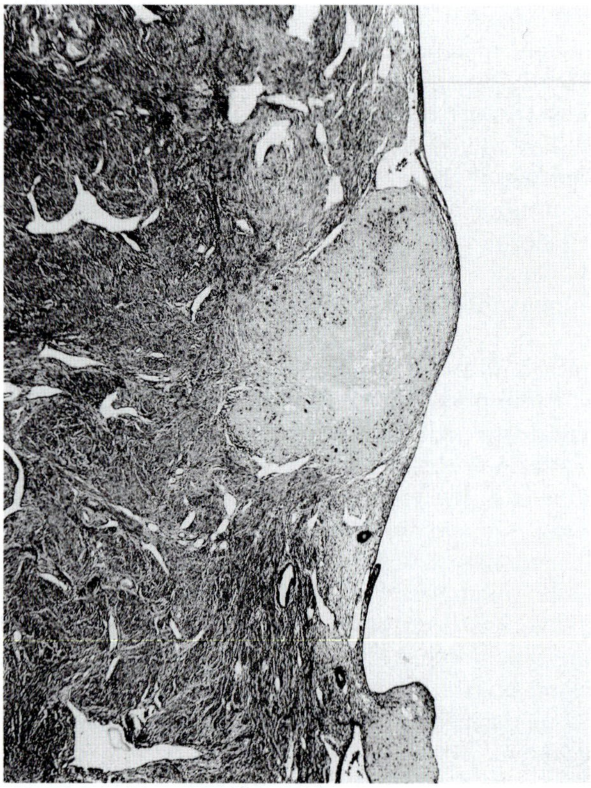

Fig. 24.50. **Placental site nodule.** The lesion is well circumscribed and contains acellular material in the center.

large, irregular and hyperchromatic nuclei (Fig. 24.52). Multinucleated cells are occasionally present. The cytoplasm of the larger trophoblastic cells is abundant and eosinophilic to amphophilic whereas the smaller cells contain glycogen-rich clear cytoplasm (Fig. 24.53). The chorionic-type intermediate trophoblastic cells in placental site nodules are arranged in a haphazard pattern, dispersed singly, in small clusters and cords, or occasionally diffusely throughout the nodule (Figs. 24.50–24.52). Mitotic figures are absent or rare.

Based on the histologic and immunohistochemical features as well as the intimate association of some epithelioid trophoblastic tumors with placental site nodules, we have speculated that the epithelioid trophoblastic tumor represents the neoplastic counterpart of the placental site nodule. This view is supported by our observations of placental site nodules that have features intermediate between typical placental site nodules and epithelioid trophoblastic tumors. Specifically, these lesions we have provisionally designated "atypical placental site nodules" are intermediate in size between placental site nodules, which rarely exceed 4 mm in diameter, and the larger epithelioid trophoblastic tumors, which are a few centimeters. These placental site nodules tend to have higher cellularity, and the trophoblastic cells are arranged in more cohesive nests and cords than the typical placental site nodules.[188] The Ki-67 labeling index in atypical placental site nodules is higher than the usual placental site nodules but lower than epithelioid trophoblastic tumor. These findings suggest that atypical placental site nodules are intermediate between a placental site nodule and an epithelioid trophoblastic tumor. The few cases for which we have follow-up information have behaved in a benign fashion.

The trophoblastic cells in the placental site nodule exhibit an immunophenotype similar to that of trophoblastic cells in the chorion laeve but distinct from the implantation site intermediate trophoblast. They react with antibodies against cytokeratin, epithelial membrane antigen (EMA), pregnancy-specific SP-1, placental alkaline phosphatase (PLAP), and inhibin-α.[95,190,196] Most placental site nodules also express the "classical" intermediate tropho-

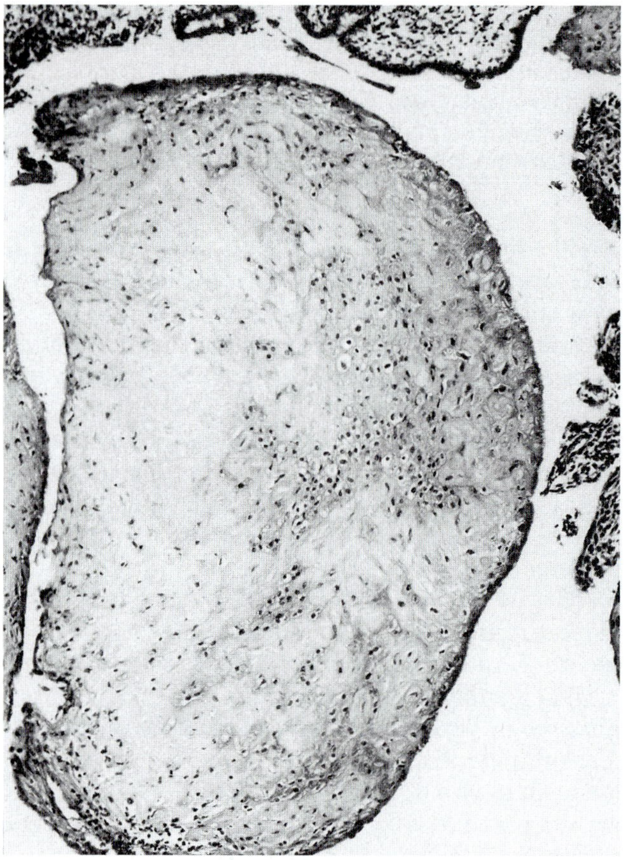

Fig. 24.51. **Placental site nodule.** The nodule is composed of hyalin material that contains scattered chorionic-type intermediate trophoblast. The remainder of the endometrium had a proliferative-phase pattern. (Reprinted by permission of Silverberg and Kurman, ref. 198.)

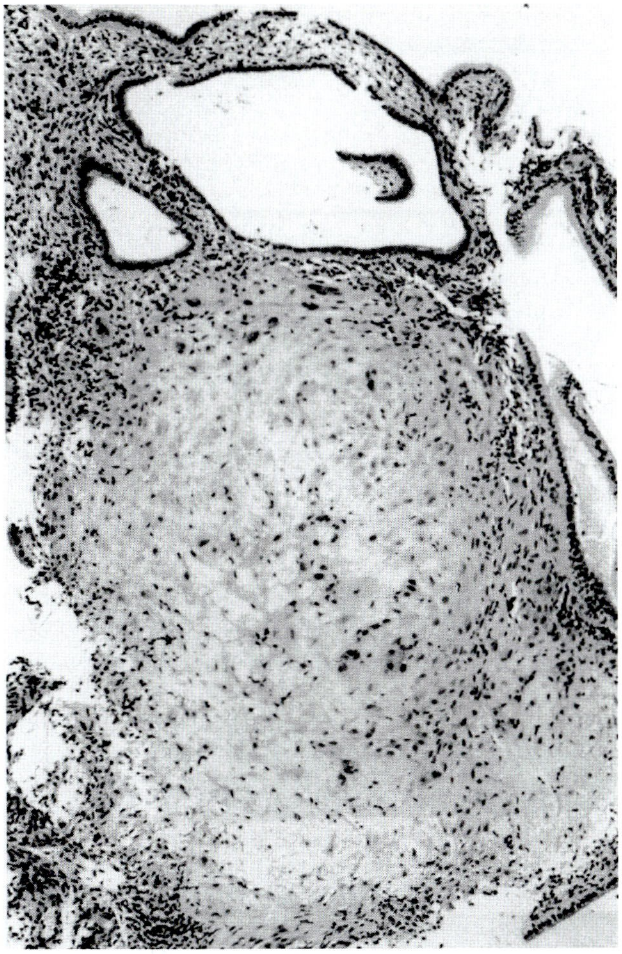

Fig. 24.52. **Placental site nodule.** The chorionic-type intermediate trophoblastic cells disperse singly and in small clusters and cords throughout the nodule.

blastic markers including hPL, Mel-CAM (CD 146), and oncofetal fibronectin although only in a small number of cells.[194] The trophoblastic cells in a placental site nodule exhibit mild proliferative activity with a Ki-67 labeling index of about 5%, which is similar to that in the intermediate trophoblastic cells in the chorion laeve (3%–6%).[194] This finding is in contrast to the absence of Ki-67 labeling trophoblastic cells in the normal implantation site as well as in the exaggerated placental site.[187,189]

A placental site nodule may be confused with a placental site trophoblastic tumor (PSTT), epithelioid trophoblastic tumor, and a nontrophoblastic lesion, notably invasive squamous cell carcinoma of the cervix.[194,218] Their microscopic size, circumscription, extensive hyalinization, and paucicellularity are features that separate them from PSTT. In difficult cases, immunostaining is helpful (see Fig. 24.5 and Table 24.9). Placental site nodules are positive for placental alkaline phosphatase but only focally positive or negative for Mel-CAM (CD 146) and hPL. In contrast, PSTTs demonstrate diffuse staining for Mel-CAM (CD 146) and hPL but show only scattered and faint staining for placental alkaline phosphatase. The differential diagnosis between placental site nodule and cervical squamous cell carcinoma is particularly difficult in cervical biopsies of patients who are being evaluated for cervical neoplasia.[194] Circumscription of the lesion, abundant eosinophilic extracellular deposit, and lack of mitotic activity favor a placental site nodule. Immunoreactivity for inhibin-α, cytokeratin 18, high molecular weight cytokeratin, and Ki-67 are particularly useful in the differential diagnosis (see Fig. 24.5). The majority of placental site nodules express inhibin-α and cytokeratin 18 but intraepithelial squamous lesions and squamous cell carcinomas do not.[194] In contrast, placental site nodules are focally positive or negative for high molecular weight cytokeratin but cervical squamous cell carcinomas are diffusely positive. The Ki-67 labeling index is low (<10%) in placental site nodule in contrast to the generally high Ki-67 labeling index in cervical carcinoma (>50%).[194] The immunoreactivity of beta-hCG is not helpful in these cases because both placental sites nodule and cervical carcinomas can be focally reactive to β-hCG.[85]

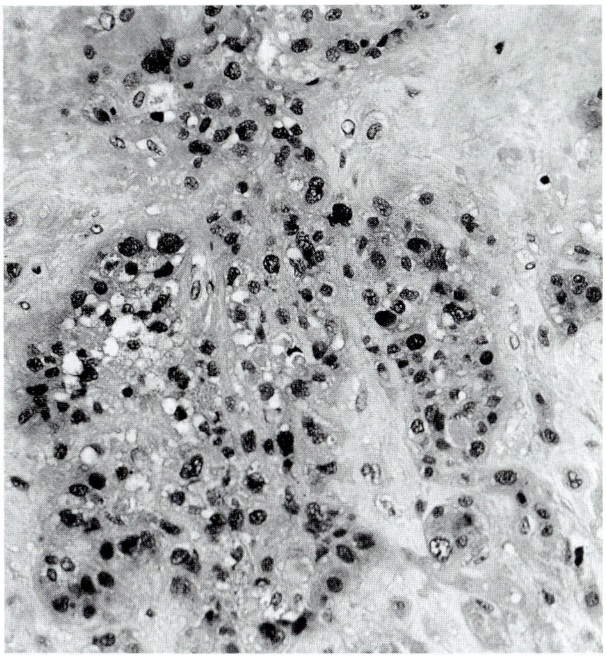

Fig. 24.53. **Placental site nodule.** Chorionic-type intermediate trophoblastic cells appear degenerate with smudged nuclei and indistinct cell borders. Mitotic figures are absent. (Reprinted by permission of Silverberg and Kurman, ref. 198.)

The differential diagnosis of the placental site nodule versus epithelioid trophoblastic tumor is considered in the discussion of epithelioid trophoblastic tumor.

Placental site nodules are benign nonneoplastic lesions. Because of their small size and circumscription, the lesions are usually removed completely by the surgical procedure that led to their discovery. Neither local recurrence nor progression to persistent GTD has been documented in placental site nodules.[194,230] Accordingly, no specific treatment or follow-up is necessary for this lesion.

References

1. Alsat E, Guibourdenche J, Luton D, et al (1997) Human placental growth hormone. Am J Obstet Gynecol 177:1526–1534
2. Aplin JD (1991) Implantation, trophoblast differentiation and haemochorial placentation: mechanistic evidence in vivo and in vitro. J Cell Sci 99: 681–692
3. Axe SR, Klein VR, Woodruff JD (1985) Choriocarcinoma of the ovary. Obstet Gynecol 66:111–114
4. Azuma C, Saji F, Nobunaga T, et al (1990) Studies on the pathogenesis of choriocarcinoma by analysis of restriction fragment length polymorphisms. Cancer Res 50:488–491
5. Babury RA, Moscovic EA (1993) Selective immunolabeling of early gestational cytotrophoblast and its neoplastic counterpart by the monoclonal antibody Ber-EP4. Histol Histopathol 8:323–328
6. Bagshawe KD (1984) Treatment of high-risk choriocarcinoma. J Reprod Med 29:813–820
7. Bagshawe KD, Lawler SD, Paradinas FJ, et al (1990) Gestational trophoblastic tumours following initial diagnosis of partial hydatidiform mole. Lancet 335:1074–1076
8. Bell KA, Van Deerlin V, Addya K, et al (1999) Molecular genetic testing from paraffin-embedded tissue distinguishes nonmolar hydropic abortion from hydatidiform mole. Mol Diagn 4:11–19
9. Benirschke K, Kaufmann P (1995) Early development of human placenta. In: Benirschke K, Kaufmann P (eds) Pathology of the human placenta, 3rd Ed. Springer, New York, pp 49–56
10. Benirschke K, Kaufmann P (1995) Nonvillous parts of the placenta. In: Benirschke K, Kaufmann P (eds) Pathology of the human placenta, 3rd Ed. Springer, New York, pp 182–267
11. Berger G, Verbaere J, Feroldi J (1984) Placental site trophoblastic tumor of the uterus: an ultrastructural and immunohistochemical study. Ultrastruct Pathol 6:319–329
12. Berkowitz RS, Bernstein MR, Harlow BL, et al (1995) Case-control study of risk factors for partial molar pregnancy. Am J Obstet Gynecol 173:788–794
13. Berkowitz RS, Cramer DW, Bernstein MR, et al (1985) Risk factors for complete molar pregnancy from a case-control study. Am J Obstet Gynecol 152:1016–1020
14. Berkowitz RS, Goldstein DP, Bernstein MR (1985) Natural history of partial molar pregnancy. Obstet Gynecol 66:677–681
15. Berkowitz RS, Im SS, Bernstein MR, Goldstein DP (1998) Gestational trophoblastic disease. Subsequent pregnancy outcome, including repeat molar pregnancy. J Reprod Med 43:81–86
16. Berkowitz LW, Lage JM (1990) Persistent gestational trophoblastic tumor after partial hydatidiform mole. Gynecol Oncol 36:358–362
17. Bracken MB, Brinton LA, Hayashi K (1984) Epidemiology of hydatidiform mole and choriocarcinoma. Epidemiol Rev 6:52–75
18. Brewer CA, Adelson MD, Elder RC (1992) Erthrocytosis associated with a placental-site trophoblastic tumor. Obstet Gynecol 79:846–849
19. Bryant-Greenwood GD (1998) The extracellular matrix of the human fetal membranes: structure and function. Placenta 19:1–11
20. Burrows TD, King A, Loke YW (1993) Expression of integrins by human trophoblast and differential adhesion to laminin or fibronectin. Hum Reprod 8:475–484
21. Burrows TD, King A, Loke YW (1994) Expression of adhesion molecules by endovascular trophoblast and decidual endothelial cells: implications for vascular invasion during implantation. Placenta 15:21–33
22. Cameron B, Gown AM, Tamimi HK (1994) Expression of c-erb B-2 oncogene product in persistent gestational trophoblastic disease. Am J Obstet Gynecol 170:1616–1621; discussion 1621–1612
23. Campello TR, Fittipaldi H, O'Valle F, et al (1998) Extrauterine (tubal) placental site nodule. Histopathology 32:562–565
24. Caniggia I, Grisaru-Gravnosky S, Kuliszewsky M, et al (1999) Inhibition of TGF-beta 3 restores the invasive capability of extravillous trophoblasts in preeclamptic pregnancies. J Clin Invest 103:1641–1650
25. Carinelli SG, Verdola N, Zanotti F (1989) Placenta site nodule: a report of 17 cases. Pathol Res Pract 185:30–34
26. Chang YL, Chang TC, Hsueh S, et al (1999) Prognostic factors and treatment for placental site trophoblastic tumor: report of 3 cases and analysis of 88 cases. Gynecol Oncol 73:216–222
27. Chassin D, Benifla JL, Delattre C, et al (1994) Identification of genes overexpressed in tumors through preferential expression screening in trophoblasts. Cancer Res 54:5217–5223
28. Chen CA, Chen YH, Chen TM, et al (1994) Infrequent mutation in tumor suppressor gene p53 in gestational trophoblastic neoplasia. Carcinogenesis (Oxf) 15:2221–2223
29. Cheung AN, Ngan HY, Collins RJ, Wong YL (1994) Assessment of cell proliferation in hydatidiform

mole using monoclonal antibody MIBI to Ki-67 antigen. J Clin Pathol 47:601–604
30. Cheung AN, Shen DH, Khoo US, et al (1998) p21WAF1/CIP1 expression in gestational trophoblastic disease: correlation with clinicopathological parameters, and Ki67 and p53 gene expression. J Clin Pathol 51:159–162
31. Cheung AN, Srivastava G, Chung LP, et al (1994) Expression of the p53 gene in trophoblastic cells in hydatidiform moles and normal human placentas. J Reprod Med 39:223–227
32. Cheville JC, Greiner T, Robinson RA, Benda JA (1995) Ploidy analysis by flow cytometry and fluorescence in situ hybridization in hydropic placentas and gestational trophoblastic disease [see comments]. Hum Pathol 26:753–757
33. Cheville JC, Robinson RA, Benda JA (1996) p53 expression in placentas with hydropic change and hydatidiform moles. Mod Pathol 9:392–396
34. Chew SH, Perlman EJ, Williams R, et al (2000) Morphology and DNA content and analysis in the evaluation of first trimester placentas for partial hydatidiform mole (PHM). Hum Pathol 31:914–924
35. Chilosi M, Piazzola E, Lestani M, et al (1998) Differential expression of p57kip2, a maternally imprinted cdk inhibitor, in normal human placenta and gestational trophoblastic disease. Lab Invest 78:269–276
36. Cole LA (1998) hCG, its free subunits and its metabolites. Roles in pregnancy and trophoblastic disease. J Reprod Med 43:3–10
37. Cole LA, Kohorn EI, Kim GS (1994) Detecting and monitoring trophoblastic disease. J Reprod Med 39:193–200
38. Conran RM, Hitchcock CL, Popek EJ, Norris HJ (1993) Diagnostic considerations in molar gestations. Hum Pathol 24:41–48
39. Coukos G, Makrigiannakis A, Chung J, et al (1999) Complete hydatidiform mole. A disease with a changing profile. J Reprod Med 44:698–704
40. Coutifaris C, Kao LC, Sehdev HM, et al (1991) E-cadherin expression during the differentiation of human trophoblasts. Development (Camb) 113: 767–777
41. Craighill MC, Cramer DW (1984) Epidemiology of complete molar pregnancy. J Reprod Med 29:784–787
42. Crescimanno C, Marzioni D, Paradinas FJ, Schrurs B, et al (1999) Expression pattern alterations of syndecans and glypican-1 in normal and pathological trophoblast. J Pathol 189:600–608
43. Cross JC, Werb Z, Fisher SJ (1994) Implantation and the placenta: key pieces of the development puzzle. Science 266:1508–1518
44. Curry SL, Blessing JA, SiSaia PJ (1989) A prospective randomized comparison of methotrexate, dactinomycin and chlorambucil versus methotrexate, dactinomycin, cyclophosphamide, doxorubicin, melphalan, hydroxyurea, and vincristine in poor-prognosis metastatic gestational trophoblastic disease: a Gynecologic Oncology Group study. Obstet Gynecol 73:357
45. Czernobilsky B, Barash A, Lancet M (1982) Partial moles: a clinicopathologic study of 25 cases. Obstet Gynecol 59:75–77
46. Damsky CH, Fisher SJ (1998) Trophoblast pseudo-vasculogenesis: faking it with endothelial adhesion receptors. Curr Opin Cell Biol 10:660–666
47. Damsky CH, Librach C, Lim KH, et al (1994) Integrin switching regulates normal trophoblast invasion. Development (Camb) 120:3657–3666
48. Davis JR, Surwit EA, Garay JP, Fortier KJ (1984) Sex assignment in gestational trophoblastic neoplasia. Am J Obstet Gynecol 148:722–725
49. Daya D, Sabet L (1991) The use of cytokeratin as a sensitive and reliable marker for trophoblastic tissue. Am J Clin Pathol 95:137–141
50. Denny LA, Dehaeck K, Nevin J, et al (1995) Placental site trophoblastic tumor: three case reports and literature review. Gynecol Oncol 59:300–303
51. Dessau R, Rustin GJ, Dent J, et al (1990) Surgery and chemotherapy in the management of placental site tumor. Gynecol Oncol 39:56–59
52. Disaia PJ, Creasman WT (1993) Clinical gynecologic oncology, 4th Ed. Mosby, St. Louis, pp 210–237
53. Dougherty CM, Cunningham C, Mickal A (1978) Choriocarcinoma with metastasis in a postmenopausal woman. Am J Obstet Gynecol 132:700–701
54. Duncan DA, Mazur MT (1989) Trophoblastic tumors: ultrastructural comparison of choriocarcinoma and placental-site trophoblastic tumor. Hum Pathol 20:370–381
55. Eckstein RP, Paradinas FJ, Bagshawe KD (1982) Placental site trophoblastic tumour (trophoblastic pseudotumour): a study of four cases requiring hysterectomy including one fatal case. Histopathology (Oxf) 6:211–226
56. Eckstein RP, Russell P, Friedlander ML, Tattersall MHN (1983) Metastasizing placental site trophoblastic tumor: a case study. Hum Pathol 16:632–636
57. Elston C (1995) Gestational trophoblastic disease. In: Fox H (ed) Haines and Taylor: Textbook of obstetrical and gynecological pathology, 4th Ed. Churchill Livingstone, New York, pp 1597–1639
58. Evans AC, Soper JT, Clarke-Pearson DL, et al (1995) Gestational trophoblastic disease metastatic to the central nervous system. Gynecol Oncol 59:226–230
59. Feinberg RF, Kliman HJ, Lockwood CJ (1991) Is oncofetal fibronectin a trophoblast glue for human implantation? Am J Pathol 138:537–543
60. Feltmate F, Genest DR, Wise L, Bernstein MR, Goldstein DP, Berkowitz RS. Placental site trophoblastic tumor: a 17-year experience at the New England Trophoblastic Disease Center. Gyn Oncol 2001;82:415–419
61. Finkler NJ, Berkowitz RS, Driscoll SG, et al (1988) Clinical experience with placental site trophoblastic tumors at the New England Trophoblastic Disease Center. Obstet Gynecol 71:854–857

62. Fisher SJ, Damsky CH (1993) Human cytotrophoblast invasion. Semin Cell Biol 4:183–188
63. Fisher RA, Lawler SD, Povey S, Bagshawe KD (1988) Genetically homozygous choriocarcinoma following pregnancy with hydatidiform mole. Br J Cancer 58:788–792
64. Fisher RA, Newlands ES (1998) Gestational trophoblastic disease. Molecular and genetic studies. J Reprod Med 43:87–97
65. Fisher RA, Paradinas FJ, Newlands ES, Boxer GM (1992) Genetic evidence that placental site trophoblastic tumours can originate from a hydatidiform mole or a normal conceptus. Br J Cancer 65: 355–358
66. Fraser GC, Blair GK, Hemming A, et al (1992) The treatment of simultaneous choriocarcinoma in mother and baby. J Pediatr Surg 27:1318–1319
67. Fukunaga M, Ushigome S (1993) Malignant trophoblastic tumors: immunohistochemical and flow cytometric comparison of choriocarcinoma and placental site trophoblastic tumors. Hum Pathol 24:1098–1106
68. Fukunaga M, Ushigome S (1993) Metastasizing placental site trophoblastic tumor. An immunohistochemical and flow cytometric study of two cases. Am J Surg Pathol 17:1003–1010
69. Fulop V, Colitti CV, Genest D, et al (1998) DOC-2/hDab2, a candidate tumor suppressor gene involved in the development of gestational trophoblastic diseases. Oncogene 17:419–424
70. Fulop V, Mok SC, Genest DR, et al (1998) c-myc, c-erbB-2, c-fms and bcl-2 oncoproteins. Expression in normal placenta, partial and complete mole, and choriocarcinoma. J Reprod Med 43:101–110
71. Fulop V, Mok SC, Genest DR, et al (1998) p53, p21, Rb and mdm2 oncoproteins. Expression in normal placenta, partial and complete mole, and choriocarcinoma. J Reprod Med 43:119–127
72. Gardner HA, Lage JM (1992) Choriocarcinoma following a partial hydatidiform mole: a case report. Hum Pathol 23:468–471
73. Genbacev O, Gerdner K, Miller R (1993) Human cytotrophoblastic cell islands from first trimester placentae: proliferative and functional activity in vitro. Placenta 14:A25
74. Genest DR, Laborde O, Berkowitz RS, Goldstein DP (1991) A clinicopathologic study of 153 cases of complete hydatidiform mole (1980–1990): histologic grade lacks prognostic significance. Obstet Gynecol 78:402–409
75. Giwa-Osagie MO, Okwerekwu G (1999) Epidemiology of molar pregnancies in Northern Ireland. Int J Gynaecol Obstet 66:175–177
76. Gloor E, Dialdas J, Hurlimann J, et al (1983) Placental site trophoblastic tumor (trophoblastic pseudotumor) of the uterus with metastases and fatal outcome. Clinical and autopsy observations of a case. Am J Surg Pathol 7:483–486
77. Goldstein DP (1991) Gestational trophoblastic neoplasia in the 1990s. Yale J Biol Med 64:639–651
78. Goldstein DP, Berkowitz RS (1994) Current management of complete and partial molar pregnancy. J Reprod Med 39:139–146
79. Goto S, Yamada A, Ishizuka T, Tomoda Y (1993) Development of postmolar trophoblastic disease after partial molar pregnancy. Gynecol Oncol 48: 165–170
80. Graham CH (1997) Effect of transforming growth factor-beta on the plasminogen activator system in cultured first trimester human cytotrophoblasts. Placenta 18:137–143
81. Graham CH, Connelly I, MacDougall JR, et al (1994) Resistance of malignant trophoblast cells to both the anti-proliferative and anti-invasive effects of transforming growth factor-beta. Exp Cell Res 214:93–99
82. Grimes DA (1984) Epidemiology of gestational trophoblastic disease. Am J Obstet Gynecol 150:309–318
83. Haining RE, Cameron IT, van Papendorp C, et al (1991) Epidermal growth factor in human endometrium: proliferative effects in culture and immunocytochemical localization in normal and endometriotic tissues. Hum Reprod 6:1200–1205
84. Hamazaki S, Nakamoto S, Okino T, et al (1999) Epithelioid trophoblastic tumor: morphological and immunohistochemical study of three lung lesions. Hum Pathol 30:1321–1327
85. Hameed A, Miller Ds, Muller CY, et al (1999) Frequent expression of beta-human chorionic gonadotropin (beta-hCG) in squamous cell carcinoma of the cervix. Int J Gynecol Pathol 18:381–386
86. Hando T, Ohno M, Kurose T (1998) Recent aspects of gestational trophoblastic disease in Japan. Int J Gynaecol Obstet 60(suppl 1):S71–S76
87. Hartenbach EM, AKS, Zachary CB, et al (1996) Placental site trophoblastic tumor presenting with scalp metastases. Int J Gynecol Cancer 6:333–336
88. Hayashi K, Bracken MB, Freeman DH Jr, Hellenbrand K (1982) Hydatidiform mole in the United States (1970–1977): a statistical and theoretical analysis. Am J Epidemiol 115:67–77
89. Heifetz SA, Czaja J (1992) In situ choriocarcinoma arising in partial hydatidiform mole: implications for the risk of persistent trophoblastic disease. Pediatr Pathol 12:601–611
90. Hertig AT (1956) Tumors of the female sex organs. Part 1. Hydatidiform mole and choriocarcinoma, Atlas of tumor pathology, sec 9, fasc 33. Armed Forces Institute of Pathology, Washington, DC
91. Hopkins M, Nunez C, Murphy JR, Wentz WB (1985) Malignant placental site trophoblastic tumor. Obstet Gynecol 66:95S–100S
92. Hou PC, Pang SC (1956) Chorioepithelioma: an analytical study of 28 necropsied cases with special reference to the possibility of spontaneous retrogression. J Pathol Bacteriol 72:95–104
93. How J, Scurry J, Grant P, et al (1995) Placental site trophoblastic tumor. Report of three cases and review of the literature. Int J Gynecol Cancer 5:241–249

94. Howat AJ, Beck S, Fox H, et al (1993) Can histopathologists reliably diagnose molar pregnancy? J Clin Pathol 46:599–602
95. Huettner PC, Gersell DJ (1994) Placental site nodule: a clinicopathologic study of 38 cases. Int J Gynecol Pathol 13:191–198
96. Ichikawa N, Zhai YL, Shiozawa T, et al (1998) Immunohistochemical analysis of cell cycle regulatory gene products in normal trophoblast and placental site trophoblastic tumor. Int J Gynecol Pathol 17: 235–240
97. Ilancheran A (1998) Optimal treatment in gestational trophoblastic disease. Ann Acad Med Singapore 27:698–704
98. Jacobs PA, Hunt PA, Matsuura JS, et al (1982) Complete and partial hydatidiform mole in Hawaii: cytogenetics, morphology and epidemiology. Br J Obstet Gynaecol 89:258–266
99. Janni W, Hantschmann P, Rehbock J, et al (1999) Successful treatment of malignant placental site trophoblastic tumor with combined cytostatic-surgical approach: case report and review of literature. Gynecol Oncol 75:164–169
100. Jauniaux E (1999) Partial moles: from postnatal to prenatal diagnosis. Placenta 20:379–388
101. Jeffers MD, O'Dwyer P, Curran B, et al (1993) Partial hydatidiform mole: a common but underdiagnosed condition. A 3-year retrospective clinicopathological and DNA flow cytometric analysis. Int J Gynecol Pathol 12:315–323
102. Jeffers MD, Richmond JA, Smith R (1996) Trophoblast proliferation rate does not predict progression to persistent gestational trophoblastic disease in complete hydatidiform mole. Int J Gynecol Pathol 15:34–38
103. Jokimaa V, Inki P, Kujari H, et al (1998) Expression of syndecan-1 in human placenta and decidua. Placenta 19:157–163
104. Jones WB, Romain K, Erlandson RA, et al (1993) Thoracotomy in the management of gestational choriocarcinoma. A clinicopathologic study. Cancer (Phila) 72:2175–2181
105. Kalousek DK, Robinson W, Harrington B, Lestou VS (1999) Molecular biology of the placenta with focus on special placental studies of infants with intrauterine growth retardation. In: Lewis SH, Perrin E (eds) Pathology of the placenta, 2nd Ed. Churchill Livingstone, Philadelphia, pp 343–365
106. Keep D, Zaragoza MV, Hassold T, Redline RW (1996) Very early complete hydatidiform mole. Hum Pathol 27:708–713
107. Kim SJ, Bae SN, Kim JH, et al (1998) Epidemiology and time trends of gestational trophoblastic disease in Korea. Int J Gynecol Obstet 60(suppl): S33–S38
108. Kim JH, Park DC, Bae SN, et al (1998) Subsequent reproductive experience after treatment for gestational trophoblastic disease. Gynecol Oncol 71:108–112
109. King LA, Okagaki T, Twiggs LB (1992) Resolution of pulmonary metastases with chemotherapy in a patient with a placental site trophoblastic tumor. Int J Gynecol Cancer 2:328–331
110. Kodama S, Kase H, Aoki Y, et al (1996) Recurrent placental site trophoblastic tumor of the uterus: clinical, pathologic, ultrastructural, and DNA fingerprint study. Gynecol Oncol 60:89–93
111. Kohorn EI (1993) Evaluation of the criteria used to make the diagnosis of nonmetastatic gestational trophoblastic neoplasia [see comments]. Gynecol Oncol 48:139–147
112. Kohorn EI, McGinn RC, Gee JBL, Goldstein DP (1978) Pulmonary embolization of trophoblastic tissue in molar pregnancy. Obstet Gynecol 51(suppl): 16S
113. Kotylo PK, Michael H, Davis TE, et al (1992) Flow cytometric DNA analysis of placental-site trophoblastic tumors. Int J Gynecol Pathol 11:245–252
114. Kurman RJ (1991) The morphology, biology, and pathology of intermediate trophoblast: a look back to the present. Hum Pathol 22:847–855
115. Kurman RJ, Main CS, Chen HC (1984) Intermediate trophoblast: a distinctive form of trophoblast with specific morphological, biochemical and functional features. Placenta 5:349–370
116. Kurman RJ, Scully RE, Norris HJ (1976) Trophoblastic pseudotumor of the uterus: an exaggerated form of "syncytial endometritis" simulating a malignant tumor. Cancer (Phila) 38:1214–1226
117. Kurman RJ, Young RH, Norris HJ, et al (1984) Immunocytochemical localization of placental lactogen and chorionic gonadotropin in the normal placenta and trophoblastic tumors, with emphasis on intermediate trophoblast and the placental site trophoblastic tumor. Int J Gynecol Pathol 3:101–121
118. Lage JM, Bagg A (1996) Hydatidiform moles: DNA flow cytometry, image analysis and selected topics in molecular biology. Histopathology (Oxf) 28:379–382
119. Lage JM, Mark SD, Roberts DJ, et al (1992) A flow cytometric study of 137 fresh hydropic placentas: correlation between types of hydatidiform moles and nuclear DNA ploidy. Obstet Gynecol 79:403–410
120. Lage JM, Popek EJ (1993) The role of DNA flow cytometry in evaluation of partial and complete hydatidiform moles and hydropic abortions. Semin Diagn Pathol 10:267–274
121. Lage JM, Weinberg DS, Yavner DL, Bieber FR (1989) The biology of tetraploid hydatidiform moles: histopathology, cytogenetics, and flow cytometry. Hum Pathol 20:419–425
122. Lala PK, Hamilton GS (1996) Growth factors, proteases and protease inhibitors in the maternal-fetal dialogue. Placenta 17:545–555
123. Lane SA, Taylor GR, Ozols B, Quirke P (1993) Diagnosis of complete molar pregnancy by microsatellites in archival material. J Clin Pathol 46: 346–348
124. Hui P, Parkash V, Perkins AS, Carcangiu ML. Pathogenesis of placental site trophoblastic tumor

may require the presence of a paternally derived X chromosome. Lab Invest 2000;80:965–972

125. Leiserowitz GS, Webb MJ (1996) Treatment of placental site trophoblastic tumor with hysterotomy and uterine reconstruction. Obstet Gynecol 88:696–699
126. Libshitz HI, Baber CE, Hammond CB (1977) The pulmonary metastases of choriocarcinoma. Obstet Gynecol 49:412–416
127. Loke YW, King A (1995) Trophoblast interaction with extracellular matrix. In: Loke YW, King A (eds) Human implantations: cell biology and immunology, 1st Ed. Cambridge University Press, Cambridge pp 151–179
128. Lurain JR, Brewer JI (1985) Treatment of high-risk gestational trophoblastic disease with methotrexate, actinomycin D, and cyclophosphamide chemotherapy. Obstet Gynecol 65:830–836
129. Lurain JR, Brewer JI, Torok EE, Halpern B (1982) Gestational trophoblastic disease: treatment results at the Brewer Trophoblastic Disease Center. Obstet Gynecol 60:354–360
130. Lurain JR, Sand PK, Brewer JI (1986) Choriocarcinoma associated with ectopic pregnancy. Obstet Gynecol 68:286–287
131. Maddox DE, Kephart GM, Coulam CB, et al (1984) Localization of a molecule immunochemically similar to eosinophil major basic protein in human placenta. J Exp Mol 160:29–41
132. Marchand F (1895) Uber die sogenannten "decidualen" Geschwulste im Anschloss an normale Geburt, Abort, Blasenmole, und Extrauterin Schwangerschaft. Monatsschr Geburtsh Gynaekol 1:419
133. Martin DA, Sutton GP, Ulbright TM, et al (1989) DNA content as a prognostic index in gestational trophoblastic neoplasia. Gynecol Oncol 34:383–388
134. Massenkeil G, Crombach G, Dominik S, et al (1996) Metastatic choriocarcinoma in a postmenopausal woman. Gynecol Oncol 61:432–437
135. Matsuda T, Sasaki M, Kato H, et al (1997) Human chromosome 7 carries a putative tumor suppressor gene(s) involved in choriocarcinoma. Oncogene 15:2773–2781
136. Matsui H, Iizuka Y, Sekiya S (1996) Incidence of invasive mole and choriocarcinoma following partial hydatidiform mole. Int J Gynaecol Obstet 53: 63–64
137. Mazur MT (1989) Metastatic gestational choriocarcinoma. Unusual pathologic variant following therapy. Cancer (Phila) 63:1370–1377
138. Mazur MT, Lurain JR, Brewer JI (1982) Fatal gestational choriocarcinoma. Clinicopathologic study of patients treated at a trophoblastic disease center. Cancer (Phila) 50:1833–1846
139. McFadden DE, Pantzar JT (1996) Placental pathology of triploidy. Hum Pathol 27:1018–1020
140. McKenzie PP, Foster JS, House S, et al (1998) Expression of G_1 cyclins and cyclin-dependent kinase-2 activity during terminal differentiation of cultured human trophoblast. Biol Reprod 58:1283–1289
141. McMaster MT, Librach CL, Zhou Y, et al (1995) Human placental HLA-G expression is restricted to differentiated cytotrophoblasts. J Immunol 154: 3771–3778
142. Menczer J, Girtler O, Zajdel L, Glezerman M (1999) Metastatic trophoblastic disease following partial hydatidiform mole: case report and literature review. Gynecol Oncol 74:304–307
143. Messerli ML, Lilienfeld AM, Parmley T, et al (1985) Risk factors for gestational trophoblastic neoplasia. Am J Obstet Gynecol 153:294–300
144. Messerli ML, Parmley T, Woodruff JD, et al (1987) Inter- and intra-pathologist variability in the diagnosis of gestational trophoblastic neoplasia. Obstet Gynecol 69:622–626
145. Mi S, Lee X, Li X-P, et al (2000) Syncytin is a captive retroviral envelope protein involved in human placental morphogenesis. Nature (Lond) 403:785–789
146. Moll UM, Lane BL (1990) Proteolytic activity of first trimester human placenta: localization of interstitial collagenase in villous and extravillous trophoblast. Histochemistry 94:555–560
147. Montes M, Roberts D, Berkowitz RS, Genest DR (1996) Prevalence and significance of implantation site trophoblastic atypia in hydatidiform moles and spontaneous abortions. Am J Clin Pathol 105:411–416
148. Morrow CP (1984) Postmolar trophoblastic disease: diagnosis, management, and prognosis. Clin Obstet Gynecol 27:211–220
149. Mortakis AE, Braga CA (1990) "Poor prognosis" metastatic gestational trophoblastic disease: the prognostic significance of the scoring system in predicting chemotherapy failures. Obstet Gynecol 76:272–277
150. Mortakis AE, Brage CA (1990) Poor prognosis metastatic gestational trophoblastic disease: the prognostic significance of the scoring system in predicting chemotherapy failures. Obstet Gynecol 76:272–276
151. Mosher R, Goldstein DP, Berkowitz R, et al (1998) Complete hydatidiform mole. Comparison of clinicopathologic features, current and past. J Reprod Med 43:21–27
152. Muhlhauser J, Crescimanno C, Kaufmann P, et al (1993) Differentiation and proliferation patterns in human trophoblast revealed by c-erbB-2 oncogene product and EGF-R. J Histochem Cytochem 41: 165–173
153. Mungan T, Kuscu E, Dabakoglu T, et al (1996) Hydatidiform mole: clinical analysis of 310 patients. Int J Gynaecol Obstet 52:233–236
154. Muto MG, Lage JM, Berkowitz RS, et al (1991) Gestational trophoblastic disease of the fallopian tube. J Reprod Med 36:57–60
155. Nagamani M, Kaspar HG, Van Dinh T, et al (1990) Hyperthecosis of the ovaries in a woman with a placental site trophoblastic tumor. Obstet Gynecol 76: 931–935

156. Nayar R, Snell J, Silverberg SG, Lage JM (1996) Placental site nodule occurring in a fallopian tube. Hum Pathol 27:1243–1245
157. Newlands ES, Bower M, Fisher RA, Paradinas FJ (1998) Management of placental site trophoblastic tumors. J Reprod Med 43:53–59
158. Newlands ES, Bower M, Holden L, et al (1998) Management of resistant gestational trophoblastic tumors. J Reprod Med 43:111–118
159. Nisula BC, Taliadouros GS (1980) Thyroid function in gestational trophoblastic neoplasia: evidence that the thyrotropic activity of chorionic gonadotropin mediates the thyrotoxicosis of choriocarcinoma. Am J Obstet Gynecol 138:77–85
160. Ober WB, Maier RC (1981) Gestational choriocarcinoma of the fallopian tube. Diagn Gynecol Obstet 3:213–231
161. O'Connor DM, Kurman RJ (1988) Intermediate trophoblast in uterine curettings in the diagnosis of ectopic pregnancy. Obstet Gynecol 72:665–670
162. Osada H, Kawata M, Yamada M, et al (1991) Genetic identification of pregnancies responsible for choriocarcinomas after multiple pregnancies by restriction fragment length polymorphism analysis. Am J Obstet Gynecol 165:682–688
163. Palmer JR (1994) Advances in the epidemiology of gestational trophoblastic disease. J Reprod Med 39:155–162
164. Paradinas FJ, Browne P, Fisher RA, et al (1996) A clinical, histopathological and flow cytometric study of 149 complete moles, 146 partial moles and 107 non-molar hydropic abortions. Histopathology (Oxf) 28:101–110
165. Parazzini F, LaVecchia C, Pampallona S, Franceschi S (1985) Reproductive patterns and the risk of gestational trophoblastic disease. Am J Obstet Gynecol 152:866–870
166. Polyak K, Lee MH, Erdjument-Bromage H, et al (1994) Cloning of p27Kip1, a cyclin-dependent kinase inhibitor and potential mediator of extracellular antimitogenic signals. Cell 78:59–66
167. Qiao S, Nagasaka T, Harada T, Nakashima N (1998) p53, Bax and Bcl-2 expression, and apoptosis in gestational trophoblast of complete hydatidiform mole. Placenta 19:361–369
168. Qiao S, Nagasaka T, Nakashima N (1997) Numerous vessels detected by CD34 in the villous stroma of complete hydatidiform moles. Int J Gynecol Pathol 16:233–238
169. Qin X, Garibay-Tupas J, Chua PK, et al (1997) An autocrine/paracrine role of human decidual relaxin. I. Interstitial collagenase (matrix metalloproteinase-1) and tissue plasminogen activator. Biol Reprod 56:800–811
170. Randall TC, Coukos G, Wheeler JE, Rubin SC (2000) Prolonged remission of recurrent, metastatic placental site trophoblastic tumor after chemotherapy. Gynecol Oncol 76:115–117
171. Redline RW, Hassold T, Zaragoza MV (1998) Prevalence of the partial molar phenotype in triploidy of maternal and paternal origin. Hum Pathol 29:505–511
172. Rice LW, Lage JM, Berkowitz RS, et al (1989) Repetitive complete and partial hydatidiform mole. Obstet Gynecol 74:217–219
173. Rinne K, Shahabi S, Cole L (1999) Following metastatic placental site trophoblastic tumor with urine β-core fragment. Gynecol Oncol 74:302–303
174. Roberts DJ, Mutter GL (1994) Advances in the molecular biology of gestational trophoblastic disease. J Reprod Med 39:201–208
175. Rodabaugh KJ, Bernstein MR, Goldstein DP, Berkowitz RS (1998) Natural history of postterm choriocarcinoma. J Reprod Med 43:75–80
176. Rosenshein NB, Wijnen H, Woodruff JD (1980) Clinical importance of the diagnosis of trophoblastic pseudotumors. Am J Obstet Gynecol 136:635–638
177. Rotmensch S, Cole LA (2000) False diagnosis and needless therapy of presumed malignant disease in women with false-positive human chorionic gonadotropin concentrations. Lancet 355:712–715
178. Rustin GJ, Newlands ES, Lutz JM, et al (1996) Combination but not single-agent methotrexate chemotherapy for gestational trophoblastic tumors increases the incidence of second tumors. J Clin Oncol 14:2769–2773
179. Rutgers JL, Baergen RN, Young RH, Scully RE (1995) Placental site trophoblastic tumor: clinicopathologic study of 64 cases. Mod Pathol 8:96A
180. Saji F, Tokugawa Y, Kimura T, et al (1989) A new approach using DNA fingerprinting for the determination of androgenesis as a cause of hydatidiform mole. Placenta 10:399–405
181. Schink JC, Singh DK, Rademaker AW, et al (1992) Etoposide, methotrexate, actinomycin D, cyclophosphamide, and vincristine for the treatment of metastatic, high-risk gestational trophoblastic disease. Obstet Gynecol 80:817–820
182. Schulte AM, Lai S, Kurtz A, et al (1996) Human trophoblast and choriocarcinoma expression of the growth factor pleiotrophin attributable to germline insertion of an endogenous retrovirus. Proc Natl Acad Sci USA 93:14759–14764
183. Scully RE, Bonfiglio TA, Kurman RJ, et al (1994) Histologic typing of female genital tract tumors, 2nd Ed. Springer, New York
184. Sharkey AM, King A, Clark DE, et al (1999) Localization of leukemia inhibitory factor and its receptor in human placenta throughout pregnancy. Biol Reprod 60:355–364
185. Shi Y-F, Xie X, Zhao C-L, et al (1996) Lack of mutation in tumour-suppressor gene p53 in gestational trophoblastic tumours. Br J Cancer 73:1216–1219
186. Shih IM (1999) The role of CD146 (Mel-CAM) in biology and pathology. J Pathol 189:4–11
187. Shih IM, Kurman RJ (1996) Expression of melanoma cell adhesion molecule in intermediate trophoblast. Lab Invest 75:377–388

188. Shih I-M, Kurman RJ (1998) Epithelioid trophoblastic tumor: a neoplasm distinct from choriocarcinoma and placental site trophoblastic tumor simulating carcinoma. Am J Surg Pathol 22:1393–1403
189. Shih IM, Kurman RJ (1998) Ki-67 labeling index in the differential diagnosis of exaggerated placental site, placental site trophoblastic tumor, and choriocarcinoma: a double immunohistochemical staining technique using Ki-67 and Mel-CAM antibodies. Hum Pathol 29:27–33
190. Shih IM, Kurman RJ (1999) Immunohistochemical localization of inhibin-alpha in the placenta and gestational trophoblastic lesions. Int J Gynecol Pathol 18:144–150
191. Shih IM, Kurman RJ. Distribution of cytokeratin subtypes in human trophoblast (unpublished)
192. Shih IM, Kurman RJ. Placental site trophoblastic tumor–past as prologue. Gynecol Oncol 82:413–414, 2001
193. Shih IM, Schnaar RL, Gearhart JD, Kurman RJ (1997) Distribution of cells bearing the HNK-1 epitope in the human placenta. Placenta 18:667–674
194. Shih IM, Seidman JD, Kurman RJ (1999) Placental site nodule and characterization of distinctive types of intermediate trophoblast. Hum Pathol 30:687–694
195. Shih I, Wang T, Wu T, et al (1998) Expression of Mel-CAM in implantation site intermediate trophoblastic cell line, IST-1, limits its migration on uterine smooth muscle cells. J Cell Sci 111:2655–2664
196. Shitabata PK, Rutgers JL (1994) The placental site nodule: an immunohistochemical study. Hum Pathol 25:1295–1301
197. Silva EG, Tornos C, Lage J, et al (1993) Multiple nodules of intermediate trophoblast following hydatidiform moles. Int J Gynecol Pathol 12:324–332
198. Silverberg SG, Kurman RJ (eds) (1992) Tumors of the uterine corpus and gestational trophoblastic disease. Atlas of tumor pathology, 3rd Ed. Armed Forced Institute of Pathology, Washington, DC
199. Smith DB, Holden L, Newlands ES, Bagshawe KD (1993) Correlation between clinical staging (FIGO) and prognostic groups with gestational trophoblastic disease. Br J Obstet Gynaecol 100:157–160
200. Somers GR, Bradbury R, Trute L, et al (1999) Expression of the human P2Y6 nucleotide receptor in normal placenta and gestational trophoblastic disease. Lab Invest 79:131–139
201. Song HZ, Yang XY, Xiang Y (1998) Forty-five year's experience of the treatment of choriocarcinoma and invasive mole. Int J Gynaecol Obstet 60(suppl 1):S77–S83
202. Soper JT, Evans AC, Conaway MR, et al (1994) Evaluation of prognostic factors and staging in gestational trophoblastic tumor. Obstet Gynecol 84: 969–973
203. Soto-Wright V, Bernstein M, Goldstein DP, Berkowitz RS (1995) The changing clinical presentation of complete molar pregnancy. Obstet Gynecol 86: 775–779
204. Stahle-Backdhal M, Inoue M, Zedenius J, et al (1995) Decreased expression of Ras GTPase activating protein in human trophoblastic tumors. Am J Pathol 146:1073–1078
205. Stanhope CR, Stuart GCE, Curtis KL (1983) Primary ovarian hydatidiform mole: review of the literature and report of a case. Am J Obstet Gynecol 145:886–889
206. Su YN, Cheng WF, Chen CA, et al (1999) Pregnancy with primary tubal placental site trophoblastic tumor: a case report and literature review. Gynecol Oncol 73:322–325
207. Surani MA, Barton SC, Norris ML (1984) Development of reconstituted mouse eggs suggests imprinting of the genome during gametogenesis. Nature (Lond) 308:548–550
208. Suzuki T, Goto S, Nawa A, et al (1993) Identification of the pregnancy responsible for gestational trophoblastic disease by DNA analysis. Obstet Gynecol 82:629–634
209. Swisher E, Drescher CW (1998) Metastatic placental site trophoblastic tumor: long-term remission in a patient treated with EMA/CO chemotherapy. Gynecol Oncol 68:62–65
210. Takeuchi S (1982) Nature of invasive mole and its rational management. Semin Oncol 9:181–186
211. Tomoda Y, Arii Y, Kaseki S, et al (1980) Surgical indications for resection in pulmonary metastasis of choriocarcinoma. Cancer (Phila) 46:2723–2730
212. Thomsen BM, Clausen HV, Larsen LG, et al (1997) Patterns in expression of insulin-like growth factor-II and of proliferative activity in the normal human first and third trimester placenta demonstrated by non-isotopic in situ hybridization and immunohistochemical staining for MIB-1. Placenta 18:145–154
213. Tsukamoto N, Iwasaka T, Kashimura Y, et al (1985) Gestational trophoblastic disease in women aged 50 or more. Gynecol Oncol 20:53–61
214. Twiggs LB, Hartenbach E, Saltzman AK, King LA (1998) Metastatic placental site trophoblastic tumor. Int J Gynaecol Obstet 60(suppl 1):S51–S55
215. Twiggs LB, Okagaki T, Phillips GL, et al (1981) Trophoblastic pseudotumor: evidence of malignant disease potential. Gynecol Oncol 12:238–248
216. Van de Kaa CA, Hanselaar AG, Hopman AH, et al (1993) DNA cytometric and interphase cytogenetic analyses of paraffin-embedded hydatidiform moles and hydropic abortions. J Pathol 170:229–238
217. van de Kaa CA, Schijf CP, de Wilde PC, et al (1996) Persistent gestational trophoblastic disease: DNA image cytometry and interphase cytogenetics have limited predictive value. Mod Pathol 9:1007–1014
218. Van Dorpe J, Moerman P (1996) Placental site nodule of the uterine cervix. Histopathology (Oxf) 29:379–382
219. Vanderpuye OA, Labarrere CA, McIntyre JA (1993) Predominant expression of the beta subunit of pro-

lyl 4-hydroxylase (disulfide isomerase) in human extravillous trophoblasts. Histochemistry 100:241–246
220. Vassilakos P, Ritton G, Kajii T (1977) Hydatidiform mole: two entities. Am J Obstet Gynecol 127:167–170
221. Veridiano NP, Gal D, Delke I, et al (1980) Gestational choriocarcinoma of the ovary. Gynecol Oncol 10:235–240
222. Wang PH, Yuan CC, Tseng JY, Chao HT (1998) High-risk gestational trophoblastic disease: analysis of clinical prognosis. Eur J Gynecol Oncol 19:302–305
223. Weed JC Jr, Hammond CB (1980) Cerebral metastatic choriocarcinoma: intensive therapy and prognosis. Obstet Gynecol 55:89–94
224. Wong SYY, Ngan HYS, Chan CCW, Cheung ANY (1999) Apoptosis in gestational trophoblastic disease is correlated with clinical outcome and Bcl-2 expression but not Bax expression. Mod Pathol 12:1025–1033
225. Wurzel J, Brooks JJ (1981) Primary gastric choriocarcinoma: immunohistochemistry, postmortem documentation and hormonal effects in a postmenopausal female. Cancer (Phila) 48:2765–2761
226. Xu B, Lin L, Rote NS (1999) Identification of a stress-induced protein during human trophoblast differentiation by differential display analysis. Biol Reprod 61:681–686
227. Yagel S, Parhar RS, Jeffrey JJ, Lala PK (1988) Normal nonmetastatic human trophoblast cells share in vitro invasive properties of malignant cells. J Cell Physiol 136:455–462
228. Yeh IT, O'Connor DM, Kurman RJ (1989) Vacuolated cytotrophoblast: a subpopulation of trophoblast in the chorion laeve. Placenta 10:429–438
229. Young RH, Kurman RJ, Scully RE (1998) Proliferations and tumors of intermediate trophoblast of the placental site. Semin Diagn Pathol 5:223–237
230. Young RH, Kurman RJ, Scully RE (1990) Placental site nodules and plaques. A clinicopathologic analysis of 20 cases. Am J Surg Pathol 14:1001–1009
231. Young RH, Scully RE (1984) Placental-site trophoblastic tumor: current status. Clin Obstet Gynecol 27:248–258
232. Young RH, Scully RE, McCluskey RT (1985) A distinctive glomerular lesion complicating placental site trophoblastic tumor: report of two cases. Hum Pathol 16:35–42
233. Yuan CC, Wang PH, Ng HT (1999) High hCG level is a risk factor for predicting the occurrence of brain and/or liver metastases from gestational choriocarcinoma. Int J Gynaecol Obstet 65:67–69
234. Yuen BH, Callegari PB (1986) Occurrence of molar pregnancy in patients undergoing elective abortion: comparison with other clinical presentations. Am J Obstet Gynecol 154:273–276
235. Zalel Y, Dgani R (1997) Gestational trophoblastic disease following the evacuation of partial hydatidiform mole: a review of 66 cases. Eur J Obstet Gynecol Reprod Biol 71:67–71
236. Zanetta G, Maggi R, Colombo M, et al (1997) Choriocarcinoma coexistent with intrauterine pregnancy: two additional cases and a review of the literature. Int J Gynecol Cancer 7:66–77
237. Zhou Y, Fisher SJ, Janatpour M, et al (1997) Human cytotrophoblasts adopt a vascular phenotype as they differentiate: A strategy for successful endovascular invasion? J Clin Invest 99:2139–2151

PART TWO

Adjunctive Techniques in Gynecologic Pathology

25

Immunohistochemistry

Norio Azumi, M.D., Ph.D. and Bernard Czernobilsky, M.D.

In recent years, immunohistochemistry has largely replaced histochemical "special stains" and electron microscopy as an adjunctive method to assist in the differential diagnosis of tumors and in the identification of infectious agents. This technique permits visualization of immunologically detectable markers (antigens) in tissue sections; thus, the pathologist can observe both the morphology and the immunophenotype of a given tissue or neoplasm. To exploit this technique fully, the pathologist must not only be acquainted with the distribution of various antigens in different tumors and tissues but also have sufficient knowledge of the methodology to avoid pitfalls in interpretation. Accordingly, this chapter is divided into a section describing various aspects of the methodology of this technique and a section describing application of immunohistochemistry in the identification of a variety of antigens, including intermediate filaments, hormone receptors, oncofetal antigens, and gene products, which can be useful in the differential diagnosis and prognosis of tumors of the female genital tract. This latter section is organized by antigens and is intended to complement the individual (organ) chapters. Finally, the last section lists important differential diagnoses in which immunohistochemical markers are useful.

Methodology

Because an antigen is morphologically not identifiable, it is necessary to visualize and localize the antigen in tissue sections. There are two major techniques that can accomplish this: the *immunoenzyme technique* (*immunohistochemistry*) and *immunofluorescence*. Because immunofluorescence is only used in kidney biopsies and in exceptional circumstances in research settings, the following discussion is limited to immunohistochemistry.

The contemporary immunoenzyme technique has two major components: (1) a primary antibody and (2) a detection system to identify the resulting antigen–antibody complex. The detection system has two subcomponents, a color development system and a bridging component or secondary antibody that connects the primary antibody and the color development system. The following sections are brief discussions of each component of the immunohistochemical technique providing the relevant information to understand the pitfalls in the interpretation of immunophenotype. More detailed technical details as well as application of immunohistochemistry to general surgical pathology can be found in monograms dedicated to the subject.[142]

Antigen and Heat-Induced Antigen Retrieval

Antigens are usually proteins, although other substances such as carbohydrates can also be antigens. Antibodies react with a part (in case of monoclonal antibodies) or parts (in case of polyclonal antibodies) of antigens, which are called *epitopes*. An antigen usually has multiple potential epitopes that can be detected by antibodies. Fixation and embedding may alter the structure of an epitope to such a degree that it is not recognized by the antibody. To overcome this problem, a mixture (cocktail) of multiple antibodies that detect the same antigen but recognize different epitopes are used to enhance the sensitivity. Because some epitopes are more resistant to routine tissue processing, it is possible to select antibodies that detect an epitope resistant to fixation. To unmask epitopes, the heat-induced antigen retrieval method (HIAR) has mostly replaced traditional proteolytic enzyme pretreatment. HIAR uses nontoxic buffer solutions. The source of heat can be a microwave, hot plate, Bunsen burner, steamer, or pressure cooker.

Almost all antigens benefit from HIAR without deterioration of antigen detection, in contrast to enzyme digestion, which may have a detrimental effect. Proteolytic enzyme pretreatment (for example, detection of epidermal growth factor receptor) or sonication by ultrasound (for example, cyclin D1 or bcl1) may be effective in retrieving specific antigens. Coagulative fixatives, specifically alcohol, preserve some antigens such as intermediate filaments as well as RNA and DNA better than formalin. A few exceptions are estrogen and progesterone receptors and S-100 protein, which are better preserved by a cross-linking, as compared to coagulative, fixative. Recently, it has been reported that alcohol and specialized fixatives are better for extraction of RNA and DNA, but more extensive study of the effects of these fixatives is needed.

Antibodies

Although any subclass of immunoglobulins can be used in immunohistochemistry, the majority that are used belong to either the IgG or, less frequently, the IgM class. Antibodies that react with antigens are called *primary antibodies*. Depending on how these antibodies are produced, two kinds of antibodies are available: polyclonal and monoclonal antibodies.

Polyclonal antibodies are produced by immunization of an animal with a specific antigen. Because the immunized animal produces antisera that include a variety of antibodies to the specific antigen as well as other nonspecific antibodies, it may be necessary to purify the antisera by removing unwanted antibodies. A polyclonal antibody recognizes multiple different and overlapping epitopes of the same antigen. Polyclonal antibodies are easier to produce and are often more sensitive as compared to monoclonal antibodies, probably because of the larger and multiple epitopes that they recognize. Polyclonal antibodies, however, have several significant disadvantages: (1) even after affinity purification, polyclonal antibodies may include antibodies that react with unwanted antigens, resulting in nonspecific staining; (2) there is a tendency to produce high background staining; and (3) batch-to-batch variation makes interlaboratory comparison impossible. Because of these shortcomings, highly specific monoclonal antibodies have largely replaced polyclonal antibodies. Certain polyclonal antibodies are still in use for diagnostic immunohistochemistry because of their superb sensitivity or for reasons of difficulty in obtaining monoclonal antibodies.

Monoclonal antibodies are produced by a hybridoma, which is a hybrid of mouse plasmacytoma cells and splenic B lymphocytes from the immunized animal (mouse or rat). Because a single clone of hybridoma cells produces the antibody, it recognizes a single epitope (monospecific). The hybridoma cells provide a constant and almost limitless supply of exactly the same antibody.

The primary antibodies can be monoclonal, polyclonal, or a cocktail of monoclonal antibodies. Although sensitivity of monoclonal antibodies is usually less than the equivalent polyclonal antibody, newly developed monoclonal antibodies and cocktails (mixtures of monoclonal antibodies that react with the same antigen but each of which detects different epitopes) provide sensitivity surpassing that of polyclonal antibodies without sacrificing specificity.

Detection System

Because an antigen–antibody complex is invisible by conventional light microscopy, a detection system is needed to generate a visible product at the site of the antigen–antibody reaction. The detection system is composed of two subcomponents: *a secondary or bridging antibody* and *a color development system*. Because the secondary antibody must connect (bridge) the primary antibody to the color development system, it is an antibody against the immunoglobulin of the primary antibody. For example, if the primary antibody is mouse IgG, the secondary antibody is rabbit or goat antimouse IgG.

Although many detection systems have been developed, the most commonly used is the avidin–biotin–complex method (ABC) with peroxidase–DAB (diaminobenzidine) system. With the ABC, the secondary antibody is biotinylated, meaning biotin molecules are bound to the secondary antibodies by covalent chemical bonds. The enzyme, peroxidase, is also biotinylated and mixed with avidin to form a complex (ABC) based on the strong chemical affinity between avidin and biotin. Because of the presence of excess biotin-binding sites on avidin, the resulting ABC has free binding sites for biotin. The biotinylated secondary antibody binds to the ABC via the free biotin-binding sites on avidin. Thus, the enzyme, peroxidase, is localized at the anigen–antibody complex. When the substrate, hydrogen peroxide, and the chromogen, DAB, are added, the peroxidase catalyzes the substrate to create oxygen radicals. These, in turn, change the colorless chromogen, DAB, to a brown-colored product that permits identification of the antigen by light microscopy.

Two enzymes that are most commonly used in modern immunoenzyme techniques are horseradish peroxidase and alkaline phosphatase, with appropriate substrates and chromogens. Many normal tissues have endogenous peroxidase activity, which results in nonspecific positivity. In many tissues, the endogenous peroxidase activity is totally suppressed after formalin fixation. For example, epithelial cells of breast and secretory endometrium do not show endogenous peroxidase activity after fixation; however, neutrophils, eosinophils, basophils, histiocytes, and red blood cells may show endogenous peroxidase activity that survives the conventional fixation process. When endogenous peroxidase activity interferes with interpretation such as when a heavy acute inflammatory infiltrate is present, it can be suppressed by incubating sections with a 0.5% H_2O_2 in absolute methanol for 30 minutes. Unfortunately, it is difficult to completely suppress the endogenous peroxidase activity without adversely affecting preservation of the antigen.

In recent years, most laboratories are using autoimmunostainers with commercial reagents and immunohistochemical detection systems. New and more sensitive detection systems, including those with additional amplification steps (such as tylamid-catalyzed signal amplification), have recently become available. Although these automated systems are superior to the manual method because of their consistent quality and superior sensitivity, it is important to familiarize oneself with the new systems because increased sensitivity may bring heretofore undetected and unexpected positivity.

Pitfalls in Interpretation

Besides knowing the antigen expression of different lesions, the pathologist must be aware of *false-positive and false-negative results* to avoid misinterpretation. Causes of false-positive results (nonspecific staining) are multiple and may occur at different stages of the immunostaining procedure. False-negative results may be caused by loss of activity of the primary antibodies or loss of antigenicity resulting from tissue processing, especially fixation. Using appropriate controls and multiple antibodies (a "panel") rather than a single antibody will reduce the chance of misinterpretation. Sources of erroneous interpretation may be multiple and may occur at any step in the immunohistochemical procedure. Sources of false results (positive or negative) can be divided into (1) tissue, (2) primary antibody, (3) secondary antibody, and (4) detection system.

Tissue

Antibodies may bind to other proteins in a nonimmunologic fashion. This phenomenon is secondary to excessive concentration of primary antibodies and/or certain types of tissue. For example, collagenous tissue and tissue fixed with a heavy metal salt solution (such as B5) can cause background staining by means of nonimmunological and nonspecific binding. Covering the tissue section with a blocking serum such as normal horse serum before applying the primary antibodies as well as appropriate titration of the primary antibodies reduces this type of nonspecific (background) staining. Tissue processing at high temperature and/or fixation may produce a loss of antigenicity. Vimentin is well known to be very sensitive to prolonged formalin fixation and can be used as a general indicator of antigen loss with the formalin fixation.

Some antigens such as p53 protein may be heat sensitive, and thus processing tissues and baking slides at high temperature should be avoided. HIAR usually does not deteriorate antigenicity even when it does not enhance it; however, it is possible that HIAR may produce false-negative and even false-positive results. One such rare example of the latter phenomenon is keratin reactivity in gliomas only in fixed tissue after HIAR. Because the effect of fixation, processing, and antigen retrieval differs from tissue to tissue, the only sure way of knowing that the antigenicity was properly preserved or recovered is to check so-called built-in, internal controls. Internal controls are tissue components in the immunostained section that are expected to be positive or negative for a particular antibody. The examples of positive internal controls are squamous epithelium for keratin and peripheral nerve for S-100 protein. When internal controls are not present and there is no immunostaining in the lesion, it cannot be determined whether this is a "true" negative immunostain or a false negative.

Primary Antibody

When a primary antibody is not specific for the antigen of interest, immunologic nonspecific binding will ensue. This phenomenon is especially common within polyclonal antibodies because they may contain a mixture of several antibodies that recognize large or multiple epitopes, and one of these epitopes may be shared by other unwanted antigens; even quality-controlled commercial antibodies may have this problem. Among the markers used frequently in gynecologic pathology, commercially available polyclonal anticarcinoembryonic antigen (CEA) antibodies may cross react with nonspecific cross-reacting antigen (NCA) contained in polymorphonuclear leukocytes.

Monoclonal antibodies are much less likely to have this problem. Shared epitopes could be, in some instances, used to advantage. For example, the antibody to an isotype of alkaline phosphatase specific to the placenta (placental alkaline phosphatase) cross-reacts with germ cell-specific alkaline phosphates. Thus, in the differential diagnosis of surface epithelial neoplasm versus germ cell neoplasm of the ovary, reactivity with placental alkaline phosphatase supports the diagnosis of a germ cell tumor.

Antibodies may become denatured depending on how diluted they are and how long they have been stored. As a rule, primary antibodies should be freshly prepared the day these antibodies are used. Stock antibodies should be immediately aliquoted into multiple vials when they are received. Commercially available concentrated antibodies tend to be stable, with a shelf life of approximately 1 year or more at 4°C. Frozen or lyophilized antibodies may have a much longer shelf life, although some antibodies cannot be frozen. Multiple freeze–thaw cycles may also destroy antibody activity. Addition of proteins, such as normal calf serum, to diluted antibodies may prolong their shelf life. Many of the antibodies from commercial sources are prediluted and stabilized. So long as one follows the specified storage conditions and expiration date, the reactivity of the antibody is assured. Even in this situation, however, it is essential to use a positive control for every run of immunostaining to ensure proper antibody reactivity.

Secondary Antibody

As in the primary antibody, the secondary antibody can show nonimmunological and/or immunologic nonspecific staining. A most common situation in which immunologic nonspecific staining becomes problematic is when staining experimental animal tissues, especially rats and mice; this occurs because the secondary antibody (either antirat or antimouse IgG antibody raised in other animals) will react with any mouse or rat tissue that is bathed in the animal's own serum.

False-negative staining may result from failure of the secondary antibody. Because the majority of commercially available secondary antibodies are so-called universal secondary antibodies that react with mouse, rat, and rabbit primary antibodies, most of the primary antibodies that are in use can be detected. When the primary antibodies are raised in unusual animals such as goat, horse, or guinea pig, appropriate secondary antibodies must be used.

Enzymes and Labels

Enzymes used in the color development system may be present in the tissue itself (endogenous activity). Although fixation usually suppresses most of the endogenous peroxidase activity, it may remain in macrophages, red blood cells, and polymorphonuclear leukocytes. When this endogenous peroxidase activity interferes with the interpretation, incubation with hydrogen peroxide–alcohol solution can be used. Alkaline phosphatase activity may be also seen in macrophages even after fixation. In frozen sections, bladder mucosa and vascular endothelial cells may show strong positivity because of endogenous alkaline phosphatase activity. In systems using avidin and biotin, the presence of biotin and/or cross-reactivity of avidin with lectin-like substances in tissues such as liver may theoretically cause false-positive staining; however, in practice, this type of nonspecific reaction produces only weak background staining in fixed tissue.

Controls Used to Avoid Misinterpretation

It is important to use appropriate negative and positive controls for validating the specificity of immunostaining. For a negative control, the primary antibody should be replaced with an irrelevant antibody of the same animal species and of the same immunoglobulin class as the primary antibody. In practice, separate negative controls may not be necessary because a panel of antibodies should be always used in diagnostic immunohistochemistry and these different antibodies act as negative controls to each other. For example, if the differential diagnosis includes carcinoma and lymphoma, a panel of antibodies consisting of keratin and leukocyte common antigen (LCA or CD 45) should be used. If the tumor is a carcinoma, LCA will serve as a negative control for keratin.

As a positive control, one should use tissue that is positive in the best of conditions (i.e., positive when your system is most sensitive); this will allow detection of the slightest decrease in sensitivity of the immunohistochemical method. For this purpose, multitumor or multitissue blocks are very useful. Multiple tumor tissues that show various degrees of positivity could be included, and disappearance of some of the weakly positive samples may be an indication of deterioration of the sensitivity in the immunostaining system. In addition, it is important to check internal controls, as discussed earlier. Because the internal positive controls are subjected to exactly the same tissue fixation, processing, and immunostaining as the lesion under investigation, the presence of positive staining in the internal control is the best assurance of the validity of the immunostaining.

Markers Useful in Gynecologic Pathology

Although immunohistochemical markers, especially lineage-specific markers, are useful in establishing the diagnosis, it cannot be overemphasized that diagnostic immunohistochemistry should be used in differentiating a narrow morphologic differential diagnosis. The pathologist must know aberrant expression of certain markers, such as keratin (epithelial marker) expression in normal myometrium, uterine smooth muscle tumors, endometrial stromal tumors, and some sarcomas. Furthermore, it must be understood that no marker is completely specific and therefore diagnostic immunohistochemistry must be employed in conjunction with the morphologic and clinical findings. The diagnostic application of immunophenotyping is based on the same principle as morphologic diagnosis, specifically, that neoplastic tissues largely preserve the immunophenotype of the putative parent normal tissue.

In this section, individual immunohistochemical markers are organized into six major categories: (1) lineage-specific markers, (2) tumor-associated and oncofetal antigens, (3) hormone receptors, (4) prognostic markers including proliferation markers and oncogene/suppressor gene proteins, (5) infectious agents including human papillomavirus (HPV), and (6) other markers useful in gynecologic pathology.

Lineage-Specific Markers

Epithelial Markers

Keratin

Keratin[93] is one of the intermediate filaments (IFs) that constitute the major cytoskeltons of epithelial cells. Twenty subtypes (excluding hard keratins such as those in nails and hair) that differ in their isoelectric pH values and their molecular weight have been characterized. Some antikeratin antibodies detect a wide range of keratin subtypes and others detect a very narrow range of subtypes or just one keratin subtype. Because epithelial cells almost always express one or more subtype of keratin, wide-spectrum antikeratin antibodies and cocktails are used as universal epithelial markers. In addition, some keratin subtypes (such as keratin 8 and 18) are present in a variety of normal and neoplastic tissues, but some show a narrower distribution.

Because expression of the keratin subtypes differs in different types of epithelia, it is possible to produce a "keratin profile" by using multiple narrow-spectrum antikeratin antibodies (Table 25.1). The keratin profiles may be helpful in arriving at a more specific diagnosis for epithelial tumors. The antikeratin antibodies that are most widely used and most relevant in gynecologic pathology are listed in Table 25.2 with the keratin classes that they detect.

Table 25.1. Keratin subtypes

Basic keratin	*Molecular weight (kDa)*	*Typical distribution in normal tissue*	*Acidic keratin*	*Molecular weight (kDa)*
		Epidermis of palm and sole	K9	64
K1	67	Epidermis, keratinizing squamous epithelia	K10	56.5
K2	65	Epidermis, keratinizing squamous epithelia	K11	56
K3	63	Cornea	K12	55
K4	50	Nonkeratinizing squamous epithelia of internal organs	K13	51
K5	58	Basal cells of squamous and glandular epithelia, myoepithelia, mesothelium	K14	50
		Squamous epithelia	K15	50
K6	56	Squamous epithelia, especially hyperproliferative	K16	48
K7	54	Basal cells of glandular epithelia, myoepithelia	K17	46
K8	52	Simple epithelia	K18	45
		Simple epithelia, most glandular and some squamous epithelia (basal)	K19	40
		Simple epithelia of intestines and stomach; Merkel cells	K20	46

From Miettinen.[93]

Keratin is abbreviated as "K" in the following section.

Keratins 20 and 7 Although initially K20[27] was considered as a possible breakdown product of other keratins, it is a distinctive keratin subtype (type I, MW 46 kDa). K20 is present in normal colonic epithelia, Merkel cells of skin, and umbrella cells of the urothelium. It is absent in skin, breast, and respiratory epithelium. Colonic adenocarcinoma is almost always K20+.

K7[27] (type II, MW 54 kDa) is characteristically present in simple epithelia in a narrower distribution as compared with K8 and K18. K7 is absent in normal colonic epithelium, hepatocytes, acinic cells of the prostate, and squamous epithelium. K7 is almost always negative in colonic adenocarcinoma. Among gynecologic neoplasms, endometrial carcinoma of

Table 25.2. Antikeratin antibodies

Antibody/clone	*Recognized keratin type(s)*	*Commercial source*[a]
AE1	10, 11, 13, 14, 15, 16, 19	Many sources
AE3	1, 2, 3, 4, 5, 6, 7, 8	Many sources
AE8	13	Research Diagnostics, NJ, USA
CAM5.2	8	Becton Dickinson, Mountain View, CA, USA
DE-K10	10	Dako, Carpinteria, CA, USA
D5/16 B4	5, 6	Mannheim Boehringer, Germany
E3	17	Dako
LP34	5, 6, 18	Novo Castra, UK
LL002	14	Novo Castra
CK 18	18	Novo Castra
CK 20	20	Novo Castra
CK 8	8	Novo Castra
OV-TL12/30	7	Zymed Labs, South San Francisco, CA, USA
34βE12	16, 14?	Dako
3βH11	8	Dako

[a]Multiple commercial sources may be available for the antibody from the same clone, and antikeratin antibodies from different clones may show similar reactivity.

the uterus and endometrioid and serous carcinoma of the ovary are K7+ and K20−. The majority of mucinous carcinomas of the ovary, especially those of colonic type, are K7+ and K20+, which contrast with primary colonic adenocarcinomas, which are K7− and K20+.[7] In mixed germ cell tumors, K7 is selectively expressed by trophoblastic components.[34]

Keratin 8, 18, and 19 K8 (type II, MW 52 kDa) and 18 (type I, MW 45 kDa) are sometimes referred to as low molecular weight keratins and appear as a pair. K19 is the lowest molecular weight keratin (type I, MW 40 kDa). These keratins are widely distributed among various simple epithelia. Most adenocarcinomas of gynecologic origin and germ cell tumors (except for dysgerminoma) are positive with K8 and K18. In granulosa cell tumors, keratin staining is negative (especially in formalin-fixed tissue). When positive, it is very focal and subtle, predominantly for K8 and K18 in the granulosa and theca cell components. Although keratin is negative in Leydig cell and steroid tumors not otherwise specified (NOS), Sertoli cell tumors often are positive with K8 and K18. K8, as detected by antibody CAM5.2, is also useful in detecting Paget cells.

K8, K18, and K19 are expressed in Paget cells but are negative in surrounding normal squamous cells. It should be also noted that the K8 and K18 pair, among all the keratins, is most commonly positive in nonepithelial tissues. K8, K18, and K19 are detected focally in a perinuclear, inclusion-like, intracytoplasmic pattern in normal myometrium as well as in smooth muscle and stromal tumors of the uterus.

Keratin 4 and 13 K4 (type II, MW 58 kDa) and K13 (type I, MW 51 kDa) are present in nonkeratinizing squamous epithelium of the internal organs and can be used to detect squamous differentiation in otherwise poorly differentiated carcinomas or adenocarcinomas because tumor cells of pure glandular differentiation lack K4 and K13. K4 and K13 expression in otherwise poorly differentiated adenocarcinoma may indicate immunophenotypic squamous differentiation and suggests the diagnosis of poorly differentiated endometrioid carcinoma. The cells in Brenner tumors as well as those that comprise transitional carcinoma predominantly express K13. K13 expression disappears, however, in poorly differentiated transitional cell carcinoma, which diminishes its value as a transitional cell marker (see description of uroplakins, following).

Keratin 5 and 6 Keratin 5 and 6 are expressed in basal cells, myoepithelial cells, and squamous cells. Because they are negative in many adenocarcinomas but positive in mesotheliomas, they can be useful in this differential diagnosis. (See the following section, "Mesothelial markers.")

Mesothelial Markers

The differential diagnosis between malignant mesotheliomas and metastatic carcinomas in the pleura has been extensively investigated. In gynecologic pathology, the differential between papillary (epithelioid) mesothelioma and ovarian-type papillary serous tumor of the peritoneum is important because of the differences in prognosis and response to treatment. Many of the immunohistochemical markers that were utilized in this differential diagnosis in the past are positive in carcinomas but negative in mesotheliomas.[112] Thus, immunohistochemical diagnosis of mesotheliomas was that of exclusion, not a positive identification of mesotheliomas. In recent years, makers that are predominantly expressed by mesothelial cells and their neoplastic counterparts have become available; these include calretinin,[26] keratin 5 and 6,[94] and thrombomodulin.[32,97] These mesothelioma markers should be used in conjunction with markers that are usually positive in adenocarcinomas and negative in mesotheliomas such as CD15 (LeuM-1), CEA, B72.3, BerEP4, and MOC-31. It should be noted that none of these markers are 100% specific and most of the published studies have presented pleural, not peritoneal, mesotheliomas and metastatic adenocarcinomas. Although peritoneal mesotheliomas including papillary mesotheliomas are expected to show an immunophenotype similar to that of pleural mesotheliomas, further studies are needed specifically addressing the immunophenotypic differential diagnosis of peritoneal papillary mesotheliomas versus ovarian-type papillary serous carcinomas versus metastatic carcinomas of gynecologic origin involving the peritoneum.

Calretinin

Calretinin is one of the calcium-binding proteins. Although calretinin was originally isolated from and is present in various neuronal tissues, it is frequently positive in reactive mesothelial cells and mesotheliomas but negative in the majority of adenocarcinomas. Among adenocarcinomas, poorly differentiated colonic adenocarcinomas have been reported to show frequent calretinin positivity in contrast to much less frequent calretinin expression by adenocarcinomas from other sites, including those of gynecologic origin. Thus, calretinin is a sensitive marker for mesotheliomas but its specificity is not as high as reported initially. Although more studies are needed, the majority of metastatic adenocarcinomas of a gynecologic origin as well as ovarian-type serous papillary carcinoma of the peritoneum are expected to be negative for calretinin.

Keratin 5 and 6

K5 (MW 58 kDa) is expressed predominantly in normal basal cells and myoepithelial cells but usually not in glandular cells. K5 is expressed in squamous cell carcinomas as well as areas of squamous differentiation in adenocarcinomas. K6 (MW 56 kDa) is expressed in normal squamous cells, salivary gland, and breast duct epithelia. K6 is also postive in squamous cell carcinomas. Both normal mesothelial cells and mesothelioma cells express K5 and K6 frequently, but pulmonary adenocarcinomas almost never do.

Virtually all cases of squamous cell carcinomas and a significant percentage of large cell undifferentiated carcinomas of the lung and transitional cell carcinomas are positive for K5 and K6. A small percentage of ovarian and uterine adenocarcinomas has been reported to show focal positivity for K5 and K6; this is particularly true when there is focal squamous differentiation. Thus, although K5 and K6 are excellent markers to separate mesotheliomas of the pleura and pleural metastasis of lung adenocarcinomas, their usefulness in differentiating metastatic adenocarcinoma of a gynecologic origin, ovarian-type serous papillary carcinomas of the peritoneal primary, and papillary mesotheliomas requires further study.

Thrombomodulin

Thrombomodulin is a cell-surface glycoprotein and an important component in the regulation of intravascular coagulation. It complexes with thrombin and activates protein C, which, in turn, modulates intravascular coagulation. Thrombomodulin is normally produced in vascular endothelial cells. In addition to normal vascular endothelial cells, it is also detected by immunochemistry in mesothelial cells and mesotheliomas whereas it is generally negative in adenocarcinomas. Thrombomodulin may be positive in adencarcinoma from the lung and kidney. Specificity and sensitivity for the differential diagnosis of mesothelioma versus carcinoma varies in different studies.

Mesenchymal Markers

Vimentin

Vimentin, one of the five IFs, is predominantly expressed by normal mesenchymal cells and tumors of mesenchymal derivation.[4] Although the antigenicity of vimentin is sensitive to fixation, heat-induced antigen retrieval makes detection of vimentin reliable and sensitive even in formalin-fixed tissue. With the use of more sensitive antibodies and antigen retrieval, increasing numbers of epithelial neoplasms are reported to express vimentin in addition to keratin. Thus, although still useful in certain circumstances, especially as a part of a panel of antibodies, vimentin is not a specific mesenchymal marker. Coexpression of vimentin and keratin is seen almost always, or very frequently, in certain types of carcinoma; these include renal cell carcinoma, papillary carcinoma of thyroid, endometrial carcinoma, and serous tumors of the ovary. Vimentin coexpression is rare in endocervical adenocarcinoma and colonic adenocarcinoma.[33] Sex cord stromal tumors such as granulosa cell tumors are also vimentin positive but keratin negative.

Muscle Markers

Desmin

Desmin, one of the IFs, is expressed by both skeletal and smooth muscle tissues. In smooth muscle tumors, desmin is not as strongly or diffusely expressed as actin. In rhabdomyoblastic cells such as in malignant mixed müllerian tumor (MMMT), desmin is a very sensitive marker.

Actin

Actin, a ubiquitous fibrillary protein thinner than desmin, is present in many epithelial and nonepithelial cells as a cytoskeletal protein. Actin forms a heterodimer that is composed of a combination of α-, β-, and δ-chains. α- and δ-chains are specific to muscle cells. Two antiactin antibodies that are specific for muscle differentiation are most useful in diagnostic immunohistochemistry: muscle-specific actin (MSA; HHF-35)[147] and α-smooth muscle actin (SMA).[122] MSA recognizes α- and δ-chains and reacts with both skeletal and smooth muscle cells, whereas α-SMA is specific for smooth muscle tissue.

In addition to normal smooth and skeletal muscle tissue, myoepithelial cells and myofibroblasts also express desmin and actin especially detectable by SMA and, to a lesser extent, by MSA. Myofibroblasts are quite ubiquitous and are postulated to be induced from mesenchymal stem cells or fibroblasts in reparative or reactive processes, such as granulation tissue and nodular fasciitis, and are believed to contribute to contraction of the scar tissue. Thus, positive SMA, MSA, and desmin must be carefully compared with the morphology before one can assume that the neoplastic cells of interest are indeed expressing these muscle markers.

h-Caldesmon

Caldesmon is a protein widely distributed in smooth and skeletal muscle cells and is thought to regulate cellular contraction in conjunction with actin and topomyosin. A high molecular weight isotype, h-caldesmon,[155] was demonstrated to be specific for smooth muscle cells and smooth muscle tumors. Although it may be expressed in myoepithelial cells, it is not expressed in myofibroblasts and vascular pericytes. In gynecologic tumors, h-caldesmon is more specific for smooth muscle differentiation as compared with actins and desmin.

Myoglobin, MyoD1, Myogenin

These three markers are specific for skeletal muscle differentiation or rhabdomyoblasts. Myoglobin is an oxygen-binding protein and is very specific for skeletal muscle tissue; however, because it is present only in well-differentiated skeletal muscle cells, its utility in the diagnosis of rhabdomyosarcoma is very limited. Myogenin and MyoD1, transcription factors of the myogenic determination family, are expressed within the nucleus in rhabdomyosarcomas but not in normal skeletal muscle tissue.[31]

Sex Cord Markers

Inhibin

Inhibin is a 32-kDa heterodimeric glycoprotein composed of α- and β-subunits. In conjunction with activin, it regulates reproductive functions. α-Inhibin is widely accepted as a marker for sex cord tumors, especially for granulosa cell tumors. It is also expressed in normal granulosa cells, luteinized thecal cells, and hilus cells in the normal ovary. Adnexal tumors of probable wolffian origin are also reported to be positive for inhibin. Because ovarian sex cord tumors may show epithelial-like patterns and ovarian adenocarinoma may have areas simulating a sex cord tumor, positive staining for inhibin is helpful in establishing the diagnosis of sex cord–stromal tumors.[71] Variable inhibin expression in other tumors with sex cord-like areas is reported. For example, uterine stromal tumors resembling sex cord–stromal tumors are reported to be inhibin positive.[74] Uterine adenomyosis with sex cord-like areas are reported to be inhibin negative.[42] High-stage granulosa cell tumors are reported to be less frequently positive with inhibin. Inhibin distribution among these lesions requires further study.

Urothelial Marker

Uroplakins

Uroplakins are specific markers for the urothelial cell and its neoplastic counterparts. They are the characteristic integral membrane proteins in the terminally differentiated, superficial urothelial asymmetric unit membrane. In ovarian tumors, so-called transitional cell carcinoma is negative for uroplakins, but Brenner tumor including malignant Brenner tumors, are uroplakin positive.[119,134] Thus, it is most likely that so-called transitional cell carcinoma of the ovary is a variant of poorly differentiated müllerian-type carcinoma and only Brenner tumors represent ovarian tumors of true urothelial differentiation.

Glial Marker

Glial Fibrillary Acidic Protein

Glial fibrillary acidic protein (GFAP) is one of the IFs and, as such, is a major component of cytoplasmic protein in glial cells. It is composed of a 51-kDa polypeptide. Although GFAP is most frequently expressed in astrocytes, ependymal cells, Schwann cells, and satellite cells of human sensory ganglia, GFAP expression in other nonglial tissues and tumors has been observed. Among gynecologic tumors, glial components of teratoma, peritoneal gliomatosis, and rare primary glial tumors express GFAP. For example, "glial polyps (or gliomas)" of the uterine cervix[81] and uterine corpus[78] express GFAP. Additionally, nonglial müllerian-derived tumors express seemingly ectopic GFAP. For example, occasional examples of endometrial adenocarcinoma show positive GFAP in scattered tumor cells that otherwise are morphologically indistinguishable from adjacent GFAP-negative carcinoma cells.[95] In MMMT, GFAP positivity is observed in the sarcomatous component showing a high-grade stromal sarcoma-like appearance as well as in occasional epithelial tumor cells.[78]

In ovarian carcinomas, GFAP may be occasionally detected in subpopulations of tumor cells of serous (ovarian and extraovarian) and endometrioid adenocarcinomas but not in mucinous or clear cell carcinomas.[95] Thus, the presence of GFAP in a metastatic adenocarcinoma might warrant the consideration of a müllerian-type primary tumor, because no other tumors, with the exception of occasional renal cell carcinomas, and salivary gland tumors, have been shown to express GFAP.[95] In ovarian teratomas, GFAP positivity has been reported in cartilaginous components as well as glial components.[107] The GFAP expression is adversely correlated with their morphologic "maturity" and expression of S-100 protein in cartilaginous tissue. Therefore, GFAP in the cartilaginous components of ovarian teratomas may indicate immature cartilage as well as its similarity to the cartilage of the respiratory tract in which GFAP-positive chondrocytes are always present.

Neuroendocrine and Melanocytic Markers

Previously, it was thought that neuroendocrine cells present in the gastrointestinal tract, lung, and other organs were derived from the neural crest, but subsequent studies have revealed they are derived from the same anlage as other epithelial cells. Thus, the designation "neuro" is not really appropriate; however, the term *neuroendocrine* is still widely used and is therefore also used in this chapter. Neoplasms with certain characteristic morphologic features such as small round cells with salt-and-pepper nuclear chromatin pattern and that display a particular immunophenotype are regarded as showing neuroendocrine differentiation. Several immunohistochemical markers are available for the detection of neuroendocrine differentiation.

Chromogranin

Chromogranin is one of the 40 acidic soluble proteins present in the dense cores of secretory granules. At least three classes of chromogranins have been isolated: chromogranin A, B, and C. Chromogranin A is the most abundant and is widely present in neuroendocrine cells. Chromogranins are present regardless of the specific types of peptide hormones produced by the tumor. Thus, it is a good universal marker for neuroendocrine differentiation. Most of the commercially available antibodies recognize both chromogranin A and B.

Neuron-Specific Enolase

Neuron-specific enolase (NSE) is an isoenzyme of 2-phospho-D-glycerate hydrolase. Although different types of enolases exist in the liver, glial cells, and skeletal muscle cells, the γ-chain is thought to be specific for neural tissue and neuroendocrine cells. Currently available commercial antibodies usually detect both $\alpha\gamma$ heterodimers and $\gamma\gamma$ homodimers. Significant numbers of apparently nonneuroendocrine tissues and tumors are positive for NSE. This nonspecificity of NSE limits its diagnostic usefulness, and therefore it should be used in conjunction with other neuroendocrine markers.

CD57

CD57 is a marker for T cells and natural killer cells. Leu-7 is the most widely used and commercially available antibody (Becton-Dickinson) to detect CD57. An epitope which Leu-7 identifies is known to be shared by a variety of molecules including myelin-associated glycoprotein and neural cell adhesion molecules. Thus, CD57 as detected by Leu-7 can be used as a neuroendocrine marker.

Synaptophysin

Synaptophysin, a 38-kDa acidic protein originally extracted from bovine presynaptic vesicles, is a universal neuroendocrine marker similar to chromogranin. Although there is a functional similarity, synaptophysin and chromogranin are believed to be different gene products.

S-100 Protein

S-100 protein was first purified from bovine brain tissue. It is a homodimer or heterodimer composed of α- or β-chains or both. Three subtypes exist in human tissue: S-100ao ($\alpha\alpha$), S-100a ($\alpha\beta$), and S-100b ($\beta\beta$). Commercially available antibodies recognize both α- and β-chains. S-100 protein is present both in the cytoplasm and in nuclei, but there is a difference in the distribution of α- and β-chains. Although S-100 protein was thought to be specific for neural, melanocytic, and Schwann cells, many other normal cells such as chondrocytes, lipocytes, Langerhans' cells of skin, and myoepithelial cells also express S-100 protein. Despite its widespread distribution, S-100 is still an important diagnostic marker when it is used as part of a panel for specific differential diagnosis. One peculiar feature of S-100 protein is the excellent preservation of its antigenicity in formalin-fixed tissue and poor antigenic preservation in alcohol-fixed tissue.

HMB45

HMB45, a more specific melanocytic marker, is present in the membrane component of melanosomes. Although its positivity indicates melanocytic origin of a given cell, negative HMB45 does not rule out melanoma. For example, spindle cell melanoma is almost always HMB45 negative.

Many otherwise typical carcinomas such as mammary, colonic, endometrial, and ovarian carcinomas may show the presence of focal neuroendocrine differentiation. This type of focal neuroendocrine differentiation must be distinguished from tumors showing almost exclusive neuroendocrine differentiation, such as strumal carcinoids in the ovary, and undifferentiated tumors showing neuroendocrine differentiation, such as small cell undifferentiated carcinomas of the cervix. So-called agyrophil cell carcinomas in the endometrium (reported frequency ranging from 20% to 50%) have been described in which variable numbers of agyrophilic carcinoma cells are present.[149] These agyrophil cell carcinomas often display chromogranin positivity in the agyrophil-positive cells. In the majority of these cases, they are morphologically indistingushable from conventional endometrial carcinomas. Neuron-specific enolase (NSE) is also reported to be positive in agyrophil cell endometrial carcinomas, although, unlike the chromogranin positivity, NSE-positive cells are apparently not agyrophilic.

The neuroendocrine differentiation in otherwise conventional endometrial carcinomas does not have prognostic significance. In contrast, small cell undifferentiated carcinomas in the endometrium (either in a pure form or as a component of a malignant mixed müllerian tumor) have been reported to be positive with Leu-7, chromogranin, and NSE.[84] These small cell undifferentiated carcinomas have an aggressive clinical behavior. Intestinal-type mucinous tumors of the ovary, heterologous elements in Sertoli–Leydig cell tumors such as intestinal-type epithelium and carcinoids, and strumal carcinoids are positive with chromogranin and NSE.[138,159] In teratomas, occasional normal tissues such as intestinal tissue, bronchial epithelium, melanocytes, glial cells, and neuronal cells may show chromogranin or NSE positivity.

In anogenital lesions, S-100 protein and HMB45 are useful in the differential diagnosis of pagetoid malignant melanoma and Paget disease. S-100 protein is almost always positive in pagetoid melanomas and is negative in Paget disease.[47] Immunostaining for S-100 should be combined with staining for keratins, especially low molecular weight keratins such as those detected by antibody CAM5.2. These keratins are expressed selectively by Paget cells but not by epidermal squamous cells in the background or pagetoid melanoma cells.[101] S-100 can be used to identify Langerhans' cells in the cervix. In early invasive squamous cell carcinomas of the cervix, the density of Langerhans' cells is significantly reduced as compared with that of the normal cervical epithelium.[140] This phenomenon may indicate a host immune response to the invasive carcinoma.

S-100 protein positivity is found in many epithelial tumors, especially in carcinoms that show partial myoepithelial differentiation such as breast carcinoma and salivary gland tumors. The distribution of S-100 positivity in the ovarian surface neoplasms is very similar to CA-125. Serous carcinoma of the ovary shows a high frequency of S-100-positive cells. S-100 positivity is especially common in borderline and malignant serous tumors. Endometrioid and clear cell carcinoma may be also S-100 positive; in contrast, mucinous tumors are rarely positive.[79] In teratomas, various tissues such as glial, melanocytes, and chondrocytes are positive for S-100.[21]

Trophoblastic Markers

Keratins and Keratin 7

Keratins are expressed by trophoblastic cells, which is useful in distinguishing them from decidua. Keratins, in general, are universal epithelial markers and are not a specific marker for trophoblastic cells. Among keratins, K7 is particularly useful as a trophoblastic marker in mixed germ cell tumors because the other components of germ cell tumors do not express K7.[34]

Human Chorionic Gonadotropin

Human chorionic gonadotropin (hCG) is a polypeptide hormone composed of α- and β-subunits. The β-subunit is specific for gonadotropin of trophoblastic origin, and antibodies to the β-subunit are used for immunoassays of serum hCG and in pregnancy tests. In the normal first-trimester placenta, hCG is localized in the syncytiotrophoblast. The degree of positivity decreases dramatically and at term is only focally present in syncytial trophoblast.[12] In ovarian germ cells tumors including embryonal carcinoma, mixed germ cell tumors containing choriocarcinoma, and dysgerminomas with syncytiotrophoblastic giant cells, hCG is demonstrated in trophoblastic cells.[54] Other tumors including rare examples of endometrial carcinomas and carcinomas of other organs such as adenocarcinoma of the lung, squamous cell carcinoma of the esophagus, and transitional cell carcinoma of the bladder[40] rarely produce hCG.

Human Placental Lactogen

Human placental lactogen (hPL)[77] is a 19-kDa glycoprotein similar to prolactin (50% homology) that is produced by syncytial and intermediate trophoblast in the normal placenta. Cytotrophoblast is devoid of hPL. In contrast to hCG, hPL increases as pregnancy progresses, and levels peak in the third trimester. Thus, in the first-trimester placenta, hPL is only focally distributed in syncytiotrophoblast. By term, hPL is diffusely distributed throughout the syncytiotrophoblast. Intermediate trophoblast tends to be hPL positive and hCG negative. Accordingly, detection of hPL in conjunction with keratin is helpful in distinguishing intermediate trophoblast from decidua and smooth muscle cells because decidua and smooth muscle do not express hPL. Placental site trophoblastic tumor is diffusely positive for keratin and hPL and focally positive for hCG because most of the cells are intermediate trophoblast. In curettage specimens, immunohistochemical demonstration of hPL, hCG, and keratin-positve trophoblastic cells rules out an ectopic pregnancy, except for rare cases in which there is a simultaneous pregnancy in the uterus and the fallopian tube.

Human Placental Alkaline Phosphatase

Human placental alkaline phosphatase (hPLAP) is one of the six organ-specific alkaline phosphatases produced by syncytiotrophoblast in the normal placenta. It is a glycoprotein molecule consisting of two subunits with a molecular weight of 64 kDa. hPLAP is detected in the serum of pregnant women and in patients with certain malignancies such as germ cell tumors, carcinomas of lung, stomach, pancreas, breast, and ovary. Specific immunohistochemical demonstration of hPLAP in tissue is difficult because of the cross-reactivity with other isoenzymes of alkaline phosphatase, such as liver, bone, and intestinal types that show extensive homology of the epitopes. Although the staining patterns of various antibodies to hPLAP and/or hPLAP-like enzymes differ somewhat, recent development of monospecific antibodies makes uniform immunohistochemical demonstration of hPLAP more feasible.[51,150] It has been reported that when antibodies specific to true hPLAP are used, only rare germ cell tumors are positive, suggesting yet another type of alkaline phosphatase, which is hPLAP-like but distinctive, that is, germ cell alkaline phosphatase.[51]

Because commercially available antibodies to hPLAP also react with hPLAP-like enzyme (placental-like alkaline phosphatase), the following discussion is based on reactivity to both hPLAP and hPLAP-like enzymes, and both types of enzymes are simply referred as hPLAP. hPLAP is also present in normal nontrophoblastic tissues and their neoplastic counterparts such as the thymus, bronchial, alveolar, endocervical, fallopian tube, and colonic epithelium. Because hPLAP is almost always expressed by germ cell tumors, it is a sensitive but only moderately specific marker for these tumors because other carcinomas especially carcinomas of müllerian-type also express hPLAP. For example, hPLAP can be immunohistochemically demonstrated in normal cervical squamous and glandular epithelium, cervical intraepithelial neoplasia (CIN), invasive cervical squamous cell carcinoma, and endocervical adenocarcinomas.[91] Endometrial carcinomas are also positive with hPLAP. In the ovary, hPLAP is positive in the epithelium of inclusion cysts. Serous tumors including serous cytoadenomas are most frequently positive with hPLAP, followed by endometrioid and poorly differentiated carcinomas.[36]

Inhibin

Inhibin[125] was discussed as a sex cord marker previously. Inhibin is also expressed by syncytial trophoblastic cells, especially in the first-trimester placenta, but remains negative in cytotrophoblast throughout gestation. Inhibin expression in syncytial trophoblast decreases as the gestation progresses to term. Nonneoplastic intermediate trophoblast in the implantation site, either normal or exaggerated, also is negative or only weakly positive. In neoplastic trophoblastic lesions including complete and partial hydatidiform moles, placental site nodule, placental trophoblastic tumors, and choriocarcinoma, inhibin is positive.

CD146

CD146[124,126] (or Mel-CAM, MUC18, A32 antigen, or S-Endo-1) is a membrane glycoprotein that functions as a cell adhesion molecule. CD146 is thought to be a member of the immunoglobulin gene superfamily. The relative narrow lineage-specific expression of CD146 can be useful in the differential diagnosis of melanomas and various types of gestational trophoblastic lesions. CD146 has been suggested to play an important role in tumor progression, implantation, and placentation. During implantation and placentation, CD146 expressed in intermediate trophoblast is believed to limit trophoblastic invasion of the myometrium. Because neoplastic intermediate trophoblast may assume an epithelioid appearance, positive CD146 and inhibin help in differentiating these tumors from carcinomas.

Hematolymphoid Markers

In addition to being useful in the diagnosis of malignant lymphoma or leukemia (granulocytic sarcoma) involving the female genital tract, hematolymphoid markers may be useful in studying the host response to various gynecologic premalignant and malignant neoplasms. Although precise subclassification of hematolymphoid cells is best accomplished with frozen tissue or flow cytometric immunophenotyping, ever-increasing numbers of the T-cell, B-cell, myelomonocytic, and macrophage markers can be used in routinely processed tissue sections. A partial list of these markers include CD1a (Langerhans' cell marker), CD2, CD4 (OPD4), CD5, CD10 (CALLA), CD15 (LeuM-1), CD20, CD23, CD43, CD45 (LCA or leukocyte common antigen), CD45RO (UCHL-1), CD68 (KP1), lysozyme (macrophage), and S-100 protein (Langerhans' cell marker).

In the cervix, natural killer cells (NK cells) are reported to be increased in CIN, suggesting a possible protective effect of NK cells against HPV infection and subsequent development of CIN.[141] In CIN and invasive squamous cell carcinoma, lysozyme-positive macrophages are significantly increased in the subjacent stroma.[49] CD15 (LeuM-1) is occasionally positive in adenocarcinomas. When positive, CD15 is helpful in differentiating adenocarcinoma from mesothelioma.

Basement Membrane Markers

Collagen Type 4 and Laminin

Among the components of basement membrane, antibodies to laminin and collagen type 4 are commercially available and can be applied to routinely processed tissue. Although it is thought that the distinction of invasive and in situ carcinoma can be established by the presence or absence of basement membrane, it is worth noting that many invasive carcinomas of the vulva, cervix, and endometrium may produce, albeit incomplete, basement membrane.[39] VIN3 and CIN3 maintain a complete basement membrane. Formation of basement membrane has also been reported around metastatic tumor cell nests in lymph nodes.[39] Endocervical adenocarcinoma is similar to squamous cell carcinoma in this regard. Although superficially invasive adenocarcinomas may show some defect in the basement membrane, some of the deeply invasive nests of adenocarcinoma may show basement membrane formation.

Normal endometrial glands are surrounded by a well-developed basement membrane, as demonstrated by laminin and collagen type 4 positivity. It is reported that the basement membrane becomes discontinuous and defective in invasive endometrial carcinomas, and, in some instances, even in endometrial hyperplasia.[152] As in the cervix, deeply invasive nests of adenocarcinoma may produce basement membrane, albeit incomplete.[158]

Tumor-Associated Antigens and Oncofetal Markers

CA-125 (OC125) and CA-19-9

Carbohydrate antigen 125 (CA-125) is a glycoprotein that is detected by a murine monoclonal antibody, OC125, raised against a serous ovarian cancer cell line OVCA 433. OC125 is used in a radioimmunoassay for detecting serum CA-125 levels. Elevated serum CA-125 levels are reported in more than 80% of ovarian cancer patients. The serum CA-125 levels are useful in monitoring ovarian cancer patients, but CA-125 is not specific for ovarian cancer. OC125 also can be used in immunohistochemistry on either frozen or paraffin-embedded tissue (with enzyme digestion). CA-125 is demonstrated by immunohistochemistry in the fetal coelomic epithelium and, consequently, it can be detected in almost all coelomic epithelium-derived tissues in adults such as endocervical, endometrial, and fallopian tube-lining epithelium but not in normal ovarian surface epithelial cells.

Immunohistochemical application of OC125 is less useful than serum CA-125 levels because of its lack of specific staining. For example, other adenocarcinomas such as colonic, gastric, and lung, as well as squamous cell carcinomas, may be positive. CA-125 is frequently positive in normal secretory endometrium. CA-125 is also positive in atypical hyperplasia and endometrial carcinomas of all grades. Although CA-125 positivity is not helpful in separating atypical hyperplasia from endometrial adenocarcinoma, CA-125 positivity in endometrial carcinoma is reported to be associated with increased metastatic potential.[6] In ovarian carcinomas, CA-125 is most frequently positive in serous tumors (more than 80%) including benign and borderline tumors and carcinomas. Mucinous tumors show much less frequent positivity (about 20% or less).[83,105,128] Thus, there is a reverse distribution of OC125 positivity compared to CEA among the different types of ovarian tumors. The CA-125-related monoclonal antibody SH-9 was reported to detect a different epitope of a CA-125-bearing molecule and is much more frequently positive in mucinous tumors as compared to OC125. CA-125 is positive in approximately 30% of clear cell and endometrioid carcinomas.

CA-19-9 is also a glycoprotein cancer-associated antigen similar to CA-125. It is reported to be positive in almost all endometrial carcinoma, especially well-differentiated carcinomas, in contrast to CEA and CA-125, which show more frequent positivity in poorly differentiated carcinomas. CA-19-9, however, cannot be used to separate atypical hyperplasia from well-differentiated carcinoma because atypical hyperplasia is positive for CA-19-9 in almost 70% of cases.[104]

TAG72 (B72.3)

Monoclonal antibody B72.3 recognizes the high molecular weight mucin-like glycoprotein complex known as "tumor-associated glycoprotein" (TAG-72). Many monoclonal antibodies against purified TAG-72 have been developed. Among those, B72.3 is the most widely used. B72.3 is frequently positive in epithelial malignancy, including many ovarian carcinomas as well as colorectal and breast carcinomas. Although, as a rule, normal mature cells, sarcomas, melanomas, and hematopoietic neoplasm are negative for B72.3,[143] it has been reported to be positive in nonneoplastic epithelia such as benign endometrial cells.[143] The most useful application of this antibody is the detection of malignant cells in peritoneal fluid and washings. With a few exceptions, benign mesothelial cells and histiocytes are negative for B72.3. Szpak et al. reported that more than 90% of morphologically recognizable malignant cells of ovarian, endometrial, and endocervical adenocarcinoma were positive with B72.3.[139] In contrast, only 6% of cases that were originally interpreted as morphologically benign peritoneal washings were positive for B72.3. After reexamination, all these cases were interpreted as either atypical or unequivocally positive for malignant cells.

Although a positive B72.3 reaction in peritoneal cytologic specimens warrants further careful examination, the diagnosis of malignancy has to be based on the morphologic findings, not merely on the localization of B72.3 . Many factors are known to influence expression of TAG-72 in cultured cell lines, including products of the normal cycling human endometrium. Normal secretory endometrium expresses this antigen whereas proliferative endometrium does not. In fact, an inverse correlation with progesterone and estrogen receptors and TAG-72 expression in the normal cycling endometrium has been reported. These findings suggest hormonal regulation of TAG-72 expression. Although most (90%) endometrial carcinomas express TAG-72 as detected by B72.3, no prognostic correlation has been found.[132] The majority of ovarian carcinomas are positive with B72.3. In serous borderline tumors, hormonal milieu appears to greatly influence TAG-72 expression.[20] For example, tumors in patients who are pregnant or receiving progesterone, show significantly prominent TAG-72 expression as compared to serous borderline tumors in nonpregnant patients.

Carcinoembryonic Antigen

Carcinoembryonic antigen (CEA) was first described as a tumor-specific antigen of colon cancers. Later, however, CEA was found to be positive in many other epithelial malignancies including ovarian carcinoma. CEA is a high molecular weight glycoprotein containing 50–60% carbohydrates and is the oldest and most widely used carcinoma marker. Because of the heterogeneity of CEA extracted from colonic and noncolonic carcinomas, the exact biochemical and immunologic characterization of CEA is problematic. Colonic carcinoma-derived CEA and ovarian cyst fluid-derived CEA are reported to be biochemically and immunologically almost identical. Many polyclonal and some monoclonal antibodies to CEA are available with different specificity and sensitivity.

When using anti-CEA antibodies, it is important to know their reactivity to other CEA-like proteins. The most common CEA-like protein is nonspecific cross-reacting antigen (NCA), which is present in many tissues, especially in leukocytes. Because of the different sensitivity and specificity of various anti-CEA antibodies utilized in published studies, the exact percentages of CEA positivity in specific types of tumors are difficult to determine. Studies showing a higher positivity in a given type of carcinoma than generally reported also report more than expected positivity in normal tissue, which may be the result of the detection of CEA-like proteins such as NCA in addition to "true" CEA. Using anti-CEA antibodies that do not react with other CEA-related antigens provides more useful information. Accordingly, the following discussion is based mainly on the studies that used specific anti-CEA antibodies.

In normal endocervical glandular cells, CEA is frequently positive. Metaplastic squamous epithelium in the cervix is CEA positive, but normal squamous cells of the cervix are negative. Endocervical adenocarcinomas are positive for CEA in 80% of cases.[33] CEA is reported to be positive in about half of CIN 1; however, CEA positivity is not correlated with the progression of CIN.[80] Both CIN 3 and invasive squamous cell carcinoma are positive for CEA[90] with a difference in staining pattern, namely, diffuse staining in CIN 3 compared to CEA-positive tumor cells at the stromal interface in invasive carcinoma. In normal endometrium, CEA is almost always negative. CEA is much less frequently positive in endometrial carcinomas (less than 20%) compared to endocervical carcinomas.[33] When CEA is combined with vimentin expression, CEA may be helpful in distinguishing endocervical from endometrial carcinoma. A vimentin-positive and CEA-negative carcinoma is most likely of endometrial origin whereas a CEA-positive and vimentin-negative carcinoma is likely of endocervical origin. It should be noted that CEA is frequently positive in metaplastic squamous epithelium, which may be present in endometrial carcinomas. This type of CEA positivity does not indicate endocervical origin.

CEA is negative in all normal ovarian tissues. In ovarian carcinomas, CEA is most frequently positive in mucinous carcinomas (70–80%), including mucinous tumors of low malignant potential and, less frequently, in mucinous cystoadenomas. Mucinous tumors showing intestinal-type epithelium almost always express CEA.[52,144] Because metastatic gastrointestinal carcinoma shows strong and diffuse staining as opposed to patchy and focal staining of primary mucinous carcinomas, the pattern of CEA positivity may be helpful in differentiating primary from metastatic carcinomas.[41] In serous tumors, CEA is much less frequently positive (about 20%). Endometrioid carcinomas (especially in the areas of squamous differentiation), undifferentiated carcinomas, and Brenner tumors are also frequently CEA positive. Clear cell carcinoma is less frequently CEA positive.[67] The CEA staining pattern does not correlate with tumor grade or virulence.[52] Although CEA has been evaluated as a discriminating marker between papillary mesothelioma and papillary ovarian carcinoma, its low positivity in papillary serous carcinoma of the ovary hampers its use in differential diagnosis.[129]

Human Milk Fat Globule and Epithelial Membrane Antigen

Many antibodies to human milk fat globules (HMFG) have been developed. This antigen is a high molecular weight glycoprotein found in human milk (milk mucin). Epithelial membrane antigen (EMA)[56] is also derived from milk mucin. The most widely used antibodies in this group are HFMG-1, HFMG-2, and EMA. Other antibodies, such as SM-3[46] and anti-Mam 3[118] have been also applied in gynecologic tumors. Although initially these antibodies were developed in the hope that they would specifically react with breast carcinomas, other carcinomas, including many gynecologic carcinomas, also react with these antibodies. HFMG-1 is reported to show cytoplasmic staining in cervical adenocarcinomas and atypical cervical glandular hyperplasia in contrast to predominantly luminal staining of benign endocervical glands and glands showing microglandular hyperplasia.[14]

HFMG-1, HFMG-2, and anti-Man 3 antibodies all show luminal staining in normal and hyperplastic endometrium,[98,118] including cases of atypical hyperplasia. The latter shows cytoplasmic staining in addition to luminal staining. Endometrial adenocarcinomas are frequently positive for these antibodies, showing both luminal and cytoplasmic patterns. Although this pattern of staining may help distinguish benign and malignant endometrial glands, they are not specific enough to be practical.

Antibodies to HMFG and EMA react with virtually all epithelial tumors of the ovary including both benign and malignant types. EMA staining, however, is significantly less in nonmucinous tumors.[11] There is no correlation between EMA positivity and tumor differentiation.[11] Expression of HMFG-1 and HMFG-2 has been reported to be more pronounced in well-differentiated ovarian carcinomas than in those that are poorly differentiated.[154]

Alpha Fetoprotein

Alpha fetoprotein (AFP) is an albumin-like protein that is present in the fetal serum. Detectable levels of serum AFP in adults have been observed most commonly in patients with hepatocellular carcinomas and germ cell tumors, although other carcinomas, such as lung, stomach, and pancreas, are also associated with high serum AFP levels. A case of poorly differentiated endometrial carcinoma showing AFP in the tumor cells has been reported.[89] In ovarian germ cell tumors, such as yolk sac tumor (endodermal sinus tumor) and embryonal carcinoma, AFP can be immunohistochemically demonstrated in different staining patterns; that is, yolk sac tumor shows clusters of AFP-positive cells whereas embryonal carcinoma shows individual positive cells.

For the differential diagnosis between clear cell carcinoma and yolk sac tumors, a combination of AFP (mostly positive in yolk sac tumor) and LeuM1 (mostly positive in clear cell carcinoma) may be of help.[161] Ovarian hepatoid carcinoma,[61] which should be differentiated from hepatoid yolk sac tumor, is also AFP positive in the tumor cells. Pure teratomas without germ cell carcinoma or yolk sac tumor components may show elevated serum AFP, and immunohistochemical demonstration of AFP in yolk sac-like vesicles, intestinal-type glands, tissue resembling liver, and immature ectodermal component has been documented.[115] Rare examples of common epithelial ovarian tumors such as a mucinous cystoadenoma may also be AFP positive.[72]

Hormone Receptors

Estrogen and Progesterone Receptors

Although the importance of estrogen (ER) and progesterone (PR) receptors is not as well established as in breast carcinomas, it has been suggested that the ER/PR status in gynecologic tumors especially in endometrial carcinomas has prognostic significance.[30] Both ER and PR are present in nuclei and cytoplasm. ER binds with ligand (estradiol), which then binds and regulates transcription of a number of proteins including PR. PR binds to DNA and is activated when it is bound with its ligand (progesterone). In the past, the standard way of measuring tissue ER/PR was the biochemical assay, which requires fresh-frozen tissue. Although this receptor function is quite labile, immunologically detectable epitopes of ER/PR are often preserved even after formalin fixation and paraffin embedding. Thus, development of monoclonal antibodies to ER and PR in conjunction with immunohistochemical techniques and heat-induced antigen retrieval now make it possible to use routinely processed tissue sections to assess ER and PR status,[25] and this is now considered the standard method of ER/PR assessment. Both ER and PR show predominantly intranuclear staining. Immunohistochemical ER and PR assays have the added advantage that the distribution in the tumor tissue as well as in the surrounding normal tissue can be evaluated.[116]

In some cases, the biochemical assay may give false-positive results when normal myometrium is included in the sample.[17,133,160] In some series, imunohistochemically determined ER was the most significant predictor of survival and was superior to the biochemical ER assay.[24,160] A good correlation between the biochemical and immunohistochemical ER/PR assay has been reported.[17,24,100,116] Normal vaginal, cervical, and endocervical epithelia show ER expression.[76,106] In normal exocervical epithelium, basal cells are ER+, PR− regardless of the phase of the menstrual cycle; parabasal cells are ER+, PR− in follicular phase and ER−, PR+ in luteal phase.[73,99] CIN and invasive squamous cell carcinoma cells are also PR positive whereas ER is generally negative. These findings suggest reduced ER and increased PR expression is related to a proliferative activity of normal, human papilloma viral-infected, and neoplastic squamous cells.[55,73,96,106] There is no significant correlation with ER/PR and prognosis in cervical squamous cell carcinoma.[35,86,121]

ER/PR density in endometrial glands depends on the hormonal milieu. ER/PR is more strongly expressed in proliferative as compared to secretory endometrium,[18] which is the inverse of B72.3 reactivity.[132] ER/PR staining pattern may be helpful for endometrial dating,[18,43] especially in a scanty tissue sample. ER expression similar to that seen in cycling endometrial tissue is also observed in foci of endometriosis.[18] PR is reported to be more frequently positive in endometrial hyperplasia without atypia than in hyperplasia with atypia.[8] Compared to hyperplasia, PR is more heterogenously distributed and is expressed at much lower levels in endometrial carcinoma.[8] Discordant ER/PR expression has also been reported between primary and metastatic endometrial carcinoma which may have some significance in terms of response to hormonal therapy.[120] ER/PR status, especially PR, correlates best with histologic differentiation and survival; that is, positive ER/PR is more frequent in well-differentiated carcinoma[44] and is associated with a better prognosis.[10,22,60,69,133]

Another study indicated that endometrial adenocarcinoma associated with hyperplasia (group 1) is most likely to be estrogen dependent and have a significantly higher incidence of PR expression and better prognosis.[37] Although there is a suggestion that ER/PR-positive endometrial carcinoma is more likely to respond to hormonal therapy, more well-controlled studies are necessary. Normal endometrial stroma and myometrial cells are positive for ER/PR. Leiomyomas of the uterus are also ER/PR positive.[102] In endometrial stromal sarcoma, ER is frequently expressed by low-grade stromal sarcoma but is seldom expressed in high-grade stromal sarcoma[103,145] providing the rationale for hormonal treatment of low-grade stromal sarcomas.

As many as 80% of normal ovarian tissues (surface epithelium and stroma),[62] benign neoplastic lesions, and carcinomas,[1] especially endometrioid carcinoma,[137] express ER/PR. Differentiation of tumors is correlated with ER expression but not with PR expression.[63] Similar to endometrial carcinoma, significant heterogeneity of ER/PR occurs within the primary tumor and between the primary and metastatic tumors.[117] PR and ER expression suggest better survival,[9,53,131] although further studies to confirm this observation are needed.[1,87] There appears to be no correlation of proliferative activity as measured by Ki-67 scores and by flow cytometric DNA analysis and ER/PR status.[62] Nevertheless, in combination with other prognostic factors such as ploidy, S-phase, and proliferation markers, ER shows significant correlation with the prognosis. A Tamoxifen trial did not show any correlation between ER/PR status and response for patients with recurrent ovarian carcinoma.[156] Rare examples of malignant Brenner tumor[75] and ovarian ependymoma[3,23] showing PR but not ER positivity have been reported. A yolk sac tumor has been reported to be negative for ER/PR by immunohistochemistry.[70]

Prognostic Markers

Ki-67 and PCNA

Ki-67 and proliferating cell nuclear antigen (PCNA; cyclin) are two independent intranuclear proteins related to cellular proliferation. Ki-67 requires frozen tissue, but newly developed antibodies such as MIB1 can be used on formalin-fixed tissue. PCNA can be also applied to paraffin-embedded tissues. Although both are apparently related to cell proliferation, positivity of Ki-67 and PCNA does not always correlate and therefore they may be used as two independent indicators of cell proliferation. In normal cervical epithelium, Ki-67 is positive in parabasal cells during the luteal phase associated with PR expression.[73] Ki-67 shows variable positivity in cervical squamous cell carcinoma (a range of 10–50%) but has no correlation with other conventional histologic parameters.[13] In ovarian carcinoma, Ki-67 ranged from 1% to 59% and showed correlation with advanced stage and patient survival but not with ER/PR status in one study.[62]

P53

p53 is a tumor suppressor gene. The *p53* gene is located on the short arm of chromosome 17. Wild-type *p53* has a very short half-life and has an inhibitory effect on cell proliferation and transformation. Mutation of this gene results in a mutant p53 protein, which has a much longer half-life than that of wild-type p53 and does not have the suppressor function. Molecular genetic studies have shown allelic deletion of chromosome 17p resulting in a mutated p53 product in many malignant tumors including ovarian and endometrial carcinomas.[109,146] The mutated p53 protein accumulates in the tumor cells intranuclearly which can be detected by immunohistochemistry.

Overexpression of mutant p53 is a very common occurrence in many carcinomas. Wild-type p53 can also accumulate and lose its suppressor function by complexing with other proteins such as the oncoprotein of certain human papillomavirus types. Therefore, accumulation of p53 protein, regardless of wild or mutant type, which is detectable by immunohistochemistry (most of the commercially available antibodies detect both wild and mutant p53) is expected in malignant cells but not in normal tissues. Initially, p53 was only detectable by immunohistochemistry on frozen tissue. Now, paraffin-embedded tissue can be used for the detection of p53 quite reliably with new polyclonal and monoclonal antibodies.[66] A significant percentage of endometrial adenocarcinomas and malignant mixed müllerian tumor (MMMT) are p53 positive. There is correlation with p53 and histologic type; p53 is most commonly positive in serous papillary adenocarcinoma. Furthermore, among the patients who died of adenocarcinoma or had persistent and recurrent carcinoma, p53 was frequently positive in the tumor cells, suggesting that p53-positive endometrial carcinoma may behave in a more aggressive fashion.[19] Serous adenocarcinomas of ovary have a high frequency of positive p53 especially in advanced-stage serous adenocarcinomas[38]; however, no significant correlation with p53 and survival has been noted.[85] Benign tumors and borderline tumors are usually negative for p53.[38,85]

HER2/NEU (C-ERBB-2)

Her2/neu is among more than 50 different proto-oncogenes (the normal cellular homologue of an oncogene) that code for proteins which function as growth factors, growth factor receptors, and cytoplasmic second messengers. *Her2/neu* is believed to play an important role in carcinogenesis of the breast and ovary. Although the function of the *Her2/neu* gene product is unknown, its similarity to the epidermal growth factor receptor suggests its involvement in cell growth and differentiation. Overexpression and amplification of the *Her2/neu* gene and accumulation of the corresponding protein usually correlate with each other and are best detected by demonstration of mRNA by Northern blot or fluorescent in situ hybridization (FISH) and by immunohistochemistry, respectively.[130] *Her2/neu* protein is well studied in breast carcinoma in that its positivity indicates more aggressive behavior. A similar correlation with *Her2/neu* protein and biologic behavior of ovarian and endometrial carcinomas has been suggested.[130]

Recently, an antibody to *Her2/neu* oncoprotein has been developed (Herceptin) that has been approved by the FDA as a treatment for end-stage breast cancer patients with *Her2/neu*-positive tumors. Use of Herceptin for the treatment of gynecologic malignancies is currently under investigation. Thus, detection of *Her2/neu* in gynecologic tumors is important not only as a prognostic marker but to qualify for Herceptin treatment. Although controversy still exist as to whether detection of *Her2/neu* should be performed by FISH or by immunohistochemistry on archival paraffin-embedded tissue, especially as screening for Herceptin treatment, the following discussion is based mainly on immunohistochemical demonstration of *Her2/neu* protein in various gynecologic tumors.

About one-third of vulvar Paget disease is reported to be positive, albeit less frequently than in mammary Paget disease,[157] thus suggesting a similar genetic alteration may be involved in mammary and vulvar Paget disease. One of the *Her2/neu*-positive cases of vulvar Paget disease in this series was associated with endocervical adenocarcinoma that was also *Her2/neu* positive. In the normal cervix, the basal layer of squamous cell epithelium and reserve cell layer of endocervical glands are only weakly positive for *Her2/neu*.[16] In CIN 3, a more pronounced *Her2/neu* positivity was demonstrated. In invasive squamous cell carcinoma, the degree of differentiation was not correlated with *Her2/neu* positivity.[16]

Normal endometrial glands are weakly to moderately positive for *Her2/neu*, which is not influenced by the phase of the menstrual cycle.[5] A small percentage (9%) of endometrial adenocarcinomas are reported to show much stronger positivity as compared to the normal endometrium. *Her2/neu* positivity in endometrial carcinomas is more frequently associated with metastatic disease and is correlated with negative estrogen receptors, suggesting that positive *Her2/neu* is associated with more aggressive behavior.[5]

Her2/neu is negative or only rarely and weakly positive in the normal ovary.[58] Strongly positive *Her2/neu* is reported in ovarian carcinomas with similar frequency as in breast carcinoma, that is, approximately one-third.[50,58,130] Although it was suggested that *Her2/neu* overexpression in the ovarian carcinoma is associated with more aggressive behavior and with poor survival,[15] another study did not confirm this correlation.[50]

Infectious Agents

Immunohistochemical demonstration of infectious agents may be useful in gynecologic pathology, especially in cervical lesions. Antibodies against viral protein such as human papillomavirus (HPV), herpes simplex virus (HSV-1 and HSV-2), and cytomegalovirus (CMV) can be used to demonstrate these viral proteins in cervical smears and paraffin-embedded tissue sections. Recent development of DNA probes and use of in situ hybridization allows more precise typing of viral DNA, especially in the case of HPV.

Human Papillomavirus

Only 30% to 40% of cases showing morphologic findings for human papillomavirus (HPV) changes are reported to be immunohistochemically positive. The frequency of HPV positivity decreases as the degree of CIN increases. This finding supports the view that HPV changes and CIN are part of a morphologic continuum in which the cytopathic effect of HPV is expressed mainly in low grades of dysplasia.[136] Type-specific analysis of HPV is best performed by in situ hybridization.

Herpesvirus Type 2

Herpesvirus type 2 (HSV-2) has been reported to be associated with CIN and squamous cell carcinoma of the cervix. Commercially available antibodies can be applied to either cervical smears or routine tissue sections. Using such antibodies, more frequent HSV-2 positivity was reported as CIN progressed.[123] Invasive squamous cell carcinoma shows the highest frequency of HVS-2 antigens. Immunocytochemical application of HSV-2 and HSV-1 antibodies can also be used for the detection of herpes in vaginal smears in which clinical genital herpes infection is suspected. Using viral culture as a gold standard, immunocytochemical detection of HSV antigens is reported to have an accuracy of 91%, which is better than that achieved by morphology alone (81%).[88]

Chlamydia, Trichomonads, and *Mycoplasma*

Immunofluorescent method can be used to detect these organisms on cervicovaginal smears.

Cytomegalovirus (CMV)

Antibodies against both cytoplasmic and intranuclear viral proteins can be used for the immunohistochemical detection of CMV. The sensitivity is only slightly better than the morphologic identification of the viral inclusions. In situ hybridization using a DNA probe is better suited for more precise detection of CMV genomes.

Other

Hyaluronan Receptor CD44

CD44s (standard form) and variant isoforms (v4, v5, v6, v7, v7–8, v9, v10) are receptors for hyaluronan, which is a ubiquitous extracellular matrix protein. CD44 has been investigated for predicting the prognosis of some neoplasms especially in regard to tumor cell–stromal interactions. In the diagnostic arena, at least one study indicates that CD44v5 is expressed in in situ and invasive endocervical adenocarcinomas whereas only reserve cells are positive in normal squamous and glandular cells of cervix.[59]

Blood Group Antigens

Blood group-related carbohydrate antigens change their phenotypic expression during normal development and during neoplastic transformation. Therefore, it is expected that immunohistochemical detection of these antigens in the preneoplastic and neoplastic cells may provide useful information. Blood group isoantigen A, B, H, and other minor blood group antigens as well as precursor antigens can be detected using immuohistochemical techniques and appropriate antibodies. The loss of blood group isoantigens has been reported in tumor cells involving many organs. Although transitional carcinomas of the urinary bladder have been the most extensively studied in this regard, many gynecologic tumors also have been reported to show this phenomenon. Blood group-related carbohydrates such as Lewisa (Lea) and Lewisb (Leb) are also detected in many carcinoma cells.

Although some antibodies against blood group antigen-related carbohydrates are reported to show affinity to certain gynecologic tumors, none is specific for gynecologic tumors and their usefulness in diagnosis and prediction of prognosis is still unproven. In cervical smears, the loss of isoantigens is associated with higher grades of CIN. The loss of isoantigen was seen in the cytologically normal squamous cells that are associated with dysplastic cells. It has been suggested that the loss of isoantigen may indicate greater risk of disease progression.[57] Minimal deviation adenocarcinoma of the cervix is reported to show inappropriate expression of blood group isoantigens based on the patient's known blood type.[135] Normal endometrial cells do not or infrequently express A, B, H, Lea, or Leb; however, endometrial carcinoma cells express these antigens frequently.[64,127,148] Loss or inappropriate expression of blood type isoantigens is also reported in ovarian carcinomas.[92] Lea and Leb are expressed by ovarian carcinomas frequently, especially in the mucinous carcinomas (approximately 80%). Serous and endometrioid carcinomas are also frequently positive with Lea and Leb.[68,111] Thomsen–Friedenreich (T) antigen, which is the immediate precursor antigen of the human blood group MN system, is expressed by ovarian tumors, especially mucinous carcinomas. T-antigen expression is correlated with increasing grades of mucinous carcinoma and is therefore believed to be a useful prognostic marker.[45]

Differential Diagnosis by Immunohistochemistry

In the following section, differential diagnoses and immunohistochemical marker panels that help establish the diagnosis are listed. It cannot be overemphasized that these immunohistochemical profiles must be interpreted in conjunction with morphologic findings. In the description of markers, "Keratins" means a cocktail of antikeratin antibodies that react with almost all 20 classes of keratin (wide spectrum). "Keratin" or "K" followed by a number indicates a narrow-spectrum keratin detecting a particular class of keratin denoted by the number. All the listed markers should be used as a panel and are listed in order of usefulness in a given differential.

Paget Disease Versus Malignant Melanoma with Pagetoid Spread[65]

Paget disease: keratins+ (especially CAM5.2 detecting K8), vimentin−, S-100−, HMB45−.
Malignant melanoma: keratins−, vimentin+, S-100+, HMB45+
Note: K7 and K8 are best in highlighting Paget cells because the background squamous cells are negative.

Endocervical Versus Endometrial Adenocarcinoma[33,59,82]

Endocervical adenocarcinoma: keratins+, vimentin−, CEA+, GFAP−, CD44+
Endometrial adenocarcinoma: keratins+, vimentin+, CEA−, GFAP+, CD44−
Note: CEA is usually positive in areas of squamous differentiation in endometrial carcinoma, which may reduce the usefulness of CEA in this differential.

Benign Endocervical Hyperplasia Versus Endocervical Adenocarcinoma In Situ[59]

Benign endocervical glands: Keratin+, CEA−, CD44−
Endocervical adenocarcinoma in situ: keratin+, CEA+, CD44+

In Situ Versus Microinvasive Endocervical Adenocarcinoma[28,140]

In situ endocervical carcinoma: CD44+, S100+, and CD1a+ Langerhans' cells in the stroma not increased; SMA− in the stroma.
Microinvasive endocervical carcinoma: CD44+, S-100+, and CD1a+ Langerhans' cells in the stroma increased, SMA+ in the stroma.

Poorly Differentiated Endometrial Adenocarcinoma Versus Malignant Mixed Müllerian Tumor (MMMT)[2,29]

Poorly differentiated carcinoma: keratin+, vimentin+/−, SMA−, desmin−, S-100−.
MMMT: keratin+, vimentin+, SMA+, desmin+ and S-100+ (in heterologous elements).

Stromal Sarcoma Versus Leiomyosarcoma[108,155]

Stromal sarcoma: h-caldesmon−, SMA+/−, MSA+/−, desmin−, keratin+/−.
Leiomyosarcoma: h-caldesmon+, SMA+, MSA+, Desmin+/−, keratin+.
Note: In leiomyosarcoma, keratin shows a paranuclear inclusion-like pattern.

Ovarian Endometrioid Carcinoma Versus Serous Carcinoma

Endometrioid carcinoma: Keratin 4/5+.
Serous carcinoma: Keratin 4/5−.
Note: Because endometrioid carcinoma of the ovary shows frequent squamous differentiation, the detection of subtle squamous differentiation favors the diagnosis of endometrioid carcinoma. Expression of K4 and K5 (high molecular weight keratins) may precede morphologically identifiable squamous differentiation.

Ovarian Endometrioid Carcinoma Versus Metastatic Carcinoma of Gastrointestinal (GI) Tract[7,27,34]

Ovarian endometrioid carcinoma: keratin 7+, keratin 20−
Metastatic carcinoma from GI: Keratin 7−, Keratin 20+
Note: K7−, K20+ is most characteristic for colonic adenocarcinomas. Gastric carcinomas are frequently K7+, K20+ or K7−, K20+. Pancreatic carcinoma is usually K7+, K20+.

Ovarian Endometrioid Carcinoma with Sertoliform Features Versus Sex Cord–Stromal Tumor[48,110]

Ovarian endometrioid carcinoma: keratin 7+, inhibin−
Sex cord–stromal tumor: keratin 7−, inhibin+

Ovarian Mucinous Carcinoma Versus Metastatic Mucinous Carcinoma from Gastrointestinal Tract[7]

Ovarin mucinous carcinoma: keratin 7+, Keratin 20+/−.
Metastatic mucinous carcinoma from colon: Keratin 7−, Keratin 20+.
Note: K7−, K20+ is characteristic for colonic adenocarcinoma. Gastric carcinoma is frequently K 7+, K 20+ or K 7−, K 20+. Pancreatic carcinoma is usually K 7+, K 20+.

Ovarian Serous Carcinoma Versus Epithelial Peritoneal Mesothelioma[32,74,94]

Ovarian serous carcinoma: keratin 5/6−, thrombomodulin−, calretinin−
Peritoneal mesothelioma: keratin 5/6+, thrombomodulin+, calretinin+

Ovarian Clear Cell Carcinoma Versus Dysgerminoma[151]

Ovarian clear cell carcinoma: keratin+, EMA+
Dysgerminoma: keratin−, EMA−
Note: Both could show predominantly clear cell features with intracytoplasmic glycogen. Although there are few reports describing dysgerminoma and keratin expression, the foregoing keratin profile is based on our experience and is extrapolated from studies on testicular seminomas.

Ovarian Clear Cell Carcinoma Versus Metastatic Renal Cell Carcinoma[153]

Ovarian clear cell carcinoma: keratin+, vimentin−.
Metastatic renal cell carcinoma: keratin+, vimentin+.

Ovarian Clear Cell Carcinoma Versus Yolk Sac Tumor

Ovarian clear cell carcinoma: α-fetoprotein-, LeuM-1 (CD15)+.
Yolk sac tumor: α-fetoprotein+, LeuM1− (mostly).

Ovarian Transitional Cell Carcinoma (Ovarian Carcinoma with TCC Features) Versus Metastatic Transitional Cell Carcinoma[113]

Ovarian TCC: keratin 20−, uroplakin−, thrombomodulin−.
Metastatic TCC: keratin 20+, uroplakin+, thrombomodulin+.

Granulosa Cell Tumor Versus Poorly Differentiated Carcinoma[71,114]

Granulosa cell tumor: inhibin+, keratin− (or +/−), vimentin+.
Poorly differentiated carcinoma: inhibin−, keratin+, vimentin+/−.

Ovarian Germ Cell Tumors: Dysgerminomatous Elements Versus Embryonal Carcinoma and Yolk Sac Tumor

Dysgerminoma: keratins−, α-fetoprotein−, hPLAP+.
Embryonal carcinoma and yolk sac tumor: keratins+, α-fetoprotein+, hPLAP+.
Note: Although there are few reports describing ovarian germ cell tumors and keratin expression, the foregoing keratin profile is based on our experience and is extrapolated from studies on testicular seminomas.

Ovarian Germ Cell Tumors: Nontrophoblastic Versus Trophoblastic Elements[34]

Trophoblastic elements: keratin 7+, βHCG+, hPLAP+.
Nonseminomatous, nontrophoblastic elements: keratin 7−, βHCG−, hPLAP+.

Decidua Versus Intermediate Trophoblast[125,126]

Decidua: keratins−, inhibin−, CD146−, hPL−. Intermediate trophoblast: keratins+, inhibin+, CD146+, hPL+.

References

1. Al-Timimi A, Buckley CH, Fox H (1985) An immunohistochemical study of the incidence and significance of sex steroid hormone binding sites in normal and neoplastic human ovarian tissue. Int J Gynecol Pathol 4:24–41
2. Auerbach HE, LiVolsi VA, Merino MJ (1988) Malignant mixed müllerian tumors of the uterus. An immunohistochemical study. Int J Gynecol Pathol 7:123–130
3. Auerbach R, Mittal K, Schwartz PE (1988) Estrogen and progestin receptors in an ovarian ependymoma. Obstet Gynecol 71:1043–1045
4. Azumi N, Battifora H (1987) The distribution of vimentin and keratin in epithelial and nonepithelial neoplasms. A comprehensive immunohistochemical study on formalin- and alcohol-fixed tumors. Am J Clin Pathol 88:286–296
5. Berchuck A, Rodriguez G, Kinney RB, Soper JT, Dodge RK, Clarke-Pearson DL, et al (1991) Overexpression of HER-2/neu in endometrial cancer is associated with advanced stage disease. Am J Obstet Gynecol 164:15–21
6. Berchuck A, Soisson AP, Clarke-Pearson DL, Soper JT, Boyer CM, Kinney RB, et al (1993) Immunohistochemical expression of CA 125 in endometrial adenocarcinoma: correlation of antigen expression with metastatic potential. Cancer Res 49:2091–2095
7. Berezowski K, Stastny JF, Kornstein MJ (1996) Cytokeratins 7 and 20 and carcinoembryonic antigen in ovarian and colonic carcinoma. Mod Pathol 9:426–429
8. Bergeron C, Ferenczy A, Toft DO, Shyamala G (1988) Immunocytochemical study of progesterone receptors in hyperplastic and neoplastic endometrial tissues. Cancer Res 48:6132–6136
9. Bizzi A, Codegoni AM, Landoni F, Marelli G, Marsoni S, Spina AM, et al (1988) Steroid receptors in epithelial ovarian carcinoma: relation to clinical parameters and survival. Cancer Res 48:6222–6226
10. Borazjani G, Twiggs LB, Leung BS, Prem KA, Adcock LL, Carson LF (1989) Prognostic significance of steroid receptors measured in primary metastatic and recurrent endometrial carcinoma. Am J Obstet Gynecol 161:1253–1257
11. Bradgate MG, Redman CW, Rollason TP, Williams A, Byrne P, Kelly K (1989) Binding of anti-EMA, AGF 4:48 and the lectin UEA-1 to human ovarian carcinomas: histological and clinical correlations. Br J Obstet Gynaecol 96:854–860
12. Brescia RJ, Kurman RJ, Main CS, Surti U, Szulman AE (1987) Immunocytochemical localization of chorionic gonadotropin, placental lactogen, and placental alkaline phosphatase in the diagnosis of complete and partial hydatidiform moles. Int J Gynecol Pathol 6:213–229
13. Brown DC, Cole D, Gatter KC, Mason DY (1988) Carcinoma of the cervix uteri: an assessment of tumour proliferation using the monoclonal antibody Ki67. Br J Cancer 57:178–181
14. Brown LJ, Griffin NR, Wells M (1987) Cytoplasmic reactivity with the monoclonal antibody HMFG1 as a marker of cervical glandular atypia. J Pathol 151:203–208
15. Brresen AL (1992) Oncogenesis in ovarian cancer. Acta Obstet Gynecol Scand Suppl 155:25–30
16. Brumm C, Rivière A, Wilckens C, Loning T (1990) Immunohistochemical investigation and northern blot analysis of c-erB-2 expression in normal, premalignant and malignant tissues of the corpus and cervix uteri. Virchows Arch [A] 417:477–484
17. Budwit-Novotny DA, McCarty KS, Cox EB, Soper JT, Mutch DG, Creasman WT, et al (1986) Immunohistochemical analyses of estrogen receptor in endometrial adenocarcinoma using a monoclonal antibody. Cancer Res 46:5419–5425
18. Bur ME, Greene GL, Press MF (1987) Estrogen receptor localization in formalin-fixed, paraffin-embedded endometrium and endometriotic tissues. Int J Gynecol Pathol 6:140–151
19. Bur ME, Perlman C, Edelmann L, Fey E, Rose PG (1992) p53 expression in neoplasms of the uterine corpus. Am J Clin Pathol 98:81–87
20. Cajigas HE, Fariza E, Scully RE, Thor AD (1991) Enhancement of tumor-associated glycoprotein-72 antigen expression in hormone-related ovarian serous borderline tumors. Cancer (Phila) 68:348–354
21. Carbone A, Poletti A, Manconi R, Sulfaro S, Volpe R (1987) S-100 protein immunostaining in teratomatous well-differentiated tissues. Histopathology. 11:980–983
22. Carcangiu ML, Chambers JT, Voynick IM, Pirro M, Schwartz PE (1990) Immunohistochemical evaluation of estrogen and progesterone receptor content in 183 patients with endometrial carcinoma. Part I: Clinical and histologic correlations. Am J Clin Pathol 94:247–254
23. Carr KA, Roberts JA, Frank TS (1992) Progesterone receptors in bilateral ovarian ependymoma presenting in pregnancy. Hum Pathol 23:962–965
24. Chambers JT, Carcangiu ML, Voynick IM, Schwartz PE (1990) Immunohistochemical evaluation of estrogen and progesterone receptor content in 183 patients with endometrial carcinoma. Part II: Correlation between biochemical and immunohistochemical methods and survival. Am J Clin Pathol 94:255–260
25. Charpin C, Martin PM, Lavaut MN, Pourreau-Schneider N, Toga M (1986) Estrogen receptor

immunocytochemical assay (ER-ICA) in human endometrium. Int J Gynecol Pathol 5:119–131
26. Chhieng DC, Yee H, Schaefer D, Cangiarella JF, Jagirdar J, Chiriboga LA, et al (2000) Calretinin staining pattern aids in the differentiation of mesothelioma from adenocarcinoma in serous effusions. Cancer (Phila) 90:194–200
27. Chu P, Wu E, Weiss LM (2000) Cytokeratin 7 and cytokeratin 20 expression in epithelial neoplasms: a survey of 435 cases. Mod Pathol 13:962–972
28. Cintorino M, Bellizzi de Ma E, Leoncini P, Tripodi SA, Xu LJ, Sappino AP, et al (1991) Expression of alpha-smooth-muscle actin in stromal cells of the uterine cervix during epithelial neoplastic changes. Int J Cancer 47:843–846
29. Costa MJ, Morris RJ, Wilson R, Judd R (1992) Utility of immunohistochemistry in distinguishing ovarian sertoli-stromal cell tumors from carcinosarcomas. Hum Pathol 23:787–797
30. Creasman WT (1993) Prognostic significance of hormone receptors in endometrial cancer. Cancer (Phila) 71:1467–1470
31. Cui S, Hano H, Harada T, Takai S, Masui F, Ushigome S (1999) Evaluation of new monoclonal anti-MyoD1 and anti-myogenin antibodies for the diagnosis of rhabdomyosarcoma. Pathol Int 49:62–68
32. Cury PM, Butcher DN, Fisher C, Corrin B, Nicholson AG (2000) Value of the mesothelium-associated antibodies thrombomodulin, cytokeratin 5/6, calretinin, and CD44H in distinguishing epithelioid pleural mesothelioma from adenocarcinoma metastatic to the pleura. Mod Pathol 13:107–112
33. Dabbs DJ, Geisinger KR, Norris HT (1986) Intermediate filaments in endometrial and endocervical carcinomas. The diagnostic utility of vimentin patterns. Am J Surg Pathol 10:568–576
34. Damjanov I, Osborn M, Miettinen M (1990) Keratin 7 is a marker for a subset of trophoblastic cells in human germ cell tumors. Arch Pathol Lab Med 114:81–83
35. Darne J, Soutter WP, Ginsberg R, Sharp F (1990) Nuclear and cytoplasmic estrogen and progesterone receptors in squamous cell carcinoma of the cervix. Gynecol Oncol 38:216–219
36. Davies JO, Davies ER, Howe K, Jackson P, Pitcher E, Randle B, et al (1985) Practical application of monoclonal antibody (NDOG2) against placental alkaline phosphatase in ovarian cancer. J R Soc Med 78:899–905
37. Deligdisch L, Holinka CF (1986) Progesterone receptors in two groups of endometrial carcinoma. Cancer (Phila) 57:1385–1388
38. Eccles DM, Brett L, Lessells A, Gruber L, Lane D, Steel CM, et al (1992) Overexpression of the p53 protein and allele loss at 17p13 in ovarian carcinoma. Br J Cancer 65:40–44
39. Ehrmann RL, Dwyer IM, Yavner D, Hancock WW (1988) An immunoperoxidase study of laminin and type IV collagen distribution in carcinoma of the cervix and vulva. Obstet Gynecol 72:257–262
40. Ersev A, Ersev D, Simsek F, Taga Y, Küllü S, Akdas A (1990) Ectopic production of human chorionic gonadotropin in transitional cell carcinoma of the bladder. An immunohistochemical study. Eur Urol 18:227–230
41. Fleuren GJ, Nap M (1988) Carcinoembryonic antigen in primary and metastatic ovarian tumors. Gynecol Oncol 30:407–415
42. Fukunaga M (2000) Adenomyosis with a sex cord-like stromal element. Pathol Int 50:336–339
43. Garcia E, Bouchard P, De Brux J, Berdah J, Frydman R, Schaison G, et al (1988) Use of immunocytochemistry of progesterone and estrogen receptors for endometrial dating. J Clin Endocrinol Metab 67:80–87
44. Geisinger KR, Marshall RB, Kute TE, Homesley HD (1986) Correlation of female sex steroid hormone receptors with histologic and ultrastructural differentiation in adenocarcinoma of the endometrium. Cancer (Phila) 58:1506–1517
45. Ghazizadeh M, Oguro T, Sasaki Y, Aihara K, Araki T, Springer GF (1990) Immunohistochemical and ultrastructural localization of T antigen in ovarian tumors. Am J Clin Pathol 93:315–321
46. Girling A, Bartkova J, Burchell J, Gendler S, Gillett C, Taylor-Papadimitriou J (1989) A core protein epitope of the polymorphic epithelial mucin detected by the monoclonal antibody SM-3 is selectively exposed in a range of primary carcinomas. Int J Cancer 43:1072–1076
47. Glasgow BJ, Wen DR, al-Jitawi S, Cochran AJ (1987) Antibody to S-100 protein aids the separation of pagetoid melanoma from mammary and extramammary Paget's disease. J Cutan Pathol 14: 223–226
48. Guerrieri C, Franlund B, Malmstrom H, Boeryd B (1998) Ovarian endometrioid carcinomas simulating sex cord-stromal tumors: a study using inhibin and cytokeratin 7. Int J Gynecol Pathol 17: 266–271
49. Hachisuga T, Fukuda K, Hayashi Y, Iwasaka T, Sugimori H (1989) Immunohistochemical demonstration of histiocytes in normal ectocervical epithelium and epithelial lesions of the uterine cervix. Gynecol Oncol 33:273–278
50. Haldane JS, Hird V, Hughes CM, Gullick WJ (1990) c-erbB-2 oncogene expression in ovarian cancer. J Pathol 162:231–237
51. Hamilton-Dutoit SJ, Lou H, Pallesen G (1990) The expression of placental alkaline phosphatase (PLAP) and PLAP-like enzymes in normal and neoplastic human tissues. An immunohistological survey using monoclonal antibodies. APMIS 98:797–811
52. Hammond RH, Bates TD, Clarke DG, Grant AG, Haines AM, Eustace DL, et al (1991) The immunoperoxidase localization of tumour markers in ovarian cancer: the value of CEA, EMA, cytokeratin and DD9. Br J Obstet Gynaecol 98:73–83
53. Harding M, Cowan S, Hole D, Cassidy L, Kitchener

H, Davis J, et al (1990) Estrogen and progesterone receptors in ovarian cancer. Cancer (Phila) 65:486–491
54. Harms D, Janig U (1986) Germ cell tumours of childhood. Report of 170 cases including 59 pure and partial yolk-sac tumours. Virchows Arch [A] 409:223–239
55. Henry RJ, Goodman JD, Godley M, Raju KS, Coffer AI, King RJ (1988) Immunohistochemical study of cytoplasmic oestradiol receptor in normal, dysplastic and malignant cervical tissue. Br J Obstet Gynaecol 95:927–932
56. Heyderman E, Steele K, Ormerod MG (1979) A new antigen on epithelial membrane: its immunoperoxidase location in normal and neoplastic tissue. J Clin Pathol 32:35–39
57. Himes TR, Ernst CS, Koprowska I (1986) Loss of blood isoantigens in exfoliated cells during the progression of CIN demonstrated by monoclonal antibody staining. Acta Cytol 30:461–469
58. Hung MC, Zhang X, Yan DH, Zhang HZ, He GP, Zhang TQ, et al (1992) Aberrant expression of the c-erbB-2/neu protooncogene in ovarian cancer. Cancer Lett 61:95–103
59. Ibrahim EM, Blackett AD, Tidy JA, Wells M (1999) CD44 is a marker of endocervical neoplasia. Int J Gynecol Pathol 18:101–108
60. Ingram SS, Rosenman J, Heath R, Morgan TM, Moore D, Varia M (1989) The predictive value of progesterone receptor levels in endometrial cancer. Int J Radiat Oncol Biol Phys 17:21–27
61. Ishikura H, Scully RE (1987) Hepatoid carcinoma of the ovary. A newly described tumor. Cancer (Phila) 60:2775–2784
62. Isola J, Kallioniemi OP, Korte JM, Wahlstrom T, Aine R, Helle M, et al (1990) Steroid receptors and Ki-67 reactivity in ovarian cancer and in normal ovary: correlation with DNA flow cytometry, biochemical receptor assay, and patient survival. J Pathol 162:295–301
63. Iversen OE, Skaarland E, Utaaker E (1986) Steroid receptor content in human ovarian tumors: survival of patients with ovarian carcinoma related to steroid receptor content. Gynecol Oncol 23:65–76
64. Iwamori M, Sakayori M, Nozawa S, Yamamoto T, Yago M, Noguchi M, et al (1989) Monoclonal antibody-defined antigen of human uterine endometrial carcinomas is Leb. J Biochem (Tokyo) 105:718–722
65. Kerner H, Gal D, Friedman M, Moll R (1988) An immunohistochemical and biochemical study of cytokeratin polypeptides in a non-Paget type adenocarcinoma of the vulva. J Obstet Gynecol 8:294–298
66. Kerns BJ, Jordan PA, Moore MB, Humphrey PA, Berchuck A, Kohler MF, et al (1992) p53 overexpression in formalin-fixed, paraffin-embedded tissue detected by immunohistochemistry. J Histochem Cytochem 40:1047–1051
67. Khalifa MA, Sesterhenn IA (1990) Tumor markers of epithelial ovarian neoplasms. Int J Gynecol Pathol 9:217–230
68. Kiguchi K, Takamatsu K, Tanaka J, Nozawa S, Iwamori M, Nagai Y (1992) Glycosphingolipids of various human ovarian tumors: a significantly high expression of I3SO3GalCer and Lewis antigen in mucinous cystadenocarcinoma. Cancer Res 52:416–421
69. Kleine W, Maier T, Geyer H, Pfleiderer A (1990) Estrogen and progesterone receptors in endometrial cancer and their prognostic relevance. Gynecol Oncol 38:59–65
70. Kommoss F, Franklin WA, Talerman A (1989) Estrogen and progesterone receptors in endodermal sinus (yolk sac) tumor. Evaluation of immunocytochemical and biochemical methods. J Reprod Med 34:943–945
71. Kommoss F, Oliva E, Bhan AK, Young RH, Scully RE (1998) Inhibin expression in ovarian tumors and tumor-like lesions: an immunohistochemical study. Mod Pathol 11:656–664
72. Konishi I, Fujii S, Kataoka N, Noda Y, Okamura H, Yamabe H, et al (1988) Ovarian mucinous cystadenocarcinoma producing alpha-fetoprotein. Int J Gynecol Pathol 7:182–189
73. Konishi I, Fujii S, Nonogaki H, Nanbu Y, Iwai T, Mori T (1991) Immunohistochemical analysis of estrogen receptors, progesterone receptors, Ki-67 antigen, and human papillomavirus DNA in normal and neoplastic epithelium of the uterine cervix. Cancer (Phila) 68:1340–1350
74. Krishnamurthy S, Jungbluth AA, Busam KJ, Rosai J (1998) Uterine tumors resembling ovarian sex-cord tumors have an immunophenotype consistent with true sex-cord differentiation. Am J Surg Pathol 22:1078–1082
75. Kuhnel R, Rao BR, Stolk JG, van Kessel H, Seldenrijk CA, Willig AP (1987) Estrogen synthesizing rare malignant Brenner tumor of the ovary with the presence of progesterone and androgen receptors in the absence of estrogen receptors. Gynecol Oncol 26:263–269
76. Kupryjánczyk J, Moller P (1988) Estrogen receptor distribution in the normal and pathologically changed human cervix uteri: an immunohistochemical study with use of monoclonal anti-ER antibody. Int J Gynecol Pathol 7:75–85
77. Kurman RJ, Young RH, Norris HJ, Main CS, et al (1984) Immunohistochemical localization of placental lactogen and chorionic gonadotropin in the normal placenta and trophoblastic tumors, with emphasis on intermediate trophoblast and the placental site trophoblastic tumor. Int J Gynecol Pathol 3:101–121
78. Liao SY, Choi BH (1986) Expression of glial fibrillary acidic protein by neoplastic cells of müllerian origin. Virchows Arch B Cell Pathol 52:185–193
79. Lin M, Hanai J, Wada A, Ozaki M, Nasu K, Okamoto S, et al (1991) S-100 protein in ovarian tumors. A comparative immunohistochemical study of 135 cases. Acta Pathol Jpn 41:233–239

80. Lindgren J, Vesterinen E, Purola E, Wahlstrom T (1986) Prognostic significance of tissue carcinoembryonic antigen in mild dysplasia of the uterine cervix. Tumour Biol 6:465–470
81. Luevano-Flores E, Sotelo J, Tena-Suck M (1985) Glial polyp (glioma) of the uterine cervix, report of a case with demonstration of glial fibrillary acidic protein. Gynecol Oncol 21:385–390
82. Maes G, Fleuren GJ, Bara J, Nap M (1988) The distribution of mucins, carcinoembryonic antigen, and mucus-associated antigens in endocervical and endometrial adenocarcinomas. Int J Gynecol Pathol 7:112–122
83. Mainguene C, Aillet G, Kremer M, Chatal JF (1986) Immunohistochemical study of ovarian tumors using the OC 125 monoclonal antibody as a basis for potential in vivo and in vitro applications. J Nucl Med Allied Sci 30:19–22
84. Manivel C, Wick MR, Sibley RK (1986) Neuroendocrine differentiation in müllerian neoplasms. An immunohistochemical study of a "pure" endometrial small-cell carcinoma and a mixed müllerian tumor containing small-cell carcinoma. Am J Clin Pathol 86:438–443
85. Marks JR, Davidoff AM, Kerns BJ, Humphrey PA, Pence JC, Dodge RK, et al (1991) Overexpression and mutation of p53 in epithelial ovarian cancer. Cancer Res 51:2979–2984
86. Martin JD, Hahnel R, McCartney AJ, De Klerk N The influence of estrogen and progesterone receptors on survival in patients with carcinoma of the uterine cervix. Gynecol Oncol 23:329–335
87. Masood S (1988) Use of monoclonal antibodies in immunocytochemical localization of estrogen receptors in ovarian cancer. Cancer Detect Prev 12: 283–290
88. Masood S, Hosein I, Pitcher M, Graf W (1990) Potential value of immunoperoxidase technique in assessment of genital herpes. J Fla Med Assoc 77:516–519
89. Matsukuma K, Tsukamoto N (1988) Alpha-fetoprotein producing endometrial adenocarcinoma: report of a case. Gynecol Oncol 29:370–377
90. McDicken IW, Rainey M (1983) The immunohistological demonstration of carcinoembryonic antigen in intra-epithelial and invasive squamous carcinoma of the cervix. Histopathology (Oxf) 7:475–485
91. McLaughlin PJ, Warne PH, Hutchinson GE, Johnson PM, Tucker DF (1987) Placental-type alkaline phosphatase in cervical neoplasia. Br J Cancer 55: 197–201
92. Metoki R, Kakudo K, Tsuji Y, Teng N, Clausen H, Hakomori S (1989) Deletion of histo-blood group A and B antigens and expression of incompatible A antigen in ovarian cancer. J Natl Cancer Inst 81: 1151–1157
93. Miettinen M (1993) Keratin immunohistochemistry: update of applications and pitfalls. Pathol Annu 28:113–143
94. Moll R, Dhouailly D, Sun TT (1989) Expression of keratin 5 as a distinctive feature of epithelial and biphasic mesotheliomas. An immunohistochemical study using monoclonal antibody AE14. Virchows Arch [B] 58:129–145
95. Moll R, Pitz S, Levy R, Weikel W, Franke WW, Czernobilsky B (1991) Complexity of expression of intermediate filament proteins, including glial filament protein, in endometrial and ovarian adenocarcinomas. Hum Pathol 22:989–1001
96. Monsonego J, Magdelenat H, Catalan F, Coscas Y, Zerat L, Sastre X (1991) Estrogen and progesterone receptors in cervical human papillomavirus related lesions. Int J Cancer 48:533–539
97. Moran CA, Wick MR, Suster S (2000) The role of immunohistochemistry in the diagnosis of malignant mesothelioma. Semin Diagn Pathol 17:178–183
98. Morris WP, Griffin NR, Wells M (1989) Patterns of reactivity with the monoclonal antibodies HMFG1 and HMFG2 in normal endometrium, endometrial hyperplasia and adenocarcinoma. Histopathology (Oxf) 15:179–186.
99. Mosny DS, Herholz J, Degen W, Bender HG (1989) Immunohistochemical investigations of steroid receptors in normal and neoplastic squamous epithelium of the uterine cervix. Gynecol Oncol 35: 373–377
100. Mutch DG, Soper JT, Budwit-Novotny DA, Cox EB, Creasman WT, McCarty KS Sr, et al (1987) Endometrial adenocarcinoma estrogen receptor content: association of clinicopathologic features with immunohistochemical analysis compared with standard biochemical methods. Am J Obstet Gynecol 157:924–931
101. Nagle RB, Lucas DO, McDaniel KM, Clark VA, Schmalzel GM (1983) New evidence linking mammary and extramammary Paget cells to a common cell phenotype. Am J Clin Pathol 83:431–438
102. Navarro D, Cabrera JJ, Falcón O, Jiménez P, Ruiz A, Chirino R, et al (1989) Monoclonal antibody characterization of progesterone receptors, estrogen receptors and the stress-responsive protein of 27 kDa (SRP27) in human uterine leiomyoma. J Steroid Biochem 34:491–498
103. Navarro D, Cabrera JJ, Leon L, Chirino R, Fernandez L, Lopez A, et al (1992) Endometrial stromal sarcoma expression of estrogen receptors, progesterone receptors and estrogen-induced srp27 (24K) suggests hormone responsiveness. J Steroid Biochem Mol Biol 41:589–596
104. Neunteufel W, Breitenecker G (1989) CA 19-9, CA 125 and CEA in the endometrial mucosa during the menstrual cycle, in atypical hyperplasia and endometrial carcinoma. Cancer Lett 48:77–83
105. Neunteufel W, Breitenecker G (1989) Tissue expression of CA 125 in benign and malignant lesions of ovary and fallopian tube: a comparison with CA 19-9 and CEA. Gynecol Oncol 32:297–302
106. Nonogaki H, Fujii S, Konishi I, Nanbu Y, Ozaki S,

Ishikawa Y, et al (1990) Estrogen receptor localization in normal and neoplastic epithelium of the uterine cervix. Cancer (Phila) 66:2620–2627
107. Notohara K, Hsueh CL, Awai M (1990) Glial fibrillary acidic protein immunoreactivity of chondrocytes in immature and mature teratomas. Acta Pathol Jpn 40:335–342
108. Nucci MR, O'Conell JT, Cviko A, Sun D, Uade BJ (2000) h-Caldesmon expression distinguishes endometrial stromal neoplasms from smooth muscle tumors [abstract]. Mod Pathol 13:129A
109. Okamoto A, Sameshima Y, Yamada Y, Teshima S, Terashima Y, Terada M, et al (1991) Allelic loss on chromosome 17p and p53 mutations in human endometrial carcinoma of the uterus. Cancer Res 51: 5632–5635
110. Ordi J, Schammel DP, Rasekh L, Tavassoli FA (1999) Sertoliform endometrioid carcinomas of the ovary: a clinicopathologic and immunohistochemical study of 13 cases. Mod Pathol 12:933–940
111. Ordoñez NG, Freedman RS, Herlyn M (1987) Lewis and related tumor-associated determinants on ovarian carcinoma. Gynecol Oncol 26:1–10
112. Ordoñez NG (1998) Role of immunohistochemistry in distinguishing epithelial peritoneal mesotheliomas from peritoneal and ovarian serous carcinomas. Am J Surg Pathol 22:1203–1214
113. Ordoñez NG (2000) Transitional cell carcinomas of the ovary and bladder are immunophenotypically different. Histopathology (Oxf) 36(5):433–438
114. Pelkey TJ, Frierson HFJ, Mills SE, Stoler MH (1998) The diagnostic utility of inhibin staining in ovarian neoplasms. Int J Gynecol Pathol 17:97–105
115. Perrone T, Steeper TA, Dehner LP (1987) Alphafetoprotein localization in pure ovarian teratoma. An immunohistochemical study of 12 cases. Am J Clin Pathol 88:713–717
116. Pertschuk LP, Beddoe AM, Gorelic LS, Shain SA (1986) Immunocytochemical assay of estrogen receptors in endometrial carcinoma with monoclonal antibodies. Comparison with biochemical assay. Cancer (Phila) 57:1000–1004
117. Quinn MA, Rome RM, Cauchi M, Fortune DW (1988) Steroid receptors and ovarian tumors: variation within primary tumors and between primary tumors and metastases. Gynecol Oncol 31:424–429
118. Ravn V, Jensen H, Hilgers J (1989) Human milkfat globule membrane antigens (Mam-3 group) in normal cycling endometrium and endometrial carcinomas—an immunohistochemical study. A preliminary report. APMIS 97:452–458
119. Riedel I, Czernobilsky B, Lifschritz-Mercer B, et al (2001) Brenner tumors but not transitional cell carcinoma of the ovary show urothelial differentiation: immunohistochemical staining of urothelial markers. Virchows Arch 438:181–191
120. Runowicz CD, Nuchtern LM, Braunstein JD, Jones JG (1990) Heterogeneity in hormone receptor status in primary and metastatic endometrial cancer. Gynecol Oncol 38:437–441
121. Scambia G, Panici PB, Baiocchi G, Battaglia F, Ferrandina G, Greggi S, et al (1990) Steroid hormone receptors in carcinoma of the cervix: lack of response to an antiestrogen. Gynecol Oncol 37:323–326
122. Schruch W, Skalli O, Seemayer TA, Gabbiani G (1987) Intermediate filament proteins and actin isoforms as markers for soft tissue tumor differentiation and origin. I. Smooth muscle tumors. Am J Pathol 128:91–103
123. Setzu A, Puligheddu P, Marcello C, Parodo G, Liguori C, Zucca A, et al (1987) Immunoperoxidase localization of HSV2 antigens in cervical dysplasia and carcinoma. Eur J Gynaecol Oncol 8:616–618
124. Shih IM, Kurman RJ (1996) Expression of melanoma cell adhesion molecule in intermediate trophoblast. Lab Invest 75:377–388
125. Shih IM, Kurman RJ (1999) Immunohistochemical localization of inhibin-alpha in the placenta and gestational trophoblastic lesions. Int J Gynecol Pathol 18:144–150
126. Shih IM, Nesbit M, Herlyn M, Kurman RJ (1998) A new Mel-CAM (CD146)-specific monoclonal antibody, MN-4, on paraffin-embedded tissue. Mod Pathol 11:1098–1106
127. Shiozawa T, Tsukahara Y, Nakayama J, Ishii K, Katsuyama T (1991) Immunohistochemical localization of blood group substances in normal and neoplastic endometrial tissues—with special reference to type 1 core chain expression. Gynecol Obstet Invest 32:185–188
128. Shishi J, Ghazizadeh M, Oguro T, Aihara K, Araki T (1986) Immunohistochemical localization of CA 125 antigen in formalin-fixed paraffin sections of ovarian tumors with the use of Pronase. Am J Clin Pathol 85:595–598
129. Silcocks PB, Herbert A, Wright DH (1986) Evaluation of PAS-diastase and carcinoembryonic antigen staining in the differential diagnosis of malignant mesothelioma and papillary serous carcinoma of the ovary. J Pathol 149:133–141
130. Slamon DJ, Godolphin W, Jones LA, Holt JA, Wong SG, Keith DE, et al (1989) Studies of the HER-2/neu proto-oncogene in human breast and ovarian cancer. Science 244:707–712
131. Slotman BJ, Nauta JJ, Rao BR (1990) Survival of patients with ovarian cancer. Apart from stage and grade, tumor progesterone receptor content is a prognostic indicator. Cancer (Phila) 66:740–744
132. Soisson AP, Berchuck A, Lessey BA, Soper JT, Clarke-Pearson DL, McCarty KS Jr, et al (1989) Immunohistochemical expression of TAG-72 in normal and malignant endometrium: correlation of antigen expression with estrogen receptor and progesterone receptor levels. Am J Obstet Gynecol 161:1258–1263
133. Soper JT, Christensen CW (1986) Steroid receptors and endometrial cancer. Clin Obstet Gynaecol 13: 825–842
134. Soslow RA, Rouse RV, Hendrickson MR, Silva EG,

Longacre TA (1996) Transitional cell neoplasms of the ovary and urinary bladder: a comparative immunohistochemical analysis. Int J Gynecol Pathol 15:257–265
135. Steeper TA, Wick MR (1986) Minimal deviation adenocarcinoma of the uterine cervix ("adenoma malignum"). An immunohistochemical comparison with microglandular endocervical hyperplasia and conventional endocervical adenocarcinoma. Cancer (Phila) 58:1131–1138
136. Sterrett GF, Alessandri LM, Pixley E, Kulski JK (1987) Assessment of precancerous lesions of the uterine cervix for evidence of human papillomavirus infection: a histological and immunohistochemical study. Pathology 19:84–90
137. Sutton GP, Senior MB, Strauss JF, Mikuta JJ (1986) Estrogen and progesterone receptors in epithelial ovarian malignancies. Gynecol Oncol 23:176–182
138. Sweeney EC, Barry-Walsh C, Robinson A (1983) Sertoli-Leydig cell tumor of the ovary with heterologous elements and carcinoid: an immunohistochemical and ultrastructural study. Ultrastruct Pathol 5:185–194
139. Szpak CA, Soper JT, Thor A, Schlom J, Johnston WW (1989) Detection of adenocarcinoma in peritoneal washings by staining with monoclonal antibody B72.3. Acta Cytol 33:205–214
140. Tay SK, Jenkins D (1989) Langerhans cell population in early invasive squamous cell carcinoma of the uterine cervix. Aust NZJ Obstet Gynaecol 29: 38–40
141. Tay SK, Jenkins D, Singer A (1987) Natural killer cells in cervical intraepithelial neoplasia and human papillomavirus infection. Br J Obstet Gynaecol 94:901–906
142. Taylor CR, Cote RJ (2000) Immunomicroscopy: a diagnostic tool for the surgical pathologist, 2nd Ed. Saunders, Philadelphia
143. Thor A, Ohuchi N, Szpak CA, Johnston WW, Schlom J (1986) Distribution of oncofetal antigen tumor-associated glycoprotein-72 defined by monoclonal antibody B72.3. Cancer Res 46:3118–3124
144. Tohya T, Iwamasa T, Maeyama M (1986) Biochemical and immunohistochemical studies on carcinoembryonic antigen of ovarian mucinous and serous tumors. Gynecol Oncol 23:291–303
145. Tosi P, Sforza V, Santopietro R (1989) Estrogen receptor content, immunohistochemically determined by monoclonal antibodies, in endometrial stromal sarcoma. Obstet Gynecol 73:75–78
146. Tsao SW, Mok CH, Oike K, Muto M, Goodman HM, Sheets EE, et al (1991) Involvement of p53 gene in the allelic deletion of chromosome 17p in human ovarian tumors. Anticancer Res 11:1975–1982
147. Tsukada T, Tippens D, Gordon D, Ross R, Gown AM (1987) HHF35, a muscle-actin-specific monoclonal antibody. I. Immunocytochemical and biochemical chracterization. Am J Pathol 126:51–60
148. Tsukazaki K, Skayori M, Arai H, Yamaoka K, Kurihara S, Nozawa S (1991) Abnormal expression of blood group-related antigens in uterine endometrial cancers. Jpn J Cancer Res 82:934–941
149. Ueda G, Yamasaki M (1992) Neuroendocrine carcinoma of the uterus. Curr Top Pathol 85:309–335
150. Vengerov YY, Gudima SO, Voronov AV, Votrin II (1988) Immunochemical studies of human placental alkaline phosphatase in normal and neoplastic tissues. Adv Enzyme Regul 27:345–354
151. Viale G, Gambacorta M, Dell'Orto P, Coggi G (1988) Coexpression of cytokeratins and vimentin in common epithelial tumours of the ovary: an immunocytochemical study of eighty-three cases. Virchows Arch A Pathol Anat 413:91–101
152. Vogel HP, Mendelsohn G (1987) Laminin immunostaining in hyperplastic, dysplastic, and neoplastic lesions of the endometrium and uterine cervix. Obstet Gynecol 69:794–799
153. Waldherr R, Schwechheimer K (1985) Co-expression of cytokeratin and vimentin intermediate-sized filaments in renal cell carcinomas. Comparative study of the intermediate-sized filament distribution in renal cell carcinomas and normal human kidney. Virchows Arch A Pathol Anat Histopathol 408:15–27
154. Ward BG, Lowe DG, Shepherd JH (1987) Patterns of expression of a tumor associated antigen, defined by the monoclonal antibody HMFG2, in human epithelial ovarian carcinoma. Comparison with expression of the HMFG1, AUA1 and F36/22 antigens. Cancer (Phila) 60:787–793
155. Watanabe K, Kusakabe T, Hoshi N, Saito A, Suzuki T (1999) h-Caldesmon in leiomyosarcoma and tumors with smooth muscle cell-like differentiation: its specific expression in the smooth muscle cell tumor. Hum Pathol 30:392–396
156. Weiner SA, Alberts DS, Surwit EA, Davis J, Grosso D (1987) Tamoxifen therapy in recurrent epithelial ovarian carcinoma. Gynecol Oncol 27:208–213
157. Wolber RA, Dupuis BA, Wick MR (1991) Expression of c-erbB-2 oncoprotein in mammary and extramammary Paget's disease. Am J Clin Pathol 96: 243–247
158. Yavner DL, Dwyer IM, Hancock WW, Ehrmann RL (1990) Basement membrane of cervical adenocarcinoma: an immunoperoxidase study of laminin and type IV collagen. Obstet Gynecol 76:1014–1019
159. Young RH, Prat J, Scully RE (1982) Ovarian Sertoli-Leydig cell tumors with heterologous elements. I. Gastrointestinal epithelium and carcinoid: a clinicopathologic analysis of thirty-six cases. Cancer (Phila) 50:2448–2456
160. Zaino RJ, Clarke CL, Mortel R, Satyaswaroop PG (1988) Heterogeneity of progesterone receptor distribution in human endometrial adenocarcinoma. Cancer Res 48:1889–1895
161. Zirker TA, Silva EG, Morris M, Ordoñez NG (1989) Immunohistochemical differentiation of clear-cell carcinoma of the female genital tract and endodermal sinus tumor with the use of alpha-fetoprotein and Leu-M1. Am J Clin Pathol 91:511–514

26

Molecular Biology

Kathleen R. Cho, M.D. and Lora Hedrick Ellenson, M.D.

Understanding the etiology and pathogenesis of human tumors has been a goal of investigators in diverse fields including pathology, oncology, epidemiology, virology, and radiation biology. Their research has provided significant insight into the properties of neoplastic cells and has laid the foundation for our current understanding and future investigations of human tumorigenesis. The application of molecular biologic techniques to cancer research has added a new dimension to our study of the neoplastic process, as molecular tools have made it possible to directly address the mechanisms that lead to the altered properties of neoplastic cells. During the past two decades molecular studies have confirmed many well-accepted hypotheses of tumorigenesis, revealed many new facts about tumor cells, and opened the door to a more thorough understanding of the pathogenesis of human cancer. It is now clear that molecular biology will enhance our basic understanding of tumorigenesis, and have great impact on the diagnosis and treatment of cancer patients.

The aim of this chapter is to provide an overview of some basic principles and techniques to build a framework for understanding molecular studies of human tumorigenesis. We also review several major concepts underlying our current knowledge of the pathogenesis of human tumors. The specific genetic alterations associated with some of the most common gynecologic malignancies are reviewed in other chapters throughout this text. To assist the reader with unfamiliar terms, a glossary appears at the end of the chapter. Terms within the text indicated in italics are defined in the glossary.

Basic Principles of Molecular Biology

Cells have the capacity to simultaneously synthesize thousands of molecules required for normal cellular function. These molecules include deoxyribonucleic and ribonucleic acids (DNA and RNA), which encode genetic information, and proteins, which are the primary effector molecules within cells. A gene can be defined as the segment of DNA involved in producing a protein. The exact number of human genes remains unknown, with estimates ranging from 28,000 to 120,000. Based on the nearly completed sequence of the entire human genome, it is now thought that the number is closer to 50,000.[38] Nucleic acids are constructed from smaller building blocks called *nucleotides*, which are linked end to end through phosphodiester bonds. The arrangement of these nucleotides in various sequences is ultimately responsible for the tremendous variety of proteins encoded by the nucleic acids of a given organism. Human chromosomes are composed of two major components: DNA and small basic proteins called histones. Although the DNA within a given chromosome encodes only a subset of the roughly 50,000 genes represented in the human genome, it is important to keep in mind that, on average, each chromosome or chromosomal arm encodes several thousand genes. Furthermore, individual genes are distributed throughout the genome, typically separated by large expanses of DNA that do not contain genes. Thus, identification of specific genes altered in various tumor types can be a monumental task.

Primary genetic information is encoded by DNA, a double helical molecule formed by two intertwined DNA strands joined by hydrogen bonds between complementary nucleotide base pairs (Fig. 26.1). Adenine (A) can pair only with thymine (T), and cytosine (C) can pair only with guanine (G). On each strand, nucleotides are joined end to end by covalent linkage of a phosphate group connecting the 5′-carbon atom of the sugar residue on one nucleotide to the 3′-carbon atom of the sugar residue in the adjacent nucleotide. This 5′–3′ linkage is responsible for setting the direction of the nucleic acid chains such that each strand has a 5′-end and a 3′-end. All nucleic acid chains are extended in the 5′ → 3′ direction. In a double-stranded DNA molecule, the two strands are complementary and opposite in orientation. The sequence of nucleotides in DNA is critical because the coding regions (*open reading frames*) of genes are read in sequential groups of three base pairs known as *codons*. Codons specify the beginning and end of proteins as well as the order of amino acids in the proteins encoded by each gene. It follows that critically placed nucleotide substitutions at the DNA level (i.e., *point mutations*) can lead to changes in the amino acid sequence of the protein encoded by that gene. These substitutions can have grave consequences on protein function.

Although chromosomal DNA is contained within the cell nucleus, protein synthesis takes place in the cell cytoplasm. One form of RNA (*messenger RNA, mRNA*) serves as an intermediate molecule for delivery of genetic information from the DNA in the nucleus to the cytoplasmic machinery responsible for the synthesis of proteins. The RNA sequence and signals for starting and stopping the synthesis of specific RNA molecules are encoded within DNA sequences. RNA is synthesized by enzymes called *RNA polymerases*, which bind to sequences in the DNA upstream (toward the 5′-end) of coding regions called *promoters*. The synthesis of RNA from a DNA template occurs by a process known as *transcription* (see Fig. 26.1), in which an RNA copy of the coding, or "sense," DNA strand of a gene is created by linking ribonucleotides end to end (using the noncoding, or "antisense," strand as a template). The sequence of nucleotides in this initial form of RNA (*heteronuclear RNA*) is identical to that of the coding DNA strand except that ribonucleotides rather than deoxyribonucleotides form the chain and RNA-specific uracil (U) residues are substituted for thymine residues.

The heteronuclear RNA subsequently undergoes

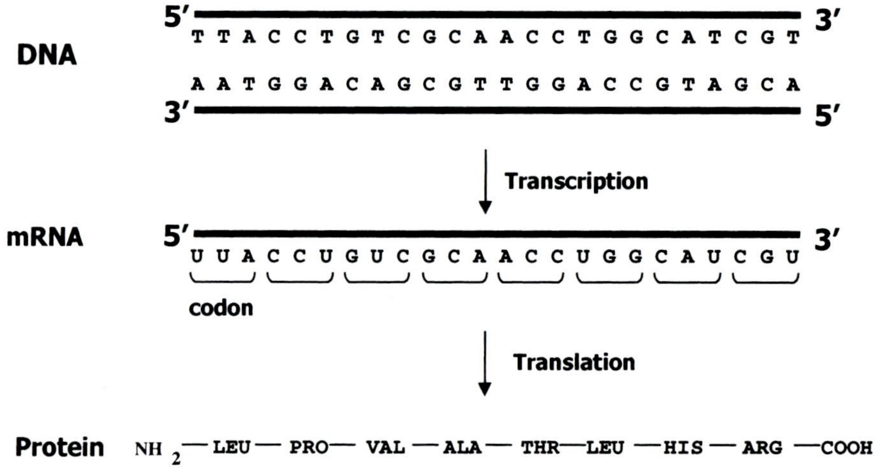

Fig. 26.1. The genetic code. DNA encodes the primary genetic information. DNA is a double-stranded molecule formed by complementary base pairing between nucleotides on strands of opposite orientation. An unwound (nonhelical) segment of *DNA* is shown. An *RNA* copy of the coding DNA strand is synthesized by a process known as *transcription*. Triplets of nucleotides (called *codons*) specify individual amino acids that are joined together to form proteins in the process known as *translation*. DNA, RNA, and protein are synthesized in a unidirectional fashion, DNA and RNA in the 5′ to 3′ direction and protein from the amino (NH_2) to carboxyl (COOH) terminus.

several modifications, including *capping*, *polyadenylation*, and *splicing*, which result in messenger RNA (Fig. 26.2). After transcription, eukaryotic mRNAs undergo "capping," in which a methylated guanosine residue is joined by triphosphate linkage to the 5′-end of the RNA molecules. The 5′-cap is believed to guide the translation machinery to the correct translation initiation codon. In addition, long runs of approximately 200 (A) residues are added to the 3′-ends of mRNAs in a process known as polyadenylation. The poly(A) sequence is not coded in the DNA but is added to the RNA after transcription. Although the function of the poly(A) tail is not understood completely, it may help protect mRNA from RNA-degrading enzymes. In the process known as splicing, the *exons*, or expressed portions of genes (including the coding regions), are joined together, and intervening noncoding regions called *introns* are removed. The mature spliced RNA (messenger RNA, mRNA) is transported to the cytoplasm, where it serves as a template to order amino acids during the process of protein synthesis known as *translation* (see Fig. 26.1). One end of a newly translated protein has an amino acid with a free amino group whereas the other end bears an amino acid with a free carboxyl group. Translation starts with the amino-terminal residue and ends with the carboxyl-terminal residue.

Clearly, only a small portion of the genome is ultimately expressed as mRNA or protein. Although cells from virtually every tissue within an individual contain the same DNA, specific genes are expressed variably in different tissues. Tissue-specific *gene expression* can be controlled at the level of DNA transcription to RNA, at the level of RNA translation to protein, or through mechanisms regulating protein turnover. A thorough discussion of these control mechanisms is beyond the scope of this chapter, but it is important to emphasize that many tumors develop and progress, at least in part, as a result of alterations of gene expression in tumor cells in comparison to their normal counterparts. Many of the molecular biologic techniques used in cancer research laboratories today are aimed at studying gross and subtle alterations of DNA, changes in gene expression at the RNA and protein levels, and alterations of protein function within tumor cells.

Commonly Used Molecular Biologic Techniques

The human genome is extremely complex, containing approximately 3 billion base pairs (bp). This complexity poses significant problems for investigators interested in studying individual genes or even smaller portions of the genome. The development and progression of many human cancers involves alterations of specific genes at the DNA level. Many different types of alterations have been iden-

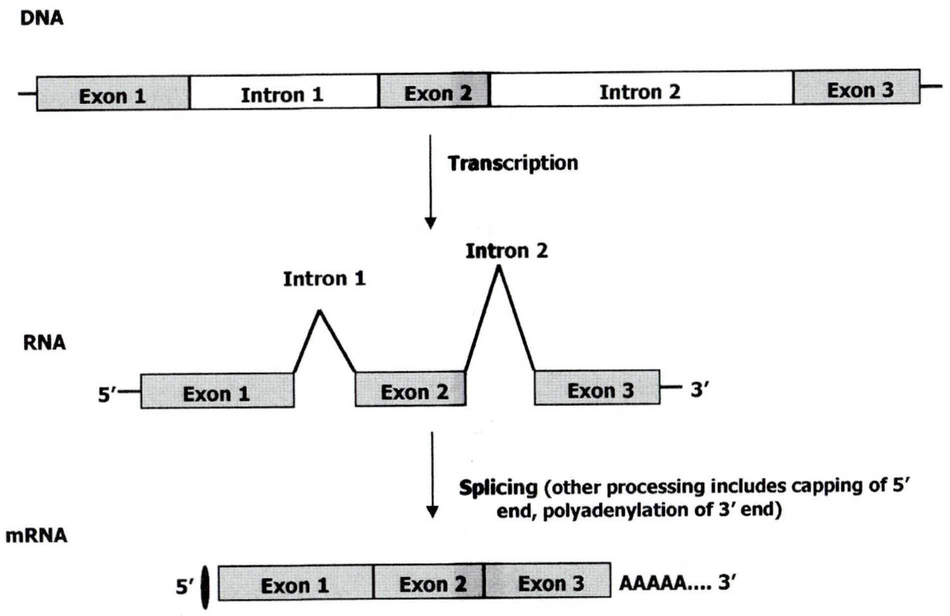

Fig. 26.2. RNA synthesis and processing. Genes are composed of alternating *exons* and *introns*. After *transcription*, introns are removed from the heteronuclear *RNA* by a process called *splicing* to produce messenger RNA (*mRNA*). The splicing machinery is directed by sequences surrounding the junctions of the exon–intron boundaries. Most eukaryotic mRNAs are modified further at the 5′-end by addition of 7-methyl guanosine residues (*capping*) and at the 3′-end by addition of several adenosine residues (*polyadenylation*).

tified, including (1) *gene amplification*, in which tumor cells contain multiple copies of a gene normally present in only two copies per somatic cell; (2) *gene rearrangement*, in which a gene is broken and one or both segments are joined to other parts of the genome; (3) *gene deletions*, in which part or all of a gene is deleted from tumor cells; (4) *insertions*, in which new genetic material is inserted into a gene; and (5) *point mutations*, in which single nucleotide substitutions at the DNA level result in proteins with amino acid substitutions (*missense mutations*) or truncated proteins (*nonsense mutations*).

More recently, it has been recognized that gene expression can be silenced as a consequence of aberrant methylation of gene promoters (*promoter hypermethylation*), an epigenetic mechanism for gene inactivation.[2,19] All the alterations just described typically cause changes in gene expression. Gene amplification results in overexpression, whereas underexpression is the usual consequence of gene deletions, insertions, or promoter hypermethylation. Rearrangements and point mutations may cause either overexpression or underexpression of the target gene depending on the specific nature of the genetic lesion. Several laboratory tools have been developed that allow detection of these abnormalities in DNA isolated from tumor cells.

Methods of DNA Analysis

Southern Blotting

This technique, developed in 1975 by E.M. Southern,[47] is an extremely powerful tool with which to analyze gene structure (Fig. 26.3). First, genomic DNA is cut with one or more *restriction endonucleases*, enzymes that cut the DNA at specific recogni-

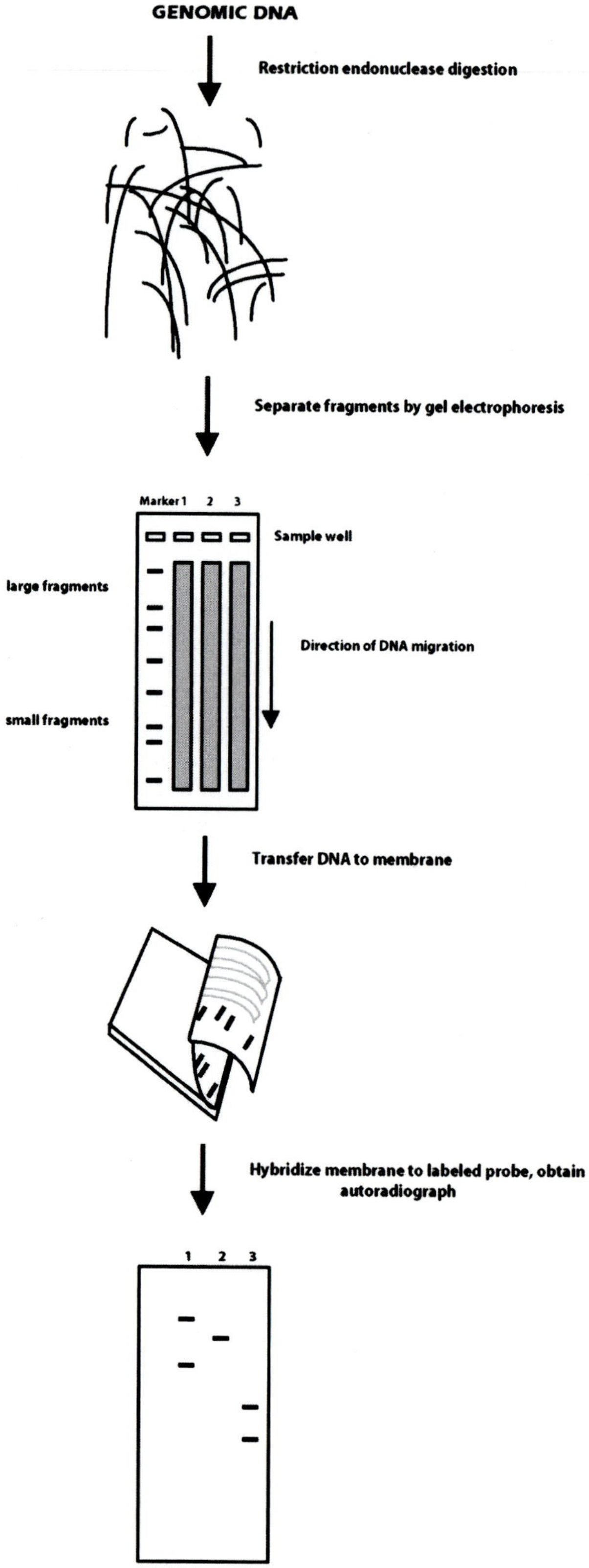

Fig. 26.3. Southern blot. This technique is used frequently to detect structural alterations of genes in human tumors. High molecular weight *genomic DNA* is cut with a *restriction endonuclease*, and the resultant DNA fragments are size fractionated by *gel electrophoresis*. The DNA is denatured in alkali, transferred from the gel, and bound to a nylon membrane. The DNA on the membrane is *hybridized* to a radiolabeled probe under conditions that allow complementary sequences to stick to each other. *Autoradiography* yields a discrete pattern of bands whose pattern, number, intensity, and size confer information about the status of a particular gene in each sample. Southern blotting can be used to detect gene amplification, gene insertions, gene deletions, and gene rearrangements and for restriction fragment length polymorphisms (RFLP) analysis (see Fig. 26.4).

tion sequences distributed throughout the genome. The resultant DNA fragments range in size from very small (a few base pairs) to very large (several thousand or more base pairs). These fragments subsequently are separated according to size by electrophoresis through an agarose gel such that smaller molecules migrate faster. The DNA in the gel is denatured in alkali to separate the strands of the double helix; the gel is then overlaid with a solid substrate (usually nylon membrane), and capillary action in an appropriate buffer is used to transport DNA out of the gel toward the membrane. The DNA fragments bind to the membrane, resulting in transfer of the DNA from the gel to the membrane. A radiolabeled probe, specific for the gene under study, is then hybridized to the DNA on the membrane under conditions that allow complementary sequences to stick to each other.

Autoradiography of the membrane results in discrete bands whose pattern, number, intensity, and size confer information about the status of the evaluated gene in that particular sample. The size of the bands is altered if there is a change in the position of the restriction endonuclease sites relative to one another. This change can occur if one of the restriction endonuclease recognition sites within or around the region of interest is changed such that the endonuclease no longer cleaves the DNA at that site, thereby changing the distance between intact recognition sites. The distance between restriction endonuclease sites also can be affected by DNA rearrangement or insertions or small deletions of DNA sequences in or around the gene under study. Therefore, when compared with the same patient's nontumor DNA, size alterations of one or more bands in tumor DNA usually indicate gene rearrangement, insertions, or small deletions; increased intensity of bands represents gene amplification; and loss of bands indicates gene deletion.

Southern hybridization to probes detecting *restriction fragment length polymorphisms* (*RFLPs*) can be used to detect *losses of heterozygosity* (*LOH*), which reflect losses of specific chromosomal regions in tumor DNA. As described in greater detail next, nonrandom losses of heterozygosity frequently occur in chromosomal regions containing *tumor suppressor genes*, genes that normally regulate cellular growth and/or differentiation and are inactivated in tumors. The term RFLP refers to single base-pair substitutions in the germline DNA of different individuals that either destroy or create new recognition sites for a given restriction enzyme. Most of these changes are without consequence because most do not affect gene products in any way. Normal cells contain two copies of each chromosome, one inherited from each parent. If the paternal and maternal copies of a given *locus* can be distinguished by RFLP analysis of DNA from normal cells, that individual is considered *heterozygous* (or *informative*) at that locus. If the two copies cannot be distinguished from one another, the individual is referred to as *homozygous* (or *uninformative*) at that locus. Therefore, if one copy of the specific chromosomal region containing that locus is lost in an individual's tumor cells, RFLP analysis will detect this loss because the individual's DNA from normal cells will be heterozygous at that locus but the tumor cell DNA will be homozygous (Fig. 26.4). Thus, the tumor cells have undergone LOH for the region of the chromosome detected by the probe. As an example, the recognition site for the restriction enzyme *Eco*RI is (. . . G-A-A-T-T-C . . .).

Although the maternally derived copy of an individual's DNA may contain this sequence at a given locus, the paternally inherited *allele* may have substituted a (T) residue for an (A) residue, such that this copy of the DNA will contain the sequence (. . . G-A-T-T-T-C . . .) at the same locus. When this individual's DNA is cut with *Eco*RI, one allele will cut at this site and the other will not, resulting in two distinguishable bands following Southern hybridization to a probe detecting the region containing the polymorphic *Eco*RI restriction site. When the patient's tumor DNA is compared with his or her own normal DNA, a loss of heterozygosity at the lo-

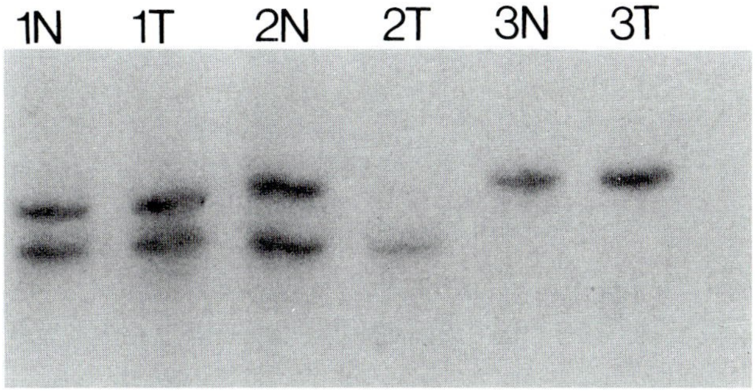

Fig. 26.4. RFLP analysis. Southern blot hybridization of paired normal and endometrial carcinoma DNAs to a RFLP probe. Each case is represented by the patient's normal DNA (*N*) in the *left lane* and tumor DNA (*T*) in the *right lane.* Case 1 is informative (heterozygous) because two bands are distinguishable in the normal DNA lane. The tumor shows no loss of heterozygosity at the locus detected by the probe because both bands are retained. Case 3 is uninformative (homozygous) because only one band is present in the normal DNA lane. In case 2, the larger band is missing in the tumor DNA; i.e., the tumor has undergone loss of heterozygosity at this locus.

cus detected by the probe shows up as a loss of one of the bands detected in the normal DNA. Southern blotting can also detect deletion of both copies of a given locus in tumor cells, a phenomenon known as *homozygous deletion*.

Although deletion of both copies of a given chromosomal region in tumors is rather rare, the finding is important, as it can effectively localize tumor suppressor genes, because homozygous deletions of large expanses of DNA are usually lethal to tumor cells. Clearly, the success of such efforts depends largely on the isolation of tumor DNA from tumors that are relatively free of contaminating normal tissue, which can mask allelic loss events. Although an individual patient may be uninformative at the locus detected by one probe, it does not render their DNA samples useless for further study because they may be informative at other loci. In addition, the development of polymerase chain reaction- (PCR-) based methods for detecting highly polymorphic regions in human DNA has made LOH studies substantially less difficult (see following). LOH analysis with probes distributed throughout the genome can be used to look for regions of chromosomes that are frequently and specifically deleted in various tumor types to identify tumor suppressor genes that are inactivated in those tumors.

DNA Cloning

DNA isolated from primary tumors and normal tissues usually is available in rather limited quantities. It is frequently desirable to obtain large amounts of specific portions of these DNAs. One method used to generate unlimited quantities of specific DNA fragments is called *cloning*. Cleavage of DNA with restriction endonucleases generates cut ends of DNA that can later be reconnected with enzymes known as DNA ligases. DNA fragments with specific cohesive ends can be ligated to *vectors* cut in a fashion generating complementary cohesive ends (Fig. 26.5). The vector containing the inserted DNA can then be introduced into bacteria by a process known as *bacterial transformation*. Using the bacterial host replication machinery, the recombinant vector can be propagated in essentially unlimited quantities. The cloned insert DNA subsequently can be excised and separated from the vector DNA using appropriate restriction enzymes. The most commonly used cloning vectors for relatively small inserts are plasmids (circular autonomously replicating bacterial minichromosomes) and bacteriophages (small viruses that replicate in bacteria). Phage vectors typically can accommodate inserts up to 23 kilobases in length. Vectors that can accommodate significantly larger DNA fragments include cosmids, yeast

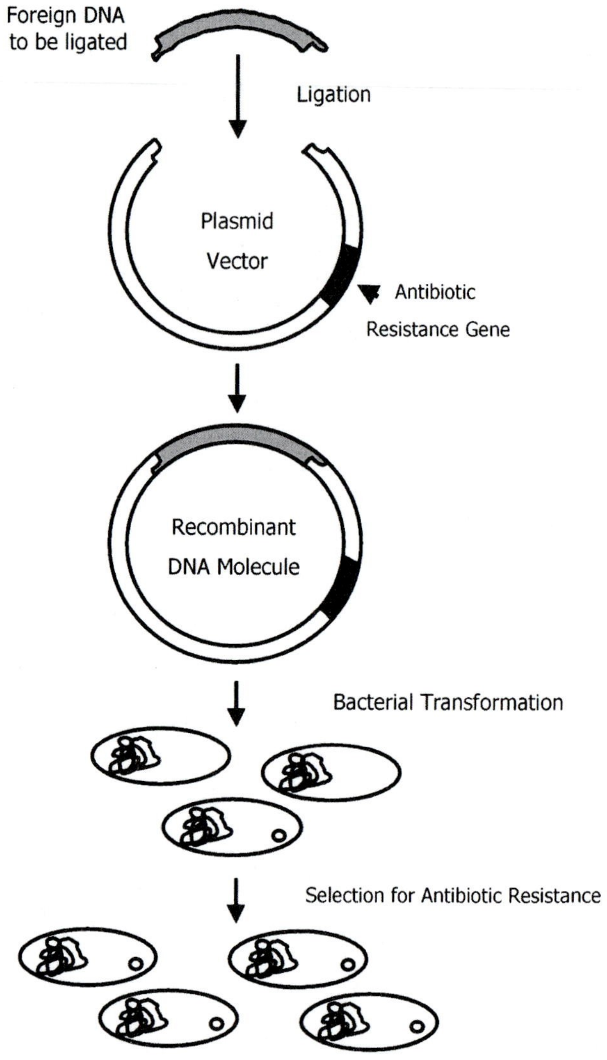

Fig. 26.5. DNA cloning. A process known as cloning allows the generation of essentially unlimited quantities of specific DNA fragments. Several different types of cloning vectors are available, each capable of accommodating DNA of specific size ranges. As an example, *plasmid vectors* are used typically to clone DNA fragments no larger than several kilobase pairs. First, the selected DNA fragment is joined to the plasmid vector using specialized enzymes called *DNA ligases.* Often, the ligation is facilitated by the presence of complementary cohesive ends on the vector and foreign fragment to be ligated. After ligation, the recombinant DNA molecule is introduced as a circular plasmid into a host strain of bacteria by a process known as *bacterial transformation.* Inside the bacteria, the plasmid replicates independently from the bacterial DNA. Because the plasmids contain a selectable marker (*antibiotic resistance gene*), bacteria that have received the plasmid can be selected for with the appropriate antibiotic, allowing growth only of transformants. Large quantities of plasmid DNA can then be isolated from the transformed bacteria and the foreign fragment reexcised from the vector.

artificial chromosomes (YACs), bacterial artificial chromosomes (BACs), and P1-based artificial chromosomes (PACs).

Polymerase Chain Reaction

Although cloning is an extremely effective method with which to generate large quantities of specific DNA fragments, the process can be quite time consuming, tedious, and difficult. In the mid-1980s, Kary Mullis developed a technique called the polymerase chain reaction (PCR) that allows production of large quantities of specific DNA sequences in a single tube within a few hours.[34,42,43] This technique has revolutionized molecular genetics and spawned the development of numerous new approaches for the identification and characterization of genes involved in tumorigenesis and for studying some particular aspects of tumor phenotype.

The reaction exploits several features of DNA replication (Fig. 26.6). The template for synthesis of a new complementary DNA strand is a single-stranded DNA molecule. Single-stranded templates can be generated simply by heating double-stranded DNA to near boiling temperature (95°C). DNA polymerases require a small section of double-stranded DNA to initiate or "prime" synthesis of the new strand. New DNA synthesis is unidirectional, incorporating nucleotides in the 5′ → 3′ direction on the new strand. Consequently, the starting point for new DNA synthesis can be specified by choosing a short

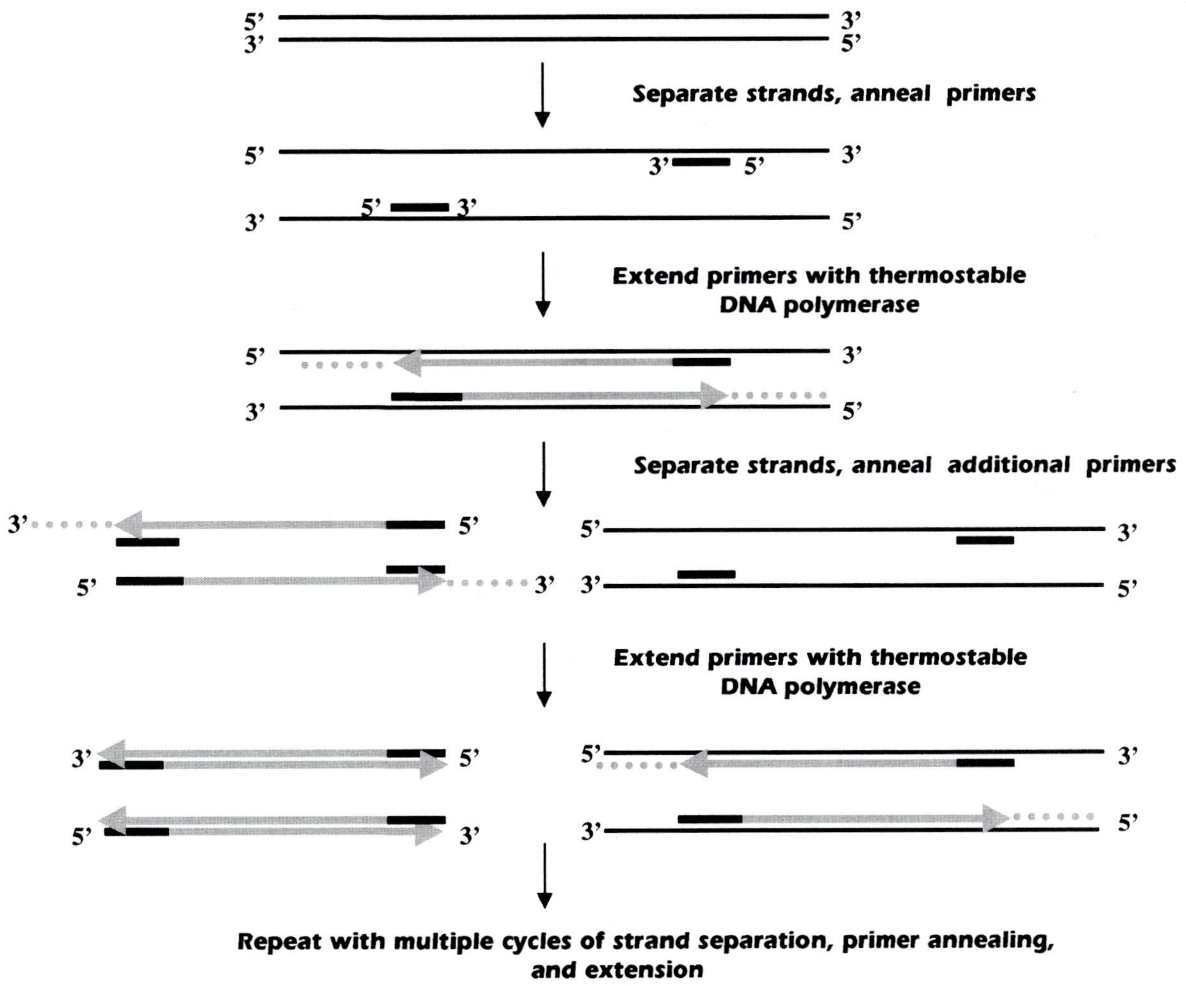

Fig. 26.6. The polymerase chain reaction. PCR provides another method with which to generate essentially unlimited quantities of specific DNA fragments. In a basic PCR experiment, the DNA template is denatured by heating at near-boiling temperature to *separate* the two strands. The temperature of the reaction in then reduced to allow short oligonucleotide primers (15–25 nucleotides) to *anneal* to each individual strand through complementary *base pairing.* The primers must be of opposite orientation with their 3′-ends facing each other. A thermostable DNA polymerase is then used to *extend* the DNA sequence from each primer in the 5′ to 3′ direction. The newly synthesized double-stranded DNA molecules can then be denatured again and subjected to multiple cycles of PCR, such that the desired DNA fragment is synthesized in an exponential fashion.

complementary oligonucleotide *primer* (usually 15–25 base pairs) that, at lower temperatures, anneals to the single-stranded DNA template at the specific initiation site. Because both strands of the melted double-stranded DNA can serve as templates for new DNA synthesis, primers can be chosen such that new double-stranded DNA molecules are formed in the region of DNA between the two-oligonucleotide primers. These new double-stranded molecules can be melted with high temperature and the cycle repeated, allowing synthesis of the specific segment of DNA in an exponential fashion. In other words, the net result of PCR is that at the end of n cycles the reaction tube will contain a theoretical maximum of 2^n double-stranded molecules representing copies of the sequence specified by the two primers.

Identification of heat-stable DNA polymerases, such as the *Taq* polymerase isolated from the bacterium *Thermus aquaticus*, greatly simplified PCR because it eliminated the need to add polymerase during the synthesis of each new DNA strand. As with other techniques, PCR is not without some drawbacks, which include: (1) limitation of the size of the amplified products to a maximum of several thousand base pairs, (2) occasional incorporation of incorrect nucleotides into the newly synthesized DNA, (3) nonspecific priming from regions of DNA partially complementary to the PCR primers, and (4) extreme sensitivity, which can cause difficulties in distinguishing between low signal and sample-to-sample contamination.

Nevertheless, PCR has opened the door to myriad new lines of laboratory investigation, certainly not limited to studies of tumor genetics. Of particular relevance to pathologists is that template DNA for PCR can be obtained from a variety of sources, including fresh and frozen tissues, blood and body fluids containing cellular material (e.g., urine, ascites, cerebrospinal fluid), and fixed, paraffin-embedded archival material. PCR also obviates the need for large quantities of template DNA: even DNA from single cells can serve as a template for PCR.

PCR-based methods have largely supplanted Southern blot analyses for the detection of losses of heterozygosity in tumors. *Microsatellites* consist of approximately 10–50 copies of 1- to 6-bp motifs that can occur in perfect tandem repetition, or less frequently, as imperfect (interrupted) repeats or together with another repeat type.[49] There are an estimated 100,000+ microsatellites distributed throughout the human genome, many of which have been mapped to specific chromosomal regions. Microsatellites typically demonstrate a high level of polymorphism or allelic variation in the number of repeat units. Hence it is relatively easy to identify microsatellite loci in specific chromosomal regions for which a given patient is informative.

With the human genome project nearing completion, even more microsatellite loci and other types of genetic polymorphisms will be characterized. For LOH analyses, forward and reverse PCR primers flanking a specific microsatellite are used to amplify DNA from a given patient's tumor and matched nonneoplastic tissues. The length of the PCR products (typically radio- or fluorescent labeled) are then evaluated by manual or automated electrophoresis. If the patient is informative at the locus, the PCR products generated from the maternally and paternally derived alleles present in DNA from their nonneoplastic cells will be of different lengths. Matched tumor DNA shows loss of one of the two alleles if LOH is present (Fig. 26.7).

PCR-based amplification of microsatellites can also be used to demonstrate a phenotype of some tumors, referred to as *microsatellite instability*, which is discussed in greater detail later. In short, microsatellite instability is a type of genomic instability that is reflected, in part, as alterations in the length of microsatellite sequences in tumor DNA when compared to matched normal DNA. Microsatellite instability is scored as upward or downward shifts in the size of PCR products generated with primers flanking the microsatellite sequence (Fig. 26.8).

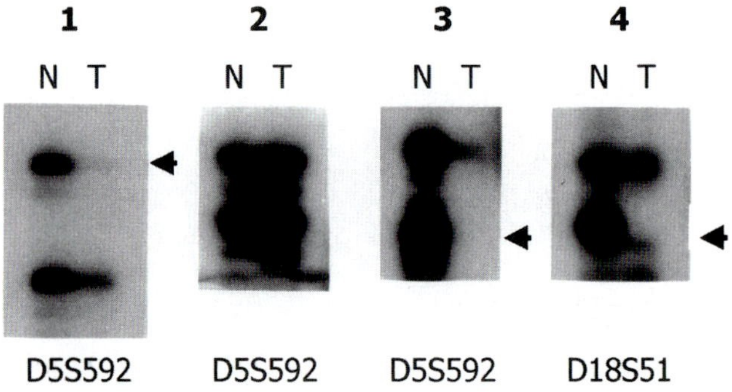

Fig. 26.7. Analysis of loss of heterozygosity (LOH) by PCR. Representative cases (1–4) were analyzed at microsatellite loci *D5S592* and *D18S51*. In each case, PCR was used to amplify the indicated microsatellite locus in DNA isolated from matched normal tissue (*N*) and tumor tissue (*T*). Radiolabeled PCR products were then evaluated by gel electrophoresis and autoradiography. All cases are informative at the loci shown because two alleles are distinguishable in normal tissue. Tumors from cases 1, 3, and 4 show loss of heterozygosity at the indicated microsatellite locus (*arrows*), whereas case 2 shows retention of both D5S592 alleles in the tumor DNA.

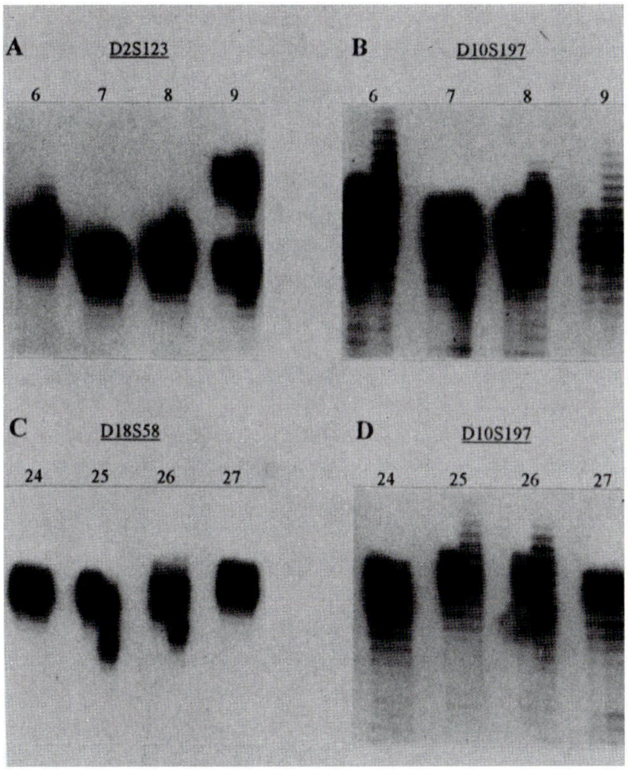

Fig 26.8. Microsatellite instability. Microsatellite instability is manifested as alterations in the length of microsatellite DNA sequences in tumor DNA when compared to matched normal DNA. Representative cases (*6–9* and *24–27*) were analyzed at the microsatellite loci specified above each panel. Each case is represented by paired sample lanes, normal (*left*) and tumor (*right*). PCR was used to amplify the indicated microsatellite locus in DNA isolated from matched normal and tumor tissue, and radiolabeled PCR products were then analyzed by gel electrophoresis and autoradiography. *Cases 6, 8,* and *9* (**A, B**) show tumor DNA with upward shifts (larger alleles) at both the *D2S123* and *D10S197* loci. Cases *25* and *26* (**C, D**) show tumor DNA with downward shifts (smaller alleles) at locus *D18258* and larger alleles at locus *D10S197*. (Reproduced with permission from Oncogene, ref. 4.)

Sequencing

Some genetic alterations that occur during tumorigenesis are subtle, involving only single nucleotide insertions, deletions, or substitutions at critical positions within a gene. Such mutations may occur in the coding region (missense and nonsense mutations), whereas others affect sequences that direct splicing of the initial RNA transcript (*splice site mutations*) or portions of the gene that regulate transcription. Both *oncogenes* and *tumor suppressor genes* can be altered by point mutations, and it is often desirable to characterize the specific mutations that occur within tumors. To sequence the region of interest, large quantities of the specific region are first generated through cloning or with PCR.

The most commonly used sequencing methods today are modifications of the one originally described by Sanger.[44] This technique capitalizes on several of the same features of DNA replication described for PCR. Again, double-stranded DNA is melted to single strands under the appropriate conditions, followed by annealing of a specific oligonucleotide primer to the strand to be sequenced. DNA polymerase is then added to the reaction and allowed to incorporate radiolabeled nucleotides into the newly synthesized strand in the $5' \rightarrow 3'$ direction. However, the nucleotides in a single reaction tube include small quantities of individual modified nucleotides (dideoxy A, C, G, or T) that terminate DNA chain elongation at the corresponding nucleotide. On inactivation of the polymerase, the reaction tube contains a series of radiolabeled DNA strands terminated at various positions along the DNA template determined by the specific chain terminator chosen. For example, a reaction containing dideoxy ATPs will contain a distribution of newly synthesized strands of varying lengths, each terminated at different (A) residues. For every template, the products of four separate reactions, each containing a different dideoxy nucleotide, can be analyzed on high-resolution polyacrylamide gels. After autoradiography, a ladder of bands is identified that displays the DNA sequence of the original template read from bottom to top (Fig. 26.9, right panel).

When analyzing gene mutations in DNA isolated from primary tumors, it is important to keep in mind that, unlike cultured tumor cell lines, primary tumors are invariably "contaminated" with normal cells. In addition, an individual gene mutation usually affects only one of the two alleles present in a given tumor cell. The other allele may be *wild type* (the "normal" genotype typically found in nature), may be deleted, or may have sustained a separate independent mutation. An individual clone of a segment of DNA can, by definition, represent only one allele. For example, if the original sample contains 80% tumor cells and 20% normal cells, and only one allele of the target gene is mutated in the tumor cells, only 40% of the target sequence clones will be derived from mutant alleles. Thus, most sequence analyses are performed on templates that reflect the relative contribution of all alleles in a given sample (e.g., PCR products or pools of cloned products: Fig. 26.9, left panel) rather than on individual clones, which may have been derived from normal rather than mutant alleles. Sanger's original sequencing method has been modified to allow both partially

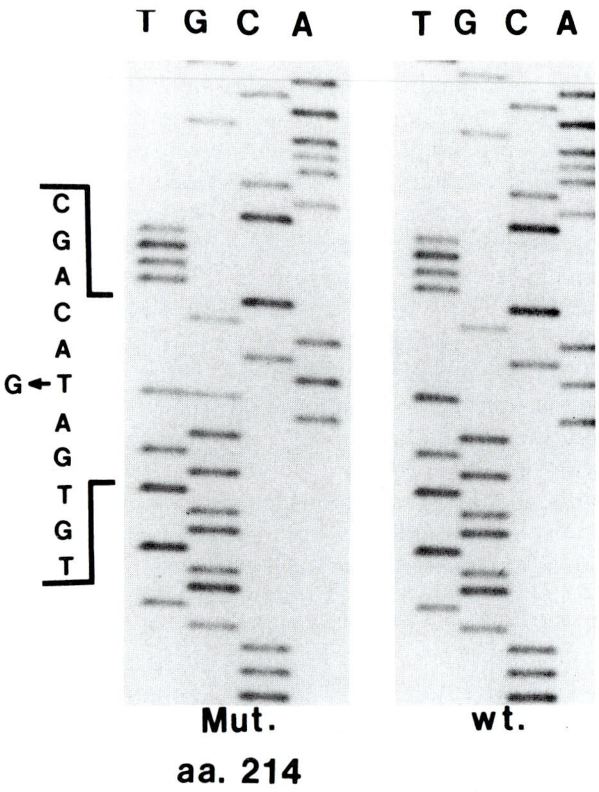

Fig. 26.9. DNA sequencing (Sanger method). DNA sequence analysis is used often to detect subtle sequence alterations such as gene mutations in human tumors. Most mutations are acquired somatically (are not present in the patient's normal/germline DNA). *Right panel* (wild type, *wt.*): Sequence of the p53 gene in DNA isolated from the patient's normal myometrium. *Left panel* (mutant, *Mut.*): Sequence of the *p53* gene in DNA isolated from the same patient's cervical carcinoma. In addition to the band in the *T* lane seen in normal DNA, the tumor DNA contains a new parallel band in the *G* lane, indicating a T to G point mutation at codon 214 of the *p53* gene. The residual band in the *T* lane may represent the contribution of DNA from normal cells contaminating the original sample or from the wild-type copy of *p53* in the tumor cells. (Reprinted with permission from the American Journal of Pathology, ref. 21.)

and fully automated PCR-based sequencing of fluorescent rather than radiolabeled DNA. As a consequence, high-throughput sequencing efforts are now commonplace.

Methods of RNA Analysis

Mutations in the DNA of tumor cells are of consequence only if they affect the function of the proteins encoded by the mutant genes. Many gene mutations lead to alterations of gene expression reflected at the RNA as well as protein level. For example, amplification of the *HER-2/neu* oncogene frequently identified in ovarian carcinomas results in its overexpression, with increases in both *Her-2/neu* RNA and protein.[46] In contrast, deletions of the FHIT gene in many cervical carcinomas is often associated with marked reduction of FHIT RNA and protein levels in the tumor cells.[3,14,50,51] Several techniques have been developed with which to analyze RNA levels in normal and neoplastic tissues. A few commonly used methods are described next.

Northern Blotting

Using straightforward extraction techniques, total cellular RNA can be isolated from the tissues to be studied. Total cellular RNA consists of ribosomal, transfer, and messenger RNA. As only 2–5% of total RNA is mRNA, it may be desirable to enrich the total RNA sample for mRNA. This enrichment may be accomplished by selection for RNA molecules with polyadenylated 3′-ends [poly(A) RNA], which are added only to mRNA molecules after transcription. The total cellular or poly(A)-enriched RNA is then size separated by electrophoresis through agarose gels. As in a Southern blot, the RNA is transferred from the gel to a solid matrix such as nylon membrane, then hybridized to a gene-specific probe (DNA, RNA, or oligonucleotide). Autoradiography results in bands whose relative intensity reflects levels of RNA specific for the gene detected by the probe (Fig. 26.10). When comparing signal intensity between two or more samples, it is important that equal quantities of RNA are loaded in each lane. To control for RNA integrity and equal loading, Northern blot analyses often include hybridization to probes detecting highly expressed genes, such as actin or glyceraldehyde phosphate dehydrogenase (GPDH), whose expression remains relatively constant, regardless of tissue type or other factors.

Reverse Transcriptase PCR

Northern blotting is an effective method to study expression of specific genes. However, the technique is limited to analysis of genes with relatively high expression levels and requires fairly large quantities of fresh tissue as a source of intact, undegraded RNA. Again, the discovery of PCR has led to the development of gene expression assays that capitalize on the tremendous sensitivity of PCR and its applicability to even minute tissue samples. The *reverse transcriptase PCR* (*RT-PCR*) method takes advantage of normal mRNA processing. As discussed earlier, the initial RNA transcript is an RNA copy of the DNA-coding strand. However, gene-specific expression is reflected in RNA molecules that have undergone splicing (joining of exons with removal of

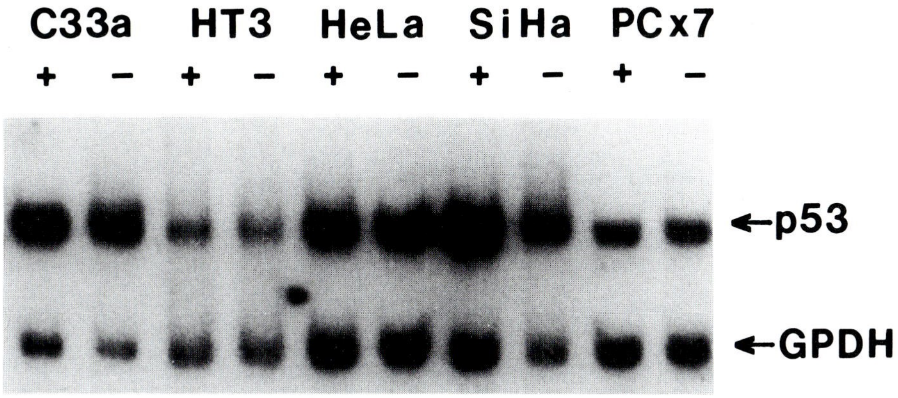

Fig. 26.10. Northern blot. Northern blot analysis is a method used to analyze gene expression and alterations of gene expression in tumor cells. An example is shown in which a blot of total RNA isolated from several cervical carcinoma cell lines has been hybridized to a radiolabeled *p53* gene probe and a *GPDH* (glyceraldehyde phosphate dehydrogenase) gene control probe. *Lanes labeled* (+) represent RNA from irradiated tumor cells, whereas *lanes labeled* (−) represent RNA from untreated cells. Irradiation does not appear to alter *p53* gene expression at the RNA level because the intensity of bands detected by the *p53* probe is the same in the irradiated and untreated samples when normalized to the intensity of the signal from the control probe.

intronic sequences). Using an enzyme called reverse transcriptase isolated from certain RNA tumor viruses, DNA copies (*complementary DNAs* or *cDNAs*) of the RNA molecules present in total RNA can be synthesized in vitro. This cDNA can be used as a template for PCR using primers specific for the gene of interest. If primers are chosen from two different exons within the target gene, the size of the PCR product generated by amplification of spliced templates (expressed sequences) will be smaller than that generated from unspliced templates or from genomic DNA (Fig. 26.11). In fact, primers may be spread out so far on genomic DNA that amplification cannot occur at all. As with Northern blotting, it is helpful to amplify the same samples using primers for genes with little variation of gene expression to control for quantity and integrity of the starting material.

In Situ Hybridization

When applied to the study of primary tissues, Northern blotting and RT-PCR evaluate specific gene expression in pools of cells that usually reflect some combination of tumor cells and associated nonneoplastic cells. Furthermore, these methods are not easily applied to studying variations of gene expression within a given lesion or within different cell types of a tissue sample. A method called in situ hybridization allows detection of specific gene expression in individual cells within the context of the tissue as a whole. The principles of this method are straightforward. Sections of the tissue to be studied are cut and mounted on glass slides. The sections are then hybridized to labeled nucleic acid probes specific for the gene being studied, under conditions that allow the probes to anneal to complementary mRNA anywhere in the tissue section. Subsequent detection of hybridized probes (autoradiography for radiolabeled probes or colorimetric or fluorescence detection for nonradioactive probes) with counterstaining of the tissue sample allows microscopic localization of the signal to individual cells. The in situ hybridization method also can be used to detect DNA in tissues. For example, type-specific DNA probes can be used to detect human papillomavirus DNA in cervical biopsies and exfoliated cervical cells.

Methods of Protein Analysis

Gene mutations and alterations of RNA expression in tumor cells achieve significance only through their effects on the function of the proteins that they encode. As a result of genetic alterations, proteins may be overexpressed, underexpressed, or expressed as mutant forms with aberrant function. Several laboratory techniques have been developed that allow detection of specific proteins in neoplastic and normal cells. Essentially all these techniques use antibodies directed at the target protein as part of the detection scheme.

Immunohistochemistry

To most pathologists, immunohistochemical staining is the most familiar assay of protein detection in tissues. A detailed discussion of the technique and

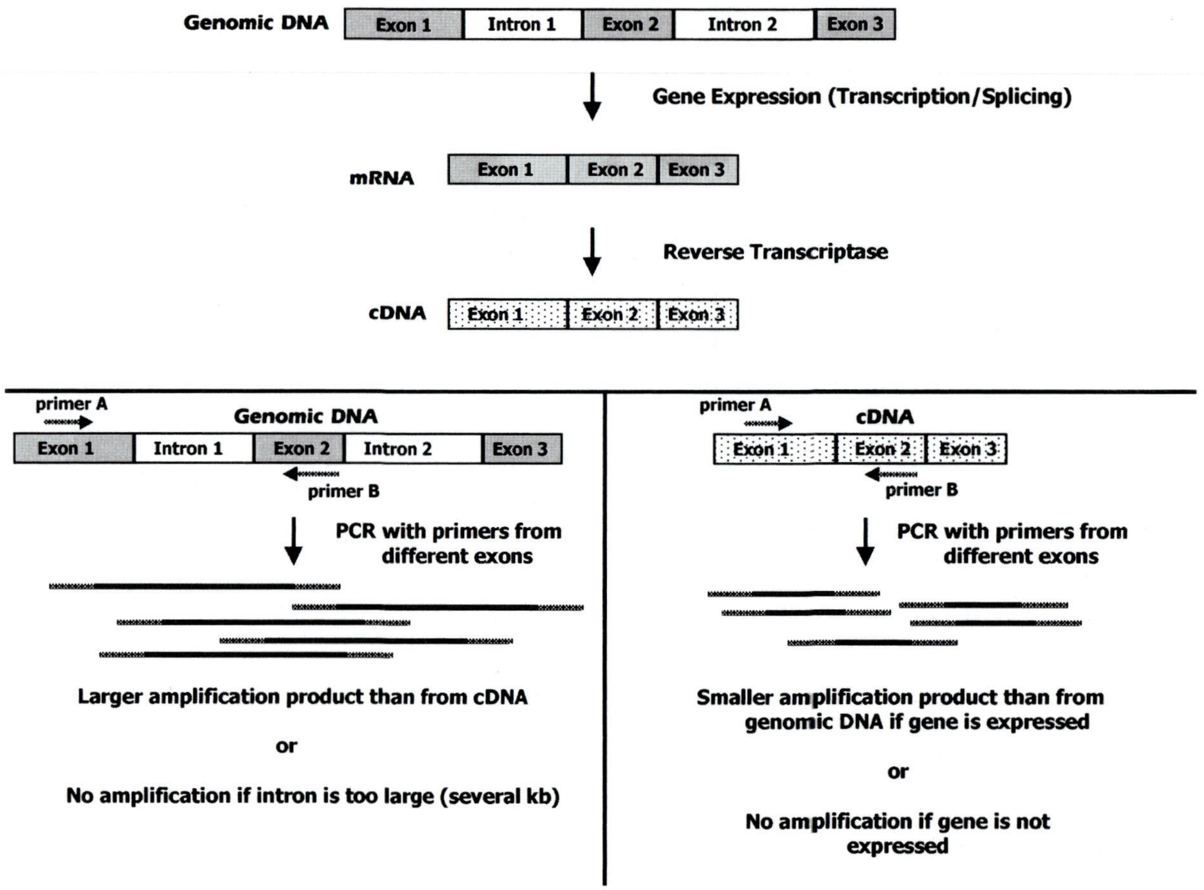

Fig. 26.11. Reverse transcriptase PCR. RT-PCR is an extremely sensitive assay for gene expression. After *transcription* of a gene, the initial RNA transcript undergoes *splicing*. Thus, in mRNA, exons are spliced together and intronic sequences are excluded. A complementary DNA molecule (cDNA) can be synthesized by the enzyme *reverse transcriptase*, using mRNA as the template. This cDNA, which also excludes introns, can then be used as a template for PCR in which primers are chosen from within different exons. If the gene is expressed, the two exons should be close enough together in the cDNA to allow amplification of a sequence of predicted size. Because genomic DNA contains introns, the PCR product will be longer than that from cDNA. Alternatively, the primers may be spread so far apart (introns can be several hundred kilobases [*kb*] or more) that amplification cannot occur at all. The size of the PCR products can be determined by gel electrophoresis.

its many applications to gynecologic pathology is well beyond the scope of this chapter. Immunohistochemistry is used widely as a diagnostic and research tool. Like in situ hybridization, immunohistochemistry allows detection of specific molecules in individual cells within the context of the tissue as a whole as well as their subcellular localization (e.g., nuclear, cytoplasmic, or membrane bound). Furthermore, it does not require the use of radioactive reagents. The technique is based on the formation of specific antigen–antibody complexes and their subsequent detection within the tissue section. The method can provide important information about the expression of specific proteins in tissue samples, from which one can infer a great deal about the phenotype and, in some cases, genotype of the cells of interest.

Although pathologists are accustomed to using immunohistochemical detection of specific proteins to characterize the type and extent of cellular differentiation, aberrant levels of protein expression can also reflect alterations of the corresponding gene within tumor cells. For example, overexpression of *Her-2/neu* often reflects gene amplification, and diffuse overexpression of *p53* often correlates with the presence of a missense mutation of the gene.[46,48] Not surprisingly, the technique has some limitations. Immunohistochemical staining does not yield more than semiquantitative protein expression data, and available antibodies may lack sensitivity or specificity in immunohistochemical applications. Some antibodies may be suitable for only fresh-frozen rather than formalin-fixed tissues. Hence, in some circumstances, other methods of protein detection may be more appropriate.

Immunoblotting (Western Blotting)

This technique combines the specificity of immunochemical detection with the resolution of gel electrophoresis. Immunoblotting can be used to determine the presence, quantity, and size of a target protein. Thus, tumors can be analyzed for changes in protein levels or the presence of mutant (e.g., truncated) forms. Typically, an unlabeled solution of proteins (usually an extract of cells or tissue) is prepared in gel electrophoresis sample buffer. The proteins are then size fractionated by electrophoresis through a polyacrylamide gel, followed by electrophoretic transfer of the proteins to a membrane. Nonspecific binding sites are first blocked, then the location of specific antigens is determined using a labeled antibody specific for the target. In some cases, specific protein is detected with unlabeled primary antibody followed by incubation with radiolabeled secondary antibody or secondary antibody conjugated to moieties allowing nonradioactive colorimetric or chemical detection. These latter methods often result in signal amplification and enhanced detection sensitivity. A major factor determining the success of an immunoblotting assay is the nature of the epitopes recognized by the antibodies. The high-resolution gel electrophoresis techniques required to separate proteins typically involve denaturation of the proteins in the sample. Thus, only epitopes resistant to denaturation are recognized by the antibodies. In addition, the target protein must be present in sufficient quantities for detection (approximately 1 part per 150,000).[17]

Immunoprecipitation

This method also combines the specificity of the antigen–antibody interaction with the resolution of gel electrophoresis. Both immunoblotting and immunoprecipitation evaluate protein expression in pools of cells rather than in individual cells. Typically, the target protein and other cellular proteins are radioactively labeled in vivo by growing cells in the presence of a labeled precursor such as a radioactive amino acid. The labeled proteins are then extracted from cells in an appropriate buffer and incubated with specific antibodies under conditions that allow formation of immune complexes between the antibody and antigen of interest. A solid-phase matrix containing staphylococcal protein A (which binds the Fc portion of antibodies) is added and allowed to adsorb the immune complexes. Unbound proteins are removed by washing the solid phase, leaving the purified antibody–antigen complex bound to the matrix. The purified complexes can be eluted from the matrix, then analyzed by gel electrophoresis to determine protein presence, size, and quantity.

Variations of this method also may be used to study the rate of synthesis or degradation of specific proteins, interactions with other cellular macromolecules, and the presence or absence of some posttranslational modifications. The appropriate choice of protein detection methods is determined by several factors, including the type of information sought, the nature of the specific antigen–antibody interaction, and availability of reagents. In practice, the best method of analyzing specific proteins in specific cell types often is determined empirically.

Methods for the Molecular Profiling of Tumors

Although studies of specific genetic alterations in human cancers have led to tremendous insights into the process by which tumors develop and progress, most have been time-consuming and often tedious analyses focused on only a few of the most common gene mutations. More recently, a number of tools allowing comprehensive molecular profiling of tumors have been developed that allow more global evaluation of the DNA, RNA, and protein of tumor cells. In addition to providing important information on the molecular basis of cancer, it is expected that comprehensive molecular analyses may lead to the development of new tumor classification schemes that are more clinically informative than those that are based on morphologic assessment alone. At the very least, one can expect that molecular information will be used to augment existing tumor classification systems, with the hope of allowing better prediction of the clinical course of an individual cancer patient. A selection of molecular profiling tools is briefly described next. The purpose of the discussion is to provide the reader with a sense of the type of information these tools can provide rather than a comprehensive review of what is currently available, particularly in light of the remarkable rapidity with which these technologies are evolving.

Comparative Genome Hybridization

Comparative genome hybridization (CGH) is a powerful cytogenetic technique that allows comprehensive and simultaneous analysis of an entire genome for changes in DNA sequence copy number.[11,20] CGH analysis of DNA from an individual tumor specimen results in a map of those chromosomal regions that are over- and/or underrepresented compared to normal DNA. Because DNA copy number changes (i.e., gains and losses of specific chromosomal regions) are known to contribute to the pathogenesis of cancer, CGH has emerged as an important tool in cancer research.

The technique is based on a modification of in situ hybridization, in which differentially labeled sample and reference DNAs are cohybridized to normal metaphase spreads. For example, tumor DNA can be labeled for green fluorescence while normal DNA is labeled for red fluorescence. Following cohybridization to normal metaphase chromosomes, copy number differences between the tumor and normal DNA samples are scored as green–red fluorescence intensity differences on each chromosome using a digital image analysis system. DNA gains (such as extra chromosomes or amplification of specific chromosomal regions) result in increased fluorescence ratios (more green) and losses of whole or portions of chromosomes result in reduced ratios (more red). In general, the technique can detect changes when the size of the affected chromosomal region is larger than 5–10 megabases, although smaller regions can be detected if highly amplified.

Expression Profiling Using cDNA and Oligonucleotide Microarrays

The nearly completed sequence of the human genome has yielded important information about the composition of the genome in human cells. However, it is important to keep in mind that only a subset (approximately 10,000) of the roughly 50,000 genes are expressed in a cell at any given time.[36] As discussed earlier, gene expression differences are largely responsible for the vast array of phenotypes displayed by both normal and neoplastic cells. The traditional gene-by-gene approach to studying expression differences between cell populations is clearly insufficient for understanding the complexities of gene expression patterns responsible for the incredible diversity displayed by cells of complex organisms. Array technologies offer the means with which to conduct genome-wide expression analyses of individual samples and are likely to become standard tools for both research and clinical diagnostics.[1,6,7,22,23,28,39] These technologies have been made possible by the public availability of expressed sequence tag (EST) or cDNA sequences corresponding to a large fraction of the total number of human genes, the ability to generate high-density sequence arrays on solid substrates ("chips") such as glass slides, and improved technologies for fluorescence labeling of cDNAs.

Two basic types of microarrays have been described. In the first, an "arrayer" is used to robotically spot cloned cDNAs or ESTs onto a glass slide so that each position in the array grid is occupied by a specific sequence. At present, as many as 25,000 cDNAs can be deposited on a single slide. In the second approach, a process called photolithography is used to synthesize oligonucleotides representing specific expressed sequences directly onto a glass slide in a predesignated array. Oligonucleotide arrays can be made at even higher density, with as many as 300,000 oligonucleotides arrayed in an area greater than 2 cm^2.[22] In both cases, the microarrays are hybridized to probes made from fluorescently labeled cDNA generated from the mRNA of the tissue or cell population being studied. Differentially labeled probes made from two samples being compared (e.g., tumor versus normal tissue) can be cohybridized to the microarray and the resulting relative fluorescence at each location on the microarray measured using a computer-controlled laser confocal fluorescent microscope.

Powerful computer packages are then used to formulate and integrate quantitative data from the huge numbers of hybridizations performed on a single slide, ultimately yielding comprehensive gene expression profiles of the samples. A series of samples can be sequentially analyzed and compared to one another by normalization to the same reference probe. Clearly, a major challenge to those employing these technologies has been the development of data management tools capable of handling these vast quantities of data and identifying effective strategies with which to mine the data for biologically important information. One commonly used strategy employs statistical algorithms such as pairwise average-linkage cluster analysis to arrange genes and/or samples according to similarity in the pattern of gene expression.[9] This type of analysis yields a hierarchical clustering of genes or samples based on similarity of their expression patterns.

Proteomics

As noted earlier, proteins, and not nucleic acids, are the primary effector molecules in cells. Notably, mRNA expression levels are not always predictive of corresponding protein expression, and posttranslational modifications such as phosphorylation, glycosylation, and acetylation can have major effects on protein function. Needless to say, there is a great deal of interest in elucidating the function of individual proteins as well as understanding the complex patterns of protein expression in different cell populations. Proteomics, or the analysis of global protein expression profiles in cells, has been in existence since the late 1970s.[36] To date, protein expression profiling has relied primarily on the use of two-dimensional gel electrophoresis (2D-GE) to simultaneously display a large number (well over 1000) of the most abundantly expressed proteins in a given cell population, followed by the identification of individual protein spots. Proteins are typically separated along a pH gradient in the first dimension and by size in the second dimension. One of the unique features of proteomics is the ability to analyze posttranslational modifications of proteins. Comparison of normalized spot intensity in gels from different samples allows assessment of relative protein expression in the samples being analyzed. Over the years, many spots have been catalogued into shared databases of expressed proteins; however, the general approach has been hampered by relatively poor reproducibility of 2D-GE conditions between laboratories and lack of sensitive and rapid analytical methods for protein identification.

Several major factors have resulted in a resurgence of interest in proteomics. The near-completion of the human genome project is allowing genes (and hence proteins) to be predicted from genomic data. In addition, advanced mass spectrometric methods have been developed that can rapidly identify small quantities of proteins with relative ease. Finally, bioinformatics tools comparable to those used for analysis of huge microarray data sets can be applied to protein expression profiling data, allowing researchers to mine the data for biologically important relationships between groups of proteins and samples. High-throughput methods for protein expression profiling that obviate the need for 2D-GE are currently in development and will likely be widely available in the next few years.

Tissue Microarrays

As described earlier, a great deal of effort is being expended toward identifying proteins that are differentially expressed among different types of cells, tumors, or tumor subsets to identify those that can serve as useful markers of specific cellular phenotypes. With respect to cancer, there is great interest in identifying biomarkers with diagnostic, prognostic, or therapeutic importance. Validation of the utility of such markers may require evaluation of that marker's expression in hundreds, or even thousands, of appropriately selected tumors at different stages of disease. Unlike immortalized cells in culture, primary tissue resources are limited and must be used more judiciously.

Recently, methods have been developed for arraying large numbers of tissue samples on a single glass slide to allow high-throughput molecular profiling of primary tumor specimens.[27] These tissue microarrays, which can include as many as 1000 individual tumors, are suitable for both in situ hybridization and immunohistochemical staining. To generate a tissue microarray, a morphologically representative cylindrical core "biopsy" (usually 6 mm in diameter) is taken from a paraffin block of fixed tissue from each tumor and arrayed into a new "recipient" paraffin block. Sections can then be cut from the microarray block for parallel detection of specific DNA, RNA, or protein in all specimens represented in the array. Consecutive sectioning of the microarray block can allow rapid analysis of many biomarker candidates (potentially hundreds) in the same set of specimens. Although the very small tissue samples may not be completely representative of heterogeneous tumors, arrays can be designed that include multiple core biopsies from any given tumor. This technology is likely to prove quite powerful for candidate biomarker validation.

Transferring Genes into Mammalian Cells (Transfection)

Research on the genetic basis of cancer has led to the identification and cloning of several cancer-related genes, including numerous oncogenes and tumor suppressor genes. However, many studies aimed at determining the function of altered genes and their normal counterparts require introduction of these genes into living cells. For instance, the effects of activated oncogene expression in normal cells and tumor suppressor gene expression in tumor cells can be studied with gene transfer experiments. Several techniques have been developed that allow expression of exogenous genes in living cells maintained in cell culture. More recently, sophisticated methods have been devised that permit investigators to introduce new genes or alter existing genes in intact animals. These advances have greatly enhanced our ability to model numerous human diseases in the laboratory.

The most common means of introducing exogenous genes into mammalian cells involves cloning the gene of interest into a plasmid vector that is then delivered into the cytoplasm of recipient cells using any of several techniques. Alternatively, viral vectors containing the gene of interest are used to infect host cells. Most vectors contain a selectable marker such as antibiotic resistance, which allows efficient selection of cells that have received the exogenous construct. Expression of the cloned gene is typically driven by an upstream promoter present in the vector. The choice of promoter can determine whether the exogenous gene is constitutively expressed or expressed only in certain cell types or under certain conditions. Depending on the transfection method used, the type of vector, and the type of recipient cells, exogenous DNA can be introduced into a large percentage of host cells. However, for many vectors, only a few (1 in 10^3–10^6) transfected cells incorporate (integrate) the exogenous DNA stably into the host genome. The remaining cells fail to integrate the DNA, which disappears from these cells in a matter of days. During this period, the transfected cells transiently express the exogenous gene using the host's transcriptional machinery. Selection for appropriate antibiotic resistance yields clones of cells that have stably integrated the expression construct and which are capable of expressing the exogenous gene indefinitely. More specialized gene delivery systems have been developed that allow tightly regulated conditional expression of exogenous genes. Such systems are particularly useful for studying genes that are lethal or toxic when constitutively expressed or for studying the immediate consequences of expression of a particular gene.

Genetic Linkage and Mapping

Inherited predispositions to particular tumor types result from germline mutations in specific genes. For example, the genes responsible for some forms of familial ovarian cancer, breast cancer, endometrial cancer, neurofibromatosis, retinoblastoma, Wilms' tumor, adenomatous polyposis coli, hereditary nonpolyposis colorectal cancer, and several other cancer types already have been identified and cloned. To localize disease genes to particular chromosomes, researchers often study families with an inherited predisposition to that disease using a method called linkage analysis. Linkage describes the tendency of genetic loci to be inherited together as a result of their location on the same chromosome. When homologous chromosomes pair during meiosis, they exchange segments in a process called recombination. The farther apart on a chromosome two loci are, the greater the chance that recombination will occur between them. In contrast, if two loci are close together recombination between them will be rare. Loci on different chromosomes would be expected to segregate independently. As part of a linkage analysis, coinheritance of polymorphic markers and disease genes (manifested by the phenotype of individuals) are followed within a family, and the odds of their being inherited separately (unlinked or not on the same chromosome) versus together (linked or on the same chromosome) are calculated.

In short, evaluation of the inheritance patterns of multiple polymorphic markers with respect to each other, and to disease phenotype, can allow the assignment of disease genes to particular chromosomes and the generation of a map of marker order along that chromosome. Identification of markers more and more closely linked to a disease phenotype can lead ultimately to localization of genes responsible for specific diseases. The DNA of individuals affected by the particular disease can then be examined for the presence of germline mutations in the disease gene.

Basic Concepts of Cancer Genetics

Although our understanding of the molecular basis of human cancer has developed at a phenomenal pace over the past decade, it is now evident that this has been a mere prologue for what will transpire over the next several years. With the human genome project near completion and the rapid speed of technologic advances in both the academic and private sectors, there undoubtedly will be an explosion of information about the molecular foundation of human cancer. In response, this section of the chapter does not attempt to provide a detailed overview of cancer genetics. Instead, it summarizes some basic principles, as presently understood, in an attempt to provide a foundation for understanding molecular cancer genetics as it unfolds over time. For specific genetic alterations involved with individual tumor types, the reader can refer to the organ-based chapters found earlier in this volume.

There are two fundamental properties of most human tumors that are inextricably linked. First, tumors develop and progress through a multistep process, and second, they evolve from the clonal expansion of a single cell. Many lines of evidence have clearly demonstrated that human cancers arise through a series of independent events. Early epidemiologic studies of age-dependent tumor incidence indicated that the kinetics were dependent on the fifth or sixth power of elapsed time, suggesting that the tumors arose secondary to at least five or six independent and successive rate-limiting steps.[16] Not only did these studies highlight that multiple events were necessary to produce the neoplastic phenotype, but they also hinted at the second fundamental feature of human tumors, clonality.

These important features of tumors can be understood easily if an assumption is made about the growth of normal cells. To ensure homeostasis, the cell mass of normal tissues must be exquisitely regulated by complex cellular pathways controlling both cell proliferation and cell death; aberrations in these pathways may result in neoplastic transformation. Thus, the cell and its progeny that accumulate sufficient alterations in such pathways have a selective growth advantage compared to cells with intact regulatory pathways (Fig. 26.12). Although

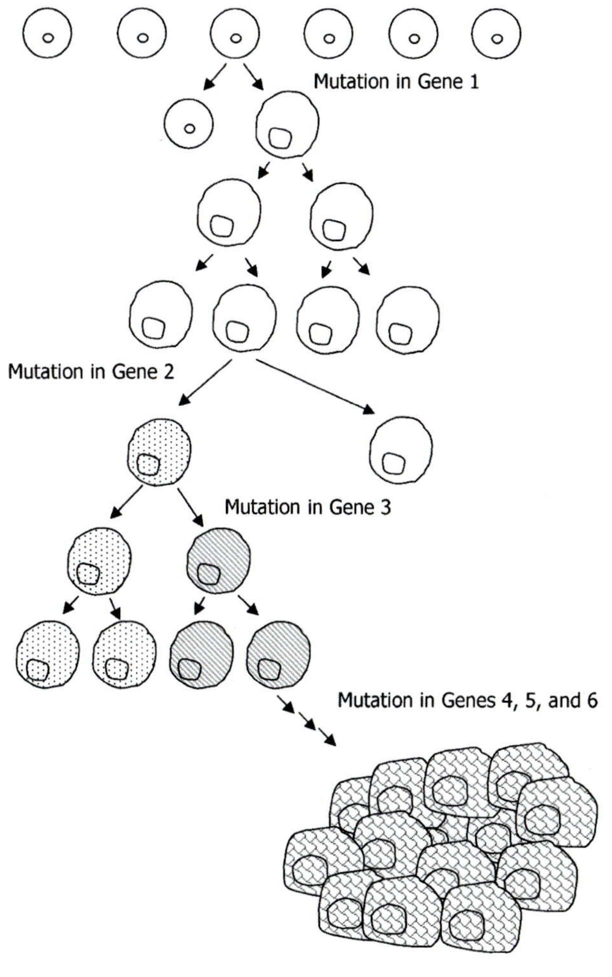

Fig. 26.12. Accumulation of genetic alterations and clonal selection during tumorigenesis. A single normal cell sustains a mutation in a gene that gives it a growth advantage over its normal counterparts. This cell continues to divide and one of its progeny undergoes a mutation in a second gene, which provides a further growth advantage. In a subsequent cell division, one of the daughter cells sustains a third mutation. Each mutation may confer a different type of selective advantage such as increased growth rate, loss of contact inhibition, decreased apoptosis, ability to invade, etc. The mutational process continues until a subpopulation of cells accumulates enough mutations in oncogenes and tumor suppressor genes to result in the fully transformed phenotype.

clonal selection was a reasonable hypothesis, until the molecular revolution that took place in cancer genetics, the nature of the biologic events underlying this multistep process of cell growth deregulation largely remained a mystery.

During the past two decades, molecular studies have confirmed both the clonal and multistep nature of human cancer. Specifically, studies have shown that the independent events critical in cancer development correspond to mutations in particular genes. As a result of successive mutations in these genes, there is a progressive loss of growth control within a single cell that ultimately, through clonal expansion, becomes a tumor. Most recently, cancer-causing genes have been divided into two major categories, (1) gatekeepers and (2) caretakers, albeit with some overlap.[24] The first category is by far the largest and consists of the widely recognized oncogenes and tumor suppressor genes. The products of these genes are involved in the regulation of cellular proliferation by controlling either cell renewal or cell death. Alterations in oncogenes and tumor suppressor genes are now thought to be involved in the development of the vast majority of human tumors.

In general, oncogenes result in an increase in cell growth while tumor suppressor genes, not surprisingly given their name, inhibit cell growth. The second class, which currently consists of a more limited number of genes, controls the rate of mutations. Thus, the products of these genes function as "caretakers" of the genome. Loss of a caretaker gene hastens the development of the transformed phenotype by accelerating the rate of mutations in gatekeeper genes. Clearly understanding the normal function of the proteins encoded by cancer-causing genes and how they contribute to the neoplastic process is critical to unraveling the etiology and pathogenesis of cancer.

For historical reasons, oncogenes are discussed first, as they were the first genes identified to play a role in the pathogenesis of human tumors. The term *oncogene* was initially coined for genes that are responsible for the transforming capabilities of cancer-causing viruses. Subsequently, normal human cells were found to contain genes that are very similar in sequence to the viral oncogenes. These cellular genes are referred to as *proto-oncogenes*, because they are not capable of transforming cells in their normal or wild-type state.[37] The proteins encoded by proto-oncogenes are thought to positively regulate normal cell growth. Typically, these genes cycle "on" and "off" in such a manner that the "on" state promotes cellular proliferation or inhibits cell death. Proto-oncogenes play a role in tumorigenesis when they are "activated" by a mutational event that alters the function of the gene product. When they are mutated to an active form, they become oncogenes.

The most common molecular mechanisms for activating proto-oncogenes are gene amplification, point mutation, and gene rearrangement. The activating mutations basically lead to the constant "on" state of the gene product, which provides the constant proliferative stimulus necessary in tumorigenesis. For this reason, oncogenes tend to behave in a "dominant" fashion, requiring the activation of only one copy of the gene while leaving the other copy of the gene in its wild-type state. Both amplification and rearrangement of oncogenes often lead to an increase in the number of their protein products, with a concomitant increase in protein functional activity. Gene amplification is created by overreplication of a specific portion of a chromosome such that multiple copies of the amplified gene are retained either on the chromosome or as extrachromosomal fragments. Gene amplification thus results in numerous copies of the proto-oncogene from which the product can be expressed. Chromosomal rearrangements increase gene expression by different mechanisms than gene amplification. For example, a chromosomal rearrangement can alter the expression of a proto-oncogene by replacing its normal regulatory region with one from a gene that is highly expressed, leading to increased expression of the proto-oncogene. In addition, chromosomal rearrangements can join the coding portions of two genes together, resulting in a hybrid product that is functionally overactive. Point mutations also can create products that are constitutively active by causing substitutions in critical amino acids of the protein.

Proto-oncogenes have been found to encode proteins that fall into four major classes based on their functions: these include *growth factors*, *growth factor receptors*, *cytoplasmic signal transduction molecules*, and *nuclear transcription factors* that regulate transcription of specific genes. Growth factors are secreted molecules that interact with growth factor receptors that are expressed on the cell surface. The interaction of these molecules sets in motion the transmission of a signal, via cytoplasmic signal transduction molecules, that ultimately reaches transcription factors in the cell nucleus. The transcription factors then activate transcription of the genes necessary for cellular proliferation, including those required for DNA synthesis. For any one of these classes it is easy to imagine how aberrations that lead to a constitutively active product would influence cellular proliferation. This classification also emphasizes the fact that normal cells have a variety of mechanisms operative throughout the cell to ensure growth control.

Tumor suppressor genes have been defined as genes whose protein products normally regulate cell proliferation in a negative manner; that is, it is loss of the normal function of their gene products that allows cells to escape growth regulation. Before tumor suppressor genes were identified and cloned, their possible existence was proposed based on the results of experiments in which tumor cells were fused with normal cells.[18] These studies demonstrated that tumor–normal hybrid cells lost many features of the transformed cells, suggesting that the normal cells provided functions that the tumor cells had lost. In addition, epidemiologic studies of retinoblastoma, a childhood eye tumor, led Knudson to propose what is now known as the "two-hit hypothesis," in which he suggested that the development of retinoblastoma requires two separate mutational events.[25,26] He posited that, in the dominantly inherited form of the disease, one mutation is inherited in the germline and the second occurs in somatic cells. In the nonhereditary form, both mutations occur in somatic cells. Cytogenetic studies of retinoblastomas revealed a consistent loss of genetic material on the long arm of chromosome 13, suggesting the presence of a gene responsible for the development of retinoblastoma.[12,31,35] The commonly deleted region was analyzed carefully, and a specific gene from within the deleted region was identified and named the retinoblastoma (Rb) gene.[13,30] In those tumors with 13q deletions removing one copy of the *Rb* gene, molecular studies showed that the second "hit" was the inactivation of the remaining normal copy of *Rb*. Hence, the other Rb allele usually is not lost by gross chromosomal deletion but is "functionally lost" by more subtle mutations that inactivate the gene product.[8] It is now recognized that deletion of the Rb-containing region of chromosome 13 is actually the second hit and the first hit is the inactivation of the other allele by intragenic mutation. Thus, the loss event typically follows, rather than precedes, the mutation. As predicted by Knudson's two-hit hypothesis, patients with early-onset or bilateral retinoblastomas have *Rb* gene mutations in their germline DNA, and in all of their somatic cells, one copy of the gene is mutant. These individuals require only one additional hit in the cell that will ultimately give rise to the tumor, and hence patients who inherit a mutant copy of the *Rb* gene inherit a predisposition to retinoblastoma. In contrast, the development of sporadic tumors requires two hits (each inactivating one copy of *Rb*) in a single cell, which is statistically much less likely. Knudson's hypothesis provides a plausible explanation for the early onset and bilaterality of retinoblastoma in the inherited form of the disease and the rarity of retinoblastoma in the general population. The finding that the target of the "second hit" was the other copy of the *Rb* gene correlated with the cell fusion studies suggesting that some cancer-causing genes behave in a "recessive" manner, requiring inactivation of both copies of the gene for the effects of the mutation(s) to be manifested.

Since the identification of the *Rb* gene, experimental studies have shown that its gene product plays a critical role in the regulation of the cell cycle and apoptosis.[15,33] Therefore, the loss of normal Rb function contributes to uncontrolled cell proliferation, an important feature of neoplastic cells. These molecular studies thus validated Knudson's hypothesis and provided important evidence for the existence of a class of genes whose "loss of function" contributes to the neoplastic phenotype. In addition, these experiments provided a paradigm that could be used to search for other candidate tumor suppressor genes. As mentioned earlier, during the development of retinoblastomas, one copy of the *Rb* gene typically is inactivated through deletion of the portion of chromosome 13 that contains the *Rb* gene. The example provided by retinoblastomas suggests that such regions of loss would target the location of tumor suppressor genes. In other words, identification of chromosomal regions frequently deleted in a specific tumor type presumably would allow localization of suppressor gene candidates important in the development of those tumors. Although the functions of most tumor suppressor gene products remain incompletely characterized, it is apparent that they will, like oncogenes, have diverse roles in the control of cell proliferation. In addition, it is important to recognize that many tumor suppressor genes are inherited in a mutant form and are responsible for a number of inherited cancer predisposition syndromes.

The second class of cancer-causing genes, the caretaker genes, consists of a number of different types of genes with the unifying function of preventing cells from fixing mutations in the genome created by either endogenous or exogenous mechanisms. Many of the genes in this class are also associated with inherited diseases in which the early onset of tumors is a prominent feature. Although the function of many of these gene products is not well understood, it is clear that their loss of function leads to genomic instability. DNA mismatch repair (MMR) genes are included in this class and their functions are relatively well understood. In addition, MMR genes are responsible for hereditary nonpolyposis colorectal cancer (HNPCC), a relatively common family cancer syndrome. For these reasons, MMR genes are briefly discussed as an example of this class of genes. MMR genes were first identified in humans based on a phenotype displayed by colorectal tumor cells in affected patients from HNPCC kindreds. DNA extracted from these tumor cells revealed alterations in the size of microsatellites when compared to the same microsatellites from matched normal DNA.

As discussed earlier in this chapter, microsatellite DNA sequences are short tandem repeats most commonly composed of di- and trinucleotides that are distributed throughout the human genome. Through an elegant series of experiments, it was shown that the genes responsible for "microsatellite instability" were involved in a normal cellular process called DNA mismatch repair.[10,29] Alterations of these genes interfere with the ability of affected cells to repair mistakes generated during DNA replication. Thus, cells with altered DNA mismatch repair genes replicate DNA errors more frequently than normal cells, including those in gatekeeper genes, allowing fixation of such alterations in daughter cells. Consequently, mutations occur at an increased rate throughout the genome accelerating the onset of cancer.

DNA mismatch repair genes, like tumor suppressor genes, require biallelic inactivation for the phenotype to develop. In sporadic tumors with microsatellite instability, both copies of the gene are inactivated somatically, whereas in HNPCC one mutant copy is inherited and the loss of the second copy occurs somatically. As in inherited retinoblastoma, the presence of one mutant MMR gene in all somatic cells explains the development of tumors at an early age in HNPCC. In some other family cancer syndromes associated with caretaker genes, such as xeroderma pigmentosum and ataxia-telangiectasia, both inherited copies are often mutated in the affected individuals.[5,32,40,41,45] Mutations of these genes are typically uncommon in sporadic tumors.

To pathologists it is clear that cancer is a complex disease with numerous aberrations in what were once normal cells. Molecular biology has allowed us to begin to dissect the critical changes that drive the cellular transformation ultimately responsible for cancer development. However, as with many things in biology and medicine, it is only when the pieces become available do we realize the enormity and complexity of the puzzle. It is now clear that cell growth is controlled by numerous pathways that converge or diverge depending on the specific cell type and its environment. Mutations in cancer-causing genes in any single cancer tend to alter a number of different pathways, thus disrupting many avenues of growth control. Some pathways are altered in a large number of tumors whereas others are limited to specific tumor types. In addition, the alterations in cancer-causing genes are only a launch pad for the multitude of cellular changes that occur during tumorigenesis. Many of the cancer-causing genes lead to changes in expression of numerous other genes that play an important role in tumor behavior and, in turn, response to cancer therapy. As outlined earlier in this chapter, new molecular biologic techniques have been developed to ascertain global changes in gene expression in human tumors. Such approaches not only will add another level of sophistication to our understanding of cancer and tumor classification but may also provide specific targets for the development of more effective cancer treatment.

The application of molecular biologic techniques to the investigation of human tumorigenesis has rapidly elevated our level of understanding of this complex process. During the past two decades, molecular studies have provided keen insights into the cellular mechanisms responsible for characteristics of neoplastic cells that had long been observed in vivo and in vitro. Further molecular studies undoubtedly will result in the discovery of additional target genes and a greater understanding of how such alterations contribute to the development and progression of human cancer.

Summary

Many long-standing questions concerning the molecular pathogenesis of gynecologic tumors can now be addressed using recently developed molecular tools. Many, if not most, of the experimental methods routinely employed in molecular biology laboratories today are straightforward and potentially accessible to diagnostic laboratories. Despite the wide availability of these powerful techniques, the importance of the contributions of clinicians and pathologists cannot be overemphasized. Simply stated, the quality of the results is only as good as the question asked and the materials and methods used. Ultimately, the knowledge gained from many molecular biologic studies will be applicable to improving the care and management of patients with gynecologic malignancies. Identification of specific genetic alterations in these tumors could potentially form the basis of new screening programs to detect early, and therefore curable, cancers. Patients with strong family histories of endometrial or ovarian cancer could be screened for inherited mutations in relevant tumor suppressor genes. Finally, this type of knowledge could be exploited in the development of new and more effective treatment strategies for cancer patients. Possible examples include gene therapy to replace defective copies of tumor suppressor genes, development of drugs that interfere with the interaction of viral oncoproteins with cellular tumor suppressor proteins, and reagents that can specifically reduce expression of overexpressed oncogenes. Like many other solid tumors, the common gynecologic malignancies appear to develop and progress, at least in part, as a result of activational mutation of oncogenes coupled with inactivation of tumor suppressor genes. Many of the specific genetic alterations within these genes have already been characterized in gynecologic tumors. High-throughput molecular profiling of tumors is also likely to identify clinical useful biomarkers and may ultimately allow development of new tumor classification schemes that are more clinically informative than those based on morphology alone.

Glossary

Allele: Alternative forms of the same gene. These alternative forms are not considered mutant genes because they are found in normal individuals and encode proteins with normal function.

Bacterial transformation: A method to introduce foreign DNA into bacterial cells, usually for the purposes of cloning.

Capping: The addition of 7-methylguanosine residues to the 5′-end of most eukaryotic mRNAs.

Cloning: An in vivo (in living cells) method to produce unlimited quantities of specific DNA fragments from as little as a single DNA molecule.

Codons: A group of three nucleotides within an open reading frame that specify either the amino acid to be incorporated into the protein or a translation termination signal.

Complementary DNA (cDNA): DNA synthesized from a mRNA template such that the DNA sequence is complementary to the mRNA.

Exons: The expressed portion of genes, including the coding regions. After transcription, portions of heteronuclear RNA encoded by exons are joined together by splicing to produce mRNA.

Gene amplification: The presence of multiple copies of a gene within a cell that is normally present in only two copies per somatic cell.

Gene deletion: The deletion of part or all of a gene through removal of DNA sequences by any of several molecular mechanisms.

Gene expression: The active transcription of a gene into an RNA molecule, followed by translation of the protein product.

Gene rearrangement: The process by which part or all of a gene is moved from its normal location in the genome to another site within the genome.

Growth factors: Secreted proteins that initiate a signaling cascade for stimulation of cell growth.

Growth factor receptors: Proteins that interact with growth factors and transmit the growth signal to the cell.

Heteronuclear RNA: A form of RNA, a pre-mRNA, that exists before splicing and consists of both introns and exons.

Heterozygous: A term used to describe the situation when the two homologous chromosomes from an individual can be distinguished from one another at a given locus; informative is an alternative term.

Homozygous: A term used to describe the situation when the two homologous chromosomes from an individual are identical at a given locus; uninformative is an alternative term.

Homozygous deletion: Deletion of both copies of a given chromosomal region. Homozygous deletions tend to occur in regions harboring tumor suppressor genes.

Informative: A term used to describe the situation when the two homologous chromosomes from an individual can be distinguished from one another at a given locus; heterozygous is an alternative term.

Insertion: The addition of DNA sequence into the genome.

Introns: Portions of genomic DNA that are interspersed between exons and are transcribed along with the exons into heteronuclear RNA. After transcription, the introns are removed during splicing so that they are not represented in mRNA.

Locus: A general term to describe a defined chromosomal region.

Loss of heterozygosity (LOH): Losses of specific regions of DNA from one copy of a given chromosome that can be distinguished from the region retained on the other chromosome; alternative terms are allelic loss or allelic deletion.

Messenger RNA (mRNA): The mature form of processed RNA used as a template for directing translation of proteins.

Microsatellite: DNA sequences with approximately 10–50 copies of 1- to 6-base-pair motifs that can occur in perfect tandem repetition, or less frequently, as imperfect (interrupted) repeats or together with another repeat type.

Microsatellite instability: Alterations in the length of microsatellite DNA sequences in tumors when compared to matched normal DNA.

Missense mutation: A nucleotide substitution (point mutation) in a codon of the open reading frame of a gene that results in the replacement of one amino acid for another in the protein product.

Nonsense mutation: A nucleotide substitution that results in a truncated protein product by generating a stop codon specifying premature cessation of translation within an open reading frame.

Nuclear transcription factors: Proteins involved in regulating the expression of genes by controlling transcription. Some factors enhance and others repress gene expression and others can do both, depending on the intracellular environment.

Oncogenes: Genes that regulate cell growth in a positive fashion, i.e., to promote cell growth. Oncogenes include transforming genes of viruses and normal cellular genes (proto-oncogenes) that are activated by mutations to promote cell growth.

Open reading frame: A sequence of DNA, representing at least some of the coding portion of a gene, that is transcribed and subsequently translated into a protein because it does not contain any internal translation termination codons.

Point mutation: The replacement of one nucleotide in the DNA sequence of the wild-type gene with another nucleotide.

Polyadenylation: A process by which a stretch of adenosine residues are added to the 3′-end of most eukaryotic mRNA molecules.

Primers: Short DNA sequences (oligonucleotides) that are complementary to portions of specific DNA sequences and are used to prime DNA synthesis.

Promoter: The DNA sequence of a gene to which RNA polymerase binds and initiates transcription. This sequence is found 5′ to the coding portion of the gene and is responsible for regulating the expression of the gene at the transcriptional level. Promoter sequences are typically rich in C and G nucleotides.

Promoter hypermethylation: Increased methylation at CG dinucleotides within gene promoters can result in gene silencing (loss of expression).

Proto-oncogenes: Cellular genes that are the normal counterparts of transforming viral oncogenes.

Restriction endonucleases: Enzymes that cleave DNA at specific DNA sequences.

Restriction fragment length polymorphism (RFLP): Variations in the DNA of different individuals that create or destroy cleavage sites for a given restriction endonuclease.

Reverse transcriptase-PCR (RT-PCR): A PCR-based method for detecting transcription of a specific gene. The mRNA sample is reverse transcribed to generate cDNA, which is then amplified using gene specific primers within two different exons.

Splice site mutations: Nucleotide substitutions that occur in the sequences adjacent to intron–exon boundaries of genes. These mutations result in aberrant RNA splicing, which in turn results in aberrant (or nonexistent) protein products.

Splicing: The process by which introns are removed from heteronuclear RNA and the exons are joined together to maintain the open reading frame of the mRNA.

Transcription: The process by which RNA is synthesized from the DNA template.

Translation: The process by which specific amino acids are incorporated into a protein as determined by the sequence of the mRNA template.

Tumor suppressor gene: Normal cellular gene that encodes a protein thought to normally regulate growth in a negative fashion or promote cellular differentiation.

Uninformative: The term used to describe the situation when the two homologous chromosomes from an individual cannot be distinguished from one another at a given locus; homozygous is an alternative term.

Vector: A DNA vehicle that can be propagated in living cells (e.g., bacteria and yeast) into which foreign DNA can be inserted and propagated with the vector DNA. Examples of vectors include bacterial plasmids, cosmids, bacteriophage, yeast artificial chromosomes, bacterial artificial chromosomes, and P1-based artificial chromosomes.

Wild type: The term used to describe the normal gene or gene product. In contrast, a gene that has had its DNA sequence altered is referred to as a mutant gene and its resultant product is a mutant protein.

References

1. The Chipping forecast (1999) Nat Genet Supp 21:1–60
2. Baylin SB, Herman JG (2000) DNA hypermethylation in tumorigenesis: epigenetics joins genetics. Trends Genet 16:168–174
3. Birrer MJ, Hendricks D, Farley J, Sundborg MJ, Bonome T, Walts MJ, Geradts J (1999) Abnormal Fhit expression in malignant and premalignant lesions of the cervix. Cancer Res 59:5270–5274
4. Burks RT, Kessis TD, Cho KR, Hedrick L (1994) Microsatellite instability in endometrial carcinoma. Oncogene 9:1163–1166
5. Cleaver JE, Thompson LH, Richardson AS, States JC (1999) A summary of mutations in the UV-sensitive disorders: xeroderma pigmentosum, Cockayne syndrome, and trichothiodystrophy. Hum Mutat 14: 9–22
6. DeRisi JL, Iyer VR (1999) Genomics and array technology. Curr Opin Oncol 11:76–79
7. DeRisi JL, Iyer VR, Brown PO (1997) Exploring the metabolic and genetic control of gene expression on a genomic scale. Science 278:680–686
8. Dunn JM, Phillips RA, Becker AJ, Gallie BL (1988) Identification of germline and somatic mutations affecting the retinoblastoma gene. Science 241:1797–1800
9. Eisen MB, Spellman PT, Brown PO, Botstein D (1998) Cluster analysis and display of genome-wide expression patterns. Proc Natl Acad Sci USA 95: 14863–14868
10. Fishel R, Lescoe MK, Rao MRS, et al (1993) The human mutator gene homolog MSH2 and its association with hereditary nonpolyposis colon cancer. Cell 75:1027–1038
11. Forozan F, Karhu R, Kononen J, Kallioniemi A, Kallioniemi OP (1997) Genome screening by comparative genomic hybridization. Trends Genet 13: 405–409
12. Francke U (1976) Retinoblastoma and chromosome 13. Cytogenet Cell Genet 16:131–134
13. Friend SH, Bernards R, Rogelj S, et al (1986) A human DNA segment with properties of the gene that predisposes to retinoblastoma and osteosarcoma. Nature (Lond) 323:643–646

14. Greenspan DL, Connolly DC, Wu R, et al (1997) Loss of FHIT expression in cervical carcinoma cell lines and primary tumors. Cancer Res 57:4692–4698
15. Hamel PA, Gallie BL, Phillips RA (1992) The retinoblastoma protein and cell cycle regulation. Trends Genet 8:180–185
16. Hansen MF, Cavanee WK (1987) Genetics of cancer predisposition. Cancer Res 47:5518–5527
17. Harlow E, Lane DP (1988) Antibodies: a laboratory manual, 1st Ed. Cold Spring Harbor Laboratory, Cold Spring Harbor, New York
18. Harris H (1988) The analysis of malignancy in cell fusion: the position in 1988. Cancer Res 48:3302–3306
19. Herman JF, Baylin SB (2000) Promoter-region hypermethylation and gene silencing in human cancer. Curr Top Microbiol Immunol 249:35–54
20. Kallioniemi A, Kallioniemi OP, Sudar D, et al (1992) Comparative genomic hybridization for molecular cytogenetic analysis of solid tumors. Science 258: 818–821
21. Kessis TD, Slebos RJC, Han S, et al (1993) p53 gene mutations and mdm2 amplification are uncommon in primary carcinomas of the uterine cervix. Am J Pathol 143:1398–1405
22. Khan J, Bittner ML, Chen Y, Meltzer PS, Trent JM (1999) DNA microarray technology: the anticipated impact on the study of human disease. Biochim Biophys Acta 1423:M17–M28
23. Khan J, Saal LH, Bittner ML, Chen Y, Trent JM, Meltzer PS (1999) Expression profiling in cancer using cDNA microarrays. Electrophoresis 20:223–229
24. Kinzler KW, Vogelstein B (1996) Lessons from hereditary colorectal cancer. Cell 87:159–170
25. Knudson AG (1971) Mutation and cancer: statistical study of retinoblastoma. Proc Natl Acad Sci USA 68:820–823
26. Knudson AG (1985) Hereditary cancer, oncogenes, and antioncogenes. Cancer Res 45:1437–1443
27. Kononen J, Bubendorf L, Kallioniemi A, et al (1998) Tissue microarrays for high-throughput molecular profiling of tumor specimens. Nat Med 4:844–847
28. Kozian DH, Kirschbaum BJ (1999) Comparative gene-expression analysis. Trends Biotechnol 17: 73–78
29. Leach FS, Nicolaides NC, Papadopoulos N, et al (1993) Mutations of a mutS homolog in hereditary nonpolyposis colorectal cancer. Cell 75:1215–1226
30. Lee WH, Bookstein R, Hong F, Young LJ, Shew JY, Lee EY (1987) Human retinoblastoma susceptibility gene: cloning, identification, and sequence. Science 235:1394–1399
31. Lele KP, Penrose LS, Stallard HB (1963) Chromosome deletion in a case of retinoblastoma. Ann Hum Genet 27:171–174
32. Meyn MS (1999) Ataxia-telangiectasia, cancer and the pathobiology of the ATM gene. Clin Genet 55: 289–304
33. Meyn MS (1999) Ataxia-telangiectasia, cancer and the pathobiology of the ATM gene. Clin Genet 55: 289–304
34. Mullis KB, Faloona F (1987) Specific synthesis of DNA in vitro via a polymerase catalyzed chain reaction. Methods Enzymol 55:335–350
35. Orye E, Delbeke MJ, Vandenabeele B (1974) Retinoblastoma and long arm deletion at chromosome 13: attempts to define the deleted segment. Clin Genet 5:457–464
36. Pandey A, Mann M (2000) Proteomics to study genes and genomes. Nature (Lond) 405:837–846
37. Parada LF, Tabin CJ, Shih C, Weinberg RA (1982) Human EJ bladder carcinoma oncogene is homologue of Harvey sarcoma virus *ras* gene. Nature (Lond) 297:474–478
38. Pennisi E (2000) Finally, the book of life and instructions for navigating it. Science 288:2304–2307
39. Roberts-Thomson IC, Ryan P, Khoo KK, Hart WJ, McMichael AJ, Butler RN (1996) Diet, acetylator phenotype, and risk of colorectal neoplasia. Lancet 347:1372–1374
40. Rotman G, Shiloh Y (1999) ATM: a mediator of multiple responses to genotoxic stress. Oncogene 18: 6135–6144
41. Rotman G, Shiloh Y (1998) ATM: from gene to function. Hum Mol Genet 7:1555–1563
42. Saiki RK, Gelfand DH, Stoffel S, et al (1988) Primer-directed enzymatic amplification of DNA with a thermostable DNA polymerase. Science 239:487–491
43. Saiki RK, Scharf SJ, Faloona F, et al (1985) Enzymatic amplification of beta-globin sequences and restriction site analysis for diagnosis of sickle cell anemia. Science 230:1350–1354
44. Sanger F, Nicklen S, Coulson AR (1977) DNA sequencing with chain-terminating inhibitors. Proc Natl Acad Sci USA 74:5463–5467
45. Sarasin A (1999) The molecular pathways of ultraviolet-induced carcinogenesis. Mutat Res 428:5–10
46. Slamon DJ, Godolphin W, Jones LA, et al (1989) Studies of the HER-2/neu proto-oncogene in human breast and ovarian cancer. Science 244:707–712
47. Southern EM (1975) Detection of specific sequences among DNA fragments separated by gel electrophoresis. J Mol Biol 98:503–506
48. Tashiro H, Isacson C, Levine RU, Kurman RJ, Cho KR, Hedrick L (1997) p53 gene mutations are common in uterine serous carcinoma and occur early in their pathogenesis. Am J Pathol 150:177–185
49. Weber JL (1990) Informativeness of human (dC-dA)n.(dG-dT)n polymorphisms. Genomics 7:524–530
50. Wistuba II, Montellano FD, Milchgrub S, et al (1997) Deletions of chromosome 3p are frequent and early events in the pathogenesis of uterine cervical cancer. Cancer Res 57:3154–3158
51. Yoshino K, Enomoto T, Nakamura T, et al (2000) FHIT alterations in cancerous and non-cancerous cervical epithelium. Int J Cancer 85:6–13

27

Epidemiology

Mark Schiffman, M.D.

Most pathologists are part-time epidemiologists as well. The two medical disciplines are more closely allied than many realize. Epidemiologists study the distribution and determinants of diseases in human populations. In current medical practices, diseases are often defined by histopathologic diagnoses or by clinical pathologic test values. Thus, whenever a pathologist shifts intellectually from the level of the individual slide or specimen to thinking about a group of diagnoses, an informal epidemiologic question is being raised. For example, "How common is this diagnosis?" is a question of prevalence or incidence. "Why am I seeing so many cases of this type of tumor?" is a question of time trends. "How would my colleague interpret these slides compared with me?" is a question of interpathologist agreement. And, "What causes this disease I am seeing every week?" is a question of etiology that can be addressed by pathologists working as epidemiologists, or with them.

This chapter is meant to introduce the major epidemiologic concepts of greatest use to pathologists who are considering a research project, or who wish to think more formally at the population level about their case material or diagnostic criteria. The review is certainly not exhaustive; rather, it is meant to be quite informal and readable and to encourage the pathologist to pursue epidemiologic projects and collaborations. The first section, accordingly, is organized around types of possible epidemiologic studies that a pathologist might wish to pursue. The next section outlines nonmathematically a few basics of statistical thinking that pathologists need to know if they wish to do more formal epidemiologic research. The third section discusses a few problem issues that usually emerge when epidemiologists and pathologists work together.

Applications of Epidemiology to Pathology Studies

This section illustrates the types of epidemiologic projects that a pathologist may undertake, either informally or formally. The examples are drawn mainly from the author's experience conducting etiologic and screening studies of gynecologic neoplasia, especially cervical neoplasia.

Throughout this section, epidemiologic terms will be introduced and simply defined. There is a useful dictionary of epidemiology for readers interested in learning more terminology.[7] For a more complete understanding of basic epidemiologic concepts, the reader is referred to one of several introductory texts.[2,5,10]

Prevalence, Incidence, and Mortality Rates of Disease

One of the first questions that an expert or novice epidemiologist is likely to ask about a disease under study is "How common is it?" The pathologist at the microscope is interested in how common various conditions are, as one element of differential diagnosis (witness the maxims, "Rare diseases occur rarely." and "If you hear hoofbeats, think of a horse not a zebra.")

For the pathologist considering a research study, the frequency of disease occurrence is crucial for two reasons. On the practical level, very rare conditions are difficult to study epidemiologically because the statistical principles underlying epidemiology require moderately large numbers to deal with chance, which is the unavoidable and defining characteristic of observational studies in humans.

More importantly, the amount of disease in a population is the starting point for epidemiologic thought, leading to all the major epidemiologic comparisons, such as "How much disease occurs in population A compared to population B, and what does the difference tell us? Why is the amount of disease changing over time? What risk factors are associated with groups having the most disease?"

Because measuring the occurrence of disease is so important to epidemiologists, they find it important, like skiers discussing snow, to define terms carefully using a resultant epidemiologic jargon (in the good sense of the word). A few key terms related to the frequency of disease occurrence are essential and worth memorizing by anyone interested in epidemiology.

The *prevalence* of a disease is the number of occurrences of the disease in a given population at a given time, for example, "Twenty percent of the patients seen in this clinic have at least reactive changes on their Papanicolaou smears." Often, prevalence is discussed with reference to a single point in time, as in a screening program, yielding a *point prevalence*: "Two percent of the screening smears last month showed changes suggestive of CIN."

The *incidence* of disease is the number of new cases that develop in a given time period. Accordingly, *incident disease* refers to new disease whereas *prevalent disease* refers to all the cases in the population, whether new or chronic. The connection between prevalence and incidence is the *duration* of the condition (Prevalence = Incidence × Duration). Therefore, the prevalence of rabies in a given week is close to the incidence because duration is short, whereas the prevalence of a long-duration disease, such as rheumatoid arthritis much exceeds the incidence for any time period. A more subtle and relevant example of how incidence and prevalence relate via duration is the following. In studies of young women, we noted about 10 years ago that the point prevalence of human papillomavirus (HPV) infection was about the same as the yearly incidence, suggesting a duration of infection of approximately 1 year. In follow-up studies, we have now confirmed that HPV infections do last about a year.

Incidence is most often defined as a yearly rate, as in "36,000 incidence cases of uterine corpus cancer were diagnosed in the United States in 2000." However, *lifetime cumulative incidence* is also an intuitively useful term, meaning the estimated risk of occurrence of a disease over a woman's life: "About 1% of women in the United States will develop cervical cancer in their lifetime." For chronic diseases such as endometriosis, genital herpes, or specific gynecologic cancers, incidence is usually thought of as a one-time phenomenon; that is, second primaries rarely occur. (In contrast to second primaries, recurrences of the same disease imply that it is prevalent, not incidence.) For acute, self-limited, or curable conditions such as gonorrhea, incidence must be defined over a narrow range of time appropriate to the duration of the illness.

Rates of death from a disease are measured as the *mortality rate*. The connection between incidence and mortality is, of course, survival, measured often by the *case:fatality ratio*.

In summary, the epidemiologist is interested in the prevalence, incidence, and mortality rates of a disease as the fundamental basis of further study. These terms can be applied to any study population, whether that population is a single gynecologic practice or hospital, a city, a country, or the world.

National incidence and mortality data are most often cited when discussing the scope of a medical problem. Where can national data be obtained? In the United States, pathologists are probably aware that mortality rates from all causes are compiled and available from a variety of sources, most notably and simply from the National Center for Health Statistics (6525 Belcrest Road, Room 1064, Hyattsville, MD 20782; 301-458-4636).

Mortality rates are usually the most reliable gauge of disease occurrence for highly fatal diseases when comparing different populations worldwide or time periods. Of course, there are obvious uncertainties and errors in ascribing causes of death, but mortality rates are reasonably well recorded and useful for many cancers. Mortality is not useful as a measurement of disease occurrence in regions where the diagnostic workups are lacking or the case: fatality ratio has been altered sharply by improved treatment.

In contrast, if a condition is not often fatal, mortality rates may not be useful at all for disease surveillance. It is often more difficult to obtain reliable incidence data, and the researcher must rely on data from voluntary registries, published surveys, or occasionally government-mandated registries. For cancer, fortunately, the National Cancer Institute's Surveillance, Epidemiology, and End Results (SEER) Program compiles incidence rates for a (nonrandom but stable) 10% sample of the U.S. population. The most accessible source of SEER cancer incidence and survival data (as well as national cancer mortality data) is *CA–A Cancer Journal for Clinicians*, published annually by the American Cancer Society and mailed free on request.[4] More detailed cancer data can be obtained from other American Cancer Society publications, such as *Cancer Facts and Figures*, or from the SEER program itself (National Cancer Institute, Bethesda, MD 20892, or http://seer.cancer.gov). The International Agency for Research on Cancer compiles international incidence and mortality rates derived from cancer registries of varying quality.[9,18]

Geographic Differences and Time Trends in Disease Occurrence

Pathologists may wish to go beyond descriptions of disease occurrence at a place and time to compare rates between geographic areas or over time. The usual hope is that the comparisons may yield clues to etiology and pathogenesis. A cautious approach is critical because of the omnipresent effects of chance on observational data. How can one tell if the amount of disease in one place or time is truly different from the amount found earlier or elsewhere? Disease rates fluctuate over time and place. Many geographic differences and temporal trends do not persist over time, appearing random (to the limit of our understanding!).

Hence, there is a need for statistics as one of the disciplines underlying epidemiology. Distinguishing chance differences from true differences requires statistical thinking and an appreciation of the types of differences that arise by chance. This point is important, because overinterpretation of chance differences is one of the most common errors that novice epidemiologists make when comparing disease rates from one place or time to another. For example, many cancer "outbreaks" where several neighbors get similar tumors turn out to be quite explainable as chance clusterings of events, expected for common malignancies such as breast cancer. A good bit of advice might be to treat health statistics like the monthly economic news: it takes a long-term trend or a persistent difference to trust that something important is happening.

When comparing one place to another, or analyzing time trends, the cardinal rule is to make sure that the comparison is valid. A checklist of commonsense questions should be asked:

1. Are the rates being compared truly comparable (incidence, prevalence, mortality)? In particular, are the sources of data comparable (for example, a mandatory registry cannot be compared to a voluntary reporting system because of differences in the completeness of reporting).
2. Are the diagnostic criteria the same in both comparison groups? This particular problem has plagued the interpretation of time trend data regarding minor cervical cytologic abnormalities because increased recognition by pathologists of subtle koilocytotic changes cannot be easily distinguished from increased incidence of koilocytotic atypia.
3. Are the two populations comparable in age and other factors affecting risk of disease? No one would think of comparing the prevalence of cervical epithelial neoplasia (CIN) in a gynecologic referral practice to the prevalence in a screening clinic because, of course, the prevalence would be higher in the referral clinic. Some researchers, however, make the analogous mistake of comparing populations that differ with regard to age, socioeconomic status, or other more subtle characteristics related to the risk of disease (called *confounding variables* in epidemiologic jargon). Most importantly, almost all diseases vary in incidence and prevalence by age, and thus almost all comparisons should take age into account. The section on error and bias (following) mentions simple meth-

ods of adjustment for age and other confounding variables. The statistical bases of making geographic and temporal comparisons are covered in the sections on descriptive data and measures of risk.

Validating New (or Old) Histopathologic Diagnostic Distinctions

The creation and refinement of pathologic classifications can be aided by epidemiologic corroboration. For example, the Bethesda System of cervical cytology combines koilocytotic atypia and CIN 1 as low-grade squamous intraepithelial lesion (LSIL). This combination was supported by epidemiologic data. The two diagnoses, which are not reliably distinguishable on morphologic grounds, share the same epidemiologic profiles of younger average age and varied human papillomavirus (HPV) types, as compared to the older average age and restricted HPV types found in higher-grade lesions. As another example, a recent pathologic study of squamous vulvar cancer, which proposed new pathologic subtypes, was strengthened by a separate epidemiologic analysis showing that the new subtypes had different epidemiologic characteristics.[6] Pathologists and epidemiologists can work iteratively to refine disease classifications, asking each other "Do categories X and Y look the same or different from your point of view?"

Judging Intra- or Interpathologist Agreement

Pathology agreement studies have been motivated by the needs of both disciplines. Pathologists are obviously concerned with the reliability of the diagnoses they make. Epidemiologists are concerned with uniform case definition in their studies. When comparisons of intra- and interpathologist agreement are performed, the epidemiologist can serve the role of scientific organizer, ensuring independence of the reviews by *masking* the reviewers (also called *blinding*) to each other's diagnoses until after the data are complete. It is the widespread opinion of epidemiologists that unmasked comparisons, in which reviewers have access to each other's diagnoses, have limited scientific value. Like all human beings, pathologists tend to agree much more in public than in private, and masking provides a guarantee that a comparison rather than a consensus is being achieved. In the area of cervical pathology, the diagnosis of CIN by either cytology or histology has proven much more variable among experts when masked comparisons were performed than initially expected. Surprisingly, the extensive histologic reviews of specimens from loop electrosurgical excision procedures (LEEP) exhibit almost as much interpathologist variability as cytology.[17] Many morphologic judgments that pathologists make regarding cancer precursor lesions are clearly difficult, regardless of tissue type and quantity.

Epidemiologic Studies of Disease Etiology

Epidemiologists attempt to find the determinants of disease by statistically correlating the presence or absence of possible *exposures* (often called *risk factors*) with the presence or absence of disease. Epidemiologic studies attempting to relate exposures and disease are called *analytic studies*, as distinguished from *descriptive studies* that yield rates of disease without directly addressing etiology.

A description of the many types of analytic studies is beyond the scope of this chapter. At the simplest level, *prospective* or *cohort studies* start with the measurement of an exposure in a group of study participants who are followed over time. The investigators then compare incidence rates or *absolute risk* of disease in the exposed versus the unexposed groups. The ratio of the incidence rate in exposed subjects divided by the incidence rate in the unexposed is called the *incidence rate ratio*. The reader might correctly expect that there are as many types of rate ratios as there are types of rates (e.g., *prevalence rate ratio, lifetime cumulative risk ratio*). Many epidemiologists casually refer to the entire group as the *relative risk* of exposed versus nonexposed subjects and use the abbreviation *RR* as a general shorthand.

Prospective studies are the most appealing type of analytic study because they most directly determine how commonly disease occurs in exposed versus unexposed individuals. The relative risk, directly measured, is an intuitively clear answer to the question: "If a woman has this characteristic (the exposure), how much more likely is she to develop the disease, compared to a similar unexposed woman?" The absolute risk translates as "How likely to get disease is an exposed woman?" (see later: "Measures of Risk"). The problem with prospective studies of cancer is that they are expensive, usually take years to organize and complete, and must be very large to generate enough cases of cancer for reliable estimates of risk, even for common tumors including in situ neoplasia.

Other analytic study designs try, in general, to estimate the relative risk estimates that might be obtained in the ideal prospective study, while saving time and money. Analytic studies that start by collecting a series of *cases* (women diagnosed with a given disease) and appropriate *controls* (women without that disease who are measured for comparison) are called *case-control* studies. The exposures of interest are ascertained for both groups and the relative risk (RR) of disease among the exposed versus the unexposed is estimated by calculating the ratio of the odds of exposure in cases versus controls (for more explanation, see the statistical section on measures of risk).

The estimation of the prospective relative risk by the case-control *odds ratio* (*OR*) is one of the most important statistical concepts in epidemiology, and one of the most subtle. For this statistical approximation to be valid, incident case and controls must be chosen to be strictly comparable. The control group must represent the group of women at risk of developing disease at the time the incident case was diagnosed, otherwise the estimation of the relative risk can be grossly mistaken because of *bias* (a nonrandom or systematic error in estimation of a statistic, to be distinguished from *random error*).

In practice, it is very difficult to define and recruit an unbiased sample of the general population of women that gave rise to the cases appearing in one hospital or clinic. Thus, all kinds of compromises of convenience and practicality must be made, and it becomes difficult to avoid bias in choosing controls. For example, smoking causes or worsens so many kinds of illness that it is very difficult to use hospitalized controls to estimate the relative risk of a disease associated with smoking (such as many cancers). The exposure to smoking in the hospitalized controls is elevated compared to the general at-risk population; thus, the odds ratio obtained in a naively conducted hospital-based study tends to provide too low an estimate of the relative risk.

Because case-control studies are so commonly used as an analytic design, choosing proper controls is one of the two most important aspects of epidemiology. The other is assuring proper measurements of exposure and disease. The mark of a good epidemiologist is a dedicated attention to control selection and measurement error, whereas many novices tend to focus more on the cases and data analysis while relying on a *convenience sample* of whichever controls are most easily available.

Besides prospective and case-control studies, another common analytic study design is the *cross-sectional* study, in which exposure and disease status are ascertained concurrently for a study population. An example would be a screening study of HPV infection and abnormal cervical cytology, in which all women attending a clinic are tested for viral DNA at the same time the cytologic smear is taken. The analysis of a cross-sectional study is somewhat similar to that of a case-control study, but the researcher must be careful because the cases are a combination of incident and prevalent disease. The odds ratio that is computed in a cross-sectional study is a good estimation of the prospective relative risk only if certain conditions are met, including an assumption that the disease under study is rare (an assumption not met for cervical cytologic abnormalities in many clinics).

The pathologist collaborator should play a key role in all analytic studies of diseases whose definitions rely on nonroutine pathologic expertise. Misclassification of disease status can be very damaging to a study because the result of misclassification on correlative statistics, like the relative risk and odds ratio, is, generally, to reduce the apparent strength of the association between disease and exposure. If the disease is defined poorly enough, no epidemiologic risk factors may be found even if they exist.[13] Moreover, it is often very difficult to measure the risk factors (exposures) without substantial error, whether laboratory testing or interviews are being used. The combination of multiple errors in measuring both exposure and disease can literally make a study worthless. For example, early studies correlating HPV DNA detection and CIN revealed only a moderate association, in that less than 50% of cases were found to be HPV positive. Moreover, HPV infection was not apparently associated with sexual activity, an established strong risk factor for CIN. These weak associations were a result of misclassification. Subsequent studies with better HPV tests and expert review of pathology revealed that virtually all cases of CIN contain HPV DNA and that HPV is the sexually transmitted agent explaining the association of sexual activity and risk of CIN.

As the result of the strong, damaging effects of misclassification on epidemiologic studies, epidemiologists pay careful attention to the pathologic classifications that define their study cases and controls and often establish formal collaborations with reviewing pathologists as part of epidemiologic studies.

Follow-Up Studies of Patients with the Same Pathologic Diagnosis

Clinicians, pathologists, and epidemiologists are all interested in learning what happens to patients diagnosed with a given disease. For a possibly fatal disease, survival rates are critical, whereas for other chronic diseases progression rates are often estimated. It is often of interest to divide the patients into groups, to determine whether subtypes of disease follow different courses, or whether different treatments influence outcome. The *randomized clinical trial* (see following) is a specialized version of such a follow-up study, in which subjects are randomly assigned to various treatment groups to maximize the comparability of the groups. The hope is that the randomization will minimize differences in both known and unknown confounding variables that could bias the comparison.

Follow-up studies almost invariably involve the concept of *time to an event*. In other words, it is important *when* incidence, progression, or death occur, not just *if* they occur. Let us discuss this issue in the context of studies of disease outcome (as opposed to disease incidence). Clearly, all participants in any follow-up study or clinical trial eventually die; the question is when (and why). A good treatment prolongs time to death whereas a bad type of disease shortens it. Because of the critical notion of "time to event" in epidemiologic follow-up studies, such studies depend heavily on actuarial methods, such as survival curves and life-table analyses, when comparing exposed to unexposed patients or treated to untreated patients. The central statistical concept in such studies is a kind of rate called a *hazard*, which refers to the risk of an outcome occurring in a unit of follow-up time. A hazard is computed as the number of *events* (e.g., death, cure, or progression) divided by the amount of *person-time* of follow-up. Person-time is computed individually for each participant as the observation time between her entry into the study and her exit. The total person-time for a study group is the sum of all the individual observation periods. For example, 10,000 women followed for a year or 100 women followed for 10 years both yield 1,000 person-years of follow-up time. Twenty deaths arising during that follow-up would yield an estimated hazard of 20 deaths per 1,000 person-years in both situations.

A hazard is a special kind of rate because it is conceived of as the rate of an outcome (disease incidence, progression, mortality, or whatever) at a single moment in time, as the mathematical "limit" of the rate as time "goes to zero." Accordingly, the hazard of disease can change from moment to moment as conditions change. An HPV-infected woman lights up a cigarette and her hazard for progression to invasive cervical cancer probably increases. She quits smoking the next day and her hazard decreases.

Moreover, the computation of the denominator of hazards, person-time of follow-up, requires some training and thought. For each successive time interval during follow-up, the denominator of women at risk for an event changes. For example, women are lost to follow-up as they drop out of the study, or they die for other reasons, or they experience the event itself (because one can only progress for the first time or die once). Thus, computing the proper amount of person-time during which the events occurred requires some knowledge of *censoring*, which is the proper deletion of irrelevant follow-up time during which the subject was not truly at risk of the outcome.

It is useful to compute the hazard of conditions like death that happen once and do not reverse. Life-table methods are more confusing when a condition can come and go. For example, say we want to study "HPV infection" without defining specific types. However, the term "HPV infection" is like "a cold." Multiple types can present a confusing picture of clearance and "recurrence," with ambiguous meaning. Proper counting of events and censoring of person-time are very difficult in this context, making simpler analyses more appealing, such as the computation of cumulative incidence rate ratios (ever infected versus not infected over the course of study).

Usually, researchers are not content to describe the simple survival or progression curve of a disease after diagnosis. They wish to determine which factors affect the hazard, that is, what the relative or *proportional hazard* of death, etc., might be for women in different groups defined by pathologic differences or treatment types. The proportional hazard is almost identical to the incident rate ratio already discussed, but the denominator is person-time of follow-up, not just time. Proportional hazard analyses are too complex to be described here, and pathologists performing follow-up studies might consider consulting an epidemiologist or biostatistician early in the design phase of such projects. Data collection must be organized carefully to permit a correct determination of person-time.

Randomized Clinical Trials

Randomized clinical trials are conceptually simple prospective analyses, with eligible women divided into treatment arms. Randomization serves to balance known and unknown biases in the arms. There is a placebo or standard treatment arm, compared to one or more new treatment arms. These trials are very appealing as a court of judgment regarding best medical practice when "equipoise" exists, that is, we do not know which practice is best. Such trials are highly influential. However, they are surprisingly difficult and should not be undertaken as quickly as observational studies. The maxim "Do no harm" is applicable because the participants' fate is influenced by the randomization. Clinician judgment as to the individual's optimal treatment must explicitly be set aside. The stakes are always high when a trial is under way. We want a result quickly and definitively, but the two objectives are in conflict. The time-honored rules used to ensure fairness can seem bureaucratic and rigid. "Clinical trialists" are statisticians, epidemiologists, and others who specialize in randomization, data monitoring, intermediate analyses ("data peeks" before the scheduled end of follow-up), and stopping rules (in case the intermediate analyses reveal an especially good or bad outcome). Pathologists contribute expert review of entry diagnoses and outcomes. Often, the burden of pathology review is large, reproducibility is paramount, and the review process is highly controlled by central administration. Of all collaborations with epidemiologists, pathologists should be most wary of clinical trials because of the inevitable attendant requirements. Still, the rewards are vital.

Screening for Gynecologic Malignancies

Screening is inherently epidemiologic; thus, the pathologist involved in screening programs (e.g., cervical cytologic screening or CA-125 testing) needs to understand the interrelated concepts of sensitivity, specificity, and predictive value. The basics are outlined later in a statistical section on screening.

A common mistake in evaluating the results of a screening trial is to ignore the clinical setting. The *sensitivity* of a screening technique (percentage of diseased women who test positive) and its *specificity* (percentage of disease-free women who test negative) theoretically do not change when the test is taken out of a high-risk hospital clinic to be applied to the general population. But most clinicians are more interested in the *positive predictive value* and *negative predictive value*, two statistics that are highly dependent on the clinical setting. The positive predictive value is the percentage of women testing positive who truly have disease. The negative predictive value is the reassurance that disease does not exist given a negative test result.

Here is an important practical point: Given the same sensitivity and specificity (i.e., the same assay accuracy), positive predictive value decreases sharply as the prevalence of the disease decreases. True positives can be swamped by false positives once the test is applied to many normal women. Therefore, the same screening test that looks promising because of high sensitivity in a high-risk clinic will often perform poorly in the general population, producing so many false positives compared to the disease yield that the costs outweigh the benefits. As a general rule, specificity is perhaps surprisingly important as a requirement for a screening test. A screening test such as a tumor marker must be highly specific (negative in virtually all nondiseased women, certainly more than 90%) to be cost-effective for general population screening.

Basic Statistical Concepts

Hopefully, the preceding discussion has firmly established the relevance of epidemiology to gynecologic pathology research and even daily practice. Epidemiologic work requires an understanding of biostatistics. This section presents the bare basics of what the author believes pathologists collaborating in epidemiologic research might wish to know about biostatistical methods. Introductory biostatistics texts are available and easy to read for the pathologists wishing to work independently or for those who want computational formulae for chi-square or other commonly used tests.

Variability as a Fundamental Principle of Pathology

Virtually all measurements that one could make about a human population are variable. Height, weight, fine points of anatomy, metabolic patterns, serum levels of hormones, and nutrients are all commonly recognized to be variable. The same variability is seen by pathologists at the tissue and cellular levels and by research pathologists at the molecular biologic level (e.g., varying tissue levels of DNA adducts given equivalent carcinogenic exposures, genetic polymorphisms in human genes, and varying molecular responses to infection with viral DNA). Even the intricate, multistep molecular pathways to cancer demonstrate substantial variability between individuals who develop the same type of malignancy.

Variability in pathology is mainly described by *categorical* or *discrete* data and statistics, as compared with *continuous* data and statistics (the province of the mean, median, and standard deviation). Similar (but not identical) histologic and cytologic appearances are categorized and named. More attention is paid to the borderlines and overlaps of the categories, rather than subtler differences within the categories (unless splitting into finer categories is being considered). Categorical data analysis relies on *contingency tables*, which are discussed in a following section. Contingency tables such as the common *2 × 2 table* are frequently counts of categorical data; for example, how many (not what percent of) CIN 2 lesions demonstrated aneuploidy or not, compared with how many CIN 3 lesions demonstrated aneuploidy or not.

The variability in categorical data such as pathology categories shows up in diagnostic error, that is, the misassignment of a patient to the wrong category. In general, error cannot be avoided. To the epidemiologist, categorization of variable biologic continuua virtually dictates that there will be error. If two categories blend into each other with regard to a characteristic (even one as complex and general as microscopic appearance), they cannot be perfectly separated based on that characteristic. Thus, pathologists search for additional characteristics to discriminate difficult-to-distinguish indeterminate cases, such as immunocytochemistry, but these ancillary measurements also have error and overlap. There is a field of statistics called *discriminant analysis* in which the goal is to determine how many characteristics must be measured to maximize correct assignment to overlapping categories. This complicated set of statistical methods underlies the development of computer-assisted cytology screening.

Error Versus Bias

Error is inevitable, but epidemiologists hope that it is mainly random, not systematically pushing the data in one way or the other. *Random error* reduces the *reliability* of repeated measurements, affecting their *precision*, and reduces the perceived strength of correlations, but the average measured value still becomes increasingly true or *accurate* as the study size increases. Systematic error, called *bias*, impacts directly on the accuracy of the measurement; no matter how large a study based on biased measurements is, the answer will be wrong. Thus, epidemiologists struggle to reduce random measurement error, but they have an even stronger dislike of biased measurements. If the exact direction and magnitude of a fixed bias were known, the data could be adjusted (like a scale that always reads three pounds too heavy), but adjustments for bias are not usually possible.

Epidemiologists combat error and bias in a few standard ways. To quantify and reduce random error, reliability is measured by repeating data collection, whether that involves reasking a question, rerunning an assay, or submitting a pathology slide for rereview.

For continuous variables, statistics of reliability begin with the *variance*. It is the sum of the squared deviations of measurements from their arithmetic average or *mean*, divided by the number of data points minus one. The *standard deviation* is the square root of the variance, and is commonly used to indicate the "spread" of a group of numbers. The standard deviation of a measurement can be computed for individual members of the overall study population or for repeated samplings of a study statistic such as the mean (in which case it is called the *standard error* of the mean). Standard errors are important in making *confidence intervals* around the mean, when we compare different populations to see whether they are statistically significantly different regarding the characteristic under study.

When epidemiologists assess laboratory assays, they often consider the *coefficient of variation* (*CV*), which is the ratio of the standard deviation to the mean. Low CVs (under 10% is excellent) indicate high assay reproducibility, although they do not ensure accuracy. Remember that a reproducible assay can still be biased.

For categorical variables such as pathology interpretations, statistics of reliability include the simple percentage of agreement and more complicated statistics mentioned below in the section on measures of interpathologist agreement. Epidemiologists would like to compare the pathology diagnoses to a reference standard of truth, but such reference standards virtually never exist. Certainly, there is no source of absolute truth in pathology, only advancing degrees of expertise correlated with decreasing amounts of diagnostic error. Therefore, to reduce bias in pathology, researchers are limited to the comparison of different experts. To the extent that truly independent experts agree (without consideration of each other's opinion), the possibility that either one is biased is reduced. To reduce the possibility of bias, epidemiologists try to ensure that all study measurements are made independent of each other so that knowledge of one variable cannot bias a decision about another. The difficulties of masking are discussed in a later section.

Descriptive Data

The terms used most often to describe and summarize descriptive data, such as prevalence and incidence, were defined earlier in the section on geographic differences and time trends and are not repeated. A few additional statistical concepts critical to the interpretation of descriptive data should be mentioned.

First, there is an important choice of scale in the plotting of descriptive data. The scale of the y or vertical axis greatly affects the appearance of the data and must always be noted when examining plotted data. A log scale flattens curves and reduces the apparent strength of trends and differences whereas an arithmetic scale does the opposite. On a log scale, an increasing, straightline trend implies an exponential, not linear rate of increase.

A common error in inference when interpreting descriptive data is the *ecologic fallacy*, the attribution of causality to an association seen only in descriptive data. For example, the international risk of colon cancer (mortality rates for each country plotted on a graph) correlates with the average dietary intake of those countries for fat, meat, and sugar and with the average amount of sunlight (the major determinant of vitamin D levels). To assume automatically that all four variables are true risk factors for colon cancer at the level of the individual would be an example of the ecologic fallacy, confusing descriptive data for analytic (individual level) data.

In the interpretation of time trend data, the possibility of a *cohort effect* must be kept in mind. A cohort effect, familiar by analogy to anyone who studies the sociology of baby-boomers, is the variation in disease occurrence that occurs in a population over time, as successive birth cohorts (persons of the same age) experience the unique environment that typifies their life course. For example, based on cross-sectional prevalence data compiled in Portland, Oregon, in 1991, the prevalence rates of koilocytotic atypia of the cervix decreases sharply with increasing age from a peak at about 20–25 years. This age trend might represent a biologic phenomenon, the result of immunity, with many women becoming infected with HPV at the time of initiation of sexual intercourse, then becoming increasingly immune and having fewer new sexual partners as they age. Or, the age trend could also reflect a cohort effect, with changing sexual practices and increasing prevalence of HPV infection over the past decades placing younger women today at higher risk for koilocytotic changes compared with their older sisters and mothers.

To distinguish cohort effects from simple age trends requires a *cohort analysis*, a type of descriptive graphing in which the age-specific prevalence rates are graphed separately for each birth cohort. These analyses are usually difficult enough in interpretation to merit a statistical consultation.

The Basic Contingency Table

The pathology slide of epidemiology is the contingency table, the basic form of which is the 2 × 2 table (Table 27.1). Most important epidemiologic findings, relating an exposure to risk of a disease, have been derived and can be expressed in this simple form. Extension of the table to more rows or columns does not change the concepts, only the statistical complexity.

The most common statistics computed from a contingency table are simple proportions or percentages (proportions of 100%), which can then be compared: "Ninety percent of the group with disease were smokers [$(a/a + c) = 0.90$] compared with 20% of the nondiseased [$(b/b + d) = 0.20$]. These proportions could be compared statistically using the well-known *t-test* or another test of the difference between independent proportions. More often, the *chi-square statistic* is computed, which gives equivalent interpretations but has a slightly different intent.

The chi-square test is meant to determine whether the disease categories and the exposure categories are associated or independent; that is, does being exposed affect the probability of having disease? Chi-square values are derived by comparing the expected counts of a, b, c, and d, to the values that would be expected if disease and exposure were totally independent. For example, the expected value of a is the cross product of $(a + b) \times (a + c)$ divided by n. The divergence of observed from expected values for all the *cells* of the table (a, b, c, d) are summed to derive the chi-square statistic. The larger the statistic, summarizing how much observed counts differ from expected, the more likely disease and exposure are associated by more than chance.

The chi-square statistic obtained is compared to the tabled values of the *chi-square distribution* to yield a *p-value*, the probability of observing such a chi-square value if disease and exposure are not related. In other words, this is the probability of concluding that an association exists in error. To falsely

Table 27.1. The basic contingency table

	Disease	*No disease*	*Total*
Exposed or test positive	a	b	a + b
Unexposed or test negative	c	d	c + d
Total	a + c	b + d	a + b + c + d = n

accept an association, when the *null assumption* would be correct, is considered a type 1 error. This name was chosen perhaps because it is generally considered a more important scientific error than failing to detect a true association (a type 2 error). If the p-value is less than an appropriate cutpoint, such as 0.05 or 0.01, then convention dictates that chance is unlikely to explain the degree of association seen in the table and the association is considered *statistically significant*.

Thanks to many published cautions, most clinicians and researchers know that a strict dependence on p-values is incorrect because the magnitude of the p-value is dependent on the size of the study. Smaller studies require stronger associations to achieve the same level of statistical significance; thus a p-value of 0.06 in a small study by no means rules out a true exposure–disease association whereas a highly statistically significant difference from a huge study may be so small as to be clinically irrelevant.

Contingency tables larger than 2×2 should be analyzed in a methodical and hierarchical fashion, not restricting the analysis to the most "significant looking" internal comparisons. First, the evidence for association in the full table should be assessed and, if there is none, then the analysis should stop. A common mistake some novices make is to look at a large contingency table, choose the most interesting difference seen, then test the significance of that extracted comparison. Given a large enough contingency table, some subtables will yield statistically significant results by chance alone. Permitting a prescreening of the data before applying a statistical test to the most divergent data points is wrong. If one wishes to define the likely source of the association when the overall contingency table indicates statistical significance, the proper approach is to analyze smaller subtables in a complete and hierarchical manner. A formal description of the proper approach to contingency table analyses can be found in standard biostatistics texts.

When the number of study subjects is very small, such that the expected count in any cell is less than about five, then chi-square analyses are unreliable and should be replaced by a test called *Fisher's exact test*. Of course, if the study is too small, no result will be statistically significant.

One other key point about contingency tables is that the two measurements (disease status and exposure, for example) must be assumed to be independent as one embarks on statistical testing. Although a significant chi-square statistic indicates that the measurements are not independent, the initial or *null hypothesis* of independence is what the test is designed to reject. Thus, standard chi-square analyses should not be performed to test tables where the measurements are explicitly correlated, as in interpathologist agreement studies (see later) or comparisons of the efficacy of two cell collection techniques used in the same group of patients. For these *paired-sample comparisons*, the *McNemar's test* is easy to use. The test ignores the points of agreement of the two measurements and tests the statistical significance of the amount of divergence.

It would also be wrong to include more than one measurement per subject in a standard contingency table. Measurements from a given person tend to be "auto-correlated," that is, more alike than random measurements. A difficult and evolving field of epidemiology explicitly considers multiple measurements from subjects. For example, in a prospective cohort study, it may be very interesting to study the patterns of mildly abnormal cytologic interpretations over time that indicate a risk of subsequent severe neoplasia. The level of study remains the woman, not the slide, and a simple contingency table cannot be used as it would lump together all the interpretations naively.

Measures of Risk (Absolute, Relative, and Attributable Risks)

The chi-square provides limited information regarding the strength of an association (yes/no). Therefore, epidemiologists often prefer instead to compute the more informative statistic, the relative risk (or odds ratio estimate of the relative risk). These key terms were defined in the section on epidemiologic studies of disease etiology. In this section, the relation of the terms to the contingency table are explained, with a brief discussion of ancillary topics such as statistical adjustment of confounding variables, interaction, and confidence intervals.

Suppose a prospective study started by defining an exposed group and an unexposed group of women, then followed the two groups for disease occurrence. The absolute risk of disease following exposure can be represented as an incidence rate $a/(a + b)$. The time period for this incidence rate is implicitly the duration of follow-up. The absolute risk of disease in the unexposed group, analogously, would be the incidence rate $c/(c + d)$. The ratio of these absolute risks would be the relative risk (specifically, the incidence rate ratio) in exposed versus nonexposed women, $a/(a + b)$ divided by $c/(c + d)$. A relative risk of approximately 1.0 implies the exposure is not related to risk of the disease. A relative risk greater than 1.0 implies an increased risk. For example, a relative risk of 2.0 means that the risk of disease in exposed women is twice that of unexposed women. In contrast, a relative risk between 0.0 and 1.0 indicates a protective association (a relative risk of 0.5 implies a halving of risk associated with the exposure). Prospective studies permit the computational directness and intuitive quality of the relative risk calculation, and the ability to decompose the relative risk into the absolute risks among the exposed and unexposed groups.

In contrast, absolute risks cannot usually be calculated in case-control studies, because the true numbers of exposed women ($a + b$) and unexposed women ($c + d$) are not known. In fact, in 2×2 tables from case-control studies the values $a + b$ and $c + d$ are meaningless and should never be computed. The numbers of cases ($a + c$) and controls ($b + d$) are chosen first, and not in proportion to the true ratio of cases to controls in the population. Cases are almost always sampled in excess; in fact, oversampling cases to overcome the limitation of rarity is the major reason to perform a case-control analysis.

As mentioned earlier, although case-control data do not permit direct calculation of the relative risk, the odds ratio provides a valid estimate of it if the following assumptions are met. The cases and controls must represent an unbiased sample of all women with and without disease in the population. The disease in question must be rare if prevalent cases are studied. If the cases are all incident, the rare disease assumption is not as important, unless the disease is so common that a nonnegligible percentage of the population is developing it at any given time.

To understand these points more intuitively, again consider a prospective study. The odds of disease in exposed women is a/b, very close to the risk of disease $a/(a + b)$ if a, the occurrence of disease among the exposed, is very infrequent. Similarly, the odds of disease in nonexposed women is c/d, close to the risk of the disease if uncommon in the nonexposed women, $c/(c + d)$. With a little algebra, it is easy to see that the relative odds or odds ratio for a rare disease (a/b divided by c/d, often computed as the cross-product ad/bc) is quite close to the relative risk.

The important point is that the cross-product ad/bc can be computed from a case-control study without knowing the total number of exposed and unexposed women. So long as the odds a/c and b/d are unbiased with regard to the entire population, then a/c divided by b/d equals ad/bc equals the prospective odds ratio of a/b divided by c/d. The key is to select an unbiased sample of cases and controls. Because epidemiologists usually try to recruit all cases occurring in a population, bias among cases is not usually an issue unless participation rates are poor. The place where bias is a major concern is among the controls. Epidemiologists spend most of their intellectual energy attempting to ensure that the ratio b/d in controls (also thought of as the percentage of controls exposed to the risk factor) is unbiased compared to the same ratio in the whole population that gave rise to the cases. Without the elimination of bias, the odds ratio does not estimate the relative risk, and the case-control design will yield a false result.

Confounding is the type of bias that concerns epidemiologists the most, particularly when they are conducting case-control studies or nonrandomized prospective studies. *Confounding variables* are factors that influence both the risk of disease and the likelihood of exposure to a risk factor under study. The relationship between exposures, confounding variables, and disease outcome is illustrated in Fig. 27.1.

When assessing whether an exposure, such as genital herpes infection causes cervical cancer, the researcher must consider and adjust for the confounding influence of HPV infection, the sexually transmitted agent that is the central cause of cervical cancer. Women who have more sexual partners are more likely to be both herpes type 2 and HPV infected (i.e., the confounding variable HPV is linked to the likelihood of the study exposure, herpes). The apparent influence of herpes type 2 on risk of cervical cancer is reduced by statistically adjusting for HPV infection status. In summary of this important point, epidemiologic analyses must adjust statistically for the influence of confounding factors to generate unbiased risk estimates. Note that confounding factors are true risk factors for disease, despite the name that suggests confusion; it is the exposure–disease association that is under question.

Adjustment for confounding is commonly undertaken by one of three methods: *exclusion*, *stratification*, or *regression modeling*. Exclusion is exem-

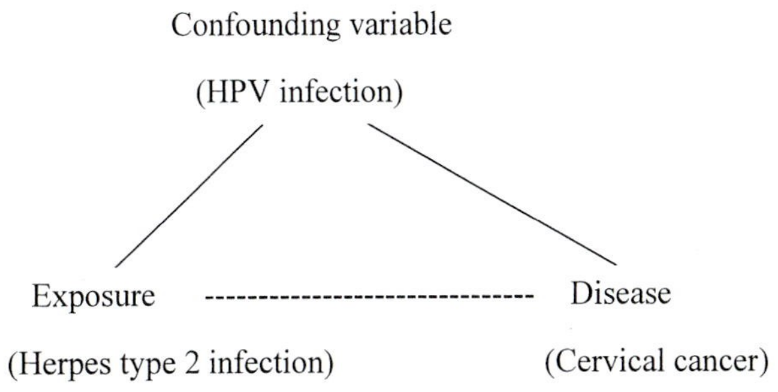

Fig. 27.1. Confounding

plified in the foregoing example by restricting the analysis to women known to be infected with HPV. Using stratification, rather than excluding any subjects, the association of sexual behavior with cervical cancer could be examined separately in each of the two strata (HPV−/HPV+), providing two unconfounded estimates akin to those derived by exclusion. The risk estimates could then be pooled to obtain a global estimate for the risk of genital herpes adjusted for HPV. This kind of stratified analysis is commonly performed using a group of procedures called a *Mantel–Haenszel analysis* in recognition of its developers.

A more conceptually difficult approach that is widely used is *logistic regression analysis*, a multivariable regression technique available in the major statistical software packages such as SAS, STATA, and BMDP. Logistic regression is especially well suited to calculation of the odds ratio as an estimate of the relative risk in case-control studies. This technique permits the simultaneous estimation of the relative risks for multiple risk factors, adjusted for each other's confounding influences. A discussion of this technique, and its uses and misuses, is beyond the scope of this chapter. The commercially available statistical packages offer multivariable regression packages in a seductively simple format that might inspire some novice epidemiologists to perform complicated analyses. However, to master the art of multivariable regression analysis takes statistical training and apprenticeship. Moreover, the results cannot be "checked" easily. It is wise to both avoid and distrust complicated analyses, especially because the bulk of what can be learned from most data sets can be expressed using simple tables and intuitively approachable statistics. In short, all modeling should be checked against simple tables for commonsense agreement.

Adjustment for confounding is often not perfectly achieved, particularly when the confounding variable cannot be measured well or when variables under study are highly correlated. In fact, it is sometimes virtually impossible using statistical methods to adjust for the confounding influences of correlated variables. For example, the most conceptually difficult areas of chronic disease epidemiology relate to time. In all data analyses involving time, the correlated effects of age at first exposure, duration of exposure, and latency (time since first exposure) are among the most difficult to figure out.

Sometimes the risk of an exposure varies by the level of another exposure. For example, the risk of esophageal cancer associated with smoking is much higher among alcohol drinkers than among nondrinkers. This effect modification is often called *interaction*. Extreme positive effect modification is sometimes called synergy, but that term is inexact and probably is worth avoiding. Effect modification is different from confounding, in that no global adjustment to arrive at a single correct risk estimate for the exposure is possible. The risks truly vary by levels of the effect modifier. The proper approach is to present the risk estimates for the exposure separately for each level.

It is common to place *confidence intervals* around relative risk estimates to indicate the likely range of the true risk that we are trying to estimate. Confidence intervals take into account only random error, not bias, and are conceptually somewhat similar to p-values though more informative. Thus, a 95% confidence interval and a p-value of 0.05 are both commonly chosen as standard and have analogous interpretations. For example, if the relative risk of an exposure for a disease is 1.8 with a 95% confidence interval of 1.1 to 3.0, this implies that given random error, the true relative risk has a 95% chance of falling within that range. If the confidence interval for a relative risk excludes 1.0, the result is conventionally considered statistically significant. A relative risk with confidence intervals including 1.0 indicates no statistically significant association between exposure and disease. As with p-values, confidence intervals should be used as a guide but not followed slavishly in interpreting data.

Most analytic epidemiologic research centers on estimation of relative risks. Another very useful concept, especially for public health applications of epidemiologic results, is the *attributable risk*, also known as the *attributable proportion* or *etiologic fraction*. These terms subsume several computational forms and subtle differences in meaning, but the general meaning is clear: how much of the disease (from 0 to 100%) is due to the exposure and would theoretically disappear if the exposure were eliminated. One useful computational formula for the attributable risk, using the notation in Table 27.1, is Attributable risk $= [(a/a + c) \times (1 - 1/\text{RR})] \times 100\%$. In words, the fraction of disease attributable to the risk factor is equal to the percentage of cases of the disease who are exposed, adjusted for the strength of the estimated relative risk. Although the formula may appear a bit complicated, it is very easy to use. The adjustment part of the formula $(1 - 1/\text{RR})$, goes to 0 as the relative risk goes to 1.0 and goes to 1 as the relative risk goes to infinity. Thus, even if all cases are exposed, the attributable risk will be 0% if all controls are also exposed because the RR is 1.0 and the adjustment term is 0.

Causal Intermediates and Surrogate Endpoints

Increasingly, many pathology and epidemiology studies of gynecologic neoplasia do not include invasive tumors. There is a keen interest in the validation of biomarkers and intermediate/surrogate endpoints for screening, diagnosis, and etiologic research. Cancers arise as multistep processes. An exposure can become a biologically effective internal dose, resultant genetic alteration can lead to a subtle lesion, and the precursor can progress to cancer. Each step might be reversible and influenced by the genetic susceptibility of the individual. The earliest *intermediate endpoints* are often common and reversible, such as HPV infection. Later steps are less common and more fixed, such as progression of a simple HPV infection to CIN 3. Although molecular biologists may view oncogenesis as a series of "molecular hits," epidemiologists may discuss "conditional probabilities." For example, conditional on a woman being infected with an oncogenic type of HPV, what is the probability of progression to CIN 3? Conditional on having CIN 3, what is the probability of invasion? If the CIN 3 lasts for 5 years without regression, how does that affect the probability of invasion?, and so on. Oncogenesis occurs mechanistically but, lacking all the details, epidemiology presumes that events will happen by useful measurements of "chance."

The importance of a biomarker or intermediate endpoint can be evaluated using the relative risk of cancer when positive compared to when negative. A high relative risk implies importance. A *surrogate endpoint* is a more stringent term. Many studies examining the associations between biomarkers are not clinically relevant because no association with attributable risk of disease is directly made. If a biomarker is a valid surrogate endpoint, then reducing its occurrence should proportionately reduce the occurrence of the cancer itself. CIN 3 is a good surrogate endpoint for invasive cervical cancer.

The statistical evaluation of possible intermediate endpoints is linked to the analysis of confounding algebraically, but there are important differences of interpretation. When a biomarker or preinvasive lesion is proposed as an intermediate endpoint for a cancer, it should share the general risk factor profile of that cancer. In fact, its consideration by statistical adjustment should "explain" the association of known epidemiologic risk factors for that cancer. If not, the validity of the intermediate endpoint as a surrogate for the cancer is in question. As an example, the risk of ovarian cysts detected by transvaginal ultrasound is not reduced by multiparity and oral contraceptive use. These are two very powerful protective factors in the etiology of ovarian cancer, casting doubt on the etiologic relevance of most of the cysts found by ultrasound.[3] On the other hand, HPV infection almost completely explains the strong association of sexual behavior and risk of cervical cancer, as befits a central causal intermediate.[11]

Measures of Interpathologist Agreement

Simply put, there is no universally accepted statistical measure of interrater agreement. The problem is adjustment for the influence of chance agreement, which varies with the numbers of categories and the composition of the study population. All currently available statistical methods have limitations and, therefore, it is best when possible to present the actual data to the reader, in addition to any percentage or statistic.

Consider a study of interpathologist agreement for the categories of the Bethesda System of cervical cytology. A group of 100 smears was given to pairs of pathologists, who were asked to rate them as normal or benign reactive changes, atypical squamous cells of undetermined significance (ASCUS), LSIL, or HSIL (high-grade squamous intraepithelial lesion).[14,15] The trouble with simply calculating percent agreement is not only that some agreement is expected by chance. The results are strongly dependent on how the smears are chosen. If mainly normal smears were submitted, the percentage of agreement would be high. If a wide range of changes were equally represented, then agreement would undoubtedly decrease. In general, the most information is obtained by choosing a wide range of smears, oversampling the rarer grades to achieve a balanced study group.

The most widely used, more sophisticated statistic of agreement of use to pathologists is the *kappa statistic*. The kappa statistic computes the proportion of agreement in excess of the expected chance agreement. Kappa values can range from 1.0 (perfect agreement) to less than 0.0 (zero implies only chance agreement). The statistic has some limitations.[8] Only tables of identical size can be compared, and the statistic is slightly dependent on the prevalence of disease. Also, the interpretation of kappa values is not absolutely clear cut, in that researchers disagree as to what defines good agreement. In general, values greater than 0.75 represent excellent agreement beyond chance, 0.40 to 0.75 is fair to good, and less than 0.40 indicates poor agreement beyond chance.[1] An asymmetry chi-square, analogous to a multicategory McNemar's test, is often calculated with the kappa statistic. The purpose is to test whether one rater is yielding systematically more severe interpretations than the other, or whether disagreements are randomly distributed.

Many pathologists are willing to admit how difficult it is to distinguish grades of intraepithelial neoplasia as assessed by cytology. Objective molecular measurements such as HPV DNA testing are useful in clarification of equivocal cytology.[14] However, as mentioned earlier, much less is said about the irreproducibility of histologic diagnoses or intraepithelial neoplasia. Interpathologist agreement based on cytology or histology tends to be moderate, not excellent,[16] which is a sobering thought given the importance of the interpretations in guiding patient management. To the knowledgeable epidemiologist, misclassification of pathology is inevitable and not a matter of fault in most instances.

Screening Terms

Screening is a special area of epidemiology distinct from descriptive or analytic studies. It is rare to find a useful screening test. Finding a strong risk factor for a disease does not imply that we should screen for that risk factor, because the factor is often too common in the general population to permit its use as a trigger for clinical action.

Screening terms have very exact meanings, which may vary from other common uses of the same terms. In Table 27.1, the women in cell "a" have *true-positive* screening tests, in that they have the disease and tested positive. The women in cell "c" have *false-negative* results, because they have the disease but tested negative. The *sensitivity* of a test, also called the true-positive rate, is the percentage of diseased women who test positive [$a/(a + c)$ in Fig. 27.1]. The screening sensitivity must be clearly distinguished from the analytic sensitivity of a laboratory assay, which has a different meaning. Typically, the more analytic sensitivity the better. However, increasing screening sensitivity can lead to decreasing specificity, as indicated in the following section on ROC curves.

The *true-negative* results are in cell "d"; the *false-positive* results are in cell "b". The *specificity*, also called the true negative rate, is the percentage of women without the disease who test negative [$d/(b + d)$]. The concept of specificity is more important in screening than most realize. Because the overwhelming majority of women in a population do not have the disease under study, as the specificity percentage falls even slightly, the absolute numbers of false-positive screening tests rise dramatically in comparison to the number of true positives.

Therefore, decreased specificity leads to low *positive predictive value*, the percentage of women with a positive test who truly have the disease [$a/(a + b)$]. Positive predictive value is, for many diseases, the major screening statistic of interest. Clinicians ask: If a woman tests positive, what is the likelihood that she will have disease confirmed on referral to the next clinical step (e.g., colposcopically directed biopsy, laparoscopy, or more major surgery). Low positive predictive value leads to overreferral and overtreatment.

For grave diseases, where overtreatment of normal women is less of a concern than not missing any cases, the *negative predictive value* is a very important concept of reassurance. The negative predictive value is the percentage of women who test negative who are truly disease free [$d/(c + d)$]. A clinician may ask, accordingly, "If the test is negative, what is the percentage assurance that the disease is not present and that I can safely stop the diagnostic workup?" The sensitivity of the test is usually the key determinant of negative predictive value.

When screening is mentioned, there is always an implicit notion of a *reference standard* or *gold standard* of disease. The performance of screening tests is described statistically in relation to this reference standard, and if it is flawed, then the screening statistics will be flawed. For example, colposcopically directed biopsy with pathologic diagnosis is often taken as the reference standard of cervical intraepithelial neoplasia (CIN), but the colposcopic biopsy may be misdirected or the histopathologic diagnosis may be in error. Thus, the true performance of screening tests such as cytology, cervicography, or HPV testing may be misinterpreted when compared with the results of colposcopically directed biopsies.[17]

Screening tests may detect prevalent disease or predict the future diagnosis of disease, and the two time frames may be confused. If some type of HPV test could truly predict incipient cervical neoplasia, even when biopsies were still negative, it would be misleading to compare the HPV screening result only to prevalent (same-day) disease defined by biopsies.

Another mistake is the following: Researchers who wish to compare the sensitivity of two screening tests double-test a research population, referring for a definitive diagnostic procedure those women who are positive for either screening test. If they then compute and report the "sensitivity" of each test, an error of circular reasoning has been made.

Because both screening tests could have missed disease (double false-negatives), the true sensitivity of either test cannot be known without referring all women in the study population for the definitive workup. Sometimes, in large studies, it suffices to refer a random sample of the women who screen negative on both tests, as a way of correcting (or of verifying, to think optimistically) the estimates of sensitivity.

The point of this discussion is that, when screening terms such as sensitivity or specificity are mentioned, then the reference standard must be explicitly stated and, if necessary, questioned.

The Receiver–Operating Characteristic (ROC) Curve

Some of the current controversy regarding the proper clinical management of inconclusive cervical cytologic smears centers on the competing needs for good negative predictive value (assurance that we are not missing any high-grade disease) and good positive predictive value (desire to not overtreat). This problem highlights an inescapable feature of screening (or more fundamentally of trying to categorize overlapping distributions): increased sensitivity virtually always leads to decreased specificity and, as a corollary, increasingly reassuring negative predictive value can only be obtained at the price of decreased positive predictive value.

There is a formal method for choosing the proper screening *cutpoint* (e.g., the viral load threshold of a DNA-based assay meriting colposcopic referral to detect CIN 2–3 or cancer) to achieve an optimal compromise between sensitivity and specificity. The technique is called the *receiver–operating characteristic* (*ROC*), because the approach was developed to test how well an electronic receiver could distinguish signals from electrical noise. The concepts are useful and well explained in a few key articles that are recommended to anyone wishing to evaluate a screening test.[12,19]

In brief, most test measurements range from zero to some high value. It is conceivable to set a series of cutpoints that define a positive screening test result demanding further attention. Lower cutpoints may detect more cases of disease but refer more women. In a ROC curve, sensitivity for detection of the target disease is plotted against 100% specificity. The expression 100% minus specificity is very close to percent referred. A very good screening test will have very high sensitivity and specificity. In other words, it will detect women with disease but refer few extra women. The quality of screening or diagnostic tests is easy to compare using ROC curves.

Problem Areas

The major goal of including an introduction to epidemiology in a textbook on gynecologic pathology was to encourage pathologists to do epidemiologic studies and to work with epidemiologists. Accordingly, it may be worth alerting the pathologist to recurrent problem areas that exist at the juncture of the two disciplines. This section quite informally catalogs a few practical problems that appear to arise most commonly.

Dividing a Spectrum of Disease into Categories

Unfortunately, some epidemiologists may seek out pathologists to perform a service function of "making sure the cases are right," without understanding much about pathology (just as pathologists might seek out statisticians to do a rote data analysis or to figure "How many cases are needed for statistical significance?"). Providing rote pathology review may prove a difficult collaboration, because epidemiologists are prompted by their statistical methods to seek overly simplistic and discrete categorization of disease outcomes. Because the statistical methods for considering a spectrum of disease are difficult to perform and understand, epidemiologists tend to simplify disease measurements into a few (ideally two) reliably distinguished categories, such as "invasive cervical cancer" versus "normal." But, as the example of cervical neoplasia demonstrates, diseases may exist as a spectrum of changes that are impossible to divide perfectly into a few categories.

When an epidemiologist asks a pathologist to state whether a slide shows disease (i.e., defines a case) or not (i.e., rejects the case), an uncertain or heavily qualified diagnosis is difficult to force into the study dichotomy. Often, the epidemiologist must subsequently exclude the uncertain diagnoses from the analyses. It is possible to perform a "malicious analysis" in which the uncertain cases are added to the analysis as cases, then reanalyzed as controls, to see whether the uncertainty in pathologic definition affects the comparisons being made. However, too large a proportion of uncertain diagnoses can make an analytic study unreliable.

The collaborating epidemiologist must be willing to understand diagnostic error as a fact of nature and not a failing of pathologists. The pathologist must be willing to sacrifice absolute truth to simplify the statistical data to the point of understanding. The limitations of epidemiology should be recognized. As a great physician-epidemiologist once said: "Epidemiology is a butcher shop; don't try to use a scalpel." In other words, epidemiology can only study strong risk associations, because even strong associations are made to appear weak by unavoidable measurement errors and biases. Truly weak associations will probably be missed by all but the largest and luckiest studies. With this in mind, the routine use of pathologic qualifiers such as "consistent with" and "cannot exclude" should be abandoned for epidemiologic studies, with the recognition that diagnostic errors will exist (the extent of which should be measured by reliability studies and reported).

The Need for Masking

Epidemiologists tend to mask all data collection as an automatic part of good research technique to avoid the influence of possible subtle biases that could distort risk estimates. Thus, they do not routinely tell interviewers the disease status of the subjects to minimize bias in questioning, they do not tell laboratory collaborators the identity of specimens until the results are obtained, and they ask pathologists to make their diagnoses with a minimum of information regarding the patients. Pathologists working together (panel reviews) tend to agree more readily than if the independent opinions are compared. The social tendency to promote consensus may be the cause. Epidemiologists are seeking a completely independent decision from pathologists, without influence from previous diagnoses or clinical tests, which often are being studied as risk factors for the current condition. All common statistical tests assume that the study measurements are completely independent of each other; thus, using any piece of data to influence a decision on another piece of data is wrong.

Pathologists, however, realize that diagnoses are best made in the context of complete information regarding the patient, and that asking for a microscopic diagnosis out of context, as one would demand a lab result from a machine, risks error. Some pathologists incorrectly view the request for masking as a sign of distrust of their intellectual integrity or ability to make an independent decision. The request is actually a sign of epidemiologists' belief that everyone is biased about every decision unless masked. As a revealing example, an epidemiologists' wine tasting group in Maryland covers all labels from the bottles before tasting and unmasks the results only after the "data" (opinions) are in. Fortunately, it is usually easy for good collaborators to achieve a balance between automatic demands for complete masking and the kind of complete disclosure of study information that could lead to serious biases.

Standardization of the Scientific Art of Pathology

A more thorny problem arises when epidemiologists challenge the accuracy and reliability of pathologic diagnoses, either as part of a formal pathology agreement study or as part of a larger epidemiologic project. This challenge takes the form of calculation and publication of rates of (dis)agreement between experts or between the expert and himself/herself on different days. The epidemiologist is trained to believe that all biological phenomena are variable and that all measurements of biologic phenomena are prone to random error. The pathologist has the weighty daily task of being the final arbiter of disease definition, a responsibility that does not mesh well with error.

The epidemiologist author has learned something about the world of gynecologic pathology only because of the intellectual humility of expert gynecologic pathologists (responsible for several of the chapters in this text) whose curiosity outweighed their urges to preserve their national reputations for infallibility. Most of the comparisons performed have related to the cytopathology and histopathology of cervical intraepithelial neoplasia and benign "look-alikes." Agreement rates between expert pathologists have been only fair at best but have led to a greatly increased understanding of the diagnoses.

A pathologist may feel irritated at the demands for reliability studies from new epidemiologist colleagues. If so, it might help to ask the eager-beaver epidemiologist when they had last compared their design or analytic performance in a masked comparison with other epidemiologists. Because such painful comparative exercises are almost never perpetrated by epidemiologists on themselves, mutual humility and curiosity should reign.

Specimen Adequacy Versus the Bias of Convenience Samples

Epidemiologists seeking to minimize bias are loath to permit exclusions from a complete series. They suspect that the excluded members of the set will differ from those included in a systematic (biased), rather than random, way. Thus, epidemiologists working with pathologists wish to start their analyses by considering the entire collection of pathologic specimens available, winnowing out as needed to usable specimens but always with an eye to possible biases of exclusion that could affect the general applicability of the results. Epidemiologists distrust *convenience samples*, groups of specimens that happen to be available for testing or for review. Pathologists may view the task of defining and retrieving all relevant specimens from their center to be unnecessary. It may be difficult to decide in advance when a convenience sample is sufficient and when a more definitive collection is required. In general, convenience samples are useful for preliminary methodologic work, such as checking if genomic DNA can be amplified from the paraffin blocks available, but such studies cannot be used to reach definitive, generalizable conclusions.

Deciding How Large a Study to Do: Statistical Significance Versus Practicality

Bigger is better for the epidemiologist. It is not much more difficult to do a statistical analysis of 1000 patients than 100; in fact, it is methodologically easier because the numbers are clearly sufficient. However, the pathologist collaborator may view it differently. The question of study size is almost always negotiable, in that bigger studies permit the detection of smaller differences, but the critical difference that needs to be detected is usually open to discussion.

There are minimum numbers of subjects that permit epidemiologic analyses. It is impossible to generate a statistically significant result with fewer than 5 subjects, regardless of how strong an association is. Thirty subjects is another breakpoint. Thirty subjects is a common minimum number in that common statistics such as means start to "behave" more reliably when there are about 30 or more data points. About 200 cases and 200 controls are needed to find reliably a relative risk of about 2.0 (a doubling of risk), given typical prevalences of common exposures. Case-control studies of more than 1000 subjects are relatively rare. Cohort studies, however, often require thousands or even tens of thousands of subjects to generate enough disease endpoints for analysis. Clinical trials range from small (20 subjects) to large (thousands of subjects) based on the size of the difference being sought. In general, small studies miss weak associations, do not permit adequate adjustment for confounding, and generate less reliable estimates of risk. Still, many landmark studies of new topics have been small.

The key to defining the proper size of the study is to agree on the hypothesis and the range of expected results. Sample size calculations are very assumption dependent and usually demand information not available until the study is completed. Most epidemiologists choose a reasonable number based on cost and time available, then compute the *statistical power* of such a study to detect associations of various strengths. It is standard to require the study to have an 80% or greater chance of finding (as statistically significant) the key disease–exposure association under study, assuming the association truly exists. Epidemiologists therefore commonly accept a 20% chance of making a type 2 error (failing to "observe" a true association) whereas they restrict themselves to approximately a 5% chance of making of a type 1 error (falsely declaring a null association to be significant). As scientific skeptics, epidemiologists stack the deck against themselves to avoid being rash. When they are making multiple comparisons, they often reduce the required level of significance below 1% to even tougher standards of evidence.

For the pathologist, boredom and time commitment can be real problems in big epidemiologic collaborations. Pathology quality assurance group members can easily spend 10 hours a week on review work of fairly monotonous, unchallenging cases. Of course, the friendly epidemiologic collaborator will be monitoring to avoid any drift in diagnostic interpretations over time. There will be cases sent back with relabeling to assess intrapathologist reproducibility. The situation requires dedication, trust, and scientific interest. In truth, to answer big questions often takes big studies by a cooperative team.

Incorporating Research into Pathology Practice

The value of well-characterized pathology collections is increasing. The field of molecular diagnostics is being powered at the speed of molecular biology. The clinical relevance of new findings and potential assays, however, can only be evaluated at the restraining speed of clinical studies and epidemiology. A few new themes are emerging.

In this volume, there are discussions of genomics, RNA microarrays, and proteomics. However, venerable old histology collections are usually not useful for archival studies of DNA and especially RNA because of the destructive nature of acidic fixatives. Even neutral buffered formalin is not nucleic acid "friendly." Pathologists who wish to conduct a lot of molecular work come under pressure to perform frozen sections or to use ethanol or other fixatives favoring the molecular analysis as well as the morphology. As a very pragmatic point, will pathologists keep tissues past the regulatory requirements to promote science, at the expense and risk that accompany archived materials?

As another issue of practicality and trust, institutions need to work together more than ever before to further new leads into the origins of relatively rare tumors and new subdivisions of neoplasia. Issues of relabeling, confidentiality, and ambiguities of informed consent can stop conceptually appealing multiinstitutional collaborations.

For those readers who have actually displayed exceptional interest by completing this chapter, a good question might be "Where do we interdisciplinary types go from here?" Journals of common general interest to pathologists and epidemiologists are rare. Funding committees often are not composed to evaluate our jointly conceived projects. Interdisciplinary meetings for pathologists and epidemiologists are difficult to imagine and virtually nonexistent. For now, we meet in response to specific research questions, in ad hoc meetings and collaborations.

For the future, however, consider this. I am in a research group that previously contained only epidemiologists and clinicians. Then we added molecular biologists. Starting this year, we will have our first full-fledged pathologist epidemiologist. Laser capture microdissection and microarrays are beginning to replace questionnaires and abstracts as the "meat and potatoes" of cancer epidemiology.

References

1. Fleiss JL (1981) Statistical methods for rates and proportions, 2nd Ed. Wiley, New York
2. Gordis L (2000) Epidemiology, 2nd Ed, Saunders, Philadelphia
3. Hartge P, Hayes R, Reding D, et al (2000) Complex ovarian cysts in postmenopausal women are not associated with ovarian cancer risk factors. Preliminary data from the PLCO cancer screening trial. Am J Obstet Gynecol 183: 232–1237
4. Greenlee RT, Murray T, Bolden S, Wingo PA (2000) Cancer statistics, 2000. CA A Cancer J Clin 50:7–33
5. Knapp RG, Miller MC (1992) Clinical epidemiology and biostatistics. National medical series for independent study. Williams & Wilkins, Baltimore
6. Kurman RJ, Toki T, Schiffman MH (1993) Basaloid and warty carcinomas of the vulva. Am J Surg Pathol 17: 33–145
7. Last JM, Abramson JH (1995) A dictionary of epidemiology, 3rd Ed. Oxford University Press, New York
8. Maclure M, Willett W (1987) Misinterpretation and misuse of the kappa statistic. Am J Epidemiol 126: 161–169
9. Pisani P, Parkin DM, Bray F, Ferlay J (1999) Estimates of the worldwide mortality from 25 cancers in 1990. Int J Cancer 83:18–29 (see erratum Int J Cancer (1999) 83:870–873)
10. Sackett DL, Haynes RB, Tugwell P, Guyatt GH (1991) Clinical epidemiology: a basic science for clinical medicine. Lippincott, Philadelphia
11. Schiffman MH, Bauer HM, Hoover RN, et al (1993) Epidemiologic evidence showing that human papillomavirus infection causes most cervical intraepithelial neoplasia. J Natl Cancer Inst 85:958–964
12. Schiffman M, Herrero R, Hildesheim A, et al (2000) HPV DNA testing in cervical cancer screening: results from women in a high-risk province of Costa Rica. JAMA 283:87–93
13. Schiffman MH, Schatzkin A (1994) Test reliability is critically important to molecular epidemiology: an example from studies of human papillomavirus infection and cervical neoplasia. Cancer Res 54:1944s–1947s
14. Sherman ME, Schiffman MH, Lorincz AT, et al (1994) Towards objective quality assurance in cervical cytopathology: correlation of cytopathologic diagnoses with detection of high-risk HPV types. Am J Clin Pathol 102:182–187
15. Smith A, Sherman ME, Scott DR, et al (2000) Review of the Bethesda System Atlas does not improve reproducibility or accuracy in the classification of atypical squamous cells of undetermined significance. Cancer Cytopathol 90:201–206
16. Stoler MH, Schiffman M, ALTS Group (2001) Interobserver reproducibility of cervical cytologic and histologic diagnoses: realistic estimates from the ASCUS-LSIL triage study (ALTS). JAMA 285:1500–1505
17. Wacholder S, Armstrong B, Hartge P (1993) Validation studies using an alloyed gold standard. Am J Epidemiol 137:1251–1258
18. Whelan SL, Parkin DM, Masuyer E (1991) Patterns of cancer in five continents, IARC scientific publication no. 102. Oxford University Press, New York
19. Zweig MH, Campbell G (1993) Receiver-operating characteristic (ROC) plots. Clin Chem 39:561–577

28

Gross Description, Processing, and Reporting of Gynecologic and Obstetric Specimens

Stanley J. Robboy, M.D., Frederick T. Kraus, M.D., and Robert J. Kurman, M.D.

The surgical pathology report provides the histopathologic diagnosis and specific information relating to prognosis and treatment. Accordingly, the surgical pathologist must have sufficient familiarity with the management of gynecologic and obstetric disorders to assure that a major focus of the report is to communicate the clinically relevant information. This chapter provides an approach to the processing of gynecologic and obstetric tissue specimens. The techniques of the gross examination and the method of reporting the pathologic findings are guided by the clinical principles on which patient management is based.

The types of gynecologic tissue specimens that are submitted to the surgical pathology laboratory can be divided generally into two categories: biopsy specimens and therapeutic resections. Obstetric tissue specimens include placentas and sometimes uterine curettings. The main purpose of the biopsy is to provide a histologic diagnosis that will guide management. Biopsy specimens should, therefore, be processed expeditiously. The gross description must be precise and brief. There should be correlation between the microscopic tissue section and the gross specimen with regard to the number of specimens and the approximate site of each or aggregate site of the total. This is especially important when it appears that a slide or block may have been mislabeled. Two examples of appropriate description are "3 ovoid fragments 2 to 4 mm in diameter," "multiple shreds of tissue 5 cm in aggregate size," or the exact size given in three dimensions. When the case may need review later, only the tissue slides themselves are used.

For operative specimens, particularly those containing a tumor, information in the surgical pathology report should include a description of the extent of the tumor and specific features that are related to prognosis. The adequacy of the surgical treatment as well as the need for additional therapy depend on these findings. Because the gynecologic surgeon has seen the pathology in vivo, it is important that he communicate the operative findings as these will bear directly on how the pathologist processes the specimen. For example, adequacy of resection margins requires an appreciation of the orientation of the specimen to certain anatomic landmarks that are obvious to the surgeon but cannot always be reconstructed by the pathologist in the laboratory.

The gross description and final diagnosis must be clearly written. A good gross description enables the reader to reconstruct an image that corresponds to the specimen and its lesion. Because the histologic diagnosis for many tumors has been made by biopsy before the operative procedure, the gross description of the specimen should focus on the site and extent of the lesion and its relationship to adjacent structures. In this sense the gross description is analogous to the provisional anatomic diagnosis of a postmortem examination in which the microscopic examination confirms the gross anatomic findings. Key findings should be suggested from the gross examination of the specimen. Microscopic findings should be complementary to those identified grossly, and it should be uncommon for them to be in conflict. A careful gross examination and description are mandatory to ensure that the appropriate microscopic sections are obtained.

The final diagnosis of a tumor should include its cell type, grade, location, and extent as well as the adequacy of the resection margins, presence of lymphatic or vascular invasion, and status of the regional lymph nodes. It is one thing to report an "endometrial adenocarcinoma" but far better to report "serous carcinoma of the endometrium with vascular invasion, penetrating to within 0.2 mm of the margin, with metastases to 2 of 24 lymph nodes" with a detailed listing to follow of which lymph nodes, and how many in each group, are involved. The former merely reaffirms what was known before the operation, whereas the latter presents information that helps to predict prognosis and plan further treatment.

It is common today to perform ancillary tests that will influence the final diagnosis rendered. Examples include special stains, immunocytochemical determinations, molecular diagnostic techniques, and ultrastructural examination. The fact that the test was performed and the results of each should be clearly identified in some area of the report. Common locations include a special section in the report or in a "comment" following the diagnosis.

General Procedures

Gross Description

Specimens received in the fresh state should be described before fixation because formalin alters the natural color and consistency of tissue. The opening sentence of the gross description should indicate whether the tissue is received fresh or fixed and how it is labeled. Note whether the specimen received corresponds with how it is labeled. For example, "Received fresh is a specimen labeled 'uterus, tubes, and ovaries'; however, only the uterus and right ovary and tube are identified." The overall measurements and weight of the entire specimen are useful, but those of the individual components are critical.

The gross description should proceed in an orderly fashion, with the focus on the primary lesion. For example, in a radical hysterectomy, the cervical cancer should be described before the normal ovaries, incidentally removed appendix, and multiple lymph nodes. Emphasize the pathology and avoid elaborate descriptions of normal anatomy. For example, a normal appendix can be described as "5 cm long" and "normal" rather than as a "5 cm long, 4 mm in diameter, vermiform appendix with a tan, unremarkable serosa, 1-mm-thick wall, and a lumen without identifiable abnormality." The gross description, especially of small specimens, should conclude with a statement of whether all the tissue has been processed for microscopic examination or whether tissue remains. All descriptions should include an inventory listing the number of blocks sampled and from where they were obtained.

Drawings and Photographs

The description of a specimen with complicated relationships may be simplified by including a drawing or photograph as part of the surgical pathology report. This method permits orientation of the tumor to the remainder of the specimen, especially surgical resection margins, and visual identification of section codes.

Synoptic Checklists

As the complexity of information contained in reports increases and tumor cases are accessioned into trials with specific entry criteria, checklists are being used with increasing frequency to record and evaluate the details of operative and pathologic findings. The checklists we have developed for each organ and which detail areas of importance are included in an appendix at the end of this chapter.[1] In recent years, the College of American Pathologists has also developed checklists for most organs, including the genital tract. Although checklists are useful, it is important they be employed with care and full understanding of their purpose. They help highlight features that are of known importance or are being currently investigated as of potential import, thus serving as an aid to foster issuance of more complete reports. In particular, they should not be slavishly adopted, for "pigeonholing" according to the checklist may hinder rather than foster open-mindedness as specimens are examined.

In emphasizing its philosophy of use, the College of American Pathologists has added the following statement, advice which should be well remembered:

"The College recognizes that this document may be used by hospitals, attorneys, managed care organizations, insurance carriers, and other payers. However, the document was developed solely as a tool to assist pathologists in the diagnostic process by providing information that reflects the state of relevant medical knowledge at the time the protocol was first published. It was not developed for credentialing, litigation, or reimbursement purposes. The College cautions that any uses of the protocol for these purposes involve considerations that are beyond the scope of this document."[3]

Sections Codes

Many operations result in two or more separate specimens being submitted to the pathology department. Cervical examinations often produce 2 or 3 colposcopically directed biopsies plus endocervical curettage. Twenty or more specimens from a staging laparotomy are also common. As a first step, each specimen received should be numbered and checked against the clinical manifest to ensure that all specimens removed have in fact reached the pathologist. This information is usually listed on the requisition sheet. Each specimen should be uniquely labeled.

It is important that every department agree on a numbering system that is clear and used consistently throughout the specimen. The most common systems in use today are computer generated, providing the accession number for the overall case, the container number for each portion of the specimen when it is received in multiple segments, each paraffin block, the level within each paraffin block, and the type of stain used with any given slide.

Most systems use a one- or two-letter prefix to identify the general type of case received (S = surgical, C or P = cytology, and A = autopsy), followed by a 2-digit number designating the year (00 = 2000), followed by a sequential 5- or 6-digit number. One system, in common use worldwide, then assigns a unique letter to each container received starting at the beginning of the alphabet, i.e., "A". Each block sampled from that specimen/container than receives a sequential number, e.g., A1, A2, . . . A*n*. Each subsequent specimen/container receives the next additional letter, e.g., B, with multiple blocks from the container having sequential numbers, B1 . . . B*n*. If multiple levels of a single paraffin block are made (a practice for cervical biopsies in many institutions), the letter "L" is appended to designate the slide level, e.g., -L2 for the second level of the block. Thus, a typical specimen number might be SG-00-02167 B4-L2, which translates to "Surgical specimen of a gynecologic nature, received in year 2000, accession number 2167, container B, 4th block taken from the specimen B, and 2nd slide prepared from that paraffin block." Variants of this system typically utilize letters in upper and lower case, Roman numerals, and Arabic numbers, usually in some combination and defined sequence.

In departments where numbers are assigned manually, some systems label all blocks consecutively regardless of the parent container. The block numbers may be in alphabetical order, e.g., A, B, C . . . Z, proceeding thereafter to AA; after AZ, proceed to BA, and so forth. Another method common in manual systems is to label organs with letters, e.g., RO and LO for right and left ovaries. Although this method has the advantage of providing an intuitive link to the organ sampled, it may lead to ambiguities when dealing with margins and relations with other organs and sometimes leads to overly complex lettering schemes. This method is usually only practical in a group of one or two pathologists who can agree on the abbreviations chosen.

A key at the end of the gross description is used more often and clearly seen than a key included in the text of the gross description. However, inclusion of the key, or at least portions of the key within the text of the gross description, often leads to greater clarity. For example, it is easier in describing a probable leiomyosarcoma to state that the borders in one region are irregular (Block B10) and in another area appear to blend into the surrounding myometrium (Block B11) than to repeat the finding in detail in the key summary.

Regardless of the section code method used, it is critical that the reader can link the tissues received to the sections processed and both to the final diagnoses. For example, four cervical biopsies from the same patient are received in separate containers, but from the same operation. Information on the requisition slip indicates the colposcopically directed specimens are from 3, 6, 9, and 12 o'clock, respectively. In this example, the accession number might be SG-00-02167 and the containers are labeled A, B, C, and D, respectively. Because the paraffin block usually is identified solely by the code, then this same code should appear throughout. Thus, the gross might read "A. 3:00 bx" (the wording exactly replicating what the clinician wrote on the container itself) while the final diagnosis would include "A. Cervix, Biopsy at 3 o'clock: Diagnostic finding." Obviously, the label on the slide must provide all the necessary identifiers.

Formalin Fixation

Formalin-based fixatives are generally the most practical and commonly used today. A specimen that is submitted for tissue processing should be less than 3 mm thick. Thicker sections do not get adequately fixed and are difficult to dehydrate; this inhibits paraffin infiltration, leading to poorly prepared slides that are difficult to interpret. It is much easier and efficient to cut blocks from tissue that have been fixed for several hours instead of attempting to cut 3-mm blocks directly from the fresh specimen. Large specimens should be bread-loafed or alternatively cut into slabs, about 1 cm in thickness, to permit adequate penetration by formalin and then trimmed to 3-mm blocks after about 3 hours of fixation. For large specimens, such as uteri removed for leiomyomata, fixation is facilitated by allowing the tissue blocks that have been placed into cassettes (with all labeling complete) to fix for an extra 24 hours.

With the advent of a large number of immunocytochemical reagents that are effective on paraffin-embedded tissue, it is not necessary to snap-freeze tissues for immunocytochemical analyses. Similarly, because electron microscopy now plays a small role in diagnostic surgical pathology, it is no longer necessary to routinely fix some tissue from tumors in gluteraldehyde except for selected cases involving sarcomas, lymphomas, and pediatric and pituitary tumors.

Specific Procedures

Biopsies and Curettings

Vulvar Biopsy

Excisional biopsies should be handled like skin biopsies. Several methods are in common use to assess both deep as well as lateral resection margins. Orientation is aided if the surgeon places a suture for orientation. In one method, India ink is used to facilitate their recognition on microscopic examination. Sections should be perpendicular to the surface and should be obtained from the longitudinal axis and perpendicular to it across the shorter axis. A second method uses two ink colors, commonly black and alcian blue. Black is used on one lateral margin and alcian blue on the other lateral and entire deep margin. Sections are then taken sequentially from the cranial to caudal end of the specimen. In each method, the color code used needs to be recorded in the section on Gross Description.

Small punch biopsies are submitted totally. Specimens large enough to bisect may be cut perpendicular to the mucosal surface, and the cut surface inked. It is useful also to request at the time of submission that the paraffin block be cut at multiple levels. This step shortens the turnaround time, because small biopsies frequently are sectioned inadequately the first time they are cut. Remounting the block and cutting again takes more time than obtaining multiple levels at the outset and not infrequently exhausts the specimen.

Vaginal Biopsy

Most vaginal biopsies are small punch biopsies and should be handled in a manner similar to vulvar punch biopsies.

Cervical Punch Biopsy

Colposcopically directed punch biopsies should be handled in the same manner as small vulvar and vaginal biopsies. A technique to facilitate orientation is to sandwich the biopsy specimen between blue Gelfoam sponges that fit into the cassette. Another effective technique is to have the gynecologist place the biopsy on its side on a piece of paper towel and then place the specimen and attached paper into fixative (Fig. 28.1). The paper must be removed by the surgical pathologist before processing.

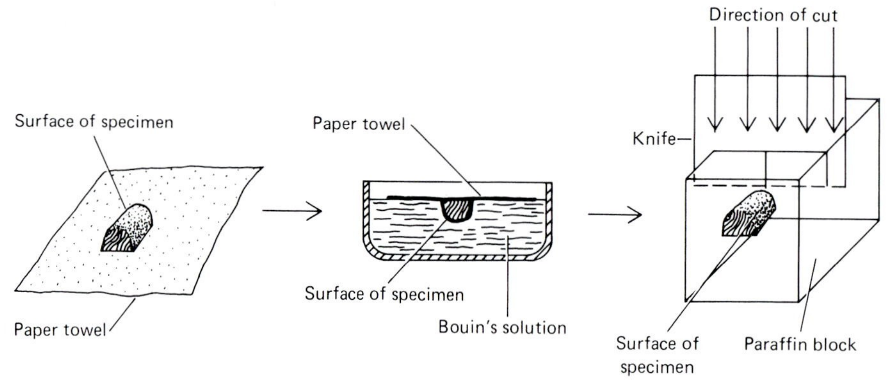

Fig. 28.1. Cervical punch biopsy. Orientation, fixation, and microtome sectioning of a cervical punch biopsy. (Courtesy of Alex Ferenczy, M.D., Montreal, Quebec, Canada.)

Endocervical Curettings

The endocervical curettage is performed to evaluate the presence of endocervical neoplasms, cervical neoplasia in the endocervical canal, or to determine whether endometrial carcinoma has spread into the cervix. Clinical management depends on the presence or absence of disease in the curettings and, therefore, considerable care must be exercised in handling these specimens, which are typically scant and composed mostly of blood and mucus.

The specimen should be transferred directly from the curette by the gynecologist to a Telfa pad. Sponges should be avoided as tissue becomes enmeshed in the sponge and is difficult to retrieve. After the curettage is completed, the curette can be passed through the fixative to dislodge small fragments of tissue that otherwise might remain adherent to the curette. In the laboratory, the entire specimen should be wrapped in a Shandon mesh bag or a tea bag before placing it into a cassette so as to avoid losing small fragments of tissue during processing. Filter paper should be avoided as it is difficult to handle.

Cervical Cone Biopsy and Loop Electrosurgical Excision Procedure (LEEP)

This procedure can be diagnostic or therapeutic. In either case, the information desired is the microscopic diagnosis, depth of invasion if microinvasive cancer is present, and status of margins.

The gynecologist should remove the cone biopsy intact, if possible. If a laser is used, the endocervical margin should be resected with scissors so that the tissue at this crucial site can be evaluated microscopically in the absence of cautery artifact. Another method to assess the endocervical margin is to amputate the endocervical margin and send it as a separate specimen labeled "apical margin." Avoid manipulation of the surface epithelium because it is easily denuded. The specimen, wrapped in saline-soaked gauze, should be transported immediately to the surgical pathology laboratory.

The surgical pathologist can limit the gross description to the measurements of the specimen and any obvious lesion. The endocervical margin is marked with alcian blue ink, and pinned on a corkboard with the mucosa facing up (Fig. 28.2). Three hours of fixation before cutting is adequate. The specimen should be sectioned serially at 1- to 3-mm intervals. Each block should be marked with India ink or eosin to orient embedding. Serially cut blocks should be submitted in separate cassettes numbered consecutively, and the entire specimen should be submitted. When there are many blocks, and especially if the blocks are small, it is often more convenient and economical to place two to three blocks in each cassette.

The LEEP biopsy uses a low-voltage diathermy loop to excise a lesion or the entire transformation zone. The specimen should be serially sectioned at 1- to 3-mm intervals as with a cone biopsy. The cautery artifact that results from the procedure is comparable to that of the laser. Surgical margins may be difficult to evaluate.

Endometrial Biopsy and Curettings

All tissues should be submitted from diagnostic procedures, whereas selected samples should be submitted from therapeutic procedures in which a large volume of tissue is received, for example, curettage performed to remove products of conception. Endometrial biopsies and diagnostic curettings should be processed in the same manner as endocervical curettings. The gross description should include a measurement of the aggregate specimen. The specimen should be wrapped in fine Shandon mesh bags or tea bags, or equivalent, and submitted in its entirety.

For abortion specimens, evaluate the completeness of removal of the fetus and placenta when possible. Single small samples of fetal parts and placenta should suffice for sectioning. If fetal parts are not identified grossly, then particular attention should be given to find the feathery papillations diagnostic of chorionic villi. A dissecting scope or hand lens may be helpful in this regard. Soft, tan, solid tissue often is decidua, and in itself is insufficient to diagnose the presence of an intrauterine pregnancy. When a fetus or fetal parts can be identified grossly, usually only a single slide is sufficient if there is no gross abnormality. Note the length of the fetus and, if possible, obtain the weight. As a routine, we find that submission of three cassettes is sufficient to identify the presence of chorionic villi in most cases, if villi are present. If microscopic examination does not reveal any tissues of fetal origin, only then should additional tissue be processed. At times, extensive amounts of tissue must be processed to find even a small focus of villi or trophoblast. In contrast to an ectopic pregnancy in the fallopian tube where blood clots typically contain chorionic villi, blood clots from intrauterine pregnancies rarely contain chorionic villi and therefore generally are not sampled. If no tissues of fetal origin are found after examination of all tissues, it is important that the clinician be notified immediately about the possibility of an ectopic pregnancy or a failed therapeutic abortion.

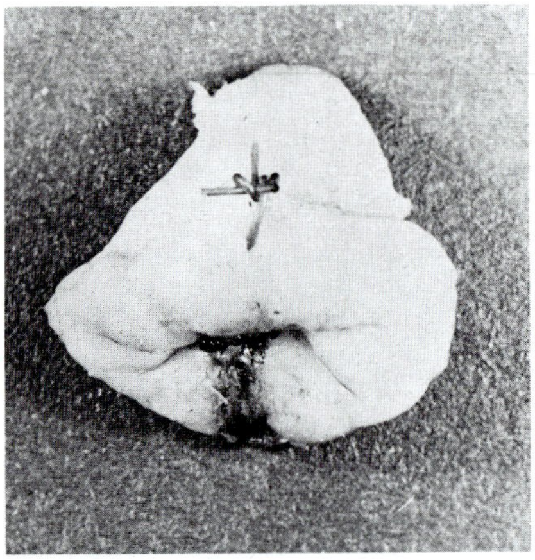

Cone of cervix

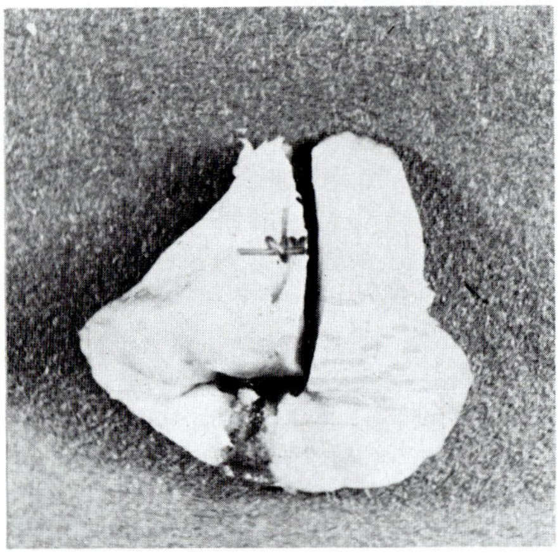

Incised at 12 o'clock

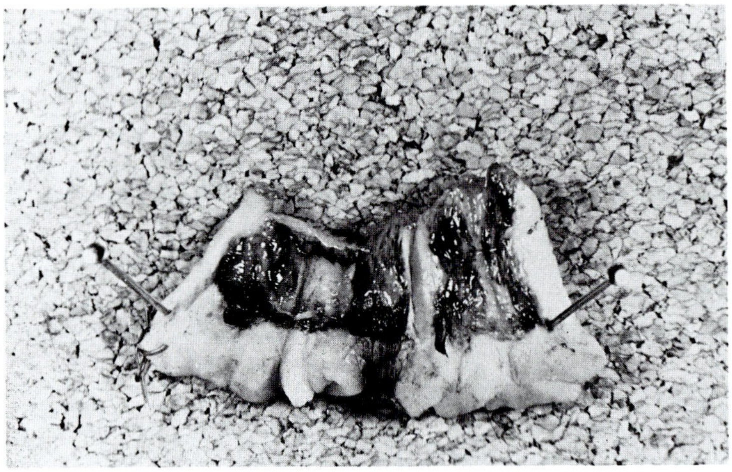

Opened cervix

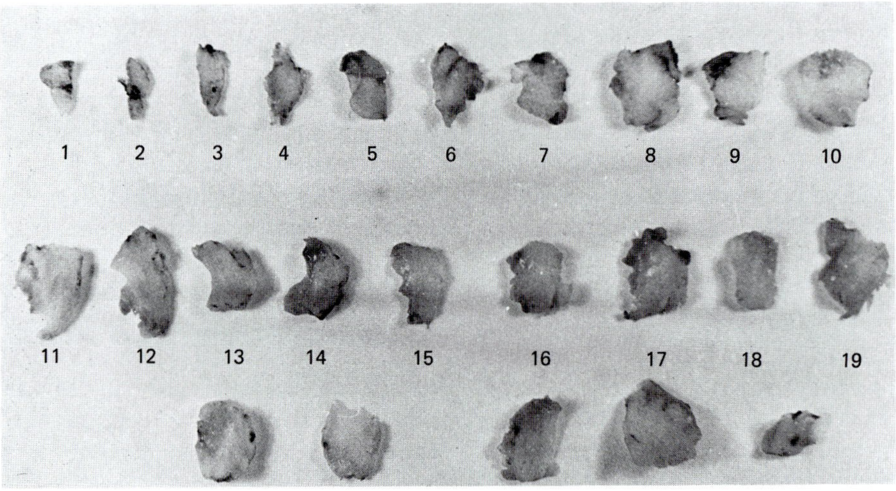

20 21 22 23 24

Fixation

Fig. 28.2. Method of sectioning a cone biopsy of the cervix. In this case, the specimen has been opened at 12 o'clock.

Curettings from a hydatidiform mole come in two parts: the suction curettage and the sharp curettage. The former should be examined carefully for the presence of fetal parts. Tissue from the sharp curettage should be processed entirely, since it must be evaluated for the presence of myometrial invasion. It should also be remembered that, with suction curettage, most vesicles have been forcibly disrupted and thus the classic gross appearance will not be present.

Large Operative Specimens

Wide Local Excision and Superficial Vulvectomy

Most specimens are highly variable in their composition because these procedures are tailored to the extent of the lesion. Recently, wide local excision has been performed for superficially (<1 mm) invasive tumors, whereas laser techniques often are used to treat vulvar intraepithelial neoplasia (VIN 3). The operative specimens include the labia minora, labia majora, clitoris, perineal body, and perianal tissue without subcutaneous fat.

The gross description should specify the features and extent of the lesion as well as the anatomic structures involved. Because intraepithelial lesions are subtle, careful attention must be paid to coloration and surface texture. The lesions typically are red, brown, or white and often are roughened. They should be measured, and distances from the lesion to the resection margin should be recorded.

Because the disease process often is multifocal and difficult to discern with the naked eye, all surgical resection margins must be examined microscopically; this requires sections through all obvious lesions to rule out invasive carcinoma and sections from all the peripheral resection margins. Sections parallel to the surgical margins (shave biopsies) often are taken to evaluate the excision lines. Although this method uses fewer sections to evaluate margins than those taken perpendicular to the line of resection, often the number of slides needed to evaluate the specimen overall is greater. Multiple perpendicular sections, however, have the advantage that the central lesion, margin, and intervening areas can be included in one slide and tumor "close to" the margin is much easier to evaluate. To facilitate sectioning, pin the specimen on a corkboard or a block of paraffin and fix for 2–3 hours before sectioning. When pinned to a corkboard, the specimen can then be floated upside down in a tub of formalin, which avoids compression that gravity otherwise introduces.

The surgical pathology report should include the microscopic diagnosis, extent of the involvement, and adequacy of the surgical resection margins.

Total Vulvectomy (Appendix, Table 28.1)

The specimen includes the entire vulva and subcutaneous fat, since the surgical dissection is carried down to the deep fascia. This procedure usually is performed only for vulvar Paget disease.

The gross description is similar to that outlined for the superficial vulvectomy. Although Paget disease of the vulva usually is an intraepithelial lesion, at times it may be invasive. The specimen should be pinned, fixed, and then sectioned at approximately 0.5-cm intervals to evaluate adequately the underlying dermis for an invasive carcinoma. Typically, microscopic involvement of Paget disease substantially exceeds the visible extent of the lesion on gross examination. Occult foci of Paget disease also may be present within normal-appearing skin, and consequently the entire deep and peripheral resection margins must be thoroughly evaluated in a similar manner as that described for the superficial vulvectomy specimen.

The surgical pathology report should include the microscopic diagnosis, extent of involvement, adequacy of the resection margins, and whether an underlying carcinoma is present.

Radical Vulvectomy, with Lymphadenectomy (Appendix, Table 28.1)

The specimen consists of the vulva, inguinal skin, subcutaneous tissue, femoral and inguinal lymph nodes, and portions of the saphenous veins. The procedure is performed for invasive squamous carcinoma.

The gross description should include the size, location, and depth of penetration of the primary lesion, and all resection margins, including the perirectal and vaginal margins. Examination often is aided if the specimen is first pinned out and fixed for a short period. Sections should include the tumor, showing the maximum depth of invasion, labia majora and minora, distal urethra, clitoris, resection margins including the vaginal margin, and all lymph nodes. Sections should evaluate the status of the skin immediately adjacent to the primary lesion, as preinvasive disease often is present. Separation of lymph nodes into superficial and deep groups requires communication with the gynecologic surgeon. Invasive vulvar neoplasms, in contrast to intraepithelial lesions, tend to be solitary and, consequently, evaluation of resection margins can be limited to the margins near the tumor. Because the specimen contains a considerable amount of fatty tissue, identification of lymph nodes may be difficult. In the fresh state, lymph nodes are recognized by palpation. Alternatively, xerography (Fig. 28.3) may assist in locating lymph nodes. The fatty tissue should be bread-loafed at 1- to 2-cm intervals to allow adequate penetration of the fixation. Location of lymph nodes is facilitated by an understanding of the lymphatic drainage of the vulva (Fig. 28.4).

The surgical pathology report should include the microscopic diagnosis, tumor grade, dimensions, location and maximum depth of invasion, presence of lymphatic invasion, number and location of the involved lymph nodes, and status of resection margins.

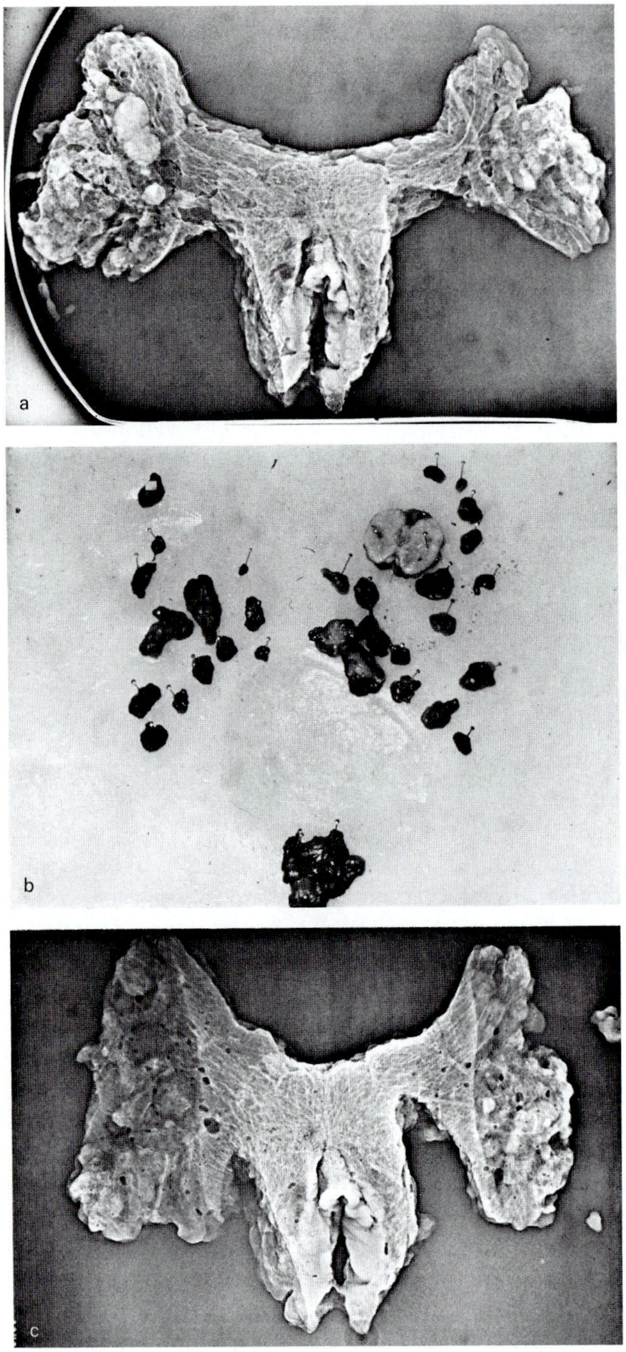

Fig. 28.3. Lymph nodes in vulvar cancers. **a**: Xerogram of radical vulvectomy specimen before dissection. Nodes can be clearly seen. **b**: Lymph nodes dissected from specimen. **c**: Xerogram of postdissection specimen. (Courtesy of J. Milbrath, M.D., and Edward J. Wilkinson, M.D., Gainesville, FL.)

Vaginectomy and Pelvic Exenteration

The vaginectomy specimen consists of the vagina as well as the cervix and uterus as the procedure is an en bloc resection for invasive carcinoma of the vagina. Depending on the location and extent of the tumor, the urinary bladder and rectum also may be removed. The procedure is termed an *anterior exenteration* if the urinary bladder is included and a *posterior exenteration* if the rectum is included. Pelvic exenteration is performed infrequently today. The most common indication is for a central recurrence of a cervical carcinoma.

The vagina should be opened longitudinally on the side opposite the tumor. The total length of the vagina is measured and the distances between the tumor, the cervix, and the resection margins are recorded. The tumor mass should be described and measured and the maximum depth of invasion noted. The extent of involvement should be de-

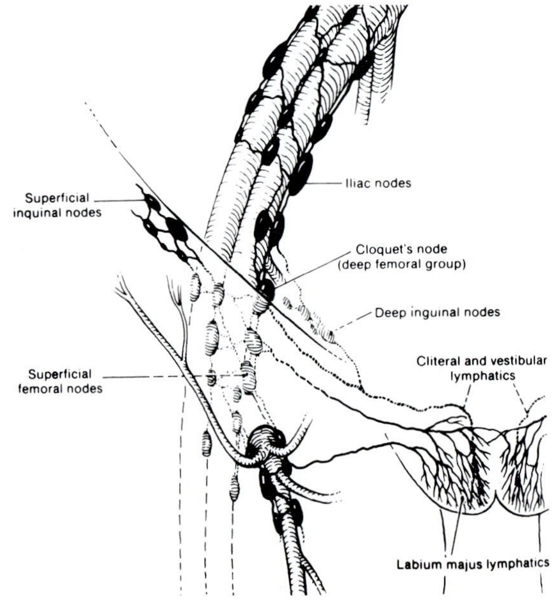

Fig. 28.4. Lymphatics of the vulva. (Reprinted by permission of Schmidt WA (1983) Principles and techniques of surgical pathology. Butterworth-Heinemann, Stoneham.[2])

scribed, in particular, the relationship of the tumor to the cervix and the urinary bladder or rectum if the latter organs have been removed. To evaluate these features, the rectum and bladder must be opened, the specimen fixed, and sections taken perpendicular to the mucosa directly overlying the tumor in the vagina. A good method that provides excellent orientation of the tumor to adjacent structures for exenteration specimens is to inflate the urinary bladder and rectum with formalin and fix the specimen for several hours. The entire specimen can then be hemisected through the neoplasm, and the appropriate sections can be obtained (Fig. 28.5). Sections from the surgical resection margins and any lymph nodes identified in the attached soft tissue should be obtained. India ink marking of all resection margins and a diagram describing the specimen, tumor, and section code are useful for orientation and correlation of the microscopic sections and the gross findings.

The surgical pathology report should include the microscopic diagnosis, tumor grade, dimensions, location and relationship to adjacent structures, presence of lymphatic invasion, number of involved lymph nodes, and adequacy of the surgical resection margins.

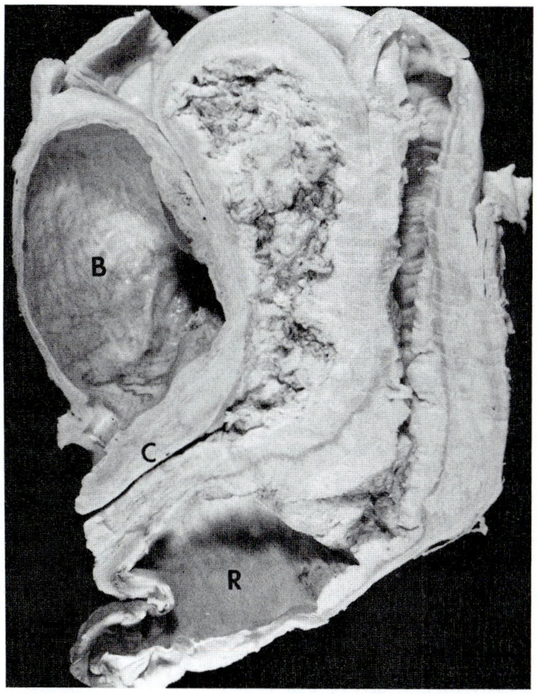

Fig. 28.5. Pelvic exenteration for cervical cancer. Hemisection of bladder (*B*), uterus with cervix (*C*), rectum (*R*), and sigmoid colon. (Courtesy of Dennis O'Connor, M.D., Washington, D.C.)

Total Hysterectomy

The total hysterectomy specimen consists of the cervix and the uterine corpus. Supracervical hysterectomy, a procedure in which the uterus is amputated at the internal cervical os, is now rarely performed. Removal of the cervix and uterus is treatment for a variety of benign and malignant diseases. Because of the diverse nature of the disease processes for which a hysterectomy is performed, the approach to processing the specimen as well as the hysterectomy procedure itself vary accordingly. The different pathologic techniques used, therefore, are considered according to the surgical indication.

Hysterectomy for Benign Uterine Disease

Included in this category are hysterectomies for persistent abnormal bleeding, uterine prolapse, or intractable pelvic pain. The last sometimes may result from unrecognized organic causes, such as adenomyosis or endometriosis, that are recognized only after thorough pathologic examination.

Begin the description by listing the specimens received, including whether the cervix or adnexae are attached or separate. The specimen is oriented (Fig. 28.6) by identifying the round ligaments that insert anterior to the fallopian tubes. One easy method to determine laterality is to lift the specimen by the two ovaries, which will be posterior to the fallopian tubes. In addition, on the posterior surface of the uterus the peritoneum covers a larger area and extends farther down toward the cervix than anteriorly, where it is reflected high over the bladder (Fig. 28.7). The specimen should then be weighed after the adnexae have been removed or the weight estimated if the ovaries and tubes are small and the weight inconsequential. The parous uterus is heavier (premenopausal adult, 75–100 g) than the nulliparous uterus (premenopausal adult, 30–40 g), and weight increases with increasing parity. After eight pregnancies, a weight of 240 g is normal. The postmenopausal uterus, because of the diminished amount of muscle, weighs 20–40 g. The following measurements should be taken: (1) top of the fundus to the exocervix (premenopausal adult, 5–8 cm), (2) cornu to cornu (premenopausal adult, 3–5 cm), (3) thickness from anterior to posterior surface (premenopausal adult, 2–4 cm), and (4) length and diameter of the cervix (premenopausal adult, 3 cm each).

The uterine serosa, particularly the posterior surface, should be examined carefully for adhesions and brown hemosiderin deposits, so-called powder burns, if endometriosis is suspected, and small vesicles or gritty foci for endosalpingiosis, ovarian im-

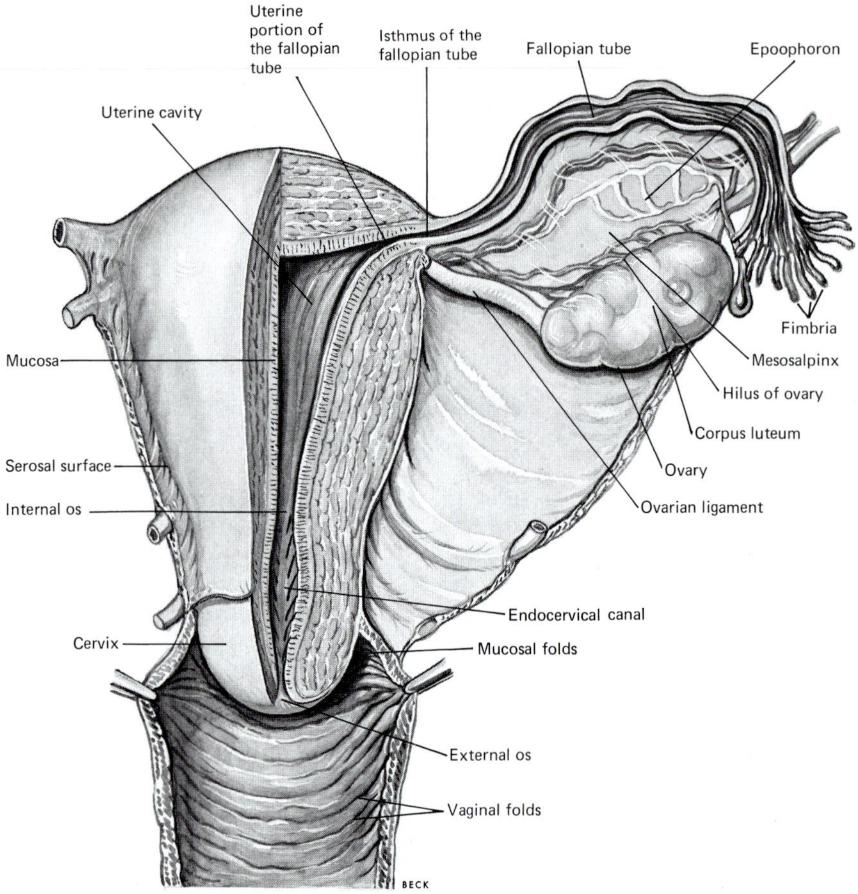

Fig. 28.6. The uterus, vagina, and adnexa. (Modified from Gray's Anatomy, 30th Ed. (C.D. Clemente, ed.), 1985. Courtesy of Lea & Febiger.)

plants, and psammoma bodies. The exocervix should be examined for lacerations, scarring, ulcerations, and cysts.

Before opening of the uterus, the cervical canal and endometrial cavity should be probed; this establishes the patency of the endocervical canal and facilitates opening the uterus. An incision is made with a scalpel or scissors along the probe extending from the cervical os to the cornu along one lateral margin to the fundus and then along the other lateral margin (Fig. 28.8). The average thickness of the endometrium should be measured and a statement made whether it is atrophic, polypoid, or hemorrhagic. Polyps should be measured and their location specified. The myometrium is evaluated with sections through the full thickness of the anterior and posterior walls. The maximum thickness of the myometrium should be measured. A thickened myometrium showing small cystic or focal areas of hemorrhage is suggestive of adenomyosis. The minimum number of sections to be examined in a uterus remains a subject of debate and personal preference. If the disease process is obvious, such as a polyp, even one section may be sufficient, if it includes the polyp, endometrium at some distance from the polyp, the wall, and serosa. On the other hand, menorrhagia, a common preoperative sign, often has no obvious gross lesions seen in the specimen. In this case, usually a minimum of four sections is useful, each full thickness through the wall. Each should be from an anterior and posterior wall with one each of the pair sampling toward the right and left sides. Adenomyosis is often focal and not uncommonly is found in only one of the four sections. It is important that the sections include serosa, for often the significant pathology in these cases is endometriosis or adhesions. If the cervix is normal, a section including the endocervix and portio is adequate. The section of the cervix should include the entire wall to involve the endocervix, squamocolumnar junction, and exocervix. The section through the endometrium, if the lesion is benign, should be up to

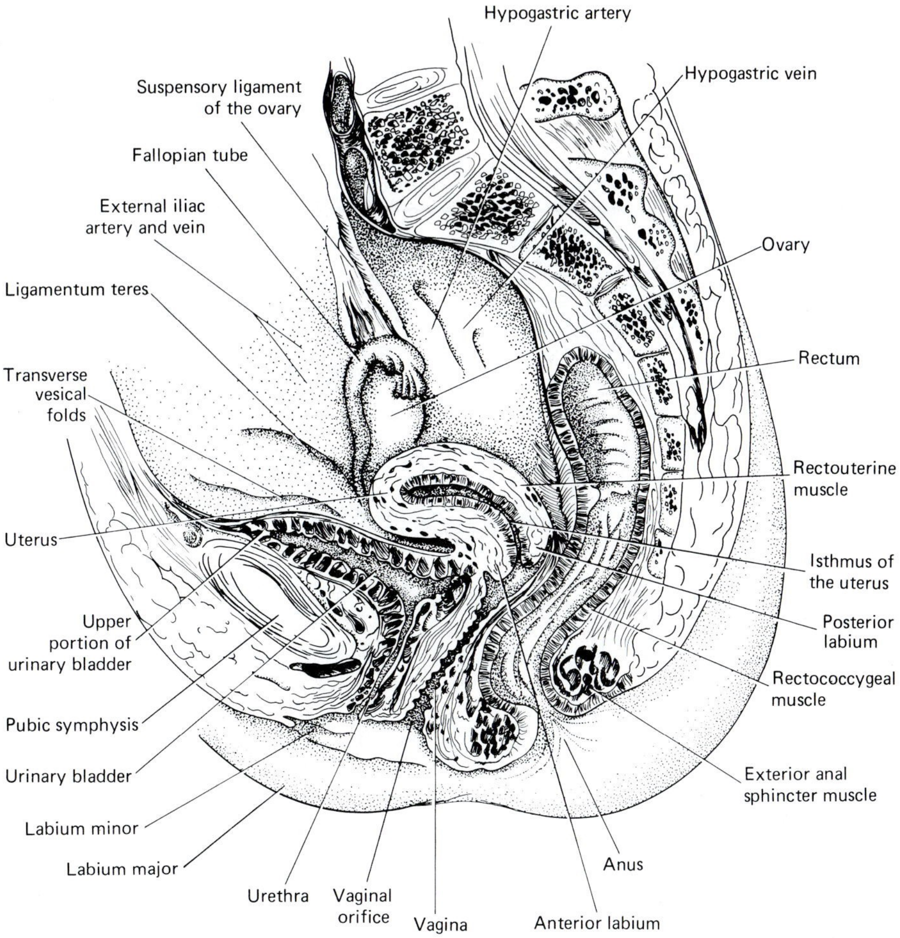

Fig. 28.7. Sagittal section through the pelvis illustrating the anterior and posterior peritoneal reflections on the uterus. (Modified from Gray's Anatomy, 30th Ed. (C.D. Clemente, ed.), 1985. Courtesy of Lea & Febiger.)

2 cm long and should include the full thickness of the endometrium and a wedge of myometrium.

Hysterectomy for Benign Organic Uterine Disease

This procedure includes hysterectomies performed for leiomyomas and endometrial hyperplasia. In addition to the routine processing described previously, more detailed examination is required in these cases.

In a specimen removed for leiomyomas, the number of leiomyomas present, their location (submucosal, intramural, subserosal) and size (e.g., "ten less than 1 cm and two measuring 13 and 18 cm in diameter") should be noted. If submucous, whether the tumor distorts the endometrial cavity or whether it protrudes into the lower uterine canal or cervix should be stated. Each leiomyoma should be sectioned and examined grossly but not necessarily microscopically. Usually one to two blocks in total are sufficient if all the leiomyomas are small, white, firm, whorled, have well-circumscribed margins, and do not contain areas that are soft, necrotic, or hemorrhagic. Because smooth muscle tumors less than 5 cm in size virtually never metastasize regardless of microscopic appearance, routine microscopic examination of every typical leiomyoma is considered unnecessary. Conversely, as leiomyomas tend to be multiple and leiomyosarcomas single, solitary tumors that are soft, degenerating, or in any way suspicious must be sampled thoroughly. From general experience, we have found that one block for each 2 cm of tumor is sufficient to sample a tumor. Of far greater importance than the number of blocks taken, however, is the areas from which the blocks are taken. Sections taken for variation of color, soft or hemorrhagic areas, or some other specific finding yield much greater information than "random" sections. For myomectomy specimens, each leiomyoma should be transected and a section

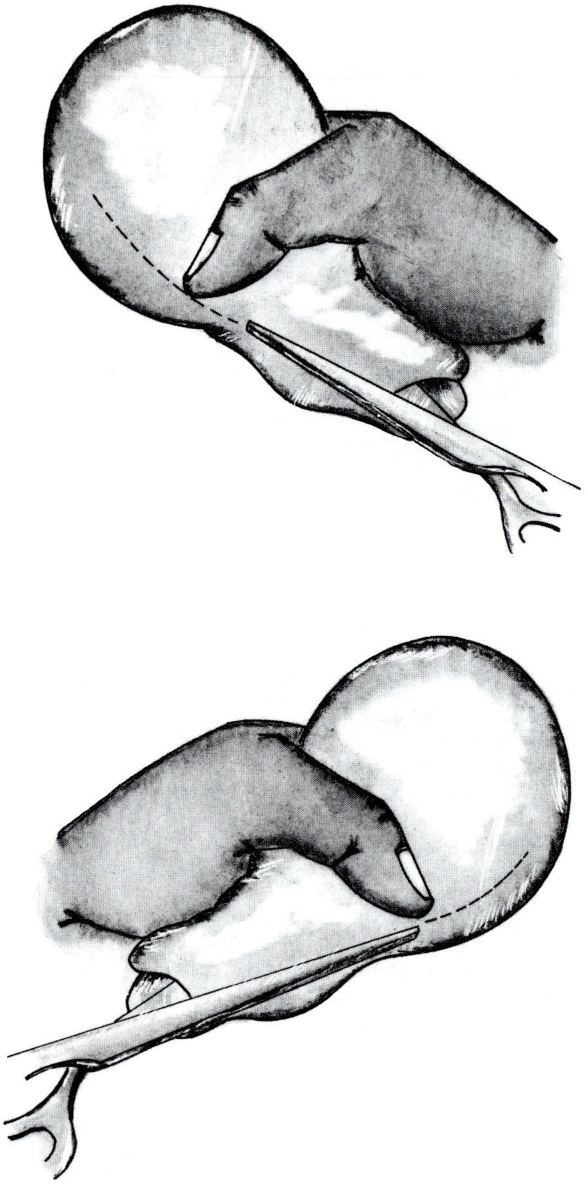

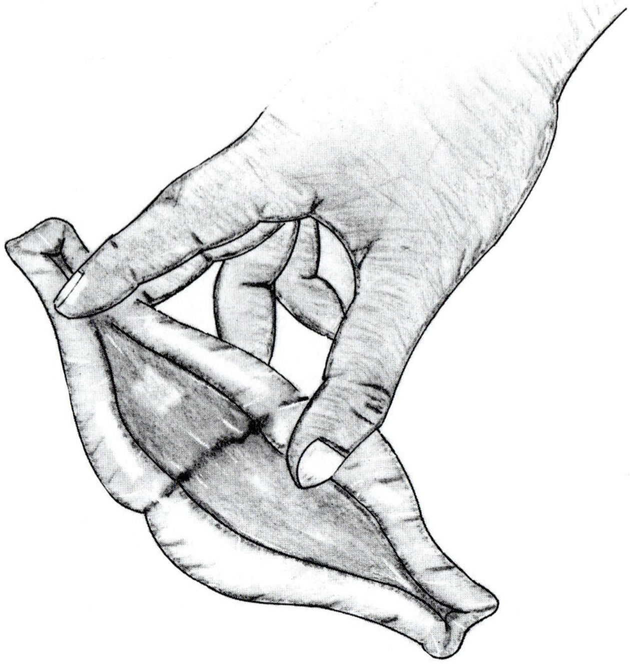

Fig. 28.8. Bivalve opening of the uterus. The specimen is opened to best demonstrate the uterine lesion present.

taken from each. Additional sections should be taken if problematic areas are encountered on histologic sections.

Uteri removed for endometrial hyperplasia should have multiple full-thickness sections of the endomyometrium to rule out the presence of carcinoma. Four sections (two sections, each 2 cm long, of each wall) should adequately sample the endometrium in most cases, which may represent 25–50% of the endometrium.

Hysterectomy for Malignant Cervical Disease (Appendix, Table 28.2)

For intraepithelial neoplasms, a simple hysterectomy often with a vaginal cuff is performed. For microinvasive squamous carcinoma, a simple hysterectomy or a modified radical hysterectomy (inclusion of some paracervical soft tissue) is performed depending on the depth of invasion and the institutional criteria, which vary. For stage I squamous carcinomas, depending on size and configuration of the tumor in the endocervical canal, and for stage IIa tumors, depending on the extent of vaginal involvement, a radical hysterectomy (Wertheim hysterectomy) and pelvic lymphadenectomy is performed. Paraaortic lymph nodes also are frequently sampled.

The extent of the workup for uteri removed for intraepithelial neoplasia depends on the information sought from the pathologic examination. For example, a patient may have had a prior cone biopsy where the intraepithelial neoplasia was completely excised, but close to the section margin. In this case, an extensive microscopical workup is not always cost efficient. Often, one generous full-thickness section through each of the four quadrants is sufficient. On the other hand, there are certainly many instances where extensive analysis is important and it is useful to examine the cervix as if it were a giant conization specimen. In these instances, it may be useful to amputate the cervix no less than 0.5 cm above the level of the external os and then proceed to process it as a cone biopsy. Preferably the amputation should include the maximum amount of endocervix that will fit into the cassette. If a vaginal cuff has been submitted, the distance from the exocervix to the line of resection should be measured. Sections should be obtained from the surgical resection line to determine the adequacy of the margin. As with the vulva, sections may be circumferential or perpendicular so long as the blocking process is thorough and complete. Complete, however, does not require that 100% of the margin be examined with perpendicular specimens so long as the intervening space between sections is not overly generous and the tumor mass is not grossly near the margin. Sections perpendicular to the line of resection, as stated earlier, permit assessment of the cervical lesion and margins together in context. This information, along with the microscopic diagnosis, should appear in the surgical pathology report.

A radical hysterectomy differs from a simple hysterectomy by virtue of the presence of attached paracervical tissues, which extend to the ureter and iliac artery and vein. Accompanying the specimen is a cuff of vagina and pelvic lymph nodes. The gross description should include the dimensions of the tumor, its location, relation to the vaginal margin, depth of invasion, and an impression of whether the lymph nodes appear normal or contain metastases. The cervix can either be processed as a cone biopsy or selectively sampled to demonstrate the maximum depth of invasion and relationship to the surgical margins. The vaginal resection margin is evaluated as described previously. In addition, because the lymphatic drainage of the uterus is lateral toward the parametrium, these areas are especially important in defining the spread of disease. The parametrial tissue should be completely processed because this represents the lateral and most significant resection margin. The outer surface of the cervix overlying the tumor anteriorly and posteriorly should be marked with India ink to delineate the extent of the tumor in relationship to the bladder and rectum. Lymph nodes should be grouped according to areas. Right and left should be separated and internal iliac, external iliac, obturator, and so on should be separately grouped. Lymph nodes often can be evaluated better when they are fresh, at which time they are firm and nodular.

The surgical pathology report should include the microscopic diagnosis, maximum size, location, extension, and depth of invasion of the tumor. In addition, the presence of lymphatic invasion, number of involved lymph nodes, and adequacy of the resection margins, especially lateral margins, adjacent to the uterine arteries should be noted.

Hysterectomy for Malignant Uterine Disease (Appendix, Table 28.3)

This procedure includes uteri removed for endometrial carcinoma and sarcomas of the uterus. Hysterectomy specimens received with a preoperative diagnosis of carcinoma or sarcoma must be evaluated for residual tumor. The gross evaluation should be the same as for uteri removed for benign organic disease. In addition, the description should include whether the tumor is focal or diffuse, sessile, or polypoid. The uninvolved endometrium should be described and sampled microscopically, including the lowermost margin of the neoplasm. The dimensions and location of the tumor including involvement of the cervix should be noted, and the gross depth of myometrial invasion recorded. Microscopic sections should be obtained to determine the maximum depth of myometrial invasion and involvement of the cervix.

The surgical pathology report should include the tumor type and grade, depth of myometrial invasion, thickness of the involved myometrium, involvement of the cervix, presence of vascular invasion, and the number of positive lymph nodes with their location specified, that is, pelvic or para-aortic, and the size of the larger metastases (if substantial) in the nodes.

Hysterectomy Performed During Obstetric Procedures

Hysterectomy at the time of delivery is performed for intractable hemorrhage, placenta accreta, uterine rupture, or cervical neoplasia. For the last, processing of the specimen should be as described previously. For the other conditions, the gross description and sectioning should focus on the relationship of the placenta and membranes to the uterus. Lacerations should be described carefully as to location, extent, and depth of penetration. Sections should be obtained from these sites. If the patient has had a previous cesarean section, the old scar, usually in the anterior lower uterine segment, should be sampled. In instances of placenta previa, the zone of the internal os should be sampled carefully to identify associated placenta accreta.

Salpingectomy

Removal of the fallopian tube (salpingectomy) often accompanies removal of the ovary (oophorectomy). Removal of both fallopian tubes and ovaries (bilateral salpingo-oophorectomy) often is performed in conjunction with a hysterectomy, especially in older women in whom it is no longer necessary to preserve fertility. In these cases, there is typically no pathologic condition in the fallopian tubes, and the gross examination and sampling are routine. The overall length and diameter of the tube should be measured. The patency of the fimbriated end can be determined with a blunt-tipped probe. If a lesion is present, it should be measured, its location (cornual, isthmic, infundibular, or ampullary) noted, and its relationship to the lumen and serosa described. If no lesion is present, transverse sections from the isthmic, infundibular, and ampullary portions of the tube can be placed into one cassette and labeled "right" or "left" (Fig. 28.9).

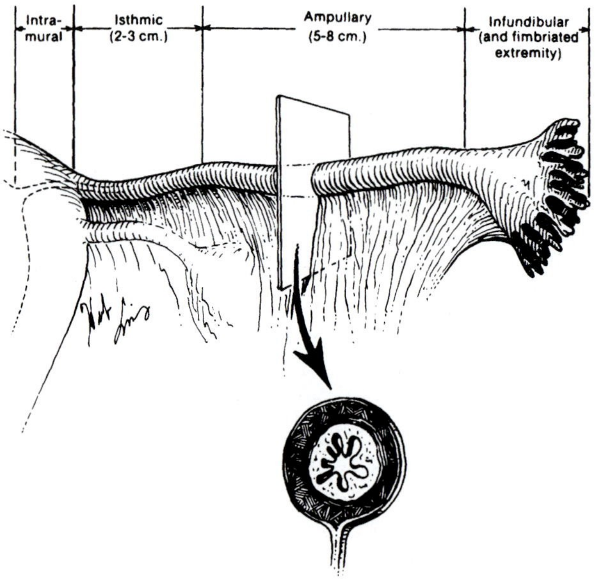

Fig. 28.9. Technique for sectioning the fallopian tube in the absence of abnormalities. Representative transverse sections are obtained from the isthmic, infundibular, and ampullary regions. (Modified from Robboy SJ, Anderson MC, Russell P (2001) Pathology of the Female Genital Tract. Churchill Livingstone, New York.)

Total or Partial Salpingectomy for Tubal Ectopic Pregnancy or Sterilization

If the tubal pregnancy is apparent, its site and location should be noted as described previously. A rupture site if present should be described and sampled. If the ectopic pregnancy is not obvious, a focal enlargement or swelling of the tube should be sought. Blood distending the lumen of the fallopian tube is so unlikely to result from any other cause that it is worth documenting. It may be necessary to section the area extensively. Even a tubal abortion leaves foci of trophoblast at the implantation site. Blood clot in the tube, sometimes submitted as a separate specimen, should be examined carefully for gray-white tissue and sampled for microscopic examination to identify trophoblastic cells or chorionic villi.

When removed for ligation, the single most important finding is that the tube has been ligated; this requires that a complete cross section of the tube, which includes the lumen, be identified and differentiated from round ligament. Measure the length and the diameter of each tube. One method for sampling is to slice the tube into sections, 1–3 mm in length and to submit all for microscopic examination, each piece being cut on end. Even if per chance some sections are cut tangentially, usually at least some will be intact to document that the lumen is present; this step saves substantial time and effort by not having to request additional recuts. Another technique that saves effort is to place the specimens into agar, which aligns the specimen for embedding.

Salpingectomy for a Tubal Neoplasm

Tubal carcinoma is rare, and its behavior and management are similar to ovarian carcinoma. Typically, a total abdominal hysterectomy and bilateral salpingo-oophorectomy are performed. The size of the tumor, location, and extent, with reference to other pelvic structures, should be described. Transverse sections through the full thickness of the tube permit determination of the depth of penetration. All this information as well as the grade of the tumor should be included in the microscopic diagnosis of the surgical pathology report.

Oophorectomy

The ovaries, like the fallopian tubes, frequently are removed at the time of hysterectomy in older women even if there is no apparent pathology. Routine processing of this type of specimen includes weighing and measuring the ovary in three dimensions. The normal ovary in the reproductive years weighs ap-

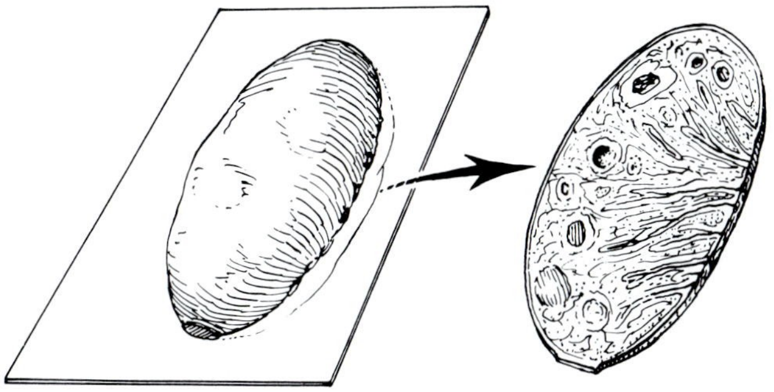

Fig. 28.10. Technique for sectioning the ovary in the absence of abnormalities. The cross section contains cortex, medulla, and hilum. (Reprinted by permission of Schmidt WA (1983) Principles and techniques of surgical pathology. Butterworth-Heinemann, Stoneham.[2])

proximately 12 g, is ovoid, and measures approximately $4 \times 2.5 \times 1.5$ cm. The external surface should be inspected for stigmata of ovulation, adhesions, excrescences hemorrhage, or hemosiderin (powder burns), indicative of possible endometriosis. The hilus and broad ligament should be examined, and any suspicious lesion should be submitted for microscopic examination. Each ovary should be sectioned sagittally through its greatest dimension to include the hilus and submitted in a single cassette labeled "right" or "left" (Fig. 28.10).

Cystectomy or Oophorectomy for a Neoplasm

Cystectomy usually is performed for a dermoid cyst. After weighing and measuring the specimen in three dimensions, the external surface should be examined and the cyst opened. The sebum within the cyst can be removed by washing with hot water. The water must be hot to liquefy the sebum. Short exposure to hot water does not destroy the epithelial lining. Identify and serially block the knobby protuberance in the wall, so-called Rokitansky's tubercle, teat, or mammilla, and any other areas where the wall is thickened.

Except for obvious benign paraovarian and functional ovarian cysts, all other cystic and solid ovarian neoplasms are treated by a unilateral salpingo-oophorectomy or a hysterectomy and bilateral salpingo-oophorectomy. The hysterectomy specimen and normal-appearing contralateral ovary and fallopian tube should be processed and reported as described previously. The ovarian tumor should be weighed and measured in three dimensions. The fallopian tube generally is removed with the ovary but it may be draped over the tumor and difficult to identify. If present, it should be measured and its relationship to the ovary noted. Similarly, if a tumor appears to have largely replaced the ovary, any residual ovary should be identified and its relationship to the tumor noted. Not uncommonly, the only portion of residual ovary in a tumor is that portion of the gonad immediately adjacent to the fallopian tube. Therefore, it is useful to take sections transversely through the fallopian tube to include a wedge of ovary.

The gross description should state whether the specimen is received intact or fragmented. The capsule should be examined for rents, adhesions, implants, or extension and penetration of the underlying tumor. The tumor is then hemisected, and the cut surfaces are examined. Each cyst of a cystic tumor should be examined for papillary excrescences and solid foci, because these may reveal areas of low malignant potential or frankly malignant tumor on microscopic examination. In about 5% of mucinous tumors, evidence of a dermoid cyst, for example, hair, will be found in a mucinous locule. If a solid ovarian tumor is small, identify its location as cortical, medullary, or hilar.

Microscopic sections should be obtained from the external surface of the neoplasm, especially in areas of adhesions, to document whether tumor involves the surface or if the adherence is the result simply of a chemical reaction. In particular, penetration of underlying tumor through the surface should be documented because this plays a role in staging. Surgeons should be asked to place a stitch in the adhesions noted during the operative procedure. It is important to demonstrate invasion microscopically. Blocks cut to show the interface between the tumor and the adjacent tube are especially useful. All solid and hemorrhagic areas should be sampled thoroughly. It is commonly stated that the pathologist should submit a minimum of one block per 1–2 cm of the greatest tumor dimension. However, this dictum is clearly to be applied with judgment. For example, serous tumors tend to be relatively uniform throughout. Other tumors, in contrast, such as mucinous tumors, vary greatly such that large areas may appear grossly and microscopically benign, whereas only a few areas are typically of borderline or frank malignancy. Solid areas need to be more thoroughly sought grossly, and those should be sampled extensively microscopically. Unilocular cysts with a smooth lining of the inner wall, in contrast, may be large, but require fewer sections for microscopic examination. The microscopic diagnosis should include the cell type and, for epithelial tumors, whether benign, of low malignant potential, or frankly malignant. For frankly malignant tumors, include tumor grade, whether the surface is involved, the extent of the tumor, and the site and number of involved lymph nodes.

Placental Examination

Routine Processing

Because most newborns and their mothers are normal and healthy, detailed pathologic examination of all placentas is not warranted. The obstetrician must select for examination those placentas that may help in the diagnosis of illness in parent or newborn. The pathologist must respond with an informative report.

Examination of the placenta can provide information useful in patient management, especially infections, and identify instances in which karyotyping is indicated. Furthermore, in the current litigious environment, placental examination may define types of birth injury that lie outside the control of the obstetrician. Documentation of twinning relationships may be useful in later life, for example, in patients evaluated for organ transplantation.

Placentas selected for examination should be sent fresh to the laboratory with a requisition that states the questions the pathologist is requested to answer. Placentas not selected can be labeled and stored in plastic bags, either frozen or refrigerated, for retrieval if problems develop in the neonatal period.

Indications for placental examination and a format suitable for transmission of the placenta and necessary data to the laboratory are listed in Table 28.5 (see Appendix). The list begins with the mother's name and age. It can be used as a checklist sufficient to provide the pathologist with enough clinical data to start the examination. The membrane of the specimen should be translucent and the fetal surface should be shiny, dark purple. Reconstruct the membranous sac, noting its narrowest margin between placental edge and site of rupture. The absence of a margin may explain bleeding; any margin excludes placenta previa. Record tears or bands. Cut a strip of membrane about 5 cm wide, roll it toward the placental margin, and affix it with a pin (Fig. 28.11). Cut away the rest of the membranes from the rest of the placental margin with scissors. Next, examine the fetal surface. Note exudate, discoloration (green-brown) from meconium staining, and adherent extraneous material that does not easily wipe away. The umbilical cord must be carefully examined and measured. Record knots, hemorrhages, and number of vessels on cross section cut away from the placenta near the fetal surface. Insertion of the cord near the narrowest membrane margin may be a cause of intrapartum fetal distress (vasa previa). The inspection should conclude with an examination of the maternal surface. Cotyledons should be intact. Note any adherent clot, especially clots that compress the placenta or have become indurated and laminated.

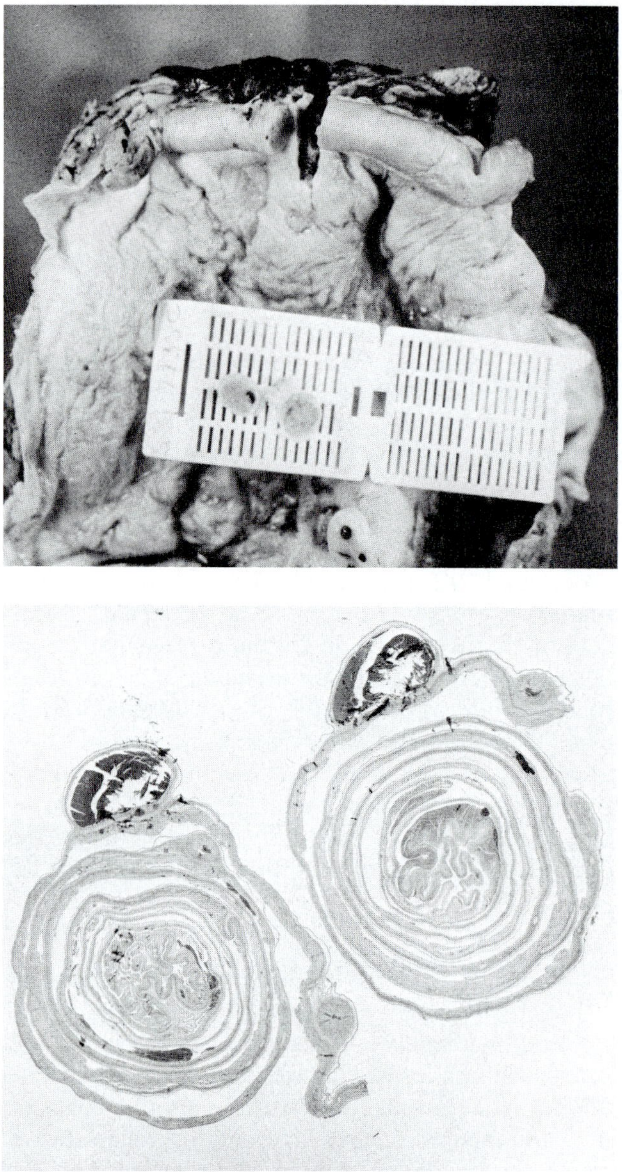

Fig. 28.11. Placental examination. *Top*: A placenta with membrane roll attached at top before fixation. The resulting spiral in cassette retains its tight coil after the block has been processed. *Bottom*: Margin of membrane opening is always at the center of the spiral. This consistent orientation helps demonstrate the ascending route of infections.

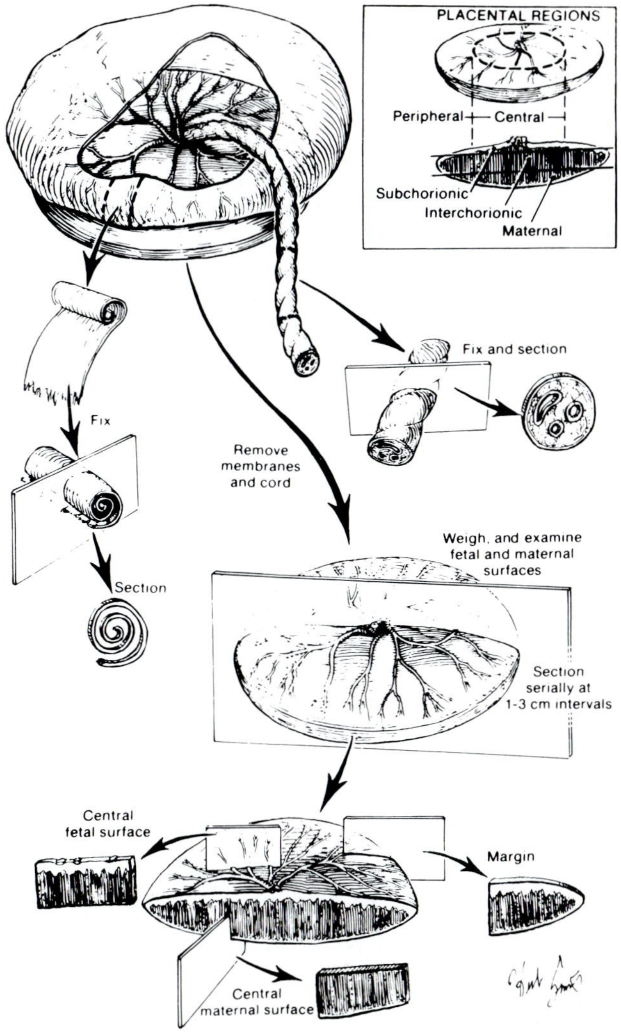

Fig. 28.12. Placental examination. Adequate sampling for histologic study includes membrane roll, cross section of cord, and specific placental regions, specifically cut to display fetal and maternal surfaces. (Reprinted by permission of Schmidt WA (1983) Principles and techniques of surgical pathology. Butterworth-Heinemann, Stoneham.[2])

Weigh the placenta and record the maximum dimensions. Cut sections at 1- to 20-cm intervals with a sharp knife; this is accomplished most easily with the maternal surface up. The cut surface should have a uniform granular surface and a bright red color. Record clots, infarcts, and other lesions.

After the specimen has been fixed for several hours in 10% buffered neutral formalin, blocks can be cut for histologic sections (Fig. 28.12) to include a cross section of the cord, membrane roll, fetal surface with amnion attached, and lesions identified on cross section.

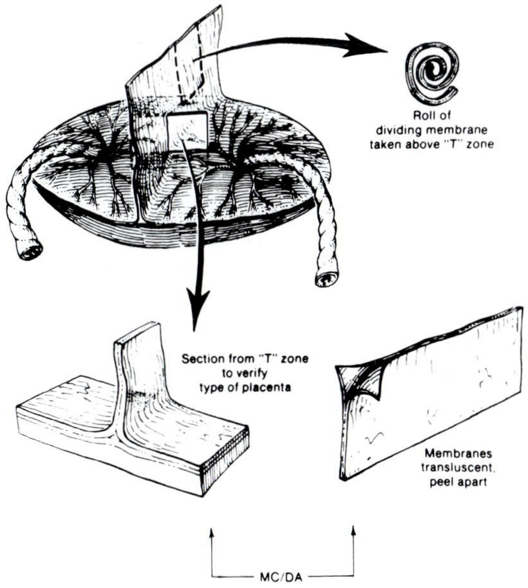

Fig. 28.13. Examination of placenta of twins. Sampling of a twin placenta includes a section of septal membrane dividing the amnionic cavities, cut to display the T-zone, where the septal membrane attaches to the placental surface. (Reprinted by permission of Schmidt WA (1983) Principles and techniques of surgical pathology. Butterworth-Heinemann, Stoneham.[2])

Twins and Other Multiple Gestations

The amnionic septum between two amnionic cavities serves to define identical or fraternal relationships insofar as placental examination allows. The dividing membrane of dichorionic placentas is thicker and opaque because of the intervening chorionic tissue. Attach a roll of this membrane as described for single placentas, affixing it to the placental surface with a pin. After fixation, cut a cross section from this roll and the T-zone, where it attaches to the fetal surface of the placenta (Fig. 28.13). When both amnions are stripped away, a ridge or layer of chorion persists in fused dichorionic twin placentas. In monochorionic twin placentas the septal site vanishes, and the only visible traces are vascular connections on the fetal surface.

Culture Methods

Aerobic and anaerobic bacterial cultures, when performed by swabbing the fetal surface, introduce so many contaminants that the procedure has little value. To reduce the frequency of contaminants the subchorionic zone is best cultured with a swab af-

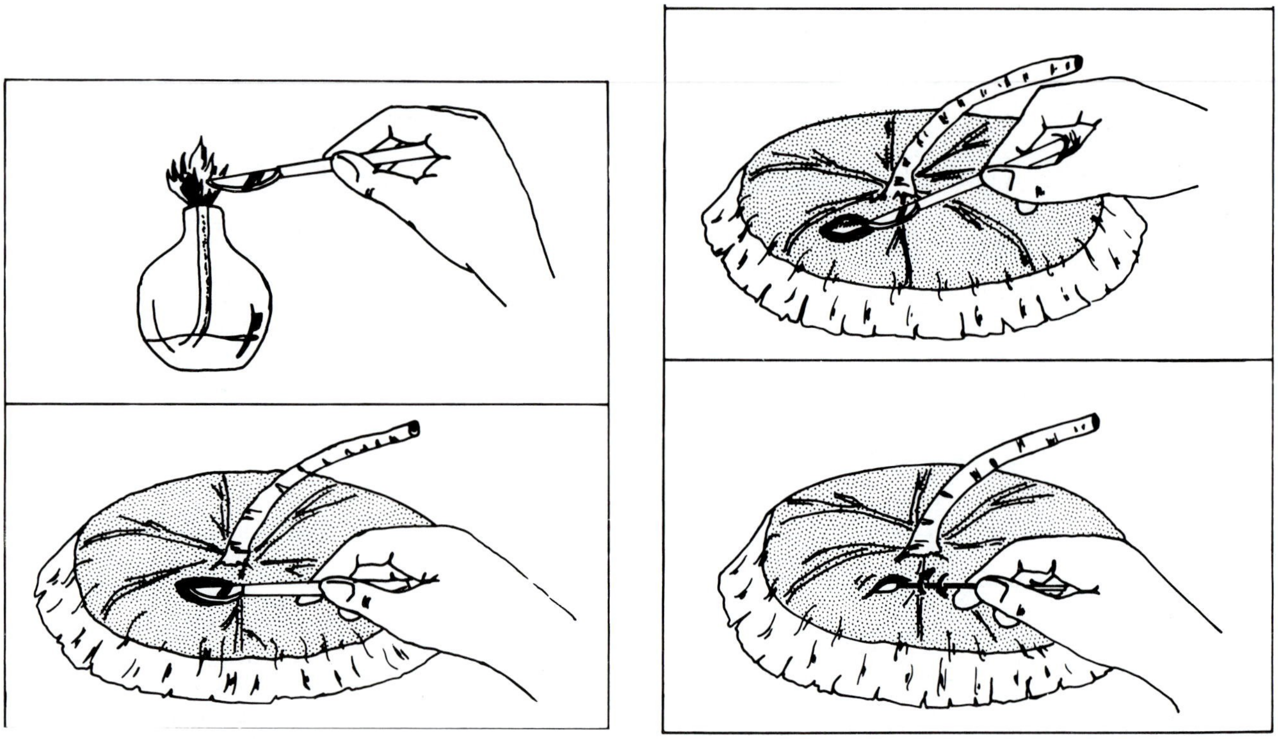

Fig. 28.14. Culture technique to sample subchorionic fibrin layer. This method reduces surface contamination.

ter the surface has been seared and incised with a heated or sterile scalpel (Fig. 28.14).

Cytogenetic Studies

These studies require a fragment of villous tissue or skin or pericardium if perinatal death has occurred. Death of the fetus does not necessarily preclude successful culture. The tissue should be placed in sterile media containers provided by the cytogenetics laboratory. Tissue obtained properly may be shipped to a distant facility if desired.

Dissecting Microscope

A dissecting microscope should be available for adequate study of many small abortuses. Some anomalies, including fusion defects of the facial clefts, fused or supernumerary digits, partial limb reduction, and such ocular defects as coloboma, are too minute to evaluate adequately with the unaided eye, but alone or in combination they may be sufficiently suggestive of trisomy to indicate the need for karyotypes of the conceptus and possibly the parents.

References

1. Robboy SJ, Bentley RC, Krigman H, Silverberg SG, Norris HJ, Zaino RJ (1994) Synoptic reports in gynecologic pathology. Int J Gynecol Pathol 13:161–174
2. Schmidt WA (1983) Principles and techniques of surgical pathology. Butterworth-Heinemann, Stoneham
3. Scully RE (1999) Protocol for the examination of specimens from patients with carcinoma of the vagina: a basis for checklists. Arch Pathol Lab Med 123:62–67

Appendix

Table 28.1. Vulvar carcinoma

Operative Procedure: CASE: ________________

Diagnosis:
VULVA: ________________ (histology), measuring ___ × ___ × ___ cm depth
with extension into ________________ .
and metastases to ________________ lymph nodes
and ________________ (other sites).
Resection margins ________________

1	Degree of differentiation Squamous cell	Well, moderately, poorly differentiated
2	Size of tumor	___ × ___ cm
	Tumor thickness:	___ mm (FM granular layer (surface if no keratin to deepest point of invasion)
	Depth of invasion:	___ mm (Fm epithelial stromal junction of adjacent most supfl dermal papillae to deepest point of invasion)
	Uninvolved zone to deep margin:	___ mm
3	Location & Gross configuration	Unifocal Multifocal
		Left Right Cross_Midline
		Labia: Minora Majora
		Ant Post
		Clitoral PeriUrethral
		PeriVaginal Bartholin Gland
		Post Fourchette
		PeriAnal Perineum
4	Margins, distance to:	If uninvolved, closest distance ___ mm
	Surface margin	Involved, which: Ant Post L_Lat R_lat
	Deep margin	Involved
5	Depth invasion For melanoma	*Levels* / *Invasive in -mm*
		1 (In epidermis/In situ) 0 mm
		2 (Into papillary dermis) <1 mm
		3 (To pap/reticular interface) 1–2 mm
		4 (Into reticular dermis) >2 mm
		5 (Into subcutaneous fat) In fat
6	Extravulvar tumor:	
	Anus:	No Wall Mucosa
	Rectum:	No Wall Mucosa
	Vagina:	No Wall Mucosa Lower Upper
	Urethra:	No Wall Mucosa Lower Upper
	Bladder:	No Wall Mucosa
	Pelvic bone attachment:	No Yes
	Other	________________ where
7	Vascular involvement:	No Yes_type_Uncertain
		Lymphatics Blood_vessel Both
8	Associated changes	
	Squamous	None VIN-I II III
	Appendages involved	No Yes

Adapted from
INTERNATIONAL SOCIETY
OF GYNECOLOGICAL
PATHOLOGISTS

Squamous Lesions
Squamous cell carcinoma
Basaloid carcinoma
Verrucous carcinoma
Basal cell carcinoma

Glandular Lesions
Paget disease
Bartholin gland tumors
Breast CA & others of ectopic origin
Carcinomas of sweat gland origin
Other adenocarcinomas

Mesenchymal Tumors
Embry. rhabdomyosarc (sarc botryoid)
Aggressive angiomyxoma
Leiomyosarcoma
Dermatofibrosarcoma protuberans
Malignant fibrous histiocytoma
Epithelioid sarcoma
Malignant rhabdoid tumor
Malignant schwannoma
Angiosarcoma
Kaposi sarcoma
Hemangiopericytoma
Liposarcoma
Alveolar soft-part sarcoma

Miscellaneous Tumors
Malignant melanoma
Malignant lymphoma
Tumors of germ cell type
Yolk sac (endodermal sinus tumor)
Neuroectodermal tumors
Merkel cell tumor

9 Special studies:			
DNA ploidy:	Euploid Tetraploid Aneuploid		
HPV type:	6/11 16/18 31/33/35		
10 Non-neoplastic changes			
Lichen sclerosus	No Yes		
Hyperplasia	No Yes		
Hyperkeratosis	No Yes		
Koilocytosis	No Yes		
Other:	Yes, ________________ Specify		
11 Lymph nodes: NOS	None ___ of ___ contain metastases		
	Left	*Right*	
Inguinal, NOS	None ___/___ w Mets	None ___/___ w Mets	
Superficial	None ___/___ w Mets	None ___/___ w Mets	
Deep	None ___/___ w Mets	None ___/___ w Mets	
Pelvic, NOS	None ___/___ w Mets	None ___/___ w Mets	
External iliac	None ___/___ w Mets	None ___/___ w Mets	
Obturator (Med Ext Iliac)	None ___/___ w Mets	None ___/___ w Mets	
Internal iliac (Hypogastr)	None ___/___ w Mets	None ___/___ w Mets	
Aortic, NOS	None ___/___ w Mets	None ___/___ w Mets	

Reprinted by permission of Robboy et al., ref. 1.

Table 28.2. Cervical carcinoma

Operative Procedure: CASE: ________________

Diagnosis:
CERVIX: ________________ (histology)
FIGO grade ___, measuring ___ × ___ × ___ cm depth
with extension into ________________
and metastases to ________________ lymph nodes
and ________________ (other sites).
Resection margins ________________.

1	Grade	
	If Squamous cell	Non-keratinizing; Keratinizing
	If glandular	
	Architectural grade (% solid growth)	G1-Well differentiated (5% or less solid growth) G2-Moderately differentiated (6–50% solid growth) G3-Poorly differentiated (over 50% solid growth)
	.Solid excludes squamous growth	
2	Size of tumor	___ × ___ cm (length/width)
	Depth invasion:	___ mm
	Uninvolved zone to deep margin:	___ mm
3	Location:	Left Right Ant Post Exocervix SQ_junction Endocervix Confined to polyp Parametrium
4	Shape of cervix:	Normal, Cylindrical, Barrel shaped (>4 cm)
5	Extracervical tumor:	No ________________ (where)
	Uterine corpus:	No Yes Lower uter segment Endomet Myomet
	Vagina:	No Upper 2/3rds Lower 3rd Mucosa Wall
	Parauterine:	No Yes Left Right
	Ureter:	No Yes L/R Hydronephrosis Non-function kidney
	Bone Pelvic Side wall:	No Yes L/R
	Bladder:	No Wall Mucosa
	Rectum:	No Wall Mucosa
	Abdomen/peritoneum:	No Yes
	Liver:	No Yes
6	Vascular involvement:	No Yes type Uncertain Lymphatics Blood vessel Both
7	Associated premalignant changes	
	Squamous	None CIN-I II III
	Glandular	None AIN-I/Atyp II III/In-situ
	If involved	Multifocal
8	Margins, distance to:	If uninvolved, closest distance ___ mm
	Surface margins:	Involved, which: Cranial Caudal L_Lat R-lat
	Depth:	Involved:
9	Special studies:	
	DNA ploidy:	Euploid Tetraploid Aneuploid
	HPV type:	6/11 16/18 31/33/35
10	Non-Neoplastic cervix	
	Koilocytosis (Condyloma)	No Yes
	Other:	Yes, ________________ Specify

Adapted from
INTERNATIONAL SOCIETY OF GYNECOLOGICAL PATHOLOGISTS

Squamous Lesions
Squamous cell carcinoma
Keratinizing Non-keratinizing
Verrucous
Warty (condylomatous)
Papillary (transitional)
Lymphoepithelioma-like

Glandular Lesions
Adenocarcinoma
Mucinous adenocarcinoma
Clear-cell adenocarcinoma
Minimal deviation (adenoma malignum)
Villoglandular adenocarcinoma

Other Epithelial Tumors
Adenosquamous carcinoma
Glassy cell carcinoma
Adenoid basal carcinoma
Adenoid cystic carcinoma
Carcinoid tumor
Small cell carcinoma
Wolffian duct (mesonephric)

Mesenchymal Tumors
Leiomyosarcoma
Endocervical stromal sarcoma
Sarc botryoidese (embry rhabdomyosarc)
Alveolar soft-part sarcoma
Osteosarcoma

Mixed Epithelial & Mesenchymal Tumors
Adenosarcoma
Malig mixed mesodermal tumor (MMMT)
Wilms tumor

Miscellaneous Tumor
Malignant melanoma
Lymphoma and leukemia
Germ cell type
Yolk sac tumor

11 Lymph nodes: NOS	None ___ of ___ contain metastases	
	Left	*Right*
Parauterine	None ___/___ w Mets	None ___/___ w Mets
Obturator (Med Ext Iliac)	None ___/___ w Mets	None ___/___ w Mets
External iliac	None ___/___ w Mets	None ___/___ w Mets
Sacral	None ___/___ w Mets	None ___/___ w Mets
Internal iliac (Hypogastric)	None ___/___ w Mets	None ___/___ w Mets
Common Iliac	None ___/___ w Mets	None ___/___ w Mets
Pelvic, NOS	None ___/___ w Mets	None ___/___ w Mets
Aortic, NOS	None ___/___ w Mets	None ___/___ w Mets
Inguinal, NOS	None ___/___ w Mets	None ___/___ w Mets

Reprinted by permission of Robboy et al., ref. 2.

Table 28.3. Endometrial cancer[a]

Operative Procedure: CASE: ___________________

Diagnosis:
UTERUS: ___________________ (histology) (___ % each major cell type)
FIGO grade ___, measuring ___ × ___ × ___ cm
with extension into ___________________
and metastases to ___________________ lymph nodes
and ___________________ (other sites).
Tumor penetrates ___ mm into ___ thick myometrium.

1	Architectural grade:	G1-Well differentiated (5% or less solid growth)
	% solid growth	G2-Moderately differentiated (6–50% solid growth)
		G3-Poorly differentiated (over 50% solid growth)
	.Solid excludes squamous growth	
	.Notable nuclear atypia, inappropriate for architectural grade, raises the nuclear grade by 1.	
	.Nuclear grade takes precedence for clear cell, squamous & serous CA.	
2	Special_Attributes	
	Nuclear grade:	1 (Uniform nuclei, small nucleoli, rare mitoses)
	(glandular)	2 (More variability, larger nucleoli, more mitoses)
	(controversial)	3 (Pleomorphic, many mitoses)
	Squamous differentiation	___ % total neoplasm
3	Size of uterus	Weight ___ gm; ___ × ___ × ___ cm
	Size of tumor	___ × ___ cm (length/width)
	Thickness of myometrium:	___ mm
	Deepest invasion:	None ___ mm Serosa involved
4	Location:	Unifocal Multifocal
		Ant Post Cornua
		Fundus Body Lower_uterine segment
		Polyp (involves limited to)
5	Extrauterine tumor:	
	Ovary:	No Left Right Histology: ___________________
		Synchronous v metastasis
	Fallopian tube:	No Left Right
	Broad Ligament:	No Left Right
	Cervix:	No Yes Supfl/glands Wall/stroma
		Endocervix Exocervix
	If endocervix curetted:	No Tumor_only (No stroma) EC with implant
		EC with invasion into stroma
	Parauterine:	No Yes Left Right
	Vagina:	No Yes
	Pelvic Peritoneum:	No Yes
	Cul-de-sac:	No Yes
	Omentum:	No Yes
	Large intestine:	No Yes
	Other:	No ___________________ (where)
6	Vascular involvement:	No Yes type Uncertain
		Lymphatics Blood vessel Both
7	Tissues adjacent to cancer	
	Non-hyperplastic	Prolif Secretory Atrophy Disordered_prolif
	Hyperplasia	Simple Complex Atypical
8	Ascites (>100cc)	Absent Neg Pos
	Pelvic washing:	Neg Pos
9	Special studies:	
	DNA ploidy:	Euploid Tetraploid Aneuploid
	Estrogen-receptor:	Neg Pos
	Progesterone-receptor:	Neg Pos
	S-Phase fraction:	
	Other:	Yes, ___________________ Specify

Adapted from
INTERNATIONAL SOCIETY
OF GYNECOLOGICAL
PATHOLOGISTS

Epithelial Tumors
Adenocarcinoma
(endometrioid)
Secretory Ciliated cell
Adenoca with Squamous
differentiation
Adenoacanthoma
Adenosquamous CA
Serous adenocarcinoma
Clear cell adenocarcinoma
Mucinous adenocarcinoma
Squamous cell carcinoma
Mixed
Undifferentiated

10 Non-Neoplastic endometrium/uterine			
Metaplasia:			
	Squamous Mucinous Ciliary Clear cell		
	Eosinophilic-cell Surface syncytial		
Adenomyosis	Papillary Other, Specify		
Arias-Stella:	No Yes W tumor		
Other:	No Yes		
	Yes, ________________ Specify		
11 Lymph nodes: NOS	None ___ of ___ contain metastases		
	Left	*Right*	
Parauterine	None ___/___ w Mets	None ___/___ w Mets	
Internal iliac (Hypogastric)	None ___/___ w Mets	None ___/___ w Mets	
Obturator (Med Ext Iliac)	None ___/___ w Mets	None ___/___ w Mets	
External iliac	None ___/___ w Mets	None ___/___ w Mets	
Common iliac	None ___/___ w Mets	None ___/___ w Mets	
Pelvic, NOS	None ___/___ w Mets	None ___/___ w Mets	
Aorotic, NOS	None ___/___ w Mets	None ___/___ w Mets	
Inguinal, NOS	None ___/___ w Mets	None ___/___ w Mets	
12 Serum blood levels			
CA-125			

Reprinted by permission of Robboy et al., ref. 2.
[a]FIGO staging incorporates pathologic findings.

Table 28.4. Ovarian carcinoma[a]

Operative Procedure: CASE: ___________________

Diagnosis:
OVARY: __________________ (histology) (___ % each major cell type)
FIGO grade ___, measuring ___ × ___ × ___ cm
with extension into ___________________
and metastases to ___________________ lymph nodes
and ___________________ (other sites).

1 Architectural grade: (% solid growth) (Common epith tumors) — G1-Well differentiated (5% or less solid growth); G2-Moderately differentiated (6–50% solid growth); G3-Poorly differentiated (over 50% solid growth)

2 Size of tumor & Location — Left: ___ gm; ___ × ___ × ___ cm (___ Check if normal); Right: ___ gm; ___ × ___ × ___ cm (___ Check if normal)

3 Tumor characteristics

Capsule	
Adhesions	Inflammatory Tumor
Ruptured	Spontaneous Surgically
Surface tumor	Benign Borderline Malig
Implants on ovary	No Yes
Parenchyma	
Solid	None Minimal (<10%) Extensive All
Necrosis	None Minimal (<10%) Extensive All
Cysts/locules	None Single Rare (<5) Many Hundreds

4 Staging bx, Peritoneum:

Under diaphragm:	Neg Pos
Liver:	Neg Supfl Parenchymal
Stomach:	Neg Pos
Omentum:	Neg Invasive Non-invasive
Abdominal peritoneum:	Neg Invasive Non-invasive
Gutter:	Neg Pos
Pelvic peritoneum:	Neg Pos
Side-wall:	Neg Pos
Cul-de-sac, Ant Post:	Neg Pos
Falciform ligament:	Neg Pos
Uterosacral ligament:	Neg Pos
Serosal bowel implants:	Neg Pos
Mesentery:	Neg Pos
Small:	Neg Pos
Large:	Neg Pos
Rectosigmoid:	Neg Pos
Appendix:	Neg Pos
Vagina, apex:	Neg Pos
Misc _________	
Pelvis: staging	
Fallopian tube:	No Yes L/R Mucosa Wall Serosa/Mesosalpinx
Uterus:	Neg Pos Serosa Endocervix Endometrium
Broad ligament:	Neg Pos Left Right
Retroperitoneum:	No Yes _________________ (where)

5 Possible 2nd primary: No Yes _________________ (where)
Possible synchronous primary
If endometrium involved ___________________ Histology, _________ Grade

Adapted from
WORLD HEALTH
ORGANIZATION

Common epithelial tumor
Serous
  Borderline malignancy (LMP)
    Cystadenoma/papillary cystadenoma
    Surface papilloma
    Adenofibroma and cystadenofibroma
  Malignant
    Adenocarcinoma
    Surface papillary carcinoma
    Malignant adeno/cystadenofibroma
Mucinous
  Borderline malignancy (LMP)
    Cystadenoma
    Adenofibroma and cystadenofibroma
  Malignant
    Adeno/cystadenocarcinoma
    Malignant adeno/cystadenofibroma
Endometrioid
  Borderline malignancy (LMP)
    Cystadenoma
    Adenofibroma and cystadenofibroma
  Malignant
    Carcinoma
      Adenocarcinoma
        W squamous differentiation
      Malignant adenofibroma
    Endometrioid stromal sarcoma
    Mesodermal (mullerian) mixed turn
Clear-cell
  Of borderline malignancy (LMP)
  Malignant
Brenner
  Prolif (borderline malignancy)
  Malignant
  Transitional cell
Undifferentiated carcinoma
Mixed (specify)

Sex-cord-stroma
Granulosa-cell tumor
  Adult
  Juvenile
Tumors in thecoma-fibroma group

	If myometrium involved	Invade from Endomet Invade from Serosa
	Possible peritoneal primary	
	If peritoneum involved	If borderline: ___ Type & Locations
		If carcinoma: ___ Type & Locations
6	Effusions/fluids:	
	Ascites (>100cc)	Absent Neg Pos
	Washing, peritoneal, NOS	Neg Pos
	Washing, diaphragm	Neg Pos
	Washing, left abdomen	Neg Pos
	Washing, right abdomen	Neg Pos
	Washing, pelvis	Neg Pos
	Scraping (Pap) diaphragm	Neg Pos
	Pleural:	Absent Neg Pos
7	Vascular involvement:	No Yes_type Uncertain
		Lymphatics Blood_vessel Both
8	Non-neoplastic changes	
	Stromal luteinization	No Yes
	Endometriosis:	Ovary Elsewhere (___ sites)
	Endometrium:	Atrophy Prolif Secretory Hyperplasia Carcinoma
	Peritoneum:	Common epithelial changes:
		Benign ("endosalpingiosis"): ___ Locations
9	Lymph nodes: NOS	None ___ of ___ contain metastases
		Left *Right*
	External iliac	None ___/___ w Mets None ___/___ w Mets
	Obturator (Med Ext Iliac)	None ___/___ w Mets None ___/___ w Mets
	Common Iliac	None ___/___ w Mets None ___/___ w Mets
	Pelvic, NOS	None ___/___ w Mets None ___/___ w Mets
	Aortic, NOS	None ___/___ w Mets None ___/___ w Mets
	Inguinal, NOS	None ___/___ w Mets None ___/___ w Mets
10	Special studies:	
	DNA ploidy:	Euploid Tetraploid Aneuploid
	Oncogenes	_______________ Specify
	Receptors	_______________ Specify
	Other:	_______________ Specify
11	Serum blood levels	
	CA-125	

Fibroma-fibrosarcoma
  Cellular fibroma
  Fibrosarcoma
Sertoli-stromal cell tumors
Sertoli-Leydig cell tumor
  Gynandroblastoma
  Sex-cord tumor with annular tubules

Steroid (lipid-lipod)-cell tumors
  Leydig-cell tumor
  Steroid-cell tumor, NOS

Tumors of rete ovarii

Tumors of uncertain cell type
  Of probable wolffian origin
  Small cell carcinoma

Reprinted by permission of Robboy et al., ref. 2.
[a]FIGO staging incorporates pathologic findings.

Table 28.5. Request for placental examination

Circle appropriate indications
Mother's name ___________________ Age ____ M.D. ___________________
Cesarean section/vaginal delivery

1. Specific maternal disease: Diagnosis ___________________
2. High-risk pregnancy: Diagnosis ___________________
3. Death: Antepartum Intrapartum–Neonatal
4. Baby small for date: Baby anemic
5. Postmature
6. Premature rupture of membranes
7. Possible intrauterine infection: viral (specify) ___________________
   toxoplasma ___________________ chorioamnionitis ___________________ other ___________________
8. Isoimmunization: Rh ___________________ Other ________________
9. Malformations of baby or placenta ___________________ Single umbilical artery ___________________
10. Evaluate antepartum intrauterine procedures (specify) ___________________
11. Gestational bleeding: 1st 2nd 3rd trimester ___________________
12. Placenta previa-vasa previa ___________________
13. Premature separation ___________________
14. Toxemia, eclampsia ___________________
15. Maternal diabetes mellitus ___________________
16. Maternal anemias (sickle cell, megaloblastic, other)
17. Other disease ___________________
18. History of habitual abortion ___________________
19. Cord entanglements, amniotic bands, or adhesions. Membrane tears, defects

Index

ISBN 0-387-95203-9

EAN

9 780387 952031